Coté, Lerman *and* Anderson's

A Practice of Anesthesia for Infants and Children

Coté, Lerman and Anderson's

Seventh Edition

A Practice of Anesthesia for Infants and Children

Charles J. Coté, MD, FAAP

Professor of Anaesthesia (Emeritus)
Harvard Medical School
Division of Pediatric Anesthesia
MassGeneral Hospital for Children
Department of Anesthesia, Critical Care and Pain Management
Massachusetts General Hospital
Boston, Massachusetts

Jerrold Lerman, MD, FRCPC, FANZCA

Clinical Professor of Anesthesiology
Jacobs School of Medicine and Biomedical Sciences
Pediatric Anesthesiologist
John R. Oishei Children's Hospital
Buffalo, New York

Brian J. Anderson, CNZM, MB ChB, Dip Obstet, PhD, FANZCA, FCICM

Professor of Anaesthesiology
University of Auckland
Auckland, New Zealand;
Paediatric Anaesthetist and Intensivist
Auckland Starship Children's Hospital
Auckland, New Zealand

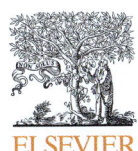

ELSEVIER

Elsevier
1600 John F. Kennedy Blvd.
Ste 1800
Philadelphia, PA 19103-2899

A PRACTICE OF ANESTHESIA FOR INFANTS AND CHILDREN,
SEVENTH EDITION

ISBN: 978-0-323-82560-3

Notice

Practitioners and researchers must always rely on their own experience and knowledge in evaluating and using any information, methods, compounds, or experiments described herein. Because of rapid advances in the medical sciences, in particular, independent verification of diagnoses and drug dosages should be made. To the fullest extent of the law, no responsibility is assumed by Elsevier, authors, editors, or contributors for any injury and/or damage to persons or property as a matter of products liability, negligence or otherwise, or from any use or operation of any methods, products, instructions, or ideas contained in the material herein.

Previous editions copyrighted 2019, 2013, 2009, 2001, 1993 and 1986.

Content Strategist: Kayla Wolfe
Content Development Specialist: Joanie Milnes
Publishing Services Manager: Julie Eddy
Project Manager: Julie Taylor
Design Direction: Renee Duenow

Printed in India

Last digit is the print number: 9 8 7 6 5 4 3 2 1

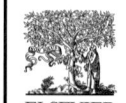

Working together
to grow libraries in
developing countries

www.elsevier.com • www.bookaid.org

DEDICATION

We dedicate this book to the children to whom we provide anesthesia daily and to their parents/guardians to assure them that their children will receive the highest standard of care and will be safe from harm. Our specialty continues to investigate the possible adverse effects of anesthetics on the developing brain to determine whether the findings in newborn animals are simply laboratory curiosities or are in fact translatable and potentially harmful to infants and children. Currently, the evidence neither confirms nor refutes meaningful injury to the developing human brain.

We also dedicate the seventh edition of *A Practice of Anesthesia for Infants and Children* to the memory of Dr. John F. Ryan, the founding editor of this textbook, who passed on January 2, 2020.

We hope that physicians around the world who have the pleasure and responsibility to care for children in the operating room, ICU, or other venues where anesthesia and sedation services are provided find this text a rich and comprehensive reference. In particular, we acknowledge those practitioners who take care of children and deliver the best possible care with limited resources and at times antiquated equipment, limited drugs, undependable electricity, and even limited availability of oxygen. Our specialty has grown exponentially in the past 35 years and as a result of new licensing laws, medications are now more thoroughly investigated before they are released for use in children. Ultrasound technology has made regional anesthesia and invasive line insertion far safer than in the past. The quality of airway devices continues to improve. Noninvasive continuous cardiac output devices and cerebral EEG devices may provide the next generation of monitors to safeguard the care of our children. Depth of anesthesia monitors continue to evolve; we hope that advances will ensure greater reliability in the infant and young child to assess the depth of anesthesia and differentiate sedation from general anesthesia.

This seventh edition of *A Practice of Anesthesia for Infants and Children* highlights key advances and questions in our specialty that we hope will continue to inspire anesthesiologists worldwide through the text, the web-based videos and illustrations, as well as the pocket reference card.

LIST OF CONTRIBUTORS

Rania K. Abbasi, MD, FASA
Anesthesiologist in Chief and Vice Chair of Pediatric Anesthesia
Riley Hospital for Children
Associate Professor of Clinical Anesthesia
Indiana University School of Medicine
Indianapolis, Indiana
Mechanical Circulatory Support

Trevor L. Adams, MD
Associate Professor
Anesthesiology and Pain Medicine
Seattle Children's Hospital
University of Washington
Seattle, Washington
Essentials of Hematology

Adam C. Adler, MS, MD, FAAP, FASE
Associate Professor of Pediatric Anesthesiology
Baylor College of Medicine
Department of Anesthesiology, Perioperative and Pain Medicine
   Texas Children's Hospital
Houston, Texas
Mechanical Circulatory Support

Warwick A. Ames, MBBS, FRCA
Associate Professor
Pediatric Anesthesiology
Duke University Medical Center
Durham, North Carolina
Essentials of Nephrology

Brian J. Anderson, CNZM, MB ChB, Dip Obstet, PhD, FANZCA, FCICM
Professor of Anaesthesiology
University of Auckland
Auckland, New Zealand;
Paediatric Anaesthetist and Intensivist
Auckland Starship Children's Hospital
Auckland, New Zealand
Growth and Development; Pharmacology of Drugs Used in Children; Total Intravenous Anesthesia and Target-Controlled Infusion; Orthopedic and Spine Surgery

Dean B. Andropoulos, MD, MHCM
Anesthesiologist in Chief
Pediatric Anesthesiology
Texas Children's Hospital
Houston, Texas;
Professor
Anesthesiology and Pediatrics
Baylor College of Medicine
Houston, Texas
Cardiopulmonary Bypass and Management

William Anninger, MD
Associate Professor
Ophthalmology
Childrens Hospital of Philadelphia
Perelman School of Medicine at the University of Pennsylvania
Philadelphia, Pennsylvania
Ophthalmologic Surgery

Philip Arnold, BM, FRCA
Consultant Anaesthetist
Anaesthesia
Alder Hey Children's Hospital
Liverpool, United Kingdom;
Honorary Lecturer
University of Liverpool
Liverpool, United Kingdom
Medications for Hemostasis

Motaz Awad, MD
Assistant Professor of Anesthesiology
University of Kentucky
Lexington, Kentucky
Chronic Pain

Philip D. Bailey, Jr., DO, MBA
Professor
Anesthesiology and Critical Care Medicine
The Children's Hospital of Philadelphia
Philadelphia, Pennsylvania
Ophthalmologic Surgery

M.A. Bender, MD, PhD
Director, Odessa Brown Sickle Cell Clinic
Pediatric Hematology
University of Washington
Seattle, Washington
Essentials of Hematology

Laura K. Berenstain, MD, FASA, ACC
Certified Leadership Coach
Volunteer Professor of Anesthesiology
University of Cincinnati College of Medicine
Cincinnati, Ohio
Mechanical Circulatory Support

Adrian T. Bösenberg, MB ChB, FFA(SA)
Professor
Anesthesiology and Pain Management
University Washington
Seattle, Washington;
Pediatric Anesthesiologist
Anesthesiology and Pain Management
Seattle Children's Hospital
Seattle, Washington
Pediatric Anesthesia in Developing Countries

Daniel Braunold, MBBS
Department of Anesthesiology
Rambam Health Care Campus
Affiliated with Technion - The Ruth and Bruce Rappaport
    Faculty of Medicine
Haifa, Israel
Trauma and Mass Casualties

Yitzhak Brzezinski Sinai, MD
Division of Anesthesia, Pain and Intensive Care
Tel Aviv Sourasky Medical Center Ichilov
Affiliated with Tel Aviv University School of Medicine
Tel Aviv, Israel
Trauma and Mass Casualties

Alyssa M. Burgart, MD, MA
Clinical Associate Professor
Anesthesiology, Perioperative, and Pain Medicine
Stanford University
Palo Alto, California
Ethical Issues in Pediatric Anesthesiology

Carolyn G. Butler, MD
Instructor in Anaesthesia
Harvard Medical School;
Associate in Perioperative Anesthesia
Department of Anesthesiology, Critical Care, and
    Pain Medicine
Boston Children's Hospital
Boston, Massachusetts
Pediatric Neurosurgical Anesthesia

Michele M. Carr, DDS, MD, MEd, PhD, FRCSC
Professor, Department of Otolaryngology
Jacobs School of Medicine and Biomedical Sciences at
The University at Buffalo
Buffalo, New York
Otorhinolaryngologic Procedures

Harmony F. Carter, MD
Associate Professor of Anesthesiology
Loma Linda University School of Medicine
Department of Anesthesiology
Loma Linda, California
*Preoperative Evaluation, Premedication, and Induction
    of Anesthesia*

Luciana Cavalcanti Lima, PhD (Anesthesiology)
Professor
Medicine
Faculdade Pernambucana de Saúde
Recife, Pernambuco, Brazil;
Pediatric Anesthesiologist
Instituto de Medicina Integral Prof. Fernando Figueira
Recife, Pernambuco, Brazil;
Director of Residence Program for Pediatric Anesthesia
Instituto de Medicina Integral Prof. Fernando Figueira
Recife, Pernambuco, Brazil
Infectious Disease Considerations for the Operating Room

Vidya Chidambaran, MD, MS
Professor of Anesthesiology
Cincinnati Children's Hospital Medical Center
Cincinnati, Ohio
Pharmacogenomics

Annabelle N. Chua, MD
Associate Professor
Pediatrics, Division of Nephrology
Duke University Medical Center
Durham, North Carolina
Essentials of Nephrology

Jeffrey B. Cooper, PhD
Professor of Anaesthesia (Emeritus)
Harvard Medical School
Department of Anesthesia, Critical Care and Pain Medicine
Massachusetts General Hospital
Executive Director Emeritus
Center for Medical Simulation
Boston, Massachusetts
Simulation in Pediatric Anesthesia

Charles J. Coté, MD, FAAP
Professor of Anaesthesia (Emeritus)
Harvard Medical School
Division of Pediatric Anesthesia
MassGeneral Hospital for Children
Department of Anesthesia, Critical Care and Pain Management
Massachusetts General Hospital
Boston, Massachusetts
*Growth and Development; Preoperative Evaluation, Premedication,
    and Induction of Anesthesia; Pharmacology of Drugs Used in
    Children; Strategies for Blood Product Management, Reducing
    Transfusions, and Massive Blood Transfusion; The Pediatric
    Airway; Burn Injuries; Sedation for Diagnostic and Therapeutic
    Procedures Outside the Operating Room; Procedures for Vascular
    Access; Pediatric Equipment and Monitoring*

Joseph P. Cravero, MD
Senior Associate in Perioperative Anesthesia
Anesthesia, Critical Care, and Pain Medicine
Boston Children's Hospital
Boston, Massachusetts;
Professor of Anaesthesia
Harvard Medical School
Boston, Massachusetts
*Anesthesia Outside the Operating Room; Sedation for Diagnostic
    and Therapeutic Procedures Outside the Operating Room*

Daniela Damian, MD
Assistant Professor of Anesthesiology and Perioperative Medicine
University of Pittsburgh School of Medicine
Director of Pediatric Transplant Anesthesiology
UPMC Children's Hospital of Pittsburgh
Pittsburgh, Pennsylvania
Essentials of Hepatology

Andrew J. Davidson, MBBS, MD, FANZCA, FAHMS
Staff Anaesthetist
Anaesthesia and Pain Management
Royal Children's Hospital
Melbourne, Victoria, Australia;
Medical Director
Melbourne Children's Trials Centre
Murdoch Children's Research Institute
Melbourne, Victoria, Australia;
Professor
Department of Paediatrics
University of Melbourne
Melbourne, Victoria, Australia
Surgery, Anesthesia, and the Immature Brain

James A. DiNardo, MD, FAAP, FASA
Professor of Anaesthesia
Harvard Medical School
Senior Associate in Cardiac Anesthesia
Boston Children's Hospital
Boston, Massachusetts
Cardiac Physiology and Pharmacology

Marie-Agnès Docquier MD, PhD
Service d'Anesthésiologie
Cliniques universitaires Saint-Luc
UCLouvain
Bruxelles, Belgium
Essentials of Neurology and Neuromuscular Disorders

Timothy M. Earley, DO
Assistant Professor
Department of Anesthesiology
Children's Hospital at Dartmouth
Lebanon, New Hampshire
The Postanesthesia Care Unit and Beyond

Michael J. Eisses, MD
Associate Professor of Anesthesia
Anesthesiology and Pain Medicine
Seattle Children's Hospital, University of Washington
    Medical School
Seattle, Washington
Essentials of Hematology

Marla B. Ferschl, MD
Health Sciences Clinical Professor of Anesthesia
Department of Anesthesia and Perioperative Care
University of California
San Francisco, California
Fetal Intervention and the EXIT Procedure

John E. Fiadjoe, MD
Associate Professor of Anaesthesia
Harvard Medical school
Executive Vice-Chair
Department of Anesthesia Critical Care & Pain Medicine
Boston, Massachusetts
The Pediatric Airway; Plastic and Reconstructive Surgery

Paul G. Firth, MB ChB, BA
Pediatric Anesthesiologist
Department of Anesthesia, Critical Care and Pain Medicine
Massachusetts General Hospital
Boston, Massachusetts;
Associate Professor of Anaesthesia
Harvard Medical School
Boston, Massachusetts
Essentials of Pulmonology

Kaitlin M. Flannery, MD, MPH
Clinical Assistant Professor
Department of Anesthesiology, Perioperative and Pain Medicine
Stanford University
Stanford, California
Organ Transplantation

Ralph Gertler, MD, PhD
Executive Senior Physician
Department of Anaesthesiology and Intensive Care
Helios Klinikum München West
München, Germany
Essentials of Cardiology; Cardiopulmonary Bypass and Management

Elizabeth A. Ghazal, MD
Associate Professor of Anesthesiology
Loma Linda University School of Medicine
Department of Anesthesiology
Loma Linda, California
Preoperative Evaluation, Premedication, and Induction of Anesthesia

Kenneth Goldschneider, MD
Professor, Clinical Anesthesia and Pediatrics
Department of Anesthesiology
Cincinnati Children's Hospital Medical Center
Cincinnati, Ohio
Chronic Pain

Erin A. Gottlieb, MD, MHCM
Associate Professor
Department of Surgery and Perioperative Care
The University of Texas at Austin Dell Medical School
Austin, Texas;
Chief of Pediatric Cardiac Anesthesiology
Dell Children's Medical Center
Austin, Texas
Cardiopulmonary Bypass and Management

Eric F. Grabowski, MD, ScD
Associate Professor of Pediatrics
Harvard Medical School
Director,
Massachusetts General Hospital Comprehensive Hemophilia
    Treatment Center
Co-Director,
Pediatric Stroke Services
Director,
Cardiovascular Thrombosis Laboratory
Department of Pediatrics
Hematology/Oncology
Massachusetts General Hospital
Boston, Massachusetts
*Strategies for Blood Product Management, Reducing Transfusions,
    and Massive Blood Transfusion*

A. Rebecca L. Hamilton, MD, MSc
Assistant Professor in Anesthesia
University of Toronto
Division of Cardiac Anesthesia
Department of Anesthesiology and Pain Medicine
The Hospital for Sick Children
Toronto, Ontario, Canada
Simulation in Pediatric Anesthesia

Gregory B. Hammer, MD
Professor, Department of Anesthesiology, Perioperative and Pain
    Medicine
Professor, Department of Pediatrics
Stanford University School of Medicine
Stanford, California
Anesthesia for Thoracic Surgery

Tom G. Hansen, MD, PhD
Consultant Pediatric Anesthesiologist
Anesthesiology & Intensive Care
Akershus University Hospital
Lørenskog, Norway;
Professor
Institute of Clinical Medicine, Faculty of Medicine
Oslo University
Oslo, Norway
General Abdominal and Urologic Surgery

Jeana E. Havidich, MD, MS
Associate Professor
Monroe Carell Jr. Children's Hospital at Vanderbilt
Vanderbilt University Medical Center
Nashville, Tennessee
The Postanesthesia Care Unit and Beyond

James Houghton BSc(hons), MB ChB, FANZCA
Paediatric Anaesthetist
Paediatric Anaesthesia
Starship Children's Hospital
Auckland, New Zealand
Total Intravenous Anesthesia and Target-Controlled Infusion

Samuel A. Hunter, MD
Assistant Professor
Anesthesiology and Critical Care Medicine
Children's Hospital of Philadelphia, University of Pennsylvania
Philadelphia, Pennsylvania
Ophthalmologic Surgery

Jared R.E. Hylton, MD, MS
Assistant Professor
Department of Anesthesiology
University of Wisconsin
Medical Director of Pediatric Pain Management
American Family Children's Hospital
Madison, Wisconsin
Acute Pain

Andre L. Jaichenco, Sr., MD
Head Chief
Anesthesia
National Pediatric Hospital "Dr. Prof. J. P. Garrahan"
Ciudad Autónoma de Buenos Aires
Buenos Aires, Argentina;
Associate Director
Anesthesia Specialist Career
Universidad de Buenos Aires
Buenos Aires, Argentina;
Cardiac Anesthesia Fellowship Director
Anesthesia
National Pediatric Hospital "J. P. Garrahan"
Buenos Aires, Argentina
Infectious Disease Considerations for the Operating Room

Cathie T. Jones, MD
Senior Associate in Anesthesia
Anesthesiology, Critical Care & Pain Medicine
Boston Children's Hospital
Boston, Massachusetts;
Instructor in Anaesthesia
Harvard Medical School
Boston, Massachusetts
Fluid Management

Siri Kanmanthreddy, MD
Assistant Professor
Anesthesiology and Pain Medicine
Seattle Children's Hospital,
University of Washington
Seattle, Washington;
Pediatric Anesthesiologist
Anesthesiology and Pain Medicine
Seattle Children's Hospital
University of Washington
Seattle, Washington
Essentials of Hematology

Manoj Kumar Karmakar, MD, FRCA, FHKCA
Professor
Department of Anaesthesia and Intensive Care
The Chinese University of Hong Kong
Prince of Wales Hospital
Shatin, NT, Hong Kong
China
Regional Anesthesia

T. Bernard Kinane, MD
Associate Professor of Pediatrics
Harvard Medical School
Department of Pediatrics
Massachusetts General Hospital
Boston, Massachusetts
Essentials of Pulmonology

Reeti Kumar, MD
Assistant Professor
Pediatrics, Division of Nephrology
Duke University Medical Center
Durham, North Carolina
Essentials of Nephrology

Vasco Laginha Rolo, MD
Paediatric Consultant Anaesthetist
Anaesthetic Department
Birmingham Children's Hospital
Birmingham, United Kingdom
Anesthesia for Children Undergoing Heart Surgery

Jennifer E. Lam, DO
Associate Professor
Anesthesiology
Cincinnati Children's Hospital Medical Center
Cincinnati, Ohio
The Extremely Premature Infant (Micropremie) and Common Neonatal Emergencies

Mary Landrigan-Ossar, MD, PhD
Senior Associate in Perioperative Anesthesia
Anesthesia, Critical Care, and Pain Medicine
Boston Children's Hospital
Boston, Massachusetts;
Assistant Professor of Anaesthesia
Harvard Medical School
Boston, Massachusetts
Anesthesia Outside the Operating Room; Sedation for Diagnostic and Therapeutic Procedures Outside the Operating Room

Gregory J. Latham, MD
Professor
Anesthesiology and Pain Medicine
Seattle Children's Hospital, University of Washington
Seattle, Washington
Essentials of Hematology; Perioperative Management of the Oncology Patient

Amit Lehavi, MD, FANZCA
Department of Anesthesiology
Rambam Health Care Campus
Affiliated with Technion - The Ruth and Bruce Rappaport Faculty of Medicine
Haifa, Israel
Trauma and Mass Casualties

Jerrold Lerman, MD, FRCPC, FANZCA
Clinical Professor of Anesthesiology
Jacobs School of Medicine and Biomedical Sciences
Pediatric Anesthesiologist
John R. Oishei Children's Hospital
Buffalo, New York
Growth and Development; Pharmacology of Drugs Used in Children; General Abdominal and Urologic Surgery; Otorhinolaryngologic Procedures; Plastic and Reconstructive Surgery; Malignant Hyperthermia

Andreas W. Loepke, MD, PhD, FAAP
Professor of Anesthesiology & Critical Care
Perelman School of Medicine
University of Pennsylvania
Philadelphia, Pennsylvania;
Chief, Cardiac Anesthesiology
Department of Anesthesiology & Critical Care Medicine
Children's Hospital of Philadelphia
Philadelphia, Pennsylvania;
Endowed Chair in Pediatric Cardiac Anesthesiology
Children's Hospital of Philadelphia
Philadelphia, Pennsylvania
Surgery, Anesthesia, and the Immature Brain

Christine L. Mai, MD, MS-HPEd
Assistant Professor of Anaesthesia
Harvard Medical School
Department of Anesthesia, Critical Care and Pain Medicine
Massachusetts General Hospital
Boston, Massachusetts
Simulation in Pediatric Anesthesia

Iris Mandell, MD
Assistant Professor
Pediatrics/Pediatric Critical Care Medicine
Cohen Children's Medical Center
New Hyde Park, New York
Cardiopulmonary Resuscitation

Lizabeth D. Martin, MD
Associate Professor
Anesthesiology and Pain Medicine
Seattle Children's Hospital
Seattle, Washington
Essentials of Endocrinology

J.A. Jeevendra Martyn, MD, FTCA, FCCM
Professor of Anaesthesia
Harvard Medical School
Hellman Endowed Chair in Anesthesia
Director, Clinical & Biochemical Pharmacology Laboratory
Massachusetts General Hospital
Anesthetist-in-Chief
Shriners Hospital for Children
Boston, Massachusetts
Burn Injuries

Nuria Masip, MD, DESA
Consultant Anaesthetist
Alder Hey Children's Hospital,
Liverpool, United Kingdom
Medications for Hemostasis

Linda J. Mason, MD, FASA, FCAI
Professor of Anesthesiology and Pediatrics
Loma Linda University School of Medicine
Loma Linda, California;
Director of Pediatric Anesthesia
Department of Anesthesiology
Loma Linda University Children's Hospital
Loma Linda, California
Preoperative Evaluation, Premedication, and Induction of Anesthesia

Craig D. McClain, MD, MPH
Associate Professor of Anaesthesia
Department of Anesthesiology, Critical Care and Pain Medicine
Harvard Medical School
Boston, Massachusetts;
Senior Associate in Anesthesia
Department of Anesthesiology, Critical Care and Pain Medicine
Boston Children's Hospital
Boston, Massachusetts
Fluid Management; Pediatric Neurosurgical Anesthesia

Angus McEwan, MB ChB, FRCA
Department of Anaesthesia
Great Ormond Street Hospital
London, United Kingdom
Anesthesia for Children Undergoing Heart Surgery

Michael L. McManus, MD, MPH
Associate Professor of Anaesthesia (Pediatrics)
Harvard Medical School
Boston, Massachusetts;
Senior Associate and Vice-Chair
Department of Anesthesia, Critical Care, and Pain Medicine
Boston Children's Hospital
Boston, Massachusetts
Fluid Management

Julianne Mendoza, MD
Clinical Associate Professor
Department of Anesthesiology, Perioperative and Pain Medicine
Stanford University
Stanford, California
Organ Transplantation

Wanda C. Miller-Hance, MD, FACC, FASE
Adjunct Professor of Anesthesiology and Pediatrics
University of Texas Health Sciences Center at Houston,
    McGovern Medical School
Department of Anesthesiology, Critical Care, and Pain Medicine
Division of Pediatric Cardiology, Children's Heart Institute
Staff Physician, Memorial Herman Hospital
Houston, Texas
*Essentials of Cardiology; Anesthesia for Noncardiac Surgery in
    Children with Congenital Heart Disease*

Kimmo Murto, MD, FRCPC
Associate Professor
Department of Anesthesiology and Pain Medicine
University of Ottawa Faculty of Medicine,
Ottawa, Ontario, Canada;
Director of Research
Department of Anesthesiology and Pain Medicine
Children's Hospital of Eastern Ontario
Ottawa, Ontario, Canada
Otorhinolaryngologic Procedures

Marie-Cécile Nassogne, MD, PhD
Neurologie Pédiatrique et Maladies héréditaires du Métabolisme
Cliniques Universitaires Saint-Luc
UCLouvain
Bruxelles, Belgium
Essentials of Neurology and Neuromuscular Disorders

Pooja Nawathe, MD
Associate Professor
Pediatrics
Cedars-Sinai Medical Center
Los Angeles, California;
Cardiology
Smidt Heart Institute
Los Angeles, California;
Medical Director, Simulation
Pediatrics
Cedars-Sinai Medical Center
Los Angeles, California
Cardiopulmonary Resuscitation

Olivia Nelson, MD
Assistant Professor
Department of Anesthesiology and Critical Care Medicine
The Children's Hospital of Philadelphia and the Perelman School
    of Medicine at the University of Pennsylvania
Philadelphia, Pennsylvania
Plastic and Reconstructive Surgery

John H. Nichols, MD
Instructor in Anaesthesia
Chief, Division of Pediatric Anesthesia
Medical Director of Procedural Services
MassGeneral Hospital for Children
Department of Anesthesia, Critical Care, and Pain Medicine
Massachusetts General Hospital
Boston, Massachusetts
Burn Injuries

Bukola Ojo, MD
Assistant Professor
Anesthesiology and Pain Medicine
Seattle Children's Hospital
University of Washington
Seattle, Washington
Perioperative Management of the Oncology Patient

Vanessa A. Olbrecht, MD, MBA, FASA
Chair, Department of Anesthesiology and Perioperative Medicine
Nemours Children's Hospital, Delaware
Wilmington, DE;
Professor of Anesthesiology
Sidney Kimmel Medical College – Thomas Jefferson University
Philadelphia, PA
*Anesthesia Outside the Operating Room; Sedation for Diagnostic
and Therapeutic Procedures Outside the Operating Room*

Senthil Packiasabapathy, MD, MS
Assistant Professor of Clinical Anesthesia
Riley Hospital for Children
Indiana University School of Medicine
Indianapolis, Indiana
Pharmacogenomics

Stephanie J. Pan, MD
Clinical Assistant Professor
Department of Anesthesiology, Perioperative and Pain Medicine
Stanford University School of Medicine
Stanford, California
Anesthesia for Thoracic Surgery

David M. Polaner, MD, FAAP
Professor of Anesthesiology and Pain Medicine
University of Washington
Attending Pediatric Anesthesiologist
Seattle Children's Hospital
Seattle, Washington
Regional Anesthesia; Acute Pain

Casey A. Quinlan, MD
Assistant Professor
Anesthesiology and Pain Medicine
Seattle Children's Hospital
Seattle, Washington
Essentials of Endocrinology

Ellen Rawlinson, MA, MB, BChir, MRCP, FRCA, LLM
Doctor
Anaesthesia
Great Ormond Street Hospital
London, United Kingdom
Interventional Cardiology

Erinn T. Rhodes, MD, MPH, MS, MA
Director of Endocrinology Healthcare Research, Quality,
and Safety
Division of Endocrinology
Boston Children's Hospital
Boston, Massachusetts;
Assistant Professor of Pediatrics
Department of Pediatrics
Harvard Medical School
Boston, Massachusetts
Essentials of Endocrinology

Mark D. Rollins, MD, PhD
Professor
Department of Anesthesia and Perioperative Medicine
Mayo Clinic
Rochester, Minnesota
Fetal Intervention and the EXIT Procedure

Echo Rowe, MD
Clinical Associate Professor
Pediatric Anesthesiology
Stanford University
Stanford, California
Essentials of Endocrinology

Faith J. Ross, MD, MS
Associate Professor
Anesthesiology and Pain Medicine
Seattle Children's Hospital
University of Washington
Seattle, Washington
Perioperative Management of the Oncology Patient

Senthil Sadhasivam, MD, MPH, MBA, FASA
Executive Vice-Chair of Clinical Quality, Patient Safety and
Clinical Research
Tenured Professor, Department of Anesthesiology and
Perioperative Medicine
University of Pittsburgh Medical Center
Director of Perioperative Research, University of Pittsburgh
Director of Perioperative Genomics, University of Pittsburgh
Pittsburgh, Pennsylvania
Pharmacogenomics

Charles L. Schleien, MD, MBA
Philip Lanzkowsky Professor and Chair of Pediatrics
Pediatrics and Anesthesiology
Zucker School of Medicine at Hofstra/Northwell
New Hyde Park, New York;
Senior Vice President
Pediatrics
Cohen Children's Medical Center
New Hyde Park, New York
Cardiopulmonary Resuscitation

Annette Y. Schure, MD, DEAA
Senior Associate in Cardiac Anesthesia
Program Director Pediatric Cardiac Anesthesiology Fellowship
Department of Anesthesiology, Critical Care and Pain Medicine
Boston Children's Hospital;
Assistant Professor of Anaesthesia
Harvard Medical School
Boston, Massachusetts
Cardiac Physiology and Pharmacology

Luis Sequera-Ramos, MD
Assistant Professor of Anesthesiology and Critical Care
Perelman School of Medicine at the University of Pennsylvania
The Children's Hospital of Philadelphia
Philadelphia, Pennsylvania
The Pediatric Airway

Nadav Sheffy, MD
Department of Anesthesia and Pain Medicine
Rabin Medical Center, Beilinson Hospital
Affiliated with Tel Aviv University School of Medicine
Petah Tikva, Israel
Trauma and Mass Casualties

Eliahu Simhi, MD
The Anesthesia Department and Surgical Suite
Schneider Children's Medical Center of Israel
Affiliated with Tel Aviv University School of Medicine
Petah Tikva, Israel
Trauma and Mass Casualties

Justin J. Skowno, MBChB, DA, FCA(SA), FANZCA, PhD
Associate Professor
Discipline of Child and Adolescent Health, Faculty of Medicine
    and Health
University of Sydney
Sydney, Australia;
Department of Anaesthesia
The Children's Hospital at Westmead
Sydney Children's Hospital's Network
Sydney, Australia
Pediatric Equipment and Monitoring

Steven R. Sloan, MD, PhD
Associate Professor, Harvard Medical School
Blood Bank Medical Director, Boston Children's Hospital
Now Clinical Program Director, Hematology, CSL Behring,
Boston, Massachusetts
*Strategies for Blood Product Management, Reducing Transfusions,
    and Massive Blood Transfusion*

Sulpicio G. Soriano, MD
Professor of Anaesthesia
Department of Anaesthesia
Harvard Medical School
Boston, Massachusetts;
Endowed Chair in Pediatric Neuroanesthesia
Anesthesiology, Perioperative and Pain Medicine
Boston Children's Hospital
Boston, Massachusetts
Pediatric Neurosurgical Anesthesia

James P. Spaeth, MD
Chief, Pediatric Anesthesia
Children's Hospital New Orleans
Professor of Anesthesiology, Tulane University School of Medicine
Clinical Professor of Anesthesiology
LSU Health New Orleans
New Orleans, Louisiana
*The Extremely Premature Infant (Micropremie) and Common
    Neonatal Emergencies*

James E. Squires, MD, MS
Associate Professor of Pediatrics
Director, Pediatric Transplant Hepatology Fellowship Program
Associate Director of Hepatology
Division of Gastroenterology, Hepatology and Nutrition
Children's Hospital of Pittsburgh,
Pittsburgh, Pennsylvania
Essentials of Hepatology

Abhinash Srivatsa, MBBS
Attending Physician
Endocrinology
Boston Children's Hospital
Boston, Massachusetts;
Assistant Professor
Pediatrics
Harvard Medical School
Boston, Massachusetts
Essentials of Endocrinology

Mary Lyn Stein, MD, FAAP
Department of Anesthesiology, Critical Care, and Pain Medicine
Boston Children's Hospital
Assistant Professor of Anaesthesia
Harvard Medical School
Boston, Massachusetts
The Pediatric Airway

Daniel Stocki, MD
Division of Anesthesia, Pain and Intensive Care
Tel Aviv Sourasky Medical Center Ichilov
Affiliated with Tel Aviv University School of Medicine
Tel Aviv, Israel
Trauma and Mass Casualties

Paul A. Stricker, MD
Professor of Anesthesiology and Critical Care
Department of Anesthesiology and Critical Care Medicine
The Children's Hospital of Philadelphia and the Perelman School
    of Medicine at the University of Pennsylvania
Philadelphia, Pennsylvania
The Pediatric Airway; Plastic and Reconstructive Surgery

Rani Sunder, MD, DNB
Associate Professor
Anesthesiology and Pain Medicine
Seattle Children's Hospital
Seattle, Washington
Regional Anesthesia

Santhanam Suresh, MD, MBA, FAAP
Arthur C. King Professor & Senior Vice-President
Pediatric Anesthesiology
Ann & Robert H Lurie Childrens Hospital of Chicago
Chicago, Illinois;
Professor
Anesthesiology & Pediatrics
Northwestern Feinberg School of Medicine
Chicago, Illinois
Regional Anesthesia

Alexandra Szabova, MD, MEd
Associate Professor
Clinical Anesthesia and Pediatrics
Department of Anesthesiology
Cincinnati Children's Hospital Medical Center
Cincinnati, Ohio
Chronic Pain

Andreas H. Taenzer, MD
Associate Professor
Department of Anesthesiology
Children's Hospital at Dartmouth
Lebanon, New Hampshire
The Postanesthesia Care Unit and Beyond

Carol Vetterly, PharmD, BCPPS
Director of Pharmacy
Department of Pharmacy
UPMC Children's Hospital
Pittsburgh, Pennsylvania
Essentials of Hepatology

Francis Veyckemans, MD
Honorary Professor, Faculty of Medicine
UCLouvain
Bruxelles, Belgium
Essentials of Neurology and Neuromuscular Disorders

David B. Waisel, MD
Professor of Anesthesiology
Chief Division of Pediatric Anesthesia, Anesthesiology
Yale School of Medicine
New Haven, Connecticut
Ethical Issues in Pediatric Anesthesiology

Benjamin Walker, MD
Professor (CHS) and Division Chief, Pediatric Anesthesiology
Department of Anesthesiology, UWSMPH
Medical Director of Perioperative Services, American Family
    Children's Hospital
Madison, Wisconsin
Acute Pain

Jue Teresa Wang, MD
Instructor in Anaesthesia
Harvard Medical School;
Associate in Perioperative Anesthesia
Department of Anesthesiology, Critical Care, and Pain Medicine
Boston Children's Hospital
Boston, Massachusetts
Pediatric Neurosurgical Anesthesia

John C. Welch, DNP, MS, CRNA
Senior Nurse Anesthetist
Department of Anesthesiology, Critical Care, & Pain Medicine
Boston Children's Hospital
Boston, Massachusetts;
Associate Clinical Professor & Director of Nurse Anesthesia
    Program
College of Nursing
The Ohio State University
Senior Director of Flagships & Special Projects
Partners In Health
Boston, Massachusetts
Infectious Disease Considerations for the Operating Room

Niall C. Wilton, MB ChB, MRCP, FRCA
Department of Paediatric Anaesthesia
Starship Children's Hospital
Auckland, New Zealand
Orthopedic and Spine Surgery

Joseph I. Wolfsdorf, MB, BCh
Boston Children's Hospital Chair in Endocrinology
Division of Endocrinology
Boston Children's Hospital
Boston, Massachusetts;
Professor of Pediatrics
Harvard Medical School
Boston, Massachusetts
Essentials of Endocrinology

Peggy Yip, BHB, MB ChB, FANZCA
Paediatric Anaesthesia
Starship Children's Hospital
Auckland, New Zealand
Procedures for Vascular Access

PREFACE

A Practice of Anesthesia for Infants and Children, Seventh Edition, has continued to evolve from its humble beginnings in 1986 with only 304 pages in the first edition to more than 1100 pages in this, the seventh edition. Of the founding coeditors, Dr. Nishan Goudsouzian has retired from practice and Dr. I. David Todres and Dr. John F. Ryan have passed. Two new coeditors joined to fill the vacancies left by these giants in our field: Dr. Jerrold Lerman joined for the fourth edition and Dr. Brian J Anderson for the fifth edition.

The current edition includes 115 authors from five continents, 53 of whom are new contributors. The book continues to be a highly respected, evidence-based synopsis of the practice of pediatric anesthesia reflecting a broad perspective of reasoning and practice from a host of international experts. As in past editions, many of the current authors are board certified in pediatrics and anesthesiology, surgery, nursing, and a number of pediatric subspecialties, enhancing our understanding of hematology, pulmonology, cardiology, nephrology, hepatology, and neurology. All chapters are meticulously referenced with up to a dozen annotated references that reflect pivotal publications on the topic of the chapter in the printed version with the full list of references at Elsevier eBooks+ with hypertext links to PubMed.org.

To navigate this edition more easily, we have continued several notable changes that we introduced in the last edition. The book is divided into 10 color-coded sections: Introduction, Drug and Fluid Therapy, The Chest, The Heart, The Brain and Glands, The Abdomen, Other Surgeries, Emergencies, Pain, and Special Topics. This format allows the reader to identify sections under broad headings and then within each section, to find specific subjects of interest. We have again sought contributions from pediatric subspecialists who share their perspectives and insights and paired them with a pediatric anesthesiologist to ensure that the basic science is intertwined with a practical anesthesiology clinical perspective. These are the "Essentials" chapters.

Our text is accompanied by a website that contains many supplemental pictures, tables, figures, and video clips that will enhance the readers' experiences, particularly for performing regional anesthesia and vascular access procedures. A pocket reference card provides general recommendations for doses of commonly used medications by weight and other useful guides such as appropriately sized airway devices, and other quick references.

As with previous editions of our textbook, the current revision involved quite a journey reflecting a microcosm of the world and life in general with many contributors having experienced challenges such as loss of loved ones, personal crises, illness, and others including the stress of the COVID-19 pandemic during the writing of their chapters. Despite these obstacles, our authors have succeeded in crafting masterful chapters to create what we hope you will agree is an up-to-date state of the art text in pediatric anesthesia; the entire text and E-only content is also available for purchase as an eBook.

Once again, while assembling this new edition, the editors spent many days, evenings, and weekends debating controversial issues and crafting the language of the chapters such that all chapters were edited and reviewed by all three editors and common ground reached. This is an especially useful exercise since it improves the readability of the text and represents a fusion of the USA, Canadian, and New Zealand approaches to pediatric anesthesia that combines our global experience and understanding.

We believe that *A Practice of Anesthesia for Infants and Children, Seventh edition*, continues to provide a framework for residency and fellowship training in pediatric anesthesia globally and will continue to be a valuable resource for passing the subspecialty boards in pediatric anesthesiology as well as a resource for practicing pediatric anesthesiologists and other pediatric care providers around the world. When we look back to the first edition of Leigh and Belton's Pediatric Anesthesia (1948), the editors stated that *"This book ....discusses many of the methods which the authors have employed satisfactorily over a period of years"*. Similarly, Smith stated in his first edition of Smith's Anesthesia for Infants and Children (1959) that *"My intention in writing this book is to organize and evaluate this information and to add what I can from first-hand experience and observation."* Dripps, Eckenhoff, & Vandam's Introduction to Anesthesia (1977), the first anesthesia textbook CJC used as a resident, stated that *"Much of the teaching of anesthesia is by word of mouth....This is the lore of anesthesia that must be passed on from individual to individual."*

We hope that with this edition you will appreciate that as pediatric anesthesiologists there are many important aspects of our practice that set us aside from other specialists:

We love children.
We are not bothered by the sound of a crying child.
We are happy to pick up and comfort the crying child.
We enjoy families.
We empathize and provide them comfort.
We provide them with guidance during this stressful time.
We protect their child from harm.
We provide their child with analgesia and amnesia.
We enjoy teaching those who will carry our specialty into the future and further advance the care of our most vulnerable population.

This is what we do and what makes us pediatric anesthesiologists. In this book, we continue the mantra of the early texts on pediatric anesthesia and pass forward the lore and the tricks of the trade, and teach the needed skills to our students and colleagues.

ACKNOWLEDGMENTS

We wish you think our wives, husbands, significant others, children, friends, secretaries, and fellow staff members who lent their support to this wonderful international family of experts that has come together to produce the seventh edition of *A Practice of Anesthesia for Infants and Children*. It is also important to recognize and thank the departments of anesthesiology, pediatrics, surgery, and internal medicine around the world who supported the academic endeavors of their staff and thus made it possible for them to contribute to this seventh edition.

We thank Elsevier for their continued support of international education in less medically advanced countries by providing copies of *A Practice of Anesthesia for Infants and Children* on a yearly basis to the pediatric anesthesia fellows participating in the World Federation of Societies of Anaesthesiologists pediatric anesthesia fellowship programs. This continued effort helps to support young pediatric anesthesia fellowships around the world. It is through such international endeavors that we ensure the global availability of the most recent advances in our specialty, especially in the less medically advanced venues.

Charles J. Coté
Jerrold Lerman
Brian J. Anderson

CONTENTS

SECTION I: INTRODUCTION

1. **Growth and Development** — 1
   Charles J. Coté, Brian J. Anderson, and Jerrold Lerman
2. **Preoperative Evaluation, Premedication, and Induction of Anesthesia** — 22
   Elizabeth A. Ghazal, Harmony Carter, Linda J. Mason, and Charles J. Coté
3. **Ethical Issues in Pediatric Anesthesiology** — 65
   David B. Waisel and Alyssa M. Burgart

SECTION II: DRUG AND FLUID THERAPY

4. **Pharmacogenomics** — 79
   Senthil Packiasabapathy, Vidya Chidambaran, and Senthilkumar Sadhasivam
5. **Pharmacology of Drugs Used in Children** — 100
   Brian J. Anderson, Jerrold Lerman, and Charles J. Coté
6. **Total Intravenous Anesthesia and Target-Controlled Infusion** — 190
   Brian J. Anderson and James Houghton
7. **Fluid Management** — 216
   Cathie T. Jones, Craig D. McClain, and Michael L. McManus
8. **Essentials of Hematology** — 236
   Trevor L. Adams, Siri Kanmanthreddy, Michael J. Eisses, M.A. Bender, and Gregory J. Latham
9. **Perioperative Management of the Oncology Patient** — 261
   Bukola Ojo, Faith J. Ross, and Gregory J. Latham
10. **Strategies for Blood Product Management, Reducing Transfusions, and Massive Blood Transfusion** — 278
    Charles J. Coté, Eric F. Grabowski, and Steven R. Sloan

SECTION III: THE CHEST

11. **Essentials of Pulmonology** — 307
    Paul G. Firth and T. Bernard Kinane
12. **The Pediatric Airway** — 324
    Mary Lyn Stein, Luis Sequera-Ramos, John E. Fiadjoe, Paul A. Stricker, and Charles J. Coté
13. **Anesthesia for Thoracic Surgery** — 370
    Gregory B. Hammer and Stephanie J. Pan

SECTION IV: THE HEART

14. **Essentials of Cardiology** — 391
    Wanda C. Miller-Hance and Ralph Gertler

15. **Anesthesia for Children Undergoing Heart Surgery** — 433
    Angus McEwan and Vasco Laginha Rolo
16. **Cardiac Physiology and Pharmacology** — 468
    Annette Y. Schure and James A. DiNardo
17. **Cardiopulmonary Bypass and Management** — 504
    Ralph Gertler, Erin A. Gottlieb, and Dean B. Andropoulos
18. **Medications for Hemostasis** — 529
    Philip Arnold and Nuria Masip
19. **Mechanical Circulatory Support** — 549
    Adam C. Adler, Rania K. Abbasi, and Laura K. Berenstain
20. **Interventional Cardiology** — 573
    Ellen Rawlinson
21. **Anesthesia for Noncardiac Surgery in Children With Congenital Heart Disease** — 587
    Wanda C. Miller-Hance

SECTION V: THE BRAIN AND GLANDS

22. **Essentials of Neurology and Neuromuscular Disorders** — 619
    Marie-Agnès Docquier, Marie-Cécile Nassogne, and Francis Veyckemans
23. **Surgery, Anesthesia, and the Immature Brain** — 650
    Andreas W. Loepke and Andrew J. Davidson
24. **Pediatric Neurosurgical Anesthesia** — 678
    Craig D. McClain, Jue Teresa Wang, Sulpicio G. Soriano, and Carolyn G. Butler
25. **Essentials of Endocrinology** — 705
    Lizabeth D. Martin, Erinn T. Rhodes, Casey A. Quinlan, Abhinash Srivatsa, Echo Rowe, and Joseph I. Wolfsdorf

SECTION VI: THE ABDOMEN

26. **Essentials of Nephrology** — 729
    Reeti Kumar, Annabelle N. Chua, and Warwick A. Ames
27. **General Abdominal and Urologic Surgery** — 745
    Tom G. Hansen and Jerrold Lerman
28. **Essentials of Hepatology** — 768
    James E. Squires, Carol Vetterly, and Daniela Damian
29. **Organ Transplantation** — 775
    Julianne Mendoza and Kaitlin M. Flannery

SECTION VII: OTHER SURGERIES

30. **Orthopedic and Spine Surgery** — 809
    Niall C. Wilton and Brian J. Anderson

31. Otorhinolaryngologic Procedures   841
Kimmo Murto, Michele M. Carr, and Jerrold Lerman

32. Ophthalmologic Surgery   900
*Samuel A. Hunter, William Anninger, and
Philip D. Bailey, Jr.*

33. Plastic and Reconstructive Surgery   914
*Olivia Nelson, Paul A. Stricker, John E. Fiadjoe, and
Jerrold Lerman*

34. Burn Injuries   932
*John H. Nichols, Charles J. Coté, and
J.A. Jeevendra Martyn*

SECTION VIII: EMERGENCIES

**35. The Extremely Premature Infant (Micropremie) and
Common Neonatal Emergencies**   953
James P. Spaeth and Jennifer E. Lam

36. Fetal Intervention and the EXIT Procedure   982
Marla B. Ferschl and Mark D. Rollins

37. Trauma and Mass Casualties   1000
*Daniel Stocki, Daniel Braunold, Yitzhak Brzezinski Sinai,
Nadav Sheffy, Eliahu Simhi, and Amit Lehavi*

38. Cardiopulmonary Resuscitation   1016
Pooja Nawathe, Iris Mandell, and Charles L. Schleien

39. Malignant Hyperthermia   1030
Jerrold Lerman

SECTION IX: PAIN

40. Regional Anesthesia   1053
*David M. Polaner, Manoj Kumar Karmakar,
Rani Sunder, Santhanam Suresh, and Charles J. Coté*

41. Acute Pain   1134
*Jared R. E. Hylton, Benjamin Walker, and
David M. Polaner*

42. Chronic Pain   1181
*Alexandra Szabova, Kenneth Goldschneider,
and Motaz Awad*

SECTION X: SPECIAL TOPICS

43. Anesthesia Outside the Operating Room   1195
*Vanessa A. Olbrecht, Joseph P. Cravero, and
Mary Landrigan-Ossar*

**44. Sedation for Diagnostic and Therapeutic Procedures
Outside the Operating Room**   1215
*Vanessa A. Olbrecht, Charles J. Coté, Joseph P. Cravero, and
Mary Landrigan-Ossar*

45. The Post Anesthesia Care Unit and Beyond   1238
*Timothy M. Earley, Jeana E. Havidich, and
Andreas H. Taenzer*

46. Procedures for Vascular Access   1255
Peggy Yip and Charles J. Coté

**47. Infectious Disease Considerations for the
Operating Room**   1278
*Andre L. Jaichenco Sr., Luciana Cavalcanti Lima, and
John C. Welch*

48. Pediatric Anesthesia in Developing Countries   1299
Adrian T. Bösenberg

49. Pediatric Equipment and Monitoring   1314
Justin J. Skowno and Charles J. Coté

50. Simulation in Pediatric Anesthesia   1347
*A. Rebecca L. Hamilton, Jeffrey B. Cooper, and
Christine L. Mai*

Index   1357

VIDEO CONTENTS

CHAPTER 2 PREOPERATIVE EVALUATION, PREMEDICATION, AND INDUCTION OF ANESTHESIA

Video 2.1   Inhalation Induction of Anesthesia With Parents
Video 2.2   Inhalation Induction of Anesthesia Without Parents
Video 2.3   Inhalation Induction of Anesthesia With a Child-Life Specialist
Video 2.4   Single-Breath Induction

CHAPTER 5 PHARMACOLOGY OF DRUGS USED IN CHILDREN

Video 5.1   Nystagmus After Ketamine Administration

CHAPTER 12 THE PEDIATRIC AIRWAY

Video 12.1   The Pediatric Airway
Video 12.2A   Effects of Jaw Thrust on Airway
Video 12.2B   Effects of Jaw Thrust at the Pinna vs Jaw Thrust at the Angle of the Mandible
Video 12.3   Laryngeal Web
Video 12.4   Laryngeal Edema
Video 12.5   Stretching of the Trachea
Video 12.6   Continuous Ventilation During Intubation With Air-Q LMA
Video 12.7   Traditional Insertion Technique for the Laryngeal Mask Airway
Video 12.8   Nontraditional Laryngeal Mask Airway Insertion Technique
Video 12.9   Complete Tracheal Rings
Video 12.10   Modified Nasal Airway
Video 12.11   Awake Laryngeal Mask Insertion
Video 12.12   Fiberoptic Intubation
Video 12.13   Fiberoptic Intubation in Child With Cri du Chat Syndrome
Video 12.14   GlideScope Intubation
Video 12.15   Intubation With Airtraq
Video 12.16   Shikani Optical Stylet
Video 12.17   Laryngeal Mask Airway as a Conduit for Intubation
Video 12.18   Pilot Balloon Reconstruction After Fiberoptic Intubation Through Classic Laryngeal Mask Airway

CHAPTER 14 ESSENTIALS OF CARDIOLOGY

Video 14.1   Bicuspid Aortic Valve (Short-Axis View)
Video 14.2   Ventricular Septal Defects (Four-Chamber View)
Video 14.3   Secundum Atrial Septal Defect (Four-Chamber View)
Video 14.4A   Dilated Cardiomyopathy (Long-Axis View)
Video 14.4B   Dilated Cardiomyopathy (Short-Axis View)
Video 14.5A   Hypertrophic Cardiomyopathy (Long-Axis View)
Video 14.5B   Hypertrophic Cardiomyopathy (Short-Axis View)
Video 14.6A   Asymmetric Septal Hypertrophy (Long-Axis View)
Video 14.6B   Asymmetric Septal Hypertrophy (Short-Axis View)
Video 14.7   Restrictive Cardiomyopathy (Four-Chamber View)
Video 14.8A   Bacterial Endocarditis of Mitral Valve (TEE, Four-Chamber View)
Video 14.8B   Fungal Endocarditis of Tricuspid Valve (TEE, Four-Chamber View)
Video 14.9   Left Atrial Myxoma (Four-Chamber View)
Video 14.10   Atrioventricular Septal Defect (TEE, Four-Chamber View)
Video 14.11   Two-Dimensional Echocardiogram (Left Ventricular Long-Axis View)
Video 14.12   Doppler Echocardiography (Color and Spectral Doppler)
Video 14.13   Assessment of Right Ventricular/Pulmonary Artery Systolic Pressure (Doppler Echocardiography)
Video 14.14   Magnetic Resonance Imaging-Aortic Coarctation
Video 14.15   Magnetic Resonance Imaging-Total Anomalous Pulmonary Venous Return
Video 14.16   Transcatheter Closure of Secundum Atrial Septal Defect (TEE)
Video 14.17A   Angiogram-Aortic Coarctation (AP Projection)
Video 14.17B   Angiogram-Aortic Coarctation (Lateral Projection)

CHAPTER 24 PEDIATRIC NEUROSURGICAL ANESTHESIA

Video 24.1   Endoscopic Fenestration of Cyst and Ventriculostomy

CHAPTER 27 GENERAL ABDOMINAL AND UROLOGIC SURGERY

Video 27.1   Robotic-Assisted Laparoscopic Ureteral Reimplantation
Video 27.2   Robotic-Assisted Laparoscopic Pyeloplasty

CHAPTER 30 ORTHOPEDIC AND SPINE SURGERY

Video 30.1   Patient Positioning for Scoliosis Surgery

CHAPTER 34 BURN INJURIES

Video 34.1   Tangential Excision
Video 34.2   Skin Harvest
Video 34.3   Full-Thickness Excision
Video 34.4   Saline with Epinephrine Injection to Reduce Blood Loss for Both Excision and Skin Harvest
Video 34.5   Music Therapy During Preparation for Anesthesia

CHAPTER 35 THE EXTREMELY PREMATURE INFANT (MICROPREMIE) AND COMMON NEONATAL EMERGENCIES

Video 35.1   Microlaryngoscopy/Bronchoscopy of Subglottic Hemangioma in Infant With PHACES Syndrome
Video 35.2   Microlaryngoscopy/Bronchoscopy of Tracheoesophageal Fistula Near the Carina With Placement of Catheter Into the Fistula
Video 35.3   Video of a Laparoscopic Pyloromyotomy

CHAPTER 40 REGIONAL ANESTHESIA

Video 40.1   Popliteal Block with Nerve Stimulator Showing Movement of Toes
Video 40.2   Sonoanatomy of the Sacrum Relevant for Caudal Epidural Injection in Children
Video 40.3   Ultrasound-Guided Caudal Epidural Injection: In-plane Approach
Video 40.4   Spinal Sonographic Changes During a Single-Shot Caudal Epidural Injection in a Neonate
Video 40.5   Single Shot Caudal Epidural Block
Video 40.6   Caudal Catheter Insertion
Video 40.7   Caudal Catheter Dressing Application
Video 40.8   Ultrasound Localization of a Lumbar Epidural Catheter in Children
Video 40.9   Supraorbital Nerve Block
Video 40.10   Greater Occipital Nerve Block
Video 40.11   Infraorbital Nerve Block
Video 40.12   Great Auricular Nerve Block
Video 40.13   Nerve of Arnold Block
Video 40.14   Ultrasound-Guided Ilioinguinal and Iliohypogastric Nerve Block
Video 40.15   Ultrasound-Guided Ilioinguinal Nerve Block
Video 40.16   Ultrasound-Guided Transverse Abdominis Plane (Lateral-TAP) Block
Video 40.17   Ultrasound-Guided Quadratus Lumborum Block
Video 40.18   Thoracic Paravertebral Sonography: The Transverse Scan Sequence
Video 40.19   Ultrasound-Guided Thoracic Paravertebral Block
Video 40.20   Ultrasound-Guided Brachial Plexus Block: Axillary Approach
Video 40.21   Ultrasound-Guided Radial Nerve Block at the Axillary Plexus
Video 40.22   Ultrasound- and Nerve-Stimulator–Guided Subgluteal Sciatic Nerve Block
Video 40.23   Finger Motions of Each Branch of the Brachial Plexus with Nerve Stimulator
Video 40.24   Ultrasound-Guided Brachial Plexus Block: Infraclavicular Approach
Video 40.25   Ultrasound-Guided Selective Upper Extremity Nerve Block: Median and Ulnar Nerve
Video 40.26   Ultrasound-Guided Sciatic Nerve Block at the Subgluteal Space
Video 40.27   Subgluteal Sciatic Ultrasound Nerve Block
Video 40.28   Ultrasound-Guided Mid-Thigh Saphenous Nerve Block
Video 40.29   Ultrasound-Guided Rectus Sheath Block
Video 40.30   Lateral Femoral Cutaneous Nerve Block
Video 40.31   Ultrasound-Guided Femoral Nerve Block

CHAPTER 44 SEDATION FOR DIAGNOSTIC AND THERAPEUTIC PROCEDURES OUTSIDE THE OPERATING ROOM

Video 44.1   Minimal Sedation (Axiolysis)
Video 44.2   Moderate Sedation
Video 44.3   Deep Sedation
Video 44.4   Anesthesia (Not Sedation)
Video 44.5   Sedation Documentation Using Children's National Medical Center Electronic Medical Record

CHAPTER 45 THE POSTANESTHESIA CARE UNIT AND BEYOND

Video 45.1   Emergence Delirium (Before Treatment)
Video 45.2   Emergence Delirium (After Treatment)

CHAPTER 46 PROCEDURES FOR VASCULAR ACCESS

Video 46.1   Central Venous Cannulation of Internal Jugular Vein Using Ultrasound
Video 46.2   Ultrasound-Guided Central Line Placement
Video 46.3   Arterial Line

CHAPTER 47 INFECTIOUS DISEASE CONSIDERATIONS FOR THE OPERATING ROOM

Video 47.1   Extubation Over Face Mask in COVID-19 Patient

CHAPTER 48 PEDIATRIC ANESTHESIA IN DEVELOPING COUNTRIES

Video 48.1   DiaMedica Portable Anesthesia (DPA) O_2 + ISO Vaporizer
Video 48.2   Glastovent Anesthesia Machine
Video 48.3   DiaMedica Portable Anesthesia Machine
Video 48.4   Helix Portable Ventilators
Video 48.5   Glostavent Helix Anesthesia Machine
Video 48.6   Oxygen Reservoir System Description

CHAPTER 50 SIMULATION IN PEDIATRIC ANESTHESIA

Video 50.1   Simulation Technologies
Video 50.2   Elements of High-Fidelity Simulation

Growth and Development

1

CHARLES J. COTÉ, BRIAN J. ANDERSON, AND JERROLD LERMAN

Normal and Abnormal Growth and Maturation
Gestational Age Assessment
Weight and Length
Head Circumference
Face
Teeth
Airway and Respiratory System
Upper Airway Development
Respiratory System Development
Transition to Air Breathing
Mechanics of Breathing
Airway Dynamics
Cardiovascular System
Heart Rate
Blood Pressure
Cardiac Output
Normal Electrocardiographic Findings

Renal System
Digestive and Endocrine System
Hepatic System
Gastrointestinal Tract
Pancreas
Hematopoietic and Immunologic System
Hemoglobin
Leukocytes and Immunology
Platelets
Coagulation
Polycythemia
Neurologic Development and Cognitive Development Issues
Neurologic Development
Interactions With the External World During Growth and Development
The Skin and Thermoregulation
Annotated References

HUMAN GROWTH IS A COMPLEX succession of phenomena that begins with the fusion of two cells and matures by 9 months into a complex organism known as a neonate that is capable of existing outside the mother. This complex process not only produces a human being; it also traces the history of species with each and every fetus through embryology. Development is more than a simple increase in the number of cells; it includes interactions between the cells and interactions between the fetus and the environment, effects that are modulated by intracellular and intercellular signaling.[1]

It is incumbent upon the physician to understand the developmental changes that occur to the fetus and infant over time, and how these changes affect both responses to diseases and to drug pharmacokinetics and pharmacodynamics.

Normal and Abnormal Growth and Maturation

Growth is the quantitative increase in size of the body, whereas maturation is the genetic, biologic, and physical development of the child. Both phenomena continue throughout pregnancy and after birth. Prenatal growth is the most important phase in development, comprising organogenesis in the first 8 weeks (embryonic growth), followed by the functional development of organ systems and maturation of the fetus (fetal growth). Rapid growth occurs particularly in the second trimester; a major increase in weight from subcutaneous tissue and muscle mass occurs in the third trimester. The duration of gestation and the weight of an infant are important correlates that vary with ethnicity, maternal environment, and pathology (Table 1.1).[2,3]

By convention, the term *prematurity* has been applied to neonates who weigh less than 2500 grams at birth. However, the designation *preterm neonate* may be more appropriate, defined as an infant born before 37 completed weeks of gestation. A *term or full-term neonate* is an infant born between 37 and 42 completed weeks of gestation. *A post-term neonate* is one born after 42 completed weeks of gestation.

Preterm neonates are further classified according to their actual birth weight. A low-birth-weight (LBW) neonate weighs less than 2500 grams regardless of the duration of the pregnancy. A very-low-birth-weight (VLBW) neonate weighs less than 1500 grams, and an extremely low-birth-weight neonate weighs less than 1000 grams. Neonates that weigh less than 750 grams at birth are referred to as "*micropremies*." The Tiniest Babies Registry has recorded 291 survivors with birth weights 212 to 399 grams but long-term outcomes are unavailable.[4] Very limited information has been published regarding the anesthetic management of this vulnerable micropremie subpopulation of neonates (see Chapter 35).[5] Common neonatal problems as they relate to age and birth weight are presented in Table 1.2.

After birth, the rapid physical growth continues during the first 6 months of extrauterine life, and slows by 2 years of age. Physical growth then accelerates a second time during the pubertal period. Assessment of growth is measured by changes in weight, length, and head circumference. Percentile charts[6,7] are valuable for monitoring the child's growth and development. A simple way to remember how rapidly infants grow is that birth weight doubles by 6 months of age and triples by 1 year; length doubles by 4 years of age. This scale, however, does not consistently affect all organs or organ functions. It is important to correctly assess the child's stage of development because any substantial deviations warrant an investigation of the cause. For example, height and weight are important metrics of maturity, although other factors may also impact maturity,[8] including those that cause excessive weight gain or prevent normal weight gain (Figs. 1.1 and 1.2).

Gestational Age Assessment

The gestational age (GA) of an infant may be assessed in one of three ways. The most accurate means of assessing gestational age is by measuring the crown-rump length of the fetus during a first-trimester ultrasonographic examination.[9] A second method involves calculating gestational age from the first day of the mother's last menstrual period, but this is commonly inaccurate and can result in errors. Alternately, the Dubowitz scoring system is a well-accepted method that combines neurologic and physical criteria of the neonate to provide an accurate assessment of gestational age. Compared with ultrasound, the Dubowitz score rated 95% of gestational age within 2.6 weeks, whereas the Ballard score overestimated gestational age by 0.4 weeks and dated pregnancies within ± 4.2 weeks.[10–12] A summary of the significant neurologic and physical signs of maturity is presented in Table 1.3.

TABLE 1.1	The Relationship of Gestational Age to Weight
Gestation (weeks)	**Mean Weight (g)**
28	1165 ± 109
32	1760 ± 128
36	2621 ± 274
40 (full term)	3351 ± 448

Data from Naeye RL, Dixon JB. Distortions in fetal growth. *Pediatr Res*. 1978;12:987-991.

TABLE 1.2	Common Neonatal Problems With Respect to Weight and Gestation	
Gestation	**Relative Weight**	**Neonatal Problems at Increased Incidence**
Preterm (<37 weeks)	SGA	Respiratory distress syndrome
		Apnea
		Perinatal depression
		Hypoglycemia
		Polycythemia
		Hypocalcemia
		Hypomagnesemia
		Hyperbilirubinemia
		Viral infection
		Thrombocytopenia
		Congenital anomalies
		Maternal drug addiction
		Fetal alcohol syndrome
	AGA	Respiratory distress syndrome
		Apnea
		Hypoglycemia
		Hypocalcemia
		Hypomagnesemia
		Hyperbilirubinemia
	LGA	Respiratory distress syndrome
		Hypoglycemia: infant of a diabetic mother
		Apnea
		Hypocalcemia
		Hypomagnesemia
		Hyperbilirubinemia
Normal (37–42 weeks)	SGA	Congenital anomalies
		Viral infection
		Thrombocytopenia
		Maternal drug addiction
		Perinatal depression
		Hypoglycemia
	AGA	—
	LGA	Birth trauma
		Hyperbilirubinemia
		Hypoglycemia: infant of a diabetic mother
Postmature (>42 weeks)	SGA	Meconium aspiration syndrome
		Congenital anomalies
		Viral infection
		Thrombocytopenia
		Maternal drug addiction
		Perinatal depression
		Aspiration pneumonia
		Hypoglycemia
	AGA	—
	LGA	Birth trauma
		Hyperbilirubinemia
		Hypoglycemia: infant of a diabetic mother

AGA, Appropriate for gestational age; *LGA*, large for gestational age; *SGA*, small for gestational age.

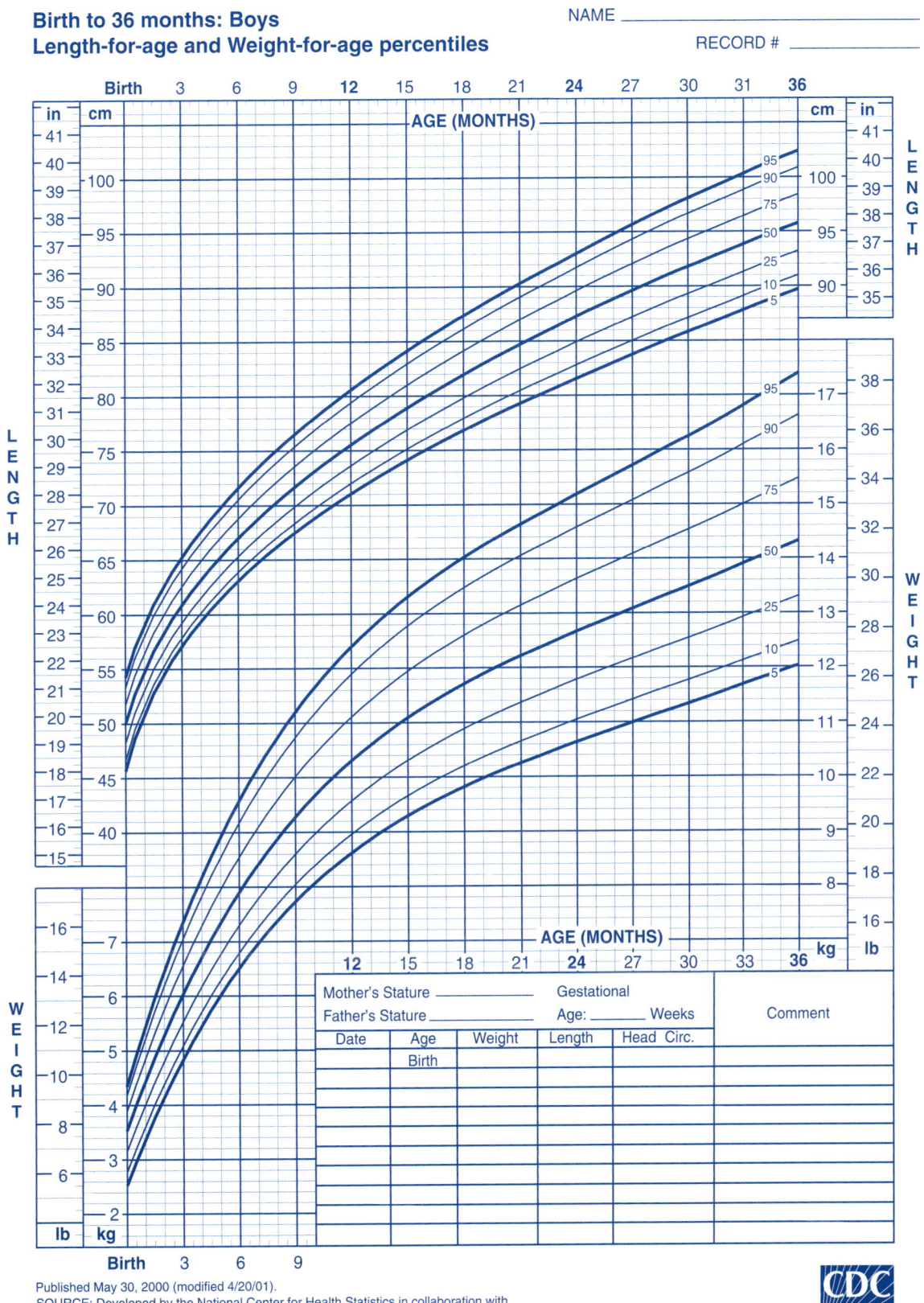

Birth to 36 months: Boys
Length-for-age and Weight-for-age percentiles

NAME _____

RECORD # _____

Published May 30, 2000 (modified 4/20/01).
SOURCE: Developed by the National Center for Health Statistics in collaboration with
the National Center for Chronic Disease Prevention and Health Promotion (2000).
http://www.cdc.gov/growthcharts

FIGURE 1.1 Growth Chart for Boys. (From the National Center for Chronic Disease Prevention and Health Promotion. 2000. https://www.cdc.gov/growthcharts.)

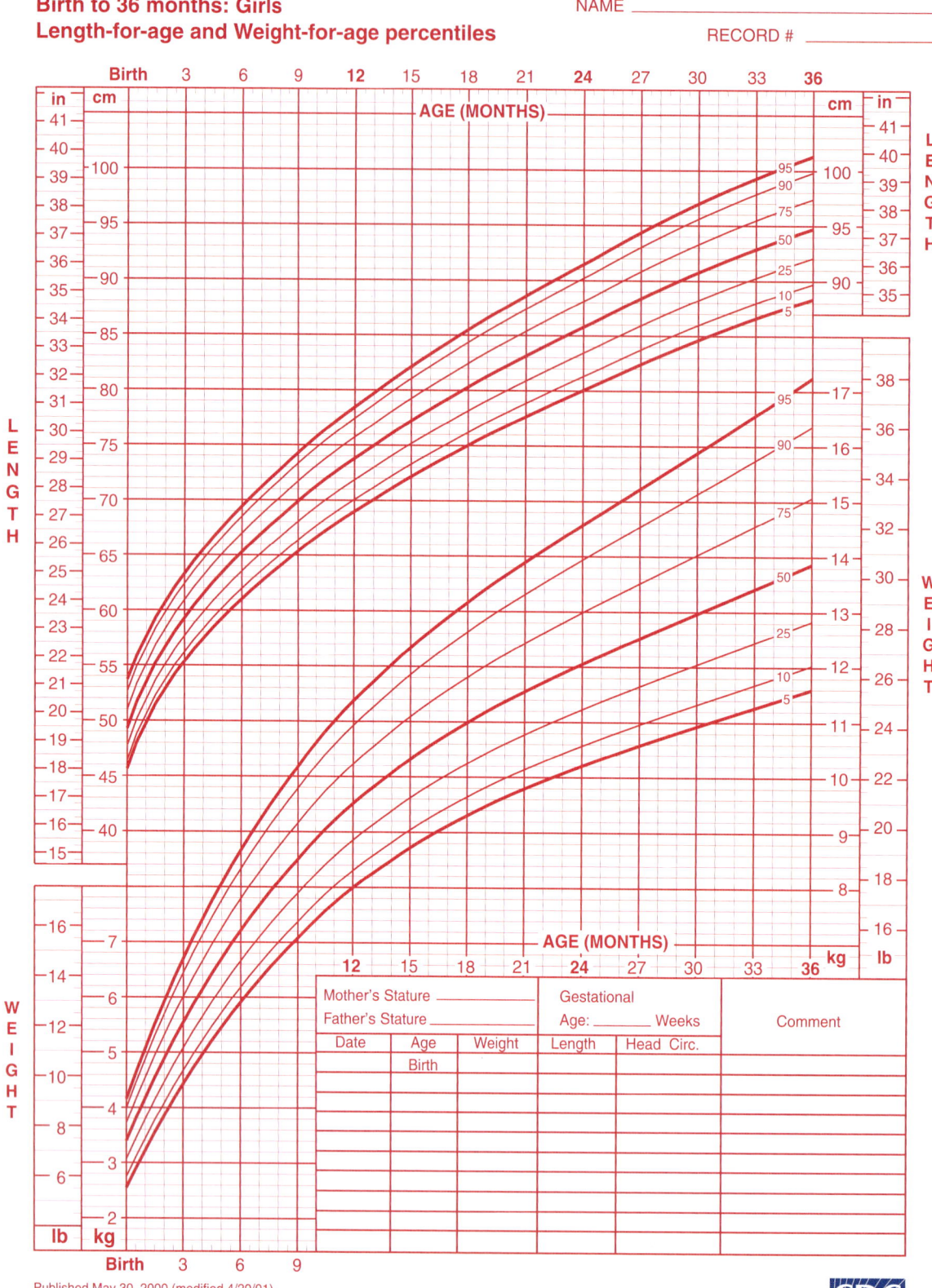

FIGURE 1.2 Growth Chart for Girls. (From the National Center for Health Statistics in collaboration with the National Center for Chronic Disease Prevention and Health Promotion 2000. https://www.cdc.gov/growthcharts.)

TABLE 1.3	Neurologic and External Physical Criteria to Assess Gestational Age	
Physical Examination	**Preterm (<37 weeks)**	**Term (≥37 weeks)**
Ear	Shapeless, pliable	Firm, well formed
Skin	Edematous, thin skin	Thick skin
Sole of foot	Creases on anterior third	Whole foot creased
Breast tissue	<1-mm diameter	>5-mm diameter
Genitalia		
Male	Scrotum poorly developed	Scrotum rugated
	Testes undescended	Testes descended
Female	Large clitoris, gaping labia majora	Labia majora developed
Limbs	Hypotonic	Tonic (flexed)
Grasp reflex	Weak grasp	Can be lifted by reflex grasp
Moro reflex	Complete but exhaustible (>32 weeks)	Complete
Sucking reflex	Weak	Strong, synchronous with swallowing

WEIGHT AND LENGTH

Growth is assessed by changes in weight, length, and head circumference. Percentile charts are valuable for monitoring a child's growth and development over time. Deviations in growth from the past percentile are more important than any single measurement (Figs. 1.3 and 1.4). Weight is a more sensitive index of well-being, illness, or poor nutrition than length or head circumference and is the most commonly used measurement of growth. Changes in weight reflect changes in muscle mass, adipose tissue, skeleton, and body water; as a result, weight is a nonspecific metric of growth. Measurement of length provides the best indicator of skeletal growth because it is not affected by changes in adipose tissue or water content.

Term neonates may lose 5% to 10% of their body weight during the first 24 to 72 hours after birth from loss of body water, and preterm infants lose slightly more, ~15%.[3] However, by 7 to 10 postnatal days, they return to their birth weight. An average daily increase of 30 grams (210 g/week) is expected during the first 3 months after birth, after which an increase of 70 grams each week is expected for the subsequent 10 to 12 months (Table 1.4).

When graphing the weight of a preterm infant on a growth chart, it is common to use the infant's corrected gestational age (postmenstrual age; the postconceptional age is the number of weeks since conception and is approximately 2 weeks less than the postmenstrual age) instead of the chronologic age (postnatal age [i.e., from birth]) during the first 2 years of the infant's life to correct for prematurity.

Weight and length are important metrics of growth, although other changes affect the composition of the body itself, especially total body water, which decreases at the expense of the extracellular compartment during infancy. Adult proportions are achieved by approximately 1 year of age (see Fig. 5.9).[13,14] These changes in the distribution of water throughout the body have important implications for drug dosing and distribution in the neonate and infant. Male infants have a greater percent of water,

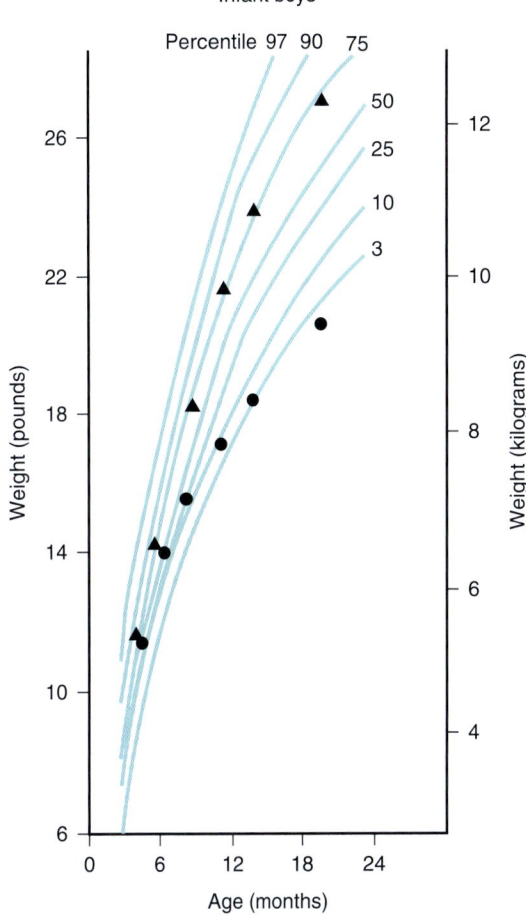

FIGURE 1.3 Postnatal Growth Curve (Weight) for Term Male Infants. This figure represents normal growth curves. *Triangles* indicate a normal child. *Circles* demonstrate failure to thrive in a child with severe renal failure.

whereas female infants have a slightly greater percent of fat. The percent decrease in extracellular water is greater than the decrease in total body water because of the simultaneous increase in intracellular water (Table 1.5).[15]

Another, more precise metric to assess development is to calculate the body surface area (BSA).[16] BSA can also be described using an allometric equation with an exponent of two-thirds (see Chapter 5):

$$BSA \propto weight^{2/3}$$

HEAD CIRCUMFERENCE

Head size reflects the growth of the brain and correlates with intracranial volume and brain weight. Changing head circumference reflects head growth and is a part of the total body growth process; it may or may not reflect underlying involvement of the brain. An abnormally large or small head may indicate abnormal brain development, which must alert the anesthesiologist to possible underlying neurologic problems. A large head may indicate a normal variant, familial feature, or pathologic condition (e.g., hydrocephalus or increased intracranial pressure), whereas a small head may indicate a normal variant, familial feature, or pathologic condition such as craniosynostosis or abnormal brain development.

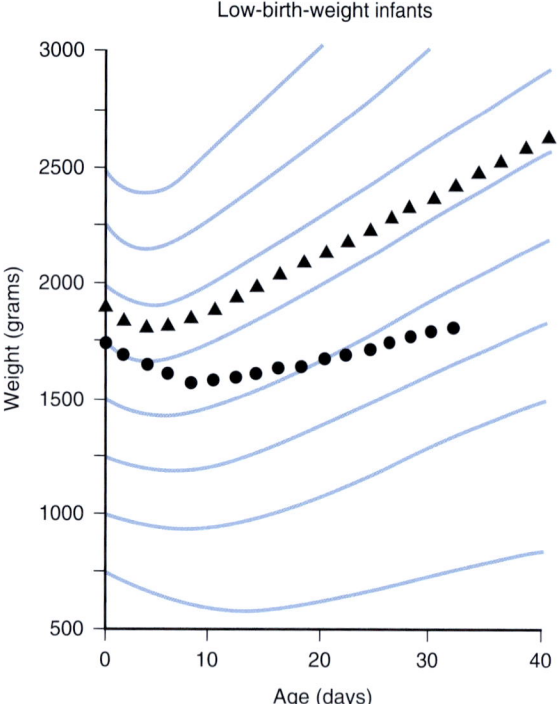

FIGURE 1.4 Postnatal Growth Curve (Weight) for Preterm Infants. This figure represents normal growth curves for preterm infants. *Triangles* indicate a normal preterm infant. *Circles* demonstrate failure to thrive in an infant with bronchopulmonary dysplasia.

TABLE 1.4	Approximate Relationship of Age to Weight
Age (years)	**Weight (kg)**
1	10
3	15
5	19
7	23

Corresponding equation for 18 months to 8 years of age is: Weight (kg) = 2 × Age (years) + 9.
For age >8 years: Weight (kg) = 3 × Age (years).

TABLE 1.5	Relationship of Age to Body Water		
Age	**Body Water (%)**	**Extracellular**	**Intracellular**
Fetus	90	60	25
Preterm	80	55	30
Full-term	70	50	35
6–12 months	60	30	40

During the first year of life, head circumference increases on average 10 cm, and in the second year, 2.5 cm. By 9 months of age, head circumference reaches 50% of adult size, and by 2 years, it reaches 75%. Head circumference is closely followed on standard percentile growth curves. As with weight, deviations in the growth of the head from its past percentile are more significant than an isolated measurement.

The anterior fontanel should be palpated to assess whether it is sunken (dehydration) or bulging abnormally (suggesting increased intracranial pressure as in hydrocephalus, infection, hemorrhage, or increased partial pressure of carbon dioxide in the arterial blood [$PaCO_2$]). If it is bulging, the sutures should be palpated for abnormal separation because of increased intracranial pressure. The anterior fontanel closes between 9 and 18 months of age; the posterior fontanel closes by 2 to 4 months of age (Fig. 1.5). Cranial molding occurs particularly in low-birth-weight neonates and is usually of no clinical importance; the head circumference/chest circumference ratio at birth in very-low-birth-weight infants can be used to predict later physical growth at 6 years.[17]

FACE

Although the cranial vault increases rapidly in size, the face and base of the skull develop at a slower rate. At birth, the mandible is small; but as a child develops, forward growth occurs, reducing the obliquity of the mandibular angle. The first three pharyngeal arches give rise to the maxilla, mandible, and hyoid bone with their accompanying nerves and muscles, whereas arches four to six give rise to the laryngeal cartilages with their associated muscles and are supplied by branches of the vagus nerve. An interruption of mandibular development leads to micrognathia and retrodisplacement of the tongue base (also known as glossoptosis)[18] (e.g., Pierre Robin sequence, Treacher Collins, or Goldenhar syndromes). These syndromes often have other associated anomalies. After 2 years of age, the size of the cranial vault increases only marginally, whereas the facial configuration undergoes substantive changes. The maxilla grows rapidly to accommodate the developing teeth. In addition, the frontal sinuses develop by 2 to 6 years of age, and the maxillary, ethmoidal, and sphenoidal sinuses appear after 6 years of age.

TEETH

The first tooth, usually a lower incisor, erupts at approximately 6 months after birth (deciduous dentition). Thereafter, one tooth usually erupts each month until all 20 primary deciduous teeth are present by 28 months of age. Preterm infants may show severe enamel hypoplasia in their primary dentition.[19,20]

Permanent teeth begin to appear by 6 years, with the shedding of the deciduous teeth; this process continues over the next 6 to 8 years. Some hereditary disorders[21] such as Down syndrome, and other disorders including cerebral palsy, as well as medications (e.g., tetracycline,[22] glucocorticoids[23]), microcephaly,[24] and nutritional defects can lead to abnormally developed teeth.[25]

Airway and Respiratory System

Airway development includes a large number of structures: the cranial vault and base, craniovertebral growth, face, branchial apparatus, larynx, and oral cavity.

These structures ensure the integrity of the respiratory system (to provide enough oxygen and to remove carbon dioxide) including separating breathing from the swallowing of liquid and food. The anesthesiologist must consider these developmental changes because they have implications for how most effectively to manage the airway and ensure adequate ventilation.

UPPER AIRWAY DEVELOPMENT

During development, the upper airway of the infant undergoes major anatomic modifications that include changes in size, shape, and interrelationships; this is particularly prominent during the first few years of life.

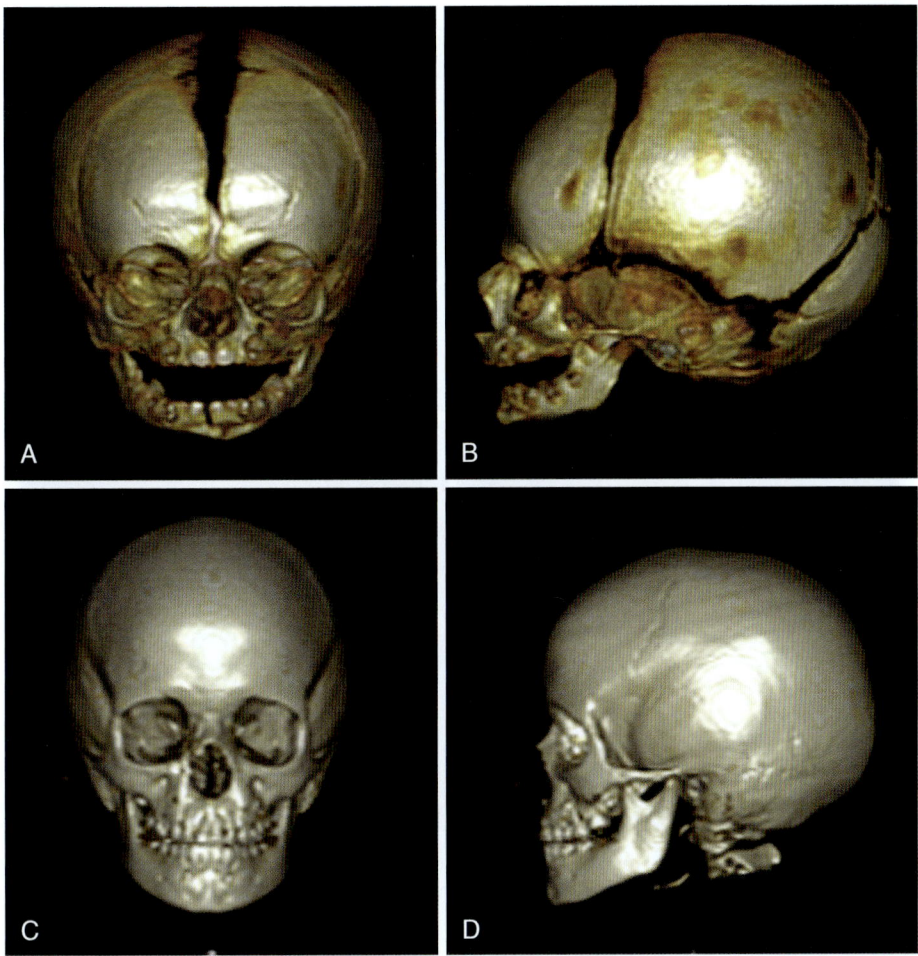

FIGURE 1.5 Cranial Development. **(A)** and **(B)** depict the skull of a neonate with wide-open suture. **(C)** and **(D)** depict the skull of a 7-year-old boy with fused sutures.

The face and the nasal chamber, the oropharynx with the tongue, and the laryngotracheal lumen are the three main components of the upper airway. Development of the neurocranium leads to maturation of the cranial vault and skull base, whereas development of the viscerocranium leads to the skeletal portions of the face. The primordial areas involved in forming the covering of the tongue appear early in the second month of development.

The skull base grows rapidly until the age of 6 years, with relatively slower growth thereafter. The cranial base flexes postnatally in a rapid growth trajectory that is complete by 2 years of age. The palate is formed from lateral palatine processes that project medially on each side of the tongue and fuse with the nasal septum; cleft lips and palates result from failure of this fusion process. The depth of the nasopharynx increases as a result of remodeling of the palate and changes in the angulation of the skull base. During childhood, the soft tissues of the pharyngeal structures surrounding the upper airway increase proportionally to the skeletal structures. After birth, the dimensions of the nasal cavity increase very rapidly. During the first year of life, the total minimal cross-sectional area increases by 67% and the volume of the anterior 4 cm of the nasal airways by 36%.[26,27]

The tongue is derived from the first four pharyngeal arches, which explains its complicated innervation via the trigeminal, glossopharyngeal, and vagus nerves. The anterior two-thirds of the tongue is derived mostly from the first arch and the posterior one-third from the third and fourth arches. At birth, the entire tongue lies within the mouth and the posterior third descends into the oropharynx over the first 4 years of life. The volume of the oral cavity in the neonate is proportionally less than that in the adult, primarily because of the shorter mandibular ramus, but its volume greatly increases during the first 12 months of life because of rapid growth in the height of the mandibular ramus. In the neonate, the tongue contains considerably less fat and soft tissue compared with that in the adult, but it is large relative to the dimensions of the mouth. It has greater extrinsic musculature and a less developed superior longitudinal muscle, resulting in a flat dorsal surface with poor lateral mobility (see also Chapter 12).

The larynx is developed embryologically from ectodermal, endodermal, and mesodermal tissues that are derived from the third, fourth, and sixth branchial arch and pouch apparatus. The development of the larynx and airway in the neonate is outlined in detail in Chapter 12. The laryngeal opening (epiglottis and vocal cords) in a neonate and 2-year-old boy are shown in Fig. 1.6. Note the long, omega-shaped epiglottis and the pearly white vocal cords in the neonate.

RESPIRATORY SYSTEM DEVELOPMENT

The lung develops in five stages: embryonic, pseudoglandular, canalicular, saccular, and alveolar.[28] Embryonic development

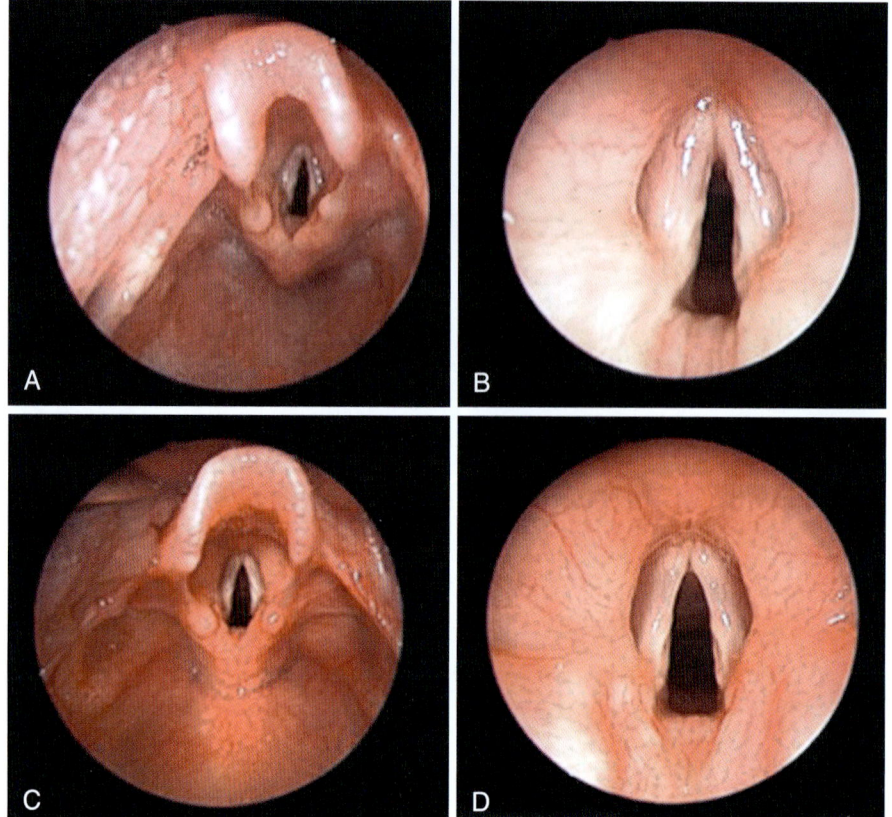

FIGURE 1.6 Larynx Development From Neonate to 2 Years Old. The larynx in the neonate (**A** and **B**), with the long epiglottis (**A**) and the vocal cords (**B**, close-up). The larynx in a 2-year-old (**C** and **D**) with a shorter epiglottis (**C**) and the vocal cords (**D**, close-up).

starts at ~3 weeks with primary lung buds that further grow into a mass of mesodermal cells later to form blood vessels, smooth muscle, and cartilage. Pseudoglandular development (weeks ~5 to 16) involves formation of the bronchial tree and birth of the acinus. The canalicular stage (weeks ~17 to 27) involves development of distal airway with branching, appearance of surfactant, and acini. The saccular stage (weeks ~28 to 36) involves expansion of the future air spaces. The alveolar stage (~36 weeks to young adulthood) involves formation of alveoli that continue to develop until 2 years of age (Fig. 1.7).[28,29]

Airways: The bronchial tree down to and including the terminal bronchioles forms by week 16 of gestation. The acinus, consisting of all the airway structures distal to the terminal bronchiole and the entire gas-exchanging apparatus, develops throughout the remainder of gestation.

Alveoli: Alveoli develop mainly after birth, increasing in number until approximately 3 years of age and in size until growth of the chest wall ceases, which occurs in young adulthood.[29]

Pulmonary vessels: Arteries and veins accompanying the bronchial tree form by week 16 of gestation. Those vessels lying within the acinus follow the development of the alveoli. Both the appearance and growth of arterial smooth muscle lag behind the sprouting of new vessels; microvascular development is not completed until young adulthood.[29]

TRANSITION TO AIR BREATHING

Fetal breathing movements have been detected as early as 11 weeks of gestational age; they are interspersed with long periods of apnea and produce little tidal movement of lung fluid.[30–32] The critical event in the change from placental to pulmonary gas exchange is the first inspiration, which initiates pulmonary ventilation, promotes the clearance of lung fluid, and triggers the change from the fetal to the neonatal pattern of circulation. Air entering the lungs increases pulmonary blood flow via vasodilation thus reducing pulmonary vascular resistance (PVR), especially to well-ventilated lung regions (matching of blood flow with aeration).[33,34] A burst of cortisol supports development of a variety of physiologic responses such as endogenous catecholamine release, maturation of surfactant production, increasing thyroid hormone, and others.[35] A catecholamine burst (endogenous epinephrine and norepinephrine) increases the blood pressure and supports substrate metabolism of glucose, fatty acids, and initiating thermogenesis through brown fat metabolism.[35] These bursts of catecholamines, cortisol, and angiotensin II are smaller in preterm infants and those born by cesarean section.

The first breath is a gasp that generates a transpulmonary distending pressure of 40 to 80 cm H_2O.[36] This moves the tracheal fluid (100 times more viscous than air), overcomes surface forces that develop as the air-fluid interface reaches the small airways, and overcomes tissue resistance. The hydrostatic pressure gradient, which develops primarily during inspiration, drives the tracheal fluid from the airways to the interstitium.[34] Much of the fluid is cleared from the airways during the first four to five breaths after birth, although clearance from the interstitial lung tissue takes up to several hours.[34] In some neonates, removing the lung fluid is delayed, resulting in the syndrome known as *transient tachypnea of the newborn.*[37–39] Tachypnea lasts for 24 to 72 hours and is associated with a characteristic chest radiographic appearance consisting

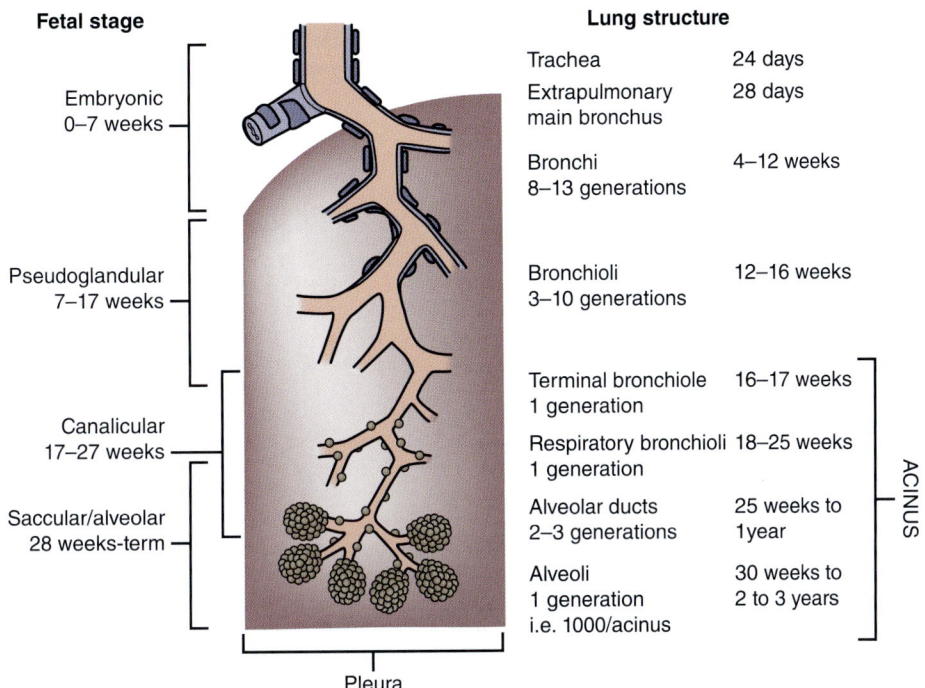

FIGURE 1.7 Development of the Bronchial Tree. (Adapted from that used by Dr Alison Hislop, personal communication.)

of increased perihilar markings, fluid in the interlobar fissures, and streaky linear opacities in the parenchyma. The incidence of *transient tachypnea of the newborn* is inversely proportional to gestational age (~10% 33 to 34 weeks GA, ~5% 35 to 36 weeks GA, ~1% ≥37 weeks GA).[39,40]

With the onset of pulmonary ventilation, pulmonary blood flow sharply increases. Decreased pulmonary vascular resistance and increased peripheral systemic vascular resistance (loss of the umbilical circulation) are the two crucial events involved in the immediate transition from the fetal circulation to the normal postnatal pattern.[41] The increase in systemic afterload causes an immediate closure of the flap valve mechanism of the foramen ovale and reverses the direction of shunt through the ductus arteriosus. There is some evidence that cord clamping should be delayed until the onset of respirations so as to improve cardiac filling to optimize pulmonary blood flow and venous return.[34,42,43] Until these fetal shunt pathways close anatomically, the pattern of circulation is unstable. Increased pulmonary vascular reactivity in response to hypoxia and acidosis may precipitate a reversal to right-to-left shunting ("flip-flop" circulation) (see also Chapter 16).[44]

In the first few minutes after birth, a state of "normal" asphyxia exists because of the impaired placental blood flow during labor. The partial pressure of oxygen in arterial blood (PaO_2) and pH are reduced, whereas the $PaCO_2$ is increased immediately after birth, but these partial pressures change rapidly in the first hours after birth. Extrapulmonary shunting through fetal channels and intrapulmonary shunting, probably through unexpanded regions of the lung, persist for some time after birth, so that in neonates the physiologic right-to-left shunt is about three times that in adults.[45]

MECHANICS OF BREATHING
Chest Wall and Respiratory Muscles
The accessory muscles of inspiration are relatively ineffective in infants because of an unfavorable configuration of the rib cage. In infancy, the ribs extend horizontally from the vertebral column, moving little with inspiration.[46] Hence, the cross-sectional area of the thoracic cage remains fairly constant throughout the breathing cycle. In fact, inspiration depends almost exclusively on the descent of the diaphragm. These factors increase the workload on the diaphragm, rendering it at risk for fatigue, particularly in the preterm infant.

The chest wall of a neonate is three times more compliant than lung compliance and becomes similar to adult compliance by 1 year of age.[47] The chest wall is floppy because it consists of noncalcified cartilage, its musculature is poorly developed, and the ribs are incompletely calcified.[48,49] As the work of breathing increases, diaphragmatic displacement must also increase to overcome these deficiencies and maintain the tidal volume. The increased workload may lead to diaphragmatic fatigue and respiratory failure or apnea, especially in preterm infants.[50,51]

Muscle strength depends on the presence of an adequate number of type I (slow twitch, high oxidative capacity) muscle fibers to respond to an increased workload. The diaphragm of the neonate and more critically, the preterm infant, has limited numbers of type I (slow twitch, high oxidative capacity)(~10%) muscle fibers (see Fig. 12.11).[52] This compounds the risk for respiratory failure in the developing infant because any degree of airway obstruction increases the work of breathing (see Figs. 2.13 and 2.14).

Elastic Properties of the Lung
Changes in the static pressure/volume relationship of the lungs during growth are caused by increases in volume and changes in the elastic properties of lung tissue. Volume is the principal factor that determines lung compliance, which increases throughout childhood; specific lung compliance remains relatively constant throughout childhood.[53,54] In contrast, specific compliance of the chest wall declines throughout childhood and adolescence, reflecting the progressive calcification of the ribs and the increasing bulk of the thoracic muscles.

TABLE 1.6	Age-Dependent Respiratory Variables						
	Newborn	**6 months**	**12 months**	**3 years**	**5 years**	**12 years**	**Adult**
F (breaths/minute)	50 ± 1	30 ± 5	24 ± 6	24 ± 6	23 ± 5	18 ± 5	12 ± 3
TV (mL)	21	45	78	112	270	480	575
(mL/kg)	6–8						6–7
VE (mL/minute)	1050	1350	1780	2460	5500	6200	6400
(mL/kg per minute)	200–260						90
VA (mL/minute)	665		1245	1760	1800	3000	3100
(mL/kg per minute)	100–150						60
VD/VT	0.3						0.3
VO₂ (mL/kg per minute)	6–8						3–4
VC (mL)	120			870	1160	3100	4000
FRC (mL)	80			490	680	1970	3000
(mL/kg)	30						30
TLC (mL)	160			1100	1500	4000	6000
(mL/kg)	63						82
pH	7.3–7.4		7.35–7.45				7.35–7.45
PaO₂ (mm Hg)	60–90		80–100				80–100
PaCO₂ (mm Hg)	30–35		30–40				37–42

F, frequency; *FRC*, functional residual capacity; *PaCO₂*, arterial carbon dioxide concentration; *PaO₂*, arterial oxygen concentration; *TLC*, total lung capacity; *TV*, tidal volume; *VA*, alveolar ventilation; *VC*, vital capacity; *VD/VT*, dead space to tidal volume ration; *VE*, minute ventilation; *VO₂*, oxygen consumption.

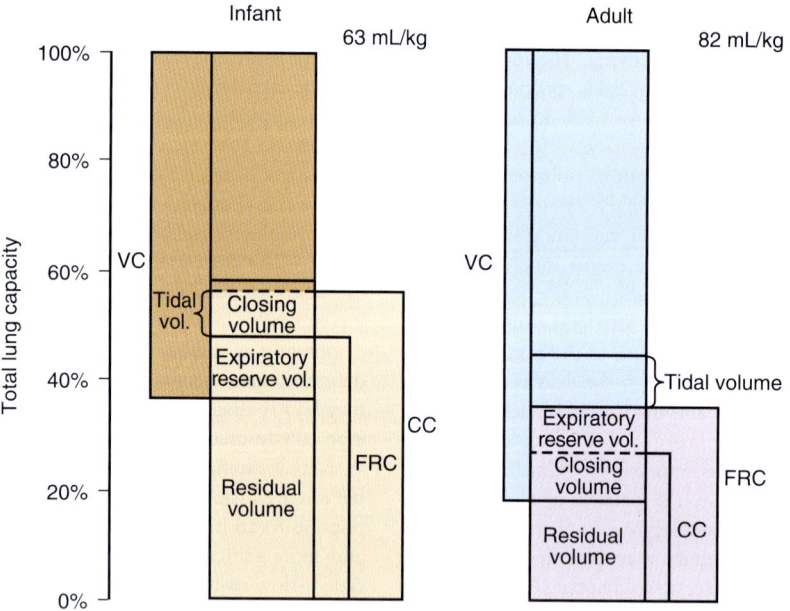

FIGURE 1.8 Lung Volumes in Infants and Adults. Note that in infants, tidal volume breathing occurs at the same volume as closing volume. *CC*, Closing capacity; *FRC*, functional residual capacity; *VC*, vital capacity. (Modified from Nelson NM. Respiration and circulation after birth. In: Smith CA, Nelson NM, eds. *The Physiology of the Newborn Infant*. Springfield, IL: Charles C Thomas; 1976: 207.)

Static Lung Volumes

A detailed description of static lung volumes based on body weight is presented in Table 1.6.

Total Lung Capacity

Adults have a much greater total lung capacity than infants (Fig. 1.8). This difference reflects the fact that total lung capacity is an effort-dependent variable, dependent on the strength and efficiency of the inspiratory muscles, which can be estimated by the maximum inspiratory pressure at functional residual capacity. An adult can generate negative pressures greater than 100 cm H₂O; a neonate can generate pressures as great as 70 cm H₂O, a surprisingly large value considering the weaknesses cited earlier. This has been attributed to the small radius of curvature of the infant's rib cage, which by the Laplace relationship converts a small tension into a large pressure gradient.[55]

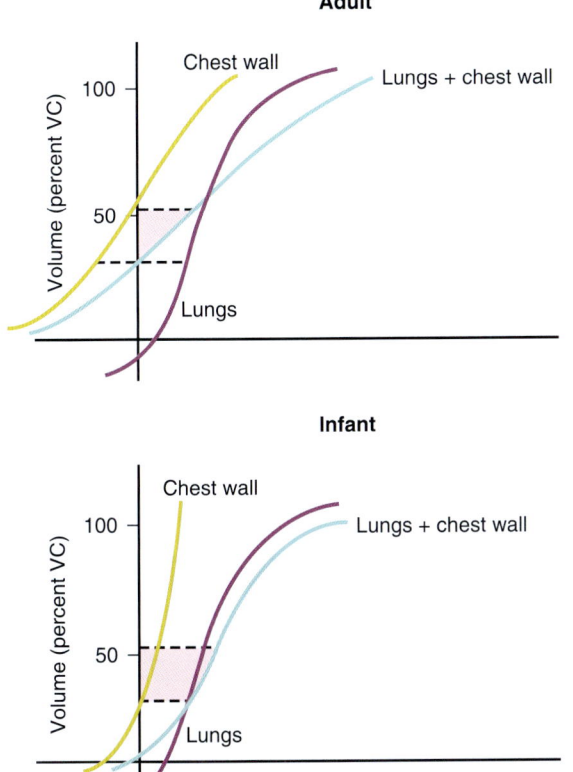

Adult

Infant

FIGURE 1.9 Compliance curves for the chest wall *(yellow)*, lungs *(purple)*, and thorax (combination of chest wall and lungs *[blue]*) in infants and adults. (Modified and reproduced with permission from Pérez Fontán JJ, Haddad GG. Respiratory physiology. In: Behrman RE, Kliegman RM, Jenson HB, eds. *Nelson Textbook of Pediatrics.* 17th ed. Philadelphia: WB Saunders; 2003:1363.)

Functional Residual Capacity
Functional residual capacity normalized to weight (per kilogram) is constant throughout development, although the mechanical factors on which it is based differ in infants and adults.[56] Functional residual capacity is the volume of gas within the lungs at end-expiration, when the outward forces of the chest wall are balanced against the inward, elastic recoil of the lungs (Fig. 1.9). In the supine neonate, functional residual capacity is small, in part because the weak outward forces of the compliant chest wall are more than offset by the elastic recoil of the lungs. In addition, the large abdomen pushes the diaphragm upward. The neonate may increase the functional residual capacity by exhaling against a closed glottis (glottic braking).

An important clinical implication of the dynamic control of functional residual capacity is that an apneic infant has a disproportionately smaller reserve of intrapulmonary oxygen on which to draw than a similarly affected adult. This, combined with their increased metabolic rate, contributes to the rapid development of hypoxemia if the airway becomes compromised.

Closing Capacity
As exhalation proceeds to completion, small airways in dependent regions of the lung close, leading to air trapping in the affected areas. Closing capacity is closely related to age; it decreases throughout childhood and adolescence but increases thereafter through adult life (see Fig. 1.8). This pattern of change has been

related to the development of and deterioration in lung elastic tissue and its effect on recoil pressure. The latter is the principal determinant of transmural pressure and therefore patency of the smallest airways, which lack intrinsic stability because they contain no cartilage.

Closing volume is within the range of tidal breathing in many older adults and some children younger than 10 years of age (see Fig. 1.8). It is not possible to measure closing volume in children younger than 5 years, but because the elastic recoil pressure is small in infancy (see Fig. 1.9), some airways likely remain closed throughout tidal breathing. This notion is supported by the finding that infants have a large "trapped gas volume" that is not in free communication with the conducting airways. Age-related changes in PaO_2, which parallel the changes in the difference between functional residual capacity and closing volume, may also be related in part to airway closure.[57]

AIRWAY DYNAMICS
Resistance and Conductance
Airway resistance decreases markedly with growth from 19 to 28 cm H_2O/L per second in neonates to less than 2 cm H_2O/L per second in adults.[56,57] Airway resistance is greater in preterm than in full-term infants. On the other hand, specific airway conductance (reciprocal of resistance) is greater in preterm infants but decreases steadily during the first 5 years of life.[58,59]

Distribution of Resistance
The distribution of airway resistance changes markedly at approximately 5 years of age. Airway resistance per gram of lung tissue is constant at all ages in the "central airways" (trachea to the 12th to 15th bronchial generation), whereas it decreases markedly at approximately 5 years of age in the "peripheral airways" (i.e., distal to the 12th to 15th generation to the alveoli).

Inspiratory and Expiratory Flow Limitation
Tracheal compliance in neonates is twice that of adults; it is even greater in preterm infants and appears to be a consequence of cartilaginous immaturity. The functional importance of this finding is that dynamic collapse of the trachea may occur with inspiration and expiration (see Figs. 12.11 and 12.12). The normal inspiratory time for preterm infants is 0.3 to 0.35 seconds and in a term infant 0.35 to 0.40 seconds.[60]

Regulation of Breathing
In neonates as in adults, PaO_2, $PaCO_2$, and pH control ventilation, with PaO_2 acting mainly through peripheral chemoreceptors in the carotid and aortic bodies and $PaCO_2$ and pH acting on central chemoreceptors in the medulla. In contrast to the adult, an infant's response to hypercapnia is not potentiated by hypoxia, but the latter may actually depress the hypercapnic ventilatory response in term and preterm infants.[61,62] Neonates of smoking mothers and substance abuse mothers have a blunted response to hypercarbia compared with those of nonsmoking mothers and an increased risk for sudden death.[63–65] They also have a blunted response to hypoxemia that may be related to nicotine exposure causing cholinergic stimulation.[66] These may be contributing factors to sudden infant death syndrome.[67,68]

High concentrations of oxygen depress respiration in the neonate, whereas low concentrations stimulate it. The hypoxic response, however, is not consistent. Initially, hypoxia restores respiration to baseline but thereafter it depresses it. This pattern of response persists in normal term infants throughout the first week of life but may persist longer in preterm neonates. After this initial period, the response to persistent hypoxia gradually transitions to the adult response, which is a sustained increase in ventilation.[69,70]

Periodic breathing commonly occurs in neonates. This should be distinguished from clinical apnea, which occurs in as many as 25% of all preterm infants, especially in the most severely preterm infant. Apnea of prematurity may be a life-threatening condition. In this situation, the apneas may be prolonged and associated with desaturation of arterial oxygen, bradycardia, and loss of muscle tone.

Prematurity is an important risk factor for life-threatening apnea in neonates and infants undergoing general anesthesia.[71] The risk of postanesthetic respiratory depression is inversely related to gestational age and postconception age at the time of anesthesia (see Fig. 2.12 and E-Fig. 2.7).[72] There is a general consensus that infants may be at risk for postoperative apnea up to 60 weeks after conception.[72,73]

The reduced PaO_2 of neonates is offset by the greater oxygen-carrying capacity that results from the increased hemoglobin (Hb) concentrations. Hb concentrations decline during the first several weeks of life. At birth, the Hb content of the blood is 50% fetal Hb. The position of the oxyhemoglobin dissociation curve depends on the ratio of adult to fetal Hb. At birth, the increased fetal Hb content shifts the curve to the left of the adult curve (from a P_{50} of 27 for Hb A to a P_{50} of 19 for Hb F). During the first week after birth, the curve shifts to the right, reflecting the transition from fetal to adult Hb formation.[53] Normal $PaCO_2$ and pH are somewhat reduced in the neonatal period compared with later infancy (see Table 1.6). Studies that sought to define the optimal target SpO_2 in premature infants reported no difference in composite death or disability between SpO_2 85% to 89% versus 91% to 95%, but that the 85% to 89% range was associated with a greater risk of death and necrotizing enterocolitis (NEC) but a lesser risk for retinopathy of prematurity.[74–76] Therefore, an SpO_2 target range of 91% to 95% is recommended.[77]

Cardiovascular System

Understanding the developmental changes in the cardiovascular system from birth is critical for anesthesiologists. This section briefly considers the developmental changes in heart rate, blood pressure, cardiac output, and the electrocardiogram that occur after birth; for more detailed descriptions, refer to Chapters 14 and 16.

The neonatal myocardium differs from the adult myocardium histologically, in that it contains fewer muscle cells (poorly organized rather than in parallel) and more connective tissue. Furthermore, the neonatal myocardium depends to a great extent on free cytosolic ionized calcium for contractility.[78,79] These differences result in a limited effect of an augmented preload on cardiac output (stroke volume), greater sensitivity to an increased afterload and decreased ionized calcium levels compared with the adult myocardium. Immature autonomic regulation is also a feature of the neonate with a dominant parasympathetic system.[80]

HEART RATE
Autonomic control of the heart in utero is mediated predominantly through the parasympathetic nervous system. It is only shortly after birth that sympathetic control begins to appear, although the parasympathetic nervous system continues to dominate in childhood, waning only as adolescence is reached. In neonates, the heart rate may have a wide variation that is within normal limits. The mean heart rate in neonates in the first 24 hours of life is ~120 beats per minute.[81] It increases to a mean of 160 beats

per minute at 1 month of age, after which it gradually decreases to 75 beats per minute at adolescence (Table 1.7).[82,83]

BLOOD PRESSURE
Mean systolic blood pressure in neonates and infants increases from 65 mm Hg in the first 12 hours of life to 75 mm Hg at 4 days and 95 mm Hg at 6 weeks. There is little change in mean systolic pressure between 6 weeks and 1 year of age and even between 1 year and 6 years of age; thereafter, systolic pressure gradually increases with age.[84,85] These measurements apply to infants and children who are awake and calm. The blood pressure in preterm infants in the first 12 hours is less than that in full-term infants; a gradual increase in blood pressure occurs after birth (~68/43 mm Hg on day 1 of life compared with 90/55 mm Hg on day 90 of life) (Table 1.8).[86,87] Blood pressure measured in the lower extremity may be less than in the upper extremity in children.[88,89] Some report mean arterial pressure differences between the upper and lower extremities in neonates as great as 20 mm Hg in favor of the upper extremity.[90] Another study of children 0 to 8 years of age that compared standard noninvasive and invasive blood pressure measurements reported a mean difference of 10 mm Hg.[91]

TABLE 1.7 The Relationship Between Age and Heart Rate[a]

Age	Mean Heart Rate in Beats per Minute (range)
Premature	120–170
0–3 months	100–150
3–6 months	90–120
6–12 months	80–120
1–3 years	70–110
3–6 years	65–110
6–12 years	60–95
>12 years	55–85

Data from Hartman ME, Cheifetz IM. Pediatric emergencies and resuscitation. In: Kliegman RM, Stanton BF, St Geme III JW, Schor NF, Behrman RE, eds. *Nelson Textbook of Pediatrics.* 19th ed. Philadelphia: Elsevier; 2011:280.
[a]Note that the heart rate will be lower during sleep or during anesthesia.

TABLE 1.8 The Relationship Between Age and Blood Pressure[a]

Age	NORMAL BLOOD PRESSURE (MM HG)	
	Mean Systolic	Mean Diastolic
Premature	55–75	35–45
0–3 months	65–85	45–55
3–6 months	70–90	50–65
6–12 months	80–100	55–65
1–3 years	90–105	55–70
3–6 years	95–110	60–75
6–12 years	100–120	60–75
>12 years	110–135	65–85

Data from Hartman ME, Cheifetz IM. Pediatric emergencies and resuscitation. In: Kliegman RM, Stanton BF, St Geme III JW, Schor NF, Behrman RE, eds. *Nelson Textbook of Pediatrics.* 19th ed. Philadelphia: Elsevier; 2011:280.
[a]Note that the blood pressure will be lower during sleep or during anesthesia.

TABLE 1.9 | Normal Ranges for Cardiovascular Indices Approximated to Two Significant Figures

Age (years)	Stroke Volume Index (mL/m²)	Cardiac Index L/min/m²	Systemic Vascular Resistance Index (dynes sec/cm⁵/m²)	Mean Arterial Pressure (mm Hg)	Heart Rate (beats per minute)
1–2	31–55	3.5–6.5	750–1600	48–83	93–140
3–4	37–67	3.6–7.1	750–1700	52–86	78–130
5–12	42–76	3.3–6.9	910–2000	61–94	62–110

From Cattermole GN, Leung PY, Ho GY, et al. The normal ranges of cardiovascular parameters in children measured using the Ultrasonic Cardiac Output Monitor. *Ped Crit Care.* 2010;38:1875.

CARDIAC OUTPUT

Determination of cardiac output and blood pressure allows calculation of systemic vascular resistance. It provides important information relating to the left ventricular afterload and allows rational application of vasoactive (e.g., vasoconstrictor, vasodilator) and inotropic drugs. Measurement of cardiac output may be carried out by the Fick method (using oxygen extraction) or thermodilution using a pulmonary artery flow-directed catheter. In neonates, the latter technique is rarely used because shunts at the atrial and ductal levels introduce errors when interpreting the results. Pulsed Doppler determinations of cardiac output provide excellent noninvasive estimates of cardiac output for clinical application in neonates. Cardiac output, normalized for body weight, in neonates between 780 and 4740 grams at birth, increased linearly with advancing birth weight and gestational age.[92] The range of cardiac output in both full-term and preterm neonates is 220 to 350 mL/kg per minute, proportionally 2- to 3-fold greater than in adults.[92,93] Between birth and the end of the first year of life, mean cardiac output (normalized for body weight or surface area) remains fairly constant at 204 ± 45 mL/kg per minute.[94] The relatively large cardiac output (in milliliters per minute per kilogram) in neonates reflects their greater metabolic rate (on a weight basis) and oxygen consumption compared with adults[95] (see Chapter 5).

Pulsed Doppler estimation of cardiac output has also been found useful in assessing left ventricular myocardial dysfunction in neonates after perinatal asphyxia and acidosis, and older children in circulatory shock, to assess responses to therapeutic interventions.[96–98] A large study of 1197 Chinese children 1 to 12 years of age estimated normative values for cardiac index, stroke volume index, heart rate, and mean arterial pressure versus age (Table 1.9).[99] New noninvasive techniques using changes in bioimpedance or bioreactance (simple surface ECG electrodes) correlate very closely with other methods such as transthoracic ECHO and cardiac MRI.[100–102] A meta-analysis of 25 studies that compared measurements using ultrasound, bioimpedance, MRI, and other measures of cardiac output reported no significant differences between devices except in neonatal stroke volume studies, suggesting that these devices hold great promise for the future (see Chapter 49; Figs. 49.11 and 49.12).[103]

NORMAL ELECTROCARDIOGRAPHIC FINDINGS

The P wave reflects atrial depolarization and varies little with age. The PR interval increases with age (mean value for the first year of life is 0.10 seconds, increasing to 0.14 seconds at 12 to 16 years of age).[104] The duration of the QRS complex increases with age, but prolongation greater than 0.10 second is abnormal at any age.

At birth, the QRS axis is right sided, reflecting the predominant right ventricular intrauterine development. It shifts leftward in the first month as left ventricular muscle hypertrophies. Thereafter, the QRS follows a gradual change toward a left-sided axis. In addition,

T waves are upright in all chest leads. Within hours, they become isoelectric or inverted over the left chest; by the seventh day, the T waves are inverted in V_4R (V_4 position under the right clavicle), V_1, and across to V_4. From then on, the T waves remain inverted over the right chest until adolescence, when they become upright over the right side of the chest again. Failure of T waves to become inverted in V_4R and V_1 to V_4 by 7 days may be the earliest electrocardiographic evidence of right ventricular hypertrophy (see also Chapter 14).[105,106]

Renal System

The complex development of the human kidney begins in week 4 of gestation and continues into adulthood. Serious renal malfunction is usually associated with growth retardation. Urine production begins in utero at 10 to 12 weeks of gestation and is excreted into the amniotic cavity, helping to maintain amniotic fluid volume. The fetus maintains its metabolic homeostasis through the placenta. It is only after birth that the kidney assumes this responsibility. More than 90% of neonates void urine within the first 24 hours after birth. All normal neonates should void by 48 hours after birth; otherwise, they should be investigated for anomalies including posterior urethral valves.[107]

Tubular function begins to develop after 34 weeks of gestation and reaches adult levels by ~2 years of age.[108] The number and function of the Na^+/K^+-ATPase transporters are reduced at birth, although their activity increases 5- to 10-fold in the postnatal period. All transporters that rely on the Na^+ gradient are also reduced in function. The renal tubular threshold for resorption of Na^+, glucose, and bicarbonate are decreased in the neonatal period; hence, neonates are at increased risk for hyponatremia, osmotic polyuria, and metabolic acidosis, respectively.

Nephrogenesis is complete by 36 weeks of gestation. Renal blood flow and glomerular filtration rate (GFR) are reduced and correlate with gestational age. GFR is 20% to 25% of adult rates at term. GFR increases rapidly in the postnatal period as the result of an increase in cardiac output and a decrease in renal vascular resistance. Adult GFR is achieved by ~2 years of age[109] (see Fig. 5.13). A reduced GFR affects the ability of the neonate to excrete saline and water loads, as well as drugs that are cleared by the kidney (e.g., aminoglycosides, cephalosporins). At birth, the serum creatinine concentration reflects the maternal concentration, but this value decreases during the first days after birth with a plateau reached between 65 to 220 days of life.[110,111] Thereafter, the serum creatinine concentrations increase with age, and are greater in males, from the rapid growth and increase in muscular mass. Creatinine clearance slowly increases in neonates, reaching adult values between 1 and 2 years of age (Fig. 1.10).[109–111]

In utero, the fetus maintains a mild respiratory acidosis, with a similar plasma bicarbonate concentration, but a greater $PaCO_2$

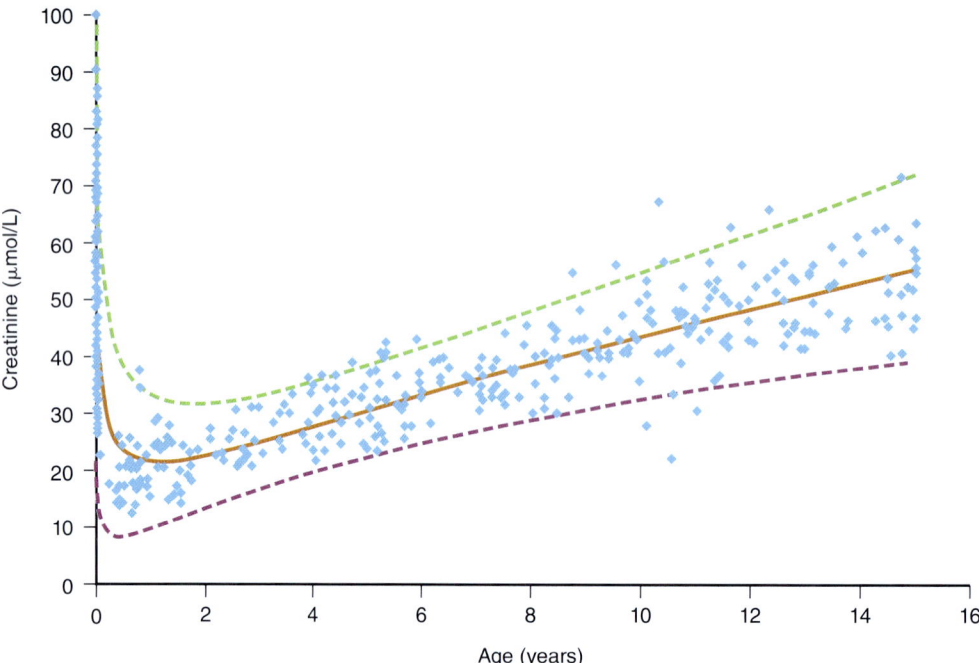

FIGURE 1.10 Age-adjusted pediatric reference intervals: Creatinine values are plotted vs age, the mean creatinine fitted from fractional polynomials is indicated by the solid line, and the dashed lines indicate the upper and lower reference limits (2.5th and 97.5th percentiles). Ceriotti F, Boyd JC, Klein G, et al. Reference intervals for serum creatinine concentrations: assessment of available data for global application. *Clin Chem.* 2008;54(3):559-566.

than its mother. After birth, plasma bicarbonate concentration and PaCO$_2$ are reduced in neonates and infants compared with older children and adults. In addition, the basal acid production in neonates is comparatively greater than in adults and they are less able to respond to an acid load. Endogenous acid production in small children is between 50% and 100% greater per kilogram than adults. This is primarily due to the deposition of Ca^{2+} in bone, a process that produces 0.5 to 1 mEq/L of acid per day. Bicarbonate absorption from the gastrointestinal tract is an important source of base to neutralize acid, and in part, explains the tendency of infants to become profoundly acidotic when suffering from gastroenteritis. The neonate or infant is living near its limit of acid compensation and is therefore prone to develop acidosis during the course of an acute illness or starvation.[112,113]

Neonates and preterm infants are obligate salt losers and as such, have limited ability to tolerate hypotonic IV fluids.[114] Immaturity of distal tubular function and relative hypoaldosteronism explain why preterm infants are at increased risk for hyperkalemia.[114,115] Neonatal hypernatremia (mild = serum Na$^+$ 146 to 149 mmol/L, moderate = Na$^+$ 150 to 169 mmol/L, severe = Na$^+$ > 170 mmol/L) may be due to poor breastfeeding and dehydration.[116]

Digestive and Endocrine System

HEPATIC SYSTEM

Organogenesis begins during the fourth week of embryogenesis.[117] Development of the liver and bile ducts begins as an outgrowth of the foregut; by 10 weeks of gestation, the biliary tract has completed its development. The vitelline veins give rise to the portal and hepatic veins. The hepatic acinus is developed by the third month of gestation.[117] Hepatic sinusoids form the ductus venosus, the bridge between the hepatic vein and the inferior vena cava. Most umbilical venous blood from the placenta passes through the ductus venosus to the inferior vena cava, supplying

~75% of total liver blood flow.[117] The remainder passes via the portal vein through the liver to the hepatic veins. The portal venous drainage to the left lobe is less than to the right lobe, leading to a relative underdevelopment of the left lobe. The ductus venosus closes soon after birth.[118]

At 12 weeks of gestation there is evidence of gluconeogenesis and protein synthesis; at 14 weeks, glycogen is found in liver cells. Although by late gestation liver cell morphology is similar to that of adults, the functional development of the liver is immature in neonates and more so in preterm infants. Zone 1 hepatocytes (close to the portal triad) receive the greatest oxygen supply and thus perform the majority of gluconeogenesis, protein synthesis, and lipid metabolism.[117] Zone 3 hepatocytes, located near the central veins, perform biotransformation reactions, glycolysis, and urea synthesis (see also Chapters 5 and 28).[117] The fetal and neonatal liver account for a greater percent of body weight than the adult counterpart (3.6% of body weight vs. 2.4% in adults).[119] Hepatic organ blood flow in the neonate is 0.58 L/minute per kilogram tissue, and is reduced to 0.4 L/minute per kilogram tissue by 12 months postnatal age. Adult rates of 0.25 L/minute per kilogram tissue are reached in teenage years.[120] The neonatal liver contains approximately 20% fewer hepatocytes than adult livers, and the cells are nearly half the size of adult hepatocytes.

The liver has a major role in metabolism, controlling carbohydrate, protein, and lipid delivery to the tissues. Toward the end of pregnancy, large amounts of glycogen appear in the liver, and, as a result, preterm and small-for-gestational-age (SGA) infants accrue smaller stores of glycogen and are prone to develop hypoglycemia. Bile acid secretion in neonates is reduced, and malabsorption of fat occurs.

The liver is the site for the synthesis of proteins; this process is active in fetal and neonatal life. In fetal life, the main serum protein is alpha-fetoprotein. This protein first appears at 6 weeks of gestation and reaches a peak at 13 weeks of gestation. Albumin synthesis starts at 3 to 4 months of gestation and approaches adult values by birth; in preterm infants, the level is reduced. Proteins involved in clotting are also formed in the liver, but their concentrations in preterm and full-term neonates are less than normal for the first few days after birth. Hematopoiesis occurs in the fetal liver, with peak activity at 7 months of gestation. After 6 weeks of age, hematopoiesis is confined to the bone marrow except under pathologic conditions, such as hemolytic anemia (see Chapter 28).[121]

The capacity to enzymatically break down proteins is reduced at birth but matures rapidly throughout the first year of life, reaching adult levels by adolescence. This is particularly important in preterm infants, in whom the intake of a large protein load can result in dangerously high levels of serum amino acid concentrations and the subsequent development of a metabolic acidosis.

Hepatic function is immature at birth, even in neonates born at term, and many of the hepatic enzyme systems responsible for drug and xenobiotic clearance develop within the first few years of postnatal life. For many drugs, the reduced metabolism in neonates relates to reduced total quantities of cytochromes P-450 (CYP) enzymes in the hepatic microsomes. CYP activity measured in hepatic microsomes obtained from term neonates approaches half of the activity found in adults. Uridine 5'-diphosphoglucuronosyltransferase (UGT), responsible for morphine, acetaminophen, and dexmedetomidine clearance is also immature, as is UGT1A1, which is responsible for the conjugation of bilirubin that contributes to the development of physiological jaundice of the newborn. (see also Chapters 4 and 5).

Physiologic Jaundice

Bilirubin has two forms: conjugated (direct bilirubin) and unconjugated (indirect, binds to albumen). Normally only 0.2 to 0.7 mg/dL is unconjugated (indirect); this form is more fat soluble and therefore more toxic (able to cross biologic membranes, e.g., central nervous system (CNS) causing kernicterus in premature neonates). Kernicterus is now called bilirubin neurotoxicity (BNTx), which results in kernicterus spectrum disorder.[122] Physiologic jaundice is unconjugated hyperbilirubinemia that may last up to 1 week.[123] Hyperbilirubinemia (defined as a total serum bilirubin level >5 mg/dL) is a particularly important problem in neonates. About 60% of term and 80% of preterm neonates develop jaundice in the first week of life, with a total bilirubin concentration exceeding 5 mg/dL.[124]

Several mechanisms account for the jaundice (Table 1.10).[125,126] In term neonates, the normal total bilirubin concentration is usually less than 5 mg/dL (86 μmol/L) and is rarely greater than 12 mg/dL without a risk factor, peaking on the third to fourth postnatal day. Values more than 17 mg/dL are abnormal.[123] In preterm infants, the bilirubin concentration peaks at 10 to 12 mg/dL on the fifth to seventh postnatal day. After this period, the concentration gradually decreases, reaching adult values (<2 mg/dL) by 1 to 2 months in both term and preterm infants. The concentration of indirect bilirubin is also increased in the first few days after birth. The cause of

nonhemolytic physiologic hyperbilirubinemia is excessive bilirubin production from breakdown of red blood cells and increased enterohepatic circulation of bilirubin with deficient hepatic conjugation resulting from decreased uridine 5'-diphosphoglucuronosyltransferase activity (UGT1A1, see Chapters 4, 5 and 28). Approximately 1% of breastfed infants develop hyperbilirubinemia, with an onset that is delayed from 6 to 14 days after birth.[123] Breastfed hyperbilirubinemia is considered to be benign. The provenance of this phenomenon remains unclear but has been attributed to the beta-glucuronidases and nonesterified fatty acids in human milk that inhibit conjugation.[123] An earlier hypothesis that ascribed this phenomenon to inhibition of UGT activity by 3α, 20β-pregnanediol activity has not been substantiated. In addition, genetic variants may affect bilirubin metabolism.[127,128]

Important pathologic causes of jaundice in neonates are presented in Table 1.11. The relative rarity of cholestasis is in sharp contrast with the very common finding of jaundice during the first weeks of life, and therefore, a false diagnosis of physiologic or breast milk jaundice is easily made. Symptoms indicative of cholestasis such as dark urine and pale stools are often unrecognized.[129]

Once the distinction between physiologic and hemolytic hyperbilirubinemia has been made, the underlying cause can then be treated and efforts can be directed at preventing bilirubin-induced encephalopathy (kernicterus spectrum disorder) by the use of phototherapy and, in selected cases, exchange transfusions.[122] Phototherapy reduces serum bilirubin concentrations by converting bilirubin through structural photoisomerization and photooxidation into excretable products.[130] There are risks and consequences to phototherapy, particularly in very-low-birth-weight infants, including hypocalcemia attributable in part to parathyroid hormone suppression,[131] skin rash, bronze baby syndrome (increased pigmentation in skin, mucous membranes, and urine),[132] and mild hemolysis.[133,134] However, phototherapy is not associated with the development of benign or malignant melanocyte lesions.[135]

Sick preterm infants are especially at risk for kernicterus (at bilirubin levels as small as 10 to 14 mg/dL) and are more aggressively treated at reduced bilirubin concentrations than full-term infants.[123] Increasingly common is a form of cholestatic jaundice in low-birth-weight infants receiving hyperalimentation for prolonged periods.[136,137] The mechanism of the jaundice is unclear, although it has been attributed to the inhibition of bile flow by amino acids.[138] Infants who were less than 750 grams at birth, and those with gastroschisis or jejunal atresia are at particular risk.[139] Promising therapies for hyperbilirubinemia in low-birth-weight infants may include the use of tin-mesoporphyrin, which inhibits the production of bilirubin and is still undergoing clinical investigation.[140–142]

TABLE 1.10	Causes of Jaundice in Neonates
Excess bilirubin production	
Impaired uptake of bilirubin	
Impaired conjugation of bilirubin	
Defective bilirubin excretion	
Increased enterohepatic circulation of bilirubin	

TABLE 1.11	Pathologic Causes of Jaundice in Neonates
Antibody-induced hemolysis (Rh and ABO)	
Hereditary red blood cell disorders (e.g., glucose-6-phosphate dehydrogenase deficiency, which gives rise to hemolysis from drugs or infection)	
Infections (e.g., neonatal hepatitis, sepsis, severe urinary tract infections)	
Hemorrhage into the body (e.g., intracerebral)	
Biliary atresia	
Metabolic (e.g., hypothyroidism, galactosemia)	

GASTROINTESTINAL TRACT

In an embryo, the digestive tract consists of the developing foregut, midgut, and hindgut.[143] These rapidly elongate so that a loop of gut is forced into the yolk sac. At 5 to 7 weeks, this loop twists around the axis of the superior mesenteric artery and returns to the abdominal cavity. The celiac artery supplies the foregut, the superior mesenteric artery the midgut, and the inferior mesenteric artery the hindgut.[143] Maturation occurs gradually from the proximal to the distal end. Blood vessels and nerves (Auerbach and Meissner plexuses) are developed by 13 weeks of gestation and peristalsis begins. However, gut motility is not propulsive until ~30 weeks of gestation with marked maturational changes between 29 and 32 weeks of gestation. This is one factor limiting tolerance of enteral feeding before 29 to 30 weeks of gestation.[143] The pancreas arises from two outgrowths of the foregut; a diverticulum of the foregut gives rise to the liver.

Enzyme levels of enterokinase and lipase increase with gestational age but are reduced at birth compared with older children. Full-term neonates and preterm neonates handle protein loads reasonably well, although preterm neonates may have difficulty with large loads. Fat digestion is limited, particularly in preterm neonates, who absorb only 65% of adult levels. CNS abnormalities will delay these maturational changes.[144]

Swallowing is a complex process under central and peripheral control. The reflex is initiated in the medulla, through cranial nerves to the muscles that control the passage of food through the pharyngoesophageal sphincter. Swallowing begins at ~11 to 12 weeks of gestation, nutritive swallowing is observed at ~18 to 24 weeks of gestation, but effective nutritive sucking not until ~34 to 35 weeks of gestation.[143] In the process, the tongue, soft palate, pharynx, and larynx all are smoothly coordinated. Any pathologic condition of these structures can interfere with normal swallowing. Neuromuscular incoordination, however, is more likely to be responsible for any dysfunction. This is particularly evident when the CNS has sustained damage either before or during delivery.

Lower esophageal sphincter pressures are reduced at birth but increase steadily, reaching adult values by 3 to 6 weeks postnatal age. Daily vomiting or "spitting up" is reported in 50% to 60% of all infants between 0 and 2 months of age and in 60% to 70% of infants 4 to 6 months of age.[145,146] Most of these infants suffer no ill effect ("happy spitters") and grow normally.[147] This condition usually begins in the first weeks after birth and resolves spontaneously by 9 to 24 months of age as solid food is introduced and the child assumes the upright position. Between 1:300 and 1:1000 infants have gastroesophageal reflux significant enough to warrant treatment to prevent complications.[148] Immaturity of the lower esophageal sphincter place preterm infants at greater risk (~22% for those born <34 week's gestational age).[146] Severe and recurrent reflux is associated with reactive airway disease,[149] recurrent pneumonia, and life-threatening apnea events.[150,151]

Meconium is the material contained in the intestinal tract before birth. It consists of desquamated epithelial cells from the intestinal tract, bile, pancreatic and intestinal secretions, and water (70%). Meconium is usually passed in the first few hours after birth; virtually all term neonates pass their first stool by 48 hours. However, passage of the first stool is usually delayed in low-birth-weight neonates, possibly because of immaturity of bowel motility and lack of gut hormones from delayed enteral feeding. Meconium ileus occurs in cystic fibrosis and Hirschsprung disease.[152]

Meconium aspiration at birth can cause severe respiratory distress due to particulate airway obstruction, atelectasis, and chemical pneumonitis with pulmonary inflammatory responses.[153,154] Inhaled nitric oxide[155,156] and steroids to reduce inflammation are the treatments of choice.[157]

The gastrointestinal transit time in the neonate is less than that in the adult but increases with age. The normal physiologic range of stool frequency varies greatly (from 10 times per day to 1 to 2 times per week)[158] and more often in breastfed infants. The frequency of bowel movements gradually decreases during the first years of life, reaching adult habits at about 4 years of age.

Necrotizing enterocolitis is an acquired gastrointestinal disease associated with significant morbidity and mortality; the major risk factors are low-birth-weight, prematurity, formula feeding, and intestinal dysbiosis.[159] The disease affects ~6% to 7% of very-low-birth-weight infants (see also Chapter 35); mortality is ~10% to 30%.[159]

PANCREAS

The placenta is impermeable to both insulin and glucagon. The islets of Langerhans in the fetal pancreas, however, secrete insulin from week 11 of fetal life[160]; the amount of insulin secretion increases with age. After birth, the insulin response is related to gestational and postnatal ages and is more mature in term infants.

Maternal hyperglycemia, particularly when uncontrolled, results in hypertrophy and hyperplasia of the fetal islets of Langerhans. This leads to increased levels of insulin in the fetus, affecting lipid metabolism and giving rise to a large for gestational age (4000 to 4500 grams), overweight neonate characteristic of a mother with diabetes (infant of a diabetic mother, IDM).[161] Infants of diabetic mothers are at risk for preterm birth.[162] Hyperglycemia alone is not instrumental in this effect; an infant of a diabetic mother may also be the result of an increase in serum amino acids in diabetic mothers. Hyperinsulinemia of the fetus persists after birth and may lead to rapid development of serious hypoglycemia. In addition to severe hypoglycemia, the incidence of congenital anomalies is increased as is the risk for birth injuries,[163] such as shoulder dystocia, Erb palsy,[164] respiratory distress, hypoglycemia,[165] asphyxia, and perinatal death.[166]

Neonates who are small for gestational age are frequently hypoglycemic, possibly because of malnutrition in utero. In addition, hepatic glycogen stores are inadequate, and deficient gluconeogenesis exists. Preterm neonates may be hypoglycemic without demonstrable symptoms, necessitating close monitoring of blood glucose levels.

Full-term neonates undergo a metabolic adjustment postnatally with regard to glucose. In 1988, a multicenter study associated a blood sugar <47 mg/dL with adverse developmental outcomes.[167] Since then conflicting recommendations have been made by the American Academy of Pediatrics[168] and the Pediatric Endocrine Society.[169,170] Studies have defined abnormal glucose concentrations as follows: plasma glucose concentrations less than 35 mg/dL in the first 3 hours after birth; less than 45 mg/dL after 12 hours.[168,171] If the blood level is less than 35 mg/dL 1 hour after feeding, initiate IV glucose treatment.[168] It is important to recognize that neonates may develop serious hypoglycemia that could lead to irreversible CNS damage, even though they may demonstrate few or no signs and symptoms. Other neonates may present with sweating, poor suck, weak cry, tremors, hypothermia, irritability, lethargy, hypotonia, seizures, coma, apnea, grunting respirations, tachypnea, or cyanosis.[170]

Hyperglycemia (plasma glucose ≥150 mg/dL) occurs in stressed neonates, particularly in low-birth-weight neonates receiving glucose-containing solutions. Hyperglycemia commonly occurs in neonates and infants during elective surgery under general anesthesia; infusion of glucose-containing solutions may increase the risk of hyperglycemia. Thus, it is advisable that intraoperative glucose concentrations be monitored. A study in infants undergoing surgery under general anesthesia showed that postsurgical plasma glucose values were significantly greater than postinduction values; insulin changes, however, were minimal.[172] The risk of hyperglycemia is considerably greater in infants weighing less than 1000 grams compared with infants 2000 grams or greater.[173] Hyperglycemia may also lead to osmotic diuresis and dehydration and has been associated with an increased incidence of intraventricular hemorrhage and a neurologic handicap. It is recommended that intraoperative glucose-containing solutions be administered with an infusion pump and only run at basal rates (see also Chapter 7); 1% to 2.5% glucose-containing solutions (not commercially available in all countries) have been recommended although a 1% solution in a balanced salt solution (not a sodium chloride solution) has garnered the most interest in neonates as it provides glucose without an increased risk of perioperative hyperglycemia and hyponatremia.[174–176]

Hematopoietic and Immunologic System

The blood volume in a full-term neonate depends on the time of cord clamping, which modifies the volume of placental transfusion. The blood volume is 93 mL/kg when cord clamping is delayed after delivery, compared with 82 mL/kg with immediate cord clamping.[177] A 1-minute delay in cord clamping transfuses ~80 mL of blood and a 3 minute delay transfuses ~100 mL into the neonate's circulation.[178] Within the first 4 hours after delivery, however, fluid is lost from the blood and the plasma volume contracts by as much as 25%. The greater the placental transfusion, the greater the loss of fluid in the first few hours after birth, resulting in hemoconcentration. The blood volume in preterm infants is greater (90 to 105 mL/kg) than in full-term neonates because of increased plasma volume.[179,180]

HEMOGLOBIN

The normal range of hemoglobin in the neonate is 14 to 20 g/dL. The site of sampling must be considered when interpreting these values for the diagnosis of neonatal anemia or hyperviscosity syndrome. Capillary sampling (e.g., heel-stick) generally overestimates the true hemoglobin concentration because of stasis in peripheral vessels that decreases the volume of plasma and causes hemoconcentration. This difference on average is ~12% greater (capillary vs. venous) on day 1 of life and these differences decrease over time (~5% to 7% up to day 28 of life); there is no difference with heel warming.[181] The average effect may be an increase in hemoglobin concentration by 2 g/dL on day 1 and 1 g/dL on day 28 of life[181]; for accuracy, venipuncture is preferred over capillary sampling.

Erythropoietic activity from the bone marrow decreases immediately after birth in both full-term and preterm infants. The cord blood reticulocyte counts of 5% persist for a few days and decline below 1% by 1 week. This is followed by a slight increase to 1% to 2% by the 12th week, where it remains throughout childhood. Preterm infants have greater reticulocyte counts (up to 10%) at birth. Neonatal reticulocyte counts vary with the type of delivery, gestational age, maternal hemoglobin values, and need for intubation.[182] Abnormal reticulocyte values generally reflect hemorrhage or hemolysis.

In term neonates, the hemoglobin concentration decreases during the 9th to 12th weeks to reach a nadir of 10 to 11 g/dL (hematocrit 30% to 33%) and increases thereafter.[183] This decrease in hemoglobin concentration is the result of a decrease in erythropoiesis and, to some extent, to a shortened life span of the

red blood cells. This "physiologic anemia of infancy" is a normal adjustment to extrauterine life. In preterm infants, the decrease in the hemoglobin concentration after birth is greater and directly related to the degree of prematurity. Furthermore, the nadir in the hemoglobin concentration is reached earlier, by weeks 4 to 6.[183,184] In infants weighing 1000 to 1500 grams, the decrement may reach 8 g/dL and for preterm infants less than 1000 grams to approximately 7 g/dL.[183] Despite these reductions in hemoglobin, the oxygen delivery to the tissues may not be compromised because of a shift of the oxygen-hemoglobin dissociation curve (to the right), secondary to an increase in 2,3-diphosphoglycerate and replacement of fetal hemoglobin with adult hemoglobin.[185] In preterm neonates, this degree of anemia is not "physiologic" and in part is due to frequent blood sampling, as well as diminished erythropoietin responses.[183] Exogenous recombinant erythropoietin therapy has had mixed results and of limited efficacy in treating the anemia of prematurity.[183] Restrictive transfusion practice seems to be equally efficacious.[186–188] Reduced hemoglobin concentrations, especially in preterm infants, may be associated with apnea and tachycardia.[189] Vitamin E administration does not prevent anemia of prematurity; no significant difference was noted between vitamin E–supplemented and unsupplemented groups in terms of hemoglobin concentration, reticulocyte and platelet counts, or erythrocyte morphology in infants at 6 weeks of age.[190] Current views point to delayed cord clamping or umbilical cord milking at the time of cord clamping in the delivery room as the most effective means to prevent anemia of prematurity.[191,192] After the third month, the hemoglobin concentration stabilizes at 11.5 to 12 g/dL until about 2 years of age. The hemoglobin concentration in full-term and preterm infants is comparable after the first year. Thereafter, there is a gradual increase in the hemoglobin concentration to mean values at puberty of 14 g/dL for females and 15.5 g/dL for males (see also Chapter 8).

LEUKOCYTES AND IMMUNOLOGY

White blood cell counts (lymphocytes) are generally greater in venous compared with capillary sampling.[181] The white blood cell count may normally reach 21,000/mm^3 in the first 24 hours of life and 12,000/mm^3 at the end of the first week, with the number of neutrophils equaling the number of lymphocytes. The white blood cell count then decreases gradually, reaching adult values by puberty. At birth, lymphocytes are the predominate white cells, comprising about 70% of the cells. But from the first week of life through 4 years of age and into adulthood, lymphocytes progressively decrease in numbers, finally stabilizing at about 35% of white cells in adults.[193] In contrast, neutrophils comprise about 20% of white cells in the first few months but increase progressively, reaching about 69% in the elderly.[193] These proportions were similar in males and females. Similarly CD3 complex and T cells increase from infancy to adulthood.[193] Neonates have an increased susceptibility to bacterial infection, which is related in part to immaturity of leukocyte function. Sepsis may be associated with a minimal leukocyte response or even with leukopenia. Spurious increases in the white blood cell content may be due to drugs (e.g., epinephrine). The incidence of neonatal sepsis correlates inversely with gestational age and may be as great as 58% in very-low-birth-weight infants.[194]

PLATELETS

The platelet count increases throughout gestation, at about 2000/mm^3 per week.[195] Although the mean platelet count was 200,000/mm^3 even in premature infants, the lower fifth percentiles were 104,000/mm^3 in infants ≤32 weeks and 123,000/mm^3 in term neonates. Thus, platelet counts between 100,000 and 150,000/mm^3

are likely more frequent in extremely premature infants compared with full-term neonates and children.[195] Platelet counts obtained by capillary sampling are generally less than in a venous sample by ~40,000 to 50,000/mm³.[181]

Platelet hyporeactivity has been described in full-term neonates and may be more pronounced in preterm neonates.[195-198] This hyporeactivity seems to normalize by 10 to 14 days of life.[195] There appears to be an inverse correlation between gestational age or birth weight and the severity of platelet hyporeactivity. Thrombocytopenia is a common hematologic finding in neonates, occurring in 1% to 2% of healthy term neonates.[199] Mechanical ventilation has been associated with a significant decrease in the platelet count in neonates.[200] A study of neonatal thrombocytopenia and its impact on hemostatic integrity showed that thrombocytopenic infants are at greater risk for bleeding than equally sick nonthrombocytopenic infants (see Chapters 8, 18, and 35). Platelet counts normally decrease from neonatal age to adolescence.[193]

COAGULATION

At birth, vitamin K–dependent factors (i.e., II, VII, IX, and X) are 20% to 60% of adult values; in preterm infants, the values are even less. The result is prolonged prothrombin times, normally encountered in full-term and preterm neonates. Synthesis of vitamin K–dependent factors occurs in the liver, which, being immature, produces relatively small concentrations of coagulation factors, even with the administration of vitamin K. It takes several weeks for the levels of coagulation factors to reach adult values; the deficit is even more pronounced in preterm neonates. The American Academy of Pediatrics (AAP) recommends intramuscular administration of vitamin K to all neonates who weighed more than 1500 grams as a single dose (1 mg) within 6 hours of birth and a reduced dose (0.3 to 0.5 mg) in infants less than 1500 grams; intravenous vitamin K is not recommended for prophylaxis in preterm infants.[201,202] The majority of cases of neonatal vitamin K deficiency occur in normal neonates with parental refusal a major factor for vitamin K deficiency bleeding. Omission of vitamin K can lead to serious and life-threatening consequences, especially if surgery is undertaken. Breastfeeding, especially in mothers not taking vitamin supplements, may also be associated with severe vitamin K deficiency; exclusively breastfed infants should receive vitamin supplementation. The AAP guideline specifically admonishes that vitamin K deficiency bleeding be considered *"in the first 6 months of life, even in infants who received prophylaxis, and especially in breast fed infants."*[201]

However, in theory, the increasing risk of bleeding is balanced by the protective effects of physiologic deficiencies of coagulation inhibitors, as well as by the decreased fibrinolytic capacity. Developmental hemostasis should be considered, as well as laboratory variations of coagulation tests that may render any diagnosis of bleeding disorder in infants difficult to establish.[203,204] Infants of mothers who have received anticonvulsant drugs during pregnancy may develop a serious coagulopathy similar to that encountered with vitamin K deficiency.[205] Other risk factors include maternal use of drugs such as warfarin, rifampin, and isoniazid.

POLYCYTHEMIA

Neonatal polycythemia (central hematocrit ≥65%) occurs in 3% to 5% of full-term neonates.[206] This may be associated with post-term delivery, small-for-gestational-age infants, twin-to-twin transfusion, and chromosomal abnormalities.[207] Using M-mode echocardiography, a study of neonates demonstrated an increase in both pulmonary and systemic vascular resistance with hyperviscosity.[208] Partial exchange transfusion to reduce the hematocrit

and decrease the blood viscosity improves systemic and pulmonary blood flow and oxygen transport, although one review questioned the efficacy when the exchange transfusion was conducted after 6 hours of life in asymptomatic infants.[209] The increased organ blood flow should prevent the cardiovascular and neurologic symptoms associated with the hyperviscosity syndrome.

Neurologic Development and Cognitive Development Issues

NEUROLOGIC DEVELOPMENT

The brain weighs about 335 grams at birth and grows rapidly in the first year of life, doubling in size by 6 months and reaching adult size by 12 years of age.[210] Brain development starts with the formation of the neural tube (neurulation) and forebrain (prosencephalon) in the third week of gestation.[211] Intensive growth and proliferation of the brain cells then follow, during which time the cells migrate to genetically programmed areas, gradually forming the layers and structures of the brain. The nervous system is anatomically complete at birth; functionally it remains immature with the continuation of myelination and synaptogenesis. Myelination is usually complete by 7 years of age. An infant's normal mental development depends on the maturation of the CNS. This development may be affected by physical illness, inadequate psychosocial support, or poor nutrition. In a randomized trial of diet in preterm babies, a suboptimal diet resulted in reduced intelligence quotients 7 to 8 years later in life.[212]

The rate of brain growth is different from the growth rate of other body systems. The brain has two growth spurts: neuronal cell peak multiplication occurs between 15 and 20 weeks of gestation and neuronal development and cortical organization commences at ~22 to 24 weeks of gestation.[213] Failure of closure of the neural tube may result in various forms of deformity (encephalocele, meningomyelocele, meningocele).[213] Many other CNS defects are due to abnormal dorsal or ventral neural tube closure and genetic abnormalities.[213] Myelination proceeds from deep to superficial brain regions at different rates and can be assessed with MRI.[214] Myelination in most rapid during the first 2 years of life but remodeling may continue into adulthood, explaining in part brain plasticity and strategies for treating traumatic brain injuries.[215,216] Malnutrition during the first 2 years of neural development may have profound handicapping effects.

Plasma membrane transport selectively promotes the passage of essential substrates such as glucose, organic acids, and amino acids across the blood-brain barrier. The blood-brain barrier is composed of pericytes, neurons, glia, and endothelial cells lining CNS blood vessels all held together with "tight junctions;" cross-talk and molecular signaling between them regulate the blood-brain barrier.[217] Hypoxemia and ischemia may lead to a breakdown in this barrier, with resulting edema and increased intracranial pressure. Injury to the blood-brain barrier may result from abnormal entry of calcium or formation of free radicals causing neuroinflammation. Further studies of the mechanism of this breakdown will lead to rational approaches to therapy.[218,219] In preterm neonates stressed by hypoxia, the blood-brain barrier may become particularly permeable to the water-soluble unbound bilirubin, with possible damage to the brain.[220] It appears that, contrary to early reports of a "leaky" blood-brain barrier in neonates, that these assumptions are incorrect and that it is the fragile cerebral blood vessels that *"render the neonatal brain more vulnerable to drugs, toxins, and pathological conditions."*[221]

TABLE 1.12	Relationship of Motor Milestones to Age
Motor Milestone	**Age**
Supports head	3 months
Sits alone	6 months
Stands alone	12 months
Balances on one foot	3 years

TABLE 1.13	Relationship of Fine Motor/Adaptive Milestones to Age
Fine Motor/Adaptive Milestones	**Age**
Grasps rattle	3 months
Passes cube hand to hand	6 months
Pincer grip	1 year
Imitates vertical line	2 years
Copies circle	3 years

TABLE 1.14	Relationship of Language Milestones to Age
Language Milestones	**Age**
Squeals	1.5–3 months
Turns to voice	6 months
Combines two words	1.5 years
Composes short sentencesç	2 years
Gives entire name	3 years

TABLE 1.15	Relationship of Personal-Social Milestones to Age
Personal-Social Milestones	**Age**
Smiles spontaneously	3 months
Feeds self crackers	6 months
Drinks from cup	1 year
Plays interactive games	2 years

Full-term neonates show various primitive reflexes including the Moro response and grasp reflex. Milestones of development are useful indicators of mental and physical development guiding expectations for both normal and abnormal development. These milestones represent the *average child,* but there is a range of maturation of different body functions that are within the normal range.[222] The Denver Developmental Screening Test is useful for assessing these milestones. The test focuses on four areas of development: (1) gross motor function, (2) fine motor and adaptive skills, (3) language, and (4) personal and social skills. Developing infants rapidly acquire motor skills beginning with control of posture in a cephalocaudal direction; this begins with head control and rapidly progresses to sitting, standing, walking, and finally running (Table 1.12).

Adaptive skills are performed through well-coordinated fine motor movements (Table 1.13). Abnormal development may be reflected in a delay in the appearance of a particular milestone or in its pathologic persistence with maturation in a child. For example, at 5 months, a child reaches and retrieves objects, frequently placing them in their mouth. As an infant matures, however, this behavior pattern usually ceases at 12 to 13 months of age; in infants with developmental delay, this oral practice may continue for a longer period of time.

Language development correlates closely with cognitive skills (Table 1.14). Personal and social skills are modified by environmental factors and cultural patterns (Table 1.15). Development of walking, speech, and sphincter control is most important. For appropriate evaluation consider familial patterns, level of intelligence, and physical illness. Deafness may cause delayed speech.

The potential adverse effects of many medications used to provide anesthesia on the developing brain of animal models and in humans are still uncertain (see Chapter 23). Several studies in humans lend support to the notion that a brief exposure to general anesthesia does not harm young children[223–225]; further studies are needed since there are so many conflicting data and unanswered questions.[226]

The incidence of cerebral palsy is estimated to be 1 to 4/1000 live births worldwide and 1/345 children in the United States, with the greatest prevalence in preterm infants and low-birth-weight infants.[227–229] Reduction of perinatal mortality during the past decade has not resulted in the expected reduction in the prevalence of cerebral palsy. The most common etiologies of cerebral palsy are perinatal ischemic stroke, white matter disorder, and intrauterine inflammation.[227,230] Less than 5% of cases of cerebral palsy result from perinatal asphyxia. The strongest predictors of cerebral palsy appear to be congenital anomaly (congenital heart disease in particular), low-birth-weight, low placental weight, multiple fetuses, preterm delivery, intrauterine infection, or abnormal fetal position before labor and delivery.[231]

INTERACTIONS WITH THE EXTERNAL WORLD DURING GROWTH AND DEVELOPMENT

The environment with all its potential toxins and pollutants may have a direct influence on growth and development, interfering with both physiologic and pathologic aspects. For the past 2 decades, we have known that programmed cell death (or apoptosis) is part of normal development[232] and that triggering factors result from both evolutionary pathways and external influences. This occurs at both anatomic and functional levels and opens the potential for many and varied investigations. Neurogenesis, particularly in specific parts of the brain such as the hippocampus, has long been thought to occur only during development, but recent evidence has shown that it continues throughout human life and both genetics and inflammation may hold the keys to neurodegenerative disorders.[233,234] Implications of an interaction between memory and its influence on degenerative neurologic diseases are now firmly established.[235] Anesthetic drugs have been shown to adversely affect the developing brain in rodents and primates, but with the discovery of neurogenesis in adults, we now know that similar changes occur in adults as well.[236–238] However, recent evidence suggests it is quite unlikely that anesthetics affect the neurobehavioral changes in human infants and toddlers (see also Chapter 23).

Evidence has confirmed that the functional aspect of brain development in the fetus is far more complex than previously thought and is not limited just to the last weeks before birth.[239] A waking-like brain state exists that is present earlier in gestation and inducible with maternal behavioral changes and external stimuli (e.g., music).[240] These factors may have long-term neurodevelopmental effects and the beginning of memorization likely occurs earlier than previously thought.[241] A mother's voice, heartbeat, speech, and language all impact the fetal neural plasticity.[242–245]

A large number of interactions between the neonate and the external world exist. The child has some direct influences on their external environment. The ethnologic concept of "baby schema" was proposed by Lorenz,[246] who suggested that some type of positive features can result in a positive response in the human.[247,248] Infantile physical features, such as a round face and big eyes, are perceived as cute and motivate caretaking behavior in the human, with the evolutionary function of enhancing offspring survival. This has been observed across animal species.[249] A baby's smile, for example, can increase the speed of the caring response[250,251] and narrow the intentional focus of the mother independently of face recognition.[252,253] Comparisons between neurophysiologic and neuropsychological studies are difficult but may prove an important confounding factor in our search to understand the complexities of human growth and development.

The Skin and Thermoregulation

Neonates and particularly preterm neonates are very susceptible to hypothermia by four possible routes: convection (34%), conduction (3%), radiation (39%), and evaporation (24%).[254] Insensible

fluid loss and heat loss from evaporation are increased in the preterm neonate because of their thin skin and minimal subcutaneous fat.[255] Conduction and convection losses are also increased because of their large surface area to mass ratio. Adults and children generate heat by shivering; however, preterm infants and neonates have minimal muscle mass for shivering. Thus nonshivering thermogenesis via brown fat, accumulated around the kidneys, adrenal glands, scapulae, and in the mediastinum during the last trimester of pregnancy is the prime source of generating body heat.[256,257] This brown adipose tissue may comprise up to 5% of the term neonate's weight.[258] In addition, regulation of skin blood flow is less efficient in the preterm neonate.[259]

Anesthesia further disrupts the normal thermoregulation by shifting blood flow peripherally. There is earlier vasoconstriction in infants during hypothermia as well as broadening of the response thresholds for compensatory mechanisms in those infants subjected to hypothermia while under anesthesia (Fig. 1.11). Hypothermia can contribute to developing a metabolic acidosis, impaired peripheral perfusion, increased risk of infection, and

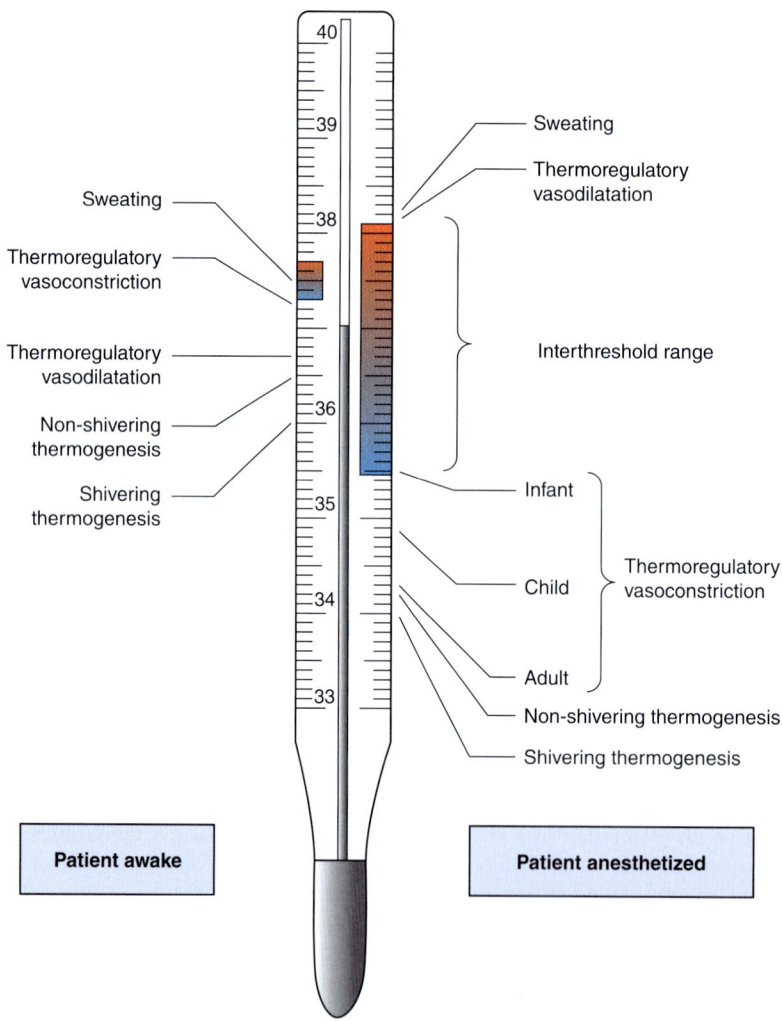

FIGURE 1.11 Schematic illustration of thermoregulatory thresholds and gains in awake and anesthetized states, demonstrating a broadening of the response thresholds for compensatory mechanisms under anesthesia but earlier vasoconstriction in infants during hypothermia. (Reproduced with permission from Luginbuehl I. Temperature regulation: physiology and pharmacology. In: Bissonnette B., ed. *Pediatric Anesthesia*. Shelton, Connecticut: PMPH-USA; 2011: 229. Adapted from Bissonnette B. Thermoregulation and paediatric anaesthesia, *Current Opinion in Anaesthesiology*. 1993;6:537-542.)

coagulation abnormalities. Hypothermia will also reduce drug clearance due to the reduced metabolic rate. The thin stratum corneum, rich skin blood flow, and relatively large body surface area, increases the potential for systemic exposure of topical drugs (e.g. corticosteroids, local anesthetic creams, antiseptics).[260–262]

Acknowledgment

We wish to thank Bruno Marciniak for his prior contributions to this chapter.

ANNOTATED REFERENCES

Ameisen JC. On the origin, evolution, and nature of programmed cell death: a timeline of four billion years. *Cell Death Differ.* 2002;9:367-393.

This paper discusses how programmed cell death is a genetically regulated process of cell suicide that is central to the development, homeostasis, and integrity of multicellular organisms. Dysregulation of mechanisms controlling cell suicide plays a role in the pathogenesis of a wide range of diseases. The author explores these processes that also have relevance to current debate concerning the effects of anesthesia on neonatal development.

Friis-Hansen B. Body water compartments in children: changes during growth and related changes in body composition. *Pediatrics.* 1961;28:169-181.

This classic paper describes body water compartments in children and their changes with age. Results still hold true and are widely used today.

Holliday MA, Segar WE. The maintenance need for water in parenteral fluid therapy. *Pediatrics.* 1957;19:823-832.

Another classic paper outlining fluid requirements in children. The paper served as a reference for many years but has come under recent criticism and a reanalysis of fluid and electrolyte requirements in children is due.

Kotecha S. Lung growth for beginners. *Paediatr Respir Rev.* 2000;1:308-313.

A great primer that can be used as a foundation for further learning.

Nowakowski RS, Hayes NL. CNS development: an overview. *Dev Psychopathol.* 1999;11:395-417.

Another classic paper that serves as a great primer.

Leibovitz Z, Lerman-Sagie T, Haddad L. Fetal brain development: regulating processes and related malformations. *Life (Basel).* 2022;12(6):809.

This paper describes the processes that regulate normal development of the embryonic-fetal CNS. The current literature on CNS malformations associated with these regulating processes are discussed. Each malformation is described with reference to the etiology, genetic causes, prenatal sonographic imaging, associated anomalies, differential diagnosis, complimentary diagnostic studies, clinical interventions, neurodevelopmental outcome, and life quality.

Schittny JC. Development of the lung. *Cell Tissue Res.* 2017;367:427-444.

This paper provides an excellent summary of neonatal lung development from early embryology to young adulthood.

Sottas C, Cumin D, Anderson BJ. Blood pressure and heart rates in neonates and preschool children; an analysis from ten years of electronic recording. *Pediatr Anesth.* 2016;26:1064-1070.

Blood pressure in children undergoing anesthesia is generally lower than that observed in healthy awake children. There is concern about what is an acceptable lower limit, particularly in the very young. The authors review observed blood pressure from a single institution involving 54,896 anesthetics in children younger than 6 years. A mean blood pressure drop of 28.6% was noted in infants 0 to 10 weeks of age.

A complete reference list can be found online at Elsevier eBooks+.

2 Preoperative Evaluation, Premedication, and Induction of Anesthesia

ELIZABETH A. GHAZAL, HARMONY CARTER, LINDA J. MASON, AND CHARLES J COTÉ

Preparation of Children for Anesthesia
Fasting
Piercings
Primary and Secondary Smoking and Vaping
Psychological Preparation of Children for Surgery
Child Development, Preoperative Anxiety,
and Behavioral Interventions
Parental Presence During Induction
Health Care Provider Interventions
Pharmacologic Interventions
Pharmacologic Interventions Versus Behavioral Interventions
History of Present Illness
Past/Other Medical History
Laboratory Data
Pregnancy Testing
Premedication and Induction Principles
General Principles
Medications
Induction of Anesthesia
Preparation for Induction

Inhalation Induction
Intravenous Induction
Intramuscular Induction
Full Stomach and Rapid-Sequence Induction
Special Problems
The Fearful Child
Autism
Anemia
Upper Respiratory Tract Infection
Obesity
Obstructive Sleep Apnea
Asymptomatic Cardiac Murmurs
Fever
Postanesthesia Apnea in Former Preterm Infants
Hyperalimentation
Diabetes
Bronchopulmonary Dysplasia
Seizure Disorders
Sickle Cell Disease

Preparation of Children for Anesthesia

FASTING

Infants and children are fasted before sedation and anesthesia to minimize the risk of pulmonary aspiration of gastric contents and pneumonitis.[1] In the fasted child, only basal secretions of gastric juice should be present in the stomach preoperatively as reflected by Digby Leigh's recommendation for a 1-hour preoperative fast after clear fluids in the first textbook on pediatric anesthesia in 1948.[2] However, Mendelson reported 66 cases of aspiration in pregnant women under anesthesia, with two deaths resulting from the aspiration of solid material, prompting anesthesiologists to focus on both the duration of fasting and the types of food ingested preoperatively to minimize the risk of aspiration pneumonitis.[1,3] Thereafter, the fasting interval before elective surgery in all patients increased to 8 hours. By the early 1980s however, children were fasted 4 hours after clear fluids preoperatively and overnight after solids. The next major change in preoperative fasting occurred in the late 1980s and early 1990s when research proved that fasting more than 2 hours after clear fluids preoperatively affected neither the risk nor the severity of pneumonitis should regurgitation and aspiration occur, regardless of the child's age.[4–12] It also became apparent that the threshold for pneumonitis after aspiration, which had always been based on a gastric fluid volume ≥0.4 mL/kg and pH ≤2.5, had never been established in humans.[1,13,14] Two studies in primates subsequently confirmed that the critical volume for pneumonitis after acid aspiration was 0.8 mL/kg, not 0.4 mL/kg.[15,16] Using these revised criteria for aspiration pneumonitis (gastric fluid volume >0.8 mL/kg and pH <2.5), studies in children again confirmed that the risks of pneumonitis after aspiration when children were fasted for 2 hours or greater after clear fluids were the same.[4–11]

The half-life to empty clear fluids from the stomach is approximately 15 minutes; as a result, 98% of clear fluids exit the stomach in children by ~1 hour. Clear liquids include water, fruit juices without pulp, carbonated beverages, clear tea, and black coffee. Fasting for 2 hours after clear fluids (excluding those with increased caloric or protein content)[17,18] ensures nearly complete emptying of the residual volume within this fasting period. Two small studies in adults suggested that gastric emptying is not appreciably changed when milk was added to either coffee or tea, although aspiration of milk products is far more likely to trigger pneumonitis than aspiration of clear fluids.[19,20] Important benefits of a 2-hour fasting interval after clear fluids in healthy children is less thirst, hunger, and improved child cooperation.[4] In addition, there is a reduced risk of hypoglycemia, which may occur in children who are debilitated, have chronic disease, are poorly nourished, have metabolic dysfunction, or are preterm or formerly preterm infants. The risks of hypotension during induction[21] and success with the first attempt at IV insertion[22] are similar whether the child is fasted for only 2 hours or for a prolonged period. Undesirable prolonged fasting in children may be lessened by electronic reminders to parents on the day before surgery in some communities.[23]

Gastric emptying studies demonstrate that solids empty from the stomach follow a zero-order elimination (i.e., empty at a constant rate) but fluids follow first-order kinetics (empty at an exponential rate), highlighting the importance of knowing both the substance type and volume ingested.[24] Gastric ultrasound has proven valuable in establishing accurate baseline gastric fluid volumes noninvasively and providing real-time examination of gastric contents preoperatively. Gastric ultrasound studies quantified the average baseline gastric volume in fasted individuals to be 0.4 to 0.6 mL/kg, with an upper limit of 1.5 mL/kg.[25–28] Point-of-care ultrasound of the gastric antrum has demonstrated both interrater reliability in assessing gastric volume and stratifying aspiration risk when fasting times are unmet or unknown.[28–33]

If elective surgery for a preterm infant or neonate is delayed, hypoglycemia or hypovolemia may occur.[21,34,35] In such circumstances, a glucose-containing intravenous fluid should be infused at maintenance rates before induction of anesthesia.[36] Alternatively, if the fasting interval is protracted, the infant should be offered clear fluids orally (up to 3 mL/kg) until 2 hours before induction.

Although some consider breast milk to be synonymous with clear liquids, this assumption has no basis in fact.[37] Breast milk can injure the lungs if aspirated, and cause much worse damage than clear fluids.[38] In addition, breast milk has a very high and variable fat content (determined by maternal diet) that delays gastric emptying.[39] Gastric emptying half times after breast milk (50 minutes) and formula (75 minutes) in full-term and preterm neonates are prolonged compared with that for clear fluids.[39,40] Subsequent studies confirmed that the order of gastric emptying half-lives is clear fluids <<breastmilk <infant formula (Fig. 2.1).[41,42] However more recent studies have questioned this relationship. In one study in preterm infants, the mean gastric emptying times after both breast milk and infant formula evaluated by ultrasound were similar, 3.5 hours, although only 28% of the antrum area could be predicted from the fasting interval.[43] In healthy term neonates, the mean gastric emptying times after infant formula were more rapid than those in preterm infants and quite variable (45 to 150 minutes), although the gastric fluid volume was measured in ≤10% of the infants beyond 2 hours, limiting interpretation of the emptying times.[44] These inconsistent results may be attributed to small sample sizes, measurements of limited duration, and unaccounted for variability.

A systemic review and meta-analysis of preoperative gum chewing in both children and adults concluded that chewing gum does not increase the risk of major morbidity from pulmonary aspiration.[45,46] Several studies reported that gum chewing increases gastric fluid volume and pH, likely due to swallowing alkaline saliva, leaving gastric emptying unaffected. Consequently, if the gum is expectorated and discarded, then elective anesthesia can proceed without additional delay. If, however, the child swallows the gum, then general anesthesia should not proceed unless the surgery is deemed to be urgent/emergent because aspirated gum may completely block the airway and at body temperature, may be very difficult to extract from the trachea or a bronchus.

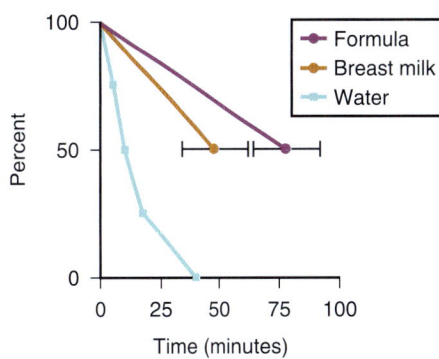

Feeding remaining in the stomach

FIGURE 2.1 Percentage of gastric feeding remaining in the stomach after water, breast milk, or formula versus time after ingestion by infants. Data are expressed as mean ± standard deviation. The time to 50% gastric emptying of water was 15 minutes, of breast milk 50 minutes, and of formula 80 minutes. Based on these data, about 95% emptying (i.e., four half-lives) of gastric feedings should occur in about 1 hour after water, about 3.5 hours after breast milk, and about 5.5 hours after infant formula. However, note the wide standard deviations for the emptying times for breast milk and formula. (From Cavell B. Gastric emptying in preterm infants. *Acta Paediatr Scand*. 1979; 68:725-730; Cavell B. Gastric emptying in infants fed human milk or infant formula. *Acta Paediatr Scand*. 1981;70:639-641.)

The incidence of pulmonary aspiration in modern elective pediatric or adult anesthesia without risk factors for aspiration is small, 0.6 to 9:10,000, with no long-term morbidity or death from respiratory sequelae reported.[47–58] This low risk may be attributed to several factors including strict adherence to preoperative fasting guidelines for solids to ensure empty stomachs and to the types of fluids that constitute clear fluids. Most patients with clinical status of American Society of Anesthesiologists (ASA) 1 or 2 who aspirate clear gastric contents have minimal to no sequelae; if clinical signs or sequelae from an aspiration in a child are going to occur, the signs will be apparent within 2 hours of the event.[47,51] The majority of reported aspirations in children occur during induction of anesthesia, although it can occur at any time during anesthesia including after extubation.[51,53,55,59] Risk factors for perianesthetic aspiration included neurologic or esophagogastric abnormality, emergency surgery, ASA physical status ≥3, gastrointestinal comorbidity, nil per os (NPO) violations, increased intracranial pressure, opioid use, inadequate anesthesia, obesity, choice of airway management, and an inexperienced intubator.[28,48,52,55,59,60] However, neither age nor gender impact this risk.[55] When the anesthesiologist suspects that the child has a full stomach or that other risk factors for aspiration are present, induction of anesthesia and airway management should be adjusted appropriately to mitigate the risk of pulmonary aspiration (see later in chapter).

Recent concerns focused on the large number of infants and children who were noncompliant with preoperative fasting guidelines, that is, they were fasted for prolonged periods preoperatively, which possibly exposed them to harm.[61–64] The evidence that prolonged fasting is either unsafe or harmful for healthy children undergoing elective general anesthesia is nonexistent.[21,22,64] In theory, prolonged fasts may be uncomfortable for children, rendering them thirsty and hungry; this may prompt them to ingest solids from their sibling or roommate and not disclose food ingestion preoperatively. Evidence holds that the majority of such children who were questioned, reported they were not "very thirsty" even after fasting >6 hours after clear fluids.[65–67] There are a multitude of reasons why parents, who are responsible for administering preoperative fluids to their children since >80% of surgeries are outpatient procedures, are noncompliant with the preoperative instructions to give oral clear fluids up to 2 hours preoperatively.[68–70] In an effort to address these concerns, the European Society of Pediatric Anaesthesia recently published guidelines reducing the fasting interval after clear fluids from 2 to 1 hour.[71] However, there is scant evidence that a 1-hour fast after clear fluids either addresses the reasons parents are noncompliant or eliminates prolonged fasting intervals; 30% of children fasted for prolonged periods after clear fluids despite implementing an abbreviated fasting regimen.[72] Two strategies have proven effective in improving parental compliance with preoperative fasting instructions; quality improvement, which is impractical to implement in most centers, and texting parent's phones on the evening before surgery, the most effective, simplest, and inexpensive strategy published to date.[23,73,74] Prolonged fasting after clear fluids can be eliminated and each institution should adopt the strategy that is most effective in this regard.

Residual gastric fluid volume and thus NPO times do not predict the risk of regurgitation and aspiration.[75,76] Moreover, residual gastric fluid volumes do not correlate with NPO times after clear fluids when the fasting interval exceeds ~2 hours.[77] However, when the fasting interval after clear fluids is <2 hours, residual gastric fluid volume increases exponentially.[77] Since the vast majority of studies include fasting intervals ≥2 hours after clear fluids, it is not surprising that the NPO times after clear fluids do not correlate with the risk of regurgitation and pulmonary aspiration. The half-time to emptying clear fluids from the stomach, 15 to 20 minutes, predicts complete emptying in ~1 hour, although recent MRI evidence reported that the half-time to emptying clear fluids is ~26 minutes.[78–80] Gastric emptying times may be greater than previously thought and depend upon the characteristics of the fluid: osmolarity, protein/fat content, volume ingested, and the presence of any underlying diseases (e.g., gastric dysmotility, gastroesophageal reflux, neurological impairment) (Fig. 2.2).[17,81] It is an insurmountable task to completely define the clear fluid a parent should administer to their child preoperatively (in terms of content and volume) as well as the timing (if different from the standard guidelines) because of the child's medical condition. To preclude a regurgitation at induction of anesthesia, we recommend a fasting interval of 2 hours after clear fluids, and that a fasting interval ≤1 hour should be proscribed. For the child who fasted 1 to 2 hours after clear fluids, the decision on whether to proceed with general anesthesia should be determined on an individual basis by the attending anesthesiologist and local guidelines (Fig. 2.3).[64] Concerns remain that the 1-hour fast advocated by the European Pediatric consortium and many pediatric anesthesia societies requires further study as does confirmation regarding the accuracy of ultrasound gastric volume to assess small gastric fluid volumes. The Task Force on Fasting of the American Society of Anesthesiologists has not changed its NPO guidelines (Table 2.1) but will revisit this issue in the near future.[64,82,83]

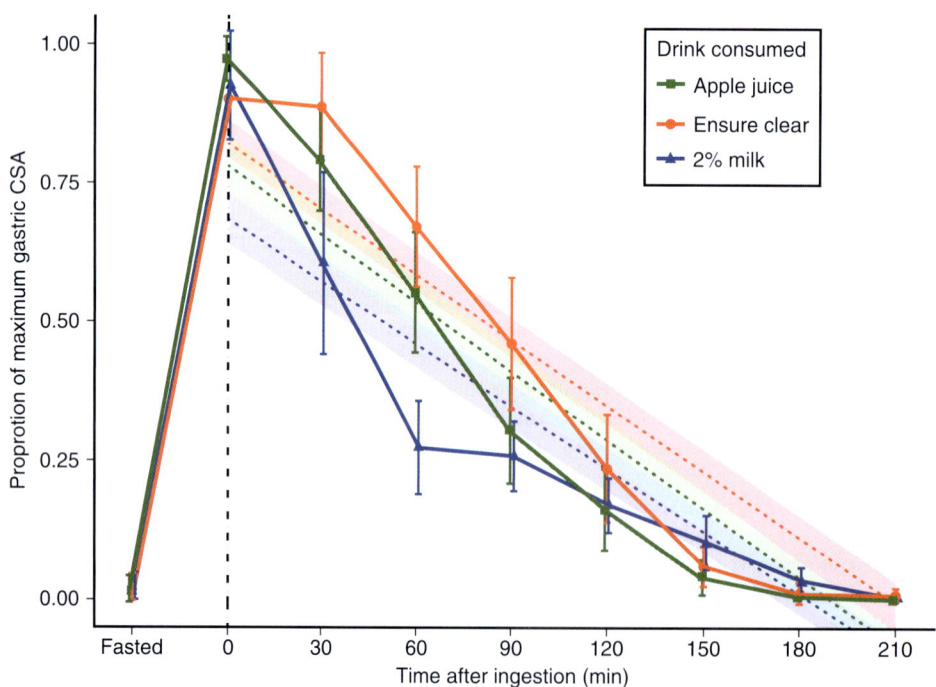

FIGURE 2.2 Time course of gastric antral cross-sectional area (CSA) as a method for assessing gastric fluid volume. Early differences were noted for apple juice, 2% milk, and a high protein drink but these difference became negligible after 3 to 3.5 hours. Error bars show 95% confidence intervals. Lineal-model ANCOVA with 95% upper and lower limits are also depicted. (From Du T, Hill L, Ding., et al. Gastric emptying for liquids of different compositions in children. *Br J Anaesth.* 2017;119(5):948-955.)

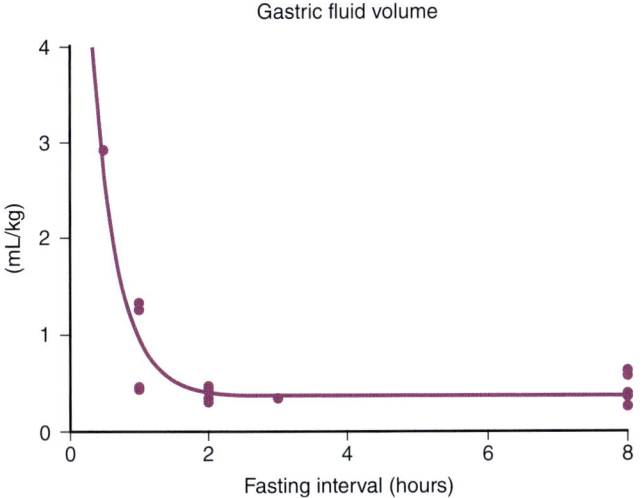

FIGURE 2.3 Gastric fluid volume versus fasting interval. (r^2 = 0.90) Based on data published in Andersson H, Schmitz A, Frykholm P. Preoperative fasting guidelines in pediatric anesthesia: are we ready for a change? *Curr Opin Anesthesiol.* 2018;31:342-348

TABLE 2.1	Preoperative Fasting Recommendations in Infants and Children
Clear liquids[a]	2 hours
Breast milk	4 hours
Infant formula, nonhuman milk, or light meal	6 hours[b]
Solids (fatty or fried foods)	8 hours

Practice guidelines for preoperative fasting and the use of pharmacologic agents to reduce the risk of pulmonary aspiration: Application to healthy patients undergoing elective procedures: An updated report by the American Society of Anesthesiologists Task Force on Preoperative Fasting and the Use of Pharmacologic Agents to Reduce the Risk of Pulmonary Aspiration. Anesthesiology. 2017;126(3):376-393.
[a]Include only fluids without pulp, clear tea, or coffee without milk products.
[b]Some centers allow plain toast (no dairy products) up to 6 hours prior to induction.

PIERCINGS

Body piercing is common practice in adolescents and young adults. Single or multiple piercings may appear anywhere on the body. To minimize the liability and risk of complications from metal piercings, their location should be documented preoperatively and, if possible, they should be removed before surgery. Complications that may occur if they are left in situ during anesthesia are listed in E-Table 2.1.[84–88]

PRIMARY AND SECONDARY SMOKING AND VAPING

Primary Smoking and Vaping

Each day, 3800 American adolescents smoke their first cigarette and of these, more than 50% will become regular smokers. The annual burden of smoking-attributable mortality remains high, with 5.6 million youth currently 0 to 17 years of age projected to die prematurely from a smoking-related illness.[89] Even though the rate of new cigarette smokers in North America has declined over the past 2 decades, this has been offset with a tremendous increase in use of other nicotine products such as electronic cigarettes (e-cigarettes) (Fig. 2.4). Vaping is a term referring to the inhalation of aerosols produced by a variety of devices that heat a liquid generally containing nicotine, flavoring, and various other chemicals. Other names for vaping devices, or electronic nicotine delivery systems, include mods (because of the ability to modify), vapes, subohms, vape pens, e-hookahs, tank systems, and e-cigarettes.[90,91] These vaping devices resemble common items such as a pen, a flashlight, or computer flash drive. Vaping is an emerging public health crisis that impacts the perioperative care of adolescents.[91,92] Since 2014, e-cigarettes have become the most commonly used tobacco-based product among youth in the United States.[93] In 2020, an estimated 3.6 million (13.1%) US middle and high school students reported using e-cigarettes within the past 30 days with more than 80% using flavored products.[94] Because of the ongoing COVID-19 pandemic, methodological changes were made in the 2021 National Youth Tobacco Survey, during which eligible students could participate in the survey in classrooms or remotely. Prior surveys were primarily conducted on school campuses thus preventing year-to-year comparison. Nonetheless, in 2021, 11.3% of 9th to 12th grade students (1.72 million) and 2.8% (320,000) of 6th to 8th grade students reported they use

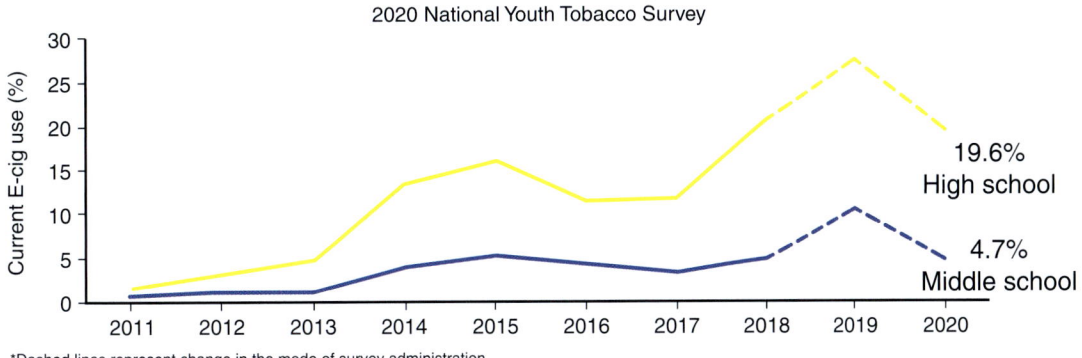

FIGURE 2.4 Use of e-cigarettes among middle school and high school students in the United States. https://digitalmedia.hhs.gov/tobacco/hosted/2020-National-Youth-Tobacco-Survey.pdf.

e-cigarettes. Among both groups, the most commonly used device type was disposables, and the most common brand was Puff Bar.[95] Many factors including ease of purchasing products at various retail outlets or online,[96,97] harmless water vapor messaging, a strong social media presence with celebrity endorsements, and flavors targeting a young audience ("Cupcake," "Alien Blood," "Cherry Crush," "Chocolate Treat," etc.) play a role in influencing initiation of e-cigarette use in this age group.[98] Marijuana products are also becoming increasingly popular among students who vape.[99] Youth e-cigarette users are 3.6 times more likely than nonusers to report subsequent initiation of conventional cigarettes within a year.[100] These findings raise concern that e-cigarettes have the potential to addict a new generation to nicotine and tobacco, slowing or reversing the decline in adolescent cigarette smoking that has occurred over the past 20 years.[101]

Smoking is known to increase blood carboxyhemoglobin concentrations,[102] decrease ciliary function,[103] decrease forced vital capacity and the forced expiratory flow in midphase ($FEF_{25\%-75\%}$),[104] and increase sputum production. There is extensive evidence that smokers undergoing surgery are more likely to develop wound infections and postoperative respiratory complications.[105] Although stopping smoking for 2 days decreases carboxyhemoglobin levels and shifts the oxyhemoglobin dissociation curve to the right, stopping for at least 6 to 8 weeks is necessary to reduce the rate of postoperative pulmonary complications.[106,107]

Current harmful effects of e-cigarette use focus on nicotine exposure, the potential for these products to be a gateway to cigarette use, and the possibility of exposure to harmful flavoring chemicals such as diacetyl (2,3-butanedione).[108] This chemical is used to give foods a buttery or creamy flavor and has been shown to cause acute-onset bronchiolitis obliterans.[109,110] Furthermore, vaping products may have greater levels of nicotine when compared with traditional cigarettes. No consensus has been reached on how the strength of nicotine is reported on these products.[111]

E-cigarette, or vaping, product use–associated lung injury (EVALI) is a newly identified lung disease caused by vaping. Initial clinical presentation varies, but most commonly includes respiratory and gastrointestinal tract symptoms along with fever and malaise.[112] The majority of patients present with respiratory symptoms, and respiratory failure can progress quickly and may even develop into adult respiratory distress syndrome.[113] Although the mechanism of injury is not well defined, EVALI is considered a diagnosis of exclusion and infectious, oncologic, and rheumatologic etiologies need to be considered and ruled out.[114] Tetrahydrocannabinol (THC)-containing products have most commonly been associated with EVALI.[115] Other compounds linked to vaping and EVALI include vitamin E acetate,[116] cinnamaldehyde,[117] propylene glycol,[117,118] diacetyl,[118] benzene, toluene, and trace metals.[119]

Fortunately, the number of EVALI cases has rapidly declined as a result of increased public awareness of the risk associated with THC-containing e-cigarettes or vaping product use, removal of vitamin E acetate from some products, and rapid public health response and law enforcement actions related to the illicit products. Data are lacking on long-term exposure and health effects of the use of e-cigarettes given the limited time span these products have been in the marketplace.

The perioperative period is the ideal time to abandon the smoking habit permanently, and anesthesiologists can play an active role in facilitating this process. Nonthreatening and non-judgmental queries into inhalant use that include nicotine and cannabis either through smoking or electronic nicotine delivery systems should routinely be obtained in this vulnerable patient group. Patients who use tobacco vaping products may be at risk for nicotine withdrawal in the perioperative period. Symptoms due to nicotine withdrawal include physical (headaches, sweating, restlessness, tremors, digestive issues) and psychological (irritability, anxiety, mood swings) symptoms.[90] Physician communication with adolescents regarding smoking cessation has been shown to positively impact their attitudes, knowledge, intentions to smoke, and quitting behaviors.[120] During the preoperative visit with adolescents, anesthesiologists should inquire about cigarette smoking and vaping, emphasizing the need to stop the habit and offering measures to ameliorate the withdrawal (e.g., nicotine patch).

Secondary Smoking

A national survey in the United States revealed the percent of children 3 to 19 years of age without asthma who were exposed to secondhand smoke decreased from 57.3% to 44.2% between 1999 and 2010 although a greater percent of children with asthma, 54.0%, were exposed to secondhand smoke.[121] Children exposed to secondhand smoke are more likely to have asthma, to have more severe asthma attacks,[122] otitis media,[123] atopic eczema, hay fever,[124] and dental caries[125]; infants are at greater risk for lower respiratory tract illnesses.[126,127] A systematic review reported the risk of hospitalization for an exacerbation of asthma in children who were exposed to secondhand smoke in westernized countries was 2-fold greater than in those asthmatic children not exposed to secondhand smoke.[128]

Several investigators have demonstrated that secondhand smoke results in increased perioperative airway complications in children. Urinary cotinine, the major metabolite of nicotine, has been used as a surrogate marker of secondhand smoke exposure.[129] A strong association has been described between urinary cotinine and airway complications during induction and emergence from anesthesia. A prospective investigation in Australia demonstrated that the risk for perioperative adverse respiratory events in children exposed to the mother or both parents smoking was greater than when only the father smoked.[130] Respiratory adverse events include laryngospasm, bronchospasm, airway obstruction, oxygen desaturation (<95%), severe or sustained cough, and stridor in the postanesthesia care unit (PACU).[131] A meta-analysis of 15 anesthetic related studies reported that children who were exposed to secondhand smoke were two and a half times more likely to experience perianesthetic respiratory adverse events than those not exposed.[132] The evidence for adverse perioperative events in children from secondhand smoke is overwhelming.[131] During the preoperative visit, the anesthesiologist should ascertain the child's exposure to secondhand smoke by asking parents or guardians about who smokes and where the smoking takes place (indoors or outdoors). This strong evidence should empower health care providers to convey the harmful effects of secondhand smoke to parents and guardians about the dangers of secondhand smoke for their children's sake.[133]

PSYCHOLOGICAL PREPARATION OF CHILDREN FOR SURGERY

Approximately 3.9 million children undergo anesthesia and surgery in the United States every year[134] and 40% to 60% of them report anxiety or develop behavioral stress before their surgery.[135,136] Many parents express more concern about the risks of anesthesia than those of the surgery. Factors that influence the ability of the child and family to cope with perioperative stress include family dynamics, the child's developmental and behavioral status, cultural biases, and our ability to explain away misperceptions and misinformation. There may be limited time to evaluate family dynamics and establish rapport. Accordingly, it is vital for the anesthesiologist to interact directly, in a child-oriented approach with the child, consistent with their age and level of development.

Although the preoperative evaluation and preparation of children are similar to those of adults from a physiologic standpoint, the psychological preparation is very different and begins when parents are first informed that the child is to have surgery or a procedure that requires general anesthesia. Parental satisfaction correlates with accessibility to care, the comfort of the environment and the trust established between the anesthesiologist, the child, and the parents.[137,138] Preparatory educational information (written and verbal), high-quality perioperative communication with the anesthesiologist, perceived respect and positive interactions with the entire health care team all contribute to establishing trust and increasing satisfaction.[137–140] Parental presence during induction, if deemed to be in the child's best interest, is also associated with greater parental satisfaction but does not impact parental state anxiety or the child's anxiety level.[141] The level of parental anxiety and the child's social functioning are important predictors of parental satisfaction with perioperative care.[142]

Informed consent should include a detailed description of what the family can anticipate and our role to protect the welfare of the child. Before surgery, the anesthetic risks should be discussed in clear terms but in a reassuring manner by describing the measures that will be taken to monitor the safety of their child. Mentioning specific details and the purpose of the various monitoring devices may help diminish parents' anxiety by demonstrating that their child will be anesthetized with the utmost safety and care. A blood pressure cuff will *"check the blood pressure,"* an electrocardiographic monitor will *"watch the heartbeat,"* a pulse oximeter will *"measure the oxygen in the bloodstream,"* a carbon dioxide analyzer will *"monitor the breathing,"* an anesthetic agent monitor will *"accurately measure the level of anesthesia,"* and an intravenous catheter will be placed *"to administer fluid and medications as needed."* Children and their parents should be given ample opportunity to ask questions preoperatively. Finally, they should be assured that our anesthetic plan will be designed specifically for their child's needs, taking into account the child's underlying medical conditions to ensure analgesia, the safety of their child, and to provide optimal conditions for surgery.

It has been shown that parents desire comprehensive perioperative information, and that discussion of highly detailed anesthetic risk information does not increase a parent's anxiety level.[143,144] In contrast, inadequate preparation of children and their families may lead to a traumatic anesthetic induction, with the possibility of postoperative psychological disturbances.[145] Numerous preoperative educational programs for children and adults have evolved to alleviate some of these fears and anxiety. They include preoperative tours of the operating rooms, educational videos, play therapy,[146] magical distractions, puppet shows, anesthesia consultations, and child-life preparation, although cost may limit the availability of these resources.[136,147] New immersive technologies, such as virtual reality exposure, have also been successfully used for education and distraction purposes.[148–150] The timing of the preoperative preparation has been found to be an important determinant of whether the intervention will be effective. For example, children older than 6 years of age who participated in a preparation program more than 5 to 7 days before surgery were least anxious during separation from their parents, those who participated in no preoperative preparation were moderately anxious, and those who received the information 1 day before surgery were the most anxious. The predictors of anxiety also correlated with the child's baseline temperament and history of previous hospitalizations.[151,152] Children of different ages vary in their response to the anesthetic experience.[153] Even more important may be the child's trait anxiety when confronted with a stressful medical procedure.[154]

CHILD DEVELOPMENT, PREOPERATIVE ANXIETY, AND BEHAVIORAL INTERVENTIONS

Understanding age-appropriate behavior in response to external situations is essential. Age-specific perioperative anxieties are outlined in E-Table 2.2 Special aspects of a child's perception of anesthesia should be anticipated; children often have the same fears as adults but are unable to articulate them. The reason and need for a surgical procedure should be carefully explained to the child. It is important to reassure children that sleep from anesthesia is not the same as the usual sleep at home, but rather a special sleep caused by the medicines we give during which they cannot be awakened and, no matter what the surgeon does, they cannot feel pain. Many children fear the possibility that they will wake up in the middle of the anesthetic during surgery. If appropriate, it is important for them to appreciate that they will feel that they were only asleep for *"as long as it takes to blink"* but they will only wake up after the operation is completed.

The words the anesthesiologist uses to describe what can be anticipated must be carefully chosen, because children think concretely and tend to interpret the facts literally. Examples of this are presented by the following anecdotes:

Example 1: A 4-year-old child was informed that in the morning she would receive a *"shot"* that would *"put her to sleep."* That night, a frantic call was received from the mother, describing a very upset child; the child thought she was going to be *"put to sleep"* like the veterinarian had permanently *"put to sleep"* her sick pet.

Example 2: A 5-year-old child admitted for elective inguinal herniorrhaphy received a heavy premedication and was deeply sedated on arrival in the operating room. After discharge, the parents frequently discovered him wandering about the house at night. On questioning, the child stated that he was *"protecting"* his family. He stated: *"I don't want anyone sneaking up on you and operating while you are sleeping."*

In the first example, the child's concrete thought processes misunderstood the anesthesiologist's choice of words. The second case represents a problem of communication: the child was never told he would have an operation.

Variation in children's behavioral responses to the perioperative experience has its origin in at least four domains:

- Age and developmental maturity
- Previous experience with medical procedures and illness
- Individual capacity for affect regulation and trait (baseline) anxiety
- Parental state (situational) and trait anxiety

Previous studies that examined the behavioral responses to induction of anesthesia in children did so in terms of these four domains.[135,153,155–157] Children between the ages of 1 and 5 years are at greatest risk for developing extreme anxiety and distress. This is not surprising because separation anxiety often does not generally occur until 9 to 12 months of age and children older than 5 years can more easily cope with new situations. A history of previous stressful medical encounters, such as previous hospitalization, affects how a child reacts to new medical encounters; these are important risk factors for preoperative anxiety. Children who are shy and inhibited, as identified by temperament tests, and those who lack good social adaptive abilities are also at increased risk for developing anxiety and distress before surgery.[152,158]

The importance of proper psychological preparation for surgery should not be underestimated. Anesthesiologists have a key role in defusing fear of the unknown if they understand a child's age-related perception of anesthesia and surgery. They can convey their understanding by presenting a calm and friendly face (smiling, looking at the child, and making eye contact), offering a warm introduction, directing your description of the anesthetic conduct to the child and being completely honest before turning your attention to the parents. Children respond positively to an honest description of exactly what they can anticipate. This includes informing them of the steps that will occur whether it is a "*small pinch*" of starting an intravenous, the possible bitter taste of oral premedication, or breathing magic laughing gas through a flavored mask. Many parents are concerned their child will awaken after the surgery in pain or with vomiting. Hence, preemptory disclosure that during the surgery you will be administering pain medication (or a regional block) commensurate with the level of pain after the specific surgery and medications to prevent nausea and vomiting during the surgery.

The postoperative process, from the operating room to the recovery room, and the risk of postoperative pain and vomiting, should be outlined. Encourage the child and family to ask questions. Strategies to maintain analgesia postoperatively should be discussed where appropriate, including the use of long-acting local anesthetics; nerve blocks; neuraxial blocks; patient-controlled, nurse-controlled, or parent-controlled analgesia or epidural analgesia; or intermittent opioids (see also Chapters 40 and 41).

As children age, they become more aware of their bodies and may develop a fear of mutilation occurring from the surgery. Adolescents frequently appear quite independent and self-confident, but as a group, they have unique problems. In a moment their mood can change from an intelligent, mature adult to a very immature child who needs support and reassurance. Coping with a disability or illness is often very difficult for adolescents. Because adolescents often compare their physical appearance with that of their peers, they may become particularly anxious if they have a physical disability. In general, they want to know exactly what will transpire during anesthesia. Adolescents are usually cooperative, preferring to be in control, and if appropriate, should participate in the decision to premedicate and administer a regional block.

Monitoring the attitude and behavior of a child is very useful. A child who clings to the parents, avoids eye contact, and does not speak may be very anxious. A self-assured, cocky child who "knows it all" may use this confident behavior to hide their apprehension or fear. They may decompensate just when cooperation is most needed, at induction of anesthesia. In some cases, nonpharmacologic supportive measures may be effective. In the extremely anxious child, supportive measures alone may be insufficient to reduce anxiety, and premedication is indicated.

Parental characteristics also have a strong influence on a child's behavior. Children of parents who are more anxious, children of parents who use avoidance coping mechanisms, and children of separated or divorced parents all appear to be at high risk for developing preoperative anxiety.[151] Because children of anxious parents are more likely to experience a great deal of preoperative anxiety, it is important to identify the predictors of increased *parental* preoperative anxiety. Parent gender (mothers are more anxious than fathers),[159] the child's age (<1 year), children with repeated hospital admissions, and the child's temperament, are all predictors of increased parental preoperative anxiety.[151,160–163] Identification of children and parents who are at the greatest risk for preoperative anxiety and distress allows for appropriate intervention for this "at-risk" population.

It is important to observe the family dynamics to better understand the child and determine who is in control, the parent or the child. Many families may be in a state of stress, particularly if the child has a chronic illness; these parents are often angry, guilt ridden, or simply exhausted. Ultimately, the manner in which a family copes with an illness largely determines how the child will cope.[164] The "veterans" or "frequent flyers" of anesthesia can range from knowing exactly what they want and demanding it in the perioperative period, especially if their previous experiences were negative, to those who are easy-going because they recall their last anesthetic went well and ask the same for this encounter. The previous anesthetic should be reviewed, the child's need for and response to premedication, and whether other measures such as a parent at induction was necessary to ensure the safe conduct of anesthesia. There is the occasional parent who is overbearing and demands total control of the situation. It is important to be empathetic and understanding but to set limits and clearly define the parent's role as well as your own in the conduct of anesthesia.

PARENTAL PRESENCE DURING INDUCTION

Although many parents may express an interest to be present during induction of anesthesia,[165–167] each child and family must be evaluated individually by the anesthesiologist who will make that decision.[168–171] Evidence to date has been ambivalent regarding routinely permitting parents to be present during induction of anesthesia.[167,171–174] Although early studies suggested that parental presence reduced anxiety and increased cooperation,[168,169] subsequent studies failed to confirm these results.[171–173,175] Characteristics of the parent and child have an impact on the effectiveness of parental presence. For example, older children (>4 years), children with a "calm" and less active baseline temperament, parents with less situational anxiety, and parents with lower external locus of control, benefit most from parental presence during induction.[163,172] The match between parent and child anxiety level also appears to be important. Calm children with anxious parents do more poorly during induction compared with calm children with calm parents or anxious children with either calm or anxious parents.[163] Allowing parental presence during induction without adequate preparation of the parent may also be counterproductive. Some parent behaviors, such as criticism, excessive reassurance, and commands are associated with greater distress for the child.[176,177] If the practice of having parents present at induction is to work well, both the anesthesiologist and the parents must be comfortable with such an arrangement. Parents must be informed about what they can anticipate in terms of the anesthetizing location, what they may observe during induction, and that they will obey the anesthesiologist when they are asked to leave the operating room, no matter what is occurring. They must also be instructed regarding their participation in the induction process such as by comforting the child, encouraging the child to trust the anesthesiologist, distracting the child, and consoling the child (Videos 2.1 and 2.2). Personnel should be immediately available to escort parents back to the waiting area at the appropriate time. Someone should also be available to care for a parent who needs to prematurely leave the induction area or who becomes lightheaded or faints.

Explaining what parents might see or hear is essential. We generally tell parents:

As you see your child fall asleep today, there are several things you might observe that you are not used to seeing. First, the eyes roll up, something that we do not generally see during sleep at home. That is expected and normal. The second thing is that as your child goes to sleep from the anesthesia medications, they may snore or make vibrating noises. Again, we expect this, and it is normal. The third thing you might see is what we call "excitement." As the brain begins to go to sleep, your child's arms and legs may twitch and move. About 30 to 60 seconds later, your child might suddenly look around or turn their head from one side to the other. To you it may appear that they are upset or awakening from anesthesia, but in reality, it indicates to us that your child is falling asleep and 15 to 30 seconds later they will stop moving and be completely anesthetized. Also, you should know that your child will not remember any of the activities that you witnessed while your child is becoming anesthetized. As soon as your child loses consciousness, we will ask you to give your child a kiss and return to the waiting room.

A child-life specialist may also prove valuable to the anesthesiologist by calming and preparing both children and parents for the operating room experience, and may accompany the child to the operating room to provide additional support through the induction of anesthesia.[178]

Occasionally, our best efforts to relieve a child's anxiety by parental presence or giving a premedication (or both) are unsuccessful, and an anticipated smooth inhalation induction does not go as planned. There are four options that may remedy the situation depending on the age of the child: (1) renegotiating (which is seldom successful); (2) allowing the child to hold the mask themself; (3) replacing the mask with your hands, holding the elbow of the breathing circuit between your fingers (Fig. 2.5); or (4) suggesting an intravenous or intramuscular induction. If the situation is totally out of control, either elective surgery can be rescheduled, or intramuscular ketamine can be used if the parents choose to proceed. These situations are particularly difficult for the parents and the caregivers and must be handled on an individual basis. The latter addresses mask phobias very effectively.

In many centers, intravenous access is completed in the preoperative holding area. In this case, premedication may be administered intravenously before entering the operating room.

Cognitively challenged adolescents fall into two groups in terms of their willingness to come to the operating room: those who come voluntarily or if accompanied by their parents and those who are unwilling to come to the operating room under any circumstances. If the child falls into the latter category, then an intramuscular sedative such as ketamine should be administered after positioning the child on a stretcher.

HEALTH CARE PROVIDER INTERVENTIONS

In addition to behavioral interventions targeting children and their parents, a promising new line of research supports the use of behavioral interventions targeting anesthesiologists and nurses. Specifically, an empirically derived intervention titled Provider-Tailored Intervention for Perioperative Stress (P-TIPS) was shown to be successful in changing anesthesiologist and nurse behaviors in the perioperative setting and represents a new clinical avenue for decreasing perioperative anxiety in children. The development of P-TIPS was based on research documenting that adult behaviors (parents and health care providers) affect children's distress during invasive medical procedures, including surgery. Specifically, the use of distraction, nonprocedural talk, and humor are conceptualized as "coping promoting" behaviors and have been shown to decrease children's distress.[179–183] Conversely, adults' use of reassurance, apology, empathy, criticism, or allowing the child too much control over the medical procedure are conceptualized as "distress promoting" behaviors and lead to increased distress in children.[179,184–187] With P-TIPS, a new behavior that affected child distress also emerged: medical reinterpretation (i.e., reconceptualizing medical experiences and equipment as nonthreatening) and was found to increase a child's coping when used with medical experiences that were in the child's immediate environment. One important benefit to the type of approach offered by P-TIPS is that it is not necessary to conduct individual training with parents of children undergoing surgery; rather, health care providers who interact with multiple children and parents are targeted, which reduces both logistical and financial constraints of behavioral interventions.

PHARMACOLOGIC INTERVENTIONS

The primary goals of administering a premedication to children are to facilitate an anxiety-free separation from their parents and a smooth, stress-free induction of anesthesia. Other effects that may be achieved by pharmacologic preparation of the child include amnesia, anxiolysis, prevention of physiologic stress (e.g., avoiding tachycardia in patients with cyanotic congenital heart disease), and analgesia.

PHARMACOLOGIC INTERVENTIONS VERSUS BEHAVIORAL INTERVENTIONS

When pharmacologic interventions are directly compared with behavioral interventions, children who are sedated are less anxious and more compliant than those who are accompanied to the operating room by a parent.[173] Parental anxiety also decreases when the child is premedicated. When premedication and parental presence during induction were compared, the combination of parental presence and sedative premedication reduced parental anxiety and improved parental satisfaction more effectively than premedication alone.[158]

Furthermore, parental presence during induction of anesthesia offered no additional anxiolysis for children who were premedicated preoperatively. Nonetheless, parents who accompanied their sedated children to the operating rooms were themselves less anxious and more satisfied both with the separation process and

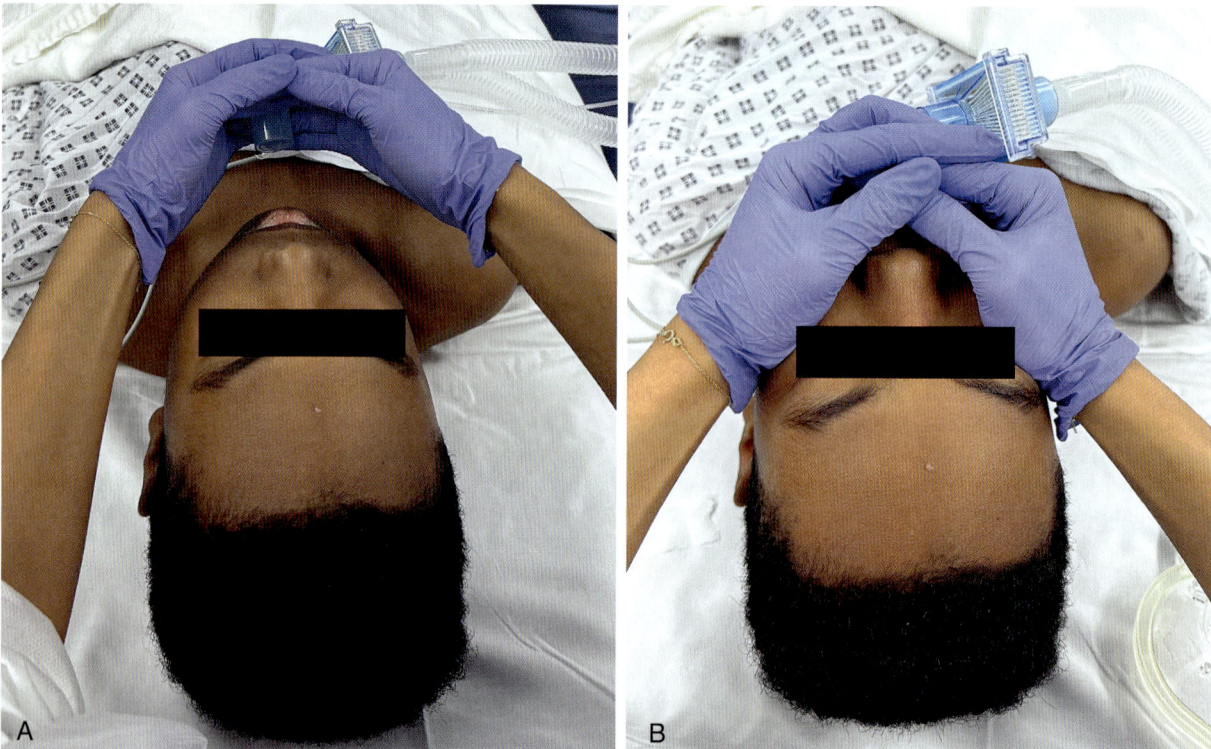

FIGURE 2.5 For children who are claustrophobic, mask phobic, or resistant to a facemask over their face, we can still perform an inhalational induction. The anesthesia facemask is removed from the breathing circuit and the elbow is placed between the anesthesiology provider's fingers of one hand. A gas mixture of 66% to 70% nitrous oxide in oxygen is set at a 6 L/minute flow. If the child picked a flavor for the mask, apply the same flavor to the gloved fingers. **A,** The fingers are interlaced, with the hands held below the chin, resting gently on the chest. It is important to position the hands in this manner as the nitrous oxide/oxygen mixture is heavier than air. A Yankauer suction is placed near the head of the bed to draw away excess gases and reduce the exposure of operating room personnel to the gases. **B,** As the child is distracted, the provider moves their hands closer and closer to the face until they completely envelope the nose and mouth. At this point, 8% sevoflurane may be added to the fresh gas flow. As soon as the child loses consciousness, the anesthesia facemask is attached to the elbow of the breathing circuit and applied to the face to seal the airway and deepen the anesthetic. The entire process should be complete within 90 seconds.

with the overall anesthetic, nursing, and surgical care provided. It is important to note that these parents had no preparation for their presence at anesthesia induction. Premedication combined with an advanced behavioral preparation resulted in similar outcomes on child and parental anxiety at induction and child compliance with induction.[188] Furthermore, children who received behavioral preparation evidenced significantly less emergence delirium and required less analgesia in the recovery room compared with those who received only premedication.

Although sedative premedications are effective for treatment of preoperative anxiety, they should *not* be used routinely in all children undergoing surgery. Their use should be directed to children who are at risk for developing preoperative and separation anxiety. Variables such as age, duration of surgery, and potential recovery delays, should also be considered. Nonetheless, it is important that premedication is not withheld if the premedication would likely benefit the child. For example, for the child who is scheduled for a very brief procedure (such as bilateral myringotomy and tubes) and who is very anxious, we would prefer that a parent is present at induction rather than give a premedication whose duration of action likely will cause a prolonged recovery and delay discharge from hospital.

HISTORY OF PRESENT ILLNESS

The medical history of a child obtained during the preanesthetic visit allows the anesthesiologist to determine whether the child has been optimized for the planned surgery, to anticipate potential problems due to coexisting diseases, to determine whether appropriate laboratory or other tests are needed, to select optimal premedication, to formulate the appropriate anesthetic plan including perioperative monitoring, and to anticipate postoperative concerns including pain management, the need for intensive care observation, and postoperative ventilatory needs. The history of the present illness is described to the physicians by the parents or caregiver and verified by the referring physician or consultant surgeon's notes. If the child is old enough, it is helpful to obtain the child's input. The history should focus on the following aspects:

- A review of all organ systems (Table 2.2) with special emphasis on the organ system involved in the surgery
- A review of patient and parental smoking history
- Medications (over-the-counter and prescribed) related to and taken before the present illness, including herbals and vitamins, and when the last dose was taken
- Medication allergies with specific details of the nature of the allergy and whether immunologic testing was performed

TABLE 2.2 | Review of Systems: Anesthetic Implications

System	Factors to Assess	Possible Anesthetic Implications
Respiratory	Cough, asthma, recent cold	Irritable airway, bronchospasm, medication history, atelectasis, infiltrate
	Croup	Subglottic narrowing
	Apnea/bradycardia	Postoperative apnea/bradycardia
Cardiovascular	Murmur	Septal defect, avoid air bubbles in intravenous line and syringes
	Cyanosis	Right-to-left shunt
	History of squatting	Tetralogy of Fallot
	Hypertension	Coarctation, renal disease
	Rheumatic fever	Valvular heart disease
	Exercise intolerance	Congestive heart failure, cyanosis
	Postcardiac surgery with prosthetic material	Bacterial endocarditis prophylaxis
Neurologic	Seizures	Medications, metabolic derangement
	Head trauma	Intracranial hypertension
	Swallowing incoordination	Aspiration, esophageal reflux, hiatus hernia
	Neuromuscular disease	Neuromuscular relaxant drug sensitivity, malignant hyperthermia
Gastrointestinal/hepatic	Vomiting, diarrhea	Electrolyte imbalance, dehydration, full stomach
	Malabsorption	Anemia
	Black stools	Anemia, hypovolemia
	Reflux	Possible need for full-stomach precautions
	Jaundice	Drug metabolism/hypoglycemia
Genitourinary	Frequency	Urinary tract infection, diabetes, hypercalcemia
	Time of last urination	State of hydration
	Frequent urinary tract infections	Evaluate renal function
Endocrine/metabolic	Abnormal development	Endocrinopathy, hypothyroid, diabetes
	Hypoglycemia, steroid therapy	Hypoglycemia, adrenal insufficiency
Hematologic	Anemia	Need for transfusion
	Bruising, excessive bleeding	Coagulopathy, thrombocytopenia, thrombocytopathy
	Sickle cell disease	Hydration, possible transfusion
Allergies	Medications	Possible drug interaction
Dental	Loose or carious teeth	Aspiration of loose teeth, bacterial endocarditis prophylaxis

- Previous surgical and hospital experiences, including those related to the current problem
- Timing of the last oral intake, last urination (wet diaper), and vomiting and diarrhea. It is essential to recognize that decreased gastrointestinal motility often occurs with an illness or injury.

A relevant family history of inherited diseases such as malignant hyperthermia, muscular dystrophy, sickle cell disease, and anesthetic complications for which there may be a genetic basis (e.g., pseudocholinesterase deficiency) should be sought.

In the case of a neonate, problems that may have been present during gestation and birth may still be relevant in the neonatal period and beyond (E-Table 2.3). The maternal medical and pharmacologic history (both therapeutic and drug abuse) may also provide valuable information for the management of a neonate requiring surgery (see Table 2.2).

PAST/OTHER MEDICAL HISTORY

The past medical history should include a history of all past medical illnesses with a review of organ systems, previous hospitalizations (medical or surgical), childhood syndromes with associated anomalies, medication list, herbal remedies, and any allergies, especially to antibiotics and latex. Whether the child was full-term or preterm at birth should be discerned; if preterm, any associated problems should be noted, including admission to a neonatal intensive care unit, duration of tracheal intubation, history of apnea or bradycardia (including oxygen treatment, home apnea monitor, intraventricular hemorrhage), and congenital defects.

Examination of previous surgical and anesthesia records greatly assists in planning the anesthesia. Particular attention should be paid to any difficulties encountered with airway management, venous access, or emergence. The response to or need for premedication and the route of administration used should be noted. Taking all the previous information into consideration an ASA Physical Status Classification has been developed for pediatric patients (E-Table 2.4).

Herbal Remedies

The use of herbal medicinal products has become increasingly popular, likely driven by the notion that natural substances have fewer side effects. A survey in five geographically diverse centers in the United States found that 3.5% of pediatric surgical patients (with significant geographical difference e.g., 7.7% in Palo Alto vs. 1.9% in Virginia and Delaware) had been given herbal supplements or homeopathic remedies 2 weeks before surgery.[189] The findings of the National Health Interview Survey confirm a similar prevalence rate in which natural product usage among children aged 0 to 17 years amounts to 3.9%.[190] Herbal medicine use is more common in adults; 32% of adult surgical patients take one or more herb-related compounds.[191] Nearly 70% of adults failed to disclose their use of herbal remedies when asked about medications during routine perioperative assessment. Herbal medicines are regulated as food supplements under the Dietary Supplement Health and Education Act of 1994 and as such, manufacturers are not required to demonstrate safety or efficacy before placing a product on the market.[192] Without Food and Drug Administration (FDA) regulation, there are no quality assurance requirements for manufacturing and labeling and much variation can occur in each preparation.[193] Anesthesiologists should include specific inquiries regarding the use of these medications because of the potential for adverse effects and drug interactions.

Herbal medicines are associated with cardiovascular instability, coagulation disturbances, potentiation of sedation, and immunosuppression.[194] The most commonly used herbal medications are garlic, ginseng, *Ginkgo biloba*, St. John's wort, and *Echinacea*,[195] with *Echinacea* and other herbal medicines for the treatment of coughs and colds taking the lead in the pediatric population.[189,196] The three "g" herbals (garlic, ginseng, *Ginkgo biloba*), together with feverfew *(Tanacetum parthenium)* and cannabidiol (CBD oil), potentially increase the risk of bleeding during surgery. The amount of active ingredient in each preparation and the dose taken may vary, thus making detection of a change in platelet function and other subtle coagulation disturbances difficult. St. John's wort is the herb that most commonly interacts with anesthetics and other medications, usually via a change in drug metabolism, because it induces cytochrome P-450 enzymes (e.g., CYP3A4) and P-glycoprotein. A potentially fatal interaction between cyclosporine and St. John's wort has been well documented.[197–200] Heart, kidney, or liver transplant recipients who were stabilized on a dose of cyclosporine experienced decreased plasma concentrations of cyclosporine with some cases resulting in acute rejection episodes after taking St. John's wort. Finally, diuretic herbs, heavily marketed to adolescents for weight loss, such as dandelion and green tea, may be associated with electrolyte disturbances. A summary of the most commonly used herbal remedies and their potential perioperative complications is shown in E-Table 2.5.

To avoid potential perioperative complications, the ASA has encouraged the discontinuation of all herbal medicines 2 weeks before surgery,[201] although this recommendation is not evidence based. Recognizing that this is not always feasible, the ASA further recommends that anesthesiologists have knowledge of herbal medications and their potential interactions (https://www.asahq.org/madeforthismoment/wp-content/uploads/2017/10/asa_supplements-anesthesia_final.pdf). Valerian and kava cause sedation although sudden discontinuation of valerian may lead to withdrawal by 48 hours that may require IV midazolam. Each herb should be carefully evaluated using standard resource texts, and a decision should be made regarding the timing of or need for discontinuation as determined on a case-by-case basis.[202]

Anesthesia and Vaccination

Children may present for surgery after having been recently immunized. The anesthesiologist and surgeon must then consider (1) whether the immunomodulatory effects of anesthesia and surgery might affect the efficacy and safety of the vaccine and (2) whether the inflammatory responses to the vaccine will alter the perioperative course.

An international survey[203] revealed that only one-third of responding anesthesiologists had the benefit of a hospital policy, ranging from a formal decision to delay surgery to an independent choice by the anesthesiologist. A scientific review of the literature associating anesthesia and vaccination in children demonstrated a brief and reversible influence of anesthesia on lymphoproliferative responses that generally returned to preoperative values within 2 days. Potential vaccine-driven adverse events (e.g., fever, pain, irritability) to inactivated vaccines such as diphtheria-tetanus-pertussis (DPT) become apparent from 2 days and to live attenuated vaccines such as measles-mumps and rubella (MMR) from 7 to 21 days after immunization.[204] Therefore, to avoid misinterpretation of vaccine-associated adverse events as perioperative complications, a reasonable approach is to delay elective surgery for 1 week after an inactive vaccine and for 3 weeks after a live attenuated vaccine.[205,206] Likewise, it seems prudent to delay vaccination *after* surgery until the child is fully recovered. Other immunocompromised patients, such as human immunodeficiency virus (HIV)-positive children, cancer patients, and transplant recipients, have distinct underlying immune impairments, and the influence of anesthesia on vaccine responses has not been comprehensively investigated. The recent COVID-19 pandemic and associated immunizations has also raised question as to the timing of elective surgery.[207] A multidisciplinary consensus statement on behalf of the Association of Anaesthetists, Centre for Perioperative Care, Federation of Surgical Specialty Associations, Royal College of Anaesthetists, Royal College of Surgeons of England recommends a delay of elective surgery within 7 weeks of infection with virulent COVID-19 variants due to a 3-fold increased perioperative mortality in adults within that time frame. These recommendations are not applicable to those infected with subsequent less virulent strains. They recommend "optimizing vaccination" before surgery and suggest that elective surgery be delayed until at least 2 weeks after the third dose; there are no pediatric recommendations.[208]

Allergies to Food, Medications, and Latex

Most electronic medical records list the medications and materials to which children are reported to be "allergic". The most common medication- and hospital-related allergies in children in the United States are penicillin and latex allergy. Food allergies are increasingly more common in children compared with adults, with up to 10% affected. Peanuts, shellfish, milk, eggs, soy, wheat, and seeds account for the majority of the latter reactions.[209] In Europe, allergic reactions to muscle relaxants are also common. Possible reasons for the difference in its frequency from elsewhere in the world is discussed later in the chapter.

The source of the vast majority of the reported allergies on patient's charts is a parent or caregiver, who in the majority of penicillin allergies, reported finding a red rash after commencing the oral antibiotic as the reason they and/or the doctor diagnosed penicillin allergy.[210] The frequency of unconfirmed penicillin allergy in children is 5% to 12%, although laboratory testing (oral or intradermal testing) has confirmed in multiple studies that 90% to 96% of these so-called allergies are not penicillin allergies and that the children could receive penicillin in the future.[211–214] Seventy-five percent of the reported allergies to penicillin occur in children before their third birthday, although age should not be a determinant of the child's risk for penicillin allergy.[212,215]

The frequency of true penicillin allergy in children is rare, 4 to 15:100,000.[212,214,216,217] True allergic reactions are manifested by either an immediate IgE-mediated (Type 1 reactions) or a delayed T-cell mediated (Type 4 reactions) according to the Gell and Coomb's classification.[218] However, most cases of penicillin allergy are unconfirmed and not immunologically-mediated, but based on low-risk evidence from a parent who reported a maculopapular rash or pruritus after an oral dose of penicillin.[212] In most instances, parents were cautioned to avoid penicillin antibiotics and its congeners in the future even though up to 7% of children who receive amoxicillin develop rashes that are benign.[219] Rarely were signs or symptoms that suggested an immune-mediated reaction present (i.e., urticaria, angioedema, anaphylaxis), and even less frequently was skin testing conducted to confirm the allergic diagnosis. Skin testing has demonstrated that >90% of these unverified histories of allergies to penicillin are in fact not allergic reactions to penicillin. The reactions such as rashes may have been associated with the underlying infectious organisms, and minor allergies to the dye in the liquid vehicle.[220] For example, skin testing for penicillin allergy was positive in 93% of patients 7 to 12 months after the original exposure but in only 22% 10 years after exposure.[221] Additional evidence confirms that positive skin testing has decreased dramatically over time from Kaiser Permanente in California with a frequency of 15% in 1995 to <1% in 2013 and from the Mayo Clinic with a frequency of 1% of 30,883 patients.[217] Penicillin allergy fades with time and may be unapparent after a period. Although skin testing is usually difficult and unpleasant to undertake in young children, it is a safe procedure. The problem we face in children is that the positive predictive value of skin testing is poor, 20%![213] Moreover, 80% of the skin tests may yield a false positive result and the sensitivity of the test in children is <10%, raising serious moral grounds about subjecting young children to skin testing to verify their possible antibiotic allergy.[213,222] Since few children are ever tested to confirm their allergy either at the time of the initial reaction or subsequently, we must accept that these unconfirmed reports of penicillin allergy are NOT true penicillin allergies. However, this notion should be framed with the knowledge that even after many years, these children may become resensitized to penicillin if they are indeed allergic and are reexposed in the future, although the rate of resensitization is very small ~5%.[221] It is also reassuring to know that the incidence of anaphylaxis to penicillin is exceedingly small, 1:95,258.[223]

Clinicians should proceed with antibiotics based upon their best understanding of the child's risk of developing an allergy to penicillin (or its derivatives) and cephalosporins (see later in the chapter) and a frank discussion with the parents. If the child has been tested immunologically for penicillin allergy and proven to be allergic, then it is best to avoid this class of antibiotics. However, in the absence of confirmatory testing, a weak and nonspecific history of penicillin allergy, a history or documentation that lacks evidence of an IgE or Type IV delayed hypersensitivity reactions such as Stevens-Johnson syndrome, serum sickness-like reactions, drug reaction with eosinophilia systemic symptoms (DRESS) syndrome, toxic epidermal necrosis (TENS), or acute generalized exanthematous pustulosis (AGEP), and a gap of at least 5 years since the initial "reaction" to penicillin, then we recommend that the child be reexposed to penicillin or one of its congeners under controlled conditions such as the operating room and with an anesthesiologist present.[213,224,225] An algorithm to stratify the risk of penicillin allergy in children has been developed to assist nonallergist physicians to delabel penicillin allergy in children.[226]

Although there is a small (2%–4%) cross-reactivity between first-generation cephalosporins and penicillin,[227,228] there is no similar cross-reactivity with second- and third-generation cephalosporins. Nonetheless, many institutions advise against using cephalosporins in children with a history of penicillin allergy, even in unconfirmed penicillin allergy. A label of penicillin allergy has been associated with a greater use of several non-beta lactam antibiotics (including macrolides and clindamycin), a greater prevalence of infections, prolonged hospitalizations, a greater frequency of readmissions and surgical site infections, and increased morbidity.[214,217] In a single center retrospective analysis of 558 cerebrospinal fluid diversion procedures, the use of clindamycin for perioperative prophylaxis and for the presence of cardiac disease was associated with surgical site infections with an odds ratio of 4.99 and 7.19 (P<0.02), respectively.[229] The authors recommended that strategies to maximize the number of children who can receive cephalosporins for surgical site infection prophylaxis and for cardiac disease and in cerebrospinal fluid diversion surgery should be sought. To address this inconsistency, some institutions have removed the restriction on using cephalosporins in children identified as allergic to penicillin. The result was an increase in the use of cephalosporins without an increase in the frequency of anaphylaxis, new allergies, or treatment failures.[230] To date, there have been no fatal anaphylactic reactions in penicillin-allergic children from a cephalosporin.[216] In aggregate, we propose that unconfirmed penicillin allergies in children should not direct antibiotic therapy away from the most appropriate antibiotics, notwithstanding the remote risk of penicillin allergy and its sequelae.

Recent evidence suggests that diagnoses of unconfirmed allergies, particularly to antibiotics, steer the choice of antibiotics in children and this may lead to substantive adverse consequences. Alternative antibiotics used as substitutes in children with unconfirmed antibiotic allergy (as in the case of avoiding cephalosporins in children with unconfirmed penicillin allergy) may lead to antimicrobial failure or resistance, adverse reactions to a broader spectrum antibiotic and increased health care costs and hospitalization.[224,228,231] Furthermore, substitute antibiotics to prevent surgical skin infections, such as clindamycin, are less effective prophylactic antibiotics and may cause a maculopapular rash and diarrhea that may be associated with Clostridium difficile.[227,232] These events have led to a global effort to delabel penicillin allergy.[224]

Latex allergy is an acquired immunologic IgE-mediated sensitivity resulting from repeated exposure to latex, usually on mucous membranes. This commonly occurs in children with neural tube defects (meningomyelocele, spina bifida) or children with congenital urologic abnormalities who have undergone repeated bladder catheterizations with latex catheters, those with more than four surgeries, or those requiring home ventilation. It occurs more frequently in atopic individuals and in those with certain fruit and vegetable allergies (e.g., banana, chestnut, avocado, kiwi, pineapple).[233–239] The incidence of latex sensitization in children is 0.3% to 4%.[239] There are at least 15 separate allergic components in latex; other fruits and vegetables have a moderate cross reactivity (apple, carrot, celery, melon, papaya, potato, tomato).[240] For a diagnosis of latex anaphylaxis, the child should have experienced an anaphylactic reaction to latex, skin-tested positive for anaphylaxis to latex, or experienced swelling of the lips after touching a toy or balloon to the lips, or a swollen tongue after a dentist inserted a rubber dam into the mouth (although dentists have recently shifted away from latex rubber dams).[239] The avoidance of latex within the hospital prevents acute anaphylactic reactions to latex in children who are at risk.[241] Latex gloves and other latex-containing products should be removed from the immediate vicinity of the child. Prophylactic therapy with histamine H_1- and H_2-receptor antagonists and steroids do not prevent latex anaphylaxis.[233,242] Latex anaphylaxis should be addressed by the immediate removal of the source of latex (oftentimes unrecognized latex surgical gloves), administration of 100% oxygen, intravascular volume expansion, and epinephrine as first line treatment (Table 2.3).[239] In some severe reactions, a continuous infusion of epinephrine alone (0.01–0.2 µg/kg per minute) or combined with other vasoactive medications may be required for several hours.[239]

Anaphylaxis is a severe, life-threatening reaction to one of four general categories: drugs, latex, foods, and Hymenoptera. The incidence is reported to be 1:10,000 (range: 1:1250–1:36,000), with a 1% fatality rate.[218,243–245] All reactions are either allergic- (IgE- or IgG-) mediated or nonallergic (pseudo allergic or anaphylactoid, old terms) anaphylaxis.[246] The mechanism by which anaphylaxis is mediated is a foreign antigen interacts with IgE antibodies on tissue mast cells and circulating basophils, releasing several vasoactive and bioactive mediators including histamine. Some drugs can directly trigger mast cell degranulation to trigger an anaphylactic presentation (as in opioids, vancomycin, and radiocontrast dye).[247] A triad of findings is diagnostic for anaphylaxis, although not all of these may occur concurrently: cutaneous, respiratory, and hemodynamic signs. Classic anaphylaxis includes all three responses, although anaphylaxis also occurs with just one or two of these signs. Hypotension was the first sign in 60% of cases in one multicenter retrospective review, followed by tachycardia and bronchospasm.[248] Perioperative anaphylaxis may be graded with treatment commensurate with the severity of the reaction.[249] The definitive treatment for anaphylaxis is epinephrine in a dose between 1 and 10 µg/kg IV or subcutaneously depending on the severity of the reaction where 1 to 2 µg/kg may suffice for mild cutaneous signs and mild bronchospasm to 10 µg/kg for severe hypotension or cardiac arrest.[218] Supplemental support with 100% oxygen, balanced salt solutions, steroids, and other interventions are often warranted (Table 2.3). Serum tryptase levels should be sent within 30 minutes of the start of a reaction to confirm an immunologic basis for the reaction (increase >20% from baseline), although normal levels do not exclude anaphylaxis.[250] The positive predictive value for tryptase to diagnose anaphylaxis is 93% with a negative predictive value of 54%.[250] Other laboratory tests may also be performed including histamine levels, IgE-specific antibodies, and others.[250]

In the operating room, the incidence of anaphylaxis ranges from 1 to 4:10,000.[251] The etiology of the anaphylaxis differs from adults to children and from country to country. The most common triggers in the 1990s in children were latex, antibiotics (cefazolin), and muscle relaxants (atracurium, rocuronium), although with the elimination of latex from the operating room, this source of anaphylaxis has all but disappeared, but others remain.[218,251]

The curious case of anaphylaxis to muscle relaxants (neuromuscular blocking drugs) drew widespread attention because of the dramatic regional variability in the incidence among countries: it was far more common in parts of Europe and Australia and virtually unheard-of in North America. Compounding this curiosity was the observation that these reactions occurred despite the patients never having been exposed to the muscle relaxants, which raised the specter of a cross-sensitivity with a nonanesthetic epitope. Indeed, quaternary ammonium and tertiary amine groups occur ubiquitously in drugs, foods, cosmetics, and industrial materials, providing clinical exposure to a nonanesthetic epitope to prime the immune system for subsequent exposure. One such compound, pholcodine is an antitussive compound present in over-the-counter cough medicines in some countries in Europe and Australia that shares a quaternary ammonium group with rocuronium, succinylcholine, and morphine.[252–254] In Norway where pholcodine was sold until 2007, the incidence of sensitization to these three anesthetics was 10-fold greater than in neighboring Sweden where pholcodine was not available.

TABLE 2.3 | Management of an Anaphylactic Reaction to Latex in Children

Primary Management
1. Remove latex and maintain anesthesia, if necessary.
2. Notify the surgical team and complete surgery as quickly as possible.
3. Call for help.
4. Secure the airway (tracheal intubation) and ventilate with 100% oxygen.
5. Special handling for severe reactions:

Grade 3 Reaction
a. Hypotension
   Using Trendelenburg position, administer balanced salt or colloid solution in 20 mL/kg bolus doses with parenteral intravenous bolus doses 1–10 µg/kg epinephrine, depending on the severity of the hypotension.
b. Bronchospasm (in association with hypotension)
   Parenteral intravenous boluses doses 1–10 µg/kg epinephrine, depending on the severity of the bronchospasm, and β_2-agonists via metered-dose inhaler or nebulized solution (the latter every 20 min).

Grade 4 Reaction
As required, repeated intravenous bolus doses of 10 µg/kg epinephrine. Consider preparing an infusion beginning at 0.1 µg/kg per min increasing up to 1 µg/kg per min.

Secondary Management*
1. Consider alternate vasopressors (titrate to effect), including glucagon (20–30 µg/kg bolus then 5–15 µg/min [1 mg maximum]), phenylephrine (0.1–1 µg/kg per min), noradrenaline (0.01–2 µg/kg per min), or vasopressin (0.3–3 mU/kg per min).
2. Corticosteroids methylprednisolone or hydrocortisone 1–2 mg/kg IV.
3. Antihistamines diphenhydramine (1.0–2.0 mg/kg [50 mg maximum]) or ranitidine (1–2 µg/kg) IV or per os.
4. Bronchodilators-metered-dose inhaler or nebulized β_2-agonists (salbutamol).

Investigation and Follow-up
1. Admit patients with grade 3 and grade 4 reactions to the intensive care unit until stable.
2. Collect blood for mast cell tryptase at 0, 2, and 24 hours postreaction (peaks at 1–2 hours).
3. Add signage noting "latex allergy" or "latex alert" on all relevant areas of patient care, including notes and databases.
4. Inform pharmacy and central supply of patient latex sensitivity so that latex can be eliminated from all preparations.
5. Refer child to allergist/immunologist for follow-up and testing.
6. Advise the parents of need for medical alert bracelet for child for latex allergy/anaphylaxis after diagnosis is confirmed.

*Secondary management is required for grade 3 and 4 reactions in which hypotension is refractory to epinephrine and above measures.
Although such reactions are unreported in children, they have occurred in adults who were β-blocked and in whom epinephrine treatment was delayed.
Reproduced with permission from Sampathi V, Lerman J. Case scenario: perioperative latex allergy in children. *Anesthesiology.* 2011;114(3):673-680.

When pholcodine was discontinued in Norway, the incidence of anaphylaxis to these compounds in Norway decreased dramatically to comparable levels in Sweden. Australia has yet to ban pholcodine. In adults, the frequency of IgE-mediated anaphylaxis to muscle relaxants in females is greater than males, suggesting that compounds such as cosmetics that are applied to mucous membranes in females may sensitize them to these same compounds but this remains to be confirmed.

A purported association between food allergy and propofol exists since the commonly used propofol formulation is in a lipid emulsion that includes egg lecithin and soybean oil. Egg lecithin, a natural emulsifier, is derived from egg yolk and contains very little egg white proteins, the source (ovalbumin) of most immunologic reactions to eggs. Although two egg yolk proteins are known to be potentially allergenic, their trace concentrations in egg lecithin are subimmunogenic.

Anaphylactic reactions to propofol are rare, occurring at a rate of 1:60,000 adults and 6:1,000,000 children.[255,256] Overwhelming evidence supports the use of propofol in patients who are allergic to peanut, soy, and/or egg as safe and unlikely to trigger allergic reactions.[257–260] In a study of 28 egg-allergic children who received 43 exposures to propofol, two of the children reported a history of egg anaphylaxis.[257] One of the children with egg anaphylaxis experienced a nonanaphylactic reaction 15 minutes after receiving a dose of propofol possibly attributable to propofol or a different trigger. A skin prick test was just positive at 3 mm and intradermal testing was not performed. The preponderance of evidence suggests that propofol is safe in children with food allergies, specifically egg and soy food allergies.[261]

Family History

It is important to inquire about a family history, particularly focusing on a number of conditions that include malignant hyperthermia, muscular dystrophy, prolonged paralysis associated with anesthesia (pseudocholinesterase deficiency), sickle cell disease, bleeding (and bruising) tendencies, and drug addiction (drug withdrawal), and HIV infection. The precise relationship to the proband must be documented.

LABORATORY DATA

Laboratory data obtained preoperatively should be appropriate to the history, illness, and surgical procedure. Routine hemoglobin testing or urinalysis is not indicated for most elective procedures; the value of these tests is questionable when the surgical procedure will not involve clinically important blood loss.[262] There are insufficient data in the literature to make strict hemoglobin testing recommendations in healthy children. A preoperative hemoglobin value is usually determined only for those who will undergo procedures with the potential for blood loss, those with specific risk factors for a hemoglobinopathy, former preterm infants, and those younger than 6 months of age. Coagulation studies (platelet count, international normalized ratio [INR], and partial thromboplastin time [PTT]) may be indicated if major reconstructive surgery is contemplated, especially if warranted by the medical history, and in some centers before tonsillectomy. In addition, collection of a preoperative type-and-screen or type-and-crossmatch sample is indicated in preparation for potential blood transfusions depending on the nature of the planned surgery and the anticipated blood loss.

In general, routine chest radiography is not necessary; routine chest radiographs are not cost-effective in children.[263,264] The oxygen saturation of children who are breathing room air is very helpful. Baseline oxygen saturations (SpO_2) of 95% or less suggest clinically important pulmonary or cardiac compromise and warrant further investigation.[265]

Selective preoperative laboratory tests, such as electrolyte and blood glucose determinations, renal function tests, blood gas analysis, blood concentrations of seizure medication and digoxin, electrocardiography, echocardiography, liver function tests, computed tomography (CT), magnetic resonance imaging (MRI), or pulmonary function tests, should be performed when appropriate. These tests may be ordered after consideration of specific information obtained from sources such as medical records, patient interview, physical examination, and the type and invasiveness of the planned procedure and anesthesia.

PREGNANCY TESTING

Although the teen pregnancy rate in the United States is at a record low, it remains substantially greater than in other western industrialized nations[266–269] and a small percentage of adolescents may still present for elective surgery with an unsuspected pregnancy. Birth rates in females aged 15 to 19 years in the United States decreased from 41.6 births per 1000 in 2003 to 16.7 per 1000 in 2019.[268–270] However, routine preoperative pregnancy testing in adolescent girls may present ethical and legal dilemmas, including social and confidentiality concerns. Coercing a patient into having a pregnancy test against her wishes violates patient autonomy. Informed consent for pre-procedure pregnancy testing should be obtained.[271,272] This places the anesthesiologist in a predicament when faced with a question of whether to perform routine preoperative pregnancy screening. Each hospital should adopt a policy regarding pregnancy testing to provide a consistent and comprehensive policy for all females who have reached menarche. It should be noted that only seven claims in the Anesthesia Closed Claims database related to undiagnosed pregnancy; three claims were paid because the test was obtained but the anesthesiologist failed to check the results.[272]

A survey of members of the Society for Pediatric Anesthesia practicing in North America revealed that pregnancy testing was routinely required by approximately 45% of the respondents regardless of the practice setting (teaching versus nonteaching facilities).[262] A retrospective review of a 2-year study of mandatory pregnancy testing in 412 adolescent surgical patients[273] revealed that the overall incidence of positive tests was 1.2%. Five of 207 patients aged 15 years and older tested positive, for an incidence of 2.4% in that age group. None of the 205 patients younger than 15 years of age had a positive pregnancy test. A prospective study of 261 menarcheal patients 10 to 34 years of age revealed three pregnancies but none in the 107 children <15 years.[274]

The most recent ASA Task Force on Preanesthesia Evaluation recognized that a history and physical examination may not adequately identify early pregnancy and issued the following statement: *"The literature is insufficient to inform patients or physicians on whether anesthesia causes harmful effects on early pregnancy. Pregnancy testing may be offered to female patients of childbearing age and for whom the result would alter the patient's management."*[275] Because of the risk of exposing the fetus to potential teratogens and radiation from anesthesia and surgery, the risk of spontaneous abortion, and the risk of apoptosis reported in the rapidly developing fetal animal brain (see Chapter 23), elective surgery with general anesthesia is not advised during early pregnancy. Therefore, if the situation is unclear, and when indicated by medical history, it is best to perform a preoperative pregnancy test. If the surgery is required in a patient who might be pregnant, then using an opioid-based anesthetic such as remifentanil and the lowest concentration of inhalational agent or propofol that provides adequate anesthesia is preferred.[276]

Premedication and Induction Principles

GENERAL PRINCIPLES

The major objectives of preanesthetic medication are to (1) allay anxiety, (2) block autonomic (sympathetic and parasympathetic) reflexes, (3) reduce airway secretions, (4) produce amnesia, (5) provide prophylaxis against pulmonary aspiration of gastric contents, (6) facilitate the induction of anesthesia, and (7) if necessary, provide analgesia. Premedication may also decrease the stress response to anesthesia and prevent cardiac arrhythmias.[277] The goal of premedication for each child must be tailored to the patient and used in combination with nonpharmacological modalities when appropriate. Factors predictive of poor behavioral compliance during induction include younger age (>8 months and <5 years), temperament (shy, inhibited, withdrawn), anxious parents, and children with a previous negative anesthesia or hospital experience.[135,172,278] Light sedation, even though it may not eliminate anxiety, may adequately calm a child so that the induction of anesthesia will be a smooth and less stressful experience. In contrast, heavy sedation may be needed for the very anxious child who is unwilling to separate from their parents.

Factors to consider when selecting a drug or a combination of drugs for premedication include the child's age, ideal body weight, drug history, and allergy status; underlying medical or surgical conditions; parent and child expectations; and the child's emotional maturity, personality, anxiety level, cooperation, and physiologic and psychological status. The anesthesiologist should also consider the proposed surgical procedure and the attitudes and wishes of the child and the parents.

The route of administration of premedicant drugs is very important. Many children can verbalize that receiving a needle puncture was their worst experience in the hospital.[279,280] In most cases, medication administered without a needle will be more pleasant for children, their parents/guardians, and the medical staff. Oral medications do not increase the risk of aspiration pneumonia unless large volumes of fluids are ingested.[281] In general, the route of delivery of the premedication should depend on the drug, the desired drug effect, and the psychological impact of the route of administration. For example, a small dose of oral medication may be sufficient for a relatively calm child, whereas an intramuscular injection (e.g., ketamine) may be best for an uncooperative, combative, extremely anxious child. Intramuscular administration may be less traumatic for this type of child than forcing them to swallow a drug, giving a drug rectally, or forcefully holding an anesthesia mask on the face.[282] The timing of administration of premedication requires clear communication with the preoperative nursing team in order to optimize its efficacy while minimizing delays to the operating room schedule. Sedative drugs should be given after the child's fasting status is confirmed and when there is reasonable certainty that surgery will proceed. Preoperative medication should be administered in a location where the patient can be observed appropriately with resuscitation equipment readily available. Special consideration should be given to the child with obstructive sleep apnea (OSA) if sedation is indicated, as sedative premedication may cause airway obstruction and/or desaturation.

Since Waters'[283] classic work on premedication of children, numerous reports have addressed this subject. Despite the wealth of studies and variety of premedicants, no single drug or combination of drugs has been found to be ideal for all children. Many drugs used for premedication confer similar effects, although any one drug may have various effects in different children or in the same child under different conditions.

MEDICATIONS

Several categories of drugs are available for premedicating children before anesthesia (Table 2.4). Selection of drugs for premedication depends on the goal desired. Drug effects should be weighed against potential adverse effects and possible drug interactions. Commonly used premedicants include benzodiazepines, opioids, ketamine, and α_2-agonists for their anxiolytic, sedative, and/or amnestic properties (see Chapter 5).

Benzodiazepines

Benzodiazepines calm children, allay anxiety, and diminish recall of perianesthetic events. In small doses, they produce minimal drowsiness and rarely depress the cardiovascular or respiratory systems even in children with systemic disease such as OSA.[284]

Midazolam, a short-acting, water-soluble benzodiazepine with an elimination half-life of approximately 2 hours, is the most widely used premedication for children.[285,286] The major advantage of midazolam over other drugs in its class is its rapid absorption and elimination.[287] It can be administered intravenously, intramuscularly, intranasally, rectally, and orally, although it leaves a bitter taste in the mouth or nasopharynx after oral or intranasal administration.[288–294] Most children are adequately sedated after

TABLE 2.4	Doses of Drugs Commonly Administered for Premedication	
Drug	**Route**	**Dose (mg/kg)**
Benzodiazepines		
Midazolam	Oral	0.25–0.75
	Intravenous	0.05–0.1
	Sublingual	0.2–0.5
	Intranasal	0.2
	Intramuscular	0.1–0.15
Phencyclidine		
Ketamine	Oral	5–10
	Intranasal	3–5
	Intramuscular	5
α_2-Adrenergic Agonist		
Clonidine	Oral	0.004
	Intranasal	0.002
	Intramuscular	0.002–0.004
Dexmedetomidine	Intranasal	0.001–0.004
Opioids		
Morphine	Intramuscular	0.1–0.2
Fentanyl	Intranasal	0.001–0.002

receiving a midazolam dose of 0.025 to 0.1 mg/kg intravenously, 0.1 to 0.2 mg/kg intramuscularly, 0.25 to 0.75 mg/kg orally, or 0.2 mg/kg intranasally.

Orally administered midazolam calms most children quickly when given in sufficient doses[295] and does not decrease gastric pH or increase gastric fluid volume.[173,296] Evidence suggests that the required dose of midazolam increases as age decreases in children, similar to that for inhaled agents and intravenous agents.[297] An increased clearance (expressed on a kilogram basis) in younger children contributes to their increased dose requirement.[298] A number of substances and medications compete with midazolam in the gastrointestinal tract wall, including grapefruit juice, erythromycin, protease inhibitors, and calcium-channel blockers, through CYP3A4, which in turn increases the bioavailability of midazolam with a greater duration of sedation.[299–305] Conversely, anticonvulsants (phenytoin[306] and carbamazepine[307]), St. John's wort,[308] glucocorticoids,[309] and other CYP3A4 inducers[310] increase hepatic clearance and decrease midazolam's duration of action. The dose of oral midazolam should be adjusted when the above medications are concurrently administered.

Concerns have been raised about possible delayed discharge after premedication with midazolam. Oral midazolam, 0.5 mg/kg, administered to children 1 to 10 years of age, did not affect awakening times, time to extubation, postanesthesia care unit, or hospital discharge times, after sevoflurane anesthesia.[311] In contrast, premedication with oral midazolam, 0.5 mg/kg, delayed spontaneous eye opening by 4 minutes and discharge from the PACU by 10 minutes compared with placebo in children 1 to 3 years of age undergoing adenoidectomy[312]; premedicated children also exhibited a more peaceful sleep at home on the first night after surgery.[312] In an escalating oral dose-finding study (0.25, 0.5, or 1.0 mg/kg, maximum 20 mg), the duration of PACU stay was similar although recovery was more rapid in infants 6 months to < 2 years old when compared with older children.[295] The true test of whether a premedication delays discharge occurs when the infants are premedicated for myringotomy and tympanotomy surgery that lasts 5 to 7 minutes. Intranasal midazolam (0.2 or 0.3 mg/kg) did not prolong the PACU stay or delay discharge compared with placebo in infants anesthetized with sevoflurane.[313] Similar results have been reported in children and adolescents after 20 milligrams of oral midazolam (max dose)[295]; however, preoperative sedation in this group of children was predictive of delayed emergence.[314]

Although anxiolysis and a mild degree of sedation occur in most children after midazolam, a few develop undesirable adverse effects. Some children become agitated after oral or intravenous midazolam (paradoxical excitation)[315]; if this occurs, intravenous ketamine or flumazenil may reverse the agitation.[316–318]

Anxiolysis and sedation usually occur within 10 minutes after intranasal midazolam[319]; nasal administration is not as well accepted as the oral route because it produces irritation, discomfort, and a burning aftertaste.[320–323] This route of administration as a nasal spray has been used to treat status epilepticus in children without intravenous access due to its lack of first pass metabolism, rapid absorption, high bioavailability, and possible central nervous system (CNS) distribution (E-Fig. 2.1).[324,325] An alternative method of delivery is nebulized midazolam as it is associated with less discomfort than liquid intranasal administration, although larger doses are needed.[326–328] Other transmucosal routes include sublingual midazolam (0.2 mg/kg) that has been reported to be as effective as, and better accepted than intranasal midazolam.[329] Oral transmucosal midazolam given

in three to five small allotments (0.2 mg/kg total dose) placed on a child's tongue (8 months to 6 years of age) was found to provide satisfactory acceptance and separation from parents in 95% of children.[330]

Nonbarbiturate Sedatives

Chloral hydrate and *triclofos* are orally administered nonbarbiturate drugs used to sedate children; both have slow onset times and are relatively long acting (see also Chapters 5 and 44). Chloral hydrate is occasionally used by anesthesiologists but it is unreliable and has a prolonged duration of action.[331] It is unpleasant to taste, and is irritating to the skin, mucous membranes, and gastrointestinal tract. Use in neonates is not recommended because of immature clearance with consequent prolonged duration of sedation.[332,333] Commercially prepared chloral hydrate is no longer available in the United States, but a powdered form can be reconstituted by the hospital pharmacy for oral administration.

Opioids

Opioids may be useful to provide analgesia and sedation in children who have pain preoperatively but may also confer adverse effects, including nausea, vomiting, respiratory depression, sedation, and dysphoria. Therefore, all children who receive an opioid premedication should be continuously observed and monitored.

Morphine, 0.05 to 0.1 mg/kg intravenously, may be given to children with preoperative pain. It is also effective when given orally; rectal administration is not recommended owing to erratic absorption.[334] Neonates are more sensitive to the respiratory depressant effects of morphine, and it is rarely used to premedicate that age group.[335]

Fentanyl was introduced in a "lollipop" delivery system known as oral transmucosal fentanyl citrate (OTFC) for premedication in children in the United States but is no longer available for that indication, in part due to the high incidence of preoperative nausea and vomiting. Its current use is to treat breakthrough cancer pain. Fentanyl has also been administered intranasally (1 to 2 µg/kg) but primarily after induction of anesthesia as a means of providing analgesia in children without intravenous access.[336]

Tramadol is a weak µ-opioid receptor agonist whose analgesic effect is mediated via inhibition of norepinephrine reuptake and stimulation of serotonin release. Tramadol is devoid of action on platelets and does not depress respirations in the clinical dose range.[337] Serum concentrations peak by 2 hours after oral dosing with clinical analgesia maintained for 6 to 9 hours. Tramadol is metabolized in part by CYP2D6 to the M1 metabolite; single nuclear polymorphisms contribute to large variability.[338] Although rarely used preoperatively, intravenous tramadol (1.5 mg/kg) given before induction of general anesthesia has been compared with local infiltration of 0.5% bupivacaine (0.25 mL/kg) for ilioinguinal and iliohypogastric nerve blocks. Tramadol was as effective as the regional blocks in terms of pain control, although the incidence of nausea and vomiting was greater in the tramadol group. Time to discharge was similar in both groups.[339]

Opioids combined with midazolam: When fentanyl or other opioids are combined with midazolam greater respiratory depression is observed than with either drug alone.[340] If opioids are used in combination with other sedatives such as benzodiazepines, the dose of each drug should be appropriately reduced to avoid serious respiratory depression. For example, if fentanyl is indicated to control pain in a child who has already received midazolam, the fentanyl dose should be titrated in small increments (0.25 to 0.5 µg/kg) to prevent desaturation and hypopnea or apnea.

Ketamine

Ketamine is a phencyclidine derivative that causes dissociation of the cortex from the limbic system, producing reliable sedation and analgesia while preserving upper airway muscle tone and respiratory drive.[341] Ketamine may be administered by the intravenous, intramuscular, oral, nasal transmucosal, and rectal routes.[342] The disadvantages of ketamine include sialorrhea, nystagmus, an increased incidence of postoperative emesis, and possible undesirable psychological reactions such as hallucinations,[343] nightmares, and delirium, although to date no psychological reactions have been reported after oral ketamine. Concomitant administration of midazolam may eliminate or attenuate these emergence reactions, although one study reported that there was no salutary relationship with midazolam premedication and hallucinations.[343–345] The addition of atropine or glycopyrrolate is recommended to decrease the sialorrhea caused by ketamine[346]; however, a meta-analysis concluded that atropine reduced hypersalivation and increased heart rate but did not affect the incidence of vomiting, desaturation, agitation, or laryngospasm.[347]

Intramuscular ketamine is an effective means of sedating combative, apprehensive, or developmentally delayed children who are otherwise uncooperative and refuse oral medication. A low dose (2 mg/kg) is sufficient to adequately calm most uncooperative children within 3 to 5 minutes so that they will accept a mask for inhalation induction and does not prolong hospital discharge times even after brief procedures.[282] However, the combination of intramuscular ketamine (2 mg/kg) and midazolam (0.1 to 0.2 mg/kg) significantly prolongs recovery and discharge times, making the ketamine-midazolam combination less suitable for brief ambulatory procedures.[348]

Larger doses of intramuscular ketamine are particularly useful for the induction of anesthesia in children in whom there is a desire to maintain a stable blood pressure and in whom there is no venous access. Larger doses (4 to 5 mg/kg) sedate children within 2 to 4 minutes,[349] and very large doses (10 mg/kg) induce deep sedation that may last from 12 to 25 minutes. Large doses and repeated doses may be associated with hallucinations, nightmares, and vomiting, as well as prolonged recovery from anesthesia.[282,350] Propriety concentrations of ketamine 100 mg/mL are available for intramuscular injection. It is imperative to label these syringes to avoid a syringe swap with others containing more dilute concentrations of ketamine.

Oral ketamine alone[351] and in combination with oral midazolam is an effective premedication and has been used to alleviate the distress of invasive procedures (e.g., bone marrow aspiration) in pediatric oncology patients.[352,353] A dose of 5 to 6 mg/kg oral ketamine alone sedates most children within 12 minutes and provides sufficient sedation in more than half of the children to permit establishing intravenous access.[348,354] A larger dose of 8 mg/kg[353] has been used but prolonged recovery from anesthesia, although by 2 hours the recovery was no different from that after 4 mg/kg.[355] Oral doses of up to 10 mg/kg have been described as a premedicant for children having procedures for burns; the relative bioavailability was 45%, and absorption was slow with an absorption half-life of 1 hour.[356] The combination of oral midazolam (0.5 mg/kg) and ketamine (3 mg/kg) provides more effective preoperative sedation than either drug alone. This oral lytic cocktail is a good alternative for children who were not adequately sedated with oral midazolam alone and did not prolong recovery after surgical procedures that lasted more than 30 minutes.[357]

Intranasal ketamine in a dose of 6 mg/kg is also an effective premedication for children, with sedation developing by 20 to 40 minutes.[358] There remain concerns that nasally administered ketamine could cause neural tissue damage if it reaches the cribriform plate. Preservative-free ketamine may be safer to administer by the nasal route, although this has not been established.[359] If ketamine is given intranasally, we recommend the 100 mg/mL concentration to minimize the volume that must be instilled.

Rectal ketamine (5 mg/kg) produces good anxiolysis and sedation within 30 minutes of administration.[360] However, the rectal route does not provide reliable absorption.

α_2-Agonists

Clonidine, an α_2-agonist, causes dose-related sedation by its effect in the locus coeruleus.[361] It acts both centrally and peripherally on α_2 receptors to decrease blood pressure, thereby attenuating the hemodynamic response to intubation.[362] Clonidine is devoid of respiratory depression, even when administered in overdoses.[361] The clonidine-sedation response relationship is shallow (high concentrations are required for deep sedation).[363] The sedative properties of clonidine decrease the minimum alveolar concentration (MAC) of sevoflurane for tracheal intubation[364] and the concentration of inhaled anesthetic required for the maintenance of anesthesia,[365–367] without prolonging emergence from anesthesia or leading to airway-related complications.[368]

During the first 12 hours after surgery, oral clonidine (4 µg/kg) reduces postoperative pain and the requirement for supplementary analgesics.[369,370] In children scheduled for tonsillectomy, those who received oral clonidine (4 µg/kg) were more anxious at the time of separation and during induction of anesthesia than those who received oral midazolam (0.5 mg/kg).[371–373] Even though discharge readiness, postoperative emesis, and 24-hour analgesic requirements were similar in both groups, midazolam was judged to be the better premedicant for children undergoing tonsillectomy.[371] Oral clonidine (4 µg/kg) reduces the incidence of vomiting after strabismus surgery compared with a placebo, clonidine (2 µg/kg), or oral diazepam (0.4 mg/kg).[374] Postoperative negative behavioral changes after midazolam and clonidine oral premedication were similar.[372] Oral clonidine offers several desirable qualities as a premedication, particularly sedation and analgesia; however, the need to administer it 60 minutes before induction of anesthesia makes its use impractical in busy outpatient settings.[371]

Dexmedetomidine is a sedative with properties that are similar to those of clonidine except that it has an ~8-fold greater affinity for the α_2-adenoreceptors than clonidine. Based on bioavailability studies in adults, it is well absorbed through the oral mucosa.[375] Dexmedetomidine is being used with increased frequency in multiple routes and doses.[376,377] The concentration-response curve for dexmedetomidine is, like clonidine, shallow.[378,379] One randomized study of 60 children 1 to 7 years of age reported equivalent preoperative sedation but improved recovery in children who received 4 µg/kg of oral dexmedetomidine compared with 0.75 mg/kg midazolam.[380]

The nasal route has had increased interest, with one study reporting a bioavailability of 84%.[381] A study of 13 children (4 to 14 years of age), of whom 9 had neurobehavioral disorders, intranasal dexmedetomidine (2 µg/kg) provided adequate sedation for a mask induction within 20 to 30 minutes of administration. It was postulated that a larger dose of 3 to 4 µg/kg might be more effective.[382] A double-blind comparison of intranasal dexmedetomidine (4 µg/kg) compared with oral midazolam (0.5 mg/kg) reported a similar rate of satisfactory separation from parents and acceptance of venipuncture as well as a reduced incidence of emergence agitation. However, they found a greater incidence of hypotension and bradycardia in the dexmedetomidine group.[383] As a result, the intranasal dose was scaled back to 1 to 3 μg/kg to achieve anxiolysis without excessive sedation, with varied results. Anxiolysis was superior with oral midazolam (0.5 mg/kg) than intranasal dexmedetomidine (2 μg/kg) although sedation was greater with the dexmedetomidine.[373] Children undergoing transthoracic echocardiography were satisfactorily sedated with 3 μg/kg intranasal dexmedetomidine in an observational study[384] as were children undergoing auditory brainstem response testing with the same dose of dexmedetomidine compared with oral chloral hydrate with a more rapid onset of sedation and return to baseline activity with the former.[385] Even a dose of 1 μg/kg intranasal dexmedetomidine sedated children significantly better than oral midazolam (0.5 mg/kg).[386] The optimal dose of intranasal dexmedetomidine for anxiolysis is approximately 2 μg/kg.

In children with burns, both intranasal dexmedetomidine (2 μg/kg) and oral midazolam (0.5 mg/kg) administered 30 to 45 minutes before induction of anesthesia provided adequate conditions for induction of anesthesia and emergence, although dexmedetomidine produced more sleep preoperatively.[387] A study of 62 children (2–6 years of age) undergoing minor elective surgery were randomly assigned to two groups to receive dexmedetomidine either 1 μg/kg buccally or 1 μg/kg intranasally for premedication 45 minutes before induction. Levels of sedation, parental separation, and mask acceptance scores in the intranasal group were significantly greater and deemed to be more effective than those in the buccal administration group.[388] Intranasal dexmedetomidine (1 μg/kg) and intranasal midazolam (0.2 mg/kg) produced equal decreases in anxiety upon separation from parents but midazolam was superior in providing satisfactory conditions during mask induction.[389]

Oral midazolam (0.5 mg/kg given 30 minutes before surgery), oral clonidine (4 μg/kg given 90 minutes before surgery), and transmucosal dexmedetomidine (1 μg/kg given 45 minutes before surgery) all produced similar preanesthetic sedation and response to separation from parents in a comparative trial, although children who received dexmedetomidine and clonidine experienced attenuated mean arterial pressure and heart rate preoperatively and reduced pain scores postoperatively compared with midazolam.[390] In a similar study using intranasal dexmedetomidine 2 μg/kg 40 minutes preoperatively, midazolam yielded more effective anxiolysis and less sedation than in those patients given clonidine or dexmedetomidine.[373]

Antihistamines

Antihistamines are rarely used for premedication in children, in part because their sedative effects are quite variable. They are rarely given to infants but may occasionally be indicated for older children, especially those who are hyperkinetic.

Hydroxyzine is mainly administered for its tranquilizing properties[391,392]; it also has antiemetic, antihistaminic, and antispasmodic properties, with minimal respiratory and circulatory effects. It is commonly administered with other classes of drugs as an intramuscular "cocktail" in a dose of 0.5 to 1.0 mg/kg.

Diphenhydramine is an H_1-receptor blocker with mild sedative and antimuscarinic effects. The dose in children is 2.5 to 5 mg/kg per day (maximum 300 mg/day) in four divided doses orally, intravenously, or intramuscularly. Although the duration of action is 4 to 6 hours, it does not appear to interfere with recovery from anesthesia.[393] The combination of oral diphenhydramine (1.25 mg/kg) and oral midazolam (0.5 mg/kg) has been used to provide sedation for healthy children undergoing MRI.[394] The combination was more effective than midazolam alone without a delay in discharge and recovery times.

Anticholinergic Drugs

In the past, anticholinergic agents were used (1) to prevent the undesirable bradycardia associated with some anesthetic agents (halothane and succinylcholine), (2) to minimize the autonomic vagal reflexes manifested during surgical manipulations (e.g., laryngoscopy, strabismus repair), and (3) to reduce secretions. The most commonly used anticholinergic drugs are atropine, scopolamine, and glycopyrrolate. Anticholinergics also provide undesirable effects, including tachycardia, dry mouth, skin erythema, and hyperthermia, as a result of inhibited sweating. Atropine and scopolamine cross the blood-brain barrier and may cause CNS excitation manifested as agitation, confusion, restlessness, ataxia, hallucinations, slurred speech, and memory loss if given in excessive doses.[395]

Because most modern inhalational anesthetics are not associated with bradycardia and succinylcholine is infrequently used in children, the routine use of an anticholinergic drug is not generally warranted. Most anesthesiologists administer these agents only when indicated, such as before intravenous succinylcholine, combined with ketamine, before laryngoscopy and intubation in neonates, and when surgery stimulates vagal reflexes, such as during strabismus repair.

The recommended doses of anticholinergics are *atropine,* 0.01 to 0.02 mg/kg, and *scopolamine,* 0.005 to 0.010 mg/kg. Atropine is more commonly used and blocks the vagus nerve more effectively than scopolamine, whereas scopolamine is a better sedative, antisialagogue, and amnestic. Infants who are at risk for or show early evidence of a slowing of the heart rate should receive the atropine before the heart rate actually decreases to ensure a prompt onset of effect to maintain cardiac output.[396] There is no minimum dose of atropine in infants.[397] *Glycopyrrolate* is a synthetic quaternary ammonium compound that does not cross the blood-brain barrier. It is twice as potent as atropine in decreasing the volume of oral secretions, and its duration of effect is three times greater. The recommended dose of glycopyrrolate (0.01 mg/kg) is half that of atropine. The routine use of an anticholinergic drug for the sole purpose of drying secretions is probably unwarranted because a dry mouth can be a source of extreme discomfort for a child. Therefore, it is best to reserve the use of glycopyrrolate for specific indications such as to limit sialorrhea associated with ketamine.

Topical Anesthetics

Needle phobia is a phenomenon well recognized by anesthesiologists and a cause of distress.[279,280,398] Untreated pain has a tremendous impact on a child throughout their life. Pain experienced in early infancy correlates with a stronger negative response to venipuncture weeks to months later; similarly older children have reported greater pain during follow-up cancer-related procedures if the pain of the initial procedure was poorly controlled.[399] Pharmacologic and nonpharmacologic measures such as virtual reality headsets[400] and distraction techniques[401] are quite useful in reducing children's acute pain and subsequent negative behaviors during venipuncture and intravenous catheter insertion.[402] Topical anesthetic creams and needle-less methods to alleviate procedural pain are attractive alternatives to intradermal infiltration and intramuscular injections.

A eutectic mixture of local anesthetics (EMLA, Astra Zeneca, Wilmington, DE) is composed of two local anesthetics, lidocaine (2.5%) and prilocaine (2.5%). An application of EMLA cream to intact skin with an occlusive dressing provides adequate topical anesthesia within 60 minutes[403] for a variety of superficial procedures, including intravenous catheter insertion, lumbar puncture, vaccination, laser treatment of port-wine stains, and neonatal circumcision.[404–407] EMLA has been used in neonates to reduce the pain of circumcision, venous catheter placement, arterial puncture, and heel lancing. A meta-analysis of 11 studies in neonates concluded that EMLA reduced the pain of circumcision but not heel lancing.[408] A recent meta-analysis of 10 randomized controlled trials of the efficacy and safety of EMLA cream for pain control during venipuncture in infants <3 months yielded little or no effect in reducing pain compared with sucrose, breastfeeding, or placebo.[409]

EMLA cream is not without side effects that further compromise its usefulness. EMLA causes venoconstriction and skin blanching that may obscure superficial veins resulting in more difficult intravenous cannulation.[410] The prilocaine in the cream may cause methemoglobinemia,[411] although methemoglobinemia did not occur after a 1-hour application at a maximum dose of 1 gram applied to intact skin in full-term neonates and infants younger than 3 months of age.[412] Methemoglobin concentrations in the EMLA group were greater than in the placebo group 3.5 to 13 hours after application, but toxic levels were not detected. Methemoglobinemia has been reported in neonates and infants when applied to mucous membranes or in chronic use.[413] Lidocaine toxicity has been reported when EMLA was applied to mucosal membranes for extended periods.[414] Toxicity (methemoglobinemia, cardiac, neurologic) from systemic absorption or accidental ingestion of both lidocaine and prilocaine has been reported when maximum surface area applications were exceeded.[415–417]

L.M.X.4 (previously ELA-max, Ferndale Laboratories, Ferndale, MI) is a topical anesthetic cream containing lidocaine (4%) that decreases the pain associated with dermatologic procedures[418] and intravenous catheter insertion after only a 30-minute application.[419] L.M.X.4 blanches the skin like EMLA, but does so to a lesser extent, and dilates the veins better than EMLA.[420] In a single study that compared L.M.X.4 to EMLA or dorsal penile block for analgesia in circumcision in neonates, L.M.X.4 compared favorably with the other two techniques.[421]

Heat-enhanced drug-delivery systems, such as the *Synera Patch* (a eutectic mixture of lidocaine and tetracaine, 70 mg each per patch, Galen Pharma, Audubon, PA), use a controlled heating system to accelerate delivery and effectiveness of the local anesthetic. After 20 to 30 minutes of application to intact skin, the pain associated with venipuncture is reduced significantly.[422] The patch causes mild and transient local erythema and edema and no blanching of the skin.[423]

Ethyl chloride, a vapocoolant spray, may be sprayed for 4 to 10 seconds at a distance of approximately 3 to 7 inches from the skin, to control minor pain associated with topical procedures[424,425] and for temporary relief of minor sports injuries. The coldness decreases the nerve conduction velocity of C and A-delta fibers, which in turn interrupts the nociceptive inputs to the spinal cord. Some children may not like the cooling effect and data on efficacy are variable.[426,427]

Needle-free pressurized delivery systems allow for rapid delivery of lidocaine before peripheral venous access or other needle-based procedures such as lumbar puncture.[428–430] One such system, the J-Tip device (National Medical Products, Irvine, CA), uses compressed carbon dioxide for drug delivery, instead of a needle, to deliver 0.25 mL of local anesthetic subcutaneously. This device must be filled with local anesthetic by the user, typically 0.25 mL of lidocaine 1%. In one study, J-Tip–delivered lidocaine was found to be no more effective than J-Tip–delivered placebo in providing local anesthesia for needle insertion and both may provide superior analgesia compared with no device use; the majority of patients receiving the jet device reported that they would request it for future needle insertions.[431] In a retrospective and a prospective study, the use of the J-Tip did not affect first-attempt success for intravenous line placement in children, but there was a significant reduction in pain scores.[432,433] Introduced after the J-Tip, Zingo (Marathon Pharmaceuticals, Northbrook, IL) is a prefilled syringe of sterile lidocaine powder (up to 2.5mg) that uses pressurized helium to enable the drug to penetrate the epidermis numbing the site within 1 to 3 minutes. The latter system is bulkier and priced significantly higher than the J-Tip.

There are many safe options for providing topical anesthesia in children for painful procedures. The choice of product should be based on patient needs, provider preference, ease of administration, time sensitivity, and/or cost (Table 2.5).

TABLE 2.5	Common Topical Anesthetic Agents			
Product	Ingredients	Time to Onset	Duration of Action	Common Adverse Effects
LMX-4	4% liposomal lidocaine	20–30 minutes	~1 hour	Erythema, blanching
EMLA	2.5% prilocaine/ 2.5% lidocaine	45–60 minutes	~4 hours	Erythema, blanching, edema
Ethyl Chloride	Ethyl chloride	Immediate	~15 seconds	Temporary alteration of pigmentation, vasoconstriction may increase difficulty of venous access
J-Tip	User fills	Specific to ingredient	Specific to ingredient	Loud popping noise may frighten some children

Data obtained from package inserts.

Nonopioid Analgesics

Acetaminophen (paracetamol) is the most common nonopioid analgesic used for treatment of postoperative pain in children. It can be administered orally preoperatively, or intravenously once intravenous access has been established.

The oral doses of acetaminophen for antipyresis (10 to 15 mg/kg) are as effective as ketorolac (1 mg/kg),[434] given 10 or more minutes postoperatively for myringotomy and tube placement.[435] Oral acetaminophen is very rapidly absorbed with a bioavailability of 0.9 to 1.[435] Neonates may be at less risk for hepatotoxicity because the hepatic enzyme systems in neonates are immature and produce smaller quantities of toxic metabolites than in older children.[436–438] When given preemptively, acetaminophen has opioid-sparing properties that enhance analgesia in children after tonsillectomy.[439,440] A relationship between concentration and analgesic effect for pain relief after tonsillectomy has been observed in children. An effect compartment concentration of 10 mg/L was associated with a reduction of pain by 2.6 units (using a visual analog scale ranging from 0 to 10).[435,441]

Excessive fasting, a very large loading dose of acetaminophen (>200 mg/kg),[442] and sevoflurane anesthesia can deplete glutathione stores and may contribute to the development of hepatic failure.[443] The coadministration of antiepileptic drugs has also been implicated in hepatotoxicity from acetaminophen.[444] *Because hepatic toxicity is a potentially fatal complication of an acetaminophen overdose, a complete medication history of acetaminophen consumption and concomitant drugs should be completed preoperatively, and the recommended maximum daily dose should not be exceeded.*

The US FDA has approved intravenous acetaminophen for use in children 2 years of age and older. The recommended dose for children 2 to 12 years old weighing less than 50 kg is 15 mg/kg every 6 hours or 12.5 mg/kg every 4 hours with a maximum of 75 mg/kg per day. Use in children younger than 2 years is considered off-label. Practitioners in the United States who choose to use intravenous acetaminophen off-label should consider reduced dosage for patients younger than 2 years of age. In infants 1 month to 2 years of age, dosing from the pharmacokinetic data suggests a dose reduction of 33%, 10 mg/kg every 4 hours or 12.5 mg/kg every 6 hours, with a maximum dose of 50 to 60 mg/kg per day. In full-term neonates up to 28 days of age, the dose of intravenous acetaminophen should be reduced by 50% to 7.5 mg/kg every 6 to 8 hours with a maximum daily dose of 30 mg/kg. This dosing regimen produces a similar pharmacokinetic profile as in children older than 2 years of age.[445,446] The major concern in this age group is accidental overdose of acetaminophen and hepatic toxicity. Three near-fatal cases of infants who received 10- and 20-fold overdoses of intravenous acetaminophen have been reported.[447,448] In some instances, overdose errors resulted for dosages calculated in milligrams, but administered in milliliters.[449,450] Careful documentation of the dose of intravenous acetaminophen is warranted in infants.[451]

Children and adolescents who are obese also present dosing challenges for acetaminophen. Adolescents (14–20 years of age) with a body mass index (BMI) >95th percentile for age and sex or a BMI >40 kg/m² undergoing laparoscopic or robotic assisted or vertical sleeve gastrectomy received intravenous acetaminophen (1000 mg) after completion of the surgical procedure. A single dose of acetaminophen (1000 mg) yielded serum concentrations less than the target concentration of 10 mg/L in all patients within 2 hours after administration (Fig. 2.6). The best size descriptor for acetaminophen dosing in obese adolescents remains uncertain although the dose that achieves a target concentration of 10 mg/L in the effect compartment is better predicted using total body weight with allometric scaling.[452] Current dosing regimen is restricted to a maximum of 1000 mg 6 hourly due to concerns of hepatotoxicity.

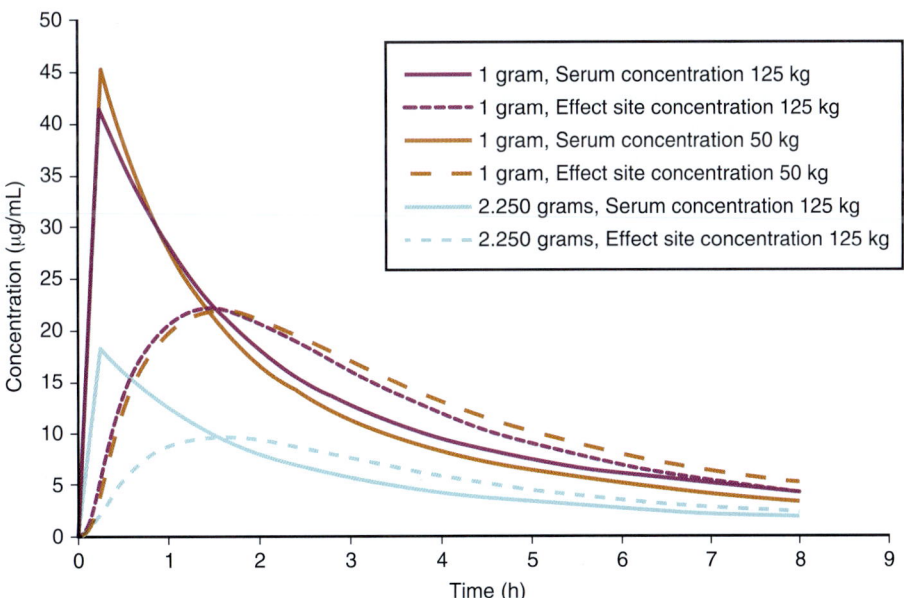

FIGURE 2.6 Simulations shows serum and effect site time-concentration profiles for a 50-kg adolescent given 1 gram (1000 mg) acetaminophen and an 125-kg adolescent given 1 gram (1000 mg) acetaminophen. An acetaminophen dose of 2.25 grams (2250 mg) is required in an obese adolescent to achieve similar concentrations to a non-obese adolescent. Effect site equilibration half-time of 0.7 hours was assumed. (From Hakim, Anderson BJ, Walla H, et al. Acetaminophen pharmacokinetics in severely obese adolescents and young adults. *Pediatr Anesth.* 2019;29:20-26.)

Several studies regarding opioid sparing with intravenous acetaminophen have been undertaken. In a study of 50 children, ages 2 to 5 years, undergoing elective adenoidectomy or adenotonsillectomy, intravenous acetaminophen (15 mg/kg) had a time to first rescue analgesic of a median of 7 hours, although few children required any rescue analgesics during the first 6 hours.[453] In children undergoing tonsillectomy, intravenous acetaminophen (15 mg/kg) yielded comparable analgesia but less sedation and earlier discharge readiness compared with intramuscular meperidine (1 mg/kg).[454] In children undergoing dental restoration with the same medications and doses, pain scores in those given acetaminophen were greater but discharge readiness occurred earlier.[455] In 45 healthy children (5 months to 5 years of age) undergoing primary cleft palate repair intravenous acetaminophen (12.5 mg/kg age <2 years) or 15 mg/kg (age 2–5 years) every 6 hours for 24 hours resulted in improved analgesia and decreased postoperative opioid requirements.[456] Administration of intravenous nonnarcotic analgesics may also decrease nausea and vomiting compared with oral medications. In children undergoing craniosynostosis correction, those who received oral ibuprofen (10 mg/kg) and acetaminophen (15 mg/kg) vomited more than those who received intravenous ketorolac (0.5 mg/kg) and acetaminophen (15 mg/kg),[457] suggesting that the route of administration impacts the risk of vomiting.

Antiemetics

Antiemetic administration should be considered in children undergoing high-risk procedures such as tonsillectomy and strabismus repair as well as those who have a history of motion sickness or prior history of postoperative nausea and vomiting. The uses of these medications are presented elsewhere in the text (see Chapters 5, 31, and 32).

Corticosteroids

Patients requiring chronic corticosteroid therapy (e.g., for treatment of asthma, Crohn's disease, lupus, acute lymphocytic leukemia), and those who have recently discontinued chronic corticosteroid therapy, may suffer from suppression of the hypothalamic-pituitary-adrenal axis and secondary adrenal insufficiency (see also Chapter 25).[458] There is no general consensus on the dose or duration of exogenous steroids required to cause adrenal insufficiency, although supraphysiological doses of glucocorticoid equivalent to >10 mg/m^2 per day of hydrocortisone increase the risk.[459] Steroid treatment courses as brief as two weeks may result in transient suppression of endogenous cortisol and the risk increases with longer duration of treatment (>4 weeks). The duration of adrenal insufficiency following discontinuation of steroids is variable and can range from 3 to 18 months.[460] The administration of stress-dose steroids in the perioperative period may prevent an adrenal crisis but the recommendations are inconsistent, and evidence is lacking. Nonetheless, many endocrinologists continue to recommend a dose of supplemental corticosteroids before or shortly after induction of anesthesia for stress corticosteroid coverage. The usual recommended dose is 1 to 2 mg/kg of hydrocortisone (maximum 100 mg) at induction of anesthesia or as soon as intravenous access is established for minor surgery. For more complicated operations, the corticosteroid dose may be repeated every 6 hours for up to 72 hours (see Chapter 25). Any dose should be tempered if steroids (dexamethasone) are administered for postoperative nausea and vomiting.

Insulin

Diabetes mellitus is the most common endocrine problem encountered in children. The perioperative management of children who are on insulin depends on their insulin regimen rather than on whether they have type 1 or type 2 diabetes. Optimal management of children with diabetes undergoing surgery entails maintaining glucose homeostasis, avoiding hyperglycemia with resultant osmotic diuresis, impaired wound healing, increased infection rate, and avoiding hypoglycemia. Anesthesiologists should work together with the endocrinologist or primary care physician to design a plan for each child's specific diabetes treatment regimen, glycemic control, and anticipated postoperative care. The preoperative fasting time should be the same as that recommended for nondiabetic children. Every attempt should be made to schedule these children as the first case of the day to minimize the fasting period. Preoperative laboratory tests generally include hematocrit, serum electrolytes, and glucose levels; blood glucose concentrations should be measured at frequent intervals during the perianesthetic period. Several protocols have been crafted to control the blood sugar in children who are diabetic[461]; these are described in more detail in Chapter 25 (see also Figs. 25.1 to 25.5), which describe a variety of management strategies). Intraoperative management of insulin pumps requires knowledge of how the pump can be reset and to protect it from pressure and exposure to ionizing radiation; hourly assessment of blood glucose values to assess possible pump failure is indicated (see also Chapter 25).[462,463]

Antibiotics

Antibiotics are frequently administered to prevent or reduce surgical site infections that occur in up to 5% of patients undergoing an inpatient surgical procedure, increasing mortality by 2- to 11-fold.[464] A retrospective review identified the overall rate of surgical site infections in children undergoing a variety of surgical procedures as ~2.4%.[465] Surgical site infections prolong hospitalizations by 7 to 10 days and cost an estimated $1 billion annually in the United States.[466] The appropriate timing of antibiotics is now a source of performance benchmarking for some insurance carriers, making communication with surgeons essential for the success of this anesthesiology-directed quality assessment measure. Current guidelines define appropriate antibiotic prophylaxis for surgical site infection as administration within 60 minutes prior to incision.[467] Compliance with these guidelines remains a concern.[468] A systematic review of available evidence failed to reach a clear benefit of surgical antibiotic prophylaxis in children as a result of the poor quality evidence.[469] Intraoperative redosing is needed if the duration of the procedure exceeds two drug half-lives or there is excessive blood loss. Pediatric doses provided in these guidelines are based on pharmacokinetic data and the extrapolation of adult efficacy data to pediatric patients. In both normal weight and obese children, total body weight may be used for dose calculation until adult dosing limits are reached; pediatric dosing should not exceed the maximum recommended adult dose (Table 2.6).[470]

Prophylaxis against infective endocarditis is only recommended in patients with cardiac conditions associated with the greatest risk of adverse outcomes from endocarditis. Antibiotics should ideally be administered either intravenously 30 to 60 minutes or orally 1 hour before the induction of anesthesia and surgery. In reality, in children these antibiotics are usually administered after induction of anesthesia and establishment of intravenous access, and may be administered up to 2 hours after the procedure if the dose was inadvertently missed.[471,472] Clindamycin is no longer recommended for prophylaxis in dental procedures[473] (see Tables 14.2 and 14.3).

TABLE 2.6	Current American Society of Hospital Pharmacists Recommendations for Surgical Antibiotic Prophylaxis (Weight-Normalized)		
Antibiotic	Recommended Child Dose (mg/kg but not to exceed adult dose)	Recommended Adult Dose	Recommended Repeat Intraoperative Dosing Interval (hours) or >15% EBV Loss
Ampicillin-sulbactam	50 (Ampicillin component)	3 grams	2
Ampicillin	50	2 grams	2
Aztreonam	30	2 grams	4
Cefazolin	30	2 grams; use 3 grams if >120 kg	4
Cefuroxime	50	1.5 grams	4
Cefotaxime	50	1 gram	3
Cefoxitin	40	2 grams	2
Cefotetan	40	2 grams	6
Ceftriaxone	50–75	2 grams	NA
Ciprofloxacin	10	400 mg	NA
Clindamycin	10	900 mg	6
Ertapenem	15	1 gram	NA
Fluconazole	6	400 mg	NA
Gentamicin	2.5; based on dosing weight	5 mg/kg; based on dosing weight single dose	Single dose
Levofloxacin	10	500 mg	NA
Metronidazole	15; neonates <1200 g: 7.5 mg/kg (single dose)	500 mg	NA
Moxifloxacin	10	400 mg	NA
Piperacillin-tazobactam	Infants 2–9 months: 80 mg/kg of piperacillin component; Children >9 months and ≤40 kg: 100 mg/kg of piperacillin component	3.375 grams	2
Vancomycin	15	15 mg/kg	NA

EBV, Estimated blood volume.
Originally published in Bratzler DW, Dellinger EP, Olsen KM, et al. Clinical practice guidelines for antimicrobial prophylaxis in surgery. *Am J Health Syst Pharm.* 2013;70(3): 195-283. Adapted with permission.

TABLE 2.7	Doses of Antacids, H_2-Receptor Antagonists, and Gastrointestinal Motility Drugs
Drug	Dose
Antacids	
Bicitra (oral)	30 mL (0.5–1 mL/kg up to 30 mL)
Prokinetic	
Metoclopramide (IV)	0.1–0.15 mg/kg
H_2-Receptor Antagonists	
Cimetidine (IV)	5–10 mg/kg
Ranitidine (PO/IV)	2–2.5 mg/kg
Famotidine (PO/IV)	0.5 mg/kg (not to exceed 40 mg/day)

Antacids, H_2-Receptor Antagonists, and Gastrointestinal Motility Drugs

The risk of aspiration during induction of or emergence from anesthesia may be increased in children who are developmentally delayed or obese, have gastroesophageal reflux, have experienced previous esophageal surgery, have a difficult airway, or those who have sustained a traumatic injury. Preanesthetic administration of drugs that reduce gastric fluid volume and acidity may decrease the risk of pulmonary acid aspiration syndrome (Table 2.7).[1,474]

Gastric fluid pH may be increased by administration of a nonparticulate antacid such as sodium citrate; particulate antacids should be avoided because they can cause severe pneumonitis if aspirated.

Cimetidine and *ranitidine* are H_2-receptor antagonists that decrease gastric acid secretion, increase gastric fluid pH, and reduce gastric residual volume.[475,476] These drugs can be given orally, intravenously, or intramuscularly.

Metoclopramide is often administered with an H_2-receptor antagonist to increase the tone of the lower esophageal sphincter, relax the pyloric sphincter and the duodenal bulb, and promote gastric emptying by increasing peristalsis of the duodenum and jejunum. The drug effect is apparent 30 to 60 minutes after oral administration and 1 to 2 minutes after intravenous administration.[477] Adverse effects such as extrapyramidal signs relate to the effect of metoclopramide on the CNS through blockade of dopaminergic receptors.

These medications should not be routinely administered for the purpose of reducing the risk of pulmonary aspiration in patients with no apparent increased risk for pulmonary aspiration.[83]

Induction of Anesthesia

PREPARATION FOR INDUCTION

An essential step in preparation for induction of anesthesia is the confirmation of the patient's identity, the planned procedure, site of surgery, and that consent for surgery has been given. Wrong site surgery is a "never event" and the surgical site should be marked in cases involving laterality. When confirmation by the patient is not possible, as in the case of children, a parent or guardian can assume this role and verify the surgical laterality. If the guardian or family member is not available, or in case of an emergency, the surgeon, anesthesiologist together with nursing personnel should be in agreement before inducing anesthesia. The formal use of a surgical safety checklist with the operating room team (nurses, surgeon, and anesthesiologist) should occur before each perioperative phase: induction, procedure start, and departure from the operating room; such checklists constitute a vital safety net in the operating room (Fig. 2.7).[478,479]

The anesthesia machine and monitoring equipment should be prepared before the child's arrival to the operating room to ensure that all necessary equipment is on hand and to minimize any last-minute delays (E-Figs. 2.2 and 2.3), see also Chapter 49). The preinduction checklist should include a variety of sizes of masks, oral airways, laryngoscope blades, tracheal tubes (one-half size larger and one-half size smaller than the anticipated size), an appropriate sized laryngeal mask airway (LMA), and functioning wall suction. Difficult airway equipment should be readily accessible, and the risk of aspiration should be evaluated as part of the airway assessment. If difficult intravenous access is anticipated, an ultrasound machine should be readily available. The need for a

blood transfusion should be anticipated in surgeries where the blood loss is expected to exceed 20% of the blood volume and commensurate fluid delivery systems and monitoring including invasive monitors prepared.

The operating room should be prepared in advance of the child's arrival. In the case of neonates and infants, the operating room should be warmed to 80 to 85°F and warming devices checked (e.g., forced air warmer, heat lamp, and warming blanket). Precordial and esophageal stethoscopes, once considered among the most essential monitors, have been supplanted by pulse oximetry and capnography.[480–482] If a parent accompanies the child to the operating room, a chair or stool for the parent to sit on may prevent the parent from having a syncopal episode. Ensuring a quiet, calm operating room environment, free of clanging instruments and loud conversations among the staff, allows for a smooth and calm induction. When available, child-life specialists can provide valuable interventions in the perioperative period.[178]

There are a variety of techniques for inducing general anesthesia. The technique selected depends on several factors, including the child's developmental age, understanding and ability to cooperate, the presence of an existing intravenous catheter, and the child's previous experiences with anesthesia; the presence of a parent; and the interaction of these factors with the child's underlying medical or surgical conditions.

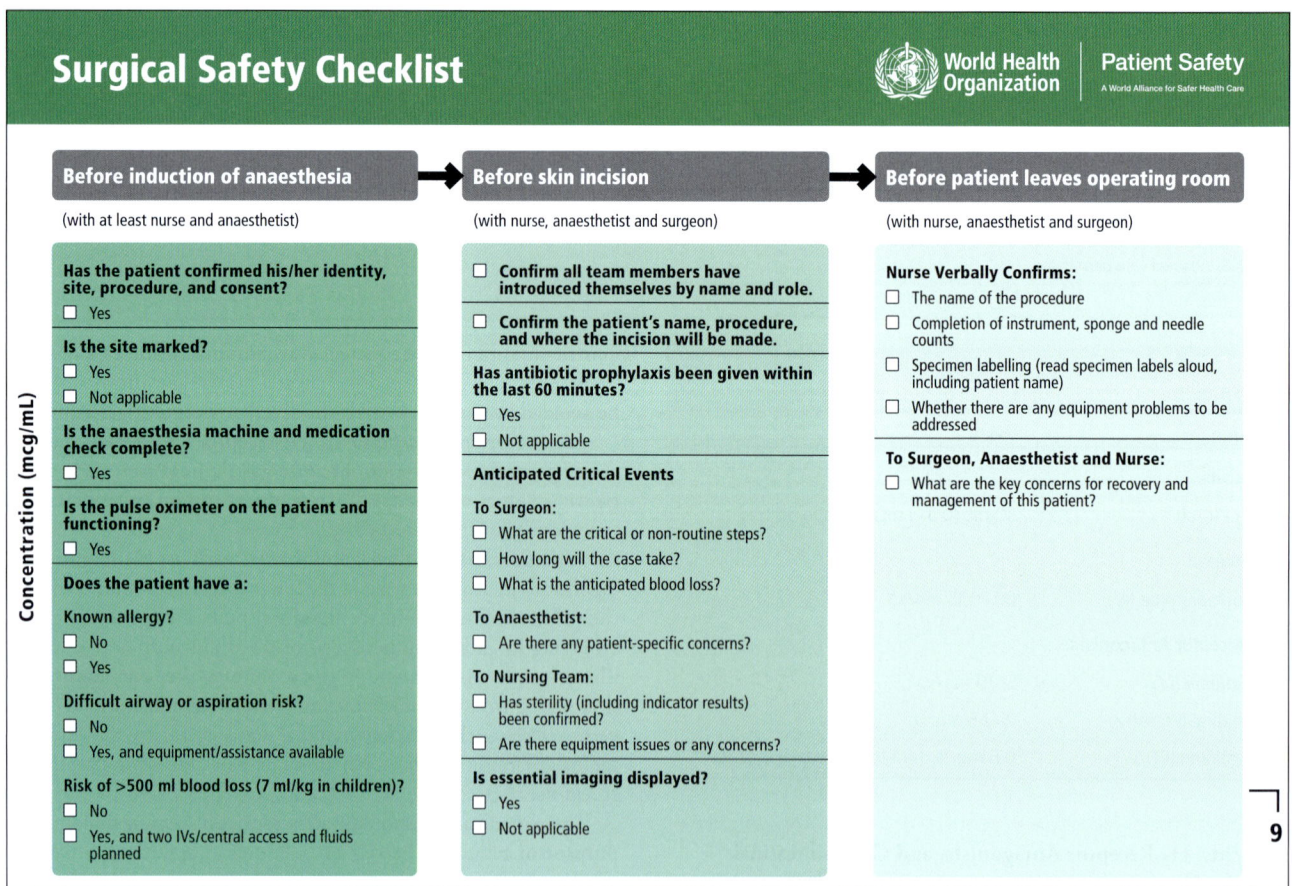

FIGURE 2.7 The World Health Organization Surgical Safety Checklist was introduced in 2008 to reduce harm and improve patient safety. The safety checklist identifies three phases during which key information is reviewed: a sign-in before the induction of anesthesia, a time-out after induction and before incision, and a sign-out before the patient leaves the operating room. A tailored version of this checklist should be a formalized part of the perioperative routine. (Available from: https://www.who.int/teams/integrated-health-services/patient-safety/research/safe-surgery/tool-and-resources.)

INHALATION INDUCTION

The most common method of inducing anesthesia in younger children without intravenous access is inhalational induction by mask using sevoflurane. The benefits of an inhalational induction and avoiding placement of an intravenous cannula awake should be weighed against clinical risk factors such as the child's cardiovascular stability, potential need for volume resuscitation, and the likelihood of perioperative adverse respiratory events. A randomized clinical trial of 300 children <9 years of age reported increased frequency of adverse respiratory events during inhalational induction in those with ≥2 risk factors for such events (e.g., an upper respiratory tract infection [URI] in the preceding 2 weeks, wheezing in the past year, and others) when compared with an intravenous induction with propofol and lidocaine.[483]

During inhalational induction, the anesthesiologist should be flexible and adapt an approach that suits the child, accounting for age, degree of sedation, and level of cooperation. After priming of the breathing circuit with nitrous oxide in oxygen, the mask is gently placed near the child's face and gradually brought closer and closer until it gently contacts the face. After the child has been breathing nitrous oxide for 1 to 2 minutes, the inspired concentration of sevoflurane is increased in a single step to 8%. Adequate monitoring should be instituted as soon as possible in the induction, with most children tolerating application of the pulse oximeter probe while they are awake.

If a parent wishes to accompany a young child to the operating room, the child may remain in the parent's lap for the induction (E-Fig. 2.4 A,B and E-Fig. 2.5). It is vital to instruct the parent that they must hold the child in a "bear hug" with the arms snugly wrapped around the child and holding the child's arms in such a way that the child cannot reach up to the face mask. It is also essential to warn the parents that as their child loses consciousness, that the child will become limp. This approach can be difficult with either an inexperienced anesthesiologist or a very strong child who vigorously evades the mask, preventing its tight application. An experienced individual should be available in front of the child and parent to hold onto the child as induction proceeds and help place the child on the operating room table after successful induction. At this point, the parent is escorted to the waiting room.

The optimal induction sequence in toddlers is to playfully engage, allowing them to choose which flavor of "candy air" or "silly air" they will breathe through the mask and having them seated (not lying supine) on the operating room bed, with the back supported by the anesthesiologist's chest or on the parent's lap (Video 2.2). They may be distracted by asking them to try to "blow up the balloon" by taking deeper and deeper breaths or watching a brief video such as "Pedi Pop", where the balloon refers to the reservoir bag. Other distraction techniques may be used, including allowing them to bring their favorite toy or security blanket into the operating room. Older children may be distracted by allowing them to watch a movie or play interactive games on a tablet.

Child-life specialists are helpful allies in preparing children and parents to cope with the stress and uncertainty surrounding anesthesia and surgery. Such specialists are trained to explain procedures and equipment to children in age-appropriate language, and to introduce coping strategies to reduce anxiety, such as therapeutic medical play. For example, children may be less afraid of an anesthesia face mask if they are allowed to hold the mask in the preoperative holding area, apply a scented flavor of their choosing, and decorate the mask with stickers. One technique often used by child-life specialists is to distract children by allowing them to play interactive games on a tablet. In this scenario, the child-life specialist accompanies the child to the operating room, with the child continuing to play their preferred game on the tablet during transport. The child-life specialist holds the device for the child so that the game may be continued as the face mask is applied and the anesthetic induction begins (Video 2.3).

Some children refuse to have the face mask placed anywhere near their face. They may have a fear of masks or may have been traumatized previously with exposure to large concentrations of sevoflurane at the outset through the face mask, without premedication or pretreatment with nitrous oxide. One solution to this problem is to remove the mask, place the elbow of the breathing circuit between one's fingers, and then cup your hands below the child's chin. Because nitrous oxide is heavier than air, cupped hands act like a reservoir. The hands are gradually brought closer and closer to the face, while the child is distracted, until they gently cover the mouth. Once the child is becoming sedated, the mask can be placed on the face and 8% sevoflurane introduced. Infants who refuse a mask may be soothed by placing one's small finger ("pinky") in the corner of the infant's mouth to suck on as the mask is gently advanced to the nose and mouth (Fig. 2.8).

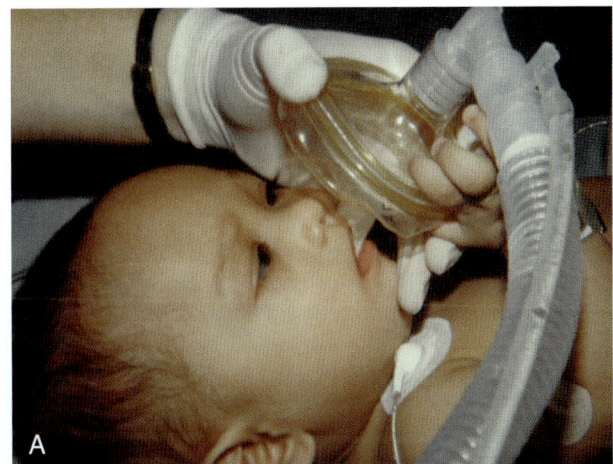

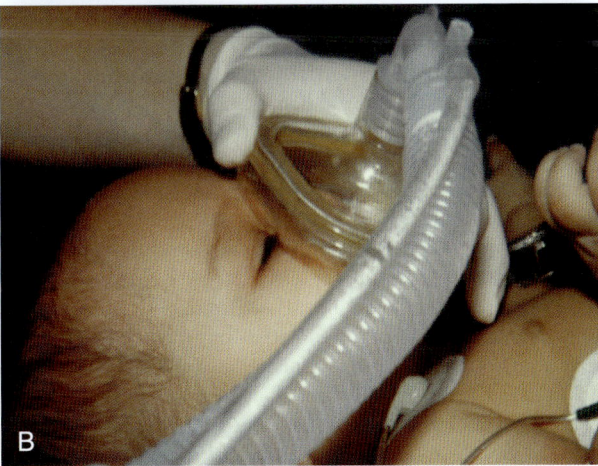

FIGURE 2.8 **A,** Infants 6 months of age or younger are often consoled during induction by placing the little finger ("pinky finger") of your hand in their mouth while you hold the face mask near their face with the rest of the hand. In general, they are so hungry that they will stop crying and eagerly suckle on your pinky finger. **B,** As the infant loses consciousness, the intensity of the suckling diminishes, the pinky finger is gently removed, and the face mask is fully applied.

Inhalation With Sevoflurane

The traditional mask induction of anesthesia is accomplished by placing the mask lightly on the child's face and administering a mixture of nitrous oxide in oxygen (2:1) for 1 or 2 minutes until the full effect of nitrous oxide is achieved. This admixture ratio has been questioned in a retrospective study of 27,258 cases in which the incidence of hypoxemia after an inhalation induction of anesthesia in children with an inspired concentration of oxygen <40% was 2.37-fold greater than the overall incidence[484]; this hypothesis warrants a prospective study to confirm as this has not been our experience. Offering children the choice of a scented mask or "sleepy air," such as bubble gum or strawberry flavor, applied to the inside of the face mask may disguise the odor of the plastic. Sevoflurane is then introduced and can be rapidly increased to 8% in a single stepwise increase, without significant bradycardia or hypotension in otherwise healthy children. After anesthesia is induced, nitrous oxide should be discontinued and sevoflurane administered in oxygen while the airway is being secured. The concentration of sevoflurane should be maintained at the maximum tolerable concentration with ventilation gently assisted as needed. The reason for continuing to deliver a high concentration of sevoflurane is to minimize the risk of awareness as well as other sequelae during the early induction period despite the purported risks of epileptiform EEG discharges (see Chapter 5).[485,486] Data from unmedicated children (aged ≥3 years) indicate that sevoflurane is usually associated with small increases in heart rate, although the heart rate does decrease to 80 to 100 beats/minute in some children after breathing sevoflurane for a period of time.[487] However, some children may develop transient tachycardia that may briefly affect cardiac filling pressures; the clinical importance of this observation is unclear.[488] In contrast to halothane,[489,490] sevoflurane does not increase the myocardial sensitivity to epinephrine.[491] In a study of three techniques for delivering sevoflurane for induction of anesthesia, minimal differences were detected among the three: incremental increases in sevoflurane (2%, 4%, 6%, and 7%) in oxygen, a high concentration of sevoflurane (7%) in oxygen, and a high concentration of sevoflurane in a 1:1 mixture of nitrous oxide in oxygen.[492] When nitrous oxide was added, there was a decreased time to loss of the eyelash reflex and a decreased incidence of excitement during the induction. Agitation or excitement in early induction (shortly after loss of eyelash reflex) with sevoflurane has been observed (Chapter 5).

During inhalation induction, if the oxygen saturation decreases and there is no mechanical cause for the desaturation (such as partial dislodgment of the oximeter probe, patient clenching of fingers or toes, or blood pressure cuff inflating), 100% oxygen should be administered until the oxygen saturation returns to normal while the cause of the desaturation is addressed. If the cause of the desaturation is not related to upper airway obstruction, the most common cause in a healthy child is a ventilation-perfusion mismatch due to segmental atelectasis. To reverse the atelectasis, a gentle recruitment maneuver may be undertaken by applying a sustained inflation pressure of 15 to 20 cm H_2O for 30 seconds or as tolerated until a tracheal tube is inserted. After intubation, persistent desaturation may be addressed by recruiting the lung with inflation of the lungs to 30 cm H_2O for 30 seconds or as tolerated.[493] Alternatively, mild to moderate upper airway obstruction from collapse of the hypopharyngeal structures or mild laryngospasm causes hypoventilation and desaturation. In general, this upper airway obstruction is readily relieved by applying a tight mask fit, closing the pop-off valve sufficiently to generate 5 to 10 cm of positive end-expiratory pressure, and allowing the distending pressure of the bag to stent open the airway. (see Figs. 12.11 and 31.8). Simultaneously, pressure should be applied to the superior pole of the condyle of the mandible bilaterally, directing the force to the hairline on the forehead.[494] Since children are not relaxed at this point, the temporomandibular joint will not sublux; pressure on the condyle at this time causes intense pain (also known as the Dokko point in martial arts), which stimulates the reticular activating system and stimulates the child to cry, which opens their vocal cords. Laryngospasm is then broken, oxygen saturation is restored to normal, and the airway is then secured (see also E-Fig. 12.1). This maneuver may supplant the need for an oral airway. It is very important to avoid applying digital pressure to the soft tissues of the submental triangle because this pushes the tongue and soft tissues into the hypopharynx, occluding the oropharynx and nasopharynx. If the child develops symptomatic bradycardia, then oxygenation and ventilation must first be established, followed by intravenous atropine (0.02 mg/kg) and, if necessary, chest compressions and intravenous epinephrine (see Chapter 38).

Inhalation Induction With Halothane

Halothane has largely been replaced by sevoflurane for inhalation induction of anesthesia because of halothane's slower wash-in and emergence and greater incidence of bradycardia, hypotension, and arrhythmias, rendering it obsolete in medically advanced countries. Halothane sensitizes the heart to catecholamines, and ventricular arrhythmias may commonly be seen, especially during periods of hypercapnia or light anesthesia.[489] If bigeminy or short bursts of ventricular tachycardia occur, then the following strategies should be considered: (1) hyperventilation (to reduce the arterial carbon dioxide tension [$Paco_2$]), (2) deepening the level of anesthesia (with halothane or propofol), or (3) changing to an alternate potent inhalation agent.[489] There is no role for intravenous lidocaine to treat these transient arrhythmias.

Inhalation Induction With Desflurane

Desflurane is very pungent, as evidenced by severe laryngospasm (49%), coughing, increased secretions, and hypoxemia (22%) during mask inductions with desflurane in nitrous oxide and oxygen.[495] When anesthesia was induced with desflurane in oxygen, however, the incidence of airway events was attenuated: moderate to severe laryngospasm (30%), hypoxemia (18%), and breath holding (50%).[496] Therefore, *desflurane is not recommended for inhalation induction in children* but may be used safely for maintenance of general anesthesia after the airway has been secured.

Hypnotic Induction

Hypnosis can reduce anxiety and pain in children with chronic medical problems and those undergoing painful procedures[497,498] as well as reduce preoperative anxiety. Hypnosis is an altered state of consciousness with highly focused attention, based on the principle of dissociation.[499] Hypnosis results in a state of inner absorption that leads to a reduction in awareness of immediate physical surroundings and experiences. Children are more likely to be absorbed in fantasy, and their natural power of play makes them more hypnotizable than adults.[500] When hypnosis was administered 30 minutes before surgery, it significantly reduced preoperative anxiety at the time of face mask application and the frequency of behavior disorders postoperatively when compared with oral midazolam (0.5 mg/kg).[501] Hypnosis provided a relaxed state of well-being and enabled children to actively participate in anesthesia, thus leaving them with a pleasant memory.[498] In an observational study of 140 children 6 years of age and older, hypnosis combined with nitrous oxide (50%) and/or midazolam was of value performing esophagogastroduodenoscopy or rectosigmoidoscopy.[502]

Although an anesthesiologist may not have training in hypnosis, they can use hypnotic suggestions or purposeful active distractions, engaging children in age-appropriate scenarios, such as going to the zoo, a fancy tea party, a baseball game, or flying a jet. Words should be spoken purposefully and rhythmically with descriptions of sights and sounds that are familiar to the child as well as repeated suggestions of "feeling good." The hypnotic suggestions distract the child so that the smell of the anesthetic agent becomes the scent of the zoo animals, the tea brewing, the aviation fuel, and so on. Any number of stories can be told with the same result as long as one remembers to repeatedly say things that can be identified by the child and that fit with what the child is experiencing at the time of induction. New immersive technology such as the use of virtual reality headsets is gaining in popularity as an alternative distraction technique, with emerging research demonstrating its safety and efficacy in alleviating preoperative anxiety through immersive distraction. Virtual reality may be used alone or in combination with other anxiety-reducing measures.[149,503,504]

Modified Single-Breath Induction

The single-breath induction technique is especially appealing to children who desire to fall asleep "really fast" with a face mask, because loss of consciousness is achieved much more rapidly than with a traditional escalating-dose technique. This technique works best for older children who can hold their breath deliberately, although some as young as 3 years of age can be anesthetized with this technique if they are cooperative. Before beginning, the child should be coached through a mock induction by instructing them to "breathe in the biggest breath possible" through the mouth (not the nose) and then "breathe all the way out until there is no more air in the lungs" (Fig. 2.9). If the child is used to swimming and holding their breath underwater, this makes the exercise much easier. Once this has been practiced a few times, then a practice run is repeated with only the mask (no circuit) on the face.

Before induction, the circuit and reservoir bag are primed with 70% nitrous oxide in oxygen and the maximum concentration of sevoflurane the vaporizer can deliver. This is achieved by running

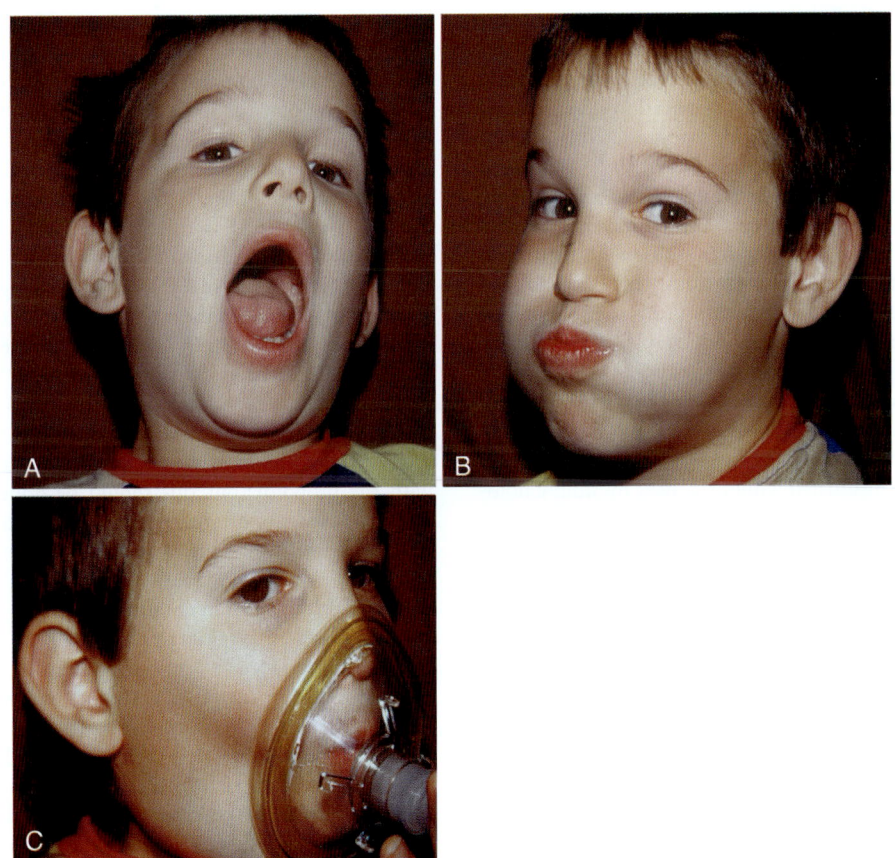

FIGURE 2.9 A single-breath induction is another useful method that is most appropriate for children 5 to 10 years of age. It is important to practice several times without the mask attached to the circuit before the actual induction (see text for details of preparing the circuit). This allows the child to become familiar with the feel of the mask as it is applied to the face and to properly time the sequence of events. **A** and **B,** Typically, we ask the child to take "the biggest breath possible and hold it." Then we ask the child to "breathe all the way out until you have no more air in your lungs and hold it" and place the face mask on the child's face. **C,** We then ask the child to take in "the biggest breath you have ever taken, hold it, then breathe normally." If a full vital capacity breath is taken with a good mask seal around the mouth and nose, most children will lose their lid reflex within 15 to 30 seconds, which is similar to IV induction agents.

modest fresh gas flows through the circuit and intermittently emptying the reservoir bag manually into the scavenger system (i.e., with the circuit Y-connector occluded). Once the circuit is primed with the maximum concentration of inhalation agent, the mask is placed on the Y-connector, then the distal end of the circuit is occluded (to avoid contaminating the operating room), and the child is instructed to take a deep breath of room air and to exhale all the air and hold expiration. The face mask is then placed securely over the child's mouth and nose while they are instructed to take in the "deepest breath ever through the mouth and hold it." Alternatively, there may be an increased success rate with a double-breath technique, altering the single-breath technique by instructing the child to inhale maximally, exhale maximally, and then inhale maximally again and hold the breath as long as possible before resuming normal breathing after the second deep breath.[505] Loss of consciousness, as noted by loss of the eyelash reflex, occurs within 15 to 30 seconds after 1 to 2 vital capacity breaths (Video 2.4).[506,507]

INTRAVENOUS INDUCTION

The topic of intravenous vs. inhalation induction has garnered much discussion.[508–511] One mode of induction may be indicated over the other in particular clinical situations and when absolute contraindications exist for inhalation agents (e.g., malignant hyperthermia, full stomach). Needle phobia is well recognized[398] but the risk of pain on cannulation can be minimized with the aid of child-life specialists, distraction,[512] and application of topical anesthetics. Similarly, mask phobia is widely appreciated, and alternative strategies should be used in these children.[513,514] Despite all efforts, vein cannulation can still be traumatic for children and caregivers if the level of anxiety is very high. Intravenous induction is usually reserved for older children, those who request an intravenous induction, those with a previously established intravenous catheter, those with potential cardiovascular instability, and those who need a rapid-sequence induction (RSI) because of a full stomach. There are many different options as far as medications that can be used for an intravenous induction in a child (Table 2.8). Ideally, all children should breathe 100% oxygen before an intravenous induction; if the face mask is met with objections, oxygen may be insufflated without a mask by simply holding the Y-connector of the circuit between your fingers over or near the child's face.

Thiopental

Thiopental (sodium pentothal) has been replaced by propofol as the most commonly used intravenous induction agent. The recommended induction dose of thiopental in healthy, unpremedicated children is 5 to 6 mg/kg[515]; neonates require a smaller dose (3 to 4 mg/kg).[516,517] Debilitated or severely ill patients,

TABLE 2.8	Doses of Commonly Used Intravenous Induction Agents
Drug	Dose (mg/kg)
Thiopental	5–8
Propofol	2.5–3.5
Etomidate	0.2–0.3
Ketamine	1–2

those who are hypovolemic, and those who have been premedicated may also require a smaller dose for induction of anesthesia. The beta-elimination half-life of thiopental in neonates is twice that in their mothers (15 vs. 7 hours), so a single dose may produce excessively prolonged effect in neonates.[518] This drug is no longer available in the United States.

Methohexital

Methohexital is an ultra-short-acting oxybarbiturate that is infrequently used for IV induction (1.0 to 2.5 mg/kg)[519]; premedicated children require a smaller dose. Recovery after IV administration is more rapid than after thiopental.[520] Larger doses cause skeletal muscle hyperactivity, myoclonic movements, and hiccups.[519] Pain at the injection site is common, necessitating pretreatment with intravenous lidocaine.

Propofol

Propofol is the most commonly used intravenous induction agent in children (see Chapter 5). The induction dose of propofol varies with age: the median effective dose (ED_{50}) for a satisfactory induction in healthy infants 1 to 6 months old is 3.0 ± 0.2 mg/kg, and in healthy children 10 to 16 years old, it is 2.4 ± 0.1 mg/kg.[521] The 95% effective dose (ED_{95}) in healthy unpremedicated children 3 to 12 years of age is 2.5 to 3.0 mg/kg.[522] The early distribution half-life is about 2 minutes, and the terminal elimination half-life is about 30 minutes.[523] Clearance is very large (2.3 ± 0.6 L/minute) and exceeds liver blood flow.[523,524] Advantages to propofol for induction of anesthesia include a reduced incidence of airway-related problems (e.g., laryngospasm, bronchospasm), more rapid emergence,[525,526] and a reduced incidence of nausea and vomiting.[527,528] The major disadvantage of propofol is pain at the site of injection, especially when administered in small veins (e.g., the back of the hand).[529] The administration of lidocaine (0.5 to 1.0 mg/kg) while applying manual tourniquet pressure proximal to the IV site (mini-Bier block) for 30 to 60 seconds before injecting the propofol effectively eliminates the pain in more than 90% of patients.[530–532] However, younger children may not tolerate even the discomfort from the mini-Bier block. Other techniques that have been met with variable success at attenuating the pain include mixing lidocaine (0.5 to 1 mg/kg) with the propofol (but this should be done within 60 seconds of administration of the propofol), refrigerating the propofol, pretreating with an opioid or ketamine, and diluting propofol to a 0.5% solution (see also Chapter 5).[533–541] A meta-analysis of 11 controlled trials in children found that lidocaine was equivalent to low-dose ketamine or alfentanil in reducing the pain of injection.[542]

In addition to its use as an induction agent, propofol can be administered by infusion for total intravenous anesthesia (see Chapters 5 and 6) because of its relatively low context-sensitive half-life.[543] It is especially useful for pediatric patients undergoing nonoperating room procedures such as CT, MRI, radiotherapy, bone marrow biopsy, upper and lower gastrointestinal endoscopy, and lumbar puncture.

Etomidate

Etomidate is a hypnotic induction agent that provides marked cardiovascular stability. Etomidate is available for use in the United States and several other countries, but it is not available in many others because of concern for adrenal suppression. It is indicated for the induction of anesthesia in children with sepsis, cardiac instability, cardiomyopathy, or hypovolemic shock. The recommended induction dose is 0.2 to 0.3 mg/kg depending on the cardiovascular status of the child. Etomidate causes pain and myoclonic movements when injected intravenously[544] and may suppress adrenal steroid synthesis (see also Chapter 5).[545]

Ketamine

Ketamine is a useful induction agent for children with cardiovascular instability, especially in hypovolemic states, or for those who cannot tolerate a reduction in systemic vascular resistance, such as those with aortic stenosis (Williams syndrome)[546,547] or congenital heart disease in whom the balance between pulmonary and systemic blood flow is vital for maintaining cardiovascular homeostasis. In children whose circulation is already maximally compensated by endogenous catecholamines, ketamine is a myocardial depressant that can result in systemic hypotension.[548] The induction dose of ketamine in healthy children is 1 to 2 mg/kg IV. The dose should be reduced in the presence of severe hypovolemia (see also Chapter 5). Smaller doses of intravenous ketamine (0.25 to 0.5 mg/kg) have also been used successfully for procedural sedation.

Ketamine causes sialorrhea, psychomimetic side effects (hallucinations, nightmares), and postoperative nausea and vomiting. The administration of an antisialagogue and midazolam is recommended to attenuate these side effects.

INTRAMUSCULAR INDUCTION

Although it is preferable to avoid intramuscular injections in children, there are occasions when this route may be indicated, such as for the uncooperative child or adolescent who refuses all other routes of sedation, those susceptible to malignant hyperthermia, those with congenital heart disease, and those who have poor venous access. In infants, but especially in older children, intramuscular ketamine is a very useful medication because it is available in a concentrated solution (100 mg/mL) (see earlier discussion and Chapter 5).[282]

FULL STOMACH AND RAPID-SEQUENCE INDUCTION

A full stomach is one of the most challenging and serious problems that pediatric anesthesiologists face. The problem we face is to anesthetize the child with a stomach that contains food who may regurgitate and aspirate after anesthesia is induced and before the airway is secured with a tracheal tube. In the neonate and infant, this problem is further compounded by the risk that hypoxia may occur before the airway is secured because it is difficult to preoxygenate infants and there may be a reluctance to ventilate the lungs after anesthesia is induced out of concern it may trigger regurgitation.

The preferred method to secure the airway in the presence of a full stomach is an intravenous rapid-sequence induction (RSI) immediately followed by tracheal intubation, although other methods have been safe and effective.[549] Before induction of anesthesia, the anesthesiologist must ensure that the proper equipment is at hand (Table 2.9). Preoxygenation is critically important as it increases the apnea time before desaturation occurs, reduces the incidence of hypoxemia during laryngoscopy and if sufficient, obviates the need for positive-pressure ventilation before tracheal intubation. Preoxygenation in infants increases the arterial oxygen tension (PaO_2) in infants more rapidly than in older children; the F_EO_2 reaches >90% in ~100 seconds in children.[550,551]

It is possible to increase the PaO_2 even in a crying child by enriching the immediate environment with high flow oxygen.

TABLE 2.9	Necessary Equipment for Rapid-Sequence Intubation
Functioning laryngoscope blades and handles (two each)
Suction (two)
Anesthetic medications
Checked anesthesia workstation and breathing circuit
Tracheal tubes of appropriate sizes
Tracheal tube stylets
Functioning monitors (including pulse oximeter, blood pressure cuff, ECG, end-tidal carbon dioxide monitor)

After preoxygenation and anesthesia/paralysis, the time to desaturate from 100% to 95% SaO_2 during apnea in infants 1 year old (140 seconds) is half that in children >10 years (>300 seconds), and is ~50 seconds less in those with a symptomatic recent URI compared with those who were asymptomatic.[552-555] Preoxygenation should not upset the child and may require premedication (e.g., intravenous midazolam, 0.05 to 0.1 mg/kg in divided doses, or remifentanil infusion if using total intravenous anesthesia [TIVA]).

Evacuating liquid and gas from the stomach before induction of anesthesia is particularly effective in pyloric stenosis and other scenarios when the stomach is suspected to be full of liquid. A large bore oral or vented nasogastric tube should be passed into the stomach and the child positioned in the left lateral decubitus position, followed by right decubitus and finally supine while the tube is suctioned.[556] The gastric tube may then be removed.

The use of cricoid pressure (Sellick maneuver) remains controversial particularly in infants and children. If used, it should be maintained until the tracheal tube has been successfully placed and carbon dioxide is detected in the tracheal tube.[557,558] The purpose of cricoid pressure is to occlude the esophageal lumen to preclude regurgitated material from passing from the stomach into the oropharynx and then the lungs. Before induction of anesthesia, the cricoid ring is palpated between the thumb and the middle finger and as soon as the child loses consciousness, pressure is steadily increased using the index finger. To prevent passive gastroesophageal reflux, a force of 30 to 40 N (3 to 4 kg of force) must be applied to the upper esophagus (in adults), which creates an intraluminal pressure of approximately 50 cm H_2O in the upper esophagus.[559] However, in infants and children, much smaller forces should be applied as 5 N force in infants may compress the lumen within the cricoid ring by 50% delaying passage of the tracheal tube through the cricoid ring or precluding its passage.[560] If active vomiting occurs while cricoid pressure is applied, esophageal pressures may increase to greater than 60 cm H_2O. This could overcome the effects of cricoid pressure, resulting in regurgitation and pulmonary aspiration or worse, rupture of the esophagus (Boerhaave syndrome) if the cricoid pressure were not immediately released.[561]

The efficacy of cricoid pressure has come under increasing scrutiny. It has been posited that visualizing the larynx while cricoid pressure is applied is more difficult, particularly in infants whose neck is short, and the larynx is more rostral. However, this issue is far from clear, particularly since most children are not placed in the "tonsil position" as Sellick described.[557] Sellick suggested that cricoid pressure may actually facilitate tracheal intubation as the larynx is displaced posteriorly.[557] Cricoid pressure is

TABLE 2.10	Contraindications to Cricoid Pressure
Contraindication	**Potential Complication**
Active vomiting	• Possible rupture of esophagus (Boerhaave syndrome)
Airway issues	• Fractured cricoid cartilage may be made worse • Sharp foreign body in larynx may result in further laryngeal injury
Esophageal issues	• Zenker diverticulum[a] • Sharp foreign body in upper esophagus may result in further esophageal injury
Vertebral/ neurologic issues	• Unstable cervical spine may result in spinal cord injury • Sharp foreign body in the neck may result in injury to other structures in the neck

[a]From Thiagarajah S, Lear E, Keh M. Anesthetic implications of Zenker's diverticulum. *Anesth Analg.* 1990;70:109-111.

contraindicated under certain circumstances; these should be carefully reviewed to avoid complications (Table 2.10). If mask ventilation is undertaken with cricoid pressure in place, peak inspiratory pressures should be less than 20 cm H_2O (preferably 10–12 cm H_2O) to preclude gastric insufflation.[562,563] The Sellick maneuver should seal the esophagus if a nasogastric tube remains in place,[564] but removing the nasogastric tube before intubation provides a better mask fit on the face and exposure for laryngoscopy and intubation. If the nasogastric tube is left in place, leaving it open to atmospheric pressure or suction will vent liquid and gas present in the stomach.

Surveys from the United Kingdom show that cricoid pressure is used in only 40% to 50% of children in whom it was indicated.[565,566] Reluctance to apply cricoid pressure may be attributed to the indications for its use and how often it is applied with the correct position and pressure.[567–569] MRI assessments in adults revealed the esophagus to be to opposed in 71% with lateral displacement in 67% and airway compression in 81%.[570] In children and young adults assessed by ultrasound, 62% had the esophagus positioned to the left of the cricoid and after cricoid pressure it was displaced to the left in in 54/55 patients.[570,571] At times, cricoid pressure may have to be released to facilitate a clear view of the larynx for successful tracheal intubation, particularly in infants.[572] Cricoid pressure also decreases the tone of the upper and lower esophageal sphincters facilitating passive regurgitation of gastric contents up the esophagus.[559,573] Despite these concerns, properly applied cricoid pressure may facilitate intubation with RSI.[574]

Rapid control of the airway in infants and children most commonly includes rapidly inducing a deep plane of general anesthesia before instrumenting the airway, ventilating gently (with low peak airway pressures (10–12 cm H_2O peak inspiratory pressure) by facemask as needed, avoiding cricoid pressure, and confirming muscle paralysis before airway manipulation and finally, rapidly securing the airway with a cuffed tracheal tube.[563,565,574,575] Avoiding or only using minimal cricoid pressure reduces distortion of the anatomy of the upper airway, particularly in neonates and infants, and allows external laryngeal pressure to aid glottic visualization.[576,577] A retrospective cohort study from 35 pediatric intensive care units (United States, Canada, Singapore, Japan, New Zealand) revealed 106 regurgitation events with equal incidence in those with or without cricoid pressure; since this was a retrospective study it is unclear how many of these patients truly had a full stomach or how many had a true indication for cricoid pressure.[578] A Cochrane review concluded that there were inadequate randomized controlled studies of cricoid pressure in children.[579] In a small randomized clinical trial of adults at risk for aspiration, cricoid pressure did not reduce the rate of aspiration or clinical sequelae compared with no pressure using pepsin as the biomarker for aspiration.[580] In the largest randomized, controlled trial on cricoid pressure to date 3,472 adult patients who required a rapid-sequence induction were randomized to either cricoid pressure or a sham procedure; noninferiority of the sham procedure in preventing aspiration was rejected primarily because the study design assumed the incidence of vomiting would be 2.8%, more than 4-fold greater than the actual incidence reported in the study, which resulted in a Type II statistical error (underpowered design).[581] Adult studies support concerns regarding the efficacy or lack of efficacy of cricoid pressure since most complications relate to inappropriate or excessive application of cricoid pressure, which can lead to impaired laryngeal visualization and interference with manual ventilation should initial attempts at intubation fail.[576] Since aspiration is still a leading cause of death related to general anesthesia in adults[60,582] we do not recommend totally abandoning the practice. Each clinician must use their clinical assessments and judgment that when cricoid pressure is applied to infants and children, that less force is required to occlude the esophagus than in adults and that this approach should be applied in select cases.[52,560] It is unlikely that a randomized controlled study could ever be carried out for cricoid pressure in children bearing in mind the need for ethics committee approval and the large number of children who would be enrolled (~25,000 per cohort).[583]

After preoxygenation, anesthesia is induced with intravenous, propofol (3–4 mg/kg),[584,585] ketamine (1–2 mg/kg), or etomidate (0.2–0.3 mg/kg), followed immediately by 2 mg/kg of succinylcholine. Succinylcholine remains a popular paralytic agent of choice for rapid onset and short duration although high-dose rocuronium is an equally effective alternative.[586] The intubating conditions 30 seconds after 1.2 mg/kg rocuronium were similar to those after 1.5 mg/kg succinylcholine.[586] The mean time to return of 25% of the twitch response was 46 ±23 minutes (range, 30–72 minutes) for rocuronium compared with 5.8 ± 3.3 minutes (range, 1.5–8.2 minutes) for succinylcholine. The availability of sugammadex to antagonize rocuronium and vecuronium reduces concern about the risks associated with a prolonged duration of action of large doses of nondepolarizing relaxants, particularly in the presence of a difficult airway or a "cannot ventilate, cannot intubate" scenario (see Chapters 5 and 12). The ability to immediately reverse nondepolarizing neuromuscular blocking agents must be weighed against the short duration of action of succinylcholine when selecting a paralytic agent for a rapid-sequence induction.

Evidence suggests that the gastric residual volume in children undergoing emergency surgery is greater if a child is anesthetized within 4 hours after hospital admission (1.1 mL/kg).[587] If, on the other hand, surgery can be delayed for at least 4 hours, then the mean gastric residual volume is on average much less (0.51 mL/kg)[587]; this gastric residual volume is in fact similar to that observed in children who have fasted for routine surgical procedures (Fig. 2.10).[1] This does not imply that these children should not be regarded as having a full stomach; rather, the risk may be somewhat reduced if surgery can be delayed several hours. In addition, evidence suggests that in emergency cases, the gastric

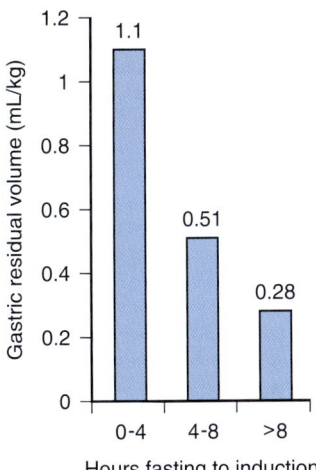

FIGURE 2.10 Mean gastric residual volume is plotted against hours of fasting before anesthetic induction in emergency pediatric cases. These data suggest that a 4-hour fast, if it does not compromise patient safety, may reduce gastric residual volume, and therefore reduce (but not eliminate) risk for aspiration. (Data abstracted from Schurizek BA, Rybro L, Boggild-Madsen NB, Juhl B. Gastric volume and pH in children for emergency surgery. *Acta Anaesthesiol Scand.* 1986;30:404-408.)

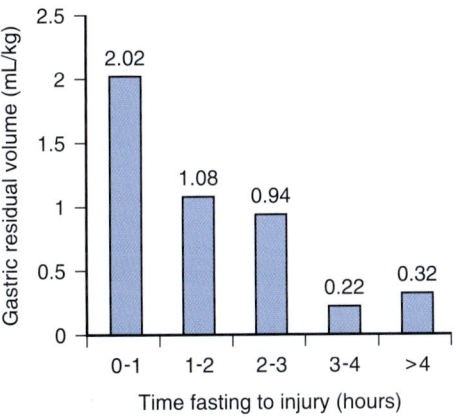

FIGURE 2.11 Mean gastric residual volume is plotted against time from last food ingestion to time of injury. These data suggest that the longer the time from ingestion to injury, the lower the risk for pulmonary aspiration of gastric contents. Also, if more than 4 hours has elapsed between the time of last food ingestion and time of injury, the risk is similar to that for patients with routine fasting. However, even with a 4-hour fasting time, these patients must still be treated as though they have a full stomach. It should be noted that these volumes also relate to the severity of injury (increased volumes with increased injury severity). (Data abstracted from Bricker SRW, McLuckie A, Nightingale DA. Gastric aspirates after trauma in children. *Anesthesia.* 1989;44:721-724.)

residual volume depends, in part, on the time interval between the last food ingestion and the time of the injury as well as the severity of the injury.[587] Children who last ate more than 4 hours before the injury have a gastric residual volume similar to those who fasted as if it were elective surgery (Fig. 2.11). *There is some comfort in these numbers, but one should never consider such children as not having a full stomach but rather as having a "less full" stomach.* Additionally, the possible value of H_2-receptor blocking agents, metoclopramide, and clear antacids may be considered, but their use in this regard is not evidence based.

A controlled rapid-sequence induction and intubation may be preferred in small infants who will likely desaturate during brief periods of apnea and will therefore require assisted ventilation before the trachea is secured.[563] A controlled rapid-sequence induction and intubation consists of gentle face mask ventilation prior to intubation (maximum peak inspiratory pressure 12 cm H_2O), avoidance of cricoid pressure and the use of nondepolarizing muscle relaxants. In a study of 1001 patients from newborns to children greater than 12 years of age, the incidence of regurgitation (1:1000) or pulmonary aspiration (0:1001) (although this number is too small to say this with certainty) was within clinical limits.[563] There was also a low incidence of moderate desaturation (SpO_2 80%–89%, n = 5) and severe desaturation (SpO_2 <80%, n = 3) during anesthesia induction; one patient was observed to regurgitate but not aspirate.[563] It should be noted that only 107 children were ≤2 years of age and of these 30 were neonates and 34 others <1 year of age. There were no episodes of bradycardia or hypotension. This was especially important in neonates, infants, and toddlers. If a nasogastric tube was in place, it was left in place during the induction while continuous suction was applied.[563] It is important to ensure that sufficient time has passed for complete muscle relaxation to occur before laryngoscopy and tracheal intubation are undertaken as aspiration is in part related to incomplete muscle relaxation at intubation in the presence of a gastrointestinal comorbidity.[51]

Neonates may also be intubated while awake if indicated; this may provide a greater margin of safety because it preserves spontaneous ventilation as well as laryngeal reflexes. Skillfully performed awake intubation in neonates that is performed rapidly is not associated with clinically significant hemodynamic instability or increased intracranial pressure beyond that which occurs during crying.[588,589]

Special Problems

THE FEARFUL CHILD

This is a difficult problem without a satisfactory solution. The child's fear is generally based on the child's developmental status, the hospital environment, and the impending surgery. This is why it is so vital that as much information as possible be presented and queries as to why the child is afraid are so important. Frequently, a few well-directed questions and honest answers will resolve most of the child's concerns. If the child will ingest a small drink, oral premedication may be effective. This may only be achieved if the parent coaxes the child to drink the medicine. As an added incentive to take the medicine, one editor (JL) lets the child know they can have a small cup of water if they drink the medication. Often, allowing a parent to hold the child during induction of anesthesia or allowing the child to hold the anesthetic mask themselves will reassure and settle the child. In other situations, one commonly practiced solution is to use intramuscular ketamine.

AUTISM

Autism spectrum disorder is a neurodevelopmental disorder characterized by variable impairment in social interactions and communication skills, restricted interests, repetitive behavior, and, for some, touch, visual, taste, or sound hypersensitivity. Children present early in life but deficits may not become fully manifest until social communication demands exceed capabilities.[590] The diagnosis, usually by age 3 years, is based on observation and assessment of behavior and cognition and is aided by validated assessment tools. The 5th edition of *Diagnostic and Statistical Manual of Mental Disorders*

(DSM-V) adopted the umbrella term autism spectrum disorder (ASD), which includes autism, Asperger syndrome, and pervasive developmental disorder.[591]

The overall ASD prevalence in the United States is currently estimated to be 1 in 44 children with a male: female ratio of 4:1; prevalence was similar across racial and ethnic groups although increased since the prior estimate (1 in 54 children). The prevalence of intelligence quotient ≤70 was 35% (50% Black, 33% Hispanic, and 30% White).[592] The increased prevalence is likely due to broader diagnostic criteria, increased public awareness, and the development of more sensitive screening tools. The global prevalence of ASD is thought to be approximately 1%.[593,594] More than 70% of children and adolescents with autism have concurrent medical (gastrointestinal, seizures, insomnia, mitochondrial disease), developmental (intellectual disability), or psychiatric problems (social anxiety disorder, attention-deficit/hyperactivity disorder [ADHD], oppositional defiant disorder).[590]

Behavior and cognitive training are the most effective therapy for ASD, but this must be initiated at an early age to achieve the best possible neurologic improvement. Existing pharmacologic management for ASD has not been promising for treating core symptoms but has been effective in decreasing the burden of emotional and behavioral problems and improved engagement in therapy.[595] Antipsychotic drugs, with risperidone as standard therapy, have been shown to effectively reduce repetitive behaviors, temper outbursts, and self-injurious behavior, but associated adverse effects limit their use to patients with severe impairment.[596] Serotonin reuptake inhibitors may reduce repetitive behaviors, although findings are inconsistent.[596–598] The effect of stimulants on symptoms of ADHD occurring in children with ASD requires more study but shows promise.[599] It is critical for the anesthesiologist to be familiar with these medications and their potential interactions with anesthetic agents (see Table 2.11).[600–602]

The perioperative period can be a stressful time for children with ASD; they do not respond well to changes in routine and may challenge the ingenuity of the anesthesiologist. They are very sensitive to stimuli such as light, sound, touch, and pain and may be unable to articulate the concerns they have. The hospital setting is anxiety-provoking and usually upsets many autistic children with some becoming disruptive and uncooperative. The anesthesiologist's approach to the autistic child depends on the severity of the disorder.

Information regarding the child's previous anesthetic experience, assessment of the child's behavior and idiosyncrasies, and bonding with parents or caregivers should be accomplished during the preanesthetic visit. The family should be encouraged to bring favorite toys, electronic devices, and other comforting items. Collecting pertinent information about baseline behavior, triggers of emotional outbursts, and signs of escalating anxiety is invaluable.[603] Sedative premedication can be very effective but the decision to administer premedication must be made on an individual basis. Oral midazolam (0.5–1 mg/kg)[604] is the most commonly used preoperative anxiolytic for children, although other choices include oral ketamine (6 mg/kg)[354] and a combination of oral midazolam (0.5 mg/kg) and ketamine (3–6 mg/kg).[357] Oral dexmedetomidine (mean dose 2.6 μg/kg) has also provided adequate sedation prior to induction of anesthesia in children with ASD.[382,605] Some may have problems with certain textures and tastes; administering oral premedication in a favorite drink should be considered in the context of NPO guidelines. The overly anxious child may be uncooperative with oral medication and may require intramuscular ketamine. In the emergency department,

TABLE 2.11	Commonly Used Pharmacologic Agents for Children With Autism Spectrum Disorder	
Medication	**Target Symptoms**	**Potential Adverse Effects**
Antipsychotics: Haloperidol[a] Risperidone Aripiprazole Quetiapine	Aggression, irritability, self-injury, temper tantrums, withdrawal, tics	Weight gain, sedation, extrapyramidal symptoms, hypotension with general anesthesia and proarrhythmic properties (risperidone) [a]Haloperidol should no longer be used because of dyskinetic side effects
Atypical Antipsychotic: Clozapine	Repetitive behaviors	Agranulocytosis, hyperthermia, cardiac conduction problems, hypotension Discontinuation can cause dystonia dyskinesia, delirium, and psychosis
Selective Serotonin Reuptake Inhibitors (SSRIs): Fluoxetine Citalopram	Depressive symptoms, repetitive behaviors, anxiety (lower dosage), obsessive compulsive disorder (higher dosage)	Agitation, gastrointestinal symptoms; reduced platelet aggregation and increased transfusion risk
Stimulants: Methylphenidate Amphetamines	Hyperactivity, inattention	Insomnia, decreased appetite, weight loss, headache, irritability, may increase anesthetic requirement, increase risk of hypertension and arrhythmias, lower seizure threshold and interact with vasopressors
Melatonin	Insomnia	No side effects recorded

[a]Haloperidol should no longer be used because of dyskinetic side effects

sedation of children with ASD who required minor procedures was achieved using IV ketamine or intranasal midazolam in 72% of children.[606] Parents can also offer insight into which strategies would make their child's life easier during this difficult time. It is important to take the time to address parental concerns and establish a trusting relationship with the family.

There is great variation in the severity of autism and the affected patients' hospital needs.[607] The focus for optimal management has been on early communication to provide a flexible and individualized admission process and anesthetic plan.[607] A quiet room, scheduling the case as early in the day as possible, minimizing the waiting period, an individualized perioperative management plan with the caregiver and child-life specialist involvement may offer an advantage.[608]

Intraoperative goals should include adequate analgesia, prophylaxis of postoperative nausea and vomiting, and optimal intraoperative hydration to allow early removal of the intravenous cannula, which may reduce negative emotional outbursts in the recovery room. Finally, the appropriate use of parents in the PACU can facilitate the transition from surgery to recovery.

Studies have shown that children who are reunited with their parents sooner require less pain medication and are discharged earlier in an ambulatory setting.[609]

ANEMIA

The minimum hematocrit necessary to ensure adequate oxygen transport in children has not been well established. Preoperative hemoglobin testing is of limited value in healthy children undergoing elective surgery when minimal blood loss is expected,[610] but anemia is an independent risk factor for postoperative apnea in former preterm infants.[611,612] Children with chronic anemia, such as those with renal failure, do not require preoperative transfusion because of compensatory mechanisms, including increased 2,3-diphosphoglycerate, oxygen extraction, and cardiac output. Elective surgery for children who are anemic should take into consideration their medical history, underlying diseases (e.g., renal failure, hemoglobinopathies, von Willebrand, sickle cell, other factor deficiencies), the nature of the surgery, and its urgency. Most pediatric anesthesiologists would recommend a hematocrit greater than 25% before elective surgery in the absence of chronic disease. If significant blood loss is anticipated and the surgery is elective, then the cause of anemia should be investigated, treated, and the surgery postponed until the hematocrit is restored to the normal range. Children with preoperative anemia undergoing noncardiac surgery may be at increased risk for in-hospital mortality.[613] It remains unknown if correction of preoperative anemia, through the development of a patient blood management program, improves patient outcomes or simply reduces the need for transfusion. *Healthy children scheduled for elective surgery that is not expected to cause substantive bleeding should not routinely receive a blood transfusion just to bring their hematocrit to an arbitrary limit such as 30%.*

Physiologic anemia of infancy occurs between 2 and 4 months of postnatal age. At this time, there is an increased production of hemoglobin A and an increase in red cell 2,3-diphosphoglycerate, which contribute to a right shift of the oxygen-hemoglobin dissociation curve (see Chapter 8). Therefore, in infants 2 to 4 months of age, a reduced hemoglobin value is acceptable. Anemia, with a hematocrit of less than 30%, in formerly preterm infants represents a special category of patients who may have an increased incidence of postoperative apnea (see discussion later in chapter), but transfusion is still not recommended.[612]

UPPER RESPIRATORY TRACT INFECTION

The child with a nonpurulent active or recent URI (within 4 weeks) often presents a conundrum, even for the most experienced anesthesiologist. Between 20% and 30% of all children have a runny nose during a substantial part of the year.[614] A differential diagnosis of a child with a runny nose is presented in Table 2.12. In the preanesthetic evaluation, we must rely on history, physical examination, and, rarely, laboratory data to decide whether to proceed with anesthesia.

A number of perioperative anesthetic risks have been studied in children with URIs.[615] The risk of postintubation croup was similar in children who had an active URI and those who did not.[616] Bronchospasm occurs more frequently in children whose tracheae are intubated and who have active URIs[617]; the incidence in children with a URI (41:1000) is 10-fold greater than it is in those without a URI (4:1000).[618] The incidence of laryngospasm in children with a URI (96:1000) is 5-fold greater than it is in children without a URI (17:1000).[618] The incidence of minor but

TABLE 2.12	Differential Diagnosis of a Child With a Runny Nose
Noninfectious Causes	
Allergic rhinitis: seasonal, perennial, clear nasal discharge; no fever	
Vasomotor rhinitis: emotional (crying); temperature changes	
Infectious Causes **Viral infections**	
Nasopharyngitis (common cold)	
Flu syndrome (upper and lower respiratory tract)	
Laryngotracheal bronchitis (infectious croup)	
Viral exanthems	
Measles	
Chickenpox	
Acute bacterial infections	
Acute epiglottitis	
Meningitis	
Streptococcal tonsillitis	

not major intraoperative hemoglobin desaturation events in children with a URI is greater than in those without a URI.[617] Lastly, the incidence of all respiratory-related adverse events combined in children with a URI was reported as 9-fold greater than in those without a URI and 11-fold greater in children who had a URI and required tracheal intubation.[619]

When a tracheal tube and supraglottic airway were compared in children with a URI, the incidence of mild bronchospasm, major desaturation events, and overall respiratory events was reduced in the presence of a supraglottic airway, although the incidence of laryngospasm was similar with either of the two airway devices.[620,621]

Prognostic factors of adverse anesthetic events in children with URIs who were scheduled for elective surgery include the type of airway management (tracheal intubation >supraglottic airway); a parent's statement that the child has a "cold"; the presence of nasal congestion, snoring, passive smoking; the induction agent (thiopental >halothane >sevoflurane ~propofol); sputum production; and whether the neuromuscular agent was antagonized.[622] Reactive airway disease and a history of prematurity have also been associated with adverse outcomes in children with URIs.[623]

Age has not been an independent predictor of adverse events in children with URIs in most studies, although one study suggested that the incidence of bronchospasm in infants younger than 6 months with active URIs was greater (20.8% vs. 4.7%, $P = 0.08$) than in older children.[624] Also in this study, the greatest incidence of adverse respiratory events occurred in children undergoing airway surgery (e.g., tonsillectomy and adenoidectomy, direct laryngoscopy, bronchoscopy). Paternal smoking history was another risk factor for overall respiratory events ($P = 0.018$).

Cancellation of cardiac surgery carries special import because of the risk that the child's heart will deteriorate, or the disease process will progress (e.g., pulmonary hypertension), as well as the extensive time, materials, and personnel committed to a planned case. In a prospective study of children scheduled for cardiac surgery, the incidences of respiratory adverse events

TABLE 2.13	Factors Affecting Decision for Elective Surgery in a Child With Upper Respiratory Tract Infection
Proceed With Caution	**Consider Cancellation**
• Child has "just a runny nose," no other symptoms, "much better"	• Parents confirm symptoms: fever, malaise, cough, poor appetite, just developed symptoms last night
• Active and happy child	• Lethargic, ill-appearing
• Clear rhinorrhea	• Purulent nasal discharge
• Clear lungs and symptoms have leveled off or have improved	• Wheezing, rales that do not clear
• Older child	• Child <1-year-old, former preterm infant
• Social issues: hardship for parents to be away from work, insurance will run out	• Other factors: history of reactive airway disease, major operation, endotracheal tube required
• No fever	• Fever >38.5°C
• Outpatient procedure that will not expose immunocompromised children to possible infectious agent	• Inpatient procedure that may result in exposure of immunocompromised children to viral/bacterial infection

From Tait AR, Malviya S. Anesthesia for the child with an upper respiratory tract infection: still a dilemma? *Anesth Analg.* 2005;100: 59-65.

(29.2% vs. 17.3%, $P < 0.01$), multiple postoperative complications (25% vs. 10.3%, $P < 0.01$), and bacterial infection (5.2% vs. 1.0%, $P = 0.01$) were greater in those with a URI than in those without.[625]

A national survey suggested that more experienced anesthesiologists are less likely to cancel surgery because of the presence of a URI.[626] Cancellation may also impose emotional and economic burdens on the parents.[627,628] Factors that should be considered when deciding whether to proceed with elective surgery in a child with a URI are summarized in Table 2.13.

Insofar as which techniques will help to prevent complications from a URI, pretreating healthy children with bronchodilators who either had a URI within the preceding 6 weeks, or had an active URI, neither inhaled ipratropium or albuterol/salbutamol, provided benefit.[629,630] In 484 children (0–8 years of age) undergoing tonsillectomy, an adverse respiratory event occurred in untreated children 2.8 times more frequently than in those given preoperative albuterol/salbutamol ($P = 0.001$); the incidence of laryngospasm (11.8% vs. 5%) and desaturation (22.7% vs. 14.9%, $P = 0.03$) also occurred more frequently.[631,632] However, 25% to 30% of the children in that study had a URI in the preceding 2 weeks, 40% were exposed to passive smoking and 18% had a history of asthma. Many clinicians would not proceed with a general anesthetic for elective surgery in children who had a URI in the preceding 2 weeks raising questions about the external validity of their results. Humidification, intravenous hydration, and anticholinergics may also decrease perioperative respiratory complications,[626] although the results of at least one study suggested that glycopyrrolate did not reduce the incidence of perioperative adverse respiratory events when it was given after induction of anesthesia to children with URIs.[633] Use of supraglottic airways coated with topical lidocaine in children with URIs was associated with less postoperative coughing[634,635] and overall perioperative

complication rates.[635] The decision to administer preoperative bronchodilators seems reasonable for children already using these medications, but it is otherwise up to the individual practitioner to make that decision on a case-by-case basis. Children who present with an exacerbation of their underlying respiratory disorder should be canceled and optimized before returning for elective surgery.

If the decision is made to postpone anesthesia because of an exacerbation of an underlying respiratory disorder, then how long should one wait before rescheduling the general anesthetic?[627] Bronchial hyperreactivity, which is associated with URIs in children, shows spirometric changes in the lungs for as long as 7 weeks after a URI.[636,637] Postponing surgery for at least 7 weeks after resolution of a URI is impractical because most children will be infected with a new URI by that time. Postponing surgery for 2 weeks after resolution of the URI is a common but as yet unproven strategy. In fact, some data suggest that the incidence of adverse respiratory events is just as great in this population as it is in those who were anesthetized during the acute phase of the URI.[638,639] Currently, there is no consensus on the optimal time interval before surgery is rescheduled. In a survey of anesthesiologists, most wait 3 to 4 weeks before proceeding with surgery.[614,626] The rationale for this time period is that the risk of respiratory complications is unchanged for 4 to 6 weeks.[624]

Key points we know are that children with a current and recent (up to 2 weeks) URI have an increased risk of perioperative respiratory adverse events (e.g., laryngospasm, bronchospasm, desaturation, and breath holding). In such children, the risk factors that further increase the risk for perioperative respiratory adverse events include age less than 2 years, prematurity, exposure to passive smoking, respiratory comorbidities, airway surgery, and the use of a tracheal tube. To reduce the risk of perioperative respiratory adverse events in children with a current or recent URI, anesthetic management can be optimized by the use of perioperative inhaled bronchodilators (albuterol/salbutamol), intravenous induction with propofol, avoidance of desflurane, use of TIVA or sevoflurane with a propofol or lidocaine bolus before manipulating the airway.[614]

Good judgment, common sense, clinical experience, a measured discussion with the surgeon, and informed consent from the parents or guardians must be used when deciding whether to proceed or postpone the surgery. All of these deliberations and discussions including the risks and benefits should be documented in the chart (see Chapter 11 for additional discussion and perspectives).

OBESITY

There are several definitions for obesity in children. The Centers for Disease Control (CDC) defines obesity in children and adolescents 2 to 19 years of age as a BMI at or greater than the 95th percentile for age, based on CDC growth charts for normal children from 2000.[640] Overweight is defined as a BMI between the 85th and 95th percentiles. A second definition is from the World Health Organization, which uses standard deviations (BMI z scores) from the mean BMI for age to define childhood overweight and obesity (see https://www.who.int/news-room/fact-sheets/detail/obesity-and-overweight). A third definition uses pooled international data to provide age-specific and gender-specific BMI cutoff points for childhood obesity.[641]

The prevalence of childhood obesity is rapidly increasing worldwide. Globally, the World Health Organization estimates that 39 million children under the age of 5 years were overweight or obese in 2020 (see https://www.who.int/news-room/fact-sheets/detail/obesity-and-overweight). In the United States, the CDC data on obesity among children and adolescents in 2017–18 reported 14.4 million individuals aged 2 to 19 years as obese (19.3%) (https://www.cdc.gov/obesity/data/childhood.html). The majority of childhood obesity cases are caused by excessive caloric intake and relative lack of physical activity, with the remainder resulting from conditions such as endocrine disorders, neurologic dysfunction, and genetic syndromes (e.g., Prader-Willi).[642]

Obesity is a complex endocrine state inducing metabolic dysregulation and metainflammation[643,644] associated with numerous comorbidities (Table 2.14). The incidences of these comorbidities increase as BMI and the duration of obesity increase.[645] Weight loss may reduce perioperative risk factors.

Children who are obese have a greater incidence of perioperative adverse respiratory events compared with normal-weight children.[646,647] Functional residual capacity, expiratory reserve volume, forced expiratory volume in 1 second, and diffusion capacity are all reduced. Increased closing volumes due to lung compression from a large abdominal girth may cause atelectasis and right-to-left intrapulmonary shunting.[648] Bronchial hyperreactivity and asthma are more prevalent among obese children. A review of over 2200 referrals to a pediatric asthma specialist in the United States found that nearly 30% of patients with physician-diagnosed asthma were obese.[649] The incidence and severity of asthma increases as BMI increases. In addition, a cross-sectional study of 1129 preadolescent children noted that the risks of developing URIs and perioperative respiratory complications in overweight children with a BMI ≥90th percentile for age was twice those for children with a reduced BMI.[650]

Obstructive sleep apnea affects 13% to 59% of obese children.[651–653] Children with OSA may display increased sensitivity to opioids.[654] Opioids should be carefully titrated to respiratory responses in these children during the perioperative period. If apnea occurs after a small dose of opioids, further doses should be reduced or not given while respirations are closely monitored. An apnea under these circumstances often indicates additional analgesic medications are not required and a change to nonopioid analgesics is needed. Similarly, caution must be used when administering benzodiazepines for premedication in obese children with OSA given the risk of respiratory depression. If the child is regularly managed with continuous positive airway pressure (CPAP) or biphasic positive airway pressure (BiPAP), this therapy should be maintained postoperatively until the child is awake and can maintain a patent airway.

Obese children have an increased blood volume, stroke volume, and cardiac output.[655] Hypertension is present in 20% to 30% and the incidence rises with increasing BMI.[656,657] Blood pressure should be measured preoperatively and exercise tolerance determined to establish whether cardiopulmonary compromise exists.

Obesity leads to insulin resistance; nearly half of obese adolescents suffer from the metabolic syndrome and are at high risk of developing type 2 diabetes.[658] For morbidly obese children, preoperative fasting blood glucose concentrations are recommended, as type 2 diabetes may be present but previously undiagnosed.[659] Adolescents with type 2 diabetes display adverse measures of cardiac structure and function positively related to BMI and blood pressure.[660] Preoperative electrocardiography and echocardiography should be considered in morbidly obese children to rule out right ventricular hypertrophy and pulmonary hypertension.[661,662]

Childhood obesity is a risk factor for gastroesophageal reflux. Up to 20% of severely obese children have symptoms of gastroesophageal reflux, compared with 2% of normal-weight children.[663] Despite the increased prevalence of symptomatic reflux, gastric fluid volumes are identical across all BMI categories (when corrected for ideal body weight) and regardless of fasting interval. Obesity is not an independent risk factor for aspiration.[664] Overweight and obese children with gastroesophageal reflux may be allowed clear liquids 2 hours before surgery, similar to nonobese children.[665]

Preoperative height, weight, blood pressure, heart rate, pulse oximetry, and fasting glucose should be documented for all obese children. A thorough airway examination must be performed. The risk of difficult mask ventilation is greater in obese children than in normal-weight children.[647,666,667] Jaw thrust and CPAP are useful in reducing upper airway collapse during spontaneous ventilation. Equipment for difficult intubation should be readily available prior to the induction of anesthesia. Vascular access may be difficult to establish in obese children.

Intravenous drug dosing is problematic as the pharmacokinetics of many anesthetics are affected by obesity.[668] Unfortunately, there are few pharmacokinetic studies of obese children and data to guide drug dosing are limited. Drug doses for anesthesia may be calculated based on the patient's total body weight, ideal body weight, or lean body weight depending on the drug (Table 2.15). In general, the per kilogram dose decreases with increasing weight.

TABLE 2.14	Comorbidities Associated With Childhood Obesity
Affected Organ System	**Obesity-Related Comorbidity**
Respiratory system	• Decreased lung and chest wall compliance • Bronchial hyperreactivity • Asthma (present in 30%) • Increased incidence of upper airway infections • Obstructive sleep apnea (OSA, present in 13%–59%)
Cardiovascular	• Systemic hypertension (present in 20%–30%) • Left ventricular hypertrophy (in adolescents) • Pulmonary hypertension in those with OSA
Endocrine	• Metabolic syndrome (present in 40%–50% of obese adolescents) • Diabetes or prediabetes • Dyslipidemia (hyperlipidemia and hypercholesterolemia) • Polycystic ovarian syndrome
Gastrointestinal	• Gastroesophageal reflux (present in 20% of severely obese children)
Hepatic	• Asymptomatic steatosis hepatis (present in 80%), may progress to hepatic fibrosis, nonalcoholic acute steatohepatitis, or rarely cirrhosis. • With every 5 cm increase in waist circumference, the odds of liver steatosis increase 1.4-fold
Neurologic/psychological	• Pseudotumor cerebri • Low self-esteem • Poor school performance
Orthopedic	• Slipped femoral epiphysis

From Mortensen A, Lenz K, Abildstrom H, Lauritsen TLB. Anesthetizing the obese child. *Paediatr Anaesth.* 2011;21:623-629; Chidambaran V, Tewari A, Mahmoud M. Anesthetic and pharmacologic considerations in perioperative care of obese children. *J Clin Anesth.* 2018;45:39-50.

TABLE 2.15 Dosage of Intravenous Anesthetics in Obese Children

Drug	Initial Dose[a] Based on	Maintenance Dose Based on
Propofol	LBW, titrate to effect	TBW
Benzodiazepines	LBW	IBW
Synthetic opioids: fentanyl, alfentanil, and remifentanil	LBW	LBW
Sufentanil	TBW	LBW
Morphine	IBW	IBW
Lidocaine	TBW	IBW
Nondepolarizing neuromuscular blockers	IBW	IBW
Succinylcholine	TBW	
Neostigmine	TBW	
Sugammadex	TBW	

[a]Not to exceed adult maximum dose
IBW, Ideal body weight; *LBW,* lean body weight; *TBW,* total body weight.
From Mortensen A, Lenz K, Abildstrom H, Lauritsen TLB. Anesthetizing the obese child. *Paediatr Anaesth.* 2011;21:623-629; Chidambaran V, Tewari A, Mahmoud M. Anesthetic and pharmacologic considerations in perioperative care of obese children. *J Clin Anesth.* 2018;45:39-50.

The loading dose depends on volume of distribution and maintenance dose on drug clearance. These two parameters change independently of each other with body size metrics. Succinylcholine should be dosed based on total body weight because the drug distributes to extracellular fluid and the effective dose is calculated based on the two-to-three times ED$_{95}$; a larger dose is given to ensure adequate neuromuscular blockade (see also Chapters 5 and 6).[669] Care must be undertaken if a TIVA anesthetic is administered to an obese child to monitor the depth of anesthesia if a prompt emergence is expected.[670]

OBSTRUCTIVE SLEEP APNEA

Sleep apnea is a sleep-related breathing disorder in children characterized by a periodic cessation of air exchange, with apnea episodes lasting longer than 10 seconds frequently associated with episodes of hypoventilation (hypopnea). The apnea-hypopnea index categorizes the total number of episodes per hour of sleep. Mild OSA has an apnea-hypopnea index of 1 to 5, moderate has an apnea-hypopnea index of 6 to 10, and severe apnea-hypopnea has an index of >10.[671] Sleep apnea may be defined as central (absent gas flow, lack of respiratory effort), obstructive (absent gas flow, upper airway obstruction, and paradoxical movement of rib cage and abdominal muscles), or mixed (due to both CNS defect and obstructive problems). Diagnosis is made by clinical assessment, nocturnal pulse oximetry, or polysomnography.

OSA is manifested by episodes that disturb sleep and ventilation. These episodes occur more frequently during rapid eye movement (REM) sleep and increase in frequency as more time is spent in REM sleep periods as the night progresses. OSA occurs in children of all ages (about 2% of all children) but is more common in children 3 to 7 years of age. It occurs equally in boys and girls, although the prevalence is greater in African American and Hispanic children compared with Caucasians.[672–675]

Signs of OSA are sleep disturbances (including daytime sleepiness, irritability, poor school attention), irritability, night terrors, nocturnal enuresis, sleeping in odd positions, sleep walking, snoring loud enough to be heard through a closed door, pauses and/or gasps during the night, failure to thrive resulting from poor intake due to tonsillar hypertrophy, speech disorders, and decreased size (decreased growth hormone release during disturbed REM sleep). With the worldwide increase in childhood obesity, the presence of obesity in children with OSA exacerbates the signs and symptoms of OSA. Parents of obese children should be specifically asked about such signs and symptoms. This syndrome can cause cardiac, pulmonary, and CNS impairment due to chronic oxygen desaturation. Indeed, both OSA and obesity are systemic inflammatory responses.[676] When they occur together in a child, the severity of the signs and symptoms are greater than if only one had occurred, and resolution of the OSA after tonsillectomy is less likely. In children with OSA and morbid obesity, the incidences of hypertension and diabetes are greater than in the absence of these disorders. Therefore, it is important to evaluate the cardiovascular status; although right ventricular dysfunction with pulmonary hypertension is classic, biventricular hypertrophy can develop. It is more likely to occur in children with severe OSA but has been reported in children with only mild OSA.[677] Cardiac evaluation is recommended for any child with signs of right ventricular dysfunction, systemic or pulmonary hypertension, or multiple episodes of desaturation below 70% (see also Fig. 31.6). Electrocardiography and chest radiography are insensitive diagnostic tests; rather, echocardiography is recommended.[678] Relief of the tonsillar/adenoidal obstruction can reverse many of these disorders and prevent progression of others (pulmonary hypertension and cor pulmonale) within 6 months after tonsillectomy, although approximately 30% of children with severe OSA will not have resolution after tonsillectomy.

Children with OSA may be premedicated with caution with oral midazolam; however, post premedication monitoring of hemoglobin saturation in these children would seem reasonable.[284] Avoidance of premedication may be more advantageous postoperatively. However, for young children with a URI in the preceding 2 weeks, a history of asthma or exposure to secondhand smoke, albuterol/salbutamol premedication may be salutary before tonsillectomy.[631]

Children who are at increased risk for postoperative upper airway obstruction after tonsillectomy and/or adenoidectomy for OSA include those aged younger than 2 years, children with craniofacial anomalies, failure to thrive, hypotonia, morbid obesity, previous upper airway trauma, cor pulmonale, a polysomnogram with a respiratory distress index greater than 40 or oxygen saturation nadir less than 70%, and a child undergoing an additional uvulopalatopharyngoplasty.[679] A more recent retrospective study reported slightly different risk factors for perioperative respiratory adverse events in these children: craniofacial, genetic, cardiac or neurologic conditions, airway anomalies, apnea-hypopnea index of >5 events per hour and oxygen saturation nadir <80% on polysomnogram.[680] *Repeated nocturnal desaturation events to less than 85% upregulates the genes responsible for control of opioid receptors, resulting in an increased sensitivity to opioids; opioid requirement is reduced by approximately 50%, making standard doses of opioids a relative overdose in children with severe OSA. This has been demonstrated in both animals and humans.*[654,681,682] To attenuate the risk of perioperative respiratory complications, opioids should be carefully titrated to the respiratory responses during surgery, and if an increased sensitivity to opioids is detected, all perioperative opioids should be reduced or avoided accordingly (see Chapter 31 for further details).[683]

There is increasing evidence of marked ethnic variations in the cytochromes responsible for drug metabolism (see also Chapters 4 and 5). In 8% to 10% of children, a single nuclear polymorphism of CYP2D6 yields poor metabolizers, rendering the children unable to convert codeine to morphine, whereas the "ultrarapid metabolizers" have multiple copies of the gene that yields a relative morphine overdose, contributing to fatalities in children with OSA.[684–687] As a result, the FDA has added a boxed warning to codeine-containing products and recommends against the use of codeine in children undergoing tonsillectomy who are ≤18 years of age (https://www.fda.gov/media/85072/download)

Some would argue that banning the drug is not the solution, but the polymorphism in each patient should be identified to tailor drug administration to those who can process the drug appropriately. Hence, St. Jude's hospital, which found codeine very effective for postoperative pain after adenotonsillectomy, determined the genotype in each child and only administered codeine to those who can convert codeine to morphine at normal rates and administered alternative analgesics to those who could not convert the codeine (poor metabolizers) or were at risk for a possible overdose (ultrarapid metabolizers).[688] By exploiting gene technology, this institution tailored the drug to children who would not be harmed by single nucleotide polymorphisms.

If nocturnal upper airway obstruction continues after tonsillectomy, ancillary strategies that have been met with variable success have been used: nasal CPAP or BiPAP, nasal steroids, oxygen therapy, and weight loss.[679]

Preoperative screening tools may be useful to determine prospectively those at risk for adverse perioperative events. Although polysomnography is the gold standard for the diagnosis of OSA (see Chapter 31), questionnaire screening tools may be helpful in identifying children with sleep-disordered breathing symptoms who may be at risk for perioperative respiratory adverse events.[689,690] The STBUR (snoring, trouble breathing, unrefreshed) questionnaire has five symptom items (Tables 2.16 and 2.17). The likelihood of perioperative respiratory adverse events is 3-fold greater in the presence of three STBUR symptoms and increased 10-fold when all five symptoms were present.[691] A study of 555 children found that a positive STBUR questionnaire was associated with a 3.5-fold increase in adverse perioperative respiratory events.[692] Another study of 6025 children found 1522 with a low threshold score and 270 with a high threshold score; positive scores were associated with need for supplemental oxygen, prolonged PACU stay, and escalation of care.[693] The tool had a high

TABLE 2.17	American Academy of Pediatrics Clinical Practice Guidelines: Risk Factors for Postoperative Respiratory Complications in Children With Obstructive Sleep Apnea Undergoing Adenotonsillectomy
Younger than 3 years of age	
Severe obstructive sleep apnea on polysomnography	
Cardiac complications of obstructive sleep apnea	
Failure to thrive	
Obesity	
Craniofacial anomalies	
Neuromuscular disorders	
Current respiratory infection	

From Clinical Practice Guideline: diagnosis and management of childhood obstructive sleep apnea syndrome. *Pediatrics.* 2012;130:576-584.

negative predictive value and the strength of the STBUR tool is its simplicity as it consists of only five items that are easy to administer in a busy perioperative clinic setting.

The ASA and others[694,695] provide recommendations for inpatient monitoring of children at high risk for postoperative complications who are at risk for having OSA and are undergoing adenotonsillectomy. These guidelines advocate that high-risk patients undergo surgery in a facility capable of treating complex pediatric patients and be hospitalized overnight for close monitoring. In addition the American Academy of Pediatrics has developed a guideline for management of children with OSA.[694] The ASA considers this such a growing problem for both adults and children that they have formulated a Practice Guideline with tables to assist in patient screening (Tables 2.18 and 2.19 modified for children).[695] The tables help to clarify the identification and assessment of children potentially at risk for OSA and offer a proposed (although as yet unvalidated) risk assessment scoring system. This system attempts to characterize those patients who are at increased risk for perioperative complications.

Despite these practice guidelines and risk identification scoring systems, a worrisome number of children with OSA have died or suffered neurologic injury as a result of apnea after tonsillectomy. A survey of Society for Pediatric Anesthesia members and review of the ASA Closed Claims Project yielded 111 reports of adverse events between 1990 and 2010 in children undergoing tonsillectomy.[696] Death or neurologic injury occurred in 77% of these cases. Nearly half of the events within 24 hours of the procedure occurred after hospital discharge. Children who fulfilled ASA criteria to be at risk for OSA were more likely to have the adverse event attributed to apnea, whereas all others were more likely to have the event attributed to hemorrhage. Two children died in the PACU after they became agitated and received additional sedating medications, but the monitors were not reapplied (one in his father's lap and the other in the stretcher with her mom).[696] These cases illustrate the insidious nature of apnea and provide a stark reminder of the increased perioperative risk secondary to OSA. These children must be closely monitored for apnea and should not be discharged from the recovery area to an unmonitored setting (i.e., home or unmonitored hospital bed) until no longer at risk of postoperative respiratory depression.[695]

Among children 1 to 18 years of age with OSA, those without complicating medical conditions such as neuromuscular disease,

TABLE 2.16	Symptom Items Comprising the STBUR Questionnaire

1. While sleeping does your child snore more than half the time?
2. While sleeping does your child snore loudly?
3. While sleeping does your child have trouble breathing or struggles to breathe?
4. Have you ever seen your child stop breathing during the night?
5. Does your child wake up feeling unrefreshed in the morning?

STBUR, Snoring, trouble breathing, unrefreshed.
From Tait AR, Voepel-Lewis T, Christensen R, O'Brien LM. The STBUR questionnaire for predicting perioperative respiratory adverse events in children at risk for sleep-disordered breathing. *Paediatr Anaesth.* 2013;23:510-516.

TABLE 2.18 | Candidate Criteria for Identification and Assessment of Obstructive Sleep Apnea[a]

A: Clinical Signs and Symptoms Suggesting Obstructive Sleep Apnea

1. Predisposing physical characteristics

a. ≥95th percentile for age and gender
b. Craniofacial abnormalities affecting the airway (e.g., Down syndrome)
c. Anatomic nasal obstruction
d. Tonsils nearly touching or touching in the midline (kissing tonsils)

2. History of apparent airway obstruction during sleep (two or more of the following are present; if patient sleep is not observed by another person, then only one of the following needs to be present)

a. Snoring (loud enough to be heard through a closed door)
b. Frequent snoring
c. Observed pauses in breathing during sleep
d. Awakened from sleep with choking sensation
e. Frequent arousal from sleep
f. Intermittent vocalizations during sleep
g. Parental report of restless sleep, difficulty breathing, or struggling respiratory efforts during sleep
h. Child with night terrors
i. Child sleeps in unusual positions
j. Child with new-onset enuresis

3. Somnolence (one of the following is present)

a. Frequent daytime somnolence or fatigue despite adequate "sleep"
b. Falls asleep easily in a nonstimulating environment (e.g., watching television, reading, riding in, or driving a car) despite adequate "sleep"
c. Parent or teacher comments that the child appears sleepy during the day, is easily distracted, is overly aggressive, or has difficulty concentrating
d. Child is often difficult to arouse at the usual awakening time

B: Determination of Severity

a. If a child has signs or symptoms in two or more of the above categories, there is a significant probability that they have obstructive sleep apnea (OSA). The severity of OSA may be determined by a sleep study (polysomnogram). If a sleep study is not available, such patients should be treated as though they have moderate sleep apnea unless one or more of the signs of symptoms above is severely abnormal (e.g., weight ≥95th percentile for age and gender, respiratory pauses that are frightening to the observer, child regularly falls asleep within minutes after being left unstimulated without another explanation), in which cases patients should be treated as though they have severe sleep apnea.

b. If a sleep study has been done, the result should be used to determine the perioperative anesthetic management of a child. (Review the polysomnogram for evidence of nocturnal desaturations <85%, which increases sensitivity to opioids). However, because sleep laboratories differ in their criteria for detecting episodes of apnea and hypoxemia, the Task Force recommends that the sleep laboratory's assessment (none, mild, moderate, or severe) take precedence over the actual apnea-hypopnea index (AHI, the number of episodes of sleep-disordered breathing per hour). If the overall severity is not indicated, it may be determined by using the following table:

Severity of OSA	Adult AHI	Pediatric AHI
None	0–5	0
Mild OSA	6–20	1–5
Moderate OSA	21–40	6–10
Severe OSA	>40	>10

Modified from Practice guidelines for the perioperative management of patients with obstructive sleep apnea: an updated report by the American Society of Anesthesiologists Task Force on Perioperative Management of Patients with Obstructive Sleep Apnea. *Anesthesiology.* 2014;120:268-286.
[a]Note: This table has been modified for children; the scoring system is intended only as a guide and has not been validated.

obesity, or craniofacial abnormalities but with mild sleep apnea may have either no or some improvement in their airway obstruction on the night of surgery.[697] Based on current literature, one may consider discharging children 3 to 12 years of age home on the day of surgery after an extended period of observation (4–6 hours) if they meet these criteria. However, those with moderate to severe OSA (particularly obese children) may actually experience worse OSA on the night of their surgery.[697,698] These children should receive reduced doses or no opioids and be admitted for overnight monitoring with pulse oximetry and an apnea monitor.[699] The American Academy of Otolaryngology Head and Neck Surgery Foundation has provided evidence-based recommendations regarding analgesia that may be provided by alternating doses around the clock of acetaminophen and ibuprofen.[700]

ASYMPTOMATIC CARDIAC MURMURS

The presence of a cardiac murmur is a common finding in children[701] and may have important anesthetic implications. A history should be obtained to delineate the nature of the murmur. In most cases, the parents will report that the murmur was detected previously by the child's pediatrician and determined to be an "innocent flow murmur" without any anatomic or physiologic abnormalities. When a pediatric cardiologist confirms the classic clinical features of an innocent murmur, an echocardiogram seldom reveals heart disease, especially if the child is older at presentation.[702] However, even an experienced cardiologist can occasionally make a misdiagnosis; the only certain means to exclude a structural defect is with an echocardiogram.[703] "Appropriate use criteria" for initial transthoracic echocardiography in outpatient pediatric cardiology have been established in a joint project with the American College of Cardiology, the American Society of Echocardiography, and the Society of Pediatric Echocardiography to support the clinical decision as to the appropriateness of care delivered to the pediatric patient.[704] A presumptively innocent murmur with no symptoms, signs, or findings of cardiovascular disease and a benign family history is rated as a "rarely appropriate" indication. In general, nonpathologic murmurs occur during systole and are soft and nongraduating with normal feel to peripheral pulses; there are normal blood pressures in both upper and lower extremities. However, if the murmur is harsh and difficult to localize, if there are bounding pulses, if the murmur is louder than grade II/VI, or if it is accompanied by other findings (Tables 2.20 and 2.21), then further evaluation is warranted.[705] If the murmur has not been detected previously, referral to a pediatric cardiologist is indicated or an echocardiogram by an experienced pediatric echocardiographer should be obtained before induction of anesthesia.[706]

TABLE 2.19	Obstructive Sleep Apnea Risk Scoring System: Example[a]

A. Severity of Sleep Apnea Based on Sleep Study (or Clinical Indicators if Sleep Study is not Available: Point Score 0–3[b,c]
Severity of Obstructive Sleep Apnea (OSA)

None	0
Mild	1
Moderate	2
Severe	3

B. Invasiveness of Surgery and Anesthesia: Point Score 0–3
Type of surgery and anesthesia

Superficial surgery under local or peripheral nerve block anesthesia without sedation	0
Superficial surgery with moderate sedation or general anesthesia	1
Peripheral surgery with spinal or epidural anesthesia (with no more than moderate sedation)	1
Peripheral surgery with general anesthesia	2
Airway surgery with moderate sedation	2
Major surgery with general anesthesia	3
Airway surgery with general anesthesia (e.g., tonsillectomy)	3

C. Requirement for Postoperative Opioids: Point Score 0–3
Opioid requirement

None	0
Low-dose oral opioids (tonsillectomy)	1
High-dose oral opioids, parenteral, or neuraxial opioids	3

D. Estimation of Perioperative Risk—Overall Score Equals the Score for "A" (Assessed from Table 2.17) Plus the Greater of the Score for "B" or "C": Possible Score 0–6[d]

Modified from Practice guidelines for the perioperative management of patients with obstructive sleep apnea: an updated report by the American Society of Anesthesiologists Task Force on Perioperative Management of Patients with Obstructive Sleep Apnea. *Anesthesiology.* 2014;120:268-286.
[a]Note: This table has been modified for children. A scoring system similar to this table may be used to estimate whether a child is at increased perioperative risk of complications from OSA.
This example has not been clinically validated, and such a scoring system is simply meant to provide guidance.
[b]One point may be subtracted if a patient has been on continuous positive airway pressure (CPAP) for noninvasive positive-pressure ventilation before surgery and will be using their appliance consistently during the postoperative period.
[c]One point should be added if a child with mild or moderate OSA also has a resting arterial carbon dioxide tension greater than 50 mm Hg.
[d]Children with a score of 4 may be at increased perioperative risk from OSA; children with a score of 5 or 6 may be at increased perioperative risk from OSA.

TABLE 2.20	Grading of Heart Murmurs
Grade I	Heard only with intense concentration
Grade II	Faint, but heard immediately
Grade III	Easily heard, of intermediate intensity
Grade IV	Easily heard, palpable thrill/vibration on chest wall
Grade V	Very loud, thrill present, audible with only edge of stethoscope on chest wall
Grade VI	Audible with stethoscope off the chest wall

Modified from Emmanouilides GC, Allen HD, Riemenschneider TA, Gutgesell HP. *Moss and Adams Heart Disease in Infants, Children, and Adolescents Including the Fetus and Young Adult.* 5th ed. Baltimore: Williams & Wilkins; 1995.

TABLE 2.21	Symptoms and Signs of Heart Disease

Feeding difficulties: disinterest, fatigue, diaphoresis, tachypnea, dyspnea

Poor exercise tolerance

Tachypnea, dyspnea, grunting, nasal flaring, and intercostal, suprasternal, or subcostal retractions

Frequent respiratory tract infections (a result of compression of airways by plethoric vessels leading to stasis of secretions and atelectasis)

Central cyanosis (involving warm mucous membranes: tongue and buccal mucosa) or poor capillary refill

Absent or abnormal peripheral pulses

Modified from Pelech AN. Evaluation of the pediatric patient with a cardiac murmur. *Pediatr Clin North Am.* 1999;46:167-188.

is usually small (0.3 minutes) and with no clinical relevance.[708] On the other hand, acetaminophen has no effect on platelet function and is an excellent antipyretic that may be administered intravenously; it is also rapidly absorbed when administered orally. In contrast, rectal administration requires at least 60 minutes to achieve effective blood concentration (E-Fig. 2.6).[709–711] There is no evidence that an existing fever predisposes to a malignant hyperthermic reaction.[712]

POSTANESTHESIA APNEA IN FORMER PRETERM INFANTS

Former preterm infants have a multitude of residual problems owing to intensive care therapy, prolonged intubation, and still-maturing organogenesis. The incidence of subglottic stenosis is increased and they are prone to perioperative respiratory complications.[713] At the time of surgery they may or may not have apnea spells, although they often appear normal for their age; a number of prospective studies have defined the population at greatest risk for postoperative apnea.[612,713–721] Former preterm infants <44 weeks postconception age are at a greater risk for apnea after general anesthesia than are those older than 44 weeks postconception age.[611] In an analysis of eight published prospective papers from four institutions conducted over 6 years, the incidence of apnea varied inversely with both the gestational age and postconception age.[611] For example, consider two infants who are now 45 weeks postconception age: one was born at 28 weeks and the other at 32 weeks of gestation. The risk of apnea in the 28-week gestational age infant is twice that in the 32-week gestational age infant (Fig. 2.12).[611] Similarly, consider two infants of the same gestational age: one anesthetized at 45 weeks postconception age

FEVER

The presence of a low-grade fever before elective surgery poses a dilemma whether to proceed or delay. In general, if a child has only 0.5°C to 1.0°C of fever and no other symptoms, this degree of fever is not a contraindication to general anesthesia. However, if the fever is associated with a recent onset of rhinitis, pharyngitis, otitis media, dehydration, or any other sign of impending illness, it is prudent to postpone the procedure. If the planned surgery is of an urgent nature, efforts should be made to reduce the fever before induction of anesthesia, primarily to reduce oxygen demands. Ibuprofen is widely used to control fever, but may be associated with an increase in bleeding time,[707] although that effect

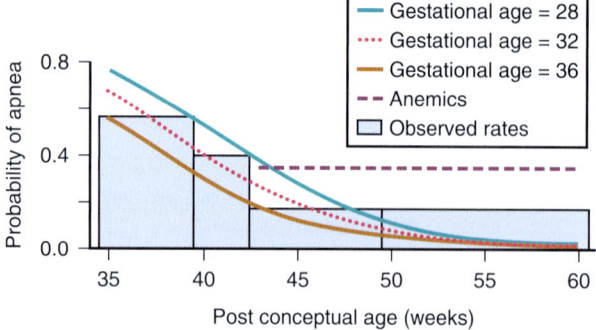

FIGURE 2.12 The predicted probability of apnea for all infants was inversely related to gestational age at the time of birth and postconception age at the time of surgery. The probability of apnea was the same regardless of postconception age or gestational age for infants with anemia (dashed magenta line). (From Coté CJ, Zaslavsky A, Downes JJ, et al. Postoperative apnea in former preterm infants after inguinal herniorrhaphy: a combined analysis. Anesthesiology. 1995;82:807-808.)

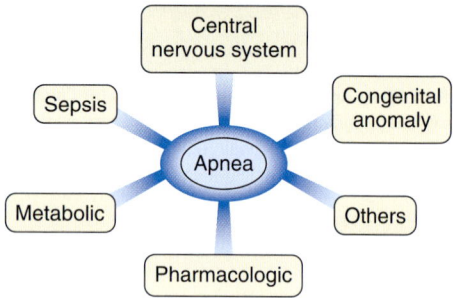

FIGURE 2.13 Apnea, defined as the absence of movement of air at the mouth or nose, may have many causes. Those that anesthesiologists are most often involved with are of metabolic, pharmacologic, or respiratory origins.

and the other at 50 weeks postconception age; the younger-postconception age infant would be at greater risk for postoperative apnea. The recognition of apnea events depends on the type of device used to monitor the infants (E-Fig. 2.7); simple observation and impedance pneumography are more likely to miss apneic events than continuous recording devices.[611,722,723] Preterm infants with anemia (hematocrit <30%) are more prone to apnea, and the incidence is unrelated to postconception age or gestational age (see Fig. 2.12).[611,612] It appears that the risk for apnea exceeds 1% with statistical certainty until approximately 56 weeks postconception age in infants with a gestational age of 32 weeks or 54 weeks postconception age in those with a gestational age of 35 weeks, if one excludes anemic infants and those with obvious apnea in the recovery room. This analysis determined that (1) apnea was strongly and inversely related to both gestational age and postconception age; (2) ongoing apnea at home is a risk factor; (3) small-for-gestational-age infants are protected from apnea compared with appropriate- and large-for-gestational-age infants; (4) anemia is a significant risk factor, particularly for infants more than 44 weeks postconception age; and (5) a history of necrotizing enterocolitis, neonatal apnea, respiratory distress syndrome, bronchopulmonary dysplasia, or operative use of opioids or muscle relaxants did not correlate with postoperative apnea.[611] Each clinician must decide how to balance the risk of an unrecognized apnea with the benefit of proceeding with the surgery in terms of cost savings and not hospitalizing the infant for overnight monitoring.[724] The most practical and appropriate plan is to admit and monitor all formerly preterm infants who are less than 60 weeks postconception age until they are free of apnea for a minimum of 12 hours.

When sevoflurane and desflurane were compared for maintenance of anesthesia in 30 infants under 37 weeks gestation and under 47 weeks postconception age undergoing inguinal hernia repair after a sevoflurane induction, the time to wakefulness in infants who received desflurane was more rapid than those who received sevoflurane, although the frequency of postoperative respiratory events in the two groups was similar.[725,726] *Although the majority of former preterm infants in the Coté et al. microanalysis were anesthetized with halothane,[611] apnea has been reported with all anesthetics, including sevoflurane, desflurane, and regional anesthesia (spinal or caudal epidural, discussed later in the chapter).[725–728]*

The preoperative evaluation of these infants requires reserving a monitored bed postoperatively and a clear discussion with the family regarding the perioperative risks of anesthesia and apnea. If the child is receiving theophylline or caffeine preoperatively, this therapy should be continued postoperatively.[729] If the child is not receiving theophylline or caffeine, there is no evidence to support the routine administration of aminophylline postoperatively, but there is weak evidence that caffeine (10 mg/kg) may reduce postoperative apnea spells in high-risk infants.[721,730] The pharmacokinetics of caffeine[731] (and theophylline[732]) in preterm and full-term neonates suggest that a single intravenous dose of caffeine will have a clinical effect that may last for several days. However, the pharmacokinetics of caffeine change dramatically with age: in older infants (e.g., those who are 60 weeks postconception age, the half-life of caffeine is reduced to approximately 5 hours (E-Fig. 2.8).[733] A Cochrane review of prophylactic caffeine in formerly preterm infants concluded that although caffeine can be used to prevent postoperative apnea, bradycardia, and episodes of oxygen desaturation, there was insufficient evidence to adopt this as routine anesthetic practice.[734] *If caffeine is administered to a former preterm infant, postoperative admission and overnight respiratory monitoring are still required, because caffeine is not 100% effective in preventing postoperative apnea.*

Apnea may be related to many causes besides prematurity (Fig. 2.13); the most common causes after surgery, however, relate to metabolic derangements, pharmacologic effects, or central nervous system immaturity. Metabolic causes of apnea such as hypothermia, hypoglycemia, hypocalcemia, acidosis, and hypoxemia should be avoided (see Chapter 35). However, pharmacologic effects on respirations cannot be avoided because most drugs used in anesthesia depress the respiratory system either directly or indirectly.[735] Respiratory depression is probably even more likely to occur in neonates who have an immature respiratory center; residual anesthetic action may contribute to the development of postoperative apnea.[736] In addition, most drugs or inhalation agents decrease muscle tone of the upper airway, thus contributing to the development of upper airway obstruction, more labored breathing, fatigue, and subsequent apnea.[719] Potent inhalation anesthetic agents also decrease intercostal muscle tone, reducing functional residual capacity and thereby increasing the propensity to develop hypoxemia (Fig. 2.14).[737]

Regional anesthesia has been used to reduce the risk of postoperative apnea.[715,738–742] A multicenter, multinational study comparing **G**eneral **A**nesthesia with **S**pinal anesthesia (the GAS study) for former preterm and full-term infants found no difference in

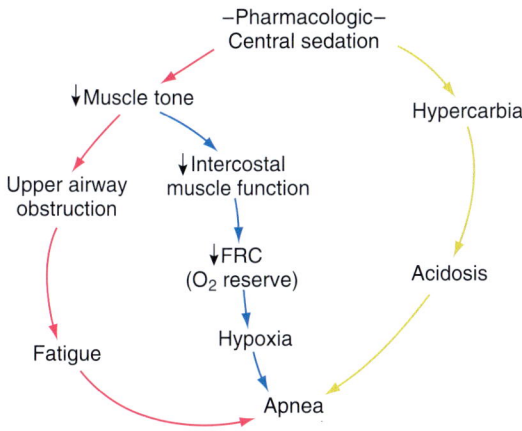

FIGURE 2.14 Pharmacologic interventions may result in several sequences of events leading to apnea. *FRC*, Functional residual capacity.

the incidence of apnea comparing spinal to general anesthesia (~6% in former preterm infants). However, the severity of the apnea was less and the incidence was lower in the first 30 minutes in the PACU following spinal anesthesia.[728,741] In addition, the GAS study did not find an association of postoperative apnea with anemia, which is at odds with previous studies.[611,741,743] Spinal anesthesia may offer potential advantages; however, several infants who had spinal anesthesia experienced life-threatening events many hours after discharge from PACU.[611,741] Although spinal anesthesia offers an advantage, it does not eliminate our need for vigilance. In addition, because all the infants in the general anesthesia group were anesthetized with sevoflurane compared with the 1995 study, in which all were anesthetized with halothane, the use of a more modern anesthetic agent did not seem to have any salutary effects on apnea as some practitioners have suggested.

A Cochrane review found *"no difference in the effect of spinal compared to general anesthesia on the overall incidence of postoperative apnea, bradycardia, oxygen saturation, need for postoperative analgesics or respiratory support."*[742] Additive drugs used to prolong the duration of a spinal or caudal block, such as clonidine, or sedatives, such as midazolam and dexmedetomidine, have been associated with postoperative or intraoperative apnea.[744–748] Spinal anesthesia is also associated with a significant failure rate (20% in some studies) and the need for multiple attempts to achieve accurate placement of the needle,[728,749,750] although in experienced hands, the success rate for placing a spinal block was 97.4% and an adequate level of spinal anesthesia was achieved in 95.4% of infants.

Anesthesia has changed over the past 30 years: new inhalation agents have replaced halothane, artificial surfactant has rescued many infants, and improved respiratory strategies have reduced barotrauma-induced chronic pulmonary disease. Although it would seem logical that these advances should have reduced the reported incidence of postanesthesia apnea in former preterm infants from 1995,[611] this belief is not substantiated. *"Despite these medical advances, former preterm infants should not be anesthetized as outpatients even when a regional technique has been used; they require admission for postoperative monitoring overnight for apnea."*[741]

With respect to full-term neonates, three reports have described infants who developed apnea after apparently uneventful general anesthesias.[751–753] Therefore, if a full-term infant who is younger than 44 weeks postconception age demonstrates any abnormality of respiration after anesthesia, we recommend that

they be admitted overnight for apnea monitoring. The algorithms in Fig. 2.15 can be used as a decision tree for outpatient surgery in term and former preterm infants. A review of postoperative complications in preterm and term infants undergoing inguinal hernia repair confirmed the risk for respiratory complications in former preterm infants ≤60 weeks postconception age but suggested that full-term infants >1 month of age and who were ASA class I or II may be candidates for same-day surgery.[754] Obviously this unique age for surgery still presents a dilemma and the decision to admit and monitor must be made on a case-by-case basis.

HYPERALIMENTATION

Anesthesiologists frequently encounter chronically ill infants and children who are unable to tolerate enteral feedings and are therefore maintained on total parenteral nutrition (TPN). It is important to identify the composition and rate of administration of these fluids so that potential intraoperative complications, such as hypo- and hyperglycemia can be avoided. Most of these solutions are hypertonic, have high glucose content, and must be administered through a centrally placed intravenous route.

The basic principles of care are:

1. Avoid contaminating the line. It is best not to puncture the line for administering medications or changing fluid.
2. Intralipid infusions may be discontinued before surgery, because of the potential to become a culture medium if contaminated. In contrast, DO NOT DISCONTINUE the glucose-containing solution, because the relative hyperinsulinemic state could induce hypoglycemia, the signs of which might be masked by general anesthesia.
3. An infusion device should be used so that the rate of infusion is constant. Accidental rapid infusion of large amounts of total parenteral nutrition fluid can cause a hypertonic nonketotic coma.[755] The 10% dextrose infusion is usually continued at the preoperative NICU rate to avoid intraoperative hypoglycemia,[756] although recent evidence albeit from a retrospective study, supports halving the dextrose infusion rates during surgery without developing either hyper- or hypoglycemia.[757]
4. Perioperative and intraoperative monitoring of glucose, potassium, sodium, and calcium, as well as acid-base status, is important for long procedures.
5. Preoperative confirmation of correct intravascular line placement (radiography or aspiration of blood) is important to avoid intraoperative complications such as hydrothorax or hemothorax.

DIABETES

The incidence of both type 1 and type 2 diabetes, one of the most common endocrine disorders in children, continues to rise in the United States.[758] Preoperative assessment should include a thorough knowledge of the child's specific treatment regimen and glycemic control. When feasible, elective surgery for children with diabetes should be delayed until metabolic control is acceptable (i.e., absence of ketonuria, normal electrolytes, and the HbA1c value within the ideal range for the child's age).[461,759] Every attempt should be made to schedule a diabetic child as the first case of the day so that prolonged fasting is avoided. Patients presenting for emergent surgeries may require collaboration with the endocrinologist. A blood glucose determination should always take place before the anesthetic is started. Several protocols have been advocated for glycemic control in diabetics depending on the

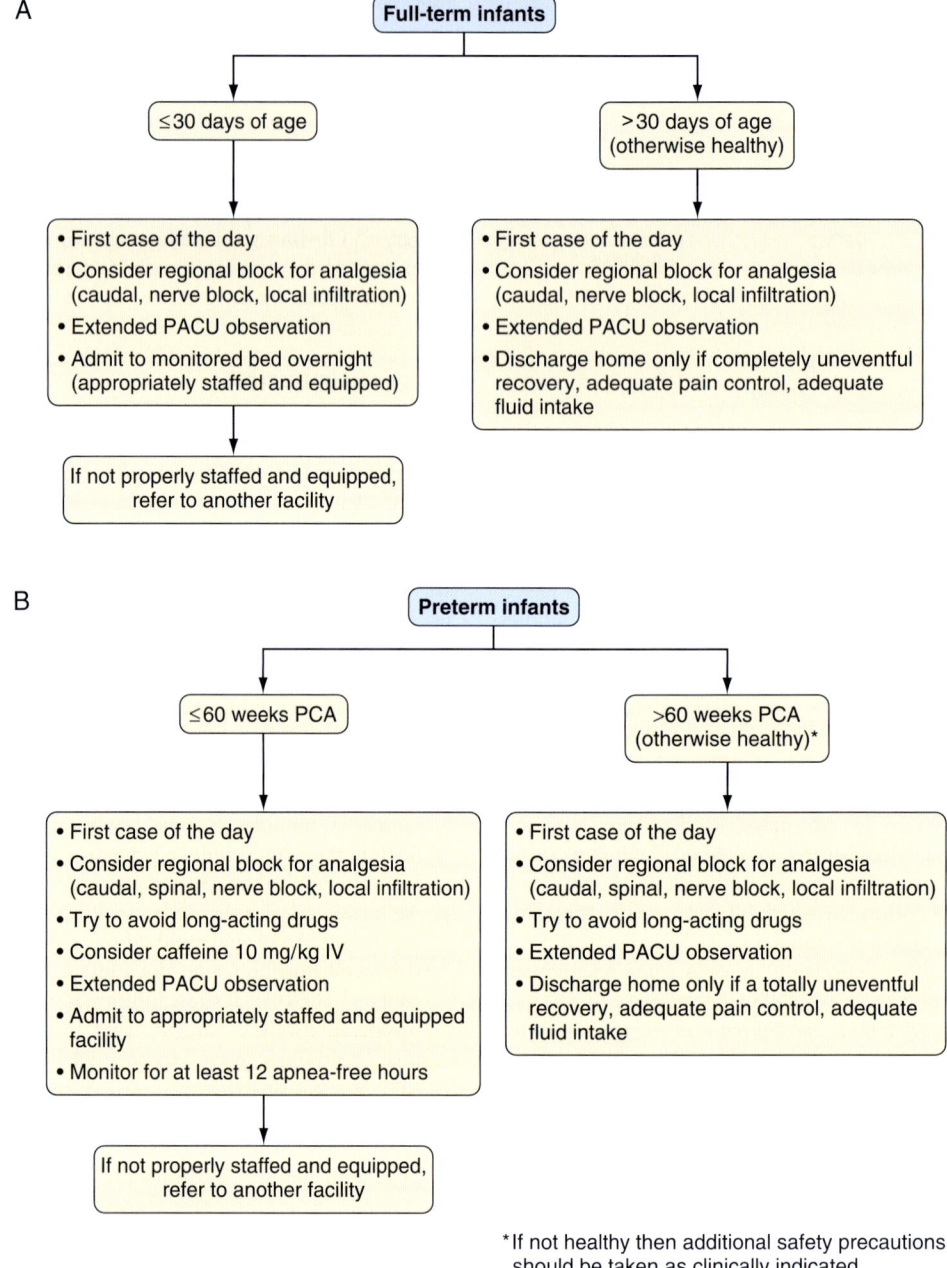

A Full-term infants

≤30 days of age

- First case of the day
- Consider regional block for analgesia (caudal, nerve block, local infiltration)
- Extended PACU observation
- Admit to monitored bed overnight (appropriately staffed and equipped)

If not properly staffed and equipped, refer to another facility

>30 days of age (otherwise healthy)

- First case of the day
- Consider regional block for analgesia (caudal, nerve block, local infiltration)
- Extended PACU observation
- Discharge home only if completely uneventful recovery, adequate pain control, adequate fluid intake

B Preterm infants

≤60 weeks PCA

- First case of the day
- Consider regional block for analgesia (caudal, spinal, nerve block, local infiltration)
- Try to avoid long-acting drugs
- Consider caffeine 10 mg/kg IV
- Extended PACU observation
- Admit to appropriately staffed and equipped facility
- Monitor for at least 12 apnea-free hours

If not properly staffed and equipped, refer to another facility

>60 weeks PCA (otherwise healthy)*

- First case of the day
- Consider regional block for analgesia (caudal, spinal, nerve block, local infiltration)
- Try to avoid long-acting drugs
- Extended PACU observation
- Discharge home only if a totally uneventful recovery, adequate pain control, adequate fluid intake

*If not healthy then additional safety precautions should be taken as clinically indicated

FIGURE 2.15 Algorithms used as a decision tree for outpatient surgery in term infants **(A)** and in former preterm infants **(B)**. *PACU*, Postanesthesia care unit; *PCA*, postconception age.

length of the procedure and the child's baseline treatment regimen. A more detailed discussion of the perioperative management of the child with diabetes is presented in Chapter 25.

BRONCHOPULMONARY DYSPLASIA

Bronchopulmonary dysplasia is a form of chronic lung disease associated with prolonged mechanical ventilation and oxygen toxicity in preterm neonates characterized by impaired alveolar growth and airway inflammation.[760] Antenatal glucocorticoids, surfactant therapy, and gentle ventilation strategies to minimize lung injury have changed the clinical characteristics of bronchopulmonary dysplasia.[761] The current definition of bronchopulmonary dysplasia has been validated in early infancy and determines three levels of

severity (mild, moderate, or severe) using gestational age, oxygen dependence at 36 weeks postconception age, total duration of oxygen supplementation, and positive-pressure ventilatory requirements.[762,763] The clinical manifestations of bronchopulmonary dysplasia include tachypnea, dyspnea, and airway hyperactivity, as well as oxygen dependence. These infants suffer from hypoxemia, hypercarbia, abnormal functional airway growth, tracheomalacia, bronchomalacia, subglottic stenosis, increased pulmonary vascular resistance, and congestive heart failure. Pulmonary function abnormalities, including a reduced functional residual capacity, reduced diffusion capacity, airway obstruction, and reduced exercise tolerance, which may persist into the school-age years.[764] Even in the postsurfactant era, retrospective studies estimate a 25% to 35%

prevalence of pulmonary hypertension among extremely low-birth-weight infants with bronchopulmonary dysplasia requiring prolonged positive-pressure ventilation, which is an important determinant of morbidity and mortality.[765] Extreme phenotypic variability exists among preterm infants of similar gestational ages, making it difficult to predict which infants are at increased risk for developing pulmonary hypertension.[766] These children are often cared for at home on oxygen therapy with diuretics, digoxin, and β2-agonists. Preoperative preparation should focus on optimizing oxygenation, reducing airway hyperactivity, and correcting electrolyte abnormalities caused by chronic diuretic therapy. These patients may benefit from the use of nebulized β2-adrenergic agonists before the induction of anesthesia. Particular attention should be paid to fluid balance. Adequate expiratory time to avoid excessive positive-pressure ventilation is important. The possibility of pulmonary hypertension and right ventricular dysfunction should be considered and, when indicated, evaluated via electrocardiogram and echocardiography. Stress-dose steroid administration is indicated in children with a history of corticosteroid use in the past 6 months.

SEIZURE DISORDERS

Management of children with seizure disorders requires a knowledge of the antiseizure medications, medication schedule, and possible interactions between these medications and anesthetic drugs. The stress of surgery and anesthesia may lower the seizure threshold and cause a seizure. Seizure medications should be continued until the time of elective surgery. Characterization of the clinical manifestations of the seizure is useful to be able to diagnose potential seizures postoperatively. If the child is expected to have a significant problem with oral intake postoperatively, then a game plan with the child's neurologist should be developed to build a transition to intravenous antiseizure medications. Preoperative and postoperative management of anticonvulsant blood concentrations may also ensure proper therapeutic effect (see also Chapter 22).

A ketogenic diet has been used as an alternative or supplementary treatment to medically refractory seizures since the early 1920s.[767] Although the ketogenic diet lost its popularity with the discovery of new anticonvulsant therapies, a recent resurgence in interest has resulted in more patients presenting to the operating room while consuming this type of diet. The classic ketogenic diet, which is high in fat and low in protein and carbohydrate, uses a 4:1 ratio of fat to carbohydrate and protein. The exact anticonvulsant mechanism of the ketogenic diet remains unknown and is probably multifactorial.[768] Production of ketone bodies by the liver is a hallmark feature, and measurement of β-hydroxybutyrate levels in the blood is often used as a clinical indicator of successful ketosis. Optimal seizure protection lags days to weeks behind ketonemia, which occurs within hours of implementing a ketogenic diet, suggesting that adaptations to ketonemia rather than the direct effects are responsible for the anticonvulsant nature of the diet.[768]

Epilepsy is the most common indication for the ketogenic diet in children. Once a patient fails a number of anticonvulsant medication classes, nonpharmacological options are considered next.[769] These include a ketogenic diet, epilepsy surgery, or placement of a vagal nerve stimulator. Contraindications to this type of diet include disorders in fat metabolism, porphyria, and inability to maintain adequate nutrition. The classic ketogenic diet is often initiated during inpatient admission to allow for stricter clinical and laboratory monitoring as ketosis is reached.[770] The patient is monitored by a neurologist and a dietician with laboratory investigations at regular intervals. Patients then test urine ketones at home several times per week. Some of the adverse effects of a ketogenic diet include gastrointestinal symptoms (abdominal pain, constipation, diarrhea), hyperlipidemia, hypoglycemia, growth failure, severe metabolic acidosis, nephrolithiasis, pancreatitis, liver transaminitis, and osteopenia.[771] Cardiac abnormalities are rare but serious; there have been reports of cardiomyopathy and prolonged QT interval with some cases related to selenium deficiency.[771]

With the resurgence of interest in ketogenic diets, the pediatric anesthesiologist is likely to encounter children presenting for various diagnostic and surgical procedures. Case reports and series have been published describing the perioperative management of children on ketogenic diets for procedures of varying lengths.[772–776] All of these publications emphasize the importance of (1) continuing ketosis, (2) avoiding medications with high carbohydrate content, and (3) monitoring the patient's serum glucose, electrolytes, and pH throughout the perioperative period (Table 2.22).

TABLE 2.22	Recommendations for the Perioperative Management of Children on a Ketogenic Diet

Preoperative Preparation
1. Consult with neurologist regarding nutritional status, efficacy of diet, and concurrent anticonvulsant therapy and side effects
2. Laboratory testing: CBC, comprehensive metabolic panel
3. Avoid prolonged fasting to decrease the risk of hypoglycemia
4. Avoid administration of carbohydrate-containing medications and intravenous fluids
5. Measure preoperative fasting serum glucose on the day of surgery
6. Avoid preoperative sedation with carbohydrate-containing oral midazolam solutions. Alternatives include intranasal midazolam or dexmedetomidine.

Intraoperative Management
1. Avoid carbohydrate-containing medications
2. Avoid high doses of propofol infusions for prolonged periods secondary to the risk of propofol infusion syndrome
3. Use isotonic crystalloid solutions (NS or LR) for volume replacement. Some authors consider LR to be relatively contraindicated; large volumes of NS result in hyperchloremic metabolic acidosis.
4. Monitor serum pH, glucose, electrolytes, and bicarbonate levels during >3 hours or major surgical procedures
5. Do not overcorrect hypoglycemia. Start with dextrose 0.25 grams/kg for serum glucose <40 mg/dL.

Postoperative Management
1. Inpatient monitoring versus same-day discharge as clinically indicated
2. Advance diet as surgically appropriate to resume a ketogenic diet; consider measuring serum or urine ketone levels

Modified from Conover ZR, Talai A, Klockau KS, Ing RJ, Chatterjee D. Perioperative management of children on ketogenic dietary therapies. *Anesth Analg.* 2020;131(6):1872-1882.

The plan for perioperative ketogenic diet management should be discussed with the patient's neurologist or nutritionist preoperatively. The anesthesiologist must carefully consider the carbohydrate content of every medication administered or the potential of the medication to cause hyperglycemia (steroids). Most oral suspensions (midazolam, ibuprofen, and acetaminophen) contain carbohydrate.[777,778] The choice of intravenous fluid is important. Lactated Ringer's solution theoretically could risk losing ketosis through gluconeogenesis and therefore, is relatively contraindicated[779]; normal saline is preferred. However, large volumes of normal saline carry the risk of developing a hyperchloremic metabolic acidosis. Glucose or carbohydrates may also be present in blood and blood products, although the impact may be limited.[780]

SICKLE CELL DISEASE

Whenever a child presents with either sickle cell disease or sickle cell trait, the anesthetic and postanesthetic management must be modified (see also Chapters 8 and 10). It is important to obtain a detailed family history, and if the child has not been previously tested, a sickle preparation should be obtained; this is especially important for children not born in the United States who may not have had neonatal screening. If a sickle test is positive and the surgery is elective, then surgery should be postponed pending hemoglobin electrophoresis to delineate the nature of the hemoglobinopathy more carefully. It must be emphasized that the status of hydration and oxygenation is critical for all children with sickle cell disease or trait. Preoperatively oral hydration up to 2 hours before surgery is encouraged. If the surgery is delayed and fasting is prolonged, intravenous fluids should be administered. A secure intravenous route with hydration of at least 1.5 times maintenance is recommended well into the postoperative period, especially after procedures in which ileus may result. Meticulous attention to detail to ensure stable cardiovascular and ventilatory status establishes adequate oxygenation to prevent sickling. Pulse oximetry is of particular value in managing these children by providing an early warning of desaturation. Children with hemoglobin SC are especially at risk because they have a relatively normal hemoglobin level yet are extremely vulnerable to sickling. Further recommendations regarding management of these children, including indications for preoperative transfusion to bring the hemoglobin concentration to 10 g/dL or exchange transfusions to decrease the percentage of hemoglobin S, are discussed in Chapter 8; continued oxygen therapy for 24 to 48 hours is recommended.

Acknowledgment

We wish to thank Marissa Vadi, and Zeev N. Kain for their prior contributions to this chapter.

ANNOTATED REFERENCES

American Society of Anesthesiologists Physical Status (ASA PS) Classification for Pediatric Patients. Available at: https://www.asahq.org/standards-and-guidelines/asa-physical-status-classification-system.
A new standard and guideline that includes the description of pediatric patients ASA Physical Status Classification.

Coté CJ, Posner KL, Domino KB. Death or neurologic injury after tonsillectomy in children with a focus on obstructive sleep apnea: Houston, we have a problem! *Anesth Analg.* 2014;118:1276-1283.
Identifies factors leading to deaths or neurologic injury after tonsillectomy caused by apparent apnea in children. Children with severe obstructive sleep apnea may have heightened analgesic and respiratory sensitivity to opioids. Respiratory monitoring continued throughout first- and second-stage recovery, as well as on the ward during the first postoperative night, reduces adverse events.

Davidson AJ, Morton NS, Arnup SJ, et al. Apnea after awake regional and general anesthesia in infants—do we have an answer? *Anesthesiology.* 2015;123:38-54.
This multicenter, multinational study comparing general anesthesia with spinal anesthesia (the GAS study) for former preterm and full-term infants found no difference in the incidence of apnea in the general anesthesia compared with the regional anesthesia group. The incidence and severity of apnea were lower in the first 30 minutes in the PACU following spinal anesthesia compared with general anesthesia.

Frykholm P, Disma N, Andersson H, et al. Pre-operative fasting in children. A guideline from the European Society of Anaesthesiology and Intensive Care. *Eur J Anaesthesiol.* 2022;39:4-25. Lerman J. New ESAIC fasting guidelines for clear fluids in children. Much ado about nothing or is it? *Eur J Anaesthesiol.* 2022;39:639-641.
Discussion for recommendation for reducing clear fluid fasting to 1 hour and breast milk fasting to 3 hours.

Jones LJ, Craven PD, Lakkundi A, et al. Regional (spinal, epidural, caudal) versus general anaesthesia in preterm infants undergoing inguinal herniorrhaphy in early infancy. *Cochrane Database Syst Rev.* 2015;(6):CD003669.
The review found "no difference in the effect of spinal compared to general anesthesia on the overall incidence of postoperative apnea, bradycardia, oxygen saturation, need for postoperative analgesics or respiratory support."

Committee on Standards and Practice Parameters, Apfelbaum JL, Connis RT, et al. Practice Advisory for Preanesthesia Evaluation: an updated report by the American Society of Anesthesiologists Task Force on Preanesthesia Evaluation. *Anesthesiology.* 2012;116(3):522-538.
An updated practice advisory for preanesthesia evaluation including preoperative testing based on "analysis of expert opinion, clinical feasibility data, open forum commentary, and consensus surveys."

Schwengel DA, Sterni LM, Tunkel DE, Heitmiller ES. Perioperative management of children with obstructive sleep apnea. *Anesth Analg.* 2009;109:60-75.
An excellent review article on the diagnosis, treatment, and anesthetic management of children with obstructive sleep apnea syndrome.

Taghizadeh N, Davidson A, Williams K, et al. Autism spectrum disorder (ASD) and its perioperative management. *Paediatr Anaesth.* 2015;25:1076-1084.
An excellent review article surveying the literature on autism spectrum disorder and its perioperative management.

Tait AR, Malviya S, Voepel-Lewis T, et al. Risk factors for perioperative adverse respiratory events in children with upper respiratory tract infections. *Anesthesiology.* 2001;95:299-306.
Several risk factors for perioperative adverse respiratory events in children were identified: use of an endotracheal tube (<5 years of age), history of prematurity, history of reactive airway disease, paternal smoking, surgery involving the airway, presence of copious secretions, and nasal congestion.

Wang Z, May SM, Charoenlap S, et al. Effects of secondhand smoke exposure on asthma morbidity and health care utilization in children: a systemic review and meta-analysis. *Ann Allergy Asthma Immunol.* 2015;115:396-401.
This review and meta-analysis found that children with asthma and secondhand smoke exposure are "nearly twice as likely to be hospitalized with asthma exacerbation and more likely to have lower pulmonary function test results."

A complete reference list can be found online at Elsevier eBooks+.

Ethical Issues in Pediatric Anesthesiology

DAVID B. WAISEL AND ALYSSA M. BURGART

Implicit and Explicit Bias
Informed Consent
The Informed Consent Process
Special Situations in Pediatric Informed Consent
The Impaired Parent
End-of-Life Issues
Forgoing Potentially Life-Sustaining Treatment

Improving Communication in Pediatric Intensive Care Units
Organ Donation After Circulatory Death
Clinical and Academic Practice Issues
Pediatric Research
Managing Potential Conflicts of Interest
Physician Obligations, Advocacy, and Good Citizenship
The Ethics Consultation Service

CLINICIANS MUST TAKE SERIOUSLY "the experience, perspective, and power of children".[1] Clinicians should treat every child and family with the grace and consideration with which they would want their own child and family treated. Taking the experience of children seriously means involving interested children in developmentally appropriate decision making. Clinicians should not solicit a child's views without intending to consider them. *Pro forma* solicitations, those taken merely as a courtesy, are harmful.

Treating every child with dignity and respect means taking time to allow premedication to work, even if it leads to criticism for a delayed anesthesia start time. It means using names and pronouns that patients and parents provide. It means rigorously following sterile practice protocols for central lines. It means patiently explaining anesthetic options to the parents as many times as needed.

Bioethics helps motivated physicians to identify and resolve ethical dilemmas. Solving ethical dilemmas is not solely a matter of being moral or ethical. Consider a child with a mild or early upper airway respiratory infection. Usually the surgery would be postponed but suppose the child has missed two previous surgical dates because of an unstable home situation. The clinician must determine what is in the child's best interest by balancing the risks of proceeding with those of not proceeding, the duty to ensure that the child receives necessary health care, the weight to be given to the parent's (or surrogate's) consent to proceed, and the duty to "do no harm." Mindful clinicians will seek to identify lurking conflicts of interest in considering whether to proceed.

Implicit and Explicit Bias

Implicit and explicit bias against individuals based on their race, disability, gender, sexual orientation, and weight remain pervasive elements in modern society, negatively impacting patients, their families, and health care workers.[2] While well-meaning clinicians may believe they are not biased against their patients or co-workers, the evidence demonstrates that bias exists in the practice of health care, including pediatric anesthesia.[3–5] Persistent evidence of health inequities demonstrate the need for critical evaluation and reassessment of biases, not only by individuals, but through

systematic education and training. The pain and anxiety experienced by Black and Hispanic children in the USA, for example, has been shown to be systematically under treated compared with White children.[6,7] A recent study of adult physicians demonstrated that despite caring for patients with disabilities, only 40% of physicians were confident they could provide the same quality of care to patients with disabilities, and only 56% claimed to welcome patients with disabilities into their practice.[8] Despite gender-affirming care being the most effective intervention to prevent suicide in gender-diverse adolescents, some clinicians refuse to provide medically indicated treatments.[9]

Such beliefs among physicians likely contribute to persistent health inequities among already marginalized communities. The just care of our patients requires that these beliefs be systematically addressed across the practice of health care to minimize or eliminate their negative effects.

Informed Consent

The American Academy of Pediatrics (AAP) bases pediatric informed consent on assent, informed permission, and the best interest standard.[1]

THE INFORMED CONSENT PROCESS

Assent: The Role of the Patient

Although most children cannot legally consent to medical care, children should share in decision making to the extent that their development permits (Table 3.1). As children grow older, participation in decision making should increase, depending on both their maturity and the consequences involved in the decision.

School-age children are developing decision-making capacity, so anesthesiologists should seek both informed permission from the parent and assent and participatory decision making from the child. School-age children can use logic and reason and are able to define and relate multiple aspects of a situation. Such situations may include whether to sedate a 6-year-old before an inhalation induction, whether to use an inhalation or intravenous induction of anesthesia in an 8-year-old, and whether to insert an epidural in a 12-year-old.

TABLE 3.1	Graduated Involvement of Minors in Medical Decision Making[a]	
Age	**Decision-Making Capacity**	**Techniques**
<6 years	None	Best interests standard
6–12 years	Developing	Informed permission/Informed assent
13–18 years	Mostly developed	Informed assent/Informed permission
Mature minor doctrine	Developed, as legally determined by a judge, for a specific decision. Although particulars vary by state, the mature minor doctrine in general requires adolescents to be at least 14 years old, to demonstrate decision-making capacity, and tends to permit decisions of lesser risk.	Informed consent
Minor Consent Laws	In some states, law allows minors to make certain medical decisions solely based on age, requiring no judicial involvement. Such decisions may include reproductive health services, mental health services, emergency medical services, and work up to diagnose child abuse.	Informed consent
Emancipated minor	Developed as determined by statutes defining eligible situations (e.g., being married, in the military, economically independent).	Informed consent

[a]This broad outline should be viewed as a guide. Specific circumstances should be taken into consideration.

Many adolescents 14 years of age and older can use abstract thought, apply complex reasoning, foresee outcomes, simultaneously evaluate multiple options, and understand concepts such as probability. Although some adolescents have cognitive abilities similar to those of adults, adolescents may be hindered by insufficient psychosocial and emotional development and they may not have developed a reasonably stable set of values.[10] Anesthesiologists should try to fulfill the ethical requirements of consent while obtaining assent. Situations involving these aspects include obtaining consent from a 16-year-old and their guardian for a sedated thoracic epidural placement for a pectus repair. In many jurisdictions, adolescent patients have the legal right to independently consent to some or all medical care.[11] Pediatric anesthesiologists must be aware of these rights and ensure they preserve patient autonomy, confidentiality, and other Health Insurance Portability and Accountability Act protections (HIPAA; US Department of Health and Human Services 1996).

Informed Permission, the Best Interest Standard, and the Harm Threshold Standard

Parents have traditionally acted as the surrogate decision makers for their children, and legally given consent. However, surrogate consent does not fulfill the spirit of consent, which is based on obtaining an individualized autonomous decision from the patient receiving the treatment. The American Academy of Pediatrics has suggested that the proper role for the surrogate decision maker is to provide *informed permission*.[1] Informed permission has the same requirements as informed consent, but it recognizes that the doctrine of informed consent cannot apply.

The *best interest standard* requires decision makers to select the objectively best care. It acknowledges that the cornerstone of informed consent, the right to self-determination, is inapplicable when it is impossible to know or surmise from previous interactions a child's likely preference or future preference. Using this standard requires determining (1) who will make the decision and (2) what is the best care. The difficulties arise in assuming that there is always one best choice, because if there is, it should not matter who makes the decision. In our society, acceptable decision making is broadly defined, and reasonable people may disagree regarding a subjective "best" decision. Parents capable of participating in the

decision-making process are the appropriate primary decision makers because of society's respect for the concept of the family and the assumption that parents care greatly for their children. Although a child's preferences cannot be known, it is reasonable to assume that because children will incorporate some of the parents' values as they mature, parental values are a good first approximation for the child's future values. A few anesthesiologists have questioned the presumption that parents are the best decision makers.[12] Objections center on the legitimacy of the parents' knowledge of the preferences of the child's future self. Although these concerns are theoretically interesting and help clinicians understand the complexities of the best interest standard, the standard is that parents or legal guardians have extensive leeway in determining what is in their child's best interest.

The best interest of a child can be defined by what choices fall outside the range of acceptable decision making. Criteria to make this determination include the extent of harm to the child from the intervention or its absence, the likelihood of success, and the overall risk-to-benefit ratio.

The best interest standard can guide treatment among acceptable options and determine the limits of parental decision-making authority, but the best interest standard can be indeterminate, particularly for the decision to attempt to limit parental authority. Given the broad reluctance to override parents, limiting parental authority is a high-stakes decision.

Some suggest using a *harm threshold standard* rather than a best interest standard to determine whether to limit parental authority. The standard for whether a decision exceeds the harm threshold is if a parental decision threatens the health and safety of the child, which is a "lower standard" than whether the decision is one of the "best" options. This harm threshold is a standard like the one in assessing for child maltreatment. Whether this concept of harm threshold is a new cognitive approach or is already used in determining best interest depends in large part about how the borders of acceptable decision making are established; some clinicians may use the harm threshold in determining acceptable decision making and others may not.[13–17]

The harm threshold standard needs further clarification. It may not help clarify the best interest standard and it may not be useful in court, given the inconsistency in how courts assess cases.[18,19]

Nonetheless, at the very least, it provides another conceptual way of evaluating whether a treatment is outside acceptable boundaries.

Communication

While communication is a daily, vital skill set in the effective practice of medicine, few anesthesiologists receive formal training in effective communication.[20] Rather than rely on a rote informed consent process, anesthesiologists should seek to satisfy the needs of the decision makers by meeting their information and decision-making needs. This approach to shared decision making may be referred to as patient-centered, family-centered, and/or relationship-centered communication. Patients and surrogates differ in the extent to which they prefer to receive information and to participate in decision making.[21,22] In general, 10% to 15% of patients prefer less information than their peers but the majority want some form of shared decision making.[23]

The consent conversation with a parent and children who have a very limited understanding of anesthesia and have no significant health concerns will necessarily differ from that with a family in which the members have experienced multiple anesthetics, have chronic health conditions, or have previously experienced perioperative complications. Once the preoperative assessment is complete, asking the patient for their agenda increases the likelihood a physician will understand the relevant concerns and more effectively address them.[23] One approach is to ask the patient and guardian, *"What questions or worries do you have today about anesthesia?"* Patients and guardians may have completely different concerns, both of which are relevant to the consent/assent process.

Addressing emotional cues is vital to the informed consent process and the relationship among the anesthesiologist, patient, and guardian.[24] By cultivating skills in empathy, physicians can identify and respond to strong emotions that negatively affect cognition. Increasing our response to emotions improves patients' ability to retain information.[25]

Performing patient-centered, family-centered, and/or relationship-centered informed consent requires communication of the anesthesiologist's opinion/recommendation along with an explanation of the supporting reasons. With this information, the decision makers are better able to determine which anesthetic approach, on balance, provides the most desired benefits.

Anesthesiologists should inform families about matters that the anesthesiologist feels must be communicated, about options that affect the perioperative experience (e.g., regional versus general anesthesia),[26] and then ask whether the decision makers wish to know more. By being attentive to the words, actions, and emotional cues of the decision makers, anesthesiologists can tailor the process effectively.

Decision makers often overrate the extent of their knowledge about risks and benefits.[27] We can increase the likelihood of the decision makers having sufficient knowledge by modifying practices. For example, informed consent documents often use poorly formatted, dense, incomprehensible text written at too high a reading level for most decision makers.[27,28] Straightforward language written at an eighth-grade reading level (verified using the Flesch-Kincaid grade level) with reader-friendly formatting permits better understanding and thus better decision making about risk, benefits, and options.[29] By assessing patient/guardian understanding using techniques such as Ask-Tell-Ask and Teach-back, clinicians can ensure that the information they believe they have conveyed was received and processed effectively.[30,31]

Patients and guardians may have difficulty understanding quantitative aspects of risk. Risks should be presented as absolute data (e.g., occurs 10% of time) rather than relative data compared with other treatments (e.g., decreases the risk by 50%).[32,33] Some decision makers may understand frequencies better, so it is wise to include both absolute and frequency data. For example, the statement *"If she has regional anesthesia, she has a 20% chance of postoperative vomiting, which means 2 of 10 people will have postoperative vomiting, and if she has general anesthesia, she has a 40% chance of postoperative vomiting, which is 4 of 10 people will have postoperative vomiting. That means that 20 more people of 100 will have postoperative vomiting if we use general anesthesia"* is better than *"She has a 100% more likely chance of postoperative vomiting with general anesthesia as compared with regional anesthesia."* Pictorial representations improve understanding. In this example, a graphic may be a picture of 10 people, with regional anesthesia having 2 people in one color and general anesthesia having an additional 2 people in a different color, showing the increased risk.

Risk perceptions may be affected by whether risks or benefits are presented last.[33] For example, oncology patients gave more weight to the last topic discussed, even though risks and benefits were presented in the same conversation.[34] Table 3.2 lists recommendations on communications.

Informed Refusal

The requirements to achieve an informed refusal of a procedure are like the requirements for informed consent such that decision makers should be substantially well versed about the risks, benefits, and alternatives before declining. When parents refuse what clinicians believe is necessary care for a child who cannot participate in the decision-making process, clinicians may invoke the best interest standard or incorporate the harm threshold standard. This situation is more complicated when the child expresses significant decision-making capacity and refuses nonemergent procedures.[35–37] Anesthesiologists should respect the right of children

TABLE 3.2	Recommendations for Risk Communication to Patients[30,31,33]
1.	Ask the patient and guardian what worries and questions they have about anesthesia. Use these concerns to set an agenda for the consent conversation.
2.	Track and respond to emotional cues from the family. This reduces cognitive load and improves information retention.
3.	Consider presenting only the information that is most critical to the patient's or parents' decision making, even at the expense of completeness.
4.	Use language at the eighth-grade level to improve understanding of written and oral communications. Always use an interpreter when participants do not have a shared language.
5.	Present data using absolute risks and frequencies.
6.	Use pictorial recommendations to communicate choices and statistics when appropriate.
7.	The order in which risks and benefits are presented may affect risk perceptions. The last topic presented has more weight in decision making.
8.	Recognize that comparative risk information (e.g., the average person's risk) is persuasive as well as informative.
9.	Assess understanding using Ask-Tell-Ask and Teach-backs (e.g., a medical procedure is explained and then it is validated that the child/family clearly understand what was told to them).

(typically those over the age of 10 years who are cognitively intact) not to assent to a procedure, and they should not coerce the child to proceed. In children, particularly adolescents, the distinction between persuasion and coercion is critical. *Persuasion,* the act of using argument and reason to influence a patient's decision, is appropriate. *Coercion,* the outright use of a credible threat, manipulation, or misleading information, is not acceptable and contributes to patient harm. Achieving the child's assent may necessitate further discussions with the child, parents, and other providers, and such discussions may best take place away from the operating room.

Consider a 15-year-old girl who is scheduled for an elective knee arthroscopy. The day before the procedure, she gave assent, and her parents gave informed permission for anesthesia and surgery. She is now crying in the preoperative area and refusing to cooperate. Rather than forcibly or surreptitiously sedating her, the anesthesiologist should discuss her concerns. If she is unable to discuss the issues, the anesthesiologist should consider removing her from the area and giving her time to regain composure before readdressing the situation. Simple actions often allow the situation to be resolved. If the withdrawal of assent was in part related to anxiety, the adolescent may assent to receiving ample premedication before returning to the holding area. Anesthesiologists must obtain her assent before administering the sedation, however, and not simply assume that forceful or surreptitious administration is justified.[38]

Legal Matters Related to Disclosure

The "reasonable person" standard—the legal standard for most of the United States, Canada, and other countries—requires that the information disclosed be sufficient to satisfy a hypothetical reasonable person. This standard does not define exactly what information should be given, and it does not consider the patient's desires and needs. The "subjective person" standard suggests that informed consent should be matched to the wants and needs of the decision makers. Although this patient-centered (or family-centered) consent better fulfills the spirit of informed consent, its ambiguity makes it difficult to use as a legal standard.

It is rare to be found liable for informed consent in malpractice issues. The standard for being liable is that there is a duty, a breach of that duty, and a harm directly related to the breach of the duty. Liability in informed consent requires that the information not shared would have affected the patient's choices. Forming a bond with the parents is more effective in reducing malpractice lawsuits.[39]

"Doctor, If This Were Your Child, What Would You Do?"

Clinicians should respond to requests for advice by using medical facts to explain how different paths support specific values so that decision makers can choose the most concordant path.[40–42] However, the question, *"If this were your child, what would you do?"* can be asked for a number of different reasons, forcing clinicians to put the question into a broader context. Do not duck this question; attempting to evade this question may frustrate and confuse decision makers.

For example, parents may be declaring that they are having difficulty comprehending the overwhelming information and need help making a reasonable decision. They may be asking what would give their child the best chance of getting better. In this situation, clinicians should explain the reasons and values underlying their personal choice. Or parents may be looking for support that they are making the right choice in an untenable situation. Clinicians should answer with their best judgment if they agree with the family. If they disagree, clinicians should lend support through comments such as *"Other parents in the same situation have made the same choice,"* or by acknowledging that it is normal to feel uncertain.[41] If the family persists in asking what they should do, clinicians may wish to acknowledge that their choice might have been different. Clinicians should emphasize, however, that parental values are more valid than clinician values when choosing for their own child.

Parents may be asking for help in making a life-altering decision. One approach to this question is to offer a process for answering the question (e.g., *"I would talk with the chaplain"*). Clinicians should feel comfortable admitting that they are unable to determine what they would do if in the same situation. Honesty reinforces the difficulty of the decision for the parents.

Disclosure and Apology of Medical Errors

Medical errors and other adverse events are important complications in health care. Ideally, all errors and complications would be avoidable, but we know they will occur in the practice of anesthesiology. Hiding medical errors and complications is indecent and breaches informed consent.[43] Physicians may avoid appropriate disclosure and apology due to a fear of consequences, inadequate support, limited trust in the institution, and lack of education.[44–48] Forthrightly disclosing medical errors, although upsetting, often strengthens the patient–physician relationship.[48,49] Learning about a hidden medical error destroys trust and may trigger legal action.

Although disclosures of errors are premised as legal evidence, physician apologies or sympathetic comments often are prohibited as legal evidence of wrongdoing.[49–51] Apologizing may influence whether patients pursue legal action and whether such action is successful.[50,52] Sincere apologies and subsequent redress to prevent future occurrences improves the patient–physician relationship, mitigating the communication problems that lead to legal action.[53]

Physicians without expertise in disclosure and apology often botch the process. Such clinicians should consider reaching out to experts in risk management and/or ethics, to gather timely advice. Disclosure is a process over time. Initial disclosure should take place as soon as possible after an event and should center on the medical implications. Do not speculate about cause or fault. When disclosing, it is wise to bring along an appropriate colleague who can help with the disclosure by providing psychological support for the patient and family. Soon thereafter, a specific, permanent liaison to the family should be identified. The liaison should be available to arrange meetings, explain the results of the investigation into the cause of the event, and describe plans to prevent future events. The liaison should be trained and experienced in apology and disclosure (e.g., a colleague in risk management).

An apology expresses regret or sorrow. Sincere apologies followed by consistent actions are priceless; insincere apologies are costly. It is always appropriate to apologize for the adverse effects of an event and although the standard teaching is that physicians should not assume responsibility for an event before an investigation is performed, it seems bizarre to dissemble about clear errors. To evade responsibility (e.g., "Somehow one drug was given when another was intended") for a clear error mocks the apology.

Different strategies are being tested to improve disclosure and apology. An approach called "disclosure, apology, and offer" shows promise.[54] Patients indicate their interest in an apology process which includes: acknowledgment of the event, expression of remorse, offer to repair damages, and plan to protect future patients from similar harm.[53] Open disclosure, prompt and fair compensation, and a vigorous defense of acceptable care leads to a transparency that reduces adversarial relationships, contributes to patient safety, and curtails legal action and costs.[54–56] Success in this program requires aligning of incentives of the clinician and hospital system. Differing incentives, such as whether to settle or not, lead to distrust and dooms the program.

SPECIAL SITUATIONS IN PEDIATRIC INFORMED CONSENT
Confidentially for Adolescents
The obligation to maintain confidentiality requires clinicians to protect patient information from unauthorized and unnecessary disclosure.[57] Confidentiality is necessary for an open flow of information.[58–60] Clinicians enhance trust by interviewing the adolescent in private, acknowledging the adolescent's concerns about confidentiality, and keeping promises. Emancipated and mature minors have a right to complete confidentiality. For other adolescents, if maintaining confidentiality entails minimal harm, clinicians should encourage adolescents to be forthright with parents but respect their decision not to be. If maintaining confidentiality may result in serious harm to the adolescent, clinicians may be ethically justified in notifying the parents. State laws vary in their extent of requirements, and anesthesiologists must be aware of these requirements to avoid inadvertent confidentiality violations and patient harm. The implementation of the 21st century CURES Act and OpenNotes (rapid access to electronic medical documentation) that ensures interoperability and information sharing, poses unique risks to adolescent confidentiality.[61] Medical records may contain information that only the adolescent is legally entitled to access, and must be appropriately designated to prevent inadvertent disclosure to parents.

Pregnancy Testing in Adolescents
Anesthesiologists face confidentially issues when an adolescent has a pregnancy test before anesthesia. Given the principles of confidentiality, it is ethically appropriate to inform only the adolescent of the result (positive or negative).[62,63] Because locales may statutorily prohibit sharing pregnancy information with anyone other than the adolescent (without their permission), anesthesiologists must share this information with the adolescent without disclosing to parents.[64] Anesthesiologists should consider involving a pediatrician, gynecologist, and/or a social worker with expertise in adolescent issues in the disclosure of a positive pregnancy test.

Matters become more complex if the clinicians and adolescent believe the case should be postponed, and the adolescent chooses not to inform their parents about a positive pregnancy test.[65] Anesthesiologists must be careful not to inadvertently inform the parents of the pregnancy test while postponing anesthesia and surgery. Nor should anesthesiologists betray the adolescent by saying, *"The case is postponed. If you want to know why, ask your child."* Although such a statement is factually true and within the letter of the law of confidentiality, terse obliqueness scorns the spirit of confidentially.

Some anesthesiologists may have an understandable desire to tell the parents or guardian. But we would suggest that such clinicians may be too narrowly applying their own experiences and expectations. Not all parents are wise and gentle, and not all homes are safe and healthy. Confidentiality statutes specifically address concerns about child abuse in pregnant adolescents.

The extent to which anesthesiologists should protect the adolescent's confidentiality is debatable, but the need to protect

patient safety is not. The use of more active deception, although less desirable, may be appropriate and necessary to protect the patient from the harms of parental disclosure. It is rare to condone deception.[66,67] Deception should not be undertaken without serious reservations. But, under certain circumstances, the obligation to the patient may supersede prohibitions on deception. At times, the harms of not deceiving outweigh the harms of deceiving. Successful deception avoids initiating unnecessary diagnostic evaluations or treatment and does not unduly worry parents. For example, do not attribute the delay to *"hearing a new murmur."* Vague, unremarkable reasons such as *"an oncoming cold"* are best.

The Adolescent and Abortion
Even though pediatric patients who are pregnant may be statutorily or by practice emancipated, numerous states require some form of parental involvement, such as parental consent or notification, before an elective abortion.[68] The rights to an abortion for any reason (e.g., maternal risks) varies[69] (https://reproductiverights.org/maps/worlds-abortion-laws/). Whether parents need to be informed about the pregnancy or for the request for an abortion in any specific country also varies. In the USA, if a state requires parental involvement, the ability of the minor to circumvent this regulation by seeking relief from a judge, known as *judicial bypass,* may be available. Requirements and enforcement of statutes vary from state to state in the USA.[68,70] The need for parental involvement in a minor's planned abortion is not always legally straightforward, and it may be best to consult with hospital counsel in determining these issues. Although this is an area in which honorable people disagree, both the American Academy of Pediatrics and the American Medical Association have affirmed the rights to *judicial bypass.*[70,71]

Children of Jehovah's Witnesses
Jehovah's Witnesses, although generally accepting medicine and medical interventions, interpret biblical scripture as prohibiting transfusion therapy because blood holds the *"life force"* and anyone who takes blood will be *"cut off from his people"* and not earn eternal salvation.[72–74] For adults, it is a *"matter of conscience"* whether they accept transfusion products. Adults may refuse potentially life-sustaining transfusion therapy as an informed decision about the risks and benefits of transfusion in the setting of their personal goals and values. However, based on the obligations of the state to protect the interests of minors, courts have uniformly intervened when parents desire to refuse transfusion therapy on behalf of their children. Based on the mature minor doctrine, older adolescents who are able to articulate significant decision-making capacity and maturity have been permitted to refuse potentially life-sustaining transfusion therapy.[11] Most clinicians start considering this option when the patient is 16 years of age, but younger children have been permitted to refuse potentially life-sustaining transfusion therapy.[75]

Obtaining informed permission and assent for the care of a ward of a Jehovah's Witness should address transfusion therapy. For non-urgent procedures, patients with underlying anemia should be referred to their pediatrician or a pediatric hematologist, to ensure they are optimized for invasive procedures to reduce the risk of transfusion. The Jehovah's Witness organization hosts a site for clinicians caring for patients who refuse transfusions, which includes selected case reports and research studies supporting the avoidance of blood products. When clinicians are aware of and have reviewed these resources, patients and their families sometimes feel more convinced of a clinicians' dedication to reduce the risk of transfusion.[76] Jehovah's Witness families sometimes present with a church-appointed hospital liaison to provide religious support for patients and serve as a resource for clinicians with questions about how to best support Witness members. Clinical information should only ever be discussed with liaisons when the patient or decision maker has given their permission to do so.

Anesthesiologists should clarify what therapy is acceptable. Synthetic colloid solutions, dextran, erythropoietin, desmopressin, and preoperative iron are usually acceptable. Note that erythropoietin is available in two forms: lyophilized and dissolved in saline with trace concentrations of albumin (to prevent adherence of erythropoietin to the glass ampoule). Jehovah's Witnesses who accept albumin will accept either formulation, whereas those who refuse albumin should be offered the lyophilized formulation. If erythropoietin is planned, the child should be pretreated with oral iron and Vitamin C for several weeks to ensure adequate iron stores when the bone marrow is stimulated to produce reticulocytes. Some Jehovah's Witnesses accept the removal and return of blood in a continuous loop (e.g., cell saver blood, acute normovolemic hemodilution) without interruption. Anesthesiologists should consider the risks and benefits of anesthetic approaches (regional anesthesia, tolerable degree of hypotension), management of anticoagulation (intraoperative antifibrinolytic agents, recombinant activated factor VII, coagulation factor concentrates, desmopressin), and establish the acceptable lower threshold for anemia before surgery. Thromboelastography can be useful intraoperatively to assess coagulopathies.

No matter how much preparation is completed, the family should understand that in a life-threatening situation, the anesthesiologist will seek a court order authorizing the administration of life-sustaining blood. When the likelihood of requiring blood is substantial or the local judiciary is not very familiar with case law for Jehovah's Witnesses, the anesthesiologist may choose to obtain a court order in advance of the operation.

A common concern is the sudden need for an emergent transfusion in a healthy child undergoing a low-risk procedure. In emergencies where the child's life is believed to be at risk, based on the obligation to protect children, anesthesiologists should take the legally correct and ethically appropriate action to protect the child by transfusing blood without a court order. A court order may then be sought if desired. Some hospital systems allow for a bypass of the court order by utilizing a special consent document that allows parents/guardians to acknowledge the legal limitations of their ability to refuse blood products for a minor. Many Jehovah's Witness families are aware of these limitations and primarily want their beliefs documented, so that it is clear they have not directly consented to blood transfusion.

Clinicians may wonder if they should change their transfusion triggers for a child of a Jehovah's Witness. It may be appropriate for clinicians to delay transfusion as compared with their usual practices to honor the parents' preferences and in recognition of our inadequate knowledge of when to transfuse. Other clinicians, while acknowledging the difficulty in knowing when to transfuse, believe it is appropriate to use their usual transfusion triggers, in the belief that the requirement is to treat this child of a Jehovah's Witness as you would treat any other child. From a communication standpoint, it is incredibly valuable to disclose to the family and document one's approach to transfusion before surgery, so that families are not surprised if a transfusion becomes necessary.

Decision makers may consider postponing a procedure that can be delayed until the child is of sufficient age and maturity to decide about transfusion therapy. The complexity is whether the delay may increase the risk or decrease the likelihood of a good outcome. This decision requires the same balancing act as for determining best interest for a child. Relevant factors include the quantitative and qualitative change in risk or benefit. Consider that it may be easier to wait on a procedure that is purely cosmetic than on a procedure for which waiting has a small chance of leading to permanent injury. If individual clinicians choose to honor the wishes of a mature minor, they must ensure the fidelity of the agreement by making certain that postoperative and on-call clinicians will also honor the mature minor's wishes.

Emergency Care

Anesthesiologists should provide necessary emergent care for minors who do not have a parent available to give legal consent.[77,78] Emergencies include problems that could cause death, disability, and the increased risk of future complications.

The right of an adolescent to refuse emergency care treatment depends on the adolescent's decision-making capacity and the resulting harm from refusal of treatment. If the harm is significant and the adolescent's rationale is decidedly short-term or filled with misunderstanding, it becomes necessary to consider whether the adolescent has sufficient decision-making capacity for this decision. In this situation, it may be appropriate to consider what is in the best interest of the adolescent. In emergency and urgent treatment, where there is lack of evidence of an informed refusal, there may be incredibly rare occasions where patients may be treated over their expressed refusal. In such a scenario, the patient should be honestly notified of what will take place, and steps should be taken to reduce the trauma of the unwanted interventions.

For example, a 15-year-old football player with a cervical fracture might refuse emergency stabilization, stating that he does not want to live life without football. Most physicians and guardians would hold that his conclusion overly values short-term implications, especially considering the suddenness of the injury, and that he should receive emergency treatment over his refusal.

THE IMPAIRED PARENT

Parents may be unable to fulfill decision-making responsibilities because of acutely impaired judgment, such as acute intoxication.[79] Clinicians have to weigh the benefits of waiting for appropriate legal consent against what is in the best interest of the child. It may be in the child's best interest to proceed with a routine procedure in the situation of an impaired parent who is unable to give legal consent. Clinicians may wish to consult legal and risk management colleagues for guidance.

End-of-Life Issues

FORGOING POTENTIALLY LIFE-SUSTAINING TREATMENT

Required Reconsideration and Perioperative Limitations on Life-Sustaining Treatment

The concept of limiting potentially life-sustaining medical treatment is the same for children as it is for adults. Decision makers choose to limit life-sustaining medical treatment because they do not consider the potential burdens worth the potential benefits.[80,81] The American Academy of Pediatrics, the American Society of Anesthesiologists, and the American College of Surgery mandate "required reconsideration" of any limitations on life-sustaining medical treatment before proceeding to the operating room.

Although the term "Do Not Resuscitate" is commonly used, the term "Life-Sustaining Medical Treatment" is increasingly common. One purpose of this shift is to emphasize that desired limitations on medical treatment are continuous rather than dichotomous. The term "potentially" is often used to modify life-sustaining medical treatment to emphasize the uncertainty about whether a therapy will be life sustaining.

Reevaluation of life-sustaining medical treatment preferences for the perioperative period starts with clarifying the patient's goals for the proposed surgery and end-of-life care (Table 3.3). Anesthesiologists should involve the patient, family, and other clinicians such as surgeons, intensivists, and pediatricians in determining what is in the best interest of the child.

Benefits of potentially life-sustaining medical treatment include an improved quality of life and prolongation of life under certain circumstances. Burdens include intractable pain and suffering, disability, and events that cause a decrement in the quality of life, as viewed by the patient.[44,82] These guidelines help in considering short- and long-term goals and putting into appropriate context specific fears such as long-term ventilatory dependency, pain, and suffering.

Legitimate procedures for a child with limitations on life-sustaining medical treatment include procedures that decrease pain, provide vascular access, enable the child to be at home, treat an urgent problem unrelated to the primary problem (e.g., appendicitis), or treat a problem that may be related but is not considered a terminal event (e.g., bowel obstruction). However, seeking these interventions does not obviate the desire to avoid potential resuscitation burdens such as need for extensive ventilator support, cognitive deficits, or physical limitations.

The goal-directed approach for perioperative limitations on life-sustaining medical treatment permits decision makers to guide therapy by prioritizing outcomes rather than procedures.

TABLE 3.3	Components of a Pediatric Perioperative Life-Sustaining Medical Treatment Discussion

- Planned procedure and anticipated benefit to child
- Advantages and opportunities of having specific, identified clinicians providing therapy for a defined period
- Likelihood of requiring resuscitation
- Reversibility of likely causes for resuscitation
- Description of potential interventions and their consequences
- Chances of successful resuscitation, including improved outcomes of witnessed arrests compared with unwitnessed arrests
- Ranges of outcomes with and without resuscitation
- Responses to iatrogenic events
- Intended and possible venues and types of postoperative care
- Postoperative timing and mechanisms for reevaluation of the limitations on life-sustaining medical treatment
- Establishment of an agreement (which may include a full resuscitation status) through a goal-directed approach
- Documentation

Adapted from Truog RD, Waisel DB, Burns JP. DNR in the OR: a goal-directed approach. *Anesthesiology.* 1999;90:289-295; and Fallat ME, Deshpande JK. Do-not-resuscitate orders for pediatric patients who require anesthesia and surgery. *Pediatrics.* 2004;114:1686-1692.
From Bosslet GT, Pope TM, Rubenfeld GD, et al. An official ATS/AACN/ACCP/ESICM/SCCM policy statement: responding to requests for potentially inappropriate treatments in intensive care units. *Am J Respir Crit Care Med.* 2015;191(11):1318-1330.

After defining desirable outcomes, decision makers ask anesthesiologists to use their clinical judgment to determine how specific interventions will affect achieving the specific goals. Predictions about the success of interventions made at the time of the resuscitation are more accurate than predictions made preoperatively when the quality and nature of the problems are unknown. Therapy may be guided by goals rather than specific procedures (as is done on the ward), because during the perioperative period children are cared for by dedicated anesthesiologists for brief, defined periods. It is helpful to define a goal-directed approach by discussing the acceptable burdens, the desirable benefits, and the likelihood of distinct outcomes. Most decision makers choose a goal-directed approach of desiring therapy if the interventions and burdens were temporary and reversible (i.e., if they could return to the present state without suffering too much).

Prior determination of acceptable postoperative life-sustaining medical treatment is less critical in pediatrics, because usually parents are available in the postoperative period to make decisions regarding therapy. Nonetheless, when a sufficiently mature child participates in discussions about life-sustaining medical treatment, anesthesiologists should ensure that the discussion incorporates the child's preferences for postoperative trials of therapy. The willingness to undergo a trial of therapy indicates a belief that the burdens of the trial (e.g., a few days of ventilator support) may be worth the benefits (e.g., extubation of the trachea) initially, but at some point, the increasing burdens may not be worth the decreasing likelihood of the benefits. Flexibly inherent in the goal-directed approach is that it promotes trials of therapy to evaluate whether said therapy achieves its desired goals. This is particularly important given our ever-changing knowledge about the outcomes of resuscitation.[83]

A time-limited trial of therapy is *"an agreement between clinicians and a patient/family to use certain medical therapies over a defined period to see if the patient's condition improves or deteriorates according to the agreed on clinical outcomes."*[84] The results of a time-limited trial can help decision makers determine whether to continue therapy or shift to comfort care measures. Knowing the results of a burdensome therapy makes withdrawing a therapy that does not achieve the identified goals more ethically stout than simply withholding the therapy and not knowing what the effects of the therapy would be.

Iatrogenic problems such as cardiac arrest do not obviate decisions to limit life-sustaining medical treatment.[85] To decision makers, the cause of the arrest is irrelevant. Decision makers care about the factors they considered in requesting limited resuscitation, including the likelihood of successful resuscitation and physical and mental status after the arrest. The benefits of continued therapy after certain types of iatrogenic arrests should be addressed as part of the perioperative discussion.[85]

The "temporary and reversible" goal-directed perioperative do not resuscitate order can be documented as *"The patient desires resuscitative efforts during surgery and in the postanesthesia care unit (PACU) only if the adverse events are believed to be both temporary and reversible, in the clinical judgment of the attending anesthesiologists and surgeons."* With the patient's permission, anesthesiologists may want to include selected family members in the reevaluation discussion to enable the best communication of the patient's preferences.

Barriers to Honoring Preferences for Resuscitation

Barriers to honoring limitations center on clinician attitudes, time pressures, and inadequate knowledge about policy, law, and ethics.[85–92] Although required reconsideration has been accepted for more than 20 years, and there has been some improvement, anesthesiologists and surgeons still have inadequate knowledge and practices about perioperative life-sustaining medical treatment.[93–95] Deficiencies include lack of knowledge about required reconsideration, infrequent preoperative determination of the presence of an advance directive, and inadequate willingness to care for patients with perioperative limitations on life-sustaining medical treatment.[96] On balance, however, it seems that the extent of knowledge and practices is institution-dependent.

Anesthesiologists may falsely believe that law or hospital policy requires full resuscitation during the perioperative period. However, any such policy would violate a patient's right to self-determination. Clinicians who act in accordance with statutory requirements are often explicitly protected from liability when they honor a child's or family's refusal of resuscitation. In an informed consent discussion, clinicians and decision makers should assess the relative risks and benefits of the procedure and anesthesia considering a risk of cardiopulmonary collapse. Given the well-established right of children and parents to refuse medical treatment and the paucity of cases finding clinicians liable for honoring limitations on life-sustaining medical treatment, the risk of liability for honoring an appropriately documented perioperative limitation on life-sustaining medical treatment is not substantive and is likely to be less than the risk of not honoring limitations.

Physician Orders for Life-Sustaining Treatment

Physician orders for life-sustaining treatment (POLST) were designed in part to improve honoring resuscitation preferences and are becoming more common in pediatric patients. POLST has two main advantages compared with other forms of advance directives.[97] A POLST document has the advantages of being a medical order that is valid across different locations beyond hospitals and clinics, such as schools. These features will likely increase compliance with the documented preferences, particularly in terms of emergency medical treatment. The POLST document defines code status and preferences for medical interventions, typically documented as full treatment, trial of treatment, and selective treatment.[98] Although clinicians feel that POLSTs limit unwanted resuscitation and that the declared preferences are durable, some clinicians report difficulty in using the form or having it honored across locations.[99–104] Systems to optimize POLST practices require further investigation.[102,104]

Potentially Inappropriate Interventions

It is more helpful to think about potentially inappropriate interventions instead of futile treatments. An intervention is futile only if it cannot accomplish a physiologic goal. A more common and difficult dilemma is how to handle potentially inappropriate interventions. Interventions may be inappropriate when *"there is no reasonable expectation that the patient will improve sufficiently to survive outside the acute care setting, or when there is no reasonable expectation that the patient's neurologic function will improve sufficiently to allow the patient to perceive the benefits of treatment."*[105] This useful concept may be less useful to pediatric decision making given the relatively sparse specific outcome data for the very young.[106,107]

Treatments with small likelihoods of success may be considered inappropriate because of the burden to the child, cost, or uncertain benefit. Discussions about inappropriate treatment should bear in mind the goals of the treatment and the likelihood of achieving a defined result. When offering the likelihood of a result, clinicians should be clear whether the information used to form the estimation is based on intuition, clinical experience, or

rigorous scientific studies. Scoring systems that are useful for population predictions in determining potentially inadvisable care should be considered as contributory but not determinative for decision making for individuals.

Parents and clinicians may disagree about therapy for a child near the end of life. Hospitals should have defined processes to help resolve conflict about applying potentially inappropriate interventions.[108]

IMPROVING COMMUNICATION IN PEDIATRIC INTENSIVE CARE UNITS

Pediatric intensivists should emphasize interdisciplinary communication, tailor the communication style to the parents, and maximize meaningful parental participation in the child's care.[109,110] The goal is to be an empathic professional who establishes compassionate relationships with the child and family by managing emotional, informational, and care needs. In almost all conversations, clinicians should explain the meaning of the conversation in terms of overall care.

Patient-centered characteristics such as asking questions, using empathic statements, increasing the amount of parental contributions to the conversation, and focusing on psychosocial and lifestyle issues as compared with medical issues, improved parent satisfaction during family conferences.[111] When wanting to convey sympathy to patients and families, wish statements, such as *"I wish things were different"* seem effective.[112] Table 3.4 lists parental desires for communication in the intensive care unit.

ORGAN DONATION AFTER CIRCULATORY DEATH

Death may be determined by two criteria: neurologic (i.e., brain death) or circulatory. In organ procurement after a declaration of death through neurologic criteria, the child is declared dead before being brought to the operating room. The organs are then retrieved while total body homeostasis is maintained through mechanical ventilation, pharmacologic therapy, and other standard resuscitative techniques.

Concern about the limited availability of organs for transplantation has resulted in the now widely accepted concept of donation after circulatory death (DCD).[91,113,114] In donation after circulatory death procurement, the parent/guardian determines that therapy should be withdrawn based on a standard benefits and burdens assessment, the child is brought to the operating room and therapy is withdrawn. No organ procurement takes place until the child is declared dead and a specified period passes (usually 2–5 minutes). If the child dies after life-sustaining therapy is withdrawn, they are declared dead by circulatory criteria and the organs are retrieved. If they do not die within this period, palliative care is continued until death occurs. Ethical issues regarding donation after circulatory death protocols center on whether the protocols seriously alter the dying process by shifting decision making away from the best interest of the dying child and by interfering with the family's ability to be with their dying child (Table 3.5). To avoid perceived or actual conflicts of interest, anesthesiologists who participate in the withdrawal of life support are prohibited from participating in the procurement of organs.

Clinical and Academic Practice Issues

PEDIATRIC RESEARCH

The anesthesiologist Henry K. Beecher was one of the first to propose that pediatric research had different requirements compared

TABLE 3.4　Parents' Desires for Communication in the Intensive Care Units

1. **Honest and complete information** should be tailored to the parents' needs and information-receiving preferences. Comprehension of the child's potential trajectories permits better participation in care and a greater chance of appropriate end-of-life care.

2. **Ready access to staff** should include periodic scheduled informal visits to the bedside and the availability of email interactions. The goal is to provide the parents with easy and frequent opportunities to have their questions answered, with sufficient repetition and clarification of the "big picture."

3. To maximize successful **communication**, clinicians should actively assess the parents' preferences for communication and decision making. This includes considering how to relate information to parents when clinicians have different management opinions. Parents frequently recognize that there are differences between options, and some prefer to hear the range of options, whereas others prefer to hear only the recommended option.

4. **Emotional expression and support by staff** are critical to parents. To do this successfully, clinicians should adapt their style to parents' preferences. Most clinicians should adopt practices that give parents more room to control the conversation, including talking less, listening more, and tolerating silence as parents gather themselves to continue communicating.

5. Parents respond and benefit from the **relational aspects of compassion, mercy, authenticity, and integrity**. More colloquially, the relational aspect is referred to as "being there"—interacting with the parents as a caring person with feelings and emotions. For example, although some clinicians may believe it is inappropriate to show emotion, parents appreciate compassion and some level of distress at the sharing of bad news, rather than cold hard professionalism.[106]

6. **Preservation of the integrity of the parent–child relationship** means enabling parents to continue in their self-identified and prominent role as decision maker and protector. Loss of this role harms parents and may impair their ability to participate in decision making for the child.

7. **Faith and spiritual matters** are highly personal, and parents may feel uncomfortable expressing their faith in an institutional setting. Spiritual matters should be accepted and integrated into the intensive care unit practice to assist those who benefit from spiritual support.

8. **Parents' lifelong views of these events** are profoundly colored by vivid memories and strong feelings about seminal discussions. How difficult discussions are handled and the quality of the communication among clinicians and families often become the basis for the family's lifelong narrative of these events.

Modified from Meyer EC, Ritholz MD, Burns JP, Truog RD. Improving the quality of end-of-life care in the pediatric intensive care unit: parents' priorities and recommendations. *Pediatrics*. 2006;117:649-657.

TABLE 3.5　Ethical Issues Surrounding Donation After Cardiac Death (DCD)

Ethical Issue	Discussion Points
Should interventions be permitted prior to withdrawal of care?	The burdens from the interventions are not in the best interests of the child. On the other hand, the burdens of the interventions are mostly theoretical and may improve the quality of the transplanted organs.
Should withdrawal of therapy occur in the intensive care unit (ICU) or in the operating room?	Withdrawing therapy in the operating room may increase the quality of the organs transplanted. Withdrawing therapy in the ICU is likely to be less jarring to the family and more consistent with the premise of withdrawing therapy for the child's benefit. In addition, it may remove some of the awkwardness that may occur if the child does not die within the defined interval.
Who should withdraw therapy?	To be consistent with the premises of withdrawal of therapy, it should be the same person who would normally withdraw therapy from the child. Even if the decision is made to withdraw therapy in the operating room, an anesthesiologist who has not been caring for the child should not be asked to withdraw therapy because of the physical location of the event.
How long should cessation of cardiac function exist for a child to be declared dead?	Proposed times may be based on the premises of how long it would take to autoresuscitate compared with how long it would take to be resuscitated through medical intervention.
What are the contents of a good DCD policy?	Acceptable interventions before withdrawing therapy Acceptable locations of withdrawing therapy Amount of time to wait until death before forgoing procurement Which individual should withdraw therapy What to do if the family will not leave after death is declared

with adult research.[115] Pediatric research is closely examined because children are incapable of consenting to experiments and because the developing child is at greater risk for long-term harm.[116] Federal guidelines describe four categories of pediatric research, with each ascending category requiring greater scrutiny of the risk-to-benefit ratio, especially in research without therapeutic benefit for the subject (Table 3.6). Whereas obtaining the assent of the child whenever possible is important for therapeutic medical procedures, it is essential in the context of research, along with the informed permission of the parents.

Minimal Risk

Minimal risks are defined as those risks that are not greater in and of themselves than those ordinarily encountered in daily life or during the performance of routine physical or psychological examinations. Most interpret this to mean the risks encountered in daily life by healthy children, such as running in the backyard, playing sports, or riding in a car.[117–119] A less favored relative interpretation uses, as a benchmark, those risks encountered in the daily lives of children who will be enrolled in the research. In other words, if a child were living in a manner that exposed the

TABLE 3.6 | Federal Classification of Pediatric Research

1. Research not involving greater than minimal risk
   a. IRB determines minimal risk
   b. IRB finds and documents that adequate provisions are made for soliciting assent from children and permission from their parents or guardians

2. Research involving greater than minimal risk but presenting the prospect of direct benefit to the individual subject
   a. IRB justifies the risk by the anticipated benefit to the subjects
   b. The relationship of the anticipated benefit to the risk is at least as favorable as that presented by available alternative approaches
   c. Adequate provisions are made for assent and permission

3. Research that involves greater than minimal risk and no prospect of direct benefit to the individual subject but is likely to yield generalizable knowledge about the subject's disorder or condition
   a. IRB determines that the risk represents a minor increase over minimal risk
   b. The intervention or procedure presents experiences to subjects that are reasonably commensurate with those inherent in their actual or expected medical, dental, psychological, social, or educational situations
   c. The intervention or procedure is likely to yield generalizable knowledge which is of vital importance for the understanding or amelioration of the subject's disorder or condition
   d. Adequate provisions are made for assent and permission

4. Research not otherwise approvable, which presents an opportunity to understand, prevent, or alleviate a serious problem affecting the health or welfare of children

Where research is covered by numbers 3 and 4 above and permission is to be obtained from parents, both parents must give their permission unless one parent is deceased, unknown, incompetent, or not reasonably available, or when only one parent has legal responsibility for the care and custody of the child.
IRB, Institutional review board.
From United States Department of Human Services: 45 CFR 46 Subpart D. Additional Protections for Children Involved as Subjects in Research.

child to risk (e.g., undergoing repeated general anesthesia), then it would be acceptable to expose the child up to that level of risk in a study.

Individuals are poor at estimating the risk levels of activities and often correlate risk to familiarity, control of the activity, and reversibility of the potential harms. Institutional review boards may reject low-risk studies because they involve unfamiliar matters whereas they may approve studies that have excessive risks.

Minor Increase Over Minimal Risk

The pediatric research category that involves *"greater than minimal risk and no prospect of direct benefit to the individual subject but is likely to yield generalizable knowledge about the subject's disorder or condition ... which is of vital importance"*[120] is based on the idea that it is acceptable to expose a child to a "minor increase over minimal risk" under certain conditions. Parsing the regulation may help clarify this somewhat unhelpful definition. One suggestion has been that "minor increase" means that the pain, discomfort, or stress must be transient, reversible, and not severe.[121] The condition of the subject should be used to mean a set of characteristics *"that an established body of scientific or clinical evidence has shown to negatively affect children's health and well-being or to increase the risk of developing a health problem in the future."* Interpreting "condition" to include "having the potential to have the condition" permits otherwise healthy children to participate in research for diseases that they may develop (e.g., cellulitis). Vital

importance implies that the evidence supporting the relevance of the study should require a higher order of proof.

Socioeconomic Concerns and Distribution of Risk

Socioeconomically disadvantaged children living in urban areas may be overrepresented in research studies because urban academic centers in disadvantaged areas perform the majority of clinical research.[118] Children living in socioeconomically disadvantaged areas are often more affected by diseases associated with their environment, such as asthma or nutritional disorders complicated by limited access to stocked grocery stores. One could argue that this unequal burden of risk, primarily manifested by greater participation of socioeconomically disadvantaged children in research studies, is reasonable because these children are more likely to develop these diseases and therefore are more likely to benefit from the research. Most reject that view and believe that in some sense, socioeconomically advantaged patients gratuitously gain the benefits of the research without sharing the risks. The disproportionate risk borne by one segment of society compared with another likely breeches the most accepted interpretation of the core ethical value of justice.

Socioeconomically disadvantaged families may be more likely to be influenced by the small gifts offered to research participants. Aside from compensating for costs (e.g., parking vouchers), gifts should not of themselves encourage participation. The problem is that gifts that represent a small expression of gratitude for some families may provide an incentive for participation for socioeconomically disadvantaged families.[122]

Imperative for Pharmacologic Research

Through the mid-1990s, more than 70% of new molecular entities were without pediatric drug labeling. Inadequate information exposed children to age-specific adverse reactions, ineffective treatment owing to inappropriate dosing, and lack of access to new drugs because physicians tended to prescribe less effective, known medications. Inadequate research into pediatric drugs forced physicians to prescribe drugs in nonstandard ways, such as sprinkled or crushed tablets. Even when there is some pediatric labeling, there is scant labeling for children younger than 2 years of age. In 2009 a survey of a Canadian pediatric tertiary hospital found that even when comparing off-label (see later in the chapter) use with contemporary pediatric references (an unofficial and very liberal interpretation), 16% of drug administrations during the perioperative period were considered off-label. Based on a more traditional standard of the *Canadian Compendium of Pharmaceutical Specialties*, 55% of drugs administered were used off-label.[123] Neonatology and pediatric intensive care units are particularly at risk for off-label use. In a study of more than 65,000 patients, drugs that were considered to have high-risk status or high priority for study by the United States Food and Drug Administration (FDA) were used off-label in 85% of patients.[124] Off-label drugs included dexmedetomidine, dopamine, hydromorphone, lorazepam, and milrinone.

The following selective history highlights the overall intent to ensure that (1) children get the same benefits of pharmacologic advances as adults and (2) research is performed in the youngest children. Readers should also learn from this history that persistent advocacy is often required before regulatory change can be successfully obtained. In 1962 the Kefauver-Harris Amendments (passed after the thalidomide disaster) required that drug companies demonstrate safety and efficacy before marketing a drug. Because most drugs did not undergo pediatric-specific investigation, this requirement led to less pediatric labeling, with the package insert (drug label) often reading, *"Safety and efficacy have not been demonstrated for children <12 years,"* because of the expense of getting this information. In 1994 the FDA began requiring sponsors to explain why pediatric labeling cannot occur but did not require sponsors to perform pediatric studies.

The 1997 FDA Modernization Act and the 1998 Final Rule were legislative initiatives designed to gain more data from drug companies through pediatric studies in exchange for the benefit of an additional 6 months of patent exclusivity. This effort was further codified with the passage of the Best Pharmaceuticals for Children Act (BPCA) in 2002. With these requirements, the FDA now had the legal power to mandate pediatric studies if a new drug might be used in a substantial number of children, if it might provide a meaningful therapeutic benefit, or if inadequate labeling could pose significant risks. The pharmaceutical industry responded with an explosion of pediatric studies. However, the exclusivity provision did not encourage study of generic drugs or drugs with insufficient sales. Further, once exclusivity was credited for older pediatric age groups, there was no incentive to conduct studies in younger groups.

In December 2003, the Pediatric Research Equity Act (PREA) required pediatric studies for all drugs and biologic products with a new indication, new dosage form, new route, new dosing regimen, or new active ingredient. Studies need to evaluate safety, efficacy, dosing, and administration for a drug intended for use in a specific pediatric subpopulation. Studies could be waived if they were impracticable, if the therapy would be ineffective or unsafe in pediatric patients, or if there would be no meaningful therapeutic benefit over existing therapies and the moiety would not be used in a substantial number of children.

In 2012 the Food and Drug Administration Safety and Innovation Act (FDASIA) made the Best Pharmaceuticals for Children Act and Pediatric Research Equity Act permanent. The FDA Safety and Innovation Act initiated new requirements such as a Pediatric Study Plan, which included an outline of the studies including study objectives, design, statistical approach, age of patients, relevant outcomes, and a timeline. An increased focus on the youngest patients included requiring that neonates be included in studies unless the disease did not affect neonates or studies were not feasible or safe. The FDA Safety and Innovation Act offered priority review for therapies for rare pediatric diseases. Through August 2016, the FDA granted pediatric exclusivity for 217 drugs.[125] In 2014 the FDA put in similar requirements for medical devices intended for use in children. Other nations have adopted similar regulatory requirements and incentives to encourage drug and medical device research.[126,127]

MANAGING POTENTIAL CONFLICTS OF INTEREST

A *conflict of interest* is *"a set of conditions in which professional judgment concerning a primary interest (such as a patient's welfare or the validity of research) tends to be unduly influenced by a secondary interest."*[128] Because these conditions in an individual are internal, they are best characterized by describing situations that may create the potential for conflicts of interest. Focusing on potential conflicts of interest moves the concept away from attacking an individual's morals and toward more uniform definitions. Potential conflicts of interest may be induced by financial, personal, and professional benefits such as prestige, promotion, and personal gratification.[129] Anesthesiologists should be mindful of these potential conflicts and attempt to identify them to better understand the likelihood of compromised judgment.

Conducting Research

Perhaps the most powerful conflict in conducting research is the loss of equipoise that can come from originating and developing an idea. Other sources of conflict related to research center on academic promotion and reputation. Research disclosures do not help identify conflicts of interest. In one study, only 80% of physicians disclosed payments related to the research, and only 50% disclosed payments from the same company but unrelated to the product being discussed. Indirect payments were just as likely to influence behavior as direct payment.[130]

In 2009 an anesthesiologist funded by a pharmaceutical agency was accused of falsifying data that had encouraged multimodal pain therapy. Concerns of an internal reviewer brought about the internal investigation that found major irregularities in the research in the form of fraud. Major journals retracted articles. The editor of *Anesthesia and Analgesia* declared, *"We are left with a large hole in our understanding of this [multimodal pain therapy]."*[131,132] The editor of the journal called the scandal *"a tragedy"* for the profession, for patients, and for the anesthesiologist involved personally. Given that the anesthesiologist's studies were *"robust"* and influential, *"the big chunk of what people have based their [multimodal] protocol on is gone."* It is important to emphasize that the anesthesiologist's coauthors were deceived by him and were not complicit. In fact, they assisted in assessing the legitimacy of articles that were not retracted.[132] Unfortunately, that investigator was not alone in perpetrating fraud in anesthesia research, with some perpetrating a host of malfeasance of similar or greater magnitude and lasting impact as the proband.[133-136]

Conflicts of interest also come from industry support of research. To be clear, the academic–anesthesia–industry research complex is necessary to continue the rapid advancement of science. Rigorous oversight minimizes these abuses.[137] Researchers need to be involved in trial development, must have access to raw data, and must be able to publish without the company's authorization. Cozy relationships between powerful members of the local academic community and industry should be examined and brought to light to minimize influence and potential conflicts of interest.[138]

Financial relationships among physicians, researchers, hospitals, and industry are publicly available through the Open Payments program in the Sunshine Act (section 6002) of the Patient Protection and Affordable Care Act.[139] This program *"collects information about the payments drug and device companies made to physicians and teaching hospitals for things like travel, research, gifts, speaking fees and meals."*[140,141] In 2021, the Open Payments Program reported payments to 533,056 physicians valued at 3.8 billion dollars.[142] The actual benefits from the Open Payments program are unclear.[143-146]

Interaction With Industry

Interaction with industry affects clinicians' prescribing behavior, often through unconscious feelings of gratitude, obligation, or fellowship.[138,147-150] Because clinicians are mostly unaware of the social dynamic industry is creating, clinicians can legitimately assert they do not consciously adjust their clinical practice, but stealthily creating familiarity and good feelings for a product or an individual is a core competency in advertising. Consequently, it is necessary to cultivate and maintain cynicism about advertisements. Clinicians should independently evaluate information supplied by industry because they commonly overstate benefits and understate risks (Table 3.7).

Risks associated with industry misrepresentation will increase as increasing clinician workload decreases time for study. For these

TABLE 3.7	Strategies Used by Drug Companies to Influence Physicians

1. Teach salespeople subtle verbal and nonverbal techniques to influence physicians.

2. Instruct salespeople to misdirect and to dissemble when questioned about possible complications.

3. Cherry-pick which data are distributed to physicians.

4. Prohibit distribution of studies that may criticize the product. (One strategy is to classify concerning studies as background studies and then prohibit distribution of background studies.)

5. Seek "opinion leaders" to speak in favor of the product.

6. Continue the well-established gift-giving strategy to subconsciously curry favor with the physician and to develop a positive association about the product and the company.

reasons, it is instructive to look more closely at this problem. Evidence published in the 2000 Vioxx Gastrointestinal Outcomes Research (VIGOR) study indicated that rofecoxib (Vioxx) dramatically increased the rate of myocardial infarction in patients. In 2001 the FDA determined that clinicians should be made aware of the cardiovascular effects of rofecoxib, and in 2004 the drug was withdrawn from the market. Congressman Henry Waxman later wrote the following[151]:

"Merck, the manufacturer of Vioxx, ... has an excellent reputation within the drug industry and supports many products, such as vaccines, that are medically essential but not very profitable. ... Yet as we learned, even a company like Merck can direct its sales force to provide clinicians with a distorted picture of the relevant scientific evidence."

On February 7, 2001 the Arthritis Drugs Advisory Committee of the FDA voted unanimously that physicians should be made aware of VIGOR's cardiovascular results. The next day, Merck sent a bulletin to its rofecoxib sales force [which] ordered, *"do not initiate discussions on the FDA arthritis advisory committee ... Or the results of the ... VIGOR study."* It advised that if a physician inquired about VIGOR, the sales representative should indicate that the study showed a gastrointestinal benefit and then say, *"I cannot discuss the study with you."*

Merck further instructed representatives to show those doctors who asked whether rofecoxib caused myocardial infarction a pamphlet called "The Cardiovascular Card." This pamphlet, prepared by Merck's marketing department, indicated that rofecoxib was associated with 1/8 the mortality from cardiovascular causes of that found with other antiinflammatory drugs.

The Cardiovascular Card did not include any data from the VIGOR study. Instead, it presented a pooled analysis of preapproval studies, in most of which small doses of rofecoxib were used for a short period. None of these studies were designed to assess cardiovascular safety. In fact, FDA experts had publicly expressed *"serious concerns"* about using preapproval studies as evidence of the drug's cardiovascular safety: *[B]ut it would be a mistake to restrict the lessons learned to a single company. The testimony we heard indicated that Merck's marketing practices may be less aggressive and more ethical than many of its competitors."*

Production Pressure

Production pressure is *"the internal or external pressure on the anesthetist to keep the operating room schedule moving along speedily."*[152] Almost half of surveyed anesthesiologists reported seeing what they considered unsafe anesthetic practices in response to this production pressure.[153] As a consequence, anesthesiologists may not want to take the time to allow a child to ask questions about the anesthetic, to adequately premedicate an anxious child, or to engage the parents in a lengthy discussion about postponing the surgery in a child with a cold. Anesthesiologists should be cognizant of their level of skill. For example, the "routine" tonsillectomy may be beyond some anesthesiologists' ability in a child with multiple congenital deficits. Anesthesiologists have an obligation to the patient and themselves to only provide care that is within their skills and to recognize when economic and administrative pressures may induce them to do otherwise.

PHYSICIAN OBLIGATIONS, ADVOCACY, AND GOOD CITIZENSHIP

An implicit social contract obligates physicians to serve society beyond direct patient caring. Society enables medical students, physicians in training, and physicians to train, perform research, and, perhaps most importantly, learn from and with patients. In return, society expects pediatric anesthesiologists to *"manage all things pediatric anesthesia"* (Table 3.8).[154–159] Clinicians should participate in relevant community advocacy, such as reducing

TABLE 3.8	Examples of Obligations of Anesthesiologists to Participate and Advocate

Obligations of Pediatric Anesthesiologists[146–154]

Treat every child with the grace and consideration you would want for your child and family

Tailor the perioperative experience to the individual

Respond to problems that may harm children (e.g., impaired colleagues)

Practice mindfulness and critical self-reflection

Actively engage in continuing medical education

Support advancement of the science

Participate in quality improvement initiatives such as Wake Up Safe

Participate in professional organizations such as the Society for Pediatric Anesthesia and the American Academy of Pediatrics Section on Anesthesiology and Pain Medicine

Prepare future generations through teaching, mentoring, creating opportunities, and developing systems to enable anesthesiologists to fulfill these obligations

Community Advocacy and Participation

Raise public awareness about a health or social issue

Participate in public advocacy and lobbying

Work toward eliminating racial disparities in care

Encourage a medical society to act on an issue that concerns the public health

Serve in a local organization, political interest group, or political organization

Topics of particular relevance to pediatric anesthesiologists:
- Pediatric obesity
- Pediatric sedation safety in hospitals and nonhospital facilities
- Child abuse
- Health care access
- Role of subspecialty training in improving care for children

variations in pediatric care secondary to issues like race, insurance status, and language barriers.[152–154]

Individual anesthesiologists do not need to fulfill every obligation. "Units" of anesthesiologists, such as private practice groups, academic departments, and state societies, should fulfill these obligations collectively.

Participating in Patient Safety Efforts

Medical errors come from human mistakes and system flaws.[160–163] Parents in particular are interested in medical errors. In one study, 39% of parents felt obligated to be vigilant for medical errors in their child's care.[164] Clinicians have an obligation to work to reduce system flaws, including participating in quality improvement activities and data collection, following policies meant to improve care in high-risk situations (e.g., nosocomial infections), and actively engaging in policies designed to reduce medical errors, such as universal standards of patient identification.[165] Clinicians should also participate in the data collection of national and international databases.

Although clinicians may not see the big picture and therefore resent doing "extra" steps, it is vital for clinicians to accept that participation in such quality improvement programs is necessary for good patient care.[158] Surreptitiously circumventing policies may harm patients, does not permit remediation of the policy, and weakens the fidelity of the entire system, encouraging others to "make their own rules."

Clinicians also have an obligation to report potential medical errors. Although the "blame-free" approach is well touted, clinicians perceive significant barriers to honestly reporting near-misses, hindering improved patient safety. Institutional barriers center on inadequate procedures and lack of trust in the administration.[166] When clinicians believe that policies are harmful or unnecessary, they are obligated to raise these questions through appropriate channels, particularly to address institutional barriers to reporting patient safety events.

Adverse Childhood Experiences and Trauma-Informed Care

Adverse childhood experiences (ACEs) encompass experiences leading to negative physical and psychological sequelae among children and adults. Trauma-informed care (TIC) is an emerging approach calling for the evaluation, assessment, and surveillance of trauma experiences, recognizing how these experiences can impact the delivery and receipt of health care.[167] Our experiences shape the way we view and interact with the world. Many children with chronic medical conditions have experienced medical trauma at the hands of health care workers. A fundamental ethos in trauma-informed care suggests that we ask, "What happened to you?" rather than "What is wrong with you?" By actively incorporating this understanding into the provision of pediatric care, we can reduce the risk of further harming children through our behavior and treatments. It is not necessary for the clinician to know the exact nature of the patient's trauma, but to approach patients with gentle curiosity, sensitive dialogue, and development of trust.[168]

Treating Suffering

Bioethicist and internist, Dr. Eric Cassel described suffering as an intensely personal feeling that can be defined as *the state of severe distress associated with events that threaten the intactness of the person.*[169] Suffering should be considered when managing pain, and adequate steps should be taken to find and alleviate sources of suffering. Factors that contribute to a child's suffering include not knowing the origin or meaning of the pain, believing that pain is

a punishment, and fearing that the pain will never be relieved. Anesthesiologists minimize suffering by clearly communicating about these issues with parents and children and affording children as much control of their care as possible.

Suspicion of Child Maltreatment

Child maltreatment includes acts of physical abuse, sexual abuse, psychological abuse, emotional abuse, and neglect.[170–173] Anesthesiologists should be particularly sensitive to bruises or burns in the shape of objects, injuries to soft tissue areas such as the upper arms, unexplained mouth and dental injuries, fractures in infants, height and weight less than the fifth percentile, and injuries that are not explained by the history (see Fig. 37.2). Children with physical or intellectual disabilities are particularly prone to abuse.[174] Anesthesiologists, like all physicians, are legally required to report the suspicion of child abuse or neglect to appropriate authorities. Indeed, in most jurisdictions, a physician can be criminally prosecuted if found liable for *failing* to report suspected child abuse. Pediatricians with specific expertise in child abuse and neglect may be available at your organization to provide additional support.

Suspicion of Medical Child Abuse

Medical child abuse (previously referred to as Munchausen syndrome by proxy) is *"a form of child maltreatment in which a child receives unnecessary and harmful or potentially harmful medical care at the instigation of a caregiver".*[175] Medical child abuse victims endure prolonged, unnecessary hospitalizations, painful procedures, significant morbidity, and even death; they are more likely to develop adult somatoform disorders and to have psychiatric comorbidities.[176] A hallmark of medical child abuse includes parental/caregiver pursuit of multiple invasive procedures in pursuit of an elusive organic diagnosis, many of which require the services of pediatric anesthesiologists. Therefore, the perioperative environment provides a unique opportunity to identify children suffering from medical child abuse. Often a significant amount of evidence must be compiled to demonstrate abuse, especially when children have underlying or induced chronic medical conditions. When a pediatric anesthesiologist suspects medical child abuse, these concerns should be shared with clinicians on the care team (such as the primary pediatrician and surgeon) and report suspicion to the appropriate authorities.

THE ETHICS CONSULTATION SERVICE

The ethical dilemmas that occur in the practice of anesthesiology may be difficult for the practitioner to resolve alone. Ethics committees and their consulting services act in an advisory role to help clinicians, patients, and families amicably resolve ethical dilemmas. Anesthesiologists may find ethics consultation helpful with questions about informed consent, decision-making capacity, and resuscitation decisions and in resolving disagreements among patients, families, and clinicians.

Although most ethics consultation services are comprised of a small group (typically three people) to perform consultations, some use the entire committee and some use a single individual.[177] Physicians, nurses, social workers, chaplains, administrators, and laypeople serve on ethics committees and perform consultations. Common characteristics of ethics consultation services are that they permit anyone to request an ethics consultation; that they require notification (not permission) of the patient, parents, and attending physician prior to the consultation; and that choosing to follow the recommendations is wholly voluntary. Ethics committees are also available to consult on policy development, organizational ethics matters, and to organize continuing educational programs.

For pediatric ethics consultations, in one study, the attending physician requested the majority of consults, but consult requests were also commonly received from nurses, social workers, nurse practitioners, and families.[178] Typical ethical concerns include end-of-life care, goals of care, prognosis, quality of life, parental decision making, pediatric assent, cultural differences, professional obligations, disagreement among professionals, communication concerns, and moral distress.[178–180] Ethics consultation seems to work efficiently, reaching consensus promptly and consistently.

The opinions of ethicists may differ from the opinions of subsets of physicians. For example, when interpreting the best interest standard for a neonate, ethicists are more likely to consider the infant's interests and the effects on the family. Neonatologists were influenced by parents' wishes, but were more likely to consider only the infant's interests and were less likely to consider the effects on the family.[181] After consultations, clinicians feel greater satisfaction in managing cases with ethical conflicts, not only because of their heightened awareness of the expert consulting services available, but also because of their increased knowledge and comfort in dealing with these issues.

ANNOTATED REFERENCES

Cassel EJ. The nature of suffering and the goals of medicine. *N Engl J Med.* 1982;306:639-646.

Physicians relieve suffering. Cassel's 30-year-old treatise is the unparalleled explanation of suffering.

Committee on Bioethics, American Academy of Pediatrics. Informed consent, parental permission, and assent in pediatric practice. *Pediatrics.* 1995;95:314-317.

This article is the basis of informed consent for children. Pay particular attention to the introduction, in which Dr. William Bartholome (in abstentia) exhorts clinicians to respect "the experience, perspective and power of children".

Gruen RL, Pearson SD, Brennan TA. Physician-citizens: public roles and professional obligations. *JAMA.* 2004;291:94-98.

Gruen et al. provide a thoughtful perspective on the public and professional obligations of physicians. They provide a path on how to fulfill these obligations.

Kon AA, Shepard EK, Sederstrom NO, et al. Defining futile and potentially inappropriate interventions: a policy statement from the Society of Critical Care Medicine Ethics Committee. *Crit Care Med.* 2016;44(9):1769-1774.

This article elegantly describes the characteristics of potentially inappropriate intervention and provides practical advice about implications.

Lang K, Dupree C, Kon A, Dudinski D. Calling out implicit racial bias as a harm in pediatric care. *Camb Q Healthc Ethics.* 2016;25(3):540-552.

A thorough, readable and nonjudgmental analysis of one of those problems we prefer not to discuss—differences in care by race.

Nato CG, Tabacco L, Bilotta F. Fraud and retraction in perioperative medicine publications: what we learned and what can be implemented to prevent future recurrence. *J Med Ethics.* 2022;48(7):479-484.

This narrative summarizes the fraud perpetrated by six anesthesiologists and critical care physicians who in aggregate, authored 421 of the 475 papers that have been retracted, the largest number of retractions of any discipline in medicine. The review describes the researchers' background and training, how their malfeasance was uncovered, their punishment if any, and the steps that should be taken to preclude repeat occurrences.

Quill TE. "I wish things were different": expressing wishes in response to loss, futility, and unrealistic hopes. *Ann Intern Med.* 2001;135(7):551.

A short paper that changes the way you think about communicating with the patient or family during difficult times. The "wish" statement initiates deeper discussion and conveys empathy and being on the "same side of the fence" with the patient and family.

Shafer SL. Tattered threads. *Anesth Analg.* 2009;108:1361-1363.

Shafer elegantly articulates the harms of false data.

Waxman HA. The lessons of Vioxx: drug safety and sales. *N Engl J Med.* 2005;352:2576-2578.

Waxman's recounting of public testimony eviscerates the reassuring murmurings of industry.

A complete reference list can be found online at Elsevier eBooks+.

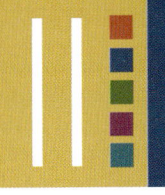

Pharmacogenomics

4

SENTHIL PACKIASABAPATHY, VIDYA CHIDAMBARAN, AND
SENTHILKUMAR SADHASIVAM

Historical Perspectives
Basic Concepts and Nomenclature
Hepatic Metabolism and Developmental Pharmacogenetics
Phase I Reactions: Cytochromes P-450
Developmental Changes of Specific Cytochromes
Phase II Reactions
Alterations in Biotransformation at Birth
Genomics of Drug Metabolism, Exposure, and Effects
Pharmacogenomics of Pain and Analgesia
Pain Perception and Genetics
Genetic Variations Affecting Opioid Pharmacokinetics
Codeine
Tramadol
Hydrocodone
Oxycodone
Morphine
Methadone
Genetic Variations Affecting Opioid Pharmacodynamics
Opioid Receptor (*OPRM1*)
Blood-Brain Barrier Transporter (*ABCB1*)
Opioid-Cannabinoid System Interactions
Genes of Addiction
Nonsteroidal Antiinflammatory Drugs and Genetics

Acetaminophen and Genetics
Acute and Chronic Postsurgical Pain – Genetics and Epigenetics
Pharmacogenomics Affecting Anesthesia
Intravenous Anesthetics
Inhalational Anesthetics
Benzodiazepines
Neuromuscular Blocking Drugs
Local Anesthetics
Perioperative Outcomes
Postoperative Nausea and Vomiting
Perioperative Bleeding
Hemodynamic Response
Effect on Other Perioperative Outcomes
Ancestry/Race and Genetics
Pharmacogenomics Methods
Common Genotyping Methods
Common Limitations of Genetic Research
Studies and Interpretation of Genetic Studies
Current Costs of Genotyping and Third-Party
Coverage for Genotyping
Genetic Counseling
Clinical Translation: Bench to Bedside: Where Are We Now?
Conclusion

UNITED STATES PRESIDENT WILLIAM CLINTON, when announcing the relative completion of the Human Genome Project in July 2000 stated, *"With this profound new knowledge, humankind is on the verge of gaining immense new power to heal. Genome science will have a real impact on all of our lives - and even more, on the lives of our children. It will revolutionize the diagnosis, prevention, and treatment of most, if not all, human disease."*[1] This marked the beginning of enhanced interest and vigor in the development of personalized medicine, which simply stated, means *"right treatment for the right patient at the right time."* This is especially relevant in anesthesia and analgesia as the perioperative period is a state of stress, inflammation, pain, and hemodynamic and metabolic shifts superimposed on chronic disease; all factors have interindividual variability in response.[2] Moreover, use of multiple drugs in a short course of time, as occurs in the perioperative period, introduces variability in metabolism and drug-drug interactions that can impact the care we deliver. This occurs because genetic factors contribute to about 50% of the variability in drug responses,[3] and 59% of drugs are involved in adverse drug reactions and metabolized by at least one gene with variants that affect its metabolism.[2,4] Hence, knowledge of pharmacogenomics and its applications for individualizing drug dosing in anesthesia is critical.[5,6] In this chapter, we discuss the basics and current understanding of pharmacogenomics relevant to the practice of pediatric anesthesia.

Historical Perspectives

The current understanding of personalized medicine is traceable to the writings of Hippocrates, the "father of Western medicine," who lived in the fifth century BCE.[7] Anecdotally, in 510 BCE, Pythagoras noted that ingestion of fava beans caused a potentially fatal reaction in some, but not all, individuals.[8] The "seeds" of modern genetics were sown by Gregor Mendel, who presented his research on experiments in plant hybridization in 1865. Multiple scientists received Nobel Prizes for ground-breaking discoveries of "nuclein" (Albrecht Kossel in 1910), the double-helical structure of the nucleic acid (Watson, Crick, and Wilkins in 1962), cracking the genetic code (Nirenberg, Khorana, Holley in 1968), and pioneering DNA sequencing methods (Sanger, Gilbert, Berg in 1980). These revolutionized the science of genetic sequencing and in 2003, the Human Genome Project successfully completed the unraveling of the approximately 3 billion DNA base pairs that make up the human genome. Anesthesia is in no way a silent bystander in the history of pharmacogenomics. Some of the initial discoveries of genetic effects on drugs related to interactions involving barbiturates in patients with porphyria (1937),[9] cholinesterase deficiency leading to succinylcholine-induced prolonged apnea (1957),[10] and malignant hyperthermia (1962).[11]

Basic Concepts and Nomenclature

The term *"pharmacogenetics,"* which was coined by Friedrich Vogel of Heidelberg, Germany, in 1959,[11] refers to the role of genetic variation affecting drug response or adverse reactions to drugs. A broader term, *"pharmacogenomics,"* was introduced in the 1990s with emergence of the Human Genome Project and the development of the genome sciences, encompassing all genes in the genome that may determine drug responses.[12] We now know that the human genome contains about 21,000 genes. The most common type of allelic variation is a *single-nucleotide polymorphism* (SNP) when two alternative bases occur at an appreciable frequency ($>1\%$ of the population).[13] On the other hand, *mutations* which occur less frequently ($<1\%$ of the population) include duplications, deletions, insertions, translocation, or inversion of DNA segments. However, since more than one *codon* (triplet of nucleotides) code for the same amino acid, not all mutations cause structural changes in the protein (called *nonsense variant*), whereas others do change the structure of the protein (called *missense variant*).

Cells use a two-step process of *transcription* (DNA to messenger RNA [mRNA]) and *translation* (mRNA to amino acid) to read each genetic code and produce amino acid sequences that make up proteins. Since proteins function as receptors, enzymes, and transporters for drugs, initially thinking held that exonic variants with "functional" roles in genes would affect protein structure and hence be of clinical significance. However, we now understand that the process is not quite as simple as previously thought. Transcription could be affected by alternative splicing and differential gene expression (depending on regulatory variants, microRNA, epigenetic factors), translation by RNA degradation, or inefficient translation. Moreover, protein formation depends on translation initiation sequences and then posttranslational modifications. Furthermore, protein expression varies in different parts of the body, affected by age, environmental conditions, and disease.[14] This complexity has given rise to various genomic technologies with exciting clinical potential for applications. Consequently, the genotype may not always correspond with a distinct phenotype in a particular individual.

Transcriptomics is the study of all mRNA molecules in the cell. For example, repeated exposure to large doses of ketamine, an *N*-methyl-D-aspartate (NMDA) receptor antagonist, can alter the expression of apoptotic relevant genes and increase NMDA receptor gene expression in developing neurons in postnatal day 7 rat pup brains.[15]

Proteomics is the large-scale study of proteins, particularly their structures and functions. Tools of proteomic research mainly involve separation and elimination of contaminants with enzymes (e.g., DNAase, RNAase, denaturing agents) followed by protein separation by size (one- or two-dimensional polyacrylamide gel electrophoresis), cleavage into peptides and analysis by mass spectrometry (MS) (commonly matrix-assisted laser desorption time of flight [MALDI-ToF], electrospray ionization, surface-enhanced laser desorption time of flight [SELDI-ToF], and tandem MS/MS).[16] This is based on the property that six or more amino acids define a peptide sequence that can be used to identify the gene that coded for them.[17] Chromatin immunoprecipitation (ChIP) is a type of immunoprecipitation experimental technique used to investigate the interaction between proteins and DNA in the cell. The technique aims to determine whether specific proteins are associated with specific genomic regions, such as transcription factors on promoters or other DNA-binding sites, and is an important investigational tool.

Proteomics has applications in identifying differential expression in the spinal cord after peripheral nerve injury in rat models,[18] including specific dorsal horn proteins involved in transmission and modulation of noxious information, cellular metabolism, plasma membrane receptor trafficking, oxidative stress, apoptosis, and degeneration under neuropathic pain conditions.[19] Proteomics has enabled identification of protein-binding sites of inhalation anesthetics.[20] After desflurane anesthesia, protein expression levels in the rat brain remained altered for at least 72 hours, which lends strength to the notion that the physiologic effects of anesthesia outlast the immediate postoperative period.[21,22] Effects on proteomic expression (proteins broadly classified into groups involved in cytoskeletal/neuronal growth, cellular metabolism, signaling, and cell stress/death responses) on the brain of rats were studied after sevoflurane and propofol anesthesia. The authors showed that proteins concerned with cell death and stress responses were downregulated by both agents, but they had variable effects on proteins in the other groups. Proteins such as ULIP-2 and dihydropyrimidinase-like 2 (DPYSL2; associated with cytoskeletal/neuronal growth) were regulated in opposite directions by propofol and sevoflurane. They also found that sevoflurane had more pronounced effects on a wider range of proteins and over an apparently greater duration than propofol. These findings revealed that sevoflurane could be considered a more disruptive anesthetic agent and suggest that the agents have different underlying mechanisms of protein regulation.[23] It is expected that in the future, proteomics will revolutionize preoperative risk stratification as well as approaches to anesthetic and analgesic drug delivery as they relate to specific protein binding.[14]

Metabolomics is the systematic study of the unique chemical fingerprints that specific cellular processes leave behind. Metabolomics of the live rodent brain differ during isoflurane and propofol anesthesia, with greater concentrations of lactate and glutamate characteristic of isoflurane anesthesia.[24] The use of high-resonance magnetic spectroscopy to measure metabolomics raises exciting avenues for noninvasive recognition of anesthesia-induced brain effects in humans and may be a way of recognizing differential anesthesia-induced apoptosis or neurotoxicity observed in the young, immature brain after exposure to anesthesia (see Chapter 23). Similarly, metabolic profiling of hearts exposed to sevoflurane and propofol in the isolated working rat heart model revealed distinct regulation of fatty acid and glucose oxidation, which could have clinical implications for the responses of a diseased heart under anesthesia.[25]

Another exciting field is *epigenetics,* which encompasses nonstructural DNA modifications that control gene expression by altering transcription via histone modification and changes of DNA methylation.[26] The concept was initially proposed as a bridge between an organism's heritable genome and environmental influences[27]; such environmental influences are evident from reports of a high frequency of epigenetic differences between aging monozygotic twins.[28]

DNA methylation involves the addition of a methyl group to the 5′ carbon of the cytosine pyrimidine ring in a DNA dinucleotide by DNA methyltransferase enzymes (DNMT1, DNMT3A, DNMT3B), converting it into 5-methylcytosine. Regions in the DNA (60% in gene promoter regions) have been identified where cytosine and guanine appear next to each other in repeating sequence, held together by phosphodiester bonds, and are called CpG islands. Methylation has been found to prevent binding of transcription factors[29] or attracting methylated DNA-binding proteins that repress transcription, leading generally to gene silencing.[30,31] DNA methylation analysis either involves pyrosequencing of bisulfite-treated DNA or use of commercial arrays. There has been immense interest in the role of epigenetics in the transition from acute to chronic pain,[32] the functional regulation of μ-opioid receptors, the main receptor for endogenous as well as exogenous opioids,[33] and neuropathic pain.[34]

Histone deacetylation refers to modification of nucleosomes (histone octamers and surrounding DNA) that involves acetylation of the exposed *N*-terminal tails of histone by histone acetyl transferases (HATs)[35]; this alters chromatin structure and makes it less compact, thus allowing transcription factors to bind more easily, resulting in increased gene expression, especially when located in gene promoter regions. This is analyzed using ChIP, and more recently, combined with sequencing (ChIP-seq).[36] An example of epigenetics as therapeutic targets for pain is provided by the study of the rat brainstem nucleus raphe magnus. This is important for central mechanisms of chronic pain, persistent inflammatory, and neuropathic pain where epigenetic suppression of *GAD2* (the gene that encodes glutamic acid decarboxylase 65 [GAD65], a γ-aminobutyric acid [GABA] synthetic enzyme that regulates pain) transcription through histone deacetylase (HDAC)-mediated histone hypoacetylation, results in impaired GABA synaptic inhibition. Importantly, histone deacetylase inhibitors strongly increased GAD65 activity, restored GABA synaptic function, and relieved sensitized pain behavior, proving to have therapeutic potential.[37]

Epigenetics has been lauded as a possible "epicenter" for future anesthesia research.[38] The 20,000 genes that code for proteins account for only 1.5% of DNA. The National Human Genome Research Institute Encyclopedia of DNA Elements (ENCODE) project was implemented to elucidate the regulatory elements affecting gene expression, with the intention of understanding the role of the unaccounted (98.5%) DNA.[39] Small nucleolar RNAs, long noncoding RNAs, small interfering RNA (siRNA), and microRNA are now included in the list along with known messenger, transport, and ribosomal RNA. *MicroRNAs* are small (19–22 nucleotides) noncoding RNA that bind to mRNA via base pairing with complementary sequences and cause gene silencing or degradation. A short sequence (5–7 nucleotides) in the mature microRNA determines the specificity of binding to mRNAs, so microRNAs can bind multiple mRNAs, and one mRNA can be bound to multiple microRNAs simultaneously. Isoflurane protects mouse hearts from ischemia-reperfusion injury by a microRNA-21–dependent mechanism.[40] Since endogenous microRNAs in tissue can be easily increased or decreased with chemical mimics and inhibitors, this finding may hold clinical relevance for future therapeutic strategies to modulate cardiac gene regulation.

Hepatic Metabolism and Developmental Pharmacogenetics

Metabolism of many drugs involves the *cytochrome P-450 (CYP) enzyme* system. Multiple isoforms of the cytochrome P-450 enzyme system exist with different substrate specificities for different drugs.[41–43] Induction and inhibition of these enzymes by different drugs and chemicals requires a thorough understanding of both the nomenclature of the cytochrome P-450 system as well as the specific isoforms responsible for metabolism of the drugs used in pediatric anesthesia. There are both genetic and ethnic polymorphisms leading to clinically important differences in the capacity to metabolize drugs; these differences can make individual drug responses unpredictable.[44–49] In the future, it may be possible to tailor drug doses to the individual's requirements by determining the child's unique metabolic capacity.[49,50]

PHASE I REACTIONS: CYTOCHROMES P-450

Cytochromes P-450 are heme-containing proteins that provide most of the phase I drug metabolism for lipophilic compounds in the body. The generally accepted nomenclature of the cytochrome P-450 isozymes begins with CYP and groups enzymes with more than 36% DNA homology into families designated with an Arabic number followed by alphanumeric letters for the subfamily of closely related proteins (>77% homology) followed by a number for the specific gene—for example, CYP3A4.[51,52] Isozymes that are important in human drug metabolism are found in the *CYP1, CYP2,* and *CYP3* gene families. Table 4.1 outlines the P-450 isozymes and their common substrates, inducers, inhibitors, and polymorphisms.

DEVELOPMENTAL CHANGES OF SPECIFIC CYTOCHROMES

For many drugs, metabolism in neonates is reduced and correlates with fewer cytochrome P-450 enzymes in the hepatic microsomes.[53] Although the concentrations of CYP enzymes increase with gestational age, some reach only 50% of adult values at term.[53] In neonates, reduced cytochrome P-450 decreases clearance for many drugs, including theophylline, caffeine, diazepam, phenytoin, and phenobarbital.[42,43,54–58] Although many isozymes are immature in the neonate, some P-450 isozymes exhibit near-adult activity, whereas others produce unique metabolic pathways that invalidate broad generalizations about drug metabolism in the neonate. Developmental patterns and clinical consequences of relevant genes are summarized in Table 4.2.

Cytochrome P4501A2 (CYP1A2) accounts for much of the metabolism of caffeine (1,3,7-trimethylxanthine)[59,60] and theophylline (1,3-dimethylxanthine)[61,62]; these methylxanthines are frequently used to treat neonatal apnea and bradycardia. *CYP1A2* activity is nearly absent in the fetal liver and remains minimal in the neonate.[63] This limits *N*-3- and *N*-7-demethylation of caffeine in this age group. Furthermore, renal clearance, the other method of elimination, is also immature,[64] hence elimination in preterm and term neonates is poor.[65,66] These developmental issues hold important clinical implications for drug dosing and the timing between serial doses for the treatment of apnea of prematurity.[67–69] *CYP1A2* activity reaches adult levels by 4 to 6 months postnatal age.[70,71] A

TABLE 4.1 Common Relevant CYP450 Enzymes, Substrates, Their Inducers and Inhibitors, and Common Polymorphisms With Effect on Enzyme Activity

P450 Enzymes	Selected Substrates	Inducers	Inhibitors	Number of Variants Identified	Examples of Variants	Effect on Enzyme Activity
CYP2B6	Ketamine Methadone Propofol Meperidine Phenobarbital	Carbamazepine (S)[a] Phenytoin Rifampin (S)[a] Efavirenz (W)[c]	Clopidogrel (W)[f] Ticlopidine (W)[f] Prasugrel (W)[f]	>28	*6(516G>T, 785A>G) *16 *5 (172H-262K-487C)	Decreased

CYP2C9	NSAIDs Diclofenac Ibuprofen, Naproxen, Indomethacin
	Others
	  Celecoxib
	  Warfarin
	  Oral hypoglycemic (tolbutamide, glipizide)
	  Phenytoin
		Carbamazepine (M)[b]
		Rifampin (M)[b]
		Phenobarbital (W)[c]
		St. John's wort (W)[c]
			Amiodarone (M)[e]
			Fluconazole (M)[e]
				>30	*2 (430C>T)
					*3 (1075A>G)
						Decreased

CYP2C19	Antiepileptics Diazepam Midazolam Phenytoin, Phenobarbitone
	Others
	  PPIs
	  TCA
	  SSRI
	  MAOI
	  Clopidogrel
		Rifampin, (M)[b]
		Efavirenz, Ritonavir
		St. John's wort
			Fluconazole (S)[d]
			Fluvoxamine (S)[d]
			Ticlopidine (S)[d]			

CYP2D6	Codeine
	Dextromethorphan
	Oxycodone
	Hydrocodone
	Tramadol
	Ondansetron
	Dolasetron
	Palonosetron
	Tropisetron
	Antidepressants
	  Amitriptyline
	  Imipramine
	  Fluoxetine
	  Duloxetine
	  Paroxetine
		None known	Bupropion (S)[d]
			Fluoxetine (S)[d]
			Paroxetine (S)[d]
			Quinidine (S)[d]
			Duloxetine (M)[e]
			Amiodarone (W)[f]
			Cimetidine (W)[f]
			Celecoxib (W)[f]
			Methadone (W)[f]
				>100	PM: two inactive alleles (*3-*8, *11-*16, *19-*21, *38, *40, *42)
					IM: two decreased-activity alleles (*9,*10, *17, *29, *36, *41) or carrying one active (*1, *2, *33, *35) and one inactive (*3-*8, *11-*16, *19-*21, *38, *40, *42) allele, or carrying one decreased-activity (*9, *10, *17, *29, *36, *41) and one inactive allele (*3-*8, *11-*16, *19-*21, *38, *40, *42)
					UM: a gene duplication in absence of inactive (*3-*8, *11-*16, *19-*21, *38, *40, *42) or decreased-activity (*9, *10, *17, *29, *36, *41) alleles	

CYP2E1	Volatile agents
	  Halothane
	  Isoflurane
	  Enflurane
	  Desflurane
	  Methoxyflurane
	  Acetaminophen
	  Caffeine
		Ethanol
		Isoniazid
			Disulfiram	13	*5 (-1293G>C, 1053C>T)	Increased

CYP3A4.5	Benzodiazepines
	  Diazepam
	  Midazolam
	  Triazolam
	  Alprazolam
	Opioids
	  Morphine
	  Meperidine
	  Fentanyl
	  Sufentanil
	  Remifentanil
	  Alfentanil
	  Methadone
	Granisetron
	Amide group (LA)
		Carbamazepine (S)[a]
		Efavirenz (M)[b]
		Nevirapine (M)[b]
		Phenobarbital
		Phenytoin (S)[a]
		Pioglitazone
		Rifabutin (W)[c]
		Rifampin (S)[a]
		St. John's wort (S)[a]
		Aprepitant (W)[c]
		Prednisone (W)[c]
			HIV antivirals (S)[d]
			Ketoconazole (S)[d]
			Clarithromycin (S)[d]
			Erythromycin (M)[e]
			Grapefruit juice (M)[e]
			Verapamil (M)[e]
			Diltiazem (M)[e]
			Aprepitant (M)[e]
			Atorvastatin (W)[f]
			Cimetidine (W)[f]
			Isoniazid (W)[f]
			Oral contraceptives (W)[f]
				>50	CYP3A4*1B
					CYP3A5*3
					CYP3A4*1G
						Increased
						Nonfunctional
						Decreased

W: Weak; M: Moderate; S: Strong

[a]Strong inducers: ≥80% decrease, [b]Moderate inducers: 50%–80% decrease, [c]Weak inducers: 20%–50% decrease in the area under the curve of a substrate, [d]Strong inhibitor: >5-fold increase, [e]Moderate inhibitor: 2- to 5-fold increase, [f]Weak inhibitor: <2-fold increase in the area under the curve of a substrate.

EM, Extensive metabolizer; *IM*, intermediate metabolizer; *LA*, local anesthetics; *MAOI*, monoamine oxidase inhibitor; *PM*, poor metabolizer; *PPIs*, proton pump inhibitors; *SSRI*, selective serotonin reuptake inhibitor; *TCA*, tricyclic antidepressant; *UM*, ultrarapid metabolizer.

From US Food and Drug Administration. Drug development and drug interactions: table of substrates, inhibitors, and inducers. https://www.fda.gov/Drugs/Development ApprovalProcess/DevelopmentResources/DrugInteractionsLabeling/ucm093664.htm#4; https://medicine.iupui.edu/clinpharm/ddis/clinical-table/.

TABLE 4.2 | Developmental Genetics for Important Hepatic Enzymes in the Neonate and Clinical Consequences

Enzymes	Developmental Patterns	Clinical Consequences

Uridine diphosphoglucuronyltransferase (UDP-GT)
Substrates
  Morphine
  Acetaminophen
  Lorazepam
	Ontogeny is isoform specific. In general, adult activity is achieved by 6–18 months of age.	Infants <3 months of age need lower morphine doses due to reduced clearance.[485]

Sulfotransferase
Substrates
  Acetaminophen
  Dopamine
	Ontogeny seems to be more rapid than UDP-GT; however, it is substrate specific. Activity for some isoforms may exceed adult values during infancy and childhood (e.g., that responsible for acetaminophen metabolism).	Higher acetaminophen-sulfate formation in neonates provides "relative protection" from glucuronide formation deficiency.[112]

CYP1A2
  Acetaminophen
  Caffeine
	Not present to an appreciable extent in human fetal liver. Adult levels reached by 4 months of age and may be exceeded in children 1–2 years of age.	

CYP2C9	Not apparent in fetal liver. Inferential data using phenytoin disposition as a nonspecific pharmacologic probe suggest low activity during the first week of life, with adult activity reached by 6 months of age and peak activity reached by 3–4 years of age.	Large interpatient variability for ibuprofen effects is due to low levels of *CYP2C9* in premature infants.[486]
CYP2C19	CYP2C19 activity can be detected by 8 weeks of gestation and remains unchanged throughout gestation and at birth. Over the first 5 months of postnatal age, CYP2C19 activity increases linearly. Adult activity is reached by 10 years of age.	Allelic variations of *CYP2C19* produce PM phenotypes, which increase systemic exposure to PPI in neonates.[487] Diazepam half-life is prolonged in PM phenotype (*CYP2C19 *2/*2, *3/*3, *2/*3*), causing delayed emergence from anesthesia.[410]
CYP2D6	Low to absent in fetal liver but uniformly present at 1 week of postnatal age. Poor activity (~20% of adult values) at 1 month of postnatal age. Adult competence reached by 3–5 years of age. Metabolism inhibited by cimetidine.	All newborns (<2 weeks) PNA are PM phenotypes, susceptible to drug toxicity, although genetic variability contributes more than ontogeny to variability at all ages.[488]
CYP3A4	CYP3A4 has low activity in the first month of life, with approach toward adult levels by 6–12 months postnatally.	Clearance of midazolam affected: adults>full-term neonates>preterm neonates.[73]
CYP3A7	CYP3A7 is functionally active in the fetus; ~30%–75% of adult levels of CYP3A4.	Cisapride accumulation in neonates due to inadequate metabolism might explain QTc prolongation on ECG due to cisapride.[489]

ECG, Electrocardiogram; *PM*, poor metabolizer; *PPI*, proton pump inhibitor.
Adapted from Leeder JS, Kearns GL. Pharmacogenetics in pediatrics: implications for practice. *Pediatr Clin North Am.* 1997; 44:55-77.[52]

similar pharmacokinetic pattern of reduced metabolism at birth occurs with theophylline in which *CYP1A2* catalyzes N-3-demethylation and 8-hydroxylation.[61] Theophylline clearance reaches adult rates by 4 to 5 months, which coincides with the changes in *CYP1A2* activity as reflected in urine metabolite patterns.[72]

Other P-450 enzymes that are reduced or absent in the fetus include *CYP2D6* and *CYP2C9*.[73–75] *CYP2D6* has minimal activity (<5% of adult activity) in the last trimester but matures quickly in the first month postnatally to 50% to 75% of adult values, albeit with large interindividual variability. *CYP2C9*, which is responsible for the metabolism of nonsteroidal antiinflammatory drugs (NSAIDs), warfarin, and phenytoin, has minimal activity antenatally[74] but develops rapidly postnatally[58,76] from 21% of adult values immediately after birth to peak (adult) activity by 3 months, when expressed as milligrams per kilogram per hour.[77] *CYP2E1* activity is minimal in utero, increasing by the third trimester, and surges within the first 24 hours postnatally.[78] *CYP2E1* activity in vitro remains decreased in infants younger than 90 days postnatal age, resulting in slower metabolism of substrates during this period compared with

older infants, children, and adults.[79] Thereafter, its activity increases steadily reaching adult activity levels by 1 year of age.[79]

CYP3A is the most important cytochrome involved in drug metabolism. It comprises the majority of adult human liver cytochrome P-450 (see Table 4.1) and metabolizes a broad range of drugs.[80] *CYP3A* is detectable during embryogenesis as early as 17 weeks, primarily in the form of *CYP3A7*,[63] and reaches 75% of adult activity by 30 weeks gestation.[73] It has been hypothesized that this is due to the potential protective role of *CYP3A7* in preventing retinoic acid–induced human embryotoxicity.[81] In vivo, *CYP3A* activity appears to be mature at birth[82]; however, there is a poorly understood postnatal transition from the fetal *CYP3A7* to the predominant adult isoform *CYP3A4*.[83,84]

CYP2D6 is involved in the metabolism of β-blockers, antiarrhythmics, antidepressants, antipsychotics, and several opioids including codeine. It is either absent or less than 1% of adult values in the fetus[85] and is eventually expressed postnatally (see Table 4.1).[73,86] O-demethylation begins postnatally with rapid maturation of this enzyme system irrespective of the gestational age at birth, although activity may remain less than 25% of adult values at 5 years of age. Interestingly, CYP2D6 is a noninducible enzyme whose activity, however, may vary with certain disease states, including malignancy, cigarette smoking, and some chronic inflammatory diseases (rheumatoid arthritis).[87] Consensus recommendations from the Clinical Pharmacogenetics Implementation Consortium and Dutch Pharmacogenetics Working Group have recently proposed standardization of CYP2D6 genotype to phenotype conversions, to enable drug dosing.[88–90]

PHASE II REACTIONS

The other major route of drug metabolism, designated phase II reactions, involves synthetic or conjugation reactions that increase the hydrophilicity of molecules to facilitate renal elimination.[91,92] The phase II enzymes include glucuronosyltransferase, sulfotransferase, N-acetyltransferase, glutathione S-transferase, and methyl transferase. The phase II enzymes also show developmental changes during infancy that influence drug clearance (see Table 5.2).[43,93–95]

Most conjugation reactions have limited activity during fetal development.[96] One of the most familiar synthetic reactions in young infants involves conjugation by uridine diphosphoglucuronosyltransferases (UGTs). This enzyme system includes numerous isoforms and is also responsible for glucuronidation of endogenous compounds, such as bilirubin (UGT1A1).[96] As with the maturation of bilirubin conjugation, UGT activity is limited immediately postnatally and the different isoforms mature at different rates postnatally.[97] Dose adjustments are often needed to avoid toxicity in neonates from drugs that require conjugation by UGT for clearance. Experience with chloramphenicol in the 1960s illustrated this lesson when neonates received standard pediatric doses of chloramphenicol without understanding the immaturity of UGT and its role in the elimination of chloramphenicol. Infants accumulated large concentrations of chloramphenicol and developed fatal circulatory collapse, a condition known as the gray baby syndrome.[98,99] Although the clearance of chloramphenicol is poor in neonates, appropriate dose adjustments and monitoring allow safe treatment of preterm and term infants with this antibiotic.[100]

Morphine, acetaminophen (paracetamol), dexmedetomidine, and lorazepam are all cleared by glucuronide conjugation. The major steps in the metabolic disposition of morphine in children and adults are glucuronidation in the 3- and 6- positions.[101] The limited ability of neonates to glucuronidate morphine necessitates dosage adjustment.[102–104] Morphine clearance,[103,105] in particular 3- and 6-glucuronide formation, is limited at birth and increases with birth weight,[104] gestational age,[41] and postnatal age.[101,102] Morphine clearance, expressed per kilogram, approaches adult values by 1 month.[102,106] However, size models such as the per kilogram model confound interpretation and clearance does not reach adult values until at least 5 to 6 months when scaled using allometry (see Chapter 5).[103,107] Overall, the maturation of UGT enzymes varies among isoforms, but, in general, adult activity is reached within the first 2 years of life.[52] The time courses of maturation of drug metabolism for morphine,[108,109] acetaminophen,[110] and glomerular filtration rate[111] are strikingly similar (see Fig. 5.11) with 50% of size-adjusted adult values reached between 8 and 12 weeks after full-term delivery. Drugs cleared predominantly by UGT that convert the parent compound into a water-soluble metabolite excreted by the kidneys have clearance maturation profiles that match the maturation in glomerular filtration.

In contrast to glucuronosyltransferase, the sulfotransferase enzyme system is well developed in the neonate, and for some compounds it may compensate for limited glucuronidation. Thus, drugs like acetaminophen, which undergoes primarily glucuronidation in

the adult, also undergo sulfate conjugation in neonates. Hence, the half-life of acetaminophen is only moderately prolonged in neonates compared with older infants and adults.[112–114] This has been attributed to its increased volume of distribution in neonates, and as explained earlier, increased sulfation, leading to a greater percent of the dose excreted as the acetaminophen-sulfate conjugate.[112,114–117] However, this does not confer safety from hepatotoxicity because the toxic metabolite is created through the oxidative pathway mediated by CYP2E1. This is detailed later in this chapter.

ALTERATIONS IN BIOTRANSFORMATION AT BIRTH

Transition from the intrauterine to the extrauterine environment is associated with major changes in blood flow. There may also be an environmental trigger for the expression of some metabolic enzyme activities, resulting in a slight increase in maturation rate above that predicted by postmenstrual age.[118–120] Many biotransformation reactions, especially those involving certain forms of cytochrome P-450, are inducible before birth through maternal drug exposure, cigarette smoke, or other inducing agents. Postnatal biotransformation reactions may also be induced through drug exposure or slowed by hypoxia/asphyxia, organ damage, and/or illness. For example, the reduced thiopental clearance estimated from data when the drug was given to control neonatal seizures caused by hypoxic-ischemic insults may not be applicable to healthy neonates undergoing anesthesia.[121,122]

Genomics of Drug Metabolism, Exposure, and Effects

Genetic variations can have impact on both pharmacokinetics and pharmacodynamics. Single-nucleotide changes or polymorphisms (SNPs) in the DNA sequence in CYP enzymes usually decrease but may also increase metabolic activity for a specific drug or drug substrate.[12] Some of the explanations for variations in drug responses within large populations described as "biologic variation" likely relate to genetic differences in drug metabolism, receptor binding, and intracellular coupling to effector mechanisms. A genetic cause for individuals who were either fast or slow acetylators (N-acetyltransferase [NAT]) of isoniazid was identified in the 1950s.[123] Pseudocholinesterase deficiency causing prolonged apnea after succinylcholine deficiency was identified around the same time, although a more obscure variant, the Cynthiana (C5) or Netlich variant that possesses much more activity that the usual plasma cholinesterase causes an extremely brief duration of action of succinylcholine.[10,124,125] After recognizing that certain individuals demonstrated exaggerated hypotensive responses to debrisoquine, the enzyme responsible for its metabolism, CYP2D6, was also one of the early drug-metabolizing enzyme deficiencies identified.[126–128]

Variability in the clinical response to codeine prompted investigations into genetic variants or polymorphisms of CYP2D6. This enzyme is mapped to chromosome 22 at 22q13.1. Fifty-five polymorphisms of CYP2D6 have been described to date with a frequency that exceeds 1% of the population.[129] These include both functional and nonfunctional polymorphisms and gene duplication. The polymorphisms are numbered with *1 denoting the normal or wild allele (the * denotes an allele) (Table 4.3). The mutant alleles, *3, *4, *5, *6, and *9, for example, confer no CYP2D6 activity.[87,129,130] These latter polymorphisms account for more than 90% of the poor metabolizers (PM). Variants *2, *10, and *17 have modestly reduced activity and are referred as intermediate metabolizers (IM).[87] To further complicate the genetic pattern, multiple copies of the same genes[130] may be present in

TABLE 4.3 | CYP2D6 Polymorphisms and Recommendations for Codeine Therapy

Likely Phenotype[a]	Activity Score[c]	Examples of Diplotypes	Implications for Codeine Metabolism	Recommendations for Codeine Therapy[b]	Classification of Recommendation for Codeine Therapy	Considerations for Alternative Opioids
Ultrarapid metabolizer (UM) (~1%–2% of patients)	>2.0	*1/*1xN, *1/*2xN	Increased formation of morphine following codeine administration, leading to higher risk of toxicity.	Avoid codeine use due to potential for toxicity.	Strong	Alternatives that are not affected by this CYP2D6 phenotype include morphine and nonopioid analgesics. Tramadol, and to a lesser extent hydrocodone and oxycodone, are not good alternatives because their metabolism is affected by CYP2D6 activity.
Extensive metabolizer (EM) (~77%–92% of patients)	1.0–2.0	*1/*1, *1/*2, *2/*2, *1/*41, *1/*4, *2/*5, *10/*10	Normal morphine formation	Use label-recommended age- or weight-specific dosing.	Strong	
Intermediate metabolizer (IM) (~2%–11% of patients)	0.5	*4/*10, *5/*41	Reduced morphine formation	Use label-recommended age- or weight-specific dosing. If no response, consider alternative analgesics such as morphine or a nonopioid.	Moderate	Monitor tramadol use for response.
Poor metabolizer (PM) (~5%–10% of patients)	0	*4/*4, *4/*5, *5/*5, *4/*6	Greatly reduced morphine formation following codeine administration, leading to insufficient pain relief.	Avoid codeine use due to lack of efficacy.	Strong	Alternatives that are not affected by this CYP2D6 phenotype include morphine and nonopioid analgesics. Tramadol, and to a lesser extent hydrocodone and oxycodone, are not good alternatives because their metabolism is affected by CYP2D6 activity; these agents should be avoided.

[a]Frequency estimates in White populations.
[b]Crews KR, Gaedigk A, Dunnenberger HM, et al. Clinical Pharmacogenetics Implementation Consortium guidelines for cytochrome P450 2D6 genotype and codeine therapy: 2014 update. *Clin Pharmacol Ther*. 2014;95(4):376-382.
[c]Some investigators define patients with an activity score of 0.5 and 1.0 as intermediate metabolizers and define patients with an activity score of 1.5 and 2.0 as extensive metabolizers. Classifying patients with an activity score of 1.0 as extensive metabolizers in this guideline is based on data specific for formation of morphine from codeine in these patients. https://www.pharmgkb.org/guideline/PA166104996

some individuals, resulting in bizarre phenotypes. The wide array of *CYP2D6* polymorphisms of codeine may be summarized into three broad categories: (1) poor metabolizers (PM), negligible morphine produced; (2) extensive metabolizers (EM), normal metabolism; and (3) ultra-extensive metabolizers (UM) rapid conversion to large amounts of morphine. Up to 10% of Caucasians and 30% of Hong Kong Chinese are PM, rendering codeine an ineffective analgesic in these children.[87] In contrast, 29% of the Ethiopian and 1% of Swedish, German, and Chinese populations are UM, rendering codeine a dangerous analgesic as excessive doses of the morphine metabolite may be rapidly produced after codeine is administered.[87] The frequency of *CYP2D6* polymorphisms, particularly in children who are PM, may be more common and more varied than previously thought. Earlier studies had shown that individuals might also possess normal or reduced metabolic activity (PM) for debrisoquine and sparteine.[128,131] The frequency of PM varies among ethnic groups, occurring in approximately 7% of Americans in the United States[44] and less than 1% of Chinese and Japanese.[132] The clinical relevance of *CYP2D6* polymorphisms on codeine metabolism are described later in this chapter. Allele frequencies in different races of the various relevant variants related to pharmacokinetics of anesthetic and analgesic drugs are given in Table 4.4.

Pharmacogenomics of Pain and Analgesia

One of the fundamental goals of a pediatric anesthesiologist is to have a comfortable patient in the postoperative period and beyond. Opioids remain the most commonly used medications to provide

TABLE 4.4 Race and Allelic Frequencies of Common Variants Affecting Drug PK/PD

Genetic Variant and Population		EU TSI	North American/CEU	AA/ASW	North African MKK/YRI LWK	Hispanic/ MXL/MEX	ME	JPT	Asian/GIH	CHD CHB	Misc.
CYP2B6*6 516G>T, rs3745274 785A>G, rs2279343		0.284 0.214	0.27	0.298 0.462	0.366 0.421 0.33 0.455	0.284 0.273		0.204	0.421 0.188	0.17 0.19	
OPRM1 A118G		0.162	0.155	0.035	0.032 0 0.009	0.198		0.469	0.416	0.426 0.361	0.210 (Ash. Jews)
COMT Val158Met rs4680 G>A		0.451	0.478	0.272	0.271 0.313 0.294				0.395 0.526		
UGT2B7, 161C/T, 802C/T[a]		C 0.51 T 0.49	C 0.46, T 0.53	C 0.68 T 0.32				C 0.73 T 0.26	C 0.73 T 0.26		
ABCB1 C3435T[b]		0.466	0.534	0.188	0.152 0.117	0.460	0.37 0.38 0.26	0.478	0.597	0.417	
CYP2D6[cd]	UM	0.08–0.1	0.043	0.049	0.29 (Oceania)	0.017	0.12–0.20			0.009	
	PM	0.01–0.09	0.077	0.019–0.073	0.018–0.19	0.022–0.066	0.032	0	0.018–0.048	<0.001	
CYP2C9*2[e]		0.13	0.015		0.016	0.057–0.07			0.024		
CYP2C19*2[e]		0.128	0.157		0.15	0.083–0.097			0.278		0.355 (AUS)
CYP3A5*3[f]		0.90			0.20				0.75		

Certain studies are region or population specific; the regions or populations are indicated in parentheses. Unless stated by references pertaining to the gene italicized in the left-hand column, the references for the frequencies noted in the table were obtained from www.pharmgkb.org (5/24/2016). Please note that since more than one reference has been used for some genetic variants, a range of frequencies has been reported. Also, the definitions of ethnic groups may not have been strictly the same among different studies.

AA, African Americans; Ash. Jews, Ashkenazi Jews; ASW, African ancestry in Southwest United States; AUS, Australia; CEU, Utah residents with Northern and Western European ancestry from the Centre d'Etude du Polymorphisme Humain (CEPH) collection; CHB, Han Chinese in Beijing, China; CHD, Chinese in Metropolitan Denver, Colorado; EM, extensive metabolizer; EU, European; GIH, Gujarati Indians in Houston, Texas; IM, intermediate metabolizer; JPT, Japanese in Tokyo, Japan; LWK, Luhya in Webuye, Kenya; ME, Middle East; MEX, Mexican; Misc, miscellaneous; MXL, Mexican ancestry in Los Angeles, California; MKK, Maasai in Kinyawa, Kenya; PK/PD, pharmacokinetics/pharmacodynamics; PM, poor metabolizer; UM, ultrarapid metabolizer; TSI, Toscani in Italia; YRI, Yoruba in Ibadan, Nigeria.

[a]Saito K, Moriya H, Sawaguchi T, et al. Haplotype analysis of UDP-glucuronosyltransferase 2B7 gene (UGT2B7) polymorphisms in healthy Japanese subjects. Clin Biochem. 2006;39(3):303-308.

[b]Ameyaw MM, Regateiro F, Li T, et al. MDR1 pharmacogenetics: frequency of the C3435T mutation in exon 26 is significantly influenced by ethnicity. Pharmacogenetics. 2001;11(3):217-221.

[c]Ingelman-Sundberg M, Sim SC, Gomez A, Rodriguez-Antona C. Influence of cytochrome P450 polymorphisms on drug therapies: pharmacogenetic, pharmacoepigenetic and clinical aspects. Pharmacol Ther. 2007;116(3):496-526.

[d]Bernard S, Neville KA, Nguyen AT, Flockhart DA. Interethnic differences in genetic polymorphisms of CYP2D6 in the US population: clinical implications. Oncologist. 2006;11(2):126-135.

[e]Sistonen J, Fuselli S, Palo JU, et al. Pharmacogenetic variation at CYP2C9, CYP2C19, and CYP2D6 at global and microgeographic scales. Pharmacogenet Genomics. 2009;19(2):170-179.

[f]Rodriguez-Antona C, Sayi JG, Gustafsson LL, et al. Phenotype-genotype variability in the human CYP3A locus as assessed by the probe drug quinine and analyses of variant CYP3A4 alleles. Biochem Biophys Res Commun. 2005;338(1):299-305.

analgesia perioperatively. However, safe and effective analgesia is still not achievable in about 50% of children[133,134] because of interindividual differences in pain perception and drug responses that are partly explained by pharmacogenomics.[135] To address this deficiency, a multicenter, randomized trial is underway to assess the efficacy of pharmacogenetic-guided opioid use as evidenced by the success of a single-center study of pharmacogenetic-guided codeine use in children after adenotonsillectomy.[136,137]

PAIN PERCEPTION AND GENETICS

Pain is both a subjective experience and a biopsychosocial phenomenon. It is well known that there is large interindividual variability in pain responses, particularly in adolescents experiencing postoperative pain. Animal studies have identified markers in more than 400 genes that affect nociception; these are presented in the Pain Genes Database, an interactive web browser of pain-related transgenic knock-out studies.[138]

Neurotransmitters such as catecholamines (epinephrine, norepinephrine, and dopamine) are vital components in the pain perception pathway. Catecholaminergic neurons in the solitary nucleus integrate visceral and somatic sensory information when inflammation is present peripherally.[139,140] One of the genes that affect this pathway is catechol-O-methyltransferase (COMT) that codes for the enzyme COMT involved in degradation of catecholamines. Decreased COMT activity increases catecholamines and leads to increased pain. Four common SNPs of COMT (rs6269, rs4633, rs4818, and rs4680) are involved. SNP rs4680 is coded by 472G>A, which causes the substitution of valine by methionine at amino acid position 158 (Val158Met). These four SNPs define low pain sensitivity (LPS: GCCG$_{val}$), average pain sensitivity (APS: ATCA$_{met}$), and high pain sensitivity (HPS: ACCG$_{val}$) haplotypes.[141,142] The presence of these haplotypes was shown to cause differences in mRNA structure, enzymatic activity, and protein levels in cells expressing COMT.[143] The low pain sensitivity haplotype exhibited the greatest enzymatic activity, whereas the high pain sensitivity haplotype exhibited the least enzymatic activity and protein levels in cells expressing COMT. Variations within COMT are associated with experimental pain responses to heat, cold, pressure, and mechanical stimuli. In addition, the COMT genotype is predictive of chronic pain in fibromyalgia, temporomandibular joint disorder,[141] and postsurgical pain.[144] Although there have been conflicting reports of Val/Val genotypes requiring larger doses of morphine in cancer patients[145] compared with Met/Met's larger pain ratings in experimental studies,[146] it is possible that population differences, haplotype differences, and other gene interactions might contribute to these conflicting observations. In a pediatric study involving 149 children undergoing tonsillectomy, associations of COMT SNPs (rs6269, rs4633, rs4818, and rs4680) and haplotypes with maximum pain scores and morphine consumption were studied. In addition to haplotype differences in morphine requirement, the authors found that minor allele carriers of COMT SNPs were approximately three times more likely to require analgesic interventions than homozygotes of major alleles.[147]

The metabolism of phenylalanine and the synthesis of serotonin, dopamine, epinephrine, norepinephrine, and nitric oxide (NO) are reliant on adequate cellular levels of tetrahydrobiopterin (BH4), an essential cofactor of enzymes involved in their synthesis (hydroxylases and nitric oxide synthases). GTP cyclohydroxylase 1 (GCH1), the rate-limiting enzyme responsible for the synthesis of BH4, is regulated by gene GCH1. GCH1 transcription is induced in the presence of inflammatory markers and nerve injury, leading to increased BH4 and nitric oxide production; nitric oxide sensitizes transient receptor potential vanilloid

subfamily type 1 (TRPV1) and subfamily ankyrin repeats type 1 (TRPA1), causing increased calcium influx into the neuron and increased pain responses.[148] Concomitantly, loss-of-function haplotype defined by three polymorphisms (rs8007267G<A, rs3783641A<T, and rs10483639C<G) was associated with decreased GCH1 activity in vitro and with pain protection in experimental pain models in volunteers[149] and in patients undergoing diskectomy for persistent radicular low back pain.[150] There have been negative association studies since, but whether the association is spurious or dependent on the effect size is not clear because of multiple confounding variables.

Combinatorial genetics likely contribute to a greater extent than single genes in predicting variability. In 201 Caucasians undergoing abdominal surgery, the authors tested associations among morphine consumption, postoperative pain, and SNPs within opioid receptor μ-1 (OPRM1), COMT, uridine-5'diphosphate glucose-glucuronosyltransferase-2B7 (UGT2B7), and estrogen receptor (ESR1) gene loci to elucidate genetic predictors of opioid consumption. Age and nine SNPs in ESR1, OPRM1, and COMT explained the greatest proportion of variance of morphine consumption (10.7%; p = 0.001). Three SNPs in ESR1, OPRM1, and COMT explained 5% of the variance (p = 0.007). There was also an interaction between rs4680 in COMT and rs4986936 in ESR1 (p = 0.007) on opioid consumption.[151]

There are also some congenital conditions that lead to insensitivity to pain, caused by pathogenic mutations in genes such as the neurotrophic tyrosine kinase receptor type 1 gene (NTRK1) and nerve growth factor-β (NGFB) with an anhidrosis phenotype.[152] Various mutations of the sodium channel voltage-gated type IX, alpha subunit SCN9A gene leading to nonfunctional alpha subunits of NaV1.7 channels inhibit the generation and transmission of nerve signals, leading to pain insensitivity along with anosmia.[65] A comprehensive overview of pharmacogenomics and pain is beyond the scope of this chapter; please refer to review articles.[135,153,154]

Genetic Variations Affecting Opioid Pharmacokinetics

Pharmacogenetics affecting enzyme activity affects both drug exposure and effect, leading to either toxic effects or decreased effectiveness. The United States Food and Drug administration (FDA) has issued warnings and guidelines for pharmacogenetics pertaining to the effects of some drugs used in pediatric anesthesia practice.

CODEINE

Codeine is a weak opioid endorsed by the World Health Organization as the second step on the analgesic ladder for cancer pain and has been used routinely for postoperative and breakthrough pain in chronic sufferers. It is a prodrug with a 200-fold weaker affinity for μ-opioid receptors than morphine. Although 80% of the administered drug is inactivated by glucuronidation to codeine-6-glucuronide by UGT2B7 and N-demethylation to norcodeine by CYP3A4, 5% to 10% of codeine undergoes O-demethylation to morphine, its active analgesic form via CYP2D6[155] (Fig. 4.1). Without O-demethylation, codeine confers a small fraction of the analgesic potency of morphine, and much of its analgesic effect is likely contributed by a metabolite, codeine 6-glucuronide.[156]

A small proportion of the population (ranging from 2%–10% in different ethnic groups) are CYP2D6 PM and thus have limited analgesia with codeine.[66,157] Alternative analgesics should be sought in children who are PM although testing for CYP2D6 polymorphisms is not undertaken routinely today before prescribing codeine.

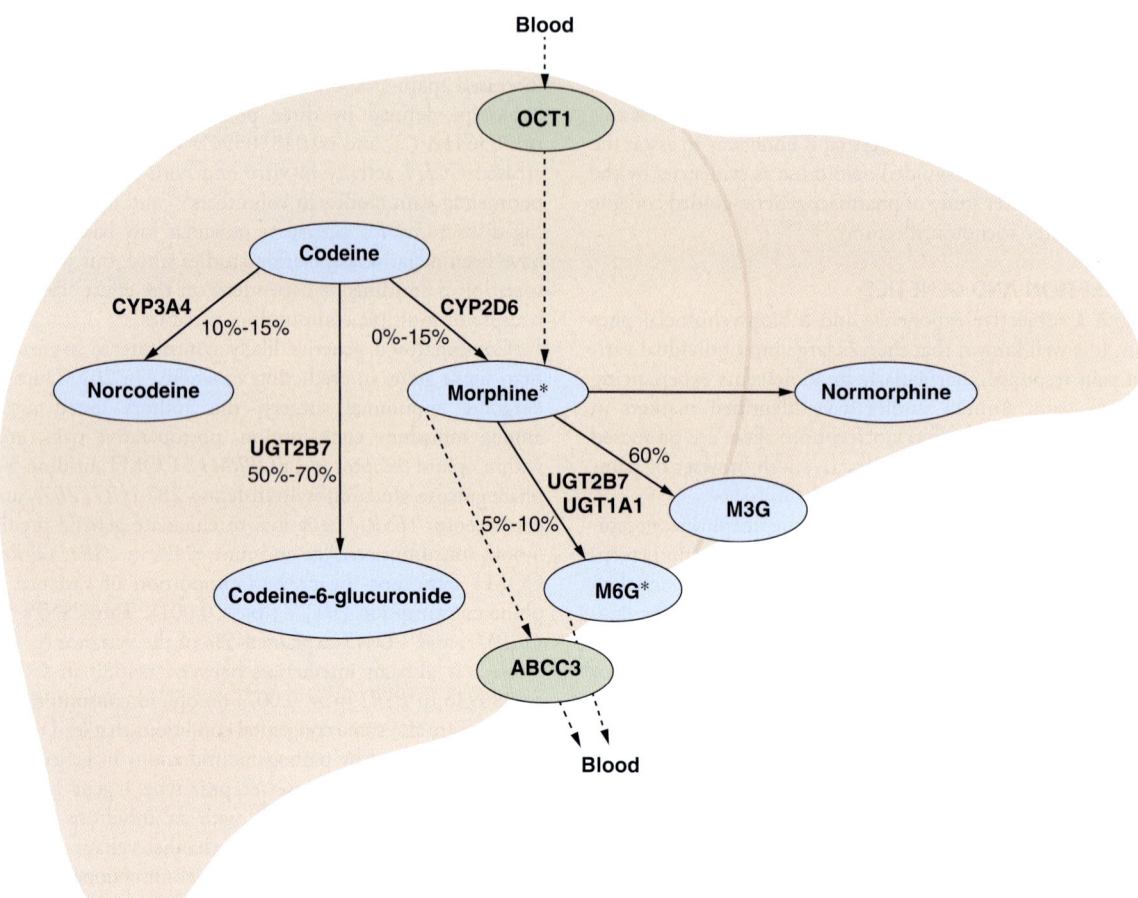

FIGURE 4.1 Diagrammatic presentation of the candidate genes involved in the pharmacokinetic pathway of codeine and morphine in the liver. Codeine, a prodrug, is converted to active form* morphine primarily by cytochrome (*CYP2D6*). Approximately 50%–70% of codeine is converted to codeine-6-glucuronide by uridine glucuronosyltransferase (*UGT2B7*); 10%–15% of codeine is *N*-demethylated to norcodeine by cytochrome P450 enzyme (*CYP3A4*). Both these metabolites have a similar affinity to codeine for the μ-opioid receptor. Between 0% and 15% of codeine is *O*-demethylated to morphine by *CYP2D6*, the most active metabolite*, which has 200-fold greater affinity for the μ-opioid receptor compared with codeine. Morphine is mainly (60%) glucuronidated to morphine-3-glucuronide (M3G), whereas 5%–10% is glucuronidated to morphine-6-glucuronide (M6G) primarily by *UGT2B7*, and to a lesser extent, *UGT1A1*. M6G is the active metabolite with a higher affinity for the μ-opioid receptor. *OCT1* is a hepatic transporter responsible for transporting morphine from blood into liver cells. *ABCC3* is a hepatic efflux transporter, and it transports morphine and morphine glucuronides from liver cells into blood.

The safety and efficacy of codeine in children who are UM have been called into question; the frequency of UM genotypes is substantive from 1% in Denmark and Finland, 10% in Greece and Portugal, and 29% in Ethiopia.[158] Children with *CYP2D6* polymorphisms who also have upregulated opioid receptors as a result of chronic intermittent nocturnal hypoxia (obstructive sleep apnea) may be particularly vulnerable to a mishap after regular codeine use.[159] Consequently, the wide clinical response to a standard (or less than standard) dose of codeine necessitates careful monitoring in those with compromised cardiorespiratory status. Several deaths or near-deaths have been reported with "standard" doses of oral codeine in children later found to be UM.[160,161] A fatality after codeine administration was reported in a healthy 2-year-old boy given weight-appropriate codeine doses after adenotonsillectomy; he died on the second postoperative day. Increased blood concentrations of morphine (32 ng/mL) and reduced codeine concentrations (0.70 ng/mL) were found. Genotyping revealed functional duplication of the *CYP2D6* allele.[160] This was followed by further reports[162,163] that

ultimately led to new regulations by the FDA, European Medicines Agency, and the UK Medicines and Healthcare Products Regulatory Agency. Restrictions were placed on pediatric use, and some centers have removed codeine from their formularies.[164] The 2012 Clinical Pharmacogenetics Implementation Consortium (CPIC) guidelines for *CYP2D6* genotype and codeine therapy were updated in 2014.[165] This guideline recommends using alternative analgesics to codeine in patients who are *CYP2D6* PM or UM (see Table 4.2). A new *black-box warning*, the FDA's strongest warning, was added to the drug label of codeine-containing products about the risk of codeine in postoperative pain management in children. The warning specifies that *"Health care professionals should prescribe an alternate analgesic for postoperative pain control in children who are undergoing tonsillectomy and/or adenoidectomy. Codeine should not be used for pain in children following these procedures"* (https://www.fda.gov/drugs/fda-drug-safety-podcasts/fda-drug-safety-podcast-fda-restricts-use-prescription-codeine-pain-and-cough-medicines-and-tramadol). It should be noted that these same concerns apply to children who require analgesia for greater than 1 day regardless of the surgical procedure, particularly obese children who may have obstructive sleep apnea.

There are also safety concerns for breastfed babies whose mothers take codeine for pain relief. This was highlighted in 2006 with the report of death in a breastfed infant after codeine was administered to the mother; she was an UM of codeine and analysis of her breast milk revealed a very large blood concentration of morphine, 87 ng/mL.[166] Hence, the safest advice is to avoid codeine in anyone whose *CYP2D6* activity is unknown; those with high levels of activity may suffer from toxicity, whereas those with low levels will suffer unnecessary pain. Others have taken a more active posture by identifying the CYP2D6 isoforms in their patients, in this case, children with sickle cell disease, and determined which children would benefit from or suffer from possible sequelae after codeine administration to treat sickle cell pain.[137] This study demonstrated that codeine is an effective and safe analgesic provided the genetic *CYP2D6* isoform is known before prescribing the drug, although the phenotype of the isoforms was not determined. Despite pharmacokinetic evidence that children with *CYP2D6* UM convert more codeine to morphine than those who are EM,[167] phenotypic variability in the 2D6 isoform, particularly the EM isoform, should be reported to provide an accurate prediction of drug responses. Variability in the phenotypic expression of the *CYP2D6* EM depends on several factors including the patient's ethnicity, diet and supplements, and unidentified sequence variations that in aggregate, may yield substantial variability in the activity of the isoform. This variability, known as the Activity Score, encompasses all these factors in a final common pathway such as the metabolism of dextromethorphan to portend whether the child with EM may behave phenotypically as an EM or as an UM. For example, Caucasian people who are EM with a 2D6*2 isoform metabolize dextromethorphan more rapidly than African American people with the same isoform.[162,168]

TRAMADOL

Tramadol is a weak opioid agonist metabolized by several pathways including *CYP2D6*-mediated oxidation to *O*-desmethyltramadol, which although a minor metabolite, has a 200-fold greater affinity for μ-opioid receptors than the parent drug.[169] Tramadol exerts its analgesic activity through complementary mechanisms: activating the μ-opioid receptor mainly by *O*-desmethyltramadol and weak inhibition of norepinephrine and serotonin reuptake (primarily by tramadol). For children who are *CYP2D6* PM, both the plasma concentrations for the active metabolite and analgesia are less than with the EM, whereas for those who are 2D6 UM, both the plasma concentrations and analgesia, and the side effects are greater than in those who are EM.[170–172] However, as with codeine, genotype may not predict phenotype in all individuals. Not all subjects who are genotype *CYP2D6 PM* (*n* = 20) have slow clearance of its active metabolite (Fig. 4.2)[173] As was the case with codeine, the FDA issued a black-box warning contraindicating the use of tramadol for pain relief in children younger than 12 years of age because of reported deaths. It also recommended against its use in children younger than age 18 years for analgesia after adenotonsillectomy and children between 12 and 18 years of age with obesity and obstructive sleep apnea. The use of tramadol is not recommended in breastfeeding mothers (https://www.fda.gov/drugs/fda-drug-safety-podcasts/fda-drug-safety-podcast-fda-restricts-use-prescription-codeine-pain-and-cough-medicines-and-tramadol).

HYDROCODONE

Hydrocodone is also metabolized by *CYP2D6* to hydromorphone, which has 10- to 33-fold greater affinity for opioid receptors than hydrocodone. *CYP2D6* polymorphisms can impact hydrocodone and the concentration of its metabolites and thus, its analgesic efficacy.[174] Although pharmacokinetic studies demonstrated that the peak concentrations of hydromorphone in children who are PM

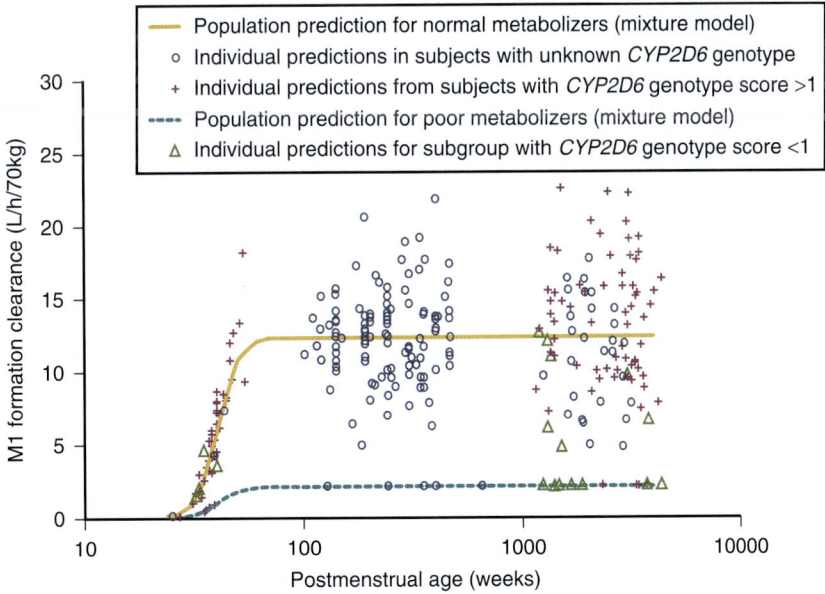

FIGURE 4.2 Maturation of tramadol formation clearance (CLPM) to *O*-desmethyl tramadol (M1 metabolite) labeled according to the availability of an individual *CYP2D6* genotype activity score. There is a distinct group of patients who are poor metabolizers identified by the phenotype *(dashed line)*. Not all subjects with a low genotype *CYP2D6* activity (*n* = 20) are included in this poor metabolizer group. (From Allegaert K, Holford NHG, Anderson BJ, et al. Tramadol and *O*-desmethyl tramadol clearance maturation and disposition in humans: a pooled pharmacokinetic study. *Clin Parmacokinet.* 2015;54(2):167-178. Used with permission from Springer.)

are less than in those with the other isoforms of 2D6, there is no clear clinical evidence how CYP2D6 genotypes affect its metabolism.[175,176] According to CPIC guidelines, hydrocodone may not be a good alternative to codeine in CYP2D6 UMs and PMs.

OXYCODONE

Oxycodone is a semisynthetic opioid agonist, that when compared with morphine, has a greater oral bioavailability, is more potent, and has a greater duration of action. Unlike morphine, it does not release histamine. As a result, oxycodone is widely used as the oral opioid of choice for postoperative analgesia in children.

The maturation pharmacokinetics of oxycodone are described.[177,178] About 11% of the drug is O-demethylated by CYP2D6 to the active metabolite oxymorphone, which has a 40-fold greater affinity and 8-fold greater opioid potency than oxycodone. The remaining 89% of the drug is N-demethylated by CYP3A to noroxycodone, a metabolite with weak antinociceptive properties. Both metabolites, oxymorphone and noroxycodone, are further degraded to noroxymorphone by CYP2D6 and CYP3A.[179] Unlike codeine, the parent compound oxycodone is responsible for more than 80% of its analgesic effect.[180] Although the impact of CYP2D6 polymorphisms on oxycodone metabolism has been well studied, information regarding the CYP3A4 variants in this context is sparse due to the low population frequency of the CYP3A4 polymorphism. In addition, there is no evidence of a CYP3A4 nonfunctional allele.[181] The greatest oxymorphone/oxycodone concentration ratios occur in CYP2D6 EM and UM and the smallest occur in CYP2D6 PM.[182] The noroxycodone/oxycodone ratio and daily oxycodone escalation rate are greater in cancer patients with the CYP3A5*3/*3 genotype.[183] Postoperative analgesic requirement is less in patients with CYP2D6 UM compared with PM.[184,185] CYP2D6 activity correlated with experimental pain assessment, impacting oxycodone pharmacodynamics and possibly the relative analgesic contribution of metabolites to the parent drug.[186] Other studies in postsurgical patients and cancer patients have demonstrated clinical differences among the genotypes.[187,188] Per the recent Clinical Pharmacogenetics Implementation Consortium, current evidence was insufficient to make firm clinical recommendations regarding genetic testing for oxycodone dose adjustment. Subsequently they concluded CYP2D6-dependent oral opioids, such as oxycodone, have the greatest potential for actionability[90] with opportunities for genotype-guided prescribing.[189]

MORPHINE

Approximately 60% of morphine is glucuronidated to morphine-3-glucuronide (M3G). Only 5% to 10% is glucuronidated to morphine-6-glucuronide (M6G), principally by UGT2B7 in the liver, and in part, by UGT1A1 and UGT1A8.[190] M6G is an active metabolite, with slower onset and more prolonged duration of action compared with morphine.[191] It is uncertain whether UGT2B7 variants affect morphine pharmacokinetics or dynamics. The UGT2B7-840G allele and the -161 C>T SNP are associated with reduced glucuronidation of morphine,[192,193] although other studies refuted this finding. There was no correlation between 12 SNPs of UGT2B7 and the morphine glucuronide/morphine serum ratios among 175 patients with normal hepatic and renal function who received long-term oral morphine therapy.[194]

In vitro studies have suggested that morphine has low transporter-independent permeability and 60% of total hepatic uptake is transporter dependent. Hence, there is an interest in the genetics of various hepatic transporters known to play a role in the disposition of morphine and its metabolites based on in vitro studies and mice.[190,195–200] OCT1, a member of the organic cation transporters (OCT), is predominantly expressed in the sinusoidal membrane of the human liver and mediates cellular uptake of morphine into hepatocytes (see Fig. 4.1). Approximately 10% of Caucasian people are compound homozygous carriers of one of the four common coding polymorphisms for OCT1 (Arg61Cys, Gly401Ser, Gly465Arg, and deletion of Met420) that result in reduced or lost OCT1 transporter activity and greater plasma concentrations of morphine.[198] OCT1 genotypes play a significant role in intravenous (IV) morphine clearance in children undergoing tonsillectomy.[201] Morphine clearance in homozygotes of loss-of-function OCT1 variants (OCT1*2–*5/*2–*5) was reduced (20%) compared with the wild type (OCT1*1/*1) and heterozygotes (OCT1*1/*2–*5).[201] The relatively common allelic frequencies of defective OCT1 variants among Caucasian people may explain their reduced morphine clearance and possibly greater frequencies of adverse events compared with Black children.

Another transporter belonging to the ATP-binding cassette (ABC) subfamily, ABCC3, is expressed in the basolateral membranes of hepatocytes and is an efflux transporter of M3G and M6G from the hepatocyte into the bloodstream (see Fig. 4.1). ABCC3 SNP -211T (rs4793665) is located in the promoter region of the gene and has been reported to alter hepatic mRNA expression[202] and contribute to reduced efflux of morphine glucuronides.[203] In children undergoing tonsillectomy, in addition to the effects of polymorphisms of OCT1 genotype on morphine pharmacokinetics, the C/C polymorphisms of ABCC3 -211C>T significantly increased the transformation of morphine-6-glucuronide and morphine-3-glucuronide by ~40% compared with the C/T+T/T genotypes.[204] Similarly, in 316 children undergoing tonsillectomy, ABCC3 variants rs4148412 (allele A) and rs729923 (allele G) caused a 2.36 (95% confidence interval [CI]=1.28–4.37, $P=0.0061$) and 3.7 (95% CI=1.47–9.09, $P=0.005$) times increased odds ratio of morphine-induced respiratory depression, leading to prolonged postoperative care unit stay. These clinical associations were supported by increased formation clearance of morphine glucuronides in children with rs4148412 AA and rs4973665 CC genotypes in this cohort, as well as an independent spine surgical cohort of 67 adolescents.[205] Homozygotes with the 3435C>T variant of another ABC efflux transporter of morphine, ABCB1, expressed large cerebrospinal fluid concentrations of morphine. This efflux transporter is responsible for removing unwanted medications and toxins from the central nervous system and gastrointestinal tract. The ABCB1 3435 C>T allele is linked to greater analgesia with morphine in cancer-related pain and reduced morphine requirements in a mixed chronic pain population.[206,207] After tonsillectomy, children with GG and GA genotypes of ABCB1 polymorphism rs9282564 have a fourfold greater risk of respiratory depression prolonging hospital stays.[208] Despite the large volume of literature on morphine pharmacogenetics, the data are contradictory, leading to a lack of consensus. Evidence associating genetic variants to morphine pharmacokinetics, and subsequently to clinical outcomes is still weak and requires further research.

METHADONE

Methadone is a long-acting opioid that has been traditionally used in the management of substance use disorders and chronic pain. The use of methadone to manage perioperative pain in children and adults has increased over the last 2 decades.[209,210] Methadone is primarily eliminated by the hepatic cytochrome P450 enzyme system. Several CYP enzymes are involved in the metabolism of methadone to its inactive metabolites: 2-ethylidene-1,5-dimethyl-3,3-diphenylpyrrolidine, and 2-ethyl-5-methyl-3,3-diphenylpyrroline. These include CYP2B6, CYP3A4, CYP3A5, CYP2C19, CYP2C9, and CYP2D6.[211]

The greatest volume of methadone is eliminated via the CYP3A4 pathway followed by CYP2B6. However, the CYP2B6 pathway is of greater interest given its stereoselectivity (S-methadone > R-methadone) and genetic variability.[211,212] Genetic polymorphisms cause the expression of CYP2B6 to vary 20- to 250-fold among individuals.[213] The most common and clinically significant variant allele is *CYP2B6*6* (516G>T, Q172H; 785A>G, K262R), which markedly reduces *CYP2B6* expression and activity.[214] Concomitantly, S-methadone concentrations were greater in *CYP2B6*6* homozygotes compared with heterozygotes and noncarriers, and these *CYP2B6*6* patients had reduced dose requirements.[215,216] *CYP2B6*4, *9* variants are also associated with reduced methadone metabolism and decreased dose requirements.[212] In fact, genetic influence is found to be greater for oral than IV methadone and S- compared to R-methadone.[212] The influence of *CYP2B6* variants on methadone related perioperative pain and adverse outcomes have also been described in the pediatric literature.[217]

Other *CYP2B6* variant alleles, namely *CYP2B6*5, *11,* have been reported to impact methadone dose requirements in disorders of opioid use; however, there are conflicting results.[218–220] Many genetic variants have also been reported for *CYP2C19, CYP2C9, CYP2D6, CYP3A4,* and *CYP3A5*.[215,218,221–223] The impact of these variants on methadone clearance and their clinical significance are unknown.

Polymorphisms in the *ABCB1* gene coding for P-glycoprotein can impact the hepatic and renal clearance of methadone. The most common variants studied include *1236C>T, 3435C>T,* and *2677G>T/A*; the *3435C>T* variant has been known to decrease S-methadone clearance.[218] The *2677G>T* polymorphism was associated with lower trough concentrations of R- and S-methadone.[224,225] The homozygous 1236C>T variant has been associated with greater methadone dose requirements.[226] *POR* and *ORM1* polymorphisms are also being studied in relation to methadone metabolism. *POR* codes for cytochrome P450 oxidoreductase.[227,228] *POR* polymorphisms can decrease CYP activity.[218,227] *ORM1* codes for alpha-1-acid glycoprotein, which serves as the primary plasma binding protein for methadone.[228]

Genetic Variations Affecting Opioid Pharmacodynamics

Genetic modulation of the density of opioid receptors, affinity, or coupling affects the variability in the intersubject responses to opioids. In a study of 121 adult twin pairs who were randomly assigned to receive alfentanil or placebo, there was significant heritability for respiratory depression (30%), nausea (59%), and drug disliking (36%), as well as significant familial effects for sedation (29%), pruritus (38%), dizziness (32%), and drug liking (26%) after alfentanil administration.[229,230]

OPIOID RECEPTOR (*OPRM1*)

This gene, located on chromosome 6q24-q25, is a member of the G protein–coupled receptor family and of major interest as it codes for the μ-opioid receptor, a molecular binding site of all clinically effective opioids and endogenous opioid peptides like

β-endorphin.[231] It is widely distributed throughout the nervous system (periaqueductal gray area, in the substantia gelatinosa area in dorsal horn of the spinal cord, in the olfactory bulb, the cerebral cortex, and the amygdala) as well as the gastrointestinal tract. This gene mediates opioid-induced analgesia and adverse effects including respiratory depression, and constipation. One of the most commonly studied SNPs of *OPRM1* is A118G (rs1799971), in which guanine (G) is substituted for an adenine (A) at base 118, which in turn causes the amino acid exchange at position 40 of the μ-opioid receptor protein from asparagine to aspartic acid (N40D), that leads to the loss of an *N*-glycosylation site in the extracellular region of the receptor.[232] The allele frequency shows a racial bias; it is greater in the Asian population (50%) than in European American (10.5%–18.8%) and African American (5%–15%) populations.[233]

In vitro studies have shown reduced cell-surface receptor binding site availability for morphine in cells expressing the G variant compared with the A variant, less efficient agonist-induced receptor signaling in postmortem human brain tissue in 118G carriers, and 1.5- to 2.5-fold increased mRNA expression in 118A human brain cells compared with the G variant.[234–236] An in vivo study investigating the effects of A118G genotype on μ-opioid receptor binding potential in human brains using carfentanil positron emission tomography, found that smokers homozygous with the wild-type AA genotype exhibited significantly greater levels of receptor binding potential than smokers carrying the G allele in the bilateral amygdala, left thalamus, and left anterior cingulate cortex.[237] In contrast, the variant receptor had a threefold greater binding affinity for endogenous β-endorphins with potentially different connotations for pain sensitivity but not analgesic response to opioids.[238]

In accordance with the mechanistic findings mentioned previously, several studies in adults have shown that the opioid requirements (morphine, M6G, fentanyl, and alfentanil) in postoperative patients and volunteers with the GG/AG genotypes were greater and the adverse effects such as nausea less compared with those with the AA genotypes at the A118G SNP.[239–246] In postsurgical Asian adult patients undergoing knee arthroplasty, hysterectomy, and Cesarean section,[239,240,244] carriers of the G allele had greater pain scores and greater morphine requirements than those with the AA genotypes. In a prospective genotype-blinded study of 88 healthy adolescents undergoing spine fusion for idiopathic scoliosis, the risk of morphine-induced respiratory depression in patients with the AA genotype was greater (odds ratio 5.6, 95% CI=1.4–37.2, P=0.03) compared with the AG/GG genotypes.[208] Similar results in human volunteers found a two to four times greater dose of alfentanil was required to produce the same level of analgesia as the wild type, and a 10- to 12-fold greater dose was needed for the same level of respiratory depression in the homozygous 118GG volunteers.[247] However, no association was found for the A118G effects on M6G-induced respiratory depression (measured by the isocapnic acute hypoxic ventilatory response) and postoperative nausea or vomiting (PONV) after fentanyl.[245,248] A meta-analysis of the OPRM1 A118G effects concluded that the evidence that homozygous GG carriers of A118G exhibited slightly greater opioid requirements and slightly less nausea was weak.[249]

In addition to the rs1799971 (A118G) variant, a novel C-T variant (rs563649) has been identified in the 5′ untranslated region of the spliced isoform MOR1K that is preferentially expressed in the medulla oblongata.[250] This variant had the strongest single contribution to measured pain sensitivity responses in 196 pain-free European and American females. The C-T variant is located within a structurally conserved internal ribosome entry site upstream of exon 13 and affects both mRNA levels and translation efficiency of MOR1K isoforms. Strong linkage disequilibrium was identified between rs563649 and rs1799971, and the minor T allele of rs563649 tagged a 6-SNP (AGTCTG) haplotype associated with great pain sensitivity. Haplotype combinations rather than single variants may be a better predictor of OPRM1 effects.

BLOOD-BRAIN BARRIER TRANSPORTER (*ABCB1*)

P-glycoprotein (P-gp), a surface phosphoglycoprotein encoded by *ABCB1* and a member of the superfamily of ABC transporters, is an ATP-dependent drug efflux transporter. P-gp is expressed on the epithelial surface at the intestinal lumen, biliary canaliculi, renal proximal tubule, and in the choroid plexus as the blood-brain barrier (BBB). Morphine, fentanyl, methadone, sufentanil, alfentanil, morphine-6-glucuronide, and loperamide are all confirmed P-gp substrates.[196,251–254] Variations in the *ABCB1* efflux transporter at the blood-brain barrier can alter cerebral penetration and pharmacokinetics of opioids.[255] The most commonly studied variants in the coding region of *ABCB1* are c.1236C>T (rs1128503), c.2677G>T/A (rs2032582), and c.3435C>T (rs1045642) and these are in strong linkage disequilibrium.[256] *ABCB1* genotypes 1236 TT, 2677TT, and 3435TT, together with the 1236TT genotype alone, were associated with early and profound respiratory suppression in adults given IV fentanyl during spinal anesthesia.[246,257] The homozygous diplotype (GG-CC at c.2677G>T/A and c.3435C>T) has a borderline association with morphine-associated PONV[256]; however, in another report of adults treated with morphine, a combined effect of 3435T of *ABCB1* and 80A of *OPRM1* was associated with increased pain relief but without influence on the incidence of adverse effects.[206]

Another SNP that has been studied is *rs9282564*, a non-synonymous polymorphism with a threefold greater maximum velocity for adenosine triphosphatase activity compared with the wild type.[258] Children with GG and GA genotypes of *ABCB1* rs9282564 have a greater risk for respiratory depression after tonsillectomy, resulting in prolonged postanesthesia care unit stays. Each additional copy of the minor allele (G) of the *ABCB1* SNP, rs9282564, increased the odds of respiratory depression that resulted in a 4.7-fold (95% CI=2.1–10.8) greater duration of stay in the postanesthesia care unit. This variant allele had also been reported to have a modest effect in reducing the trough levels of methadone.[259] Haplotypes of SNPs at positions 61, 1199, 1236, 2677, and 3435 influenced methadone requirements in opioid-dependent and nondependent patients, but they did not predict opioid dependence.[260] However, others have reported contradictory results that there was no association between *ABCB1* polymorphisms and the trough plasma concentrations, methadone dose, or methadone response.[261]

OPIOID-CANNABINOID SYSTEM INTERACTIONS

Fatty acid amide hydrolase (*FAAH*), opioid and cannabinoid systems reciprocally and synergistically modulate functions at multiple levels. *FAAH* codes for an enzyme that hydrolyzes anandamide, the "bliss" molecule. Inhibition of *FAAH* increases the bioavailability of anandamide and thereby augments analgesia; this offers a potential therapeutic target for treating pain.[262,263] Five specific *FAAH* SNPs, including a missense variant (rs324420) that affects *FAAH* stability, were reported to be associated with

more than twofold greater risk for refractory PONV in children undergoing tonsillectomy.[264]

Genes of Addiction

Alongside a multitude of environmental factors, genetic variations contribute to vulnerability and resilience to substance use. This is especially relevant in adolescence and early adulthood, which is the prime time when these addictions occur. Forty to sixty percent of the risk is genetic, regardless of the drug of addiction.[265] In a national survey in 2015 to 2016, 27.5% of the respondents, corresponding to 32.8 million individuals (including 21% adolescents and 32.2% young adults) reported using prescription opioids in the past year. The prevalence of opioid misuse was 3.8% among adolescents and 7.8% among young adults.[266] A precursor to addiction is opioid exposure, including prescription opioids, and family history, suggesting genetic vulnerability for opioid use disorder.[267]

Dopamine is an important neurotransmitter responsible for the euphoric response to opioids, leading to dependence and addiction.[268] Dopamine receptor expression in the mesolimbic area has been linked to addictive traits like pleasure seeking, impulsivity, and reward deficiency syndrome.[269] Polymorphisms in *DRD2* gene coding for D2 dopamine receptor have been associated with heroin use.[270] *DRD2* variants rs1076560 and rs1800497 have been associated with opioid use disorders.[271,272] *DRD3* variants are associated with sensation seeking and *DRD4* variants have been linked to greater vulnerability to opioid dependence.[273,274] Likewise, the dopamine D1 receptor (*DRD1*), which modulates opioid reinforcement, reward, and opioid-induced neuroadaptation, and the μ-1 opioid receptor gene (*OPRM1*), a target of opioids, also had variants that predicted opioid dependence or protection thereof, in association studies.[275] The A118G SNP of the *OPRM1* gene is the most studied and has been associated with phenotypes including opioid dependence and other substance dependencies.[276,277] A recent large genome-wide association study identified *OPRM1* rs1799971 to be significantly associated with opioid use disorder.[278] *OPRK1, OPRD1* polymorphisms are also being studied in the context of opioid use disorder.[279,280] Variants of gene coding for the dopamine metabolizing enzyme COMT have also been studied in this context.[281]

A meta-analysis of 5-hydroxytryptamine (serotonin) 2A receptor gene (*HTR2A*) genotypes at SNPs rs6313 and rs6311 from available genetic association studies from different populations showed their contribution to genetic susceptibility to substance use disorders, especially alcohol dependence.[282] Certain variants of the glutamate receptor, the NMDA 2A (*GRIN2A*) gene that encodes the 2A subunit of the NMDA receptor, were involved in the development of heroin addiction.[283] Neurotrophic factors like brain-derived neurotrophic factor (BDNF) play a role in the transition from drug use to drug dependence.[284] Variants in genes coding for neurotrophic factors such as *BDNF, NRXN3* have been implicated in genetic vulnerability to opioid use disorders.[285,286] Recent genome-wide association studies have identified other genes of interest such as *KCNC1, KCNG2,* and *CNIH3* that could play a role in opioid use disorders.[287] *KCNC1* and *KCNG2* code for voltage-gated potassium channels involved in downstream μ-opioid receptor signaling pathways, which are responsible for synaptic long-term potentiation.[288] *CNIH3* codes for an auxiliary protein on the α-amino-3-hydroxy-5-methyl-4-isoxazolepropionic acid (AMPA) receptor, which has been known to play a role in the evolution of opioid addiction.[289]

Nonsteroidal Antiinflammatory Drugs and Genetics

NSAIDs act by inhibiting cyclooxygenase enzymes (COX-1 and COX-2) coded for by the prostaglandin endoperoxide synthase genes, *PTGS I and II*. Commonly used NSAIDs such as ibuprofen and diclofenac undergo phase 1 detoxification (*CYP2C9* for S(+)-ibuprofen; *CYP2C8* for R(−)-ibuprofen; *CYP2C9* and *CYP3A4* for diclofenac)[290,291] followed by glucuronidation (mainly *UGT2B7*).[292] Multidrug resistance–associated proteins 2 (*MRP2/ABCC2*) and breast cancer resistance protein (*BCRP/ABCG2*) affect biliary excretion of diclofenac glucuronides, and *MRP3/ABCC3* was the main efflux transporter from liver to blood.[293] Dubin-Johnson syndrome is caused by acquired or hereditary deficiency of *ABCC2*, leading to increased concentration of bilirubin glucuronides.[294] As diclofenac shares the same *ABCC2* transporter pathway, it should be prescribed to those individuals with caution to avoid adverse reactions to diclofenac, particularly hepatotoxicity.[295]

There are two frequent allelic variants for *CYP 2C9*; *CYP2C9-CYP2C9*2* (430C>T Arg144Cys) and *CYP2C9*3* (1075A>C Ile359Leu) that decrease the activity in in vitro and in vivo studies. *CYP2C9*2*, *3*, and *CYP2C8*3* allelic variants reduce ibuprofen metabolism and/or clearance.[296] However, *CYP2C8*3* is in strong linkage disequilibrium with the *CYP2C9*2* variant, making it difficult to distinguish whether the effects are due to *CYP2C8* or *CYP2C9*. Investigations into the association between *CYP2C9* and *CYP2C8* polymorphisms and response to ibuprofen therapy for patent ductus arteriosus closure in extremely preterm neonates showed that greater gestational age and non-Caucasian ethnicity were associated with an ibuprofen response, but not the *CYP2C* polymorphisms.[297] Gastroduodenal bleeding was strongly associated with *CYP2C9*3* carriers as opposed to noncarriers (adjusted odds ratio 7.3) in adults given NSAIDs, including diclofenac, ibuprofen, celecoxib, and naproxen.[298] These findings were not consistent in all studies.[299,300]

Ketorolac, another nonselective COX inhibitor, is safe for use in neonates[301] although as in children and unlike adults, it does not penetrate the cerebrospinal fluid to any significant extent. The transporter gene, *MDR-1,* has been implicated in the transport of ketorolac across the blood-brain barrier and may explain its limited presence in cerebrospinal fluid.[302] Furthermore, developmental differences in COX-1 expression in the spinal cord in animals, may explain the lack of analgesic efficacy of ketorolac in 3-day-old compared with 21-day-old pups[303] and 2-week-old compared with 4-week-old rats.[304] The authors extrapolated that "*should similar deficits occur in humans, COX-1 inhibitors may exhibit reduced efficacy in infants.*"[304] However, this lack of effectiveness was not observed in clinical studies of ketorolac in neonates, in whom analgesia was achieved in 94.4%.[301]

Selective COX-2 inhibitors produce less inhibition of COX-1 and are expected to have short-term gastrointestinal safety benefits, although, their long-term benefits remain inconclusive.[305] COX-2 mRNA and protein expression are increased in the presence of gastric mucosal lesions, suggesting that they may be involved in the repair process of those lesions.[306] Thus selective COX-2 inhibition might disturb the COX-2 enzyme–mediated protective prostaglandin production.

Celecoxib, a COX-2 inhibitor metabolized by *CYP2C9,* has been investigated for *CYP2C9* variant effects on its pharmacokinetics. In a study in volunteers, those with the *CYP2C9*1/*3* and *CYP2C9*3/*3* variants experienced a greater concentration exposure (2-fold and 7.7-fold, respectively) and maximum concentration (1.5-fold and 1.8-fold, respectively) and a reduced clearance (2.3-fold and 10-fold, respectively) than those with the *CYP2C9*1/*1* variant.[307] A case report described severe drug-induced gastropathy in an IM of the *CYP2C9* gene, presumably resulting from prolonged drug exposure.[308] Children given celecoxib who had the genotype *CYP2C9*3* had less pain and improved functional recovery after tonsillectomy.[309] Celecoxib is currently on the FDA biomarker list, cautioning use in *CYP2C9* PM (dose reduction by 50% or select an alternate medication).

Acetaminophen and Genetics

Acetaminophen is primarily converted to two pharmacologically inactive conjugates: glucuronide (52%–57%) and sulfate (30%–44%), with a minor fraction undergoing oxidation to a reactive metabolite *N*-acetyl-p-benzoquinone imine (NAPQI) (5%–10%).[310] *UGT1A1, UGT1A6, UGT1A9,* and *UGT2B15* are involved in acetaminophen glucuronidation,[311] whereas a family of cytosolic enzymes, called *sulfotransferases* (*SULT*), are involved in the acetaminophen sulfation (*SULT1A1, SULT1A3*).[312] Acetaminophen is bioactivated to the reactive intermediate (NAPQI)[313] by three CYP-450 isoforms: *CYP3A4, CYP2E1,* and *CYP1A2* of which *CYP2E1* is the most important. The contribution of *CYP3A4* to the production of NAPQI is controversial.[314,315] NAPQI is then conjugated with the sulfhydryl group of glutathione to form a nontoxic conjugate. Acetaminophen overdoses initially saturate sulfation, followed by glucuronidation; increased NAPQI production depletes glutathione stores, leading the NAPQI to bind to intracellular hepatic macromolecules to produce cell necrosis and damage.

Infants younger than 90 days postnatal age express less *CYP2E1* activity in vitro compared with older infants, children, and adults,[79] *CYP3A4* appears during the first week after birth, whereas *CYP1A2* appears later.[316] *CYP3A4* and *CYP1A2* activity in 12- to 48-month-old children exceeds that of all other stages of development and could potentially increase NAPQI production in 1- to 4-year-olds,[317] but this is favorably offset by an increased capacity to conjugate the drug with sulfate in this same age group. Nonetheless, two 10-fold overdoses of acetaminophen and two reports of multiple doses from multiple caregivers who were unaware of the other doses,[318] have been reported in infants. These reports underscore the need for extreme care when administering and also documenting the dosage of IV acetaminophen[319]; both infants with these massive acetaminophen overdoses recovered fully.

UGT1A polymorphism c.2042C>G (rs8330) is associated with increased human liver acetaminophen glucuronidation, an increased *UGT1A* exon 5a/5b splice variant/mRNA ratio, and decreased risk of unintentional acetaminophen-induced acute liver failure.[320] Individuals carrying the *CYP3A5* rs776746 A allele were overrepresented among patients with acute liver failure who had intentionally overdosed with acetaminophen with an odds ratio of 2.3 (95% CI=1.1–4.9, P=0.034), although this was not significant after adjusting for multiple comparison testing.[321]

Acute and Chronic Postsurgical Pain – Genetics and Epigenetics

Acute pain thresholds depend less on genetics than do chronic pain thresholds, with estimated heritability scores of 22% to 55%.[322] Leveraging systems biology approaches, both shared and unique genetic pathways associated with acute and chronic postsurgical pain (CPSP), have been described.[323] Family and twin studies have estimated heritability of chronic pain susceptibility at ~50%.[324-326] Genetic effects account for 12% to 60% response variability to experimental pain[327] and chronic pain conditions.[328-331] Basic and clinical genetic perspectives in pediatric chronic postsurgical pain have been described in detail.[332] Recent systematic reviews describe chronic postsurgical pain–genetic associations.[333-335] In a comprehensive review of 21 gene association studies, only one study (age 14–35 years) included children with chronic postsurgical pain, without specifying the number of adolescents included.[336,337] Six variants of five genes (COMT: rs4680 and rs6269, Mu-1 opioid receptor/OPRM1: rs1799971, GTP cyclohydrolase 1/GCH1: rs3783641, potassium voltage-gated channel modifier subfamily S member 1/KCNS1: rs734784, tumor necrosis factor/TNFA: rs1800629)[338-346] were associated with this chronic pain state, but only rs734784 (A>G) of KCNS1 was found to increase the risk of chronic postsurgical pain via meta-analysis. In conjunction with single-gene variants having small effect sizes in prediction of complex pain conditions, polygenic risk profiles have also been identified in pilot studies to improve the prediction of CPSP.[347]

Chronic pain conditions of the neck and back in monozygotic versus dizygotic twins showed a heritable component of up to 60%.[348] Imbalances in β_2-adrenergic receptor (ADRβ2) function increase the vulnerability to chronic pain conditions.[349] An association between a potassium channel modulatory subunit (KCNS1, also called Kv9.1) polymorphism and pain phenotype was identified in five of six independent chronic pain cohorts (including post–limb amputation and postmastectomy pain). The KCNS1 allele missense rs734784 is one of the first described prognostic indicators of chronic neuropathic pain risk.[350]

Dramatically altered gene expression is also found in patients who subsequently develop persistent postoperative pain, with at least 10% of the transcriptome being dysregulated in traumatic injury models of neuropathic pain. These mechanisms involve sensitization of peripheral nociceptors (transient receptor potential, TRPA1/TRPV1),[351,352] central signaling systems affecting dorsal horn plasticity (for example, brain-derived neurotrophic factor, BDNF),[353] and neuroimmune mechanisms including proinflammatory mediators (interleukins, IL-6, tumor necrosis factor TNF).[354] In chronic pain conditions such as inflammatory bowel disease, abdominal pain has been associated with increased capsaicin receptor TRPV1 expressing sensory fibers in colonic biopsies.[355] The gene BDNF, a member of the neurotrophin family, also increased expression in colonic mucosa, along with structural alterations, suggesting contributions to the visceral hyperalgesia seen in these patients.[356] Systems that affect the distribution of δ- and μ-opioid receptors (OPRM1) also control heat pain, mechanical pain, opioid effects, and nerve injury–induced mechanical hypersensitivity.[357,358] Voltage-gated calcium channels control trafficking/pain conduction from the dorsal root ganglion to the presynaptic terminals at the dorsal horn[359] (CACNA1A), leading to hyperalgesia and allodynia, probably resulting from increased calcium-dependent release of pronociceptive neurotransmitters such as glutamate and substance P.

Besides genetic variants, epigenetic mechanisms have been studied with respect to postoperative pain, chronic pain, and CPSP in children. These include nonstructural processes such as DNA methylation,[360] chromatin remodeling through histone modifications (methylation and acetylation), and noncoding RNAs (e.g., microRNAs)[361-367] regulating gene expression.[362,368] They are subject to environmental changes and thus modifiable, unlike genetic structural changes. Epigenetic effects on pain are illustrated by an epigenome study in identical twins, which showed the role of the TRPA1 promoter in pain sensitivity,[369]

association of COMT methylation with socioeconomic status,[370] and DNA demethylation at specific CpG sites in the IL1B promoter in response to inflammation.[371] These mechanisms may play an important role in nociceptive priming in neonates, especially as the peripheral immune system can retain "memory" and can regulate "tolerance" and "sensitization" to repeat insults and hence neuroplasticity.[372] DNA methylation in blood has been studied in children undergoing spine surgery as a predictor of acute and CPSP. Differential DNA methylation was identified in an active regulatory region of OPRM1 gene associated with CPSP[373] at transcription sites that were also implicated in opioid and heroin addicts.[374,375] Epigenome-wide studies also identified enriched genomic pathways underlying CPSP and anxiety sensitivity in children undergoing spine fusion.[376,377] These differentially DNA methylated positions enriched γ amino butyric acid receptor and dopamine-DARPP32 feedback in cyclic adenosine monophosphate signaling pathways in children[377] and non-hispanic White and Black adults with chronic low back pain.[377,378]

Pharmacogenomics Affecting Anesthesia

Genetics influence both the pharmacokinetics and pharmacodynamics of some agents commonly used in pediatric anesthesia, and hence could affect perioperative outcomes.

INTRAVENOUS ANESTHETICS

Propofol

The main enzyme that metabolizes propofol in hepatic as well as renal cortical microsomes is UGT1A9 (53%), with secondary contribution from hydroxylation (38%), mainly through the CYP2B6 and CYP2C9 in the liver.[379] The activity levels of CYP2B6 in infants younger than 10 months are only 10% and at 1.3 years, 50% of adult levels.[380] Very little is known about the developmental changes in UGT1A9. However, there is a 100-fold interindividual variability in activity of these enzymes throughout life. Propofol clearance varies more than 300% in the neonatal period with genetics thought to exert a greater influence on its clearance than age.[119,381] SNPs of UGT1A9 affect glucuronidation: 2152C>T, -440C>T, -331T>C, -275T>A, and 98T>C.[382] In vitro studies of UGT1A9 expression from DNA isolated from Japanese volunteers showed that transversion of 766G>A in the UGT1A9 gene that results in the substitution of amino acid D256N affected propofol glucuronidation kinetics.[383]

Propofol exerts its hypnotic actions by activation of the central inhibitory neurotransmitter GABA-A controlled by the GABRE gene.[384] Adverse effects of propofol have been described, including a rare but life-threatening complication called propofol infusion syndrome,[385] but it is not clear if genetic factors predispose to this complication. Although investigators report the time to loss of verbal contact and a bispectral index less than 70 varied 6.6- and 4.3-fold, respectively; the time to emergence from propofol anesthesia in adults varied 15.5- to 111-fold and the clearance of propofol varied greatly. However, there were no associations between variations in CYP2B6 (R487C, K262R, and Q172) variants or GABRE variants (mRNA358G/T, 20118C/T, 20326C/T, and 20502A/T) and the observed interindividual variability in response.[386] To date, there is no conclusive evidence of pharmacogenomic variations affecting clinical outcomes with propofol anesthesia.

Dexmedetomidine is metabolized extensively in the liver by glucuronidation (UGT1A4, UGT2B10)[387,388] and hydroxylation, mediated by CYP2A6.[389] There is great interindividual variability in response to dexmedetomidine,[390] for which the role of CYP2A6

SNPs was evaluated for their effect on clearance. However, several studies concluded that *CYP2A6* variants did not alter dexmedetomidine pharmacokinetics.[391,392] The sedative and anxiolytic effects of dexmedetomidine are mediated by subtypes of the α_2-adrenergic receptors, mainly by α-2A (*ADRA-2A*). Since receptor sensitivity would be expected to affect dexmedetomidine pharmacodynamics, variants affecting *ADRA2A* have been studied. The effects of *ADRA2A* C1291G polymorphism on dexmedetomidine response were studied in 110 patients undergoing coronary artery bypass grafting. It was found that those with the G allele were less sedated than those with the C allele.[393] Similarly, certain SNPs were also found to be associated with statistically significant interindividual differences in blood pressure changes.[394]

INHALATIONAL ANESTHETICS

Inhalational anesthetics act through a different site on the *GABAA* receptor. Preschool-age children with the AA genotype in the *GABAγ2* nucleotide position 3145 in intron A/G exhibited a greater incidence of emergence agitation compared with the non-AA genotype after sevoflurane anesthesia.[395] The human melanocortin-1 receptor (*MC1R*) gene is expressed on the surface of melanocytes and affects melanin biosynthesis and pigmentation. Sex specificity in response to κ-opioid agonists has been demonstrated in both mice and humans. Women with two variant *MC1R* alleles displayed significantly greater analgesia from the κ-opioid, pentazocine, than all other groups.[396] Women with three particular mutations of the *MC1R* gene (R151C, R160W, and D294H) demonstrated increased desflurane anesthetic requirements.[397] Moreover, those with inactive variants had a particular phenotype of red hair and pale skin, lending credence to the perception of altered anesthetic and analgesic requirements in redheads. They are metabolized primarily by *CYP2E1* in the liver to varying degrees.[398] Although the tendency of halothane hepatitis to cluster in families points to a genetic contribution, the hereditary mechanisms involved have not been defined.[129]

Nitrous Oxide

The effects of genetic variants on nitrous oxide action are related to its inhibitory actions on methionine synthesis whose activated form, S-adenosylmethionine, is the principal substrate involved in the formation of the myelin sheath, neurotransmitters, and DNA synthesis in rapidly proliferating tissues. Nitrous oxide irreversibly oxidizes the cobalt atom of vitamin B_{12}, thereby inhibiting the activity of the cobalt-dependent enzyme methionine synthase, which is the catalyst for the formation of methionine. Hence, in a patient who has a deleterious mutation in the 5,10-methylenetetrahydrofolate reductase *(MTHFR)* gene, exposure to nitrous oxide can lead to neurologic deterioration. This occurred in a male infant whose neurologic status unexpectedly deteriorated; the infant died after two exposures to nitrous oxide for lumbar puncture.[399] Postmortem analysis showed 5,10-methylenetetrahydrofolate reductase deficiency in this infant's fibroblasts and a complex combination of mutations in his *MTHFR* gene, including C677T and A1298C SNPs associated with a reduction in the enzyme activity. Patients who were homozygote for these variants developed greater plasma concentrations of homocysteine after nitrous oxide anesthesia.[400] Although mitigated by B vitamin infusions, this was not found to be related to an increase in perioperative troponin.[401]

BENZODIAZEPINES

Midazolam exerts its primary effects by reversible interactions with the inhibitor GABA receptor in the central nervous system.

It is primarily metabolized by the *CYP3A4/CYP3A5* enzymes in the liver to its hydroxyl derivatives. Hepatic CYP3A4 activity is reduced in neonatal versus adult livers, resulting in reduced midazolam clearance in the former.[402] Midazolam is metabolized mainly by hepatic hydroxylation (*CYP3A4*), followed by glucuronidation of the hydroxymetabolites.[403] *CYP3A7* is the dominant *CYP3A* enzyme in utero; it is expressed in the fetal liver and appears to have activity from as early as 50 to 60 days after conception. There appears to be a temporal switch in the immediate perinatal period; *CYP3A4* expression increases dramatically at about 1 week of age, reaching 30% to 40% of adult expression by 1 month.[74] Foods and drugs that may interfere with the cytochrome isoforms that metabolize midazolam (*CYP3A4*) include grapefruit juice, erythromycin, calcium channel blockers, and protease inhibitors.[404–407] The net effect is to prolong the duration of action of midazolam.

Diazepam, which is mainly metabolized by the *CYP2C19* enzyme[408] to desmethyldiazepam, acts by binding to a specific subunit on the GABAA receptor.[409] *CYP2C19* polymorphisms found to affect diazepam clearance and emergence from general anesthesia in Japanese patients were classified as follows: no variants, *1/*1 (EM); one variant, *1/*2 or *1/*3 (IM); and two variants, *2/*2, *2/*3 or *3/*3 (PM).[410] The presence of a SNP (G681A) of the *CYP2C19* gene was found to be associated with impaired metabolism of diazepam in a gene-dosage effect manner (4-fold greater half-life in homozygotes and 2-fold greater half-life in heterozygotes carrying the SNP) in Chinese patients.[411] The human GABA-A receptor α-4 subunit is a unique diazepam-insensitive binding site, and it is hypothesized that variations at this site might explain differences in diazepam sensitivity among individuals.[412] A Pro385Ser (1236C>T) amino acid substitution in the human GABA-A α-6 subunit has also been found to play a role in benzodiazepine sensitivity.[413]

NEUROMUSCULAR BLOCKING DRUGS

Pseudocholinesterase deficiency and malignant hyperthermia were the first pharmacogenetic disorders recognized in anesthesia in the 1960s; the latter is discussed elsewhere (see Chapters 5 and 39).

In 1957 Werner Kalow, a pharmacologist from Toronto, Canada, investigated several cases of prolonged apnea after electroconvulsive therapy in which succinylcholine was administered.[414] After conducting meticulous interviews with family members and reviewing the blood tests, he concluded the apneas after a single dose of succinylcholine resulted from low activity of pseudocholinesterase enzyme or butyrylcholinesterase (BChE), the plasma enzyme that normally hydrolyzes neuromuscular blocking agents such as succinylcholine and mivacurium, as well as ester-local anesthetic agents very rapidly.[415] This proved to be an autosomal recessive defect. Low pseudocholinesterase activity may lead to prolonged apnea after succinylcholine of variable duration depending on the actual genetic polymorphism,[415–417] the age of the patient and comorbidities.[417–420] More than 30 variants of the gene (*BChE*, 3q26.1-q26.3) found on chromosome 3 have been described, of which the two most common are the A (atypical) (209A>G, Asp-70Gly) and the K (Kalow) variants (1615G>A, Ala539Thr).[421] The homozygosity incidence for the A variant is 3:1000 in Irish people but may be as great as 1:175 individuals in some ethnicities in Iraq, Iran, and South India.[422,423] The BChE activity is decreased by 70% in A homozygotes and about 30% in the K homozygotes (see Chapter 5). Duration of apnea after 1.0 to 1.5 mg/kg of succinylcholine increases from 5 to 10 minutes in homozygous typical pseudocholinesterase to 10 to 20, 20 to 35, and 35 to 60 minutes in heterozygous one atypical gene, heterozygous two abnormal gene, and homozygous atypical gene, accordingly, and greater if the fluoride resistant or silent gene is present (see also Chapter 5).[424] Ultrarapid metabolism of substrates of pseudocholinesterase has also been reported resulting in paralysis of only a very brief duration after succinylcholine in humans. This has been attributed to the presence of either the Cynthiana or Neitlich variant of pseudocholinesterase or comorbidities.[124,418,425]

LOCAL ANESTHETICS

The effects of pseudocholinesterases on ester local anesthetics are less relevant in modern anesthesia because ester anesthetics have been supplanted by the amide local anesthetics. The latter anesthetics, epitomized by lidocaine and bupivacaine, which are metabolized by *CYP3A4,* and ropivacaine, which is metabolized by *CYP1A2. CYP1A2* is not fully mature in children before 3 years of age, and *CYP3A4* is immature at birth, with the predominant fetal enzyme being *CYP3A7.* These developmental delays likely explain the increased risk for toxicity of amide local anesthetics in infants younger than 6 months of age.[426] Local anesthetics are sodium channel blockers; hence genetic mutations within the *sodium channel gene* are likely to cause variable binding and efficacy for these drugs. In vitro experiments have shown that the N395K mutation in the *SCN9A* gene attenuates the inhibitory effect of lidocaine on the Nav1.7 channels and produces greater resistance to lidocaine.[427] One case report indicated that bupivacaine induced electrocardiographic and arrhythmic manifestations of the Brugada syndrome were due to a silent carrier of a cardiac sodium channel SCN5A missense mutation; whole-cell patch-clamping analysis revealed a reduction in sodium current.[428] Lidocaine also acts on vanilloid receptors belonging to the *TRPA1* and *TRPV1* family on sensory neurons, whereby calcitonin gene-related peptide (CGRP), a vasodilatory and nociceptive transmitter, is released.[429,430] A point mutation induced at residue R701 of *TRPV1* led to diminished lidocaine sensitivity in mice.[430] Similar to inhalation anesthesia, *MC1R* variants (phenotypes with red hair) have been found to be more sensitive to thermal pain with reduced subcutaneous lidocaine effectiveness.[431]

Perioperative Outcomes

POSTOPERATIVE NAUSEA AND VOMITING

A genome-wide association study on motion sickness in 80,494 individuals concluded that 35 SNPs involved in balance, glucose homeostasis, and other nervous system roles played an important part in motion sickness and likely, PONV as well.[432] In addition, correlations have been reported between A2A2 alleles at the dopamine D2 receptor (*DRD2*) (Taq1A SNP)[433,434] as well as rs2165870 SNP in the promoter region of the M3 muscarinic acetylcholine receptor (*CHRM3*) gene with PONV.[435] *CYP2D6* is the enzyme that metabolizes commonly used agents for PONV, such as the 5-HT$_3$ receptor antagonists (ondansetron and dolasetron), which are less effective in *CYP2D6* UM. The incidence of vomiting (and hence ondansetron failure) in women undergoing surgery with three *CYP2D6* copies was significantly greater compared with those with two copies, but not from those with one copy. When analyzed by genotype, the incidence of vomiting in PM, IM, EM, and UM were 8%, 17%, 15%, and 45%, respectively ($P<0.01$).[436] Only granisetron is primarily metabolized by *CYP3A4* and may have a better effect in *CYP2D6* UM patients.[437] Although palonosetron is metabolized by 2D6, its duration of action is independent of its clearance because it binds allosterically

and exhibits positive cooperativity with the 5-HT$_3$ receptor, deforming the conformational structure of the receptor, which takes 36 to 48 hours to return to normal.

PERIOPERATIVE BLEEDING

Postoperative bleeding after cardiac surgery has been associated with SNPs of coagulation proteins and platelet glycoproteins (GPIaIIa-52C>T and 807C>T, GPIb alpha 524C>T, tissue factor -603A>G, prothrombin 20210G>A, tissue factor pathway inhibitor-399C>T, and angiotensin-converting enzyme [ACE] deletion/insertion).[438] Plasminogen activator inhibitor 1 (PAI-1) attenuates the conversion of plasminogen to plasmin, and the use of plasminolytic inhibitors may be subject to PAI-1 variants. In a study that evaluated the effectiveness of tranexamic acid (TXA) for reducing postoperative chest tube blood loss in adults undergoing cardiac bypass, patients with plasminogen activator inhibitor-1 5G/5G homozygotes who did not receive tranexamic acid showed more postoperative bleeding than those with other *PAI-1* genotypes. Those with 5G/5G homozygotes who received tranexamic acid showed the greatest blood-sparing benefit.[439]

HEMODYNAMIC RESPONSE

The β$_2$-adrenergic receptor (β2-ADR) is a member of the 7-transmembrane domain family of receptors that is encoded by a gene located on chromosome 5 (β2-ADR, 5q31-q32). The β2-ADR controls vascular and bronchial smooth muscle tone, and hence controls both response to bronchodilators and may contribute to vasopressor responses after laryngoscopy[440,441] and regional anesthesia. While nine β2-ADR variants have been described,[442] the most extensively studied are the Arg16Gly and the Gln27Glu variants, which are in linkage disequilibrium. Mechanistically, it appears that 16Gly variants have enhanced agonist-induced β-ADR downregulation, while the Arg16 genotype shows complete absence of downregulation,[443] which implies that Arg16 and Gln27 homozygotes will be more sensitive to β$_2$-agonist effects. In accordance, blood pressure variability after neuraxial anesthesia was found to be predicted by variant Arg16Arg (less hypotension)[444] and Glu27 (more hypotension)[445] in two different studies. Similarly, phenylephrine dose was increased by 200 μg in women with the Arg16 homozygous genotype compared with those with the Gly16 homozygous genotype while undergoing cesarean delivery under spinal anesthesia.[446] A detailed review of the β2-ADR gene can be found elsewhere.[447]

EFFECT ON OTHER PERIOPERATIVE OUTCOMES

Genetic risk factors have been identified for perioperative cardiac ischemia and arrhythmias,[448] as well as neurologic outcomes such as cognitive dysfunction/stroke,[449] which are beyond the scope of this chapter. Readers are referred to a review on perioperative outcomes for further elaboration.[6] There is a potential mechanistic pathway for perioperative cardiac ischemia and stroke influenced by inflammatory superseded thrombosis-related genes. Associations between specific genetic variants and perioperative renal compromise,[450] protection against sepsis,[451] inflammatory response, and graft rejection after heart and lung transplants[452] have also been described.

Ancestry/Race and Genetics

The "Out of Africa" theory of human migration advocates for a common origin of human races.[453] The definitions of "race" defined by physical characteristics and "ethnicity" based on sociocultural factors are complicated by genetic admixture and interracial mating.[454] Consequently, genetic studies often use ancestry information markers

(AIMs), which are a set of haploid markers (mitochondrial DNA or Y-chromosome haplotypes) or multiple unlinked autosomal markers that are diploid, that exhibit substantially different frequencies between populations from different geographic regions as a basis for race. An ideal ancestry information marker should have one allele that is fixed (i.e., allele frequency of 1.0) in one ancestral population and not present in the other,[455] but since the level of genetic variation between human populations is only 5% to 10%, there are challenges with genetic ancestry inference.[456]

The influence of race and ethnicity exists in frequency distribution of polymorphisms of genes encoding drug-metabolizing enzymes, transporters, and receptors.[457] As mentioned earlier, examples are the ethnic differences of pharmacokinetic enzymes such as *CYP2D6*; UM phenotypes, which are more prevalent among Sub-Saharan populations and low among Caucasian populations; and in *OPRM1*, where the frequency of the A118G allele is estimated to be much higher in the Asian (46%) compared with European and African American populations (5%–25%).[233] African American children clear morphine more rapidly than their Caucasian counterparts, which is likely due to differences in allele frequencies for *OCT1* variants.[201]

Race has been associated with an unequal burden of perioperative pain and opioid adverse effects in children. Caucasian children had less postoperative pain and more opioid-related adverse effects postoperatively despite fewer opioid doses after tonsillectomy.[458] African American and Hispanic patients also have less tolerance for experimentally induced pain compared with Caucasian patients.[459,460] In another cohort of children who had tonsillectomies, ethnicity affected morphine-induced outcomes; children of Latin ethnicity had more adverse effects from morphine compared with those of non-Latin ethnicity. No genetic variants examined contributed to these differences.[461] Although most studies have focused on Caucasian and African American group differences, some studies have reported reduced pain tolerance in Asian Americans compared with non-Hispanic Caucasian populations.[462] These findings assume importance as race can affect differential treatment of groups, and while this will lead to individualization, it can also lead to overtreatment or undertreatment if it is unclear whether the differences are of genetic variance versus based on race.

Racial disparities are reported in the prescription of opioid analgesics for management of postoperative pain.[463] African Americans and Hispanic Americans were prescribed fewer analgesics than their non-Hispanic Caucasian counterparts; these two groups also took their analgesics less frequently than prescribed and experienced limited pain relief from analgesic medications.[464] This has been contradicted by other studies showing decreased opioid requirements and increased sensitivity in African Americans.[465] The effects of race and ethnicity may be medication-specific and affected by numerous contextual factors and should be interpreted with care.[466]

Pharmacogenomics Methods

COMMON GENOTYPING METHODS

There are many options for genotyping. The most used for anesthesia and pain-related pharmacogenetic research and clinical practice are the candidate gene approach and SNPs testing. Other more comprehensive and expensive genotyping include genome-wide association study (GWAS) platforms with 500,000 to 5 million SNPs, whole-exome sequencing (WES), and whole-genome sequencing (WGS) with different depth of coverages. Since the turn of the century, the overall cost of genotyping has decreased significantly. With the whole-exome and whole-genome sequencing approaches, large

amounts of genetic data are typically generated per patient; analyzing and associating any clinical outcome or condition would require a large sample size and complex and robust analytical methods.

COMMON LIMITATIONS OF GENETIC RESEARCH STUDIES AND INTERPRETATION OF GENETIC STUDIES

Interpretation of genetic studies is often limited by study inadequacies (e.g., lack of adequate sample sizes needed to analyze multiple genes or polymorphisms), mostly owing to the expense of genetic testing and population stratification for different racial and ethnic backgrounds. Moreover, publication bias; the winner's curse; statistical and bioinformatics analytical challenges in adjusting for gene and environmental interactions; the lack of reproducibility of results in independent and external cohorts; and the inability to validate genetic associations with mechanistic studies also lead to inadequate proof for clinical implementation of genetic information in clinical care to personalize interventions and care. In addition to genetic risk factors, other factors may influence clinical outcome measures. Consequently, pharmacogenetic studies also need to be complemented by epigenetic, proteomic, transcriptomic, and metabolomic information to gain additional knowledge and insight to improving personalized care.

CURRENT COSTS OF GENOTYPING AND THIRD-PARTY COVERAGE FOR GENOTYPING

Currently, access to preoperative genotyping, robust evidence to change clinical practice based on underlying genetic risk factors, affordability, and payer coverage for genetic testing are limited. As compelling evidence for personalization of perioperative care based on genetic risk factors (e.g., *CYP2D6* and codeine-related deaths, *RYR1* and malignant hyperthermia) increases, there will be better adaptability of routine preoperative genotyping and coverage of such services by third-party payers. For example, many third-party payers are covering perioperative *CYP2D6* genotyping for prescription of oral opioids in our pediatric institution.

Genetic Counseling

Another ethical fallout of pharmacogenomic research, especially in pediatrics, is the need for genetic counseling. Findings need to be conveyed to children and parents. Assistance with interpretation of incidental findings from secondary analyses may be required. Genetic counselors help patients and their families understand and adapt to the medical, psychological, and familial implications of genetic contributions to clinical outcomes and/or disease, and need to be an integral part of such research efforts. Genetic counseling has been provided traditionally for single-gene conditions (e.g., malignant hyperthermia and *RYR1* gene). As we transition from single-gene testing and genetic counseling to a full genomic medicine approach, clinical implications will get more complex for most health care professionals.[467] One potential solution would be the development of clinical outcome or disease-related multigenic clinical decision-support algorithms for more effectively helping patients and health care professionals.

Clinical Translation: Bench to Bedside: Where Are We Now?

Adverse drug reactions account for up to 20% of hospital admissions, resulting in annual costs of $136 billion.[468,469] Genetic factors presumably contribute to variability in individual drug response and to about 20% of the reported adverse drug events.[470] There is evidence that pharmacogenetics-guided personalized medicine could be cost-effective.[470] Compared with the traditional "one size fits most" approach, the current paradigm of so-called "P4 medicine" embraces a more *predictive, preventive, participatory, and personalized* approach to patients, health, and diseases.[469] As we routinely use the global positioning system to navigate maps and roads, in the future, it is anticipated that we will use a genomic prescribing system (GPS) to proactively identify underlying genetic risks and guide personalized care.[471] Despite the promise of personalized medicine, there are numerous challenges and barriers to effectively implement personalized medicine, and to integrate clinical decision-support tools into electronic health record systems. Despite the many challenges, real progress is being made in the current era of big data, combined with machine learning and artificial intelligence.

Pharmacogenomics forms the centerpiece of personalized medicine. To implement pharmacogenomics-based clinical decision support, there is a need for more robust study designs, independent validations, larger study populations, and robust statistical approaches.[472,473] Existing validated pharmacogenomic markers explain only a minor part of the observed clinical variability. Extensive knowledge of rare genetic variants, epigenetics, phenoconversion as well as nongenetic factors such social, demographic data, along with the emerging "omics" knowledge base will enable clinicians to improve the precision of data-driven, artificial intelligence–powered predictive models.[469,474] Since genetic association studies do not explain causality, additional research to identify biologic and mechanistic pathways would be needed for better insight to risk stratification and targeted interventions influencing the mechanistic pathways. Coordinated international efforts, like the National Institutes of Health–funded PharmGKB platform,[213] aim to disseminate pharmacogenomic information and to overcome the barriers for clinical implementation of personalized medicine. An increasing number of drug labels now contain pharmacogenetic information.

In the field of perioperative pain management and opioid responses, pharmacogenetics-guided personalized prescription of codeine is well recognized. Apart from this, polymorphisms of genes involved in pain pathways (*COMT*[147]), opioid pharmacokinetics (*CYP2D6*,[475] *CYP2B6*,[215] *OCT1*[201]), ABC B1 and C3 genes (*ABCB1*[208] and *ABCC3*[201,204,205]), and pharmacodynamics[5,135,165,476–479] (*FAAH*[264]), and opioid μ-receptor 1 (*OPRM1*[208]) and genetics of CPSP and prescribed opioid addiction hold promise in determining postoperative clinical and economic outcomes. These genetic risk factors relevant to opioid pharmacogenetics and

surgical pain management have the potential to improve clinical and safety outcomes. To realize the promise of personalized medicine to perioperative care, we need to develop implementation science tools and infrastructure to generate and integrate better evidence to clinical practice at point-of-care, preferably in the electronic health record; engagement and education of physicians, patients, the pharmaceutical industry, health care, payers, and policy makers is also needed. Perioperative personnel should embrace the technological advances to deliver on the promise of safer, cost-effective, and patient-centered healthcare.

Conclusion

Pharmacogenetics pertaining to anesthesia is still an evolving field with exciting prospects in the future, so that anesthesia and analgesia can be individualized using a reactive rather than "trial and approach" strategy. It is important to realize that genetics needs to be combined with other factors to make an individualized approach comprehensive. Completion of the Human Genome Project, as well as rapidly accumulating data in this field from knock-in and knock-out genetic animal models, laboratory-based cell line experiments, and human studies poses a huge challenge in the understanding, education, and interpretation of results and applicability. An average proteomic experiment, for example, might generate 10,000 to 1,000,000 individual data points, with countless potential interactions between data points. Hence, a few web-enabled resources may be worth mentioning, especially given the daily updates that happen with current publications (Table 4.5).

The ultimate goal of pharmacogenetics research is clinical translation. Examples of translational potential include the proposed genomic prescribing system to guide therapy,[471] the genotype-based dosing of opioids based on *OPRM1, COMT,* and *MC1R*,[480,481] and genetic risk signatures for opioid-induced respiratory depression.[478] The Electronic Medical Records and Genomics (eMERGE) Network, announced in September 2007, is a National Institutes of Health –organized and –funded consortium of US medical research institutions with unique and valuable pioneer experience using a variety of commercial and homegrown electronic health records (https://www.genome.gov/Funded-Programs-Projects/Electronic-Medical-Records-and-Genomics-Network-eMERGE). The challenges and solutions for integrating genomic data into the electronic health record, creation of integrated genomic decision support, and the human and electronic processes, including standards required for such successful integration, are still a work in progress.[482,483]

TABLE 4.5	Online Resources for Current Pharmacogenomics Information
Online Resource	**Description and Uses**
The Pharmacogenomics Knowledgebase www.pharmgkb.org	A comprehensive resource that curates knowledge about the impact of genetic variation on drug response for clinicians and researchers. This knowledge base can be searched by gene, drug, or clinical phenotype, and provides in-depth information about pharmacogenomics, curated publications to clinical implementation guidelines.
Encyclopedia of DNA Elements (ENCODE) Consortium www.encodeproject.org	Provides a comprehensive parts list of functional elements in the human genome, including elements that act at the protein and RNA levels, and regulatory elements that control cells and circumstances in which a gene is active.
Genotype-Tissue Expression (GTEx) project www.gtexportal.org	This project provides the scientific community a resource with which to study human gene expression and regulation and its relationship to genetic variation. This project collects and analyzes multiple human tissues from donors for this purpose. By analyzing global RNA expression within individual tissues and treating the expression levels of genes as quantitative traits, variations in gene expression that are highly correlated with genetic variation can be identified as expression quantitative trait loci (eQTLs).

In conclusion, the future of precision medicine was aptly described and emphasized by President Barack Obama in his State of the Union address on January 20, 2015, "*I want the country that eliminated polio and mapped the human genome to lead a new era of medicine—one that delivers the right treatment at the right time.*"[484]

ANNOTATED REFERENCES

Andrzejowski P, Carroll W. Codeine in paediatrics: pharmacology, prescribing and controversies. *Arch Dis Child Educ Pract Ed.* 2016; 101(3):148-151.

This article highlights the safety and efficacy aspects of codeine use in children, a very contemporary and important topic. The authors discuss the developmental pharmacology, pharmacokinetics, pharmacodynamics, and pharmacogenetics of codeine in children, how this relates to prescribing, as well as the practical issues and the recent regulatory framework surrounding its use.

Bond C, LaForge KS, Tian M, et al. Single-nucleotide polymorphism in the human mu opioid receptor gene alters beta-endorphin binding and activity: possible implications for opiate addiction. *Proc Natl Acad Sci USA.* 1998;95:9608-9613.

This is one of the early studies on genetics of opioid addiction. With a sample of 152 opioid addicts and nonaddicts, this study identified association between A118G variant of OPRM1 and beta-endorphin binding and the implication for opioid use disorders.

Chidambaran V, Gang Y, Pilipenko V, Ashton M, Ding L. Systematic review and meta-analysis of genetic risk of developing chronic postsurgical pain. *J Pain.* 2020;21(1–2):2-24.

This is a meta-analysis on the role played by genetic factors on the incidence of CPSP. The authors were able to identify a few SNPs that were widely studied in this context, but these single genetic factors had small effect sizes on complex conditions like CPSP. The authors emphasized the importance of large robust studies to understand genetic factors underlying CPSP.

Chidambaran V, Mavi J, Esslinger H, et al. Association of OPRM1 A118G variant with risk of morphine-induced respiratory depression following spine fusion in adolescents. *Pharmacogenomics J.* 2015;15(3): 255-262.

This article is the first clinical study to show that the opioid receptor polymorphism A118G influences susceptibility to morphine-induced respiratory depression in children.

Chidambaran V, Venkatasubramanian R, Zhang X, et al. ABCC3 genetic variants are associated with postoperative morphine-induced respiratory depression and morphine pharmacokinetics in children. *Pharmacogenomics J.* 2017;17(2):162-169.

This article presents the first study to report association of ABCC3 variants with both morphine pharmacodynamics (opioid-related respiratory depression) and morphine pharmacokinetics (metabolite formation) in two independent surgical cohorts.

Crettol S, Déglon J-J, Besson J, et al. ABCB1 and cytochrome P450 genotypes and phenotypes: influence on methadone plasma levels and response to treatment. *Clinical Pharmacology & Therapeutics.* 2006; 80:668-681.

This study on pharmacogenetics of methadone, on 245 patients receiving methadone maintenance, analyzed multiple candidate gene polymorphisms and found associations between methadone metabolism and SNPs in CYP2B6, CYP3A4 and ABCB1.

Crews KR, Gaedigk A, Dunnenberger HM, et al. Clinical Pharmacogenetics Implementation Consortium guidelines for cytochrome P450 2D6 genotype and codeine therapy: 2014 update. *Clin Pharmacol Ther.* 2014;95(4):376-382.

This article summarizes the evidence from the literature supporting the association of CYP2D6 activity and polymorphisms, provides therapeutic recommendations for codeine based on the CYP2D6 genotype, and includes essential guidelines for prescribing pediatric providers.

Doehring A, Hentig N, Graff J, et al. Genetic variants altering dopamine D2 receptor expression or function modulate the risk of opiate addiction and the dosage requirements of methadone substitution. *Pharmacogenetics and Genomics.* 2009;19:407-414.

This prospective study comparing methadone substituted patients to a cohort of healthy controls identified DRD2 SNPs associated with both opioid addiction as well as response to methadone maintenance.

Doehring A, Oertel BG, Sittl R, Lötsch J. Chronic opioid use is associated with increased DNA methylation correlating with increased clinical pain. *Pain.* 2013;154:15-23.

This is an epigenetic study of drug-induced epigenetic modification: in this case OPRM1 methylation resulting from chronic opioid use, which may predispose chronic opioid users to increased chronic pain.

Gelernter J, Kranzler HR, Sherva R, et al. Genome-wide association study of opioid dependence: multiple associations mapped to calcium and potassium pathways. *Biological Psychiatry.* 2014;76:66-74.

One of the first and a large genome-wide association study on opioid dependence. This study identified SNPs in genes involved in potassium signaling pathways (KCNG1, KCNG2) associated with opioid dependence.

Sadhasivam S, Chidambaran V, Zhang X, et al. Opioid-induced respiratory depression: ABCB1 transporter pharmacogenetics. *Pharmacogenomics J.* 2015;15(2):119-126.

This article shows that ABCB1 polymorphisms may affect blood-brain barrier transport of morphine, and therefore individual response to its central analgesic and adverse effects in postsurgical children.

Sadhasivam S, Zhang X, Chidambaran V, et al. Novel associations between FAAH genetic variants and postoperative central opioid-related adverse effects. *Pharmacogenomics J.* 2015;15:436-442.

This study explored the interplay between opioid and cannabinoid systems. In a cohort of 259 children undergoing adenotonsillectomy surgery, the authors were able to identify SNPs of FAAH associated with opioid-related respiratory depression and PONV.

Stamer UM, Lehnen K, Höthker F, et al. Impact of CYP2D6 genotype on postoperative tramadol analgesia. *Pain.* 2003;105:231-238.

This is a large prospective genetic study that established an association between CYP2D6 metabolizer status and tramadol analgesia.

A complete reference list can be found online at Elsevier eBooks+.

5 Pharmacology of Drugs Used in Children

BRIAN J. ANDERSON, JERROLD LERMAN, AND CHARLES J. COTÉ

Pharmacokinetic Principles and Calculations
First-Order Kinetics
Half-Life
First-Order Single-Compartment Kinetics
First-Order Multiple-Compartment Kinetics
Zero-Order Kinetics
Apparent Volume of Distribution
Pharmacokinetic Example
Repetitive Dosing and Drug Accumulation
Steady State
Loading Dose
Population Modeling
Pediatric Pharmacokinetic Considerations
Size
Maturation
Organ Function
Pharmacodynamic Models
Minimum Effective Concentration
Sigmoid E_{max} Model
Quantal Effect Model
Logistic Regression Model
Linking Pharmacokinetics With Pharmacodynamics
Drug Distribution
Protein Binding
Body Composition
Regional Blood Flows
Blood-Brain Barrier
Absorption
Enteral
Cutaneous
Intramuscular
Nasal
Bioavailability
Metabolism and Excretion
Hepatic Metabolism
Phase I Reactions: Cytochrome P-450
Phase II Reactions
Alterations in Biotransformation
Extrahepatic Routes of Metabolic Clearance
Renal Excretion
Pharmacodynamics in Children
Measurement OF Pharmacodynamic Endpoints
The Target Concentration Approach
Defining Target Concentration

Drug Interactions
The Drug Approval Process, The Package Insert, and Drug Labeling
Inhalation Anesthetic Agents
Physicochemical Properties
Pharmacokinetics of Inhaled Anesthetics
Control of Anesthetic Depth
Pharmacodynamics of Inhaled Anesthetics
Clinical Effects
Nitrous Oxide
Environmental Impact
Oxygen
Intravenous Anesthetic Agents
Barbiturates
Propofol
Ciprofol
Ketamine
Etomidate
Alfaxalone
Neuromuscular Blocking Drugs
Neuromuscular Monitoring
Neuromuscular Junction
Pharmacodynamics
Pharmacokinetics
Depolarizing Neuromuscular Blocking Drugs
Succinylcholine
Intermediate-Acting Nondepolarizing Neuromuscular Blocking Drugs
Rocuronium
Cisatracurium
Atracurium
Gantacurium
Vecuronium
Clinical Implications When Using Short- and Intermediate-Acting Neuromuscular Blocking Drugs
Long-Acting Nondepolarizing Neuromuscular Blocking Drugs
Pancuronium
Antagonism of Neuromuscular Blocking Drugs
General Principles
Sugammadex
Calabadion
Neuromuscular Blocking Drugs in Special Situations
Opioids
Morphine

Diamorphine
Oliceridine
Meperidine
Hydromorphone
Oxycodone
Hydrocodone
Methadone
Fentanyl
Alfentanil
Sufentanil
Remifentanil
Butorphanol and Nalbuphine
Codeine
Tramadol
Tapentadol
Acetaminophen
Nonsteroidal Antiinflammatory Agents (NSAIDs)
Pharmacodynamics
Pharmacokinetics
Adverse Effects
Intravenous Formulations
Benzodiazepine Sedatives
Midazolam
Diazepam

Other Sedatives
Clonidine
Dexmedetomidine
Chloral Hydrate
Antihistamines
Diphenhydramine
Cimetidine, Ranitidine, and Famotidine
Antiemetics
Metoclopramide
5-Hydroxytryptamine Type 3–Receptor Antagonists
Neurokinin 1 and Other Antiemetics
Dexamethasone
Anticholinergics
Atropine and Scopolamine
Glycopyrrolate
Antagonists
Naloxone
Naltrexone
Methylnaltrexone
Flumazenil
Physostigmine

THE PHARMACOKINETICS AND PHARMACODYNAMICS of most medications in children, especially neonates, differ from those in adults.[1] *Pharmacokinetics* is defined as what the body does to the drug, whereas *pharmacodynamics* is defined as what the drug does to the body. Children exhibit different pharmacokinetics (PK) and pharmacodynamics (PD) from adults because of their immature renal and hepatic functions, different body composition, altered protein binding, distinct disease spectrum, diverse behavior, and dissimilar receptor patterns. Pharmacokinetic differences necessitate modification of the dose to achieve the desired concentration associated with a clinical response and to avoid toxicity. In addition, some medications may displace bilirubin from its protein binding sites predisposing to kernicterus in premature neonates. Pharmacodynamics may be influenced by altered capacity of the end organ, such as the heart, neuromuscular junction, and brain to respond to medications in children compared with adults. In this chapter we discuss basic pharmacologic principles as they relate to drugs commonly used by anesthesiologists.

Pharmacokinetic Principles and Calculations

Changes in drug concentrations within the body over time are referred to as *pharmacokinetics*. The principles and equations that describe these changes can be used to adjust drug doses rationally to achieve more effective drug concentrations at the site of action.[2,3] The equations in this section are intended for general and practical use, whereas the more rigorous mathematical intricacies of pharmacokinetics are covered elsewhere.[4,5]

Within the body, a drug may diffuse between body fluids and tissues at different rates, yet the consistent change in its circulating concentration may be used to characterize its kinetics and to guide dosages. The rate of removal of drug from the circulation is usually described using either first-order and/or zero-order exponential equations. The difference between these two equations has important implications for drug treatment.

FIRST-ORDER KINETICS

Most drugs are cleared from the body with first-order exponential rates in which a constant fraction or constant proportion of drug is removed per unit of time. Because the proportion of drug cleared remains constant, the greater the concentration, the greater the amount of drug removed from the body. Such rates can be described by exponential equations that fit the following form:

$$C = C_0 e^{-kt} \qquad \text{Eq. 5.1}$$

where C is the concentration at time t, C_0 is the starting concentration (a constant determined by the dose and distribution volume), e is the base of the natural logarithm (~2.71828), and k is the elimination rate constant with units of time^{-1}. First-order indicates that the exponent is raised to the first power ($-kt$ in Eq. 5.1). Second-order equations are those that are raised to the second power, such as $e^{(z)2}$. First-order exponential equations, such as Eq. 5.1, may be converted to the form of the equation of a straight line (y = mx + b, where x and y are variables [e.g., time and concentration], m is the slope parameter, and b is a constant) by taking the natural logarithm of both sides, after which they may be solved by linear regression.

$$\ln C = \ln C_0 + (-kt) \qquad \text{Eq. 5.2}$$

If ln C (i.e., natural logarithm of C) is graphed versus time, the slope is -k, and the intercept is ln C_0. If log C (i.e., common logarithm of C) is graphed versus time, the slope is -k/2.303, because ln x equals 2.303 log x. When graphed on linear-linear axes, exponential rates are curvilinear whereas when they are graphed on semilogarithmic (i.e., linear-logarithmic) axes, exponential rates produce a straight line.

HALF-LIFE

Half-life, the time for a drug concentration to decrease by one-half, is a familiar exponential term used to describe the kinetics of many drugs. *Half-life is a first-order kinetic process because the same proportion or fraction of the drug is removed during equal periods of time.* As described earlier, the greater the starting concentration, the greater the amount of drug removed during each half-life.

Half-life can be determined by several methods. If concentration is converted to the natural logarithm of concentration and graphed versus time, as described in Eq. 5.2, the slope of this graph is the elimination rate constant, k. For both accuracy and precision, at least three concentration-time points should be used to determine the slope, and they should be obtained over an interval during which the concentration decreases at least by half. In clinical practice, for infants and small children, however, k is often estimated from just two concentrations obtained during the terminal elimination phase. With multiple data points, the slope of ln C versus time may be calculated by least squares linear regression analysis. Half-life ($T_{1/2}$) may be calculated from the elimination rate constant, k (time^{-1}), as follows:

$$T_{1/2} = \frac{\text{Natural Logarithm}(2)}{k} = \frac{0.693}{k} \qquad \text{Eq. 5.3}$$

Graphic techniques may be used to determine half-life from a series of timed measurements of drug concentration. The concentration-time points should be graphed on semilogarithmic axes and used to determine the best-fitting line either visually or by linear regression analysis. This approach is illustrated in Fig. 5.1, in which the least squares regression line has been fitted to the concentration-time points and crosses a concentration of 20 μg/mL at 100 minutes and a concentration of 10 μg/mL at 200 minutes. The concentration decreased by one-half in 100 minutes, so the half-life is 100 minutes. The elimination rate constant is 0.693/100 per minute or 0.00693 per minute.

Elimination half-life is of no value for characterizing the disposition of many intravenous (IV) anesthetic drugs during dosing periods relevant to anesthesia. A more useful concept is that of the context-sensitive half-time (CSHT) where "context" refers to the duration of the infusion. This is the time required for the plasma drug concentration to decrease by 50% after terminating the infusion.[6] The context-sensitive half-time is the same as the elimination half-life for a one-compartment model that does not change with the duration of the infusion. However, most drugs in anesthesia conform to multiple compartment models and the context-sensitive half-times markedly differ from their respective elimination half-lives.

Context-sensitive half-time may be independent of the duration of the infusion (e.g., remifentanil, 2.5 minutes); be moderately affected (propofol, 12 minutes at 1 hour, 38 minutes at 8 hours); or be marked affected (e.g., fentanyl, 1 hour at 24 minutes, 8 hours

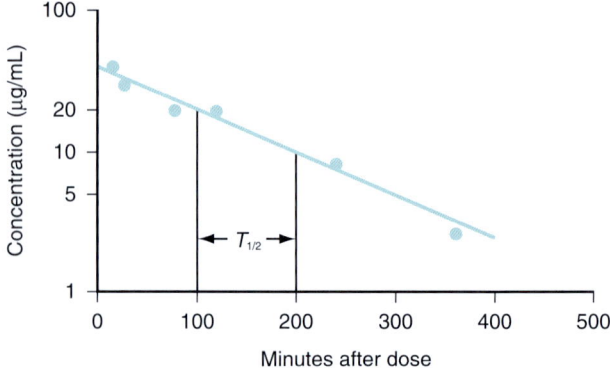

FIGURE 5.1 Graphic determination of half-life. Half-life can be determined from a series of concentration-time points on a semilogarithmic graph if the kinetics are first-order exponential. The concentrations are plotted on semilogarithmic axes; the best-fit line is drawn through the points; convenient concentrations are chosen that decrease in half, such as 20 μg/mL and 10 μg/mL, as illustrated; and the interval between those concentrations is the half-life, which is 100 minutes in the illustration.

at 280 minutes). These differences may be attributed to the varying rate of return of drug from peripheral compartments to plasma after stopping the infusion. Peripheral compartment sizes and clearances in children differ from those in adults so when the infusion is stopped, more or less drug remains in the body of children for any given plasma concentration compared with adults. The context-sensitive half-time for propofol in children, for example, is greater than that in adults.[7] The context-sensitive half-time gives insight into the pharmacokinetics of a drug, but the parameter may not be clinically relevant; the percentage decrease in concentration required for recovery from the drug effect is not necessarily 50%.

FIRST-ORDER SINGLE-COMPARTMENT KINETICS

The number of exponential equations required to describe the change in concentration determines the number of compartments. Although a drug may diffuse among several tissues and body fluids, its clearance often fits first-order, single-compartment kinetics if it quickly distributes homogeneously within the circulation and is removed rapidly from the circulation through metabolism or excretion. This may be judged visually if a semilogarithmic graph of the change in drug concentration fits a single straight line. Kinetics may appear to be single-compartment, when they are really multiple compartments, if drug concentrations are not measured early after intravenous administration to detect the initial distribution phase (α phase).

FIRST-ORDER MULTIPLE-COMPARTMENT KINETICS

If drug concentrations are measured several times within the first 15 to 30 minutes after IV administration as well as during a more prolonged period, more than one elimination phase is often present. This can be observed as a marked change in slope of a semilogarithmic graph of concentration versus time (Fig. 5.2). The number and nature of the compartments required to describe the clearance of a drug do not necessarily represent specific body fluids or tissues. When two first-order exponential equations are required to describe the clearance of drug from the circulation, the kinetics are described as first-order, two-compartment (e.g., central and peripheral compartments) that fit the following equation (see Fig. 5.2):

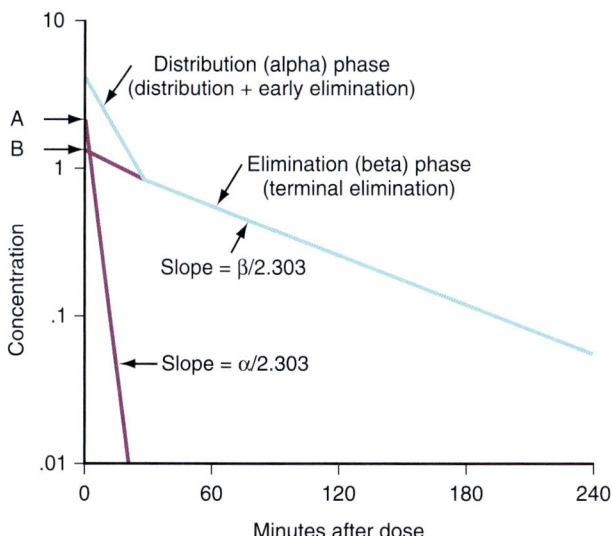

FIGURE 5.2 Two-compartment kinetics in a semilogarithmic graph. The initial rapid decrease in serum concentration reflects distribution and elimination followed by a slower decrease because of elimination. *A* is the concentration at time 0 for the distribution rate. Subtraction of the initial decrease in concentration resulting from elimination, using the concentrations from the elimination line extrapolated back to time 0 at *B*, produces the lower line with a steep slope = α (distribution rate constant)/2.303. The terminal elimination phase has a slope = β (elimination rate constant)/2.303.

$$C = Ae^{-\alpha t} + Be^{-\beta t}, \qquad \text{Eq. 5.4}$$

where concentration is C, t is time after the dose, A is the concentration at time 0 for the distribution rate represented by the purple line graph with the steepest slope, α is the rate constant for distribution, *e* is base of natural logarithm, B is the concentration at time 0 for the terminal elimination rate, and β is the rate constant for terminal elimination. Rate constants indicate the rates of change in concentration, and each corresponds to the slope of the respective line divided by 2.303 for logarithm concentration versus time.

Such two-compartment or biphasic kinetics are frequently observed after IV administration of drugs that rapidly distribute out of the central compartment (the circulation) to a peripheral compartment. In such situations, the initial rapid decrease in the drug concentration is referred to as the α or distribution phase. It represents the distribution of drug to the peripheral (tissue) compartments in addition to drug elimination. The terminal (β) phase, which begins after the inflection point in the line, signifies the beginning of the elimination phase. This phase accounts for most of the change in the drug concentration (blue line). To determine the initial change in concentration as a result of distribution (see Fig. 5.2), the change in concentration that results from elimination must be subtracted from the total change in concentration. The slope of the line representing the difference between these two rates is the rate constant for distribution.

These parameters (A, B, α, β) have little connection with underlying physiology. An alternative parameterization is to use a central volume and three rate constants (k_{10}, k_{12}, k_{21}) that describe drug distribution between compartments. Another common method is to use two volumes (central, V1; peripheral, V2) and two clearances (total body CL and Q) where Q is the intercompartment clearance,

and the volume of distribution at steady state is the sum of V1 and V2. A more detailed mathematical discussion may be found elsewhere.[2,5]

Although many drugs demonstrate multiple-compartment kinetics, for clinical estimates of dose and dosing intervals, it is often not necessary to use multiple-compartment kinetics. To minimize cost, limit blood loss, and simplify pharmacokinetic calculations, dose adjustments are often based on only two plasma concentrations (peak and trough), and linear, single-compartment kinetics (such as that of gentamicin and vancomycin). Because the elimination rate constant should be determined from the terminal elimination phase, it is important to avoid drawing the peak blood concentrations of multiple-compartment drugs prematurely, that is, during the initial distribution phase. If they are drawn too early, the concentrations will be greater than those during the terminal elimination phase (see Fig. 5.2), which will overestimate the slope and the terminal elimination rate constant. Population modeling has improved analysis and interpretation of such data.[8,9]

ZERO-ORDER KINETICS

The elimination of some drugs occurs with loss of a *constant amount of drug per time, rather than a constant fraction per time.* Such rates are termed zero-order, and because $e^0 = 1$, the change in the amount of drug in the body fits the following equation[10]:

$$-dA/dt = k_0, \qquad \text{Eq. 5.5}$$

where dA is the change in the amount of drug in the body (in milligrams), dt is the change in time, and k_0 is the elimination rate constant with units of amount per unit time. After solving this equation, it has the following form:

$$A = A_0 - k_0t, \qquad \text{Eq. 5.6}$$

where A_0 is the initial amount of drug in the body and A is the amount of drug in the body (in milligrams) at time t.

Zero-order (also known as Michaelis-Menten) kinetics may be designated as saturation kinetics because such processes occur when excess amounts of drug saturate the capacity of metabolic enzymes or transport systems. In this situation, only a constant amount of drug is metabolized or transported per unit of time. If kinetics are zero order, then the serum concentration versus time data graphed on linear-linear axes yield a straight-line relationship whereas when they are graphed on semilogarithmic axes, they yield a curved relationship. Clinically, first-order elimination may become zero order after administration of excessive doses or prolonged infusions or during dysfunction of the organ of elimination. Certain drugs administered to neonates exhibit zero-order kinetics at therapeutic doses and may accumulate to excessive concentrations including thiopental, theophylline, caffeine, diazepam, furosemide, and phenytoin. Some drugs (e.g., phenytoin, ethyl alcohol) may exhibit mixed-order kinetics (i.e., first-order at low concentrations and zero-order after enzymes are saturated at greater concentrations). For these drugs, a small increment in dose may cause disproportionately large increments in serum concentrations (Fig. 5.3).

APPARENT VOLUME OF DISTRIBUTION

The apparent volume of distribution (Vd) is a mathematical term that relates the dose to the circulating concentration observed immediately after administration. It might be viewed as the volume of dilution that can be used to predict the change in concentration after a dose is diluted within the body (i.e., a scaling factor). The

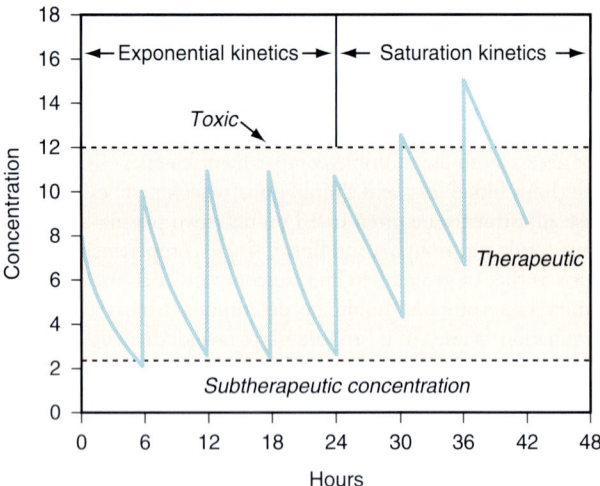

FIGURE 5.3 Transition from exponential to saturation kinetics. During every-6-hour dosing, concentrations during the first 24 hours reflect exponential kinetics with a half-life of 3 hours ($k = 0.231$/hour) followed by a change to saturation kinetics at 24 hours with elimination of 1 mg/hour, leading to drug accumulation to toxic concentrations.

volume of distribution does not necessarily correspond to a physiologic body fluid or tissue volume, hence the designation "apparent." For drugs that distribute out of the circulation or bind to tissues, such as digoxin, volume of distribution may reach 10 L/kg, a physical impossibility for a fluid compartment in the body. This illustrates the mathematical nature of the volume of distribution. The units used to express concentration are amount per unit volume, and dose is expressed as the amount per kilogram and the volume of distribution as volume per kilogram that dilutes the dose to produce the concentration as the ratio:

$$\text{Concentration (mg/L)} = \frac{\text{Dose (mg/kg)}}{\text{Vd (L/kg)}} \qquad \text{Eq. 5.7}$$

This equation serves as the basis for most pharmacokinetic calculations because it is easily rearranged to solve for volume of distribution and dose. It is also important to note that this equation represents the change in concentration after a rapidly administered IV dose of a drug.

Knowledge of the apparent volume of distribution is essential for dose adjustments. Volume of distribution may be calculated by rearranging Eq. 5.7:

$$\text{Vd (L/kg)} = \frac{\text{Dose (mg/kg)}}{\text{C (postdose)} - \text{C (predose) (mg/L)}} \qquad \text{Eq. 5.8}$$

The concentration after a drug infusion, C (post-dose), must be measured after the distribution phase to avoid overestimating the peak concentration that would, in turn, lead to an erroneously small volume of distribution. For the first dose, the predose concentration is 0.

PHARMACOKINETIC EXAMPLE
The following example illustrates the application of these pharmacokinetic principles using a four-step approach: (1) calculate volume of distribution; (2) calculate half-life; (3) calculate a new dose and dosing interval based on a desired peak and trough; and (4) check the peak and trough of the new dosage regimen.

For example, vancomycin was administered in a dose of 15 mg/kg IV over 60 minutes every 12 hours. The plasma concentrations were measured on the third day of treatment (presumed steady state). The predose or trough concentration was 12 mg/L; the peak concentration, measured 60 minutes after the *end* of the infusion, was 32 mg/L:

$$\text{Vd (L/kg)} = \frac{15 \text{ mg/kg}}{32 \text{ mg/L} - 12 \text{ mg/L}}$$
$$\text{Vd (L/kg)} = 0.75 \text{ L/kg}$$

Step 1: Substituting the data into Eq. 5.8, we calculate volume of distribution.

Step 2: At steady state, peak and trough concentrations reach the same levels after each dose. The time between the peak and trough concentrations is 10 hours—that is, 12 hours minus 1 hour infusion minus 1 hour to peak concentration. Half-life may be solved by rearranging Eq. 5.2 to solve for k (elimination rate constant) and substituting the calculated k into Eq. 5.3. In this case, the calculated elimination rate constant is 0.098/hour, which corresponds to a half-life of 7.1 hours. However, a practical and clinically applicable "bedside" approach may be used without the need for logarithmic calculations. For example, the plasma concentration decreased from 32 to 16 mg/L in one half-life and then from 16 to 12 mg/L in a fraction of the second half-life. At the end of the second half-life, the concentration would have decreased to 8 mg/L. Because 12 mg/L is the midpoint between the first and second half-lives, 1.5 half-lives have elapsed during the 10 hours between the peak and trough. Thus, if one assumes a linear decrease, the half-life is estimated as 6.67 hours (10 hours ÷ 1.5 half-lives). Note that the discrepancy between the actual half-life, 7.1 hours and the estimated half-life, 6.67 hours, is attributed to the linear assumptions between half-lives. In fact, first-order elimination is a nonlinear process with the concentration decreasing from 32 mg/L to 22.6 mg/L during the first 50% of the first half-life rather than from 32 mg/L to 24 mg/L estimated via the linear approach. The same occurs during subsequent half-lives. However, the small error associated with this method is often acceptable for rapid bedside estimates of pharmacokinetic parameters.

Step 3: A new dosage regimen must be calculated if the concentrations are unsatisfactory. Accordingly, one must decide on desired peak and trough concentrations. For example, if the desired vancomycin peak and trough concentrations were 32 mg/L (20–40 mg/L) and 8 mg/L (5–10 mg/L), respectively, then Eq. 5.8 may be rearranged to solve for the new dose:

$$\begin{aligned} \text{Dose (mg/kg)} &= \text{Vd (L/kg)} \times [\text{C (peak desired)} \\ &\quad - \text{C (trough desired) (mg/L)}] \\ \text{Does (mg/kg)} &= 0.75 \text{ L/kg} \times (32 \text{ mg/L} - 8 \text{ mg/L}) \\ \text{Dose (mg/kg)} &= 18 \text{ mg/kg} \end{aligned} \qquad \text{Eq. 5.9}$$

The current dose produces a peak concentration of 32 mg/L that is in the recommended therapeutic range, and extending the dosing interval to 2 half-lives (hours) after the peak is reached (2 hours after beginning the dose infusion) will produce a trough concentration of 8 mg/L. The dose interval should be increased to 16 hours and the dose increased to 18 mg/kg.

Step 4: Estimating peak and trough concentrations with the new regimen provides a good double-check against a mathematical error. Sixteen hours after the 15 mg/kg dose is administered (or approximately 2 half-lives after the measured peak), the trough should be approximately 8 mg/L. At this time, administration of 18 mg/kg will increase the concentration by 24 mg/L (assuming a volume of distribution of 0.75 L/kg) to a peak concentration of 32 mg/L.

REPETITIVE DOSING AND DRUG ACCUMULATION

When multiple doses are administered, the dose is usually repeated before complete elimination of the previous one. In this situation, peak and trough concentrations increase until a steady-state concentration (C_{SS}) is reached (see Fig. 5.3). The average C_{SS} ($AvgC_{SS}$) can be calculated as follows[3]:

$$AvgC_{ss} = \frac{1}{Clearance} \times \frac{f \times D}{\tau}$$

$$AvgC_{ss} = \frac{1}{k \times Vd} \times \frac{f \times D}{\tau} \qquad \text{Eq. 5.10}$$

$$AvgC_{ss} = \frac{1.44 \times T_{1/2}}{k \times Vd} \times \frac{f \times D}{\tau} \qquad \text{Eq. 5.11}$$

In Eqs. 5.10 and 5.11, f is the fraction of the dose that is absorbed, D is the dose, T is the dosing interval in the same units of time as the elimination half-life, k is the elimination rate constant, and 1.44 equals the reciprocal of 0.693 (see Eq. 5.3). The magnitude of the average C_{ss} is directly proportional to the ratio of $T_{1/2}/_T$ and D.[3]

STEADY STATE

Steady state occurs when the amount of drug removed from the body between doses equals the amount of the dose administered.[11,12] Five half-lives are usually required for drug elimination and distribution among compartments to reach equilibrium. When all tissues are at equilibrium (i.e., steady state), the mean concentrations are identical after each dose. During continuous infusions, the fraction of steady-state concentration that has been reached can be calculated in terms of multiples of the drug's half-life.[3] After 3 half-lives, the concentration is 88% of the steady state concentration. When changing doses during chronic drug therapy, the concentration should usually not be rechecked until several half-lives have elapsed, unless elimination is impaired or signs of toxicity develop.

During infusions, clearance is the main determinant of dose that achieves a target concentration at steady state:

$$\text{Infusion rate (mg/h)} = \text{Target concentration (mg/L)}$$
$$\times \text{Clearance (L/h)} \qquad \text{Eq. 5.12}$$

LOADING DOSE

If the time to reach a constant concentration by continuous or intermittent dosing is excessive (e.g., 3–5 half-lives), a loading dose may be used to reach the target concentration more rapidly. For example, propofol is usually given as a loading dose before establishing an infusion for anesthesia.[7]

Dose calculations to achieve a target concentration in plasma (Cp_{TARGET}) using a one-compartment model

$$\text{Dose} = V \times Cp_{TARGET} \qquad \text{Eq. 5.13}$$

may not be applicable to many anesthetic drugs that are characterized using multicompartment models. The use of V1 (central volume of distribution) as V results in a loading dose that is too large, whereas the use of volume of distribution at steady state results in a loading dose that is too small. Too large a dose may cause transient toxicity, although slowing the rate of administration may prevent excessive concentrations during the distributive phase. A loading dose of dexmedetomidine is usually given over 10 to 20 minutes in children because a rapid infusion causes undesired pharmacodynamic effects including an increase in blood pressure and bradycardia (see Chapter 6, Fig. 6.9).[13]

The loading dose is used to target a concentration at the effect site, not plasma, and there is a time delay between peak plasma concentration and peak concentration at the effect site. The time to peak effect (T_{PEAK}) depends on clearance and the effect site equilibration half-time. At a submaximal dose, T_{PEAK} is independent of the dose. At supramaximal doses, the maximum effect occurs earlier than T_{PEAK} and persists for a greater duration because of the shape of the pharmacodynamic sigmoidal concentration-response relationship. The T_{PEAK} concept has been used to calculate the optimal initial bolus dose.[14] The volume of distribution (Vpe) at the time of peak effect site concentration (C_{PEAK}) is calculated and used (Eq. 5 14):

$$Vpe = \frac{Dose}{Concentration (T_{PEAK})} \qquad \text{Eq. 5 14}$$

Loading dose can then be calculated as

$$\text{Loading dose} = C_{PEAK} \times Vpe \qquad \text{Eq. 5.15}$$

Population Modeling

Pediatric anesthesiologists have embraced the population approach for investigating pharmacokinetics and pharmacodynamics. This approach, achieved through nonlinear mixed-effects models, provides a means to study variability in drug responses among individuals representative of those in whom the drug will be used clinically. Traditional approaches to interpreting time-concentration profiles relied on "rich" data from a small group of subjects. In contrast, mixed effects models can be used to analyze "sparse" data (two to three samples) from each one of a large number of subjects. Sampling times are not crucial for population methods and can be fit around clinical procedures or outpatient appointments. Sampling time bands rather than exact times is equally effective and allows flexibility in children.[14,15] Interpretation of truncated individual sets of data or missing data is also possible with this type of analysis, rendering it particularly useful for pediatric studies. Population modeling also allows pooling of data across studies to provide a single robust pharmacokinetic analysis rather than comparing separate smaller studies that are complicated by different methods and analyses.

Mixed-effects models are "mixed" because they describe the data using a mixture of fixed and random effects. Fixed effects predict the average influence of a covariate, such as weight, as an explanation of some of the variability between subjects in a parameter like clearance. Random effects describe the remaining variability among subjects that are not predictable from the fixed effect average. Explanatory covariates (e.g., age, size, renal function, sex, temperature) can be introduced that explain the predictable part of the between-individual variability. Nonlinear regression is performed by an iterative process to find the curve of best fit.[16,17]

Pediatric Pharmacokinetic Considerations

Growth and development are two major aspects of children not readily apparent in adults. How these factors interact is not necessarily easy to determine from observations because they are quite highly correlated. Drug clearance, for example, may increase with weight, height, age, body surface area, and creatinine clearance. One approach is to standardize for size before incorporating a factor for maturation.[18]

SIZE

Clearance in children 1 to 2 years of age, expressed as liters per hour per kilogram, is commonly greater than that observed in older children and adolescents. This is a size effect, not because the liver is larger or hepatic blood flow is increased in that subpopulation. This "artifact of size" disappears when allometric scaling is used. *Allometry* is a term used to describe the nonlinear relationship between size and function. This nonlinear relationship is expressed as

$$y = a \times Body\ Mass^{EXP} \qquad \text{Eq. 5.16}$$

where *y* is the variable of interest (e.g., basal metabolic rate [BMR]), *a* is a scaling parameter, and *EXP* is the allometric exponent. The value of *EXP* has been the subject of much debate. BMR is the most common variable investigated, and camps advocating for a *EXP* value of two-thirds (i.e., body surface area) are at odds with those advocating a value of three-quarters. Support for a value of three-quarters comes from investigations that show the log of BMR plotted against the log of body weight produces a straight line with a slope of three-quarters across all species studied, including humans. Clearance is a metabolic process and the log of clearance plotted against the log of body weight also produces a straight line with a slope of three-quarters when different species are studied. Fig. 5.4 exemplifies this for tramadol.[19] Fractal geometry mathematically explains this phenomenon. The three-quarter–power law for metabolic rates was derived from a general model that describes how essential materials are transported

through space-filled fractal networks of branching tubes.[20] A great many physiologic, structural, and time-related variables scale predictably within and between species with weight (*W*) exponents (*EXP*) of three-quarters, 1, and one-quarter, respectively.[21]

These exponents have applicability to pharmacokinetic parameters; for example, the exponent for clearance is three-quarters, volume (*V*) is 1, and half-time ($T_{1/2}$) is one-quarter.[21] The factor for size (*Fsize*) for total drug clearance may be expressed as

$$Fsize = \left(\frac{W}{70}\right)^{3/4} \qquad \text{Eq. 5.17}$$

Remifentanil clearance, which depends on nonspecific blood esterases, in children aged 1 month to 9 years is similar to adult rates when scaled using an allometric exponent of three-quarters.[22] Nonspecific blood esterases that metabolize remifentanil are mature at birth.[23]

MATURATION

Allometry alone is insufficient to predict the clearance in neonates and infants from adult estimates for most drugs. The addition of a model describing maturation is required. The sigmoid hyperbolic or Hill model[24] has been found useful for describing this maturation process. This maturation factor (*MF*) can be described:

$$MF = \frac{PMA^{Hill}}{TM_{50}^{Hill} + PMA^{Hill}} \qquad \text{Eq. 5.18}$$

The TM_{50} describes the maturation half-time, while the Hill coefficient relates to the slope of this maturation profile. Maturation of clearance begins before birth, suggesting that postmenstrual age (*PMA*) would be a better predictor of drug elimination than postnatal age (PNA).[21] Fig. 5.5 shows the maturation profile for dexmedetomidine, expressed as both the standard per-kilogram model and by using allometry. Clearance is immature in infancy. Clearance, expressed as per kilogram, reaches its zenith at 2 years of age, decreasing subsequently with age. This "artifact of size" disappears with use of the allometric model. Appropriate size scaling shows

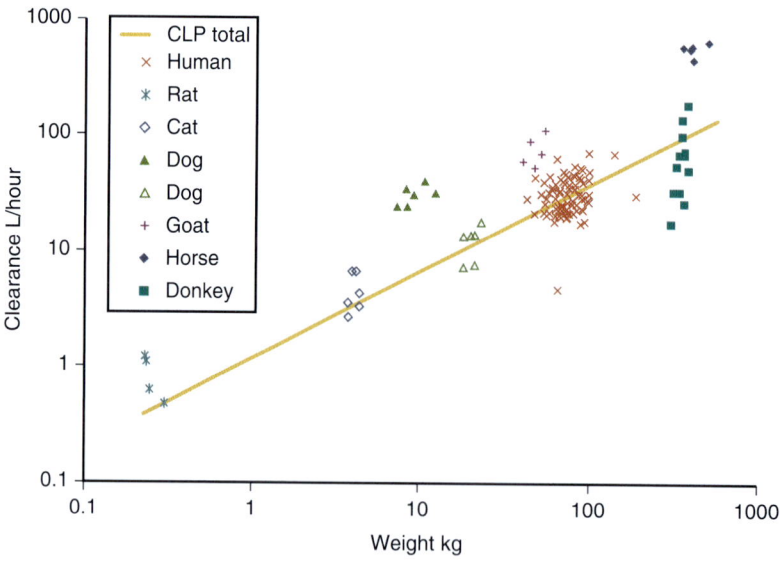

FIGURE 5.4 Weight-predicted tramadol total clearance *(CLP total)* compared with human allometric prediction *(solid line)* using a three-quarter–power exponent *(solid line)*. (From Holford SD, Allegaert K, Anderson BJ, et al. Parent-metabolite pharmacokinetic models for tramadol—tests of assumptions and predictions. *J Pharmacol Clin Toxicol.* 2014;2[1]:1023-1034, with permission.)

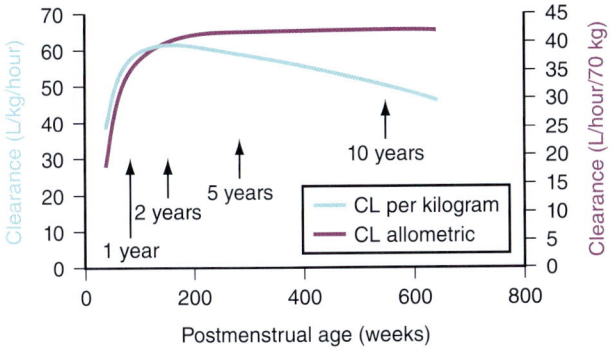

FIGURE 5.5 The clearance *(CL)* maturation profile of dexmedetomidine, expressed using the per-kilogram model and the allometric three-quarter–power model. This maturation pattern is typical of many drugs cleared by the liver or kidneys. (Data extracted from Potts AL, Anderson BJ, Warman GR, et al. Dexmedetomidine pharmacokinetics in pediatric intensive care—a pooled analysis. *Paediatr Anaesth.* 2009;19(11):1119-1129.)

that the pharmacokinetics in children (>2 years old) are similar to adults. Maturation changes are generally completed within the first 2 years of postnatal life; consequently, infants may be considered as immature children, whereas children are just small adults.[25]

ORGAN FUNCTION

Changes associated with normal growth and development can be distinguished from pathologic changes describing organ function.[18] Morphine clearance is reduced in neonates because of immature glucuronide conjugation, and even less in critically ill neonates compared with healthier cohorts,[26–28] possibly attributable to other covariates such as reduced hepatic function or perfusion. Positive-pressure ventilation may also reduce morphine clearance[29]; this is possibly attributable to a consequent reduced hepatic blood flow with a drug that has perfusion-limited clearance (e.g., propofol, morphine).

Creatinine clearance is commonly used as a measure of renal function and dictates the dose of those drugs with renal clearance. Renal function in children can be estimated using formulae that allow estimation of glomerular filtration rate from clinical characteristics.[30] These formulae use simple markers such as height, plasma creatinine concentration and body surface area. We might expect the maturation of creatinine clearance, a marker for glomerular filtration rate, to reflect the influences of size, maturation, and organ function. Estimation methods such as those of Schwartz incorporate a size factor (body length or height) and a scaling factor (k) that is age dependent (e.g., k = 0.33 for premature neonates; k = 0.45 for term infants 0–1 year; k = 0.55 for 1–12 years; k = 0.7 for 13- to 21-year-old adolescent males)[31–33]:

$$GFR = \frac{k \cdot height}{Serum\ Creatinine} \qquad \text{Eq. 5.19}$$

Dosing of drugs that are cleared renally should be based on size- and maturation-based predictions of glomerular filtration rate in children with normal renal function.[34] Creatinine clearance is used in those with abnormal function, but this estimation may overpredict glomerular filtration rate in children, possibly because of tubular secretion and reabsorption. Glomerular filtration rate will account for all kidney handling even for drugs eliminated by tubular secretion: the intact nephron hypothesis.[35] Serum creatinine changes with age and these changes have been

related to postnatal age, allowing a guide to renal function in an individual.[36,37] Pharmacokinetic parameters *(P)* can be described in an individual as the product of size *(Fsize)*, maturation *(MF)*, and organ function *(OF)* influences, where *Pstd* is the parameter value in a standard size adult without pathologic changes in organ function[18]:

$$P = Pstd \cdot Fsize \cdot MF \cdot OF \qquad \text{Eq. 5.20}$$

Pharmacodynamic Models

Pharmacokinetics is what the body does to the drug, while *pharmacodynamics* is what the drug does to the body. The precise boundary between pharmacodynamics and pharmacokinetics is ill-defined and often requires a link describing movement of drug from the plasma to the effect site and its target. Drugs may exert effects at nonspecific membrane sites, by interference with transport mechanisms, by enzyme inhibition or induction, or by activation or inhibition of receptors.

MINIMUM EFFECTIVE CONCENTRATION

The minimum effective concentration (MEC) of an analgesic can be established by titrating an analgesic to achieve an acceptable level of pain at rest or in response to a nociceptive stimulus. A blood assay for analgesic drug concentration at these times can be used to determine the effective concentration. Further blood assays when pain recurs or when further analgesics are required improve the accuracy of assessment. This technique has been used to determine the minimum effective analgesic concentration (MEAC) of oxycodone.

The minimum effective or minimum analgesic concentration is a poor target concentration measure since concentrations differ with the type of pain. An oxycodone MEC 20 to 35 μg/L and MEAC 45 to 50 μg/L for pain after laparoscopic cholecystectomy has been described.[38] Larger mean estimates of MEC 31 μg/L and MEAC 75 μg/L have been reported in adults undergoing major intraabdominal surgery.[39] Smaller values are reported after cardiac surgery in adults (MEC 6–12 μg/L, MEAC 15–25 μg/L).[40] The general therapeutic range of oxycodone is 10 to 100 μg/L; a range too large to be clinically useful. Although oxycodone metabolites have negligible contribution to analgesic effect,[41] factors such as drug interactions, sedation, or time of assessment, influence estimates. Even if patients titrate their own dose using patient-controlled analgesia to an individualized plasma opioid concentration, the veracity of such assessments have been debated extensively.[4]

SIGMOID E$_{MAX}$ MODEL

The relationship between the drug concentration and its effect may be described by the Hill equation or Emax model (see maturation model described previously)[24]:

$$Effect = E_0 + \frac{(E\max \cdot Ce^N)}{(EC_{50}^N + Ce^N)}, \qquad \text{Eq. 5.21}$$

where E_0 is the baseline response, *Emax* is the maximum effect change, *Ce* is the concentration in the effect compartment, EC_{50} is the concentration producing 50% Emax, and *N* is the Hill coefficient defining the steepness of the concentration-response curve (Fig. 5.6). Efficacy is the maximum response on a dose or concentration-response curve. EC_{50} can be considered a measure of potency relative to another drug, provided N and Emax for the two drugs are the same.

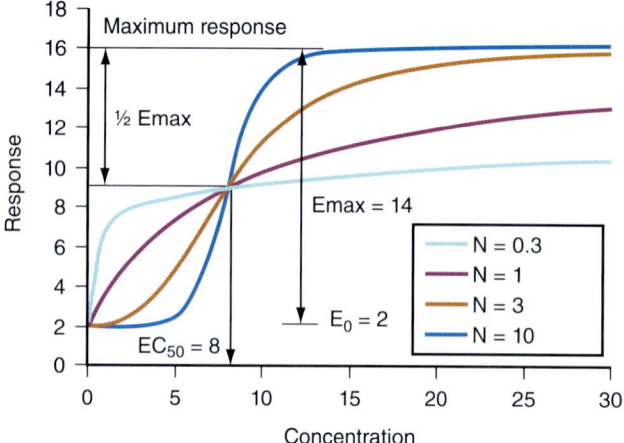

FIGURE 5.6 The sigmoid Emax model is commonly used to describe the relationship between drug response and concentration. Changing the Hill coefficient *(N)* dramatically alters the shape of the curve. E_0, Baseline response; EC_{50}, concentration producing 50% Emax; *Emax*, maximum effect change; *N*, Hill coefficient defining the steepness of the concentration-response curve.

QUANTAL EFFECT MODEL

The potency of inhaled anesthetics is expressed by minimum alveolar concentration (MAC), which is the concentration at which 50% of subjects move in response to a standard surgical stimulus. At first glance, MAC is similar to the EC_{50}; however, it is actually an expression of a quantal response rather than magnitude of effect. There are two methods of estimating MAC. Responses can be recorded over the range of clinical doses in a large number of subjects and logistic regression applied to estimate the relationship between the dose and the quantal effect; MAC can then be interpolated. However, large numbers of subjects may not be available, so an alternative method known as the "up-and-down" method described by Dixon[45,46] may be used to estimate only the MAC value, rather than delineate the entire sigmoid curve.[47] The latter method usually involves a study of only one concentration of inhaled anesthetic in each subject and, in a sequence of subjects, each receives a concentration depending on the response of the previous subject; the concentration is either decreased if the previous subject did not respond or increased if they did. The MAC is calculated either as the mean concentration of equal numbers of responses and no responses or is the mean concentration of pairs of "response–no response" (e.g., with bilateral inguinal herniorrhaphy). This technique has also been used to determine the EC_{50} of local anesthetic drugs used in central neuraxial blockade.[48–50]

This sigmoid Emax concentration-response relationship is commonly inverted to describe anesthetic drug concentration effects on the bispectral index (Fig. 5.7).[42] The model is used widely to describe pharmacodynamics in children (e.g., propofol in children 1 to 16 years who had an E_0 estimate as 93.2, Emax –83.4, EC_{50} 5.2 mg/L, and *N* 1.4).[43] The pharmacodynamics of the neuromuscular blocking drug, rocuronium, have used the same model. A train of four response using the adductor pollicis model was used to estimate an EC_{50} 1.24 mg/L with a Hill coefficient (N) of 3.97. The equilibration half-time ($T_{1/2}$ keo) was 3.25 minutes in adults.[44]

LOGISTIC REGRESSION MODEL

When the pharmacologic effect is difficult to grade, then it may be useful to estimate the probability of achieving the effect as a function of plasma concentration. Effect measures, such as movement/no movement or rousable/non-rousable, are dichotomous. Logistic regression is commonly used to analyze such data and the interpolated EC_{50} value refers to the probability of response. For example, an EC_{50} of 0.52 mg/L for arousal after ketamine sedation in children has been estimated using this technique.[51] Logistic regression was used to determine a morphine ED_{50} of 0.096 mg/kg that was associated with a 50% probability of vomiting after tonsillectomy surgery.[52]

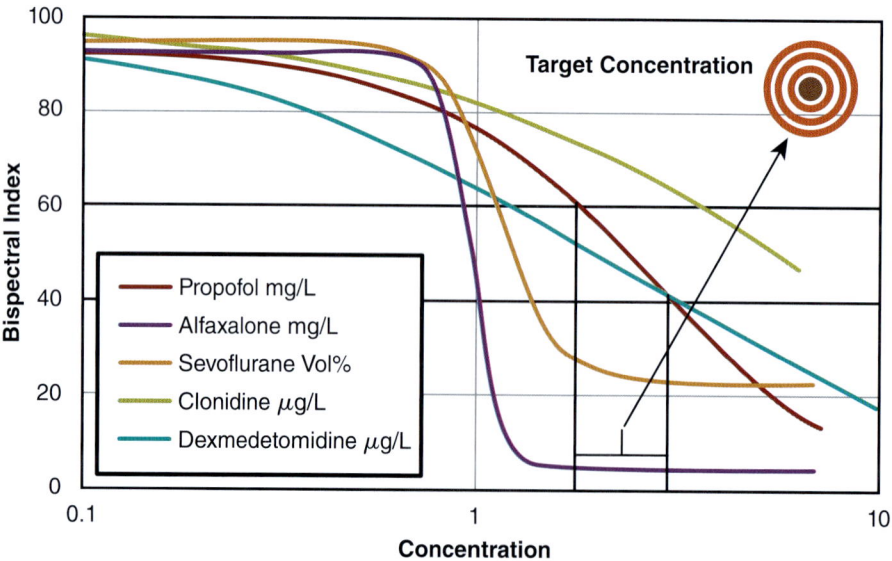

FIGURE 5.7 The concentration-response relationship, measured using the bispectral index *(BIS)*, is shown for propofol, alfaxalone, sevoflurane, clonidine, and dexmedetomidine. The target effect range for the BIS monitor is 40–60, propofol concentrations that are consistent with anesthesia. The target concentrations that achieve these BIS values can be determined from the concentration-response relationship.

Linking Pharmacokinetics With Pharmacodynamics

A simple situation in which drug effect is directly related to the concentration does not mean that the drug effects parallel the time course of the concentration. This occurs only when the concentration is small in relation to EC_{50}. In this situation the half-life of the drug may correlate closely with the half-life of drug effect. Conversely, observed effects may not be directly related to serum concentration; many drugs have a short half-life but a long duration of effect. This may be attributable to induced physiologic changes (e.g., aspirin and platelet function) or may be a result of the shape of the Emax model. If the initial concentration is very high in relation to the EC_{50}, then drug concentrations 5 half-lives later, when we might expect a minimum concentration, may still exert considerable effect.

There may also be a delay in transferring the drug to the effect site (e.g., neuromuscular blockers, a lag time (e.g., diuretics), physiologic response (e.g., antipyresis), active metabolite (e.g., valdecoxib), or synthesis of physiologic substances (e.g., warfarin). A plasma concentration-effect plot can form a hysteresis loop because of this delay in effect. Hull and Sheiner introduced the effect compartment concept for neuromuscular blockers.[53,54] A single first-order parameter ($T_{1/2}keo$) describes the equilibration half-time. This mathematical trick assumes that the concentration in the central compartment is the same as that in the effect compartment at equilibrium, but that a time delay exists before the drug reaches the effect compartment. The concentration in the effect compartment is used to describe the concentration-effect relationship.[55]

Adult $T_{1/2}keo$ values are well described (e.g., morphine, 16 minutes; fentanyl, 5 minutes; propofol, 3 minutes; alfentanil, 1 minute). This $T_{1/2}keo$ parameter is commonly incorporated into target-controlled infusion pumps to achieve a rapid effect-site concentration. The adult midazolam $T_{1/2}keo$ of 5 minutes may be prolonged in the elderly, resulting in overdose if this is not recognized during dose titration.[53]

The $T_{1/2}keo$ for propofol in children has been described. As expected, a shorter $T_{1/2}keo$ with decreasing age based on size models has been observed.[43,54,56]

$$T_{\frac{1}{2}keoCHILD} = T_{\frac{1}{2}keoADULT} \times \left(\frac{Weight}{70} \right)^{1/4} \qquad \text{Eq. 5.22}$$

Similar results have been demonstrated for sevoflurane and changes in the electroencephalogram (EEG).[57,58] If the effect site is targeted and Tpeak is anticipated to be later than it actually is because it was determined in a teenager or adult, this will result in excessive dose in a young child.

Drug Distribution

PROTEIN BINDING

Acidic drugs (e.g., diazepam, barbiturates) tend to bind mainly to albumin, whereas basic drugs (e.g., amide local anesthetic agents) bind to globulins, lipoproteins, and glycoproteins. In general, plasma protein binding of many drugs is decreased in the neonate relative to the adult in part because of reduced total protein and albumin concentrations (Fig. 5.8).[59] Many drugs that are highly protein bound in adults have less of an affinity for protein in neonates (E-Fig. 5.1).[59–63] Reduced protein binding increases the unbound (free) fraction of medications, thus providing more free medication to cross biologic membranes and cause greater pharmacologic effects.[64–68] This effect is particularly important for medications that are highly protein bound

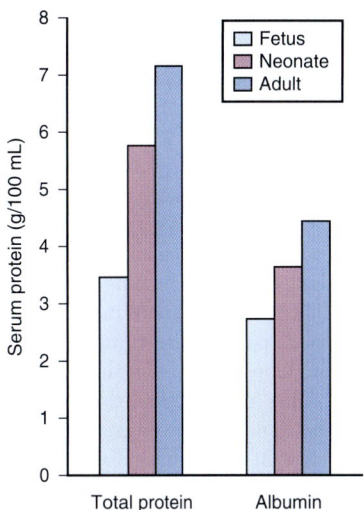

FIGURE 5.8 Changes in total serum protein and albumin values that occur with maturation. Note that total protein and albumin are less in fetuses than in neonates and less in neonates than in adults. The result may be altered pharmacokinetics and pharmacodynamics for drugs with a high degree of protein binding, because less drug is protein bound and more is available for clinical effect in the neonate and fetus. (Data from Ehrnebo M, Agurell S, Jalling B, et al. Age differences in drug binding by plasma proteins: studies on human foetuses, neonates and adults. *Eur J Clin Pharmacol.* 1971;3(4):189-193.)

because the reduced protein binding increases the free fraction of the medication to a greater extent than for low protein-bound drugs. For example, phenytoin is 85% protein bound in healthy infants but only 80% in those who are jaundiced. This equates to a 33% increase in the free fraction of phenytoin when jaundice occurs (E-Fig. 5.2). Differences in protein binding may have considerable influence on the response to medications that are acidic and are therefore highly protein bound (e.g., phenytoin, salicylate, bupivacaine, barbiturates, antibiotics, theophylline, and diazepam). In addition, some medications, such as phenytoin, salicylate, sulfisoxazole, caffeine, ceftriaxone, diatrizoate (Hypaque), and sodium benzoate, compete with bilirubin for binding to albumin (see E-Fig. 5.2). If large amounts of bilirubin are displaced in premature neonates, particularly in the presence of hypoxemia and acidosis, which increases movement across the blood-brain barrier, kernicterus may result.[60,63,69–72] Because these metabolic derangements often occur in sick neonates who are scheduled for surgery, special care must be taken when selecting medications for the anesthetic.[72]

Medications that are basic (e.g., lidocaine or alfentanil) are generally bound to plasma α_1-acid glycoprotein; α_1-acid glycoprotein concentrations in preterm and term infants are reduced but are similar to those in adults by 6 months, although between patient variability is high (e.g., α_1-acid glycoprotein 0.32–0.92 g/L).[73] Therefore, for a given dose, the free fraction of a drug is greater in preterm and term infants.[73–75] In contrast to drugs bound to plasma proteins, unbound lipophilic drugs passively diffuse across the blood-brain barrier, equilibrating very quickly. This may explain the propensity of bupivacaine to induce seizures in neonates. Decreased protein binding, as in the neonate, leads to a greater proportion of circulating unbound drug. Reduced protein binding in neonates and preterm infants increases the free fraction of drugs delivered to the kidneys and liver for metabolism; however, reduced clearance results in a greater potential for toxicity.[64,65,67,76] An important example is the immature clearance of bupivacaine, which resulted in large plasma concentrations that increased sufficiently to cause seizures in neonates treated with epidural infusions at rates greater than the rate at which it was metabolized.[77]

These binding changes in neonates differ from adults in whom protein binding changes are important for the relatively unusual case of a drug that is more than 95% protein bound, with a high extraction ratio and a narrow therapeutic index, that is given parenterally (e.g., IV lidocaine), or a drug with a narrow therapeutic index that is given orally and has a very rapid $T_{1/2}$keo (e.g., antiarrhythmic drugs; propafenone, verapamil).[78]

Maturational changes in tissue binding also affect drug distribution. Myocardial digoxin concentrations in infants are 6-fold greater than those in adults, despite similar serum concentrations. Erythrocyte/plasma concentration ratios of digoxin in infants are one-third smaller during loading digitalization than during maintenance digoxin therapy. These findings are consistent with a greater volume of distribution of digoxin in infants and may explain, in part, the unusually large therapeutic doses needed in infants.[79]

BODY COMPOSITION

Preterm and term infants have a much greater proportion of body weight as water than do older children and adults (Fig. 5.9).[80] The net effect on water-soluble medications is a greater volume of distribution in infants, which in turn increases the initial (loading) dose, based on weight, to achieve the desired target serum concentration and clinical response.[64–66,81,82] Term neonates often require a greater loading dose (milligrams per kilogram) for some medications (e.g., digoxin, succinylcholine, and aminoglycoside antibiotics) than older children.[81–85] However, neonates also tend to be sensitive to the respiratory, neurologic, and circulatory effects of many medications and therefore tend to be more responsive to these effects at reduced blood concentrations than are children and adults. Preterm infants are usually more sensitive than term neonates and in general require even smaller target blood concentrations.[64] On the other

hand, dopamine may increase blood pressure and urine output in term neonates only at doses as large as 50 μg/kg per minute. This dose, which would induce intense vasoconstriction in adults, suggests that the vascular receptors in neonates are less sensitive in their cardiovascular responsiveness.[65,83,86–89] *It is important to carefully titrate the doses of all medications that are administered to preterm and term infants to the desired clinical response.*

Compared with children and adolescents, preterm and term neonates have a smaller proportion of body weight in the form of fat and muscle mass; with growth, the proportion of body weight composed of these tissues increases (Fig. 5.10).[64,65,80,87,90–92] This may cause an increase or decrease in distribution volume, depending on drug physicochemical properties. Redistribution of barbiturates and propofol is less in neonates than that observed in adults; higher plasma concentrations are sustained because clearance is small, and prolonged undesirable clinical effects are common.

Obesity

Obesity among children and adolescents in the United States has increased 3-fold in the past 30 years with 15.5% of children and adolescents currently estimated to be obese (BMI ≥95th percentile for age).[93] The prevalence of obesity has important ethnic variations (e.g., 25.6% Hispanic, 24.2% Black, 16.1% White, and 8.7% Asian children aged 2–19 years, 2017–18).[94] In children, obesity is not easily defined numerically or clinically. Obesity must be assessed using total body weight or body mass index (BMI) referenced to standard charts that display weight or BMI distribution at each year of life. There are few guidelines for anesthesia drug dosing in obese children[95,96] and it is acknowledged as a dilemma.[97]

Size Scalers

Volume (determining loading dose) and clearance (determining maintenance dose) of some drugs are known to differ when

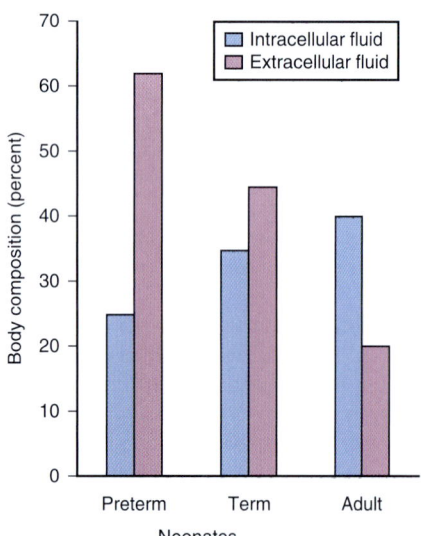

FIGURE 5.9 Changes in the intracellular and extracellular compartments that occur with maturation. Note the large proportion of extracellular water in preterm and term infants. This large water compartment creates an increased volume of distribution for highly water-soluble medications (e.g., succinylcholine, gentamicin) and may account for the large (by weight) loading dose required for some medications to achieve a satisfactory clinical response. (Data from Friis-Hansen B. Body composition during growth. In vivo measurements and biochemical data correlated to differential anatomical growth. *Pediatrics.* 1971;47(1 Suppl 2):264+.)

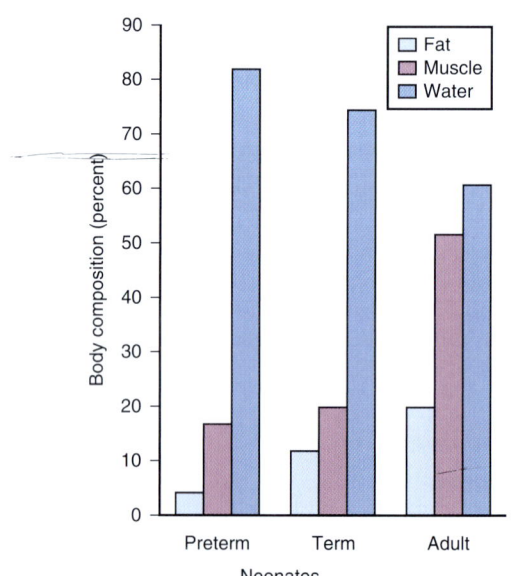

FIGURE 5.10 Changes in body content for fat, muscle, and water that occur with maturation. Note the small percentage of fat and muscle mass in preterm and term infants. These factors may greatly influence the pharmacokinetics and pharmacodynamics of medications that redistribute into fat (e.g., barbiturates) and muscle (e.g., fentanyl) because there is less tissue mass into which the drug may redistribute. (Data from Friis-Hansen B. Body composition during growth. In vivo measurements and biochemical data correlated to differential anatomical growth. *Pediatrics* 1971;47(1 Suppl 2):264+.)

obesity is present.[98] Although body fat has minimum metabolic activity, fat mass contributes to the overall body size and may have an indirect influence on both metabolic and renal clearance. Alternately, the volume of distribution of a drug depends on its physicochemical properties.[99] There are drugs whose apparent volume of distribution may be independent of fat mass (e.g., digoxin) or be extensively determined by it (e.g., diazepam). A number of size descriptors have been put forward for use in the obese patient (e.g., total body weight, lean body mass, ideal body weight, body mass index, fat-free mass, normal fat mass).[100]

Ideal body weight has been proposed as the preferred metric for maintenance dosing of benzodiazepines (diazepam,[101] midazolam[102]), morphine,[103] and neuromuscular blocking drugs such as vecuronium,[104] rocuronium,[105,106] and cisatracurium.[107] However, lean body mass (commonly used interchangeably with lean body weight or fat free mass) has also been claimed as the optimal size scalar for most drugs used in anesthesia including opioids and anesthetic induction agents.[96,108–110] The use of lean body mass that assumes a linear relationship over the mass range appears to be a good predictor of the dose of remifentanil.[111]

Formulae for lean body mass in children have been derived based on the assumption that extracellular fluid volume is proportional to estimated lean body mass in both adults and children. Estimated extracellular fluid volume (eECF) was determined from height and total body weight (TBW) (Eq. 5.23 and Eq. 5.24):

$$eECF = 0.0215 \cdot TBW^{0.6469} \cdot Height^{0.7236} \qquad \text{Eq. 5.23}$$

$$eLBM = 3.8 \cdot eECF \qquad \text{Eq. 5.24}$$

These formulae have been used to create nomograms enabling determination of the ideal body mass and lean body mass (LBM) in children.[112] Clearance was considered to be related linearly to lean body mass,[98] although when a wide range of masses was analyzed, clearance was more closely related to lean body mass in a nonlinear manner based on allometric scaling.[34,113] The issue is further confused because the size metric used for loading dose (determined by volume of distribution) may differ from that used for maintenance dose or infusion (determined by clearance).

Normal Fat Mass

The use of normal fat mass (NFM)[114] with allometric scaling as a size descriptor may prove versatile.[34,113,115,116] That size descriptor uses the notion of the fat-free mass (FFM, similar to lean body mass but excludes lipids in cell membranes, central nervous system, and bone marrow) plus a "bit more." The "bit more" differs for each drug where the maximum "bit more" added to the fat-free mass would equal the total body water.[117]

$$NFM = FFM + Ffat \cdot (TBW - FFM) \qquad \text{Eq 5.25}$$

The parameter *Ffat* is estimated and accounts for different contributions of fat mass. If *Ffat* is estimated to be zero, then fat-free mass alone predicts size whereas if *Ffat* is 1, then size is predicted by total body water. This parameter is drug specific and also specific to the pharmacokinetic parameter such as clearance or volume of distribution. It has a value of 0.211 for glomerular filtration rate, which implies that 21% of fat mass is a size driver for kidney function in addition to fat-free mass.[34] Size based on normal fat mass assumes that fat-free mass is the primary determinant of size with an extra *Ffat* factor (which may be positive or negative) that determines how fat mass contributes to size. A negative value for *Ffat* might suggest organ dysfunction; not an uncommon scenario in the morbidly obese. A negative value has been reported for dexmedetomidine in that cohort.[118]

Fat mass does have a contribution to dexmedetomidine volume (*Ffat* = 0.293), but has little contribution to clearance (Ffat =0).[119] Total body weight (Ffat = 1) can be used for propofol,[120] acetaminophen,[115] fentanyl,[121] and oxycodone.[122]

REGIONAL BLOOD FLOWS

Relative organ mass and regional blood flow change with growth and development during the first few months of life in addition to the physiologic changes that take place at birth. During this period, the brain and kidney receive an increasing proportion of the cardiac output, while the liver receives a decreasing proportion. The proportional mass of the head and liver are much greater in the infant than in the adult.[123] Mean cerebral blood flow peaks in early childhood (70 mL/minute per 100 g) at about 3 to 8 years of age[124]; flows in both neonates and adults are less (50 mL/minute per 100 g).[125] The highly lipophilic drugs used for anesthetic induction rapidly equilibrate concentrations with brain tissue, but the reduced cerebral perfusion translates into a slower onset time after an intravenous induction in neonates than in early childhood. Offset time is also delayed because redistribution to the well-perfused and deep, underperfused tissues is reduced.

BLOOD-BRAIN BARRIER

The blood-brain barrier is a network of complex tight junctions between specialized endothelial cells that restricts the paracellular diffusion of hydrophilic molecules from the blood to the brain substance. There are specific transport systems selectively expressed in the barrier endothelial cell membranes that mediate the transport of nutrients into the central nervous system and of toxic metabolites out of the central nervous system. Small molecules can cross into fetal and neonatal brains more readily than they do into adult brains.[126] Blood-brain barrier function improves throughout fetal brain development, reaching maturity at term.[126] This maturation explains why kernicterus is more common in the preterm than the term neonate. Blood-brain barrier breakdown or alterations in transport systems may occur in some diseases. Proinflammatory substances and specific disease-associated proteins often mediate blood-brain barrier dysfunction.[127]

Fentanyl is actively transported across the blood-brain barrier into the brain by a saturable adenosine triphosphate (ATP)-dependent process, whereas ATP-binding cassette proteins such as P-glycoprotein actively pump opioids such as fentanyl and morphine out of the brain.[128] P-glycoprotein modulation significantly influences brain opioid distribution and onset time and the magnitude and duration of analgesic response.[129] Modulation may occur during disease processes, increased temperature, or the presence of other substances (e.g., verapamil, magnesium).[128] Genetic polymorphisms affecting P-glycoprotein–related genes may explain some individual differences in central nervous system–active drug sensitivity (see also Chapter 4).[130]

The sensitivity of human neonates to most of the sedatives, hypnotics, and opioids may in part be related to increased brain permeability (immature blood-brain barrier or damage to the blood-brain barrier) for some medications.[131–137] However, respiratory depression, measured by CO_2 response curves or arterial oxygen tension, is similar from 2 to 570 days after birth at the same blood concentration of morphine.[138] Altered pharmacokinetics may contribute to the increased sensitivity to morphine in neonates. A reduced clearance and volume of distribution in neonates increase the plasma concentrations in this age group compared with older children given similar weight-scaled doses,[139,140] and this greater concentration contributes more to respiratory depression than the increased brain permeability in those who were not premature.

Absorption

Anesthetic drugs are mainly administered through the intravenous and inhalational routes, although premedication and postoperative analgesics are commonly administered enterally. Drug absorption after oral administration is slower in neonates than in children because of delayed gastric emptying (Fig. 5.11).

ENTERAL

Enteral absorption rates equal to those in adults may not be reached until 6 to 8 months after birth.[141,142] Congenital malformations (e.g., duodenal atresia), coadministration of drugs (e.g., opioids), and disease characteristics (e.g., necrotizing enterocolitis) may further affect the variability in enteral absorption. Delayed gastric emptying and reduced clearance may dictate reduced doses and frequency of repeated drug administration. For example, a mean steady-state target acetaminophen concentration greater than 10 mg/L at trough can be achieved by an oral dose of 25 mg/kg per day in preterm neonates at 30 weeks, 45 mg/kg per day at 34 weeks, and 60 mg/kg per day at 40 weeks postmenstrual age.[143] Because gastric emptying is slow in preterm neonates, dosing may only be required twice a day.[143]

The effects of bowel maturation on drug absorption are not yet fully understood. Gastric pH is high (~7.0) in neonates after delivery (from ingestion of amniotic fluid *in utero*) but decreases steadily to a fasting value of ~pH 3.5 within a week.[144] Bile salt and bile acid concentrations are reduced in the intestinal lumen at birth, enterohepatic bile circulation and transporter-mediated uptake is not fully functional. Intestinal enzymes are responsible for some metabolism of orally ingested drugs. Premature infants have a low first-pass effect by intestinal and hepatic metabolism by CYP3A, which increases the bioavailability of parenteral midazolam.[145]

Rectal absorption of some drugs (e.g., thiopental, diazepam) is more rapid in neonates than adults. However, the between-individual variability in absorption half time and relative bioavailability (F) after rectal administration may be more extensive compared with oral administration, making rectal administration less suitable for repeated administration.[146] The frequent passage of stools in the neonate may render the use of suppositories ineffective. Variable absorption and bioavailability has resulted in respiratory arrest when repeat opioids are administered by the rectal route to children.[147]

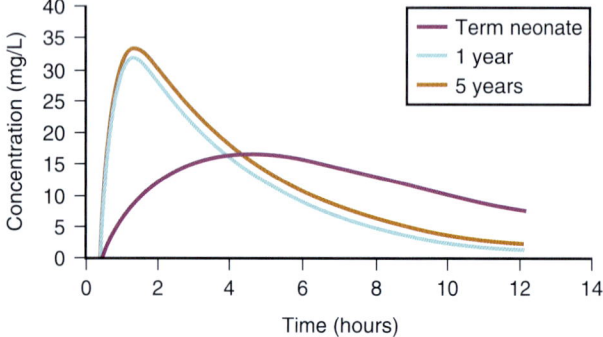

FIGURE 5.11 Simulated mean predicted time-concentration profiles for a term neonate, a 1-year-old infant, and a 5-year-old child given paracetamol elixir. The time to peak concentration is delayed in neonates because of slow gastric emptying and reduced clearance. (Reproduced with permission from Anderson BJ, van Lingen RA, Hansen TG, Lin YC, Holford NH. Acetaminophen developmental pharmacokinetics in premature neonates and infants: a pooled population analysis. *Anesthesiology.* 2002;96(6):1336-1345.)

CUTANEOUS

The larger relative skin surface area, increased cutaneous perfusion, and thinner stratum corneum in neonates increase systemic exposure of topical drugs (e.g., corticosteroids, local anesthetic creams, antiseptics). Neonates have a greater tendency to form methemoglobin because of reduced methemoglobin reductase activity compared with older children. Furthermore, fetal hemoglobin is more readily oxidized by drugs such as prilocaine compared with adult hemoglobin. Combined with an increased transcutaneous absorption, these have resulted in toxicity following repeat or large surface area application of topical local anesthetics, such as EMLA (eutectic mixture of local anesthetics [lidocaine-prilocaine]) cream, in this age group.[148,149] Similarly, cutaneous application of iodine antiseptics in neonates may result in transient hypothyroidism.[150]

INTRAMUSCULAR

The intramuscular (IM) route is frowned upon in children. Although bioavailability is high and approaches unity for most drugs, absorption is delayed compared with the intravenous route. Ketamine, however, remains popular as a premedication, with peak plasma concentrations reached within 10 minutes after 4 mg/kg (IM).[151]

NASAL

Exploration of alternative delivery routes in young children has centered on the nasal passages.[152,153] There remain concerns that intranasal drugs may pass through the posterior nasopharynx or irritate the vocal cords.[154] There is a postulated connection along perivascular and neutral structures from the nasal mucosa directly through the cribriform plate into the CNS bypassing the blood-brain barrier (E-Fig. 2.1).[153] It has been suggested that drugs administered by this route be preservative-free and free of neurotoxicity based on animal evidence,[155] although the risk is low and would depend on the preservative used. The probability of transport to CSF via this route is very small.[153,156–160] A meta-analysis of opioid overdose reported that nasal administration of naloxone is as effective as intravenous administration and this route is now standard practice for first responders caring for patients who overdosed on opioids.[161]

Nasal diamorphine 0.1 mg/kg, used in the United Kingdom for forearm fracture pain in the emergency room, is rapidly absorbed as a nasal spray in 0.2 mL of sterile water, with peak morphine plasma concentrations (Tpeak) occurring at 10 minutes.[162] Nasal S-ketamine (2 mg/kg) results in peak plasma concentrations of 355 ng/mL within 18 minutes.[163] Concentrated nasal fentanyl (150 µg/mL) 1.5 µg/kg given to children (3–17 years of age) for fracture pain resulted in good analgesia; peak concentrations occurred at 13 minutes.[164,165]

Advances in aerosol delivery devices have improved dosing accuracy. Administration of ketorolac 15 mg [weight 30–50 kg] or 30 mg [weight >50 kg]) to adolescents by the intranasal route had reduced relative bioavailability, but resulted in a rapid increase in plasma concentration (time to peak concentration was 52 ± 6 minutes) and may be a useful therapeutic alternative to intravenous injection. A target concentration of 0.37 mg/L in the effect compartment was achieved within 30 minutes and remained above that target for 10 hours.[166] The nasal passages change with age and sex, with adult dimensions achieved by 16 years. Nasal dimensions in males are greater than those in females. It would not be surprising if drug absorption by the nasal route also changes with age. Drug combinations may show benefits over single-drug therapy. Formulations containing two drugs may improve analgesia by additivity while decreasing adverse effects.[167]

Buccal and sublingual administration, like the nasal route, offer ease of administration, rapid systemic absorption, and avoidance of hepatic first-pass metabolism.[168] Midazolam administered by the buccal surface is now more popular than rectal administration for the acute management of seizures.[169]

Bioavailability

The oral bioavailability of a drug may be affected by (1) interactions with food when feeding is frequent in the neonate (e.g., phenytoin[170]), (2) use of adult formulations that are divided or altered for pediatric use (nizatidine[171]), and (3) lower cytochrome P450 enzyme activity in the intestine. The last factor may cause an increased bioavailability of midazolam because CYP3A activity is reduced.[172] Drug calculation errors are common[173] and the use of drug vials designed for adults may result in dose inaccuracy when proportioned for infants and children, causing a relative increase or decrease in assumed bioavailability.[174]

Dose accuracy is lost when buccal and sublingual administration is attempted because those routes require prolonged exposure to the mucosal surface. Infants find it difficult to hold the drug in their mouth for the requisite retention time (particularly if taste is unfavorable) and this results in more swallowed drug or drug spat out than in adults.[175] If the drug has an extensive first-pass effect, then the reduced relative bioavailability results in reduced plasma concentrations. Although many analgesics are available in an oral liquid formulation, taste is a strong determinant of compliance and unpalatable preparations may be refused.[176] Taste preferences change with age.

First-pass effect impacts bioavailability and contribution of active metabolites to effect. The oral bioavailability of clonidine is poor (F = 0.55) in children 3 to 10 years of age. Consequently, larger oral doses of clonidine (per kilogram) are required when this formulation is used to achieve concentrations similar to those reported in adults.[177] Oral absorption is slow (absorption half-time 0.45 hours), and peak concentrations are not reached until 1 hour. Dexmedetomidine also has slow absorption (absorption half-time 1 hour) and low bioavailability (F_{NASAL} 0.41).[178] Similarly, oral ketamine needs to be given in doses of up to 10 mg/kg to achieve therapeutic effect in children 1 to 8 years of age who have suffered burns.[179] Not only is bioavailability reduced (F = 0.45) but absorption is also slow; absorption half-time was 59 minutes, and between-subject variability in this cohort is substantive.[179] Analgesic effect, however, may be supplemented by the increased concentration of the active metabolite norketamine.

Metabolism and Excretion

The main routes by which drugs and their metabolites leave the body are the hepatobiliary system, the kidney, and the lung. Microsomal enzyme activity can be classified into three groups[180]:

1. Mature at birth but decreasing with age (e.g., CYP3A7 responsible for methadone clearance in neonates)
2. Mature at birth and sustained through to adulthood (e.g., plasma esterases that clear remifentanil)
3. Immature at birth

The last group accounts for the majority of enzymatic activity; the concentrations, and activities of many microsomal enzymes are reduced or absent in the neonate.

HEPATIC METABOLISM

The liver is the main organ in drug metabolism. Two types of drug biotransformation can occur: phase I and phase II reactions. Phase I reactions transform the drug via oxidation, reduction, or hydrolysis. Phase II reactions transform the drug via conjugation reactions, such as glucuronidation, sulfation, and acetylation, into more polar forms.[181,182] Hepatic drug metabolism activity appears as early as 9 to 22 weeks gestation, when the activity of the fetal liver enzymes varies from 2% to 36% of adult activity.[183] These enzyme activities are responsible for drug clearance in the neonate. However, clearance depends on enzyme activity, organ blood flow, and organ size and they change independently with age.

The ability to metabolize and conjugate medications improves considerably with age as a result of both increased enzyme activity and increased delivery of drug to the liver. Other factors influence the rate of hepatic maturation and metabolism (e.g., sepsis and malnutrition may slow maturation, whereas previous exposure to anticonvulsants, such as phenytoin or phenobarbital, may hasten maturation).[184–186] The opening or closing of a patent ductus may have profound effects on drug delivery to metabolizing organs in preterm infants.[187,188]

Half-life is often used to describe maturation. In general, the half-lives of medications that are eliminated by the liver are prolonged in neonates, decreased in children 4 to 10 years of age, and reach adult values in adolescents, mirroring clearance changes with age (Fig 5.5; E-Fig. 5.3). Half-life is determined by the clearance and volume of distribution (Vd); both change independently with age.

$$T_{1/2} = \ln(2) \cdot \frac{Vd}{CL} \qquad \text{Eq. 5.26}$$

Consequently, clearance is a better parameter to gauge maturation. Some medications are extensively metabolized by the liver and are referred to as having large extraction ratios. This extensive metabolism produces a "first-pass" effect in which a large proportion of an enteral dose is inactivated as it passes through the organ before reaching the systemic circulation (e.g., propranolol, morphine, and midazolam). Clearance of these drugs is commonly termed "perfusion limited." In contrast, drugs with poor intrinsic clearance (diazepam, phenytoin, acetylsalicylic acid [aspirin]) are termed "capacity limited."

Metabolism via cytochrome P-450 in the intestinal wall may also occur during drug absorption.[189–191] Competition between drugs for these intestinal wall enzymes may increase the bioavailability of one drug over another. The relative bioavailability of phenylephrine was increased when coadministered with acetaminophen owing to competition for gut wall sulfate conjugation.[192,193] Certain foods (e.g., grapefruit juice) may also induce or inhibit intestinal cytochromes, resulting in food-drug interactions.[194] The concentrations of these enzymes in neonates are less than in older children. These enzymes may also be affected by diseases such as cystic fibrosis or celiac disease.[195,196]

PHASE I REACTIONS: CYTOCHROME P-450

Phase I hepatic metabolism converts drugs into inactive, partially active, or active metabolites, often involving the cytochrome P-450 (CYP) enzyme system.[197] Multiple isoforms of the CYP enzyme system exist with different substrate specificities for different drugs. Induction and inhibition of these enzymes by different drugs and chemicals requires a thorough understanding of both the nomenclature of the CYP system, as well as the specific isoforms responsible for metabolism of the drugs used in pediatric anesthesia. There are both genetic and ethnic polymorphisms that may lead to clinically important differences in the capacity to metabolize drugs (e.g., the conversion of codeine to the active metabolite morphine)[198–200]; these differences can make individual drug responses in some cases unpredictable.[201–203] Epigenetics is an area of research that examines variable but heritable differences in gene expression without modifications to the DNA sequence. This subject is discussed further in Chapter 4.

The generally accepted nomenclature of the cytochrome P-450 isozymes begins with CYP, and group enzymes with more than 36% DNA homology subgrouped into families designated with an Arabic number, followed by letters for the subfamily of closely related proteins (>77% homology), followed by a number for the specific enzyme gene, such as CYP3A4.[204,205] Isozymes that are important in human drug metabolism are found in the *CYP1, CYP2,* and *CYP3* gene families. Table 5.1 outlines the CYP isozymes and their common substrates.

For many drugs, the reduced metabolism in neonates relates to reduced total quantities of CYP enzymes in the hepatic microsomes.[206] Although the concentrations of CYP enzymes increase with gestational age, they may contribute only 30% of adult clearance at term. Most isozymes are immature in the neonate, but some CYP isozymes exhibit near-adult activity, whereas others produce unique metabolic pathways in the neonatal period that invalidate broad generalizations about neonatal drug metabolism

(see Table 5.1). Developmental changes of specific cytochromes are discussed in Chapter 4.

PHASE II REACTIONS

The other major route of drug metabolism, designated phase II reactions, involves synthetic or conjugation reactions that increase the hydrophilicity of molecules to facilitate renal elimination.[181,182] The phase II enzymes include glucuronosyltransferase, sulfotransferase, *N*-acetyltransferase, glutathione *S*-transferase, and methyltransferase. The phase II enzymes also show developmental changes during infancy that influence drug clearance (Table 5.2).[207–209]

Most conjugation reactions have limited activity during fetal development.[210] One of the most familiar synthetic reactions in young

TABLE 5.1	Developmental Patterns and Activities for Important Cytochrome P-450 Enzymes (Phase I Reactions) in the Neonate			
Enzymes	Selected Substrates	Inducers	Inhibitors	Developmental Changes
CYP1A2	Acetaminophen, caffeine, theophylline, warfarin	Cigarette smoke, charcoal-broiled meat, omeprazole, cruciferous vegetables	α-Naphthoflavone	Not present to an appreciable extent in human fetal liver. Adult levels reached by 4 months of age and may be exceeded in children 1–2 years of age. Inhibited by phenobarbital and phenytoin.
CYP2A6	Warfarin, nicotine	Barbiturates	Tranylcypromine	
CYP2C9	Diclofenac, phenytoin, torsemide, *S*-warfarin tolbutamide	Rifampin	Sulfaphenazole, sulfinpyrazone	Not apparent in fetal liver. Inferential data using phenytoin disposition as a nonspecific pharmacologic probe suggests low activity during the first week of life, with adult activity reached by 6 months of age and peak activity reached by 3–4 years of age. Metabolism induced by rifampin and phenobarbital and inhibited by cimetidine.
CYP2C19	Phenytoin, diazepam, omeprazole, propranolol	Rifampin	Tranylcypromine	
CYP2D6	Amitriptyline, captopril, codeine, dextromethorphan, fluoxetine, hydrocodone, ondansetron, propafenone, propranolol, timolol	None known	Fluoxetine, quinidine	Low to absent in fetal liver but uniformly present at 1 week of postnatal age. Poor activity (approximately 20% of adult values) at 1 month of postnatal age. Adult competence reached by 3–5 years of age. Metabolism inhibited by cimetidine.
CYP3A4	Acetaminophen, alfentanil, amiodarone, budesonide, carbamazepine, diazepam, erythromycin, lidocaine, midazolam, nifedipine, omeprazole, cisapride, theophylline, verapamil, *R*-warfarin	Carbamazepine, dexamethasone, phenobarbital, phenytoin, rifampin	Azole antifungals, ethinyl estradiol, naringenin, troleandomycin, erythromycin	CYP3A4 has low activity in the first month of life, which approaches adult levels by 6–12 months postnatally.
CYP3A7	Dehydroepiandrosterone, ethinyl estradiol, various dihydropyrimidines	Carbamazepine, rifampin, phenytoin, dexamethasone, phenobarbital	Azole antifungals, erythromycin, cimetidine	CYP3A7 is functionally active in the fetus; approximately 30%–75% of adult levels of CYP3A4.

Adapted from Leeder JS, Kearns GL. Pharmacogenetics in pediatrics: implications for practice. *Pediatr Clin North Am.* 1997;44(1):55-77.

TABLE 5.2	Developmental Patterns for Important Conjugation (Phase II) Reactions in the Neonate	
Enzymes	Selected Substrates	Developmental Patterns
Uridine diphosphoglucuronyltransferase (UDP-GT)	Chloramphenicol, morphine, acetaminophen, valproic acid, lorazepam	Ontogeny is isoform specific. In general, adult activity is achieved by 6–18 months of age. May be induced by cigarette smoke and phenobarbital.
Sulfotransferase	Bile acids, acetaminophen, cholesterol, polyethylene, glycols, dopamine, chloramphenicol	Ontogeny seems to be more rapid than UDP-GT; however, it is substrate specific. Activity for some isoforms may exceed adult values during infancy and childhood (e.g., that responsible for acetaminophen metabolism).
N-Acetyltransferase 2	Hydralazine, procainamide, clonazepam, caffeine, sulfamethoxazole	Some fetal activity present by 16 weeks. Virtually 100% of infants between birth and 2 months of age exhibit the slow metabolizer phenotype. Adult activity present by 1–3 years of age.

Adapted from Leeder JS, Kearns GL. Pharmacogenetics in pediatrics: implications for practice. *Pediatr Clin North Am.* 1997;44(1):55-77.

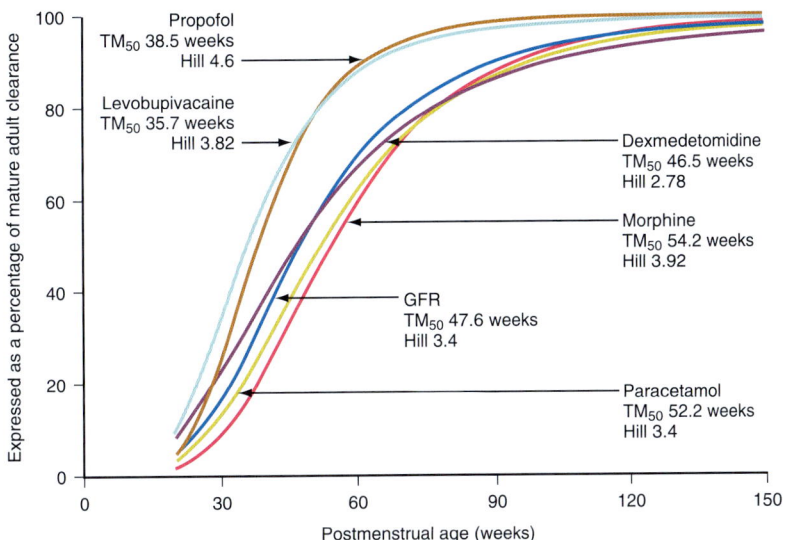

FIGURE 5.12 Clearance maturation, expressed as a percentage of mature clearance, of drugs where glucuronide conjugation (paracetamol, morphine, dexmedetomidine) plays a major role. These profiles are closely aligned with glomerular filtration rate *(GFR)*. In contrast, cytochrome P-450 isoenzymes also contribute to propofol and levobupivacaine metabolism and cause a faster maturation profile than expected from glucuronide conjugation alone. *Hill*, Hill coefficient; TM_{50}, maturation half-time. (Maturation parameter estimates from Anderson BJ, Holford NH. Mechanistic basis of using body size and maturation to predict clearance in humans. *Drug Metab Pharmacokinet.* 2009;24(1):25-36; Anand KJ, Anderson BJ, Holford NH, et al. Morphine pharmacokinetics and pharmacodynamics in preterm and term neonates: secondary results from the NEOPAIN trial. *Br J Anaesth.* 2008;101(5):680-689; Potts AL, Warman GR, Anderson BJ. Dexmedetomidine disposition in children: a population analysis. *Paediatr Anaesth.* 2008;18(8):722-730; Allegaert K, Hoon JD, Verbesselt R, Naulaers G, Murat I. Maturational pharmacokinetics of single intravenous bolus of propofol. *Paediatr Anaesth.* 2007;17(11):1028-1034; Chalkiadis GA, Anderson BJ. Age and size are the major covariates for prediction of levobupivacaine clearance in children. *Paediatr Anaesth.* 2006;16(3):275-282; Rhodin MM, Anderson BJ, Peters AM, et al. Human renal function maturation: a quantitative description using weight and postmenstrual age. *Pediatr Nephrol.* 2009;24(1):67-76; Anderson BJ, Holford NH. Tips and traps analyzing pediatric PK data. *Paediatr Anaesth.* 2011;21(3):222-237.)

infants involves conjugation by uridine diphosphoglucuronosyltransferases (UGTs). This enzyme system includes numerous isoforms and is also responsible for glucuronidation of endogenous compounds, such as bilirubin (by UGT1A1).[210] As with the maturation of bilirubin conjugation, UGT activity is limited at birth and the different isoforms mature at different rates postnatally.[211] Drugs that are conjugated by UGT for clearance often require dose adjustments to avoid toxicity in neonates. Experience with chloramphenicol in the 1960s illustrated this lesson when neonates received standard pediatric doses of chloramphenicol without understanding that UGT, which is critical to eliminate chloramphenicol, is immature in neonates. Infants accumulated large concentrations of chloramphenicol and developed abdominal distension, cyanosis, and fatal circulatory collapse, a condition known as the gray baby syndrome.[212-214] Although the clearance of chloramphenicol is poor during the neonatal period, by adjusting and monitoring the dose, preterm and term infants can be safely treated with chloramphenicol.[215]

Morphine, acetaminophen, dexmedetomidine, and lorazepam also undergo glucuronidation. The major steps in the metabolic disposition of morphine in children and adults is glucuronidation in the 3- and 6-position.[216,217] Morphine clearance,[218,219] in particular 3- and 6-glucuronide formation, is limited at birth and increases with weight,[220] postmenstrual age,[197] and postnatal age (to a minor extent).[27,217,221] The maturation of glucuronosyltransferase enzymes varies among isoforms but, in general, adult activity is reached by 6 to 18 months of age.[205,221] The time courses of maturation of drug metabolism for morphine,[26] acetaminophen,[222] dexmedetomidine,[223] and glomerular filtration rate[34] are strikingly similar (Fig. 5.12) with 50% of size-adjusted adult values reached between 8 and 12 weeks postnatally. All three drugs are cleared predominantly by UGT, which converts the parent compound into a water-soluble metabolite that is excreted by the kidneys; the clearance maturation profiles of these drugs are similar to the glomerular filtration rate maturation. Glucuronidation is also the major metabolic pathway of propofol metabolism, although multiple CYP isoenzymes, including CYP2B6, CYP2C9, and CYP2A6, contribute to its metabolism and cause a faster maturation profile than expected from glucuronide conjugation alone.[224] A phase I reaction (CYP3A4) is the major enzyme system for oxidation of levobupivacaine, and clearance through this pathway is faster than those associated with UGT maturation.[26,34,222,225-228]

In contrast to glucuronosyltransferase, the sulfotransferase enzyme system is well developed in the neonate, and for some compounds it may compensate for limited glucuronidation. In adults, the primary pathway for acetaminophen metabolism is glucuronidation, yet its half-life is only moderately prolonged in neonates compared with older infants and adults.[229-231] This is explained in part by the increased volume of distribution in neonates (Eq. 5.20) and because the neonate forms more sulfate than glucuronide conjugate, leading to a greater percent of the dose excreted as the acetaminophen-sulfate conjugate.[143,230-233] Unfortunately, this does not confer safety from hepatotoxicity. The toxic metabolite is created through the oxidative pathway mediated by CYP2E1.

ALTERATIONS IN BIOTRANSFORMATION

Transition from the intrauterine to the extrauterine environment is associated with major changes in blood flow. There may also be an environmental trigger for the expression of some metabolic enzyme activities, resulting in a slight increase in maturation rate above that predicted by postmenstrual age (E-Fig. 5.4).[224,227] Many biotransformation reactions, especially those involving certain forms of CYP, are inducible before birth through maternal exposure to drugs, cigarette smoke, or other inducing agents. Postnatally, biotransformation reactions may be induced through drug exposure (see Tables 5.1 and 5.2) and may be slowed by hypoxia, asphyxia, organ damage, and/or illness. The reduced thiopental clearance estimated from data when the drug was given to control seizures in neonates that resulted from hypoxic-ischemic insults may not be applicable to healthy neonates undergoing anesthesia.[234,235]

EXTRAHEPATIC ROUTES OF METABOLIC CLEARANCE

Many drugs undergo metabolic clearance at extrahepatic sites. Remifentanil and atracurium are degraded by nonspecific esterases in tissues and erythrocytes. Clearance, expressed per kilogram, is increased in younger children,[22,236–239] likely attributable to size, because clearance is similar when scaled to a 70-kilogram person using allometry.[22] Nonspecific blood esterases that metabolize remifentanil are mature at birth.[23]

Ester local anesthetics are metabolized by plasma butyrylcholinesterase, which is reduced in neonates. The in vitro plasma half-life of 2-chloroprocaine in umbilical cord blood is twice that in maternal blood,[240] but there are no in vivo studies of the effects of age on its metabolism. Succinylcholine clearance is increased in neonates when expressed on a weight basis, suggesting butyrylcholinesterase activity is mature at birth.[241,242]

RENAL EXCRETION

Renal function in preterm and term infants is less efficient than in adults, even after adjusting for the differences in body weight. This reduced efficiency is related to a combination of incomplete glomerular development, low perfusion pressure, and inadequate osmotic load to produce full countercurrent effects.[243–248] However, glomerular filtration and tubular function both develop rapidly during the first few postnatal months (see E-Fig. 5.4),[34] nearly mature by 20 weeks of age, and fully mature by 2 years of age (Figs. 5.12 and 5.13).[244–248] For these reasons, *drugs that are excreted primarily through glomerular filtration or tubular secretion, such as aminoglycoside and cephalosporin antibiotics, have a prolonged elimination half-life in neonates* (E-Fig. 5.5).[249–251] In cases where both the drug and its active metabolite (e.g., morphine and morphine 6 glucuronide) are renally cleared, repeat doses in the neonate should be adjusted to account for the impaired renal function. In the presence of renal failure, drugs that are excreted via the kidneys

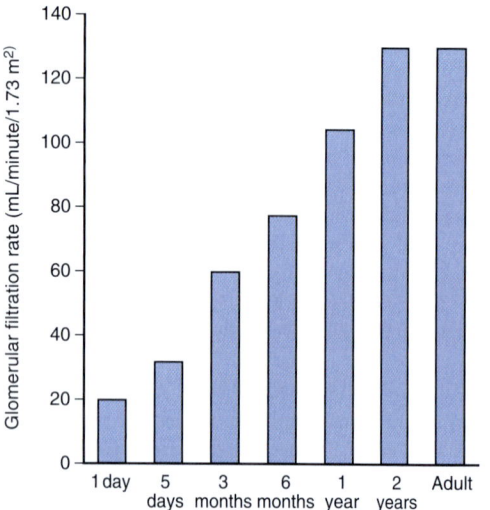

FIGURE 5.13 Changes in glomerular filtration rate versus age. Note the rapid development of glomerular function during the first year of life. Abnormal or immature renal function may delay drug excretion. (Data from Chantler C. *Clinical Pediatric Nephrology.* Philadelphia: JB Lippincott; 1976.)

often achieve and maintain prolonged therapeutic drug concentrations if there is no alternate pathway of excretion.

The pharmacokinetics and pharmacodynamics of the old muscle relaxant, curare, exemplify the complex interaction of increased volume of distribution, smaller muscle mass, and decreased rate of excretion as a result of immaturity of glomerular filtration. The initial dose (per kilogram) of curare needed to achieve neuromuscular blockade is similar in infants and adults.[83] In infants, however, this blockade is achieved at reduced serum concentrations compared with those in older children and adults, corresponding to differences in muscle mass and receptor immaturity. A larger volume of distribution (total body water) accounts for the equivalent dose for each kilogram of body weight, and the reduced glomerular function in infants compared with older children or adults accounts in part for the longer duration of action.[83] As in the case of drugs excreted by the liver, there is a triphasic developmental response to drugs excreted by the kidneys when expressed as per kilogram (see Fig. 5.5): a prolonged half-life in neonates (immature renal function), a shortened half-life in young children, and a greater elimination half-life in adolescents and adults (size-related).

Pharmacodynamics in Children

Children's responses to drugs have much in common with the responses in adults.[252] The perception that drug effects differ in children may be attributed to the patchy study of drugs in pediatric populations who have size- and maturation-related effects, as well as different diseases. Neonates and infants, however, often have altered pharmacodynamics. For example, the increased sensitivity of the neonate to morphine compared with children may be attributed, in part, to altered pharmacokinetics (reduced clearance, smaller volume of distribution), but it may also reflect the developmental regulation of opioid receptors.[253]

The MAC for most inhalational anesthetics is less in neonates than in infants, which in turn is greater than that observed in children and adults.[254] The MAC of isoflurane in preterm neonates less than 32 weeks gestation is 1.28%, and that in neonates 32 to 37 weeks gestation is 1.41%.[255] This value increases to 1.87% by 6 months of age before decreasing again throughout childhood.[255] The cause of these age-related differences is uncertain and may relate to maturational changes in cerebral blood flow, γ-aminobutyric acid (GABA) class A receptor numbers, or developmental shifts in the regulation of chloride transporters.[256–258]

Neonates have an increased sensitivity to the effects of neuromuscular blocking drugs.[83] The reason for this is unknown, but it is consistent with the observation that there is a 3-fold reduction in the release of acetylcholine from the infant rat phrenic nerve as well as a relatively reduced muscle mass.[259–262] The increased volume of distribution, however, means that a single neuromuscular blocking drug dose (calculated as milligrams per kilogram) in the neonate blocks the neuromuscular junction at a reduced plasma concentration while the decreased clearance prolongs the duration of effect.

Both the coagulation[263,264] and the fibrinolytic systems[265–268] are immature at birth. Consequently, the target plasma concentration of antifibrinolytic drugs required to achieve similar effects in neonates is less than that in adults. Although the concentration of ε-aminocaproic acid (EACA) required to inhibit fibrinolysis in adult plasma in vitro is 130 mg/L, the concentration required in neonatal plasma is much smaller, 50 mg/L.[269,270] The dose of EACA must be adjusted in neonates because of both the immaturity of their antifibrinolytic clearance pathways and the coagulation cascade.

Cardiac calcium stores in the endoplasmic reticulum are reduced in the immature neonatal heart. Exogenous calcium has greater impact on contractility in this age group than in older children and adults. Conversely, neonates may suffer cardiac arrest if given the calcium antagonist, verapamil, potent inhalation agents that have calcium channel blocking properties, e.g. halothane,[271,272] or a rapid infusion of citrated blood products such as fresh frozen plasma.[273,274] Immaturity of myocardial potassium channels prolongs the QT interval in neonates; neonates exhibit a greater sensitivity toward QTc (corrected QT) interval prolongation compared with older children. This makes them more sensitive to sotalol given for supraventricular tachycardia (SVT).[275]

Larger doses of local anesthetics are required for spinal anesthesia in neonates. In the case of amide local anesthetics in neonates and infants, the duration of spinal blocks is shorter and the weight-scaled dose is larger to achieve the same dermatomal level of block compared with blocks in older children and adults. This may be attributed, in part, to myelination, spacing of the nodes of Ranvier, the length of nerve exposed, increased relative volume of CSF (E-Fig. 40.4), as well as other size factors.

There is an age-dependent expression of intestinal motilin receptors and the modulation of gastric antral contractions in neonates. Prokinetic agents may not be useful in very preterm infants, partially useful in older preterm infants, and useful in full-term infants. Similarly, bronchodilators in infants are less effective because of the paucity of bronchial smooth muscle that can cause bronchospasm.

Drug effects in neonates may not be evident until later in life. Neonates and young children may suffer permanent effects resulting from a stimulus applied at a sensitive point in development. Examples include untreated congenital hypothyroidism causing lifelong phenotypic changes and increased risk for vaginal carcinoma in children of mothers who were treated with stilboestrol during pregnancy.[276] Corticosteroids are associated with growth restriction in children with asthma.[277] There are concerns that neonatal animal exposure to a multitude of commonly used anesthetic agents may cause widespread neuronal apoptosis and long-term memory deficits although these effects in humans have not been confirmed (see Chapter 23).

MEASUREMENT OF PHARMACODYNAMIC ENDPOINTS

Outcome measures are more difficult to assess in neonates and infants than in children or adults. Measurement techniques, disease and pathology differences, heterogeneous groups, recruitment issues, ethical considerations, inability to communicate with the neonate (e.g., pain level) and endpoint definitions for establishing efficacy and safety often confuse interpretation of the measures, resulting in the use of surrogates.[278]

Common effects measured in infancy include anesthesia depth, pain responses, depth of sedation, and intensity of neuromuscular blockade. A common effect measure used to assess depth of anesthesia is the EEG or a modification of detected EEG signals (spectral edge frequency, bispectral index [BIS], entropy). Physiologic studies in adults and children indicate that EEG-derived anesthesia depth monitors can provide an imprecise and drug-dependent measure of arousal. Although the outputs from these monitors do not closely represent any true physiologic entity, they can be used as trend guides for anesthesia, and in so doing, may improve outcomes in adults. In older children the physiology, anatomy, and clinical observations indicate the performance of the monitors may be similar to that in adults. In infants, however, their use cannot be supported in theory or in practice at this time.[279,280] During anesthesia, the EEG in infants is fundamentally different from the EEG in older children (see also Chapter 49)[281–285]; there remains a need for specific neonate-derived algorithms if EEG-derived anesthesia depth monitors are to be used in neonates.[286,287] Monitors that use

four simultaneous channels of frontal EEG waveforms, an enhanced patient state index (PSI), and a density spectral array (DSA) display may prove more helpful.[288]

The effectiveness of remifentanil when combined with propofol is also difficult to quantify using modified EEG signals. Current evidence in children confirmed that remifentanil has little effect on BIS in children. This monitor provides information mainly limited to cortical brain activity that reflects the hypnotic component of anesthesia. Although, during surgery antinociception may be required to maintain hypnosis, response to painful stimulation cannot be predicted by BIS because the analgesic component of anesthesia involves subcortical autonomic responses.[289]

Sedation scoring may also be useful though imprecise. For example the Children's Hospital of Wisconsin Sedation Scale has been used to investigate ketamine in the emergency department.[51,290] However, despite the use of such scales in procedural pain or sedation studies, few behavioral scales have been adequately validated in this setting and interobserver variability can be substantial.[291–293] Most scores are validated for the acute, procedural setting and are less robust for subacute or chronic pain or stress.

THE TARGET CONCENTRATION APPROACH

The goal of treatment is the target effect. A pharmacodynamic model is used to predict the target concentration given a target effect. Population estimates for the pharmacodynamic model parameters and covariate information are used to predict typical pharmacodynamic values in a specific patient. Population estimates of pharmacokinetic model parameter estimates and covariate information are then used to predict typical pharmacokinetic values in a typical patient. For example, a dexmedetomidine steady-state target concentration of 0.6 μg/L may be achieved with an infusion of 0.33 μg/kg per hour in a neonate, 0.51 μg/kg per hour in a 1-year-old, and 0.47 μg/kg per hour in an 8-year-old.[228] This target concentration strategy is a powerful tool for determining the clinical dose.[294] Monitoring the drug concentrations in serum and Bayesian forecasting may be used to further improve the dose in individual patients.

This target effect approach is intrinsic to pediatric anesthesiologists using target-controlled infusion systems (see also Chapter 6). These devices target a specific plasma or effect-site concentration in a typical individual and this concentration is assumed to have a typical target effect. The target concentration is one that achieves a target therapeutic effect (e.g., anesthesia) without excessive adverse effects (e.g., hypotension). These devices are in use in Europe but are not approved by the Food and Drug Administration (FDA) for use in the United States.

DEFINING TARGET CONCENTRATION

An effect-site target concentration has been estimated for many drugs used in anesthesia, analgesia, and sedation. For example, a propofol target brain concentration of 3 mg/L (or 3 μg/mL) in a typical patient can be achieved using preprogrammed target-controlled infusion devices. In teenagers, a BIS monitor can provide feedback to guide the infusion rate to achieve a desired target effect in the particular individual. The luxury of such a feedback system is not available for most drugs and unfortunately may be of little value in neonates and infants where neither the target concentration is known nor the EEG monitoring adequate.[295]

A target concentration of 10 μg/L may be used for morphine analgesia. After cardiac surgery in children, steady-state serum concentrations greater than 20 μg/L resulted in hypercarbia (PaCO$_2$ [partial pressure of carbon dioxide in arterial blood] >55 mm Hg) and flattened CO$_2$ response curves. During wash-out, morphine concentrations in excess of 15 μg/L caused hypercarbia in 46% of children, whereas concentrations less than 15 μg/L caused hypercarbia in only 13%. No age-related differences in the respiratory effect occurred at the same serum concentration of morphine.[138] Observation or self-reporting pain scales are used as part of the feedback loop for dose incremental changes.

The target concentration may vary depending on the desired target effect. The target concentration for ketamine analgesia (0.25 mg/L) differs substantially from that of anesthesia (2 mg/L), and BIS monitoring has proved completely ineffective because ketamine causes central excitation, thus increasing rather than decreasing the BIS monitoring values.[296–299]

Drug Interactions

There are many common examples of drug interactions that increase or decrease responses mediated through either pharmacokinetic or pharmacodynamic routes. Phenobarbital induction of CYP3A4 metabolism and consequent increased ketamine requirements for radiologic sedation[185] is an example of a pharmacokinetic interaction.

Drug enzyme inhibition is another example of an important pharmacokinetic interaction. The protease inhibitor, ritonavir, is a strong inhibitor of CYP 3A. The drug is used for management of the human immunovirus and is currently part of an oral antiviral drug combination (nirmatrelvir-ritonavir) for the early treatment of SARS-CoV-2 (COVID-19) positive patients aged 12 years and over who have recognized comorbidities. The CYP3A enzyme system is responsible for clearance of numerous drugs used in anesthesia (e.g., alfentanil, fentanyl, methadone, rocuronium, bupivacaine, midazolam, ketamine). Ritonavir will have an impact on drug clearances that are dependent on ritonavir concentration, anesthesia drug intrinsic hepatic clearance, metabolic pathways, concentration-response relationship and route of administration. Drugs with a steep concentration-response relationship (ketamine, midazolam, rocuronium) are mostly affected because small changes in concentration have major changes in effect response. An increase in midazolam concentration is observed after oral administration because CYP3A in the gastrointestinal wall is inhibited, causing a large increase in relative bioavailability.[300]

Pharmacokinetic interactions are often dealt with in mixed-effects modeling by including the effect of a second drug as a covariate on affected pharmacokinetic parameters such as those describing clearance, volume of distribution, or bioavailability (F). The midazolam-propofol pharmacokinetic interaction has been investigated by adjusting midazolam clearance and V using propofol plasma concentrations included in an exponential covariate model, that is:

$$CL_{IND} = CL_{POP} * exp^{(COV(C_{PROP} - Median\ C_{PROP}))},$$ Eq. 5.27

where CL is clearance from the central compartment, for the population (CL_POP) and the individual (CL_IND). Here, the effect of plasma propofol concentration (C_{PROP}) on the clearance parameter is estimated (the parameter "cov") and scaled to the population median C_{PROP}.

Interactions may also occur at entry into the effect site, for example, an increase in the equilibrium constant half-life ($T_{1/2}$keo) of *d*-tubocurarine with increasing inspired concentrations of halothane has been reported.[301] Halothane is a negative inotrope[302] and reduces skeletal muscle blood flow,[303] so it is reasonable to interpret changes in $T_{1/2}$keo as a result of changes in organ blood flow.

Competitive antagonists reduce receptor availability by competing for occupancy at the same receptor site. Drugs that elicit an effect are called agonists, while those that do not are called antagonists, so the occupancy of some receptors by the antagonists

results in less effect. In general, competitive antagonists shift the effect-concentration curve to the right by altering the C_{50}. The Emax equation (Eq. 5.21) can then be expressed as:

$$Effect = E0 + \frac{E\max \cdot Ce^{N}}{\left(\left(EC_{50}^{N} \cdot \left[1 + \frac{A}{EA_{50}}\right]\right) + Ce^{N}\right)}$$ Eq. 5.28

where Ce is the concentration in the effect site, and A and EA_{50} represent ligand A concentration and potency. Noncompetitive antagonists shift the observed maximum effect (Emax) rather than the C_{50}:

$$Effect = E0 + \frac{E\max \cdot \left(1 - \frac{A}{A + EA_{50}}\right) \cdot Ce^{\gamma}}{Ce^{\gamma} + C_{50}^{\gamma}}$$ Eq. 5.29

Pharmacodynamic interactions are not restricted to same-site binding interactions; some proteins have multiple binding sites, and ligands binding at these sites can also alter the above relationship (i.e., through changes in protein conformation that lead to downstream changes or modulate agonist-receptor affinity). These are referred to as "allosteric" interactions.

Anesthetic drug interactions traditionally have been characterized using isobolographic analysis or multiple logistic regression. Minto[304] and Greco[305] proposed models based on response-surface methodology (see Chapter 6). Computer simulations based on interactions at the effect site predicted that the maximally synergistic three-drug combination (midazolam, propofol, and alfentanil) tripled the duration of effect compared with propofol alone. The response surface for ibuprofen and acetaminophen is shown in Fig 5.14; the addition of acetaminophen to ibuprofen improved analgesia when the dose of ibuprofen was less than 100 mg (5 mg/kg) in a 5-year-old child.[306] Response surfaces can describe anesthetic interactions, even those between agonists, partial agonists, competitive antagonists, and inverse agonists.[304,307]

Inhalation anesthetic agents can prolong the duration of block, and this effect is agent specific. When compared with halothane, sevoflurane potentiates the duration of block with vecuronium to a greater extent. When compared with balanced anesthesia, both

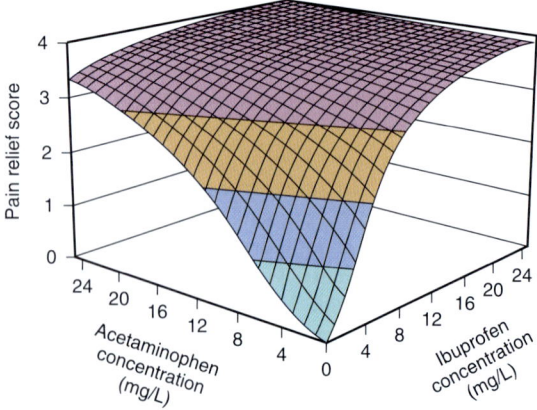

FIGURE 5.14 The response surface of analgesic effect for acetaminophen and ibuprofen. Concentrations are those in the effect compartment. The concentration response for acetaminophen is plotted on the *x-y* axis, while that for ibuprofen is on the *z-y* axis. The "surface" is that plotted between these axes. Each point on the surface is a measure of the pain relief provided by acetaminophen and ibuprofen combination. (From Hannam J, Anderson BJ. Explaining the acetaminophen-ibuprofen analgesic interaction using a response surface model. *Paediatr Anaesth.* 2011;21(12):1234-1240, with permission.)

sevoflurane and halothane decrease the dose requirements of vecuronium by 60% and 40%, respectively.[308]

Surface modeling techniques have been used to demonstrate strikingly synergistic effects from sevoflurane with alfentanil[309] and remifentanil with propofol[310,311] on respiration in adults.[309,310] It comes as no surprise that the use of three or more sedating medications is associated with significantly more adverse outcomes than the use of one or two medications.[310,312]

The Drug Approval Process, the Package Insert, and Drug Labeling

A great concern has been the general lack of regulatory approval of many of the medications for populations of pediatric patients. This is particularly ironic because most of the changes in US legislation pertaining to pharmaceuticals have been the result of adverse events in infants and children. The 1938 Federal Food, Drug, and Cosmetic Act[313] replaced the original Federal Food and Drugs Act of 1906 (Wiley Act)[314] because nearly 100 individuals, mostly children, were poisoned by diethylene glycol (an antifreeze analog for vehicles) that had been added to an elixir of sulfanilamide. This new legislation prohibited the addition of "poisonous substances" (unless they were demonstrated to be safe in small concentrations) and instituted other measures to protect the consumer. The next major piece of legislation was the Kefauver-Harris Amendments, which were passed in 1962 after the thalidomide catastrophe.[315] This legislation strengthened the safety standards by requiring the drug company to demonstrate effectiveness before marketing. The US FDA then allowed drugs to be marketed to adults as *"safe and effective,"* but now the drug label was required to indicate that *"safety and effectiveness had not been established in children"* because no trials in children had been carried out. This had an enormous negative impact on drug development for children and led Shirkey to coin the now common expression *"therapeutic orphans"* when referring to drug development for children.[316]

Until the late 1990s, nearly 80% of approved medications contained language within the drug label (package insert) that excluded children of varying ages; it should be noted that the legislation described later in the text has now resulted in some pediatric labeling in ~60% of marketed medications, which is an unequivocal victory for drug safety in children.[317] The majority of the drugs used in the operating room (OR) and the intensive care unit (ICU) today have similar language.[318] Common examples of disclaimers for drugs used in our daily practice include those for bupivacaine (*"Until further experience is gained in children younger than 12 years, administration of Sensorcaine [bupivacaine HCl] injection is not recommended"*)[319] and for fentanyl (*"The safety of SUBLIMAZE in children younger than two years of age has not been established"*).[320] Such disclaimers are placed in the package insert because the contents of the package insert must, by law, be based on *"adequate, well controlled studies involving children."*[315,321–323] Any use of a drug that is not specifically described in the package insert is considered *"unapproved"* or *"off label."* The reason for the lack of labeling for children is that the appropriate controlled clinical trials were never supported by industry and the FDA did not have the legislative power to require that the pharmaceutical companies perform studies in children.[324] In 1994, the FDA passed a new interpretation of the original Food, Drug, and Cosmetic Act[313,322,325] that allowed manufacturers to review the published medical literature and submit these data to the FDA to support revised pediatric labeling.[325] This led to additional changes in the drug label for 48 medications. Unfortunately, for drugs that were no longer under patent protection, there

was no financial incentive to force the issue, so many drugs remained unlabeled for children despite many publications that outlined their safe use in children of all ages.

During the early stages of the AIDS epidemic, there was great pressure placed on the FDA to reduce the time for the drug approval process. New legislation was passed to raise funds to pay for additional consultants and experts to help the FDA with this process (The Prescription Drug User Fee Act [PDUFA]).[326] This legislation was renewed in 1997, 2002, 2007, and 2012 and was redrafted for the sixth time (PDUFA VI) and signed into law in August 2017, thus providing "stable and consistent funding during fiscal years 2018–2022."[327,328] PDUFA VII, expected to cover 2023–27, has been the subject of many discussions with industry including premarketing, postmarketing, manufacturing and inspections, and multiple steering committees (https://www.fda.gov/industry/prescription-drug-user-fee-amendments/pdufa-vii-fiscal-years-2023-2027 [(accessed April 17, 2021]). The PDUFA regulations have three components: (1) an application fee when a new drug or biologic is submitted to the FDA, (2) an annual product fee for nongeneric marketed drugs, and (3) an annual fee for each manufacturing site for nongeneric drugs.[327] The goals of these legislative efforts are to further enhance scientific expertise and processes for regulatory decisions, improve patient perspectives in drug development, and provide longer stability of the PDUFA initiative. A report to Congress outlines the continued efforts achieved and supported, as well as planned commitments of PDUFA VI, is available at https://www.fda.gov/media/138325/download (accessed April 17, 2021). The monies from these fees greatly reduce the time from a new drug application (NDA) or biologic license application (BLA) to be marketed. The most recent iterations have expanded funding to support marketing safety and pharmacoepidemiology activities, as well as increased inspection of non–USA-based pharmaceutical manufacturing facilities. Approximately 72% of new drug applications or biologic license applications were approved on the first submission under PDUFA V compared with ~55% under PDUFA IV.[329,330] Approximately 94% of new drug applications or biologic license applications submitted in 2018 were approved on first submission and 100% approved in 2019 demonstrating the amazing efficacy of the PDUFA program in facilitating drug approvals with the majority occurring in 8 months or less.[331]

Additional changes at the FDA relating to pediatric medications occurred in the late 1990s when the Food and Drug Administration Modernization Act[332] and the Final Rule were passed.[333] Tacked onto this legislation was the Better Pharmaceutical Act for Children, which granted 6 months of patent extension in exchange for pediatric studies of drugs that were still patent protected. This was later replaced with the Best Pharmaceutical Act for Children (BPCA) in 2002, which earmarked money for the National Institutes of Health (NIH) to support study of drugs no longer patent protected.[334] This was subsequently challenged as giving excessive legal power to the FDA, but further legislation reinstituted the legal power to the FDA to now require drug companies to conduct research in children if the drug would have use in children (the Pediatric Research Equity Act).[335] In 2007, the Food and Drug Administration Amendments Act renewed PDUFA IV, the Medical Device User Fee and Modernization Act, and Best Pharmaceuticals for Children Act.[336] Of importance to researchers was the new requirement for registration of all clinical trials with an archive of thousands of trials that is easily searchable for clinicians as well as the public.[337] Many journals now will not publish clinical pharmaceutical trials that have not been registered. Since the first legislation for children passed in 1998, there has been an explosion of pediatric drug trials with thousands of drug trials (>1000 requested or carried out since 1997). Many new labels have been developed including 74 drugs, 2 vaccines, and 3 blood products between January 2019 and April 2020 (https://www.fda.gov/media/143552/download [accessed April 17, 2021]). Unfortunately, the money that was supposed to be earmarked to the NIH for generic drug trials was not fully provided, so deficiencies in labeling for older drugs persist.[338]

It is important for clinicians to appreciate that despite language on the label regarding use in children, physicians are perfectly within their medical and legal rights to use these drugs based on their best clinical judgment. *"Unapproved use does not imply an improper use and certainly does not imply an illegal use."*[339,340] The use of a drug in a child is the decision of the individual physician and may be based on the available literature, despite the fact that formal FDA approval and labeling have not been achieved.[321,322,341] The Committee on Drugs of the American Academy of Pediatrics is very clear on this issue: *"Lack of approval for a specific use should not prevent physicians from prescribing an available drug in the best interest of their patients."*[339,340] Furthermore, *"Labeling is not intended to preclude the practitioner from using his or her best medical judgment in the interest of patients or to impose liability for off-label use. Indeed, the practice of medicine will more than likely require a practitioner to use drugs off label to provide the most appropriate treatment of a patient."*[341]

Inhalation Anesthetic Agents
PHYSICOCHEMICAL PROPERTIES
The current potent inhaled anesthetics are ether-based anesthetics with either a methyl ethyl (isoflurane and desflurane) or a methyl isopropyl (sevoflurane) polyhalogenated skeleton (E-Table 5.1). The single exception in chemical structure is halothane, which is a polyhalogenated alkane. Of the methyl ethyl ether anesthetics, desflurane differs from isoflurane in the single atomic substitution of a fluoride for a chlorine atom on the α-carbon of isoflurane. Sevoflurane differs from isoflurane in the substitution of a trifluoromethyl group for the chlorine atom, resulting in a methyl isopropyl structure. Although the general chemical structures of the three ether agents are similar, the single atomic substitutions confer substantially different physicochemical and pharmacologic properties described in later text and contrasted to the properties of halothane (see E-Table 5.1).

In comparison to the potent inhaled anesthetics, nitrous oxide and xenon exist in gaseous form under atmospheric conditions. Nitrous oxide is a by-product of chemical processes, whereas xenon is a naturally occurring element (0.05 ppm in the atmosphere), produced by fractional distillation of atmospheric gas. Environmentally, nitrous oxide depletes the ozone layer, whereas xenon is environmentally inert. There is a wealth of data on the pharmacology of nitrous oxide in humans but far less on xenon in adults and none, to date, in children.[342]

PHARMACOKINETICS OF INHALED ANESTHETICS
There is a wealth of knowledge about the pharmacokinetics of inhaled anesthetics, but this information is mostly based on physiology. Pharmacodynamics are generally described in terms of the minimum alveolar concentration (MAC) of the agent, a measure of the potency of the anesthetic. However, it is possible to describe the pharmacokinetics/pharmacodynamics using both compartment

TABLE 5.3	Determinants of the Wash-In of Inhalational Agents
• Inspired concentration • Alveolar ventilation • Functional residual capacity	Delivery of agents to the lungs
• Cardiac output • Solubility • Alveolar to venous partial-pressure gradient	Uptake of agents from the lungs

models and a sigmoid Emax response (see Fig. 5.7). This technique has been used to describe the relationship between the end-tidal sevoflurane concentration and BIS response in children.[58] Size standardization using allometry explained clearance and volume changes with age. The effect site sevoflurane concentration that elicits half the maximum response at age 40 years was 1.3% (95% confidence interval [CI] 1.22, 1.42) and that decreased with increasing age from 1.6% at 3 years to 1.1% at 70 years of age. The equilibration half-time ($T_{1/2}keo$ 1.48 minutes) could be predicted using allometry in those younger than 40 years.

Physiology provides a practical and well-studied basis to explain the pharmacokinetics of inhaled anesthetics. The rate of increase or equilibration of the alveolar to inspired anesthetic partial pressure (also known as the wash-in) is a function of the rate of delivery of anesthetic to and uptake from the lungs. Six factors determine the wash-in of inhaled anesthetics (Table 5.3)[343]: the first three determine the delivery of anesthetics to the lungs, and the second three determine their rate of removal (uptake) from the lungs. The wash-in, defined as the ratio of the alveolar to inspired anesthetic partial pressures (Fa/Fi, or fractional alveolar to fractional inspired partial pressures), increases from zero to a value of unity (1), when the inspired and alveolar partial pressures have equilibrated (Fig. 5.15). Although not shown in the figure, the wash-in of xenon should be the most rapid of all inhaled anesthetics based on its physicochemical properties (see E-Table 5.1).[344] For the Fa/Fi to equilibrate, the rate of delivery of anesthetic to the lungs must substantially exceed its uptake from the lungs.

The rates of increase of Fa/Fi of halothane (as well as isoflurane, and nitrous oxide) in infants and children are more rapid than those in adults (Fig. 5.16).[345–347] The more rapid rate of increase of Fa/Fi in neonates compared with adults has been attributed to four factors (Table 5.4); the order in the table reflects their relative contributions to the rapid wash-in. Based on these factors and their physical chemical properties, we speculate that the wash-in of sevoflurane and desflurane in neonates and infants will be comparable to those in adults. This amounts to a safety factor for the latter anesthetics that was not previously afforded with halothane.

Factors Affecting Delivery of Inhaled Anesthetics to the Lungs
Inspired Concentration
The effect of the inspired concentration on the Fa/Fi of anesthetics relates only to those that are administered in large concentrations (i.e., nitrous oxide and xenon) because of their low potency (large MAC values).[348] The greater the Fi of nitrous oxide, the more rapid the increase of Fa/Fi.[349] This effect, known as the concentration effect (second gas effect), depends on both a concentrating effect and an increase in alveolar ventilation that results from the rapid uptake of nitrous oxide.[343] Hence, the wash-in of anesthetics that depend on alveolar ventilation for their delivery (i.e., the more soluble anesthetics) is more rapid when administered with nitrous oxide or xenon. This effect diminishes with anesthetics that are less soluble and with time.[350–352]

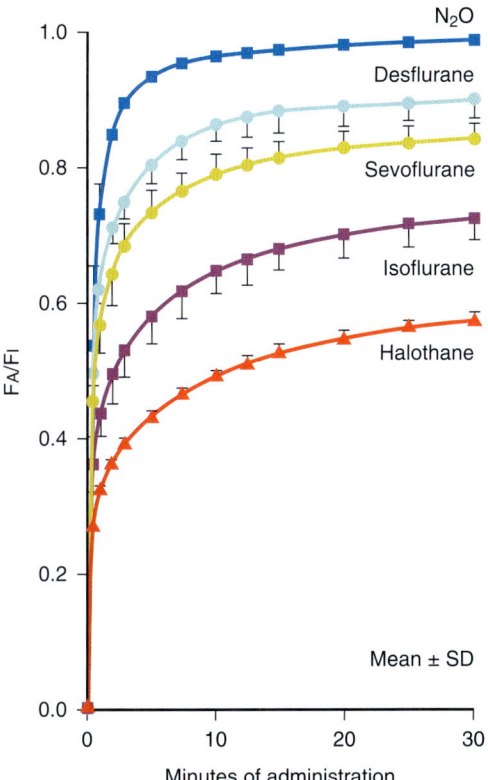

FIGURE 5.15 Wash-in (or Fa/Fi) of N₂O, desflurane, sevoflurane, isoflurane, and halothane in adults. The order of wash-in (N₂O > desflurane > sevoflurane > isoflurane > halothane) is inversely related to their solubilities in blood. *Fa*, Fractional alveolar partial pressure of anesthetic; *Fi*, fractional inspired partial pressure of anesthetic; *N₂O*, nitrous oxide; *SD*, standard deviation. (Redrawn from Yasuda N, Lockhart SH, Eger EI 2nd, et al. Comparison of kinetics of sevoflurane and isoflurane in humans. *Anesth Analg.* 1991;72(3):316-324.)

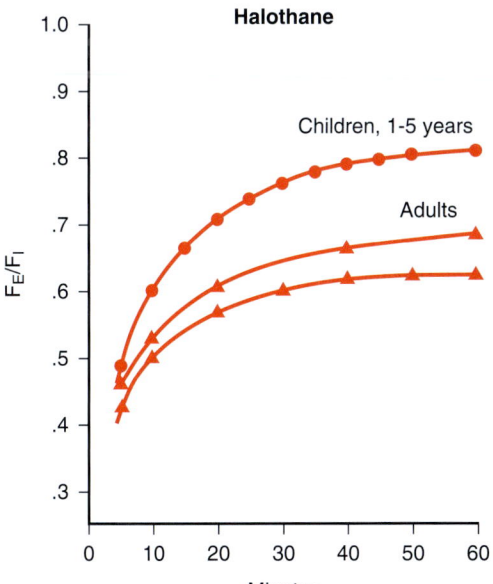

FIGURE 5.16 Rate of rise of expired to inspired fractional partial pressures (*Fᴇ/Fɪ*) of halothane in children and adults. (Redrawn from Salanitre E, Rackow H. The pulmonary exchange of nitrous oxide and halothane in infants and children. *Anesthesiology.* 1969;30(4):388-394.)

TABLE 5.4	Determinants of the Rapid Wash-In of Inhalational Agents in Infants Compared with Adults
Greater ratio of alveolar ventilation to functional residual capacity	
Greater fraction of the cardiac output distributed to the vessel-rich group	
Reduced tissue/blood solubility	
Reduced blood/gas solubility	

Alveolar Ventilation and Functional Residual Capacity

The ratio of alveolar ventilation (Va) to functional residual capacity (FRC), Va/FRC, is the primary determinant of the rate of the delivery of inhaled anesthetics to the lungs. The greater the Va/FRC ratio, the more rapidly the Fa/Fi ratio approaches equilibrium (E-Fig. 5.6). However, the ratio does not affect all anesthetics similarly: Va/FRC affects more soluble anesthetics (e.g., halothane) to a greater extent than less soluble anesthetics (e.g., sevoflurane and desflurane). In the case of soluble anesthetics (e.g., halothane), the increase in Fa/Fi depends substantively on a large Va/FRC ratio since their uptake from the lungs is rapid (because they are soluble in blood and tissues), and this slows the rate of increase in Fa/Fi. Changes in the Va/FRC directly affect the Fa/Fi of anesthetics in proportion to their blood solubilities.

In terms of age-related effects of Fa/Fi, the Va/FRC ratio accounts for most of the differences between the Fa/Fi of anesthetics in neonates and adults (see Table 5.4). The Va/FRC ratio is approximately 5 : 1 in neonates compared with only 1.5 : 1 in adults. The greater Va/FRC ratio in neonates may be attributed to the 3-fold greater metabolic rate and, therefore, 3-fold greater Va/FRC in neonates compared with adults.

Factors that Affect the Uptake (Removal) of Inhaled Anesthetics From the Lungs

Cardiac Output

The rate of increase in Fa/Fi is inversely related to changes in cardiac output; that is, the smaller the cardiac output, the more rapidly Fa/Fi equilibrates and vice versa (E-Fig. 5.7). As cardiac output diminishes, less anesthetic is removed from the lungs, thus increasing the alveolar concentration and the rate of equilibration of Fa/Fi. A patient in heart failure who receives an inhalational induction may achieve greater anesthetic concentrations in the lungs more rapidly than expected compared with a patient with a normal cardiac output. This very serious problem may be exacerbated if the "overpressure" technique has been used, because it may cause acute anesthetic-induced myocardial depression and cardiac decompensation. Conversely, in a high cardiac output state (as in the case of anxiety), the greater blood flow through the lungs removes more anesthetic from the alveoli, reducing the alveolar partial pressure of anesthetic, which slows the rate of equilibration of Fa/Fi. The impact of changes in cardiac output on Fa/Fi depends, in part, on the solubility of the anesthetic: the less soluble the anesthetic (sevoflurane and desflurane), the less the importance of this effect and vice versa.[343] This represents yet another safety feature of the less soluble anesthetics currently in use.

Paradoxically, the greater cardiac index in neonates actually speeds the increase in Fa/Fi. This has been attributed to the preferential distribution of the cardiac output to the vessel-rich group (VRG) of tissues (brain, heart, kidney, splanchnic organs, and endocrine glands) in neonates. The VRG receives a greater proportion of the cardiac output in neonates compared with adults because the VRG constitutes 18% of the body weight in the former compared with only 8% in the latter. As a result of the increased blood flow to the VRG in neonates, the partial pressures of anesthetics in the VRG equilibrate with those in the alveoli in neonates more rapidly than in adults. Because the uptake of anesthetic by tissues other than those in the VRG in neonates is small, the rapid increase in Fa/Fi in the VRG and blood suggests that the partial pressure of anesthetic in venous blood returning to the lungs rapidly equilibrates with that in the alveoli. Uptake of anesthetic from the lungs then diminishes. The net effect of the greater cardiac output in neonates is paradoxical in that it speeds the equilibration of anesthetic partial pressures in the VRG and thus speeds the equilibration of Fa/Fi. This also explains the "downward spiral" that occurs when an excessive concentration of inhaled anesthetic (particularly the soluble anesthetic, halothane) is administered to a neonate or infant during controlled ventilation, as discussed later.

Solubility

Inhalational anesthetics partition into two compartments in body fluids and tissues: (1) the aqueous phase and (2) the protein/lipid phase. This partitioning is analogous to the distribution of gases such as oxygen in blood between the aqueous phase (dissolved fraction) and hemoglobin (bound fraction). Because inhaled anesthetics move along partial pressure gradients (and not concentration gradients) within and between fluids and tissues, the rate of increase of Fa/Fi and, therefore, the anesthetic partial pressure in blood determines how rapidly anesthetics move in and out of tissues and affect organ function (e.g., central nervous and cardiac systems).

The rate of increase of Fa/Fi of inhalational anesthetics, which varies inversely with the solubility of the anesthetic in blood, follows the order: nitrous oxide > desflurane > sevoflurane > isoflurane > halothane (see E-Table 5.1 and Fig.5.15).[343,353] Although the solubilities of nitrous oxide and desflurane are similar, the rate of increase in Fa/Fi of nitrous oxide is more rapid than that after desflurane because of the concentration effect from administering 70% nitrous oxide. In theory, the wash-in of xenon should be the most rapid of all inhalational anesthetics given its very low blood solubility ($\sim$0.14–0.17)[344,354] and the concentration effect in light of its large MAC, 0.71.[348] After a stepwise increase in the inspired partial pressure of less soluble anesthetics, the alveolar partial pressure equilibrates rapidly with the new inspired partial pressure. Because the wash-out of these anesthetics is equally rapid (see below), the alveolar partial pressure can be adjusted to previous values rapidly by decreasing the inspired partial pressure. Thus, anesthetic depth can be adjusted more rapidly with a less soluble (e.g., desflurane or sevoflurane) than with a more soluble inhalational anesthetic (e.g., halothane).

Age is an important determinant of the solubility of inhalational anesthetics in blood. The blood solubilities of halothane, isoflurane, enflurane, and methoxyflurane are 18% less in neonates than in adults (E-Fig. 5.8; see also E-Table 5.1).[355] Serum cholesterol and proteins (including albumin) account for these age-related differences in blood solubilities.[355,356] In contrast, the blood solubility of the less soluble anesthetic sevoflurane is similar in neonates and adults and in theory, the same should also hold true for desflurane and xenon, although such evidence has not been forthcoming.[356] Therefore, the more rapid wash-in of these less soluble anesthetics in neonates compared with adults cannot be attributed to the reduced blood solubility in this age group.

The hemoglobin concentration, serum concentration of α_1-acid glycoprotein, and prematurity do not significantly affect the blood solubility of most inhaled anesthetics.[355,356]

The tissue/gas solubilities of the inhaled anesthetics in the VRG in neonates are approximately one-half those in adults (E-Fig. 5.9).[357] The reduced tissue solubilities in neonates are attributable to two differences in the composition of tissues: (1) greater water content and (2) decreased protein and lipid concentrations. In terms of the uptake and distribution of inhaled anesthetics in tissues, the tissue/blood solubilities determine the speed of equilibration of anesthetics in tissues. The reduced tissue solubilities of inhaled anesthetics reduce the time for partial pressure equilibration of anesthetics (see time constant discussion, later). Although the partial pressures of inhaled anesthetics in tissues cannot easily be measured in vivo, they are estimated by their concentrations in the end-tidal or alveolar gases. The solubilities of these anesthetics in the brain of adults vary approximately 50% from desflurane to halothane (see E-Table 5.1). In the case of neonates, the reduced tissue solubilities of inhaled anesthetics speed the rate of increase in Fa/Fi compared with the rates in adults. In the cases of sevoflurane and desflurane, their respectively small but similar blood solubilities and likely similar tissue solubilities in neonates and adults offer a safety factor in neonates compared with adults, because tissue equilibration of these relatively insoluble inhalational anesthetics is similar in both age groups. In contrast, the reduced tissue solubility of halothane in neonates leads to a more rapid and unexpected anesthetic effect (e.g., hypotension) compared with the time course in adults.

We can estimate the time to equilibration of the partial pressures of inhaled anesthetic in tissues using the time constant for tissue equilibration. For example, the time constant (tau τ) for equilibration of the anesthetic partial pressure in the brain is:

$$\tau_{brain} = \frac{\text{Volume of the brain (mL)} \times \text{Brain/blood solubility}}{\text{Brain blood flow (mL/minute)}}, \quad \text{Eq. 5.30}$$

where one time constant is the time for 63% equilibration of brain to blood anesthetic partial pressures. With brain blood flow at approximately 50 mL/minute per 100 g of brain tissue and brain/blood solubility ratio for an inhalational anesthetic is 2.0 (assuming the density of brain tissue is 1 g/mL), then the time constant is:

$$\tau_{brain} = \frac{100 \text{ mL} \times 2}{50 \text{ mL/minute}} = 4 \text{ minutes} \quad \text{Eq. 5.31}$$

Knowing that four time constants achieve 98% equilibration, then the time to 98% equilibration is 16 minutes (4 time constants multiplied by 4 minutes per constant). If the brain/blood solubility ratio were halved to 1.0, as in the case of the neonate, then the time to 95% equilibration would decrease by 50% to 8 minutes. *Thus, the time to equilibration of anesthetic partial pressure within the brain of the neonate (8 minutes) would be approximately one-half that in the adult (16 minutes).* This holds true for the more soluble anesthetics, such as halothane, whose tissue solubility in neonates is diminished compared with adults[357] but not for the less soluble anesthetics, such as desflurane, sevoflurane, and xenon, whose tissue solubilities may be similar in neonates and adults.

The wash-in of inhalational anesthetics during the first 15 to 20 minutes depends primarily on the characteristics of the VRG, whereas the wash-in during the subsequent 20 to 200 minutes depends primarily on the muscle characteristics.[343] The solubility of inhalational anesthetics in skeletal muscle varies directly with age in a logarithmic relationship.[357] Thus the lower solubility of inhalational anesthetics in the muscle of neonates and the smaller muscle mass speed the increase in Fa/Fi during this later period compared with adults. This effect of age on the solubility of anesthetics in muscle has been attributed to age-dependent increases in protein concentration (i.e., muscle bulk) during the first 5 decades of life and in fat content during the subsequent 3 decades of life.[357] Overall, the reduced solubility combined with the reduced muscle mass in neonates (and infants) decreases the uptake by the muscle group, hence contributing to the more rapid equilibration of Fa/Fi in neonates compared with adults.

Alveolar to Venous Partial Pressure Gradient

The difference in the anesthetic partial pressures between the alveolar and venous blood returning to the heart is a measure of the driving force of inhalational anesthetics from the alveoli into the bloodstream. As the anesthetic partial pressures in the VRG, muscle group, and others approach equilibration, less anesthetic is removed from the blood. The anesthetic partial pressure in the blood returning to the heart approximates that when it left the alveoli. This reduces the partial pressure gradient between the alveoli and blood and diminishes the uptake of anesthetic from the lungs.

Second Gas Effect

When two anesthetics are administered simultaneously, the wash-in of the inhaled anesthetic administered in a small concentration (e.g., sevoflurane) may be increased if the uptake of the second anesthetic (e.g., nitrous oxide) is relatively large.[343] Nitrous oxide and xenon are the only anesthetics for which their uptake may be relatively large compared with that of the other potent inhalational anesthetics. Although evidence has cast doubt on the clinical relevance of the second gas effect,[358,359] modeling supports a second gas effect particularly in less soluble anesthetics, when it was based on the partial pressures of inhalational anesthetics in blood rather than in expired gases.[360]

Induction

The more rapid increase in Fa/Fi of insoluble anesthetics (i.e., the wash-in or pharmacokinetics) is generally thought to induce anesthesia more rapidly than that with soluble anesthetics, although induction of anesthesia actually depends on four factors: (1) the potency or MAC of the agent, (2) the rate of increase of the inspired concentration, (3) the maximum inspired concentration, and (4) respiration (including airway irritability and the mode of ventilation [spontaneous or controlled]). It is the combination of these four factors that determines the relative rate of induction of anesthesia.

The rate of wash-in of inhalational anesthetics into the lungs (or alveoli) varies inversely with their solubilities in blood. Although anesthetics that are less soluble (e.g., sevoflurane, desflurane, and xenon) wash-in to the lungs more rapidly than more soluble anesthetics (e.g., halothane), this is offset in part, by the greater MAC values of these less soluble anesthetics (see E-Table 5.1). To ensure that induction of anesthesia is as rapid with less soluble anesthetics as it is with more soluble anesthetics, two criteria must be satisfied: (1) the inspired concentration of the less soluble anesthetic must be increased in greater increments (based on the relative MAC values and wash-in profile, where the MAC is defined as the minimum alveolar [or end-tidal or end-expiratory] concentrations of anesthetic at which 50% of subjects do not move in response to a noxious stimulus) than the more soluble anesthetic and, (2) the maximum inspired concentration of the less soluble anesthetic delivered must provide an alveolar concentration that is equipotent to or greater than that of the more soluble anesthetic. Theoretically, the overpressure technique should provide rapid and similar rates of induction of anesthesia with anesthetics of differing solubilities. However, if the maximum inspired anesthetic concentrations delivered by the vaporizers preclude the delivery of equipotent end-tidal concentrations or if airway irritability interrupts the smooth delivery of anesthetic (as in the case of desflurane), the speed of induction of anesthesia will differ.

To illustrate this, contrast the steep wash-in of Fa/Fi for sevoflurane and halothane during the first few minutes of induction of anesthesia. The Fa/Fi for halothane in adults reaches 0.35 in the first few minutes of wash-in (see Fig. 5.15), whereas that in children may reach ~0.45.[353] This latter value corresponds to an alveolar concentration of 2.25% when breathing an inspired concentration of 5% or ~2.25 MAC in a child. Contrast this to the wash-in of sevoflurane during the same time frame; the Fa/Fi for sevoflurane in adults and children both reach ~0.5. This corresponds to an alveolar concentration in children of ~4% breathing an inspired concentration of 8% or 1.6 MAC multiples, 25% less than that achieved with halothane. An 8% sevoflurane vaporizer cannot deliver anesthetic concentrations that are equipotent with a 5% halothane vaporizer (e.g., 5 × MAC); a sevoflurane vaporizer that delivers ≥10% would facilitate a more rapid induction of anesthesia but such concentrations support combustion at very high temperatures (e.g., in the presence of a laser in the airway) and has been proscribed.[361,362]

A similar but clinically more important case can be made for neonates with MAC values for halothane of ~0.87% and sevoflurane of 3.3%. In the case of halothane, the alveolar concentration reaches 2.9 MAC multiples within the first few minutes of induction breathing 5% halothane, whereas with sevoflurane it reaches only 1.2 MAC multiples breathing 8% sevoflurane, 60% less depth of anesthesia. Thus, it is difficult to rapidly induce a deep level of anesthesia with sevoflurane in spontaneously breathing neonates and infants but at the same time, more difficult to cause an anesthetic overdose during induction with sevoflurane compared with halothane increasing the margin of safety for sevoflurane in neonates.

These two examples illustrate several extremely important features of the pharmacology of sevoflurane that distinguish it from halothane. (1) It may be difficult to rapidly achieve a deep level of anesthesia with sevoflurane in children (as was previously achieved with halothane) when sevoflurane is the sole anesthetic. Hence, inserting an IV catheter or performing laryngoscopy and tracheal intubation or bronchoscopy immediately after induction of anesthesia with sevoflurane may result in a physiologic or motor (withdrawal) response or sequelae (e.g., bronchospasm), even if the inspired concentration remains at 8%. We caution against decreasing the inspired concentration of sevoflurane (and/or discontinuing nitrous oxide before undertaking a stimulating procedure) as soon as the eyelash reflex is lost or the child appears to have lost consciousness, because a deep level of anesthesia has not been achieved (despite theoretical fears of epileptiform brain activity, see later in the chapter). In such cases, supplemental IV anesthetics should be administered to rapidly deepen the level of anesthesia. (2) These examples illustrate an important safety feature of sevoflurane. With the current vaporizer design, anesthetic overdose with sevoflurane is not easily accomplished in neonates and infants because their large MAC values more than offset the reduced solubilities of sevoflurane in blood and tissues. These insights contribute to the cardiovascular safety profile of sevoflurane and explain why the morbidity and mortality associated with sevoflurane in infants and children are less than with halothane.[363]

CONTROL OF ANESTHETIC DEPTH

Two feedback responses modulate the depth of anesthesia during inhalational anesthesia: (1) a negative-feedback respiratory response and (2) a positive-feedback cardiovascular response. The feedback responses refer to the relationships between the inspired concentration of anesthetic and depth of anesthesia. After an increase in the inspired concentration, a negative-feedback response refers to a decrease in the depth of anesthesia, whereas a positive-feedback response refers to an increase in the depth of anesthesia. Two examples are used to illustrate the importance of these responses in clinical pediatric anesthesia practice.

During spontaneous respirations, as the partial pressure of inhaled anesthetics increases, alveolar ventilation decreases, thereby limiting both the wash-in of anesthetics and the depth of anesthesia achieved (E-Fig. 5.10A).[364] This negative-feedback response is a protective mechanism that permits the safe use of inspired concentrations of inhalational anesthetics that are severalfold greater than MAC (overpressure technique) during spontaneous respirations. An anesthetic overdose cannot normally be achieved during spontaneous respirations (irrespective of the inspired concentrations of anesthetics, even if multiple anesthetics are administered simultaneously) because the negative-feedback effect of such anesthetic concentrations depress minute ventilation. As alveolar ventilation decreases and the wash-in of anesthetics slows, the uptake of anesthetic by blood slows and the delivery of anesthetics to the VRG slows. When the partial pressure of anesthetics in the VRG exceeds that in blood, anesthetics move along their partial pressure gradients from the VRG into blood and other tissues, thus decreasing the depth of anesthesia. As the depth of anesthesia decreases, alveolar ventilation again increases and uptake of anesthetic from the alveoli resumes. *Thus, spontaneous ventilation protects against an anesthetic overdose by virtue of its negative feedback effect to decrease respiration.*

In contrast to the negative-feedback response of spontaneous ventilation, the positive-feedback effect of controlled ventilation relentlessly delivers inhaled anesthetic to the alveoli, increasing both Fa/Fi and the depth of anesthesia, which in turn decreases cardiac output that, if unabated, may lead to cardiac arrest (E-Fig. 5.10B).[364] For a specific minute ventilation in a neonate, the risk of profound cardiovascular collapse is reflected in part by the maximum number of MAC multiples the vaporizer can deliver; halothane and isoflurane ≫ sevoflurane and desflurane (Table 5.5). With sevoflurane and desflurane, the number of MAC multiples that can be

administered (~2.0) is less than with halothane (~6), building in a safety margin with the former two anesthetics.

The safety of spontaneous versus controlled ventilation during inhalational anesthesia is predicated on the feedback loops. This has been illustrated in anesthetized dogs that all survived when they breathed halothane at 4% to 6% spontaneously, but died in a dose response when ventilation was controlled.[364] This concept is of particular importance in neonates and small infants who are more susceptible to the cardiodepressant effects of inhaled agents, with the effect with more soluble anesthetics much greater than with less soluble anesthetics.[343]

Shunts

Two types of shunts exist in the lungs and heart: left-to-right or right-to-left. Left-to-right shunts refer to conditions in which blood recirculates through the lungs (usually via an intracardiac defect, such as a ventricular septal defect). In general, left-to-right shunts do not significantly affect the pharmacokinetics of inhalational anesthetics, provided cardiac output remains unchanged. In contrast, right-to-left shunts refer to conditions in which venous blood returning to the heart bypasses the lungs as in an intracardiac shunt (cyanotic heart disease) or intrapulmonary shunt (pneumonia or an endobronchial intubation). With these shunts, the equilibration of Fa/Fi can be markedly delayed. The magnitude of the delay depends on the solubility of the anesthetic: the Fa/Fi of less soluble anesthetics is delayed to a greater extent than that of the more soluble anesthetics.[343] These effects are independent of the location of the shunt: intracardiac or intrapulmonary.

To understand the effects of right-to-left shunts on the pharmacokinetics of inhalational anesthetics, consider a simplified model of a right-to-left shunt using an endobronchial intubation to mimic the shunt. In this model, each lung is represented by one alveolus, and each is perfused by one pulmonary artery (Fig. 5.17). When the tracheal tube is positioned with its tip at the mid-trachea level (Fig. 5.17A), ventilation is divided equally between both alveoli (lungs), thereby yielding equivalent anesthetic partial pressures in both pulmonary veins ($P\bar{v} = 1$). However, if the tip of the tracheal tube is advanced into the right main-stem bronchus (equivalent to a right-to-left shunt) (Fig. 5.17B), all of the ventilation is delivered to one alveolus (lung); that is, the ventilation to that alveolus (lung) is doubled and ventilation to the nonventilated lung is nil. Under these conditions, total ventilation remains unchanged. For the remainder of this discussion, it is important to recognize that with a right-to-left shunt, the end-tidal and blood anesthetic partial pressures will differ, with the magnitude of the difference directly dependent on the solubility of the anesthetic.

With a more soluble anesthetic (e.g., halothane), when the tracheal tube that is positioned in the right main-stem bronchus (to model a right-to-left shunt) doubling the ventilation to that lung speeds the increase in Fa/Fi (effect of changes in ventilation on the wash-in of soluble anesthetics) (see E-Fig. 5.6) such that the augmented ventilation increases the Fa/Fi sufficiently to offset, for the most part, the absence of ventilation to the contralateral lung (see Fig. 5.17B).[343] The more soluble the anesthetic, the closer the partial pressure of anesthetic in the combined pulmonary vein that drains both the ventilated and nonventilated lungs approximates the partial pressure from delivering the anesthetic to lungs without a right-to-left shunt. The net effect of a right-to-left shunt on the Fa/Fi of a more soluble inhalational anesthetic is thus minimal.

Agent	Maximum Vaporizer Output (%)	MAC (%)	Maximum Possible MAC Multiples
Halothane	5	0.87	5.75
Isoflurane	5	1.20	4.2
Sevoflurane	8	3.3	2.42
Desflurane	18	9.16	1.96

TABLE 5.5 Minimum Alveolar Concentration Multiples for a Neonate Allowed by Current Vaporizers

See text for further discussion.
MAC, minimum alveolar concentration.

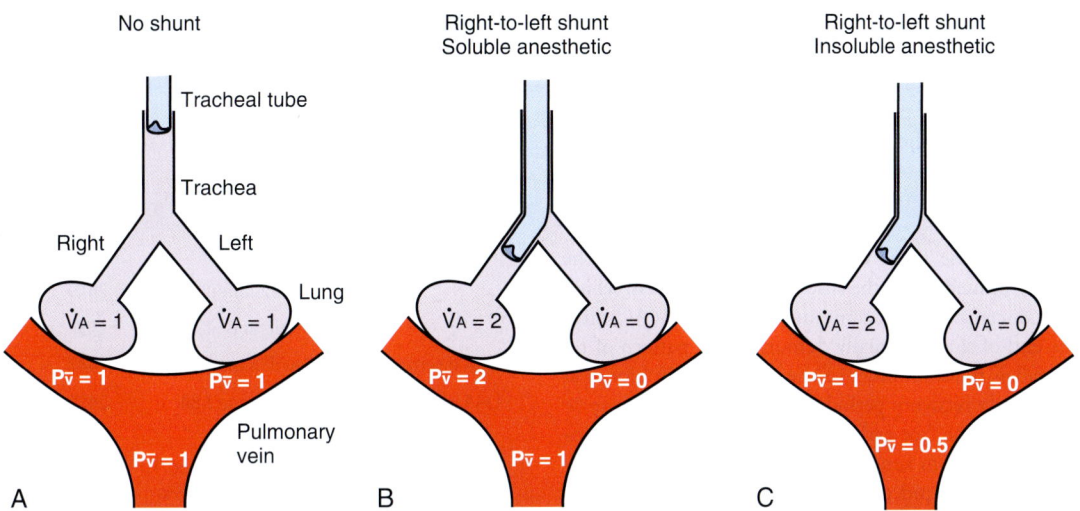

FIGURE 5.17 Effect of a shunt on the rate of increase of anesthetic partial pressure in blood using a model. **A,** Normal situation with no shunt, equal alveolar ventilation ($\dot{V}_A$) to both lungs, and normocapnia. **B,** The effect of a right-to-left shunt (via an endobronchial intubation) with a more soluble anesthetic (e.g., halothane). Ventilation and therefore normocapnia are maintained, and hypoxic pulmonary vasoconstriction is negligible. In this case, the increased ventilation to the ventilated lung speeds the increase in FA/Fi (wash-in) and offsets the effect of the shunt. Results in terms of the mixed pulmonary venous partial pressure of the anesthetic ($P\bar{v} = 1$) are similar to those in **A**. **C,** The effect of a shunt with a less soluble anesthetic (e.g., desflurane or sevoflurane). Because the increase in alveolar ventilation does not increase Fa/Fi in the ventilated lung, there is a dramatic reduction in the anesthetic partial pressure in the blood ($P\bar{v} = 0.5$). *FA,* Fractional alveolar partial pressure of anesthetic; *Fi,* fractional inspired partial pressure of anesthetic. (Redrawn from Lerman J. Pharmacology of inhalational anaesthetics in infants and children. *Paediatr Anaesth.* 1992;2:191-203.)

In contrast, with a less soluble anesthetic (e.g., sevoflurane, desflurane, or xenon) in a child with a right-to-left shunt, doubling the ventilation to the lung marginally increases the Fa/Fi, because ventilation has a limited effect on the speed of increase of Fa/Fi of less soluble anesthetics (see E-Fig. 5.6 and Fig. 5.17C).[343] Consequently, the increase in Fa/Fi in the ventilated lung is insufficient to offset the lack of anesthetic in the blood draining the nonventilated lung. The *net effect is to almost halve* the anesthetic partial pressure in the combined pulmonary vein. The less soluble the anesthetic (with xenon having the least solubility in blood), the greater the discrepancy between the anesthetic partial pressure in the pulmonary vein that drains the ventilated and nonventilated lungs and the partial pressure when the tube is in the trachea. The overall effect of a right-to-left shunt with a less soluble anesthetics is to slow induction of anesthesia and/or limit the depth of anesthesia that can be achieved.[365–367]

Two clinical situations pose challenges with these shunts: children with right-to-left cardiac shunts and infants with chronic lung disease. In the case of halothane, anesthesia remained quite effective in children with right-to-left shunts even though the ratio of arterial to inspired partial pressures lags behind the ratio when the shunt is closed.[366] The most likely explanation for this is that the 5% inspired concentration of halothane from the vaporizer permitted delivery of a 5 × MAC overpressure effect. Although the ratios of the arterial to inspired partial pressures of sevoflurane and desflurane have not been measured in children with right-to-left shunts, we theoretically expect that they will pose even greater difficulties than halothane, particularly with their limited overpressure effect (i.e., the maximal inspired concentrations of the vaporizers are limited to 3 × MAC or less [see Table 5.5]). Our experience suggests that with less soluble anesthetics in circumstances that require a deep level of anesthesia

(e.g., bronchoscopy), intravenous anesthetics are needed to achieve an adequate depth of anesthesia.

Wash-Out and Emergence

The wash-out of inhalational anesthetics follows an exponential decay (the inverse of the wash-in curves, see Fig. 5.15) and during emergence, this is achieved by setting the inspired concentration to zero.[353] The speed of the wash-out (and speed of emergence) of the inhalational anesthetics parallels their blood solubilities: desflurane > sevoflurane > isoflurane > halothane > methoxyflurane (see E-Table 5.1).[353,368] Given that the blood solubility of xenon is the least of all inhalational anesthetics, the wash-out of xenon should be even more rapid than desflurane and nitrous oxide.[369] In adults, emergence after xenon anesthesia was independent of the duration of administration up to 6.5 hours.[369] For most inhalational anesthetics, metabolism does not contribute substantively to the wash-out. Halothane is the one exception; its wash-out is as rapid as that of isoflurane, likely because its metabolism is 15- to 20-fold greater than that of isoflurane (see later discussion). The order of the wash-out of anesthetics in children should be similar to that in adults, whereas the wash-out in neonates and infants is likely to be more rapid than that in adults for the same reasons the rate of wash-in is more rapid (see Table 5.4).

Although some advocate switching from a more soluble to a less soluble inhalational anesthetic toward the end of surgery for economy and to facilitate a rapid emergence, there is a dearth of evidence to support such a practice in children. In adults, it has been suggested that switching from isoflurane to desflurane 30 minutes before the end of a 2-hour anesthetic does not speed emergence.[370]

A number of other strategies have been used to speed emergence and recovery from anesthesia. In adults, discontinuing nitrous oxide accelerates the wash-out of and emergence from inhalational anesthesia.[371] Most recently, charcoal filters added to anesthesia breathing circuits adsorb anesthetics and have been shown to speed emergence.[372] Hypercapnic hyperventilation with a charcoal filter to adsorb the inhaled anesthetic has been shown to speed emergence from isoflurane, sevoflurane, and desflurane anesthesia in adults by about 60%.[373,374] Similar data in children are lacking.

When comparing the speed of recovery after anesthesia, the results are heavily influenced by the study design. Studies in which the anesthetic concentration is maintained at a fixed MAC multiple until the end of surgery usually demonstrate a pattern of recovery that parallels the solubilities of the anesthetics in blood, at least during the early recovery period: halothane > isoflurane > sevoflurane > desflurane (see earlier).[375–379] Data from adults indicate that emergence from xenon is the most rapid of all inhalational anesthetic, more rapid than after desflurane. Comparable data in children are lacking.[342]

However, when the inspired concentrations of inhalational anesthetics are tapered toward the end of surgery, this attenuates the differences reported with the fixed MAC technique. Differences in the speed of recovery among anesthetics parallels the duration of anesthesia; for example, differences will be less for brief surgery and greater for surgery of greater duration.[376,380–382] Failure to prevent or treat pain before emergence will trigger a much more rapid and stormy emergence after less soluble than after more soluble anesthetics.[376,379] A more sophisticated approach to the wash-out of inhalational anesthetics is to use the context-sensitive half-time, which is a measure of the time required for the anesthetic partial pressure to decrease by 50%. Using a computer model and pharmacokinetic data from adults, the context-sensitive half-times of the potent inhalational anesthetics, isoflurane, sevoflurane, and desflurane were similar (<5 minutes) and were unaffected by the duration of the anesthetic.[383] The 80% decrement times were similar for desflurane and sevoflurane (<8 minutes), whereas that for isoflurane was greater (by 30 minutes). However, after 6 hours of simulated anesthesia, the 90% decrement times differed substantially: 14 minutes for desflurane, 65 minutes for sevoflurane, and 86 minutes for isoflurane. These data suggest that the early recovery (up to 80% decrement in partial pressure) after inhalational anesthesia is similar among these four anesthetics (although sevoflurane and desflurane are more rapid), but after 6 hours (i.e., prolonged anesthesia) 90% decrement is achieved much more rapidly with desflurane than with the remainder.

In animal models, recovery of motor function (a metric for more complete recovery than the expired anesthetic concentrations) parallels the speed of wash-out of inhalational anesthetics from fastest to slowest: desflurane > sevoflurane > isoflurane > halothane.[384] Notably, the time to recover increases in parallel with the duration of anesthesia.[384] In pediatric studies in which the recovery times after two or more anesthetics were compared, the end-tidal concentrations of the anesthetics were maintained at approximately 1 MAC until the conclusion of surgery, after which the anesthetics were abruptly discontinued.[375,376,385] In this paradigm, the rates of recovery paralleled the rates of wash-out, which in turn paralleled the solubilities of the inhalational anesthetics, including xenon and desflurane.[386] In clinical practice, however, anesthetic concentrations are gradually tapered as the end of surgery approaches. This practice may attenuate the differences in the speed of recovery among inhalational anesthetics.

TABLE 5.6	MAC Values in Children	
	MAC (%)	**References**
Tracheal intubation	Halothane: 1.33	2445
	Enflurane: 2.93	2446
	Sevoflurane: 2.69, 2.66, 2.83	397, 418, 2447
Tracheal extubation	Isoflurane: 1.4	2448
	Sevoflurane: 1.70, 2.3	2449, 2450
	Desflurane: 7.7	2451
LMA insertion	Sevoflurane: 2.0	2447
LMA extubation	Sevoflurane 1.84	2452
	Desflurane (with 1–1.3 µµg/kg fentanyl): 3.56%	2453
Tracheal intubation/ skin incision ratio[a]	Halothane, enflurane, sevoflurane: 1.33	Calculated from MAC data
MAC awake	Sevoflurane: 0.66 (2–5 years) and 0.43 (5–12 years)	2454
IV cannulation	Sevoflurane: 1.32% ± 1% (95%ile 3.5%)	387a

LMA, Laryngeal mask airway; *MAC*, minimum alveolar concentration.
[a]Calculated using the above MAC data.

PHARMACODYNAMICS OF INHALED ANESTHETICS
Minimum Alveolar Concentration
MAC is an acronym for the minimum alveolar (or end-tidal or end-expiratory) concentration of anesthetic at which 50% of patients do not move in response to a noxious stimulus.[387] The classic stimulus for MAC in humans is a skin incision; although the MAC or ED_{50} values for other stimuli and procedures are also highlighted including tracheal intubation, insertion of a laryngeal mask airway, tracheal extubation, intravenous cannulation,[387a] and awake responsiveness (Table 5.6). The MAC response to tracheal intubation during sevoflurane anesthesia in children is attenuated in the presence of adjuvants, such as clonidine (E-Table 5.2).[388] Conflicting evidence exists regarding the relative potencies of isomers or enantiomers of chiral inhalational anesthetics.[389–391] Studies in animals suggest that the $S(+)$ optical enantiomer may be more potent than the $R(-)$ enantiomer, as evidenced by its ability to enhance potassium conductance in neurons.[389,390] In adults, the $R(-)$ enantiomer of isoflurane was nominally (17%) more potent than the $S(+)$ enantiomer.[391]

The difference in the potency (or MAC) of inhalational anesthetics varies inversely with lipid solubility; that is, as the lipid solubility decreases, the potency decreases in parallel (i.e., MAC increases) (see E-Table 5.1).

In children, MAC varies significantly with age. For example, the MAC of halothane increases as age decreases, reaching a maximum value in infants 1 to 6 months of age (1.20% ± 0.06%) and then decreases by about 30% to (0.87 ± 0.03%) in full-term neonates.[392] Similar relationships hold true for isoflurane and desflurane (Fig. 5.18 and E-Fig. 5.11).[393,394] However, the relationship for sevoflurane differs substantively from that of

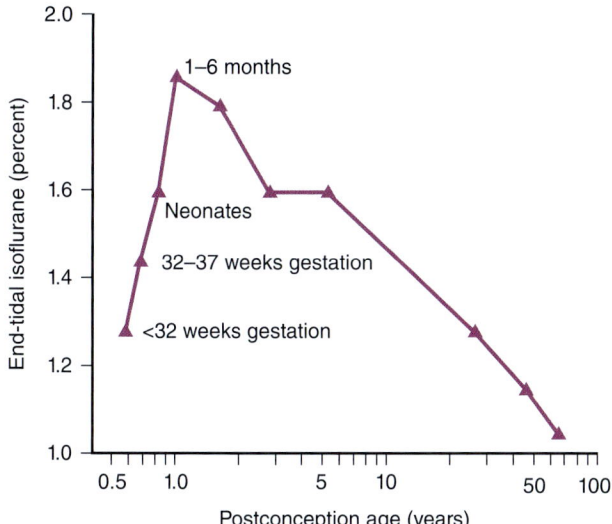

FIGURE 5.18 Minimum alveolar concentration (MAC) of isoflurane in preterm and full-term neonates, infants, and children. MAC increased with gestational age in infants younger than 32 weeks gestation (1.3%), reaching a zenith in infants 1 to 6 months of age of 1.87%, and decreased thereafter with increasing age to adulthood. Postconceptional age is the sum of the gestational age and postnatal age in years. (Data from Cameron CB, Robinson S, Gregory GA. The minimum anesthetic concentration of isoflurane in children. *Anesth Analg.* 1984;63(4):418-420; and LeDez KM, Lerman J. The minimum alveolar concentration (MAC) of isoflurane in preterm neonates. *Anesthesiology.* 1987;67(3):301-307.)

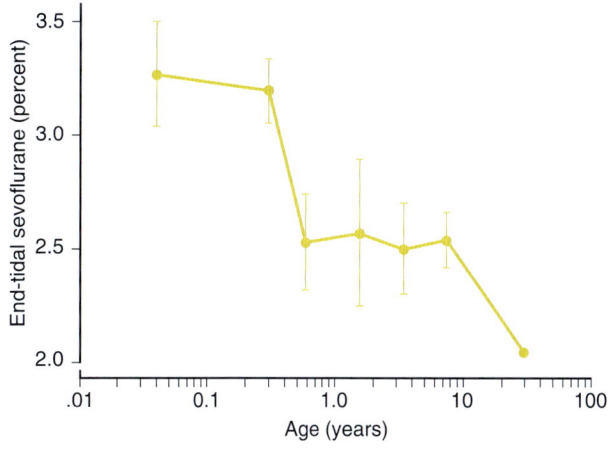

FIGURE 5.19 The minimum alveolar concentration (MAC) of sevoflurane in neonates, infants, and children. MAC is greatest in full-term neonates (3.3%), less in infants 1 to 6 months of age (3.2%), and then decreases 25%, to 2.5%, for all infants and children 6 months to 10 years of age. (The *thin vertical yellow bars* are standard deviations.) Age is postnatal age in years. The MAC of sevoflurane in adults, 30 years of age, is shown for completeness. All MAC measurements were performed with sevoflurane in 100% oxygen using a single skin incision. (Data from Lerman J, Sikich N, Kleinman S, Yentis S. The pharmacology of sevoflurane in infants and children. *Anesthesiology* 1994;80(4):814-824.)

the other inhalational anesthetics in that the MAC of sevoflurane does not increase steadily as age decreases (Fig. 5.19).[395] In fact, the MAC of sevoflurane in neonates and infants younger than 6 months of age is 3.3%, whereas in older infants and children it is 2.5%.[395–397] The explanation for this different relationship for sevoflurane remains unclear.

The MAC of inhalational anesthetics in preterm neonates has been determined only for isoflurane (see Fig. 5.18). The mean ± standard deviation MAC of isoflurane in preterm neonates younger than 32 weeks gestation (1.28% ± 0.17%) is 10% less than it is in neonates of 32 to 37 weeks gestational age (1.41% ± 0.18%), which in turn is 12% less than it is in full-term neonates (1.60% ± 0.03%).[255] The etiology of these age-dependent changes in MAC remains elusive. Several possible causes have been proposed, including maturational changes in the CNS and neurohumoral factors, but none of these have been confirmed.

Several other factors are known to affect MAC. The presence of the melanocortin-1 receptor gene affects the MAC of desflurane. That is, 90% of adults who are either homozygous or heterozygous for mutations of this gene (i.e., redheads) require 20% more anesthesia than those who have no mutations (brunettes),[398] although neither the anesthetic concentrations nor the BIS readings differed between self-reporting red-hair phenotype adults and matched controls in a secondary analysis of an awareness study.[399] Children with complex I defect in the electron transport chain require 50% less sevoflurane to achieve a BIS ≤60 during induction of anesthesia than those with complex II–IV defects or normal controls, although further research is required to validate these findings with a larger sample size.[400] Hypothermia decreases MAC; in children 4 to 10 years of age, the MAC of isoflurane decreases 5% per degree Celsius.[401]

Cerebral palsy and severe cognitive impairment reduce the MAC of halothane approximately 25% compared to those without cognitive impairment.[402] Although tetanic stimulation was used to elicit the pain response, this stimulus underestimates the MAC compared with skin incision.[403] Nonetheless, the MAC of halothane in children without cognitive impairment using tetanic stimulation was similar to published data with skin incision.[392] Chronic anticonvulsant therapy decreased the MAC of halothane in children receiving anticonvulsants by 15%, compared with those without anticonvulsants, from 0.71% ± 0.10% to 0.62% ± 0.03%.[402] Several factors may account for this decrease in MAC, including central sensory impairment, increased pain threshold or insensitivity, and a disequilibrium of inhibitory and excitatory regulatory neurons within the spinal cord in these children.[404,405] Although the acute administration of barbiturates and benzodiazepines decreases MAC,[406,407] chronic administration of similar medications does not.[408] The effects of specific anticonvulsants such as valproic acid and phenytoin, on the MAC of inhalational anesthetics in children remain unclear. Oral gabapentin decreases the MAC of isoflurane 20% in dogs although IV gabapentin exerted no effect on the MAC in cats.[409,410] Studies in humans have not been forthcoming.

The MAC for nitrous oxide has been estimated to be 104% in adults[411]; comparable data do not exist in children. The additivity of MAC fractions of nitrous oxide with inhalational anesthetics is well established. The concept of additivity has been confirmed in adults for nitrous oxide with all inhalational anesthetics, including sevoflurane and desflurane,[412,413] although in children, it holds true only for halothane and isoflurane.[414,415] When nitrous oxide is combined with sevoflurane or desflurane in children,[251,416] 60% nitrous oxide decreases the MAC of sevoflurane only 20% and that of desflurane 26% (Table 5.7).[394,395,417] Mathematical modeling of ventilation/perfusion inhomogeneity in the lungs suggests that in the presence of nitrous oxide, end-tidal gas measurements

TABLE 5.7	Percent MAC Reduced in 2-Year-Olds With 60% Nitrous Oxide		
Agent	MAC With Oxygen (%)	MAC With 60% Nitrous Oxide	Percent MAC Reduced
Halothane	0.91	0.37	65
Desflurane	8.67	6.4	26
Sevoflurane	2.5	2.0	20

MAC, Minimum alveolar concentration.
From Gregory GA, Eger EI 2nd, Munson ES. The relationship between age and halothane requirements in man. *Anesthesiology.* 1969;30(5):488-491; Taylor RH, Lerman J. Minimum alveolar concentration of desflurane and hemodynamic responses in neonates, infants, and children. *Anesthesiology.* 1991;75(5):975-979; Lerman J, Sikich N, Kleinman S, Yentis S. The pharmacology of sevoflurane in infants and children. *Anesthesiology.* 1994;80(4):814-824; Murray DJ, Mehta MP, Forbes RB, Dull DL. Additive contribution of nitrous oxide to halothane MAC in infants and children. *Anesth. Analg.* 1990;71(2):120-124; Fisher DM, Zwass MS. MAC of desflurane in 60% nitrous oxide in infants and children. *Anesthesiology.* 1992;76(2):354-356.

may underestimate the depth of anesthesia (compared with the blood partial pressures) particularly for less soluble anesthetics.[360] The MAC response to tracheal intubation during sevoflurane anesthesia in children is also attenuated by nitrous oxide.[418] The explanation for the differential additivity effect of nitrous oxide remains unclear. The MAC for xenon in middle-aged adults is about 70%[419,420]; the MAC of xenon in children has not been determined.

Central Nervous System

All potent inhalational anesthetics depress the central nervous system, as evidenced by dose-dependent decreases in the cerebral vascular resistance and the cerebral metabolic rate for oxygen ($CMRO_2$). The decrease in vascular resistance causes a reciprocal increase in cerebral blood flow that begins at approximately 0.6 MAC.[421] The extent of the increase in cerebral blood flow, however, depends on the inhalational anesthetics: halothane ~ desflurane > isoflurane > sevoflurane.[421–424] In adults, the cerebral vasculature remains responsive to CO_2 under general anesthesia but decreases with increasing MAC, disappearing at 1.5 MAC in the case of desflurane.[425] The net effect of inhalational anesthetics is a dose-dependent increase in the ratio of the cerebral blood flow to $CMRO_2$.

The effects of inhalational anesthetics on the CNS in children have not been fully elucidated. Autoregulation of cerebral blood flow does not vary with age in children up to 1.5 MAC sevoflurane.[426,427] Cerebral blood flow velocity in children varies directly with the end-tidal CO_2 ($ETCO_2$) during halothane and isoflurane anesthesia.[428] Cerebral blood flow velocity increases as the concentrations of halothane[429] and desflurane[430] increase. Compared with halothane, however, sevoflurane does not increase cerebral blood flow velocity.[431] Based on current evidence, sevoflurane and isoflurane remain the preferred inhalational anesthetics for neuroanesthesia in children at small MAC values (<1 MAC) and in the presence of mild hyperventilation (see Chapter 24).

In children, the EEG activity during halothane anesthesia differs substantially from that of sevoflurane. In the case of halothane, the EEG is characterized by slow waves superimposed on fast rhythms (α and β waves), whereas in the case of sevoflurane, the EEG is characterized by mainly sharp slow waves.[432] Furthermore, the shift of power of the EEG from low (1–4 Hz) to medium frequencies (8–30 Hz) is greater with halothane than it is for sevoflurane. The

clinical relevance of these EEG differences remains unclear but may contribute in part to the inconsistencies reported with processed EEG monitoring in children anesthetized with various inhalation anesthetics (see later discussion).

When sevoflurane was first introduced into clinical practice, three neurologic events were reported during induction of anesthesia: seizures, myoclonic/tonic clonic jerking movements, and epileptiform EEG tracings. Although frank seizures were rare, investigators cautioned that myoclonic jerking movements and epileptiform EEG tracings occurred frequently and represented a forme fruste for seizures.[433–437] The frequency of epileptiform EEG discharges during inhalational inductions with sevoflurane is 20%, although some have reported frequencies as great as 95%.[438–440] These discharges occurred more frequently at large (~8%) concentrations of sevoflurane during induction of anesthesia.[441] Since the EEG is not routinely monitored during anesthesia, several investigators recommended limiting the maximum inspired concentration during induction to 5% to 5.5% in nitrous oxide or abruptly decreasing the inspired concentration of sevoflurane to <1.5 MAC when the eyelash reflex was lost and to reduce the risk of epileptiform EEG tracings.[441,442]

The partial pressure (or alveolar concentration) of sevoflurane during induction of anesthesia exceeds that within the brain, with a lag time to equilibration estimated by the $T_{1/2}keo$, ~2 minutes, in 3-year-olds.[58,443] Hence the time to equilibrate sevoflurane in the brain with the alveolar concentration requires 4 to 5 half-lives or 8 to 10 minutes, at least 6-fold greater than the time to loss of the eyelash reflex during a sevoflurane inhalational induction, 45 seconds to 2 minutes.[376–378] Although epileptiform discharges are more frequent at deep levels of sevoflurane anesthesia during induction, limiting or reducing the concentration when the eyelash reflex is lost will result in partial pressures within the brain of a mere 1.5% to 2% sevoflurane, <1 MAC sevoflurane. Therefore, dramatically decreasing the inspired concentration of sevoflurane during induction of anesthesia as soon as the eyelash reflex is lost could result in the child moving during insertion of an IV or other procedure, or trigger an episode of laryngospasm, awareness, or hyperdynamic circulatory responses to other manipulations such as intubation. The authors strongly discourage reducing the concentration of sevoflurane after loss of the eyelash reflex.

Investigators previously recommended that the sevoflurane concentrations be decreased from 8% to ~1 MAC to reduce the frequency of major epileptiform discharges. They associated an 8% inspired concentration with major epileptiform discharges.[441] However, the frequency of epileptiform discharges during induction of anesthesia with sevoflurane at 6% and 8% are similar.[440] Moreover, investigators demonstrated that decreasing the concentration of sevoflurane even further, from 8% to 4% did not impact the frequency of epileptiform discharges, casting further doubts on the previous recommendation to dramatically reduce the inspired concentration of sevoflurane once the eyelash reflex was lost to reduce epileptiform discharges.[439] In addition, investigators determined the MAC associated with major epileptiform discharges during steady-state conditions (not during induction of anesthesia) was 4.3 ± 0.1% in 100% oxygen and 4.6 ± 0.2% in 50% nitrous oxide.[444] These MAC values that indicate the steady-state brain partial pressure at which 50% of the children develop epileptiform EEG activity are far greater than those achieved during a rapid sevoflurane induction once the eyelash reflex is lost and exceed the concentration to "prevent" epileptiform activity recommended previously. Thus, reducing the inspired concentration during induction of anesthesia is neither scientifically sound nor clinically safe. As a result, few have endorsed such a practice.

A handful of anecdotal reports described transient seizure-like or myoclonic/jerking movements of one or more extremities during induction of anesthesia with sevoflurane.[433–436] Both sevoflurane and enflurane have triggered transient seizures.[445] In the case of sevoflurane, isolated brief seizure-like motor movements of the extremities have been reported during and after anesthesia, often in combination with hyperventilation.[433–436,446] These movements appeared when sevoflurane was first introduced into clinical practice in the early 1990s. At the time, the sevoflurane concentration was increased slowly, in 1% to 2% stepwise increments, every 3 to 4 breaths until 8% (after the practice with halothane). The movements often resembled decorticate or decerebrate posturing, starting at ~1 to 2 MAC sevoflurane or 2.5% to 3%, consistent with a light plane of anesthesia.[433,434] If ventilation was controlled (causing hypocapnia) during the slow inductions, the sum of the two effects resulted in an even greater frequency of myoclonic-like movements. Nitrous oxide and spontaneous (or assisted) ventilation (maintaining an end-tidal $pCO_2 \geq 40$ mm Hg) reduced the frequency of myoclonic jerking movements as well as epileptiform EEG tracings.[437,447] When clinicians were advised to increase the sevoflurane concentration from 0% to 8% with a single turn of the vaporizer dial, the frequency of these movements all but disappeared. This may explain why we rarely witness myoclonic jerking movements during induction with sevoflurane today.

At least two single nucleotide polymorphisms have been associated with myoclonic movement during induction of anesthesia with sevoflurane in adults. The first involves N-methyl-D-aspartate (NMDA) receptors which are G-protein, cation channels that are activated by glutamate. Comprised of at least three complexes known as glutamate ionotropic receptor NMDA type (GRIN): NR1 or GRIN1 (containing a glycine binding site), NR2 or GRIN2A/B/C/D (containing a glutamate binding site, present in abundance in the CNS) and NR3 or GRIN3 (insensitive to anesthetics),[448,449] anesthetics interact primarily with the first two. In a recent study, the authors reported that women with an NMDA polymorphism, GRIN2A rs12918566 T allele, were more prone to spontaneous myoclonic/jerky movements during sevoflurane anesthesia than those without the polymorphism.[450] Furthermore, NMDA receptor gene polymorphisms (GRIN1, GRIN2A/B and GRIN2D) in children have been associated with a wide spectrum of neurodevelopmental disorders including cognitive impairment, seizures, autism spectrum, and movement disorders.[451] The second involves the methionine synthase reductase (MTRR) gene. Three single nucleotide polymorphisms predicted a greater risk of agitation/movement during induction that was associated with EEG evidence of a shift to high frequency spike activity.[452] This new evidence provides context for these infrequent reports of myoclonic jerking movements during induction of anesthesia with sevoflurane that may explain the rarity of the events despite sevoflurane-induced EEG changes.

These EEG recordings prompted widespread concern that they may herald seizures, although the evidence in support of this has not been forthcoming. In the only study in infants in whom video-EEG was monitored during sevoflurane inductions, one infant had an EEG seizure before sevoflurane was administered, one had an EEG seizure during sevoflurane, and three others had focal interictal epileptiform discharges, yielding an overall incidence of epileptiform discharges of 7.4%.[453] Epileptiform EEG tracings are characterized by spikes, polyspikes, triphasic waves, periodic epileptiform discharges, and/or burst suppression.[438] Such EEG patterns are indistinguishable from epileptic foci reported in children with epilepsy except that myoclonic or tonic/clonic movements do not occur in the vast majority of cases where the patterns were detected.[438] The epileptiform EEG tracings recorded during induction with sevoflurane may not portend frank seizures as these same tracings have been reported in nonconvulsive status epilepticus, do not evolve in a temporal manner towards seizures, occur over the entire cortex, and do not have the same pathological basis as seizures, raising questions about the nature and possible consequences of these EEG patterns.[438,454]

The relationship between interictal epileptiform discharges and epileptogenesis is far from clear: those who developed epilepsy may have had interictal epileptiform EEG discharges in their past EEG tracings, whereas those who have interictal epileptiform EEG discharges may never develop seizures or epilepsy. Moreover, hippocampus-driven interictal discharges may prevent seizures.[455] Several studies have reported interictal EEG discharges in healthy, awake children without epilepsy who were monitored with an EEG. The prevalence of these EEG epileptiform tracings was 3.5% to 6.5%.[456,457] Longitudinal follow-up and EEG monitoring of 131 children who were 6 to 18 years of age at the time of recording the initial epileptiform EEG discharges (prevalence of 3.5%) yielded no evidence of interictal discharges 8 to 9 years later. Moreover, there were no cases of epilepsy, which led the authors to conclude that these interictal epileptiform discharges do not portend long-term neurologic sequelae.[457] However, apart from the few isolated reports of seizures, seizures have not occurred during or after sevoflurane anesthesia even when epileptiform EEG tracings were recorded.[438–440] Although nonconvulsive ictal discharges resulted in neuronal damage in animals, similar findings have not been forthcoming in humans.[454] Possible explanations for the absence of seizure-like manifestations associated with the epileptiform EEG tracings during sevoflurane anesthesia include the possibilities that sevoflurane suppresses spinal cord motor neuron transmission and/or that the brain mechanism may be similar to that found in nonconvulsive status epilepticus.[454] Epileptiform EEG tracings are more frequent with increased concentrations of sevoflurane and hyperventilation (3- to 4-fold greater) but decreased in the presence of nitrous oxide and propofol.[437,440,447] Whether these epileptiform EEG tracings represent normal variants or pathological changes remains unclear. Some have suggested that these interictal epileptiform discharges are misdiagnosed and labeled as abnormal findings when in fact they are normal variants.[458,459] Currently, it remains unclear whether these interictal epileptiform EEG tracings are completely benign or pathological, although to date, general anesthesia with sevoflurane in healthy children has not been associated with substantive cognitive or neurological sequelae (see Chapter 23).[460] These laboratory findings are interesting and merit further investigation, but currently there is insufficient evidence to warrant altering our practice. We recommend that clinicians continue to induce anesthesia with sevoflurane up to 8%, in combination with nitrous oxide as desired, using spontaneous or assisted respiration only.

Awareness during inhalational anesthesia has been reported to occur with an incidence of 1:51,500 to 1:100 during sevoflurane anesthesia in children.[461–465] This wide discrepancy in frequency may be attributed to the technique used to identify the episodes (self-reporting, retrospective chart review, or direct questioning after the event),[466] a shift from halothane to sevoflurane anesthesia with anesthetic induction rooms,[414,467] and the types of surgery and anesthesia (cardiac, obesity, and TIVA).[466] In addition, a multivariate analysis in five cohort studies curiously reported that the use of nitrous oxide and tracheal intubation were independently associated with a greater frequency of awareness[463] even though the omission of nitrous oxide has been associated with awareness in adults, with a frequency ranging from 0.17% to 4%.[468] The psychological effects of perioperative awareness on children are quite variable and unpredictable from a minimal effect to severe distress.[464,469]

Concerns regarding awareness during anesthesia increased interest in the use of processed EEG monitoring in children,[470] although the incidence of awareness in children is actually exceedingly small (see earlier in this section) and in adults, the risk of awareness and more rapid recovery from anesthesia using BIS monitoring is similar to that of end-tidal gas monitoring.[471] With problems identified with using the BIS in children, its routine use has not been established. The BIS monitor displays values between 0 and 100 representing burst suppression at one extreme and wakefulness at the other (see Chapter 49). In adults, BIS readings of 40 to 60 are associated with a reduced risk of awareness and recall, whereas readings greater than 70 are associated with an increased risk of awareness and recall.

The BIS value has been studied in children to a limited degree to date, but its validity and role in the anesthetic management of infants and children younger than 5 years of age remain in question. One concern is that the EEG algorithm in the BIS is derived from adult EEG data, not from infants and children. Since the EEG evolves throughout infancy and childhood, the reliability of the processed EEG readings based on the adult EEG is dubious.[472,473] EEG recordings from children are problematic because there are few longitudinal studies of EEG throughout childhood and into adulthood in healthy, normal subjects.[474] Moreover, EEG recordings in children suffer from artifact interference and are brief in duration requiring processing to scrub out extraneous data before being suitable for analysis.[475] Despite these issues, BIS measurements that have been reported in older children for the most part, track the depth of anesthesia appropriately, and the values appear to correlate with the end-tidal concentration of the anesthetic. However, several unexplained curiosities have been reported that raise questions about the rigor of the BIS readings in children. The BIS readings for halothane in children exceed those for isoflurane, desflurane, and sevoflurane at equi-MAC values.[284,285,476] This has been attributed to the differential effects of anesthetics on the EEG. In fact, the distinct spectral features noted in the steady-state frontal EEG recordings during sevoflurane and xenon anesthesia in adults has prompted calls for anesthetic-specific algorithms for these brain-monitoring devices.[477] In addition, the BIS value decreases with increasing age for the same sevoflurane concentration.[281,284,478] Paradoxically, the BIS value actually increases as the sevoflurane concentration increases >3%, an observation that has been attributed to increased epileptiform discharges at deep concentrations of sevoflurane in children.[478,479] In contrast, BIS readings parallel the depth of anesthesia during total intravenous anesthesia including propofol and remifentanil.[479] In terms of outcomes from using the BIS monitor in pediatric anesthesia, a recent blinded study in which half of the clinicians had access to the BIS readings and the other half did not, the duration of stay in the recovery room and time to discharge from the hospital as well as the frequency of emergence delirium and severity of the pain scores did not differ between the two groups.[480] In a study of third molar extractions in sedated children with native airways breathing spontaneously,

the risk of airway obstruction increased as the BIS decreased from 77 to 64.[481]

A further concern is the enormous interindividual variability in processed EEG monitoring, making it difficult to define thresholds for awareness or lack thereof.[478] Spontaneous respirations increase the variability in the BIS readings[482] whereas ketamine, nitrous oxide, and opioids do not depress the EEG in a dose-dependent manner.[483] Discrepant BIS readings have also been reported from the right and left sides of the brain[484] as well as in the prone position.[485] Given that the BIS assesses both the level of hypnosis and electromyographic activity, low BIS readings in an awake, but paralyzed volunteer, similar to those at deep hypnotic levels without paralysis,[486] suggest a worrisome false negative rate for awareness. Alternately, if the BIS readings in an anesthetized and paralyzed patient suddenly increased to values >60, two possible scenarios may exist: either the level of hypnosis decreased, or the paralysis wore off. Many of us have identified such a false positive scenario as the neuromuscular blockade has worn off. Hence, optimal interpretation of changes in the BIS readings depends on maintaining a consistent level of anesthesia and paralysis. The BIS values in children with cognitive impairment or cerebral palsy were less than those who were unaffected at the same anesthetic concentration, although the MAC reduction for cognitive impairment was not accounted for.[487,488] Had the reduced MAC been accounted for in cognitively impaired children,[402] the BIS readings may not have differed. With the State Entropy monitor, entropy increases in the presence of nitrous oxide, rendering those readings misleading. The aggregate of this evidence undermines the validity of processed EEG monitoring during inhalational anesthesia in children. It is equally important to appreciate that the sensitivity of the BIS to detect awareness does not differ from end-tidal gas monitoring (see Chapter 49 for further details).[489]

Cardiovascular System

Inhalational anesthetics (with the exception of xenon) affect the cardiovascular system either directly (by depressing myocardial contractility [calcium channel blockade], altering the conduction system, or by dilating the peripheral vasculature) or indirectly (by affecting the balance of parasympathetic and sympathetic nervous systems and neurohumoral, renal, or reflex responses). The cardiovascular responses to inhalational anesthetics in children are further complicated by maturational changes in the cardiovascular system and responsiveness to inhalational anesthetics. In aggregate, all of these developmental changes reduce the margin of safety between adequate anesthesia and severe cardiopulmonary depression in infants and children compared with adults. The salient features of the immature cardiovascular system in infants and children at both the macroscopic and microscopic levels have been reviewed elsewhere.[490]

Assessment of cardiovascular variables in infants and children presents a challenge for clinicians. Although blood pressure and electrocardiography are standard monitors of hemodynamics in infants and children of all ages, measures of cardiac output and myocardial contractility are much more difficult to quantitate accurately. Two-dimensional echocardiography and impedance cardiometry have been used to estimate cardiac output and myocardial contractility in infants and children,[491–494] although the echocardiographic measurements are subject to variability depending on the preload and afterload. Load-independent–derived echocardiographic variables (stress-velocity and stress-shortening indexes) have improved the accuracy of echocardiographic estimates of myocardial function and are used with increasing frequency.[495] Transesophageal echocardiography is used much more frequently in children, although its use is limited to children with congenital heart disease undergoing cardiac surgery. The few studies that have examined continuous noninvasive cardiac output measurements such as electrical cardiometry and capnodynamics to date have yielded mixed results but these techniques may find their niche in the future.[496–504]

In children, several factors determine the blood pressure responses to inhalational anesthetics, including the particular anesthetic studied, the dose, the administration of a premedication, the level of preoperative anxiety, and the systemic pressure measured: systolic, diastolic, or mean. Most studies demonstrate modest, dose-dependent decreases in blood pressure with all of the inhalational anesthetics, although the magnitudes of the changes vary. In a direct comparison of sevoflurane and halothane, systolic blood pressure decreased 7.5% at 1 MAC sevoflurane and 12.5% at 1 MAC halothane, but returned to awake values at 1.5 MAC with both anesthetics.[495] In children older than 1 year of age, systolic blood pressure decreased 0% to 11% at 1 MAC sevoflurane, and 22% to 28% at 1 MAC desflurane, compared with awake values.[394,395] At 1 MAC, mean blood pressure in children decreased 15% to 25% with isoflurane and sevoflurane.[492,494] All of the inhalational anesthetics (in concentrations up to 1.5 MAC) modestly depress the systolic blood pressure in children.

Myocardial contractility decreases to a greater extent during halothane (up to 1.5 MAC) than during isoflurane or sevoflurane anesthesia, as evidenced by decreases in cardiac output and ejection fraction in healthy children.[493,494,505] Cardiac index decreases to similar extents with halothane and sevoflurane at 1 and 2 MAC: 10% at 1 MAC and 20% to 35% at 2 MAC.[494] Ejection fraction decreases 30% at 0.5 and 1.5 MAC halothane compared with awake values, but is unchanged at equipotent concentrations of isoflurane.[492] The addition of nitrous oxide to halothane or isoflurane in infants and small children depresses myocardial function to a similar extent as equipotent anesthetic concentrations of halothane or isoflurane in oxygen.[505] In children, halothane decreases myocardial contractility in a dose-dependent manner and to a greater extent than the ether anesthetics. Isoflurane and sevoflurane decrease myocardial contractility to a lesser extent than halothane and are preferred for children with limited cardiovascular reserves. Intravenous atropine restores the decrease in myocardial function, in part, associated with halothane anesthesia likely the result of its chronotropic and Bowditch treppe effects,[505–509] whereas IV balanced salt solution restores the decrease in myocardial function associated with isoflurane anesthesia likely by augmenting preload.[493]

The mechanism by which inhalational anesthetics depress myocardial function remains controversial. Studies in both animal and human myocardial cells suggest that halothane, isoflurane, and sevoflurane directly depress myocardial contractility by decreasing intracellular calcium ion (Ca^{2+}) flux and/or the sensitivity to the Ca^{2+}.[510,511] Inhalational anesthetics decrease the Ca^{2+} flux by their action on the calcium channels themselves, Na^+-Ca^{2+} exchange pumps, and the sarcoplasmic reticulum.[490] Evidence suggests that inhalational anesthetics attenuate contractility of ventricular myocytes via voltage-dependent L-type calcium channels (which are responsible for release of large amounts of calcium from the sarcoplasmic reticulum).[512,513]

That neonates and infants are more sensitive to the depressant actions of inhalational anesthetics than are older children is supported by experimental evidence of maturational differences between neonatal and adult rat, rabbit, and feline myocardium.[513–516] Structural differences that may account, in part, for the changes in myocardial sensitivity to inhalational anesthetics with age include a reduction in contractile elements including reduction in actin-myosin cross-bridge attachment and detachment,[517] immature sarcoplasmic reticulum, and functional differences in calcium sensitivity of the contractile elements, calcium channels, and the sodium-calcium exchange pump in the neonatal myocardium.[490,512–514,516,518–520] The determinants of Ca^{2+} homeostasis in neonatal ventricular myocardial cells depend on transsarcolemmic Ca^{2+} flux to a far greater extent than on the sarcoplasmic reticulum.[490] This is based on a growing body of experimental evidence that includes the finding that the concentration of the Na^+-Ca^{2+} exchange protein in the neonatal myocardium, a protein that regulates transsarcolemmic flux of Ca^{2+}, exceeds that in adult cells by 2.5-fold and that its concentration decreases with age as the concentration of L-type voltage-dependent calcium channels increases.[514] Furthermore, halothane reversibly inhibits the Na^+-Ca^{2+} exchange protein in immature myocardial cells.[514] The sarcoplasmic reticulum is poorly developed in neonatal myocardial cells, and this finding weighs heavily against the sarcoplasmic reticulum being the major source of Ca^{2+} required for myocardial contractility. Indeed, evidence suggests that inhalational anesthetics depress myocardial contractility in neonates by inhibiting Ca^{2+} influx and Na^+-Ca^{2+} exchange channels rather than by inhibiting Ca^{2+} release from sarcoplasmic reticulum.[511]

Ever since the introduction of halothane into clinical practice, clinicians have been aware of a greater incidence of hypotension and bradycardia in neonates who were anesthetized with halothane than in adults. However, this was not the case when *equipotent* concentrations (approximately 1 MAC) of halothane[392,507] were administered to neonates and older infants 1 to 6 months of age. Subsequent studies demonstrated that isoflurane,[521] sevoflurane,[395] and desflurane[394] all decreased systolic pressure in neonates to similar extents as in older infants 1 to 6 months of age. Interestingly, systolic blood pressure decreased 30% in response to 1 MAC sevoflurane in neonates and infants 1 to 6 months of age, which was substantially greater than the 5% decrease in older infants and children up to 12 years of age.[395] In the case of desflurane, systolic blood pressure decreased 30% in response to 1 MAC desflurane across all age groups.[394] These data suggest that systolic blood pressure decreases up to 30% in response to 1 MAC of all inhalational anesthetics in infants and children, and that caution should be exercised when administering these anesthetics to infants and children who are at risk for hemodynamic instability, or in whom greater concentrations of inhaled anesthetics are required. Although blood pressure decreased 30% with both halothane and sevoflurane, the decrease in myocardial contractility with halothane was greater than with sevoflurane whereas the decrease in peripheral vascular resistance with sevoflurane exceeded that with halothane.[522] On the basis of echocardiographic determinations, cardiac output and ejection fraction decrease in a dose-dependent fashion from awake to 1.5 MAC halothane and isoflurane in neonates and infants.[491] In a comparison of sevoflurane and halothane up to 1.5 MAC in infants, sevoflurane maintained cardiac index but decreased blood pressure and systemic vascular resistance.[523] Myocardial contractility decreased in a dose-dependent manner with halothane as well as with sevoflurane, although the decrease with the former exceeded that with the latter.

The baroreceptor reflex response is also depressed in infants with either halothane[524] or isoflurane,[525] albeit to a greater extent with halothane. In view of the greater incidence of hypotension in neonates and infants than older children, an intact baroreceptor reflex could offset, in part, the cardiovascular consequences. However, inhalational anesthetics blunt this response, leaving the infant vulnerable to the direct cardiodepressant actions of the anesthetics. Prophylactic anticholinergics augment the cardiac output by increasing the heart rate. The baroreceptor reflex in children is depressed equally with sevoflurane and halothane.[522]

Two studies evaluated the effects of inhalational anesthesia on the hemodynamics of children with congenital heart disease undergoing cardiac surgery.[526,527] Sevoflurane maintained cardiac index and heart rate with less hypotension and negative inotropic effect than halothane. Isoflurane maintained cardiac index and ejection fraction, increased heart rate, and caused less depression of mean arterial pressure (MAP) than halothane.[526] Sevoflurane was also associated with fewer episodes of severe hypotension and reduced need for vasopressors and chronotropes during emergence than halothane.[527]

Inhalational anesthetics vary in their effects on the cardiac rhythm. Halothane slows the heart rate, in some cases leading to junctional rhythms, bradycardia, and asystole. This response is dose-dependent. Three mechanisms have been proposed to explain the genesis of halothane-associated dysrhythmias: a direct effect on the sinoatrial node, a vagal effect, or an imbalance in the parasympathetic and sympathetic tone. It has also been suggested that the etiology of the bradycardia during halothane anesthesia may be a withdrawal of sympathetic tone. Bradycardia is particularly marked in the neonate, presumably because parasympathetic influences predominate over the sparse sympathetic innervation of the myocardium in this age group.

Arrhythmias occur more frequently during halothane anesthesia than during anesthesia with ethers because the former sensitizes the myocardium to catecholamines, particularly in the presence of hypercapnia and "light anesthesia."[528] In addition, it decreases the threshold for ventricular extrasystoles during epinephrine administration by threefold.[529–531] Most of these arrhythmias are unifocal or multifocal premature ventricular beats, nodal rhythm, bigeminy, or supraventricular arrhythmias.[381,528,532–534] Despite their appearance, most of these arrhythmias are benign and preserve the blood pressure; however, if ventricular tachycardia occurs, hypotension may ensue. Arrhythmias during halothane are more frequent during spontaneous ventilation, associated with hypercarbia and high levels of circulating catecholamines.[528]

Management of arrhythmias during halothane anesthesia includes inflating the lungs with large tidal volumes, hyperventilation to decrease the arterial CO_2 tension, increasing the concentration of halothane during "light" anesthesia (i.e., sweating, hypertension), and substituting an ether inhalational anesthetic for halothane.[528,535] Lidocaine has no role in the treatment of these arrhythmias because the myocardium is not intrinsically irritable. Moreover, a rapid IV bolus of lidocaine (2 mg/kg) may cause profound bradycardia.[528,536] In infants and children anesthetized with halothane, 10 μg/kg atropine increases the heart rate by 50% or more and promotes sinus rhythm.[537] This dose of atropine also increases blood pressure and cardiac output in infants and children 2 years of age and older during halothane anesthesia.[538]

Sevoflurane has limited effects on heart rate,[363] at 1 MAC and during induction of anesthesia, generally maintaining or increasing the heart rate.[382,496] The heart rate may slow transiently during the first few minutes of induction of anesthesia, often preceded by

a nodal rhythm. In these circumstances, the heart rate usually recovers spontaneously without treatment.[474] Heart rate is usually unaffected by the administration of desflurane[381,468] unless the inspired concentration is increased suddenly in the absence of opioids, which results in a neurosympathetic response, a phenomenon reported in adults but not in children.[479,480]

Halothane also sensitizes the myocardium to catecholamines, particularly in the presence of hypercapnia and "light anesthesia."[528] Halothane decreases the threshold for ventricular extrasystoles during epinephrine administration 3-fold.[529–531] In contrast, isoflurane, desflurane, and sevoflurane maintain or increase heart rate during the early induction period of anesthesia.[376,394,395,482,492,494,521,523,539]

When bradycardia occurs in an anesthetized child, the primary diagnosis should be hypoxia before other causes, such as a direct drug effect (i.e., high concentration of halothane) are considered. Isoflurane, desflurane, and sevoflurane do not sensitize the myocardium to catecholamines to the same extent as does halothane, and ventricular arrhythmias are rare.[529,530,540] When children with Down syndrome are anesthetized with sevoflurane, bradycardia occurs three to four times more frequently than in those without Down syndrome, irrespective of the presence of a congenital heart defect and may cause a sufficiently severe bradycardia[541] to prompt an intervention with chronotropic medications e.g., anticholinergic or CPR.[542,543]

The mechanism by which the sinus node controls automaticity is incompletely understood but may include potassium ion (K^+) currents, hyperpolarization-activated current, and T and L forms of Ca^{2+} currents.[490] Moreover, developmental changes in these channels likely account, in part, for the differential effects of inhalational anesthetics on heart rate with age.[518]

Concerns of a relationship between inhalational anesthetics and prolonged QT interval that progressed to cardiac arrest or torsades de pointes have emerged. Although the ether inhalational anesthetics including sevoflurane prolong the QTc interval (with >500 milliseconds being abnormal),[544,545] this alone appears to be insufficient to induce torsades de pointes. Torsades de pointes also requires the transmural dispersion of repolarization. This is defined as the variability in the rate of repolarization across the myocardium, from epicardium to endocardium. The rate of repolarization may be estimated by the interval in the peak to end of the T wave on a 12-lead electrocardiogram. Evidence has demonstrated that the risk of torsades de pointes during sevoflurane anesthesia is exceedingly unlikely to ever occur even in the presence of ondansetron as the dispersion of repolarization remains unchanged.[546,547]

Paroxysmal increases in blood pressure (both systolic and diastolic pressures) and heart rate have been reported in adults after a rapid increase in the inspired concentration of isoflurane or desflurane but not sevoflurane.[548] A similar response has also been observed in a child during an inhalational induction with desflurane in 50% nitrous oxide(unpublished data, CJC).[549] Increasing the concentration of desflurane from 4% to 12% suddenly may lead to a massive sympathetic response, mediated by norepinephrine and/or epinephrine, that culminates in tachycardia and hypertension.[549,550] Repetitive small increases (1%) in the inspired concentration of the anesthetic produce transient but attenuated catecholamine bursts and hyperdynamic circulatory responses compared with larger increases in concentration.[551,552] Increasing the inspired concentration of desflurane further while attempting to attenuate the tachycardia and hypertension is ineffective and is more likely to exacerbate the response. To restore vital signs to normal, the inciting anesthetic should be discontinued and replaced with another. Fentanyl (2 μg/kg), esmolol, labetalol, and clonidine have all been effective in preventing, attenuating, or eliminating these responses.[553–556] It is likely that two sites are responsible for triggering the sympathetic discharge after a rapid increase in desflurane concentrations >6%: the lung or airways and one of the VRG organs,[557] with the latter mediating the greater response.[548,558,559] Neuroexcitatory responses have not been reported in children.

Xenon offers an immense advantage over the ether-based inhalational anesthetics in that it maintains circulatory stability.[342] In the cardiac catheterization laboratory, the effects of 50% to 65% xenon in combination with sevoflurane were compared with sevoflurane alone in children <4 years of age undergoing diagnostic/interventional heart catheterization.[560] The study was terminated prematurely when the incidence of the primary outcomes, a heart rate change >20%, mean arterial pressure >20%, or an intervention to treat hemodynamic instability, was similar between the two groups. Nonetheless, children anesthetized with xenon-sevoflurane had decreased vasopressor requirements, better preserved cerebral oxygen saturation and more rapid recovery. Although the MAC of xenon in adults is very large (see E-Table 5.1), the MAC for xenon in children, which has not been determined, may be even greater. If the MAC in children actually exceeds the adult value, xenon may require an intravenous agent to be coadministered to allow for an adequate inspired concentration of oxygen. In the case of children with cyanotic congenital heart disease, this agent would present the greatest challenge for induction as its very low solubility in blood combined with its very large MAC in the presence of a right-to-left shunt will result in a very slow induction and a limited depth of anesthesia necessitating administration of a supplemental intravenous agent.[367]

Respiratory System

During spontaneous ventilation, both tidal volume and respiratory rate vary with the specific anesthetic, depth of anesthesia, and nociception. The increased respiratory rate during inhalational anesthesia in children has been attributed to sensitization of the stretch receptors within the lung as well as possible central effects. Inhalational anesthetics significantly affect respiration in infants and children in a dose-dependent fashion via effects on the respiratory center, chest wall muscles, and reflex responses. Halothane depresses minute ventilation by decreasing tidal volume and attenuating the response to CO_2.[561–564] This depression is offset, in part, by an increase in the respiratory rate.[561,564] These ventilatory responses to halothane are age dependent; minute ventilation in infants decreases to a greater extent than in children.[563] In infants and young children anesthetized with halothane, intercostal muscle activity is attenuated before the diaphragm.[561,565] This effect is most pronounced in preterm and full-term neonates and infants and when a tracheal tube is used in place of a laryngeal mask airway.[566] The movement of the chest and abdomen during the respiratory cycle is one of synchronized protrusion of the abdomen and collapse of the chest wall during inspiration (with some intercostal indrawing) and indrawing of the abdomen and flattening of the chest wall during expiration. This is commonly referred to as the "rocking horse" movement of the chest (similar to the phenomenon that occurs during upper airway obstruction in infants and children). This results in loss of FRC and is of particular concern in infants younger than 2 years of age who have decreased type I muscle fibers in both the diaphragm and intercostal muscles (see Fig. 12.12). This explains why infants fatigue easily and why positive end-expiratory

pressure is useful in this age group. Isoflurane, sevoflurane, and desflurane also depress ventilatory drive, decrease tidal volume, and attenuate the response to CO_2.[562,564,567–572] The increase in respiratory frequency that follows respiratory depression (decreased tidal volume) may not restore minute ventilation to preanesthetic levels.

Sevoflurane depresses respiration to a similar extent as halothane up to 1.4 MAC but depresses respiration to a greater extent at concentrations greater than 1.4 MAC.[567] This results from a direct effect of sevoflurane on respiratory frequency.[569] Although respiratory effort may decrease rapidly during sevoflurane or desflurane anesthesia, the low blood solubilities and rapid wash-out profiles of these drugs in part ensure that this is a self-limiting phenomenon during spontaneous respirations. Sevoflurane decreases the tone of the intercostal muscles to a lesser extent than halothane.[565,567] The compensatory changes in respiratory rate differ among the anesthetics; respiratory rate increases at 1.4 MAC or more with halothane, is unchanged with isoflurane, but decreases at 1.4 MAC or less with sevoflurane.[562,564] This inadequate compensatory response to respiratory depression with sevoflurane suggests that when children are anesthetized with those anesthetics, spontaneous ventilation must be carefully monitored to avoid hypopnea or apnea. Sevoflurane maintains or decreases airway resistance in children with normal airways and those with asthma or a recent upper respiratory tract infection. Insertion of a tracheal tube during sevoflurane anesthesia increases airway resistance without sequelae.[573,574]

Desflurane depresses respiration in children during spontaneous respirations at greater than 1 MAC by decreasing tidal volume.[572] However, desflurane increases airway resistance in children with asthma and respiratory tract infections to a greater extent than sevoflurane.[574] Desflurane is probably best avoided in these children.

Studies of the upper airway in children anesthetized with inhalational anesthesia have sought to explain the pathophysiology of airway obstruction. Sevoflurane at 1 MAC causes more upper airway obstruction than halothane.[575] In escalating doses between 0.5 and 1.5 MAC, sevoflurane decreased the cross-sectional area of the airway by one-third, predominantly in the anteroposterior dimension.[576] This effect primarily results from pharyngeal wall collapse, which can be easily offset with positive end-expiratory pressure (see Chapter 12).

Renal System

Potent inhalational anesthetics may affect renal function via four possible mechanisms: cardiovascular, autonomic, neuroendocrine, and metabolic. Although the first three mechanisms pose no direct threat to renal function, the fourth mechanism, metabolic, is a serious clinical concern that in the past has resulted in renal dysfunction after some inhalational anesthetics.

Inhalational anesthetics are metabolized in vivo by the CYP isozyme system to varying extents (E-Table 5.3). Metabolism of inhalational anesthetics may release both inorganic and organic fluoride moieties.[577] It is the inorganic fluoride that is released from ether anesthetics that has raised concern.

Isoflurane and desflurane undergo limited metabolism in vivo, resulting in very small plasma concentrations of inorganic fluoride even after 131 MAC hours of isoflurane.[578] In contrast, halothane is metabolized to a substantially greater extent but releases most of the fluoride in an organic form, trifluoroacetate. Trifluoroacetate has, however, been linked to halothane hepatitis (see later discussion). The metabolism of sevoflurane and methoxyflurane yields greater plasma concentrations of inorganic fluoride than isoflurane. The metabolism of sevoflurane yields both inorganic and organic fluoride moieties.[579] The organic form, hexafluoroisopropanol, is rapidly conjugated and excreted by the kidneys[579] and poses no threat to humans. Peak plasma concentrations of inorganic fluoride after exposure to inhalational anesthetics follow an order similar to that in E-Table 5.3: methoxyflurane > sevoflurane > isoflurane > halothane ≅ desflurane.[580–584] In the case of methoxyflurane, two metabolites are produced: inorganic fluoride and oxalic acid; both were implicated in the pathogenesis of renal dysfunction.[585] Subsequent studies demonstrated that subclinical nephrotoxicity occurred after more than 2.5 MAC hours of methoxyflurane, provided the plasma concentration of inorganic fluoride exceeded 50 μmol/L. Nephrotoxicity occurred after more than 5 MAC hours if the concentration of inorganic fluoride exceeded 90 μmol/L.[586] These clinical concerns led to the voluntary withdrawal of methoxyflurane from clinical practice.

That the plasma concentrations of inorganic fluoride in children who were anesthetized with sevoflurane were similar to or greater than those after enflurane[587–589] raised concerns about possible renal dysfunction after prolonged exposure. However, inorganic fluoride concentrations after relatively brief anesthetics in children are similar to those in adults: less than 20 μmol/L after about 1 MAC hour, which decreases to less than 10 μmol/L by 4 hours after discontinuation of anesthesia.[571] Nonetheless, the peak plasma concentrations of inorganic fluoride paralleled the MAC hour exposure to sevoflurane in both children and adults.[589] Concerns regarding the risk of renal dysfunction after sevoflurane were heightened after reports that the peak plasma concentration of inorganic fluoride in some adults exceeded the purported threshold for nephrotoxicity (50 μmol/L).[590] Despite the large plasma concentrations of inorganic fluoride after sevoflurane anesthesia, there was no evidence of renal dysfunction. These reports, together with a dearth of evidence in the toxicology literature, suggest that fluoride-mediated nephrotoxicity may be independent of the plasma concentration of inorganic fluoride.

Kharasch and colleagues postulated that inhalational anesthetic-induced nephrotoxicity might be anesthetic specific. They determined that the primary isozyme responsible for the degradation of enflurane, isoflurane, sevoflurane, and methoxyflurane anesthetics was CYP2E1,[577,591–593] with secondary isozymes including CYP2A6 and CYP3A.[594] Subsequently, they reported large quantities of CYP2E1 within the liver and kidneys.[591] They also noted that the affinity of renal CYP2E1 for methoxyflurane was 5-fold greater than it was for sevoflurane.[594] This provided further evidence that the renal dysfunction after ether inhalational anesthetics resulted from the local production of inorganic fluoride within the renal medulla rather than extrarenal production, and that certain anesthetics were more prone to release of inorganic fluoride than others (e.g., methoxyflurane much more so than sevoflurane). Because CYP2E1 has a greater affinity for methoxyflurane than sevoflurane, we now understand why renal dysfunction occurs after methoxyflurane and not after sevoflurane.[594] The lack of an association between sevoflurane, plasma inorganic fluoride concentration, and renal dysfunction in children and adults supports this new understanding of the mechanism of renal dysfunction after inhalational anesthesia. Consequently, the risk of renal dysfunction after sevoflurane is independent of the duration of exposure to sevoflurane. Sevoflurane does not pose any greater risk for perioperative renal disease than other maintenance anesthetics.[595] A second theoretical cause of sevoflurane-associated renal dysfunction is compound A, a product of alkaline hydrolysis of sevoflurane in the presence of CO_2 absorbents, whose formation is catalyzed by the presence sodium hydroxide (NaOH) and potassium hydroxide (KOH) within the CO_2 absorbent (see later discussion).[596,597]

Hepatic System

In vivo metabolism of inhalational anesthetics varies with age, increasing to adult values within the first 2 years of life. The developmental changes in metabolism may be attributed to reduced activity of the hepatic microsomal enzymes, reduced fat stores, and more rapid elimination of inhalational anesthetics in infants and children compared with adults. Postoperative liver dysfunction and/or liver failure in adults after halothane and isoflurane has been reported with a frequency of 3% and after sevoflurane and desflurane with a frequency of 4.1%.[598–600] In children, halothane and sevoflurane have been associated with transient hepatic dysfunction.[601–604] Indeed, several pediatric cases of transient postoperative liver failure and one case of fulminant hepatic failure and death have been attributed to "halothane hepatitis" that were confirmed serologically with antibodies to halothane-altered hepatic cell membrane antigens.[601] The exact mechanism of the hepatic dysfunction after halothane exposure remains unclear, although some clinicians have speculated that it is caused by an immunologic response to a metabolite of halothane. This putative toxic metabolite, a trifluoroacetyl halide compound, is produced during oxidative metabolism of halothane. It is thought that this compound induces an immunologic response in the liver by binding covalently to hepatic microsomal proteins, thereby forming an immunologically active hapten. A subsequent exposure to halothane then incites an immunologic response in the liver.[605] Hepatic enzymes may also be induced by previous administration of drugs, such as barbiturates, phenytoin, and rifampin. Although some have admonished clinicians for administering repeat anesthetics with halothane in children, it is our opinion that, in view of the millions of uneventful repeat halothane anesthetics in infants and children worldwide, and one author's experience in children with burn injuries anesthetized dozens of times with halothane (CJC), insufficient evidence exists to support such an admonition.

CLINICAL EFFECTS
Induction Techniques

Although the physicochemical characteristics of the ether series of anesthetics would predict that anesthesia could be induced smoothly and more rapidly with these agents than with halothane,[355,357] this has not proved to be the case. All of the ether anesthetics except sevoflurane irritate the upper airway in children, resulting in a high incidence of breath-holding, coughing, salivation, excitement, laryngospasm, and hemoglobin–oxygen desaturation.[532,606–615] Clinical studies with desflurane in children demonstrated a high incidence of breath-holding, laryngospasm, and desaturation during inhalational induction (~50%).[606,615] As a result, a "black box" warning was issued against the use of desflurane for induction of anesthesia in infants and children. Before the introduction of desflurane, some advocated inducing anesthesia in children with isoflurane.[609–613] For example, it has been suggested that the quality and speed of induction of anesthesia with isoflurane in oxygen in infants and children is similar to that with halothane.[610] However, airway reflexes were commonly triggered with isoflurane despite the use of a number of strategies to attenuate them,[614–616] including slowly increasing the inspired concentration and using scented masks. Given the smooth induction characteristics, economy, and availability of sevoflurane, there are no reasons to consider other anesthetics for induction of anesthesia in infants and children.

In contrast to the noxious effects of the methyl ethyl ether series of anesthetics on the airway, sevoflurane does not irritate the upper airway and is well tolerated when administered by mask to infants and children at any concentration.[376,377,380,381,385,395,539,617–621] The introduction of sevoflurane has challenged and displaced halothane as the induction agent of choice in children in most countries. The incidences of coughing, breath-holding, laryngospasm, and hemoglobin–oxygen desaturation during induction with sevoflurane, whether by slow incremental increases in concentration or a single breath, are similar to those that occur during halothane (there was a significantly greater incidence of breath holding with halothane compared with sevoflurane but a greater incidence of induction excitement with sevoflurane compared with halothane) (E-Table 5.4). The observation that the airway reflex responses are infrequent after a single-breath induction with 8% sevoflurane or 5% halothane casts doubt on the adage that large concentrations of inhalational anesthetics trigger airway reflex responses.[621–623] In fact, the induction is so smooth with sevoflurane that adjuvants, such as a premedication, concurrent use of nitrous oxide, or other strategies to prevent airway reflex responses, are generally unnecessary.

Induction of anesthesia with xenon has not been studied in children. In adults, inhalational induction with xenon at equi-MAC with sevoflurane resulted in a more rapid induction with stable respirations.[624] These data suggest that xenon may be an excellent induction anesthetic in children, provided its characteristics are upheld in clinical trials.

There is no universal approach to induce anesthesia by inhalation for all children. However, we advocate empowering children as much as possible to minimize their fears. After appropriate preoperative preparation (involving premedication or parental presence or distraction techniques), the child is seated on the bed or on a parent's lap and encouraged to breathe through a face mask scented with a favorite flavor (to disguise the plastic odor of the mask) that is held over the nose and mouth. A fresh gas composed of 70% nitrous oxide in oxygen is breathed (while the pop-off value is completely open for 1 to 2 minutes). Once the end-tidal nitrous oxide concentration reaches 50%, a single stepwise increase in the sevoflurane concentration to 8% is dialed. We wait until the end-tidal nitrous concentration reaches 50% before starting sevoflurane to minimize the risk of the child recalling the odor of sevoflurane.

Induction of anesthesia with halothane was performed by increasing the inspired concentration in stepwise increments (0.5% to 1.0% every three to four breaths) until an adequate depth of anesthesia was achieved. This slow increase in the inspired concentration of halothane was thought to attenuate the incidence of airway reflex responses, although this is not evidence-based. In fact, when a single-breath vital capacity induction was performed in children older than 6 years of age with 5% halothane, the incidence of airway reflex responses was surprisingly small.[621]

Initially, anesthesia was induced with sevoflurane by increasing the inspired concentration in slow stepwise increments of 1% to 1.5% until 8% was reached, but this frequently caused transient agitation and involuntary movement of the extremities that could be violent, particularly in adolescents.[395] These were attributed to an exaggerated excitement phase as a result of the larger MAC of sevoflurane than halothane. To minimize the excitement phase, the inspired concentration of sevoflurane can be rapidly increased

in a single step from 0% to 8%.[621] This is based on a study of single-breath induction with 8% sevoflurane and 5% halothane in which the incidence of involuntary movement and the need for restraint were significantly less with sevoflurane than with halothane.[621] Induction of anesthesia with 12% sevoflurane was reported to be more rapid than with 8%.[361] This is not a surprising finding, although 12% sevoflurane vaporizers cannot be deployed in clinical practice because inspired concentrations of sevoflurane (in a laboratory setting) of 11% in oxygen and 10% in nitrous oxide both support combustion. Hence the maximum deliverable concentration of sevoflurane is 8% or less depending on the jurisdiction.

Although some have reported that induction of anesthesia with sevoflurane is more rapid than with halothane, others have not. This inconsistency in the relative speed of induction reflects differences in study design that likely failed to take advantage of the 8% sevoflurane vaporizer and the differences in MAC. For children who are unable to perform a single-breath vital capacity induction, a rapid increase in the inspired concentration of sevoflurane has been a very effective alternative, with results comparable to the single-breath technique.[380,619–621]

Sevoflurane does not trigger airway reflex responses either alone or in combination with other agents, such as nitrous oxide. One study suggested that sevoflurane is the least irritating to the airway of all the inhalational anesthetics.[625] Previous studies suggested that airway irritability and excitement during sevoflurane anesthesia were similar whether nitrous oxide was present or absent, although others have disputed these findings.[621,626] The lack of effect of nitrous oxide on the speed of induction in the single-breath study was attributed to its concentration-reducing effect on sevoflurane.[621]

Arrhythmias are rare during anesthesia with the ether series of anesthetics, but when they occur, they are usually nodal in origin.[381,524,525,532,534,612,621,627] Arrhythmias during anesthesia with the ether anesthetics are usually self-limiting, resolving spontaneously or with parenteral administration of an anticholinergic. If the arrhythmias persist, then a cardiology consultation should be sought, particularly in a child with a history of congenital heart disease. Both IV and inhalational anesthetics have been used for induction and maintenance of anesthesia in children with congenital heart disease. (See the earlier cardiovascular section in this chapter and Chapter 21 for a more detailed discussion.)

Once an adequate depth of anesthesia has been achieved, it is prudent to maintain spontaneous respirations with the maximal inspired concentration of sevoflurane tolerated until IV access has been achieved. If hypopnea or apnea develop, then ventilation should be gently assisted so as to prevent awareness from occurring in the early induction period.[461,462] Discontinuing or decreasing the inspired concentration of nitrous oxide or sevoflurane individually or together prematurely may predispose the patient to adverse sequelae, particularly if the child is stimulated at a light plane of anesthesia, as described earlier. This may occur in situations when anesthesia is induced in one location (induction room) and the child is then transferred to another (OR) without continuously administering sevoflurane. Appreciating the limited solubility of nitrous oxide and sevoflurane and the large $T_{1/2}keo$ (~2 minutes) for the latter will help to understand how rapidly inhaled anesthetics egress from the body and the interval required to equilibrate the partial pressure in the brain. Once IV access is established, some practitioners administer propofol or another IV anesthetic before discontinuing the nitrous oxide to facilitate insertion of a laryngeal mask airway or tracheal intubation.[628,629]

The concentration of sevoflurane can then be decreased without risking adverse events.

Emergence

Emergence or recovery has been arbitrarily divided into early (extubation, eye opening, following commands) and late (drinking, discharge time from postanesthesia care unit or hospital). Although most studies have demonstrated a more rapid early recovery after less soluble anesthetics,[377–379,382,385] few have demonstrated a more rapid late recovery.[376,385,627,630] A recent systematic review of emergence times including extubation and awakening after desflurane was more rapid than after sevoflurane.[631]

The speed of emergence and recovery from anesthesia are discussed earlier in this chapter. The incidence of complications, such as airway reflex responses and vomiting during emergence from anesthesia, after either mask anesthesia or tracheal intubation, are similar with most inhalational agents.[377,379,380,382,525,609,610,630,632] However, the incidence of airway responses of any severity after desflurane was significantly greater than after isoflurane. Moreover, the incidence of airway adverse responses after removing a laryngeal mask airway (LMA) deep during desflurane anesthesia was significantly greater than was the incidence after removal of an LMA after recovery from desflurane (awake) or after isoflurane anesthesia.[633] In both a randomized controlled trial and a systematic review, the incidence of respiratory events with LMAs during desflurane anesthesia was similar to that with sevoflurane, although desaturation occurred more frequently in younger children during emergence after desflurane.[634,635]

Emergence Delirium

Emergence delirium is defined as a dissociated state of consciousness in which children are inconsolable, irritable, uncompromising, and/or uncooperative (see Videos 45.1 and 45.2).[636,637] Children who experience emergence delirium often demand that all monitors, IV lines, and bandages be removed and that they be dressed in their own clothing. Many of these children fail to recognize and respond appropriately to their parents. Parents who witness this transient state usually volunteer that this behavior is unusual and uncustomary for their child. The core behaviors identified in association with emergence delirium after anesthesia in children include nonpurposeful action and averting eyes or staring.[638]

Emergence delirium is not a new phenomenon, first reported in 1961[639] and again after the introduction of almost every new anesthetic, including most inhalational anesthetics,[375,376,379,382,632,640–642] as well as IV agents, including midazolam, remifentanil, and propofol.[642,643] The incidence of emergence delirium after inhalational anesthesia in children ranges from 2% to 80%.[377,379,382,630,636]

The incidence of emergence delirium is greatest in children 1 to 5 years of age, similar after all inhalational anesthetics except halothane, reduced in the presence of adjuvant medications (e.g., opioids, propofol), increased in the presence of pain, and quite variable when a nonvalidated assessment scale is used.[631,636,637,644–647] These episodes have an average duration of 10 to 20 minutes and resolve spontaneously without sequelae. The mechanism by which emergence delirium occurs remains unknown. To date, the only systematic review of models to predict the risk of developing emergence delirium identified one suitable scale, the Emergence Agitation Risk Scale (EARS). However, this scale has low usability and carries a high risk for bias rendering its validity questionable.[648]

Emergence delirium has been reported in adults as well as infants, although the incidence is much less in both age groups than

in children. Diagnosing emergence delirium after anesthesia and surgery has been complicated by our inability to distinguish it from pain. In one study, ketorolac decreased the incidence of emergence delirium 3- to 4-fold after myringotomy with either halothane or sevoflurane anesthesia.[632] Because ketorolac does not sedate children, it is likely that ketorolac reduced pain and not emergence delirium. Subsequent studies in children demonstrated that emergence delirium occurs after sevoflurane anesthesia even in the presence of neuraxial blocks.[636,647] The frequency of emergence delirium is independent of the speed of awakening from anesthesia,[649,650] the duration of a deep level of anesthesia,[651] the duration of general anesthesia,[652] and the presence of parents.[646]

The definitive study regarding the incidence of emergence delirium was undertaken in healthy children who required anesthesia for magnetic resonance imaging (MRI) and who did not undergo surgery.[646] The incidence of emergence delirium was 2-fold greater after sevoflurane than it was after halothane.

However, in most published studies, the metric used to diagnose emergence delirium had not been validated. To address this deficiency, the pediatric anesthesia emergence delirium (PAED) scale was developed (see Table 45.5).[637] The threshold PAED score to diagnose emergence delirium was thought to be greater than 10, but more recently a value greater than 12 was suggested.[653] When the PAED scale was compared with two nonvalidated scales,[653] the three appeared to be comparable, although the results were biased because the PAED scale was assessed in the children first, and then the same observers assessed the children with the other two scales (Table 5.8).

To understand the nature and possible origins of emergence delirium, investigators recorded the EEG during anesthesia. In the first study, EEG recordings during emergence from sevoflurane anesthesia reported that children who developed emergence delirium aroused from EEG tracings that were devoid of sleep-like patterns whereas age-matched controls who did not develop emergence delirium aroused from EEG tracings that showed sleep-like patterns.[654] Neuronal excitability indicative of interictal epileptiform discharges was associated with the absence of the sleep patterns. In a larger study of children, those who developed emergence delirium during emergence from sevoflurane anesthesia presented with greater delta (low frequency) wave activity and lower alpha and beta wave activities on the frontal EEG than those who did not develop emergence delirium.[655] The most recent study was an observational study that sought to correlate EEG findings in young children during anesthesia and emergence with emergence delirium.[656] Epileptiform (interictal) discharges

TABLE 5.8	Development and Psychometric Evaluation of the Pediatric Anesthesia Emergence Delirium Scale

1. The child makes eye contact with the caregiver.
2. The child's actions are purposeful.
3. The child is aware of their surroundings.
4. The child is restless.
5. The child is inconsolable.

Items 1, 2, and 3 are reverse scored as follows: 4 = not at all, 3 = just a little, 2 = quite a bit, 1 = very much, 0 = extremely. Items 4 and 5 are scored as follows: 0 = not at all, 1 = just a little, 2 = quite a bit, 3 = very much, 4 = extremely. The scores of each item were summed to obtain a total pediatric anesthesia emergence delirium (PAED) scale score. Emergence delirium is diagnosed if the total score is ≥10 or ≥12.

From Sikich N, Lerman J. Development and psychometric evaluation of the pediatric anesthesia emergence delirium scale. *Anesthesiology.* 2004;100(5):1138-1145.

during induction of anesthesia correlated directly with the probability of developing emergence delirium. Future studies are needed to determine whether monitoring these frontal EEG patterns can identify and prevent the development of emergence delirium or allow for prompt treatment before signs of emergence delirium are clinically manifested during awakening.

Several pharmacologic interventions have been shown to prevent and/or treat emergence delirium (see Table 45.7).[644,657] These include fentanyl,[658] ketamine,[659] a propofol infusion or a bolus at the end of anesthesia, clonidine,[660,661] and dexmedetomidine.[662] Intranasal dexmedetomidine (0.2 μg/kg) reduced emergence delirium 4-fold compared with oral midazolam and placebo.[663] In contrast, a single dose of propofol at induction of anesthesia, midazolam, and flumazenil were all ineffective.[657,664–668] Additional studies using a validated delirium scale are needed to clarify the contribution of anesthetics to emergence delirium during pain-free procedures.

Neuromuscular Junction

All inhalational anesthetics potentiate the actions of nondepolarizing muscle relaxants[669–671] and decrease neuromuscular transmission[672]; the latter, however, occurred only at increased concentrations. The mechanism of the reduced neuromuscular transmission is unknown but is likely attributable to actions of these anesthetics at the synaptic junction rather than pharmacokinetics or CNS effects. The potentiation of action of nondepolarizing relaxants follows the following order: isoflurane ~ desflurane ~ sevoflurane > halothane > nitrous oxide–opioid technique.[669,673] However, this potentiation depends upon the type of nondepolarizing relaxant studied (longer-acting relaxants are affected to a greater extent than intermediate-acting relaxants),[669,670,674] and the concentration of anesthetic (reduced concentrations may yield small or no differences between anesthetics, whereas greater concentrations may demonstrate substantive differences).[670,674,675] In adults, the duration of action of vecuronium during xenon is less than during sevoflurane[676]; the effects of xenon on the duration of action of other neuromuscular blocking agents and in comparison to other inhalational anesthetics remain to be reported. These observations suggest that inhalational anesthetics potentiate both intermediate-acting and long-acting neuromuscular blocking drugs.

Malignant Hyperthermia

All potent inhalational anesthetics, except xenon,[677] trigger malignant hyperthermia (MH) reactions in susceptible adults and children.[678–687] Studies indicate that the relative capabilities of the four inhalational anesthetics to augment caffeine-induced contractures in MH-susceptible muscle in vitro are halothane > enflurane > isoflurane > methoxyflurane.[688] Using the surrogate marker of the time interval from administration of anesthesia until a reaction was detected to estimate the relative potency of the modern anesthetics to trigger MH, the order was halothane ~ isoflurane > sevoflurane ~ enflurane.[689] All inhalational anesthetics should be avoided in children who are MH susceptible. Inhalational anesthetics should be purged from anesthetic workstations, a challenge given the varied components of the workstations, leading most to replace components and insert charcoal absorbents filters before inducing anesthesia (see Chapter 39 for a full discussion).

Stability and Toxicology of Breakdown Products

Inhalational anesthetics may be degraded via several pathways in the presence of most CO_2 absorbents to form several potentially toxic by-products. Isoflurane and desflurane (but not halothane and sevoflurane) react with desiccated soda lime to produce carbon monoxide. Halothane and sevoflurane react with soda lime to yield several organic compounds that are potentially organ toxic. In contrast, xenon is completely inert with CO_2 absorbents, thereby posing no risk from metabolites or degradation products to humans.

Two strategies to address the clinical risks associated with the degradation of ether inhalational anesthetics are molecular sieves[690] and new CO_2 absorbents.[691–695] While molecular sieves were thought to hold great promise, they have not reached the market for clinical use. In contrast, a number of new CO_2 absorbents have been developed to absorb CO_2 from the breathing circuit without degrading inhalational anesthetics to carbon monoxide and metabolites including compound A (E-Table 5.5).[691,692] The previous generation of CO_2 absorbents differed in their composition and, therefore, in their affinity to degrade inhalational anesthetics. Soda lime contained 95% calcium hydroxide, either NaOH or KOH, and the balance as water. Baralyme, which is no longer available, contained 80% calcium hydroxide, 20% barium hydroxide, and the balance as water. E-Table 5.5 compares the compositions of the older with the newer CO_2 absorbents, which do not contain a strong base (NaOH or KOH). Most recently, Amsorb Plus (Armstrong Medical, Coleraine, UK), Drägersorb Free (Dräger, Lubeck, Germany), and Yabashi lime (Yabashi product, Gifu, Japan) minimally degrade inhalational anesthetics (<1 ppm compound A) and zero carbon monoxide, while providing efficient CO_2 absorption.[696,697] Recent studies indicate that by eliminating KOH and reducing NaOH to <2%, compound A and carbon monoxide are not produced in concentrations that may be clinically toxic.[597]

Carbon monoxide may be produced when a methyl ethyl ether inhalational anesthetic is incubated with a desiccated CO_2 absorbent (most commonly soda lime or Baralyme). The absorbent within a CO_2 canister may become desiccated if dry fresh gas flows through the canister at a rate sufficient to remove most of the moisture (i.e., >5 L/minute continuously through the absorbent canister for 24 hours or longer while it is not in service) with the reservoir bag detached from the canister. This cannot occur in anesthetic machines in which the fresh gas enters distal to the inspiratory flow valve. If the fresh gas flows retrograde through the canister for a sufficient time, it desiccates the absorbent and increases the risk of degradation of subsequently administered inhalational anesthetics. If one of the methyl ethyl ether inhalational agents (desflurane, isoflurane) is administered through a desiccated absorbent, carbon monoxide may be generated.[695,698,699] The magnitude of the carbon monoxide production for a specific absorbent follows the order: desflurane ≥ isoflurane ≫ halothane = sevoflurane. Other factors that determine the magnitude of the carbon monoxide concentration produced include the concentration of the inhalational agent, the dryness of the absorbent, the type of absorbent (Baralyme > soda lime > newer absorbents), and the temperature of the absorbent.[698] The newer absorbents contain minimal or no strong alkalis which are essential for the production of carbon monoxide, virtually eliminating this risk (see E-Table 5.5).[700]

Small concentrations of carbon monoxide (up to 18 ppm) have been detected in children who were anesthetized with desflurane or sevoflurane using fresh CO_2 absorbent that included KOH and NaOH.[701] The concentration of carbon monoxide correlated closely with the fresh gas flow to minute ventilation ratio (<0.68) and weakly with the type of anesthetic agent (desflurane) and age.[701] Carbon monoxide has been detected in concentrations up to 3 ppm during and after anesthesia, even spinal anesthesia.[702] One may question whether a minimum fresh gas flow with desflurane and other non-sevoflurane anesthetics is warranted. The presence of carbon monoxide in the exhaled breath has been attributed to heme metabolism, inflammation, and sepsis, although the authors did not use fresh soda lime in their breathing circuits.[702]

Carbon monoxide is not detectable by any freestanding anesthetic agent analyzer, pulse oximetry, or blood gas analyzer (with the exception of CO-oximeters), although it is detectable by mass spectrometry. A carbon monoxide analyzer is currently marketed for use during anesthesia. The solution to this problem is prevention: turn off the anesthetic machine at the end of the day, disconnect the fresh gas hose to the absorbent canister, always have the reservoir bag connected to the canister, and avoid passing desflurane or isoflurane through a desiccated absorbent. Others have suggested that high-flow anesthesia should be avoided whenever a circle circuit is used to prevent inadvertent desiccation of absorbent. If the absorbent is desiccated, some have suggested "rehydrating" the absorbent, although this, too, is fraught with potential problems (including clumping of the absorbent).[703] If there is suspicion that the absorbent is desiccated, we strongly recommend replacing the absorbent before introducing an inhalational anesthetic. Alternatives to conventional absorbents, such as the molecular sieve and the newer absorbents, may very well obviate degradation of the ether anesthetics, provided the absorbent is not desiccated.[691,692,694,695] When methyl ethyl ether anesthetics are incubated with desiccated Amsorb, carbon monoxide is not produced, although it may be produced with other desiccated absorbents (E-Table 5.6).[691,692,695] The incidence of carbon monoxide poisoning during anesthesia remains extremely rare even when soda lime is used as the absorbent. In contrast, the potential for carbon monoxide poisoning is zero if Amsorb or one of the absorbents that does not include strong metal alkali is used. Subclinical exposure to <20 ppm carbon monoxide results in <3% carboxyhemoglobin, which has no known clinical effects.

Halothane is degraded in the presence of CO_2 absorbents to the unsaturated vinyl compound, 2-bromochloroethylene, which is lethal in mice.[704] Although 2-bromochloroethylene is potentially nephrotoxic, it poses very little risk in humans, even under low-flow conditions, because its maximal concentration in the circuit is less than 3% of its lethal concentration (LC_{50}).[705]

Sevoflurane is both absorbed and degraded via the Cannizzaro reaction in the presence of absorbent, resulting in five degradation products.[706,707] Although the degradation of sevoflurane by the absorbent was initially posited to delay its wash-in, evidence suggests that this effect is trivial.[708] Of the five degradation products produced when sevoflurane is degraded in soda lime, compounds A and B appear in the greatest concentrations. Compound A, fluoromethyl-2,2-difluoro-1-(trifluoromethyl) vinyl ether, is nephrotoxic in rats at concentrations of 100 ppm or greater and has an LC_{50} of 1100 ppm. Compound B, a methoxyethyl ether compound that is minimally volatile at room temperature, is present in closed circuits at less than 5 ppm and poses no serious risk to animals or humans. The remaining three metabolites, compounds C, D, and E, are present in such low concentrations in the breathing circuit that they are inconsequential. In a low-flow closed-circuit model with an inspired concentration of 2.5% sevoflurane, the concentration of compound A peaks at 20 to 40 ppm after several hours of anesthesia.[708–712] In children, compound A concentrations reach 16 ppm after 5.6 MAC hours of sevoflurane in a semi-closed circuit with 2-L/minute fresh

gas flow.[713] Factors that are known to increase the production of compound A include an increase in the inspired concentration of sevoflurane, Baralyme greater than soda lime, and an increase in the temperature of the absorbent.[707,708] The newer formulation of CO_2 absorbents degrade sevoflurane to a lesser degree compared with the previous absorbents (see E-Tables 5.5 and 5.6). As in the case of carbon monoxide production, monovalent bases are important ingredients for the degradation of sevoflurane to compound A and their absence reduced the extent of degradation of sevoflurane.[693,700,714] In rats under low-flow conditions, compound A is nephrotoxic.[715–717] In contrast, studies in humans have been far from conclusive.[709–712,718]

One mechanism to explain compound A–induced nephrotoxicity is the β-lyase–dependent metabolism to nephrotoxic fluorinated compounds. However, this has been the subject of intense debate.[719,720] If compound A–associated nephrotoxicity were proven to depend on the β-lyase metabolic pathway, the limited concentration of this enzyme system in the renal cytoplasm and mitochondria of humans would make nephrotoxicity an unlikely outcome. Indeed, the inconsistency in the evidence of nephrotoxicity associated with compound A between rats and humans has been attributed to an 8- to 30-fold greater concentration of β-lyase in rats compared with humans.[721] To date, there have been no reported complications related to compound A and kidney damage in humans.

At the present time, sevoflurane is the only inhalational agent for which some federal authorities have recommended a minimum fresh gas flow when it is administered in a closed circuit with soda lime or Baralyme. The minimum fresh gas flow is 1 to 2 L/minute for 2 MAC-hours in the United States, although this limitation has not been universally adopted.

NITROUS OXIDE

Nitrous oxide (N_2O) confers several properties that differ substantively from those of the potent inhalational anesthetics. Nitrous oxide has a very limited solubility in blood, with a blood/gas partition coefficient ($\lambda_{blood/gas}$) value of 0.47. The MAC for nitrous oxide is 104% in adults; MAC has not been determined in children. Its chemical structure is $N\equiv N=O$.

Nitrous oxide diffuses into gas cavities that are filled with nitrogen more rapidly than nitrogen egresses because it is 34 times more soluble in blood than nitrogen ($\lambda_{blood/gas}$ for nitrogen 0.014). Consequently, the volume of the cavity expands. However, the magnitude of the increase in the volume of the cavity depends, in part, on the concentration of nitrous oxide administered, as determined by the formula $100/(100 - \% N_2O)$. The rate at which the cavity expands also depends on the source of the blood supply: those cavities in which the blood supply decreases as the volume of the cavity increases (e.g., a loop of obstructed bowel) will expand slower and to a smaller overall volume than a cavity in which the blood supply is independent of the cavity volume (e.g., a pneumothorax). By using a model of these conditions the time to double the volume of a loop of obstructed bowel with N_2O was estimated to be 120 minutes, whereas the time to double the volume of a pneumothorax was 12 minutes.[722] Any gas-filled cavities within the body are vulnerable for expansion if N_2O is administered; expansion can occur with obstructed bowel,[722] pneumothorax, gas cavities within the eye, tracheal tube cuffs,[723] laryngeal mask airways,[724,725] bubbles in veins,[726] and pneumoencephalography.[727] Theoretically, N_2O should be avoided during laparoscopic surgery to avoid expanding CO_2 bubbles that reach the venous circulation (see Chapter 27).

All inhalational anesthetics increase the risk for early postoperative nausea and vomiting (PONV) in children and adults compared with propofol, a risk that increases very slowly with the duration of exposure.[728,729] Nitrous oxide is also generally considered emetogenic, although evidence from adults suggested that the incidence of PONV is reduced when it is omitted during emetogenic surgery (number needed to treat of six) but the incidence of PONV did not change when it was omitted in nonemetogenic surgery.[468] Hence, avoiding N_2O in surgery that is emetogenic is reasonable. Importantly, the authors of that meta-analysis also noted that the number needed to harm in the form of intraoperative awareness when N_2O was omitted from the anesthetic, was 46, or more than 2%. However, a Cochrane review failed to corroborate the impact of omitting N_2O on the incidence of awareness in adults after general anesthesia.[730] The effectiveness of N_2O to trigger PONV in adults depends on the duration of exposure; a significant increase occurs after 2 hours, with a risk ratio of 1.78 and with a number needed to treat of 9.[731]

A number of studies have investigated the contribution of N_2O to postoperative vomiting in children. Although there is some evidence that avoiding N_2O reduces the incidence of postoperative vomiting in children,[732] the preponderance of evidence failed to prove a substantial benefit.[733–737] In part, this may be attributed to the multiplicity of factors that contribute to postoperative vomiting, as well as the salutary effects of other factors, such as the use of propofol and/or antiemetics.[731] Similar data in children have not been forthcoming. In none of the studies in children where N_2O was omitted was awareness reported. The inclusion of N_2O in remifentanil-propofol anesthesia in children reduces postoperative hyperalgesia.[738]

ENVIRONMENTAL IMPACT

The National Institute for Occupational Safety and Health (NIOSH) recommendations currently limit the chronic exposure to nitrous oxide to 25 ppm and to inhalational anesthetics to 10 ppm. The basis for these recommendations is uncertain but may be attributed to the risk of teratogenicity and end-organ dysfunction. In pediatric anesthesia, mask anesthesia and/or uncuffed tracheal tubes and laryngeal mask airways in children leak inhalational anesthetics into the environment. As a result, there is local exposure to inhaled anesthetics during anesthesia in children that should be considered.

Concern over the pollution of the stratosphere and ozone layer depletion by polyhalogenated anesthetics has raised further questions for the long-term use of these agents and the need to fully recycle or adsorb the waste gases.[739] The polyhalogenated anesthetics are produced in extremely low concentrations and although they have a large molecular weight, atmospheric winds may sweep them up into the stratosphere where they can cause global warming and decrease the ozone layer. However, the most compelling data of their impact on the environment relate to their half-lives in the atmosphere and their global warming potentials. The half-lives of these polyhalogenated anesthetics in the stratosphere are approximately 5 years except for desflurane, which has an atmospheric lifetime of 14 years.[740] Nitrous oxide, a compound with a very small molecular weight, which is administered in large concentrations (50%–70%), has a half-life in the stratosphere of 114 years. Nitrous oxide is a known greenhouse gas that also depletes the ozone layer but agriculture and industry account for the vast majority of the nitrous oxide released into the atmosphere, with medical sources accounting for a trivial, unidentified fraction.[741] The global warming potentials for these anesthetics

are quite varied ranging from 20-year time horizon for halothane and 190 to 6810 years for desflurane. These global warming potentials whether for 20, 100, or 500 year time horizons follow the same pattern: desflurane>>>enflurane>isoflurane>>sevoflurane ~nitrous oxide >halothane.[740] These data identify desflurane as the greatest driver of climate change. To preserve the ozone layer, all anesthetic providers should strive to limit the fresh gas flow and concentrations of inhalational anesthetics and nitrous oxide.

Oxygen

The concentration of oxygen should be carefully titrated to the child's needs. Requirements are monitored by inspired oxygen concentration measurement, oxygen-hemoglobin saturation (pulse oximetry), and arterial blood gas determinations. Oxygen is often liberally administered in excess of the child's metabolic needs. However, potential dangers in this excess should be noted,[742] particularly in two areas. (1) Pulmonary oxygen toxicity is well documented; despite the fact that it develops slowly, general recommendations are to use an air/oxygen combination for prolonged procedures when nitrous oxide is contraindicated.[743] (2) Of additional concern is the remote possibility of adverse effects on the immature neonatal retina leading to retinopathy of prematurity (ROP).[744–755] Several early cases of ROP have been reported in infants whose only known exposure to supplemental oxygen occurred in the OR. Curiously no new cases of retinopathy associated with anesthesia have been reported since 1981![756,757] The evidence implicating hyperoxia in the development of ROP must be recognized but held in perspective. The infants who have been affected by ROP are for the most part <1000 grams in weight, although it has affected those <1500 grams at birth and ≤28 weeks gestation.[758–760] Although tight control of the oxygen saturation and minimizing the exposure to exogenous oxygen were believed to be key factors in reducing the incidence of ROP,[761] a multicenter study, the Supplemental Therapeutic Oxygen Prethreshold for Retinopathy of Prematurity study (STOP-ROP), failed to support that hypothesis.[762] The authors of that study concluded that: *"Although the relative risk–benefit of supplemental oxygen for each infant must be individually considered, clinicians need no longer be concerned that supplemental oxygen, as used in this study, will exacerbate active prethreshold ROP."*[762] In another study, continuous oxygen tension monitoring did not reduce the risk of ROP in infants weighing ≤1000 grams compared with controls.[763] It appears the major risk factor for developing ROP is extreme prematurity; *oxygen therapy represents only part of this complex problem.*[747,748,750] In sum, these studies suggest that anesthesiologists should adopt appropriate measures to protect the infant's retina from hyperoxemia without unduly endangering the infant's life.

A panoply of other factors has been implicated in the development of ROP. Retinopathy of prematurity has even been reported in children with cyanotic congenital heart disease, infants not exposed to exogenous oxygen, and in stillborn infants further obfuscating the pathophysiology of ROP.[764,765] Putative *non-oxygen related factors* have included arterial CO_2 variations, hypercarbia, hypotension, candida sepsis, inflammatory response, red blood cell transfusions, corticosteroid therapy, duration of ventilation, increased blood glucose values, low gestational age, chronic lung disease, a deficiency of insulin-like growth factor, and vascular endothelial growth factor, as well as hypoxemia and fluctuating levels of oxygen most of which have not been validated with substantive evidence.[766–789] Other factors such as exogenous bright light, maternal diabetes, maternal chorioamnionitis, and maternal antihistamine use within 2 weeks of delivery, are risk factors; the evidence for vitamin E deficiency is less convincing.[790–793]

The possibility that candidate genes and pathways for developing ROP may be identified by whole exome sequencing of preterm infants has not yielded fruitful results.[779,794–796] To date no comprehensive epidemiologic studies have examined anesthetic risk factors for ROP, but given the many cofactors that have been implicated, it may just be that anesthesia, although very important, may not be a pivotal piece of this puzzle.

It should be noted that new treatments may involve systemic administration of propranolol (which improves neovascularization)[797,798] and intravitreal injections of anti–vascular endothelial growth factors[799]; both these treatments may have anesthetic implications.[800,801]

Bearing in mind the possible role of hyperoxia and hypercarbia, intraoperative management must include careful monitoring of inspired oxygen and expired CO_2 concentrations. Maintaining the oxygen saturation at 93% to 95% results in an arterial partial pressure of oxygen (PaO_2) of approximately 70 mm Hg, with values exceeding 80 mm Hg on occasion.[749,802,803] Unfortunately, individual oximeters may vary considerably in terms of their accuracy, so practitioners must be familiar with their equipment.[804] The use of air blended with oxygen can be used to adjust the inspired oxygen concentration. A transport system equipped with an air-oxygen blender is desirable to continue the titration of oxygen therapy from the OR to the ICU. (When using portable oxygen tanks, a good rule of thumb to determine the capacity of an E-cylinder is as follows: the minutes of oxygen delivery left in the tank = pounds of pressure [in pounds per square inch] × 0.3 divided by gas flow [in liters per minute].) While avoiding hyperoxia, one must never lose sight of the importance of *avoiding hypoxemia; hypoxemia is life-threatening whereas hyperoxia is not.* One cannot be faulted if ROP should occur, provided a reasonable and safe approach to oxygen administration and ventilation has been made.

Intravenous Anesthetic Agents

The anesthetic effects of IV agents are primarily reflected by brain concentrations (the effect site). To achieve anesthesia, it is necessary to obtain an adequate cerebral blood concentration that equilibrates with the effect site. Each drug is rapidly redistributed from vessel-rich well-perfused areas (brain, heart, lung, liver, kidneys, and endocrine glands) to muscle, and finally to vessel-poor less well-perfused areas (bone, fat). Thus, termination of the effect of a single drug dose is primarily determined by redistribution. The much slower tertiary distribution to relatively underperfused tissues of the body is noted with long-term drug infusions. Protein binding, body composition, cardiac output, distribution of cardiac output, metabolism, and excretion all alter the pharmacokinetics and pharmacodynamics of IV drugs. Anesthetic depth may be altered if a constant cerebral blood concentration is not maintained. The changes in body composition and the blood-brain barrier that occur during maturation may also greatly affect the duration of action of IV drugs, especially in neonates. In addition to perinatal circulatory changes (e.g., ductus venosus, ductus arteriosus), there are maturational differences in relative organ mass and regional blood flow, while a symptomatic patent ductus arteriosus (PDA) may also result in differences in distribution. Blood flow, as a fraction of the cardiac output, to the kidney and brain increases with age, whereas blood flow to the liver decreases

through the neonatal period.[805] Cerebral and hepatic mass, as proportions of body weight in the infant, are much greater than in the adult.[123] Whereas onset times are generally faster for neonates than adults (a size effect), reduced cardiac output and cerebral perfusion in neonates means that the expected onset time after an IV induction is slower in neonates, although reduced protein binding may counter this observation for some drugs. Offset time is also delayed because redistribution to well-perfused and deep underperfused tissues is more limited.

BARBITURATES

The barbiturates, methohexital and thiopental, were once the mainstays of anesthesia induction. Their role has now been supplanted by propofol. The most likely anesthetic mechanism of action of barbiturates is via binding to $GABA_A$ receptors, which increases the duration of GABA-activated chloride channel opening.

Methohexital

Methohexital (Brevital) is a short-acting barbiturate for IV induction of anesthesia (1–2 mg/kg). Administered intravenously as a 1% solution (10 mg/mL), it produces pain at the injection site; hiccups, apnea, and seizure-like activity may also be occasionally observed.[806,807] Methohexital has minimal effects on cardiovascular function (increased heart rate) in children.[808] Methohexital may be contraindicated in children with temporal lobe epilepsy.[806] Slow IV titration averts apnea. A possible advantage of methohexital (clearance 0.76 L/minute per 70 kg) over thiopental (clearance 0.24 L/minute per 70 kg) is that its mature rate of metabolism is greater, while the volumes of distribution at steady state are similar (170 L/70 kg),[809] suggesting a more rapid recovery when large doses have been administered.[810–812] Anesthesia is achieved at plasma concentrations of 3.12 ± 0.99 mg/L.[813]

Rectal methohexital, given through a well-lubricated catheter in a 10% solution (20–30 mg/kg), is now a rarely used technique as a method of induction or for brief radiologic procedures (e.g., CT scan), despite an acceptably small incidence of undesired adverse effects (hiccups 13%, defecation 10%).[814–816] Absorption by this route is quite variable and may account for an occasional child with slow or rapid onset of sedation.[810,817] It is also an alternative for children who are still in diapers and who are not candidates for other premedicants, such as midazolam (e.g., a child taking erythromycin).[818,819]

Oxygen desaturation occurs in approximately 4% of children sedated with rectal methohexital and is usually related to airway obstruction, which is readily corrected by repositioning the head[814,820]; methohexital should be administered only under the supervision of a physician trained in airway management to ensure adequacy of the airway because airway obstruction, seizures, or apnea may rarely occur.[821] *Children must not be left unobserved after administration of this sedation.*

Thiopental

The median effective dose (ED_{50}) of intravenous thiopental varies with age: 3.4 mg/kg in neonates, 6.3 mg/kg in infants, 3.9 mg/kg in children aged 1 to 4 years, 4.5 mg/kg in children 4 to 7 years, 4.3 mg/kg in children 7 to 12 years, and 4.1 mg/kg in adolescents aged 12 to 16 years.[822,823] The ED_{95} in children is 5 to 6 mg/kg and further increased to 7 to 8 mg/kg in children recovering from burn injuries.[824–826] Although doses of 6 mg/kg have been given before intubation in term infants without physiologic consequences,[827] the mean dose required for satisfactory induction in neonates is less, at 3.4 ± 0.2 mg/kg.[822] The effect-site concentration of thiopental for induction of anesthesia in neonates may be less than that in infants because the neonate has relatively immature cerebral cortical function, rudimentary dendritic arborization, and relatively few synapses.[828] Acute tolerance to thiopental may occur.[829] A total IV dose of 10 mg/kg is generally the upper limit; however, with this dose it is common to have a prolonged period of sedation after brief procedures.

Thiopental in a 10% solution (20–30 mg/kg) may also be used for induction of anesthesia by rectal instillation when methohexital is contraindicated (temporal lobe epilepsy).[806] The period of sedation may be greater for thiopental than for methohexital, partly because of the reduced rate of metabolism.[830] Children aged 13 to 68 months given rectal thiopental (44 mg/kg) 45 minutes before surgery were either asleep or adequately sedated with plasma concentrations above 2.8 mg/L.[831]

The hypotensive response in neonates given thiopental appears not as dramatic as that associated with propofol, although it still may occur with reversion to fetal circulation.[832,833] Thiopental has little direct effect on vascular smooth muscle tone. Cardiovascular depression is centrally mediated by inhibition of sympathetic nervous activity and direct myocardial depression through effects on trans-sarcolemmic and sarcoplasmic reticulum calcium flux. Vasodilator and myocardial depressant effects may cause systemic hypotension in the *hypovolemic* state (e.g., dehydration resulting from prolonged fasting or trauma).[834]

The duration of the clinical effect of thiopental depends primarily on redistribution rather than metabolism (10% per hour). As a result, repeated doses of thiopental may accumulate, causing prolonged sedation. Children 5 months to 13 years of age, however, metabolize thiopental almost twice as rapidly as adults when expressed as per kilogram (see E-Fig. 5.3).[835–837] The elimination half-life of thiopental in neonates is greater than that in adults and children[838,839] because of reduced clearance. Clearance, expressed using a three-quarter allometric model, at 26 weeks postmenstrual age was 0.015 L/minute per 70 kg and increased to 0.119 L/minute per 70 kg by 42 weeks postmenstrual age.[234] Maturation of the CYP2C19 pathway increases rapidly after birth in term neonates,[840] and the mature clearance of 0.24 L/minute per 70 kg is achieved within 3 months of age.

Thiopental has also been used in the pediatric critical care setting as a continuous high-dose infusion (~2–4 mg/kg per hour) to control intracranial hypertension. Monitoring the blood concentration of thiopental may be useful during such therapy to avoid depressing myocardial function. The elimination of thiopental after a continuous infusion may be markedly prolonged compared with that after a single bolus (11.7 vs. 6.1 hours) because of zero-order elimination (Michaelis-Menten kinetics).[836,837] The maximum rate of metabolism (V_{max}) increased from 11 mg/hour per 70 kg at 25 weeks postmenstrual age to 172 mg/hour per 70 kg at term. The adult estimate for V_{max} was 402 mg/hour per 70 kg with a Michaelis constant of 28.3 mg/L.[234,841] Slower elimination reported in neonates may, in part, be attributed to the underlying illness (e.g., hypoxic insult) and intercurrent drug treatment.

PROPOFOL

Propofol (Diprivan) is a sedative-hypnotic agent useful for both the induction and maintenance of anesthesia.[842] Diprivan is formulated with 1% propofol, 10% soybean oil, 1.25% egg yolk phosphatide (ovolecithin), 2.25% glycerol, EDTA (ethylenediaminetetraacetic acid), and sodium hydroxide to maintain a pH of 7.0 to 8.5. This formulation has a white milky appearance because it is a lipid macroemulsion with an average droplet size of 0.15 to 0.3 μmol/L (where 5 to 7 μmol/L size is required to pass through capillaries).[843] These droplets remain distinct in suspension owing to the negative surface charges on the phosphate moieties in the ovolecithin phospholipids in the aqueous outer layer. These droplets may coalesce if the negative surface charges on the emulsion droplets dissipate, which is a slow, naturally occurring process, but which may also be precipitated by physical maneuvers (freeze-thawing, high temperatures, or agitation) or by changes in the chemical composition of the emulsion, such as by decreasing pH or the addition of electrolytes (i.e., sodium, potassium, calcium, or magnesium) or medications (i.e., lidocaine [see later discussion]).[843] Soybean oil is composed of long-chain triglycerides (LCT), defined by the 12 to 22 carbon atoms in their skeletons: linoleic acid (54%), oleic acids (26%), linolenic acid (7.8%), and stearic acid (2.6%). EDTA was added to Diprivan after 1998 as an antimicrobial agent. Generic formulations of propofol are available; these contain sulfites or metabisulfite as the antimicrobial agent.

Propofol is a very lipophilic drug that is rapidly distributed into vessel-rich organs ($T_{1/2}keo$ 2.4 minutes),[56] accounting for its rapid onset and usefulness as an induction agent. Termination of this effect is achieved by the combination of rapid redistribution and rapid hepatic and extrahepatic clearance.[844–846] The rapidity of the redistribution from vessel-rich organs accounts for its brief action and the need for repeated small boluses or a constant infusion to maintain a stable plane of anesthesia and sedation. Pharmacokinetic studies demonstrated a larger volume of distribution at steady state (9.7 L/kg) in children compared with adults, and more rapid redistribution, but a clearance (34 mL/minute per kilogram) similar to or greater than that reported in adults (see Chapter 6 for a review of pharmacokinetic parameter sets used to describe propofol disposition).[847–850] Clearance, standardized to a 70-kilogram person using allometry, is immature in preterm neonates (0.4 L/minute per 70 kg at 30 weeks postmenstrual age); there is rapid maturation around term age (1 L/minute per 70 kg), achieving 90% of mature clearance (1.8 L/minute per 70 kg) by 5 months postnatal age (see Fig. 5.12).[226,851–854] Parameters for several propofol "universal" pharmacokinetic models have been estimated; these models describe propofol clearance from neonates to adults using both a maturation model and allometric theory (see Chapter 6).[295,855]

Clearance is limited by hepatic blood flow and is consequently reduced in children in low cardiac output states.[856] Reduced clearance in neonates causes pronged recovery; maintenance dosing is also less. Propofol is conjugated to a water-soluble glucuronide in the liver and excreted in the urine.[847] Propofol also undergoes extrahepatic metabolism in the lung and kidney.[857] Hepatic metabolites include 4-sulfate conjugates of 2,6-diisopropyl-1,4 quinol. The green color of urine reflects absorption at 490 and 590 nm using liquid chromatography and mass spectrometry believed to be attributed to the presence of phenolic metabolites but they remain unconfirmed.[858,859] There is one case report of hair discoloration in an adult.[860] Crystallization of uric acid has been noted in urinary catheter collection bags. This is attributed to propofol competition for an anion transport exchanger in the renal tubule, inhibiting uric acid reabsorption.[861]

In unmedicated children, the dose of propofol (per kilogram) required for loss of the eyelash reflex generally increases with decreasing age to infants.[862–866] The ED_{50} for loss of the eyelash reflex in infants (1–6 months of age) is 3 ± 0.2 mg/kg, which decreases in children (1–12 years of age) to 1.3 to 1.6 mg/kg, and increases in older children (10–16 years of age) to 2.4 ± 0.1 mg/kg. A more linear decrease in propofol dosing with increasing age between infants and children 12 years of age was determined in Chinese children.[865] A 10% decrease in the propofol dose for the ED_{95} between children younger than age 2 years, 2 to 5 years, and 6 to 12 years was noted. The ED_{90-95} for loss of eyelash reflex for all age groups is 50% to 75% greater than the ED_{50}.[862,863] Larger doses may be required for acceptance of the face mask.[863,867]

The dose of propofol for tracheal intubation in neonates has not been clearly established but appears to be slightly less on the first day of life than later in the first month (see discussion later in the chapter); the mean dose in one study was 3.3 ± 1.2 mg/kg, although 39% of neonates developed hypotension and 15% of neonates required additional medication for intubation.[868] Hypotension has resulted in the premature termination of several other studies of propofol as the sole agent to facilitate intubation in neonates[832,869]; the severity of the hypotension when general anesthesia is induced whether using an intravenous agent such as propofol or sevoflurane in neonates is similar.[870] If the neonate is dehydrated before induction of anesthesia, the severity of the resultant hypotension is likely greater. Furthermore, extremely premature neonates have a limited ability to mobilize compensatory sympathetic responses to hypotension hence the importance of preloading with balanced salt solution *before* induction of anesthesia rather than afterward may be salutary. Hypotension may not reflect cerebral ischemia as cerebral tissue oxygenation only transiently decreases despite persistent hypotension.[871–873] Characterization of the pharmacokinetics of propofol in neonates, infants, and children led to a reduced clinical dose recommendations (see Chapter 6).[295] Further studies are needed to clarify the impact of isolated hypotension without ischemia during propofol in neonates.

In one study, a dose of 2.5 mg/kg permitted tracheal intubation in the majority of neonates, although the exact dose used was not specified.[874] In neonates, the ED_{50} for tracheal intubation ranged from 0.72 to 1.3 mg/kg, although only 58% were successfully intubated on the first attempt, prompting investigators to combine anesthetics with adjuvants for tracheal intubation.[875] In infants 1 to 4 months of age, the intubating conditions 1 minute after a (median) propofol dose of 3 mg/kg and remifentanil 2 μg/kg were poor in almost one-third[876]; the addition of rocuronium 0.2 mg/kg did not improve their success rate. After induction of anesthesia with sevoflurane and nitrous oxide, excellent conditions for tracheal intubation are achieved with 1.5 to 2 mg/kg in children.[629,877–879] In contrast to the propofol doses needed for tracheal intubation with inhalation agent, successful insertion of an LMA in unpremedicated children requires an even larger dose of propofol (5.4 mg/kg [4.7–6.8 mg/kg, 95% CI]).[880]

Although measuring the concentration of propofol in blood has been the sole means to assess its disposition in vivo, alternate noninvasive techniques have been sought to provide online measurements. Mass spectrometry of the exhaled breath from adults and children, a technique similar to end-tidal gas monitoring of inhalational anesthetics, has proven to provide stable estimates of the concentration of propofol in blood.[881–884] It may soon be possible to guide administration of propofol in the OR by the measurement of expired propofol although there are no updates as of this printing.[885–888]

There are integrated pharmacokinetic/pharmacodynamic studies using BIS as a measure of anesthesia depth in children and adults (See Chapter 6).[43,56,889,890] Integrated pharmacokinetic/ pharmacodynamic studies in neonates are lacking, partly because of a lack of consistent effect measures. The equilibration half-time ($T_{1/2}keo$) for the effect compartment is smaller (<2 minutes) than in adults (3 minutes).[891,892] Reduced $GABA_A$ receptor numbers in the neonatal brain may contribute to a reduced target concentration, but this hypothesis remains untested. A circadian night-rhythm effect has been noted in an investigation of infant propofol sedation after major craniofacial surgery,[893] but such an effect is unlikely in neonates who do not have established day-night sleep cycles.[894]

Propofol is widely used as a continuous infusion for sedation or maintenance anesthesia (see Chapter 6). Repeated sedation with propofol over a prolonged period such as radiation oncology has not demonstrated the development of tolerance.[895]

Propofol affects a number of organ system responses in vivo. Systolic blood pressure decreases approximately 15% in children,[848,867,896,897] which is similar to what occurs in adults.[898] Most studies reported similar decreases in blood pressure after propofol and thiopental in children.[897,899] A study of preterm infants (29–32 weeks gestational age) enrolled in the Intubation Surfactant Extubation (INSURE) study found unacceptable hypotension after low-dose propofol (1 mg/kg) 10 minutes after propofol administration (mean arterial pressure 38 mm Hg reduced to 24 mm Hg); the authors concluded that *"propofol should be used with caution in very preterm infants with respiratory distress during the first hours of life."*[832] The incidence of apnea after an induction bolus of either propofol or thiopental is similar.[867,896,897,899]

The major clinical disadvantage of propofol in children is pain when it is injected into a small vein.[900] This pain can be diminished by using any one of a number of strategies, including injecting propofol into a large vein; pretreatment with IV lidocaine (0.5 mg/kg) or meperidine, as well as with nitrous oxide, metoprolol, dexmedetomidine, low-dose ketamine or tramadol; and combining a small dose of lidocaine (0.5–1.0 mg/kg) with the propofol immediately before administration.[848,863,867,897,899,901–908] The most effective method to eliminate pain in adults is to apply a "mini-Bier block" by manually occluding the IV flow by squeezing the extremity or applying a tourniquet proximal to the IV site for 45 to 60 seconds and injecting IV lidocaine (0.5–1.0 mg/kg).[900] As soon as the mini-Bier block is released, the desired dose of propofol is administered painlessly (E-Fig. 5.12). The average number of patients who need to be treated to benefit from this maneuver to prevent pain *(number needed to treat)* in adults is less than two,[904] indicating that this technique is extremely effective.[900] Some advocate that the use of IV lidocaine should be routine practice[909]; a meta-analysis has confirmed the validity of this practice.[910] In children, IV lidocaine 2 mg/kg before propofol (without a tourniquet) dramatically reduced the pain.[909] In a meta-analysis, IV lidocaine effectively reduced pain before propofol, although in most of the studies, lidocaine (10–20 mg) was admixed with the propofol immediately before administration.[910] Pretreatment of lidocaine with a tourniquet may be of greater benefit to prevent injection pain of propofol LCT/medium-chain triglycerides (MCT) compared to a premixed injection with lidocaine (see Chapter 6).[911]

The mechanism by which IV propofol causes pain has been attributed to the nociceptive effects of trace concentrations of propofol (15–20 μg/mL) in the outer aqueous layer of the Diprivan soybean-oil micelles. When the concentration of propofol in the outer layer was reduced (i.e., by increasing the concentration of MCT in the formulation or IV lidocaine), irritation of the nociceptive nerve endings in the veins and the severity of the pain during injection were attenuated.[912]

In children, propofol exerts a dose-dependent effect on the airway. When propofol is given as a rapid IV bolus, apnea will occur, the duration of which will depend on the dose administered.[865,877,897] Propofol also compromises airway patency and respiration; the upper airway narrows particularly in the hypopharyngeal region, but it does remain patent.[913] If airway obstruction occurs, the chin lift maneuver augments the patency of the upper airway.[914,915] Theoretically, collapse of the upper airway increases in parallel with the dose of propofol by direct inhibition of genioglossus muscle activity, as well as an inhibition of centrally mediated airway dilatation and airway reflexes.[916] All of these upper airway changes are reversed on emergence from anesthesia.[917]

Recovery from anesthesia in terms of the times to eye opening and extubation are more rapid in children when anesthesia was induced with propofol than with thiopental.[918–923] Recovery of psychomotor function is more rapid after induction and maintenance of anesthesia with propofol compared with thiopental-isoflurane anesthesia.[924] Recovery room stay and time to hospital discharge are more rapid with propofol.[918,920] When sevoflurane was compared directly with propofol for all stages of anesthesia, one study reported that recovery after sevoflurane was more rapid than after propofol, whereas a second study found no difference.[925–927] Discrepancies in emergence may be attributed to difficulties in delivering equipotent depths of anesthesia with an intravenous and inhalational anesthetics. However, emergence agitation after sevoflurane in both studies exceeded that after propofol by several fold. Emergence delirium rarely occurs after propofol anesthesia in children, and small doses at the end of inhalation anesthesia have been shown to reduce emergence delirium.[928–930]

Propofol reduces the incidence of nausea and vomiting when it is used for induction and/or maintenance of anesthesia compared with inhalational anesthetics.[728,729] Propofol has an antiemetic effect with an EC_{50} 0.343 mg/L.[52,920,931–937] A systematic review including 558 children undergoing strabismus surgery reported that the incidence of early and late postoperative vomiting as well as discharge after either TIVA with propofol or sevoflurane with a single antiemetic were similar, although time to tolerating first oral intake occurred earlier with TIVA.[938] Vomiting may be considered a surrogate endpoint for serious adverse outcomes after surgery in children. No studies have demonstrated clinically important abbreviated times to discharge or decrease in overnight admission rate for vomiting and/or dehydration in children treated with propofol. Short-term infusions of propofol for surgical or medical procedures have shown that the depth of sedation is easily controlled by adjusting the infusion rate while still ensuring rapid and complete recovery.[939–943]

Diprivan and the current lipid-based generic formulations of propofol must be handled with aseptic techniques because the lipid is a culture medium.[944] Propofol 1% can support the growth of at least four common organisms: *Staphylococcus aureus, Pseudomonas aeruginosa, Escherichia coli,* and *Candida albicans.*[945–947] When Diprivan was first introduced, it was prepared (as are all lipid emulsions) under strict aseptic conditions, with a layer of nitrogen above the liquid emulsion in each vial.[843] Once opened, external contamination of the vials, however, resulted in severe sepsis and several deaths before bacteriostatic or bactericidal agents were mandated to be included in the propofol formulations to prevent or retard bacterial growth. In very small concentrations, EDTA inhibits bacterial growth by chelating vital trace

metals without affecting the emulsion droplet size or stability. Other formulations of propofol contain sulfite or metabisulfites, which release sulfur dioxide that prevents bacterial growth. Sulfites are more effective at reduced pH values, but there is a limit to how acidic the emulsion can become because this destabilizes the emulsion droplets. Dust covers on flip-top vials such as propofol are not infectious barriers; anesthesiologists should consider the stoppers contaminated and wipe them clean with a disinfectant such as alcohol before puncturing the stopper.[948] Patient deaths have been reported when clinicians failed to practice aseptic technique and administered propofol from vials that contained bacterial contamination. To further minimize the risk of bacterial contamination, we recommend the use of the "one vial for one patient" practice for propofol and to discard unused syringes of the drug.

When it was first introduced, propofol was infused for long-term sedation in infants and children in ICUs after recognizing that its favorable pharmacokinetics would facilitate a rapid recovery.[844] However, a report of five deaths in infants and children (4 weeks to 6 years of age) who were sedated with propofol raised serious doubts about the safety of such a practice.[949] The syndrome, known as propofol infusion syndrome (PRIS), occurs primarily, but not exclusively, in children who are sedated for prolonged periods in ICUs.[949–953] Clinical experience indicates that PRIS is most common when propofol is infused continuously at more than 5 mg/kg per hour (70 µg/kg per minute) for more than 48 hours. The children who develop PRIS are often septic as a basis for their admission, which may predispose developing a systemic inflammatory response particularly in the presence of propofol. Manifestations of PRIS include the insidious onset of lipemia, fever, hepatomegaly, metabolic acidosis, hyperkalemia, and rhabdomyolysis[954] that may precipitously transform into profound myocardial instability, and cardiovascular collapse, refractory to all resuscitative efforts. Manifesting signs may be subtle, with the sudden onset of bradycardia refractory to the usual interventions, unexplained metabolic acidosis, and rhabdomyolysis.[954] In an adult neurosurgical ICU where propofol sedation was used, a retrospective review determined that for every 1 mg/kg per hour that the infusion exceeded 5 mg/kg per hour, the odds ratio of death was 1.93.[955] After adult and pediatric deaths, the FDA cautioned against the use of propofol for long-term sedation. Predisposing risk factors include concomitant catecholamine inotrope infusions, high-dose corticosteroids, and sepsis. In addition, some have cautioned against using propofol for extended periods of time in children with mitochondrial disorders, although several reviews have demonstrated successful anesthesia with propofol in these patients.[956–958] Mortality from PRIS ranges from 30% to 80%; institution of hemodialysis, partial exchange transfusion, and extracorporeal membrane oxygenation may improve survival.[959,960] One trauma center reported their experience with adult patients and correlated PRIS with duration of infusion and increasing triglyceride levels and suggested that the latter might be a useful biomarker for PRIS.[961] Propofol sedation is not recommended in ICU patients with COVID-19.[962]

Despite PRIS risk, infusion at rates greater than 5 mg/kg per hour continue to be used in the ICU.[963,964] Unraveling factors that predispose to PRIS has proven to be difficult. Early investigations noted that during PRIS, the blood concentrations of malonylcarnitine and C5-acylcarnitine increased. These compounds are known to inhibit carnitine palmitoyl transferase and the transfer of LCT into mitochondria.[965,966] Propofol itself directly inhibits carnitine palmitoyl transferase to impede flux of LCT into mitochondria. Within the mitochondria, propofol uncouples the β-oxidation spiral at complex II in the respiratory chain, which in turn inhibits transmembrane flux of LCT into mitochondria, strangling the mitochondria from a much-needed source of energy. Recent evidence from murine cardiac mitochondria suggest that propofol induced a dose-dependent increase in proton leak resulting in substrate oxidation at coenzyme Q.[967] Administration of the quinone analog CoQ_0 blocked the propofol-induced leak while increasing respiratory chain complex II and III activities. Some have recommended replacing LCT in propofol with MCT to reduce the risk of PRIS and pain during injection. When 1% propofol with LCT was compared with MCT, both with 1 mL of 2% lidocaine, the frequency of pain and its intensity during injection were similar.[968]

The dose responses for propofol for both loss of the eyelash reflex and tracheal intubation in neonates have not been reported although if the data for thiopentone held true for propofol,[822,823] the dose for loss of the eyelash reflex in neonates should be ~60% of that in children. Nonetheless, the safety of propofol in neonates has been questioned after reports of cardiorespiratory collapse.[969–971] Precipitous and severe decreases in heart rate, systolic blood pressure, and oxygenation have been observed after a single induction dose of propofol (1–7 mg/kg) without evidence of congenital heart defects or cardiomyopathy. A myriad of causes of bradycardia associated with propofol have been proposed.[972] In a comprehensive review of bradycardia after propofol in children and adults, the authors concluded that "propofol carries a finite risk for bradycardia with potential for major harm."[973] Whether these unusual responses reflect acute right-to-left shunting, a return to fetal circulation, or another, as yet undisclosed cause in neonates, has not been confirmed. Until further evidence clarifies the pathophysiology of these events, caution should be exercised when propofol is used in doses >2 mg/kg in neonates and epinephrine should be immediately available.[833,869]

Although anaphylactoid reactions have been reported after propofol administration in children, specific causes for the allergic reaction have not been identified.[974] In some instances, the "reactions" were primarily respiratory and attributed to preservatives, such as metabisulfites.[975] Although 13 of 14 adults who developed anaphylactoid reactions after their first exposure to propofol displayed a hypersensitivity response to propofol with at least one test during immunologic testing,[976] similar findings in children have not been reported. It has been proposed that first-exposure reactions suggest a previous sensitization, possibly arising from isopropyl epitopes similar to propofol in cosmetics, detergents, and cough medicines.

Some clinicians avoid propofol in patients with egg, soy, or peanut allergies out of concern that cross-sensitivity with trace components in propofol may trigger perioperative anaphylactoid reactions. However, case series and reviews including a large retrospective review of >200,000 anesthetics in children with food allergies to egg, soy, or peanut allergies concluded that there is no association between food allergy and a perioperative reaction to propofol and thus do not recommend eschewing propofol in such children.[977–981]

The package insert for Diprivan cautions against its use in all patients with "egg allergy." However, children with egg allergy (including severe allergy) have received the measles-mumps-rubella vaccine, which is derived from eggs, without untoward experience,[982–984] although isolated reactions have been reported. In the past 3 decades, no immunologically verified anaphylactic reactions have been reported in children with egg allergy who received Diprivan.[978] In fact, Diprivan contains egg lecithin, which is derived from heated egg yolk. Egg lecithin is a phospholipid and has not been reported to trigger allergic reactions, although trace concentrations of egg yolk, of which only two of nine proteins present (Gal d 5 and Gal d 6) are possibly immunogenic. When propofol was given 43 times to 28 children with egg allergy, only 1 experienced a mild non-anaphylactoid reaction, which led to the recommendation to avoid propofol only in children with documented anaphylaxis to eggs.[978]

Soy protein allergy is primarily a gastrointestinal allergy that dissipates by 5 to 6 years of age because most foods consumed contain soy protein, resulting in natural desensitization. Very rarely is soy allergy a systemic disease. Although propofol is a soy-based emulsion, the AstraZeneca website states that all protein moieties are removed during the manufacturing process, rendering soy an exceedingly unlikely epitope to trigger an immunologically based anaphylactic reaction, although one case has been reported[985] in an adult not known to be soy-allergic. The reader should note that there is an approximately 5% cross-reactivity between soy and peanut allergy.[986]

CIPROFOL

Ciprofol (HSK3486) is a GABA receptor potentiator similar to propofol. Advantages over propofol include less injection pain and fewer incidents of hypotension. Early results from adult clinical trials suggest that its effectiveness is similar to propofol, but the same anesthesia depth is achieved with 20% to 25% of the dose. Pharmacokinetics have been characterized with a three-compartment model with half-lives of initial, second, and terminal elimination phases of 2.0, 34.9, and 6.2 hours, respectively.[987–991]

KETAMINE

Ketamine (Ketalar) is a derivative of phencyclidine that similarly antagonizes the NMDA receptor.[992] Its action is related to central dissociation of the cerebral cortex, and it also causes cerebral excitation. The latter property may be responsible for precipitating seizures in susceptible children and the reason that processed EEG monitoring devices do not work with ketamine sedation or anesthesia.[297–299,993,994]

Ketamine is available as a mixture of two enantiomers; the S(+) enantiomer has four times the potency of the R(-) enantiomer. S(+)-ketamine has approximately twice the potency of the other enantiomer. The metabolite norketamine has a potency that is one-third that of its parent compound. Plasma concentrations associated with anesthesia are approximately 3 μg/mL,[995] whereas concentrations for hypnosis and amnesia during surgery are reported to be 0.8 to 4 μg/mL; awakening usually occurs at concentrations less than 0.5 μg/mL. Pain thresholds are increased at 0.1 μg/mL.[996] The concentration-response curve for ketamine sedation is steep.[51,997] This means that small serum concentration changes will have dramatic effect on the degree of sedation observed (Fig. 5.20).

Ketamine is very lipid soluble with rapid distribution and the onset of anesthesia after IV administration is approximately 30 seconds. This is usually heralded by horizontal or vertical nystagmus (Video 5.1).[998,999] Studies separating equivalent anesthetic doses of ketamine isomers identified a reduced incidence of adverse effects, more potent analgesia and rapid onset, and fewer cardiovascular effects with the dextro isomer rather than the levo isomer[163,998,1000–1002]; acute tolerance has been reported.[1003]

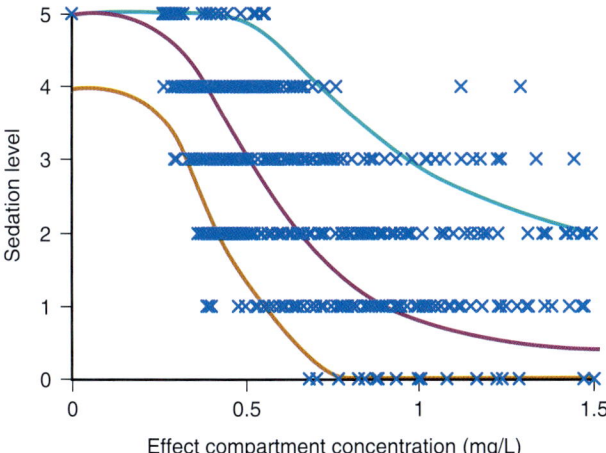

FIGURE 5.20 The relationship between effect compartment concentration and level of ketamine sedation *(purple line)*. The concentration producing 50% of the maximum effect (EC$_{50}$) was 0.562 mg/L. Categorical data are shown as crosses. The *brown* and *blue lines* demonstrate the 5% and 95% confidence intervals. (Reproduced with permission from Herd DW, Anderson BJ, Keene NA, Holford NH. Investigating the pharmacodynamics of ketamine in children. *Paediatr Anaesth.* 2008;18(1):36-42.)

TABLE 5.9	Ketamine Equivalency by Route of Administration[a]
Route	**Approximate Bioequivalence (mg/kg)**
Intravenous	2
Intramuscular	2.15
Nasal	4
Rectal	8
Oral	11.75

[a]Note that these are estimates and that there is extreme patient-to-patient variability. Extrapolated from data from Grant IS, Nimmo WS, McNicol LR, Clements JA. Ketamine disposition in children and adults. *Br J Anaesth.* 1983;55(1):1107-1111; Grant IS, Nimmo WS, Clements JA. Pharmacokinetics and analgesic effects of i.m. and oral ketamine. *Br J Anaesth.* 1981;53(8):805-810; Clements JA, Nimmo WS, Grant IS. Bioavailability, pharmacokinetics, and analgesic activity of ketamine in humans. *J Pharm Sci.* 1982;71(5):539-542.

Children require greater doses of ketamine (per kilogram) than adults because of greater clearance (per kilogram); however, there is considerable patient-to-patient variability.[296,996,998,1000]

Ketamine undergoes *N*-demethylation to norketamine. It is metabolized mainly by CYP3A4, although CYP2C9 and CYP2B6 also have a role. Elimination of racemic ketamine is complicated by the *R*(-)-ketamine enantiomer, which inhibits the elimination of the *S*(+)-ketamine enantiomer.[1004] Clearance is immature in neonates but matures to reach adult rates (80 L/hour per 70 kg; i.e., liver blood flow) within the first 6 months of life, when described using allometric size models.[1005] Clearance in neonates is reduced (26 L/hour per 70 kg),[1006–1008] whereas volume of distribution at steady state is increased (3.46 L/kg at birth, 1.18 L/kg at 4 years of age, 0.75 L/kg at adulthood).[1006] This larger volume of distribution at steady state in neonates contributes to the observation that neonates require a 4-fold greater dose than 6-year-old children to prevent gross motor movement.[1009] Pharmacokinetic parameter estimates are also published for *S*(+)-ketamine with a greater clearance of 112 L/hour per 70 kg.[1010]

Bioavailability after IM administration is approximately 93% in adults and even greater in children.[996,1011,1012] There is a high hepatic extraction ratio, and the relative bioavailability of oral, nasal, and rectal formulations is 20% to 50% (Table 5.9).[179,1012,1013] Children presenting for burn surgery had slow absorption (absorption half-time [T$_{1/2}$abs] of 59 minutes) with large between-subject variability.[179] *S*(+)-ketamine (esketamine) has been approved in some countries for nasal administration in adults for the treatment of depression; a bioavailability of ~54% of a 28-milligram spray was absorbed through the nasal cavity and the remainder swallowed with ~18.6% after first-pass metabolism reaching the systemic circulation.[1014]

Ketamine is an excellent analgesic and amnestic; the recommended dose for induction of anesthesia is 1 to 3 mg/kg intravenously or 5 to 10 mg/kg IM.[1002,1015] The duration of action of a single IV dose is 5 to 8 minutes, with an α-elimination half-life of 11 minutes and a β-elimination half-life of 2.5 to 3.0 hours.[1016–1018] Further supplementary doses of 0.5 to 1.0 mg/kg are administered

when clinically indicated. Atropine or another antisialagogue accompanying the initial dose diminishes the production of copious secretions that may occur with ketamine.[1019–1021] Ketamine may also be administered in very low doses intravenously (0.25–0.5 mg/kg) or IM (1–2 mg/kg), either alone or in combination with low-dose midazolam (0.05 mg/kg [50 μg/kg]), along with atropine (0.02 mg/kg) for sedation, for a variety of procedures, such as oncology evaluations, suture of lacerations, or radiologic interventions.[1002,1015,1022–1027] If an antisialagogue is not administered, there is a greater risk for laryngospasm,[1028] although guidelines for emergency departments suggest that supplementation with atropine or a benzodiazepine may not be necessary with doses of 1 to 1.5 mg/kg.[1029–1031] Larger doses of ketamine will produce a state of general anesthesia.[1032–1034] Even after small doses there is potential for apnea, laryngospasm, or airway obstruction, particularly when combined with other sedating medications.[1032,1035,1036]

Ketamine has also been administered orally, nasally, and rectally, both as a premedication before general anesthesia and for procedural sedation.[1037–1055] Oral ketamine is administered as a premedication in a dose of 5 to 6 mg/kg[1050] or in combination with midazolam in doses of 3 mg/kg and 0.5 mg/kg, respectively. A recent systematic review that compared oral midazolam with midazolam/ketamine combination reported low grade evidence, anxiolysis was similar but sedation and cooperation were better with the combination premedication of midazolam and ketamine.[1056] Similarly, ketamine is reported to reduce emergence delirium, although heterogeneity of the studies, and a low certainty of the evidence, limit recommendations from the systematic review.[1057] Evidence is conflicting regarding the efficacy of ketamine to reduce pain scores after tonsillectomy.[1058–1061]

There are concerns regarding both rectal and nasal drug administration. Rectal administration can result in irregular and less predictable times of onset and peak sedation, just as with rectal barbiturates. Nasal drug administration may result in drug entering directly into the CNS by tracking along neurovascular tissues (E-Fig. 2.1),[156,1062–1065] although this remains unproven in humans. Because the preservative in the preparation of ketamine made in France has been shown to be neurotoxic in rabbits, CNS toxicity is theoretically possible but unproven in humans.[155,1066] These theoretical concerns have not been evident in clinical practice. The bioavailability of both *S*(+)-ketamine and racemic ketamine administered by nasal spray was ~36% with a peak blood level occurring at ~8.5 minutes.[163,167] A ketamine-sufentanil combination nasal administration provided rapid onset of analgesia for a variety of painful procedures with few adverse effects and has promising features for use in pediatric procedural pain management.[167] Ketamine has also been combined with fentanyl, midazolam, and dexmedetomidine, for sedation and/or analgesia via the intranasal route in children.[1067–1070]

Ketamine has also been administered as a means of providing longer duration of caudal epidural analgesia.[1015,1071–1078] There is risk of neurotoxicity during neuraxial administration of ketamine: *epidural ketamine must not be administered unless it is preservative free.*

The use of ketamine is increasing for postoperative pain management when administered in small doses as an opioid-sparing drug.[1002,1015,1079–1082] Although a meta-analysis documented reduced pain scores and nonopioid-sparing effects, it failed to substantiate its efficacy in opioid-sparing (see later discussion). Ketamine has also been used topically to treat mucositis and other painful conditions.[1083–1089]

Ketamine increases heart rate, cardiac index, and systemic blood pressure; it also increases pulmonary artery pressure in adults but has a small effect on respiration.[998,1090] In children, ketamine does not affect pulmonary artery pressure provided ventilation is controlled.[1091] However, if a child is sedated with ketamine and allowed to breathe spontaneously, increases in $ETCO_2$ could increase pulmonary artery pressures.[1092] Ketamine has negative inotropic effects in those who depend on vasopressors.[1093] Ketamine sedation has been shown to maintain peripheral vascular resistance better than propofol, thus reducing intracardiac shunting during cardiac catheterization.[1094] However, the combination of ketamine and propofol[1095,1096] might be superior to either drug alone in this circumstance[1097,1098]; mixtures of 1% or 2% propofol with ketamine in a ratio of 5:1 to 6.7:1 maintain drug stability for up to 6 hours.[1099] An induction dose of ketamine (1 mg/kg) before a propofol infusion in children undergoing diagnostic MRI reduced the infusion rate of propofol and led to a more rapid postanesthetic recovery.[1100]

Ketamine has one of the best safety profiles of any anesthetic agent. After unintended overdoses as great as 56 mg/kg IM and 15 mg/kg IV,[1101] the duration of sedation persisted for 3 to 24 hours; respiratory depression occurred in four children, whereas tracheal intubation was required in two. When the children who received an overdose were monitored and their airways were maintained, recovery occurred without incident. This report, combined with the minimal effect of ketamine on airway patency may explain in part, the successful widespread use of this anesthetic by nonanesthesiologists. However, there remains a small but consistent incidence of adverse airway-related events including laryngospasm, apnea, and airway obstruction associated with ketamine, underscoring the need to ensure that the personnel responsible for administering ketamine are trained in advanced airway management. Ketamine also relaxes the smooth musculature of the airway stimulated by histamine[1102]; treatment of acute asthma with subanesthetic doses has yielded mixed results.[1103–1108]

The effect of ketamine on the musculature of the upper airway differs from that of midazolam; in adults, ketamine does not cause airway obstruction, whereas midazolam does.[1109] The most common adverse reaction to ketamine is postoperative vomiting, which occurs in up to 33% of children depending on the route of administration.[999,1037] Intraoperative and postoperative dreaming and hallucinations occur more commonly in older than in younger children.[999] The incidence of these latter adverse effects may be reduced when ketamine is supplemented with a benzodiazepine.[1110,1111] A soporific environment may reduce the incidence of emergence phenomena.[1112]

Ketamine is useful for children who have a developmentally delay or those who become combative because they are too frightened to come to the OR. Intravenous ketamine can be used in very low doses (0.25–0.5 mg/kg) for short-term procedures, such as diagnostic spinal punctures and bone marrow aspiration, and in larger doses for angiography and cardiac catheterization. Ketamine may be particularly valuable for changes of burn dressings, suture removal, induction of anesthesia in hypovolemic children, children for whom application of a face mask may prove hazardous (such as those with epidermolysis bullosa), and children who require invasive monitoring before induction of general anesthesia.[998,1000,1113–1115] Ketamine has been successfully used even in neonates with less apparent cardiovascular depression than occurs with halothane or isoflurane.[1116] Oral ketamine given to children with burns is slowly absorbed owing to burn-associated delayed gastric emptying.[1117,1118] However, formation of the active metabolite (norketamine) contributes to analgesia and facilitates IV cannulation for subsequent IV administration in the OR.[179]

The role of ketamine for postoperative pain has been reviewed in a meta-analysis. Administration of ketamine in the OR was associated with decreased postoperative pain intensity and nonopioid analgesic requirement in the postoperative care unit, but it failed to exhibit a postoperative opioid-sparing effect in the subsequent 6 to 24 hours.[1119,1120] Postoperative low-dose ketamine infusions decreased opioid consumption by 50% in children undergoing minimally invasive repair of pectus excavatum.[1121]

Ketamine may produce increases in intracranial pressure (ICP) as a result of cerebral vasodilation; it also increases cerebral oxygen consumption ($CMRO_2$). Ketamine may be contraindicated in children with intracranial hypertension.[1122,1123] This concern regarding ICP has been challenged[1124,1125]; adult patients whose lungs were mechanically ventilated and who were sedated with a ketamine infusion demonstrated a decrease in ICP after bolus doses of 1.5, 3.0, and 5.0 mg/kg.[1126] The caveat is that the tracheas were already intubated, ventilation was controlled, and they were sedated. There may be a use for ketamine sedation in the ICU, where there is meticulous attention to airway management and control of ventilation.[1125]

A 30% increase in intraocular pressure (IOP) has also been noted; thus ketamine may be potentially dangerous in the presence of a large (>4 mm) corneal laceration.[1127] In children with active upper respiratory tract infections, copious secretions caused by ketamine may well exacerbate an already irritable airway and trigger laryngospasm.[1019,1028] Ketamine may cause an incompetent gag reflex and thus should not be administered in anesthetic induction doses to children with a full stomach without appropriate airway management. Ketamine may not be useful as the sole anesthetic agent in any surgical procedure in which total control of the child's position is necessary because purposeless movements frequently occur. Ketamine may be inappropriate in any child with a history of psychiatric or seizure disorder because of its psychotropic and epileptogenic effects.[993,998]

In addition, studies in newborn rodents and nonhuman primates correlated ketamine treatment with increased neuronal apoptosis during rapid synaptogenesis.[992,1128,1129] Infusions of ketamine (20–50 µg/kg per hour) to neonatal rhesus monkeys yielded apoptosis after 24-hour but not after 3-hour infusions.[1130] The clinical importance of these findings is unclear since it is unknown if these data can be extrapolated from animals to developing humans (see Chapter 23).

Although the administration of ketamine appears simple, its adverse effects are potentially dangerous. *Ketamine, like any sedative, should be administered only by those experienced with managing a compromised airway.* We urge that it not be used as a premedication unless properly trained personnel are present to supervise the child's airway.

ETOMIDATE

Etomidate (Amidate) is a steroid-based hypnotic induction agent metabolized principally by hepatic esterases. Concentrations associated with anesthesia are 300 to 500 µg/L. As with most induction agents, offset of effect is by redistribution. Etomidate pharmacokinetics have been studied in children with a median age of 4 years (range 0.53–13.21 years) and weight 15.7 kilograms (7.5–52 kg). The estimates of pharmacokinetic parameters (standardized to a 70-kilogram adult) for typical 4-year-old children were clearance 1.50 L/minute per 70 kg; Q2 1.95 L/minute per 70 kg; Q3 1.23 L/minute per 70 kg; V1 9.51 L/70 kg; V2 11.0 L/70 kg; and V3 79.2 L/70 kg.[1131] Similar to propofol, younger children require a larger bolus dose of etomidate than older children to achieve equivalent plasma concentrations.[1132] Etomidate clearance is reduced in neonates and infants (postnatal age 0.3–11.7 months) with congenital heart disease. A two-compartment model with allometric scaling to a 70-kilogram adult revealed a clearance of 0.624 L/minute per 70 kg and Q2 0.44 L/minute per 70 kg; central (V1) and peripheral distribution volume (V2) were 9.47 L/70 kg and 22.8 L/70 kg, respectively. Children also require a 30% increased bolus dose because of an increased V1.[1133]

Etomidate is painful when administered intravenously. Concerns regarding the risks of anaphylactoid reactions and suppression of adrenal function (which lasts for ~24 hours)[1134,1135] have resulted in most anesthesiologists avoiding this agent in routine cases.[1136] However, etomidate is useful in children with head injury and those with an unstable cardiovascular status, (e.g., cardiomyopathy, aortic stenosis) because of its lack of effect on cardiac function or cerebral blood flow.[1137–1141] It is often used by emergency physicians for management of the airway.[1142–1145] Usual doses are 0.2 to 0.3 mg/kg before administration of a low-dose opioid and a neuromuscular blocking drug. Etomidate is often used to facilitate tracheal intubation in critically ill children (i.e., those in whom it would seem to offer the most advantage). Because a very large proportion of critically ill children, particularly those resistant to vasopressors, suffer from relative adrenal insufficiency, corticosteroid supplementation may be indicated in such patients in whom etomidate is deemed necessary for their airway management.[1146,1147]

New formulations of etomidate that maintain hypnosis while attenuating its negative effects (primarily adrenal suppression) are under development (Fig. 5.21).[1148–1152] Methoxycarbonyl-etomidate (MOC-etomidate) is an ester-substituted analog of etomidate that is vulnerable to rapid ester hydrolysis by nonspecific esterases (E-Fig. 5.13). With rapid degradation, adrenal suppression was transient.[1153] However, after prolonged infusions of the MOC-etomidate, the carboxylic acid metabolite of MOC-etomidate accumulated, which in turn prolonged recovery. This

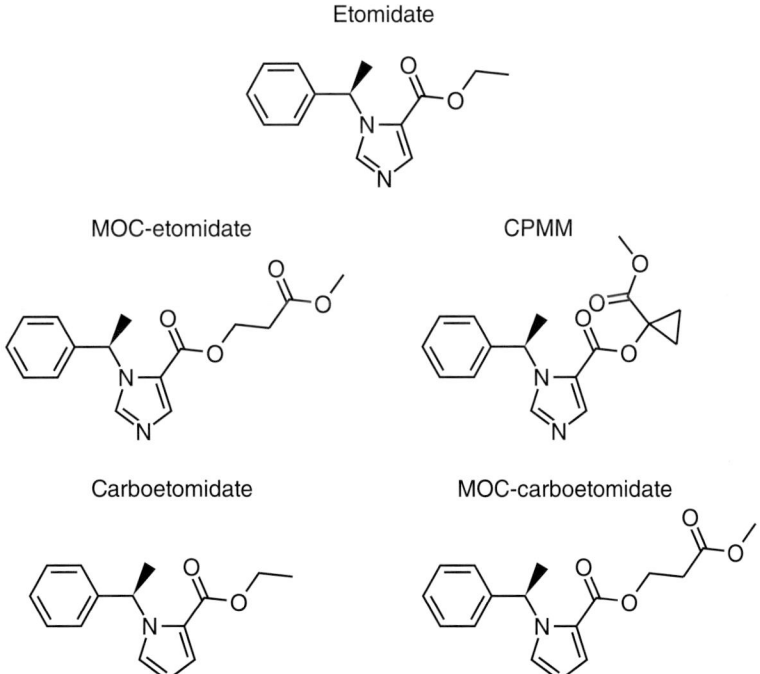

FIGURE 5.21 Molecular structures of etomidate (parent compound), cyclopropyl MOC-etomidate (*CPMM*), methoxycarbonyl-etomidate *(MOC-etomidate)* (the doubly substituted ester side chain), carboetomidate (the imidazole ring has been replaced by a pyrrole ring), and MOC-carboetomidate (in which both the double ester and the pyrrole-for-imidazole ring substitutions are present). MOC-carboetomidate has a brief duration of action, does not suppress adrenal hormone synthesis, and appears to share similar potency with etomidate. (From Chitilian HV, Eckenhoff RG, Raines DE. Anesthetic drug development: Novel drugs and new approaches. *Surg Neurol Int.* 2013;4:S2-10.)

rendered the drug unsuitable for prolonged infusions as a sedative in the intensive care unit. Carboetomidate was synthesized by substituting a pyrrole group in place of the imidazole group to preclude the binding of etomidate to 11-β-hydroxylase in the synthesis of adrenal hormones. As a consequence, carboetomidate did not bind well to 11-β-hydroxylase and therefore did not suppress adrenal hormone synthesis (E-Fig. 5.14).

To preclude prolonged recovery after infusions of these analogues, esters with greater potency were developed. These newer analogues were degraded more slowly, resulting in a slower accumulation of metabolites and thus facilitated a rapid recovery. This led to two compounds: cyclopropyl-methoxycarbonyl metomidate (CPMM or ABP-700) and dimethyl-methoxycarbonyl metomidate (DMMM).[1153,1154] The first, ABP-700, produced dose-dependent hypnosis after an infusion up to 30 minutes in duration in volunteers. Circulatory and respiratory homeostasis and adrenal function were maintained throughout. Recovery after the infusion was rapid; however, involuntary muscle movements, in some instances severe, were observed. These new formulations are potential candidates for both bolus and infusion techniques.

ALFAXALONE

Alfaxalone, (3α-hydroxy-5α-pregnane-11,20-dione) is a fast onset, short-acting anesthetic and sedative with potent anticonvulsant and neuroprotective properties[1155–1159] through actions at $GABA_A$ receptors.[1160,1161] Although it is a progesterone analogue, it is devoid of progestational, oestrogenic, glucocorticoid or mineralocorticoid, or thymolytic activity.[1162] Alfaxalone was used in clinical anesthesia from 1972–84 in many countries as Althesin or similar product name, but was withdrawn from the market because of hypersensitivity reactions caused by the Cremophor EL excipient. That drug was associated with short duration of action and fast recovery making it particularly suitable for day case anesthesia, and maintenance of anesthesia by infusion.[1163–1170]

Alfaxalone has been reformulated for human use in an aqueous solution (10 mg/mL) using 13% 7-sulfobutylether beta-cyclodextrin [SBECD; betadex] as an excipient. This formulation has been shown in preclinical[1171] and clinical[1172] studies to have the same pharmacodynamic properties as those described for Althesin following single intravenous injection; namely a fast-onset, short-duration intravenous anesthetic, with dose requirements and times to induce anesthesia and recover that are equal with those reported for Althesin.

A three-compartment model used to fit adult pharmacokinetic data with an additional compartment, linked by an equilibration half-time ($T_{1/2}keo$) to describe the effect compartment, yielded alfaxalone pharmacokinetic parameter estimates: median clearance 1.08 (95% CI 0.87, 1.34) L/minute, intercompartment clearances Q2 0.87 (95% CI 0.32, 1.71) L/minute and Q3 0.46 (95% CI 0.19, 1.03) L/minute, central volume of distribution (V1) 0.99 (95% CI 0.53, 2.05) L, peripheral volumes of distribution V2 6.36 (95% CI 2.79, 10.7) L and V3 19.1 (95% CI 8.61, 37.4) L. Pharmacodynamic interrogation assumed a baseline BIS of 96, with an estimated median fractional maximum effect (E_{MAX}) 0.94 (95% CI 0.71, 0.99), a C_{50} of 0.98 (95% CI 0.83, 1.09) mg/L, and a Hill coefficient (γ) 12.1 (95% CI 6.7, 15) (see Fig. 5.7). The T1/2keo was 8 (95% CI 4.70, 12.8) min. The mean time to a BIS 50 was 0.94 (standard deviation [SD] 0.2) minutes.[1173]

Neuromuscular Blocking Drugs

NEUROMUSCULAR MONITORING

The measurement of evoked responses after an electrical stimulus is the standard method for evaluating neuromuscular function.[1174] This method allows nearly instantaneous evaluation of the degree of neuromuscular blockade in the unconscious individual. The force of contraction of the thumb, the accelerometer, or the electromyogram may be used to make this assessment.[1175] Twitch tension measurements use the force of contraction of the adductor pollicis. This muscle is the only thumb muscle supplied by the ulnar nerve; measurements therefore approach the single-muscle precision of the experimental nerve muscle preparation.[669] The evoked tension of the adductor pollicis in response to stimulation of the ulnar nerve can be recorded by a force displacement transducer (E-Fig. 5.15A). With the electromyogram, the compound muscle action potential is recorded by surface or needle electrodes applied to any muscle, usually the adductor pollicis brevis, the abductor digiti minimi, or the first dorsal interosseous muscle of the hand (E-Fig. 5.15B). To achieve reproducibility and to ensure full activation of all stimulated nerve and muscle fibers, the stimuli should be supramaximal in intensity, square wave in nature, and no longer than 0.2 milliseconds in duration.

Clinically, three types of stimulation are used (E-Fig. 5.16):

1. Single twitch (0.1 to 0.25 Hz [cycles/second])
2. Train-of-four (2 Hz for 2 seconds)
3. Tetanus (50 Hz, usually for 5 seconds)

Single-twitch rates are useful whenever there is an observable control response. By comparing the percentage change of twitch tension before and after administration of the neuromuscular blocking agent, one can assess the degree of paralysis. Single stimuli detect relatively profound degrees of neuromuscular blockade. In fact, depression of the twitch response can be observed only if more than three-quarters of the postsynaptic receptors are blocked.[1176]

The *train-of-four* is the most commonly used method for assessing nondepolarizing neuromuscular blockade. It consists of four supramaximal stimuli applied to the ulnar nerve at a frequency of 2 cycles/second. The ratio of the amplitude of the fourth twitch to the first is an indicator of the degree of neuromuscular blockade. The main advantage of the train-of-four is that it does not require a control measurement. Furthermore, the train-of-four technique can be repeated every 10 seconds, thus allowing rapid changes in neuromuscular blockade to be closely monitored.[669] In general, when the train-of-four is zero, the conditions for tracheal intubation are satisfactory (excellent or good).[1177] Preterm infants younger than 32 weeks postconception age (PCA) have reduced train-of-four fourth-response values (83% ± 2%) compared with more mature neonates (E-Fig. 5.17).[1178] In full-term infants younger than 1 month of age, the height of the fourth evoked response of the train is about 95%.[1179] The change to the greater value during the first month of life probably indicates maturation of the myoneural junction. In children 2 months of age and older, all components of the train-of-four are nearly equal (100%).[1178]

Tetanic stimulation is usually obtained by supramaximally stimulating the nerve for 5 seconds or more. During tetanic stimulation, synthesis of acetylcholine increases; however, this increase is limited. If the duration of stimulation is too prolonged or the frequency of stimulation is too great, fade occurs (i.e., a decrement in the height of tetanus is noted). The usual explanation for the occurrence of fade is that during repetitive stimulation, the acetylcholine output-per-impulse wanes. Under normal circumstances, the diminution of acetylcholine output does not affect transmission because of the continuing excess of both acetylcholine and receptors at the myoneural junction (safety factor). During partial receptor blockade with a nondepolarizing relaxant, the progressive diminution of acetylcholine output eventually results in a decreased number of stimulated receptors and a consequent decrease in the amplitude of contraction. Alternatively, fade may not be simply the consequence of a spontaneously occurring decrease in the transmitter action but, in fact, a different and separate action of the drug. This suggests that the relaxant has a prejunctional effect.[1180] In infants and children anesthetized with halothane, the percent of fade during tetanic stimulation for 5 seconds at 20 cycles/second is 5% and at 50 cycles/second it is 9%.[1179] These values are comparable to those for adults.[1181] If the duration of stimulation is prolonged, an even greater degree of fade may be noted. In small infants, a more than 50% decrement in the height of tetanus has been observed during 15 seconds of tetanic stimulation; this decrement is even more marked in preterm infants.[1182,1183] These findings suggest that small infants can indeed sustain short periods of tetanic stimulation, but their musculature becomes fatigued more quickly than that of older children.

The integrity of the myoneural junction can also be analyzed by evaluation of post-tetanic facilitation. The increased synthesis and release of acetylcholine that occur during tetanic stimulation continue for a short interval after the stimulation has stopped. This increased production normally does not result in facilitation because all the muscle fibers are excited by the stimulus. In the presence of nondepolarizing (competitive) neuromuscular blockade, however, the increased post-tetanic acetylcholine release stimulates a greater number of muscle fibers, producing the characteristic post-tetanic facilitation.[1181]

The post-tetanic count has been used to evaluate intense neuromuscular blockade in children.[1184,1185] This is a measure obtained by applying a 50-cycle/second tetanic stimulus to the ulnar nerve for 5 seconds, followed by single-twitch stimulation at 1 cycle/second; the number of twitches observed in the post-tetanic period is known as the post-tetanic count (E-Fig. 5.18). Because tetanus and post-tetanic responses are indicators of deep neuromuscular blockade, they can usually be elicited during recovery before the reappearance of the train-of-four. At very deep levels of blockade, no tetanus or post-tetanic effect can be seen; as the patient recovers, a single post-tetanic response eventually manifests itself. The number of post-tetanic counts increases as recovery proceeds until, at post-tetanic counts of six to seven, the first twitch of the train-of-four reappears. It has been shown that during recovery, the first post-tetanic response precedes the first response of the train-of-four by 5 to 10 minutes with intermediate relaxants and by 20 to 30 minutes with long-acting relaxants.[1184,1185] In a clinical situation in which neuromuscular recording instruments are not available, the number of contractions during train-of-four is counted. This technique depends on the fact that the number of twitches in the train-of-four usually correlates well with the degree of blockade. When the height of the first twitch is about 21% of control, three contractions are usually detected during train-of-four stimulation; at a single-twitch height of 14% of control, two contractions are in evidence; when the single-twitch height is about 7%, only one contraction is detected.[1186] During procedures in which a child's hand is covered by surgical drapes, palpating the number of contractions provides a satisfactory alternative. The number of contractions during train-of-four stimulation thus yields a practical assessment of neuromuscular blockade. For more profound blockade, the post-tetanic counts can be used intermittently. However, repeated tetanic stimulation is not ideal because it is painful and can lead to post-tetanic exhaustion.

Although twitch monitoring is the standard method of evaluating neuromuscular blockade, the neuromuscular blockade in one group of muscles can differ substantively from that in another. For example, 1.7 times more relaxant is required to block the diaphragm and the vocal cords than the adductor pollicis.[1187,1188] Nonetheless, recovery of the twitch response is also approximately 50% more rapid in these central muscles. Accordingly, it is conceivable that children could cough or react during intubation in the absence of the twitch response when it is measured peripherally. Perhaps more importantly, when the peripheral twitch response has recovered at the end of the procedure, it is a clear indication that the diaphragm and the vocal cords are in a more advanced stage of recovery. Monitoring the orbicularis oculi contraction (as an estimate of the relaxation of central muscles) to predict whether the conditions for tracheal intubation are suitable is preferred because it occurs before the twitch response of the adductor muscle of the thumb.[1189] Similar comparisons have been made for rocuronium using the adductor pollicis and masseter muscles to measure effect. The masseter muscle has faster onset of blockade (1.5 vs. 2.7 minutes) and similar recovery profile compared to the adductor pollicis muscle. These findings were best explained by a faster plasma effect-site equilibration of the masseter muscle ($T_{1/2}$keo 2.86 vs.3.25 minutes) and a steeper concentration-response curve (Hill coefficient 4.68 vs. 3.97).[44]

Another method for monitoring neuromuscular blockade is acceleromyography, which uses a piezoelectric sensor to quantitate the movement of the thumb, converting this to an electrical signal. There is considerable disagreement in the published literature as to which of these techniques is most accurate.[1190–1192] Monitors based on acceleromyography are becoming more commonly available; however, these are not "user friendly" and are difficult to use in infants because of the small arc of the displaced thumb. Some consider this monitor to be more accurate than standard mechanomyography-based train-of-four monitors.[1193,1194] Others think that mechanomyography is more accurate because it is "less influenced by external disturbances" (i.e., it does not go out of calibration).[1195] Therefore, at present, for clinical purposes in infants and children, mechanomyography still seems to be the simplest and most helpful clinical monitor.

NEUROMUSCULAR JUNCTION

Adult postjunctional acetylcholine receptors possess five subunits—two α and one β, δ, and ε subunits. Preterm neonates (<31 weeks postmenstrual age) have a γ subunit instead of an ε subunit in their neuromuscular receptor.[1196] Fetal receptors have a greater opening time than adult receptors, allowing more sodium to enter the cell, with a consequent larger depolarizing potential. The resulting increased sensitivity to acetylcholine is at odds with the observed increased sensitivity to neuromuscular blockers, but may compensate for reduced acetylcholine stores in the terminal nerve endings.[1197]

Neuromuscular transmission is immature in neonates and infants until the age of 2 months.[1179,1198] Neonates deplete acetylcholine vesicle reserves more quickly than do infants older than 2 months, in response to tetanic nerve stimulation.[1179] Data from phrenic nerve–hemidiaphragm preparations from rats aged 11 to 28 days suggest this is the result of a low quantal content of acetylcholine in neonatal endplate potentials.[260] Neonates display an increased sensitivity to neuromuscular blockers. An alternative proposal to explain this increased sensitivity is based on neuromuscular blocker synergism observations.[1199,1200] Neonates display poor synergism and this has been explained on the basis that neuromuscular blockers occupy only one of the two α-subunit receptor sites in neonates as opposed to two in children and adults.[1200] If this is true, then neonates may use neuromuscular blockers more efficiently than children.

Preterm infants tolerate respiratory loads poorly. The diaphragm in the preterm neonate contains only ~10% of the slowly contracting type I fibers (see Fig. 12.12). This proportion increases to ~25% at term and to ~55% by 2 years of age.[262] A similar maturation pattern has been observed for the intercostal muscles.[262] Type I fibers tend to be more sensitive to neuromuscular blockers than type II fibers, and consequently the diaphragmatic function in neonates may be better preserved and recover earlier than peripheral muscles.[1188,1201–1203]

Total body water and extracellular fluid[1204] are greatest in preterm neonates and decrease throughout gestation and postnatal life, whereas fat as a percentage of body weight increases with postnatal age (Fig. 5.10). Muscle contributes only ~10% of body weight in neonates and ~33% by the end of childhood. Polar drugs, such as depolarizing and nondepolarizing neuromuscular blockers, distribute rapidly into the extracellular fluid, but enter cells more slowly. Consequently, a larger initial dose of such drugs is required in infants compared with children or adults. Increasing the muscle bulk contributes new acetylcholine receptors. This greater number of receptors requires a greater amount of drug to block activation of receptor ion channels.

PHARMACODYNAMICS

The pharmacokinetics of neuromuscular blocking drugs can be described using multi-compartment models. Pharmacodynamics conform to the sigmoid Emax model.[44] Both pharmacokinetics and pharmacodynamics change with age. Other drugs can alter response, as can physiological changes with blood flow.

Investigation of concentration-response relationships demonstrate that the plasma concentration required in neonates to achieve the same level of neuromuscular block as in children or adults is 20% to 50% less, consistent with immaturity of the neuromuscular junction.[83,1205–1208] In addition, duration of neuromuscular blockade is greater in neonates than in children.[1209] The increased volume of distribution (pharmacokinetics parameter) from an expanded extracellular fluid in neonates means a similar initial dose (per kilogram) is given to neonates and teenagers.

The onset time for neuromuscular blockers in neonates is faster than it is in older children and adults. Onset time (time to maximal effect) after vecuronium 70 μg/kg was most rapid for infants (1.5 ± 0.6 minutes) compared with that for children (2.4 ± 1.4 minutes) and adults (2.9 ± 0.6 minutes).[1209] These observations are similar to those reported for other intermediate- and long-acting neuromuscular blockers.[1203] The more rapid onset of these drugs in neonates has been attributed to a greater cardiac output seen with the per-kilogram model[1203] and is consistent with allometric theory (Eq. 5.22) An onset time standardized to a 70-kilogram person using an allometric one-quarter–power model is around 3 minutes for most long-acting neuromuscular blockers.

Plasma concentration requirements are reduced by inhaled anesthetic agents.[674,1210,1211] This is a function of both the muscle

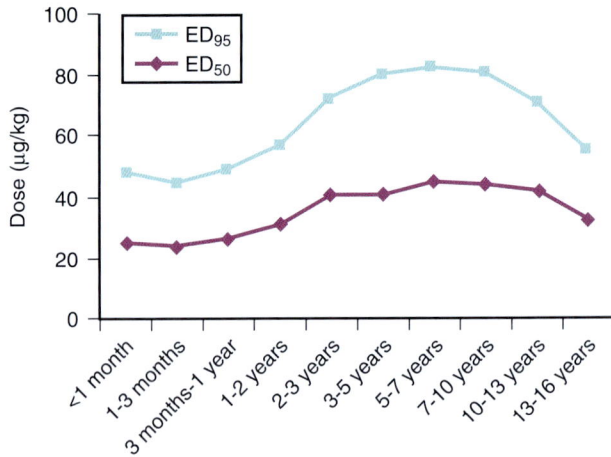

FIGURE 5.22 Dose changes with age for vecuronium during balanced anesthesia. ED_{50} is the dose that achieves 50% of the maximum response; ED_{95} is the dose that achieves 95% of the maximum response. (Data extracted from Meretoja OA, Wirtavuori K, Neuvonen PJ. Age-dependence of the dose-response curve of vecuronium in pediatric patients during balanced anesthesia. *Anesth Analg.* 1988;67(1):21-26.)

relaxant properties of inhalation agents and changes to regional blood flow. Cardiac output is used as a surrogate measure for muscle perfusion. In children with low cardiac output or decreased muscle perfusion, onset times are prolonged. The onset time of neuromuscular paralysis is proportional to $T_{1/2}keo$. An old study demonstrated an increase in the $T_{1/2}keo$ of d-tubocurarine with increasing inspired halothane concentrations[301]; a possible explanation for the delayed action of tubocurarine is that halothane is a negative inotrope[302] and decreases muscle blood flow.[303]

There is age-related variability in the dose required to achieve a predetermined level of neuromuscular blockade during balanced thiopental-N_2O-fentanyl anesthesia. The ED_{95} of vecuronium was 47 ± 11 μg/kg in neonates and infants, 81 ± 12 μg/kg in children between 3 and 10 years of age, and 55 ± 12 μg/kg in children aged 13 years or older (Fig. 5.22).[1212] Similar profiles have been reported for other neuromuscular blockers.[1188,1213–1216] Children tend to require larger doses than adults; the reason for the larger dose requirement in children is unclear but it may be the result of both increasing clearance (pharmacokinetics) and muscle bulk (pharmacodynamics) with age.

PHARMACOKINETICS

The dose of neuromuscular blockers at different ages depends on the complex interweaving of pharmacodynamic and pharmacokinetic factors. The volume of distribution mirrors extracellular fluid changes and can be predicted using either an allometric one-quarter–power model or the surface area model (two-thirds–power model), both of which approximate extracellular fluid changes with weight.[54]

The clearance of d-tubocurarine, standardized to an allometric or surface area model, is reduced in neonates and infants compared with older children and adults.[83] These age-related clearance changes follow age-related maturation of glomerular filtration in the kidney,[34] which is the elimination route of d-tubocurarine. Total plasma clearance of other nondepolarizing muscle relaxants cleared by renal (alcuronium) and/or hepatic pathways (pancuronium, pipecuronium, rocuronium, and vecuronium) are all reduced in neonates.[1205,1207,1217–1219] In contrast, the clearances of atracurium and cisatracurium are neither renal- nor hepatic-dependent but rather depend on Hofmann elimination, ester hydrolysis, and other unspecified pathways.[1220] Clearance of these drugs is increased in neonates when expressed as per kilogram.[1221-1223] When clearance is standardized using allometric three-quarter–power scaling, the clearances for atracurium and cisatracurium are similar throughout all age groups. The clearance of succinylcholine, expressed as per kilogram, also decreases as age increases.[241,242] Succinylcholine is hydrolyzed by butyrylcholinesterase. These observations are consistent with that observed for the clearance of remifentanil,[22] which is also cleared by plasma esterases. These clearance pathways are mature at birth.[23]

Conversion of d-tubocurarine half-times from chronologic time to physiologic time is revealing. $T_{1/2}\alpha$ increases with age in chronologic time, but in physiologic time it is the same at all ages, as we would expect from a distribution phase standardized by allometry. $T_{1/2}\beta$ decreases with age in physiologic time, consistent with reduced clearance in the very young. The $T_{1/2}$keo is large in neonates and infants, reduced in children, and further reduced in adults, possibly because of increased muscle bulk and concomitant increased muscle perfusion in children and young adults.

Depolarizing Neuromuscular Blocking Drugs

SUCCINYLCHOLINE

Succinylcholine is the only depolarizing neuromuscular blocker used in children. Infants are more resistant to its neuromuscular effects than adults with an ED_{95} more than double that for adults (E-Table 5.7).[1224] Early studies demonstrated that the degree of neuromuscular blockade achieved by 1 mg/kg IV in infants is about equal to that produced by 0.5 mg/kg in older children.[1225] The increase in dose requirement in younger children is thought to result, in part, from the drug's rapid distribution into the infant's large extracellular fluid volume (see E-Table 5.7 and Table 5.10).

Succinylcholine remains the neuromuscular blocker with the most rapid onset of action. The onset time of a paralyzing dose (1.0 mg/kg) of succinylcholine is 35 to 55 seconds in children and adolescents; the onset time after 3 mg/kg in neonates is faster (30–40 seconds).[1226] Onset time is dependent on both age and dose; the younger the child and the greater the dose, the shorter the onset time.

TABLE 5.10	Suggested Standard Intubating IV Doses of Commonly Used Relaxants in Infants and Children	
	Infants (mg/kg)	Children (mg/kg)
Succinylcholine	3	1.5–2
Cisatracurium	0.1	0.1–0.2
Atracurium	0.5	0.5
Rocuronium[a]	0.25–0.5	0.6–1.2
Pancuronium	0.1	0.1
Vecuronium	0.07–0.1	0.1

See text for source data.
[a]Low-dose rocuronium (0.3 mg/kg) allows tracheal intubation after 3 minutes during inhalational anesthesia in children, but then is easily antagonized in about 20 minutes. Large-dose rocuronium (1.2 mg/kg) may be used as a substitute for succinylcholine for rapid intubation in children in less than one minute.

As in adults, administration of a continuous infusion of succinylcholine in infants and children can result in tachyphylaxis (increased requirement). In addition, Phase II block may be produced, as evidenced by a train-of-four less than 50% (blockade similar to that produced by nondepolarizing muscle relaxants). In children, tachyphylaxis generally develops after administration of about 3 mg/kg of succinylcholine, and Phase II block develops during tachyphylaxis after 4 mg/kg.[242,1227]

Succinylcholine is effective when administered by the IM route; in this instance, complete paralysis is achieved in 3 to 4 minutes. Evidence of relaxation of the respiratory muscles, as manifest by decreased positive pressure required to ventilate by face mask, can be detected before the abolishment of the twitch response. A dose of 2 mg/kg IM does not achieve satisfactory relaxation in all children, whereas the larger dose of 3 mg/kg IM produces a mean twitch depression of 85%; 4 mg/kg produces profound relaxation in all children, but its effects may last up to 20 minutes.[1228] In infants younger than 6 months of age, a dose of 5 mg/kg IM is required to achieve profound relaxation; maximal twitch depression occurred at a mean of 3.3 ± 0.4 minutes.[1229] Recovery from the neuromuscular effect of IM succinylcholine is faster in infants than in children. Changes in the heart rate after IM succinylcholine are not pronounced. Consequently, routine IM administration of atropine with IM succinylcholine is not generally indicated.[1230] Succinylcholine (1.1 mg/kg) resulted in apnea in 75 ± 4 seconds when administered intralingually, in 35 ± 1 seconds when 2.2 mg/kg was administered intravenously, and in 210 ± 17 seconds when administered IM.

In an emergency, an alternate route to administer succinylcholine when an IV line is not in place should offer a fairly rapid onset of relaxation. Intralingual administration is more rapid (75 seconds) than IM (3 mg/kg) injection (336 seconds).[1229,1231,1232] Caution should be exercised, however, when administering sublingual or intralingual medications. To preclude an intralingual hematoma, it is advised that a 25-gauge needle be used and the blood vessels on the undersurface of the tongue identified to minimize the risk of puncture. The submental approach would seem to avoid the potential for causing bleeding from the tongue.

Cholinesterase Deficiency

Plasma cholinesterase (pseudocholinesterase) is a circulating glycoprotein that metabolizes succinylcholine into succinylmonocholine. The activity of plasma cholinesterase may be increased or decreased as a result of genetic inheritance (see Chapter 4).

Activity of plasma cholinesterase may decrease as a result of a congenital enzyme variant or an acquired cause. This enzyme codes at the E1 locus of the long arm of chromosome 3. Ninety-six percent of the population is homozygous for the "usual" cholinesterase enzyme and 4% are homozygous or heterozygous for the variant alleles.[1233] Five alleles code for the majority of cholinesterase enzyme: (1) normal cholinesterase enzyme, which is designated by "usual" (E^u); (2) decreased cholinesterase activity or quantity, which is designated as atypical (E^a) (homozygote in 1:3000 to 1:10,000); (3) fluoride-resistant allele (E^f) (homozygote in 1:150,000); (4) silent allele (E^s) (homozygote 1:10,000); and (5) the Cynthiana (C_5) or Neitlich variant, which is associated with an increase in (or rapid) cholinesterase activity.[1234] Variations on the silent gene have been detected in Inuit populations with three variants labeled: S for silent, T for trace, and R for residual. The duration of succinylcholine in children who are homozygous for the silent gene may be up to 6 to 8 hours. Additional genetic variants of pseudocholinesterase have been identified, including types H, J, and K, which represent a 60%, 66%, and 30% reduction in enzyme activity, respectively.[1233] Evidence suggests that the K variant (named after Werner Kalow who discovered pseudocholinesterase deficiency) occurs in 13% of the population and that the K/K homozygous variant may be present in 1:63, one of the most common variants with a duration of prolonged blockade of less than 1 hour. Moreover, the K variants have occurred in the presence of other mutations suggesting that multiple mutations may be present in the same patient.

Heterozygote atypical (E^uE^a), which occurs in 1:30 of the population, may prolong neuromuscular blockade by only a few minutes and may go undetected. In contrast, homozygote atypical (E^aE^a), which occurs in approximately 1:3000 population, may cause paralysis for up to 1 hour after a single dose of succinylcholine. Of the genetic variants of cholinesterase, the silent gene (E^s) confers the least plasma cholinesterase activity and therefore the most prolonged duration of paralysis. Homozygote (E^sE^s) occurs in 1:10,000 population and may result in 8 hours of paralysis.

Plasma cholinesterase activity is more often diminished when a genetic variant is present, but a number of clinical conditions may also reduce its activity. These include neonates and infants, severe liver disease, malnutrition, organophosphate poisoning, severe burns, renal failure, plasmapheresis, and medications (cyclophosphamide, echothiophate iodide, oral contraceptives).[240,1233,1235,1236] Several conditions are associated with increases in plasma cholinesterase activity, including thyroid disease, obesity, nephrotic syndrome, and developmentally delayed children.[1233,1237–1239]

Plasma cholinesterase activity is determined by the percent inhibition of benzyl choline degradation by the amide local anesthetic dibucaine when it is incubated with a sample of plasma. With the homozygous normal allele (E^uE^u), dibucaine profoundly inhibits plasma cholinesterase activity (approximately 80%), whereas with the homozygous atypical allele (E^aE^a), it inhibits the activity by only 20%. When fluoride is added to the plasma, fluoride inhibits E^uE^u by 60% but inhibits E^fE^f by only 36%. Thus, a low dibucaine number indicates a deficiency of plasma cholinesterase.

Adverse Effects of Succinylcholine
Temporomandibular Joint Stiffness
Intravenous succinylcholine is infrequently associated with an increase in masseter muscle tone that limits mouth opening (trismus), particularly when given during halothane anesthesia. The incidence of isolated trismus when IV succinylcholine is administered during halothane anesthesia is 0.3% to 1%; it is severalfold greater than that after IV thiopental and succinylcholine, 0/4457 (upper 95% confidence interval of 7/10,000).[1240,1241] The increase in masseter muscle tone after succinylcholine is transient, lasting for only a few minutes and occurring despite abolition of the evoked twitch response in the masseter and peripheral muscles. The increase in masseter muscle tone is usually mild and can be overcome by manually distracting the mandible.[1242] However, on rare occasions, the increase in muscle tone may be so severe that mouth opening is impossible, thus interfering with or preventing tracheal intubation. Whether this marked increased tone is related to the so-called "jaws of steel" (see Fig. 39.2) encountered in children with MH remains a matter of debate.[1243] Prospective studies designed to evaluate masseter muscle tone have failed to demonstrate a child with a marked increase in masseter tone who later developed evidence of MH.[1244,1245] In several retrospective reports, however, a number of children experienced severe trismus and did develop or have a positive test response for MH.[1246–1248] These

studies failed to clarify how best to proceed when severe trismus occurs. Some advocate canceling the surgical procedure, treating the child as susceptible to MH, and recommending a muscle biopsy.[1248,1249] This recommendation is based on a 50% incidence of positive muscle biopsies for MH in children who developed severe trismus after succinylcholine. Others advocate continuing the procedure, avoiding further exposure to triggering agents by changing the anesthetic technique to one that is free of triggers, observing for signs of MH (e.g., increased CO_2 production or tachycardia), and, if indicated, initiating arterial and central venous blood gas sampling, as well as early treatment.[1250,1251] Finally, others have advocated continuing with the original triggering anesthetic while monitoring for signs of an MH reaction (see Chapter 39 for further discussion).[1240] For the most part, this entire issue has become moot because sevoflurane has supplanted halothane as the primary inhaled anesthetic in children, and the FDA issued a black box warning regarding the routine use of succinylcholine for tracheal intubation in children. Curiously, the now widespread use of nondepolarizing relaxants has generated several purported reports of masseter muscle rigidity after use of these agents. Whether these cases actually represent nondepolarizing relaxant-induced masseter spasm or a combination of light anesthesia and incomplete muscle relaxation is unclear.[1252–1254]

Arrhythmias
The molecular structure of succinylcholine resembles that of two acetylcholine molecules joined by an ester linkage. The consequent stimulation of cholinergic autonomic receptors can be associated with cardiac arrhythmias, increased salivation, and bronchial secretions. Changes in heart rate are frequently observed after treatment with succinylcholine. Heart rate usually increases transiently, and this response appears to be more pronounced in the presence of sevoflurane than halothane.[1232,1255] The majority of children (8 of 10) given intralingual succinylcholine who did not receive concomitant atropine developed arrhythmias (primarily bradycardia), but all were induced with a barbiturate and maintained with halothane before succinylcholine was administered. Without an inhalation agent, the incidence of bradycardia after succinylcholine is small: zero (n=20) in several studies and 6% in a fourth.[1256–1259] Thiopental reduced the incidence of dysrhythmias during halothane/succinylcholine inductions by 4-fold.[1259] Atropine does not prevent all episodes of bradycardia (e.g., from hypoxia) but reduces the frequency during halothane anesthesia[1260] and may prevent the onset of new arrhythmias during intubation of children in the ICU;[1261] some have questioned the routine use of atropine before succinylcholine.[1262,1263]

Succinylcholine-associated arrhythmias are rarely a result of ventricular irritability. As in adults, the incidence and severity of these irregularities in heart rate increase after a second dose.[1232,1263] Of greater concern is the occasional bradycardia and asystole after a single dose in children. It is suggested that a vagolytic agent (≥ 10 µg/kg IV atropine) precede the IV administration of succinylcholine, particularly when a second dose of succinylcholine is needed.[1258]

Hyperkalemia
Succinylcholine-induced muscle fasciculation is also associated with mild hyperkalemia, increased intragastric and intraocular pressures, and skeletal muscle pains; rhabdomyolysis and myoglobinemia may occur in patients with neuromuscular disorders. These disorders may have subtle signs in infants and young children and be particularly challenging to diagnose in neonates.

Congenital myotonic dystrophy, for example, may present with mild respiratory dysfunction or feeding difficulty in the neonate. The response to succinylcholine in these neonates, however, remains dramatic, with sustained muscle contraction.[1264]

The serum potassium concentration increases 1 mEq/L or less after IV succinylcholine in healthy children, an increase that does not cause arrhythmias.[1265] However, life-threatening hyperkalemia can occur after a single IV dose of succinylcholine in children with burns (>8% body surface area), those who have been immobilized for prolonged periods, those with chronic infections (including intraabdominal sepsis and *Clostridium*), upper motor neuron lesions (e.g., paraplegia, encephalitis), lower motor neuron lesions (e.g., tetanus, neuropathy complicating nephropathy), crush injuries, and neuromuscular diseases (including Werdnig-Hoffmann and Duchenne muscular dystrophy disease).[1266–1273] In these situations, direct denervation injury or a pseudo-denervation state (immobilization) leads to a proliferation of extrajunctional normal acetylcholine receptors, as well as proliferation of immature (containing γ subunits) and nicotinic (neuronal) acetylcholine receptors, along the muscle membrane such that the entire muscle becomes capable of releasing potassium during depolarization.[1273] These immature and nicotinic acetylcholine receptors release more intracellular potassium, and for a longer period after the channels open, than do the usual acetylcholine receptors. The presence of extrajunctional receptors has been documented within several hours of injury, although clinically significant hyperkalemia does not seem to occur until 1 to 3 days after injury. Thus administration of succinylcholine to children with these injuries may result in a massive efflux of intracellular potassium, leading to a cardiac arrest.[1274] In contrast to these acquired conditions, children who are born spastic quadriparetic from cerebral palsy or those with a myelomeningocele respond with a normal increase in serum potassium concentration (<1 mEq/L) after IV administration of succinylcholine.[1274–1276] Another recent concern is the possible fatal interaction of β-blockade-induced hyperkalemia due to impaired potassium cellular uptake and succinylcholine.[1277,1278]

The definitive treatment of succinylcholine-induced hyperkalemia to eliminate arrhythmias is IV calcium (10 mg/kg calcium chloride or 30 mg/kg calcium gluconate or more). This restores the gap between the resting membrane potential of the cardiac cells and the threshold potential for depolarization thereby preventing arrhythmias but does not reduce the serum potassium concentration. Acute reduction in the potassium concentration is achieved only by treatment with intravenous glucose and insulin and beta-blockers. Repeated doses of calcium may be required, together with cardiopulmonary resuscitation, epinephrine, sodium bicarbonate, hyperventilation, inhaled albuterol (salbutamol) (or the IV formulation), or glucose and insulin, until the arrhythmias abate. Defibrillation of the heart has no role in this circumstance. Successful treatment of hyperkalemia might require a very prolonged resuscitation. Sodium polystyrene sulfonate by nasogastric or rectal administration may be required to leach potassium after acute redistribution between extracellular and intracellular spaces by the aforementioned measures (see Chapters 7, 10, 26, and 38).

Biochemical Changes

Serum creatinine kinase concentrations increase after administration of succinylcholine in children in the presence of inhalation agents,[1279,1280] an effect that was more pronounced in children with neuromuscular diseases.[1281] After an MH reaction, creatine kinase peaks at 12 to 20 hours after the onset of the reaction.

It may also be found in association with a jaws of steel response to succinylcholine.

Rhabdomyolysis

Rhabdomyolysis can occur after halothane or sevoflurane,[1281,1282] even in the absence of succinylcholine as in the case of Duchenne and Becker muscular dystrophy, *LPIN1* gene mutation, or Stuve-Weidemann syndrome.[1283–1285] Isolated rhabdomyolysis or rhabdomyolysis in combination with hyperkalemia, as in the case of Duchenne muscular dystrophy, requires hyperhydration and osmotic diuresis with alkalinization of the urine to prevent acute tubular necrosis from deposition of myoglobin.

Myoglobinemia

Myoglobinemia, another sensitive indicator of muscle injury, may occur after succinylcholine treatment but rarely leads to myoglobinuria (i.e., "cola"-colored urine).[1286] If it occurs, it should be aggressively treated as described previously for rhabdomyolysis.

Fasciculations

Fasciculations are usually observed in adolescents and older children[1286,1287] and less frequently in infants; in children 1 to 3 years old they are described as gross muscle movements.[1287] Pretreatment with small doses of succinylcholine (100 μg/kg), pancuronium (20 μg/kg), fentanyl (1–2 μg/kg), or alfentanil (50 μg/kg) may decrease the frequency and intensity of the fasciculations and the resulting increase in intragastric pressure.[1287–1291] This increase in intragastric pressure, however, is more than offset by the increase in skeletal muscle tone of the crura of the diaphragm, with a net effect of increasing the barrier to regurgitation.

Intraocular Pressure

Intraocular pressure increases transiently in children after IV succinylcholine independent of the presence of fasciculations.[1292] The exact mechanism of this increase in IOP is not clear. Initially, the increase in IOP was attributed to tonic contractions of extraocular muscles, but it is probably because of the cycloplegic action of succinylcholine, with deepening of the anterior chamber and increased outflow resistance. The IOP usually increases by about 10 mm Hg, peaks in 2 to 3 minutes, and then returns to baseline in 5 to 7 minutes.[1292] It is advisable to perform applanation tonometry before succinylcholine or to wait at least 7 minutes after succinylcholine before performing tonometry in children. Although the use of succinylcholine in children with open-eye injuries has not resulted in further damage to the eye,[1293] it is nonetheless prudent to refrain from its use in situations of penetrating ocular wounds unless the eye is not salvageable. High-dose rocuronium (1.2 mg/kg) is a reasonable substitute for succinylcholine rapid-sequence intubation in these circumstances (see Chapter 32 for further discussion).[1294]

Clinical Uses of Succinylcholine

The use of succinylcholine for routine surgical procedures in children has been abandoned, primarily because of the rare but life-threatening possibility of cardiac arrest in male children with undiagnosed muscular dystrophy.[1295,1296] On the other hand, succinylcholine does have the most rapid onset and the briefest duration of action of all currently available muscle relaxants. Consequently, succinylcholine is still used by some for rapid-sequence tracheal intubation, for brief procedures, and for the treatment of laryngospasm.[1226,1297,1298] Because the rapidity of onset is dose related, 1.5 to 2.0 mg/kg IV succinylcholine should be administered to children to depress the neuromuscular twitch 95% within 40 seconds; the smaller dose of 1.0 mg/kg would achieve the same degree of depression in about 50 seconds.[1226,1297] In infants younger than 1 year of age, 3 mg/kg IV would be an appropriate dose because of the larger volume of distribution. These doses provide excellent intubating conditions in all children.[1226] To decrease the incidence of arrhythmias after succinylcholine (particularly after a second dose), atropine 0.01 to 0.02 mg/kg IV should precede the succinylcholine.

In 1993 the FDA issued a black box warning against the routine use of succinylcholine in children and adolescents except for emergency airway management. This was based on several case reports of hyperkalemic cardiac arrests, primarily in children with undiagnosed Duchenne muscular dystrophy.[1299] The disturbing observation about this complication was the staggering mortality rate of 55%. Almost all of these cases, however, occurred in male children 8 years old and younger. In many instances the arrhythmias were misdiagnosed as MH and not treated with IV calcium in a timely manner. Subsequently, the FDA and the manufacturer revised the product label (package insert) to read:

"Since there may be no signs or symptoms to alert the practitioner to which patients are at risk, it is recommended that the use of succinylcholine should be reserved for emergency intubation or in instances where immediate securing of the airway is necessary, e.g., laryngospasm, difficult airway, full stomach, or for intramuscular use when a suitable vein is inaccessible."

In cases in which the child has a full stomach and is at risk for a hyperkalemic response to succinylcholine, a standard rapid-sequence intubation with equivalent intubation conditions may be performed using rocuronium (1.2 mg/kg)[1294] or a large dose of propofol with an opioid (e.g., propofol/remifentanil).[1300] The main disadvantage of using the larger dose of nondepolarizing relaxant is that the duration of blockade may exceed the duration of the planned procedure. Less likely is the disadvantage of an ensuing "cannot intubate, cannot ventilate" situation in which the dose of the relaxant cannot be antagonized. The widespread availability of sugammadex allows rapid intubation with high-dose rocuronium, even for brief emergency procedures, and full antagonism even immediately after administration, thereby obviating the use succinylcholine in such circumstances (see discussion later in the chapter).[1301–1304]

Intermediate-Acting Nondepolarizing Neuromuscular Blocking Drugs

ROCURONIUM

Rocuronium (Zemuron) is a monoquaternary steroidal muscle relaxant similar to vecuronium. It has the fastest onset of action of the intermediate-acting nondepolarizing relaxants because of its low potency and greater dose requirements.[1305] The pharmacodynamics have been described using sigmoid Emax model (EC$_{50}$ 323 µg g/L and a Hill coefficient of 3.97) for the adductor pollicis muscle. The ED$_{95}$ was 600 µg/kg. A T$_{1/2}$ keo of 3.25 minutes was estimated.[44] Onset of blockade was faster in the masseter muscle T$_{1/2}$ keo of 2.86 minutes, reflecting muscle perfusion.[44]

The time to onset of neuromuscular blockade with rocuronium is 1 to 1.5 minutes after a dose of 2 × ED$_{95}$; this is 20 to 70 seconds faster than vecuronium, although their durations of action are similar.[1306] Rocuronium is eliminated primarily by the liver; the kidney excretes only ~10%.[1307–1312] Renal failure does not affect the onset of rocuronium-induced neuromuscular blockade in adults or children although it may prolong the duration of action of rocuronium in adults, a finding not shared for children older than 1 year of age.[1307,1309,1312]

Rocuronium has an ED$_{95}$ of 303 µg/kg in children during halothane anesthesia,[1313] with slightly greater doses required during N$_2$O:O$_2$ opioid (balanced) anesthesia.[1314–1316] After the administration of 600 µg/kg rocuronium (2 × ED$_{95}$), 90% and 100% neuromuscular block occurred in 0.8 and 1.3 minutes, respectively (see E-Table 5.7 and Table 5.10). At this dose, heart rate increased by approximately 15 beats/minute in children; mean time to recover to 25% of control was approximately 28 minutes, and recovery to 90% of control was 46 minutes.[1316]

For brief cases in which children are anesthetized with 8% inspired sevoflurane, 0.3 mg/kg rocuronium yields satisfactory intubating conditions within 2 to 3 minutes.[1317] The intubating conditions after rocuronium (600 µg/kg) have been compared with those after vecuronium (100 µg/kg), atracurium (500 µg/kg), and succinylcholine (1 mg/kg). It was found that tracheal intubation could be performed within 60 seconds in all the children who had received rocuronium or succinylcholine, but not until 120 seconds after vecuronium and 180 seconds after atracurium.[1318,1319] The time for intubating conditions is shortened by increasing the dose[1320]; at a dose of 1.2 mg/kg (3 to 4 × ED$_{95}$), the intubating conditions are similar to those after treatment with succinylcholine.[1294,1316] At the larger doses, heart rate increases transiently, while systolic and diastolic pressures are unchanged.[1313,1321] It is unclear whether this increase in heart rate after rocuronium is the result of pain on injection or an inherent chronotropic effect.[1303] Dosing studies in infants 2 to 11 months of age demonstrated a slightly faster onset of neuromuscular blockade than in older children with the same dose (600 µg/kg). The times to 90% and 100% twitch depression were 37 and 64 seconds, respectively. In infants, the rate of onset of neuromuscular blockade 60 seconds after rocuronium is comparable to that after succinylcholine.[1313,1322] Neonates appear to be more sensitive to rocuronium than older infants.[1323] In neonates, the duration of action of 600 µg/kg is approximately 90 minutes, and there is marked patient-to-patient variability. Consequently, 450 µg/kg rocuronium provides adequate intubating conditions, with a duration of action of approximately 1 hour.[1323]

Rapid antagonism of rocuronium 600 µg/kg IV was evaluated with sugammadex 1 to 4 mg/kg in infants and children anesthetized with sevoflurane until TOF ≥0.9.[1324] An optimal dose of 2 to 4 mg/kg achieved full antagonism within 70 seconds.

In a pharmacokinetics study, the clearance of rocuronium in infants was less than in children (4 vs. 7 mL/kg per minute), whereas the volume of distribution was greater in infants. The mean residence time was 56 minutes in infants versus 26 minutes in children, thus explaining the prolonged duration of action of rocuronium in infants compared with children. In a steady-state target-controlled infusion study, the potency of rocuronium was greatest in infants, least in children, and intermediate in adults.[1325] The greater plasma clearance and smaller volume of distribution of rocuronium in children compared with infants and adults result in a markedly smaller mean residence time and a decreased duration of neuromuscular blockade.[1207] Consistent with the dose-response effects of curare and vecuronium in infants, smaller plasma concentrations of rocuronium are required in the effect compartment in infants than in children to produce the same degree of neuromuscular blockade.[83] Sevoflurane markedly potentiates the effects of rocuronium.[1326]

If an IV route is unavailable, the IM route for rocuronium is a reasonable alternative; IM rocuronium (1.8 mg/kg, 3× the IV intubating dose) provided poor intubating conditions 4 minutes after administration in most children. Neuromuscular blockade (>98%) was achieved in 6 to 8 minutes.[1327] The bioavailability of IM rocuronium at these doses is approximately 80%.[1328] IM rocuronium appears to be a viable alternative to IM succinylcholine, although the time of onset of neuromuscular blockade is very slow and would not be appropriate for emergent situations. The duration of IM rocuronium effect (approximately 80 ± 22 minutes) is much greater than that after IM succinylcholine.[1327]

CISATRACURIUM

Cisatracurium (Nimbex) is one of the 10 stereoisomers of atracurium (1R-cis, 1'R-cis). Cisatracurium is three times more potent than atracurium, with the same duration of action.[1329] Similar to other nondepolarizing relaxants, its onset can be accelerated by increasing the dose (see E-Table 5.7 and Table 5.10); as with the other relaxants, this will increase the duration of the action. Cisatracurium, like atracurium, is a noncumulative agent with recovery occurring during the elimination phase rather than during the distribution phase.

Cisatracurium has a slightly slower onset of action than atracurium, consistent with its relative potency. Twice the ED_{95} dose (80 µg/kg) of cisatracurium completely suppresses the twitch response in 2.5 minutes. In 40 children ≤3 years of age, the onset of neuromuscular blockade after 100 µg/kg was 2.8 (SD 0.5) and 3.3 (SD 1.0) minutes during sevoflurane and TIVA anesthesia, respectively.[1330] The duration of action was 2 (SD 0.66) and 1.2 (SD 0.5) minutes during sevoflurane and TIVA, respectively.[1330] However, of the children paralyzed with 100 µg/kg cisatracurium, 8% (with an extrapolated risk of up to 20%) of children were paralyzed (e.g., TOF <0.90) at the end of surgery. The recovery to 25% and 95% of control response occurs in 31 and 53 minutes, respectively.[1329,1331–1333] Its histamine-releasing effects are minimal; activation of the MAS-related G-protein coupled receptor member X2 protein (MRGPRX2) by atracurium or cisatracurium degranulates mast cells.[1334] The duration of clinical effect and recovery after cistracurium are similar to atracurium.

The distribution and elimination half-lives of cisatracurium in children are 3.5 and 23 minutes, respectively. The volume of distribution at steady state and the total body clearance of most drugs in children are greater (expressed as milligrams per kilogram; see the example of dexmedetomidine [Fig. 5.5]) than in adults, thus explaining the faster recovery in children.[1222] In adults with renal failure, the clearance of cisatracurium is reduced by 13%; plasma laudanosine levels were greater but were only about 10% of those reported with atracurium.[1335] The duration of action of cisatracurium in patients with renal failure is not prolonged.[1336] It should be noted that patients receiving chronic anticonvulsant therapy (carbamazepine or phenytoin) can develop a moderate resistance to the action of cisatracurium.[1337]

ATRACURIUM

Chemically, atracurium (Tracrium) is an imidazoline bisquaternary compound that undergoes spontaneous decomposition into inactive metabolites. At physiologic (alkaline) pH, it undergoes enzymatic hydrolysis independent of plasma cholinesterase (Hofmann elimination), ester hydrolysis, and other unspecified pathways.[1220] In blood and other tissue fluids, the quaternary ammonium compound breaks down primarily into laudanosine and a related quaternary acid (methyl acrylate). The elimination

half-life of atracurium is similar in infants and children (14–20 minutes). The steady-state plasma concentration resulting in 50% neuromuscular block (EC_{50}) does not differ between infants, children, or adults (363, 444, or 436 ng/mL, respectively).[1206]

For intubating purposes, two to three times the ED_{95} (300–600 µg/kg) is given to produce effective blockade in most children.[1338,1339] Such doses provide satisfactory conditions for intubation within 2 minutes. The period of absence of twitch response after an intubating dose of atracurium usually lasts 15 to 30 minutes. Hence, in clinical situations an intubating dose should provide complete neuromuscular blockade for such an interval, followed by another 20 minutes of intermediate blockade (twitch height 5%–25%); complete recovery usually occurs within 40 to 60 minutes. Comparison of data from children and adults demonstrates that children require more atracurium per kilogram and generally recover faster. This difference, however, is relatively small and is masked in most cases by the wide range of individual patient responses.

Atracurium can be administered by continuous infusion because it is degraded quickly and its metabolites do not have neuromuscular blocking properties. The infusion requirement to maintain 90% to 99% twitch depression in children is 6 µg/kg per minute during isoflurane anesthesia, 7 to 8 µg/kg per minute with halothane, and 9 µg/kg per minute with an $N_2O:O_2$ opioid technique.[674,675] Infants have a larger volume of distribution (176 vs. 139 mL/kg) and more rapid clearance (9.1 vs. 5.1 mL/kg per minute) than children; there were no significant differences in the volume of distribution. Clearance or half-lives have been detected for atracurium between healthy children and children with impaired hepatic function.[1221] The metabolite, laudanosine, concentrations tend to be greater in children with hepatic impairment than in children with normal hepatic function.[1221]

The side effects of atracurium are minimal; at doses of up to 600 µg/kg, there are no noteworthy changes in the heart rate or blood pressure in children. Mild cutaneous flushing reactions are sometimes observed.[1338] Laudanosine interactions with GABA, opioid, and nicotinic acetylcholine receptors remain poorly studied, but are probably inconsequential with the customary atracurium doses used.[1340] Extremely rare instances of anaphylactoid reactions or bronchospasm have been reported.[1341]

GANTACURIUM

Gantacurium is one of a new series of compounds, the asymmetric mixed-onium chlorofumerates.[1342] These drugs have a fast onset and rapid-to-intermediate duration of action and can be rapidly reversed by L-cysteine adduction without side effects that are commonly observed with anticholinesterase reversal drugs.[1343] Cysteine adduction replaces chlorine with cysteine forming a heterocyclic ring that cannot interact with the postjunctional acetylcholine receptor. Consequently, metabolites are inactive.[1343]

Gantacurium ED_{95} in adults is 0.19 mg/kg. The onset of blockade after the gantacurium ED_{95} is <3 minutes and may be abbreviated to ~1.5 minutes by increasing the dose to 4 × ED_{95}. At these doses, the duration of action of gantacurium (recovery to train-of-four of ≥0.90) is approximately 15 minutes.[1344] Histamine release is possible through the same mechanism as that for atracurium. Children are yet to be studied and the drug is not yet available for clinical practice.

VECURONIUM

Vecuronium is the monoquaternary homologue of pancuronium in which the methyl group of the 2β-nitrogen atom is absent.

The volume of distribution is greater in infants than in children (357 ± 70 vs. 204 ± 116 mL/kg), whereas plasma clearances are similar (5.6 ± 1.0 vs. 5.9 ± 2.4 mL/kg per minute).[1205]

Its primary advantage is the absence of any adverse cardiovascular effects even in doses several times greater than the usually recommended clinical doses (see E-Table 5.7 and Table 5.10).[1345] Vecuronium is primarily metabolized by the liver and excreted in bile.[1346] Dose requirements according to age groups are much more pronounced (>50%), with a biphasic distribution of the dose requirement and duration of action; infants younger than 1 year of age are more sensitive to the action of vecuronium than older children. As adolescence is reached, the requirement diminishes to that of adults.[1209,1212,1347,1348]

Vecuronium has been popular in critically ill children because of the absence of cardiovascular side effects and because its metabolites do not seem to have CNS effects. However, adult and pediatric patients in ICUs have had residual weakness after the discontinuation of vecuronium, possibly contributed by active 3-OH metabolite or its steroid-like structure.[1349–1351] In one study in which the rate of infusion was adjusted by accelerometry, all children recovered within 1 hour; the requirements of neonates and small infants were 45% less than those of older children.[1352] In this respect, cisatracurium may offer advantage because its recovery from prolonged infusion is faster than vecuronium.[1353] The major reason vecuronium is not widely used in the OR is that it requires reconstitution before use in contrast to rocuronium which comes formulated in an aqueous solution.

CLINICAL IMPLICATIONS WHEN USING SHORT- AND INTERMEDIATE-ACTING NEUROMUSCULAR BLOCKING DRUGS

Short- and intermediate-acting neuromuscular blockers have great utility in infants and children because of the large number of brief surgical procedures performed. Because of their short duration of action, these drugs can be given in one intubating dose: (atracurium [500 µg/kg]; cisatracurium [200 µg/kg]; vecuronium [100 µg/kg]; rocuronium [600 µg/kg]). If more than 45 minutes elapse after the last dose of these neuromuscular blockers, one may reasonably assume that neuromuscular function has nearly recovered, but safe practice would recommend confirming *recovery of neuromuscular integrity by clinical signs or by assessment with a neuromuscular blockade monitor. We recommend antagonism in all neonates and infants despite clinical signs of recovery.*

The benzylisoquinoliniums and organosteroidal neuromuscular blockers are acidic compounds (pH 3–4) that can precipitate thiopental (pH 10–11) if admixed.[1354] Consequently, when these drugs are administered in tandem, the IV tubing should be thoroughly flushed between the thiopental and these relaxants. Vecuronium and rocuronium are painful when administered intravenously in a small vein during the light stages of anesthesia. This pain is usually demonstrated by withdrawal of the hand. Pain can be attenuated by deepening the level of anesthesia prior to administration or pretreating with fentanyl, lidocaine, or ketamine.[1355,1356]

Long-Acting Nondepolarizing Neuromuscular Blocking Drugs

For almost half a century the mainstay of neuromuscular blockers was curare (*d*-tubocurarine); its use diminished because its duration of action was too great for most surgeries, and large doses released histamine. Curare is no longer available. After curare, several long-acting neuromuscular blockers with minimal adverse effects were developed including metocurine, pipecuronium, and doxacurium, which are 2, 4, and 10 times as potent as curare, respectively. The only long-acting relaxant that is still used in some institutions is pancuronium.

PANCURONIUM

Pancuronium bromide (Pavulon) is a bisquaternary ammonium steroidal compound with nondepolarizing neuromuscular blocking properties. Pancuronium undergoes partial (15%–20%) hepatic deacetylation to produce 3-OH, 17-OH, and 3,17-di-OH metabolites. A prolongation of effect can be expected in patients with renal or hepatic failure because a major proportion of pancuronium is excreted in the urine (40%–60%) and in the bile (11%). The volume of distribution (203 ± 36 mL/kg) and plasma clearance (1.7 ± 0.2 mL/kg per minute) of pancuronium are associated with a prolonged elimination half-life (103 ± 23 minutes) in children (3–6 years) under halothane anesthesia.[1357] It induces mild tachycardia by blocking presynaptic noradrenaline uptake (increased cardiac output in infants) but has no histamine-releasing properties, so systolic blood pressure tends to increase.[1358] Pancuronium (100 µg/kg) provides satisfactory conditions for tracheal intubation in 70% to 90% of infants and children within 150 seconds of administration. Increasing the initial dose to 150 µg/kg provides satisfactory intubating conditions in all children within 80 seconds (see E-Table 5.7 and Table 5.10).[1297,1359]

Pancuronium is frequently advocated for cardiac surgery and other high-risk procedures in infants and children although recently, rocuronium has supplanted pancuronium for neonatal surgery and surgeries of intermediate duration. The anesthetic combination of high-dose opioid (fentanyl) with air-oxygen-pancuronium or rocuronium maintains circulatory homeostasis and blunts the stress response in neonates and infants. The vagolytic effect (tachycardia) of pancuronium counteracts the vagotonic effect (bradycardia) of potent opioids, and its relaxant properties counteract opioid-induced chest wall and glottic rigidity.[1360]

Pancuronium has been used to facilitate ventilation in preterm infants in neonatal ICUs.[1361] Because pancuronium increases the heart rate, blood pressure, and plasma epinephrine and norepinephrine levels in premature neonates, there is some concern that it may contribute to the risk of an intracerebral hemorrhage.[1362] Accordingly, it would seem prudent to administer pancuronium with either general anesthesia or with adequate sedation to blunt adverse cardiovascular responses. Vecuronium may offer an advantage over pancuronium because it does not significantly increase the blood pressure.[1363–1367] Nasotracheal intubation or intratracheal suctioning in neonates who are paralyzed with pancuronium results in smaller increases in intracranial pressure than in neonates who are not paralyzed.[1367,1368] By abolishing fluctuations in cerebral blood flow through the use of muscle relaxants, the incidence and severity of intraventricular hemorrhages should theoretically be reduced.

Antagonism of Neuromuscular Blocking Drugs

GENERAL PRINCIPLES

In children and especially infants, oxygen consumption is greater than in adults. Therefore, a slight diminution in respiratory muscle power may lead to hypoxemia and CO_2 retention. Consequently, it is essential that neuromuscular function is returned to normal at the end of the surgical procedure. Neonates are at greater risk for residual neuromuscular blockade than adults for several reasons, including (1) immaturity of the neuromuscular system, (2) greater elimination half-life of relaxants, (3) the reduced number of type I muscle fibers in the ventilatory musculature (thus being more susceptible to fatigue [see Chapter 12, Fig. 12.12]),[262] and (4) the closing lung volume of a neonate overlaps with the tidal volume (i.e., airway closure occurs at the end of expiration) (Fig. 1.8).[1369] If respirations are mildly impaired as a result of residual muscle paralysis, even more alveoli will collapse. The result may be hypoxemia as well as hypercarbia and acidosis, which may potentiate and prolong the duration of action of the muscle relaxant, thus creating a vicious cycle (Figs. 2.13 and 2.14).

When monitoring neuromuscular blockade in infants and children, train-of-four monitoring of the adductor pollicis overestimates the degree of neuromuscular blockade in the diaphragm.[1188] Larger doses of muscle relaxants are required to block the diaphragm than the adductor pollicis train-of-four would suggest. Therefore, if the train-of-four of the adductor has fully recovered, one can assume that the diaphragm has fully recovered.

Clinical evaluation of the adequacy of antagonism in infants is more difficult than in children or adults. Neither grip strength nor voluntary head lifting can be elicited; rather, it is important when working with infants to observe the clinical conditions preoperatively (muscle tone, depth of respiration, vigor of crying) and to aim for a comparable level of activity in the postantagonism period. Useful clinical signs that the neuromuscular blockade has been antagonized include the ability to flex the hips, flex the arm, lift the legs, and the return of abdominal muscle tone.[1370] Inspiratory force may be measured; a negative force of -25 cm H_2O or greater indicates adequate antagonism.[1371] A crying vital capacity greater than 15 mL/kg indicates an adequate respiratory reserve. The train-of-four is a valuable aid because it can be used in the smallest of infants in whom the force of contraction can easily be palpated (four equal contractions indicating adequate antagonism).

Although edrophonium antagonism may establish a faster onset of effect, final recovery is invariably greater with neostigmine, which is why the latter has been recommended for routine pediatric practice until recently when sugammadex became widely available (see later).[1372,1373] The distribution volumes of neostigmine are similar in infants (2–10 months), children (1–6 years), and adults (volume of distribution at steady state 0.5 L/kg), whereas the elimination half-life is lower in children.[1374] Clearance decreases as age increases (13.6, 11.1, 9.6 mL/minute per kilogram in infants, children, and adults 29–48 years, respectively).[1374] The dose requirement of anticholinesterase agents to antagonize neuromuscular blockade in children is less than in adults.[1374] However, the speed of antagonism depends on the extent of neuromuscular blockade at the time of the antagonism, as well as the type and dose of antagonizing agent. In the presence of train-of-four responses with fade, 20 to 25 µg/kg of neostigmine, preceded by 10 to 20 µg/kg of atropine or 5 to 10 µg/kg of glycopyrrolate, is sufficient to achieve full recovery of muscle strength. This dose of neostigmine can be repeated if required (up to 70 µg/kg). Doses of neostigmine in excess of 100 µg/kg may induce a paradoxical weakness from excessive acetylcholine at the neuromuscular junction. The dose of edrophonium for children is greater than it is for adults; at least 0.3 mg/kg is needed, but 0.5 to 1.0 mg/kg is most common.[1373,1375–1378]

Some have suggested that it is not necessary to antagonize intermediate-acting neuromuscular blockers, particularly if a lengthy time interval has elapsed since the last dose. With the advent of reliable neuromuscular monitors and their use in conjunction with clinical observations and measurements of respiratory adequacy, clinicians are more confident that antagonism is not always required. This may be appropriate for healthier patients who received the short- and intermediate-acting neuromuscular blockers, particularly atracurium or cisatracurium, which are hydrolyzed in plasma. Children have the additional advantage of recovering from neuromuscular blockade more rapidly than adults.[1377,1378] In neonates, the elimination of all muscle relaxants may be delayed, necessitating antagonism of any neuromuscular blocker; if there is any concern that some degree of neuromuscular blockade persists, then the blockade must be antagonized.

Hypothermia potentiates the action of most nondepolarizing muscle relaxants and delays their elimination.[1379] This effect can create a special problem at the end of a surgical procedure when the children attempt to resume spontaneous respirations. Shivering increases oxygen consumption and augments the load on the respiratory system. If the respiratory muscles are unable to match this increased load, hypoxemia and CO_2 retention may occur, which in turn may lead to acidosis, which, again, may potentiate the relaxant. To avoid the extra cardiorespiratory load in a postsurgical infant, all neonates and infants should be warmed if their temperature is less than 35°C (95°F). Once the core temperature exceeds 35°C (95°F), neuromuscular blockade may be antagonized.

Theoretically, all antibiotics depress neuromuscular function when coadministered with neuromuscular blockers.[1380] Among the putative antibiotics, aminoglycoside derivatives, such as gentamicin, tobramycin, and neomycin, have the greatest effect. A single clinical dose of antibiotic will likely have minimal effect on the neuromuscular blockade.[1381] This factor alone does not rule out the possibility that large concentrations of antibiotics, especially in the presence of other potentiating factors, may augment the neuromuscular blockade. The clinical importance of the interaction of antibiotics with neuromuscular blockers to prolong neuromuscular blockade has diminished with the introduction of intermediate-acting neuromuscular blockers.

Magnesium also relaxes muscles and may also potentiate neuromuscular blockade. After sugammadex antagonized paralysis from rocuronium in an adult, plasma magnesium at concentrations of 2.67 mM caused recurarization that resolved after 45 minutes.[1382]

SUGAMMADEX

Sugammadex (Org 25969), a member of the cyclodextrin family, is a cyclic oligosaccharide[1383] with hydrophobic molecules within the center (Fig. 5.23).[1384,1385] This compound encapsulates rocuronium, and vecuronium to a lesser degree, and forms a stable complex that prevents further action of the relaxants. The chemical encapsulation decreases the plasma concentration of rocuronium, thus promoting the dissociation of rocuronium from the acetylcholine receptor (with a very large association rate), speeding recovery of muscle strength. The dissociation rate of relaxants from sugammadex is exceedingly small and clinically irrelevant.[1386]

Sugammadex, like rocuronium, is cleared via the kidneys, although the former depends to a greater extent on renal elimination than the latter. As a result, the elimination kinetics of both are prolonged in renal failure.[1307,1387–1390] In adults, clearance decreases and elimination half-life increases steadily as the severity of renal

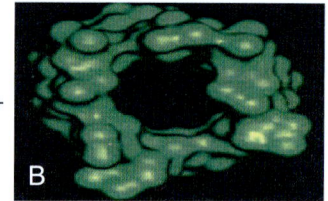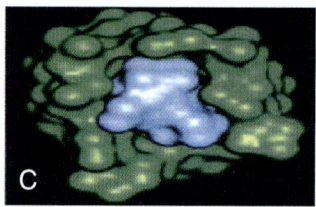

FIGURE 5.23 X-ray crystallography of **A,** the rocuronium molecule (shown in *blue*) and **B,** sugammadex *(green ring).* **C,** The 3-D conformation of the rocuronium molecule complements the conformation of the inner ring of sugammadex. The rocuronium-sugammadex complex is stable, without a dissociation constant, and is excreted unchanged via the kidneys. (Redrawn from Gijsenbergh F, Ramael S, Houwing N, van Iersel T. First human exposure of Org 25969, a novel agent to reverse the action of rocuronium bromide. *Anesthesiology.* 2005;103(4):695-703.)

insufficiency increases from mild to end-stage failure.[1387,1391] In end-stage renal failure, the changes in PK indices for sugammadex are several fold greater than for those of rocuronium.[1387] Because the dissociation constant for the rocuronium-sugammadex complex is exceedingly small,[1387] the delayed elimination of sugammadex in renal failure has neither affected its efficacy to antagonize neuromuscular blockade nor resulted in recurarization.[1392]

The dose recommendation for sugammadex is 2 mg/kg for ≥2 twitches in the TOF, 4 mg/kg for 1 to 2 post-tetanic twitches (no TOF twitches) and 16 mg/kg for 0 post-tetanic twitches (rapid reversal of profound blockade). Several studies have demonstrated that sugammadex 2 to 4 mg/kg effectively antagonized rocuronium 0.6 mg/kg to TOF ≥0.9 in 0.75 to 1.6 minutes during moderate neuromuscular blockade in infants, children, and adolescents anesthetized with sevoflurane.[1302,1324,1390,1393] In a large phase IV study, 2 mg/kg sugammadex after rocuronium or vecuronium restored TOF ≥0.9 within 3 minutes in >90% of the children,[1393] although in adults, larger doses of sugammadex may be required to completely antagonize vecuronium in a timely manner.[1394] When compared with neostigmine, sugammadex antagonizes rocuronium blockade to TOF ≥0.9 5-fold more rapidly than neostigmine.[1393,1395–1397] Other studies have similarly demonstrated much more rapid times to extubation and recovery after sugammadex compared with neostigmine in children with similar or fewer adverse effects.[1390,1396,1398] In adults, the time for T1 to 90% after sugammadex antagonizes rocuronium is almost 50% faster than the time to reach 90% T1 after succinylcholine.[1399] The FDA approved the use of sugammadex in children ≥2 years in July 2021.[1400]

Sugammadex (16 mg/kg) effectively antagonizes large doses of rocuronium (with profound neuromuscular blockade) rapidly in children and adults (to TOF ratio ≥0.9 within two minutes), even when no twitches are present.[1400–1408] The rapidity of the reversal depends on both the intensity of the block and the dose of sugammadex but at 16 mg/kg, 87% of patients recover within 3 minutes.[1301,1303,1324,1390,1399,1409] In an emergency situation of "cannot ventilate, cannot intubate" in an 850-gram infant, 16 mg/kg antagonized the effects of 1.2 mg/kg rocuronium to facilitate ventilation and restore oxygenation.[1410] Given the capability of rocuronium to restore neuromuscular function rapidly, rocuronium is supplanting succinylcholine in many circumstances including rapid-sequence intubations for brief procedures in children.[1394]

Limited data are available for the use of sugammadex in neonates,[1394,1397,1400] including several case reports.[1411–1413] The data showed prompt antagonism of rocuronium-induced neuromuscular blockade after ≥4 mg/kg, complemented by a similar or more rapid interval from antagonism to exiting the OR. A

more rapid recovery has been observed in neonates compared with older children and compared with those given neostigmine.[1397] Currently, the use of sugammadex in neonates is off-label.

A number of side effects associated with the use of sugammadex have been reported including rare cases of allergic or anaphylactic reactions, bradycardia, and recrudescence of neuromuscular blockade after antagonism.[1414-1419] Hypersensitivity and anaphylaxis has been reported in adults after the first or subsequent doses of sugammadex in healthy volunteers.[1420,1421] The frequency was independent of the dose although the mechanism remains unclear. In a retrospective review of 835,405 children in Japan who received general anesthesia, 621 developed intraoperative anaphylaxis. Using case-control matching of 1 to 4 for anaphylaxis and no anaphylaxis, sugammadex was not significantly associated with either anaphylactic shock or the sign/symptoms of anaphylaxis.[1422] In a single-center retrospective review of 19,821 adults, two anaphylactic reactions to sugammadex were reported.[1423] In studies of children who received sugammadex, hypersensitivity or anaphylaxis is rare.[1393,1424,1424a] In vitro studies in rats reported that mast cell degranulation after rocuronium is attenuated by the addition of sugammadex,[1421] suggesting that sugammadex quells mast cell degranulation in response to rocuronium and may stop allergic reactions.[1425] Bradycardia has been reported after the use of sugammadex in children,[1426] although the incidence is less than or similar to that after neostigmine.[1393–1395,1397] One prospective study of 221 children reported 18 (8%) cases of bradycardia, half of which occurred in children with congenital heart disease.[1427] A prospective study of 99 children with congenital heart disease reported that bradycardia occurred in 20% of children; older male children and those who weighed more were most likely to experience bradycardia but none required treatment.[1428] Sugammadex has been used in children after cardiac transplant to avoid possible bradycardia associated with the use of neostigmine, although bradycardia may occur in these children after sugammadex.[1429,1430]

The cost of sugammadex has decreased dramatically with the coming availability of multiple generic formulations; the cost to antagonize muscle relaxants with sugammadex will soon be comparable and may in the future be lower than with neostigmine and atropine. A multicenter study of 45,712 adult patients reported the incidence of major pulmonary complications such as pneumonia in patients whose neuromuscular blockade was antagonized with sugammadex was less than in those who received neostigmine.[1431] Sugammadex is almost the ideal drug to rescue the "cannot intubate, cannot ventilate" situation after a rapid intubating dose of rocuronium (1.2 mg/kg) within 2 minutes, possibly more rapid than the time to recover to T1 >0.9 after succinylcholine.[1399] However, in such a critical situation, simulated scenarios are crucial to preclude delays that may jeopardize a successful outcome.[1432,1433] Future developments toward the ideal antagonist for neuromuscular blockade should seek an even faster onset time and the ability to antagonize both steroidal and benzylisoquinolinium blocking drugs.

If neuromuscular blockade must be reestablished after sugammadex, the required dose of rocuronium is unclear[1357]; the most prudent approach in this situation is to switch to a benzylisoquinolinium muscle relaxant, as they are unaffected sugammadex. In adults, 0.6 mg/kg rocuronium is required to reestablish neuromuscular blockade provided the interval since the dose of sugammadex was ≥3 hours; if the interval was <2 hours, up to 1.2 mg/kg may be required.[1434] This subject has been explored and a decision-making algorithm prepared to guide clinicians who must reparalyze a patient after neuromuscular blockade was antagonized with sugammadex. Anecdotally, after antagonizing the neuromuscular blockade with 4 mg/kg sugammadex in a 2-year-old after a ventriculoperitoneal shunt procedure, the time to reestablish full blockade (T1 of 0%) with 2 mg/kg rocuronium was 6 minutes.[1435]

Interactions between sugammadex and adjunctive medications are not widely reported. In vitro, dexamethasone inhibits sugammadex-mediated antagonism of neuromuscular blockade. When dexamethasone 0.5 mg/kg was administered IV in a randomized, controlled trial to children undergoing adenotonsillectomy, the time to reverse neuromuscular blockade after sugammadex was unchanged compared with the control.[1436] One important nuance regarding the use of sugammadex in menarchal females is that sugammadex binds progesterone and may interfere with contraceptive effectiveness for 7 days after administration of sugammadex.[1437] However, two reviews demonstrated that the majority of women of childbearing age were neither questioned about their use of oral contraceptives nor counselled regarding the possible failure of this form of birth control after sugammadex by the perioperative team.[1437,1438] Anesthesiologists should document in the electronic medical record whether oral contraceptives are used preoperatively and provide counselling regarding the risks of their failure for the first week postoperatively if sugammadex is used. Alternative contraceptive measures should be considered.

CALABADION

This new compound is a an acyclic, glycoluril, tetrameric, cucurbituril container that encapsulates both steroidal and benzylisoquinolinium neuromuscular blockers (rocuronium, vecuronium, cisatracurium) irreversibly in a manner similar to sugammadex. However, calabadion-2 binds rocuronium with 89-fold greater affinity than sugammadex, which leads to a very rapid recovery of neuromuscular function. Laboratory evidence also indicates that the role of calabadion-2 in anesthesiology may extend beyond antagonizing neuromuscular blockade rapidly as it also encapsulates ketamine and etomidate. Studies are needed in humans to assess pharmacodynamic effect and adverse effects.[1343]

Neuromuscular Blocking Drugs in Special Situations

Of the many drug combinations possible, that of succinylcholine after a halothane induction seems to be most likely to trigger MH (see Chapter 39).[689,1439] Succinylcholine, especially in combination with halogenated agents, should be avoided in children at risk for MH.[1440] Total intravenous anesthesia (see Chapter 6) is now the safest general anesthetic technique for children at risk for MH, replacing opioid/benzodiazepine with N_2O/O_2 combinations, together with benzodiazepines/propofol, and a nondepolarizing relaxant. Nondepolarizing agents devoid of cardiovascular adverse effects may offer an advantage in not causing tachycardia, an early sign of MH.[1441,1442]

The use of neuromuscular blockers in children with neuromuscular and mitochondrial diseases has been the subject of debate.[1442–1444] Rhabdomyolysis has been reported after succinylcholine in children with Duchenne and Becker muscular dystrophies (see Chapters 22 and 39). It is prudent to avoid succinylcholine in any child with a suspicious neuromuscular or mitochondrial disease. There has been some concern of the potential association between mitochondrial disease and MH.[1445] An extensive review, along with evidence from pathology specimens from patients who had a family member with MH, suggests that this is not at all clear and may be a case of "fortuitous association."[1446] Because many of these children are bedridden, it would seem prudent to avoid succinylcholine, although there are *inadequate data to support the recommendation ... that the anesthetic plan for patients with mitochondrial disease should routinely include MH precautions."*[1447] Similarly, it may be prudent to minimize exposure to the potent inhalational anesthetics as there may be a greater risk for rhabdomyolysis in these children.[1448]

All general anesthetics interfere with electron transport in the respiratory chain in mitochondria to varying degrees. Since some children with mitochondrial disorders have impaired electron chain transport, it may be further impaired by administering general anesthetics.[1449,1450] However, to date, the clinical experience with both inhalational anesthetics and propofol has overwhelmingly demonstrated that they can be used to anesthetize children with mitochondrial myopathies safely.[957,1451] Although some have alluded to the entity, "Propofol infusion syndrome," when propofol is infused in children with mitochondrial disorders, propofol infusion syndrome is an exceedingly rare complication in the OR.[953]

The response of children with neuromuscular disease to nondepolarizing relaxants is variable. Most are relatively sensitive to the neuromuscular blockers, particularly those with muscular dystrophy, because of muscle wasting.[1442,1452,1453] The duration of neuromuscular blockade is often prolonged. Rarely, resistance may be evident as a result of chronic immobilization. Of all the nondepolarizing relaxants, we suggest cisatracurium because of its multiple sites of degradation that are independent of organ function.[1454–1456] The dose requirement of atracurium in children with Duchenne muscular dystrophy is similar to that in unaffected children, although the duration of action may be prolonged.[1454] The twitch response to 0.3 and 0.6 mg/kg rocuronium in children with Duchenne muscular dystrophy shows similar twitch depression but marked prolongation of both the onset and recovery times (2- to 5-fold greater) compared with healthy children.[1457] Thus, neuromuscular blockers should be administered with caution in children with severe preexisting respiratory dysfunction, because even a small dose of a neuromuscular blocker may cause profound and prolonged muscle weakness resulting in the need for ventilatory support.[1458] Similarly, it is important to antagonize any residual neuromuscular blockade at the end of surgery. *If there is any doubt about the competence of the neuromuscular junction, the trachea should remain intubated until muscle strength has recovered.* Alternatively, the use of TIVA may obviate the need for a neuromuscular blocker.

Succinylcholine can cause hyperkalemia in children with burns, which may lead to cardiac arrest.[1459] The more extensive the burn, the more likely and the greater the hyperkalemic response. An 8% burn is the smallest burn that has been associated with hyperkalemia. Although most instances of cardiac arrest have occurred 20 to 50 days after the burn injury, exaggerated increases in the plasma concentration of potassium after succinylcholine can occur within a few days of the burn. However, hyperkalemia after succinylcholine has not been reported in the first 24 hours after a burn. Hyperkalemia is thought to result from the upregulation of acetylcholine receptors along the surface of the muscle membrane in the postburn phase (see Chapter 34).[1273,1460]

Children with burns may require two to three times the usual IV dose of nondepolarizing relaxants. This resistance peaks about 2 weeks after the burn, persists for many months in those with major burns, and decreases gradually as the burns heal. The degree of resistance appears to correlate with both the extent of the burn and the period of healing. The resistance can be explained, in part, by an increase in the volume of distribution of the relaxant (including binding to an increased plasma concentration of α_1-acid glycoprotein) and an increase in number, sensitivity, and type of extrajunctional acetylcholine receptors (see Chapter 34).[1459]

Opioids

MORPHINE

Morphine is the most frequently used opioid to treat postoperative pain in children and is the standard against which all other opioids are compared.[1461] Morphine exerts its dominant analgesic effect by activating the supraspinal μ_1-receptors. The μ_2-receptor in the spinal cord conveys an important analgesic role when the opioid is administered via the intrathecal or epidural route.[1462] Morphine is soluble in water, but poorly soluble in lipids compared with other opioids.

Pharmacodynamics

Target plasma concentrations for analgesia are considered to be 10 to 20 ng/mL after major surgery in neonates and infants.[1463,1464] No concentration-response relationship has been described in children.[1465] Morphine may display similar pharmacodynamics for respiratory depression and analgesia.[1466] A $T_{1/2}keo$ estimate for the respiratory depressant effect of morphine was 16 minutes in a child,[1467] similar to that reported for analgesia. The EC_{50} for the respiratory depressant effect of morphine, 10 to 18 ng/mL,[1466–1469] is consistent with clinical observations for both analgesic concentrations (10 to 20 ng/mL)[140,1470,1471] and respiratory depression (hypercapnia in 46% children with concentration >15 ng/mL).[138]

The large pharmacokinetic and pharmacodynamic variability suggests that morphine should be titrated to effect using small incremental IV doses (0.02 mg/kg) in neonates and infants with postoperative pain.[1472,1473] Both sex and genetics have major impact on pharmacodynamics.[1474] There is polymorphism A118G of the human μ-opioid receptor gene controlling response through the OPRM1 on chromosome 6 as well as via efflux transporter proteins known as the ATP-binding cassette family.[1475,1476] Inflammatory cytokines, mood, and adrenergic response also impact on pharmacodynamics (see Chapter 4).[1477]

Morphine's hydrophilicity (i.e., its low oil-water partition coefficient of 1.4 and its pKa of 8 [10%–20% un-ionized drug at physiologic pH]) explains its delayed onset of peak action and CNS penetration. The $T_{1/2}keo$ for morphine is approximately

17 minutes in adults,[14,1478] but may be as small as 8 minutes using allometry in the full-term neonate.[1479]

Pharmacokinetics

Morphine is primarily metabolized by the hepatic enzyme UGT2B7 to morphine-3-glucuronide (60% converted to M3G) and morphine-6-glucuronide (6%–10% converted to M6G); both have pharmacologic activity. Sulfation and renal clearance are minor pathways in adults but are more dominant in neonates. Animal data suggest that morphine and M6G act via distinct μ-receptor pathways and that an additive relationship exists between morphine and M6G for analgesic effects.[1480,1481] M6G can also contribute to respiratory depression in children with renal failure.[1467] M6G has a $T_{1/2}keo$ of 6.7 hours (range 4–8 hours) for both analgesic effect and for respiratory depression.[1467] It has been suggested that M3G antagonizes morphine and contributes to the development of tolerance.[1482]

Clearance of morphine increases from 3.2 L/hour per 70 kg at 24 weeks postmenstrual age to 19 L/hour per 70 kg at term, reaching adult values (80 L/hour per 70 kg) at 6 to 12 months (see Fig. 5.12).[26,29,1483] The immaturity of the clearance at birth explains in part the prolonged duration of action in neonates. Although there is an increase in clearance initiated by the change to extrauterine life, this change is small (see E-Fig. 5.4). There is also a complex relationship between the formation and elimination clearance of metabolites that changes with age. M3G (the dominant metabolite) concentrations increase dramatically in neonates, whereas M6G concentrations increase slowly because renal clearance of metabolites is immature in neonates. Renal function is normal in a 6-year-old and a plateau concentration is achieved at steady state with infusion. It is worthwhile noting that the M6G concentration in the child is less than half that observed in the neonate (Fig. 5.24).

The maturation profile also suggests that older infants are able to exceed the reported clearance (in liters per hour per kilogram) of morphine in adults. Clearance is perfusion-limited, with a high hepatic extraction ratio. Oral bioavailability is approximately 35% because of this first-pass effect.[1484] The metabolites are cleared by the kidney and, in part, by biliary excretion; impaired renal function leads to M3G and M6G accumulation.[1485] Clearance is reduced in critically ill neonates compared with healthier cohorts and in those undergoing cardiac surgery (Fig. 5.25).[26–28,1463]

A large number of covariates also contribute to pharmacokinetic variability. For example, the incidence of opioid-related adverse effects is greater but pain is less in Caucasian children than in African American children after tonsillectomy, although morphine clearance is greater in the latter children. Variability in clearance is influenced by genetic factors controlling the UGT enzyme system[1477]; even the patient's domicile (e.g., high altitude due to chronic hypoxia) could have an impact (see also Chapter 4).[1486,1487]

Infusion regimens are based on clearance. Conjugation with glucuronide (UGT2B7) produces both active (M6G) and inactive metabolites (M3G) that are excreted by the kidneys.[139]

Routes of Administration

Although morphine is usually administered intravenously to neonates, other routes have been used. A large variability in the analgesic effect of morphine has been observed after rectal administration[1488]; however, delayed absorption with multiple doses causing respiratory arrest has been reported so **this route is not recommended.**[147] Morphine administered orally also has considerable absorption variability (relative bioavailability [F] 0.3, coefficient of variation [CV] 36%; absorption half-time [$T_{1/2}abs$] 0.71 hour;

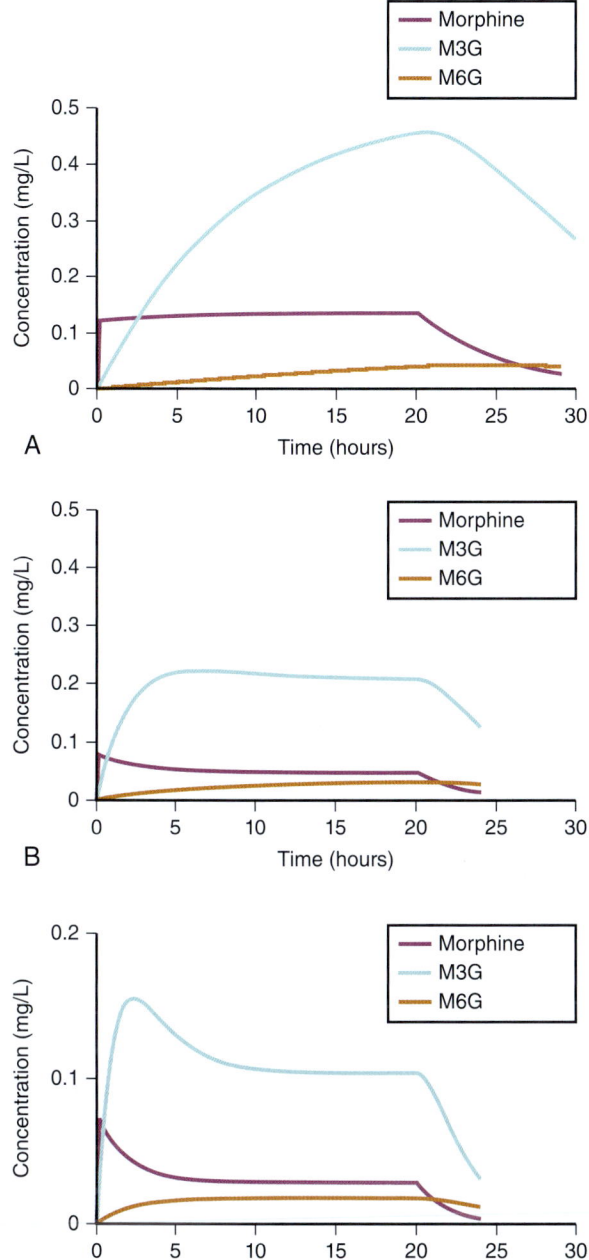

FIGURE 5.24 Morphine administered as a bolus 0.07 mg/kg with subsequent infusion 0.03 mg/kg/per hour in a neonate (A), a three month old infant (B) and a 6-year-old child (C). The concentrations of parent drug and metabolites are different in the two individuals because of the complex interplays between formation and elimination clearances. (From Anderson BJ, Holford NHG. Tips and traps analyzing paediatric PK data. *Pediatr Anesth.* 2011;21(3):222-237, with permission.)

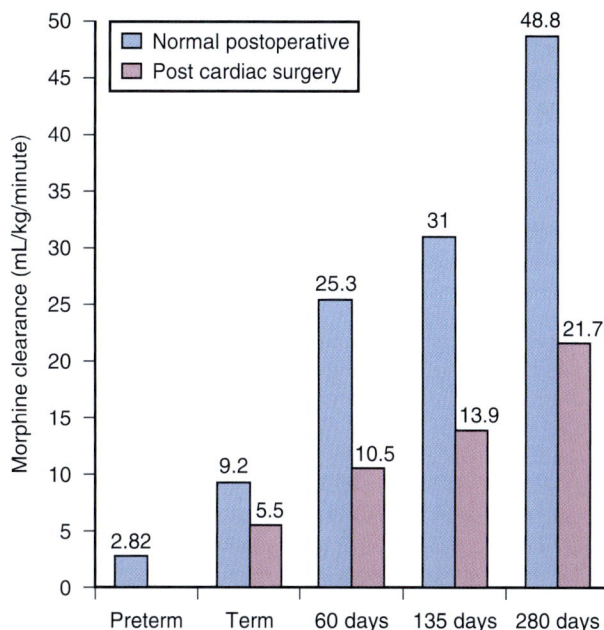

FIGURE 5.25 Morphine clearance versus postconception age in normal postoperative infants and infants undergoing cardiac surgery. Note that there is a rapid increase in an infant's ability to metabolize morphine in the first several weeks of life and that some infants achieve adult values by 1 month of age. Also note that after cardiac surgery infants have a marked impairment of morphine metabolism, which may reflect the use of vasopressors and/or decreased cardiac output to the liver. There is extreme patient-to-patient variability at all ages; preterm infants have the lowest clearance of any age group. (Data from Lynn A, Nespeca MK, Bratton SL, et al. Clearance of morphine in postoperative infants during intravenous infusion: the influence of age and surgery. *Anesth Analg.* 1998;86(5):958-963; and Mikkelsen S, Feilberg VL, Christensen CB, Lundstrøm KE. Morphine pharmacokinetics in preterm and mature newborn infants. *Acta Paediatr.* 1994;83(10):1025-1028.)

CV 55%), contributing to wide prediction intervals for observed concentrations.[1489] Morphine (25–50 µg/kg) can also be given via the caudal route and subarachnoid spaces (see Chapters 40 and 41). Although systemic absorption is slow, morphine spreads within the CSF to the brainstem, where it may cause respiratory depression lasting from 6 to more than 18 hours.[1490]

Morphine may be administered IV by intermittent bolus, continuous infusion, or patient-controlled analgesia (see Chapter 41).[1491–1493] The usual initial IV dose is 0.05–0.2 mg/kg. A reduced dose is indicated in neonates, children who are critically ill, those who are receiving supplemental analgesics or hypnotics, and/or those who have nocturnal hemoglobin desaturation (<85%) during obstructive sleep apnea (OSA).[1494–1496]

Adverse Effects

The major risk associated with opioid use in infants and children is respiratory depression.[126,1453] Morphine infusion rates of 10 to 30 µg/kg per hour provide adequate postoperative analgesia without respiratory depression in children.[1471] Postoperative analgesia is achieved at reduced infusion rates in infants 4 weeks of age or older (~5 µg/kg per hour for neonates, ~8.5 µg/kg per hour at 1 month, ~13.5 µg/kg per hour at 3 months, ~18 µg/kg per hour at 1 year, and slightly less than 16 µg/kg per hour for 1- to 3-year-olds).[138] Respiratory depression may occur at plasma concentrations of 20 ng/mL in infants and children.[138] The overall incidence of serious harm was only 1:10,000 with postoperative opioid infusions. Those at risk for harm include young infants, and those with neurodevelopmental, respiratory, or cardiac comorbidities.[1497,1498]

When morphine depresses respiration, both tidal volume and respiratory rate decrease. Whether morphine shifts the CO_2 response curve to the left or right or changes the slope as well as shifting the curve has not been clearly established. In neonates, morphine depresses respiration to a greater extent than meperidine.[1499] Although the mechanism underlying this difference remains unclear, it may relate to altered pharmacokinetics, an immature blood-brain barrier,[131] altered regional blood flow, or an increased cerebral uptake.

Alternately, reduced clearance could lead to drug accumulation in some infants given repeat doses of morphine.[1500] Another possibility is maturation of the pharmacodynamic effects on respiration rather than altered pharmacokinetics.[1501] Whether one or more of these mechanisms is involved, morphine must be used with caution in preterm infants and in infants younger than 1 year of age.

Histamine release may follow a rapid IV bolus of morphine and, on rare occasions, result in systemic hypotension.[1502] Urticaria over the course of the vein in which morphine was infused is a local, not systemic, allergic reaction and does not prohibit administering additional doses.

The incidence of PONV is related to the morphine concentration and by inference, the dose; doses >0.1 mg/kg are associated with a greater than 50% incidence of vomiting in children.[1503,1504] For unclear reasons, Latino children have a 4-fold greater incidence of pruritus and a 7-fold greater incidence of vomiting with similar morphine and morphine metabolite values.[1505] Sex may also be a factor as White females undergoing tonsillectomy experienced a greater incidence of PONV and a prolonged stay in the postanesthesia care unit than White males.[1506]

Withdrawal symptoms may be observed in neonates after cessation of a continuous morphine infusion for more than 2 weeks, and after infusion periods less than 2 weeks if the morphine infusion rate is >40 μg/kg per hour. Strategies to prevent withdrawal from morphine include the use of neuraxial analgesia, nurse-controlled sedation management protocols, ketamine or naloxone mixed with morphine infusion, and the use of alternate agents (e.g., methadone) with lower potential for tolerance.[1507,1508] Table 5.11 summarizes the relative doses of opioids administered to adults via the parenteral and oral routes. Pediatric opioid equivalence remains unquantified because pharmacokinetics change with age, complicating the dose-concentration relationship.[1509]

The use of oral morphine for tonsillectomy pain and other chronic painful conditions is increasing after the safety issues regarding codeine were promulgated by the FDA and the American Academy of Pediatrics.[1484,1510-1512] There is considerable pharmacokinetic and pharmacodynamic variability associated with morphine. Simulations of oral morphine suggest that repeat modest oral doses (e.g., 200 μg/kg 6 hourly) may yield concentrations >20 ng/mL

in some children.[1489] A starting dose of 1500 to 2000 μg/kg per day has been suggested for children with chronic pain.[1513] These doses would likely be excessive for children with acute pain, particularly those with hypoxia-induced opioid receptor sensitivity (e.g., from OSA) (See Chapter 31). Conversion from IV to oral morphine is estimated at 3 to 6 mg equivalent to 1 mg IV and oral morphine solutions are available in multiple concentrations. Extended-release tablets are also available although pediatric data are limited and oral morphine solutions are likely only effective in adolescents with chronic pain.

DIAMORPHINE

Diamorphine (diacetylmorphine, heroin) has greater fat solubility than morphine, enabling rapid transfer across the blood-brain barrier. It is rapidly deacetylated into inactive 3-monoacetylmorphine and active 6-monoacetylmorphine (6-MAM, a mu opioid agonist), and then to morphine. Morphine binds to mu opioid receptors, resulting in euphoric, analgesic, and anxiolytic effects. When given orally it undergoes extensive first-pass deacetylation metabolism, making it a prodrug for the systemic delivery of morphine.

The nasal route, which avoids first pass metabolism, has proven to be effective to manage acute pain. Nasal diamorphine 0.1 mg/kg, used in the United Kingdom for forearm fracture pain in the emergency room, is rapidly absorbed as a nasal spray in 0.2 mL of sterile water, with plasma concentrations of morphine peaking (Tpeak) at 10 minutes.[162] Nasal diamorphine 0.1 mg/kg is also described for breakthrough pain in those children undergoing palliative care.[1509,1514]

OLICERIDINE

Crystallization of the unstable membrane protein of the mu opioid receptor transformed analgesic research by allowing test binding to ligands and facilitated structure-based drug discovery.[1515] Differential activation of signaling pathways downstream of the mu receptors dissociates analgesia (G protein) from adverse effects of gut and respiratory dysfunction (β-arrestin) (Fig. 5.26).[1516,1517] Up to 3 million molecules were docked to the mu opioid receptor in a search to find a suitable analgesic drug.[1518]

Oliceridine (TRV130) is one candidate recently approved by the FDA. It is a biased μ-opioid receptor agonist that is G-protein biased such that it has antinociceptive effect without β-arrestin-dependent microopioid receptor internalization.[1519] Oliceridine is approved to treat moderate to severe pain in adults. Two randomized trials compared the analgesic efficacy and adverse effects of patient controlled analgesia boluses of 0.35 mg oliceridine with 1 mg morphine in adults undergoing bunionectomy or abdominoplasty after a loading dose.[1520] The frequency of opioid-induced respiratory depression with oliceridine was several fold less than that after morphine although gastrointestinal effects were similar.[1520-1522] Although respiratory depression is minimal,[1523,1524] other adverse effects remain common with oliceridine, including nausea (31%), constipation (11%), and vomiting (10%) in adults.[1520,1525]

MEPERIDINE

Meperidine (pethidine, Demerol) is a μ-receptor agonist that has a potency approximately one-tenth that of morphine, but it is no longer indicated to treat nociception because of adverse effects from its metabolite. Repeat doses of meperidine may result in the accumulation of normeperidine, which causes seizures.[1526,1527] We do not recommend the use of this opioid in

TABLE 5.11	Relative Comparison of Commonly Used Oral and Parenteral Opioids in an Adult		
Drug	Parenteral Dose (mg)	Oral Dose (mg)	Half-Life (Hours)
Morphine	10	30–40	2.0–3.5
Hydromorphone	1.5–2.0	6.0–7.5	2–4
Oxycodone		15–30	2–4
Methadone	7.5–10.0	15	22–25
Meperidine	75–100	300	3–5
Codeine	120–130	200	3
Fentanyl	0.1	0.1	0.5

Adapted from Lugo RA, Kern SE. Clinical pharmacokinetics of morphine. *J Pain Palliat Care Pharmacother.* 2002;16(4):5-18.

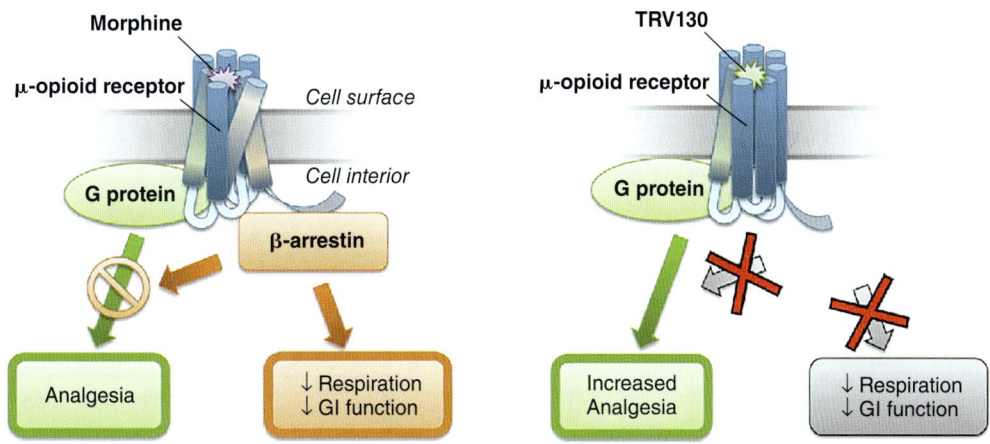

FIGURE 5.26 Morphine binding to the lμ-opioid receptor *(left panel)* engages analgesic signaling through G protein coupling to inhibit nociception by neuronal hyperpolarization, but also engages b-arrestins to the same receptor, which inhibits G protein coupling and promotes hypoventilation and gastrointestinal dysfunction. Oliceridine *(TVR130)* is a G protein–biased ligand that engages G protein coupling similarly to morphine but with less b-arrestin recruitment. (From Soergel DG, Subach RA, Burnham N, et al. Biased agonism of the mu-opioid receptor by TRV130 increases analgesia and reduces on-target adverse effects versus morphine: a randomized, double-blind, placebo-controlled, crossover study in healthy volunteers. *Pain.* 2014;155(9):1829-1835, with permission.)

infants and children other than for a single-dose administration for shivering.

Analgesic effects are detectable within 5 minutes of IV administration, and peak effect is reached within 10 minutes in adults ($T_{1/2}$keo of approximately 7–8 minutes).[1528,1529] Meperidine is metabolized by *N*-demethylation to meperidinic acid and norme-peridine. Meperidine clearance in infants and children is approximately 8 to 10 mL/minute per kilogram.[1530,1531] Elimination in neonates is greatly reduced, and elimination half-time in neonates who have received meperidine by placental transfer may be 2 to 7 times greater than that in adults.[1532] The elimination half-life of meperidine in children after IV administration is approximately 3 ± 0.5 hours,[1530] with a very variable half-life in neonates between 3.3 and 59.4 hours.[1531] The volume of distribution at steady state in infants, 7.2 (3.3–11) L/kg,[1531] is greater than that in children 2 to 8 years (2.8 ± 0.6 L/kg).[1530]

In children, meperidine is used to stop postoperative shivering, rather than for analgesia. The dose of meperidine is 1 to 2 mg/kg (see Table 5.11), although reduced doses should be used in critically ill children. Peak plasma values after IV, IM, and rectal administration are 5 minutes, 10 minutes, and 60 minutes, respectively.[1533,1534] Rectal administration of meperidine in children results in wide variations in systemic bioavailability (32%–81% of administered dose) and **is not recommended**.[1530]

In infants, respiratory depression after meperidine is less than that after morphine; the larger volume of distribution of meperidine may contribute.[1499] The LD_{50} of meperidine in the neonatal animal is only 20% less than in the adult animal, correlating with the human clinical response.[1535] As with any opioid, the use of meperidine in very young infants must be accompanied by careful observation for respiratory depression and airway obstruction.[1531] Meperidine was used for a number of years as a component of various "lytic cocktails" that provided sedation. The safety of these admixtures is dubious, and its use in sedation mixtures is not indicated.[312]

HYDROMORPHONE

Hydromorphone (Dilaudid) is a semisynthetic congener of morphine with a potency of around 5 to 7.5 times that of morphine.[1536]

A target plasma concentration for analgesia of 20 μg/L has been proposed.[1537] Hydromorphone is metabolized to hydromorphone-3-glucuronide (95%) and to other metabolites and does not appear to present added risk caused by polymorphisms.[1538] Allometrically scaled pharmacokinetic parameter estimates in children 4 to 18 years of age are systemic clearance (0.748 L/minute per 70 kg), volume of distribution (V1 33 L per 70 kg), peripheral clearance (Q 1.57 L/minute per 70 kg), and peripheral volume of distribution (V2 146 L per 70 kg); similar to reported adult parameter estimates. Sex, race, age, and type of surgery were not significant covariates.[1537] Clearance maturation has not yet been investigated, hindering dose prediction in neonates and infants.

The IV and IM dose is 10 to 20 μg/kg with a continuous IV infusion of 1 to 4 μg/kg per hour. Its bioavailability is about 55% after nasal or oral administration (30–80 μg/kg every 3–4 hours) and about 35% after rectal administration (**not recommended**)[1539–1541]; there is extensive first-pass metabolism.[1542] An initial patient-controlled analgesia loading dose of 15 μg/kg followed by a demand dose of 6 μg/kg with lockout intervals of 20 minutes is appropriate for acute pain in children.[1537]

Hydromorphone is commonly administered IV, orally, in the epidural space, and more recently through the nasal mucosa.[1543,1544] It is used when prolonged analgesia is required.[1545–1548] Morphine can be switched to hydromorphone to reduce the adverse effects or because of concern of accumulation of morphine metabolites, particularly in the presence of renal failure.[1549] Hydromorphone is commonly administered intravenously, orally, epidurally, and intranasally.[1536,1544–1546,1550–1552] Hydromorphone is used for chronic cancer pain; plasma concentrations of ~4.7 ng/mL (range 1.9–8.9 ng/mL) relieve mucositis in children given patient-controlled analgesia devices.[1536,1553] Some may require greater plasma concentrations (10–30 ng/mL) to control severe pain. Oral extended-release formulations are available but are not approved for children <17 years of age.

OXYCODONE

Oxycodone (OxyContin) is a long-acting semisynthetic opioid that can be administered IV, oral, intranasal, buccal, and epidural,[1554,1555] and is available in oral controlled-release formulations.[1556–1558]

The relative bioavailability in adults of intranasal, oral, and rectal formulations is approximately 50% that of the IV route. The buccal and sublingual absorption of oxycodone is similar in young children[1553]; the bioavailability after buccal administration was 55%; and after orogastric, 37%.[1559,1560] Oxycodone may also be administered rectally, with a similar bioavailability, although absorption can be prolonged **and is not recommended**.[1561]

Oxycodone and morphine are presumed to have similar analgesic potency (0.7:1) when used for postoperative pain.[1562,1563] An oxycodone plasma concentration of 35 μg/L has been proposed, although the therapeutic concentration range is broad: 10 to 100 μg/L.[1564,1565]

The intravenous loading and maintenance doses for oxycodone in a typical 5-year-old child are 100 μg/kg and 33 μg/kg per hour, respectively. In a typical adult the loading dose is 100 μg/kg and maintenance dose 23 μg/kg per hour.[122] Oxycodone (100 μg/kg) may cause greater ventilatory depression than comparable analgesic doses of other opioids.[1566] However, the time-course of respiratory depression in six healthy adult participants (21–30 years of age, 68–80 kg) given intravenous oxycodone (e.g., loading dose of 50 μg/kg followed by 275 μg/kg per hour infusion) and intravenous morphine (e.g., loading dose 39 μg/kg bolus followed by 215 μg/kg per hour infusion) over 2 hours were similar.[1567] Fatal consequences are reported with oxycodone concentrations greater than 200 μg/L. The IV formulation of oxycodone depresses respiration; 100 μg/kg in children after ophthalmic surgery caused greater ventilatory depression than other opioids.[1566,1568–1570] Maximum mean $ETCO_2$ concentration and minimum mean ventilatory rate occurred 8 minutes after administration of oxycodone IV in children, but the minimum mean peripheral arteriolar oxygen saturation occurred at 4 minutes.

Metabolism is through CYP3A-mediated *N*-demethylation to noroxycodone and CYP2D6 *O*-demethylation to oxymorphone and noroxymorphone; these pathways are immature in neonates.[1571,1572] Extremely preterm neonates have a median elimination half-life of 8.8 hours (range 6.8–12.5 hours); the half-life in preterm neonates is 7.4 hours (4.2–11.6 hours) and in older neonates it is 4.1 hours (2.4–5.8 hours). Infants aged 6 to 24 months have an even smaller half-life of 2.0 hours (1.7–7.2.6 hours).

A three-compartment model with first-order elimination best described the disposition of oxycodone. Population parameter estimates were clearance 48.6 L/hour per 70 kg (CV 71%); inter-compartmental clearances (Q2) 220 L/hour per 70 kg (CV 64%); Q3 1.45 L/hour per 70 kg; volume of distribution in the central compartment (V1) 98.2 L per 70 kg (CV 76%); rapidly equilibrating peripheral compartment (V2) 90.1 L per 70 kg (CV 76%); slow equilibrating peripheral compartment (V3) 28.9 L per 70 kg. Total body weight was the best size descriptor for clearances and volumes. Absorption half-times (T_{ABS}) were: 1.1 minutes for IM, 70 minutes for epidural, 82 minutes for nasogastric, and 159.6 minutes for buccal administration routes. Clearance matured with age; 8% of the typical adult value at 24 weeks postmenstrual age, 33% in a term neonate, and 90% of the adult clearance value by the end of the first year of life (Fig. 5.27).[1573] Clearance may be decreased in patients with liver dysfunction.[1574]

Although oxycodone's metabolites make a negligible contribution to its analgesic effects,[41] concerns have been expressed about CYP2D6 *O*-demethylation producing oxymorphone, which accounts for only 10% of the circulating oxycodone metabolites but is 14 times more potent than oxycodone because of its 40-fold greater affinity for the μ-opioid receptor. Consequently, "ultrarapid metabolizers" who are breastfeeding mothers may expose their

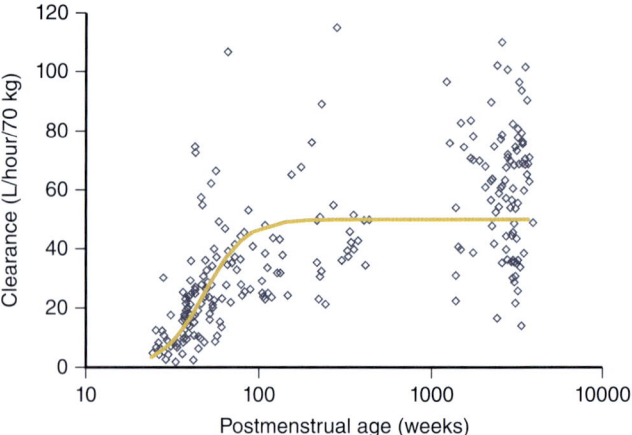

FIGURE 5.27 Maturation of oxycodone clearance with age. Changes in clearance attributed to size have been accounted for by allometric scaling of total body weight. Clearance matures over the first year of life. (From Morse JD, Sundermann M, Hannam JA, Kokki H, Kokki M, Anderson BJ. Oxycodone population pharmacokinetics: premature neonates to adults Pediatr Anesth 2021;31:1332-1339.)

infants to excessive opioids (see also Chapter 4).[1566,1575] It has been postulated that children who are rapid metabolizers and in some populations such as those with OSA may be at risk for developing excessive plasma concentrations.[1576] These concerns remain speculative; oxymorphone may be potent, but little undergoes formation metabolism and its elimination clearance is not abnormal. This opioid is commonly used to transition from patient-controlled analgesia and to treat chronic painful conditions (see Chapters 41 and 42).[1566]

HYDROCODONE

Hydrocodone is a semisynthetic hydrogenated codeine derivative and opioid agonist with analgesic and antitussive effects. The therapeutic plasma concentration is between 10 and 40 ng/mL.[1577]

Hydrocodone in a dose of 20 to 30 mg given orally has similar effectiveness as oxycodone 10 mg. The volume of distribution is 3.3 to 4.7 L/kg with a terminal half-life that averages 3.8 hours (range 3.3–4.4 hours) in adults.[1578] Clearance is 83 L/hour, but there is wide variability that depends in part, on the child's CYP2D6 metabolizer status.

Hydrocodone is metabolized through a series of enzymes (CYP2D6, CYP3A4, conjugation and keto-reduction; ~40 percent of its clearance occurs via non-CYP pathways. Two of its metabolites are active, dihydrocodeine and hydromorphone.[1579,1580] Genotype variability (see also Chapter 4) may affect the analgesic effectiveness of hydrocodone and the potential for toxicity with ultrarapid metabolism or with slow metabolism,[1581] although this remains speculative. A pediatric study of African American children treated for sickle cell disease report a genetic distribution of CYP2D6 for metabolic conversion from hydrocodone to hydromorphone,[1582] but plasma concentrations and clearance (CYP3A4) of hydromorphone were not investigated. The CYP2D6 inhibitor, quinidine, did not change the responses of extensive metabolizers.[1583] Caution is advised as inadequate analgesia and potential toxicity in some children may occur with this opioid.[1584–1586]

This drug is frequently provided in combination with acetaminophen in fixed doses (e.g., Lortab elixir); therefore, it is essential to avoid adding other acetaminophen-containing analgesics when it is prescribed. The dose should be based on the patient's ideal body weight.[1587] The dose of hydrocodone should be reduced by 33% to 50% for children with hypoxia-induced (from OSA) upregulation of opioid receptors (see Chapter 31).

METHADONE

Methadone is a synthetic opioid with an analgesic potency similar to that of morphine but with a more rapid distribution and a slower elimination. Methadone is used as a maintenance drug in opioid-addicted adults to prevent withdrawal. Methadone might have beneficial effects because it is a long-acting synthetic opioid with a very high bioavailability (80%) by the enteral route. It is also an NMDA receptor antagonist, which may be beneficial to treat chronic pain because this receptor is associated with opioid tolerance and hyperalgesia. Methadone is a racemate, but its clinical effect is mediated via the R-methadone isomer. Methadone is 2.5 to 20 times more analgesic than morphine.[1588]

The primary indication for methadone in children is to wean from long-term opioid infusions,[1589] to prevent withdrawal, and to provide analgesia when other opioids have failed or have resulted in intolerable side effects.[1590] Oral administration has been recommended as the first-line opioid for severe and persistent pain in children.[1591] Methadone is safe when administered enterally, as an alternative to IV opioids in palliative pediatric oncologic patients.[1592]

Intravenous methadone is an effective analgesic for postoperative pain relief. The minimum effective analgesic concentration of methadone in opioid-naïve adults is 58 µg/L,[1593] whereas withdrawal symptoms were not observed in any neonates with opioid withdrawal when the plasma concentration of methadone was >60 µg/L.[1594] One pediatric study reported that the perioperative administration of multiple small oral doses (0.1 mg/kg) every 12 hours for 3 to 5 doses did not result in respiratory depression and improved multimodal postoperative analgesia.[1595] The racemate of methadone, which is commonly used in pediatric and anesthetic care, is metabolized to EDDP (2-ethylidene-1,5-dimethyl-3,3-diphenylpyrrolidine) and EMDP (2-ethyl-5-methyl-3,3-diphenylpyrroline).

Methadone is cleared by the cytochrome P450 mixed oxidase (CYP3A4, CYP2B6, and CYP2D6) enzyme systems, all of which are immature at birth. CYP3A7 may contribute to clearance in the neonate.[1596,1597] Methadone has high lipid solubility with a large volume of distribution of 6 to 7 L/kg in children and adults.[1598,1599] Pharmacokinetic parameters, standardized to a 70-kilogram adult using allometry, have been estimated using a three-compartment linear disposition model. Population parameter estimates (CV, between subject variability) were central volume (V1) 21.5 (29%) L/70 kg; peripheral volumes of distribution V2 75.1 (23%) L/70 kg; V3 484 (8%) L/70 kg; clearance 9.45 (11%) L/hour per 70 kg; and intercompartment clearances Q2 325 (21%) L/hour per 70 kg, Q3 136 (14%) L/hour per 70 kg. EDDP formation clearance was 9.1 (11%) L/hour per 70 kg; formation clearance of EMDP from EDDP was 7.4 (63%) L/hour per 70 kg; elimination clearance of EDDP was 40.9 (26%) L/hour per 70 kg; and the rate constant for intermediate compartments was 2.17 (43%) per hour.[1600] These parameter estimates in neonates and children are consistent with those reported by others in neonates,[1508] children,[1599] adolescents,[1601] and adults.[1602] Clearance did not mature with age and the clearance of enantiomers of methadone in neonates was also similar to that in adults.[1600]

An intravenous regimen of 0.2 mg/kg methadone 8 hourly in neonates achieves a target concentration of 60 µg/L within 36 hours. An infusion of methadone, rather than intermittent dosing, should be considered if the goal is to achieve the target concentration in older children after cardiac surgery. Analgesic responses in adults in chronic methadone programs suggest a steep concentration-response relationship for pain relief (Hill = 4.4 ± 3.8) with very rapid equilibration between plasma methadone concentrations and the sites mediating pain relief. Consequently, the drug rapidly loses effect as concentrations decrease to less than the EC$_{50}$. A single dose of 0.2 mg/kg will provide limited analgesia after a few hours. A methadone infusion (Fig. 5.28) has been recommended to treat postoperative pain after spinal instrumentation surgery in adolescents,[1601] and after cardiac surgery in children. It should be noted that methadone, like other opioids, has large between-subject pharmacokinetic variability that could result in drug accumulation and possible fatal outcomes with long-term administration.[1603]

FENTANYL

Fentanyl (Sublimaze) offers greater hemodynamic stability than morphine, a rapid onset (T$_{1/2}$keo of 6.6 minutes in adults), and a short duration of effect. Its relative increased lipid solubility and small molecular conformation enables efficient penetration of the blood-brain barrier and redistribution. It is the most commonly used opioid during general anesthesia in infants and children. It is particularly effective in the care of high-risk preterm and term neonates, as well as in infants and children during cardiac surgical procedures. Large doses of fentanyl (10–100 µg/kg) are often administered to maintain cardiovascular homeostasis and prevent a stress response to surgery.[1360,1604–1614] Fentanyl may be administered IV, IM, intranasally, as a supplement to epidural analgesia, orally, oral transmucosal absorption, and transdermally, both passively and by iontophoresis.[1615–1622]

Fentanyl is metabolized primarily by oxidative N-dealkylation (CYP3A4) to norfentanyl and in 1% by alkyl hydroxylation to hydroxynorfentanyl.[1623] All metabolites are inactive and a small amount of fentanyl is eliminated via the kidneys unchanged. Despite extensive use in daily clinical practice, few studies have been performed.[1624] Compared with term neonates, the clearance of fentanyl in preterm infants is markedly reduced (mean elimination half-life is 17.7 ± 9.3 hours), contributing to prolonged respiratory depression in preterm neonates. Clearance matures with gestational age; 7 mL/minute per kilogram at 25 weeks postmenstrual age, 10 mL/minute per kilogram at 30 weeks postmenstrual age, and 12 mL/minute per kilogram at 35 weeks postmenstrual age.[1625] The clearance of fentanyl is 70% to 80% of adult values in term neonates and, when standardized to a 70-kilogram person, reaches adult values (~50 L/hour per 70 kg) within the first 2 weeks of life.[1005] Physiological changes increase clearance during the early postnatal period,[1626] although the impact on dosing is probably negligible.[221] Clearance of fentanyl in older infants (>3 months of age) and children is greater than that in adults when expressed per kilogram (30.6 mL/kg per minute vs. 17.9 mL/kg per minute, respectively), resulting in a reduced elimination half-life (68 minutes vs. 121 minutes, respectively).[1604,1607,1627–1629] Clearance was related to total body weight using allometry (i.e., NFM with Ffat=1).[121]

The volume of distribution at steady state of fentanyl is approximately 5.9 L/kg in term neonates and decreases with age to 4.5 L/kg during infancy, 3.1 L/kg during childhood, and 1.6 L/kg in adults.[1630] This increased volume of distribution at steady state results in a smaller blood concentration after bolus administration in neonates and infants.[1631] Administration of fentanyl 3 µg/kg by slow IV push in term infants (1–7 months of age) intraoperatively

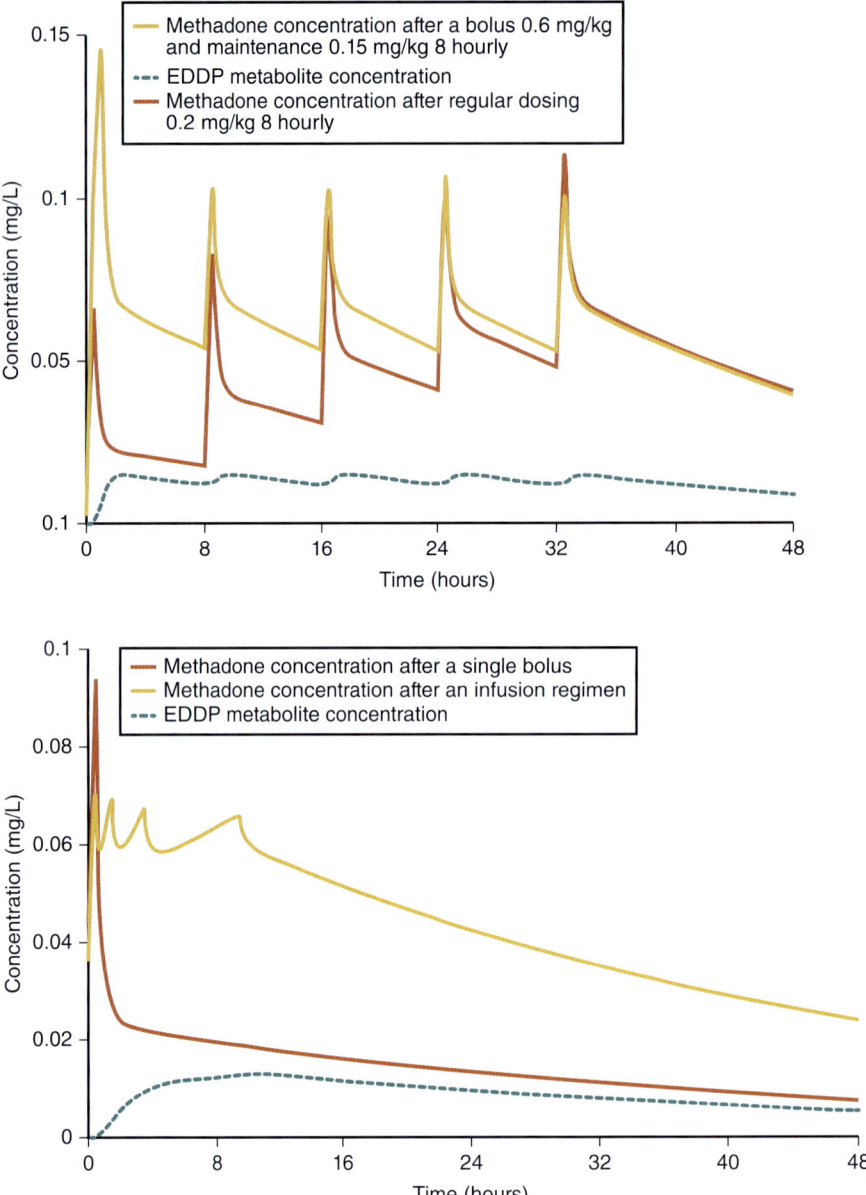

FIGURE 5.28 The *upper panel* shows a simulation for a 3.5-kg neonate given a methadone loading dose of 0.6 mg/kg followed by a maintenance dose of 0.15 mg/kg 8 hourly. EDDP concentrations track parent drug concentrations. The methadone target concentration of 0.06 mg/L is achieved rapidly compared with the neonate given 0.2 mg/kg 8 hourly without a loading dose. A single dose of methadone 0.2 mg/kg given for postoperative analgesia in a child is unlikely to achieve long duration of analgesia because concentrations are below 0.03 mg/kg within 1.5 hours *(lower panel)*. An infusion may be a better option. A regimen consisting of a methadone bolus of 0.15 mg/kg followed by 0.15 mg/kg per hour for 1 hour, 0.075 mg/kg per hour for 2 hours, and 0.025 mg/kg per hour for 6 hours maintains a concentration of 0.06 mg/L. EDDP concentrations after this infusion regimen are also shown. *EDDP*, 2-ethylidene-1,5-dimethyl-3,3-diphenylpyrrolidine. (From Ward RM. The pharmacokinetics of methadone and its metabolites in neonates, infants, and children. *Paediatr Anaesth.* 2014;24(2):591-601, with permission.)

neither depressed respiration nor caused hypoxemia in placebo-controlled trials.[1632,1633] Slow administration and both an increased volume of distribution at steady state and an increased clearance (per kilogram) in this age group contributed to these results. Fentanyl clearance may be impaired with decreased hepatic blood flow (e.g., from increased intraabdominal pressure in neonatal omphalocele repair), although a maldistribution of blood away from regions of concentrated cytochrome enzyme activity in the liver may also play a role.[1634]

Infants with cyanotic heart disease had reduced volume of distribution at steady state and greater plasma concentrations

of fentanyl with continuous infusions.[1606] Although there may be adherence to the cardiopulmonary circuit,[1606] a major contributor to greater plasma concentrations was from a reduced clearance (34 L/hour per 70 kg), which was attributed to hemodynamic disturbance and consequent reduced hepatic blood flow.[1635] Hypothermia also reduces fentanyl clearance.[1636] Profound hypotension has been reported after a bolus of midazolam in neonates in whom fentanyl was infused and vice versa.[1637] Other drugs metabolized by CYP3A4 (e.g., cyclosporine, erythromycin) may compete for clearance and result in increased fentanyl plasma concentrations.

Fentanyl is a potent μ-receptor agonist with a potency 70 to 125 times greater than that of morphine. A plasma concentration of 15 to 30 ng/mL is required to provide total IV anesthesia in adults, whereas the EC_{50}, based on EEG evidence, is 10 ng/mL.[1638,1639] Fentanyl prevents surgical stress responses and improves postoperative outcomes in preterm neonates.[1640] Single doses of fentanyl (3 μg/kg) can reduce the physiologic and behavioral measures of pain and stress associated with mechanical ventilation in preterm infants.[1641] Fentanyl has similar respiratory depression in infants and adults when plasma concentrations are similar.[1642]

The pharmacokinetics of fentanyl in critically ill children who are sedated with infusions long-term is also quite variable, with a mean terminal elimination half-life of 21 hours and a range of 11 to 36 hours.[1643,1644] The infusion rates of fentanyl that are required to achieve a similar level of sedation and analgesia may vary as much as 10-fold.[1643] This variability in pharmacokinetics and pharmacodynamics strongly reinforces the need to titrate the dose to effect and to be prepared to provide postoperative ventilatory support as needed in each child. Children who are sedated long-term with infusions of fentanyl are at risk of rapidly developing tolerance with a doubling of opioid dose more likely to occur after 7 days[1645]; on discontinuance of the infusion, these children may demonstrate signs of withdrawal.[1646,1647] Continuous infusions of fentanyl in mechanically ventilated preterm infants combined with intermittent boluses reduce acute pain compared with bolus dosing alone.[1648] All long-term infusions should be tapered slowly over days rather than discontinuing them abruptly.[1628,1646,1649]

With low-dose fentanyl, the termination of action is primarily a combination of redistribution and rapid clearance by the liver.[1628,1650] The context-sensitive half-time after a 1-hour infusion of fentanyl is approximately 20 minutes, which increases to 270 minutes after an 8-hour infusion in adults (Fig. 5.29).[6] Although the context-sensitive half-time is reduced in children, there are no data in neonates.[1629] High-dose fentanyl accumulates in muscle and fat and is therefore released (recirculated) more slowly, thus accounting in part for the prolonged respiratory depression after large doses. There is no evidence of dose-dependent kinetics (i.e., there is no tissue or enzyme saturation in the clinically used ranges).[1650] In some respects, the pharmacology of opioids is very similar to that of barbiturates: at low doses their clinical effect is terminated by redistribution, whereas at large doses their clinical effect is terminated by metabolism.[1642,1650–1653]

The usual initial intravenous dose of fentanyl is 1 to 3 μg/kg in children, a dose that may be supplemented as clinically indicated. Continuous intraoperative and postoperative infusions of fentanyl are common in children of all ages.[1606,1653,1654] Fentanyl is also used to provide patient-controlled analgesia (see Chapter 41).[1655,1656]

Chest wall and glottic rigidity have been reported after intravenous opioids, although most often after fentanyl. The reason for this is not clear.[1657–1662] Glottic rigidity may account for the inability to ventilate by bag and mask after IV fentanyl.[1662,1663] This adverse response can be minimized by administering the opioid slowly, and it can be reversed by administering either a muscle relaxant or naloxone.[1663] Another concern is the rare association of increased vagal tone with bolus administration; bradycardia may have profound effects on the cardiac output of neonates. Additionally, fentanyl markedly depresses the baroreceptor reflex control of heart rate in neonates.[1664] It is for these reasons that pancuronium (with its vagolytic effect) is often combined with high-dose fentanyl and why atropine is administered before a fentanyl-succinylcholine combination for neonatal intubation.[1665]

Oral transmucosal fentanyl (Fentanyl Oralet) was approved by the FDA for premedication of children but is no longer marketed. A new formulation (Actiq) has been approved for adults and children 16 years of age or older, but it has been used off-label in children for the treatment of cancer breakthrough pain.[1666–1668] This route of administration provides more rapid onset of analgesia than buccal immediate-release tablets but is slower in onset than nasal administration.[1668] Fentanyl is rapidly absorbed through the oral mucosa, which bypasses the liver.[1616,1617,1669–1674] Nonetheless, approximately half the absorption is gastrointestinal. Consequently, the bioavailability of this formulation in children (33%) is less than that in adults (50%).[1616,1617] Uptake continues for a period of time after consumption, which potentially can provide analgesia for several hours.[1616,1617,1674]

Transdermal fentanyl (fentanyl patch) was developed to provide an extended release of fentanyl similar to that provided with a continuous IV infusion.[1615,1675–1684] *This formulation was not designed to be administered to treat postsurgical pain, but rather for those who require opioids chronically.* This fentanyl transdermal therapeutic system (TTS) is available with a drug release rate of 12.5 μg/hour and matches the smaller dosing requirements of cancer pain control in children.[1685] An approximate conversion factor of 45 mg/day oral morphine to 12.5 μg/hour fentanyl TTS is used for initial dose estimation in children receiving long-term morphine therapy. This is conservatively low to avoid respiratory depression. In adults, uptake of fentanyl begins within 1 hour and achieves therapeutic levels within 6 to 8 hours and peak levels at 24 hours.[1681,1684,1686] In children, the peak occurs earlier, at about 18 hours.[1687] The skin acts as a reservoir, and even after removal of the patch, uptake continues for several hours, with a consequent apparent elimination half-life of 14.5 ± 6 hours.[1687] Fentanyl uptake is markedly affected by skin blood flow, skin thickness, location of the patch, and adherence to the skin.[1685,1688–1690] Alterations in skin blood flow (e.g., fever) may increase absorption.[1691] Alterations to skin blood flow caused by warming devices (increased absorption) or hypothermia (decreased absorption)

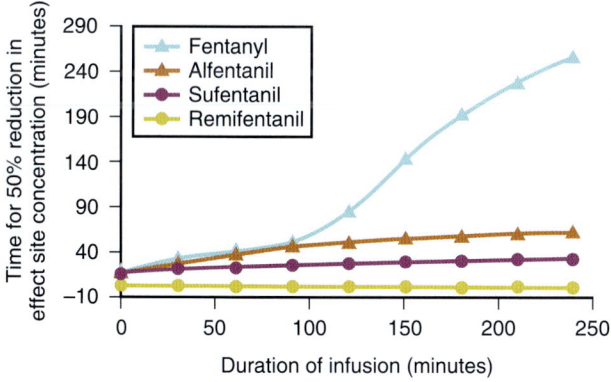

FIGURE 5.29 This figure is a simulation of the time required for a 50% reduction in the effective site concentration of remifentanil *(yellow circles)*, sufentanil *(purple circles)*, alfentanil *(brown triangles)*, and fentanyl *(blue triangles)* after an infusion (duration of 240 minutes) designed to maintain a constant effect-site concentration. Note that there is a completely flat curve for remifentanil, suggesting that a plateau effect is rapidly reached with remifentanil compared with the other opioids, such that even after a long infusion, the time to 50% reduction in effect-site concentration is still less than 4 minutes. (Redrawn and modified with permission from Westmoreland CL, Hole JF, Sebel PS, Hug CC Jr, Muir KT. Pharmacokinetics of remifentanil [GI87084B] and its major metabolite [GI90291] in patients undergoing elective inpatient surgery. *Anesthesiology.* 1993;79(5):893-903.)

during anesthesia should be considered in children with chronic pain who present with TTS fentanyl.

The use of TTS medication should be limited to pain specialists who are familiar with the unusual pharmacokinetics of this drug delivery system.[1692] One study suggests that the pharmacokinetics of fentanyl by this route in children and adult patients are similar.[1687] A multicenter study in children 2 to 16 years of age reported satisfactory long-term analgesia. However, it should be noted that the data submitted to the FDA revealed plasma concentrations of fentanyl in children 1.5 to 5 years of age that were twice those in adults.[1693] These data are consistent with another study that found a negative correlation between fentanyl concentrations and age, that is, greater concentrations in younger children.[1687] Children may be particularly vulnerable to the rapid drug absorption compared with adults because they have thinner skin and better skin blood flow.[1062] Accordingly, it seems prudent to begin with the smallest size patch and gradually increase as indicated (see Chapters 41 and 42). All patches, including those that have already been used, contain large amounts of fentanyl that may cause a fatal intoxication if accidentally or intentionally ingested or improperly applied.[1694–1696] Proper disposal of these opioid-containing patches is required.[1697]

Epidural fentanyl is often combined with an amide local anesthetic for provision of postoperative analgesia; pruritus, nausea, and vomiting may be exacerbated by the addition of fentanyl. Spread beyond the site of administration is dose dependent but limited, and respiratory depression is uncommon.[1556,1698] It should be noted, however, that plasma concentrations may increase for a period of time after cessation of epidural fentanyl, thus prolonging the potential for respiratory depression for several hours.[1622]

ALFENTANIL

Alfentanil (Alfenta) is a fentanyl analog whose main advantage is its reduced lipid solubility and smaller volume of distribution compared with fentanyl.[1699] It has a rapid onset ($T_{1/2}$keo of 0.9 minutes in adults), a brief duration of action, and one-quarter the potency of fentanyl. A target plasma concentration of 400 ng/mL is used in anesthesia. Metabolism is through oxidative N-dealkylation by CYP3A4 and O-dealkylation and then conjugation to metabolites that are excreted renally.[1700] Brain concentrations of alfentanil are 7-fold to 9-fold less, the volume of distribution is four times less, and protein binding is greater than fentanyl.[1701]

Alfentanil is eliminated more rapidly from the body than fentanyl, thus necessitating more frequent dosing. Clearance in neonates (20–60 mL/minute per 70 kg) is one-tenth that in adults (250–500 mL/minute per 70 kg) with rapid maturation.[54] In preterm neonates, the half-life is 6 to 9 hours.[1702,1703] The volume of distribution in children and adults is similar but is increased in preterm neonates (volume of distribution 1.0 ± 0.39 vs. 0.48 ± 0.19 L/kg). Clearance is greater in children when expressed per kilogram (11.1 ± 3.9 mL/kg per minute vs. 5.9 ± 1.6 mL/kg per minute). As a result, the elimination half-life in children is less (63 ± 24 vs. 95 ± 20 minutes).[1704–1707] The volume of distribution and elimination half-life in infants 3 to 12 months of age and older children are similar.[1706] With clearance markedly diminished in children with hepatic disease, the clinical effects of alfentanil are prolonged in those with reduced hepatic blood flow (e.g., children with increased intraabdominal pressure, children receiving vasopressors, and those with some forms of congenital heart disease).[1699,1708,1709] Renal failure has little effect on its elimination.[1710] Because less alfentanil is bound to α_1-acid glycoprotein in preterm infants (65%) than in term infants (79%), an increased unbound fraction of alfentanil is available for biologic effect in the former.[74]

The pharmacokinetics and pharmacodynamics of alfentanil suggest potential applications for the rapid control of analgesia and awakening from anesthesia. It can be used as an alternative to remifentanil during TIVA (see Chapter 6). Alfentanil (10 μg/kg) has been combined with propofol (2.5 mg/kg) for tracheal intubation without a neuromuscular blocking drug.[1711] High-dose alfentanil is also used for cardiac procedures. Alfentanil should be used with caution without neuromuscular blockers in neonates because of the frequency of chest wall or glottic rigidity.[1531,1712]

SUFENTANIL

Sufentanil (Sufenta) is a potent synthetic opioid that in many respects is similar to fentanyl and alfentanil. Sufentanil is 5 to 10 times more potent than fentanyl, with a $T_{1/2}$keo of 6.2 minutes in adults.[1713] A concentration of 5 to 10 ng/mL is required for total intravenous anesthesia, and 0.2 to 0.4 ng/mL for analgesia. Pharmacodynamic differences are suggested in neonates. The plasma concentration of sufentanil at the time of additional anesthetic supplementation to suppress hemodynamic responses to surgical stimulation was 2.51 ng/mL in neonates, notably greater than the concentrations of 1.58, 1.53, and 1.56 ng/mL observed in infants, children, and adolescents, respectively.[1714]

Elimination of sufentanil is by O-demethylation and N-dealkylation in animal studies. As with fentanyl and alfentanil, the CYP3A4 enzyme is responsible for the N-dealkylation.[1715] A central volume of distribution (volume of distribution 4.7, IQR 4.1–5.4 L/kg) and clearance (CL 11, IQR 7–13 mL/kg per minute) is estimated in full-term neonates, with weight and postmenstrual age as main covariates.[1716] Pharmacokinetic studies of sufentanil focused on children undergoing cardiac surgery. Sufentanil pharmacokinetics are age-dependent; neonates have a larger volume of distribution at steady state, reduced clearance, and a greater and more variable elimination half-life than older children and adults (E-Fig. 5.19).[1714,1717,1718] Clearance in neonates undergoing cardiovascular surgery (6.7 ± 6.1 mL/kg per minute) is reduced compared with values of 18.1 ± 2.7, 16.9 ± 3.2, and 13.1 ± 3.6 mL/kg per minute in infants, children, and adolescents, respectively,[1714] which is consistent with rapid development of hepatic metabolic pathways.[1716,1717] Maturation in clearance standardized to a 70-kilogram person using allometry is similar to that of other drugs that depend on CYP3A4 for metabolism (e.g., levobupivacaine, fentanyl, alfentanil) (see Fig. 5.12).[1719] Clearance rates in infants (27.5 ± 9.3 mL/kg per minute) were greater, expressed per kilogram, than those in children (18.1 ± 10.7 mL/kg per minute) in another study of children undergoing cardiovascular surgery.[1718]

Clearance in healthy children (2–8 years) was greater (30.5 ± 8.8 mL/kg per minute) than in those undergoing cardiac surgery.[1720] Decreased hepatic blood flow reduces clearance.[1720] The elimination of sufentanil is unaffected by renal failure but markedly altered by factors that influence hepatic blood flow; cirrhosis apparently has little effect on its elimination.[1699,1721,1722] The volume of distribution at steady state was 4.15 ± 1.0 L/kg in neonates, greater than the values of 2.73 ± 0.5 and 2.75 ± 0.5 L/kg observed in children and adolescents, respectively.[1714,1720] A clearance of 45 L/hour per 70 kg is reported in children (4.05 range 2.2 months–17.4 years) during long-term ventilation, when standardized for size using allometry. Reduced clearance was not reported in infants, consistent with rapid clearance maturation.[1723]

Bradycardia and asystole have been observed after a bolus administration of sufentanil, suggesting that pretreatment with a vagolytic agent (atropine, glycopyrrolate, or pancuronium bromide) may be prudent.[1724,1725]

Nasal sufentanil may have a role for sedation/analgesia in children undergoing painful procedures,[167] although data in neonates are lacking and there are concerns about the risk of respiratory depression.[1726–1731] Several studies demonstrated that children are more likely to accept nasal sufentanil compared with nasal midazolam, although there was a greater incidence of vomiting after sufentanil and several children experienced decreased chest wall compliance after or during induction of anesthesia. The dose of sufentanil that is most effective when administered intranasally is 2 to 3 µg/kg.[1727,1729] The nasal preparation has been mixed with ketamine to augment analgesia in children.[167]

Epidural sufentanil (0.7–0.75 µg/kg) has been effective in children, lasting more than 3 hours, although pruritus can be bothersome.[1732–1734] If administered as a continuous epidural infusion, it should be noted that sufentanil is slowly eliminated. Plasma concentrations may continue to increase even after discontinuation, which could potentially lead to respiratory depression.[1735] Nasal sufentanil 0.5 µg/kg had a maximum plasma concentration (C_{max}) of 0.042 µg/L at 13.8 minutes.[167]

REMIFENTANIL

Remifentanil (Ultiva) is a synthetic opioid, with a brief elimination half-life of 3 to 6 minutes that is independent of the duration of the infusion.[237,1736–1739] Blood and tissue esterases rapidly terminate its action by degrading an ester linkage in the molecule to a carboxylic acid metabolite.[1739] This brief half-life contributes to rapid recovery within about 10 minutes, independent of infusion duration.[237,1736,1739] Clearance in patients with butyrylcholinesterase deficiency is unaffected. The nonspecific blood esterases that metabolize remifentanil are mature at birth.[23]

Metabolism is unaffected by hepatic or renal function.[1740] The active metabolite of remifentanil that is eliminated by the kidneys has approximately 1/300 to 1/1000 the opioid activity of the parent compound and without clinical manifestations in children, even in those with impaired renal function.[1741] There were no residual opioid effects after a 12-hour infusion in adults with renal failure.[1742]

A target plasma concentration of 2 to 3 µg/L is adequate for laryngoscopy, 6 to 8 µg/L for laparotomy, and 10 to 12 µg/L might be sought to ablate the stress response associated with cardiac surgery (see Chapter 6 for remifentanil use in total IV anesthesia).[1743] Analgesic concentrations are 0.2 to 0.4 µg/L. The $T_{1/2}$keo is 1.16 minutes in adults,[236] but the neonatal $T_{1/2}$keo has not been reported. Analgesic alternatives should be administered when the short-duration analgesic effects from remifentanil are dissipating.

Remifentanil clearance can be described in all age groups by simple application of an allometric model.[22] This standardized clearance of 2790 mL/minute per 70 kg is similar to that reported by others in children[237,1744] and adults.[236,1745] A model that included neonates, children and adults (0–85 years, 2–106 kg) estimated a similar common clearance using allometric scaling (2580 mL per minute per 70 kg). The $T_{1/2}$keo (adult 1.09 minutes) decreased with younger ages.[1746] The smaller the child, the greater the clearance when expressed as milliliters per minute per kilogram. Clearance decreases with increasing age, with rates of 90 mL/kg per minute in infants younger than 2 years of age, 60 mL/kg per minute in children 2 to 12 years of age, and 40 mL/kg per minute in adults (Fig. 5.30 and Table 5.12).[22,237,1744]

The volume of distribution at steady state was greatest in infants younger than 2 months of age (452 mL/kg) and decreased to 308 mL/kg in children 2 months to 2 years, and to 240 mL/kg in children older than 2 years of age,[237] and the context-sensitive half-time is constant (see Fig. 5.29).[1741] For example, when the infusion rates of remifentanil differed as much as 20-fold, the time to return to spontaneous respirations varied by only 1 to 3 minutes.[1740,1747]

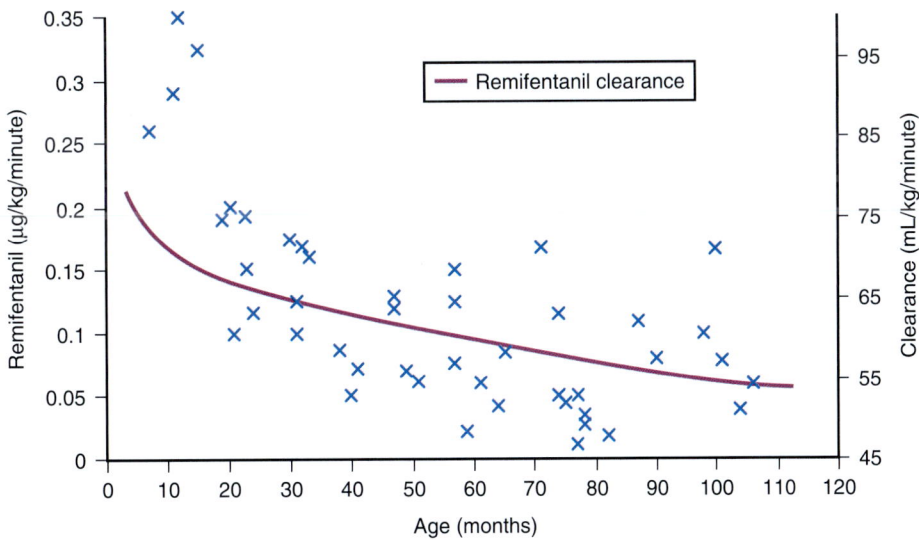

FIGURE 5.30 The effect of age on the dose (infusion rate) of remifentanil tolerated during spontaneous ventilation under anesthesia in children undergoing strabismus surgery.[290] Superimposed on this plot is the estimated remifentanil clearance determined using an allometric model.[68] There is a mismatch between clearance and infusion rate for those individuals still in infancy. The larger infusion rates recorded in those infants can be attributed to greater suppression of respiratory drive in this age group than with the older children during the study; a respiratory rate of 10 breaths/minute in an infant is disproportionately slow compared with the same rate in a 7-year-old child, suggesting excessive dose. (Reproduced with permission from Anderson BJ. Pediatric models for adult target-controlled infusion pumps. *Paediatr Anaesth.* 2010;20(3):223-232; Rigby-Jones AE, Priston MJ, Sneyd JR, et al. Remifentanil-midazolam sedation for paediatric patients receiving mechanical ventilation after cardiac surgery. *Br J Anaesth.* 2007;99(2):252-261; and Barker N, Lim J, Amari E, Malherbe S, Ansermino JM. Relationship between age and spontaneous ventilation during intravenous anesthesia in children. *Paediatr Anaesth.* 2007;17(10):948-955.)

TABLE 5.12	Remifentanil Pharmacokinetics by Age					
	0–2 Months	2 Months–2 Years	2–6 Years	7–12 Years	13–16 Years	16–18 Years
C_{max}	24.2 ± 10.2[a]	25.4 ± 3.7[a]	34.8 ± 8.2	42.5 ± 13.7	35 ± 10.2	42.7 ± 12.9
Vdss	452.8 ± 144.7[a]	307.9 ± 89.2	240.1 ± 130.5	248.9 ± 91.4	223.2 ± 30.6	242.5 ± 109.2
CL (mL/minute per kilogram)	90.5 ± 36.8[a]	92.1 ± 25.8[a]	76 ± 22.4	59.7 ± 22.5	57.2 ± 21.1	46.5 ± 2.1
Half-life (minutes)	5.4 ± 1.8	3.4 ± 1.19	3.6 ± 1.19	5.3 ± 1.4	3.7 ± 1.1	5.7 ± 0.7

CL, clearance; C_{max}, peak plasma concentration; Vdss, volume of distribution at steady state.
[a]Significantly different from other groups.
Data extracted from Ross AK, Davis PJ, Dear G, et al. Pharmacokinetics of remifentanil in anesthetized pediatric patients undergoing elective surgery or diagnostic procedures. *Anesth Analg.* 2001;93(6):1393-1401.

As an opioid, the effect of remifentanil on respiration is an excellent reflection of its pharmacodynamic effects.[1748] After 3-hour infusions of alfentanil and remifentanil in adults, the elimination half-lives were 47.3 ± 12 minutes for alfentanil, compared with 3.2 ± 0.9 minutes for remifentanil. The time to recover 50% of the minute ventilation, a pharmacodynamics effect of opioids, was 54.0 ± 48.1 minutes for alfentanil, compared with 5.4 ± 1.8 minutes for remifentanil.[1748]

Although covariate effects, such as cardiac surgery, appear to have a muted effect on pharmacokinetics, cardiopulmonary bypass does have an impact. Remifentanil dosage adjustments are required during and after cardiopulmonary bypass because of marked changes in its volume of distribution.[1749] Other pharmacokinetic changes during cardiopulmonary bypass are consistent with adult data in which a decreased metabolism occurred with a reduced temperature[1750] and with reports of greater clearance after cardiopulmonary bypass (increased metabolism) compared with during cardiopulmonary bypass.[1744]

Respiratory depression is concentration dependent.[1751,1752] This adverse effect has been used to advantage during cardiac imaging in children 1 month to 9 years of age undergoing MRI.[1753] Apnea sequences were successful in 80% of patients at a remifentanil infusion rate of 0.184 (95% CI 0.178–0.190) µg/kg per minute.[1754] Increasing age was associated with reduced remifentanil requirements, consistent with allometric expectations of reduced clearance (L/hour per kg) with increasing age.

Closure of the vocal cords, commonly interpreted as muscle rigidity, remains a concern if intravenous bolus doses exceed 3 µg/kg as may occur when intubating the trachea in neonates.[1755] Induction with propofol (4 mg/kg) and either remifentanil (3 µg/kg) or succinylcholine (2 mg/kg) for tracheal intubation was similar, without bradycardia, hypotension, or chest wall rigidity.[1756] The initial loading dose of remifentanil may cause hypotension and bradycardia,[1757] prompting some to target the plasma rather than effect-site concentration when initiating an infusion. This hypotensive response has been quantified in children undergoing cranioplasty surgery. A steady-state remifentanil concentration of 14 µg/L would typically achieve a 30% decrease in mean arterial pressure (see Fig. 6.21) This concentration is twice that required for laparotomy but is easily achieved with a bolus injection. The $T_{1/2}$keo of 0.86 minutes for this hemodynamic effect[1758] is less than remifentanil-induced spectral edge frequency changes described in adults ($T_{1/2}$keo of 1.34 minutes).[236,1759]

One unresolved concern associated with the long-term administration of remifentanil is the development of acute tolerance; activity at δ-opioid receptors may contribute.[1760] A study of adolescents undergoing spinal instrumentation for scoliosis demonstrated acute tolerance.[1761] These results are inconsistent with studies that reported no relation between the dose of remifentanil and postoperative opioid consumption.[1762] The use of fentanyl for spinal instrumentation surprisingly found a greater opioid requirement and pain scores than a remifentanil-treated cohort.[1763] A prospective randomized trial in children 1 to 5 years of age undergoing laparoscopic procedures that compared three remifentanil infusions of 0, 0.3, 0.6, and 0.9 µg/kg per minute found that those who received 0.6 or 0.9 µg/kg per minute required more postoperative fentanyl at 24 hours than those who received 0 or 0.3 µg/kg per minute, suggesting that large doses of remifentanil may cause tolerance.[1764] The rapid development of tolerance or hyperalgesia with remifentanil is as yet unsettled.

Remifentanil has an important role in providing safe analgesia to children of all ages, but particularly in very sick preterm infants and children.[1765–1769] Its main advantage is the ability to provide an intense opioid effect with cardiovascular stability during the procedure, and then transition to a less intense opioid effect, allowing for early extubation.[1765,1770] *Remifentanil is the only opioid for which there is a greater rather than a reduced clearance (per kilogram) in neonates (see Fig. 5.30), and the reason why it is so valuable in this age group.*[1771–1778] These pharmacologic differences have important clinical implications because they translate into the ability to rapidly titrate the opioid effect, without concern for prolonged sedation. *This opioid should be administered only by continuous infusion. If an IV line becomes interrupted, kinked, or disconnected, the opioid effect will rapidly dissipate, and the child will show evidence of pain.*

High concentrations of remifentanil cause hypotension (Fig. 6.21); many practitioners either avoid a loading dose before infusion or target the plasma rather than effect site.[887] As with many synthetic opioids, severe bradycardia and hypotension may occur after bolus administration, especially at large doses.[237,1779] Remifentanil may have a direct negative chronotropic effect, requiring the concomitant use of a vagolytic drug.[1780,1781] The negative chronotropic effect and the concomitant decrease in blood pressure at large concentrations (e.g., 15–20 ng/mL) may also be used to induce controlled hypotension.[1782,1783]

Remifentanil has little effect on the BIS and provides a deep analgesic effect that allows spinal cord-evoked motor and sensory monitoring.[1784,1785] Remifentanil has also been used to supplement propofol to facilitate endotracheal intubation without the use of a neuromuscular blocking drug (see Chapter 6).[1786]

BUTORPHANOL AND NALBUPHINE

Butorphanol (Stadol) and nalbuphine (Nubain) are synthetic opioid agonist-antagonist analgesics that are equianalgesic.[1787–1790] They are effective through κ-receptor agonism and partial μ-receptor antagonism, have 0.5 to 0.7 times the potency of morphine, and an antagonist effect 25 times weaker than naloxone. An appealing pharmacodynamics effect is sedation, particularly when compared with midazolam.[1787,1790–1793] The elimination half-life of nalbuphine is significantly smaller in children 1.5 to 5 years of age (0.9 hours) than in children 5 to 8.5 years of age (1.9 hours) and in adults (2.3 hours). A half-life of 4 hours has been reported in neonates, reflecting immaturity of hepatic glucuronide metabolism. The half-life of butorphanol is similar to that of nalbuphine at about 3 hours in adults.[1790,1794–1796] Nalbuphine pharmacokinetics have been reported using allometric scaling in children 1 to 10 years: clearance 130 L/hour per 70 kg, Q 75.6 L/hour per 70 kg, V1 210 L/70 kg, and V2 151 L/70 kg.[1796]

Both of these drugs can be administered orally with bioavailability in young adults of 12% to 17%, but this dramatically increases to about 80% when administered to the nasal mucosa.[1795,1797–1799] The claimed advantage of this family of drugs is adequate analgesia with a ceiling on respiratory depression.[1787,1788,1800–1802] Thus, there is some popularity for use in children,[1803–1809] although a systematic review reported that quantitative analysis of nalbuphine compared with other analgesics for postoperative pain management was lacking.[1810] The administration of butorphanol by the nasal route may offer particular advantage for children without IV access.[1803,1811–1814] One report suggested that the frequency of postoperative vomiting after butorphanol was less than with morphine.[1804] Another describes the use of rectal administration; as expected, the authors found irregular absorption, but peak blood levels were relatively rapidly achieved (25 ± 11 minutes), and the elimination half-life was 2.7 ± 0.7 hours.[1815] **We do not recommend the rectal route of administration.** What must be remembered is that these agents may reverse μ-receptor–mediated analgesic effects of the more potent opioids and should therefore be used as the initial or the sole opioid.

This family of drugs has had mixed results in reversing or preventing opioid-induced pruritus.[1816,1817] Nalbuphine does not reverse respiratory depression after morphine,[1818] but may be effective after fentanyl.[1819] Butorphanol has also been administered by the caudal epidural route (25 μg/kg).[1820,1821]

CODEINE

Codeine, or methylmorphine, is a morphine-like opium alkaloid with 10% of the potency of morphine. The affinity of codeine for opioid receptors is very weak as it is a prodrug; pain relief is effected primarily from its morphine metabolite that depends on CYP2D6 metabolism and secondarily from hydrocodone and other unclear pathways.[1822]

The primary routes for delivery of codeine are oral and IM, although the rectal route has also been advocated.[1823] The dose of codeine by all three routes is similar, 0.5 to 1.5 mg/kg. Intravenous codeine was used in the past, but serious life-threatening adverse effects, including transient but severe cardiorespiratory depression[1824–1826] and seizures,[1827] led to proscription of this route of delivery.

The popularity of codeine as a perioperative analgesic in children is based in part on its favorable pharmacokinetics. When given orally, it is rapidly and completely absorbed, with 50% undergoing first-pass hepatic metabolism. Bioavailability after oral codeine is 90%, although after surgery the bioavailability may be quite variable.[1822,1828] Blood concentrations after oral codeine reach a peak by 1 hour. Its terminal elimination half-life is 3 to 3.5 hours. When given by the IM and rectal routes, peak blood concentrations are achieved rapidly, within 0.5 hours. The duration of action after IM administration is 1 to 2 hours. A volume of distribution of 3.6 L/kg and a clearance of 0.85 L/hour have been described in adults, but there are few data detailing the developmental changes in children.

Codeine is no longer recommended for pain management in infants and children in the United States because of deaths when it was prescribed to children with CYP2D6 ultra-rapid polymorphisms (see further text and Chapters 4 and 31). Most children's hospitals have removed this drug from their formulary because of safety concerns.[1363,1829–1832] The American Academy of Pediatrics recognized the dangers of this drug and the need for alternative methods for analgesia, particularly in obese children at risk for OSA.[1510] In 2013 the US FDA issued a black box warning against the use of codeine in children after tonsillectomy and adenoidectomy surgeries after a number of deaths were attributed to overdoses associated with undiagnosed ultrarapid polymorphisms (see Chapters 4 and 31). The FDA extended this warning in 2017 to obese children and those with OSA or lung disease who are less than 18 years of age undergoing adenotonsillectomy or tonsillectomy (FDA Drug Safety Communication: FDA restricts use of prescription codeine pain and cough medicines and tramadol pain medicines in children; recommends against use in breastfeeding women) and also removed codeine from all cough preparations.[200,201,1510,1833]

Despite the safety concerns, codeine continues to be used but often in centers that perform genetic polymorphism testing. For example, since codeine was so effective for sickle crisis, one center screened the children with crisis for their CYP2D6 polymorphisms and then only prescribed codeine for those who did not have the poor and ultrarapid polymorphisms.[1834] The remainder of the children with crises were successfully managed with alternatives to codeine. This lesson illustrates that the power of exploiting genetic polymorphisms for the safe use of drugs that can have consequential complications in specific cohorts of children.

Codeine is eliminated via a number of different pathways [https://www.wikipathways.org/index.php/Pathway:WP1604#nogo2].[1822] In vivo, a minority of the drug (5%–15%) is excreted in the urine unchanged. The remaining 85% to 95% undergoes metabolism in the liver by one of three routes: glucuronidation (principal route), O-demethylation, and N-demethylation.[1822] A total of 5% to 15% of codeine undergoes O-demethylation primarily via CYP2D6 to morphine. Approximately 10% is metabolized by N-demethylation, which depends on the CYP3A enzyme system, to norcodeine, an inactive metabolite.[1835] However, a full accounting of the metabolism of codeine remains to be completed.

The wide array of CYP2D6 polymorphisms of codeine (more than 100) may be summarized into three broad categories: poor metabolizers (PM, negligible morphine produced), extensive metabolizers (EM, normal), and ultrarapid metabolizers (UM, rapid production and large amounts of morphine produced). Up to 10% of Caucasians and 30% of Hong Kong Chinese are PM, rendering codeine an ineffective analgesic for these children.[1822] Alternately, 29% of the Ethiopian and 1% of Swedish, German, and Chinese populations are UM.[1822] Children with these polymorphisms who also have upregulated opioid receptors as a result of long-term intermittent nocturnal hypoxia may be particularly vulnerable to a mishap after a usual or subclinical dose of codeine.[1511,1512] Consequently, this drug is no longer recommended for those with compromised cardiorespiratory status, obesity, and/or possible OSA since deaths and near-deaths have been reported with "standard" doses of oral codeine in children later found to be UM.[1511,1831,1836–1838]

In children who are PM, codeine confers little or no analgesia, although adverse effects persist.[1839] In UM metabolizers a large incidence of adverse effects might be expected, including apnea, because of large plasma morphine concentrations. Administration (especially of codeine preparations with an antihistamine and a decongestant) in the neonate may cause intoxication.[1510,1840] A mother, later found to be an UM, who ingested codeine while breastfeeding is thought to have transferred morphine in the breast milk, resulting in a fatality in her neonate.[1836,1841] Because of the unpredictable variability in converting codeine to morphine, we recommend alternative medications.[1833]

TRAMADOL

Tramadol (Ultram) is a weak opioid with minimal effects on respiration and causes monoaminergic spinal cord inhibition of pain.[1842–1845] This formulation is structurally related to morphine and codeine.[1845] Two enantiomers provide analgesia; one is a opioid μ-receptor agonist, and the other inhibits neuronal reuptake of serotonin and inhibits norepinephrine uptake, thus producing "multimodal antinociception."[1845] It is primarily metabolized into *O*-desmethyltramadol (M1) by CYP2D6. PMs have both reduced analgesia and nausea.[1846,1847] Unfortunately, the identification of genotype does not predict phenotype. Those classed as PM may have normal clearance (see Fig. 4.2). The active M1 metabolite has a μ-receptor affinity approximately 200 times greater than tramadol. Tramadol provides analgesia both from the parent compound (target concentration 100 ng/mL) and from its M1 metabolite (target concentration 15 ng/mL).[1848]

Tramadol clearance increases from 25 weeks PCA (5.52 L/hour per 70 kg) to reach 84% of the mature value (8.58 L/hour per 70 kg) by 44 weeks postmenstrual age.[1849] A target concentration of 300 µg/L is achieved after a bolus of tramadol hydrochloride of 1 mg/kg, and can be maintained by an infusion of tramadol hydrochloride at 0.09 mg/kg per hour at 25 weeks, 0.14 mg/kg per hour at 30 weeks, and 0.18 mg/kg per hour at 40 weeks postmenstrual age.[1849] CYP2D6 activity was observed as early as 25 weeks PCA.[1849] Clearance in children is similar to that in adults, using standardized allometric models.[1850] Tramadol was advocated for analgesia for moderate to severe pain in a variety of pediatric populations.[1851–1859] However it is no longer recommended by the FDA for obese patients at risk for OSA and those undergoing tonsillectomy because of the metabolism by CYP2D6 polymorphisms to the M1 metabolite. Indeed one 5-year-old with OSA was prescribed 1 mg/kg tramadol for postoperative pain. Eight hours after discharge, the child was found lethargic and resuscitated with naloxone. After a full recovery, his genotyping identified UM for CYP2D6.[1860] The FDA issued a contraindication for use in children younger than 18 years of age undergoing tonsillectomy or adenotonsillectomy and a warning for obese 12- to 18-year-olds (FDA Drug Safety Communication: FDA restricts use of prescription codeine pain and cough medicines and tramadol pain medicines in children; recommends against use in breastfeeding women | FDA).

Despite FDA recommendations regarding tramadol, the drug remains popular in both children[1861] and breastfeeding mothers.[1862] Apnea has been associated with a 10-fold dosing error in children (>9 mg/kg),[1863] although seizures have been reported after a minimal dose of 4.8 mg/kg.[1864–1866] One formulation (100 mg/mL) designed for adults is prescribed in drops rather than in milliliters and this confused caregivers and resulted in an accidental overdose.[1867] The three fatalities reported by the FDA occurred outside the United States in children less than 6 years of age. Increased serum tramadol concentrations were noted in all three, suggesting overdose. Tramadol was given to treat pain after tonsillectomy and clubfoot surgery, and to manage fever in these cases. All three children received tramadol oral drops (100 mg/mL). In a review of the adverse events after tramadol in infants and children, the evidence from the WHO indicates these episodes were either accidental or intentional overdoses that likely involved other drugs.[1860] Simulation of doses 0.5 to 1 mg/kg suggests M1 metabolite concentrations are 50-fold less than that associated with analgesia (15 ng/mL) because the formation of the M1 metabolite, even in ultrarapid metabolizers, is less than the elimination clearance through the renal system.[1868] A reduced strength of 10 mg/mL is recommended with a daily dose restriction of 3 mg/kg orally. The limited incidence of respiratory depression and constipation, fewer controls on use, and similar frequency of nausea and vomiting (10%–40%) compared with other opioids have made tramadol an attractive alternative to other opioid analgesics such as morphine and oxycodone.[1868]

Tramadol (1.5–2 mg/kg) has been administered rectally with peak plasma concentrations measured at approximately 2 hours.[1869] Tramadol has also been administered in the caudal epidural space[1548] with longer-lasting analgesia than when administered intravenously.[1870] Caudal epidural tramadol (5%, 2 mg/kg) was also compared with caudal epidural bupivacaine (0.25%, 2 mg/kg) and found to provide superior analgesia.[1871] *Caudal administration is not recommended until further clarification of potential neurotoxicity.*[1851,1872] Tramadol has also been very useful as a transition to oral analgesics after IV therapy (see Chapter 41).

TAPENTADOL

Tapentadol (Nucynta, Palexia, and Tapal) is an oral opioid analgesic in the benzenoid class with a dual mechanism of action that is similar to tramadol; it is a μ-opioid receptor agonist and also inhibits the reuptake of norepinephrine.[1873] Its advantage over tramadol is that it has only weak effects on the reuptake of serotonin and is a more potent opioid with no known active metabolites.[1874] We might anticipate better analgesia than occurs after tramadol in those children who are PM of CYP2D6. It is generally regarded as a weak-moderate strength opioid that can be antagonized with naloxone.

The plasma target concentration has not been identified, but a range 20 to 60 µg/L appears effective for moderate pain.[1873,1875,1876] A concentration response curve has not been published to date, but the current recommended dose to treat acute pain in children older than 2 years of age is 1 mg/kg q12 hours. Larger doses have been proposed but these are based on comparative adult areas under the curve estimations.[1877] Tapentadol is cleared by glucuronide conjugation (as is acetaminophen and morphine). A one-compartment model using allometry has been used to describe pharmacokinetics; clearance is estimated to be 64.7 L/hour per 45 kg with TM_{50} 36.7 and a Hill coefficient of 1 describing maturation. Volume was larger at birth but rapidly became smaller ($T_{1/2}$ maturation = 11 weeks, similar to that of acetaminophen) to reach an adult value 270 L per 70 kg. Oral bioavailability (F_{ORAL}) was 0.265.[1615]

All drugs that act on mu receptors have potential to depress respirations. Oral tapentadol 100 mg but not 150 mg, had a modest respiratory advantage over oxycodone 20 mg in healthy adult volunteers. Adverse effect profiles (nausea, dizziness, vomiting, and somnolence) appear similar to those described for tramadol.[1878] Tapentadol confers both nociceptive and neuropathic pain relief, but at the same time may be abused and create dependency. Tapentadol should be used cautiously within 14 days after cessation of monoamine oxidase inhibitors because a serotonin syndrome could occur.[1879]

Acetaminophen

Acetaminophen (Tylenol, paracetamol) is widely used in the management of pain but lacks antiinflammatory effects. Prostaglandin H_2 synthase (PGHS) is the enzyme responsible for metabolism of arachidonic acid to the unstable prostaglandin H_2. The two major forms of this enzyme are the constitutive PGHS-1 (COX-1) and the inducible PGHS-2 (COX-2). PGHS has two sites, a cyclooxygenase (COX) site and a peroxidase (POX) site. The conversion of arachidonic acid to prostaglandin G_2, the precursor of the other prostaglandins (E-Fig. 5.20), depends on a tyrosine-385 radical at the COX active site. Acetaminophen acts as a reducing co-substrate on the POX site. Alternatively, acetaminophen effects may be mediated by an active metabolite (*p*-aminophenol). *P*-Aminophenol is conjugated with arachidonic acid by fatty acid amide hydrolase and exerts its effect through cannabinoid receptors.[1880]

Sulfate metabolism is the dominant route of elimination in neonates, whereas glucuronide conjugation (via UGT1A6) is dominant in adults. A total body clearance of 0.74 L/hour per 70 kg at 28 weeks postmenstrual age and 4.9 L/hour per 70 kg (CV = 38%) in full-term neonates after enteral acetaminophen has been reported using an allometric three-quarter–power model.[1881,1882] Clearance increases during the first year of life (see Fig. 5.12) and reaches 80% of that in older children (16 L/hour per 70 kg) by 6 months postnatal age.[143,222] Similar clearance estimates are reported in neonates after intravenous formulations of acetaminophen.[1882,1883] The relative bioavailability of the oral formulation (F_{ORAL}) is 0.9. The volume of distribution for acetaminophen is 49 to 70 L per 70 kg. The volume of distribution decreases exponentially, with a TM_{50} of 11.5 weeks, from 109.7 L per 70 kg at 28 weeks postmenstrual age to 72.9 L per 70 kg by 60 weeks postmenstrual age, reflective of fetal body composition and water distribution changes over the first few months of life.[143] The relative bioavailability of rectal to oral acetaminophen formulations (rectal/oral) is approximately 0.5 in children but the relative bioavailability is greater in neonates and approaches unity.[143]

The $T_{1/2}$absorption of acetaminophen from the duodenum is rapid (4.5 minutes) in children who were given acetaminophen as an elixir.[52] The $T_{1/2}$absorption in infants younger than 3 months of age was delayed (16.6 minutes), consistent with delayed gastric emptying in young infants.[52,143] In contrast, rectal absorption is slow and erratic with large variability. For example, absorption parameters for the triglyceride base were a $T_{1/2}$absorption of 1.34 hours (CV = 90%) with a lag time before absorption began of 8 minutes (CV = 31%). The $T_{1/2}$absorption for rectal formulations was prolonged in infants younger than 3 months of age (1.51 times greater) compared with older children.[1881]

An Emax model has been used to describe analgesic response after acute pain. An estimate of a maximum effect was 5.17 (the greatest possible pain relief [Visual Analog Scale (VAS) 0 to 10] would equate to an Emax of 10 out of 10 pain units) and an EC_{50} of 9.98 mg/L (Fig. 5.31). A similar maximum effect is reported in adults with chronic pain.[1884] The $T_{1/2}$keo of the analgesic effect compartment was 53 minutes.[1885,1886] A target effect compartment concentration of 10 mg/L was associated with a pain reduction of 2.6/10.[1886] Time delays of approximately 1 hour between peak concentration and peak effect have been reported.[1885,1887]

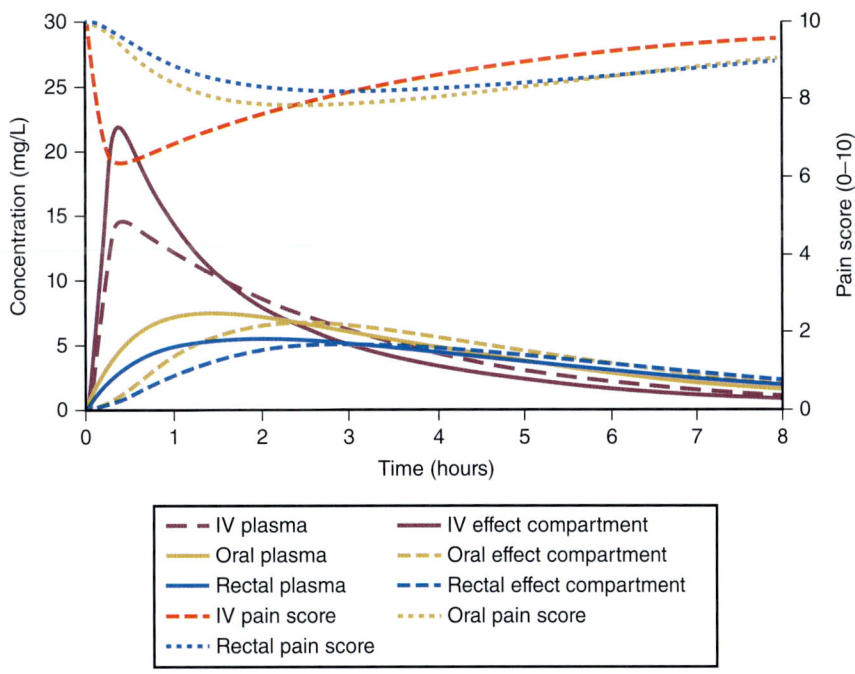

FIGURE 5.31 Profiles for acetaminophen 15 mg/kg given intravenously over 15 minutes, orally as elixir and as a rectal suppository in a 5-year-old child (20 kg). Effect compartment concentrations are delayed compared to plasma and this delay is described by $T_{1/2}$keo. Rectal formulations are absorbed more slowly than oral. A loading dose for enteral formulations is required to achieve better analgesia and that analgesia is sustained longer than that given intravenously. (Parameter estimates from Anderson BJ, Holford NHG. Mechanistic basis of using body size and maturation to predict clearance in humans. *Drug Metab Pharmacokinet.* 2009;24(1):25-36.)

Acetaminophen is commonly used to supplement postoperative analgesia from morphine infusion, but this usually only reduces morphine consumption by 10% to 20% in children and is probably insufficient to decrease morphine-related adverse effects.[1888] However, a reduction in morphine consumption of 66% is reported in postoperative infants after major noncardiac surgery.[1889] Variability in the effect of acetaminophen on pain levels may be attributed to genetic polymorphisms of the vanilloid 1 receptor (TRPV1) that is activated by AM404.[1890]

There is no evidence that acetaminophen is useful in treating adults with cancer pain, either alone or combined with an opioid. Nor is there evidence to disprove that it is useful.[1891] Similarly, there was no evidence from randomized controlled trials to support or refute a role for acetaminophen to treat chronic noncancer pain in children and adolescents. Although acetaminophen is widely used in chronic pain conditions, no conclusions could be made about efficacy or harm in the use of paracetamol (acetaminophen) to treat chronic pain in children and adolescents.[1892,1893]

The toxic metabolite of acetaminophen, N-acetyl-p-benzoquinone imine (NAPQI), is formed by CYP2E1, 1A2, and 3A4. This metabolite binds to intracellular hepatic macromolecules to produce cell necrosis and other damage. In infants less than 90 days postnatal age, expression of CYP2E1 activity in vitro is less than in older infants, children, and adults.[1894] CYP3A4 appears during the first week after birth, and CYP1A2 appears later.[1] Neonates can produce hepatotoxic metabolites (e.g., NAPQI), but the reduced activity of CYP in neonates may explain the rare occurrence of acetaminophen-induced hepatotoxicity in neonates.[1895,1896] Nonetheless, two massive 10-fold overdoses of acetaminophen reported in infants underscore the need for extreme care when administering IV forms of acetaminophen.[1897] Neither infant progressed to acute liver necrosis and both recovered fully.

Acetaminophen is useful as an adjunct to spare opioids, particularly for mild to moderate pain.[1898–1905] Acetaminophen can be administered orally before induction of anesthesia to achieve a therapeutic blood concentration at the time of emergence, even after brief surgery, such as myringotomy and tube insertion. For procedures of greater duration, rectal administration of acetaminophen at the beginning of surgery provides therapeutic blood concentrations at the time of emergence and before the child would be likely to tolerate oral medications.[1906] The ED$_{50}$ for rectal acetaminophen to reduce the need for supplemental opioids after day-stay surgery is 35 mg/kg (Fig. 5.32).[1899] However, with the introduction of IV paracetamol, the rectal route of administration has fallen by the wayside. The current maximum 24-hour dosing of oral acetaminophen varies around the world between 75 and 90 mg/kg per day in hospitalized children, although the total daily dose should be reduced in neonates.[1907] Suppository doses of 35 to 40 mg/kg followed by 20 mg/kg every 6 hours have been proposed for children for the first 24 hours,[1907] consistent with reduced bioavailability and slower absorption of rectal formulations.[1908]

The Rumack and Matthew acetaminophen toxicity nomogram[1909] is widely used to guide management of acetaminophen overdose in adults and children. Acetaminophen concentrations of more than 300 mg/L at 4 hours were always associated with severe hepatic lesions, but none were observed in adults with concentrations less than 150 mg/L. Children (1–5 years of age) with reported accidental ingestion of greater than 250 mg/kg should have serum concentration measured at 2 hours after ingestion rather than the 4-hour time point recommended in adults.[1910]

Toxicity can also occur after regular dosing for 2 to 3 days. A review of acetaminophen-associated toxicity revealed 76 children

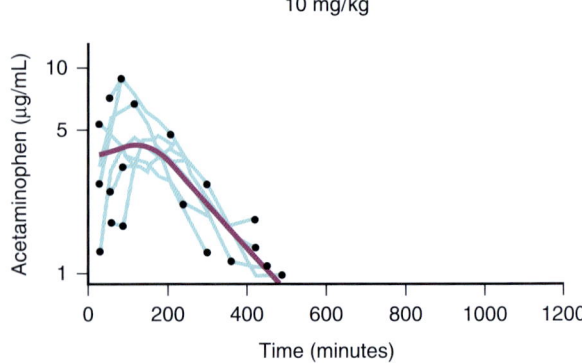

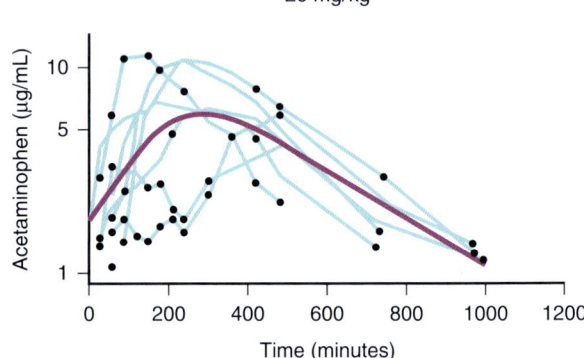

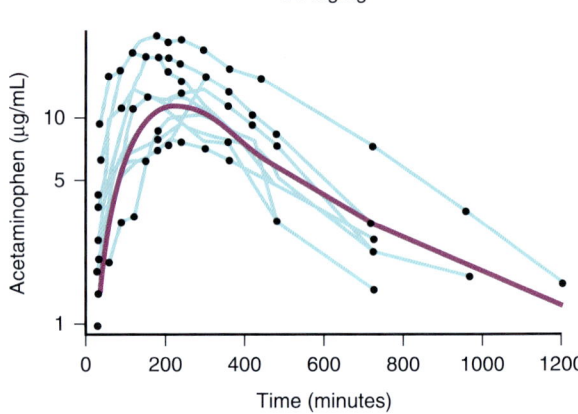

FIGURE 5.32 Acetaminophen concentrations after rectal administration of 10, 20, or 30 mg/kg were recorded. Values for serum concentration of acetaminophen (*solid circles, teal lines*) are plotted against time for each child. Thick (*magenta*) lines indicate "average" values. Note that only children who received 30 mg/kg achieved the antipyretic threshold of 10 to 20 μg/mL, but that even at this dose that range was not sustained. These data suggest the need to use a larger loading dose (approximately 40 mg/kg) followed by subsequent doses of 20 mg/kg every 6 hours; see text for details. (From Birmingham PK, Tobin MJ, Henthorn TK, et al. Twenty-four-hour pharmacokinetics of rectal acetaminophen: an old drug with new recommendations. *Anesthesiology.* 1997;87:244-252.)

with hepatic injury and 26 deaths after repeated administration in children younger than 6 years of age; no deaths or injury occurred when the total daily dose was less than 75 mg/kg.[1911] Hepatic and renal disease, malnutrition, and dehydration may increase the propensity for toxicity. Medications that induce the NAPQI formation (e.g., phenobarbitone, phenytoin, and rifampicin) may also increase the risk of hepatotoxicity. Reduced metabolism by individuals with genetic polymorphisms of the UGT2B15 and SULT1A1 may enhance NAPQI production.[1890] NAPQI binds to intracellular hepatic macromolecules to produce cell necrosis and damage. During hepatocyte lysis acetaminophen-protein adducts are released into plasma and these can be used as specific biomarkers of acetaminophen toxicity in patients with acute liver injury.[1912] It is difficult to assess those prone to hepatotoxicity after routine dosing. Liver function changes during therapy are commonly transitory and may not reflect hepatotoxicity.[1913]

Nonsteroidal Antiinflammatory Agents (NSAIDs)

The NSAIDs are a heterogeneous group of compounds that share common antipyretic, analgesic, and antiinflammatory effects. NSAIDs act by reducing prostaglandin biosynthesis through inhibition of the COX site of the PGHS enzyme (see E-Fig. 5.20). The prostanoids produced by the COX-1 isoenzyme protect the gastric mucosa, regulate renal blood flow, and induce platelet aggregation. NSAID-induced gastrointestinal toxicity, for example, is likely mediated through blockade of COX-1 activity, whereas the antiinflammatory effects of NSAIDs are likely mediated primarily through inhibition of the inducible isoform, COX-2. Relative COX-1/COX-2 specificity ratios vary from greater than 1 (aspirin, indomethacin, ibuprofen), to approximately 1 (diclofenac, naproxen), to less than 1 (celecoxib, etoricoxib).

NSAIDs are commonly used in children as antipyretics and analgesics. Additionally, the antiinflammatory properties of the NSAIDs have been used to manage diverse disorders such as juvenile idiopathic arthritis, renal and biliary colic, dysmenorrhea, Kawasaki disease, and cystic fibrosis. The NSAIDs indomethacin and ibuprofen (as is paracetamol) are also used to treat delayed closure of a patent ductus arteriosus in preterm infants.[1914–1919]

PHARMACODYNAMICS

NSAID-associated analgesia has been compared with analgesia from other analgesics or analgesic modalities (e.g., caudal blockade, acetaminophen, or morphine) in children. These data confirm that NSAIDs in children are effective analgesic drugs, improving the quality of analgesia, but the effects are poorly quantified for most NSAIDs (Fig. 5.33).[1920] Parameter estimates for acetaminophen and some common NSAIDs using a sigmoid Emax model are shown in Table 5.13. Data from adult patients given ketorolac for postoperative pain relief after orthopedic surgery revealed an Emax of 8.5/10 (VAS 0–10) and $T_{1/2}$keo 24 minutes. The reason for the higher Emax observed in elderly patients with bone fractures remains uncertain but may be attributable to the nature of the pain.[1921] Interpretation of analgesia is also complicated by active metabolites. Naproxcinod is an active metabolite of naproxen. Diclofenac's 4'-hydroxyl metabolite has 30% of the antiinflammatory and antipyretic activity of the parent compound. Approximately 20% of the parent drug is processed to this metabolite. Despite the impact of this metabolite, there are reasonable data to support the contention that diclofenac 50 mg is as effective as diclofenac 100 mg in adults.[1922] Little or no information on developmental differences in arachidonic acid release, prostaglandin formation, or COX-2 expression is available for children. It has been assumed that attaining similar adult exposure to 50 mg in children should give similar

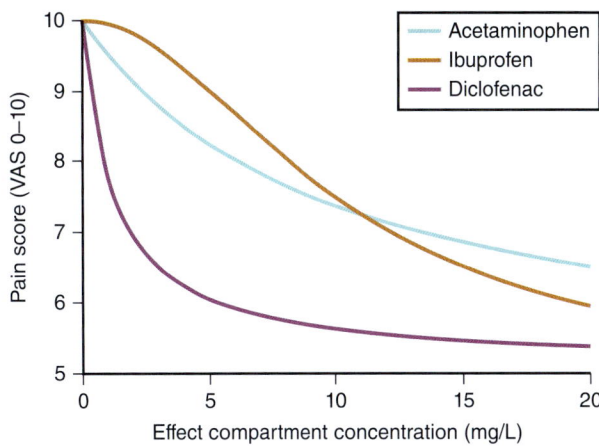

FIGURE 5.33 The effect compartment concentration-response for acetaminophen, ibuprofen, and diclofenac. A visual analogue pain score (VAS 0–10) measured effectiveness. Diclofenac achieves a "ceiling" analgesia at low concentrations, further increasing concentration has little additional effect. When the drug is given so that large concentrations are achieved, then the dosing interval can be extended.

TABLE 5.13	Parameter Estimates for the Sigmoid Emax Equation for Some Common NSAIDs and Paracetamol			
Parameter	**Paracetamol**	**Ibuprofen**	**Ketorolac**	**Diclofenac**
Emax (0–10)	5.2	6.5	8.5	4.89
EC$_{50}$	9.8 mg/L	3.95 mg/L	0.37 mg/L	1.2 mg/L
N	1	1.48	1	1
T$_{1/2}$keo	53 minutes	64 minutes	24 minutes	14 minutes
Reference	1898	1954	1921	1953

Emax, Maximum effect change; *Ce*, concentration in effect compartment; *EC$_{50}$*, concentration producing 50% Emax; *N*, Hill coefficient.

effectiveness. This argument has been used to support a single dose of diclofenac 0.3 mg/kg for intravenous, 0.5 mg/kg for suppositories, and 1 mg/kg for oral diclofenac in children aged 1 to 12 years.[1758] Pediatric intravenous parecoxib dosing is also based on effect observed in adults.[1923,1924] Preliminary evidence suggests a role for oral celecoxib to reduce pain and analgesic consumption post adenotonsillectomy. The single nucleotide polymorphism, CYP2C9*3 allele, may influence the recovery with such a regimen.[1925]

PHARMACOKINETICS

NSAIDs undergo extensive phase I and phase II enzyme biotransformation in the liver, with subsequent excretion into urine or bile. Renal elimination is not an important elimination pathway for the commonly used NSAIDs. Pharmacokinetic parameter variability is large, in part attributable to covariate effects of age, size, and pharmacogenomics. Ibuprofen, for example, is metabolized by the CYP2C9 and CYP2C8 subfamily. Considerable variation exists in the expression of CYP2C activities among individuals, and functional polymorphism of the gene coding for CYP2C9 has been described.[1926] CYP2C9 activity is low immediately after birth (21% of adult values), subsequently increasing progressively to reach a peak activity within 3 months, when expressed as milligrams per hour per kilogram.[1927]

Clearance (liters per hour per kilogram) is generally greater in children than it is in adults, as we might expect when the linear per-kilogram model is used. Ibuprofen clearance maturation, for example, follows the similar pattern to other drugs (e.g., Fig. 5.5). Maturation of clearance, standardized to a 70-kilogram person was described using the Hill equation. Mature clearance was 3.81 L/hour per 70 kg. The maturation half-time was (TM_{50}) 36.8 weeks postmenstrual age and the Hill coefficient 11.5 (95% CI 8.1, 15), reflecting rapid and early maturation.[1928] A target effect of 4 units (visual analog scale 0–10) correlated with an effect site concentration of 6.3 mg/L. These models have been used to determine dose at all ages using the target concentration strategy.[1928] Similar maturation data exist for indomethacin.[1914,1929,1930]

Many NSAIDs exhibit stereoselectivity.[1931] Ibuprofen stereoselectivity is reported in preterm neonates (<28 weeks gestation). R- and S-ibuprofen half-lives were about 10 hours and 25.5 hours, respectively. The mean clearance of R-ibuprofen (12.7 mL/hour) was about 2.5-fold greater than that of S-ibuprofen (5.0 mL/hour).[1932] Pharmacokinetics may also be influenced by chronobiology.[894]

The apparent volume of distribution (V/F) is small in adults (less than 0.2 L/kg, suggesting minimal tissue binding) but is larger in children; for example, ketorolac V/F in children 4 to 8 years old is twice that of adults.[1933,1934] Premature neonates (22–31 weeks' gestational age) given IV ibuprofen had a V/F of 0.62 (SD 0.04) L/kg.[1935] A dramatic reduction in ibuprofen central volume following closure of the PDA in premature neonates (0.244 vs. 0.171 L/kg) is reported.[1936]

The NSAIDs, as a group, are weakly acidic, lipophilic, and highly protein bound. The bound fraction in children and premature neonates is slightly less than in adults. The impact of this reduced protein binding is probably minimal with routine dosing because NSAIDs cleared by the liver have a low hepatic extraction ratio and they have a long equilibration time between plasma and effect compartments.[78] There is relatively little transfer from maternal to fetal blood. Excretion of NSAIDs into breast milk of lactating mothers is small.[1937]

NSAIDs are rapidly absorbed in the gastrointestinal tract after oral administration in children. The relative bioavailability of oral preparations approaches unity. The rate and extent of absorption after rectal administration of NSAIDs, such as ibuprofen, diclofenac, flurbiprofen, indomethacin, and nimesulide, are less than after the oral routes.

ADVERSE EFFECTS

NSAIDs undergo drug interactions through altered clearance and competition for active renal tubular secretion with other organic acids. A large fractional protein binding has been proposed to explain drug interactions between NSAIDs and oral anticoagulant agents, oral hypoglycemics, sulfonamides, bilirubin, and other protein-bound drugs. The classic example is that of the coadministration of warfarin and phenylbutazone (an NSAID). Both the plasma warfarin concentration and the prothrombin time were increased.[1938] However, even though phenylbutazone displaces warfarin from its albumin binding sites in vitro, this observation does not explain the changes in prothrombin time. The increased prothrombin time has been attributed to increased serum warfarin concentrations, which stems from its reduced clearance, and not from changes in protein binding.[78] Both warfarin and phenylbutazone compete for similar protein binding sites; they also compete for similar clearance pathways. NSAIDs have the potential to cause gastrointestinal irritation, blood clotting disorders, renal impairment, neutrophil dysfunction, and bronchoconstriction,

effects attributed to COX-1/COX-2 ratios, although this concept may be an oversimplification.

Ibuprofen reduces the glomerular filtration rate by 20% in preterm neonates, affecting aminoglycoside clearance, an effect that appears to be independent of gestational age.[1939] No significant difference in the change in cerebral blood volume, change in cerebral blood flow, or tissue oxygenation index was found between administration of ibuprofen or placebo in neonates.[1940] The risk of acute gastrointestinal bleeding in children given short-term ibuprofen was estimated to be 7.2/100,000 (CI 2–18 per 100,000), a prevalence not different from children given acetaminophen.[1941–1943] The incidence of clinically significant gastropathy in children with juvenile arthritis given NSAIDs is comparable with that in adults given long-term NSAIDs, but the prevalence of gastroduodenal injury may be greater, depending on the assessment criteria applied (e.g., abdominal pain, anemia, endoscopy).[1944,1945] Aspirin- or NSAID-exacerbated respiratory disease (ERD) occurs more frequently in adults, although instances in children and teenagers have been reported.[1946] These cases are countered by reports that the symptoms of asthma improved when ibuprofen was administered for antipyresis. One study concluded that a benefit is likely to occur in younger children with mild episodic asthma and that aspirin-ERD is a concern in one in three teenagers with severe asthma and coexistent nasal disease.[1946,1947] COX-2 inhibitors are reported to be safe in NSAID-ERD.[1947]

The commonly used NSAIDs have reversible antiplatelet effects, which are attributable to the inhibition of thromboxane synthesis. Bleeding time is usually slightly increased, but remains within normal limits in children with normal coagulation systems. Neonates given prophylactic ibuprofen to induce PDA closure did not have an increased frequency of intraventricular hemorrhage.[1948] A Cochrane review has established that even after pediatric tonsillectomy, NSAIDs did not cause any increase in bleeding that required a return to the OR. There was significantly less nausea and vomiting with NSAIDs compared with alternative analgesics, suggesting their benefits outweigh their negative aspects.[1949,1950]

Recent concerns with OSA-associated deaths from opioids for postoperative pain management have resulted in several studies examining alternating doses of ibuprofen and acetaminophen; this regimen provided adequate analgesia with no increase in the incidence of post-tonsillectomy bleeding requiring surgical intervention.[1951,1952] Combination therapy achieves the same maximal response (Emax), but this response is achieved using smaller doses of each drug, and the duration of effect is greater.[306,1953,1954]

INTRAVENOUS FORMULATIONS

There are few IV NSAID formulations that are commonly used.

Ketorolac

Ketorolac (Toradol) is an NSAID with very potent analgesic properties,[1933,1955–1958] reflected in an Emax of 8.5 reported when used for bony fractures.[1921] The drug is available in a number of formulations. Ketorolac may also be administered nasally, although pediatric perioperative data are limited.[166,1959,1960] Although the dose of ketorolac that the FDA approved for use in adults was 40 mg IV, recent evidence confirmed that ketorolac, like most NSAIDs, had a ceiling effect and the ceiling is achieved at 15 mg in adults. Doses >15 mg IV yielded no further analgesia and may risk adverse events.[1961–1965] Based on these data, we administer a weight-proportional dose in children based on a 15-mg dose in 70 kg adults although this may underestimate the dose in infants and young children (see racemate).

The pharmacokinetics for the racemate, ketorolac, using allometry in children and adults are similar (E-Table 5.8). The EC_{50} for analgesia is 0.36 mg/L ketorolac with an effect-site equilibration time estimated to be 24 minutes (based on adult data).[1921] The terminal elimination half-life in children 4 to 8 years of age is approximately 6 hours, although there is considerable variability.[1934,1966–1968] Using allometry to analyze a pool of 64 children between 2 months and 16 years of age who received ketorolac, the volume of distribution decreased in the first year after birth and stabilized from 1 year of age through adulthood, whereas clearance, size standardized using allometry remained unchanged throughout the same period.[1968]

Ketorolac has also been administered via the intranasal route to adolescents. The pharmacokinetics of intranasal ketorolac are similar to that in adults (using the same delivery device), described by a one-compartment model.[166] Plasma concentrations peak rapidly (52 minutes), rendering it an alternative to IV injection. Allometry predicted the clearance better than weight.[166]

Ketorolac is supplied and administered as a racemic mixture that contains a 1:1 ratio of the $R(+)$ and $S(-)$ stereoisomers.[1968] Pharmacologic activity resides almost exclusively with the $S(-)$ stereoisomer.[1931,1969] The $S(-)$ enantiomer is cleared four times more rapidly than the $R(+)$ enantiomer (6.2 vs. 1.4 mL/minute per kilogram) in children 3 to 18 years of age.[1970] The terminal half-life of $S(-)$-ketorolac is 40% that of the $R(+)$ enantiomer (107 vs. 259 minutes), and the volume of distribution of the $S(-)$ enantiomer is greater than that of the $R(+)$ form (0.82 vs. 0.50 L/kg). Recovery of $S(-)$-ketorolac glucuronide is 2.3 times that of the $R(+)$ enantiomer. Because of the greater clearance and shorter half-life of $S(-)$-ketorolac, pharmacokinetic predictions based on racemic assays may overestimate the duration of pharmacologic effect.[1970] The ED_{50}-racemate, 0.37 mg/L, in adults corresponds to a mean concentration of the active enantiomer, S-ketorolac, of 0.057 mg/L. However, in a recent pharmacokinetics pooled analysis of data from infants to adults, enantiomer-specific age-related differences were identified; the concentration of S-ketorolac in infants was almost 20% less than that in adults, 0.046 mg/L.[1971] This suggests that when maturational pharmacodynamic differences are taken into account, infants require a larger dose on a weight basis than that predicted from adults, by approximately 20%.

One of the major concerns regarding the use of ketorolac in the perioperative period is that it inhibits platelet function, which may cause postsurgical bleeding. Ketorolac has minimal effect on prothrombin and partial thromboplastin times but causes modest increases in the bleeding time.[1956,1972–1975] Unlike aspirin however, the antiplatelet effect of ketorolac is short-lived.[1976] This effect on platelet function limited its use during adenotonsillectomy.[1977–1980] In the studies that reported bleeding post-adenotonsillectomy, ketorolac was administered at the beginning of or during surgery, before hemostasis was achieved. In addition, the incidence of increased bleeding occurred primarily during the first 24 hours, which corresponds to the several half-lives it would take to eliminate ketorolac from the body; the incidence of bleeding after the first 24 hours did not appear to differ.[1981] It would therefore be reasonable to withhold ketorolac until the end of surgery, after hemostasis is achieved. Some practitioners eschew this issue altogether and administer ketorolac only when the potential for a life-threatening hemorrhage is less.[1813] Concerns regarding the possibility of postoperative hemorrhage appear to be valid, but the true frequency of life-threatening bleeding exclusively the result of ketorolac administration is quite small.[1982–1986]

There is a dose-response relationship for this bleeding propensity; the risk associated with the drug was larger and clinically important when ketorolac was used in larger doses, in older subjects, and for more than 5 days.[1987] A systematic review found an increased risk for bleeding in adults but not in children younger than 18 years of age after tonsillectomy.[1988] Safety assessments showed no changes in renal or hepatic function tests, surgical drain output, or continuous oximetry between groups given placebo, 0.5 mg/kg, or 1 mg/kg ketorolac at 6 to 18 hours after surgery.[1931,1969] Many clinicians discuss the possible use of ketorolac with the surgeon before administering it and document the conversation in the anesthesia record. Ketorolac can be used to treat pain after congenital heart surgery without an increased risk of bleeding complications.[1984] A retrospective report of 1451 pediatric neurosurgical patients reported no increase in the incidence of bleeding with short-term therapy.[1989] Ketorolac has been safely used to provide analgesia for preterm and term infants, but the pharmacokinetics in this age group has not been described.[1990]

Another concern is the potential for adverse effects on bone healing, particularly spinal fusion.[1991,1992] Evidence suggests that nonunion of the spine is associated only with large-dose and not small, clinical doses of ketorolac.[1993] However, ketorolac has been used safely to provide analgesia for other types of orthopedic conditions with no evidence of delayed union or nonunion of fractures.[1993–1996] One concern is a single report of sudden and profound bradycardia after rapid IV administration of ketorolac among the millions of doses administered to children in the perioperative period[1997]; the mechanism of this response remains unclear.

Parecoxib

Parecoxib sodium is an intravenous NSAID with increased use in pediatric practice despite limited data concerning pharmacokinetics and pharmacodynamics in this population.[1998–2000] Parecoxib is a prodrug that is rapidly and completely converted to valdecoxib (the active metabolite) within 0.5 to 1 hour. Valdecoxib acts by specifically inhibiting COX-2–mediated prostaglandin synthesis. Onset of analgesia in adults was 7.14 minutes with a peak effect within 2 hours and duration of analgesia that ranged from 6 to 24 hours. Valdecoxib is extensively metabolized by the liver through the cytochrome P450 pathways (CYP3A4 and CYP2C9). The volume of distribution of most NSAIDs is small in adults (<0.2 L/kg) but larger in children.

A three-compartment parent and one-compartment metabolite model with first-order elimination has been used to describe parecoxib pharmacokinetics. Parameter estimates were Clearance$_{PARECOXIB}$ 19.1 L/hour per 70 kg, V1$_{PARECOXIB}$ 4.2 L per 70 kg, Q2$_{PARECOXIB}$ 6.29 L/hour per 70 kg, V2$_{PARECOXIB}$ 130 L per 70 kg, Q3$_{PARECOXIB}$ 6.02 L/hour per 70 kg, and V3$_{PARECOXIB}$ 2.03 L per 70 kg. All parecoxib was assumed to be metabolized to valdecoxib with Clearance$_{VALDECOXIB}$ 9.53 L/hour per 70 kg and V$_{VALDECOXIB}$ 51 L per 70 kg. There was no maturation of clearance over the age span studied (4–15 years).[1924] Intravenous drug doses that achieve similar plasma concentrations to adults given parecoxib 40 mg were: parecoxib 0.9 mg/kg in a 2-year-old, 0.75 mg/kg in a 7-year-old, and 0.65 mg/kg in a 12-year-old child. Parecoxib doses above 1 mg/kg added no additional analgesia.[1924]

Benzodiazepine Sedatives

These drugs produce anxiolysis, amnesia, and hypnosis. They are commonly used as adjuncts to both local and general anesthesia. Benzodiazepines bind to $GABA_A$ receptors, resulting in increased cellular chloride entry. This renders these receptors resistant to excitation because they are hyperpolarized.

MIDAZOLAM

Midazolam is a water-soluble benzodiazepine that offers clinical advantages over diazepam. It is not painful when administered IV or IM. Midazolam is only one of a few medications that are approved as premedicants in children, and it is the only benzodiazepine approved by the FDA for use in neonates including preterm infants.

Midazolam is metabolized mainly by hepatic hydroxylation (CYP3A4).[2001] These hydroxylated metabolites undergo glucuronide conjugation and are excreted in the urine. CYP3A7 is the dominant CYP3A enzyme in utero and in the neonate; it is expressed in the fetal liver and appears to have activity from as early as 50 to 60 days after conception. CYP3A4 expression increases dramatically after the first week of life, reaching 30% to 40% of adult expression by 1 month of age.[1719] Midazolam has a hepatic extraction ratio in the intermediate range of 0.3 to 0.7. Metabolic clearance depends on both liver perfusion and enzyme activity.

Clearance is reduced in neonates (0.8–2.2 mL/minute per kilogram, 60 mL/minute per 70 kg) (E-Fig. 5.21),[2002–2009] but increases rapidly (Hill = 3) after 39 weeks postmenstrual age,[2006] to reach 90% mature clearance at 1 year of age.[2009] Mature clearance was 523 mL/minute per 70 kg. The TM_{50} was 73.6 weeks.[2007,2009] Central volume of distribution is related to weight (V1 = 0.591 ± 0.065 L/kg), whereas peripheral volume of distribution remained constant (V2 = 0.42 ± 0.11 L) in 187 neonates weighing 0.7 to 5.2 kilograms.[2006] Total body weight is an inappropriate size scaler for midazolam in obese adolescents[2010]; ideal body weight is a more appropriate scalar.[102]

It has been suggested that midazolam induces its own clearance.[2011] The latter observation, from infants after cardiac surgery, likely results from the improved hepatic function after the insult of cardiopulmonary bypass. Neonates have an increase in volume of distribution at steady state during extracorporeal membrane oxygenation therapy (0.8 L/kg–4.1 L/kg), caused by sequestration of midazolam by the circuitry, although clearance (1.4 ± 0.15 mL/minute per kilogram) was unchanged.[2012]

Gut enzymes (CYP4) are capable of metabolizing the drug as it crosses the intestinal mucosa. The oral bioavailability of midazolam, reflecting the intestinal and hepatic CYP3A activity, was on average less than the reported 49% to 92% for preterm neonates, and greater than the reported 21% for children >1 year of age and 30% for adults.[2013] Hepatic clearance may be reduced in the presence of critical illness.[2014,2015] The clearance of midazolam is reduced after circulatory arrest for cardiac surgery.[2016] Covariates, such as hypothermia,[2017] renal failure, hepatic failure,[2018] and concomitant administration of CYP3A inhibitors,[818,819] are important predictors of altered midazolam and metabolite pharmacokinetics in pediatric intensive care patients.[2019] The clearance of midazolam is reduced by 30% in neonates who are given sympathomimetic amines, probably as a consequence of the underlying compromised hemodynamics.[2006]

One further concern relates to the administration of drugs that interfere with the cytochrome isoforms that metabolize midazolam (CYP3A4). Examples of such drugs and foods are grapefruit juice, erythromycin, calcium channel blockers, and protease inhibitors. The net effect is that the duration of action of midazolam may be prolonged. There are pharmacokinetic and pharmacodynamic interactions between propofol and midazolam.[2020] In addition, hypotension induced by propofol can decrease clearance of midazolam through reduced hepatic blood flow.[2021]

Pharmacokinetic/pharmacodynamic relationships have been described for intravenous midazolam in adults. When an EEG signal is used as an effect measure, the EC_{50} is 35 to 77 ng/mL, with a $T_{1/2}keo$ of 0.9 to 1.6 minutes.[53,2022,2023] Duration of effect persists despite decreasing plasma concentrations. Simulation using adult pharmacodynamic and neonatal pharmacokinetic parameter estimates demonstrates impact of effect in the very young (Fig. 5. 34). The $T_{1/2}keo$ is increased in the elderly and in low cardiac output states. Pharmacokinetic/pharmacodynamic relationships are more difficult to describe after oral midazolam because the active metabolite, 1-hydroxymidazolam, has approximately half the activity of the parent drug.[2024]

Sedation in children is more difficult to quantify. No pharmacokinetic/pharmacodynamic relationship was established in children, age 2 days to 17 years, who were given a midazolam infusion in the ICU. Midazolam dosing could, however, be effectively titrated to the desired level of sedation, assessed by the COMFORT distress scale (see Table 41.5).[2025] Consistent with this finding, desirable sedation in children after cardiac surgery was achieved at mean serum concentrations between 0.1 and 0.5 mg/L.[2011,2018,2026] Plasma concentrations of 0.3 to 0.4 mg/L are associated with anesthesia in adults.[2027,2028] A target concentration for sedation (arouses to command) in adults is 0.1 mg/L.[223]

The desired clinical effects for anesthesia include antegrade amnesia (approximately 50%),[2029–2031] as well as sedation and anxiolysis before induction of anesthesia or a medical procedure.[1054,2032–2037] Amnestic properties may be superior to those of diazepam.[2038] The clinical pharmacodynamic endpoints with midazolam may differ somewhat when compared with diazepam. Midazolam produces a general calming effect with minimal sedation and little effect on speech. In contrast, diazepam frequently causes obvious sedation and slurring of speech.

The recommended infusion rate of midazolam is 0.5 µg/kg per minute for preterm infants younger than 32 weeks gestational age and 1.0 µg/kg per minute for infants more than 32 weeks gestational age. Fixed rates such as these fail to account for clearance maturation. Plasma concentration would be above target in a neonate weighing less than 1 kilogram and below target for a neonate bigger than 2 kilograms,[2039] although the target concentration remains unknown in premature neonates. Any factor that impairs hepatic blood flow (e.g., increased intraabdominal pressure, cardiopulmonary bypass, vasopressors) may decrease midazolam elimination, although cirrhosis only minimally affects its elimination in adults.[2016,2019,2040,2041] Midazolam offers the best pharmacokinetic profile for neonates because the active metabolite has a half-life similar to the parent compound, but with minimal clinical activity.[1629] *Bolus administration to preterm and term neonates has been associated with profound hypotension; the likelihood may be greater if fentanyl is also administered.*[1638] *Likewise, a neonate who is receiving a midazolam infusion is more likely to suffer profound hypotension with a bolus of fentanyl.* Rapid intravenous and nasal administration have also been associated with myoclonic activity.[2042] Midazolam has been administered as a continuous infusion, both in the OR as an adjunct to general anesthesia and in the ICU.[1007,2043–2045] Prolonged administration leads to tolerance, dependency, and benzodiazepine withdrawal.[2046,2047] Long-term infusions, particularly

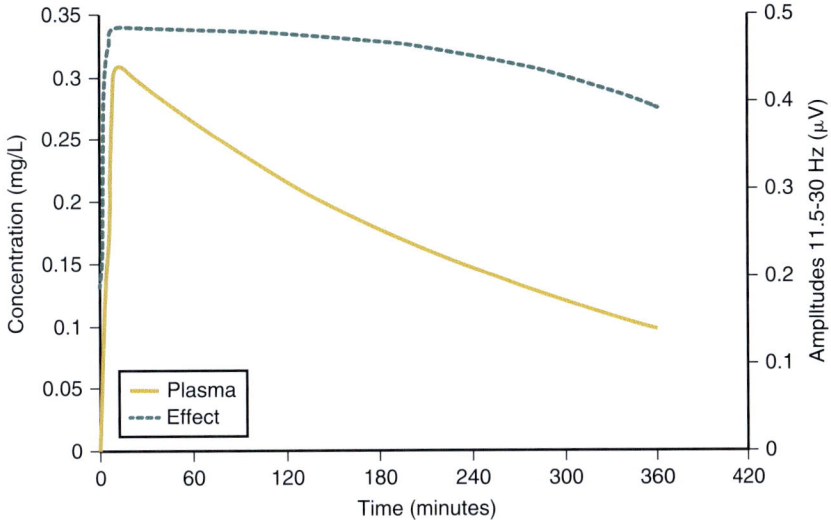

FIGURE 5.34 Plasma concentrations and effect in a neonate given midazolam bolus (0.1 mg/kg) on two early occasions (5-minute interval) to achieve sedation. Plasma concentration declines slowly because of immature clearance. Sedation recovery lags way behind the decline in plasma concentration even though a maintenance infusion was not even given. (Pharmacodynamic parameter estimates are from Mandema J, Tuk B, van Steveninck AL, Breimer DD, Cohen AF, Danhof M. Pharmacokinetic-pharmacodynamic modeling of the central nervous system effects of midazolam and its main metabolite alpha-hydroxymidazolam in healthy volunteers. *Clin Pharm Ther.* 1992;51(6):715-728.) (From Wolf A, Blackwood B, Anderson BJ. Tolerance to sedative drugs in PICU: can it be moderated or is it immutable? *Intensive Care Med.* 2016;42(2):278-281.)

in neonates should be tapered over days while carefully monitoring for signs of withdrawal (vomiting, agitation, sweating, bowel distention, seizures, change in neurologic status).[1649,2048,2049] A theoretical concern associated with midazolam is benzyl alcohol toxicity with the development of metabolic acidosis and gasping respirations.[2050,2051] The 24-hour dose of benzyl alcohol in midazolam when administered according to recommended dosing guidelines should not cause toxicity.

When midazolam was first introduced, a number of deaths were attributed to respiratory depression. These deaths likely resulted from combining large doses of midazolam with other medications, particularly opioids. An important pharmacologic difference between the benzodiazepines is that the time to achieve peak CNS effect with IV midazolam (4.8 minutes) is almost 3-fold greater than with diazepam (1.5 minutes) (see Fig. 44.7).[53,2052] This is because of the greater fat solubility of diazepam and therefore a more rapid transit into the CNS.[2053] Accordingly, one must wait sufficient time between doses of midazolam (3–5 minutes) to achieve the peak CNS effects before considering supplemental doses or other medications.[2054] Intravenous midazolam depresses the response to hypoxemia, an effect that is exaggerated in the presence of a potent opioid, such as fentanyl. This combination (0.1 mg/kg midazolam and 6 µg/kg fentanyl IV) has been associated with a respiratory arrest in an infant.[2055,2056] Children with sleep-disordered breathing who were premedicated with oral midazolam (0.5 mg/kg) experienced only a small incidence (1.5%) of transient desaturation.[2057] However, IV midazolam (0.1 mg/kg) has been shown to cause both central apnea as well as upper airway obstruction, the latter by reducing pharyngeal muscle tone.[2058] In addition, the combination of oral midazolam (0.5 mg/kg) and nitrous oxide (50%) may cause partial upper airway obstruction four times more frequently in children with large tonsils than in those with normal-sized tonsils.[2059] Interestingly, mouth opening may increase upper airway collapse,

thus increasing the airway obstruction in children sedated with midazolam for dental procedures.[2060]

Midazolam is the most commonly used benzodiazepine in pediatric anesthesia. It is administered orally, nasally, buccally, rectally, IV, and IM. Buccal and sublingual administration (0.3 mg/kg [maximum 10 mg]), like the nasal route, offer ease of administration, rapid systemic absorption, and avoidance of hepatic first-pass metabolism. The buccal route is popular for emergency seizure control. It is better than rectal diazepam (relative risk 1.14; 95% CI, 1.06–1.24).[169]

Midazolam has been used as an induction agent, but it is not as satisfactory as other agents.[2061,2062] Pharmacokinetic/pharmacodynamic variability, titration of dose, delayed effect, and hypotension are unfavorable for rapid induction.[2063] Commonly used doses and routes of administration are presented in Table 5.14. The buccal and nasal routes have advantages because they avoid first pass metabolism and are now being used to deliver antiseizure medication by non–health care providers.[2064–2066] It also has been

TABLE 5.14	Dosing and Onset Times of Midazolam in Infants and Children (Excluding Neonates)		
Route	**Dose (mg/kg)**	**Time of Onset (minutes)**	**Time to Peak Effect (minutes)**
Intravenous	0.05–0.15	~1	3–5
Intramuscular	0.1–0.2	3–5	10–20
Oral	0.25–0.75	5–30	10–30
Nasal	0.1–0.2	3–5	10–15
Rectal	0.75–1.0	5–10	10–30
See text for details.			

used as a method of sedation and anxiolysis combined with opioids and dexmedetomidine for the emergency department procedures and prior to anesthesia.[1067,1068,2032,2067–2070] Onset of sedation is more rapid than the oral route.[2071] In addition, 85% of children who receive nasal midazolam cry and complain of a bitter aftertaste.[175,1731]

Remimazolam

Many new drugs are structural modifications of existing drugs that offer fewer adverse effects or shorter duration of effect; ester moieties, for example offer rapid metabolism by blood esterases.[2072,2073] Remimazolam, a short acting benzodiazepam, may be an alternative to propofol or midazolam, depending on whether it is marketed as a sedative or induction agent. In adults undergoing colonoscopy or flexible bronchoscopy, remimazolam (5 mg intravenously, with supplementary doses of 2.5 mg) achieved better success rates and earlier recovery than intravenous midazolam.[2074–2076] Propofol remains popular for these procedures and comparisons with propofol are not yet available. Preliminary studies suggest that remimazolam may be a useful hypnotic component of general anesthesia and as an anticonvulsant and for intensive care sedation.[2077] Mean arterial blood pressure decreased by 24% and heart rate increased by 28%.[2078] The use of remimazolam as either an induction agent or as a target controlled infusion is not yet established, but pharmacokinetic/pharmacodynamic models have been described.[2078,2079]

Remimazolam is metabolized (CESI gene) to CNS7054, an inactive metabolite. In adults, clearance was rapid (1.15 L/minute), steady-state volume of distribution (Vss) 35.4 L and a brief terminal half-life (70 minutes).[2078] The simulated context-sensitive half-time after an infusion of 4 hours was 6.8 ± 2.4 minutes. Pharmacodynamics using the Modified Observer's Assessment of Alertness and Sedation score (0–5) was best described by a sigmoid probability model with effect site compartment. The half-maximum effect site concentration for a score ≤ 1 (deep sedation) was 695 ± 239 µg/L. The $T_{1/2}$keo is 2.7 minutes. Remimazolam can be reversed by flumazenil, although recovery occurs within 10 minutes without requiring reversal.

DIAZEPAM

Diazepam (Valium) has been used extensively as a premedication, as an adjunct to balanced anesthesia, and for sedation, amnesia, and control of seizures, although use has now been overshadowed by midazolam. It is highly plasma bound, with a serum half-life varying from 20 to 80 hours. Its half-life is reduced in younger adults and children (~18 hours).[2080] There was no relationship between diazepam plasma concentration and recall at induction in children,[2080] reflecting active metabolite effects.

Diazepam has capacity limited clearance with low first-pass effect; hepatic disease may decrease the elimination of diazepam.[2081,2082] Neonates who received diazepam transplacentally just before delivery demonstrate prolonged drug effects and serum half-lives (40–100 hours) as a result of immature hepatic excretory mechanisms and reduced hepatic blood flow (see E-Fig. 5.21).[2083–2085] Diazepam undergoes oxidative metabolism by demethylation (CYP 2C19). Its active metabolite, desmethyldiazepam, has potency similar to the parent compound and a half-life as great or greater than the parent compound, thus emphasizing that caution is required when administering this benzodiazepine to neonates.[2083,2086,2087]

Diazepam (0.2–0.3 mg/kg) is rapidly absorbed after oral administration, with peak plasma concentrations at 30 to 90 minutes; the absorption rate is more rapid in children than in adults.[2083,2088] The recommended intravenous dose is 0.1 to 0.2 mg/kg; its main

disadvantage when given intravenously is pain. The greater fat solubility of diazepam compared to midazolam results in faster onset of peak EEG effect (1.5. minutes vs. 4.8 minutes) due to a more rapid transit into the CNS (see Fig. 44.7).[2089–2092] Rectal diazepam (0.2–0.5 mg/kg) is used for prehospital treatment of pediatric status epilepticus and for sedation in doses ranging from 0.3 to 1.0 mg/kg.[2080,2093–2095] There is more rapid absorption when given in liquid rather than suppository form, attributable to greater rectal surface area exposure.[2080] Bioavailability after nasal administration in adults is 70% to 90% with maximal blood concentrations at ~45 minutes.[2096] Intramuscular administration is painful and results in irregular absorption; plasma concentrations are only 60% of those obtained with a similar oral dose.[2097–2099] The IM route is not recommended because of the pain and erratic absorption.

The preservative benzyl alcohol is present in many formulations of diazepam. This preservative should be avoided in neonates because it is difficult to metabolize, is associated with kernicterus, and can cause a metabolic acidosis.[2100–2102] However, the amount of benzyl alcohol that accompanies a usual dose of diazepam would likely be insufficient to cause harm to the neonate.[2103] Diazepam has respiratory depressant effects that are quite variable, especially when combined with opioids.[2104]

Other Sedatives

CLONIDINE

Clonidine is commonly used in pediatric anesthesia practice as a premedicant, as an adjunct to anesthesia and analgesic agents,[2105,2106] to reduce emergence delirium,[2107–2109] as an antiemetic, to prevent postoperative shivering, to supplement regional blockade,[2110–2112] to reduce the stress response secondary to tracheal intubation and surgery, to sedate in the ICU,[2113,2114] and as an adjuvant to treat opioid withdrawal.[2115–2118] Clonidine can be administered by multiple routes including IV, intranasal, IM, transdermal, oral, rectal, and epidural.[177,2119,2120]

Population parameter estimates (between subject variability) for a two-compartment model were clearance 14.6 (CV 35.1%) L/hour per 70 kg; central volume of distribution (V1) 62.5 (71.1%) L per 70 kg; intercompartment clearance (Q) 157 (77.3%) L/hour per 70 kg; and peripheral volume of distribution (V2) 119 (22.9%) L per 70 kg.[2120,2121] Clearance at birth was 3.8 L/hour per 70 kg and matured with a half-time of 25.7 weeks to reach 82% of the adult rate by 1 year of age. Clearance in neonates is approximately one-third that described in adults, consistent with immature elimination pathways.[2120] The volume of distribution, but not clearance, were increased after cardiac surgery (V1 123%, V2 126%). There was a lag time (T_{LAG}) of 2.3 (CV 73.2%) minutes before rectal absorption began. The absorption half-life (T_{abs}) from the epidural space is slower than that from the rectum (0.98 hours CV 24.5% vs. 0.26 hours CV 32.3%). The relative bioavailability of epidural, nasal, and rectal clonidine was unity (F = 1).[2119,2120] Oral bioavailability is reduced in children (F = 0.55).[177] The reduced clearance in neonates dictates a greater steady-state concentration than that in infants,[2122] explaining why neonates had better sedation during mechanical ventilation than infants when given the same clonidine intravenous infusion rate (µg/kg per hour) for sedation.[2123]

Approximately 50% of clonidine is eliminated unchanged by the kidney. The exact amount of clonidine that undergoes hepatic biotransformation is uncertain, but has been reported to be between 40% and 60%.[2124–2127] The major metabolite of clonidine is p-hydroxyclonidine, formed by hydroxylation of the phenol ring, which accounts for less than 10% of the concentration in the urine.[2125] Cytochrome P450 2D6 is involved in this process.

The target clonidine concentration depends on the effect sought. A plasma clonidine concentration range of 0.3 to 0.8 μg/L has been estimated as satisfactory for preoperative sedation in children 1 to 11 years of age.[2128] Fifty percent of children achieve a modified Ramsay sedation score of 3 (appears sleepy but retains purposeful responses to verbal commands at conversation level) at a concentration of 0.79 μg/L, and 90% of children achieve this at 0.95 μg/L. The concentration required for 50% of children to achieve a sedation scale of 4 (appears to be asleep, purposeful responses to verbal commands but at louder than usual conversation level or requiring light glabellar tap) is slightly more at 0.85 μg/L, and 90% of children achieve this at 1.15 μg/L.[2129] A BIS of less than 60 in adults is associated with adequate anesthesia, and this is achieved with a concentration of 4 μg/L[2130]; the target concentration for analgesia in adults is greater than that for sedation. Such information[2131–2133] has been used to construct a concentration-response relationship for adults and children (see Fig. 5.7)[2113] that can be used to determine dose, based on the target concentration strategy.[2114] The equilibration half time ($T_{1/2}$keo) was ~7 minutes.[2113] Deep sedation is difficult to achieve with clonidine, and large concentrations are more likely to cause hypotension and bradycardia. Augmentation with opioids or benzodiazepines is required to achieve such a state.

Morphine use is reduced up to 30% when clonidine is added to analgesic regimens[2130,2134] with a plasma clonidine concentration of 1.5 to 2 μg/L.[2135,2136] The biphasic hypotensive/hypertensive blood pressure response, reported with dexmedetomidine (Fig. 5.35),[2137] has also been demonstrated with clonidine. Decreases in blood pressure were related to plasma concentrations of 1.5 to 2 μg/L, but at greater concentrations the hypotensive effect

was attenuated.[2124] Intensive care studies have concluded that clonidine is safe, but a valid characterization of the safety profile remains challenging due to limited, biased and heterogeneous data, and missing investigation of long-term effects.[2117]

A single caudal/epidural dose of clonidine combined with various local anesthetics range from 1 to 2 μg/kg[2112,2138–2143]; continuous epidural infusions combined with various local anesthetics have also been used and concentrations range from 0.6 to 1 μg/mL (see Chapters 40 and 41).[2144]

DEXMEDETOMIDINE

Dexmedetomidine (Precedex), the *dextro* optical isomer of medetomidine, is a pharmacologically selective α2-agonist with sedative, anxiolytic, and analgesic properties. Dexmedetomidine is in the same class as clonidine but differs from clonidine in its 8-fold greater affinity for α2- compared with α1-receptors than with clonidine. In anesthesia and intensive care, dexmedetomidine is currently being administered for procedural sedation and as an anesthetic adjunct.[2145] Dexmedetomidine has been administered orally,[2146–2148] nasally,[2149–2152] IM,[2153,2154] IV, subarachnoid,[2155] and as an adjunct to regional anesthesia techniques.[2111,2156–2159] Dexmedetomidine provides an interesting quality of sedation that permits arousal with gentle stimulation.[2160] The lack of respiratory depression distinguishes this sedative from opioids, benzodiazepines, and other sedatives.[2161–2164] Dexmedetomidine provides a modest degree of analgesia, reducing the need for, but not supplanting, opioids and other analgesics.[2165–2167]

Dexmedetomidine is metabolized extensively in the liver (UGT1A4 and UGT2B10), with 40% metabolized by aliphatic hydroxylation (CYP 2A6), and N–methylation (CYP2D6).[2165] After metabolism to methyl and glucuronide conjugates, 95% of dexmedetomidine is eliminated via the kidneys.[2168] There is no

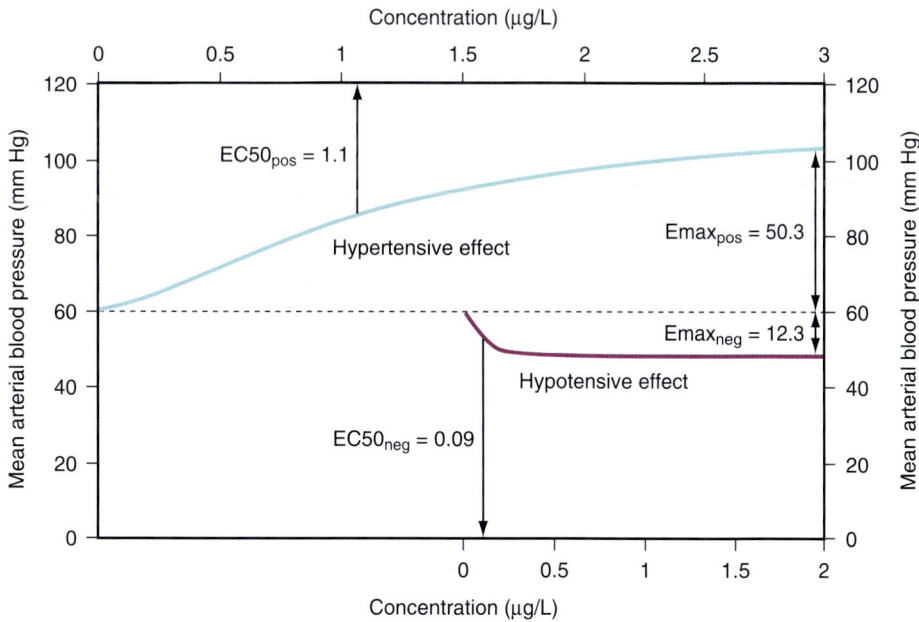

FIGURE 5.35 Composite Emax model showing the hypertensive and hypotensive effect of dexmedetomidine on mean arterial blood pressure in children after cardiac surgery. The vasoconstrictor effect occurred with minimal time delay, whereas an equilibration half-time ($T_{1/2}$keo) of 9.66 minutes was estimated for the sympatholytic response.[2444] *EC50*, Concentration that produces half the maximal effect. (Reproduced with permission from Potts AL, Anderson BJ, Holford NH, Vu TC, Warman GR. Dexmedetomidine hemodynamics in children after cardiac surgery. *Pediatr Anesth.* 2010;20(5):425-433.)

evidence that dexmedetomidine interferes with the pharmacokinetics of other medications that are substrates for CYP2D6 metabolism.[2168] Dexmedetomidine is 93% protein-bound in children.[2160,2165]

A universal pharmacokinetic model has developed from pooled pediatric and adult data (40.6 postmenstrual weeks to 70.8 years of age, 3.1–152 kg).[119] This three-compartment pharmacokinetic model with first-order elimination was superior to a two-compartment model to describe these pooled dexmedetomidine data. Population parameter estimates (CV %) were clearance 0.9 L/minute per 70 kg (36%); intercompartmental clearances (Q2) 1.68 L/minute per 70 kg (63%); Q3 0.62 L/minute per 70 kg (90%); volume of distribution in the central compartment (V1) 25.2 L per 70 kg (103.9%); rapidly equilibrating peripheral compartment (V2) 34.4 L per 70 kg (41.8%); slow equilibrating peripheral compartment (V3) 65.4 L per 70 kg (62%).[119] Obesity was best described by fat free mass for clearances and normal fat mass for volumes with a factor for fat mass (FfatV) of 0.293. Lean body weight is a better size descriptor for dexmedetomidine clearance than total body weight.[119]

Clearance increases from 18.2 L/hour per 70 kg at birth in a full-term neonate to reach 84.5% of the mature value by 1-year postnatal age (see Figs 5.5 and 5.12). Cardiopulmonary bypass reduces the clearance in infants and children compared with those not undergoing cardiopulmonary bypass.[2169] The clearance of dexmedetomidine infusion after cardiac surgery was also reduced by 27% compared with the clearance after a bolus in a noncardiac surgical population.[2170] Similar parameter estimates, including a reduced clearance in children who received a dexmedetomidine infusion after cardiac surgery, have been described by others[2171]; this trend has also been described for morphine, fentanyl, and midazolam.

The pharmacokinetics of dexmedetomidine have also been studied after parenteral (IM), buccal, and oral administration.[2172] Parenteral delivery yielded kinetics similar to the IV route; buccal administration yielded an 82% bioavailability, and orogastric delivery yielded only a 16% bioavailability. Intranasal bioavailability was estimated to be 40.6% (95% clearance 34.7, 54.4%) and 40.7% (95% clearance 36.5, 53.2%) for atomization and drops respectively.[178] The absorption half-time for dexmedetomidine when delivered intranasally is 0.5 to 1 hour.[178] Data from adults indicate limited effects of renal failure on the kinetics of dexmedetomidine.[2173]

Context-sensitive half time is increased in obese children (see Fig. 6.23) and in neonates. Clearance in a 1-year-old child is similar to that described in an adult (0.013 L/minute per kg) but body fat composition differs. Clearance, expressed on a per kilogram basis is increased in children 5 to 12 years of age, the years when muscle mass increases and context-sensitive half-time is smaller than adult estimates. Although age does influence context-sensitive half-time, its influence on recovery time may not be as obvious as Fig. 5.36 suggests because the variability in the predicted context-sensitive half-time at each age is considerable; neonates however, have an increased context-sensitive half-time.[2174]

Dexmedetomidine exerts its effects on numerous organ systems via α-adrenoceptors. These sympathetic adrenoceptors are categorized as either α_1- or α_2-receptors, based on receptor selectivity.[2175] The latter are further subdivided into three subtypes: α_{2A}-, α_{2B}-, and α_{2C}-adrenoceptors according to ligand binding. The α_2-agonists, such as dexmedetomidine, bind all three receptor subtypes, although the receptor subtype binding may vary with the dose of dexmedetomidine. The α_2-adrenoceptors trigger responses by activating G proteins. The common path for the effector response to dexmedetomidine is sympatholysis (suppression of the sympathetic nervous system). Depending on the specific receptor that is activated, α_2-agonists may cause hypotension, bradycardia, sedation, analgesia, attenuation of shivering, and a number of other physiologic responses. Consequently, dexmedetomidine use in neonates and children has expanded to include prevention of emergence delirium, as an adjuvant for postoperative pain management,[2111,2156–2159] invasive and noninvasive procedural sedation,[2070,2148–2151,2176] ICU sedation,[2170,2177] and the management of opioid withdrawal.[2161,2162,2178–2186]

The α_2-adrenoceptors are located ubiquitously throughout the body. In the CNS, they are located primarily in the locus coeruleus, spinal cord, and autonomic nerves. The CNS manifestations of α_2-agonists include sedation and anxiolysis, both of which are mediated through the locus coeruleus. Sedation may also be

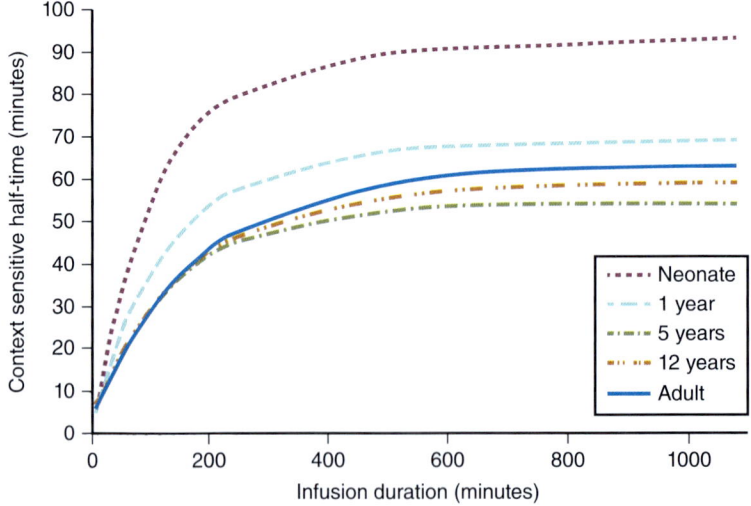

FIGURE 5.36 Context-sensitive half-time changes of dexmedetomidine with age. (Pharmacokinetic parameters from Morse and colleagues. From Morse J, Cortinez LI, Anderson BJ. Pharmacokinetic concepts for dexmedetomidine target-controlled infusion pumps in children. *Pediatr Anesth.* 2021;31. Used with permission.)

mediated by α_2-agonist inhibition of the ascending norepinephrine pathways. Analgesia is mediated primarily via the spinal cord, although there is evidence that supraspinal and peripheral nerves may contribute to this effect as well. Cardiovascular manifestations of α_2-adrenoceptors include actions on the heart and the peripheral vasculature. The primary cardiac action of α_2-adrenoceptors is a chronotropic effect in which it slows heart rate by blocking the cardioaccelerator nerves as well as by augmenting vagal activity. In infants, dexmedetomidine-induced bradycardia may be exacerbated by the coadministration of digoxin; decreasing the dose of dexmedetomidine restores the heart rate to normal values.[2187] The α_2-agonist action on the autonomic ganglia includes decreasing sympathetic outflow, which can lead to hypotension and bradycardia. Actions on the peripheral vasculature depend on the dose of dexmedetomidine: vasodilatation is the result of sympatholysis, which occurs at low doses, and vasoconstriction is the result of direct action on smooth muscle vasculature at large doses (see Fig. 5.35).

In the peripheral nervous system, α_2-adrenoceptors are located at both the presynaptic and postsynaptic junctions.[2175] The presynaptic and postsynaptic effects of α_2-agonists diminish norepinephrine release and inhibit sympathetic activity. Other manifestations of α_2-adrenoceptors include inhibiting shivering as well as promoting diuresis, although their mechanisms remain elusive.[2165,2175]

The CNS effects of dexmedetomidine have been addressed in animals and, in part, in humans.[2188] Dexmedetomidine decreases cerebral blood flow directly by vasoconstricting the smooth muscle of the cerebral blood vessels and indirectly by reducing arterial blood pressure and cardiac output. In humans, dexmedetomidine decreases cerebral blood flow by 30%, as determined by positron emission tomography, as well as Doppler measurements of the middle cerebral artery. Interestingly, using Doppler measurements of the cerebral blood vessels in adult volunteers, both the CO_2 response and autoregulation of cerebral blood flow were preserved. When dexmedetomidine was infused before introducing an inhalational anesthetic, dexmedetomidine attenuated the cerebral vasodilatation induced by the inhalational anesthetic. Regional brain oxygenation and cerebral blood flow velocity were similar during propofol and dexmedetomidine sedation in adults.[2189]

A plasma concentration >0.6 μg/L is thought to produce satisfactory sedation in adult ICU patients,[2190] and similar target concentrations are estimated in children who require sedation in the ICU after cardiac surgery.[2170] The target concentration required for sedation in radiology is greater (approximately 1 μg/L), consistent with concentration-response relationship for sedation described in adults.[178,2191,2192] Blood pressure[2137] and heart rate[2193] effects have been described in children using sigmoid Emax models. The delay between plasma and effect is the effect site equilibration half-time ($T_{1/2}$keo) and is 3 to 6 minutes for sedative effect[178,2194] and 9.9 minutes for central vasodilation.[2137]

Adverse effects due to the biphasic blood pressure response (see Fig. 5.35) or bradycardia are well described. A bolus dose of dexmedetomidine 0.49 μg/kg intravenously given over 5 seconds in children (5–9 years of age) caused a maximum median decrease in heart rate of 20 beats per minute and a maximum median mean arterial pressure increase of 12.5 mm Hg which occurred at 100 seconds after bolus dose administration. The heart rate in 15 of 21 children was <60 beats per minute, whereas 1 subject had a rate <40 beats per minute for 60 seconds after the bolus of dexmedetomidine.[2195] Slowing the rate of administration or administration in a series of fractional doses may prevent excessive

concentrations during the early distributive phase. Dexmedetomidine is commonly administered slowly over 10 to 20 minutes in children to maintain cardiovascular stability and avoid rapid change in blood pressure or pulse (see Chapter 6).[13]

The decrease in heart rate after dexmedetomidine[2160–2163,2196–2198] has been attributed to a centrally mediated sympathetic withdrawal, which resulted in unregulated cholinergic activity. With doses of dexmedetomidine (2–3 μg/kg over 10 minutes followed by 1.5–2 μg/kg per hour), 12 children <6 years of age experienced heart rates <50 beats per minute although their blood pressures were maintained.[2198] Administration of anticholinergics or other medications to increase the heart rate during dexmedetomidine-induced bradycardia has not generally been required and may be problematic with glycopyrrolate.

Dexmedetomidine 0.5 μg/kg IV has resulted in several episodes of bradycardia 30 seconds or longer with an unrecordable systolic blood pressure in two children during strabismus surgery (without anticholinergic pretreatment) when the surgeon pulled gently on the extraocular muscle (personal communication, JL, 2017). Vital signs were restored after administration of ephedrine 0.1 to 0.2 mg/kg IV. At the other extreme, reports of severe and in some cases persistent hypertension after giving anticholinergics to treat dexmedetomidine-induced bradycardia[2185,2199,2200]; the mechanism for this interaction remains unclear at this time but we caution against using glycopyrrolate in this setting.

Both sinus and atrioventricular node function are depressed by dexmedetomidine. Use of dexmedetomidine during electrophysiology studies may be associated with adverse effects in patients at risk for bradycardia or atrioventricular nodal block.[2201] However, dexmedetomidine did not interfere with the conduct of pediatric electrophysiologic studies for supraventricular tachycardia and the successful ablation of such arrhythmias, this despite a greater need for isoproterenol when dexmedetomidine was used.[2202] A meta-analysis of nine studies involving 1851 children reported a reduction in junctional ectopic tachycardia in children undergoing cardiac surgery.[2203,2204] Dexmedetomidine is increasingly used in the management of children with congenital heart disease.

One of the major advantages of dexmedetomidine over other sedatives is its minimal respiratory depression in adults and children.[2160,2163,2196,2197,2205–2207] Although dexmedetomidine blunts the CO_2 response curve,[2208] it does not lead to extreme hypoxia or hypercapnia. Indeed, respiratory rate, CO_2 tension, and oxygen saturation are generally maintained during dexmedetomidine sedation in children.[2160,2161,2164] In children without obstructive sleep apnea, increasing doses of dexmedetomidine (1–3 μg/kg) results in small changes in the upper airway and are not associated with clinical signs of airway obstruction. Even though these changes are small, all precautions to manage airway obstruction should be taken when dexmedetomidine is used for sedation.[2209] In children with suspected OSA, less frequent artificial airway support was required when dexmedetomidine (2 μg/hour per kilogram) was used for sedation for MRI sleep studies, compared with propofol for sedation.[2210] One report using dexmedetomidine sedation determined that the addition of ketamine did not affect airway patency compared with dexmedetomidine alone.[2211]

When compared with propofol for sedation during MRI, dexmedetomidine provides adequate sedation during the scan but has a slower onset and recovery profile (see Fig. 5.36).[2212,2213] Sedation may require the addition of other sedatives, such as midazolam or propofol,[2214,2215] for a child to remain motionless for a procedure such as an MRI.[2161,2216,2217] However, characterization of nasal absorption pharmacokinetics with its slow uptake, reduced relative bioavailability (F 0.4),[2218] the larger dose required for intranasal delivery (2–3 µg/kg) and subsequent slow recovery has made this route increasingly popular for radiological sedation.[2219]

Quantifying the MAC-sparing effect of dexmedetomidine has proven difficult. Three studies have estimated the MAC of isoflurane or sevoflurane in adults at two concentrations of dexmedetomidine, high (0.6–0.7 ng/mL) and low (0.36–0.3 ng/mL).[2197,2220,2221] The MAC-sparing effect of large-dose dexmedetomidine concentration ranged from 17% to 50% and that of low-dose dexmedetomidine concentration from 0% to 35%. Accordingly, it is difficult to predict the exact MAC-reducing effect of dexmedetomidine on sevoflurane and isoflurane in adults. Premedication with intravenous dexmedetomidine, 1 and 2 µg/kg in children 3 to 7 years undergoing adenotonsillectomy decreased the MAC for extubation by 41% and 64%, respectively.[2222]

Dexmedetomidine depresses sensory-evoked potentials but, for the most part, the potentials are adequate for evaluations.[2223] Similarly, motor-evoked potentials are reduced in a dose-dependent manner during dexmedetomidine infusion but are measurable nonetheless.[2224] There are contrasting reports about the degree of evoked potential suppression, but most report successful spinal cord monitoring during scoliosis surgery (see also Chapter 30).[2225–2228]

Emergence delirium occurs in 15%–30% of children after most inhalational anesthetics particularly in the 3–5 year age range.[2205] A number of medications attenuate the incidence of delirium after anesthesia, including dexmedetomidine.[2182] Dexmedetomidine decreases the incidence of emergence delirium after sevoflurane anesthesia: after an infusion of dexmedetomidine (0.2 µg/kg per hour), recovery was not prolonged,[2229] whereas after a single dose of 0.5 µg/kg administered 5 minutes before the end of surgery, emergence was prolonged.[2230] Dexmedetomidine was superior to placebo, midazolam, and opioids but did not differ noticeably from propofol, ketamine, or clonidine among other sedatives.[2231,2232] Children undergoing strabismus surgery benefit from an infusion of dexmedetomidine rather than a bolus at the end of surgery and a reduced incidence of the oculocardiac reflex compared with placebo.[2233] Nasal dexmedetomidine, 2 µg/kg, was superior to midazolam 0.5 mg/kg or placebo in reducing emergence delirium in children undergoing strabismus repair.[663]

The interaction between dexmedetomidine and neuromuscular blockade has been studied during balanced anesthesia with propofol and alfentanil.[2234] In adults, dexmedetomidine decreased the twitch response after sevoflurane 7%, although this was not deemed to be clinically important. Current evidence does not substantiate any clinically significant interaction between dexmedetomidine and neuromuscular blockade.

Dexmedetomidine has had extensive use for ICU sedation, although trial design to prove benefit over conventional sedation has proven difficult.[2235] A systematic review and meta-analysis of 32 studies including 3267 children revealed that infusion rates were quite varied (0.1–2.5 µg/kg per hour with a duration of 15 to 549 hours. The incidence of bradycardia was 2.6% and hypotension 6.1%. The authors concluded that dexmedetomidine sedation should be considered safe but that there was need for study of dosing and withdrawal.[2236]

Dexmedetomidine has also been used as an adjuvant for prolonging caudal analgesia. Block duration of postoperative analgesia was longer but increased bradycardia and prolonged postoperative sedation with higher sedation scores 2 hours after surgery noted.[2237]

One reservation concerning dexmedetomidine is the fear of a withdrawal from dexmedetomidine itself after prolonged use (>24 hours). Up to 80% of children (0–17 years of age) in intensive care experienced withdrawal symptoms after infusion (0.42 ± 0.17 µg/kg per hour).[2177,2238] Withdrawal symptoms may occur after 4 days in children receiving on average 1 µg/kg per hour.[2239]

CHLORAL HYDRATE

Chloral hydrate is one of the oldest and, in the past, most widely used sedatives in infants and children, exerting its sedation effect by enhancing the GABA receptor complex. Like many other sedatives, it has no analgesic properties. Its primary use in pediatrics is for sedation for noninvasive procedures and as a premedication. Its principal advantage is that it may be administered orally or rectally, with excellent absorption and relatively good sedation, within 30 to 45 minutes, and the infrequent need to supplement the sedation with other sedatives. The usual dose is 20 to 75 mg/kg orally or rectally, although total doses up to 100 mg/kg (maximum 2 grams) have been used alone or in combination with other sedatives.

Chloral hydrate used to be the most commonly used sedative for infants undergoing a variety of nonpainful procedures[2240–2244]; however, chloral hydrate liquid production ceased in the United States in May 2017. Since this drug is no longer commercially available in the United States, individual hospital pharmacies continue to prepare the drug[2245] and must reformulate it with reconstituted crystals. One study reported that for unexplained mechanisms, the duration of sedation was less, the frequency of supplemental sedatives greater, and the incidence of sedation failures greater with compounded chloral hydrate compared with the commercial preparation.[2246]

Chloral hydrate has minimal effects on respiration[2247]; however, it has caused airway obstruction and desaturation, particularly in children with enlarged tonsils.[2248–2250] In addition, apnea, airway obstruction, bradycardia, and hypotension have been reported in a series of infants younger than 6 months of age who were sedated for echocardiograms; this report emphasized that this is not the benign drug that many previously thought.[2251] Arrhythmias have been reported after chloral hydrate, attributed to its primary metabolite, trichloroethanol. After a single dose of 30 mg/kg, sedation was evident for up to 12 hours after administration in former premature nursery graduates. Bradycardia (as slow as 60 beats/minute) was also observed in these neonates.[2252] Deaths after chloral hydrate overdose when given for sedation have also been reported.[1526,2253–2255]

Chloral hydrate has several disadvantages. It has a bitter taste and is known to cause vomiting.[2256] This drug should not be administered for long periods of time because theoretically (1) its metabolites may be carcinogenic, (2) it may cause severe gastritis (possibly related to its metabolism to trichloroacetic acid), and (3) drug metabolites may accumulate.[2257,2258] In addition, it may interfere with the binding of bilirubin to albumin and toxic metabolites may accumulate, leading to metabolic acidosis, renal failure, and hypotonia in neonates.[2259]

Chloral hydrate is metabolized in the liver and erythrocytes by alcohol dehydrogenase to an active metabolite, trichloroethanol, which has a half-life of 9.7 ± 1.7 hours in toddlers but 39.8 ± 14.3 hours in preterm infants (see Fig. 44.3).[2260] Trichloroethanol is cleared by UGT (see the sections on morphine, acetaminophen, and dexmedetomidine), which is immature in neonates. The long half-life implies that residual drug effect will be present long after any procedure requiring sedation.[2261–2263] Because of the long half-life, there is risk for prolonged sedation and death after leaving medical supervision.[2241,2254,2264-2266] It is for this reason that *chloral hydrate is not generally recommended for premedication before surgery* and that a prolonged period of observation is recommended after sedation for a procedure. If nitrous oxide is administered to children who have received chloral hydrate, a state of deep sedation or general anesthesia may occur.[2267]

Antihistamines

DIPHENHYDRAMINE

Antihistamines are often used in pediatric anesthesia both for their histamine 1 (H_1)-receptor inhibition and for their sedative properties. Diphenhydramine (Benadryl) is one of the more commonly used antihistamines. It is rapidly absorbed when administered orally (at a dose of 1.25 mg/kg) with a duration of effect that lasts anywhere from 3 to 6 hours. Clearance is through CYP2D6. It is often administered as a premedicant or as an in-hospital sedative. Caution is advised for children with respiratory problems because diphenhydramine dries secretions, causing difficulty expectorating. The IV dose to treat an allergic reaction is 0.5 mg/kg.

CIMETIDINE, RANITIDINE, AND FAMOTIDINE

Cimetidine (Tagamet) was the first generation of potent, very hydrophilic, competitive inhibitors of H_2-receptor-mediated histamine reactions, which was later followed by ranitidine and famotidine. This class of drugs increases gastric-fluid pH and reduces gastric fluid residual volume.[2268] Indications for an H_2-receptor antagonist include a history of gastroesophageal reflux, hiatus hernia, previous esophageal surgery, obesity, or an anticipated difficult intubation that will require prolonged laryngoscopy, as well as, perhaps, high-risk patients (American Society of Anesthesiologists classes 3 and 4). Cimetidine is likely the most studied of this category of drugs, but its use has diminished because of serious drug interactions through its effects on the cytochrome oxidase system. Cimetidine partially inhibits numerous CYP enzymes (CYP1A2, CYP2C9, CYP2C19, CYP2D6, CYP2E1, and CYP3A4), which prolongs the half-lives of many drugs, including phenytoin, phenobarbital, theophylline, cyclosporine, carbamazepine, benzodiazepines that do not undergo glucuronidation, calcium channel blockers, propranolol, quinidine, sulfonylureas, mexiletine, warfarin, and tricyclic antidepressants, such as imipramine.[2269] The elimination half-life of cimetidine is prolonged in neonates and infants compared with older children.[2270] The kidney is the primary clearance organ in children. Renal clearance in children 4 to 13 years of age constituted 70% of total body clearance, more than double that of adults. As expected, children have a greater total body clearance (11.6 mL/minute per kilogram) than do adults (7.0 mL/minute per kilogram), a larger volume of distribution (1.24 vs. 0.80 L/kg), and a shorter elimination half-life (83 vs. 122 minutes).[2271]

Although ranitidine (Zantac) also weakly reduces CYP activity, *it does not increase the half-life of other medications significantly* when administered at the usual therapeutic doses.[2272-2275] As a result it supplanted cimetidine in clinical practice. Ranitidine may be administered by intermittent bolus (2–4 mg/kg in four divided doses), or as a loading dose (0.5 mg/kg) followed by an infusion of 0.05 mg/kg per hour.[2276-2278] The peak effect occurs between 2 and 4 hours after administration.[1789] The elimination half-life of ranitidine is 3 ± 1.35 hours. When a dose of 1.5 mg/kg per 8 hours was administered, ranitidine maintained the gastric fluid

pH greater than 4.[2277] Reduced doses have met with less success in controlling the gastric fluid pH.[2276]

Famotidine (Pepcid) is ~8 times more potent than ranitidine and about 40 times more potent than cimetidine.[2279] Famotidine has been well studied, including in neonates. Because famotidine is primarily excreted by the kidneys, dosing depends on the maturity of the renal function. Infants younger than 3 months of age have reduced clearance and require 24 hours between doses (0.25 mg/kg IV or 0.5 mg/kg orally), whereas infants older than 3 months of age are similar to older children and adults and require 12 hours between doses.[2270,2280,2281] There is some evidence to suggest decreased responsiveness to famotidine (a weaker effect in altering gastric acid pH and volume) with long-term administration.[2282] Famotidine increases gastric fluid pH, although it does not reduce gastric residual volumes when administered before anesthesia.[2283]

Antiemetics

METOCLOPRAMIDE

Metoclopramide (Reglan) has been used in children for its antiemetic and gastric emptying properties.[2284] Its antiemetic properties result from its direct effects on the chemoreceptor trigger zone. Gastric emptying results from the antagonism of the neurotransmitter dopamine, which stimulates gastric smooth muscle activity.[2285,2286] A dose of 0.15 mg/kg at the end of surgery effectively reduces emesis after strabismus surgery and tonsillectomy, although the magnitude of its effectiveness may be limited.[2287] Metoclopramide is less effective than 5-hydroxytryptamine type 3 (5-HT_3) receptor inhibitors as an antiemetic, but is an alternative rescue medication.[2288] As with many other medications, it is cleared by sulfate and glucuronide conjugation, the elimination half-life in neonates is prolonged compared with older children, thus necessitating a 6-hour interval between oral doses (0.15 mg/kg).[2289] Clearance in infants (0.9–5.6 months of age) was 0.67 ± 0.13 L/hour per kg with volume of distribution at steady state 4.4 ± 0.6 L/kg.[2290]

The use of metoclopramide in children has been limited in part, by its reduced effectiveness for antiemesis compared with other drugs (e.g., ondansetron and dexamethasone) and its side effects, most notably extrapyramidal signs. In a systematic review of the safety of metoclopramide in children from 108 studies of which 58 were prospective, 9% of the children developed extrapyramidal signs, 6% developed diarrhea, and 6% became sedated.[2291] Side effects occurred more commonly when repeat doses of metoclopramide were administered.

5-HYDROXYTRYPTAMINE TYPE 3–RECEPTOR ANTAGONISTS

Drugs that antagonize the 5-HT_3 receptor including ondansetron (Zofran), granisetron (Kytril), dolasetron (Anzemet), tropisetron (Navoban), and palonosetron (Aloxi), are very effective at preventing and treating PONV in children. Although all of them are widely used, identifying which has the most cost-effective profile, has the best side-effect profile, has the greatest duration of action, is most effective when combined with other agents, and costs the least remain a subject of debate.[2292-2304] Because ondansetron was the first in this class of serotonergic receptor antagonists that effectively reduced the incidence of nausea and vomiting in children, it forms the basis for discussion of measures to prevent PONV after pediatric surgery.[2305-2314] Some studies report that ondansetron (0.1 mg/kg) is superior to metoclopramide (0.15 mg/kg) for the prophylactic control of postoperative vomiting in children undergoing tonsillectomy.[2315] Most pediatric anesthesiologists limit their routine use to children undergoing procedures known to have a substantial incidence of PONV, such as strabismus repair, tonsillectomy, or middle ear surgery, and to children with a known history of motion sickness or previous nausea and vomiting after surgery.[2316–2324] Ondansetron is effective in preventing nausea and vomiting, as well as in reducing the severity of established nausea and vomiting. The usual recommended dose is 100 to 150 μg/kg every 6 hours or a single dose of 50 to 100 μg/kg when combined with dexamethasone for prophylaxis against PONV. One clinical trial found efficacy in children as young as 1 month of age; however, the pharmacokinetics were different in the infants younger than 4 months of age, suggesting the need for a greater interval between dosing.[2325] This is not surprising, given that clearance is by hydroxylation, followed by glucuronide or sulfate conjugation in the liver. A mature clearance of 541 mL/minute per 70 kg is reported, but ondansetron clearance was reduced by 31%, 53%, and 76% for the typical 6-, 3-, and 1-month-old infant, respectively. Clearance matured with a maturation half-time (TM_{50}) of 4 months. Simulations showed that an ondansetron dose of 0.1 mg/kg in children younger than 6 months of age produced exposure similar to a 0.15-mg/kg dose in older children.[2326] Pharmacodynamically, the indication for antiemetics in children <2 years of age are limited as postoperative vomiting is uncommon in this age group. One final concern with this class of drugs (dolasetron in particular) is the potential for ventricular tachyarrhythmias (e.g., torsades de pointes) in patients with long QT syndrome, especially when they are anesthetized with potent inhalation agents such as sevoflurane.[2327,2328] However, concentrations reached after routine dosing are well below the inhibitory concentration of 50% (IC_{50}) reported for inhibition of Na channels in healthy individuals.[2294] Nonetheless, cases of sustained supraventricular and ventricular tachycardia, myocardial infarction and one fatal cardiac arrest were reported in 2006 in association with the use of dolasetron in both children and adolescents that led to its withdrawal from the market in some countries.

A number of studies in children demonstrated that the antiemetic effect of drugs from this class can be improved if they are combined with dexamethasone or other anesthetic techniques known to reduce vomiting.[2309,2310,2312,2329,2330] An oral disintegrating tablet of ondansetron is also available.[2331]

Other agents in this class (e.g., granisetron, dolasetron, tropisetron) have all been shown to be effective in ameliorating PONV, which is further improved when combined with other antiemetic modalities.[2305,2323,2332–2339] Granisetron and tropisetron have greater half-lives (7.8 hours) and coincident duration of action than ondansetron (4 hours); the former may be better suited to chemotherapy-induced nausea and vomiting. Dolasetron and tropisteron are metabolized primarily by CYP2D6, which renders their termination susceptible to polymorphisms and an extended elimination half-life of 40 hours is reported in PMs. CYP3A4 is the predominant enzyme pathway for ondansetron and granisetron metabolism with CYP2D6 a secondary pathway.[2294]

Palonosetron differs from the 5-HT_3 receptor antagonists described previously[2340] in that it allosterically inhibits the receptor rather than physically binding to the receptor.[2341] Because it takes 30 to 40 hours for the receptor to restore its normal conformation, the agent may be metabolized (and is susceptible to polymorphisms of CYP2D6), but that does not affect its antiemetic effect as the receptor remains deformed for the duration. Palonosetron

effectively reduces PONV in adults.[2342] In a dose-finding study in children, palonosetron (0.5 μg/kg) was as effective as 1 and 1.5 μg/kg for PONV for 48 hours after strabismus surgery.[2343] A double-blind, double dummy study of 502 pediatric patients undergoing emetogenic chemotherapy found noninferiority for 20 μg/kg 6 hourly compared with ondansetron 150 μg/kg 8 hourly; it is approved for this indication in children as young as 1 month of age.[2344]

NEUROKININ 1 AND OTHER ANTIEMETICS

Despite the introduction of 5-HT_3 receptor antagonists along with dexamethasone to treat PONV, PONV has continued. It has been known that the receptor for substance P, the neurokinin 1 (NK1) receptor, in the brainstem (area postrema and nucleus tractus solitarius) may hold the key to persistent PONV.[2345,2346] NK1 receptors likely prevent PONV by downregulating receptor activity at several sites: the chemoreceptor trigger zone, the gastrointestinal tract, and the dorsal motor nucleus of the vagus. The first NK1 receptor antagonist released for clinical use was aprepitant (Emend), which has proven effective in reducing nausea and vomiting in adults after chemotherapy and surgery and in children after chemotherapy.[2347,2348] Aprepitant is an oral drug, fosaprepitant is the parenteral formulation of aprepitant, and several others are under development for use (and dosing) in PONV in combination with 5-HT_3 receptor antagonists and dexamethasone.[2349,2350] Preliminary study of aprepitant pharmacokinetics, safety, and efficacy support further clinical evaluation of this drug for PONV prophylaxis in children.[2351] All NK1 antagonists undergo hepatic metabolism and biliary excretion.

Several analogues of aprepitant are current under development.[2291] Rolapitant, casopitant, and vestipitant are NK1 antagonists that may be administered orally or intravenously. Only rolapitant is FDA licensed for use in chemotherapy-induced nausea and vomiting; casopitant and vestipitant remain unlicensed. Rolapitant has 91% bioavailability when given orally with a half-life of 5 to 8 days after a single dose. Casopitant has a 60% bioavailability when given orally with a half-life of 2.5 to 7 days. Vestipitant has a relatively short half-life of 5 to 9 hours rendering it least likely of the three to reach market. Amisulpride (Barhemsys), a dopamine antagonist is another new agent shown to be effective in several double-blind placebo controlled studies for prevention and treatment of vomiting in adult patients but it has not yet been approved for pediatric patients under age 18 years of age.[2352,2353]

DEXAMETHASONE

Dexamethasone is a glucocorticoid with minimal mineralocorticoid activity that is used ubiquitously in anesthesia for prevention of postoperative nausea and vomiting (see Chapters 2, 31 and 45). The steroid undergoes extensive hepatic metabolism to 6-hydroxy-dexamethasone and side-chain cleaved metabolites with CYP3A4 responsible for the formation of 6-hydroxylated products. It has a plasma half-life of 4 to 5 hours but prolonged duration of effect (36–54 hours). Dexamethasone is commonly administered via IV but can be given IM or enterally.

A single intraoperative dose of dexamethasone reduces the incidence of emesis during the first 24 hours after adenotonsillectomy[2354] with the number of children needed to treat only four. The combination of antiemetic and morphine-sparing advantages of a single dose of dexamethasone, its low cost and safety profile, suggest that routine use of dexamethasone reduces morbidity after adenotonsillectomy in children.[2354,2355] The smallest effective dose remains somewhat unclear. The frequency of postoperative vomiting, pain scores, time to first liquid intake, and time to first analgesics did not differ between doses of 0.0625 and 1.0 mg/kg IV.[2329,2356]

Complications of dexamethasone that have been associated with chronic steroid use such as aseptic necrosis of the hip have not been reported after a single dose in children. However, acute tumor lysis syndrome with hyperkalemic cardiac arrest has been reported in children and adults after a single dose was administered to a patient with an unrecognized hematopoietic cancer such as leukemia or lymphoma.[2357,2358] In patients with known or suspected hematopoietic disorders, steroids should not be given before consulting an oncologist. Any patient who becomes unstable after even a single dose of steroids should be investigated and treated for possible acute tumor lysis syndrome.

Anticholinergics

ATROPINE AND SCOPOLAMINE

Atropine (0.02 mg/kg) and scopolamine (0.01 mg/kg) both have CNS effects, although the sedating effect of scopolamine is 5 to 15 times greater than atropine. Scopolamine possesses two to three times more potent antisialagogue action than atropine. Atropine and scopolamine decrease the ability to sweat, and thus may cause a slight increase in temperature.[2359] Atropine and scopolamine have equipotent cardiovascular accelerator properties. The dose for both anticholinergics in infants to speed the heart rate is greater per kilogram than in adults.[2360]

Anticholinergics are appropriate in specific situations, such as to diminish secretions preoperatively, to block laryngeal and vagal reflexes, to treat or prevent the bradycardia associated with succinylcholine, to treat the bradycardia of anesthetic-induced myocardial depression, the muscarinic effects of neostigmine, and the oculocardiac reflex. Atropine is painful when administered IM. When it is administered as a premedicant, it does not block laryngeal reflexes; it is more effective in blocking laryngeal reflexes when it is given IV. Although some data suggest that children with trisomy 21 are more susceptible to the cardiac effects of atropine,[2361] this notion is not supported by clinical experience.[2362,2363] Because some children with trisomy 21 have narrow-angle glaucoma, atropine must be administered cautiously because it might worsen their glaucoma.[2362,2363]

Atropine may be administered orally, rectally, and via the trachea. Oral atropine may blunt the hypotensive response to potent inhalation agents during induction of anesthesia in infants younger than 3 months of age.[538] When administered via the trachea, atropine is rapidly absorbed, producing physiologic effects.[2364–2367]

Atropine is metabolized in the liver by N-demethylation followed by conjugation with glucuronic acid[2368]; both processes are immature in the neonate. Half the drug is also eliminated by the kidneys. An old technique to diagnose atropine poisoning was to place a small aliquot of the victim's urine into the eye of a cat and observe for mydriasis!

It is anticipated that clearance is reduced in the neonatal age range because of an immaturity of renal and hepatic function, but data remain elusive. Children younger than 2 years of age have an increased volume of distribution at steady state compared with those older than 2 years of age (3.2 ± 1.5 vs. 1.3 ± 0.5 L/kg).[2369] Clearance was similar in those younger than 2 years of age (6.8 ± 5.3 mL/minute per kg) and those older than 2 years of age (6.5 ± 1.6 mL/minute per kg). The elimination half-life in healthy adults is 3 ± 0.9 hours, whereas that in term neonates is 4 times longer.[2369,2370]

Pharmacodynamic characterization is similarly lacking in neonates. Some have held that the minimum dose of atropine in neonates and infants is 0.1 mg. Infants younger than 6 months require a larger dose to increase heart rate than older children.[537] A dose of 5 µg/kg had no impact on heart rate and does not cause bradycardia in young infants 4 to 6 months age.[2371] Systolic blood pressure did not change for any dose of atropine (5–40 µg/kg) in this neonatal cohort.[537]

In clinical practice, scopolamine is usually limited to those situations in which its sedative effect, combined with that of morphine, will be most advantageous, such as during cardiac surgery. It is also very useful as an adjuvant to ketamine anesthesia because of its antisialagogue and central sedative effects. The central sedative effects of both atropine and scopolamine may be antagonized with physostigmine. Most centers no longer routinely administer anticholinergic medications as part of the premedication because they are painful, the optimal effect may not coincide with induction of anesthesia, and current potent inhalation agents produce fewer secretions and infrequent bradycardia.

Scopolamine is a tertiary amine with greater CNS effects than atropine, causing sedation and amnesia. It has moderate antiemetic activity.[2372] To minimize the relatively large incidence of side effects, the transdermal dosage form has been developed for nausea and vomiting; however, its use is generally limited to teenagers to avoid potential toxicity.[2373–2375] A placebo controlled study demonstrated reduced PONV and the need for rescue antiemetics.[2376,2377] Scopolamine patch–induced delirium has been reported and is more likely in younger patients.[2374] Unequal pupils have also been reported,[2378] but scopolamine is not more likely to induce drowsiness, blurring of vision, or dizziness compared with other agents.[2376] Scopolamine withdrawal has been reported in children on long-term treatment with scopolamine patches to reduce salivary secretions.[2379]

Scopolamine has a distribution volume of 1.4 L/kg in adults.[2365] Glucuronide conjugation, sulfate conjugation, and hydrolysis by the CYP3A family are involved in its clearance.[2373] Both glucuronidation and the CYP3A enzyme systems are immature at birth and clearance is anticipated to be reduced.[2365]

GLYCOPYRROLATE

Glycopyrrolate (0.005–0.01 mg/kg) is a synthetic quaternary ammonium compound with potent anticholinergic properties. It offers some advantage over atropine and scopolamine because it minimally penetrates the blood-brain barrier and thus causes few CNS effects. Glycopyrrolate's anticholinergic effects last several hours.[2380,2381] The heart rate changes minimally after IV administration, causing fewer arrhythmias and offering an advantage when tachycardia might be detrimental.[2382,2383] It should be noted that prolonged and severe hypertension has been reported when glycopyrrolate was used to treat dexmedetomidine-induced bradycardia[2199]; the mechanism for the hypertension is unknown. Further pretreatment of children before administration of dexmedetomidine demonstrated no value in blunting bradycardia and resulted in greater increases in systolic blood pressure compared with no pretreatment (~20% vs. ~10%).[2200] In some children, gastric fluid volume and acidity are reduced after glycopyrrolate administration.[2384,2385] The drug remains popular for antagonizing the parasympathomimetic effects of neostigmine and is as effective as atropine for preventing the oculocardiac reflex.[2386]

There is poor absorption from the gastrointestinal tract (10%–25%).[2387] Clearance in infants younger than 1 year of age (n = 8) was 1.01 (range 0.32–1.85) L/kg per hour and volume of distribution at steady state of 1.83 (range 0.70–3.87) L/kg,[2387] but there are no neonatal data available. However, the renal system accounts for 85% of elimination,[2380] and clearance is anticipated to be reduced in neonates because renal function is immature.[34]

Antagonists

NALOXONE

Naloxone (Narcan) is a pure opioid antagonist with a greater affinity for the μ-receptor compared with the κ- and δ-receptors. When given intravenously, naloxone has a very rapid onset of antagonism of the opioid receptors (within 30 seconds to 1 minute). Naloxone undergoes glucuronidation in the liver, with minimal bioavailability after oral administration. The plasma clearance of naloxone is large (~3.5 L/minute), the volume of distribution moderate (~110 L) and the elimination half-time brief ($T_{1/2}$ 1–1.5 hours) in adults.[2388] When administered IM, the apparent elimination half-life is prolonged from 80 minutes to 6 hours in adults because of the depot effect.[2389] It is for this reason that after IV reversal of opioid-induced respiratory depression with naloxone, the same dose of naloxone should be administered IM to preclude a recrudescence of the respiratory depression (see later in this chapter).

There are few pharmacokinetic studies of naloxone in children, but neonates have prolonged elimination ($T_{1/2}$ 3 hours), presumably due to their reduced clearance due to glucuronide conjugation.[2390] Naloxone has a relatively short duration of action (30–45 minutes) and supplementary doses (IV or IM) may be required to maintain antagonism after an initial dose 5 to 10 μg/kg IV.

Naloxone has a fast reversal capacity, which is explained by rapid receptor association and dissociation kinetics and a small effect-site equilibrium half-life ($T_{1/2}keo$) of approximately 5 to 7 minutes.[2388] The speed of reversal, however, depends on the opioid-receptor kinetics. Opioids with slow receptor kinetics such as morphine limit the ability of naloxone to rapidly disperse the receptor's opioid agonist. Therefore, increasing the dose will not speed the onset of action, but will increase the duration of effect. This does not apply to fentanyl or other phenylpiperidines that have fast receptor kinetics. The pharmacokinetic/pharmacodynamic relationship remains unknown in children.[2391]

Naloxone is effective for reversing opioid-induced adverse effects, including respiratory depression, chest-wall and glottic rigidity, nausea and vomiting, pruritus,[2392] urinary retention, and constipation. It may be administered via any route, including parenteral, nasal, IM, neuraxial, tracheal, and oral. For children who are ventilating and not in extremis, but in whom opioid-induced respiratory depression needs antagonism in the perioperative period, it is reasonable to initiate antagonism with a very small dose of IV naloxone (0.25–0.5 μg/kg). This is similar to the dose recommended in one large review of 10 to 20 μg of naloxone in children in the perioperative period.[2393] If the response is inadequate, the same dose may be repeated until ventilation improves. The same cumulative total IV dose of naloxone can then be administered as an IM injection to ensure that recrudescence of the respiratory depression does not occur. *For children in extremis or in whom a potential opioid overdose has occurred (including neonatal resuscitation), a larger dose of 10 to 100 μg/kg IV of naloxone may be indicated.*

The American Academy of Pediatrics simplified the naloxone dosing for infants and children up to 5 years of age, recommending 100 μg/kg, and for children older than 5 years of age (20 kg) (2 mg naloxone).[2394] This is based, in part, on concerns that smaller doses of naloxone may not be uniformly effective. However, it is equally important to recognize that overzealous dosing of naloxone will not only reverse the opioid analgesic effect but could also lead to profound systemic hypertension, cardiac arrhythmias (including ventricular fibrillation), and pulmonary edema (noncardiogenic).[2395] Evidence suggests that pulmonary edema may not be a dose-dependent response to naloxone, because it has been reported after as little as a single dose of 100 μg. A retrospective review of the management of 195 children and adolescents who received naloxone postoperatively, in the emergency department, or in the pediatric ICU revealed an IV dosing range of 1 to 500 μg/kg; this resulted in resolution of the respiratory depression, systolic hypertension in 17% of children, and one case (incidence of 0.5%) of pulmonary edema.[2393] A continuous infusion of naloxone may be required to treat severe opioid-induced respiratory depression.[2396] *Any child who receives naloxone for antagonism of opioid-induced respiratory depression must be observed in a monitored environment for a minimum of 2 hours to ensure that there is no recrudescence of the respiratory depression.*

Intramuscular and nasal naloxone is now being administered by firefighters, emergency medical technicians, and other emergency providers to treat acute opioid overdose.[2397–2400] The absorption profile of intranasal naloxone (0.4 mg/mL) in children (n = 20; 6 months to 10 years of age) given 20 μg/kg (maximum 0.4 mg) has been investigated.[2401] A maximum concentration (C_{MAX} 2–6 ng/mL) and time to maximum concentration (T_{MAX}) were reached in more than half of children within 20 minutes.[2401]

The recommended dose of naloxone during neonatal resuscitation far exceeds that in older children. Doses as great as 400 μg/kg IM have been used without ill effects.[2402] In a systematic review of naloxone use in neonates, evidence demonstrated that naloxone increased alveolar ventilation, although there was no evidence that outcome, in terms of assisted ventilation or admission to a neonatal ICU, was affected by the use of naloxone.[2403] Caution is recommended when administering naloxone to an infant of a mother who has chronically abused opioids because seizures have been reported.[2404]

Naloxone has also been administered via intravenous infusion at low doses (≥ 1 μg/kg per hour)[2405] concomitantly to ameliorate adverse effects from opioids, including nausea and vomiting, pruritus, urinary retention, and constipation.[2406] Evidence is mixed regarding the beneficial effect of such a practice,[2407,2408] although double-blind, randomized controlled trials have provided a significant reduction in morphine-associated nausea and pruritus during patient-controlled analgesia when administered as a separate infusion.[2409] When administered for this indication, there is a need to balance antagonism of the opioid-induced side effects with the antagonism of the pain relief.

NALTREXONE

Naltrexone (Depade, ReVia) is an oral opioid antagonist that also has a greater affinity for the μ- rather than κ- and δ-receptors. The activity of naltrexone is thought to be a result of both the parent and its 6β-naltrexol metabolite (via hepatic dihydrodiol dehydrogenase). The mean elimination half-lives for naltrexone and 6β-naltrexol in adults are 4 hours and 13 hours, respectively. Naltrexone has a good oral bioavailability, with an elimination half-life of up to 8 hours in children, which is similar to that in adults.[2410] This opioid antagonist has also been used in the management of autism.[2411,2412] Children displaying self-injurious behavior or hyperactivity have been noted to have high CSF endorphin concentrations and decreased pain sensitivity. Some opioid-induced behavior in animals and people with opioid addiction resembles that seen in autistic children. Naltrexone reduces self-injurious behavior.[2411]

Although naltrexone reverses opioid-associated adverse effects, its use for this purpose has not become popular.[2403,2413] Naltrexone and its primary metabolite, 6β-naltrexol, are excreted, albeit in low concentrations, in breast milk from a lactating female.[2414] Care should be taken when managing infants of opioid-addicted mothers.

METHYLNALTREXONE

Methylnaltrexone (Relistor) is the first quaternary ammonium opioid antagonist that has very limited ability to penetrate the blood-brain barrier.[2415] It is prepared in an oral as well as in a parenteral formulation for subcutaneous and IV administration. Doses of 0.45 mg/kg have been administered intravenously to adults. Because methylnaltrexone does not cross the blood-brain barrier, it is suited to reverse the peripheral adverse side effects of opioids without attenuating the central analgesic effect. Opioid-induced side effects, including gastric emptying, urinary retention, postoperative ileus, and chronic constipation,[2416] improve after administration of methylnaltrexone.[2417–2421] There are few pediatric data available.[2422] If the preliminary adult safety and efficacy data are also demonstrated in children, this drug may offer the benefit of improving our ability to provide opioid-induced analgesia, while eliminating many of the peripheral adverse effects, thus improving the comfort of children. The drug is used currently for opioid-induced constipation in children with cancer and those in palliative care.[2423]

FLUMAZENIL

Flumazenil (Romazicon) is a specific $GABA_A$ receptor-competitive antagonist that reverses the effects of benzodiazepines. Flumazenil has been administered by rectal, nasal, IM, and IV routes.[2424–2427] After a single IV dose, flumazenil shows limited protein binding (40%) with an elimination half-life of approximately 1 hour in adults, owing primarily to rapid and extensive metabolism by hepatic carboxylesterases.[2428–2430] In adults with severe liver disease, elimination of flumazenil is reduced.[2431] In children, the elimination half-life after a single IV dose of 10 μg/kg flumazenil followed by an infusion of 5 μg/kg per minute is 35 minutes.[2432] The rectal dose required is greater (e.g., 50 μg/kg). The pharmacokinetics of intranasal flumazenil (40 μg/kg) were determined in healthy children with a median age of 4 years. The elimination half-life was 2 hours.[2424] Plasma concentrations after nasal flumazenil were similar to those after intravenous administration,[2424] hence the intranasal route has been utilized in emergency room patients.[2433] Oral flumazenil is also available, but its bioavailability is poor, 16%, owing to the first-pass effect in the liver.[2430]

In adults, 17 μg/kg flumazenil effectively antagonized benzodiazepine-induced sedation, whereas in studies in children, 24 μg/kg was required to antagonize the same sedation without evidence of re-sedation.[2432] There is a limited role for flumazenil in clinical pediatric anesthesia, although specific indications are warranted, including benzodiazepine overdose,[2434] wake-up test during scoliosis surgery, treatment of a comatose child, and paradoxical response to benzodiazepines.[2435,2436] *With its brief elimination half-life, re-sedation after the initial response has been reported in children 1 to 5 years of age, thus necessitating close observation for at least 2 hours after antagonism of benzodiazepine-induced sedation.*[2437,2438] Caution should be taken in administering larger doses of flumazenil because seizures have been reported.[2439]

PHYSOSTIGMINE

This tertiary ammonium is a reversible cholinesterase inhibitor used to treat central cholinergic syndrome and delirium, and to antagonize the actions of atropine and scopolamine in the peripheral nervous system and CNS.[2440–2442] It is not generally used to antagonize neuromuscular blockade because its nonionized ammonium group facilitates transfer across the blood-brain barrier, causing CNS effects. After an IV dose, its elimination half-life is 20 to 30 minutes with a duration of action that may exceed 1 hour, depending on the cholinesterase activity. Physostigmine is hydrolyzed at the ester linkage by cholinesterase. The usual single IV dose of physostigmine in children is 10 to 30 μg/kg.[2443] To treat intoxication by long-acting drugs, an infusion of physostigmine may be required at an infusion rate of 30 μg/kg per hour. Side effects of physostigmine include cardiac arrhythmias (bradycardia), cholinergic crisis, and seizures.[2443] Accordingly, physostigmine should be administered with electrocardiographic monitoring.

ANNOTATED REFERENCES

Anderson BJ, Holford NHG. Mechanism-based concepts of size and maturity in pharmacokinetics. *Annu Rev Pharmacol Toxicol.* 2008; 48:303-332.
A review explaining the fundamentals of allometric theory and its application to pharmacology.
Görges M, Zhou G, Brant R, Ansermino JM. Sequential allocation trial design in anesthesia: an introduction to methods, modeling, and clinical applications. *Paediatr Anaesth.* 2017;27(3):240-247.
Sequential allocation trial design is commonly used in anesthesia to determine the MAC of inhalation agents, impact of other drugs, and minimal effective dose. The authors explain the theory behind this methodology and its limitations and offer practical examples.
Hannam JA, Anderson BJ. Pharmacodynamic interaction models in pediatric anesthesia. *Paediatr Anaesth.* 2015;25:970-980.
A review paper explaining interpretation of drug interaction models commonly used in anesthesia.
Kearns GL, Abdel-Rahman SM, Alander SW, et al. Developmental pharmacology—drug disposition, action, and therapy in infants and children. *N Engl J Med.* 2003;349(12):115-167.
This article explains the complex interactions that come into play to shape developmental pharmacology.
Morse JD, Cortinez LI, Anderson BJ. A Universal pharmacokinetic model for dexmedetomidine in children and adults. *J Clin Med.* 2020; 9(11):3480.
Allometric theory, normal fat mass and maturation are used to explore clearance from premature neonates to adults. Such information, when used in conjunction with models describing effects (sedation, pulse, and blood pressure changes), can be used to determine target concentration, loading dose duration, maintenance dose, context sensitive half-time changes with age, and duration of effect. "Universal" models like these can be incorporated into target-controlled pumps for total intravenous anesthesia at any age.
Upton RN, Foster DJ, Abuhelwa AY. An introduction to physiologically-based pharmacokinetic models. *Paediatr Anaesth.* 2016;26(11):1036-1046.
Physiological-based pharmacokinetic models can be used to predict pediatric PK. PBPK models require detailed physiological data. Data on the ontogeny of individual clearance pathways, derived from measurements of enzyme expression and activity in postmortem livers, and from in vivo data from drugs that are cleared by similar pathways are useful. Information concerning genetic, physiological, organ and tissue size and composition, protein binding, demographic, and clinical data has progressively improved their prediction ability.

A complete reference list can be found online at Elsevier eBooks+.

6 Total Intravenous Anesthesia and Target-Controlled Infusion

BRIAN J. ANDERSON AND JAMES HOUGHTON

Pharmacokinetic and Pharmacodynamic Principles
Pediatric Pharmacokinetic Parameter Sets
The Target Concentration
Linking Pharmacokinetics With Pharmacodynamics
Pharmacodynamic Interaction Models
Traditional Methods
Response Surface Models
Depth of Anesthesia Monitoring
Common TIVA Drugs
Achieving the Target Concentration in a Multicompartment Model
Fixed Infusion Rate and a Three-Compartment Model
Bolus And Variable Rate Infusion in a Three-Compartment Model
The Target-Controlled Infusion

A Practical Approach in Children
Drug Delivery
Manual Infusion Regimens
Induction
Establishing TIVA After an Inhalational Induction
Spontaneously Breathing With TIVA
Intubation
Recovery
Ready Mixes
Special Cases
The Obese Child
A Neonate Having Combined Anesthesia and Regional Blockade
The Future

THE MOST COMMON INDICATIONS for total intravenous anesthesia (TIVA) techniques in children are: those at risk for malignant hyperthermia (in whom inhalational agents are contraindicated); children with a high risk of postoperative nausea and vomiting; brief radiologic or painful procedures when rapid recovery is needed (e.g., magnetic resonance imaging, bone marrow aspiration, gastrointestinal endoscopy); frequent repeated anesthesia (e.g., radiation therapy); major surgery to control the stress response; neurosurgical procedures to assist with control of intracranial pressure and for cerebral metabolic protection; spinal instrumentation requiring evoked motor and auditory brain potentials; and children in need of airway procedures (e.g., bronchoscopy).[1–3] Total intravenous (IV) sedation and anesthesia are used in pediatric intensive care, but propofol use is relatively contraindicated for prolonged use in very sick or young children because of concerns regarding propofol infusion syndrome (PRIS, see Chapter 5).[4–13] Guidelines for the safe use of IV drug infusions for general anesthesia have been published.[14]

Pharmacokinetic and Pharmacodynamic Principles

The goal of pharmacologic treatment is a desired response, known as the target effect. An understanding of the concentration-response relationship (i.e., pharmacodynamics [PD]) can be used to predict the target concentration required to achieve this target effect in a typical child.[15] Pharmacokinetic (PK) knowledge (e.g., clearance [CL], volume [V]) then determines the dose that will achieve the target concentration. Calculation of the dose for a drug where the PK disposition can be described using a one-compartment model with first-order elimination can be readily calculated:

$$\text{Loading Dose} = \text{V} \times \text{Target Concentration}$$
$$\text{Maintenance Dose} = \text{CL} \times \text{Target Concentration}$$

However, most drugs used in anesthesia require two or more compartments to describe their disposition and although the principles for drug dosing calculation are the same, calculations are complicated by two or more clearances and volumes (see later in the chapter).

Although the parameters used in PK and PD equations (known as models) for many drugs are published, the individual parameter estimates may vary substantively from child to child. Several covariates have been identified to better predict the dose for a particular child. These include weight, age, sex, pathology, drug interactions, and pharmacogenomics. Current pumps used for TIVA incorporate weight and age to predict the typical drug dose and infusion rate for a specific patient.[16]

The use of TIVA for propofol is a good example of "pharmacology in action." The target effect (e.g., level of general anesthesia) for propofol has been defined (e.g., bispectral index [BIS] 50–55), the target (plasma) concentration to achieve this level of anesthesia is known (e.g., propofol 4 mg/L) and its PK in children is well described. Advanced concepts in PK modeling and computer technology have led to sophisticated delivery systems that facilitate anesthesia given by the IV route. Further advances involving feedback from receptor organs have also been developed for children.[17,18] Target-controlled infusion (TCI) devices or "smart pumps" are an example of a sophisticated delivery system that may be directed at either plasma (Cp) or effect-site (Ce) drug concentration. These computerized pumps are a considerable advance over earlier manual techniques for children[19,20] that targeted only the Cp of the drug. However, they require input of both PK and PD parameters and a lack of robust PK-PD estimates and variability in the parameter estimates have, until recently, limited the current accuracy of TCI in children under 3 years of age.[21]

Commercial TCI systems (Smart Pumps) programmed with pediatric PK–PD parameters are unavailable for anesthesia practice in the USA, although use is possible by employing research software in Institutional Review Board (IRB)–approved research studies.[22]

PEDIATRIC PHARMACOKINETIC PARAMETER SETS

TCI techniques use propofol and remifentanil as the principal drugs for induction and maintenance of anesthesia. Popular pediatric programs used for propofol infusion targeting a plasma concentration are based on data from Marsh[23] and Gepts,[24] Kataria,[20] Short,[25] Rigby-Jones,[26] Schuttler,[27] Murat,[28] Saint-Maurice,[29] Coppens,[30] or Absalom (Paedfusor).[31] These parameter sets are commonly termed "models" and named after the author who reported them (e.g., the Kataria model). Parameter estimates

(e.g., CL; intercompartment clearance [Q]; central volume of distribution [V1]; peripheral volume of distribution [V2]) are different for each parameter set (Table 6.1). Although parameter estimates are different for each author, most predict similar concentrations for the same infusion regimen (Fig. 6.1).

Several covariates that contribute to the variability in the parameters, such as the severity of illness, are often unaccounted for; for example, the volume of the central compartment is increased in children after cardiac surgery.[26] Even weight or age, the most common sources of variability,[32] may be omitted from parameter estimates. Both the administration method (IV bolus or infusion)[33] and the collection of venous blood for assay rather than arterial blood will influence the PK parameter estimates in the early phase when the drug is moving into the effect-site compartment. Time-concentration profiles and context-sensitive half-lives will differ depending on which parameter set is used.[34]

There is a paucity of validation studies for these differing parameter sets.[30] The Paedfusor model[31] is reported to have a median performance error, bias (MDPE) of 4.1% and a median absolute performance error, precision (MDAPE) of 9.7% in children between 1 and 15 years of age.[31] Others concluded that

TABLE 6.1	Propofol Parameter Estimates for a 20-kg Child									
Parameter	Kataria et al.[20]	Marsh[23] & Gepts[24]	Paedfusor[31]	Short et al.[25]	Schuttler & Ihmsen[27]	Rigby-Jones et al.[26]	Murat et al.[28]	Saint-Maurice et al.[29]	Coppens et al.[30]	Morse et al.[42]
V1 (L)	10.4	4.56	9.16	8.64	7.68	11.68	20.6	14.44	3.48	5.28
V2 (L)	20.2	9.28	18.98	10.8	20.74	26.68	19.4	35.6	4.68	11.74
V3 (L)	164	58.04	116.58	69.4	264.82	223.86	121.74	168	19.02	65.71
CL (L/minute)	0.68	0.542	0.568	0.836	0.56	0.444	0.98	0.62	0.78	0.75
Q2 (L/minute)	1.16	0.51	1.044	1.22	1.036	0.32	1.34	1.24	2.04	1.49
Q3 (L/minute)	0.52	0.192	0.384	0.34	0.46	0.268	0.4	0.22	0.66	0.33

Performance of these models differed markedly during the different stages of propofol administration. Most models underestimated propofol concentration 1 minute after the bolus dose, suggesting an overestimation of the initial volume of distribution. Not all models tested were within the accepted limits of performance (median performance error, bias <20% and median absolute performance error, precision <30%). The model derived by Short and colleagues performed best[34] in children aged 3–26 months during infusion durations greater than 1 hour.
SHORTFORMS ARE NOT DEFINED

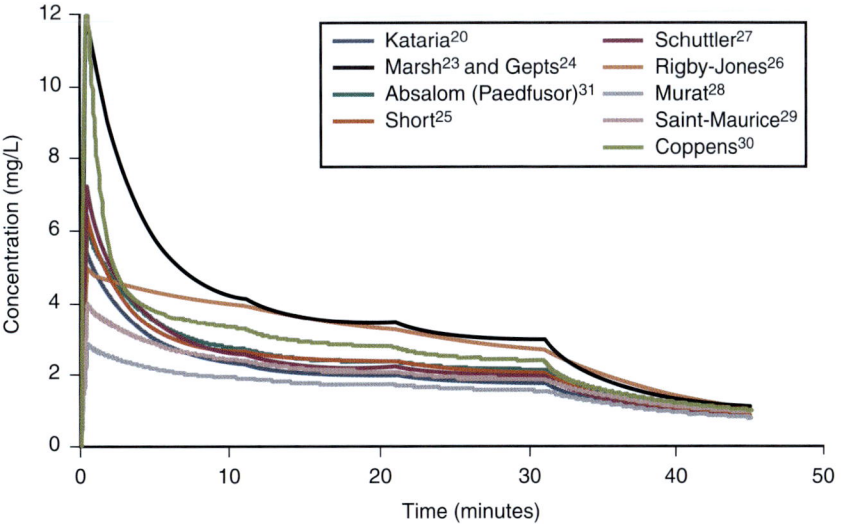

FIGURE 6.1 Simulated time-concentration profiles for propofol using differing parameter sets are shown. A 3-mg/kg bolus was administered, and the infusions were administered as for an adult (10-8-6 regimen, see text). (From Anderson BJ. Pharmacology of pediatric TIVA. *Rev Colomb Anestesiol.* 2013;41:205-214. Used with permission.)

all parameter sets except the Marsh model performed acceptably in children between 3 and 26 months of age,[34] whereas some described a poor fit for the Kataria model, despite it being the most widely used model.[35] However, clearance (expressed as liters per hour per kilogram) decreases with age and MDPE is minimized at low CL and exaggerated at greater CL. The Short model[25] for children, and the Schuttler[36] general-purpose model[36] had acceptable performance in children aged 3 to 11 years when used over a prolonged period, up to 6 hours.[37] Applying models outside the age range in which their parameter sets were determined increases their bias and reduces their ability to predict the correct dose for that child.

Using the Kataria model, reduced clearance (expressed as per kilogram) in older children decreases the effect-site target concentration (Ce) for propofol displayed on the smart pump compared with the concentration measured in plasma. This has led to the suggestion that the propofol Ce differs with age (e.g., Ce_{50} 5 μg/mL in children aged 3 years and Ce_{50} 1.6 μg/mL at 11 years of age).[38,39] Age-related changes also contribute to confusion interpreting BIS values when the Ce is calculated and displayed by the TCI pump because of this link with age for reduced plasma concentrations.[40]

Covariate effects due to size can be accounted for by using allometry (see Chapter 5). Propofol parameter estimates, standardized for size in children 1.3 to 11.9 years, are reported.[41] Those covariate effects attributable to age (27 weeks postmenstrual age to 12 years) and size have been reviewed by determining the maturation of propofol clearance in children ("Morse" model, Fig. 6.2).[42] Plasma propofol concentrations determined using these "Morse" parameter estimates[42] are similar to those determined in an even larger cohort that extends from neonates to adults ("Eleveld" universal model).[43,44] Investigators anticipate that when these PK models are programmed into smart pumps dose precision will improve although approximately 50% of concentrations still lay outside of the target range in a simulation study using these models.[42] Variability that cannot be explained using age and size alone remains considerable.

Adult remifentanil PK parameters ("Minto" model)[45] continue to be used in TCI devices for patients of all ages. There is an element of safety with this approach because both volume of distribution[46] and clearance (expressed as milliliter per minute per kilogram)[47] decrease with increasing age and the elimination half-life is small with a constant context-sensitive half-time (CSHT). The greater volume of distribution in children reduces the peak concentrations of remifentanil after bolus dosing; the increased clearance in children decreases the plasma concentration when infused at adult rates and expressed in milligram per minute per kilogram.

Remifentanil PK can be described in all age groups by simple application of an allometric size model.[47] A standardized clearance of 2970 mL/minute per 70 kilograms is similar to that reported by others in children[46,48] and adults.[45,49] Remifentanil clearance estimation in patients aged 5 days to 85 years (2.5–106 kilograms) that scaled size using allometry was 2580 mL/minute per 70 kilograms.[50] The smaller the child, the greater the clearance when expressed as milliliters per minute per kilogram. Owing to these enhanced clearance rates, smaller (younger) children will require larger infusion rates of remifentanil than larger (older) children and adults to achieve equivalent blood concentrations. As a rule of thumb, children less than 5 years of age or 20 kilograms will require up to twice the dose of remifentanil (μg/kg) to produce the same clinical effect as older children and adults.[51,52]

THE TARGET CONCENTRATION

The target concentration is the concentration desired at the effect site. The plasma and effect-site concentrations are the same at steady state. The target concentration depends on the desired effect. This effect is determined by an understanding of the concentration–response relationship of the drug. This will differ with age, pathology, drug interactions, and stimulus. The target concentration may vary depending on the magnitude of the desired effect. A remifentanil target of 2 to 3 μg/L is adequate for laryngoscopy, 6 to 8 μg/L for laparotomy and 10 to 12 μg/L might be sought to ablate the stress response associated with cardiac surgery.[53]

A propofol concentration of 2 to 3 mg/L is an appropriate target for sedation and 4 to 6 mg/L is adequate for anesthesia. The target effect-site propofol concentrations for both the loss and return of consciousness in children, 2.0 ± 0.9 mg/L and 1.8 ± 0.7 mg/L,

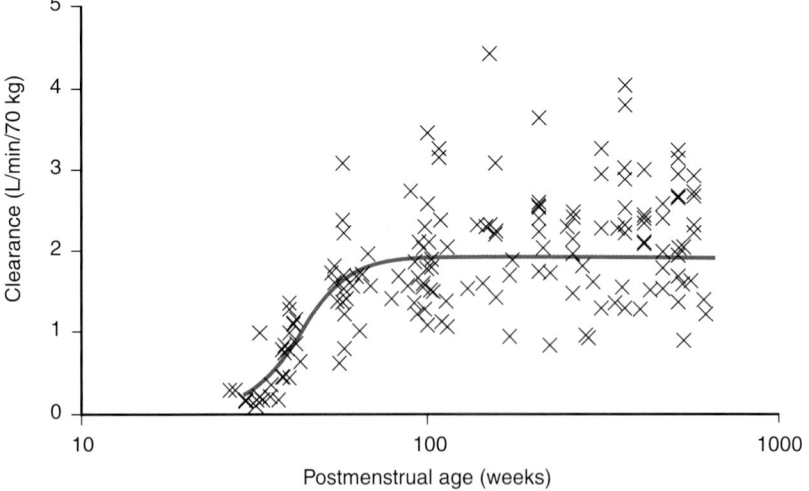

FIGURE 6.2 Maturation of propofol clearance with age in children. The population prediction is shown as a solid line. Individual estimates (×) demonstrate variability evident despite correction for the covariates of age and size. (From Morse J, Hannam JA, Cortinez LI, et al. A manual propofol infusion regimen for neonates and infants. *Pediatr Anesth.* 2019;29:907-914. Used with permission.)

respectively (mean ± standard deviation), are similar to those reported in adults.[54,55] The relationship between drug concentration and effect is commonly described by the Hill equation[56]:

$$Effect = E0 - \frac{Emax \cdot Ce^N}{(EC_{50}^N + Ce^N)} \qquad \text{Eq. 6.1}$$

where $E0$ is the baseline level of consciousness (e.g., BIS = 100), $Emax$ is the maximum response, EC_{50} the concentration at half this maximum response, Ce the concentration in the effect compartment, and N defines the steepness of the slope.

Jeleazcov et al.[57] have described propofol PD in children 1 to 16 years using BIS where $E0$ was estimated as 93.2, $Emax$ 83.4, EC_{50} 5.2 mg/L, and N 1.4. This relationship is very similar to that described in obese children.[58] The equilibration rate constant (keo) between the plasma and effect compartment was 0.6/minute ($T_{1/2}keo$ 1.15 minutes). Children may have a slightly reduced sensitivity to propofol than adults (Fig. 6.3),[35] although this difference may be due to PK rather than PD factors.[59] The Kataria parameter set does not standardize size using allometry and underpredict concentration as age increases. When this parameter set is used to estimate PD parameters, older children appear to require a smaller concentration to maintain anesthesia[60]; this is a PK effect and not a PD effect.[61]

Maintenance infusion requirements for propofol in neonates differ substantively from those in older infants and children. These may be attributed to differences in PK and/or PD. In terms of the kinetics, the clearance of propofol in neonates is reduced compared with older infants; clearance decreases with decreasing postmenstrual age owing to immature enzyme clearance systems (see Fig. 6.2).[62] Propofol infusion rates in infants and children have been estimated using empiric methodology in infants younger than 3 years of age (Table 6.2).[63] The predicted infusion rates for the first 10 minutes in neonates are large (24 mg/kg per hour; 400 μg/kg per minute), values that should be used cautiously because of the danger of an overdose if the infusion continues beyond 10 minutes. Delayed awakening, hypotension, and an increased incidence of bradycardia

TABLE 6.2	Propofol Dose Requirements in Children Younger Than 3 Years of Age				
Time (minutes)	0–3 months	3–6 months	6–9 months	9–12 months	1–3 years
0–10	24.3	19.7	15.3	14.8	12.1
10–20	20.4	15.2	12.3	11.9	9
20–30	15.1	12	9	9	6
30–40	12	9	6	6	6
40–50	9	6	6	6	6
50–60	6	6	6	6	6

Infusion rates are expressed as milligrams per kilogram per hour.
Adapted from Steur RJ, Perez RS, De Lange JJ. Dosage scheme for propofol in children under 3 years of age. *Paediatr Anaesth.* 2004;14:462-467.

have been reported in neonates and infants using this dosing regimen.[63]

Propofol infusion rates in infants and children have also been estimated using a target concentration strategy[15,64] that encompassed information about clearance maturation from 27 weeks postmenstrual age.[42] However, PK-PD relationships in this age group remain elusive[65] and the target concentration used is assumed the same as that estimated in adults. Consequently, the manual infusion regimen shown in Table 6.3 includes target concentrations of 2 μg/mL and 3 μg/mL.

LINKING PHARMACOKINETICS WITH PHARMACODYNAMICS

A simple situation in which drug effect is directly related to concentration does not mean that drug effects parallel the time course of concentration. This occurs only when the concentration is low in relation to EC_{50}. In this situation, the half-life of the drug may correlate closely with the half-life of drug effect.

A plasma concentration-effect plot can form a hysteresis loop because of a delay in effect. Hull et al.[66] and Sheiner et al.[67] introduced the effect compartment concept for muscle relaxants. A

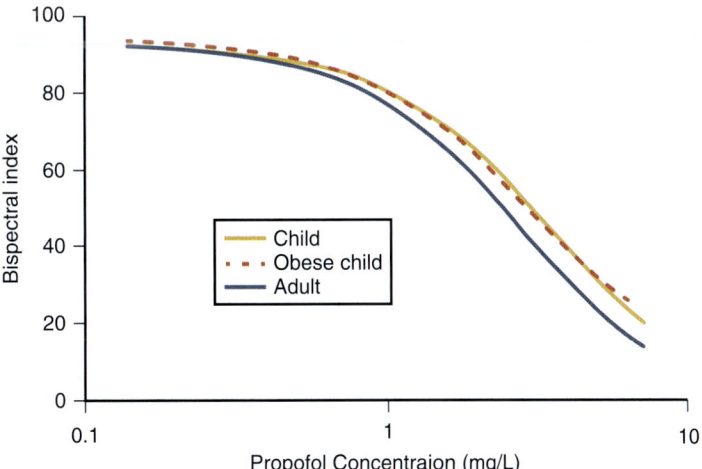

FIGURE 6.3 The propofol concentration and its relationship with bispectral index in children and adults. (Data from Coppens MJ, Eleveld DJ, Proost JH, et al. An evaluation of using population pharmacokinetic models to estimate pharmacodynamic parameters for propofol and bispectral index in children. *Anesthesiology.* 2011;115:83-93; and Chidambaram V, Venkatasubramanian R, Sadhasivam S, et al. Population pharmacokinetic-pharmacodynamic modeling and dosing simulation of propofol maintenance anesthesia in severely obese adolescents. *Pediatr Anesth.* 2015;25:911-923.)

TABLE 6.3	Manual Propofol Infusion Rates Recommended for Propofol in Neonates and Infants Under 3 Years to Target a Propofol Plasma Concentration of Either 2 μg/mL or 3 μg/mL. Infusion Rates are Shown in Milligrams Per Kilogram Per Hour				
Age	Induction dose (mg/kg)	0–15 min	15–30 min	30–60 min	60–120 min
Target Plasma Concentration 2 μg/mL					
27–44 PMA weeks	1.5	6	5	4	3
44–52 PMA weeks	1.5	8	7	6	6
3–12 months	1.5	9	8	7	6
1–3 years	1.5	10	8	8	7
Target Plasma Concentration 3 μg/mL					
27–44 PMA weeks	2	9	7	6	5
44–52 PMA weeks	2.5	11	10	9	8
3–12 months	2.5	12	11	10	9
1–3 years	2.5	13	12	11	10

PMA, Postmenstrual age.
From Morse J, Hannam JA, Cortinez LI, Allegaert K, Anderson BJ. A manual propofol infusion regimen for neonates and infants. *Pediatr Anesth.* 2019;29:907-914.

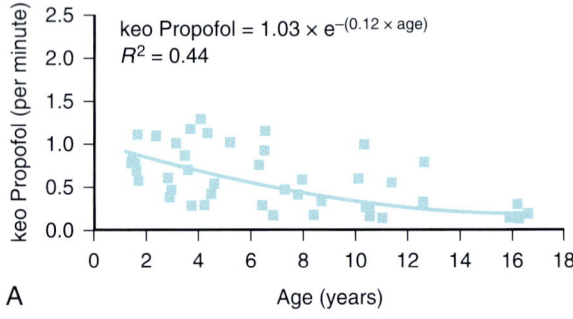

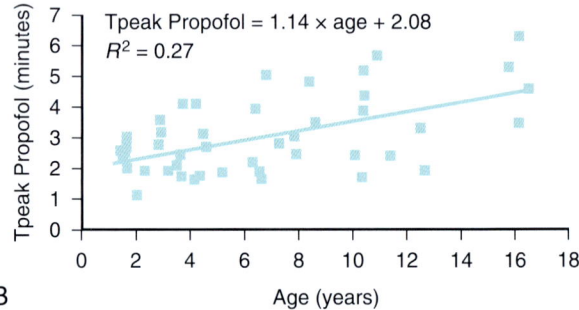

FIGURE 6.4 This figure shows the equilibration rate constant of propofol and time to peak propofol concentration as a function of age. The keo decreases with age; that is, the $T_{1/2}$keo increases with age. This results in a later time to peak concentration (Tpeak) as age (and weight) increases. *keo,* Site equilibration constant; $T_{1/2}$keo, time taken to achieve 50% effect-site concentration. (Data from Jeleazcov C, Ihmsen H, Schmidt J, et al. Pharmacodynamic modelling of the bispectral index response to propofol-based anesthesia during general surgery in children. *Br J Anaesth.* 2008;100:509-516.)

single first-order parameter ($T_{1/2}$keo) describes the equilibration half-time:

$$T_{1/2}keo = \frac{Ln(2)}{keo} \qquad Eq.\ 6.2$$

This mathematical trick assumes the concentration in the central compartment is the same as that in the effect compartment at equilibrium, but that a time delay exists before the drug reaches the effect compartment. The concentration in the effect compartment is used to describe the concentration-effect relationship.[68]

Adult $T_{1/2}$keo values are well described; for example, in the case of morphine it is 16 minutes; for fentanyl it is 5 minutes; alfentanil, 1 minute; and for propofol, it is 3 minutes. This $T_{1/2}$keo parameter is commonly incorporated into TCI pumps to achieve a rapid effect-site concentration.

There are estimates of the $T_{1/2}$keo for propofol in children using simultaneous PK-PD modeling. In healthy children 2 to 12 years of age, the $T_{1/2}$keo for propofol has been estimated at 1.86 min (95% confidence interval [CI] 1.16–2.31),[69] and in obese children at 1.2 minutes (95% CI 0.85–2.1).[58] We might expect a smaller $T_{1/2}$keo with decreasing age based on size models.[70] Faster half-times in children can be accounted for by considering the physiologic time that scales to a power of $1/4$[71]:

$$T_{1/2}keo_{CHILD} = T_{1/2}keo_{ADULT} \times \left(\frac{WT}{70}\right)^{1/4} \qquad Eq.\ 6.3$$

An increasing $T_{1/2}$keo with age (linked to weight) has been described for propofol in children (Fig. 6.4).[57] An allometrically standardized $T_{1/2}$keo (i.e., $T_{1/2}$keo$_{ADULT}$) of 2.38 minutes (95%CI 1.84, 3.16) for propofol is described.[41] If this allometric change is unrecognized, this will result in excessive dose in a young child if

the effect site is targeted and peak effect (Tpeak) is anticipated to be later than it actually is because it was determined in a teenager or adult (Fig. 6.5).

When both PK and PD data are collected simultaneously and parameters for both models are estimated together, then the model is described as "integrated." PK estimates should not be used in conjunction with PD estimates from a different data set without a few "fudge factors." Tpeak methodology (see Chapter 5) is commonly used to estimate $T_{1/2}$keo that then links separate PK and PD data sets. Tpeak will increase with age. Model dependence of the $T_{1/2}$keo was demonstrated by an estimate of 1.7 minutes with the Kataria[20] parameter set and 0.8 minute with the Paedfusor model (Graseby Medical Ltd., Hertfordshire, UK) parameter set.[31]

Pharmacodynamic Interaction Models

Drugs may interact with each other at multiple levels (see Chapter 5). Drug interactions for those drugs used in TIVA are commonly described using PD interaction models.

TRADITIONAL METHODS

Traditional methods of evaluating PD interactions include using isoboles (graphs illustrating equi-effective combinations of drugs), shifts in dose (or concentration) response curves (see Chapter 5), or interaction indexes based on parameters of potency derived from separate monotherapy and combination therapy analyses. Such methods provide an estimation of the magnitude of effect for dose or concentration combinations, but they do not inform us on the time course of that effect or its associated variability.

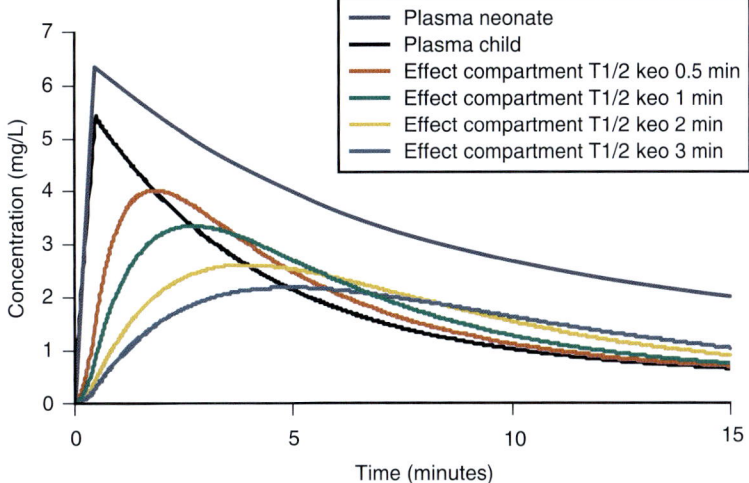

FIGURE 6.5 This figure shows simulated plasma time-concentration profiles for a typical 20-kg child given propofol 3 mg/kg using the Kataria parameter set. The $T_{1/2}$keo used will affect predicted effect-site concentrations—that is, the greater the $T_{1/2}$keo, the longer it takes to achieve the target concentration. $T_{1/2}$keo, Time taken to achieve 50% effect-site concentration.

Competitive antagonists reduce receptor availability by competing for occupancy at the same receptor site. Drugs that elicit an effect are called agonists, whereas those that do not are called antagonists, so the occupancy of some receptors by the antagonists results in less effect. In general, competitive antagonists shift the effect-concentration curve to the right by altering the EC_{50}. Noncompetitive antagonists shift the observed maximum effect (Emax) rather than the EC_{50}.

RESPONSE SURFACE MODELS

Emax models for individual drugs can be combined and extended to incorporate PD interactions between two or more drugs. The "response surface" models are an extension of empirical, single-drug models that can be used to describe and predict the combined effects between two or more drugs (Fig. 6.6). Horizontal lines within the response surface hold equivalent information to that given by isoboles. Surface parameters are estimated using data points pertaining to all areas of the concentration and effect range for both drugs simultaneously (as opposed to considering individual concentration pairs or effect levels in isolation, as is done with isobolographic analyses). Resulting PD models can be used to characterize the type of interaction across the entire range of concentrations and responses and make predictions about response (effect) for any ratio of the studied drugs.[72]

Two equations are commonly used: those of Greco et al.[73] and Minto and Vuyk[74] (see Chapter 5). The Greco equations have been used to describe additive effects for propofol, remifentanil, and fentanyl on BIS response in children aged 1 to 16 years undergoing general surgery.[57] These authors reported EC_{50} estimates of propofol 5.20 μg/mL, remifentanil 24.1 ng/mL, and fentanyl 8.6 ng/mL, and suggested a propofol and remifentanil pair of 2.3 μg/mL and 4.3 ng/mL, respectively, to maintain hemodynamic parameters and sedation scores within ranges suitable for surgery. The Greco model has also been used to describe loss of response to various noxious stimuli under propofol-remifentanil anesthesia[75]; synergistic surfaces for sedation and response to laryngoscopy were reported.

The Minto equations have been used to assess synergy for hypnosis among three commonly combined drugs for anesthesia: propofol, midazolam, and alfentanil.[76] Computer simulations based on interactions at the effect site predicted that a synergistic three-drug combination (midazolam, propofol, and alfentanil) tripled the duration of effect compared with propofol alone. Response surfaces can describe anesthetic interactions, even those among agonists, partial agonists, competitive antagonists, and inverse agonists.[76]

Synergism between propofol and alfentanil has been demonstrated using response-surface methodology. Remifentanil alone had no appreciable effect on response to shaking and shouting or response to laryngoscopy, whereas propofol could ablate both responses. Modest remifentanil plasma concentrations dramatically reduced the concentrations of propofol required to ablate both responses.[77] When comparing the different combinations of midazolam, propofol, and alfentanil, the responses varied markedly at each endpoint assessed and could not be predicted from the responses of the individual agents.[78] Similar response-surface methodology has been used to investigate the combined administration of sevoflurane and alfentanil[79] and remifentanil and propofol[80] on control of ventilation. These combinations have a strikingly synergistic effect on respiration, resulting in severe respiratory depression in adults.

The concurrent administration of opioids during TIVA techniques in children has a noteworthy "propofol-sparing" effect while providing analgesia and stress control.[81,82] It is sensible to take advantage of this synergism to avoid excessive propofol dosing and long-chain triglyceride loads, particularly with concerns about propofol infusion syndrome during prolonged surgeries or sedations. *Remifentanil provides the most effective propofol-sparing effect, but fast recovery means alternative techniques of analgesia must be well established before the remifentanil is discontinued.* Other analgesics and anesthetics are also effective in reducing the propofol dose required. Fentanyl, alfentanil, and sufentanil are effective, as are local and regional analgesia techniques, once the block becomes established. Nitrous oxide and low concentrations of inhalational anesthetics also act synergistically with propofol and opioids to attenuate the dose required.

The Propofol-Remifentanil Interaction

The ability of propofol to ablate responses to noxious stimuli has been studied in children between 3 and 10 years of age undergoing

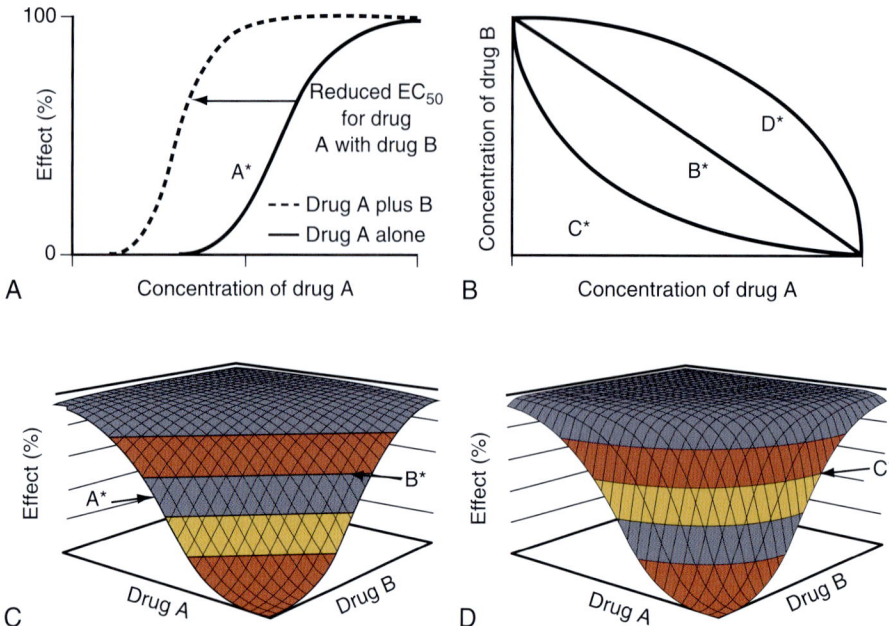

FIGURE 6.6 Methods of investigating interactions. **A,** Shift in response curve analyses involve plotting the concentration- (or dose-) effect relationship for one drug alone (A*) and in the presence of steady-state concentrations of a second drug. **B,** Isoboles are constructed using iso-effect lines with curves derived from observations assessed against the expected (or "additive") response line (B*). Supra-additivity is depicted by curves bowing toward the plot origin (C*), while infra-additivity is shown with outward curves (D*). Information from both methods is represented within response surfaces with isoboles displayed as horizontal planes and individual concentration–response curves as vertical slices (indicated by *arrows* on surfaces for A* single concentration–response curve drug A, B* additive isobole, and C* supra-additive isobole). **C** shows the additive response surface for two drugs. **D** shows the synergistic response surface for two drugs, with synergy depicted through outward bowing of the surface. (Data from Hannam JA, Anderson BJ. Pharmacodynamic interaction models in pediatric anesthesia. *Pediatr Anesth.* 2015;25:970-980.)

esophagogastroduodenoscopy.[81] The EC_{50} for 50% probability of no response was reduced from a propofol concentration of 3.7 μg/mL to 2.8 μg/mL when it was combined with a remifentanil infusion at 0.025 μg/kg per minute. Remifentanil infusions at greater infusion rates did not further reduce the propofol requirements, but they did increase the risk of remifentanil-related adverse respiratory events. There is additivity of anesthetic effect when used with propofol described in adults[83,84] and in children aged 1 to 11 years,[41] although effects such as apnea appear synergistic.[83]

A PD model describing the propofol and remifentanil additive interaction for anesthesia in children 1 to 12 years of age using BIS as an effect measure is similar to that reported in adults. The EC_{50} for remifentanil of 21 ng/mL and an EC_{50} for propofol of 2.99 μg/mL was reported.[41] Remifentanil, delivered at clinically relevant concentration ranges in children, has little effect on BIS. This monitor provides information mainly limited to cortical brain activity that reflects the hypnotic component of anesthesia. Although, during surgery, antinociception may be required to maintain hypnosis, response to painful stimulation cannot be predicted by BIS because the analgesic component of anesthesia involves subcortical autonomic responses.[85]

When used as an adjunct, remifentanil adds a degree of "propofol smoothing" even in those children who require sedation only (e.g., during radiological imaging).[86] The addition of remifentanil to a propofol anesthetic reduces movement in response to surgical stimulation since propofol is not an analgesic[51]; there is approximately 30% more movement with propofol alone compared with an inhalational anesthetic at the same anesthetic

depth. Remifentanil reduces pain during limb procedures where a tourniquet is used, even if a regional block is used. Most procedures can be rendered pain-free by a remifentanil Ce of between 3 and 8 ng/mL; it is unusual to require a concentration in excess of 6 ng/mL.

Depth of Anesthesia Monitoring

A common effect measure used to assess the depth of anesthesia is the electroencephalogram (EEG) or a modification of detected EEG signals (spectral edge frequency, BIS, entropy). Physiologic studies in adults and children indicate that EEG-derived anesthesia depth monitors provide an imprecise and drug-dependent measure of arousal. Although the outputs from these monitors do not closely represent any true physiologic entity, they can be used as guides for anesthesia and in so doing have improved outcomes in adults. In older children the physiology, anatomy, and clinical observations indicate the performance of the monitors may be similar to that in adults. The BIS showed a close relationship with the modeled effect-site propofol concentration and serves as a measure of anesthetic drug effect in children older than 1 year of age.[57]

The anesthetic requirement in children with cognitive impairment may be reduced. Processed EEG use may better dictate dose than clinical assessment. BIS readings in children with cognitive impairment were 28 points less than unaffected peers at the same inhalational anesthetic partial pressure, although the minimum alveolar concentration reduction for cognitive impairment was not accounted for in that study.[87] A lower minimum alveolar concentration was described in cognitively impaired children.[88] Noncommunicative/nonverbal children with cerebral palsy required less propofol to obtain the same BIS values (e.g., 35–45) than otherwise healthy children.[89] The BIS may be a useful monitor in this cohort of children because their anesthetic requirements are reduced.

The use of processed EEG in infants anesthetized with propofol cannot yet be supported in theory or in practice,[90,91] although the Narcotrend shows promise for infants older than 4 months of age given sevoflurane[92] and may prove useful for propofol in that cohort. During anesthesia, the EEG in infants is fundamentally different from that in older children; there remains a need to develop specific neonate-derived algorithms if EEG-derived anesthesia depth monitors are ever to be used in this age group.[93,94] The ability of three methods (Neonatal Pain, Agitation and Sedation Scale; amplitude-integrated electroencephalogram; and Bispectral Index), and their combination, have been used to detect different levels of sedation in neonates. Although none alone was satisfactory to discriminate between degrees of sedation, the combination was useful to distinguish between light and deep sedation.[95] The use of EEG waveforms and processed parameters involving spectral edge frequency (SEF), density spectral array (DSA), and waveform patterns may assist TCI dosing in individual infants.[96]

Depth of anesthesia monitors were used in 1% of all general anesthetics in the United Kingdom in 2015. Routine or frequent use occurred in only 28% of cases in a repeat survey in 2018.[97] The main indications for using BIS were avoiding awareness (47%), avoiding under- or over-dosage (43%), and when TIVA was used with a neuromuscular-blocking drug (33%). Despite limitations in infants, BIS is useful in older children, particularly when neuromuscular-blocking drugs are used in conjunction with TIVA[98]; modified EEG has also been successfully used for closed-loop anesthesia.[17,21] These systems may prove superior to open-loop systems that rely on a calculated effect Ce that are associated with large variability.

Awareness has been more commonly reported after TIVA than after inhalational anesthesia. However, many reports of awareness occur after the switch from inhalational anesthesia to TIVA where a loading dose was not given.[99] The clearance of inhalational anesthetics occurs before attainment of effective steady-state concentrations of propofol. A better understanding of the sevoflurane–propofol interactions,[100] depth of anesthesia monitoring, and point-of-care propofol assay using either breath[101,102] or plasma[103–105] concentrations may be useful to reduce this complication.

Common TIVA Drugs

The commonly used medications for TIVA include propofol, remifentanil, alfentanil, and sufentanil; ketamine is occasionally used but has a long CSHT with consequent delayed awakening.[53] Dexmedetomidine use is increasing as its pharmacokinetic profile is characterized[106] and pharmacodynamics clarified.[107–109]

Drug delivery can be achieved using either a manual infusion scheme (Table 6.4) or PK model–driven infusion devices with software developed specifically for use in children. Unfortunately, current commercially available software packages usually limit the applicable age to 1 to 3 years of age or older or weight to 10 to 15 kilograms or greater, and the PK parameters are derived from studies of a relatively few healthy children. Propofol programs that allow for age-, weight-, and sex-related changes in central compartment volume, clearance, and distribution have been developed and perform well in healthy children.[34,110] However, there are considerable gaps in knowledge for some drugs, for ill children, and for young children, infants, and neonates. Consequently, caution is needed when applying such programs to these populations. The anesthesiologist can use these preprogrammed devices as a basis for initiating a TIVA technique but must also use skill, knowledge, and experience to titrate the IV agents to effect to avoid awareness, pain, and adverse effects.

TABLE 6.4	Manual Infusion Schemes		
Drug	**Loading Dose**	**Maintenance Infusion**	**Notes**
Propofol[196]	1 mg/kg	10 mg/kg per hour for 10 minutes, then 8 mg/kg per hour for 10 minutes, then 6 mg/kg per hour thereafter	Adult regimen to achieve blood concentration of 3 μg/mL
			Underdelivers to children and achieves lower blood concentration of 2 μg/mL
Propofol[82]	1 mg/kg	13 mg/kg per hour for 10 minutes, then 11 mg/kg per hour for 10 minutes, then 9 mg/kg per hour thereafter	Concurrently with alfentanil infusion
Alfentanil[197]	10–50 μg/kg	1–5 μg/kg per minute	Results in blood concentration of 50–200 ng/mL
Remifentanil[117]	0.5 μg/kg per minute for 3 minutes	0.25 μg/kg per minute	Produces blood concentrations of 6–9 ng/mL
Remifentanil[117]	0.5–1.0 μg/kg over 1 minute	0.1–0.5 μg/kg per minute	Produces blood concentrations of 5–10 ng/mL
Sufentanil[117,125]	0.1–0.5 μg/kg	0.005–0.01 μg/kg per minute	Results in blood concentration of 0.2 ng/mL for sedation and analgesia
Sufentanil[117,125]	1–5 μg/kg	0.01–0.05 μg/kg per minute	Results in blood concentrations of 0.6–3.0 ng/mL for anesthesia
Fentanyl[197]	1–10 μg/kg	0.1–0.2 μg/kg per minute	
Ketamine[197]	1–2 mg/kg	0.1–2.5 mg/kg per hour	Smaller dose and infusion rate for analgesia and sedation. Larger dose and infusion rate for anesthesia titrated to effect
Midazolam[197]	0.05–0.1 mg/kg	0.1–0.3 mg/kg per hour	

Achieving the Target Concentration in a Multicompartment Model

For a fixed infusion rate in a single-compartment model, it takes five half-lives to reach a steady-state concentration (>96% of the target) in the blood (Fig. 6.7). A loading dose is required to more rapidly achieve the target concentration. This dose rapidly fills the volume of distribution, after which the calculated infusion maintains the blood concentration (Fig. 6.8). Calculation of the loading dose is relatively easy for a simple one-compartment model. Unfortunately, drugs such as propofol require two- or three-compartment models to describe their disposition. A loading dose may be too large if calculated using the volume of distribution at steady state (Vss, where Vss = V1 + V2 + V3 for a three-compartment model) for a drug that is described by multiple compartments because it is initially administered into the smaller central compartment (V1) to affect the desired response: loss of consciousness. A loading dose based on the Vss will cause adverse effects, hemodynamic instability, and/or toxicity. Even a remifentanil bolus should be administered over several minutes to reduce the risk of bradycardia, hypotension, and/or difficult mask ventilation. An anticholinergic drug may prove useful if remifentanil 3 μg/kg is used for rapid-sequence intubation.

The loading dose and duration over which that loading dose is given depends on both the volume the drug distributes to and adverse effects that are related to effect-site concentration. Rapid administration of dexmedetomidine 0.49 μg/kg in a 5-year-old (20 kg) child can achieve acceptable sedation but it is at a cost of rapid hemodynamic changes associated with pulse reductions and blood pressure increases.[111] When infusion time is over 15 minutes, a larger dose (0.57 μg/kg) is required for the same level of sedation but cardiovascular changes are less variable (Fig. 6.9).[112] The loading dose is used to target a concentration at the effect site, not plasma, and there is a time delay between peak plasma concentration and peak concentration at the effect site. This delay between plasma and effect is the effect-site equilibration half-time ($T_{1/2}$keo) and is 3 to 6 minutes for sedative effect[107,113] and 9.9 minutes for central vasodilation.[114] The time to peak effect (Tpeak) depends on clearance (CL) and the effect-site equilibration half-time. At a submaximal dose, Tpeak is independent of the dose. At supramaximal doses maximal effect will occur earlier than Tpeak and persist for longer because of the shape of the PD sigmoidal concentration-response relationship. The Tpeak concept has been used to calculate optimal initial bolus dose.[115] The volume of distribution (Vpe) at the time of peak effect-site concentration (C_{PEAK}) is calculated and used:

$$Vpe = \frac{Dose}{Concentration(T_{PEAK})} \qquad \text{Eq. 6.4}$$

Loading dose can then be calculated as

$$Loading\ Dose = C_{PEAK} \times Vpe \qquad \text{Eq. 6.5}$$

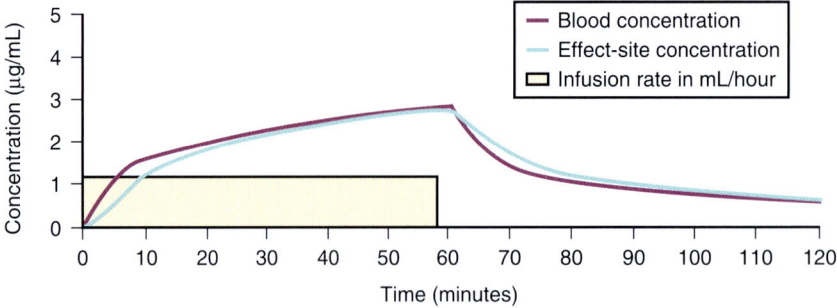

FIGURE 6.7 A fixed-rate infusion of propofol at 10 mg/kg per hour with no bolus dose in a healthy 10-kg, 1-year-old infant. Note that a steady state is not reached even after 1 hour. There is a lag of effect-site concentration behind blood concentration both during infusion and after stopping infusion. Effect-site concentration reaches blood concentration at about 1 hour. The context-sensitive half-time is 9 minutes (simulated using Tivatrainer; available at http://www.eurosiva.eu).

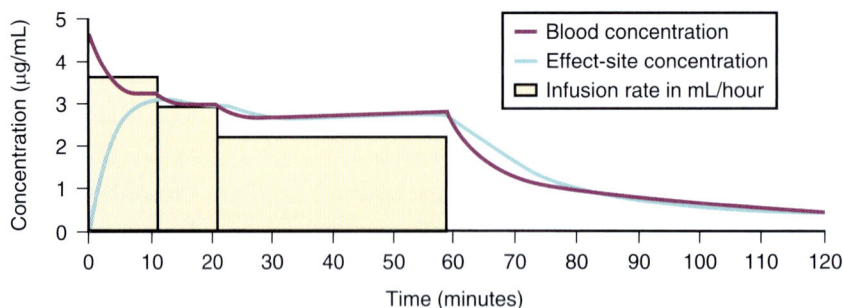

FIGURE 6.8 This figure illustrates the manual infusion technique in a healthy 70-kg 40-year-old. Note the importance of the early higher initial infusion rates to ensure that the target concentration is more constant. (Data from the Diprifusor pharmacokinetic data set.) Bolus dose (propofol 1%) was 1 mg/kg, then 10 mg/kg per hour for 10 minutes, 8 mg/kg per hour for 10 minutes, then 6 mg/kg per hour thereafter until 60 minutes when the infusion is discontinued. The maximum blood concentration is 4.5 μg/mL. Effect-site concentration reaches 3 μg/mL after around 10 minutes but drifts down to around 2.6 μg/mL and then very gradually rises. The context-sensitive half-time after 1-hour infusion is 7 minutes.

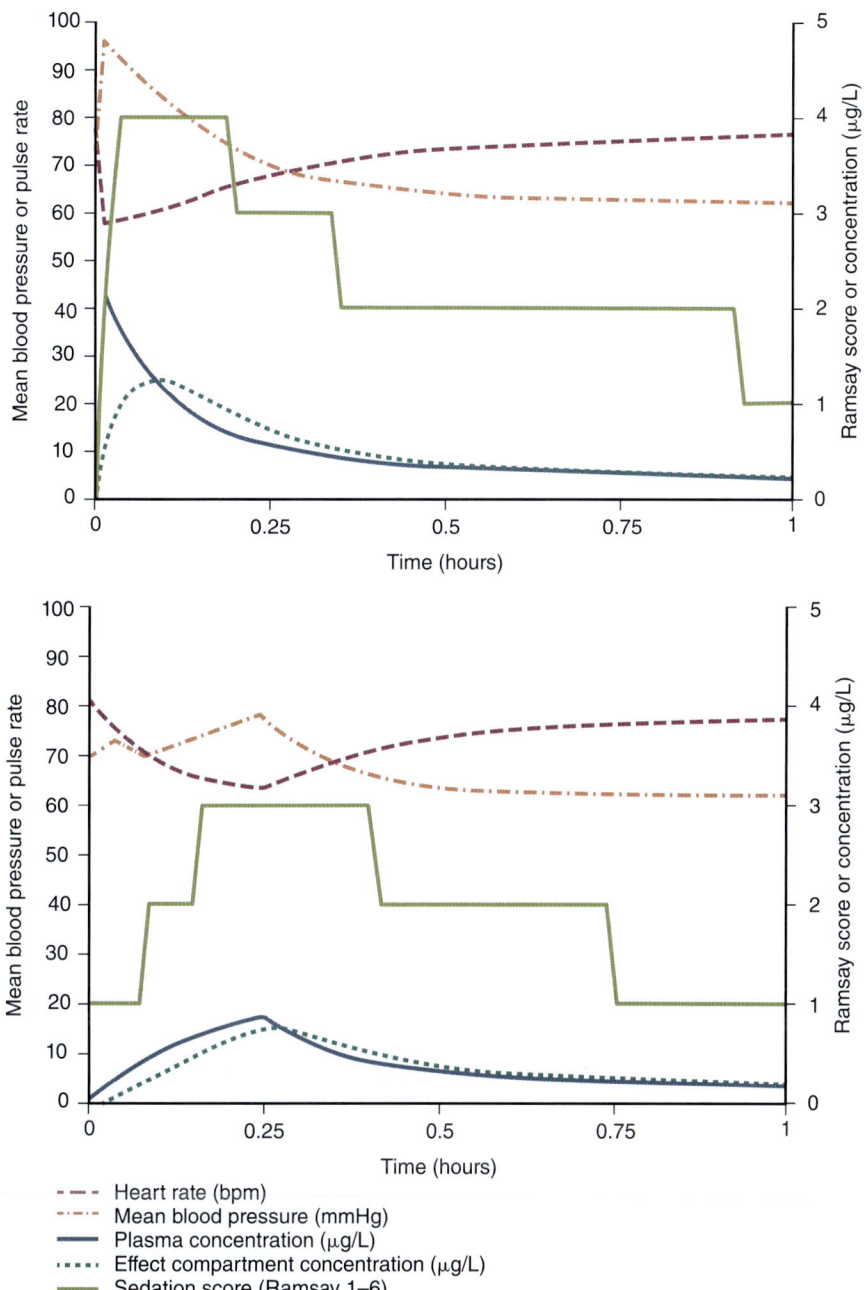

FIGURE 6.9 Simulation of dexmedetomidine hemodynamic effects when given intravenously to a 5-year-old child. Drug in the upper panel was given as a rapid bolus (0.49 µg/kg). The lower panel shows hemodynamic changes after a larger dose (0.57 µg/kg) administered as an infusion over 15 minutes. A similar level of sedation is achieved at 15 minutes, but a slow infusion is without the major changes in blood pressure and heart rate observed with a rapid infusion. (From Morse J, Cortinez LI, Anderson BJ. Pharmacokinetic concepts for dexmedetomidine target-controlled infusion pumps in children. *Pediatr Anesth.* 2021;31 (9):924-931. Used with permission).

To more clearly understand the disposition of drugs after an IV dose, it is useful to consider a three-compartment model (Fig. 6.10, Table 6.5). The drug is delivered and eliminated from a central compartment V1 (which includes the blood) but also distributes to and redistributes from two peripheral compartments, one representing well-perfused organs and tissues (fast compartment, V2) and the other representing more poorly perfused tissues such as fat (slow compartment, V3). The transfer of the drug between V1 and the two peripheral compartments (V2, V3), in addition to eliminating the drug from V1, is described by

a series of clearances (CL, Q2, Q3) indicating the distribution back and forth between paired compartments, such as V1 to V2 and then V2 back to V1. The primary target organ that intravenous anesthetic agents affect is the brain. Therefore, an additional rate constant is added to describe the equilibration between the central compartment and the effect site in the brain (keo = k1e at equilibrium). This compartment is not represented by a volume but rather by the time required to equilibrate. Consequently, there is a time lag before changes in the blood concentration are reflected in the effect site (shown on Figs. 6.7 and 6.8).

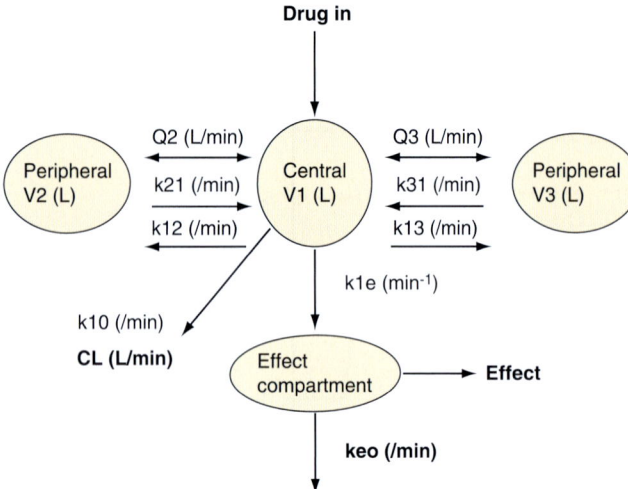

Drug in

FIGURE 6.10 A three-compartment model with an additional compartment used to describe concentration in the effect compartment. A single first-order parameter (k_{1e} = keo at steady state) describes the equilibration rate between the central (V_1) and effect compartment. This compartment model is conceptualized in Fig. 6.11, where hydraulics are used to illustrate compartment interactions. The *arrows* in this figure could be considered "pipes" that deliver drug into the central compartment, out rapidly to V_2 (and back to V_1) and out more slowly to V_3 (and back to V_1) and are then eliminated through simultaneous clearance. k_{1e} is the rate constant describing drug movement from compartment V_1 to the effect compartment. *CL*, Clearance.

TABLE 6.5	Nomenclature for TCI Systems	
Term	**Meaning**	**Units**
TCI	Target-controlled infusion	
Vc or V1	Central compartment volume	L
V2	Fast compartment volume (vessel-rich group) = V1 × k_{12}/k_{21}	L
V3	Slow compartment volume (vessel-poor group) = V3 × k_{13}/k_{31}	L
Cl 1 or CL	Elimination clearance = V1 × k_{10}	L/hour
Cl 2 or Q2	Clearance between V1 and V2 = V2 × k_{21}	L/hour
Cl 3 or Q3	Clearance between V1 and V3 = V3 × k_{31}	L/hour
Cp	Blood concentration	
Ce	Effect-site concentration	
T	Target concentration	
CALC	Concentration calculated by TCI software	
MEAS	Concentration measured	
k_{10}	Elimination rate constant	/minute
keo	Rate constant for equilibration between blood and effect-site	/minute
$T_{1/2}$keo	Half-time for equilibration between blood and effect site $$T_{1/2}keo = \frac{L_N(2)}{keo}$$	minutes
k_{12}, k_{21}	Rate constants for movement between V1 and V2	/minute
k_{13}, k_{31}	Rate constants for movement between V1 and V3	/minute

A hydraulic model is useful for understanding these concepts. The central compartment is connected to the peripheral compartments and effect site by a series of pipes of different diameters and a drainage pipe to represent elimination (Fig. 6.11A–F). The height of the columns of fluid, which represents the concentration of drug, illustrates the gradient down which the drug travels between the central and peripheral compartments; this can be animated over time to show filling and emptying of compartments relative to each other. The diameter of the interconnecting pipes between the central and peripheral compartments represents the intercompartment clearances (Q2, Q3), and the size of the drainage channel represents elimination (CL). This hydraulic analogy is used in the TIVA Trainer simulation program.[116]

FIXED INFUSION RATE AND A THREE-COMPARTMENT MODEL

When a fixed infusion rate is started (see Fig. 6.7), the blood concentration will increase but, almost simultaneously, distribution of the drug to the fast compartment and elimination both begin. Distribution of drugs throughout the body contributes more to the removal of drug from blood than to its elimination for most medications. Remifentanil is an exception; it has rapid esterase clearance and elimination of this drug is far greater than redistribution from the central compartment. As the concentrations within each compartment equilibrate, the concentration gradient between compartments lessens (slowing drug transfer between compartments) but distribution to the slow compartment continues along with elimination. The net effect is that the blood concentration continues to increase, albeit at a slower rate. As the blood concentration increases toward equilibrium, elimination becomes relatively more important; Fig. 6.7 illustrates how far behind the effect-site concentration lags. Eventually, after several hours (or in some cases, days), a steady state is reached where the infusion rate is directly proportional to clearance.

BOLUS AND VARIABLE RATE INFUSION IN A THREE-COMPARTMENT MODEL

The infusion begins with a loading dose that starts to fill the central compartment to achieve a specific target concentration in the effect-site without overshoot. The infusion rate is then decreased in a stepwise manner to maintain a constant effect-site concentration until a steady state is reached. As drug is delivered into the central compartment, it continuously distributes to the peripheral compartments while it is also continuously eliminated. The infusion rate has to vary to compensate for the concurrent changes in the contribution of distribution and elimination with time (Figs. 6.12 and 6.13). When the infusion is stopped, elimination will continue to remove the drug from the central compartment, although the drug will continue to distribute to V2 and V3 along concentration gradients from V1 for some time. Once equilibrium is reached, the drug begins to move back from the peripheral compartments into the central compartment, to maintain the drug concentration in the central compartment. This can continue for a protracted period, particularly for highly lipid-soluble drugs that have a very large compartment V3 contributing a reservoir or depot effect (e.g., fentanyl; see Fig. 6.11F). Eventually the central compartment concentration will decrease. For most anesthetics, the longer a drug is infused, the more the drug distributes into the peripheral compartments and the larger the reservoir of drug that must be redistributed back into the central compartment and eliminated once the infusion ceases. The half-time of the decrease in drug concentration in blood is related to

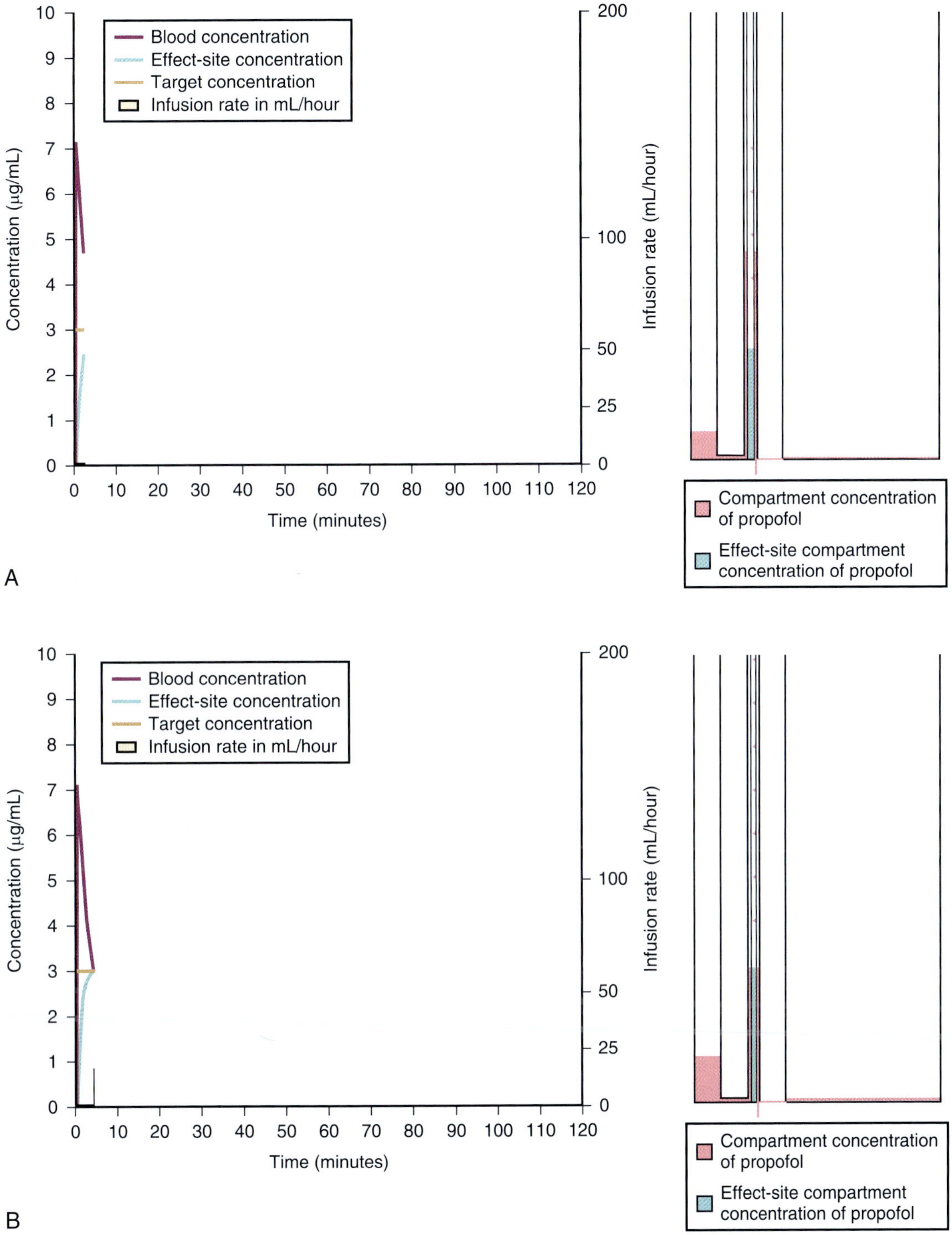

A

B

FIGURE 6.11 A, Hydraulic model representation of effect-site TCI. Compartment volumes and intercompartmental clearance values for the Paedfusor model in a healthy 10-kg, 1-year-old infant. In the first few minutes the central compartment to effect-site concentration gradient is marked to "overpressure" the transfer of propofol to the effect site. The peak blood concentration is 7.1 μg/mL. Distribution from the central compartment (C1) to the first peripheral compartment (C2) occurs rapidly also, which slows the rise in effect-site concentration and blood concentration. Elimination from C1 and distribution from C1 to the second peripheral compartment (C3) is also occurring. **B,** At 4.5 minutes, the effect-site concentration has reached the target of 3 μg/mL and has equilibrated with the concentration in C1. The infusion device, which has been off after the initial loading infusion, now switches back on to maintain the effect-site target concentration at 3 μg/mL.

Continued

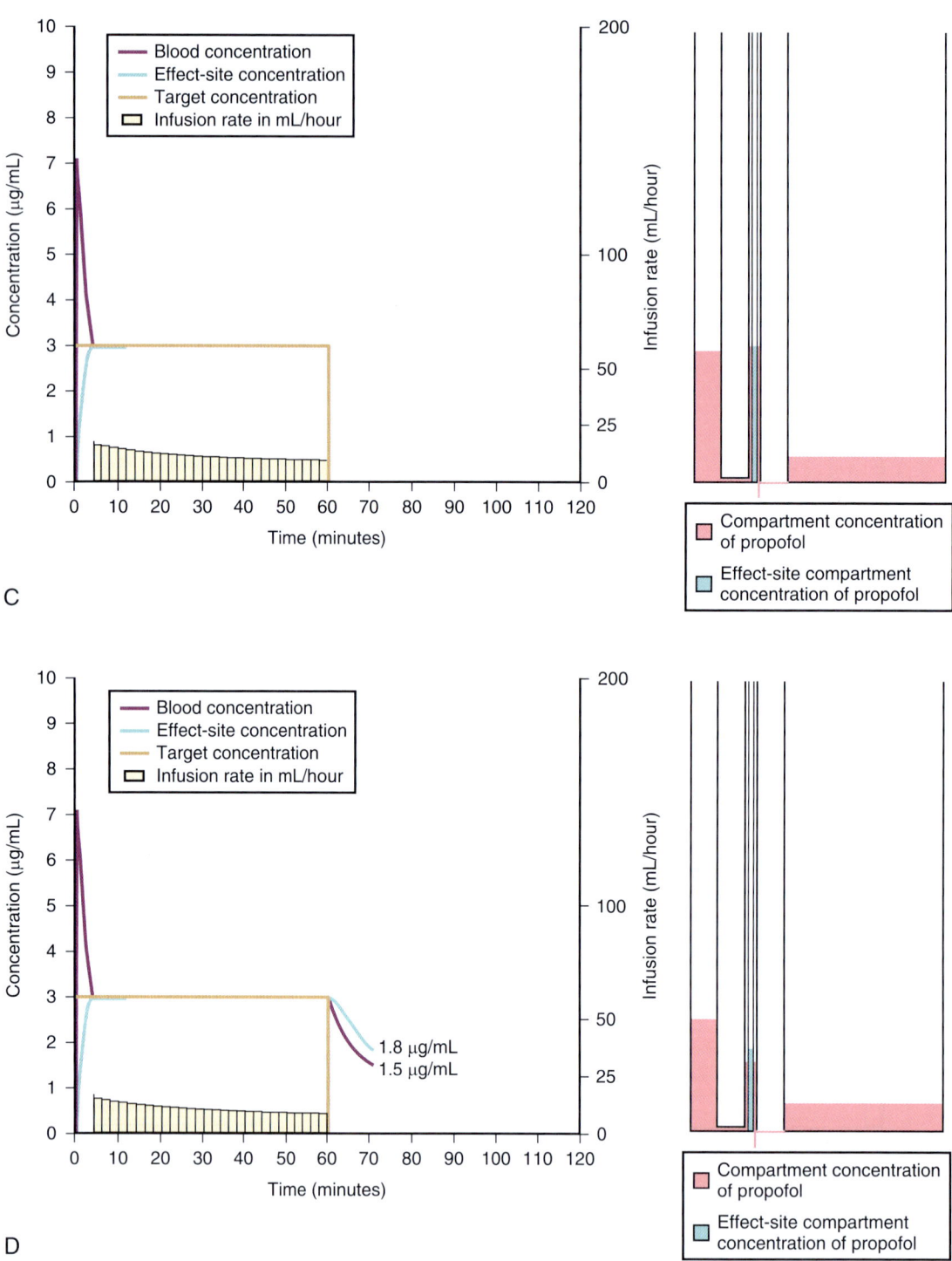

C

D

FIGURE 6.11, cont'd C, After 1 hour of maintenance at an effect-site concentration of 3 μg/mL, the target is set to 0 μg/mL and the pump switches off. A total of 14 mL of propofol (1%) has been administered, or 14 mg/kg. There is now a considerable accumulation of propofol in C_2 and C_3, whereas C_1 and the effect site are still in equilibrium. **D,** Approximately 10 minutes after the effect-site target concentration is set to zero, the blood concentration has halved; thus, the context-sensitive half-time is 10 minutes. The lag in the decline in effect-site concentration is clearly seen, and there is now a gradient between effect site and C_1. There is now also a concentration gradient from C_2 to C_1 and to C_3 and this slows the decline in the concentration in C_1.

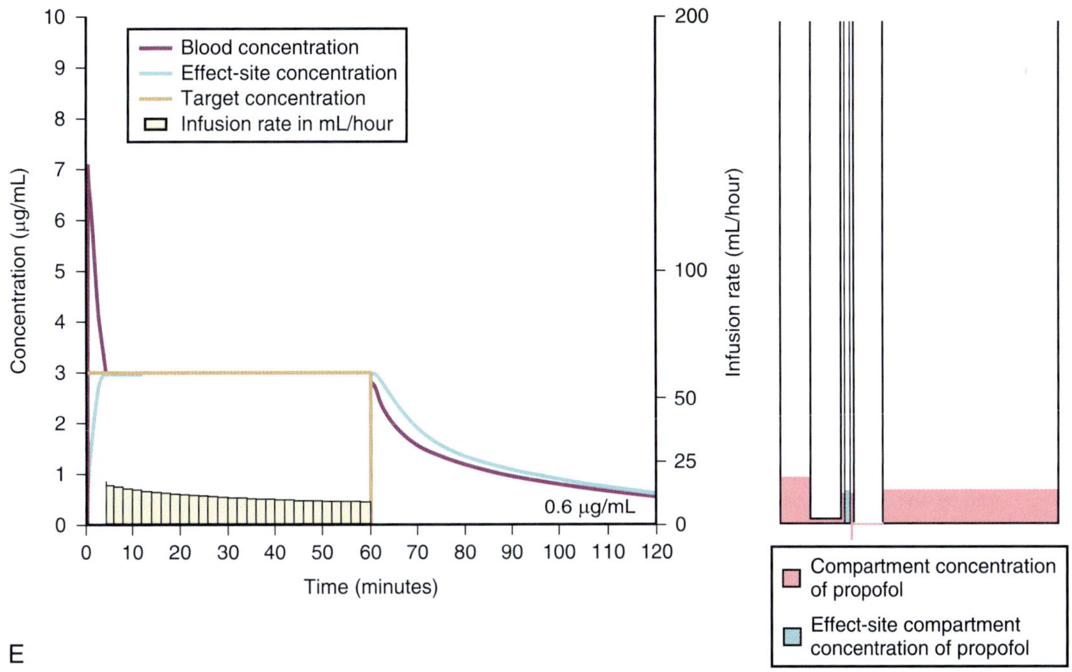

E

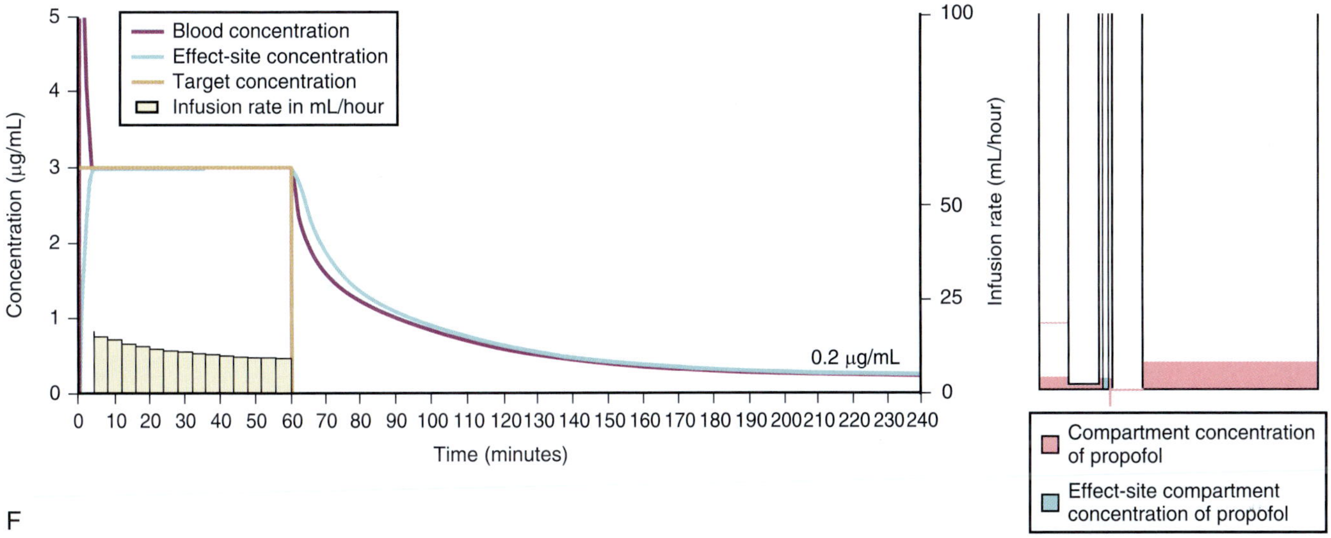

F

FIGURE 6.11, cont'd E, One hour after the infusion is stopped, the blood and effect-site concentrations have fallen to 1/5 of the maintenance effect-site concentration. There are still large quantities of propofol in compartments C2 and C3 that slow the decline of the concentration of C1 and effect-site concentrations. **F,** Even after 4 hours, the depot of propofol in C2 and C3 is considerable, although blood and effect-site concentrations are extremely low. However, these low concentrations may still be exerting significant antiemetic and anxiolytic effects (data from the Paedfusor pharmacokinetic data set).

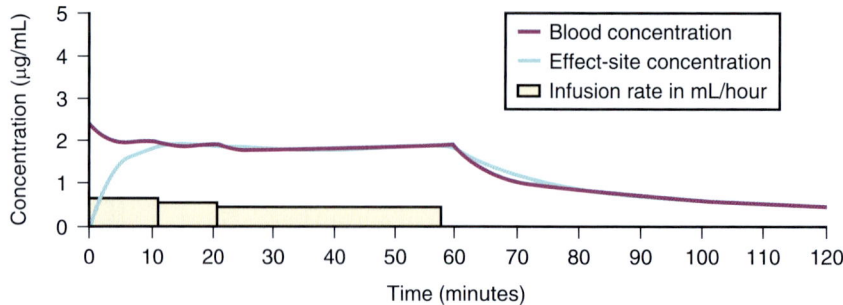

FIGURE 6.12 This figure illustrates the manual infusion technique of propofol in a healthy 1-year-old, 10-kg child. Note the importance of the early higher initial infusion rates to ensure that the target concentration is more constant. The adult dose regimen is illustrated. The figure shows a bolus dose of 1 mg/kg, then 10 mg/kg per hour for 10 minutes, then 8 mg/kg per hour for 10 minutes, then 6 mg/kg per hour thereafter. The infusion was stopped at 60 minutes. The effect-site concentration dose does not equilibrate until 11 minutes. The blood and effect-site concentrations stabilize around 1.8 μg/mL. However, this is unlikely to represent a sufficient depth of anesthesia for surgery. The context-sensitive half-time after 1 hour infusion is 9 minutes (data from the Paedfusor pharmacokinetic data set).

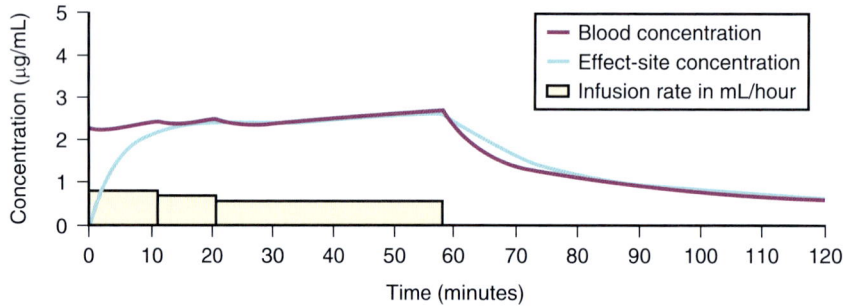

FIGURE 6.13 Manual infusion of propofol in 1-year-old, 10-kg child. The figure shows a bolus dose of 1 mg/kg, then 13 mg/kg per hour for 10 minutes, then 11 mg/kg per hour for 10 minutes, then 9 mg/kg per hour thereafter. The infusion was stopped at 60 minutes. The effect-site concentration does not equilibrate until 20 minutes. The blood and effect-site concentrations stabilize around 2.4 μg/mL but gradually rise over the next hour to 2.6 μg/mL. This concentration is larger than that achieved using the adult 10-8-6 regimen but may still be inadequate. Larger infusion doses are required in a 1-year-old child. (Data from the Paedfusor pharmacokinetic data set.)

the duration of the infusion for most drugs (except remifentanil). This is termed the *context-sensitive half-time, or CSHT,* where the context is the duration of the infusion and relates to a pseudo-steady state maintained by a TCI. For an individual drug in an individual patient, CSHTs can be plotted against the duration of the infusion (Fig. 6.14A,B). The CSHT will eventually asymptote and this is when the pseudo-steady state becomes a true steady state. At that time, the infusion has become context *in*sensitive. This pattern is observed for nearly all IV anesthetics. In the case of propofol, the slope of the CSHT with time increases from adults to children to infants to full-term and then preterm neonates, with preterm neonates having the greatest half-life of all age groups. The exception is remifentanil for which the half-time becomes context insensitive almost immediately after initiation of the infusion because its elimination is rapid and complete; the capacity of the red cell, plasma, and tissue esterase enzyme systems are enormous.

PK parameters for remifentanil, alfentanil, and sufentanil are summarized in Table 6.6.[117] The differences in CSHTs are illustrated in Table 6.7 and Fig. 6.14A,B. Fentanyl has a small CSHT when given by infusion for a short time, but this dramatically increases as the duration of the infusion increases. Alfentanil's CSHT reaches a plateau after approximately 90 minutes.

CSHT is smaller in children, mainly because CL is greater. However, fat mass also has an effect on CSHT if a drug has lipophilicity that affects its distribution volume. The CSHTs for oxycodone (Fig. 6.15) are smaller in neonates (immature CL) and obese children, but greater in infants (greater CL).[118]

THE TARGET-CONTROLLED INFUSION

A TCI is accomplished by a computer that performs rapid sequential calculations every 8 to 10 seconds to estimate the infusion rate required to produce a user-defined drug concentration in the blood or at the effect site of action of the drug in the brain in an open-loop system.[117] *Thus TCI may be blood targeted or effect-site targeted.* The standard nomenclature for TCI systems is listed in Table 6.5. Modern TCI systems are computer-controlled syringe drivers capable of infusion rates up to 1200 mL/hour with a precision of 0.1 mL/hour. They incorporate a user interface and display a range of safety alarms, monitoring functions, and warning systems. For most programs, the user has to choose a drug and its concentration from a menu and also select a PK parameter set (referred to as a model).

Experience with the different models may be gained by running the simulation programs such as Tivatrainer (http://eurosiva.eu/; European Society for Intravenous Anaesthesia [EuroSIVA];

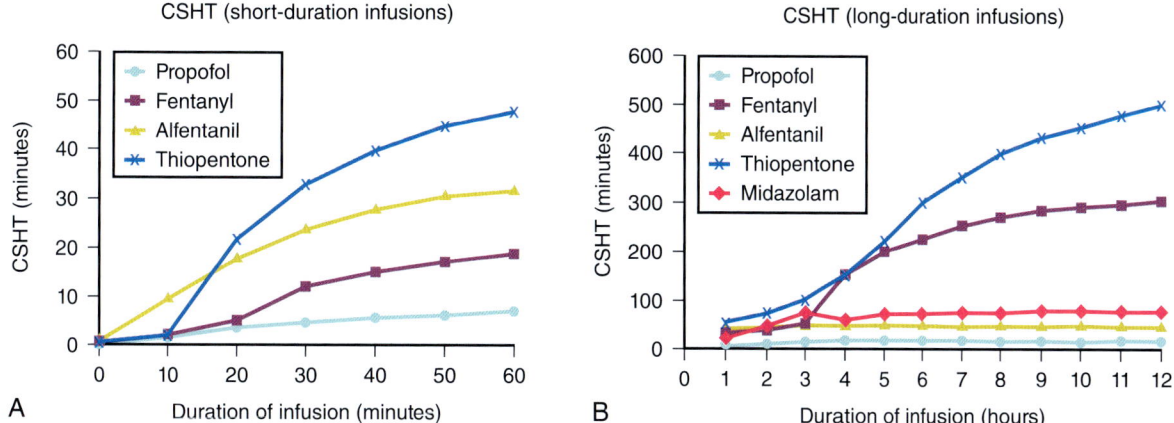

FIGURE 6.14 A, Context-sensitive half-times *(CSHTs)* after short-duration infusions. **B,** CSHTs after longer-duration infusions. For very lipid-soluble drugs such as fentanyl and propofol, V3 is very large compared with V1. Intercompartmental clearance between V1 and V3 is given by the equation V1 χ k_{13} = V3 χ k_{31}, which implies that if V1 is much smaller than V3, rapid distribution from V1 to V3 is associated with very slow redistribution from V3 to V1. This is indeed seen with propofol and fentanyl, which have a slow offset of effects after prolonged infusions. Propofol has a CSHT that varies between approximately 3 minutes for a short-duration infusion to approximately 18 minutes after a 12-hour infusion. This is because elimination is quite rapid compared with the rate of redistribution from V3. For alfentanil, the concentration of the unionized form is 100 times greater than that of fentanyl (pKa alfentanil 6.4, fentanyl 8.5). Alfentanil therefore has a more rapid onset time and shorter half-life *keo*, a smaller V1, lower volume of distribution at steady state, and lower clearance than fentanyl. Fentanyl does, however, have a shorter CSHT than alfentanil after a short-duration infusion lasting less than 2 hours **(A)**; but for longer-duration infusions, alfentanil reaches a maximum CSHT after about 90 minutes, whereas for fentanyl the CSHT continues to increase after 12 hours **(B)**. This is because fentanyl has a huge V3, and redistribution back to V1 maintains the blood concentration when the infusion stops. *keo,* Site equilibration constant. (Simulated using Tivatrainer; available at www.eurosiva.eu/.)

TABLE 6.6	Pharmacokinetic Parameters for Short-Acting Opioids		
	Remifentanil[45,198]	**Alfentanil**[199]	**Sufentanil**[200]
V1	5.1–0.0201 × (age − 40) + 0.072 × (LBM − 55)	Male: 0.111 × weight Female: 1.15 × 0.111 × weight	0.164 × weight
V2	9.82–0.0811 × (age − 40) + 0.108 × (LBM − 55)	12.0	0.359 × weight
V3	5.42	10.5	1.263 × weight
k_{10}	2.6–0.0162 × (age − 40) + 0.0191 × (LBM − 55)/V1	0.356/V1	0.089
k_{12}	2.05–0.0301 × (age − 40)/V1	0.104	0.35
k_{21}	2.05–0.0301 × (age − 40)/V2	0.067	0.16
k_{13}	0.076–0.00113 × (age − 40)/V1	0.017	0.077
k_{31}	0.076–0.00113 × (age − 40)/5.42	0.0126	0.01
keo	0.595–0.007 × (age − 40)	0.77	0.12

Age in years; weight in kilograms.

k_{10}, Elimination rate constant; k_{12} and k_{21}, rate constants for movement between V1 and V2; k_{13} and k_{31}, rate constants for movement between V1 and V3; *keo*, effect-site equilibration rate constant; *LBM*, lean body mass; *V1*, central compartment volume; *V2*, fast compartment volume; *V3*, slow compartment volume (in liters).
From Absalom AR, Struys MMRF. *An Overview of TCI and TIVA*. Ghent, Belgium: Academia Press; 2005.

TABLE 6.7	Context-Sensitive Half-Times (minutes) of Opioids in Children				
	INFUSION DURATION (MINUTES)				
Opioid	**10**	**100**	**200**	**300**	**600**
Remifentanil	3–6	3–6	3–6	3–6	3–6
Alfentanil	10	45	55	58	60
Sufentanil		20	25	35	60
Fentanyl	12	30	100	200	

Amsterdam, The Netherlands) or Rugloop (http://www.demed.be/rugloop.htm; Demed, Temse, Belgium) on a personal computer. Tivatrainer now allows uploading of new models via a central website and server and contains details and simulations of pediatric models for propofol and neonatal and pediatric models for sufentanil, in addition to a wide range of adult models for propofol, alfentanil, remifentanil, fentanyl, ketamine, and midazolam. The simulation shows animated graphs of blood and effect-site concentrations against time, infusion rates, volumes, compartment sizes, and many other features.

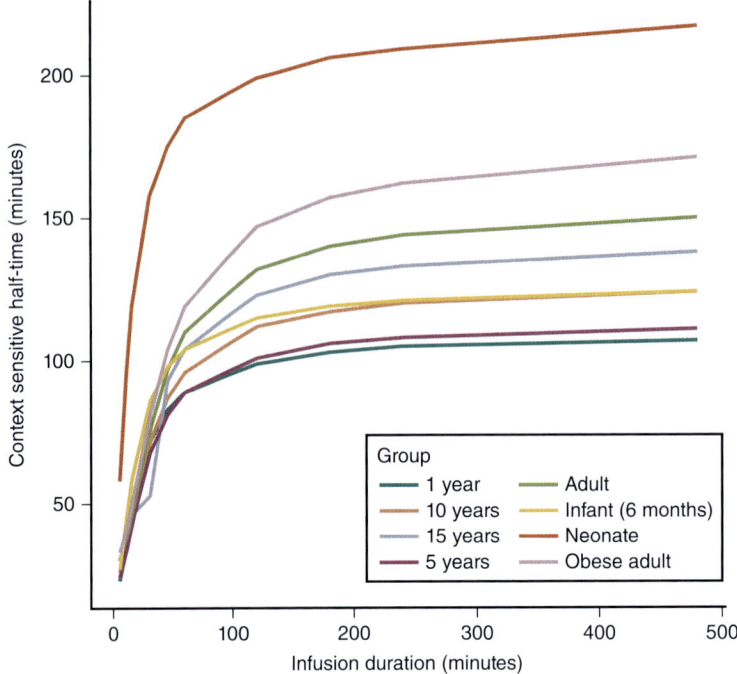

FIGURE 6.15 Context-sensitive half-time (CSHT) changes with age. These age-related changes mirror those observed for clearance changes. Obese adults and neonates have greater CSHT values. `(From Morse JD, Hannam JA, Anderson BJ, Kokki H, Kokki M. Oxycodone target concentration dosing for acute pain in children. *Pediatr Anesth.* 2021;31(12):1325-1331, with permission.)

The models within TCI systems serve only as a guide to drug administration for an individual patient.[34] Parameter estimates determined in healthy children may not be applicable to children with pathology (e.g., intensive care patients or children with neuromuscular disease undergoing scoliosis surgery).[105] The accuracy of TCI propofol has been assessed in children[23,34] for the Paedfusor,[119] (Table 6.8)[23,120,121]; the model performed well in children, even those undergoing cardiac surgery.[31,119,122] Parameter estimates for the Kataria model (Table 6.8) also performed reasonably well,[20,34] but all models have shortcomings.[123] Experience shows that clinicians need to learn how to use each model to optimize levels of anesthesia, ensure stability during induction and maintenance phases, and enhance recovery speed and quality. Most pediatric models overestimate the initial volume of distribution, which risks too large an initial bolus dose.[34] The Paedfusor model makes an allowance for the increased clearance with age (per kilogram) in younger children; particularly those below 30 kilograms in weight (see Tables 6.8 and 6.9, Fig. 6.16). The minimum age and weight limits for each model also differ with age: 1 year and 5 kilograms for the Paedfusor system and 3 years and 15 kilograms for the Kataria system. Below a weight of 12.5 kilograms and age 2 years, the second compartment becomes negative with the Kataria model, which means that model cannot be used clinically in such young patients. For simulation using the Paedfusor data set, the adult value for keo of 0.26/minute (T$_{1/2}$keo 2.7 minutes) can be used (see Table 6.9). This means effect-site targeting may be simulated with the Paedfusor model (Table 6.10), and it may be possible to display an effect-site predicted concentration while using a pump in blood-targeted TCI mode, as with Diprifusor. Attempts have been made to define a more accurate keo for children in an ingenious study using auditory evoked responses with both the Paedfusor and Kataria models.[124] For children aged 3–11 years, the median extrapolated keo values for the Paedfusor models was 0.91/minute (T$_{1/2}$keo 0.8 minutes) and for the

TABLE 6.8 | **Paedfusor Propofol Pharmacokinetic Parameters**

1–12 years	V1 = 0.4584 × weight; V2 = V1 × k_{12}/k_{21}; V3 = V1 × k_{13}/k_{31}
	k_{10} = 0.1527 × weight$^{-0.3}$
	k_{12} = 0.114; k_{21} = 0.055
	k_{13} = 0.0419; k_{31} = 0.0033
	keo = 0.26
13 years	V1 = 0.400 × weight
	k_{10} = 0.0678
	(other constants as above)
14 years	V1 = 0.342 × weight
	k_{10} = 0.0792
	(other constants as above)
15 years	V1 = 0.284 × weight
	k_{10} = 0.0954
	(other constants as above)
16 years	V1 = 0.22857 × weight
	k_{10} = 0.119
	(other constants as above)

Weight in kilograms k_{10}, Elimination rate constant; k_{12} and k_{21}, rate constants for movement between V1 and V2; k_{13} and k_{31}, rate constants for movement between V1 and V3; *keo*, effect-site equilibration rate constant; *V1*, central compartment volume; *V2*, fast compartment volume; *V3*, slow compartment volume.

Note: The k_{10} value in the age group 1–12 years is a negative power function of weight that reflects the increasing clearance values in younger children.

Data from Marsh B, White M, Morton N, Kenny GN. Pharmacokinetic model driven infusion of propofol in children. *Brit J Anaesth.* 1991;67:41-48; Rigby-Jones AE, Nolan JA, Priston MJ, et al. Pharmacokinetics of propofol infusions in critically ill neonates, infants, and children in an intensive care unit. *Anesthesiology.* 2002;97:1393-1400; Murat I, Billard V, Vernois J, et al. Pharmacokinetics of propofol after a single dose in children aged 1–3 years with minor burns. Comparison of three data analysis approaches. *Anesthesiology* 1996;84:526-532.

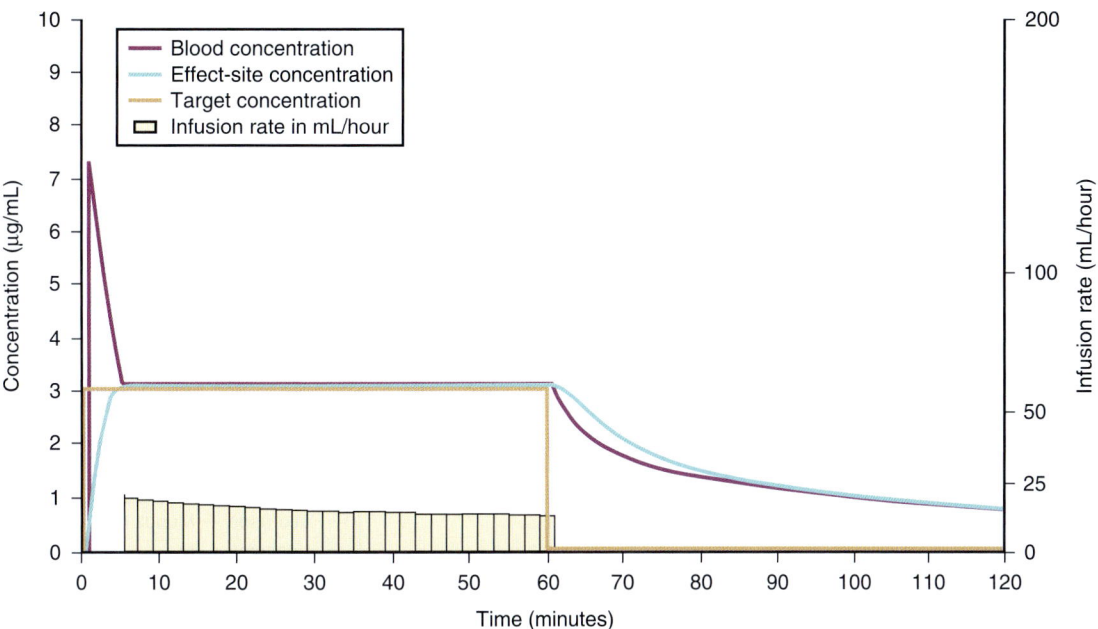

FIGURE 6.16 Target-controlled infusion modeled using the Paedfusor pharmacokinetic data set. Effect-site–targeted infusion of propofol in a healthy 1-year-old, 10-kg child. The effect-site target is 3 μg/mL. The figure shows a bolus dose of 3.4 mg/kg delivered at 45.5 mL/hour to accentuate the gradient from blood to effect site, then the infusion switches off for 4 minutes. Peak blood concentration after bolus dose is 7.1 μg/mL. Stepwise-reducing the infusion from 15.7 mg/kg per hour to 9.5 mg/kg per hour for 1 hour was done. The infusion was stopped at 60 minutes (i.e., effect-site target is set for zero μg/mL). The effect-site concentration reaches 3 μg/mL at 3 minutes 39 seconds. The total dose of propofol is 14 mg/kg. The context-sensitive half-time is 10 minutes 37 seconds.

TABLE 6.9	Comparison Between Paedfusor and Kataria Models for Propofol in Children	
	Paedfusor[23,31,119,122]	**Kataria[20]**
V1	0.458 × weight	0.41 × weight
V2	0.95 × weight	0.78 × weight + 3.1 × age
V3	5.82 × weight	6.9 × weight
k_{10}	0.1527 × weight^{-03}	0.085
k_{12}	0.114	0.188
k_{21}	0.055	0.102
k_{13}	0.0419	0.063
k_{31}	0.0033	0.0038
keo	0.26[a]	N/A[a]

Age in years; weight in kilograms.
[a]This is the value for adults, but Munoz et al.[124] have studied these two models to define a more accurate keo for children aged 3–11 years, and the values are 0.91 for the Paedfusor model and 0.41 for the Kataria model. Jeleazcov et al.[57] have derived age-related keo values by the formula $keo = 1.03 * e^{-0.12 \times age}$.

TABLE 6.10	Example of Target-Controlled Infusion (Propofol Target 5 μg/mL) Based on Calculated Blood-Concentration Targeting Compared with Calculated Effect-Site Concentration Targeting for a Healthy 1-Year-Old (10 kg), Using the Paedfusor Pharmacokinetic Data Set	
	Blood-Concentration Targeting	**Effect-Site Concentration Targeting**
Loading dose	1.7 mg/kg	5.7 mg/kg[a]
Maximum blood target reached	5 μg/kg	12 μg/kg[a]
Total propofol infused after 60 minutes	23.2 mg/kg	23.3 mg/kg
Time to achieve effect-site target of 5 μg/mL	17.5 minutes	4.5 minutes[b]

[a]Potential for hemodynamic changes due to high peak blood concentration from larger bolus dose.
[b]Very much shorter time to achieve effect-site target.

Kataria model 0.41/minute ($T_{1/2}$keo 1.7 minutes). The BIS was used to derive a value for the time to peak effect, and hence, keo.[27,57,125] It was concluded that the time to peak effect after a bolus dose in children was less than in adults as the extrapolated $T_{1/2}$keo values were considerably smaller (see Eq. 6.3).[123] Similar findings were reported by Hahn et al. using state entropy monitoring.[126] This approach has enabled calculation of an age-specific range of values for the keo (see Fig. 6.4), which should allow more accurate effect-site targeting using propofol in the future. It must be stressed that compartmental values are highly specific to a single

model and are not interchangeable.[34,123] It can be argued that these calculations and extrapolations are a trick to sidestep imperfect PK values.[34,123] Integrating pharmacokinetic and pharmacodynamics into models appropriate for use in children is challenging, not the least because of doubts about the sensitivity and specificity of the depth of anesthesia monitoring in children.[30,35,126,127]

Some pumps display predicted plasma or effect-site concentrations from the programmed PK model and are valuable as an educational tool for demonstrating the intricacies of TIVA. Effect-site

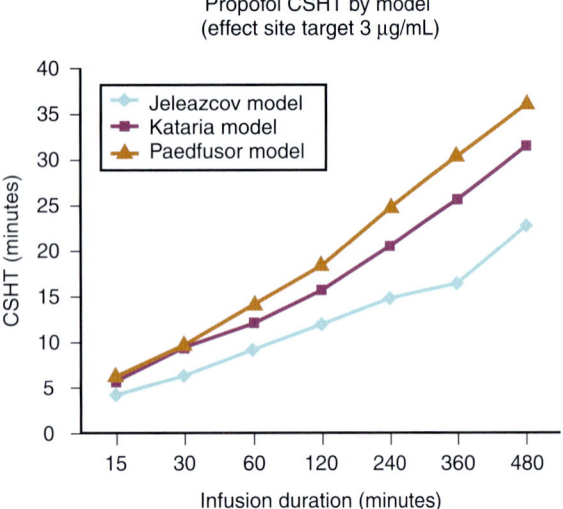

FIGURE 6.17 The predicted context-sensitive half-time *(CSHT)* of propofol depends on the pharmacokinetic model. Effect-site targeting can result in higher propofol doses if the keo is incorrect. The Jeleazcov model uses age-appropriate keo values and this results in the shortest predicted CSHTs for all infusion durations. This has clinical importance as it predicts a shorter recovery time for a given target concentration. *keo,* Site equilibration constant. (Data from Limb J, Morton NS. Age specific effect-site TCI in children; modelling using Tivatrainer. *Anaesthesia.* 2010;65:542; and Absalom A, Vereecke HE, Eleveld DJ. A hitch-hiker's guide to the intravenous PK/PD galaxy. *Paediatr Anaesth.* 2011;21:915-918.)

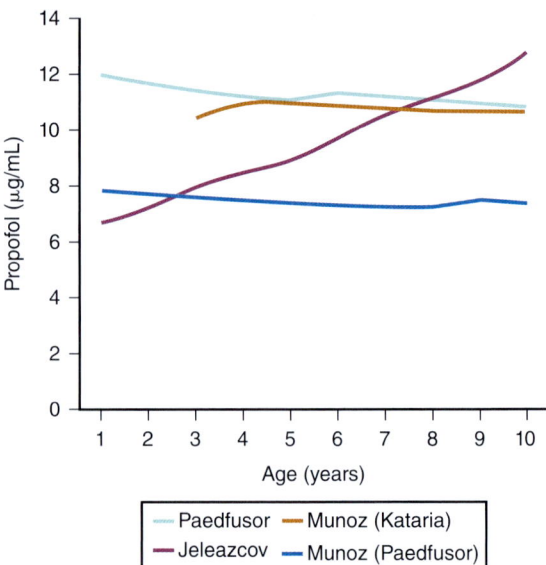

FIGURE 6.18 The peak plasma concentrations attained in simulations in Fig. 6.17 for an effect-site target of 5 μg/mL are shown. A large bolus dose does not necessarily equate to high peak plasma concentrations because of the variable volumes of distribution in the pediatric models at different ages. Even though more drug may be administered when using effect-site targeting if the keo is inappropriate, this may not mean an increase in peak plasma concentration because the peripheral volumes of distribution may be increased in any one model. More drug is redistributed. *keo,* Site equilibration constant. (Data from Limb J, Morton NS. Age specific effect-site TCI in children; modelling using Tivatrainer. *Anaesthesia.* 2010;65:542; and Absalom A, Vereecke HE, Eleveld DJ. A hitch-hiker's guide to the intravenous PK/PD galaxy. *Paediatr Anaesth.* 2011;21:915-918.)

targeting offers the advantages of more rapid achievement of desired depth of anesthesia and less titration of the target depth in practice, but while it has been used in research in children, it has yet to become a clinical tool.[128] Table 6.10 shows how the behavior of the TCI infusion differs between blood and effect-site targeted infusion using the adult keo of 0.26/minute ($T_{1/2}$keo 2.7 minutes). It can be expected that effect-site targeting may have more profound cardiovascular and respiratory effects than blood targeting owing to the larger initial bolus doses with resultant larger peak propofol blood concentrations attained.[128] It is known that the slower propofol is administered, the better spontaneous respiration is preserved in children,[129] and the use of an age-appropriate $T_{1/2}$keo value and careful titration from a low initial target value may ameliorate some adverse effects. Without such titration, adverse effects may be greater in infants (Fig. 6.17).[57,128] Although the use of BIS remains uncertain in children,[40] particularly those younger than 1 year of age, the use of age- or weight-appropriate $T_{1/2}$keo values in TCI systems provides the prospect of more accurate and efficient propofol delivery to children.[128] This has safety implications in terms of reducing lipid load and clinical utility by increasing speed of recovery (Fig. 6.18).

A Practical Approach in Children

Mastery of TIVA requires familiarity with the technique. Such familiarity can be gained by practice with older children before progressing to younger children and infants and beginning with children who present for elective, nonurgent surgery where a known stimulus will be applied. Cooperation from surgical colleagues is always advantageous when mastering the use of TIVA.

DRUG DELIVERY

Secure intravenous access is essential with infusion lines sited as close as possible to the venous cannula.[130] One-way, nonreturn valves prevent retrograde flow in intravenous fluid lines.[131] Combined infusions into a single vein run the risk of inadvertent bolus of a companion drug unless proximal dead space is minimized. The infusion site is not always readily accessible in small children when the limbs are covered with surgical drapes. As a consequence, unrecognized and inadvertent disconnects, kinked tubing or subcutaneous tissue infiltration may occur, which in the case of a disconnect may result in awareness and/or movement during surgery. Central venous access with a multilumen catheter should be considered for major surgery because it allows a dedicated port for TIVA and diminishes the risk of undisclosed subcutaneous infusion. Pump performance characteristics (e.g., lag time), intravenous tubing dead space, and syringe size and type all contribute to the observed response. The more dilute the solution is, the faster the syringe movement with a more matched delivery to change of prescription.[130] Common drug delivery problems are listed in Table 6.11.

Pumps should be serviced regularly. Unrecognized pump failures can occur with subsequent patient awareness or overdose, so vigilance is required. If problems with anesthesia occur, then the prudent thing to do may be to convert to an inhalational anesthetic technique if clinically appropriate.

MANUAL INFUSION REGIMENS

Before TCI systems were available, anesthesiologists used manual infusion regimens to administer TIVA. These regimens comprised an intravenous propofol loading dose and then a subsequent

TABLE 6.11	Potential Problems with Drug Delivery From Intravenous Anesthesia Pumps[a]
Problem	**Prevention/Detection/Solution**
IV cannula disconnect/out of vein	Venous access should be visible and accessible during procedure
Disconnection of infusion tubing from pump or cannula	Pump and tubing connections should be visible
	Use Luer-lock syringes
Pump power supply failure or pump paused	Ensure pump has an audible alarm
Occlusion of IV cannula or tubing	Pump high-pressure alarm
Occlusion alarm because of small cannula or long infusion tubing (e.g., PICC)	Ability to alter alarm threshold
"Backtracking" of propofol into intravenous fluid infusion tubing	Use of one-way valves
Drug disparity between settings and drug used (e.g., different concentration)	Keep only one concentration of propofol in hospital. Double-check drug dilution concentrations (or dispense from pharmacy premixed)
	A dedicated IV with a constant carrier solution for TIVA is the ideal
Wrong drug programmed into pump (remifentanil rather than propofol)	Prominent pump displays with the drug name
	Color coding of the pump LCD displays and syringe labels
	Bar coding

IV, Intravenous; *PICC*, percutaneous intravenous central catheters; *TIVA*, total intravenous anesthesia.
[a]Adapted from Nimmo AF, Cook TM. Accidental awareness during general anesthesia in the United Kingdom and Ireland. In: Pandit JJ, Cook TM, eds. *National Audit Project*, 5th ed. Royal College of Anaesthetists and the Association of Anaesthetists of Great Britain and Ireland, 2014:151-158.

decreasing infusion rate to maintain a target plasma concentration (e.g., Cp 3 μg/mL). The first such regimen in adults was the "10-8-6 rule" from Bristol, UK.[132] This comprised a loading dose of propofol 1 mg/kg followed immediately by an infusion of 10 mg/kg per hour for 10 minutes, 8 mg/kg per hour for the next 10 minutes and 6 mg/kg per hour thereafter.[132] When this 10-8-6 regimen is modeled and verified using the Marsh model for an adult patient, the estimated blood concentration slightly exceeds 3 μg/mL but remains reasonably stable.[23] Adolescents can generally be grouped as small adults and this 10-8-6 regimen used.

Children require larger infusion rates of propofol than adults to maintain clinical anesthesia (Fig. 6.19) because clearance (expressed per kilogram) is greater in children than in adults (Table 6.12). A popular manual pediatric infusion is that of McFarlan et al.[133] based on the Kataria pharmacokinetic parameter estimates[134] for children between the ages of 3 and 11 years. Subsequent clinical assessment of the infusion regimen's performance proved acceptable.[135] The CSHT in children was greater than in adults, increasing from 10.4 minutes at 1 hour to 19.6 minutes at 4 hours compared with adult estimates of 6.7 minutes and 9.5 minutes, respectively.[19] This increased dose requirement for propofol in children can cause concerns because it is formulated as a lipid emulsion and the lipid load can be considerable (Fig. 6.20). Propofol formulations are now available in some countries in concentrations varying from 5 mg/mL to 20 mg/mL (0.5%–2%); the most effective "lipid-sparing" strategy for infusions is to use 20 mg/mL propofol (2%) as this immediately halves the lipid load.

The Steur regimen[63] was adapted from clinical observations in children under the age of 3 years (see Table 6.2). Few adverse effects were recorded (bradycardia [12%], blood pressure decrease [8%], oxygen saturation decrease [1%]) and all were easily countered by routine measures.[63] However, neonates are susceptible to hypotension with propofol[65] and it is advisable to gradually increase the infusion rate until anesthesia is achieved rather than starting at a large infusion rate.[136] The Morse regimen (see Table 6.3),[42] based on propofol clearance maturation in neonates and infants, has recently been introduced and may obviate the need for large initial infusion rates.

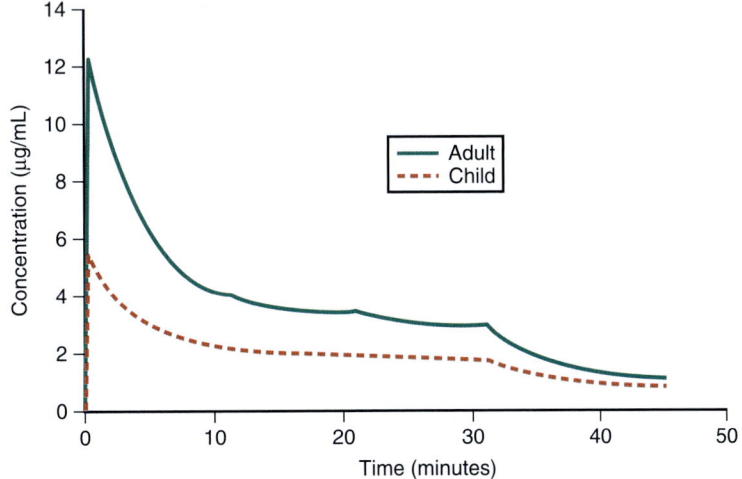

FIGURE 6.19 Simulated time-concentration profiles for propofol using a pediatric parameters set and an adult set. A 3 mg/kg bolus was administered, and the infusions were administered as for an adult (10-8-6 regimen). Peak concentrations in the child are smaller because of an increased volume of distribution. Increased clearance (expressed per kilogram) in children means subsequent concentrations also remain smaller.

TABLE 6.12	Differences Between Adult and Pediatric Propofol Pharmacokinetic Parameters		
Age	Vd (mL/kg)	Elimination Half-Life (minutes)	Clearance (mL/minute per kg)
1–3 years	9500	188	53
3–11 years	9700	398	34
Adult	4700	312	28

Notes: The apparent volume of distribution *(Vd)* of propofol in the child is twice that of adults. The clearance of propofol in young children is twice that of adults and elimination is much more rapid.

Data from Absalom A, Struys MMRF. *An Overview of TCI and TIVA.* Gent, Belgium: Academia Press; 2005.

TABLE 6.13	Possible Weight-Based Propofol Regimens in Children
Weight	Infusion Scheme
>35 kg	Schnider effect-site concentration model
15–35 kg	Kataria and Paedfusor plasma concentration model *or*
	McFarlan manual plasma concentration regimen
<15 kg	Steur manual infusion regimen
	Morse manual infusion regimen

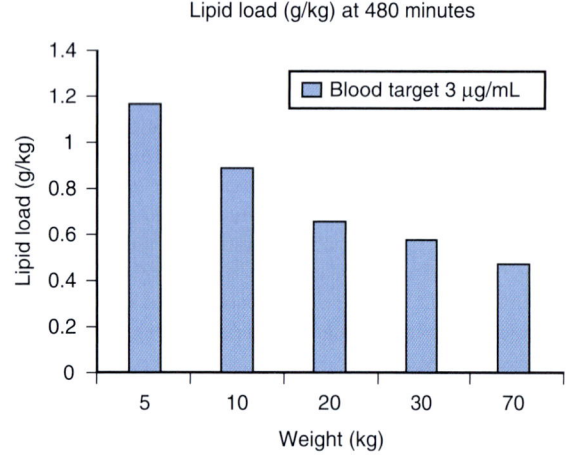

FIGURE 6.20 Lipid load after 480 minutes of a blood-targeted propofol 1% infusion (formulated in vehicle containing 0.1 grams/mL lipid) with target concentration of 3 μg/mL. Note the smaller infants have almost twice the lipid load and so 2% propofol is recommended to halve the relative lipid exposure and other propofol-sparing and lipid-sparing measures should be used. (Simulated using Tivatrainer; available at http://www.eurosiva.eu.)

Both TCI devices and manual infusion regimens provide similar depth of anesthesia and hemodynamic stability when titrated against traditional clinical signs in adults.[137] However propofol administration in children using manual infusion guided by clinical assessment of depth of anesthesia (change in heart rate and/or blood pressure, movement) was associated with greater risks of over- or under-dosage when compared with BIS-guided administrations.[138] When propofol infusion was guided by the BIS, no major difference was found between use of different pharmacokinetic parameter sets.[138]

The adult Schnider[139] model may be more accurate than either the pediatric Kataria,[20] pediatric Marsh,[23] or Schuttler[27] models in children weighing more than 35 kilograms.[35] The Kataria TCI model is plasma targeted and is valid for children from 3–15 years of age weighing 15–65 kilograms. One approach to the use of propofol regimens in children for TIVA is shown in Table 6.13.

Remifentanil as an Adjunct

Most children will maintain spontaneous respirations with a remifentanil-propofol combination. Fig. 5.30 demonstrates the remifentanil infusion rates that will maintain a spontaneous respiration rate of 10 breaths/minute. Use of the adult Minto parameter set for remifentanil infusion in children confers a degree of safety because concentrations measured will be less than those predicted because of the greater clearance (expressed as per kilogram) in children. Occasionally some respiratory support may be required; that is easily done using the pressure support ventilation mode. Controlled ventilation is required when large target concentrations of remifentanil are used. Large effect-site remifentanil concentrations (>10 ng/mL) are associated with hypotension (Fig. 6.21) and this property can be used advantageously during some neurosurgical procedures or spinal instrumentation.[140]

Fixed propofol-remifentanil combinations (mixed together in the same syringe) are frowned upon because (1) drug mixing results in a new unlicensed drug; (2) drugs may not be a homologous mix in the syringe; (3) they do not allow separate titration of analgesia and sedation; and (4) targeting a propofol concentration can result in a relatively large accompanying bolus of remifentanil.[141] However, they remain widely used by practitioners in some countries[142–144] (e.g., propofol 10 mg/mL with remifentanil 5 μg/mL) for brief painful procedures such as endoscopy. If a combination is used with a TCI pump, then a propofol target concentration of 3 μg/L usually allows spontaneous breathing, whereas a propofol target of 6 μg/mL requires ventilation support. Although such mixtures are widely used, remifentanil in such mixtures may become unstable and has a limited life span in the syringe. The weaker the mixture, the less stable it is. This is due to a pH effect on the rate of ester hydrolysis of the remifentanil.[145]

Reports of a rapid development of μ-receptor tolerance with remifentanil are conflicting; activity at δ-opioid receptors may contribute.[146–148] It has been suggested that longer acting opioids (e.g., morphine) be administered approximately 40 minutes before the end of surgery to allow time for it to bind to opioid receptors occupied by remifentanil.[149] This morphine dose timing is consistent with the equilibration half-time between central and effect compartments for morphine (T1/2keo) of 16 minutes.[150,151]

INDUCTION

To achieve an adequate effect-site concentration at induction, propofol needs to be administered as a bolus. This can be accomplished either manually or using a variable rate infusion from the TCI smart pump. An initial target concentration of 4 to 6 μg/mL is adequate to anesthetize a child and avoid unwanted adverse effects such as hypotension.

Smart pumps inject propofol at a large default rate (usually 1200 mL/hour) unless the patient weighs less than 18 kilograms, or the duration of the pump bolus dose is increased more than the default 10 to 20 seconds. The pain associated with IV injection of propofol is problematic. This is especially common when given through the small veins in the hands or feet. Perhaps the best approach to reduce the pain on injection of propofol is to site a larger bore cannula in a proximal (e.g., basilic vein) rather than a distal limb vein. Lidocaine 1 mg/kg placed in the IV with a

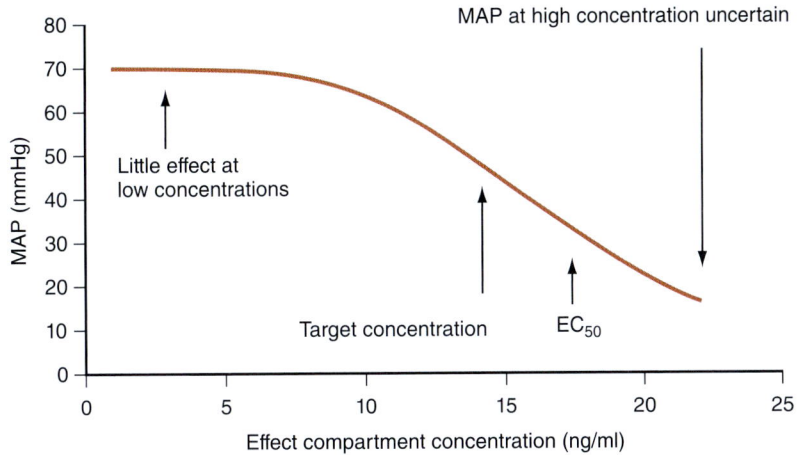

FIGURE 6.21 The relationship between remifentanil concentration and mean arterial blood pressure *(MAP)* in an individual undergoing cranioplasty surgery. A steady-state remifentanil concentration of 14 μg/L would typically achieve a 30% decrease in mean arterial blood pressure. *EC50,* Concentration is that at half maximum response. (From Anderson BJ, Holford NH. Leaving no stone unturned, or extracting blood from stone? *Paediatr Anaesth.* 2010;20:1-6. Used with permission.)

proximal tourniquet (or just manual compression of the arm to stop the IV from flowing) applied for 30 to 60 seconds is one of the most effective strategies to attenuating the pain when propofol is administered through a small vein,[152] but the tourniquet can cause discomfort in children. Intravenous lidocaine 2 mg/kg without a tourniquet can reduce the pain associated with propofol injection[153] and a premixed propofol/lidocaine injection may be equally effective with long-chain triglyceride propofol emulsion provided the admixture is administered within 30 seconds of preparation or when a medium-chain triglyceride propofol emulsion is used.[154–157] Opioid or ketamine administered IV before propofol injection is also helpful. This can be best done by beginning the remifentanil infusion first and running it at a Cp of approximately 4 ng/mL for 2 minutes before starting the propofol infusion or waiting for similar Ce[158]; most children will continue to maintain spontaneous respirations through this short period. Alternatively, a bolus of fentanyl 1 μg/kg or remifentanil 1 μg/kg through the IV cannula is effective.

ESTABLISHING TIVA AFTER AN INHALATIONAL INDUCTION

Propofol TIVA can start once an inhalational induction has been performed and IV access established. The use of a fixed infusion rate only is discouraged because it requires three to four elimination half-lives to establish steady-state concentrations (see Fig. 6.7). While the end-tidal inhalational agent partial pressure decreases, it is reasonable to target a reduced propofol concentration of 3 μg/mL as an initial target and then titrate against the clinical response. If a manual regimen is used, then the initial bolus should be reduced, especially if spontaneous respirations are required; a bolus of propofol 1 mg/kg is usually satisfactory in children.[159]

SPONTANEOUSLY BREATHING WITH TIVA

If it is desirable to keep a child breathing during anesthesia (e.g., during bronchoscopy), then some changes to technique are usually required. Avoidance of remifentanil as the opioid is perhaps the easiest way to keep the child breathing spontaneously and dexmedetomidine infusion can be substituted. Remifentanil causes apnea after bolus doses or large infusion rates and consequent large Ce. Substituting fentanyl or alfentanil for remifentanil often allows the patient to continue to breathe spontaneously,

although neither provides such a profound degree of analgesia and therefore patient movement is more likely, unless coupled with a local anesthetic agent to supplement analgesia. Remifentanil infusions of up to 0.15 μg/kg per minute used with propofol in patients over 3 years of age or up to 0.3 μg/kg minute in those less than 3 years of age may allow spontaneous breathing to continue.[160] These infusion rates reflect changing clearance with age and achieve similar target concentrations of 1 to 1.5 μg/L.[161] Monitoring the child's respiratory rate may give an indication of impending apnea, with a rate below 10 breaths per minute often indicating that apnea is imminent.[162] A tail to the end-tidal carbon dioxide trace, suggesting prolonged expiration often precedes apnea, as does an observed tidal volume reduction.

INTUBATION

A target remifentanil concentration of 2 to 3 ng/mL combined with propofol 3 to 4 μg/mL modulates the sympathetic response associated with laryngoscopy when accompanied by a neuromuscular-blocking agent. Tracheal intubation without the use of a neuromuscular-blocking agent can be facilitated using combinations of propofol and remifentanil.[163] Dose-response studies concluded that remifentanil 3 μg/kg combined with propofol 3–4 mg/kg provided the best intubating conditions similar to those with a neuromuscular-blocking agent. Remifentanil 2 μg/kg did not produce satisfactory intubating conditions.[164] Resumption of spontaneous respirations after a remifentanil–propofol combination was similar to that after succinylcholine.[165–167]

Age also influences the dose of remifentanil. Children (0–3 years of age) who were given propofol 5 mg/kg required a remifentanil ED50 for intubation of 3.1 (95% CI 2.5–3.8) μg/kg at 0 to 3 months of age, 3.7 (95% CI 2.0–5.4) μg/kg at 4 to 12 months of age, and 3.0 (95% CI 2.1–3.9) μg/kg at 1 to 3 years age.[168]

RECOVERY

Whether propofol should be stopped before the remifentanil to speed recovery remains uncertain. The propofol infusion can be reduced to a target Ce of 2 μg/mL at the time of skin closure, provided a local block is being used or the remifentanil is continued at an analgesic dose (0.1–0.2 μg/kg per minute or Ce 1.5–2.5 ng/mL). Recovery after propofol in children takes longer than in adults due to the increased CSHT of propofol in children.[133] The mean time from discontinuing propofol (mean rate 14.8 mg/kg per hour, 246 μg/kg per minute, duration 30 minutes) and remifentanil (mean rate 0.11 μg/kg per minute) infusions to purposeful spontaneous movement in children (3 months–10 years of age) was 17 minutes and occurred at a propofol Ce of 2 (SD 0.5) μg/mL.[54]

Most children will awaken at an estimated *plasma* concentration (Cp) of propofol calculated by the smart pump of 1.2 to 1.8 μg/mL. The variability associated with this Cp for purposeful spontaneous movement depends on the PK model used in the smart pump and age of the child,[34,38] adjunct drugs used, between patient variability of PK and PD parameters, and $t_{1/2}$keo estimates. Opioids potentiate the sedative, hypnotic, and anesthetic effects of propofol. For example, if remifentanil is continued after cessation of a propofol infusion, purposeful spontaneous movement is achieved at reduced propofol concentrations. This variability dictates that clinical signs and not just the Cp or Ce predicted by the smart pump be used to assess anesthesia depth. Processed EEG signals are also useful, particularly in the presence of neuromuscular blockade.

Return of consciousness after prolonged anesthesia with propofol and remifentanil is determined primarily by the CSHT of propofol. CSHT is greater in children than adults because children accumulate proportionally greater amounts of propofol in peripheral tissues due to the greater dose requirements. Opioids with a longer duration of action (e.g., sufentanil) delay recovery.[169]

Ready Mixes

Individual anesthesia practitioners, like good chefs, often have their own recipes using fixed drug mixes for some clinical scenarios. These have the advantage of simplicity but lack the versatility of separate infusions. Sterile infusions are prepared by the pharmacy in some centers, although there can be reluctance to prepare such infusions because of concerns about stability and the lack of clinical studies documenting the safety and efficacy of these mixtures. A common example used for endoscopy is shown in Table 6.14.

Ketofol is a mixture of ketamine and propofol (1:1) that is finding a niche for procedural sedation in the emergency room.[170] Stable hemodynamics, analgesia, and good recovery are reported.[171] The additive interaction for anesthesia induction in adults has been reported.[172] These data have been used to simulate effect in children[173]; an optimal ratio of racemic ketamine to propofol of

TABLE 6.14	Recipe for Gastrointestinal Endoscopy Using a Propofol–Remifentanil Mixture
Age >10 Years	
50 μg remifentanil in 19 mL propofol (2.5 μg/mL remifentanil)	
Start propofol mix at 175 μg/kg per minute	
Age <10 Years	
100 μg remifentanil in 18 mL propofol (5 μg/kg remifentanil)	
Start propofol mix at 150 μg/kg per minute	
If a higher remifentanil concentration is used in teenagers, then they breathe at 2–4 breaths/minute and have systolic blood pressure of approximately 75 mm Hg. If a lower remifentanil concentration is used, they breathe at 8–10 breaths/minute and have a systolic blood pressure of 76–84 mm Hg. Those aged <10 years generally do not usually require any up or down change in the rate of infusion and breathe at normal rates.	

1:5 for 30 minutes of anesthesia and 1:6.7 for 90 minutes of anesthesia was suggested (Fig. 6.22).[173] The "ideal mix" for sedation depends on the duration of sedation and the degree of analgesia required. The CSHT of ketamine increases with the duration of the infusion, resulting in delayed recovery.[174]

Special Cases

There are a number of situations where it may be more challenging to use TIVA in children; these include neonates and obese children.

THE OBESE CHILD

Investigation of propofol PK in obese adults[175] and children[176,177] suggests that using total body weight scaled as per kilogram in the models will lead to a relative overdose of propofol. Scaling using total body weight and allometry was a better option.[178–180] There are also parameter sets (bespoke models) available for propofol that only apply to obese adults.[181]

Remifentanil infusions scale better using lean body mass.[50,182] There are problems implementing lean body mass into anesthesia practice because the formula[183] programmed into many common infusion pumps in adults for intravenous anesthesia is inconsistent at extremes of size, particularly in those adults of short stature where a reduction of lean body mass is predicted as total body weight increases.[184] Methods used to circumvent this problem in pumps used for adults include calculation of a fictitious height,[185] creating a new metric,[186] or by placing limits on maximum programmable weight allowed.[187] The addition of 40% of the excess weight to the ideal body weight[188] for propofol infusion calculation has been suggested.[189]

An approach to circumvent this dosing difficulty in children is to use actual body weight, deliver generous amounts of remifentanil, and adjust the propofol Ce according to either BIS values[190] or clinical response.[191] A similar clinical result can be achieved by reducing the prescribed target concentration (e.g., propofol 4 μg/mL rather than 6 μg/mL) and then titrating to effect, while ideally avoiding neuromuscular blockade.

The use of normal fat mass (NFM) (see Chapter 5) as a size standard in conjunction with allometry to describe PK parameters offers a solution to dosing in obese adults and children. These models have been used to describe PK for propofol,[44] remifentanil,[50] and dexmedetomidine.[106] Fat mass has no contribution to clearance but does have a contribution to dexmedetomidine volume.[106] Concentration in an obese child will be greater than that in a nonobese child after a similar dose given as an infusion over 10 minutes. While dose is normalized to total body weight, volume is aligned with normal fat mass and increases with weight as a curvilinear function.[179] Simulation of dexmedetomidine concentration in plasma and effect compartments using parameter estimates that use normal fat mass[106] are shown in Fig. 6.23 for a normal weight, obese (BMI 20 kg/m^2; Grade I, 95th centile) and morbidly obese (BMI>30 kg/m^2; Grade III, 140% of 95th centile) 8-year-old child administered dexmedetomidine 0.75 μg/kg. Peak concentration in the effect compartment (Ce) is smaller in a normal weight child compared with the Grade I obese and Grade III morbidly obese child (2.6 μg/L, 2.8 μg/L, 3.2 μg/L, respectively). The influence of obesity on CSHT is shown in Fig. 6.24 where a normal weight (25 kg) and an obese (50 kg) 8-year-old child are compared. After a 2-hour infusion there is greater disposition in "deep" compartments in the obese child with return to the plasma after infusion cessation. An understanding of CSHT is

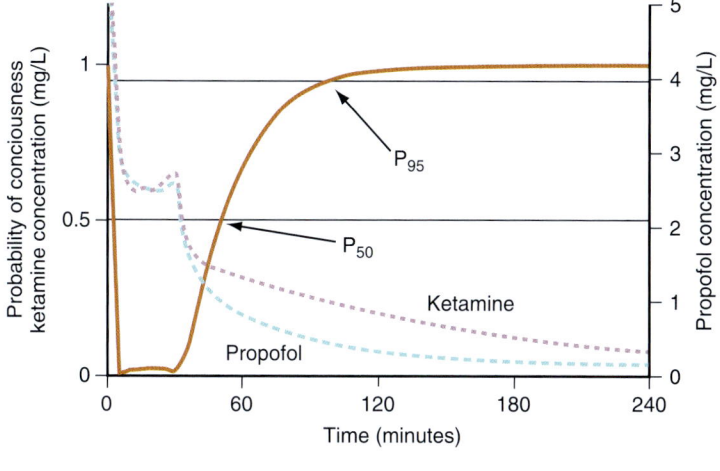

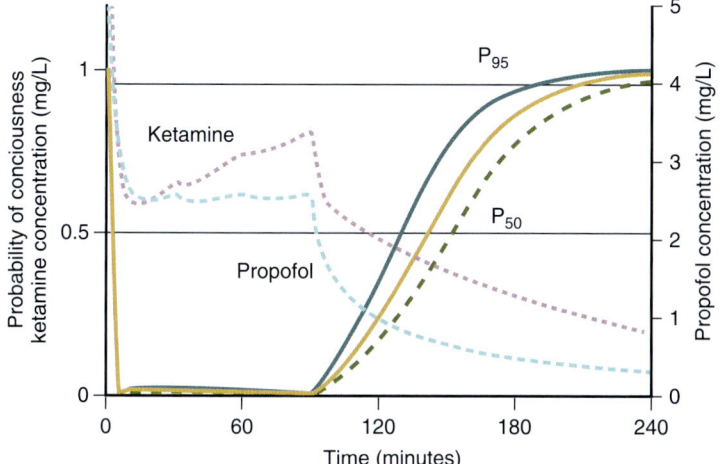

FIGURE 6.22 The upper panel shows the probability of consciousness during anesthesia using a propofol/ketamine ratio of 5:1. The loading dose for induction of anesthesia was 2.5 mg/kg propofol and 0.5 mg/kg of ketamine. The infusion rate was 67% of that suggested by McFarlan, Anderson, and Short[19] for propofol alone. Ketamine time-concentration profile is shown as a *purple dotted line*. Propofol time-concentration profile is shown as a *blue dotted line*. The lower panel shows simulation results for a 90-minute infusion. This panel also shows the probability of consciousness as age increases from a 2-year-old *(solid blue line)*, to a 5-year-old *(solid orange line)*, and a 10-year-old *(green dashed line)* child. The younger children have greater clearance and regain consciousness earlier than older children. P_{50} is the probability of consciousness in 50% of children; P_{95} is the probability of consciousness in 95% of children. (From Coulter FL Hannam JA, Anderson BJ. Ketofol simulations for dosing in pediatric anesthesia. *Pediatr Anesth.* 2014;24:806-812. Used with permission.)

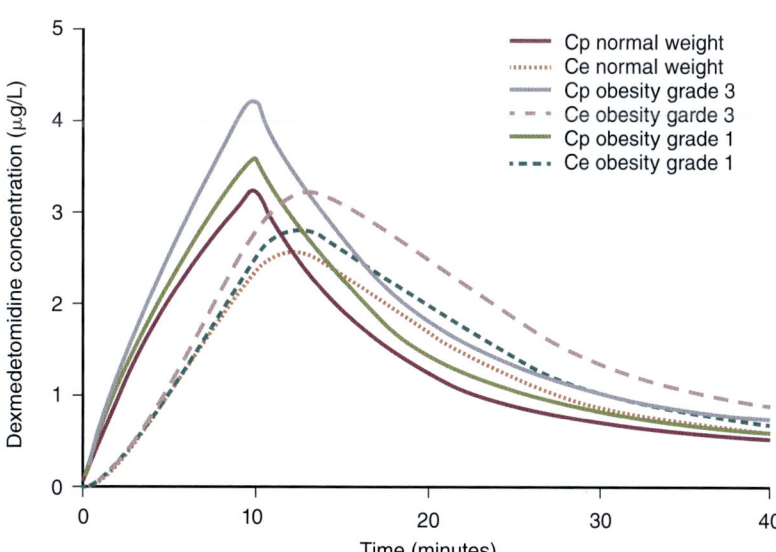

FIGURE 6.23 Time-concentration profiles for both the plasma concentration *(Cp)* and effect-site concentration *(Ce)* for a normal weight, obese (BMI 20 kg/m²; Grade I, 95th centile) and morbidly obese (BMI>30 kg/m²; Grade III, 140% of 95th centile) 8-year-old child administered dexmedetomidine 0.75 µg/kg over 10 minutes. (From Morse J, Cortinez LI, Anderson BJ. Pharmacokinetic concepts for dexmedetomidine target-controlled infusion pumps in children. *Pediatr Anesth.* 2021;31(9):924-931. Used with permission.)

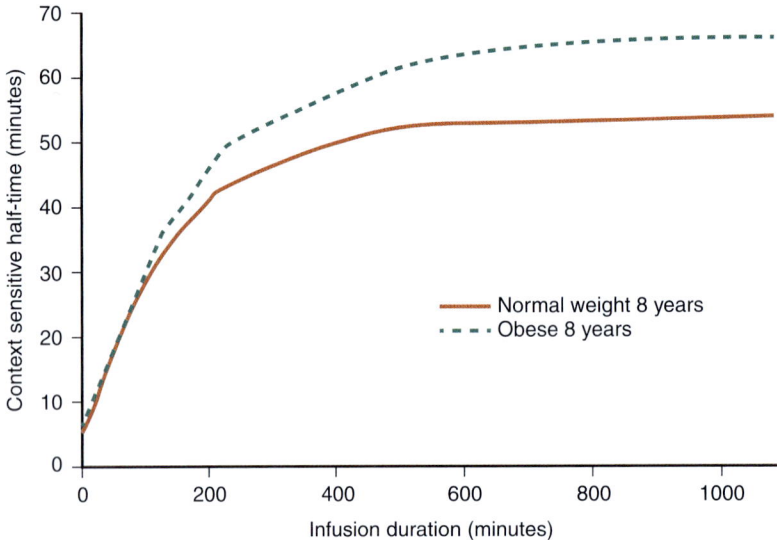

FIGURE 6.24 Context-sensitive half-time changes with a normal body weight (25 kg) and an obese (50 kg) 8-year-old child. After a 2-hour infusion duration there is greater disposition in peripheral compartments with delayed equilibration to the plasma after infusion cessation, demonstrating why delayed emergence is likely in obese children. (From Morse J, Cortinez LI, Anderson BJ. Pharmacokinetic concepts for dexmedetomidine target-controlled infusion pumps in children. *Pediatr Anesth.* 2021;31(9):924-931. Used with permission.)

useful because this confounded parameter can be used to estimate a concentration associated with sedation recovery after infusion. Time to recovery will be slower in obese patients.

A NEONATE HAVING COMBINED ANESTHESIA AND REGIONAL BLOCKADE

Dexmedetomidine[192,193] and remifentanil[192,193] may be alternative drug options if concerns that some anesthetic drugs may cause neuronal apoptosis in the developing brain of a human neonate are confirmed (see Chapter 23). One regimen consists of IV premedication of glycopyrrolate 5 µg/kg followed by a loading dose of dexmedetomidine 0.6 µg/kg and 1 µg/kg remifentanil followed by an infusion rate of dexmedetomidine 1 to 1.5 µg/kg per hour. The dexmedetomidine infusion can be titrated up or down within 50% of starting doses as needed, although it is crucial to appreciate that dexmedetomidine is not a complete general anesthetic.[194] Similarly, a remifentanil infusion 0.1 µg/kg per minute can be titrated up or down (maximum infusion 0.5 µg/kg per minute). Airway management may require a tracheal tube or supraglottic airway and ventilation assisted to maintain normocapnia.

The Future

The field of TIVA continues to develop and evolve. The introduction of PK models that extend from premature neonates to elderly patients will simplify smart pump use. Perhaps the major obstacle to it becoming more widely adopted in routine clinical practice is the absence of a reliable feedback to indicate that the patient is receiving an appropriate quantity of drug. The introduction of processed EEG as a surrogate measure has gone some way to achieving this, but lack of validation in infants means it is yet to become the routine standard of care.[195] An accurate "closed-loop" system based on depth of anesthesia monitoring, proportional correction or exhaled propofol concentration will be developed in the future and this will allow us to titrate our intravenous agents more accurately.[17]

ANNOTATED REFERENCES

Absalom A, Amutike D, Lal A, et al. Accuracy of the "Paedfusor" in children undergoing cardiac surgery or catheterization. *Br J Anaesth.* 2003;91:507-513.
A widely used parameter set (children 1–15 years) programmed into target-controlled infusion pumps is the Paedfusor model. This parameter set is one of the few whose performance has been validated.

Anderson BJ, Bagshaw O. Practicalities of total intravenous anesthesia and target-controlled infusion in children. *Anesthesiology.* 2019;131: 164-185.
This review outlines the practicalities of delivering total intravenous anesthesia to children. It is important to understand the drug pharmacology that underlines this anesthetic type; it is equally important to appreciate PK-PD variability and clinical solutions and practice skills that experienced anesthesiologists use in day-to-day delivery of these drugs.

Eleveld DJ, Colin P, Absalom AR, Struys M. Pharmacokinetic–pharmacodynamic model for propofol for broad application in anaesthesia and sedation. *Brit J Anaesth.* 2018;120:942-959.
This model describes The PK of propofol from 27 weeks postmenstrual age to 88 years of age, and the weight range was 0.68–160 kg. The final model uses age, postmenstrual age, weight, height, sex, and presence/absence of concomitant anesthetic drugs as covariates. It predicts the BIS for this broad population, suitable for TCI applications. Allometric theory is used to standardize for size. It is not yet used in commercial TCI pumps, but future pumps may only require this one parameter set that can account for all ages, obesity, and concomitant anesthetic drugs.

Holford NHG, Sheiner LB. Understanding the dose-effect relationship: clinical application of pharmacokinetic-pharmacodynamic models. *Clin Pharmacokinet.* 1981;6:429-453.

This classic study describes the use of the Hill equation to explain the concentration-response relationship. The equation and its variants are used to relate both vapors and drugs to anesthesia depth using such monitors as BIS.
Kataria BK, Ved SA, Nicodemus HF, et al. The pharmacokinetics of propofol in children using three different data analysis approaches. *Anesthesiology.* 1994;80:104-122.

Population modeling was used to determine a propofol parameter set in children 3–11 years of age. This parameter set is known as the Kataria model and is programmed into many target-controlled infusion pumps.

A complete reference list can be found online at Elsevier eBooks+.

6

7

Fluid Management

CATHIE T. JONES, CRAIG D. McCLAIN, AND MICHAEL L. McMANUS

Regulatory Mechanisms: Fluid Volume, Osmolality, and Arterial Pressure
Maturation of Fluid Compartments and Homeostatic Mechanisms
Body Water and Electrolyte Distribution
Circulating Blood Volume
Maturation of Homeostatic Mechanisms
Fluid and Electrolyte Requirements
Neonatal Fluid Management
Intraoperative Fluid Management
Intravenous Access and Fluid Administration Devices
Choice And Composition of Intravenous Fluids
Colloid Solutions
Hydroxyethyl Starches
Glucose Solutions
Hyperalimentation
Fasting Recommendations

Ongoing Losses and Third-Spacing
Assessment of Intravascular Volume
Postoperative Fluid Management
General Approach
Postoperative Physiology and Hyponatremia
Postoperative Fluid Overload
Pathophysiologic States and Their Management
Fluid Overload and Edema
Dehydration States
Septic Shock
Hypernatremia and Hyponatremia
Disorders of Potassium Homeostasis
Syndrome of Inappropriate Antidiuretic Hormone Secretion
Diabetes Insipidus
Hyperchloremic Acidosis
Hypochloremic Metabolic Alkalosis
Cerebral Salt Wasting

ELECTROLYTE DISTURBANCES ARE COMMON in children because of their small size, large ratio of surface area to volume, and immature homeostatic mechanisms. As a result, fluid management can be challenging. On the ward, in the operating room, or in the intensive care unit, additional difficulties may result when fluid management is not tailored to the individual or when therapeutic decisions are based on extrapolations from adult data. To better understand the former and to limit the latter, this chapter reviews the basic mechanisms underlying fluid and electrolyte regulation, the developmental anatomy and physiology of fluid compartments, and the management of selected pediatric disease states relevant to anesthesia and critical care.

Regulatory Mechanisms: Fluid Volume, Osmolality, and Arterial Pressure

Water is in thermodynamic equilibrium across cell membranes, and it moves only in response to the movement of solutes (E-Fig. 7.1). Movement of water is described by the Starling equation:

$$Q_f = K_f[(P_c - P_i) - \sigma (\pi_c - \pi_i)],$$

where Q_f is fluid flow; K_f is the membrane fluid filtration coefficient (a proportionality constant); subscripts c and i refer to capillary and interstitial; P_c and P_i are hydrostatic pressures and π_c and π_i are osmotic pressures on either side of the membrane; and σ is the reflection coefficient for the solute and membrane of interest. The reflection coefficient gives a measure of a solute's permeability and, consequently, its contribution to osmotic force after equilibration. Across the blood-brain barrier, for example, the σ for sodium approaches 1.0,[1] whereas in muscle and other cell membranes, σ is on the order of 0.15 to 0.3.[2] Therefore, when isotonic sodium-containing solutions are given intravenously, usually only 15% to 30% of administered salt and water remains in the intravascular space, whereas the remainder migrates to the interstitium.[3,4] In contrast, hypertonic solutions permit greater expansion of circulating blood volume with smaller fluid loads and less fluid in the interstitium (e.g., as edema).[5–7]

Both the amount and the concentration of solutes are tightly regulated to maintain the volumes of intravascular and intracellular compartments. Because sodium is the primary extracellular solute, this ion is the focus of homeostatic mechanisms concerned with maintaining intravascular volume. When osmolality is held constant, water movement follows sodium movement. As a result, total body sodium (although not necessarily serum Na^+) and total body water (TBW) generally parallel one another. Because sodium "leak" across membranes limits its contribution to the support of intravascular volume, this compartment also critically depends on large, impermeable molecules such as proteins. In contrast to sodium, albumin molecules, for example, follow the Starling equilibrium with a reflection coefficient in excess of 0.8.[8] Soluble proteins create the so-called *colloid oncotic pressure,* approximately 80% of which is comprised of albumin.

Although the presence of albumin supports intravascular volume, protein leak into the interstitium (and consequent water movement) may limit its effectiveness. It has been observed that

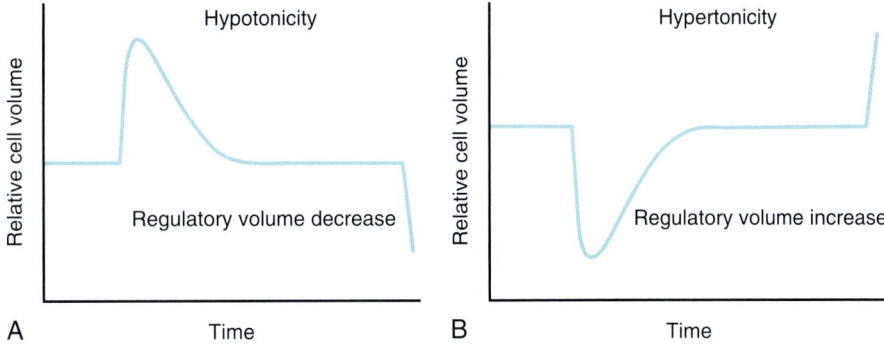

FIGURE 7.1 Activation of mechanisms regulating cell volume in response to volume perturbations. Volume-regulatory losses and gains of solutes are termed *regulatory volume decrease* **(A)** and *regulatory volume increase* **(B),** respectively. The course of these decreases and increases varies with the type of cell and experimental conditions. Typically, however, a regulatory volume increase mediated by the uptake of electrolytes, or a regulatory volume decrease mediated by the loss of electrolytes and organic osmolytes occurs over a period of minutes. When cells that have undergone a regulatory volume decrease **(A)** or increase **(B)** are returned to normotonic conditions, they swell above or shrink below their resting volume. This is caused by volume-regulatory accumulation or loss of solutes, which effectively makes the cytoplasm hypertonic or hypotonic, respectively, as compared with normotonic extracellular fluid. (From McManus ML, Churchwell KB, Strange K. Regulation of cell volume in health and disease. *N Engl J Med.* 1995;333:1260-1266.)

the reflection coefficient for albumin decreases by as much as one-third after mechanical trauma.[9] Furthermore, because of ongoing leakage, a slow continuous infusion of albumin is superior to bolus administration for increasing the serum albumin concentration (as a short term measure) in critically ill individuals.[10]

Potassium is the primary intracellular solute, with approximately one-third of cellular energy metabolism devoted to Na^+/K^+ exchange. Sodium continuously leaks into cells along its concentration gradient, yet it is rapidly extruded in exchange for potassium. As the cell is exposed to varying osmolarity, water movement occurs, causing cell swelling or shrinkage. Because stable cell volume is critical for survival, complex regulatory mechanisms have evolved to ensure that stability is maintained.[11,12] The processes by which swollen cells return to normal size are collectively termed *regulatory volume decrease* processes, and those returning a shrunken cell to normal are termed *regulatory volume increase* processes (Fig. 7.1). With sudden, brief changes in osmolality, regulatory volume increase or decrease processes are activated after small (1%–2%) changes in cell volume, returning cell volume to normal primarily through transport of electrolytes. If anisosmotic conditions persist, chronic compensation occurs through the accumulation or loss of small organic molecules once termed "idiogenic osmoles" and now referred to collectively as *osmolytes*. Many of these agents are cytoprotective under stress and include polyols, sorbitol, myoinositol, amino acids and their derivatives (e.g., taurine, alanine, proline), and methylamines (e.g., betaine, glycerylphosphorylcholine).

Like intracellular volume, circulating blood (intravascular) volume is also tightly controlled. Increases in intravascular volume result from increases in sodium and water retention, whereas decreases in intravascular volume result from increases in excretion of sodium and water. As noted earlier, serum osmolality must be maintained within a very narrow range if serum sodium is to be an effective focus of intravascular volume control. Serum osmolality is usually maintained between 280 and 300 mOsm/L, with compensatory mechanisms triggered by osmolarity changes as small as 1%.

Serum osmolality is primarily regulated by arginine vasopressin, thirst, and renal concentrating ability. Because the indirect

aim of osmolar control is actually volume control, these same osmoregulatory mechanisms are also influenced by factors such as blood pressure, cardiac output, and vascular capacitance.[13,14] In pathologic conditions such as ascites or hemorrhage, intravascular volume preservation takes precedence over osmolality and osmoregulatory mechanisms operate to restore intravascular volume, even at the expense of disrupting solute balance.

Arginine vasopressin is released from neurons within the supraoptic and paraventricular nuclei of the hypothalamus.[15] Microelectrode recordings suggest that different subpopulations of neurons are responsive to osmotic input, baroreceptor-mediated input, or both. Osmoresponsive cells react to osmolar fluctuations in cell size, so solutes that readily permeate cell membranes (such as urea) increase the serum osmolality without triggering the release of antidiuretic hormone (ADH). Infusion of solutes with large actual or effective cell membrane reflection coefficients (σ) (e.g., sodium, mannitol) elicit a robust arginine vasopressin release. Typically, arginine vasopressin release begins when the serum osmolality reaches a threshold of approximately 280 mOsm/L. In keeping with our understanding of cell volume regulation, rapid increases in osmolality lead to greater release of arginine vasopressin than slow increases. Meanwhile, baroreceptors on the arterial side of the circulation (left ventricle, carotid sinus, aortic arch, and juxtaglomerular apparatus) provide tonic inhibition of nonosmotic arginine vasopressin release. Hypovolemia and hypotension diminish this inhibition, release arginine vasopressin stores, and increase the overall "gain" of the system (E-Fig. 7.2). Thus, in a volume-depleted or hypotensive child, brisk arginine vasopressin release can occur even in the presence of plasma osmolality as low as 260 to 270 mOsm/L. On balance, baroreceptor signals always override osmotic signals so that water is retained as needed to maintain circulatory homeostasis.

Intravascular fluid volume, salt and water intake, electrolyte balance, and cardiovascular status are interrelated at several levels.[16] For example, as the veins and arteries distend with fluid and the systemic blood pressure increases, arginine vasopressin release decreases, and both *pressure diuresis* and *natriuresis* begin.[17] The resulting relationship between urine output and arterial pressure is termed the *renal function curve* and its intersection with salt and water intake determines the *equilibrium point* at which arterial blood pressure ultimately stabilizes (Fig. 7.2). Equilibrium (chronic) blood pressure is influenced only by shifts of the renal function or fluid intake curves. Transient changes in arterial pressure secondary to peripheral vascular resistance changes are always resolved by opposing shifts in total body salt and water.

In response to a decreasing arterial pressure, the renin-angiotensin system is also activated. With decreased renal perfusion, juxtaglomerular cells release renin, which in turn converts renin substrate (angiotensinogen) to angiotensin I. Angiotensin I is then rapidly converted to angiotensin II by angiotensin-converting enzyme present in lung endothelium. Angiotensin II supports arterial pressure in three ways: (1) direct vasoconstriction, (2) increased salt and water retention (via renal vasoconstriction and decreased glomerular filtration), and (3) stimulation of aldosterone secretion (Fig. 7.3).

Arginine vasopressin, pressure diuresis, and the renin-angiotensin system permit wide ranges in salt and water intake while maintaining the blood pressure and volume status within narrow ranges; all serve to support the systemic circulation when threatened and to complement the more immediate activity of the sympathetic nervous system. In addition to high-pressure sensors

such as aortic arch and carotid sinus baroreceptors, intravascular volume information is provided by low-pressure thoracic sensors. For this reason, effective increases or decreases in intrathoracic blood volume may mimic changes in whole-body volume status and produce natriuresis, diuresis, or fluid retention. Intravascular volume may also be sensed by atrial muscle fibers; as the fibers stretch, atrial natriuretic peptide is released.[18] Atrial natriuretic peptide may then serve to "fine-tune" the volume status by vasodilating modestly, gently increasing the glomerular filtration rate (GFR), and decreasing reabsorption of sodium. The combination of complex autoregulatory mechanisms with complementary actions operating on varying time scales, and all responding to different, interrelated effector stimuli, yields an elegant system by which the mature individual may maintain circulation amid a variety of challenges. In this context, it is interesting to observe that successful heart transplant recipients typically manifest fundamental derangements in body fluid homeostasis, despite general cardiovascular stability.[19]

Maturation of Fluid Compartments and Homeostatic Mechanisms

BODY WATER AND ELECTROLYTE DISTRIBUTION

Much of our understanding of the development of body water compartments is derived from deuterium oxide dilution studies performed in the 1950s.[20] In a series of 21 neonates, TBW was found to be approximately 78% ± 5% of body weight. Subsequent measurements in fewer subjects showed that TBW decreased to approximately 60% of body weight in the second 6 months of life with most of the loss being extracellular. A smaller decrease (to about 57%) is observed late in childhood (Fig. 7.4).

The importance of the extracellular compartment, its relationship to the intracellular space, and much of the chemical anatomy of both were first described by Gamble in educational monographs issued during the first part of the 20th century (E-Fig. 7.3).[21,22] The chemical compositions of mature body fluid compartments are provided in Table 7.1.

CIRCULATING BLOOD VOLUME

The blood volume in neonates was determined to be 82 ± 9 mL/kg using an iodine-121–labeled human serum albumin technique, although substantial variability may result from the degree of placental-fetal transfusion.[23] In low–birth-weight (LBW), preterm, or critically ill infants, values as high as 100 mL/kg have been measured.[24] Blood volume increases slightly during the first few months of life, reaching its zenith at 2 months of age

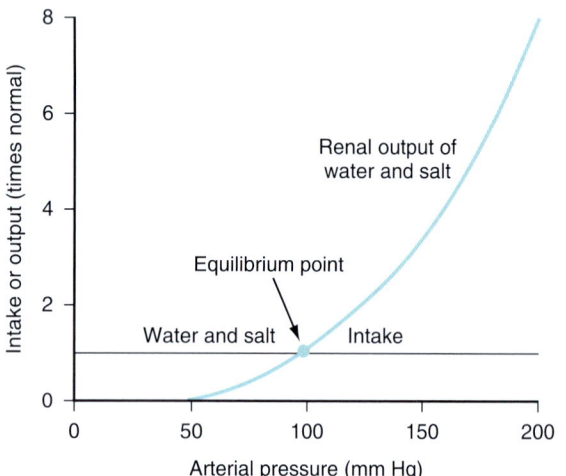

FIGURE 7.2 Analysis of arterial pressure regulation by equating the renal output curve with the salt and water intake curve. The equilibrium point describes the level to which the arterial pressure will be regulated. (That portion of the salt and water intake that is lost from the body through nonrenal routes is ignored in this figure.) (From Guyton AC, Hall JC, eds. *Textbook of Medical Physiology*. Philadelphia: WB Saunders; 1996;221-237.)

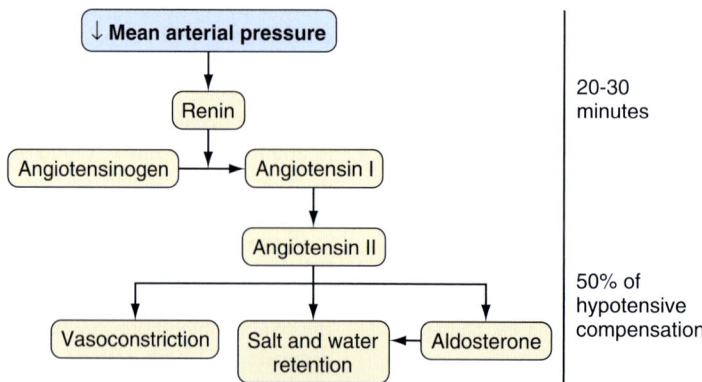

FIGURE 7.3 Physiologic responses to hypotension.

Body Water Compartments

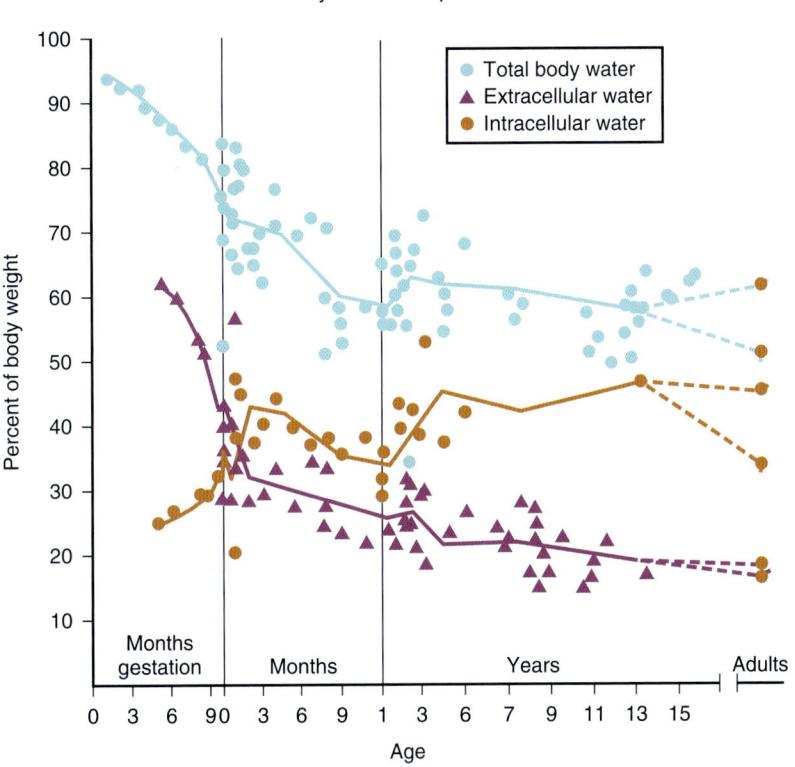

FIGURE 7.4 Total body water *(blue circles)*, extracellular water *(purple triangles)*, and intracellular water *(orange circles)* as percentages of body weight in infants and children, compared with corresponding values for the fetus and adults. (With permission: Friis-Hansen B. Changes in body water compartments during growth. In: Die Physiologische Entwicklung des Kindes. Linneweh F (Ed). Springer-Verlag oGH. Berlin 1959. pp 196-203.)

TABLE 7.1	Composition of Body Fluid Compartments	
	Extracellular Fluid	**Intracellular Fluid**
Osmolality (mOsm)	290–310	290–310
Cations (mEq/L)	**155**	**155**
Na^+	138–142	10
K^+	4.0–4.5	110
Ca^{2+}	4.5–5.0	—
Mg^{2+}	3	40
Anions (mEq/L)	**155**	**155**
Cl^-	103	—
HCO_3^-	27	—
HPO_4^{2-}	—	10
SO_4^{2-}	—	110
PO_4^{2-}	3	—
Organic acids	6	—
Protein	16	40

TABLE 7.2	Estimate of Circulating Blood Volume
Age	**Estimated Blood Volume (mL/kg)**
Preterm infant	100
Full-term neonate	90
Infant	80
School age (5 years)	70
Adults	70

MATURATION OF HOMEOSTATIC MECHANISMS

Renal development begins at approximately 5 weeks gestation and continues in a centrifugal pattern until the full complement of nephrons is present by about the 38th week. In the outermost regions of the renal cortex, differentiation of nephrons continues postnatally for several weeks to months. In the early stages of gestation, renal blood flow is approximately one-fifth of adult values. Initially, this is related to structural immaturity, and later it is caused by increased renovascular resistance. By 38 weeks gestation, renal blood flow is approximately one-third of adult values; high renovascular resistance protects the developing nephron from both pressure and volume overload. The resulting renal contribution to metabolic homeostasis in utero is limited.

As in the pulmonary vascular bed, renal vascular resistance decreases after birth, abruptly increasing renal blood flow. At that time, renal function increases only marginally above that predicted by postmenstrual age.[26] In utero, urine output is brisk despite a low GFR, owing to the poor reabsorption of salt and water.

(approximately 86 mL/kg), then returns to near 80 mL/kg and finally stabilizes at ~70 mL/kg by the end of the first year of life. In general, the ratio of blood volume to weight decreases with growth. The lean body mass is the most accurate basis to predict the blood volume, a measurement that is independent of the variation in sex even into adulthood.[25] Estimates of the circulating blood volume for each age are presented in Table 7.2.

Plasma renin activity is increased in utero, decreases immediately after birth, and then increases again as excess extracellular water is mobilized and excreted. Aldosterone concentrations are increased in cord blood and are maintained at this concentration for the first 3 days of life. The increased aldosterone may be necessary for sodium retention during periods of increased anabolism early in life.

Intrarenal gradients of sodium chloride (NaCl) and urea are less steep in the immature kidney, and full nephron growth has yet to be achieved. Consequently, urine-concentrating ability is limited in neonates, with maximum urine osmolality being about half that of the adult (700–800 mEq/L vs. 1300–1400 mEq/L). In part, this also relates to low circulating concentrations of ADH and decreased renal responsiveness to ADH. Although overall ADH production is not impaired, excessive secretion may occur in some disease states. Limited urine-concentrating ability necessitates large urine volumes for elimination of large solute loads.

Renal plasma flow and GFR (based on body surface area or allometry) are 30% of adult values in neonates. Both increase during the first year, reaching 50% of adult values by 6 months of age, 350 and 70 mL/minute per meter squared, respectively, and 90% by approximately 1 year[27] (see Figs. 5.12 and 5.13).[28] At birth, the serum creatinine reflects the maternal concentration of creatinine, which may be increased in term and preterm infants, but normalizes in the second month after birth,[29] reflecting creatinine production/elimination ratios. Fractional excretion of sodium (FE_{Na}) is markedly increased in preterm infants, decreases somewhat by term, and stabilizes at adult rates by the second month of life. Although the adult kidney may easily achieve FE_{Na} values as small as 0.5%, the 34-week-gestation infant is limited to no less than 2%.

These maturational features limit the ability of the preterm or young infant to handle large fluctuations in fluid and solute loads. Both sodium conservation and regulation of extracellular fluid volume are impaired when compared with the older child and adult. Limited GFR makes excretion of a fluid challenge difficult. Excessive urinary sodium loss leads to increased maintenance requirements; hyponatremia is common. Conversely, diminished concentrating ability increases free water losses during excretion of a solute load, whereas the high ratio of surface area to volume increases evaporative water loss. Consequently, fluid requirements are relatively large, and dehydration is common. Errors in fluid management are poorly tolerated. As a rule, the most severe impairment exists in preterm infants, and the majority of homeostatic mechanisms are fully developed after the first year of life.

Fluid and Electrolyte Requirements

Holliday has summarized the evolution of contemporary hydration therapy.[21] In 1831, the use of intravenous (IV) fluids to resuscitate patients dehydrated by cholera was described.[30] In 1918, nine infants were successfully treated by intraperitoneal injection of IV fluids[31] and then in 1923, Gamble and associates detailed the anatomy of fluid and electrolyte compartments, introducing the use of milliequivalents to clinical practice.[22] This paved the way for the development of the "deficit therapy" regimen of Darrow.[32]

In subsequent decades, various recipes to replace the extracellular and intracellular fluid losses were suggested. For the most part, they failed because of excessive potassium and insufficient sodium content. When the focus of the treatment shifted to replacing the extracellular fluid deficit, rapid restoration of extracellular fluid volume using solutions with sodium concentrations similar to those in blood became commonplace. This, along with oral rehydration, is the preferred method of treatment today.

The concept of "maintenance fluids" is a complex subject. Although water and salt are required to sustain life, it is fair to say that for any individual child at any particular time, the precise amounts necessary are unknown. Instead, fluids and electrolytes, like anesthetics, are titrated to effect with general guidelines provided by clinical assessment, basic physiologic principles, and limited published data. The term *maintenance fluids* is often more limiting than helpful, and in all cases, it is less precise than other terms familiar to anesthesiologists, such as *minimum alveolar concentration* (MAC) or *median effective dose* (ED_{50}).

Holliday and Segar provided calculations for a first approximation of *"the maintenance need for water in parenteral fluid therapy"* in 1957.[33] Integrating the relevant known physiology at that time, these authors observed that *"insensible loss of water and urinary water loss roughly parallel energy metabolism and do not parallel weight."* However, because water utilization parallels energy metabolism, energy metabolism has a curvilinear relationship to weight, commonly characterized using body surface area in humans. Body surface area can be described allometrically using an exponent of 2/3.[34] Consequently, it is possible to derive an estimated water requirement from weight alone using "diminishing returns" as the curvilinear relationship plateaus. The authors then proceeded under a series of assumptions to extrapolate from limited data to a *"relationship between weight and energy expenditure that might easily be remembered."*

Assuming energy requirements of *"hospitalized patients"* to be *"roughly midway between basal and normal levels,"* they constructed a curve of caloric requirement versus weight.[33] This curve could be seen as consisting of three linear sections: 0 to 10 kilograms, 10 to 20 kilograms, and 20 to 70 kilograms (Fig. 7.5). Viewing the curve in this manner, the authors reasoned that *"fortuitously, the average need for water, expressed in milliliters, equals energy expenditure in calories"*: 100 mL/kg per day for weights to 10 kilograms, an additional 50 mL/kg per day for each kilogram

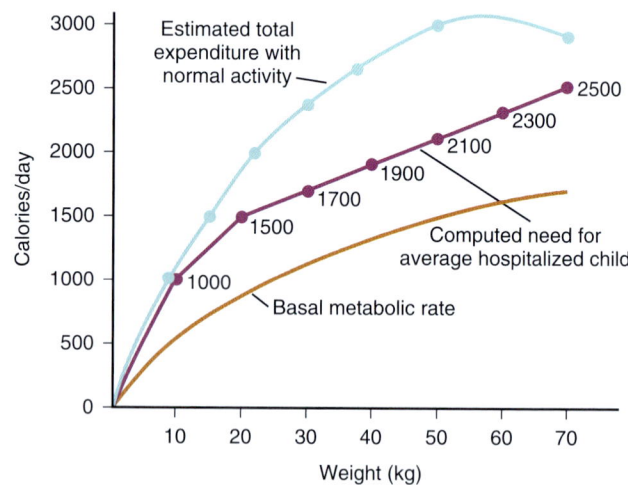

Comparison of Energy Expenditure in Basal and Ideal State

FIGURE 7.5 The upper and lower curves were plotted from data from the study by Talbot.[262] Weights at the 50th percentile level were selected for converting calories at various ages to calories related to weight. The computed line for the average hospitalized child was derived from the equations:
- 0–10 kg: 100 kcal/kg.
- 10–20 kg: 1000 kcal + 50 kcal/kg for each kg over 10 kg
- ≥20 kg: 1500 kcal + 20 kcal/kg for each kg over 20 kg

(From Holliday MA, Segar WE. The maintenance need for water in parenteral fluid therapy. *Pediatrics.* 1957;19:823-832.)

TABLE 7.3 | Relationship Between Weight and Hourly or Daily Maintenance Fluid Requirements of Children as per the 4-2-1 Rule

Weight (kg)	MAINTENANCE FLUID REQUIREMENTS	
	Hour	Day
<10	4 mL/kg	100 mL/kg
10–20	40 mL + 2 mL/kg for every kg >10 kg	1000 mL + 50 mL/kg for every kg >10 kg
>20	60 mL + 1 mL/kg for every kg >20 kg	1500 mL + 20 mL/kg for every kg >20 kg

TABLE 7.4 | Normal Water Losses for Infants and Children

Cause of Loss	Volume of Loss (mL/100 kcal)
Output	
• Urine	70
• Insensible loss	
Skin	30
Respiratory tract	15
Hidden intake (from burning 100 calories)	15
Total	100

TABLE 7.5 | Perioperative Causes of Increased Antidiuretic Hormone Release

Nonosmotic
Pain
Inflammation
Stress, catecholamines
Surgery; laparoscopic surgery
Vomiting
Hypoxia
Hypercapnia
Medications (e.g., opioids, amiodarone, vincristine)
Respiratory diseases (e.g., asthma, pneumonia, atelectasis)
Central nervous system disorders (e.g., head injury, tumors)
Osmotic
Fasting
Hypovolemia
Hypertonicity
Hypotension
Renal insufficiency
Hepatic insufficiency

from 11 to 20 kilograms, and 20 mL/kg per day more for each kilogram beyond 20 kilograms. In anesthetic practice, this formula has been further simplified, with the hourly requirement referred to as the "4-2-1 rule" (4 mL/kg per hour for the first 10 kilograms of weight, 2 mL/kg per hour for the next 10 kilograms, and 1 mL/kg per hour for each kilogram thereafter; Table 7.3).

For decades, the simplicity and elegance of the Holliday and Segar formula made it the starting point for fluid management in healthy children. At the beginning of this century, many anesthesiologists used the Holliday and Segar estimate to guide administration of hyponatremic glucose-containing solutions to children undergoing elective surgery.[35] However, the uncritical use of these solutions was never intended, and broad application to replace fluid loss during surgery eventually led to instances of hyponatremia, aspiration, and death in children.[36–38] Further, as Holliday has since pointed out, the original approach did not consider near-isotonic solutions[39] or acute illness and surgery in which physiologic stress and increased ADH are present. Thus, *"understanding of the limitations and of exceptions to the system [is] required. Even more essential is the clinical judgment to modify the system as circumstances dictate."*[39] General water losses for infants and children are summarized in Table 7.4.

Holliday and colleagues ultimately revised the approach to fluid therapy that they had originally offered.[40] In a related commentary, they pointed out the pitfalls in applying the original 4-2-1 rule to acutely ill children undergoing surgery.[41] Chiefly, ADH secretion is upregulated by a host of nonosmotic factors (pain, stress, mechanical ventilation, medications) common in acute illnesses (Table 7.5).[42] As a result, the choice of intravenous fluid and the rapidity of deficit replacement must be approached with care. The authors recommended a relatively simple strategy for healthy children undergoing elective surgery (including outpatients) to turn off ADH secretion and prevent perioperative water retention with subsequent hyponatremia beginning with using

isotonic rather than hypotonic solutions.[43] When a child without significant heart or kidney disease presents with marginal to moderate hypovolemia (e.g., after fasting for surgery), 20 to 40 mL/kg of isotonic fluids can be given during the surgery and postanesthesia care unit stay, at rates of 10 to 20 mL/kg per hour.[42] There is even some evidence that super-hydration (as much as 30 mL/kg per hour) with isotonic solutions in healthy children undergoing outpatient surgery may decrease the incidence of postoperative nausea and vomiting.[44,45] Clinical judgment must always allow for modification of these recommendations if indicated for an individual child.[39,46] If hypovolemia is more severe (e.g., after an extensive bowel preparation), 40 to 80 mL/kg may be necessary during the perioperative period. Some have expressed concern that such volumes of fluid could cause volume overload even in healthy children. However, children handle crystalloid volumes much more efficiently than adults.[47]

Postoperative IV fluid therapy should consist of an isotonic solution infused to replace ongoing fluid losses plus about half the rate described in the original 4-2-1 fluid regimen (i.e., 2 mL/kg for the first 10 kilograms, 1 mL/kg for the next 10 kilograms, and 0.5 mL/kg for each additional kilogram thereafter).[39] Historically, when a child is unable to tolerate oral intake postoperatively, routine maintenance fluid therapy has been resumed 6 to 12 hours postoperatively with hypotonic saline solution (e.g., 0.45% saline).[40] Although this regimen may effectively blunt the ADH response and reduce the risk of postoperative hyponatremia and hypernatremia,[39,40,46] persistent pain and surgical stress can maintain upregulated ADH levels, increasing the risk of hyponatremia with seizures and encephalopathy.[37,38,48–50] In the postoperative setting, therefore, an isotonic salt solution is a better choice for maintenance[51] at a rate of 2-1-0.5 rule for the first 12 hours then returning to the 4-2-1 rule with a hypotonic glucose-containing solution thereafter, until the child tolerates oral fluids.[38,52,53] Regardless of the fluids administered, it remains prudent to serially monitor plasma electrolyte concentrations until the child is drinking fluids normally and homeostasis is restored.[51,54,55]

NEONATAL FLUID MANAGEMENT

In the first few postnatal days, isotonic losses of salt and water cause the healthy neonate to lose 5% to 15% of body weight. Although GFR increases rapidly, urine output is initially minimal, and renal losses are modest. Day 1 fluid requirements of the wrapped neonate, therefore, are relatively small. Over the next few postnatal days, losses and fluid requirements increase. In the poorly feeding infant, progression to hypernatremia and dehydration are common. When intake is appropriate, the term infant will regain body weight during the first week.

Three distinct phases of fluid and electrolyte homeostasis have been described in low–birth-weight[56] and very low–birth-weight (VLBW)[57] infants. In the first postnatal day, there is minimal urine output, and body weight is stable despite limited fluid intake. In the second phase, days 2 and 3 of life, diuresis occurs irrespective of the amount of fluid administered. By days 4 and 5, urine output begins to vary with changes in fluid intake and state of health.

Prematurity increases neonatal fluid requirements substantively. Fluid requirements are therefore estimated and then titrated to the infant's changing weight, urine output, and serum sodium concentration.

No less important is glucose homeostasis. In the ninth month of gestation, the fetus begins to form glycogen stores at a rate of more than 100 kcal/day. In the unstressed, term infant, hepatic glycogen stores are ~5% of body weight. Immediately after birth, glycogenolysis depletes most of these stores within the first 24 to 48 hours. Gluconeogenesis must then proceed to yield glucose at a rate of approximately 4 mg/kg per minute.

At birth, the serum glucose concentration in the fetus is 60% to 70% of the maternal value. This may decrease within the first postnatal hours before recovering but should exceed 45 mg/dL (2.5 mmol/L) to avoid neurologic injury. Symptoms of hypoglycemia may include jitteriness, lethargy, temperature instability, and seizures. 10% dextrose in water ($D_{10}W$) may be given as a bolus of 2 to 4 mL/kg followed by a continuous infusion (using a pump) at 4 to 6 mg/kg per minute. The serum glucose concentration is then analyzed frequently, and the infusion adjusted as necessary to prevent hypoglycemia and hyperglycemia. Alternately, a 40% dextrose gel may be applied to the buccal mucosa for rapid absorption and resolution of hypoglycemia.[58,59] This obviates the need for IV access if not established by this time. It is important that the amount of glucose being provided be calculated in milligrams per kilogram per minute to avoid errors during fluid changes and to facilitate the diagnosis of persistent hypoglycemia.

Typical *day 1* infant fluid orders recommend 70 to 80 mL/kg of $D_{10}W$. Because $D_{10}W$ contains 10 g of glucose per deciliter, this regimen provides:

$$10 \text{ g/dL} \times 70 \text{ to } 80 \text{ mL/kg per day} = 7 \text{ to } 8 \text{ g/kg per day}$$
$$= 0.33 \text{ g/kg per hour}$$
$$= 5 \text{ mg/kg per minute}$$

On *day 2,* fluids are routinely increased to at least 100 mL/kg per day, and sodium is added at 2 to 3 mEq/dL. After urine output is established, potassium is added at 1 to 2 mEq/dL. The final solution, containing 30 mEq Na^+ and 10 to 20 mEq K^+ per liter, approximates the 0.2% saline "maintenance" solution commonly used in older children.

In the neonatal intensive care unit (ICU), fluid management focuses on provision of adequate nutrition, maintenance of electrolyte balance, and limitation of fluid overload. The last factor is of particular concern because plasma oncotic pressure is reduced in premature infants and the whole-body protein reflection coefficient is less than that in adults.[60] VLBW infants are at particular risk for fluid and electrolyte imbalances.[61] Even modest fluid overload may exacerbate pulmonary edema, prolong ductal patency, and more readily produce congestive heart failure. This perspective typically accompanies the infant to the operating room, where the primary considerations are routinely quite the opposite: restoration of circulating blood volume after third-space accumulation, maintenance of intravascular volume amid ongoing blood loss, replacement of potentially massive evaporative losses, and maintenance of blood pressure despite anesthetic-induced vasodilatation and increased venous capacitance. During surgery, these concerns must take precedence, yet unnecessary administration of fluid is best avoided.

Intraoperative Fluid Management

INTRAVENOUS ACCESS AND FLUID ADMINISTRATION DEVICES

In infants and children, the first step toward intraoperative fluid management is often the most challenging: establishing IV access. In general, simple procedures in healthy children are successfully approached using a single peripheral IV line. Although preferences vary among anesthesiologists, establishing IV access is most easily accomplished after induction of anesthesia. In young children, anesthesia is often induced by inhalation, and a catheter is inserted by an assistant into a hand or foot vein. In older children, or when IV access is desirable before anesthesia is induced, IV access may be facilitated by using topical anesthesia (e.g., EMLA [eutectic mixture of local anesthetics] cream, Synera patches [lidocaine & tetracaine], lidocaine via J-Tip or via infiltration), sedation, or both.[62]

Complex surgery in sicker children usually requires at least two large-bore catheters. In pediatrics, however, "large-bore" is a relative term, with 22-gauge catheters typically providing adequate access in infants. Preferred sites for larger catheters include the antecubital and saphenous veins (see Fig. 46.1). Ultrasound-guided IV access is preferred to improve first pass success rates in children with a history of difficult placement.[63]

In cases where access to the central circulation is required (as for pressure monitoring, infusion of vasoactive medications, or prolonged access), longer catheters may be placed using the femoral, subclavian, or internal jugular vein (the latter usually via a cephalad, anterior approach; see Figs. 46.2–46.7).[64] Although secure access may also be obtained via the external jugular vein, it is often difficult to negotiate the J-wire or catheter tip into the central circulation.[65] Peripherally inserted central catheter (PICC) lines have become common in hospitalized children. Although they represent a long-term means of delivering IV fluids and medications, their intraoperative utility is very limited for several reasons. First, patient safety practices prohibit repeated access to central lines and practitioners must maintain strict sterile technique whenever entering them. Second, flow resistance is great within long, small-diameter catheters, precluding their use for large-volume resuscitation. Finally, PICCs are often placed for delivery of hyperalimentation or other solutions, which may be incompatible with anesthetic medications. For these reasons and others, separate IV access is often required and secure larger-bore shorter IV catheters with much less resistance must be placed if large fluid shifts or blood loss is anticipated.

When selecting the appropriate IV catheter, it is useful to consider the relative effects of catheter length and diameter on solution flow rates.[66] Longer catheters offer more resistance to flow than shorter ones and are therefore less desirable when rapid infusion of a large volume of fluids is necessary (see E-Figs. 49.2 and 49.3, and Fig. 49.1). In vitro, catheters designed for peripheral venous access had 18% to 164% greater flow rates compared with the same-gauge catheters designed for central venous use. Under pressure, as might be used during emergent volume resuscitation, flow rates differed up to 17-fold.[67] Although this seems to suggest that short peripheral catheters should be preferred, in vivo data are more complex. In animal models, overall catheter flow rates are less than in vitro rates, and central access can sometimes present somewhat less resistance to flow than peripheral access.[68] Finally, when the risks and benefits of central versus peripheral access are compared, central administration of resuscitation medications may provide little practical advantage compared with peripheral administration.[69]

Intraosseous devices are now commonly used in the initial resuscitation of critically ill or injured children (see Figs. 46.3 and 46.4).[62,70,71] Flow rates via these devices depend less on needle diameter than on resistance in the marrow compartment.[72] In the operating room, the intraosseous route has been used for both induction and maintenance of anesthesia.[73–75] However, onset of drug effect is less predictable and the device is more easily dislodged than an IV catheter. Potential complications include compartment syndrome[76–78] and, very rarely, growth plate injury.[71,79] On balance, therefore, intraosseous devices are still best considered as emergency secondary options (see Chapter 46).[74]

To prevent accidental volume overload, particularly in infants and very small children, the volume of fluid directly available for infusion should not exceed the child's calculated hourly requirement; a volumetric chamber should be used to accomplish this. Similarly, a microdrip infusion set limits the rate of fluid administration and permits much greater control. Although a fluid infusion pump provides the most precise mode of regulating the rate of fluid administration (and is therefore very useful in providing supplemental fluids or medications), such devices are impractical on primary access lines because they hinder the ability to administer drugs and fluids rapidly. In addition, the clinician should be mindful that pumps may continue to infuse through dislodged catheters, giving misleading reassurance that adequate IV access is secure, and fluids are being administered.

In neonates and small infants, when rapid infusion of resuscitation solutions or blood products is anticipated, many practitioners include a stopcock manifold in the IV setup. With a manifold in place, fluid may be prepared in syringes and prewarmed for rapid infusion during periods of sudden blood loss. In prolonged surgeries, or when volume replacement is great, all IV infusions should be warmed to maintain thermal homeostasis. In younger infants and children in whom communication exists between the right and left sides of the circulation (e.g., patency of the foramen ovale), an in-line "bubble" filter is appropriate.

CHOICE AND COMPOSITION OF INTRAVENOUS FLUIDS

In the early 1960s,[80] simultaneous measurements of intravascular and interstitial fluid volumes demonstrated that intravascular volume is initially supported by fluid shifts from the extravascular space during surgery. At the same time, it was also observed that IV resuscitation fluids redistributed from the intravascular space to a nonfunctional "third" space, which was unavailable to the circulation. This "third space" is now understood as simply expansion of the interstitial space due to disruption of the endothelial glycocalyx. The escape rate of albumin from capillaries to interstitium is normally ~5% of the plasma albumin per hour. However, during surgery this rate can double and further increase to more than four-fold in septic shock.[81] Because of the differences in fluid distribution and renal function in infants compared with older children, at first it was unclear that these findings could be extended to infancy. Thus fluid restriction remained the standard of care in infants until careful studies conclusively demonstrated that fluid and electrolyte requirements are often extremely large in neonates undergoing major surgery.[82–84]

Historically, hypotonic fluids were the preferred inpatient maintenance solutions but, as suggested earlier, this is no longer practice. Isotonic solutions are preferred intraoperatively for several reasons.[43] First, most ongoing volume losses are isotonic, consisting of shed blood and interstitial fluids. Second, large volumes of hypotonic solutions may rapidly diminish serum osmolality, producing very low concentrations of electrolytes (in particular, sodium) and undesirable fluid shifts. Indeed, even large volumes of "isotonic" fluids significantly decrease the serum osmolality in adult volunteers.[85] As a result, there is a risk of hyponatremia after an infusion of hypotonic fluids in hospitalized children after only 12 hours of use.[86] Third, plasma volume expansion that is necessary to diminish vascular tone under anesthesia may be difficult to achieve even with isotonic fluids. Finally, increases in ADH concentrations and other elements of intraoperative physiology will persist and retain free water in excess of sodium if the intravascular volume has not been restored to euvolemia with an infusion of isotonic fluids.[50]

The compositions of commonly used intravenous solutions are presented in Table 7.6. Assuming that normal plasma osmolality is 275 to 290 mOsm/L, 0.9% NaCl (normal saline [NS]) is

TABLE 7.6	Composition of Extracellular Fluid and Common Intravenous Solutions								
		CATIONS (mEq/L)			ANIONS (mEq/L)				
	mOsm/L	Na+	K+	Ca2+	Mg2+	NH4+	Cl−	HCO3−	HPO4−
Extracellular fluid	280–300	142	4	5	3	0.3	103	27	3
Lactated Ringer's (LR) solution	273	130	4	3			109	28	
0.45% NaCl	154	77					77		
0.9% NaCl (normal saline)	308	154					154		
Plasma-Lyte A[a]	294	140	5		3	1.6	98	98	
3% NaCl	1024	513					513		

[a]Plasma-Lyte is a trademark of Baxter International Inc., its subsidiaries or affiliates. (Plasma-Lyte also contains acetate 27 mEq/L and gluconate 23 mEq/L.)

theoretically hypertonic to plasma but is effectively isotonic when the in vivo activities of its constituents are considered.[87] For dextrose-containing solutions, the osmolality decreases rapidly as sugar is metabolized, resulting in increased volumes of free water. Therefore, administration of 5% dextrose in water is ultimately equivalent to administering free water and should be avoided.

COLLOID SOLUTIONS

Colloids consist of natural protein colloids (albumin) and synthetic colloids (gelatins, dextrans, and hydroxyethyl starches). Colloids carry theoretical benefits over crystalloid solutions in their ability to rapidly expand intravascular volume and remain longer in the intravascular space. They hold promise for maintaining circulation more effectively than crystalloid, preserving intravascular oncotic pressure, and reducing pulmonary edema related to dilutional hypoalbuminemia.[88] Crystalloid solutions, however, are much less expensive, are easier to store, have few general adverse effects, and do not carry colloid's potential for anaphylaxis. These competing risks and benefits have fueled decades of research.

There have been many studies comparing colloids and crystalloids without clear benefit in adults.[89] Subgroup analyses from later trials suggested that some patients, such as those with head injury,[90] may be harmed by albumin, whereas others, such as those with septic shock,[91] may realize some benefit. In adult ICU patients with hypovolemia, there was no difference seen in 28-day mortality between colloid- and crystalloid-treated groups. Mortality was slightly improved at 90 days in patients who received colloids but the study could not determine efficacy.[92] A Cochrane review in critically ill adults showed that mortality was not affected whether colloids or crystalloids were infused.[93] In adults undergoing major abdominal surgery, the use of colloids and crystalloids in a closed loop system for goal-directed therapy using stroke volume and a stroke volume variation to direct fluid management demonstrated that patients treated with colloids experienced fewer postoperative complications than those given crystalloids, which may be related to a reduced fluid balance.[94]

Several studies in children have been forthcoming evaluating these fluids. Albumin is the colloid used most often in neonates and infants.[95] The choice of solution may depend on the underlying medical conditions and remains a matter of clinical judgment. The first study of 20 mL/kg modified 4% gelatin in either balanced salt solution or saline in children less than 12 years of age undergoing major surgery reported that both solutions were safe and effective, although the acid-base balance was superior with a balanced salt solution with the 4% gel.[96] In a retrospective study of 86 children <5 years of age undergoing neurosurgery with a blood loss >10% of their blood volume, the children received either hydroxyethyl starch or human albumen. Both fluids were effective with minor clotting differences and trends to differences in length of stay suggested that a randomized trial with these fluids is warranted.[97]

HYDROXYETHYL STARCHES

Hydroxyethyl starches (HES) are synthetic colloids that are simply modified polysaccharides. Circulating amylases quickly degrade natural polysaccharides, but HES solutions are not quickly degraded because the solutes contain hydroxyethyl groups in place of hydroxyl groups at carbon positions C-2, C-3, and C-6, rendering the molecules resistant to hydrolysis. These compounds are characterized by three attributes: average mean molecular weight (MW), molar substitution (MS), and the C-2/C-6 ratio, which relates to the relative positions of hydroxyethyl groups on the polysaccharide molecule.

HES solutions with a greater MW/MS ratio remain in the intravascular space for longer periods than those with smaller ratios. However, they also are prone to more adverse effects including hypocoagulability. Newer, smaller MW/smaller MS solutions have much less effect on hemostatic mechanisms than older, greater MW/greater MS solutions. The precise mechanism by which HES compounds affect coagulation remains unclear, although it has been attributed to interference with von Willebrand factor, factor VIII, thrombin formation, and platelet function.[98–103] A greater C-2/C-6 ratio is responsible for a slower degradation of the starch by amylase with fewer adverse effects.[95] When renal function is normal, newer HES solutions (e.g., HES 130/0.42/6:1) are safe for children undergoing elective surgery, since they maintain hemodynamic stability and produce only mild to moderate changes in acid-base status.[104] Synthetic colloids such as these can therefore be considered in surgical patients who demonstrate the need for aggressive intraoperative fluid resuscitation (see also Chapter 10).

In recent years, HES solutions have fallen out of favor in the adult population.[105] A review in adults that examined the effects of HES on kidney function compared with other fluid therapies in critically ill patients reported that HES products were associated with a 59% increased risk of kidney failure and a 32% increased risk of dialysis.[106,107] Other studies have not found these effects in adult patients at risk of postoperative kidney injury undergoing major abdominal surgery.[108] Concerns have also been raised over the increased risk of death in septic patients who receive HES solutions.[105] Lastly, a large number of trials on HES were retracted because of malfeasance by a single investigator, J. Boldt, which pitched the literature on HES into disarray.[109] One-third of the randomized controlled trials were withdrawn and the remaining 28 trials had low power. The net effect of the remaining publications failed to prove HES is safer than other volume expanders.[110,111]

Use of these solutions in cardiac surgery remains controversial. A meta-analysis showed that HES solutions increased blood loss, reoperation for bleeding, and blood product transfusion after cardiopulmonary bypass in adults. There was no evidence that these risks could be mitigated by lower molecular weight and substitution,[112] given the effects on coagulation factors and platelet function induced by the cardiopulmonary bypass circuit. A study in pediatric cardiac surgery patients did not find that HES solutions were associated with postoperative kidney injury.[113] Although these studies may not all be fully applicable to the general pediatric population, the findings warrant caution when considering the use of HES solutions.

The US Food and Drug Administration (FDA), which originally approved HES solutions for the treatment of hypovolemia, recently added a black box warning.[114] The warning highlights the risk of mortality, kidney injury, and excess bleeding. There is also a statement that HES products should not be used unless adequate alternative treatment is unavailable.[114] Similar concerns and warnings have also been raised in the United Kingdom and other countries.[105]

GLUCOSE SOLUTIONS

The routine intraoperative use of glucose-containing solutions has also been a subject of debate. As a rule, operative stress evokes physiologic responses that increase serum glucose. In practice, therefore, hypoglycemia is seldom a problem in healthy, fasted children when glucose is omitted from perioperative IV fluids.[115,116] The risk should be particularly small if the period of fasting is limited to less than 10 hours.[116] At the same time, rapid administration of dextrose solutions may produce acute hypergly-cemia and hyperosmolality.[115,116] Therefore, glucose-containing electrolyte solutions should not be used to replace fluid deficits, third-space losses, or blood losses, but may be used for background maintenance.[117] Some populations, such as debilitated infants,[118] children who are malnourished, neonates and infants younger than 6 months of age,[115,119,120] and those undergoing cardiac surgery, are at risk for intraoperative hypoglycemia.[121,122] In such cases, glu-cose-containing solutions (1%–2.5% dextrose)[115,117,119,123] along with intraoperative glucose monitoring are advised.

Concerns regarding the routine intraoperative use of dextrose-containing solutions increased with recognition that hyperglyce-mia may exacerbate neurologic injury after an ischemic or hypoxic event.[124,125] As a result, many clinicians now elect to avoid dex-trose-containing solutions during routine surgery. When dextrose-containing solutions are used, appropriate monitoring is advised to avoid serum glucose extremes. Many practitioners administer glucose-containing solutions as a separate piggyback infusion us-ing an infusion pump or other rate- or volume-limiting device to avoid accidental bolus administration. Alternatively, evidence in-dicates that isotonic solutions containing reduced glucose concen-trations (e.g., 1% or 2.5% vs. 5%) are safe alternative solutions for intraoperative use.[126]

An adult study with tight glucose control in the surgical ICU showed reduced morbidity and mortality with blood glucose in the range of 81 to 110 mg/dL (4.5–6.1 mmol/L).[127] However, another multicenter study showed that intensive glucose control increased mortality in adult ICU patients.[128] A similar study was conducted in pediatrics, which found that critically ill children with hyperglycemia did not benefit from tight glycemic control. An upper-end level for treatment is a glucose level of 150 to 180 mg/dL (8.3–10 mmol/L).[129]

In the United States, several FDA–approved solutions contain-ing 2.5% dextrose are available, but none with concentrations lower than 2.5%. In Europe, 1% dextrose electrolyte solutions are available.[117,119,126] Because intraoperative administration of solu-tions containing 5% dextrose (D_5 lactated Ringer's solution) fre-quently causes hyperglycemia, anesthesiologists should selectively administer dextrose-containing solutions to those who are at particular risk for intraoperative hypoglycemia (i.e., neonates, chronically malnourished children, and cachectic children). In these instances, it may be sensible to administer solutions with a reduced dextrose concentration.[95,117,119]

HYPERALIMENTATION

It is now common practice that critically ill children arrive in the operating room with hyperalimentation solutions infusing. Common contents of hyperalimentation solutions are shown in Table 7.7. In general, children require 0.5 to 3.0 mg/kg per day of protein, 6 to 9 mg/kg per minute of glucose, and 0.5 to 3 g/kg per day of fat. Children receiving parenteral nutrition preoperatively should continue to receive those infusions separately, and a cor-responding volume should be deducted from isotonic operative fluids. Hyperalimentation typically consists of two infusions: fat (e.g., Intralipid, Omegaven, SMOFlipid from Fresenius Kabi; Nutrilipid from B. Braun) and a concentrated glucose/protein solution. Lipid-containing lines carry high risk for infection, so it is prudent to discontinue the lipid solutions during surgery. When this is not possible, lipid ports should not be accessed, and great care must be taken to avoid contamination.

Conversely, preoperative infusions of concentrated glucose/protein solutions should be continued, since circulating insulin

TABLE 7.7	Common Contents of Parenteral Nutrition Solutions[a]
Carbohydrates	
10%, 12.5%, 20%, 25%, 30% Dextrose	
Limited to D_{10} or $D_{12.5}$ if through a peripheral catheter	
Protein	
In the form of amino acids	
0.5, 1.0, 1.5, 2.0, 2.5, or 3.0 g/kg per day	
Lipids[b]	
10%, 20% Lipids	
Oil Sources: Soybean, Fish, Olive, MCT (Medium Chain Triglycerides)	
Standard Additives	
Sodium: 30 mEq/L	
Potassium: 20 mEq/L	
Calcium: 15 mEq/L	
Magnesium: 10 mEq/L	
Phosphorus: 10 mmol/L	
Heparin	

[a]Common contents of parenteral nutrition solutions containing dextrose, protein, lipids, and standard additives such as electrolytes. These values represent standard starting points that may be modified based on individual patient needs.
[b]Lipid composition may vary based on brand used. Brands include Intralipid, Nutrilipid, Omegaven, and SMOFlipid.

levels have equilibrated. However, reduced metabolism under anesthesia and anticipated hyperglycemic responses to surgical stress led some practitioners to empirically decrease hyperalimen-tation infusion rates by one-third to one-half. If this practice is followed, it is prudent to measure serum glucose concentrations at regular intervals. Under no circumstances should concentrated glucose solutions (such as D_{10} or D_{20}) be abruptly discontinued, since high concentrations of circulating insulin may cause a pre-cipitous and profound decrease in the serum glucose concentration.

FASTING RECOMMENDATIONS

The goal of fasting is to minimize the volume of gastric contents and thereby lessen the risk of vomiting and aspiration during in-duction of anesthesia. In children, as opposed to adults, this is a particular concern since inhalation inductions are common and there are longer periods of vulnerability to regurgitation. Particu-larly in very small children, the effectiveness of fasting in reducing aspiration risk must be weighed against the potential stress and discomfort of dehydration. Numerous studies of gastric volume and pH have convincingly demonstrated that clear liquids are rapidly emptied from the stomach and the stimulated peristalsis actually serves to decrease gastric volume and acidity. Fasting 2 hours after clears ensures an empty stomach, whereas the risk of dehydration is unlikely. The benefits of improved hydration and mental status after a brief fast render prolonged *nil per os* (NPO) unwarranted and possibly deleterious to children. Clear fluids are emptied from the stomach with a half-life of ~20 minutes,[130] depending, in part, on the volume of sugar and other osmotic moieties in the fluid ingested.[131] A number of investigators have asserted that a 1 hour fast after clear fluids reduces the risk of prolonged fasts without increasing the risk of pneumonitis in healthy children presenting for elective anesthesia.[132,133] However, a large study from the Pediatric Sedation Consortium showed no association between NPO status and risk of aspiration; however, these patients generally did not undergo any airway manipulation as part of their sedation management.[134] NPO guidelines currently in use in many institutions are included in Table 2.1.[135] Some pediatric anesthesia societies in Europe have adopted fasting for 1 hour for clear fluids before elective anesthesia,[136] although the small number of or zero infants and children who actually fasted only 1 hour does not justify this shift in policy.[133,136–138]

Historically with longer fasting intervals, it was recommended to replace the fluid "deficit" that resulted from fasting. This was accomplished by providing an extra volume of "maintenance" fluids corresponding to the volume "missed" during fasting. For example, a 20 kg child fasted for 8 hours would have a calculated deficit of ~160 mL (60 mL/hour × 8 hours NPO). This "missed" volume would be replaced over 3 hours, with half in the first hour. In adults, circulating blood volumes after fasting has been shown to be normal,[139] and the need to replace a fluid deficit in all patients has been questioned.[140] In children, one study found no effect of clear fluid fasting on postinduction blood pressure, but prolonged clear fluid fasting times did increase the risk of hypotension during surgical preparation.[141] As described earlier, 20 to 40 mL/kg of lactated Ringer's solution given intraoperatively will provide adequate replacement for the vast majority of children.

ONGOING LOSSES AND THIRD-SPACING

During all surgical procedures, fluid loss from the vascular space is primarily the result of three simultaneous physiologic processes. First, whole blood is shed at various rates and must be replaced. Second, capillary leak and surgical trauma result in extravasation of isotonic, protein-containing fluid into interstitial compartments (the so-called third space). Third, anesthetic-induced relaxation of sympathetic tone produces vasodilatation (increased capacitance) and relative hypovolemia (a virtual loss). In very small infants, a fourth source of losses, direct evaporation, must also be considered. These ongoing losses are often difficult to quantitate or even estimate. Although these losses occur in children of all sizes, the small circulating blood volume of an infant (e.g., for a 5-kg infant, 80 mL/kg × 5 kg = 400 mL) leaves little room for error. Faced with uncertainty, the prudent response is constant vigilance, careful titration, and reliance on general principles.

As a rule, 1 mL of shed blood is initially replaced with 1 mL of colloid (5% albumin or blood) or about 1.5 to 3 mL of isotonic crystalloid such as lactated Ringer's solution.[89,123] Isotonic crystalloid is also used to replenish third-space losses. Surgical procedures that involve only mild tissue trauma may entail third-space losses of 3 to 4 mL/kg per hour. More extensive surgical procedures involving moderate trauma may require replacement equivalent to 5 to 7 mL/kg per hour to adequately support intravascular volume. In small infants undergoing very large abdominal procedures, the losses may approach 10 mL/kg per hour or more.[82,84] In neonates, fluid requirements for emergent abdominal surgery for necrotizing enterocolitis have been estimated at up to 50 mL/kg per hour.[123] These "losses" include both evaporation and redistribution of fluid to the interstitium. The latter must be considered most carefully because it is exacerbated by the hemodilution and increased capillary pressures that result from excessive fluid administration.

Although necessary intraoperatively, third-space accumulation represents whole-body salt and water overload that will need to be mobilized postoperatively. The price of unchecked fluid administration is generalized anasarca, pulmonary edema, bowel swelling, and laryngotracheal edema. In the healthy child, this relative fluid overload is well tolerated, with most excess fluid excreted over the first 2 postoperative days. In children with impaired pulmonary, cardiac, or renal function; however, such fluid excess may result in clinically important postoperative morbidity.

The enhanced recovery after surgery (ERAS) initiative has focused attention on the advisability of restricting intraoperative fluids. Many adult centers aim for intraoperative euvolemia[142] but there is concern that this practice cannot be extrapolated to children. A review of pediatric ERAS pathways did not show noteworthy benefits for children[143] and a study of restrictive fluid strategy during major pediatric abdominal surgery showed higher heart rates and more negative intraoperative base excess than controls. Children in the restrictive group had the same total fluid requirement and showed no differences in postoperative kidney function, chest x-ray, variation of body weight, or postoperative outcomes.[144] A meta-analysis of adult studies found no difference in severe postoperative complications between liberal and restrictive fluid groups, but patients receiving liberal fluids had fewer major renal events.[145] Taken together, ERAS studies suggest that fluids should be tailored to the individual patient, with careful monitoring, frequent reassessment, and careful titration to intraoperative needs.

ASSESSMENT OF INTRAVASCULAR VOLUME

Traditional clinical clues to volume status are often lost or confounded by operative events. Tachycardia, for example, may be a reasonable marker of volume status in the quietly resting child, but more related to anesthetic depth intraoperatively. Systolic blood pressure may be normal in the hypovolemic, but compensated, awake child and then plummet dramatically with induction. It is the challenge of the anesthesiologist to view the entire clinical picture, consider the possibilities, integrate them into a hypothesis, and then test the hypothesis.

Assessment of intravascular volume begins with knowledge of age-related norms for heart rate and blood pressure (see Tables 1.7 and 1.8). Is the heart rate persistently increased or does it vary only with surgical stimulation? Is the pulse pressure narrow or, more ominously, is the blood pressure reduced for age? Does it vary with positive-pressure breaths? Are the extremities warm? Is capillary refill brisk? What is the urine output? Are these variables changing? What is the rate of the change?

Measurement and continuous monitoring of central venous pressure (CVP) is commonly taken as both a direct measure of cardiac preload and an indirect measure of circulating volume (see Figs. 46.5 to 46.7). In addition to traditional central lines introduced into the superior vena cava or left atrium, animal[146] and limited clinical[147] data suggest that femoral lines that terminate in the abdominal vena cava may also be useful. In one study of infants and children, mean end-expiratory pressure measurements of venous pressure in the right atrial and inferior vena cava differed by less than 1 mm Hg.[147] Unfortunately, CVP as a static measure of volume status is confounded by many factors, including right ventricular compliance, positive end-expiratory pressure, abdominal pressure, and so on. In sum, these confounders may in some cases render the CVP a relatively poor predictor of preload and volume status.[148]

Dynamic assessments best reflect the volume status and "volume responsiveness" (>10%–15% increase in stroke volume after a bolus) best indicate the volume for administration.[149] The respiratory cycle produces cyclic changes in stroke volume that are augmented when the ventricle is underfilled. This is particularly true under positive-pressure ventilation. As a result, systolic blood pressure, diastolic blood pressure, and pulse pressure variation are readily apparent on the arterial waveform of a hypovolemic child (see Fig. 10.12). Pulse pressure variation may be quantified as $([PP_{max} - PP_{min}]/[PP_{max} + PP_{min}/2]) \times 100$, and volume responsiveness inferred from decreasing pulse pressure variation. With this guidance, volume has been administered by some in 5- to 10-mL/kg test challenges until systolic blood pressure and pulse pressure variation no longer respond.[148] However, the usefulness of variability to determine volume status in children continues to be debated and should be performed carefully.[150–152]

Goal-directed fluid management is one of the important components of ERAS programs. Technologies like esophageal Doppler or plethysmography variability index have been evaluated as a means of determining fluid responsiveness.[153] In a study of pediatric patients under 6 years of age who were spontaneously ventilating under anesthesia, Pleth Variability Index values were higher in patients who responded to fluid than those who did not. Pleth Variability Index also decreased predictably with passive leg raise, volume centralization, and increased stroke volume. The routine clinical utility of this technique remains uncertain as there appears to be some overlap between fluid responsive and nonfluid responsive patients; this monitor remains under study.[154] Similarly, ultrasound assessment of the inferior vena cava is routinely used for volume assessment in emergency departments and ICUs, but utility in the operating room is limited by case-type and access.[155,156] Other noninvasive methods for assessing continuous cardiac output even in preterm infants include bioimpedance and bioreactance which require simple ECG electrodes (see Figs. 49.11 and 49.12) and no other special equipment. Considerable data indicate a good correlation with other methods of assessment such as echocardiography and Fick calculations, but these have not yet been adopted into routine practice.[157–161]

Postoperative Fluid Management

GENERAL APPROACH

Well-planned postoperative fluid management complements the intraoperative plan and accounts for evolving physiology as the child recovers from anesthesia. Fluid deficits and ongoing losses are replaced, and the child is repeatedly reassessed, adjusting the intake until normal fluid and electrolyte homeostasis are present. To aid in decision making, trends in vital signs are identified, all sources of fluid intake and output quantitated, urine specific gravity is monitored, daily weights obtained, and serum electrolytes are measured.

In simple outpatient surgeries, discharge from the hospital is possible after fluid deficits have been replaced. In complex cases, replacement fluids may require hourly readjustment based on the prior hour's intake and output. Rather than reacting to isolated variables, such as low urine output, the overall pattern must be discerned. High urine output and low urine specific gravity may indicate overhydration or diabetes insipidus. Oliguria may suggest hypovolemia when it is accompanied by high urine specific gravity and clinical signs of dehydration or low cardiac output when it is accompanied by signs of poor perfusion. In the well-hydrated child, oliguria may represent renal failure if the urine specific gravity is normal (or dilute) but increased concentrations of ADH if the urine is concentrated. A careful physical examination is always necessary and, in challenging cases, certainty in diagnosis may require simultaneous measurement of serum and urine electrolytes.

Frequently, losses via surgical or gastric drains are large in both real and relative terms. For example, a neonate with a nasogastric tube may lose more than 100 mL/kg per day (normally 20–40 mL/kg per day) in gastric fluid. Therefore, in determining the volume and composition of replacement fluids, it is sometimes helpful to consider the electrolyte content of various losses (Table 7.8).

POSTOPERATIVE PHYSIOLOGY AND HYPONATREMIA

Children retain salt and water postoperatively, in part because of neuroendocrine activation by stress, continued capillary leak with third-space accumulation, nonosmotic stimulation of ADH (see Table 7.5) and hypovolemia-induced renin secretion. As outlined earlier, depleting the intravascular volume is a potent nonosmotic signal to retain fluid that may override osmotic signals under a variety of clinical circumstances.

At the same time, ongoing fluid and electrolyte losses after surgery via chest tubes, nasogastric suction, weeping incisions, and even continued slow bleeding may be substantial. Children often depend entirely on IV fluids to replace these and other postoperative losses. Unless isotonic, sodium-containing fluids are provided and the child is rendered euvolemic, children in the postoperative phase of recovery are universally at risk for developing hyponatremia.[50,86,162,163] In an older retrospective review of 24,412 surgical admissions to a large children's hospital, the incidence of postoperative hyponatremia was 0.34%, with a substantial mortality rate (8.4%) in these previously healthy children.[36] A more recent study using data from the American College of Surgeons National Surgical Quality Improvement Program–Pediatric

TABLE 7.8	Composition of Body Fluids					
Source	Na$^+$ (mEq/L)	K$^+$ (mEq/L)	Cl$^-$ (mEq/L)	HCO$_3^-$ (mEq/L)	pH	Osmolality (mOsm/L)
Gastric	50	10–15	150	0	1	300
Pancreas	140	5	0–100	100	9	300
Bile	130	5	100	40	8	300
Ileostomy	130	15–20	120	25–30	8	300
Diarrhea	50	35	40	50		
Sweat	50	5	55	0	Alkaline	
Blood	140	4–5	100	25	7.4	285–295
Urine	0–100[a]	20–100[a]	70–100[a]	0	4.5–8.5[a]	50–1400[a]

[a]Varies considerably with fluid intake.
From Herrin J. Fluid and electrolytes. In: Graef JW, ed. *Manual of Pediatric Therapeutics*. 6th ed. Philadelphia: Lippincott-Raven; 1997:63-75.

(2014 to 2015) reported preoperative hyponatremia to be present in ~15% of children (N = 5422) with an increased 30 day mortality (~0.8%), particularly in preterm infants (those with necrotizing enterocolitis and congenital diaphragmatic hernia).[164] This study suggests that the association of hyponatremia with adverse outcomes is not limited to postoperative care. Although postoperative mortality rates as great as 40% to 60% have been reported after hyponatremia, hyponatremia remains a surrogate marker for a disease with a poor prognosis rather than the actual cause of the death.[53,165,166]

In reviewing the etiology of hyponatremia, two factors stand out: extensive extrarenal loss of electrolyte-containing fluid and IV replacement with hypotonic fluids.[36,86] In addition, delay in recognition often plays a major role in associated morbidity. The solutions are simple: (1) administration of hypotonic fluids without a specific indication should be avoided postoperatively; only isotonic solutions should be administered during recovery, (2) ongoing losses should be replaced with balanced salt solutions in a timely fashion, and (3) serum electrolytes should be measured serially in children who exhibit potential symptoms of hyponatremia (see later discussion).

POSTOPERATIVE FLUID OVERLOAD

Children who receive large volumes of fluid intraoperatively are at risk for development of pulmonary edema as operative fluids are mobilized.[167] Usually, fluid begins to be mobilized on the second postoperative day and continues through day 3 or 4. Although this is less common in children than in the elderly, it occurs occasionally in children with burn injuries[168] or in pediatric patients receiving large amounts of fluid during resuscitation from trauma or sepsis. In one review,[169] 13 patients (11 adults and 2 children) developed postoperative pulmonary edema; all began to exhibit symptoms within 36 hours after surgery and had total net fluid retention in excess of 67 mL/kg postoperatively.

Fluid overload can contribute to more than pulmonary edema.[170] A recent study looking at fluid resuscitation in pediatric colectomy patients found that high-volume fluid administration intraoperatively was associated with longer length of stay, longer time to first meal >4 days, and need for supplemental oxygen requirement over 24 hours.[171] In pediatric cardiac surgery, higher fluids on the day of surgery contributed to fluid overload in the early postoperative period, and was associated with higher mortality and morbidity. Risk factors for fluid overload include underlying kidney dysfunction, hemodynamic instability, and higher blood loss on the day of the surgery.[172]

Pathophysiologic States and Their Management

FLUID OVERLOAD AND EDEMA

Edema is essentially a "sodium disease," representing sodium and water overload with excessive fluid residing in the extracellular space. Although intracellular volume changes can sometimes be substantial, prolonged cell swelling represents failure of essential volume-regulatory functions and is possibly a preterminal event. In fluid-overload states, plasma volume is generally increased unless the balance of Starling forces is disturbed, as in nephrotic syndrome or lymphatic obstruction. Edema formation is opposed by (1) low compliance of the interstitial compartment, (2) increased lymphatic flow, (3) osmotic washout of interstitial proteins, and (4) impedance and elasticity of the proteoglycan gel. The differential diagnosis of fluid overload and

TABLE 7.9	Differential Diagnosis of Fluid Overload and Edema Formation
Condition	**Differential Diagnosis**
Imbalance of intake and output	Salt poisoning
	Formula dilution errors
	Intravenous infusion errors
	Drugs given as sodium salts
Steroid excess with normal sodium intake	Congenital adrenal hyperplasia
	Exogenous steroids
Perceived decreases in effective plasma volume	↓ MAP → baroreceptors → ↑ sympathetic tone, ADH, renin, aldosterone
	Vasodilators
	Congestive heart failure
	Cirrhosis
	Nephrotic syndrome
Impaired sodium excretion	Chronic renal failure
	Acute glomerular disease (↓ GFR with normal tubular function)
	Nonsteroidal antiinflammatory drugs (↓ PGE_2 and RBF)
Water excess	SIADH
	Hypotonic infusion
	Stress (↑ ADH)

ADH, Antidiuretic hormone; *GFR*, glomerular filtration rate; *MAP*, mean arterial pressure; *PGE₂*, prostaglandin E₂; *RBF*, renal blood flow; *SIADH*, syndrome of inappropriate antidiuretic hormone secretion.

edema formation is presented in Table 7.9. Principles of therapy for fluid overload states include:

- Fluid restriction
- Salt restriction
- Diuresis, dialysis
- Salt-poor albumin for diminished plasma volume

DEHYDRATION STATES

Dehydration states are common in children. The extent of dehydration is best assessed by weight, because clinical signs such as tachycardia, capillary refill, and skin elasticity[173] may be influenced by factors other than hydration status. A capillary refill time of 1.5 to 3.0 seconds, for example, suggests a fluid deficit of between 50 and 100 mL/kg, yet this sign is extremely dependent on ambient temperature.[174] Capillary refill time is generally assessed by squeezing the child's nailbed for 5 seconds; an abnormal time is ≥3 seconds and normal ≤2 seconds.[175,176] A systematic review of 21 studies in 1915 children confirmed that a capillary refill time of ≥3 seconds should be considered abnormal; use of a stop watch improves the accuracy of assessment.[177] Similarly, poor skin elasticity reflects significant volume loss, yet elasticity may be well preserved in children with hypernatremic dehydration.[173] Sunken eyes and a weak pulse are other signs of severe dehydration.[178] Clinical signs associated with varying levels of dehydration are presented in Table 7.10.

As a first approximation, correction of dehydration states in older children is most readily achieved with administration of a simple bolus of NS, lactated Ringer's solution, or Plasma-Lyte 148

TABLE 7.10	Clinical Signs and Symptoms for Estimation of Severity of Dehydration in Infants		
	DEGREE OF DEHYDRATION		
Clinical Signs	**Mild**	**Moderate**	**Severe**
Weight loss (%)	5	10	15
Behavior	Normal	Irritable	Hyperirritable to lethargic
Thirst	Slight	Moderate	Intense
Mucous membranes	May be normal	Dry	Parched
Tears	Present	Normal to reduced	Absent
Anterior fontanel	Flat	Possibly sunken	Sunken
Skin turgor	Normal	Slightly increased	Increased
Urine output	Normal	Oliguric	Anuric

Modified in part from Herrin J. Fluid and electrolytes. In: Graef J, ed. *Manual of Pediatric Therapeutics*. 6th ed. Philadelphia: Lippincott-Raven; 1997:63-75.

(balanced crystalloid solution). In infants or children with unusual, prolonged, or severe dehydration, however, management must be more precise. A 5-point questionnaire to assess the severity of dehydration may help develop an appropriate treatment strategy[179]:

1. *Does a volume deficit exist and, if so, how great is it?*
   As noted previously, assessment of volume deficit is best made by weight, yet rough estimates of 5% (mild), 10% (moderate), and 15% (severe) may be made in infants based on clinical signs (see Table 7.10).
2. *Does an osmolar disturbance exist and is it acute or chronic?*
   An osmolar imbalance is determined by measuring the serum sodium concentration. The majority of clinically encountered dehydration states (~80%) are isotonic (Na^+ = 130–150 mEq/L). These isotonic losses are easily managed by almost any strategy.
   Approximately 15% of dehydrated children present with hypertonic dehydration (Na^+ >150 mEq/L). These children are at greatest risk and have usually experienced the greatest fluid losses for a given set of clinical signs.[180] If the condition is chronic, they may require extensive, slow rehydration over prolonged periods.[181]
   Five percent of children present with hypotonic dehydration (Na^+ <130 mEq/L). For a given fluid deficit, these individuals are often more symptomatic than others, and their requirement for sodium replacement is greatest. Surprisingly, rapid improvement in clinical condition often results after the first fluid bolus.
   In general, states of acute dehydration (<24 hours) may be corrected rapidly, whereas states of chronic dehydration must be corrected slowly. This difference in treatment plan is attributed to the speed at which the cell volume equilibrates: acutely through gain or loss of electrolytes (which are transported rapidly across membranes) or chronically through gain or loss of organic osmolytes (which are transported more slowly).[11] Equilibration of brain cell volume during correction of hypertonicity can be very slow, mandating patience in correction of chronic fluid deficits.

Similarly, rapid correction of hyponatremic disturbances can be hazardous,[36] even when seemingly safe isotonic solutions are infused.[182]

3. *Does an acid-base abnormality exist?*
   Quantitation of the child's acid-base status gives useful, although limited, information in terms of the severity of dehydration. When evaluating acid-base status, it is important to recall that bicarbonate reabsorption and urine acidification are limited in preterm and young infants, leaving even the normal infant in a state of mild metabolic acidosis (pH, 7.3; serum bicarbonate 20–21 mEq/L [normal 22–26 mEq/L]). Although slow, spontaneous correction of acid-base status is typically observed on rehydration, rapid fluid boluses in poorly perfused children may result in a transient "reperfusion acidosis" as returning circulation washes the products of anaerobic metabolism out of the tissues. In this setting, or when renal insufficiency exists, blood-buffering capacity is such that children with serum bicarbonate concentrations less than 8 mEq/L or pH less than 7.2 may benefit from administration of supplemental base (sodium bicarbonate) (Fig. 7.6).[179]
   Rapid bedside evaluation of acid-base status uses the following general relationships: a pH decrease of 0.1 unit accompanies a base excess (BE) of approximately 6 mEq/L or an increase in carbon dioxide tension (PCO_2) of 10 to 12 mm Hg. The

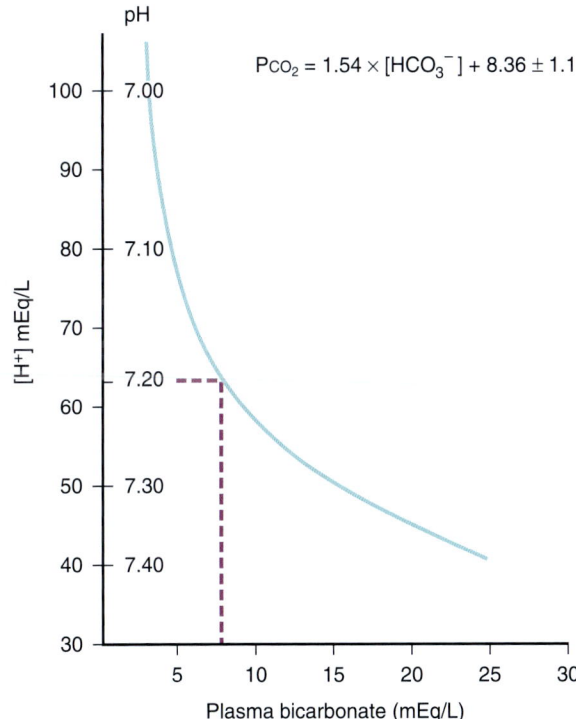

$$PCO_2 = 1.54 \times [HCO_3^-] + 8.36 \pm 1.1$$

FIGURE 7.6 Data from children with metabolic acidosis[263] were used to depict the displacement of pH as serum bicarbonate declines. The zone of rapid pH displacement (pH <7.20) has a slope that is several times greater than the zone of gradual pH displacement (pH ≥7.20). As the pH moves through the zone of rapid pH displacement, a further decline of serum bicarbonate of as little as 1 or 2 mEq/L produces a highly leveraged further decrease of pH. *[H⁺]*, Hydrogen ion concentration; *[HCO₃⁻]*, bicarbonate ion concentration; *PCO_2*, carbon dioxide tension. (From Kallen RJ. The management of diarrheal dehydration in infants using parenteral fluids. *Pediatr Clin North Am*. 1990;37:265-286.)

total replacement base required is then determined by the following equation:

$$\text{Dose (mEq)} = 0.3 \times \text{weight (kg)} \times \text{BE (mEq/L)}$$

Clinically, a smaller sodium bicarbonate dose (1–2 mEq/kg) is given initially, the response is verified by blood gas analysis, and the remaining doses are titrated to effect.

4. *Is renal function impaired?*

Initial evaluation includes the timing of the last urine void and recent urine output, measurement of urine specific gravity, and serum levels of blood urea nitrogen and creatinine. If uncertainty persists, measurement of serum and urine electrolytes for comparison and calculation of the FE_{Na} are indicated (see Chapter 26).

FE_{Na} values of less than 1% imply prerenal conditions causing renal dysfunction, whereas FE_{Na} values greater than 2% to 3% suggest renal insufficiency. In prematurity, however, values as large as 9% have been recorded in otherwise normal infants.[183]

5. *What is the state of potassium balance?*

Potassium homeostasis is critical to life, and serum potassium concentrations are generally maintained within a very narrow range. Nonetheless, serum potassium concentrations do not reflect whole-body stores and substantial potassium depletion may exist in the presence of modest changes in serum potassium concentration (K^+_{serum}). Gastrointestinal losses or metabolic acidosis is usually accompanied by a potassium deficit, whereas other dehydration states are not. Rapid fluid boluses or pH correction, or both, may acutely reduce K^+_{serum},[184] and refractory hypokalemia may occur in children deficient in magnesium.[185] In all cases, adequate renal function should be present before administration of potassium, and complete repletion should span 48 to 72 hours.

Once the nature and severity of dehydration have been determined, the clinician may proceed using any of a variety of correction strategies. In one approach, moderate to severe dehydration deficits may be estimated, as in Table 7.10. Fluid and electrolyte repair may then proceed according to a three-phase approach wherein circulating plasma volume, perfusion, and urine output are restored rapidly using isotonic crystalloid or colloid solution and remaining deficits are corrected over 24 hours[186]:

- Emergency Phase: 20 to 30 mL/kg isotonic crystalloid/colloid bolus
- Repletion Phase 1: 25 to 50 mL/kg over 6 to 8 hours. Anions: Cl^- 75%, acetate 25%
- Repletion Phase 2: remainder of deficit over 24 hours (isotonic) or 48 hours (hypertonic). Include calcium replacement as necessary.

SEPTIC SHOCK

Both the pediatric advanced life support (PALS) recommendations from the American Heart Association and the "Surviving Sepsis" campaign from the Society of Critical Care Medicine have long emphasized fluid administration as the cornerstone of successful resuscitation. As an Ib recommendation, the original "Surviving Sepsis" campaign called for "a minimum of 30 mL/kg of crystalloid".[187–189] Since these guidelines have been promulgated, fluid overload has been increasingly recognized as associated with poor outcome in a variety of settings including certain populations of children with sepsis.[190–194]

Current therapies for sepsis and cardiac arrest suggest that rapid administration of large crystalloid volumes (20–30 mL/kg) is unphysiologic and counterproductive since only a small fraction remains in the circulation, saltatory effects dissipate rapidly, and resulting edema can exacerbate circulatory and respiratory derangements.[195–197] PALS 2020 recommends an initial fluid bolus of 20 mL/kg for infants and children with shock, with subsequent patient reassessments.[198] Surviving Sepsis guidelines for pediatrics currently divide fluid therapy based on the available resources.[199] If intensive care is available a fluid bolus of 10 to 20 mL/kg per bolus is recommended, with up to 40 to 60 mL/kg in bolus fluid over the first hour. These boluses are given while monitoring for signs of fluid overload. In low resource settings, a fluid bolus is not recommended, and maintenance fluids alone should be started if the patient is not hypotensive. Crystalloids are recommended for initial resuscitation.[189] Anesthesiologists are accustomed to continually reassessing circulatory homeostasis, and in the setting of septic shock, should feel comfortable pursuing standard physiologic endpoints with judicious fluid administration complemented with inotropes and vasopressors.

HYPERNATREMIA AND HYPONATREMIA

As previously detailed, disorders of sodium equilibrium are primarily marked by disturbances of fluid balance and are corrected according to the principles outlined earlier. Serious hypernatremia or hyponatremia is accompanied by neurologic symptoms whose severity is determined by the degree and rate of change of Na^+_{serum}.

Hypernatremia

In contrast to its rareness in adults, acute hypernatremia is common in children. A mortality rate greater than 40% for the acute disorder and 10% for the chronic disorder has been reported (serum sodium >160 mEq/L).[165,200] Mortality and permanent neurologic injury are even more common in infants. Depending on the degree and duration, neurologic findings include irritability and coma; seizures may be a presenting symptom but are more commonly encountered after the start of therapy. Children with acute conditions are usually symptomatic, whereas those with chronic conditions (acclimated individuals) are typically asymptomatic. General principles for treatment of hypernatremia are:

- In the setting of circulatory collapse, colloid or NS bolus should be administered. Although the assertion is debatable, a colloid bolus provides the theoretical benefit of sustained hemodynamic support with a smaller fluid load. Saline, in contrast, rapidly re-equilibrates, necessitating repeated boluses while adding to the total salt burden.
- Once a stable circulation has been restored, fluid deficit should be assessed as accurately as possible and corrected over 48 to 72 hours. Cautious correction of the serum sodium concentration is required. The serum sodium concentration and osmolality should be continuously reassessed during fluid administration, aiming for a correction of no more than 1 to 2 mOsm/L per hour. After as little as 4 hours of hypernatremia, idiogenic osmoles (e.g., trimethylamines) appear in the brain to prevent cerebral volume depletion. Rapid administration of free water could induce cerebral edema, seizures, and death. Free water should therefore be administered cautiously so as to reduce serum sodium levels no more than 0.5 mEq/L per hour.[201] Because of possible associated hypoglycemia, some solutions should be glucose-containing, and serum glucose levels should be monitored.

- Vigilance for seizures, apnea, and cardiovascular compromise is essential because appropriate and timely treatment of such complicating factors can be the primary determinants of successful outcome.

Hyponatremia

Hyponatremia is also common in infants and children; increasing prevalence owing to erroneous formula dilution has intermittently been reported.[202,203] In the practice of anesthesiology, mild hyponatremia is a common postoperative condition after surgery of any severity[204–206]; in neurosurgical patients, hyponatremia may represent cerebral salt wasting or syndrome of inappropriate antidiuretic hormone secretion (SIADH).[207] In general, symptomatic patients are acutely hyponatremic and asymptomatic individuals are chronically hyponatremic.[208] After surgery, acutely hyponatremic children may present with nonspecific symptoms that are often erroneously attributed to other causes. Early central nervous system symptoms include headache, nausea, weakness, and anorexia. Advancing symptoms include mental status changes, confusion, irritability, progressive obtundation, and seizures.[209] Respiratory arrest (or irregularity) is a common manifestation of advanced hyponatremia.

When planning to correct hyponatremia, the presence of symptoms must be considered a medical emergency, whereas asymptomatic children do not require rapid intervention. Chronic hyponatremia must be corrected slowly and by no more than 0.3 to 0.5 mEq/L per hour to avoid neurologic complications that include central pontine myelinolysis.[210] The best treatment for acute hyponatremia is early recognition and intervention. Because hypoxia exacerbates any neurologic injury, the simple ABCs of resuscitation are attended to first, and the airway is secured in any child who has seizures or respiratory irregularity. Hyponatremic seizures are refractory to traditional anticonvulsants but readily respond to relatively modest (3–6 mEq/L) increases of serum sodium.[211] In several series,[203,212,213] such limited, rapid correction of symptomatic hyponatremia with hypertonic saline (514 mEq/L NaCl) was well tolerated. It should be emphasized that complete correction is unnecessary and unwise.[214] Initial therapy is aimed at increasing the Na^+_{serum} no more than is necessary to stop seizure activity (usually 3–5 mEq/L). Further correction should take place over several days. Hypertonic saline may be used for the correction until the Na^+_{serum} increases to greater than 120 mEq/L. Remembering that TBW may range from 75% in infancy to 60% or less in older children, total sodium deficit is estimated as:

$$\text{sodium change (mEq/L)} \times \text{fraction TBW (L/kg)} \times \text{weight (kg)}$$
$$= \text{mEq sodium}$$
$$\text{desired } Na^+_{serum} - \text{observed } Na^+_{serum} \times 0.6 \times \text{weight (kg)}$$
$$= \text{mEq sodium required}$$

For example, in a 25-kg child, to correct a serum sodium concentration of 110 mEq/L to 125 mEq/L using hypertonic saline (514 mEq/L), infuse

$$(125 \text{ mEq/L} - 110 \text{ mEq/L}) \times 0.6 \times 25 = 225 \text{ mEq total}$$

or

$$225 \text{ mEq/514 mEq} = 0.44 \text{ L over 48 hours} = 9 \text{ mL/hour}$$

Because such calculations involve estimates, frequent measurement of the Na^+_{serum} is necessary during correction. As with hypernatremia, much of the morbidity and mortality associated with hyponatremia relates to complicating factors such as seizures and hypoxia that may occur prior to and during correction therapy.

Therefore, children undergoing therapy should be cared for in a monitored setting. When overzealous correction has occurred, there may be value in acutely relowering Na^+_{serum} using hypotonic fluids,[208] although such therapy is not without its own hazards.

General principles for treatment of hyponatremia are:
- Asymptomatic hyponatremia in and of itself need not be rapidly corrected. Associated cardiovascular compromise caused by volume depletion may be addressed by colloid bolus or administration of isotonic saline (1 L/m² per day). Provision of sodium is accompanied by free water restriction.
- Symptomatic hyponatremia is a medical emergency and may sometimes bring irreversible neurologic injury. Correction should be rapid, yet limited, as discussed above. A dose of 2 to 3 mL/kg of 3% saline (514 mEq/L) may be administered over 20 to 30 minutes to halt seizures. When hypertonic saline is not immediately available, standard 8.4% sodium bicarbonate resuscitation solutions contain 50 mEq sodium in 50 mL, or 1000 mEq/L.
- Subsequent correction is accomplished through calculation of the sodium deficit and provision of sodium to slowly correct at a rate not to exceed 0.3 to 0.5 mEq/L per hour or 8 to 12 mEq/L (total) in 24 to 48 hours.
- If the attendant fluid load is excessive or if oliguria is present, diuretics may be useful.

DISORDERS OF POTASSIUM HOMEOSTASIS

Hyperkalemia

Hyperkalemia is occasionally the presenting finding in conditions such as congenital adrenal hyperplasia. More commonly, it results from acute renal insufficiency, massive tissue injury, acidosis, or iatrogenic mishaps. In the operating room, acute hyperkalemia may follow the use of succinylcholine in children with myopathies,[215] burns, upper and lower motor neuron lesions, chronic sepsis, or disuse atrophy,[216] transfusion of irradiated red blood cells,[217] and occasionally during massive, rapid transfusion of red blood cells or whole blood (see Chapter 10) in neonates and small children.[218–222] Hyperkalemia has been a cause of cardiac arrest during rapid transfusion for craniosynostosis repair.[223] It may also occur with rhabdomyolysis or as a late sign in malignant hyperthermia (see Chapter 39).[224]

Although neurologic status is the main concern for children with abnormal Na^+_{serum}, cardiac status (rate and rhythm) determines the care of children with hyperkalemia. In children with hyperkalemia, peaked T waves appear at K^+ concentrations of 5.5 to 6.5 mEq/L, followed by lengthening of the PR interval and widening of the QRS complex until P waves are lost. Finally, the QRS complex merges with its T wave to produce a sinusoidal pattern (Fig. 7.7). Successful treatment traditionally uses the approach:
- Emergent therapy is first directed toward antagonism of the cardiac effects of potassium through cautious administration of IV calcium (chloride 20 mg/kg, or 60 mg/kg of calcium gluconate as a 10% solution) over 3 to 5 minutes to avoid bradycardia. Calcium does not decrease the serum potassium concentration but rather reestablishes the gradient between the resting membrane potential, which is increased in the presence of hyperkalemia, and the threshold potential, which is determined by the calcium concentration. It also increases the refractory period of the action potential, the net effect being the prevention of spontaneous depolarization. Calcium administration should continue until sinus rhythm is restored.[225]
- Serum potassium is then reduced by returning potassium to the intracellular space. This is achieved by correcting the

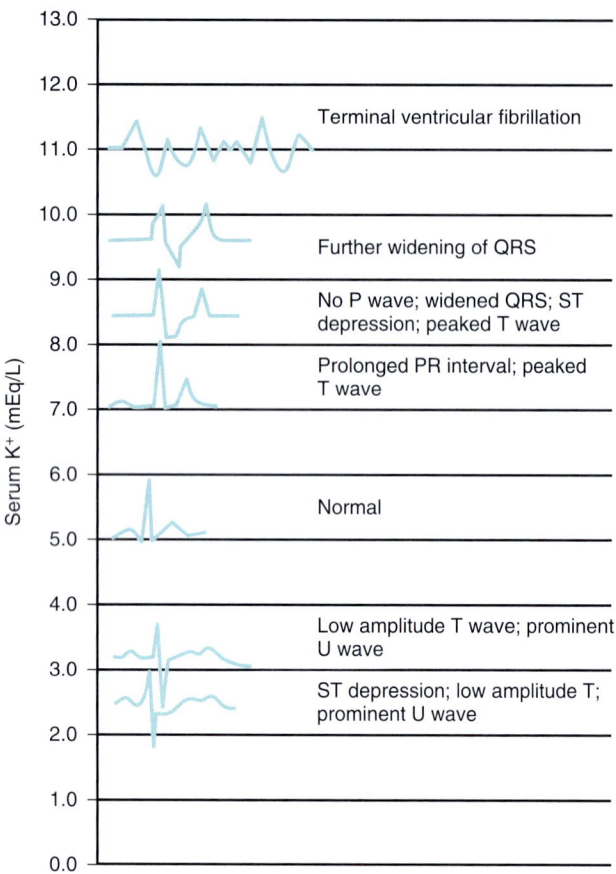

FIGURE 7.7 Electrocardiographic changes associated with hypokalemia and hyperkalemia. (From Williams GS, Klenk EL, Winters RW. Acute renal failure in pediatrics. In: Winters RW, ed. *The Body Fluids in Pediatrics: Medical, Surgical, and Neonatal Disorders of Acid-Base Status, Hydration, and Oxygenation.* Boston: Little, Brown; 1973;523-557.)

acidosis through administration of sodium bicarbonate (1–2 mEq/kg) intravenously, a β-agonist, and mild to moderate hyperventilation.

■ To maintain potassium in the intracellular space, glucose and insulin are administered by infusion (0.5–1.0 grams/kg glucose with 0.1 U/kg insulin over 30 to 60 minutes).

■ After stabilizing the K^+_{serum}, attention is directed toward removal of the whole-body potassium burden (sodium polystyrene sulfonate [Kayexalate], furosemide, dialysis) and correction of the underlying cause (Fig. 7.8).

The knowledge that β-adrenergic stimulation modulates the translocation of potassium into the intracellular space[226,227] first prompted the consideration of β-agonists in the treatment of acute hyperkalemia.[228–231] In children, a single infusion of an IV β-agonist such as salbutamol (5 µg/kg over 15 minutes) effectively reduces serum potassium concentrations within 30 minutes. Because of the rapidity, efficacy, and safety of salbutamol in children, it has become a common emergency room treatment for hyperkalemia.[228] In addition to IV therapy, salbutamol[232] (also known as albuterol)[231] by inhalation effectively reduces the serum potassium concentration. The inhalation route has the advantages of being readily available in emergency departments and not requiring IV access. Since paradoxical exacerbation of hyperkalemia may occur on initiation of treatment[232] and associated arrhythmias can occur,[233] other measures should be undertaken simultaneously.

However, β-agonist inhalation during an acute event may be an extremely useful temporizing measure. Oral medications such as patiromer (Veltassa, Vifor Pharma Redwood City, CA)[234] (which exchanges potassium for calcium) and sodium zirconium cyclosilicate (Lokelma, AstraZeneca, Wilmington, DE)[235] (which selectively attracts potassium) are inorganic orally administered polymers that attract potassium from the distal colon, increasing fecal excretion[236]; there are no pediatric data. These new modalities would most likely only be of value to treat chronic hyperkalemia not acute hyperkalemia, and neither is currently approved for use in children.

Hypokalemia

Hypokalemia is most common in children as a complication of diarrhea or persistent vomiting associated with gastroenteritis. Muscle weakness is the most common sign in hypokalemia and has been correlated with the serum potassium concentration.[237,238] In the operating room or ICU, hypokalemia may also accompany a wide variety of other conditions, including diabetes, hyperaldosteronism, pyloric stenosis, starvation, renal tubular disease, chronic steroid or diuretic use, β-agonist therapy, and a variety of syndromes.[238,239] Severe hypokalemia can also be accompanied by electrocardiographic changes, including QT prolongation, diminution of the T wave, and appearance of U waves (see Fig. 7.7).

As noted previously, the K^+_{serum} does not accurately reflect total potassium homeostasis, and low serum concentrations may or may not be associated with depletion of total body potassium. Indeed, the extracellular fraction of potassium is only a tiny proportion (approximately 3%) of the entire body store. For these reasons, the precise point at which to begin replacement therapy is controversial, and total replacement requirements are impossible to calculate. In general practice, K^+_{serum} between 2.0 and 2.5 mEq/L are corrected before surgery on the assumption that further decreases may predispose the child to muscular weakness, arrhythmias, and hemodynamic instability.

Potassium replacement is best accomplished orally over an extended period while the underlying cause is evaluated and treated. When IV correction is required, concentrations up to 40 mEq/L should be given slowly (*not to exceed 1 mEq/kg per hour*) in a monitored setting. Because such solutions can cause phlebitis, large-bore or central catheters are preferred. In the setting of hypochloremia and hypokalemia, chloride deficits must first be replaced, usually by administration of NS.

SYNDROME OF INAPPROPRIATE ANTIDIURETIC HORMONE SECRETION

Many nonosmotic factors are capable of stimulating ADH release, and these can occasionally override osmotic control priorities. When this occurs, clinicians have historically deemed the increased ADH concentrations "inappropriate" because control of the serum osmolarity is lost (see Chapter 26). As detailed earlier, however, intravascular depletion is the most potent stimulus for vasopressin release, and it is hardly *inappropriate* that defense of circulation takes priority over defense of serum sodium levels. Moreover, pain, surgical stress, critical illness, sepsis, pulmonary disease, central nervous system injury, drugs, and a variety of other factors may also stimulate ADH release above and beyond that necessary to maintain osmolar balance (see Table 7.5).[209,240]

SIADH is common in children, yet it is often overlooked. Minor head trauma, for example, may elicit spikes in ADH concentrations, although infrequently to the extent that it produces serious hyponatremia and seizures.[241] Urine output after spinal

Treatment Algorithm for Hyperkalemia

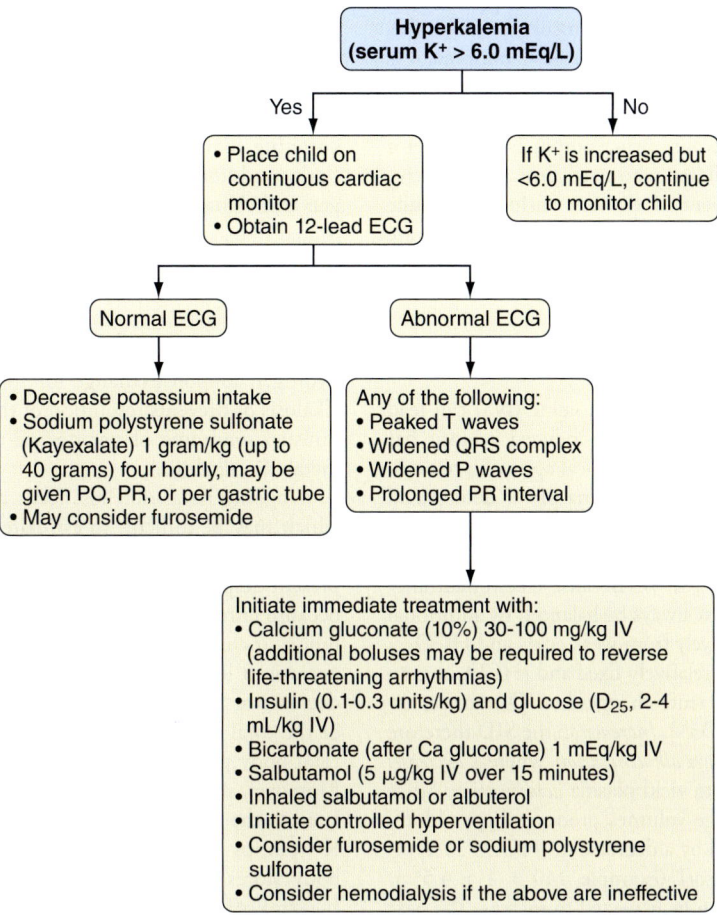

FIGURE 7.8 Algorithm for treatment of hyperkalemia. After stabilization, attention is directed toward removal of the whole-body potassium burden (Kayexalate, dialysis) and correction of the underlying cause. D_{25}, 25% Dextrose; *ECG*, electrocardiogram; *IV*, intravenous; *PO*, orally; *PR*, per rectum.

fusion is often reduced because of increased concentrations of ADH, which usually return to normal within 24 hours without therapy.[242] Infants with bronchiolitis and hyperinflated lungs frequently demonstrate markedly increased plasma ADH concentrations and exhibit fluid retention, weight gain, urinary concentration, and plasma hypoosmolality until their illness begins to resolve.[243] Hyponatremia to the point of seizures, however, is only occasionally observed.

The diagnosis of SIADH rests on the identification of impaired urinary dilution in the setting of plasma hypoosmolality. Hyponatremia (Na^+ <135 mEq/L), serum osmolality less than 280 mOsm/L, and urine osmolality greater than 100 mOsm/L in the absence of volume depletion, cardiac failure, nephropathy, adrenal insufficiency, or cirrhosis are generally considered sufficient for diagnosis. Therapeutic principles are similar to those for hyponatremia and depend on:

- Restriction of free water
- Repletion of sodium deficits (if present)
- Administration of diuretics to offset the effects of vasopressin

DIABETES INSIPIDUS

In the operating room and the ICU, diabetes insipidus is most commonly associated with the care of neurosurgical patients.[244–246]

Diabetes insipidus is also caused by neuroendocrine failure in brain death and management may be necessary if organ donation is planned.[247,248] Diabetes insipidus results from decreased secretion of, or renal insensitivity to, vasopressin (see Chapter 26). Manifestations include massive polyuria, volume contraction, dehydration, and plasma hyperosmolality.[249] Dilute polyuria (<250 mOsm, >4 mL/kg per hour) in the presence of hypernatremia (Na^+ >145 mEq/L) with hyperosmolality (>300 mOsm/L) is the hallmark. In central diabetes insipidus, administration of desmopressin concentrates the urine although water deprivation does not. Postoperative diabetes insipidus may initially be difficult to distinguish from mobilization of operative fluids.

Children with craniopharyngioma or a similarly situated pathologic lesion may not manifest vasopressin deficiency early in the disease but become symptomatic preoperatively after steroid administration or intraoperatively during surgical manipulation. Postoperative diabetes insipidus typically begins on the evening after surgery and may resolve in 3 to 5 days if osmoregulatory structures have not been permanently injured. An often-confusing triphasic response may also occur wherein postoperative diabetes insipidus appears to resolve, fluid status normalizes, or SIADH appears and then vasopressin secretion ceases and diabetes insipidus returns. It is hypothesized that this pattern reflects nonspecific vasopressin release from degenerating neurons in the hypothalamic supraoptic and paraventricular nuclei.

Attempts have been made to develop protocols for perioperative management of diabetes insipidus.[250] Because vasopressin is difficult to titrate to urine output, our practice involves maximal antidiuresis and fluid restriction. In this setting, volume status must be monitored closely, because urine output is no longer a marker of renal perfusion. Children who need close perioperative monitoring for the development of diabetes insipidus include those with preexisting diabetes insipidus as well as those who are undergoing resection of craniopharyngiomas or pituitary lesions or other procedures that involve resection or manipulation of the pituitary stalk.[251]

HYPERCHLOREMIC ACIDOSIS

Administration of large amounts of normal saline (NS) can lead to excess serum chloride.[252] Normal saline-induced acidosis has been explained by the Stewart physicochemical approach to acid-base balance.[253,254] In this framework, plasma pH is determined by its "strong ion difference" (SID), or the concentration differences between dominant cations and anions ($[SID] = [Na^+] + [K^+] + [Ca^{+2}] + [Mg^{+2}] - [Cl^-]$). Because electroneutrality must be preserved, the SID must always be balanced by additional negative charges arising collectively from weak acids and HCO_3^-. Since the mass of weak acids is relatively fixed and $[HCO_3^-]$ is an immediately responsive buffer, acute changes in SID translate directly to acute changes in $[HCO3^-]$. *Increases* in the SID therefore *increase* $[HCO3^-]$ to yield plasma *alkalinization,* whereas *decreases* in the SID *decrease* $[HCO3^-]$ to yield plasma *acidification.* Since administration of saline in large volumes produces hyperchloremia, this must be accompanied by a decrease in $[HCO3^-]$. Typically, the SID is ~40 to 42 mEq/L (example, 140 + 4 + 4.5[a] + 2[b] − 110). Increasing $[Cl^-]$ can be expected to increase the base deficit by an equivalent amount.

A simpler explanation of NS-induced acidosis is that it arises through dilution of $[HCO_3^-]$. When plasma volume is expanded by saline, its primary buffer system ($CO_2/[HCO_3^-]$) is diluted. Because it is an open system, respiration holds the buffer acid (CO_2) constant while the buffer base ($[HCO_3^-]$) decreases. This physicochemical behavior and the resulting base deficit acidosis can be reproduced in model systems.[255]

Regardless of the source, it is clinically apparent that administration of large NS volumes is accompanied by metabolic acidosis related to both the amount and rate of infusion. In healthy women undergoing gynecologic surgery, 35 mL/kg NS over 2 hours produced acidosis, whereas similar infusions of lactated Ringer's solution did not.[252] In a study of children undergoing craniofacial surgery, 80% of those who received NS (39% to pH ≤7.25) and 37% of those who received Ringer's lactate solution (8% to pH ≤7.25) developed an acidosis.[256] The clinical significance of the saline-associated acidosis and a reduced incidence with Ringer's lactate solution is uncertain, but one large study observed less postoperative morbidity in adults receiving nonsaline balanced solutions for replacement of losses during abdominal surgery.[257] Historically NS was given during renal transplants to avoid the potassium load from lactated Ringer's

solution; however, recent studies have shown lower potassium concentrations and less acidosis when lactated Ringer's solution is given.[258,259]

HYPOCHLOREMIC METABOLIC ALKALOSIS

Infants with pyloric stenosis and other children with chronic vomiting may develop a hypochloremic metabolic alkalosis. In both conditions, chronic vomiting results in large losses of hydrogen and chloride ions and water. This leads to an alkalotic, dehydrated state. In the absence of IV fluid therapy, the renal response is to conserve water by retaining sodium through upregulation of aldosterone, in which hydrogen ions (which are already in short supply because of the vomiting), and potassium ions are excreted in the urine in exchange for sodium. Excretion of the remaining hydrogen ions in exchange for sodium exacerbates the existing alkalosis or prevents resolution of the alkalosis. It also leads to the unusual syndrome of paradoxical aciduria in the presence of a metabolic alkalosis.

Ongoing potassium loss leads to hypokalemia, the extent of which may be difficult to estimate. As discussed earlier, normal serum potassium levels (i.e., between 3.4 and 4.4 mEq/L) may be present despite significant total body potassium depletion. This is because chronic hypokalemia equilibrates throughout all bodily fluids, including the intracellular fluid volume where normal potassium levels are 135 to 145 mEq/L. As a result, a chronic decrease of 1 mEq/L in extracellular potassium (only 1% to 2% of the total body potassium) may reflect enormous depletion of total body potassium stores (100 to 200 mEq K^+ in an adult). Moreover, since extracellular potassium levels are nonlinearly related to the total body potassium (due to interference from Na^+/K^+ pumps and other electrolyte-stabilizing mechanisms) total body stores may be even lower. Thus, even mild hypokalemia (<3 mEq/L) may signal very significant total body potassium depletion.

In infants and children with chronic hypokalemic or hypochloremic metabolic alkalosis, correction of the electrolyte abnormalities and hypovolemia is optimally achieved using NS with 20 mEq/L K^+ infused at a rate of 10 to 20 mL/kg per hour through a peripheral IV line until the potassium level is greater than 3.0 mEq/L, the chloride concentration is greater than 100 mEq/L, serum bicarbonate is less than 30 mEq/L, and the clinical signs of hypovolemia are resolved. In the case of pyloric stenosis, this may take 24 to 48 hours depending on the severity of the electrolyte and fluid imbalance.

CEREBRAL SALT WASTING

Cerebral salt wasting (also known as renal salt wasting) is a hyponatremic syndrome of unclear etiology.[260] Most commonly recognized in neurosurgical patients, it is a primary natriuresis, probably related to dysregulation of brain or atrial natriuretic peptides. The condition has been increasingly recognized, and an incidence as great as 5% has been reported in children with brain tumors.[261] Cerebral salt wasting can sometimes be difficult to distinguish from SIADH but the former is marked by hyponatremia, natriuresis, and *hypovolemia,* while the latter features *hypervolemia.* Thus, cerebral salt wasting should be suspected in neurosurgical patients exhibiting hyponatremia and hypovolemia. With this in mind, intervention is straightforward: fluid resuscitation with isotonic solutions and ongoing correction of intravascular volume depletion with sodium-containing solutions. Although spontaneous resolution is the norm, persistent cases may require mineralocorticoid therapy.

---

[a]Normal Ca = 8 to 10 mg/dL = 4 to 5 mEq/L (mg/dL × 10 × 2 Eq/mol × 1/40 g/mol, so multiply by 0.5).
[b]Normal Mg = 2 mg/dL = 1.6 mEq/L (mg/dL × 10 × 2 × 1/24 g/mol, so multiply by 0.83).

7

ANNOTATED REFERENCES

Arieff AI, Ayus JC, Fraser CL. Hyponatraemia and death or permanent brain damage in healthy children. *BMJ.* 1992;304:1218-1222.

Much concern has been displayed about iatrogenic hyponatremia caused by administration of hypotonic solutions. This study highlights the grave consequences of such errors.

Benzon HA, Bobrowski A, Suresh S, Wasson NR, Cheon EC. Impact of preoperative hyponatraemia on paediatric perioperative mortality. *Br J Anaesth.* 2019;123(5):618-626.

Although preoperative hyponatremia is an independent risk factor for postoperative mortality in adults, this risk factor has not been investigated in children. The authors reviewed data from the 2014 and 2015 data sets of the American College of Surgeons National Surgical Quality Improvement Program–Pediatric (NSQIP-P), we conducted a retrospective study of children undergoing surgery and identified a clear association between preoperative hyponatremia and perioperative mortality and length of stay in pediatric patients.

Constable PD. Hyperchloremic acidosis: the classic example of strong ion acidosis. *Anesth Analg.* 2003;96:919-922.

This review is an excellent description of alternative methods of evaluating acid-base status. The focus of this paper is on the physiology behind the acidosis created by large volume, rapid administration of normal saline.

Holliday MA, Friedman AL, Segar W, et al. Acute hospital-induced hyponatremia in children: a physiologic approach. *J Pediatr.* 2004;145:584-587.

This update to the authors' classic 1957 article addresses the problems associated with applying the original formula (4-2-1 rule) to perioperative fluid management. The authors present an alternative approach to perioperative fluid management with a focus on attenuating the antidiuretic hormone response to perioperative stress.

Oh GJ, Sutherland SM. Perioperative fluid management and postoperative hyponatremia in children. *Pediatr Nephrol.* 2016;31:53-60.

This thorough review traces the history of fluid management in the perioperative period with a focus on the development of postoperative hyponatremia. The review is evidence-based, analyzing how the composition of common perioperative electrolyte solutions may contribute to hyponatremia in the face of perioperative upregulation of ADH.

Sümpelmann R, Becke K, Brenner S, et al. Perioperative intravenous fluid therapy in children: guidelines from the Association of the Scientific Medical Societies in Germany. *Pediatr Anesth.* 2017;27(1):10-18.

The Scientific Working Group for Paediatric Anaesthesia updated its 2006 guidelines for perioperative intravenous fluid therapy in children. The recommendations highlighted as brief a fasting interval as possible preoperatively, balanced isotonic electrolyte solution with 1% to 2.5% glucose as a background maintenance solution and a glucose-free balanced electrolyte solution to maintain circulatory homeostasis. Colloid solutions may be administered in place of balanced electrolyte solution to replace ongoing fluid losses when blood products are not indicated. Monitoring electrolyte concentrations should be undertaken serially when intravenous fluids are continued postoperatively to ensure electrolyte and glucose homeostasis.

A complete reference list can be found online at Elsevier eBooks+.

8 Essentials of Hematology

TREVOR L. ADAMS, SIRI KANMANTHREDDY, MICHAEL J. EISSES, M.A. BENDER, AND GREGORY J. LATHAM

The Basics
Laboratory Values and Diagnostic Tests
Guidelines for Transfusion
Hemolytic Anemias
Hereditary Spherocytosis
Glucose-6-Phosphate Dehydrogenase Deficiency
Hemoglobinopathies
Sickle Cell Disease
Thalassemias
Thrombocytopenia
Platelet Disorders and Bleeding
Idiopathic Thrombocytopenic Purpura

Coagulation Disorders
Screening
Von Willebrand Disease
Hemophilia
Hypercoagulability
Hematologic malignancies
Acute Lymphoblastic Leukemia
Acute Myelogenous Leukemia
Hodgkin Lymphoma
Non-Hodgkin Lymphoma
Langerhans Cell Histiocytosis
Myelodysplastic and Myeloproliferative Disorders

HEMATOLOGIC DISORDERS IN CHILDHOOD may present to an anesthesiologist in many ways. They may be the primary cause for a surgical procedure, such as hereditary spherocytosis (HS) in a child requiring splenectomy, or a factor complicating a common surgical procedure, such as sickle cell disease in a child undergoing tonsillectomy. Questions about hematologic problems such as anemia, thrombocytopenia, decreased or increased coagulation, childhood cancer, and hematopoietic stem cell transplantation (HSCT) are often raised in the perioperative setting.

In this chapter, we address hematologic diseases and considerations that are of significance and interest to pediatric anesthesiologists. We highlight priorities of the hematologist that the anesthesiologist should incorporate in the care of a child during the perioperative period.

The Basics

LABORATORY VALUES AND DIAGNOSTIC TESTS

What is a normal hematocrit or platelet count for an infant or child who comes to the operating room? Red blood cell (RBC), white blood cell, platelet, and coagulation indices evolve in various ways through late gestation, the neonatal period, infancy, and childhood (Table 8.1).

A term neonate has relative polycythemia, reticulocytosis, and leukocytosis compared with an older child. Neonatal platelet counts are similar to those of adults. Although in vitro function may be impaired for the first postnatal month, most in vivo assays of platelet function indicate normal or accelerated function. Both the prothrombin time (PT) and activated partial thromboplastin time (aPTT) are prolonged in preterm and term neonates because of a relative deficiency in vitamin K–dependent and contact activation factors, respectively; however, concentrations of factor VIII and von Willebrand factor (vWF) are increased.[1] The average international normalized ratio (INR), a normalized PT, is 1.0 for all age groups. Fibrinogen concentrations are comparable between term neonates and adults, although neonatal fibrinogen is qualitatively dysfunctional. The plasma concentrations of many anticoagulant factors (i.e., tissue factor pathway inhibitor, antithrombin, vitamin K–dependent glycoproteins, and proteins C and S) are decreased in preterm and term neonates. The quantity and quality of plasminogen are decreased in neonates.[1,2] Despite these differences, the neonatal hemostatic system should be viewed as functionally balanced, wherein procoagulant properties effectively counteract anticoagulant properties and ultimately confer no tendency toward either coagulopathy or thrombosis. Therefore, although laboratory values may imply impaired hemostasis when compared with normal adolescent and adult indices, this does not necessarily reflect an increased risk of hemorrhage.[1,3]

After the immediate neonatal period, preterm and term infants experience physiologic anemia, presumably due to the downregulating effect of increased oxygen supply in extrauterine life on erythropoiesis and to the dilutional effect of a rapidly increasing blood volume. Preterm infants reach their nadir hemoglobin of 7 to 9 g/dL at 3 to 6 postnatal weeks, and term infants reach their nadir hemoglobin concentration of 9 to 11 g/dL at 8 to 12 postnatal weeks.

Most hematologic values reach adult norms by the end of infancy (i.e., first postnatal year), although some continue to change gradually into the second decade. All of these changes underscore the importance of age-adjusted standards accompanying laboratory results for infants and children.

There is no ideal single screening test to assess the *bleeding risk* of a child in the perioperative period. *Bleeding time* appears to be greater in the infant and child (and less in the neonate) than it is

TABLE 8.1 | Hematology Values at Different Ages

Measurement*	Preterm 28–32 Weeks	Preterm 32–36 Weeks	Term Neonate	1-Year-Old	Child	Adult
Hemoglobin (g/dL)	12.9	13.6	16.8	12	13	15
Hematocrit (%)	40.9	43.6	55	36	38	45
Reticulocyte count (%)	—	—	5	1	1	1.6
White blood cell count (/mm³)	5160	7710	18,000	10,000	8000	7500
Platelet count (/mm³)	255,000	260,000	300,000	300,000	300,000	300,000
Prothrombin time (seconds)	15.4	13	13	11	11	12
International normalized ratio (INR)	—	1	1	1	1	1
Activated partial thromboplastin time (seconds)	108	53.6	42.9	30	31	28
Fibrinogen (mg/dL)	256	243	283	276	279	278
Bleeding time (minutes)	—	3.5	3.5	6	7	5

*All values expressed as the mean.
Data from Andrew M. The relevance of developmental hemostasis to hemorrhagic disorders of newborns. *Semin Perinatol.* 1997;21:70-85; Andrew M, Vegh P, Johnston M, et al. Maturation of the hemostatic system during childhood. *Blood.* 1992;80:1998-2005; Goodnight SH, Hathaway WE. *Disorders of Hemostasis and Thrombosis, a Clinical Guide,* 2nd ed. New York: McGraw-Hill; 2001: 31-38; Ohls RK, Christensen RD. Development of the hematopoietic system. In: Behrman RE, Kliegman RM, Jenson HB, eds. *Nelson Textbook of Pediatrics,* 17th ed. Philadelphia: WB Saunders; 2004: 1599-1604.

in the adult, but the range of values is wide and overlapping (see Table 8.1). Although bleeding time is potentially helpful in predicting posttonsillectomy and adenoidectomy hemorrhage,[4] as well as hemorrhage after percutaneous renal[5] and liver[6] biopsy, there is little evidence to support its use as a screening test to predict bleeding in the presence of a careful, inclusive clinical history.[7–9]

In contrast to the standard historical laboratory tests, point-of-care testing using viscoelastic tests, such as the thromboelastogram (TEG), rotational thromboelastometry (ROTEM), and Sonoclot, allow the practitioner to receive data about the bleeding patient more quickly. The advantage of point-of-care viscoelastic testing is that it provides information of the entire clotting process from fibrin formation to clot retraction and fibrinolysis at the bedside. These tests also use whole blood, which allows the interaction of plasma-derived coagulation factors with red cells and platelets, thereby providing information on platelet function. Viscoelastic point-of-care coagulation devices require trained personnel to maintain strict quality control procedures as well as strict standardization procedures, in order to ensure optimal accuracy and reliability.[10] The TEG has been used to investigate the coagulation status of children undergoing spinal fusion,[11] neurosurgical procedures,[12] cardiopulmonary bypass for cardiothoracic procedures[13,14] and trauma,[15] as well as in critically ill neonates with both surgical and nonsurgical problems.[16] Although the thromboelastogram may provide useful information to evaluate fibrinolysis, hypercoagulability, and other coagulation perturbations, its use is usually limited to clinical scenarios with dynamic coagulation changes, such as open-heart surgery with cardiopulmonary bypass and liver transplantation.

The platelet function analyzer (PFA-100) is increasingly used to assess platelet abnormalities. It has the benefit of avoiding some of the difficulties of obtaining a bleeding time in children. Although several studies suggest PFA-100 analysis is equivalent or superior to the bleeding time for detecting bleeding abnormalities, there is no consensus about its role in preoperative screening.[17] Current evidence does not identify a single screening tool

sensitive or specific enough to predict bleeding disorders or surgical bleeding risk in children. However the PFA-100 analysis had the greatest probability of detecting a bleeding disorder in children.[18] With the increasing use of newer agents that modify platelet function (e.g., platelet G protein–coupled receptor P2Y12 antagonists, glycoprotein GPIIb-IIIa complex antagonists), clinicians must understand that the thromboelastogram, PFA-100, and other methods that assess platelet function may vary in their ability to monitor the effects of these agents and those of cyclooxygenase inhibitors.[19]

GUIDELINES FOR TRANSFUSION
Critical analyses of the risks and benefits of transfusions in infants and children in the perioperative period have resulted in fewer transfusions. Even for infants and children in intensive care, a restrictive transfusion threshold (i.e., 7 g/dL) reduces transfusions without increasing morbidity compared with a liberal threshold (i.e., 9.5–10 g/dL).[20,21] Data from the United Kingdom's national audit of clinical transfusion, the Serious Hazards of Transfusion (SHOT), indicate that infants and children younger than 18 years of age are at greater risk for adverse transfusion-related reactions (37 and 18 in 100,000, respectively) than are adults (13 in 100,000). Most events were error related, including administrative, laboratory, clinical judgment, and handling errors.[22]

Guidelines for RBC transfusion in infants and children in the perioperative setting should be consistent with those established by the American Society of Anesthesiologists Task Force on Blood Component Therapy, which proposed that transfusion is not indicated for hemoglobin concentrations greater than 10 g/dL but is indicated for concentrations less than 6 g/dL.[23,24] When the concentration is between 6 and 10 g/dL, packed red blood cells (PRBCs) should be transfused based on the child's vital signs, adequacy of oxygenation and perfusion, acuity and degree of blood loss, and other physiologic and surgical factors.[25,26] The revised pediatric guidelines from the British Committee for Standards in Haematology (BCSH) recommend a perioperative transfusion threshold of 7 g/dL be used in stable patients without major comorbidity or bleeding.[27] In a neonate or infant, one should also take into account increased baseline concentrations of hemoglobin in this population; increased oxygen consumption; increased affinity of residual fetal hemoglobin for oxygen; and absolute blood volume (i.e., 85 mL/kg for a term neonate and 100 mL/kg for a preterm neonate). The threshold for transfusing a healthy neonate may be 7 g/dL in some clinical settings, but it may be 12 g/dL or greater for a neonate in other settings, such as extreme prematurity and significant lung disease requiring mechanical ventilation.[25,28,29] For a preterm infant, the risks of hypovolemia, hypotension, acidosis, and postoperative apnea are magnified in the setting of operative blood loss and anemia. The precise transfusion thresholds used will depend on the clinical situation. It is impossible to address all of the guidelines in this chapter, but many pediatric hematology and oncology consultants have clearly defined transfusion thresholds for their patient populations that should be reviewed preoperatively.

Consensus committees from France, the United Kingdom, and the United States have published guidelines for platelet transfusion; these reports are based on available evidence that has been gathered and critically reviewed (Table 8.2).[23,24,27,30–36] Without evidence that platelet function is significantly different in the healthy infant and child, these guidelines should be applicable to these patients. The decision to transfuse platelets must take into account underlying medical conditions, platelet transfusion history, current medications, surgical bleeding, surgical interventions (e.g., cardiopulmonary bypass), and all other factors that may affect platelet function and turnover.[37–41] Sevoflurane and propofol have been reported to both suppress[42] and enhance platelet aggregation in vitro.[43] Despite these effects on platelet aggregation, no change in the bleeding time has been reported, suggesting that the possible inhibitory effects of these agents do not impair hemostasis in vivo.[44]

Transfusion guidelines for other blood products, including fresh frozen plasma (FFP) and cryoprecipitate, have been established,[23,24,27,40,45] and are discussed later in the context of coagulation disorders. Indications[46] for transfusing FFP are usually limited to:

1. Replacement of documented congenital or acquired coagulation factor deficiency when a specific sterilized or combined factor concentrate is unavailable, especially in the setting of anticipated or active bleeding
2. Acquired coagulopathy resulting from massive transfusion
3. Immediate reversal of warfarin's effect when prothrombin complex concentrate (PCC) is unavailable
4. Coagulation support in disease processes such as disseminated intravascular coagulation (DIC) and thrombotic thrombocytopenic purpura
5. A source of antithrombin III for children deficient of this inhibitor who require heparin

Cryoprecipitate should be administered only for anticipated or active bleeding in children with congenital fibrinogen deficiencies or von Willebrand disease who are unresponsive to desmopressin acetate (DDAVP) or for patients with acquired hypofibrinogenemia (less than 80–100 mg/dL) associated with massive transfusion.

Guidelines have been established by the College of American Pathologists and other transfusion study groups for leukocyte reduction of RBC units,[28] and irradiation (x-ray or γ-ray) of cellular blood components (Tables 8.3 and 8.4).[47,48] These guidelines are valuable when determining the specific choice of blood components that should be ordered and administered in the perioperative setting. For hematologic patients receiving chronic RBC transfusions,

TABLE 8.2	Commonly Used Triggers for Platelet Transfusion
Medical Condition or Procedure	**Platelet Count (/mm³)**
Stable hematology-oncology or chronically thrombocytopenic patient	10,000–20,000
Lumbar puncture in stable leukemic child	10,000
Bone marrow aspiration or biopsy	20,000
Gastrointestinal endoscopy in cancer patient	20,000–40,000
Disseminated Intravascular Coagulopathy (DIC)	20,000–50,000
Fiberoptic bronchoscopy in hematopoietic stem cell transplantation patient	20,000–50,000
Neonatal alloimmune thrombocytopenia	30,000
Major surgery	50,000
Dilutional thrombocytopenia with massive transfusion	50,000
Spinal anesthesia	50,000
Cardiopulmonary bypass	50,000–60,000
Liver biopsy	50,000–100,000
Nonbleeding preterm infant	60,000
Obstetric epidural anesthesia	70,000–100,000
Neurosurgery	100,000

DIC, Disseminated intravascular coagulation.
Data from references[35–37,40,41]

TABLE 8.3	Indications for Leukocyte-Reduced Red Blood Cell Units
Prevention of Alloimmunization	
Congenital hemolytic anemias (including sickle cell disease and thalassemia)	
Hypoproliferative anemias likely to need multiple transfusions	
Aplastic anemia	
Myelodysplasia/myeloproliferative syndrome	
Plasma cell dyscrasias	
Hematopoietic stem cell transplants	
Hematopoietic malignancies	
Therapy for Preexisting Conditions	
Recurrent, severe febrile hemolytic transfusion reactions	
Known HLA alloimmunization	
Possible Uses	
Alternative to cytomegalovirus-seronegative components (see Table 8.5)	
Human immunodeficiency virus–infected patients	

HLA, Human leukocyte antigen.
Copyright College of American Pathologists, used with permission from Simon TL, Alverson DC, AuBuchon J, et al. Practice parameter for the use of red blood cell transfusions: developed by the Red Blood Cell Administration Practice Guideline Development Task Force of the College of American Pathologists. *Arch Pathol Lab Med.* 1998;122:130-138.

TABLE 8.4 | Indications for Irradiation of Cellular Blood Components

Well-Defined Indications

Hematopoietic stem cell transplantation

Actual or anticipated congenital cell-mediated immunodeficiency

Intrauterine transfusion or after intrauterine transfusion

Directed donation from blood relative or HLA-matched donor

Hodgkin disease

Acute lymphocytic leukemia

Immunocompromised organ transplant recipient

Probable Indications

Malignancy and organ transplantation treated with immunosuppressive therapy

Exchange transfusion in neonate

Extracorporeal membrane oxygenation in neonate

Low–birth-weight neonate (<1200 grams)

Human immunodeficiency virus–infected patient with opportunistic infection

Possible Indications

Term neonate (<4 months)

Human immunodeficiency virus–infected patient

Modified from Simon TL, Alverson DC, AuBuchon J, et al. Practice parameter for the use of red blood cell transfusions: developed by the Red Blood Cell Administration Practice Guideline Development Task Force of the College of American Pathologists. *Arch Pathol Lab Med.* 1998;122:130-138; Treleaven J, Gennery A, Marsh J, et al. Guidelines on the use of irradiated blood components prepared by the British Committee for Standards in Haematology blood transfusion task force. *Br J Haematol.* 2010;152:35-51.

TABLE 8.5 | Indications for Cytomegalovirus-Seronegative or Leukocyte-Reduced Red Blood Cells for Prevention of Virus Transmission

Well-Defined Indications

Low–birth-weight neonate (<1200 grams)

Human immunodeficiency virus–infected patient

Recipient of seronegative allogeneic organ or hematopoietic stem cell transplant or prospective recipient

Pregnant woman

Intrauterine transfusion

Possible Indications

Hodgkin disease or non-Hodgkin lymphoma

Recipient of immunosuppressive therapy

Candidate for autologous hematopoietic stem cell transplantation

Hereditary or acquired cellular immunodeficiency

Probable Absence of Indications

Seronegative term infant

Seropositive pregnant woman

Copyright College of American Pathologists, used with permission from Simon TL, Alverson DC, AuBuchon J, et al. Practice parameter for the use of red blood cell transfusions: developed by the Red Blood Cell Administration Practice Guideline Development Task Force of the College of American Pathologists. *Arch Pathol Lab Med.* 1998;122:130-138.

an extended phenotypic crossmatch and leukocyte reduction can decrease the risk of developing alloantibodies and transfusion reactions, especially in children of African descent if the local donor pool is primarily derived from Caucasian populations of Northern European descent.[49] For oncology patients, updated specific requirements for blood products including leukocyte reduction and irradiation are often indicated and should always be reviewed with oncology specialists. To reduce the risk of cytomegalovirus (CMV) transmission in susceptible patients, donated seronegative CMV blood, leukoreduced blood, or both can be used.[50] However, the risk cannot be completely eliminated because supposed seronegative donors could be in the initial stages of viremia at the time blood is collected (Table 8.5).[51]

Hemolytic Anemias

Hemolytic syndromes are a group of disorders in which lysis of erythrocytes often leads to anemia. Although RBCs in these disorders may be characterized by abnormal morphology and shorter life span, these parameters may be normal at baseline. Clinical signs of a hemolytic syndrome include anemia, splenomegaly, and jaundice, signs that may be apparent chronically or only during acute exacerbations of a disease process. Hemoglobinuria may be a late finding if massive hemolysis has occurred. Although not well studied, in theory any hemolytic disorder may alter nitric oxide (NO) metabolism.

Many of the hemolytic anemias important to the anesthesiologist result from intracellular defects and can be classified as erythrocyte membrane defects, such as hereditary spherocytosis (HS); enzymatic defects, such as glucose-6-phosphate dehydrogenase (G6PD) deficiency; and qualitative and quantitative defects of hemoglobin, such as sickle cell disease and thalassemia. Other hemolytic anemias that may be encountered in the operating room are largely extracellularly mediated, such as transfusion-related hemolysis and other immune-mediated anemias (alloimmune or autoimmune); this group of anemias is not reviewed here.

HEREDITARY SPHEROCYTOSIS

Hereditary spherocytosis (HS), the most common cause of inherited chronic hemolysis in North America and Northern Europe, has a prevalence of approximately 1 to 2 cases per 5000 people, if mild forms of the disease are included.[52,53] First described in 1871, HS is present in many ethnic populations, but rare in African Americans. Because 75% of children inherit the disease in an autosomal dominant pattern, there is often a family history of the disorder, although autosomal recessive mutations, de novo mutations, and incomplete penetrance have been reported.[53]

Pathophysiology

Abnormalities in any of several erythrocyte membrane proteins, including the β subunit of spectrin, ankyrin, and band 3, can lead to HS. The variety of proteins affected and mutations observed in each gene account for the clinical heterogeneity of the disorder.[52] When the erythrocyte loses surface area, it changes from a biconcave disk to a sphere, which alters its stability and flow pattern through the capillaries. The deformity leads to a more rigid membrane, which predisposes it to rupture, a condition that is worsened if the membrane surface area decreases by more than 3%.[53]

Damaged erythrocytes are sequestered in the splenic capillaries, which can lead to splenomegaly. The combination of intravascular and extravascular hemolysis can result in anemia, which induces extramedullary erythropoiesis. The life span of the erythrocyte is reduced from 120 days to just a few days when the RBC membrane has been deformed. If large numbers of damaged erythrocytes are lysed, unconjugated bilirubin is released, which causes jaundice and possibly gallstones in as many as 60% of children.[52] Membrane fragments from hemolytic reactions can lead to DIC. Pulmonary hypertension may occur in the HS population, presumably as a result of hemolysis-induced alterations in NO metabolism.

Clinical and Laboratory Features

Children may present at any age with the triad of anemia, splenomegaly, and jaundice that often is aggravated by concomitant viral infection. HS can manifest soon after birth and should be considered in infants who are jaundiced after the first postnatal week: resulting hyperbilirubinemia can sometimes necessitate an exchange transfusion. Mild, moderate, and severe forms of HS occur and are characterized by variations in laboratory results and clinical correlates. Mild disease occurs in 20% of children with HS; these children only occasionally present with symptomatic bilirubinate gallstones before adolescence. Approximately 5% of children have severe HS characterized by chronic anemia (hemoglobin concentration less than 8 g/dL) and need for chronic transfusions. The course of this disease may be complicated by viral infections such as parvovirus B19 infection, which can suppress reticulocyte production[53] and precipitate aplastic crises.

HS is most commonly suspected when numerous spherocytes with loss of central pallor appear on a peripheral smear. A complete blood cell count usually reveals a reduced hemoglobin and increased reticulocyte count. Osmotic fragility (OF) was regarded as the gold standard for the diagnosis of HS, but this test produces age-related results and must be performed by experienced laboratory technicians in a timely fashion. The OF test is known to give false negatives in 10% to 20% of patients, as well as false positives in autoimmune hemolytic anemia patients. The guidelines for the diagnosis and management of HS no longer recommends the OF test as a first-line screening tool.[54] Increasingly, flow cytometry using eosin-5′-maleimide is employed to confirm the diagnosis because it requires little blood and can be performed after overnight storage.[55] In addition, as a direct result of chronic hemolysis, unconjugated bilirubin and serum lactate dehydrogenase concentrations increase, and serum haptoglobin concentrations decrease. Thrombocytopenia may develop because of hypersplenism.

Perioperative Considerations

Anemia, thrombocytopenia, and splenomegaly are the major considerations for a child with HS undergoing surgery. The most common disease-related operations performed in children with HS are splenectomy and cholecystectomy, individually or in combination, and these procedures may be performed by laparotomy or laparoscopy.

Splenectomy significantly increases red cell survival in most cases and reduces the severity of the anemia and jaundice. Correlation with clinical symptoms or presence of complications such as severe anemia that require frequent RBC transfusions, poor growth, chronic fatigue, or evidence of extramedullary hematopoiesis (e.g., frontal bossing) can help determine whether to proceed with surgery, which is usually reserved for moderate to severe cases of HS. Splenic enlargement in a child interested in participating in

contact sports is another indication.[53,54] Splenectomy is ideally performed after the age of 6 years because of the increased risk of overwhelming infection by encapsulated organisms such as *Streptococcus pneumoniae*, *Neisseria meningitidis*, and *Haemophilus influenzae* type B in splenectomized younger children.[56] Preoperative vaccination against these organisms is essential unless surgery is required emergently.[57] Guidelines for the indications and duration of postoperative penicillin prophylaxis vary among institutions.[52]

Splenectomy in children is more frequently performed laparoscopically than by open laparotomy because the former is associated with decreased blood loss, less pain, shorter hospital stay, and improved cosmesis. Conversion from laparoscopic to open splenectomy is necessary in fewer than 1% of cases.[58,59] If anemia recurs after splenectomy, it may indicate the presence of accessory splenic tissue that was unrecognized initially.[60] Partial splenectomies are increasingly performed, especially in younger children with severe disease, because they reduce the sequestration of spherocytes and subsequently improve anemia while theoretically allowing retention of some immune function against bacterial infections. However, symptomatic anemia can recur and necessitate total splenectomy at a later time.[61,62] Transient postsplenectomy thrombocytosis marked by dramatic increases in platelet counts may also occur in children,[63] in addition to a general increase in the risk of thromboembolic disease.

Gallstones occur in 21% to 63% of children with HS, but cholecystectomy is usually performed only when children are symptomatic with cholelithiasis. Children who undergo splenectomy and who also have radiographically identified gallstones may undergo concurrent cholecystectomy, whether or not the stones are symptomatic.[64–66] Table 8.6 summarizes the clinical features and important perioperative considerations

TABLE 8.6	Perioperative Concerns for Patients With Hereditary Spherocytosis
Preoperative Considerations	
Hemoglobin, reticulocyte count, platelet count	
History of transfusions and special blood requirements (e.g., extended phenotypic matching, leukocyte reduction)	
History of infections, aplastic crises, and presplenectomy vaccinations	
Presplenectomy antibiotic prophylaxis and immunization when indicated	
Intraoperative Considerations	
Appropriate antibiotic coverage	
Attention to physiologic effects of laparoscopy on circulatory and respiratory function	
Potential for significant blood loss (unusual in splenectomy and cholecystectomy)	
Judicious use of regional anesthesia, intramuscular medications, nasogastric tubes, nasal intubation, and other methods when platelet count is low	
Limited use of medications with potential bleeding risk (e.g., ketorolac)	
Postoperative Considerations	
Sequential hemoglobin determinations and platelet counts	
Potential thrombocytosis: management as recommended by hematology consultants	
Infection risk	

for the child with HS undergoing incidental or disease-related surgical procedures.

GLUCOSE-6-PHOSPHATE DEHYDROGENASE DEFICIENCY

G6PD deficiency causes hemolysis in the presence of oxidative stressors. It is the most common enzyme deficiency in humans, affecting approximately 400 million people worldwide. This enzyme deficiency is inherited in an X-linked, recessive fashion. Although males are most commonly affected, females (heterozygous or homozygous for the gene) may have clinical manifestations of the disease. More than 400 variants have been described, including a relatively mild form that affects about 10% of African American males (i.e., G6PD A−) and a more severe form that affects Italians, Greeks, and other populations in the Mediterranean, African, and Asian regions (i.e., G6PD Mediterranean).[67–70] This deficiency is prevalent in geographic areas where the incidence of malaria is high, presumably because G6PD deficiency may attenuate the severity of malarial infections.

Pathophysiology

G6PD plays an important role in the hexose monophosphate/pentose phosphate shunt, which is essential for normal energy metabolism in erythrocytes. G6PD generates the reduced form of nicotinamide adenine dinucleotide phosphate (NADPH). NADPH maintains glutathione in the reduced form (GSH), which reduces peroxides and protects cells from oxidative damage in the course of normal biochemical events or in the event of excess free oxygen radical generation. Superoxide ion or hydrogen peroxide, or both, can oxidize hemoglobin, which then precipitates as insoluble membrane inclusions. These inclusions, together with the oxidative damage to cell membranes, lead to cell damage in the G6PD-deficient child. Erythrocytes are particularly sensitive to oxidative damage because of their lack of synthetic activity. In the presence of oxidants and free radicals (e.g., produced by infection or by ingestion of certain medications and foods), this cascade of events may precipitate hemolysis in the G6PD-deficient child.[67,69]

Clinical and Laboratory Features

Clinical symptoms of G6PD deficiency may be deceptively variable, and they may occur in the neonatal period or in older age groups. Presenting signs include anemia and jaundice; in severe cases, these signs can be followed by lumbar and abdominal pain and by renal failure. It is important to recognize that in the majority of individuals with G6PD deficiency, there is no anemia in the steady state.[71] However, episodic exacerbations triggered by acute illness such as diabetic acidosis or ingestion of a variety of substances may precipitate a hemolytic event (Table 8.7). Fava beans, also known as broad beans, contain high concentrations of vincine and convincine, which are nonvolatile glucosides that can trigger hemolysis.[72] On a global basis, favism is likely the most common form of acute hemolytic anemia associated with G6PD deficiency.[73] Hemolysis may range from benign and transitory to severe and life threatening; the latter situation is more likely if the triggering agent is not eliminated or controlled. In a small minority of cases, G6PD deficiency can be associated with a chronic hemolytic process. Laboratory findings include normocytic anemia, increased reticulocyte count and serum bilirubin concentration, and presence of Heinz bodies in the peripheral blood smear.

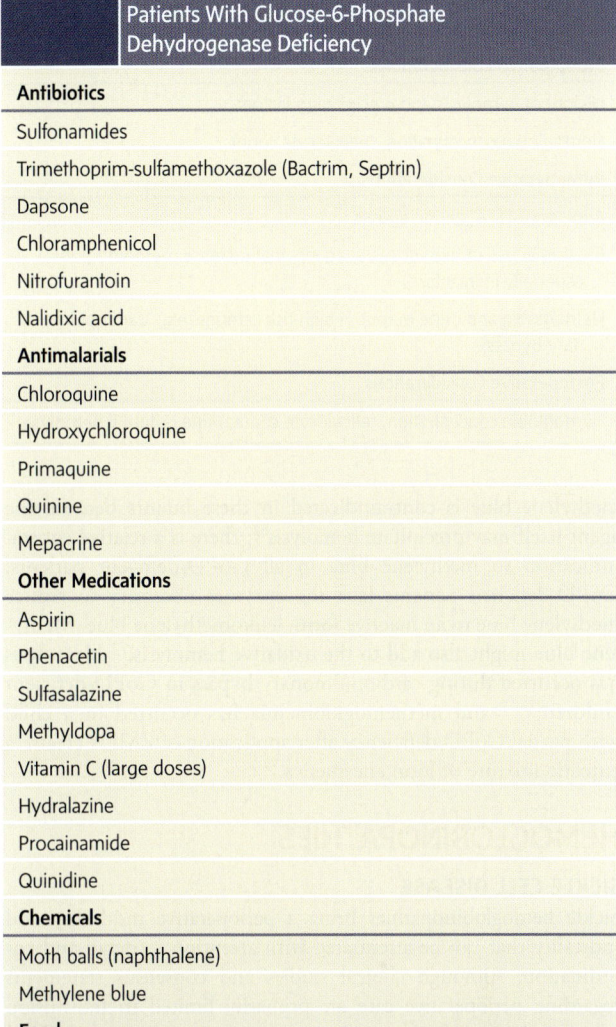

TABLE 8.7	Agents That May Precipitate Hemolysis in Patients With Glucose-6-Phosphate Dehydrogenase Deficiency
Antibiotics	
Sulfonamides	
Trimethoprim-sulfamethoxazole (Bactrim, Septrin)	
Dapsone	
Chloramphenicol	
Nitrofurantoin	
Nalidixic acid	
Antimalarials	
Chloroquine	
Hydroxychloroquine	
Primaquine	
Quinine	
Mepacrine	
Other Medications	
Aspirin	
Phenacetin	
Sulfasalazine	
Methyldopa	
Vitamin C (large doses)	
Hydralazine	
Procainamide	
Quinidine	
Chemicals	
Moth balls (naphthalene)	
Methylene blue	
Food	
Fava (broad) beans	

Perioperative Considerations

In the perioperative setting, G6PD deficiency does not usually cause problems. The most effective management strategy centers on avoiding oxidative stressors (such as pain and anxiety) and avoiding the triggering agents (Table 8.8). Treating or eliminating precipitating causes such as infection is also paramount in safely anesthetizing G6PD-deficient patients. Monitoring for and treatment of possible complications are appropriate; transfusion is rarely required.[74]

Administration of large or excessive doses of medications such as prilocaine, benzocaine, and sodium nitroprusside may trigger hemolysis in G6PD-deficient children in the perioperative setting.[67,69,75,76] Although these children can reduce methemoglobin that is normally produced by these agents, G6PD-deficient children may not tolerate large amounts of potent oxidizing agents (i.e., superoxide ion and hydrogen peroxide) produced by methemoglobin. Infants may be particularly susceptible to symptomatic methemoglobinemia (because of their low NADPH dehydrogenase activity) and to methemoglobin-induced hemolysis if they are G6PD deficient. Treatment of methemoglobinemia with

TABLE 8.8	Perioperative Concerns for Patients With Glucose-6-Phosphate Dehydrogenase Deficiency
Preoperative Considerations	
History of hemolysis and precipitating factors	
Hemoglobin concentration, reticulocyte count	
Intraoperative Considerations	
Avoidance of triggering agents	
Caution in use of high doses of agents that increase methemoglobin, especially in infants	
Hemoglobin and urine output in high-risk settings (e.g., cardiopulmonary bypass)	
Postoperative Considerations	
Hemoglobin concentration, reticulocyte count, urine output if hemolysis	

methylene blue is contraindicated in these infants because the agent itself may precipitate hemolysis[62]; there is a relative contraindication to methylene blue in all G6PD-deficient patients. G6PD-deficient patients lack the enzymes necessary to reduce methylene blue to an inactive form, leukomethylene blue. Methylene blue might also add to the oxidative hemolysis.[77] Hemolysis has occurred during cardiopulmonary bypass in G6PD-deficient children,[76,78] and methemoglobinemia has occurred in a child with partial G6PD deficiency after application of EMLA cream, a eutectic mixture of local anesthetics.[79]

HEMOGLOBINOPATHIES

SICKLE CELL DISEASE

Sickle hemoglobinopathies bring a perioperative morbidity and mortality that can be attenuated with attention to detail and coordination. Although clinical studies and consensus statements regarding perioperative care are primarily limited to transfusion practices, logic and other studies suggest than an awareness of and addressing the complex pathophysiology of sickle cell disease (SCD) would be practical and effective in decreasing complications.

First identified by Herrick about 100 years ago, SCD is a group of inherited hemoglobinopathies with a diverse worldwide prevalence. The disease affects about 1 in 365 African American and 1 in 16,300 Hispanic births.[80] The spectrum of the disease includes sickle cell anemia (HbSS), which accounts for about 70% of the American sickle cell disease population; sickle cell/hemoglobin C disease (HbSC), accounting for about 20%; sickle cell/β-thalassemia (HbSβ-thalassemia), accounting for about 10%; and a host of other, uncommon sickle variants whose prevalence is increasing over time.[81] HbSβ-thalassemia includes HbSβ⁰- and HbSβ⁺-thalassemias; the distinction between the two is the absence of normal HbA in the former versus decreased amount of HbA in the latter, even a small amount of HbA present in the latter partially mitigates the severity of disease. Although there are large phenotypic variations within each form of sickle cell disease, in general HbSS and HbSβ⁰-thalassemia are clinically similar and more severe than HbSC and HbSβ⁺-thalassemia. Sickle cell trait (HbAS), in which approximately 40% of hemoglobin is hemoglobin S, occurs in about 8% of African Americans and in a much smaller percentage of Hispanic and other subpopulations.[80] The sickle gene is found commonly in sub-Saharan Africa, the Mediterranean, the Arabian Peninsula, and India, where sickle cell trait provides a significantly increased fitness in malaria-endemic regions.[82] Its spread to the United States was primarily due to the forced migration of enslaved people.

Pathophysiology

Hemoglobin A is composed of two α- and two β-globin chains. Hemoglobin S results from a single base pair mutation in the β-globin gene on chromosome 11, which results in the replacement of a negatively charged, hydrophilic glutamate residue with a noncharged, hydrophobic valine residue. This hydrophobic valine is exposed when HbS is deoxygenated and is stabilized by binding the same hydrophobic valine pocket on other HbS molecules, thereby leading to polymerization of HbS, precipitation, and hemolysis.[83]

In contrast to prior simplistic models in which sickled cells were simply thought to block flow through the microcirculation, the pathophysiology of sickle cell disease is now understood to be considerably more complex. This understanding is, in turn, leading to more therapeutic interventions.[83] Any factor that promotes hemoglobin crystallization (e.g., hypoxia, acidosis, and cellular dehydration) or prolongs capillary transit time (e.g., dehydration, hypothermia, leukocytosis, thrombosis, and inflammation) increases HbS polymerization and formation of sickled cells. Inflammation, vascular endothelial adhesion abnormalities, platelets, and coagulation cascade activation all contribute to vasoocclusive episodes. The sickle red cell membrane becomes compromised due to exposure to destructive oxidizing effects of precipitated HbS, thereby leading to altered permeability to sodium, potassium, and calcium, causing dehydration of the cell and irreversible sickling.[83] Membrane abnormalities of phospholipid content also contribute to its deformability, and exposure of phosphatidyl serine facilitates activation of the clotting cascade. These and other factors lead to entrapment of irreversibly sickled red cells in the microcirculation, activation of coagulation and inflammatory pathways, ischemia, and infarction of tissue. At the same time, chronic intravascular hemolysis decreases production of NO, whereas increased scavenging decreases the bioavailability of NO. The resulting NO deficiency causes endothelial dysfunction and disease complications, such as pulmonary hypertension, priapism, and skin ulceration.[83]

Clinical and Laboratory Features and Treatment

Sickle cell disease is a multisystem process involving most organs of the body and at times necessitating surgical intervention. Although there is considerable variation in disease severity, all patients have a progressive clinical course. Therapeutic interventions, genetic factors and critically, access to expert sickle cell care account in large part for the differences in outcome. Children with persistence of hemoglobin F (which itself protects against the effects of deoxygenation on red cells) and those with HbSC or HbSβ⁺ have fewer complications than those with HbSS or HbSβ⁰.

Early diagnosis and treatment of sickle cell disease have been facilitated by the universal neonatal screening. An eluate from a dried blood spot is analyzed by isoelectric focusing and/or high-performance liquid chromatography. As not all children with sickle cell disease are African American (i.e., Native American, Hispanic, and Caucasian),[84] since 2006 all neonates have been screened for sickle hemoglobinopathies. The parents of infants diagnosed with sickle trait (HbAS) during neonatal screening may not be informed of the diagnosis, although perioperative complications associated with sickle cell trait are exceedingly rare. Affected children born in the United States before universal neonatal screening and those born outside the United States without routine health care may not have been diagnosed with a hemoglobinopathy and managed appropriately preoperatively. Notwithstanding the controversy over the utility of nonselective preoperative screening, children at risk whose hemoglobin status is unknown preoperatively should be tested with a sickle-screening test followed by a hemoglobin electrophoretic evaluation if the screening yields a positive result.[85] Caution should be used in interpreting screening tests as both false positive (e.g., from profound anemia or some variants), and false negative (e.g., high fetal hemoglobin) results have been reported. Electrophoresis and high-performance liquid chromatography (HPLC) are diagnostic at all ages, though turnaround times can be prolonged. Children older than 10 years of age with a normal hemoglobin value, standard peripheral blood smear, and unremarkable clinical history have a low risk of a clinically significant hemoglobinopathy.[86]

Common clinical symptoms of sickle cell disease in children include episodes of excruciating pain secondary to recurrent vasoocclusive episodes, chronic hemolytic anemia, acute chest syndrome (ACS), infection, renal insufficiency, osteonecrosis, and cholelithiasis.[83] Pulmonary hypertension, priapism, and skin ulcerations may also occur and are related to the degree of red cell hemolysis.[87] Chronic pulmonary and neurologic disease (e.g., stroke) are additional causes of significant morbidity and mortality.[83] In the perioperative period, the most common complications in sickle cell children include ACS (about 10%), fever or infection (about 7%), vasoocclusive episodes (about 5%), and transfusion-related events (about 10%).[88]

Chronic hemolytic anemia is a hallmark of HbSS disease. It is characterized by a baseline hemoglobin concentration of 5 to 9 g/dL, reticulocytosis (5%–10%), and a distinctive red cell morphology observed on a peripheral blood smear.[83,89] In contrast, the hemoglobin concentration in those with HbSC disease usually exceeds 9 g/dL. Red cell fragility and chronic hemolysis in HbSS are associated with anemia, increased red cell turnover, a propensity to form biliary stones, and critically, altered NO metabolism. The anemia may be complicated by other events such as acute splenic sequestration, that typically occurs in infants and young children after a viral illness; or an acute cessation of red cell production, the equivalent of transient erythroblastopenia of childhood and typically associated with parvovirus B19 infection. In some children, chronic and acute severe anemia are managed with RBC transfusions, which may lead to them developing alloantibodies to RBC antigens, and iron overload if untreated. The latter can progress to life-threatening cirrhosis and cardiac failure. Most children receive chronic folic acid therapy to prevent megaloblastic erythropoiesis from increased demands for purine synthesis from red cell production. Of note, a newly approved drug, voxelotor increases the baseline hemoglobin concentration notably by binding hemoglobin, which increases oxygen affinity and decreases its ability to crystallize.[90]

Vasoocclusive episodes in HbSS occur as a result of episodic microvasculature occlusions at one or more sites. The occlusive process occurs most commonly in the phalanges (i.e., dactylitis or hand-foot syndrome), long bones, ribs, sternum, spine, and the pelvis; it also can occur in the mesenteric microvasculature, producing abdominal pain that may mimic a surgical acute abdomen. Pain from vasoocclusive episodes should be managed using a multifaceted approach including reversal of potential triggers (via warming, hydration, and ambulation), distraction, psychological and behavioral interventions, and complementary modalities in addition to analgesic medications. Initial pharmacologic management often entails scheduled antiinflammatory agents because inflammation is central to the vasoocclusive process, and these agents are synergistic with opioids. It is essential to foster an ideal environment for pain control (e.g., calm, pleasant distractions, supportive personnel and objects). Hydroxyurea is used to prevent vasoocclusive episodes and end-organ damage. Currently, it is widely recommended for all patients with HbSS and HbSβ⁰.[91] Although underutilized, hydroxyurea is a safe and effective component of chronic management in decreasing the frequency of events through several mechanisms; inhibiting hemoglobin precipitation by increasing fetal hemoglobin concentrations; reducing white blood cell count; modifying the inflammatory response; and facilitating NO metabolism.[83,91,92] Inhaled NO or precursors of NO may prove to be effective therapy for vasoocclusive episodes.[83,93–95]

ACS is characterized by a new infiltrate on chest radiograph. ACS frequently occurs 2 to 3 days after a vasoocclusive episode, and both physical examination and symptoms can vary widely.[96–98] Although presentation may include fever, tachypnea, cough, or hypoxemia, at times none are present, and it is not uncommon to present with a normal physical examination. As such, one must maintain a high index of suspicion, especially perioperatively. ACS, which may have a relatively benign course or may progress to respiratory failure and even death, is the most common cause of death in children with HbSS.[81] The inconsistent presentation in part reflects the complex and variable pathogenesis of ACS. An episode may have a single or multiple causes, including infection (i.e., bacteria or atypical bacteria [often *Chlamydia* or *Mycoplasma*], viruses or a combination of agents), pulmonary fat embolism, pulmonary infarction, and pulmonary hemorrhage.[96] Acute management includes supportive care and oxygen, antibiotics that treat encapsulated and atypical organisms, bronchodilators, pain control, ventilatory support as needed, and transfusion. Incentive spirometry or continuous positive airway pressure can be helpful, especially in the perioperative setting.[99] Hydroxyurea therapy and chronic transfusion therapy decrease the frequency of ACS, whereas inhaled NO, NO precursors and antioxidants (e.g., arginine and glutamine) may attenuate the process acutely.[83,91,93,100,101] Airway reactivity is also common in children with sickle cell disease, in part due to NO deficiency, and is responsive to bronchodilator therapy.[102,103] NO regulation and deficiency, the result of decreased production, increased consumption, or altered metabolism, contributes to the development of restrictive lung disease and pulmonary hypertension, also potentially contributed to by repeated ACS-induced lung injury and chronic inflammation.[83,87,104]

Susceptibility to infections and sepsis increase dramatically after the first few months of life. This has been attributed to repeated splenic infarcts that led to splenic atrophy. In the absence of a spleen, the child becomes a vulnerable target for infections.[83] In children less than 6 years of age, infections from encapsulated pathogens such as *S. pneumoniae*, *H. influenzae* type B, and meningococcus are common. To prevent these infections, penicillin prophylaxis is given to children until 6 years of age along with additional immunizations. In older children and adults, infections from Gram-negative organisms (e.g., *Salmonella* osteomyelitis and *E. coli* urosepsis) are common.[83,96]

Stroke is a devastating complication of sickle cell disease. Historically, overt stroke, which peaks in children 2 to 9 years of age, is reported in approximately 10% of children.[105–108] However, silent infarcts, which are generally underappreciated, occur in an additional 30% with associated neurocognitive deficits.[105] One-fourth of children have motor or cognitive deficits at the time of surgery.[106,107] Risk factors include reduced hemoglobin concentration, increased concentration of HbS, hypertension, increased leukocyte count, and a history of dactylitis, whereas greater HbF and alpha thalassemia concentrations provide some protection.[108] Pain episodes, ACS, and infection may precipitate strokes.[109] Emergent exchange transfusion to reduce the concentration of HbS to less than 30% is the center piece of acute management, followed by chronic transfusions and hydroxyurea administration to minimize the risk of recurrence.[91,110] The thrust of the current management of stroke is prevention. Yearly screening with transcranial doppler (TCD) starting at age 2 identifies most children at high risk, and subsequent management with chronic transfusion and hydroxyurea therapy may minimize the risk of a future stroke.[80,91,111,112]

Renal abnormalities can include proteinuria, hematuria, hyposthenuria, and renal tubular acidosis.[113] Acute and chronic renal failure may develop, and ACE inhibitors may be of benefit for resulting hypertension.[113,114] Renal dialysis and transplantation have proven successful interventions for renal complications of the disease.[115]

HbAS is usually benign, although it may be characterized by microhematuria and hyposthenuria, and sickling or sudden death may occur under extremely altered physiologic circumstances (e.g., cardiopulmonary bypass, extreme exercise, or cell-salvage).[115–118] There is also a small but significant risk of pulmonary embolism. An increased risk of rhabdomyolysis with exercise, as well as sudden death with extreme exertion in individuals with HbAS, has led to the controversial mandate to offer trait testing to all National Collegiate Athletic Association (NCAA) division one athletes.[119]

Children with HbSC disease usually have a greater baseline hemoglobin concentration and fewer complications than those with HbSS disease. Because splenic function is often preserved, the risk for infection in early childhood is reduced.[86] Children with HbSC disease are more likely to have proliferative retinopathy and avascular necrosis of long bones.

Children with HbSβ⁰ (i.e., one sickle globin allele and one thalassemic allele expressing no β-globin) have a course identical to that of HbSS, whereas those with HbSβ⁺ (i.e., one sickle globin allele and one thalassemic allele expressing β-globin at a reduced level) tend to have a more benign course that is proportional to the amount of normal β-globin expression. The coexistence of hemoglobin S with α-thalassemia produces a variable clinical picture that includes a greater risk of pain but a reduced risk of stroke, renal complications, and gallstones.[82,86]

Many additional approaches to sickle cell care are being investigated and are notable for targeting multiple aspects of the complex physiology.[83,120–123] These include administration of short-chain fatty acids such as butyrate or demethylating agents such as decitabine to induce production of hemoglobin F; small molecules to interfere with polymerization; antibodies to alter cell adherence ion channel inhibitors to decrease cellular dehydration; NO-related compounds and precursors, modifying heme excess, altering hemoglobin oxygen affinity, and manipulation of inflammatory pathways. New therapeutic targets such a

BCL11A, a zinc finger protein that plays a key role in the silencing of fetal globin genes, are being targeted by multiple mechanisms.[124] HSCT is increasingly used as a curative intervention for sickle cell disease.[125,126] Although cure rates with HLA-matched sibling donors exceed 85%, the lack of such donors for most patients has led to the increasing use of unrelated and haploidentical donors. To circumvent many complications of transplantation, gene therapy protocols using a child's own modified stem cells are underway, and multiple gene editing approaches are being pursued.[127–130]

Perioperative Considerations

Perioperative morbidity and mortality are greater in children with sickle cell disease than in the general population, and as clinical trial data are scant, a focus on addressing the complex physiology of SCD, as well as multidisciplinary coordination are key.[85,131–133] Children with SCD often require surgical procedures, the most common being cholecystectomy,[134] ear, nose, and throat procedures,[135] and orthopedic procedures (especially hip procedures for osteonecrosis).[136] Placement of long-term vascular access for transfusions, antibiotics, analgesia, and other therapies is frequently performed. The Cooperative Study of Sickle Cell Disease reported that 7% of all deaths among children with this disease were related to surgery.[81] Early reviews reported perioperative mortality rates as great as 10% and morbidity rates as great as 50% for children with sickle cell disease.[137–140] Studies published in the 1990s indicated that the 30-day mortality rate was about 1%.[141] In a group of more than 600 patients managed according to standard guidelines of care and prospectively studied, the incidence of any complication was about 30%, and the incidences of ACS and vasoocclusive pain episodes were 10% and 5%, respectively.[88] Patient factors (e.g., age, history of pulmonary disease, number of prior hospitalizations) and surgical factors (i.e., invasive vs. superficial) affect the incidence of complications. The impact of newer interventions and technologies (e.g., laparoscopic and robotically assisted cholecystectomy and splenectomy)[142–144] on perioperative morbidity and mortality rates is unclear, although more recent reports cite reduced rates of complications than in the past.[145] Given the high risk of pain and ACS, and the dearth of comparative studies identifying optimal perioperative care in SCD, it is paramount to remain aware of and attempt to address the pathophysiology leading to these sequalae.

The principles of optimal perioperative care are based on maintaining optimal physiologic parameters throughout the perioperative period, avoiding and prospectively attenuating factors that may precipitate acute sickle related complications. This requires close communication and planning between hematologists, surgeons, and anesthesiologists (Table 8.9).[146] One approach is to have the child with sickle cell disease who is undergoing surgery be viewed and managed primarily as a hematology patient whose care is being shared with, rather than assumed by, the surgeon and anesthesiologist during the perioperative period. Avoiding unnecessary and potentially dangerous surgical procedures (e.g., exploratory laparotomy to rule out appendicitis in a child who is experiencing an abdominal pain crisis) and minimizing perioperative complications by avoiding known triggers of vasoocclusion should be the focus of the multidisciplinary care team. Based on a survey of perioperative management of sickle cell disease among anesthesiologists in North America, most anesthesiologists consult with hematologists in all cases or on a case-by-case basis.[147]

TABLE 8.9	Perioperative Concerns for Patients With Sickle Cell Disease

Preoperative Considerations

Screening if unknown status in at-risk children

Primary management by hematology service (in most circumstances)

History of acute chest syndrome, vasoocclusive pain crises, hospitalizations, transfusions, transfusion reactions

Neurologic assessment (e.g., strokes, cognitive limitations)

History of analgesic and other medication use

Hematocrit

Oxygen saturation (on room air), chest radiograph

Pulmonary function tests (when appropriate)

Practice incentive spirometry at home

Work with child life specialist if indicated

Echocardiography (when appropriate)

Neurologic imaging (for recent changes)

Renal function studies

Transfusion crossmatch (e.g., antibody-matched, leukocyte-reduced, sickle negative)

Transfusion to correct anemia (in most circumstances)

Parenteral hydration for *nil per os* (NPO) status

Pain management

Aggressive bronchodilator therapy

Appropriate antibiotic therapy, including presplenectomy antibiotics and immunizations (as indicated)

Intraoperative Considerations

Maintenance of oxygenation, perfusion, normal acid–basis status, temperature, hydration

Availability of appropriately prepared blood (as indicated)

Replacement of blood loss

Anesthetic technique appropriate for procedure and postoperative analgesic requirements

Attention to physiologic effects of laparoscopy on circulatory and respiratory function

Appropriate antibiotic therapy

Judicious use of tourniquets, cell saver, and cardiopulmonary bypass

Postoperative Considerations

Management by hematology service

Monitoring for complications, especially acute chest syndrome and vasoocclusive pain crises

Maintenance of oxygen saturation monitoring and supplementation as needed, including prophylactic supplemental oxygen the first 24 hours regardless of oxygen saturation

Appropriate hydration (oral plus parenteral)

Appropriate antibiotic therapy

Aggressive pain management: must assure ability to breathe deeply and do incentive spirometry

Early mobilization

Incentive spirometry (possibly with continuous or bilateral positive airway pressure) and bronchodilator therapy

Although there is no evidence to support or refute many of the long-standing guidelines for perioperative care and individual practices vary widely,[147] it seems prudent to avoid those factors that may promote intravascular sickling: hypoxia, acidosis, hyperthermia, hypothermia, and dehydration.[131] Meticulous attention to pain management is essential as in addition to perioperative vasoocclusive pain being common, it can interfere with deep-breathing and incentive spirometry, increasing the risk of ACS. Monitoring vital signs throughout the perioperative period is mandatory, especially monitoring oxygenation with pulse oximetry. Oxygen saturation as determined by pulse oximetry may underestimate measured oxygen saturation in patients with sickle cell disease, although this is usually clinically insignificant.[148,149] Because ACS, a common (10%) and potentially life-threatening complication of surgery, occurs 1 to 3 days postoperatively, it is important to extend adherence to guidelines of care into the postoperative period, regardless of the apparent well-being of the child.[88] In light of the renal concentrating defect found in these patients, perioperative hydration is important to maintain and may require in-hospital preoperative care, although one must be aware that over-hydration may compromise vulnerable cardiovascular and respiratory physiology.

Transfusion in the perioperative period remains a controversial subject despite several studies suggesting its benefit, in part as some argue with improved anesthesia techniques, and being provided in a controlled environment, that transfusion is not needed.[88,131,150–152] Transfusion of non-HbS RBCs to a child with sickle cell disease has several beneficial effects: correction of anemia; dilution of HbS red cells; compensation for blood loss; and prevention of some complications (e.g., ACS and stroke). However, transfusion is not without risks, including alloimmunization,[49,153] transfusion reactions (about 7% in the perioperative period),[88] infection, iron overload, time, and expense. Although there have been many reports of surgery performed safely in children with sickle cell disease without preoperative transfusion,[154,155] uncontrolled studies indicate that preoperative transfusion does decrease the rate of perioperative complications.[134,141] The Preoperative Transfusion in Sickle Cell Disease Study Group demonstrated prospectively in 604 operations (70% were cholecystectomies and otolaryngologic and orthopedic operations) that simple transfusion (i.e., correction of preoperative anemia to 10 grams/dL with simple transfusion) was as effective as aggressive transfusion (i.e., lowering the preoperative HbS level to less than 30%, often with exchange transfusion) in preventing perioperative complications and was associated with less alloimmunization and fewer transfusion-related complications in children.[88]

To directly determine if transfusion prevents perioperative complications in the current era of surgical and anesthesia practices, an international randomized trial was initiated, the Transfusion Alternatives Preoperatively in Sickle Cell Disease (TAPS) trial. This trial was halted early due to an excessive number of complications in the nontransfusion group. In addition, transfusion was found to be cost-effective.[156] This led to the continued recommendation of transfusion for moderate and complicated operations in sickle cell patients.[91,151,157] It is currently recommended that most children with HbSS undergoing all but the most minor surgical procedures (e.g., bilateral myringotomy and tubes) receive preoperative correction of anemia with a "simple" (i.e., direct) transfusion targeting a hemoglobin concentration of 10 g/dL. Children in chronic transfusion programs (e.g., for stroke prevention or acute chest) should continue such management preoperatively, and common-sense dictates performing surgery soon after a scheduled transfusion.

Recommendations for children with baseline hemoglobin concentrations close to 10 g/dL are more complicated and have not been investigated.[152] Patients with HbSC, S/B+ thalassemia or who due to therapeutic interventions (e.g., hydroxyurea or voxelotor), or other genetic factors often have these relatively high hemoglobin values. For sickle cell patients with a hemoglobin concentration greater than 8.5 to 9 g/dL or who have a history of ACS, frequent pain crises, underlying pulmonary disease, or other severe end-organ complications, a preoperative exchange transfusion to reduce the HbS and ending with a hemoglobin of 10 g/dL is often recommended.[91,155,158] As arranging vascular access and obtaining a sufficient number of compatible units can take time, hematology should be consulted well in advance.

Although a retrospective review suggests children with sickle cell disease undergoing MRI and other examinations under sedation/anesthesia without prior transfusion do not have increased complications, there are case reports of deaths during such procedures.[159] Thus it is prudent to work with families and support staff to avoid sedation when possible.[160]

Because of the high risk of alloimmunization in SCD, the local blood bank should be consulted as it may take significant time to acquire appropriate units. Red cells should undergo extended genotypic, and/or phenotype matching, including Rh, Cc, D, Ee, and Kell antibodies in addition to ABO and to any antigens for which alloantibodies have developed.[91,161] Red cells should be leukocyte-reduced and sickle negative, but there is no need for irradiation unless it is days before a stem cell transplant. Directed donation of blood from family members should be avoided if the child is a HSCT candidate because it can lead to alloimmunization and later graft rejection.

Although the goal of perioperative management is to avoid triggering pathways that may lead to vasoocclusion and ACS, sadly the focus of research has been limited to whether to transfuse or not. That said, it is important to evaluate other interventions. That direct transfusion is as effective as exchange transfusion in many situations suggests the total Hgb may be more important than the percent of HbS.[88] Voxelotor is an FDA approved drug for SCD that binds to α-globin, shifting the oxygen dissociation curve left and decreasing HbS crystallization and hemolysis, resulting in a higher hemoglobin, often over 10 g/dL, the target of a direct transfusion.[90] Whether voxelotor will provide as good protection from perioperative complications as transfusion, or if these patients should receive an exchange transfusion is unknown. An additional approach to evaluate is positive pressure ventilatory support (CPAP/BiPAP). ACS is a major postoperative complication; incentive spirometry helps prevent ACS, whereas CPAP/BiPAP are useful to treat it. A retrospective review of laparoscopic cholecystectomies in untransfused patients with sickle cell disease showed that when oxygen and CPAP were administered for at least 24 hours postoperatively, the frequency of complications was not excessive.[155] Hence, the goal of blocking or attenuating the pathophysiology to decrease complications can be undertaken through multiple approaches, potentially avoiding transfusion.

Anesthetic agents and techniques do not have a clear effect on perioperative outcomes for children with sickle cell disease.[162] Inhalational anesthetics do not affect the sickling process, although there is experimental evidence suggesting that halothane may increase the viscosity of sickled blood.[163] Pharmacokinetics of some agents commonly used with general anesthesia such as atracurium may be altered in this population.[164] Regional anesthesia is controversial as it has been associated with an increased risk of postoperative complications in one retrospective study, but it has not been shown to affect perioperative outcome in others, despite increasing case reports.[134,133,136,141] The vasodilatory and analgesic properties of regional anesthesia can minimize the risk of or treat vasoocclusive episodes and priapism as well as reduce perioperative pain.[165,166]

Other aspects of anesthetic care of SCD patients merit consideration. Hyperventilation should be avoided because of its potential to reduce cerebral perfusion in children at increased risk for stroke.[167] The use of a tourniquet in HbSS and HbAS diseases remains debated.[168–170] However, tourniquets have been applied intraoperatively for up to 2 hours without complication, and the predominance of evidence supports their safe use as long as they are used carefully and selectively in combination with general guidelines of perioperative care.[171–174] Intraoperative blood salvage with cell saver devices has been used safely in sickle cell patients,[175] although there are concerns that the salvage device itself may produce sickling in the processed blood, even sickle trait blood.[176] Although it has never been studied and there is no official consensus regarding sickling in trait, salvage should be avoided in sickle cell disease unless absolutely necessary. Cardiopulmonary bypass presents conditions that are favorable toward sickling, given the cold, hypoxic, acidotic, and stagnant environment created even in sickle trait patients. Although there are reports of bypass surgery conducted in children with HbAS or even HbSS with standard bypass procedures without transfusion,[177–181] patients with severe sickle hemoglobinopathies are better managed with aggressive exchange transfusion before bypass.

In spite of the absence of comparative studies that specifically address optimal postoperative care, understanding of the pathophysiology of the disease and studies of sickle cell pain suggest that efforts to minimize postoperative pain should be sought to facilitate deep inspirations, and encourage the use of incentive spirometry, and early ambulation in order to prevent ACS.[85,132,133] The aggregate of maintaining euvolemia, normothermia, and sufficient oxygenation should minimize the risk of vasoocclusive pain at this time of increased risk due to anesthesia and postoperative inflammation.

THALASSEMIAS

Although thalassemia is common, there is a lack of clinical studies on perioperative practices, and the literature is primarily filled with case reports. Thalassemia disorders are among the most common genetic disorders worldwide. They are characterized by a perturbation of the normal 1:1 ratio of α to β globin polypeptide chains, usually due to reduced synthesis of one polypeptide, but also possibly due to excess genes (e.g., triplicated α-globin genes).[182–184] The clinical severity of the disease is proportional to the degree of chain imbalance, which ranges from an asymptomatic carrier state to profound ineffective erythropoiesis with transfusion dependence to fetal death due to hydrops fetalis. Both α-thalassemia and β-thalassemia primarily affects children of Mediterranean, African, and Southeast Asian descent. Whereas neonatal assay screening for HbS can detect many forms of α-thalassemia, these tests typically detect only profound forms of β-thalassemia. The concomitant presence of qualitatively abnormal hemoglobins (e.g., HbS, HbE) affects the clinical course of thalassemia disorders. The primary ineffective erythropoiesis and hemolytic anemia, as well as resultant disease therapy, may affect perioperative care.

Pathophysiology

Anemia in thalassemia is the result of hemolysis and ineffective erythropoiesis; the latter results in turn, from accelerated cell apoptosis triggered in part by excess deposition of unpaired globin chains in erythroid precursors.[182,183] Unpaired globin subunits are oxidized and form hemichromes, whose degree of formation affects the degree of hemolysis. Precipitation of hemichromes leads to a complex process that includes release of toxic agents and formation of reactive oxygen species; alteration of red cell membranes causes cells to aggregate, which in turn lead to embolic complications and activation of the coagulation cascade. As a result of chronic anemia and ineffective erythropoiesis, bone marrow expansion and extramedullary hematopoiesis (EMH) may develop in the liver and spleen and lead to paraspinous pseudo tumors (which can make epidurals difficult). Marrow space expansion may occur at sites such as the cranium and paravertebral areas, which could result in pathologic fractures, disfiguring bony changes and pain, which can impact intubation.[185] Erythroid hyperplasia and ineffective erythropoiesis reduce hepcidin expression (a polypeptide that inhibits iron absorption by binding to the ferroportin in the gut wall and macrophages), which may increase iron absorption from the gastrointestinal tract and cause iron overload, even in the absence of transfusion iron overload. Iron overload and deposition lead to fibrosis and cirrhosis with concomitant organ dysfunction and eventual failure. The most relevant target organs for iron overload are the liver, pancreas, heart, and pituitary; the extent of iron deposition in each can be accurately and sequentially monitored by MRI.[186]

Clinical and Laboratory Features and Treatment

Disease severity in α-thalassemia typically reflects the complete loss of expression of between one and all four of the α-globin genes.[184] A four-gene globin deletion typically results in hydrops fetalis with in utero or perinatal death unless diagnosed early and supported with in utero transfusions. A three-gene deletion, or hemoglobin H (HbH) disease, is relatively benign, characterized by chronic hemolytic anemia, which may be exacerbated by exposure to stress and oxidants.[187,188] The few patients with profound anemia or requiring intermittent transfusion therapy often have a two-gene deletion along with a hemoglobin Constant Spring (HbCS) mutation (HbH-Constant Spring) or other unstable α-chains.[187,188] A two-gene deletion alone is benign, manifest by a mild, clinically insignificant microcytic anemia. A one-gene deletion results in a silent carrier state with no anemia or microcytosis.

In contrast to α-thalassemia, β-thalassemia reflects partial or complete loss of expression of the β-globin genes. The broad spectrum of disease results from the number of genes affected and the degree to which each gene is affected. When only one β-globin gene is affected (i.e., β-thalassemia trait), mild microcytic anemia is the primary clinical manifestation. When both β-globin genes are affected, the clinical picture may be mild to moderate, potentially requiring intermittent, but not chronic transfusions (thalassemia intermedia), or severe, requiring chronic transfusions (thalassemia major or Cooley's anemia). Children with hemoglobin E (HbE)/β-thalassemia manifest a dramatic range of severity ranging from very mild to severe and transfusion dependent.

The clinical problems in thalassemia relate to chronic anemia, the physiologic response to ineffective erythropoiesis, iron overload

from transfusions and paradoxical increased iron absorption, as well as chelation therapy.[182,183] Clinical problems include transfusion-associated alloimmunization and infection, splenomegaly, bone abnormalities (due to extramedullary hematopoiesis, chelation therapy, and other factors), endocrine dysfunction (including hypogonadism, hypopituitarism, and diabetes mellitus), short stature, pulmonary hypertension, venous thrombosis and thromboembolism, and cardiomyopathy (primarily due to iron overload). Thalassemia patients also may be hypercoagulable, a condition that may be exaggerated after splenectomy.[189–191]

The approach to moderate to severe disease is to balance transfusion to treat the underlying anemia and suppress erythropoiesis while minimizing and aggressively treating iron overload. Phenotypic matching as in sickle cell, and leukocyte reduction of transfused blood can reduce immune complications, and careful surveillance for end-organ damage and endocrine management is essential.[182,183,192] When an appropriate donor is available, hematopoietic stem-cell transplantation (HSCT) is recommended before severe liver damage occurs because it provides a potential cure for thalassemia. To ameliorate the course of the disease, other therapies are being investigated, including administration of erythropoietin, fetal hemoglobin modifiers (e.g., hydroxyurea, butyrate), and antioxidants. Most recently, the modulation of ineffective erythropoiesis by manipulating erythropoietin gene signaling via inhibition of the Jak2-Stat5 pathway has garnered a great deal of attention.[193] Increasing numbers of trials of gene therapy are currently underway and early indicators are that they are proving successful.[194]

Perioperative Considerations

Children with thalassemia may require surgeries including cholecystectomy related to gallstones, vascular access placement to facilitate transfusions, removal of pseudo tumors related to extramedullary hematopoiesis, treatment of fractures or ulcers and splenectomy. Although splenectomy can aid transfusion support, it is avoided if possible because of the increased risk of thromboembolic disease.[195–197] Due to the high risk of sepsis and death, all attempts should be made to fully vaccinate for encapsulated organisms (e.g., pneumococcus) including boosters before splenectomy.[198] If splenectomy is performed, short-term antithrombotic prophylaxis with unfractionated or low molecular weight heparin should be considered during and after surgery. In addition, severe hypertension, resistant to medical management, and thrombocytosis can occur post splenectomy.[196,197] Pneumococcal and other encapsulated organism vaccination protocols, as well as prophylactic antibiotic protocols for asplenic patients should be followed.[198,199] Thalassemia patients who have been splenectomized should be considered at high risk for thrombosis and given appropriate prophylaxis therapy when exposed to transient thrombotic risk factors such as surgery, pregnancy, and immobilization.[190,196,197,200] Demineralized long bones may be prone to fracture, and older children may require osteotomies for bony deformities.

Perioperative management of children with thalassemia has not been extensively studied but should be co-managed with a thalassemia specialist to review and address transfusion support, airway abnormalities, and medical consequences of iron overload and chelation therapy.[196] It is important to consult with a hematologist to define transfusion parameters and the optimal preoperative hemoglobin level. Bony abnormalities of the maxillofacial area may render securing the airway challenging.[185,196,201] Multiple strategies to address this have been reported.[196] Similarly, extramedullary erythropoiesis can lead to paravertebral masses potentially interfering with epidural or other nerve blocks. In addition, one should be aware of the risk of the possible complications of iron overload

TABLE 8.10	Perioperative Concerns for Patients With Thalassemia

Preoperative Considerations

Hemoglobin concentration

Transfusion crossmatch if appropriate (antibody-matched, leukocyte-reduced source for frequently transfused children)

Evaluation for endocrine dysfunction (e.g., diabetes mellitus, hypopituitarism)

Cardiac function, including echocardiogram (when appropriate)

Hepatic function, awareness of risk of cirrhosis and iron- or virus-induced damage

Airway evaluation

Presplenectomy antibiotics and immunizations (when appropriate)

Preparation for possible difficult airway

Intraoperative Considerations

Careful positioning of demineralized extremities

Attention to cardiovascular function, including postsplenectomy hypertension

Attention to physiologic effects of laparoscopy on circulatory and respiratory function

Prophylaxis for thromboembolism

Postoperative Considerations

Monitoring of cardiac function

Prophylaxis for thromboembolism

in these patients: liver dysfunction; diabetes; pituitary dysfunction; and cardiac dysfunction. There should be a low threshold for a preoperative electrocardiogram and ECHO.[196,197] Additional chelation may be required before surgery to improve cardiac function, and consultation with cardiology to develop strategies to avoid cardiac depression. Renal function should be evaluated as chelation may impair function. Similarly, there should be a low threshold to evaluate for pulmonary hypertension and restrictive lung disease.[196,197]

Although there is no consensus on the optimal perioperative hemoglobin, many accept a hemoglobin of at least 10 g/dL, but this should be discussed with hematology on a case-by-case basis. Patients are hypercoagulable, thus deep vein thrombosis precautions should be taken.[191,196,197] The risk of thromboembolic phenomenon is greater after splenectomy, and in thalassemia intermedia compared with thalassemia major. No clinical trials or standards exist for antiplatelet therapy in this setting.[191,196] Patients with α-thalassemia can show dramatic hemolysis when exposed to oxidants. Thus, a perioperative drug review should be undertaken, and oxidants should be avoided or used with extreme caution as in G6PD deficiency (e.g., sodium nitroprusside).

Perioperative considerations and concerns for children with thalassemia, especially for those with thalassemia major, are listed in Table 8.10.

Thrombocytopenia

PLATELET DISORDERS AND BLEEDING

Platelets are an essential component of hemostatic regulation. Platelets are distributed between the bloodstream and spleen in a ratio of 2:1 with a life span of 7 to 10 days. In children, a decreased number of platelets may be attributed to decreased production or increased consumption, or they may have abnormal function. Bleeding typical of platelet disorders often involves skin and mucous membranes. Although there are many causes of primary and secondary thrombocytopenia in infants and children, this discussion focuses on idiopathic thrombocytopenic purpura (ITP).

IDIOPATHIC THROMBOCYTOPENIC PURPURA

Idiopathic thrombocytopenic purpura (ITP) is the most common cause of acute-onset thrombocytopenia in the otherwise healthy child, and it commonly manifests in the operative setting. ITP has an estimated incidence of about 4 per 100,000 children, and is usually a benign, self-limited disorder affecting children between the ages of 2 and 10 years.[63] Primary ITP has no clear predisposing etiology, but secondary ITP is triggered by a drug or medical disorder. Diagnosis is often by exclusion, the differential list is extensive, and response to ITP-specific treatment usually solidifies the diagnosis.

Pathophysiology

ITP is characterized by antibody-mediated clearance of platelets by tissue macrophages, resulting in thrombocytopenia (platelet count less than $100,000/mm^3$) and shortened platelet survival. Antibodies may also suppress megakaryocytes and platelet development. Platelet autoantibodies may exist alone or as part of immune complexes, and they usually are immunoglobulin G (IgG) in type. They often show specificity for platelet membrane glycoproteins IIb-IIIa and Ib-IX.[202] Thrombocytopenia develops when the reticuloendothelial system, typically the spleen, destroys the antibody-covered platelets.

Clinical and Laboratory Features and Treatment

Typically, ITP in children is a benign disorder that occurs after a viral illness or immunization. It is manifested as petechiae of mucosal surfaces or purpura over bony prominences, thrombocytopenia, and a normal to increased mean platelet volume with increased megakaryocytes in the marrow. This process resolves within weeks or months regardless of therapy. ITP is classified as newly diagnosed (less than 3 months in duration), persistent (3–12 months), and chronic (more than 12 months).[203]

Although platelet counts in children with ITP may be significantly reduced, guidelines suggest that treatment be initiated only if there is associated bleeding, regardless of platelet count.[204,205] Observation with avoidance of activity that may lead to trauma is an increasingly accepted management treatment plan. When indicated, medical treatment most commonly consists of agents that decrease monocyte/macrophage-mediated destruction of antibody-coated platelets (e.g., steroids, intravenous immunoglobulin, anti-D immunoglobulins, vinca alkaloids). Agents that decrease antibody production (e.g., cyclophosphamide, anti-CD20 antibody) and investigational agents that stimulate the thrombopoietin receptor are reserved for those who demonstrate an inadequate response to initial therapy.[206] Platelet transfusions are recommended only for life-threatening emergencies. Splenectomy removes a major site of platelet destruction and is recommended as an option only in chronic, symptomatic ITP or acute, life-threatening ITP unresponsive to medical treatment.[207,208] This procedure, which is commonly performed noninvasively, has a success rate of about 75%.[208–210]

Perioperative Considerations

In view of the clinical and laboratory features of ITP, the anesthesiologist providing care for the child with ITP who is undergoing

TABLE 8.11	Perioperative Concerns for Patients With Idiopathic Thrombocytopenia Purpura

Preoperative Considerations

Hemoglobin concentration, platelet count

History of platelet transfusions

History of corticosteroid use

History of infections

Presplenectomy antibiotic prophylaxis and immunizations (when appropriate)

Discussion with a hematologist regarding medical therapy and platelet transfusion for a platelet count <30,000/mm³

Discontinuation of any platelet-inhibiting medication (e.g., aspirin)

Intraoperative Considerations

Appropriate antibiotic coverage

Stress corticosteroid coverage

Medical therapy and platelet transfusion as above (platelets ideally administered after clamping of the splenic artery during splenectomy)

Judicious use of regional anesthesia, intramuscular medications, nasogastric tubes, nasal intubation, and other methods

Limited use of medications with potential bleeding risk (e.g., ketorolac)

Attention to physiologic effects of laparoscopy on circulatory and respiratory function

Postoperative Considerations

Hemoglobin concentration, platelet count

Infection

Corticosteroid coverage

Pain management

splenectomy or incidental surgery should consider the concerns listed in Table 8.11. A hematologist should be consulted to assess the need for medical therapy, including platelet transfusion, before surgery.

Coagulation Disorders

Children may present for surgery with a personal or family history suggesting a bleeding disorder. The anesthesiologist must decide expeditiously whether to postpone surgery to further evaluate or treat the child. A careful medical history, physical examination, and family history, followed by laboratory evaluation in consultation with a hematologist, are important elements in screening for, diagnosing, and treating a bleeding disorder in the perioperative setting.

SCREENING

The clinical history of the child and family is the most essential screening tool. The family history should identify family members who have been labeled as "bleeders", who have required blood transfusion unexpectedly during surgery, or who returned to surgery for unexpected postoperative bleeding. A history of maternal menorrhagia may also be significant. Suggestive signs and symptoms in a child's medical history are easy bruising, mucosal bleeding, and in older girls, menorrhagia. Although diagnosing easy bruising is subjective, the clinician should suspect bleeding tendencies if skin bruising occurs in nontraumatized sites (e.g., trunk)

or is unusually large without evidence of previous trauma. Mucosal bleeding includes epistaxis and gingival bleeding. Occasional nosebleeds can be common in children, but their clinical significance is enhanced by increased frequency, duration, bilaterality, and coexistence with abnormal bleeding from other sites. Gingival bleeding is common after tooth brushing or flossing, but its clinical significance is enhanced by spontaneous occurrence or chronicity, especially in the presence of good dental hygiene.[211] A history of prolonged or excessive bleeding is important when associated with umbilical cord stump dehiscence, dental work (especially extractions), and circumcision. Although mouth injuries can produce impressive blood loss acutely in any individual, recurrent or persistent bleeding from such an injury may indicate an underlying disorder.

Consultation with a hematologist and laboratory evaluation should be considered for children with a clinical history and physical examination result that suggest a bleeding diathesis, especially for children scheduled to undergo procedures associated with large blood loss or that make particular demands on hemostasis, such as tonsillectomy. Laboratory evaluation of all children, regardless of history or type of surgery, may result in false-positive results that lead to costly workups and potentially unnecessary cancellation of operations, both of which can contribute to greater health care inefficiencies and expense. Bleeding due to medications should be distinguished from an actual bleeding disorder.

When a bleeding disorder is strongly suspected, a set of laboratory tests that include a platelet count, PT, INR, aPTT, thrombin time (TT), and fibrinogen concentration should be ordered. The PT test is most sensitive to deficiencies in factors II, V, VII, and X, and it is useful for differentiating a vitamin K deficiency from other causes. The PT is most often used to monitor the anticoagulant effects of warfarin; it is not sensitive to the effects of heparin. The aPTT test is most sensitive to deficiencies in factors VIII, IX, and XI and less sensitive to deficiencies of factor V, factor X, prothrombin, and fibrinogen. The aPTT is also prolonged in deficiencies of the contact or kallikrein/kinin system proteins, factor XII, prekallikrein, and high-molecular-weight kininogen, but these deficiencies are not associated with bleeding. Because aPTT reagents vary in sensitivity for detection of deficiencies of each factor, it is inappropriate to make a general statement about the ability of this test to detect a specific abnormality; abnormal results require discussion with a hematologist or laboratory medicine physician. Although a prolonged aPTT may be caused by a deficiency in one or more factors, it can also result from inhibition by heparin or a plasma inhibitor, such as lupus anticoagulant. Correction of a prolonged aPTT after mixing the child's plasma with normal plasma (1:1 mix) suggests a factor deficiency. The TT test, which determines the amount of time it takes for blood to clot, is useful for determining deficiencies or abnormalities in fibrinogen and is very sensitive to heparin contamination. Bleeding time, a thromboelastogram, and platelet function screens (e.g., PFA-100) are probably not appropriate as first-line screening tests.

Children with an upper limit of normal aPTT test result and a strongly suspicious personal or family history for a bleeding disorder may have an abnormality (e.g., von Willebrand disease [vWD]). These children require further evaluation in consultation with a hematologist. Whether a procedure should be delayed for the consultation depends on several factors, including the patient's history, site and urgency of surgery, potential bleeding risks associated with the planned procedure, and results of previously discussed set of screening tests.

VON WILLEBRAND DISEASE

vWD is one of the most common bleeding disorders, affecting up to 1% of the population, although studies suggest that the prevalence may be as low as 0.1%.[212] Initially named *pseudohemophilia* because of an inheritance pattern that is different from that of hemophilia, vWD is the result of an abnormal amount, structure, or function of the vWF.[213]

Pathophysiology and Classification

The glycoprotein vWF serves two main roles in the coagulation cascade: adhering platelets to damaged subendothelium and carrying factor VIII in plasma. vWD exists as small and large multimers. Large multimers play a more active role in the binding of platelets to subendothelium than do small ones and are, therefore, necessary for platelet adhesion, whereas binding to factor VIII is independent of multimer size. The two aspects of vWF make it an essential part of primary hemostasis (through platelet binding) and secondary hemostasis (as carrier of factor VIII to sites of injury).

Classification of vWD is essential for understanding and management of this disorder. The current classification was developed by a subcommittee on vWD through the International Society on Thrombosis and Haemostasias.[214] vWD is classified qualitatively into two general types; quantitative abnormalities (types 1 and 3) and qualitative abnormalities (type 2, including subtypes A, B, M, and N). All types are inherited in an autosomal dominant pattern, except types 2N and 3, which are autosomal recessive.

Because vWD is heterogeneous, clinical definitions have been proposed using categories such as mild, moderate, and severe, categories that are based on bleeding history (i.e., number of bleeding episodes), and laboratory measurement of factor concentration and activity.[215] As the molecular basis of vWD becomes better understood, classification of this disease likely will change to reflect the new data. For example, Rodeghiero and colleagues proposed a practical approach to diagnosing and categorizing patients with vWD to provide optimal management.[215] Their approach includes a standardized bleeding history score, focused laboratory analysis, and a trial infusion of DDAVP in certain subtypes.[216] Better categorization of patients with vWD may predict clinical outcomes and allow better management in the perioperative setting.[217]

Clinical and Laboratory Features and Treatment

Children with vWD may exhibit many of the clinical features associated with bleeding disorders in general, although there is a notable absence of joint bleeding. The typical symptoms of vWD reflect poor platelet adhesion and include bruising, epistaxis, and menorrhagia.

Children with vWD have traditionally been described as having prolonged bleeding times and aPTTs, but those with mild disease often have normal values. The aPTT is prolonged only if factor VIII activity is equal to or less than a concentration that is determined by the sensitivity of the particular assay at an institution (often below 30%–35%). The platelet functional assay (PFA-100) has better sensitivity and specificity (both near 90%) for diagnosis of the disease.[218] The PFA-100 test, which measures closure time of an aperture on a membrane coated with collagen and adenosine diphosphate (ADP) or epinephrine, depends on vWF activity and platelet function. Because this test has some variability, its interpretation should be used in conjunction with results of other tests.[219] Platelet count is typically normal in all types of vWD except type 2B.

Other laboratory tests used to delineate vWD include: vWF antigen (vWF:A), which is a measure of the total level of vWF; vWF activity, often measured as a ristocetin cofactor activity (vWF:R), itself a measure of vWF binding to platelets through GPIb receptors; factor VIII coagulant activity; and vWF multimer analysis. Certain disease states have been associated with "acquired vWD" and include lymphoproliferative disorders or gammopathies (marked by antibodies to vWF), chronic renal failure, hypothyroidism, Wilms tumor, and certain types of congenital heart disease (characterized by proteolysis of vWF multimers).[220,221] Treatment focuses on increasing concentrations of endogenous vWF with administration of DDAVP when possible or on replacement of factors with factor concentrates.[222] DDAVP is usually effective in type 1 but less so in types 2A and 2M. DDAVP may have little or even undesired effects in some children: it may increase abnormal vWF in types 2A, 2M, and 2N; it can exacerbate thrombocytopenia in type 2B; its repeated administration may lead to tachyphylaxis. DDAVP usually is not administered to very young children because of the risk of free water retention, hyponatremia, and central nervous system (CNS) pathology, including seizures. Similarly, intravenous fluids may need to be limited after its administration to any child. Factor concentrates (including factor VIII and vWF [Humate-P or Alphanate]) typically are required for types 2B, 2N, and 3. Cryoprecipitate may be used when vWF-containing concentrates are unavailable, but it is not recommended as first-line therapy because it is not virus free, and vWF in solvent or heat-treated cryoprecipitate may be abnormal.[223] Because of the complexity of response to therapies in this disease and the ever-changing availability of replacement products, determination of appropriate treatment in conjunction with a hematologist before surgery is crucial.[216,224]

Perioperative Concerns

The major preoperative concerns in children with confirmed vWD are directed toward appropriate preoperative treatment, avoidance of medications that may interfere with coagulation, and anticipation of intraoperative and postoperative bleeding (Table 8.12).[225,226] Regarding neuraxial anesthesia, a recent analysis in patients with hemorrhagic disorders suggests that its use can be performed safely in patients with vWD by maintaining appropriate hemostatic thresholds.[227]

HEMOPHILIA

Hemophilia was first reported in the *Talmud,* in which there are descriptions of 8-day-old boys exsanguinating after ritual circumcision. Widespread public attention was drawn to this disease after members of Queen Victoria's family developed sequelae from hemophilia in the late 19th and early 20th centuries. The discovery of multiple forms of hemophilia was first made in 1944 when blood from two hemophiliacs was mixed and found to clot. In 1952, hematologists explained their earlier finding by noting that a 10-year-old boy, Stephen Christmas, exhibited a type of hemophilia, factor IX deficiency, which differed from the classic form, factor VIII deficiency.

Hemophilia is a group of congenital bleeding disorders caused by deficiency in factor VIII (i.e., hemophilia A, or classic hemophilia), factor IX (i.e., hemophilia B, or Christmas disease), or factor XI (i.e., hemophilia C). Prevalence of hemophilia as a group is 13 to 18 per 100,000 men, with hemophilia A generally four times more prevalent than hemophilia B.[228] Because of X-linked recessive inheritance of hemophilia A and B, family history is very important in establishing the diagnosis. Although boys are usually affected, girls may rarely inherit the disorder if their fathers are affected, and their mothers are carriers or in instances of extreme lyonization (inactivation of an X chromosome). The daughter of an affected father is an obligate carrier with a 50% chance of passing it on to any of her sons. De novo mutations are relatively

TABLE 8.12	Perioperative Considerations for Patients With von Willebrand Disease

Preoperative Considerations

Consultation with hematologist: establish correct diagnosis and response to desmopressin (DDAVP); administer DDAVP *or* viral attenuated factor concentrates containing factor VIII and von Willebrand factor (vWF) such as Humate-P for severe vWD or for those types not responsive to DDAVP[219]

Determination of actual and desired factor concentrations and expected duration of postoperative therapy[225]

Discontinuation of any platelet-inhibiting medication (e.g., aspirin)

Intraoperative Considerations

Judicious use of regional anesthesia, intramuscular medications, nasogastric tubes, nasal intubation, and other procedures that may cause bleeding

Limited use of medications with potential bleeding risk (e.g., ketorolac)

Coagulation profiles, including platelet counts for more invasive surgeries

Treatment of bleeding with appropriate blood products

Consider use of antifibrinolytic agents (i.e., ϵ-aminocaproic acid, tranexamic acid)[224]

Possible use of recombinant factor VIIa for severe bleeding episodes in severe vWD type 3 or patients with inhibitors

Postoperative Considerations

Follow factor concentrations (i.e., factor VIII and vWF)

Availability of blood products and factors

Appropriate treatment of bleeding episodes

Monitor for thromboembolism in children receiving multiple concentrates or antifibrinolytic agents, or both[219]

vWD, von Willebrand disease.

common (about one-third of hemophilia A and B cases) and suspected in male patients lacking a family history.[211] Hemophilia C, affecting primarily Ashkenazi Jews, is a mild form of hemophilia. It is also known as plasma thromboplastin antecedent (PTA) deficiency or Rosenthal syndrome. In the United States, its incidence is 1:100,000 adults, or 10% the incidence of hemophilia A. It is distinguished from the other two forms of hemophilia by an autosomal recessive inheritance pattern (the gene for factor XI is located on chromosome 4), lack of joint bleeding, and infrequent need for treatment. Affected female patients may notice heavy menses and affected male patients may have frequent nosebleeds and occasionally have excessive bleeding during surgery.

Pathophysiology

Normal in vivo hemostasis initiates at sites of endothelial disruption through interaction of activated factor VII (FVIIa) and tissue factor (TF) to form a complex that activates factor IX and factor X directly. Activated factor IX in conjunction with factor VIII further activates factor X, which, with factor V, converts prothrombin to thrombin. Both factor VIII and factor IX are required for sufficient hemostasis, as evidenced by the severe bleeding that occurs if either is completely deficient. Factor XI activates factor IX, but its precise role in the hemostatic pathway is not completely understood.

Clinical and Laboratory Features and Treatment

The wide range of clinical features is similar for hemophilia A and B (Table 8.13). The severity of bleeding in these children directly relates to the degree of their deficiency.[229] Children with mild or moderate hemophilia may bleed excessively only after a hemostatic challenge such as trauma or surgery, whereas children with severe hemophilia may bleed spontaneously (e.g., hemarthroses).[230] Female carriers on average have 50% of normal factor concentrations and usually are asymptomatic, although they occasionally present with a clinical picture similar to that of mild cases of hemophilia.[229]

Results of a general coagulation screen are typically normal except for the aPTT, which is prolonged in proportion to the concentration of factors in the blood. The diagnosis is confirmed by measuring the specific factor concentrations.[231] If hemophilia is suspected but there is no family history, testing for vWD is

TABLE 8.13	Clinical Manifestations of Hemophilia A		
Clinical Manifestations	Mild (>10%)[a]	Moderate (2%–10%)[a]	Severe (<2%)[a]
Age at first hemorrhage	3–14 years or older	<2 years	<1 year
Signs in neonatal period	None	Postcircumcision bleeding	Postcircumcision bleeding, intracranial hemorrhage
Musculoskeletal bleeding	Unusual except with severe trauma	Joint and muscle bleeding with minor trauma	Spontaneous
Central nervous system bleeding	Rare except with severe trauma	Less prevalent than severe	Prevalence, 3% Mean age, 14 years
Postsurgical bleeding	Hematomas and oozing	Wound hematomas and oozing	Usually frank bleeding
Trauma-related bleeding	Hematomas and deep bleeding with significant trauma	Muscle and joint bleeding with minor trauma	Common with minor trauma
Dental bleeding	Often	Common	Usual
Inhibitors present	Rarely	<3%	Prevalence, 15%–20%

[a]Percent factor VIII activity.
Modified from DiMichele D. Hemophilia A (FVIII deficiency). In: Goodnight SH Jr, Hathaway W, eds. *Disorders of Hemostasis and Thrombosis*. New York: McGraw-Hill; 2001: 127-139.

prudent, especially for the types that may mimic hemophilia (i.e., types 2N and 3). Because of the variable sensitivity of the aPTT to specific factor deficiencies, the ability of this test to detect carriers varies between laboratories; diagnosis of a carrier state usually requires specific factor assays.

Hemophilias A and B are treated by replacing the deficient factor concentrations. These factor concentrations should be maintained at specified levels to prevent sequelae (Table 8.14). Exposure to plasma products should be minimized. The duration of treatment should be tailored to the severity of disease. DDAVP may be effective in selected mild cases by increasing factor VIII concentrations through the release of endogenous stores. Because tachyphylaxis limits the prolonged use of DDAVP, it is typically recommended only for minor operations, although its use may be worth considering in more moderate hemophilia cases since it will not result in inhibitor formation.[232] For most cases, especially for those who require increased factor concentrations to be maintained for effective hemostasis, factor concentrates should be used. Although recombinant forms are preferable because they do not carry infectious risk, substitution with plasma-derived forms may be needed when supplies are limited.[229,232] For the rare patient with hemophilia C who has excessive surgical bleeding, treatment with recombinant factor XI or FFP may be required. It is essential to consult with a hematologist to determine a customized factor treatment plan for every child with hemophilia.

Children who have developed inhibitors to factor concentrates pose a challenge in the perioperative period. For years, they were denied surgery unless it was absolutely necessary, at which point they were often managed with increased concentrations of factors or a desensitization regimen. However, recently there has been improved management in these patients with the use of bypassing agents, which are agents that treat bleeding by stimulating thrombin generation through pathways that do not require the missing factors (VIII or IX). Such agents include recombinant factor VIIa (rfVIIa, Novoseven RT, NovoNordisk) and activated prothrombin complex concentrates, such as FEIBA, which have shown efficacy greater than 80%. Specific factor concentrates are preferred, however, unless patients have significantly increased levels of inhibitors.[233]

Perioperative Concerns

The perioperative concerns in hemophilia focus on prevention and treatment of bleeding, similar to the management of patients with vWD (Table 8.15). Many consider regional anesthesia to be contraindicated for patients with hemophilia, but there are reports of its use without complications as long as factor concentrations are maintained.[234]

HYPERCOAGULABILITY

A hypercoagulable state is a condition in which the development of thrombus is favored (i.e., thrombophilia). The condition results in an increased risk for abnormal clot formation and venous thromboembolic events (VTEs), which often are the presenting symptoms at the time of diagnosis. Thrombophilia can be acquired or congenital. The incidence of VTE among children is less

TABLE 8.14	Treatment Targets for Hemophilia A and B			
Type of Hemorrhage	Desired Plasma Factor Levels (IU/DL) for Hemophilia A[a]	Desired Plasma Factor Levels (IU/DL) for Hemophilia B[a]	Duration (days)[b]	
Muscle				
Superficial	40–60	40–60	2–3	
Deep (initial)	80–100	60–80	1–2	
Deep (maintenance)	30–60	30–60	3–5	
Joint	40–60	40–60	1–2	
Gastrointestinal Tract				
Initial	80–100	60–80	7–14	
Maintenance	50	30		
Oral mucosa	30–50	30–50	2–3	
Epistaxis	30–50	30–50	2–3	
Renal	50	40	3–5	
Surgery (major)				
Pre op	80–100	60–80	1–3	
Post op	30–80	30–80	4–14	
Surgery (minor)				
Pre op	50–80	50–80	1–5	
Post op	30–80	30–80	1–5	
Central Nervous System				
Initial	80–100	60–80	1–7	
Maintenance	50	30	8–21	

[a]Recommended targets when there are no product constraints. Targets may be adjusted lower when products are constrained.
[b]May be increased or reduced depending on clinical circumstances and severity of disease.
Modified from Brown DL. Congenital bleeding disorders. *Curr Probl Pediatr Adolesc Health Care.* 2005;35:38-62; Srivastava A, Brewer AK, Mauser-Bunschoten EP, et al. Treatment Guidelines Working Group on behalf of the World Federation of Hemophilia. Guidelines for the management of hemophilia. *Haemophilia.* 2013;19:e1-e47.

TABLE 8.15	Perioperative Concerns for Patients With Hemophilia
Preoperative Considerations	
Consultation with hematologist, establishment of correct diagnosis	
Determination and testing of treatment plan, including use of desmopressin or factors (concentrates or recombinant)	
Consideration of multiple procedures performed together to reduce factor exposure	
Discontinuation of any platelet-inhibiting medication (e.g., aspirin)	
Intraoperative Considerations	
Judicious use of regional anesthesia, intramuscular medications, nasogastric tubes, nasal intubation, and other procedures that may cause bleeding	
Limited use of medications with potential bleeding risk (e.g., nonsteroidal antiinflammatory drugs)	
Follow coagulation profiles, especially factor levels (factors VIII and IX)	
Anticipate and treat bleeding with appropriate blood products	
Consider recombinant activated factor VII (rFVIIa) for severe bleeding	
Postoperative Considerations	
Maintain factor concentrations for specified time period as recommended by the hematologist	
Ensure availability of blood products and factors from the blood bank	
Anticipate and treat bleeding episodes	

than adults, even in those with known congenital thrombophilic conditions, although neonates and adolescents are at relatively high risk in the pediatric population.[235] Congenital thrombophilic conditions include factor V Leiden disorder, prothrombin gene mutation, protein C and S deficiencies, and antithrombin III deficiency.[236] Risk factors for acquired thrombophilia include the presence of a central venous catheter, infection, malignancy, surgery, or trauma.[237] Preoperative screening of nonoperative children with suspected hypercoagulability is controversial and not recommended for those who are asymptomatic, even those with a positive family history.[238]

Evidenced-based guidelines for children with respect to screening and prophylactic treatment of those with suspected hypercoagulability are lacking. Current evidence suggests pharmacologic prophylaxis in the nonoperative setting is recommended only in children on long-term home total parenteral nutrition (TPN) and those with specific complex cardiac lesions (e.g., Fontan patients).[239] However, children who present for surgery with a strong family history of thromboses may benefit from screening and referral to a hematologist for management and consideration of pharmacologic prophylaxis, such as enoxaparin administered postoperatively. The use of nonpharmacologic prophylaxis, including early mobilization after surgery, adequate hydration, and compression stockings, is left to the discretion of individual providers and to institutional practice based on the child's medical history, family history, and risk factors for VTE.

Studies on the use of antifibrinolytic medications for preventing blood loss in high-risk surgeries (e.g., scoliosis, craniosynostosis) for patients with thrombophilia or a family history of thrombophilia are lacking. A risk/benefit discussion with the patient, family, and surgeon for each individual patient and surgery is recommended.

Hematologic Malignancies

In contrast to adults, hematologic malignancies in children are very common, accounting for over 40% of all new cancer diagnoses; the majority of these are leukemias.[240] Childhood malignancy occurs within any blood cell lineage. Each of the hematologic malignancies are heterogeneous diseases with multiple distinct biological subtypes and thus multiple treatment options and survival rates. The hematologic malignancies are often categorized as listed in Table 8.16, which lists the groups and most common

subtypes. However, recent advances have demonstrated overlapping pathogenesis and features between some subgroups, leading to recent changes to some categorizations.[241] Fig. 8.1A illustrates the incidence of pediatric hematologic cancers by age. The incidence of acute lymphoblastic leukemia (ALL) spikes between 1 and 4 years of age and then quickly decreases thereafter (see Fig. 8.1A), whereas the incidence of acute myelogenous leukemia (AML) decreases from a zenith of younger than 1 year of age and decreases to a minimum by 5 to 9 years of age. The incidence of lymphoma increases steadily throughout childhood and adolescence, with Hodgkin lymphoma increasing at twice the rate as non-Hodgkin lymphoma between 5 and 19 years of age (see Fig. 8.1A). Fig. 8.1B illustrates the incidence of pediatric hematologic cancers during the past 4 decades: the incidence of Hodgkin lymphoma and ALM have remained constant, lymphoid lymphoma and CNS neoplasms have increased very gradually and the incidence of non-Hodgkin lymphoma and reticuloendothelial neoplasm, which remained constant until 2008, saw its rate almost double in the next decade (Fig. 8.1B). Hence, children of all ages are at risk for a newly diagnosed hematologic malignancy, and each can present unique and challenging considerations during anesthetic care.

All hematologic malignancies stem from genomic alterations within a specific blood cell lineage in either the immature progenitor stage or mature stage of cellular differentiation. Leukemia is a malignant transformation of lymphoid or myeloid progenitor cells in the bone marrow, whereas lymphoma is a malignant transformation of progenitor lymphoid cells (or less commonly, mature lymphocytes) in lymph nodes or other lymphatic tissues. Several subtypes of leukemia and lymphoma are very closely related and thus it is challenging to differentiate both clinically and histologically, especially if marrow and lymph involvement are both present at diagnosis. Histiocytoses comprise a group of malignant disorders characterized by abnormal function of dendrocytes, monocytes, or macrophages. Myelodysplastic syndromes and myeloproliferative neoplasms are rare malignant disorders of pluripotent hematopoietic stem cells that result in aberrant proliferation of one or more hematopoietic cell lineages and suppression of the rest.

ACUTE LYMPHOBLASTIC LEUKEMIA

ALL is the most common childhood malignancy, accounting for 25% of all pediatric cancers and 76% of all leukemias.[242] Continued evolution of treatment protocols has led to an overall survival rate of 90% in children and adolescents in Western countries, with some subgroups reaching survival rates as high as 95%.[243,244] Subgroups with lower 5-year survival rates include infant diagnosis (53% survival), adolescent diagnosis (76%), T-cell immunophenotype (82%), and so called "high-risk" categorization group (83%).[243]

Pathophysiology

ALL is a heterogeneous malignancy caused by mutation of lymphocyte progenitor cells at an early phase of differentiation, called lymphoblasts. The mutation arises either in B-cell or T-cell lymphoblasts in the bone marrow. Approximately 85% of ALL cases arise from the pre-B-cell lineage (B-ALL), and the remaining 15% originate from the progenitor T-cell lineage (T-ALL).[245] Both B-ALL and T-ALL can be further classified into several distinct genetic subtypes that influence the approach to treatment and subsequent outcomes. Leukemic potential commonly arises from a series of gene alterations that include chromosomal translocations and changes to chromosomal number. Subsequent additional genetic alterations then trigger the ultimate conversion to

TABLE 8.16	Incidence of Hematologic Malignancies in Childhood (0–14 years of age)	
Cancer	Incidence per 1,000,000	5-Year Survival (%)
Leukemias	54.1	85
Acute lymphoblastic leukemia	41.2	89
Acute myelogenous leukemia	8.4	65
Lymphomas	16.7	93
Hodgkin lymphoma	6.0	98
Non-Hodgkin lymphoma	7.5	89
Histiocytosis	–	–
Langerhans cell histiocytosis	5	85–100
Myelodysplastic syndromes	2	50

Data from references:[271,353,357,368]

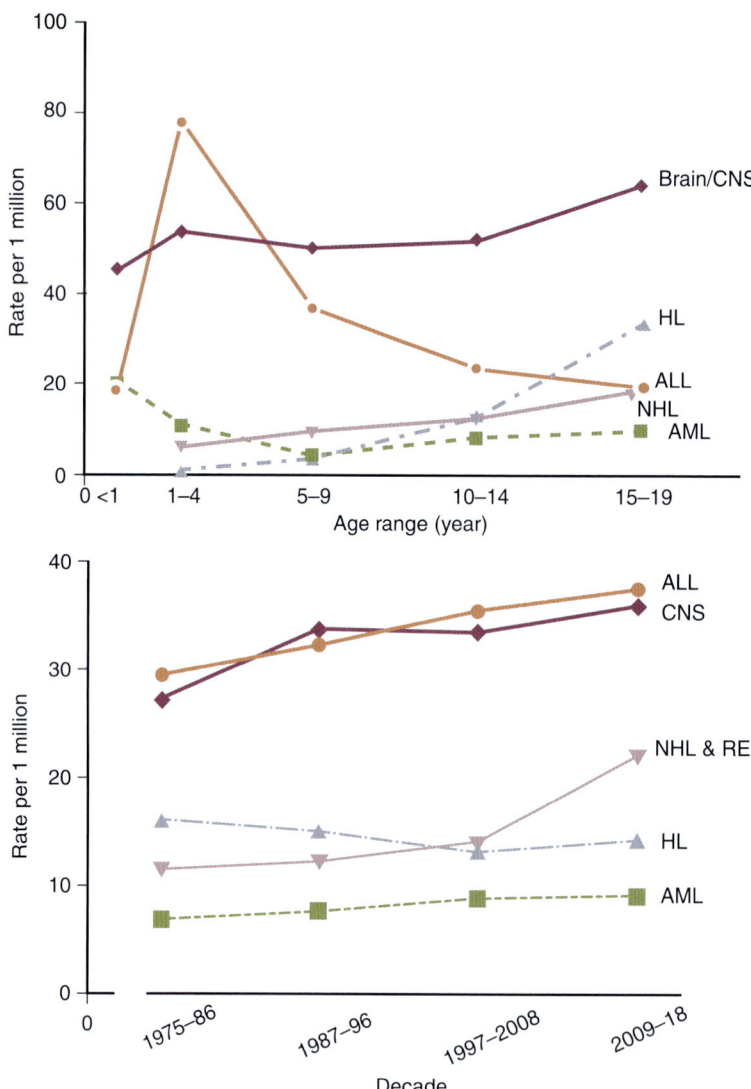

FIGURE 8.1 A, Age-specific incidence rates for childhood cancer by ICCC group, all races, both sexes, Surveillance, Epidemiology, and End Results Program, National Cancer Institute (SEER) 1975–2018. **B,** Incidence of childhood cancer by ICCC group, all races, both sexes per decade, SEER 1975–2018. **ALL,** Acute lymphoid leukemia; **AML,** acute myeloid leukemia; **CNS,** central nervous system malignancies; **HL,** Hodgkin lymphoma; **NHL,** non-Hodgkin lymphoma; **RE,** reticuloendothelial neoplasms; **ICCC,** International classification of childhood cancer. (Data from Howlader N, Noone AM, Krapcho M, et al. SEER Cancer statistics Review, 1975-2018, National Cancer Institute. Bethesda, MD, https://seer.cancer.gov/csr/1975_2018.)

leukemia via inappropriate suppression or activation of regulatory proteins. These acquired genetic alterations lead to clonal proliferation and accumulation of immature blast cells in the bone marrow.[246–248] Rapid expansion of blast cells crowds the marrow space and leads to ineffective hematopoiesis and peripheral cytopenias. Over time, leukemic cells invade other organs and tissues.

There are few risk factors that are known to predispose to developing ALL. Generally accepted risks include prior exposure to radiation (including in utero), inherited genetic polymorphisms, and genetic syndromes (e.g., Trisomy 21, Bloom syndrome, ataxia telangiectasia, and Fanconi anemia).[249,250] Children with Trisomy 21 have an 18-fold increased risk of developing leukemia during childhood, and two-thirds of the leukemic diagnoses are ALL. Historically, survival of children with Trisomy 21 and ALL was less than in the non-Trisomy 21 population because of the frequencies of relapse and treatment-related mortality, but recent overall mortality may be approaching parity.[251–253]

Clinical and Laboratory Features and Treatment

The presenting signs and symptoms of childhood ALL are usually nonspecific in the early stages. The extent of bone marrow suppression and cytopenias influences the severity of presenting symptoms, which often include frequent upper respiratory infections, fevers, fatigue, malaise, pallor, petechiae, easy bruisability, lymphadenopathy, hepatosplenomegaly, pain in extremities, and refusal to walk.[254] When a complete blood count (CBC) is first obtained, it is often suggestive of leukemia. The initial CBC will typically show leukocytosis in half of children, anemia in 80% of children, neutropenia, and thrombocytopenia.[254–256] Often, the child will appear pale and tired but otherwise healthy. However, children with advanced disease and a large tumor burden with extramedullary spread at diagnosis might be decidedly sicker; they can present with hyperuricemia, renal insufficiency, calcium and phosphorus abnormalities from skeletal invasion, liver dysfunction from leukemic infiltration, and mild coagulopathy.[256] At the time of diagnosis, the presence of CNS leukemia or an anterior mediastinal mass is uncommon in children with B-ALL. In contrast, half of children have an anterior mediastinal mass, one-half have hyperleukocytosis and risk for vascular stasis, and 10% to 15% have CNS leukemia at the time of diagnosis of T-ALL.[254,255,257] A bone marrow aspirate provides the definitive diagnosis, and immunophenotyping and cytogenetic studies confirm the ALL subtype and genetic characteristics that guide the child's therapy. Usually under the same anesthetic, a lumbar puncture is performed to assess the presence of lymphoblasts in the cerebrospinal fluid (CSF).

Because ALL is a heterogeneous disease, genomic data from the child's specific leukemia cells guide estimates of survival probability, response to treatments, and optimal treatment protocol. Massive advances in genetic sequencing have led to the identification of novel subtypes of ALL, also spurring research in new therapeutic targets.[258] In most pediatric oncology centers, treatment occurs in five phases: induction, consolidation and CNS preventive therapy, interim maintenance, delayed intensification, and maintenance. The intensity and time interval of each therapy is tailored to the child's risk category, which in turn is determined by the risk of relapse of the specific tumor subtype. Of note, cranial radiation is seldom used for newly diagnosed ALL in children; outcomes are similar without it, and radiation risks chronic neurocognitive dysfunction and secondary tumors.[259,260]

Induction begins soon after diagnosis, and the goal is to administer intensive systemic and intrathecal chemotherapy to eradicate >99% of leukemic cells and restore normal hematopoiesis. In standard-risk ALL, a three-drug regimen that includes a glucocorticoid, vincristine, and asparaginase is used. Those at increased risk typically receive a fourth agent such as an anthracycline.[244,261] Remission at the end of the 4- to 6-week induction is defined as <5% blasts in the marrow and recovery of normal blood counts. Submicroscopic depth of remission can be further quantified by minimal residual disease (MRD) detection, typically by flow cytometry. The child's rapidity of response to induction and degree of MRD at the end of this cycle are important predictors of outcome and influence therapy in subsequent stages.[262] Although most children achieve remission at the end of induction, relapse is inevitable without continued therapy.[244] The overall health of the child during this phase is variable.[263]

Thereafter, consolidation, interim maintenance, and delayed intensification are employed for 6 to 9 months depending on the treatment protocol. This phase uses high-dose intrathecal and intravenous chemotherapy to continue leukemic cytoreduction in all tissues and maintain remission. The pharmacologic regimen, duration, and intensity vary per treatment protocol but will often include cyclophosphamide, cytarabine, mercaptopurine, and methotrexate.[261] The recent addition of targeted antitumor agents (e.g., imatinib for Philadelphia chromosome positive leukemia) has improved the outcomes for children who are at increased risk during this phase of treatment.[264] Significant myelosuppression and toxicities of therapy are common during this period and often limit and delay chemotherapy dosages, particularly the presence of severe neutropenia. Alopecia, mucositis, anorexia, vomiting, significant infections, and fatigue are common during this period.[257] Although most children are treated as outpatients, hospitalization is often required during intensive stages or at any time to manage sequelae of this aggressive phase. Supportive care with blood transfusions, nutritional support, infection precautions, and medications to counter toxicity are crucial.[265] The final phase is maintenance for 1.5 to 2.5 years, and this phase is managed with oral chemotherapy (daily mercaptopurine and weekly methotrexate with or without vincristine and steroid pulses) in the outpatient setting.[261] Children at this stage often lead near normal lives outwardly. However, some may require short-term hospitalization for neutropenic infections or deterioration of their clinical status, and many continue to suffer chronic therapy-related dysfunction, including pain, neuropathies, depression, and psychosocial dysfunction.[263]

Up to 20% of children will relapse; survival rates are significantly reduced with relapse, especially if it occurs during treatment rather than after treatment.[266] Because of increasingly poor outcomes in relapsed disease, therapies with greater toxicity or investigative therapies are often employed. HSCT is a frequently used modality in relapsed children, whereas HSCT is uncommonly used during initial diagnosis, save for those at greatest risk.[267] Investigational therapies, such as adoptive T-cell therapies discussed in Chapter 9, are showing considerable promise as well.[268] The overall clinical status of children during relapse is broad, ranging from outpatient to intensive care management.

Perioperative Considerations

The newly diagnosed child with ALL will present soon after diagnosis for long-term central venous access under anesthesia to facilitate frequent intravenous chemotherapy and blood draws. Before the first anesthetic, the presence of an anterior mediastinal mass must be ruled out (see also Chapter 13), given that more than half of children with T-ALL will have a mass at the time of diagnosis, although only a minority will be symptomatic.[255] During induction and consolidation stages of therapy (in the first 6 to 9 months), children undergo multiple bone marrow aspirations and lumbar punctures, the latter often including intrathecal methotrexate. Some now argue that in those children receiving methotrexate, there may be compelling circumstantial evidence to avoid nitrous oxide in these children due to concerns for possible neurotoxicity. Other surgical procedures during ALL treatment are not particularly common, with the exception of revision of malfunctioned or infected central venous access. Before any anesthetic, a CBC should be reviewed. Table 8.2 lists commonly recognized minimal safe platelet counts before invasive procedures, but institutional protocols may vary for lumbar puncture and bone marrow aspiration. Strict adherence to aseptic protocols is imperative, especially for neutropenic children, as is attention to friability of oral mucosal tissue during laryngoscopy in patients with mucositis. Indiscriminate use of parenteral steroids should be avoided, especially before the diagnosis is confirmed and a treatment plan is prescribed, as it may: (1) complicate the diagnosis by inducing tumor cell necrosis[269]; (2) precipitate tumor lysis syndrome[270]; and/or (3) affect treatment randomization. Table 8.17 lists general perioperative considerations for all children with hematologic malignancies, and additional detailed anesthetic considerations are discussed in Chapter 9.

ACUTE MYELOGENOUS LEUKEMIA

Although far more prevalent in older adults, AML is the second most common leukemia in childhood, representing 18% of pediatric leukemias but 50% of all leukemic deaths in children.[271,272] The incidence of AML in children is biphasic, with the greatest incidence before age 3, reaching a nadir at 5 to 9 years of age and then increasing very slowly thereafter until 19 years of age (see Fig. 8.1). The increasing incidence in adolescence reflects the gradual increased prevalence throughout all of adulthood.[271] The 5-year survival of childhood AML has improved dramatically in

TABLE 8.17	Perioperative Concerns in Pediatric Cancer and Hematopoietic Stem Cell Transplantation

Preoperative Considerations

Consultation with service primarily responsible for child's care

Complete blood cell count (when appropriate)

Echocardiogram or chest radiograph, or both (when appropriate)

Transfusion crossmatch with specifications (e.g., cytomegalovirus seronegativity, leukocyte reduction, irradiation) determined in consultation with oncology service

Determination of blood typing requirements for all stem cell transplant recipients

History of acute and chronic pain medication use

Infection prophylaxis with antibiotics

Avoidance of *any* marrow-suppressive medications in stem cell transplant patients

Observation of indicated isolation precautions

Sterile technique with central line access

Intraoperative Considerations

Attention to skin, teeth, eyes, and joints; careful positioning and padding

Careful airway instrumentation in the setting of mucositis

Sterile technique with all vascular catheter placements (arterial, central venous, peripheral)

Full-stomach precautions (when appropriate, as in graft-versus-host disease)

Appropriate hydration and maintenance of urine output

Continuation of total parenteral nutrition (and other parenteral fluids with high glucose concentration)

Avoidance of high fraction of inspired oxygen (FiO_2) and restriction of hydration if prior treatment with bleomycin

Judicious use of cardiac depressants in patients with compromised cardiac function

Nausea and vomiting prophylaxis: avoid corticosteroids for antiemesis unless discussed with oncology

Administer stress dose steroids when indicated, after consultation with oncology

Regional anesthesia when safe and indicated

Postoperative Considerations

Patient-appropriate opioid and other analgesic administration

Sterile technique with central line access

Observation of indicated isolation precautions

---

the past several decades to 65% to 70%, but survival is less, 50% to 60%, in the 15- to 39-year-old group.[273] Despite the optimistic 5-year survival, nearly half of all children diagnosed with AML eventually relapse and die from the disease. AML remains one of the major groups of childhood cancer with the worst overall survival rates, and the mortality rate increases with increasing age at diagnosis.[271,272,274]

Pathophysiology

AML is a heterogenous malignancy of undifferentiated myeloid precursor cells. AML can arise as a de novo disease or secondary to previous cytotoxic exposures (e.g., previous cancer therapy) or myelodysplastic syndromes. Like ALL, AML is categorized based on the subtype of tumor cytology, and as such, treatment protocols and outcomes differ among the subtypes.[275] AML arises from a series of genetic mutations that lead to rapid clonal proliferation and accumulation of maturation-arrested myeloid cells.[276] Marrow crowding and eventual infiltration of extramedullary sites lead to the array of symptoms at presentation.[275]

Inherited risks are important in the development of childhood AML. Some of the more common risk factors include Trisomy 21, Fanconi anemia, Bloom syndrome, ataxia telangiectasia, Shwachman-Diamond syndrome, and familial monosomy 7.[277] Trisomy 21 is the most common of these syndromes, with a 10- to 20-fold increased risk of developing AML.[278] Environmental risks are not well understood in childhood AML, with the exception of the greatly increased risk in children exposed to high doses of radiation (e.g., survivors of atomic bombs in the 1940s in Japan). Prior exposure to chemotherapeutics, especially topoisomerase inhibitors, and acquired marrow suppression conditions are important causes of secondary AML.[275]

Clinical and Laboratory Features and Treatment

Clinical symptoms before the diagnosis are usually nonspecific but often include pallor, bleeding, easy bruising, and infections, all resulting from pancytopenia. Depending on the degree of marrow suppression at the time of diagnosis, anemia and thrombocytopenia are present in the majority of patients.[275,279] The white blood cell count may range from low to high, but neutropenia, which predisposes to severe infections, is common. Hyperleukocytosis ($>100,000/mm^3$) is present in 20% of patients with AML at diagnosis.[280] Approximately 14% of children are at risk of bleeding and thrombosis due to thrombocytopenia, platelet dysfunction, and anti- or procoagulant factors released from tumor cells; this is particularly an issue in acute promyelocytic leukemia.[281] Extramedullary manifestations are uncommon, found in about 10% of children at diagnosis, and they most commonly occur in skin (leukemia cutis), head, neck, brain (leptomeningeal), and spinal cord.[282] When AML is suspected, a bone marrow aspiration and biopsy is diagnostic. Cytogenetic evaluation of leukemic cells in the marrow influences the treatment protocol and estimation of survival.[283]

The goal of induction is to induce remission of the leukemic cell burden, for which cytarabine and daunorubicin are standard treatments. Compared with ALL induction, AML induction is significantly more intense with a much greater risk of life-threatening complications including infection. Intensification chemotherapy during both induction and consolidation is highly toxic, and evidence-based supportive care guidelines have been developed to assist the child throughout intensification.[284] Although postinduction remission rates have risen over time to approximately 85% to 90%, treatment-related morbidity and mortality continue to present problems.[285] Substantial myelosuppression is usual, and supportive care is crucial, including hospitalization through induction therapy and aggressive management of neutropenic infections.[286] Tumor lysis syndrome is also a risk in children with a large tumor burden.[287] Up to 4% of children develop significant cardiomyopathy early after daunorubicin or other anthracycline therapy.[288] CNS involvement is present in 10% to 30% of children; thus, lumbar punctures with intrathecal chemotherapy are routine.[289,290] Like ALL, additional therapy is required after induction to avoid universal relapse of disease. Many treatment protocols use three to four cycles of intensification therapy after induction, which attempt to balance optimal tumor suppression with avoidance of severe toxicity. The role of HSCT in newly diagnosed childhood AML is typically reserved for children with high-risk AML in postremission therapy.[262] 55% of survivors of AML have chronic health conditions, particularly those treated with HSCT.[291] With the high risk of relapse in pediatric AML, many children will then undergo more intensive treatment protocols, including HSCT. Thus, these children are at risk for greater morbidity and mortality with this treatment.[292]

There are several important subtypes of AML. Acute promyelocytic leukemia (APL), which occurs in 5% to 10% of AML cases, is a subtype in which the predominant cells are promyelocytes with a specific mutation to the retinoic acid receptor gene.[293] When APL cells were found to be exquisitely sensitive to all-trans-retinoic acid (ATRA), ATRA was added to the treatment protocols, increasing the survival rate in childhood to approximately 90%, which is significantly better than that of AML overall.[294] The current therapy for APL omits all chemotherapy other than ATRA and arsenic trioxide; thus the toxicity profile and chronic morbidity are dramatically different than that of other AML therapy. Of note, severe coagulopathy is often present at the time of diagnosis. The risk of bleeding and thrombosis is multifactorial, in part due to the frequency of DIC and hyperleukocytosis.[281,295,296]

Children with Trisomy 21 are at significant risk of myeloid malignancies. De novo AML in Trisomy 21 has an excellent overall survival, allowing reduction of chemotherapy intensity.[297] This reduced intensity chemotherapy attenuates the risk of treatment-related morbidity in children with Trisomy 21 that occurred in the past, specifically a 17% incidence of early, symptomatic cardiomyopathy and 3% mortality from cardiomyopathy.[298] Transient abnormal myelopoiesis (TAM), which is currently classified as a myeloproliferative disorder rather than a myeloid leukemia, is present in at least 4% to 10% of Trisomy 21 neonates. TAM shares some similarities with AML, yet it usually undergoes spontaneous remission. Progressive cases can require chemotherapy to achieve remission and survival. Approximately 16% to 20% of these children will subsequently develop AML after remission of the myelopoietic disorder.[299,300]

Therapy-related AML (t-AML) comprises 10% to 20% of childhood AML. It occurs in 1% to 2% of children treated with chemotherapy or radiotherapy for a malignant or nonmalignant condition. The onset of t-AML occurs 2 to 10 years after exposure to the causative chemotherapy drug. Prognosis is very poor overall, although the use of HSCT in early remission may improve outcomes.[301]

Perioperative Considerations

As in ALL, children with AML present soon after their diagnosis is confirmed for a surgically placed central venous access and serial bone marrow aspirates and lumbar punctures. Newly diagnosed children should be screened for hyperleukocytosis, retinoic acid syndrome, an anterior mediastinal mass, and the sequelae of pancytopenia. Because anthracycline chemotherapeutics are routine during AML therapy, the presence of cardiomyopathy must be assessed, and serial echocardiograms should be performed throughout the course of treatment. Aseptic technique should always be observed. In children with mucositis, care should be taken during laryngoscopy to minimize any trauma to friable oral mucosal tissue. Indiscriminate use of parenteral steroids should be avoided, especially before the diagnosis and treatment determination, as it may: (1) cause tissue necrosis thereby impairing diagnosis; (2) cause tumor lysis syndrome; and (3) affect the treatment randomization. Additional detailed anesthetic considerations are

discussed in detail in Chapter 9, including recommendations for those with cardiomyopathy and post-HSCT.

HODGKIN LYMPHOMA

Hodgkin lymphoma (HL) is the 8th most common pediatric cancer and constitutes 40% to 50% of all pediatric lymphoma cases. In economically advantaged countries, the incidence of HL has a bimodal age distribution, with the first peak 15 to 35 years of age and the second beyond 55 years of age. As such, infantile HL is rare, but the steady increase in incidence with age leads to HL being the most common childhood cancer among 15- to 19-year-olds. Onset of the disease in earlier childhood is more prevalent in developing countries.[271,302,303] Survival rates for pediatric HL are excellent, with 5-year survival exceeding 97% in the United States.[271] Given the excellent survival, the current focus of treatment protocols has shifted to minimizing lifelong morbidity while maintaining these survival rates.[304,305]

Pathophysiology

HL is a B-cell lineage malignancy characterized by clonal proliferation of malignant Hodgkin/Reed-Sternberg (HRS) cells. The HRS cells accumulate within lymph nodes and other lymphatic tissues and are joined by a significant infiltrate of variable inflammatory cells, which constitute 99% of the tumor volume.[306] Established risk factors for childhood HL include immunodeficiency states, infection with Epstein-Barr virus (EBV), and family history of HL. Depending on the age of diagnosis and geographic location, up to 40% to 50% of pediatric HL cases are associated with latent EBV infection, as determined by EBV+ tumor cells.[307,308] HL is subclassified into classical HL and nodular lymphocyte predominant HL; although the prevalence of each subtype varies across age groups, with classical HL constituting approximately 80% to 90% of pediatric cases with slightly less favorable outcomes compared with the nodular lymphocyte predominant subclass.[309]

Clinical and Laboratory Features and Treatment

Splenomegaly and painless lymphadenopathy of the cervical, supraclavicular, axillary, and occasionally inguinal lymph nodes are the presenting signs in 80% of children. Mediastinal involvement is common; 55% to 65% have a mediastinal mass with the possibility of cardiopulmonary compromise (see also Chapter 13), and 5% have pericardial involvement with the possibility of effusion at presentation. Up to 10% of children present with constitutional "B" symptoms, which include fever, drenching night sweats, and >10% weight loss within 6 months before diagnosis. The presence of "B" symptoms has important implications for staging and prognosis.[310–312] Laboratory evaluation at diagnosis is often nonspecific, including leukocytosis, lymphopenia, eosinophilia, and monocytosis. RBC and platelet counts are usually normal except in the setting of severe metastatic disease. However, immune suppression is often already present at the time of diagnosis.[311]

Diagnostic evaluation includes physical examination and imaging studies; however, many children require general anesthesia to undergo these studies (such as MRI) which may pose challenges particularly in those with anterior mediastinal masses. A chest x-ray rapidly screens for mediastinal disease, and CT of neck, chest, abdomen, and pelvis evaluates the extent of adenopathy. Diagnostic staging and interim assessment with positron emission tomography (PET) is increasingly used.[313] Definitive diagnosis requires a lymph node biopsy to provide the scarce HRS cells for histologic confirmation.[314]

The treatment protocol depends on the child's risk stratification from the biopsy and imaging studies. Decades ago, treatment protocols with high-dose radiation therapy and chemotherapy led to excessive chronic toxicity in survivors of childhood HL. Current strategies focus on less toxic combined modality therapy that includes low doses of multiple chemotherapeutics and low-dose or even elimination of radiation therapy.[314,315] When used, radiation is low-dose and conformed to the tumor site, greatly limiting radiation of extraneous normal tissues. Most acute affects are transient and reversible.[315] More prevalent use of fluorodeoxyglucose (FDG)-PET allows identification of adequate responders to chemotherapy for whom radiation therapy may safely be omitted.[316] Outcomes in relapsed HL remain favorable, and as such, children with low-risk relapse can often be cured with conventional-dose chemotherapy and radiation therapy. However, high-risk relapse often requires high-dose chemotherapy and HSCT.[317,318]

Perioperative Considerations

Lymph node biopsy and long-term central venous access are usually performed under anesthesia soon after presentation. At least two-thirds of children will have mediastinal lymphadenopathy at the time of diagnosis, and one-half of those will have a symptomatic anterior mediastinal mass >30% of the cardiac silhouette,[310,312,319] which places them at risk of cardiopulmonary collapse during anesthesia.[320] Any child with significant lymphadenopathy should be suspected of having a lymphoma and be assessed for the presence of an anterior mediastinal mass before beginning anesthesia, as discussed in Chapters 9 and 13. With large, compressive mediastinal masses, the risks of general anesthesia even for minor procedures such as lymph node biopsy may warrant that the procedure be performed under local anesthesia with or without sedation.

Although chemotherapy protocols vary, most patients will be treated with a 4- to 7-drug combination of a vinca alkaloid (e.g., vincristine), anthracycline (e.g., doxorubicin), bleomycin, cyclophosphamide, corticosteroid, methotrexate, procarbazine, and etoposide, as well as possible radiation therapy.[318,321] Thus, significant myelosuppression and toxicities of therapy may occur during treatment. Children who receive bleomycin are at risk for developing pulmonary dysfunction and acute respiratory failure, particularly after high concentrations of oxygen. Recent evidence has questioned the role of oxygen in the pathogenesis of bleomycin-induced lung injury, although the risk in children has never been confirmed (see also Chapter 9).[322–324] Among survivors of childhood cancer, those with HL have one of the greatest burdens of chronic disease, especially those treated with both chemotherapy and radiation. The rate of cardiac disease during and after treatment with anthracyclines and chest radiation is of particular concern, and survivors must be screened for cardiac disease; however, most cardiac-related mortality does not occur until years later.[325–328] As usual, attention to sterile technique, awareness of possible friability of oral mucosal tissue during laryngoscopy, and indiscriminate use of parenteral steroids should be avoided. Additional detailed anesthetic considerations are discussed in Chapter 9.

NON-HODGKIN LYMPHOMA

Non-Hodgkin lymphoma (NHL) accounts for 7% of all childhood cancers, making it the 5th most common pediatric cancer. It is rarely diagnosed in infancy; the incidence increases steadily throughout childhood. It occurs predominantly in males, especially in the preadolescent age group. Among the lymphomas, NHL is more common in children less than 10 years of age, whereas HL is more common in those greater than 10 years of

age. The 5-year survival of children 0 to 19 years old at the time of diagnosis of NHL is 87%, which is considerably less than HL but almost equal to ALL.[271,329]

Pathophysiology

NHL is a heterogeneous group of neoplasms that derive from lymphocyte B-cell progenitors, T-cell progenitors, mature B cells, or mature T cells and accumulates predominantly in lymph nodes and lymphoid tissues. However, up to 40% of NHL tumors arise in nonlymphatic extranodal tissues, which may create a diagnostic challenge.[330,331] Compared with HL, NHL is a more systemic malignancy that disseminates from lymphoid tissues to extranodal tissues (and vice versa) and is more aggressive at the time of diagnosis.[314,332] Multiple subtypes of NHL occur in children, the most common being Burkitt lymphoma, lymphoblastic T-cell or B-cell lymphoma, diffuse large B-cell lymphoma, and anaplastic large cell lymphoma; other subtypes are rare.[314,333] A congenital or acquired immunodeficiency state is the leading risk factor for the development of NHL, which include Wiskott-Aldrich syndrome, ataxia telangiectasia, X-linked lymphoproliferative syndrome, AIDS, and post-transplant or other iatrogenic immunosuppressed states. Inherited conditions, however, account for <2% of pediatric cases.[334,335]

Clinical and Laboratory Features and Treatment

Clinical presentation is similar to that of HL; most children present with painless but rapidly expanding masses, which can produce symptomatic mass effect of surrounding tissues and structures. As such, clinical emergencies from compression of vital structures are common in NHL, including an anterior mediastinal mass, spinal cord compression, CNS involvement in 6% of children, pericardial tamponade, thromboembolism, and intestinal intussusception or obstruction.[332,336] The most common sites of primary tumor in all children with NHL are the abdomen, mediastinum, and peripheral lymph nodes, especially of the head and neck.[337] In Burkitt lymphoma, which is the most common form of pediatric NHL, the most common primary sites of disease are the head, neck, and then abdomen; however, tumor masses may also be found in bone, bone marrow, skin, testes, and CNS. Advanced disease with bone marrow and CNS involvement is present in 25% of children.[332,338]

Results of initial laboratory evaluation are variable. The CBC can be normal, but pancytopenia is present when there is extensive marrow invasion. Thrombocytopenia and anemia are signs of splenic sequestration and internal bleeding, respectively. About 20% of children experience tumor lysis syndrome at induction of treatment as a result of the high metabolic rate of rapidly proliferating NHL tumor cells. A significant percentage of these children may require dialysis.[339,340] Initial CT imaging of the neck, chest, abdomen, and pelvis evaluates the extent of disease. Because extranodal spread of noncontiguous tumor is common in childhood NHL, PET scan has become an integral part of baseline, interim, and post-treatment staging; however, the role of PET to influence treatment protocols remains under investigation.[313,341,342] MRI scans are usually limited to evaluation of specific tissue involvement, such as bone or brain.[333] Definitive diagnosis is made by histologic and subcellular evaluation of affected tissue (commonly a lymph node), and then bilateral bone marrow aspiration and biopsy and CSF cytology provide further disease staging.[332]

Treatment of pediatric NHL is primarily chemotherapy with protocols that vary with the subtype of NHL and clinical staging. Common chemotherapeutic agents often include cyclophosphamide, vincristine, prednisone, doxorubicin, etoposide, and methotrexate.[343]

Targeted therapies are increasingly utilized for some subtypes of NHL, particularly rituximab, which markedly improves survival in children with high-risk NHL.[329,344,345] As opposed to the treatment of ALL, treatment cycles of many stages of pediatric NHL are very brief, utilizing high-dose pulses of chemotherapy drugs with intensive supportive care. The use of prophylactic radiation therapy has become exceedingly uncommon in pediatric NHL as it risks life-long toxicity and has not appreciably improved outcomes in most subtypes. As such, radiation therapy has been relegated to those with documented CNS involvement at the time of diagnosis or incomplete response to chemotherapy.[346-348] The usual sequelae of chemotherapy are seen during treatment, including myelosuppression, infections, mucositis, nausea and vomiting, cardiac toxicity, and neurobehavioral complications.

Perioperative Considerations

Like most pediatric hematologic malignancies, surgery during therapy is mostly limited to the initial diagnostic biopsy, placement of central venous access, and treatment of any complications of therapy. Complete resection of localized tumors is rare, and debulking surgery of large tumor masses is no longer indicated.[349] However, tumor invasion and destruction of the bowel or other vital organs may require urgent surgical attention. Lumbar punctures with cerebrospinal cytology and intrathecal methotrexate may be indicated as prophylaxis in some subtypes of NHL and in children with CNS disease at diagnosis.[332]

The primary anesthetic considerations specific to children with newly diagnosed NHL include anterior mediastinal mass, mass effect of tumor on the upper airway, and tumor lysis syndrome. Because of the considerable risks of anesthesia in the presence of an anterior mediastinal mass, all children with suspected NHL must receive a thorough physiologic and radiographic evaluation (in particular, echocardiography) before undertaking an anesthetic (see also Chapter 13). NHL lesions of the upper airway may obstruct the airway or bleed during airway management.[350,351] Although tumor lysis syndrome most frequently occurs during chemotherapy induction, it can occur spontaneously, during anesthesia and surgery, or with a dose of corticosteroids.[352] A single dose of dexamethasone may prove fatal in an undiagnosed hematologic cancer.[270] Additional discussion of anterior mediastinal mass, tumor lysis syndrome, and anesthetic considerations not specific to NHL are discussed in detail in Chapter 9.

LANGERHANS CELL HISTIOCYTOSIS

Histiocytosis is a category of disorders of "histiocytes," which is an archaic term for dendrocytes, macrophages, and monocytes. Histiocytosis is generally divided into Langerhans cell histiocytosis (LCH) and non-Langerhans histiocytosis. Given the rarity of the non-Langerhans subtypes, the subsequent focus of this section will be on LCH only.

The etiology and epidemiology of LCH remain poorly understood. It is an uncommon but predominantly childhood disorder with an incidence of 4 to 9 cases per million children per year, similar to that of HL and AML. The usual age at diagnosis is 1 to 6 years old.[353-356] The spectrum of childhood LCH ranges from single-system focal lesions to life-threatening multisystem disease. The overall survival rate of the more common low-risk focal disease is 99%, but high-risk disseminated disease has a survival of only 85%.[353,357]

Pathophysiology

LCH is an inflammatory neoplasia of myeloid dendritic cell precursors. Although the etiology is poorly understood, malignant transformation of dendritic cells leads to clonal proliferation and accumulation into lesions. The lesions are accompanied by a host of inflammatory cells that release a local cytokine storm, leading to the symptomatic destruction of surrounding tissues.[358]

Clinical and Laboratory Features and Treatment

The majority of children with LCH (70%) present with single-system focal lesions. A minority, 30%, present with multisystem disease, occurring most commonly in the youngest children.[354,356,359] The lesions can form in any organ, although nearly 80% present with lytic bone lesions, followed by papular skin lesions in 40%.[360] Involvement of bone marrow, liver, lung, or spleen portends a poor prognosis. Physical symptoms depend on the site and extent of tissue lesions. Laboratory values are most notable for evidence of an inflammatory state, although anemia is common.[354,356]

LCH can be difficult to diagnose because its clinical presentation is often insidious and representative of a broad differential diagnosis. The exception is in the subset of neonates who present with a rapidly progressive disseminated disease.[353] Biopsy of a lesion, usually skin or bone, confirms the diagnosis. The histology demonstrates LCH cells surrounded by a substantial volume of inflammatory cells. Subsequent radiologic imaging with skeletal survey, CT, and PET confirm the extent of disease and influence the approach to treatment.[361] Unless the liver, spleen, or pituitary gland is directly involved, laboratory analysis is usually normal.

Treatment of childhood LCH is widely variable depending on the extent of disease and organs involved. Isolated bone lesions may be treated with surgical curettage and intralesional steroids with excellent results, but reactivation of disease can occur. Isolated cutaneous disease can be resolved with topical medications only or may regress on its own, but subsequent progression to multisystem disease may be fatal in young children. Thus, most children with multifocal or CNS-involved LCH are treated with a combination of corticosteroids and relatively low-dose chemotherapy, such as vinblastine and prednisone for 1 year. For those with high-risk LCH, mercaptopurine may be added to the regimen. Surgical removal of lesions may be indicated in some cases, but radiation is sparingly used for invasion of critical organs or structures (e.g., CNS).[357,362-365]

Perioperative Considerations

Depending on the clinical staging, treatment administered, and presence of disease relapse, 3% to 50% of children will have diabetes insipidus before, during, or especially after treatment.[354,360] Children with polyuria and polydipsia should be fully evaluated before elective surgery. Those with diabetes insipidus should be managed in consultation with oncologists, as optimal treatment with desmopressin and fluid management varies among children.[366] Chemotherapy protocols are generally less toxic than in other childhood hematologic cancers, and major toxicity is less common. However, liver and lung fibrosis can occur and can be at least mildly symptomatic.[367]

MYELODYSPLASTIC AND MYELOPROLIFERATIVE DISORDERS

Myelodysplastic and myeloproliferative disorders are rare hematologic malignancies that are categorized into three distinct groups: myelodysplastic syndromes (MDS), juvenile myelomonocytic leukemia (JMML), and Trisomy 21-specific diseases. Transient abnormal myelopoiesis of Down syndrome and myeloid leukemia of Trisomy 21 were discussed under AML and will not be discussed here.

The MDSs are a rare form of myeloid malignancy in children, accounting for just 4% of hematologic malignancies, the median age at the time of diagnosis being 7 years old.[241,368] Recognition of MDS is important because of its frequent evolution to pediatric AML. The 5-year survival is variable (~50%) and depends on the disease characteristics.[369] JMML is a rare myeloid malignancy of young children, with an average age of onset at 2 years old.[241] Approximately 13% of patients with JMML eventually progress to AML.[370] The 5-year survival is ~40% but specific survival is highly variable based on disease characteristics.[369]

Pathophysiology

MDSs are clonal hematologic disorders, characterized by abnormal proliferation and differentiation of hematopoietic stem cells. Mutation of hematopoietic stem cells early in the cell line leads to chronic cytopenia of all cell lines but with varying severity, and as such, MDS may appear similar to aplastic anemia or bone marrow failure disorders. MDS is subclassified into three groups: refractory cytopenia, refractory anemia with excess blasts (RAEB), and refractory anemia with excess blasts in transformation (RAEB-t).[241,371] Inherited bone marrow failure syndromes are associated with childhood MDS in 20% of children, including Fanconi anemia, Kostmann syndrome, Shwachman-Diamond syndrome, Diamond-Blackfan anemia, Trisomy 8 mosaicism, familial MDS, severe congenital neutropenia, and aplastic anemia. Prior chemotherapy and radiation are important acquired factors.[241,370,372]

JMML is also a potentially lethal malignant disorder of myeloid stem cell proliferation, but in this disorder differentiation and maturation of monocytes is not blocked, leading to isolated monocytosis.[373] Neurofibromatosis type 1 (NF1) is the primary risk factor for JMML; over 10% of children with JMML have NF1, and another 20% have mutation of the tumor suppressor *NF1* gene.[374]

Clinical and Laboratory Features and Treatment

Children presenting with MDS are typically pancytopenic, and hepatosplenomegaly is very common.[370] Initial treatment is dependent on the severity of cytopenia. Some children, especially those with refractory cytopenia or mild RAEB, have mild disease for months or even years with only infrequent need for blood transfusions, whereas others present with severe disease. Regardless of presentation, progression is inevitable, and the best chance for survival is HSCT.[375] Recent data suggest that outcomes improve in children who do not receive pre-HSCT chemotherapy and who advance to HSCT shortly after diagnosis.[376,377] Preconditioning regimen-related mortality and HSCT-related mortality are high, and survival rates in children who relapse after HSCT are dismal.[241]

In children with JMML, anemia, thrombocytopenia, and monocytosis are seen on initial laboratory studies; RBC evaluation demonstrates Hgb F in a majority of children.[370,373] Clinical presentation usually includes fever, respiratory symptoms, skin rash, adenopathy, and hepatosplenomegaly, which may be severe in advanced disease. Peripheral blood tests can confirm the diagnosis, but bone marrow studies are usually performed.[378] The clinical course can be rapidly progressive or indolent; regardless, JMML is resistant to treatment with chemotherapy, and without HSCT, survival is short with only 6% surviving 10 years.[379] Thus all patients are treated with HSCT. Despite advances in HSCT and supportive care, half of these children will not survive 5 years, and within that time period, up to 15% will progress to AML.[380,381]

Perioperative Considerations

Anesthetic considerations for children with MDS or JMML are similar to those discussed previously for children with AML. As most of these children will undergo HSCT, Chapter 9 details the anesthetic considerations for children pre- and post-HSCT.

ANNOTATED REFERENCES

Allen CE, Kelly KM, Bollard CM. Pediatric lymphomas and histiocytic disorders of childhood. *Pediatr Clin North Am.* 2015;62(1):139-165.
This review article summarizes the biology, treatment, and complications of pediatric lymphomas and histiocytic disorders.

Cooper SL, Brown PA. Treatment of pediatric acute lymphoblastic leukemia. *Pediatr Clin North Am.* 2015;62(1):61-73.
This review article summarizes the risk stratification, treatment, and complications of pediatric ALL.

Guzzetta NA, Miller BE. Principles of hemostasis in children: models and maturation. *Paediatr Anaesth.* 2011;21:3-9.
This review article summarizes the fundamentals of hemostasis and highlights the differences in thrombosis and coagulopathy from the preterm neonate through childhood. The impact of disease states on hemostasis are also discussed.

Inaba H, Mullighan CG. Pediatric acute lymphoblastic leukemia. *Haematolgica.* 2020;105(11):2524-2539.
This comprehensive review summarizes the contemporary role of genomic studies, risk stratification, treatment, and outcomes of pediatric ALL.

Kato GJ, Piel FB, Reid CD, et al. Sickle cell disease. *Nat Rev Dis Primers.* 2018;4:18010.
This review article summarizes sickle cell disease including etiology, diagnosis, complications and disease management.

Key NS, Derebail VK. Sickle-cell trait: novel clinical significance. *Hematology.* 2010;2010:418-422.
This review discusses sickle cell trait as a risk factor for adverse outcomes, focusing on its impact on exercise, renal function, and venous thromboembolism.

Latham GJ, Greenberg RS. Anesthetic considerations for the pediatric oncology patient—part 1: a review of antitumor therapy. *Paediatr Anaesth.* 2010;20:295-304.
This review discusses sickle cell trait as a risk factor for adverse outcomes, focusing on its impact on exercise, renal function, and venous thromboembolism.

Latham GJ, Greenberg RS. Anesthetic considerations for the pediatric oncology patient—part 2: systems-based approach to anesthesia. *Paediatr Anaesth.* 2010;20:396-420.
This article briefly reviews the current principles of cancer therapy and the general mechanisms of toxicity to the child, focusing on the impact to perioperative care and decision making.

Monagle P, Newal F. Management of thrombosis in children and neonates: practical use of anticoagulants in children. *Hematology Am Soc Hematol Educ Program.* 2018;2018(1):399-404.
A systems-based approach is used to assess the impact of the tumor and its treatment on children, and relevant anesthetic considerations are discussed.

Morley SL. Red blood cell transfusions in acute paediatrics. *Arch Dis Child Educ Pract Ed.* 2009;94:65-73.
This review is a practical reference for managing anticoagulation therapies in children and neonates; these therapies are being used increasingly often in our operating rooms, and on the wards.

Vichinsky EP, Haberkern CM, Neumayr L, et al. A comparison of conservative and aggressive transfusion regimens in the perioperative management of sickle cell disease. The Preoperative Transfusion in Sickle Cell Disease Study Group. *N Engl J Med.* 1995;333:206-213.
The risks and benefits of blood product transfusion in children are considered on the basis of current evidence from adult and pediatric studies.
This multicenter study found that a conservative transfusion regimen was as effective as the aggressive strategy in patients with sickle cell disease, and the conservative regimen resulted in one-half as many transfusion-associated complications.

A complete reference list can be found online at Elsevier eBooks+.

Perioperative Management of the Oncology Patient

BUKOLA OJO, FAITH J. ROSS, AND GREGORY J. LATHAM

Principles of Cancer Therapy
Conventional Chemotherapeutics
Targeted Antitumor Agents
Adoptive T-Cell Therapies in Children
Radiation Therapy
Preoperative Considerations by Organ System
Airway
Cardiac
Anterior Mediastinal Mass
Pericardial Effusion
Pulmonary
Renal
Hepatic
Gastrointestinal
Central Nervous System
Endocrine
Hematology
Coagulation
Pain

Neuropsychology
Tumor Lysis Syndrome
Retinoic Acid Syndrome
Hematopoietic Stem Cell Transplant
Background
Clinical Features And Treatment
Graft-Versus-Host Disease
Preoperative Laboratory Testing and Evaluation
Perioperative Considerations
Children With Cancer
Hematopoietic Stem Cell Transplantation Recipients
Transfusion Considerations
Red Blood Cells
Thrombocytopenia
Coagulation Factor Deficiency
Blood Product Preparation
Effects of Anesthetic Agents on Perioperative Immunomodulation

ALTHOUGH CHILDHOOD CANCER is not particularly common, it is the second most common cause of death in children aged 5 to 14 years.[1–3] The most common malignancies affecting children differ from those affecting adults. Leukemia, brain tumors, lymphomas, and sarcomas of tissue and bone are the most common pediatric cancers[4] and account for over 50% of all pediatric malignancies with an incidence of 19.1 per 100,000 population 2014–18 (https://cancerstatisticscenter.cancer.org/#!/childhood-cancer) (Table 9.1). Embryonal tumors (e.g., neuroblastoma, Wilms tumor, retinoblastoma, medulloblastoma) are unique to early childhood, which underscores the need for these children to be cared for in pediatric centers with sufficient expertise in their management. Survival rates for most pediatric cancers have improved significantly in the past several decades; more than 80% of children diagnosed with a childhood malignancy in developed countries will become 5-year survivors of their cancers,[5,6] and 5-year survival rates for acute lymphoblastic leukemia (ALL) have now increased to nearly 90%.[7] The great improvements in survival for many malignancies of childhood are directly related to advances in diagnostic modalities and the large percentage of children treated in cooperative clinical trial protocols.[7,8] Treatment options in these protocols include chemotherapy, radiation therapy, biologic modifiers, hematopoietic stem cell transplantation (HSCT), and adoptive T-cell therapies.

Children with cancer typically undergo many surgical procedures that require anesthesia. The procedures may occur before or during the cancer therapy, years into remission, or during terminal stages of the disease. Certain considerations apply to this population, including the direct effects of the tumor, effects of the chemotherapy and radiation therapy, impact of the surgical procedure, pain syndromes, and psychological vulnerabilities of the child and family. Children undergoing active treatment for cancer range from gravely ill to relatively healthy with excellent functional capacity. Survivors of childhood cancer experience various long-term and often debilitating sequelae after completion of cancer therapy. In one report, 62% of survivors of childhood cancer reported at least one chronic health condition from cancer, one-third reported impaired task efficiency and memory and 28% reported a severe or life-threatening condition.[6,9] Active (93%) versus passive (67%) screening of survivors after childhood cancer revealed a much greater incidence of chronic health conditions.[10] These chronic health conditions may impact nearly every organ system and have considerable bearing on any anesthetic plan years into remission. The field of pediatric oncology is extensive, complicated, and ever-changing. Multidisciplinary communication in the perioperative period is crucial to ensure the safe care of these complex patients.

Principles of Cancer Therapy

Most pediatric cancers are treated with an aggressive multimodal approach that may include surgical resection, radiation therapy,

TABLE 9.1 | Pediatric Cancer Incidence by Age and 5-Year Survival Rates From 2009–2015

Primary Cancer Site	RELATIVE INCIDENCE BY AGE GROUP[a]					5-year survival, all ages (%) (2014)[b]
	0–4 years (%)	5–9 years (%)	10–14 years (%)	15–19 years (%)	0–19 years (%)	
Leukemias	36.1	33.4	21.8	12.4	25.2	86.6
Central nervous system tumors	16.6	27.7	19.6	9.5	16.7	74.9
Lymphomas	3.9	12.9	20.6	25.1	15.5	98.6 (Hodgkin) 90.9 (Non-Hodgkin)
Carcinomas and other malignant epithelial tumors	0.9	2.5	8.9	20.9	9.2	–
Soft-tissue sarcomas	5.6	7.5	9.1	8.0	7.4	75.6
Germ cell, trophoblastic, and other gonadal tumors	3.3	2.0	5.3	13.9	7.0	97.0 (Testicular)
Malignant bone tumors	0.6	4.6	11.3	7.7	5.6	74.0
Sympathetic nervous system tumors	14.3	2.7	1.2	0.5	5.4	–
Renal tumors	9.7	5.4	1.1	0.6	4.4	88.9
Retinoblastoma	6.3	0.5	0.1	0.0	2.1	100.0
Hepatic tumors	2.2	0.4	0.6	0.6	1.1	76.1

[a]Data from: Ries LAG, Percy CL, Bunin GR. Introduction. In: Ries LAG, Smith MA, Gurney JG, et al., eds. *Cancer Incidence and Survival Among Children and Adolescents: United States SEER Program 1975–1995.* NIH Pub. No. 99-4649 ed. Bethesda, MD: National Cancer Institute, SEER Program, 1999: 1-16.
[b]SEER*Explorer: An interactive website for SEER cancer statistics [Internet]. Surveillance Research Program, National Cancer Institute. https://seer.cancer.gov/statistics-network/explorer/.

and chemotherapy for control of local and metastatic disease. Equally important is supportive care to ensure minimization of toxicity from the tumor and treatment therapy, including nutritional, emotional, and psychological support. A brief review of these therapies with pertinence to the perioperative period follows, but additional sources are available concerning the current indications, side effects, and precautions of the available chemotherapeutic drugs.[11–13]

CONVENTIONAL CHEMOTHERAPEUTICS

Conventional chemotherapeutics, along with radiation therapy, have been the mainstay of pediatric antitumor treatment for decades. In the modern era of multidrug combination chemotherapy, molecularly targeted therapies, radiation therapy, rescue therapies, and hematopoietic stem cell transplantation (HSCT), anticipation of precise toxicities from any given therapy in an individual patient is difficult. However, treatment protocols include a potentially vast array of antitumor agents with widely divergent mechanisms of action and toxicity profiles, and the average child with cancer will be at risk for focal or widespread toxicity to nearly every organ system.[14] Most chemotherapeutic agents are cytotoxic to rapidly dividing cells via several mechanisms. Because these agents lack specificity to tumor cells alone, the impact to healthy tissues is unavoidable and often limits effective chemotherapy dosing schedules. Concurrent administration of several chemotherapeutics with nonoverlapping toxicity profiles and at reduced doses lessens the additive toxicity while increasing the simultaneous cytotoxic attack on tumor cells.[15] Regardless, bone marrow suppression, immunosuppression, myocardial toxicity, pulmonary toxicity, and dysfunction of nearly every other organ system are possible in children with cancer[16] and must be thoroughly considered when evaluating and caring for these children. These toxicities range from short-term to lifelong effects.

Several chemotherapeutic agents are of specific interest to the anesthesiologist caring for a child with cancer. Anthracycline chemotherapeutics (e.g., doxorubicin, daunorubicin, idarubicin, and epirubicin) and mitoxantrone cause cardiomyopathy in a dose-dependent fashion, an effect exacerbated by mediastinal irradiation. L-Asparaginase is associated with a 1% to 2% risk of hemorrhage or thrombosis owing to deficiencies in fibrinogen, plasminogen, antithrombin III, and von Willebrand factor, as well as hepatic dysfunction and acute hemorrhagic pancreatitis.[17–19] Bleomycin may cause acute pneumonitis with progression to pulmonary fibrosis.[20] Cisplatin and ifosfamide may cause renal tubular damage that can lead to Fanconi syndrome with electrolyte wasting.[21,22] In large doses, methotrexate (>1 gram/m^2) may cause renal failure.[23,24] Corticosteroids may be directly cytotoxic to some hematopoietic tumors by inducing apoptosis and acute tumor lysis syndrome, as well as causing adrenal suppression, hypertension, thromboembolism, and obesity. Specific toxicities of chemotherapeutic agents pertinent to anesthesia are discussed in detail later in the chapter; Table 9.2 provides a brief list of major toxicities of the traditional chemotherapy agents. E-Table 9.1 provides a comprehensive list of traditional chemotherapeutic agents, molecularly targeted agents, and adjuvant medications used in children, with their corresponding toxicities.

Several nonchemotherapy adjunct medications and therapies are used to provide supportive care and to attenuate the toxicities of chemotherapy. With adequate treatment of toxic adverse effects, larger doses and/or additional chemotherapeutic agents can enhance the rate of remission. Such therapies include antiemetics, hematopoietic growth factors, HSCT, transfusion of blood products, and several medications that lessen or block organ-specific toxicity. Many of these therapies also pose acute and chronic risks to children; these risks must be balanced against their benefits.[15]

TABLE 9.2 | Therapy-Related Adverse Effects and Toxicity

Drug	Adverse Effects
L-Asparaginase	Hyperglycemia, hypersensitivity, hepatic dysfunction (secondary hypoalbuminemia and coagulopathies), pancreatitis, thrombosis, stroke
Bischloroethyl nitrosourea (BCNU)	Encephalopathy, hepatotoxicity, pulmonary toxicity
Bleomycin	Anaphylactoid reactions, fever, hyperpigmentation, nausea, vomiting, oxygen toxicity, pulmonary fibrosis
Busulfan	Encephalopathy, hepatotoxicity, pulmonary toxicity
Carboplatin	Myelosuppression, nausea, vomiting, nephrotoxicity, neurotoxicity, ototoxicity
Cisplatin	Nausea/vomiting, nephrotoxicity, ototoxicity, peripheral neuropathy
Corticosteroids	Adrenal suppression, avascular necrosis, cataracts, edema, gastritis, hyperglycemia, hypertension, myopathy, osteoporosis, obesity, osteopenia, tumor lysis syndrome, tumor necrosis, psychosis
Cyclophosphamide (Cytoxan)	Cardiotoxicity, hemorrhagic cystitis, myelosuppression, nausea, vomiting, syndrome of inappropriate secretion of antidiuretic hormone (SIADH)
Cyclosporine	Cortical blindness, electrolyte disturbances, encephalopathy, gingival hyperplasia, hemolytic uremia, hepatotoxicity, hyperlipidemia, hypertension, hirsutism, myositis, paresthesias, tremor
Cytarabine	Myelosuppression, mucositis, hepatitis, nausea/vomiting, neurotoxicity
Dactinomycin (Actinomycin D)	Nausea/vomiting, mucositis, myelosuppression, radiation recall?[a]
Daunorubicin (Daunomycin) Doxorubicin (Adriamycin) Idarubicin (Idamycin)	Cardiomyopathy, mucositis, myelosuppression, red-orange urine
Etoposide	Hypotension, mucositis, myelosuppression, nausea, vomiting
Ifosfamide	Hemorrhagic cystitis, myelosuppression, nephrotoxicity, neurotoxicity
Melphalan	Mucositis
Methotrexate	Hepatotoxicity, mucositis, myelosuppression, renal failure, neurotoxicity
Mercaptopurine (6-MP)	Hepatotoxicity, myelosuppression
Mycophenolate mofetil (CellCept)	Electrolyte disturbance, gastrointestinal toxicity, hypercholesterolemia, myelosuppression, rash
Procarbazine	Myelosuppression
Sirolimus	Hyperlipidemia, myelosuppression
Tacrolimus (Prograf)	Anemia, anorexia, back pain, encephalopathy, diarrhea, hyperglycemia, nephrotoxicity, pleural effusion, rash
Thiotepa	Neurotoxicity, mucositis
Thioguanine (6-TG)	Hepatotoxicity, myelosuppression
Total body irradiation	Dental/bony maldevelopment, gastrointestinal toxicity, hepatotoxicity, pulmonary toxicity
Vinblastine (Velban)	Myelosuppression, neurotoxicity, SIADH
Vincristine (Oncovin)	Neurotoxicity, SIADH

[a]Radiation recall: the "recalling" by skin of previous radiation exposure in response to the administration of certain response-inducing drugs.
Modified from Carpenter PA, Mielcarek M, Woolfrey AE. Hematopoietic cell transplantation. In: Irwin S, Rippe JM, eds. *Intensive Care Medicine*. 6th ed. Philadelphia: Lippincott Williams & Wilkins; 2008:2150-2168.

TARGETED ANTITUMOR AGENTS

Commensurate with the growing understanding of cancer biology is the relatively recent development of chemotherapeutics with a more focused target that achieve enhanced tumoricidal effects while reducing cytotoxic effects to healthy cells. These therapies may be broadly categorized as those that boost the host immune system to enhance its attack on tumor growth ("immunotherapy") or those that inhibit tumor-specific molecular pathways necessary for tumor cell growth and survival ("targeted therapy"). Immunotherapeutics, which have shown great promise in several pediatric cancers, include drugs that activate the host immune response (e.g., checkpoint inhibitors) and those that immunomodulate via tumor-expressed targets (e.g., monoclonal antibodies and adoptive T-cell therapies).[25]

Few molecular targeted therapies are approved for use in children, despite several gaining adoption into pediatric cancer treatment protocols. Importantly, the relatively recent addition to pediatric therapy means that long-term efficacy and toxicity are not fully understood.[26] However, several show considerable promise, for example the use of tyrosine kinase inhibitors (e.g., imatinib) in BCR-ABL (Philadelphia chromosome)–positive leukemia. Other targeted agents include antiangiogenic therapies, immunomodulatory therapies, gene therapies, and humanized antibodies.[27,28] Monoclonal antibodies are targeted to specific, unique tumor cell surface antigenic proteins. Small-molecule drugs, which are designed to target specific genetic signatures and biologic pathways critical to cancer growth and progression, have been developed that target tumor cell apoptotic pathways, histone deacetylation, protein farnesyltransferases, proteasome action, angiogenesis, and inhibition of the epidermal growth factor receptor tyrosine kinase.[27,29,30]

Although toxicities of these agents as a whole appear to be far less than those of traditional chemotherapeutic agents, rash, fatigue, alterations to skeletal growth plates (antiangiogenic agents), nausea, diarrhea, hypotension, and anaphylaxis have been reported.[31] The use of investigational and novel targeted antitumor agents amplifies the importance of reviewing cases with the oncologist.

ADOPTIVE T-CELL THERAPIES IN CHILDREN

There have been rapid and dramatic advances in adoptive immunotherapy using an infusion of T cells genetically engineered to express a single chain antibody targeting a specific tumor antigen (e.g., CD19 in ALL or CD30 in Hodgkin lymphoma). The most widely studied therapy is chimeric antigen receptor (CAR) T-cell therapy, with an incidence of complete remission of up to 90% in some cohorts.[32] Pediatric indications are expanding, but most applications in children are associated with relapsed cancer or residual tumor after HSCT. Briefly, autologous T cells are removed through a central venous catheter, genetically engineered ex vivo to express a single chain antibody to the desired antigen, and then reinfused into the proband. After infusion, the cells engraft, multiply, and eradicate tumor cells for months or years.[33–35] However, sufficient engraftment and expansion depend on prior lymphodepletion, which requires significant immunosuppression with total body irradiation (TBI) and chemotherapy, with all the associated risks.[36] The process of production of autologous CAR-T cells can be cumbersome, and new clinical trials have demonstrated the feasibility of off-the-shelf, allogeneic CAR-T cell products.[37] These are genetically engineered T cells, with disrupted endogenous T-cell receptors to mitigate incompatibility, from healthy donors that can be given to any patient. Some key points should be understood when caring for these children before and after T-cell infusions.

Perioperative team care: T-cell and other cellular forms of adoptive cellular therapy constitute a rapidly changing field that requires effective communication between the oncologist and the perioperative team to ensure the safe and optimal management of the child. There is consensus agreement that critical care assessments should be considered as early as possible in patients with high-grade toxicities.[38]

Infectious risk: Akin to children receiving HSCT, these children are immunosuppressed and at significant risk for infections and death from neutropenic sepsis. Isolation and meticulous use of sterile technique must be observed.

Toxicity: This therapy is accompanied by potentially significant morbidity and mortality. In addition to the toxicity of the preconditioning regimen, the modified T cells occasionally trigger an autoimmune response. Cytokine-release syndrome (CRS), the most serious toxicity, is a result of supraphysiologic levels of immune cell activation and the subsequent massive release of inflammatory cytokines. Mild cases manifest as rash, fevers and myalgias, but severe cases may lead to cardiorespiratory failure, multiorgan dysfunction, and possible death if not treated early.[33–35] Symptoms may manifest within 7 days of therapy to up to 10 to 14 days of infusion. Symptoms of neurotoxicity are also common, with an incidence of 21.7%.[39] They range from tremors and expressive aphasia to delirium and seizures.[40] Management of CRS may include supportive care, corticosteroids, and the interleukin-6 receptor inhibitor, tocilizumab.[41]

Cardiac: A high incidence of systolic dysfunction, with hypotension requiring inotropic support, has been reported in pediatric CAR-T cell patients.[42] The mechanism of this acute cardiac toxicity is unclear.

Pulmonary: Pulmonary capillary leak predisposes these patients to noncardiogenic pulmonary edema, which may progress to acute respiratory distress syndrome. Judicious fluid administration is important as these patients often receive aggressive hydration to prevent tumor lysis syndrome and manage fevers.

Hematology: Severe CRS may be associated with coagulopathy and hypofibrinogenemia. Empiric guidelines for fibrinogen replacement in CAR-T trials suggest a target fibrinogen level of ≥1.5 g/L.[43] Patients undergoing CAR-T therapy may present with bleeding sequalae including pulmonary hemorrhage, thus fibrinogen levels should be monitored in patients with moderate or severe CRS to prevent potentially fatal bleeding events.

RADIATION THERAPY

One-quarter of all children newly diagnosed with cancer will require radiation as frontline therapy.[44] Photons (e.g., x-rays) and particle radiation (e.g., electrons, protons, neutrons) are the two major types of ionizing beam radiation. Regardless of the particle source, ionizing radiation leads to cell death by damaging cellular DNA. Toxicity from the effects of radiation therapy to surrounding healthy tissues is unavoidable, and the developing tissues of children are particularly susceptible to the acute and late effects of irradiation. The susceptibility of normal tissues depends on the total and fractional dose received, the inherent sensitivity of the tissue to the dose of radiation, the volume of tissue irradiated, and time course of treatment (Table 9.3).[45] Overall, normal host cells have a greater capacity to repair the damaging effects of radiation than cancer cells but require time to recover. To allow sufficient time for the healthy tissue to repair, the total dose of radiation is usually divided into a series of fractional doses over time.[46] Recent technological advances have led to three-dimensional conformal radiotherapy, which closely conforms the radiation dose to the tumor shape and minimizes radiation to the surrounding tissues.[47–49] Despite these advances to reduce the toxicity of radiation therapy to healthy tissues, children remain at risk for acute and chronic complications. Furthermore, concurrent chemotherapy may potentiate the radiation toxicity, increasing the tissue damage.

Proton radiation therapy (PRT) is a newer modality in pediatric radiation oncology and has become an established alternative to traditional photon therapy; however, PRT centers remain relatively uncommon (38 in the United States in 2022 [http://www.proton-therapy.org/map.htm]), which limits rapid access to frontline PRT for many children worldwide. In contrast to the destructive impact to all tissues in the path of a traditional photon beam, the specifically charged velocities of the proton beams are targeted to the calculated depth and shape of the tumor. By modulating the energy of the proton beam to become maximally energized at a specific depth of tissue, the relative dose to the healthy tissues in the plane of entry is as low as 20% to 30%, increases to 100% at the depth of tumor, and then decays to nearly no further penetration beyond the tumor (Fig. 9.1).[50] As such, the advantages of PRT include limited damage to healthy tissues surrounding the tumor and enhanced cell killing of the targeted tumor tissues.[51] Despite these beneficial physical properties, the overall advantage of PRT over conventional radiation therapy is not yet uniformly supported by clinical trials, randomized pediatric trials are lacking, and long-term outcomes are yet to be realized.[52] However,

TABLE 9.3	Late Effects of Radiation Therapy	
Radiation Field	**Late Effects**	**Risk Factors**
Cranial	Neurocognitive deficits	>18 Gy, IV/IT methotrexate
	Leukoencephalopathy	>18 Gy with IT methotrexate
	Growth hormone deficiency	>18 Gy
	Panhypopituitarism	>40 Gy
	Large vessel stroke	>60 Gy
	Second cancers	Variable
	Dental problems	>10 Gy
	Cataracts	>2–8 Gy single dose, 10–15 Gy fractionated dose
	Ototoxicity	>35–50 Gy
Chest	**Cardiac disease**	
	Coronary artery disease	>30 Gy
	Cardiomyopathy	>35 Gy, >25 Gy with anthracyclines
	Valvular disease	
	Pericardial disease	>40 Gy
	Arrhythmias	>35 Gy
		Unknown
	Thyroid disease	
	Hypothyroidism	>20 Gy local, >7.5 Gy TBI
	Hyperthyroidism	>20 Gy local, >7.5 Gy TBI
	Thyroid nodules, cancer	Any dose
	Pulmonary disease	
	Pulmonary fibrosis	>15–20 Gy
	Restrictive lung disease	Unknown
	Obstructive lung disease	Unknown
Abdomen/ Pelvis	Chronic enteritis	>40 Gy
	Gastrointestinal malignancy	Unknown
	Hepatic fibrosis/cirrhosis	>30 Gy
	Renal insufficiency	>20 Gy
	Bladder disease	
	Fibrosis	>30 Gy prepubertal, >50 postpubertal
	Hemorrhagic cystitis	Enhances cyclophosphamide and ifosfamide effect
	Bladder cancer	Unknown
	Gonadal dysfunction	
	Ovarian failure	4–12 Gy
	Testicular failure	>1–6 Gy
Any Radiation	Skin cancer	
	Musculoskeletal changes	
	Bone length discrepancy	>20 Gy
	Pathologic fractures	>40 Gy
TBI	All the above	

Gy, Gray; *IT*, intrathecal; *IV*, intravenous; *TBI*, total body irradiation.
From Latham GJ, Greenberg RS. Anesthetic considerations for the pediatric oncology patient—part 1: a review of antitumor therapy. *Pediatr Anesth.* 2010;20:295-304. Used with permission.

there is increasing evidence that the purported advantages of PRT are clinically actualized, including decreased neurotoxicity, improved health-related quality of life, and reduced neuroendocrine deficits with PRT compared with historical data with conventional photon radiation therapy.[53–55]

Preoperative Considerations by Organ System

AIRWAY

Though primary tumors of the airway are rare in children,[56,57] various cancer treatment regimens can cause airway changes that challenge the anesthesiologist. Both chemotherapy and radiation treatment can cause mucositis and xerostomia, first appearing soon after initiating treatment.[58,59] Severe mucositis causes painful and friable oral mucosa and may threaten the airway as a result of pseudomembrane formation, supraglottic edema, bleeding, or aspiration of blood and secretions.[60,61] Graft-versus-host disease (GVHD) after HSCT may also cause significant mucositis, with up to 30% of those children developing a difficult airway.[61] Chronic radiation therapy to the head and neck may cause fibrosis, which distorts facial tissues and renders them less mobile.[62] Children who have undergone chronic radiation therapy may present a challenge during laryngoscopy, with difficult glottic visualization, poor laryngeal mask airway seal, and subglottic stenosis.[62,63]

Anesthesiologists caring for children who have undergone chemotherapy, HSCT, or radiation therapy should perform a thorough preoperative airway history and physical examination focusing on symptoms of airway compromise, prior anesthetic history, visualization of oral mucosa, and external assessment of the degree of distortion and immobility of face and neck tissues.

CARDIAC

Primary cardiac tumors (most commonly rhabdomyomas, fibromas, teratomas, or myxomas) are uncommon in children, but when they occur (e.g., in children with tuberous sclerosis), they are usually benign with a long-term mortality rate of 8%.[64,65] Cardiac tumors that are not diagnosed in utero typically present with dyspnea (14%), arrhythmias (14%), or heart failure (19%) but can occasionally cause left ventricular outflow tract obstruction and cardiogenic shock.[65–67] Benign tumors may regress spontaneously or with medical treatment with the mTOR inhibitor everolimus. Malignant cardiac tumors are extremely rare and associated with significant mortality.[68]

Noncardiac cancers can also cause cardiovascular compromise in children secondary to anterior mediastinal mass (AMM), pericardial effusion, hypertension, cardiomyopathy, or heart failure as sequelae of the tumor itself or as side effects of therapy. Chronic cardiac disease in cancer survivors is common, with a 10-fold increased risk of coronary artery disease, 15-fold increased risk of heart failure, and a 9-fold increased risk of cerebrovascular events within 30 years of diagnosis.[69,70] Recent research has focused on prevention and mitigation of acute and chronic cardiovascular complications of cancer treatment.

Anthracycline chemotherapeutic agents (doxorubicin, daunorubicin, idarubicin, and epirubicin) as well as the unrelated agent mitoxantrone, are well known for their dose-dependent cardiotoxic effects on the myocardium, which range from subclinical myocardial dysfunction to arrhythmias to fulminant heart failure.[71,72] Half of children receiving moderate-dose anthracycline ($\geq$100 to <250 mg/m^2) for ALL have troponin elevation during

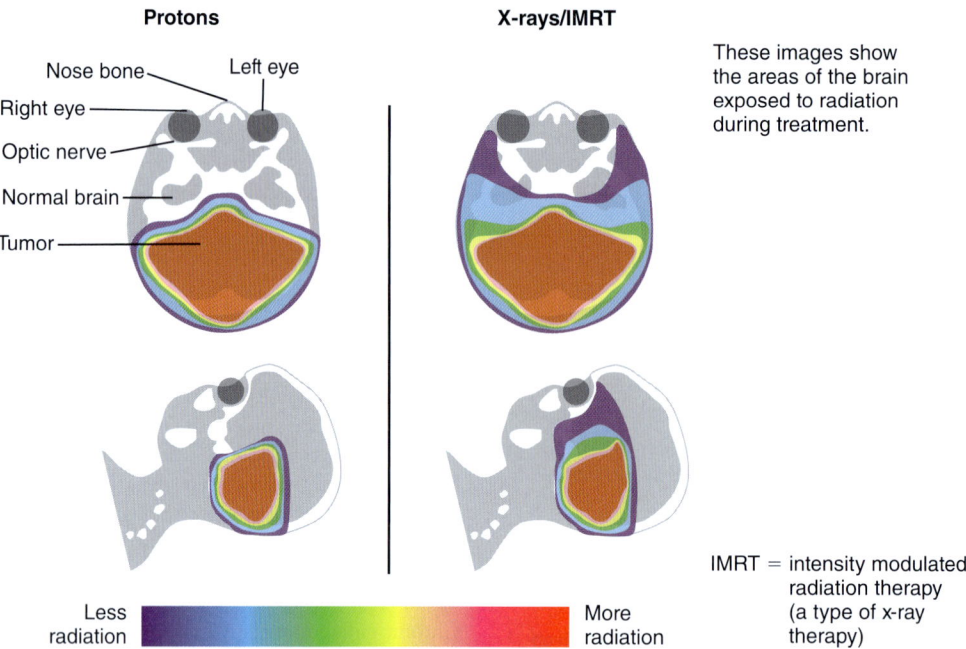

FIGURE 9.1 Rendering of the difference between photon (x-ray) and proton beam therapies for posterior fossa radiation. As radiation passes from posterior to anterior, the entry dose of radiation to healthy tissues of the posterior skull is similar. However, the exit radiation dose is markedly different: the protons lose their energy at a calculated depth, resulting in no radiation to sensitive tissues beyond the tumor (eyes, pituitary, and so on). (From Fred Hutchinson Cancer Center – Proton Therapy.)

treatment, and there is some evidence that even subclinical myocardial dysfunction during acute treatment may predispose children to early cardiac disease in adulthood.[73] Twelve percent of children receiving larger doses of anthracycline (>250 mg/m^2) experience acute cardiac toxicity with left ventricular (LV) systolic dysfunction, and 4% have cardiomyopathy with hypotension, heart failure, or arrhythmias.[74] Most children recover from acute toxicity with supportive therapy, but chronic progressive dilated or restrictive cardiomyopathy may develop within a year of treatment. The onset of symptoms can be delayed, and children may present with cardiac failure 20 or more years after treatment.[75–77] Overall, more than half of patients treated with anthracyclines will eventually develop evidence of chronic subclinical heart disease, and up to 16% exhibit symptomatic chronic cardiac dysfunction.[78] Although the risk of cardiotoxicity increases with increasing anthracycline doses, especially when the cumulative dose exceeds 250 to 360 mg/m^2,[77] there is no "safe" threshold dose for anthracyclines, as doses less than 240 mg/m^2 have resulted in cardiac damage.[79] Preventive measures include the use of newer anthracycline analogs, antioxidants, iron chelators, and alterations in the chemotherapeutic dose.[75] The cardiotoxic effects of chemotherapy are compounded (perhaps tripled) by concurrent chest irradiation. One in eight survivors of childhood cancer who received both anthracyclines and chest radiation develop a serious, chronic cardiac disease.[77,80,81] Other traditional chemotherapeutics such as cyclophosphamide, fluorouracil, vinca alkaloids, cytarabine, cladribine, L-asparaginase, paclitaxel, trastuzumab, etoposide, teniposide, and pentostatin have also been associated with cardiac toxicity.[72,82]

Unlike traditional chemotherapeutic agents that primarily affect the myocardium, radiation therapy can damage all components of the cardiovascular system. Complications from mediastinal radiation include cardiomyopathy, pericardial effusions, pericarditis, valvular fibrosis, conduction disturbances, and accelerated arteriosclerosis.[75,81] Radiation-related myocardial fibrosis can induce a progressive restrictive cardiomyopathy, leading to pulmonary vascular disease and pulmonary hypertension. Systolic and/or diastolic dysfunction may be present. Premature arteriosclerosis affects the coronary arteries as well as the carotid arteries, pulmonary arteries, renal arteries, and aorta.[80] Fatal myocardial infarction has been reported in children 6 to 22 years of age after mediastinal radiation.[83] Valvular heart disease is predominately characterized by progressive mitral and aortic stenosis and insufficiency. Conduction disturbances range from atrial and ventricular arrhythmias to right bundle branch block, and occasionally complete heart block requiring pacemaker placement. Radiation damage to autonomic nerves in proximity to the heart can result in tachycardia and loss of phasic respiratory variability similar to the presentation of a denervated heart. Autonomic denervation can attenuate the perception of anginal pain, so providers should have a low threshold for suspicion of myocardial ischemia in those who have undergone mediastinal radiotherapy in infancy and childhood. With low doses of radiation ($<25–30$ Gy), short-term radiation toxicity is limited, but late toxicity occurs even at these low doses.[80,81,84,85]

Newer targeted cancer therapies inhibit specific pathways necessary for tumor cell survival and growth and may reduce cardiac toxicity from traditional chemotherapeutics either intrinsically or due to dose reduction of more toxic agents, but these agents have also been reported to have some cardiotoxic effects.[86] For example, tyrosine kinase inhibitors, which preferentially inhibit the enzymatic activity necessary for the proliferation of certain tumor cells, can also affect the vascular endothelium, leading to hypertension, thromboembolism, and myocardial dysfunction.[87,88] Immunotherapy with CAR-T cells can also cause acute cardiac dysfunction.

In one study, 24% of pediatric CAR-T cell recipients developed hypotension that required inotropic support, and 41% of these children had echocardiographic evidence of cardiac dysfunction at discharge.[42] Given the novelty of these agents, data on the long-term effects of targeted antitumor drugs and immunotherapy in children are still limited.

Treatment of heart failure related to cancer treatment is similar to treatment of heart failure from other etiologies including angiotensin-converting enzyme (ACE) inhibitors, diuretics, beta blockers, and statins.[89] Long-term hypertension is common and is treated in the standard manner.

Even in patients without clinical evidence of chronic heart failure, the potential for cardiovascular compromise in the setting of major surgical stress and anesthesia should be considered. Patients who require more thorough clinical evaluation include those who have received:[90]

- Cumulative anthracycline dose >240 mg/m^2
- Any dose of anthracycline during infancy
- Chest irradiation >40 Gy (or >30 Gy with concomitant anthracycline treatment)
- Unknown doses of chemotherapy and radiation

There are no data supporting a specific protocol for preoperative risk stratification in cancer survivors, but preoperative ECG should be considered in select cases. Major ECG changes are associated with larger cumulative dose of anthracyclines or radiation and are predictive of cardiac and all-cause mortality; however, the clinical relevance of abnormal ECG in the perioperative period is unclear as there is poor correlation between abnormal ECG and echocardiographic evidence of cardiac dysfunction.[91,92] Children with subclinical cardiomyopathy typically do not experience serious complications of anesthesia and minor surgery.[93]

ANTERIOR MEDIASTINAL MASS

Anterior mediastinal masses (AMM) are of great concern to the anesthesiologist as they can result in cardiovascular and respiratory collapse during anesthesia. The most common causes of AMM are Hodgkin and non-Hodgkin lymphoma and children with these malignancies typically have mediastinal involvement at the time of diagnosis.[94] Less common oncologic causes of AMM include neuroblastoma, germ cell tumors, and ALL.[95] Children with AMM may require anesthesia for biopsy or resection of the mass, intravenous line placement, or radiologic procedures.

Masses in the anterior mediastinum overlie the great vessels, superior vena cava, and the tracheobronchial tree, which may become compressed with changes in respiratory patterns and thoracic muscle tone under anesthesia. Children with clinical findings of superior vena cava syndrome or airway compression from AMM are at the greatest risk for life-threatening perioperative complications (Table 9.4). Symptoms of orthopnea, upper body edema, stridor, nighttime cough, the need to sleep on one preferred side or position, or wheezing should alert the anesthesiologist of the need for further evaluation. Radiographic or ultrasound evidence of airway or great vessel compression, pulmonary artery outflow obstruction, ventricular dysfunction, or pericardial effusion are particularly concerning findings that necessitate a discussion about the utility of preoperative treatment to reduce the size of the mass.[96] Pretreatment is controversial because either corticosteroids or radiation may alter the tumor histology by causing tumor necrosis and render the precise diagnosis more difficult. In such cases, the diagnosis may require both tissue and subcellular analyses. However, diagnosis may still be possible in 95% of children after a 5-day course of corticosteroids.[97]

TABLE 9.4	Risk Stratification of Children With Anterior Mediastinal Mass Undergoing Anesthesia/Sedation

Low risk
  Mild respiratory symptoms without orthopnea
  No airway/cardiac compression on imaging
Intermediate risk
  Mild orthopnea or other respiratory symptoms
  Tracheal compression <50% cross-sectional area
High risk
  Orthopnea
  Stridor, wheeze, or cyanosis
  Upper body edema (signs of SVC syndrome)
  Tracheal compression >50%
  Tracheal compression <50% with any bronchial compression
  Tamponade physiology
  Right atrial collapse
  Pulmonary artery outflow obstruction
  Ventricular dysfunction
  Pericardial effusion

SVC, Superior vena cava.

Perioperative complications develop in 10% to 20% of children with AMM, so multidisciplinary risk stratification and procedural planning involving oncology, surgery, anesthesia, interventional radiology, and critical care is essential to clarify the optimal management for these children (Fig. 9.2). Anesthetic considerations for children with an anterior mediastinal mass are presented in detail in Chapter 13. In brief, local anesthesia and sedation are preferred. However, if general anesthesia is required, crucial perioperative considerations include maintaining spontaneous ventilation (i.e., avoiding paralysis) and being prepared to secure the airway with a tracheal tube and turn the child to the left lateral decubitus or prone position to resuscitate in the face of cardiopulmonary collapse.[98,99]

PERICARDIAL EFFUSION

Pericardial effusions in children with cancer may arise from venous or lymphatic obstruction, hematogenous metastases to the pericardium, or opportunistic infection. They are most common in children who have a mediastinal tumor or who are undergoing HSCT.[99a,99b] Patients with pericardial tamponade are at increased risk for cardiovascular collapse under anesthesia. Anesthetic goals for these patients are similar to those for patients with AMM including maintenance of spontaneous ventilation and avoidance of neuromuscular blockade.

PULMONARY

Primary and metastatic lung malignancies are uncommon in children.[100] Pulmonary compromise as a direct effect of pediatric tumors is more often the result of a pleural effusion, pulmonary infiltrates, pulmonary embolus, chylous effusions, anterior mediastinal mass, or hyperleukocytosis-induced pulmonary leukostasis.[101]

Therapy-related symptomatic pulmonary dysfunction or abnormal pulmonary function tests occur in 6% of children treated with chemotherapy alone, 20% treated with both chemotherapy and radiation, and 25% after HSCT.[75] Several chemotherapeutic agents—most notably bleomycin—have the potential to cause acute or chronic lung injury, including pneumonitis, pulmonary fibrosis, or noncardiogenic pulmonary edema.[20,102] Pneumonitis presents insidiously with nonproductive cough, progressive dyspnea, and rales. Although the symptoms usually resolve with completion of the

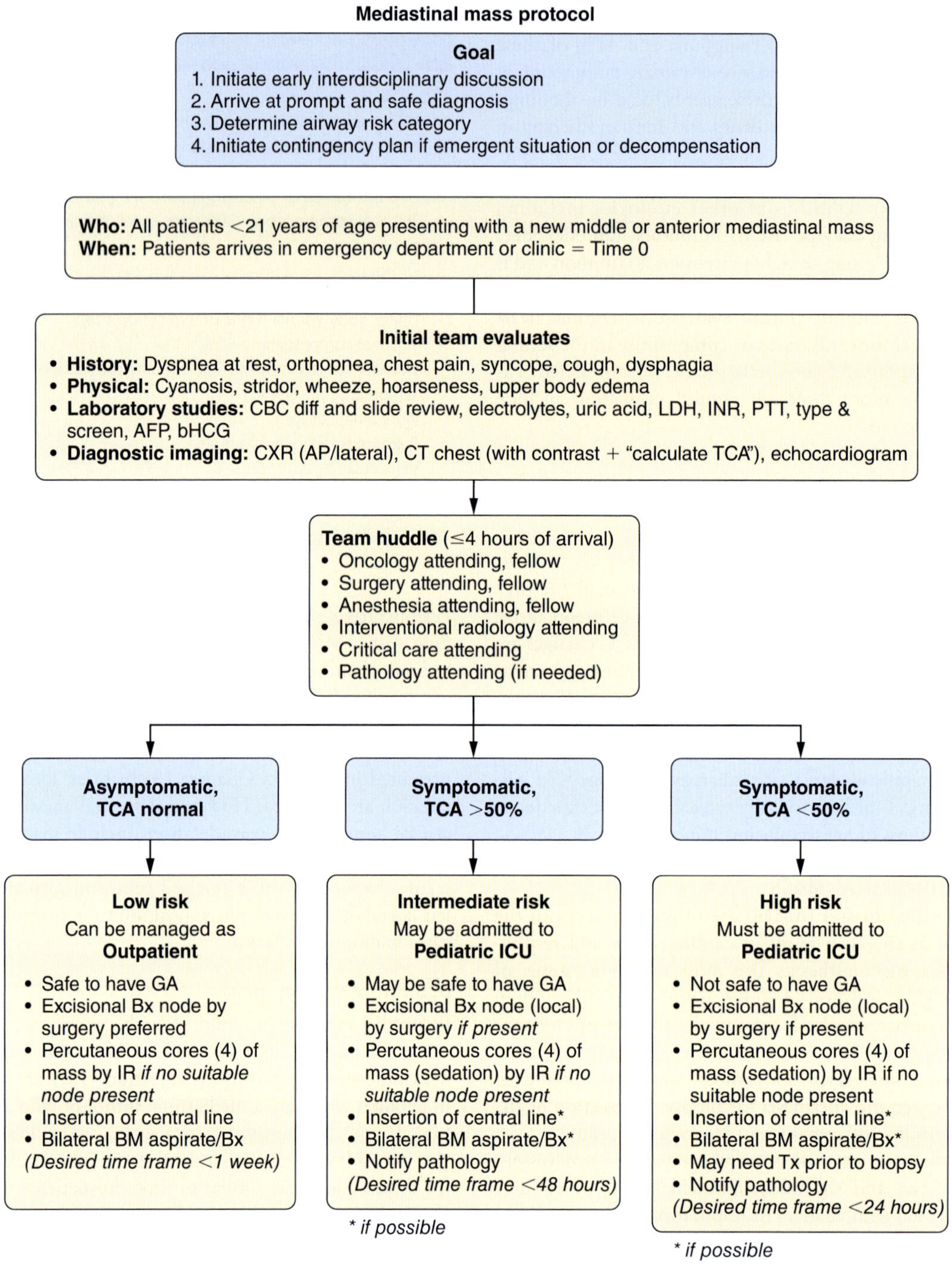

Mediastinal mass protocol

Goal
1. Initiate early interdisciplinary discussion
2. Arrive at prompt and safe diagnosis
3. Determine airway risk category
4. Initiate contingency plan if emergent situation or decompensation

Who: All patients <21 years of age presenting with a new middle or anterior mediastinal mass
When: Patients arrives in emergency department or clinic = Time 0

Initial team evaluates
- **History:** Dyspnea at rest, orthopnea, chest pain, syncope, cough, dysphagia
- **Physical:** Cyanosis, stridor, wheeze, hoarseness, upper body edema
- **Laboratory studies:** CBC diff and slide review, electrolytes, uric acid, LDH, INR, PTT, type & screen, AFP, bHCG
- **Diagnostic imaging:** CXR (AP/lateral), CT chest (with contrast + "calculate TCA"), echocardiogram

Team huddle (≤4 hours of arrival)
- Oncology attending, fellow
- Surgery attending, fellow
- Anesthesia attending, fellow
- Interventional radiology attending
- Critical care attending
- Pathology attending (if needed)

| **Asymptomatic, TCA normal** | **Symptomatic, TCA >50%** | **Symptomatic, TCA <50%** |

Low risk

Can be managed as **Outpatient**

- Safe to have GA
- Excisional Bx node by surgery preferred
- Percutaneous cores (4) of mass by IR *if no suitable node present*
- Insertion of central line
- Bilateral BM aspirate/Bx
(Desired time frame <1 week)

Intermediate risk

May be admitted to **Pediatric ICU**

- May be safe to have GA
- Excisional Bx node (local) by surgery *if present*
- Percutaneous cores (4) of mass (sedation) by IR *if no suitable node present*
- Insertion of central line*
- Bilateral BM aspirate/Bx*
- Notify pathology
(Desired time frame <48 hours)

* if possible

High risk

Must be admitted to **Pediatric ICU**

- Not safe to have GA
- Excisional Bx node (local) by surgery if present
- Percutaneous cores (4) of mass (sedation) by IR if no suitable node present
- Insertion of central line*
- Bilateral BM aspirate/Bx*
- May need Tx prior to biopsy
- Notify pathology
(Desired time frame <24 hours)

* if possible

FIGURE 9.2 Example algorithm for initial management of children with new diagnosis of anterior mediastinal mass and presumptive malignancy. *AFP,* Alpha-fetoprotein; *AP,* anterior-posterior; *bHCG,* beta-human chorionic gonadotropin; *BM,* bone marrow; *Bx,* biopsy; *CBC,* complete blood count; *CT,* computed tomography; *CXR,* chest x-ray; *GA,* general anesthesia; *ICU,* intensive care unit; *INR,* international normalized ratio; *IR,* interventional radiology; *LDH,* lactate dehydrogenase; *PTT,* prothrombin time; *TCA,* tracheal cross-sectional area; *Tx,* treatment.

treatment, in some children pneumonitis progresses to irreversible pulmonary disease.[20,103] In adults, bleomycin-induced pneumonitis occurs in up to 46%, with a 3% mortality. The incidence of pneumonitis in children is less well established.[104,105]

Pulmonary fibrosis may present acutely during treatment or as a late sequela of chemotherapy, radiation treatment, or GVHD and may be associated with severe morbidity and mortality.[76] The administration of large concentrations of oxygen to children with bleomycin-induced pulmonary fibrosis can acutely or chronically exacerbate their restrictive lung disease.[106,107] Thus the concentration of inhaled oxygen should be adjusted to the minimum concentration required to ensure adequate tissue oxygen delivery in the perioperative period. Overall, it is important to assess the clinical and functional status of these children for symptomatic or occult pulmonary disease before administering anesthesia.[96] A thorough assessment of baseline pulmonary status is particularly important to assess the need for postoperative ventilatory support or tolerability of thoracoscopy. It is reasonable to seek preoperative pulmonary function testing in those with clinical evidence of pulmonary dysfunction, bearing in mind that formal pulmonary function testing may be a challenge in young children.

RENAL

Wilms tumor is the most common primary renal tumor in children, followed by clear cell sarcoma of the kidney, malignant rhabdoid tumor, congenital mesoblastic nephroma, and renal cell carcinoma.[108,109] Each of these tumors can directly impact renal function. Similarly, extrarenal tumors, such as neuroblastoma, can impact the renal system by infiltrating the kidneys, obstructing urinary flow, or compressing the renal vasculature.[109]

Most chemotherapeutic drugs are directly nephrotoxic in a dose-dependent manner or lead to physiologic conditions that impair renal function (e.g., sepsis, dehydration, tumor lysis syndrome [TLS]). Cisplatin, carboplatin, and ifosfamide are notorious nephrotoxic chemotherapeutic agents in children and adults, especially when combined.[110] Cisplatin causes a dose-dependent nephrotoxicity and hypomagnesemia.[22] Ifosfamide causes subclinical glomerular toxicity in up to 90% of patients, with clinically apparent toxicity occurring in 30%. Ifosfamide can also induce Fanconi syndrome in up to 7% of children, with a delayed presentation possible up to 18 months after therapy.[21,110] Methotrexate has the potential to cause severe acute renal failure in children.[23] Many other chemotherapeutic drugs cause nephrotoxicity at large doses. The syndrome of inappropriate antidiuretic hormone (SIADH) is associated with multiple chemotherapeutic agents. Many nonchemotherapeutic drugs (such as antibiotics and diuretics) commonly used in children with tumors also contribute to nephrotoxicity.[109]

Focal abdominal radiation or total body irradiation as preconditioning for HSCT can cause radiation nephritis, which presents with azotemia, proteinuria, anemia, and hypertension.[111] The cumulative dose that leads to renal damage in children has not been established.[112] After HSCT, the incidence of acute renal failure in children is as great as 40%, with chronic renal failure in 18% to 54%.[113–115]

Anesthesia providers should be aware of the size and location of renal or juxtarenal tumors to determine the risk of intraoperative bleeding or great vessel obstruction, particularly in tumors that involve the renal vasculature. Preoperative evaluation of children who have undergone chemotherapy or abdominal radiation treatment should focus on identifying clinical and subclinical renal dysfunction, electrolyte disturbances (hypomagnesemia, hypophosphatemia), fluid overload, anemia, and hypertension. The need for preoperative dialysis should be considered in those with profound renal dysfunction. Nonsteroidal antiinflammatory drugs (NSAIDs) should be used with caution in children with renal dysfunction as NSAID-related restriction of renal perfusion may exacerbate any preexisting renal dysfunction.

HEPATIC

Primary liver tumors comprise only 1% of childhood cancers, and up to 20% of these are associated with a genetic syndrome, such as Beckwith-Wiedemann syndrome. In young children, hepatoblastomas are the most prevalent primary hepatic tumor, followed by sarcomas, germ cell tumors, and rhabdoid tumors. Hepatocellular carcinoma is occasionally found in older adolescents.[116]

Methotrexate, actinomycin D, 6-mercaptopurine, and 6-thioguanine are associated with acute hepatic toxicity, which can present hours to weeks after a chemotherapeutic dose. Hepatic impairment is typically transient and reversible.[96] Radiation typically causes self-limited acute toxicity, but chronic hepatic fibrosis may follow large doses of radiation (>40 Gy).[76] Most concerning is the potential to develop sinusoidal obstruction syndrome (SOS) in children after HSCT. SOS is characterized by portal hypertension, liver failure, and multiorgan system failure affecting the heart, lungs, and kidneys. Up to 60% of children develop SOS after HSCT, with an associated mortality rate of 19% to 50%.[117,118]

Both acute and chronic liver disease may be found in children with cancer, associated with a coagulopathy and/or impaired drug metabolism. The dose and timing of drugs that undergo significant hepatic elimination should be adjusted accordingly. Potentially hepatotoxic medications (e.g., acetaminophen) should be used with caution in children who are particularly vulnerable to further hepatic insult. Children exhibiting chronic liver failure may have coexisting genetic syndromes, such as Beckwith-Wiedemann syndrome, which present additional anesthetic challenges.[96]

GASTROINTESTINAL

Primary gastrointestinal (GI) tumors are uncommon in children; however, various intraabdominal malignancies can affect the GI tract by intestinal obstruction, intussusception, erosive perforation, intraabdominal hemorrhage, biliary obstruction, venous or arterial obstruction, and massive hepatomegaly.[96,119] The most common GI concern in children with cancer pertains to adverse effects of the chemotherapy and radiation treatment.

As chemotherapy and radiation treatments target rapidly proliferating tissues, the gastrointestinal mucosa is particularly vulnerable. Chemotherapeutic agents are well known to cause nausea and vomiting but may also cause more serious GI pathology such as diarrhea, mucositis, stomatitis, and neutropenic enterocolitis.[120] These adverse effects may exacerbate the malnutrition and dehydration that are often found in children with cancer. Similarly, radiation doses in excess of 20 to 30 Gy can cause inflammation and edema of GI tissues.[121] Importantly, acute and chronic GVHD after HSCT (discussed in detail later in the chapter) commonly impacts the GI tract, although the majority of cases are mild in the current era of prophylaxis with calcineurin inhibitors plus methotrexate or mycophenolate. The incidence of moderate to severe gut GVHD after HSCT is approximately 10%, and the mortality rate is substantial without prompt treatment.[122]

Before induction of anesthesia, children who have been treated for their cancer may have chronic nausea and vomiting or delayed gastric emptying, both of which are exacerbated by opioids. These children may be at increased risk for aspiration and should be managed accordingly. Children with GI dysfunction may also present with malnutrition, dehydration, and electrolyte imbalances that warrant correction before embarking on elective surgical procedures.

CENTRAL NERVOUS SYSTEM

Primary intracranial tumors such as astrocytomas, ependymomas, primitive neuroectodermal tumors, and gliomas represent 17% of all childhood malignancies.[2] Signs and symptoms of the tumor itself depend on the size and location of the tumor and the local mass effect on adjacent neurologic structures. Symptoms may include irritability, lethargy, macrocephaly, and vomiting. Increased intracranial pressure, herniation, stroke, seizure, or leukemic meningitis may herald acute decompensation.[95] Primary spinal tumors are uncommon but may present with acute spinal cord compression requiring immediate surgical treatment.[123] Furthermore, 3% to 5% of children with metastatic disease have some degree of spinal cord compression, often at initial diagnosis.[124,125] Detailed discussion and perioperative management of children with brain tumors is covered in Chapters 22 and 24.

Platinum chemotherapeutic agents (cisplatin, carboplatin, oxaliplatin), L-asparaginase, ifosfamide, methotrexate, cytarabine, etoposide, vincristine, and cyclosporine A may cause neurologic toxicity.[126,127] Acute toxicity is characterized by altered mental status, seizures, stroke, encephalopathy, ototoxicity, and peripheral nerve dysfunction.[15] These symptoms are often reversible with cessation of the drug. Chronic toxicity usually manifests as neurocognitive and psychiatric dysfunction, which are discussed later in the chapter. Brain irradiation can also have profound neurologic effects. Radiation doses in excess of 50 Gy can cause severe focal tissue damage, myelitis, stroke, and optic toxicity. Smaller doses, less than 18 Gy, are associated with subtler neurocognitive dysfunction.[121]

As discussed in detail in Chapters 22 and 24, children who present for resection of an intracranial tumor should undergo a thorough neurologic evaluation focusing on the signs and symptoms of increased intracranial pressure (ICP) and existing neurologic deficits. The benefits of sedative premedications must be balanced against their risks in children with increased ICP. As timely postoperative neurologic examination is important in these children, the choice of anesthetic agents and timing of extubation should be tailored to facilitate as early an assessment as circumstances allow.

ENDOCRINE

Primary endocrine tumors account for less than 5% of childhood cancers.[128] Gonadal germ cell tumors (testicular, ovarian, and extragonadal tumors), thyroid adenomas and carcinomas, and pituitary tumors (craniopharyngiomas and pituitary adenomas) account for the vast majority of these childhood endocrine tumors.[129]

Most chemotherapeutic agents have minimal effect on endocrine function, and chronic endocrine dysfunction is very uncommon in survivors of childhood cancer.[130,131] However, the use of glucocorticoids leads to a dose-dependent adrenal suppression. Studies in children with cancer have demonstrated that although a majority of children with ALL recover adrenal function in 2 weeks after cessation of chronic steroid therapy, some remain suppressed to various degrees of severity for 2 to 8 months.[132] It has thus been recommended that stress-dose steroids be administered before stressful procedures in the first 1 to 2 months after cessation of therapy.[132] If the anesthesiologist considers intraoperative stress-dose steroids or steroids for antiemesis, this must first be discussed with the child's oncologist; steroids are active anticancer drugs that, in some tumors, may cause tumor necrosis or tumor lysis syndrome, immune suppression, impact the cancer treatment protocol, and constitute grounds for a study violation.[96]

Unlike the minimal chronic endocrine suppression of chemotherapy drugs, total body irradiation preconditioning for HSCT and focal cranial radiotherapy, especially to regions in proximity to the hypothalamus, can cause, chronic neuroendocrine dysfunction.[130] Cumulative radiation doses as small as 18 to 20 Gy can cause growth hormone and gonadotropin deficiency, and doses greater than 35 to 40 Gy can cause panhypopituitarism.[133] Hypothyroidism can occur at doses of 20 Gy, typically manifesting 2 to 4.5 years after therapy.[134]

HEMATOLOGY

Myelosuppression is commonplace during pediatric cancer treatment, both as a consequence of the tumor effect itself and subsequent treatment of disease. Several cancers present with anemia at first diagnosis, including neuroblastoma, rhabdomyosarcoma, Hodgkin disease, Ewing sarcoma, osteosarcoma, and leukemia.[135,136] Thrombocytopenia is common in children with hematologic cancers as well as solid tumors invading the bone marrow.[137] The presenting leukocyte count in children with leukemia is variable. Neutropenia is typical at presentation in some children with ALL, but hyperleukocytosis ($>100,000/mm^3$) may be present in 20% of children with acute myelogenous leukemia. Hyperleukocytosis can cause hyperviscosity and potentially fatal leukostasis as tissue perfusion is impaired by plugging of leukocytes in the vasculature.[138]

Both chemotherapy and radiation therapy can have profound effects on myeloid cell production. Chemotherapy-related myelosuppression is common and is often dose limiting. Although radiation has the potential to completely suppress myeloid cell production, this typically requires exposure of a large percentage of marrow sites to cause clinically significant suppression. However, total body irradiation for HSCT preconditioning, by design, results in complete destruction of the host hematopoietic cells to prepare the marrow space for new cells. Doses for total body irradiation of only 3 to 5 Gy to all marrow sites are fatal if new cells are not transplanted. Recovery of hematopoiesis after HSCT follows a predictable pattern: granulocytes recover first, followed by platelets, lymphocytes, and lastly erythrocytes. During recovery, the child is susceptible to infections, bleeding, and anemia.[139] Reducing the dose of chemotherapy or stopping radiation allows cell counts to recover; however, owing to the life span of hematologic cells and the time to produce new cells, pancytopenia typically requires 4 weeks to resolve.[140,141] For prophylaxis or chronic treatment of cytopenia, both erythropoietin and recombinant human granulocyte-macrophage colony-stimulating factor may minimize anemia and neutropenia.[142]

Children with neutropenia are at increased risk for life-threatening infections. Providers should be vigilant about patient isolation and strict aseptic technique during invasive procedures or access of existing lines. Administration of medications and placement of temperature probes in the rectum can cause bacteremia and should be avoided. Similarly, catheterization of the urinary tract should also be used sparingly.[143]

COAGULATION

Abnormal bleeding in cancer patients may result from a number of factors, including thrombocytopenia, clotting factor deficiency, circulating anticoagulants, and defects in vascular integrity.[144] Even in the presence of adequate platelet numbers and function, the presence of any of these other coagulopathic defects may increase the risk of procedural bleeding. Hematologic cancers, especially any of the subsets of leukemia, often present with unexplained bleeding and a coagulopathy.[145] Disseminated intravascular coagulation may be present at the time of diagnosis of acute promyelocytic leukemia and less commonly with acute myelogenous leukemia and T-cell ALL. Patients may have lupus anticoagulant syndrome with subsequent thrombophilia or factor VIII inhibitors, leading to acquired hemophilia. Up to 8% of children with Wilms tumor have acquired von Willebrand syndrome at the time of diagnosis.[146,147]

Chemotherapy can cause a major coagulopathic response. L-Asparaginase may be associated with up to a 2% risk of hemorrhage or thrombus via induced deficiencies in plasminogen, fibrinogen, antithrombin III, and von Willebrand factor.[17] Vitamin K deficiency in the setting of hepatic dysfunction or severe malnutrition also contributes to coagulopathy.[148] Sepsis, disseminated intravascular coagulation, hepatic failure, acute or chronic anticoagulant usage, platelet sequestration with splenomegaly, and the burden of chronic disease may also contribute to the increased risk of perioperative hemorrhage.

Venous thromboembolism (VTE) is rare in children in general but considerably more common in those with malignancy as a result of coagulation dysfunction and frequent use of long-term indwelling vascular access. Nearly 8% of children with cancer experience VTE, with the greatest incidence among those with sarcoma and hematologic malignancies.[149] The optimal timing to stop anticoagulants before surgery in children with VTE warrants discussion with both the surgical and hematology-oncology teams. These children are at risk for perioperative thrombosis,[150] and their management must strike a delicate balance between provoking additional thrombus formation and an increased risk of surgical bleeding.

PAIN

Both acute and chronic pain are common sequelae of cancer and cancer therapy.[151] In one survey of 160 children undergoing cancer treatment, 87% of inpatients and 75% of outpatients rated their pain as moderate to severe.[152] In a survey of survivors of pediatric cancer, the single most painful experience during their treatment was a painful medical procedure or surgery.[153]

The use of general anesthesia for painful procedures, such as lumbar puncture and bone marrow biopsies, is one of the most effective techniques for reducing pain; anesthesiologists have a central role in optimizing patient comfort and parental stress during this difficult period.

Just as with other sources of chronic pain, children with cancer are often opioid tolerant and may benefit from a multimodal approach to analgesia. Regional anesthesia can be advantageous, but the benefits must be carefully weighed against the risks in those with a coagulopathy or significant chemotherapy-induced neuropathy. A multidisciplinary discussion with anesthesia, surgery, oncology, and pain service providers is essential to ensure an optimal balance between comfort and safety for these complex patients.

NEUROPSYCHOLOGY

Up to 40% of childhood cancer survivors suffer neurocognitive impairment in at least one of several areas, including academic achievement and executive function.[154,155] Intrathecal methotrexate and cranial irradiation appear to be particularly detrimental; thus children with ALL, central nervous system (CNS) tumors, and head and neck sarcomas are at the greatest risk for cognitive impairment.[156] The increasing availability of proton beam radiotherapy and its precise targeting of malignant tissue has been shown to reduce collateral tissue injury, and it may result in improved neurocognitive outcomes.[157–160]

The psychological response to cancer diagnosis and treatment is extremely age and individual dependent. Young children are often distressed by parental separation and anticipation of painful procedures. Many of these children benefit from an honest discussion of upcoming procedures to allow them a greater sense of control in their treatment. The placement of central access devices and topical anesthetic creams have greatly reduced the anxiety associated with many interventions required in their treatment.

Role-playing and desensitization can be particularly helpful in this age group.[161] Older children and adolescents are in many ways more profoundly affected by the psychosocial stress associated with cancer treatment. Compliance with medical treatment can be problematic in adolescents, who have difficulty coping with their diagnosis. To the extent that it is possible, adolescents should be actively involved in their own care, and assent from adolescent patients should be sought for anesthesia and invasive procedures.[90,161] Children and adolescents with cancer become isolated from peers because of school absences and the rigors of the treatment schedule, despite the natural need for peer interactions for healthy coping and adjustment. Feeling "alone" with their disease can worsen the sense of isolation from their healthy peers. As such, opportunities for peer engagement and interactions should be encouraged and provided. Peer interactions may include the child's choice of peers, as well as formal socialization or mentorship from other children with cancer or cancer survivors. Camps, group interventions, or formal coaching by childhood cancer survivors are highly effective.[162]

TUMOR LYSIS SYNDROME

Children with rapidly proliferating cancers, particularly ALL and non-Hodgkin lymphoma, are at risk for developing potentially fatal TLS. TLS has been reported in more than 40% of patients with non-Hodgkin lymphoma, although the rate of serious tumor lysis syndrome was only 6% in one study.[163] Nonhematologic malignancies with rapid proliferation, large tumor burden, and high sensitivity to chemotherapy are also subject to TLS after initiation of therapy. TLS occurs when rapid destruction of tumor cells yields a massive release of intracellular contents, resulting in hyperuricemia, hyperkalemia, hyperphosphatemia, hypocalcemia, and acid-base derangements. The cellular outpouring most commonly precipitates acute renal failure, but arrhythmias, cardiac failure, seizures, multiorgan failure, and death may occur. TLS can present suddenly with induction of chemotherapy, radiotherapy, fever, surgery, or anesthesia but most often occurs 1 to 3 days after initiation of cytotoxic therapy.[163,164] The incidence of severe TLS has decreased with the institution of appropriate preventative measures in high-risk children. The occurrence of perioperative TLS requires prompt and aggressive management, including hydration and diuresis, rasburicase (a uric acid–reducing agent), and allopurinol to ameliorate organ damage as well as aggressive measures to treat life-threatening arrhythmias owing to hyperkalemia (see Chapter 7; see also Fig. 7.7).[163] The cytotoxic effects of corticosteroids such as dexamethasone have been associated with tumor lysis, and alternative perioperative antiemetics should be used in those at risk.

RETINOIC ACID SYNDROME

Retinoic acid syndrome (also referred to as differentiation syndrome) is a potentially life-threatening complication found in 2% to 27% of children treated for acute promyelocytic leukemia with all-*trans* retinoic acid. The exact mechanism of this condition is unknown but is believed to be related to the release of inflammatory cytokines from acute promyelocytic leukemia cells during all-*trans* retinoic acid treatment. Retinoic acid syndrome typically occurs around 7 days after beginning treatment and is characterized by respiratory distress, fever, pulmonary infiltrates, and weight gain. Pericardial effusion, hypotension, cardiac failure, and renal failure can also occur. Thus children who were recently managed with induction therapy with all-*trans* retinoic acid for acute promyelocytic leukemia should be screened for pulmonary, cardiac, and renal abnormalities before undertaking general anesthesia.[165,166]

Hematopoietic Stem Cell Transplant

BACKGROUND

The first attempts to use bone marrow to treat malignancy took place over 50 years ago,[167] and the first successful pediatric transplant occurred almost 40 years ago.[168] HSCT is a potentially curative treatment for a wide range of malignant and nonmalignant pediatric disorders. HSCT is used in the treatment of many forms of leukemia, Hodgkin and non-Hodgkin lymphoma, and many types of solid tumors, including germ cell tumors, some sarcomas, neuroblastoma, Wilms tumor, and some malignant brain tumors. Additionally, it is used to treat many nonmalignant diseases, including myelodysplasia, aplastic anemia, hemoglobinopathies (including sickle cell disease and thalassemia), and congenital immune and metabolic deficiencies.[169–172] Because of the prevalence of ALL in the pediatric population, it is the primary indication for HSCT in many centers.

Hematopoietic stem cells used for transplantation can be obtained from bone marrow, "mobilized" peripheral blood, or umbilical cord blood. The source of the cells may be the child (autologous), an identical twin (syngeneic), or another individual (allogeneic). Allogeneic donor cells are commonly derived from human leukocyte antigen (HLA)–identical siblings (available in about 25% to 30% of patients), but advances in matching and supportive care have improved outcomes with HLA-matched unrelated and mismatched donors.[173,174]

CLINICAL FEATURES AND TREATMENT

The process of HSCT involves several steps:

1. The preparative or conditioning regimen, during which high-dose chemotherapy with or without irradiation or immuno-modulating agents eradicates malignancy (where present), clears marrow space for incoming stem cells, and suppresses the recipient's immune system
2. Transplantation through infusion of hematopoietic stem cells
3. Transplant engraftment (>30 days after transplantation)
4. Early engraftment (30–100 days after transplantation)
5. Late engraftment (>100 days after transplantation)

Cumulative toxicity associated with HSCT is the result of the underlying illness and complications of past therapy, the transplant-conditioning regimen, complications from long-term myelosuppression, and GVHD and its treatment. The incidence of transplant-related morbidity and mortality depends on the child's age, primary disease, comorbidities, and histocompatibility between donor and recipient.[175] Overall, 100-day mortality is 5% to 20% from sibling donors and 10% to 40% from unrelated donor allogeneic HSCT.[176]

HSCT-related toxicity can involve every organ of the body through the direct and indirect effects of irradiation and chemotherapy, as discussed previously. Immunologic and physical host defenses are impaired throughout the transplantation process. Infections are among the most important causes of transplant-related morbidity and mortality.[177] Children are vulnerable to a wide range of routine and opportunistic pathogens, including bacteria, fungi, and viruses. Mucositis is common and may increase the risks of aspiration and airway compromise.[61,178] Sinusoidal obstruction syndrome (SOS), previously called venoocclusive disease, occurs in 10% to 60% of children after HSCT. Mortality rates in the setting of SOS-induced hepatorenal failure and subsequent multiple-organ

failure range from 19% to almost 50%.[179] Hepatorenal syndrome and fluid retention associated with SOS mandate careful attention to fluid balance, sodium administration, and the presence of acquired coagulopathy, including thrombocytopenia that is refractory to platelet transfusions.[117,179,180] Other GI complications include hemorrhage, infections, and opioid-induced abdominal pain and distention (i.e., opioid-associated bowel syndrome).[181] Acute pulmonary complications, which occur in 30% to 60% of children after HSCT, include infection, hemorrhage, edema, bronchiolitis obliterans, acute respiratory distress syndrome, and idiopathic pneumonia syndrome, a noninfectious inflammatory lung process.[182–184]

In the early phase after HSCT, cardiomyopathy and arrhythmias are uncommon (5%), but sepsis, heart failure, and cardiovascular collapse are common admitting diagnoses in 10% to 40% of children who require intensive care after HSCT.[182,185,186] Late cardiac complications depend on the dose of radiation and the cardiotoxic chemotherapeutic agents used during the conditioning regimen. Acute renal failure occurs in 30% to 50% of children and warrants judicious use of fluids[113,114,187]; hemorrhagic cystitis is also common.[188] A process of thrombotic microangiopathy similar to hemolytic uremic syndrome may occur in as many as 25% of children who were treated with cyclosporine or the calcineurin inhibitor, tacrolimus.[189] CNS complications may include infection, hemorrhage, encephalopathy, and peripheral neuropathy owing to metabolic and chemotherapeutic effects.[190]

In contrast to the myeloablative procedures described previously, pediatric centers are increasingly using reduced-intensity preconditioning regimens and even nonmyeloablative preconditioning to reduce morbidity and mortality after hematologic malignancies.[191,192] Use of these regimens is based on the observation that in some instances, minimal myelotoxicity in conjunction with profound and prolonged immunosuppression leads to successful donor engraftment.[193] This modality is mostly used in children with nonmalignant hematologic conditions, marrow failure, and immunodeficiency syndromes but is increasingly used in pediatric hematologic malignancies.

GRAFT-VERSUS-HOST DISEASE

GVHD is the clinical manifestation that donor T cells recognize recipient alloantigens. Acute GVHD occurs in 20% to 80% of children within the first 100 days after HSCT. The incidence depends on the histocompatibility of the donor and recipient, as well as the stem cell source.[194] It is characterized by inflammatory dermatitis, enteritis, and hepatitis. Chemoprophylaxis (cyclosporine or tacrolimus with short-course methotrexate) is crucial as the outcomes after the onset of acute GVHD are disappointing. Treatment includes continuation of immunosuppression, the addition of corticosteroids, and the introduction of salvage therapy with profound immunosuppression. These children are at very high risk of succumbing to opportunistic infections.[194]

Chronic GVHD occurs in 6% to 50% of children 100 days or more after HSCT. This broad range of incidence depends on the age of the donor and recipient, gender matching, and degree of matching between donor and recipient.[195] Chronic GVHD has many features of autoimmune diseases, impacting nearly every organ of the body (e.g., sclerodermatous changes; dry mouth and conjunctivae; esophagitis; pulmonary dysfunction, including bronchiolitis obliterans; contractures or fasciitis of extremities and soft tissue; liver dysfunction; alopecia; thrombocytopenia). The pulmonary system is involved in 30% to 60% of children. Significant cardiac and renal disease is rare in chronic GVHD.

Opportunistic infections are common during chronic GVHD, in part, because of the immunosuppression associated with GVHD. Hemolysis is an additional manifestation of alloantigenicity, the result of major and minor blood group incompatibilities between donor and recipient.[196]

Preoperative Laboratory Testing and Evaluation

As is the case for children without cancer, there is insufficient evidence to recommend any routine preanesthetic testing in children with cancer. Instead, preoperative laboratory or radiologic testing should be based on the child's history, physical examination, concurrent illnesses, and surgical procedure. Tests should be ordered only if they have the potential to influence the surgical risk or the child's perioperative management.[197] In complex patients, these tests should be ordered in advance to (1) permit corrective action to be taken and satisfactory responses recognized and (2) allow communication with the oncology team before commencing the anesthetic plan. It is helpful for the oncology service to provide up-to-date information regarding hemoglobin, platelet counts, absolute neutrophil counts, coagulation studies, the most recent echocardiogram and pulmonary test results, as well as any other information that might affect anesthetic management. Possible factors that may require preoperative laboratory testing in the child with cancer are further discussed in the chapter.

A complete blood cell count is not routinely required before anesthesia in children with cancer. However, it may be warranted based on the condition of the child, presence of comorbidities, proposed surgical procedure and potential blood loss, potential thrombocytopenia, attendant risk of prolonged bleeding, and known or suspected anemia (Table 9.5).[90]

Preoperative coagulation testing is not routinely indicated in children with cancer. A preoperative platelet count is frequently obtained for children who are scheduled for lumbar puncture, neuraxial anesthesia, surgical procedures with risk of significant blood loss, or neurosurgical procedures. If the platelet count is sufficient for the surgical procedure and the regional anesthetic plan and there is no further clinical evidence of bleeding, then additional coagulation studies are probably unwarranted. However, any history of abnormal coagulation in the setting of an appropriate platelet count does warrant further investigation.[90]

TABLE 9.5	Risk Factors for Hematologic Abnormalities in Children With Cancer

Children at Risk for Anemia

- New diagnosis of leukemia (50%–80% incidence) or lymphoma
- Recent chemotherapy, radiation therapy, or hematopoietic stem cell transplant
- Children with cancer and age less than 6 months

Children at Risk for Hyperleukocytosis Include any New Diagnosis of Leukemia (>20% Incidence)

Children at Risk for Leukopenia and Neutropenia Include any Child Receiving Aggressive Chemotherapy or Irradiation

Children at Risk for Thrombocytopenia Include:

- New diagnosis of leukemia
- Any child receiving aggressive chemotherapy or irradiation
- Disseminated intravascular coagulation
- Splenomegaly

From Latham GJ, Greenberg RS. Anesthetic considerations for the pediatric oncology patient—part 3: pain, cognitive dysfunction, and preoperative evaluation. *Pediatr Anesth.* 2010;20(6):479-489. Used with permission.

The International Late Effects of Childhood Cancer Guideline Harmonization Group has published recommendations for chronic cardiotoxicity screening.[198] Cardiac surveillance should be considered for childhood cancer survivors who were treated with anthracyclines, mitoxantrone, or chest radiation (Table 9.6). Testing intervals in high-risk patients include within at least 2 years following treatment, again within 5 years post-treatment, and every 5 years thereafter. Surveillance is reasonable for those at moderate risk and may be considered for those at low risk.[198]

Perioperative Considerations

CHILDREN WITH CANCER

The perioperative complication rate after anesthesia in 177 children undergoing 3833 radiotherapy sessions was 1.3%, an incidence comparable to that for children without cancer anesthetized with propofol.[199] However, many children with cancer who present to the operating room are gravely ill with limited physiologic reserves and susceptible to relatively small changes to their physiology. Most

TABLE 9.6	Cardiomyopathy Surveillance Recommendations for Childhood Cancer Survivors					
Cardiomyopathy Risk Group	Anthracycline Dose (mg/m²)	Chest Radiation Dose (Gy)	Combined Anthracycline + Chest Radiation	Surveillance	Surveillance Frequency	Surveillance Before or During Pregnancy
High risk	≥250	≥35	≥100 mg/m² + ≥15 Gy	Recommended	<2 years PT ≤every 5 years after	Reasonable
Moderate risk	100 to <250	≥15 to <35	–	Reasonable	<2 years PT Every 5 years after	Reasonable
Low risk	<100	–	–	May be reasonable	<2 years PT Every 5 years after	Reasonable

PT, Post treatment.
Data adapted from Armenian SH, Hudson MM, Mulder RL, et al. Recommendations for cardiomyopathy surveillance for survivors of childhood cancer: a report from the International Late Effects of Childhood Cancer Guideline Harmonization Group. *Lancet Oncol.* 2015;16(3):e123-136.

children with standard risk leukemia in clinical remission receiving maintenance chemotherapy live a near normal lifestyle with good physical capacity; however, a number of children with cancer, especially those immediately before and after HSCT, can have multiorgan dysfunction and require intensive support in the hospital. It is imperative that the anesthesiologist carefully stratifies the risk of each child with cancer who presents for surgical or procedural intervention. The previously described considerations regarding the possible effects of pediatric cancer and its treatment on each organ system must be considered preoperatively. Prior anesthesia experiences, plus current information regarding the child's treatment protocol, cumulative chemotherapy or radiation therapy doses, major side effects, recent echocardiogram, current laboratory values, and organ dysfunction must be readily available. When current information is not readily available to the team preparing to anesthetize the child, the authors recommend that an updated data summary sheet be provided by the oncology team to the anesthesiologists before commencing anesthesia (E-Fig. 9.1).

Children with cancer undergo a host of procedures that require anesthesia during acute and chronic phases of disease. Included among these are diagnostic tumor or lymph node biopsy, tumor resection, placement and replacement of chronic indwelling venous catheters for treatment and nutrition, diagnostic and monitoring procedures (e.g., lumbar puncture, bone marrow aspirate and biopsy, lung and liver biopsy, skin biopsy, bronchoalveolar lavage, esophagogastroduodenoscopy), radiologic procedures, radiation therapy, and placement of pain management devices (e.g., indwelling epidural catheters). Splenectomy is performed as part of staging or management of some pediatric malignancies, and the procedure may be associated with increased risk of postoperative infection, postoperative thrombocytosis, and thrombocytopenia.[200]

Lumbar puncture and bone marrow aspiration procedures are commonly performed in children with cancer, especially those with hematologic malignancies. The use of short-acting medications for a brief general anesthetic ensures complete comfort during the procedure while permitting a rapid recovery and discharge from the hospital. Propofol and a short-acting opioid or low-dose ketamine, for instance, are commonly used to achieve this goal.[201–205] The anesthesiologist must be fastidious with sterile technique when accessing central venous sites, regardless of whether the child is immunosuppressed, to avoid catheter-related infections. *It is of paramount importance that systems are in place to avoid the inadvertent administration of vincristine chemotherapy into the intrathecal space during lumbar punctures.* Intrathecal vincristine causes severe neurologic consequences and may have contributed to nearly 100 fatalities in children with otherwise curable hematopoietic tumors.[206] *Intravenous chemotherapy should be excluded from any procedure room where lumbar punctures and intrathecal chemotherapy are performed.*

Radiation beam therapy is used in frontline treatment of many pediatric brain tumors and some extracranial solid tumors. The duration of radiation therapy varies depending on tumor type but typically occurs daily over 4 to 8 weeks, frequently concurrent with chemotherapy.[45] The goal of modern radiation therapy—both conventional photon beam and the newer proton beam therapies—is to accurately conform radiation to the tumor while minimizing radiation of healthy surrounding tissues. As such, immobility is crucial and requires general anesthesia in younger children.

Radiation treatment planning begins with a simulation, which requires anesthesia in those who will need anesthesia for the subsequent treatments. The child is ideally positioned as they will be for treatment, computed tomographic imaging of the tumor is obtained, and appropriate custom-made molds or masks are formed that will allow reproducible positioning during daily treatments (Fig. 9.3). For PRT, custom brass and/or acrylic molds are later fabricated that will be used to tightly shape and focus the proton beam as required to conform precisely to the tumor mass (Fig. 9.4). Provision of anesthesia in the radiation oncology suite presents key challenges. Many radiation therapy centers, especially PRT centers, are freestanding outpatient facilities separate from a hospital or children's hospital; it is therefore obligatory that all necessary equipment and medications are available to handle any potential anesthesia-related emergency, including rapid transport to a pediatric hospital. Children may suffer physical and emotional stress from daily anesthetics, procedures, diagnostics tests, chemotherapy, and previous or upcoming surgery. As much as possible, parent and child education, peer-to-peer support, distraction techniques, and reward systems may be used to ease the child's anxiety.[162,207] The parents and anesthesia team cannot remain in the treatment vault during irradiation; therefore, multiple video feeds of the child and anesthesia equipment/monitor are essential for the safe care of the child under anesthesia (see Fig. 9.5).

Most children will have an indwelling central venous catheter, which facilitates intravenous induction and maintenance of anesthesia. Strict aseptic technique is mandatory to avoid sepsis and the need for catheter removal, both of which risk morbidity and delays in treatment.[208] Port-a-catheters may be accessed on Monday (topical anesthetic cream may be used) and left accessed until Friday to lessen the anxiety of daily percutaneous port access. A standing anesthesia consent is used in some centers to ease the burden of daily consents, but such consent does not negate the need to evaluate the child before each anesthetic. The risk of anesthetizing a child with mild to moderate respiratory infection must be considered in conjunction with the risk of missing a treatment. A key consideration in choosing the anesthetic regimen includes the use

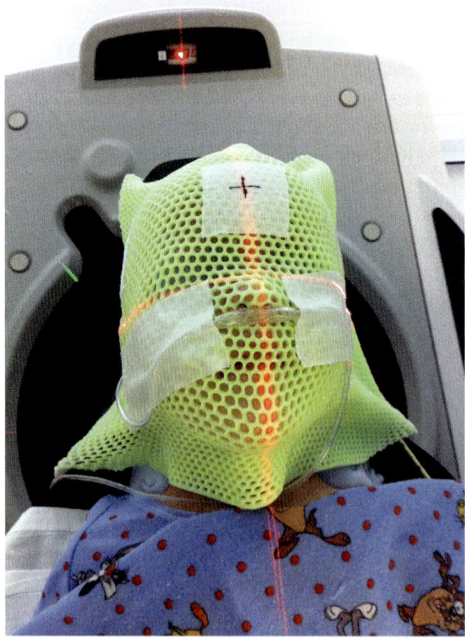

FIGURE 9.3 A custom-made mask holds this anesthetized child's head in the repeatable, exact position required for cranial radiation therapy. A nasal canula provides supplemental oxygen and end-tidal CO_2 monitoring during a total intravenous anesthetic with propofol. (Photo courtesy Andrew Pittaway, BM, BS.)

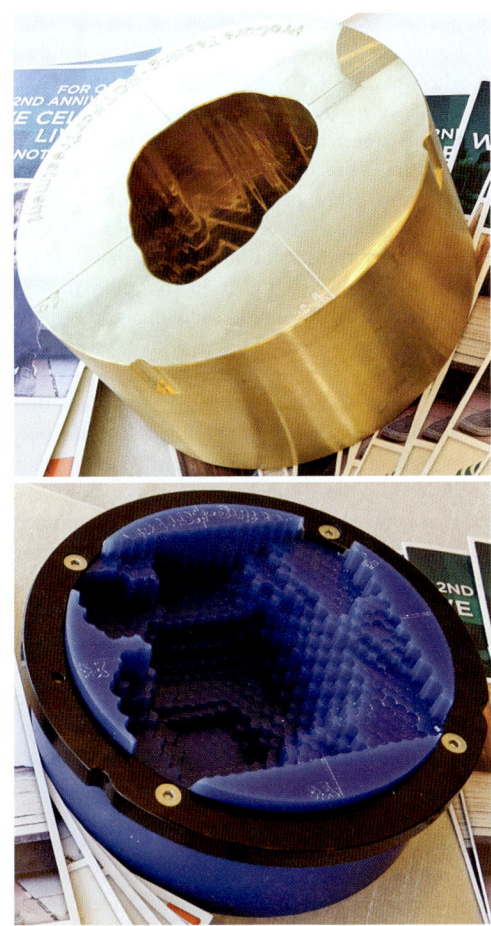

FIGURE 9.4 Upper image: an aperture made from brass composite shapes the lateral borders of the proton beam to shield healthy tissues lateral to the tumor. Lower image: a compensator made of wax or acrylic is used to control the active depth of the protons along the distal border of the tumor. Use of the aperture and compensator together shapes the lateral and distal treatment field accurately, leaving primarily entry path radiation to healthy tissues. (Photo courtesy Fred Hutchinson Cancer Center – Proton Therapy. Used with permission.)

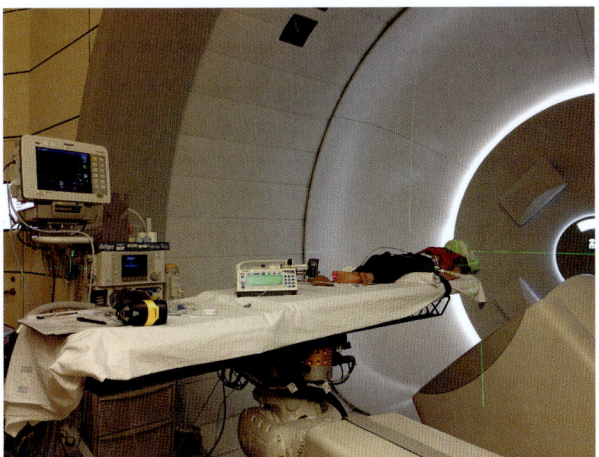

FIGURE 9.5 An anesthetized child in a proton therapy vault. The head mold positions the child's head, and a nasal cannula provides oxygen and CO₂ monitoring. Propofol total intravenous anesthesia is used, and an anesthesia machine and rescue medications are immediately available. Video feeds in a shielded control room allow the anesthesia and radiation teams to view the patient, the propofol pump, and vital signs continuously. (Photo courtesy Karen Wong, MB, BS.)

of short-acting medications to allow quick recovery from anesthesia, and to this end, various anesthetic techniques have been described in the literature.[199,208–210] Total intravenous anesthesia with propofol is commonly used as it provides rapid onset of anesthesia, excellent immobility during radiation, rapid emergence from anesthesia, and theoretic antiemetic properties. Although adjunct medications such as opioids and benzodiazepines can be added, they are often unnecessary and may increase respiratory events.[199,211] A nasal cannula provides supplemental oxygen and the ability to monitor end-tidal CO₂ as a surrogate of effective ventilation via remote monitoring (see Fig. 9.5). Sevoflurane anesthesia with a laryngeal mask airway is another option with a low rate of complications.[209] If an invasive airway is needed routinely in a child receiving cranial radiation, then the head mold must be modified to allow access to the airway.

Surgical intervention may be required for acute and potentially life-threatening emergencies in children with cancer, and the effects of specific tumors may complicate the anesthesia care. Wilms tumor may be accompanied by an acquired von Willebrand condition,[146] and anterior mediastinal masses may produce superior vena cava obstruction, pulmonary artery compression, and tracheal obstruction.[212] Neuroblastoma may be accompanied by pheochromocytoma-like signs and symptoms (3% of cases),[213] venous obstruction, and in advanced stages, it may cause massive hepatic enlargement, making the potential for massive rapid blood loss a significant risk. Spinal tumors may cause acute spinal cord compression, and tumor or hemorrhage in the brain may cause acute intracranial hypertension. In view of the complexity of pediatric oncologic disease, there are many considerations for the perioperative period[96] (Table 9.7).

HEMATOPOIETIC STEM CELL TRANSPLANTATION RECIPIENTS

Surgical and procedural interventions are common throughout the transplantation process and are similar to those described previously for children with cancer. Harvesting of hematopoietic stem cells from the recipient or another individual is an integral component of HSCT. Harvesting of bone marrow in children usually requires general anesthesia, although the procedure can be performed safely with the child under spinal anesthesia if required.[214] The donor is usually placed in a prone position to extract approximately 10 mL/kg (recipient weight) of marrow from the posterior iliac crests. When stem cells are obtained from peripheral blood, sedation or general anesthesia is usually required to establish vascular access. There is little evidence to support the avoidance of nitrous oxide for harvesting procedures, a concern raised in the past because nitrous oxide affects methionine synthase activity and DNA synthesis.[215]

In view of the wide range of possible complications at the time of HSCT, the many issues outlined earlier for children with cancer must be considered for children undergoing HSCT (see Table 9.7). Radiation, glucocorticoids, mucositis, and chronic GVHD may contribute to an airway that is friable and a neck that is scarred, thereby increasing the risks of airway trauma, dental injury, and difficult tracheal intubation. Chemotherapy and GVHD may affect the skin and make venous access difficult. Chronic GVHD can lead to sclerodermatous changes, which can profoundly restrict range of motion, and sicca syndrome, which may necessitate use of artificial tears. GVHD may alter gut motility and delay gastric emptying. Immune compromise increases the risk of infection from vascular access lines, and therefore, mandates meticulous technique at all times. Chemotherapy may

TABLE 9.7	Perioperative Concerns in Pediatric Cancer and Hematopoietic Stem Cell Transplantation

Preoperative Considerations

Consultation with service primarily responsible for child's care

Complete blood cell count, serum electrolytes (when appropriate)

Echocardiogram or chest radiograph, or both (when appropriate)

Transfusion cross-match with specifications (e.g., cytomegalovirus seronegativity, leukocyte reduction, irradiation) determined in consultation with oncology service

Determination of blood typing requirements for all stem cell transplant recipients

History of acute and chronic pain medication use

Anxiolytic and analgesic therapy (when appropriate)

Infection prophylaxis with antibiotics

Avoidance of *any* marrow-suppressive medications in stem cell transplant patients

Observation of indicated isolation precautions

Sterile technique with central line access

Use of support services (when appropriate)

Intraoperative Considerations

Attention to skin, teeth, eyes, and joints; careful positioning and padding

Sterile technique with central line access

Full-stomach precautions (when appropriate, as in graft-versus-host disease)

Appropriate hydration and maintenance of urine output

Continuation of total parenteral nutrition (and other parenteral fluids with high glucose concentration)

Avoidance of high fraction of inspired oxygen (FiO_2) and restriction of hydration if prior treatment with bleomycin

Judicious use of cardiac depressants in patients with compromised cardiac function

Nausea and vomiting prophylaxis

Stress corticosteroids (when appropriate)

Regional anesthesia when safe and indicated

Postoperative Considerations

Patient-appropriate opioid and other analgesic administration

Sterile technique with central line access

Observation of indicated isolation precautions

compromise cardiac and pulmonary function, alter hepatic metabolism of medications, and limit renal excretion of medications and fluids. Immune compromise and modifications resulting from transplantation require special processing of blood components, as recommended by hematology and blood bank consultants, as described in the following text and in E-Tables 10.1 and 10.2. It is critical to coordinate the choice of blood products with the transplant service.

Transfusion Considerations

RED BLOOD CELLS

Anemia is very common in children with cancer, with an incidence that ranges from 51% to 74% in children with solid tumors

or Hodgkin disease, greater than 50% of children with Wilms tumor and osteosarcoma,[135] greater than 80% of children receiving chemotherapy, and 97% of children with leukemia.[216] There is limited evidence regarding the optimal transfusion thresholds for children with cancer, and guidelines have not been established. Accordingly, current practice patterns stem from adult oncology studies, data from other pediatric populations (e.g., intensive care), and individual institutional practice patterns.[217] The threshold for red blood cell transfusion in adults with cancer is a hemoglobin concentration of 7 to 9 g/dL in asymptomatic individuals and 8 to 10 g/dL in symptomatic individuals.[218] Whether these thresholds are appropriate for children with cancer, who range in age from infancy to adolescence and with conditions ranging from leukemia to brain tumors, is unknown. Nonetheless, these values have been adopted empirically in children.[219] In practice, pediatric oncology patients usually receive transfusions when their hemoglobin concentrations decrease to 5.5 to 8 g/dL.[216]

Several factors should be considered when determining the need for blood transfusion, including the overall clinical condition of the child, symptoms of anemia, the presence of cardiopulmonary dysfunction, the stress and anticipated blood loss of the surgical procedure, the risk of increased intraoperative hemorrhage owing to coexisting coagulopathy, and the ability of the child to tolerate a volume load. Finally, blood products should be administered cautiously in those with hyperleukocytosis as the added viscosity can trigger leukostasis.[220] Thus, sound clinical judgment and attention to the greater clinical context are warranted in each case.[221]

THROMBOCYTOPENIA

Thrombocytopenia occurs commonly in association with marrow suppression from chemotherapy, radiation, or even marrow replacement by hematologic malignancy. Additional effects on platelets include consumption during infections or disseminated intravascular coagulation, platelet sequestration with splenomegaly, and platelet dysfunction from medications.[219] The platelet count is not the sole indicator of the risk of bleeding in children with cancer, as evidenced by the occurrence of major bleeding at any platelet count[222]; treatment- or cancer-induced damage to vascular epithelium and alterations anywhere in the coagulation cascade pose additive risks for hemorrhage. Regardless, platelet transfusions play an important role in avoiding the risk of catastrophic hemorrhage in children.[223] Of note, the risk/benefit of perioperative platelet transfusion in the immediate post-HSCT period must be discussed with the oncology team, as transfusions during this time may impact the transplant engraftment.[223]

The optimal prophylactic platelet transfusion strategy in pediatric oncology remains complicated and controversial. As noted previously, the risk of bleeding is neither solely dependent on nor inversely proportional to the platelet count.[222] However, in the absence of adequate prospective trials, most practice guidelines continue to recommend a platelet count >50,000/μL for invasive procedures to >100,000/μL for CNS procedures, and 10,000 to 20,000/μL for lumbar punctures.[224] Despite the knowledge that these thresholds may not be appropriate for every age of child and cancer diagnosis, they remain our best guide at this time for children presenting for surgery.[223]

COAGULATION FACTOR DEFICIENCY

Perioperative administration of fresh frozen plasma or factor components is reasonable if the child with cancer has documented prolongation of prothrombin or partial thromboplastin time, verified factor deficiency, or surgical bleeding despite normal platelet levels and function. The invasiveness of the surgical procedure also should be considered. Cryoprecipitate and coagulation factor concentrates may also be necessary in the setting of abnormal laboratory studies and clinical coagulopathy.[221] It should be noted that fresh frozen plasma is ineffective in reversing the coagulopathy associated with L-asparaginase.[225]

BLOOD PRODUCT PREPARATION

Immunocompetent white blood cells in donor blood can elicit a profound immune response and other complications in the recipient, especially immunocompromised children. Leukoreduction by filtration eliminates greater than 99% of donor leukocytes. Most blood products in the United States and all blood products in Canada and Europe are routinely leuko-reduced,[219] and leuko-reduced products should be used in children with cancer. (Table 8.3 and E-Tables 10.1 and 10.2 provide a complete list of indications for leuko-reduced products. Leukoreduction reduces the rate of platelet alloimmunization, transfusion-related immunomodulation, febrile transfusion reactions, and transfusion-related infections, including cytomegalovirus (CMV) infection.[226,227] Although leukoreduction may be sufficient to prevent donor-related CMV infection, CMV-negative donor blood is recommended for CMV-negative infants and children with cancer, especially children undergoing HSCT (Table 8.5 and E-Table 10.1).[228]

Donor lymphocytes contained in the component blood products can replicate and engraft in the host, leading to a transfusion-associated graft-versus-host disease (TA-GVHD), especially in immunocompromised patients. TA-GVHD manifests days to weeks after transfusion, is resistant to treatment, and is often fatal. Leukoreduction alone is insufficient to eliminate the risk of TA-GVHD. As a result, irradiation of platelets and red blood cells is mandatory for immunosuppressed patients, including children with cancer (Table 8.4 and E-Table 10.2).[226,229,230] Irradiation of blood products can lead to cell membrane destabilization, leading to ongoing leakage of intracellular potassium and a shortened shelf life; thus irradiation optimally occurs immediately before use of the blood to avoid hyperkalemia.[229]

Children who have undergone HSCT may represent a challenge for blood typing. Major and minor ABO mismatch, as occurs in the setting of allogeneic HSCT, potentiates a shift in the ABO/Rh status of the recipient, the degree of which depends on the timing and engraftment status of the transplant. Preoperative communication with the blood bank and oncologist is warranted for all children who have recently undergone HSCT and are at risk for requiring perioperative transfusion of blood products.[231]

Effects of Anesthetic Agents on Perioperative Immunomodulation

Recent research has focused on the potential impact of multiple perioperative factors on immunomodulation and the risk of tumor recurrence. To date, research has been in vitro or in retrospective adult studies; thus some or all of the findings may not be directly applicable to children.[232,233] Theoretically, a host of perioperative factors could potentially suppress the host immune system or even directly augment the cancer cells, leading to the growth of minimally residual tumor cells and recurrence of cancer.[233,234] Some studies have reported potentially harmful immunosuppression or cancer cell augmentation after anesthesia with volatile anesthetics, ketamine, opioids (particularly morphine), and benzodiazepines.[232–234] Propofol has shown mixed results, and nitrous oxide, although harmful in vitro, has not been linked to cancer recurrence in adults. The use of regional anesthesia has been shown to confer protection against recurrence in some but not all studies.[233,235] Multiple other factors have shown intermittent association with poor outcomes, including surgical stress response, hypotension, hypothermia, hyperglycemia, blood transfusions, glucocorticoids, and NSAIDs.[232] In summary, data are insufficient to support altering the anesthetic plan in children on the basis of reducing the risk of tumor recurrence.

ANNOTATED REFERENCES

Bindra RS, Wolden SL. Advances in radiation therapy in pediatric neuro-oncology. *J Child Neurol.* 2016;31(4):506-516.
This paper presents an update of the recent advances in radiation technology and treatment protocols for children with cancer.

Ketterl TG, Latham GJ. Perioperative cardiothoracic and vascular risk in childhood cancer and its survivors. *J Cardiothorac Vasc Anesth.* 2021; 35(1):162-175.
This review focuses on the unique risks factors, prevention strategies, and treatment of cardiovascular toxicities of the child with cancer, with an emphasis on the perioperative period.

Latham GJ, Greenberg RS. Anesthetic considerations for the pediatric oncology patient—part 1: a review of antitumor therapy. *Paediatr Anaesth.* 2010;20:295-304.
This article briefly reviews the current principles of cancer therapy and the general mechanisms of toxicity to the child, focusing on the impact to perioperative care and decision-making.

Latham GJ, Greenberg RS. Anesthetic considerations for the pediatric oncology patient—part 2: systems-based approach to anesthesia. *Paediatr Anaesth.* 2010;20:396-420.
A systems-based approach is used to assess the impact of the tumor and its treatment on children; relevant anesthetic considerations are discussed.

Latham GJ, Greenberg RS. Anesthetic considerations for the pediatric oncology patient—part 3: pain, cognitive dysfunction, and preoperative evaluation. *Paediatr Anaesth.* 2010;20:479-489.
This paper discusses the psychosocial impact of cancer and pain syndromes that should be considered in the perioperative period. A discussion of preanesthetic testing and evaluation in children with cancer follows.

Mackall CL, Merchant MS, Fry TJ. Immune-based therapies for childhood cancer. *Nat Rev Clin Oncol.* 2014;11(12):693-703.
This review excellently summarizes the rapidly growing field of immunotherapeutics used in the common forms of pediatric cancer.

A complete reference list can be found online at Elsevier eBooks+.

10 Strategies for Blood Product Management, Reducing Transfusions, and Massive Blood Transfusion

CHARLES J. COTÉ, ERIC F. GRABOWSKI, AND STEVEN R. SLOAN

Blood Volume
Blood Components and Alternatives
Packed Red Blood Cells
Whole Blood
Platelets
Special Processing of Cellular Blood Components
Plasma
Cryoprecipitate
Pathogen Inactivation/Reduction
Plasma-Derived Factor Concentrates and Recombinant Factors
Prothrombin Complex Concentrates
Desmopressin
Albumin, Dextrans, Starches, and Gelatins
Red Blood Cell Substitutes
Massive Blood Transfusion
Coagulopathy

Dilutional Thrombocytopenia
Factor Deficiency
Disseminated Intravascular Coagulation and Fibrinolysis
Hyperkalemia
Hypocalcemia and Citrate Toxicity
Acid-Base Balance
Hypothermia
Monitoring During Massive Blood Transfusion
Infectious Disease Considerations
Methods to Reduce Patient Exposure to Allogeneic Blood Components
Erythropoietin
Preoperative Autologous Blood Donation
Intraoperative Blood Recovery and Reinfusion: Autotransfusion
Controlled Hypotension
Normovolemic Hemodilution

DESPITE ADVANCES IN PEDIATRIC SURGERY, infants and children may sustain major operative blood loss, but scant information is available about when coagulation defects first appear in children.[1–5] Most studies of massive blood transfusions involved adult patients, although national data regarding massive transfusions in children are currently being gathered and some pediatric data from combat zones are emerging.[4,6–10] A rational blood transfusion strategy is imperative in children because transfusions can cause complications[11] that potentially can last for decades. In countries with sophisticated health care systems, the most common fatal hazards of transfusion are hemolytic transfusion reactions related to ABO incompatibility (usually as a result of a transfusion error), transfusion-associated circulatory overload (TACO), and transfusion-related acute lung injury (TRALI).[12–14] In developing countries, the risk of infectious disease transmission may be greater because of endemic infections (e.g., Dengue, Chikungunya, malaria) and the technical or logistic limitations of donor screening.[15,16] The neurotropic Zika virus with its marked association with microcephaly in the neonate[17] and arthrogryposis in infants is a good example; in adults it is associated with Guillain-Barré syndrome and cognitive dysfunction.[18] RNA testing of blood donors in areas with high prevalence rates such as Brazil and Puerto Rico and in the United States was instituted in 2016,[19] but this resulted in a low positive yield.[20] Thus, in nonendemic areas such as the United States, the Food and Drug Administration's (FDA) ZIKA guidance was withdrawn in 2021 due to insufficient prevalence to merit testing of the donor population. In fact, the last ZIKA RNA-positive donation occurred in March 2018.

Regarding the SARS-CoV-2 virus, the Association for the Advancement of Blood and Biotherapies (AABB) International Task Force issued two statements in 2022:

- Individuals are not at risk of contracting COVID-19 through the blood donation process or a blood transfusion, since respiratory viruses are generally not known to be transmitted by donation or transfusion. The US FDA has reported zero confirmed or suspected cases of transfusion-transmitted COVID-19 to date. In addition, no cases of transfusion-transmission were ever reported for the other two coronaviruses that emerged during the past 2 decades (SARS, the severe acute respiratory syndrome coronavirus, and MERS-CoV, which causes Mideast respiratory syndrome).
- Routine blood donor screening measures, which may include travel deferrals, are already in place to prevent individuals with clinical respiratory infections from donating blood and ensuring the safety of the blood supply.

Therefore, there is no current testing of blood donors for the SARS-CoV-2 coronavirus.

Nothing changed the use of blood products more than AIDS.[21–23] Fortunately, the risk of infection today with human immunodeficiency virus (HIV), hepatitis C virus (HCV), and hepatitis B virus (HBV) by blood transfusion is extremely rare. An exciting new development is the introduction of pathogen-reducing technology (INTERCEPT, Mirasol and THERSAFLEX, see later) which can remove viruses, bacteria, and parasites by targeting their genetic makeup; such pathogen clearing systems could replace the need for pathogen testing in the future.[24–27] Such

TABLE 10.1	Current Blood Screening Tests Used on Donated Blood in the United States

Hepatitis B surface antigen (HBsAg)

Hepatitis B core antibody (anti-HBc)

Nucleic acid amplification testing for HBV DNA

Hepatitis C virus antibody (anti-HCV)

Nucleic acid amplification testing for HCV RNA

Human immunodeficiency virus (HIV) type 1 & 2 RNA by nucleic acid amplification testing

HIV antibodies (anti-HIV-1 and anti-HIV-2)

Human T-lymphotropic virus type 1 (HTLV-I) antibody (anti-HTLV-I)

HTLV-II antibody (anti-HTLV-II)

Serologic test for syphilis (Treponema pallidum)

Nucleic acid amplification for West Nile virus (WNV) RNA[a]

Trypanosoma cruzi antibody (Chagas disease)[b]

Babesia[c]

Screen for bacterial contamination—platelets only

[a]This test sensitivity depends on the incidence in the geographic area.
[b]At first donation or after residence in endemic area.
[c]In states where testing is required by FDA guidance
From American Association of Blood Banks. Blood FAQ. https://www.aabb.org/tm/Pages/bloodfaq.aspx.

TABLE 10.2	Estimated Frequency of Complications per Number of Units Transfused	
Category	**Complication**	**Frequency**
Noninfectious	Allergic (urticarial)	1:100
	Febrile, nonhemolytic	1:100
	Transfusion-associated circulatory overload	1:1000
	Delayed hemolytic	1:1600
	Transfusion-related acute lung injury	1:10,000
	Acute hemolytic	1:50,000
	Fatal acute hemolytic	1:500,000
Infectious	Hepatitis B virus	1:1,000,000
	Hepatitis C virus	1:1,700,000
	Human T-lymphotropic virus type I	1:2,700,000
	Human immunodeficiency virus type 1	1:1,900,000
	Bacterial contamination of red blood cells	1:50,000
	Bacterial sepsis of red blood cells	1:500,000
	Bacterial contamination of platelets	<1:2000[a]
	Bacterial sepsis of platelets	1:1000–2500

[a]Starting in October, 2021, an FDA guidance required pathogen reduction methods or increased bacterial detection methods for platelet units. This has reduced the rate of transfusion-transmitted bacteria but the exact effect has not yet been published.
Data from Galel SA. Infectious disease screening. In: Fung MK, Grossman BJ, Hillyer CD, Westhoff CM, eds. Technical Manual, 18th ed. Bethesda, MD: AABB Press; 2014:194; Mazzei CA, Popovsky MA, Kopko PM. Non-infectious complications of transfusion. In: Fung MK, Grossman BJ, Hillyer CD, Westhoff CM, eds. Technical Manual, 18th ed. Bethesda, MD: AABB press; 2014:684; and Levy JH, Neal MD, Herman JH: Bacterial contamination of platelets for transfusion: strategies for prevention. Crit Care. 2018;22;271.[868]

pathogen reduction techniques likely will further improve the safety of transfusions particularly during evolving pandemics.[25,26] Implementation of donor education programs, improved health history screening, new tests, and new test technologies (Table 10.1) have markedly altered the spectrum of transfusion-transmitted infectious agents in the developed world. The risks of some of the infectious and noninfectious hazards of transfusion are summarized in Table 10.2.

Despite marked reductions in the transmission of HIV, HCV, and HBV, transfusions can produce other deleterious effects.[28,29] Every transfusion must be medically justified and its benefits weighed against the potential infectious, immunologic, and metabolic risks.[30–32] It is in the child's best interest to transfuse with a clear clinical goal and in the anesthesiologist's best interest to document the reason for each transfusion. It is not acceptable medical practice to administer a transfusion when it is of questionable benefit. One of the most effective ways to avoid transfusion reactions is to avoid unnecessary transfusions.[33] A review of 1902 incident reports from 1,100,000 transfusions revealed a 3-fold greater rate of transfusion-related adverse incidents in children (192 reports in 128,560 transfusions (15:10,000)) compared with adults (183 in 377,563 transfusions (5:10,000)) between 2010 and 2017 (P<0.00001).[34] Interestingly, the adverse events reported in children included wrong patient, expired unit, excessively large volume of blood, blood too rapidly transfused, inappropriate preparation, incorrect order/consent, transfusion reaction protocol not followed, and inadequate documentation of the transfusion.[34] This study indicates the need for increased vigilance when administering blood products to pediatric patients, particularly neonates. The results from a second study of 133,671 transfusions confirmed the almost 3-fold greater risk of adverse events in children (62:10,000) compared with adults (24:10,000) with the most frequent reactions (in children compared with adults) being allergic (2.7 vs. 1.1/1000), febrile (1.9 vs. 0.47/1000) and hypotensive (0.29 vs. 0.078/1000). Although reactions occurred equally in male and female adults, reactions occurred twice as frequently in male (79:10,000) compared with female (43:10,000) children.[35] Transfusion reactions were most common after platelet transfusions followed by packed red blood cells (PRBCs) and then plasma transfusions.[35] A meta-analysis and systematic review that reported 319,884 transfusions in children versus 1,068,479 transfusions in adults noted the relative risk for adverse blood transfusion reactions was significantly greater in children (RR 1.75, confidence limits 1.27–2.41, P=0.006)[36]; these events were primarily related to transfusion of red blood cells and platelets, but were similar for plasma and cryoprecipitate.

Blood Volume

The circulating blood volume of the child should be estimated before induction of anesthesia. The blood volume of a child varies by age: a micropremie (born weighing ≤800 grams) has a blood volume of 110 milliliters per kilogram; a preterm infant, 90–100 milliliters per kilogram; a term neonate, 80–90 milliliters per kilogram; an infant between 3 months and 1 year of age, 70–80 milliliters per kilogram; and an older child, 70 milliliters per kilogram. Body habitus affects the blood volume calculation since the latter is normalized to body weight. For example, an obese teenager has a smaller blood volume per kilogram (60–65 mL/kg) than a nonobese child of the same weight. Using the estimated blood volume, the initial hemoglobin or hematocrit, and the minimum acceptable hematocrit, we can *estimate* the maximum allowable blood loss (MABL) before red blood cell (RBC) transfusion is indicated as described below.

The minimum acceptable hematocrit varies according to an individual child's need. The balance between oxygen supply and demand depends on several factors, including the oxygen content of blood, cardiac output and its regional distribution, and metabolic needs. Rheologic considerations (e.g., ensuring adequate hepatic artery blood flow in liver transplant recipients) may also affect the optimal hematocrit. A child with severe pulmonary disease or cyanotic congenital heart disease often requires a greater hematocrit than a healthy child to satisfy oxygen demands. However, in sickle cell syndromes, optimal oxygen delivery is a product of oxygen content (hematocrit) and blood flow rate, where the latter decreases with hematocrits above 30% owing to increased whole blood viscosity.[37] Therefore, the hematocrit in sickle cell syndromes should never exceed 31% to 33%. A similar argument applies to infants with cyanotic congenital heart disease and to infants of a diabetic mother, when the hematocrit exceeds about 60%. These situations are distinct from that of the term newborn, whose hematocrit may normally be 50% without compromise to blood flow due to the greater flexibility (deformability) of newborn red cells that lowers whole blood viscosity.[38] Although earlier studies suggested that preterm infants may require a greater hematocrit to prevent apnea, reduce cardiac and respiratory work, and possibly improve neurologic cognitive outcomes,[39,40] a large prospective randomized trial has not shown any benefit from transfusing at higher hematocrits.[41–45] If there is uncertainty about the need to transfuse these infants, the neonatologist should be consulted.[39,46–48] A healthy child readily tolerates a hematocrit well below 30%. It is our practice not to transfuse otherwise healthy infants up to about 3 months old until their hematocrits have decreased to ~25% and hematocrits of older children have decreased to ~20% if there is little risk of postoperative bleeding.[49,50] *The circulating blood volume must be maintained in every case.* Observing the operative field to estimate blood loss is essential; if a procedure is expected to result in significant blood loss or fluid shifts, the use of a urine catheter, a central venous line, and invasive arterial monitoring should be considered. The child's size or age should not deter one from the use of a central venous catheter (Table 10.3). The introduction of noninvasive cardiac output monitors and pulse contour analysis may further clarify the need for and response to transfusion and volume replacement (see also Chapter 49).[51]

There are three approaches to estimate the MABL: an approximation of circulating RBC mass, a modified logarithmic equation, and a simple proportion.[52,53] All three approaches yield clinically similar estimates of the MABL. The most straightforward method is to estimate the MABL by simple proportion.[52] For purposes of discussion, we use a hematocrit of 25% as the minimum acceptable hematocrit:

$$MABL = \frac{EBV \times (\text{Child's hematorcit} - \text{Minimum acceptable hematocrit})}{\text{Child's hematocrit}}$$

TABLE 10.3	Estimated Predicted Blood Loss and Recommended Monitoring and Equipment
Predicted Blood Loss	**Recommended Monitors or Equipment**
<0.5 blood volume	Routine monitoring
0.5–1.0 blood volumes	Routing monitoring + urine catheter
1.0 blood volume or more	Routine monitoring + urine catheter + CVP + arterial line
1.0 blood volume or more with potential for rapid blood loss	Routine monitoring + urine catheter + CVP + arterial line + large-bore IV line + rapid-infusion device
Severe head injury	Routine monitoring + urine catheter + CVP + arterial line + large-bore IV line
Major trauma with unknown severity	Routine monitoring + urine catheter + CVP + arterial line + large-bore IV line (preferably in upper extremity or central) + rapid-infusion device

CVP, Central venous pressure; *IV*, intravenous.

For example, a 10-kilogram child has an estimated blood volume of 10 kilograms × 70 milliliters per kilogram, or ~700 milliliters. If the child's hematocrit is 42, the MABL is calculated as:

$$MABL = \frac{700 \times (42 - 25)}{42}$$
$$= \frac{700 \times 17}{42}$$
$$= \sim 285 \text{ mL}$$

These calculations only estimate the MABL. The actual hematocrit varies with the child's preexisting medical conditions, the rapidity of the blood loss, and the rate of crystalloid or colloid replacement.

It should be noted that commonly used crystalloid solutions for volume replacement actually consist of two different solutions: normal saline and balanced electrolyte solutions. Normal saline is slightly hyperosmolar (sodium concentration of 154 mEq/L [308 mOsm/L]) and may produce a nonanion gap hyperchloremic metabolic acidosis when given in large quantities (pH is 4.5–7.0).[54–56] Balanced electrolyte solutions comprise a group of solutions that are slightly hypoosmolar (273 mOsm/L), contain one of several bases (lactate, gluconate, or acetate) and have a pH of 5 to 8 (see also Chapter 7).

One must always be prepared for possible massive blood loss, but initial therapy is directed at replacing fluid deficits and providing maintenance requirements. Additional fluid administration is directed at replacing blood loss and third space fluid losses. There seems to be little danger in replacing the entire MABL with crystalloid, provided that the child is healthy, and that postoperative oozing will not exceed the MABL. Historically, the consensus has been to replace each milliliter of shed blood with 2 to 3 milliliters of crystalloid.[57,58] However, more recent evidence suggests to replace each milliliter of shed blood with a smaller volume of crystalloid (i.e., 1–2 mL).[59,60] The implication is that 1 milliliter of crystalloid can never be as effective as 1 milliliter of blood, which stays in the intravascular space, in restoring blood volume. Colloid replacement is expensive and without clear evidence that it is superior to crystalloid,[61] but it may be used to replace blood loss as 1 milliliter of 5% albumin per milliliter of shed blood.[62,63] The long-term and short-term safety implications of starch-based volume expanders in children are unclear[64–68]; a meta-analysis found a reduction in platelet counts and increased length of ICU stay.[69]

In our example of the 10-kilogram child with a 700-milliliter blood volume and a 285-milliliter MABL, the child's blood volume can be restored by administering either ~570 milliliters of isotonic crystalloid or ~285 milliliters of 5% albumin. However, if the blood loss exceeds the MABL or if the hematocrit decreases to 20% to 25% (particularly if additional blood loss is expected during or after surgery), then transfusion with packed red blood cells (PRBCs) or whole blood (WB) (if available) is indicated. If postoperative bleeding is likely to occur (e.g., posterior spinal fusion, open heart operations, burn wound excision and grafting), it is reasonable to transfuse to a level greater than the minimum acceptable hematocrit. This is especially true if a greater hematocrit can be achieved without exposing the child to additional units of blood postoperatively. If a unit of red blood cells or whole blood has been started, it is reasonable to give the child an additional 5% to 10% volume. It is our practice to administer as much of the unit as can be safely tolerated rather than expose the child to another unit of a blood component postoperatively. Blood banks often prepare several aliquots from one unit of red blood cells for neonates; this allows a particular child to receive aliquots from a single donor unit infused as needed at different times.

If PRBCs are used to replace the shed RBCs, then the volume of PRBCs needed to restore a specific hematocrit may be calculated quite simply. For example, if the hematocrit of a 10-kilogram child has decreased to 23% and the intraoperative blood loss is expected to continue postoperatively, then the anesthesiologist can use the formula to estimate the volume of PRBCs needed to achieve a final hematocrit of 35%:

$$\text{Volume of PRBCs} = \frac{(\text{Desired Hct} - \text{Present Hct}) \times \text{Estimated Blood Volume (70 mL/kg} \times 10 \text{ kg)}}{\text{Hematocrit of PRCBs}}$$

$$= \frac{(35 - 23) \times (70 \times 10)}{60}$$

$$= \sim 140 \text{ mL PRBCs}$$

Alternately, some clinicians rely on a simpler rule of thumb to estimate the volume of blood to transfuse: to increase the Hb 1 gram per deciliter, transfuse 4 milliliters per kilogram PRBCs or 6 milliliters per kilogram whole blood. In the above example, to increase the Hb from ~8 grams per deciliter to ~12 grams per deciliter in a 10-kilogram infant, we would require 4 milliliters per kilogram (PRBC) × 10 kilograms × 4 grams per deciliter (12–8 g/dL difference) or ~160 milliliters PRBC.

Because these volumes are less than 1 unit, transfusing a greater volume than estimated; that is, up to a hematocrit of 40% (~200 mL PRBCs) to allow an additional margin of safety for postoperative blood loss seems reasonable. A prospective study by the American College of Surgeons National Quality Improvement Program—Pediatrics involving 50 institutions found that there were significant differences in transfusion practices among institutions and that transfusions were more likely in infants and children 2 years of age or younger (odds ratio [OR] 5.9–3.4), American Society of Anesthesiologists (ASA) class IV (OR 3.2), those with preoperative septic shock (OR 14.5), and those requiring preoperative cardiopulmonary resuscitation (OR 8.1).[70] The most common surgical procedures associated with pediatric blood transfusion are cardiac surgery, craniosynostosis, and spinal instrumentation for scoliosis.[71]

Blood Components and Alternatives

In countries with well-developed health care systems, most whole blood collected from donors is fractionated into components soon after collection. A unit of whole blood provides 1 unit of PRBCs, 1 unit of whole blood–derived platelets, and 1 unit of fresh frozen plasma (FFP). Apheresis technology is also used to collect any one of these three components selectively. Separating the individual components of blood allows each to be stored under conditions that optimally preserve their function; for example, PRBCs are stored at refrigerator temperature (4°C to 10°C), FFP at less than −18°C, and platelets at room temperature (20°C to 24°C). Most children with specific disease states (e.g., anemia, clotting factor deficiencies, thrombocytopenia) require only one of these fractions, which is why component therapy is ubiquitous.

PACKED RED BLOOD CELLS

Blood components containing RBCs are indicated to treat symptomatic deficits of oxygen-carrying capacity.[72,73] PRBCs are the most widely available RBC-containing blood component, although in settings where facilities are incapable of fractionating blood into components, whole blood may be the only component available. Donor whole blood is collected in a preservative-anticoagulant solution that contains citrate, phosphate, dextrose (glucose), and adenine (CPDA) or just citrate, phosphate, and dextrose (CPD). In the latter case, the platelet-rich plasma is removed after centrifugation of the whole blood unit, and a solution containing adenine, dextrose, and occasionally mannitol is added to the PRBCs. The additive-solution systems permit storage for 42 days (compared with 35 days for CPDA) and better preservation of 2,3-diphosphoglycerate (DPG) levels. The characteristics of the CPDA and additive-solution PRBCs and of whole blood at the time of outdate are shown in Table 10.4; the hematocrit is reduced in the additive-solution PRBCs and the total volume is increased, but the red cell mass remains the same.

RBCs carry glycoconjugate antigens of the ABH histo-blood group system on the cell surface that are determined by three common alleles at the ABO locus on chromosome 9.[74] Infants

Parameter	CPDA-1 Whole Blood[a]	CPDA-1 RBC[a]	Additive-Solution RBC[b]
Storage time (days)	35	35	42
Volume RBC (mL)[c]	226	226	226
Residual plasma (mL)[c,d]	275	50	30
Hematocrit (%)	40	72	53
pH	6.98	6.71	6.6
Adenosine triphosphate (% of day 1)	56	45	60
2,3-DPG (% of day 1)	<10	<10	<10

TABLE 10.4 Composition of Components Containing Red Blood Cells at Outdate

CPDA, Citrate, phosphate, dextrose, and adenine solution; *DPG*, 2,3-diphosphoglycerate; *RBC*, red blood cell.
[a]Outdated at 35 days.
[b]Outdated at 42 days.
[c]Based on collection of 500 mL of whole blood with a hematocrit of 45%.
[d]The concentration of factors V and VIII is reduced to 20% to 50% of normal levels (0.2 to 0.5 units/mL). The other clotting factors are quite stable.

TABLE 10.5	ABO Compatibility of Blood Components			
	ACCEPTABLE COMPONENT ABO GROUPS: (SECOND CHOICE)			
Recipient ABO Group	Whole Blood	PRBC	FFP/Cryo	Platelets
O	O	O	O (A, B, AB, plasma)	O (A, B, AB)
A	A	A (O)	A (AB)	A (AB)[a]
B	B	B (O)	B (AB)	B (AB)[a]
AB	AB	AB (A, B, O)	AB	AB[a]

Cryo, Cryoprecipitate; FFP, fresh frozen plasma; PRBC, packed red blood cells.
[a]Can come from group apheresis platelets (or whole blood–derived platelets for a small child).

TABLE 10.6	Rh(D) Compatibility of Blood Components			
	ACCEPTABLE COMPONENT RH(D) TYPES (SECOND CHOICE)			
Recipient Rh(D) Type	Whole Blood or PRBCs	FFP/ Cryo	Apheresis Platelets	Whole Blood– Derived Platelets
Positive	Rh-positive (Rh-negative)	Any	Any	Rh-positive (Rh-negative)
Negative	Rh-negative (Rh-positive)[a]	Any	Any[c]	Rh-negative (Rh-positive)[a,b]

Cryo, Cryoprecipitate; FFP, fresh frozen plasma; PRBCs, packed red blood cells.
[a]Depending on inventory, the blood bank may switch to Rh(D)-positive, particularly for male patients or postmenopausal females if patient has no anti-Rh(D) antibodies.
[b]Consider Rh immune globulin for females with childbearing potential receiving whole blood–derived platelets from Rh(D)-positive donors.
[c]Very low risk of Rh alloimmunization with apheresis platelets but immunocompetent patients may be at risk.

TABLE 10.7	Common Initial Doses of Blood Components and Expected Effects in Children	
Component	Dose	Effect
Packed red blood cells (PRCBs)	10–15 mL/kg	Increase hemoglobin by 2–3 g/dL[a]
Platelets[b]	5–10 mL/kg	Increase platelet count by 50,000–100,000/mm³
Fresh frozen plasma	10–15 mL/kg	Factor levels increase by 15%–20%
Cryoprecipitate	0.1–0.2 units/kg	Increase fibrinogen by 60–100 mg/dL
Fibrinogen concentrate	70 mg/kg	Increase in fibrinogen level of 120 mg/dL

[a]Note that the hematocrit of PRBCs varies from ~60% to 70% for packed red blood cells in citrate, phosphate, dextrose (glucose), and adenine (CPDA) versus ~55% for packed red blood cells in additive-solution systems; the total volume of packed red blood cells is, however, the same.

begin to elaborate alloantibodies to whichever A or B antigens they lack in the first year of life. These isoagglutinins are invariably present after a few months and constitute a formidable immunologic obstacle to transfusion or transplantation across this ABO barrier. The RBCs for transfusion must be compatible with the ABO isoagglutinins of the intended transfusion recipient. Similarly, plasma components must be compatible with the A or B surface antigens expressed on the recipient's RBCs. Whole blood and platelet units also contain large amounts of plasma but transfusions of ABO-incompatible plasma from these units are generally safe if the amount of relevant antibodies is minimized by transfusing small doses or using units with low titers of relevant antibodies. Alternatively, some blood banks provide platelet units stored in platelet additive solution that contains minimal amounts of plasma. PRBCs must be ABO *compatible* with the recipient, whereas whole blood must be ABO *identical* because of the larger volume of donor plasma and, hence, AB isoagglutinins. Table 10.5 summarizes the permissible combinations.

Only RBCs express the Rh(D) antigen. Rh(D)-positive patients may receive Rh(D)-positive or Rh(D)-negative RBCs. Rh(D)-negative patients are routinely given Rh(D)-negative RBCs for any elective transfusions, but in the setting of massive transfusion it may be necessary to switch to Rh(D)-positive RBCs to preserve the supply of Rh(D)-negative RBCs. The blood bank usually determines when to make this substitution based on the inventory and does so more quickly for a patient who is a male or a postmenopausal female (Table 10.6). The objective is to avoid exposing a female with childbearing potential to Rh(D)-positive RBCs and possibly triggering the production of the anti-D alloantibody, which is responsible for the most severe forms of hemolytic disease of the newborn. Table 10.7 shows the common initial volume of PRBCs needed to increase the hemoglobin level by 2 to 3 grams per deciliter.

The changes that occur to RBCs during storage under conventional blood bank conditions have been well described.[75] These observations have generated physiologically plausible hypotheses about how such changes may impair the function of the banked RBCs in vivo. The reduced hemoglobin level of 2,3-DPG and its corresponding decrease in the P50 value may reduce the ability of stored RBCs to relinquish bound O_2 compared with 2,3-DPG–replete RBCs. The depletion of nitric oxide (NO) may reduce the vasodilatory properties of the RBCs, hence impairing their ability to maintain the patency of small vessels in the microcirculation and blood flow to tissues.[76] Numerous changes in the composition and behavior of the RBC plasma membrane,

including the loss and oxidation of membrane lipids and proteins and the rearrangement of some membrane constituents,[77] correlate with changes in the shape and elasticity of the RBC membrane.[78–81] The loss of elasticity in particular can impede the rapid movement of the RBCs through the microcirculation.

These hypotheses and some supportive data from animal models[82] have led to a number of observational clinical studies (mostly in trauma, critical care, colorectal surgery, and cardiac surgery) of outcomes after using stored PRBCs. Most prospective randomized studies have shown no differences in patient outcomes associated with the age of RBC units.[83–92] A retrospective study of 357 children with respiratory failure reported that RBC transfusions were independently associated with a greater duration of mechanical ventilation.[93] One prospective, observational study from 30 North American centers of 296 children younger than 18 years of age, who received blood stored 14 days or longer, reported increased multiple-organ dysfunction (OR 1.87) and increased pediatric intensive care unit (PICU) stay (~3.7 days), but no difference in mortality.[94] A small study of pediatric cardiac surgical patients found that children who received blood older than 3 days required additional RBC and FFP transfusions but this study was underpowered.[95] About half of such observational studies found a statistical association between the transfusion of RBCs that had been stored for a greater time and an unfavorable clinical outcome measure. However, no such association was reported in the other half of the studies, including two that were extensions of previous studies with positive findings. A small number of randomized, controlled trials (RCTs) addressed this issue without differences in outcomes between patients receiving RBCs stored for different amounts of time,[96] although two of them were underpowered.[97,98] Knowing that RBCs change during storage raises the question of whether these changes affect children in a clinically meaningful way, a question that remains unanswered by the observational studies.[99] A Cochrane review of 22 trials with 42,835 participants, both adult and pediatric, found *"no evidence of an effect on mortality that is related to length of storage of PRBCs....but the quality of evidence in neonates and children is low"*.[100]

Several RCTs have addressed these issues in four different patient populations, two of which were in pediatric cohorts. A multicenter RCT conducted in Canada randomized low–birth-weight neonates in ICUs to receive PRBCs stored 8 days or less or the standard of care, which was to provide aliquots from one unit of PRBCs to each infant until transfusion was no longer required or the donor unit was depleted.[95] There were no differences in the incidence of infections, bronchopulmonary dysplasia, necrotizing enterocolitis, death, or the composite between the two groups. Children in Uganda between 6 months and 6 years of age who presented with severe anemia (hemoglobin <5 g/dL) and lactic acidosis (lactate >5 mmol/L) were randomly assigned to receive PRBCs stored 10 days or less or 35 days or longer.[96] There were no differences in lactate clearance, left ventricular strain, as assessed by β-naturietic peptide or, in a subset of patients, correction of cerebral tissue oxygen saturation as measured by near-infrared spectroscopy. Two studies in adults[97,98] compared clinical outcomes after transfusion with PRBCs stored for different periods of time. Patients 12 years of age or older undergoing complex cardiac surgery and very likely to require PRBC transfusion were randomly assigned to receive PRBCs stored <8 days or longer than 28 days. No differences were observed in the change in the multiple-organ dysfunction score (MODS) or mortality at 7 or 28 days, in length of ICU or hospital stay, or in the frequency of serious adverse events. Adult patients in ICUs in Canada were randomly assigned to receive PRBCs stored 8 days or less versus the standard of care, which was to issue the oldest units first. No differences were found for 30- or 90-day mortality, ICU or hospital length of stay, changes in MODS, or several other clinical endpoints.[97,98] There is no apparent clinical benefit derived by transfusing units of PRBCs, which have been stored for a period of time that is substantially shorter than that of the PRBCs routinely supplied by our current inventory practices for these vulnerable populations.[100]

WHOLE BLOOD

Although for many years donated blood has been fractionated into its components for efficiency of blood management, a return to the use of whole blood and fresh whole blood where available is now being reexamined for patients who experienced a rapid and massive blood loss, as in some trauma patients. A small cohort-matched study of pediatric trauma patients involving 28 who received uncrossmatched, low titer group O, cold-stored whole blood (<14 days old) compared with a propensity-matched cohort of 28 pediatric trauma patients who received component therapy revealed a more rapid resolution of hypotension, a lower international normalized ratio (INR), and decreased component transfusions in those who received whole blood.[101] A single center study examined the use of low titer (A & B) whole blood in 47 pediatric patients who were transfused with up to 40 milliliters per kilogram of whole blood,[102] of whom 21 were group O and 26 were nongroup O. There were no adverse events recorded and no evidence of post-transfusion hemolysis. Another study in children with head injury in Afghanistan and Iraq reported increased survival with warm fresh whole blood but this cohort is too small and use of such blood would be impractical in civilian practice.[103] Overall, there is an increasing use of whole blood in adult and pediatric trauma as evidenced by several randomized controlled trials.[102–105]

In children undergoing craniofacial reconstruction, 52 received whole blood and 59 received component therapy; the children who received whole blood were less likely to require additional blood component exposures although there was no difference in postoperative coagulopathy.[106] In a retrospective study of 4111 children <2 years of age who underwent cardiac surgery, those who received whole blood had reduced donor exposures.[107] Because whole blood contains all of the clotting factors, although at reduced concentrations of factor V and VIII, whole blood is expected to reduce the exposure to other blood components such as FFP but not the need for platelets to treat dilutional thrombocytopenia (see section on massive transfusion).

PLATELETS

Platelets may be obtained from a unit of whole blood or collected by apheresis. Several varied approaches can be undertaken to reduce the risk of bacterial contamination of a unit of platelets including culturing, rapid bacterial detection, and pathogen reduction. If pathogen reduction is used, the plasma portion of the platelet unit is replaced by a plasma additive solution. The unit is treated to prevent replication of pathogens containing DNA or RNA before being made available for transfusion as described later in the section on pathogen inactivation/reduction. Alternatively, bacteria could be detected with cultures or a culture and a rapid bacteria detection method. With these methods, a bacterial culture is performed at the time of collection; ~1:5000 units are contaminated at the time of donation (https://www.fda.gov/regulatory-information/search-fda-guidance-documents/bacterial-risk-control-strategies-blood-collection-establishments-and-transfusion-services-enhance) (see section on pathogen reduction later). Then, if the platelets are not transfused soon after collection, a second culture is performed, or a rapid bacterial antigen test can be used in the blood bank before issuing the platelets for transfusion.

Platelets from whole blood are separated by centrifugation and suspended in 40 to 60 milliliters of plasma at a concentration that is two to four times greater than that in the circulation. Each unit contains a minimum of 5.5×10^{10} platelets and is stored at 20°C to 24°C with gentle continuous agitation for a maximum of 5 days. One unit of whole blood—derived platelets can be expected to increase the platelet count in an 18-kilogram child by ~15,000 per cubic millimeters and in a 70-kilogram adult by ~5000 to 10,000 per cubic millimeters.[79,108] A unit of platelets obtained by apheresis contains at least 3×10^{11} platelets in 200 to 350 milliliters of plasma, or the equivalent of approximately 5 to 6 units of whole blood—derived platelets. A common dose for children is 0.1 to 0.3 unit of whole blood–derived platelets per kilogram of body weight, or 10 to 15 milliliters per kilogram (see Table 10.7); this dose usually increases the platelet count by ~30,000 to 90,000 per cubic millimeter. However, in several prophylactic platelet dose trials for medical causes of bleeding, doses equivalent to the standard dose of 1 pheresis unit (or 6 units of whole blood—derived platelet concentrates) per meter squared, half of this dose and double this dose were compared in 1272 adult and children who received at least one platelet transfusion.[109,110] Blood losses were determined with the World Health Organization (WHO) bleeding scale: grade 0 = no bleeding, grade 1 = petechiae, grade 2 = mild blood loss, grade 3 = gross blood loss, and grade 4 = debilitating blood loss. The three doses yielded no differences in bleeding outcomes (WHO grade ≥2). The subset of 198 children were found to have a greater risk for bleeding than adults for unknown reasons,[111] but bleeding in this age group also did not differ by platelet dose received and was seemingly unrelated to platelet counts. This trial assessed the use of platelets to prevent bleeding events and did not address patients undergoing surgical procedures with ongoing bleeding.[112–115]

In the setting of dilutional thrombocytopenia during surgery or after trauma, with ongoing blood loss or a consumptive coagulopathy (e.g., disseminated intravascular coagulation), larger doses (up to 0.3 units/kg) may be required to boost the platelet count above 50,000 per cubic millimeter.[116] Because platelets are suspended in plasma that contains the anti-A and anti-B isoagglutinins, they should be ABO compatible with the recipient's RBCs. Some blood donors have high-titer isoagglutinins that can produce hemolysis in transfusion recipients if a large enough volume of plasma is given.[117] The transfusion of plasma-incompatible, whole blood–derived platelets to adult recipients does not produce clinically significant hemolysis because the volume of plasma given is so small relative to the plasma volume of an adult. However, apheresis platelets (and whole blood–derived platelets for small children) should be ABO compatible or have low titer anti-ABO antibodies with the recipient's RBCs. Matching for Rh(D) antigen is not necessary for apheresis platelets because platelets do not express Rh antigens and they contain virtually no RBCs. However, whole blood–derived platelets may contain enough RBCs to provoke Rh alloimmunization, so platelets from Rh(D)-negative donors are given preferentially to Rh(D)-negative recipients with childbearing potential. If a premenopausal female receives whole blood–derived platelets from an Rh(D)-positive donor, Rh immune globulin (RhoGAM) can be administered within 72 hours to prevent alloimmunization. Platelets should never be withheld in an emergency because of Rh(D) incompatibility.

Platelets are essential to achieve hemostasis associated with the vascular injury of surgery and are necessary to control surgical bleeding. Platelets are also required to maintain an intact endothelial barrier to spontaneous blood loss. The number of platelets required to provide adequate hemostasis in the surgical setting is much greater than that required to provide prophylaxis against spontaneous hemorrhage. In the absence of controlled studies, a platelet count of 40,000 to 50,000 per cubic millimeter is considered adequate to prevent spontaneous bleeding or bleeding from minor invasive procedures (e.g., lumbar puncture, line placement) in an otherwise stable child. If overt signs of bleeding are present or a more significant hemostatic challenge in the form of a surgical procedure is imminent, sustaining a level of 30,000 to 50,000 per cubic millimeter for several days may be recommended.[118–122] A target level of 50,000 per cubic millimeter is appropriate in the setting of massive transfusion.[116,119,123–125] Platelets may also be required for children with adequate counts, but in whom platelet function is impaired, such as in some forms of congenital heart disease and after cardiopulmonary bypass.[126–128] Many medications (e.g., aspirin; other nonsteroidal antiinflammatory agents, including ibuprofen and naproxen; dipyridamole; platelet P2Y12 receptor blockers such as clopidogrel or prasugrel; or glycoprotein IIa/IIIb receptor inhibitors such as abciximab, eptifibatide, or tirofiban; serotonin uptake antagonists such as sertraline [Zoloft]) and some medical conditions (e.g., renal failure with blood urea nitrogen levels above 60 mg/dL) cause abnormal platelet function.

This dysfunction may interfere with surgical hemostasis, in which case it may be necessary to maintain the platelet count at a somewhat greater concentration, at least until the effect of the medication dissipates.[129,130] In a few settings, such as intracranial, ophthalmic, spinal cord, and otologic surgery, even greater concentrations (100,000/mm^3) may be sought, although the appropriate threshold in these settings is unclear.

There is no clearcut threshold value below which the platelet count predicts clinical bleeding in the perioperative period. Each child must be individually assessed by constantly observing the surgical field for evidence of abnormal bleeding.[131] Currently, we lack a well-validated bedside tool to assess platelet function. Thromboelastography and other approaches to measure platelet function under controlled flow conditions, such as microfluidic flow devices[132,133] and the platelet function analyzer (PFA-100),[134] cannot predict the risk for hemorrhage.[135–141] The standard technique for diagnosis and evaluation of thrombocytopathies remains Born-O'Brien platelet aggregometry, but it is not useful in the intraoperative or intensive care setting owing to prolonged turnaround times. In the neonate, it simply requires too much blood: 15 milliliters.[142] Most commonly, dilutional thrombocytopenia rather than a newly acquired platelet function defect is the cause in the operative setting and in massive transfusions.

A child occasionally presents for surgery with a previously characterized platelet dysfunction that may be associated with bleeding. If the child has a normal platelet count, it is reasonable practice to ensure that the blood bank has an adequate platelet supply available for the operating room and to withhold transfusion of platelets until pathologic bleeding occurs.

Several additional points should be considered[143]:

1. Not all hospitals have platelets in the blood bank inventory. Unless the need is anticipated before surgery, platelets may not be available when they are required. Therefore, a preemptive request for platelets may have to be arranged.

2. For children who are thrombocytopenic before surgery, platelets should be infused just before the surgical procedure to ensure the greatest concentrations during the time of peak demand. The start of the procedure should *not* be delayed to obtain the results of a posttransfusion platelet count.

3. Platelets should be filtered only by large-pore filters approved for blood transfusions (≥150 μm) or leukocyte-reduction filters (if indicated).

4. Traditionally, platelets are suspended in plasma, which may help to replenish coagulation factors other than factors V and VIII, which are labile, and factor VII, which has an especially brief half-life. Platelet additive solutions (PAS) instead of plasma can be used to resuspend some platelet units. Units of platelet additive solution do not supply clotting factors and have a reduced risk of allergic reactions and transfusion-related acute lung injury. In addition, platelet additive solution suspended platelets are used for pathogen reduction treatment.

In general, platelets should not be refrigerated or placed in a cooler with ice before administration because cold-exposed platelets are rapidly cleared from the circulation. However, chilled platelets are FDA approved and do provide for rapid hemostatic activity.[144–148] These have generally been used in the military for traumas and are not currently used in many civilian hospitals.

SPECIAL PROCESSING OF CELLULAR BLOOD COMPONENTS

Leukocytes collected with whole blood donations partition into both the platelet and the PRBC components; few intact leukocytes are present in FFP. "Passenger leukocytes" are responsible for most febrile, nonhemolytic transfusion reactions, human leukocyte antigen (HLA) alloimmunization, and transmission of cytomegalovirus (CMV). To reduce the incidence of complications from these leukocytes, blood components should be passed through leukocyte-reduction filters that effectively remove leukocytes (by a 2–3 log reduction) immediately after collection (prestorage leukoreduction) or at the bedside (pretransfusion). Even with leukoreduction, some febrile reactions occur, especially to platelet units because platelets can release inflammatory mediators.[149]

CMV transmission can also be reduced by screening donors for CMV exposure (testing for antibodies to CMV), although leukocyte reduction is the more widely used approach. Even though primary CMV infection is benign in children with intact immune systems, some children are at risk of developing systemic disease and should be protected from blood-borne CMV transmission. Only patients who have never been infected with CMV (i.e., CMV-seronegative) are at risk; those who are particularly vulnerable to systemic CMV infections are listed in E-Table 10.1.

Transfused lymphocytes may mediate a graft-versus-host process in some recipients with impaired cellular immunity. Because this process involves the bone marrow as well as the usual targets (i.e., skin and gastrointestinal tract), the fatality rate is substantial. Transfusion-associated graft-versus-host disease (TA-GVHD) can be prevented by exposing cellular blood components to gamma irradiation that disables the donor lymphocytes.[150–152] Alternatively, the most widely available pathogen reduction systems eliminate the risk of TA-GVHD.[153] Children who are considered to be at risk for TA-GVHD and who should receive irradiated cellular components are listed in E-Table 10.2. This complication can also occur in children with intact immune systems in the unusual circumstance when the transfusion donor is homozygous for an HLA haplotype that is shared with the recipient. In this case, the recipient's immune system, although fully functional, cannot recognize the donor lymphocytes as foreign. The donor lymphocytes mount a GVHD attack on the recipient's tissues, recognizing the mismatched haplotype. This situation is more likely to occur when the donor is a blood relative of the recipient. It is for this reason that blood and HLA-matched platelets donated by family members are routinely irradiated.

Because irradiation damages the cell membrane, irradiated RBCs lose potassium (K^+) at a greater rate than usual. As a result, the shelf life of irradiated RBCs, 28 days, is one-third less than nonirradiated RBCs, 42 days. The problem of increased amounts of circulating K^+ can be obviated by irradiating units close to the time of donation[154] as well as time of issue[155] or washing the unit if it was irradiated early in the storage period.[150]

PLASMA

Plasma preparations are available that vary in the timing of freezing and storage after thawing. FFP represents the fluid portion of whole blood that is separated and frozen within 8 hours of collection. After thawing at 37°C, which usually requires 30 minutes, it may be administered within 24 hours if stored at 1°C to 6°C. Other plasma preparations that have been frozen within 24 hours and thawed for up to 5 days have similar therapeutic effects as FFP. The volume of 1 unit varies from 180 to 300 milliliters and represents 7% to 10% of the coagulation factor activity in a 70-kilogram patient. It contains all the clotting factors and regulatory proteins at approximately the native concentration, but after 6 hours at 1°C to 6°C, the concentrations of the labile factors V and VIII begin to diminish, as does that of the short-lived factor VII. FFP does not provide functional platelets, nor does it contain leukocytes or RBCs. Thawed FFP may be used for transfusion up to 7 days after thawing; however, it must be labeled as thawed plasma to indicate that it has reduced levels of factors V, VII, VIII, and protein S.

FFP should be ABO compatible with recipient red cells because it contains the anti-A and anti-B isoagglutinins appropriate to the donor's ABO blood group. If the recipient's blood type is not known, plasma from a donor with blood type AB, which contains neither anti-A nor anti-B, may be administered. Because the citrate anticoagulant is present in the plasma at the greatest concentration of any other blood component, rapid administration of FFP is more likely to be associated with citrate toxicity than the transfusion of components with smaller volumes of plasma (e.g., PRBCs or whole blood) (see later).

FFP is often administered without justification by evidence-based medicine.[156,157] One major surgical indication for FFP is to correct the coagulopathy associated with massive blood transfusion (see Table 10.7). Other indications include correction of a prolongation in the prothrombin time (PT) before surgery or in the setting of bleeding, the emergency reversal of warfarin, or the presence of a specific congenital or acquired coagulation protein deficiency for which a factor concentrate or a recombinant factor is not available (e.g., for factor X deficiency). Four-factor prothrombin complex concentrates (4-PCC), which contain concentrated amounts of factors II, VII, IX, and X, are often preferred for emergency reversal of warfarin but their use in children is off-label. Administration of vitamin K should be considered for children with hepatic insufficiency, those who have been exclusively breastfed,[158–160] those treated with warfarin, broad-spectrum antibiotics (which often eliminate normal vitamin K–producing gastrointestinal flora), or total parenteral nutrition for inadequate oral caloric intake, or who have had a prolonged hospitalization. Correction of a mild increase in the PT (e.g., INR <1.5) is rarely necessary. Fig. 10.1 shows the relationship between the level of coagulation factors and the in vitro clotting time; in this case, the PT. Relatively modest levels of coagulation factors can support normal hemostasis, even though the PT is prolonged. When the PT is markedly increased (see Fig. 10.1, point A), the transfusion of 1 unit of FFP, which increases the coagulation factor levels by 7% to 10% in an adult, dramatically decreases the PT. When the PT is only mildly prolonged, as at point C, where factor levels are already adequate for hemostasis, infusion of 1 unit of FFP (in an adult) decreases the PT to a much smaller extent. This small decrease in the PT does not clinically improve hemostasis.

CRYOPRECIPITATE

Cryoprecipitate is prepared by thawing FFP at 4°C to 10°C and removing most of the plasma, leaving behind precipitated protein that is then resuspended in a small volume of residual plasma (15–25 mL) and refrozen. This component contains 20% to 50% of the factor VIII from the original unit of plasma as well as von Willebrand factor (vWF), fibrinogen (approximately 250 mg), factor XIII, and a disintegrin and metalloprotease with thrombospondin type 1 repeats-13 (ADAMTS13).[161,162] Cryoprecipitate is indicated to treat factor XIII deficiency, dysfibrinogenemia, and hypofibrinogenemia (see Table 10.7),[163–170] as well as ongoing bleeding; its use in trauma patients still lacks robust clinical trials,[171,172] although there is anecdotal information regarding its usefulness in combat in-field treatment.[173] It may also be used in rare cases such as congenital deficiency in ADAMTS13, the prothrombotic condition known as Upshaw-Schulman syndrome. It has not been used for the treatment of von Willebrand disease or hemophilia A since the advent of clotting factor concentrates and recombinant factor VIII; plasma concentrates of factor XIII and

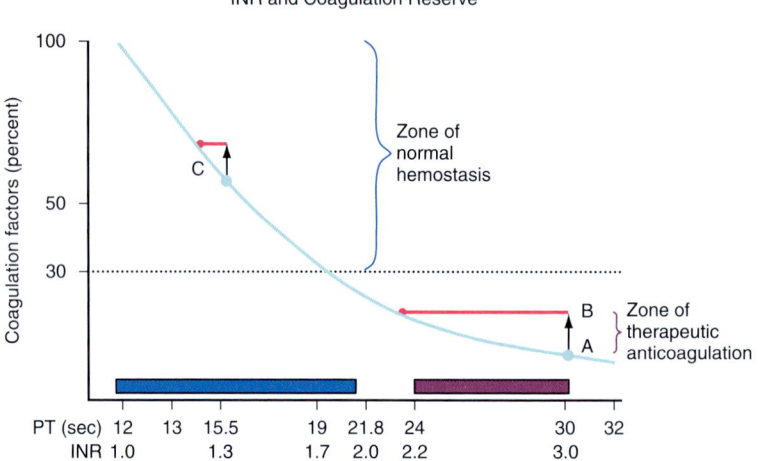

FIGURE 10.1 Nonlinear relationship between levels of coagulation factor and clotting test results. Decreases in clotting factor levels to about 30% of normal prolong the clotting test times but still support normal hemostasis. Treating an adult or child at point *A* with fresh frozen plasma to raise the level of coagulation factors to point *B* has a marked effect on the prothrombin time *(PT)* and the international normalized ratio *(INR)*. The same amount per kg of fresh frozen plasma administered to an adult or child at point *C*, however, has only a minor effect on the PT. (Modified from Dzik WH, Stowell CP. Transfusion and coagulation issues in trauma. In: Sheridan RL, ed. *The Trauma Handbook of Massachusetts General Hospital*. Philadelphia: Lippincott Williams & Wilkins; 2004:139.)

fibrinogen are licensed in the United States for use in patients with these congenital deficiencies. Fibrinogen concentrates have also been used to treat acquired hypofibrinogenemia in adult cardiac patients and found to be noninferior to crypecipitate.[174] A systematic review concluded that further well controlled trials are needed to define its role in trauma-induced coagulopathy.[175]

PATHOGEN INACTIVATION/REDUCTION

Techniques to inactivate or reduce the level of infectious agents have been in place for plasma derivatives such as intravenous (IV) immunoglobulin and plasma-derived clotting factors for over 25 years. More recently, pathogen inactivation technologies have been applied to RBCs, FFP, cryoprecipitate, and platelets[176] with the goal of eliminating a wide range of infectious organisms.[177] There are several potential advantages of these technologies over screening by donor history and testing for specific organisms, particularly for those pathogens that frequently cause asymptomatic infection, have a long serologic "window" period before screening tests become positive, are newly emerging[178,179] or are completely new and unrecognized.[180] These techniques may also allow for a longer storage period, in particular for platelets[178,181]; however, use of pathogen reduction technologies may increase the number of platelet transfusions over shorter intervals but there is no increase in bleeding events.[176]

There are two general approaches to pathogen inactivation[182]: methods that disrupt lipid membranes (solvent detergent treatment[183] and methylene blue plus visible light exposure[184]) and methods that target RNA and DNA (or nucleic acid techniques [amotosalen[185] or riboflavin[186]]) plus ultraviolet (UV) light exposure (INTERCEPT, Cerus, Concord CA; Mirasol Pathogen Reduction Technology [PRT] [now approved in the United States for platelets, cryoprecipitate, and cryopoor plasma]; Caridian-BCT, Lakewood, CO), or UV light exposure alone (THERAFLEX, Macopharma, Tourcoing France; not yet approved in the United States).[187] The nucleic acid–targeted techniques also inactivate leukocytes and eliminate the risk of transfusion-transmitted graft-versus-host disease, which may preclude the need for gamma irradiation of cellular components in vulnerable patients.[188]

However, inactivation techniques do have limitations even though they can achieve a 5 or 6 log reduction in infectious particles, particularly enveloped viruses and parasites.[189–191] They may not be completely effective in components with high pathogen loads.[192] (*Log reduction refers to the ratio of the infectious particles before and after an intervention. If 10^6 particles existed before and 10^3 particles after an intervention, the log reduction of $10^6/10^3$, is 3, which represents a 99.9% reduction in particles.*) In addition, the lipid-targeted techniques do not inactivate nonlipid enveloped viruses such as hepatitis A virus, hepatitis E virus, and parvovirus B19, and none of the techniques inactivate prions. These procedures also damage or deplete plasma proteins[193,194] and platelets, which may reduce their effectiveness.[195] The INTERCEPT system is mandatory for pathogen reduction of platelets in Switzerland and is currently approved for use in the United States and Canada.[196] Although to date, there is no evidence of major adverse effects after more than 500,000 platelet transfusions,[197,198] the potential for toxicity such as the formation of plasma or membrane protein neoantigens,[183] need for a greater number of platelet transfusions, possible increased systemic inflammatory response syndromes (SIRS, ARDS noted in adults but not children),[199] or from long-term effects of exposure to amotosalen exist.[200] A Cochrane review suggests that pathogen reduction treated platelets are not associated with increased mortality or morbidity but are associated with platelet refractoriness.[201,202] In the United States, several pathogen-inactivated component systems have been licensed by the FDA: plasma[203] and platelets[204] treated with amotosalen and UV-A light (INTERCEPT) and plasma treated with riboflavin and UV light (Mirasol)(not yet approved in the United States).[183,186] Several studies have enrolled pediatric patients including neonates with no apparent adverse effects.[205–208] Currently, there are no licensed systems for pathogen inactivation of RBCs; several are under investigation. Although expensive, these techniques may eventually replace the need for pathogen detection with pathogen elimination in donated blood and may reduce the need for wasting outdated components by extending their shelf life.[209] These techniques may be particularly effective in cleansing the blood pool in low-income countries such as those in sub-Saharan Africa with currently inadequate methods for blood screening.[210]

PLASMA-DERIVED FACTOR CONCENTRATES AND RECOMBINANT FACTORS

The most administered factor concentrate is factor VIII, used to treat hemophilia A. Children with hemophilia may present with splenomegaly, abnormal liver function, and joint disease related to hemarthrosis. In the past, the use of pooled plasma products was associated with very high rates of transmission of viral hepatitis (especially HCV) and HIV.[211–213] However, more rigorous inactivation processes and strategies to remove viruses, and the introduction of recombinant factor VIII and IX products[214–218] have greatly reduced these problems.[163–168,219–222] Initial concerns that recombinant therapy increased the incidence of inhibitors in children compared with plasma-derived factor therapy have been confirmed by the SIPPET trial (survey of inhibitors in plasma-product exposed toddlers),[223] which showed that the incidence of inhibitors in toddlers who were treated with plasma-derived factor VIII containing vWF was nearly 2-fold less than those treated with recombinant factor VIII. However, the study failed to show a significant difference regarding high-titer inhibitors and did not include any of the newer concentrates that have appeared since the trial started in 2010. More importantly, the study has had little impact on current practices insofar as newer recombinant factor VIII products, that have different structures than recombinant products available during SIPPET trial enrollment (2010 through 2014); these products have not shown any greater risk of developing inhibitors than plasma-derived factor VIII products in the past. Mild hemophilia A usually responds well to desmopressin (1-deamino-8-D-arginine vasopressin [DDAVP]) therapy.[224,225]

New extended half-life factor concentrates that are available for both hemophilia A and B appear to be well tolerated, do not increase the risk of inhibitors, and may reduce factor consumption.[226,227] For factor VIII and factor IX concentrates, the new technology includes fusion to either albumin or the monomeric Fc fragment of immunoglobin G1 (IgG1), conjugation with polyethylene glycol (glycosylation),[228] or binding to the neonatal Fc receptor. Most patients who received a standard rFVIII product have now switched to an extended half-life product. The benefit of extended half-life rFVIII products is an approximate 1.5-fold increased half-life (e.g., ~13–15 hours in children 1–11 years of age and ~16–20 hours in patients 12 years of age to adulthood for Eloctate),[229] whereas the benefit of extended half-life rFIX products has been much more substantial at 4.7-fold (~90–93 hours in children 0 to <12 years of age, 87–118 hours for people 12 years of age to adulthood for Idelvion).[230]

von Willebrand disease is routinely treated with DDAVP or plasma-derived factor VIII concentrates that are also rich in vWF, such as Humate-P, Alphanate, Koate DVI, and Wilate,[231] with dosing in ristocetin cofactor units per kilogram, not factor VIII units. In adults, recombinant vWF (VONVENDI, Baxalta, Lexington MA),[232,233] is able to correct vWF deficiency as well as secondary vWF:C deficiency.[234,235] However, it is only approved for those 18 years of age or older, although it is widely used in children.[236,237] In children who have von Willebrand disease and are resistant to DDAVP or for whom DDAVP is contraindicated (e.g., central nervous system [CNS] bleeding, allergic reaction, brain tumor, recent CNS surgery, age under 2 years), it is reasonable to withhold treatment with blood-derived products until surgery has begun unless surgery is performed in an area where even minor bleeding can produce serious complications. These children often do not demonstrate pathologic bleeding. As Vonvendi does not

contain rFVIII, it should be given 12 to 24 hours before surgery to allow time for circulating levels of endogenous factor VIII, often low in vWD, to increase to normal values. Adjunctive therapies that can further limit hemorrhage include the use of the antifibrinolytic agent ε-aminocaproic acid (Amicar) and tranexamic acid (Lysteda), a competitive inhibitor of plasminogen, both being administered orally or intravenously, and topical hemostatic agents, including topical collagen and fibrin glues.

Children with hemophilia B (i.e., Christmas disease or factor IX deficiency) are managed with standard half-life recombinant human factor IX[238,239] and newer extended half-life recombinant factor IX products (see earlier). The use of highly purified factor IX (preparations with various amounts of factors VII, X, and prothrombin) to inactivate or remove viruses is decreasing.[163,166,221,240–253] The pharmacokinetics of recombinant human factor IX may differ perioperatively compared with nonoperative indications.[254] Further, factor IX distributes into the interstitial space as well as the intravascular space, unlike factor VIII, which may affect factor IX levels in edematous states. Careful planning of any surgical procedure for these children includes close communication with the child's hematologist to ensure optimal therapy while reducing unnecessary transfusions (see Chapter 8).

Emicizumab (Hemlibra),[255] a factor VIII mimetic that binds to factors IXa and Xa on activated phospholipid membranes, is especially effective and widely used treatment for hemophilia A patients with high-titer inhibitors, and also hemophilia A patients who prefer its once every 2 to 4 week subcutaneous (SC) injections to multiple factor infusions each week and the need for intravenous access.[256] An alternative bypassing agent for hemophiliacs with inhibitors is SEVENFACT,[257] a new recombinant coagulation factor VIIa (coagulation factor VIIa [recombinant]), that has an action of 12 hours and that is approved for ages 12 years and above.

A new, truly long-acting recombinant factor VIII, Altuviiio (efanesoctocog alfa),[258] approved in 2023,[162] owes its half-life of 42 to 48 hours to its structural and binding independence from the vWF.[259]

Other newer therapies include the so-called hemostasis rebalancing agents that block or inhibit the naturally occurring inhibitors of coagulation: Alnylam (fitusiran), a therapy based on siRNA (small interfering RNA) technology to lower levers of antithrombin III; concizumab and marstacimab, agents that inhibit the K2 domain of tissue factor pathway inhibitor; and other agents that block the activated protein C pathway or protein S.[259,260]

PROTHROMBIN COMPLEX CONCENTRATES

Prothrombin complex concentrates (PCC) have been used to rapidly reverse vitamin K antagonist anticoagulants in the setting of significant hemorrhage, especially in the CNS or for cardiac surgery.[261,262] They consist of either three-factor (II, *low VII*, IX, and X, proteins C and S) or four-factor (KCENTRA,[263] II, *high VII*, IX, and X, proteins C and S (additional products available outside the United States) human plasma-derived products.[264] These have been primarily used in adults; pediatric experience is increasing.[265–268] The advantages appear to be a more rapid reversal than the administration of FFP or vitamin K (without, however, any difference in clinical outcomes) and for some patients, reduced volume of administration.[269–272] One systematic review concluded that four-factor PCC more reliably corrected the INR than three-factor PCC, whereas another suggested that protocols based on body weight offer an advantage over individual physician decisions.[273,274] However, in the setting of intracranial bleeding in patients taking warfarin, four-factor PCC has not proven superior to FFP. The efficacy of PCCs in the operating room setting to treat

TABLE 10.8	Emergency Reversal of Anticoagulation		
Generic Name	Trade Name	Activated 4-Factor Reversal (Kcentra) (25–50 Units/kg)	Other Reversal Agents
apixaban	Eliquis	Yes	Andexanet alfa (AndexXa)
betrixaban	Bevyxxa	Yes	Andexanet alfa (AndexXa)
dabigatran	Pradaxa	Yes	Idarucizumab (Praxbind)
edoxaban	Savaysa	Yes	Andexanet alfa (AndexXa)
fonda-parinux	Arixtra	Yes	rFVIIa (NovoSeven), Andexanet alfa (AndexXa)
rivaroxaban	Xarelto	Yes	Andexanet alfa (AndexXa)
warfarin	Coumadin	Yes	Vitamin K, FFP

Kcentra can reverse all of the anticoagulants listed in column 1 and column 4 lists alternatives. See package insert for recommended doses.

perioperative coagulopathy is unclear.[275] Some of the newer anticoagulants now increasingly administered to children with congenital heart disease, such as apixaban, betrixaban, dabigatran, edoxaban, fondaparinux, and rivaroxaban may be antagonized with four-factor concentrates.[276–285] A specific antagonist, andexanet alfa, is also effective in antagonizing apixaban, rivaroxaban, and edoxaban; idarucizumab (Praxbind) may be used to reverse dabigatran.[286] Fondaparinux has been antagonized with rFVIIa (NovoSeven) (Table 10.8).[282,287]

DESMOPRESSIN

DDAVP, a synthetic analog of vasopressin, can increase the levels of factor VIII:C (i.e., coagulant activity) and factor VIII:vWF in children with mild hemophilia A or von Willebrand disease.[225,288–295] An IV dose of 0.3 micrograms per kilogram (maximum 20 μg; a subcutaneous preparation is available in Europe) increases the levels of both factors 2-fold to 3-fold within 30 to 60 minutes, with a half-life of 3 to 6 hours.[289] Intranasal DDAVP is also effective, but it has a slower onset and, in younger children for whom a sustained inhalation may be more difficult, part of the dose may find its way into the gastrointestinal tract, bypassing nasal blood vessels. Between 80% and 90% of children with von Willebrand disease respond to DDAVP,[296,297] and affected children should be tested for their responsiveness to IV DDAVP. This treatment is best suited to treat bleeding from surgical procedures, which ceases within 2 to 3 days. When bleeding continues beyond this period, as is the case with some orthopedic procedures, daily IV Humate-P (or Alphanate or Koate DVI) can obviate possible tachyphylaxis with DDAVP. Products rich in the vWF allow better control over peak concentrations of factor VIII. When more than 200%, factor VIII predisposes to postoperative deep venous thrombosis and pulmonary embolism.

DDAVP has been used to treat the coagulopathy associated with antiplatelet therapy, platelet dysfunction, uremia, and cirrhosis.[298–301] It may reduce elective surgical bleeding when the potential for blood loss is substantial, such as in cardiac surgery, tonsillectomy,[302] and spinal fusion.[225,303–309] Although initial reports apparently demonstrated a benefit in patients who did not have a preexisting coagulopathy, other controlled studies failed to show an effect despite increases in factor VIII:C and vWF, and its use for these indications has largely been abandoned.[310–312] Because of the potential for hyponatremia from water retention, use of DDAVP is avoided in children younger than 2 years of age, and in children with CNS lesions, including a brain tumor, history of CNS irradiation, or recent neurosurgery or CNS trauma.[313] It is also avoided in the elderly.

ALBUMIN, DEXTRANS, STARCHES, AND GELATINS

Solutions of several high-molecular-weight molecules (i.e., colloids) have been used for volume replacement, although a systematic review has determined they offer no advantage over crystalloid solutions.[314] These colloids include albumin, dextrans, starches, and gelatins.[315]

Albumin has the longest track record and the fewest adverse effects.[316,317] In the past, dextrans (i.e., high- and low-molecular-weight glucose polymers) were administered for volume expansion and hemodilution in children,[318,319] but currently their primary use is for antithrombosis, although their value for even this indication is questionable.[320]

Starches are branched polysaccharide polymers available in high-, medium-, and low-molecular-weight ranges (480,000–70,000 Da). Although they expand blood volume, they also alter hemostasis by diluting clotting factors and impairing platelet function and the coagulation cascade.[321,322] In addition, starches accumulate in the reticuloendothelial system and carry the potential for unknown long-term adverse effects.[323] Minor coagulation changes have been reported when the dose exceeded 20 milliliters per kilogram.[324–326] A 6% hydroxyethyl starch (HES 130/0.4) yielded clinical and physiologic profiles similar to those for 5% albumin in volumes up to 16 milliliters per kilogram in noncardiac surgery and in volumes up to 50 milliliters per kilogram in cardiac surgery, although at smaller cost.[327,328] One meta-analysis of randomized controlled trials of hydroxyethyl starch concluded that 6% hetastarch significantly decreased the platelet count and increased the length of ICU stay and also may have had adverse effects on renal function; the authors recommend against their use in pediatric patients.[329] Another meta-analysis concluded that 6% hydroxyethyl starch did not alter renal function or blood loss in the perioperative period in children, although overall the studies were of low quality.[314] Several major reviews regarding the use of starches and gels in adult patients who are critically ill have raised substantive concerns regarding adverse effects on coagulation[330,331] and renal function,[332–334] and they found inadequate overall safety data, even for the third-generation products.[59,335] There seems to be limited advantage in terms of mortality in adults.[315] If these concerns have been raised in adult populations, we should hold even greater concern regarding their use in children.

Gelatins are polypeptides derived from bovine collagen that seem to have a minimal effect on coagulation and provide reasonable plasma volume expansion. However, life-threatening anaphylactic or anaphylactoid reactions have been reported, and their use in children remains limited.[316,336–341] A systematic review identified a lack of safety and efficacy data in neonates and children.[342]

RED BLOOD CELL SUBSTITUTES

Blood substitutes offer the promise of agents with universal compatibility, minimal infectious risks, and prolonged shelf life (years rather than days) to carry oxygen to vital organs.[343,344] Early efforts to develop these products involved human, bovine, and genetically engineered hemoglobin polymer solutions, perfluorocarbons, and lipid-encapsulated hemoglobin. Most failed in clinical trials because of severe complications such as renal failure, stroke, and vasoconstriction.[345,346] The majority of hemoglobin-based oxygen carriers (HBOC) under investigation, the most recent Hemospan (Sangart, Inc., San Diego CA), failed in clinical trials and are no longer being investigated.[347–349] Liposome-encapsulated hemoglobin[350] is another investigational means to carry oxygen to compromised tissues such as cerebral or myocardial infarction.[351–354] Another approach to hemoglobin-based oxygen carriers is a bovine-based hemoglobin (hemoglobin glutamer-250, HBOC-201) that has been on a 25-year journey but remains under investigation.[355,356] This product has a similar oxygen-carrying capacity as human hemoglobin (1.26 mL/g) and has been safely administered in several case series of adults with severe anemia where standard transfusion was not feasible (e.g., Jehovah's Witnesses).[357,358] One paper reported 1701 patient exposures as well tolerated[359]; clearly additional study is required given the variety of adverse events associated with this blood substitute.[360] One perfluorocarbon formulation (Vidaphor) has recently achieved orphan drug status and is undergoing investigation.[361] Many other blood substitutes (Hemolink, PolyHeme, Hemospan, Hemopure, Sanguinate, Hemo2Life, and Oxvida Hb) are at various stages of investigation (preclinical, phase I, II, or III).[356]

Massive Blood Transfusion

Massive blood transfusion may be defined as replacement of a patient's entire blood volume one or more times or as more than 30 milliliters per kilogram PRBCs transfused in less than 4 hours with ongoing uncontrolled bleeding (see https://www.facs.org/media/zcjdtrd1/transfusion_guildelines.pdf).[362,363] Various scoring schemes have been developed regarding the initiation of massive transfusion protocols; most have been developed in war zones or in the adult trauma population. In a retrospective study of 1113 combat trauma injuries in children younger than 18 years of age, the mortality in those who received 40 milliliters per kilogram or more in the first 24 hours was greater than in those who received less than 40 milliliters per kilogram.[5,10] Another prospective study of 633 pediatric patients who received at least 40 milliliters per kilogram reported an overall mortality rate of ~22%, regardless of the mechanism triggering the need for transfusion.[364] There was no transfusion threshold that predicted mortality, although some authors report a greater mortality than in massively transfused adults.[365] This suggests that a well-transfused pediatric patient in whom factors and platelets are replenished and circulating blood volume adequately maintained, will tolerate and survive massive transfusion. There are few other published pediatric data and no randomized prospective studies.[366,367] There are potential advantages of whole blood compared with blood component transfusions. Although both have equivalent amounts of citrate for anticoagulation, RBC units are usually diluted with additional preservative solution. This dilution may represent a liability for those who require a massive transfusion. However, blood components are stored under conditions that maximally preserve each of the components. Hence, whole blood must be fresher than RBCs or frozen plasma, contributing to potential whole blood supply limitations. One propensity-matched study of 56 children suggests that transfusion with whole blood resulted in a reduced INR (P=0.01) and transfusion of smaller plasma volumes and platelets in the whole blood–treated group compared with the component-treated group (P=0.03 and 0.04).[101] Data regarding potential advantages of initial transfusion with whole blood rather than

component therapy are increasing.[101,368,369] One study reported reduced chest tube bleeding and improved outcomes in infants who were transfused with fresh whole blood compared with standard blood components.[370] Conversely, a retrospective single center study compared outcomes in 602 adult patients transfused with standard PRBCs versus 749 who received whole blood; there was no difference in 24 hour, 30 day survival, or nonlethal adverse outcomes.[371]

In children, the anesthesiologist must think in terms of percent of the child's blood volume or blood volumes lost rather than units of blood transfused.[3] The composition of each blood component must be considered to anticipate problems and determine at which stage of a massive transfusion these problems may occur (see Table 10.3). Transfusion of large quantities of blood components may seriously affect coagulation, K^+ and calcium concentrations, acid-base balance, body temperature, oxygen-hemoglobin dissociation, and hematocrit (i.e., oxygen-carrying capacity).

Most blood banks have a system for the expedited or "emergency" release of blood products, when there is inadequate time to perform complete serologic testing, including the crossmatch. Group O Rh-negative blood can be transfused into any child without the need for a crossmatch; group O Rh-positive blood may be transfused into male patients. These uncrossmatched RBC units have a minimally increased risk over crossmatched units for most patients. After the blood bank has a sample of the child's blood, then the switch is made to group-specific blood and then to blood that has completed standard compatibility testing.[372] This switch usually occurs "behind the scenes" in the blood bank but underscores the critical importance of getting a properly labeled patient specimen to the blood bank as quickly as possible, before the patient's blood is substantially diluted by banked group O RBCs after which accurate testing is compromised. Many institutions also have developed massive transfusion protocols that incorporate the mechanism in place for abbreviated serologic testing as well as the expedited provision of specific blood components (see E-Fig. 10.1).

With massive blood loss, infusing crystalloid solutions alone or in large quantities may worsen the underlying coagulopathy, such as from trauma-induced bleeding, and may result in increased ICU stay.[373,374] Protocols using fixed ratios of PRBCs, FFP, and platelets (1:1:1) have been used in combat situations[375] as well as civilian trauma patients, but have not been systematically examined or proven to offer advantage compared with standard component approaches in noncombat-associated adults or children.[3,376–379] Systematic reviews regarding pediatric patients found that "evidence supporting an optimal blood product ratio of 1:1:1 is lacking".[380–382] Additionally there are likely differences between controlled massive bleeding over time compared with massive rapid bleeding which add to the difficulty of controlled trials.[383] The volume of transfusion is not predictive of mortality in pediatric patients regardless of the cause of hemorrhage.[384] The approach to trauma patients has been termed "damage control," which means correcting hypothermia, maintaining adequate perfusion, and early administration of clotting factors and platelets to correct coagulopathy; systematic pediatric trauma studies are lacking.[382,385]

COAGULOPATHY

The coagulation system involves platelets, coagulation proteins, and localized tissue factor, which initiate all steps of hemostasis. Fig. 10.2 shows that an initial step is platelet adhesion to a wound or site of vessel wall injury, with adhesion being mediated by the vWF through its receptor on the platelet, the glycoprotein Ib–glycoprotein IX complex (GPIb-IX), and fibrinogen through

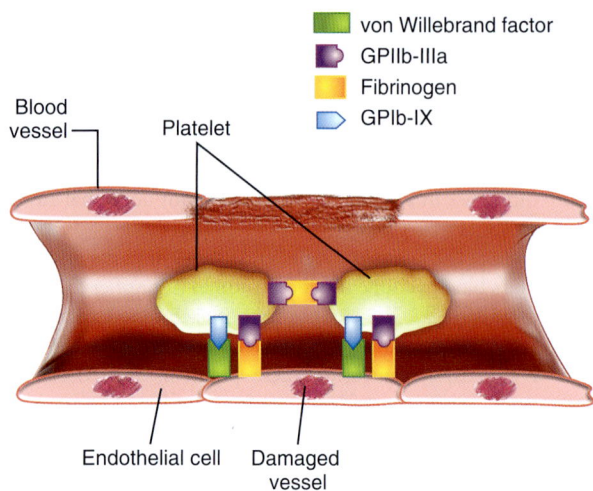

von Willebrand factor
GPIIb-IIIa
Fibrinogen
GPIb-IX

FIGURE 10.2 A blood clot forms when platelets adhere to one another through the GPIIb-IIIa complex *(purple)*, which serves as a receptor for the adhesive protein fibrinogen *(orange)*. Platelet interaction with an injured vessel wall requires synergy between the GPIb-IX *(blue)* and GPIIb-IIIa complexes and the adhesive proteins of von Willebrand factor *(green)* and fibrinogen, respectively. In high-velocity gradients, the efficacy of GPIb-IX interaction with the von Willebrand factor is impaired.

the fibrinogen receptor on the platelet, the glycoprotein IIb–glycoprotein IIIa complex (GPIIb-IIIA). In flowing blood, initial platelet attachment is facilitated by vWF, whereas platelet spreading, and more secure (shear stress-resistant) platelet-platelet aggregation is driven by fibrinogen and by the GPIIa-GPIIIa complex. However, there is also evidence that platelets attach even to intact endothelium, which has an activated phenotype, as after inflammatory cytokine exposure or sepsis.[386,387] Platelets attach to the endothelium through high-molecular-weight von Willebrand multimers. Fibrinogen is attached to endothelium through upregulated integrins and selectins.

Initial platelet hemostasis (i.e., platelet plug formation) is accompanied by the local generation of fibrin, which is the end-product of at least three surface-active enzyme complexes.[388] Clotting is initiated by the tissue factor/factor VIIa surface-active enzyme complex and amplified by the factor VIIIa/IXa/X and factor II/Va/Xa complexes. A mural platelet thrombus, which includes platelets and fibrin, then forms a scaffold on which healing of the vessel wall can take place. The fibrin component of a platelet thrombus forms beneath, not above, aggregating platelets[389] as was previously thought. The scaffold is removed when it is no longer needed by thrombolysis and the effects of macrophages.

The surface-active enzyme complexes (Fig. 10.3) are active on the phospholipid surfaces provided by platelets, leukocytes, and

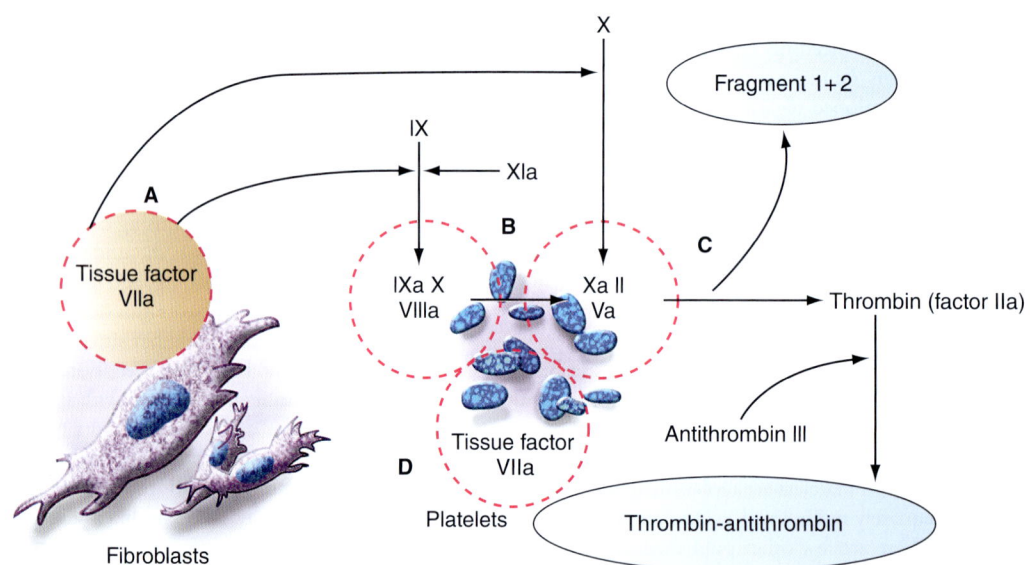

FIGURE 10.3 The key clotting factor enzyme complexes in coagulation. Tissue factor **(A)** (shown on the surface of a fibroblast) initiates coagulation, leading to the activation of clotting factors IX and X (shown on the surface of a platelet) and the processing of prothrombin (factor II) to form thrombin (factor IIa). Factor XIa has a contributory role in factor IX activation. Key to this cascade are three surface-active enzyme complexes: **A,** the complex of tissue factor and factor VIIa; **B,** the complex of factor IXa, factor VIIIa, and factor X; and **C,** the complex of factor Xa, factor Va, and factor II (where the letter "a" denotes the activated form of a factor). Prothrombin fragment 1 + 2 and thrombin-antithrombin complexes are markers of the generation of thrombin. Fragment 1 + 2 is an inactive fragment formed during the processing of prothrombin; thrombin-antithrombin complex is formed when antithrombin III binds to thrombin, resulting in the inactivation of thrombin. In addition, **D,** high doses of rFVIIa are able to generate thrombin in the presence of platelet-associated recombinant FVIIa and recombinant FVIIa can contribute to the assembly of the IXa-X-VIIIa complex via the activation of factor IX. Not shown in this diagram is the important influence of blood flow; for example, arteriolar and arterial velocity gradients, along with the presence of red cells, promote collisions between platelets and, consequently, platelet aggregation. (Modified with permission from Grabowski EF. The hemolytic-uremic syndrome toxin, thrombin, and thrombosis. *N Engl J Med.* 2002;346:58-64.)

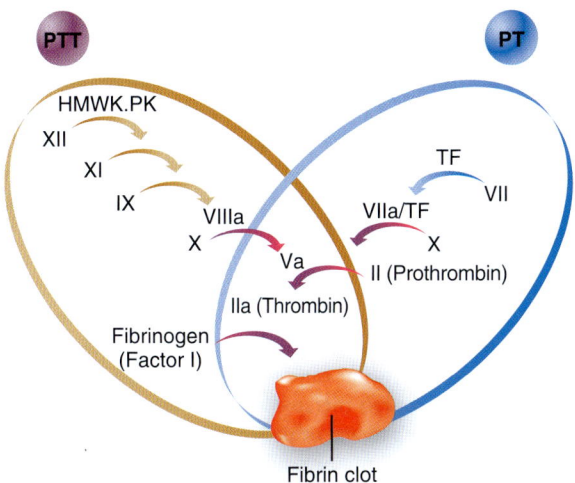

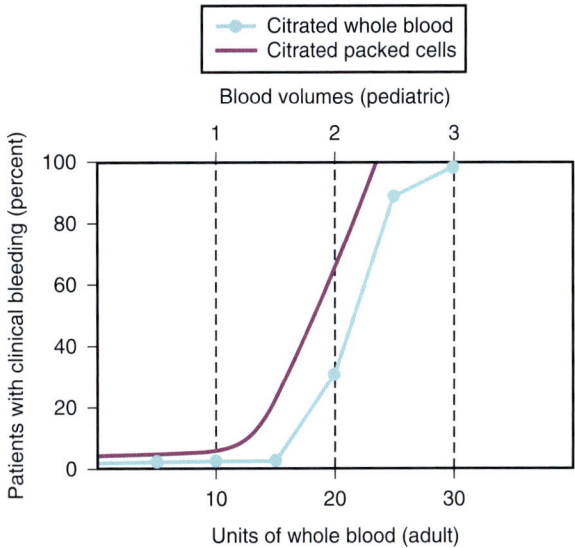

FIGURE 10.4 The conventional activated partial thromboplastin time (aPTT) is a measure of the intactness of the intrinsic coagulation system, which includes clotting factors XII, XI, IX, VIII, V, X, II, and I (fibrinogen). The prothrombin time *(PT)* is a measure of the intactness of the extrinsic coagulation system and encompasses tissue factor–bearing membrane surfaces and microparticles and factors VII, V, X, II, and I. In the PTT test, the blood does not need an exogenous agent to clot and comprises an *intrinsic* or complete clotting system. In practice, an agent such as diatomaceous earth is added to speed the reaction in the laboratory, and the term *activated* is added to the designation (aPTT). In the PT test, the blood clots by virtue of an *extrinsic* activator (i.e., tissue factor). This view in the diagram obscures the central role of tissue factor in clot initiation. Tissue factor *(TF)* circulates in an inactive form in the blood and is no longer considered only an extrinsic factor to the blood itself. *HMWK,* High-molecular-weight kininogen; *PK,* prekallikrein; *PTT,* partial thromboplastin time.

FIGURE 10.5 A study that considered the use of citrated whole blood *(blue line)* in adults found that bleeding in most cases resulted from dilutional thrombocytopenia. The *magenta line* represents estimated points of dilutional clotting factor deficiency if solely citrated packed cells are transfused. (Modified from Miller RD. Transfusion therapy and associated problems. *ASA Refresher Courses in Anesthesiology.* 1973;1:107.)

endothelial cells but not in the bulk of the blood. Initially it was believed that formation of the tissue factor/factor VIIa complex,[390] as shown, was critical for the action of recombinant FVIIa (rFVIIa) and for activation of factors IX and X. However, the high doses of rFVIIa necessary to achieve clinical hemostasis are far in excess of those required to saturate available tissue factor, suggesting that rFVIIa must also operate in large part independent of tissue factor,[391] especially in view of the observation that rFVIIa can bind to platelets directly via platelet anionic phospholipid[392] or via platelet GPIb.[391] In this regard, the conventional coagulation cascade shown in Fig. 10.4 is oversimplified, although it is a convenient approach to understanding the PT and partial thromboplastin times (PTT). All of the steps must be considered in the milieu of flowing blood, such that the high-velocity gradients of arterioles (i.e., mucous membranes of the uterus, gastrointestinal tract, upper respiratory tract, oral cavity, and gums) favor thrombi with a greater proportion of platelets (i.e., white thrombi), and low-velocity gradient states, such as those found in stasis or blood accumulation within a body cavity, favor a greater proportion of red cells (i.e., red thrombi). This explains why a patient with von Willebrand disease, characterized by a defect in the protein that allows blood platelets to adhere to a wound, tends to bleed from mucous membranes, sites of high-velocity (arteriolar) gradients, whereas a hemophiliac tends to bleed into joint spaces and muscle planes, sites of low- or near-zero–velocity gradients.

The coagulopathy associated with massive blood transfusions is usually attributable to the dilution of clotting factors or platelets, or both. The point at which the deficiency in clotting factors is sufficient to produce a coagulopathy depends on the volume of

blood lost and the type of blood component transfused (i.e., PRBCs or whole blood). Dilutional thrombocytopenia sufficient to cause clinical bleeding depends on the starting platelet count and the volume of blood replaced (Fig. 10.5). In some cases, the cause of bleeding is a consumptive coagulopathy such as fibrinolysis or disseminated intravascular coagulation (DIC).[123,393–413] In other scenarios, bleeding is caused by hypothermia, severe metabolic acidosis, poor tissue perfusion, and the release of tissue factors. Body temperature should be maintained by using efficient blood-warming devices, acidosis should be treated, and normovolemia and cardiac output should be restored to prevent a coagulopathy from developing.[400,414–417]

DILUTIONAL THROMBOCYTOPENIA

To formulate a plan to manage children who require massive blood transfusions, we must rely on our clinical experience, data extrapolated from adults and limited data from pediatric studies. A study of adult trauma patients during the Vietnam War reported that the onset of clinical bleeding occurred after about 15 units of *whole blood* or 1.5 blood volumes had been transfused (70 mL/kg in ideal 70-kg adult males). The incidence of coagulopathy was unrelated to an abnormal PT or PTT but correlated closely with a platelet count of less than 65,000 per cubic millimeter.[123,418] Studies of massive blood loss that was replaced with *whole blood* also support the notion that the associated coagulopathy results from thrombocytopenia rather than a deficiency in clotting factors.[123,400–409] Fig. 10.6 compares the calculated reduction in platelet count with the observed decline in platelet count in adults and children; when normalized for blood volumes shed, the observed changes were nearly identical. The observed and calculated decrements differ because platelets are mobilized from the bone marrow, spleen, lungs, and lymphatic tissues. The platelet count usually does not decrease to concentrations that may cause bleeding in children until 2.0 to 2.5 blood volumes have been shed[116] or until 20 to 25 units of *whole blood* have been transfused in adults.[116,407,419] Clinical bleeding does not usually

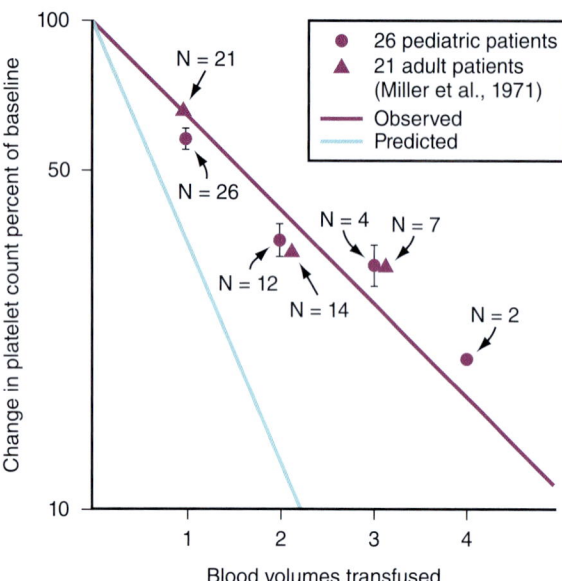

FIGURE 10.6 Percent of change in platelet count versus blood volumes transfused in young healthy adults and children.[116,123] The adult estimates assumed that these were ideal 70-kg men with a blood volume of 70 mL/kg such that 10 units of whole blood was estimated to be equivalent to 1 blood volume. The *magenta line* represents observed values, whereas the *blue line* represents calculated values. This difference suggests increased bone marrow production and/or splenic recruitment of platelets during massive transfusion. (From Miller RD, Robbins TO, Tong MJ, Barton SL. Coagulation defects associated with massive blood transfusions. *Ann Surg.* 1971;174:794-801; Coté CJ, Liu LM, Szyfelbein SK, et al. Changes in serial platelet counts following massive blood transfusions in pediatric patients. *Anesthesiology.* 1985;62:197-201.)

occur in children whose platelet counts exceed 50,000 per cubic millimeter, despite blood losses as great as 5.0 blood volumes (Fig. 10.7A).[116] Consequently, children should be monitored for thrombocytopenia and possible transfusion of platelets or clotting factor deficiency (see further) after the loss of the first 1.0 to 1.5 blood volumes. After the platelet count has decreased to 50,000 per cubic millimeter, it is likely that approximately one platelet dose (i.e., 6 units for an adult or 10–15 mL/kg for a child) will be required for each blood volume replaced. If a coagulopathy develops earlier than expected (i.e., before a 1.0-blood volume loss replaced with PRBCs and no platelets), a search should be initiated for other causes of bleeding, such as increased arterial or venous pressure in the surgical field or DIC.

Our study suggests that approximately 40% of the baseline platelet count is lost after 1.0 blood volume, 20% after the second, and an additional 10% after the third blood volume such that after 3.0 blood volumes are shed and replaced, the platelet count is generally ~30% of baseline. The starting platelet count is therefore exceedingly important to estimate how much blood loss can be tolerated before critical thrombocytopenia occurs. For example, with a starting platelet count of 600,000 per cubic millimeter, dilutional thrombocytopenia is unlikely to occur until 4.0 or more blood volumes have been shed, whereas with a starting count of 100,000 per cubic millimeter, dilutional thrombocytopenia should be anticipated after 1.0 blood volume has been shed (see Fig. 10.7B).

Although the primary platelet defect in massive transfusion is thrombocytopenia, some data suggest that platelets may not function normally (i.e., thrombocytopathy) after massive trauma, after cardiopulmonary bypass,[420] or in the presence of hypothermia.[416,421,422] This has not been our experience in the children we studied whose temperature remained within the normal range.[116,401] The only simple test to assess platelet function is the bleeding time. However, this test is also sensitive to thrombocytopenia and its predictive value is of equivocal utility.[396,421,423,424] The PFA-100 test shows less potential as a rapid screening tool than it once did because the device uses citrated blood warmed to 37°C and is relatively insensitive to milder defects in platelet-vessel wall interaction, such as that in mild von Willebrand disease. There remains a critical need for a point-of-care device or simple test to assess platelet function, as noted previously. Currently, the platelet count is our best indication for the need for platelet transfusions in situations involving rapid blood loss.[425] Other approaches such as thromboelastography to measure whole blood clotting have been used to guide transfusion therapy, but their efficacy in improving outcomes in trauma patients or patients undergoing major operative procedures has had mixed results.[426–439]

In several in vitro and animal model systems, recombinant factor VII (rFVIIa) activates factors IX and X on the surface of activated platelets, probably through the binding of rFVIIa to the platelet membrane (from which rFVIIa can also be taken up into storage sites within the platelet) and subsequent recruitment of circulating tissue factor. Although this has improved hemostasis in hemophiliacs with inhibitors to factor VIII,[440] there is limited evidence that rFVIIa reduces mortality for off-label use, as in cardiovascular surgery, trauma, and intracerebral hemorrhage.[433,441] Dosing in children appears to be greater than in adults, although this impression is anecdotal and has not been systematically investigated. rFVIIa is used increasingly in pediatric cardiac surgery although there is also an increased incidence of intravascular thrombosis,[442–447] hence its use should also consider the possibility of this sequela.

Basic clotting studies (e.g., PT, PTT, fibrinogen, platelet count) should be performed before elective surgery when major blood loss can be anticipated to determine the cause of underlying coagulopathies and provide adequate quantities of blood components.

FACTOR DEFICIENCY

Laboratory results for developing deficiencies in clotting factors are integral when managing component therapy in massive transfusions. The PT (for the extrinsic system) measures the adequacy of factors VII, X, V, prothrombin, and fibrinogen,[123] whereas the PTT (for the intrinsic system) measures the adequacy of factors XII, XI, IX, VIII, X, V, prothrombin, and fibrinogen (see Fig. 10.4). Banked *whole blood* contains normal plasma concentrations of all the clotting factors and regulatory proteins, except for factors V and VIII (which are 20%–50% of normal at the time of outdate), and factor VII. For a coagulopathy to develop with exclusive whole blood transfusion because of a clotting factor deficiency, the concentration of factor VIII must be less than 30% of normal and factor V less than 20%.[401] For these to occur, at least 3.0 blood volumes must be exchanged with *whole blood*. In this scenario, the first coagulation test that will be abnormal is the PTT because the concentration of factor VIII will be less than 30%.[397]

If blood loss is replaced exclusively with PRBCs during the initial treatment of a massive hemorrhage, as sometimes occurs, the amount of plasma that is transfused is minimal because ~70% was sequestered in the FFP fraction when it was separated. Massive replacement of blood loss with PRBCs and no other blood products quickly dilutes all of the clotting factors, including fibrinogen (see Fig. 10.4).[6,396–400,406,408,409,448–451] Hence, when a massive transfusion is anticipated, modern practice includes early transfusion of plasma and platelets along with RBCs, or alternatively whole blood.

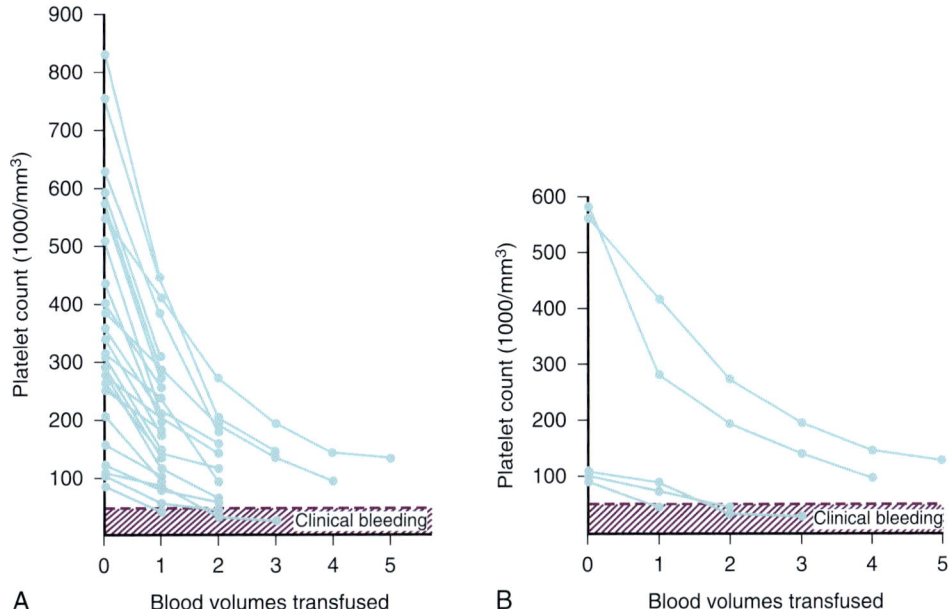

FIGURE 10.7 A, Serial changes in platelet counts are plotted for 26 pediatric patients whose blood loss was 1 to 5 blood volumes. Most of the children suffered from severe thermal injuries and many had relatively large platelet counts at baseline. Clinically evident signs of coagulopathy appeared when the platelet count decreased to less than 50,000/mm³. **B,** Platelet counts of five children abstracted from **A.** The baseline platelet count is invaluable in estimating potential platelet needs in relation to blood volumes transfused. A low initial count suggests the need for early exogenous platelet transfusion, whereas a high initial platelet count indicates that exogenous platelets may not be required until several blood volumes or more have been shed. The three children who developed a coagulopathy began surgery with a relatively low platelet count, whereas the two children with a very high platelet count did not require platelet transfusion despite losing 4 and 5 blood volumes. It should be noted that these children received sufficient fresh frozen plasma to maintain the prothrombin time and partial thromboplastin time within a normal range. (Reproduced with permission from Coté CJ, Liu LMP, Szyfelbein SK, et al. Changes in serial platelet counts following massive blood transfusions in pediatric patients. *Anesthesiology.* 1985;62:197-201.)

The PT and PTT are prolonged in children with multiple clotting factor deficiencies (e.g., during massive transfusion) at concentrations of clotting factors that are greater than in children with single clotting factor deficiencies (e.g., congenital coagulopathies).[408,409] This was also documented in adult patients who were transfused exclusively with PRBCs and crystalloid; the dilution of multiple clotting factors correlated with the volume of blood and crystalloid transfused.[345] Replacing 1.0 to 1.5 blood volumes exclusively with PRBCs and crystalloid dilutes clotting factors to approximately 30% of normal. Because moderately prolonged PT and PTT values exist without overt signs of clinical bleeding,[408] administration of FFP should be initiated with the onset of a clinical coagulopathy. However, the anesthesiologist should anticipate that PRBCs and crystalloid solutions or albumin will dilute the concentration of clotting factors so that FFP is begun after ~1.0 blood volume of blood loss has been replaced to avoid falling behind in the clotting indexes. A deficiency of fibrinogen (<80 mg/dL) may also be corrected by transfusing FFP, but marked deficiency, particularly in the presence of a consumptive coagulopathy (e.g., DIC, fibrinolysis), may require cryoprecipitate (0.2 to 0.4 unit/kg).[6,450,452-454]

Our experience includes a small study of 26 children (12 ± 4 years old, weight of 41.9 ± 15.8 kg) who underwent 22 Harrington rod procedures, three tumor excisions, and one Whipple procedure. These children received no FFP or whole blood, just PRBCs, despite losing between 0.5 and 1.0 blood volume. They exhibited no clinical signs of coagulopathy. Slight prolongations

of the PT or PTT occurred when the blood loss was equal to 1.0 blood volume or less (Table 10.9). Two children who lost 1.5 to 2.0 blood volumes exhibited prolonged PT and PTT values and one child who lost 2.0 blood volumes developed signs of a clinical coagulopathy.[455,456]

The magnitude of the increase in PT or PTT that is predictive of a clinical coagulopathy is not well defined. However, consensus panels suggest that when either clotting index exceeds 1.5 times normal (or INR >2.0),[457] it should be considered pathologic.[131,403,407,458-462] Our study suggests that the PT and PTT will be prolonged to more than 1.5 times normal when the blood loss is 1.5 blood volumes or more and the blood loss has been replaced with only PRBCs and crystalloid or 5% albumin.[455,456] Our clinical practice is to initiate FFP after losing 1.0 blood volume (Table 10.10). At that point, FFP should be administered in a ratio of 1 unit volume for every 2 units of PRBCs transfused. The indications for and timing of FFP depend on which blood product has been transfused, the volume of that transfusion as it relates to the child's blood volume, and whether the blood loss will continue perioperatively. The PT, PTT, fibrinogen concentration, and platelet count should be measured after each blood volume has been replaced and used to guide the need for additional FFP, platelets, and possible cryoprecipitate.

Recombinant factor VIIa (rFVIIa; NovoSeven)[463] is approved for use in the United States for hemophiliac patients with high-titer inhibitors and congenital factor VII deficiency. Anecdotal reports describe its effectiveness in controlling hemorrhage in a

TABLE 10.9 Changes in Prothrombin and Partial Thromboplastin Times During Massive Blood Transfusions in Children

PT and PTT Times (sec)	Baseline[a] (n = 26)	0.5 BV Loss (n = 16)	0.75 BV Loss (n = 12)	1.0 BV Loss (n = 10)
Prothrombin Time				
Mean ± SD	10.9 ± 0.96	12.5 ± 0.77	13.2 ± 0.76	13.6 ± 0.98
Range	9.3–12	11.4–14.0	11.4–14.2	11.9–15.8
Partial Thromboplastin Time				
Mean ± SD	31.8 ± 4.4	38.0 ± 4.9	40 ± 5.4	45.1 ± 13.1
Range	25–45.9	28.1–59.6	33–51.5	25.6–60.0

BV, Blood volume loss; *PT*, prothrombin; *PTT*, partial thromboplastin.
[a]Baseline normal values for blood volume may be greater in infants younger than 3 months.
NOTE: Not all children in this subset lost a half blood volume or more.

TABLE 10.10 Minimal Fresh Frozen Plasma Recommendations According to the Type of Blood Product Transfused and the Volume of Blood Lost

Type of Blood Replaced	FFP Indicated	Volume FFP to Be Transfused
Whole blood	After 2.0–3.0 blood volumes lost and each blood volume thereafter	25%–33% of each blood volume lost
PRBCs	After 1.0 blood volume lost and each blood volume thereafter	1 unit FFP/2 units PRBCs

FFP, Fresh frozen plasma; *PRBCs*, packed red blood cells.

variety of other settings including congenital heart disease.[1,2,464–469] However, in several randomized clinical trials during partial hepatectomy, liver transplantation, prostate surgery, pelvic (orthopedic) surgery, trauma, and upper gastrointestinal tract bleeding, rFVIIa failed to confer any benefit.[470–475] In a large randomized clinical trial of rFVIIa in children with intracranial hemorrhage, the largest-dose group showed only a small improvement in hematoma expansion, and 10% also experienced thromboembolic complications. In adults who received rFVIIa, the frequency of major thromboembolic complications was 1.4% to 10%, including acute myocardial infarction and stroke[476,477]; similarly thromboembolic events have been reported in children undergoing congenital cardiac surgery.[440,444,445,478] Until controlled trials demonstrate a clear benefit for its use, rFVIIa should be used with great caution for off-label indications,[465,470–475,479,480] and even then only for life-threatening bleeding.

Transfusion strategies in adult combat casualties have used fixed blood product ratios.[475,481] A consensus conference recommended an integrated approach to managing massive transfusion that included a foundation ratio of blood components directed by the results of standard coagulation testing (e.g., PT, PTT, platelet count, fibrinogen) or clot viscoelasticity, or both.[481] Some have proposed use of fixed ratios of blood components to start treating massive hemorrhages. Although civilian noncombat trauma studies of fixed ratio protocols have produced mixed results,[8,369,383] and

the largest prospective randomized controlled trial of civilian trauma patients found overall 24-hour and 30-day mortality was not impacted by the transfusion ratio. That trial found fewer deaths due to exsanguination in patients transfused initially at a 1:1:1 ratio of RBCs:plasma:platelets compared with those transfused initially at a ratio of 2:1:1.[482] Additionally, there is mounting evidence regarding reduced blood loss and improved outcomes supporting the early use of an antifibrinolytic medication (e.g., tranexamic acid; see also Chapter 18).[376–379,385,481,483–487]

The dilutional coagulopathy associated with massive blood transfusion is reasonably predictable. Fresh whole blood contains platelets but depending on the filters used during preparation, whole blood might may have reduced concentrations of platelets. However, some filters allow platelets to remain in whole blood and those platelets which have been in chilled whole blood still function soon after being transfused in pediatric trauma patients.[147] When using exclusively whole blood, dilutional thrombocytopenia can develop first and this may occur as early as after the first blood volume has been replaced (if the initial platelet count is <100,000 cubic millimeters or less). In most cases, clotting factors (particularly factors V and VIII) are not diluted until the blood loss exceeds 3.0 blood volumes. On the other hand, when PRBCs are exclusively used to replace shed blood, all the clotting factors and platelets may be diluted after as little as 1.0 blood volume is lost. However, the predictable coagulopathy of dilution is only an approximate guide. The PT, PTT, fibrinogen, and platelet count should be assessed during massive transfusions to guide replacement therapy.

DISSEMINATED INTRAVASCULAR COAGULATION AND FIBRINOLYSIS

DIC and fibrinolysis are frequently associated with shock, trauma, and other forms of tissue damage, with release of procoagulants (e.g., tissue factor) and fibrinolytics (e.g., tissue plasminogen activator). In the presence of massive blood loss, these processes must be differentiated from dilutional coagulopathy. Differentiation may be difficult, because both are associated with pathologic oozing of blood in the surgical field and each may result in prolongation of the PT and PTT, as well as thrombocytopenia.[488–492] With massive replacement using whole blood or PRBCs and *adequate* FFP, the fibrinogen concentration should remain normal; with uncompensated (acute) DIC, it may be decreased. However, replacing the blood loss with PRBCs, albumin, and crystalloid also reduces the fibrinogen concentration.

The most helpful test for DIC and fibrinolysis is documentation of an increased concentration of D-dimer, a small peptide fragment generated during the digestion of fibrin by ongoing thrombolysis (i.e., through plasmin), along with evidence on the peripheral blood smear of schistocytes and helmet cells (i.e., microangiopathic hemolytic anemia).[492–495] Abnormal RBCs and RBC fragments arise from the slicing action of immobilized fibrin strands in the microcirculation, although the precise mechanism remains unknown. A scoring system to screen for potential DIC has been developed but not evaluated in the operating room setting.[496,497] If pathologic oozing in the surgical field is observed and 1.0 blood volume or less has been lost in a child who had a normal platelet count and PT and PTT values preoperatively, the child may have developed a consumptive coagulopathy.

The most effective treatment for DIC is to eliminate the cause, such as correcting shock, acidosis, or sepsis.[490–492] Heparin therapy remains controversial even in children with thrombotic manifestations of DIC. It is not advisable in children with active bleeding, especially in the operative setting.[489,494,495,498]

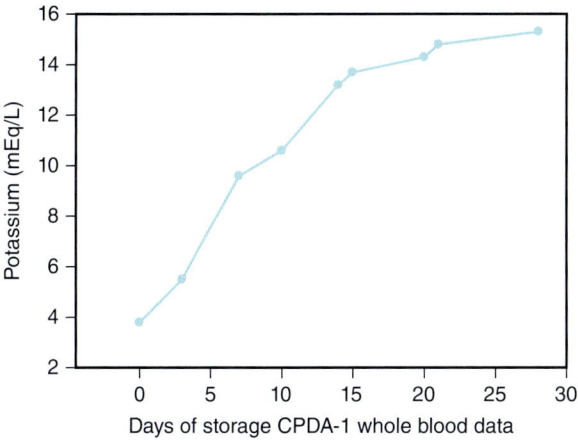

FIGURE 10.8 Changes in potassium concentrations (mEq/L) (mEq/L = mmol/L) over time in citrate, phosphate, dextrose, and adenine solution (CPDA-1) whole blood. (Data abstracted from: Antwi-Baffour S, Adjei JK, Tsyawo F, Kyeremeh R, Botchway FA, Seidu MA. A study of the change in sodium and potassium ion concentrations in stored donor blood and their effect on electrolyte balance of recipients. *Biomed Res Int.* 2019;2019:8162975; Namjoshi A, Bhatia GM, Chaudhari AS, Trimbake S. Effect of blood storage on electrolyte levels. *Int J Res Med Sci.* 1921;9:438-442.)

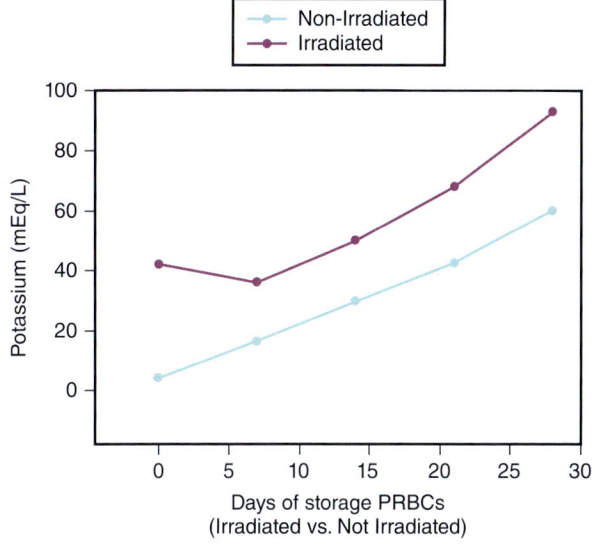

FIGURE 10.9 Changes in potassium values in packed red blood cells *(PRBCs) (purple line)* and irradiated PRBCs *(blue line)* over time (mEq/L = mmol/L). (Data extracted from: Balasubramanyam P, Basavarajegowda A, Hanumanthappa N, Negi VS, Harichandrakumar KT. Irradiating stored blood and storing irradiated blood: is it different? - A study of serial changes in biochemical parameters of red blood cell units. *Asian J Transfus Sci.* 2021; 15(2):172-178.)

HYPERKALEMIA

RBCs leak K^+ into the extracellular fluid during storage, particularly as the units of blood age (Fig. 10.8).[499–504] The concentration of adenosine triphosphate (ATP) decreases, and the ATPase-driven sodium (Na^+)/K^+ pump activity decreases. One study examined the changes in K^+ over time with 30 units of CPDA-1 preserved whole blood; the K^+ blood concentration increased from 3.53 millimole per liter (3.53 mEq/L) on day 1 to 15.36 millimole per liter (15.35 mEq/L) on day 28 (see Fig. 10.8).[500,501] Another study of stored whole blood found that the serum K^+ values increased from 7.31 millimole per liter (7.31 mEq/L) on day 1 to 20.14 millimole per liter (20.14 mEq/L) on day 35.[502] Since the volume of extracellular fluid is different for whole blood and packed RBCs collected in CPDA-1 or Additive-Solution systems, the concentration of K^+ is the greatest in CPDA-1 packed RBCs and least in CPDA-1 whole blood units (E-Table 10.3). The K^+ leak from blood that has been irradiated is doubled and more rapid than from untreated RBCs and increases further with the duration of blood storage (Fig. 10.9).[150,501,505–507] Irradiated RBCs may be stored for a maximum of 28 days compared with 35 or 42 days for whole blood or PRBCs respectively.

Clinically important hyperkalemia has not been reported when blood is slowly transfused (50–150 mL/hour) through peripheral IV lines in children 1 to 14 years of age,[508] but has occurred in children after a rapid transfusion, particularly through a central venous line.[509–516] In a summary of published studies of cardiac arrests, electromechanical dissociation and ventricular tachycardia in children from neonates to 17 years of age, 15 were neonates and 9 were 1 to 12 months of age.[517] The maximum K^+ concentration reported posttransfusion was 14.2 milliequivalents per liter in a neonate after resection of a posterior-fossa mass; 12 died, 19 survived, and in 8, the outcome was not described. The rate of increase in extracellular K^+ is estimated to be ~1 milliequivalent per liter per day of storage,[84,518] thus, the older the blood the greater the K^+ concentration; concentrations as great as 40 to 90 milliequivalents per liter have been reported

in PRBCs.[518–520] A retrospective study of children undergoing massive intraoperative, but slow transfusions with PRBCs documented transient, but not life-threatening, hyperkalemia.[521] It appears that clinically important hyperkalemia does not usually occur when PRBCs are administered *at normal, slow infusion rates through peripheral IV access.*[508,522–524] This may be explained by the combination of the small absolute amount of K^+ (~6 mEq), its rapid reabsorption into the K^+-depleted, transfused RBCs, the large volume of distribution, and dilution with crystalloid or albumin during administration. Hyperkalemic cardiac arrest in the setting of massive transfusion is usually the consequence of extensive tissue injury, an extremely rapid transfusion (e.g., rapid-infusion devices),[517] acidemia resulting from inadequate tissue perfusion (low cardiac output state), transfusing blood directly into the heart without time for electrolyte equilibration,[517] hypovolemia, hypothermia, and hypocalcemia.[525] In a retrospective single institution review of 16 patients, of whom two-thirds were adults and one-third children who experienced transfusion-associated hyperkalemic cardiac arrest, the cardiac arrest occurred after 1 unit of PRBCs in a 2-day-old neonate up to 54 units of PRBCs in an adult. The presenting cardiac rhythm was pulseless electrical activity, ventricular fibrillation, ventricular tachycardia, or asystole. Serum K^+ concentrations at the time of these events ranged from 5.9 to 9.2 milliequivalents per liter, with a 12.5% hospital survival rate.[525] A K^+ adsorption filter is under investigation in Japan and may hold promise for reducing the risk for hyperkalemia in neonates and infants or during rapid transfusions in the future.[526–529]

The need to relate the size of the patient to the rate of blood transfusion is infrequently a problem in adults, but it is vitally important to consider in an infant or small child. An alert from the Society for Pediatric Anesthesia[530] described four deaths among 11 children who developed hyperkalemia during transfusion; 8 were younger than 1 year of age, and 6 were younger than 6 months old. The Perioperative Cardiac Arrest Registry reported eight hyperkalemic cardiac arrests related to blood transfusion.[530,531] Hyperkalemia may become a problem when large volumes of whole blood or PRBCs are administered very rapidly in adults (rates ≥120 mL/minute) and in infants and children undergoing rapid blood transfusion, particularly through a central venous catheter.[532] A rapid-transfusion rate of 120 milliliters per minute in a 70-kilogram adult is equivalent to 1.5 to 2 milliliters per kilogram per minute of blood, which is relatively easy to infuse in an infant or small child using a pressure bag or a rapid-transfusion device. An adult sustained a cardiac arrest and died after receiving Adsol-preserved PRBCs with a supernatant K⁺ concentration of 24 to 34 milliequivalents per liter at a transfusion rate of 6.4 milliliters per kilogram per minute through a rapid-infusion device (see Chapter 49).[533] Similar and greater transfusion rates are possible in infants and children without such devices.[514,521,534,535]

The principle to prevent hyperkalemia-associated cardiac arrest is to avoid falling behind when replacing blood loss and a situation in which a rapid and massive infusion of blood is required. Warming the blood and administering it through a peripheral IV line (rather than a central venous catheter) reduces the risks of hyperkalemia on the cardiac conduction system.[516] When the rate of infusion of whole blood or PRBCs exceeds 1.5 to 2.0 milliliters per kilogram per minute, the electrocardiogram (ECG) must be closely monitored.[536,537] If ventricular arrhythmias occur with peaked T waves in the setting of hyperkalemia (see Fig. 7.7), appropriate treatment should be instituted (e.g., calcium chloride or calcium gluconate), hyperventilation, sodium bicarbonate, albuterol/salbutamol, glucose and insulin (see Table 26.6); Kayexalate is the slowest and least effective intervention in this situation and is not recommended as an acute intervention. Preoperative washing of PRBCs with autotransfusion devices has been recommended to avoid hyperkalemia in pediatric patients who require rapid, massive blood transfusion.[538]

Rapid, massive transfusion of whole blood or PRBCs to a neonate, particularly blood that has been stored for several weeks, can cause hyperkalemic cardiac arrest.[509–516] It is common practice to administer RBC-containing components that are relatively young to avoid hyperkalemia in neonates requiring massive blood transfusion. If relatively young units are not available and time permits, it may be possible to wash the PRBCs to reduce the K⁺ concentration.[539] However, RBC transfusion to an actively bleeding infant should not be delayed to obtain PRBCs that are less than 7 days old or to wash the units. Similarly, blood for intrauterine transfusion, exchange transfusion, or for neonates should be relatively young (usually <7 days).

These practices are consistent with the recommendations from the Society for Pediatric Anesthesia Wake Up Safe quality improvement initiative, which suggests that anesthesiologists anticipate large blood losses, transfuse early, and thus transfuse the hypovolemic child slowly through a peripheral IV catheter rather than rapidly through a central venous catheter.[516,530] If the infant requires irradiated RBC blood components, it is preferable to transfuse them soon after irradiating the blood or to wash the PRBCs to minimize the K⁺ concentration.

HYPOCALCEMIA AND CITRATE TOXICITY

Citrate works as an anticoagulant for stored blood components by chelating ionized calcium (iCa^{2+}). As citrate in the blood component is transfused, it is rapidly taken up and metabolized by nucleated cells in the body, although the primary site for clearance is the liver. During massive transfusion, particularly of whole blood or FFP, the influx of citrate may temporarily overwhelm

the child's capacity to clear it, resulting in its accumulation, which causes the plasma concentration of iCa^{2+} to rapidly decrease.[366,540–546] The residual plasma fraction in a unit of PRBCs, which contains the citrate, is a much smaller volume than in a unit of whole blood or FFP. Clinically, it is rare for the iCa^{2+} level to decrease unless the transfusion rate is very rapid; in adults, this rate is 1.0 or more units of whole blood (≥7 mL/kg) or FFP (≥4 mL/kg) in 3 to 4 minutes (or 2 mL/kg/minute whole blood or 1 mL/kg/minute FFP).[540] This effect on the iCa^{2+} concentration has been reported in neonates undergoing exchange transfusion and is more likely to occur in more-premature and lower-weight infants.[544] Pulseless electrical activity has been reported in two preterm infants who developed hypocalcemia during dilutional transfusion with FFP.[544,547] In adult cardiac surgical patients who received whole blood at 1.5 milliliters per kilogram per minute, the ventricular function curve did not improve (i.e., cardiac output did not increase although the iCa^{2+} decreased). When a similar volume of heparinized blood was administered at the same rate, the Frank-Starling response to volume loading was normal (i.e., cardiac output increased, but iCa^{2+} level did not change).[548] These case reports and the adult cardiac surgical study confirm that a decrease in iCa^{2+} concentration of clinical importance (i.e., decreased cardiac contractility) may be expected when the rate of infusion of citrated whole blood or FFP exceeds 1.5 to 2.0 milliliters per kilogram per minute.[540,548]

The change in the iCa^{2+} concentration after transfusion of large volumes of PRBCs is much less than that observed with whole blood or FFP since only ~30% of the plasma containing citrate remains in PRBCs. Although measurable decreases in the iCa^{2+} concentration have been observed during rapid transfusion, they have only rarely been associated with cardiac toxicity in adults. The rates of infusion of citrated whole blood that produce hypocalcemia and hyperkalemia are almost identical, whereas the cardiac electrophysiologic effects produced by hypocalcemia and hyperkalemia are opposite. It is important to observe the ECG for abnormalities (see Fig. 7.7), especially widening of the QRS complex, prolonged QT interval, and peaking of the T wave.[401,549] With the renewed interest in using whole blood during rapid transfusion, this complication must be anticipated.[101,106,368,550,551]

Both hypocalcemia and hyperkalemia are treated by the administration of exogenous calcium. Evidence from healthy animals and children with extensive thermal injuries demonstrated that calcium chloride and calcium gluconate dissociate at similar rates; *hepatic metabolism of the gluconate moiety is not necessary* (Fig. 10.10).[552] Studies during the anhepatic phase of liver transplantation reported a similar degree of ionization of calcium chloride and calcium gluconate, confirming that hepatic metabolism is not required to ionize calcium from calcium gluconate.[553] Calcium chloride and calcium gluconate are both indicated to treat acute ionized hypocalcemia, with the caveat that calcium gluconate, which contains one-third of the ionizable calcium of calcium chloride (by weight), be administered at a 3-fold greater dose (milligrams per kilogram) than the latter. Frequent, small boluses are as effective as single large boluses and result in smaller fluctuations in plasma iCa^{2+} values.[552] Ideally, both forms of calcium should be slowly administered through a large peripheral or central vein, because both are sclerosing medications.

The volume of plasma and therefore the absolute amount of citrate in a unit of FFP are slightly less than the amounts in a unit of whole blood but the concentration of citrate per unit volume is greater. Therefore, the citrate load can be more rapidly delivered with FFP because it can be infused more rapidly owing to its low

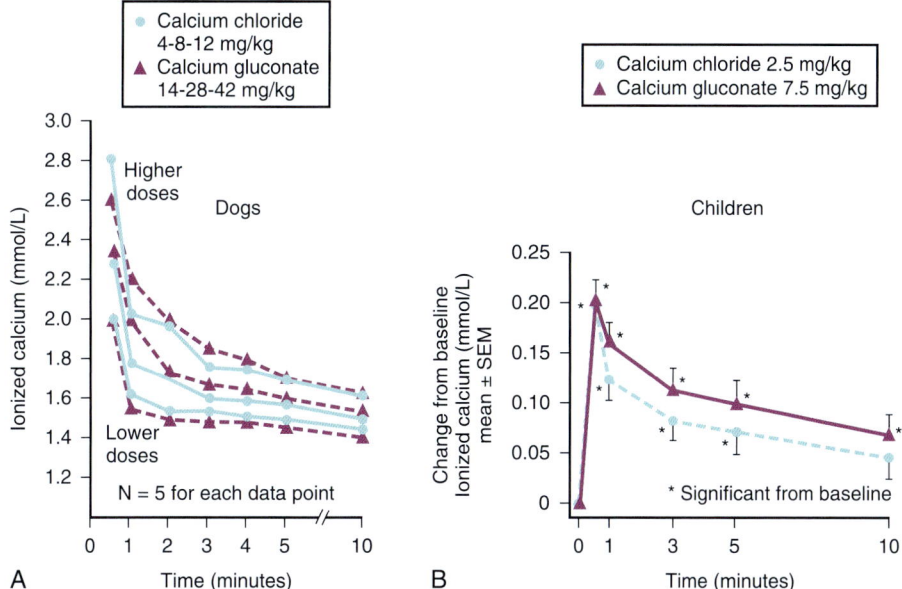

FIGURE 10.10 A, Changes in arterial ionized calcium (iCa²⁺) levels in dogs after three equal elemental calcium doses of calcium chloride (4, 8, and 12 mg/kg) or calcium gluconate (14, 28, and 42 mg/kg). The rate of change in the iCa²⁺ concentration was identical for each form of calcium at each dose. There was no significant difference between the largest and smallest doses after 2 minutes, suggesting that frequent small doses are equally effective and perhaps safer than large boluses of exogenous calcium. **B,** Changes in arterial iCa²⁺ levels in children who received equal elemental doses of calcium chloride and calcium gluconate. At 30 seconds, both forms of calcium dissociated equally; these data indicate that hepatic metabolism of the gluconate moiety is not required to liberate ionized calcium from calcium gluconate. *SEM,* Standard error of mean. (From Coté CJ, Drop LJ, Daniels AL, Hoaglin DC. Calcium chloride versus calcium gluconate: comparison of ionization and cardiovascular effects in children and dogs. *Anesthesiology.* 1987;66:465-470.)

viscosity; it is easy to give a large citrate load in a brief period. Caution is urged when FFP or whole blood is rapidly infused, especially if the child already has a low iCa²⁺ concentration or impaired hepatic function (e.g., neonates and children undergoing liver transplantation).[547] Fig. 10.11A shows the changes in iCa²⁺ concentrations that occurred in children who had extensive thermal injuries and who received rapid FFP infusions at 1.0 to 2.5 milliliters per kilogram per minute for 5 minutes. The maximum decrease in iCa²⁺ levels occurred between the fourth and fifth minutes with a similar nadir in the iCa²⁺ concentration in the three fastest rates of FFP infusion.[554] It should be noted that children with burn injury are hypermetabolic and likely to metabolize the citrate more rapidly than children without a burn injury (see further).

If exogenous calcium is administered *during* rapid FFP transfusion, large decreases in the iCa²⁺ level can be avoided (see Fig. 10.11B). We transfused FFP at 2 milliliters per kilogram per minute for 10 minutes (equivalent to an average adult receiving 1400 mL FFP over 10 minutes) in six children with extensive burn injuries and despite decreases in iCa²⁺ levels, found no consistent adverse circulatory changes. However, because these children had extensive burn injuries, we presumed they were hypermetabolic with a high cardiac output and therefore able to metabolize the excess citrate more rapidly. This would ameliorate the effect on iCa²⁺ values resulting in a more rapid recovery after the transfusion is stopped in the burn population compared with children without burn injury or those who are hypothermic or in a low cardiac output state. Although this has not been systematically examined in a nonburn population, we would expect a more profound decrease in iCa²⁺ at similar FFP infusion rates.[554]

Another issue of concern is the combined effects of inhalation agents and low iCa²⁺. In dogs anesthetized with halothane, we determined that citrate-induced ionized hypocalcemia caused greater cardiovascular depression as the expired concentration of halothane increased.[555] These findings are consistent with the combined myocardial depression caused by ionized hypocalcemia and calcium channel blockade caused by the halothane.[556,557] Although halothane exerts the greatest calcium channel blocking activity of the inhalational anesthetics, all inhalational anesthetics including sevoflurane depress the myocardium through this mechanism to some extent as well as through other mechanisms involving calcium flux, which augments the myocardial dysfunction associated with citrate-induced ionized hypocalcemia.[558–561] Thus the combination of inhalation anesthetic agent and the need for rapid administration of citrated blood products can produce an additive depression of cardiac function.

The adverse cardiac effects of citrate-induced hypocalcemia may be increased if FFP is rapidly administered through a central venous catheter because there is less time to dilute the FFP and metabolize the citrate before it enters the heart and coronary vessels. FFP may be more safely administered through a peripheral IV line. Calcium should be administered *during* rapid transfusion of FFP or whole blood (>1 mL/kg per minute) to attenuate this transient but potentially dangerous citrate toxicity, especially in the presence of potent inhalational anesthetics.[555–559] Neonates and small infants are particularly vulnerable to developing citrate toxicity because it is easier to administer a relatively large volume of FFP, whole blood, or platelets over a brief period and because citrate may not be eliminated as rapidly (i.e., first-pass effect through the liver) in infants.[547,562] In addition to thermally injured patients, children undergoing liver transplantation and

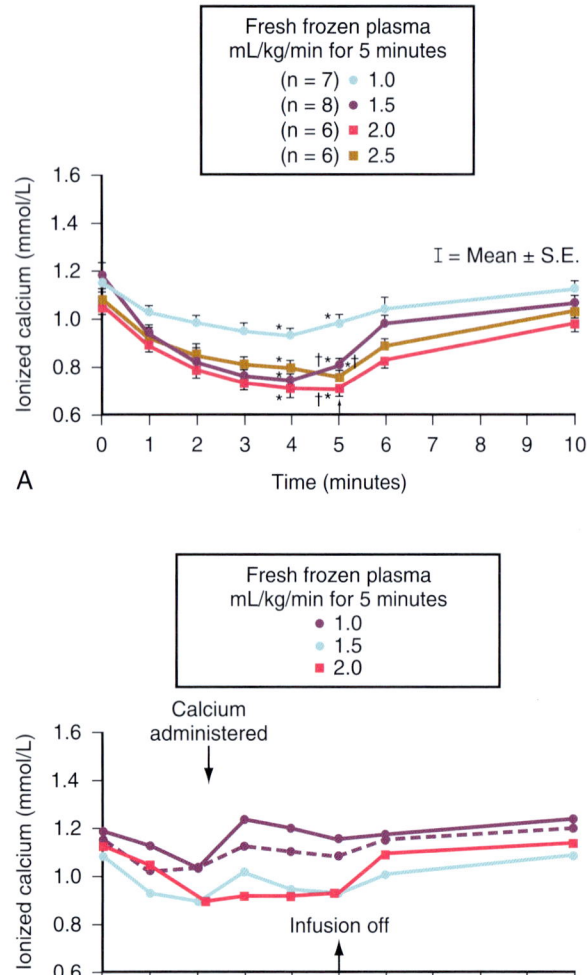

FIGURE 10.11 A, Changes in arterial ionized calcium (iCa²⁺) levels in children with severe thermal injuries during infusions of fresh frozen plasma at a rate of 1.0 to 2.5 mL/kg per minute for 5 minutes using an infusion pump. Notice the dangerous although transient decrease in the iCa²⁺ concentration, with the nadir occurring between the fourth and fifth minutes. Ionized hypocalcemia occurs when the infusion rate equals or exceeds 1 mL/kg per minute. **B,** Changes in iCa²⁺ levels occurred in four thermally injured children who received calcium chloride *(arrow)* after 2 minutes of fresh frozen plasma infusion. There were no sharp increases or decreases in iCa²⁺ levels. *SE,* Standard error. (From Coté CJ, Drop LJ, Hoaglin DC, et al. Ionized hypocalcemia after fresh frozen plasma administration to thermally injured children: effects of infusion rate, duration, and treatment with calcium chloride. *Anesth Analg.* 1988;67:152-160.)

cardiac surgery are likely to require FFP and develop hypocalcemia.[563,564] Liver transplantation recipients and patients with hepatic failure[565] are particularly susceptible to decreased iCa²⁺ levels during the anhepatic phase and the preanhepatic phase of surgery because of impaired hepatic blood flow and the reduced ability to metabolize citrate.[566–570] An IV preparation of calcium should always be available when a major transfusion with whole blood or FFP is anticipated.

ACID-BASE BALANCE

Massive transfusions usually occur in one of two situations: severe trauma with shock or major surgery with massive blood loss. In the first situation, severe metabolic acidosis may occur because of low cardiac output, hypothermia, and diminished oxygen delivery. Correction of the acidosis may be a necessary part of the resuscitation, along with blood volume replacement.[367,571] In this situation, impaired coagulation may occur because of the acidosis.[398,414,572–574] In the operating room, intravascular volume is usually maintained, and because most instances of massive blood loss are anticipated, replacement of acute blood loss is more controlled, thus avoiding metabolic acid production.[575–577] After a massive blood transfusion, a moderate to severe metabolic alkalosis[578] caused by the large volume of transfused citrate and its conversion to bicarbonate is common.[541,564,579–581] Thus it is important to determine the acid-base status *before* administering sodium bicarbonate to avoid overcorrecting the pH and shifting the oxyhemoglobin dissociation curve further to the left.

HYPOTHERMIA

Hypothermia may contribute to problems associated with major blood loss and its replacement. Although hypothermia decreases oxygen consumption and reduces oxygen demand, it may also increase oxygen consumption if the child shivers and decrease tissue delivery of oxygen by a leftward shift of the oxygen-hemoglobin dissociation curve as well as induce a refractory ventricular tachycardia in the presence of severe hypothermia (about 32°C).[401,582] Hypothermia may also profoundly compromise platelet function and impair the coagulation cascade.[398,414–416,572,573,583–585]

Prevention of hypothermia by all available means is considered an essential part of neonatal care[586] and damage-control resuscitation of trauma patients.[587–590] Hypothermia (<34°C in adults) by itself is an independent risk factor for mortality.[591] Banked blood products are stored between room temperature (21°C) and 4°C, depending on the blood component. In the setting of large transfusion volumes, all blood products should be infused through a blood warmer. No other method should be considered (e.g., storing blood in a warming cupboard, immersing in hot water, microwave) because RBCs hemolyze readily with prolonged warming or overheating (>42°C). Warming blood and all other IV infusions with a high-capacity blood warmer, using hot air warming blankets and radiant warmers, placing plastic wrap around extremities, inserting a heated humidifier in the anesthesia circuit, covering the child's head, and maintaining a warm to hot operating room contribute to maintaining thermal neutrality. Rapid-transfusion devices markedly improve the rapidity of warming blood products and other life-saving fluids.[592–598] In one case, one author (CJC) and two nurses transfused more than 50 liters of blood products and crystalloid in less than 1 hour to a 60-kilogram 12 year old, while maintaining the child's temperature at 34.5°C or greater using the Rapid-Infusion System (Haemonetics Corp., Braintree, MA) which is equivalent to two Belmont Rapid Infuser devices (Belmont Medical Technologies, Billerica, MA).[592]

MONITORING DURING MASSIVE BLOOD TRANSFUSION

If massive blood loss can be anticipated, adequate monitoring should be instituted *before* surgery begins so that baseline information can be recorded. Large-bore peripheral IV access is preferable (E-Fig. 10.2) because these catheters have reduced resistance and they deposit blood products into the peripheral circulation (avoiding hypothermia and hyperkalemia in the heart), unlike a high resistance central venous pressure (CVP) line. If a child arrives in the operating room in shock (e.g., trauma patient), the physician must be careful to differentiate hypovolemia from other causes of shock (e.g., tension pneumothorax, cardiac tamponade) (see Chapters 37 and 38); invasive monitoring may assist in diagnosing the cause of the child's volume status. Our philosophy is one of aggressive invasive monitoring to provide maximum data to evaluate and manage a critically hypovolemic child.

1. Routine ASA monitors; a pulse oximeter placed on the tongue may be particularly valuable in a child who is vasoconstricted, hypothermic, or without peripheral pulses.[599,600] Hypovolemia may occasionally manifest as pulsus paradoxus, identified with a pulse oximeter.[601]

2. A urinary catheter quantifies the urine output and assesses organ perfusion and intravascular volume status in the presence of normal renal function.

3. An arterial catheter continuously monitors systemic blood pressure, allows for serial arterial blood gas sampling for analysis as well as hematocrit, glucose, calcium, K^+, and clotting parameters. The adequacy of the circulating blood volume may be inferred from the shape of the arterial waveform, the presence of the dicrotic notch, and the absence of exaggerated respiratory variation (Fig. 10.12).

4. A CVP line provides critical data on the child's volume status, and its ease and safety of insertion have been demonstrated in children of all sizes[602]; ultrasound improves the success and safety of insertion.[603,604] CVP readings vary depending on the location of the catheter tip and whether there is rapidly infusing fluid in the same catheter.[605,606] In the latter case, the infusions should be interrupted intermittently to obtain accurate readings. It is our clinical impression that in healthy, anesthetized, supine children, a very small but sustained change in CVP (2–3 mm Hg) may represent a

change of as much as 10% to 15% of a child's blood volume. In most children, right-sided pressures correlate closely with left-sided pressures; the right atrial CVP usually is an accurate indicator of cardiac filling pressures of both ventricles. A CVP line provides access for blood sampling and a reliable site for IV administration of medications, fluid, and blood. However, a CVP line cannot always be relied on as a volume administration line because resistance is large if using a narrow lumen for central access. A centrally placed introducer is a reliable volume line; however, it is preferred to give rapid transfusions through a peripheral catheter so as to reduce the potential for hyperkalemic, hypocalcemic, or hypothermia-induced cardiac arrest.[516,530]

5. Continuous noninvasive cardiac output devices may provide further clinical guidance (see Figs. 49.11 and 49.12).[51,607,608]

Monitors and the data they generate are helpful, but anesthesiologists must rely on more than numbers. It serves no purpose to have sophisticated monitoring if the data provided cannot be interpreted and related to clinical events. The final monitor is ultimately the anesthesiologist's vigilance and judgment.

Viscoelastography such as thromboelastography (TEG), rotational thromboelastometry (ROTEM), and sonorheometry, provide standardized means for quantitating the rapidity and quality of clot formation.[429,432,435–439,609] TEG and ROTEM use stirring rods and the timing of resistance to the stirring rods generate tracings that then can be used to provide guidance regarding factor deficiencies (dilutional coagulopathy), platelet dysfunction or deficiency (dilutional thrombocytopenia), hypercoagulation (over administration of clotting factors and platelets), and fibrinolysis.[610–612] Figs. 10.13 and 10.14 illustrate classic thromboelastograms. A new device, the *Quantra sonic estimation of elasticity via resonance* uses changes in ultrasound measurement of clot formation with results comparable to TEG and ROTEM.[435–439] All three now use cartridges, which greatly simplifies their use and reduces the volume of blood needed.

These devices are used primarily during massive blood transfusions related to liver transplantation, trauma, and cardiac surgery.[430,587,589,610,611,613–622] Some studies have found that thromboelastographic screening was not useful in predicting bleeding after cardiac surgery whereas others have demonstrated reduced transfusion requirements.[623–626] The use of heparinase improves the accuracy of the results by eliminating the effects of heparin.[627] A systematic review of 17 adult studies found the proportion of patients receiving RBCs, FFP, and platelets was reduced, but without a difference in surgical reinterventions or mortality.[431] One Cochrane study, limited to ROTEM use in adult trauma patients, found inadequate predictive value to diagnose trauma-induced coagulopathy[628]; another systematic review of both TEG and ROTEM in adult trauma patients found limited positive data suggesting the early diagnosis of trauma-induced coagulopathy but inadequate data regarding transfusions and mortality.[629] These monitors have also been used to guide the effectiveness of antifibrinolytic therapy.[618,619,630] The exact role of thromboelastography, thromboelastometry, or sonorheometry in the routine care of pediatric cardiac surgical patients,[625] liver transplant recipients, and children who have had massive blood loss with ongoing coagulopathy has not been fully established but some studies suggest that TEG might be of value in assessing the coagulation defect in massive transfusion.[426,434,631,632] It should be noted that there are several subtypes of ROTEM available that modify these tests such as INTEM, for the intrinsic pathway; EXTEM, for the extrinsic pathway; HEPTEM, using heparinase to guide protamine

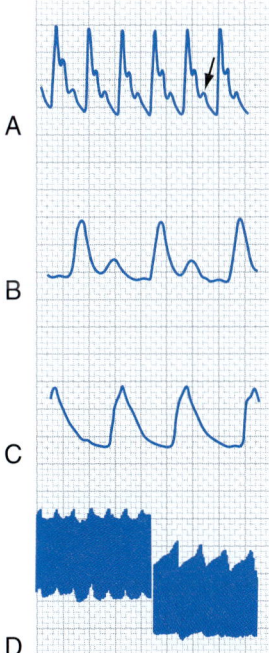

FIGURE 10.12 Changes in the contour of an arterial tracing with hypovolemia. **A,** The normal tracing shows a sharp upswing of the arterial pulse wave and position of the dicrotic notch *(arrow)*. **B,** There is movement of the dicrotic notch and widening of the pulse wave. **C,** The pulse wave widens further. **D,** There is further widening of the pulse wave and loss of the dicrotic notch. An exaggerated ("picket fence") respiratory variation of pulse wave is shown in the *right* tracing compared with the *left*. Factors other than hypovolemia, such as hypothermia, deep anesthesia, vasodilator therapy, or damped tracing (e.g., clot, air bubble), may produce artifactual changes in the shape of the arterial waveform.

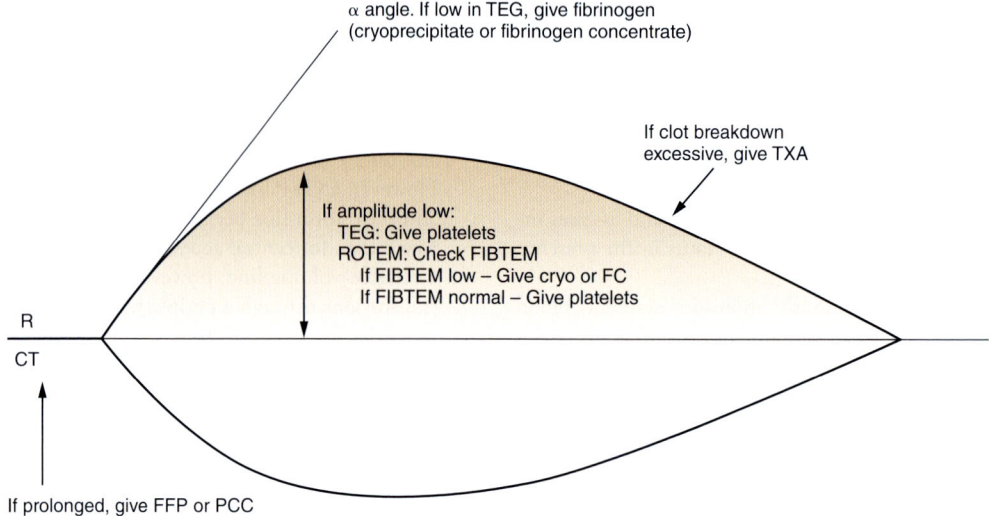

α angle. If low in TEG, give fibrinogen
(cryoprecipitate or fibrinogen concentrate)

If clot breakdown
excessive, give TXA

If amplitude low:
TEG: Give platelets
ROTEM: Check FIBTEM
If FIBTEM low – Give cryo or FC
If FIBTEM normal – Give platelets

R

CT

If prolonged, give FFP or PCC

FIGURE 10.13 General transfusion guidance based on viscoelastic analysis. Notice the need for the additional *FIBTEM* analysis if using a rotational thromboelastometry *(ROTEM)* viscoelastic analyzer. Therapeutic options are the same for both thromboelastography *(TEG)* and ROTEM. cryo, Cryoprecipitate; *CT,* clotting time; *FC,* fibrinogen concentrate; *FFP,* fresh frozen plasma; *PCC,* prothrombin complex concentrate; *R,* reaction time; *TXA,* tranexamic acid. (Reproduced with permission from Abdelfattah K, Cripps MW. Thromboelastography and rotational thrombo-elastometry use in trauma. *Int J Surg.* 2016;33:196-201.[867])

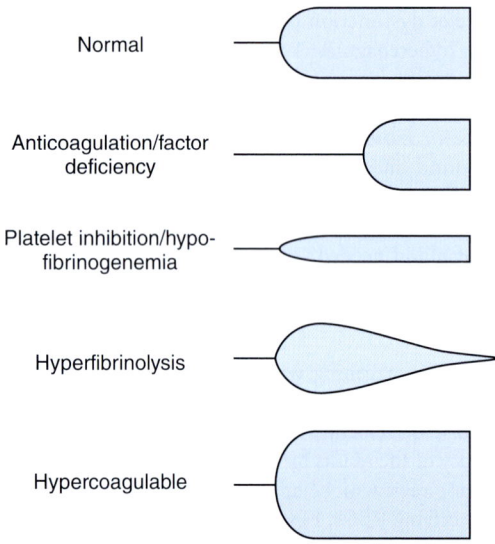

Normal

Anticoagulation/factor
deficiency

Platelet inhibition/hypo-
fibrinogenemia

Hyperfibrinolysis

Hypercoagulable

FIGURE 10.14 Typical graphical viscoelastic analysis which are similar for both rotational thromboelastometry (ROTEM) and thromboelastography (TEG) devices. (Reproduced with permission from Abdelfattah K, Cripps MW. Thromboelastography and rotational thromboelastometry use in trauma. *Int J Surg.* 2016;33:196-201.[867])

therapy; APTEM, aprotinin to measure the effect of fibrinolysis inhibitors mimicking treatment with tranexamic acid (TXA); FIBTEM, to differentiate between platelet deficiency and hypofibrinogenemia; and NATEM, using whole blood without reagents.[428] One study that compared TEG, ROTEM, and Quantra found comparable results but on average a more rapid result with Quantra (136 seconds with Quantra vs. 205 seconds with ROTEM and 450 seconds with TEG).[633] Each of these variations should still be considered investigational and a complete discussion is not possible for pediatric indications until further research

is undertaken. Tables 10.9 and 10.10 summarize the expected changes in various blood components when administered on a per kilogram basis and the estimated FFP requirement.

INFECTIOUS DISEASE CONSIDERATIONS

It is important to use basic precautions when administering blood products or contacting body fluids to minimize the risk to anesthesiologists. Blood and body fluids, even in infants, may transmit hepatitis B, hepatitis C, and HIV through parenteral exposure (e.g., cuts, needlestick), mucous membrane contact, or exposure to nonintact skin.[21,634–643] Accidental needlesticks are the most common means of exposure to anesthesiologists in the operating room. The introduction of safe IV needles, a needleless IV system, the use of stopcocks, and never recapping used needles has reduced the incidence of this problem.[644–647] The incidence of HIV seroconversion after needle puncture is estimated to be 0.2% to 0.5% (~1 in 300), although the conversion rate is much greater after a needlestick injury from individuals with hepatitis[648] (up to 30% in unvaccinated health care workers).[21,634,640–642,649,650] All institutions should have needlestick, mucous membrane, or nonintact skin exposure to blood protocols to immediately evaluate and institute treatment (see also Chapter 47).[651–655]

Anesthesiologists must practice universal blood and body fluid precautions (e.g., gloves, goggles) and should minimize the use of needles, especially the practice of recapping needles. The management of infants may be less than optimal with the use of three-way stopcocks because of the volume of fluid required to flush the system and the ease of introducing air into the IV line. In these infants, single-use needles without recapping or needleless systems are recommended. If an anesthesiologist is exposed to an HIV-positive patient or is punctured by a needle of unknown origin, the need for immediate institution of prophylactic medical therapy should be determined.[647,650] Early institution of drug therapy is recommended to reduce the potential for seroconversion (see E-Tables 47.4 and 47.5).[655,656]

Methods to Reduce Patient Exposure to Allogeneic Blood Components

Public awareness of the infectious hazards of transfusion, particularly from HIV and the hepatitis viruses, generated considerable interest in the 1980s and 1990s in developing techniques to avoid allogeneic transfusion. These techniques can minimize transfusions and the associated risks, assuaging the fears of parents and sparing the blood supply for patients for whom these options were not suitable. Within the medical community, awareness of the hazards of transfusion prompted a more thoughtful approach to transfusion, greater tolerance of asymptomatic anemia, more attention to medical treatment of anemia, and greater focus on surgical hemostasis. The amount of blood transfused for many surgical procedures has decreased steadily over time. The risks associated with transfusions have also dramatically decreased. After the HIV and hepatitis C viruses were identified, sensitive tests were developed to screen the donor population.

Transfusions are associated with other deleterious effects, but one of the most significant risks, mistransfusion,[657] does not differ materially between banked allogeneic and autologous blood; clear protocols and careful team work in patient matching with blood product is essential.[658] Additionally, electronic matching of units to identifiers attached to a patient such as those on a wrist band reduces risks of mistransfusion.[659] As the risk differential between allogeneic transfusion and its alternatives narrows, a balanced appraisal of the benefits and untoward effects of each is appropriate.

ERYTHROPOIETIN

Use of recombinant erythropoietin (combined with supplemental oral iron therapy) to promote endogenous RBC production can reduce the need for allogeneic RBC transfusions and has proved useful in many populations, including preterm infants, children receiving chemotherapy, children with renal failure, children of Jehovah's Witnesses, and children undergoing elective major reconstructive surgery, spinal surgery, liver transplantation, or cardiac surgery.[660–672] In general erythropoietin preoperatively is combined with intraoperative tranexamic acid.[669]

Coordination with the hematology department, blood banking, and the primary patient care team is required to take full advantage of this form of therapy.[661,669,673–691] A meta-analysis confirmed the efficacy of preoperative erythropoietin reduction of transfusions for infants undergoing craniosynostosis repair.[670] Although usually well tolerated, erythropoietin should be used with careful monitoring in patients with hypertension. Erythropoietin is available in a lyophilized (freeze-dried form for reconstitution) that contains no albumin or in a dilute albumin solution; some members of the Jehovah's Witness faith prefer the lyophilized formulation.

PREOPERATIVE AUTOLOGOUS BLOOD DONATION

Donation and storage of blood before elective surgery have reduced the use of allogeneic RBCs.[674,687,692–706] Banked units of PRBCs may be stored for 35 to 42 days in the liquid state,[707,708] permitting the donation of several units and the time required for the patient (usually teenagers) to regenerate the RBC mass before surgery. Children unable to mount an erythropoietic response to phlebotomy may only succeed in making themselves anemic, so administration of iron, vitamin C, and folate is important, as is monitoring for reticulocytosis to ensure that the bone marrow

is replenishing the donated RBCs. Autologous donation should not be attempted in children with cardiac ischemic disease (e.g., hypertrophic cardiomyopathy) or those with an active infection because bacteria can seed the collected unit and overgrow during storage. Autologous donation should be discouraged before procedures for which RBC transfusion is unlikely. Autologous blood donation that is not used by the donor is usually discarded rather than entered into the general blood bank inventory.

Patients or family of pediatric patients may wish to obtain blood from family members or friends (i.e., directed donation) but this is not offered by many hospital blood banks. Despite the perception that directed blood donations are safer than the pool of volunteer allogeneic donors, there is no evidence to confirm or reject this perception.[709] Directed donor blood products are screened and tested in the same manner as those from any volunteer allogeneic donors. Because there is a greater risk of TA-GVHD with cellular components from a donor who is a blood relative, these units are irradiated to eliminate the possibility of this fatal complication of transfusion.[710–713]

INTRAOPERATIVE BLOOD RECOVERY AND REINFUSION: AUTOTRANSFUSION

Recovery of blood from an operative site and reinfusion after some form of processing has been applied to major vascular, cardiac, and multiple trauma situations for many years.[698,703,704,713–725] The common techniques used a 150-micron filter and wash of the recovered blood, removing extraneous cellular debris (e.g., bone fragments, fat, etc.), excess citrate or heparin, free hemoglobin, K^+, activated clotting factors, and clotted blood are almost completely removed. This results in the child's RBCs suspended in saline at a hematocrit of 50% to 60%.[715,722] The use of 40-micron filters further removes any other debris prior to transfusion. Autotransfusion avoids the infectious and immunologic risks of allogeneic transfusion and, if reinfusion is carried out in the operating room, minimizes the opportunity for mistransfusion.[714,722,723,726]

Intraoperative blood recovery is not widely used in infants and children,[673,674,725,727–731] although pediatric-sized equipment has made this technique more cost-effective even in smaller children.[732–734] Blood recovery in conjunction with preoperative autologous blood donation and intraoperative antifibrinolytic medications are useful to minimizing allogeneic blood transfusion during scoliosis surgery.[713,718,719,728,735] One study reported no important benefit in children undergoing idiopathic scoliosis repair but a positive benefit for those with neuromuscular scoliosis.[736] The capital investment for the devices and the costs for the disposables and a trained operator, however, are substantial.[737,738] Nonetheless, these expenses can be offset if 2 to 3 fewer units of allogeneic RBCs are transfused.

Indications

Indications include any major surgical procedure in which the use of banked PRBCs is likely or in which massive blood loss is occurring or in children with rare blood types. Some institutions may require that it is likely that a minimum number of RBC units be needed to use intraoperative blood recovery.

Contraindications

Major contraindications to blood-recovery devices include contamination of the operative field by bacteria (e.g., bowel trauma, abscess), malignancy, and sickle cell disease (e.g., sickling in the device).[739,740] Recovered blood should not be processed for reinfusion if the surgical field contains topical clotting agents, some topical antibiotics (e.g., polymyxin, neomycin), or other foreign materials (e.g., methyl methacrylate).[740] Surgery for a malignancy is a relative contraindication because of the theoretical concern that malignant cells may be recovered and reinfused.[741–744]

CONTROLLED HYPOTENSION

Controlled hypotension has commonly been used in the past to reduce intraoperative blood loss or to provide a relatively bloodless operating field but is less commonly used today than in the past.[673,729,745–757] Hypotensive anesthesia may be accomplished with many techniques, including continuous infusion of vasodilators, β-adrenergic blockade, deep inhalational anesthesia, and large-dose opioid infusions (e.g., remifentanil).[746,757–762] Controlled hypotension is generally reserved for older children and teenagers undergoing major reconstructive (e.g., craniofacial surgery) or orthopedic surgery (spinal instrumentation). The choice of technique and the degree of induced hypotension depend on the surgical procedure. For procedures in which a dry surgical field is the endpoint with little potential for rapid blood loss, a technique that may take some time for recovery is acceptable (e.g., deep inhalational agent with or without β-blockade). If surgery carries the possibility of rapid or massive blood loss, a technique that is rapidly reversed (e.g., nitroprusside, nitroglycerin, remifentanil) is probably safer. *Controlled hypotension with a mean arterial pressure (MAP) of 55 to 60 mm Hg is no longer recommended especially for patients cared for in the prone position.* Moderate hypotensive techniques with a MAP of 65 to 70 mm Hg are likely associated with less risk, although no studies have been published in this regard.[691] The main concern regarding the use of this technique is reported cases of blindness after surgery performed with the patient in the prone position[763–767]; risk factors for blindness include duration of anesthesia, extensive blood loss, anemia, hypotension, and large crystalloid fluid administration (see also Chapters 30 and 33).[768] Dexmedetomidine has been used in large doses but this is associated with bradycardia and a long recovery period.[769]

General Concepts

All potent inhalational anesthetics decrease the cerebral metabolic rate for oxygen consumption ($CMRO_2$) and increase cerebral blood flow; isoflurane appears to offer the greatest advantage because it induces the greatest depression of $CMRO_2$.[770–776] Brain ischemia has been documented in adults when a MAP of 55 mm Hg is combined with hypocarbia; *we do not recommend this degree of hypotension or hypocarbia in any pediatric patient particularly if in the prone position.* Maintenance of normal arterial carbon dioxide tension ($PaCO_2$) is vitally important to ensure adequate cerebral blood flow (see Chapter 24).[777] To optimize cerebral blood flow, we typically maintain the MAP at 65 to 70 mm Hg or greater and the $PaCO_2$ at 35 to 45 mm Hg using strategies (e.g., vasodilating agents, remifentanil) that provide more precise control of blood pressure without depressing the heart.[778–787]

Pharmacology

Sodium Nitroprusside

Sodium nitroprusside has a very rapid onset of action (seconds), brief duration of action (minutes), and minimal side effects when used in the recommended dose range.[788,789] This agent must be administered by an infusion pump through a separate IV site and with a second pump to provide a continuous, uninterrupted, and stable infusion rate.[790]

Dose. The initial infusion rate is 0.3 to 1.0 micrograms per kilogram per minute[789,791,792] which is increased as needed to achieve the desired MAP.[793,794] Children can be separated into two groups that differ in response sensitivity, characterized by a high half maximal effective concentration (EC50) and low EC50; this explains the variability in blood pressure responses often observed.[789] A satisfactory reduction in systemic perfusion pressure can usually be obtained well below the recommended maximum rate of 10 micrograms per kilogram per minute, even in those with a high EC50.

Toxicity. Cyanide toxicity is characterized by an unexplained metabolic acidosis, increased blood lactate, and an increased mixed venous oxygen content.[790,794,795] The nitroprusside radical interacts with the sulfhydryl groups of erythrocytes, releasing cyanide. If the amount of cyanide released overwhelms the capacity of the rhodanese system, cyanide toxicity (i.e., binding to the cytochrome electron transport system) results. This produces a change to anaerobic metabolism, metabolic acidosis, an increase in mixed venous oxygen content, and eventually death.[794,796–800]

Reported safe doses of sodium nitroprusside are a maximum of 50 micrograms per kilogram per minute for 30 minutes and 8 to 10 micrograms per kilogram per minute for 3 hours, with frequent blood gas analyses.[794,801–803] Cyanide toxicity is heralded by three responses: (1) more than 10 micrograms per kilogram per minute required for a response, (2) tachyphylaxis developing within 30 to 60 minutes, and (3) immediate resistance to the drug.[795] Hydroxocobalamin (70 mg/kg)(Cyanokit)[804] is the antidote of choice in acute poisoning.[805] Sodium nitrite (0.2 mL/kg) or sodium thiosulfate (7 g/m²) have also been used.[805] Hydroxocobalamin may prevent toxicity by formation of cyanocobalamin (see also Chapter 16).[806]

Nitroglycerin

The main advantages of nitroglycerin are its relatively rapid onset of action (minutes), brief duration of action (minutes), and lack of tachyphylaxis and toxicity; the major disadvantage is the limited achievable reduction in blood pressure.

Dose. A nitroglycerin infusion of 1 microgram per kilogram per minute is increased until the desired response is obtained. Resistance to its hypotensive effects may occur; however, in view of the reduced potential for toxicity compared with nitroprusside, nitroglycerin is a reasonable alternative.

Toxicity. Nitroglycerin-induced methemoglobinemia is possible.[753,807–811] However, if this occurs, pulse oximetry may be of value in making the initial diagnosis (i.e., decreased saturation), but accurate saturation determinations are not possible because of the interference in light absorbance caused by methemoglobin at both ends of the absorbance spectrum used by pulse oximeters.[812,813] The use of other adjuncts (e.g., potent inhalation agents, β-adrenergic blockade, or opioids) reduces the total dose of nitroglycerin administered.

Remifentanil

Remifentanil-induced hypotension is increasing in popularity because of its relative safety, ease of administration, and titratability, particularly if a patient must be awakened during spinal fusion. Administration should be the same as for any other vasoactive drug; it requires dedicated IV access, with the infusion as close to the IV catheter as possible and with a separate pump to avoid fluctuations in the administration rate. Interruptions in infusion while changing IVs or boluses when giving other medications need to be avoided. We have found that the combination of a low-dose inhalational agent, low-dose propofol, and a remifentanil infusion provides excellent operating conditions.[814] Systemic arterial pressure can be controlled by the rate of opioid infusion, targeted to a plasma concentration,[762] and this combination does not interfere with sensory and motor potential monitoring. If an intraoperative wake up is needed, a longer-acting opioid such as fentanyl should be administered before awakening.[762,791,815] At the end of surgery, analgesic doses of a long-acting opioid such as morphine or hydromorphone should be administered to provide adequate analgesia on awakening.

General Concepts of Hypotensive Anesthesia

Before using controlled hypotension, it is important to understand the rationale for using this technique,[816] e.g., to reduce surgical blood loss or for reducing the perfusion pressure to improve operating conditions such as microsurgical techniques. In the former case, direct assessment of circulating blood pressure and volume with an arterial line and central venous catheter is important, whereas in the latter case, only a direct means of measuring blood pressure (an arterial line) is needed.

Anesthetic Management

The following baseline physiological variables are monitored: oxygen saturation and expired carbon dioxide, ECG, temperature, hematocrit, blood glucose, arterial blood gases, acid-base status, MAP, and CVP.

When the desired MAP has been attained, a new baseline CVP should be measured and maintained at this level or a slightly greater level than the new reduced CVP value throughout the procedure. To use any hypotensive technique safely, normovolemia must always be maintained. This means that even small (1 mm Hg or 2 mm Hg) decreases in the CVP prompt an appropriate fluid response. A small change in cardiac filling pressures in a healthy, supine, anesthetized pediatric patient may represent an important reduction in circulating blood volume. Even during hypotensive anesthesia, the kidneys should produce 0.5 to 1.0 milliliter per kilogram of urine per hour; if the urinary catheter is patent, an IV fluid challenge should be considered.

After hypotension has been induced and the surgical field is bloodless, the MAP should be slowly increased in increments of 5 mm Hg to 10 mm Hg until increased bleeding is observed in the surgical field. At that time, the MAP can be again reduced by approximately 5 mm Hg to achieve optimal conditions; it is sometimes necessary to reduce the MAP by only 10% to 20% from baseline to achieve satisfactory hemostasis.

POSITION. Make the operative field the highest point of the child's body to take advantage of gravitational forces to help reduce blood pressure and minimize any possible impedance to venous drainage that may contribute to blood loss. If the head is the surgical site, the arterial transducer must be calibrated at head level (usually even with the tragus of the ear) rather than heart level to ensure adequate cerebral perfusion pressure.[808,817]

LABORATORY MONITORING. An adequate hemoglobin must be maintained to have sufficient oxygen-carrying capacity; we maintain the hemoglobin at 9 to 10 grams/dL during controlled hypotensive anesthesia. This is important for children undergoing spinal instrumentation, in which traction on the spinal cord may alter spinal cord blood flow and to prevent possible blindness.

Arterial blood gases must be carefully evaluated on a 30- to 60-minute basis to diagnose changes in oxygenation, ventilation, or perfusion or the development of drug toxicity (e.g., metabolic acidosis with nitroprusside) or adverse anesthesia events.[818–820] A large difference between arterial and expired carbon dioxide values may indicate a pulmonary shunt or air embolization. An increase in mixed venous oxygen content may signal cyanide toxicity. An adequate PaO_2 and normocarbia should be maintained to ensure cerebral perfusion.[788,821,822] Although we do not advocate the routine use of β-adrenergic blockade, blood glucose values should be measured serially because β-adrenergic blockade inhibits glycogenolysis and has resulted in unsuspected hypoglycemia in children.[751,823,824]

Contraindications

The risks of hypotensive anesthesia are worrisome.[825] The risk/benefit ratio must always be considered on an individual basis, particularly with neurosurgical patients and those undergoing spinal instrumentation; any systemic disease compromising the function of a major organ is a relative contraindication. Most complications are related to inexperience of the practitioner, inappropriate patient selection, unfamiliarity with the drugs involved, or inattention to details such as blood volume status, pH, $PaCO_2$, blood glucose, or not using infusion pumps to carefully titrate medications. If a child is healthy and meticulous attention is paid to all the physiologic variables, the benefits of improved surgical technique, reduced surgical time, and decreased need for blood transfusion may outweigh the potential risks.

NORMOVOLEMIC HEMODILUTION

Intentional isovolemic hemodilution is a useful strategy for reducing allogeneic blood transfusions.[673,674,698,729,826–837] Two basic methods can be applied:

1. Allow the surgical blood loss to continue until the child's hematocrit value is in the high teens and maintain that hematocrit value until near the end of the procedure. At that time, the hematocrit can be increased to the desired value by transfusing PRBCs. This technique allows surgical bleeding to occur at a reduced hematocrit value, resulting in reduced loss of RBC mass.

2. Blood can be removed at the beginning of the operation while replacing the volume with crystalloid solution and then returning the blood at the end of the procedure or when significant bleeding occurs.

The latter technique is preferable because it reserves a quantity of the child's own blood with viable platelets, which can be returned at the end of the surgical procedure. For a Jehovah's Witness, this technique often conforms to religious guidelines if direct continuity is maintained with the child's circulation.[827,838–846]

During acute normovolemic hemodilution under anesthesia, the distribution of blood flow improves; improved blood rheology is the major compensatory mechanism for maintaining oxygen delivery despite a reduced hematocrit. Oxygen extraction increases in the presence of an inadequate circulating blood volume or when the hematocrit decreases to less than 20%. If the hematocrit decreases to less than 15%, subendocardial myocardial ischemia may develop.[847–850] At this extreme level of anemia, dissolved oxygen begins to assume a more important role in oxygen delivery.[851] In several reports, extreme acute normovolemic hemodilution (hemoglobin as low as 2 grams/dL) was well tolerated[847,852–855]; we cannot endorse the use of this technique in children because it is impossible to assess the effects of such an extreme hemoglobin concentration on the long-term cognitive ability. Nonetheless, these reports[847,855] indicate that healthy children can tolerate these extreme hematocrit concentrations provided they are anesthetized, normovolemic, slightly hypothermic, and ventilated with 100% oxygen. We prefer to maintain the hematocrit close to 20% at all times; if the surgery involves the prone position, then a greater hematocrit might be safer.[763–767]

Technique and Key Concepts

Blood is collected from the arterial line into sterile blood bags that contain the appropriate anticoagulant. Each bag is weighed before any blood is transferred and then continuously during filling by placing it on a scale. The bag is frequently but gently agitated to ensure an even distribution of the anticoagulant. The total volume of blood to be withdrawn should be calculated preoperatively to reduce the hematocrit to the range of 20% to 25%. Care must be taken to replace the blood removed with 5% albumin milliliter for milliliter or 1.5 to 2 milliters of lactated Ringer solution for each milliliter of blood removed. Sometimes, an even greater volume of replacement fluid is needed.[834] A reasonable estimate of the adequacy of replacement is to obtain a baseline CVP and then maintain the same CVP as blood is withdrawn and replaced. It is preferable to hemodilute before the surgical incision to monitor changes in hemodynamic indices, although it can be performed during the initial phases of surgery. The major concern is to maintain a normal circulating blood volume and provide adequate oxygen-carrying capacity. It is important to make an educated guess about how much blood loss is anticipated during the surgery so that autologous blood can be reinfused in place of homologous blood. Because a small-pore filter (20-μm) traps many more platelets than a large-pore filter (≥150 μm), the former is best avoided at this juncture.

Indications

Hemodilution may be indicated in any procedure in which blood loss is expected to exceed one-half of the child's blood volume.

Contraindications

Hemodilution is contraindicated in children with sickle cell disease, septicemia, cyanotic cardiac disease, or compromised function of any major organ that may be significantly affected by changes in perfusion and oxygenation. We do not recommend combining hemodilution (hematocrit <25%) with controlled hypotension or use in patients cared for in the prone position.

Complications

The major complications of hemodilution are related to blood volume status, hemoglobin content (i.e., removing too much blood), and coagulopathy (i.e., dilution of clotting factors). Anesthesiologists must pay meticulous attention to blood volume replacement. As long as normovolemia is maintained and the hematocrit exceeds 20% (preferably 25%–30% in prone patients), problems with organ perfusion or oxygenation should not occur. Sepsis becomes a concern if strict sterile techniques are not followed during the collection process.

Advantages

The benefits of normovolemic hemodilution are that the units of blood collected at the beginning of the procedure pose no risk of infection (unless contaminated by bacteria during the collection process) or mistransfusion (if they are not removed from the operating room) when they are returned to the child at a later time. It yields a net saving in loss of RBC mass because the surgical losses occur at a hematocrit of 20% rather than 40% to 45%. Fewer anesthesiologists feel comfortable with this technique for teenagers undergoing spinal instrumentation because of the association of blindness and anemia.

The Jehovah's Witness Patient

The children of Jehovah's Witnesses present a particular medical and legal dilemma.[856–859] Transfusion management of anyone with a religious objection to transfusion depends in part on the urgency of the surgical procedure and underlying medical condition of the child. If not emergent, a meeting with the patient (or the parents or guardian if a minor), the patient's spiritual adviser (if the child so chooses), and representatives of the team that will be caring for the child should be held to allow the child to clearly articulate their wishes with respect to the refusal of transfusion and its consequences and to discuss possible alternatives, including the use of erythropoietin, iron therapy, acute normovolemic hemodilution, intraoperative cell recovery and reinfusion, and the use of antifibrinolytic medications.[853,854,860–863] Specific inquiries should be made about each child's beliefs regarding the use of albumin, plasma, cryoprecipitate, platelets, and intraoperative cell recovery and reinfusion if the circuit is not continuously connected to the child and, in particular, what the child's response would be if a life-threatening event occurred while they were under anesthesia.[838,864] These discussions should be carefully documented in the child's record and informed consent signed beforehand. Not all hospitals or physicians are willing to participate in these cases, in which case arrangements should be made to transfer the child to the care of institutions or physicians who are willing to work within these constraints.

The courts have consistently ruled that the adult patient or emancipated minor has a right to refuse transfusion.[839,865] Physicians have the moral and legal obligations to respect those beliefs if an adult or teenager has made an informed decision and understands that they may die or suffer permanent injury without a transfusion if a life-threatening situation occurs. However, in the case of a minor child, the Supreme Courts in the United States and Canada have ruled that the fate of the minor child cannot be determined by the parents' religious convictions. The most important issue is full and open discussion of the effort that will be made to respect religious beliefs and avoid blood transfusions. In the case of minor children about whom a mutual understanding cannot be reached on avoiding blood transfusions, a court order can be obtained to save the child's life. The parents should be informed about this possibility beforehand.[866] The ethics related to this issue are discussed in Chapter 3.

Acknowledgment

The authors wish to thank Christopher P. Stowell for his prior contributions to this chapter.

ANNOTATED REFERENCES

Demailly Z, Wurtz V, Barbay V, et al. Point-of-care viscoelastic hemostatic assays in cardiac surgery patients: comparison of thromboelastography 6S, thromboelastometry Sigma, and Quantra. *J Cardiothorac Vasc Anesth.* 2023;37(6):948-955.

This paper compares three viscoelastic methods for assessing coagulation and points out possible advantages and disadvantages of each.

Dhabangi A, Ainomugisha B, Cserti-Gazdewich C, et al. Effect of transfusion of red blood cells with longer vs shorter storage duration on elevated blood lactate levels in children with severe anemia: the TOTAL randomized clinical trial. *JAMA.* 2015;314:2514-2523.

This study of children with severe anemia demonstrated that longer-stored RBCs were just as efficacious in delivering option and correcting lactic acidosis as RBCs stored for a short time and thus complements the ARIPI study that showed equivalent clinical outcomes (see Fergusson paper later in list).

Fergusson DA, Hébert P, Hogan DL, et al. Effect of fresh red blood cell transfusions on clinical outcomes in premature, very low-birth-weight infants: the ARIPI randomized trial. *JAMA.* 2012;308:1443-1451.

This RCT is one of four demonstrating that the duration of RBC storage does not affect patient outcomes.

Josephson CD, Granger S, Assmann SF, et al. Bleeding risks are higher in children versus adults given prophylactic platelet transfusions for treatment-induced hypoproliferative thrombocytopenia. *Blood.* 2012; 120(4):748-760.

This analysis of pediatric patients in a randomized controlled trial found that children with thrombocytopenia have a higher bleeding risk than adults but that bleeding was related to the treatment with children receiving autologous bone marrow transplant being at the highest increased bleeding risk compared to adults.

Kirpalani H, Bell EF, Hintz SR, et al. Higher or lower hemoglobin transfusion thresholds for preterm infants. *N Engl J Med.* 2020; 383:2639-2651.

This randomized controlled study found that a relatively conservative RBC transfusion strategy is safe.

Lacroix J, Hébert PC, Hutchinson JS, et al. Transfusion strategies for patients in pediatric intensive care units. *N Engl J Med.* 2007;356:1609-1619.

This landmark multicenter clinical trial compared outcomes in pediatric patients randomly assigned to red blood cell transfusion thresholds of 9.5 g/dL or 7 g/dL. There were no differences with respect to new or progressive multiple-organ failure, mortality, or other clinical outcomes between the two groups, which highlights the capacity of even acutely ill pediatric patients to tolerate anemia.

Ness PM, Cushing MM. Oxygen therapeutics: pursuit of an alternative to the donor red blood cell. *Arch Pathol Lab Med.* 2007;131:734-741.

This review provides a comprehensive and balanced summary of the development of synthetic oxygen carriers and the current challenges they face in making the transition from the laboratory to the clinic.

Schriner JB, Van Gent JM, Meledeo MA, et al. Impact of transfused citrate on pathophysiology in massive transfusion. *Crit Care Explor.* 2023;5(6):e0925.

This paper reviews the pharmacokinetics and pharmacodynamics of citrate load during massive transfusion explaining that hypothermia, hypotension, and acidemia delay the metabolism of citrate and therefore prolong its effects on ionized calcium. The authors describe this as the "Diamond of Death": bleeding, coagulopathy, acidemia, hypothermia, and hypocalcemia.

Slichter SJ, Kaufman RM, Assmann SF, et al. Dose of prophylactic platelet transfusions and prevention of hemorrhage. *N Engl J Med.* 2010;362:600-613.

This paper presents data regarding platelet transfusion for nonoperative, thrombocytopenic patients including 200 children.

A complete reference list can be found online at Elsevier eBooks+.

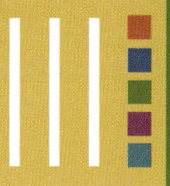
Essentials of Pulmonology

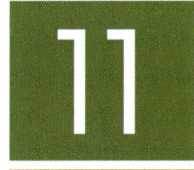

PAUL G. FIRTH AND T. BERNARD KINANE

Respiratory Physiology
Preoperative Assessment
Pulmonary Function Tests
Perioperative Etiology and Epidemiology

Upper Respiratory Tract Infection
Lower Respiratory Tract Infection
Cystic Fibrosis
Sickle Cell Disease

RESPIRATORY PROBLEMS ARE COMMON in children. The anesthesiologist often encounters pulmonary complications ranging from mild acute respiratory tract infections to chronic lung disease with end-stage respiratory failure during perioperative consultations, intraoperatively, or in the intensive care unit. This chapter discusses the basics of respiratory physiology, how to assess pulmonary function, and the practical anesthetic management of specific pulmonary problems. Airway and thoracic aspects pertinent to ventilation are discussed in Chapters 12 and 13; pulmonary issues specific to neonates, intensive care, various disease states, and infection control are addressed in the relevant chapters.

Respiratory Physiology

The morphologic development of the lung begins at several weeks after conception and continues into the first decade of postnatal life.[1] Intrauterine gas exchange occurs via the placenta, but the respiratory system develops in preparation for extrauterine life, when gas exchange transfers abruptly to the lungs at birth.

Development of the lung, which begins as an outgrowth of the foregut ventral wall, can be divided into several stages (Fig. 11.1). During the embryonic period, in the first few weeks after conception, lung buds form as a projection of the endodermal tissue into the mesenchyme. The pseudoglandular period extends from the 5th to the 17th week of life,[2] during which rapid lung growth is accompanied by formation of the bronchi and branching of the airways down to the terminal bronchioli. Further development of bronchioli and vascularization of the airways occurs during the canalicular stage (16th to 26th week)[2] of the second trimester. The saccular stage, which begins at approximately 24 weeks when terminal air sacs begin to form, extends until the 38th week.[2] During this period, two types of alveolar cells or pneumocytes form. Type 1 pneumocytes are ultrathin squamous cells devoid of organelles with basement membranes that are contiguous with the capillary endothelium, creating an air/blood interface for gas exchange. These cells cover 70% of the internal surface of the alveoli. In addition, type 1 pneumocytes are joined together by tight junctions that limit the translocation of fluids into the alveoli. Type 2 pneumocytes, which are cuboid in shape, cover only 7% of the alveolar surface area but outnumber type 1 cells by 2-fold. Type 2 pneumocytes produce surfactant, a lipoprotein that consists primarily of dipalmitoylphosphatidylcholine and several glycoprotein components, that reduce surface tension to prevent alveolar collapse during this growth period. The capillary networks surrounding air spaces proliferate, allowing sufficient pulmonary gas exchange for extrauterine survival of the premature neonate by 26 to 28 weeks; microvascular development continues into young adulthood.[2] Alveoli form from the saccules that lengthen and thin in a process that begins by the 36th week after conception in most human fetuses. Most alveoli develop after birth, typically continuing until 8 to 10 years postnatally. At birth, the neonatal lung usually contains 10 to 20 million terminal air sacs (many of which are saccules rather than alveoli), one-tenth the number in the mature adult lung; alveolar size continues to increase into young adulthood after chest wall growth is completed.[2]

The abrupt transition to extrauterine gas exchange at birth involves the rapid expansion of the lungs, increased pulmonary blood flow, and initiation of a regular respiratory rhythm. The development of a respiratory rhythm, detectable initially by intermittent rhythmic fetal thoracic movements, begins well before birth and may be necessary for normal anatomic and physiologic lung development.[3] Interruption of umbilical blood flow at birth initiates continuous rhythmic breathing. Amniotic fluid is expelled from the lungs via the upper airways with the first few breaths, with residual fluid draining through the lymphatic and pulmonary channels in the first days of life. Changes in the partial pressures of oxygen (PO_2) and carbon dioxide (PCO_2) and in hydrogen ion concentration (pH) cause an acute decrease in pulmonary vascular resistance and a consequent increase in pulmonary

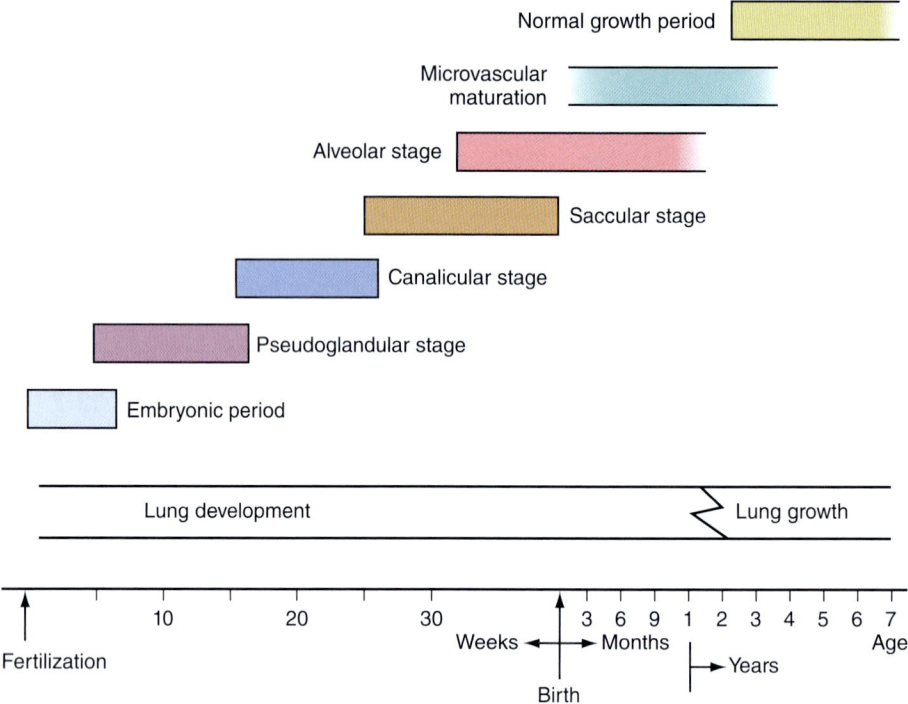

FIGURE 11.1 Timetable for lung development. (Modified with permission from Guttentag S, Ballard PL. Lung development: embryology, growth, maturation, and developmental biology. In: Taeusch HW, Ballard RA, Gleason CA, eds. *Avery's Diseases of the Newborn.* 8th ed. Philadelphia: WB Saunders; 2004:602.)

blood flow. Increased left atrial and decreased right atrial pressures reverse the pressure gradient across the foramen ovale, causing functional closure of this left-to-right one-way flap valve. Ventilatory rhythm is augmented and maintained in part by the increased arterial oxygen relative to the prior intrauterine levels.

Breathing is controlled by a complex interaction involving input from sensors, integration by a central control system, and output to effector muscles.[4] Afferent signaling is provided by peripheral arterial and central brainstem chemoreceptors, upper airway and intrapulmonary receptors, and chest wall and muscle mechanoreceptors.

The peripheral arterial chemoreceptors consist of the carotid and aortic bodies, with the carotid bodies playing the greater role in arterial chemical sensing of both arterial O_2 tension (PaO_2) and pH. The central chemoreceptors, responsive to arterial CO_2 tension ($PaCO_2$) and pH, are thought to be located at or near the ventral surface of the medulla.

The nose, pharynx, and larynx have a wide variety of pressure, chemical, temperature, and flow receptors that can cause apnea, coughing, or changes in ventilatory pattern. Pulmonary receptors lie in the airways and lung parenchyma. The airway receptors are subdivided into the slowly adapting receptors, also called pulmonary stretch receptors, and the rapidly adapting receptors. The stretch receptors, found in the airway smooth muscle, are thought to be involved in the balance of inspiration and expiration. These receptors may be the sensors in the Hering-Breuer reflexes, which prevent overdistention or collapse of the lung.[5] The rapidly adapting receptors lie between the airway epithelial cells and are triggered by noxious stimuli such as smoke, dust, and histamine. Parenchymal receptors, also known as juxtacapillary receptors, are located adjacent to the alveolar blood vessels; they respond to hyperinflation of the lungs, to various chemical stimuli in the

pulmonary circulation, and possibly to interstitial congestion. Chest wall receptors include mechanoreceptors and joint proprioceptors. Mechanoreceptors in the muscle spindle endings and tendons of respiratory muscles sense changes in length, tension, and movement.

Central integration of respiration is maintained by the brainstem (involuntary) and by cortical (voluntary) centers. Although the precise mechanism of the neural ventilatory rhythmogenesis is unknown, the pre-Bötzinger complex and the retrotrapezoid nucleus/parafacial respiratory group, neural circuits in the ventrolateral medulla, are thought to be the respiratory rhythm generators.[6] These neuron groups fire in an oscillating pattern, at an inherent rhythm that is moderated by inputs from other respiratory centers. Involuntary integration of sensory input occurs in various respiratory nuclei and neural complexes in the pons and medulla that modify the baseline pacemaker firing of the respiratory rhythm generators. The cerebral cortex also affects breathing rhythm and influences or overrides involuntary rhythm generation in response to conscious or subconscious activity, such as emotion, arousal, pain, speech, breath-holding, and other activities.[4]

The effectors of ventilation include the neural efferent pathways, the muscles of respiration, the bones and cartilage of the chest wall and airway, and elastic connective tissue. Upper airway patency is maintained by connective tissue and by sustained and cyclic contractions of the pharyngeal dilator muscles. The diaphragm produces most of the tidal volume during quiet inspiration, with the intercostal, abdominal, and accessory muscles (sternocleidomastoid and neck muscles) providing additional negative pressure. The elastic recoil of the lungs and thorax produces expiration. Inspiration is an active and expiration a passive action in normal lungs during quiet breathing. During vigorous breathing or with airway obstruction, both inspiration and expiration become active processes.

Another effect of age is a change in chest wall compliance. In adults the end-expiratory volume is equivalent to the functional residual capacity (FRC). In infants the chest wall is more compliant, so the tendency of the lung to collapse is not adequately counterbalanced by chest wall rigidity. Infants stop expiration at a lung volume greater than FRC, with the inspiratory muscles braking expiration. When this braking mechanism is impaired, as occurs with general anesthesia, the infant is prone to developing atelectasis.

Preoperative Assessment

The preoperative assessment of the respiratory system in a child is based on the history, physical examination, and evaluation of vital signs. Because ventilation is a complex process involving many systems besides the lung, the pulmonary appraisal must also include an assessment of airway, musculoskeletal, and neurologic pathology that might affect pulmonary mechanics and gas exchange under anesthesia or in the postoperative period. The potential impacts of esophageal reflux and cardiac, hepatic, renal, or hematologic disease on gas exchange and pulmonary function should be considered. Investigations, such as laboratory, radiographic, echocardiographic, and pulmonary function studies may be indicated if there is doubt regarding the diagnosis or severity of the pulmonary disease.

Because children may be unwilling or unable to give a reliable history, parents or caregivers are often the sole source or an important supplemental source of information during initial evaluation. Patient risk factors in the history that are associated with an increased risk of perioperative events include younger age, prematurity, obesity, congenital abnormalities, syndromes, a respiratory tract infection within the preceding 2 weeks, wheezing during exercise, more than three wheezing episodes in the past 12 months, nocturnal dry cough, eczema, a family history of asthma, rhinitis, or eczema, exposure to tobacco smoke, sleep-disordered breathing, neuromuscular diseases, and cardiac disorders.[7–10] Viral upper respiratory tract infections (URIs) are common in children, and the time, frequency, and severity of infection should be established. If wheezing is present, the precipitating causes, frequency, severity, and relieving factors should be determined. Chronic pulmonary diseases often have a variable clinical course, and the details of acute exacerbations of chronic problems should be elicited.

In younger children the gestational age at birth, the current postmenstrual age, neonatal respiratory difficulties, and prolonged intubation in the neonatal period are particularly important to ascertain. Apneic episodes, subglottic stenosis, and tracheomalacia are possible complications of prematurity and prolonged intubation that may be exacerbated in the perioperative period. Whereas congenital lesions often manifest at birth, symptoms of airway collapse or stenosis may become evident only later in life.

The physical examination begins with observation. With young children in particular, one's best opportunity to observe them before they react to your presence is from across the room; inspection from a distance can provide useful information. The respiratory rate is a sensitive marker of pulmonary problems, and scrutiny of the rate before a young child becomes agitated is an important metric. Conversely if the child develops symptoms when crying, that also provides valuable information. Pulse oximetry is a useful baseline indicator of oxygenation. Nasal flaring, intercostal retractions, and the marked use of accessory respiratory

muscles are all signs of respiratory distress. General appearance is also important. Apathy, anxiety, agitation, cyanosis, or persistent adoption of a fixed posture may indicate profound respiratory or airway difficulties; intense cyanosis can also be detected from a distance. Weight may relate to pulmonary function; children with chronic severe pulmonary disease are often underweight owing to restricted growth or malnourishment, whereas severe obesity can produce airway obstruction and sleep apnea. Inspection of the chest contour may reveal hyperinflation or thoracic wall deformities.

Closer physical examination adds further information. Atopy and eczema may be associated with hyperreactive airways (the so-called "allergy, atopy, asthma triad").[11–13] Auscultation may reveal wheezes, rales, fine or coarse crepitus, transmitted breath sounds from the upper airway, altered breath sounds, or cardiac murmurs. Chest percussion can provide an estimate of the position of the diaphragm and serve as a useful marker of hyperinflation. Patience, a gentle approach, and warm hands improve diagnostic yield and patient satisfaction.

Pulmonary Function Tests

Further pulmonary investigations include chest imaging, measurement of hematocrit, arterial blood gas analysis, pulmonary function tests, and sleep studies. Special investigations are not routinely indicated preoperatively and should be reserved for cases in which the diagnosis is unclear, the progression or treatment of a disease needs to be established, or the severity of impairment is not evident. In most cases a comprehensive history and careful physical examination are adequate to establish an appropriate anesthetic plan. Before requesting a new investigation, the clinician should have a clear idea of the question the test is expected to answer and how the answer will modify anesthetic management and outcome. Many tests are difficult to perform in children who have short attention spans and who cannot sit still for any length of time. Judgment must be exercised when ordering these tests for young children, and consideration given to the child's age, level of maturity, and the influence of the parents.

Pulmonary function tests include dynamic studies, measurement of static lung volumes, and diffusing capacity. Pulmonary function tests enable clinicians to (1) establish mechanical dysfunction in children with respiratory symptoms, (2) quantify the degree of dysfunction, and (3) define the nature of the dysfunction as obstructive, restrictive, or mixed obstructive and restrictive.[14] Table 11.1 presents common indications for pulmonary function testing in children.

The dynamic studies, which are the most used tests, include spirometry, flow-volume loops, and measurement of peak expiratory flow. Spirometry measures the volume of air inspired and expired as a function of time and is by far the most frequently performed test of pulmonary function in children. With a forced exhalation after a maximal inhalation, the total volume exhaled is known as the forced vital capacity (FVC), and the fractional volume exhaled in the first second is known as the forced expiratory volume in 1 second (FEV_1). Fig. 11.2 illustrates a normal pulmonary function test (normal flow-volume loop and spirometry parameters).

An obstructive process is characterized by decreased velocity of airflow through the airways (Fig. 11.3), whereas a restrictive defect produces decreased lung volumes (Fig. 11.4). Examination of the ratio of airflow to lung volume assists in differentiating these components of lung disease. Normally, a child should be able to

| TABLE 11.1 | Uses of Pulmonary Function Studies in Children |

- To establish pulmonary mechanical abnormality in children with respiratory symptoms
- To quantify the degree of dysfunction
- To define the nature of pulmonary dysfunction (obstructive, restrictive, or mixed obstructive and restrictive)
- To aid in defining the site of airway obstruction as central or peripheral
- To differentiate fixed from variable and intrathoracic from extrathoracic central airway obstruction
- To follow the course of pulmonary disease processes
- To assess the effect of therapeutic interventions and guide changes in therapy
- To detect increased airway reactivity
- To evaluate the risk of diagnostic and therapeutic procedures
- To monitor for pulmonary side effects of chemotherapy or radiation therapy
- To aid in predicting the prognosis and quantitating pulmonary disability
- To investigate the effect of acute and chronic disease processes on lung growth

Modified with permission from Castile R. Pulmonary function testing in children. In: Chernick V, Boat TF, Wilmott RW, Bush A, eds. *Kendig's Disorders of the Respiratory Tract in Children.* 7th ed. Philadelphia: Elsevier Saunders; 2006:168. Reproduced from National Asthma Education and Prevention Program. Full report of the expert panel: guidelines for the diagnosis and management of asthma (EPR-3). Bethesda, MD: National Heart, Lung, and Blood Institute, National Institutes of Health; 2007.

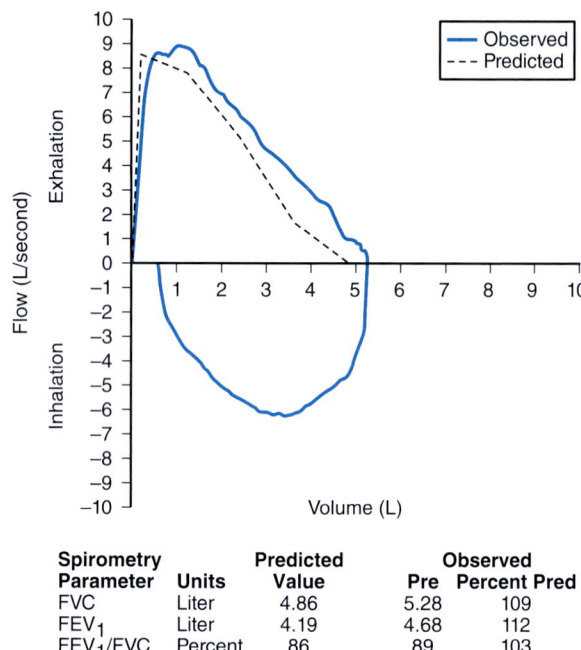

Spirometry Parameter	Units	Predicted Value	Observed Pre	Observed Percent Pred
FVC	Liter	4.86	5.28	109
FEV$_1$	Liter	4.19	4.68	112
FEV$_1$/FVC	Percent	86	89	103

FIGURE 11.2 Normal pulmonary function test. The normal flow-volume curve obtained during forced expiration rapidly ascends to the peak expiratory flow (highest point on curve), then descends with decreasing volume, following a reproducible shape that is independent of effort. In this normal flow-volume curve, the forced vital capacity *(FVC)*, forced expiratory volume in 1 second *(FEV$_1$)*, and FEV$_1$/FVC ratio are all within the normal range for this child's age, height, gender, and race. The shapes of both the inspiratory and expiratory limbs are normal as well. *Pre,* Prebronchodilator; *Pred,* predicted value.

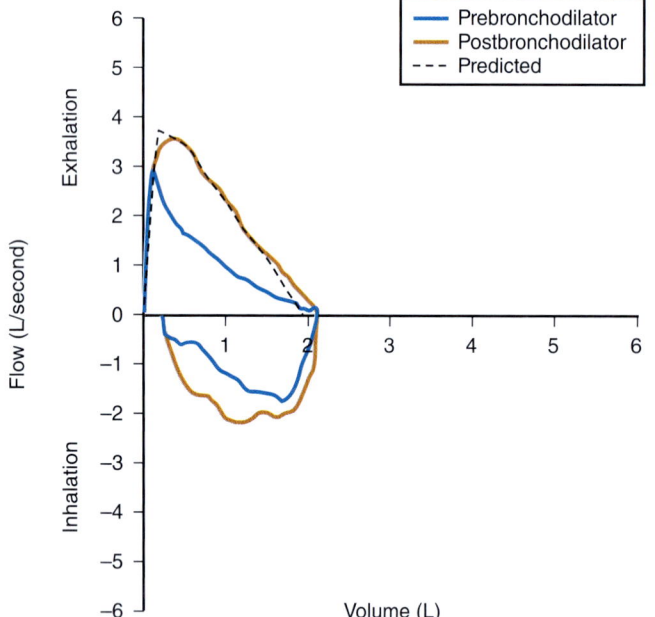

Spirometry Parameter	Units	Predicted Value	Observed Pre	Observed Percent Pred	Observed Post	Observed Percent Pred	Percent Change
FVC	Liter	1.94	2.15	111	2.14	110	0
FEV$_1$	Liter	1.71	1.30	76	1.82	106	40
FEV$_1$/FVC	Percent	90	60	67	85	94	42

FIGURE 11.3 This flow-volume curve demonstrates a reversible obstructive defect. The forced expiratory volume in 1 second *(FEV$_1$)* as a percentage of forced vital capacity *(FVC)*, or total volume exhaled, is decreased in patients with airway obstruction. The observed curve shape before bronchodilator use *(blue curve)* is scooped. After administration of a short-acting bronchodilator, the observed curve shape *(brown)* appears normal, and there is an increase in both FEV$_1$/FVC and FEV$_1$. This child has asthma and demonstrates a marked (40%) increase in FEV$_1$ after treatment with a short-acting bronchodilator. Reversible airflow obstruction is one of the hallmarks of asthma. *Post,* Postbronchodilator; *Pre,* prebronchodilator; *Pred,* predicted value.

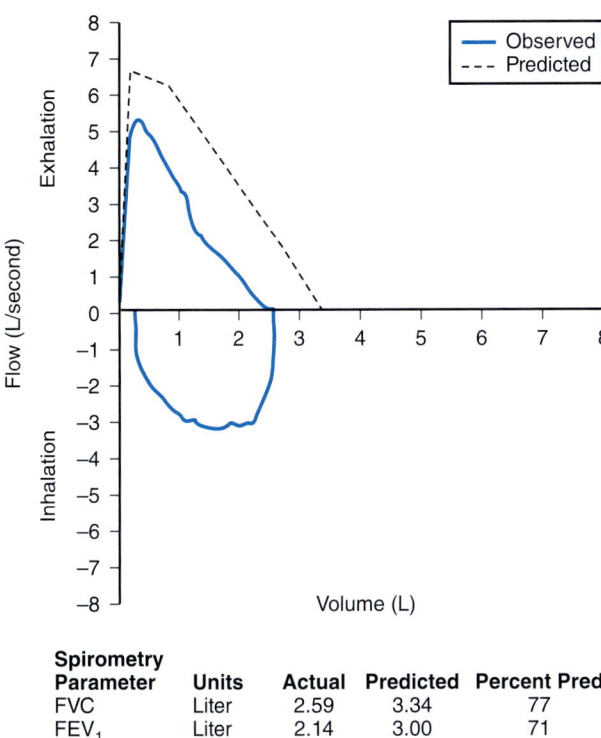

Spirometry Parameter	Units	Actual	Predicted	Percent Pred
FVC	Liter	2.59	3.34	77
FEV$_1$	Liter	2.14	3.00	71
FEV$_1$/FVC	Percent	83	92	90

FIGURE 11.4 Flow-volume curve demonstrating a restrictive defect. The flow-volume curves in children with restrictive defects are near-normal in configuration but smaller in all dimensions. The ratio of forced expiratory volume in 1 second *(FEV$_1$)* to forced vital capacity *(FVC)* is normal, but both FEV$_1$ and FVC are reduced. The curve shape appears normal. This child has interstitial lung disease. *Pred,* Predicted value.

TABLE 11.2	Characteristics of Obstructive and Restrictive Patterns of Lung Disease

	DISEASE CATEGORY	
Measurement	**Obstructive**	**Restrictive**
FVC	Normal/decreased	Decreased
FEV$_1$	Decreased	Decreased
FEV$_1$/FVC	Decreased	Normal

FEV$_1$, Forced expiratory volume in 1 second; *FVC,* forced vital capacity.

exhale more than 80% of the FVC in the first second. Children with obstructive lung disease have decreased airflow in relation to exhaled volume. If the volume exhaled in the first second divided by the volume of full exhalation (FEV$_1$/FVC) is less than 80%, then airway obstruction is present (Table 11.2; Fig. 11.3).

The FEV$_1$ needs to be interpreted in the context of the FVC. A small FEV$_1$ alone is insufficient evidence on which to make a diagnosis of airflow obstruction. Those with restrictive lung disease have both decreased FEV$_1$ and FVC: decreased flow rate and reduced total exhaled volume. Restrictive lung disease is associated with a loss of lung tissue or a decrease in the lung's ability to expand. A restrictive defect is diagnosed when the FVC is less than 80% of normal with either a normal or an increased FEV$_1$/FVC (see Table 11.2 and Fig. 11.4).

Most children with respiratory problems have an obstructive pattern; an isolated restrictive disease is far less common. Asthma is the most common obstructive pulmonary disease in children. The Center for Disease Control and Prevention (CDC, USA) estimated that 5.8% (4,226,659) of children younger than 18 years of age have asthma; the rate varies from 2% in those <4 years old, increasing to 9.1% in teenagers.[15] Rare causes of obstruction include airway lesions, congenital subglottic webs, and vocal cord dysfunction. Restrictive lung disease can arise from limitations to chest wall movement, such as chest wall deformities, scoliosis, or pleural effusions, or from space-occupying intrathoracic pathology such as large bullae or congenital cysts. Alveolar filling defects (e.g., lobar pneumonia) also reduce lung volume and can be considered as restrictive processes. Although the diseases arise from specific isolated genetic disorders, children with cystic fibrosis (CF) and sickle cell disease (SCD) can have highly variable pulmonary pathologic processes with both obstructive and restrictive components of lung disease. Bronchopulmonary dysplasia may also result in both obstructive and restrictive pathology.

Pulmonary function tests can also be used to differentiate fixed from variable airway obstruction and to localize the obstruction as above or below the thoracic inlet (Figs. 11.5–11.7, E-Fig.11.1). This information can be gleaned from distinctive changes in the configuration of the flow-volume loop, a graphic representation of inspiratory and expiratory flow volumes plotted against time. A fixed central airway obstruction, such as a tumor or stenosis, may obstruct both inspiration and expiration, flattening the flow-volume curve on both inspiration and expiration (see Video 12.1). The child with tracheal stenosis, for example, has flattening of both inhalation and exhalation curves (see Fig. 11.6). A variable obstruction tends to affect only one part of the ventilatory cycle. On inhalation, the chest expands and draws the airways open. On exhalation, as the chest collapses, the intrathoracic airways collapse. Variable extrathoracic lesions tend to obstruct on inhalation more than exhalation, whereas variable intrathoracic lesions tend to obstruct more on exhalation. This produces the characteristic flow-volume patterns.

In addition to diagnostic uses, spirometry is used to assess the indication for, and efficacy of, treatment. For example, the obstruction in patients with asthma is usually reversible, either gradually over time without intervention or much more rapidly after treatment with a short-acting bronchodilator. An improvement in FEV$_1$ of 12% and 200 mL in adults or approximately 3 mL per kg is considered a positive response. In addition to confirming the diagnosis of asthma, the degree of airflow obstruction, as indicated by the FEV$_1$, is one measure of asthma control. A low FEV$_1$ or an acute decrease from baseline may indicate a child whose asthma is not under good control and therefore who potentially is at greater risk for a perioperative exacerbation (see Fig. 11.3).

Because it measures the amount of air entering or leaving the lung rather than the amount of air in the lung, spirometry cannot provide data about absolute lung volumes. Information about FRC and lung volumes calculated from FRC, such as total lung capacity and residual volume, must be obtained by different means, such as gas dilution or body plethysmography. Gas dilution is based on measuring the dilution of nitrogen or helium in a circuit in closed connection to the lungs, whereas body plethysmography calculates lung gas volumes based on changes in thoracic pressures.

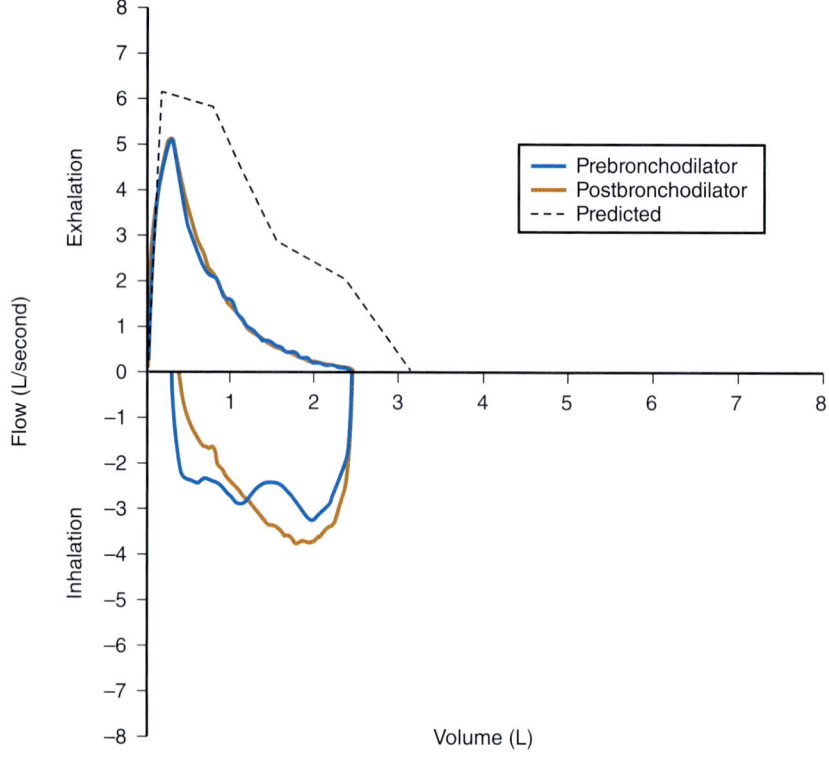

Spirometry Parameter	Units	Predicted Value	Observed Pre	Percent Pred	Observed Post	Percent Pred	Percent Change
FVC	Liter	3.16	2.50	79	2.45	78	−2
FEV$_1$	Liter	2.82	1.56	55	1.56	55	0
FEV$_1$/FVC	Percent	91	62	68	64	70	3

FIGURE 11.5 Pulmonary function test demonstrating a nonreversible obstructive defect. The ratio of forced expiratory volume in 1 second *(FEV$_1$)* to forced vital capacity *(FVC)* is decreased, as is the FEV$_1$. After administration of a short-acting bronchodilator, there is no significant improvement in the FEV$_1$, in contrast to the pattern in Fig. 11.3. This child has cystic fibrosis with a nonreversible obstructive defect. *Post,* Postbronchodilator; *Pre,* prebronchodilator; *Pred,* predicted value.

Perioperative Etiology and Epidemiology

Respiratory problems account for most of the perioperative morbidity in children[9,16–19] and cause almost one-third of perioperative pediatric cardiac arrests.[20] Adverse events include: laryngospasm, airway obstruction, bronchospasm, hemoglobin oxygen desaturation, prolonged coughing, atelectasis, pneumonia, and respiratory failure.[7–9,21,22] The incidence of perioperative adverse respiratory events in one study of 755 children was 34%,[21] whereas in another observational study of 9297 children it was 15%.[7] A multinational observational study documented critical respiratory events in 3.1% of 31,127 procedures.[9] The triggers of these problems included airway manipulation, alteration of airway reflexes by anesthetic drugs, surgical insult, and depression of breathing caused by anesthetic and analgesic medications.

Studies have consistently reported greater respiratory morbidity among younger compared with older children.[7–9,16–18,23–26] In particular, neonates are sensitive to respiratory problems for many reasons. Although the FRC approaches adult capacity (in liters per kilogram) within days after birth, a persistently large closing capacity increases the likelihood of alveolar collapse and intrapulmonary shunt. Residual patency of the ductus arteriosus

can also contribute to shunting. The greater metabolic rate of the infant increases oxygen requirements and decreases the time to arterial desaturation after an interruption to ventilation and gas exchange; as brief as 14 seconds in preterm infants.[27] The work of breathing is also greater in young infants because of high-resistance, small-caliber airways, increased chest wall compliance, and reduced lung parenchymal compliance.

UPPER RESPIRATORY TRACT INFECTION

Upper respiratory tract infections (URIs) in young children are very common, typically being infected several times a year, possibly even more frequently if they are in day care. Viruses cause the majority of URIs, with rhinoviruses constituting one-third to one-half of etiologic species.[28,29] The remainder are caused by coronaviruses, adenoviruses, and paramyxoviruses such as respiratory syncytial virus and parainfluenza viruses.[30]

Although most URIs are short-lived, self-limited infections, and, by definition, limited to the upper airway, they may increase airway sensitivity to noxious stimuli or secretions for several weeks after the infection has cleared and involve the lower airways. A meta-analysis of 23 trials and 25 observational studies found that the duration of symptoms in 90% of children was 21 days for bronchiolitis, 25 days for an acute cough, 15 days for the

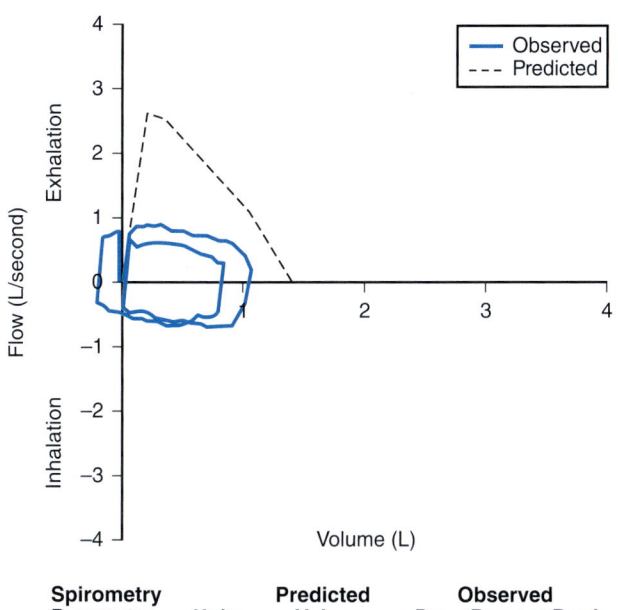

Spirometry Parameter	Units	Predicted Value	Observed Pre	Percent Pred
FVC	Liter	1.41	1.19	84
FEV$_1$	Liter	1.22	0.83	68
FEV$_1$/FVC	Percent	91	70	77

FIGURE 11.6 Pulmonary function test showing an extrathoracic airway obstruction; both the inspiratory and expiratory limbs of the flow-volume curve are flattened. This child has subglottic stenosis that developed at the site of her tracheotomy 2 years after the tracheostomy tube was removed. *FEV$_1$*, Forced expiratory volume in 1 second; *FVC*, forced vital capacity; *Pred*, predicted value.

common cold, and 16 days for nonspecific URI.[31] The mechanisms probably involve a combination of mucosal invasion, chemical mediators, and altered neurogenic reflexes.[28] URIs may also impair pulmonary function by decreasing FVC, FEV$_1$, peak expiratory flow, and diffusion capacity.[32,33]

Children with a recent or current URI have an increased incidence of perioperative laryngospasm, bronchospasm, arterial hemoglobin desaturation, severe coughing, and breath-holding compared with uninfected children (Table 11.3).[7,9,24,25,34–39] However, most complications can usually be predicted and successfully managed without long-term sequelae by suitably experienced and prepared clinicians.[9,26,28,35,37,40–43] An approach to the child with a URI is to detect the pathologic process and associated comorbidity, establish the acuteness and severity of the URI, and then decide whether to modify the anesthetic technique or to postpone surgery (Table 11.4, Fig. 11.8).

The basis for diagnosing a URI is a careful history and physical examination, with further investigations in limited situations. Because they are usually familiar with their child's state of health, the parents or caregivers can provide helpful insight into the presence and severity of a URI. The child should be evaluated for fever (defined as a temperature >100.4°F [38°C]), change in demeanor or behavior, dyspnea, productive cough, purulent sputum production, nasal congestion, rales, rhonchi, and wheezing. A chest radiograph may be considered if the pulmonary examination is questionable, but because the radiographic changes lag behind clinical symptoms, it is typically of limited value. Approximately 25% of children screening positive by polymerase chain reaction (PCR) testing will have multiple pathogens.[44] Although laboratory tests may confirm the diagnosis of a viral or

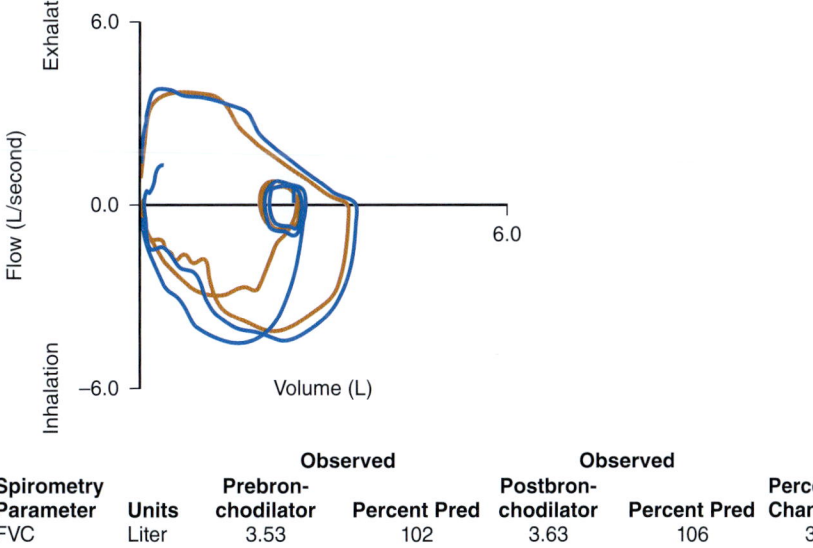

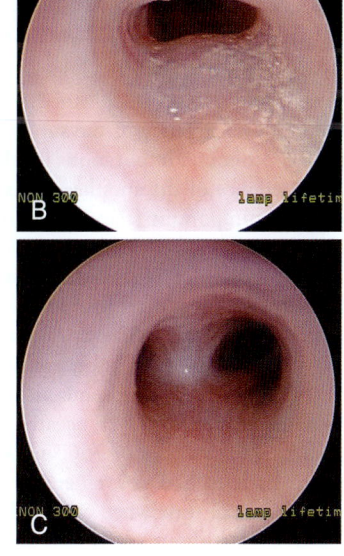

Spirometry Parameter	Units	Observed Prebronchodilator	Percent Pred	Observed Postbronchodilator	Percent Pred	Percent Change
FVC	Liter	3.53	102	3.63	106	3
FEV$_1$	Liter	2.63	89	2.65	90	0
FEV$_1$/FVC	Percent	74.7		72.8		−3

FIGURE 11.7 A, Pulmonary function test from a child with an intrathoracic airway obstruction (vascular ring). The flow-volume curves suggest a fixed expiratory obstruction. The shape of the inspiratory link is normal; the expiratory flow limb is flattened on both the prebronchodilator *(brown)* and postbronchodilator *(blue)* flow-volume curves. **B,** Slit-like tracheal compression before repair. **C,** Marked improvement in the tracheal lumen after division of the vascular ring. (See E-Fig. 11.1 for a magnetic resonance imaging angiogram of a vascular ring.) *FEV$_1$*, Forced expiratory volume in 1 second; *FVC*, forced vital capacity; *Pred*, predicted value. (Photographs **B** and **C** courtesy Christopher Hartnick, MD.)

TABLE 11.3 | Incidence of Common Upper Respiratory Tract Infection–Associated Perioperative Adverse Events

Study	LARYNGOSPASM (%)		BRONCHOSPASM (%)		HEMOGLOBIN DESATURATION (%)	
	URI	No URI	URI	No URI	URI	No URI
Tait and Knight, 1987[196]	1.3	1.2				
DeSoto et al., 1988[197]					(<95%) 20.0	0[a]
Cohen et al., 1990[23]	2.2	1.7				
Levy et al., 1992[198]					(<93%) 63.6	59.0
Rolf and Coté, 1992[37]	5.9	3.3	13.3	0.6[a]	(<85%) 13.3	10.5
Tait et al., 1998[199]	7.3		12.2		(<90%) 17.1	
Tait et al., 2001[35]	4.2	3.9	5.7	3.3	(<90%) 15.7	7.8[a]
von Ungern-Sternberg et al., 2007[25]	7.6	3.1[a]		0.9[a]	19.3	11.4[a]

[a]$P < 0.05$ versus corresponding URI group.
URI, Upper respiratory tract infection.
Data in parentheses under hemoglobin desaturation are the limits for desaturation in each study.
Modified from Tait AR. Anesthetic management of the child with an upper respiratory tract infection. *Curr Opin Anaesthesiol.* 2005;18:603-607.

bacterial URI, they are not cost-effective or practical in a busy surgical setting.

For children with symptoms of an uncomplicated URI who are afebrile with clear secretions and who are otherwise healthy, anesthesia may proceed as planned, because the problems encountered are typically transient and easily managed.[7,28,35,37,40–42] Elective surgery is usually postponed for children with more severe symptoms that include at least one of the following: *mucopurulent secretions*; *lower respiratory tract signs* (e.g., wheezing) that do not clear with a deep cough; *pyrexia* >100.4°F (38°C); or a *change in sensorium* (e.g., not behaving or playing normally, has not been eating properly).[26,28,42]

The decision to proceed with surgery becomes much more difficult when the signs of the URI are between the extremes of mild and severe. For these intermediate URIs, other considerations play a greater role in assessing the risk/benefit ratio. These include the presence of comorbidities such as asthma, cardiac disease, or obstructive sleep apnea; a history of prematurity; the frequency of URIs; prior cancellations; the type, complexity, duration, and urgency of the surgery; the age of the child; and the socioeconomic implications for the family. The comfort level and experience of the anesthesiologist may also be an underestimated but important factor in the decision to proceed with or postpone surgery, because less experienced anesthesiologists have a greater incidence of complications.[7,9,26] The need to admit a child postoperatively because of anesthetic complications or an exacerbation of the URI may expose other children to a contagious illness. An international observational registry found a greater incidence of hypoxemia in COVID-19 positive children compared with COVID-19 negative patients (24 of 329 positive children [7%] vs. 214 of 7567 negative children [3%]); symptomatic patients had an even greater rate (19%).[39]

The optimal time when an anesthetic can be given to a child after a URI without increasing the risk of adverse respiratory events remains contentious, but many clinicians wait 2 to 4 weeks after resolution of the URI before proceeding.[7,25,26,45] This reflects a balance of three critical factors: the time interval to diminish both upper and lower airway hyperreactivity; the perioperative respiratory risk, which includes a recurrence of the URI; and the need to perform the procedure. The yearly infection rate in children in the first 2 years of life is two to eight episodes per year

and in children attending day care up to 14; older children experience three to six infections per year.[46]

If the decision is to proceed with general anesthesia, management is directed toward minimizing stimulation of the potentially sensitized airway. Avoidance of the use of a tracheal tube (TT) should be considered when possible, because intubation is associated with increased complication rates, especially in younger children.[7,26,35] Although managing the airway with a face mask holds the smallest frequency of airway complications,[7] it may be inappropriate for certain cases. The use of supraglottic devices is associated with fewer episodes of respiratory events than with TTs, but their use may similarly be contraindicated by the type of surgical procedure and the need to protect the airway from pulmonary aspiration of gastric contents.

Whichever airway technique is chosen, it is essential that the depth of anesthesia be adequate to obtund airway reflexes during placement of an airway device. The optimal depth of anesthesia at which to remove an airway device is less clearly defined, with a broad variation in practice.[9] The frequency of emergence complications overall after awake and deep extubation appears to be similar in children with and without a URI.[7,25,35,47] In contrast, the incidence of arterial oxygen desaturation and coughing after removal of the TT or supraglottic airway in awake children was greater.[19,48–50]

Intravenous induction may reduce the rate of respiratory events on induction, although practical issues of needle phobia or difficult venous canulation may limit this strategy.[9,51] The incidence of laryngospasm after maintenance of anesthesia with propofol was less than with sevoflurane in an observation study of more than 9000 children[7]; this finding may be attributable to differential effects of propofol versus sevoflurane on airway reflexes.[52] The effects of spraying the vocal cords with lidocaine on the incidence of laryngospasm and bronchospasm are unclear.[7] However, after applying topical lidocaine gel lubricant to the laryngeal mask airway in children with URIs, the frequency of adverse airway events was less than without lidocaine lubricant.[53,54] Prophylactic treatment with glycopyrrolate, ipratropium, or albuterol does not affect the incidence of URI-related adverse events,[55,56] although one observational study reported that prophylactic albuterol (salbutamol) reduced perioperative airway sequelae in children with URIs.[57] Albuterol premedication also

Study	URI Status	Factors	RR/OR
TABLE 11.4	**Risk Factors for Perioperative Adverse Events in Children With Upper Respiratory Tract Infections**		
Tait et al., 2001[35]	URI	Copious secretions	3.9 RR
		TT in child <5 years	1.9
		Prematurity (<37 weeks)	2.3
		Nasal congestion	1.4
		Passive smoker	1.6
		Reactive airway disease	1.8
		Surgery of airway	1.8
Bordet et al., 2002[24]	URI and no URI	Age <8 years	1.8 OR
		LMA	2.3
		Respiratory infections	3.7
Mamie et al., 2004[21]	No URI	Nonpediatric anesthesiologist	1.7 OR
		ENT procedure	1.8
		TT without relaxants	1.2
von Ungern-Sternberg et al., 2010[7]	URI and no URI	Positive respiratory history	3.05–8.46 RR
		Symptomatic URI	2.05
		URI within previous 2 weeks	2.34
		Family history of asthma, atopy, or smoking	
		Anesthetic agent	
		Nonpediatric anesthesiologist	
Habre et al., 2017[9]	URI and no URI	Sensitized airway (URTI, wheezing, asthma, passive smoking)	2.23 RR
		Physical condition	1.21
		Induction type (intravenous versus inhalational	0.78
		TT versus facial mask	3.36
		Supraglottic airway versus facial mask	2.0
		Other versus facial mask	2.65
Michel et al., 2018[26]	URI present	Age <58 months	4 OR
		Tracheal intubation	2.5
		Use of midazolam premedication	0.6

ENT, Ear, nose, and throat; *TT*, tracheal tube; *LMA*, laryngeal mask airway; *OR*, odds ratio; *RR*, relative risk; *URI*, upper respiratory tract infection.
Modified from Tait AR. Anesthetic management of the child with an upper respiratory tract infection. *Curr Opin Anaesthesiol.* 2005;18:603-607.

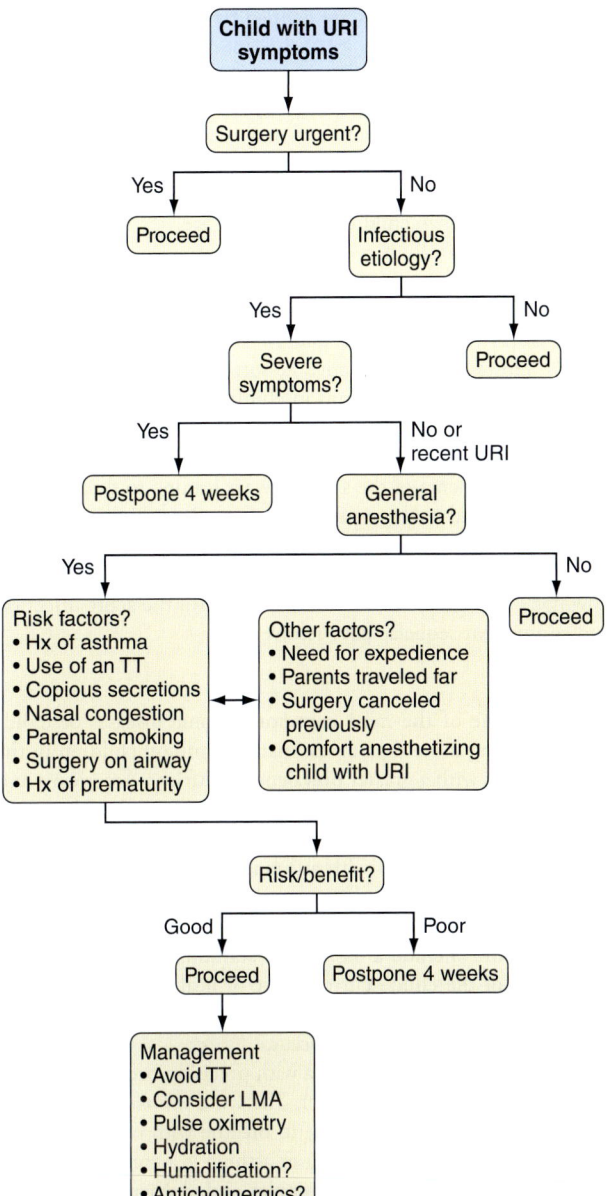

FIGURE 11.8 Suggested algorithm for assessment and management of the child with an upper respiratory tract infection *(URI). TT,* tracheal tube; *Hx,* history; *LMA,* laryngeal mask airway. (Modified from Tait AR, Malviya S. Anesthesia for the child with an upper respiratory tract infection: still a dilemma? *Anesth Analg.* 2005;100:59-65.)

reduced perioperative respiratory complications in children undergoing tonsillectomy.[58] Nasal vasoconstrictors (such as phenylephrine or oxymetazoline nose drops) have been recommended for reducing oropharyngeal secretions in children with URIs, but their efficacy remains anecdotal.[42] It should be noted that several cases of systemic toxicity resulting in hypertension and tachycardia have been reported with excessive dosing of oxymetazoline or phenylephrine nasal drops.[59–61]

LOWER RESPIRATORY TRACT INFECTION

Acute lower respiratory tract infections in infants and children may result in rapid deterioration necessitating aggressive intervention, including tracheal intubation and admission to the intensive care unit. These infections are defined by a respiratory illness of acute onset with a fever (>101.3°F [38.5°C]) and clinical and radiological evidence of pulmonary infiltrates.[62] In infants and children up to 18 months of age, syncytial virus is a common cause of respiratory infections and may produce serious complications.[62,63] Other viruses that also infect the lower respiratory tract include parainfluenza virus, rhino and adenovirus, and human metapneumovirus in children <5 years of age.[62,64] Many children are treated with antibiotics on the presumption that the infection is bacterial, which it may be. In fact, school age children may be infected with bacteria including *Mycoplasma pneumoniae, Chlamydia, Streptococcus, Pertussis,* and *Tuberculosis,* as well as rhinoviruses.[62] However, a prospective cohort study of antibiotics for uncomplicated chest infections in children neither shortened the duration nor reduced the symptoms of the infection.[65]

Acute inflammation of the small airways may result in bronchiolitis with edema of the small airways leading to desaturation, hypercapnia, and acute respiratory failure. Bronchiolitis management, especially common in children <2 years of age, can involve several days of continuous positive airway pressure (CPAP), high-flow nasal prongs, or tracheal intubation until the acute infection and consequent sequelae have resolved.[66]

Asthma

Asthma is one of the most common chronic diseases of childhood, affecting more than an estimated 6 million children in the United States with a greater prevalence in African Americans and Hispanics.[67–69] A history of wheezing is associated with an increased risk of perioperative bronchospasm.[7] Rare perioperative complications associated with asthma include anaphylaxis, adrenal crisis, and ventilatory barotrauma such as pneumothorax or pneumomediastinum.[70] An anesthetic approach to children with asthma should include a basic understanding of the disease, an assessment of the child's current state of health, modification of anesthetic technique as appropriate, and recognition and treatment of complications if they occur.

It is difficult to define asthma with precision because the exact pathophysiology remains unclear. The word *asthma* derives from the Greek *aazein,* which means "to breathe with open mouth or to pant".[71] A working definition of asthma is a common chronic disorder of the airways that is complex and characterized by variable and recurring symptoms, airway obstruction, inflammation, bronchospasm, and hyperresponsiveness of the airways.[68]

Clinical expressions of asthma include wheezing, chest tightness or discomfort, persistent dry cough, and dyspnea on exertion. Severe respiratory distress can occur during acute exacerbations and may be characterized by chest wall retraction, use of accessory muscles, prolonged expiration, pneumothorax, and progression to respiratory failure and death. In some children the development of chronic inflammation may be associated with permanent airway changes, referred to as *airway remodeling*, that are not prevented by or fully responsive to current available treatments. There is a strong association between asthma and atopy, or immunoglobulin E (IgE)-mediated hypersensitivity.[11,13,68]

The diagnosis of asthma can be challenging because cough, wheezing, and bronchospasm may arise from many disease processes. Asthma itself is unlikely to be a single disease entity, and the disease process is markedly modified by various genetic and environmental factors.[67,68,71] Many young children wheeze, and there is no definitive confirmatory blood, histologic, or radiographic diagnostic test. Given the difficulty with diagnosis, the label "preschool wheezers" may be a more appropriate description for young children with reversible airway obstruction than a diagnosis of "asthma".[71]

The Tucson birth cohort study was the largest longitudinal study in the United States to attempt to differentiate wheezing or asthma phenotypes in children who did not subsequently develop asthma.[72–74] This study examined 826 children at ages 3 and 6 years from a cohort of 1246 neonates. By the age of 6 years, 48.5% of the children had experienced at least one documented episode of wheezing and were categorized into three groups. "Transient wheezers" were children who wheezed only in response to viral infections, typically during the first 3 years of life. "Nonatopic wheezers" were children who wheezed beyond the first few years of life, often in response to viral infections, but who were less likely to persistently wheeze in later childhood. "Atopy-associated wheezers" were children who had a reversible wheeze together with a tendency toward IgE-mediated hypersensitivity; they had the greatest risk of persistent symptoms into late childhood and adulthood.[72]

The development of asthma is a complex process that probably involves the interaction of two crucial elements: host factors (specifically genetic modifiers of inflammation) and environmental exposures (e.g., viral infections, environmental allergens, pollution, secondhand smoke)[75] that occur during a crucial time in the development of the immune system.[68] Therefore, the population of young children who wheeze includes a spectrum of disorders rather than one specific pathologic process.

Asthma must be differentiated from other distinct causes that produce similar symptoms (Table 11.5). Tracheomalacia or bronchomalacia may produce wheezing, but this tends to be present from birth (which is unusual for asthma), and the wheezing is commonly of a single pitch heard loudest in the central airways, whereas asthma typically produces polyphonic sounds from the lung periphery. Breathing difficulties owing to chronic aspiration are often related to feeding times. Unremitting wheeze or stridor is often caused by a fixed obstruction or foreign body.

Chronic cough is the most common manifestation of asthma in children. Many children who cough may never be heard to wheeze but still have asthma. A cough with or without wheeze

TABLE 11.5	Causes of Wheezing in Children
Acute	
Bronchiolitis	Pneumothorax
Asthma	Endobronchial intubation
Foreign body	Herniated tracheal tube cuff
Inhalation injury	Aspiration
	Anaphylaxis
Recurrent or Persistent	
Bronchiolitis	Mediastinal mass
Asthma	Tracheomalacia/bronchomalacia
Foreign body	Vascular ring
Bronchopulmonary dysplasia	Tracheal web/stenosis
Cardiac failure	Bronchial stenosis
Cystic fibrosis	Roundworm infestation
Recurrent aspiration	
Sickle cell disease	

may be caused by a viral infection, whereas a persistent, productive cough may suggest suppurative lung disease such as CF.[70] A positive response of the cough to asthma medications suggests the diagnosis of asthma.

The exact incidence of perioperative complications in the pediatric asthma population is difficult to ascertain because of variations in the definition of asthma, the definition and detection of complications, the presence of coexisting diseases, overlap with adult populations, and changing anesthetic management techniques.

A retrospective review of 706 adults and children with a rigorous definition of asthma reported an incidence of documented bronchospasm in the perioperative period of 1.7% and no instances of pneumonia, pneumothorax, or death.[76] Of 211 children younger than 12 years of age, none developed bronchospasm at the time of surgery. A retrospective review of more than 136,000 computer-based anesthesia records found a 0.8% incidence of bronchospasm in patients with asthma.[77] By contrast, older studies from the 1960s reported that 7% to 8% of asthmatic patients wheezed.[78,79] A blinded, prospective study of 59 asthmatic patients detected transient wheezing after tracheal intubation in 25% of cases; however, most events were brief and self-limited.[80] An observational study of 9297 children reported an overall incidence of 2% for bronchospasm; in the subgroup of 2256 children with a history of respiratory problems, the incidence was 6%.[7,70] An editorial review of the subject of asthma and anesthesia concluded that, although the true incidence of major complications is small, severe adverse outcomes do result from bronchospasm, and children with asthma are at heightened risk for severe morbidity.[81]

Both the severity and the control of asthma must be established preoperatively (Table 11.6). These two aspects of the current disease state should be clearly differentiated.[82] For example, asthma may be severe yet well controlled, whereas even mild asthma may be poorly controlled. Both situations may present a heightened potential for perioperative complications, because even the child with intermittent but poorly controlled asthma can have a severe exacerbation.[50]

Severity and control of asthma may be assessed by the frequency of symptoms, limitation of effort tolerance, night awakenings, medication use, emergency department attendance, hospitalizations, and need for ventilatory support. An approach to assessment of severity and control in children aged 5 to 11 years is outlined in E-Tables 11.1 through 11.3. A history of a nocturnal dry cough, more than three wheezing episodes in the past 12 months, or a history of past or present eczema is associated with an increased risk of bronchospasm.[7]

Maintenance treatment of asthma is based on a stepwise approach, with the type of therapy often reflecting the severity of the asthma. Treatment is based on nonpharmacological and pharmacological strategies, which are augmented by education and self-management.[83] The global approach to the treatment of asthma follows the guidelines published by two committees, one from the World Health Organization,[84] and the other under the US National Heart, Lung, and Blood Institute of the National Institutes of Health from the National Asthma Education and Prevention Program (NAEPP).[85] Overall the two guidelines for the treatment of asthma in children are congruent, and depend on the age of the child and the severity of the symptoms, but they differ slightly.[83,86,87] Severity has been categorized into three age groups, 0 to 4 years, 5 to 11 years, and >12 years, and four steps in severity: intermittent, mild but persistent, moderate persistent, and severe persistent asthma (E-Fig. 11.2).[85]

Short-acting inhaled β-agonists may be first-line therapy, with inhaled corticosteroids for those patients with persistent but intermittent mild symptoms poorly managed by bronchodilators as the preferred second step. Alternative treatments at this step include a leukotriene receptor antagonist, a mast cell stabilizer such as cromolyn sodium or nedocromil, and a methylxanthine bronchodilator such as theophylline. Recently budesonide-formoterol as needed has been shown to be as effective as daily medication and has been adopted by The Global Initiative for Asthma (GINA) as an appropriate approach.[88]

The third step in therapy involves increasing the dose of inhaled corticosteroid or adding an alternative treatment to a smaller dose of corticosteroid; a long-acting β-agonist, a leukotriene receptor antagonist, or theophylline may be considered. Step 4 involves a medium dose of corticosteroid together with a long-acting β-agonist. The final steps of therapy involve a high dose of inhaled corticosteroid or commencing an oral corticosteroid (see E-Fig. 11.2). Biologics directed at the basic pathophysiology of asthma offer the hope of personalized medicine.[89] Such medicines include omalizumab which is directed against IgE,[90,91] mepolizumab and benralizumab[92] directed against interleukin 5, dupilumab against IL4 and IL13 and tezepelumab directed against thymic stromal lymphopoietin.[93,94]

Most children with asthma have disease that is intermittent or persistent but mild and will be treated with inhaled short-acting β-agonists on an as-needed basis, alone or in combination with low-dose inhaled corticosteroids or an adjunctive therapy. Poor control may relate to poor compliance with medication, inadequate inhaler technique, or incorrect diagnosis. Severe asthma is diagnosed when symptom control is poor despite high doses of corticosteroids (see steps 5 or 6 in E-Fig. 11.2). A small group of children have "brittle asthma" that is difficult to control despite optimal therapy and may lead to life-threatening respiratory compromise. A history of severe attacks or admission to intensive care is particularly ominous.

Special investigations are not routinely indicated but may be useful in specific circumstances. A chest radiograph is not usually helpful to assess the severity of asthma but can help diagnose a superimposed infection, pneumothorax, or pneumomediastinum during an acute exacerbation. Pulmonary function tests are important in monitoring long-term responses to therapy but are of little use in the immediate, routine preoperative workup of cases at a stable clinical baseline. Measurements of nitric oxide and various inflammatory markers are primarily of use as research tools at present, but their role in asthma management is evolving.[95]

Although an assessment of disease severity is essential, an important caveat is that many asthma deaths in the community setting occur not in those with severe disease but in those with what was thought to be mild or moderate disease. Asthma is often undertreated,[82] so the sensitivity of medication prescription as a marker of disease activity must be viewed with some caution. Some studies have found a poor correlation between assessment of disease severity and the occurrence of perioperative bronchospasm. However, disease *activity*, as noted by recent asthma symptoms, use of medications for symptom treatment, and recent therapy in a medical facility for asthma, is significantly associated with perioperative bronchospasm.[76]

Children should continue their regular medications before anesthesia. Midazolam has been reported to be a safe premedication for asthmatics.[96] Corticosteroids may help prevent postintubation bronchospasm in adults,[97] although controlled clinical data to substantiate this practice in children are lacking.[70] Inhaled β-agonists before or shortly after induction of anesthesia attenuate the increases in airway resistance associated with tracheal intubation.[98,99] Ketamine is the traditional choice of intravenous (IV)

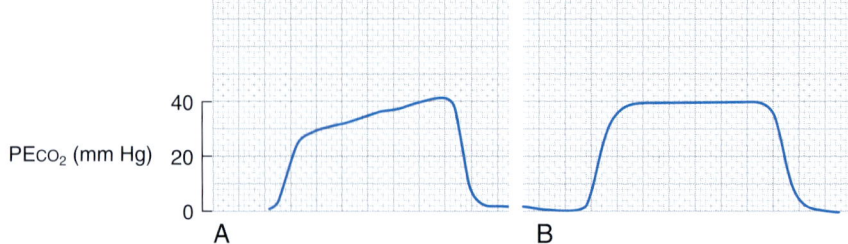

FIGURE 11.9 **A,** Tracing of expired carbon dioxide (PECO$_2$) in a child with acute bronchospasm. Notice the slowly rising PECO$_2$ value. **B,** Tracing from the same patient after administration of inhaled albuterol. Note that the PECO$_2$ waveform now has a flat plateau, indicating relief of the bronchospasm and efficient elimination of CO$_2$ from all areas of the lungs.

induction agent in children with severe asthma, although its superiority over other agents has not been substantiated in clinical trials.[100,101] Propofol is typically preferred over thiopentone because it causes less bronchoconstriction.[80,102] Desflurane is associated with an increased risk of bronchospasm compared with sevoflurane or isoflurane, and because it can increase airway resistance in children, should be avoided in asthmatics.[7]

Tracheal intubation is a potent stimulus for bronchospasm, particularly during a light level of anesthesia.[7] In children with a URI, in whom the airways may be acutely hyperactive, avoiding tracheal intubation reduces the frequency of pulmonary complications.[7,34] There are inadequate clinical outcome data on the perioperative management of asthma to make definitive recommendations about airway management. Nonetheless, avoidance of tracheal and vocal cord stimulation by use of a face mask or a supraglottic device instead of a TT whenever possible seems a sensible approach.[50] However, tracheal intubation has specific indications and it should be undertaken when those are present, such as a child with a full stomach. It would be considered reckless to not intubate the trachea in a child with a full stomach and asthma solely to avoid irritating the airway. If tracheal intubation is mandatory, a deep plane of anesthesia is preferred to blunt airway hyperreactivity.[50] Similarly, unless contraindicated by other factors, deep extubation is preferred for the same reason. Surgical stimulation is another trigger of bronchospasm, and anesthetic depth and analgesia should be adequate to prevent this response.[50]

Intraoperative bronchospasm is characterized variously by polyphonic expiratory wheeze, prolonged expiration, active expiration with increased respiratory effort, increased airway pressures, a slow upslope on the end-tidal CO$_2$ monitor waveform (Fig. 11.9), increased end-tidal CO$_2$, and hypoxemia. Other causes of wheezing must be excluded, such as partial obstruction of the TT (secretions or herniation of the cuff causing obstruction), mainstem intubation (deep endobronchial intubation), aspiration, pneumothorax, or pulmonary edema. Mechanical obstruction of the circuit or TT must also be excluded.

First-line treatment for bronchospasm involves removing the triggering stimulus if possible, deepening anesthesia, increasing the fraction of inspired oxygen (FiO$_2$) if appropriate, decreasing the positive end-expiratory pressure (PEEP), and increasing the expiratory time to minimize alveolar air trapping (I:E ratio 1:3 to 1:4 rather than 1:2).[50] In severe status asthmaticus, ventilation strategy focuses primarily on achieving adequate oxygenation, rather than attempting to normalize PaCO$_2$ at the potential cost of inducing pulmonary barotrauma. All children who experience anything more than minor bronchospasm should also receive corticosteroids, if they have not already done so.

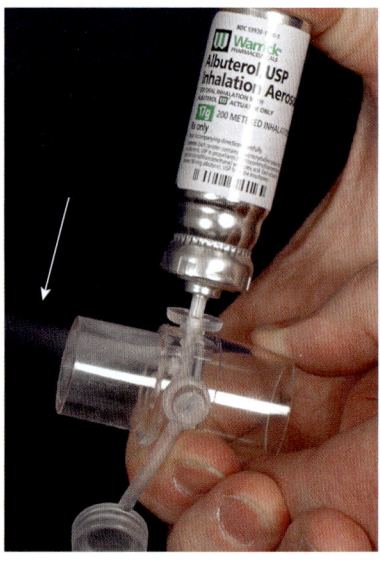

FIGURE 11.10 Adapter that allows administration of albuterol through a tracheal tube (TT) and timing of that dose with inspirations to provide maximum delivery; notice that the nebulized albuterol is directed down the TT *(arrow).* Use of a long intravenous catheter that extends to the tip of the TT is an alternative method to further improve drug delivery.

Inhaled β-agonists can be delivered by nebulizer or by a metered-dose inhaler down the airway device with specially designed adapters (Fig. 11.10). Alternatively, a 60-mL syringe can be used to deliver doses of the nebulizer into the breathing circuit (E-Fig. 11.3). However, the efficiency of delivery through an inhaler that is actuated at the elbow of the breathing circuit is poor, especially in a small-diameter TT.[103] To improve the delivery efficiency of the aerosol in pediatric-size TT, the inhaler may be actuated 10 to 20 times at the elbow or once or twice into a narrow-gauge catheter that is passed to the end of the endotracheal tube.[103,104] A limitation of these techniques, however, is that the dosage delivered cannot be accurately quantified.[105] Bioavailability is also reduced in those with severe bronchospasm.

If IV salbutamol (albuterol) is available, the IV route is preferred over tracheal administration. Onset of bronchodilation in a child with acute symptoms should be rapid with good effect at a plasma salbutamol concentration of 1 μg/L.[106] Salbutamol (10 μg/kg IV) may be repeated, followed by an infusion of 5 to 10 μg/kg per minute for the first hour until there is an improvement in the bronchospasm. Thereafter, salbutamol is commonly infused at 1 to 2 μg/kg per minute until the bronchospasm resolves. This regimen is, however, associated with a high incidence of adverse effects.[107] A pediatric pharmacokinetic-pharmacodynamic (PKPD) model for salbutamol has been described and used as a basis for dosing. An infusion of 0.5 µg/kg per minute after bolus achieves effective bronchodilation. Higher rates contribute minimal improvement of asthma symptoms, but are associated with greater tachycardia and hyperglycemia.[108]

Epinephrine (0.05 to 0.5 µg/kg per minute) is also an effective bronchodilator.

The anesthesiologist may be involved in the management of status asthmaticus when consulted to assist a child in the emergency department or on the wards. A drowsy, silent child with a quiet chest on auscultation despite therapy is in imminent danger of respiratory arrest and requires emergent tracheal intubation by an experienced practitioner. Signs and symptoms to assess the severity of an asthma exacerbation are outlined in Table 11.6, and an algorithm for management issued by the American National Heart, Lung, and Blood Institute is presented in E-Fig. 11.4.

Oxygen is recommended for most children to maintain the oxygen saturation at greater than 90%. Repetitive or continuous administration of short-acting β-agonists is first-line therapy for all children and is the most effective way of reversing airflow obstruction. The addition of ipratropium to a β-agonist may produce additional bronchodilation and may have a modest effect to improve outcome. Systemic corticosteroids should be given to those who do not respond completely and promptly to β-agonists. For severe exacerbations unresponsive to the treatment listed earlier, IV magnesium may decrease the likelihood of intubation, although the evidence is limited.[50,109] Current recommended drug doses are listed in E-Table 11.4.

There is much debate about the role of methylxanthines such as aminophylline in the management of acute exacerbations of asthma. In some countries, aminophylline is considered a first-line treatment for asthma, whereas in others it is considered second line or used less frequently. The difference in practice may be attributed to its equivocal clinical efficacy in the treatment of acute exacerbations of asthma and to complications from toxicity (including vomiting).[110–113]

Antibiotics are not recommended except for comorbid conditions. Aggressive hydration is not recommended in adults or older

TABLE 11.6	Formal Evaluation of Asthma Exacerbation Severity			
	Mild	**Moderate**	**Severe**	**Subset: Respiratory Arrest Imminent**
Symptoms				
Breathlessness	While walking Can lie down	While at rest (infant—softer, shorter cry, difficulty feeding) Prefers sitting	While at rest (infant—stops feeding) Sits upright	
Talks in	Sentences	Phrases	Words	
Alertness	May be agitated	Usually agitated	Usually agitated	Drowsy or confused
Signs				
Respiratory rate[a]	Increased	Increased	Increased	
Use of accessory muscles; suprasternal retractions	Usually not	Commonly	Usually	Paradoxical thoracoabdominal movement
Wheeze	Moderate, often only end expiratory	Loud; throughout exhalation	Usually loud; throughout inhalation and exhalation	Absence of wheeze
Pulse per minute[b]	Slightly increased	Increased	Tachycardia	Bradycardia
Pulsus paradoxus	Absent <10 mm Hg	May be present 10–25 mm Hg	Often present >25 mm Hg (adult) 20–40 mm Hg (child)	Absence suggests respiratory muscle fatigue
Functional Assessment[c]				
PEF (% of predicted or of personal best)	≥70%	Approx. 40%–69% or response lasts <2 hours	<40%	<25% (PEF testing may not be needed in very severe attacks)
PaO_2 (while breathing room air)	Normal (test not usually necessary)	≥60 mm Hg (test not usually necessary)	<60 mm Hg: possible cyanosis	
PCO_2	<42 mm Hg (test not usually necessary)	<42 mm Hg (test not usually necessary)	>42 mm Hg: possible respiratory failure (see text)	
SaO_2% (while breathing room air) at sea level	>95% (test not usually necessary)	90%–95% (test not usually necessary)	<90%	

[a]Guide to rates of breathing in awake children: at age <2 months, normal rate is <60 breaths/minute; at 2–12 months, <50/minute; at 1–5 years, <40/minute; at 6–8 years, <30/minute.
[b]Guide to normal pulse rates in children: at age 2–12 months, normal rate is <160 beats/minute; at 1–2 years, <120/minute; at 2–8 years, <110/minute.
[c]PaO_2 or PCO_2 or both may be tested. Hypercapnia (hypoventilation) develops more readily in young children than in adults and adolescents.
PaO_2, Arterial oxygen tension; PCO_2, partial pressure of carbon dioxide; PEF, peak expiratory flow; SaO_2, oxygen saturation.
Modified from National Asthma Education and Prevention Program. Full report of the expert panel: guidelines for the diagnosis and management of asthma (EPR-3). Bethesda, MD: National Heart, Lung, and Blood Institute, National Institutes of Health, 2007.

children, although it may be indicated in younger children who become dehydrated as a result of decreased oral intake and increased respiratory rate. In general, chest physical therapy and mucolytics are also not recommended.

Children with severe atopy-associated asthma are possibly at greater risk for developing anaphylaxis in response to neuromuscular blocking drugs, antibiotics, and latex.[70,114] Bronchospasm caused by anaphylaxis is differentiated from that due to asthma; it produces additional systemic signs such as angioedema, flushing, urticaria, and cardiovascular collapse.

Adrenal crisis during major surgical stress is a potential complication associated with severe asthma caused by iatrogenic suppression of the hypothalamic-pituitary-adrenal axis.[70] Adrenal suppression should be considered in any child who is taking corticosteroids for a prolonged period. Short courses of prednisolone used to treat acute flares of asthma may affect function for up to 10 days, but prolonged dysfunction is unlikely. Large doses, prolonged therapy for more than a few weeks, and evening dosing may suppress adrenal function for up to 1 year. Prophylactic corticosteroid administration may be indicated for those receiving prolonged systemic corticosteroids, when their corticosteroid regimen is interrupted by the surgical schedule, or for those who have received high-dose inhaled corticosteroids in the recent past (see Chapter 25).

CYSTIC FIBROSIS

CF is an autosomal recessive disorder that is caused by one of more than 1500 mutations in the gene coding for the CF transmembrane conductance regulator (located on chromosome 7), a protein that regulates chloride and other ion fluxes at various epithelial surfaces.[115,116] The different gene defects may variously impact the protein's translation or cellular processing, or function as a chloride channel gating. The incidence of CF is approximately 1 of every 2000 births in Caucasians, making it the most common fatal inherited disease in this population. The ethnicity distribution in the United States is ~85% Caucasian, ~10% Hispanic, and ~5% African American.[117]

The disruption of electrolyte transport in the epithelial cells of the sweat ducts, airways, pancreatic ducts, intestine, biliary tree, and vas deferens causes increased sweat chloride concentrations, viscous mucus production, lung disease, intestinal obstruction, pancreatic insufficiency, biliary cirrhosis, and congenital absence of the vas deferens. The clinical outcome is widely variable, even among children with identical mutations at the CF locus. Absence of the gene influences expression of several other gene products, including proteins important to the inflammatory response, ion maturational processing, transport, and cell signaling. These other proteins are potential modifiers of the phenotype and may help explain the substantial differences in clinical severity.

Lung disease is the main cause of morbidity and mortality in CF, and consequently it is the focus of anesthetic concern. The pathophysiology involves mucus plugging, chronic infection, inflammation, and epithelial injury.[118–120] Mucus clearance defends the lung against inhaled bacteria. The mucociliary transport system requires two fully functioning layers to be effective. The base layer of ciliary epithelia bathed in a watery liquid (sol) is overlaid by a more viscous gel (mucus) that is responsible for transporting particles along the tips of the cilia. Normally, mucus is transported at about 10 mm per minute, expelling foreign particles and pathogens from the lungs. The efficacy of clearance depends on adequate hydration of the mucus.[121] Lack of regulation of sodium absorption and chloride secretion decreases liquid on the airway luminal surfaces, slows mucus clearance, and promotes the formation of adherent plugs in the airway.[122] Increased secretions, viscous mucus, and impaired ciliary clearance contribute to airway impaction, providing a nidus for infection.

At birth, the lung structure is almost normal.[115] However, chronic and recurrent bacterial infections occur early in life, assisted by the pooling of secretions and impaired neutrophil bacterial killing on airway surfaces.[118,123] Repeated and persistent infections stimulate a chronic neutrophilic inflammatory response, ultimately destroying the airway walls. Early pathogens include *Staphylococcus aureus* and *Haemophilus influenzae*. *Pseudomonas aeruginosa* typically invade later in life, acquire a mucoid phenotype, and form a biofilm in the lung, an event that is associated with accelerated decline in pulmonary function. The invasion of the lung by antibiotic-resistant pathogens such as certain strains of *Burkholderia cepacia* is often devastating, markedly increasing the death rate from lung disease.

Various insults such as bacteria, viruses, and airborne irritants can cause acute exacerbations of respiratory symptoms of cough and sputum production. This is often accompanied by systemic manifestations such as weight loss, anorexia, and fatigue. These changes from baseline are termed *pulmonary exacerbations*.[124]

Recurrent exacerbations are associated with progressive airway obstruction, bronchiectasis, emphysema, ventilation/perfusion mismatching, and hypoxemia. Growth of blood vessels with advancing bronchiectasis predisposes to hemoptysis. Bronchial hyperreactivity and increased airway resistance are common, whereas bullae formation can lead to pneumothorax.

Pulmonary function abnormalities typically have an obstructive pattern[125] and include increased FRC, decreased FEV_1, decreased peak expiratory flow rate, and decreased vital capacity (see Fig. 11.5). Compensatory hyperventilation typically produces a reduced $PaCO_2$, although hypercapnia may supersede in end-stage pulmonary pathology. End-stage cor pulmonale may lead to cardiomegaly, fluid retention, and hepatomegaly.

Malnutrition is a common problem in CF that follows from pancreatic insufficiency, failure of enzyme secretion, impaired gastrointestinal motility, abnormal enterohepatic circulation of bile, increased caloric demand owing to severe lung disease, and anorexia of chronic disease.[115] Low weight and body mass index are closely associated with, and can predict, poor lung function.

CF-related diabetes arises from progressive pancreatic disease and scarring that compromises the pancreatic islets. More than 12% of teenagers older than 13 years with CF have insulin-dependent diabetes, and the incidence increases with age.[126] Evidence is accumulating that diabetes contributes to the lung disease and worse outcome.[118–120] In addition, classic diabetic complications occur in older CF patients. Hepatic dysfunction decreases plasma cholinesterase and clotting factors II, VII, IX, and X, whereas malabsorption of vitamin K may also contribute to coagulation issues.[127]

When CF was first distinguished from celiac syndrome in 1938, life expectancy was approximately 6 months. Since then, substantial advances in CF care has resulted in dramatic improvements survival; for individuals born between 2017 and 2021, the median predicted survival age is 53.1 years.[127,128]

The pillars of treatment include nutritional repletion, relief of airway obstruction, antibiotic therapy for lung infection, and corrector and potentiator therapies. Organ transplantation, and in particular lung transplantation, has been used in an attempt to improve quality of life and prolong survival, but a clear benefit remains to be demonstrated.[129] A review of 1885 lung transplants from 1983 to 2016, of whom 364 were for CF, reported the following survival rates: 94% at 1 year, 70% at 5 years, and 53% at 10 years; the average age at transplant was 29.5 (SD 9.7) years (E-Fig. 11.5).[130]

Corrector and potentiator therapies are recently developed treatments that are directed at the molecular defects in the CF transmembrane conductance regulator.[88,131,132] Correctors are principally targeted at cellular misprocessing, whereas potentiators aim to correct a channel's function. Ivacaftor was the first developed drug in this area, and it is a potentiator that targets several mutations in the cystic fibrosis transmembrane conductance regulator (CFTR) gene, including the G551D mutation. Elexacaftor-tezacaftor-ivacaftor, a small-molecule cystic fibrosis transmembrane conductance regulator (CFTR, a chloride channel) modulator regiment, has revolutionized the care of CF patients and targets even the most common mutation, *Phe508del*.[133] Use of this drug in children as young as 6 years of age, before chronic damage inflicted by the disease process occurs, offers considerable hope for better outcomes.

The multisystem nature of the disease and changing demographics mean that children present for a wide variety of surgical procedures. The most common indications for anesthesia in children are nasal polypectomy and ear, nose, and throat surgery, as a result of the frequency of upper airway pathologic processes such as chronic sinusitis and nasal polyps (Table 11.7).[134,135] The investigation or correction of gastrointestinal disorders is the next most common procedural category that requires anesthesia in the CF population. Other indications for anesthesia include bronchoscopy and pulmonary lavage, computed tomogram for respiratory assessment,[136] gastrointestinal endoscopy, sclerosing injection of varices resulting from portal hypertension, insertion of venous access devices, and incidental surgical problems.[135,137,138]

Because of the increasing longevity of this population, the pediatric anesthesiologist may also be involved in the care of adults.[127] Surgical procedures in adults typically include treatment of recurrent pneumothorax, cholecystectomy, and lung or cardiac transplantation. Consultation may also be requested for obstetric cases as increasing numbers of patients survive to adulthood.

Pulmonary disease is the predominant concern when planning anesthesia for these patients. Historically, morbidity and mortality from pulmonary complications were significant—for example, in 1964, a retrospective study reported a perioperative mortality rate of 27%,[139] but by 1972, this incidence had decreased to 4%.[134] More recent studies have confirmed low mortality but an appreciable rate of morbidity after general anesthesia for lung lavage; bronchoscopies; and ear, nose, and throat surgery in children with CF. With a combined cohort of 700 children, the frequency of perioperative complications was between 5% and 13%.[135,140–143] In a study of 18 patients with CF undergoing anesthesia for pleural surgery, the risks for this surgery were considered substantial, although the anesthetic hazards of CF could be minimized with careful management.[144] The effects of anesthesia on pulmonary function in children with CF are unclear. In a small study of children undergoing injection of esophageal varices, pulmonary function test results deteriorated 48 hours after general anesthesia.[145] In contrast, in almost 100 children in two studies, no difference in pulmonary function tests measured before compared with after a variety of surgical procedures was observed.[135,146] Although acute pulmonary morbidity may pose challenges, the effects of the anesthetic management techniques on pulmonary function tests are difficult to predict.[147]

An assessment of the severity, current state, and progression of pulmonary disease should guide anesthetic planning. Fitness is a positive predictor of survival,[115] and exercise tolerance is a useful marker of pulmonary function. The quality and quantity of secretions, recent and chronic infections, use and effectiveness of bronchodilators, and number of hospitalizations are also important points to elucidate in the history. Examination of the cardiopulmonary systems should aim to detect compromise of cardiac, pulmonary, and hepatic function. Special investigations are not routinely indicated but may quantify organ dysfunction in end stages of the disease. Arterial blood gas analysis, chest radiography, pulmonary function tests, electrocardiography, echocardiography, and liver function tests may assist the planning of anesthetic technique in selected children.[138,147]

Children are often emotionally vulnerable, not simply because of the usual preoperative anxieties but because of the psychological consequences of progression of an ultimately fatal disease. A preoperative visit should aim to allay distress; oral benzodiazepines have been successfully used as anxiolytics.[135,143] Prophylactic use of osmotic laxatives may be indicated if opioid-induced ileus is anticipated.[138]

Because desiccation of mucous secretions is a central pulmonary issue in CF, general anesthesia poses specific problems. During spontaneous ventilation under normal conditions, inspired gases are warmed to body temperature and saturated with water vapor, reaching this state at the isothermic saturation point just distal to the carina.[148,149] This ensures that the lower airways are kept moist and warm. The alveolar environment in optimal circumstances has a saturated water vapor pressure of 47.1 mm Hg and an absolute humidity of 43.4 g/m³ at 98.6°F (37°C).

The inspiration of cold, desiccated anesthetic gases and vapors can impair the warming and humidification of the airways. The use of any airway device (oropharyngeal airway, laryngeal mask, or endotracheal tube) bypasses the nasal and oropharyngeal passages and delivers cold, dry gas farther down the airway.[150] This shifts the isothermic saturation point distally, forcing bronchi that normally function in optimal conditions to take part in heat and gas exchange.[149] These parts of the airway are less adapted to moisture exchange and tend to dehydrate more rapidly, thereby impairing the mucociliary escalator and predisposing to impaction of secretions.[151,152] By directly impairing mucociliary motion as well as blunting the cough response and ventilatory drive, inhalational anesthetics can exacerbate this problem.

TABLE 11.7	Most Frequent Indications for Anesthesia in Cystic Fibrosis		
Neonates	**Children/Teenagers**	**Adults**	
Meconium ileus	Nasal polypectomy	Esophageal varices	
Meconium peritonitis	Intravenous access	Recurrent pneumothorax	
Intestinal atresia	Ear/nose/throat surgery	Cholecystectomy	
		Lung (liver) transplantation	

Modified from Della Rocca G. Anaesthesia in patients with cystic fibrosis. *Curr Opin Anaesthesiol.* 2002;15:95-101.

It is therefore particularly important to minimize mucus desiccation in the perioperative period. Inhalation of hypertonic saline (7% sodium chloride) accelerates mucus clearance, increases lung function, and improves quality of life[153–155]; this is now typically part of the routine maintenance management of CF.[156] Nebulized saline treatments should continue up to the start of anesthesia and recommence after the procedure. Inhaled gases should be humidified, or an artificial "nose" should be inserted into the circuit to conserve airway moisture and minimize the risk of inspissating secretions. Although removal of pulmonary secretions is considered important in principle, a small prospective trial of intraoperative bronchial wash-out and physical therapy reported an acute increase in airway resistance with no significant long-term benefit in measures of lung function.[157]

At the conclusion of surgery, complete reversal of neuromuscular blockade should be confirmed. Whenever possible, the trachea should be extubated, and the child encouraged to breathe spontaneously. A 30- to 40-degree head-up position assists movement of the diaphragm and ventilation. Postoperatively, physiotherapy, airway humidification, carefully titrated analgesics, and early mobilization should enhance clearance of secretions and minimize atelectasis. The use of neuraxial, regional, or local anesthesia, as well as nonopioid analgesics, are useful strategies to avoid respiratory depression.[158,159] Ambulatory surgery is optimal, if feasible, because it minimizes disruption to the patient's schedule and decreases exposure to nosocomial infection.

SICKLE CELL DISEASE

Sickle cell disease (SCD) is an inherited hemoglobinopathy that results from a point mutation on chromosome 11 (see also Chapter 8). The mutant gene codes for the production of hemoglobin S, a mutant variant of the normal hemoglobin A. This leads to widespread and progressive vascular damage.[160,161] Clinical features of the disease include acute episodes of pain, acute and chronic pulmonary disease, hemorrhagic and occlusive stroke, renal insufficiency, and splenic infarction, with mean life expectancy shortened to just over 3 decades.[162] Perioperative problems and management are covered in more detail in Chapter 8; the discussion here is limited to a brief review of the pulmonary pathology of SCD.

Acute chest syndrome (ACS) is an acute lung injury caused by SCD.[163] Diagnostic criteria include a new pulmonary infiltrate involving at least one lung segment on the radiograph (excluding atelectasis) combined with one or more symptoms or signs of chest pain, pyrexia greater than 101.3°F (38.5°C), tachypnea, wheezing, or cough.[164–166] Precipitants include infection, fat embolism after bone marrow infarction, pulmonary infarction, and surgical procedures.[166–168] Potential risk factors for the development and severity of perioperative ACS may include a history of lung disease, recent clustering of acute pulmonary complications, pregnancy, increased age, and the invasiveness of the surgical procedure.[160] ACS was associated with younger-age patients, reduced body temperature, and greater blood loss in a study of 60 children with SCD undergoing laparoscopic surgery.[169]

The risk of ACS is small (<5%) after minor surgeries such as inguinal hernia repair and distal extremity surgery, whereas it is severalfold greater (10% to 15%) after intraabdominal and major joint surgery.[168,170,171] Although the overall perioperative mortality from SCD is quite small, <1%,[168,172] ACS can prolong postoperative hospitalization, and cause respiratory failure and death. ACS typically develops about 3 days postoperatively and persists for approximately 8 days, with a 3.3% mortality.[167] The incidence of ACS is greatest in children who have had prior events in the first 3 years of life, those with reduced fetal hemoglobin concentration, and greater steady state hemoglobin and white blood cell counts.[173]

SCD also causes chronic lung damage, known as sickle cell lung disease (SCLD).[174] Because lung function has not yet been assessed longitudinally in a cohort from early childhood to adulthood, the precise pathology of and relationship between the obstructive and restrictive patterns of lung disease is unclear.[175] Children appear to develop a predominantly obstructive pattern,[176] whereas adults develop a more restrictive pulmonary defect.[174,177,178] In the later stages of lung damage, both vital and total lung capacities decrease, gas diffusion is impaired, and pulmonary fibrosis, pulmonary artery hypertension, right-sided cardiomyopathy, and progressive hypoxemia may occur.[174,178] The development of pulmonary artery hypertension, which can precede clinically apparent lung damage, is a particularly ominous sign of disease progression and is associated with a heightened risk of sudden death.[173,177] Recurrent ACS is an independent risk factor for the development of end-stage SCLD, but subtle evidence of parenchymal and vascular damage commonly precedes clustered episodes of ACS.[174]

Assessment of lung function should include a history of the occurrence, frequency, severity, and known precipitants of ACS and a search for progression of chronic lung damage. A recent chest radiograph can serve as a baseline for comparison if postoperative radiographs are needed and can also delineate lung pathology. Early features of lung damage include decreased distal pulmonary vascularity and diffuse interstitial fibrosis, whereas later stages are characterized by pulmonary fibrosis, pulmonary hypertension, and right ventricular hypertrophy.[174,179] Pulmonary function testing can reveal the need for bronchodilators and the presence of obstructive or restrictive lung disease.

Although the risk of developing ACS in the perioperative period is increased, distinct genotypes, wide variation in disease severity, differing chronic treatment protocols, varied surgical procedures, and logistical complexities have made research into the optimal perioperative management difficult.[180] Well-delivered anesthetic and postoperative care may be the best guarantor of a good outcome.[160,161]

Perioperative management frequently includes red blood cell transfusion to decrease the risk of perioperative ACS. The Transfusion Alternative Perioperatively in Sickle Cell Disease study prospectively enrolled 67 patients undergoing low- and medium-risk surgery with or without preoperative transfusion.[181] Although limited by early closure of the study, the small sample size, and too few patients enrolled in the low-risk surgery group to allow for subgroup analysis, the prevalence of clinically important events, including ACS, in the nontransfused group was significantly greater than in the transfused group (odds ratio 3.8). The authors concluded that preoperative transfusion may reduce the risk of ACS in patients with a homozygous HbSS genotype.

If preoperative transfusion is performed to attenuate SCD exacerbations, an exchange transfusion aimed at decreasing the concentration of hemoglobin S to 30% is no more effective than simply correcting the anemia to a hematocrit of 30%. However, exchange transfusion is more likely to lead to transfusion-related complications including the development of uncommon antibodies such as Kell and Duffy antibodies.[167] Consequently, if a decision is made to transfuse in the hope of preventing ACS, the target should be a hematocrit of 30% rather than a specific dilution of hemoglobin S.

The risk of ACS after low-risk surgeries or procedures without transfusion appears to be small.[182] A study of patients undergoing magnetic resonance imaging (MRI) with deep sedation reported an incidence of ACS of 1.2% within 1 month of the MRI,[183] whereas nontransfused patients undergoing minor surgery in the Cooperative Study of Sickle Cell Disease had a similar incidence of ACS of 1.4%.[167] In two retrospective reviews of the NSQIP-Pediatric database of 357 and 813 children with SCD undergoing semielective abdominal surgery of whom 52% to 56% were transfused, preoperative transfusions did not improve clinical outcomes.[184,185] However, perioperative complications were 2.5-fold greater in those undergoing urgent/emergent surgery.[185] In a recent retrospective review of children with SCD with different hemoglobinopathies (SS, SC, Sβ_{thal}) undergoing low and medium-risk surgeries, postoperative complications were significantly more common in those with a preoperative Hb <9 g/dL compared with those with an Hb 9 to 10 g/dL, both groups nontransfused.[186] A simple preoperative transfusion in those with an Hb 9 to 10 g/dL resulted in more postoperative complications (odds ratio 3.0) but not in those with an Hb <9 g/dL (odds ratio 0.64). In the multivariable regression, complications after medium-risk surgery were significantly more common (odds ratio 2.3).[186] A survey of North American pediatric anesthesiologists in 2011 found that most clinicians do not transfuse children who are at low risk for perioperative complications after minor procedures, whereas a greater number transfuse sicker children undergoing more invasive procedures.[187]

The one group of children with SCD who are at high risk for complications are those who have experienced or are at risk for a stroke. Risk factors for strokes include low hemoglobin, hypertension, and male gender as well as three single-nucleotide polymorphisms.[188,189] Serial transcranial Doppler ultrasound and MRI of the brain have been used to detect pathologic changes in blood flow or subclinical strokes, respectively, and in these children blood transfusion has been effective in reducing subsequent strokes.[190,191] Silent cerebral strokes have been detected in up to 30% of asymptomatic children with SCD.[188] To reduce the risk of stroke, these children have transfusions at regular intervals, based on the results of the serial investigations. However, this approach raises concern about iron overload and other complications associated with repeated blood transfusions. A study to limit the number of transfusions in those at risk for a stroke had to be stopped prematurely because two strokes occurred despite serial transcranial Doppler monitoring.[192] Chronic hydroxyurea therapy has also been shown to be effective in reducing the risk of stroke.[193] The perioperative management of children with a history of stroke continues to evolve.

Children with SCD frequently develop postoperative atelectasis. It is unclear whether this relates to an underlying sickle cell lung disease, difficulty with analgesia, other causes, or a combination of factors. Pain management can be difficult in these children. Large doses of opioids can depress ventilation and cause atelectasis.[180,194] ACS tends to involve the lower segments of the lung,[166] suggesting an association between atelectasis and ACS; incentive spirometry can prevent the development of atelectasis and pulmonary infiltrates.[195] Regional analgesia, supplemental nonopioid analgesics, prophylactic incentive spirometry, early mobilization, and good pulmonary toilet may decrease the incidence of atelectasis and ACS.

Treatment of ACS is focused on supporting gas exchange. Supplemental oxygen, noninvasive ventilatory support such as CPAP, or intubation and mechanical ventilation are indicated by the degree of dysfunction. Bronchodilators, incentive spirometry,

and chest physiotherapy may be useful in preventing disease progression. In the presence of a significant ventilation/perfusion mismatch, correction of anemia can improve arterial oxygenation. Erythrocyte transfusion increases oxygen-carrying capacity, decreases fractional peripheral tissue extraction, and increases returning venous oxygen levels. Because the mean arterial oxygen content in the presence of a shunt is significantly affected by the oxygenation of blood returning from nonventilated parts of the lung, increasing venous oxygen levels can improve arterial oxygen content. Although transfusion has not been directly linked to improved outcomes, both exchange and simple transfusions can improve oxygenation.[166,180]

ANNOTATED REFERENCES

Bishop MJ, Cheney FW. Anesthesia for patients with asthma: low risk but not no risk. *Anesthesiology*. 1996;85:455-456.
A thoughtful editorial on the implications, dangers, and practical implications of asthma.
Davis PB. Cystic fibrosis since 1938. *Am J Respir Crit Care Med*. 2006; 173:475-482.
A succinct discourse on the evolution of management of cystic fibrosis.
Firth PG, Head CA. Sickle cell disease and anesthesia. *Anesthesiology*. 2004;101:766-785.
A comprehensive review of anesthetic management of sickle cell disease.
Howard J, Malfroy M, Llewelyn C, et al. The Transfusion Alternatives Preoperatively in Sickle Cell Disease (TAPS) study: a randomised, controlled, multicentre clinical trial. *Lancet*. 2013;381(9870):930-938.
A prospective randomized trial of the effect of perioperative red blood cell transfusion.
Huffmyer JL, Littlewood KE, Nemergut EC. Perioperative management of the adult with cystic fibrosis. *Anesth Analg*. 2009;109:1949-1961.
An updated review of anesthetic implications of advanced cystic fibrosis.
National Asthma Education and Prevention Program. *Full Report of the Expert Panel: Guidelines for the Diagnosis and Management of Asthma (EPR-3)*. Bethesda, MD: National Heart, Lung, and Blood Institute, National Institutes of Health; 2007.
An extensive review of current evidence on the pathophysiology, diagnosis, and management of asthma.
Reddel HK, Bacharier LB, Bateman ED, et al. Global Initiative for Asthma Strategy 2021: executive summary and rational for key changes. *Eur Resp J*. 2022;59;2102730.
Executive summary of the recommendations of the GINA Strategy Report from 2021 for stratification of asthma therapy in children.
Tan LD, Alismail A, Ariue B. Asthma guidelines: comparison of the National Heart, Lung, and Blood Institute Expert Panel Report 4 with Global Initiative for Asthma 2021. *Curr Opin Pulm Med*. 2022;28; 234-244.
The report from the National Asthma Education and Prevent Program yielded guidelines for stratifying treatment in children. This guideline is compared with the Global Initiative for Asthma guideline to better understand the basis for their recommendations and treatment.
Templeton TW, Sommerfield D, Hii J, Sommerfield A, Matava CT, von Ungern-Sternberg BS. Risk assessment and optimization strategies to reduce perioperative respiratory adverse events in pediatric anesthesia-part 2: anesthesia-related risk and treatment options. *Paediatr Anaesth*. 2022;32(2):217-227.
A broad review of the data on perioperative upper respiratory tract infections and suggested approaches to management.
von Ungern-Sternberg BS, Boda K, Chambers NA, et al. Risk assessment for respiratory complications in paediatric anaesthesia: a prospective cohort study. *Lancet*. 2010;376:773-783.
A large prospective observational study of perioperative adverse respiratory events and predictive risk factors.

A complete reference list can be found online at Elsevier eBooks+.

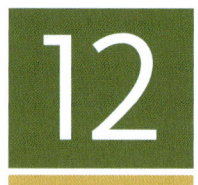

12

The Pediatric Airway

MARY LYN STEIN, LUIS SEQUERA-RAMOS, JOHN E. FIADJOE, PAUL A. STRICKER, AND CHARLES J. COTÉ

Developmental Anatomy of the Airway
Tongue
Position of the Larynx
Epiglottis
Subglottis
The Larynx
Anatomy
Function
Physiology of the Respiratory System
Obligate Nasal Breathing
Tracheal and Bronchial Function
Work of Breathing
Airway Obstruction During Anesthesia
Evaluation of the Airway

Clinical Evaluation
Diagnostic Testing
Airway Management: The Normal Airway
Mask Ventilation
Oropharyngeal Airways
Nasopharyngeal Airways
Tracheal Intubation
Supraglottic Airways
Airway Management: The Abnormal Airway
Classifying The Abnormal Pediatric Airway
Management Principles
Special Techniques for Ventilation
Special Techniques for Intubation

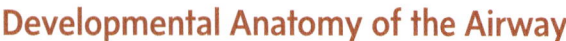

DIFFERENCES BETWEEN PEDIATRIC AND ADULT AIRWAYS are important determinants of anesthetic and airway management techniques. Knowledge of normal developmental anatomy and physiologic function is required to understand and manage both the normal and the pathologic airways of infants and children (Video 12.1). Techniques and principles to assist in this management are reviewed in this chapter.

Developmental Anatomy of the Airway

The classic works by Negus, Eckenhoff, Wilson, Fink, and Demarest form the foundation of our knowledge about the structure and function of the pediatric and adult airways.[1–4] They suggest several major anatomic differences between the neonatal and adult airways that inform the approach to managing the pediatric airway. These differences include (1) relative macroglossia, (2) cephalad position of the glottis, (3) long, angled, omega-shaped epiglottis, (4) relatively angled vocal cords, and (5) a funnel-shaped larynx with the narrowest portion at the cricoid ring. In addition to these differences, the relatively large head in infants compared with adults creates the situation where the infant's neck in the supine position is relatively flexed and may require gentle extension to allow alignment of the oral, pharyngeal, and tracheal axes.[5–7] Older children have airway features that represent a transition between the features in the neonate and those in the adult.

TONGUE

It is generally held that the tongue of the neonate and infant is relatively large in proportion to the volume of the oral cavity and therefore more easily obstructs the upper airway.[8] Furthermore, because the larynx is more cephalad in the neck of the neonate and oropharyngeal structures are closer together, the tongue rests against the roof of the mouth during quiet respiration, resulting in oral airway obstruction.[9] Magnetic resonance imaging (MRI) studies demonstrated that in children 1 to 11 years of age, there is proportional growth of the tongue and other soft tissues in relation to the bony structures that support the oral cavity[5]; however, this study did not examine neonates and infants (<12 months of age). Imaging studies indicate that the contribution of the tongue to upper airway obstruction during sedation or induction of anesthesia is relatively minor, with much of the obstruction in older children attributable to the collapse of the pharyngeal walls, lymphoid tissue, and posterior displacement of the epiglottis by the base of the tongue.[10,11] The tongue may still contribute to obstruction in all age groups and may be particularly problematic in children with conditions associated with macroglossia such as Trisomy 21 and Beckwith-Wiedemann syndrome.[12,13]

POSITION OF THE LARYNX

The larynx in the infant is more cephalad than in the adult, classically described at the level of C3–4 in infants moving rostral to C4–5 in adults (Fig. 12.1).[1–4] MRI and computed tomography (CT) have confirmed the more cephalad position of the larynx in children and demonstrated that the hyoid bone is at the level of C2–3 in infants and children up to 2 years of age.[14] The proximity of the tongue base to the more cephalad larynx produces a more acute angle between the plane of the tongue and the plane of the glottic opening making visualization of laryngeal structures more challenging. It is for this reason that when a straight laryngoscope blade is used to lift the epiglottis during laryngoscopy, the neonate's larynx is easily visualized.

In children with mandibular and midface hypoplasia (e.g., Treacher Collins, Goldenhar syndromes, see E-Table 12.1 for a more complete list), the tongue is displaced more caudally (glossoptosis). The reduced distance from the base of tongue to the glottic opening may lead to airway obstruction, making visualization of the

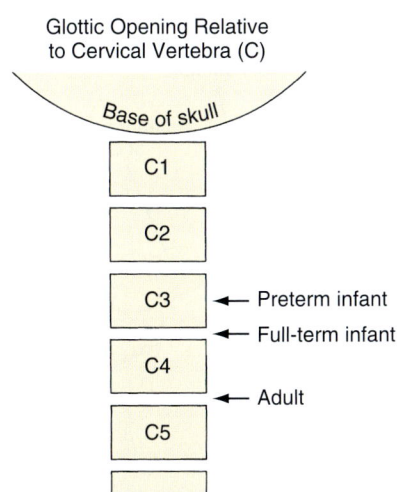

Glottic Opening Relative
to Cervical Vertebra (C)

Base of skull

C1

C2

C3 ← Preterm infant
← Full-term infant

C4
← Adult

C5

FIGURE 12.1 In a preterm infant, the larynx is located at the middle of the third cervical vertebra (C3); in a full-term infant, it is at the C3–4 interspace; and in an adult, it is at the C4–5 interspace. (Adapted from Negus VE. *The Comparative Anatomy and Physiology of the Larynx.* Oxford: Butterworth-Heinemann; 1949.)

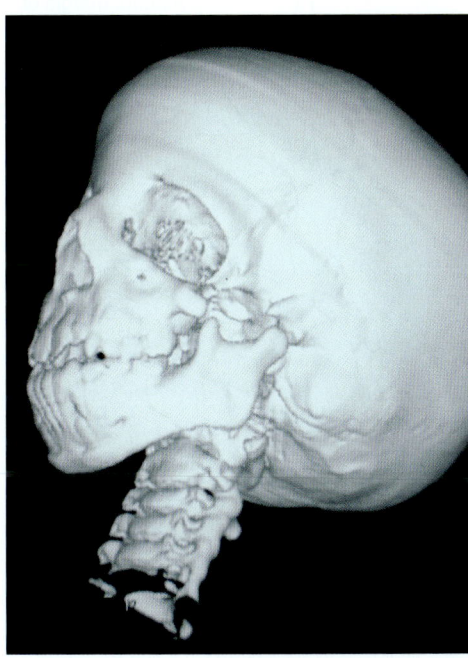

FIGURE 12.2 Three-dimensional reconstruction of a child with the Treacher Collins anomaly demonstrates the retrognathic and more posterior position of the mandible, the midfacial hypoplasia, and the closer proximity and exaggerated angle between the base of the tongue and the laryngeal inlet (almost 90 degrees), which makes direct visualization of the larynx difficult.

glottis difficult and sometimes impossible with direct laryngoscopy (Figs. 12.2 and 12.3). In this situation, conventional laryngoscopy provides excellent visualization of the esophageal inlet rather than the laryngeal inlet, necessitating the use of special equipment or special techniques to intubate the trachea.

EPIGLOTTIS

The epiglottis in the infant is narrow, omega-shaped, and angled away from the axis of the trachea, which contrasts with that in the adult, where the epiglottis is flat and broad, and its axis is parallel to the trachea (Figs. 12.4 and 12.5). This shape allows the epiglottis to approach the uvula during infant breastfeeding, separating breath from fluid and allowing respiration at the same time as swallowing. Based on these differences, the epiglottis may still obstruct the view of the glottic opening when a laryngoscope blade is placed in the vallecula. Using the tip of a straight blade to directly lift the epiglottis may yield a better view.

Vocal Folds

The vocal folds (cords) in an infant are angled such that the anterior insertion is more caudad than the posterior insertion, whereas the axis of the folds in the adult is perpendicular to that of the trachea (compare Fig. 12.4A with Fig. 12.5A). This anatomic feature alters the angle at which the tracheal tube approaches the laryngeal inlet and occasionally leads to difficulty with tracheal intubation, especially with the nasal approach. In the latter case, the tip of the tracheal tube may be held up at the anterior commissure of the vocal folds.

SUBGLOTTIS

Classic teaching based on study of autopsy specimens[6,15–21] reveals that infants have a funnel-shaped larynx, narrowest at the cricoid cartilage[22] (below the glottic opening); whereas adults have a cylindrical larynx with the narrowest part of the upper airway at the rima glottidis. Imaging studies in sedated, spontaneously breathing patients have yielded conflicting results with regard to the narrowest regions in both the pediatric[14,23,24] and adult larynges.[21,25] These conflicting findings likely arise from the dynamic movements of the vocal cords, vestibular, and aryepiglottic folds, as well as the collapse of soft tissue during the phases of respiration. In aggregate, these result in an apparent narrowing of the larynx in the proximal glottis when assessed radiologically.[22–24] Subsequent cadaveric measurements have corroborated the historical findings that the cricoid outlet is nearly circular and the narrowest part of the pediatric larynx.[22] The cricoid cartilage is *functionally* and *anatomically* the narrowest portion of the pediatric upper airway (Fig. 12.6).

Knowledge of the location of the narrowest point of the airway is important in selecting an appropriately sized tracheal tube. The cricoid is the only complete ring of cartilage in the laryngotracheobronchial tree and as such, it is nondistensible.[22] When a tracheal tube is inserted into the glottic aperture, the tube readily passes through the distensible vocal cords but may meet resistance or become "stuck" below the cords (e.g., at the level of the cricoid ring) (Fig. 12.7; see Video 12.1). Growth of the subglottic airway occurs rapidly throughout the first 2 years of life but slows thereafter, becoming linear over time.[21] The cricoid and thyroid cartilages reach adult proportions by 10 to 12 years of age, thus eliminating both the angulation of the vocal cords and decreasing the importance of the narrow subglottic area. In adults, the rima glottidis is the narrowest part of the airway,[21] and a tracheal tube that traverses the glottis generally passes into the trachea without resistance. However, in about 70% of adult cadavers, the narrowest portion of the airway has been identified in the subglottic region.[25] The range in diameter for adult females is 10 to 16 mm, and for adult males it is 13 to 19 mm. The likely reason that a tracheal tube easily passes through the rima glottidis into the trachea of an adult is that overall, the narrowest portion of the airway is still larger than the most commonly used tracheal tube sizes.

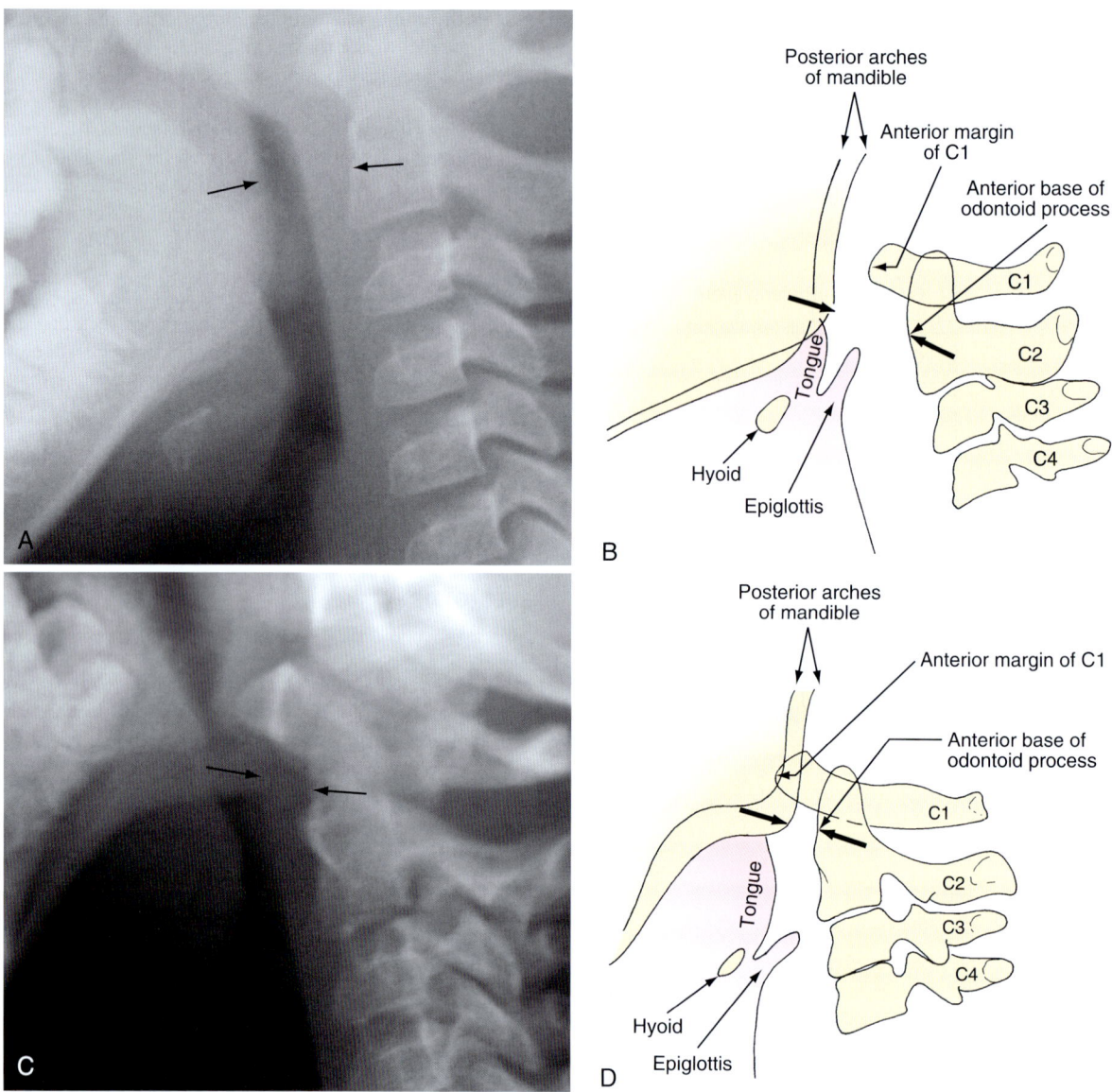

FIGURE 12.3 The larynx in children with mandibular hypoplasia is located more posteriorly than in children with normal anatomy. **A,** Lateral radiograph of the upper airway including the base of the skull and cervical spine of a normal 7-year-old child; the *arrows* denote the posterior border of the ramus of the mandible and the anterior border of the second cervical vertebra. **B,** Diagrammatic representation of the normal anatomy in **A. C,** The same radiographic projection in a 6-year-old child with Treacher Collins syndrome; the *arrows* again denote the posterior border of the ramus of the mandible and the anterior margin of the second cervical vertebra. **D,** Diagrammatic representation of the anatomy in **C.** Notice the significantly smaller space (indicated by *thick arrows* in **B** and **D**) between the ramus of the mandible and the second cervical vertebra, compared with the normal anatomy; the anterior margin of the first cervical vertebra overlaps the posterior margin of the mandible. This extreme posterior location of the tongue and larynx makes direct visualization of the laryngeal inlet almost impossible in many children with this anomaly because of the acute angulation between the base of the tongue and the laryngeal inlet. (Radiographs courtesy Donna J. Seibert, MD; John A. Kirkpatrick, Jr., MD; and Robert H. Cleveland, MD.)

The mucosa that lines the upper airway is loose-fitting pseudostratified columnar epithelium.[26,27] Pressure on the mucosa may cause reactive edema that encroaches on the diameter of the lumen. A tight-fitting tracheal tube that compresses the tracheal mucosa at this level may cause inflammation and edema when it is removed, reducing the luminal diameter and increasing the airway resistance at the time of extubation, resulting in postextubation croup or stridor and increased work of breathing. Given the subglottic region in the infant is smaller than in the adult, the same degree of airway edema increases the resistance to air flow in the infant at a much faster rate. For example, assuming that the diameter of the cricoid ring in the infant is 4 mm (radius is 2 mm) and the diameter of the adult cricoid ring is 8 mm (radius is 4 mm), 1 mm of edema circumferentially within the cricoid ring reduces the radius in the infant airway by one-half, which would reduce the cross-sectional area of the ring (Area = $\pi \times r^2$) by ~75%, whereas the cross-sectional area in the adult would decrease by only ~44%.

12

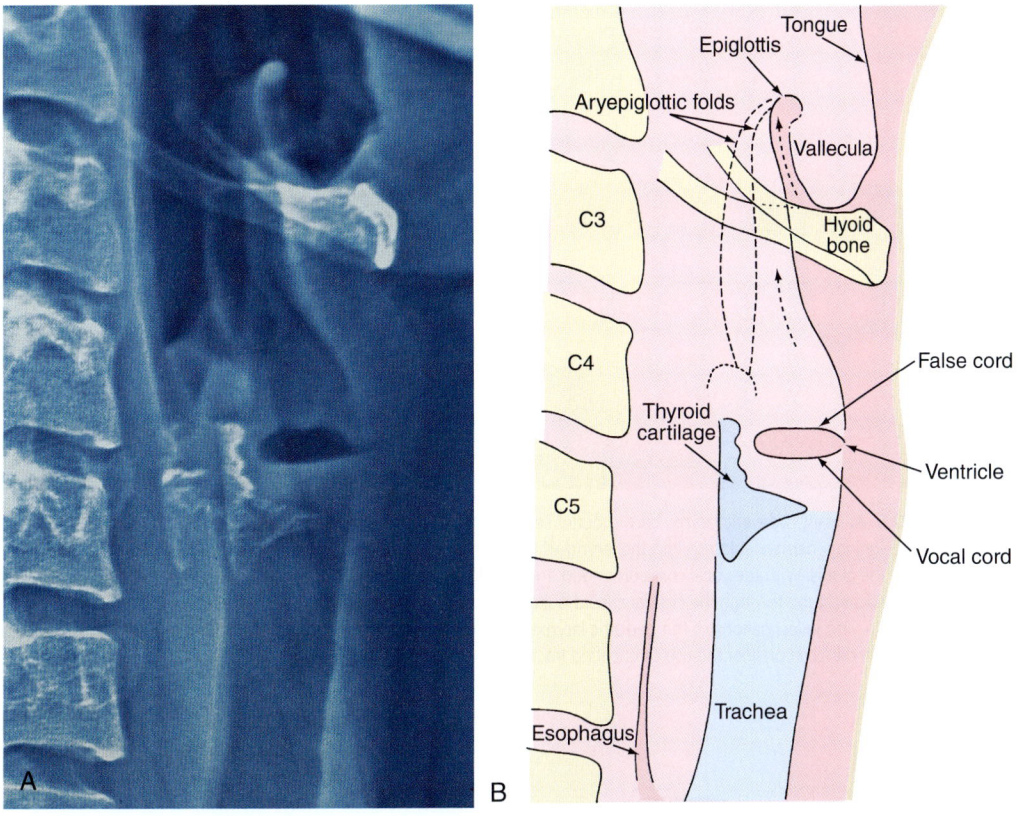

FIGURE 12.4 A, Lateral neck xerogram and **B,** schematic diagram of the larynx in an adult. Notice the relatively thin, broad epiglottis, the axis of the epiglottis which is parallel to the trachea. The hyoid bone "hugs" the epiglottis; there is no subglottic narrowing. Also note how the vocal cords are perpendicular to the axis of the trachea.

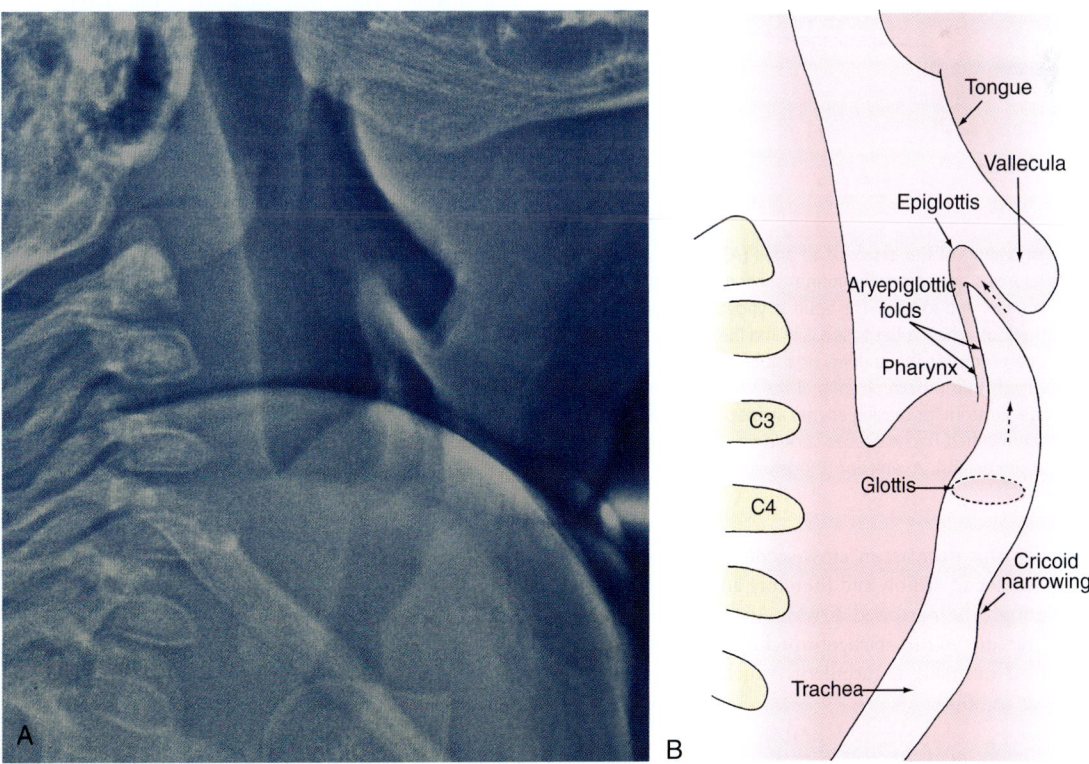

FIGURE 12.5 A, Lateral neck xerogram and **B,** schematic diagram of an infant's larynx. Notice the angled epiglottis and the narrow cricoid cartilage. Also note that the vocal cords are angled with a higher attachment anteriorly than posteriorly, compared with the perpendicular position of the vocal cords in adults.

3-month old infant

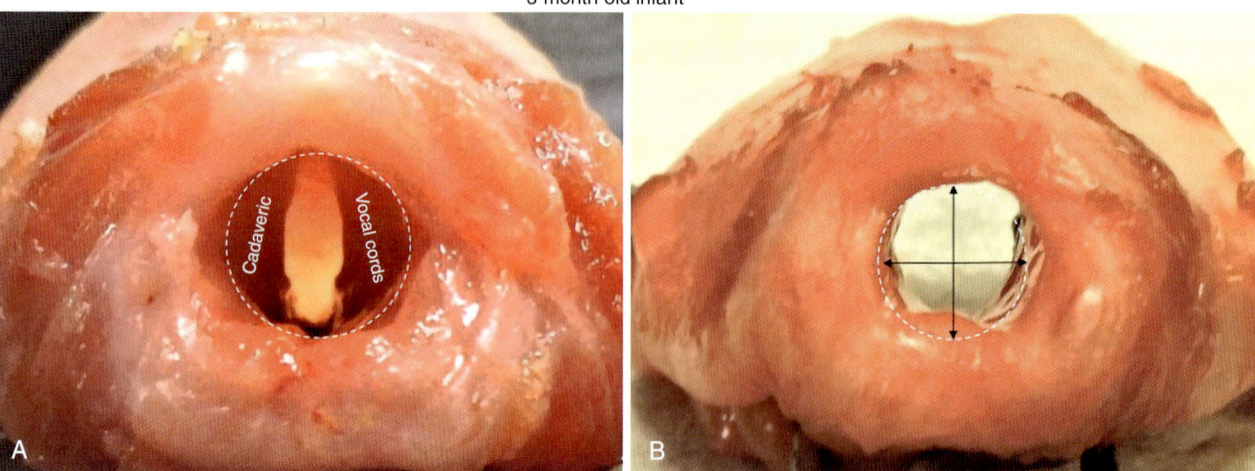

FIGURE 12.6 **A,** Infant cadaveric larynx, cricoid outlet seen from below. Note that the vocal cords are in the cadaveric position, feigning a narrow entrance into the laryngeal lumen. **B,** The same cricoid outlet also seen from below, after distending the glottis. With the vocal cords distended, the subglottic space is wide open and shows no hindrance for an advancing tracheal tube through the circular cricoid outlet. (From Isa M, Holzki J, Hagemeier A, Rothschild MA, Cote CJ. Anatomical in vitro investigations of the pediatric larynx: a call for manufacturer redesign of tracheal tube cuff location and perhaps a call to reconsider the use of uncuffed tracheal tubes. *Anesth Analg.* 2021;133(4):894-902.)

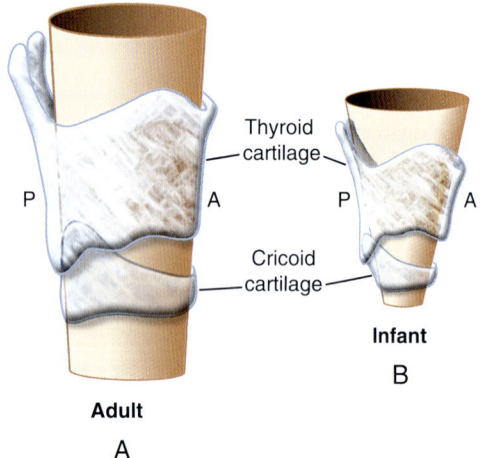

FIGURE 12.7 Configuration of the larynx of an adult **(A)** and an infant **(B)**. Notice that both larynxes are somewhat funnel shaped, but this shape is exaggerated in the infant and toddler. The adult laryngeal structures are of such size that most endotracheal tubes pass easily into the trachea. In infants and toddlers, it is common for the endotracheal tube (ETT) to pass easily through the vocal cords but to become snug at the level of the nondistensible cricoid cartilage. Concern for causing edema at this point resulted in the classic teaching that uncuffed tracheal tubes should be used in young children (see text for more details). A, Anterior; P, posterior.

Physiologically, this decrease in cross-sectional area results in an increased resistance to airflow and therefore an increased work of breathing through the narrowed airway. Airflow in the upper airway (and as far down the tracheobronchial tree as the fifth bronchial division) normally is turbulent, which is defined as a Reynolds number > 4000.

$$Reynolds\ number = \frac{DV\rho}{\mu}$$

Reynolds number is defined above as the ratio of the product of the diameter of the tube (D) and the velocity (V) and density

(ρ) of the gas or fluid, to the viscosity (μ) of the gas or fluid, resulting in a dimensionless number. Airflow beyond the fifth bronchial division in the tracheobronchial tree is laminar, which is defined by a Reynolds number < 2000.

During turbulent flow, the resistance to flow is inversely proportional to *the fifth power of the decrease* in the *radius*. In the examples presented earlier, in neonates and infants, decreasing the radius by half increases the resistance to flow by 2^5 or 32-fold compared with that in adults where decreasing the 4 mm radius to 3 mm (one-quarter) increases the resistance only ~4-fold (Fig. 12.8).[2]

The Larynx

Understanding the anatomy and function of the larynx is critical to knowledgeable, safe, and successful airway management.

ANATOMY
Structure

The larynx is composed of one bone (hyoid) and 11 cartilages (the single thyroid, cricoid, and epiglottic cartilages and the paired arytenoid, corniculate, cuneiform, and triticeal cartilages) (Fig. 12.9). These cartilages are suspended by ligaments from the base of the skull. The body of the cricoid cartilage articulates posteriorly with the inferior cornu of the thyroid cartilage. The paired triangular arytenoid cartilages rest on top of, and articulate with, the superiorposterior aspect of the cricoid cartilage. The arytenoid cartilages are thus protected by the thyroid cartilage (see Fig. 12.9). The triticeal cartilages are rounded nodules of cartilage, approximately the size of a pea in adults, located in the margins of the lateral thyrohyoid ligament.

Tissue folds and muscles cover these cartilages. In contrast to adults, but comparable to most mammals, the cartilaginous glottis accounts for 60% to 75% of the length of the vocal folds in children younger than 2 years of age.[21] Contraction of the intrinsic laryngeal muscles alters the position and configuration of these tissue folds, thus influencing laryngeal function during respiration, forced voluntary glottic closure (Valsalva maneuver), reflex laryngospasm, swallowing, and phonation.

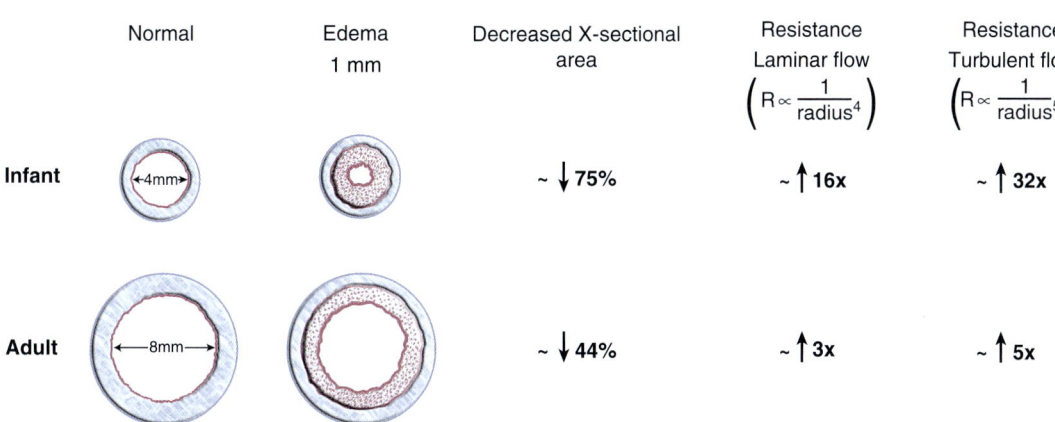

FIGURE 12.8 Relative effects of airway edema in an infant and an adult. The dimensions of the normal airways of infants and adults are presented on the left side of the graphic. Resistance to airflow is inversely proportional to the fifth power of the radius of the lumen for turbulent flow, which occurs in the upper airway between the vocal cords to the fifth bronchial division. During upper airway obstruction (e.g., croup) in an infant whose airway is 4 mm in diameter, 1 mm of circumferential edema reduces the diameter of the lumen to a diameter of 2 mm. The net effect is an ~75% reduction in the cross-sectional area and a ~32-fold increase in the resistance to air flow (or the work of breathing). In contrast, in the adult airway (8 mm diameter), 1 mm of circumferential edema reduces the diameter of the lumen to 6 mm. This reduces the cross-sectional area by ~44% and increases the resistance of air flow (work of breathing) ~4-fold.

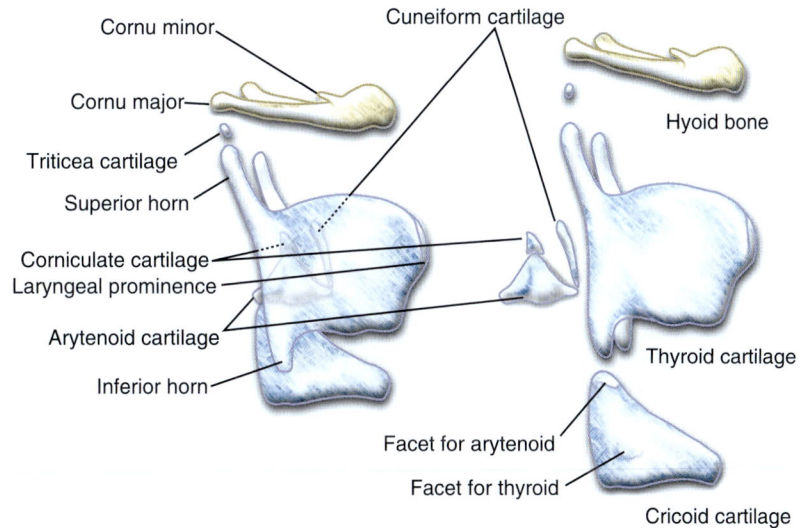

FIGURE 12.9 Laryngeal cartilages. The natural positions of the laryngeal cartilages are presented on the left, with the individual cartilages separated on the right. (Reprinted by permission from Fink BR, Demarest RJ. *Laryngeal Biomechanics.* Cambridge, MA: Harvard University Press; 1978.)

The laryngeal tissue folds (Fig. 12.10) consist of:

- Paired aryepiglottic folds extending from the epiglottis posteriorly to the superior surface of the arytenoids (the paired cuneiform and corniculate cartilages lie within for support and reinforcement).
- Paired vestibular folds (false vocal cords) extending from the thyroid cartilage posteriorly to the superior surface of the arytenoids.
- Paired vocal folds (true vocal cords) extending from the posterior surface of the thyroid plate to the anterior projection or vocal process of the arytenoids.
- A single interarytenoid fold (composed of the interarytenoid muscle covered by tissue) bridging the arytenoid cartilages.

- A single thyrohyoid fold extending from the hyoid bone to the thyroid cartilage.

Histology

The highly vascular mucosa of the mouth is continuous with that of the larynx and trachea. This mucosa consists of squamous, stratified, and pseudostratified ciliated epithelium.[26,27] The vocal cords are covered with stratified epithelium. The mucosa and submucosa are rich in lymphatic vessels and seromucous-secreting glands, which lubricate the laryngeal folds. The submucosa consists of loose fibrous stroma; therefore, the mucosa is loosely adherent to the underlying structures in most areas. However, the submucosa is scant on the laryngeal surface of the epiglottis and the vocal cords, so the mucosa

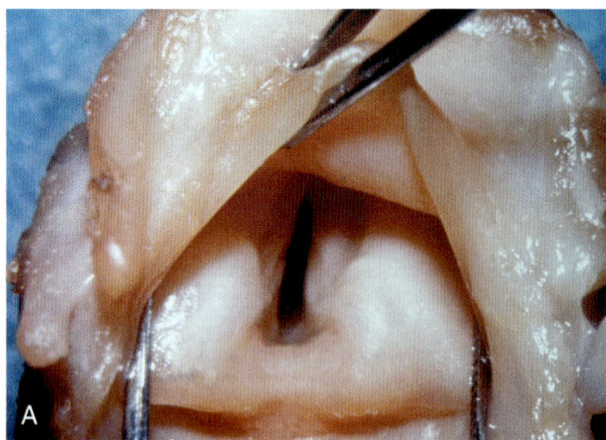
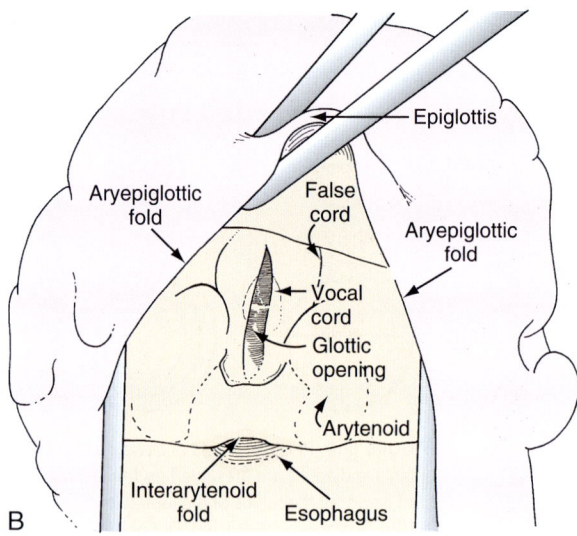

FIGURE 12.10 Photograph **(A)** and schematic diagram **(B)** of the larynx of a premature infant.

is tightly adherent in these areas.[26–28] Most inflammatory processes of the airway above the level of the vocal cords are limited by the barrier formed by the firm adherence of the mucosa to the vocal cords.[28] For example, inflammation of the epiglottitis (acute epiglottitis) is usually limited to the supraglottic structures, and the loosely adherent mucosa explains the ease with which localized swelling occurs (see Figs. 31.25A–C and 31.26 A,B).[29] In a similar manner, an inflammatory process of the subglottic region (laryngotracheobronchitis [croup]) results in subglottic edema in the loosely adherent mucosa of the airway below the vocal cords, but it does not usually spread above the level of the vocal cords (see Fig. 31.27C).[28]

Sensory and Motor Innervation

Two branches of the vagus nerve, the recurrent laryngeal and the superior laryngeal nerves, supply both sensory and motor innervation to the larynx. The superior laryngeal nerve has two branches: the internal branch, which provides sensory innervation to the supraglottic region, and the external branch, which supplies motor innervation to the cricothyroid muscle. The recurrent laryngeal nerve provides sensory innervation to the subglottic larynx and motor innervation to all other laryngeal muscles.[28,30] Local anesthetic agents administered to block the superior laryngeal nerve result in anesthesia of the supraglottic region down to the inferior margin of the epiglottis and motor blockade of the cricothyroid muscle, which causes relaxation of the vocal cords. Translaryngeal injection of local anesthetic through the cricothyroid membrane or specific superior laryngeal nerve and glossopharyngeal nerve blocks are required for subglottic and tracheal anesthesia.[31–34]

Blood Supply

Laryngeal branches of the superior and inferior thyroid arteries provide the blood supply to the larynx. The recurrent laryngeal nerve and artery lie in close proximity to each other, thus the recurrent laryngeal nerve may be injured during attempts to control bleeding during thyroidectomy.[35,36]

FUNCTION

Inspiration

During inspiration, the larynx is pulled caudad by the negative intrathoracic pressure generated by the descent of the diaphragm and contraction of the external intercostal muscles. The larynx is stretched longitudinally, increasing the distance between the aryepiglottic and vestibular folds as well as between the vestibular and vocal folds. When the intrinsic muscles within the larynx contract, the arytenoids move laterally and posteriorly (rocking backward and rotating laterally), increasing the interarytenoid distance and separating as well as stretching the paired aryepiglottic, vestibular, and vocal folds. Overall, inspiration enlarges the laryngeal inlet, both longitudinally (like opening a telescope) and laterally, allowing the passage of greater quantities of air through the airway per unit time.

Exhalation

At the end of exhalation, the larynx reverts to its resting position, with longitudinal shortening of the distance between the aryepiglottic, vestibular, and vocal folds (like closing a telescope). The arytenoids return simultaneously to their resting position by rotating medially and rocking forward, decreasing the interarytenoid distance and reducing the tension on the paired aryepiglottic, vestibular, and vocal folds and causing them to thicken.

Forced Glottic Closure and Laryngospasm

Glottic closure during forced exhalation (forced glottic closure or Valsalva maneuver) is voluntary laryngeal closure and is physiologically similar to involuntary laryngeal closure (laryngospasm). Forced glottic closure occurs at several levels. Contraction of the intrinsic laryngeal muscles results in (1) marked reduction in the interarytenoid distance; (2) anterior rocking and medial rotation of the arytenoids that cause apposition of the paired vocal, vestibular, and aryepiglottic folds; (3) longitudinal shortening of the larynx that obliterates the space between the aryepiglottic, vestibular, and vocal folds (like complete closing of a telescope). Contraction of an extrinsic laryngeal muscle, the thyrohyoid, pulls the hyoid bone caudad and the thyroid cartilage upward (cephalad), leading to further closure.[1,3,4,37–40]

Closure of the larynx during laryngospasm is similar, but not identical, to that described for voluntary forced glottic closure. There are two important differences. First, laryngospasm is accompanied by an inspiratory effort, which longitudinally separates the vocal folds from the vestibular folds. This inspiratory effort against a closed glottis may lead to pulmonary edema. Second, in contrast to forced glottic closure, neither the thyroarytenoid muscle (an intrinsic muscle of the larynx) nor the thyrohyoid muscle contract; thus, apposition of the aryepiglottic folds and median thyrohyoid folds is minimal. These two differences allow the upper portion of the larynx to be left partially open during mild laryngospasm, resulting in the hallmark high-pitched inspiratory stridor (see Video 12.1).[4,37] Anterior and upward displacement of the mandible (jaw thrust applied at the condyle of the ascending ramus of the mandible) longitudinally separates the base of the tongue, the epiglottis, and the aryepiglottic folds from the vocal folds, establishing a patent airway above the vocal cords (Videos 12.2 A & B). The pain from pressing on the condyles stimulates the child to take a breath and break the laryngospasm (see E-Fig. 12.1).[38,41–44]

Swallowing

Glottic closure during swallowing is similar to voluntary forced closure of the glottis described above. Protection of the glottic opening is achieved primarily by apposition of the laryngeal folds and secondarily by upward (cephalad) movement of the larynx. The upward movement of the larynx brings the thyroid cartilage closer to the hyoid bone, resulting in folding of the epiglottis over the glottic opening.[4,37,39,40] With loss of consciousness or deep sedation, the normal protective mechanism of the larynx may be diminished or completely lost, thus allowing pulmonary aspiration of pharyngeal contents.

Phonation

Phonation is accomplished by alteration of the angle between the thyroid and cricoid cartilages (the cricothyroid angle) and by medial movement of the arytenoids during exhalation.[4,30,45] These movements result in fine alterations in vocal fold tension during movement of air, causing vibration of the vocal folds. Lesions or malfunctions of the vocal folds (e.g., inflammation, papilloma, paresis) therefore affect phonation. Phonation is the only laryngeal function that alters the cricothyroid angle.[4] Despite significant airway obstruction during inspiration, it may still be possible to phonate.

Physiology of the Respiratory System

OBLIGATE NASAL BREATHING

Although infants are often referred to as obligate nasal breathers[9,46]; this is relative, not absolute. Although obstruction of their anterior or posterior nares (nasal congestion, stenosis, choanal atresia) can cause asphyxia,[47–49] many infants will breathe through their mouths if the nose is obstructed.[50–52] Immaturity of coordination between respiratory efforts and oropharyngeal motor and sensory input accounts in part for "obligate" nasal breathing and obstruction may occur at multiple sites.[53–58]

The ability to coordinate breathing and swallowing improves as the infant matures. The larynx enlarges and moves more caudad in the neck as the cervical spine lengthens and the infant begins to consistently breathe through the mouth by age 3 to 5 months.[59] Studies of relatively healthy preterm infants have shown that the ability to breathe through the mouth when the nares are obstructed improves with increased gestational age: 8% of preterm infants of 31 to 32 weeks' postconception age, 28% of more mature preterm infants of 35 to 36 weeks' postconception age,[60] and 40% of full-term infants were able to convert from nasal to oral breathing.[51] In another small cohort of preterm neonates, all infants switched from nasal to oral breathing within 30 seconds.[52] The presence of medical support devices such as a nasogastric tube may partially or completely obstruct one nasal passage and affect the infant's breathing.

TRACHEAL AND BRONCHIAL FUNCTION

Tracheal and bronchial diameters are a function of elasticity and of distending or compressive forces (Fig 12.11). The larynx, trachea, and bronchi in the infant are quite compliant compared with those in the adult, and therefore are more subject to distention and compression forces.[46,61,62] The intrathoracic trachea is subject to stresses that are different from those in the extrathoracic portion.[61] During exhalation, intrathoracic pressure remains slightly negative, maintaining patency of the intrathoracic trachea and bronchi (see Fig. 12.11B). During inhalation, a greater negative intrathoracic pressure dilates and stretches the *intrathoracic* trachea and bronchi.[63] The *extrathoracic* trachea at the thoracic inlet is slightly narrowed by dynamic compression (dynamic collapse) that results from the differential between intratracheal and atmospheric pressures. However, the cartilages of the trachea, along with the muscles and soft tissues of the neck, maintain patency of the airway (see Fig. 12.11A).

Obstruction of the extrathoracic upper airway that can occur with epiglottitis, laryngotracheobronchitis, or an extrathoracic foreign body alters normal airway dynamics. Inhalation against an obstruction results in greater negative intrathoracic pressure, further dilating the intrathoracic airways. Clinically, the net effect is a dynamic collapse of the extrathoracic trachea below the level of the obstruction. This collapse is maximal at the thoracic inlet, where the greatest pressure gradient exists between negative intratracheal and atmospheric pressures. As a result, inspiratory stridor is prominent (see Fig. 12.11C and Video 12.1).[61–68] With intrathoracic tracheal obstruction (e.g., foreign body, vascular ring) (see Video 12.1), stridor may occur during both inspiration and expiration.[69–72] In lower airway obstruction (e.g., asthma, bronchiolitis, anaphylaxis), intrathoracic tracheal and bronchial collapse may occur as a result of the prolonged expiratory phase and greatly increased positive extraluminal pressure resulting in wheezing (see Fig. 12.11D).[73] In addition, because the airways in children are very compliant, they may be more susceptible to closure during bronchial smooth muscle contraction (e.g., with reactive airway disease). Preterm and term infants may experience airway closure even during quiet respiration as closing capacity exceeds functional residual capacity (see Fig. 1.8).[74]

Avoiding dynamic airway collapse is particularly important. The very compliant trachea and bronchi of an infant or child are prone to collapse, particularly at the extremes of transluminal pressures that may occur when a child is crying vigorously. The susceptibility of a child to these dynamic forces on the airway is inversely related to age, with preterm infants being most susceptible and adults being least susceptible.[75] Thus, keeping the child calm is a key aspect of management for a child with impending or partial airway obstruction whether intra- or extrathoracic. Skill and understanding are required on the part of the parents, nursing staff, and physicians. *Sedatives and opioids should be used with caution as they may depress or ablate the life-sustaining voluntary efforts to breathe, resulting in major morbidity or mortality. Personnel and equipment for advanced airway management techniques including rigid bronchoscopy and surgical airway should be available to manage a child with acute or impending complete airway obstruction.*

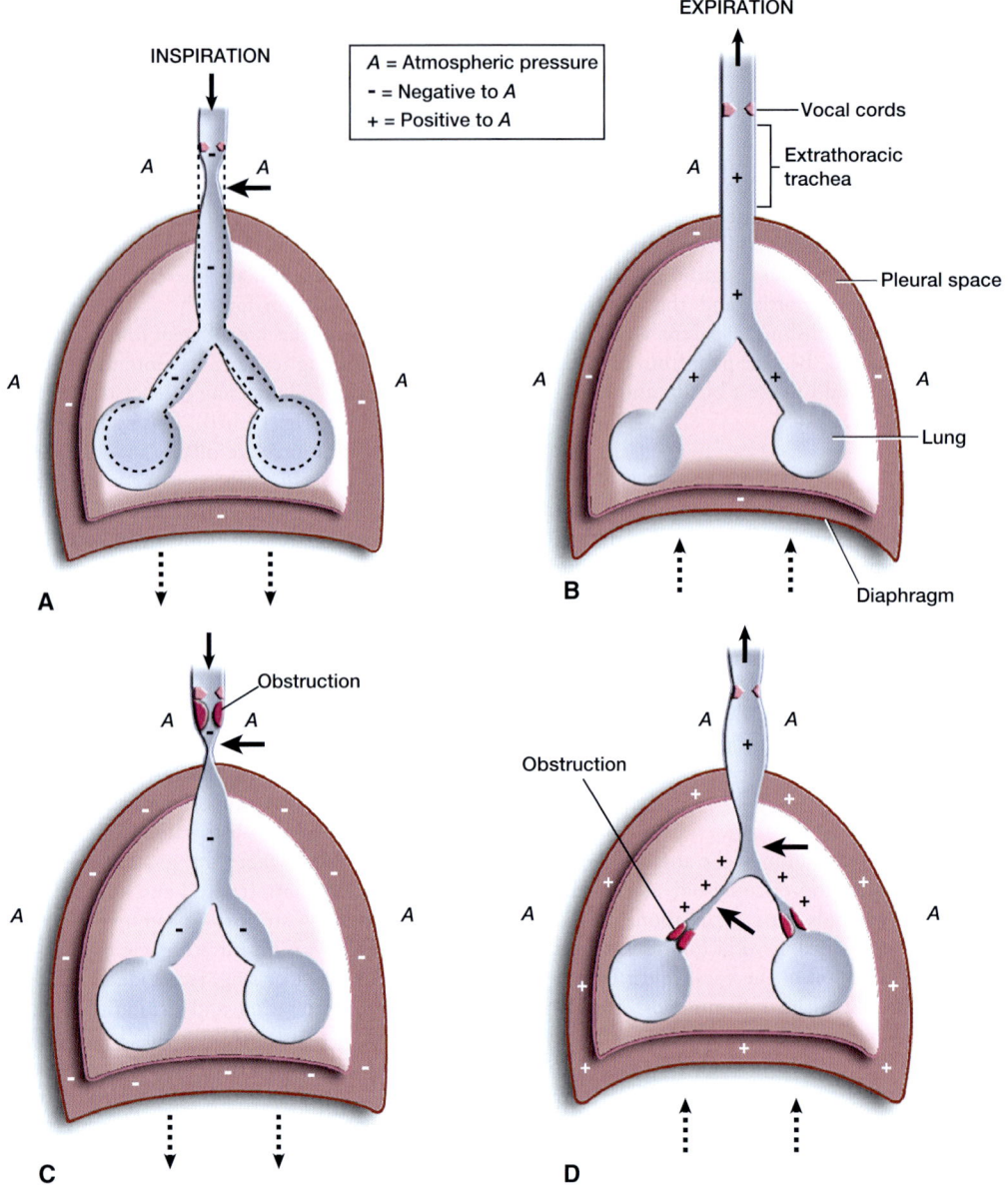

FIGURE 12.11 A, With descent of the diaphragm and contraction of the intercostal muscles, a greater negative intrathoracic pressure relative to intraluminal and atmospheric pressure is developed. The net result is longitudinal stretching of the larynx and trachea, dilatation of the intrathoracic trachea and bronchi, movement of air into the lungs, and some dynamic collapse of the extrathoracic trachea *(thick arrow)*. The dynamic collapse is due to the highly compliant trachea and the negative intraluminal pressure in relation to atmospheric pressure. **B,** The normal sequence of events at end-expiration is a slight negative intrapleural pressure stenting the airways open. In infants, the highly compliant chest does not provide the support required; therefore, airway closure occurs with each breath. Intraluminal pressures are slightly positive in relation to atmospheric pressure, with the result that air is forced out of the lungs. **C,** Obstructed extrathoracic airway. Notice the severe dynamic collapse of the extrathoracic trachea below the level of obstruction. This collapse is greatest at the thoracic inlet, where the largest pressure gradient exists between negative intratracheal pressure and atmospheric pressure *(thick arrow)*. (Extrathoracic upper airway obstruction is characterized by inspiratory stridor.) **D,** Obstructed intrathoracic trachea or airways. Notice that breathing against an obstructed lower airway (e.g., bronchiolitis, asthma) results in greater positive intrathoracic pressures, with dynamic collapse of the intrathoracic airways (prolonged expiration or wheezing *[thick arrows]*).

WORK OF BREATHING

Work of breathing may be defined as the product of pressure and volume. It may be analyzed by plotting transpulmonary pressure against tidal volume. The work of breathing per kilogram body weight is similar in infants and adults. However, the oxygen consumption of a full-term neonate (5 to 9 mL/kg per minute) is several times greater than that of an adult (2 to 3 mL/kg per minute).[76,77] This greater oxygen consumption (and greater carbon dioxide production) in infants requires increased alveolar ventilation, accomplished primarily via increased respiratory rate compared with older children.

The location of airway resistance within the tracheobronchial tree differs between infants and adults. The nasal passages account for 25% of the total resistance to airflow in a neonate, compared with 60% in an adult.[9,78] In infants, most resistance to airflow occurs in the bronchi and small airways. This results from the relatively smaller diameter of the airways and the greater compliance of the supporting structures of the trachea and bronchi.[46,79,80] In particular, the soft cartilaginous chest wall of a neonate is very compliant; the ribs provide less support to maintain negative intrathoracic pressure. This lack of negative intrathoracic pressure combined with the increased compliance of the bronchi can lead to functional airway closure with every breath (see Fig. 1.8).[81–83] In infants and children, therefore, small-airway resistance accounts for most of the work of breathing.[9,81,82,84–89]

In the presence of increased airway resistance or decreased lung compliance, an increased transpulmonary pressure is required to produce a given tidal volume, and therefore the work of breathing is increased. Any change in the airway that increases the work of breathing may lead to respiratory failure. Recall that the resistance to air flow is inversely proportional to the fifth power of the radius during turbulent flow, which occurs from the upper airway to the fifth bronchial division, and to the fourth power of the radius of the lumen during laminar flow, which occurs beyond the fifth bronchial division. Because the diameter of the airways in infants is smaller than in adults, pathologic narrowing of the airways in infants exerts a greater adverse effect on the work of breathing. Increase in the work of breathing (or pressure required to generate a given tidal volume) may also occur with a long tracheal tube of small diameter, an obstructed tracheal tube, or a narrowed airway. All of these situations increase oxygen consumption, which in turn increases oxygen demand.[90] The increased oxygen demand is initially addressed by an increase in respiratory rate, but the increased respiratory effort may not be sustainable. The end result may be exhaustion, leading to respiratory failure with CO_2 retention (hypercarbia) and eventual hypoxemia (see Figs. 2.13 and 2.14).

The difference in histology of the diaphragm and intercostal muscles of preterm and full-term infants compared with older children contributes to increased susceptibility of infants to respiratory fatigue or failure. Type I muscle fibers permit repetitive movement for prolonged periods; for example, long-distance runners through repeated exercise increase the proportion of type I muscle fibers in their legs. The percentage of type I muscle fibers in the diaphragm and intercostal muscles increases with age (preterm infants < full-term infants < 2-year-old children) (Fig. 12.12). Any condition that increases the work of breathing in preterm and full-term neonates may fatigue the respiratory muscles and precipitate respiratory failure more readily than in an older child or adult.[91–93]

AIRWAY OBSTRUCTION DURING ANESTHESIA

There are multiple sites of upper airway relaxation that may contribute to airway obstruction in infants after sedation or after induction of anesthesia.[54–58] Airway obstruction during anesthesia or loss of consciousness appears to be most frequently related to loss of muscle tone in the pharyngeal and laryngeal structures rather than apposition of the tongue to the posterior pharyngeal wall.[54,55,94,95] The progressive loss of tone with deepening anesthesia results in progressive airway obstruction primarily at the level of the soft palate and the epiglottis.[54,55,58,94,96,97] In children, the pharyngeal airway space decreases in a dose-dependent manner with increasing concentrations of both sevoflurane and propofol anesthesia.[98–100] This reduction in pharyngeal space has been observed mainly in the anteroposterior dimension. As the depth of propofol anesthesia in children increases, upper airway narrowing

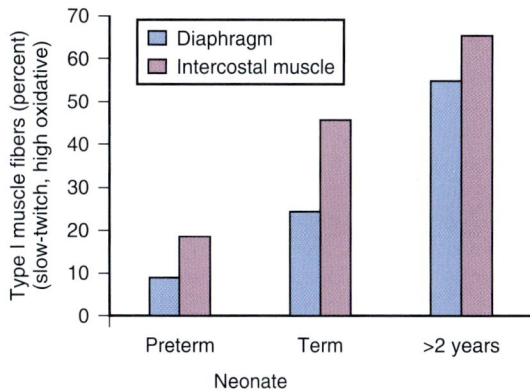

FIGURE 12.12 Muscle fiber composition of the diaphragm and intercostal muscles related to age. Note that a preterm infant's diaphragm and intercostal muscles have fewer type I fibers compared with term newborns and older children. The data suggest a possible mechanism for early fatigue in preterm and term infants when the work of breathing is increased. (Data from Keens TG, Bryan AC, Levison H, Ianuzzo CD. Developmental pattern of muscle fiber types in human ventilatory muscles. *J Appl Physiol.* 1978;44:909-913.)

occurs throughout the entire upper airway but is most pronounced in the hypopharynx at the level of the epiglottis. Extension of the head at the atlantooccipital joint with anterior displacement of the cervical spine (sniffing position) improves hypopharyngeal airway patency but does not necessarily change the position of the tongue. This observation supports the concept that upper airway obstruction is not primarily caused by changes in tongue position but rather by collapse of the pharyngeal structures.[56–58]

Pharyngeal airway obstruction also occurs during obstructive sleep apnea in children and adults.[53,101–104] The sniffing position increases the cross-sectional area and decreases the closing pressure of both the retropalatal and the retroglossal space in anesthetized adults with obstructive sleep apnea.[105] The application of continuous positive airway pressure (CPAP) is a common method to overcome such airway obstruction (see Figs. 31.8 and 31.9). During propofol anesthesia in children, CPAP works primarily by increasing the transverse dimension of the airway.[99] This occurs despite the fact that administration of anesthetic agents leads to obstruction of the airway mostly by narrowing the anteroposterior dimension. Chin lift and jaw thrust also improve airway patency in anesthetized children with adenotonsillar hypertrophy.[106–108] Lateral positioning (also known as the "recovery or tonsillectomy position") dramatically enhances the effects of these airway maneuvers[107,108]; lateral positioning alone improves airway dimensions.[10] Compared with chin lift and CPAP, the jaw thrust maneuver is the most effective means to improve airway patency and ventilation in children undergoing adenotonsillectomy (Video 12.2 A & B).[106]

Dexmedetomidine is a sedative that confers minimal changes to the upper airway dimensions during sedation with a natural airway in children[109]; however, children with underlying obstructive sleep disorders are still at risk for obstruction requiring intervention with its use,[110] as evidenced by its role in drug-induced sleep endoscopy.[111,112]

Evaluation of the Airway

A history and physical examination with specific reference to the airway should be performed in all children who require sedation or anesthesia. In particular, a history of a congenital syndrome or physical findings of a congenital anomaly (e.g., microtia, which has been associated with difficult laryngoscopy)[113] should alert the practitioner to the possibility of difficulties with airway management.

In special situations, radiologic and laboratory studies are required to further evaluate and clarify a disorder revealed by the history and physical examination. Many methods exist for evaluating and predicting the difficult airway in adults.[114–118] A meta-analysis of 35 adult studies involving 50,760 adult patients found Mallampati classification, thyromental distance, mouth opening, and other techniques individually to have moderate to fair sensitivity and specificity; however, the combination of Mallampati classification and thyromental distance provided a 95% confidence interval.[119] No comparable methods have been forthcoming in children[120,121]; however, a multinational study (NECTARINE [**NE**onate and **C**hildren audi**T** of **A**naesthesia p**R**actice **IN** **E**urope]) collected data on airway management of 4683 procedures in infants newborn to 60 weeks' postconceptional age.[122] They reported difficult intubation (defined as two failed attempts) in 266 children (271 procedures), ~5.8%. There was no attempt to predict risk factors before intubation, but hypoxemia was a common sequela; the most common solution was a change in blade or use of a stylet rather than video laryngoscopy. A call for help was an additional factor emphasizing the value of having experienced colleagues nearby. Another European multinational study (APRICOT [**A**naesthesia **PR**actice **I**n **C**hildren **O**bservational **T**rial]) prospectively examined critical incidents during 32,227 pediatric anesthesia cases in children from birth to 15 years of age and found an incidence of critical respiratory events of ~3.1%.[123] Three or more tracheal intubation attempts were reported in 120 children and in 40 for supraglottic device placement.[124] As one would expect, difficulty in securing the airway was associated with critical events such as hypoxemia (odds ratio [OR] 2.1 for tracheal intubation and 4.3 for supraglottic device placement). Reported risk factors for hypoxemia included a history of reactive airway disease, active wheezing, upper respiratory tract infection, and history of snoring or passive smoke exposure. This study additionally observed a low rate of using video-assisted laryngoscopy devices but also reported a 1% per year decrease in such events with years of practice; experience makes a difference.

The US–based Pediatric Difficult Airway Registry prospectively collected data from 13 children's hospitals and reported 1018 difficult intubation encounters.[125] Approximately 20% (204 cases) had at least one complication, with 15 cardiac arrests and 94 experiencing hypoxemia; there were five deaths within 7 days but only one was related to the difficult intubation (hypoxemia). The greatest incidence was in children weighing <10 kilograms; patients with three or more attempts at direct laryngoscopy had more complications.

Large neck circumference correlates with other issues, such as snoring, asthma, hypertension, and diabetes in children, as well as adverse perioperative respiratory events, but not with difficult laryngoscopy.[126] Routine evaluation of the airway in all children often sheds insight into the risk of a difficult airway. Characteristics that portend a difficult laryngoscopy and intubation include diagnosis of a specific syndrome associated with a difficult intubation (e.g., Treacher Collins syndrome, see E-Table 12.1), the inability to open the mouth (e.g., temporomandibular joint ankylosis, micrognathia, Pierre Robin syndrome, or first arch syndrome), massive glossoptosis (e.g., Beckwith-Wiedemann syndrome), fused cervical spine (e.g., Klippel-Feil syndrome), or oropharyngeal space occupying lesions (e.g., cystic hygroma or glossopharyngeal tumors). For some syndromes, the airway improves with age (e.g., Pierre Robin syndrome), whereas with others (e.g., Treacher Collins), the airway becomes progressively more difficult with age. A single center study found a 14% resolution of difficult airway status in pediatric patients over a 5-year period.[127]

Pierre Robin syndrome (in contrast to mandibular hypoplasia) is defined by three findings: mandibular hypoplasia, glossoptosis,

and respiratory distress in the first 24 hours after birth. Mandibular hypoplasia also occurs in children with a variety of other syndromes such as Treacher Collins, Goldenhar, and hemifacial microsomia. In a radiological investigation of 42 children with syndromic mandibular hypoplasia and an equal number of children without hypoplasia who were matched for demographics, facial metrics on CT scan were determined and differences between the two groups of children were correlated with a difficult intubation.[128] The findings indicated significant differences in growth patterns between the two groups in terms of the relative tongue position, hyoid distance, and mandibular measurements. Those with smaller hyoid anterior distances (i.e., a smaller thyromental distance) and larger inferior pogonial angle (the angle subtended by lines that join the gonia i.e., the "angle" of the mandible or the posterior mandible at the angle where the body joins the ramus) to the pogonion (lowest anterior point under the symphysis of the jaw) were at increased risk for a difficult intubation with Odds Ratios of 0.79 and 1.1, respectively.

CLINICAL EVALUATION
Medical History
The *medical history* (both present and past) should investigate the following signs and symptoms; a positive history should alert the practitioner to the potential problems noted in parentheses.

- Presence of an upper respiratory tract infection (predisposition to coughing, laryngospasm, bronchospasm, desaturation during anesthesia, or, predisposition to postintubation subglottic edema or postoperative desaturation).[129–134]
- Snoring, noisy breathing, obesity (adenoidal hypertrophy, upper airway obstruction, obstructive sleep apnea, pulmonary hypertension).[135]
- Presence and nature of cough ("croupy" cough may indicate subglottic stenosis or previous tracheoesophageal fistula repair; productive cough may indicate bronchitis or pneumonia; chronicity affects the differential diagnosis [e.g., the sudden onset of a persistent cough may indicate foreign-body aspiration; a night cough may indicate tracheal compression from a thoracic mass]).
- Past episodes of croup (postintubation croup, subglottic stenosis).
- Inspiratory stridor, usually high-pitched (subglottic narrowing [see Video 12.1], laryngomalacia [see Video 12.1], macroglossia, laryngeal web [Video 12.3], extrathoracic foreign body, or extrathoracic tracheal compression).
- Hoarse voice (laryngitis, vocal cord palsy, papillomatosis, granuloma [see Video 12.1]).
- Asthma and bronchodilator therapy (bronchospasm).
- Repeated pneumonias (incompetent larynx with aspiration, gastroesophageal reflux, cystic fibrosis, bronchiectasis, residual tracheoesophageal fistula, pulmonary sequestration, immune suppression, congenital heart disease).
- History of foreign-body aspiration (increased airway reactivity, airway obstruction, impaired neurologic function).
- History of aspiration (laryngeal edema [Video 12.4], laryngeal cleft)
- Previous anesthetic problems, particularly related to the airway (difficult intubation, difficulty with mask ventilation, failed or problematic extubation)
- Atopy, allergy (increased airway reactivity).[134]
- History of smoking or vaping by primary caregivers (increased airway resistance, increased propensity to desaturation).[123,134,136,137]
- History of a congenital syndrome (many are associated with difficult airways).
- History of prematurity (subglottic stenosis, bronchopulmonary dysplasia, apnea, desaturation).

Physical Examination

The *physical examination* should include:

- Facial expression
- Presence or absence of nasal flaring
- Presence or absence of mouth breathing
- Color of mucous membranes
- Presence or absence of retractions (suprasternal, intercostal, subcostal [see Video 12.1])
- Respiratory rate
- Presence or absence of voice change
- Mouth opening (Fig.12.13A) and ability to prognathy the mandible (move the lower teeth ahead of upper teeth)
- Size of mouth
- Size of tongue and its relationship to other pharyngeal structures (Mallampati score)[138,139]
- Loose or missing teeth (see Fig. 12.13B)
- Size and configuration of palate
- Size and configuration of mandible
- Location of larynx in relation to the mandible (see Fig. 12.13C)
- Presence of stridor and, if present:
  - Is stridor predominantly inspiratory, suggesting an upper airway (extrathoracic) lesion (epiglottitis, croup, extrathoracic foreign body)?
  - Is stridor both inspiratory and expiratory, suggesting an intrathoracic lesion (aspirated foreign body, vascular ring, or large esophageal foreign body)? (see Video 12.1)
  - Is the expiratory phase prolonged or stridor predominantly expiratory, suggesting lower airway disease (asthma), intrathoracic foreign body, heart failure, allergic reaction
- Baseline oxygen saturation in room air
- Mobility of cervical spine and any restrictions in neck extension
- Microtia (hypoplastic external ear): Microtia means *little ear* because the external ear is generally smaller than normal in size. There are four types of microtia: Type 1, a smaller than normal external ear lobe but otherwise normally functioning ear; Type 2, known as "conchal microtia" where some features of the external ear are absent and the external auditory canal may be narrowed; Type 3, the most common defect known as "lobular type microtia", where only a peanut-shaped remnant of the lobe remains and the ear canal is absent (aural atresia); and Type 4, the rarest form, where there is complete absence of the ear known as anotia. Unilateral microtia occurs in 90% of cases of microtia, bilateral in only 10%.
- Bilateral, but not unilateral, microtia is associated with difficulty in visualizing the larynx (grade 3 or 4 in the Cormack-Lehane classification, Fig. 12.14).[113] Five (42%) of 12 children

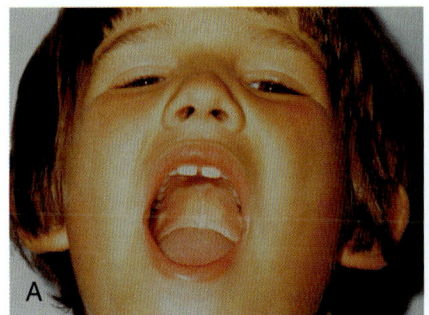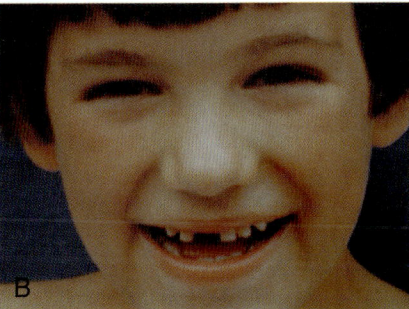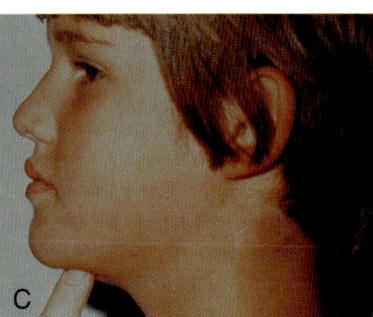

FIGURE 12.13 A, How far can a child open their mouth? Are there any abnormalities of the mouth, tongue, palate, or mandible? **B,** Are any teeth loose or missing? **C,** Is the mandible of normal configuration? How much space is there between the genu of the mandible and the thyroid cartilage? This space is an indication of the extent of the superior and posterior displacement of the larynx; there should normally be at least one finger breadth in a newborn and three finger breadths in an adolescent.

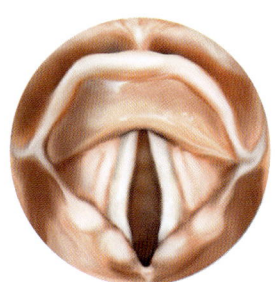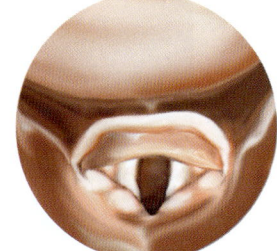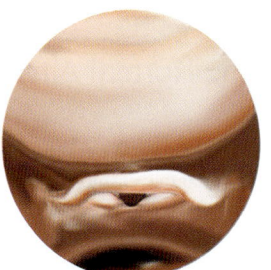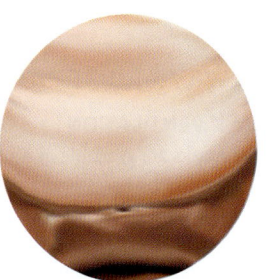

Grade I   Grade II   Grade III   Grade IV

FIGURE 12.14 The laryngoscopic grading system of Cormack and Lehane offers a reasonable means of describing visualization of the larynx. It is useful to grade the degree of visualization during laryngoscopy and how that visualization was achieved (e.g., external cricoid pressure or laryngeal manipulation, the size and configuration of the laryngoscope blade). This provides useful information for the next person attempting laryngoscopy so that they have some degree of knowledge regarding what to expect. Grade I is visualization of the complete laryngeal opening; grade II, visualization of just the posterior area; grade III, visualization of just the epiglottis; and grade IV, visualization of just the soft palate. (Reproduced with permission from Cormack RS, Lehane J. Difficult tracheal intubation in obstetrics. *Anaesthesia.* 1984;39:1105-1111.)

with bilateral microtia had a difficult laryngeal view compared with 2 (2.5%) of 81 children with unilateral microtia and 0 of 93 children without microtia.[113] Microtia may represent a mild form of hemifacial microsomia that is commonly associated with mandibular hypoplasia. Knowing that this association exists prepares the clinician to anticipate finding mandibular hypoplasia if they also observe microtia, which is often more readily diagnosed than mandibular hypoplasia, during the preoperative examination.

- Global appearance: Are there congenital anomalies that may fit a recognizable syndrome? *The finding of one anomaly mandates a search for others.* If a congenital syndrome is diagnosed, specific anesthetic implications must be considered (see E-Table 12.1).

DIAGNOSTIC TESTING

Routine evaluation of the airway usually requires only a careful history and physical examination. In the presence of airway pathology, however, radiologic evaluation can be extremely valuable. Radiographs of the upper airway (anteroposterior and lateral films and fluoroscopy) may provide evidence about the site and cause of airway obstruction. When necessary, MRI, CT, and three-dimensional (3-D) modeling provide more detailed information.[140–161] *Radiologic airway examination in a child with a compromised airway may be undertaken only if there is no immediate threat to the child's safety and only in the presence of skilled and appropriately equipped personnel able to manage the airway with careful considerations to the relative benefits of the examination compared with risks of sedation or anesthesia if required. Securing the airway through tracheal intubation must not be postponed to obtain a radiologic diagnosis when the child has severely compromised air exchange.*

Blood gas analysis is occasionally of value for assessing the degree of physiologic compromise, especially with chronic airway obstruction and compensated respiratory acidosis. Performing an arterial (or venous) puncture for blood gas analysis may provide helpful information, but it is often upsetting to the child and may risk aggravation of the underlying airway obstruction through dynamic airway collapse. Candidates for blood gas analysis must be carefully selected and the procedure skillfully performed.

Endoscopic evaluation (flexible fiberoptic endoscopy) of the airway before tracheal intubation can be useful in infants and in cooperative older children if a glottic pathologic process is suspected or if difficulty visualizing the glottis is anticipated. Ultrasound can also be used to examine the airway to estimate the internal diameter of the trachea, which can help with the selection of the optimal tracheal tube size (see later in the chapter for further details).[162–165]

Airway Management: The Normal Airway

MASK VENTILATION

Face masks are available in many sizes and shapes. We commonly use disposable, clear plastic masks with an inflatable cushioned rim. The inflatable rim molds to the contour of the face to provide an atraumatic seal. The use of clear plastic in the cone of the mask allows visualization of humidity (indicating air exchange), secretions, vomitus, and lip color. The appropriately sized mask should rest on the bridge of the nose (avoiding the eyes) and extend to the mandible. Although mask anesthesia may appear simple, it is one of the most difficult skills to master. A common mistake made by inexperienced trainees during mask ventilation is to press their fingers into the submental triangle, thereby partially occluding the airway. Minimal pressure is required, and the long finger should rest across the body of the mandible (Fig. 12.15). Another common problem arises when the mouth is completely closed while the face mask is being applied.

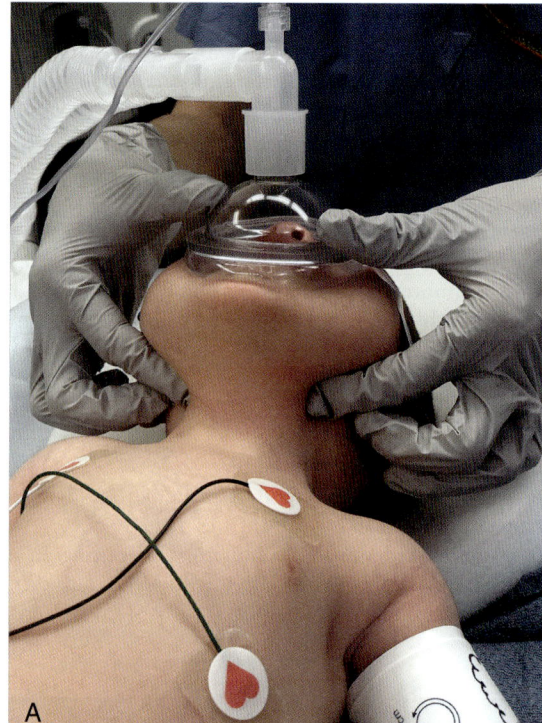

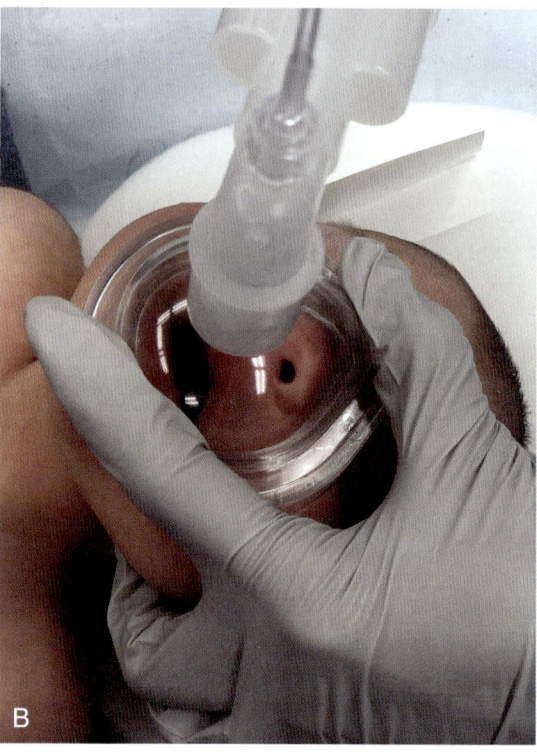

FIGURE 12.15 A, mask ventilation technique in an infant. Although mask anesthesia may appear simple, it is one of the most difficult skills to master. **A,** demonstrates two-handed technique with both thumbs on the edge of the mask and the middle fingers used to open the mouth and lift the jaw at the angle of the mandible to create the mask seal. **B,** demonstrates one-handed technique with the thumb and second finger creating a C on the mask and the third finger used to open the mouth and lift the jaw at the angle of the mandible to create the mask seal. In both techniques, there is no pressure on the submental triangle below the mandibular ridge. (*Photo credit: James M. Peyton, Mb ChB.*)

The upper airway may become completely obstructed. In such a circumstance, the fingers should be removed from the mandible and face, and a single digit applied gently to the condyles of the mandible bilaterally (for a brief period) while lifting toward the frontal hairline, until a patent upper airway is established (see Video 12.2 A & B).[44] This maneuver subluxes the temporomandibular joint, thereby opening the mouth and pulling the tongue and other soft tissues off the posterior pharyngeal wall. Admonitions against extreme positions of the infant's head during bag-and-mask ventilation are intended to minimize the risk of stretching and thus narrowing and obstructing the very compliant infant trachea. However, a study of 18 healthy, full-term infants younger than 4 months of age showed that the tracheal dimensions did not change when the head position changed.[166] Therefore, stretching of the trachea, as previously thought, may not narrow the tracheal lumen in otherwise healthy full-term infants (Video 12.5). Another study investigated the incidence of unanticipated difficult mask ventilation in 484 children from birth to 8 years of age and reported an incidence of 6.6%.[167] The incidence of difficult mask ventilation was greater in critically ill children (9.5%) based on a retrospective analysis of the National Emergency Airway Registry for Children and was associated with a two-fold greater rate of tracheal intubation and oxygen desaturation events compared with those without difficult bag-mask ventilation in this high-risk population.[168]

During spontaneous ventilation through a circle circuit, a hand on the reservoir bag can monitor respiratory rate and, with partial closure of the adjustable pressure valve, apply CPAP to maintain a patent airway. Care should be taken to provide a pressure that is appropriate for the child's pulmonary compliance. Insertion of an appropriately sized oral airway (see later) may relieve upper airway obstruction Figs.12.16A,B); however, an oral airway that is too large or too small may exacerbate the upper airway obstruction (see Figs. 12.16C,D,E,F). If these maneuvers do not improve ventilation and relieve upper airway obstruction, alternative explanations should be considered including laryngospasm; additional interventions may then be required.

We cannot overstate the importance of mask ventilation as a critical skill in caring for pediatric patients. The APRICOT study, described earlier, reported that anesthetics delivered via facemask were associated with a smaller incidence of severe critical events than those delivered via a tracheal tube, supraglottic airway (SGA), or other airway devices.[123] However, it is important to recognize that there may be other factors contributing to the choice of airway management as well as the risk for critical events.

OROPHARYNGEAL AIRWAYS

An infant's tongue may obstruct the airway during induction of anesthesia or loss of consciousness. An oropharyngeal airway of appropriate size (or an SGA such as the laryngeal mask airway [LMA; LMA North America, San Diego, CA]) may be inserted to relieve the obstruction. By holding the oral airway as shown in Fig. 12.16 from the incisors to the angle of the mandible, one can estimate the appropriate size for the child (e.g., <3 years of age ~70 mm, 3 to 8 years ~80 mm and ≥8 years ~90 mm)[169]; airways one size larger and one size smaller should be readily available as well. A tongue depressor may be inserted to prevent downfolding of the tongue when the oropharyngeal airway is inserted, which could obstruct venous and/or lymphatic drainage causing the tongue to swell and the airway to obstruct. If the airway device is too long, it may push the epiglottis into the glottic aperture, creating an additional site of airway obstruction or traumatize the epiglottis, or the tip may impinge on the

uvula causing uvular swelling and airway obstruction (see Fig. 12.16C,D).[170,171] If the airway device is too short, it may rest against the base of the tongue, forcing it posteriorly against the roof of the mouth, further aggravating airway obstruction (see Fig. 12.16E,F). Oral airways should not be considered panaceas for upper airway obstruction. Care must be taken to avoid trauma to the lips and tongue, which may be caught between the teeth and the flange of the airway. During emergence, inserting an oral airway can prevent the child from biting and obstructing the tracheal tube and to separate the mandible from the maxilla to facilitate oropharyngeal suctioning.

NASOPHARYNGEAL AIRWAYS

Nasopharyngeal airways are occasionally used in children to relieve upper airway obstruction; the distance from the naris to the angle of the mandible approximates the proper length. Commercial airways are available in sizes 12 Fr to 36 Fr. Some have an adjustable flange that enables manipulation of the airway to the appropriate length. Additionally, the nasopharyngeal airway can be used for active ventilation or passive oxygen insufflation using a simple modification such as inserting a 15-millimeter tracheal tube adapter into the proximal end.[172] Alternatively, for infants and small children, a shortened tracheal tube may be used, although this is not as soft and pliable as a commercially available nonlatex nasopharyngeal airway and may be more likely to cause trauma with insertion. Softening the tip of the tracheal tube by immersion in hot water before insertion has not been shown to reduce the incidence of bleeding during nasotracheal intubation in children.[173] The nasopharyngeal airway may be better tolerated in the lightly anesthetized child than an oropharyngeal airway. Anatomic or surgical considerations may lead to avoidance of nasopharyngeal airways to prevent trauma and bleeding as in the setting of adenotonsillar hypertrophy. In our experience, nasopharyngeal airways are most commonly used to relieve residual airway obstruction on emergence from anesthesia.

TRACHEAL INTUBATION
Technique

The techniques used to intubate the trachea in infants and children differ from those in adults due to the anatomic and physiologic differences described earlier.[1–4,8,38–40,145,174] There are several approaches to exposing the glottis in infants with a Miller blade. Robert Miller, who invented the blade, used the paraglossal approach to intubate the trachea in young infants and children,[174,175] although he did not describe it as such.[176] This approach involves inserting the blade into the mouth at the right commissure over the lateral bicuspids/incisors. The blade is advanced along the right gutter of the mouth, aiming the blade tip toward the midline while keeping the tongue to the left of the blade. The blade remains at the right commissure throughout. Once the blade tip is under the epiglottis, the epiglottis is lifted, exposing the glottic aperture. The tracheal tube is inserted lateral to the blade, helped by an assistant retracting the cheek. By introducing the blade at the right commissure, damage to the maxillary central incisors is precluded. Had Miller described inserting his blade over the central incisors, he would have recommended molding a lead plate to protect the central incisors in children as he had in adults (see E-Fig. 12.2 for full explanation).[177] Another approach consists of advancing the laryngoscope blade under constant vision along the surface of the tongue, placing the tip of the blade directly in the vallecula, and then pivoting or rotating the blade to the right to sweep the tongue to the left and adequately lifting the

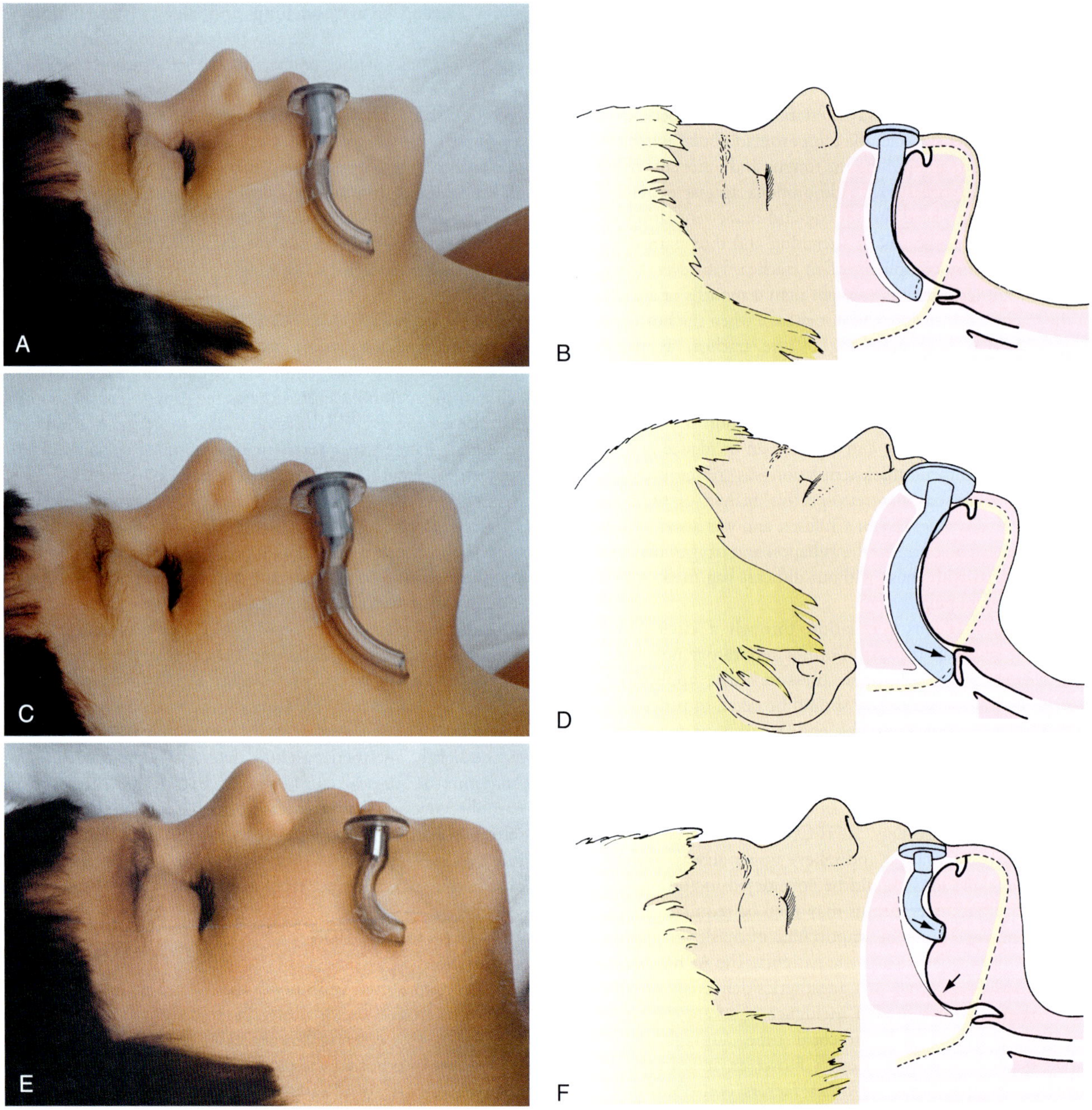

FIGURE 12.16 Correct airway selection. An artificial airway of proper size should relieve airway obstruction caused by the tongue without damaging laryngeal structures. The appropriate size can be estimated by holding the airway against the child's face: the tip of the airway should end just cephalad to the angle of the mandible (**A**). Use of the correct size should result in proper alignment with the glottic opening (**B**). If too large an oral airway is inserted, the tip will line up posterior to the angle of the mandible (**C**) and obstruct the glottic opening by pushing the epiglottis down (**D**, arrow). If too small an oral airway is inserted, the tip will line up well above the angle of the mandible (**E**) and exacerbate airway obstruction by kinking the tongue (**F**, arrows).

tongue to expose the glottic opening. This technique avoids trauma to the arytenoid cartilages although it may lacerate mucosa in the vallecula because unlike the Macintosh blade, the Miller blade does not have a rounded bulbous tip to prevent trauma to the tissue in the vallecula. Lifting the base of the tongue lifts the epiglottis, exposing the glottic opening. If this technique is unsuccessful, the epiglottis may be lifted directly with the tip of the blade (see Video 12.1). Whichever approach is used, care must be taken to avoid using the laryngoscope blade as a fulcrum to apply pressure to the teeth or alveolar ridge. If there is a substantive

risk that pressure will be applied to the teeth, a plastic tooth guard may be applied to cover the teeth at risk (the central incisors). Trainees are often instructed to insert the blade into the esophagus and then withdraw slowly to visualize the larynx; this is a technique that is best avoided. *This maneuver may traumatize tissues when the tip of the blade scrapes the esophageal mucosa, arytenoids, and aryepiglottic folds.* Optimal positioning for laryngoscopy changes with age. The trachea of older children (≥6 years) and adults is most easily exposed when a folded blanket or pillow is placed beneath the occiput of the head (5- to 10-centimeter

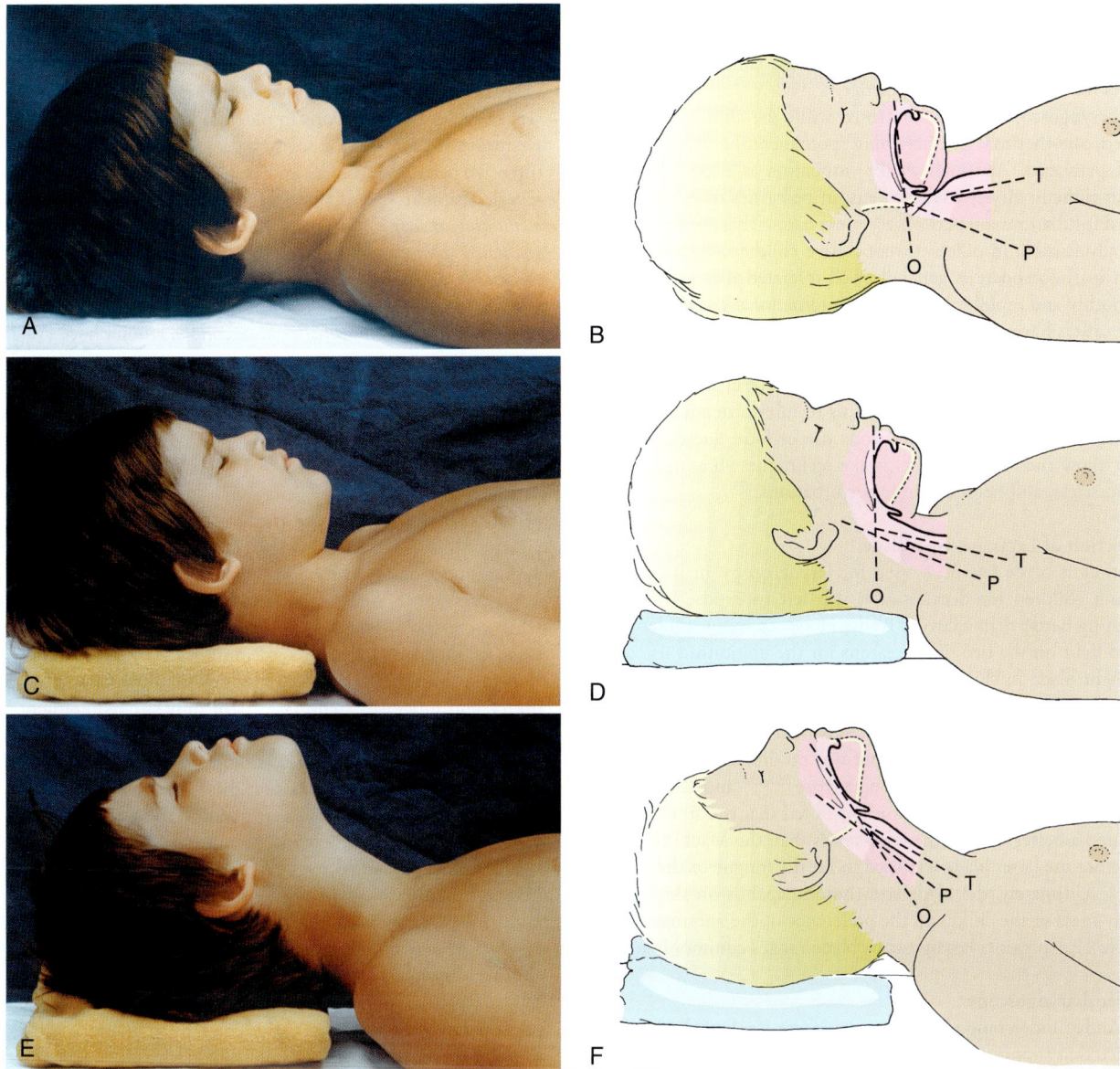

FIGURE 12.17 Correct positioning for ventilation and tracheal intubation. When a patient is lying flat on the bed or operating table **(A)**, the oral *(O)*, pharyngeal *(P)*, and tracheal *(T)* axes pass through three divergent planes **(B)**. A folded sheet or towel placed under the occiput of the head **(C)** aligns the *P* and *T* axes **(D)**. Extension of the atlantooccipital joint **(E)** results in alignment of all three axes **(F)**.

elevation), displacing the cervical spine anteriorly.[178] Extension of the head at the atlantooccipital joint produces the classic sniffing position.[145,179,180] These movements align three axes: those of the mouth or oral (O), pharynx (P), and trachea (T). Once aligned, these three axes permit direct visualization of laryngeal structures. They also result in improved hypopharyngeal patency.[56,58,94,105,179,180] Fig. 12.17 demonstrates maneuvers for positioning the head during airway management. In infants and younger children, it is usually unnecessary to elevate the head because the occiput is large in proportion to the trunk, resulting in adequate anterior displacement of the cervical spine; head extension at the atlantooccipital joint alone aligns the airway axes. If the occiput is displaced excessively, exposure of the glottis may be hindered. In neonates, it is helpful for an assistant to hold the patient's shoulders flat on the operating room table with the head slightly extended. Some clinicians have adopted the practice of placing a 2-inch rolled towel under the shoulders of neonates to facilitate tracheal intubation.[181]

The validity of the three-axis theory (alignment of the oral, pharyngeal, and laryngeal axes) to describe the optimal intubating position in adults has been challenged.[182–185] Some authors question the notion that elevation of the occiput improves conditions for visualization of the laryngeal inlet based on evidence from both MRI and clinical investigations.[182,184] However, an MRI study in children with an LMA in place found that slight head extension improved the alignment of the glottic and pharyngeal axes but worsened the alignment of the pharyngeal and laryngeal axes.[186] In a study of adults, neck extension alone was adequate for visualization of the larynx in most patients, but for obese patients and those with limited neck extension, an optimal intubating position was not determined.[182] Others favor the sniffing position but with varying support for the three-axis theory.[187–193] Even if the tracheas of only a few patients are intubated more easily when placed in the sniffing position compared with simple head extension, the current routine application of the sniffing position appears to be the best clinical practice.[194]

Laryngoscopy can be performed while the child is awake, sedated, anesthetized, and breathing spontaneously, or anesthetized and paralyzed. Although awake intubation is a cornerstone of adult difficult airway management, in pediatrics most awake tracheal intubations are performed in neonates. This approach is not usually feasible in older, uncooperative children. Awake intubation in the neonate is generally well tolerated if it is performed smoothly and rapidly; however, an international consensus group and others have cautioned against this practice unless intravenous (IV) access is not available or there is a life-threatening situation.[195–198] In most situations, preterm and term infants are best managed with sedation and paralysis to minimize adverse hemodynamic responses.[199–205] Judicious use of local anesthetics may also allow the benefits of an awake technique while minimizing pain, stress, and hemodynamic perturbations.[206]

Selection of Laryngoscope Blade

A straight blade has been used for laryngoscopy in infants and young children for decades as it was felt to expose the glottic opening better than a curved blade. However, recent evidence has shed light on the two likely reasons for the ubiquitous use of the straight blade in children over the past decades: (1) in lifting the floppy epiglottis in young children, clinicians appreciated that the straight blade exposed the vocal cords better than the Macintosh blade for lifting the epiglottis, but was no different than the Macintosh blade for lifting the tongue base,[207,208] and (2) in lifting the epiglottis in neonates, clinicians noted that the straight blade yielded a better view of the vocal cords than the Macintosh blade whether the latter blade was used to lift the tongue or the epiglottis.[209] Ultimately, the blade size chosen depends on the age and body mass of the child and the preference of the anesthesiologist; Table 12.1 presents laryngoscope blade ranges commonly used.

Video Laryngoscopy

In adults undergoing elective surgery, there is a large body of evidence that supports the routine use of video laryngoscopy for tracheal intubation to achieve greater first-attempt success rates and reduce the incidence of failed intubations.[210,211] Recent international consensus guidelines recommend the routine use of video laryngoscopy "whenever feasible."[212] In infants and children, appropriate sized blades for video laryngoscopy have become increasingly available.[213] The **V**ideo laryngoscopy **i**n **S**mall **I**nfants (VISI) trial was a randomized controlled trial of standard Macintosh or Miller blade video laryngoscopy versus direct laryngoscopy in

infants.[214] First-attempt success rates were greater, and esophageal intubations and severe complications fewer in infants intubated with video laryngoscopy.[214] A systemic review of 46 randomized trials in children reported that video laryngoscopy reduced the risk of major complications in older children as well as infants.[215] Retrospective analyses of registry data in neonatal and pediatric intensive care units (ICUs) and pediatric emergency departments revealed similar trends.[204,216–222] [*Editors' Note: The challenge in evaluating airway equipment studies in children is that many studies evaluated trainees who had limited experience with laryngoscopy and specifically with video laryngoscopy. Therefore, the conclusions hold validity for that population of trainees, but do they hold true for more experienced clinicians?*][223,224] Secondly, studies have evaluated the number of repetitions required to become proficient with a skill and in the case of tracheal intubation, that number is 50.[225] [*Authors' opinion: video laryngoscopy should be readily available for all pediatric intubations (see later)*].

Tracheal Tubes

Selection of the proper size tracheal tube depends on the individual child.[226] The goal is to select a tracheal tube with a large enough inner diameter to allow adequate gas exchange, minimize airway resistance, and facilitate airway clearance and suctioning when necessary. A second goal is to select a tracheal tube with a small enough outer diameter to minimize mucosal pressure and hopefully minimize the risk of postextubation stridor, mucosal injury, and subglottic stenosis.[26,27] The only size requirement for a manufacturer is a standardized inner diameter (ID). The external (outer) diameter (OD) varies among manufacturers, depending on the material used to construct the tube; this variation in OD mandates checking for proper tracheal tube size and leakage around the tube after every intubation.

To evaluate uncuffed tracheal tube size and leakage, first ensure that the tube passes the subglottic region without meeting resistance. Next, apply a sustained inflation pressure of 20 to 25 cm H_2O while auscultating over the glottis for an audible air leak. An air leak at this pressure is recommended because it approximates the capillary pressure of the adult tracheal mucosa.[227] Whether a similar pressure range preserves mucosal blood flow in infants and children is unknown. Excess lateral wall pressure may contribute to ischemic damage to the subglottic mucosa.[26,27,227,228] Thus, if no leak is detected at 20 to 25 cm H_2O peak inflation pressure, the tracheal tube size is excessive, and should be exchanged for one with a smaller ID. In some situations, particularly planned short-term intubation for a procedure, clinicians may choose to leave a tracheal tube in place with a detectable leak at a greater threshold (e.g., 35 cm H_2O), believing that the risks of changing the tube exceed the risks of the short-term intubation with the relatively tight tube. There may be situations in which there is laryngeal edema or even laryngospasm around the tracheal tube which prevents any gas leak and mimics a tight-fitting tracheal tube.[229] Changes in head position may also increase or decrease the leak.[229] These maneuvers are important for making the occasional diagnosis of unrecognized subglottic stenosis (see Figure 35.8, and Video 12.1).

Multiple methods of approximating the appropriate sized tracheal tube for a child have been suggested and studied including formulas based on a child's age, weight, or height (Table 12.2).[230] Some authors advocate selecting a tracheal tube of similar diameter to a child's index or pinkie (2nd or 5th) finger.[231] None of these methods is entirely reliable and, if choosing an uncuffed tracheal tube, we recommend ensuring tracheal tubes sized 0.5-millimeter ID greater or lesser than the anticipated size be

TABLE 12.1	Laryngoscope Blades Used in Infants and Children		
	BLADE SIZE		
Age	**Miller**	**Wis-Hipple**	**Macintosh**
Preterm	0	—	—
Neonate	0	—	—
Neonate–2 years	1	—	—
2–6 years	—	1.5	1 or 2
6–10 years	2	—	2
>10 years	2 or 3	—	3

TABLE 12.2	Tracheal Tubes Used in Infants and Children	
Age	Size (mm ID) Uncuffed	Size (mm ID) Cuffed
Preterm		
1000 grams	2.5	
1000–2500 grams	3.0	2.5
Neonate–6 months	3.0–3.5	3.0–3.5[a]
6 months–1 year	3.5–4.0	3.0–4.0
1–2 years	4.0–5.0	3.5–4.5
>2 years	(Age in years + 16)/4	(Age in years/4) +3

[a]In some neonates, a cuffed tracheal tube may not have a leak below 30 cm H_2O, and therefore an uncuffed tracheal tube may be more appropriate.
ID, Inner diameter.

immediately available so as to assure proper fit. Children with Trisomy 21 often require a tracheal tube with a diameter smaller than that predicted by the child's age.[232]

Cuffed tracheal tubes have greater variability in functional OD compared with uncuffed tubes because of differences in cuff shape, size, thickness, and inflation characteristics.[233] In general, compared with an uncuffed tracheal tube, a smaller diameter cuffed tracheal tube should be chosen to allow space for the cuff. We generally will downsize by 0.5 millimeters of internal diameter compared with an uncuffed tracheal tube. One study found a 99% rate of appropriate cuffed tube size selection for full-term infants through children 8 years of age using the formula[234]:

$$ID\ (mm) = (age\ [years]/4) + 3$$

Children with cardiac disease often require a larger size cuffed tube than that predicted by the child's age.[235] An investigation of tracheal tubes for children with a high-volume, low-pressure polyurethane cuff (MICROCUFF) (Fig. 12.18) used the following guidelines to select cuffed tracheal tube sizes[236]: neonates weighing ≥3 kilograms and infants ≤1 year of age, ID 3.0 millimeters; children 1 to 2 years of age, ID 3.5 millimeters; and for children ≥2 years of age, ID (mm) = (age [years]/4) + 3.5. Use of these formulas resulted in a 1.6% frequency of reintubation in children to change the tube size (6/500).[236] The incidence of postintubation croup was 0.4% (2/500 children).

Traditional teaching has advocated the use of uncuffed tracheal tubes for children younger than 8 years of age because an uncuffed tracheal tube with an air leak exerts minimal pressure on the internal surface of the circular cricoid cartilage and thus poses potentially less risk for postextubation edema resulting in croup or stridor.[228] An uncuffed tracheal tube also allows insertion of a tube with a larger ID, which may be valuable for airway clearance or to reduce airway resistance in children breathing spontaneously.[237] However, clinical data and current clinical practice have challenged these assumptions.[234,238–246] A number of studies demonstrated no differences in the incidence of postextubation complications following use of cuffed and uncuffed tubes after general anesthesia.[234,238,247] A major advantage of cuffed tracheal tubes is reduced need for multiple laryngoscopies and intubations to place an appropriate sized tube as the effective outer diameter and leak can be changed by inflating or deflating the cuff. Other advantages include improved seal and protection against aspiration, ability to change the leak with changing pulmonary compliance, more reliable gas flows and measurements allowing improved measurement and control of carbon dioxide tension (PCO_2),

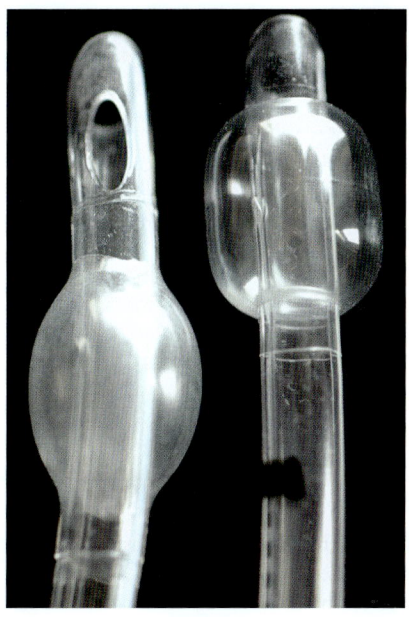

FIGURE 12.18 The MICROCUFF tracheal tube (MTT) (MICROCUFF, PET, I-MPEDC; MICROCUFF GmbH, Weinheim, Germany) *(right)* is designed with an ultrathin polyurethane (10 μm) high-volume/low-pressure cuff that has a more distal position along the shaft of the tube to better accommodate pediatric anatomy. In contrast to more traditional pediatric cuffed tracheal tubes *(left)*, the elimination of a Murphy eye from the MTT allows a more distal position of the upper cuff border. The location of the cuff on the shaft of the tube helps to ensure cuff placement below the subglottis; perhaps with the advantage of less risk for endobronchial intubation or intralaryngeal cuff position. An anatomically based depth mark on the surface of the MET helps to guide correct placement.

reduced fresh gas flows, reduced operating room pollution, less pollution of the environment, and reduced costs of anesthetic agents.[234,236,238–250] *In our practice, low-pressure, high-volume cuffed tracheal tubes are used preferentially for infants and children.[246] Uncuffed tracheal tubes are reserved for extremely low–birth-weight neonates or other children whose anatomy precludes use of a cuffed tracheal tube.[251–255] [The Editors recommend uncuffed tubes for neonates weighing <3 kilograms].*

As a rule, if a cuffed tracheal tube is chosen, the cuff should be inflated to the minimal pressure that seals the air leak; with the Microcuff tracheal tube, this is approximately 10 cm H_2O.[236,250,256,257] The cuff pressure should be reevaluated throughout the anesthetic if nitrous oxide is used because the latter may diffuse into the cuff, and with the Microcuff tracheal tube, the ultrathin-walled cuff has greater permeability for nitrous oxide than conventional tracheal tube cuffs. The net effect may be excessive tracheal mucosal pressure. Routinely checking cuff pressure,[258] use of a pressure relief valve on the cuff pilot balloon, or filling the pilot balloon with nitrous oxide[259] may reduce potential mucosal injury.[243]

Distance to Insert the Tracheal Tube

The length of the trachea (distance from vocal cords to carina) in neonates and infants up to 1 year of age varies from 5 to 9 centimeters.[63] In practice, for infants approximately 3 months of age and up to year, if the 10-centimeter mark of the tracheal tube is placed at the alveolar ridge, the tip of the tube rests above the carina. In preterm and full-term neonates, the distance is less. In children 2 years old, 12 centimeters is usually appropriate. An easy

TABLE 12.3	Distance for Insertion of an Oral Tracheal Tube by Patient Age
Age	**Approximate Distance of Insertion (cm) Even With Alveolar Ridge**
Preterm <1000 grams	6–7
Preterm 1000–2000 grams	7–9
Term newborn	9–10
1 year	11–12
2 years	12–13
6 years	15–16
10 years	17–18
16 years	18–20
20 years	20–22

rule of thumb to remember these lengths is **10** centimeters for a neonate (zero on the 10 for zero years of age), **11** centimeters for a 1-year-old (1 on the 11 for one year of age), and **12** centimeters for a 2-year-old (2 on the 12 for two-year-olds). After 2 years of age, the correct length of insertion (in centimeters) for oral intubation may be approximated by formulas based on age, weight, or tracheal tube internal diameter (see also Table 12.3)[260–263]:

$$\text{Age (years}/2 + 12)$$

$$\text{Weight (kg)}/5 + 12$$

$$\text{ID of tracheal tube} \times 3$$

Some suggest using anatomic markers to choose the appropriate depth for the tube in the trachea in neonates; however, as described earlier, these markers are most useful for uncuffed tracheal tubes.[22,264,265] An advantage of anatomic measurements is that the infant's weight may not be available immediately after birth or in sick neonates who present to the emergency department with urgent respiratory or cardiac compromise. The nasal-tragus length (the distance from the base of the nasal septum to the tip of the tragus) or the sternal length (the distance from the suprasternal notch to the tip of the xiphoid process) predicted the depth of insertion of the tracheal tube. Either distance plus 1 centimeter accurately estimated oral tracheal tube insertion distance; either distance plus 2 centimeters accurately estimated nasotracheal tube insertion distance.[264] Another formula uses body surface area as a predictor.[266] Both methods compared favorably with weight-based formulas when tube position was verified by chest radiography.

Preformed oral and nasal tracheal tubes (also known as RAE tubes for their original designers – **R**ing, **A**dair, and **E**lwyn)[267] allow improved surgical access for craniofacial and dental procedures while maintaining a secure airway. Care must be taken in using these tubes, as their length may not match a child's anatomy.[268] A comparison of oral preformed tracheal tubes from multiple manufacturers found that the distance from the bend to the tip varied by up to 1 centimeter for cuffed tubes and up to 4 centimeters for uncuffed tubes. Of greater concern, the distance from the bend to the tip of preformed nasal tubes varied by up to 5.5 centimeters for cuffed tubes and from 2 to 9 centimeters for uncuffed tubes.[268]

After the tracheal tube has been inserted, while it is being held in position by an assistant or after the first strip of adhesive tape has been applied to secure it, we observe for symmetry of chest expansion and auscultate for equality of breath sounds in the axillae and apices (not on the anterior chest wall). The anterior chest wall in the child is not used to verify tracheal intubation because breath sounds may reverberate across the precordium in small children, obscuring the diagnosis of an endobronchial intubation. Lung sliding on ultrasound,[269,270] chest x-ray, fluoroscopy, or flexible bronchoscopy can also be used to confirm appropriate positioning. An end-tidal CO_2 monitor confirms intratracheal positioning but does not preclude an endobronchial position. Unexpectedly elevated airway pressures or decreased compliance, persistent desaturation, and asymmetrical chest wall movement all suggest an endobronchial intubation. Once a satisfactory position is achieved, a second strip of tape ensures secure fixation (Fig. 12.19).

It is common for a tracheal tube to move into a mainstem bronchus after initial correct placement after repositioning for the surgical procedure; in a study of pulse oximetry, this manifested as a slight but persistent decrease in oxygen saturation (e.g., from 100% to a range of 93% to 95%).[271] Tracheal tube position can also change when a patient's head or neck position changes.[271–275] Neck extension (commonly achieved with placement of a shoulder roll) may cause the tracheal tube to move more cephalad, toward the vocal cords, resulting in inadvertent extubation, whereas neck flexion may cause it to move more caudad, predisposing to mainstem intubation. A study of 16- to 19-month-old toddlers found a mean displacement of the tracheal tube tip of 2.5 cm when moving from full flexion to full extension of the neck.[276] Clinically, we confirm appropriate tracheal tube positioning as described above both when the tracheal tube is initially inserted and then again after the patient is positioned. *When a small but persistent decrease in oxygen saturation is noted, rather than increase the inspired oxygen concentration (FiO_2), one must first investigate the cause and reassess the position of the tracheal tube to rule out a possible complete or partial endobronchial position.[271]*

Continuous Waveform Capnography

Continuous waveform capnography provides essential information to clinicians in the operating room, in nonoperating room locations, during transport, and in ICUs.[277] In an intubated patient, the presence of an appropriate exhaled carbon dioxide trace is the best confirmation of ventilation.[212] A capnogram that diminishes during the first few breaths suggests an esophageal intubation.[278] During cardiopulmonary resuscitation continuous waveform capnography can also provide valuable information on the adequacy of resuscitation efforts including chest compressions[279] and ventilation.[280,281]

Complications of Tracheal Intubation

Postintubation Croup

Perioperative postintubation croup (also referred to as postextubation croup or stridor) occurs in 0.1% to 1% of children.[233,236,243,282,283] Factors associated with an increased risk of croup include: a tracheal tube with an OD that is too large for the child's airway (no leak at >25 cm H_2O pressure or resistance at the time of insertion), changes in position during the procedure, a position other than supine, repeated attempts at intubation, traumatic intubation, patient age between 1 and 4 years, duration of surgery greater than 1 hour, coughing on the tracheal tube, and a previous history of croup.[282–284] Concurrent upper respiratory infection has been variously reported as a risk factor and as unrelated.[129,283]

Treatment of postintubation croup consists of cool, humidified mist, nebulized epinephrine and dexamethasone.[285,286] The rationale for this treatment is based primarily on experience with

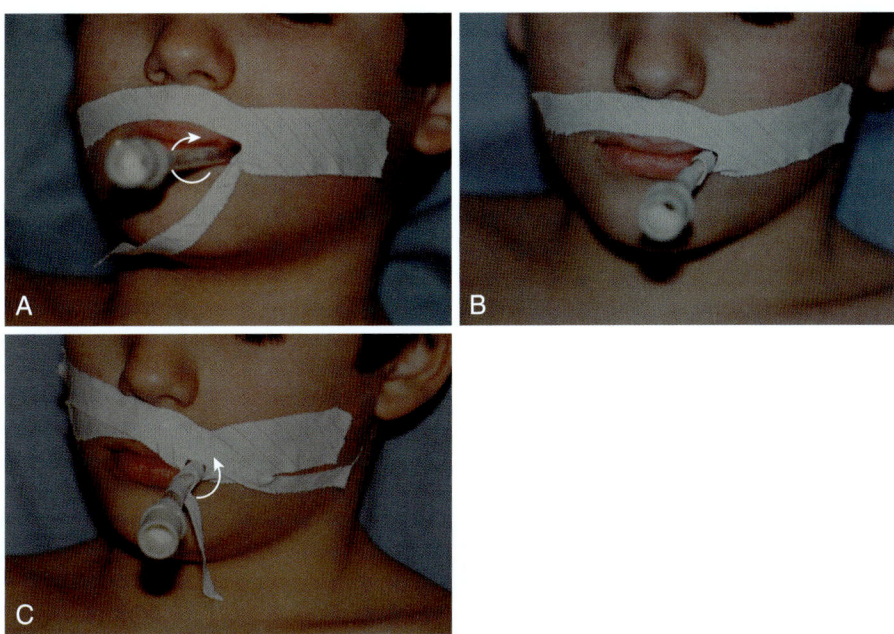

FIGURE 12.19 Securing the endotracheal tube. After insertion of the oral tracheal tube and examination for proper position, the area between the nose and upper lip and both cheeks is coated with tincture of benzoin. **A,** After the benzoin is dry, tape that has been split up the middle is applied to the cheek, and the tracheal tube is placed at the division of the split tape. **B,** One-half of the tape is wrapped circumferentially around the tube, and the other half is applied to the space above the upper lip. **C,** A second piece of tape is applied in similar fashion from the opposite direction. A nasal tracheal tube may also be secured with this technique.

the treatment of infectious croup[287–296] but the benefits of cool humidified mist remain unproven. A Cochrane review of 45 randomized controlled trials found no difference between prednisolone and dexamethasone but supports the use of glucocorticoids to treat infectious croup with low dose dexamethasone (0.15 mg/kg) apparently as effective as high dose (0.6 mg/kg).[297] Studies on the prophylactic use of dexamethasone to prevent postextubation stridor are conflicting, although the onset of clinical effect may take several hours.[286,298–301] A Cochrane review of eight trials (only three randomized) concluded that nebulized epinephrine transiently reduced symptoms.[302] Clinicians should also be aware of the potential for rebound following treatment with epinephrine and the need for extended monitoring and observation. Caution should be exercised when translating treatments from one type of croup to another.

Laryngotracheal (Subglottic) Stenosis
Subglottic stenosis is a serious complication of tracheal intubation. Although the incidence of congenital subglottic stenosis has not changed over time, the incidence of postintubation subglottic stenosis has decreased over the past several decades from 8% to a current incidence of ~0.6%.[303–306] A single center prospective study of older children requiring intubation in the ICU reported a greater incidence of postextubation tracheal injury and development of subglottic stenosis.[307] 90% of acquired subglottic stenoses are the result of tracheal intubation, particularly prolonged intubation (see Video 12.1).[308–313] An early study found that the incidence of subglottic stenosis after prolonged intubation in preterm neonates is reduced because the cricoid cartilage is relatively immature. At this age, the cartilage structure is hypercellular and the matrix has a large fluid content, making the structures more resilient and less susceptible to ischemic injury.[314]

The pathogenesis of acquired subglottic stenosis is ischemic injury secondary to lateral wall pressure from the tracheal tube or over-inflated cuff. Ischemia results in edema, necrosis, and ulcerations of the mucosa.[315] Secondary infection results in exposure of the cartilage.[315] Within 48 hours, granulation tissue begins to form within these ulcerations. Ultimately, scar tissue forms, resulting in narrowing of the airway (Fig. 12.20).[305,306,316–318] Specimens obtained from partial cricotracheal resection in children were found to have severe sclerotic scarring[319] with squamous metaplasia of the epithelium, loss of mucus glands and elastic mantle fibers (tunica elastica), and dilation of the remaining glands with formation of cysts.[318,320] The cricoid cartilage was affected on the internal and external side, with irreversible loss of perichondrium on the inside and resorption by macrophages of cartilage on both sides.[320]

Factors that predispose to subglottic stenosis include use of a tracheal tube that is too large, a high cuff pressure, laryngeal trauma (e.g., traumatic intubation, chemical or thermal inhalation, external trauma, surgical trauma, gastric reflux),[321–323] prolonged intubation (particularly greater than 25 days), repeated intubation,[324] hypotension, sepsis and infection, chronic illness, and chronic inflammatory disease.[311,325,326]

The mainstay of therapy for severe subglottic stenosis has been tracheostomy and open laryngotracheal reconstruction. In recent years, there has been a shift away from tracheostomy and a renewed interest in endoscopic approaches including balloon dilation[327–330] for the management of severe subglottic stenosis.[331–333]

SUPRAGLOTTIC AIRWAYS
Archie Brain developed the LMA, the first supraglottic airway (SGA) device, in the 1980s. Commercially produced supraglottic airways became available in the United Kingdom in 1988 and in the United States in 1992 (Fig. 12.21).[334–340] Supraglottic airways

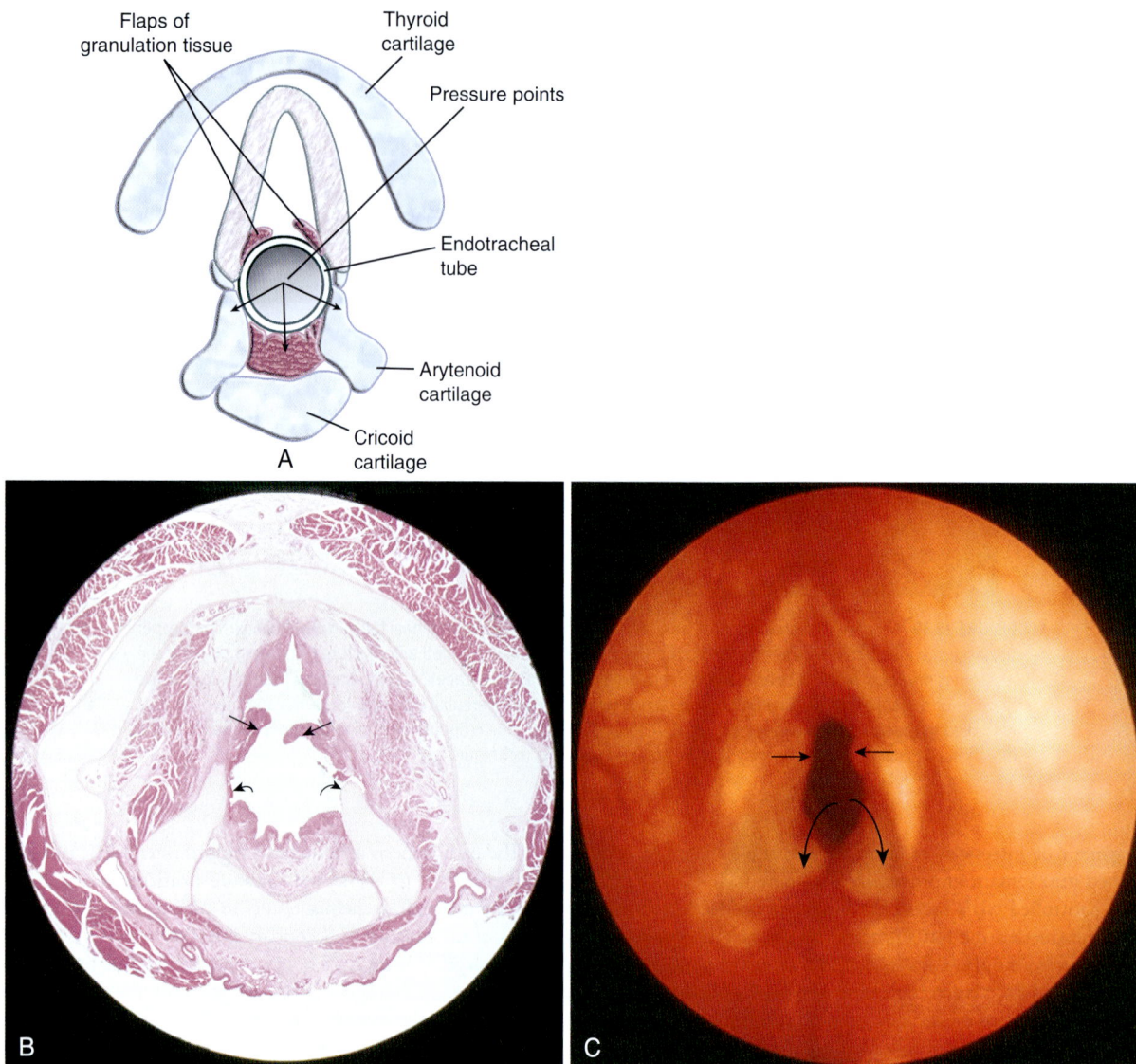

FIGURE 12.20 The pathogenesis of intubation injuries. **A,** Schemata of a cross section through the glottis. Pressure necrosis causes ulcerations at the vocal processes of the arytenoids with exposed cartilage. Flaps of granulation tissue are present anterior to these ulcerations. **B,** Cross section of the glottis at this same level; *straight arrows* indicate flaps of granulation tissue, and *curved arrows* indicate the absence of mucosa and ulcerations with exposed cartilage on the vocal processes of the arytenoids. **C,** Intubation injury to a 2-month-old infant; *straight arrows* indicate granulation tissue, and *curved arrows* indicate an area of ulcerations *(white area)*. The most severe area of injury is usually at the level of the cricoid cartilage, resulting in subglottic stenosis. (Reproduced with permission from Holinger LD, Lusk RP, Green CG. *Pediatric Laryngology and Bronchoesophagology.* Philadelphia: Lippincott-Raven; 1997.)

were developed to replace the face mask in adults during maintenance of anesthesia[341,342]; however, their use has expanded greatly. Supraglottic airways have become a standard option for airway management during general anesthesia as well as an important rescue option in cases of difficult mask ventilation or intubation for children and adults.[334–340,342–345] Supraglottic airways offer additional advantages such as freeing the anesthesiologist's hands for other tasks and reducing operating room pollution.[346,347] The use of controlled ventilation with a SGA as a means for providing positive end-expiratory pressure (PEEP) has also been described.[348–351] However, some raise concerns that this practice risks insufflation of the stomach and subsequent regurgitation of gastric contents.[350,352–355]

Insufflation of gas into the stomach is more likely to occur when high ventilation pressures are used or required.[348,350,356] Clinically undetected malpositioning is a risk factor for gastric air insufflation, especially at peak inspiratory pressures greater than 17 cm H_2O.[352] It should be further noted that given their supraglottic location, SGAs cannot be depended upon to protect against pulmonary aspiration of gastric contents.[349,353,354]

Flexible diagnostic and therapeutic bronchoscopy, radiation therapy, radiologic procedures, ear/nose/throat surgeries, and ophthalmologic procedures are the most commonly described pediatric indications for SGAs.[339,344,357–360] Supraglottic airways are also commonly used for orthopedic, plastic, and general surgery,

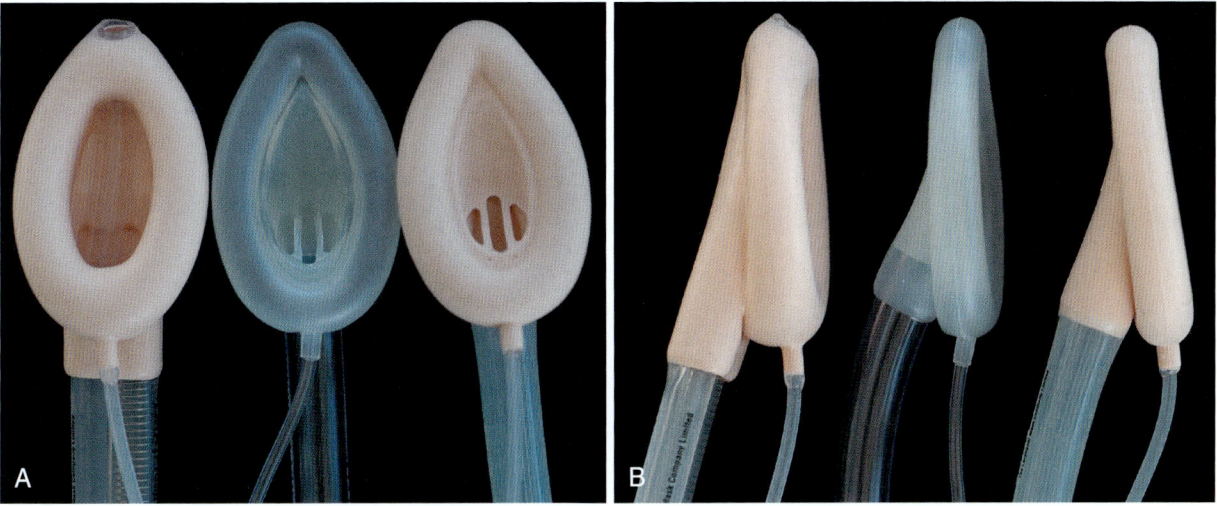

FIGURE 12.21 There are now a variety of supraglottic airway devices available in pediatric sizes. Displayed are pediatric size 2 of the reusable LMA Classic, the disposable LMA Unique, and the ProSeal LMA (PLMA). **A,** The transparent material of the disposable LMA Unique *(center)* is medical-grade polyvinylchloride (PVC), whereas the reusable PLMA *(left)* and LMA Classic *(right)* are made of medical-grade silicone. Notice the differences in structure. The drainage tube outlet of the PLMA can be seen at the most distal tip of the cuff. The PLMA uses the drain tube to elevate the epiglottis away from the larynx, whereas the Classic and Unique have aperture bars. In contrast to the Classic and Unique LMAs, the PLMA cuff is softer, has a special shape, and has a deeper mask bowl. These features of the PLMA allow for improved sealing for positive-pressure ventilation. **B,** In profile, the distinct shape of the PLMA *(left)* can be appreciated. The dual-tube structure (drainage and airway lumens) creates a larger tube profile (**A,** *left*) that incorporates a bite block and improves stability. Other commonly used devices are the air-Q and the Ambu Aura.

particularly for procedures involving extremities or superficial structures of the trunk, head, and neck. Supraglottic airways may be advantageous for certain ophthalmologic procedures as there is no associated increase in intraocular pressure with SGA placement, in contrast to tracheal intubation.[361] The advantage of the SGA for diagnostic and therapeutic flexible bronchoscopy, even in preterm infants,[362] is that it provides a conduit for oxygenation and ventilation while allowing a larger bronchoscope to be used than can be passed through an age-appropriate tracheal tube.[358,359,363–366] It also allows visualization and evaluation of the laryngeal structures. Some SGAs may provide better bronchoscopic conditions than others owing to their material or preconfigured shape.[367] For children who require frequent anesthetics over a brief period, as in radiation therapy, the SGA provides an airway without the trauma of repeated intubation.[339] The SGA has also been advocated for use in place of intubation in children who are at increased risk for bronchial airway reactivity (e.g., upper respiratory tract infection, history of reactive airway disease)[368-371]; a systematic review and meta-analysis that compared SGAs with tracheal intubation found no difference in the incidence of laryngospasm, breath holding or desaturation events but did find a reduced incidence of coughing when using an SGA.[372] Supraglottic airways also have an important role in rescue of difficult intubation and mask ventilation[342]; when the proper size tracheal tube is matched with an SGA this will serve as a conduit for fiberoptic intubation (Video 12.6).[373–375]

Styles of Supraglottic Airways

The LMA Classic was the original SGA introduced for pediatric patients, available in eight sizes designed to fit all size patients (neonates to adults >100 kg). Guidelines for selecting the appropriately sized SGA for children for multiple brands are based on weight (Table 12.4). The LMA Classic is made of medical-grade silicone and consists of a large-bore tubular structure (barrel) with

a 15-millimeter adapter at its proximal end and an elliptical, mask-like device that fits over the laryngeal inlet at its distal end. The mask is inflated by means of a valved pilot tube and balloon. A number of second-generation devices have important modifications such as an additional channel for gastric decompression or suctioning, no grill within the mask that inhibits passage of tracheal tubes, as well as superior sealing pressures.[334]

Second-generation devices include the LMA Supreme (Teleflex Incorporated, Morrisville, NC), the ProSeal LMA (PLMA) (Teleflex Incorporated, Morrisville, NC), I-gel (Intersurgical, Woking-ham, Berkshire, UK), and Ambu AuraGain (Ambu, Inc., Columbia, MD). The ProSeal LMA, which comes in seven sizes, was designed to improve sealing pressures[376,377] and to provide a conduit for evacuation of stomach contents[378,379]; these features make it more appealing compared with other SGAs for use with positive-pressure ventilation,[380] even in neonates,[381] and as an improved rescue device.[382,383] In sizes 3 and larger, there is a second dorsal cuff to increase the seal pressure of the glottic mask. The dorsal and ventral cuffs communicate, allowing simultaneous inflation by a single pilot balloon. In the smaller sizes, there is no second dorsal cuff, but the profile of the mask has been altered to improve sealing. The ProSeal LMA is easy to insert, allows greater airway pressures with positive-pressure ventilation, and better protects against gastric insufflation.[334,376,377,384] A number of studies support the efficacy of the ProSeal LMA in children for both spontaneous and controlled ventilation.[376,380,381,385–388] In children, the ProSeal LMA and the Classic LMA are similarly easy to insert, have their proper position confirmed by fiberoptic visualization, and yield similar frequencies of mucosal trauma. The advantage is that oropharyngeal leak pressure is greater and gastric insufflation is less common with the ProSeal LMA.[376,385–388] In children, the ability to provide pressure support ventilation with the ProSeal LMA during anesthesia also improves gas exchange

TABLE 12.4 | Commonly Used Pediatric Supraglottic Airways and Suggested Maximum Cuffed Tracheal Tube

Supraglottic Airway	NEONATAL/INFANT			PEDIATRIC			TEEN		
	Wt (kg)	Size	TT	Wt (kg)	Size	TT	Wt (kg)	Size	TT
LMA Unique	<5	1	3.0[a]	10–20	2	4.0[a]	50–70	4	6.0
	5–10	1.5	3.5[a]	20–30	2.5	5.0[b]	70–100	5	7.0
				30–50	3	6.0			
air-Q Intubating Laryngeal Airway	<4	0.5[c]	4.0	7–17	1.5	5.0	50–70	3.5	7.5
	4–7	1.0	4.5	17–30	2.0	5.5	70–100	4.5	8.5
				30–50	2.5	6.5			
I-gel supraglottic airway	2–5	1	3.0[a]	10–25	2	5.0[b]	50–90	4	7.0
	5–12	1.5	4.0[a]	25–35	2.5	5.0[b]	>90	5	8.0
				35–60	3	6.0			
Ambu AuraGain Laryngeal Mask	<5	1	3.0[a]	10–20	2	4.5[a]	50–70	4	6.0
	5–10	1.5	3.5[a]	20–30	2.5	5.0[b]	70–100	5	7.0
				30–50	3	6.0	>100	6	7.5

TT, Trachea tube; *Wt*, weight.
Commonly used pediatric supraglottic airways and suggested maximum cuffed tracheal tube based on the tracheal tube's internal diameter (millimeters). Tracheal tube sizes are for those with a low profile cuff. As the air-Q is designed to allow pilot balloons to pass thought it, it will also allow larger tracheal tubes than would be routinely used for a child of the indicated weight.
[a]Pilot balloon will not fit through the SGA conduit.
[b]Pilot balloon may not fit through the SGA conduit.
[c]New product air-Q R3 has sizes 0 (<2 kg) and 0.5 (2–4 kg), previously smallest was a reusable product size 0.5 for <4 kg.

and reduces the work of breathing compared with the application of CPAP.[389,390] The greater sealing pressure may also protect against aspiration in the event of regurgitation of gastric contents.[391]

The LMA Fastrach (Teleflex Incorporated, Morrisville, NC) was specifically designed to allow the blind passage of a tracheal tube in an emergent situation in which direct laryngoscopy is not possible or in patients with cervical spine immobilization.[264,392–394] This is a rigid device with a fixed angulation designed primarily for adults (available in sizes 3, 4, and 5). It requires special, flexible tracheal tubes with an ID of 6.0 to 8.0 millimeters.

The LMA Supreme is a single-use, curved SGA with an elliptical airway tube and an integrated gastric drain tube that extends to the tip of the mask bowl.[395–400] The proximal end includes a bite block, which should lie between the teeth. A fixation tab allows the LMA Supreme to be secured to the face (Fig. 12.22). The deflated mask is held at the fixation tab and is inserted along the palate into the pharynx in a fashion similar to that used for the LMA Classic (see later). An appropriately positioned mask forms a leak-free seal with the glottis, and the mask tip is embedded in the upper esophageal sphincter. Once in place, the cuff is inflated, and the mask position confirmed to be appropriate with the use of several simple maneuvers. An easy test to confirm that the position of the mask is the suprasternal notch test, whereby a small amount of water-soluble lubricant is applied to the drain tube of the airway. Application of slight pressure in the suprasternal notch should result in a slight up-and-down movement of the applied lubricant on the drain tube. This confirms that the drain tube is contiguous with and adequately sealed in the upper esophageal sphincter. The ability to easily place a gastric tube through the drain tube further confirms correct positioning. Suction should not be applied to the gastric tube until it has been advanced into the stomach; this prevents collapse of the drain tube and potential injury to the upper esophageal sphincter. The LMA Supreme is available in pediatric sizes. A study comparing the LMA Supreme with the ProSeal LMA and the Classic LMA in a neonatal manikin model demonstrated higher inflation pressures and shorter insertion times with the LMA Supreme.[401] One study found that neck flexion and extension alter device seal.[402] The curve

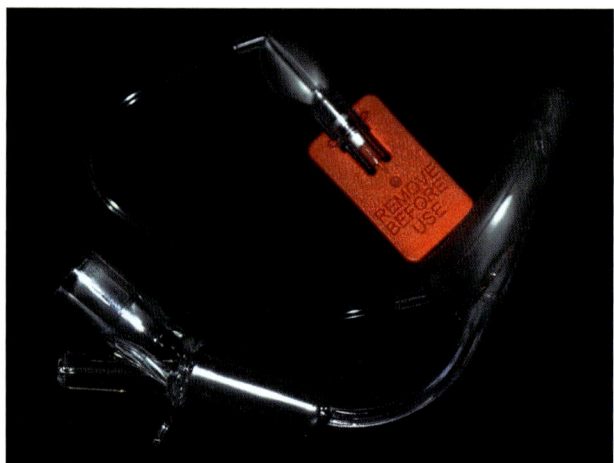

FIGURE 12.22 The LMA Supreme offers the advantages of a built-in suction port and a built-in bite block.

of the LMA Supreme makes it impractical to intubate through this device.

The Laryngeal Tube (LT; VBM Medizintech GmbH, Sulz, Germany) is designed to secure a patent airway during either spontaneous breathing or controlled ventilation. This device is available with a single lumen for ventilation only or with a double-lumen tube that also allows suction of gastric contents. This system seals the esophagus at the distal end with a small cuff attached at the tip (distal cuff), and a larger balloon cuff at the middle part of the tube (proximal cuff) stabilizes the device and blocks the oropharynx and nasopharynx. The two openings that lie between the cuffs are positioned so that the more distal opening faces the glottis. The cuffs are inflated through a single pilot tube and balloon, through which cuff pressure can be monitored. There are three black lines on the tube near a standard 15-millimeter connector that indicate adequate depth of insertion when aligned with the teeth. The nondisposable device is

TABLE 12.5	Size Selection and Recommended Cuff Volumes for the Laryngeal Tube		
Tube Size	Body Weight or Height	Recommended Cuff Volume (mL)	Connector Color
0 Newborn	<5 kg	10	Clear
1 Infants	5–12 kg	20	White
2 Children	12–25 kg	35	Green
3 Adults: small	<155 cm	60	Yellow
4 Adults: medium	155–180 cm	80	Red
5 Adults: large	>180 cm	90	Purple

made of silicone (latex-free) and is reusable up to 50 times after autoclave sterilization. There are four variations: (1) standard single-lumen, reusable (LT); (2) single-lumen, disposable (LT-D); (3) double-lumen with drain tube, reusable (LT-suction II, or LTS II); and (4) double-lumen with drain tube, disposable (LTS-D) (E-Fig. 12.3).[403] It is available in six sizes, suitable for neonates up to large adults (Table 12.5).

The Laryngeal Tube should be inserted while the child's head and neck are placed in the sniffing or neutral position. The tip of a well-lubricated Laryngeal Tube is placed against the hard palate behind the upper incisors. The device is then slid down the center of the mouth until resistance is felt or the device is almost fully inserted. After connection to the anesthesia circuit, proper placement is confirmed by assessing ease of ventilation. Some adjustment (usually slight withdrawal) may be required to provide optimal ventilation. Care should be taken not to push the tongue backward into the posterior pharynx. Ease of insertion of the standard Laryngeal Tube is reported to be comparable to that of the LMA Classic, although the Laryngeal Tube may require more readjustments of its position to obtain a clear airway.[404,405] The incidence of complications with the two devices appears to be similar.[404] The Laryngeal Tube may provide a better seal than the Classic LMA.[406] Compared with the ProSeal LMA, the Laryngeal Tube may be less effective and more difficult to insert.[407-409] Although the LT-suction device may have similar success to the ProSeal LMA,[410] there are scant data in children.[411-415] An initial report of its use in children aged 2 to 12 years found a successful placement rate of 96% (77/80 children). Complications occurred in two children: one had laryngospasm that resolved with deepening of the anesthetic and the other complained of mild difficulty with swallowing postoperatively.[412] A study that compared the Laryngeal Tube with the LMA Classic found the former to be less effective for either spontaneous or assisted ventilation and for fiberoptic evaluation of the airway in children younger than 10 years of age.[411] A study of 70 children using sizes 0 to 3 reported failure to place the Laryngeal Tube in 12% of children. Failures were caused by inability to ventilate, hypoxemia, gastric insufflation, cough, and laryngospasm or stridor, particularly for children weighing less than 10 kilograms; therefore, the Laryngeal Tube was not recommended for children of this size.[413] Although the manufacturer states that a flexible fiberoptic bronchoscope (FOB) may be passed through the device, the openings are of insufficient size to permit passage of a tracheal tube. A randomized study of 70 children 1 to 12 years of age found a lower incidence of coughing during deep anesthesia but an increased incidence of airway obstruction.[416]

The I-gel SGA (Intersurgical, Liverpool, NY) is a second-generation device that consists of a dual-channeled, noninflatable laryngeal mask made from a gel-like thermoplastic elastomer (Fig. 12.23). It has a built-in bite block and is available in pediatric sizes (Table 12.6). One channel functions as the airway tube whereas the second channel exits at the tip of the device and provides gastric access when seated properly. The lubricated posterior surface of the I-gel is inserted along the palate into the posterior pharynx. An observational study in 50 children reported easy insertion in all patients with a mean leak pressure of 25 cm H_2O; gastric access was successfully obtained in all children.[417] Sealing pressures have been found to be similar to the ProSeal LMA but there may be a lower incidence of blood staining and sore throat.[377,418–420] Some have noted a tendency for the I-gel to slide out and recommended taping it in place to prevent dislodgment intraoperatively.[421]

The air-Q Mask Laryngeal Airway (Mercury Medical, Clearwater, FL) is an oval-shaped laryngeal mask with a shortened, wide, hypercurved airway tube (Fig. 12.24). The air-Q intubating laryngeal mask is available in smaller sizes for younger children and offers some advantages over other supraglottic airways when used as an intubation conduit. It has a wider airway tube that accommodates cuffed tracheal tubes, and its length is shorter, facilitating removal of the mask after tracheal intubation. The air-Q performs well as a conduit for tracheal intubation and has been successfully used in children with difficult airways.[373,422–425] The air-Q is supplied with a red tag attached to the pilot balloon of the mask. This tag equalizes the pressure in the mask to atmospheric pressure, and the mask should be inserted with the tag attached. The manufacturer recommends light lubrication of the back of the mask and the tip of its inner surface. The air-Q was compared with the LMA Unique in a cohort of 50 children aged 6 to 36 months. The air-Q had higher airway leak pressure and a superior fiberoptic grade of view than the LMA Unique.[426] In another study that evaluated the air-Q as a conduit for tracheal intubation in infants, the mean oropharyngeal leak pressure was 18.5 ± 1.8 cm H_2O, and the mean insertion time was 13.3 ± 3.9 seconds; tracheal intubation was successful in 19 of 20 infants.[427] Another study compared the air-Q with an I-gel; the I-gel provided a greater leak pressure but the air-Q provided better fiberoptic views in children.[428] The successful use of the air-Q as a conduit for tracheal intubation has also been reported in infants with difficult direct laryngoscopy.[373,429] There are numerous studies comparing one device with another, and many clinicians find that they prefer different SGAs for different clinical scenarios.[382,430–437] Some devices also offer advantages in terms of cost.[438–440]

Insertion Technique

The recommended insertion technique for the Classic LMA is the same for children as for adults (see Video 12.7) and mimics deglutition or swallowing of food.[441] The cuff is completely deflated, and the posterior surface of the mask is well lubricated. These actions mimic lubrication of a food bolus with saliva and formation of a soft, flattened, wedge-shaped bolus. The child is placed in the age-appropriate intubating position. Following induction of anesthesia and ensuring adequate anesthetic depth, the nondominant hand is used to tilt the head to sniffing position, mimicking the anatomic movements of swallowing.[344,442,443] The SGA is inserted with the mask aperture facing anteriorly (toward the tongue). The index finger of the insertion hand may be placed in the cleft between the mask and the barrel. With the index finger, the SGA is pushed upward and backward, toward the top of the child's head. This flattens the mask against the palate. Continued backward pressure (toward the top of the child's head) guides the

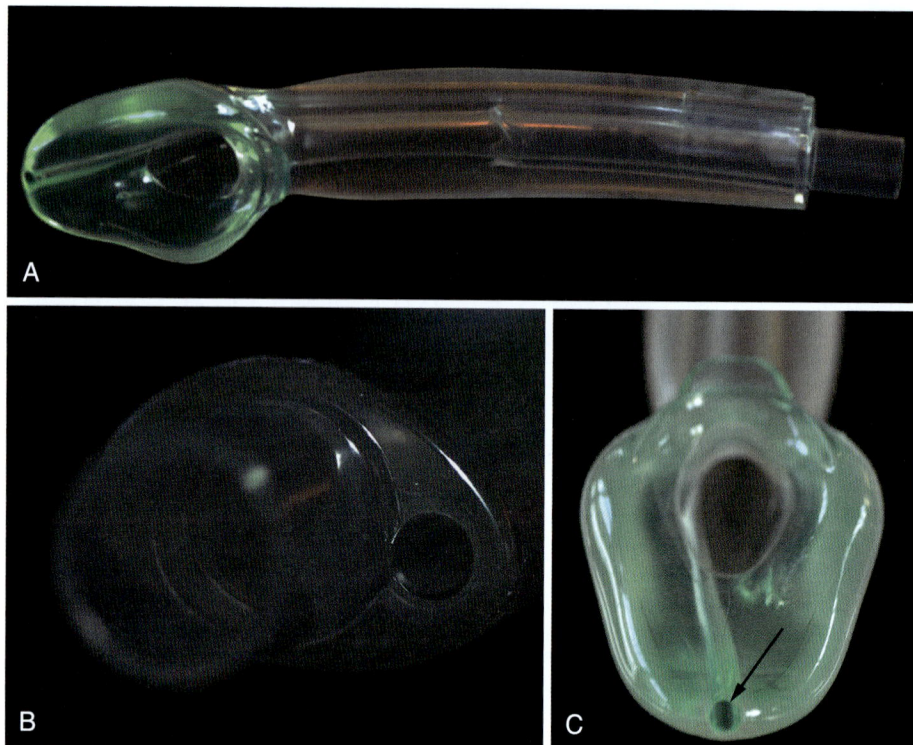

FIGURE 12.23 The I-gel supraglottic device **(A)** consists of a malleable non–latex-containing, noninflatable cuff that is designed to seal over the laryngeal inlet after insertion. The stem of the I-gel contains a "buccal cavity stabilizer," which is designed to resist accidental rotation after insertion and is made from a hard polymer that resists biting. The I-gel also contains a gastric suction channel next to the 15-mm connector **(B)**, with which practitioners may evacuate gastric contents when the device is in the correct inserted position. **C,** The distal position of the suction port *(arrow)*.

TABLE 12.6	Suggested I-gel Supraglottic Device Size, Inner Diameter, Endotracheal Tube Size, and Nasogastric Tube Size			
Size	Patient Weight (kg)	ID (mm)	Maximal Size of Tracheal Tube (mm ID)[a]	Maximal Size of Nasogastric Tube (Fr)
1	2–5	5.6	3	
1.5	5–12	6.8	4	10
2	10–25	8.8	5	12
2.5	25–35	10.2	5	12
3	30–60	11.2	6	12
4	50–90	12.3	7	12
5	>90	12.5	8	14

[a]May depend on outer diameter specifications of endotracheal tube manufacturer.
ID, Inner diameter.

SGA along the palate and down to the upper esophageal sphincter. It is essential that pressure be applied to force the SGA against the roof of the mouth. The mask is advanced along the palate until some resistance is felt. These actions mimic the propulsion of a food bolus into the hypopharynx caused by tongue pressure, first upward and backward, then downward in an arc. When resistance is felt, air is injected into the mask cuff (see Table 12.4 for size recommendations and maximum recommended inflation volumes).

Inflation of the cuff causes the end of the airway to move out of the mouth about 1 centimeter and forms a loose seal around the esophageal inlet, thereby directing gas flow into the trachea. *If no outward movement is observed with inflation of the mask, the SGA may not be properly positioned.* Proper position can be ascertained further by movement of the anesthesia bag, measure of expired CO_2, the ability to provide gentle assisted ventilation, and, if necessary, by direct visualization with a flexible bronchoscope. If the lungs cannot be gently ventilated (peak airway pressure <20 cm H_2O) or no breath sounds are heard, the SGA must be immediately removed because it has not been properly positioned, or the child's airway might be obstructed. *Remember, children may experience laryngospasm or severe bronchospasm requiring immediate treatment to restore oxygenation and ventilation!*

Several reports claim that when the above described insertion technique is used in children, the SGA frequently hangs up in the posterior pharynx, making proper positioning difficult.[444,445] Therefore other insertion techniques have been described. The rotational or reverse technique for children has been advocated to be simpler and more successful.[446,447] The SGA is placed in the mouth with the cuff facing the hard palate (the opposite of the traditional technique). It is then advanced and rotated into position simultaneously (Video 12.8).[444–448] A partial mask inflation technique has also been advocated.[443,448–450] The SGA is left partially inflated to smooth the edges of the mask and then is inserted in the usual manner,[443,449] or in a lateral manner and then rotated and advanced,[450] or with a complete 180-degree rotation.[448] For placement of the ProSeal LMA, the rotational technique was found to have no advantage over the standard technique in

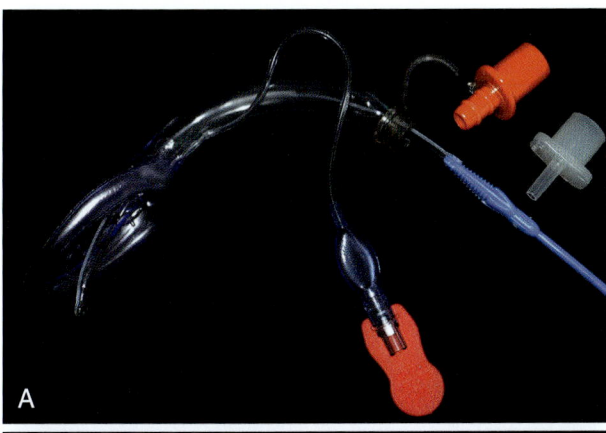

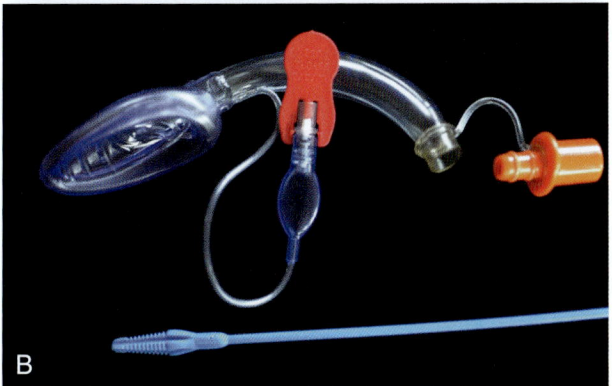

FIGURE 12.24 A, The air-Q Intubating Laryngeal Airway (Mercury Medical, Clearwater, FL) offers some advantages over traditional laryngeal masks when used as an intubation conduit in children. It has a wider airway tube that accommodates cuffed endotracheal tubes, and its length is shorter, which facilitates removal of the mask after tracheal intubation. Before the intubation attempt, one should check that the tracheal tube and its cuff will easily pass through the laryngeal airway size to be used. The 15-mm adapter of the air-Q is removed, the trachea is intubated with a bronchoscope, and the tracheal tube is advanced into the trachea. **B,** To correctly position the tracheal tube, a special stylet (coudé-tip Tracheal Tube Introducer, available in three sizes for pediatric-sized tracheal tubes) is inserted into the lumen of the tracheal tube, the cuff of the air-Q is deflated, and with slight advancing pressure the tracheal tube is held in place while the air-Q is gently withdrawn.

children.[451] A jaw thrust maneuver and the use of a rigid laryngoscope have also been advocated to assist in placement of the LMA Classic.[452] We find that a jaw thrust is often sufficient to overcome barriers to proper positioning of an SGA.

Regardless of insertion method, the most common cause of failure is use of an inappropriate size SGA. An SGA that is too large will not pass beyond the posterior pharynx. An SGA that is too small will pass easily but may not seal against the laryngeal inlet. Another common mistake when using the traditional insertion method is to try to press the SGA *down* into the pharynx. Pressure should be directed *back,* toward the pharyngeal wall, so that the airway will follow the natural curve of the pharynx and seat correctly in the esophageal sphincter without kinking. Attempting to place the SGA when the child is inadequately anesthetized may also make advancement impossible or result in laryngospasm.

Supraglottic airway use can result in injuries to upper airway structures[453–455]; damage to the recurrent laryngeal,[456] hypoglossal, lingual, inferior alveolar, or infraorbital nerves has occurred.[457–459]

The incidence of sore throat may be equal to or greater than that seen with tracheal intubation.[460–463] Supraglottic airway use in infants requires special caution. A review of the use of the size 1 SGA in 50 infants found that the SGA sometimes migrated over time, even after apparent correct initial placement; delayed airway obstruction occurred in 12 infants after apparent successful placement.[464] Constant vigilance is required. Evaluation of a large dataset revealed factors associated with SGA failure in children include: prolonged surgical duration, procedures of the head and neck, non-outpatient admission status, congenital airway abnormalities, and a category the authors called "patient transport," which consisted primarily of moving a patient's position or anesthetizing location with the laryngeal mask in situ.[465,466]

The ideal timing for removal of the SGA in children is frequently debated. Both "awake" and "deep" removal has been advocated.[467–471] Awake removal ensures return of protective reflexes but with the attendant problems of airway reactivity. Deep removal avoids excessive airway reactivity and potential laryngospasm but may increase the risk of aspiration or airway obstruction (or both) as the child emerges from anesthesia later in the recovery room. One author suggested leaving the cuff inflated until the child begins swallowing or is able to open the mouth on command as a means for reducing the potential for laryngospasm. The proposed mechanism is that secretions are swept away from the larynx, reducing the stimulus for laryngospasm.[472] Lubrication of the cuff with 2% lidocaine jelly or the addition of an IV administered opioid to the anesthetic may reduce coughing and laryngeal stimulation on emergence.[443] A systematic review that examined removal awake versus anesthetized found a reduced incidence of complications with deep (cough, desaturation) but an increased incidence of airway obstruction.[473] Another study found a lower incidence of laryngospasm compared with tracheal intubation (cuffed or uncuffed tracheal tubes vs. ProSeal LMA) in 120 infants 1 to 24 months of age undergoing lower abdominal procedures.[474]

Supraglottic Airways for Resuscitation

Given the recognition that chest compressions are the most important factor in successful outcomes after cardiac arrest and the need to avoid interrupting compressions during cardiopulmonary resuscitation,[281,475] the SGA will likely assume a greater role in airway management of cardiac arrest.[476] Supraglottic airway placement has been used successfully for neonatal resuscitation[477–481]; it may be an easier skill to acquire than bag-and-mask ventilation.[476,482–486] The SGA has also been used to deliver surfactant to neonates with respiratory distress syndrome[487,488] with one study reporting a reduced need for intubation or mechanical ventilation,[489] for longer-term intensive care management of neonates with difficult airways,[490–492] and for intrahospital transport of neonates with difficult airways.[493]

Airway Management: The Abnormal Airway

CLASSIFYING THE ABNORMAL PEDIATRIC AIRWAY

It is important to recognize circumstances that may cause airway obstruction or difficult laryngoscopy. Conditions that predispose to airway problems may be grouped according to anatomic location and may result from congenital, inflammatory, traumatic, metabolic, or neoplastic disorders. Tables 12.7 and 12.8 list the more common pediatric airway problems according to anatomic

TABLE 12.7 | Pediatric Airway Pathology Related to Anatomic Site

Anatomic Site	Etiology	Clinical Condition
Nasopharynx	Congenital	Choanal atresia, stenosis,[47,48,826–830] encephalocele[831–837]
	Traumatic	Foreign body, trauma[838–840]
	Inflammatory	Adenoidal hypertrophy,[838–840] nasal congestion[49]
	Neoplastic	Teratoma[841–843]
Tongue	Congenital	Hemangioma, Trisomy 21, glossoptosis[844]
	Traumatic	Burn, laceration, lymphatic/venous obstruction[170,171,838,845–851]
	Metabolic	Beckwith-Wiedemann syndrome[756,852–858] hypothyroidism,[859] mucopolysaccharidosis,[800,860–881] glycogen storage disease,[882–892] gangliosidosis,[893–896] congenital hypothyroidism
	Neoplastic	Cystic hygroma,[897–901] cystic teratoma
Mandible/ maxilla	Congenital hypoplasia	Pierre Robin syndrome,[595,643,725,727,902–919] Treacher Collins syndrome,[538,726,757,920–934] Goldenhar syndrome,[503,638,783,935–942] Apert syndrome,[943–945] achondroplasia,[729,946–950] Turner syndrome,[951–955] Cornelia de Lange syndrome,[956–959] Smith-Lemli-Opitz syndrome,[960–962] Hallermann-Streiff syndrome,[963] Crouzon syndrome[964,965]
	Traumatic	Fracture,[966–968] neck burn with contractures[850,851]
	Inflammatory	Juvenile rheumatoid arthritis[969–975]
	Neoplastic	Tumors, cherubism[976–978]
Pharynx/larynx	Congenital	Laryngomalacia (infantile larynx) (see Video 12.1),[838,979–982] Freeman-Sheldon syndrome (whistling face),[983–996] laryngeal stenosis,[838,997] laryngocele,[979] laryngeal web,[979,998–1000] hemangioma[1001,1002]
	Traumatic	Dislocated/fractured larynx,[838,968,1003–1009] foreign body,[69,70,838,1010–1019] inhalation injury (burn),[845–848,850,1020] postintubation edema/granuloma/stenosis,[1021–1035] swelling of uvula,[170,1036] soft palate trauma, epidermolysis bullosa[1037–1049]
	Inflammatory	Epiglottitis,[65–67,1050–1055] acute tonsillitis,[1056] peritonsillar abscess,[1057,1058] retropharyngeal abscess,[1059] diphtheritic membrane, laryngeal papillomatosis[1060–1068]
	Metabolic	Hypocalcemic laryngospasm[62]
	Neoplastic	Tumors
	Neurologic	Vocal cord paralysis, Arnold-Chiari malformation[1069–1072]
Trachea	Congenital	Vascular ring,[71,72,1073,1074] tracheal stenosis or complete tracheal rings (Video 12.9),[1075–1077] tracheomalacia (see Video 12.1)[979,997,1031,1078–1080] congenital tracheal web, hemangioma[1081–1084]
	Inflammatory	Laryngotracheobronchitis (viral),[64,67,68,283,1085–1087] bacterial tracheitis
	Neoplastic	Mediastinal tumors: neurofibroma,[1088] paratracheal nodes (lymphoma)[1089–1095]

TABLE 12.8 | Cervical Spine Anomalies.[a]

Etiology	Clinical Condition
Congenital	Trisomy 21,[1096–1105] Klippel-Feil malformation,[1106–1111] Goldenhar syndrome,[503,638,783,935–941,1112] Pierre Robin syndrome,[1113] torticollis
Traumatic	Fracture, subluxation,[967,968,1003–1007,1114–1117] neck burn contracture[851]
Inflammatory	Rheumatoid arthritis[969–975]
Metabolic	Mucopolysaccharidosis (Morquio syndrome)[860–875,1118]

[a]Abnormalities of the cervical spine may limit extension and flexion, thereby contributing to the difficulties of airway management; a significant percentage of children with Trisomy 21 have atlantoaxial instability.[1119]

location. E-Table 12.1 lists the more common pediatric syndromes and associated anesthetic considerations; more complete information may be obtained elsewhere.[494–497]

MANAGEMENT PRINCIPLES

For any laryngoscopy, but in particular for the difficult airway, an extensive array of equipment to assist with the difficult airway must be available in a difficult airway cart; suggestions for contents are listed in Table 12.9. The approach to a difficult airway, as described earlier, must include a careful history and physical examination and, when indicated, radiologic evaluation. In the past, lateral neck xerograms were useful in delineating anatomic aberrations; however, ultrasound, MRI, and CT imaging have supplanted this modality.[141–143,145–156,180,498–503] Ultrasound can be useful in the identification of subglottic stenosis; there may also be a role for use of ultrasound to help with the prediction of difficult tracheal intubations and for the examination of children with known difficult airways.[504–507] Ultrasound can also be used to intubate the trachea quickly as it can be used as a visualization tool for the lighted stylet technique and may be particularly beneficial when blood or secretions impair visualization with traditional methods.[508]

In addition to the airway pathology, the pathophysiology of the congenital syndrome or associated disease process must be fully evaluated. The safest approach to managing a difficult airway is to formulate a plan that includes several contingencies for failure or loss of the airway and to have skilled help available, especially a surgeon who is experienced in establishing a surgical airway. To maximize success and safety, a skilled assistant should help

TABLE 12.9   Items to Consider for an Emergency Intubation Cart

Drawer 1	
LMA Classic (disposable); sizes 1, 1.5, 2, 2.5, 3, 4, 5	Lens paper
air-Q Laryngeal masks; sizes 0.5, 1, 1.5, 2, 2.5, 3.5, 4.5	Surgical lubricant
LMA ProSeal (disposable); sizes 1.5, 2, 2.5, 3, 4, 5	2% Lidocaine jelly[a]
Tracheal tube stabilizers or laryngeal forceps	4% Lidocaine solution[a]
Size or weight charts for LMA	Atomizer to spray topical lidocaine
Drawer 2	Suction catheters; sizes 8, 10, 14 Fr
Transtracheal jet-ventilation catheters[a] (VBM); infant (16 ga), child (14 ga), adult (13 ga)	Yankauer suction tubes; pediatric and adult sizes
Emergency Transtracheal Airway Catheter (Cook)	Defogger
Magill forceps; adult and pediatric sizes	Silicone spray
Aillon tube bender	Halogen light bulb
Miller blades; sizes 0, 1, 2, 3, 4	Disposable teeth guards
Macintosh blades; sizes 1, 2, 3, 4	**Drawer 4**
Phillips blades; sizes 1, 2	Face masks; neonate, infant, toddler, child, adult (small/medium/large)
Wis-Hipple blades; sizes 1, 1.5	Frie endoscopy mask; infant, child, adult
Oxyscope blades; sizes 0, 1 (with oxygen tubing)	Bronchoscopy airways[a]; infant, child, adult
Handles (Medium and Short)	Bite blocks; infant, child, adult
C batteries × 2	Ovassapian airways (2)
Oxygen Y-connector	Nasal trumpets[a]; sizes 2 to 34F
Albuterol adapters for metered-dose administration (3)	Oral airways; sizes 90, 80, 70, 60, 50, 00, 000
Syringes (5 each); 5 mL, 10 mL	**Drawer 5**
Intravenous catheters, 10 of each commonly used sizes (24 ga, 22 ga, 20 ga, 18 ga, 16 ga)[a]	Self-inflating bag (Ambu) with reservoir
Swivel adapters (Portex, Sontex)	Enk Oxygen Flow Modulation set (Cook, Inc.)
No. 3 straight connectors × 2	Jet ventilator
Drawer 3	Stylets; pediatric and adult
Preparation forceps or tongue-grabbing forceps	Tracheal tube exchange catheters with both Luer-Lok and 15-mm OD adapters; sizes (mm OD) 3, 4, 5, 7
Safety glasses	Retrograde catheter with extra guidewire
	Extension cord with converter from Hubble to three-prong plug
	Other equipment to consider: lighted stylets and optical stylets (see text)

[a]Items with outdates.
Cook, Cook Critical Care, Bloomington, IN; *ETT,* endotracheal tube; *F,* French; *ga,* gauge; *ID,* inner diameter; *LMA,* laryngeal mask airway, LMA North America, San Diego, CA; *OD,* outer diameter; *VBM,* VBM Medizintechnik GmbH, Sulz, Germany.
Modified from Department of Pediatric Anesthesiology. The difficult airway cart. Lurie Children's Hospital, Chicago.

to position the child, facilitate airway management, and observe the monitors and the child's vital signs; there should be clear communication about the airway management plan and specific details about maneuvers needed to facilitate the process. Familiarity with difficult airway algorithms and difficult airway management reviews can help the practitioner formulate a reasonable plan and ensure that no viable management options are missed.[172,342,509–518]

Certain principles apply to the care of any child in whom difficulty with airway management is anticipated. In most circumstances, an awake or mildly sedated approach would be the primary management strategy for the anticipated difficult airway if airway concerns were considered in isolation. However, because of a lack of cooperation in children, assisted ventilation during general anesthesia is the preferred technique when abnormal airway anatomy is present and difficulty with patient cooperation

is anticipated; it provides adequate oxygenation while the airway is evaluated for the appropriate approach to tracheal intubation.

Traditionally, spontaneous ventilation under general anesthesia has been the approach of choice.[120,342] If specialized airway management equipment is unavailable, shaping the tracheal tube tip into a 90-degree angle with a stylet (Fig. 12.25), placing the tip behind the epiglottis (or the center of the base of the tongue if the epiglottis is not visible), and then listening for breath sounds with the ear near the proximal end of the tracheal tube or tracking the capnogram often allows the practitioner to "blindly" locate the glottic opening and trachea. Despite the rich history of the "spontaneous ventilation" approach to the difficult airway, there has recently been a shift in practice in favor of paralyzing children with difficult airways with nondepolarizing neuromuscular blocking drugs, particularly with rocuronium because of the fast onset

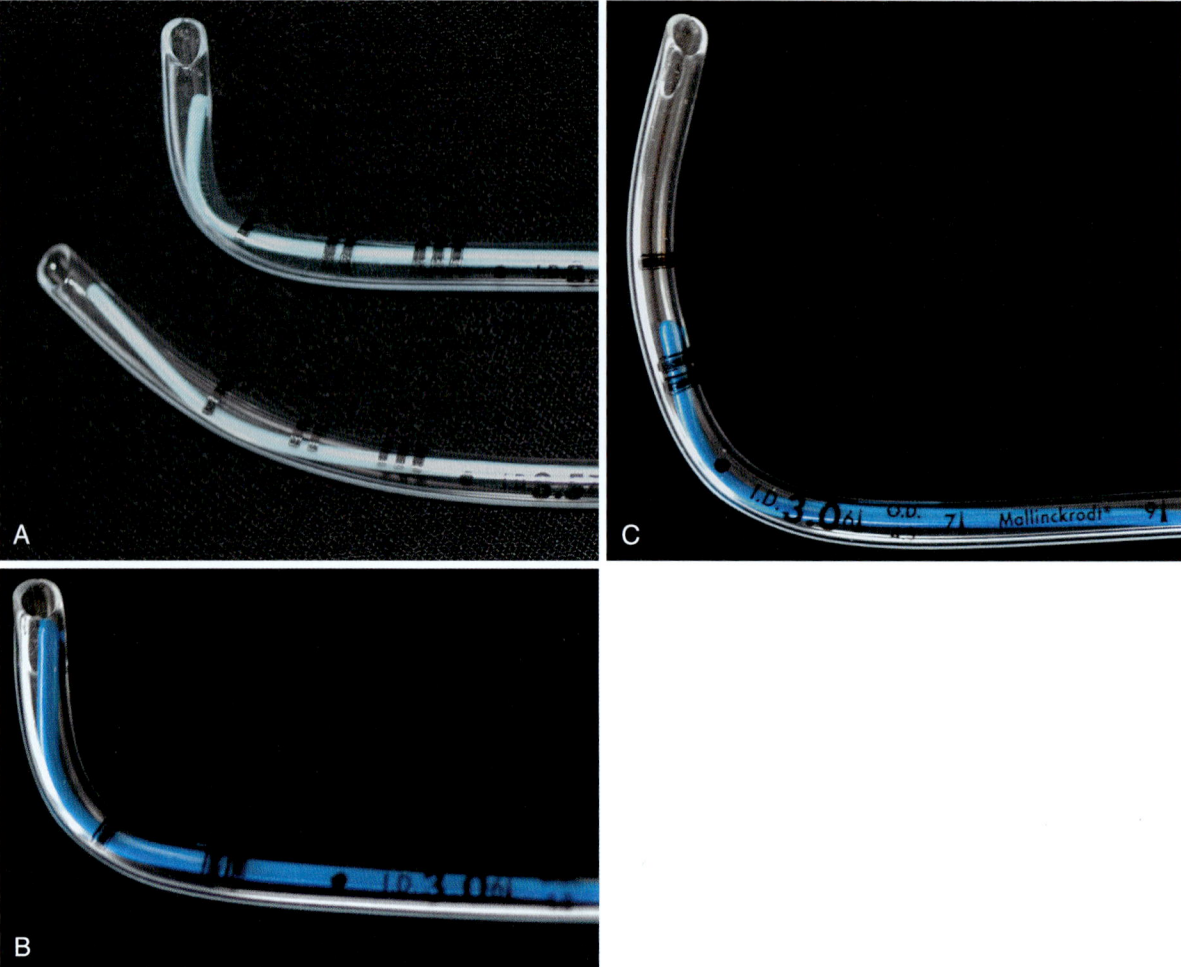

FIGURE 12.25 A stylet placed within an endotracheal tube often facilitates placement. **A,** The "hockey-stick" configuration. **B,** In children with midfacial hypoplasia syndromes, in which the anatomic relation of the base of the tongue to the laryngeal inlet is abnormal, a stylet with a 90-degree bend 1 to 2 centimeters from the tip allows placement of the tracheal tube behind the epiglottis and at the laryngeal inlet. Breath sounds audible at the 15-mm connector confirm appropriate location. **C,** Maintaining the position of the stylet while advancing the tracheal tube frequently allows successful "blind" endotracheal intubation around the base of the tongue even without the use of special airway equipment.

of blockade and availability of sugammadex to reverse the paralysis should an emergency situation arise (see airway registry later). Studies of patients with normal and difficult airways suggest that ventilation may be improved after administering a neuromuscular blocking drug,[125] and there has been a shift in practice with clinicians administering neuromuscular blocking drugs such as rocuronium with induction. The availability of rapid reversal of neuromuscular blockade has further bolstered this practice.[519]

However, there are few reports and no large studies of success in these circumstances; there is one report of reversal of neuromuscular blockade in a preterm 850-gram infant who received 1.2 mg/kg of rocuronium, failed intubation and successful antagonism with 16 mg/kg of sugammadex.[520] There remain rare reports of "cannot intubate cannot oxygenate" after administering neuromuscular blocking drugs in children with difficult airways, making it prudent to consider spontaneous ventilation in some patients (e.g., patients with space occupying lesions, neck radiation, and mucopolysaccharide disorders).

Regardless of the approach chosen when a "can't intubate can't oxygenate" situation occurs, clinicians should administer a neuromuscular blocking drug if not already given to rule out functional obstruction. One study reviewing data from the Pediatric Difficult Intubation (PeDI) registry examined airway management practices in 1289 children with difficult airways.[521] They found that 39% were managed with spontaneous ventilation, 35% controlled ventilation with a neuromuscular blocking drug, and 26% controlled ventilation without a neuromuscular blocking drug. Using propensity score matching to compare groups, spontaneous ventilation was associated with less severe complications than controlled ventilation (OR = 2.07 95% CI, 1.36–3.15; $P = 0.001$). This study suggested that the depth of anesthesia was more important than whether a neuromuscular blocking drug was used because the complication rates of children in the controlled ventilation with and without paralysis were similar.

If the child is able to cooperate while mildly sedated, there are several options for airway management. An opioid-benzodiazepine combination blunts airway reactivity, decreases discomfort, and provides anxiolysis and amnesia. Combination regimens such as midazolam and fentanyl are effective to sedate adolescents and mature preteens[515]; with the dosing guided by clinical parameters including preexisting medical conditions. However, benzodiazepine-opioid sedation may not suffice for a frightened young child because the dose requirement for sedation may exceed that which causes apnea. Alternatively, ketamine, which provides both hypnosis and analgesia, may be used alone or in conjunction with midazolam or with dexmedetomidine.[515,522,523] Ketamine usually preserves adequate spontaneous ventilation and upper airway patency[524] while preventing laryngeal reactions to airway manipulation. Ketamine and midazolam should be slowly titrated to effect to avoid oversedation and apnea.[525,526] Midazolam takes almost 5 minutes to achieve peak electroencephalographic effects, necessitating adequate time between incremental doses (see Fig. 44.7).[527,528] Ketamine is usually titrated in doses of 0.25 to 0.5 mg/kg IV every 2 minutes or by infusion, beginning with a loading dose of 0.5 to 1 mg/kg IV followed by an infusion of 10 to 15 µg/kg per minute.[529,530]

Although psychomimetic emergence reactions commonly occur in adults, these reactions are less common in children, particularly if ketamine is combined with midazolam. Ketamine may increase secretions that enhance airway reactivity and interfere with video-based airway management; antisialogogue administration may mitigate these effects. In addition, the anticholinergic effect of atropine or glycopyrrolate will blunt reflex bradycardia that can occur with airway manipulations. Dexmedetomidine has been administered as the sole sedating agent or combined with reduced doses of other sedatives or opioids for sedation while maintaining spontaneous respirations during fiberoptic intubation in adults and children.[531–541]

The Pediatric Difficult Intubation Registry compared children who were sedated to those who received general anesthesia for airway management.[125] They found no difference in first attempt success of tracheal intubation between the two groups (48.3% vs. 47.9%) and complications were similar. Although 16 of the 58 sedation cases were transitioned to general anesthesia for intubation, none of the children who were sedated failed tracheal intubation. This multicenter research and quality improvement registry[125] was developed to examine the risk factors for a difficult intubation, examine the success rates of various intubation techniques, and assess the complications that occur in children with difficult tracheal intubations. Data from this registry demonstrate that children with difficult airways were often paralyzed for airway management after confirming easy mask ventilation, likely because of concerns to prevent airway reactivity (laryngospasm, bronchospasm, coughing). Anecdotally it has been observed that performing a 5-second jaw[44] thrust in an unparalyzed anesthetized child is a useful test to assess the risk of airway reactivity when the airway is instrumented. Absence of movement, or an increase in breathing rate or heart rate in response to a jaw thrust or squeezing of the trapezius muscle has been used to assess depth of sedation prior to placement of an SGA in adults and children, and may be associated with a reduction in airway reactivity during airway instrumentation.[542–545] The depth of anesthesia, however, needs to be maintained during intubation attempts, particularly if prolonged.

Topical anesthesia may be used in conjunction with sedation or general anesthesia to blunt airway reactivity in those children in whom spontaneous ventilation is preserved.[206] Useful methods for providing topical anesthesia to the airway include (1) nebulized lidocaine (up to 10 mg/kg) [546]; (2) topical application of local anesthetic sprays, jellies, or ointments; (3) trans laryngeal delivery of lidocaine; (4) "spray as you go" with lidocaine[34] injected onto the surface of the larynx and vocal cords through the channel of a flexible bronchoscope usually used for suctioning or administering oxygen; and (5) superior laryngeal nerve block.[547]

Caution is required to avoid delivering a toxic dose of local anesthetic. Maximum doses of the local anesthetic are based on the patient's weight and should be calculated in advance (see Table 40.2). Lidocaine seems to have the best safety profile; we limit our maximum dose to 4 mg/kg.[206] We do not recommend the use of benzocaine (Cetacaine) local anesthetic spray in children weighing less than 40 kg, because it is associated with methemoglobinemia and it is difficult to titrate or limit the administered dose.[120,548–550]

Strategies to maintain oxygenation vary according to the technique (spontaneous respiration vs. paralyzed).[551,552] For infants who are breathing spontaneously, the Oxyscope (Heine Optotechnik, Herrsching, Germany) is a Miller 1 laryngoscope blade with an insufflation channel along its length so that it may be attached to an oxygen source (E-Fig. 12.4).[553–555] Other strategies include the use of a high-flow nasal cannula,[556] insufflation into the hypopharynx via a nasal trumpet or shortened preformed airway (RAE tracheal tube), or intubation through a SGA. For the nonbreathing patient, preoxygenation with 100% oxygen is vital.

Many techniques and devices for managing a difficult airway have been recommended; these are reviewed in detail later. Previous experience in normal airways can render these devices valuable adjuncts in difficult airway management. *If one is unable to secure tracheal intubation, it is important to recognize the limits of one's ability. Do not hesitate to seek assistance from a colleague or request the surgeon to perform a tracheostomy or bronchoscopy. As an alternative, the child can be awakened and referred to a major pediatric center. In an urgent, life-threatening situation, placement of a SGA device or percutaneous cricothyroidotomy can be lifesaving* (see "The Unexpected Difficult Intubation").[337,363,364,557–560]

Cognitive biases may play a role in airway management and knowledge of these thinking patterns may help clinicians select the appropriate choices when things go wrong. Some examples of biases that may occur with airway management include *loss aversion, anchoring*, and *framing*. *Loss aversion* is the idea that we dislike a loss more than we like an equivalent gain, which leads us to make irrational choices. An example would be a patient with a recognized difficult airway and a known history of difficult mask ventilation. A clinician may recognize the need for an awake or sedated approach but because of a lack of familiarity with performing the awake technique and fear of failure and the associated negative perception from peers, they may decide to proceed with inhaled induction. The loss of reputation and negative perception (loss aversion) influenced the clinician to make an inappropriate choice for the patient. *Anchoring* occurs when a starting point influences or biases subsequent decisions; an example would be a patient who is easy to mask ventilate after induction of anesthesia but subsequently becomes impossible to ventilate. A clinician may fixate on the fact that ventilation was easy before and continue to try interventions to improve ventilation and delay definitive treatment such as a surgical airway because of anchoring to the previous condition. The *cognitive frame* of the clinician plays a critical role in their next steps and framing has been shown to influence choices in many situations. A lay example is labeling of food as 90% fat-free versus 10% fat. Though both labels communicate the same information, the former is more desirable, and consumers choose that option more often. In the patient described earlier who went from being easy to mask ventilate to becoming impossible to ventilate, two thinking patterns are common in the clinician's mind. One frame could be *"This is very bad, this patient may need a surgical airway, I will be sued."* Another frame could be *"This patient needs a surgical airway, this will be lifesaving."* Clearly the latter frame results in the most favorable action, whereas the former may lead to inaction or delays.[561]

Documentation

Documentation of the difficult airway and its management is essential to provide useful information for the next time the child requires sedation or anesthesia. A note in the anesthesia record should clearly indicate:

1. Whether mask ventilation was attempted, and if so, whether there was any difficulty.
2. Special maneuvers that were required for successful mask ventilation.
3. Special maneuvers that were not helpful with mask ventilation.
4. Any difficulty with tracheal intubation.
5. Special techniques that were required for successful intubation.
6. Special techniques that were not helpful for intubation.
7. Grade of the laryngoscopic view of laryngeal structures during direct laryngoscopy (see Fig. 12.14).

In addition to discussion with the family and the child (when age appropriate), a letter should be given to the family and child outlining the difficulties with the airway, describing how the airway was managed, and referring them to the MedicAlert Foundation registry (https://www.medicalert.org/). This should be copied and circulated to the medical record and to the MedicAlert registry. In the United States, the MedicAlert registry for difficult airway/difficult intubation can be reached by telephone at 1-800-432-5378; similar registries are also being formed internationally. The MedicAlert registration form asks for clinical details about the type of airway difficulty, as well as which maneuvers were successful in management and those which were not. Any practitioner who provides airway management to the registered patient can update this information at any time. Although scoring systems used in adults[114–118] have not been thoroughly investigated in all age groups,[119,122,124] it is useful to describe in detail the view of the larynx that was achieved and how it was achieved (e.g., blade type, size, external laryngeal manipulation, SGA, video laryngoscope, etc.).

The Unexpected Difficult Intubation

With careful preoperative evaluation and planning, the unexpected pediatric difficult airway should be a rare occurrence. However, the practitioner should always be prepared for this potentially life-threatening event. Because the unexpected difficult airway occurs after the anesthesia (plan A) has been initiated, many of the management decisions required for the anticipated difficult airway have already been made. Of primary importance is maintaining adequate oxygenation while a definitive course of action is pursued (i.e., plan B, plan C, and so on).

The American Society of Anesthesiologists published updated practice guidelines for the management of the difficult airway that included the pediatric difficult airway (Fig. 12.26).[342] A 15-member international task force updated the existing guidelines emphasizing the importance of delivering oxygen during airway management, limiting the number of attempts at tracheal intubation, and paying attention to human factors. A new pediatric infographic accompanies the guidelines and begins with a time out before airway management to identify roles, including someone available to help if assistance is needed. During the time out, clinicians should consider whether to have extracorporeal membrane oxygenation (ECMO) available or a surgeon to perform invasive access. The infographic diverges after induction of anesthesia into three sections depending on whether mask ventilation is easy, marginal, or impossible. Maintaining adequate anesthetic depth and continuously providing passive oxygenation is highlighted throughout the airway management. In patients with easy ventilation, the task force suggests a maximum of four attempts using an

SGA, video laryngoscope, or flexible intubation scope. When oxygenation is marginal or impossible, the infographic directs the clinician to make their best attempts to oxygenate using a face mask or an SGA, or attempt at tracheal intubation. If attempts fail and ventilation is marginal, the patient should be awakened; however, advanced techniques such as rigid bronchoscopy, invasive airway, or ECMO should be considered if ventilation is impossible. The infographic ends with a debrief at the end of airway management to discuss lessons learned and review opportunities for improvement.

A reasonable pediatric decision tree, from the difficult airway algorithm of the American Society of Anesthesiologists (ASA), is presented in Fig. 12.26. An important difference between infants and adults should be noted in this scenario. Because infants have an increased metabolic rate and decreased functional residual capacity, the time interval between the loss of the airway and resultant hypoxemia with the associated potential secondary neurologic injury is diminished compared with adults.[76,77,562] In a mathematical model, the approximate time interval from an FiO_2 of 90% to 0% oxygen saturation is 4 minutes in a 10-kilogram child, whereas the same interval in a healthy 70-kilogram adult is almost 10 minutes.[563,564] Clinical data from premature infants, term infants, and children validated these models.[551,565–567] Once positive-pressure ventilation with oxygen has ceased, tracheal intubation should be performed as quickly and efficiently as possible. The editors recommend completing intubation in 15 seconds, which would prevent most desaturations, even in premature infants.

The Pediatric Difficult Airway Registry demonstrated that more than two direct laryngoscopy attempts in children with difficult tracheal intubation was associated with a high failure rate and an increased incidence of severe complications.[125] These findings suggest that the following strategies should be considered: (1) minimize the number of direct laryngoscopy attempts and transition to an indirect technique (video laryngoscope/fiberoptic bronchoscope) when direct laryngoscopy fails, and (2) consider a means for passive oxygenation of the lungs during tracheal intubation attempts such as high-flow nasal cannula and the modified nasal trumpet (Video 12.10).[517] A similar registry of pediatric intensive care units confirmed the association between multiple tracheal intubation attempts and associated adverse events.[218]

The use of the SGA is often a key initial step for safe management of the difficult airway. The pediatric airway guidelines published by the Difficult Airway Society/Association of Paediatric Anaesthetists of Great Britain and Ireland (APAGBI) suggest the use of an SGA, if feasible, when failed tracheal intubation occurs in the pediatric difficult airway population.[516,568] A retrospective study that examined the elective use of SGAs as the primary airway management in children with difficult airways concluded that they could be effectively used.[345] In that study, children received general anesthesia at a pediatric institution; 459 of these patients (0.6%) were reported to have a difficult airway (defined as either a history of a difficult direct laryngoscopy, a history of difficult mask ventilation, or both) and 109 of those patients received general anesthesia with an SGA for primary management with a success rate of 96% (4 patients required an alternative airway).[345]

Extubation of the Child With the Difficult Airway

Preparation for extubation begins shortly after the airway is secured. Equipment used to secure the airway should be rechecked, quickly returned to functional status, and then left in the operating room until successful safe extubation. Children who had

Difficult Airway Infographic: Pediatric Patients

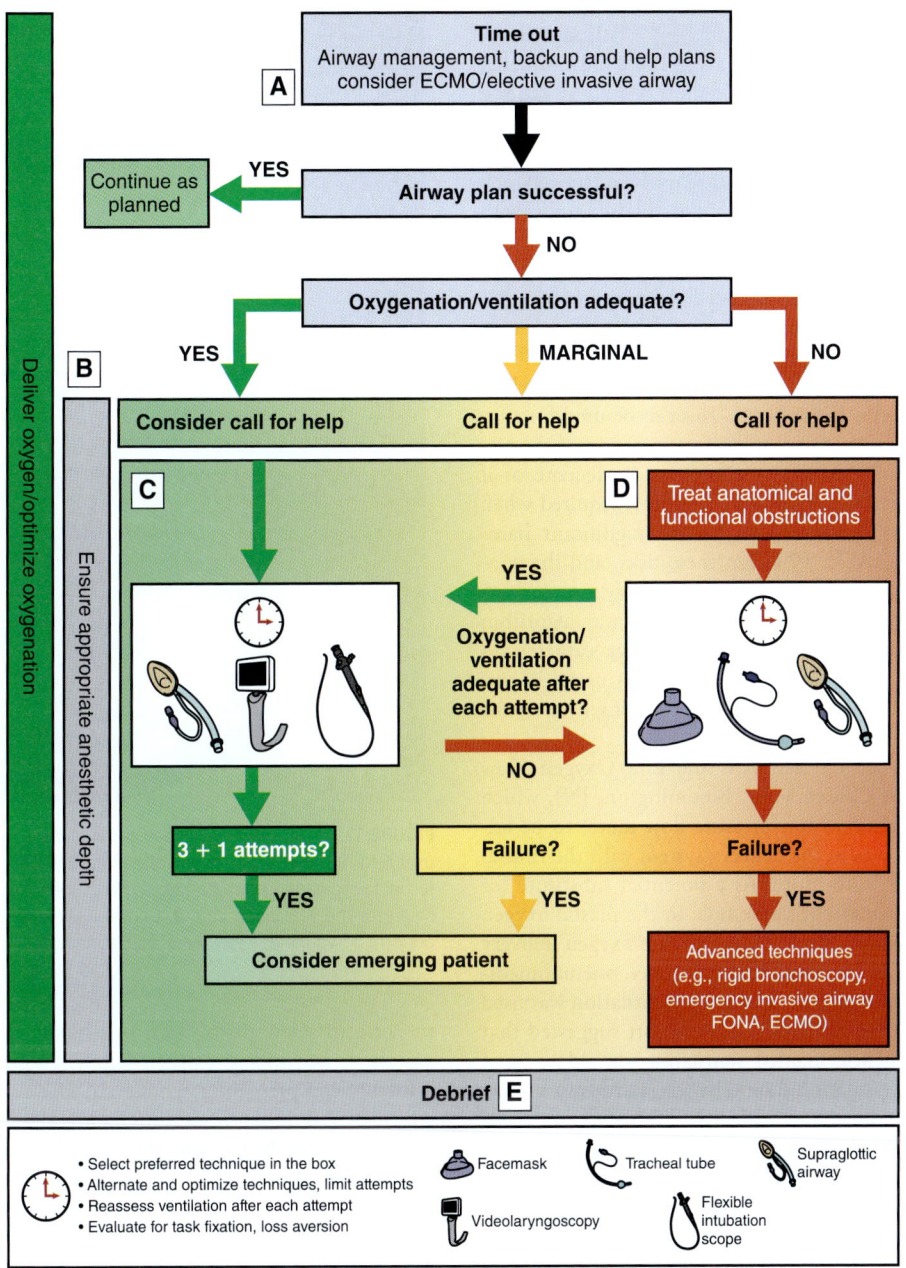

FIGURE 12.26 Difficult airway infographic: Pediatric patient example. **A,** Time Out for identification of the airway management plan. A team-based approach with identification of the following is preferred: the primary airway manager and backup manager and role assignment, the primary equipment and the backup equipment, and the person(s) available to help. Contact an ECMO team/otolaryngologic surgeon if noninvasive airway management is likely to fail (e.g., congenital high airway obstruction, airway tumor, etc.). **B, Color scheme.** The colors represent the ability to oxygenate/ventilate: *green,* easy oxygenation/ventilation; *yellow,* difficult or marginal oxygenation/ventilation; and *red,* impossible oxygenation/ventilation. Reassess oxygenation/ventilation after each attempt and move to the appropriate box based on the results of the oxygenation/ventilation check. **C, Nonemergency pathway** (oxygenation/ventilation adequate for an intubation known or anticipated to be challenging): deliver oxygen throughout airway management; attempt airway management with the technique/device most familiar to the primary airway manager; select from the following devices: supraglottic airway, video laryngoscopy, flexible bronchoscopy, or a combination of these devices (e.g., flexible bronchoscopic intubation through the supraglottic airway); other techniques (e.g., lighted stylets or rigid stylets may be used at the discretion of the clinician); optimize and alternate devices as needed; reassess ventilation after each attempt; limit direct laryngoscopy attempts (e.g., one attempt) with consideration of standard blade video laryngoscopy in lieu of direct laryngoscopy; limit total attempts (insertion of the intubating device until its removal) by the primary airway manager (e.g., three attempts) and one additional attempt by the secondary airway manager; after four attempts, consider emerging the patient and reversing anesthetic drugs if feasible. Clinicians may make further attempts if the risks and benefits to the patient favor continued attempts. **D, Marginal/emergency pathway** (poor or no oxygenation/ventilation for an intubation known or anticipated to be challenging): treat functional (e.g., airway reflexes with drugs) and anatomical (mechanical) obstruction; attempt to improve ventilation with facemask, tracheal intubation, and supraglottic airway as appropriate; and if all options fail, consider emerging the patient or using advanced invasive techniques. **E, Consider a team debrief after all difficult airway encounters:** identify processes that worked well and opportunities for system improvement and provide emotional support to members of the team, particularly when there is patient morbidity or mortality. (Developed in collaboration with the Society for Pediatric Anesthesia and the Pediatric Difficult Intubation Collaborative: John E. Fiadjoe, Thomas Engelhardt, Nicola Disma, Narasimhan Jagannathan, Britta S. von Ungern-Sternberg, and Pete G. Kovatsis.) FONA, front of neck airway.

prolonged attempts at intubation or who will have procedures that may lead to airway edema may benefit from IV dexamethasone (0.5 to 1 mg/kg, up to 20 mg).[296,297,299–301] If significant airway edema is suspected, consider leaving the child intubated postoperatively until it resolves. The child must be fully awake and have full return of strength and adequate ventilatory effort before extubation is attempted.

A Cook airway exchange catheter with Rapi-Fit adapter (Cook Critical Care, Bloomington, IN) is a hollow plastic guide with holes on its distal end so as to administer oxygen[569] that may be useful as a bridge to extubation because the adapter on its proximal end allows the placement of either a Luer-Lok connector for connection to a jet ventilator or a 15-millimeter adapter for connection to a standard anesthesia ventilating system (E-Fig. 12.5)[569–574] It is available in a variety of sizes to allow the exchange of tracheal tubes with 3.0-millimeter ID or larger. This can be used for oxygenation and ventilation and as a guide to reinsertion of the tracheal tube if the child's ventilatory efforts are inadequate or if airway obstruction occurs.[575] However, caution is required when using this device for jet ventilation, because significant barotrauma has been reported.[576–578] Given these risks, and the concern that placing an exchange catheter too deeply can cause a pneumothorax, the most recent ASA difficult airway algorithm recommended against the use of airway exchange catheters in children[342]; we still find airway exchange catheters useful in certain situations being cautious about the depth of insertion of the exchange catheter.[579,580]

An alternative to jet ventilation is the Enk Oxygen Flow Modulation set (Cook Critical Care, Bloomington, IN), which allows flow from a standard low-pressure flow meter to be adjusted by occluding holes in the delivery system with the thumb and forefinger (E-Fig. 12.6, Top). As a potential substitute for the Enk device, one could cut a side hole in the plastic oxygen delivery tubing to create a similar low-pressure oxygen delivery system (see E-Fig. 12.6, Bottom). Pneumothorax, pneumomediastinum, and deaths have occurred when jet ventilation was used with an airway exchange catheter.[581] One report suggested that only insufflation or gentle manual ventilation should be used initially and that jet ventilation should be reserved for situations in which these techniques are ineffective. These authors also recommended that the optimal management was reintubation.[569] Ventilation through small bore catheters may be safer with a novel device called the Ventrain.[582,583] With this device the expiration of gases through small bore catheters is increased by a jet flow generated suction theoretically providing a higher margin of safety than traditional jet ventilators.[584–586] If the child remains intubated for a prolonged period of time after surgery, it is advisable to return the child to the operating room for extubation. A surgeon who is prepared to perform rigid bronchoscopy and tracheostomy and an anesthesiologist who is familiar with the techniques used for the previously successful airway management should be in attendance.

SPECIAL TECHNIQUES FOR VENTILATION

Multi-Handed Mask Ventilation Techniques

Multi-handed mask ventilation techniques can provide an effective temporizing measure until the airway is secured or the child is awakened. One person uses both hands to maintain an adequate mask fit, and a second person compresses the reservoir bag (Fig. 12.27). This can also be accomplished by having a single provider use two hands on the mask while the anesthesia ventilator is activated.[587] Occasionally, a second person is required

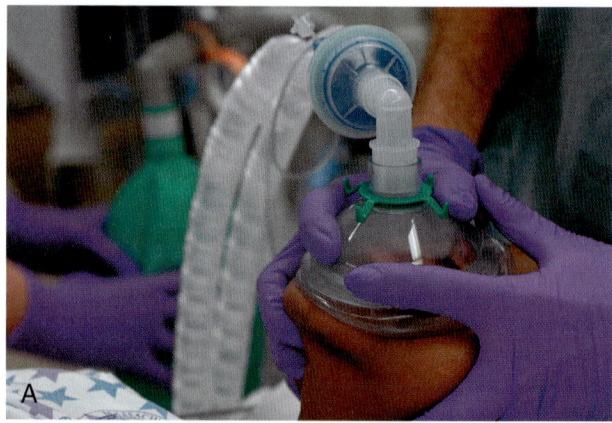
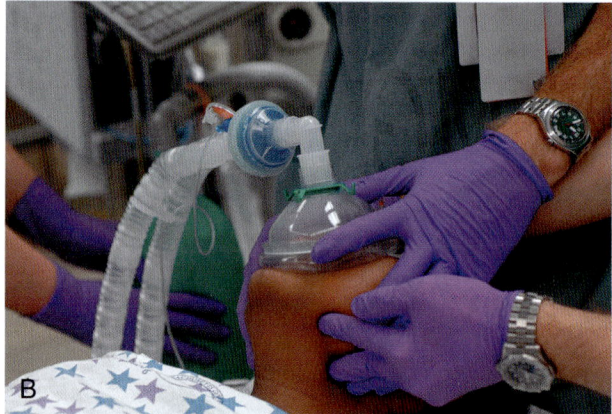

FIGURE 12.27 **A,** The two-handed technique for mask ventilation may be useful to improve mask fit and therefore ventilation when the traditional technique is inadequate. One person holds the mask while a second person squeezes the ventilation bag. **B,** Occasionally, a third person is required to perform a two-handed jaw thrust (see text for details).

to perform a jaw thrust with one hand while compressing the anesthesia bag with the other. Rarely, a third person may be required to compress the reservoir bag with two hands (to generate a greater peak inflation pressure) while the first person holds the mask with two hands and the second person performs a two-handed jaw thrust.[587,588]

Supraglottic Airways

The SGA has revolutionized difficult airway management in children. Numerous case reports and extensive clinical experience attest to the value of the SGA for establishing an airway when both ventilation and intubation are extremely difficult or impossible.[511,589–592] The SGA has been described as a tool for use in both the nonemergency pathway (*cannot intubate, can ventilate*) and the emergency pathway (*cannot intubate, cannot ventilate*) of the ASA difficult airway algorithm.[511,580] The use of multiple SGA devices has been described in the awake child (e.g., SGA insertion in awake infants with Pierre Robin syndrome)[593–596] (Video 12.11) and in the anesthetized child with a known or suspected difficult airway. It can be used as the definitive airway in some circumstances, as a conduit for intubation, or as a temporizing airway while other options are pursued (e.g., a surgical airway). There are now many SGA devices reported to be useful in the management of the child with a difficult airway (see earlier discussion), but comparative studies in pediatrics are lacking.[597,598]

Percutaneous Needle Cricothyroidotomy

The American Heart Association changed its recommendations for emergency airway management to a percutaneous needle cricothyroidotomy over a surgical cricothyroidotomy in 1992 because it was believed that the former entails less risk of injury to vital structures such as the carotid arteries or jugular veins, particularly in the hands of nonsurgical trained practitioners. In addition, most practitioners can more rapidly perform a percutaneous procedure. However, the cricothyroid membrane has a relatively small width in infants and children younger than 5 years of age. Attempts at cricothyroidotomy may readily damage cricoid and thyroid cartilages, resulting in laryngeal stenosis and permanent damage to the speech mechanism. Therefore, this procedure should be reserved for use only under emergency circumstances.[559,599,600] More studies are needed but at this time, needle cricothyroidotomy is still the technique of choice in the "cannot intubate, cannot oxygenate" situation in infants (APAGBI Pediatric Airway Guidelines [see discussion later] available from https://www.apagbi.org.uk/guidelines).

Because percutaneous needle cricothyroidotomy is rarely used in infants and children, it is recommended that experience be gained with patient simulators or in animal models, because success in the hands of the inexperienced is not assured.[560,600–604] A schema of this procedure is presented in Fig. 12.28. A commercial product called the Jet Ventilation Catheter (VBM Medizintechnik GmbH) is available in three sizes: 16, 14, and 13 Fr gauge. It consists of a slightly curved puncture needle within a Teflon, kink-resistant cannula nearly identical to an IV catheter (Fig. 12.29A). This cannula has two lateral eyes at its distal end and a combined Luer-Lok and 15-millimeter adapter at its proximal end (see Fig. 12.29B). It also has a fixation flange and foam neck tape to secure the airway.

Percutaneous needle cricothyroidotomy provides only a means for oxygen insufflation and does not reliably provide adequate ventilation. In the spontaneously breathing patient, simple delivery of intratracheal oxygen (1 to 2 L/minute) may be sufficient in the short term, because hypercarbia is generally well tolerated by healthy children.[559,605,606] A number of children with arterial carbon dioxide values well above 150 mm Hg have survived neurologically intact when adequate oxygenation was maintained.[606] Therefore, simple oxygenation without attempts at ventilation may be all that is required to sustain life (Fig. 12.30). For the child without respiratory effort, there is a need to provide ventilation in addition to oxygenation. An Ambu bag with the pop-off disabled can provide limited ventilation through a percutaneous catheter, but these devices will be ineffective at standard pop-off pressures.[559,607] Extremely high ventilating pressures are required, but midtracheal pressures are notably less (10 to 16 cm H_2O).[560] A percutaneous cricothyroidotomy catheter can also be used with a jet ventilation system. Jet ventilation via a catheter passed through a narrow glottic opening has also been described.[608–612]

If upper airway obstruction is present (e.g., after multiple unsuccessful attempts at rigid laryngoscopy), there will be a limited pathway for the egress of air and oxygen, and barotrauma may result from insufflation of oxygen or attempts at ventilation. Very serious morbidity and mortality may result from massive subcutaneous emphysema or tension pneumothorax.[581,613,614] Therefore, jet ventilation must be used with extreme caution in infants and children.[615]

Another IV catheter–type emergency airway device is the Emergency Transtracheal Airway Catheter (Cook Critical Care), which consists of a 6 Fr reinforced catheter that is advanced over

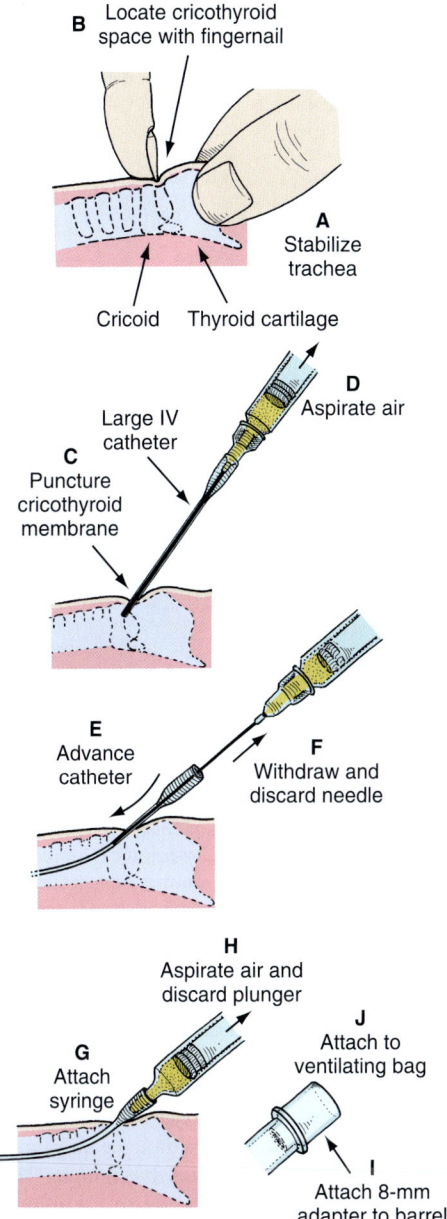

FIGURE 12.28 Percutaneous cricothyroidotomy. Extend the head in the midline with a rolled towel or folded sheet beneath the shoulders. **A,** Standing to the left of the child, stabilize the trachea with the right hand. **B,** The cricothyroid membrane is located with the index fingertip of the left hand between the thyroid and cricoid cartilages. This space is so narrow (1 mm) in an infant that only a fingernail can discern it. The trachea is then stabilized between the middle finger and thumb of the left hand while the fingernail of the index finger marks the cricothyroid membrane. **C,** A large intravenous (IV) catheter (12- to 14-gauge) is then inserted through the cricothyroid membrane, and air is aspirated **(D).** The catheter is advanced into the trachea through the membrane, and the needle is discarded; an intraluminal position is reconfirmed by attaching a 3-mL syringe **(E)** and aspirating for air **(F).** A 3-mm adapter from a pediatric endotracheal tube can be attached to any intravenous catheter **(G).** Ventilation is accomplished by attaching to a breathing circuit with a standard 22-mm connector **(H).** An alternative would be to leave the barrel of the 3-mL syringe attached to the IV catheter, insert an 8-mm endotracheal tube adapter to the syringe barrel **(I),** and then attach to a ventilating system with a standard 22-mm adapter **(J).** (From Coté CJ, Eavey RD, Todres ID, Jones DE. Cricothyroid membrane puncture: oxygenation and ventilation in a dog model using an intravenous catheter. *Crit Care Med.* 1988;16:615-619.)

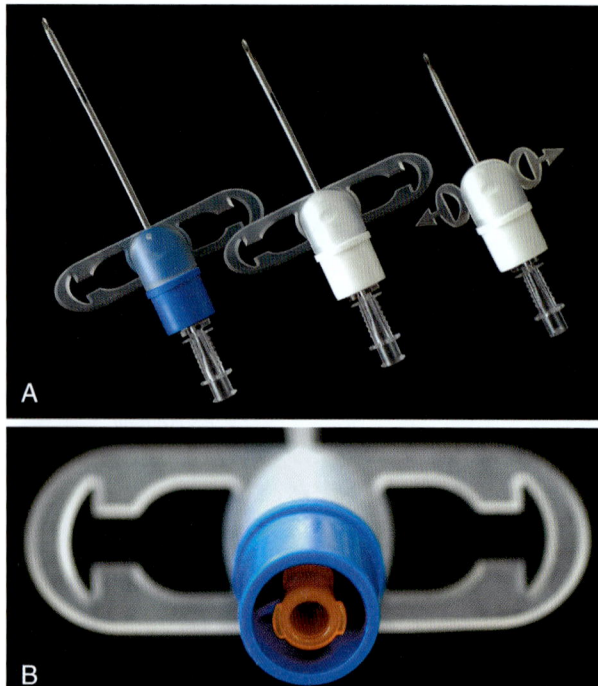

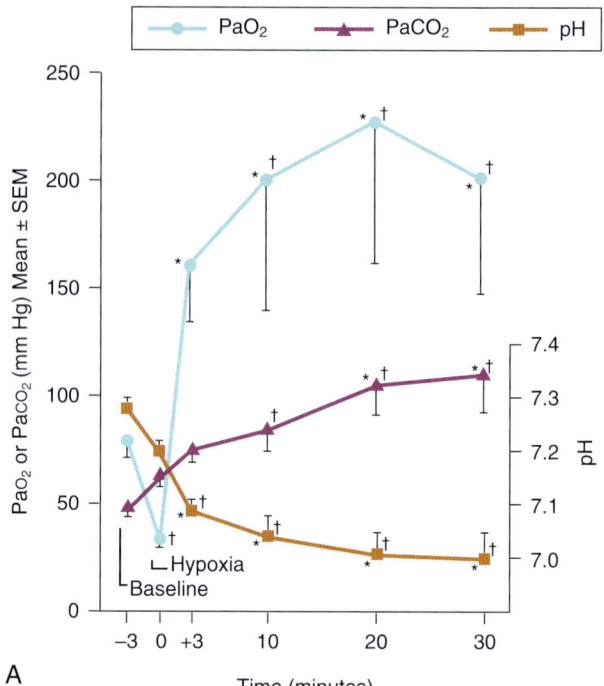

FIGURE 12.29 A, The Jet Ventilation Catheter (VBM Medizintechnik GmbH, Sulz, Germany) is available in three sizes: From left to right: 13 gauge (adult), 14 gauge (child), and 16 gauge (infant). It consists of a slightly curved puncture needle within a Teflon, kink-resistant cannula. The procedure for insertion is similar to that described in Fig. 12.28. **B,** This cannula has two lateral eyes at its distal end and a combined Luer-Lok and 15-mm adapter (surrounding the Luer-Lok) at its proximal end, allowing either jet or standard ventilation. It also has a fixation flange and foam neck tape to secure the airway.

a 15-gauge needle, similar to the devices described earlier (see E-Fig. 12.7). Another device is the Enk Oxygen Flow Modulation set (see E-Fig. 12.6). This device was studied with a variety of IV cannulae and the Emergency Transtracheal Airway Catheter. The investigators concluded that the device worked best when all holes on the Enk device were occluded simultaneously, and that minimum flow should never be less than 1 L/minute. They also suggested that initial fresh gas flow be set to 1 L/minute and then adjusted up or down as needed.[616] Another study in a rabbit model suggested a similar low oxygen flow rate.[617] Successful ventilation with uncuffed devices may depend on the patency of the upper airway (i.e., the greater the patency, the less the effectiveness of ventilation in the nonbreathing patient).[618] None of these devices has been examined in controlled trials to confirm efficacy, in part because such events are so rare. Therefore, we recommend training on simulators so that each practitioner can determine what device is best for themself.

Several percutaneous emergency airway devices are available that use a short but large-diameter needle, or a needle, guidewire, and dilator to aid insertion of a percutaneous airway.[559,619–621] The Quicktrach (Rüsch, Duluth, GA) is a device that consists of a tapered 2- or 4-millimeter catheter with a fixation flange for securing with cloth tape. A removable plastic stopper is designed to limit the depth of needle insertion. This device requires several steps: puncture of the skin, aspiration for air, removal of the stopper, removal of the needle/syringe, and attachment to standard 22-millimeter connector. A flexible connector is also provided (E-Fig. 12.8). A rabbit model to simulate infant cricothyroidotomy

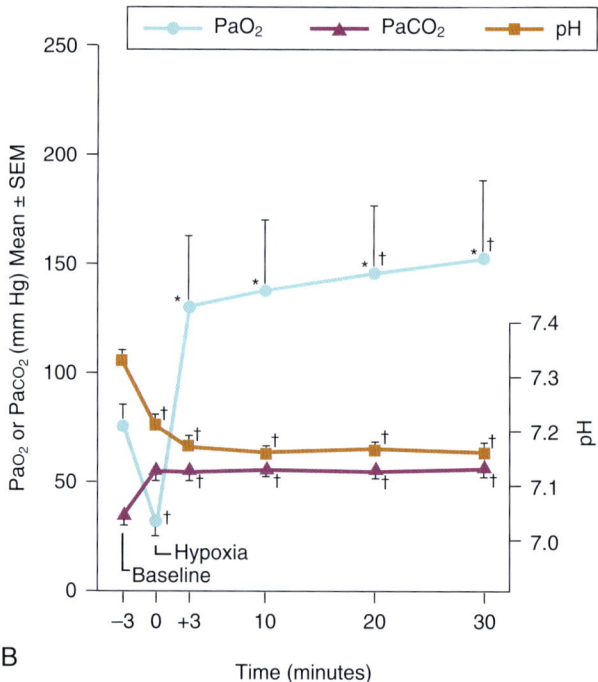

FIGURE 12.30 A, Changes in arterial blood gases and pH are plotted over time for six dogs with spontaneous ventilation; baseline values in room air are plotted at time −3; values after 2 to 3 minutes of hypoxemia as a result of airway obstruction are plotted at time 0. Marked, sustained increases in arterial oxygen tension *(PaO₂)* follow cricothyroid membrane puncture with delivery of only 1.0 L/minute oxygen. **B,** Changes in arterial blood gases and pH are plotted over time for five dogs that were not making spontaneous ventilatory efforts. Both oxygenation and ventilation were achieved with a self-inflating bag attached via a 3.0 mm ID adapter to an IV cannula introduced through the cricothyroid membrane. *PaCO₂,* Carbon dioxide tension; *SEM,* standard error of the mean; *Sig.,* significant difference. (From Coté CJ, Eavey RD, Todres ID, Jones DE. Cricothyroid membrane puncture: oxygenation and ventilation in a dog model using an intravenous catheter. *Crit Care Med.* 1988;16:615-619.)

found success in all attempts, but 2 of 10 attempts resulted in fracture of the cricoid cartilage and 1 resulted in damage to the mucosa of the posterior tracheal wall.[622] Conversely, this device has been shown to allow more rapid establishment of an airway than other devices that use a Seldinger technique[623,624]; a larger, cuffed adult model is available (E-Fig. 12.9).

Other devices that use the Seldinger technique (i.e., needle, guidewire, scalpel incision of the skin, and passage of a dilator and tracheostomy tube) are the Arndt and Melker devices (Cook Critical Care, Bloomington, IN, Bartlett, TN).[625] These devices provide a 3.0-millimeter ID airway that is sufficient for ventilation as well as oxygenation (E-Fig. 12.10). However, the time required to insert such devices may be longer than for simpler devices and may be inappropriate for immediate rapid establishment of an airway.[560,623,624] In contrast, a porcine cadaver study found greater physician comfort with this technique compared with a scalpel technique.[626] These devices are useful for elective percutaneous tracheostomy.[627]

Another device, Pertrach (Engineered Medical Systems, Bartlett, TN), uses a split needle on a syringe to puncture the cricothyroid membrane (E-Fig. 12.11). A skin incision is made, and an introducer with tracheostomy tube (3.0-mm ID) is directed into the trachea, splitting the needle, which is removed. The introducer is then removed, and the airway secured with tracheostomy tape. There are no case reports in the literature to determine the ease or difficulty of insertion in children, but the multiple steps required suggest that it may be a device for elective tracheostomy rather than emergent establishment of a surgical airway.

Another percutaneous tracheostomy device is the Bivona Pedia-Trake kit (Smiths Medical, Minneapolis, MN) (E-Fig. 12.12). A skin incision is made with a scalpel, and a large needle is introduced with a skin dilator, which in theory opens the incision sufficiently to allow passage of an obturator and a 3.0-, 4.0-, or 5.0-millimeter ID tracheostomy tube (with or without cuff). This device appears sufficiently complicated to not be useful in a *"can't intubate, can't ventilate"* emergency; it might be better suited when there is an urgent but not emergent need to establish surgical access to the airway.

Other devices with limited pediatric use[619] are kits designed to place a full-sized tracheostomy tube, such as the Nu-Trake (International Medical Devices, Northridge, CA)[628] and Abelson (Gilbert Surgical Instruments, Bellmawr, NJ) devices. They may potentially cause tracheal or laryngeal injury in small patients because of the relatively large size of the needle; again, little experience in children has been published.[620,621,627]

Supraglottic Airway Versus Percutaneous Needle Cricothyroidotomy and Transtracheal Jet Ventilation

The LMA Classic has proved to be an extremely useful device in airway emergencies. In contrast to percutaneous needle cricothyroidotomy, it is an effective device for ventilation as well as a conduit for intubation.[629] The LMA is easily inserted and requires a relatively limited skill level, as demonstrated in numerous studies, comparing this technique with other airway management skills (e.g., mask ventilation, tracheal intubation). More importantly, in contrast to transtracheal jet ventilation, the complication rate with the LMA Classic is exceedingly low.[630] However, if glottic or subglottic obstruction to ventilation is present, the SGA will be ineffective and a surgical airway with or without transtracheal jet ventilation is still the emergency technique of choice. Since the introduction of the LMA, clinical experience suggests that if glottic or subglottic pathology is not suspected, placing an LMA to establish ventilation may be appropriately attempted as the first step at airway rescue.

Surgical Airway

An emergent surgical airway is viewed by some as an alternative to needle cricothyroidotomy.[560,631] It previously fell under the purview of the surgeon, in particular the pediatric otolaryngologist.[600–602,631,632] However, with training, it can be performed quickly by anesthesiologists.[633,634] A *"can't intubate, can't oxygenate"* situation event in children is extremely rare. Very few practitioners have ever performed a surgical cricothyroidotomy in a child or an adult; there is very little clinical evidence to support any specific surgical versus needle technique. Randomized trials are ethically impossible and case series in children are not available because of underreporting and the rarity of such events. Guidelines are based largely on animal studies and expert opinion. Both needle cricothyroidotomy and the surgical scalpel bougie technique are difficult in infants because the trachea is small and mobile.[631] In nonemergent airway management for children, a tracheostomy is preferred to a cricothyroidotomy because of fewer long-term complications and better results with later decannulation of the airway.[560,635]

Although needle cricothyroidotomy has been recommended for rescue of children by nonsurgeons, several studies have shown that anesthesiologists are very poor at identifying the cricothyroid membrane in adults and children. Clinicians correctly identify the membrane about 30% of the time in children and cannulation is fraught with complications in small children.[636] For this reason an increasing number of clinicians are favoring tracheotomy in small children for the *"can't intubate, can't oxygenate"* situation. One study in a porcine model found that emergency tracheotomy was superior to transtracheal needle techniques using a jet-ventilation catheter and an IV catheter. The needle techniques were successful in 65.6% and 68.8% of attempts, whereas emergency tracheotomy was successful in 97% of attempts.[602] Another study in a porcine model compared transtracheal catheter to tracheotomy. They observed the tracheal lumen from above the access site using a bronchoscope and found a higher success rate with tracheotomy. They observed several problems with the transtracheal catheter approach including kinking of the catheter, compression of the tracheal lumen, and puncture of the posterior tracheal wall.[601] Surgical tracheotomy may be necessary in a *"can't intubate, can't oxygenate"* scenario. We encourage clinicians to become familiar with the equipment necessary to perform the procedure and engage in deliberate practice to develop confidence when this rare situation occurs.[637]

Anterior Commissure Scope and Rigid Ventilating Bronchoscope

Two pieces of equipment used by otolaryngologists that can assist in visualizing the larynx and providing a method of ventilation are the anterior commissure scope and the rigid ventilating bronchoscope. The anterior commissure scope is a rigid, tubular, straight-blade laryngoscope with a light at the tip. The technique to place the anterior commissure scope and the advantages for visualization are similar to those described later for the straight blade used with the retromolar approach.[176]

SPECIAL TECHNIQUES FOR INTUBATION
Rigid Laryngoscopy

The rigid laryngoscope is the most familiar and most universally available piece of airway equipment; therefore, it is critical for the practitioner to become familiar with its use and to know a variety of techniques. Some suggestions are reviewed here. It is reasonable to take a second look with the rigid laryngoscope after an unexpected failed intubation; however, a good rule is to always change something about the approach that may improve visualization. In the past, awake rigid intubation was the traditional approach to the problematic neonatal airway, but this approach should be used only in an extreme emergency or when IV access is not available.[196–198] Some anatomic features are unfavorable for success with the rigid laryngoscope, regardless of technique. Repeated unsuccessful attempts should be avoided because this can lead to airway trauma and edema. Because infants and children already have smaller airway structures, they are uniquely susceptible to a rapid progression from "*can't intubate,* can't *oxygenate*" to the "*can't intubate, can't ventilate*" scenario. Whether the child has a normal or an abnormal airway, it is essential to ensure correct positioning and to use age-appropriate equipment. The following maneuvers have been found to be helpful in achieving successful intubation of the child with a difficult airway.

Optimal External Laryngeal Manipulation

Pressure can be applied externally to the larynx during the intubation to maximize visualization of the larynx.[638] Optimal external laryngeal manipulation (OELM) is particularly helpful for children with immobile or shortened necks and for infants. Either an assistant or the laryngoscopist can perform external manipulation. When the laryngoscopist performs the maneuver, the assistant either can pass the tracheal tube into the glottis while the laryngoscopist maintains the external pressure or external pressure can be assumed by the assistant to allow the laryngoscopist to pass the tracheal tube.[639] Optimal external laryngeal manipulation may also be used in conjunction with other, more advanced airway devices.[638,640,641]

Intubation Guides

Intubation guides include plastic-coated, flexible metal stylets and the gum elastic bougie. These can be used for blind placement of the tracheal tube under the epiglottis. A flexible stylet is placed inside the tracheal tube and preformed to shape the tracheal tube tip to one that will optimize intubation success (see Fig. 12.25). A hockey-stick configuration is frequently useful, particularly if only the epiglottis or the most posterior portion of the glottis can be visualized. The gum elastic bougie has a preformed, angled tip. It is placed alone and then the tracheal tube is threaded over it and into the trachea (E-Fig. 12.13). When the bougie is successfully placed in the trachea, one can detect the subtle "bumpy" feel of the bougie making contact with the anterior tracheal rings. This device may also be used to facilitate intubation through an SGA or as an adjunct to other airway devices.[642–645]

Dental Mirror

The authors of one report used a short-handled dental mirror (no. 3, Storz Instrument Company, Manchester, England) to assist in the indirect visualization of the larynx of a 10-week-old infant. Laryngoscopy was impossible with a size 1 Miller blade. The infant was returned to spontaneous ventilation, a size 1 Macintosh blade was used to expose the pharynx, and the mirror was used to visualize the larynx. A styleted tracheal tube was then passed into the glottis under indirect vision.[646]

Retromolar, Paraglossal, or Lateral Approach Using a Straight Blade

Use of a straight blade in a retromolar approach may allow glottic visualization when the classic rigid intubation technique fails,

particularly if the difficulty is secondary to a large tongue or small mandible (Fig. 12.31).[176,640,643,647–651] With the child's head turned slightly to the left, a size 1 Miller blade is introduced into the extreme right side of the mouth. It is advanced in the space between the tongue and the lateral pharyngeal wall; the tongue is swept completely to the left and is essentially bypassed. It is very helpful to have an assistant pull back the right corner of the mouth with a small retractor (e.g., Senn retractor) to increase the space for tracheal tube placement. The blade is advanced while staying to the right, overlying the bicuspids and lateral incisors until the epiglottis or the glottis is visualized. When the epiglottis comes in view, it is lifted with the tip of the Miller blade to expose the glottic aperture. In contrast to possibly dislodging the central maxillary incisors when the laryngoscope blade applies excessive and direct pressure on those teeth, similar pressure on the bicuspids and lateral incisors cannot dislodge them because these teeth have either two roots or their roots are deeper than the central incisors (see E-Fig. 12.2); the bicuspids and lateral incisors are extracted only by a rotational force and not by direct pressure.

At this juncture in the laryngoscopy, the proximal end of the blade may be moved toward the midline of the mouth to increase room to insert the tracheal tube into the mouth (the cheek can be retracted in lieu of moving the blade) and manipulation, although care must be taken to avoid applying pressure on the central incisors of the maxilla lest the teeth are loosened or dislodged. Pressure on the maxillary incisors can be avoided by the laryngoscopist directing the axis of the handle of the laryngoscope toward the junction of the ceiling and the wall opposite the operator rather than flexing the wrist joint to expose the glottic aperture. If the glottis is not visualized, the head can be rotated farther to the left and the blade can be kept lateral to improve visualization. The tracheal tube should be styleted and formed into a 90-degree bend configuration to assist in placement (see Fig.12.25), particularly if the view of the glottis is only partial. A shorter-length blade (usually a size 1 Miller, even in older children) than that used in the traditional midline approach is chosen because the distance to the glottis with this method is greatly shortened.

Several mechanisms are responsible for the improved view of the glottis with the retromolar approach to laryngoscopy. First, there is a reduced need for soft tissue displacement and compression because the lateral placement of the blade bypasses the tongue. This approach to an improved view of the glottic opening is particularly useful for children with micrognathia.[640,643,648,650,651] In such children, the space available to displace the tongue is reduced, compared with the traditional midline approach to rigid laryngoscopy. Second, there is an improved line of visualization because the incisors and maxillary structures are bypassed by lateral blade placement and by shifting the head to the left. Third, the use of a straight blade avoids the possible intrusion of a curved blade into the line of sight.[176,647–649] Finally, both the angle and the distance from the insertion of the straight blade at the right commissure of the mouth are reduced, facilitating an easier view of the glottic opening, particularly during a difficult intubation, compared with inserting the blade in the midline.

Flexible Laryngoscopy/Flexible Intubation Scope

An advantage of using a flexible intubation bronchoscope for intubation of the child with a difficult airway is that it does not require extensive head or neck manipulation and is therefore useful in children who have cervical inflexibility (e.g., Klippel-Feil syndrome) or cervical instability (e.g., Down syndrome, achondroplastic dwarfism, trauma) (Videos 12.12 and 12.13). The

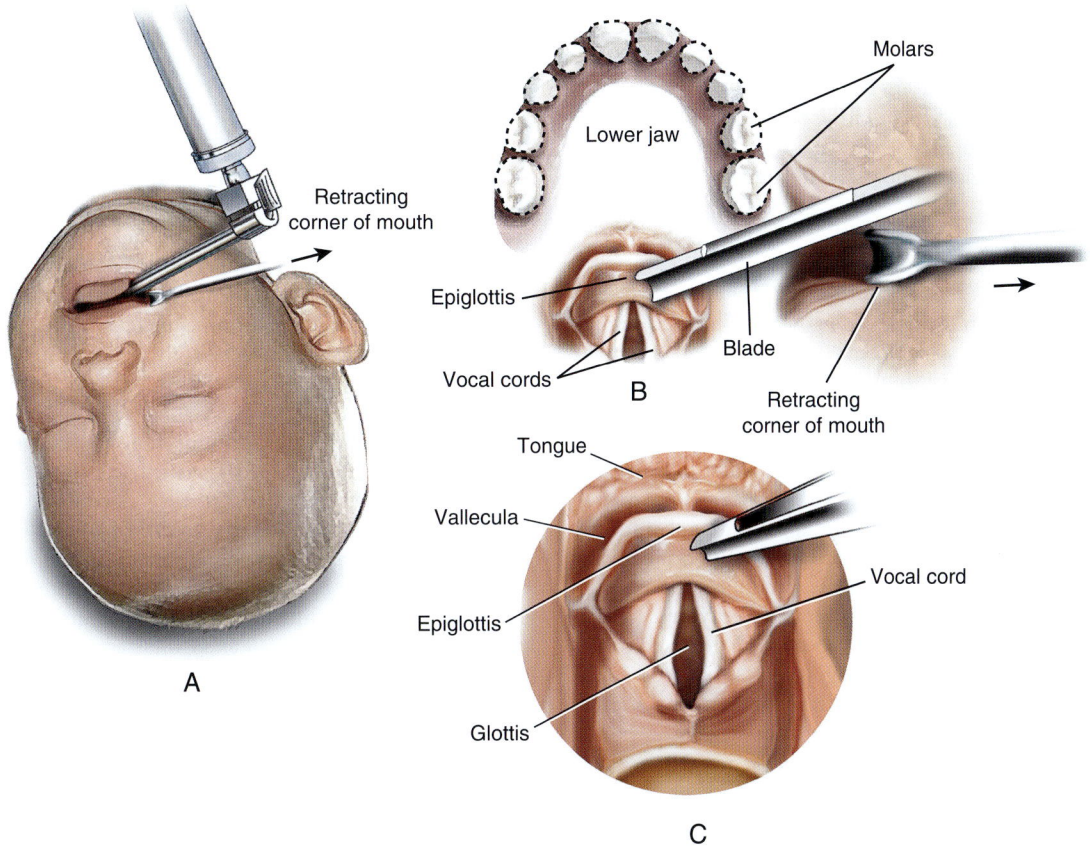

Molars

Lower jaw

Retracting
corner of mouth

Epiglottis

Vocal cords

Blade

B

Retracting
corner of mouth

Tongue

Vallecula

Epiglottis

Vocal cord

Glottis

A

C

FIGURE 12.31 A through **C,** The retromolar, paraglossal, or lateral approach to rigid laryngoscopy using a straight blade. Notice that the child's head is turned to the left and that the laryngoscope blade is inserted over the molars toward the glottic opening (see text for details).

technique is also versatile because the flexible instrument conforms to a variety of abnormal airways; it is well tolerated by the sedated, spontaneously breathing child.[515,652–654]

Its disadvantage is that the presence of blood or copious secretions may render the camera of the flexible bronchoscope ineffective. In addition, the use of the flexible intubation bronchoscope requires extensive experience and practice in normal airways first. Our experience suggests that each size of available flexible intubation bronchoscope should be used in at least 20 normal airways before attempting to use it in an abnormal airway.[655] Practice with all available sizes of flexible intubation bronchoscopes is important because the manual skills required for each size differ. Also, flexible intubation bronchoscopes are fragile and expensive. Great care must be taken when using and storing flexible intubation bronchoscopes to prevent breakage. They must also be sterilized between uses to maintain the patency of the working channel and clear, bright vision through the scope and to avoid transmission of infection.

Equipment
Flexible intubation bronchoscopes with directable tips are available in various sizes; the smallest, 2.2 millimeters in diameter (Olympus LFP; Olympus, Tokyo), can fit through a 2.5-millimeter ID tracheal tube with or without the 15-millimeter adapter removed. However, unlike most of the larger flexible intubation bronchoscopes, this scope has no working channel for suctioning or administration of oxygen or topical anesthesia. Flexible intubation

bronchoscopes with the light source incorporated into the body of the scope increases ease of portability, making its use both outside and inside the operating room simpler and more convenient.

Ancillary Equipment
Endoscopy masks can be used to provide oxygen to the spontaneously breathing child and to ventilate the paralyzed child. The Frei endoscopy mask (VBM Medizintechnik GmbH [E-Fig. 12.14]) and the Patil-Syracuse endoscopy mask (Anesthesia Associates, San Marcos, CA) are commercially available.[656,657] Patil-Syracuse masks are available in a child size but are too large for most children younger than age 4 years.[120] The Frei mask allows the flexible intubation bronchoscope to be placed in a central position, overlying the nose and mouth, which is more favorable for tracheal intubation. The clear membrane with the hole for the bronchoscope can be rotated to allow either oral or nasal approaches. Alternatively, a disposable facemask can be combined with a bronchoscopic swivel adapter.[658] The flexible intubation bronchoscope can then be passed through the diaphragm of the adapter while ventilation is maintained via the anesthesia circuit. There are two types of commercially available adapters. One type attaches directly to an anesthesia mask. The other type is designed to attach to the tracheal tube and can be modified to fit on the anesthesia mask using a 15- to 22-millimeter adapter.

Commercial oral airways designed for use in bronchoscopy are available for pediatric patients (International Medical Development Inc., Huntsville, UT); however, there are only three sizes (infant, child, and adult), and no studies have evaluated their usefulness in assisting flexible laryngoscopy/bronchoscopy in children. Guedel airways can also be modified for use as oral intubation guides.[658] A strip is cut from the convex surface of the airway to create a channel for placement of the flexible intubation bronchoscope. This modified airway may be used to maintain a midline approach to the glottis; however, it is ineffective as a bite block.

Direct Technique

The optimal position of the child for flexible bronchoscopy is different from the position for rigid laryngoscopy. The head should be flat on the table and slightly extended at the atlantooccipital joint to prevent the epiglottis from obstructing a view of the glottic opening.[659] If an oral approach is selected, it is vital that the flexible intubation bronchoscope pass in the midline. A nasal approach may make midline placement simpler and avoids the risk of the child biting the flexible intubation bronchoscope or tracheal tube. One useful technique is to apply a topical vasoconstrictor (e.g., oxymetazoline) to the naris, place a lubricated nasal trumpet into the naris, and then insert a 15-millimeter connector from a tracheal tube into the nasal trumpet (see Video 12.10). This allows oxygen and an inhalation agent to be delivered to the child while performing flexible laryngoscopy (see Videos 12.12 and 12.13). However, the oral approach offers several advantages over the nasal approach, including avoidance of shearing adenoidal tissue and nasal bleeding. If nasal intubation is chosen in a young child, a topical vasoconstrictor will reduce the risk of bleeding. With both approaches, an assistant should perform a jaw thrust to open the posterior pharyngeal and supraglottic spaces. Alternatively, a bite block or intubating airway may be used. Occasionally, the best view is obtained by direct traction on the tongue, which optimally opens the posterior pharynx. This can be accomplished by grasping the tongue with a gauze, plastic forceps, a stitch through the tongue, or application of suction to the underside or tip of the tongue (Fig. 12.32).[660]

The tip of the flexible intubation bronchoscope should be introduced behind the tongue and gradually advanced in the

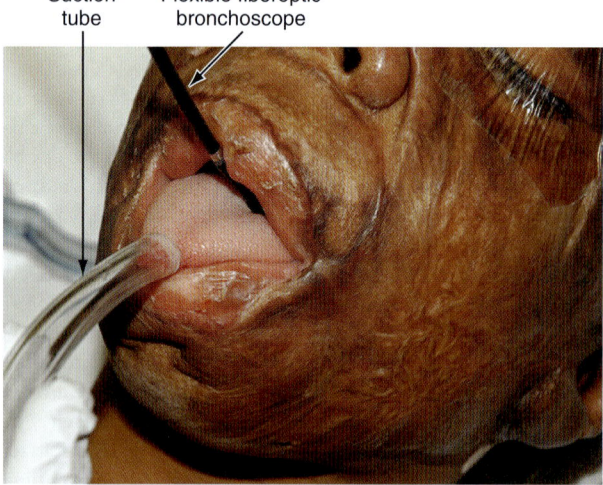

FIGURE 12.32 Suction can be applied to the tip of the tongue to facilitate pulling it forward to improve glottic visualization. This technique is particularly useful when the tongue is slippery from secretions or if the mouth opening is small and prevents direct grasping of the tongue with a dry gauze.

Suction tube   Flexible fiberoptic bronchoscope

midline under direct vision until a recognizable structure is observed. It is essential that the flexible intubation bronchoscope be kept straight so that when the direction of the tip is altered, it remains in the same plane as the handle of the flexible intubation bronchoscope. When the flexible intubation bronchoscope is rotated, the tip should be slightly bent to provide a panoramic view. In general, the tip of the flexible intubation bronchoscope is passed into the trachea before any attempts are made to pass the tracheal tube through the nose or oropharynx. Because the distances in the oropharynx in children are less than in adults, the most common initial error when using this technique is to advance the flexible intubation bronchoscope too deeply and into the esophagus. To avoid this pitfall, the flexible intubation bronchoscope should be advanced only toward identifiable airway structures.

Once the flexible intubation bronchoscope is introduced into the airway, a common problem is resistance to passage of the tracheal tube. To minimize this occurrence, the tracheal tube should be loaded onto the scope with the bevel facing down (Murphy eye up) for oral intubation and bevel facing up for nasal intubation.[661,662] This can be remembered by the mnemonic **UNDO**: bevel **U**p for **N**asal intubation, **D**own for **O**ral intubation.[663] If persistent resistance is encountered while attempting to pass the tracheal tube past the glottic opening, the tracheal tube should be rotated 90 to 180 degrees to place the bevel in a more favorable orientation for passage through the vocal cords. One study demonstrated that a 90-degree counterclockwise rotation of the tracheal tube before advancement resulted in a smooth passage of the tracheal tube into the larynx.[664] The depth of anesthesia or sedation as well as oxygen saturation (pulse oximetry) must be carefully monitored throughout the procedure. Arrhythmias may be avoided by providing an adequate depth of analgesia/anesthesia and ensuring a patent airway.

Flexible laryngoscopy techniques should be perfected on manikins and on children with normal anatomy before such techniques are attempted on children with difficult airways.[665–672] In a study that compared the time to intubation and complications in 40 infants with the Miller size 1 laryngoscope blade or the Olympus LFP flexible intubation bronchoscope, the time to intubation was slightly greater with the flexible intubation bronchoscope (22.8 vs. 13.6 seconds), whereas the complication rate was similar.[673] The authors concluded that routine use of the flexible intubation bronchoscope for intubation in normal infants is a safe and reasonable method to gain and maintain skills with this technique.[673] For children, video-assisted flexible intubation appears to offer advantages over fiberoptic intubation using a traditional eyepiece. These include faster mastering of this skill and an overall improved success rate when compared with the traditional method.[655,674]

Staged Techniques

Staged methods of flexible intubation can be used in infants and small children when the available flexible intubation bronchoscopes are too large to pass through the appropriately sized tracheal tube.[675] One method requires a flexible intubation bronchoscope with a working channel and a cardiac vascular catheter with guidewire. The guidewire is passed through the working channel of the bronchoscope to within 1 inch of its tip. The bronchoscope is then introduced into the mouth and positioned above the vocal cords. The guidewire is advanced under direct observation through the glottis into the trachea. The bronchoscope is then removed, leaving the guidewire in place. The lungs are ventilated by mask while an assistant passes the cardiac catheter over the guidewire (to stiffen the guidewire and facilitate passage of the tracheal tube). The tracheal tube is threaded over the catheter/guidewire combination, which is then removed, leaving the tracheal tube in place.[675–677] Some authors report that threading of the cardiac catheter over the guidewire is unnecessary. A modification of this technique when the flexible bronchoscope has no working channel has also been described.[678] An 8 Fr red rubber catheter was attached with waterproof tape to the bronchoscope proximal to the tip. The larynx was visualized with the flexible bronchoscope, and a guidewire was threaded through the rubber catheter into the trachea. With the guidewire in position, the bronchoscope (with the red rubber catheter) was withdrawn, and a tracheal tube was passed over the guidewire into the trachea.

Another alternative for intubation when the flexible bronchoscope is too large to pass through the appropriately sized tracheal tube is intubation under flexible scope guidance.[679–681] The bronchoscope is introduced through one naris to visually aid the placement of the tracheal tube that is passed through the other naris and manipulated into the glottis. Alternatively, if the observed tracheal tube is not easily passed into the glottis, a small catheter may be more easily manipulated into the glottis and used as a stylet to pass the tracheal tube into the trachea. Spontaneous ventilation is preserved, and oxygen can be administered via the tracheal tube during intubation. This technique was used successfully in two neonates, one with congenital fusion of the jaws and a second with Dandy-Walker syndrome associated with Klippel-Feil syndrome, micrognathia, hypoplasia of the soft palate, and anteversion of the uvula.[679,680] Another example was the use of an adult video-flexible intubation bronchoscope to guide intubation of a toddler with temporomandibular joint ankyloses.[681,682] If the available bronchoscope is both too large and lacks a working channel, another staged fiberoptic intubation technique can be used. The bronchoscope is loaded with a tracheal tube that is larger than the larynx of the infant. The larynx is visualized with the bronchoscope, and the tracheal tube is advanced and positioned just above the vocal cords. The bronchoscope is then removed, and a tracheal tube exchanger or catheter is advanced into the trachea through the larger tracheal tube. The larger tracheal tube is then removed, and the appropriately sized tracheal tube for the child is threaded over the tube changer or catheter into the trachea. This technique was used successfully in a 6-month-old infant whose operation had previously been canceled because of failure to intubate.[683]

Lighted Stylet

A lighted stylet (Light Wand) is a useful adjunct for managing the pediatric difficult airway (E-Fig. 12.15).[684–688] A number of these devices are available: Surch-Lite Lighted Intubation Stylet (Bovie Medical Corporation, Purchase, NY), Light Wand (Vital Signs, Mexicali, Mexico), and Trachlite (Rüsch, Tuttlingen, Germany).[689–691] These devices essentially comprise a malleable stylet with a high-intensity light at the tip; the stylet is shaped into a curve similar to that anticipated for successful passage into the laryngeal inlet (45 to 90 degrees). To begin, a tracheal tube is passed over a well-lubricated lighted stylet. The tip of the stylet should remain within the tip of the tracheal tube to minimize the potential for airway trauma. The room lights should be dimmed to ensure that the stylet is visible when the wand is in the mouth. The lighted stylet is then introduced into the mouth while the proximal end of the stylet is flat against the cheek. As the stylet is inserted into the mouth, the proximal end of the handle is rotated

counterclockwise until it is upright. The stylet continues to pass through the oropharynx, following the curvature of the tongue. If the tip of the lighted stylet is not in the proper position (e.g., in the esophagus), a diffuse light or no light will be observed on the surface of the neck. Proper position is usually ensured when a sharp, well-defined, bright circle or cone of light is observed trans-illuminating the neck directly in the midline at the level of the cricothyroid membrane (see E-Fig. 12.15). Once proper position is ensured, the tracheal tube is gently advanced and the stylet is removed.[687,692]

This technique is useful in those children in whom there is no intrinsic laryngeal or airway pathology but in whom visualization is anticipated to be difficult. The lighted stylet may also be of value in children with a fracture of the cervical spine, because tracheal intubation can be accomplished with minimal movement of the neck.[693] The hemodynamic response to intubation with this technique is similar to that observed with rigid laryngoscopy.[686] The limitations of this technique are that it is a blind technique, the diameter of the device limits its use to larger-sized tracheal tubes, and it may require multiple attempts; however, the success rate markedly increases with experience.[687,692] The most common cause of difficulty in passing the tracheal tube is that the tube hangs up on the epiglottis. When this occurs, the lighted stylet may be withdrawn, and its position slightly adjusted more posterior to allow passage behind and beyond the epiglottis. Alternatively, the tracheal tube can be rotated along the long axis of the stylet so that the bevel is facing up. Our advice for using this technique is similar to that for bronchoscopy: it should be used in children with normal anatomy to gain the necessary experience required for managing children with abnormal airway anatomy. This adjunct has also been combined with an LMA to guide the stylet into the trachea.[694]

Bullard Laryngoscope

The Bullard laryngoscope is now rarely used for direct visualization of the laryngeal inlet in children with airway pathology (E-Fig. 12.16). It is available in three sizes: adult, pediatric, and pediatric long. This instrument combines fiberoptic bundles and mirrors. It is positioned within the larynx like a laryngoscope blade, and the direction of force used to displace the tongue is similar to that used with a standard laryngoscope, although this is not intuitively obvious from its configuration. It is designed to provide visualization around a 90-degree bend at the tip (i.e., around the base of the tongue). This configuration may be helpful for direct visualization of the larynx in children with mandibular hypoplasia syndromes (e.g., Pierre Robin, Treacher Collins,[695] and Goldenhar syndromes), or cervical fracture restricting motion, when the acute angulation of the base of the tongue to the glottic opening is exaggerated, and in children with congenital trismus (Hecht syndrome).[696] The technique used in children is different from that used in adults. Once the laryngeal inlet is visualized, a styleted tracheal tube, with a bent configuration similar to the curve of the Bullard laryngoscope (see Fig. 12.25B), is inserted just to the side of the Bullard laryngoscope blade and advanced under direct vision into the trachea. Success with this instrument is directly proportional to the experience of the anesthesiologist, because the perspective seen through this laryngoscope, the method of visualization, and the indirect method of tracheal tube placement are so different from standard laryngoscopy.[697,698]

Despite the availability of pediatric Bullard laryngoscopes,[698] adult scopes have also been successfully used in children.[699,700] Although tracheal intubation in children 1 to 5 years of age with a Bullard laryngoscope takes more time than with a Wis-Hipple 1.5 blade, the adult Bullard laryngoscope complements the Wis-Hipple 1.5 blade. Occasionally, the Bullard laryngoscope provides a superior laryngeal view and thus allows successful intubation when a failure with the Wis-Hipple blade occurs. When multiple passes of the tube off the adult Bullard laryngoscope are required, this is usually because of contact with the right aryepiglottic fold or anterior vocal cord. The latter appears to be more problematic when the adult laryngoscope is used in children.[699,700]

Additional limitations of the Bullard laryngoscope are that the tracheal tube can partially obstruct the view of the larynx during insertion and that it can be used only for oral intubation.[701,702] An advantage is that there appears to be minimal motion of the cervical spine in patients with cervical spine disarticulations.[702–704] However, a randomized trial of 40 children (2 to 10 years of age) with simulated neck stabilization found that a short-handled Macintosh blade provided greater success than the Bullard scope.[697] A manikin study of inexperienced anesthesiologists found that the Bullard scope provided better success and shortened intubation time compared with conventional Macintosh blades.[705]

Retrograde Wire-Guided Intubation

The technique of retrograde wire-guided intubation uses transtracheal passage of an IV catheter through the cricothyroid membrane into the larynx and retrograde passage of a guidewire from a Seldinger vascular cannulation set to create a guide for intubation.[555,706–712] A commercial kit is available for use with tracheal tubes that are 5 millimeter ID or larger (Cook Critical Care). This technique is rarely used in children because of the greater compressibility of the trachea and the increased risk of posterior tracheal wall perforation by the catheter in children compared with adults.

Video and Indirect Intubating Devices

Advances in technology have led to the reduction in size of video cameras and optical lenses. The integration of these devices into various laryngoscopes and stylets has produced several enhanced tools for securing the airway in children.[713] Several of these new scopes improve visualization of the glottic aperture compared with direct laryngoscopy.[714–722] and perform better in children with difficult airways.[723–729] However, they are often associated with prolonged time to intubation compared with direct laryngoscopy, and their utility is limited in the presence of blood and secretions. These devices can be categorized as (1) video laryngoscopes, which incorporate a video camera into the tip of the device; (2) optical laryngoscopes, which use a series of mirrors, prisms, or both to transmit the image from the tip of the device; and (3) optical stylets, which incorporate video or optical systems into a rigid or malleable stylet.

Video Laryngoscopes

Video laryngoscopes are quickly becoming ubiquitous in anesthesia practice and will inevitably become the standard of care.[730,731] They offer unique advantages over standard direct laryngoscopy such as an improved view of the glottis, a shared view of the airway that facilitates guidance of a trainee and less force required to perform the intubation. Although the term video laryngoscope is loosely used to describe a large number of laryngoscopes with video and optical cameras, these devices can be very different with unique design characteristics. Video laryngoscopes can be classified in two broad categories: those with angulated blades and those with standard curved blades. The video laryngoscopes with angulated blades may perform better in patients with difficult airways, while those with standard blades may be best suited for patients with normal airways. Although angulated blades offer a better view of an "anterior" airway, passing the tube may be more challenging because of the acute angles made between the camera line of sight and the plane of the trachea. Video laryngoscopes with standard blades are less likely to be associated with this difficulty but may not offer as optimal a view as angulated blades in the difficult airway patient. Video laryngoscopes with conventional blades can be used to teach traditional laryngoscopy and therefore help trainees to maintain their skill with that technique while having the advantage of direct feedback from an instructor monitoring the camera screen. Video laryngoscopes have been associated with greater first-attempt success and success rates in adults compared with direct laryngoscopy and have been shown to have improved views of the vocal cords in children as well.[714,727,732–734] A retrospective cohort study in a pediatric emergency department compared video laryngoscopy with the C-MAC video laryngoscope (Karl Storz GmbH & Co. KG, Tuttlingen, Germany) with direct laryngoscopy and found no differences in first-attempt intubation success (adjusted Odds Ratio = 1.23, 95% CI = 0.78 to 1.94), complication rates, or intubation success rates.[735] A meta-analysis of randomized controlled trials in children (993 participants) that compared video laryngoscopes with direct laryngoscopes concluded that video laryngoscopy improved glottic visualization but prolonged the time to intubation and was associated with increased failures. They found similar first-attempt success between video laryngoscopy and direct laryngoscopy (relative risk 0.96; 95% CI 0.92 to 1.00; $I^2 = 67\%$).[736] The report of increased failures is not consistent with our experience and is most likely doubtful with currently available video laryngoscopes. A careful examination of their meta-analysis shows that most of the failures occurred in a single study that examined the Bullard laryngoscope in which 50% of first attempts failed in a cohort of 2- to 10-year-old children with simulated restricted neck mobility.[736] Curiously, in a single center trial comparing the view of the vocal cords with the Miller, Wis-Hipple and C-MAC blades (size 1 straight blade), the C-MAC video laryngoscope yielded better views than either blade during direct laryngoscopy.[714] When the C-MAC straight blade was used for direct laryngoscopy, the view of the glottic aperture was significantly inferior to those of the C-MAC via the monitor and the Miller blade during direct laryngoscopy. Many evaluations of video laryngoscopes are conducted in manikins; although this should be the first step to evaluate a new device, we encourage researchers to conduct clinical studies to expand our knowledge about the real-world performance of these devices. One study demonstrated that although trainees performed tracheal intubation with a variety of video laryngoscopes expeditiously in a manikin, they took significantly more time to intubate children less than 2 years of age.[737] A meta-analysis of 14 studies concluded that video laryngoscopes improved glottic visibility although they were associated with a decreased success rate and greater times to tracheal intubation compared with standard direct laryngoscopy.[736]

GLIDESCOPE. The GlideScope (Verathon, Bothell, WA) (E-Fig. 12.17) consists of a hypercurved blade that incorporates a high-resolution camera with a built-in antifog system. It is available in six sizes (0, 1, 2, 2.5, 3, 4) that accommodate all sizes of patients, including those weighing as little as approximately 1 kilogram. Before using the GlideScope, it should be powered on to allow the antifog system to warm up. A styleted tracheal tube should be used to ensure a successful intubation, and the stylet's curvature should mimic that of the selected GlideScope blade. The manufacturer markets a GlideScope-specific rigid stylet whose effectiveness has yielded conflicting efficacy when compared with a standard malleable stylet and a stylet with a tip that can be modified.[738–741] Unlike traditional direct laryngoscopy, sweeping the tongue to the left of the blade is unnecessary because of the distally located camera. The GlideScope blade is ideally placed in the midline or slightly to the left in the pharynx (Video 12.14). This position maximizes the space available for introduction of the tracheal tube. The blade tip is placed in the vallecula, and slight elevation of the blade exposes the glottis. The epiglottis may be elevated if placing the blade tip in the vallecula does not optimize the view of the glottic aperture. A poor view may occur if the blade size is inappropriate or if the blade is inserted too deeply in the pharynx. External laryngeal manipulations may also be used to facilitate laryngeal visualization.[716,734]

Once the best view is obtained, the styleted tracheal tube is inserted under direct vision alongside the GlideScope blade until the tube just passes the palatoglossal arches and is in full view on the GlideScope monitor. The technique of sequentially visualizing the tracheal tube directly and then on the monitor and creating space by inserting the GlideScope slightly to the left in the pharynx helps minimize the risk of injury to the soft tissues of the airway during advancement of the tracheal tube.[742–746] Children with severely obstructing tonsils may be vulnerable to injury if the laryngoscopist focuses their attention only on the screen and ignores the styleted tube as it is brought into view.[747] Success seems to be lower in children with difficult airways who weigh <10 kilograms.[748]

When the tracheal tube is visible on the monitor, the tip is directed into the glottic inlet. The stylet should be pulled back once the tracheal tube tip is inserted through the cords, because this facilitates the advancement of the tracheal tube down the trachea. Despite a good view of the glottic opening using the GlideScope and other video and optical laryngoscopes, inserting the tracheal tube between the vocal cords may prove to be difficult in some patients. This has been attributed to the indirect approach to intubation and the need for good eye-hand coordination. These skills can be acquired by using the device frequently in children with normal airways.[749–753] The GlideScope Cobalt was used to intubate the airways in a cohort of 121 infants yielding a 95% success rate on the first two attempts with an average time for successful tracheal intubation of 30 seconds.[754] It has also been used to facilitate tracheal intubation in children with craniofacial abnormalities.[638,755–757] When compared with direct laryngoscopy, the GlideScope provided superior laryngeal views in children with baseline limited views of the glottic opening.[758]

STORZ VIDEO LARYNGOSCOPE. The Storz Video Laryngoscope (Karl Storz GbmH, Tuttlingen, DE) integrates a camera into Miller- and Macintosh-type blades. This design allows the operator to perform laryngoscopy in the traditional fashion as the Miller-type blade with the video view available if necessary. The video view has been shown to provide one Cormack-Lehane grade improvement over the direct line-of-sight view because of the angulation of the video camera at the tip.[759] Since the device has no antifog mechanism, an antifog solution needs to be applied to optimize tracheal visualization. Intubation with the Miller video blade can be performed without a stylet, although a styleted tracheal tube with a slight bend at the tip facilitates intubation (E-Fig. 12.18). The Storz Video Laryngoscope is inserted into the mouth in a fashion similar to the GlideScope. The tip of the blade can be placed in the vallecula; however, because of the magnified lens of the camera, the epiglottis often obstructs the camera view.

If this occurs, the blade tip is best used to lift the epiglottis to expose the glottis. Once optimal visualization is obtained, the tracheal tube is placed directly along the shaft of the video blade, which guarantees immediate visualization of the tracheal tube in the magnified field of view of the camera and avoids injury to airway soft tissues.

When the Storz Video Laryngoscope was compared with the GlideScope in a pediatric manikin model with normal and difficult airway configurations, the times to intubation and the visual analog scale scores for field of view and ease of use of the two devices were similar.[760] In a small trial of 10 children younger than 2 years of age, the time to successful tracheal tube intubation with the Storz instrument was greater than with the Airtrach (Prodol Meditec, Guecho, Spain) although the success rates were similar.[761] In another infant manikin study, the glottic views and the intubation times with the Storz Video Laryngoscope were similar to the standard Miller laryngoscope, although the rates of intubation were more successful with the former laryngoscope.[759] The Storz Video Laryngoscope has been successfully used to intubate infants and neonates with difficult and normal airways[759,762] As with all video laryngoscopes, good hand-eye coordination is necessary for successful intubation. In addition, the operator must develop the skills necessary to manipulate the tracheal tube indirectly and on a magnified scale. This magnification effect makes subtle movements of the tracheal tube appear large on the video monitor and adds an additional challenge to intubation with these devices. Practice on children with normal airway anatomy is recommended before use on children with abnormal airways.[713]

MULTIVIEW SCOPE. The MultiView Scope (Medical Products International, Tokyo, JP) is a video laryngoscope system that integrates a camera into Miller- and Macintosh-style blades (E-Fig. 12.19). The handle of the device has a mounted video screen that displays the image from the blade tip. The image from the screen can be transmitted to an external monitor wirelessly, using a manufacturer-supplied attachment (AirView). Aside from being magnified, the direct line-of-sight view is identical to the camera view, making this an ideal tool for teaching direct laryngoscopy. The MultiView Scope also comes with a malleable stylet attachment that provides the ability to insufflate oxygen through the mounted tracheal tube. A manikin simulation found less force applied to the incisors and improved view compared with a Miller 1 blade.[763]

Optical Laryngoscopes

AIRTRAQ. The Airtraq (Prodol Meditec SA, Vizcaya, Spain) is a single-use, curved plastic laryngoscope that uses lenses and prisms to transmit the image from its distal tip to an eyepiece. It may reduce the incidence of esophageal intubation and may offer greater success rates, particularly in the hands of the inexperienced laryngoscopist.[764] It has a molded channel into which the tracheal tube is inserted (Fig. 12.33), thereby eliminating the need to manipulate the tracheal tube independently during intubation as is required with the GlideScope, Truview (Teleflex Medical, Netanya, Israel), and Storz Video Laryngoscopes. The manufacturer offers a wireless monitor for use with the device. The device should be turned on 30 seconds before use to allow the built-in antifog system to warm up. A disadvantage is that a minimum mouth opening of 16 millimeters is required to insert the Airtraq.

The selected tracheal tube and guide channel of the Airtraq are lubricated, and the cuff of the tracheal tube is fully deflated to avoid cuff damage when advancing the tube in the channel.[765,766] The appropriately sized tracheal tube is loaded into the guide

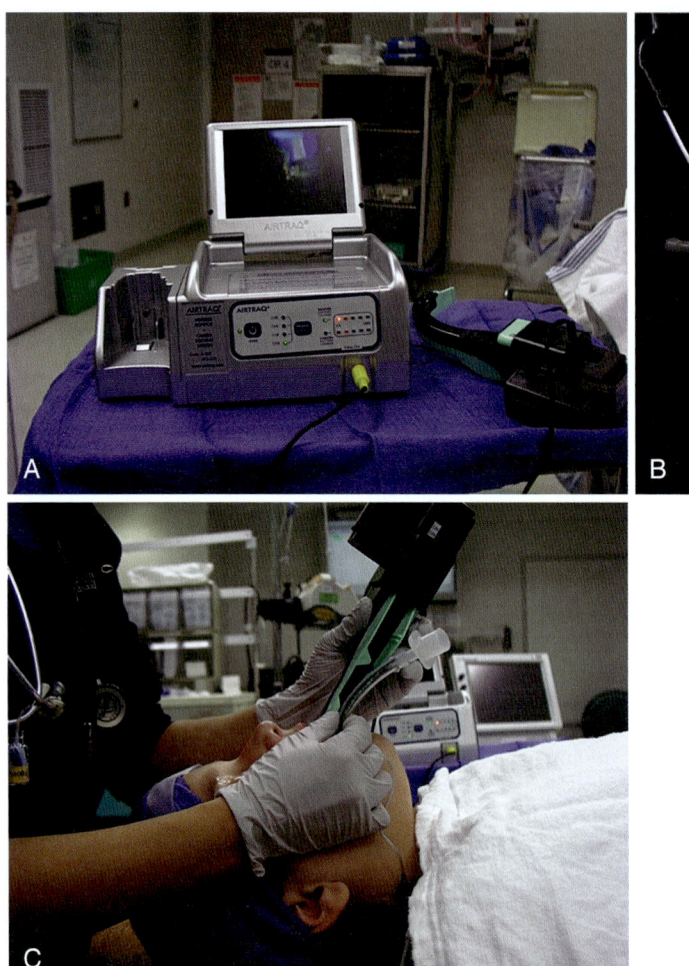

FIGURE 12.33 **A,** The Airtraq optical laryngoscope (Prodol Meditec SA, Vizcaya, Spain) is a plastic, curved laryngoscope with a distal video camera that allows improved laryngeal views. It is supplied with a portable monitor. **B,** The Airtraq with the tracheal tube (ETT) loaded into the molded channel is inserted in the midline of the pharynx. **C,** The tracheal tube is held laterally from the Airtraq after intubation, and the Airtraq is then rotated away from the operator and out of the pharynx.

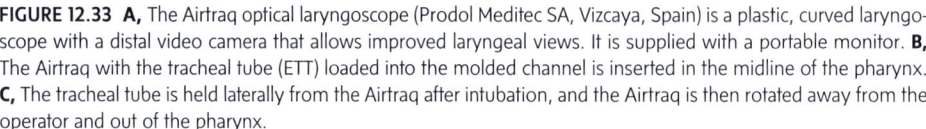

channel of the device, and the child's head is placed in a neutral position. The Airtraq is inserted in the midline in the pharynx and is advanced along the tongue base into the vallecula (Video 12.15). The epiglottis may be elevated to optimize the view, if necessary. Once in position, the Airtraq is gently lifted to obtain optimal glottic exposure, the glottis is centered in the viewfinder by rotating the entire device slightly clockwise or counterclockwise as necessary, and the tracheal tube is advanced after the optimal centered view is obtained. On occasion, the tracheal tube is directed below the glottic opening; if this occurs, the Airtraq should be withdrawn slightly, and the advancement attempted again. The guide channel deflects the tracheal tube slightly leftward (an effect that is more pronounced in infants and neonates); this tendency may be countered by rotating the device slightly clockwise as needed.[766,767] Once the trachea is intubated, the Airtraq is separated from the tracheal tube by holding the tube at the mouth and moving it laterally from the guide channel. The Airtraq is then rotated gently out of the oropharynx.

A suboptimal view with the Airtraq may result from inserting the device past the glottis. In this case, the device should be withdrawn slowly until the larynx comes into view. As with other optical and video-enhanced laryngoscopes, the Airtraq has been associated with airway soft tissue injury. A tonsillar injury in a 4-year-old child was attributed to the width of the guide channel.[715] Care should be taken when using the device in small children, given its size relative to the pharyngeal space. An Airtraq devoid of the guide channel is available for nasal intubations; the intubation may be facilitated with the use of Magill forceps or a gum elastic bougie.[768] The Airtraq has been successfully used for intubation in children with normal and difficult airways; however, despite its having a guide channel, some reports have noted difficulty with properly directing the tracheal tube in neonates and infants.[595,642,717–719,769,770] The Airtraq is easy to learn and use.[771,772] As with many optical and video devices, there remains a learning curve to using the device,[773] particularly the manipulation of the tracheal tube into the glottis in small patients.[713]

TRUVIEW. The Truview EVO2 Infant device (Teleflex Medical, Netanya, Israel) is an optical laryngoscope with an angulated, stainless-steel blade that transmits a magnified image from the tip of the device to an eyepiece (E-Fig. 12.20). A camera is available for connection to the eyepiece to allow the image to be viewed on a monitor. A side port is integrated into the blade to allow oxygen insufflation to clear the lens during intubation; however, caution should be exercised when insufflating oxygen in neonates and infants because of the rare risk of gastric insufflation and rupture.[773–776] Because of the indirect view afforded by the device, a stylet is necessary for successful intubation; a preformed stylet is available from the manufacturer. As with the GlideScope, the tracheal tube should be shaped in a curve similar to the Truview blade. The blade is placed centrally along the tongue in the pharynx to the vallecula, and slight elevation should expose the vocal cords. The tracheal tube is then passed alongside the device, taking care to look in the mouth during initial insertion to make sure the airway soft tissues are not injured. When compared with a Miller blade in children, the Truview EVO2 revealed improved views of the larynx but greater intubation times.[721] If the patient's head is in the neutral position, as for cervical spine instability, application of external laryngeal manipulation will improve the view.[777] In adults, the laryngeal view with the Truview was improved compared with standard laryngoscopy without the need to align the oral, pharyngeal, and tracheal axes.[778] As with all these devices, there is a learning curve so practicing should shorten intubation times and minimize injury to soft tissues.[713] The Truview PCD Pediatric is the most recent iteration of the original Truview design; it is available with four pediatric blade sizes (0, 1, 2, 3) for newborns weighing from 800 grams to large teenagers. In a recent study of the Truview PCD in 86 consecutive children with normal airways, 79 were successfully intubated on the first attempt and 4 children required two attempts. The average tracheal intubation time was 30 (27.9 to 37) seconds.[779]

Optical Stylets

Use of optical stylets, unlike flexible intubation bronchoscope intubation, allows the operator to visualize the tracheal tube as it enters the glottis. This is because the stylet is located just within the distal tip of the tracheal tube, providing the operator with a view of the leading edge of the tracheal tube. This view allows immediate recognition of impediments to tracheal tube advancement such as the right arytenoid and enables negotiation of the stylet around these obstacles. The Shikani and the Bonfils are two optical stylets available for pediatric use. Secretions, fogging, and airway soft tissues can impede intubation with optical stylets because of their small lenses and limited depth of view. Impairment of visualization by airway soft tissues can be addressed by combining these devices with direct laryngoscopy. The direct laryngoscope allows the creation of space for visualization with the optical stylet but may require two operators for successful intubation. Optical stylets may be easier to learn and maneuver than flexible intubation bronchoscopes, although some have questioned the utility of these devices in the pediatric population, particularly in the presence of copious secretions.[780,781]

SHIKANI OPTICAL STYLET. The Shikani Optical Stylet (SOS; Clarus Medical, Minneapolis, MN) is a malleable, J-shaped fiberoptic stylet that transmits the image from its distal tip to an eyepiece (E-Fig. 12.21). It has an adjustable tube stop to secure the tube and a port for oxygen insufflation, which should be used with caution in small children.[776,782] The nondominant hand is used to perform a jaw thrust, elevating the epiglottis from the posterior pharyngeal wall, and the stylet is then inserted in the midline in the pharynx (Video 12.16). The tongue base, uvula, and epiglottis are visualized in succession, and the tip is placed just above or just into the glottic inlet. The tracheal tube is then advanced while the scope is held steady. The Shikani optical stylet is a useful adjunct in the management of the pediatric difficult airway.[783,784]

STORZ BONFILS OPTICAL STYLET. The Bonfils Optical Stylet (Karl Storz, Tuttlingen, DE) is a rigid fiberoptic stylet with a fixed 40-degree curvature (E-Fig. 12.22). It delivers a higher-quality image than the Shikani optical stylet but is not malleable. Although the manufacturer recommends a retromolar approach to intubation, a midline approach similar to that of the Shikani optical stylet has been found to be successful in children.[785] The Bonfils is available in pediatric and infant sizes and can be coupled to a portable monitor (available from the manufacturer). The use of an antisialogogue and suctioning greatly improves visualization when intubating with optical stylets. When the Bonfils was compared with direct laryngoscopy in a cohort of children with normal airways, the Bonfils yielded better views but had a greater incidence of intubation failure.[780,781,786] In a comparison of the Bonfils, standard direct laryngoscopy, and GlideScope, the Bonfils significantly improved the laryngeal views and provided shorter intubation times.[787] Another study that compared the Bonfils with a standard flexible intubation bronchoscope found a shorter time to intubation (52 ± 22 seconds vs. 83 ± 24 seconds) and better image quality with the Bonfils, although all children were successfully intubated.[788] A case report describes its successful use in an infant with massive macroglossia and multiple hemorrhagic lymphangiomata compressing the airway, wherein it converted a grade 4 laryngoscopic view to a grade 1 view.[789]

SHIKANI VERSUS BONFILS OPTICAL STYLETS. Both devices consist of a metal stylet containing a fiberoptic illumination fiber and a fiberoptic vision fiber that are connected to an eyepiece or a video monitor. The light source may be external or battery powered and attached to the housing at the base of the eyepiece; the latter version allows easy transport in an emergency outside the traditional operating room location (see E-Figs. 12.20 and 12.21).[790,791] These devices are described for use either with or without rigid laryngoscopy. There are slight differences between them. Both provide an adapter to hold the tracheal tube that allows delivery of oxygen through the tip of the tracheal tube, but the Shikani optical stylet requires removal of the 15-millimeter adapter, whereas the Storz Bonfils device uses the 15-millimeter adapter to hold the tube in place. The pediatric Shikani optical stylet is slightly malleable and can accommodate a 3.0-millimeter ID tracheal tube; a 2.5-millimeter ID tracheal tube fits but is tight. The Storz device is not at all malleable but readily accommodates a 2.5-millimeter ID tracheal tube.[783,790,792,793] One further difference is that the quality of light (on battery mode) seems a bit brighter with the Storz device.

Supraglottic Airway as a Conduit for Intubation

Numerous case reports affirm the usefulness of the SGA as a conduit for intubation.[629,751,794–796] Multiple methods for placing the tracheal tube through the SGA have been described including blind, flexible intubation bronchoscope–assisted, stylet- or bougie-assisted, and retrograde-assisted.[558,794,797–802] Because the epiglottis frequently overlies the laryngeal inlet in children,[803] even with seemingly correct placement of the SGA as determined by the ability to ventilate the lungs easily, visual confirmation of correct tracheal tube placement (i.e., flexible intubation bronchoscope–assisted) may be the best method. However, all intubation methods are complicated by the inability to stabilize the tracheal tube as the laryngeal mask is withdrawn because the SGA and conventional tracheal tubes have similar lengths. As a result, removing the SGA over the tracheal tube may cause simultaneous withdrawal of the tracheal tube (extubation).[804–807] Several solutions have been proposed, including leaving the LMA in situ until the end of the anesthetic,[807–809] splitting the SGA,[392] cutting and shortening the SGA,[795,806,810] using uncut tracheal tubes,[811] and using a second tracheal tube telescoped into the first. Each technique has disadvantages that should be assessed by the individual operator. Leaving the SGA in place makes securing the tracheal tube difficult and precarious. Modifying the SGA may adversely affect its function, and removing a split SGA can easily dislodge the tracheal tube. Longer tracheal tubes may not be readily available. When a flexible intubation bronchoscope is used to place the tracheal tube, the SGA may be withdrawn first over the scope. The tracheal tube is then grasped, passed through the SGA, and threaded over the flexible intubation bronchoscope into the trachea.[800,812,813] An alternative is to telescope a second identical tracheal tube into the first or to use two tubes that differ in size by 0.5-millimeter ID, either larger or smaller (E-Fig. 12.23 and Video 12.17).[814–816] These tracheal tubes would then be threaded onto a flexible intubation bronchoscope. The upper tube maintains the position of the lower tube as the SGA is withdrawn.[809,817] The upper tracheal tube is then removed, the 15-millimeter adapter is then inserted onto the lower tube, and the correct position is confirmed by exhaled CO_2 and auscultation. Placing two tracheal tubes on the flexible intubation bronchoscope allows removal of the SGA, but the 15- millimeter adapter needs to be replaced, which can be difficult if the tracheal tube is covered with lubricant. The apnea time from insertion of the fiberscope into the SGA until the tracheal tube has been advanced into the trachea can be minimized by using continuous ventilation through a swivel adapter attached to the SGA or tracheal tube.[804,818,819]

It has been suggested that smaller-sized, cuffed tracheal tubes should be used for easier passage and then the cuff can be inflated to eliminate leaks. However, the pilot balloon of a cuffed tracheal tube does not pass through the internal lumen of pediatric SGA sizes of 1.0 to 2.5 (Video 12.18). In larger SGAs, the tracheal tube pilot balloon connection may be too short, so that the pilot balloon can become stuck within the SGA during withdrawal.[820] The largest tracheal tube that will pass through each size of SGA is listed in Table 12.4.

For the pediatric-sized LMA Unique and PLMA, even smaller tracheal tubes must be used. The LMA Fastrach is available only in sizes 3, 4, and 5. The air-Q offers a larger working channel particularly for smaller patients and devices and is our preferred device for planned intubation via a supraglottic airway. When the air-Q is used as a conduit for intubation, the tracheal tube and its cuff should be checked before the intubation attempt to be sure they will easily pass through the size to be used. The external surface of the tracheal tube should be liberally lubricated. The 15-millimeter adapter of the air-Q is removed, the trachea is intubated with a flexible bronchoscope, and the tracheal tube advanced into the trachea. When correct tracheal position is ensured, a special stabilizer (available in three sizes for pediatric-sized tracheal tubes) is inserted into the lumen of the tracheal tube. The cuff of the air-Q is deflated, and with slight advancing pressure the tracheal tube is held in place with the stabilizer while the air-Q is gently withdrawn (Video 12.6). Proper tracheal tube position is then reconfirmed, and the tracheal tube is taped in place.

Combined Techniques
Video Laryngoscopy and the Flexible Intubation Scope
Standard and nonstandard blade video laryngoscopes can be combined with the flexible intubation scope to intubate the trachea. The video laryngoscope is used to create space in the pharynx and guide the flexible intubation bronchoscope into the glottis. Once the flexible intubation bronchoscope is advanced beyond the view of the video laryngoscope the laryngoscopist switches their view

to that of the flexible intubation bronchoscope. This is a critical step because blind insertion of the flexible intubation bronchoscope may cause airway injury.

Retrograde Wire and the Flexible Intubation Scope
A case series reported the use of a combined retrograde wire and flexible intubation bronchoscope technique in 20 children aged 1 day to 17 years.[821] Equipment required includes a ventilating endoscopic mask, equipment for retrograde wire intubation, a flexible intubation bronchoscope with a working channel, and grasping forceps. The technique begins similarly to retrograde wire-guided intubation. A venous cannula is passed through the cricothyroid membrane in a cephalad manner. The needle is removed, and lidocaine is injected to provide topical anesthesia. Aspiration is done first; detection of air confirms correct placement of the cannula within the lumen of the trachea. A guidewire of suitable length is passed through the cannula and advanced cephalad into the pharynx until it can be retrieved from the mouth with forceps. The wire is then passed into the working channel of a flexible intubation bronchoscope in a retrograde manner starting at the tip of the flexible intubation bronchoscope (some flexible intubation bronchoscopes may require removal of tip components to allow the wire to pass). An appropriately sized tracheal tube should already be threaded onto the flexible intubation bronchoscope. The flexible intubation bronchoscope is then advanced along the wire while the laryngoscopist looks for familiar anatomic structures. After placement of the flexible intubation bronchoscope tip below the vocal cords is confirmed, the wire is removed in the caudad direction from the IV cannula. The flexible intubation bronchoscope is further advanced to the midtrachea, and the tracheal tube is threaded into place.

Tips for success with this technique are to preserve spontaneous ventilation and to remove the guidewire in the caudad direction, because this tends to pull the flexible intubation bronchoscope farther into the airway rather than out of the airway, which might occur if it is removed in the opposite direction. This technique may improve success over retrograde techniques alone because the flexible intubation bronchoscope allows direct visualization and is a stiffer guide for the tracheal tube than the wire alone. It also may improve success over the flexible intubation bronchoscope alone because the glottis is more readily identified even in the presence of blood or secretions.

Rigid Laryngoscopy and the Flexible Fiberoptic Bronchoscope
The rigid laryngoscope blade may be used to facilitate exposure so that a flexible intubation bronchoscope can be used to visualize the larynx.[822]

Flexible Fiberoptic Bronchoscope Used in a Retrograde Manner
A flexible intubation bronchoscope has been used to intubate the trachea in a 4-year-old child with Nager syndrome who presented for tracheocutaneous fistula closure after decannulation of a tracheostomy using a retrograde approach. After failed attempts at rigid and direct fiberoptic tracheal tube placement, a flexible intubation bronchoscope was placed in a retrograde fashion, using direct vision, through the fistula, past the vocal cords, into the nasopharynx, and out the naris. It was then used as a stylet for tracheal tube placement.[823] The clinical scenario was unusual, but the technique was successful for this child.

Retrograde Light–Guided Laryngoscopy
Retrograde light–guided laryngoscopy describes a method by which a light-emitting diode flashlight is placed externally in the

area of the cricothyroid membrane. Direct laryngoscopy is then performed with a laryngoscope blade with the light source switched off. The glottis is illuminated by the retrograde transmission of light and the vocal cords glow red. This bright intense light provides a discrete target for the laryngoscopist to insert the breathing tube. When compared with traditional direct laryngoscopy, use of retrograde light–guided laryngoscopy improved first-attempt intubation success rate, time to successful intubation, and the incidence of sore throat.[824,825]

Acknowledgments

Many manufacturers have graciously provided us samples of airway devices so that we could illustrate examples of commonly available equipment. There is insufficient room to illustrate all available devices. Lack of illustration of a device should not be construed as lack of efficacy, nor should illustration of a device be interpreted as endorsement. Practitioners are encouraged to use all equipment available and to make their own educated decision about what devices provide the greatest safety and efficacy in their hands.

We wish to acknowledge Julia Serber and, postuhumously thank, Ronald S. Litman for their contributions to this chapter in the previous edition.

ANNOTATED REFERENCES

2022 American Society of Anesthesiologists Practice Guidelines for Management of the Difficult Airway. *Anesthesiology.* 2022;136:31-81.
The most recent guidelines from the American Society of Anesthesiologists for management of the patient with a difficult airway, whether anticipated or unanticipated and the first version to include a pediatric-specific algorithm.
Crawford MW, Arrica M, Macgowan CK, Yoo SJ. Extent and localization of changes in upper airway caliber with varying concentrations of sevoflurane in children. *Anesthesiology.* 2006;105:1147-1152.
Crawford MW, Rohan D, Macgowan CK, et al. Effect of propofol anesthesia and continuous positive airway pressure on upper airway size and configuration in infants. *Anesthesiology.* 2006;105:45-50.
These two papers by Crawford and colleagues clarify how anesthetics produce airway obstruction in children. Airway obstruction during anesthesia or loss of consciousness appears to be primarily related to loss of muscle tone in the pharyngeal and laryngeal structures rather than apposition of the tongue to the posterior pharyngeal wall. This reduction in pharyngeal airway space decreases in a dose-dependent manner with increasing concentrations of either sevoflurane or propofol anesthesia.
Disma N, Virag K, Riva T, et al. Difficult tracheal intubation in neonates and infants. Neonate and Children audiT of Anaesthesia pRactice IN Europe (NECTARINE): a prospective European multicentre observational study. *Br J Anaesth.* 2021;126(6):1173-1181.
This is a prospective observational cohort study that included more than 5000 infants up to 60 weeks' postmenstrual age undergoing anesthetics from March 2016 to January 2017 in 165 centers in 31 European countries. Difficult intubation, defined as two failed attempts at direct laryngoscopy, occurred in 5.8% of cases. Severe hypoxemia occurred in 40% of cases of difficult intubation and was accompanied by bradycardia in 8%. In this cohort, difficult intubation was not associated with morbidity or mortality at 30 or 90 days.

Fiadjoe JE, Nishisaki A, Jagannathan N, et al. Airway management complications in children with difficult tracheal intubation from the Pediatric Difficult Intubation (PeDI) registry: a prospective cohort analysis. *Lancet Respir Med.* 2016;4(1):37-48.
This registry reviewed 1018 difficult intubation encounters in children. Complications were associated with more than two attempts at tracheal intubation, weight less than 10 kilograms, short thyromental distance, and three direct laryngoscopy attempts before an indirect technique. The most frequent complication was temporary hypoxemia, but 15 children suffered cardiac arrest. The authors concluded that limiting the number of direct laryngoscopy attempts and quickly transitioning to an indirect technique when direct laryngoscopy fails would enhance patient safety.
Fiadjoe JE, Stricker P. Pediatric difficult airway management: current devices and techniques. *Anesthesiol Clin North Am.* 2009;27:185-195.
This review paper is a comprehensive summary of the newer devices and techniques with which to manage the difficult pediatric airway.
Garcia-Marcinkiewicz AG, Kovatsis PG, Hunyady AI, et al. First-attempt success rate of video laryngoscopy in small infants (VISI): a multicentre, randomised controlled trial. *Lancet.* 2020;396(10266):1905-1913.
This randomized control trial of video laryngoscopy versus direct laryngoscopy in 564 infants with anticipated normal airway anatomy found that standard blade video laryngoscopy resulted in improved first-attempt success rates (93% vs. 88%) and decreased incidence of severe complications (2% vs. 5%). These results were particularly striking for infants weighing less than 6.5 kilograms.
Peyton J, Park R, Staffa SJ, et al. A comparison of videolaryngoscopy using standard blades or non–standard blades in children in the Paediatric Difficult Intubation Registry. *Br J Anaesth.* 2021;126(1):331-339.
In this analysis of standard Mac/Miller blade versus nonstandard hyperangulated blade video laryngoscopy in children with difficult intubations from the PeDI registry, there was no difference in first or eventual success rates by video laryngoscopy type for patients weighing more than 5 kilograms; however, in patients weighing less than 5 kilograms, standard blade video laryngoscopy was much more likely to be successful (51% vs. 26% first attempt, 81% vs. 58% eventual).
Rolf N, Coté CJ. Diagnosis of clinically unrecognized endobronchial intubation in paediatric anaesthesia: which is more sensitive, pulse oximetry or capnography? *Paediatr Anaesth.* 1992;2:31-35.
This paper determined that pulse oximetry is more sensitive than capnography in detecting endobronchial intubation. It recommends that when a small but persistent change in oxygen saturation is noted, rather than increase the inspired oxygen concentration, one must first investigate the cause and reassess the position of the endotracheal tube.
Shi F, Xiao Y, Xiong W, et al. Cuffed versus uncuffed endotracheal tubes in children: a meta-analysis. *J Anesth.* 2016;30(1):3-11.
This meta-analysis of two randomized controlled trials and two prospective cohort studies including 1979 children intubated with cuffed endotracheal tubes versus 1803 with uncuffed endotracheal tubes. Cuffed endotracheal tubes reduced the need for tracheal tube exchanges and did not increase the risk for postextubation stridor.
Wheeler M, Roth AG, Dsida RM, et al. Teaching residents pediatric fiberoptic intubation of the trachea: traditional fiberscope with an eyepiece versus a video-assisted technique using a fiberscope with an integrated camera. *Anesthesiology.* 2004;101:842-846.
Lack of proficiency using fiberoptic equipment for pediatric airway management remains a concern. This paper supports two important points: (1) one can achieve a satisfactory proficiency with a pediatric fiberoptic system with relatively few intubations, and (2) a video system can both improve the speed of skill acquisition and shorten the time required for successful intubation.

A complete reference list can be found online at Elsevier eBooks+.

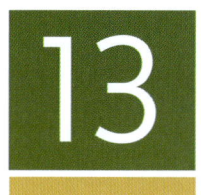

13 Anesthesia for Thoracic Surgery

GREGORY B. HAMMER AND STEPHANIE J. PAN

General Perioperative Considerations
Ventilation and Perfusion During Thoracic Surgery
Thoracoscopy
**Techniques for Single-Lung Ventilation in Infants
and Children**
Use of a Single-Lumen Endotracheal Tube
Use of Balloon-Tipped Bronchial Blockers
Use of a Univent Tube
Use of Double-Lumen Tubes

General Considerations in the Management
of Single-Lung Ventilation
Surgical Lesions of the Chest
Neonates and Infants
Childhood
Point-of-Care Ultrasound Pulmonary Exam
Introduction to the Lung Exam
Tracheal Diameter For Tracheal Tube Sizing
Tracheal Tube Positioning With Ultrasound

General Perioperative Considerations

A THOROUGH PREOPERATIVE EVALUATION is essential when caring for a child who is scheduled for thoracic surgery. Appropriate imaging and laboratory studies should be performed according to the lesion involved. Guidelines for fasting, choice of premedication, and preparation of the operating room are the same as for other infants and children scheduled for major surgery. Arterial catheterization should be considered for children undergoing thoracotomy as well as those with severe lung disease who are having thoracoscopic surgery, after induction of anesthesia, placing an intravenous (IV) catheter if not already in place, and intubating the trachea. An arterial catheter may not be required for thoracoscopic procedures of relatively brief duration in children without significant lung disease. The arterial catheter facilitates monitoring of systemic blood pressure during manipulation of the lungs and mediastinum as well as arterial blood gas tensions during single-lung ventilation (SLV). Central venous catheter placement is generally not indicated if peripheral IV access is adequate for projected fluid and blood administration.

Inhalational anesthetic agents are commonly administered in 100% oxygen during the induction of anesthesia. During maintenance of anesthesia, delivering high oxygen concentrations may have deleterious effects, including the formation of free radicals.[1] Although it is prudent for the practitioner to target a range of oxygen saturation values (e.g., 90% to 95%) and minimize the fraction of inspired oxygen (FiO_2) accordingly, higher concentrations may be appropriate in anticipation of surgical maneuvers that are likely to increase intrapulmonary shunting and decrease oxygen saturation. To prevent atelectasis during induction of anesthesia, 60% oxygen and 7 cm H_2O positive end-expiratory pressure is preferred but depends on the ability to maintain an acceptable hemoglobin oxygen saturation.[2,3] Isoflurane may be preferred because it attenuates hypoxic pulmonary vasoconstriction to a lesser extent than other inhalational agents, although this has not been studied in children[4]; nitrous oxide is avoided. IV

opioids have a sparing effect on the concentration of inhalational anesthetics required and may therefore limit the attenuation of hypoxic pulmonary vasoconstriction. Alternatively, total IV anesthesia may be used (see Chapter 6).

Various approaches have been described to prevent and treat pain after videoscopic procedures. Pain after thoracoscopic and thoracic surgery is greater than that after abdominal laparoscopic surgery.[5] Infiltration of the incision sites with bupivacaine before skin incision decreases postoperative pain[6,7] and is superior to IV fentanyl and nonsteroidal antiinflammatory drugs for reducing postoperative pain.[8] Regional anesthesia provides even better postoperative analgesia and is particularly desirable for thoracotomy but may also be beneficial for thoracoscopic procedures.[9,10] This is especially true when thoracostomy tube drainage, a source of major postoperative pain, is used after surgery. In addition, regional blockade for postoperative analgesia facilitates deep breathing and coughing, which may limit atelectasis and pneumonia. A variety of regional anesthetic techniques have been described for intraoperative anesthesia and postoperative analgesia, including ultrasound-guided peripheral nerve blocks (e.g., intercostal nerve blocks, paravertebral nerve blocks, serratus anterior plane blocks, pectoralis plane blocks, erector spinae plane blocks, and retrolaminar blocks), intrapleural infusions, and epidural anesthesia (see Chapter 40). Cryoablation of the intercostal nerves has been effective in attenuating both acute and long-term pain after thoracoscopic surgery including pectus excavatum.[11] The characteristics of the most frequently used regional techniques for thoracic surgeries are summarized in Table 13.1.[12]

VENTILATION AND PERFUSION DURING THORACIC SURGERY

Ventilation is normally distributed preferentially to the dependent regions of the lung so that there is a gradient of increasing ventilation from the least to the most dependent lung segments. Because of gravitational effects, perfusion normally follows a similar distribution, with increased blood flow to dependent lung

TABLE 13.1	Common Regional Blocks for Thoracic Surgeries				
Regional Technique	Catheter	Advantages		Disadvantages	Physiologic Effects
Epidural	• Well suited	• Well studied • Proven efficacy • Reduced mortality		• Risk of hematoma • Risk of dural puncture	Somatic and sympathetic blockade
Paravertebral Block	• Well suited	• Lower incidence of minor complications compared with neuraxial techniques • Equivalent analgesia to neuraxial anesthesia • Improved safety profile with ultrasound guidance		• Risk of hematoma • Risk of pneumothorax • Risk of epidural migration	Somatic and sympathetic blockade
Erector Spinae Plane (ESP) Block	• Well suited	• Less invasive compared with neuraxial and paravertebral techniques • Potentially opioid-sparing • Lower risk of hematoma and other major complications		• Effectiveness not well studied • Higher risk of muscle spasm • Large studies are lacking	Somatic blockade Possible sympathetic blockade
Intercostal Nerve Block	• Poorly suited, potentially in the surgical field	• Potentially opioid-sparing		• Short duration • Risk of pneumothorax • Risk of local anesthetic toxicity	Somatic blockade only
Pectoralis (PECS) 1 & 2 BLOCK	• Poorly suited, potentially in the surgical field	• Lower risk of hematoma and other major complications • Opioid-sparing		• Effectiveness not well studied • Large volume and dose of anesthetic needed for analgesic effect	Somatic blockade only
Serratus Anterior Plane (SAP) Block	• Poorly suited, potentially in the surgical field	• Lower risk of hematoma and other major complications • Potentially opioid-sparing		• Effectiveness not well studied • Large volume and dose of anesthetic needed for analgesic effect	Somatic blockade only

segments; therefore, ventilation and perfusion are typically well matched. In infants, however, ventilation is normally distributed to the nondependent areas of the lung, and perfusion is more evenly distributed because their smaller chest diameter mitigates the effect of gravity. These two effects increase ventilation/perfusion ($\dot{V}/\dot{Q}$) mismatch. During thoracic surgery, several factors further increase $\dot{V}/\dot{Q}$ mismatch.

General anesthesia, neuromuscular blockade, and mechanical ventilation may decrease the functional residual capacity of both lungs. Compressing the dependent lung in the lateral decubitus position may cause atelectasis. Surgical retraction and/or single-lung ventilation cause collapse of the operative lung. Although hypoxic pulmonary vasoconstriction diverts blood flow away from the under-ventilated lung to minimize $\dot{V}/\dot{Q}$ mismatch, its effects may be diminished by inhalational anesthetic agents and other vasodilating drugs. These factors apply equally to infants, children, and adults. The overall effect of the lateral decubitus position on $\dot{V}/\dot{Q}$ mismatch in infants, however, differs from that of older children and adults.

In adults with unilateral lung disease, oxygenation is optimal when the patient is placed in the lateral decubitus position with the healthy lung in the dependent ("down") position and the diseased lung in the nondependent ("up") position.[13] Presumably, this is related to an increase in blood flow to the dependent, healthy lung and a decrease in blood flow to the nondependent, diseased lung because of the hydrostatic pressure (or gravitational) gradient between the two lungs. This phenomenon promotes $\dot{V}/\dot{Q}$ matching in the adult patient undergoing thoracic surgery in the lateral decubitus position.

In infants with unilateral lung disease, however, oxygenation is improved with the healthy lung "up."[14,15] Several factors account for this discrepancy between adults and infants. Infants have a soft, easily compressible rib cage that cannot fully support the underlying lung. Therefore, functional residual capacity is closer to residual volume, making airway closure more likely in the dependent lung even during tidal breathing.[16] When the adult is placed in the lateral decubitus position, the dependent diaphragm has a mechanical advantage because it is "loaded" by the abdominal hydrostatic pressure gradient. This pressure gradient is decreased in infants, thereby reducing the functional advantage of the dependent diaphragm. The infant's small size also reduces the hydrostatic pressure gradient between the nondependent and dependent lungs. Consequently, the favorable increase in perfusion to the dependent, ventilated lung is attenuated in infants.

Finally, the infant's increased oxygen requirement and small functional residual capacity predispose them to hypoxemia. Infants normally consume 6 to 8 mL O_2/kg per minute compared with adult rates of 2 to 3 mL O_2/kg per minute (see Chapter 5 for allometric scaling laws in biology)[17]; for these reasons, they are at an increased risk of hemoglobin desaturation particularly during surgery in the lateral decubitus position.

A modest increase in partial pressure of carbon dioxide in arterial blood ($PaCO_2$) may be beneficial in children during thoracoscopic procedures. In a study of 12 children undergoing video-assisted thoracoscopic surgery for patent ductus arteriosus closure, hypercapnia targeting $PaCO_2$ values between 50 and 70 mm Hg increased cardiac output and central venous and arterial oxygen tensions.[18] Ventilating patients during single lung ventilation to a greater target partial pressure of carbon dioxide ($PaCO_2$) also results in less volutrauma and barotrauma (i.e., lung injury related to the use of large tidal volumes and increased inflating pressures; see later).

THORACOSCOPY

With the miniaturization of instruments, progress in video technology, and growing experience among pediatric surgeons, video endoscopic surgery of the chest, or thoracoscopy, is being performed for an increasing number of pediatric indications

TABLE 13.2	Thoracoscopic Procedures in Infants and Children
Diagnostic inspection	
Lung biopsy	
Lobectomy	
Sequestration resection	
Cyst excision	
Lung decortication	
Foregut duplication resection	
Thymectomy	
Patent ductus arteriosus ligation	
Thoracic duct ligation	
Esophageal atresia repair	
Sympathectomy	
Aortopexy	
Mediastinal mass excision	
Anterior spinal fusion	

TABLE 13.3	Advantages of Thoracoscopic Versus Open-Chest Surgery
Improved surgical visualization	
Decreased pain	
Decreased surgical stress	
Decreased ileus/earlier return to feeding	
Quicker return to normal activity (parents and child)	
Shorter hospitalization	
Fewer long-term complications	
Cosmetically superior	

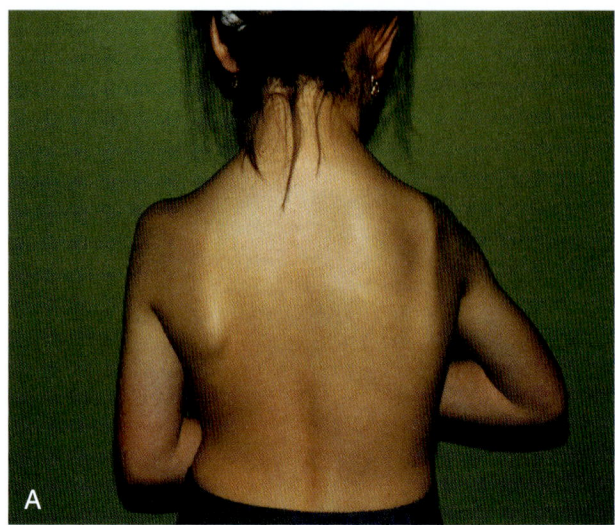

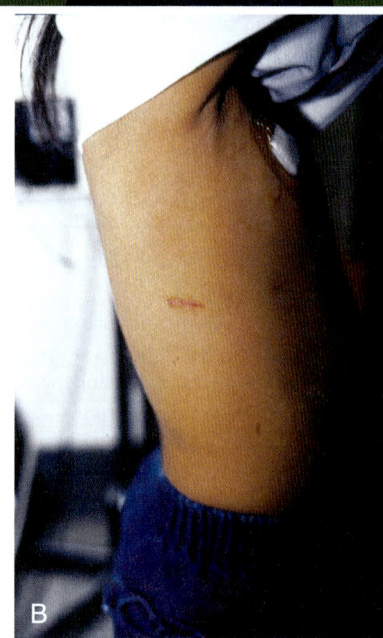

FIGURE 13.1 A, Chest deformity may occur with growth after thoracotomy. **B,** Smaller incisions associated with thoracoscopic surgery result in minimal musculoskeletal changes.

(Table 13.2). Advantages of thoracoscopy include smaller chest incisions, reduced postoperative pain, and more rapid postoperative recovery compared with thoracotomy (Table 13.3, Fig. 13.1).[19,20] Endoscopes can be passed through a needle and trocar system and digital video signals can be electronically modified to yield sharp, detailed, color images with minimum light intensity. Digital cameras are designed to maintain an image in an upright orientation regardless of how the endoscope is rotated. They are also equipped with an optical or digital zoom to magnify the image or give the illusion of moving the telescope closer to the object of interest. The smallest telescopes use fiberoptics and are less than 2 mm in diameter (Fig. 13.2). Two-millimeter disposable ports, mounted on a Veress needle, are used to introduce these small instruments. Larger instruments and ports are used in larger children and for more complex cases.

A second area of major advancement in video endoscopic surgery is the development of the endoscopic suite, in which all necessary cables and wiring are located within equipment booms, ceilings, and walls. The manipulation of digital images is controlled by voice or touchscreen command either from the operative field or at a conveniently located station nearby. High-quality digital images are displayed on flat-panel monitors that can be positioned within a comfortable viewing range. Remote-controlled cameras can direct any view in the room to any of the monitors or to a remote site. Digital radiographs can be routed from the radiology department to the operating room, and consultants in remote locations can be viewed on monitors in the operating room so that the surgeon can see to whom they are speaking. An additional feature of newer endoscopy suites is voice-controlled bed positioning. Robotic tools can be vocally directed to position telescopes in the surgical field for optimal viewing; these surgical "telemanipulators" facilitate microsurgery in confined spaces, even for small infants. Other endoscopic robots are being developed for a wide range of surgical applications.

Thoracoscopy can be performed while both lungs are being ventilated using CO_2 insufflation and placement of a retractor to displace lung tissue in the operative field. However, single-lung ventilation is extremely desirable during thoracoscopy because lung deflation improves visualization of thoracic contents and may reduce lung injury caused by surgical retractors.

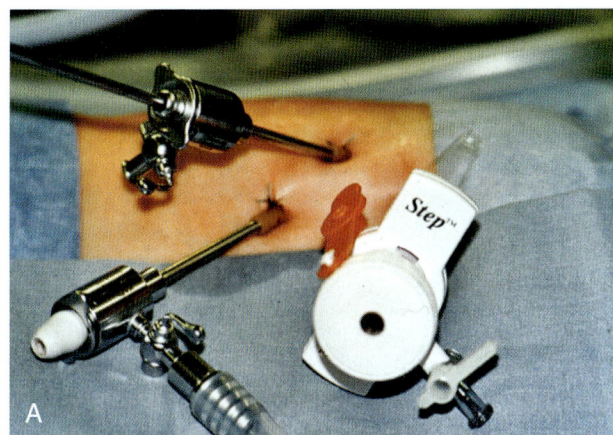

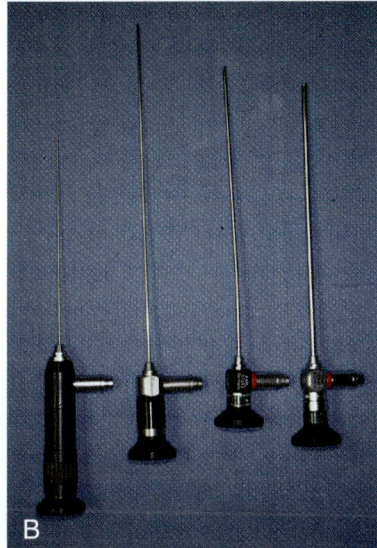

FIGURE 13.2 A, Thoracoscopic instruments in situ in an infant. **B,** Telescopes for use in infants range from 1.2 to 4.0 mm in diameter.

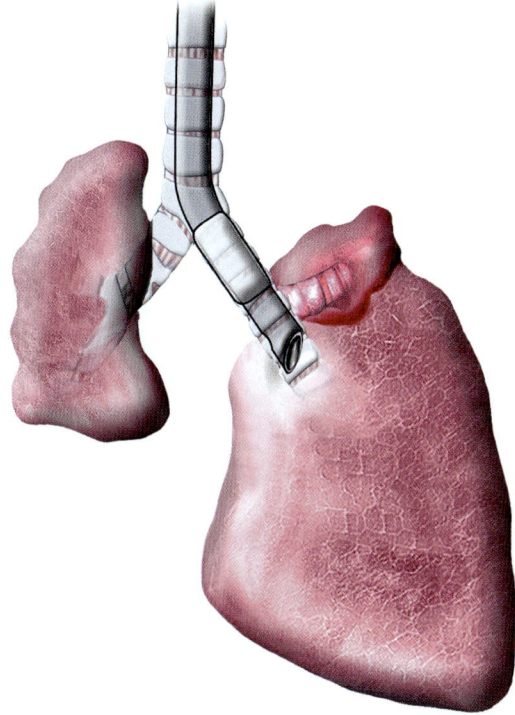

FIGURE 13.3 Placement of a single-lumen tracheal tube for left-sided single-lung ventilation results in obstruction of the upper lobe orifice if the distance from the proximal cuff to the tip of the endotracheal tube is longer than the mainstem bronchus.

Techniques for Single-Lung Ventilation in Infants and Children

USE OF A SINGLE-LUMEN ENDOTRACHEAL TUBE

The simplest means of providing single-lung ventilation is to intentionally intubate the nonsurgical mainstem bronchus with a conventional single-lumen tracheal tube (TT).[15,21] When the left bronchus is to be intubated, the bevel of the TT can be rotated 180 degrees and the child's head turned to the right.[22] The TT is advanced into the bronchus until breath sounds on the operative (right) side disappear. A fiberoptic bronchoscope (FOB) may be passed through or alongside the TT to confirm or guide placement. Alternate techniques to selectively intubate the left bronchus include passing a single-lumen tube shaped into a left-sided double-lumen tracheal tube using a stylet, with the bevel facing right has proven very successful in young children although the sample size was small;[23] a second technique uses fluoroscopy to guide and position the TT.[24] When a cuffed TT is used, the length of the cuff must be less than the length of the mainstem bronchus, and the proximal cuff must be placed just beyond the carina so that the right upper lobe orifice is not occluded (Fig. 13.3).[25] This technique is simple and requires no special equipment. This may be the preferred technique of single-lung

ventilation in emergency situations, such as airway hemorrhage or contralateral tension pneumothorax.

Problems can occur when using a single-lumen TT for single-lung ventilation. If a smaller, uncuffed TT is used, it may be difficult to provide an adequate seal of the intended bronchus. This may prevent the operative lung from adequately collapsing or fail to protect the healthy, ventilated lung from contamination by purulent material or blood from the contralateral lung. Also, one is unable to suction the operative lung using this technique. Hypoxemia may occur due to obstruction of the upper lobe bronchus, especially when the shorter right mainstem bronchus is intubated.

Variations of this technique have been described, including intubation of both bronchi independently with small TTs.[26–29] One mainstem bronchus is initially intubated with a TT, after which another TT is advanced over a FOB into the opposite bronchus. The disadvantages of this technique include technical difficulties and trauma to the vocal cords and subglottic and bronchial mucosa, although in tracheotomized children, trauma to the upper airway is obviated.[30] Even after successful bilateral bronchial intubation, the inner diameters of the tubes must be small, limiting gas flow and impeding suctioning of the airways.

USE OF BALLOON-TIPPED BRONCHIAL BLOCKERS

A Fogarty embolectomy catheter or an end-hole, balloon wedge catheter (e.g., 5 Fr Arndt Endobronchial Blocker [AEB; Cook Medical, Bloomington, IN]) may be used for bronchial blockade to provide single-lung ventilation (Fig. 13.4).[31–34] Placement of a Fogarty catheter is facilitated by bending the tip of its stylet toward the bronchus on the operative side. A FOB may be used to reposition the catheter and confirm appropriate placement.

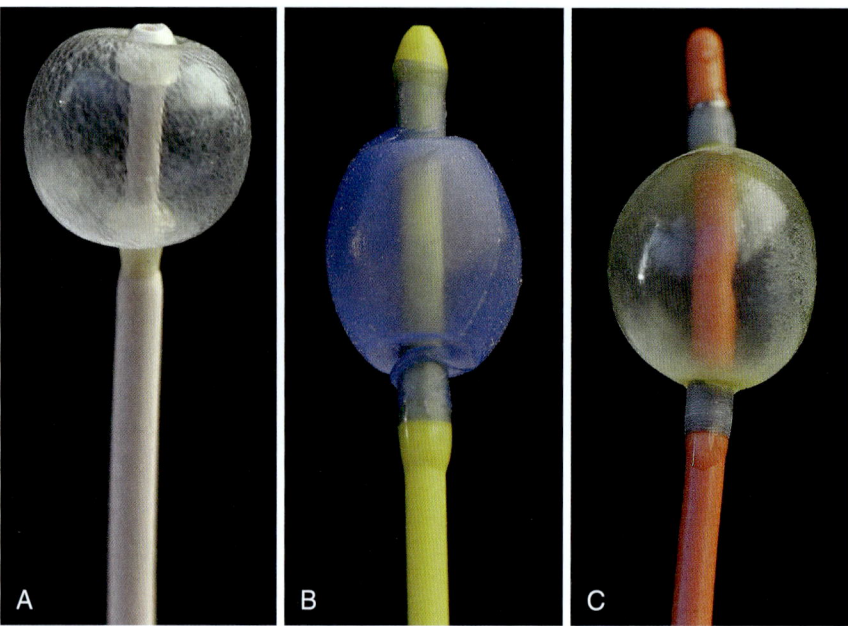

FIGURE 13.4 A variety of balloon-tipped catheters have been used for single-lung ventilation, including an Arrow balloon wedge catheter **(A)** (Arrow International, Inc., Reading, PA), a Cook pediatric bronchial blocker **(B)** (Arndt blocker, Cook Medical, Inc., Bloomington, IN), and a Fogarty embolectomy catheter (Edwards Lifesciences Corp, Irvine, CA) **(C)**. (Photographs by Michael Chen, MD.)

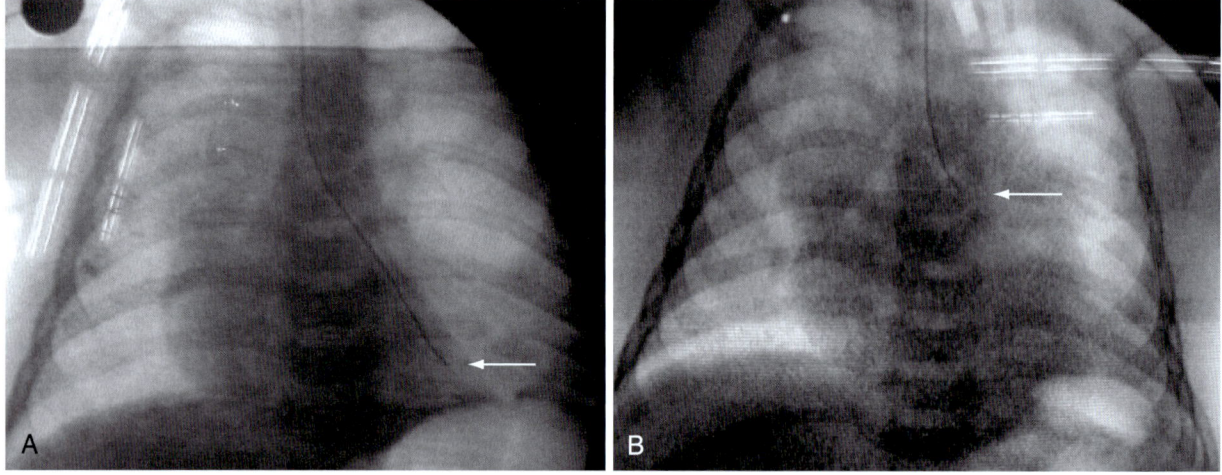

FIGURE 13.5 A bronchial blocker *(arrow)* is placed in a distal left bronchus **(A)** and withdrawn into the proximal left mainstem bronchus **(B, arrow)** under fluoroscopic guidance.

Bronchial blockers may be placed inside the TT (intraluminal) or alongside the TT (extraluminal). An advantage of placing the blocker outside the TT is that the lumen of the TT is available for passage of a suction catheter or FOB, which is often not feasible when the blocker catheter is inside the TT lumen. A variety of other techniques for placing the blocker outside the TT have been described.[35] Using one such method, the bronchus on the operative side is initially intubated with a TT[31]; a guidewire is then advanced into that bronchus through the TT, the TT is removed, and the blocker advanced over the guidewire into the bronchus. A TT is then reinserted into the trachea alongside the blocker catheter. The catheter balloon is positioned in the proximal mainstem bronchus under fiberoptic guidance. The guidewire may be removed to allow oxygen insufflation via the catheter lumen.

If a FOB small enough to pass through the indwelling TT is not available, fluoroscopy may be used to visualize the blocker balloon and facilitate placement just distal to the carina (Fig. 13.5). With an inflated blocker balloon, the airway is completely sealed, providing more predictable lung collapse and better operating conditions than with a TT in the bronchus.

One potential problem with the use of a bronchial blocker is dislodgment of the blocker balloon into the trachea, blocking ventilation to both lungs and/or preventing collapse of the operative lung. The balloons of most catheters currently used for bronchial blockade have low compliance properties (i.e., low volume, high pressure). They require 1 to 3 mL of air or saline to fully inflate. Overdistention of the balloon can damage or even rupture the airway.[36] One study, however, reported that bronchial blocker cuffs produced lower "cuff-to-tracheal" pressures than double-lumen tubes.[37] The operative lung cannot be suctioned and continuous positive airway pressure (CPAP) cannot be provided to the operative lung if needed when closed-tip bronchial blockers are used.

When a bronchial blocker is placed outside the TT, care must be taken to avoid injury caused by compression and resultant ischemia of the tracheal mucosa. The sum of the catheter diameter and the outer diameter of the TT should not exceed the tracheal diameter. Outer diameters for pediatric-size TTs are shown in Table 13.4. These numbers provide an estimate of the predicted tracheal diameter, which should approximate the size of the uncuffed TT predicted to produce a seal in the trachea. It should be noted, however, that the external diameters of TTs vary among manufacturers (~5%) as only the internal diameter is standardized.[38,39]

Bronchial blockers may be placed intraluminally according to the method described by Arndt et al. (https://www.youtube.com/watch?v=Tru-vVO6s3w) or by intubating the operative bronchus with a TT and subsequently passing the blocker through the TT before withdrawing the TT into mid-tracheal position. The blocker balloon can be positioned under FOB or fluoroscopic guidance. Adapters have been developed to ventilate the lungs while inserting a bronchial blocker through an indwelling TT.[40,41]

A 5 Fr endobronchial blocker with a multiport adapter has been designed for use with a FOB in children (Cook Medical, Bloomington, IN).[42] The balloon is elliptical so that it conforms to the bronchial lumen when inflated. The blocker catheter has a maximum outer diameter of 2.5 mm (including the deflated balloon), a central lumen with a diameter of 0.7 mm, and a distal balloon with a capacity of 3 mL. The balloon has a length of 1.0 cm, corresponding to the length of the right mainstem bronchus in children approximately 2 years of age.[43] The blocker is placed coaxially through a dedicated port in the adapter, which also has a port for passage of a FOB and ports for connection to the anesthesia breathing circuit and TT (Fig. 13.6). The FOB port has a plastic sealing cap, whereas the blocker port has a Tuohy-Borst connector (B. Braun, Bethlehem, PA) that locks the catheter in place and maintains an airtight seal. Because oxygen can be administered during passage of the blocker and FOB, the risk of hypoxemia during blocker placement is diminished. Insufflation of oxygen via the blocker lumen decreases intrapulmonary shunt, improves oxygenation, and therefore allows delivery of a lower FiO_2 to the ventilated lung to minimize oxygen toxicity. The blocker may be repositioned with FOB guidance during surgery.

When a FOB is used to place a bronchial blocker, both the blocker catheter and FOB must pass through the indwelling TT. The smallest TT through which the catheter and FOB can be passed must be larger than the sum of the outer diameters of the two. The 5 Fr Cook bronchial blocker and a FOB with a 2.2-mm diameter, for example, may be inserted through a TT with an

TABLE 13.4	Single-Lumen Uncuffed Tracheal Tube Diameters	
ID (mm)[a]	OD (mm)	Equivalent French Size[b]
3.0	4.3	13
3.5	4.9	15
4.0	5.5	17
4.5	6.2	19
5.0	6.8	21
5.5	7.5	23
6.0	8.2	25
6.5	8.9	27
7.0	9.6	29
7.5	10.2	31
8.0	10.8	32

Note: Cuffed tubes have approximately 0.5-mm additional outer diameter. The external diameter may also vary by manufacturer.
[a]Sheridan tracheal tubes (Hudson Respiratory Care Inc., Arlington Heights, IL).
[b]French (Fr) gauge is $\pi \times OD$ (~3 × OD) (mm).
ID, Internal diameter; *OD,* outer diameter.

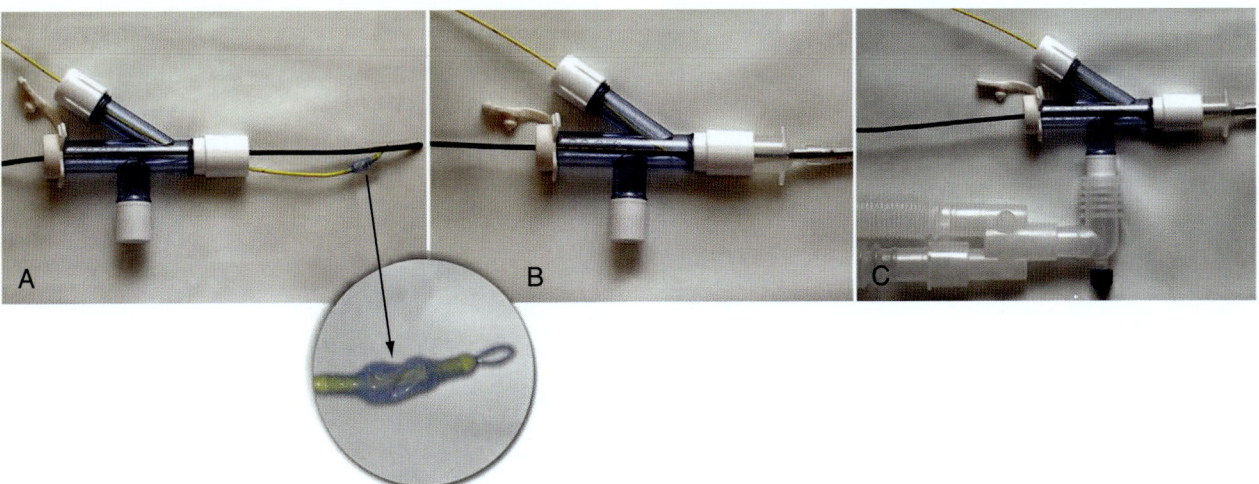

FIGURE 13.6 The Cook 5 Fr endobronchial catheter is shown inserted in the multiport adapter. **A,** The adapter has four ports for connection to the breathing circuit, fiberoptic bronchoscope (FOB), endobronchial catheter, and endotracheal tube. After the FOB and endobronchial catheter have been inserted through the multiport adapter, the FOB is placed through the monofilament loop at the distal end of the catheter *(arrow)*. The multiport adapter is then attached to the indwelling endotracheal tube **(B)** and the breathing circuit **(C)**. The FOB is directed into the mainstem bronchus on the operative side. The catheter is then advanced until the monofilament loop slides off the end of the FOB into the bronchus. (Photographs by Elliot Krane, MD.)

internal diameter as small as 5.0 mm; for children with an indwelling TT smaller than this, a blocker catheter can be positioned under fluoroscopy (see Fig. 13.5).[44]

Regardless of the method used to place a bronchial blocker, it should be noted that the right mainstem bronchus may be quite short, with a length typically one-third that of the left mainstem bronchus; the diameter of the left mainstem bronchus is generally smaller than that of the right mainstem bronchus.[45] It may be difficult or impossible to position the blocker balloon so that it does not obstruct the right upper lobe bronchial orifice.

USE OF A UNIVENT TUBE

The Univent tube (Fuji Systems Corporation, Tokyo, JP) is a conventional TT with a second lumen containing a small blocker catheter that can be advanced into a bronchus (Fig. 13.7).[46,47] A balloon located at the distal end of this small tube serves as a blocker. Univent tubes generally require a FOB to be placed successfully. Univent tubes are available in sizes with internal diameters as small as 3.5 and 4.5 mm for use in children older than 6 years of age.[48] Because the blocker tube is firmly attached to the main TT, the Univent blocker balloon is less likely to be displaced than when other blocker techniques are used. The blocker tube has a small lumen that allows egress of gas and can be used to insufflate oxygen or suction the operated lung.

One disadvantage of the Univent tube is the large cross-sectional area occupied by the blocker channel, especially in the smaller size tubes. Therefore, Univent tubes have a large outer diameter with respect to their inner (luminal) diameters (Table 13.5). Smaller Univent tubes have a disproportionately high resistance to gas flow.[49] The Univent tube's blocker balloon has low-volume, high-pressure characteristics, that predisposes to potential mucosal injury during normal inflation.[50,51]

USE OF DOUBLE-LUMEN TUBES

Double-lumen tubes are essentially two tubes of unequal length molded together. Although the bronchial lumen of a double-lumen tube appears to be round, both the bronchial and tracheal lumens are D-shaped (Fig. 13.8). The shorter tube ends in the

TABLE 13.5	Univent Tube Diameters
ID (mm)	OD (mm)[a]
3.5	7.5/8.0
4.5	8.5/9.0
6.0	10.0/11.0
6.5	10.5/11.5
7.0	11.0/12.0
7.5	11.5/12.5
8.0	12.0/13.0
8.5	12.5/13.5
9.0	13.0–14.0

[a]Sagittal/transverse.
ID, Internal diameter; *OD*, outer diameter.

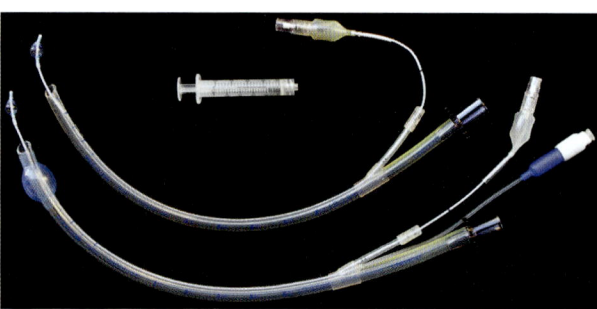
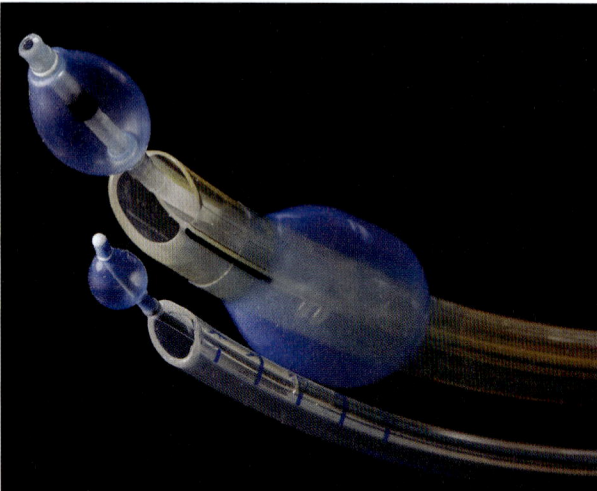

FIGURE 13.7 The Univent tube is available in a variety of adult sizes, as well as 3.5-mm internal diameter and 4.5-mm internal diameter sizes for use in children *(top)*. The adult tubes have a tracheal cuff and an end-hole bronchial blocker, allowing administration of oxygen and suction *(bottom)*. The pediatric tubes are uncuffed and have a closed-tip blocker. (Photographs by Michael Chen, MD.)

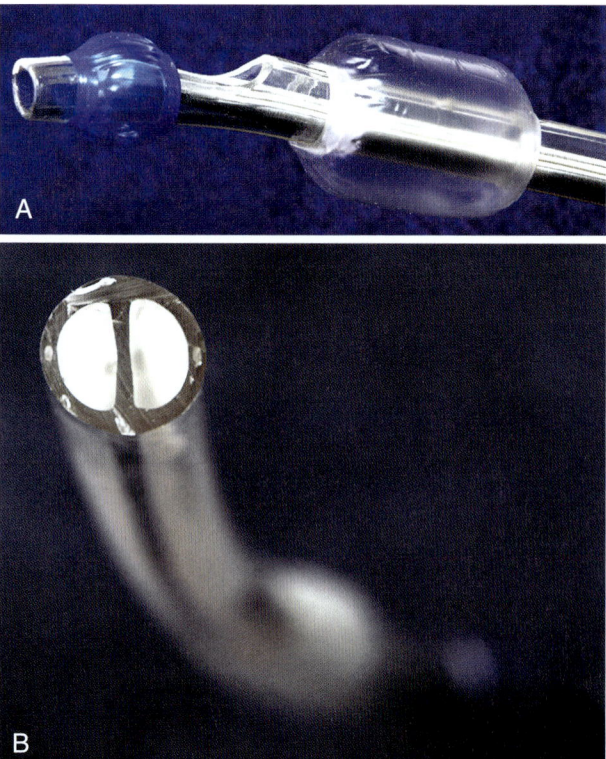

FIGURE 13.8 Although the bronchial lumen of a double-lumen tube appears to be round **(A)**, both the bronchial and tracheal lumens are D-shaped as evident in a cross-sectional view **(B)**. Their actual lumens have restricted limiting diameters. (Photograph by Michael Chen, MD)

trachea, and the longer tube ends in the bronchus. Double-lumen tubes for older children and adults have cuffs located on the tracheal and bronchial lumens. The tracheal cuff, when inflated, allows positive-pressure ventilation. The inflated bronchial cuff allows ventilation to be diverted to either or both lungs and protects each lung from contamination from secretions, purulent material, or blood originating from the contralateral side.

A bilumen tube has been described for infants[52]; it consists of two separate uncuffed tracheal tubes of different lengths attached longitudinally. This tube is not available in the United States. The smallest cuffed double-lumen tube commercially available in the United States is a 26 Fr size (Teleflex Medical, Research Triangle Park, NC). This double-lumen tube may be used in children as young as 8 years old. Double-lumen tubes are also available in sizes 28 Fr and 32 Fr (Nellcor brand, Covidien, Mansfield, MA); these are suitable for children 10 years of age and older. Numerous manufacturers produce clear, disposable, polyvinyl chloride Robertshaw-design (P³ Medical, Briston, England) double-lumen tubes, which are available in sizes 35 Fr to 41 Fr (Table 13.6) that consist of similar features with small modifications in cuff shape and location. The bronchial cuff is usually colored blue for easy identification during fiberoptic bronchoscopy. In general, the cuffs used in double-lumen tubes are high-compliance cuffs that are designed to exert less pressure on the tracheal and bronchial mucosa compared with low-compliance cuffs. For right-sided double-lumen tubes, the endobronchial cuff is donut shaped, positioned at the right upper lobe orifice to permit ventilation of the right upper lobe. Despite this design, right upper lobe occlusion may occur because of the shorter length of the right mainstem bronchus.[4,53] Therefore right-sided double-lumen tubes are used infrequently.

A novel mechanism to determine whether the child's airway is large enough to accommodate a double-lumen tube and, if so, the associated optimal double-lumen tube size, is through printed three-dimensional (3D) airway modeling.[54,55] It is now possible to create a full-scale, anatomically accurate, transparent model of the tracheobronchial tree on a 3D printer using data from computed tomography (CT) scanning. A variety of approaches to single-lung ventilation can be tested on the model, including placing the bronchial blocker inside or outside of a TT as well as a double-lumen tube. For the former approach, the appropriate size TT and bronchial blocker may be selected. If a recent CT scan has been obtained, as is common among patients for whom thoracic surgery is planned, there may be no additional imaging cost or radiation exposure required to create a 3D printed model. As 3D printers become more widely available and the cost of creating 3D printed models of an individual patient's tracheobronchial tree decreases, this technique may be more widely used for planning single-lung ventilation as well as for training anesthesiologists on how to perform these procedures more effectively.

Double-lumen tubes are inserted in children using the same technique as in adults, and left-sided tubes are used almost exclusively.[56] The tip of the tube is inserted just past the vocal cords, and the stylet is withdrawn. The double-lumen tube is rotated 90 degrees to the appropriate side and then advanced into the bronchus. After intubation, the tracheal cuff is inflated first and equal breath sounds should be confirmed. To prevent mucosal damage from excessive pressure applied by the bronchial cuff, the cuff is inflated with incremental volumes to seal air leaks around the bronchial cuff into the trachea. Inflating the bronchial cuff seldom requires more than 2 mL of air. After inflating the bronchial cuff, bilateral breath sounds should be rechecked to confirm that the bronchial cuff has not herniated across the carina to impede contralateral lung ventilation. FOB can be used to directly visualize the proximal edge of the bronchial cuff in the left bronchus, just distal to the carina. One simple way to verify that the tip of the bronchial lumen is located in the designated bronchus is to clamp the tracheal lumen at the level of the connector and then observe and auscultate left and right lungs. Usually, inspection will reveal unilateral movement of the ventilated hemithorax. With the tracheal lumen clamped, auscultation of the chest will demonstrate air entry in the left lung and no ventilation in the right lung. After auscultation and release of the tracheal clamp, the bronchial lumen is clamped, and the tracheal lumen is ventilated to confirm movement and breath sounds of the right lung. Whenever a right-sided double-lumen tube is used, ventilation of the right upper lobe must be verified. This can be accomplished by careful auscultation over the right upper lung field or, more accurately, by fiberoptic bronchoscopy. When a left-sided double-lumen tube is used, the risk of occluding the left upper lobe bronchus by advancing the bronchial tip into the distal left main bronchus should be considered.

Double-lumen tubes may be malpositioned in up to 48% of cases despite careful inspection and auscultation.[57] The simplest way to evaluate proper positioning of a left-sided double-lumen tube is to perform fiberoptic bronchoscopy through the tracheal lumen. The carina is then visualized, and only the proximal edge of the bronchial cuff should be identified just distal to the carina. Herniation of the bronchial cuff over the carina to partially occlude the contralateral mainstem bronchus should be excluded. Fiberoptic bronchoscopy should then be performed via the bronchial lumen to identify the patent left upper lobe orifice. When a right-sided double-lumen tube is used, the right upper lobe bronchial orifice must be identified while the bronchoscope is passed through the right upper lobe ventilating slot.

The use of a FOB to facilitate positioning of double-lumen tubes in children depends on the availability of small instruments.

TABLE 13.6	Double-Lumen Tube Dimensions		
Size (Fr)	Main Body OD (mm)	Limiting Diameter Tracheal Lumen (mm)	Limiting Diameter Bronchial Lumen (mm)
26[a]	8.7	N/A	N/A
28[b]	9.4	3.1	3.2
32[b]	10.6	3.5	3.4
35[b]	11.7	4.5	4.3
37[b]	12.4	4.7	4.5
39[b]	13.1	4.9	4.9
41[b]	13.7	5.4	5.4

Note: The limiting diameters correspond to the largest suction catheter or fiberoptic bronchoscope that can be placed via the lumen under ideal circumstances (e.g., adequate lubrication).
French (Fr) gauge is $\pi \times OD$ (~3 × OD) (mm). Comparing data in this table to those in Table 13.4, the OD of the double-lumen tubes corresponds to the following tracheal tubes: 26 Fr double-lumen tube is equivalent to that of a 6.0- to 6.5-mm ID tracheal tube; a 28 Fr is equivalent to a 6.5- to 7.0-mm ID; and a 32 Fr is equivalent to an 8.0-mm ID. Cuff thickness is 0.049 mm; therefore, a cuff adds 0.10 mm to overall OD of tube.
[a]Teleflex Medical, Research Triangle Park, NC.
[b]Covidien, Mansfield, MA.
ID, Internal diameter; OD, outer diameter.

FOBs with an external diameter of 3.6 mm are commonly available and will pass through a 35 Fr double-lumen tube. Smaller FOBs are needed when 26 Fr, 28 Fr, and 32 Fr double-lumen tubes are used (see Table 13.6 for "limiting diameters").

In the adult population, the depth of insertion of the double-lumen tube is directly related to the height of the patient.[58] No equivalent measurements are available as yet in children. Fortunately, there are very few reports in children of airway damage from double-lumen tubes.

The high-volume, low-pressure cuffs should not damage the airway, provided that the cuffs are not overinflated with air or distended with nitrous oxide. Alternatively, saline may be used to inflate the cuffs. Nonetheless, double-lumen tubes are more likely to cause trauma to the airway compared with a bronchial blocker.[59,60]

Another disadvantage of double-lumen tubes is the need to change to a single-lumen TT if mechanical ventilation is required after surgery. This is a particular problem for children in whom tracheal intubation was initially difficult because of anatomic or functional limitations. Even when an airway was not classified as difficult preoperatively, it may become difficult secondary to facial and supraglottic edema, the presence of secretions and/or blood in the airway, and laryngeal trauma from the initial intubation. The use of a TT exchange catheter may facilitate the exchange of a double-lumen tube for a single-lumen TT.[61] These devices are commercially available in a variety of sizes (Cook Medical) and allow oxygen insufflation and jet ventilation (see E-Fig. 12.4A–H).

Several important caveats should be considered before using a TT exchange catheter. First, it must be small enough to pass through the tracheal lumen of the double-lumen tube. This should be tested in vitro before the procedure is performed in vivo. Second, it should never be advanced against resistance, and the clinician must always be cognizant of the depth of insertion as perforations of the tracheobronchial tree have been reported.[62] Third, a jet ventilator should be immediately available in case the new TT does not follow the exchange catheter into the trachea and oxygenation via the exchange catheter is needed. The jet ventilator should be preset to a peak inspiratory pressure of 25 psi (172 kPa) by an inline regulator. When passing a TT over a TT exchange catheter, a laryngoscope should be used to facilitate passage of the TT into the trachea. It should be noted that the tip of the TT may hang up on the laryngeal inlet and may require a 90-degree rotation clockwise or counterclockwise to successfully pass, should this occur.

GENERAL CONSIDERATIONS IN THE MANAGEMENT OF SINGLE-LUNG VENTILATION

Once the TT, bronchial blocker, or double-lumen tube is in place, airway pressures should be confirmed during single-lung ventilation.[15] If the peak airway pressure is 20 cm H_2O during double-lung ventilation at a given tidal volume, the inflating pressure might increase to 40 cm H_2O at the same tidal volume as during single-lung ventilation. To minimize airway pressures, smaller tidal volumes at increased respiratory rates are delivered. The minute ventilation with two-lung ventilation is reduced compared with that during single-lung ventilation. Some degree of permissive hypercapnia is targeted to minimize lung trauma and the target oxygen saturation by pulse oximetry (SpO_2) may be less than when both lungs are ventilated (e.g., 90%–92%).

If the child is turned from the supine to the lateral decubitus position, proper position of the TT, bronchial blocker, or double-lumen tube should be reconfirmed because the tube may become displaced when the patient is turned. Two-lung ventilation should be maintained for as long as possible before switching to single-lung ventilation. When single-lung ventilation is required, the minimum FiO_2 needed to maintain an acceptable oxygen saturation should be used. Assuming an intact hypoxic pulmonary vasoconstriction response, the arterial partial pressure of oxygen (PaO_2) during single-lung ventilation with an FiO_2 of 1.0 should be between 150 and 210 mm Hg.[63] The lungs should be initially ventilated with a tidal volume of 4 to 6 mL/kg at a ventilatory rate that maintains the $PaCO_2$ between 45 and 65 mm Hg, unless this degree of hypercapnia cannot be tolerated because of other physiologic factors (e.g., concomitant metabolic acidosis, intracranial hypertension). Inadequate tidal volumes may lead to atelectasis in the ventilated lung (reduced functional residual capacity) with increased intrapulmonary shunting, resulting in hypoxemia. Large tidal volumes may force blood to the nondependent lung (similar to the application of positive end-expiratory pressure), thereby increasing the intrapulmonary shunt and exacerbating hypoxemia (Fig. 13.9).[64,65]

After the institution of single-lung ventilation, PaO_2 may continue to decrease for up to 45 minutes. Should hypoxemia develop, proper positioning of the indwelling blocker or tube should be reconfirmed by fiberoptic bronchoscopy, if possible. Several techniques can be used to improve oxygenation. The most effective maneuver for improving PaO_2 is the application of CPAP to the nondependent lung.[66] Insufflation of oxygen to achieve a CPAP of 10 cm H_2O, for example, produces alveolar inflation and decreases intrapulmonary shunt fraction. Usually this can be accomplished without significant expansion of the lung or interference with surgical conditions. If the PaO_2 continues to decrease despite the application of CPAP to the deflated lung, a malpositioned bronchial blocker or tube should be considered. This may be signaled by a sudden increase in the inflation pressure, a decrease in tidal volume, and/or a change in the capnograph. When a double-lumen tube is in place, the surgeon may aid repositioning. The surgeon can palpate the bronchi and manually occlude the main bronchial lumens, thereby guiding the tip of the double-lumen tube into the correct position. When the cause of the hypoxemia and/or hypercarbia cannot be readily identified, the balloon or cuff should be deflated and both lungs ventilated after informing the surgeon of the problem.

Single-lung ventilation may be associated with substantial lung injury, and measures should be undertaken to minimize adverse effects on the lung.[67] Collapse and subsequent reexpansion of lung tissue during single-lung ventilation has been associated with an increase in proinflammatory markers and alveolar damage.[68,69] In a study of 28 children undergoing single-lung ventilation for thoracic surgery, a preoperative dose of methylprednisolone 2 mg/kg IV decreased both interleukin-6 levels and respiratory resistance, and increased the serum concentrations of tryptase and the antiinflammatory cytokine, interleukin-10.[67] Three of 15 children in the placebo group and none of the 13 in the treatment group experienced intraoperative and postoperative respiratory complications.

A potentially therapeutic intervention to mitigate lung injury associated with single-lung ventilation is the administration of surfactant. Surfactant instilled into the subsequently deflated lung reduced the concentration of inflammatory cytokines in a piglet model of single-lung ventilation.[70] A more clinically practical method of reducing lung injury during single-lung ventilation is to minimize the FiO_2 and use a lung protective strategy during the procedure. An FiO_2 of 0.5 caused less lung injury in animals

Pulmonary blood flow during two-lung ventilation in lateral decubitus position

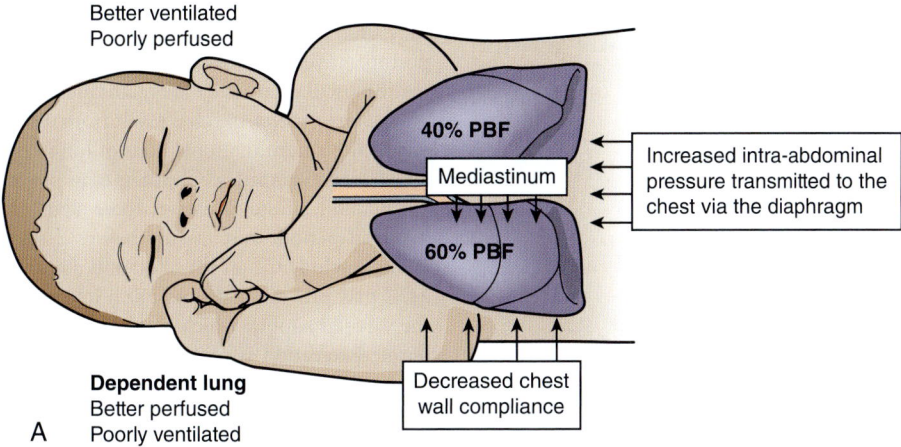

Pulmonary blood flow during single-lung ventilation in lateral decubitus position

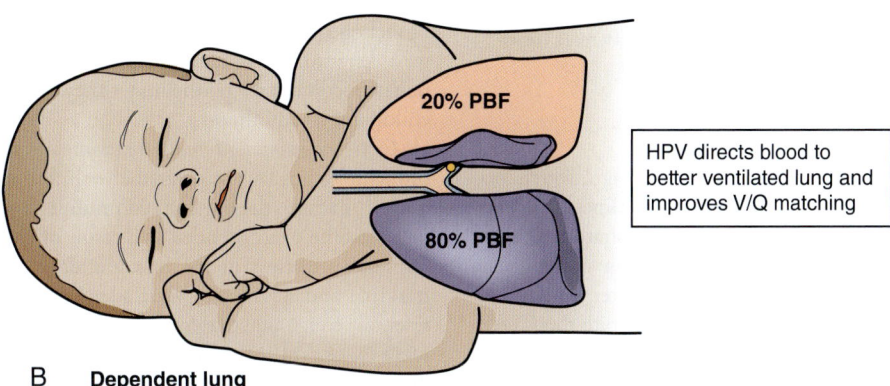

FIGURE 13.9 Lung perfusion in the lateral decubitus position before **(A)** and after **(B)** single-lung ventilation is instituted. Effects of lateral positioning on the redistribution of pulmonary blood flow and $\dot{V}/\dot{Q}$ mismatch in an anesthetized patient. In the lateral position **(A)**, there is a decrease in compliance and functional residual capacity in the dependent lung from external compression by the mediastinum, an increase in intraabdominal pressure transmitted to the chest via the diaphragm, and a decrease in chest wall compliance. Lateral positioning also leads to an increase in perfusion to the dependent lung, which receives 60% of the pulmonary blood flow and the nondependent lung receives 40% of the pulmonary blood flow. With single-lung ventilation **(B)**, collapse and atelectasis in the nondependent lung activate hypoxic pulmonary vasoconstriction, directing blood toward the better-ventilated lung, thereby improving $\dot{V}/\dot{Q}$ matching. *HPV*, Hypoxic pulmonary vasoconstriction; *PBF*, pulmonary blood flow; $\dot{V}/\dot{Q}$, ventilation/perfusion. (Reprinted with permission from Templeton TW, Piccioni F, Chatterjee D. An update on one lung ventilation in children. *Anesth Analg.* 2021;132(5):1389-1399).

subjected to single-lung ventilation for 3 hours than an FiO_2 of 1.[71] Young pigs that were mechanically ventilated with a lung protective strategy using a tidal volume of 5 mL/kg and a positive end-expiratory pressure (PEEP) of 5 cm H_2O demonstrated less lung injury than those ventilated with a tidal volume of 10 mL/kg and no PEEP.[72] Anesthesiologists should consider the use of the minimum FiO_2 needed to maintain an acceptable oxygen saturation, as well as small tidal volumes and adequate levels of PEEP, in the ventilated lung during single-lung ventilation to minimize lung injury. Preoperative administration of corticosteroids should also be considered.

Guidelines for selecting appropriate tubes (or catheters) for single-lung ventilation in children are shown in Table 13.7. There is considerable variability in overall size and airway dimensions in children, particularly in adolescents. The recommendations

shown in Table 13.7 are based on average values for airway dimensions. Larger double-lumen tubes may be safely used in large adolescents.

Surgical Lesions of the Chest

NEONATES AND INFANTS

A variety of congenital intrathoracic lesions for which surgery is required may occur in the neonatal or infancy period. These include lesions of the trachea and bronchi, lung parenchyma, and diaphragm, as well as vascular abnormalities.

Tracheal stenosis may be acquired or congenital. Tracheal stenosis occurs most commonly because of prolonged tracheal intubation, often in preterm infants with respiratory distress syndrome. Ischemic injury of the tracheal mucosa may occur as a result of a

TABLE 13.7 Tube Selection for Single-Lung Ventilation in Children

Age (years)	ETT (ID)[a]	BB (Fr)	Univent[b]	DLT (Fr)
0.5–1	3.5–4.0	2[c]		
1–2	4.0–4.5	3[c]		
2–4	4.5–5.0	5[d]		
4–6	5.0–5.5	5[d]		
6–8	5.5–6.0	5[d]	3.5	
8–10	6.0 cuffed	5[d]	3.5	26[e]
10–12	6.5 cuffed	5[d]	4.5	26[e]–28[e]
12–14	6.5–7.0 cuffed	5[d]	4.5	32[e]
14–16	7.0 cuffed	5, 7[d]	6.0	35[e]
16–18	7.0–8.0 cuffed	7, 9[d]	7.0	35, 37[e]

[a]Sheridan tracheal tubes, Hudson Respiratory Care Inc., Arlington Heights, IL.
[b]Fuji Systems Corporation, Tokyo, JP.
[c]Edwards Lifesciences LLC, Irvine, CA.
[d]Cook Medical, Inc., Bloomington, IN.
[e]Covidien, Mansfield, MA.
BB, Bronchial blocker; *DLT,* double-lumen tube; *ETT,* endotracheal tube; *Fr,* French size; *ID,* internal diameter.

tight-fitting TT at the level of the cricoid cartilage, which becomes scarred and constricted after a period of time. *Subglottic stenosis* may develop, resulting in stridor and respiratory distress after a trial extubation. Nasal CPAP with high-flow oxygen may be used to maintain the oxygen saturation early after extubation. If oxygen desaturation and hypercarbia persist despite the CPAP, tracheal reintubation may be required.

Tracheal and/or esophageal compression may occur because of a variety of lesions in the chest, including vascular rings and slings (see also Chapters 12 and 31).

A FOB is used to evaluate the severity of the stenosis and exclude other causes of stridor (e.g., vocal cord paralysis or laryngomalacia). When general anesthesia is required, inhalational anesthesia may be administered via a face mask, with the FOB inserted through an adapter; this is usually performed with the infant breathing spontaneously.[73] Alternatively, spontaneous ventilation can be maintained during FOB evaluation through the use of total intravenous anesthesia (TIVA) and supplemental oxygen (e.g., nasal cannula, high-flow nasal cannula, or blow-by oxygen). Noninvasive imaging studies are increasingly used for the diagnosis of a variety of congenital airway lesions, including vascular rings.[73] Bronchography and "virtual" CT or MRI scanning may also be useful.[74,75]

A cricoid split procedure may be performed for infants with acquired subglottic stenosis. After diagnostic bronchoscopy, the trachea is either intubated with a TT or a rigid bronchoscope is left in place during the operation. Anesthesia may be maintained with inhalational agents or an IV anesthetic technique, such as with propofol and remifentanil.[76] Typically, a TT with an internal diameter of 0.5 mm larger than the original TT is placed after the repair.

Congenital tracheal stenosis is often associated with other malformations, most commonly cardiac abnormalities.[77,78] For infants with severe congenital tracheal stenosis, a laryngotracheoplasty may be performed. This procedure involves the placement of a costal, auricular, or laryngeal cartilage graft into the anterior and/or posterior trachea.[79] In some cases, a stent may be positioned within the trachea. These infants may require a tracheal tube and mechanical ventilation for a variable period of time postoperatively. In these cases, sedation, analgesia, and at times neuromuscular blockade are maintained after surgery.

Pulmonary sequestrations result from disordered embryogenesis, producing a nonfunctional mass of lung tissue supplied by anomalous systemic arteries. Children may present with cough, pneumonia, and failure to thrive; these signs often occur during the neonatal period, and usually before 2 years of age. Diagnostic studies include CT of the chest and abdomen, and arteriography. MRI may provide high-resolution images, including definition of the vascular supply, which may obviate the need for angiography. Surgical resection is performed once the diagnosis is confirmed. Nitrous oxide should be avoided in these cases. Positive-pressure ventilation does not usually expand pulmonary sequestrations.

Congenital cystic lesions in the thorax may be classified into three categories.[80] *Bronchogenic cysts* result from abnormal budding or branching of the tracheobronchial tree. They may cause respiratory distress, recurrent pneumonia, and/or atelectasis because of lung compression. *Dermoid cysts* are clinically similar to bronchogenic cysts but differ histologically because they are lined with keratinized, squamous epithelium rather than respiratory (ciliated columnar) epithelium. They usually manifest later in childhood or adulthood.

Cystic adenomatoid malformations are structurally similar to bronchioles but lack associated alveoli, bronchial glands, and cartilage.[81] Because these lesions communicate with the airways, they may become overdistended as a result of gas trapping, leading to respiratory distress in the first few days of life. When they are multiple and air filled, cystic adenomatoid malformations may resemble congenital diaphragmatic hernias radiographically. Treatment is surgical resection of the affected lobe. As with congenital diaphragmatic hernias, prognosis depends on the amount of remaining lung tissue, which may be hypoplastic because of compression in utero.[82]

Congenital lobar emphysema often manifests with respiratory distress shortly after birth.[83] This lesion may be caused by "ball-valve" bronchial obstruction in utero, causing progressive distal overdistention with fetal lung fluid. The resultant emphysematous lobe may compress lung tissue bilaterally, resulting in a variable degree of hypoplasia. Congenital cardiac deformities are present in about 15% of children with congenital lobar emphysema.[84] Radiographic signs of hyperinflation may be misinterpreted as tension pneumothorax or atelectasis on the contralateral side (Fig. 13.10). Positive-pressure ventilation may exacerbate lung hyperinflation.[85] Nitrous oxide is contraindicated, and isolation of the lungs during anesthesia is desirable (see also Chapter 35, Fig. 35.10).

Congenital diaphragmatic hernia is a life-threatening condition that occurs in approximately 1 in 2000 live births. Failure of a portion of the fetal diaphragm to develop allows abdominal contents to enter the thorax, interfering with normal lung growth. In 80% to 90% of diaphragmatic defects, a portion of the posterior diaphragm fails to close, (80%–85% of cases on the left side), forming a triangular defect known as the *foramen of Bochdalek.*[86] Hernias through the foramen of Bochdalek that occur early in fetal life usually cause respiratory failure immediately after birth owing to pulmonary hypoplasia. The diagnosis is often made prenatally, and fetal surgical repair has been described.[87–89] Neonates present with tachypnea, a scaphoid abdomen, and absent breath sounds over the affected side. Chest radiography typically shows bowel in the

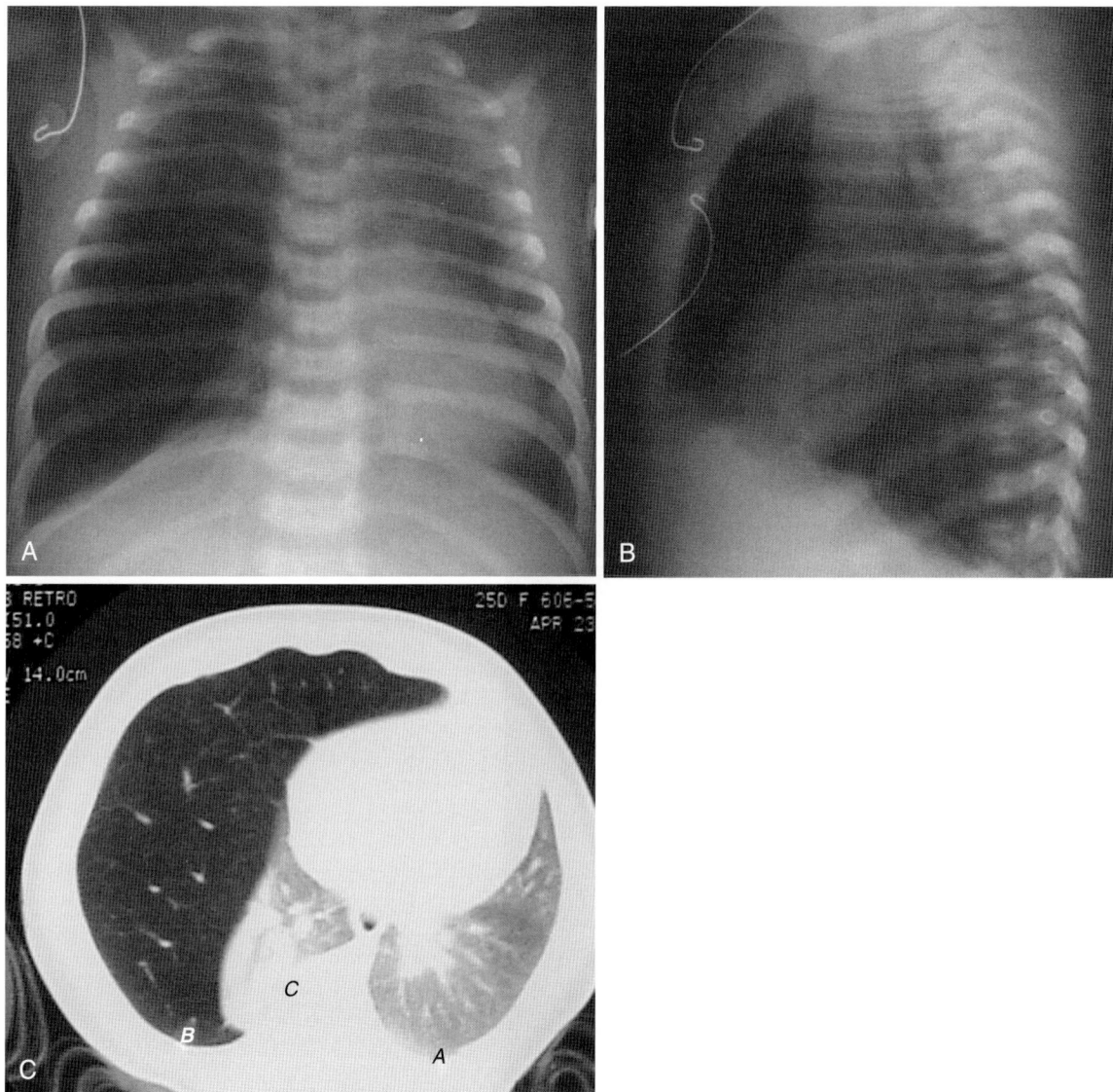

FIGURE 13.10 Congenital lobar emphysema of the right lower lobe. Plain radiography illustrates hyperlucency of the right lung on the anteroposterior image **(A)** and posterior displacement of the heart and mediastinum on the lateral image **(B)**. The computed tomography scan **(C)** demonstrates compression of the left lung *(A)* and right upper lobe *(C)* as well as hyperinflation of the right lower lobe *(B)*.

left hemithorax, with deviation of the heart and mediastinum to the right and compression of the right lung (Fig. 13.11). Right-sided hernias (see Fig. 13.11C) may occur late and manifest with milder signs. In the presence of significant respiratory distress, bag-and-mask ventilation should be avoided, and immediate tracheal intubation performed (see also Chapter 35). Distention of the thoracic gut postnatally with aggressive bag-valve-mask ventilation further compresses the inflated lungs, rendering ventilation and oxygenation more difficult.

Because pulmonary hypertension with right-to-left shunting contributes to severe hypoxemia in neonates with congenital diaphragmatic hernia, a variety of pulmonary vasodilators have been used to increase oxygenation. These include tolazoline, prostacyclin, dipyridamole, and nitric oxide.[90-94] High-frequency oscillatory ventilation has been used in conjunction with vasodilator therapy to improve oxygenation before surgery.[95] Occasionally, prostaglandin E_1 is used to maintain a patent ductus arteriosus

and reduce right ventricular afterload. In cases of severe lung hypoplasia and pulmonary hypertension refractory to these therapies (e.g., PaO_2 <50 mm Hg with FiO_2 of 1.0), extracorporeal membrane oxygenation (ECMO) should be initiated early to avoid progressive lung injury. Improved outcomes have been associated with early use of ECMO followed by delayed surgical repair.[96]

A particularly poor prognosis is predicted if congenital diaphragmatic hernia is associated with cardiac deformities, preoperative alveolar-to-arterial oxygen gradient greater than 500 mm Hg, or severe hypercarbia despite aggressive ventilation strategies.[97,98] Prognosis has also been correlated with pulmonary compliance and radiographic findings.[99,100] In a more recent analysis of outcomes, lung-to-head ratio >45% was most associated with survival, avoidance of ECMO, and primary repair, whereas total fetal lung volume correlated with mortality and patch repair.[101]

Surgical correction via a subcostal incision with ipsilateral chest tube placement may be performed before, during, or immediately

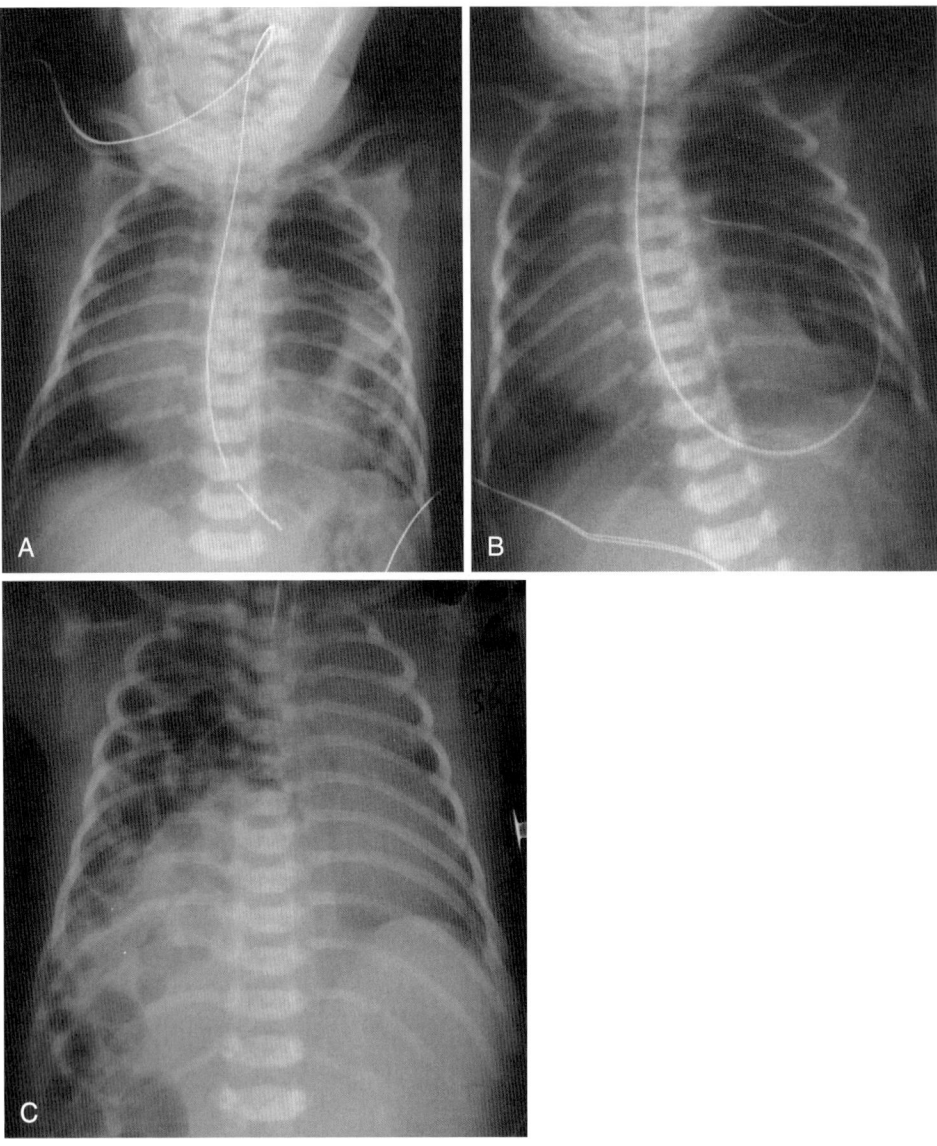

FIGURE 13.11 The majority of congenital diaphragmatic hernias are left sided. **A,** Chest radiography demonstrates the presence of bowel in the left hemithorax. **B,** A nasogastric tube has been advanced into the stomach. **C,** Congenital diaphragmatic hernias may also occur on the right side.

after ECMO.[102,103] In neonates undergoing surgical repair without ECMO, pulmonary hypertension is the major cause of morbidity and mortality. Hyperventilation to induce a respiratory alkalosis and 100% oxygen may be administered to decrease pulmonary vascular resistance. The anesthetic should be designed to minimize sympathetic discharge, which may exacerbate pulmonary hypertension (e.g., a high-dose opioid technique, use of neuraxial catheter). The lungs of these infants should be ventilated with small tidal volumes and low inflating pressures to avoid a pneumothorax on the contralateral (usually right) side. Both nitric oxide and high-frequency oscillatory ventilation have been used during surgical repair.[104,105] A high index of suspicion of right-sided pneumothorax should be maintained, and a thoracostomy tube should be placed in the event of acute deterioration of respiratory or circulatory function. It is also imperative that normal body temperature, intravascular volume, and acid-base status be maintained. Mechanical ventilation is continued postoperatively in nearly all

infants because lung compliance is markedly reduced after surgery (a consequence of returning the thoracic gut to the abdomen and the increased abdominal pressure on the diaphragm).

Failure of the central and lateral portions of the diaphragm to fuse, comprising 10%–15% of cases of diaphragmatic hernias, results in a retrosternal defect known as the foramen of Morgagni.[86] This usually manifests as signs of bowel obstruction rather than respiratory distress. Repair is usually performed via an abdominal incision (see also Chapter 35).

Tracheoesophageal fistula and/or esophageal atresia occur in approximately 1 in 4000 live births. In 80% to 85% of afflicted infants, this lesion includes esophageal atresia with a distal esophageal pouch and a proximal tracheoesophageal fistula.[106,107] The fistula is usually located one to two tracheal rings above the carina. Affected neonates present with spillover of pooled oral secretions from the pouch and may develop progressive gastric distention and tracheal aspiration of acidic gastric contents via the fistula.

A common association is the VACTERL complex, consisting of **v**ertebral, **a**norectal, **c**ardiac, **t**racheal, **e**sophageal, **r**enal, and/or **l**imb defects.[108] The diagnosis of VACTERL complex, which requires at least three features, occurs in 1:10,000 to 1:40,000 live births.[109] Esophageal atresia is confirmed when an orogastric tube passed through the mouth cannot be advanced more than about 7 cm (Fig. 13.12). The proximal pouch tube should be secured, and continuous suction applied, after which a chest radiograph is diagnostic (see also Chapter 35).

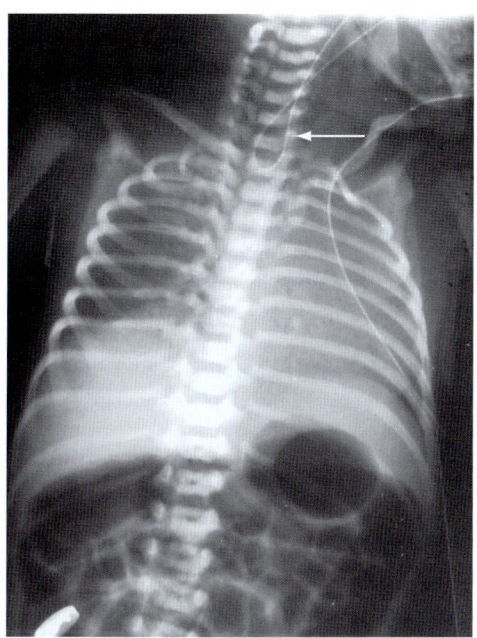

FIGURE 13.12 Tracheoesophageal fistula with esophageal atresia. Note the feeding tube coiled in the esophageal pouch *(arrow)* and the presence of a large volume of gas in the abdomen.

Mask ventilation and tracheal intubation are avoided before surgery, if possible, because they may exacerbate gastric distention and further compromise respirations. Once the trachea is intubated, it is occasionally necessary to occlude the tracheal orifice of the fistula with the tracheal tube. The tip of the tracheal tube is positioned just above the carina by auscultation of diminished breath sounds over the left axilla as the tube is advanced into the right mainstem bronchus, after which the tube is retracted until breath sounds are increased over the left chest (Fig. 13.13A). A small FOB may be passed through the tracheal tube to confirm appropriate placement. Rarely, an emergency gastrostomy is performed because of massive gastric distention. Placement of a balloon-tipped catheter in the fistula via the gastrostomy may be performed under guidance with a FOB, to prevent further gastric distention and/or enable effective positive-pressure ventilation in cases of significant lung disease or very large fistulas (see Fig. 13.13B).[110] "Antegrade" occlusion of a tracheoesophageal fistula has also been reported with a balloon-tipped catheter advanced through the trachea into the fistula (see Fig. 13.13C).[111] Preoperative evaluation should be performed to diagnose associated anomalies, particularly cardiac, musculoskeletal, and gastrointestinal defects, which occur in 30% to 50% of affected infants.[112] A poor prognosis for infants with tracheoesophageal fistula and esophageal atresia has been associated with prematurity and underlying lung disease, as well as the coexistence of other congenital anomalies.[113]

Surgical repair has generally involved a right thoracotomy and extrapleural dissection of the posterior mediastinum, although a thoracoscopic approach has become more common. In most cases, the fistula is ligated, and primary esophageal anastomosis is performed ("short gap atresia"). In cases in which the esophageal "gap" is long, the proximal segment is preserved for subsequent staged anastomosis, with or without intestinal interposition.[107] The trachea may be intubated with the infant breathing spontaneously, or during gentle positive-pressure ventilation with small tidal volumes to avoid gastric distention. If a gastrostomy tube is in place, occlusion

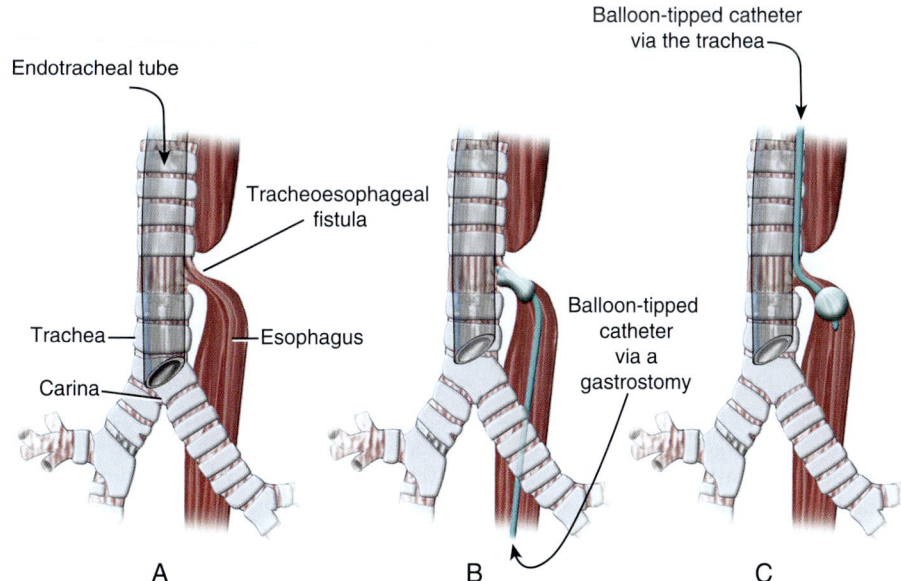

FIGURE 13.13 Methods for minimizing gastric insufflation in infants with a tracheoesophageal fistula. The tip of the endotracheal tube (ETT) may be placed distal to the fistula in cases in which the fistula is well proximal to the carina **(A)**. Alternatively, a balloon-tipped catheter may be placed in the fistula via a gastrostomy **(B)** or via the trachea **(C)**.

of the fistula may be confirmed by cessation of bubbling via underwater tubing connected to the gastrostomy or the normalization of CO_2 in the end-tidal gas. Alternatively, the tracheal tube may be positioned in the mainstem bronchus, opposite the side of the thoracotomy incision, until the fistula is ligated.

Esophageal atresia without connection to the trachea occurs much less commonly. These lesions are generally diagnosed by radiography after inability to pass an orogastric tube, at which time an absence of gas in the abdomen may be noted (see Fig. 35.9). So-called H-type tracheoesophageal fistula without esophageal atresia is relatively rare. Infants with H-type lesions may present later in childhood or adulthood with recurrent pneumonias or gastric distention during positive-pressure ventilation (see E-Fig. 35.1).[114,115]

Persistent symptoms associated with aspiration and respiratory distress after fistula ligation warrant investigation. Radiographic investigations including a barium swallow and/or rigid bronchoscopy with a 30-degree scope may be needed to identify a persistent fistula or a second fistula.[116]

CHILDHOOD

Some of the lesions described earlier may not be diagnosed until childhood. These include pulmonary sequestration, cystic lesions, and lobar emphysema. Other disorders for which thoracic surgery is performed in children, either for definitive treatment or diagnostic purposes, include neoplasms, infectious diseases, and musculoskeletal deformities.

Anterior mediastinal masses include neoplasms of the lung, mediastinum, and pleura. These tumors may be primary or metastatic. The most common primary tumors are *lymphoblastic lymphoma,* a form of non-Hodgkin lymphoma, and *Hodgkin (or Hodgkin's) disease.* Less commonly, teratomas (germ cell tumors), thymomas, as well as thyroid, parathyroid, and mesenchymal tumors may manifest as anterior mediastinal masses.[117–119] Signs and symptoms that result from vascular and/or airway compression may include dyspnea, orthopnea, pain, coughing, pleural effusion, and/or superior vena cava syndrome (swelling of the upper arms, face, and neck).[120,121]

Preoperative evaluation should include CT, echocardiography, and flow-volume studies whenever feasible (see Fig. 11.7). Tracheal, bronchial, and/or vascular (superior vena cava or pulmonary outflow tract) compression, as detected by CT, is associated with a high incidence of serious complications during induction of anesthesia.[121] However, CT scans are static pictures that may not identify dynamic compression of an airway or vascular outflow tract. These tumors may occur as extrathoracic or intrathoracic, with variable or fixed obstruction. Echocardiography identifies compression of the superior vena cava or pulmonary outflow tract. Flow-volume loops may be effective in detecting dynamic compression of the airways, although their utility in adult patients has been questioned[122] (see Chapter 11 and Figs. 11.6 and 11.7). An algorithm to manage anterior mediastinal masses from diagnosis to surgery has been published for clinicians.[119]

Establishing the correct diagnosis often requires a tissue biopsy. More often than not, there is an urgency to secure the tissue for diagnosis, because T-cell–type non-Hodgkin lymphoblastic lymphomas, which constitute 30% to 40% of non-Hodgkin lymphoma, may have a doubling time of as little as 12 hours.[119] A rapid diagnosis and chemotherapy prescription may prevent widespread dissemination of the tumor. The 5-year survival of Hodgkin lymphoma that is localized is more than 90%,[123] whereas that of non-Hodgkin lymphoblastic lymphoma is lower, but still exceeds 70%.[124] Every effort should be made to secure a

tissue diagnosis by lymph node or bone marrow biopsy using local anesthesia or sedation, thereby precluding the need for general anesthesia and facilitating early treatment.[118,125] If peripheral tissue diagnosis cannot be obtained and signs of severe airway and/or circulatory compromise are present, careful consideration should be given to administering a 12- to 24-hour burst of corticosteroids, initiating chemotherapy, and/or treating with limited radiation to decrease the size of the tumor and reduce the risk of life-threatening compression of the airway or major vessels under anesthesia. However, these interventions may cause involution of the tumor and compromise the tissue diagnosis; thus, oncologists prefer to avoid such interventions prebiopsy.[126,127] Corticosteroids cause a reduction in tissue mass (i.e., tumor lysis) of lymphomas by inducing apoptosis in the tumor via a number of mechanisms.[128] One study found that four features were predictive of perianesthesia complications in these children: orthopnea, upper body edema, great vessel compression, and mainstem bronchial compression (odds ratio of 5.1 to 8).[129] In another review, high risk for perianesthetic complications included symptoms (orthopnea and stridor or cyanosis) and signs (tracheal compression >70%, tracheal cross-sectional area <70%, great vessel compression, and tamponade by ECHO studies).[118] The extent of vascular and airway compression, according to radiologic investigations, is predictive of perianesthesia complications.[125] There may be increased risk with thoracoscopic biopsies associated with the use of inhalation anesthesia rather than sedation.[130] It must be emphasized that adolescents and adults have different risk factors than children younger than 8 years of age. In adults, for example, intraoperative complications have been associated with pericardial effusions diagnosed by CT scans, whereas postoperative respiratory complications have been associated with greater than 50% tracheal compression on preoperative CT.[131] Great care must be taken to properly prepare these children and families for general anesthesia, together with the attendant risks.

Induction of anesthesia in children with anterior mediastinal masses may be associated with severe airway obstruction and circulatory collapse.[125] This may occur even in children without signs or symptoms of respiratory or cardiovascular compromise.[132,133] Therefore a preoperative assessment of the position that provides the most reliable and consistent optimal gas exchange should be sought from the child or the parents (i.e., nocturnal sleep position). Recommended anesthetic techniques for children with anterior mediastinal masses include inhalation induction or a slow IV induction (with ketamine or propofol), with maintenance of spontaneous respirations. Inducing anesthesia in the sitting position minimizes the effect of gravity compared with the supine position, which may cause collapse of the tumor onto the pulmonary artery, superior vena cava, and/or tracheobronchial tree, causing life-threatening cardiopulmonary consequences.[119,127,134] Maintaining the sitting position as the child loses consciousness is very difficult as it is hard to stabilize the head; most prefer to induce anesthesia in such cases in the left lateral decubitus position, a position that facilitates laryngoscopy and tracheal intubation with right-handed laryngoscope blades.[119] The use of CPAP while maintaining spontaneous respirations maintains functional residual capacity that is otherwise reduced under anesthesia and prevents oxygen desaturation. In adolescents and adults, neuromuscular blockade is sometimes used to facilitate tracheal intubation and prevent coughing associated with TT placement; in general, however, neuromuscular blockade is avoided. Keeping the head of the bed elevated may decrease the deleterious effects of supine positioning, including cephalad

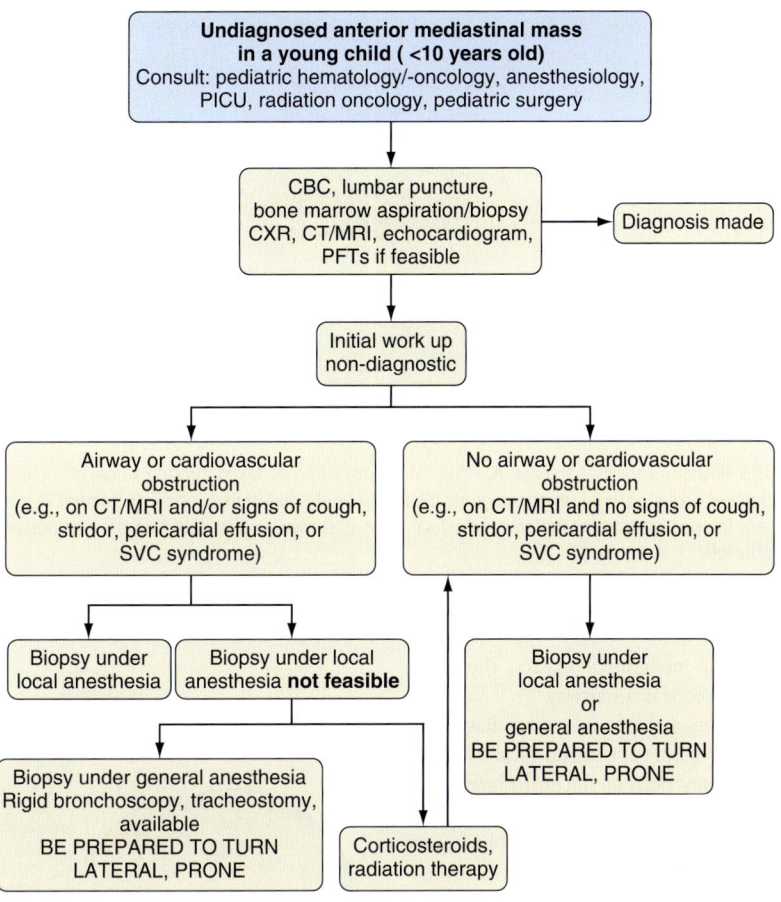

FIGURE 13.14 Algorithm for management of a child with a mediastinal mass. *CBC,* Complete blood cell count; *CPB,* cardiopulmonary bypass; *CT,* computed tomography; *CXR,* chest radiograph; *LP,* lumbar puncture; *MRI,* magnetic resonance imaging; *PFTs,* pulmonary function tests; *PICU,* pediatric intensive care unit; *SVC,* superior vena cava.

displacement of the diaphragm and secondary reduction of thoracic volume.[135] Placing the child in a partial or even full left lateral decubitus position may help to maintain airway patency and reduce cardiovascular and/or tracheal compression.[119] Performing tracheal intubation while the patient is deeply anesthetized without the use of muscle relaxants and positive-pressure ventilation preserves the normal transpulmonary pressure gradient and improves flow through conducting airways.[119,136–138] The loss of negative intrathoracic pressure associated with neuromuscular blockade increases the risk of severe airway compression and reduction in pulmonary blood flow (i.e., cardiac output).[139] As an alternative to tracheal intubation, use of a laryngeal mask airway has been described.[140] However, this could be a hazardous airway should the child need to be turned prone to restore cardiac output. The use of a helium-oxygen (70% to 30%) mixture has been recommended to decrease the resistance to breathing and to increase hemoglobin saturation when an anterior mediastinal tumor compresses the trachea and/or bronchi (i.e., where turbulent gas flow exists).[140] It should be remembered that at least 70% helium is needed to substantively increase the flow in the airway; this concentration limits the inspired concentration of oxygen. In the event of tracheal or bronchial collapse or the sudden disappearance of the capnograph (signaling a loss of pulmonary blood flow) under anesthesia, lateral or prone positioning provided the airway is secured with a tracheal tube and/or rigid bronchoscopy may be lifesaving.[119] Alternatively, towel clips or similar devices

may be placed in the xiphoid cartilage and sternal notch to lift the sternum and restore patency of the collapsed structure while a longer-term solution is planned.[141] Performing a median sternotomy and cardiopulmonary bypass in this situation has been recommended but is impractical unless access for partial bypass has been established before induction of anesthesia.[127] Institutions should have an algorithm in place for evaluating children with anterior mediastinal masses that includes a multidisciplinary approach (Fig. 13.14).[119]

Posterior mediastinal masses uncommonly present concerns for anesthesiologists. These masses, which comprise 51% of all mediastinal tumors, present with spinal cord or nerve root symptoms.[142] However, when these masses are silent and achieve a very large size, they will directly compress or erode into the lumen of the trachea and/or bronchus, which may become life-threatening very quickly. In such cases, a nonproductive cough and orthopnea will be the primary presenting symptoms. Unlike the age of presentation of anterior mediastinal masses, these masses usually present in younger age children (<5 years).[143,144] The tissue is usually neurogenic in origin, primarily neuroblastoma (the most common extracranial solid malignant tumor in children), followed by benign tumors such as ganglioneuroblastomas, ganglioneuromas, neurofibromas, or Schwannomas, and infrequently, abscesses (as in tuberculosis), meningoceles and aortic, esophageal, or lymphatic anomalies.[143,144] Rarely, lymphoma presents in the posterior mediastinum.[145,146] Like anterior mediastinal masses, only 6% of mediastinal tumors cause

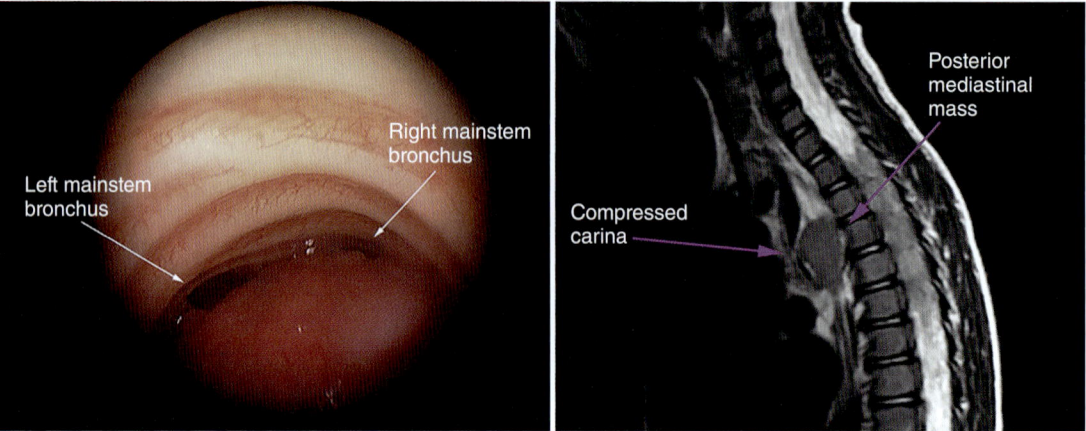

FIGURE 13.15 Posterior mediastinal mass. **A,** Photo of the distal trachea taken through a rigid bronchoscope. Note the distal tracheal occlusion, with slit openings for the left and right mainstem bronchi. **B,** Sagittal T2-weighted MRI image where the prevertebral (posterior) mediastinal mass is shown on the right and the compressed carina is shown on the left.

complications, but unlike anterior mediastinal masses, the main structure affected besides the spinal cord is the airway.[143,147] In a case of near complete airway obstruction, a child underwent diagnostic rigid bronchoscopy in preparation for a neurosurgical workup for foot drop (Fig. 13.15).[145] Ninety percent tracheal obstruction was diagnosed, a tracheal tube was positioned, after which an MRI and tissue biopsy were performed. B-cell Burkitt lymphoma was diagnosed and treated with chemotherapy that led to a complete recovery.

Point-of-Care Ultrasound Pulmonary Exam

INTRODUCTION TO THE LUNG EXAM

Point-of-care ultrasound (POCUS) is particularly well suited for use in children due to the accessibility and portability of the ultrasound machine, lack of radiation exposure, and ability to perform accurate, minimally invasive, dynamic assessments in real time. Ultrasound visualization of internal structures is often more clearly delineated in children than in adults due to their smaller size and differences in body composition (e.g., water, fat, organs). As a result, the diagnostic capabilities of pulmonary ultrasound demonstrate excellent sensitivity and specificity (e.g., pneumothorax, pleural effusion, interstitial disease) compared with chest radiography and chest CT in all age groups while avoiding radiation exposure.[148,149]

A variety of ultrasound transducers can be used for the pulmonary ultrasound examination depending on the patient's size and the goal of the examination. The microconvex transducer (4–7 MHz) is ideal for scanning between the ribs in the intercostal space with good penetration. The curvilinear transducer (2–5 MHz) is better suited for patients with thicker chest walls, such as teenagers and adults. The linear transducer (6.5–14 MHz) is optimal for visualizing the pleura and imaging multiple rib levels in neonates and infants.

The supine position is typically used for examination of the anterior and lateral chest for diagnoses including pneumothorax or pleural effusion. However, assessment for pediatric acute respiratory distress syndrome (PARDS) may necessitate the use of the sitting and lateral decubitus positions to fully appreciate full disease involvement.

The "batwing sign" is often used as a reference point in pulmonary ultrasound (Fig. 13.16). It represents the contour of two ribs

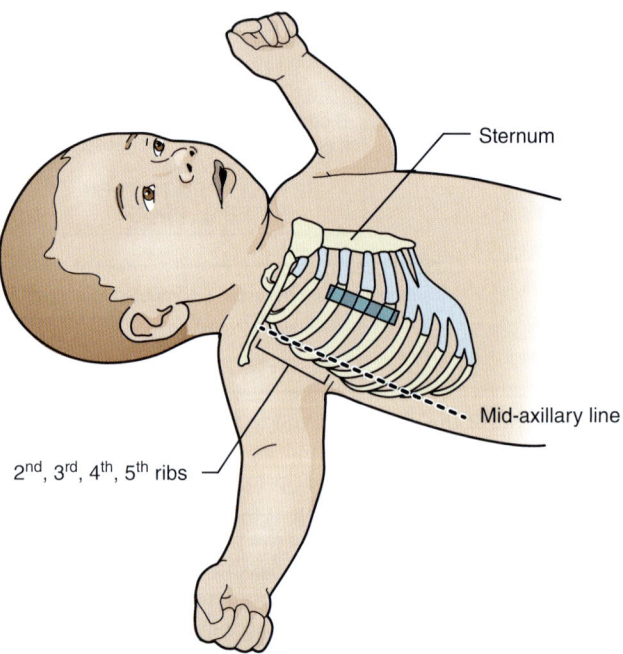

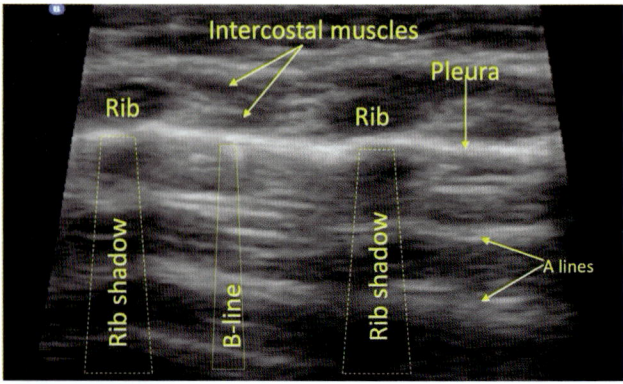

FIGURE 13.16 The "batwing" sign is the reference point in pulmonary ultrasound. The hyperechoic pleura is seen between two ribs. This image of a normal lung shows "A-lines" and a single "B-line."

with hyperechoic pleura in between. Because ultrasound waves travel poorly through calcified osseous structures, the ribs generate shadows seen as hypoechoic areas beneath each rib. However, it is common to see the pleura as a contiguous structure beneath the rib shadows as the ribs in children are less calcified. Although the ribs are seen as static hyperechoic structures, the pleura can be seen as a shimmering surface. The shimmering surface is generated by the sliding of the visceral pleura, which covers the lungs, against the parietal pleura that lines the inside of the chest wall with each inspiration and exhalation. This normal sonographic finding is known as "lung sliding" or "pleural sliding." Another sonographic finding in healthy lungs is the "A-line." A-lines are caused by reverberation artifacts from the insonation of an aerated lung. They can be seen as repeating parallel horizontal lines equidistant from the pleura.

Pneumothorax

Pulmonary ultrasound is excellent at identifying a pneumothorax (especially compared with the success rate of a chest x-ray, which fails to diagnose a pneumothorax 30%–60% of the time).[150] Because air prevents the visceral pleura from directly sliding against the parietal pleura, the absence of pleural sliding can signify a pneumothorax. Similarly, the presence of a "lung pulse" can be a sign of a possible pneumothorax. The lung pulse is caused by the absence of lung sliding such that cardiac activity is perceived at the pleural line. Despite the lack of pleural sliding or the presence of a lung pulse, the diagnosis of pneumothorax cannot be made without confirmation of a "lung point," the transition between normal lung sliding and the collapsed lung.

Lung sliding may be absent due to other reasons such as pleural adhesions, apnea, or large lung bullae. In thoracic surgery, ultrasound imaging for lung sliding can confirm successful lung isolation. M-mode lung examination, a one-dimensional time recording along a single ultrasound beam, can also be used to visualize a pneumothorax. M-mode of the normal lung has been described as the "seashore sign." Motion within the lung parenchyma creates a speckled appearance like grains of sand beneath the bright pleura line. The soft tissues superficial to the pleura do not move and thus have a linear appearance. In the presence of a pneumothorax, the M-mode image is better described by the "stratosphere sign" whereby the static structures create a linear appearance resembling a barcode.

Pleural Effusion

Ultrasound is excellent at identifying the presence of a pleural effusion and can detect amounts of fluid as small as 5 mL.[151] In comparison, a chest radiograph may be insensitive at detecting fluid volumes less than 150 mL.[152] Both the "curtain sign" and the "spine sign" can be used to detect a pleural effusion. Unlike adults, there has been no validated method to estimate the size of a pleural effusion through ultrasound examination for pediatric patients.[153]

The ultrasound transducer should be placed along the posterior axillary line in a rib interspace between the tenth and twelfth ribs to visualize the curtain and spine signs. The curtain sign is seen in healthy and aerated lungs such that the aerated lung acts like a curtain, sweeping down and over the diaphragm and either the liver on the right or the spleen on the left during inhalation. The diaphragm, liver, or spleen should reappear during exhalation.

The spine can be seen up to the edge of the diaphragm without passing the diaphragm as the air in the lungs prevents the transmission of ultrasonic waves. However, in pleural effusions, sound waves can pass through pleural fluid such that the spine can be seen above the diaphragm, thus generating the spine sign.

Pediatric Acute Respiratory Distress Syndrome

Unlike adult acute respiratory distress syndrome (ARDS), the preferred modality of imaging to diagnose PARDS remains unspecified.[154] Lung ultrasound can be used to diagnose PARDS.

The sonographic signs often found in PARDS include numerous "B-lines" in multiple lung sections bilaterally, disrupted and thickened pleura, consolidated lung tissue, and air bronchograms. These findings are usually seen in the supine position although visualization of the posterior areas may yield improved diagnostic sensitivity. Because these sonographic signs can be found in other diagnoses such as cardiogenic and noncardiogenic pulmonary edema, upper respiratory infection, or pneumonia,[155] classification systems based on combined lung and cardiac ultrasound findings with arterial blood gas analysis and the child's clinical history have been proposed to improve diagnostic clarity.[156]

B-lines occur in the presence of accumulated fluid in the interlobular septa. The accumulated fluid generates ultrasound reverberation artifacts that appear as transient, hyperechoic vertical lines that extend from the pleura to the bottom of the ultrasound screen. These vertical lines resemble searchlights or comet tails. Although the presence of one or two B-lines can be a normal finding, especially around the base of the lungs, multiple B-lines result from increasing fluid accumulation and decreasing air content. As fluid continues to build up and the air content further decreases, such as in the case of a pneumonia, the appearance of the lung under ultrasound takes on the echogenic characteristics of a solid organ such as the liver. These changes are therefore appropriately termed "hepatization of the lung." Occasionally air bronchograms, or pockets of trapped air, can also be seen as tiny hyperechoic specks within areas of consolidation.

Hemidiaphragmatic Paralysis

Ultrasonography can detect hemidiaphragmatic paralysis by visualizing diaphragmatic motion and thickening through M-mode scanning. One common approach uses the zone of apposition to visualize diaphragmatic movement by using the liver on the right side and the spleen on the left side as acoustic windows. Once the diaphragm is visualized, M-mode is used to measure the motion of the diaphragm during various respiratory maneuvers such as quiet breathing, sniffing, and deep breathing. The amplitude and velocity of the diaphragmatic excursion are measured from the baseline to the point of maximum height of inspiration. The accuracy of this approach is often difficult as the entire excursion may not be captured with deep breathing. In addition, finding and maintaining the hepatic and splenic acoustic windows can be challenging, especially through the spleen.[157] An alternative approach, called the ACBD approach, relies on a more systematic approach and uses basic visualization of the pleura without hepatic or splenic windows.[158,159] In short, the ultrasound transducer is placed at the **A**nterior axillary line such that **B**reaths or lung sliding are identified. The transducer is slid **C**audally to identify the **D**iaphragm for **E**xamination by observing for diaphragmatic muscle thickening without the involvement of

ABC Diaphragm Evaluation

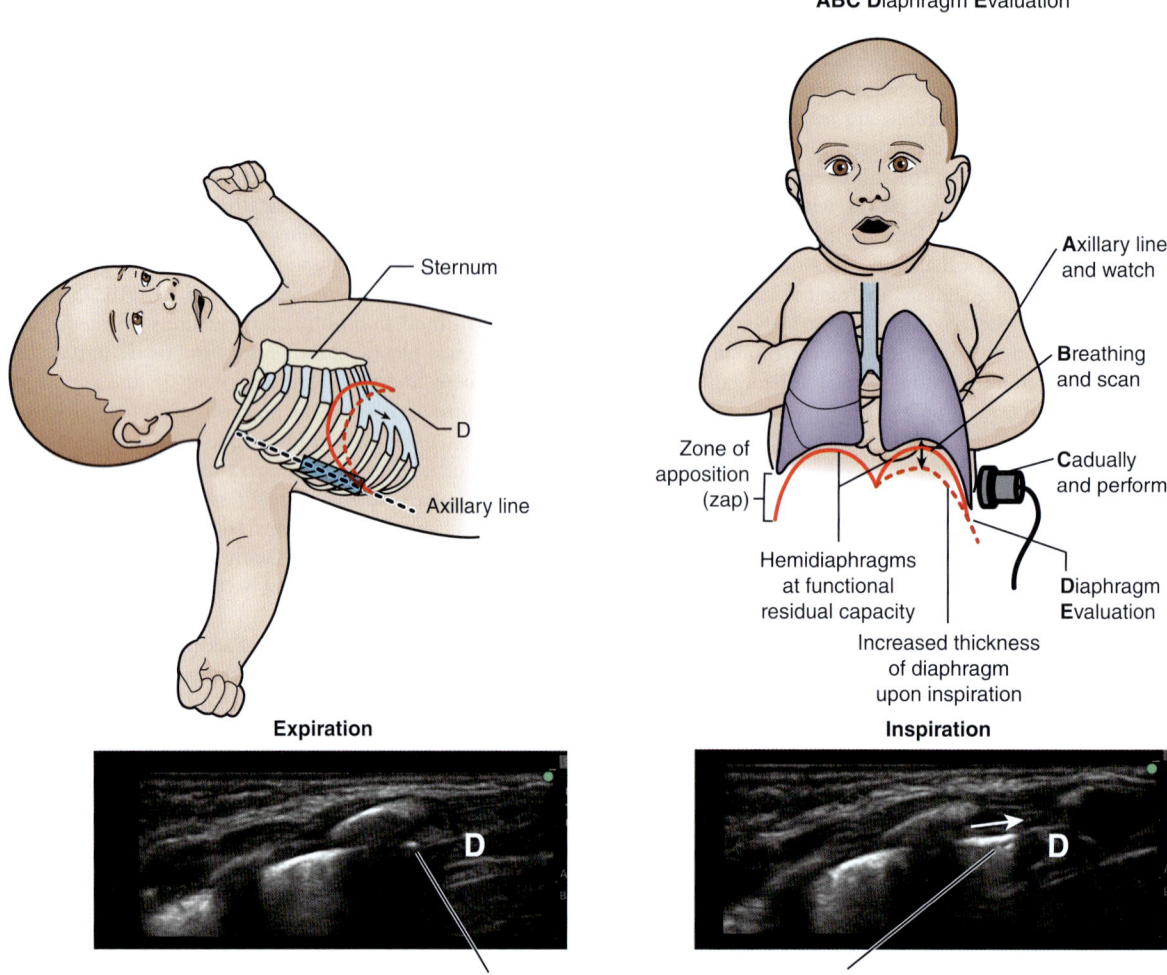

FIGURE 13.17 Diaphragmatic motion through the visualization of the pleural sliding down a rib level seen under ultrasound using the ABCDE approach. *D*, Diaphragm. During single-lung ventilation, pleural sliding pushes down the nonthickening diaphragm on the ventilated side, but not on the nonventilated side.

the pleura, as pleural motion can result from the paradoxical movement generated by the contralateral lung and diaphragm (Fig. 13.17). During spontaneous ventilation, the thickening fraction, calculated as the difference in the thickness on inspiration and at expiration divided by the thickness at expiration, is used to determine the presence of diaphragmatic paralysis.[160,161] During single-lung ventilation, the ventilated lung pushes the nonthickening diaphragm in a caudal direction with each positive-pressure breath, whereas on the nonventilated side, there is minimal lung sliding and diaphragmatic movement.

TRACHEAL DIAMETER FOR TRACHEAL TUBE SIZING

Appropriate TT size selection in the pediatric patient minimizes the need for multiple intubations that can lead to laryngeal trauma and swelling. Although age-based calculations for TT size are commonly used, ultrasound measurement provides a more accurate estimation of airway size (27.5% accuracy in age-based calculation vs. 87.8% accuracy with ultrasound) with lower frequencies of tube exchange (52% in age-based calculation vs. 12%

in ultrasound).[162,163] Ultrasound can also be used to measure the size of the trachea to facilitate appropriate selection of double-lumen tube, Univent, or bronchial blocker size, especially when other imaging of the trachea is unavailable.

To estimate the size of the appropriate TT with ultrasound, the child's head should be placed in the extended position. With the linear transducer in the transverse position across the midline of the neck, identify the vocal cords. Slide the transducer caudally until the cricoid cartilage comes into view. Measurement of the transverse air-column diameter at the level of the cricoid cartilage can be used to estimate the maximum size for the outer diameter of the TT (Fig. 13.18).[164] The transverse diameter is used because it is smaller than the anteroposterior diameter and acoustic air shadowing often obscures the posterior wall of the trachea.

Using the transverse subglottic diameter as the outer diameter of the TT without any conversion factors assumes that the cricoid is the narrowest portion of the airway. However, the narrowest part of the pediatric larynx actually occurs at the level of the vocal cords,

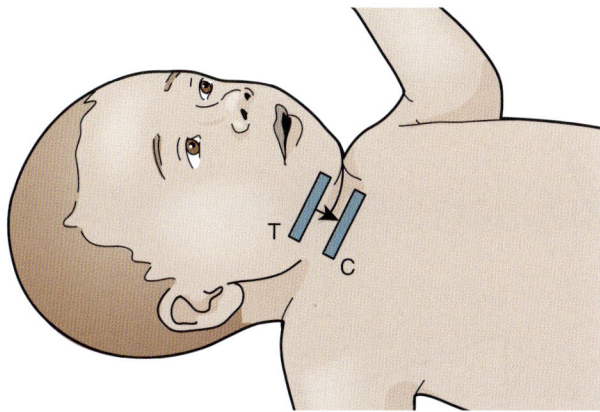

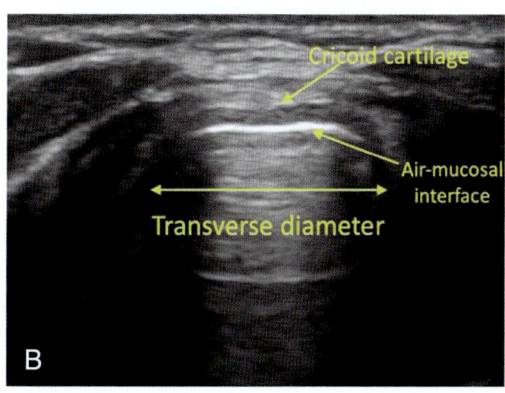

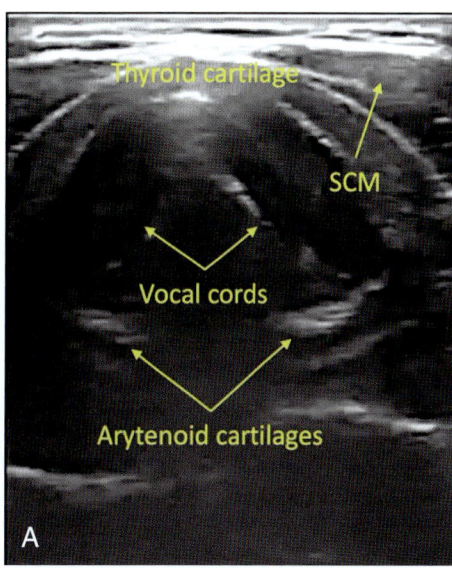

T: Thyroid cartilage

C: Circoid cartilage

FIGURE 13.18 Ultrasound images of the trachea at the level of the vocal cords **(A)** and at the level of the thyroid cartilage **(B)**. The transverse diameter below the level of the cricoid cartilage is used to estimate the size of the endotracheal tube. *SCM*, Sternocleidomastoid muscle.

followed by the subvocal cords and the cricoid.[165,166] This is in part due to measurements made during various parts of respirations (e.g., with inspiration the easily distended laryngeal structures [vocal cords, false cords, and aryepiglottic folds] move laterally [larger lumen] then move medially during expiration [smaller lumen]).[167] However, the narrowest portion of the airway is in fact the rigid nondistensible cricoid cartilage since all the other structures are easily distended with TT placement.[168] Therefore, it is not surprising that multiple conversion factors taking these varying observations into account would have various success rates.[169–173]

TRACHEAL TUBE POSITIONING WITH ULTRASOUND
Ultrasound can identify the appropriate positioning of a TT without exposure to radiation or risk of destabilizing a patient through changes in ventilation. The sensitivity and specificity for identifying an esophageal versus a tracheal intubation by ultrasound are both 100%. In contrast, the sensitivity and specificity for identifying an endobronchial mainstem intubation versus a tracheal intubation are 85.7% and 98.3%, respectively.[174]

The first step is to rule out an esophageal intubation by placing the transducer horizontally across the anterior neck to visualize the trachea. In an endotracheal intubation, a hyperechoic shadow can be seen within the hyperechoic cartilage of the trachea creating parallel hyperechoic arcs, or the "railroad sign" (Fig. 13.19). In an esophageal intubation, a hyperechoic circular structure can be seen adjacent to the trachea, often with a hyperechoic shadow within the lumen of the esophagus ("double trachea sign").

The second step is to determine the presence of an endotracheal versus endobronchial intubation. This method involves scanning the bilateral anterior lungs to assess for pleural sliding. Unilateral pleural sliding (usually on the right side) indicates an endobronchial position. Bilateral pleural sliding demonstrates an endotracheal position. Although the original intention of this sequence of assessments was to ensure an endotracheal intubation, this secondary step is equally helpful in determining whether appropriate lung isolation has been achieved or continues to be present after repositioning of the patient.

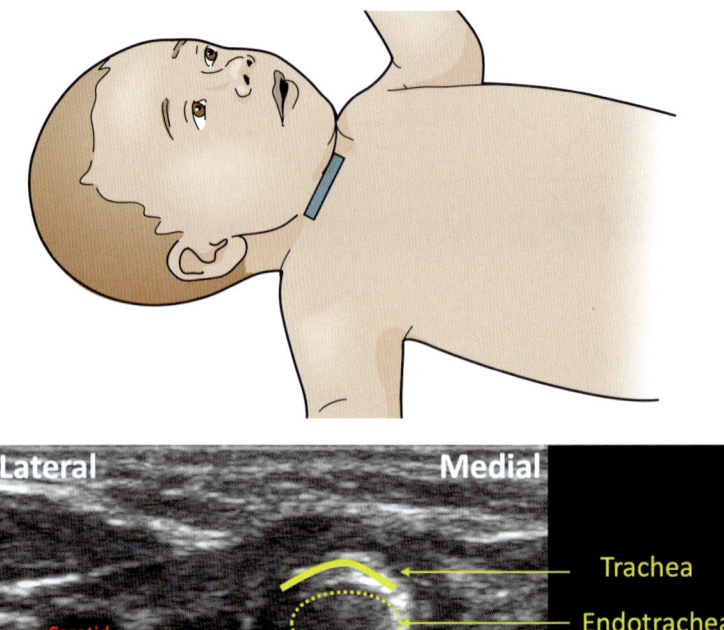

FIGURE 13.19 Ultrasound image of an endotracheal intubation where a hyperechoic shadow can be seen within the hyperechoic cartilage of the trachea creating parallel hyperechoic arcs, or the "railroad sign."

ANNOTATED REFERENCES

Capan LM, Turndorf H, Patel C, et al. Optimization of arterial oxygenation during one-lung anesthesia. *Anesth Analg.* 1980;59:847-851.
This article shows how the application of PEEP to the dependent and non-dependent lungs in one-lung ventilation can affect arterial oxygenation.

Fisher AO, Hussain K, Wolfson MR, et al. Hyperoxia during one lung ventilation: inflammatory and oxidative responses. *Pediatr Pulmonol.* 2012;47(10):979-986.
This is an important article describing the adverse effects (e.g., inflammation) caused by using high concentrations of oxygen for single-lung ventilation in a piglet model.

Hammer GB, Harrison TK, Vricella LA, et al. Single-lung ventilation in children using a new paediatric bronchial blocker. *Paediatr Anaesth.* 2002;12:69-72.
This article is the first to describe the use of the Cook 5 Fr pediatric endobronchial blocker. This is now the most commonly used bronchial blocker in children. The characteristics of the catheter and the details of the methodology for insertion and proper placement are highlighted.

Heaf DP, Helms P, Gordon MB, Turner HM. Postural effects on gas exchange in infants. *N Engl J Med.* 1983;28:1505-1508.
Changes in ventilation and perfusion of the lung associated with body position were first described in adults. This paper describes such relationships in infants, highlighting the important differences in this population that have significant clinical relevance during thoracic anesthesia.

Potter SK, Griksaitis MJ. The role of point-of-care ultrasound in pediatric acute respiratory distress syndrome: emerging evidence for its use. *Ann Transl Med.* 2019;7:507.

This review article presents the emerging evidence demonstrating that lung point-of-care ultrasound can be used to support the diagnosis of PARDS and to assess for complications, monitor progression, and guide management.

Rees DI, Wansbrough SR. One-lung anesthesia and arterial oxygen tension during continuous insufflation of oxygen to the nonventilated lung. *Anesth Analg.* 1982;61:507-512.
This article describes the maneuvers of choice for increasing oxygenation in patients during single-lung ventilation. Oxygen desaturation is common during single-lung ventilation, especially in children. It is essential that practitioners have an algorithm for addressing this problem promptly during surgery.

Templeton TW, Piccioni F, Chatterjee D. An update on one-lung ventilation in children. *Anesth Analg.* 2021;132:1389-1399.
This review provides a practical update to practicing pediatric anesthesiologists to further their understanding of the modern practice of single-lung ventilation for thoracic surgery in children. The development of new bronchial blockers, extraluminal blocker techniques, and improved understanding of the relevant anatomic constraints of the lower pediatric airway have driven changes in practice.

Wilson CA, Arthurs OJ, Black AE, et al. Printed three-dimensional airway model assists planning of single-lung ventilation in a small child. *Br J Anaesth.* 2015;115(4):616-620.
Although published as a single case report, this article highlights the utility of using 3D printing for planning the use of single-lung ventilation in an individual child. This may become an important technique going forward as 3D printing becomes more widely available and cost-effective.

A complete reference list can be found online at Elsevier eBooks+.

Essentials of Cardiology

14

WANDA C. MILLER-HANCE AND RALPH GERTLER

Congenital Heart Disease
Incidence
Segmental Approach to Diagnosis
Physiologic Classification of Pediatric Heart Disease
Acquired Heart Disease
Cardiomyopathies
Myocarditis
Rheumatic Fever and Rheumatic Heart Disease
Infective Endocarditis
Kawasaki Disease
Cardiac Tumors
Heart Failure in Children
Definition and Pathophysiology
Etiology and Clinical Features
Treatment Strategies
Anesthetic Considerations
**Syndromes, Associations, and Systemic Disorders:
Cardiovascular Disease and Anesthetic Implications**
Chromosomal Syndromes
Gene Deletion Syndromes
Single-Gene Defects
Associations
Other Disorders
**Selected Vascular Anomalies and Their
Implications for Anesthesia**
Aberrant Subclavian Artery

Persistent Left Superior Vena Cava to the Coronary Sinus
Evaluation of the Child with a Cardiac Murmur
Basic Interpretation of the Electrocardiogram in Children
**Essentials of Cardiac Rhythm Interpretation and Acute
Management of Arrhythmias in Children**
Basic Rhythms and Conduction Disorders
Cardiac Arrhythmias
**Pacemaker and Defibrillator Therapy in the
Pediatric Age Group**
Pacemaker Nomenclature
Permanent Cardiac Pacing
Diagnostic Modalities in Pediatric Cardiology
Chest Radiography
Barium Esophagram
Echocardiography
Cardiovascular Magnetic Resonance Imaging
Computed Tomography
Cardiac Catheterization and Angiography
**Perioperative Considerations for Children with
Cardiovascular Disease**
General Issues
Clinical Condition and Status of Prior Repair

Congenital Heart Disease

INCIDENCE

Congenital heart disease (CHD), defined as a structural abnormality in the heart or major blood vessel existing from birth, is the most common major congenital anomaly in humans. In the most recent Global Burden of Disease Study, the global prevalence of CHD at birth was estimated to be that of approximately 1.8 cases per 100 live births.[1] The prevalence of CHD in preterm infants is even greater than that in full-term infants.[2] It is estimated that nearly 40,000 births per year in the United States are affected by CHD.[3] Approximately one in four neonates with CHD have severe or critical disease requiring a surgical intervention or other procedure in their first year of life. Although CHD represents the leading cause of neonatal mortality, advances in medical and surgical management over the past several decades, including significant contributions related to anesthesia care, have led to increasing survival rates among affected infants.[4] This progress accounts for the substantial global increase in the prevalence of CHD in both children and adults over time.[5]

A bicuspid aortic valve, the most common congenital cardiac defect, occurs in approximately to 1% to 2% of the general population (Video 14.1).[3] In a neonatal population, the prevalence of bicuspid aortic valve was reported to be ~4.6 per 1000 live-born neonates, with a greater prevalence in males.[6] Communications such as ventricular septal defects (VSDs; Video 14.2), atrial septal defects (ASDs; Video 14.3), and patent ductus arteriosus (PDA) represent the next most common congenital pathologies.[5] Among cyanotic lesions, tetralogy of Fallot (TOF) predominates, affecting ~4.4% of children with CHD (Fig. 14.1).[5] This defect may not be detected until later in life because cyanosis is absent or only mild arterial desaturation is present in some infants. In the first week of life, D-transposition of the great arteries is the most frequently encountered cause of cardiac cyanosis (Fig. 14.2).

SEGMENTAL APPROACH TO DIAGNOSIS

The *segmental, sequential approach* is the essence of diagnostic assessment in CHD.[7–9] It assumes a stepwise, systematic examination of all cardiac structures or segments and their relationships (i.e., connections or alignments between segments) by navigating through the heart in the direction of blood flow. The fundamental principle of this scheme is that specific cardiac chambers and vascular structures have characteristic morphologic properties that determine their identities, rather than their positions within the body.[10]

The approach starts by determining the cardiac position within the thorax, the direction of the cardiac apex, and the arrangement or situs of the thoracic and abdominal organs. The cardiac position can be described as the spatial location of most of the cardiac mass within the thorax, using the sternum as the midline reference (Fig. 14.3). The cardiac orientation refers to the alignment from the base (great arteries) to the apex (ventricular apex). In most cases, the cardiac position and base-to-apex orientation agree, namely, both are aligned in the same direction. Thus, for simplicity the following terms are frequently used in clinical practice: *levocardia* if the heart is in the left hemithorax and the ventricular apex is directed toward the left (as is the case of the normal heart); *dextrocardia* if the heart is in the right hemithorax and the apex is toward the right; and *mesocardia* if the heart and apex are in midline position. An abnormal location of the heart within the thorax into the right or left thoracic cavity is referred to as *dextropositioning* or *levopositioning*, respectively. This can result from displacement of the heart by adjacent structures or underlying noncardiac malformations (e.g., diaphragmatic hernia, lung hypoplasia, scoliosis).

The visceral situs, or sidedness, of the abdominal organs (i.e., liver and stomach) and atrial situs are considered independently (Fig. 14.4). Visceral situs is classified as *solitus* (i.e., normal

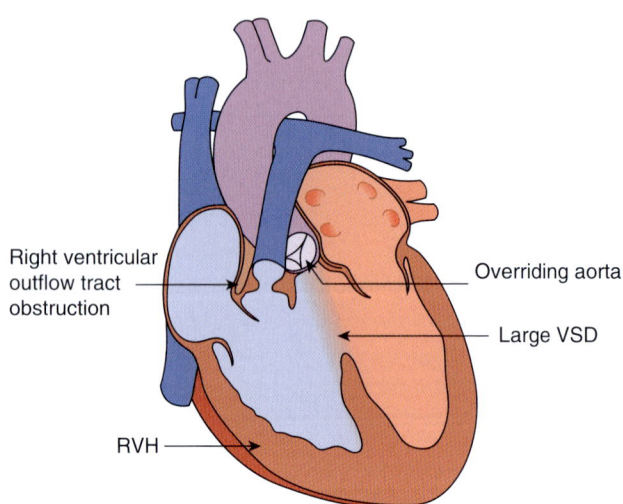

FIGURE 14.1 The anatomic features of tetralogy of Fallot are depicted, consisting of right ventricular outflow tract obstruction (may occur at any or a combination of valvar, subvalvular, and supravalvular levels), a large ventricular septal defect *(VSD)*, aortic override, and right ventricular hypertrophy *(RVH)*. The *purple color* in the aorta represents arterial desaturation from intracardiac right-to-left shunting. Note the infundibular narrowing and the hypoplastic pulmonary arteries.

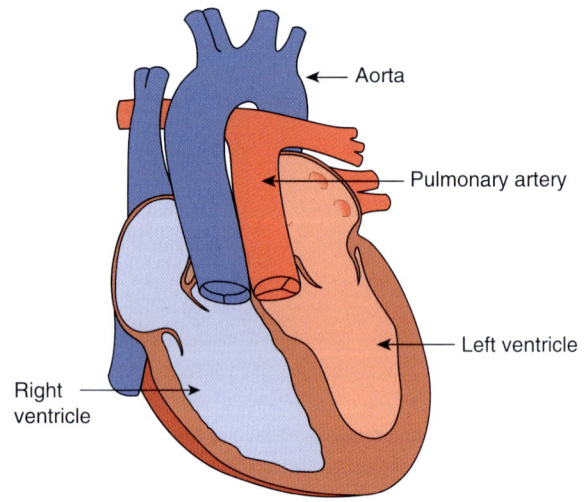

FIGURE 14.2 Diagrammatic representation of D-transposition of the great arteries displaying the discordant ventriculoarterial connections. In this lesion, the right ventricle ejects blood into the aorta and the left ventricle ejects blood into the pulmonary artery. Intercirculatory mixing is essential for survival in this anomaly.

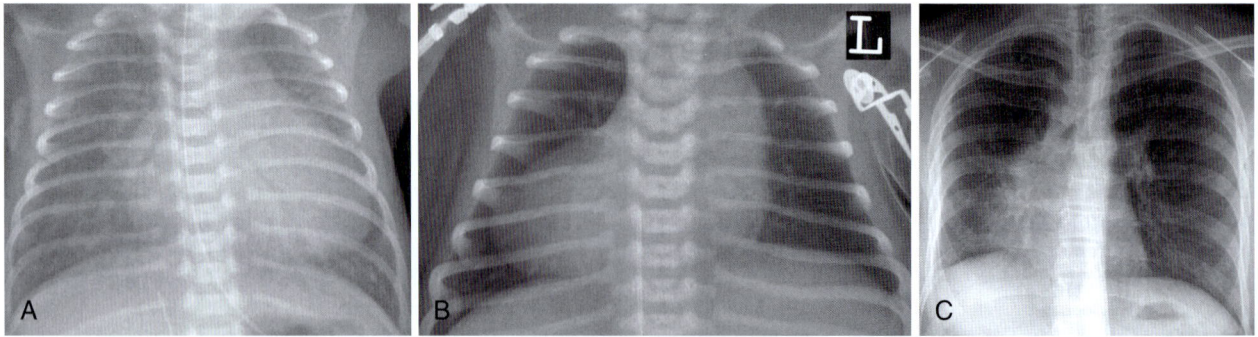

FIGURE 14.3 Chest radiographs demonstrate various cardiac positions within the thorax. **A,** Levocardia (left-sided position). **B,** Dextrocardia (right-sided position). **C,** Mesocardia (centrally located cardiac mass).

Types of visceroatrial situs: atrial localization

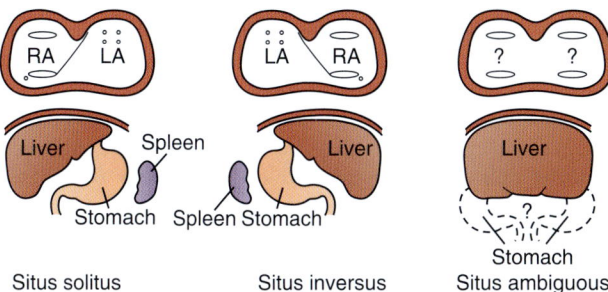

Situs solitus   Situs inversus   Situs ambiguous

FIGURE 14.4 Three types of visceroatrial situs are shown. *Situs solitus* indicates a normal arrangement of the viscera and atria, with the right atrium *(RA)* on the right side and the left atrium *(LA)* on the left side. The stomach and spleen are on the left, and the liver is on the right. *Situs inversus* indicates inverted arrangement of viscera and atria, with the RA on the left side and the LA on the right side, as in a mirror image of *situs solitus*. In visceral *situs inversus*, the stomach and spleen are on the right, and the liver is on the left. *Situs ambiguous* denotes that the visceroatrial situs is anatomically uncertain or indeterminate because the anatomic findings are ambiguous. (Reproduced with permission from Park MK, Salamat M. *Park's Pediatric Cardiology for Practitioners.* 7th ed. Philadelphia, PA: Elsevier, 2021:243-246.)

arrangement of viscera, with the liver on the right, stomach on the left, and a single spleen on the left), *inversus* (i.e., inversion of viscera, with the liver on the left and stomach on the right), or *ambiguous* (i.e., indeterminate visceral position). Abnormal arrangements or sidedness of the abdominal viscera, heart, and lungs, as seen in *heterotaxy syndromes*, also referred to isomerism, are associated with a high likelihood of complex cardiovascular disease (Fig. 14.5). The atrial situs or arrangement, atrioventricular (AV) connections, ventricular looping (i.e., position of the ventricles from the direction of bending of the straight heart tube during early development), ventriculoarterial connections, and the relationship between the great vessels are then delineated. Additional goals of the complete morphologic evaluation in CHD include, among other aspects, interrogation of structures such as the branch pulmonary arteries, aortic arch, and coronary arteries.

Associated malformations are described, including number, size, and location of septal defects, valvar pathology, and great vessel abnormalities. Whereas many types of congenital defects fall neatly into well-known classification schemes, others, such as those associated with heterotaxy syndromes where there may be malposition of the heart and abdominal organs and complex arrangements, are often more difficult to precisely define.

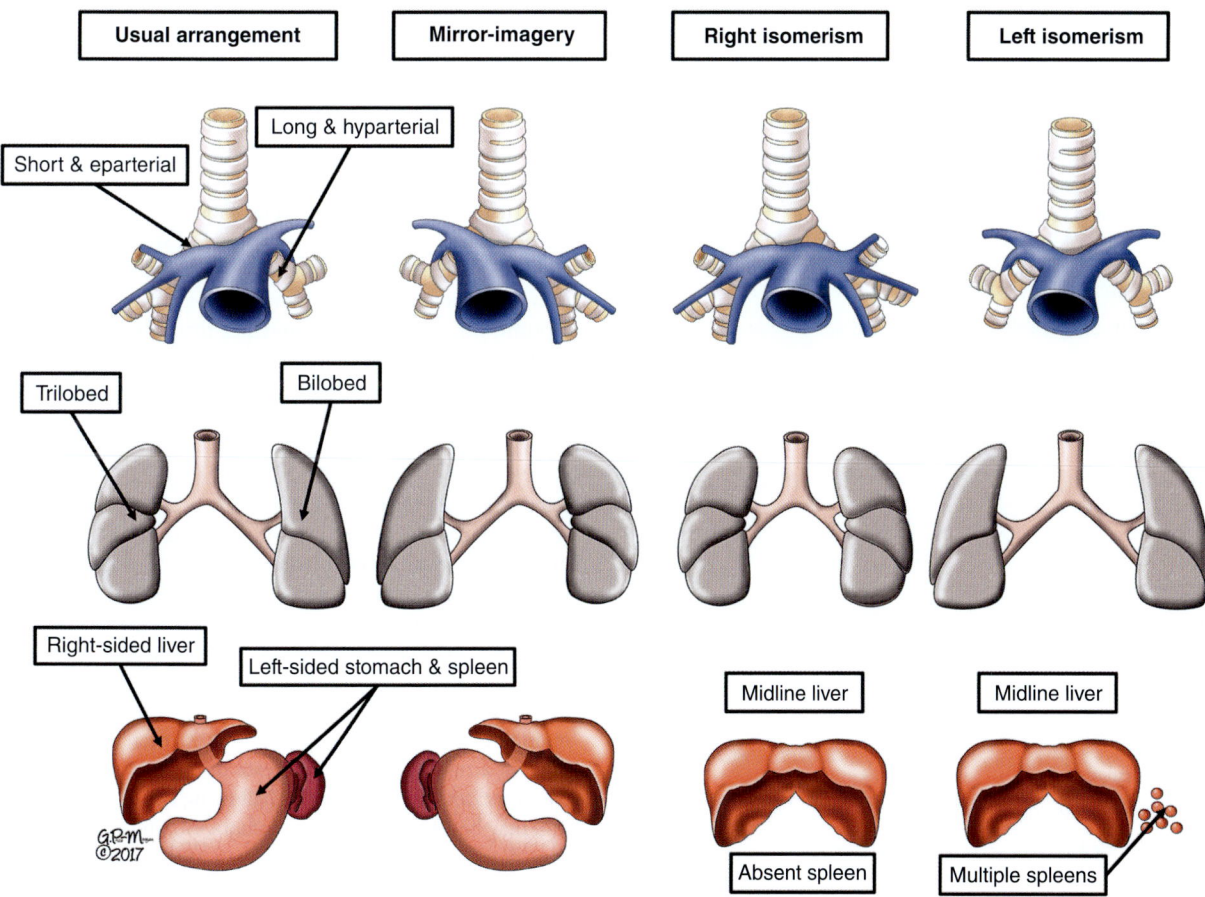

FIGURE 14.5 The graphic depicts variations of the bodily organs. The lateralized (left two columns) and isomeric (right two columns) arrangements of the bodily organs in the clinical settings are shown. The *upper panels* show the bronchial morphology, and the relations of the bronchi to the pulmonary arteries. The *middle panels* show the pulmonary (lobar) morphology. The *lower panels* show the arrangement of the abdominal organs. (Reproduced from Anderson RH, Spicer DE, Loomba R. Is an appreciation of isomerism the key to unlocking the mysteries of the cardiac findings in heterotaxy? *J Cardiovasc Dev Dis.* 2018;5:1-11. Used under Creative Commons Attribution (CC BY) license).

PHYSIOLOGIC CLASSIFICATION OF PEDIATRIC HEART DISEASE

The wide spectrum of cardiovascular malformations in the pediatric age group presents a challenge to the clinician who does not specialize in the care of these children. Even for those with a focus or interest in cardiovascular disease, the wide range of structural defects and the varied associated physiologic perturbations can be overwhelming (see Chapter 21). These barriers may be less of a case when acquired conditions that affect the cardiovascular system in children are considered, but nevertheless, they may also impact patient care.

Several classification schemes have been proposed to broadly categorize the various congenital cardiac defects, including some that catalog the malformations into simple or complex lesions, consider the presence or absence of cyanosis, or recognize whether pulmonary blood flow is increased or decreased.[11–13] A physiologic classification system, as displayed in Table 14.1, can also facilitate understanding of the basic hemodynamic abnormalities common to a group of congenital lesions or acquired conditions and assist in patient management.[13,14] The following approach sorts pediatric heart disease into these six broad categories according to the underlying physiology or common features of the pathologies.

Volume Overload Lesions

Volume overload lesions typically are caused by left-to-right shunting at the level of the atria, ventricles, or great arteries. If the location of the shunt is proximal to the mitral valve (e.g., ASD, partial anomalous pulmonary venous return, unobstructed total anomalous pulmonary venous return), right heart dilation occurs. Lesions distal to the mitral valve (e.g., VSD, PDA, truncus arteriosus) lead to left heart dilation. Children with AV septal defects, also referred to as AV canal or endocardial cushion defects, also fit into this category. The magnitude of the shunt and resultant pulmonary-to-systemic blood flow ratio ($\dot{Q}_{pulm}/\dot{Q}_{sys}$) dictate the presence and severity of the symptoms and guide medical and surgical therapies. Diuretic therapy and afterload reduction are beneficial in controlling pulmonary over-circulation and ensuring adequate systemic cardiac output. Surgical interventions or transcatheter approaches may be considered to address the primary pathology associated with ventricular volume overload (see Chapter 20).

Obstruction to Systemic Blood Flow

Several lesions are associated with systemic outflow tract obstruction. Conditions characterized by ductal-dependent systemic blood flow in the neonate include critical aortic stenosis, severe aortic coarctation, aortic arch interruption, and hypoplastic left heart syndrome. Prostaglandin E_1 therapy maintains ductal patency and ensures adequate systemic blood flow until a surgical or transcatheter intervention is performed to relieve the outflow obstruction. Inotropic and/or mechanical ventilatory support are often necessary in the affected neonate/small infant. These children frequently also have increased pulmonary blood flow with a large $\dot{Q}_{pulm}/\dot{Q}_{sys}$ ratio, requiring diuretic therapy and balancing of the systemic and pulmonary circulations to control blood flows, favor cardiac output, and ensure tissue oxygen delivery.

Obstruction to Pulmonary Blood Flow

Defects with pulmonary outflow tract obstruction include those with ductal-dependent pulmonary blood flow. Critical pulmonary valve stenosis and pulmonary atresia with intact ventricular septum, for example, are anomalies that rely on patency of the ductus arteriosus for pulmonary blood flow. Affected infants frequently require prostaglandin E_1 infusions for management of their cyanosis until the pulmonary outflow obstruction is relieved or bypassed.

Parallel Circulation

In the neonate with D-transposition of the great arteries, the pulmonary and systemic circulations operate in parallel rather than in the normal configuration in series. In this condition, the right ventricle ejects deoxygenated blood into the aorta, and the left ventricle ejects oxygenated blood into the pulmonary arteries. Mixing of blood in this setting can occur at the atrial, ventricular, or ductal levels (see Fig. 14.2). Although prostaglandin E_1 therapy maintains ductal patency and enhances intercirculatory mixing, balloon atrial septostomy to create or enlarge an existing restrictive interatrial communication, allowing for or augmenting mixing, may be necessary in some infants. Mixing at the atrial level is considered much more effective than at the ventricular or ductal levels.

Single-Ventricle Lesions

This category is the most heterogeneous group, consisting of defects associated with AV valve atresia (i.e., tricuspid atresia), heterotaxy syndromes, and many others.[15] In some cases, both atria empty into a dominant ventricular chamber (i.e., double-inlet left ventricle), and although a second rudimentary ventricle can be

TABLE 14.1	Physiologic Classification of Congenital Heart Disease (Representative Lesions)
Volume Overload Lesions	
Atrial septal defect	
Ventricular septal defect	
Atrioventricular septal defect	
Patent ductus arteriosus	
Truncus arteriosus	
Obstruction to Systemic Blood Flow	
Aortic stenosis	
Coarctation of the aorta	
Interrupted aortic arch	
Hypoplastic left heart syndrome	
Obstruction to Pulmonary Blood Flow	
Pulmonary stenosis	
Tetralogy of Fallot	
Pulmonary atresia	
Parallel Circulation	
D-Transposition of the great arteries	
Single-Ventricle Lesions	
Tricuspid atresia	
Double-inlet left ventricle	
Unbalanced atrioventricular septal defect	
Intrinsic Myocardial Disorders	
Cardiomyopathy	
Myocarditis	

present, the physiology is that of a single-ventricle or univentricular heart. Other cardiac malformations with two distinct ventricles (i.e., unbalanced AV septal defect) can also be considered in the functional single-ventricle spectrum because of associated defects that may preclude a biventricular repair. A common feature of these lesions is complete mixing of the systemic and pulmonary venous blood at the atrial or ventricular level prior to palliation. Another frequent finding is aortic or pulmonary outflow tract obstruction.

An important goal in single-ventricle management involves optimization of the balance between the pulmonary and systemic circulations early in life. This is a critical issue because low pulmonary vascular resistance, limitation of ventricular volume overload, and preserved ventricular function are prerequisites for later palliative strategies and optimal outcomes in these children. These considerations are also relevant for anesthesia management during noncardiac surgery given that children with single-ventricle physiology represent a high-risk group for adverse perioperative events (see Chapter 21).[16–24]

Intrinsic Myocardial Disorders

Children with primary cardiomyopathies or myocarditis have intrinsic diseases of cardiac muscle. They frequently have impaired systolic and/or diastolic ventricular function and benefit from therapies tailored to their disease process.

Acquired Heart Disease

CARDIOMYOPATHIES

The term *cardiomyopathy* refers to diseases of the myocardium associated with cardiac dysfunction.[25–27] They have been classified as primary and secondary forms.[28] Primary forms are those predominantly involving the heart owing to genetic mutation, including ion channelopathies, acquired disease, or mixed. The most common types in children are dilated, hypertrophic, and restrictive cardiomyopathies. Other less common forms include left ventricular noncompaction cardiomyopathy (LVNC)[29–31] and arrhythmogenic right ventricular cardiomyopathy.[32] Secondary forms of cardiomyopathies are those with systemic involvement in other organ systems as seen in association with neuromuscular disorders such as Duchenne muscular dystrophy, glycogen storage diseases (e.g., Pompe disease), hemochromatosis or iron overload, and mitochondrial disorders. Chemotherapeutic agents such as anthracyclines can result in dilated cardiomyopathy. It is important to understand the hemodynamic processes behind the myocardial disease and implications for acute and chronic management.

Dilated cardiomyopathy (DCM), also known as congestive cardiomyopathy, is characterized by thinning of the left ventricular myocardium, dilation of the ventricular cavity, and systolic functional impairment.[33] The broad number of etiologies range from genetic or familial forms to those caused by infections, metabolic derangements, toxic exposures, and degenerative disorders.[34] Chronic tachyarrhythmias can also lead to dilated cardiomyopathy that may or may not improve after control of the rhythm disturbance.

Most children with dilated cardiomyopathy present with signs and symptoms of congestive heart failure (e.g., tachypnea, tachycardia, gallop rhythm, diminished pulses, hepatosplenomegaly). The chest radiograph (CXR) typically demonstrates cardiomegaly, pulmonary vascular congestion, and in some cases, atelectasis (Fig. 14.6). The electrocardiogram (ECG) can identify the likely

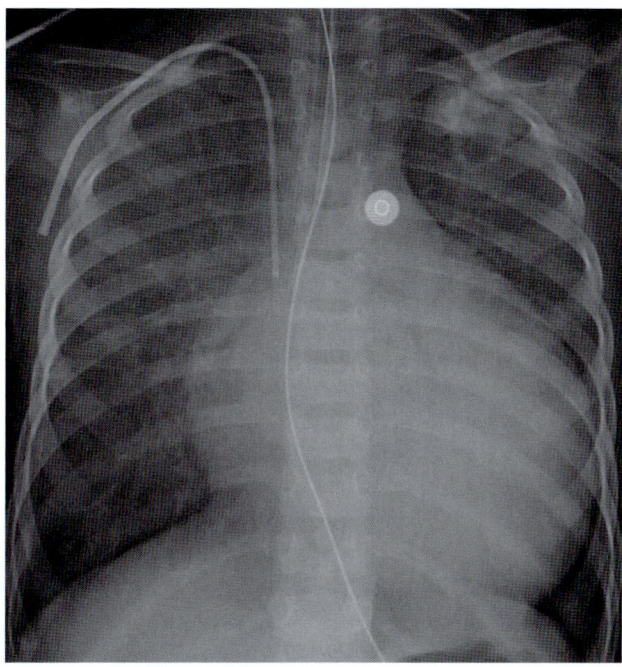

FIGURE 14.6 The chest radiograph of a young child with dilated cardiomyopathy in the posteroanterior projection depicts moderate to severe cardiomegaly and pulmonary vascular congestion. Note the presence of a central venous catheter with its tip appropriately positioned at the junction of the superior vena cava and right atrium, as well as a feeding tube.

etiology of the cardiac dysfunction in those with cardiomyopathy caused by rhythm disorders or anomalous origin of the left coronary artery from the pulmonary artery (ALCAPA). The echocardiogram can confirm the suspected diagnosis by demonstrating a dilated left ventricle with decreased systolic function (Video 14.4 A,B). The use of brain natriuretic peptide (BNP) and N-terminal pro-brain natriuretic peptide (NT-proBNP) in the evaluation and treatment of children with CHD in general has been widely demonstrated, including in those with dilated cardiomyopathy.[35–37] Therapy in the acute setting is supportive and aimed at stabilization. Management includes afterload reduction, inotropic support, and mechanical ventilation. Children with dilated cardiomyopathy have a volume-loaded, poorly contractile ventricle; gentle diuresis may be beneficial. The infusion of large fluid boluses is poorly tolerated and can result in hemodynamic decompensation and cardiovascular collapse. Several options have been considered for long-term management of heart failure in children, including drug therapy (e.g., angiotensin-converting-enzyme inhibitors, β and other cardiac channel blockers), cardiac resynchronization therapy, palliative pulmonary artery banding, and cell therapy.[38] New medical therapies are also emerging for chronic heart failure (refer to section on Heart Failure in Children).[39,40] The outcomes of children with dilated cardiomyopathy vary. For most, either the extent of cardiac dysfunction remains unchanged or recovery of left ventricular systolic function occurs, but others eventually require cardiac transplantation.[41] A subset of children with severe disease may require mechanical circulatory support as a bridge to recovery or cardiac transplantation (Fig. 14.7A,B) (see Chapter 19).[42–46]

Hypertrophic cardiomyopathy (HCM) is characterized by ventricular hypertrophy without an identifiable hemodynamic cause that results in increased myocardial wall thickness.[47–49] This

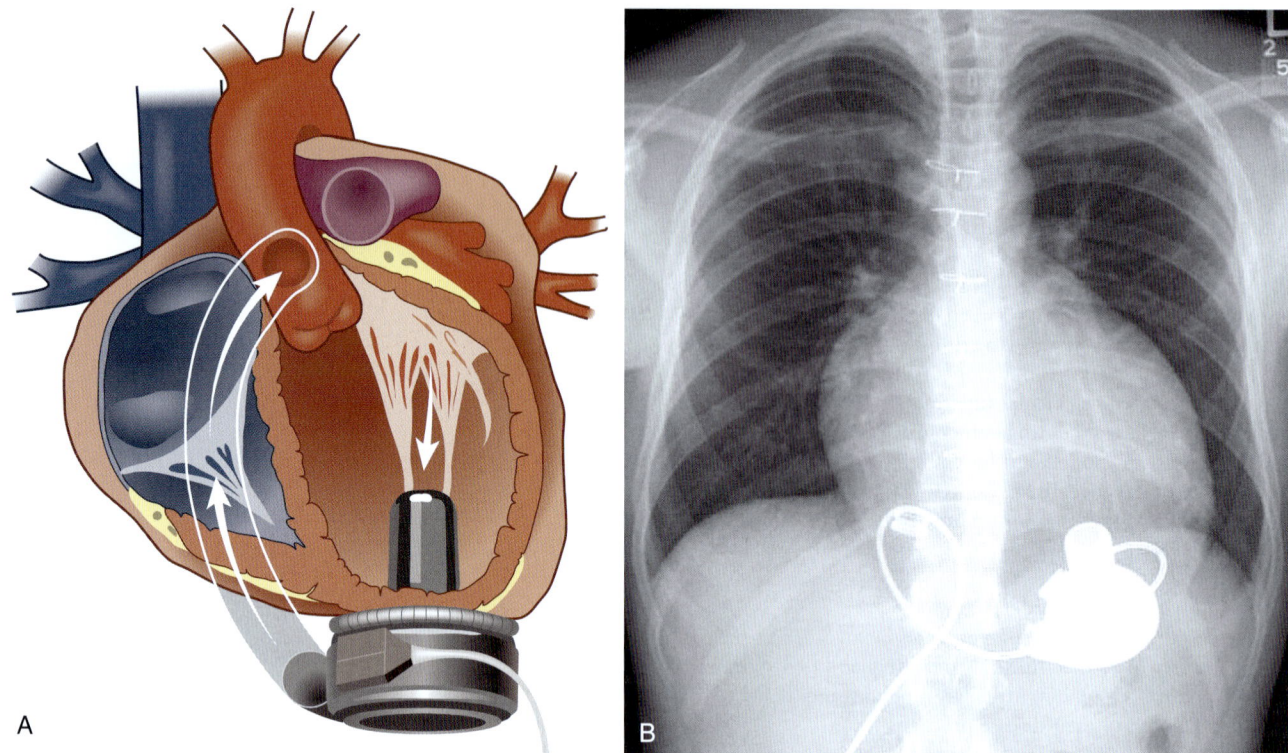

FIGURE 14.7 Mechanical circulatory support may be required in children with dilated cardiomyopathy (DCM) and severe cardiac dysfunction. **A,** A ventricular assist device system consists of a small continuous-flow pump with integrated inlet cannula placed in the left ventricle, an outflow graft placed in the aorta (not radiopaque), and a driveline that connects to an external controller with a power source. **B,** Chest radiograph of a child with end-stage dilated cardiomyopathy after placement of a ventricular assist device for circulatory support as a bridge to cardiac transplantation. (Illustration **A** reproduced with permission from Texas Children's Hospital.)

accounts for almost 40% of cardiomyopathies in children.[50–52] The condition represents a heterogeneous group of disorders, and most of the identified genetic defects exhibit autosomal dominant inheritance patterns.[53] This is the most common cause of sudden cardiac death (SCD) in athletes. Some children with hypertrophic cardiomyopathy have left ventricular outflow tract obstruction (i.e., obstructive cardiomyopathy). Risk factors for heart failure and sudden cardiac death in children appear to differ from those documented in the adult population and efforts to define them continue to be the objective of ongoing investigations.[54] It is unclear whether those with hypertrophic obstructive cardiomyopathy, previously known as idiopathic hypertrophic subaortic stenosis, are at increased risk for sudden cardiac death compared with children without obstruction or if obstruction may be protective.[54–57]

Most children with hypertrophic cardiomyopathy present for evaluation of a heart murmur, syncope, palpitations, or chest pain. Occasionally, an abnormal ECG leads to referral. A detailed family history is essential. Upon physical examination, palpation of an apical impulse is often prominent; auscultation may reveal a systolic ejection outflow murmur that becomes louder with maneuvers that decrease preload or afterload (e.g., standing, Valsalva maneuver) or increased contractility. The murmur decreases in intensity with squatting and isometric hand grip. A mitral regurgitant murmur can also be present. The ECG meets criteria for left ventricular hypertrophy in most children (Fig. 14.8). In some, the electrocardiographic findings can be striking (Fig. 14.9). A hypertrophied, nondilated left ventricle is a diagnostic feature as determined by two-dimensional echocardiography (Video 14.5 A,B). In many children, the hypertrophy can be asymmetric

(Video 14.6 A,B). Echocardiography is the preferred imaging tool for long-term assessment of ventricular wall thickness, chamber dimensions, presence and severity of obstruction, systolic and diastolic function, valve competence, and response to therapy. Other diagnostic approaches such as cardiac catheterization and cardiovascular magnetic resonance imaging can add helpful information in some cases.

The care of children with hypertrophic cardiomyopathy includes maintenance of adequate ventricular preload, particularly in those with dynamic obstruction. Diuretics are not indicated and can be detrimental to the hemodynamic state by reducing left ventricular volume and increasing the outflow tract obstruction. Drugs that augment myocardial contractility (e.g., inotropic agents, calcium infusions) are not well tolerated. β-Blockers and calcium channel blockers are the primary drugs for outpatient therapy. Therapies in the pediatric age group range widely and include longitudinal observation with medical management of heart failure and arrhythmias, implantation of a cardioverter-defibrillator (potential option in older children/young adults), surgical myotomy or myectomy, and cardiac transplantation. The limited published experience indicates that when affected pediatric patients undergo anesthetic care at specialized centers there is a relatively low perianesthetic mortality (0.6%) and prevalence of minor complications (12% of cases).[58] With careful balancing of preload and afterload, these cases can be undertaken with inhalational anesthesia and a vasoconstrictor even for complex noncardiac surgery.[59]

Restrictive cardiomyopathy (RCM) is the least common of the major types of cardiomyopathies (5%) and portends a poor

14

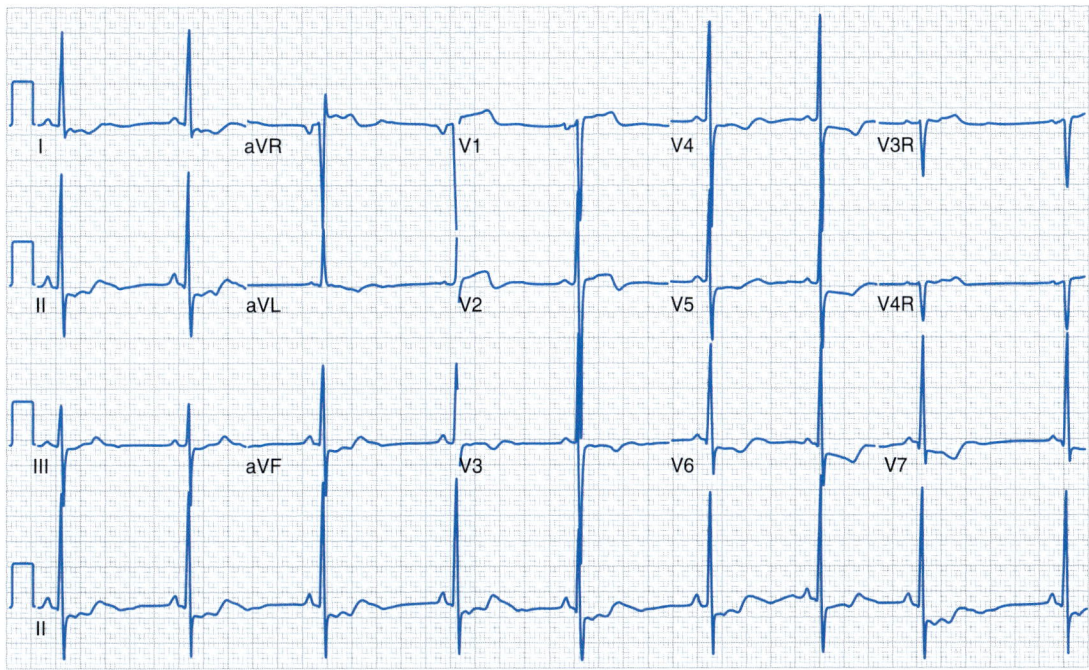

FIGURE 14.8 The electrocardiogram from an adolescent with hypertrophic cardiomyopathy demonstrates left ventricular hypertrophy (i.e., deep S wave in lead V₁ and tall R waves over the left precordial leads). The ST-segment depression and T-wave inversion over the left precordial leads are related to repolarization changes associated with left ventricular hypertrophy, also known as a *strain pattern*. Reciprocal ST-segment elevation can be seen over the right precordial leads. This recording is consistent with sinus bradycardia (heart rate average of 50 beats/minute).

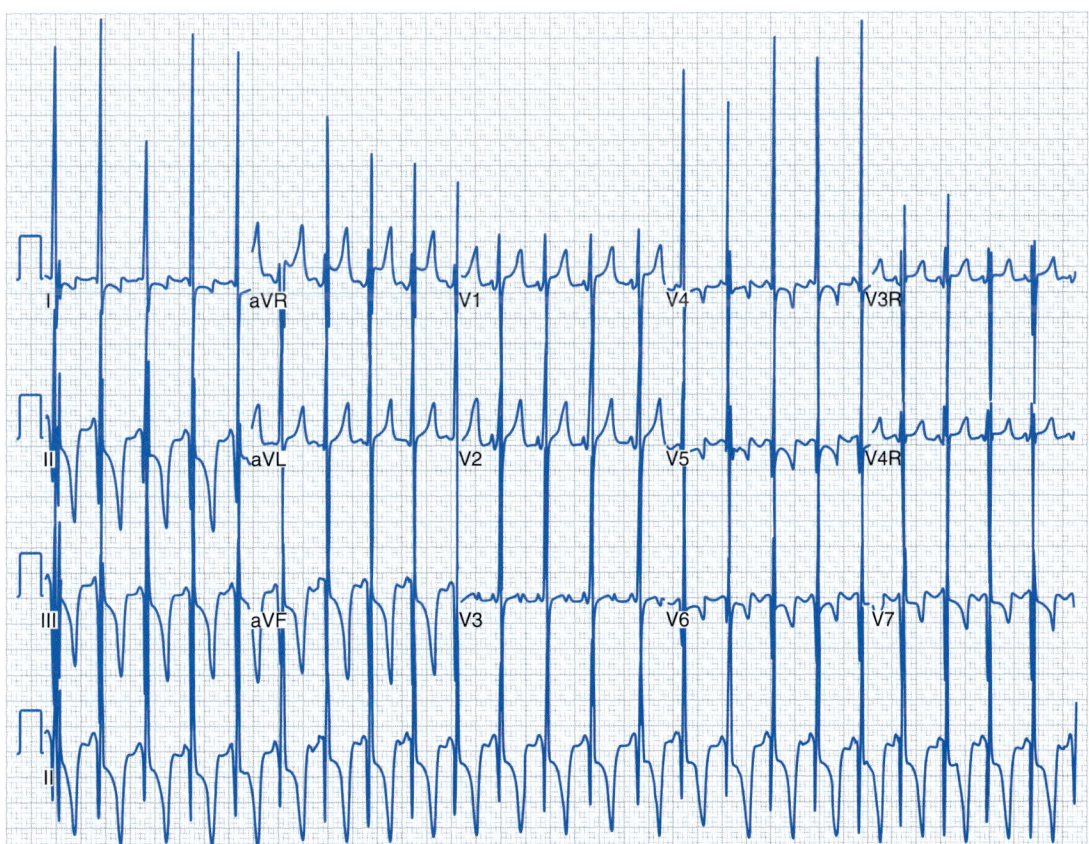

FIGURE 14.9 Pompe disease is an inherited disorder characterized by the accumulation of glycogen in cells. The electrocardiographic tracing for an infant with this glycogen storage disease and a severe form of hypertrophic cardiomyopathy displays dramatic right and left ventricular voltages, in addition to ST-segment and T-wave abnormalities. The recording is displayed at full standard (10 mm/mV), meaning that the electrocardiogram was not reduced in size to fit on the paper.

prognosis when it manifests during childhood.[60–62] The disorder is characterized by diastolic dysfunction related to a marked increase in myocardial stiffness resulting in impaired ventricular filling; most cases are thought to be idiopathic.[63] Presenting symptoms are nonspecific and primarily respiratory. Occasionally, the diagnosis is made after a syncopal or sudden near-death event. The physical examination can demonstrate hepatosplenomegaly, peripheral edema, and ascites.

The echocardiographic hallmark of restrictive cardiomyopathy is that of severe atrial dilation and normal- or small-sized ventricles (Video 14.7). The marked diastolic dysfunction leads to increased end-diastolic pressures, left atrial hypertension, and secondary pulmonary hypertension. Children with restrictive cardiomyopathy are prone to thromboembolic complications and anticoagulation therapy is frequently recommended.[64] This is an important consideration during perioperative care because adjustments in the anticoagulation regimen may be necessary. Atrial and ventricular tachyarrhythmias can also occur. Optimal medical treatment is controversial because no specific agents or strategies have been shown to alter outcomes. As in the case of hypertrophic cardiomyopathy, diuretics often cause a decrease in the needed preload with detrimental effects on hemodynamics. The administration of intravenous fluids can also lead to hemodynamic decompensation due to the underlying already elevated left atrial pressure. Inotropic agents are not indicated because systolic function is preserved and the arrhythmogenic properties of inotropic drugs can create hemodynamic instability and even induce a terminal event. In many centers, cardiac transplantation has been effectively used. In recent years others have favored heart failure and arrythmia treatments to delay or possibly prevent the need for cardiac transplantation.[65]

MYOCARDITIS

Myocarditis is defined as an inflammation of cardiac muscle, often associated with necrosis and myocyte degeneration.[66,67] Among infectious agents, viral infections predominate. Over the past 20 years, the spectrum of viral pathogens causing myocarditis has changed, such that adenovirus, enteroviruses (e.g., coxsackievirus B), and parvovirus have become the most frequent causes of fulminant disease.

The overall true incidence of myocarditis is unknown because it is frequently underdiagnosed and unrecognized as a nonspecific viral syndrome. However, according to the Global Burden of Disease Study the incidence of myocarditis was that of approximately 3.0 million cases worldwide in 2017.[68] A large, 10-year, population-based study on cardiomyopathy found an annual incidence of 1.24 cases per 100,000 children younger than 10 years of age; only a fraction of cases represented those with myocarditis.[69] As the COVID-19 pandemic evolved, an inflammatory syndrome became evident in children following SARS-CoV-2 infection/exposure. This was termed multisystem inflammatory syndrome in children or MIS-C by the US Centers for Disease Control (CDC) and the World Health Organization (WHO).[70] Since then, numerous publications have reported on the clinical features, treatment, and outcome of the condition.[71] The syndrome is characterized by an inflammatory vasculopathy, somewhat similar to Kawasaki disease, that can affect various organ systems including the heart.[72] The spectrum of cardiac manifestations in MIS-C includes myocarditis, coronary artery dilation as well as aneurysms, conduction abnormalities, and cardiac rhythm disturbances.[73] Some children exhibit cardiac dysfunction that if severe may cause hemodynamic instability and even frank shock.

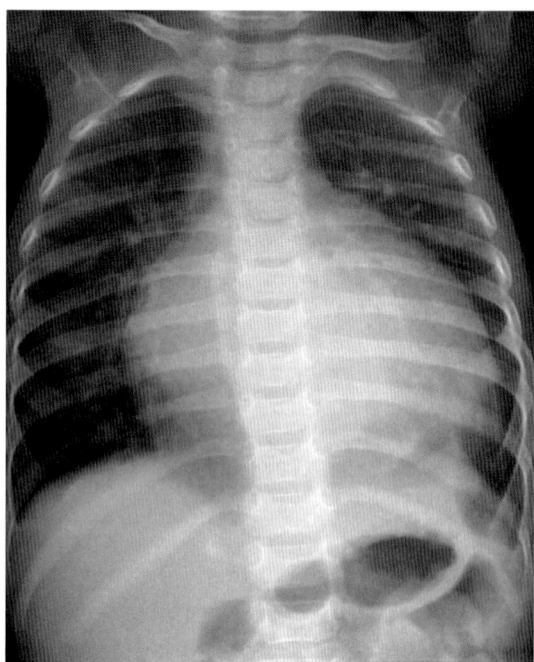

FIGURE 14.10 The chest radiograph of a child with acute myocarditis shows severe cardiomegaly and mildly increased pulmonary vascularity.

It is also of interest that myocarditis has been reported in a small number of children (usually males with a median age of 15 years) after receiving the COVID-19mRNA vaccine. This, however, should be considered a rare occurrence.[74]

In general, the diagnosis of myocarditis is made using clinical history, physical examination, and cardiac testing.[75] The condition is highly suspected when a child presents with new-onset congestive heart failure or ventricular arrhythmias without evidence of structural heart disease.[76] The ECG typically demonstrates low-voltage QRS complexes with tachycardia, which sometimes is ventricular in origin. The CXR often shows cardiomegaly with pulmonary vascular congestion (Fig. 14.10). Echocardiography displays ventricular dilation and dysfunction, similar to dilated cardiomyopathy, and it is useful in the exclusion of alternative diagnoses, such as pericardial effusion or coronary artery anomalies. CMRI has been increasingly used during presentation and surveillance of children with myocarditis.[77] This condition represents a clinical diagnosis because definitive confirmation requires the analysis of tissue obtained through myocardial biopsy, which is rarely performed.

Many children with myocarditis have subclinical or mild clinical disease, whereas others may progress to overt heart failure, hemodynamic compromise, and/or life-threatening arrhythmias. Among children with heart failure, approximately one-third will have restoration of full ventricular function, one-third will recover but continue to demonstrate impaired systolic function, and one-third will require cardiac transplantation. A subset of children, not all of whom initially manifest severe symptoms in the acute period, will progress to develop dilated cardiomyopathy.

Although no specific therapies have been identified to directly treat the myocardial injury, a variety of strategies have been used.[76] The current paradigm includes diuresis and afterload reduction to improve myocardial performance without placing a large burden on an already failing heart. Rhythm disturbances are treated appropriately. Therapy with immune modulation or suppression with intravenous immunoglobulin is the standard of care at many centers. Mechanical circulatory support may be required in fulminant disease (see Chapter 19).[75] In the case of MIS-C the treatment is generally supportive and, depending on the extent of cardiac involvement, additional therapies may be considered that include immunomodulatory medications.[78] Thrombotic risks in these children may also require antiplatelet agents or anticoagulants.[79]

RHEUMATIC FEVER AND RHEUMATIC HEART DISEASE

Acute rheumatic fever and rheumatic heart disease are leading causes of death related to acquired cardiac disease in developing countries and still occur, albeit infrequently, in developed countries.[1,80] The availability of antibiotic therapy for streptococcal tonsillopharyngitis (strep throat) has markedly reduced the incidence of this disease in the United States, but sporadic cases still occur.[81] The peak incidence in children occurs between 5 and 14 years of age.

Rheumatic fever results from infection by particular strains of group A β-hemolytic *Streptococcus* or *Streptococcus pyogenes* leading to a multisystemic inflammatory disorder. The incubation period for most strains of group A β-hemolytic *Streptococcus* is typically 3 to 5 days, although some children present with a more remote history of pharyngitis.

The clinical diagnosis of rheumatic fever is based on the *Jones criteria*. The combination of manifestations (major and minor) necessary to meet these criteria, which were developed in 1944, has been modified several times over the years. The 2015 revised Jones criteria considered the contributions of echocardiography in the diagnosis of cardiac involvement.[82] The most common manifestations of acute rheumatic fever are carditis and arthritis; thus, these represent major criteria for diagnosis. Cardiac involvement or carditis occurs in 50% of children with their first attack of rheumatic fever. Rheumatic heart disease is a sequela of the acute process, and it most frequently affects the mitral and aortic valves. The polyarticular arthritis has a migratory pattern, typically affecting large joints.

Primary prevention of rheumatic fever and rheumatic heart disease begins with prompt recognition and appropriate treatment of the initial streptococcal infection.[83] Penicillin (or amoxicillin) is the treatment of choice for most patients with group A streptococcal pharyngitis. Secondary prevention with antibiotic prophylaxis is aimed at avoiding recurrences in individuals with a known history of rheumatic fever as they are considered at high risk. Intramuscular injections of penicillin every 3 to 4 weeks is recommended. The duration of prophylaxis depends on several factors including echocardiographic findings. The American Heart Association (AHA) guidelines do not recommend infective endocarditis prophylaxis for patients with rheumatic heart disease, except in those few instances where a prosthetic valve has been inserted or prosthetic material has been used in valve repair (refer to next section).[84] In these cases, an alternate to penicillin is recommended because of the potential to develop drug resistance.

Elective or emergent surgery may be required in a subset of children with severe cardiac involvement.[85] Mitral valve regurgitation is often the cause of congestive symptoms; medical management therefore has limited efficacy. Valve repair is always preferred to replacement.

INFECTIVE ENDOCARDITIS
Causes and Treatment
Congenital heart disease is a major risk factor for infective endocarditis in children in developed countries.[86–88] The risk is largely based on the nature of the cardiac condition. The infection results from deposition of bacteria or other pathogens on tissues in areas of abnormal or turbulent blood flow. The diagnosis of infective endocarditis is made clinically by applying the *modified Duke criteria*.[89] Major criteria include demonstration of microorganisms (two positive blood cultures) and evidence of pathologic lesions by echocardiography. The presentation of the disease can be acute or subacute. New or changing heart murmurs can indicate the development of regurgitation or obstruction on an affected valve. Physical findings of systemic embolization (i.e., minor criteria) include splinter hemorrhages (i.e., linear streaks under the nail beds), Janeway lesions (i.e., painless macules on the hands or feet), Osler nodes (i.e., small, painful nodules on the fingers), and Roth spots (i.e., retinal hemorrhages with clear centers). Inflammatory markers, such as erythrocyte sedimentation rate and C-reactive protein, are typically increased, albeit nonspecific. Microscopic hematuria, as a manifestation of renal involvement, is frequently seen.

Acute bacterial endocarditis is most commonly caused by *Staphylococcus aureus*.[90] The clinical presentation includes high fevers, chills, myalgias, fatigue, and lethargy. Some children present in a critically ill state or in shock. Both left- and right-sided infective endocarditis can occur in children with CHD. Children with indwelling venous catheters have an expanded spectrum of pathogens known to cause acute infective endocarditis, including coagulase-negative staphylococcal species or other nonbacterial organisms.

Subacute bacterial endocarditis (SBE) often has a more indolent course and presentation. Children display a low-grade fever, malaise, anemia, and somatic complaints such as fatigue or weakness. Most frequently, one of the *Viridians streptococcus* group and *Enterococcus* species is the underlying pathogen.

Initial evaluation for bacterial endocarditis includes serial blood cultures obtained from separate sites before initiation of antimicrobial therapy. The temporal frequency of cultures depends on the clinical scenario and stability of the child. In up to 20% of children with evidence of infective endocarditis, a pathogen cannot be isolated (i.e., negative-culture endocarditis), requiring empirical treatment throughout. Transthoracic echocardiography is routinely performed to evaluate for evidence of vegetations or other abnormalities. *Although visualization of a vegetation establishes the diagnosis, a negative echocardiographic study does not exclude endocarditis.* Depending on how strongly the diagnosis is suspected, further imaging, including transesophageal echocardiography (TEE), may be necessary (Video 14.8 A,B). These imaging modalities are also valuable during follow-up.

Parenteral antibiotics are initiated after blood cultures are collected. Broad-spectrum agents are used initially, and after a pathogen has been identified, the antibiotic regimen is narrowed. Usually, repeat blood cultures are obtained until they remain sterile, confirming the adequacy of treatment. A prolonged course of antibiotics (i.e., 4–6 weeks) is required in most children. This can be facilitated by placing a peripherally inserted central catheter (PICC). Home therapy for infective endocarditis might be feasible in some children, but it depends on many factors, including clinical status, initial response to antibiotics, sensitivity of the organism to antimicrobial therapy, and the ability of infrastructure to support outpatient treatment of a serious infection (e.g., parental or family member's ability, home health care provider). Overall mortality is less than in adults without CHD (7.1% vs. 14.1%),[91] although the incidence up to 18 years of age is greater than in adult controls.[92]

Roughly 40% of hospitalized children with infective endocarditis require surgical intervention.[91] Failure of medical therapy (i.e., inability to clear the bacteremia), abscess formation, refractory heart failure, large vegetation, and serious embolic phenomenon are indications for early surgery. Typically, the procedures involve resection of a vegetation, tissue debridement, or repair of consequent cardiac abnormalities. These children should subsequently receive endocarditis prophylaxis for at-risk procedures for the rest of their lives. With that in mind, recurrence rates are low.[93]

A high level of suspicion for infective endocarditis must be maintained when evaluating a child with known heart disease and persistent bacteremia (or fungemia) or a fever of unknown origin. The same holds true for any child with foreign material in the heart or vascular tissue, such as indwelling central venous catheters, transvenous pacemakers or defibrillators, and closure devices.

Endocarditis Prophylaxis

The risk for developing infective endocarditis from transient bacteremia is extremely small in children with normal cardiac anatomy; however, as previously discussed, certain cardiac conditions are predisposed to acquiring endocarditis. Guidelines of the AHA do not recommend antibiotic prophylaxis based exclusively on an increased lifetime risk of endocarditis. It is proposed that prophylaxis should be restricted to those at greatest risk for an adverse outcome resulting from infective endocarditis. Children in this category include those with specific congenital heart defects or after certain interventions, prosthetic cardiac valves or material, a history of infective endocarditis in the past, and cardiac transplant recipients with valvular disease (Table 14.2).[84] Since the implementation of the 2007 endocarditis guidelines,[94] which limited the underlying conditions for which antibiotic prophylaxis was recommended, some studies have shown an increased incidence of endocarditis whereas others have shown no change.[95] In the 2021 AHA scientific statement only minor changes to the 2007 guidelines were recommended in terms of prophylaxis and patients considered at high risk.[84] This document underscores: (1) a lack of convincing evidence that the frequency, morbidity, or mortality of *Viridians streptococcus* group endocarditis has increased since the 2007 guidelines in the United States or Canada, and (2) the need for randomized controlled studies to determine the effectiveness of antibiotic prophylaxis to further refine their recommendations. For the most part, the 2015 European Society of Cardiology published guidelines are in agreement with the recommendations by the AHA on antibiotic prophylaxis for the prevention of bacterial endocarditis.[96]

Transient bacteremia can occur during dental procedures that involve the gingival tissues or the periapical region of teeth or perforation of the oral mucosa.[97] Although several respiratory tract procedures are associated with transient bacteremia, no definitive data demonstrate a cause-and-effect relationship between these and infective endocarditis. Caution may be warranted for children at high risk undergoing invasive procedures of the respiratory tract that involve incision or biopsy of the mucosa. Routine prophylactic administration of antibiotics solely to prevent infective endocarditis is not recommended for those undergoing genitourinary or gastrointestinal tract procedures. However, for specific clinical scenarios, antibiotic prophylaxis may be considered.[98] Routine endoscopy or TEE does not merit routine antibiotic administration. Prophylaxis is not considered necessary for cardiac catheterization; and although many practitioners routinely administer antibiotics during transcatheter placement of devices, there is insufficient evidence to support this practice.

The AHA guidelines recommend the administration of antibiotic prophylaxis 30 to 60 minutes before the procedure to achieve

TABLE 14.2	Antibiotic Prophylaxis for a Dental Procedure: Underlying Conditions for Which Antibiotic Prophylaxis Is Suggested
Prosthetic Cardiac Valve or Material	
Presence of cardiac prosthetic valve	
Transcatheter implantation of prosthetic valves	
Cardiac valve repair with devices, including annuloplasty, rings, or clips	
Left ventricular assist devices or implantable heart	
Previous, Relapse, or Recurrent Infective Endocarditis	
Congenital Heart Defect	
Unrepaired cyanotic congenital CHD, including palliative shunts and conduits	
Completely repaired CHD with prosthetic material or device, whether placed by surgery or by transcatheter during the first 6 months after the procedure	
Repaired CHD with residual defects at the site of or adjacent to the site of a prosthetic patch or prosthetic device	
Surgical or transcatheter pulmonary artery valve or conduit placement such as Melody valve and Contegra Conduit	
Cardiac Transplant Recipients Who Develop Cardiac Valvulopathy	
AP for a Dental Procedure not Suggested	
Implantable electronic devices such as a pacemaker or similar devices	
Septal defect closure devices when complete closure is achieved	
Peripheral vascular grafts and patches, including those used for hemodialysis	
Coronary artery stents or other vascular stents	
CNS ventriculoatrial shunts	
Vena cava filters	
Pledgets	

AP, Antibiotic prophylaxis; *CHD*, congenital heart disease; *CNS*, central nervous system.
From American Heart Association, Inc.

adequate tissue concentrations of antibiotics before bacteremia occurs (Table 14.3). In the case that antibiotic prophylaxis is inadvertently not given, the recommendation is for administration up to 2 hours after the procedure. The standard prophylactic regimen for children is for oral amoxicillin. For the child who is allergic to penicillin, oral alternatives include cephalexin, azithromycin, clarithromycin, or doxycycline. In children who are unable to ingest oral medications, alternative antibiotics include ampicillin, cefazolin, or ceftriaxone by an IV or intramuscular route. Since IV access is obtained in most children who present for elective surgery or medical procedures after induction of anesthesia, it is prudent to administer the antibiotics as soon as IV access has been established to achieve adequate tissue levels of antibiotic before skin incision or other sources of bacteremia. In contrast to prior recommendations, because clindamycin may be associated with more frequent and severe reactions (e.g., *Clostridioides difficile* infection), this drug is no longer recommended for antibiotic prophylaxis.[84]

KAWASAKI DISEASE

Kawasaki disease (i.e., mucocutaneous lymph node syndrome) is a fairly common and potentially serious form of systemic vasculitis of unknown origin.[99] It is a condition that occurs primarily in

TABLE 14.3	American Heart Association Guidelines for Prevention of Infective Endocarditis: Antibiotic Regimens		
		DOSE[a]	
Situation	Antibiotic	Children	Adults
Able to take oral medication	Amoxicillin	50 mg/kg	2 grams
Unable to take oral medication	Ampicillin	50 mg/kg IM or IV	2 grams IM or IV
	or		
	Cefazolin or ceftriaxone	50 mg/kg IM or IV	1 gram IM or IV
Allergic to penicillin or ampicillin and able to take oral medication	Cephalexin[b,c]	50 mg/kg	2 grams
	or		
	Azithromycin or clarithro-mycin	15 mg/kg	500 mg
	or		
	Doxycycline	<45 kg, 2.2 mg/kg >45 kg, 100 mg	100 mg
Allergic to penicillin or ampicillin and unable to take oral medication	Cefazolin or ceftriaxone[c]	50 mg/kg IM or IV	1 gram IM or IV

IM, Intramuscular; *IV,* intravenous
Clindamycin is no longer recommended for antibiotic prophylaxis for a dental procedure.
[a]Single dose to be administered 30 to 60 minutes before the procedure. The total pediatric dose should not exceed the adult dose.
[b]Alternatively, another first- or second-generation oral cephalosporin can be administered in an equivalent pediatric or adult dosage.
[c]Cephalosporins should not be used in an individual with a history of anaphylaxis, angioedema, or urticaria to penicillin or ampicillin.
From American Heart Association, Inc.

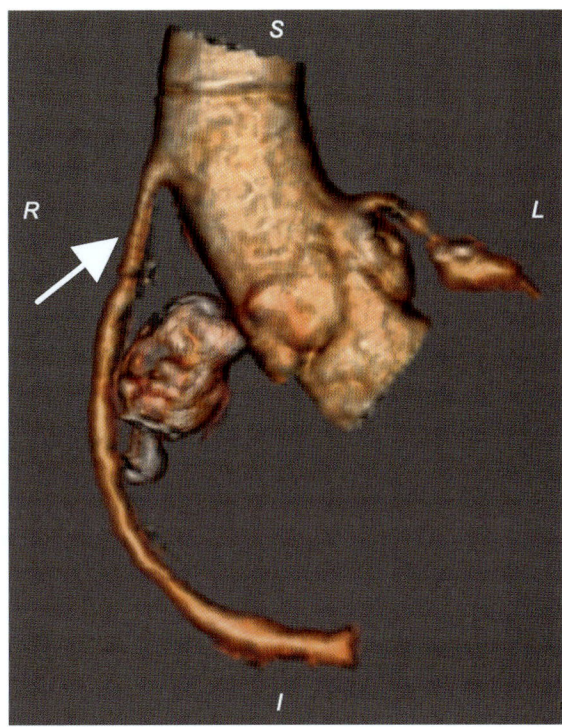

FIGURE 14.11 Computed tomography in a child with Kawasaki disease demonstrates large, fusiform coronary artery aneurysms in both the right and left main coronary arteries. *I,* Inferior; *L,* left; *R,* right; *S,* superior. Note the coronary bypass graft well above the level of the right coronary artery origin *(arrow).*

infants and young children. The disease can affect the coronary arteries resulting in dilation and aneurysm formation.[100,101] Kawasaki disease is considered the most common cause of acquired heart disease in developed countries.

The diagnosis relies on clinical features. To meet criteria, a child must have persistent fevers (>5 days) and at least four of the following findings:[102]

- Rash (polymorphous exanthem)
- Peripheral extremity changes (e.g., erythema, desquamation, edema of the hands or feet)
- Conjunctivitis (bilateral, nonexudative)
- Cervical lymphadenopathy (often unilateral)
- Oral changes (i.e., strawberry tongue; red, dry, or cracked lips)

Nonspecific findings can include irritability, hydrops of the gallbladder, sterile pyuria, arthritis, and aseptic meningitis. Acute-phase reactants and thrombocytosis are usually present.

Intravenous gamma globulin (IVIG) and high-dose aspirin are recommended during the acute phase of the disease. In some cases, antiinflammatory adjunctive therapy may be used (e.g., corticosteroids, interleukin receptor antagonists, and others). The incidence of coronary artery aneurysms is reduced if high-dose

IVIG is administered within the first 10 days of the illness. The presence of coronary artery aneurysms is considered diagnostic for Kawasaki disease. In children with coronary artery aneurysms, low-dose aspirin therapy is administered, in some cases in combination with anticoagulants or antiplatelet agents. Myocardial ischemia and infarction, although uncommon, are important potential complications. Anesthetic care in these children requires careful consideration regarding myocardial oxygen demand and supply; on rare occasions, coronary revascularization may be necessary (Fig. 14.11).[103]

CARDIAC TUMORS

Cardiac tumors are rare in children and more commonly benign in nature. The natural history and optimal treatment strategies are often determined from limited case series and small studies.[104–109] In adults, atrial myxomas comprise more than 90% of primary cardiac tumors; in children, rhabdomyomas comprise 90% of primary cardiac tumors.[108,110] Less common tumors in children include hemangiomas, myxomas (Video 14.9), Purkinje cell tumors, and teratomas. In adults, most cardiac tumors are found in the left atrium, whereas in children, they can occur in any cardiac chamber. Malignant primary tumors such as sarcomas are rare, and data on their outcomes are limited. Other nonprimary or metastatic cardiac tumors, such as Wilms tumor, can invade vascular structures and extend into the heart.

Rhabdomyomas often involve the ventricular septum and left ventricle, and in most cases multiple tumors are present (Fig. 14.12). Although they are considered benign, children can present with cardiomegaly, congestive heart failure, arrhythmias, or sudden death. The complications from a rhabdomyoma are determined primarily by its size and the obstruction it may cause.

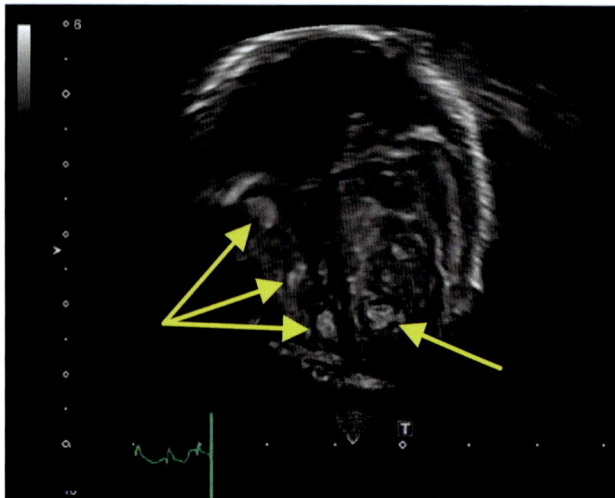

FIGURE 14.12 The apical four-chamber echocardiographic image displays multiple rhabdomyomas *(arrows)* in a child with tuberous sclerosis.

Tumors of this type tend to regress over time or completely resolve in early childhood. Current therapy of symptomatic patients is usually supportive; surgery is not indicated unless symptoms are present. In recent years mammalian target of rapamycin (mTOR) inhibitors (everolimus or sirolimus) have been used in children with symptomatic cardiac rhabdomyomas with reported clinical improvement.[111,112] These agents suppress the activity of the mTOR signaling pathway, which regulates cell growth and proliferation. Many children with cardiac rhabdomyomas have associated tuberous sclerosis, a multiorgan genetic disease.[113]

Cardiac fibromas are the second most common type of primary pediatric cardiac tumors.[114,115] They are typically single and involve the ventricular free wall. In a subset of fibromas, the tumor can invade the conduction system.[116] Surgery, or rarely cardiac transplantation, may be required. The tumors can be very large, and complete surgical resection can impact cardiac function.

The primary concerns in the perioperative care of children with cardiac tumors are the impact of the mass on hemodynamics and the associated abnormalities of cardiac rhythm.[117]

Heart Failure in Children
DEFINITION AND PATHOPHYSIOLOGY
Heart failure continues to be major field of interest and investigation in pediatric cardiology and the subject of various publications, scientific meetings, and several textbooks.[118–122] The cellular basis of heart failure, compensatory mechanisms, and therapeutic strategies in children have received the most attention. The following discussion highlights key concepts as they relate to anesthetic practice.

Heart failure is considered to be a pump and circulatory failure involving neurohumoral aspects of the circulation. Several conditions may ultimately compromise the ability of the cardiovascular system to generate an adequate cardiac output to meet the systemic circulatory demands. This disease state does not necessarily imply impairment of ventricular systolic function. For example, diastolic heart failure is an increasingly recognized clinical entity.

ETIOLOGY AND CLINICAL FEATURES
Pediatric heart failure results from markedly different etiologies from those reported in adults.[123] The causes of heart failure in children vary with age. In the perinatal period, cardiac dysfunction can be related to birth asphyxia or sepsis or constitute an early presentation of CHD. The neonate with heart failure frequently presents with clinical signs of a low cardiac output state. Causes include left-sided outflow obstruction (e.g., aortic stenosis, aortic coarctation, hypoplastic left heart syndrome), severe valve regurgitation (e.g., Ebstein anomaly), or absent pulmonary valve syndrome.

During the first year of life, heart failure is predominantly caused by congenital heart disease. Other causes include severe anemia,[124] cardiomyopathies owing to inborn errors of metabolism, or acute events such as myocarditis. In infants with heart failure, tachypnea, dyspnea, tachycardia, feeding difficulties, and failure to thrive are prominent features.[125] The physical examination can display grunting respirations, rales, intercostal retractions, a gallop rhythm, and hepatosplenomegaly. Frequently, a mitral regurgitant murmur is present.

Beyond the first year of life, heart failure is usually a consequence of previous surgical interventions, unpalliated or unrepaired cardiovascular disease, cardiomyopathies, myocarditis, or anthracycline therapy for a malignancy.[126] Occasionally, a child may present with severe ventricular systolic impairment related to ongoing myocardial ischemia due to a coronary artery anomaly, or rarely, because of acquired pathologies such as Kawasaki disease. Older children with heart failure exhibit exercise intolerance, fatigue, and growth failure, whereas adolescents have symptoms like those of adults (Table 14.4).

TREATMENT STRATEGIES
Clinical features in acute decompensated heart failure such as the presence/absence of congestion and perfusion status have been used to classify patient status into four categories: warm and dry, warm and wet, cold and dry, and cold and wet. Treatment is thus instituted accordingly. The main goal of therapy for acute heart failure is to lessen congestion, when present, and to maintain organ perfusion. In general, therapy is tailored to the cause of the cardiac dysfunction and may include supportive care, mechanical ventilation, afterload reduction, inotropic support, prostaglandin E_1 therapy to maintain pulmonary or systemic blood flow, maneuvers to balance the systemic and pulmonary circulations, catheter-based interventions, and/or surgery.[122,127,128] Pharmacologic agents include inotropes

TABLE 14.4	Symptoms Characteristic of Heart Failure in Children	
	Commonly Encountered	**Less Commonly Encountered**
Infants and young children	• Tachypnea • Feeding difficulty (reflux, vomiting, feeding refusal) • Diaphoresis • Pallor	• Cyanosis • Palpitations • Syncope • Facial edema • Dependent edema • Ascites
Older children and adolescents	• Fatigue • Effort intolerance • Dyspnea • Orthopnea • Abdominal pain • Nausea • Vomiting	• Palpitations • Chest pain • Dependent edema • Ascites

Reproduced with permission from Kantor PF, Lougheed J, Dancea A, et al. Presentation, diagnosis, and medical management of heart failure in children: Canadian Cardiovascular Society guidelines. *Can J Cardiol.* 2013;29(12):1535-1552.

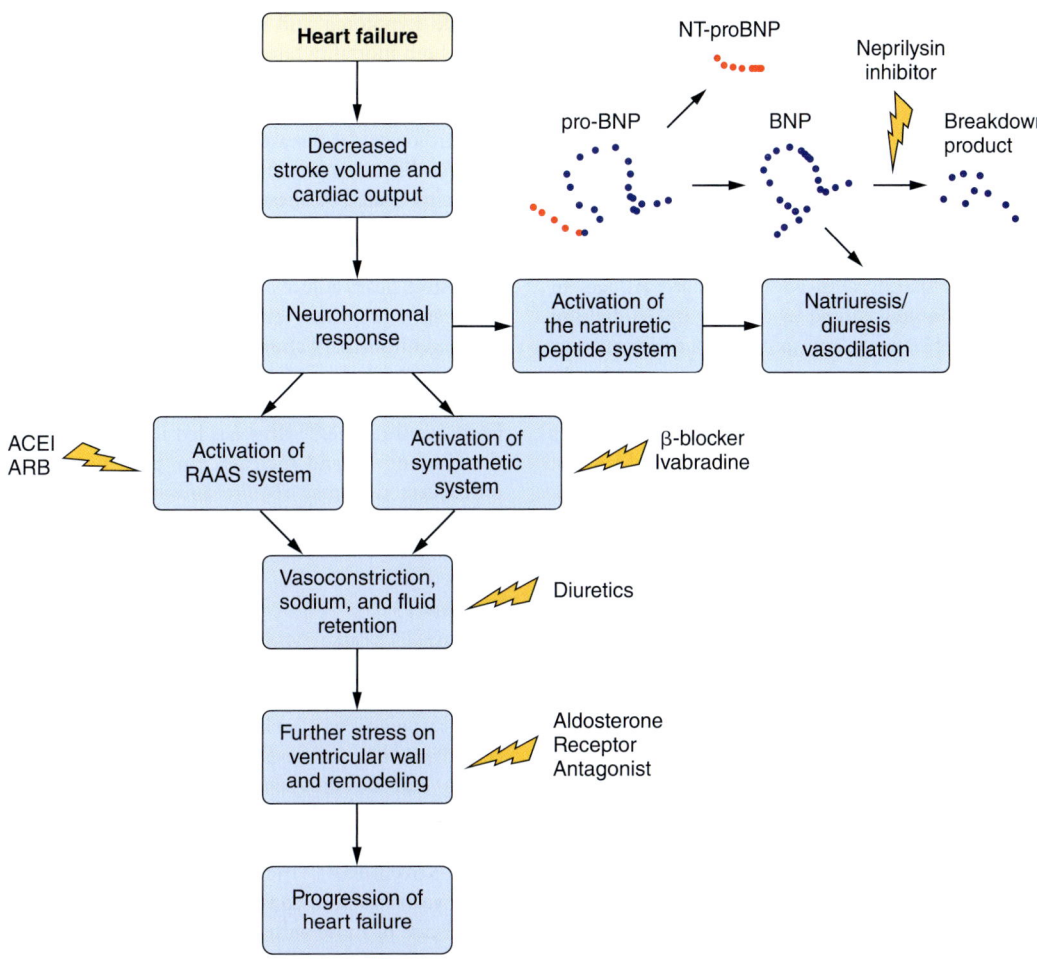

FIGURE 14.13 The figure depicts the pathophysiology of heart failure with respective medication targets. *ACEI*, Angiotensin-converting-enzyme inhibitor; *ARB*, angiotensin receptor blocker; *BNP*, brain natriuretic peptide; *NT-proBNP*, N-terminal pro-brain natriuretic peptide; *pro-BNP*, pro-brain natriuretic peptide. (Reproduced with permission from Watanabe K, Shih R. Update of pediatric heart failure. *Pediatr Clin North Am.* 2020;67:889-901.)

(used on a very-short-term basis, if necessary) and inodilators (e.g., milrinone). Favored drugs for chronic therapy in children are diuretics, aldosterone receptor antagonists, and angiotensin-converting enzyme inhibitors.[40,122,129] Other agents that have been used to manage chronic pediatric heart failure include nesiritide (a recombinant form of human B-type natriuretic peptide), carvedilol (a third-generation β-blocker), and ivabradine (a heart rate–reducing agent that functions via selective inhibition of the "funny current" responsible for spontaneous depolarization of cardiac pacemaker cells).[40,130,131] In recent years, a combination drug for heart failure (valsartan and sacubitril, brand name of Entresto, Novartis Pharmaceuticals, Cambridge MA) has received increasing attention. The drug relies on angiotensin receptor blockade (valsartan) while also targeting neurohormonal regulation (sacubitril, a neprilysin inhibitor).[132] The drug received FDA approval to treat symptomatic heart failure in children with systemic ventricular dysfunction based on early findings of a randomized trial; however, studies are ongoing.[133] An overview of the pathophysiology of heart failure and medication targets can be found in Fig. 14.13.

ANESTHETIC CONSIDERATIONS

Anesthesia for children with heart failure can be quite challenging. The severity of the condition and degree of baseline decompensation can influence the likelihood of an untoward event and the potential for hemodynamic instability and a poor outcome. Several publications have addressed the risks associated with anesthesia in this setting.[134–137] It is important to first reexamine the risk/benefit ratio in these patients before going forward with the planned procedure. In most surgical settings, tracheal intubation and mechanical ventilation are indicated. The need for invasive monitoring should be based on the clinical situation, anticipated nature of the procedure, and impact on hemodynamic state. The preemptive initiation of inotropic/vasoactive support just before or at the induction of anesthesia might be considered in some cases given that blunting of an underlying high catecholamine state with anesthetic agents can lead to hemodynamic decompensation and/or associated cardiovascular collapse.

Syndromes, Associations, and Systemic Disorders: Cardiovascular Disease and Anesthetic Implications

Many disorders, including those resulting from chromosomal abnormalities, single-gene defects, gene deletion syndromes, known associations (i.e., nonrandom occurrence of defects), and teratogenic exposure, can manifest as cardiovascular disease. The coexistence of frequently associated multiple organ system comorbidities with cardiovascular disease presents several challenges to the anesthesia care provider.

CHROMOSOMAL SYNDROMES

Trisomy 21

Trisomy 21 (Down syndrome) is the most common chromosomal anomaly, occurring with a frequency of 1 per 800 live births.[138,139] The incidence increases sharply with advanced maternal age. In most cases, Down syndrome is caused by an error in cell division resulting in three full copies of chromosome 21, but it may occur from a balanced or unbalanced chromosomal translocation or mosaicism. The phenotypes are indistinguishable. Affected children are typically smaller than normal for age. Craniofacial features include microbrachycephaly, short neck, oblique palpebral fissures, epicanthal folds, Brushfield spots, small and low-set ears, macroglossia, and microdontia with fused teeth. Mandibular hypoplasia and flattened facial features are common. A narrow nasopharynx with hypertrophic lymphatic tissue (e.g., tonsils, adenoids) and macroglossia in combination with generalized hypotonia frequently leads to obstructive sleep apnea.[140] Other conditions include developmental delay, cervical spine disorders with vertebral and ligamentous instability (i.e., subluxation risk), hypothyroidism, leukemia, obesity, subglottic stenosis, and gastrointestinal problems, particularly duodenal atresia.

The preoperative assessment of children with Down syndrome should include a comprehensive evaluation and management plan to minimize risks.[141,142] The intellectual disability of these children may require the use of premedication or sedatives. Specific issues of concern include the potential for upper airway obstruction caused by a large tongue, subglottic stenosis,[143] postextubation stridor, and cervical spine instability.[144–146]

Vascular access can be challenging. Subjectively, children have small and abnormal radial vessels, vascular hyperreactivity, fragile tissue consistency, and a documented increased risk for complications after arterial cannulation.[147]

Cardiovascular defects occur in 40% to 50% of children with Down syndrome, and it has been recommended that they all should undergo screening for CHD in early infancy.[148] The most common lesions include AV septal defects (Video 14.10), VSDs, TOF, and PDA. Bradycardia under anesthesia occurs commonly, although the mechanism is poorly understood.[149,150] This may represent a manifestation of autonomic dysfunction in these children.[151] Pulmonary hypertension can result from the cardiac pathology and/or from chronic hypoxemia caused by upper airway obstruction (i.e., obstructive sleep apnea) and should be considered in their management. Reduced nitric oxide bioavailability has been reported in patients with Down syndrome, leading to endothelial cell dysfunction, possibly explaining the observed increased pulmonary vascular reactivity.[152]

Trisomy 18

Trisomy 18 (Edwards syndrome) is recognized as the second most common chromosomal trisomy (1 per 3500 live births). Most children exhibit microcephaly, delayed psychomotor development, and developmental delay.[153] Characteristic craniofacial features include micrognathia or retrognathia and microstomia, which can affect airway management, as well as malformed ears, and microphthalmia.[154–157] An increased incidence of obstructive sleep apnea has also been reported.[158] Skeletal anomalies include clenched fingers and severe growth delay. Neurologic problems include hypotonia and central nervous system malformations. Their high mortality rate is related to cardiac and renal problems, feeding difficulties, sepsis, and apnea caused by neurologic abnormalities.

Cardiovascular disease, consisting primarily of VSD and polyvalvular disease, is present in most children with trisomy 18.[159,160] Problems related to anesthetic management primarily encompass difficult mask ventilation and intubation as well as difficult intravenous access[157]; additional concerns include the increased risk of congestive heart failure and aspiration pneumonia.[154] These children can require interventions to address associated gastrointestinal or genitourinary anomalies.

Over the last several years an increasing number of cardiac interventions are being performed as the paradigm has shifted from comfort care.[161] This has led to improved survival rates beyond infancy[162] and increases the potential need for additional procedures that may require anesthesia. Surveillance guidelines have been developed to facilitate the care, monitoring of complications, and treatment.[163]

Trisomy 13

Trisomy 13 (Patau syndrome) is an uncommon autosomal trisomy with an incidence that ranges from 1 per 5000 to 12,000 live births. Major features include cleft lip and palate, holoprosencephaly, polydactyly, rocker-bottom feet, microphthalmia, microcephaly, and severe developmental delay.[164,165] As in the case of Down and Edwards syndromes, sleep disordered breathing is common. Almost all affected children have associated cardiovascular defects, including PDA, septal defects, valve abnormalities, and dextrocardia.[159] The overall prognosis for these children for many years has been considered extremely poor. However, similar to the case of those with trisomy 18, the care of these children is evolving to the point where this condition is no longer considered uniformly fatal.[162]

Turner Syndrome

Turner syndrome is a genetic disorder characterized by complete or partial absence of an X chromosome.[166] The estimated incidence is 1 per 5000 live-born female infants. Spontaneous miscarriages occur commonly in affected fetuses. Features of this syndrome include webbed neck, low-set ears, multiple pigmented nevi and micrognathia, lymphedema, short stature, and ovarian failure.[167] Systemic manifestations include cardiac defects (notably bicuspid aortic valve and left heart obstruction),[168,169] hypertension, hypercholesterolemia, renal anomalies, liver disease, and inflammatory bowel disease. Aortic dilation and the potential for aortic dissection are concerns in the long term.[170] Obesity is common in older children, together with an increased incidence of endocrine abnormalities such as hypothyroidism and diabetes.[171,172]

GENE DELETION SYNDROMES

Williams Syndrome

Williams syndrome (also known as Williams-Beuren Syndrome) is a congenital disorder with an incidence of 1 per 10,000 to 20,000 live births. In most cases, it results from a deletion in the long arm of chromosome 7, altering the elastin gene.[173] Features of Williams syndrome are elfin facies, hypersocial personality, endocrine abnormalities (including hypercalcemia and hypothyroidism), developmental delay, growth deficiency, and altered neurodevelopment.[174] Dental abnormalities can lead to airway difficulties. The spectrum of disease severity in elastin arteriopathy is broad ranging from minimal vascular involvement to severe

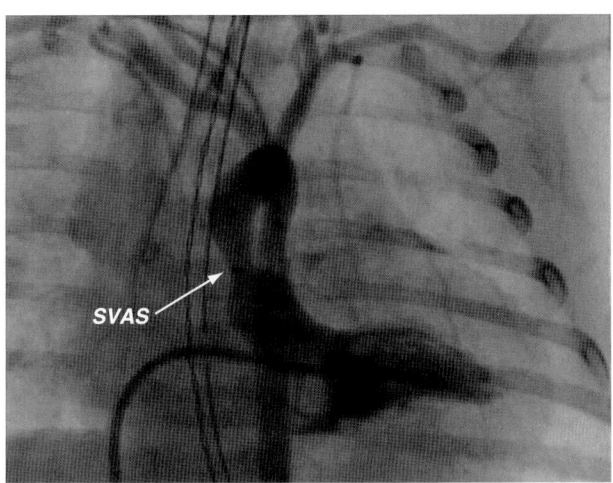

FIGURE 14.14 The angiogram displays the classic angiographic appearance of supravalvular aortic stenosis *(SVAS, arrow)* in a child with Williams syndrome.

vascular disease. Structural cardiovascular abnormalities, which occur in 80% of these children, most commonly involve valvar and supravalvular aortic stenosis (Fig. 14.14) and aortic coarctation.[175] The arteriopathy, manifested as stenosis, can also involve the pulmonary arteries, origins of the coronary arteries, or other vessels (e.g., aortopathy). Diffuse narrowing of the abdominal aorta can be associated with renal artery stenosis. Other structural cardiac abnormalities are relatively common in these patients, including VSD, mitral valve prolapse, and aortic insufficiency. A prolonged corrected QT (QTc) period on ECG is present in 13% of patients with Williams syndrome and has been considered a risk factor for sudden death.[176,177]

Several reports have described acute hemodynamic deterioration, cardiovascular collapse, and death during anesthesia in children with Williams syndrome.[178–181] Two conditions can increase morbidity and the potential for anesthesia and sedation-related cardiac arrest: coronary artery abnormalities, leading to myocardial ischemia, and severe biventricular outflow tract obstruction. In fact, in the literature most children who suffered a cardiac arrest or complication were under 3 years of age and had biventricular outflow tract obstruction. A comprehensive cardiac evaluation of all children is advisable because the spectrum of disease and the potential for devastating implications in affected individuals vary.[182,183] Children undergoing sedation or anesthetic care occasionally require further studies and even management changes before proceeding with a planned procedure. Even asymptomatic children and those without evidence of clinical cardiovascular disease might be at risk for major morbidity and death during situations associated with hemodynamic stress. Extreme vigilance and particular attention to signs of myocardial ischemia is warranted, as is a plan of action in the event of acute decompensation. This syndrome was one of the leading causes of cardiac arrest in the Pediatric Perioperative Cardiac Arrest (POCA) registry and requires the consideration of specific management issues.[184]

In view of these concerns and the fact that resuscitative efforts are frequently unsuccessful and refractory to aggressive efforts in children with elastin arteriopathy, the following measures have been proposed: (1) careful risk/benefit assessment of the planned procedure, (2) care of children by personnel with expertise in this patient population and familiarity with potential challenges that may be encountered, and (3) care to be delivered at institutions with available resources to support the need for an acute intervention and an aggressive resuscitation.[180] Given the challenges involved in the care of these children as outlined above, a periprocedural risk stratification scheme has been proposed that considers factors such as age, severity of cardiac pathology, and ECG findings, among several other parameters.[185] With careful planning and modifications in the standard anesthesia management, the high risk in this patient group can be mitigated.[186,187]

Children with Williams syndrome can exhibit some degree of muscular weakness, and the cautious use of neuromuscular blocking drugs has been recommended.[188] Associated neurodevelopmental delay, attention-deficit disorder, and autistic behavior often require a premedication. Subclinical hypothyroidism is common.[189] Renal manifestations include renovascular hypertension, reduced function, and hypercalcemia-induced nephrocalcinosis.

Chromosome 22q11.2 Deletion Syndrome: DiGeorge and Velocardiofacial Syndrome

The 22q11.2 deletion syndrome, with an estimated incidence of approximately 1 per 3000 live births, encompasses DiGeorge, conotruncal face, and velocardiofacial syndromes. This represents the most common microdeletion syndrome in children resulting from impaired development of the pharyngeal pouch system. The syndrome is also known as CATCH 22, a mnemonic for **c**ardiac defects, **a**bnormal facies, **t**hymic hypoplasia, **c**left palate, and **h**ypocalcemia, all of which are commonly present. Cardiac malformations, speech delay, and immunodeficiency are the most common features of the chromosome 22q deletion syndromes.[190,191] Because no single feature is overwhelmingly associated with the deletion, the diagnosis should be considered for any child with a conotruncal anomaly, neonatal hypocalcemia, or any of the less common manifestations when seen in association with facial dysmorphism.[192]

Cardiac malformations are often described as conotruncal anomalies; however, outflow tract problems are also common.[193,194] The remainder of the cardiac defects encompass an enormous spectrum, leaving only a minority of children with a normal cardiovascular system. Because of thymic hypoplasia, children can have diminished T-cell numbers and function.[191] Their immunodeficiency requires the use of irradiated blood products and strict aseptic precautions during vascular access. Neurodevelopmental features include primarily speech delay and attention-deficit disorders. Psychiatric disorders are well described in these individuals.[195,196]

SINGLE-GENE DEFECTS
Noonan Syndrome

Noonan syndrome, an autosomal dominant disorder of variable expression, occurs in 1 per 1000 to 2500 live births. The syndrome is one of a group of related conditions, collectively known as RASopathies or developmental syndromes of RAS/mitogen-activated protein kinase (MAPK) pathway dysregulation. Dysmorphic features in Noonan syndrome include neck webbing, low-set ears, chest deformities, hypertelorism, and short stature. The diagnosis is suspected from key clinical features.[197] In neonates, the facial features may be less apparent; however, generalized edema and excess nuchal folds can be present as in Turner syndrome. The facial features are more difficult to detect in later adolescence and adulthood.

The disorder is associated with a high incidence of cardiovascular involvement (about 80% to 90%); pulmonary valve dysplasia or stenosis is the most common feature.[198,199] Hypertrophic cardiomyopathy can develop during the first few years of life in some children.[200,201] Clinical problems can also include developmental delay and bleeding diathesis.[202]

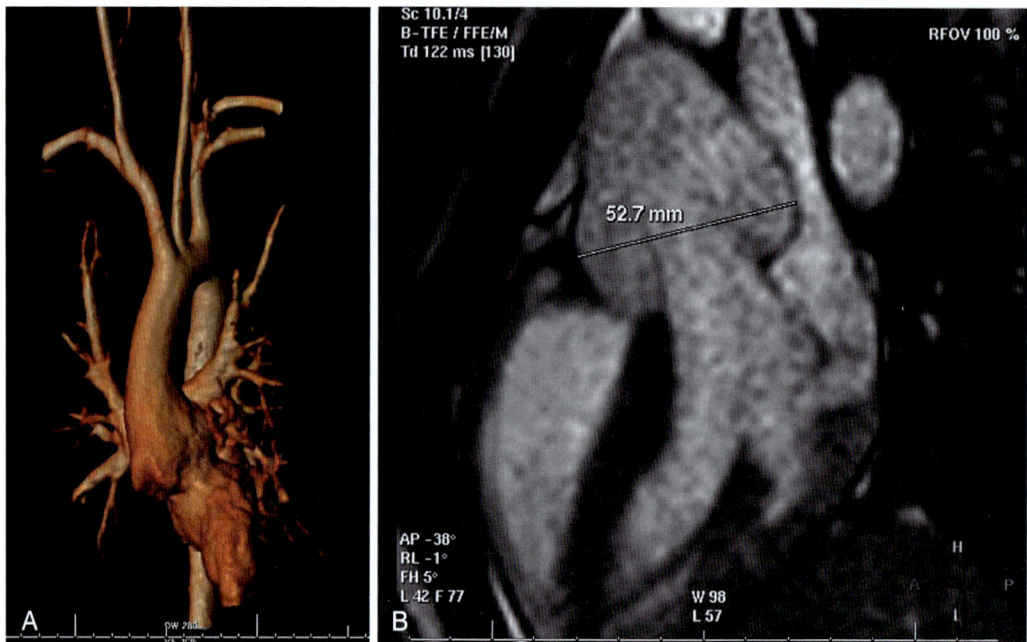

FIGURE 14.15 A severely dilated aortic root as displayed by magnetic resonance imaging in a patient with Marfan syndrome. The three-dimensional reconstruction **(A)** and sagittal view **(B)** demonstrate the aneurysmal appearance of the aortic root.

Marfan Syndrome

Marfan syndrome is a multisystem connective tissue disorder with variable expression resulting in most cases from a mutation in the fibrillin gene, located on chromosome 15. The estimated incidence of Marfan syndrome is 1 in 5000 individuals.[203] The condition is inherited in an autosomal dominant pattern with variable penetrance. Clinical manifestations typically involve the cardiovascular, skeletal, and ocular systems.[204,205] Cardiovascular manifestations include mitral valve prolapse and regurgitation, ascending aortic dilation (Fig. 14.15), and main pulmonary artery dilation. The risk of aortic dissection increases considerably as the aortic size increases, but it can occur at any point in the course of the disease.[206] Cardiac arrhythmias can be related to valvular heart disease, cardiomyopathy, or congestive heart failure.

Medical therapy with either β-blocker or angiotensin receptor blocker is considered standard therapy in slowing progression of aortic disease.[207] Blood pressure control in children with aortic root dilation should be continued perioperatively. Aortic root replacement in Marfan syndrome has been associated with a greater risk of repeat dissection and recurrent aneurysm compared with other children who have undergone similar interventions.[208] It is wise to maintain hemodynamics near baseline values in the perioperative period. After aortic root surgery, some individuals may require chronic anticoagulation therapy. Bridge outpatient therapy usually with low-molecular-weight heparin or preoperative hospitalization may be necessary to adjust the anticoagulation regimen in anticipation of surgery. In emergency cases, administration of coagulation factors and other blood products may be required. In addition to vascular pathology, children with Marfan syndrome have a predisposition for ventricular dilation and abnormal systolic function.[209,210]

Several factors can result in pulmonary disease in these children.[211] Chest wall deformities and progressive scoliosis can contribute to restrictive lung disease. The fibrillin defect can affect lung development and homeostasis, impairing pulmonary function. Development of a spontaneous pneumothorax is relatively common.

A nationwide study addressing perioperative events during spinal fusion for scoliosis in children with Marfan syndrome reported that nearly 60% of patients experienced at least one complication and a high rate (10%) of 90-day hospital readmission, supporting the need for careful perioperative management of this cohort.[212]

CHARGE Syndrome

CHARGE syndrome is a genetic disorder that is characterized by congenital anomalies including **c**oloboma, **h**eart defects, choanal **a**tresia, **r**etardation of growth and development, **g**enitourinary problems, and **e**ar abnormalities.[213,214] Most affected patients have mutations on the *CHD7* gene (chromodomain helicase DNA-binding protein), located on chromosome 8q12. The syndrome is estimated to occur at a rate of 1 per 8000 to 10,000 live births. Cardiac defects occur in many children and commonly include conotruncal malformations, septal defects, and aortic arch anomalies.[215] Delayed growth and development usually result from cardiac disease, nutritional problems, and/or growth hormone deficiency. Most children have some degree of cognitive impairment. The anesthetic implications, in addition to those related to the cardiac defects, focus on the airway. In a retrospective review, upper airway abnormalities other than choanal atresia and cleft lip and palate were reported in 56% of children.[216] A high risk of postoperative airway events has also been reported in affected patients.[217]

ASSOCIATIONS

VACTERL (or VATER) Association

VACTERL association is an acronym given to describe a series of nonrandom anomalies that include **v**ertebral, **a**nal, **c**ardiovascular, **t**racheo**e**sophageal, **r**enal, and **l**imb defects.[218] There is strong evidence for a genetic basis for this condition in some children but not as much in others.[219] Up to 75% of children with VACTERL association have CHD. The most common lesions include VSDs, ASDs, and TOF. Complex pathology such as truncus arteriosus and transposition of the great arteries occur less frequently.

Approximately 70% of children with VACTERL have vertebral anomalies, usually consisting of hypoplastic vertebrae or hemivertebra, that predispose to scoliosis. Anal atresia or imperforate anus is reported in about 55% of cases. These anomalies often require surgery in the first days of life and/or during infancy. Esophageal atresia with tracheoesophageal fistula occurs in a significant number of affected infants. Vertebral and tracheal anomalies can complicate airway management and regional anesthesia. Low birth weight (<1500 grams) and associated cardiac pathology are independent predictors of mortality in infants undergoing surgery for esophageal atresia or tracheoesophageal fistula (see Chapter 35). The presence of a ductal-dependent cardiac lesion further increases perioperative morbidity and mortality.[220] Renal defects occur in about 50% of children. Limb defects occur in most children, potentially affecting vascular access and monitor placement.

As in the case of other children with complex or severe congenital malformations, these individuals may require repeated diagnostic procedures and/or surgical interventions. In addition to the anesthetic considerations specific to each of these, it is important for the provider to be aware of potential fears that children may have related to the procedure and/or anesthesia and consider strategies aimed at comfort and support.[221]

OTHER DISORDERS

Tuberous sclerosis complex (TSC) is a rare genetic disease with an autosomal dominant inheritance pattern and an incidence of approximately 1 per 25,000 to 30,000 births. It can be attributed to spontaneous mutations in most children. The disorder is caused by defects, or mutations, on two genes known as TSC1 and TSC2, which produce proteins thought to act as growth suppressors and regulate cellular hyperplasia. The TSC1 gene is on chromosome 9 and produces a protein called *hamartin*, whereas the TSC2 gene is on chromosome 16 and produces the protein *tuberin*.[222,223] This systemic disease primarily manifests as cutaneous and neurologic symptoms, but cardiac and renal lesions are frequent findings.

The presence of upper airway nodular tumors, fibromas, or papillomas in affected children can interfere with airway management. Developmental delay, autism, attention-deficit disorder, and aggressive behavior are common. Brain and renal tumors (60% to 80%) can produce important comorbidities.[224,225] Seizures are relatively common in affected individuals. Cardiac pathology includes rhabdomyoma in 60% of children (refer to section on Cardiac Tumors) and coexisting CHD in 33% of cases.[226–228] Cardiac abnormalities with obstruction to blood flow, heart failure, arrhythmias, conduction defects, or preexcitation can affect the selection of anesthetic agents. Preoperative evaluation in most cases should include an ECG to evaluate for arrhythmia, conduction defects, or preexcitation.[229,230] Blood pressure and renal function should also be assessed. Anticonvulsants should be optimized and continued until the morning of surgery. Baseline medical treatment should be resumed as soon as possible because seizures are the most common postoperative complication.

Selected Vascular Anomalies and Their Implications for Anesthesia

ABERRANT SUBCLAVIAN ARTERY

An aberrant or anomalous subclavian artery in the classic setting arises from the descending aorta as a separate vessel distal to the usual last subclavian artery, in a posterior location. In a left aortic arch, this arrangement is: the first branch is the right carotid artery, the second is the left carotid artery, and the third is the left subclavian artery. The aberrant right subclavian artery, rather than arising proximally from the innominate artery as the first arch vessel, originates distal to the left subclavian artery as the fourth branch and courses behind the esophagus toward the right arm. This branching variant is one of the most common aortic arch anomalies, occurring in 0.4% to 2% of the general population. It may or may not be associated with CHD.[231] This anomaly has a high incidence among children with Down syndrome and is associated with VSDs, TOF, and other cardiac lesions. In a right aortic arch, the anomalous left subclavian artery originates distal to the origin of the right subclavian artery (Fig. 14.16). This anomaly can be seen in the context of conotruncal malformations. The diagnosis of an aberrant subclavian artery is made by most currently available imaging modalities.

This variant has several implications:

- It can influence vessel selection during creation of a systemic-to-pulmonary artery shunt.
- It should be considered in the selection of a site for arterial line placement if TEE is planned during surgery. The aberrant vessel can be compressed along its retroesophageal course by the imaging probe, resulting in inaccurate arterial blood pressure recordings.[232] Regardless of the site of arterial line placement, it may be wise to monitor the arm supplied by the anomalous vessel by pulse oximetry or other methods during esophageal instrumentation.
- It is sometimes a component of a vascular ring.
- Rarely, older children with an aberrant subclavian artery and without the findings of a complete vascular ring can complain of mild dysphagia (i.e., dysphagia lusoria).

PERSISTENT LEFT SUPERIOR VENA CAVA TO THE CORONARY SINUS

A persistent left superior vena cava (LSVC) is a variant or form of anomalous systemic venous drainage identified in 4.4% of children with CHD, most frequently those with septal defects.[233] It represents a venous remnant that typically involutes during development. If it persists, it remains patent and usually drains through an enlarged coronary sinus into the right atrium. Bilateral superior vena cavae can be present (Fig. 14.17), or the right superior vena cava can be absent. Bilateral superior vena cavae can communicate through an innominate or bridging vein. This anomaly has several implications:

- In the absence of an innominate vein, a catheter placed in the left arm or left internal jugular vein and advanced into the central circulation can rest within the coronary sinus, a potentially undesirable location in a small infant. On CXR, an unusual course is identified as the catheter courses along the left aspect of the mediastinum and can be mistaken for intracarotid, intrapleural, or mediastinal locations.
- An LSVC can be of relevance during venous cannulation for cardiopulmonary bypass to ensure adequate venous drainage and optimal surgical conditions.
- The presence of an LSVC is important in patients with single-ventricle physiology undergoing surgical palliation. In these cases, instead of a single cavopulmonary (Glenn) connection (right superior vena cava to right pulmonary artery anastomosis), two cavopulmonary connections or bilateral bidirectional Glenn shunts (each superior vena cavae anastomose to ipsilateral pulmonary artery) may be undertaken.
- The anomaly can be associated with a dilated coronary sinus. On echocardiography, it can be confused with other defects, including an ostium primum ASD (i.e., one that lies in the inferior aspect of the atrial septum) or anomalous pulmonary venous return to the coronary sinus.

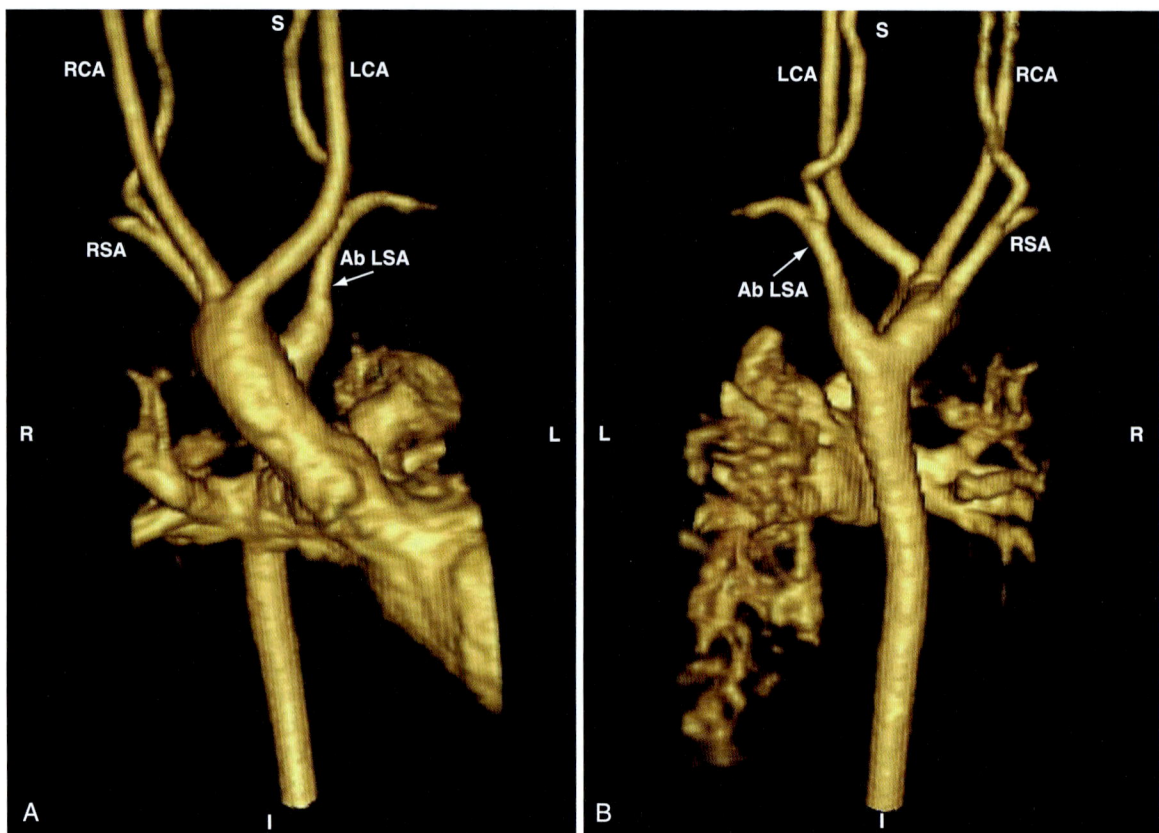

FIGURE 14.16 Three-dimensional reconstruction of a vascular ring obtained by magnetic resonance imaging. The images display anterior **(A)** and posterior **(B)** views of a right aortic arch with an aberrant left subclavian artery *(Ab LSA)*. The first arch vessel is the left carotid artery *(LCA)*, followed by the right carotid artery *(RCA)*, and right subclavian artery *(RSA)*. The Ab LSA is the most distal branch originating from the descending aorta and coursing posterior to the esophagus toward the left arm. This vessel can be compressed by a transesophageal echocardiographic probe when used. *I*, Inferior; *L*, left; *R*, right; *S*, superior.

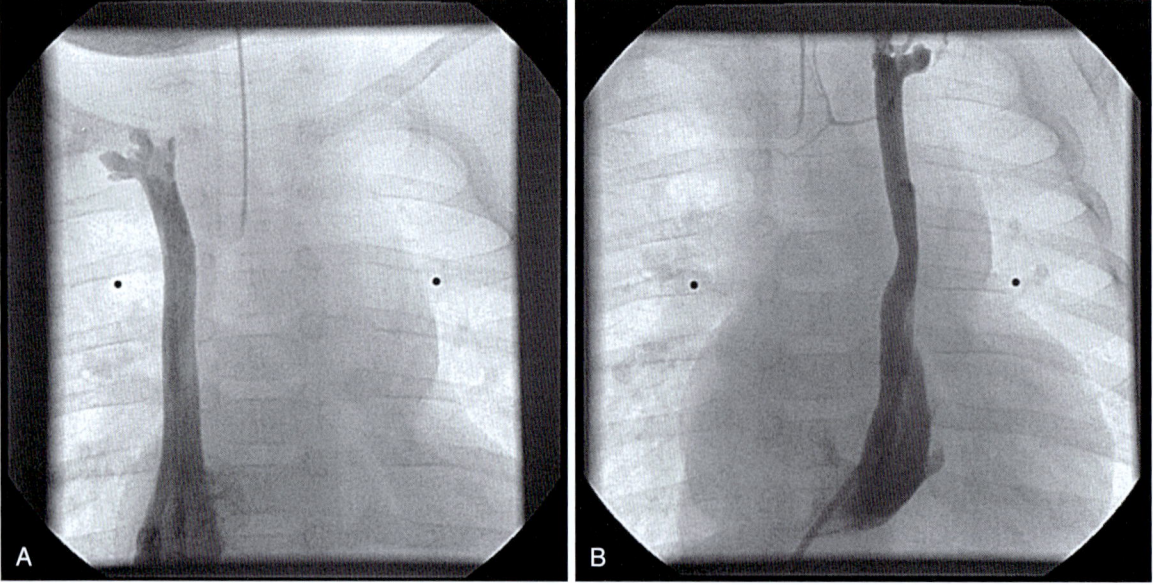

FIGURE 14.17 Bilateral superior vena cavae can exist separately or communicate through an innominate or bridging vein. **A,** The angiogram depicts the superior vena cava, normally a right-sided structure, as it drains into the right atrium. **B,** In the same patient, an angiogram shows drainage of a large left superior vena cava into the coronary sinus. The catheter courses from the inferior vena cava into the right atrium, coronary sinus, and left superior vena cava. Contrast injection into the left superior vena cava demonstrates no innominate vein between the two cavae. The coronary sinus is dilated as it receives the systemic venous blood from the left superior vena cava.

- On occasion, an LSVC can drain to an unroofed coronary sinus or directly into the left atrium, in which case a cardiac shunt is present with shunt direction depending on hemodynamics. It can be identified by injection of agitated saline into a left arm or left neck vein while performing an echocardiogram, and it can be associated with systemic arterial desaturation. This constitutes a risk for paradoxical systemic embolization.
- During cardiac surgery, an enlarged coronary sinus can interfere with the administration of retrograde cardioplegia.
- It can confound transvenous placement of a pulmonary artery catheter in some cases.

Evaluation of the Child With a Cardiac Murmur

The finding of an incidental murmur during the perioperative period can result in distress to the child or family; trigger additional diagnostic studies, including a cardiology consultation; and has the potential to delay the scheduled procedure when identified preoperatively. Although cardiac auscultation is a challenging skill that takes many years of practice to master,[234] it is important for the anesthesiologist who routinely cares for children to recognize the main physical findings that may distinguish an innocent cardiac murmur from a pathologic one.[235] Knowledge of several core concepts and red flags can help avoid overlooking potentially important diagnoses.

About 90% of normal children have a murmur at some point in their lives. This commonly occurs during the neonatal period and early school years. Most murmurs are functional, considered innocent in nature, and require no special treatment. This diagnosis is based on physical findings consistent with the benign nature of the specific murmur.

Although a complete discussion of cardiac murmur evaluation is beyond the scope of this chapter, it is important to review those findings that help to distinguish innocent from pathologic murmurs.[236,237] The basic systematic approach to assessing a heart murmur is the same as when evaluating any child's cardiovascular system.[238] The chest should be auscultated with both the diaphragm and bell of the stethoscope in the positions of the four primary cardiac valves in a quiet environment. Innocent murmurs in infancy and childhood include pulmonary flow murmur, a Still murmur, physiologic pulmonary branch stenosis, venous hum, and carotid bruit.[239] These murmurs are usually of low intensity (grades I and II of VI) and associated with a normal cardiovascular examination (e.g., normal precordial activity, first and second heart sounds, peripheral pulses, capillary refill). Innocent murmurs, such as those associated with peripheral pulmonary branch stenosis, right ventricular outflow murmurs, and Still murmurs, are usually soft, systolic ejection type, and not holosystolic in duration. Physiologic murmurs often resolve by changing the child's hemodynamic state with maneuvers such as lying down, sitting up/standing,[240] or with temporal changes such as resolution of fever and improvement in anemia. Diastolic or continuous murmurs are typically pathologic, except for a venous hum. This murmur is thought to be related to turbulent flow of systemic venous return in the jugular veins and superior vena cava and is best heard at the base of the neck. *Murmurs accompanied by a palpable thrill are always pathologic.*

When there is doubt regarding the benign or pathologic nature of a murmur, consultation with a pediatric cardiologist is indicated. A CXR and ECG, although thought by some to add minimal value in the initial diagnostic assessment of a cardiac murmur and to not be cost-effective, can be helpful when considering if further consultation is indicated.[241]

Basic Interpretation of the Electrocardiogram in Children

Despite the increasing applications of imaging modalities in the structural and functional assessment of pediatric heart disease, electrocardiography continues to play an important role in the diagnosis and management of these children.[242] An ECG is considered an integral part of the evaluation of most children with congenital or acquired cardiovascular pathology.

Although the characteristic features of a normal ECG in infants and children were described many decades ago, it is surprising that it continues to be one of the most often misinterpreted screening tests in pediatric medicine.[243] This is largely because of the developmental changes that occur in the normal individual as they progress from the neonatal period through childhood, adolescence, and adulthood.[244] Normal values for children of different ages have been established.[245] Knowledge of normal configurations and values for various ages of children is essential for accurate interpretation. Immediately after birth, there is a predominance of right ventricular forces represented by tall R waves in the right precordial leads (V_1 and V_2) (Fig. 14.18). Over the first childhood years, the ECG changes to a more familiar left heart–dominant configuration with larger S waves in the right precordial leads and a gradual RS progression with tall R waves in the left precordial leads (V_5 and V_6) (Fig. 14.19). The predominance of right heart forces and the need to evaluate for dextrocardia are the primary reasons that pediatric ECGs should include the V_3R and V_4R leads, which are not routinely obtained in adult studies. These electrodes are placed in the corresponding V_3 and V_4 locations over the right hemithorax.

Clinical information of relevance in the interpretation of an ECG includes the child's age, gender, suspected or documented diagnosis, and indications for the examination. Several requirements are essential for accurate interpretation, including appropriate skin preparation, electrode placement, and an artifact-free recording. The approach to the pediatric ECG should be systematic and organized. *Determination of the rate and rhythm, with evaluation of the P-wave vector and the relationship between each P wave and QRS complex, is the first step.* It is important to consider the influences of age, autonomic nervous system, level of physical activity, medications, pain, and temperature on the child's heart rate. The P wave should be upright or positive in leads I and aVF, consistent with the sinus node being the pacemaker of the heart (i.e., sinus rhythm) (see Fig. 14.19). Normally, the P wave should precede the QRS complex. *Next, the QRS electrical axis should be determined.* The QRS frontal plane axis is assessed by identifying the most isoelectric lead, which is perpendicular to the direction of ventricular depolarization. Alternatively, the direction of depolarization in leads I and aVF can be examined to roughly estimate the axis. As with all other components of the evaluation, the physiologic changes that occur with growth are responsible for the change in normal values for the QRS axis based on age. Regardless of age, QRS axes that lie in the northwest quadrant (between 180 and 270 degrees with an S-wave–dominant pattern in leads I and aVF) are always abnormal and merit further investigation. This is a classic finding in children with AV septal defects. *Evaluating the T wave, or repolarization axis, is also important*, because a difference of greater than 90 degrees between the QRS and T-wave axes

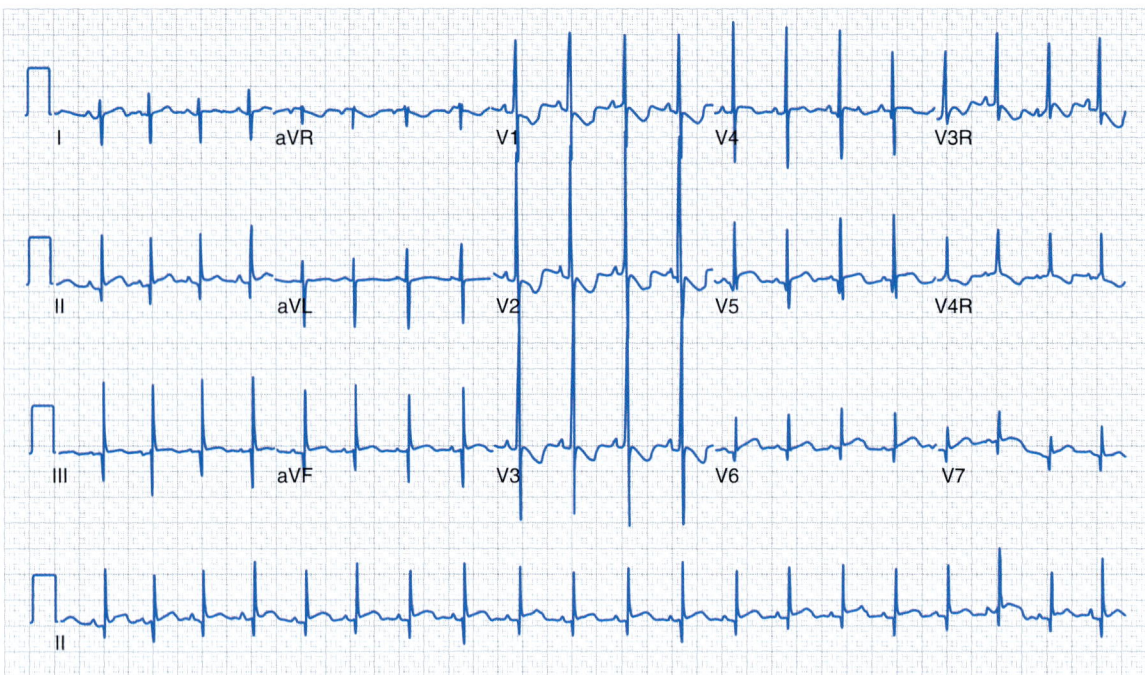

FIGURE 14.18 Normal electrocardiogram for a 2-day-old neonate shows the expected predominance of right ventricular forces during this age period (i.e., tall R waves in the right precordial leads, V₁, and V₂). The inverted T waves in V₁₋₃ are normal for this age.

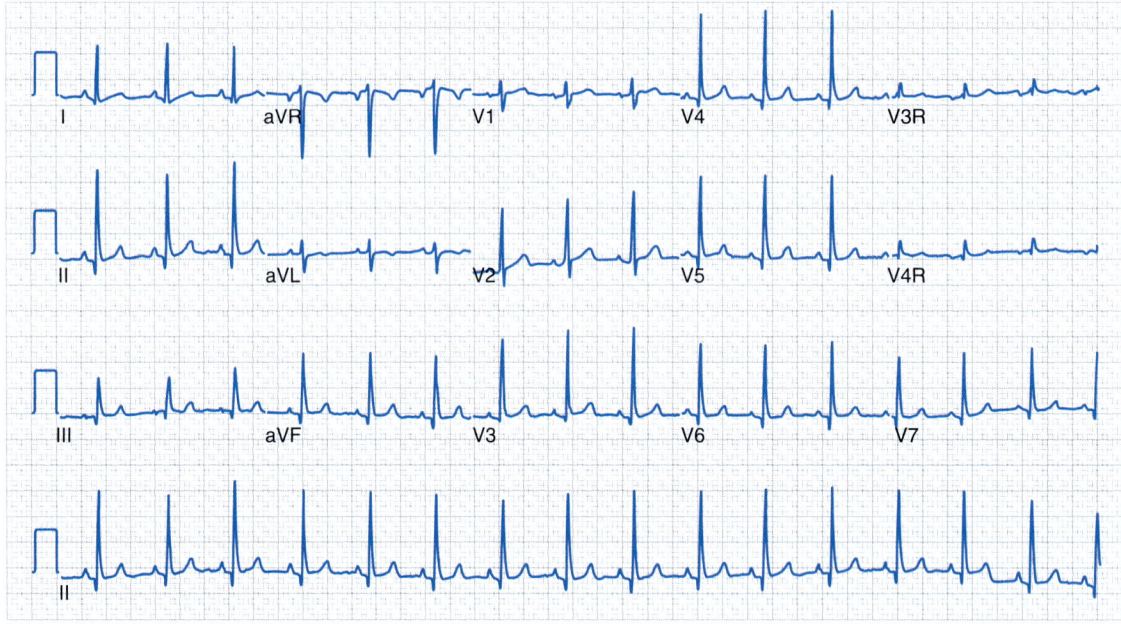

FIGURE 14.19 The normal electrocardiographic tracing was recorded for a 10-year-old child. The typical left heart–dominant configuration of children this age is characterized by gradual RS progression with tall R waves in the left precordial leads (V₅ and V₆). This contrasts with the right ventricular–dominant pattern seen during infancy and early childhood. The tracing demonstrates normal sinus rhythm as indicated by positive P waves in leads I and aVF.

can represent strain on the ventricle, a potential finding in ventricular hypertrophy (see Fig. 14.8).

After the evaluation of rhythm and axes is complete, *each component of the cardiac cycle as reflected by the ECG should be examined.*[246] The P wave represents atrial systole, and its morphology, with particular interest in leads II and V₁, can demonstrate right atrial (P-wave amplitude >2.5 mm or 3.0 mm based on age)

or left atrial (P-wave duration >100–120 msec based on age) enlargement (Fig. 14.20). The PR interval represents the time required for passage of an impulse from the sinoatrial node until ventricular depolarization and is largely composed of the AV nodal delay. A prolonged PR interval, which is age specific, indicates first-degree AV block. A short PR interval should prompt evaluation of the QRS duration for signs of preexcitation

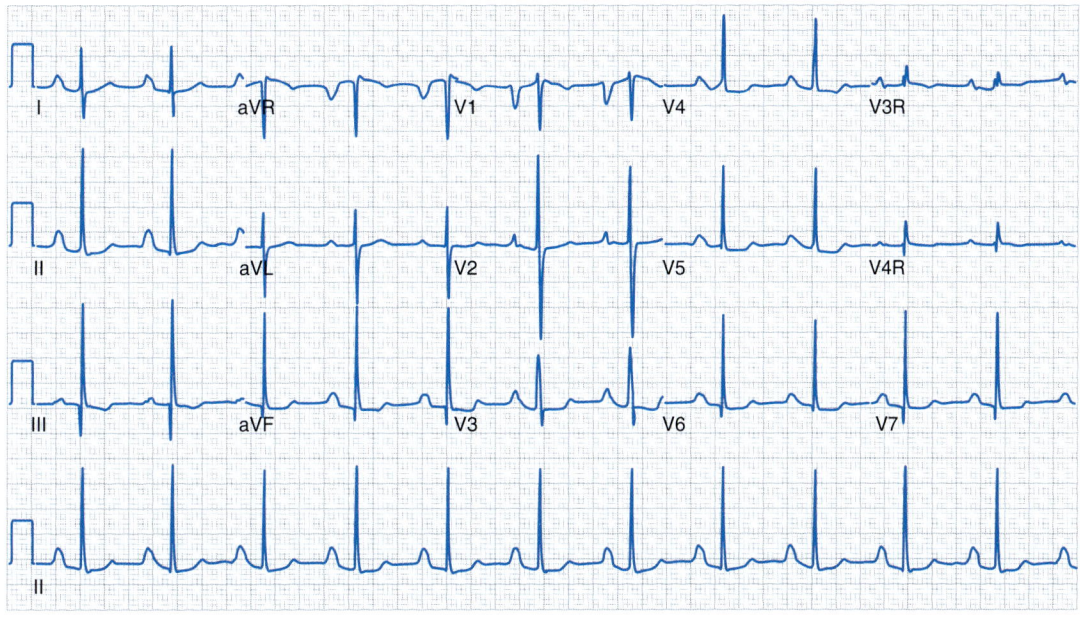

FIGURE 14.20 The tracing was obtained in the emergency room for a patient subsequently found to have restrictive cardiomyopathy. Biatrial enlargement is reflected by the tall and wide P waves in leads II and V₁, respectively.

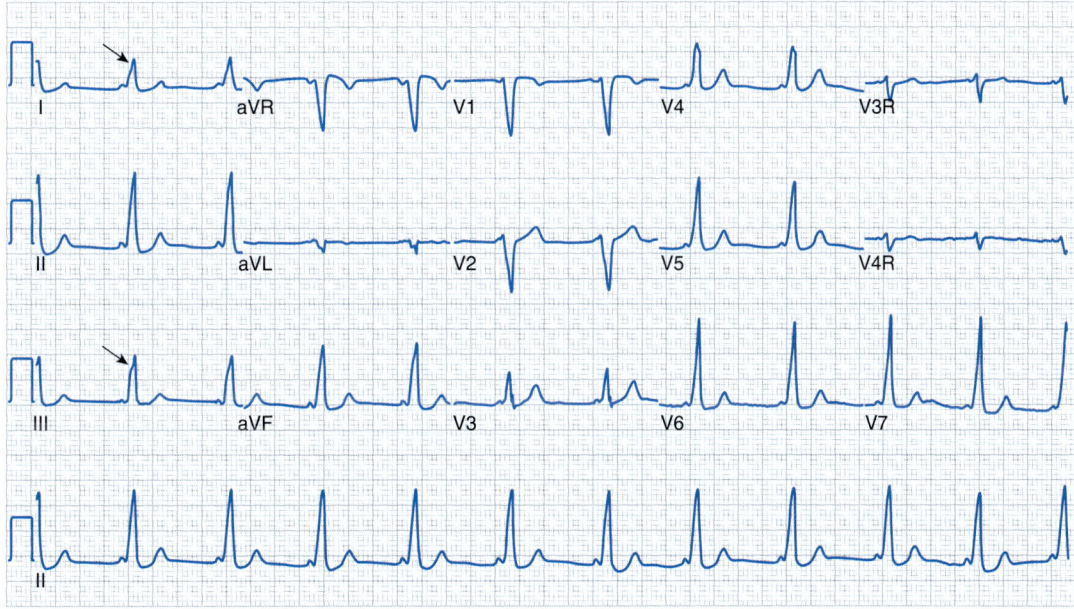

FIGURE 14.21 The tracing demonstrates the typical electrocardiographic features of Wolff-Parkinson-White syndrome: short PR interval, delta wave *(arrows)*, and prolongation of the QRS interval.

(i.e., Wolff-Parkinson-White syndrome), although a short PR interval can also reflect a low right atrial pacemaker (Fig. 14.21).

The QRS complex represents ventricular depolarization. The QRS duration should be examined in a lead with a Q wave present (often lead V_5 or V_6) for signs of conduction delay. Age-dependent normal values are important because the upper limit of normal QRS duration is only 80 milliseconds in neonates. The presence of a wide QRS complex with an RSR′ pattern in V_1 indicates a right bundle branch block, whereas a QS pattern in V_1 and a tall, notched R wave in V_6 is consistent with a left bundle branch block. Other conditions associated with prolongation of the QRS duration include ventricular preexcitation and ventricular pacing.

In addition to the QRS duration, the components of the QRS complex should be examined. The Q waves are often present in the lateral and inferior leads and in lead aVR, but they should be narrow (<40 msec) and shallow (age-dependent but usually <5-mm deep). Deep or wide Q waves suggest myocardial ischemia and require further evaluation. An uncommon but crucial finding occurs in infants with anomalous origin of the left coronary artery from the pulmonary artery (ALCAPA). Classically, the ECG in this lesion demonstrates deep, wide Q waves in leads I and aVL with ST-segment and T-wave changes in the anterior distribution (V_2 to V_4) consistent with compromised myocardial blood flow (Fig. 14.22). The QRS amplitudes are also important in assessing left and right

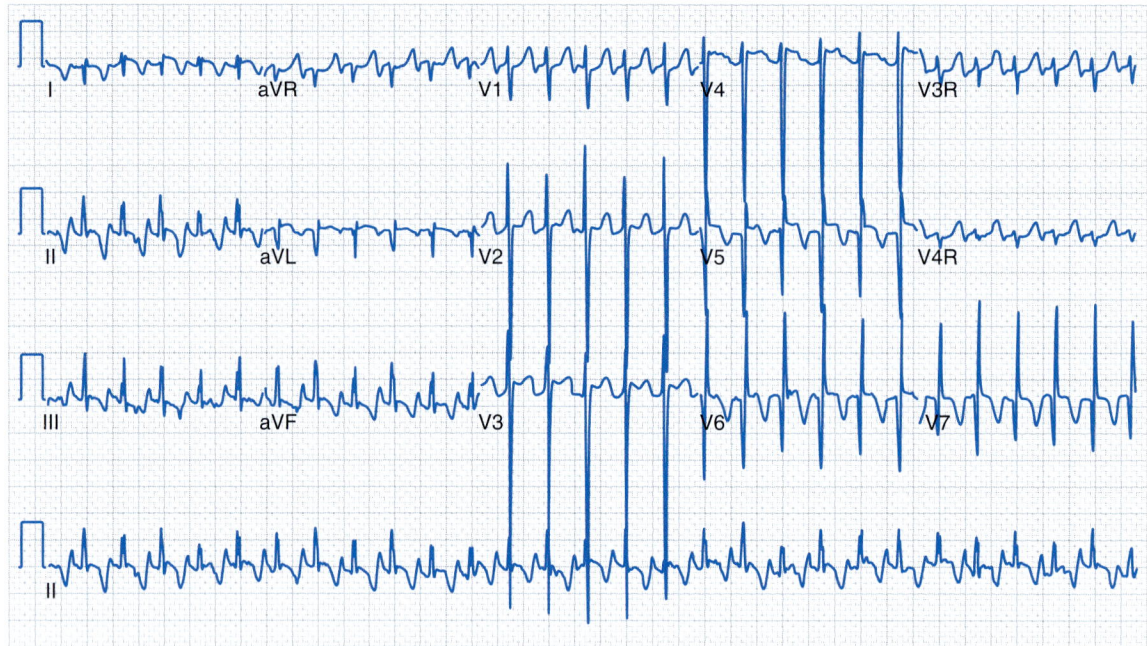

FIGURE 14.22 Electrocardiographic tracing for an infant with poor systolic ventricular function who was found to have anomalous origin of the left main coronary artery from the pulmonary root. The presence of Q waves in the aVL lead and the diffuse ST-T wave changes suggest ischemia and are classic findings in this anomaly.

ventricular hypertrophy. Conditions associated with increased QRS voltages that likely require echocardiographic assessment include HCM, LVNC, and Pompe disease (see Figs. 14.8 and 14.9).

ST segments should be flat and should not be depressed more than 0.5 mm or elevated more than 1 mm in any lead. The major exception to this rule is when there is gradual upsloping of the ST segment in the mid-precordial leads, as seen in early repolarization. T waves represent ventricular repolarization and should all be upright in the precordial leads at birth. Within 1 to 3 days they become inverted, initially in V_1 and eventually in V_2, V_3, and sometimes in V_4. Starting at several years of age, the T waves return to the upright position in the reverse order. In normal adolescents and adults, the T wave in lead V_1 can be upright or inverted. The only limb lead that typically displays an inverted T wave is aVR.

An aspect of the cardiac cycle that must be examined on any ECG is the QT interval, the time from the onset of ventricular depolarization (marked by the onset of the QRS complex), until the completion of repolarization (marked by the end of the T wave). It represents the duration of electrical activation and recovery of the ventricular myocardium, and it is measured as:

$$\text{Corrected QT (QTc)} = \frac{\text{Measured QT interval}}{\text{Square root of preceding R-R interval}}$$

A QTc that exceeds 470 milliseconds is considered abnormal, regardless of age. All QTc values that exceed normal values for age merit further investigation. Medications that prolong the QT interval should be avoided until the child has been evaluated by a cardiologist.[247]

Although a detailed organized approach to interpretation of a pediatric ECG is necessary, there are occasions when particular conditions or circumstances cause global changes that must be quickly recognized. One such case that can occur in the operating room is related to the ECG changes associated with hyperkalemia.

As the potassium level increases acutely, the T-wave amplitude increases. This is followed by widening of the QRS duration (Fig. 14.23 A,B) (see also Fig. 7.7) and owing to an intraventricular conduction delay and by AV block and arrhythmias, including ventricular tachycardia and fibrillation. Other electrolyte disturbances can result in characteristic changes on the ECG:

- Hypokalemia: decreased T-wave amplitude, ST-segment depression, and the presence of U waves
- Hypercalcemia: shortening of the QT interval, sinus rate slowing, and sinoatrial block
- Hypocalcemia: lengthening of the QT interval
- Hypomagnesemia: enhanced effects of hypocalcemia

Essentials of Cardiac Rhythm Interpretation and Acute Management of Arrhythmias in Children

Rhythm abnormalities can be seen during the preoperative assessment, in the operating room, or in the postoperative period. Considerations usually include identification of the rhythm disorder, establishing the need for acute therapy, deciding whether to consult a pediatric cardiologist, and conveying pertinent information to the consultant to assist in the characterization of the rhythm disturbance and to establish a management plan. The following principles should be considered in addressing these issues:

- Operating room, bedside, or transport monitors and strip recordings facilitate the recognition of rhythm disorders, but in most cases, they are inadequate for definitive diagnosis. A 15-lead surface ECG and rhythm strip should be obtained for all children when feasible.
- Clinicians caring for children should have a basic knowledge of cardiac rhythm interpretation. Although a comprehensive discussion of arrhythmia interpretation is beyond the scope of this

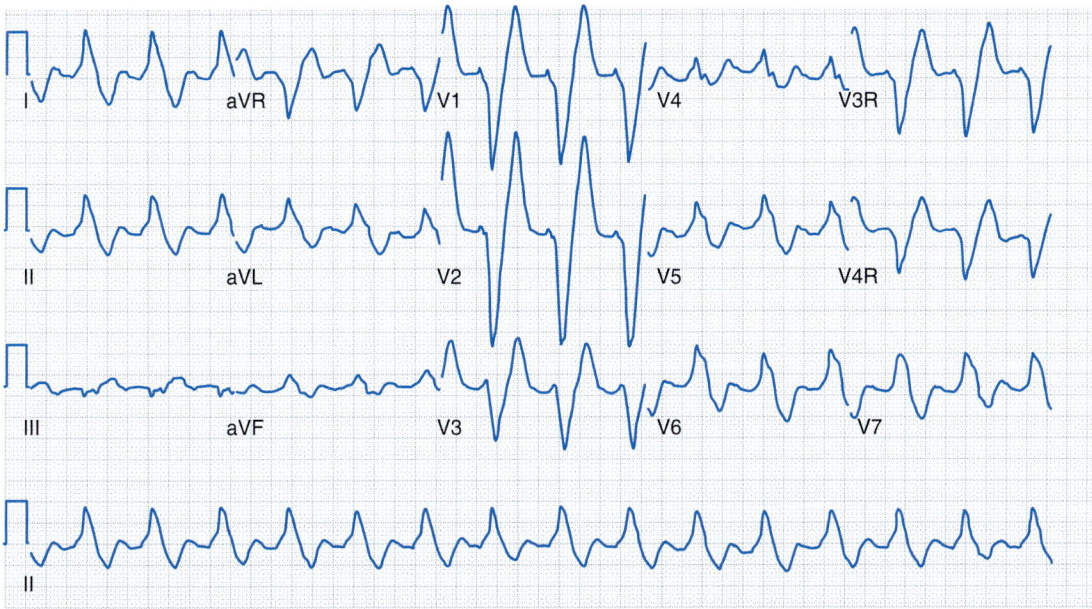

A   25 mm/sec 10 mm/mV 100 Hz

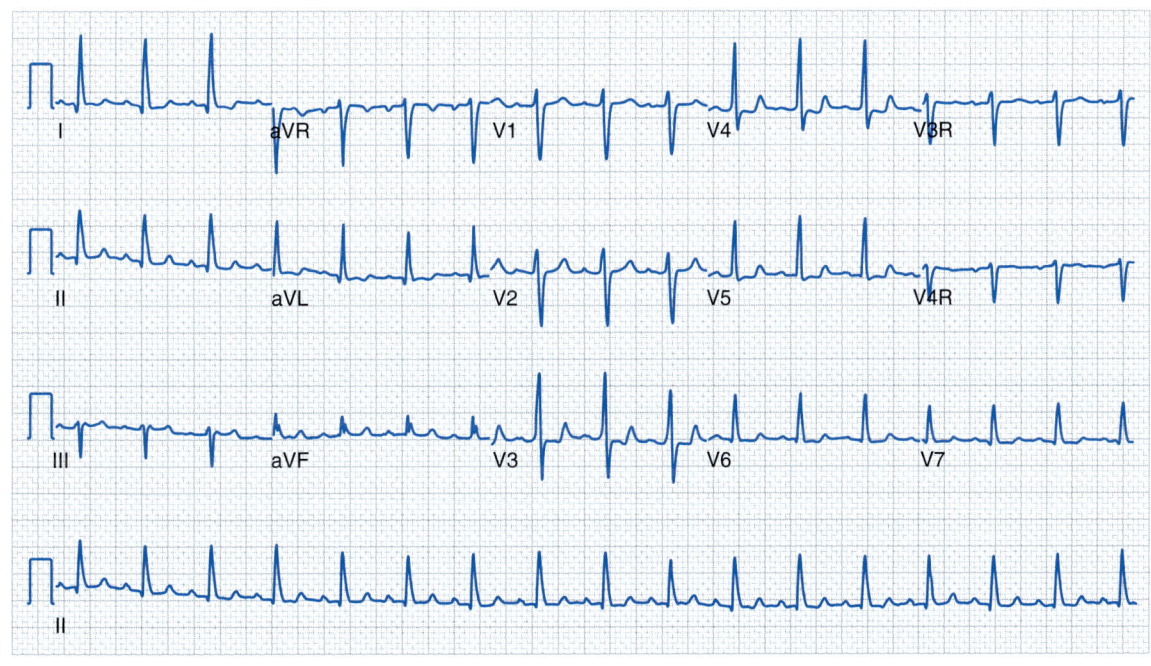

B

FIGURE 14.23 These electrocardiographic changes can result from hyperkalemia. **A,** Marked widening of the QRS complexes is associated with peaked T waves. If untreated, this condition may progress to ventricular fibrillation and asystole. **B,** A tracing obtained several hours after treatment of the electrolyte disturbance in the same patient demonstrates resolution of the electrocardiographic changes.

chapter, a brief overview of the characteristic features of normal and abnormal cardiac rhythms in the pediatric age group is presented in the next section.

- The need for acute therapy for a rhythm disturbance should be based primarily on the nature of the disorder, urgency of the situation, and the likelihood that this abnormality would or would not be tolerated beyond the immediate short-term period. The guidelines established by the American Heart Association for Pediatric Advanced Life Support should be followed in all patients.[248] In otherwise healthy children and in contrast to ventricular arrhythmias, supraventricular tachyarrhythmias are rarely life-threatening.

- The degree of comfort in the characterization and management of pediatric cardiac arrhythmias is likely to be quite variable among anesthesia care providers. For arrhythmias caused by respiratory compromise, electrolyte imbalance, or metabolic derangements, consultation with a pediatric cardiologist is probably not required. This is also the case for variants or benign rhythm disturbances such as sinus arrhythmia, low atrial rhythms, or occasional premature atrial beats (Fig. 14.24).

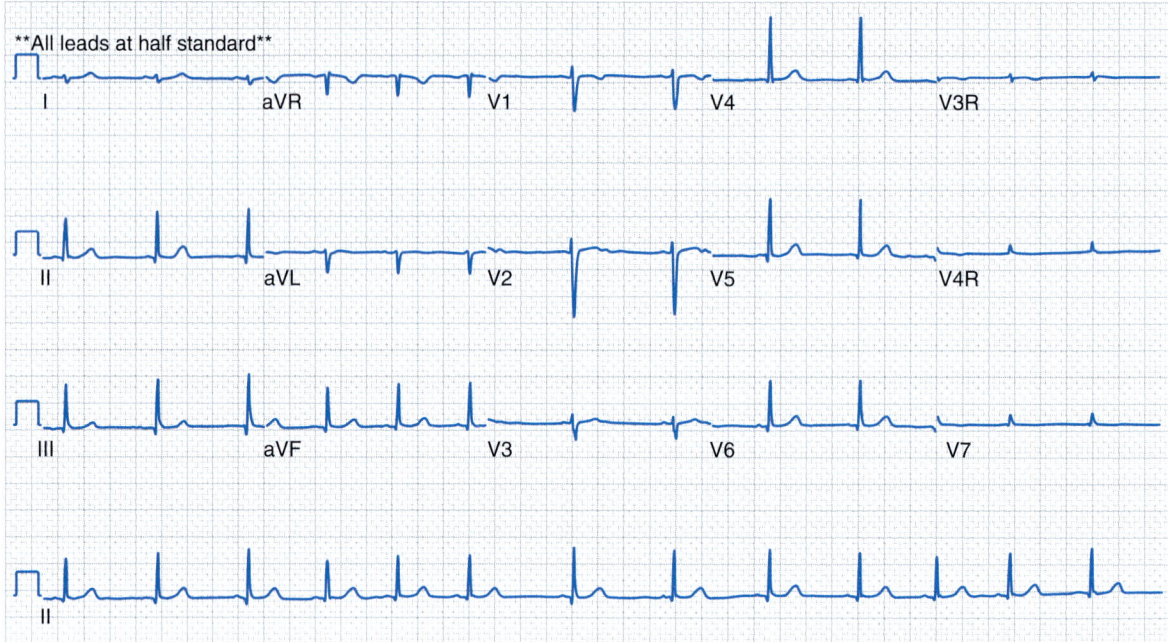

FIGURE 14.24 The rhythm tracing displays the normal heart rate variability with respiration. There is a normal increase in heart rate during inspiration. This sinus arrhythmia is a natural response and is more commonly seen in children than adults.

Consultation is appropriate for most children with known congenital or acquired cardiovascular pathology, in those with a history of a cardiac rhythm disorder under the care of a cardiologist, and in most of those with acute arrhythmias, particularly when initiation of antiarrhythmic drug therapy is contemplated.

- Information that may be helpful to a consultant includes pertinent details regarding the child's history, diagnosis, nature of the procedure/intervention, relevant laboratory values, description or characterization of the rhythm abnormality, associated hemodynamic parameters, circumstances surrounding the event (including the presence or absence of an intracardiac catheter), review of the pharmacologic agents administered (including anesthetic agents), and other therapies if applicable. The specialist should assist in the characterization of the rhythm disorder, advise about whether further evaluation is indicated, make recommendations for treatment, and facilitate diagnostic/therapeutic interventions as necessary.

BASIC RHYTHMS AND CONDUCTION DISORDERS

Tables 14.5 and 14.6 with associated figures (Figs. 14.8, 14.19, 14.24, 14.25, 14.26, 14.27) highlight common cardiac rhythms and conduction disorders, their characteristic features, and management.

CARDIAC ARRHYTHMIAS

Supraventricular Arrhythmias

Premature Atrial Contractions or Beats

Isolated premature atrial contractions (PACs) are relatively common in infants and small children. On the ECG, the early P waves exhibit a morphology and axis that are different from those in normal sinus rhythm. Premature atrial contractions can be conducted to the ventricles normally, blocked at the AV node, or conduct aberrantly (i.e., abnormal QRS morphology). They are usually benign and require no therapy. If a central venous catheter is present, the tip position should be evaluated.

Supraventricular Tachycardia

Supraventricular tachycardia (SVT) is the most common concerning arrhythmia in infants and children.[249–251] It is characterized by a regular tachyarrhythmia (tachycardia heart rate is age dependent but typically exceeding 230 beats/minute in children) with a narrow or usual complex QRS morphology. Supraventricular tachycardia can occur in structurally normal hearts and in various forms of CHD. *Usual complex* implies that the QRS morphology in tachycardia is similar to that in normal sinus rhythm (Fig. 14.28). Occasionally, widening of the QRS in SVT can result from bundle branch block or related to the tachycardia mechanism (i.e., SVT with aberrancy). A wide QRS complex can make the distinction between supraventricular and ventricular tachycardia difficult.

The two types of SVT are automatic and reentrant. They can be differentiated by assessing characteristics of the tachycardia, usually assisted by the input from a specialist. The evaluation of a tachyarrhythmia should include a surface 15-lead ECG and continuous rhythm strip to document onset and termination. If a medication such as adenosine has been administered, a recording of the response to the drug or pacing/electrical cardioversion maneuvers should be obtained. The management of SVT depends on the clinical status of the child, type of tachycardia, and precise electrophysiologic mechanism.

General management principles include:

- Hemodynamic stability should be determined. Synchronized direct current cardioversion (0.5–1.0 J/kg) should be performed for hemodynamic instability.
- Antiarrhythmic therapy is based primarily on the clinical condition and suspected tachycardia mechanism. Vagal maneuvers can be considered but should not delay treatment. Adenosine is the drug of choice in the acute setting for diagnosis and

TABLE 14.5 | Basic Rhythms

BASIC RHYTHMS

Rhythms	Characteristic Features	Management
Sinus rhythm	• P wave that precedes every QRS, QRS follows every P wave, and upright P wave in leads I and aVF (see Fig. 14.19)	• No treatment (normal rhythm)
Sinus arrhythmia	• Cyclic changes in the heart rate during breathing (see Fig. 14.24)	• No treatment • Normal finding in healthy children
Sinus bradycardia	• Refers to sinus rhythm with heart rate below normal for age (see Fig. 14.8) • Can be observed during sleep or at times of high vagal tone • If significant, may lead to a slow junctional escape rhythm or a slow atrial rhythm originating from an ectopic focus • Certain forms of CHD are prone to slow heart rhythms (i.e., heterotaxy syndromes) • Can occur with laryngoscopy, tracheal intubation, suctioning, drug administration (i.e., opioids), or increased parasympathetic tone • Can result from hypoxemia, hypothermia, acidosis, electrolyte imbalance, or increased intracranial pressure	• Rarely poses significant hemodynamic compromise and, if necessary, can be easily treated with removal of the stimulus, administration of a vagolytic agent (e.g., glycopyrrolate and atropine), or with chronotropic drugs (e.g., epinephrine) • If due to hypoxemia, should be treated promptly with the administration of supplemental oxygen and appropriate airway management • Approach to other secondary forms should focus on addressing the underlying cause • For worrisome slow heart rates, particularly in small infants, or for clinical evidence of compromised hemodynamics, initiate chest compressions and pharmacologic therapy (i.e., epinephrine, atropine, or isoproterenol infusion) or temporary pacing should be considered
Sinus tachycardia	• Heart rate above normal for age (see Fig. 14.25) • Often the result of surgical stimulation, stress, pain, hypovolemia, anemia, fever, medications (i.e., inotropic agents), or a high catecholamine state • May impair diastolic filling time, reduce ventricular preload, and compromise cardiac output (children at risk include those with significant degrees of ventricular hypertrophy or diastolic dysfunction, aortic stenosis, and HCM)	• Treatment directed at the underlying cause
Junctional rhythm	• QRS complexes of morphology identical to that of sinus rhythm without preceding P waves (see Fig. 14.26) • Usually slower than the expected sinus rate (junctional bradycardia) • When it completely takes over the pacemaker activity of the heart, retrograde P waves and AV dissociation can be seen • During cardiac surgery is frequently the result of manipulation or dissection near the right atrium • Central venous pressure contour typically demonstrates prominent cannon *a* waves (i.e., right atrial pressure wave at the end of systole) owing to the loss of AV synchrony • Lack of atrial contribution to ventricular filling can result in hemodynamic changes	• Observation in most cases if transient

AV, Atrioventricular; *CHD*, congenital heart disease; *HCM*, hypertrophic cardiomyopathy.

TABLE 14.6 | Conduction Disorders

CONDUCTION DISORDERS

Disorder	Characteristic Features	Management
Bundle branch block	*Incomplete right bundle branch block* • rSR' in the right precordial leads with near-normal QRS duration • Occurs in children with right ventricular volume overload (e.g., those with ASDs) *Complete right bundle branch block* • QRS complex >100 msec for infants, 120 msec for older children • Characterized by an rSR' wave pattern in V_1, an inverted T wave, and a wide and deep S (slurred) wave in V_6 • Frequently seen after right ventricular outflow tract surgery *Left bundle branch block* • Uncommon finding in the pediatric age group • Can result from cardiac interventions along the left ventricular outflow tract • Criteria include a prominent QS or rS complex in lead V_1 and tall, wide, and often notched R wave in leads I, aVL, and V_6	• None

Continued

TABLE 14.6 | Conduction Disorders—cont'd

CONDUCTION DISORDERS

Disorder	Characteristic Features	Management
Atrioventricular block	*First degree* • Prolongation of the PR interval beyond the normal range for age • Each P wave is followed by a conducted QRS complex • May be found in healthy individuals but can also be seen in various disease states	• Benign condition requiring no specific treatment

	Second degree
	• Characterized by a periodic failure to conduct atrial impulses to the ventricle (i.e., P wave without following QRS complex)
	• Several forms, Mobitz type I (Wenckebach) and Mobitz type II are the two predominant types
	• Type I:
	  • There is a gradual lengthening of the PR interval with eventual failure of conduction of the next atrial impulse to the ventricle; the RR intervals concomitantly shorten
	  • Degree of block expressed as the ratio of P waves to QRS complexes (i.e., 2:1, 3:2)
	  • Can occur during periods of high vagal tone or in the postoperative setting
	• Type II:
	  • There is a relatively constant PR interval before an atrial impulse that fails to conduct
		• Type I usually a benign phenomenon that requires no therapy
		• Type II is considered a more serious conduction disturbance and merits further investigation

	Third degree • Characterized by total failure of conduction of atrial impulses to the ventricle • There is complete AV dissociation, with more atrial than ventricular contractions, and the ventricular rate is usually slow and regular (see Fig. 14.27) • It can be congenital or acquired	• Temporary pacing may be indicated in the acute setting

ASD, Atrial septal defect; *AV,* atrioventricular.

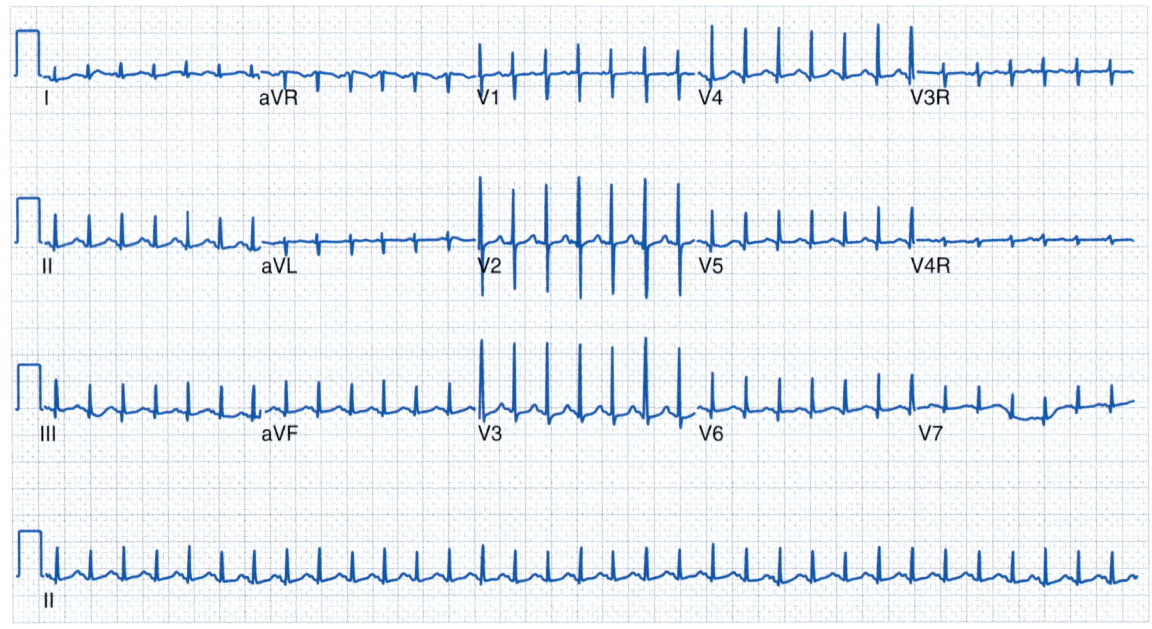

FIGURE 14.25 Electrocardiogram for a febrile infant with sinus tachycardia, characterized by a heart rate above normal for age and QRS complexes of normal appearance preceded by P waves, which are upright in leads I and aVF.

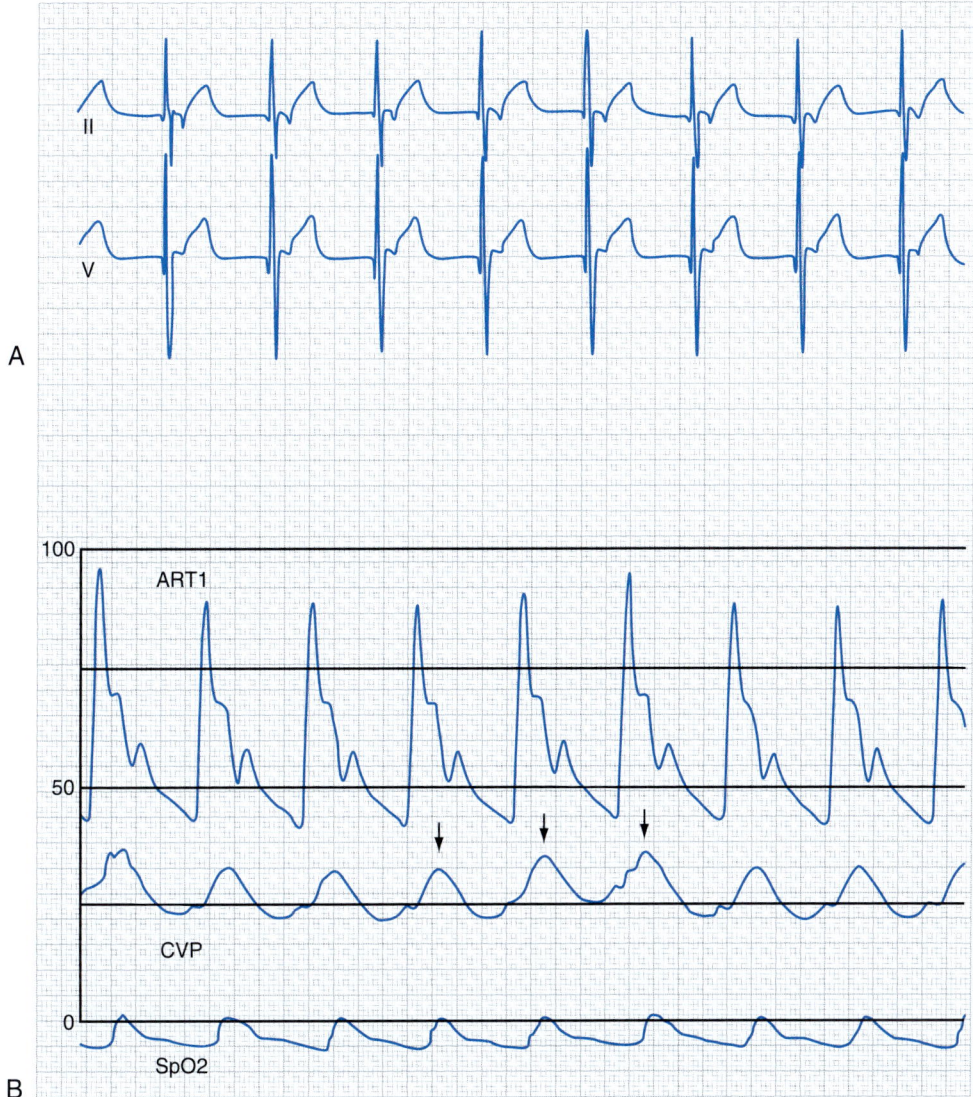

FIGURE 14.26 A, The tracing obtained during cardiac surgery at the time of right atrial dissection demonstrates the features of a junctional rhythm. Retrograde P waves are identified after the QRS complexes. **B,** The central venous pressure *(CVP)* tracing demonstrates prominent cannon a waves *(arrows)* related to the loss of atrioventricular synchrony and right atrial contraction against a closed tricuspid valve (scale of 0–30 mm Hg for CVP).

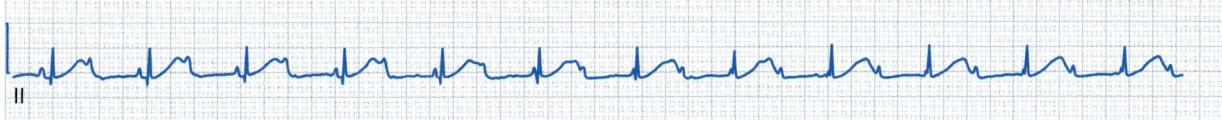

FIGURE 14.27 Rhythm strip demonstrates independent atrial and ventricular activity (i.e., atrioventricular dissociation) and failure of any atrial impulses to conduct to the ventricles. These features characterize a complete atrioventricular block.

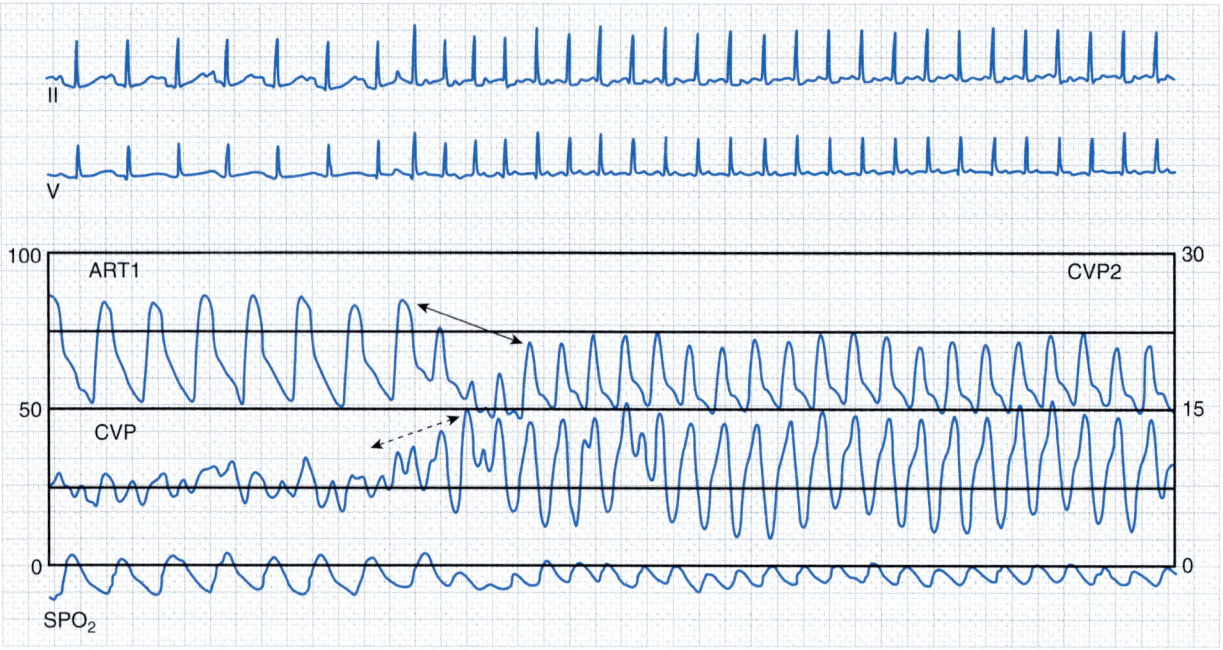

FIGURE 14.28 The initial portion of the intraoperative recording demonstrates normal sinus rhythm. A premature atrial beat initiates a narrow complex tachycardia (i.e., QRS morphology is the same as in sinus rhythm). The supraventricular tachycardia is associated with hemodynamic changes such as a decrease in the systemic arterial pressure (*ART 1*, scale of 0–100 mm Hg) *(solid arrow)* and increase in the central venous pressure (*CVP*, scale of 0–30 mm Hg) *(broken arrow)*. SpO₂, Oxygen saturation.

termination of most supraventricular tachycardias. β-blockers are most often used for chronic therapy.

- Other measures include treatment of fever (if present), sedation, correction of electrolyte disturbance, and decreasing or withdrawing medications associated with sympathetic stimulation (i.e., inotropic agents) or with vagolytic properties.
- In addition to pharmacologic therapy, atrial pacing or cardioversion may be required.

Ventricular Arrhythmias

Premature Ventricular Contractions or Beats

Premature ventricular contractions (PVCs) are characterized by prematurity of the QRS complex, a QRS morphology different from that in sinus rhythm, usually a prolongation of the QRS duration for age, abnormalities of the ST segment and T wave, and premature ventricular activity not preceded by a premature atrial beat. PVCs of a single QRS morphology (i.e., uniform), without associated symptoms, and in children with structurally normal hearts are considered benign. An ECG during sinus rhythm should allow careful measurement of the QT interval. Further investigation and consultation are warranted in the presence of PVCs of multiple morphologies (i.e., multiform), if they occur with moderate frequency or in succession (i.e., couplets or runs) and are associated with symptoms or a structurally abnormal heart.

Ventricular ectopy in the perioperative period can be the result of profound hypoxemia, electrolyte disturbances, or metabolic derangements. Other causes include the use of recreational drugs, myocardial injury, poor hemodynamics, and prior cardiac surgical intervention.

Ventricular Tachycardia

Ventricular tachycardia (VT) is relatively uncommon in children. It is defined as three or more consecutive ventricular beats occurring at a rate greater than 120 beats/minute (Fig. 14.29). The QRS morphology in VT is different from that in sinus rhythm, and the QRS duration is typically prolonged for age. ECG features that support this diagnosis include AV dissociation, intermittent fusion (i.e., QRS complex of intermediate morphology between two other distinct QRS morphologies), QRS morphology of VT similar to that of single PVCs, and tachycardia rate in children usually below 250 beats/minute.

Acute onset of VT in pediatric patients can be caused by hypoxia, acidosis, electrolyte imbalance, or metabolic problems. Ventricular tachycardia can also occur in the context of depressed ventricular function, inhalation anesthesia (particularly halothane) with or without hypercarbia,[252] poor hemodynamics, prior surgical interventions, cardiomyopathies, myocardial tumors, acute injury (e.g., inflammation, trauma), and prolonged QT syndromes.[253]

Long QT Syndrome

Long QT syndrome (LQTS) (Fig. 14.30) is an electrical cardiac disturbance that can predispose children to arrhythmias that include torsades de pointes ventricular tachycardia (Fig. 14.31), ventricular fibrillation, and bradyarrhythmias; any of these can result in syncope, cardiac arrest, or sudden death.[254,255] It occurs with an incidence of 1 per 2500 births; congenital and acquired forms have been described. The congenital varieties are likely the result of genetic defects in the ion channel proteins responsible for maintaining electrical homeostasis.[256] The Romano-Ward form of LQTS accounts for 90% of pediatric cases; it has an incidence of 1 per 10,000 births and an autosomal dominant pattern of inheritance. The Jervell and Lange-Nielsen syndrome has an incidence of 1 per 1,000,000 births, an autosomal recessive pattern of inheritance, and an association with deafness. Diagnostic criteria for LQTS include ECG findings, clinical history (e.g., deafness, syncope), and family history. Prolongation of the QTc on the resting ECG is the hallmark of this syndrome but may not always be present.

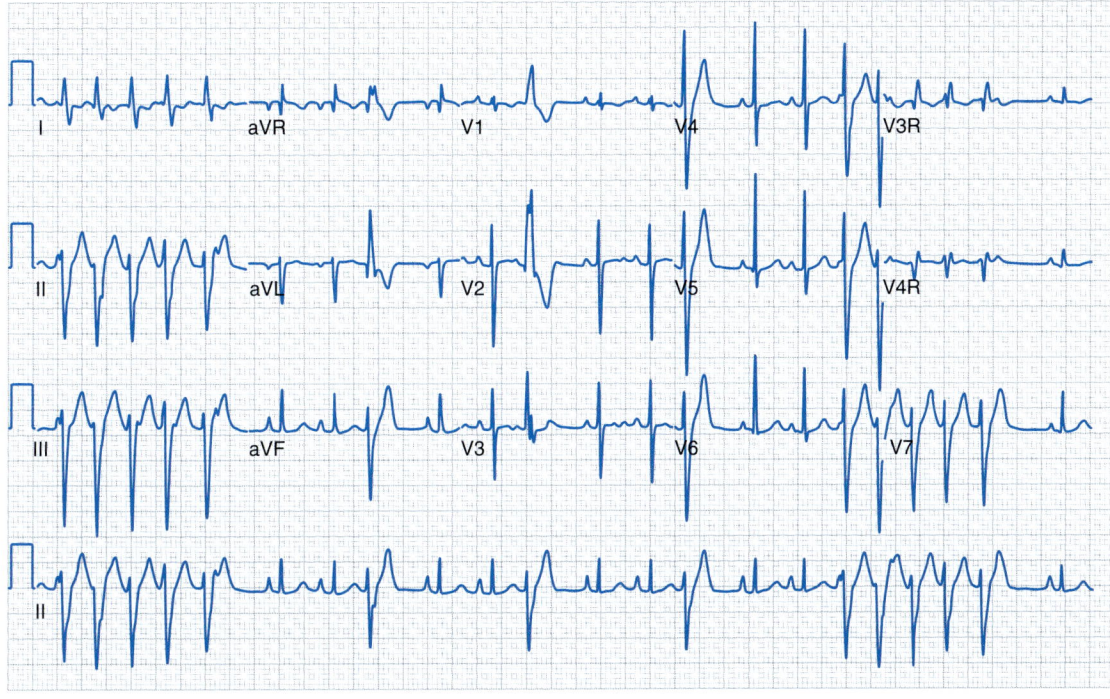

FIGURE 14.29 The tracing demonstrates frequent, uniform premature ventricular beats and episodes of non-sustained, monomorphic ventricular tachycardia.

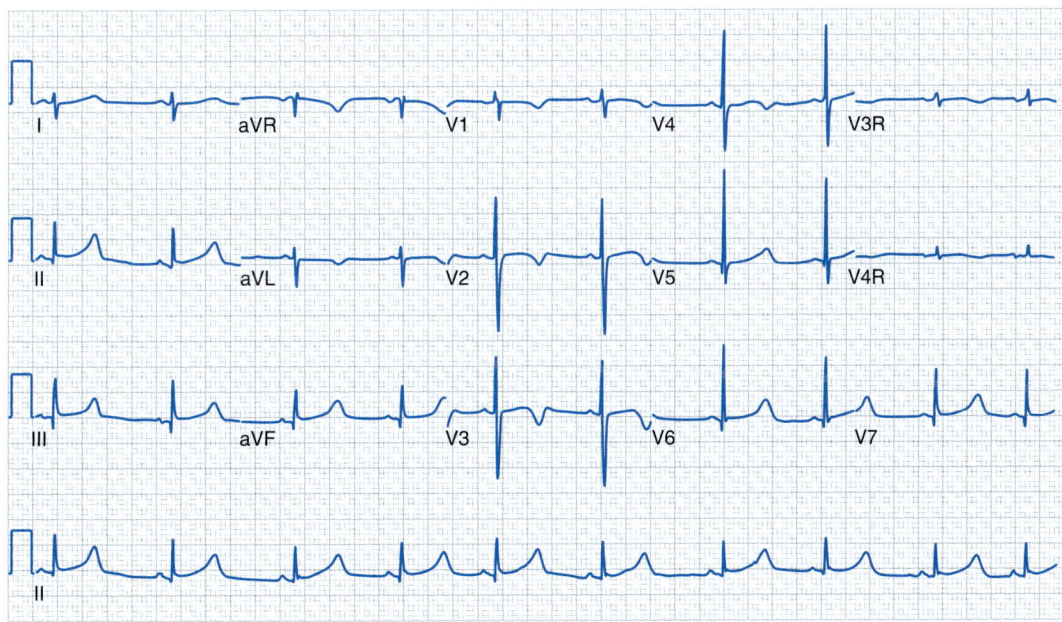

FIGURE 14.30 For a patient with long QT syndrome, the electrocardiogram demonstrates prolongation of the QT interval.

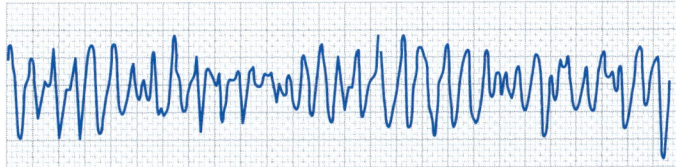

FIGURE 14.31 The rhythm strip displays positive and negative oscillation of QRS complexes, which is characteristic of torsades de pointes ventricular tachycardia.

Torsades is a rare but potentially life-threatening arrhythmia. To trigger torsades, increased dispersion of repolarization must also occur. This phenomenon refers to the variance in the rate of repolarization; in this case, it is a circumscribed region in the heart muscle (i.e., transmurally from the epicardium to the endocardium). There is much debate over how to quantify an increased dispersion of repolarization from surface ECGs. Some suggest the dispersion is the QTc-max to QTc-min, whereas others recommend measuring the duration of the T wave from its peak to the end; in both instances the upper limit of normal is 65 milliseconds and abnormal values exceed 100 milliseconds.

Prolongation of the QT interval and genesis of torsades occur more commonly in the presence of several conditions and drugs: electrolyte derangements (e.g., hypokalemia, hypocalcemia, hypomagnesemia), combination drug therapies (e.g., antibiotics, antiarrhythmic agents, class III antiarrhythmics such as amiodarone and procainamide), antipsychotic drugs, neurologic or endocrine abnormalities (e.g., hypothyroidism), 5-HT$_3$ receptor–blocking drugs (except palonosetron), neostigmine, stress (including induction of and emergence from anesthesia and laryngoscopy), female gender, bradycardia, and other conditions.[257] The risk for developing torsades from the many drugs known to trigger it is almost unpredictable. A comprehensive list of drugs that prolong the QT interval or may induce torsades can be found in the frequently updated website of The Arizona Center for Education and Research on Therapeutics (https://crediblemeds.org/index.php/login/dlcheck).

Although many anesthetics prolong the QT interval, few affect the dispersion of repolarization (as in the case of sevoflurane), and the risk of torsades during general anesthesia in children is rare. The perioperative risk of torsades in neonates and infants who require urgent procedures after failed first-line management of their underlying long QT syndrome is greater than that in older children.[258] An important consideration in the care of children with LQTS is ensuring adequate β-adrenergic blockade preoperatively and minimizing adrenergic stimulation.

In a retrospective study of children with LQTS, three adverse events were reported during emergence from anesthesia immediately after administration of ondansetron and anticholinesterase medications; one was described as torsades.[259] These arrhythmias resolved quickly with IV β-blockers, lidocaine, or the administration of both agents. The report suggests that children with LQTS are at risk for arrhythmias during periods of enhanced sympathetic activity (i.e., during emergence), particularly in the presence of drugs that prolong the QT interval. Conditions (e.g., hypothermia) and drugs that are known to prolong the QT interval should not be combined if possible.

Management of ventricular tachycardia requires the following considerations:

- Although some atypical forms of supraventricular tachyarrhythmias may mimic VT, a wide QRS tachycardia should in its origin, always be attributed to the ventricle.
- The initial approach in the setting of an acute ventricular rhythm disturbance consists of prompt evaluation of clinical status and hemodynamic stability. Sustained ventricular arrhythmias are poorly tolerated and require immediate attention. In the unstable child, cardiopulmonary resuscitation should be instituted while preparing for cardioversion. Expert consultation is advisable when advanced drug therapy is contemplated. Potential pharmacologic interventions include lidocaine, amiodarone, and procainamide.
- Magnesium sulfate is considered the first-line treatment of torsades. Procainamide and amiodarone are contraindicated

owing to prolongation of the QT interval. Correction of electrolyte disorders is also appropriate. Isoproterenol and overdrive pacing can be effective to increase heart rate in the case of bradycardia. Electrical cardioversion (1–2 J/kg) should be performed only if the arrhythmia is refractory to pharmacologic treatment.

- LQTS should be treated with β-blockade (not overdrive pacing); some forms of the LQTS may require the implantation of a cardioverter-defibrillator.

Ventricular Fibrillation

Ventricular fibrillation (VF) is an uncommon arrhythmia in children. It is characterized by chaotic, asynchronous ventricular activity that fails to generate an adequate cardiac output. The ECG during VF demonstrates low-amplitude, irregular deflections without identifiable QRS complexes. A loose electrode can mimic these surface ECG features, therefore immediate clinical assessment should be performed, and adequate pad contact ensured when VF is suspected.

Management of VF includes the following considerations:

- This is a lethal arrhythmia if untreated.
- Immediate defibrillation (initial dose of 2 J/kg) is the definitive therapy. Cardiopulmonary resuscitation, beginning with chest compressions per Pediatric Advanced Life Support protocols, should be immediately instituted and continued for 2 minutes. If defibrillation is unsuccessful, the energy dose should be doubled (4 J/kg) and repeated. Pediatric paddles (2.2 cm in diameter) are recommended for children weighing less than 10 kilograms or less than a year of age. Adult paddles (8–9 mm in diameter) are suggested for children weighing more than 10 kilograms to reduce impedance and maximize current flow.
- Adequate airway control and chest compressions should be rapidly instituted while preparing for defibrillation or between shocks if several defibrillation attempts are needed. Resuscitative drugs and amiodarone should be considered without delaying defibrillation.

Pacemaker and Defibrillator Therapy in the Pediatric Age Group

PACEMAKER NOMENCLATURE

Pacemaker nomenclature follows the guidelines of the North American Society of Pacing and Electrophysiology and the British Pacing and Electrophysiology Group (Table 14.7)[260]:

- First letter: chamber(s) paced (A = atrium, V = ventricle, D = dual or both, O = none)
- Second letter: chamber(s) sensed (A = atrium, V = ventricle, D = dual or both, O = none)
- Third letter: pacemaker response to sensing (I = inhibited, T = triggered, D = dual response, O = none)
- Fourth letter: rate modulation (R = rate modulation, O = none)
- Fifth letter: multisite pacing (A = atrium, V = ventricle, D = dual or both, O = none)

The most common pacing modes are listed in Table 14.8.

PERMANENT CARDIAC PACING

Indications

The updated guidelines for device-based therapy of cardiac rhythm abnormalities in children were recently published.[261] In general terms, indications for permanent cardiac pacing in children include symptomatic sinus bradycardia, bradycardia-tachycardia

TABLE 14.7	The Revised NASPE/BPEG Generic Pacemaker Codes[a]				
POSITION NUMBER AND CATEGORY					
I	II	III		IV	V
Chamber(s) Paced	Chamber(s) Sensed	Response to Sensing		Rate Modulation	Multisite Pacing
A = Atrium	A = Atrium	I = Inhibited		R = Rate modulation	A = Atrium
V = Ventricle	V = Ventricle	T = Triggered			V = Ventricle
D = Dual (A + V)	D = Dual (A + V)	D = Dual (I + T) response restricted to dual-chamber devices			D = Dual (A + V)
O = None	O = None	O = None		O = None	O = None

[a]The pacemaker mode, specified by a code, describes the mode in which the pacemaker is operating.
Reproduced with permission from Bernstein AD, Daubert JC, Fletcher RD, et al. The revised NASPE/BPEG generic code for antibradycardia, adaptive-rate, and multisite pacing. *Pacing Clin Electrophysiol.* 2002;25:260-264, with minor modifications.

14

TABLE 14.8	Most Common Pacing Modes

Single-Chamber Pacing

AAI: atrial demand pacing (atrial pacing and sensing, inhibited on sensed beat)

AAIR: atrial demand pacing (atrial pacing and sensing, inhibited on sensed beat), rate responsiveness

VVI: ventricular demand pacing (ventricular pacing and sensing, inhibited on sensed beat)

VVIR: ventricular demand pacing (ventricular pacing and sensing, inhibited on sensed beat), rate responsiveness

Asynchronous Pacing (No Sensing)

AOO: fixed-rate atrial pacing

VOO: fixed-rate ventricular pacing

DOO: fixed-rate AV pacing

Dual-Chamber Pacing

DDD: paces and senses both chambers

DDDR: paces and senses both chambers, sensor-driven rate responsiveness

syndromes, congenital third-degree AV block, and advanced second- or third-degree AV block.

Perioperative Considerations

It is essential for anesthesia providers involved in the care of patients with a cardiac implantable electronic device (CIED) to understand basic aspects such as indications for placement, functionality, and potential issues that may be encountered perioperatively.[262,263] Although device interrogation has been considered an essential part of the preoperative evaluation in all patients with an implanted pacemaker, which seems a reasonable recommendation, the need for interrogation in all patients has been questioned.[264] Results of a recent 15-lead ECG should be reviewed if available. Familiarity with unit type, settings, date of and indications for implantation, device location, and underlying cardiac rhythm is highly recommended. If records are not available and there is no identification card providing details about the unit implanted, a radiopaque marker on a CXR can assist in the identification of the device. Major pacemaker manufacturers can also be readily contacted because they maintain computerized records of all implanted devices.

Reprogramming may be required before the planned procedure to avoid potential problems with pacemaker malfunction related to electrocautery. This represents one of the most common potential sources of electromagnetic interference in children with implanted cardiac devices. Recommendations for the perioperative management of the patient with a cardiac pacemaker include the use of bipolar cautery instead of a unipolar configuration if possible, avoiding cauterization near the site of the generator, and positioning the indifferent plate (dispersive pad) for electrocautery as far away as possible from the pacemaker so that the device is not between the electrocautery electrodes.[264] Devices such as the harmonic scalpel and battery-operated, hot wire, handheld cautery units do not interfere with implanted cardiac devices. Rate-responsive features of pacemakers should be deactivated in most cases.

Chronotropic drugs and alternate pacing modalities should be readily available in the event of pacemaker malfunction and compromising underlying rate. Although inserting a transvenous pacemaker has been recommended for children with complete AV block who were undergoing pacemaker implantation, no benefit to routine preoperative temporary pacing has been reported.[265] Capture thresholds can be affected by pharmacologic agents, and this should be considered if pacing is required in the child receiving antiarrhythmic drug therapy.

Perioperative conditions can also influence pacing thresholds. A magnet should be accessible to allow asynchronous pacing if required. Most generators respond to magnet application by pacing at a fixed rate asynchronously (i.e., AOO, VOO, or DOO). A potential problem is that the specific magnet rate, as determined by the manufacturer for the device, can be different from the desirable or optimal pacing rate. The use of a magnet should not be considered a substitute for preoperative pacemaker interrogation/programming when deemed necessary. In addition to perioperative electrocardiographic monitoring, additional modalities that confirm pulse generation during pacing (e.g., pulse oximetry, invasive arterial blood pressure monitoring) are strongly encouraged. The device should be tested and reprogrammed after the procedure is completed.

Transcutaneous Pacing

Several devices that combine defibrillation and cardioversion capabilities with external pacing features are available. Emergency transthoracic pacing can be considered as a temporizing measure for children with symptomatic bradycardia unresponsive to pharmacological therapy,[266] but this has not been effective in the treatment of asystole in children.[267] Suitable pacing electrodes should be selected according to patient size. Device settings typically include pacing rate and power output. Sedation may be necessary for tolerance of discomfort originating from soft tissue and skeletal contractions.[268] Prolonged periods of transcutaneous pacing can result in local cutaneous injury. In addition to monitoring for pacemaker capture by ECG, ongoing clinical assessment of the adequacy of cardiac output and oxygen delivery should be undertaken.

Implantable Cardioverter-Defibrillators

The primary goal of an implantable cardioverter-defibrillator (ICD) is the prevention of sudden death. Children with channelopathies such as LQTS, hypertrophic cardiomyopathy, history of near-death events, arrhythmogenic right ventricular dysplasia, and operated CHD with a history of malignant arrhythmias represent potential candidates for device implantation.[261] The capabilities of these units include pacing and defibrillation. It may be feasible to terminate tachyarrhythmias by pacing.

Although implantation of these devices is less common in pediatrics as compared with adult medicine, hardware advances have resulted in more children receiving implantable devices over time, and an increasing number of them requiring anesthetic care. The main considerations associated with intraoperative care of patients with these devices relate to monitoring, managing issues related to potential for electromagnetic interference, and performing emergent defibrillation, cardioversion, or heart rate support.[263] Perioperative consultation with a cardiologist or electrophysiologist is essential in most, if not all, cases. These devices should be interrogated and likely require programming before (deactivation of defibrillatory/antitachycardia modes) and at the conclusion of the planned procedure (reactivation of modes).

Diagnostic Modalities in Pediatric Cardiology

The most frequently used imaging modalities in the assessment of CHD and acquired heart disease in the pediatric population are briefly reviewed in the sections that follow. Although each of these is discussed independently, they are in fact complementary to each other and frequently are used in combination.[269] A comparison of these modalities is summarized in Table 14.9.

CHEST RADIOGRAPHY

The standard posteroanterior and lateral CXRs provide clues to a child's underlying cardiovascular anatomy; however, these are an insensitive screening tool for cardiac disease. Children with numerous types of significant CHD can have an initially normal-appearing CXR; alternatively, an infant with a poor inspiratory effort and the presence of a large thymus can give the appearance of cardiomegaly and have normal intracardiac anatomy (Fig. 14.32).

Interpretation of a CXR begins with identification of the patient's name and ensuring that the right-left orientation of the image is correct. All catheters and tubes should be followed to verify their location, course, and likely site of termination. The bones and soft tissues should be inspected for evidence of sternal wires, fractures, vertebral anomalies, or wide intercostal spaces, suggesting a prior thoracotomy. Sidedness, including the location of the gastric bubble, liver, and position and orientation of the cardiac mass, should be observed. The lung parenchyma should be examined for evidence of focal consolidation, such as pneumonia or atelectasis, and for pulmonary vascularity.

The cardiac silhouette and great vessels should be assessed. In young children, the thymus can obscure the superior portions of the cardiac shadow. Careful inspection of the cardiac silhouette includes an assessment of overall size and evidence of individual chamber or vessel dilation. The size of the main pulmonary artery segment can provide further evidence of the degree of pulmonary over circulation in children with left-to-right shunt lesions. The tracheal indentation can usually be seen and is useful in determining aortic arch sidedness, although in a young child with a prominent thymus, this can be difficult to assess.

More useful than an individual CXR as a diagnostic tool are serial chest films obtained to monitor a child's cardiovascular status over time. In a young child with a defect that results in ventricular volume overload, the physical examination and somatic growth parameters coupled with the degree of cardiomegaly and pulmonary over circulation are more helpful than more advanced imaging techniques. A plain CXR can also guide initiation and titration of pharmacologic therapy and the timing of a surgical intervention.

TABLE 14.9	Characteristics of Different Imaging Modalities.					
	2D echo	**3D echo**	**Cardiac catheterization**	**CT**	**CMR**	
Radiation	−	−	++	+(+)	−	
Temporal resolution	<5 ms	20–200 ms	1–10 ms	50–135 ms	20–50 ms	
Spatial resolution	0.5–2.0 mm		0.3–1.2 mm	0.5 mm	0.8–2.0 ms	
Quantitative ventricular function	++	++	+	++	+++	
Ventricular volumetric	+	++	−	+	+++	
Flow in vessels	+	−	+	−	+++	
3D whole heart imaging	−	++	++	+++	+++	
Atrioventricular valve assessment	++	+++	+	+	++	
Semilunar valve assessment	++	+++	+	++	+++	
Myocardial tissue characterization	++	+	+	+	+++	
Pressure measurements/estimation	+++	−	+++	−	++	

CMR, cardiovascular magnetic resonance imaging; *CT*, computed tomography.
Reproduced from Pushparajah K, Duong P, Mathur S, Babu-Narayan SV. Cardiovascular MRI and CT in congenital heart disease. Echo Research & Practice. 2019;6(4):R121-R38.
Used under a Creative Commons Attribution-NonCommercial 4.0 International License. (http://creativecommons.org/licenses/by/4.0/), no changes made.

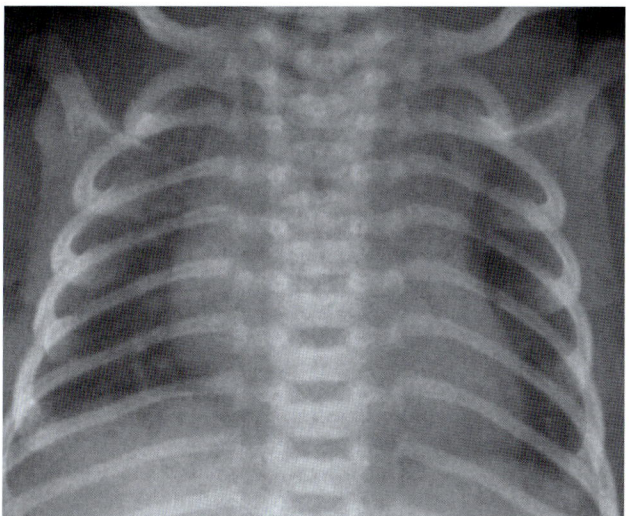

FIGURE 14.32 For a neonate with apneic episodes undergoing evaluation for potential cardiac disease, the chest radiograph demonstrates a poor inspiratory effort resulting in a large cardiothymic silhouette, making interpretation of cardiac size difficult. No evidence of cardiac disease was identified in this child.

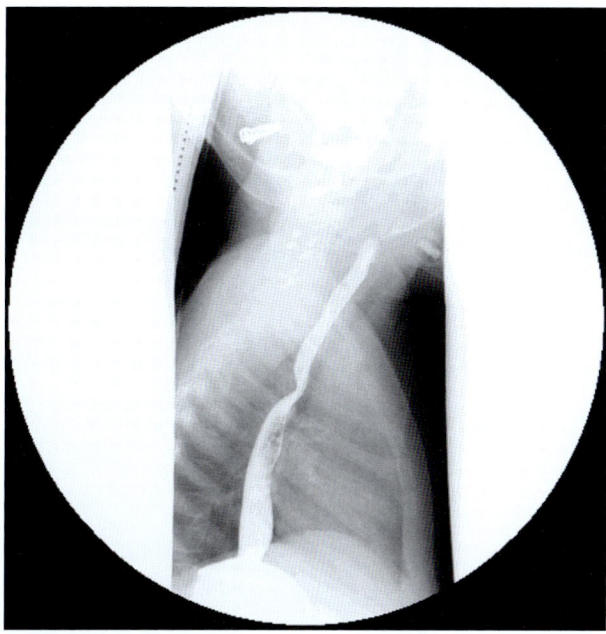

FIGURE 14.33 Barium swallow in a child with respiratory symptoms demonstrates an indentation posteriorly in the mid-esophagus, which is consistent with a vascular ring (in this particular case was caused by an aberrant subclavian artery with a retroesophageal course).

BARIUM ESOPHAGRAM

The current applications and uses of barium esophagram (swallow) studies in the diagnosis of CHD are limited. This modality has been largely replaced by chest computed tomography (CT) and CMRI. In some cases, a barium esophagram may be used as an initial screening tool when there is concern about the presence of a vascular ring, usually because of airway symptoms or, less likely, feeding or swallowing difficulties.[270] Most common types of vascular rings in children are (1) a double aortic arch and (2) a right aortic arch with aberrant left subclavian artery and left-sided ligamentum arteriosus. The indentation pattern in the barium column is suggestive of the specific vascular anomaly (Fig. 14.33).

ECHOCARDIOGRAPHY

Echocardiography is the preferred imaging tool for the initial evaluation and serial assessment in most types of pediatric heart disease.[269] Numerous echocardiographic modalities are available, including transthoracic, transesophageal, fetal, epicardial, intracardiac, and intravascular ultrasound. Each plays an important role in the evaluation and management of children with suspected or known cardiovascular disease.

Advantages of echocardiography include its noninvasive nature, provision of excellent temporal and spatial resolution, generation of portable real-time images, cost-effectiveness, and ease of use (Table 14.10).[271] As with any type of ultrasound, these waves are well-transmitted through homogeneous tissues and fluid but poorly through air and bone. Another limitation of echocardiography is related to limited acoustic windows in certain patient groups, such as those who have undergone prior cardiothoracic procedures, individuals beyond the pediatric age group, or those with a significant amount of soft tissue or body fat. For this reason, chest CT and CMRI are being increasingly used for noninvasive imaging. Additional challenges of two-dimensional echocardiography include the need to obtain serial tomographic images by sweeping the transducer scan in multiple planes to reconstruct these into three-dimensional structures in one's mind and to achieve expert interpretation. Despite these limitations, echocardiography remains

TABLE 14.10	Echocardiography
Advantages of Echocardiography	
a. Portability	
b. Noninvasive	
c. No radiation	
d. Excellent temporal resolution	
e. Good spatial and contrast resolution	
f. Invaluable in rapid hemodynamic assessment	
g. Most suitable for valve anatomy and function	
Limits of Echocardiography	
a. Limited in its ability to visualize extracardiac structures	
b. Poor spatial resolution with limited acoustic windows in the setting of obesity or after surgery	
c. Less accurate for cardiomyopathies, acute myocarditis, and ischemia	
d. Less accurate quantification for artery anomalies	
e. Less accurate quantification of volumes and masses	
f. Doppler angle dependence for quantification	

Reproduced from Gupta-Malhotra M, Schaaf W, Kutty S. A primer on multimodal imaging and cardiology-radiology congenital heart interface. *Children (Basel)*. 2019;6(4):61.

the main diagnostic imaging modality for most children. Many medical and surgical management strategies are primarily based on the findings allowed by this imaging approach.

A standard transthoracic study consists of a two-dimensional examination, M-mode imaging, and Doppler evaluation (i.e., color flow, pulsed-wave, or continuous-wave modalities). Two-dimensional imaging provides structural assessment of the heart and vasculature. Cross-sectional images are obtained from

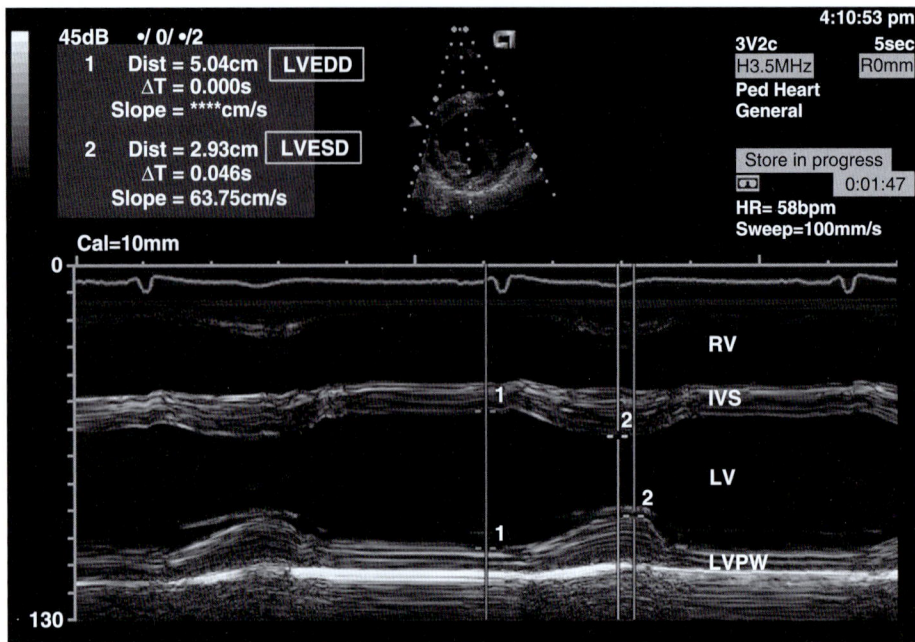

FIGURE 14.34 An M-mode echocardiogram enables determination of left ventricular dimensions and calculation of left ventricular shortening fraction. *IVS*, Interventricular septum; *LV*, left ventricle; *LVEDD*, left ventricular end-diastolic dimension; *LVESD*, left ventricular end-systolic dimension; *LVPW*, left ventricular posterior wall; *RV*, right ventricle.

several windows that allow excellent anatomic detail in multiple planes (Video 14.11). In most cases, this is adequate for a detailed segmental evaluation of the cardiac anatomy as described earlier. M-mode echocardiography allows one-dimensional imaging of the heart with excellent temporal resolution (Fig. 14.34). It is known as an "ice pick view" of the heart in real time and is primarily used in the assessment of ventricular dimensions and function.

Color flow Doppler techniques allow evaluation of directionality and velocity of blood flow. In addition to detecting flow across cardiac valves and vessels, color flow imaging allows demonstration of subtle lesions such as small septal defects that can be difficult to identify by standard two-dimensional imaging alone. Traditionally, flow toward the transducer is displayed in the red color, and flow away is represented as blue color. Turbulent blood flow is associated with increased Doppler velocities and can be readily identified as a mosaic of colors; it typically has a greenish tint (Video 14.12).

Pulsed- and continuous-wave Doppler represent spectral modalities that complement the color flow data and provide quantitative information. Pulsed-wave interrogation localizes specific sites of stenosis or turbulence but is limited in the magnitude of velocities it can detect. Continuous-wave Doppler allows quantification of much higher velocities (see Video 14.12). Velocities obtained with spectral Doppler provide estimates of pressures within various cardiac chambers by applying the simplified Bernoulli equation. It states that the difference in pressure between two locations is approximately four times the square of the velocity (V) of the jet of flow between them:

$$\text{Pressure gradient (in mm Hg)} = 4 \times V^2$$

Other echocardiographic techniques include Doppler tissue imaging (DTI) and strain imaging.[272,273] The former measures the velocity of myocardial motion using Doppler principles and the latter, also known as myocardial deformation imaging, allows for regional and global left and right ventricular function to be quantified.

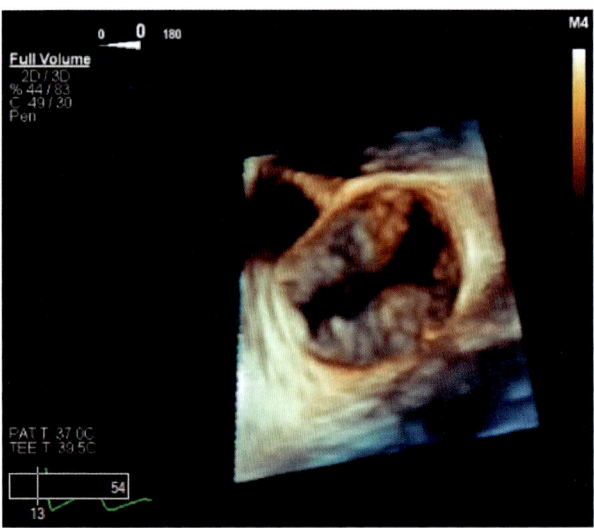

FIGURE 14.35 Three-dimensional transesophageal echocardiogram displays an en-face view of the mitral valve

The applications of three-dimensional echocardiography continue to evolve in patients with CHD.[274] An important advantage of this modality is that it can display cardiovascular structures and their interrelationships in detail, in many cases facilitating the understanding of pathologic conditions better than two-dimensional imaging. The technology is particularly helpful in cases of valvar pathology and complex anatomy. This approach can provide clear and useful volumetric and functional assessments when the images are adequate. Three-dimensional echocardiography can also be invaluable when surgical or catheter-based interventions are planned (Fig. 14.35).

Interpretation of an Echocardiographic Report
Measurements of Cardiac Chambers and Vessel Dimensions
Several measurements are routinely obtained during an echocardiographic examination. They include left ventricular end-diastolic (LVED) and left ventricular end-systolic (LVES) dimensions, thickness of the interventricular septum and left ventricular posterior wall, measurements of valve annular sizes and great artery dimensions, and left atrial volume. To determine whether these are appropriate for the child being examined, the measurements are referenced to values obtained in normal children matched for body surface area. This is accomplished in most cases by reporting the measured value and a Z score, representing standard deviations of measured values from the mean in a comparative population or the normal range values for age.

Assessment of Ventricular Function
Several echocardiographic techniques provide information regarding ventricular performance. Two of the most reported indexes of ventricular systolic function are shortening fraction (SF) and ejection fraction (EF). Shortening fraction represents the percent of change in left ventricular diameter during the cardiac cycle. This is calculated using the equation:

$$SF\,(\%) = \frac{(LVEDD - LVESD) \times 100}{LVEDD}$$

Normal values range from 28% to 44%, with a normal mean value of 36%. This parameter, however, depends on ventricular preload and afterload.

EF is the fraction of blood ejected by the ventricle (stroke volume) relative to its end-diastolic volume. This represents the percentage of blood ejected from the left ventricle with each heartbeat. EF is commonly derived by volumetric analysis of the left ventricle by means of the equation:

$$EF\,(\%) = \frac{(LVEDV - LVESV) \times 100}{LVEDV}$$

In the equation, LVEDV is the left ventricular end-diastolic volume, and LVESV is the left ventricular end-systolic volume. Normal values range between 56% and 78%. A low EF is associated with impaired systolic function; however, cardiac dysfunction can also occur in the presence of a normal EF, as in the case of diastolic heart failure.

Although these functional indexes are routinely and easily obtained, they have limitations. EF estimates are based on geometric assumptions for the elliptical left ventricle, which may not be applicable to a systemic right ventricle or other types of ventricular geometries (e.g., single ventricle). This spurred an ongoing interest in alternative approaches that may provide more sensitive and comprehensive information regarding ventricular performance, even in the absence of clinical disease. These techniques include DTI, used to evaluate intramural myocardial velocities, and strain and strain rate imaging, used to quantitate the rate of segmental myocardial deformation. Although values in normal children have been established for these imaging modalities and alterations in the presence of pathologic conditions have been described, additional clinical applications of these techniques continue to evolve. Three-dimensional echocardiography also facilitates functional assessment.

Estimation of Pressures
The peak velocity of a tricuspid regurgitant jet can be used to estimate right ventricular systolic pressure, which should equal pulmonary artery systolic pressure in the absence of pulmonary stenosis or outflow tract obstruction (Video 14.13). For example, if a peak regurgitant velocity of 3 m/second is recorded across the tricuspid valve, using the simplified Bernoulli equation or $\Delta P = 4(V^2)$, the pressure gradient or difference between the right atrial and right ventricular systolic pressures can be estimated to be $4 \times 3^2 = 36$ mm Hg. If a normal right atrial pressure is assumed (4–6 mm Hg), it would predict a right ventricular systolic pressure of approximately 40 mm Hg (36 + 4). Similarly, if the peak or maximal flow velocity across a VSD is measured at 4.5 m/second, it predicts a pressure gradient of $4 \times 4.5^2 = 81$ mm Hg between the ventricles, implying that the defect is pressure restrictive, and the right ventricular and pulmonary artery systolic pressures are relatively low.

Evaluation of Gradients
Estimation of a peak instantaneous gradient is the most clinically useful method for quantifying the severity of obstruction across a semilunar valve and/or outflow tract. It is derived by application of the simplified Bernoulli equation. When these gradients are measured across the pulmonary valve, they tend to correlate more closely with catheterization peak-to-peak gradients than with those measured across the aortic valve, for which mean gradients (obtained by automated integration of the velocities under a spectral Doppler tracing) correlate more closely. The mean rather than peak gradient determined by Doppler echocardiography is considered a better metric of the severity of the obstruction across AV valves and other low-flow venous pathways.

Evaluation of Regurgitant Lesions
Evaluation of the severity of regurgitant lesions in most pediatric cardiac centers remains largely a qualitative assessment. It is usually characterized as mild, moderate, severe, or a combination thereof when there is overlap among these categories. Serial echocardiographic assessments and comparative data are clinically more meaningful than an isolated report.

CARDIOVASCULAR MAGNETIC RESONANCE IMAGING
Cardiovascular magnetic resonance imaging (also referred to as cardiac MRI or CMRI) is considered a complementary tool to the other cardiovascular imaging modalities (Videos 14.14 and 14.15).[275] Indications for this type of study are listed in Table 14.11.[271] In addition to anatomic information, the modality provides information on hemodynamics.[276] Reported benefits include the assessment of complex cardiovascular anatomy and characterization of pathology, delineation of systemic and pulmonary vascular anomalies/variants, evaluation of global and regional ventricular function, assessment of myocardial viability, and characterization of pulmonary blood supply in children with structural alterations of the pulmonary vascular tree.[277,278] Additional applications that further expand the utility of CMRI include the quantification of volumes and shunts, visualization of blood flow within the heart or vessel(s) of interest,[279,280] and quantification of myocardial tissue-specific magnetic relaxation[281] among many others. The use of CMRI in patients with CHD and heart failure has also increased as advantages over alternate imaging approaches have been identified.[282] CMRI has also been shown to be beneficial for guiding cardiac catheterization and interventions in pediatric heart disease and pulmonary hypertension.[283–285]

Although the temporal resolution of CMRI is inferior to that of echocardiography, advances in sequence planning and techniques allow real-time acquisition similar to that of fluoroscopy. An important aspect in the acquisition of CMRI data with

TABLE 14.11	Indications for Cardiac Magnetic Resonance Imaging in Pediatric Cardiology

1. Congenital heart defects
2. Myocarditis
3. Coronary artery anomalies/Kawasaki disease
4. Extracardiac anatomy in heterotaxy syndromes
5. Pulmonary venous and arterial assessment
6. Pericardial disease
7. Cardiac tumor/mass
8. Fabry disease during enzyme replacement
9. Cardiomyopathy (hypertrophic, dilated, restrictive, and arrhythmogenic dysplasia)
10. Ventricular function and ventricular mass
11. Aortopathy
12. Cardiac stress perfusion study

Reproduced from Gupta-Malhotra M, Schaaf W, Kutty S. A primer on multimodal imaging and cardiology-radiology congenital heart interface. *Children (Basel).* 2019;6(4):61.

high spatial resolution is the use of gating to allow sampling during only specific portions of the cardiac and respiratory cycles. Slow heart rates and low respiratory rates facilitate this process. In contrast to CT, CMRI does not expose the child to radiation; this makes it preferable for serial examinations that many young children with cardiovascular disease require. However, this may be associated with the need for multiple encounters that require procedural sedation/anesthesia and their inherent risks.

Cardiac MRIs require that the child remains immobile for the duration of the scan. For small children, this usually necessitates the use of deep sedation or general anesthesia.[286,287] Specialists are often asked to provide care to infants with complex and often cyanotic CHD, during these radiologic procedures. The severity of the cardiovascular disease and the need for breathholding sequences can add to the challenges presented to the anesthesia care provider in a remote location.[288,289] Breathholding sequences require tracheal intubation to ensure apneas are achieved. The usual lengthy nature of the studies and the lengthy time to perform postprocessing of the images cause CMRI to be much more time intensive for the interpreting physician than other noninvasive imaging modalities.

Because of the nature of the magnetic fields generated in CMRI, the presence of several types of metal, including pacemakers, ICDs, cerebrovascular clips/coils, and recently implanted intracardiac or intravascular coils and devices, in general with few exceptions are considered contraindications (relative or absolute). Titanium hardware can minimize the artifact produced by the foreign material; stainless steel generates significant artifacts within the CMRI study.

As CMRI technology improves with faster scans, increasing availability, and decreasing cost, it will continue to play an increasing role in the diagnosis and longitudinal follow-up of congenital and acquired pediatric heart disease.

COMPUTED TOMOGRAPHY

Computed tomography of the chest represents an option among the various cardiovascular imaging modalities (Fig. 14.36).[290,291] Indications are listed in Table 14.12.[271] The major advantage of CT over CMRI is the very rapid scan times, and for most children, sedation is minimal or not required. Electrocardiographic gating may be needed in some cases.

Cardiac CT is not as accurate as CMRI to delineate intracardiac anatomy, but it provides excellent spatial resolution and information on extracardiac structures. CT has been beneficial in the evaluation of aortic arch anomalies and vascular rings and for defining systemic and pulmonary venous returns. Additional applications of this technology include assessing abnormalities of the coronary arteries (congenital and acquired) and evaluating cardiovascular disorders associated with airway pathology where dynamic recordings and three-dimensional reconstructions provide detailed information.

A significant drawback of CT is the radiation burden, although with modern scanners the study can be optimized to limit dosing, and in fact may cause much less exposure to ionizing radiation as compared to diagnostic cardiac catheterization. It should be noted that the radiation dose may vary among institutions. Optimizing the dose of radiation while maintaining an adequate diagnostic image quality continues to be an ongoing effort.[292] An advantage of CT imaging over cardiac catheterization is that it avoids the likely need for iodinated contrast agents and their concomitant risks.

CARDIAC CATHETERIZATION AND ANGIOGRAPHY

Cardiac catheterization invasively measures intracardiac and vascular pressures and blood oxygen saturation coupled with angiography to assess cardiac anatomy and hemodynamics (Figs. 14.37 and 14.38). Before the era of two-dimensional echocardiography,

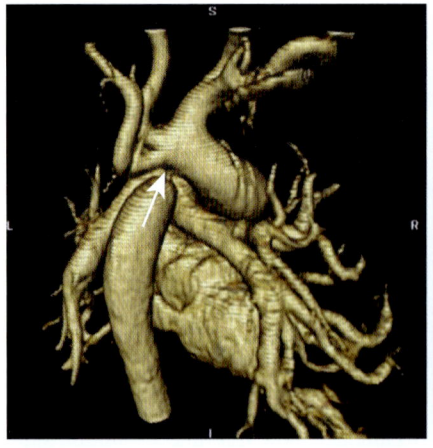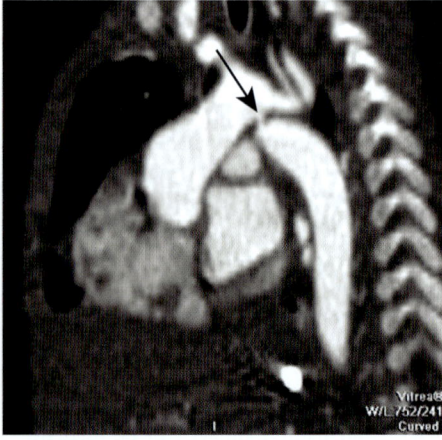

FIGURE 14.36 Computed tomography images show the detailed anatomy in an infant with severe aortic arch obstruction *(arrows)*.

TABLE 14.12	Indications for Computed Tomography in Pediatric Cardiology

1. Coronary artery anomalies
2. Kawasaki disease and other vasculitis
3. Congenital heart defect
4. Extracardiac anatomy in heterotaxia
5. Pulmonary venous and arterial assessment
6. Aortopathy
7. Pericardial disease
8. Cardiac thrombosis
9. Cardiomyopathy (hypertrophic, dilated, restrictive, and ischemic)
10. Extracardiac anatomy in heterotaxy syndromes
11. Pulmonary sequestration to check arterial supply and venous drainage

Reproduced from Gupta-Malhotra M, Schaaf W, Kutty S. A primer on multimodal imaging and cardiology-radiology congenital heart interface. *Children (Basel).* 2019;6(4):61.

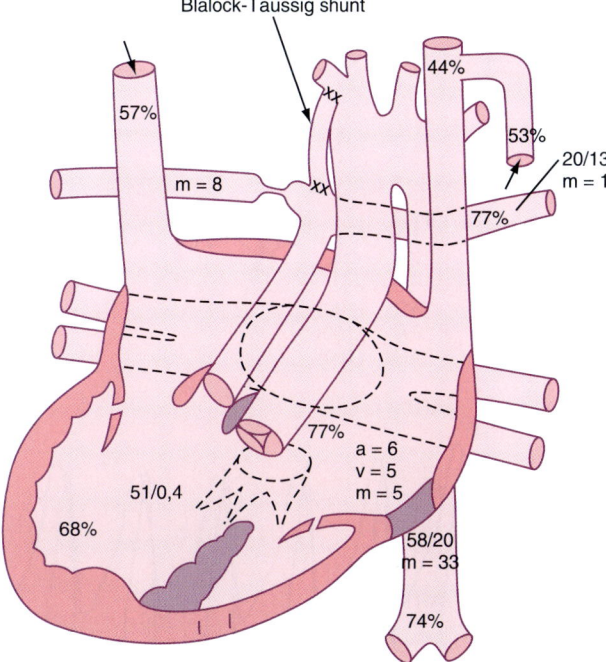

Weight 3.3 kg

Diagnosis
1. Heterotaxy
2. Dextrocardia
3. Complete atrioventricular canal
4. Double-outlet right ventricle
5. Pulmonary stenosis, severe
6. L-Transposition of the great arteries
7. Interrupted inferior vena cava with azygous continuation
8. After innominate to main pulmonary artery shunt
9. Right pulmonary artery isolation

FIGURE 14.37 A cardiac catheterization diagram is valuable when caring for patients with structural anomalies, such as this child with complex congenital heart disease. Data routinely obtained at cardiac catheterization are shown, including oxygen saturation determinations (in %) and pressure measurements (in mm Hg). Catheter courses are indicated by *unlabeled arrows*. The atrial pressures are given for the *a* wave *(a)*, which is generated during atrial systole; *v* wave *(v)*, which results from passive filling of the atrium before atrioventricular valve opening; and mean *(m)* (all in mm Hg). Refer to section titled Interpretation of a Cardiac Catheterization Report.

cardiac catheterization was frequently used for diagnostic purposes. With the advances in noninvasive imaging, diagnostic procedures represent a relatively small proportion of these studies. Current indications for cardiac catheterization at most centers include the assessment of physiologic variables such as pressure and resistance data, measurements of shunt ratios, anatomic definition when other diagnostic modalities are inadequate, need for electrophysiologic testing or treatment, and when catheter-based interventions are anticipated.

Most cardiac catheterization procedures are performed for interventions including endomyocardial biopsies; angioplasties and stenting of stenotic vessels, dilation of valves, and conduits; and occlusion techniques for native defects (Video 14.16), fistulous connections, and surgically created communications no longer considered necessary (Fig. 14.39) (see also Chapter 20). In some cases, such as critically ill neonates with complex heart disease, catheter-based interventions such as balloon atrial septostomy and other procedures (e.g., ductal stenting) can be lifesaving.

Access to the central circulation is usually accomplished percutaneously through a femoral approach, although depending on a variety of factors and guided by the nature of the intervention, alternate sites may be used. Most examinations involve hemodynamic evaluation with recording of pressure data through catheters positioned at various sites of interest. Oxygen saturation data and blood gas measurements from various cardiac chambers and vessels are obtained using point-of-care devices that allow for a short analysis time. In contrast to the oxygen saturation calculations derived from a blood gas analysis, reflectance/co-oximetry provides measured values of oxygenated and deoxygenated hemoglobin that are then used by a machine to provide a percent of hemoglobin saturation. This also allows for determination of oxygen content (i.e., total amount of hemoglobin in the blood) and, when combined with values of oxygen consumption, assessment of blood flows and other calculations (e.g., shunts).[293] Additional data that can be obtained include pressure gradients, cardiac output, and parameters for deriving vascular resistances and valve areas. Although basal measurements would ideally be performed under conditions that mimic an awake state or with light sedation, this may not be feasible in young children and in most cases requires the use of deep sedation or general anesthesia.[294] Baseline hemodynamic assessment and

oximetric data calculations are optimally obtained under conditions of normocarbia while the inspired oxygen concentration is kept low (room air if feasible) and relatively constant.

Fluoroscopy and cineangiography are essential components of most cardiac catheterization studies. Of the two, cineangiography accounts for most of the radiation exposure as images are recorded during the injection of contrast material, typically at 15 or 30 frames per second. Consequently, there is concern about radiation dose and risk during cardiac catheterization.[295,296] Most angiograms are obtained during biplane imaging by positioning the equipment to obtain optimal views allowing for delineation of the pathology in question (i.e., axial angiography) (Video 14.17 A,B).

Although cardiac catheterization has evolved over the years, providing an improved margin of safety, it remains an invasive procedure involving challenges and risks.[297–302] These include excessive blood loss, vascular complications, infection, arrhythmias, vascular or cardiac perforation, systemic air embolization, myocardial ischemia, hemodynamic decompensation, and issues associated with the administration of contrast agents. These

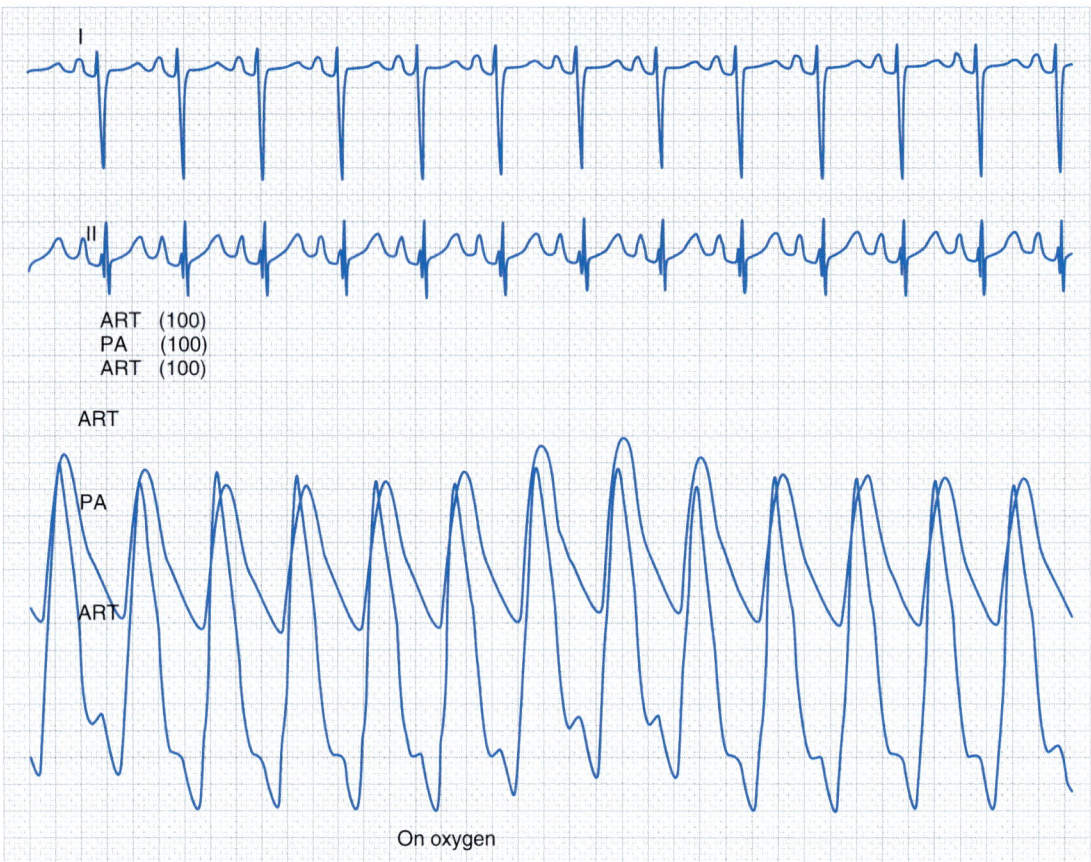

FIGURE 14.38 In the hemodynamic tracing obtained during cardiac catheterization, notice that the pulmonary artery systolic pressure (100 mm Hg) is at systemic levels in this child with multiple, left-sided obstructions. *ART*, Systemic arterial pressure; *PA*, pulmonary artery pressure.

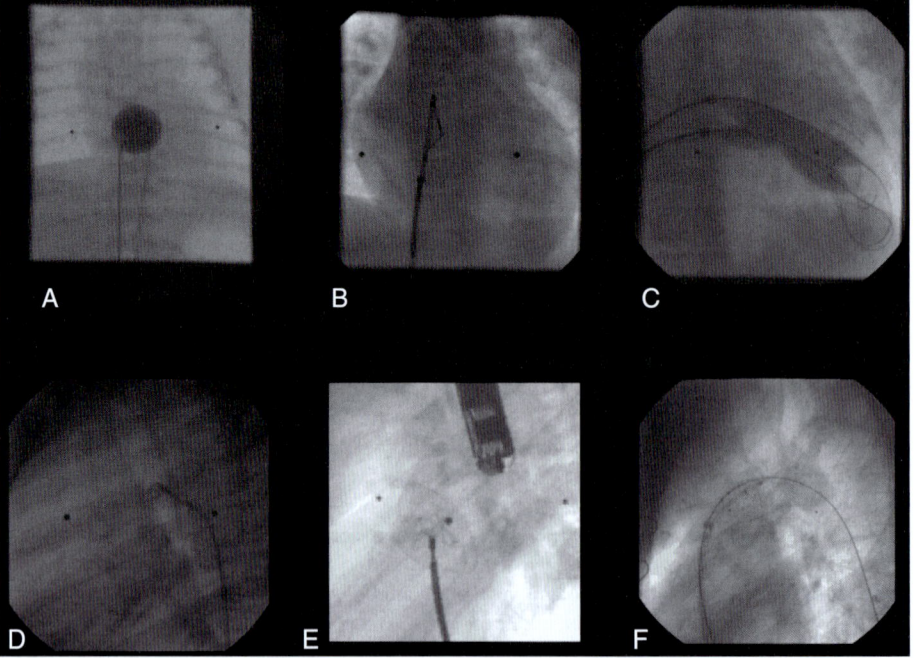

FIGURE 14.39 Several types of interventions are performed in a pediatric cardiac catheterization laboratory as depicted. **A,** Balloon atrial septostomy. **B,** Blade atrial septostomy. **C,** Double-balloon mitral valvuloplasty. **D,** Placement of a ductal coil occluder device. **E,** Transcatheter closure of a secundum atrial septal defect. **F,** Pulmonary artery dilation with stent placement.

complications are more likely to occur in neonates and infants rather than the older child. Interventional catheterizations, by the nature of the procedures, are associated with a greater rate of complications and potential for morbidity and mortality.[299] However, as transcatheter interventions become safer and more effective, an increasing number of infants and children may obviate the need for surgery, often undergoing procedures on an outpatient basis. Evolving approaches in this field include percutaneous implantation of valves, strategies that combine cardiac catheterization and surgical intervention (hybrid procedures), and catheter-based interventions during fetal life.[302–304]

Interpretation of a Cardiac Catheterization Report

Pressure Data

Atrial pressure tracings are characterized by several waves (*a*, *c*, and *v* waves) and descents (*x* and *y*). Reported values correspond to the *a* and *v* waves and the mean pressures. The right atrial pressure is typically *a*-wave–dominant. The mean right atrial pressure is normally less than 5 mm Hg. The left atrial pressure tracing is typically *v*-wave–dominant. The mean left atrial pressure rarely exceeds 8 mm Hg. Abnormal pressure waveforms are often associated with AV valve stenosis, regurgitation, rhythm disturbances, and pericardial disease.

Ventricular pressures are recorded and reported during systole, at end systole, and at end diastole. For the right ventricle, systolic pressure is normally 25 to 30 mm Hg, with end-diastolic pressures of 5 to 7 mm Hg. The systolic pressure in the left ventricle increases with age and should equal the systolic arterial pressure. The end-diastolic pressure is typically less than 10 mm Hg.

The pulmonary artery pressure is reported in terms of systolic, diastolic, and mean pressures. The systolic pulmonary artery pressure in a normal child should be equal to the right ventricular systolic pressure, and the mean pulmonary artery pressure should not exceed 20 mm Hg. The pulmonary artery wedge pressure is obtained by advancing a catheter into a distal vessel until it is temporarily occluded, reflecting the left atrial pressure.

The aortic pressure and contour of the tracing depend on the site of interrogation. Typically, there is an increase in the systolic pressure as a catheter navigates toward the peripheral circulation. This phenomenon is known as *pulse wave amplification*.

Pressure gradients, or the pressure differences between two distinct sites, can be measured in several ways (i.e., mean gradient and peak gradient). It is important to consider that several factors may affect their determination. This is significantly influenced by the severity of the obstruction and the ventricular function. Smaller gradients than those observed in the awake child can be seen in patients under sedation or anesthesia.

Shunt Calculations

Shunts are characterized in terms of their direction (e.g., left-to-right, right-to-left, bidirectional) and magnitude. Left-to-right shunts can be quantified based on the pulmonary ($\dot{Q}_{pulm}$) to systemic ($\dot{Q}_{sys}$) blood flow ratio.

$$\frac{\dot{Q}_{pulm}}{\dot{Q}_{sys}} = \frac{(S_{sys}aO_2 - S\overline{v}O_2)}{(S_{pulm}vO_2 - S_{pulm}aO_2)}$$

In the equation, $S_{sys}aO_2$ is the systemic arterial O_2 saturation, $S\overline{v}O_2$ is the mixed venous O_2 saturation, $S_{pulm}vO_2$ is the pulmonary venous O_2 saturation, and $S_{pulm}aO_2$ is the pulmonary arterial O_2 saturation. A $\dot{Q}_{pulm}/\dot{Q}_{sys}$ shunt ratio that exceeds 3 : 1 is considered significant, although smaller ratios can be associated with considerable symptoms.

Cardiac Output Determinations

The volume of blood ejected by the heart into the systemic circulation, or cardiac output, can be derived in several ways. Thermodilution measurements use saline as an indicator to measure pulmonary blood flow. In the absence of intracardiac shunts, this is equivalent to cardiac output (expressed as liters per minute). In the Fick method, oxygen is used as an indicator, and cardiac output is obtained by the application of the formula:

$$\dot{Q}_{sys} \text{ (L/minute)} = \frac{\dot{V}O_2}{C_{sys}O_2 - C\overline{v}O_2}$$

In the equation, $\dot{V}O_2$ is the oxygen consumption (assumed or measured), $C_{sys}O_2$ is the systemic arterial O_2 content, and $C\overline{v}O_2$ is the mixed venous O_2 content.

The O_2 content = O_2 saturation × (1.36 × 10 × hemoglobin concentration).

Vascular Resistances

Resistance represents the change in pressure in the systemic or pulmonary circulation with respect to flow. It is expressed in Wood units (mm Hg/L per minute) and is usually normalized for body surface area. The systemic vascular resistance (SVR) and pulmonary vascular resistance (PVR) are derived as follows:

$$SVR = \frac{\text{mean AoP} - \text{mean RAP}}{\dot{Q}_{sys}}$$

$$PVR = \frac{\text{mean PAP} - \text{PCWP (or mean LAP)}}{\dot{Q}_{pulm}}$$

Where in the above equations, AoP is the aortic pressure, LAP is the left atrial pressure, PAP is the pulmonary artery pressure, PCWP is the pulmonary artery wedge pressure, and RAP is the right atrial pressure.

Perioperative Considerations for Children With Cardiovascular Disease

GENERAL ISSUES

Anesthesia for children with heart disease can be both challenging and daunting because of:

- The wide spectrum of disease
- The remarkable range of congenital lesions and their underlying physiologic consequences
- The numerous interventional and surgical options in CHD (Table 14.13), in addition to their hemodynamic implications
- The fact that many parents are unaware of the full extent or details of the child's cardiovascular lesion(s) or abnormalities

To optimally care for these children, the following objectives should be met:

- Familiarity with the underlying cardiovascular defect(s)
- Understanding of the physiologic abnormalities and available therapies (medical, catheter-based, and surgical)
- Recognition of signs of limited reserve, compensatory mechanisms, and perioperative risks
- Ability to identify the potential impact of the proposed intervention/surgical procedure on the child's underlying condition, anticipate if/how it will be tolerated, and be prepared to manage any problems that may arise

This combination of demanding objectives and potential challenges can be intimidating even for the most experienced clinician. When caring for children with complex cardiovascular

TABLE 14.13	Surgical Procedures for Congenital Heart Disease	
Procedure	**Description**	**Goal or Result**
Arterial switch (Jatene) operation	Arterial trunks transected above the level of the semilunar valves, relocated to their appropriate respective ventricles, coronary arteries reimplanted into the neoaortic root	Establishes the normal ventriculoarterial connection (right ventricle to pulmonary artery and left ventricle to aorta) in D-transposition of the great arteries
Atrioventricular septal defect (atrioventricular canal/ endocardial cushion defect) repair	Patch closure of atrial and ventricular communications, reconstruction of atrioventricular valves, closure of cleft in left-sided atrioventricular valve	Eliminates the intracardiac shunts, repair of atrioventricular valve(s)
Blalock-Taussig shunt	Communication between innominate or subclavian artery and pulmonary artery; "modified" implies placement of a graft	Allows for or augments pulmonary blood flow
Central shunt, Waterston shunt, Potts shunt, Mee shunt	Communication between the systemic and pulmonary circulations	Allows for or increases pulmonary blood flow
Closure of septal defect	Patch or primary closure of communication at the atrial or ventricular level	Eliminates an intracardiac shunt
Coarctation repair	Relief of aortic arch obstruction (various approaches)	Addresses the obstruction and establishes patency across the aortic arch
Damus-Kaye-Stansel procedure	End-to-side anastomosis of main pulmonary artery onto the aorta; necessitates reestablishing pulmonary blood flow through an alternative route (graft from a systemic artery into the pulmonary artery or a right ventricular to pulmonary artery conduit)	Allows unobstructed systemic outflow in the context of single-ventricle anomalies associated with obstruction to aortic flow or other settings
Division or ligation of patent ductus arteriosus	Obliteration of the communication at the level of the ductus arteriosus	Eliminates shunting at the level of the great arteries
Fontan procedure	Connection that directs inferior vena cava blood into the pulmonary circulation	Separates the pulmonary and systemic circulations in patients with single-ventricle physiology; usually the final step in the single-ventricle palliation pathway
Glenn anastomosis (cavopulmonary connection or shunt)	Anastomosis between superior vena cava and pulmonary artery (bidirectional implies flow from superior vena cava into both pulmonary arteries)	Provides pulmonary blood flow while unloading the single ventricle; may be the first or intermediate step in the single-ventricle palliation pathway
Konno-Rastan procedure (aortoventriculoplasty)	Enlargement of the left ventricular outflow tract and aortic annulus; defect created in the ventricular septum to enlarge the outflow tract, which is then repaired with a large patch	Alleviates subvalvar and valvar aortic obstruction; when the aortic root is replaced by an autologous pulmonary root, it is referred to as a Ross-Konno procedure; Alternatively, cryopreserved homograft tissue can be used in the form of an extended aortic root replacement
Nikaidoh procedure	Involves reconstruction of left ventricular outflow tract with translocation of aortic root after division of outlet septum and excision of the pulmonary valve, patch closure of ventricular communication, and completion of right ventricular to pulmonary artery anastomosis with pericardial patch; May or may not include coronary artery translocation	For management of transposition of the great arteries with pulmonary stenosis and a ventricular septal defect
Norwood procedure (stage I palliation)	Involves aortic reconstruction, an atrial septectomy, and placement of a systemic-to-pulmonary artery shunt (modified Blalock-Taussig shunt) or right ventricular to pulmonary artery conduit (Sano modification)	Addresses systemic outflow tract obstruction by allowing the right ventricle to eject into a reconstructed aorta; Atrial septectomy provides unobstructed drainage of the pulmonary venous return into the right atrium; The systemic-to-pulmonary artery connection supplies the pulmonary blood flow
Pulmonary artery banding	Constrictive band placed around the main pulmonary artery	Limits excessive pulmonary blood flow
Rastelli operation	Creation of an intracardiac tunnel that allows left ventricular output into the aorta while closing a ventricular septal defect, and placement of a right ventricular conduit to pulmonary artery	Allows the left ventricle to eject solely into the aorta, abolishes intracardiac shunting at the ventricular level, and provides unobstructed pulmonary blood flow; The procedure results in separation of the pulmonary and systemic circulations

TABLE 14.13	Surgical Procedures for Congenital Heart Disease—cont'd	
Procedure	**Description**	**Goal or Result**
Sano modification of the Norwood procedure	Placement of graft between the right ventricle and main pulmonary artery as an alternative to a modified Blalock-Taussig shunt in the Norwood operation	Provides pulmonary blood flow
Senning or Mustard procedure (atrial switch)	Intraatrial baffle procedure	Allows pulmonary venous blood to be rerouted through the tricuspid valve into the right ventricle (as the systemic chamber that ejects into the aorta); Systemic venous return is channeled across the mitral valve into the left ventricle, which pumps into the main pulmonary artery
Tetralogy of Fallot repair	Closure of ventricular septal defect and relief of right ventricular outflow tract obstruction	Eliminates intracardiac shunting at the ventricular level and addresses right ventricular outflow tract obstruction (often at several levels)
Truncus arteriosus repair	Closure of the ventricular septal defect, detachment of main pulmonary artery or branched pulmonary arteries from common arterial trunk, and establishment of right ventricular to pulmonary artery continuity (usually with a homograft); May need repair of associated anomalies (e.g., truncal valve)	Abolishes intracardiac shunting and restores the normal connection between the ventricles and great arteries
Valvectomy	Valve excision	Relieves valvar obstruction
Valvotomy	Opening of stenotic valve	Relieves valvar obstruction
Valve replacement	Placement of bioprosthetic or mechanical valve	Addresses valvar pathology (obstruction and regurgitation)
Valvuloplasty	Valve repair	Relieves valvar regurgitation and/or stenosis
Yasui operation	Channels blood from the left ventricle across the ventricular septal defect into a reconstructed aorta (using the native pulmonary valve as the neoaortic valve); Establishes right ventricular to pulmonary artery continuity by means of a conduit	Provides for a biventricular repair in infants with two adequately sized ventricles and obstruction to systemic outflow

disease, a multidisciplinary approach is recommended, allowing for the formulation and execution of optimal individualized management plans. If available, consultation with the child's cardiologist or primary care physician should include inquiries about the details of the child's disease, overall clinical status, past and current medical treatment(s), prior catheterization or surgical interventions, and presence of residual pathology. The interaction between members of the perioperative team should allow an exchange of information, discussion of concerns, and recommendations that can facilitate patient care and the development of comprehensive management plans.[305] This is particularly important in the care of children with complex pathology.

A complete medical history and focused examination is essential during the preoperative assessment. In addition to evaluating the child's disease processes, overall clinical status, and functional reserve, this allows appraisal of issues that may affect anesthesia management (e.g., limited vascular access, difficult airway, gastroesophageal reflux, manipulations of pulmonary and systemic blood flow and pressures). Available studies (e.g., ECG, CXR, echocardiogram, Holter monitor, cardiac catheterization, CMRI, CT) should be reviewed. Depending on the nature of the procedure, complexity of the disease, and potential impact on perioperative outcome, additional evaluation and diagnostic studies may be warranted. In many cases, the anesthesiologist as a perioperative physician plays a major role in determining whether the available information is adequate.

An important goal in the preoperative evaluation is the identification of children who are at increased risk because of cardiac and pulmonary limitations imposed by their cardiovascular disease. The anesthesiologist caring for a child with CHD should understand the pathophysiology of the cardiac defect and implications of any previous interventions. Abnormal indexes that should raise potential concerns include hypoxemia (SpO_2 <75%), $\dot{Q}_{pulm}/\dot{Q}_{sys}$ exceeding 3:1, outflow tract gradients greater than 50 mm Hg, pulmonary hypertension (i.e., mean pulmonary artery pressure >20 mm Hg), increased pulmonary vascular resistance (index >2 Wood units/m^2), or polycythemia (i.e., hematocrit >60%). Several clinical states may place children at significant risk for severe cardiopulmonary decompensation during anesthesia and surgery: recent history of congestive heart failure, uncontrolled arrhythmias, severe ventricular dysfunction, cardiomyopathies, unexplained syncope, substantial exercise intolerance, single-ventricle physiology, supravalvular aortic stenosis (Williams syndrome), or any condition associated with significantly impaired cardiac or pulmonary function.[306,307] At times there may be a need to delay an elective procedure to perform an intervention (catheter-based or surgical) to improve a hemodynamic state or lessen perioperative risks on a future anesthetic. For some children, a planned admission to the intensive care unit following the procedure should be discussed with the care team preoperatively, parents, and child (if appropriate).

CLINICAL CONDITION AND STATUS OF PRIOR REPAIR

Children with CHD may require anesthesia care before or after palliation or following definitive procedures. Corrective interventions are those that result in a normal life expectancy and full cardiovascular reserve, and children undergoing these procedures usually require no further medical or surgical treatment. In the strict sense, only a few procedures fulfill these criteria: ligation, division, or occlusion of a PDA and closure of an isolated secundum ASD. Other interventions or surgical procedures can result in repair or correction but not necessarily in normal hemodynamics or life expectancy. The clinician should assume potential limitation in cardiovascular reserve, a need for follow-up, further medical management, and in some cases, additional catheter-based interventions, or surgical therapies. In other cases, as in children with palliated CHD, the circulation may still be abnormal. These individuals are known to be at greater risk for adverse perioperative events.[16,20–22,306,308–315] Published data from the POCA registry examined anesthesia-related cardiac arrests in children.[184] Cardiac arrests occurred more frequently in children with heart disease than in those children without heart disease. Causes were primarily cardiovascular in nature. These events occurred more frequently in the general operating room, usually during the surgical maintenance phase. The most common anatomic substrate in this setting was that of a single ventricle, particularly those early in the palliation pathway. The overall mortality rate for children with heart disease was greater than those without heart disease, with the greatest mortality rate occurring in children with aortic stenosis (Williams syndrome) and cardiomyopathy.

The effects of previous procedures on the heart and other systems require careful consideration. Problems that can remain or develop after surgical intervention include residual shunts, valvar stenoses or outflow tract obstruction, valvar regurgitation, pulmonary hypertension, arrhythmias, and ventricular dysfunction. Children who require a detailed appraisal of perioperative risks are those with residual significant pathology, suspected or known pulmonary hypertension, single-ventricle physiology, and those after outflow conduit placement, valve replacement, or cardiac transplantation (see Chapters 15, 16, 20 and 21).

Several efforts have addressed the issue of risk assessment in the patient with CHD undergoing noncardiac surgery to develop risk stratification algorithms.[20,24,185,307,315–319] This topic is discussed in further detail in Chapter 21. Although there has been an increasing number of children with CHD presenting for noncardiac surgical procedures over time, it is reassuring that this has been accompanied by a significant decline in perioperative mortality rates with the most recent reported incidence of 1.06% in 2019.[320] This has been attributed to careful patient selection and medical optimization combined with expertise of the perioperative team. A recent study exploring the question of the type and location of medical facilities where patients with CHD undergo noncardiac procedures documented that these individuals/their families were more likely to travel to a hospital with a cardiac program than to a hospital without; especially patients with single-ventricle disease, other complex cardiac malformation, and with ≥6 chronic conditions.[321] Additional studies are currently ongoing assessing clinical outcomes of patients with cardiac disease based on parameters such as institutional patient volume, as well as type of perioperative provider (pediatric anesthesiologist versus pediatric cardiac anesthesiologist).

ANNOTATED REFERENCES

Brown ML, Nasr VG, Toohey R, DiNardo JA. Williams syndrome and anesthesia for non-cardiac surgery: high risk can be mitigated with appropriate planning. *Pediatr Cardiol.* 2018;39:1123-1128.

The study reviews the experience of a large academic center where all patients with Williams syndrome undergoing noncardiac surgical, interventional, or imaging studies are cared for by main operating room pediatric anesthesiologists with consultative input from cardiac anesthesiologists. A very low rate of cardiovascular adverse events was reported in this cohort. Despite the known high risk of this patient population for anesthesia, the findings suggest that the risk can be mitigated by appropriate planning and carefully following a goal-oriented hemodynamic plan.

Choudhry S, Puri K, Denfield SW. An update on pediatric cardiomyopathy. *Curr Treat Options Cardiovasc Med.* 2019;21:36.

The article is an update that summarizes the clinical characteristics and contemporary outcomes of primary cardiomyopathies in children including dilated, hypertrophic, and restrictive cardiomyopathy. The document also briefly addresses left ventricular noncompaction and arrhythmogenic right ventricular cardiomyopathy.

Loss KL, Shaddy RE, Kantor PF. Recent and upcoming drug therapies for pediatric heart failure. *Front Pediatr.* 2021;9:681224.

This is a review of the clinical presentation and management of acute and chronic pediatric heart failure. The article focuses on systolic dysfunction in patients with a biventricular circulation and a systemic left ventricle. An in-depth discussion of available and upcoming pharmacological agents in the care of children with heart failure is presented.

Son MBF, Newburger JW. Kawasaki Disease. *Pediatr Rev.* 2018;39:78-90.

This is an excellent comprehensive review addressing important aspects of Kawasaki disease including clinical findings, laboratory abnormalities, role of echocardiography, and primary treatment of this disorder.

Wilson WR, Gewitz M, Lockhart PB, et al. Prevention of viridans group streptococcal infective endocarditis: a scientific statement from the American Heart Association. *Circulation.* 2021;143:e963-e978.

This article is the most recent American Heart Association scientific statement on the prevention of viridans group streptococcal infective endocarditis. The update addresses interval evidence of the acceptance and impact of prior recommendations.

A complete reference list can be found online at Elsevier eBooks+.

Anesthesia for Children Undergoing Heart Surgery

ANGUS McEWAN AND VASCO LAGHINA ROLO

Preoperative Evaluation
The Preoperative Visit and Evaluation
Upper Respiratory Tract Infection and Cardiac Surgery
Perioperative Challenges in Pediatric Cardiac Anesthesia
Cyanosis
Intracardiac Shunting
Impaired Hemostasis
**Anesthesia Management for Surgery Requiring
Cardiopulmonary Bypass**
Monitoring
Induction of Anesthesia
Maintenance of Anesthesia
Institution and Separation From Bypass
**Control of Systemic and Pulmonary Vascular
Resistances During Anesthesia**
Anesthetic Drugs Used in Pediatric Cardiac Anesthesia
Inhalational Agents
Intravenous Induction Agents

Opioids
Neuromuscular Blocking Drugs
Long-Term Neurocognitive-Developmental
Outcomes Associated with Anesthesia
Regional Anesthesia and Analgesia
Fast Track and Enhanced Recovery After Surgery
Stress Response to Cardiac Surgery
Reducing The Stress Response to Surgery and Bypass
Anesthesia Considerations for Specific Cardiac Defects
Simple Left-to-Right Shunts
Simple Right-to-Left Shunts
Complex Shunts
Aortic Stenosis
Coarctation of the Aorta
Interrupted Aortic Arch
Transport and Transfer to a Pediatric Intensive Care Unit

CONGENITAL HEART DISEASE (CHD) is the commonest birth defect, accounting for nearly one-third of major congenital abnormalities, with an estimated worldwide birth prevalence of up to 9.4 cases per 1000 live births.[1,2] According to the National Center on Birth Defects and Developmental Disabilities (NCBDDD), this represents the birth of 40,000 babies with CHD each year in the United States.[3,4] There has been a gradual rise in birth prevalence of congenital heart disease over the last few decades, with the disproportionate increase in numbers of mild forms of CHD suggesting an improvement in the postnatal diagnosis of such milder lesions.[1] Improvements in cardiovascular medicine, surgery, and perioperative care have resulted in a dramatic decrease in mortality rates since the 1950s, when CHD was almost universally fatal; most patients now survive into adulthood.[5,6] This represents a drastic change in scenario, altering the contribution of CHD to the global burden of disease, which led to necessary adjustments in healthcare systems in order to be able to continue to provide adequate care for this often complex, challenging population of patients.[7]

Preoperative Evaluation

Although congenital heart disease can occur in isolation, it is often associated with other cardiovascular and extracardiac malformations.[8] The incidence of CHD is increased in the presence of other congenital abnormalities, in children with chromosomal disorders such as trisomy 21 or 22q11.2 chromosome deletion, as well as in siblings of children with CHD.[9] With the increase in diagnostic ability, the majority of children with CHD are now diagnosed antenatally or early postnatally in high-income countries.[10–12] In association with improvements in diagnosis, surgical techniques, and perioperative care, most centers have shifted their practice toward performing definitive repair of the defects earlier, in contrast with the previous tendency toward performing initial palliative surgery and staged repairs, with many children presenting with CHD now undergoing corrective surgery as neonates.[13–15] Overall, about one-half of all children with CHD undergo cardiac surgery in the first year of life, and about 25% undergo surgery in the first month of life.[16–18]

The perioperative management of children with complex cardiac defects requires a dedicated, specialized team of surgeons, cardiologists, anesthesiologists, perfusionists, intensivists, and nurses. Professionals caring for these children are challenged by some of the greatest physiologic aberrations encountered in clinical medicine. The anesthesiologists responsible for the care of these children require a comprehensive understanding of cardiac anatomy, physiology, and pathophysiology and must be able to adapt to each nuance of rapidly changing pathophysiology as it is encountered.

In addition to treating children with CHD, the pediatric cardiac anesthesiologist may also be responsible for the care of adults with CHD, whose underlying cardiac problems differ substantially from those in children.[19–21] The success of pediatric cardiac surgery has resulted in an ever-increasing population with adult congenital heart disease ("grown-up CHD"), as most children with CHD are now expected to survive into adulthood.[22–24] The ideal approach for this group of patients is to care for them in specialist units.[25–28] Although these adult congenital heart disease centers are increasing in number and capacity, they are currently unable to provide universal coverage. In the meantime, the care of these patients falls to the most qualified physicians, including the pediatric cardiac anesthesiologist. Along with their underlying CHD, these patients often present with comorbidities of old age and their additional challenges.

When assessing children with complex cardiac defects, we rely to a large extent on echocardiography and magnetic resonance imaging (MRI) to acquire diagnostic data. Although fewer children are subjected to diagnostic angiography today, more interventional cardiac catheterization procedures are being performed.[29] Many conditions such as patent ductus arteriosus (PDA), atrial septal defects (ASDs), and ventricular septal defects (VSDs) that would previously have been treated surgically are now treated in the angiography suite by interventional cardiologists. Other interventions include dilating arteries with balloon catheters with and without stents and coiling of aberrant or excessive collateral vessels. The pulmonary artery or the right ventricular outflow tract are commonly balloon dilated and stented, and coarctation of the aorta is similarly treated by balloon dilation. Stenotic valves are also commonly dilated.[30] These procedures have increased the risk of patients being transferred emergently from the angiography suite to the operating room.[31,32] For the individual child, there has been a dramatic decrease in morbidity as increasing numbers of conditions are treated in the angiography suite, but the risk of complications has increased as more complex procedures are performed (see Chapter 20).

THE PREOPERATIVE VISIT AND EVALUATION

The preoperative visit is an important aspect of the overall management of anesthesia for children with CHD.[33,34]

Creating Rapport With the Child and Family

By creating a good relationship with the family, the anesthesiologist can reduce both the child's and parents' anxiety. This fosters a sense of trust, which may improve their overall hospital experience. A good rapport with the child may also facilitate a smoother anesthetic induction, and the use of specific nonpharmacologic techniques to reduce perioperative anxiety can be tailored to the child's individual preferences and previous experiences.

Providing Information

Providing information to the parents and the child in a manner that is nonthreatening and appropriate to the child's age and developmental stage is a key element of the preoperative visit.[35] This information includes the possible use of sedative premedication, appropriate fasting times, the type of induction, the type and likely position of invasive lines, the need for a stay in an intensive care unit (ICU) postoperatively, as well as the expected length of that stay. The use of other monitors such as transesophageal echocardiography (TEE), arterial and central venous lines, urinary catheter, postoperative tracheal intubation, etc., should be outlined and potential common complications identified, along with the probability that a blood transfusion may be necessary. Questions about the risk of anesthesia and surgery should be addressed to the satisfaction of the parents (see Chapter 2).

Performing a Medical Assessment

The anesthesiologist must have a clear and detailed understanding of the cardiac anatomy and pathophysiology, the planned surgery, as well as any associated congenital abnormalities or medical conditions. The medical assessment includes collation of information

from the history, prior surgical or catheterization interventions, a careful physical examination, and review of imaging and laboratory data. Most diagnostic information is obtained from the medical record. Particular attention should be paid to the echocardiographic, angiographic, MRI, and other imaging data, the chest radiograph, and the electrocardiogram. Many centers have joint cardiac conferences where decisions about treatment are discussed in a multidisciplinary forum. Reports from these meetings are valuable in the preoperative assessment.

In addition to gathering this specific diagnostic information, a directed history and physical examination should be performed to assess the overall condition of the child. Attention should focus on assessing the presence and degree of cardiac failure, cyanosis, and the presence or risk of pulmonary hypertension. Information about previous surgical procedures that may alter access to the central circulation and placement of invasive monitors should also be sought. The general nutritional state of the child should be assessed; poor growth and development may be a sign of severe CHD. Other information should be sought that may have a bearing on the anesthetic plan. For example, repeat surgery and redo sternotomy may indicate the need to establish peripheral cardiopulmonary bypass (CPB) before surgically accessing the heart and great vessels for central CPB cannulation. This has a bearing on line placement because either jugular-carotid or femoral-femoral bypass may be required; the appropriate area should be preserved for cardiopulmonary bypass cannulation and avoided for line placement. If the child received aprotinin within the preceding 12 months, another dose should not be given because the risk of anaphylaxis is increased within this period (see Chapter 18).[36]

The type of surgery to be performed is important. For example, if a Blalock-Taussig shunt is placed on the left side, the arterial line should not be placed in the left arm because the trace will be lost or distorted during subclavian cross-clamping. If a superior cavopulmonary anastomosis (Glenn shunt) is planned, a short internal jugular catheter can be useful to monitor pulmonary artery pressure, but it should be removed early in the postoperative period to reduce the risk of developing a thrombus in the superior vena cava (SVC), with its potential disastrous consequences.

Good veins should be sought and marked for the application of local anesthetic cream. This is useful in sick children even if an inhalational induction is planned because it allows a venous cannula to be placed to administer analgesic, anesthetic, neuromuscular blocking agents, or emergency drugs during a very light plane of anesthesia without the risk of a hyperreactive response to the stimulus. The early administration of anesthetic adjuvants during the induction phase allows the concentration of inhaled anesthetics to be quickly reduced, thereby avoiding myocardial depression from high partial pressures of inhalation anesthetics.

Prescribing Premedication

Sedative premedication can reduce anxiety and uncooperative or combative behavior during induction of anesthesia setting the stage for a smoother induction, although this practice varies widely. Numerous medications and routes of administration may be used, and ample recommendations exist, but the final decision on premedication is usually dictated by local preferences that are not always evidence-based. The availability of anesthetic induction rooms and parental presence during induction may also influence the decision whether to prescribe sedative premedication to the individual child. There is heightened awareness and increasing concerns about the possibility of postoperative behavioral problems resulting from inadequate preparation and handling the uncooperative child preoperatively.[37,38] It is important for the pediatric anesthesiologist to reduce perioperative anxiety in children by both nonpharmacologic and pharmacologic methods.[39,40]

Although prescribing premedication is best assessed on an individual basis, some general considerations apply to most children who present for pediatric heart surgery. Premedication for infants younger than 6 months of age is usually unnecessary. Premedication for older, healthy children who show little anxiety and with whom good preoperative rapport can be established is also often unnecessary. However, older children, particularly those who have undergone previous surgery, may have fears about anesthesia and surgery and would benefit from a premedication. Although it is important to address their fears, sedative premedication may play a pivotal role in achieving adequate anxiolysis for parental separation and a smooth induction. For children in severe congestive heart failure, the decision to premedicate must be made cautiously, if at all, as the effects of the usually prescribed doses may be unpredictable. In contrast, children with dynamic obstruction to the left or right ventricular outflow tracts often benefit from sedative premedication because crying and struggling during induction may worsen obstruction. Cyanotic children (e.g., those with tetralogy of Fallot) may further desaturate if agitated during induction. However, it is important to monitor cyanotic children after premedication and provide supplemental oxygen as needed because their ventilatory response to hypoxia is blunted.[41,42] In the USA, supplemental premedication is sometimes administered under the direct supervision of the anesthesiologist in the preoperative facility, providing for a calm child and gentle separation from the parents. In the United Kingdom, where induction of anesthesia takes place in a dedicated anesthesia room, parents are present until after the induction, often making premedication unnecessary.

The most common premedication used in children without IV access is oral midazolam (0.5–1.0 mg/kg).[43] However, the effect of midazolam may be unpredictable as it may cause paradoxical reactions, with agitation and dysphoria instead of anxiolysis and sedation. Numerous other medications including ketamine, clonidine, temazepam, chloral hydrate, and dexmedetomidine have also been effective for anxiolysis and sedation at the time of separation from parents and during anesthesia induction in children with CHD.[44,45]

Formulating an Anesthetic Plan

After assessing the child, it is possible to formulate a detailed anesthetic plan. The anesthesiologist should have acquired a complete understanding of the child's heart defect and its hemodynamic consequences, as well as the state of any comorbidities. The detailed anesthetic plan consists of a choice of anesthetic agents, techniques, ventilatory management, and inotropic/vasoactive support to attain a set of appropriate hemodynamic goals for the individual patient.

UPPER RESPIRATORY TRACT INFECTION AND CARDIAC SURGERY

Healthy children with an upper respiratory tract infection (URI) who are scheduled for elective noncardiac surgery are more likely to incur perioperative respiratory complications (Table 15.1). These complications typically are minor, easily managed, and usually result in minimal morbidity[46–49]; the decision to proceed with noncardiac surgery in a child with CHD and a URI should be made on an individual basis (see Chapter 2).[50–53]

The decision to proceed with cardiac surgery in children with a URI may be difficult. Although children with cardiac failure are

TABLE 15.1	Diagnosis of Upper Respiratory Tract Infection

At least two of the following signs plus confirmation by a parent:
   Rhinorrhea
   Sore or scratchy throat
   Sneezing
   Nasal congestion
   Malaise
   Cough
   Fever >100.4°F (38°C)

Data from Schreiner MS, O'Hara I, Markakis DA, Politis GD. Do children who experience laryngospasm have an increased risk of upper respiratory tract infection? *Anesthesiology* 1996;85:475-480.

prone to multiple URIs, they may also have signs that can mimic URIs. Surgery may be relatively urgent, so postponing surgery because of a URI could result in an increased risk to the child. Cardiac surgery in children with URIs likely increases the duration of stay in the ICU and prolongs the duration of mechanical ventilation, although overall hospital stay is not prolonged. Proceeding with surgery increases the incidence of perioperative atelectasis and postoperative bacterial infections.[46] However, neither the mortality rates (4.2% with URIs vs. 1.6% without URIs, P = NS) nor long-term sequelae in children with URIs who undergo cardiac surgery are necessarily increased.[54] The children with URIs were notably younger and smaller, which may account in part for the insignificantly increased mortality rate; this should be taken into consideration when contemplating whether to proceed with surgery. Children who are scheduled for a Glenn shunt or completion of the Fontan circulation may be at particular risk because a respiratory tract infection can increase the pulmonary vascular resistance (PVR), which can negatively affect surgical outcome. In summary, it is prudent to postpone cardiac surgery in a child with a URI who is scheduled for elective cardiac surgery. If the surgery is urgent, the risks and benefits to the child of proceeding with surgery should be discussed with the surgeons and parents to reach a consensus.

Perioperative Challenges in Pediatric Cardiac Anesthesia

CYANOSIS

Cyanotic children compensate for chronic hypoxia with increased erythropoiesis, increased circulating blood volume, vasodilation, and metabolic adjustments of factors such as the circulating concentration of 2,3-diphosphoglycerate (2,3-DPG). These changes facilitate greater delivery of oxygen to tissues. The increase in blood viscosity with polycythemia increases vascular resistance and sludging, which may result in renal, pulmonary, and cerebral thromboses, especially in dehydrated children.[55–58] Long periods without oral intake preoperatively and postoperatively should be avoided in children with polycythemia, unless adequate intravenous (IV) hydration is provided.

PVR increases more than systemic vascular resistance (SVR) when the hematocrit increases, further decreasing pulmonary blood flow in children who already have a compromised pulmonary circulation. Coagulopathies are common in children with cyanotic CHD and may adversely affect surgical hemostasis.[59–61] Furthermore, chronic hypoxemia can cause important changes in vascular function and structure, some of which are maladaptive and probably contribute to impaired cardiovascular performance.[62] When the hematocrit exceeds 65%, excessive viscosity impairs microvascular perfusion and outweighs the advantages of increased oxygen-carrying capacity, with thrombocytopenia inversely related to the increasing hematocrit.[63] Long-standing hypoxemia exerts a complex effect on blood viscosity and coagulation, the pathophysiology of which continues to be investigated. Reduction of red blood cell volume can correct the coagulopathy and improve hemodynamics when increases in hematocrit are extreme.[64] However, treatment of hyperviscosity in patients with cyanotic heart disease is controversial[65,66]; guidelines for managing adults with CHD suggest the judicious use of phlebotomy and address the issue of potential complications.[26]

INTRACARDIAC SHUNTING
Much of the pathophysiology in congenital heart disease involves communications between chambers or vessels that are normally separate, resulting in shunting of blood between ventricles, atria, the great arteries, or a combination of these, depending on the nature of the lesion. Management of shunting during anesthesia is a major concern that requires an understanding of the factors that control shunting.

Restrictive and Unrestrictive Shunts
When communications between chambers are small, the size of the defect limits shunting and considerations of relative PVR and SVR become correspondingly less important in determining the degree of shunting. When there is a large pressure differential at the same level of the circulation on either side of a communication, the communication is restrictive. Flow is limited across the defect, and other factors that determine shunt flow become less important. This is usually the situation in children with mild heart disease that is asymptomatic or minimally symptomatic, such as small ASDs and VSDs or a small PDA.

Dependent Shunting During Anesthesia
In children with dependent shunts, the direction and degree of intracardiac shunting are determined by the circulatory dynamics. Control of circulatory dynamics to minimize the shunt is a major goal of anesthesia management. Because shunting depends on the relationship between SVR and PVR, anesthesia management often revolves around control of relative vascular resistances.

In children with dependent right-to-left shunts, the shunt increases when SVR decreases or PVR increases. In children with dependent left-to-right shunts, the shunt increases when SVR increases and PVR decreases. In children with bidirectional or balanced shunting, changes in vascular resistance increase the net shunt away from the side with increased vascular resistance.

For practical purposes, acute increases in left-to-right shunts during anesthesia are of clinical importance in several situations. A substantial steal of systemic blood flow by the pulmonary circulation can occur in conditions with unrestrictive, significant, left-to-right shunting such as atrioventricular (AV) canal, truncus arteriosus, and hypoplastic left heart syndrome. Left-to-right shunting is well tolerated, except when pulmonary steal leads to systemic hypotension, increasing acidosis from poor systemic end-organ perfusion or insufficient coronary perfusion. Shunting from right-to-left, because it is accompanied by at least some degree of arterial oxygen desaturation, is more frequently a problem during anesthesia.

IMPAIRED HEMOSTASIS
Hemostasis is impaired after bypass in infants and children to a greater extent compared with adults (see Chapters 8 and 18). The initiation of CPB triggers contact activation of the hemostatic systems, with ongoing coagulation and fibrinolysis, as well as the initiation of a systemic inflammatory response, both contributing to the coagulopathy. In infants and children, these effects are further compounded by a larger size of the CPB circuit relative to patient's size. In this patient population, impaired hemostasis after bypass results from a combination of immature coagulation factor synthesis, hemodilution after bypass, and a complex interaction involving consumption of clotting factors and platelets. At birth, the levels of vitamin K–dependent coagulation factors in healthy, full-term neonates are only 40% to 66% of adult values. During the first month of life, these levels increase to 53% to 90% of adult values (see also Chapter 8).[67,68] However, in children with CHD, especially those with cyanosis or systemic hypoperfusion, coagulation factors often continue to be depressed owing to impaired hepatic protein synthesis. Although antithrombin III levels are also low, true heparin resistance is rare in infants because of parallel decreases in coagulation factors.

At the onset of CPB, the introduction of the prime volume, which can be up to two to three times greater than the child's blood volume, dilutes the clotting factors, particularly fibrinogen to 50% and platelets to 30% of their pre-bypass values. This degree of dilution occurs even when the pump circuit is primed with whole blood. Greater dilution may occur when packed red blood cells (PRBCs) are used in the priming volume. At the conclusion of neonatal bypass, the activity of clotting factors is often extremely low, the fibrinogen concentration is frequently less than 100 mg/dL, and the platelet count is only 50,000 to 80,000/mm^3.[69–71] In addition to these quantitative changes, functional changes in the platelets occur during bypass. Extracorporeal circulation causes a loss of platelet adhesion receptors, activation of platelets, and formation of leukocyte-platelet conjugates. Platelet adhesion receptors in cyanotic children are depressed to a greater extent than in those with acyanotic cardiac defects. Heparin also impairs platelet function independent of CPB.[72,73]

Cardiac surgery is associated with activation of the fibrinolytic system.[74,75] Inadequate heparin concentrations during CPB may also contribute to postoperative bleeding because inadequate anticoagulation may allow continued activation of the hemostatic pathways. Ongoing activation of the coagulation cascade causes the consumption of platelets and clotting factors. The standard measurement of anticoagulation for bypass, the activated clotting time (ACT), correlates poorly with heparin concentrations (usually measured using the surrogate, anti-Xa) in children undergoing CPB.[76] Individualized heparin monitoring and heparin titration was associated with larger doses of heparin but smaller doses of protamine for antagonism.[77] Activation of the clotting cascade using that heparin-protamine regimen is also reduced, thus potentially decreasing bleeding in the postoperative period.[77–79] As a result of this multifactorial coagulopathy, blood loss is a greater problem in children than in adults and is a particular problem in neonates and small infants (see Chapter 18).[80]

Strategies to Reduce Bleeding After Bypass
In an effort to normalize factors and platelets to effective concentrations, some medical centers use fresh whole blood in the cardiopulmonary circuit prime. In adult patients and in an in vitro aggregation study, transfusion of fresh whole blood provided equal to or greater hemostatic and functional benefit when compared with transfusion of platelet concentrates. In children, transfusion with fresh whole blood less than 48 hours from harvest reduced the blood loss compared with transfusion of reconstituted whole blood (e.g.,

packed erythrocytes, fresh frozen plasma, and platelets).[81] Other studies have shown that fresh whole blood in the prime in neonatal and pediatric cardiac surgery reduced transfusion requirements[82,83] and improved outcomes.[84] However, the benefits of using fresh whole blood to prime the CPB circuit have been questioned in at least one study, which showed not only no benefit but an increased length of stay in the ICU, as well as increased perioperative fluid overload in the group given fresh whole blood.[85] It is possible that specific pediatric patient populations (e.g., age, cyanotic vs. noncyanotic CHD) may derive greater benefit from the use of fresh whole blood than others. Until this issue is clarified, it is difficult to know in which children undergoing cardiac surgery fresh whole blood is most beneficial. Moreover, fresh whole blood is often difficult to obtain. The units must be refrigerated for 24 to 48 hours while donor screening is performed, and storage causes significant platelet injury. Insistence on fresh whole blood places tremendous pressures on the transfusion service and donor center to coordinate the matching of donor types with recipient needs. Furthermore, in the presence of suitable, simpler alternatives to this management strategy, it is likely that most centers worldwide will continue to use individual blood components in a variety of combinations, often dictated by institutional preferences, to prime the CPB circuit. It is also likely that most centers will continue to rely on the use of individual blood components to treat bleeding and coagulopathy in children undergoing heart surgery.

As a result, individual component therapy remains the standard of practice in most institutions. In neonates and small infants with dilutional coagulopathy, platelets should be given in combination with cryoprecipitate to correct the defect in clotting. An initial dose of platelets (10 mL/kg) may need to be repeated if bleeding persists and the platelet count is less than 100,000/mm³.[60] Cryoprecipitate contains high concentrations of fibrinogen, factor VIII, von Willebrand factor, and factor XIII. Fibrinogen and von Willebrand factor are required for platelet adhesion and aggregation, the fundamental first steps in primary hemostasis (see Chapters 8 and 10). The subsequent step of platelet degranulation switches on the entire coagulation cascade and cannot commence without adhesion and aggregation occurring first.[86] Administration of fresh frozen plasma (FFP), which is not evidence-based for this type of coagulopathy, may excessively dilute the red cell mass and platelets.[87]

In recent years, the use of synthetic or purified factors and factor combinations have increased to prevent or treat bleeding in children undergoing heart surgery out of concerns for exposure to allogenic blood products and the increased difficulties in procuring blood components and blood product shortages. Recombinant activated factor VII (rFVIIa) is a synthetic coagulation factor manufactured by recombinant technology and is nearly identical to the human plasma coagulation factor VIIa.[88–90] In the USA, it is approved by the Food and Drug Administration (FDA) for use in hemophilia A or B and factor VII deficiency; in Europe it is licensed for hemophilia home treatment, Glanzmann thrombasthenia, and postsurgical bleeding.[91,92] Although it has been used to treat bleeding after cardiac surgery in both adults and children, the safety of rFVIIa and its potential for thrombotic complications, without any clear benefit associated with its use, have been raised.[93,94] Hence, the routine use of rFVIIa in children undergoing heart surgery cannot currently be recommended due to ongoing uncertainties about its overall benefit-to-risk balance.[95,96]

Prothrombin complex concentrates (PCCs) are highly purified concentrates with hemostatic activity prepared from pooled plasma.[97] They contain four vitamin K–dependent clotting factors: factors II, VII, IX, and X. Depending on the concentration of factor VII, they are classified as three-factor (3F) PCCs or four-factor (4F) PCCs, with the former having low levels of factor VII and the latter therapeutic levels of all four factors. Some concentrates also contain small amounts of the anticoagulant proteins C and S and antithrombin. Most contain a minimum amount of heparin to prevent activation. The vast majority of commercially available PCC formulations are exclusively composed of inactivated factors. The only activated PCC in the USA is Factor eight inhibitor bypassing activity (FEIBA), which contains FVIIa and small amounts of FXa. These hemostatic agents have been used in children undergoing cardiac surgery, with one prospective study showing less chest drain output and fewer units of PRBCs transfused within the first postoperative 24 hours after prophylactic nonactivated 4F PCC, but with similar FFP transfusions.[98] Until today, the use of PCCs has not been associated with an increase in adverse events, although ongoing concerns about the potential thrombotic risk associated with their use, in particular in children undergoing heart surgery with prosthetic material such as conduits, grafts, or valves persist. In the absence of further evidence and well-designed studies, PCCs cannot be recommended for routine use, but should probably be relegated to use for bleeding refractory to conventional therapies.[99–103]

Fibrinogen concentrate is a virally inactivated purified plasma derivative supplied as a lyophilized powder with no other factors. Despite sparse objective data about its efficacy and safety, its use has expanded in many European countries, where cryoprecipitate is no longer available. This concentrate offers some clear advantages over cryoprecipitate itself, such as a smaller volume for an equivalent dose of fibrinogen, briefer preparation times, and ease of storage. Since it is only licensed for use as a treatment of bleeding episodes in patients with congenital fibrinogen deficiency in some countries, it cannot be recommended as an alternative to cryoprecipitate where this is currently available. However, the fact that it has become a standard treatment in many European countries with a very good safety track record suggests that its use should be strongly considered for fibrinogen replacement in children undergoing cardiac surgery.[104,105]

Transfusion guidelines have been described for adults and have been shown to reduce postoperative bleeding and transfusion requirements.[106,107] Although similar guidelines have not been as forthcoming in children in whom the practice frequently seems to be more empirical, there is a growing body of evidence that point-of-care (POC) monitoring of hemostasis is useful to guide specific blood component therapy.[108] In a surgical context, the time it takes to return routine coagulation tests is often too long for clinical decision making. Consequently, point-of-care platelet count (or, less frequently, platelet aggregometry) and viscoelastic monitoring of coagulation such as thromboelastography and thromboelastometry are being used increasingly to make timely informed decisions about blood product administration.[109,110] The use of transfusion algorithms in pediatric cardiac surgery has reduced blood product requirements and bleeding.[111–113] Blood product shortages and ongoing concerns about complications associated with transfusions make a compelling case for routine use of coagulation monitoring and directed blood component administration, in order to avoid unnecessary or excessive exposure to blood products. This tailored approach to monitoring and treating bleeding in children undergoing heart surgery, often by the use of specifically designed algorithms applicable to the pediatric population, has currently become a standard of practice in many centers worldwide.[114,115]

Antifibrinolytics

The antifibrinolytics used in pediatric cardiac surgery include aprotinin, ϵ(Epsilon)-aminocaproic acid (EACA) and tranexamic acid (TXA). Epsilon-aminocaproic acid and tranexamic acid are lysine analogs that reduce bleeding after cardiac surgery in adults and children,[116,117] with apparent similar efficacy and safety.[118-120] Doses of epsilon-aminocaproic acid and tranexamic acid for pediatric cardiac surgery have yet to be clearly established. Furthermore, in view of the disproportion between circulating blood volume and CPB prime volume, a drug target concentration that differs between neonates and children, as well as other differences in pharmacokinetics, suggests that different dosing schemes should be used in neonates and smaller children compared with older children.[121-123]

Aprotinin is a serine protease inhibitor no longer available in many countries, and with only very limited availability in others, after its marketing license was withdrawn because of safety concerns in adults. Early evidence demonstrated that aprotinin reduced bleeding, reduced the time taken to extubation, shortened ICU stay, and reduced overall mortality rates.[124] However, subsequent studies contradicted these initial findings.[125] The same volume of evidence has not been published in children, although several studies suggest that it is effective in reducing bleeding and that it reduces the duration of postoperative mechanical ventilation.[60,126-128] An increased risk of renal failure or stroke in adults undergoing revascularization surgery has been reported.[129] The same investigators reported an increase in the 5-year mortality rate for adults after the use of aprotinin in revascularization surgery, mostly resulting from stroke and myocardial infarction.[130] The 30-day mortality rate after aprotinin is increased by as much as one-third compared with epsilon-aminocaproic acid and tranexamic acid.[125] However, it appears that the early data regarding increased death rates have not been supported by a subsequent study. On balance, its benefits may outweigh the risks in specific populations, but which populations have not been defined.[131] Although the use of aprotinin in adults remains controversial, it is reasonable to assume that the increased mortality from stroke and myocardial infarction in adults have only limited relevance in children given the differences in pathophysiology and underlying risk factors. Similarly, it appears unlikely that the adverse effects of aprotinin on kidney function in adults also holds true for infants and children undergoing cardiac surgery.[132-134] An important additional safety consideration relates to the risk of severe hypersensitivity reactions. The reported incidence of adverse effects in children varies. Even though anaphylaxis seems to be infrequent in pediatric patients after primary exposure, the risk of such a severe reaction is increased after re-exposure, particularly if it occurs within 12 months of aprotinin exposure.[36,135] This has led the manufacturer to issue a black box warning for the possibility of a hypersensitivity reaction to aprotinin if the child is re-exposed within 1 year of a previous exposure. The FDA has also recommended that aprotinin should be administered only in the operative setting when CPB can be started quickly, in the event of a severe reaction. Uncertainty about the relative safety profiles of aprotinin and the lysine analogs has been met with similar considerations about the effectiveness of these different drugs. Although there is some evidence that epsilon-aminocaproic acid and tranexamic acid are at least as effective as aprotinin,[136,137] research has also suggested that aprotinin use may decrease the output of chest drains,[138] have stronger blood-sparing effects,[139] as well as confer differences in other outcomes such as cytokine activation or early indexes of postoperative recovery.[140] In fact, it appears that aprotinin may have unique antiinflammatory properties, which may benefit pediatric patients.[141] Further research is needed to clarify issues concerning safety and relative effectiveness of the two classes of drugs, as well as proving benefits and improve effective dosing schemes in specific patient populations (see Chapter 18).

Topical Agents

The use of topical agents to promote clot formation and reduce bleeding after cardiac surgery is common. The most frequently used topical agents are fibrin sealants. Fibrin sealants mimic the stages of the blood coagulation process. Unlike the synthetic adhesives, they are biocompatible.[142] Fibrin sealants are usually sourced from plasma components, and most contain virally inactivated human fibrinogen and thrombin with different quantities of factor XIII, antifibrinolytic agents, and calcium.[143] When the fibrinogen and thrombin are mixed during the application process, the fibrinogen is converted to fibrin monomers. This results in the formation of a semirigid fibrin clot. By mimicking the later stages of the coagulation process, these sealants stop bleeding and assist in wound healing.[142] They have reduced bleeding in children undergoing heart surgery.[144]

Ultrafiltration

Ultrafiltration is a process that results in the production of an ultrafiltrate by means of convection forces and a hydrostatic pressure gradient across a semipermeable membrane. As such, free water and low–molecular-weight substances are removed from a child during and after CPB. It provides many benefits, including increasing the hematocrit, concentrating the clotting factors and platelets, increasing blood pressure, reducing PVR, and removing inflammatory mediators in the ultrafiltrate. It has reduced bleeding after cardiac surgery in children.[145-147]

Desmopressin

Desmopressin is a synthetic analog of vasopressin which increases the plasma concentrations of factor VIII and von Willebrand factor (see also Chapters 8, 10 and 18). It reduces bleeding after CPB in adult cardiac surgery[148] and its use is indicated in specific subgroups of patients.[149-151] Unfortunately, studies in children failed to demonstrate a similar effectiveness in reducing bleeding or transfusion requirements.[152]

Anesthesia Management for Surgery Requiring Cardiopulmonary Bypass

MONITORING

Noninvasive monitoring during pediatric cardiac surgery includes pulse oximetry, five-lead electrocardiography, an automated blood pressure cuff, a precordial or esophageal stethoscope, continuous airway manometry, inspired and expired capnography, anesthetic gas and oxygen analysis, multiple-site temperature measurement, and volumetric urine collection. The pulse oximeter is particularly important when managing children with congenital cardiac disease. At least two probes should be placed on different limbs in the event that one fails during the procedure. In children with cyanotic heart disease, conventional pulse oximetry overestimates arterial oxygen saturation as saturation decreases[153-156]; this error tends to be exacerbated in the presence of severe hypoxemia.[157] When monitoring children with a shunt across the ductus arteriosus, a probe should be placed on the right upper limb to measure preductal oxygenation, and a second probe should be placed on a toe to measure postductal oxygenation (children with a right-sided aortic arch or variations in the usual ductal anatomy may require the preductal probe to be placed on a left upper limb). Children undergoing repair of coarctation of the aorta should be monitored with a pulse oximeter on the right upper limb because it may be the only reliable monitor during the repair, and blood pressure cuffs should be placed before and after the coarctation. These two cuffs may be cycled, and the differential documented before and after surgical repair.

Monitoring end-tidal carbon dioxide tension (PetCO$_2$) is of value in most children. However, in children with cyanotic-shunting cardiac lesions, the PetCO$_2$ measurement may be less reflective of PaCO$_2$ because of ventilation-perfusion mismatching.[158-160] Arterial blood gases are the most accurate measure of the adequacy of ventilation and oxygenation. To provide rapid decision making, it is helpful to have the blood gas analysis machine located in or near the cardiac operating room.[161,162]

Monitoring ionized calcium concentrations is essential during surgical procedures in which large quantities of citrated blood products are infused rapidly or when entire blood volumes are replaced. Neonates are particularly prone to disturbances in their ionized calcium concentration when citrated whole blood, fresh frozen plasma, or platelets are infused. Those with limited cardiac reserve tolerate ionized hypocalcemia poorly because of their greater sensitivity to the myocardial effects of citrate infusion (see Chapter 10, Figs. 10.10 and 10.11).[163] In isolation, the total serum calcium concentration is misleading.

Temperature monitoring during CPB is a critical guide to adequate brain cooling and appropriate rewarming before separation from bypass. Because it is not practical to measure brain temperature directly, surrogate measuring sites including the tympanic membrane, nasopharyngeal, and rectum have been used. The nasopharyngeal site most closely matches true brain temperature and is the site at which temperature is most often monitored. The tympanic and rectal sites tend to overestimate the brain temperature.[164] Measurement of skin temperature gives an indication regarding peripheral perfusion and provides information about adequate peripheral rewarming.

After induction of anesthesia, an arterial catheter should be placed in children who will undergo CPB. In older, cooperative children with very severe congenital heart disease, it may be prudent and safer where feasible to establish invasive blood pressure monitoring before induction of anesthesia using an adequate premedication and topical and local anesthesia of the site. The radial artery may be percutaneously cannulated with relative ease, even in infants. In neonates, the femoral arteries are frequently used for arterial access, and the axillary arteries may also be used. The radial, femoral, and axillary arteries all seem to constitute suitable sites for arterial cannulation and invasive blood pressure monitoring, with complication rates similar to those in adults.[165,166] The brachial artery is generally avoided because it is an end artery, lacking collateral circulation, although one retrospective series of 200 children reported complication rates similar to other arterial sites.[167] Catheters placed in the dorsalis pedis or posterior tibial artery often provide inaccurate hemodynamic data, especially after separation from bypass, and it may become difficult to sample blood for laboratory testing. In the rare circumstance that peripheral arterial cannulation cannot be achieved percutaneously, the cutdown method should be considered; alternatively, the surgeon may place a catheter in the internal mammary artery after sternotomy with a sterile monitoring line passed over the drapes to the anesthesiologist to transduce the pressure. The use of ultrasound to assist in arterial cannulation improves the success rate; it is likely that the widespread availability and increasing experience with this method will make it routine practice in many centers.[168-170]

Central venous catheters are very useful for both central venous pressure monitoring and as a safe, reliable route to administer inotropes, vasopressors, and potentially veno-irritant solutions. For cardiac surgery, there are two commonly used methods to obtain central access. Which method depends in part on institutional bias. In the first method, the cardiac surgeons expose the heart quickly and have it available for inspection and estimation of filling pressures. Central lines can be readily established from the surgical field and handed off to the anesthesia team. These transthoracic central lines are useful but carry a small risk.[171,172] The second method is percutaneous insertion of central venous lines via the subclavian, internal jugular, or femoral vein.[173-175] This route is particularly useful for long, complex procedures, as well as redo operations, especially when access to the infant is limited or the heart is not exposed. It is important to appreciate that the internal jugular or subclavian route may fail or be associated with pneumothorax, hemorrhage, and hematoma formation after puncture of major vessels.[176,177] Cannulation of the external jugular vein may avoid some of these serious complications when the catheter can be successfully threaded into the central circulation.[178] Increasingly, ultrasound-guided techniques are being used to establish central venous access (see also Chapter 46). In the United Kingdom, the use of ultrasound for the placement of these lines is recommended by the National Institute of Clinical Excellence (NICE); ultrasound is used routinely for the placement of central lines, with currently good evidence that it increases successes and decreases complications.[179-181]

In children with unrestrictive VSDs or ASDs, including hearts with a single ventricle or single atrium, central venous pressure is identical to left ventricular filling pressure. Cannulation of vessels that drain into the SVC should be approached with caution in children with univentricular anatomy who may undergo the Fontan procedure, because thrombosis of the SVC can be a devastating complication. In these children, the femoral veins may be the preferred sites for central venous access. Left-sided central venous lines in the SVC territory should also generally be avoided in cardiac patients; there is a greater risk of erosion and perforation from central venous catheters placed through the left internal jugular or left subclavian veins. Furthermore, in up to 10% of patients with CHD, these veins join a persistent left SVC that most often drains into the coronary sinus or left atrium, both undesirable locations for a central venous catheter tip.[182-184]

Percutaneously inserted pulmonary arterial catheters in children with intracardiac defects usually provide information that is not substantively different from that of a simple central line, are difficult to insert without fluoroscopy, and may not provide meaningful measurements of cardiac output. As a result, they are rarely used in pediatric cardiac patients. In circumstances that would be deemed useful, it is probably preferable to insert them surgically. In some complex CHD and procedures in which postoperative left ventricular dysfunction is expected, it may be valuable to have continuous monitoring of pressures in the left heart. Such measurements are usually obtained via a left atrial (LA) pressure monitoring line inserted by the surgical team.[185-187]

Transesophageal Echocardiography

Use of perioperative echocardiography has become the standard of care in the United States for both adults[188-191] and children undergoing heart surgery.[192-194] In adult practice, anesthesiologists usually perform the TEE, but in children the TEE is more commonly performed by a pediatric cardiologist. This may reflect the increased complexity of congenital lesions and the difficulty in accurately assessing these lesions and their repairs. TEE is cost-effective[195] since its use can have an important impact on surgical and medical management.[196–198] In one study, a second bypass run was undertaken in 7.3% of cases based on the findings of the TEE, surgical alteration in the management in 12.7% and medical alteration in 18.5% of cases. Pediatric cardiac anesthesiologists usually can perform TEE before and after bypass if they have received adequate training.[199]

The introduction of small probes with multiplane capability has greatly increased the use of TEE, even in infants and neonates.[200,201] In 1999, a survey of centers in the United States indicated that 93% used intraoperative echocardiography and that all but one used TEE.[202] The American Society of Echocardiography and the Society of Cardiovascular Anesthesiologists have published guidelines for performing a comprehensive intraoperative TEE in adults[191] and children.[193]

Although the use of TEE in children is generally safe, complications do occur and may be more common in small infants and neonates.[198,203] Complications include damage to the mouth, tongue, oropharynx, esophagus, and stomach. Other complications include hemodynamic disturbance because of compression of the left atrium or other structures; erroneous invasive blood pressure monitoring may result if the compressed structure is an artery proximal to the arterial line insertion site. Airway complications have also occurred in a small number of cases including inadvertent extubation, right main-stem bronchus intubation, and compression of the tracheal tube. However, the overall incidence is small, 2.4% with airway complications comprising almost half, at 1%.[204] Information gathered from the TEE examination takes place before and after bypass and may be divided broadly into two categories: hemodynamic assessment with monitoring and structural diagnostic information. Hemodynamic information includes information about ventricular function and filling.[205] Diagnostic information relates to confirmation of preoperative findings and assessment of the surgical repair. An alternative to perioperative TEE is epicardial echocardiography, which involves placing a probe such as the ones regularly utilized to perform transthoracic ultrasound imaging of the heart, covered by a sterile sheath, directly over the heart and blood vessels. This can be performed by surgeons, with the support of pediatric cardiologists, the latter also assessing and interpreting the images and data acquired during the examination. Depending on center preference and the surgeons' experience in manipulating the probe, it may also be performed by pediatric cardiologists, who will then scrub in and perform the examination themselves. Epicardial echocardiography can be used when the child's size would make the insertion of a TEE probe too difficult or risky; it is, however, used routinely in some centers as the standard method for intraoperative echocardiography.[206–208]

Near-Infrared Spectroscopy

Near-infrared spectroscopy (NIRS) allows real-time monitoring of tissue oxygenation. This technology is based on the principle of optical spectrophotometry, making use of the fact that body tissues are relatively transparent to light in the near-infrared wavelength range. The majority of NIRS monitors use reflectance-mode NIRS, in which a region underlying the sensor is interrogated by a transmitter optode and a receiving sensor. The value obtained is a reflection of the underlying heterogeneous tissue area, composed of arteries, veins, and capillaries, as well as other nonvascular tissues. Even though there are several reports of the applicability of this technology to monitor other tissue beds[209,210] such as the renal and splanchnic circulations, cerebral NIRS has received the most attention in the context of pediatric cardiac surgery. This noninvasive monitoring is becoming widely used during CPB in children to assess the adequacy of oxygen delivery to the brain.[211–213] This may lead to improved neurologic outcomes after cardiac surgery, although there is no clear evidence for target-based NIRS values in humans. One algorithm suggested that a 20% decrease from the baseline reading bilaterally was important and should trigger efforts to increase the cerebral saturation, such as optimizing the neck position, increasing mean arterial pressure, increasing $PaCO_2$, or increasing the hematocrit. If the decrease was unilateral, it may be related to incorrect aortic cannula positioning.[214] To be most accurate, baseline readings should be undertaken before induction of anesthesia as anesthesia itself may cause changes in the NIRS values (see Chapter 49).

INDUCTION OF ANESTHESIA

In the United Kingdom, most children are anesthetized in an anesthesia induction room, which is a small room immediately adjacent to the operating room, and in most cases, the parents are present at the induction. Anesthesia is commonly induced while the child is sitting with or being held by a parent. It is possible to engage some older children to hold the mask themselves during the first stages of induction; alternatively, some parents can hold the mask for the child as they are anesthetized. After the child is asleep, they are transferred to the anesthetic trolley, where venous and arterial access is secured and the trachea is intubated. This contrasts with the practice in most centers in North America, where induction of anesthesia usually occurs in the operating room after the child is premedicated and separated from the parents.

The method of induction, either intravenously or by inhalation, should be tailored to the child and the cardiac defect. When an IV induction is selected (e.g., mask induction is refused), but IV access appears to be difficult, an anxiolytic/sedative premedication may be prescribed, ideally to be taken by the child in advance of inducing anesthesia to ensure there was adequate time to sedate the child. This requires anticipation of the need for a premedication during the preanesthetic visit and clear communication with parents and the healthcare professionals looking after the child about the ideal timing for its administration before the scheduled procedure. If a premedication is ineffective or refused and the child is distressed and uncooperative to taking medications via the oral route upon arrival in theater, either the intranasal or the intramuscular route can be used for sedation while venous cannulation is performed. Alternatives that can be used via the intranasal route include a combination of ketamine and midazolam and, more recently, dexmedetomidine. All of them are safe and effective, administered via a nasal mucosal atomization device with an onset time of effect between 10 to 30 minutes.[215–217] Application of a local anesthetic cream such as EMLA (eutectic mixture of local anesthetics; AstraZeneca, Wilmington, DE) or Ametop Gel (Smith-Nephew, Mississauga, ON, Canada) also reduces the pain of injection. However, this requires identifying suitable veins during the preoperative assessment and clear instructions to the parents or nursing staff regarding where and when the cream should be applied (1 hour for EMLA and 30 minutes for Ametop). When IV access is already present, an IV induction is preferred. In severely ill children, it is generally advisable to secure IV access before induction of anesthesia.

Sevoflurane is the most commonly used inhalational induction agent in children. Sevoflurane is very rapid acting and should be used with care in the child with CHD because high concentrations can produce bradycardia, hypotension, and apnea if not titrated carefully. Concentrations should be rapidly reduced after an adequate depth of anesthesia is achieved (remembering that the minimum alveolar concentration [MAC] in children is 2.5%) to limit myocardial depression. To facilitate establishing IV access when the concentration of sevoflurane must be restricted, a topical local anesthetic cream is helpful because it permits venous cannulation at a much lighter plane of anesthesia. In children who are cyanotic with a right-to-left shunt and reduced pulmonary blood flow, inhalational inductions are slow. Moreover, in neonates and young infants with large right-to-left shunts, the desired depth of anesthesia may not be achieved; the end-tidal concentration does not accurately reflect the blood and brain partial pressures. Many include nitrous oxide during inhalational inductions for two reasons. First, it is odorless; therefore it can be started before the introduction of the sevoflurane to sedate the child before the stronger-smelling anesthetic is introduced. Second, it allows a smoother and more rapid induction compared with sevoflurane alone. Concentrations up to 70% nitrous oxide can be used to smooth induction of anesthesia even in cyanotic children, but the nitrous oxide should be replaced with air and oxygen or 100% oxygen as soon as IV access is obtained and a muscle relaxant is given. Some children do not want an inhalational induction out of fear of the mask. To address this problem, we put the mask aside and begin the induction by cupping our hands with the elbow of the breathing circuit between two fingers and slowly bringing our hands toward the face from under the chin (this gas mixture is heavier than air). It is important to warn the child about each event before it occurs (such as a mask applied to the face) and, when possible, to demonstrate the action on yourself, a parent, or a toy animal to avoid startling or scaring the child. Some children prefer to hold the mask themselves, or if the child is accompanied by a parent and unable to hold the mask, the parent may hold it. Good premedication often facilitates this process (see also Chapter 2).

For sick children in whom an IV induction is preferable, several options are available. In neonates, for example, those with severe coarctation of the aorta or with hypoplastic left heart syndrome who are not ventilated before coming to the operating room, one approach is to administer fentanyl in a dose of 2 to 3 μg/kg, followed by a neuromuscular blocking drug (NMBD) and a low dose (i.e., sedative dose) of sevoflurane or isoflurane. Fentanyl obtunds the hypertensive response to intubation, and the NMBD (e.g., pancuronium) maintains cardiac output by maintaining the heart rate. The very-low-dose inhalational agent provides the sedation or general anesthesia. In the event that pancuronium is unavailable, a combination of fentanyl, rocuronium, and inhalational agent seems to be equally effective and safe, although pancuronium is particular in its ability to maintain heart rate and therefore cardiac output, especially in younger children. In older children, etomidate is an excellent choice as an induction agent, providing stable hemodynamics, although it does cause pain on injection. Ketamine is also widely used for IV induction in neonates and older children. Ketamine maintains or increases blood pressure, heart rate, and cardiac output. The exact mechanism of these effects of ketamine is unknown; ketamine may stimulate the release of endogenous stores of catecholamines, although it has a negative inotropic effect in the denervated heart.[218] This negative inotropic effect may make ketamine a poor choice in children in whom the catecholamine response has

already been maximized, such as in severe cardiomyopathy.[219] It may also be a poor choice if tachycardia is undesirable, such as in the case of aortic stenosis or other forms of ventricular outflow tract obstruction.

Monitors should ideally be applied before induction begins, although applying monitors can upset the child, which can be detrimental (e.g., the child with TOF who begins to cry and precipitates a hypercyanotic spell). In some cases, a pulse oximeter probe may be the only monitor applied before induction of anesthesia. Sevoflurane and other halogenated agents may provide another advantage by offering a degree of ischemic preconditioning to the heart and to other organs, particularly the brain and kidney. In fact, sevoflurane use has been shown to decrease biochemical markers for myocardial and renal injury in coronary artery bypass grafting in adults.[220] Current evidence suggests a role of inhalational anesthetic agents in improving outcomes after cardiac surgery, in particular for some subsets of patients.[221–223] Further research is needed to clarify their protective role in different organs and systems, in noncoronary and noncardiac surgery, as well as recommended doses and timing of administration.[224] It is thought that the same effect is observed in children. Sevoflurane, but also midazolam and propofol, protect against myocardial injury in pediatric cardiac surgery when using cardiac troponin T as a marker of such damage.[225] One study has demonstrated definite cardioprotective effects from inhalational agents in children,[226] although these effects do not seem to be universally applicable to all children undergoing heart surgery, suggesting the need for further investigations.[227]

MAINTENANCE OF ANESTHESIA

Maintenance of anesthesia in children with CHD depends on the preoperative status and the response to induction of anesthesia. Whether inhalational agents, additional opioids, or other IV agents are used for maintenance depends on the tolerance of the child and postoperative plans for ventilation. If a primary opioid-based anesthetic is chosen, additional opioid should be administered before sternotomy, to blunt the adrenergic response to this intense surgical stimulation, as well as on initiation of CPB to offset dilution from the pump prime, to maintain adequate opioid plasma concentrations. Awareness during adult cardiac surgery has been reported when amnestic agents were not used. Although small children may be unable to describe such events, the potential for awareness during pediatric cardiac surgery should not be underestimated. In effect, although it is unclear whether the incidence of awareness in children is more or less than in adults,[228,229] anesthesiologists should be cognizant of the possibility of intraoperative awareness in pediatric anesthesia, and mindful of the potential short- and long-term psychological effects of such a complication.[230–232] Recently, a national audit project in the United Kingdom (NAP5) suggested strategies to minimize the risk of awareness in pediatric cardiac surgery[233] that in part may depend on several factors, including the child's age, hemodynamic stability, predicted duration of surgery and CPB, and plans for postoperative ventilation. The choice of a specific strategy is often dictated by institutional or personal preferences. Different agents, singly or in combination, may prevent awareness while on CPB: an inhalational agent may be administered through the membrane oxygenator with an anesthetic vaporizer, IV midazolam (0.2 mg/kg) may be administered at the initiation of CPB, and/or propofol may be given by infusion during the bypass period. More recently, the use of a dexmedetomidine infusion has been used to attenuate awareness as it attenuates the hemodynamic and neuroendocrine responses to surgical stress and CPB in pediatric cardiac surgery.[234] Other benefits include decreased intraoperative anesthetic requirements and postoperative opioid consumption,[235] which suggest it may have a role in reducing the possibility of awareness. However, dexmedetomidine is *not* a general anesthetic (conferring 0.5 MAC equivalence) and its effectiveness in preventing awareness has not been definitively established.[236] In one study, dexmedetomidine conferred a protective effect in the heart, brain, kidney, and lungs; the administration of dexmedetomidine may contribute to improved outcomes, a decrease in postoperative mortality, and a reduced incidence of complications and delirium in adults undergoing cardiac surgery.[237] Dexmedetomidine also slows sinus and AV node conduction[238]; this may prove useful in those with junctional ectopic tachycardia (JET). In fact, among other potential advantages in regard to outcomes, it has already demonstrated unequivocal benefit in preventing JET, decreasing length of mechanical ventilation and length of stay in intensive care and in hospital after congenital cardiac surgery.[239,240]

INSTITUTION AND SEPARATION FROM BYPASS

Before cannulation of the vessels and initiation of CPB, the surgeon requests heparin to be given; after administration (preferably flushed through a central venous catheter) but *before the initiation of bypass*, the ACT should be determined. By convention, the ACT measurement should be at least three times greater than the baseline value or greater than 480 seconds, although some variations in practice between centers regarding anticoagulation levels for CPB are common. Despite interindividual differences in heparin dose requirements and multiple problems associated with its use, heparin remains the anticoagulant of choice for CPB.[241,242] In fact, achieving an adequate balance between the appropriate amount of heparin to minimize the risk of thrombosis and platelet activation while reducing the risk of bleeding from excessive anticoagulation may be particularly challenging in children.[76] Similarly, the use of the ACT as the sole metric of anticoagulation may hold a number of inaccuracies, based on the inconsistent relationships between plasma heparin concentrations, thrombin inhibition, and coagulation tests.[243] Individualized management of anticoagulation and its reversal seem to result in less activation of the coagulation cascade, less fibrinolysis, and reduced blood loss and transfusion requirements. However, until further research defines the clinical impact of these findings, it is likely that the use of heparin and ACT measurement for anticoagulation management will remain the standard of care in most centers (see also Chapter 18).[77] When bypass is started, additional anesthetic drugs should be administered to counteract the effects of dilution and adsorption by the CPB circuit. Ventilation should cease when CPB machine has attained full flow (the predicted cardiac output according to the child's age and body surface area). Both hypertension and hypotension may complicate bypass. Blood pressure should be controlled within an appropriate range to ensure end-organ perfusion and avoid complications, most commonly by using α-adrenergic agonists or blockers such as phenylephrine and phentolamine. The child is usually cooled at this stage, guided by the nasopharyngeal temperature. If the heart is to be stopped (either to facilitate surgical exposure or to avoid entraining air into the circulation), cardioplegia is given by the perfusionist after the aorta is cross-clamped to provide myocardial protection during the period of ischemia.[244,245] Most cardioplegia solutions require repeat administrations every 20 to 30 minutes, with the exception of Custodiol cardioplegia (or Bretschneider's or histidine-tryptophan-glutarate [HTK]), which confers myocardial protection after a single dose

for up to 180 minutes, this likely explains its increasing popularity in many centers for complex procedures.[246] Cardioplegia is not required if the surgery is performed while the heart is beating. Myocardial damage is related to the duration of the aortic cross-clamping and the effectiveness of the myocardial protection.[247]

At an appropriate time during the surgery, the cross-clamp is removed, and perfusion to the heart is restored. The heart usually starts to beat in normal sinus rhythm, although this is not always the case. In the early phase of reperfusion, it is possible for various degrees of heart block to occur. However, these are usually short-lived and as the effects of cardioplegia wear off, normal sinus rhythm usually resumes. Persistent heart block may result from damage to the conducting system during surgery. It is also possible, although less often than in adult heart surgery, for the heart to restart its activity in an abnormal rhythm after removal of the aortic cross-clamp, such as ventricular fibrillation or ventricular tachycardia. In congenital cardiac surgery, such a development should raise suspicion that flow to the coronary arteries may be compromised by the presence of air, compression by other structures, or direct damage.[248]

After release of the cross-clamp, vasopressors, inotropes, and/or vasodilators that are required are usually started. Rewarming may have begun before release of the cross-clamp, but more commonly, the child is rewarmed after release of the clamp. Although it is beyond the scope of this chapter to discuss which inotropes and vasoactive agents are used in children undergoing cardiac surgery, it is worth mentioning that although the choice of specific vasopressors, inotropes, or vasodilators (or combinations thereof) is very often dictated by institutional preferences, there has been a shift in practice away from the use of dopamine in favor of epinephrine and norepinephrine (see Chapters 16 and 17). The potential reno-protective effects of dopamine have never been confirmed, and concerns have been raised about its potential to increase arrhythmias and mortality in adults with cardiogenic shock.[249] Recent guidelines for pediatric resuscitation by the European Resuscitation Council specifically discourage its use in circulatory shock.[250]

When the child has: (1) adequately rewarmed, as reflected by a normal core and minimal core-peripheral temperature gradient, (2) vasoactive infusions have been initiated as needed, (3) satisfactory heart function is restored, and (4) adequate ventilation of the child's lungs achieved, the child is ready to be weaned from CPB. If a TEE probe is in place, the heart should be scanned for the presence of air. If air is present, additional attempts to de-air the heart should be initiated before separating from bypass. In the early stages after separation from bypass, the perfusionist can infuse additional volume through the aortic cannula, usually under the direction of the surgeon or anesthesiologist. Many centers institute modified ultrafiltration at this point, which involves taking arterial blood from the aortic cannula and passing it through an ultrafine filter. This blood, which is oxygenated and warm, is then reinfused into the right atrium. As previously discussed, reported benefits from the use of modified ultrafiltration include increasing the hematocrit, concentrating the clotting factors and platelets, increasing blood pressure, reducing PVR, and removing inflammatory mediators from the patient. When this process is complete, a thorough TEE examination can be undertaken.

When the team is satisfied with the TEE (or epicardial echocardiogram) result, the perfusionist and the surgical team should be informed that protamine will be administered soon. The surgeon should remove any pump suckers from the field, and the perfusionist should stop all pump suction. This is done to ensure that no protamine enters the bypass circuit in case it is necessary to reestablish bypass for any reason, especially if this needs to be done emergently. Once these preliminary activities are complete, the surgeon requests that protamine is administered to antagonize the circulating heparin. At this point, a blood gas analysis is performed and the ACT repeated; the ACT should return to pre-bypass levels (with an accepted ~10% deviation). Required blood products may be given during modified ultrafiltration or after the administration of protamine, usually while the surgeons are achieving hemostasis. As soon as reasonable stability is achieved and the chest is closed (or the decision to leave the chest open has been made), the child can be transferred to the ICU.

Control of Systemic and Pulmonary Vascular Resistances During Anesthesia

In some children with hypoplastic left heart syndrome (HLHS) who present for a Norwood procedure, excessive blood flow to the lungs resulting from a relatively low PVR and a relatively high SVR steals blood from the systemic circulation, leading to hypotension, poor tissue oxygen delivery, myocardial ischemia, and progressive acidosis. However, when the reverse occurs and the PVR is greater than the SVR, the child develops progressive excessive desaturation.[251,252] Similar pathophysiology exists with other duct-dependent circulations and to some extent with other shunting lesions. It may prove difficult to manipulate the SVR and PVR predictably because control of PVR is poorly understood, vasoactive drugs usually are distributed on both sides of the circulation, and pharmacologic attempts to modify the degree and direction of shunting have produced unpredictable results.[253,254] Despite these problems, several techniques have proved useful in manipulating the relative PVR and SVR. Increasing inspired oxygen to 100% and hyperventilation to a pH of 7.6 or greater decreases the PVR in children. Positive end-expiratory pressure, acidosis, hypothermia, and the use of 30% or less inspired oxygen can increase PVR. Potent inhalational anesthetics reduce SVR more than PVR. Etomidate does not change pulmonary blood flow in children with TOF, whereas ketamine increases the flow in children with limited cyanosis (presumably by dilating the pulmonary artery) and decreases the flow in children with moderate cyanosis (by constricting the pulmonary artery).[255] Because vasoconstrictors such as phenylephrine increase SVR more than PVR, they are effective acutely in reducing right-to-left shunting and increasing left-to-right shunting in the operating room.

During cardiac surgical procedures, a direct method of selectively increasing PVR or SVR is to have the surgeon place partially obstructing tourniquets around pulmonary arteries or the aorta to increase resistance so that flow to the opposite side of the circulation increases. Although these are only temporary measures, they may reestablish a better relative balance of resistances and a more normal physiology in a deteriorating clinical situation.

Anesthetic Drugs Used in Pediatric Cardiac Anesthesia

INHALATIONAL AGENTS

Sevoflurane

Sevoflurane is the induction agent of choice for inhalational inductions in pediatric anesthesia.[256,257] It is associated with little myocardial depression or dysrhythmias,[258–260] and there is a reduced likelihood of precipitating airway hyperreactivity than that observed with other inhalational agents. It has specific advantages over halothane when used in children with CHD, particularly in children younger than 1 year of age and in cyanotic children.[261,262] In contrast to halothane, sevoflurane does not reduce heart rate at 1.0 and 1.5 MAC in healthy children compared with awake values.[263] However, at greater concentrations, it can slow the heart rate and depress respiration. Both features are important in children with CHD because a slow heart rate reduces cardiac output and hypoventilation leads to hypercarbia and hypoxia, which can increase PVR. In the absence of nitrous oxide, sevoflurane depresses myocardial contractility to a lesser extent than halothane during induction of anesthesia. However, it does decrease left ventricular systolic function to a limited extent as well as SVR, but in common with halothane and isoflurane, it does not alter the degree of left-to-right shunting through an ASD or VSD at concentrations of ~1 MAC in 100% oxygen.[264] Sevoflurane causes bradycardia in specific subsets of patients (e.g., trisomy 21)[265,266] and conduction abnormalities in susceptible children,[267] which may be clinically important in children with marginal cardiovascular reserve. Sevoflurane should also be used with great caution in children with severe ventricular outflow tract obstruction.[268]

Isoflurane

Isoflurane is not recommended for induction of anesthesia because the frequency of laryngospasm is greater than 20%.[269] The inability to ventilate whether due to laryngospasm or other causes quickly leads to hypoxemia and hypercarbia, both of which increase PVR. This increase in PVR and the resulting pulmonary hypertension is poorly tolerated in small children with heart disease, especially in the presence of right-to-left shunting (see Chapter 5). Even though isoflurane depresses the hemodynamics in healthy neonates and infants to a similar extent as halothane at equipotent concentrations,[270,271] isoflurane may hold an advantage in children with CHD, as it depresses myocardial contractility to a lesser extent than halothane.[272,273]

Halothane

In the United States, Canada, and the United Kingdom, the use of halothane has all but ceased, but it is still widely used in other parts of the world. It is included here for completeness. Uptake of halothane in infants younger than 3 months of age is more rapid than it is in adults. This also is the case for the uptake of halothane by the myocardium.[274] Although the precise effects of halothane on the human neonatal myocardium are unknown, young rodents have a reduced cardiovascular tolerance for halothane but require greater amounts for anesthesia.[275] Studies in infants with normal cardiovascular systems have demonstrated hypotension with bradycardia during induction with halothane.[276] During induction of anesthesia in normal infants, halothane decreases the cardiac index to 73% of awake values at 1.0 MAC and to 59% at 1.5 MAC.[271] The MAC for halothane in infants 1 to 6 months of age is the greatest of any age group.[277] This increased anesthetic requirement in infants, combined with the immaturity of their cardiovascular system, explains in part the relative cardiovascular intolerance of halothane by infants. In fact, hemodynamic depression associated with halothane has been shown to be inversely related to age in pediatric patients.[278] When compared with induction of anesthesia with sevoflurane, halothane decreased heart rate and systolic blood pressure in children of different age groups.[256] As such, atropine intramuscularly before induction and

IV atropine during anesthesia partially offset the myocardial depression by halothane by attenuating the severity of the bradycardia and hypotension and increasing cardiac output. Despite the hypotension caused by halothane, it increases the arterial saturation in children with cyanotic CHD.[279]

A careful induction with sevoflurane is usually well tolerated in children with mild to moderate heart disease. However, large concentrations of potent inhalational agents may be an unwise choice for induction in young infants with severe cardiac disease. In children of any age with marginal cardiovascular reserve and in those with severe desaturation of systemic arterial blood due to right-to-left shunting, inhalational anesthetic-induced myocardial depression and systemic hypotension are poorly tolerated. A more appropriate use of these anesthetic agents in children with severe heart disease is the addition of low concentrations of the inhalational agent to provide amnesia and hypnosis, as well as to control possible hypertensive responses after an IV induction (see Chapter 5).

Nitrous Oxide

Nitrous oxide should be avoided for maintenance of anesthesia in children with CHD because of the risk of enlarging intravascular air emboli and the potential to increase the PVR. Nitrous oxide may expand microbubbles and macrobubbles, increasing obstruction to blood flow in arteries and capillaries. In all children with right-to-left shunts, there is a potential for these bubbles to be shunted directly into the systemic circulation and coronaries, a phenomenon designated as paradoxical embolization. The passage of air bubbles from the right-to-left sides is possible even in patients with predominantly left-to-right shunts, as the direction of shunting may transiently change under the influence of multiple factors during anesthesia and surgery. Consequently, care must be taken to ensure that no air bubbles are accidentally injected into the veins. Adverse outcomes after coronary air embolism are exacerbated by nitrous oxide.[280] The hemodynamic effects of venous air embolism are increased by nitrous oxide, even without paradoxical embolization.[281] In children with preexisting right-to-left shunts, paradoxical air embolism is clearly a potential problem; but even those with large left-to-right shunts can transiently reverse their shunts, as mentioned previously. This is particularly true during coughing or a Valsalva maneuver, when the normal transatrial pressure gradient is reversed. Right-to-left shunting of microbubbles of air after injection of saline into the right atrium has been demonstrated during these maneuvers.[282–284] Because coughing and Valsalva maneuvers may occur during anesthesia induction, even the most rigorous attention to removing air bubbles from IV lines may not prevent small amounts of air from reaching the systemic circulation. Microbubbles have also been observed after CPB.[285]

Nitrous oxide can increase PVR in adults.[286,287] However, in a 50% inspired concentration, it does not affect the PVR or pulmonary artery pressure in infants.[288] Nitrous oxide mildly decreases cardiac output at this concentration.[289] Avoidance of its use has been suggested in children with limited pulmonary blood flow, pulmonary hypertension, or depressed myocardial function. In the well-compensated child who does not require 100% inspired oxygen, nitrous oxide (usually at concentrations of 50%) may be used during induction of anesthesia but discontinued before tracheal intubation. If a reduced inspired oxygen concentration is required to maintain an appropriate balance between PVR and SVR after tracheal intubation, air may be added to the inspired gas mixture.

Despite all the discussion regarding the use of nitrous oxide, the benefits of adding it to the inspired gas mixture up to a concentration of 50% in oxygen, followed by the gradual introduction of sevoflurane, may offset its potential adverse effects, if by doing so a smoother anesthetic induction is achieved, without agitation, coughing, or breath-holding and Valsalva maneuvers.

INTRAVENOUS INDUCTION AGENTS

Ketamine

Ketamine is a dissociative anesthetic agent that is a good analgesic. It increases blood pressure, heart rate, and cardiac output. Although the mechanism responsible for these responses is incompletely understood, it is thought to result from its ability to stimulate the release of endogenous catecholamines.[290–292] Ketamine exerts a negative inotropic effect on isolated human myocardium in vitro,[293–295] which is dependent on the underlying adrenergic tone.[296,297] Consequently, the net effects of ketamine in vivo are likely to reflect the balance between its direct myocardial depressant effects and its ability to cause sympathetic stimulation. As such, it may be a poor choice for children in whom sympathetic stimulation may already be maximal, such as in those with severe cardiomyopathy. It is also a poor choice if tachycardia is undesirable, such as in a child with aortic stenosis. Ketamine is thought to have minimal effects on PVR in children with CHD as long as the airway and ventilation are well preserved.[298,299] These likely clinically insignificant effects on PVR seem to be applicable to children with normal[300,301] and increased[255,302,303] pulmonary artery pressures, although it has been shown to occasionally cause an increase in PVR, as well as a decrease in pulmonary blood flow in certain subsets of patients with CHD.[304] Ketamine is quite a versatile anesthetic that may be administered intramuscularly and orally when IV access is difficult or an inhalational induction is contraindicated. The usual IV dose of 1 to 2 mg/kg produces a very predictable response, and an intramuscular dose of 4 to 10 mg/kg (possibly combined with intramuscular midazolam) is less predictable. The oral dose of ketamine is 5 to 6 mg/kg. The use of ketamine varies greatly from one institution to another, with some units using it extensively and others using it rarely (see Chapter 5).

Etomidate

Etomidate is an imidazole derivative short-acting anesthetic without any analgesic properties. It is a very safe drug, with a median lethal dose (LD_{50})/median effective dose (ED_{50}) ratio of 26 in animal models,[305] which indicates that the lethal dose (LD) is 26 times greater than the effective dose (ED). Etomidate has little effect on systemic blood pressure, heart rate, and cardiac output after a single dose in healthy children[306]; it also appears to have minimal hemodynamic effects in children with CHD.[306,307] It has a favorable hemodynamic profile even when used in children in shock and appears to have a low risk of clinically important myoclonus or status epilepticus, pain on IV injection, and nausea and vomiting.[308,309] The major concern regarding etomidate is the increased mortality rates reported when it is administered as a continuous infusion. This adverse effect has been attributed to adrenal suppression.[310–312] The effect of etomidate to inhibit steroid synthesis has been confirmed after both a single IV dose and prolonged infusions, resulting in concerns regarding its use as an anesthetic agent, particularly in critically ill patients in ICUs in some jurisdictions.[313–315] The decrease in plasma cortisol and ACTH concentrations in children undergoing heart surgery after etomidate may persist for 24 hours or greater and may be potentiated by the use of other anesthetic agents.[316] The notion that etomidate causes adrenal suppression is well established, but what remains unclear is whether patient outcomes differ after a single bolus dose for induction of anesthesia.[317] Newer analogs of etomidate have addressed these deficiencies and may lead to a surge in its use in the future (see also Chapter 5).

Propofol

Propofol is a rapidly acting IV hypnotic agent that may be administered as a single dose or by continuous infusion. It has no analgesic activity, but it possesses antiemetic properties, even in subhypnotic doses.[318–322] It is effective for prophylaxis against emergence agitation in young children.[323,324] Its short duration of action is the result of rapid redistribution and metabolism, which also allows the drug to be given by continuous infusion with limited accumulation. Induction doses decrease SVR, blood pressure, and cardiac output; the effect on heart rate varies. The ED_{50} for propofol in infants and small children is greater than it is in adults.[310–313,318,325–327] If propofol is given very slowly, smaller doses are required to achieve the anesthetic state, although the induction time increases. A slower infusion also results in more stable hemodynamics.[328] Pain on injection and involuntary movement after IV propofol have been concerns that have been overcome (see Chapter 5). However, there remain concerns that it can trigger propofol infusion syndrome (PRIS) after continued use in the presence of a systemic inflammatory response. This rare but potentially lethal syndrome is characterized clinically by acute bradycardia progressing to asystole; it is frequently associated with progressive metabolic acidosis, hemodynamic instability, myocardial failure, and rhabdomyolysis.[329–332] The symptoms of PRIS may develop rapidly and often are refractory to aggressive pharmacologic treatment, requiring hemodialysis or hemoperfusion; cardiorespiratory support with extracorporeal membrane oxygenation has been utilized in some cases.[333–335] These concerns about propofol have led to recommendations to maintain close vigilance for developing signs reflective of PRIS, as well as limiting continuous infusion rates and their duration when it is given continuously.[336] Although propofol can be used safely in children with CHD, it is typically avoided as an induction agent in those with severe CHD, especially in those with a fixed cardiac output such as severe aortic or mitral stenosis; in these patients, it may cause severe hypotension due to its effects on SVR and blood pressure. It can be used by continuous infusion during CPB to reduce awareness and may be particularly useful if an early tracheal extubation is planned (see also Chapters 5 and 6).[337,338]

OPIOIDS
Fentanyl

As in adults with severe cardiac disease, an IV induction with fentanyl combined with pancuronium and 100% oxygen or air and oxygen provides hemodynamic stability even in very sick children with CHD, although it is not amnestic. Inclusion of IV midazolam or another amnestic agent is strongly urged to avoid awareness. In neonates and infants, the use of high-dose opioid anesthesia provides excellent hemodynamic stability, with suppression of the hormonal and metabolic stress responses.[339,340] When fentanyl or other opioids are combined with nitrous oxide, the negative inotropic effects of nitrous oxide may be evident, particularly in sicker children.[341] The high-dose fentanyl technique is effective in preterm neonates undergoing ligation of a PDA.[342] In high-risk, full-term neonates and in older infants with severe CHD, the high-dose fentanyl technique in doses of up to

75 µg/kg, combined with pancuronium, maintains stable hemodynamics during induction, tracheal intubation, and surgical incision.[343] Oxygen saturation is well maintained and often improves during induction, even in cyanotic children.[344] The cardiac index, SVR, and PVR in infants given 25 µg/kg of fentanyl do not change substantively.[345] Combining pancuronium with fentanyl is desirable because the vagolytic effects of pancuronium offset the potential vagotonic effects of fentanyl. The hemodynamic stability reported in infants with the combination of high-dose fentanyl and pancuronium may not be replicated when other muscle relaxants are used (see Chapter 5).[346] However, if such an anesthetic regimen is applied to toddlers and older children, amnestic agents such as midazolam and an inhalational agent should be included.

Sufentanil

Sufentanil (5–20 µg/kg), an alternative to fentanyl, is 5 to 10 times more potent than fentanyl but has a large margin of safety.[347,348] It is highly lipophilic and is rapidly distributed to all tissues. It is infrequently used in infants and children with CHD, although it is the preferred opioid in some countries due to its apparent shorter elimination half-life when compared with fentanyl, particularly when high doses are used, either by repeated boluses or continuous infusions. This might be of clinical relevance if an early tracheal extubation is planned, as there is some evidence that extubation can be achieved earlier with the use of sufentanil rather than fentanyl.[349–351]

Remifentanil

Remifentanil is an ultra-short-acting opioid that is rapidly metabolized in the plasma and tissue by nonspecific esterases to an inactive metabolite. It has a very brief elimination half-life, with a context-sensitive half-life of only 3 minutes, independent of the duration of infusion (see Fig. 5.29). In pediatric cardiac surgery, it is an attractive alternative to fentanyl that provides intense analgesia during the most stimulating parts of surgery but facilitates rapid awakening and weaning from mechanical ventilation without residual opioid effect. Its pharmacodynamics are unaffected by CPB.[352] It provides stable hemodynamic conditions in children, although there is a tendency toward bradycardia and systemic hypotension.[353–355] It has no negative inotropic effect, even in the failing heart.[356]

The development of acute tolerance with increasing analgesic requirements after discontinuing remifentanil is debated.[357–359] One study suggested that this is not clinically important.[360] Strategies to prevent tolerance to remifentanil have included nitrous oxide as well as IV magnesium infusion.[361,362] Remifentanil is also used for prolonged sedation of children in the ICU. Many units have moved toward early extubation and discharge from the ICU after cardiac surgery (i.e., fast tracking), and remifentanil is a useful drug in this setting (see also Chapters 5 and 6). Consideration must be given to transitioning to a longer-acting opioid before discontinuation of remifentanil.

NEUROMUSCULAR BLOCKING DRUGS

Pancuronium has been studied in depth in children with CHD.[363] When administered over a 60- to 90-second interval, pancuronium maintains heart rate and blood pressure.[364,365] An intubating bolus dose of pancuronium may produce tachycardia and increase cardiac output. This bolus dose effect is sometimes desirable to support cardiac output in infants in congestive heart failure because their stroke volume is fixed. Pancuronium may be the neuromuscular blocking drug of choice when high-dose opioid techniques are used to offset the vagotonic effects of opioids such as fentanyl. Other neuromuscular blocking drugs are also widely used, particularly if patients are to be extubated in the operating room or early in the ICU.

LONG-TERM NEUROCOGNITIVE-DEVELOPMENTAL OUTCOMES ASSOCIATED WITH ANESTHESIA

Concerns have been raised about the possibility that many of the anesthetic agents such as inhalational anesthetics, propofol, ketamine, and midazolam may cause long-term neurocognitive-developmental problems in neonates and young infants.[366–369] This effect is thought to result from the neuronal apoptosis caused by these agents in newborn rodents and primates. Neither opioids nor dexmedetomidine have been implicated in these changes up until today.[370,371] There is no evidence to directly link anesthetic exposure in infancy to long-term neurocognitive defects.[372] There is much ongoing research in this area (see Chapter 23), including an interest in elucidating the potential contributive role of different anesthetic techniques in determining neurodevelopmental outcomes in children undergoing heart surgery.[373–375] In fact, many full-term children with CHD have been shown to have widespread brain abnormalities with small brain volumes similar to those of preterm infants before any surgery, CPB, or anesthesia.[376–378]

Regional Anesthesia and Analgesia

The use of regional anesthetic or analgesic techniques to provide pain relief during and after cardiac surgery in adults also reduces the stress response to surgery and may reduce morbidity and mortality. In adults undergoing cardiac surgery, the benefits of regional analgesia or anesthesia techniques, whether in isolation or combined with general anesthesia, include earlier extubation, fewer respiratory complications, a reduction in renal failure, fewer strokes, and less myocardial damage after CPB.[379–384] In animals, thoracic epidural anesthesia reduces myocardial damage after coronary occlusion.[385] Similar effects in improving blood flow, thus reducing coronary ischemia and myocardial damage, have been shown by the use of thoracic epidural anesthesia in adults undergoing coronary bypass graft surgery.[386,387] The same benefits may be achieved by using intrathecal (spinal) analgesia.[388] For example, high spinal anesthesia using bupivacaine reduces the stress response to CPB and β-adrenergic dysfunction and improves cardiac performance after cardiac surgery in adults.[389]

Research into regional anesthesia and analgesia in pediatric cardiac surgery is limited. Caudal morphine has been used to provide postoperative analgesia and has produced good analgesia for about 6 hours while reducing analgesic requirements for up to 24 hours.[390] Two retrospective studies in children[391,392] included a variety of neuraxial regional anesthetic techniques. Most children were extubated in the operating room, although approximately 4% required reintubation within 24 hours. Adverse effects included emesis (39%), pruritus (10%), urinary retention (7%), postoperative transient paresthesia (3%), and respiratory depression (1.8%). The rate of adverse effects was less with a thoracic epidural catheter approach compared with various caudal, lumbar epidural, and spinal approaches.[392] Hospital duration of stay was unaffected by the presence of regional anesthesia complications. The number of children enrolled in the study is too small to conclude that regional analgesia is safe for pediatric cardiac surgery.

The use of neuraxial regional anesthesia in children undergoing heart surgery remains controversial.[393,394] The main concern is the risk of bleeding and the potential for disastrous neurologic complications. The risks may be greater in children than in adults because of the presence of collateral vessels, increased venous pressure, coagulopathy related to cyanosis, and the use of aspirin or other antiplatelet agents and anticoagulants. There still remain many unanswered questions regarding neuraxial block in children, such as the true incidence of epidural hematoma, the time delay required between placement of the epidural catheter and full anticoagulation, and the correct management of a bloody tap, even though a considerable research effort has been made to address these issues.[391,395–397] The estimated risk of epidural hematoma during cardiac surgery in adults is 1 case per 1000 patients and 1 case per 2400 patients for spinal and epidural block, respectively.[398] Whether the risks are similar or greater in children cannot be determined because the numbers of children reported thus far are too small. A large, randomized, prospective study to evaluate a true risk/benefit ratio without bias is needed; until such data are available, various commentators have advised great caution with the use of regional analgesia for cardiac surgery, and some have suggested that it may not be possible to perform the study required because of ethical considerations.[393]

More recently, there has been an increasing interest in bilateral thoracic paravertebral blocks as a means of providing good-quality regional analgesia while possibly minimizing complications associated with neuraxial techniques. Although their use in thoracic surgery has been shown to result in equally effective pain control and a better adverse-effect profile compared with thoracic epidurals in both adults[399,400] and children,[401,402] their use in cardiac surgery remains controversial. Similar considerations about anticoagulation and neuraxial analgesia techniques in cardiac bypass procedures may apply to paravertebral blocks, although the risk of serious neurologic complications resulting from bleeding and subsequent hematoma formation is, at least theoretically, reduced by the use of non-neuraxial analgesia. These concerns have been addressed in the literature in adult cardiac surgery,[403,404] and although paravertebral blocks have been used for analgesia in children undergoing heart surgery and recommended by some authors, the evidence for their use in children is limited.[405–407] They are, however, routinely and widely used in some centers as a means of providing multimodal analgesia for congenital heart disease surgery, in particular in instances where early extubation of the trachea is planned. It is likely, though, that hesitations in their routine use by some clinicians will persist until concerns about safety are completely clarified by a methodologically sound, large, randomized, prospective study.

There has been a surge in interest in a novel analgesic block, first described in 2016, to provide analgesia for thoracic neuropathic pain. It is an interfascial block that consists of an ultrasound-guided injection of local anesthetic immediately superior to the transverse process at the level of intended analgesia, thereby separating the erector spinae muscle group from the transverse process by creating a local anesthetic pocket with caudad and cephalad spread.[408] Its use in children who are undergoing congenital heart surgery has been described, either as a single-shot or a continuous catheter infusion. Both its analgesic effects and safety track record appear promising, and there is a general perception that it should carry less risk of neurological complications than deeper blocks (such as paravertebral blocks) or neuraxial techniques, in patients who will be anticoagulated shortly after the performance of the block.[409,410] Due to its advantages and potential lack of serious adverse effects, it shows promise as a useful block when part of a multimodal analgesia plan in cardiac surgery; its opioid-sparing effects seem particularly interesting as contributing toward facilitating early tracheal extubation and promoting rapid recovery from surgery. Until more evidence about its safety becomes available, its routine use cannot yet be recommended for children undergoing heart surgery.

Fast Track and Enhanced Recovery After Surgery

Although often used interchangeably, the terms "fast track" and "enhanced recovery after surgery" (ERAS) do not mean exactly the same. Fast track was the term originally used in the early 1990s to describe the approach developed by Kehlet, whose initial goal was to promote earlier discharge from hospital after surgery through a comprehensive program to improve perioperative care. This consists of a multimodal package of techniques that aim to reduce physiologic stress, decrease postsurgical organ dysfunction and complications, and to improve postoperative recovery, thereby abbreviating the perioperative period of children undergoing cardiac surgery.[411–413] The original concept of fast track has evolved into what are currently referred to as ERAS programs, which share many of the early principles with fast track. The term ERAS puts more emphasis into a holistic approach to recovery, with a broader focus on outcomes that are important for the patients and their families, which include expediting return to health and functional status.[414] Enhanced recovery protocols are the implementation strategies used to institute an ERAS guideline. The goal of enhanced recovery protocols is to ensure that an evidence-based and standardized approach is applied to all patients undergoing surgery. Enhanced recovery protocols involve all multidisciplinary team members and engage patients and their families in their care.[414] Although initially fast track programs were designed for colorectal surgery, their application to other areas of surgical care has rapidly expanded. The implementation of enhanced recovery protocols in cardiac surgery has been shown to result in improved outcomes and lower health care costs.[415–418] Enhanced recovery programs for children undergoing heart surgery should include every phase of the child's journey from referral and preoperative evaluation and optimization, to less invasive surgery, early weaning from respiratory support, extubation, and discharge from the ICU and hospital. In this context, the term "fast tracking" is generally used to designate extubation shortly after arrival to the intensive care unit, most commonly in the first 6 hours, whereas the term "ultra-fast" tracking usually refers to extubation of the trachea in the operating room immediately after surgery.[419]

Early extubation of pediatric patients after cardiac surgery offers advantages in terms of cost and reduced morbidity associated with longer ICU stays.[405–407,420–424] The success of this approach depends on the close teamwork of a multidisciplinary team, with every member of the team working toward the same goal. Successful fast tracking usually requires the development of care pathways to ensure that the quality of patient care is not compromised.[425] Early extubation and discharge from the ICU requires preplanning and the adoption of a technique that facilitates this goal. The use of very large doses of fentanyl is not appropriate; alternative techniques have been used, including smaller doses of fentanyl in combination with inhalational agents[426,427] or the use of remifentanil or, more recently, dexmedetomidine in combination with inhalational agents or with propofol. Others have advocated regional anesthesia as a means of speeding extubation, but this approach remains controversial. It is important to choose a neuromuscular blocking drug with a duration of action that matches

surgical time to ensure that it is easy to reverse the neuromuscular block at the end of surgery. Other important considerations to ensure that early extubation is a success include adequate pain relief, patient-controlled or nurse-controlled analgesia, and antiemetics because nausea appears to be more of a problem in children who are extubated early.

Some clinicians advocate extubating the trachea in the operating room, whereas others advocate waiting until the child is in the ICU. Delaying the extubation until the child is in the ICU may save operating room time and may reduce the risks of cardiovascular instability, bleeding, and hypothermia.[428] Despite these concerns, the tracheas of many children are extubated in the operating room with good outcomes. Although currently available evidence does not allow for a definitive evidence-based recommendation about early extubation in children undergoing heart surgery, data available at the present date attest its role in improving outcomes and reducing hospital length of stay. It is safe to conclude that enhanced recovery after surgery programs, possibly including tracheal extubation in the operating room, have now demonstrated their efficacy, safety, and feasibility in low- to medium-risk pediatric congenital cardiac surgery patients.[429–432] The fact that ERAS programs have shown to be feasible, safe, and effective at promoting early recovery, reducing costs and possibly improving outcomes as well as patient and family satisfaction has led the American Association for Thoracic Surgery (AATS), through the Congenital Cardiac Surgery Working Group, to publish a consensus document on a comprehensive perioperative approach to enhanced recovery after pediatric cardiac surgery.[433]

Stress Response to Cardiac Surgery

Cardiac surgery and CPB are altered physiologic conditions associated with an amplified stress response characterized by the release of numerous hormonal and metabolic substances. This constitutes part of the systemic reaction to injury, which consists of a broad variety of hematologic, immunologic, and neuroendocrine effects. Substances released as part of the stress response include catecholamines, cortisol, growth hormone, glucagon, glucose, insulin, prostaglandins, complement, β-endorphins,[339,340,434,435] as well as oxidative stress mediators[436–438] and many others.[439–441] The cause of the elaboration of these substances is likely to be multifactorial: contact of blood with foreign surfaces, nonpulsatile flow, low perfusion pressure, anemia, hypothermia, myocardial ischemia, and possibly deep anesthesia. Other factors that contribute to the increase in stress hormones are delayed renal and hepatic clearance and exclusion of the pulmonary circulation during extracorporeal circulation.[442]

Neonates of all gestational ages, older infants, and children have nociceptive systems that are sufficiently developed and integrated with brainstem cardiovascular control centers to trigger humoral and circulatory responses to pain and stress.[443–446] Substantial humoral, metabolic, and cardiovascular responses to painful and stressful stimulation during surgery have been documented in neonates of all gestational ages and in older infants.[447,448] Hormonal stress responses in neonates subjected to cardiac and noncardiac operations are 3- to 5-fold greater than those in adults after similar surgeries. Circulatory responses to stressful stimuli in children include systemic and pulmonary hypertension.

Humoral stress responses are particularly extreme during and after cardiac surgery. These responses are characterized by increases in a number of circulating regulatory substances, including catecholamines, cortisol, insulin, glucagon, growth hormone, and β-endorphins; circulating concentrations of catecholamines may increase by as much as 400% over baseline preoperative concentrations. This is evidence of a massive activation of sympathetic outflow in response to surgical stimulation. Some of these responses may continue for several days postoperatively.[449]

It has been suggested that such extreme stress responses and neuroendocrine activation may be associated with greater morbidity and mortality. In adults, intraoperative adrenergic levels 50% above baseline are associated with postoperative alterations in β-adrenergic receptor function, including increased β-receptor density and decreased receptor affinity. Mortality among adults with severe congestive failure is associated with increased levels of hormones regulating cardiovascular function, including aldosterone, epinephrine, and norepinephrine.[450] In neonates undergoing cardiac surgery, increased concentrations of stress hormones may be associated with increased mortality rates.[449]

The metabolic response to stress in children includes increased oxygen consumption, glycogenolysis, gluconeogenesis, and lipolysis, which cause substantial intraoperative and postoperative catabolism. The metabolic response is usually related to changes in plasma cortisol, catecholamines, and other counter regulatory hormones such as glucagon and growth hormone. The most prominent clinical effects that result from activation of these processes are perioperative hypoglycemia and hyperglycemia, lactic acidemia, and negative nitrogen balance extending well into the postoperative period. Neonates and infants tolerate such metabolic derangements poorly. Their impaired tolerance is the result of a relative lack of endogenous reserves of carbohydrates, fat, and proteins; the large metabolic cost of rapid growth; a high obligate requirement for glucose by the relatively large brain; the immature hormonal control of intermediary metabolism; and the limited functional capabilities of immature enzyme systems in the metabolic organs. Severe stress responses superimposed on the normal neonatal and infant physiology may be poorly tolerated. However, it remains unclear whether these metabolic alterations may provide some beneficial effects by mobilizing the bodily resources to provide a metabolic milieu for healing tissues or they are purely maladaptive, resulting in detrimental effects on postoperative outcome.

Another factor is the potential effect of stress-induced hyperglycemia on the neurologic outcome. Neonates and young infants are capable of substantial rates of glucose production, mainly from glycogenolysis and gluconeogenesis during surgical stress that can result in hyperglycemia. Such hyperglycemic responses may be associated with poorer neurologic outcomes, particularly after a period of cerebral ischemia.[451] The use of high doses of fentanyl (>50 μg/kg) has reduced the hormonal stress response and resultant hyperglycemia and may lessen the risk of neurologic injury.[452]

In sufficient doses, opioids can blunt the stress responses in neonates, infants, and adults.[442,453,454] This blunting results in a more normal, homeostatic humoral and metabolic milieu in the circulation by reducing neuroendocrine activation and levels of regulatory hormones. In infants, the use of high-dose opioids for major surgical procedures and postoperative sedation substantially attenuates the neuroendocrine response to surgically induced pain and stress. Catecholamine release from intraoperative stress responses may predispose the vulnerable myocardium to dysrhythmias. In neonates with HLHS, sudden ventricular fibrillation occurred in 50% during surgical manipulation under halothane anesthesia. This incidence was dramatically reduced when high doses of fentanyl were introduced as the primary analgesic/sedative.[455] With the use of high-dose opioids, intraoperative ventricular fibrillation has virtually disappeared as a problem in this group of neonates.[456] Opioids increase the ventricular fibrillation threshold in isolated cardiac Purkinje fibers and alter action potential duration similar to that with class III antiarrhythmic agents.[457] Even electrophysiologic events in the neonatal heart, in addition to humoral and hemodynamic responses, may be altered by using high-dose fentanyl anesthesia to attenuate the effects of pain and stress.

There has been a growing interest in the use of dexmedetomidine, a new generation highly selective alpha2-adrenergic receptor (α2-AR) agonist to blunt the stress response to cardiac surgery and CPB in adults, children, and infants. In fact, its effects on perioperative outcomes such as postoperative complications and mortality[458] are likely related to the decrease in levels of mediators of the systemic response to injury, which has been the object of a considerable number of studies.[459] Dexmedetomidine has demonstrated its efficacy and safety at maintaining hemodynamic stability in pediatric cardiac surgery.[460] Due to its ability to blunt the stress response by inducing a favorable mix of beneficial physiologic actions and a limited adverse-effect profile, it appears very promising as an anesthetic adjuvant agent for pediatric cardiac surgery, with an established role in the perioperative pediatric cardiac setting, despite the fact that evidence for its potential cardioprotective, neuroprotective, and renoprotective effects is still limited.[461] The other alpha2-adrenergic receptor agonist, clonidine, remains popular and there are no comparative studies between the two drugs.[462]

REDUCING THE STRESS RESPONSE TO SURGERY AND BYPASS

Corticosteroids

Corticosteroids are used in many centers in an attempt to reduce the inflammatory response to surgery and bypass and improve outcomes after cardiac surgery.[463] There is huge variability in the formulation of the corticosteroids used, the doses administered, the timing of administration, and the indications for their use. Although several small studies in humans and animals suggest that prophylactic corticosteroids in cardiac surgery may confer a benefit,[464,465] their routine use in children undergoing heart surgery is not supported by currently existing evidence.[466,467] Many investigators have called for a large multicenter study to determine the benefit of corticosteroids before bypass and the optimal dose and timing.[468]

Aprotinin

Aprotinin, which was originally used to reduce bleeding after CPB, is now also appreciated to confer antiinflammatory effects.[469–473] In adults, it has been shown to reduce mortality and length of ICU stay,[474] even though these effects were not replicated by later studies. In children, it improves pulmonary function in the postoperative period and reduces the time to extubation and ICU stay.[140] However, aprotinin is no longer available for routine use in the United States or continental Europe, because some grave concerns have been raised about its use increasing complications and mortality rates in adult cardiac surgery. In the United Kingdom, it is available for use on a named patient basis, but its use has been dramatically reduced as a result.

Allopurinol

Allopurinol is thought to provide protection against oxygen free radicals during reperfusion by inhibiting xanthine oxidase. It reduces oxygen free radical production and may reduce neurologic and cardiac damage after deep hypothermic circulatory arrest.[475] Analogously, it has been used in trials to prevent mortality and morbidity in neonates with hypoxic-ischemic encephalopathy.[476] This strategy does not appear to have developed widespread use, probably because of insufficient evidence that it has clinically important benefits, and uncertainties about its effects on mortality and long-term neurodevelopmental outcomes.

Ischemic Preconditioning

The heart is capable of short-term rapid adaptation to brief ischemia such that during a subsequent, more severe ischemic insult, myocardial necrosis is delayed. Numerous animal studies have been conducted to further characterize this property of the myocardium, which could have very important clinical applications. The infarct-delaying properties of ischemic preconditioning have been observed in all species studied. An ischemic period of 5 minutes is sufficient to initiate preconditioning, and the protective period lasts for 1 to 2 hours. Laboratory experiments have demonstrated that the stimulation of adenosine receptors initiates preconditioning and the intracellular signal transduction mechanisms involve protein kinase C and adenosine triphosphate (ATP)-dependent potassium channels, although there may be some differences between species. An analysis of studies of myocardial infarction in humans has demonstrated that some adults who report having had angina in the days before infarction have a better outcome after their infarction in part owing to the ischemic preconditioning. More direct evidence has come from an investigation of adults undergoing percutaneous transluminal angioplasty in whom the ST-segment changes induced by balloon inflation were more marked during the first inflation than the second. In adults undergoing coronary artery bypass grafting, the decline in ATP content during the first 10 minutes of ischemia was reduced in those subjected to a brief preconditioning protocol.[477–481]

It may be possible to protect organs other than the heart by ischemic preconditioning. It may even be possible to protect organs remotely by producing a period of ischemia in one area such as a limb, which then confers protection to remote organs.[482] One study demonstrated that the use of a blood pressure cuff to produce short periods of limb ischemia can produce beneficial effects on the heart, lungs, and generalized inflammatory response.[483] The effects of remote ischemic preconditioning on children undergoing heart surgery have been inconsistent, likely reflecting heterogeneity between different studies developed to evaluate its ischemia-delaying properties.[484]

A wide variety of anesthetic agents and anesthesia adjuvants have also been found to offer protection against ischemia to the heart and other organs, particularly the brain and kidney, by ischemic preconditioning mechanisms. Inhalational anesthetics, but also midazolam and propofol, among others, protect against myocardial injury in pediatric cardiac surgery. Other studies have shown definite cardioprotective effects from inhalational agents in children, although these do not seem to be universally applicable to all children undergoing heart surgery. Further research is needed to clarify their protective role for different patient populations, to different organs and systems, as well as recommended doses and timing of administration.

Glucose-Insulin and Potassium

The use of glucose-insulin and potassium has been advocated for more than 40 years in adult cardiac surgery. It is thought to

protect the myocardium from the effects of ischemia caused by aortic cross-clamping.[485–488] Its effects have not been studied in children undergoing cardiac surgery.

Anesthesia Considerations for Specific Cardiac Defects

Discussion of anesthesia considerations for repair of every form of CHD is beyond the scope of this chapter. However, a brief discussion of the problems that may be encountered during repair of the more common congenital heart lesions is presented. It is useful to group lesions together because the management principles can be applied more generally within groups (Table 15.2). Moreover, the general physiological and pharmacological considerations regarding the anesthetic management of obstructive and regurgitant valvular lesions in adults undergoing heart surgery also apply to children undergoing heart surgery for the repair of similar lesions. A useful review of the general principles pertaining to the management of children with congenital heart disease (and some forms of acquired cardiac disease in children), as well as the recommended approach and hemodynamic goals for different groups of lesions, is available elsewhere.[489]

SIMPLE LEFT-TO-RIGHT SHUNTS

Simple left-to-right shunts increase pulmonary blood flow. If the shunt is large, blood flow to the lungs can be as much as 3- to 4-fold greater than normal, resulting in volume loading of the right heart. This can lead to right atrial and right ventricular enlargement that is potentially associated with tricuspid and pulmonary valve regurgitation. The combination of these pathophysiologic consequences of large left-to-right shunts results in cardiac failure (Table 15.3).

Medical management is primarily achieved with diuretics. If pulmonary blood flow is large and left untreated, pulmonary

TABLE 15.2	Classification of Congenital Heart Disease

Simple Left-to-Right Shunt: Increased Pulmonary Blood Flow
Atrial septal defect (ASD)
Ventricular septal defect (VSD)
Patent ductus arteriosus (PDA)
Endocardial cushion defect (e.g., atrioventricular septal defect [AVSD])
Aortopulmonary window (AP window)

Simple Right-to-Left Shunt: Decreased Pulmonary Blood Flow With Cyanosis
Tetralogy of Fallot (TOF)
Pulmonary atresia
Tricuspid atresia
Ebstein anomaly

Complex Shunts: Mixing of Pulmonary and Systemic Blood Flow With Cyanosis
Transposition of the great arteries (TGA)
Truncus arteriosus
Total anomalous pulmonary venous connection (TAPVC)
Double-outlet right ventricle (DORV)
Hypoplastic left heart syndrome (HLHS)

Obstructive Lesions
Aortic Stenosis
Mitral Stenosis
Pulmonary Stenosis
Coarctation of Aorta
Interrupted Aortic Arch

TABLE 15.3 Clinical Features of Cardiac Failure in Children

Failure to thrive	Cardiac murmur
Difficult feeding	Hepatomegaly
Breathlessness	Cardiomegaly
Recurrent chest infection	Pulmonary plethora
Tachycardia	Wheezing

vascular disease begins to develop, resulting in pulmonary hypertension.[490–495] In the early stages, the changes are reversible, but in time, the changes may become irreversible. Eisenmenger syndrome refers to severe pulmonary hypertension that leads to suprasystemic pulmonary artery pressures that cause the shunt to reverse, leading to cyanosis. The previous left-to-right shunt reverses to become a right-to-left shunt. At this point, the child's condition becomes inoperable.

Increasingly, definitive surgery is being performed at a younger age to reduce the risk of developing pulmonary vascular disease. If early definitive surgery is not possible, a pulmonary artery band may be applied through a sternotomy incision, to reduce pulmonary blood flow. This provides the infant the opportunity to grow, postponing the need for definitive surgery without increasing the risk of developing pulmonary hypertension. In the presence of substantively increased pulmonary blood flow, pulmonary vascular disease is often severe and irreversible by 1 year of age. Definitive surgery should be performed between 3 and 6 months of age to avoid this complication.

Atrial Septal Defect

ASD is a common heart defect in children, occurring in 1 of 1500 live births and accounting for approximately 10% of all CHD.[2,4] Several types of ASDs exist.

- Patent foramen ovale (PFO) is a normal fetal communication between the two atria that usually closes soon after birth. The PFO remains patent in up to 30% of people. PFO is usually left untreated in children.
- Primum ASD (Fig. 15.1A) is located in the inferior part of the atrial septum close to the AV valve and may be associated with a cleft mitral valve. This is a variant of AV septal defect (AVSD).
- Secundum ASD (see Fig. 15.1B) is found in the region of the fossa ovalis and results from a deficiency in the septum secundum.
- Sinus venosus ASD (see Fig. 15.1C) can be of the superior or inferior sinus venosus types, close to the opening of the SVC or inferior vena cava (IVC), respectively. It may be associated with anomalous pulmonary venous drainage.
- Coronary sinus ASD (i.e., unroofed coronary sinus) is a defect in the atrial wall that allows blood to flow from the left atrium to right atrium through the coronary sinus.
- Common atrium has a complete absence of the atrial septum. The AV valves may be abnormal or unaffected.

Many ASDs can be closed using a percutaneous, transcatheter device. PFO and secundum ASDs are most commonly closed using this technique.

Anesthesia Considerations

- These children can frequently be extubated on the operating table or early in the ICU, and smaller doses of opioids can be used. Alternatively, short-acting drugs (e.g., remifentanil

or dexmedetomidine) administered by infusion and possibly in combination with propofol are useful if early extubation is planned.
- The problems of postoperative pulmonary hypertension are seldom encountered.

Ventricular Septal Defect

VSD is the most common congenital defect in children, occurring in 1.5 to 3.5 of 1000 live births and accounting for more than 20% of CHD (Fig. 15.2A).[496,497] Four types are described: subarterial (5%), perimembranous (80%), inlet (5%), and muscular (10%). If the flow through the VSD is small, it is referred to as *restrictive*, but if the flow is large, it is called *unrestrictive*. A significant proportion of VSDs close spontaneously during the first few years of life. It is possible to close a small percent of VSDs in children using percutaneous, transcatheter devices.

Anesthesia Considerations

- Children who are asymptomatic preoperatively and undergo a predictably uncomplicated VSD surgical closure should be considered for fast tracking, and anesthetic management should aim to facilitate early extubation.
- Inotropic support may be required postoperatively for children in cardiac failure.
- Postoperative pulmonary hypertension may be a problem if the left-to-right shunt has been significant preoperatively or if the surgery is undertaken late.

Atrioventricular Septal Defect

AVSDs are also known as AV canal defects or endocardial cushion defects. They arise from a defect in the AV septum, with inadequate fusion of the superior and inferior endocardial cushions with the atrial septum and muscular ventricular septum, respectively. Their incidence is approximately 0.2 cases per 1000 live births, and they account for about 3% of CHD. They are commonly associated with trisomy 21, TOF, and DiGeorge syndrome (Table 15.4). It is worth noting that with a common AV valve annulus, the two separate valve orifices are referred to as the left and right AV valves, not the mitral and tricuspid valves. Three types of AVSD exist:

- Incomplete or partial AVSD usually consists of a primum ASD with a cleft in the anterior mitral valve leaflet; two separate AV valves are present and there is no VSD (see Fig. 15.1A).
- Complete AVSD consists of a large septal defect with atrial and ventricular components and a large common AV valve (see Fig. 15.2A).
- With transitional AVSD an ASD is present, and the left and right AV valves may be only partially separated; the VSD may be small or moderate in size (see Fig. 15.2B).

Other descriptions of AVSD refer to balanced or unbalanced conditions, depending on the relative contributions of the two sides of the heart to the circulation. This in turn may depend on relative sizes of the two sides of the heart, but also on whether the AV valve is stenotic or atretic or if there is significant AV valve overriding (i.e., one AV valve emptying into two ventricles) or some of the valve chordae or papillary muscles are straddling (i.e., crossing to the other side of the ventricular septum). The hemodynamic effects associated with AVSD vary according to the type of defect and AV valve morphology and include shunting at the atrial or ventricular level and AV valve stenosis and/or regurgitation.

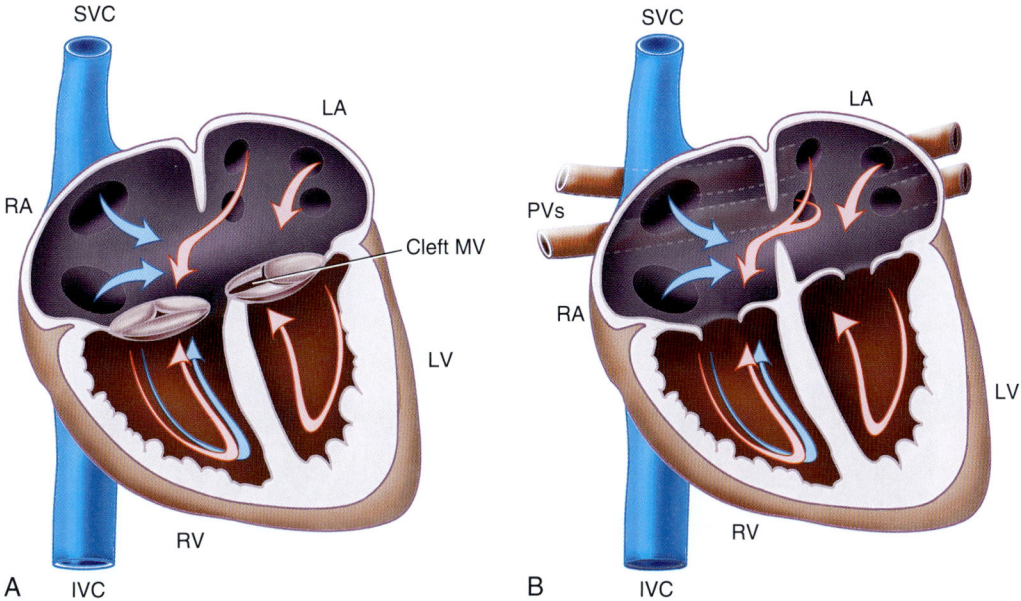

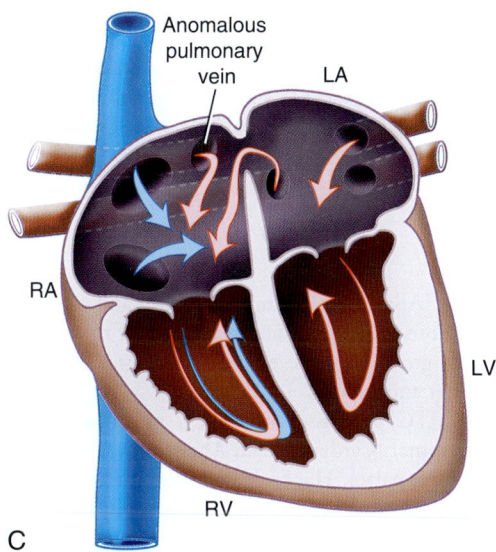

FIGURE 15.1 A, Diagram of a primum atrial septal defect (ASD) with the great vessels removed to show the left-to-right shunt through the defect and a cleft of the mitral valve *(MV)*, also called a partial atrioventricular septal defect. **B,** Diagram of a secundum ASD with the great vessels removed to show the left-to-right shunt through the defect. **C,** Diagram of a sinus venosus ASD shows the left-to-right shunt through the defect close to the superior vena cava *(SVC)* and an anomalous pulmonary vein *(PV)* draining to the right atrium *(RA)*. *IVC,* Inferior vena cava; *LA,* left atrium; *LV,* left ventricle; *RV,* right ventricle. (Modified from May LE. *Pediatric Heart Surgery: A Ready Reference for Professionals.* Milwaukee, WI: Maxishare; 2005.)

Anesthesia Considerations
- If the child has trisomy 21 or DiGeorge syndrome, the anesthesia implications of the associated comorbidities need to be managed.
- Inotropes are frequently required.
- Postoperative pulmonary hypertension may occur.
- There is often postoperative stenosis and/or regurgitation of one or both AV valves, with potential implications for hemodynamics and anesthesia management.
- TEE is particularly helpful in assessing the repair of the left AV valve.
- Heart block and dysrhythmias may occur postoperatively.

Aortopulmonary Window
Aortopulmonary window is a rare CHD defect in which there is a communication between the main pulmonary artery and the ascending aorta, and it accounts for 0.1% of CHD (Fig. 15.3). Four types are classified according to the size and exact position of the defect.[498] A left-to-right shunt is usually present. These children present with heart failure and are at risk for pulmonary vascular disease if not treated early. Aortopulmonary window is frequently associated with other cardiac and noncardiac anomalies:
- VACTERL: **V**ertebral anomalies, **A**nal atresia, **C**ardiac defect, **T**racheo**E**sophageal atresia or fistula, **R**enal anomalies, and **L**imb abnormalities

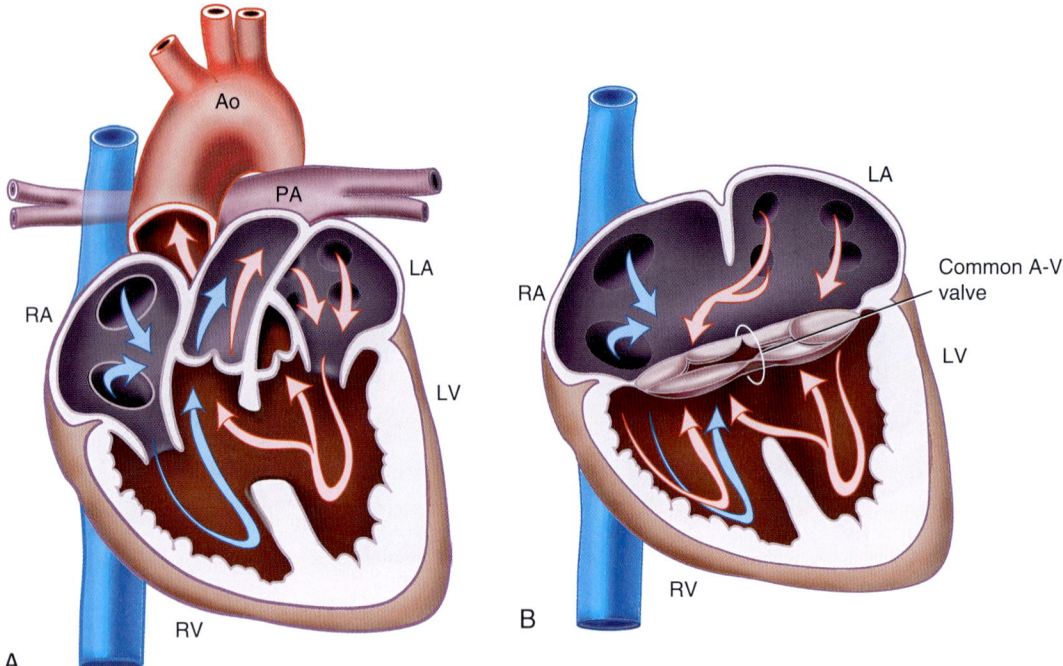

FIGURE 15.2 A, Diagram of a ventricular septal defect shows a left-to-right shunt. **B,** Diagram of a complete atrio-ventricular septal defect with the great vessels removed to show the left-to-right shunt through both atrial and ventricular components of the defect and a single common atrioventricular *(A-V)* valve. *Ao,* Aorta; *LA,* left atrium; *LV,* left ventricle; *PA,* pulmonary artery; *RA,* right atrium; *RV,* right ventricle. (Modified from May LE. *Pediatric Heart Surgery: A Ready Reference for Professionals.* Milwaukee, WI: Maxishare; 2005.)

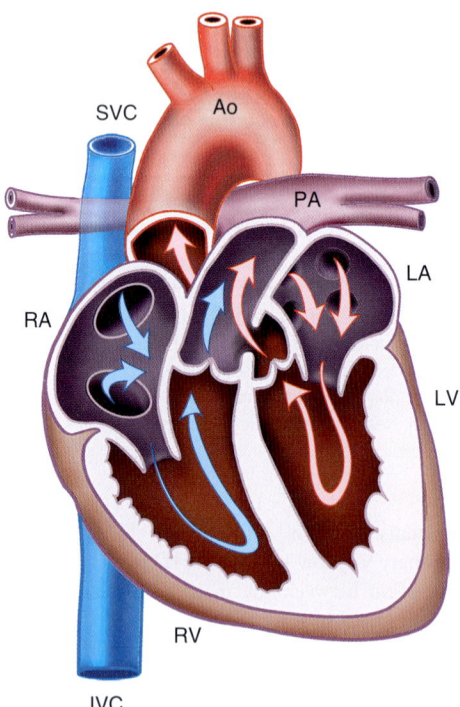

FIGURE 15.3 Diagram of an aortopulmonary window shows a left-to-right shunt through the defect. *Ao,* Aorta; *IVC,* inferior vena cava; *LA,* left atrium; *LV,* left ventricle; *PA,* pulmonary artery; *RA,* right atrium; *RV,* right ventricle; *SVC,* superior vena cava. (Modified from May LE. *Pediatric Heart Surgery: A Ready Reference for Professionals.* Milwaukee, WI: Maxishare; 2005.)

- CHARGE: **C**oloboma of the eye and central nervous system anomalies, **H**eart defects, **A**tresia of the choanae, **R**etardation of growth and development, **G**enital or urinary defects, and **E**ar anomalies
- CATCH-22 association (i.e., mnemonic for DiGeorge syndrome): **C**ardiac defect, **A**bnormal facies, **T**hymic hypoplasia, **C**left palate, **H**ypocalcemia (velocardiofacial syndrome), with 22q11 chromosome microdeletion (see Table 15.4)

Anesthesia Considerations
- Inotropes may be required.
- Postoperative pulmonary hypertension may be problematic.

Patent Ductus Arteriosus
The ductus arteriosus, a remnant from the fetal circulation, most frequently extends from the undersurface of the descending aorta, distal to the origin of the left subclavian artery, to the main pulmonary artery and usually closes soon after birth (see Fig. 16.1).

TABLE 15.4	Clinical Features and Concerns of DiGeorge Syndrome
Absent or small thymus	
T-cell abnormality with associated immunodeficiency	
Hypoparathyroidism with associated hypocalcemia	
Dysmorphic features, particularly a small mouth	
Increased surgical morbidity and mortality	
Irradiated blood products needed to prevent graft-versus-host disease	

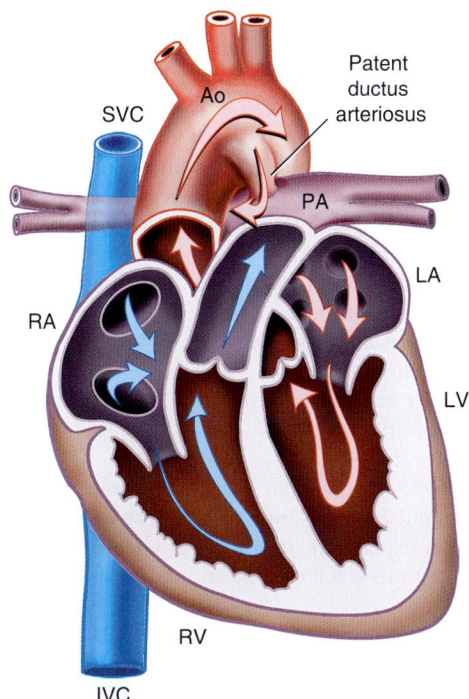

FIGURE 15.4 The diagram of a patent ductus arteriosus shows a left-to-right shunt. *Ao,* Aorta, *IVC,* inferior vena cava; *LA,* left atrium; *LV,* left ventricle; *PA,* pulmonary artery; *RA,* right atrium; *RV,* right ventricle; *SVC,* superior vena cava. (Modified from May LE. *Pediatric Heart Surgery: A Ready Reference for Professionals.* Milwaukee, WI: Maxishare; 2005.)

However, it remains patent in approximately 1 of 2500 live births and accounts for about 10% of all CHD (Fig. 15.4). In the fetus, blood from the right ventricle is directed into the pulmonary artery, but because of the high PVR, it flows into the descending aorta through the ductus arteriosus. After birth, the PVR decreases, and blood flows from the aorta to the lungs. PDA is common in preterm infants, in whom it is associated with respiratory distress syndrome (RDS), intraventricular hemorrhage (IVH) and necrotizing enterocolitis (NEC); its presence may explain an ongoing requirement for mechanical ventilation. In these infants, should medical treatment fail to close the PDA, surgery is required to ligate or divide it, most often via a left thoracotomy approach, even though minimally invasive approaches are possible. The presence of a PDA may also only be detected in older children; but at this age, where size no longer constitutes a limitation for the use of endovascular devices, percutaneous closure by an interventional cardiologist is the preferred approach. The anesthesia implications are similar to those of other lesions described with left-to-right shunts preoperatively.

In many centers, the PDA closure in preterm infants who weigh less than 1000 grams and who are already mechanically ventilated is performed in the neonatal intensive care unit. This avoids the need to transfer these very small infants to the operating room and the associated problems, particularly hypothermia.

Preoperative requirements include:

- Crossmatched blood
- Antibiotics (risk of endocarditis)
- Vitamin K
  Particular perioperative risks include:
- Difficulty ventilating or oxygen desaturation because of lung retraction

- Inadvertent ligation of the aorta or pulmonary artery
- Tearing the PDA with massive hemorrhage
- Endocarditis
- Paradoxical air embolism

Monitoring

Monitoring includes the use of all standard monitors, including end-tidal carbon dioxide assessment, and two pulse oximeters, one on the right hand and one on a lower limb, thus monitoring preductal and postductal saturations. If the pulse is lost from the lower limb during a test clamping of the duct, it may indicate that the aorta has been clamped inadvertently. In many institutions, all the operative requirements are stipulated in a protocol and monitoring and other requirements are in place before the arrival of the operating room team.

Invasive blood pressure monitoring is helpful if already established but is not usually placed if not already established. Monitors used in non–operating room sites may not be compatible with the electrocautery equipment, resulting in loss of monitoring whenever the cautery is used.

Anesthesia Considerations

- A dedicated IV line for fluids and drugs with a long (100 to 150 cm), low-caliber extension to allow access from a distance (space around the cots in NICU is limited)
- High-dose opioids
- Neuromuscular blockade
- The uncuffed tracheal tube should have only a small air leak. A large leak may prevent adequate ventilation during lung retraction (recheck tube size and position before the start of the procedure, as well as security and correct position of the tip of the tube after repositioning in the decubitus position, before starting surgery)
- Intercostal nerve block can be placed by surgeon at the completion of surgery or a paravertebral or an erector spinae plane block may be used, depending on the child's age and weight
- Glucose-containing fluids maintained at basal rates

SIMPLE RIGHT-TO-LEFT SHUNTS

Tetralogy of Fallot

Tetralogy of Fallot (TOF) is the most common cyanotic CHD defect accounting for 6% to 11% of all CHD. Its hallmark is the anterocephalad deviation of the outlet septum, resulting in four features (Fig. 15.5):

- VSD
- Overriding aorta
- Right ventricular outflow tract obstruction (RVOTO)
- Right ventricular hypertrophy

The RVOTO ranges from mild to severe, and the level of the obstruction also varies. Subvalvular, valvular, or supravalvular obstruction can occur in any combination, which will determine whether the obstruction is exclusively or mostly fixed and/or dynamic. Commonly, a dynamic subpulmonary infundibular obstruction is present. Dynamic narrowing of the infundibulum is frequently the cause of hypercyanotic episodes, also known as "*tet spells,*" in which there is an increase in the shunting of blood from right-to-left. However, the RVOTO may also be at the level of the pulmonary valve or main or branch pulmonary arteries (PAs). There are four main variants of TOF:

- TOF with pulmonary stenosis—the stenosis may be subvalvular, valvular, supravalvular, or any combination of the three; this represents the most common subtype of TOF.

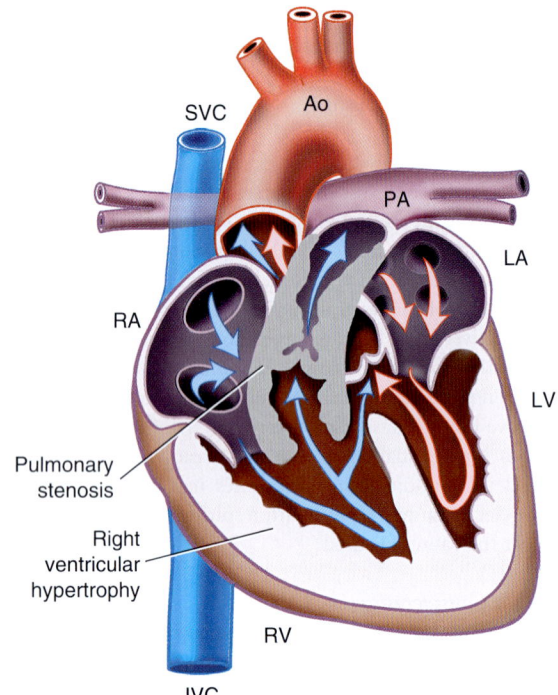

FIGURE 15.5 The diagram shows the features of the tetralogy of Fallot: ventricular septal defect, overriding aorta, right ventricular hypertrophy, and pulmonary stenosis. Pulmonary and subpulmonary obstructions are shown *(gray area).* The result is right-to-left shunting leading to cyanosis. *Ao,* Aorta; *IVC,* inferior vena cava; *LA,* left atrium; *LV,* left ventricle; *PA,* pulmonary artery; *RA,* right atrium; *RV,* right ventricle; *SVC,* superior vena cava. (Modified from May LE. *Pediatric Heart Surgery: A Ready Reference for Professionals.* Milwaukee, WI: Maxishare; 2005.)

- TOF with pulmonary atresia—severe variant, with no antegrade flow from the right ventricle into the pulmonary artery; it is commonly associated with hypoplastic pulmonary arteries with major aortopulmonary collateral arteries (MAPCAs); if the pulmonary arteries are well developed, pulmonary blood flow is usually derived from a PDA.
- TOF with absent pulmonary valve—the pulmonary valve is dysplastic and incompetent, resulting in dilatation of the pulmonary arteries, potentially causing bronchial compression and, if severe enough, breathing difficulties.
- TOF with AVSD—the rarest form of TOF, in which ASD and TOF coexist, making complete surgical repair particularly challenging.

The right-to-left shunt and cyanosis observed in children with TOF results from a combination of the RVOTO and VSD. The degree of hypoxemia depends on the relationship between the RVOTO and the SVR that determines the degree of right-to-left shunting across the ventricular septal defect. TOF may be associated with a large number of other cardiac and extracardiac anomalies. Extracardiac anomalies most commonly include DiGeorge syndrome (see Table 15.4) and trisomy 21.

Hypercyanotic Episodes

Hypercyanotic spells are episodes of cyanosis that occur in most untreated children. They result in increased right-to-left shunting, with the resulting increase in oxygen desaturation, most commonly after a precipitating event. They may be initiated by crying, exercise, feeding or straining, and may even occur during anesthesia. The cause and exact pathophysiology of these spells is unclear, but metabolic acidosis, increased $PaCO_2$, circulating catecholamines, and surgical stimulation have all been implicated, with infundibular spasm and an increase in right ventricular outflow tract obstruction being the most likely culprit.

Management of a tet spell requires urgent intervention. Simple measures (e.g., Valsalva maneuver or legs-to-knee chest position to increase SVR, morphine to reduce infundibular spasm) may be effective. Early and aggressive use of a vasoconstrictor is essential (e.g., metaraminol or phenylephrine). Management may require any of several interventions:

- 100% oxygen and hyperventilation
- IV fluid bolus
- Sedation or analgesia (e.g., fentanyl, morphine) and paralysis
- Sodium bicarbonate
- Vasoconstriction
    - Phenylephrine is given as a 1-μg/kg bolus and doubled at 1-minute intervals until a satisfactory response is achieved (doses required in small preterm infants may be up to 30 μg/kg); this is followed by an infusion at 1 to 5 μg/kg per minute
    - Norepinephrine is given at a rate of 0.01 to 0.2 μg/kg per minute, if central venous access is available
- β-Blockers are administered to relax infundibular spasm and reduce the heart rate
    - Propranolol 15 to 20 μg/kg is given as a slow intravenous injection (max 100 μg/kg), and repeated depending on clinical effect
    - Esmolol is given as a 500-μg/kg loading dose administered over 1 minute, followed by a continuous infusion at a rate of 50 to 250 μg/kg per minute

Surgical Management

The optimal surgical management of children with TOF remains controversial. The choice is between initial palliation with a systemic-to-pulmonary shunt followed by a complete repair when the infant is older and complete repair during the neonatal or early infant period. The current trend is toward early complete repair.[499,500] Complete repair involves closure of the VSD and relief of the RVOTO. Relief of the RVOTO may require a transannular patch (i.e., a patch extending from the right ventricular outflow tract across the pulmonary valve annulus into the supravalvular area), which involves a right ventriculotomy. If this is the case, pulmonary regurgitation is inevitable. Right ventricular dysfunction is a particular problem after repair, and it usually manifests as RV restrictive physiology in the immediate postoperative period; compliance of the RV is greatly reduced, resulting in severe diastolic dysfunction. The echocardiographic hallmark of restrictive RV physiology is antegrade flow in the pulmonary artery in diastole, reflecting the fact that the RV has lost its ability to relax enough to accommodate a volume load during diastole and has started to act like a passive conduit for blood during this phase of the cardiac cycle, due to very poor compliance and severe diastolic dysfunction. Long-term follow-up of patients with TOF repair has revealed the consequences of pulmonary regurgitation after a transannular patch technique to be more serious than previously anticipated. In fact, late RV dilatation and dysfunction with reduced tolerance to exercise, hemodynamic compromise, dysrhythmias, and an increased risk of sudden death have led surgeons to avoid a transannular patch whenever possible, often accepting a degree of pulmonary stenosis as a trade-off.[501–503] In the immediate postoperative period, junctional ectopic tachycardia (JET) is a particular risk after complete correction. JET is a self-limiting, narrow QT tachycardia, arising from increased automaticity from the AV node region, which does not predispose to more severe dysrhythmias. Its importance resides in the fact that it usually occurs postoperatively in the first 24 to 48 hours, when a degree of already existing cardiac dysfunction may be further aggravated by the rapid heart rate and loss of the contribution of atrial contraction to ventricular filling.

Anesthesia Considerations

SYSTEMIC-TO-PULMONARY SHUNT. The systemic-to-pulmonary shunt typically is a modified Blalock-Taussig shunt. This is a connection between the innominate artery (or brachiocephalic trunk) or subclavian artery to a branch pulmonary artery via the interposition of a synthetic tube graft.

- The patient is usually a neonate or small infant.
- Sedative premedication is useful to prevent crying during induction, which may provoke a hypercyanotic spell.
- There is a risk of a hypercyanotic spell during induction and surgery.
- Inhalational or IV induction are both appropriate.
- Surgery is most often performed through a thoracotomy (left or right) but may occasionally be performed through a sternotomy.
- CPB is not usually required.
- Arterial and central venous access are required.
- The tracheal tube should be snug (or use a cuffed tracheal tube), with no or minimal air leak because lung retraction during surgery can make ventilation difficult.
- The arterial line should not be in the arm on the side that the shunt will be placed because the subclavian artery will be clamped, and the arterial pressure will be lost.
- Hemodynamic and respiratory disturbance can be problematic during surgery.
- The surgeon may request a small dose of heparin.
- Bleeding may occur after clamps are released; be prepared for a blood transfusion.
- Postoperatively, the pulmonary blood supply predominantly depends on the size of the shunt. If the shunt is too small, the infant may have a low saturation level; if the shunt is too large, the infant may develop heart failure or pulmonary edema and hypotension.
- Pulmonary blood flow also depends on systemic blood pressure; the greater the blood pressure, the more blood flows to the lungs and the higher the saturation.
- Milrinone is often combined with norepinephrine because norepinephrine increases the low diastolic pressure created by the shunt by systemic-to-pulmonary artery runoff in diastole, but does not produce the unwanted tachycardia seen with epinephrine.
- Postoperative ventilation may be required.

COMPLETE REPAIR. If the child is scheduled for early complete correction with no previous palliation by a systemic-to-pulmonary shunt, the child is likely to be a neonate or small infant. These children remain at risk for hypercyanotic spells. However, if the child has had a shunt placed previously, they are likely to be older and much less likely to have a hypercyanotic episode. Some children with less severe disease may not require a shunt and may be operated on when they are a bit older because they remain asymptomatic. Good sedative premedication is important in those at risk for hypercyanotic episodes.

- Both IV and inhalational induction agents are appropriate.
- CPB is required.
- Right ventricular dysfunction and pulmonary regurgitation may be postoperative problems.
- Intense inotropic support may worsen RVOTO postoperatively by dynamic narrowing of the RVOT; norepinephrine may be preferable to epinephrine in this setting, considering its predominant α-adrenergic effects.
- Milrinone may be particularly useful owing to its lusitropic properties, promoting diastolic relaxation of the stiff right ventricle.
- Surgeons frequently measure right ventricular pressure to assess the quality of the repair.
- Perioperative echocardiography is useful in assessing repair and right ventricular function.
- Excessive β-adrenergic stimulation and pyrexia, such as other stimuli that may induce a catecholamine surge may contribute to triggering JET postoperatively.

COMPLEX SHUNTS

In complex shunts (i.e., mixing shunts), there is mixing of pulmonary and systemic blood flow, with resulting cyanosis.

Transposition of the Great Arteries

Transposition of the great arteries (TGA) is common and accounts for about 6% of all CHD. It frequently occurs as an isolated lesion and is rarely associated with extracardiac anomalies. The operation most commonly performed in these infants is the arterial switch operation, the short- and long-term results of which have improved to such an extent that children with a good repair can expect a normal life.[504]

TGA refers to the situation in which the aorta arises from the morphologic right ventricle and the pulmonary artery arises from the morphologic left ventricle (Fig. 15.6). In this ventriculoarterial (VA) discordance, the atria are related to the ventricles in the normal way (i.e., AV concordance). This results in two circulations that run in parallel rather than in series, which is the normal anatomic arrangement. Without some mixing of the two circulations, the systemic circulation would remain completely deoxygenated. However, some mixing does occur through the PDA or through a VSD that is present in approximately 25% of cases. If there is no VSD and mixing is inadequate, ductal patency is maintained after birth with an IV prostaglandin E_1 infusion, and a balloon atrial septostomy is performed urgently in the neonatal period.

In TGA with an intact ventricular septum, the arterial switch operation should be performed early in the neonatal period, preferably in the first 2 to 3 weeks of life, because the left ventricle is exposed only to the pressure of the pulmonary circulation. The longer this situation is allowed to continue, the less the left ventricle will be able to adapt to the work required to pump blood at systemic pressure after corrective surgery. However, if there is an unrestrictive VSD, the left and right ventricle pressures equalize and both ventricles are exposed to systemic blood pressure, and the left ventricle is better conditioned to perform the work of the systemic ventricle after the arterial switch operation.

If untreated, most infants with TGA die in the first year of life of hypoxia and heart failure. Pulmonary vascular disease develops early and contributes to this high mortality rate.[505,506] The mechanism for the early development of pulmonary vascular disease is complex and not simply related to high pulmonary blood flow. However, the presence of a VSD further accelerates this process.

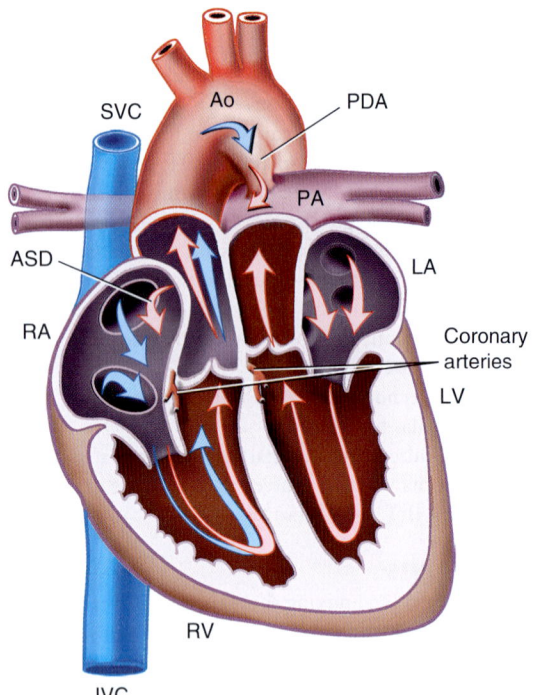

FIGURE 15.6 Diagram of transposition of the great arteries shows an intact ventricular septum. The aorta *(Ao)* arises from the right ventricle *(RV)*, and the pulmonary artery *(PA)* arises from the left ventricle *(LV)*. The coronary arteries arise from the aorta. These children are cyanotic. *ASD,* Atrial septal defect; *IVC,* inferior vena cava; *LA,* left atrium; *PDA,* patent ductus arteriosus; *RA,* right atrium; *SVC,* superior vena cava. (Modified from May LE. *Pediatric Heart Surgery: A Ready Reference for Professionals.* Milwaukee, WI: Maxishare; 2005.)

These infants are at risk for pulmonary hypertensive crises in the postoperative period.[507]

Surgical Options

ARTERIAL SWITCH OPERATION. An arterial switch is the operation of choice if the intracardiac anatomy is appropriate. The switch repair involves transecting the two main arterial trunks distal to their respective valves and switching them to produce VA concordance (Fig. 15.7). It also involves disconnecting the coronary arteries from the "old" aorta and reconnecting them to the neoaorta. This restores anatomic and physiologic normality. The coronary anatomy varies widely in TGA but must be well assessed preoperatively because moving the coronary arteries to the neoaorta is difficult but crucial to a successful outcome. In some cases, the coronary arteries run in the wall of the aorta (intramural), and this poses particular difficulties for the surgeon. Ventricular function after surgery depends largely on unrestricted flow in the coronary arteries.

MUSTARD AND SENNING PROCEDURES. The Mustard and Senning procedures are atrial switch operations. They involve the use of intraatrial baffles to redirect deoxygenated blood from the venae cavae to the left atrium, left ventricle, and pulmonary artery, and oxygenated pulmonary venous blood to the right atrium, right ventricle, and aorta. They create AV discordance, restore physiologic but not anatomic normality, and leave the morphologic and physiologic right ventricle as the systemic ventricle. These procedures were performed as definitive procedures before the arterial switch became successful but are rarely used today as

definitive repairs. They are still used as palliation in children with TGA, VSD, and pulmonary vascular disease.[508] In these cases, the VSD is left open. Atrial switch operations are also used as definitive repairs in congenitally corrected transposition of the great arteries (ccTGA or L-TGA), a rarer form of TGA with both AV and VA discordance. In these cases, an atrial switch is combined with an arterial switch repair, thus restoring AV and VA concordance, as components of what is denominated a double-switch procedure.[509–511]

RASTELLI PROCEDURE. The Rastelli procedure is used in children with TGA, VSD, and left VOTO (LVOTO). The procedure closes the VSD in a way that directs blood from the left ventricle to the aorta. The pulmonary artery is ligated just distal to the pulmonary valve, and a valved conduit is inserted from the right ventricle to the pulmonary artery. The result is continuity between the left ventricle and aorta and between the right ventricle and the pulmonary artery, and the LVOTO (i.e., subpulmonary area) is bypassed. In the past, the Rastelli procedure was performed at 2 to 3 years of age, following palliation in the neonatal period by a Blalock-Taussig shunt. However, as with other forms of CHD, there is currently a trend toward neonatal Rastelli repair, thus eliminating the need for previous palliation.

Anesthesia Considerations for the Arterial Switch Procedure

- The patient is a neonate in the first few weeks of life.
- Inhalational or IV induction is possible.
- Invasive arterial and central venous lines are required.
- Myocardial ischemia occurring after the cross-clamp is removed may be related to coronary air emboli or inadequate coronary anastomoses. A generous perfusion pressure after removal of cross-clamp encourages flushing air from coronary arteries. If ischemia results from an anatomic problem with the transferred coronary arteries, they may need to be revised with a second bypass run.
- TEE or epicardial echo is useful in assessing adequate de-airing, myocardial function, and adequacy of coronary anastomoses.
- Post-CPB myocardial dysfunction may result from one or more of:
  - Coronary air
  - Poor coronary transference
  - Poor myocardial protection
  - Inherently poor left ventricle
- The anesthesiologist should anticipate pulmonary hypertension.
- Inotropes are almost always required. Epinephrine or norepinephrine can be used, and milrinone is a particularly useful agent in these cases because it is an inodilator.
- After the repair, the pulmonary artery is anterior to the aorta. Any dilation of the pulmonary artery as a result of pulmonary hypertension can lead to coronary artery compression and myocardial ischemia.
- The left ventricle is frequently noncompliant, and volume should be increased with care and in small amounts. LA pressure can rise quickly if fluid is given injudiciously.
- Coagulopathy after bypass is common.
- Antifibrinolytics are often used.

Truncus Arteriosus

Truncus arteriosus is a rare congenital heart defect that occurs in about 0.7 of 1000 live births and accounts for about 1% of all CHD. The basic lesion is that of a common arterial outlet for the aorta and pulmonary artery associated with a single valve with

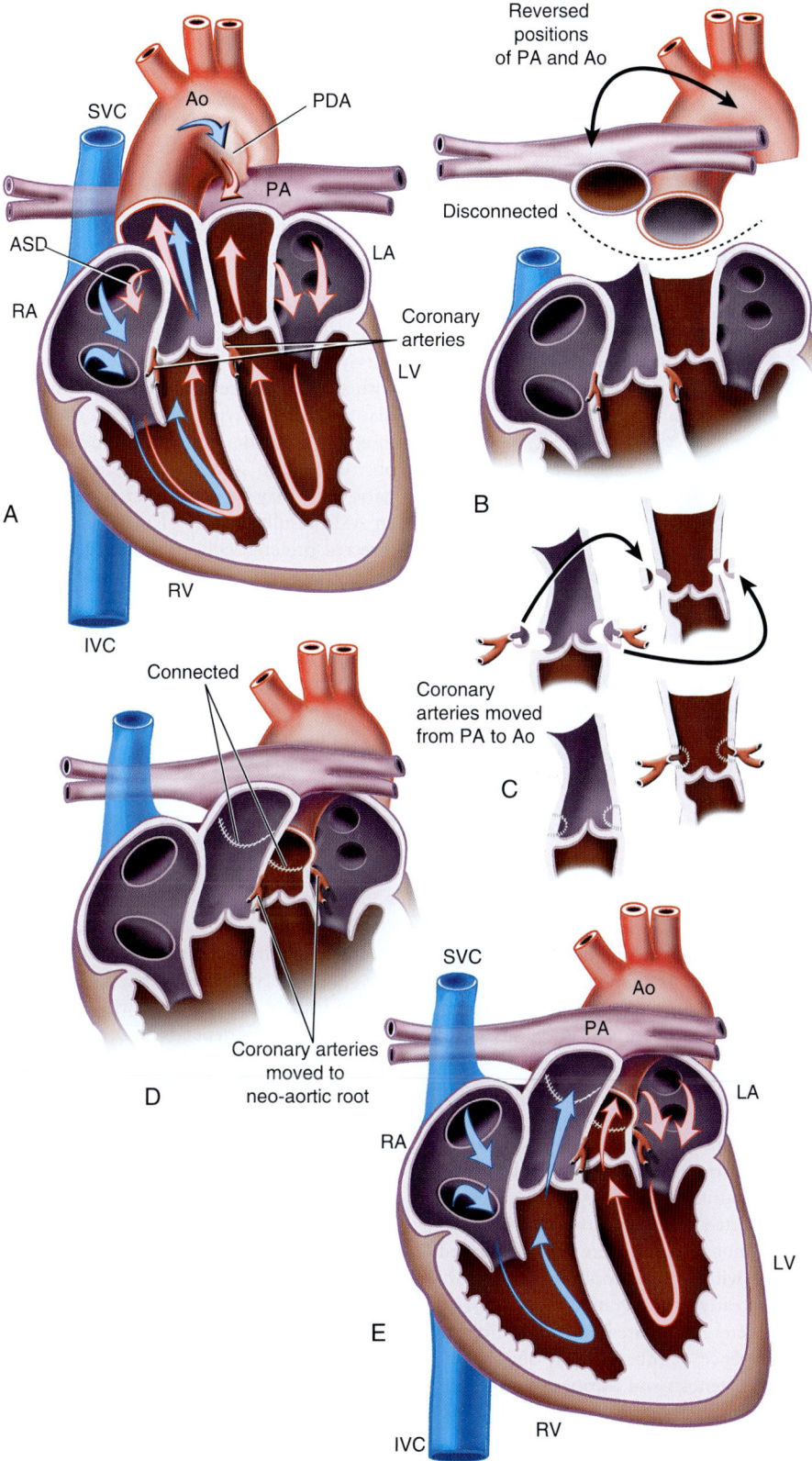

FIGURE 15.7 Diagram of an arterial switch operation. **A,** The original anatomy. The aorta *(Ao)*, pulmonary arteries *(PA)*, and coronary arteries are disconnected from their origins. **B,** The PA is moved anterior to the Ao. **C,** The Ao is connected to the left ventricle, and the PA is connected to the right ventricle. **D,** The coronary arteries are connected to the neoaortic root. **E,** Final configuration. *IVC,* Inferior vena cava; *LA,* left atrium; *LV,* left ventricle; *RA,* right atrium; *RV,* right ventricle; *SVC,* superior vena cava. (Modified from May LE. *Pediatric Heart Surgery: A Ready Reference for Professionals.* Milwaukee, WI: Maxishare; 2005.)

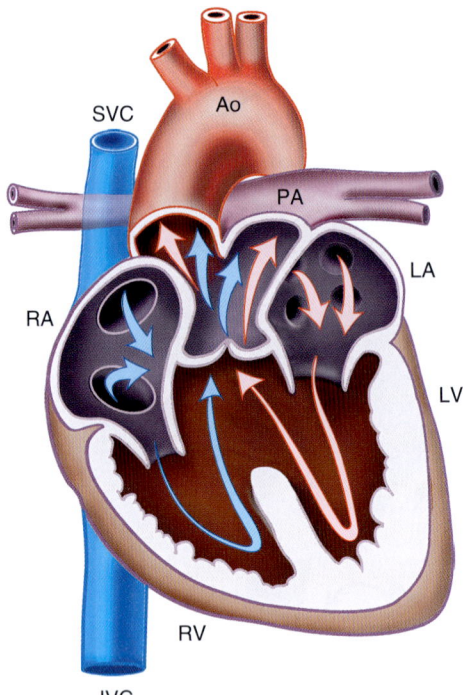

SVC

Ao

PA

LA

RA

LV

RV

IVC

FIGURE 15.8 The diagram of a truncus arteriosus shows the common truncal valve and mixing of red and blue blood. *Ao,* Aorta; *IVC,* inferior vena cava; *LA,* left atrium; *LV,* left ventricle; *PA,* pulmonary artery; *RA,* right atrium; *RV,* right ventricle; *SVC,* superior vena cava. (Modified from May LE. *Pediatric Heart Surgery: A Ready Reference for Professionals.* Milwaukee, WI: Maxishare; 2005.)

variable morphology (called a truncal valve) and a VSD (Fig. 15.8). The different subtypes depend on how the pulmonary arteries arise from the aorta and on the size of the aorta. Blood mixes at the arterial level with a resultant high pulmonary blood flow. This leads to heart failure and early development of pulmonary hypertension. Surgery must be performed early in life to prevent pulmonary hypertension from becoming irreversible. Truncus arteriosus has a known association with DiGeorge syndrome (see Table 15.4). In the presence of this syndrome or uncertainty about an existing 22q11 deletion, irradiated blood products should be used, and calcium concentrations carefully monitored.

Surgical repair involves separating the systemic and pulmonary circulations as well as closing the VSD. The pulmonary artery or arteries are disconnected from the aorta, and the truncal valve is repaired. The pulmonary arteries are then connected to the right ventricle, usually with a valved conduit. Circulatory arrest may be required. The early postoperative mortality rate ranges from 5% to 25%. Several factors are known to influence mortality, including the presence of other cardiac abnormalities, particularly truncal valve stenosis and coronary abnormalities, as well as chromosomal anomalies and low birth weight.[512,513]

Anesthesia Considerations
- The patient is a small neonate.
- The airway may already be intubated, the lungs ventilated, and the patient already managed with inotrope support.
- If the lungs are not ventilated, premedication is probably best avoided.
- Heart failure is possible.

- Repair is a high-risk procedure.
- Risks include a postoperative pulmonary hypertensive crisis.
- Invasive lines are required.
- Circulatory arrest may be required.
- Coagulopathy may occur after bypass.
- Antifibrinolytics are often used.

Anomalous Pulmonary Venous Drainage
Anomalous pulmonary venous drainage comprises about 2.5% of CHD and may be total (TAPVD) or partial (PAPVD). In TAPVD, all four pulmonary veins insert into an anomalous site, and in PAPVD, a subset of the veins insert into an anomalous site and the remaining veins insert into the left atrium. Survival is usually good but depends on the site of insertion, with survival poorer for the infracardiac than for the supracardiac and cardiac types; the size of the venous confluence at the insertion into the left atrium; and the presence or absence of obstruction. In some circumstances, even though the pulmonary veins may be appropriately connected to the left atrium, an ASD results in part of the pulmonary venous return being directed preferentially to the right atrium. It is probably more appropriate to refer to these forms of CHD as anomalous pulmonary venous drainage or return, even though the term anomalous pulmonary venous connection is also used. Four types of TAPVD exist:
- In supracardiac TAPVD, the pulmonary veins drain to the SVC territory via the left brachiocephalic vein through an ascending vertical vein (Fig. 15.9A).
- In cardiac TAPVD, the pulmonary veins connect to the right atrium through the coronary sinus (see Fig. 15.9B).
- In infracardiac TAPVD, the pulmonary veins drain to the IVC territory through a common vein, which traverses the diaphragm (see Fig. 15.9C).
- In mixed TAPVD, any combination of the previously mentioned three types may occur (see Fig. 15.9C).

Infants with obstructed anomalous pulmonary venous drainage, pulmonary hypertension, and reduced pulmonary blood supply usually present early with cyanosis and tachypnea. The degree of cyanosis depends on the size of an existing ASD and the associated right-to-left shunt, as well as on the degree of mixing of systemic and pulmonary venous blood. Children without pulmonary venous obstruction and pulmonary hypertension usually have few symptoms.

Anesthesia Considerations
- The patient may be a neonate.
- Heart failure can occur.
- Pulmonary edema may be present.
- There is a risk of pulmonary hypertension preoperatively and postoperatively; nitric oxide may be required.
- Circulatory arrest may be used, and profound hypothermia may be required.
- Coagulopathy may occur after bypass.
- Antifibrinolytics are often used.

As previously mentioned, there is a risk of pulmonary hypertension, for which inhaled nitric oxide may be necessary. However, it should be used with caution in these patients. In fact, children with obstructive lesions at the atrial level before surgery or patients with a poorly compliant left ventricle may be unable to tolerate an acute increase in pulmonary venous return; the use of inhaled nitrous oxide could thus result in paradoxical pulmonary hypertension.[514,515]

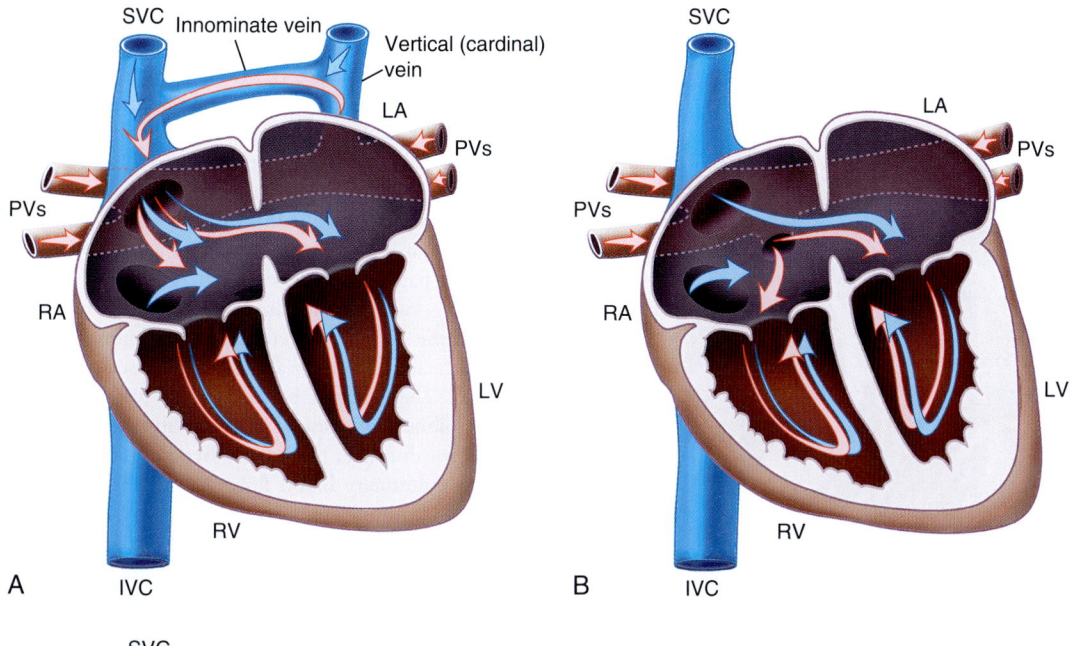

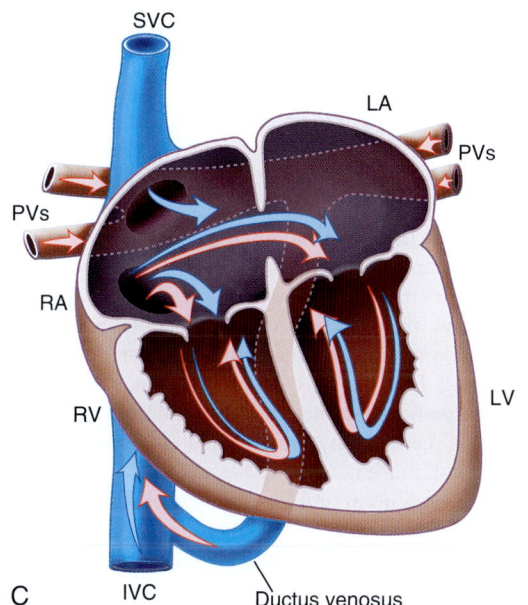

FIGURE 15.9 **A,** In the diagram of a supracardiac total anomalous pulmonary venous connection (TAPVC), the main arteries are removed. The pulmonary veins *(PVs)* drain through the innominate vein to the right atrium *(RA)*, and there is an atrial septal defect (ASD). The result is a left-to-right shunt. These children are cyanotic. The veins may also be obstructed, leading to pulmonary hypertension. **B,** In the diagram of an intracardiac TAPVC, the PVs drain to the RA. There is a ventricular septal defect, and the effect is to create a left-to-right shunt. The veins may also be obstructed, which can lead to pulmonary hypertension. **C,** In the diagram of an infracardiac TAPVC, the PVs drain through the ductus venosus to the RA. An ASD exists, and the circulation results in a right-to-left shunt; the child is blue. The veins may also be obstructed. *IVC,* Inferior vena cava; *LA,* left atrium; *LV,* left ventricle; *RA,* right atrium; *RV,* right ventricle; *SVC,* superior vena cava. (Modified from May LE. *Pediatric Heart Surgery: A Ready Reference for Professionals.* Milwaukee, WI: Maxishare; 2005.)

Hypoplastic Left Heart Syndrome

The incidence of HLHS in the United States is about 2 cases per 10,000 live births. In Europe, this figure is probably less because many mothers with a prenatal diagnosis of HLHS opt to terminate the pregnancy *in utero.*

The anatomic features of HLHS (Fig. 15.10) include:

- Hypoplastic left ventricle
- Mitral stenosis or atresia
- Aortic stenosis or atresia
- Hypoplastic aortic arch
- Duct-dependent circulation

The prognosis for infants who are born with HLHS has improved dramatically. Previously, virtually all of these infants died of this condition, but in some centers, most children now survive at least into childhood, with many surviving into adulthood.[516] The longer-term outlook has not been fully determined, and many hurdles remain.

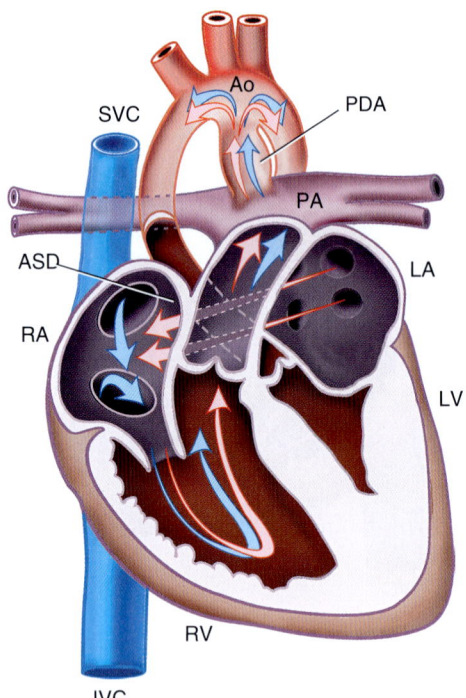

FIGURE 15.10 Diagram of hypoplastic left heart syndrome shows a very small left ventricle *(LV)*, mitral valve, aortic valve, and aortic arch. Pulmonary venous blood drains to the left atrium *(LA)*, then through an atrial septal defect *(ASD)* to the right atrium *(RA)*, and from there through the right ventricle *(RV)* to the pulmonary artery *(PA)*. A patent ductus arteriosus *(PDA)* provides blood to the systemic circulation. *Ao,* Aorta; *IVC,* inferior vena cava; *SVC,* superior vena cava. (Modified from May LE. *Pediatric Heart Surgery: A Ready Reference for Professionals.* Milwaukee, WI: Maxishare; 2005.)

The diagnosis of HLHS is usually made in the prenatal period, although it can be difficult and is sometimes missed. At birth, neonates present with tachypnea, tachycardia, cyanosis, and a systolic murmur.

Surgical Palliation

The aim of surgery is to convert the anatomy of the HLHS into a single-ventricle–type circulation in which the right ventricle becomes the single systemic ventricle, and the pulmonary blood flow is supplied passively from the SVC and IVC (i.e., Fontan circulation). This is done by a series of three operations known as Norwood stage I, Norwood stage II (also called superior cavopulmonary connection, bidirectional Glenn, or hemi-Fontan), and Norwood stage III (total cavopulmonary connection or Fontan).

NORWOOD STAGE I. The Norwood stage I operation is performed in the neonatal period. It involves reconstructing the aortic arch so that it arises from the pulmonary trunk. The pulmonary valve becomes the neoaortic valve. The branch pulmonary arteries are disconnected from the pulmonary trunk, and a new source of pulmonary blood supply is provided by a shunt from the subclavian artery (i.e., Blalock-Taussig shunt) or from the right ventricle (i.e., Sano modification) (Fig. 15.11).[517] If the ASD is restrictive, it is enlarged to allow for unobstructed pulmonary venous return into what becomes a common atrium, then draining across the interatrial septum through the right side into the right ventricle. The important physiologic principles of the Norwood stage I operation are unobstructed pulmonary venous return with unrestrictive interatrial communication; unobstructed

systemic blood flow and adequate coronary perfusion; and controlled source of pulmonary blood flow.

NORWOOD STAGE II. The Norwood stage II (superior cavopulmonary connection, bidirectional Glenn or hemi-Fontan) operation takes place at about 6 months of age. It involves taking down the shunt that was created at the first operation and creating a new connection from the SVC to the pulmonary arteries (i.e., a bidirectional or Glenn shunt). The result is a pulmonary blood supply that is provided by systemic venous blood from the SVC. Flow is passive and depends on pulmonary artery pressures remaining low, since its driving force is the pressure gradient between the SVC (connected to the pulmonary arteries, upstream from the lungs) and atrial pressure (pressure downstream from the lungs). The gradient between these two pressures is called the transpulmonary gradient, and any obstruction between these two sites (for example, pulmonary hypertension) will result in inadequate pulmonary blood flow. The infants remain cyanotic with arterial saturations in the mid-80s because desaturated blood from the IVC continues to flow into the heart and the systemic circulation (Fig. 15.12).

NORWOOD STAGE III. The Norwood stage III (Fontan) operation converts the anatomy into a Fontan circulation. The surgery involves connecting the IVC through an extracardiac or intracardiac conduit to the pulmonary artery. This creates a single-ventricle or Fontan circulation (Fig. 15.13). The single right ventricle pumps blood to the systemic circulation, and the pulmonary blood supply is provided by passive flow by systemic venous blood from the SVC and IVC. The PVR must remain low because any increase will dramatically reduce pulmonary blood flow. It is common for a small hole (i.e., fenestration) to be created between the conduit and the right atrium so that if the PVR rises, blood will be directed to the right atrium and allow cardiac output to be maintained. In this situation, the child becomes cyanotic, but cardiac output is maintained, a much safer situation than a state of low cardiac output. Later, if PVR remains consistently low, the fenestration can be closed with a transvenous device. Postoperatively, increased systemic venous pressure may cause pleural effusions, an enlarged liver, or protein-losing enteropathy.

The long-term problem for these children is that the morphologic right ventricle, which then becomes the systemic ventricle, fails over time. The only recourse is heart transplantation.[518,519]

Anesthesia Considerations
NORWOOD STAGE I
- The anesthesiologist must understand the anatomy and physiology of HLHS.
- Balance between systemic and pulmonary circulations is maintained by balancing PVR and SVR. If the PVR decreases, blood flow will be directed away from the systemic circulation and there will be pulmonary over-circulation. This results in hypotension and systemic hypoperfusion with increasing acidosis. If PVR increases, cyanosis will increase. Before anesthesia, these infants are best managed spontaneously breathing in room air with a prostaglandin E_1 infusion to maintain ductal patency. However, if mechanical ventilation is required, it is important to maintain normal to high $PaCO_2$ and very low FiO_2, usually with air. Even though oxygen saturations as read by pulse oximetry have traditionally been used as a guide to balance the circulation, there is evidence that, when considered in isolation, they are a poor reflection of such a balance. As such, systemic venous saturations should also be used to provide an estimate of tissue oxygen delivery.[252,254,520,521] NIRS

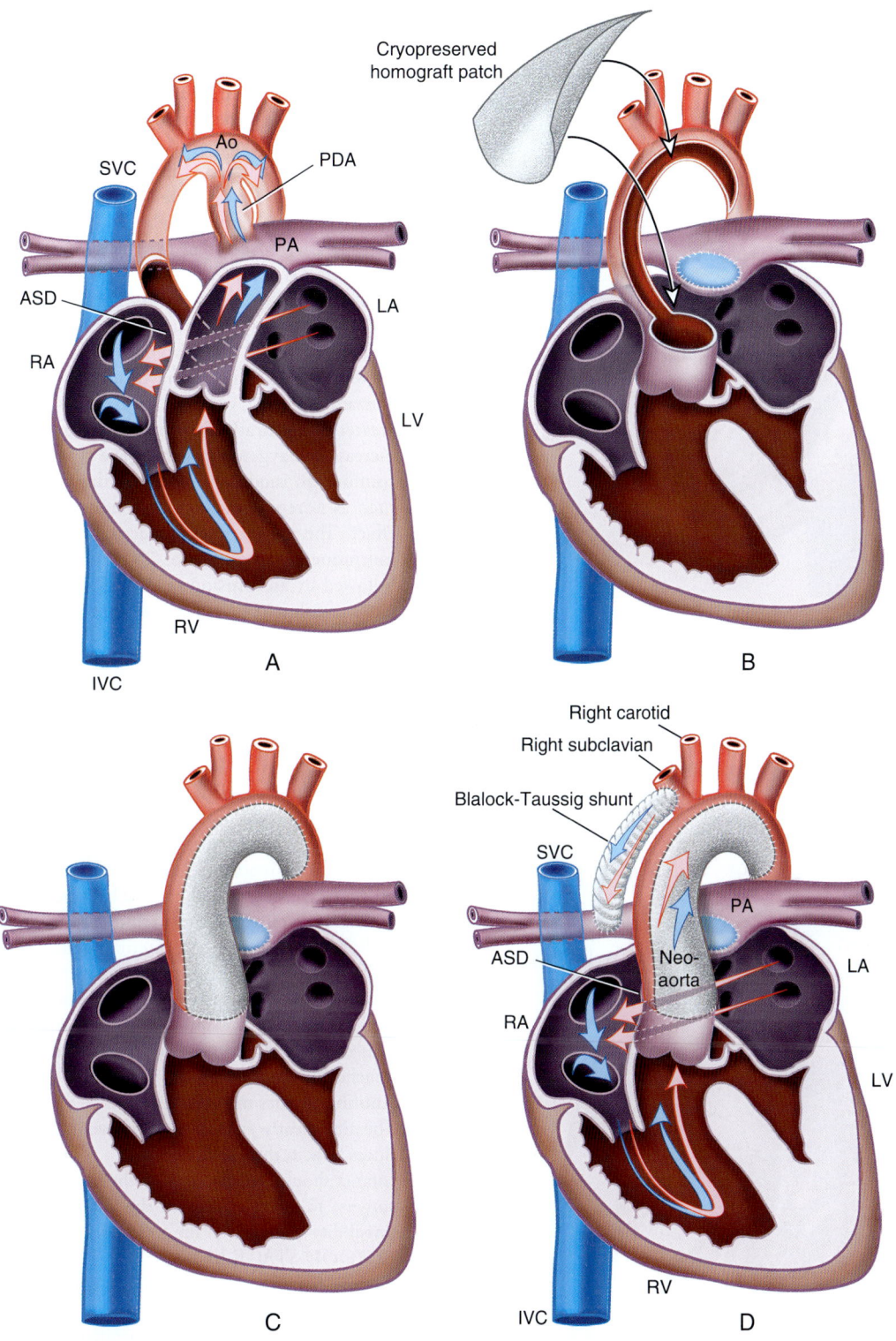

FIGURE 15.11 Diagram of the Norwood stage I operation. **A,** The main pulmonary artery *(PA)* is disconnected from the right ventricle *(RV)*. **B** and **C,** The aortic arch is reconstructed with homograft and connected to the RV, which becomes a single ventricle. **D,** Pulmonary blood is then supplied by a Blalock-Taussig shunt from the subclavian artery to the PA. The children remain cyanotic. *Ao,* Aorta; *ASD,* atrial septal defect; *IVC,* inferior vena cava; *LA,* left atrium; *LV,* left ventricle; *PDA,* patent ductus arteriosus; *RA,* right atrium; *SVC,* superior vena cava. (Modified from May LE. *Pediatric Heart Surgery: A Ready Reference for Professionals.* Milwaukee, WI: Maxishare; 2005.)

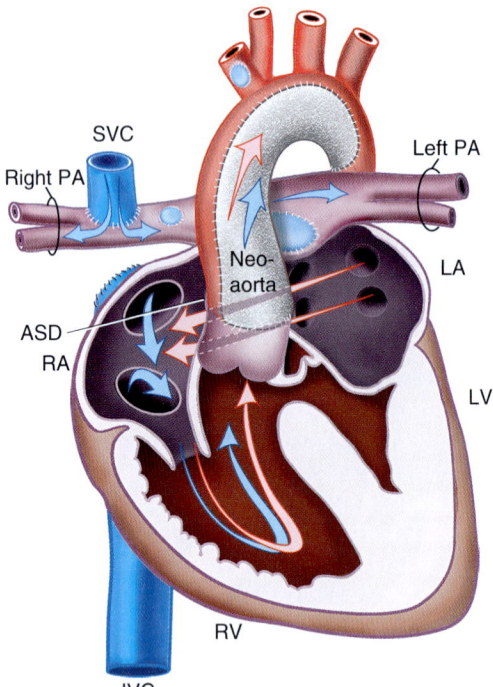

FIGURE 15.12 Diagram of Norwood stage II (hemi-Fontan) operation. The Blalock-Taussig shunt is disconnected, and a Glenn shunt is created by connecting the superior vena cava *(SVC)* to the pulmonary artery *(PA)*. *ASD,* Atrial septal defect; *IVC,* inferior vena cava; *LA,* left atrium; *LV,* left ventricle; *RA,* right atrium; *RV,* right ventricle. (Modified from May LE. *Pediatric Heart Surgery: A Ready Reference for Professionals.* Milwaukee, WI: Maxishare; 2005.)

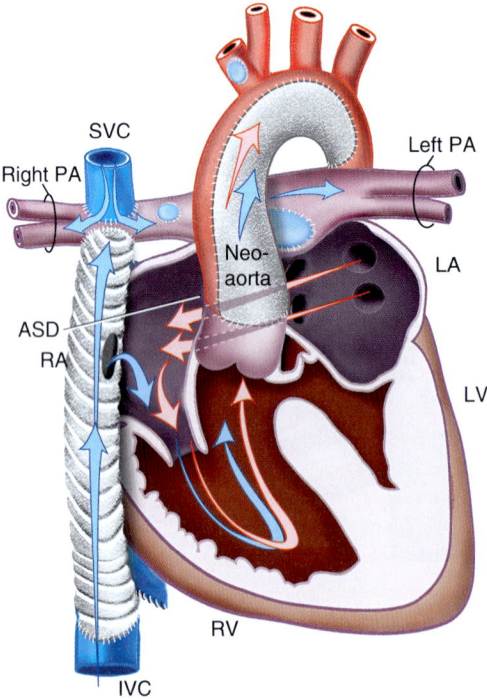

FIGURE 15.13 Diagram of Norwood stage III (Fontan) operation. The Fontan circulation is created by connecting the inferior vena cava *(IVC)* to the pulmonary artery *(PA)* with a conduit. A fenestration is shown between the conduit and the right atrium *(RA)*. *ASD,* Atrial septal defect; *LA,* left atrium; *LV,* left ventricle; *RV,* right ventricle; *SVC,* superior vena cava. (Modified from May LE. *Pediatric Heart Surgery: A Ready Reference for Professionals.* Milwaukee, WI: Maxishare; 2005.)

monitoring can also be used as a continuous indicator of the adequacy of oxygen delivery to the brain.

- Air should be available for transfer to and from the ICU; alternatively, a self-inflating bag can be used.
- Venous access is gained through the femoral or umbilical veins. The internal jugular vein is avoided because narrowing of the SVC would jeopardize a future Glenn shunt.
- High-dose opioid technique is preferred.
- Profound hypothermia may be required.
- Postoperative myocardial dysfunction is common, and inotropes are required.
- Balancing systemic and pulmonary blood flow remains an issue after bypass and estimating the relative systemic and pulmonary blood flows is not always straightforward. Some centers use the long-acting α-adrenergic blocker phenoxybenzamine after bypass to reduce SVR variability, allowing greater concentrations of oxygen to be used and an overall increase in oxygen delivery.[522] The alternative approach is to combine an inodilator such as milrinone with a vasopressor such as norepinephrine or epinephrine to achieve a similar effect. The authors' preference is to deliver a bolus dose of milrinone (0.5 µg/kg over 20 minutes during rewarming), followed by an infusion of 0.3 µg/kg per minute, in combination with a continuous infusion of epinephrine, 0.05 to 0.1 µg/kg per minute.
- Coagulopathy is likely to occur after bypass.
- Antifibrinolytics are often used.
- The sternum is frequently left open, and closure may be delayed for several days.

NORWOOD STAGE II

- The procedure is carried out with CPB.
- Cardioplegia is not used. The heart remains beating, and inotropes are seldom required.
- Venous access is achieved through the femoral veins. However, only a single side should be used because femoral bypass is occasionally required. A short temporary cannula is useful as an additional monitor in the internal jugular vein. It reflects the pulmonary artery pressure after anastomosis of the SVC to the pulmonary artery. It is removed early in the postoperative period to avoid any possibility of thrombosis in the SVC.
- This is repeat surgery, and external defibrillator pads should be attached.
- Antifibrinolytics may be used.
- The aim is early extubation; positive intrathoracic pressure reduces flow in the Glenn shunt.
- Infants should be nursed with the head up at 30 degrees after surgery, to improve flow in the Glenn shunt and reduce the possibility of edema in the SVC territory.

NORWOOD STAGE III

- Surgery is carried out with CPB but usually without cross-clamping the aorta.
- PVR must remain low postoperatively, careful management of the lungs is important to minimize atelectasis, and inhaled nitric oxide is occasionally required.[523]
- Milrinone is a good choice if inotropes are needed because of its beneficial effects on PVR.
- Early extubation is beneficial in terms of hemodynamics.
- Large amounts of fluid may be required in the early postoperative period.

HYBRID PALLIATION APPROACH

In an effort to avoid the high-risk initial surgical palliation for HLHS, in particular the serious physiological consequences and potential adverse effects of a complex operation performed in the neonatal period, a hybrid surgical and transcatheter-based approach has been devised as an alternative to the Norwood Stage I operation. Also known as the Giessen approach, it consists of surgical banding of both pulmonary arteries (without the use of CPB), a transcatheter atrial septostomy, and maintaining ductal patency via the endovascular deployment of a stent (or a prostaglandin infusion).[524] This initial palliation aims to achieve a balanced circulation with adequate and controlled pulmonary and systemic blood flow, allowing the child to grow until completion of the second stage, at about 6 months of age. The second stage operation involves reconstructing the aortic arch so it comes from the pulmonary trunk, transecting the pulmonary artery (similarly to what is performed in the Norwood Stage I procedure), removing the pulmonary artery bands (a pulmonary artery reconstruction might be necessary at this stage), creating a superior cavopulmonary connection, as well as ligating the previously stented duct. The second stage in the hybrid palliation approach pathway thus becomes the most complex procedure of the staged repair, as opposed to the major operation performed in the Norwood Stage I, in the neonatal period. Both approaches then converge to a common end result with the completion of the Fontan procedure.

Despite the initial enthusiasm for the hybrid approach and the promising prospect of delaying major surgery until the age of 6 months, with the potential for improving outcomes and avoiding the potential effects of surgical stress and anesthesia on a fragile neonate, the literature has failed to consistently show any significant morbidity or mortality differences between the two approaches.[525–528] It is likely that a fair comparison between the two strategies will never be feasible, as the hybrid palliation approach tends to be selected for higher-risk patients in many centers, therefore introducing an important bias.[529] However, it is worth noting that a potential advantage of the hybrid palliation is the possibility of a successful future biventricular repair (BVR), when the initial operation is performed as a salvage procedure in very sick patients; as the initial palliation in patients with uncertain feasibility of single-stage biventricular repair due to severe left ventricular outflow tract obstruction; or as part of a LV recruitment strategy in patients with a borderline LV.[530–532] Further research is needed to clarify the roles of the hybrid approach and the classic Norwood Stage I operations, with some evidence suggesting that a tailored approach, taking into account the patient characteristics, risk factors, and comorbidities, could help decide which strategy to use in the individual patient, with the hybrid strategy being an acceptable alternative in higher-risk patients.[533,534] In the future, it is possible that the development of a bespoke flow restrictor that can be percutaneously inserted into both branches of the pulmonary artery to limit pulmonary blood flow will be an integral part of an entirely nonsurgical stage I procedure, which could alter the balance towards performing a totally transcatheter technique in a fragile neonate, as opposed to major surgery in the neonatal period.[535]

Anesthesia Considerations
HYBRID PALLIATION
- As previously mentioned, the anesthesiologist must understand the anatomy and physiology of HLHS.
- Considerations about the balance between the pulmonary and systemic circulations, blood flow, and pulmonary and systemic vascular resistances apply to patients undergoing a hybrid palliation, before, during and after the procedure.

- The patient might be relatively stable before the procedure, but most likely will be a very sick neonate with multiple risk factors and comorbidities, in which case the approach to transfer between ICU and theaters should be as previously described for Norwood Stage I.
- Despite a preoperative fragile state, patients undergoing the hybrid procedure have relatively stable intraoperative and early postoperative hemodynamics.
- The procedure is performed without CPB and with minimal narcotic and anesthetic exposure.
- Patients typically do not require blood transfusions or inotropic support and are extubated at either the end of the procedure or within 24 h of ICU admission.
- In summary, anesthetic management is fairly straightforward and requires relatively few interventions compared to traditional neonatal repairs.[536,537]

COMPREHENSIVE STAGE II
- The procedure is carried with CPB, moderate or deep hypothermia, circulatory arrest (possibly with selective antegrade cerebral perfusion).
- Venous access is achieved through the femoral veins. However, only a single side should be used because femoral bypass is occasionally required. A short temporary cannula is useful as an additional monitor in the internal jugular vein. It reflects the pulmonary artery pressure after anastomosis of the SVC to the pulmonary artery. It is removed early in the postoperative period to avoid any possibility of thrombosis in the SVC.
- This is repeat surgery, and external defibrillator pads should be attached.
- Antifibrinolytics may be used, and bleeding may be an issue, as it is an extensive repair.
- Immediate postoperative care should focus on minimizing systemic and myocardial oxygen consumption, reducing systemic vascular resistances, optimizing pulmonary perfusion and ventricular preload.
- Cornerstones of intensive therapy are early extubation and noninvasive respiratory support, balanced fluid management, avoiding excessive edema and controlling heart rate.
- In this pathophysiological situation, tissue oxygen delivery cannot be further increased, so every effort should be made to minimize oxygen consumption and avoid stress.[538]

NORWOOD STAGE III
- Surgery is carried out with CPB but usually without crossclamping the aorta.
- PVR must remain low postoperatively, careful management of the lungs is important to minimize atelectasis, and inhaled nitric oxide is occasionally required.[523]
- Milrinone is a good choice if inotropes are needed because of its beneficial effects on PVR.
- Early extubation is beneficial in terms of hemodynamics.
- Large amounts of fluid may be required in the early postoperative period.

AORTIC STENOSIS
Obstruction to the LVOT can occur at the valvular, subvalvular, or supravalvular areas or in various combinations, and it occurs commonly, accounting for up to 10% of CHD.[539,540] Congenital valvular aortic stenosis is frequently associated with a bicuspid valve. Severe critical aortic stenosis in neonates occurs in approximately 10% of cases and requires urgent treatment. Supravalvular aortic stenosis may be associated with Williams syndrome.[541]

Despite the many anatomic varieties of aortic stenosis, the resulting pathophysiology remains essentially the same. There is an increasing imbalance between myocardial oxygen supply and demand. Coronary blood flow is impaired due to low coronary perfusion pressure, whereas workload on the left ventricle is increased, leading to subendocardial ischemia, left ventricular hypertrophy, and a risk of left ventricular failure. The risk of sudden death is always present, especially with Williams syndrome.[542] The age at which the child presents is a risk factor; younger children are most at risk. Two-thirds of those presenting in the first 3 months of life will require inotropic or ventilatory support before treatment of the stenosis.[543] *Approximately 5% of Williams syndrome patients may suffer a cardiac arrest during anesthesia.*[544]

Treatment Options

Treatment options depend on the patient's age and the type and severity of the lesion. In neonates with critical aortic stenosis, an urgent valvuloplasty is required. It can be performed surgically using CPB, but it typically is performed using transluminal balloon angioplasty in the cardiac catheterization laboratory.[545] Complications in this age group include ventricular fibrillation, aortic incompetence, or residual aortic stenosis.

In the older child, several surgical approaches may be used, depending on the anatomy. Transluminal balloon valvuloplasty commonly is performed in older patients. The most common complications of valvuloplasty are aortic incompetence and residual aortic stenosis. Valve replacement with a mechanical valve or bioprosthetic valve is delayed as long as possible because of the long-term problems associated with the anticoagulation needed with a mechanical valve and because of the inevitable calcification of the bioprosthetic valve. An alternative surgical option is the Ross procedure, which involves moving the pulmonary valve into the aortic valve position and using a homograft in the pulmonary position. The need for reoperation with the Ross procedure is reduced because the systemic valve (i.e., neoaortic valve) grows with the child and calcification of the homograft in the pulmonary position is slow. There is no need for anticoagulation.[546–548] More recently, there has been an interest in the possibility of aortic valve repair for aortic stenosis (rather than replacement) by use of a reconstruction technique with pericardial patch, thus avoiding the potential problems associated with valve replacement.[549–551]

Anesthesia Considerations

- A crucial aim of anesthesia is to maintain the balance of oxygen supply and demand. This involves maintaining a normal heart rate (no tachycardia or bradycardia), maintaining SVR and diastolic blood pressure to preserve coronary perfusion, avoiding hypertension, and avoiding myocardial depression.
- Anesthesia for neonates with aortic stenosis having surgery with CPB is similar to other neonatal cardiac surgery.
- For transluminal balloon valvuloplasty:
  - The catheter crossing the aortic valve and inflation of the balloon can lead to dramatic cardiovascular changes. Cardiac output decreases, myocardial ischemia occurs, and bradycardia is common. In neonates, ventricular fibrillation may occur after passing the wire across the valve. The anesthesiologist must be prepared to resuscitate the neonate quickly, and drugs, particularly epinephrine, should be immediately available.

- It is possible the child will remain ventilated after the procedure because ventricular function can remain poor for some time.
- Arterial access is needed by the cardiologist for the procedure, but pressure is not always displayed. An independent arterial line is very useful.
- Occasionally, adenosine is given to slow or stop the heart at the time of balloon inflation to prevent damage to the valve by the inflated balloon being expelled through it. However, this practice is not universal.

COARCTATION OF THE AORTA

Coarctation of the aorta is a discrete narrowing of the aorta, and it accounts for about 5% of CHD. The lesion is often isolated with no other associated abnormalities. This type of lesion, however, may occur in association with other CHD, such as aortic arch, valve abnormalities, or VSD. The coarctation may be preductal, juxtaductal, or postductal, depending on the relationship to the ductus arteriosus. The most common form presenting in the neonatal period is the preductal type. Preductal coarctation is associated with minimal collateral circulation below the coarctation and requires prostaglandin to maintain ductal patency. Juxtaductal and postductal coarctations are characterized by the development of collateral vessels that supply the area below the coarctation. This is important because the spinal cord is supplied by these collaterals, which will provide blood flow to the spinal cord during aortic cross-clamping.

In practical terms, children with coarctation of the aorta can be classified in two groups. One group presents in the neonatal period with preductal coarctation with few collaterals, very poor left ventricular function, and possible heart failure. The second group of children (usually older than 1 year of age) have well-developed collaterals and better left ventricular function. Femoral pulses are often weak, and patients usually have a progressive acidosis. Differences between the systolic systemic blood pressures in the right arm (proximal to the stenosis) and legs (distal to the stenosis) may indicate the presence of a coarctation of the aorta.

Anesthesia Considerations

NEONATAL REPAIR

- These infants are sick, with poor left ventricular function. They should be treated very carefully, and the anesthesiologist should not be misled by an infant who looks reasonably well.
- In some infants, the tracheas are already intubated, the lungs ventilated, and they require inotropic support.
- IV access often is established to give prostaglandin E1; this IV line can also be used to administer induction agents. The authors' preference is to give incremental doses of fentanyl (up to 5 µg/kg) and then a muscle relaxant and to supplement this with a very low dose of inhalation agent (e.g., isoflurane [0.3%–0.5%]). This can be omitted if hypotension ensues.
- Inotropes may be required before surgery, and they should be available.
- Ideally, the arterial line should be placed in the right arm (right radial or axillary arteries) to allow continuous blood pressure measurement during arterial cross-clamping. The left subclavian may be partially obstructed during the repair. Some have advocated an arterial line below the coarctation to measure perfusion pressure during cross-clamping, but this may be very difficult in practice because femoral pulses are usually absent.
- A central venous line should be placed.

- Surgery usually takes place through a left thoracotomy without the use of CPB. The lung is retracted, and ventilation may be problematic. The endotracheal tube must fit snugly and have a minimal leak because a tracheal tube with a large leak may make ventilation very difficult. Alternatively, a cuffed endotracheal tube can be used.
- Paraplegia occurs in about 1% of cases and is thought to result from hypoperfusion during aortic cross-clamping.[552,553] To reduce the chance of spinal cord damage, infants should be cooled to 34°C or 35°C before the cross-clamp is applied, although this approach is not evidence-based. Normocarbia and upper limb blood pressure should be maintained, and the anesthesiologist should resist the temptation to lower blood pressure while the cross-clamp is applied. Low-dose anticoagulation may be requested. A short cross-clamp time is thought to be important.
- Epidural anesthesia is occasionally used but controversial, especially if anticoagulation is to be used, owing to the risk of neurologic injury.
- Postoperative hypertension may be a problem, since ventricular remodeling after relief of the obstruction is not immediate; a degree of left ventricular hypertrophy is to be expected for some weeks to months; in the immediate postoperative period, a vasodilator such as sodium nitroprusside may be required.

ANESTHESIA FOR THE OLDER CHILD

- These children usually are not as sick as the neonates with this heart defect.
- Issues about intravascular lines are similar to those in neonatal repair.
- Careful IV induction with a combination of fentanyl and an induction agent of choice is standard. Etomidate is a good anesthetic because of its cardiovascular stability.
- Although a collateral blood supply is present, the spinal cord remains at risk during the cross-clamping, and the same precautions taken with neonates should be taken with these children.
- An oral cuffed tracheal tube is useful because early extubation is the norm.
- Postoperative hypertension is a common problem, and good analgesia combined with sodium nitroprusside and β-blockers are usually required. Up to 30% of children eventually develop long-term hypertension that will require therapy.

Some of these children are managed in the catheterization laboratory with balloon angioplasty, with or without stent placement. Rupture of the aorta is a risk in these patients, and the institution in which the procedure is undertaken should be in a position to deal with this possibility, with a rescue plan clearly established.

INTERRUPTED AORTIC ARCH

Interrupted aortic arch is a rare anomaly, accounting for less than 1% of CHD. In this condition, disruption occurs between the ascending aorta and descending aorta (Fig. 15.14). The three types depend on where the disruption takes place. It is a duct-dependent systemic circulation, since a PDA is required to supply the descending aorta. A VSD is also common. An interrupted aortic arch is frequently associated with chromosome 22q11 deletion and results in the aforementioned DiGeorge syndrome (see Table 15.4).[554]

These children are often small for gestational age and are started on a prostaglandin infusion to maintain ductal patency. They are often sick with progressive acidosis and poor cardiac output. There

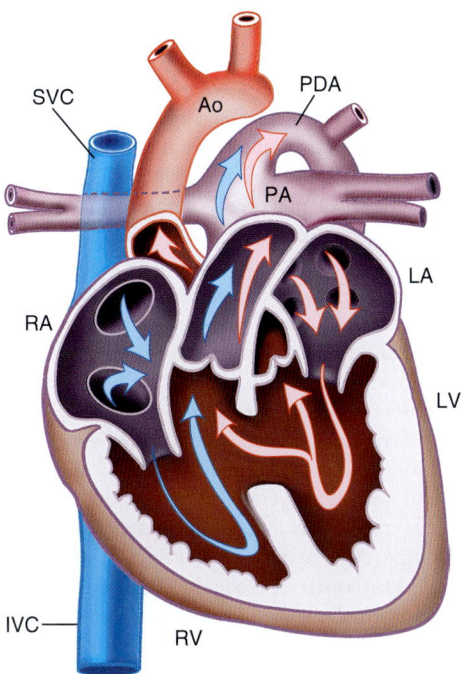

FIGURE 15.14 Diagram of an interrupted aortic arch. The patent ductus arteriosus *(PDA)* supplies the body below the interruption. *Ao,* Aorta; *IVC,* inferior vena cava; *LA,* left atrium; *LV,* left ventricle; *PA,* pulmonary artery; *RA,* right atrium; *RV,* right ventricle; *SVC,* superior vena cava. (Modified from May LE. *Pediatric Heart Surgery: A Ready Reference for Professionals.* Milwaukee, WI: Maxishare; 2005.)

is increasing pulmonary blood flow as the duct closes. Surgical repair depends on the presence of associated lesions, particularly a VSD. In the single-stage repair, the arch is reconstructed and the VSD is closed. The two-stage repair involves repair of the aortic arch and banding of the pulmonary artery to limit blood flow to the lungs. The VSD is closed at a later date. Either way, deep hypothermic circulatory arrest is likely to be used. Some centers use selective antegrade regional (cerebral) perfusion (SACP) to try and limit neurologic injury.[555] The early and late mortality rates are high. Greater mortality rates correlate with small size, preoperative acidosis, and associated cardiac lesions.[556]

Anesthesia Considerations

- The patient is a small, sick neonate.
- DiGeorge syndrome should be identified preoperatively, especially regarding the potential for hypocalcemia and the need for irradiated blood products; in case of uncertainty about 22q11 deletion status, it is prudent to proceed as if it is present.
- High-dose opioid technique is standard.
- Ideally, blood pressure should be monitored above and below the interruption, but this is often difficult in practice.
- Deep hypothermic circulatory arrest may be used.
- Coagulopathy is likely to occur after bypass.
- An antifibrinolytic is frequently used.
- Anticipate poor renal function postoperatively.
- There is a risk of postoperative pulmonary hypertensive crises.

These infants are likely to require repeat operations to deal with recurrent LVOTO, which may occur at any level. Restenosis of the repaired aortic arch can often be diagnosed and immediately treated in the catheterization laboratory by transluminal balloon dilation.

Transport and Transfer to a Pediatric Intensive Care Unit

After surgery is completed, cardiac surgical patients need a period of intensive care. The first phase of this care is transport of the children from the operating room to the pediatric intensive care unit (PICU). This is a potentially hazardous time and requires good organization, teamwork, and appropriate equipment. Guidelines exist for the safe transport of these children.[557]

Transport to the PICU can be subdivided into a preparatory phase, transport phase, and stabilization phase.[558] During the preparatory phase, the estimated time of arrival in the PICU is communicated with the PICU. The bed space is prepared, ventilator and monitors are configured in an appropriate way, and any additional interventions that may be required are made ready. In many institutions, a form is sent to the PICU that indicates the child's age and weight, the ventilator settings that will be required, the number of transducers that will be required, and the infusions that are running. After arrival in the PICU, two basic tasks need to be completed: transfer of technology and transfer of information. It is better to allow the technology transfer to occur before the information handover. This includes ensuring that all the monitors are connected and working appropriately, that the ventilator is connected and delivering adequate ventilation, that all infusions are working, and that drains and urinary catheter are all in place with baseline readings documented. After this has been accomplished, a single handover of information should be done with all the appropriate personnel present, and it should include information given by the anesthesiologist and surgeon. In many centers, a checklist is followed to ensure that no important information is omitted. It is important to avoid a large number of information handovers between individuals rather than a single, comprehensive handover with all the relevant personnel present.

ANNOTATED REFERENCES

Finucane E, Jooste E, Machovec KA. Neuromonitoring modalities in pediatric cardiac anesthesia: A review of the literature. Journal of Cardiothoracic and Vascular Anesthesia 34 (2020) 3420-3428.

Transcranial Doppler ultrasound, electroencephalography, near-infrared spectroscopy, and processed electroencephalography are the neuromonitoring modalities commonly used. Each modality has merits, but no single modality is able to reliably guide changes to management that improve neurologic outcomes. Combinations may prove useful in some circumstances. This review provides a brief overview of current neurodevelopmental outcomes in children with congenital heart disease and summarizes the evidence for the use these four neuromonitoring modalities.

Faraoni D, Van der Linden P. Factors affecting postoperative blood loss in children undergoing cardiac surgery. *Journal of Cardiothoracic Surgery.* 2014;9:32-32.

In this retrospective study, the authors hypothesized that the influence of cyanotic disease on postoperative blood loss is closely related to age in children undergoing heart surgery. It is known that hemodilution, surgical, and patient-related risk factors predispose to the development of postoperative coagulopathy in this patient population. This study demonstrated that the presence of cyanotic disease is associated with increased blood loss in children aged 1 to 6 months. The authors also observed that the use of fresh frozen plasma significantly decreased bleeding in children aged <1 month.

Vogt W. Evaluation and optimisation of current milrinone prescribing for the treatment and prevention of low cardiac output syndrome in paediatric patients after open heart surgery using a physiology-based pharmacokinetic drug-disease model. Clin Pharmacokinet 2014; 53: 51-72.

The author developed a physiologically-based pharmacokinetic drug-disease model for milrinone in in children with and without low cardiac output syndrome after open heart surgery. Age, disease and surgery differently impact the pharmacokinetics of milrinone. Current milrinone dosing for low cardiac output syndrome was suboptimal to maintain the therapeutic target range across the entire pediatric age range. The authors proposed dosing regimens to ensure safe and effective prescribing. These still remain rarely used.

Kamra K, Russell I, Miller-Hance WC. Role of transesophageal echocardiography in the management of pediatric patients with congenital heart disease. *Paediatr Anaesth.* 2011;21(5):479-493.

The role of transesophageal echocardiography for congenital heart surgery is reviewed, highlighting its role in routine management of the pediatric cardiac patient population, with a focus on indications, views, applications and technological advances.

Mangano DT, Tudor IC, Dietzel C. The risk associated with aprotinin in cardiac surgery. *N Engl J Med.* 2006;354:353-365.

Mangano and associates reported a large observational study in adult patients undergoing revascularization surgery. They reported an increase in renal failure, myocardial infarction, heart failure, stroke, and encephalopathy. This study has been criticized for not being randomized and subsequent review of data questions findings. These effects have not been shown in children, but created an unease about the use of aprotinin in children. It is important that well-designed, independent, large studies are carried out in children to establish the role and safety of drugs used in adults that are borrowed for pediatric use.

Arnold P. Treatment and monitoring of coagulation abnormalities in children undergoing heart surgery. Pediatr Anesth 2011; 21:494-503.

The author outlines causes and management of coagulaopathy during congenital heart surgery. The role of laboratory and point of care tests, which aim to identify the cause of bleeding in the individual patient, is discussed. An attempt is made to examine the current evidence for available therapies, including use of blood products and, more recently proposed, approaches based on human or recombinant factor concentrates. Although further coagulation factors and substitutes have become available since publication of this paper, their efficacy during cardiac surgery is not yet fully assessed. This paper remains a solid framework for concepts and treatments.

Pasquali SK, Li JS, He X, et al. Comparative analysis of antifibrinolytic medications in pediatric heart surgery. *J Thorac Cardiovasc Surg.* 2012;143:550-557.

An observational study in children concerning aprotinin and demonstrating the usefulness of national data collection. The Society of Thoracic Surgeons Congenital Heart Surgery Database (2004–2008) was linked to medication data from the Pediatric Health Information Systems Database. A total of 22,258 children were included in the study. Aprotinin (vs. no drug) was associated with a reduction in combined hospital mortality/ bleeding requiring surgical intervention overall (odds ratio [OR], 0.81; 95% confidence intervals [CI], 0.68–0.91) and in the redo sternotomy subgroup (OR, 0.57; 95% CI, 0.40–0.80). There was no benefit in neonates and no difference in renal failure requiring dialysis in any group. In comparative analysis, there was no difference in outcome for aprotinin versus aminocaproic acid recipients. Tranexamic acid (vs. aprotinin) was associated with significantly reduced mortality/bleeding requiring surgical intervention overall (OR, 0.47; 95% CI, 0.30–0.74) and in neonates (OR, 0.30; 95% CI, 0.15–0.58). These observational data suggest aprotinin is associated with reduced bleeding and mortality in children undergoing heart surgery with no increase in dialysis. Comparative analyses suggest similar efficacy of aminocaproic acid and improved outcomes associated with tranexamic acid.

Murphy T, Sale SM, Gonzalez Barlatay F, et al. Initial results from an enhanced recovery program for pediatric cardiac surgical patients. Pediatr Anesth 2022;32:647-53.

Enhanced recovery programs are of interest for the perioperative management in children, as is "fast track" management for congenital heart surgery. The authors describe their management approach in a "Level 1" pediatric cardiac surgical center. A total of 89% of patients met the target extubation time of 6 h after administration of protamine. Median postoperative intensive care unit length of stay was 23.5 h (range 15.2-89.5). This represented a 22% reduction in median intensive care unit stay, although the total hospital length of stay remained unchanged. There were 83% of patients who met the target hospital discharge target of the fifth postoperative day. These preliminary results suggest that enhanced recovery pathway implementation for selected pediatric cardiac surgical patients is feasible, with acceptable outcomes.

Williams GD, Ramamoorthy C. Brain monitoring and protection during pediatric cardiac surgery. *Semin Cardiothorac Vasc Anesth.* 2007;11:23-33.

This article reviews brain monitoring modalities available during pediatric cardiac surgery. Its emphasis is on ways of reducing brain injury during cardiopulmonary bypass and deep hypothermic circulatory arrest in children. Neuroprotective strategies are discussed, including selective cerebral perfusion during deep hypothermic circulatory arrest, management of acid-base balance, the degree of hemodilution, blood glucose management, and antiinflammatory therapy.

Zhou G, Feng Z, Xiong H, et al. A combined ultrafiltration strategy during pediatric cardiac surgery: a prospective, randomized, controlled study with clinical outcomes. *J Thorac Cardiovasc Surg.* 2013;27:897-902.

The combined use of ultrafiltration of the prime solution, zero-balance ultrafiltration, and a modified ultrafiltration (MUF) strategy was associated with modest improvements in pulmonary function compared with the combination of conventional and MUF strategies in the early postoperative period, but the principal clinical outcomes are similar.

A complete reference list can be found online at Elsevier eBooks+.

15

Cardiac Physiology and Pharmacology

ANNETTE Y. SCHURE AND JAMES A. DINARDO

Cardiovascular Physiology
Fetal Circulation
Transitional Circulation
Neonatal Cardiovascular System
Pulmonary Vascular Physiology
Incidence and Prevalence of Congenital Heart Disease
Pathophysiologic Classification of Congenital Heart Disease
Shunting
Intercirculatory Mixing
Single Ventricle Physiology
Special Situations
Exercise Physiology in the Child with
Repaired Congenital Heart Disease

Fontan Physiology
Physiology of the Transplanted Heart
Cardiovascular Pharmacology
Rational Use of Vasoactive Drugs
Practical Considerations for the Use of Vasoactive Agents
Vasoactive Drugs
Calcium
Triiodothyronine (Thyroxine)
Calcium-Sensitizing Agents
B-type Natriuretic Peptide and Nesiritide (Natrecor)
β-Blocking Agents
Vasodilators
Antiarrhythmic Agents

THE CARDIOVASCULAR SYSTEM plays a dominant role within the human body: a centrally located "powerhouse" provides oxygen and nutrients via an extensive network of vessels and capillaries throughout the body. All other organ systems depend on its normal development and function. At birth, and especially in the first few hours of life, the heart and the vascular system must adapt to the extrauterine conditions. Prematurity, congenital defects, complications during labor and delivery, and many other factors can prevent or delay the necessary changes and cause significant morbidity.

A thorough understanding of the fetal circulation, the changes at birth, and the age-specific characteristics is important for the safe management of neonates, infants, and especially the growing number of preterm and small-for-gestational-age infants who come to our diagnostic suites and operating rooms. Given the complex embryology and difficult transition from fetal to extrauterine life, it is amazing that more than 90% of neonates are delivered without any special interventions and that congenital heart defects occur in only 7 to 10 of every 1000 live births.[1] (A detailed discussion of the embryologic development is beyond the scope of this chapter; the interested reader is referred to the excellent review by Van Praagh[2] or Langman's medical embryology text.[3])

Congenital heart defects are among the most common birth defects. In the United States, approximately 32,000 infants are born every year with congenital heart disease (CHD); a number require urgent interventions in the catheterization laboratory or surgical procedures during the neonatal period. In addition, CHD is often associated with other, noncardiac anomalies, and many of these children will present for procedures outside the cardiac operating room. Pediatric anesthesiologists must be able to classify and recognize the pathophysiologic effects of CHD on the neonate or infant and the potential impact of anesthesia and surgical manipulations.

With recent advances in surgical techniques, critical care, and anesthesia management, 85% of all infants with CHD are now expected to reach adulthood. Anesthesiologists will increasingly encounter children with "repaired" or "palliated" CHD presenting for noncardiac procedures. Chapter 21 addresses specific long-term problems and anesthetic considerations for various repaired heart defects, but a few conditions deserve additional discussion: the basic changes in the exercise physiology of repaired heart defects, the characteristics of the Fontan physiology after single ventricle palliation, and the altered physiologic responses in the transplanted heart.

Many conditions require pharmacologic support with cardiovascular drugs, some of which can have noteworthy age-specific effects. Pediatric drug dosing is often based on long-standing experience in children with CHD, with unrepaired, repaired, or palliated defects, or extrapolation from adult data rather than clinical pharmacological studies. Understanding the basic pharmacology of the most commonly used cardiovascular drugs and the special considerations for infants and children is essential for successful perioperative care. This chapter will help the pediatric anesthesiologist understand the complexity of the neonatal cardiovascular system, the implications of CHD, basic pharmacologic considerations, and will provide the necessary tools to develop a safe management plan.

Cardiovascular Physiology

FETAL CIRCULATION

In utero, the placental gas exchange provides the fetus with poorly oxygenated blood; the partial pressure of oxygen (PO_2) in the umbilical vein is approximately 30 mm Hg, and in the umbilical arteries it is approximately 16 mm Hg. The fetal lungs are fluid filled and only minimally perfused (10% to 15% of the cardiac output). The normal postnatal circulation is described as a serial circuit: two pumps, the right ventricle (RV) and left ventricle (LV), supporting two distinct resistance systems, the pulmonary and systemic. In contrast, the fetal circulation is best described as a parallel circuit: both ventricles provide systemic blood flow and a variety of fetal shortcuts or connections allow for mixing of oxygenated and deoxygenated blood (Fig. 16.1).[4,5] Oxygenated blood from the placenta returns via the umbilical vein to the portal venous system, where 30% to 50% of the blood flow is shunted across the *ductus venosus* to the inferior vena cava (IVC), bypassing the liver and thereby maintaining higher oxygenation and velocity. The rest of the umbilical venous blood passes through the hepatic microcirculation into the suprahepatic IVC.

The IVC blood entering the right atrium (RA) is a mixture of bloodstreams with different velocities and saturations: the low-velocity, deoxygenated venous return from the lower body and hepatic veins and the high-velocity, oxygenated umbilical venous blood from the ductus venosus. Valve-like tissue in the RA (eustachian valve) and the Chiari network preferentially direct the high-velocity bloodstream from the IVC across the *foramen ovale* into the left atrium (LA), bypassing the RV and pulmonary vessels. In the LA, the oxygenated blood mixes with the minimal amount of venous return from the pulmonary circulation and is then ejected by the LV into the ascending aorta and the major vessels of the aortic arch. This blood, with a maximum

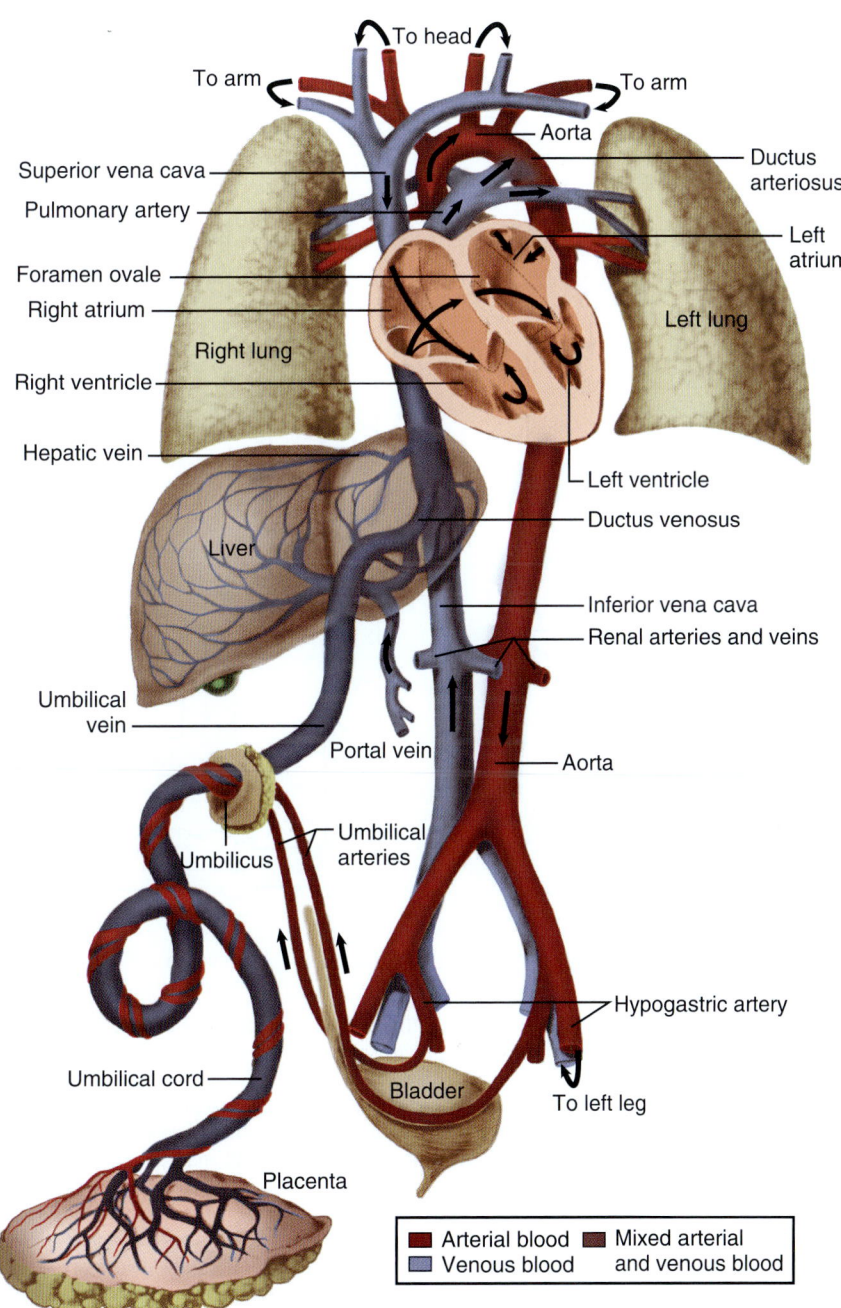

| Arterial blood | Mixed arterial |
| Venous blood | and venous blood |

FIGURE 16.1 Course of the fetal circulation in late gestation. Notice the selective blood flow patterns across the foramen ovale and the ductus arteriosus. (From Greeley WJ, Berkowitz DH, Nathan AT. Anesthesia for pediatric cardiac surgery. In: Miller RD, ed. *Anesthesia*. 7th ed. Philadelphia: Churchill Livingstone; 2010, Fig. 83.1.)

hemoglobin oxygen saturation (SaO$_2$) of 65% to 70%, provides oxygen to the growing heart and brain.

Most of the venous return from the superior vena cava (SVC) and about 20% of the IVC blood flow (mainly the low-velocity, deoxygenated part) reach the RV and are pumped into the pulmonary artery (PA), where the high pulmonary resistance in the nonexpanded lung redirects 90% of the blood flow into the descending aorta via the *ductus arteriosus*. The bulk of the blood flow in the descending aorta is generated by the RV, with minor contributions from the LV. The blood has a saturation of only 55% to 60%; two-thirds of it returns to the placenta for oxygenation, and the rest is distributed to the intestines, kidneys, and lower part of the body (Fig. 16.2).

The fetal circulation supports a growing fetus in a relatively cyanotic atmosphere (SaO$_2$ in utero is 65% to 70%). This difficult task is further complicated by the parallel circuit, which creates increased workload for the RV, and the limitations of the fetal shortcuts,

which add additional volume load by incomplete shunting of oxygenated and deoxygenated blood. Initially, our understanding of the fetal circulation was based mainly on experimental animal data, but recent advances in ultrasound technology have facilitated assessment and monitoring of fetal cardiovascular parameters, especially stroke volume and cardiac output, under various conditions throughout the gestational period. RV stroke volume has been found to increase from about 0.7 mL at 20 weeks to 7.6 mL at 40 weeks, and LV stroke volume increases from 0.7 to 5.2 mL. The combined fetal cardiac output of both ventricles is estimated to be 400 to 425 mL/kg per minute, with an RV dominance because of the increased volume load. At 38 weeks, the RV provides approximately 60% of the combined cardiac output (E-Table 16.1).[6–8] Intrauterine growth restriction and placental compromise are associated with redistribution of cardiac output and relative changes in the size of the foramen ovale.[9] A functional placenta, the fetal cardiovascular high-output state, greater hemoglobin concentrations,

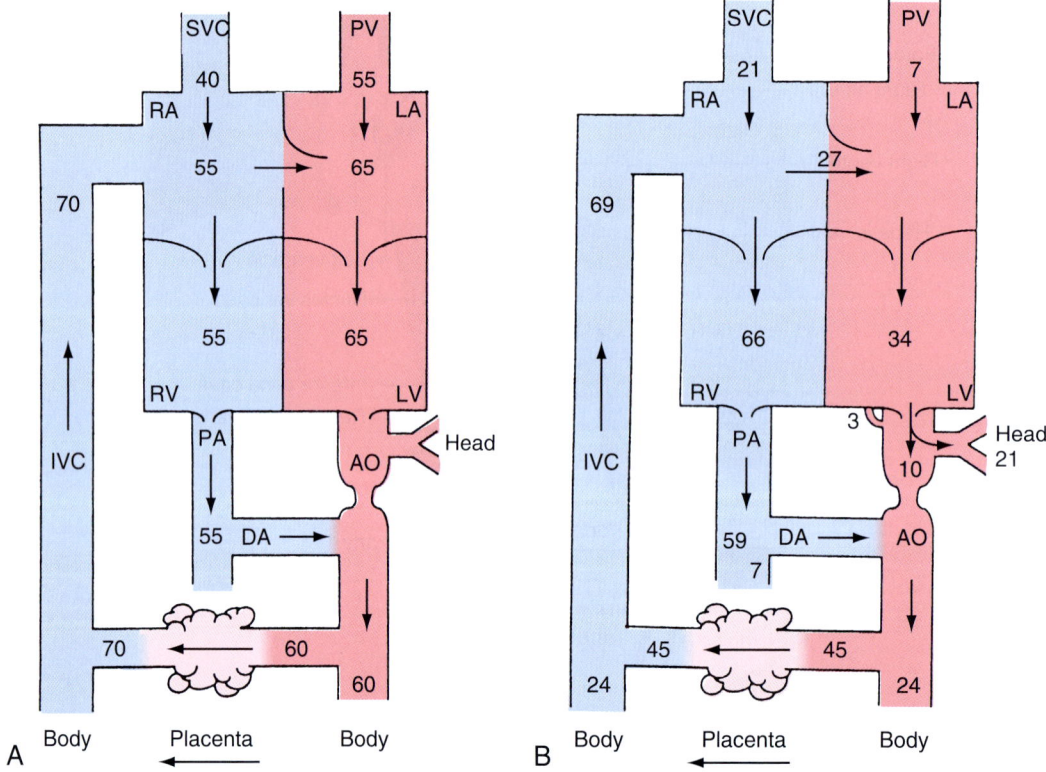

FIGURE 16.2 Fetal circulation in the late-gestation lamb. **A,** The numbers indicate the percentage of oxygen saturation. Oxygen saturation is greatest in the inferior vena cava *(IVC)*, representing flow that is primarily from the placenta. The saturation of the blood in the heart is slightly greater on the left side than on the right side. **B,** The course of the circulation. The numbers represent the percentage of combined ventricular output. Some of the return from the IVC is diverted by the crista dividens in the right atrium *(RA)* through the foramen ovale into the left atrium *(LA)*, where it meets the pulmonary venous return *(PV)*, passes into the left ventricle *(LV)*, and is pumped into the ascending aorta. Most of the ascending aortic flow goes to the coronary, subclavian, and carotid arteries, with only 10% of combined ventricular output passing through the aortic arch (indicated by the narrowed point in the aorta) into the descending aorta *(AO)*. The remainder of the IVC flow mixes with return from the superior vena cava *(SVC)* and coronary veins (3%), passes into the RA and right ventricle *(RV)*, and is pumped into the pulmonary artery *(PA)*. Because of the increased pulmonary resistance, only 7% of the blood passes through the lungs *(PV)*, with the rest passing through the ductus arteriosus *(DA)* to the AO and then to the placenta and lower half of the body. (Modified from Rudolph AM. *Congenital Diseases of the Heart.* Chicago: Year Book Publishers; 1974:1-48; and from Freed MD. Fetal and transitional circulation. In: Fyler DC, ed. *Nadas' Pediatric Cardiology.* Philadelphia: Mosby-Year Book; 1992:57-61.)

and additional alterations in oxygen binding and release (hemoglobin F, increased 2,3-diphosphoglycerate) are all necessary to provide adequate tissue oxygenation for the developing fetus.

Congenital heart disease, even in utero, can compromise other organ function; fetal cardiovascular defects induce intrinsic autoregulatory changes in cerebral perfusion and thereby compromise brain development.[10–12] Ultrasound and magnetic resonance imaging demonstrate that 25% to 40% of neonates with CHD have neurologic abnormalities before any surgical intervention.[13,14]

TRANSITIONAL CIRCULATION

Humoral, biochemical, and physiologic changes occur abruptly at birth. First, the placental circulation is eliminated soon after the lungs expand. Second, the lungs expand to a normal functional residual capacity (FRC) that results in an optimal geometric relationship for the pulmonary microvasculature. Third, air that expands the lungs decreases the alveolar PCO_2 and increases the alveolar PO_2. These three factors act in concert to markedly reduce the pulmonary vascular resistance (PVR).[5,15,16] The net effect is a substantial increase in pulmonary blood flow, which in turn augments pulmonary venous return to the left heart. Along with elimination of the placenta and the low-resistance umbilical circulation, the LV is suddenly subjected to increased volume and afterload (Table 16.1). Typically, LV end-diastolic pressure, and thus LA pressure, increases enough to exert hydrostatic pressure on the septum primum, resulting in functional closure of the foramen ovale. In contrast to the increased stress for the LV, the RV is relatively unloaded by the transition to extrauterine life.

The three fetal connections (ductus arteriosus, ductus venosus, and foramen ovale) close over a variable period after birth. The ductus arteriosus functionally (but not anatomically) closes in 58% of normal full-term infants by day 2 after birth and in 98% by day 4.[17] Although many substances (such as eicosanoids) have been implicated in initiating the ductus to constrict, the increase in arterial oxygen tension[18,19] and reduction in circulating prostaglandins that follow the separation of the placenta are likely the primary triggers of this initial constriction.[20] The response to oxygen is age dependent: term neonates usually demonstrate effective constriction of the smooth muscles in the ductal tissue when exposed to oxygen, whereas preterm infants respond poorly and may require medical (prostaglandin inhibitor) or even surgical therapy if respiratory function is compromised. Additional catecholamine-induced changes in PVR and systemic vascular resistance (SVR) and other substances such as acetylcholine contribute to ductal closure. Within 2 to 3 weeks, functional constriction is followed by a process of ductal fibrosis, leaving a band-like structure, the ligamentum arteriosum.[21,22] With ligation of the umbilical vein, the portal pressure falls, triggering functional closure of the ductus venosus. This process rarely requires more than 1 to 2 weeks; by 3 months only fibrous tissue, the ligamentum venosum, is left.

The foramen ovale is functionally closed when the LA pressure exceeds the RA pressure, but it remains anatomically patent in most infants, in 50% of children younger than 5 years of age, and in 25% to 30% of adults.[23] Echocardiographic studies have confirmed right-to-left shunting via the foramen ovale in healthy infants emerging from general anesthesia, and this can be a significant cause of persistent arterial desaturation at that time despite ventilation with 100% oxygen.[24]

NEONATAL CARDIOVASCULAR SYSTEM

Compared with the adult, the neonatal myocardium is immature and incompletely developed (Table 16.2). Differences in cytoarchitecture and metabolism account for many of the functional limitations. The neonatal heart contains fewer muscle

TABLE 16.1	Hemodynamic Changes at Birth	
Right Ventricle	**Left Ventricle**	
Decreased Afterload:	**Increased Afterload:**	
Decreased pulmonary vascular resistance	Placenta eliminated	
Ductal closure	Ductal closure	
Decreased Volume Load:	**Increased Volume Load:**	
Eliminated umbilical vein return	Increased pulmonary venous return	
Output diminished 25%	Output increased almost 50%	
	Transient left-to-right shunt at ductus	

TABLE 16.2	Characteristic Differences Between the Immature and the Adult Myocardium	
	Immature Myocardium	**Adult Myocardium**
Cytoarchitecture	Fewer mitochondria and SR Poorly formed T tubules Limited contractile elements and increased water content Dependence on extracellular calcium for contractility	Organized mitochondrial rows, abundant SR Well-formed T tubules Increased number of myofibrils with better orientation Rapid release and reuptake of calcium via SR
Metabolism	Carbohydrates and lactate as primary energy sources Increased glycogen stores and anaerobic glycolysis for ATP Decreased nucleotidase activity, retained ATP precursors Better tolerance to ischemia with rapid recovery of function	Free fatty acids as primary source for ATP Limited glycogen stores and glycolytic function Increased 5′-nucleotidase activity, rapid ATP depletion Less tolerance to ischemia
Function	Decreased compliance Limited CO augmentation with increased preload Decreased tolerance to afterload Immature autonomic innervation: parasympathetic dominance, incomplete sympathetic innervation	Normally developed tension Able to improve CO with increased preload and to maintain CO with increasing afterload

ATP, Adenosine triphosphate; *CO*, cardiac output; *SR*, sarcoplasmic reticulum.

Data from Mossad EB, Farid I. Vital organ preservation during surgery for congenital heart disease. In: Lake CL, Booker PD, eds. *Pediatric Cardiac Anesthesia.* 4th ed. Philadelphia: Lippincott, Williams & Wilkins; 2005:266-290; and DiNardo J, Zwara DA. Congenital heart disease. In: DiNardo J, Zwara DA, eds. *Anesthesia for Cardiac Surgery.* 3rd ed. Malden, MA: Blackwell Publishing; 2008:167-251.

cells and more connective tissue than the adult myocardium: contractile elements represent only 30% of the total cardiac mass in the neonate compared with 60% in the adult.[25] The ratio of surface area to mass and water to collagen content are greater in the neonate than the older child. There are fewer myofibrils that are less organized (i.e., not parallel to the long axis of the cell) within the muscle cells. The sarcoplasmic reticulum and the T-tubule network, both important components of rapid and effective calcium regulation, are incompletely developed, and the immature myocardium relies substantially on the calcium flux through the sarcolemma to initiate and terminate contraction.[26–28] One practical consequence of this disorganized and immature myocardium is a greater degree of contractile dysfunction in the infant when exposed to substances that decrease extracellular ionized calcium, such as citrate (blood products) and albumin; there is also increased sensitivity to inhalational anesthetics (due to calcium channel blocking properties) and calcium channel blockers.

Reduced numbers of underdeveloped mitochondria and maturational differences in various signaling pathways and related messenger systems are also characteristic of the neonatal myocardium. Immature mitochondrial enzyme activity for fatty acid transport may explain the primary use of carbohydrates and lactates as energy sources and might be a reason for the greater anaerobic tolerance and faster recovery after periods of ischemia. A variety of developmental changes in contractile proteins occur from fetal through early postnatal life, including changes in pH, calcium sensitivity, and adenosine triphosphate (ATP) hydrolyzing activity. The key features of the immature cardiac function are summarized in Table 16.2.

The increased amount of noncontractile tissue in the neonate decreases ventricular compliance and limits the response to an increased preload. Compliance of both ventricles progressively increases during fetal life and the postnatal period, so that the maximum stroke volume occurs at a lower atrial pressure in the neonate than in the fetus (Figs. 16.3 and 16.4).[29–31] The high metabolic rate of the neonate (oxygen consumption, 6–8 mL/kg per minute, compared with 2–3 mL/kg per minute in the adult) requires a proportional increase in cardiac output. The neonatal heart meets this demand, in part, by a greater heart rate (HR).[32,33] The cardiac output is commonly described as depending primarily on HR owing to a fixed stroke volume, but echocardiographic studies in human fetuses and neonates have demonstrated the capacity to increase stroke volume (Fig. 16.5).[34] To meet metabolic demand, the neonate increases cardiac output using a combination of tachycardia and increases in stroke volume. Alternately, neonates exhibit exquisite sensitivity to pharmacologic agents that produce negative inotropic or chronotropic effects. At birth, the mass of the two ventricles is equal. Increases in pressure in one ventricle shifts the common septum, thus decreasing the compliance of the other ventricle. The net result is that cardiac output is reduced. Neonates and infants often present with biventricular failure as a result of this interventricular dependence.

Immature autonomic regulation of cardiac function persists throughout the neonatal period. Both sympathetic and parasympathetic innervation of the heart is present at birth. However, the sympathetic nervous system is incompletely developed at both the postganglionic nerve-receptor and receptor-effector levels.[35] The sympathetic system reaches maturity by early infancy, whereas the parasympathetic system reaches maturity within a few days after birth.[36] The relative imbalance of these two components of the autonomic nervous system at birth may account

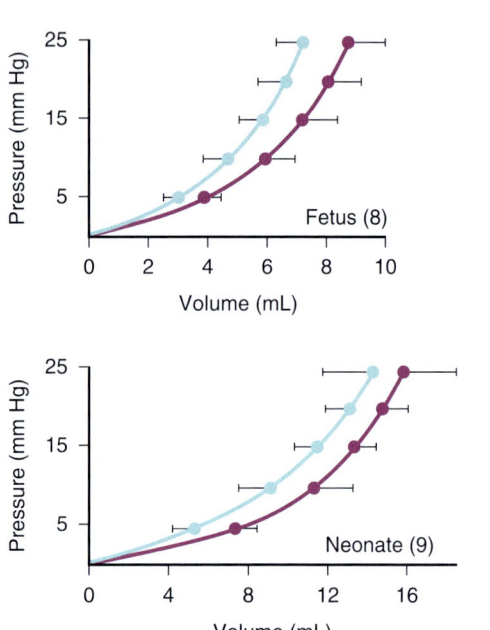

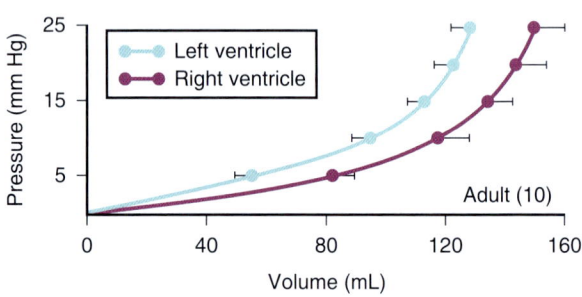

FIGURE 16.3 Comparison of ventricular pressure-volume curves for fetal, neonatal, and adult sheep. Differences between ventricles are significant only in adult sheep. Notice that the right and left ventricles have similar compliance curves in the neonates, making the physiologic relationship between ventricles more intimate (i.e., infants tend to develop biventricular failure). (From Romero T, Covell J, Friedman WF. A comparison of pressure-volume relations of the fetal, newborn and adult heart. *Am J Physiol.* 1972;222:1285-1290.)

for the clinical observation that neonates are predisposed to marked vagal responses to a variety of stimuli.

PULMONARY VASCULAR PHYSIOLOGY

At birth, pulmonary vascular development is incomplete. Lung sections demonstrate a diminished number of arterioles, and the arterioles exhibit thick medial muscularization (Fig. 16.6).[37–39] The pulmonary vasculature matures during the first few years of life. During this period, arterioles proliferate faster than alveoli, and the medial smooth muscle thins and extends more distally in the vascular tree. PVR continues to decrease as long as pulmonary mechanics and alveolar gas composition remain favorable, with an important decrease occurring immediately after birth as the result of lung expansion and oxygenation. Progressive remodeling of the pulmonary vasculature facilitates further decreases in PVR (assuming normal physiology) during the first 2 to 3 months of life; by 6 months of age, the PVR has almost reached adult levels.[39]

The fetal pulmonary vasculature is extremely reactive to a number of stimuli. Hypoxia, acidosis, increased levels of leukotrienes, and mechanical stimulation (e.g., coughing on an endotracheal

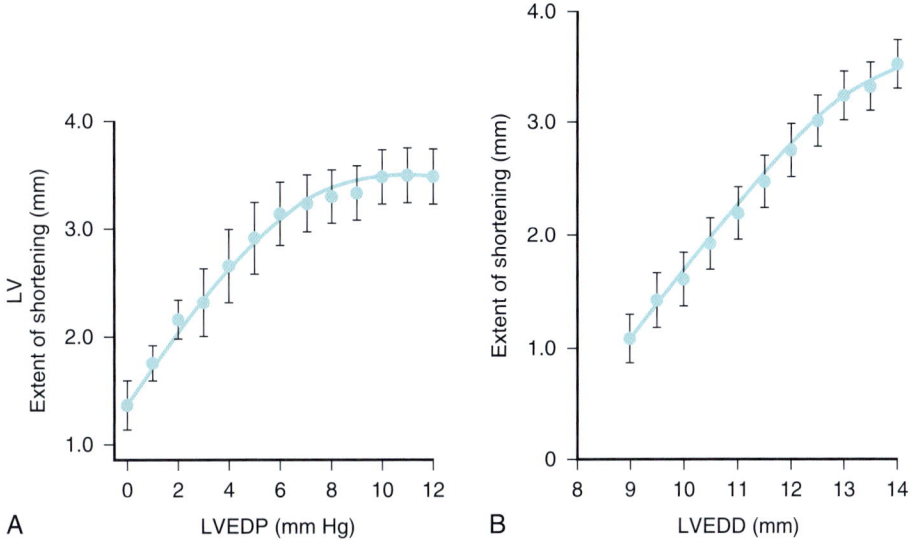

FIGURE 16.4 Frank-Starling relationship in fetal lamb model (gestational age, 135 ± 5 days). **A,** The relationship between left ventricular end-diastolic pressure *(LVEDP)* and shortening in a chronically instrumented fetal lamb model. Although myocardial performance improves with increasing LVEDP, the effect achieves a plateau at 10 mm Hg. **B,** In the same model, the relationship between left ventricular end-diastolic diameter *(LVEDD)* and left ventricular shortening. Taken together, these experiments support the capacity, albeit blunted, of the fetal heart to change stroke volume based on volume loading conditions. Each point and vertical bars represent mean ± standard error. (From Kirkpatrick SE, Pitlick PT, Naliboff J, et al. Frank-Starling relationship as an important determinant of fetal cardiac output. *Am J Physiol.* 1976;231:495-500.)

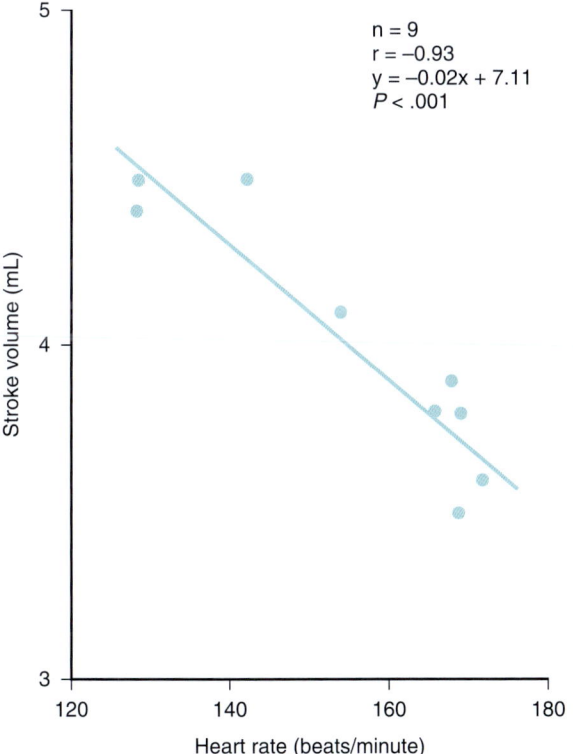

FIGURE 16.5 Doppler echocardiographic comparison of the effect of spontaneous changes in heart rate on stroke volume in a normal human fetus in utero, illustrating decreased stroke volume with increased heart rate. These observations confirm the ability of the fetal heart to change stroke volume under normal physiologic conditions. (From Kenny J, Plappert T, Doubilet P, et al. Effects of heart rate on ventricular size, stroke volume, and output in the normal human fetus: a prospective Doppler echocardiographic study. *Circulation.* 1987;76:52-58.)

tube) can increase PVR (e.g., reactive pulmonary hypertension) for prolonged periods. Alternately, acetylcholine, histamine, bradykinin, prostaglandins, β-adrenergic catecholamines, and nitric oxide (NO) are strong vasodilators.[40] In the first days after birth, many pathophysiologic conditions can trigger severe and sustained increases in PVR[41,42] and prevent the normal adjustment to extrauterine life (E-Table 16.2). The acute load this imposes on the RV may cause diastolic dysfunction and shunt blood right-to-left via the foramen ovale. Once PVR exceeds the SVR, a right-to-left shunt develops through both the ductus arteriosus and the foramen ovale. This situation is called *persistent fetal circulation,*[43] and it can result in a life-threatening hypoxemia that may require inhaled NO,[44–48] sildenafil,[49] and/or extracorporeal support (i.e., extracorporeal membrane oxygenation)[50,51] (see Chapter 19) to provide adequate oxygenation and sustain life.

Pulmonary arterial hypertension is associated with structural changes in the pulmonary vasculature after prolonged exposure to increased pressures and flow patterns in utero and postnatally. Lung biopsies demonstrate thickened muscle layers in the small pulmonary arteries, intimal hyperplasia, scarring, and thrombosis as well as a decreased number of distal (intra-acinar) arteries.[38] Over time, these changes progress and ultimately irreversibly obstruct pulmonary blood flow with increases in PVR and PA pressures. The very muscularized pulmonary arteries are also extremely sensitive to pulmonary vasoconstrictors, which can easily trigger a pulmonary hypertensive crisis.

Many cardiac defects are associated with abnormal pulmonary flow patterns and can be categorized into three basic groups:

- *Exposure of the pulmonary vasculature to systemic arterial pressures and high flow:* The classic example is a large, nonrestrictive ventricular septal defect (VSD) with rapid progression of pulmonary vascular obstructive disease (PVOD).
- *Exposure of the pulmonary vasculature to high flow without increased pressure:* Large atrial septal defects (ASDs) and small,

Alveoli to Artery Ratio

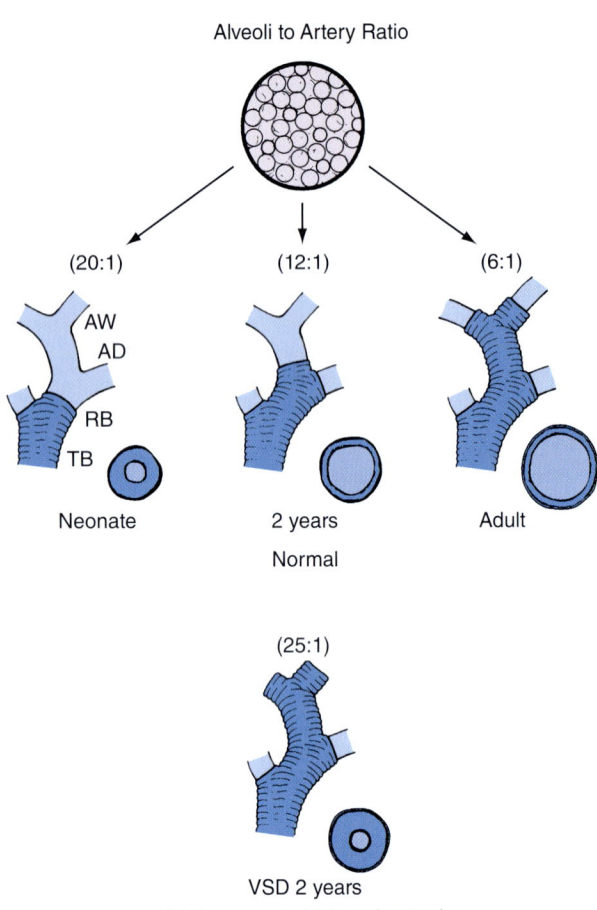

VSD 2 years
(high pressure, high resistance)

FIGURE 16.6 Peripheral pulmonary artery development. The normal pattern of pulmonary vascular development and that of a 2-year-old child with pulmonary vascular changes accompanying a large ventricular septal defect *(VSD)*. Rabinovitch and colleagues characterized the pulmonary vasculature morphometrically in three respects: vessel thickness, muscular extension, and the ratio of alveoli to arteries seen on lung biopsy specimens. The normal neonate exhibits thick vascular smooth muscle, but this extends only as far as the arterioles accompanying the respiratory bronchiole. In neonates, the alveoli/artery ratio is 20:1. In the first few months of life, the vessels thin substantially and proliferate relative to the alveoli, so that by the age of 2 years, the normal child has an alveoli/artery ratio of 12:1 and thin muscles extending to the arteries associated with alveolar ducts. In the normal adult, the alveoli/artery ratio is 6:1 and muscle extends all the way to the arteries in the alveolar wall. In contrast, in the 2-year-old child with a large VSD, the vessel numbers are markedly diminished (alveoli/artery ratio, 25:1), and persistent neonatal muscle thickness extends all the way to the alveolar wall. *AD,* Artery at alveolar duct; *AW,* artery at alveolar wall; *RB,* respiratory bronchiole; *TB,* artery at terminal bronchiole. (From Steven JM, Nicolson SC. Congenital heart disease. In: Miller RD, series editor. *Atlas of Anesthesia.* Vol 7. In: Greeley WJ, volume editor. *Pediatric Anesthesia* Orlando, FL: Harcourt Publishers; 1998:6.6; modified from Rabinovitch M, Haworth SG, Castaneda AR, et al. Lung biopsy in congenital heart disease: a morphometric approach to pulmonary vascular disease. *Circulation.* 1978;58:1107-1122.)

restrictive patent ductus arteriosus (PDA) defects are in this category. PVOD develops much more slowly in this setting.

- *Obstruction of pulmonary venous drainage resulting in increased PA pressures:* Pulmonary vein stenosis (e.g., total anomalous pulmonary venous return [TAPVR], cor triatrium) or increased LA pressures (e.g., mitral atresia, congenital aortic stenosis, severe coarctation) can cause backpressure in the pulmonary vasculature and induce PVOD.

TABLE 16.3 | Manipulations of Pulmonary Vascular Resistance

Increasing PVR	Decreasing PVR
PEEP	No PEEP
High airway pressures	Low airway pressures
Atelectasis	Lung expansion to FRC
Low FiO_2	High FiO_2
Respiratory and metabolic acidosis	Respiratory and metabolic alkalosis
Increased hematocrit	Low hematocrit
Sympathetic stimulation	Blunted stress response (deep anesthesia)
Direct surgical manipulation	Nitric oxide
Vasoconstrictors: phenylephrine	Vasodilators: milrinone, prostacyclin, others

FiO_2, Fraction of inspired oxygen; *FRC,* functional residual capacity; *PEEP,* positive end-expiratory pressure; *PVR,* pulmonary vascular resistance.

The muscle tone in the pulmonary arteries is regulated by numerous factors. Several therapeutic interventions can influence the PVR (Table 16.3)[16]:

- *Arterial oxygen tension (PaO_2):* Alveolar as well as arterial hypoxia increases PVR. A PaO_2 value less than 50 mm Hg, especially when associated with an acidic pH (<7.4), leads to significant pulmonary vasoconstriction. On the other hand, increased inspired oxygen can lead to pulmonary vasodilation and overcirculation.
- *Arterial carbon dioxide tension ($PaCO_2$):* Hypercapnia increases PVR, independent of the blood pH. In contrast, hypocapnia induces an alkalosis and decreases PVR. Reliable pulmonary vasodilation can be achieved with a $PaCO_2$ of 20 to 33 mm Hg and a pH of 7.5 to 7.6.
- *pH:* Respiratory and metabolic acidosis increase PVR; alkalosis reduces PVR.
- *Lung volumes:* PVR is optimized at a lung volume close to the FRC; larger volumes compress small intraalveolar vessels, and smaller volumes can cause atelectasis and vascular collapse.
- *Stimulation of the sympathetic nervous system:* Catecholamine surges from stress, pain, or light anesthesia can trigger significant increases in PVR.
- *Vasodilators:* Most intravenous (IV) agents used for pulmonary vasodilation also affect the systemic circulation and induce hypotension. Alternatively, inhaled substances such as NO or prostacyclin can provide a more selective pulmonary vasodilation (see the section on "Cardiovascular Pharmacology").

The pulmonary vasculature undergoes a complex maturation process that can be influenced by a multitude of external factors and congenital heart defects. Persistent fetal circulation and PVOD are examples of inadequate adaptation and development. If PVR increases, ventilator strategies including greater concentrations of inspired oxygen, lung volumes close to the FRC, and interventions that target a PaO_2 greater than 60 mm Hg, a $PaCO_2$ of 30 to 35 mm Hg, and a pH of 7.5 to 7.6 can all increase pulmonary blood flow.

Incidence and Prevalence of Congenital Heart Disease

CHD can be defined as *"a gross structural abnormality of the heart or intrathoracic great vessels that is actually or potentially of functional significance."*[52] This definition covers a wide array of defects, which are among the most common congenital malformations. However, the precise incidence of CHD, both collectively and by individual anatomic subset, varies depending on definition, method of case identification, and epoch (E-Table 16.3). Including all categories of CHD, large epidemiologic surveys place the prevalence between 4 and 50 cases per 1000 live births.[53–56] When stratified according to trivial, moderate, and severe forms, the incidence for moderate and severe forms of CHD has been relatively consistent, at about 6 per 1000 live births.

The incidence of anatomic diagnoses in infants with CHD vary according to the methodology used to identify cases. In 2002, Hoffman and Kaplan compiled 62 epidemiologic studies published since 1955 and investigated the potential causes for the wide variability in the incidence of CHD.[57] Subsequent studies based mainly on prenatal and postnatal echocardiographic screening data often include a large number of trivial lesions (e.g., tiny VSDs, nonstenotic bicuspid aortic valve, "silent" PDA) for which no interventions were required. Other data collections, such as the New England Regional Infant Cardiac Program (NERICP), a registry of children with CHD who died or required catheterization or surgery during the first year of life, were biased toward more severe forms of CHD.[1] Inclusion criteria based on the incidence of VSDs, the severity of the cardiac defects, and when the defects were first diagnosed, explain the variability in the frequency of CHD in infants in the literature but also confirm a lack of variability in their incidence among countries or over time.

The increasing availability of prenatal diagnostic methods may influence the relative prevalence of reported lesions as well as their outcome. When fetal echocardiography is used, the apparent shift toward more complex lesions may reflect technical limitations in identifying simple defects.[58] In addition, evaluation in utero skews the results because it includes fatally malformed fetuses that will not survive to term. The prevalence of CHD among spontaneous abortions reaches 20% and remains as large as 10% among stillborn infants.[55] In one study, 50% of women whose children were given a prenatal diagnosis of CHD elected to terminate the pregnancy, particularly when presented with complex heart lesions.[58]

On the other hand, female infants with severe CHD have a mortality rate that is 5% less than similarly affected male infants,[1] and with increased survival rates, more females will reach childbearing age, where they continue to have reduced mortality.[59] The recurrence risk of CHD for their offspring is about 3% to 4%.[60,61]

A study from Canada examined the changing epidemiology of CHD with respect to prevalence and age distribution in the general population between 1983 and 2010.[62] The prevalence of all categories of CHD in 2010 was ~13 per 1000 in children (<18 years of age) and ~6 per 1000 in adults. For the subcategory of severe CHD, the prevalence was ~1.8 per 1000 in children and ~0.62 per 1000 in adults. In 2010, 60% of all patients with severe CHD were adults, compared with 49% in 2000 and 35% in 1985. Between 1983 and 2010 the prevalence of CHD has been steadily increasing for both children and adults but at a different pace: from 1985 to 2000 the increase for severe CHD was 85% in adults and 22% in children compared with 57% for adults and 11% for children from 2000 to 2010. The median age of all patients with severe CHD was 11 years in 1985, 17 years in 2000 and 25 years in 2010, reflecting the fact that more children with CHD were surviving to adulthood (E-Fig. 16.1). Improved survival may be attributed to improved prenatal care, early diagnostic imaging, and major advances in pediatric cardiac care, particularly for those with severe CHD; these improved outcomes will continue to influence the future demographic profile. The growing number of adolescents and adults with CHD will require long-term follow-up with experienced cardiologists and access to specialized care facilities; this will require a thorough understanding of their underlying pathophysiology by all members of the adult care team, including anesthesiologists.[63]

Pathophysiologic Classification of Congenital Heart Disease

CHD consists of an almost endless array of anatomic and functional variants. Many different classification systems have been introduced, some using a segmental approach to anatomic features, others by examining the amount of pulmonary blood flow (cyanotic versus acyanotic) or the common physiologic characteristics (e.g., volume versus pressure overload).[64–74] Several of these classifications are discussed in Chapter 14. However, certain defects are better described using the concepts of shunting (physiologic, anatomic, simple, or complex), intercirculatory mixing, and single ventricle physiology, which are presented in the following sections.

SHUNTING

Shunting occurs when the blood return from one circulatory system (systemic or pulmonary) is recirculated to the same system, completely bypassing the other circulation. For example, if deoxygenated blood from the systemic veins flows directly to the aorta, the result is a right-to-left shunt with recirculation of deoxygenated blood in the systemic circulation. In contrast, redirection of oxygenated blood from the pulmonary veins to the PA causes a left-to-right shunt with recirculation of oxygenated blood within the pulmonary circulation. The terms *physiologic* and *anatomic* are often used to describe shunting. Basically, any kind of recirculation of blood within one circulatory system is called *physiologic shunting*. In most cases, physiologic shunting is caused by an anatomic shunt (i.e., a communication between the cardiac chambers or the great vessels), but physiologic shunting can also exist by itself, as in the classic transposition physiology.

To really understand the pathophysiology of shunting and its implications, it is important to introduce the concepts of effective and total systemic/pulmonary blood flows. *Effective blood flow* is the quantity of venous blood from one circulatory system that reaches the arterial system of the other circulatory system. Effective *pulmonary* blood flow is the volume of systemic venous blood reaching the pulmonary circulation, whereas effective *systemic* blood flow is the volume of pulmonary venous blood reaching the systemic circulation. Effective pulmonary blood flow and effective systemic blood flow are always equal, no matter how complex the lesions. *Total blood flow*, on the other hand, is the sum of recirculated and effective blood flow and a measure of the workload of the circulatory system. Total systemic and pulmonary blood flows are not equal. Even in healthy patients there is a small amount of normal physiologic shunting (e.g., thebesian cardiac veins, bronchial vessels), but with CHD the difference can be quite substantial. Physiologic shunting or recirculation should be viewed as a noneffective, superfluous load added to the essential nutritive blood flow (effective blood flow).

Anatomic shunts are communications between the two circulatory systems, either within the heart or at the level of the great vessels. They can be divided into simple and complex shunts, depending on the presence of additional outflow obstructions. In *simple shunts* without any additional outflow obstruction, the size of the communication (the so-called shunt orifice) determines the flow characteristics. For small orifices (restrictive shunts) with large pressure gradients across the communication, the size of the opening essentially regulates the amount of shunting. Changes in SVR or PVR have little influence. In contrast, for large orifices or nonrestrictive shunts (also classified as *dependent shunts*), the quantity and direction of blood flow are controlled by the respective outflow resistances (i.e., the ratio of SVR to PVR) (Table 16.4 and Fig. 16.7).

Complex shunts are defined by an additional outflow obstruction, which can be at various levels within the ventricle, valves, or great vessels and is often described as subvalvular, valvular, or supravalvular. These obstructions can be fixed (e.g., valvular stenosis) or variable (e.g., dynamic infundibular obstruction by muscle bundles). Shunt flow and direction are determined by the combined resistance across the outflow obstruction and the pulmonary/systemic vascular beds. For severe obstructions downstream, SVR or PVR will have little influence on the shunt. Tetralogy of Fallot (TOF) is a good example of a complex shunt lesion. The amount of right-to-left shunt and therefore the amount of cyanosis are influenced by the degree and type of right ventricular outflow tract obstruction. This is especially evident in the setting of a dynamic infundibular obstruction, where changes in preload, contractility, and HR can lead to significant decreases in pulmonary blood flow and increased shunting (Table 16.5).

INTERCIRCULATORY MIXING

The concept of intercirculatory mixing is often used to explain the unique physiology in children with transposition of the great arteries (TGA). In this cardiac defect, the aorta arises from the RV, transporting deoxygenated blood back to the right heart, and the PA originates from the LV, returning oxygenated blood to the

TABLE 16.4	Characteristics of Simple Shunts (Without Additional Outflow Obstruction)	
	Restrictive (Small Shunt Orifice)	**Nonrestrictive (Large Shunt Orifice)**
Examples	Small ASD, VSD, or PDA; modified Blalock-Taussig shunt	Large VSD, PDA, CAVC
Pressure gradient across shunt	Large	Small or none
Direction and magnitude of shunt	Independent of PVR/SVR	PVR/SVR dependent
Influence of pharmacologic and ventilatory interventions	Minimal	Large

ASD, Atrial septal defect; *CAVC*, common atrioventricular canal; *PDA*, patent ductus arteriosus; *PVR*, pulmonary vascular resistance; *SVR*, systemic vascular resistance; *VSD*, ventricular septal defect.
Modified from DiNardo J, Zwara DA. Congenital heart disease. In: DiNardo J, Zwara DA, eds. *Anesthesia for Cardiac Surgery*. 3rd ed. Malden, MA: Blackwell Publishing; 2008:167-251.

pulmonary circulation (see Fig. 15.6). Unless there is some mixing of blood via an ASD, VSD, or PDA, this defect will result in a complete separation of the two systems, a parallel circulation with 100% physiologic shunting, or recirculation of oxygenated and deoxygenated blood that is incompatible with life once the fetal ductus arteriosus has closed. Effective pulmonary blood flow (i.e., deoxygenated blood reaching the pulmonary vascular bed for

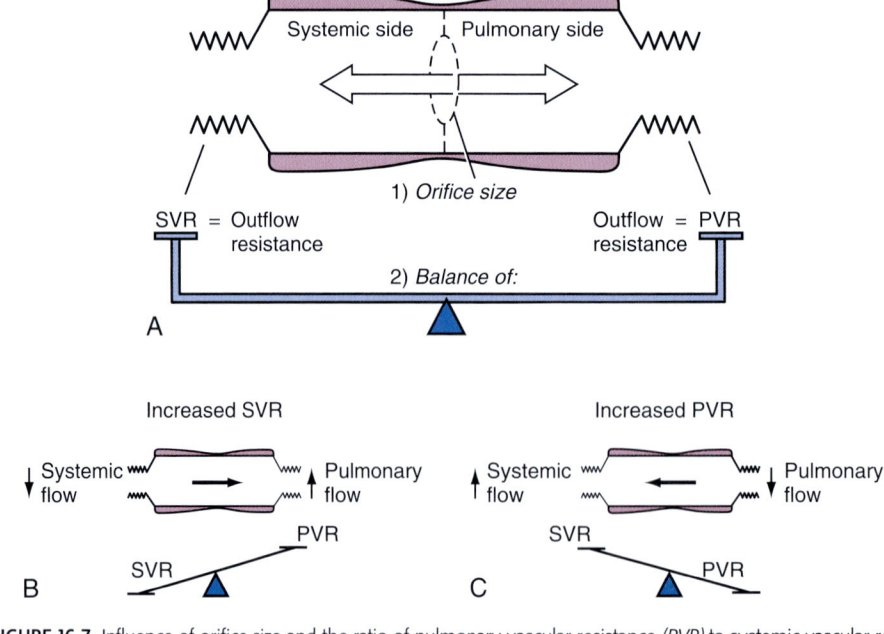

FIGURE 16.7 Influence of orifice size and the ratio of pulmonary vascular resistance *(PVR)* to systemic vascular resistance *(SVR)* on the magnitude and direction of a simple shunt. **A,** PVR and SVR are balanced, resulting in equal pulmonary and systemic blood flows. **B,** PVR is reduced relative to SVR, resulting in an increase in pulmonary blood flow and a decrease in systemic blood flow. **C,** PVR is elevated relative to SVR, resulting in a decrease in pulmonary blood flow and an increase in systemic blood flow. (Modified from DiNardo J, Zwara DA. Congenital heart disease. In: DiNardo J, Zwara DA, eds. *Anesthesia for Cardiac Surgery*. 3rd ed. Malden, MA: Blackwell Publishing; 2008:167-251.)

TABLE 16.5	Characteristics of Complex Shunts (With Additional Outflow Obstruction)	
	Partial Outflow Obstruction	**Complete Outflow Obstruction**
Examples	TOF, VSD/PS, VSD/coarctation	Tricuspid or mitral atresia, Pulmonary or aortic atresia
Shunt magnitude and direction	Relatively fixed	Totally fixed
Dependence on PVR/SVR ratio	Inversely related to obstruction	Independent
Pressure gradient across shunt	Dependent on shunt orifice and degree of obstruction	Dependent only on shunt orifice

PS, Pulmonary stenosis; *PVR,* pulmonary vascular resistance; *SVR,* systemic vascular resistance; *TOF,* tetralogy of Fallot; *VSD,* ventricular septal defect.
Modified from DiNardo J, Zwara DA. Congenital heart disease. In: DiNardo J, Zwara DA, eds. *Anesthesia for Cardiac Surgery.* 3rd ed. Malden, MA: Blackwell Publishing; 2008:167-251.

and pulmonary total blood flows consists of recirculated blood (Fig. 16.8). Usually the total blood flow and the volume in the pulmonary system are two to three times greater than in the systemic circulation.

The arterial saturation (SaO_2) is influenced by the volumes and saturations of recirculating and effective systemic blood flows and can be calculated using the equation:

$$\text{Aortic saturation} = [(\text{Systemic venous saturation} \times \text{Recirculated blood flow}) + (\text{Pulmonary venous saturation} \times \text{Effective blood flow})] \div [\text{Total systemic venous blood flow}$$

Increasing the intercirculatory mixing will improve the arterial saturations, and in severely cyanotic neonates with TGA, intact ventricular septum, and inadequate atrial communication, a balloon atrial septostomy (balloon dilation of an existing patent foramen ovale or small ASD, either echo-guided at the bedside or under fluoroscopy in the catheterization laboratory) can be lifesaving. Additional measures to improve systemic and pulmonary venous saturations (e.g., blood transfusion, inotropic support, ventilatory strategies) can help to stabilize the arterial saturation.

oxygenation) must be provided by some form of right-to-left shunt; effective systemic blood flow (i.e., oxygenated blood returning to the systemic circulation) must be achieved by a left-to-right shunt. Intercirculatory mixing is the combined systemic and pulmonary effective blood flow and is only a small portion of the total blood flow. The bulk of the respective systemic

SINGLE VENTRICLE PHYSIOLOGY

Single ventricle physiology defines the circulation present in a wide variety of complex cardiac defects. It is characterized by complete mixing of systemic and pulmonary venous blood return at either the atrial or the ventricular level; the mixed blood is then distributed to both systemic and pulmonary circulations in parallel. The

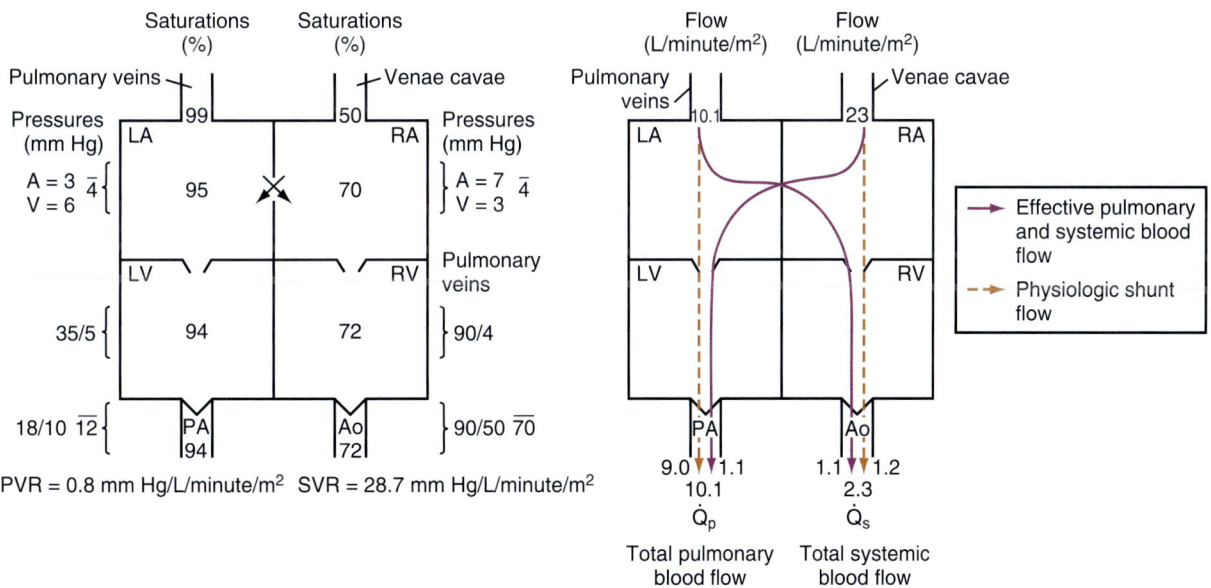

FIGURE 16.8 Saturations, pressures, and blood flows in transposition of the great arteries with a nonrestrictive atrial septal defect and a small left ventricular *(LV)* outflow tract gradient. Intercirculatory mixing occurs at the atrial level. Effective pulmonary and effective systemic blood flows are equal (1.1 L/minute per m²) and are the result of a bidirectional anatomic shunt at the atrial level. The physiologic left-to-right shunt is 9.0 L/minute per m²; this represents blood recirculated from the pulmonary veins to the pulmonary artery *(PA)*. The physiologic right-to-left shunt is 1.2 L/minute per m²; this represents blood recirculated from the systemic veins to the aorta *(Ao)*. Total pulmonary blood flow $(\dot{Q}_P = 10.1$ L/minute per m²) is almost five times greater than the total systemic blood flow $(\dot{Q}_S = 2.3$ L/minute per m²). The bulk of pulmonary blood flow is recirculated pulmonary venous blood. In this depiction, pulmonary vascular resistance *(PVR)* is low (approximately 1/35 of systemic vascular resistance [*SVR*]) and there is a small (17 mm Hg peak to peak) gradient from the LV to the PA. These findings are compatible with the high pulmonary blood flow depicted. *LA,* Left atrium; *RA,* right atrium; *RV,* right ventricle. (From DiNardo J, Zwara DA. Congenital heart disease. In: DiNardo J, Zwara DA, eds. *Anesthesia for Cardiac Surgery.* 3rd ed. Malden, MA: Blackwell Publishing; 2008:167-251.)

defects can consist of one anatomic single ventricle with severe hypoplasia and inflow or outflow obstruction of the other one (hypoplastic left heart syndrome [HLHS] or pulmonary atresia with intact ventricular septum) or even two well-developed ventricles with atresia of the outflow tract or severe obstruction (TOF with pulmonary atresia, interrupted aortic arch). In some lesions, a PDA is the only source of systemic or pulmonary blood flow; these are called duct-dependent circulations. In others, intracardiac communications provide adequate blood flow to both circulations (Table 16.6).

Irrespective of the anatomic features, in single ventricle physiology the ventricular output (delivered by one or two ventricles) is the sum of the pulmonary and systemic blood flows. The distribution of the respective flows depends on the relative outflow resistances into the two parallel circulations. Oxygen saturations in the aorta and PA are equal. The severity and location of anatomic obstructions and the ratio of PVR to SVR determine the balance of flows to the two circulations.

The following equation illustrates the factors that influence the arterial saturation (SaO_2) in a single ventricle physiology:

Aortic blood saturation = [(Systemic venous saturation × Total systemic venous blood flow) + (Pulmonary venous saturation × Total pulmonary venous blood flow)] ÷ [Total systemic venous blood flow + Total pulmonary venous blood flow)]

Accordingly, three major variables determine arterial saturation and the initial management options for patients with single ventricle physiology:

- *The ratio of pulmonary to systemic blood flow ($\dot{Q}_{pulm}/\dot{Q}_{sys}$)*. With high $\dot{Q}_{pulm}/\dot{Q}_{sys}$, a greater percentage of the blood in the ventricle (or ventricles) is oxygenated because more fully saturated pulmonary venous blood is entering the heart to mix with

desaturated systemic venous return. Saturations greater than 85% can be achieved only by significant pulmonary overcirculation. $\dot{Q}_{pulm}/\dot{Q}_{sys}$ can be influenced by careful manipulations of the PVR/SVR ratio.

- *Systemic venous saturation ($S_{sys}vO_2$)*: For a given $\dot{Q}_{pulm}/\dot{Q}_{sys}$ and pulmonary venous saturation ($S_{pulm}vO_2$), any decrease in $S_{sys}vO_2$ causes a decrease in arterial saturation. Oxygen delivery and consumption are the basic determinants for SvO_2. Adequate oxygen delivery depends on cardiac output and arterial oxygen content and thus on hemoglobin levels and arterial saturation. All measures that increase oxygen delivery (e.g., transfusion to increase the hematocrit to 0.45–0.50) or decrease oxygen consumption (e.g., adequate analgesia and sedation during painful procedures) improve arterial saturations.

- *Pulmonary venous saturation ($S_{pulm}vO_2$)*: Normally the blood in the pulmonary veins should be fully saturated ($S_{pulm}vO_2 = 100\%$) on room air, but lung disease, $\dot{V}/\dot{Q}$ mismatch, or large intrapulmonary shunts can cause pulmonary venous desaturation. $\dot{V}/\dot{Q}$ mismatch usually responds to therapy with increased inspired oxygen, whereas intrapulmonary shunts are refractory to oxygen therapy. Pulmonary venous desaturation will decrease arterial saturations.

Special Situations

EXERCISE PHYSIOLOGY IN THE CHILD WITH REPAIRED CONGENITAL HEART DISEASE

Children with CHD, including those with lesions considered repaired, exhibit an array of abnormalities elicited during exercise testing consistent with reduced exercise capacity (E-Table 16.4). It is worthwhile reviewing the possible abnormalities in exercise testing to understand the limitations imposed by the presence of congenital heart lesions.

Oxygen consumption ($\dot{V}O_2$) is equal to the product of cardiac output and O_2 extraction. O_2 extraction is equal to the arterial-venous oxygen content difference. Peak $\dot{V}O_2$ is the greatest measure of $\dot{V}O_2$ obtained during a progressively more difficult exercise test. $\dot{V}O_2$ at rest is defined as 1 metabolic equivalent energy expenditure unit or 1 MET (approximately 3.5 mL O_2/kg per minute).[75] A typical elite endurance athlete can reach 20 to 22 METs, or 70 to 77 mL O_2/kg per minute, at peak exercise. Activities of daily living require at least 4 METs or 14 mL O_2/kg per minute. Peak $\dot{V}O_2$ is the best overall assessment of the capabilities of the cardiovascular system, but determination of normal values is difficult owing to the effects of age, gender, effort, and body composition (e.g., adipose tissue) on peak $\dot{V}O_2$. Nonetheless, peak $\dot{V}O_2$ is a reliable predictor of hospitalization and mortality in patients with a wide variety of congenital heart lesions.[76]

During exercise, the HR normally increases with increases in $\dot{V}O_2$. Maximum HR used in clinical exercise testing has been defined (in beats per minute [beats/minute]) as 220-age (years), although the evidence behind creating the formula was generally flawed.[77] Two subsequent studies reported relationships that yielded greater maximum HR values particularly in the elderly,[78,79] although some advocate discarding age-predicted maximal heart rate norms in favor of alternative age-specific metrics to be determined.[80] In children with chronotropic incompetence, which is defined as the inability to increase HR to greater than 80% of the predicted value at peak exercise, the relationship between HR and $\dot{V}O_2$ is depressed. Chronotropic incompetence is an indicator of poor prognosis and is most commonly the result of sinus node dysfunction. By comparison, well-trained endurance athletes have

TABLE 16.6	Examples of Single Ventricle Physiology	
Congenital Heart Defect	Aortic Blood Flow From	Pulmonary Blood Flow From
Hypoplastic left heart syndrome	PDA	RV
Neonatal critical aortic stenosis	PDA	RV
Interrupted aortic arch	Proximal LV, distal PDA	RV
Tetralogy of Fallot with pulmonary atresia	LV	PDA, MAPCAs
Pulmonary atresia with intact septum	LV	PDA
Tricuspid atresia 1B (VSD and PS)	LV	LV through VSD to RV
Truncus arteriosus	LV and RV	Aorta
Double-inlet left ventricle, no TGA	LV	LV through VSD to bulboventricular foramen

LV, Left ventricle; *MAPCAs*, major aortopulmonary collateral arteries; *PDA*, patent ductus arteriosus; *PS*, pulmonary stenosis; *RV*, right ventricle; *TGA*, transposition of the great arteries; *VSD*, ventricular septal defect.
Modified from DiNardo J, Zwara DA. Congenital heart disease. In: DiNardo J, Zwara DA, eds. *Anesthesia for Cardiac Surgery*. 3rd ed. Malden, MA: Blackwell Publishing; 2008:167-251.

a normal peak HR and a depressed HR/$\dot{V}O_2$ relationship, because they can generate a larger-than-normal stroke volume increase as exercise progresses. The inability to increase stroke volume (discussed later in the chapter) during exercise results in an increased HR/$\dot{V}O_2$ relationship as a compensatory mechanism.

The *oxygen pulse* is the quantity of oxygen delivered per heartbeat. The peak O_2 pulse is calculated by dividing the peak $\dot{V}O_2$ by the peak HR. Because peak $\dot{V}O_2$ = cardiac output × O_2 extraction and because O_2 extraction remains remarkably constant over a wide range of exercise, O_2 pulse is proportional to stroke volume. Determination of normal peak O_2 pulse is hampered by the same factors that confound determination of normal peak $\dot{V}O_2$. In addition, O_2 pulse overestimates stroke volume in the presence of erythrocytosis and underestimates it in the presence of anemia or reduced arterial O_2 saturation. O_2 pulse is reduced in patients with impaired ventricular function, severe valvular regurgitation, or pulmonary vascular disease.[76] It is also uniformly reduced in those with Fontan physiology as a consequence of the inability of this circulation to augment systemic ventricular preload during exercise.[81]

The *respiratory exchange ratio* (RER) is defined as the ratio $\dot{V}CO_2/\dot{V}O_2$ (ratio of the volume of CO_2 produced per minute to the volume of oxygen consumed per minute). A normal resting RER is between 0.67 and 1.0, depending on the precise composition of protein, carbohydrates, and fat in the diet. As exercise intensifies, anaerobic metabolism commences and the lactate threshold is reached; buffering of lactic acid with bicarbonate causes the carbon dioxide production ($\dot{V}CO_2$) to increase out of proportion to oxygen consumption ($\dot{V}O_2$), resulting in an increased RER. An RER of 1.09 or greater is thought to indicate the onset of anaerobic metabolism and to be consistent with a good effort.[75,76] Because RER increases only if anaerobic metabolism occurs, exercise limitation and low $\dot{V}O_2$ owing to musculoskeletal problems or poor effort are associated with an RER less than this threshold.

The *ventilatory anaerobic threshold* (VAT) is used to identify the onset of anaerobic metabolism that occurs before $\dot{V}O_2$ peaks and is relatively effort and motivation independent. As aerobic exercise progresses, minute ventilation ($\dot{V}_E$) increases in direct proportion to $\dot{V}CO_2$ and $\dot{V}O_2$. When anaerobic metabolism commences and CO_2 production increases as lactic acid is buffered, $\dot{V}_E$ increases accordingly. VAT is the point at which $\dot{V}_E/\dot{V}O_2$ and $\dot{V}_E/\dot{V}CO_2$ diverge, with $\dot{V}_E$ increasing in proportion to $\dot{V}CO_2$ but out of proportion to $\dot{V}O_2$. An important characteristic of successful endurance athletes is the ability to reach and sustain effort at an anaerobic threshold that is a large percentage (80%–85%) of peak $\dot{V}O_2$.

Ventilation efficiency can be assessed with the use of the $\dot{V}_E/\dot{V}CO_2$ slope. This relationship is defined as 863 • $\dot{V}CO_2/[PaCO_2 • (1 − V_D/V_T)]$, where V_D/V_T is the ratio of physiologic dead space to tidal volume.[82] The $\dot{V}_E/\dot{V}CO_2$ slope can be thought of as the number of liters of ventilation required to eliminate 1 L of CO_2. Normal children have a $\dot{V}_E/\dot{V}CO_2$ slope of less than 28.[76] To maintain a normal $PaCO_2$ during exercise, children with increased V_D/V_T and reduced ventilatory efficiency have a greater than normal increase in $\dot{V}_E$ and therefore a steeper $\dot{V}_E/\dot{V}CO_2$ slope. Increased V_D/V_T is the consequence of either reduced V_T in the setting of a normal V_D or pulmonary flow maldistribution and subsequent $\dot{V}/\dot{Q}$ mismatch that increases V_D. The latter is the major source of inefficient ventilation and steepening of the $\dot{V}_E/\dot{V}CO_2$ slope in children with cardiac disease.

In children with PA stenosis, (e.g., repaired TOF), pulmonary hypertension, or increased LA pressure from any cause (e.g., LV systolic or diastolic dysfunction, mitral valve disease), an increase in the $\dot{V}_E/\dot{V}CO_2$ slope is associated with increased mortality. When pulmonary stenosis is corrected in children with TOF, the $\dot{V}_E/\dot{V}CO_2$ slope and peak $\dot{V}O_2$ improve.

Children with Fontan physiology also exhibit an increase in $\dot{V}_E/\dot{V}CO_2$ slope. These children have inherent nonhomogeneous pulmonary perfusion at rest owing to the lack of pulsatile pulmonary blood flow. In addition, there is poor recruitment of the distal pulmonary vasculature during exercise. The presence of a Fontan fenestration further increases the $\dot{V}_E/\dot{V}CO_2$ slope by allowing mixed venous blood high in CO_2 to be shunted into the systemic circulation. This produces, via central chemoreceptor stimulation, an increase in $\dot{V}_E$ out of proportion to $\dot{V}CO_2$.[83] Fontan fenestration closure eliminates this right-to-left shunt and reduces the $\dot{V}_E/\dot{V}CO_2$ slope but does not improve the peak $\dot{V}O_2$.[83] The reason is that the primary limitation to increases in $\dot{V}O_2$ during exercise in Fontan patients is the inherent inability of the pulmonary vascular bed to substantially increase surface area, flow, and preload delivery to the systemic ventricle.

FONTAN PHYSIOLOGY

In 1971, Francis Fontan, a French cardiac surgeon, described a new treatment for complex cardiac malformations with only one ventricle.[84] To decrease the chronic volume overload for the single ventricle and normalize oxygenation, he separated the systemic and pulmonary circulations by directly connecting the systemic venous return (SVC and IVC) to the PA, without a pumping chamber. This created a circulation wherein pulmonary blood was driven solely by a nonpulsatile pressure gradient across the pulmonary vascular bed, with the single ventricle being the sole source of kinetic energy. All other shunt connections were interrupted. The original indication was tricuspid atresia, but over the years the classic Fontan technique has been modified in many ways and is now used for various complex cardiac lesions with single ventricle physiology, such as HLHS, double-inlet RV, and pulmonary atresia with intact septum (see also Chapters 15 and 21).[85–90]

It is impossible to create a Fontan circulation at birth; high PVR and small vessel sizes prevent adequate pulmonary blood flow. In the neonatal period, palliative procedures such as stage I Norwood operation with aortic arch reconstruction, atrial septostomy, and aortopulmonary shunts (modified Blalock-Taussig shunt) or the Sano modification of the Norwood procedure (RV-to-PA conduit) aim for balanced systemic and pulmonary blood flows, allowing the infant to grow for several months despite cyanosis and volume load on the ventricle. At the age of 3 to 6 months, an intermediate procedure called the bidirectional Glenn operation or superior cavopulmonary anastomosis is performed. The SVC is connected directly to the PA, providing nonpulsatile pulmonary blood flow, whereas the IVC remains connected to the heart. As a result, the volume load on the ventricle is significantly reduced, but oxygenated and deoxygenated blood still mix and the saturations remain in the low 80% range. By the age of 1 to 5 years, most of these children are ready for the Fontan circulation.[91] With adequate growth and maturation of the pulmonary vascular bed, the resistance should be small enough to allow the complete separation of the systemic and pulmonary flows. The IVC is now also connected to the PA, most often via a lateral tunnel in the atrium or an extracardiac conduit, with or without a small fenestration (small opening in the baffle or conduit connecting the systemic venous return with the common atrium of the single ventricle). The fenestration can provide a residual right-to-left shunt in case of sudden increases in PVR,

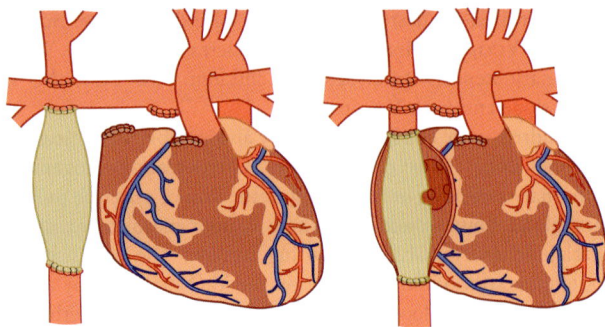

FIGURE 16.9 Fontan modifications: extracardiac conduit *(left)* and lateral tunnel with fenestration *(right)*. (Courtesy of Children's Hospital of Boston.)

maintaining ventricular preload and function. This seems to facilitate the adaptation to the new loading conditions, shorten the recovery time, and decrease the incidence of early complications. The fenestration often occludes spontaneously, or it is closed during a cardiac catheterization and hemodynamic evaluation with a special device (Fig. 16.9; see also Figs. 15.11 through 15.13).[92–95]

The Fontan operation has dramatically improved the mortality rates for children with single ventricles, but the success comes at a price: chronic systemic venous hypertension and congestion have been implicated in a multitude of potential early and long-term complications, including arrhythmias, residual right-to-left shunts, coagulopathies with increased risk for thrombosis and stroke, lymphatic dysfunction with pleural effusions, and protein-losing enteropathy.[96–102] Late cardiac failure and poor functional outcome remain risks for patients with Fontan circulations.[103] The anatomy of the single ventricle and the type of Fontan connection influence the duration of freedom from complications. Children with systemic RVs and the classic atriopulmonary Fontan procedure (RA directly anastomosed to the PA) tend to have a shorter duration of freedom from complications than those with systemic LVs and newer Fontan modifications (E-Figs. 16.2 and 16.3).[104]

Inherent limitations of the Fontan circulation, such as altered control of cardiac output with decreased hemodynamic response to stress and reduced exercise tolerance, have been documented (Fig. 16.10).[105–114] Even at rest, cardiac output is usually only 70% (range, 50%–80%) of normal for body surface area. Cardiac output is classically determined by four factors: preload, contractility, HR, and afterload. Over a physiologic range, cardiac output improves with increased preload, contractility, and HR and with decreased afterload. For the Fontan circulation, the determinants of cardiac output are more complex (Fig. 16.11).[109,115,116] The classic determinants of cardiac output are important; however, other factors, such as transpulmonary gradient and PVR, may be equally or more important. Several mechanisms regulate cardiac output in children with Fontan physiology:

- *Preload:* The RV usually provides the kinetic energy to distend the pulmonary vasculature and create a preload reservoir for the LV, thereby enabling an increase in cardiac output up to 5-fold or greater with exercise.[115,117] The lack of a prepulmonary pump leads to a significant decrease in available pulmonary blood volume and, consequently, reduced or absent LV preload reserve.[109,118,119]
- *Contractility:* During the staged palliation, the single ventricle typically develops from a volume-overloaded and dilated ventricle to a hypertrophied, underfilled ventricle.[120,121] Although the contractile response to β-adrenergic stimulation seems to

be preserved, the resulting increase in cardiac output is diminished, most likely owing to limited preload reserve.[112,119]

- *Heart rate and rhythm:* Within the physiologic range, atrial pacing at different HRs does not alter cardiac output because there is a simultaneous decrease in stroke volume.[122] Normalization of HR increases the reduced cardiac output associated with severe bradycardia or tachycardia.[123] During exercise testing, Fontan patients demonstrate chronotropic incompetence, a blunted HR response to exercise. This is likely the result of autonomic dysfunction or abnormal reflex control. In contrast to the HR, cardiac rhythm is of utmost importance. Ectopy or loss of AV synchronization compromises ventricular filling and decreases the transpulmonary gradient.[120]
- *Afterload:* The Fontan circulation is characterized by increased afterload, which is a physiologic response to decreased cardiac output and occurs because a single ventricle is ejecting into two large resistance beds (systemic and pulmonary vascular) arranged in series.[109,119,124,125] Autonomic regulation and activation of various endocrine systems increase the systemic venous resistance and help to maintain adequate perfusion pressures and venous tone. Because of the limited preload reserve, attempts at afterload reduction often result in significant hypotension. On the other hand, excessive afterload, such as that which occurs with residual aortic arch obstruction, is poorly tolerated.
- *Transpulmonary flow:* Transpulmonary flow is directly proportional to the gradient between the systemic venous pressure (usually between 10 and 15 mm Hg, rarely >20 mm Hg) and the preventricular atrial pressure, which is determined by the functional status of the AV valve, the ventricle, the rhythm, and the potential presence of outflow obstruction. Transpulmonary flow is inversely proportional to the resistance over the Fontan circuit. This resistance is largely determined by PVR, but mechanical obstruction such as stenosis or thrombosis may also play a role. The geometry of the cavopulmonary connections is also important in that turbulent flow produces energy loss and a reduction in effective driving pressure. It has been suggested that PVR is the key determinant of transpulmonary flow, delivery of pulmonary venous flow to the systemic ventricle, and, consequently, cardiac output (Fig. 16.12).[109,118,126–135]

The role of selective pulmonary vasodilators to enhance preload and thereby cardiac output in Fontan patients is still under investigation.[136–138] Future studies with new technologies like wave intensity analysis, speckle tacking echocardiography or volume pressure loop recordings via micro conductance catheters will further clarify these complex hemodynamic interactions and guide individualized therapeutic and surgical strategies.[139–141]

The Fontan circulation can be described as a serial circulation with a single kinetic energy pump. Increased systemic venous pressures are necessary to create the transpulmonary pressure gradient that drives flow across the pulmonary vascular bed; however, these increased pressures simultaneously increase the ventricular afterload. Cardiac output depends on an adequate preload and low PVR. Decreased cardiac output at rest, saturations of 92% to 93%, and limited exercise tolerance, are characteristics of the Fontan circulation.

PHYSIOLOGY OF THE TRANSPLANTED HEART

According to the International Society for Heart and Lung Transplantation (ISHLT), children younger than 18 years of age account for about 14% of all heart transplantations. Approximately

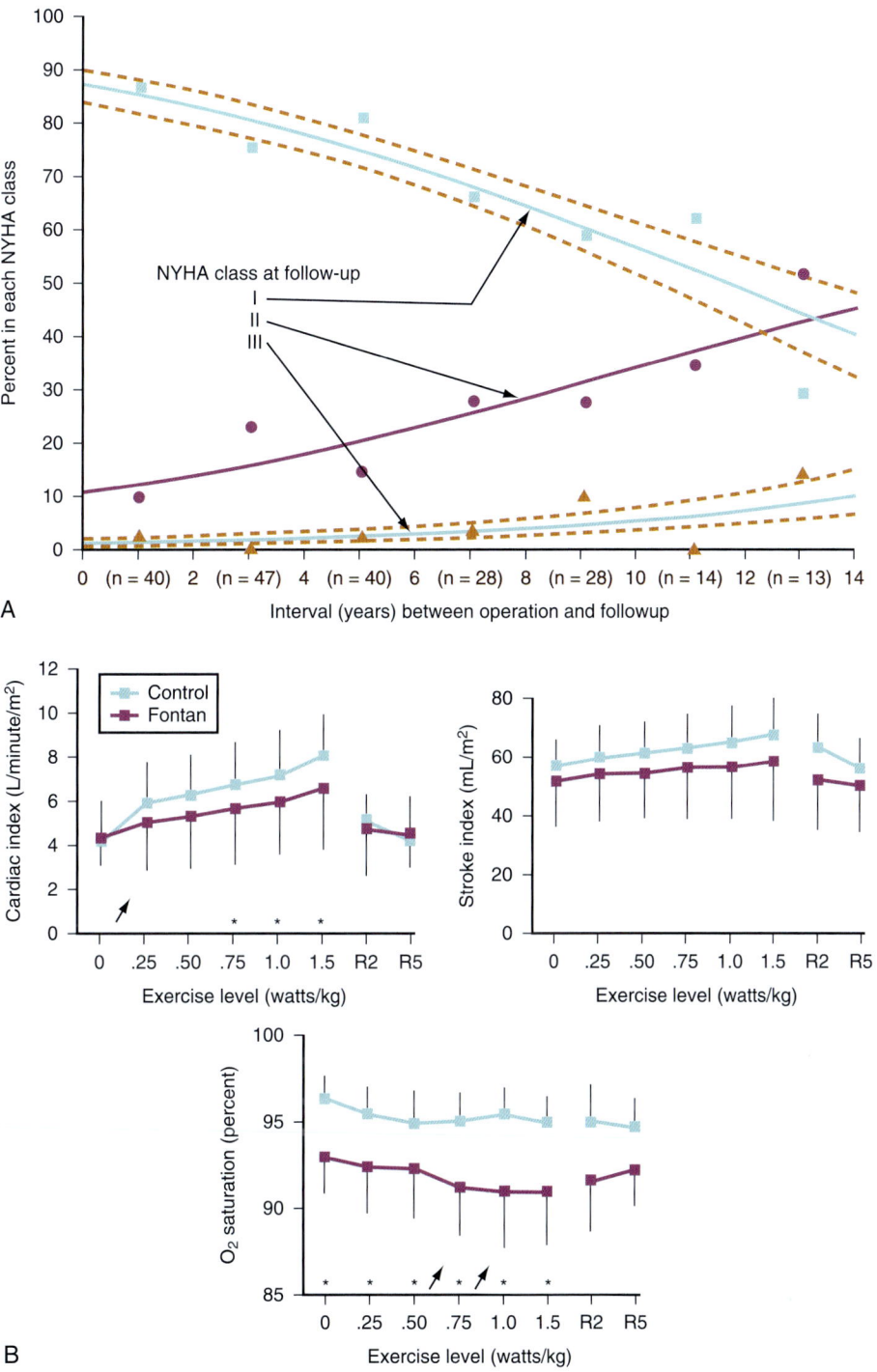

FIGURE 16.10 A, Symptomatic outcomes of 334 survivors of Fontan operations who were monitored for 1 month to 20 years. The graph illustrates the changes since surgery in patients assessed as New York Heart Association *(NYHA)* classification I *(blue squares),* II *(purple circles),* or III *(brown triangles).* Although most children exhibited good functional status (NYHA class I) immediately after surgery, mild functional limitations evolved over time. Broken lines indicate 70% confidence intervals. **B,** Results of exercise studies (cardiac index, stroke index, and oxygen saturation vs. exercise level) of 42 children after Fontan operation *(purple squares)* compared with normal control subjects *(blue squares).* Although the protocol was designed to achieve modest targets, significant differences emerged in the capacity of Fontan children to increase cardiac output with exercise, and systemic arterial oxygen saturation remained below normal throughout. The primary reason for the inability to increase cardiac output appears to be an inability to increase pulmonary blood flow and, consequently, systemic ventricular filling. Potential reasons for decreased arterial saturation include intrapulmonary shunting owing to arteriovenous malformations and ventilation/perfusion imbalance. *Arrows* indicate a significant difference ($P < 0.05$) in values between consecutive exercise levels. (**A** from Fontan F, Kirklin JW, Fernandez G, et al. Outcome after a "perfect" Fontan operation. *Circulation* 1990;81:1520-1536; **B** from Gewillig MH, Lundstrom UR, Bull C, et al. Exercise responses in children with congenital heart disease after Fontan repair: patterns and determinants of performance. *J Am Coll Cardiol.* 1990;15:1424-1432. Reprinted with permission from the American College of Cardiology.)

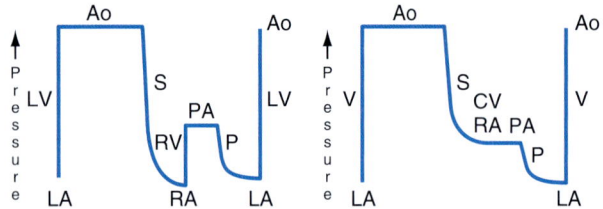

FIGURE 16.11 In the normal cardiovascular circulation *(left)*, the pulmonary circulation *(P)* is connected in series with the systemic circulation *(S)*. The right ventricle *(RV)* maintains a right atrial *(RA)* pressure that is lower than the left atrial *(LA)* pressure and provides enough energy for the blood to pass through the pulmonary resistance. In the Fontan circuit *(right)*, the systemic veins are connected to the pulmonary artery *(PA)* without a subpulmonary ventricle or systemic atrium (the RV is not present on the right). In the absence of a fenestration, there is no admixture of systemic and pulmonary venous blood, but the systemic venous pressures are markedly increased. *Ao,* Aorta; *CV,* caval veins; *LV,* left ventricle; *V,* single ventricle. (From Gewillig M, Brown SC, Eyskens B, et al. The Fontan circulation: who controls cardiac output? *Interact Cardiovasc Thorac Surg.* 2010;10:428-433.)

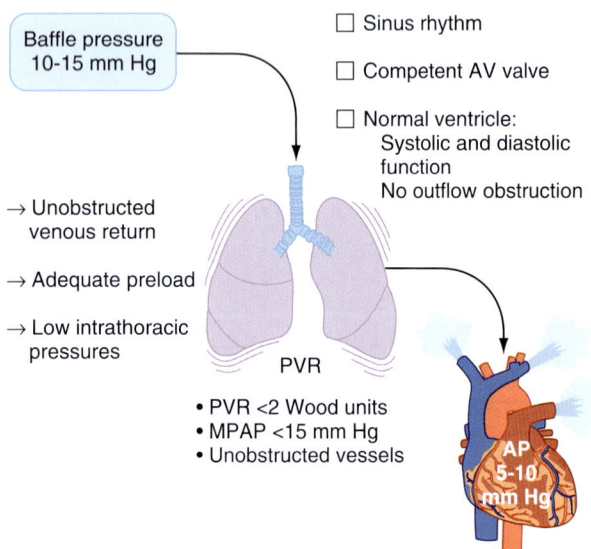

FIGURE 16.12 Several factors determine the transpulmonary gradient in the Fontan circulation. These include unobstructed venous return, adequate preload, and low intrathoracic pressure on the venous side; low pulmonary vascular resistance *(PVR)*, and unobstructed pulmonary vessels; and, on the atrial side, adequate ventricular function, competent atrioventricular valves, normal sinus rhythm, and no evidence of outflow obstruction. *AP,* Atrial pressure; *MPAP,* mean pulmonary arterial pressure. (Courtesy A. Schure.)

590 children undergo cardiac transplantation annually, primarily from centers in Europe and North America.[142] Major indications for transplantation include cardiomyopathies, CHD, and a growing number of repeat transplantations, especially in older children. The median survival time (the time at which 50% of recipients are still alive) has improved over the years, mainly because of reduced early posttransplant mortality. Survival time is currently 24.5 years for infants, 20.2 years for children aged 1 to 5 years, 15.9 years for children aged 6 to 10 years, and 14.3 years for teenagers. Over 80% of transplant recipients describe a normal functional status with no limitations during physical activity.[142]

As survival continues to improve, more and more children with transplanted hearts will present to operating rooms and sedation suites for diagnostic studies and general procedures. A basic understanding of the physiologic changes in the transplanted heart and the implications of current immunosuppressive therapy are important for their safe management.

Physiology of the Denervated Heart

After transplantation, the function of the surgically denervated heart depends primarily on an intact Frank-Starling mechanism and stimulation from circulating catecholamines. The classic Frank-Starling mechanism describes the ability of the cardiac muscle to increase contractility in response to stretch or tension (e.g., increasing cardiac output with increases in venous return). Afferent and efferent denervation has multiple effects on circulatory control mechanisms and leads to physiologic changes, including an increase in the resting HR and a blunted response to stress and exercise. Despite excellent physical activity, exercise testing easily demonstrates that heart transplant recipients can usually achieve only 60% to 70% of normal capacity. In the transplanted heart, exercise-induced increase in cardiac output is initially caused by an increase in stroke volume, a highly preload-dependent process. Tachycardia occurs only later, in response to circulating catecholamines.[143] Further details of the altered physiology are summarized in Fig. 16.13.[143] The incidence, timing, and extent of sympathetic reinnervation are still being investigated, but the positive effects on cardiac performance have been clearly demonstrated.[144] During standardized exercise testing, transplant recipients with evidence of reinnervation show improved endurance with greater peak HRs and better contractile function.[145]

Chronic denervation also causes an altered response to many medications. Atropine, glycopyrrolate, digoxin, and pancuronium have no chronotropic effect on the denervated heart. Sympathomimetics that act indirectly, such as ephedrine and dopamine, have a blunted response, whereas adrenergic agents that act directly, such as epinephrine, isoproterenol, and dobutamine, can cause exaggerated effects that should be carefully titrated.[146] A single-center retrospective study did not find any negative effects of neostigmine in patients with heart transplants,[147] although several case reports have described profound bradycardia and even cardiac arrest after neostigmine was used to antagonize neuromuscular blockade.[148–151] Neostigmine has been shown to produce an atropine-sensitive, dose-dependent bradycardia in both recent (<6 months) and remote (>6 months) cardiac transplants. Direct stimulation of postganglionic nicotinic cholinergic receptors with denervation hypersensitivity, a direct effect of the old sinoatrial node on the pacemaker cell of the new sinoatrial node, and parasympathetic reinnervation have been postulated as potential mechanisms.[152–155] Avoidance of neuromuscular blockade, use of short-acting neuromuscular-blocking agents without reversal, and use of edrophonium for reversal have all been suggested.[150,151] Edrophonium seems to have less effect on the HR in this population than neostigmine.[153]

Sugammadex has been increasingly used as an alternative to neostigmine to antagonize rocuronium and vecuronium in children (see Chapter 5).[156–158] However, profound bradycardia has been reported in several cases, including in one pediatric heart transplant recipient.[159–161] The exact mechanism for the bradycardia remains unknown but may involve encapsulating endogenous catecholamines. It seems that the reversal of a neuromuscular blockade in patients with denervated hearts requires the same vigilance and risk/benefit discussion as for other reversal agents.[161]

The denervated heart is also very sensitive to adenosine. The magnitude and duration of the effects on the AV node are three to five times greater than in native hearts. The initial and subsequent doses should be reduced by 50% to attenuate these

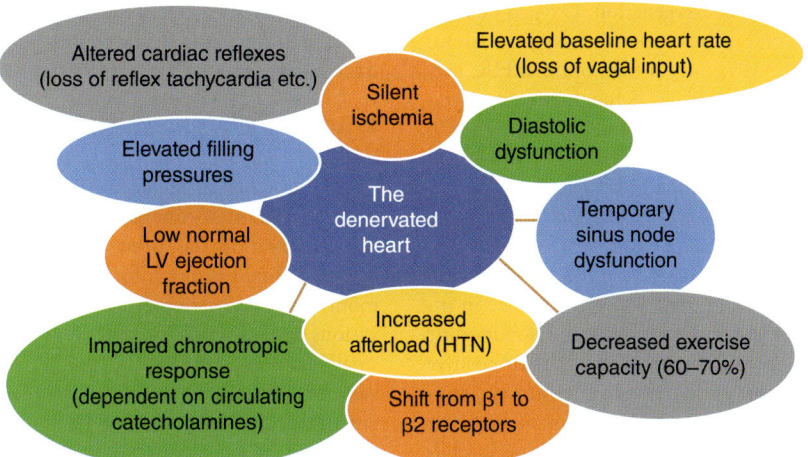

FIGURE 16.13 Physiology of the transplanted heart. *HTN*, hypertension; *LV*, left ventricle. (Modified from Cotts WG, Oren RM. Function of the transplanted heart: unique physiology and therapeutic implications. *Amer J Med Sci.* 1997;314:164-72; published in: Burbano-Vera N and Schure Y. Pediatric heart transplantation. In: Lalwani K, Cohen IT, Choi EY, Raman VT, eds. *Pediatric Anesthesia – A Problem-Based Learning Approach.* Oxford University Press; 2018:111-186.)

TABLE 16.7	Altered Response of the Denervated Heart to Medications	
Decreased Response	**Exacerbated Response (Supersensitivity)**	
Indirect acting sympathomimetics Dopamine, ephedrine - depleted NA storage in cardiac nerve endings	**Direct-acting sympathomimetics Epinephrine, norepinephrine** - Lack of presynaptic uptake	
Atropine and glycopyrrolate - No heart rate response	**Ca-channel or β-blocker, Adenosine** - Profound bradycardia/ asystole	
Digitalis	**Direct vasodilators Nitroprusside, nitroglycerine, hydralazine** - Lack of reflex tachycardia	

Modified from Cotts WG, Oren RM. Function of the transplanted heart: unique physiology and therapeutic implications. *Amer J Med Sci.* 1997;314:164-172. Published in: Burbano-Vera N and Schure Y. Pediatric heart transplantation. In: Lalwani K, Cohen IT, Choi EY, Raman VT, eds. *Pediatric Anesthesia – A Problem-Based Learning Approach.* Oxford University Press; 2018:111-186.

effects.[162,163] Calcium channel blockers and β-blocker drugs are associated with exaggerated bradycardia and hypotension. The lack of reflex tachycardia can also lead to profound hypotension with the use of direct vasodilators such as nitroglycerine, nitroprusside, or hydralazine; therefore, initial doses of these medications should also be reduced (Table 16.7).

Transplant Morbidity

Children who have undergone cardiac transplantation continue to experience morbidity associated with immunosuppressive therapy. Rehospitalization to treat infections and rejection is common, especially during the first year after transplantation (~42%). Acute rejection episodes are a major threat. With the latest immunosuppressive regimens, the incidence of rejection during the first year has decreased from ~24% in 2005–2009 to ~13% in 2010–2018.[142] Rejection is thought to be associated

with the development of cardiac allograft vasculopathy (CAV) or coronary artery disease, which is a major cause of morbidity and graft failure. Indeed, 10 years after transplantation, ~16% of infants, ~25% of children 1 to 10 years of age, and ~43% of adolescents have CAV.[142] Most centers include annual coronary angiography or intravascular echocardiography as a part of regular rejection surveillance.[164,165] Children with CAV present the same anesthetic challenges as adults with severe coronary artery disease and ischemic heart disease. Aggressive immunosuppressive therapy with induction and maintenance regimens carries its own risks.[166,167] A detailed discussion is beyond the scope of this chapter but, in general, monoclonal or polyclonal T-cell antibodies (OKT3, ATG) and specific interleukin-2 receptor antagonists (basiliximab, daclizumab) are used for the induction phase and various combinations of corticosteroids, calcineurin inhibitors (cyclosporine, tacrolimus, FK506), mechanistic target of rapamycin inhibitors (mTOR inhibitors: sirolimus, everolimus) and antiproliferative agents (azathioprine, mycophenolate mofetil) are used for maintenance. Adverse effects, which are common, include neurotoxicity with seizures, hypertension, liver and renal dysfunction, hyperlipidemia, diabetes, gingival hypertrophy, hypertrichosis, bone marrow suppression, and posttransplantation lymphoproliferative disease.[168]

Several excellent review articles describe the anesthetic management of children with heart transplants (see also Chapter 21).[169–172] A thorough preoperative evaluation with attention to episodes of rejection, presence of coronary artery disease, and organ dysfunction; a detailed medication history with investigation of major side effects; consideration of the denervated physiology; and appropriate choice of anesthetic drugs and other medications are essential components of a sensible anesthetic plan for those with a transplanted heart.

Cardiovascular Pharmacology

RATIONAL USE OF VASOACTIVE DRUGS

Many factors influence the selection of appropriate inotropic and vasopressor therapies, including the clinical situation, underlying cardiac abnormalities, and perfusion requirements of other organs.

The major goal is to improve tissue oxygenation. Oxygen delivery to tissues depends primarily on cardiac output and oxygen content. In addition to an increased cardiac output (i.e., optimal HR, preload, contractility, and afterload), adequate hemoglobin concentration and oxygen saturation values are important components. On the other hand, a careful balance of pulmonary and systemic blood flows can be crucial for certain congenital heart defects.

Catecholamines and catecholamine-like agents remain the most used inotropic and vasoconstrictor drugs. It is likely that dopamine and dobutamine increase cardiac output in neonates because they increase both HR and contractility. Evidence in infants and young children suggests that dopamine and dobutamine increase cardiac output after cardiac surgery through their positive chronotropic effects rather than an increase in the intrinsic contractility.[173–175] With few exceptions, drugs that primarily increase afterload, such as α-adrenergic agonists, have limited use in children. Large increases in afterload without corresponding increases in the contractile state are often poorly tolerated by infants and children, particularly in the context of significant underlying contractile dysfunction.

PRACTICAL CONSIDERATIONS FOR THE USE OF VASOACTIVE AGENTS

Commonly used drugs, their doses, and a summary of their effects on selected cardiac functions are presented in Table 16.8; most of this information has been empirically derived from studies in adults. Limited direct information regarding the effects of commonly used vasoactive drugs in children at different ages and in various pathophysiologic states is available. Neonates, infants, and small children demonstrate unique responses to inotropic and vasoactive drugs primarily because of age-specific pharmacokinetics; differences in receptor types, number, and function; and a variability in drug delivery. Important variations in the volume of distribution and measured plasma concentrations have been

TABLE 16.8	Inotropics and Vasopressors	
Agent	**Intravenous Dose**	**Comments**
Dopamine	2–20 µg/kg per minute infusion	Primary effects at β_1, β_2, and dopamine receptors, somewhat related to dose; lower doses (2–5 µg/kg per minute) can increase contractility and can also have a direct dopaminergic receptor effect to increase splanchnic and renal perfusion; increasing doses increase contractility via β-effects and increase likelihood of α-mediated vasoconstriction; effects depend on endogenous catecholamine stores.
Dobutamine	2–20 µg/kg per minute infusion	Relatively selective β_1 stimulation; also potential β_2 stimulation, tachycardia, and vasodilation, especially at higher doses (>10 µg/kg per minute); may be less potent than dopamine, especially in immature myocardium; no significant α-adrenergic effects; tachydysrhythmias perhaps more likely than with dopamine; effects are independent of endogenous catecholamine stores.
Epinephrine	0.02–1.0 µg/kg/min infusion	Primary β-effects to increase contractility and vasodilation at doses (<0.1 µg/kg per minute); increasing doses (>0.1 µg/kg per minute) are accompanied by increased contractility and increased α-mediated vasoconstriction; may be best choice to augment contractility and perfusion, especially in situations of severely compromised ventricular function, shock, or anaphylaxis.
Isoproterenol	0.05–2.0 µg/kg per minute infusion	Pure, nonselective β-agonist; significant inotropic, chronotropic (β_1 and β_2), and vasodilatory (β_2) effects; may be an effective pulmonary vasodilator in some children; tachycardia and increased myocardial oxygen consumption may be dose limiting; tachydysrhythmias may also occur; bronchodilator.
Norepinephrine	0.05–2 µg/kg per minute infusion	Primary effects on α_1-, α_2-, and β_1-receptors, no significant clinical effects on β_2. Increased systemic blood pressure and cardiac output (α_1 and β_1) as well as improved pulmonary blood flow (α_2). Less tachycardia. Mainly used for treatment of septic shock and pulmonary hypertension.
Phenylephrine	2–10 µg/kg bolus, 0.1–0.5 µg/kg per minute infusion Preterm and term infants may require as much as a 30 µg/kg bolus (see Chapter 15)	Pure α-mediated vasoconstriction; no increase in contractility.
Vasopressin	0.0003–0.002 U/kg per minute	Induces intense vasoconstriction via V_{1a} receptors in the vascular endothelium. May cause vasodilation via V_2 receptors in specific tissues (release of nitric oxide and vasodilating prostaglandins). Used for the treatment of vasodilatory shock, refractory hypotension, and pulmonary arterial hypertension. Careful when programming syringe pumps: multiple dosing forms (U/minute, U/kg per hour, U/kg per minute, or mU/kg per minute).
Amrinone	0.75–1 mg/kg repeated twice, maximum 3 mg/kg Neonates and infants may require loading doses of 2–4 mg/kg and infusions of 10 µg/kg per minute	Increases cyclic adenosine monophosphate by phosphodiesterase inhibition; positive inotropy, positive lusitropy, and smooth muscle vasorelaxation; hypotension; reversible thrombocytopenia.
Milrinone	50–75 µg/kg loading dose, 0.5–1.0 µg/kg per minute infusion	Similar to amrinone (antiplatelet effects may be less).

TABLE 16.8	Inotropics and Vasopressors—cont'd	
Agent	**Intravenous Dose**	**Comments**
Calcium chloride Calcium gluconate	10–20 mg/kg per dose (slowly) 30–60 mg/kg per dose (slowly)	Positive inotropic and direct vasoconstricting effects; inotropy is significant only if ionized calcium is low and/or ventricular function is depressed by other agents; can slow sinus node; increases electrophysiologic abnormalities from hypokalemia and digoxin.
Digoxin	Total digitalizing dose (TDD)[a]: Premature: 15–25 µg/kg Neonate (<1 month): 20–30 µg/kg Infant (<2 years): 30–50 µg/kg Child (2–5 years): 25–35 µg/kg Child (>5 years): 15–30 µg/kg Child (>10 years): 8–12 µg/kg	TDD given in divided doses: ½ TDD followed by ¼ TDD q8–12 hours × 2; slows sinus node and decreases AV node conduction; used to slow ventricular response in atrial flutter and fibrillation and may also treat junctional tachycardia or SVT; variable effect on accessory pathways; long half-life (24–48 hours) that is prolonged by renal dysfunction; numerous drug interactions; toxicity includes SVT, AV block, ventricular dysrhythmias; toxicity symptoms include drowsiness, nausea, vomiting; toxicity exacerbated by hypokalemia.

observed in children who received inotropic agents. The plasma concentrations for a given infusion rate are reported to vary by as much as 10-fold.[176–178]

Substantial pharmacodynamic variability (i.e., variability in the serum concentration required to produce the desired effect) can also be observed. Some of these differences are related to receptor maturation and function. For example, it appears that β-adrenergic receptors have a high density in the term neonate and young infant but their coupling to adenyl cyclase may be incomplete.[35,179] In addition to developmental changes, which are to some extent controlled by thyroid hormone, β-receptor, and adenyl cyclase activities are diminished in response to sustained administration of exogenous β-agonists and also as a result of increased endogenous catecholamine concentrations, which are often identified as a complication of moderate to severe heart failure and other forms of severe stress (e.g., sepsis).[180–182]

In the neonatal myocardium, chronic catecholamine exposure may upregulate adrenergic receptor number or function, or both, perhaps mimicking the normal developmental program of increasing sympathetic nervous system activity as term approaches.[183] With further maturation in early postnatal life, β-adrenergic receptor density decreases. The impacts of various pathophysiologic states on these processes have been incompletely identified. For example, β-receptor and adenyl cyclase expression and activity all decrease in children with congestive heart failure, cardiopulmonary bypass (CPB), and ischemic reperfusion.[184–187] On the other hand, β-receptor density increases and receptor-stimulated adenyl cyclase activity is greater with increased gene and protein expression in the myocardium of infants with tetralogy of Fallot.[188,189]

Attention must be paid to the technical issues when administering vasoactive infusions to infants. Infusions for infants are often very concentrated, and prepared in nonstandardized solutions to minimize the amount of volume to be infused; hence, the potential for dose or concentration error is substantial.[190] Because these drugs are concentrated compared with the child's size, small errors (either in calculation or in infusion pump flow rate) will have an enormous impact on the actual amount of drug delivered. The extremely small infusion rates can also lead to a delay in drug delivery and effect (see Chapters 6 and 49). Confirming that the pump drive mechanism is actually delivering drug at the distal end of the infusion tubing, connecting the infusion tubing as close to the child as possible, and using a carrier infusion to "push" the medication at a constant rate are important steps to ensure the safety and effectiveness of drug infusions. The rate of the carrier infusion is also crucial. Most standard infusion setups require rates in excess of 5 mL/hour to effect rapid (less than ~10 minutes) changes in the concentration of drug delivered to the infant and therefore may offset attempts to restrict fluids.

VASOACTIVE DRUGS

Dopamine

Dopamine, the most frequently used inotropic agent in neonates, infants, and children, exerts its actions via α-, β-, and dopaminergic receptors. Dopamine augments cardiac contractility through two mechanisms. It directly stimulates cardiac β1-receptors and provokes norepinephrine release from cardiac sympathetic nerve terminals. Circulating concentrations of endogenous epinephrine and norepinephrine increase during dopamine infusions, leading to the suggestion that at least some of the effects of a dopamine infusion are indirectly mediated via induced release of endogenous catecholamines.[191] Because of its indirect effects, particularly the release of myocardial norepinephrine stores, the response to dopamine may be diminished in children with congestive heart failure or other relatively long-standing forms of hemodynamic stress.

Activity at dopaminergic receptors in the kidney and gastrointestinal tract may improve the perfusion of these organ systems. The evidence that dopamine specifically and selectively improves renal perfusion via stimulation of renal dopaminergic receptors (i.e., as opposed to a nonspecific and generalized improvement in cardiac output that might occur with any positive inotrope) is conflicting.[192–196] Regardless of the mechanism, most evidence indicates that dopamine increases renal blood flow and perfusion, even at very large infusion rates.

As with other inotropes, the pharmacokinetics of dopamine show large variability in the serum concentrations in neonates and children.[197,198] Because the plasma concentration is so variable for a given infusion rate, as well as the wide range of serum concentrations necessary to produce a given effect, doubling or halving a dopamine infusion rate may be a logical approach to bracketing the optimal infusion rate. The frequent practice of changing the infusion rate by small proportions (i.e., 5%–10%) may be inconsistent with our current understanding of the pharmacokinetics and pharmacodynamics of most inotropes.

Cardiac output in neonates has classically been understood to depend to a greater extent on HR, less on myocardial compliance, and to be relatively resistant to the inotropic effects of exogenous catecholamines. Nonetheless, there is substantial echocardiographic evidence that small dopamine infusion rates

(≤5 µg/kg per minute) increase myocardial contractility before it increases HR.[199,200] Evidence regarding the effects of dopamine in sick preterm infants is also somewhat controversial.[193,201–205] There may be a relative dissociation between its effects on the renal and mesenteric beds in these infants, such that a portion of the increase in arterial blood pressure during a dopamine infusion may result from mesenteric vasoconstriction and an actual decrease in mesenteric blood flow.

Although it is generally accepted that large infusion rates (>10–15 µg/kg per minute) of dopamine cause substantive vasoconstriction, both cardiac output and renal blood flow improve, even at infusion rates ≥20 µg/kg per minute in neonates and infants.[206,207]

The effects of dopamine on PVR vary; both a minimal effect and an increase in PVR have been reported.[175,208–214] The effects of dopamine on PVR most likely depend on the dose as well as the underlying state of the vascular endothelium and smooth muscle. Vasoconstriction may be more likely after ischemia-reperfusion and in the presence of hypoxia. Conversely, the presence of vasodilators, such as nitroprusside, or α-adrenergic blockers, such as phenoxybenzamine, can prevent the increases in PVR in response to dopamine.[215,216] Overall, dopamine remains the drug of choice in most infants and children, owing to its beneficial effects on mesenteric and renal blood flow, lesser chronotropic effects than some other agents, and a somewhat reduced arrhythmogenic potential.

Dobutamine (Dobutrex)

Dobutamine is a structural analog of isoproterenol that was developed to stimulate relatively selective β-adrenergic receptors. Its inotropic and α-adrenergic effects are somewhat less potent than those of dopamine. Dobutamine does possess significant β₂-adrenergic receptor agonist properties, accounting for its peripheral vasodilatory properties. Substantial vasodilation and tachycardia occur at larger infusion rates (≥10 µg/kg per minute).[174,217–220] Its tendency to produce tachycardia and tachyarrhythmia may be greater in neonates than in older children or adults. There is some evidence from immature animal models that the efficacy of dobutamine is reduced, possibly the result of greater circulating catecholamine concentrations and alterations in β-receptor expression and function.[173,174,221–223]

Because the actions of dobutamine are independent of endogenous catecholamine stores, it may be more effective in increasing cardiac output in patients with severe congestive heart failure or cardiogenic shock.[224,225] In children with normal LV function, dobutamine increases LV relaxation. It also improves diastolic relaxation by decreasing end-systolic wall stress.[226] Evidence indicates that dobutamine improves LV contractility in neonates with LV dysfunction, dispelling the notion that there is relative resistance in neonates.[227] Dobutamine does not selectively improve renal or mesenteric blood flow independently of its effect on increasing cardiac output. The improvement in cardiac output with dobutamine depends on both an increase in contractility and a decrease in SVR via vasodilation.[228] Pulmonary vasodilation in the presence of an increased PVR may also occur.[223]

As is the case with dopamine, exponential increases in serum concentrations are required to produce linear improvements in cardiac index. There is also substantial pharmacokinetic variability in the plasma concentrations of dobutamine.[177,217,229–233] Tolerance may occasionally develop.[234] In one animal study, high-dose dobutamine infusion was associated with significant dysfunction of platelet aggregation after hypoxia and reoxygenation.[235]

Isoproterenol (Isuprel)

Isoproterenol is a pure, nonselective β-adrenergic agonist.[236] It increases HR and contractility and vasodilates mesenteric and renal vessels and skeletal muscle. Isoproterenol is also a fairly effective vasodilator of the pulmonary circulation.[237] The tachycardia, which almost always accompanies its use, and greater contractility, increase myocardial oxygen consumption, which is usually well tolerated. However, these changes may be limiting in compromised hearts. The pulmonary vasodilation produced by isoproterenol may be useful in settings in which tachycardia is either unimportant or somewhat beneficial.[238] Systemic vasodilation induced by isoproterenol can be sufficiently profound as to cause systemic hypotension.[213,239] The positive chronotropic effects of isoproterenol may be useful in children with bradycardia.[240] The drug is increasingly used in electrophysiology suites to facilitate the detection of abnormal conduction pathways in infants and children under general anesthesia.[231,241–243] and occasionally to unmask borderline aortic coarctation for interventional procedures.[244] Isoproterenol is also a potent bronchodilator. Prolonged use or large doses of isoproterenol and other catecholamines may be associated with the development of myocardial fibrosis.[245]

Epinephrine (Adrenaline)

Epinephrine has α-, β₁-, and β₂-adrenergic agonist effects. Data derived mainly from studies in adults indicate that smaller doses, 0.02 to 0.1 µg/kg per minute, are associated with predominantly β-adrenergic effects. In this range, increases in HR and systolic blood pressure and reduced diastolic blood pressure owing to skeletal muscle vasodilation predominate. Doses between 0.1 and 0.2 µg/kg per minute have mixed α- and β-effects. At larger doses, α-adrenergic–induced vasoconstriction is noticeable, and hence there is reduced skin, muscle, renal, and mesenteric blood flow. Compared with pure α-agonists, epinephrine provides greater inotropic effect. The effects of epinephrine do not depend on endogenous tissue catecholamine stores. Epinephrine may be effective in children who do not respond to dopamine or dobutamine, particularly those with dysfunction of the systemic ventricle in the immediate postoperative period. The addition of moderate vasoconstriction to increased contractility may be advantageous to maintain myocardial perfusion and may also increase both systemic and pulmonary blood flow in children with shunt-dependent circulations. Important adverse effects include dysrhythmias (usually ventricular) and, at larger doses, regional ischemia and hypoperfusion as the result of vasoconstriction.

Inotropes display linear kinetics with considerable parameter variability. There is also considerable pharmacodynamic parameter variability resulting in a variable individual dose-response relationship; dose should be titrated to effect.[246,247] In infants and children with postoperative low cardiac output syndrome, increased concentrations of glucose and of lactate have been reported after 1 to 2 hours of an epinephrine infusion of 0.1 µg/kg per minute.[246]

Norepinephrine (Levophed, Noradrenaline)

Norepinephrine is often indicated as a first- or second-line treatment for severe hypotension associated with septic shock, but it has also been used in the treatment of persistent pulmonary hypertension of the newborn and other forms of pulmonary hypertension.[248–255] This endogenous adrenergic agent activates both α- and β-receptors. Compared with epinephrine, it seems to be equally effective on β₁-receptors, slightly less on α₁-receptors, and has no clinically significant effects on β₂-receptors. Norepinephrine increases systemic blood pressure as well as cardiac output, oxygen delivery, and splanchnic perfusion in animal models and clinical studies.[256,257] It causes less tachycardia than epinephrine. Norepinephrine reduces PVR and can improve pulmonary blood flow by activating α_2-receptors and release of nitric oxide.[208,258-261] Norepinephrine has a very rapid onset of action with a duration of effect of only 1 to 2 minutes. It is metabolized by catechol-O-methyltransferase and monoamine oxidase; the inactive metabolites are eliminated in the urine. Pharmacokinetic data are mainly derived from adult studies; the few available pediatric reports emphasize the large variability between individual parameters and the need to titrate the rate carefully. The initial rate of 0.05 to 0.1 µg/kg per minute is increased slowly until the desired effect is reached, usually in a range of 0.1 to 2 µg/kg per minute. In a small prospective observational study in term neonates, the majority of neonates responded to a mean dose of 0.5 ± 0.4 µg/kg per minute, with a range of 0.2 to 7.1 µg/kg per minute.[252] A retrospective study in children in septic shock reported mean initial doses of 0.5 ± 0.4 µg/kg per minute to 2.5 ± 2.2 µg/kg per minute, with a maximum individual dose of 10.5 µg/kg per minute.[250] Norepinephrine may be administered via peripheral venous access (and is recommended to avoid delays in treatment) until central access can be established, but some institutions report IV infiltrates in up to 15% of children on vasoactive infusions especially during transport. Accordingly, ongoing vigilance is important.[262-264] Other side effects include arrhythmias and hypertension, which usually respond to dose reductions.

Phenylephrine (Neosynephrine)

Phenylephrine is a pure α-adrenergic agonist. As such, its major function is to cause peripheral vasoconstriction. It is devoid of β-adrenergic and inotropic effect and therefore does not increase contractility. It may be used temporarily to improve afterload, systemic blood pressure, and, therefore, critical organ blood flow. But without concurrent inotropic support, an isolated acute increase in afterload is often poorly tolerated, particularly by a compromised ventricle. There are at least three situations in which phenylephrine can be extremely useful. The first is to increase systemic afterload and decrease right-to-left shunting in children with TOF and dynamic right ventricular outflow tract obstruction (TOF or tet spell). This pure α-adrenergic effect is particularly important in this situation, since any additional increase in contractility would worsen the outflow obstruction. Second, phenylephrine is also beneficial in cyanotic children who depend on a systemic-to-PA shunt for pulmonary blood flow and adequate oxygenation. The increased afterload may increase flow across the shunt and improve pulmonary blood flow. Third, acute hypotension in children with hypertrophic obstructive cardiomyopathy or critical aortic stenosis increases the outlet obstruction; phenylephrine increases afterload attenuating the severity of the obstruction.[265-268]

Vasopressin (Pitressin)

Arginine vasopressin is a peptide secreted by the pituitary gland. Secretion is promoted by angiotensin II and increased stimulation from hypothalamic osmoreceptors; increased activity from cardiopulmonary baroreceptors and increased levels of natriuretic peptide inhibit the secretion of vasopressin. Vasopressin acts at the tissue level by binding to specific receptors, i.e., the vasopressin$_{1a}$ (V_{1a}) receptors that mediate vasoconstriction and the vasopressin$_2$ (V_2) receptors that mediate renal reabsorption of water, renal secretion of renin, and synthesis of renal prostaglandins. In addition, vasopressin may mediate vasodilatation via V_2 receptors by increasing the release and synthesis of NO and vasodilating

prostaglandins. Vasopressin also sensitizes baroreceptors and therefore may vasodilate by decreasing sympathetic activity. Normally, vasopressin acts primarily via V_2 receptors in the kidney to promote water retention. However, during extreme hypotension, vasopressin may act via V_{1a} receptors in the vascular endothelium to induce intense vasoconstriction.

In adults, vasopressin is beneficial in treating vasodilatory shock and during cardiopulmonary resuscitation.[269] A few pediatric case reports and small observational studies have demonstrated improved blood pressure and accelerated weaning of inotropic support with low-dose vasopressin.[270-273] However, a multicenter, randomized, controlled trial in children with vasodilatory shock did not confirm these findings. Low-dose vasopressin (0.0005–0.002 U/kg per minute) had no beneficial effects compared with placebo; there was even a suggestion of increased mortality.[37] Further studies are necessary to determine the effectiveness and safety of vasopressin in children. Currently its role as a "rescue" medication to treat catecholamine-resistant vasodilation in septic shock,[248] during or after congenital cardiac surgery,[274,275] and for refractory hypotension in extremely low–birth-weight (ELBW)[276] infants has been suggested. In 2013, a Cochrane Review found no eligible studies to evaluate the effects of vasopressin and its analogues on refractory hypotension in neonates.[277] All available evidence for a role of vasopressin in children is based on case reports, small case series, and three randomized controlled trials in older children.[251,278,279] A small pilot study in 20 infants, published in 2015, compared vasopressin and dopamine as the primary treatment for hypotension in ELBW infants. Vasopressin appeared to be safe and effective, but this interpretation must be tempered by the small sample size.[256,280,281] The prophylactic use of low-dose vasopressin (0.0003 U/kg per minute) in the early postoperative phase after the Norwood or arterial switch procedure decreased catecholamine and fluid requirements.[282] Refractory pulmonary hypertension is another potential indication for vasopressin and its analogues. In animal studies and in vitro experiments with human tissue, vasopressin causes pulmonary vasodilation via endothelium-dependent release of NO or by direct activation of smooth muscle receptors.[283-286] This vascular response appears to depend on the child's age and the specific disease, which could explain the conflicting results in the literature. Several case reports and case series describe the successful use of vasopressin for this indication, but further studies are necessary to assess appropriate dosing and safety.[287-290] Pediatric dosing algorithms extrapolated from adult data range from 0.0003 to 0.002 U/kg per minute. Careful attention to the infusion rate is important, especially when programming syringe pumps. The literature and common reference tools often cite the doses in units per minute (U/minute), units per kilogram per hour (U/kg per hour), units per kilogram per minute (U/kg per minute), or even milliunits per kilogram per minute (mU/kg per minute), which can be quite confusing and readily lead to dosing errors.

Phosphodiesterase Inhibitors

Phosphodiesterase inhibitors, which include amrinone, milrinone, and enoximone, are the most commonly used non–catecholamine-mediated inotropic agents. Their mechanism of action is also relatively straightforward. Phosphodiesterases degrade cyclic adenosine monophosphate (cAMP) to 5'-AMP. Phosphodiesterase inhibitors prevent this degradation and therefore increase levels of cyclic nucleotides, primarily cAMP. The increased concentration of this secondary messenger leads to an increase in calcium availability and thus increased contractility. Because the response is related to an increase in cAMP and not purely to inhibition of phosphodiesterase, the greatest effect occurs if initial levels of cAMP exceed normal values. In this way, synergy exists with β-agonists.[291] The absence of adrenergic stimulation minimizes effects on HR, rhythm, and dependency on endogenous tissue catecholamine stores. In addition to positive inotropic effects, these drugs also have significant lusitropic properties (i.e., diastolic relaxation) and promote peripheral vasodilation.[292–294] Phosphodiesterase drugs may also have substantial antiinflammatory properties that are currently not well understood.[295–297]

Amrinone (Inocor, Wincoram, Cordemcura)

Amrinone increases myocardial contractility and reduces ventricular afterload.[293,298,299] As with all phosphodiesterase inhibitors, debate continues regarding the relative contribution of systemic vasodilation and afterload reduction relative to the increased cardiac contractility as the primary underlying mechanism for improving cardiac output. Amrinone improved cardiac performance in neonates and infants after cardiac surgery such as the arterial switch procedure and in older children after the Fontan operation.[294,298,300] Pharmacokinetic data in children suggest that the loading and infusion doses for amrinone need to be approximately twice those reported for adults.[301] In addition to differences in volume of distribution and clearance (both greater in infants), binding of amrinone to the oxygenator membrane needs to be considered if the loading dose is administered during CPB.[302] Overall, these data suggest that loading doses of 2 to 4 mg/kg and infusion rates starting in the range of 10 μg/kg per minute may be indicated in the neonate and infant.[302] Large bolus doses of amrinone can cause systemic hypotension, particularly in the period immediately after cardiac surgery. From a practical standpoint, it may be best to administer the loading dose of amrinone slowly over 1 hour. Caution is also indicated because the elimination half-life of amrinone is large (3–15 hours). Other side effects include thrombocytopenia, which is reversible, occasional drug-related fever, and increased hepatic enzymes.[303]

Milrinone (Primacor)

The use of milrinone after cardiac surgery improves cardiac output and outcome in neonates and infants as well as with other states associated with ventricular dysfunction.[228,304–309] Renal clearance is the primary route of elimination; the maturation of milrinone clearance parallels the glomerular filtration rate.[310,311] Milrinone has a larger volume of distribution and greater clearance (expressed per kilogram) in children compared with adults; adjustments to bolus dosing and infusion rates have therefore been recommended.[304,309] Unlike amrinone, milrinone does not bind to the CPB circuit and has less deleterious effect on platelet function. Loading doses of 50 to 100 μg/kg (typically 75 μg/kg) and initial infusion rates of 0.5 to 1.0 μg/kg per minute have been recommended,[304,307] although more precise dosing that relates to age and renal function using a target concentration range (100–300 ng/mL) strategy have been proposed.[312] Neonates with HLHS who underwent stage I palliation exhibited reduced renal clearance in the immediate postoperative period, and dose adjustments should be considered (i.e., infusion rates of 0.2 μg/kg per minute).[313] Milrinone increases cardiac output, reduces cardiac filling pressures, and reduces afterload; its effects are typically not associated with tachyphylaxis and are independent of β-adrenergic receptor density or activity. An initial multicenter, double-blind, placebo-controlled trial demonstrated that prophylactic use of high-dose milrinone significantly reduced the development of low cardiac output syndrome relative to placebo after cardiac surgery in high-risk pediatric subjects.[306] In 2018, a survey of members of the Pediatric Cardiac Intensive Care Society (PCICS) showed that 97% of the respondents used milrinone in the perioperative period.[314] Several limited small studies reported that milrinone and the calcium sensitizer, levosimendan, were equally effective in preventing low cardiac output syndrome.[315–317] In addition, a Cochrane Review that included only five eligible studies, found that prophylactic milrinone did not reduce mortality.[318] Milrinone is also used increasingly to improve oxygenation in neonates with persistent pulmonary hypertension who are unresponsive to therapy with NO.[319–322] Animal studies have shown that IV or inhaled milrinone enhances the response of the pulmonary vasculature to iloprost and prostacyclin.[323,324] Potential side effects of milrinone include hypotension, tachycardia, tachyarrhythmias, and platelet dysfunction.[325]

Enoximone (Perfan)

Enoximone is a phosphodiesterase inhibitor that has been used extensively in Europe but is not currently available in the United States. Its properties are similar to those of the other members of its class. Infants treated with enoximone after cardiac surgery show improved indirect indexes of cardiac function such as mixed venous oxygen saturation, ventricular filling pressures, and systemic arterial blood pressure. In addition, the length of hospital stay was reduced.[326] Enoximone was also useful to support cardiac function and potentially reduce PVR in children after cardiac transplantation.[327]

Digoxin (Digitek, Digox, Lanoxicaps, Lanoxin)

Digoxin can act as an inotropic agent; however, its effectiveness in children with congestive heart failure from large left-to-right shunts has been questioned. The clinical picture in such children often improved without echocardiographic evidence of increased contractility; frequently progressive ventricular dilatation was observed.[328,329] The role of digoxin to improve RV dysfunction associated with pulmonary hypertension or as part of a multimodal therapy during the interstage phase for infants with single ventricle physiology has also been debated.[330] A retrospective cohort study using data from the Pediatric Heart Network Single Ventricle Reconstruction Trial showed that 31% of eligible infants were discharged from the hospital with prescriptions for digoxin. The interstage mortality in these infants was 2.9% compared with 12.3% for those who were not prescribed digoxin (hazard ratio 3.5).[331] A recent analysis of the Pediatric Health Information (PHIS) database demonstrated an increased trend to prescribe digoxin to patients after the Norwood procedure.[332,333]

Digoxin has both direct and indirect physiologic effects. Its direct effects are mediated by inhibition of the membrane sodium-potassium ATP and thereby outward sodium ion flux. The resulting increased intracellular sodium concentration stimulates the membrane sodium-calcium exchanger, producing increased intracellular calcium and positive inotropic effect. The indirect effects of digoxin are mediated by stimulating the parasympathetic nervous system. The parasympathetic effects of digoxin slow the atrial and AV node conduction. The drug can also be used to slow down the ventricular response in atrial flutter and atrial fibrillation and to treat supraventricular tachycardia (SVT) (see discussion later in chapter).

A loading dose is usually administered (see Table 16.8) to achieve target concentrations because the volume of distribution is large and clearance, particularly in neonates and infants, is reduced and follows renal function maturation. Renal dysfunction can significantly prolong its elimination half-life. Therapeutic digoxin concentrations are between 0.5 and 2.0 ng/mL. Intravenous and oral dosing regimens are similar, although the onset of electrophysiologic effects from IV dosing are rapid (5–20 minutes).

Many drugs interact with digoxin and influence its pharmacokinetics. It should be assumed that almost any drug administered along with digoxin can affect the absorption and clearance, usually requiring the dose to be reduced.[334,335] The likelihood of digoxin toxicity increases with serum concentrations greater than 3 ng/mL.[336,337] Symptoms of toxicity include drowsiness, nausea, and vomiting. Various conduction abnormalities and SVT are the most frequent cardiac rhythm manifestations of digoxin toxicity in infants and young children. Older children and adults are more likely to experience AV block, ventricular dysrhythmias, junctional tachycardia, and premature ventricular contractions. Hypokalemia, specifically intracellular potassium depletion (often a result of long-standing diuretic use), exacerbates the proarrhythmogenic effects of digoxin.

CALCIUM

The role, mechanisms of action, and potential for deleterious consequences of IV calcium continue to be controversial.[338] It is the ionized calcium concentration that is important for myocardial function. Calcium is a positive inotrope, particularly when administered in the presence of hypocalcemia. It may also improve ventricular contractility when LV function is depressed by inhalational agents, β-adrenergic blockade, or disease (e.g., sepsis).[339,340] In the presence of a normal myocardium and normal ionized calcium concentrations, the effects of IV calcium on contractility are much more modest.[341] Extracellular calcium concentrations also play an important role in the regulation of peripheral vascular resistance. A calcium-sensing receptor has been identified on vascular cell walls.[342]

There is evidence in adults that the primary effect of calcium administered after cardiac surgery is to increase SVR and mean arterial pressure with little or no effect on intrinsic myocardial contractility.[338,343] In fact, the increase in afterload, if not accompanied by a corresponding increase in contractility, may only serve to decrease stroke volume and cardiac output. Calcium may cause or exacerbate reperfusion injury and cellular damage by mechanisms that include activation of calcium-dependent proteases and phospholipases and organelle damage caused by cellular calcium overload.[344–346] These concerns are particularly relevant in children immediately after cardiac surgery. IV calcium may also attenuate the β-adrenergic effects of concurrently administered epinephrine.[338]

The role of IV calcium administration in neonates and young infants, both alone and after cardiac surgery, is more complicated. Preterm and term neonates have erratic calcium handling and are prone to ionized hypocalcemia.[347,348] The neonatal myocardium is more sensitive to ionized hypocalcemia than the adult myocardium, owing to reduced intracellular calcium stores, immaturity of sarcoplasmic reticulum calcium-handling mechanisms, and greater dependency on transmembrane calcium flux for excitation-contraction coupling.[349] Furthermore, the need to administer substantial volumes of citrated and albumin-containing blood products (both of which bind calcium) and other fluids after CPB increases the likelihood of ionized hypocalcemia.[350] The most prudent approach includes awareness of the greater dependency of the immature myocardium on extracellular calcium, monitoring

of ionized calcium concentrations, and careful administration to maintain normal, or at most mildly increased, ionized calcium concentrations. This approach is particularly needed in neonates and in those with diminished LV function. Administration of large bolus doses of calcium immediately on reperfusion of the heart after a period of ischemia is probably ill-advised because of the potential to exacerbate reperfusion injury and even to cause myocardial contracture.

Extravasation of calcium can cause local venous irritation and local tissue necrosis.[351,352] Although it has been suggested that calcium gluconate may cause less venous harm than calcium chloride, we recommend that both forms be administered via a centrally positioned catheter whenever possible. Both forms of calcium increase ionized calcium concentrations similarly when equal amounts of elemental calcium are administered (3 : 1 calcium gluconate to calcium chloride).[353] Calcium may cause slowing of AV conduction and should be administered cautiously in children with sinus bradycardia or junctional rhythm. Care must also be exercised when administering calcium to children who are receiving digoxin, particularly in the presence of concurrent hypokalemia, because IV calcium exacerbates the potential for digoxin-induced dysrhythmias in this setting.

TRIIODOTHYRONINE (THYROXINE)

Triiodothyronine hormone (T_3) is essential for the maturation of sarcolemmal calcium channels, myosin, actin, and troponin. In addition, hypothyroid rats demonstrate reduced numbers of β-receptors and reduced density of stimulatory secondary messenger protein with an increase in inhibitory secondary messenger protein density. T_3 is mostly produced by monodeiodination of thyroxine. This process is inhibited by surgery, hypothermia, catecholamines, propranolol, and amiodarone; therefore, postoperative T_3 concentrations are often reduced.[354–356]

T_3 replacement therapy acts via two pathways, intranuclear and extranuclear. Intranuclear effects include an increase in mitochondrial density and respiration, an increase in contractile protein synthesis, and an upregulation in β-adrenoceptors. Extranuclear effects include an improvement in glucose transport, increased stimulation of L-type calcium channels with subsequent calcium mobility, and increased efficiency in calcium reuptake with subsequent improvement in diastolic relaxation.

Endocrine function is compromised after cardiac surgery. Infants younger than 3 months of age with low T_3 concentrations on intensive care admission after cardiac surgery have a more complicated intensive care course. Low cortisol concentration is common in the early postoperative period but is not associated with postoperative complications.[357] A randomized, double-blind, placebo-controlled study of T_3 administration in children undergoing simple or complex cardiac surgery demonstrated that myocardial function was better and length of stay in the intensive care unit was decreased in the T_3 group.[358] T_3 improved contractility without any associated increase in oxygen consumption. In addition, the T_3 group demonstrated no delay in recovery of thyroid function secondary to exogenous administration. The dose of T_3 used was 2 µg/kg on day 1 followed by 1 µg/kg on days 2 through 12. A randomized, double-blind, placebo-controlled study of T_3 administration in neonates undergoing the Norwood procedure or repair of interrupted aortic arch and VSD closure demonstrated only more rapid achievement of negative fluid balance.[359] Many follow-up studies have been flawed by small numbers and patient heterogenicity; thus, routine postoperative T_3 replacement therapy remains controversial.[360–364]

CALCIUM-SENSITIZING AGENTS

Levosimendan (Simdax, Simendan)

Calcium-sensitizing agents represent a relatively new class of drugs with inotropic properties. Levosimendan has been in clinical use since 2000 and is one of the best studied drugs in this class. It provides positive inotropy, lusitropy, vasodilation, and cardioprotection via two distinct mechanisms: calcium sensitizing and opening of K^+ channels. Levosimendan binds to troponin C and seems to maintain the calcium-binding site of troponin C in its active conformation. This shifts the calcium-binding–concentration relationship toward increased binding (i.e., more binding at reduced intracardiac calcium concentrations). Contraction is thereby enhanced for a given cytosolic calcium concentration. In contrast to other types of inotropic agents, myocardial contractility is greater with minimal increase in oxygen demand. The concept of increasing the sensitivity to calcium rather than the cellular calcium concentration is also attractive because it reduces the deleterious effects of increased calcium concentrations on oxygen consumption, mitochondrial function, and activation of various calcium-dependent proteases and phospholipases (e.g., during ischemia-reperfusion).

Levosimendan has also been shown to stimulate membrane and mitochondrial ATP-sensitive potassium (K_{ATP}) channels; the former dilates the coronary, pulmonary, and the systemic vasculature. Opening mitochondrial K_{ATP} channels is likely to be an important mechanism of pharmacologic (and anesthetic) preconditioning and potential cytoprotection. Interestingly, and for reasons that are not entirely clear, levosimendan has either no effect or a positive effect on lusitropy (diastolic relaxation). At much larger doses than clinically used, it does inhibit phosphodiesterase III. Compared with other inotropic agents (e.g., dopamine, amrinone, milrinone), its effectiveness as a positive inotrope is maintained in the depressed myocardium.[325,365,366] The safety of levosimendan has been well established in adults; headaches, hypokalemia, and tachycardia are the most common side effects. A reported possible increased incidence of atrial fibrillation is controversial.[367,368]

Clinical effects include improved cardiac output, reduced ventricular filling pressures, and decreased PVR during the acute treatment of adult patients with either stable or decompensated heart failure.[367–370] However, initial mortality studies failed to show any improvements in short- or long-term prognosis for acute heart failure with levosimendan compared with dobutamine or placebo[371]; a meta-analysis of 45 studies in a wide variety of settings reported potential advantages.[372] Other investigations reported improved cardiac performance after cardiotomy and bypass, including beneficial responses in adult patients who appeared to be poorly responsive to other inotropes.[373–378] Beneficial effects were also found with levosimendan pretreatment directly before bypass,[379] but a large multicenter randomized controlled trial (LICORN) failed to demonstrate any major advantage of prophylactic levosimendan for adult patients with decreased ventricular function undergoing cardiac surgery.[380]

Current recommendations suggest a 6- to 12-µg/kg loading dose followed by an infusion of 0.05 to 0.2 µg/kg per minute for 24 hours. Although the elimination half-life is approximately 1 hour, effects are mediated through changes in structural calcium sensitivity that may last for 7 to 9 days. At least one metabolite (OR-1896) has prolonged (approximately 80 hours) effects and this may, in part, account for observations of sustained benefit after drug discontinuation.[381]

There are limited data available regarding the use of levosimendan in children or immature animal preparations. Most of the evidence in children stems from retrospective and observational studies, case reports, or registry inquiries.[315,382–395] These reports suggest that levosimendan is well tolerated, improving cardiac output and reducing afterload in children with low cardiac output syndrome.[383] Only a few randomized controlled trials have been published: two studies compared levosimendan with milrinone in children after congenital cardiac surgery and concluded that levosimendan is safe and at least as effective as milrinone.[315,316] Another study compared levosimendan with a standard treatment with milrinone and dopamine and came to the same conclusion.[396] In one study, the effect of levosimendan on pulmonary artery pressures was superior to dobutamine during pediatric cardiac surgery.[397] A Cochrane review in 2017 and subsequent small controlled trials failed to demonstrate any benefits from the prophylactic use of levosimendan compared with standard preventive measures.[398–400] The most recent comparison of milrinone and levosimendan on myocardial function using transthoracic echocardiography failed to identify any important differences.[401] The current data suggest the need for further studies to clearly define a role for levosimendan in infants and children with decreased myocardial performance from cardiac surgery, myocarditis, and sepsis.[325,383,402] It may have a role in inotrope rotation for children suffering cardiomyopathy. Its widespread clinical application is limited due to the high cost of the drug and the restricted availability. Currently levosimendan is still in phase III trials in North America and only approved in Europe, Asia, South America, and Australia. Its use in children (<18 years of age) is off-label, under compassionate care, and requires informed consent.[325]

B-TYPE NATRIURETIC PEPTIDE AND NESIRITIDE (NATRECOR)

B-type natriuretic peptide (BNP) and its N-terminal precursor are members of the natriuretic peptide family. These peptides are released from the heart in response to pressure and volume overload and play an important role in maintaining fluid balance and hemodynamic stability. BNP is secreted from cardiac ventricles in response to increased stimulation of cardiac stretch receptors and increased wall tension. It acts mainly via natriuretic peptide receptors that are present in large vessels and kidneys. Once stimulated, natriuretic peptide receptors promote diuresis, natriuresis, and vasodilation and inhibit the renin-angiotensin-aldosterone system. BNP is used as a marker for heart failure in adults and as a monitor for the response to anticongestive heart failure therapies.[403] These markers are also increasingly used to diagnose cardiovascular disease in neonates, infants, and children. The concentrations of N-terminal precursor-BNP are often dramatically increased immediately after birth and then wane during the first week of life. Age-adjusted cut points and reference values have been suggested.[404,405] Post hoc analysis of a large multicenter heart failure trial (Pediatric Carvedilol Trial) tried to establish prognostic cutoff values. In children with moderately symptomatic heart failure from cardiomyopathy or CHD, a BNP greater than or equal to 140 pg/mL was associated with worse outcomes.[406] Disease-specific cutoff points and their prognostic value, especially for congenital heart defects and perioperative risk assessment, are still under investigation.[407–412]

Nesiritide is a recombinant form of BNP and therefore acts via natriuretic peptide receptors to promote diuresis, natriuresis, and vasodilation. Early investigations in the adult population suggested that nesiritide may be beneficial for patients with decompensated heart failure; it seemed to improve cardiac output, reduce pulmonary capillary occlusion pressure, and dilate arterial and venous vessels with only minimal increase in HR or myocardial oxygen consumption.[413–415] However, a large multicenter study found no advantages of nesiritide and only recommended its use as an individualized case-based therapy.[416] Empirical perioperative nesiritide or milrinone infusions were not associated with improved early clinical outcomes after Fontan surgery.[417] Although nesiritide reduces mean arterial pressure in children after cardiac surgery and has been used as adjunct therapy in children with biventricular failure, more extensive studies are required before its usefulness and safety in children can be determined.[418–427]

β-BLOCKING AGENTS

There are several indications for the use of β-blockers in children, including control of systemic hypertension (both acutely in the perioperative period and chronically), treatment of cyanotic spells and right ventricular outflow tract obstruction in TOF, reduction of left ventricular outflow tract obstruction in hypertrophic cardiomyopathy, and control of HR in thyrotoxicosis, pheochromocytoma, and SVT (see discussion later in the chapter).[428–432] In contrast to the situation in adults, the use of β-blockers to treat chronic heart failure in children is controversial.[433] It seems that nonselective β-blockers are less effective than selective types due to age-related differences in receptor downregulation.[434,435] In pediatric heart failure both β_1 and β_2 adrenergic receptors are downregulated, as opposed to only the β_1 receptors in adults. Other important distinctions include β-receptor subtype selectivity, variability in half-life and metabolism, and intrinsic sympathomimetic activity. Even "selective" β-blockers lose their selectivity at increased plasma concentrations. Although the mechanism is incompletely understood, β-blocker use in children is associated with hypoglycemia.[436] Consequently, vigilance should be exercised during periods of fasting and illness as reflex adrenergic responses to hypoglycemia may be blunted.

Propranolol (Inderal, InnoPran)

Propranolol is one of the most frequently used β-blockers in children. Typical oral doses start at 0.25 to 0.5 mg/kg every 6 hours, titrated every 3 to 5 days; the usual dose is 2 to 4 mg/kg per day. A sustained-release form is available for older children who are able to swallow pills. IV propranolol is administered at doses of 0.01 to 0.1 mg/kg over several minutes; this may be increased if necessary (maximum dose 1 mg in infants, 3 mg in children). Sinus bradycardia and hypotension can be serious complications, particularly in infants or after IV administration. Propranolol may also cause conduction disturbances at the AV node and worsen pump function in congestive heart failure. Other important adverse effects include fatigue, depression, and lethargy. Interactions with the β_2-receptor may also exacerbate bronchospasm.[437] Propranolol is primarily metabolized in the liver; significant population variability in its kinetics has been noted. Metabolism is also affected by factors that alter hepatic blood flow because it has perfusion limited clearance. Its major metabolite, 4-hydroxypropranolol, is also active.[429]

Atenolol (Tenormin)

The use of atenolol has been increasing in children.[432,438,439] Compared with propranolol, it is more selective for the β_1-adrenergic receptor subtype; the elimination half-life is 8 to 12 hours. There is little hepatic biotransformation, and there are no active metabolites. The typical starting dose is 0.8 to 1.5 mg/kg per day in 1 or 2 doses daily, with an upper limit in the range of 2 mg/kg per day. No IV form is available. Atenolol does not cross the bloodbrain barrier, so some of the limiting adverse effects common to

propranolol are absent. At large doses, β_1 selectivity is probably lost, leading to the potential to exacerbate bronchospasm and hypoglycemia.

Esmolol (Brevibloc)

Esmolol is a relatively selective β_1-adrenergic blocker with several unique features. These features include its rapid onset of action, the ease of titratability to a desired endpoint, and its rapid termination via metabolism by red blood cell and plasma esterases.[440,441] The drug has been particularly useful to control perioperative hypertension acutely and to treat SVT (see discussion later in the chapter). Loading doses between 100 and 500 μg/kg given over 1 to 5 minutes are followed by maintenance infusions of 50 to 100 μg/kg per minute. If the desired response is not achieved, the infusion rate is then doubled every 5 minutes until a desired response is achieved.

Specific data on pediatric dosing are limited.[442] One study investigated the pharmacokinetics of esmolol therapy after an episode of stimulated or spontaneous SVT; the results were similar to the findings in the adult population.[443] Esmolol has been investigated to control blood pressure immediately after coarctation repair using 3 different bolus doses: 125 μg/kg, 250 μg/kg, and 500 μg/kg IV infused over 10 to 20 seconds, each followed by an infusion that consisted of the same dose as in the bolus every minute.[444] Blood pressure response and adverse events were similar among the groups. Clearance in neonates was twice that in older children (281 mL/kg per minute vs. 126 mL/kg per minute), consistent with other drugs cleared by plasma esterases (e.g., remifentanil).[444] The current maximum loading dose recommended is 500 μg/kg followed by an infusion rate of 25 to 300 μg/kg per minute.[445] A major potential adverse effect of esmolol is hypotension, particularly during bolus therapy. As noted earlier, esmolol rapidly distributes and has a very small elimination half-life (7–10 minutes) that is unaffected by organ blood flow or disease. Therefore, hypotension is usually shortlived, but therapy with vasopressors may occasionally be required until it resolves.[446,447]

Labetalol (Normodyne, Trandate)

Labetalol has nonselective β-adrenergic blocking properties and is also a selective α-adrenergic receptor blocker. The ratio of α- to β-blockade efficiency is 1:3 and 1:7 after oral and IV administration, respectively. The primary use of labetalol in children is to control hypertension. The drug has been given by IV to treat hypertensive crisis, to control hypertension after aortic coarctation repair, and as an adjunct to induce controlled hypotension during surgery.[448–451] Typical doses are 0.1 to 0.4 mg/kg given every 5 to 10 minutes until the desired effect is achieved with infusions of 0.25 to 1 mg/kg per hour. The elimination half-life of labetalol is 3 to 5 hours.

Carvedilol (Coreg)

Carvedilol is a nonselective β-blocker with additional vasodilator and some antioxidant properties.[452,453] The ratio of α_1 to β_1 blockade is 1:1.7; it is primarily used to treat heart failure. In adults, benefits include reduced mortality, reduced hospital stay, improved New York Health Association (NYHA) functional class, and a somewhat reduced progression of the clinical disease.[454] However, a randomized, double-blind, placebo-controlled, multicenter study of children and adolescents with symptomatic systolic heart failure found no differences in outcome between carvedilol and placebo during an 8-month follow-up period and a

Cochrane review found insufficient evidence to support its use.[456] These findings could be explained by the age-related differences in receptor downregulation.[434,435] Nevertheless, carvedilol is often prescribed after an episode of acute decompensation in patients with cardiomyopathy[457] and is part of the pediatric heart failure management guidelines published by the International Society for Heart and Lung Transplantation.[458] Carvedilol may have differential effects based on ventricular morphology, and further studies are necessary.[459–462] A retrospective review of the initial experience with carvedilol therapy in children showed that adverse effects— mainly dizziness, headaches, and hypotension—were common (>50%) but well tolerated.[463,464] The ideal dose in children has not yet been determined. Pharmacokinetic studies suggest a faster elimination in young patients, especially in children less than 3.5 years of age, and the need for more frequent dosing as well as larger doses per kg.[465,466] The clinical experience in small patient populations favors smaller doses and gradual dose adjustments with frequent echocardiographic and BNP monitoring.[462] The usual starting dose is 0.05 mg/kg per day divided in 2 doses, with slow increases every 2 weeks.

Ivabradine (Corlanor)

Ivabradine selectively blocks the I_f (funny) current in the sinoatrial node and can effectively lower heart rate. It has been recommended for the management of refractory heart failure or angina in specific groups of adult patients.[467,468] It has also been used in children with dilated cardiomyopathy and to treat junctional ectopic tachycardia.[469,470]

VASODILATORS

Vasodilators are used in children to control blood pressure during and after surgery, to treat systemic and pulmonary hypertension, and to decrease afterload on either the systemic or the pulmonary ventricle to improve pump function. Vasodilators are also administered during CPB to reduce SVR, improve regional perfusion, and facilitate rapid and even core cooling and rewarming. Tobias et al. provide a detailed overview of frequently used medications, typical indications, dosing, and common side effects.[471]

Vasodilators can be divided into pharmacologic groups. Direct-acting nitrosovasodilators such as sodium nitroprusside (SNP) and nitroglycerin are the most commonly used cardiovascular medications. These drugs relax vascular smooth muscle to cause vasodilation by directly (SNP) or indirectly (nitroglycerin), releasing NO that subsequently activates smooth muscle soluble guanylyl cyclase to form cyclic guanosine monophosphate (cGMP). Nicardipine is a dihydroxypyridine calcium channel blocker that is highly selective for calcium channels in the coronary and peripheral vasculature. It is an effective vasodilator with minimal effects on HR and contractility and is often used as a longer-acting alternative to SNP. Clevidipine is a short-acting, intravenous calcium channel blocker of the dihydroxypyridine class that is frequently used in adult patients as an alternative to SNP; it is currently not approved for children. Hydralazine is another direct-acting smooth muscle vasodilator that is occasionally given to children to reduce blood pressure. Selective α-adrenergic blockers, such as phentolamine and phenoxybenzamine, are occasionally used perioperatively to reduce blood pressure and SVR. The classic indication is the treatment of pheochromocytoma, but they are also frequently given during hypothermic CPB.

Ventricular "remodeling" and long-term blood pressure control is often achieved with angiotensin-converting enzyme (ACE) inhibitors. Prostaglandin E_1 (PGE_1) is a direct-acting vasodilator primarily used to maintain the patency of the ductus arteriosus in duct-dependent circulations. In contrast, prostacyclin and inhaled NO are vasodilators with relatively selective effects on the pulmonary vasculature. Commonly used vasodilators and antihypertensive agents are summarized in Table 16.9.

TABLE 16.9	Antihypertensives and Vasodilators[a]	
Drug	**Intravenous Dose**	**Comments**
Propranolol	0.01–0.1 mg/kg slowly	Nonselective β-blockade; bradycardia, hypotension, worsening of myocardial pump function; atrioventricular block; hypoglycemia; bronchospasm; depression; fatigue.
Labetalol	0.1–0.4 mg/kg per dose; 0.25–1.0 mg/kg per hour infusion	Nonselective β-blockade; selective α-blockade; ratio of α- to β-blockade is 1:7 for intravenous form; doses (0.1 mg/kg) can be repeated every 5–10 minutes until desired effect is achieved; side effects are similar to those of propranolol.
Esmolol	100–500 µg/kg loading dose (over 5 min); 50–250 µg/kg per minute infusion	Relatively selective β-blockade; short elimination half-life (7–10 minutes); hypotension, especially during bolus administration; if less than desired response after 5 minutes, can repeat or double bolus dose, followed by doubling infusion rate; non–organ-based metabolism by plasma and red blood cell esterases; infusion concentrations >10 mg/mL may predispose to venous sclerosis; dilute infusion at high rates increases risk of volume overload.
Sodium nitroprusside	Start at 0.3–1.0 µg/kg per minute infusion; maximum 6–10 µg/kg per minute	Potent direct smooth muscle relaxation; dilates both arteriolar resistance and venous capacitance vessels; hypotension potentiated by hypovolemia, inhalation anesthetics, other antihypertensives; variable pulmonary vasodilation; potential cyanide toxicity; reflex tachycardia; check cyanide and thiocyanate levels if >4 µg/kg per minute is infused or drug is used longer than 2–3 days.
Nitroglycerin	0.5–10 µg/kg per minute infusion	Direct smooth muscle relaxation; predominantly dilates venous capacitance vessels, modest effects on arterial resistance at larger doses; weak antihypertensive effects; variable pulmonary vasodilation; used to facilitate cooling and rewarming during cardiopulmonary bypass.

TABLE 16.9	Antihypertensives and Vasodilators—cont'd	
Drug	**Intravenous Dose**	**Comments**
Nicardipine	Start at 0.5–1 µg/kg per minute infusion; maximum 4–5 µg/kg per minute	Dihydroxypyridine calcium channel blocker: primary effects on coronary and peripheral vasculature, predominantly vasodilation, minimal effects on heart rate and contractility. Hypotension potentiated by inhalational agents. Potentiation of neuromuscular blockers. Prolonged effects after discontinuation.
Phentolamine	0.05–0.1 mg/kg dose; 0.5–5 µg/kg per minute infusion	Selective α-blocker, produces mainly arteriolar vasodilation; some direct vasodilation with mild venodilation.
Enalaprilat	5–10 µg/kg per dose q8–24 hours	Long duration of effect; angioedema, renal failure, hyperkalemia; potential problematic hypotension with anesthetic agents (see text).
Hydralazine	0.1–0.2 mg/kg bolus q6 hours	Maximum 20 mg/dose; direct-acting smooth muscle (predominantly arteriolar) vasodilation; long effective half-life; tachyphylaxis; reflex tachycardia; lupus-like syndrome; drug fever; thrombocytopenia.
Prostaglandin E$_1$	0.05–0.1 µg/kg per minute infusion	Direct smooth muscle relaxation, relatively specific for ductus arteriosus; variable pulmonary and systemic vasodilation; apnea in neonates.

^{a}All drugs should be started in the lower dose range and titrated to effect.

Sodium Nitroprusside (Nipride, Nitropress)

The primary indication for SNP is to reduce afterload and blood pressure rapidly and consistently before, during, and after a wide variety of procedures. For example, it is used to control intraoperative and postoperative hypertension in children with aortic coarctation and other forms of left ventricular outflow tract obstruction. The reduction in afterload may improve performance of a dysfunctional ventricle, particularly when combined with a positive inotropic agent.[472,473] The ability of nitroprusside to successfully treat pulmonary hypertension is variable and may be age dependent.[474–478]

SNP is an extremely potent vasodilator that acts directly on smooth muscle to cause dilation.[479,480] Its effects reduce cardiac preload as well as afterload. Onset of effect is fast (within minutes), and offset is similarly rapid; the effect ends within 1 to 2 minutes after termination of the infusion. Because of its potency, it should always be administered using an infusion pump in conjunction with continuous direct arterial pressure monitoring. The initial infusion rate is 0.3 to 1 µg/kg per minute. This rate can be titrated to achieve the desired effect. The titration of nitroprusside to achieve specific blood pressure goals can be rather frustrating and often results in large blood pressure swings.[481] Population-based pharmacokinetic-pharmacodynamic models have been used to produce dosing guidelines. A starting dose of 0.3 µg/kg per minute, small dose adjustments, and slow weaning are recommended to avoid hypotension or rebound hypertension.[482,483] The hypotensive effects of nitroprusside are potentiated by hypovolemia, inhalation anesthetics, and drugs that inhibit the reflex responses to direct vasodilation (e.g., increase in sympathetic tone, renin release), such as propranolol and ACE inhibitors.

Adverse effects of SNP include cyanide and thiocyanate toxicities, rebound hypertension, inhibition of platelet function, and increased intrapulmonary shunting via attenuation of hypoxic pulmonary vasoconstriction. Rebound hypertension is most likely caused by activation of the reflex mechanisms. This effect is minimized by slowly tapering the infusion rather than abruptly discontinuing it. Toxicity may occur when more than 10 µg/kg per minute of SNP is administered, if tachyphylaxis develops within 30 minutes, or if there is immediate resistance to the drug. A blood cyanide concentration of approximately 500 µg/dL has been linked to a pediatric death,[484] but subsequent studies showed that increased concentrations of cyanide were not necessarily associated with the clinical signs of cyanide toxicity.[485,486] Cyanide and thiocyanate toxicities are rare but may be more likely in neonates and young infants and in those with impaired hepatic or renal function.[487]

Cyanide is produced from the metabolism of SNP. Free cyanide is then conjugated with thiosulfate by rhodanase in the liver to produce thiocyanate. A major mechanism of cyanide toxicity is binding to cytochrome oxidase in the mitochondrial electron transport chain, which prevents mitochondrial respiration and ATP production. Signs of toxicity include tachyphylaxis, an increase in mixed venous oxygen saturation, and metabolic acidosis. For children who have received prolonged (>24 hours) or large-dose infusions of nitroprusside and in those with organ dysfunction, it may be prudent to measure blood cyanide concentrations periodically.[486,488–491] Serum thiocyanate concentrations may also be measured. Thiocyanate concentrations may increase if renal function is abnormal. Central nervous system (CNS) dysfunction can occur when thiocyanate concentrations reach 5 to 10 mg/dL. Treatment of cyanide toxicity consists of IV infusion of sodium nitrite, 6 mg/kg (maximum dose 300 mg) over 5 minutes, and sodium thiosulfate, 250 mg/kg or 7 g/m^2 (maximum dose 12.5 g) over 15 minutes. In children with abnormal renal function in whom stimulating the production of thiocyanate from thiosulfate may be contraindicated, administration of hydroxocobalamin has been recommended.[492,493]

Nitroglycerin (Nitronal, Nitro-Bid)

Nitroglycerin is primarily a venodilator that acts on venous capacitance vessels. It has a substantially smaller effect on arteriolar smooth muscle, and its ability to attenuate an increased PVR is variable. Compared with nitroprusside, it is a poor antihypertensive agent. It has a brief half-life and no toxic metabolites. Like nitroprusside, nitroglycerin may increase intrapulmonary shunting and cause platelet dysfunction. Nitroglycerin is typically infused at rates between 0.5 and 3.0 µg/kg per minute. The onset of clinical effects occurs within 2 minutes of starting the nitroglycerin and resolves within 5 minutes after it is discontinued. Mild decreases in blood pressure may be observed at infusion rates exceeding 2 to 3 µg/kg per minute. If nitroglycerin or nitroprusside are infused for prolonged periods, methemoglobin and cyanmethemoglobin levels can accumulate.[494]

Nitroglycerin is frequently used during CPB to facilitate rapid and effective cooling and rewarming and to improve tissue blood flow. Nitroprusside and nitroglycerin differ substantially with regard to their effects on the microcirculation. Because nitroprusside primarily reduces arteriolar tone and dilates precapillaries, it decreases microvascular blood flow and tissue perfusion more than nitroglycerin does, particularly in the presence of reduced arterial blood pressure (e.g., during CPB).[495] In contrast, nitroglycerin dilates precapillaries and postcapillaries with equal efficacy, thereby maintaining stable or enhanced capillary perfusion.[496,497]

Nicardipine (Cardene)

Nicardipine was the first IV dihydroxypyridine calcium channel blocker available for clinical use to treat hypertension in children of all ages, for over 20 years. Compared with nifedipine, nicardipine has a greater selectivity for calcium channels in the coronary and peripheral vasculature, resulting in predominant vasodilation and only minimal effects on HR and contractility.[498,499] Many adult studies investigated nicardipine for perioperative blood pressure control,[500–503] but only limited pediatric data are available, derived mainly from small case series and observational reports.[504–508] Nicardipine has been successfully used to control hypertension in preterm infants and neonates.[505,509,510] Given as a continuous infusion at an initial rate of 0.5 to 1 µg/kg per minute, the rate is slowly increased every 15 to 30 minutes until the target blood pressure is reached. Usual doses range from 1 to 3 µg/kg per minute, with a maximum dose of 4 to 5 µg/kg per minute[504,511,512]; 50% of the maximum change occurs within 45 minutes. In one retrospective study in children, it took an average of 2.7 ± 2.1 hours (range 0.5–9 hours) to achieve blood pressure control with this dosing regimen.[504] An alternative high-dose approach has been described, starting with an initial dose of 5 to 10 µg/kg per minute and followed by a smaller maintenance dose of 2 to 3 µg/kg per minute (range 1–5 µg/kg per minute) once the blood pressure is well controlled.[513,514] Nicardipine is extensively metabolized in the liver (cytochrome P450, isoenzyme CYP3A4) and excreted in urine and feces. An adult two-compartment pharmacokinetic model revealed an α-half-life of 2.7 minutes, a β-half-life of 44.8 minutes, and a slow terminal phase (γ-half-life) of 14.4 hours, contributing to the prolonged effects of nicardipine. After discontinuing the infusion, the antihypertensive effects decrease by 50% within the first 30 minutes but persist for up to 50 hours. Clearance is reduced by hepatic dysfunction. Common adverse effects include mild reflex tachycardia, flushing, nausea and vomiting, or phlebitis at the infusion site.[504] In contrast to nitroprusside, there is no tachyphylaxis, and nicardipine can be administered for extended periods of time without concern for accumulating toxic metabolites. Interactions with inhalational anesthetic agents and neuromuscular-blocking drugs should be considered during intraoperative use.[513] Inhalational anesthetics blunt the baroreflex-mediated increase in HR and increase the hypotensive effects of nicardipine[515]; the effects of depolarizing and nondepolarizing neuromuscular-blocking drugs will be potentiated and should be closely monitored.[516] In the United States, nicardipine is increasingly used as a substitute for nitroprusside due to the limited availability and high costs of nitroprusside.

Clevidipine (Cleviprex)

Clevidipine was introduced in 2007 as a short-acting intravenous L-type dihydropyridine calcium channel antagonist to treat acute hypertension. It is currently only approved for adults in the USA where it is often an alternative to SNP for tight blood pressure control in the perioperative period. Due to its rapid metabolism by nonspecific blood and tissue esterases, the half-life is only 1 to 3 minutes. Initial studies using infusion rates from 0.4 to maximal 8 µg/kg per minute, noted that the target blood pressure was achieved in a median time of 5 to 6 minutes and returned to baseline in 5 to 15 minutes after discontinuation.[517–519] Pediatric experience remains limited to small case series, retrospective reviews, and observational studies.[520–525] Clevidipine seems to be effective for the control of blood pressure in various clinical situations (e.g., spinal fusions, renal failure, postoperative period after cardiac surgery). In most cases the infusion was started at 0.5 to 1 µg/kg per minute and titrated up by 0.5 to 1 µg/kg per minute every 2 minutes as needed to achieve the target pressures. At the larger dosing ranges (5–7 µg/kg per minute) reflex tachycardia was occasionally observed that required treatment with β-blockers. Otherwise, the infusion was well tolerated. In the spinal fusion series, 40% of patient were back at their baseline pressures within 10 minutes after discontinuation of the infusion.[521]

Interestingly, clevidipine was ineffective during cooling on CPB, possibly due to hypothermia induced inactivation of the receptors and required additional direct-acting agents to control mean arterial pressure. Adverse effects are similar to nicardipine and include mild increase in intracranial pressure and impairment of hypoxic pulmonary vasoconstriction; reflex tachycardia may be more pronounced. Clevidipine is prepared in a lipid solution with disodium EDTA to suppress bacterial growth. To avoid contamination, infusions should be changed every 12 hours. Concerns have been expressed regarding administering clevidipine to patients with allergies to eggs and soy products or disorders of lipid metabolism, although these concerns are likely carried over from those associated with propofol and its carrier medium (i.e., unlikely).[526] When used in combination with propofol infusions, it can result in mild elevations of triglyceride concentrations.[524]

Phentolamine (Regitine, OraVerse) and Phenoxybenzamine (Dibenzyline)

Both phentolamine and phenoxybenzamine are α-adrenergic blocking agents with little selectivity for α-receptor subtypes. Their primary effect is to decrease resistance on the arterial side of the circulation, although both possess weak venodilating capabilities. Phentolamine is usually administered by infusion at 0.5 to 5 µg/kg per minute, whereas phenoxybenzamine is administered orally initially 0.2 mg/kg once daily, then slowly increased every 4 days by 0.2 mg/kg per day. The usual maintenance dose is 0.4 to 1.2 mg/kg per day divided in three doses. Phentolamine in a dose of 0.2 mg/kg is often used to facilitate even cooling during CPB.[527] In an animal model phentolamine has been shown to decrease cerebral metabolic rate of oxygen and vascular resistance index but without any effect on apoptosis.[528] The elimination half-life of phenoxybenzamine is much greater than that of phentolamine. Some cardiovascular centers have found the long-acting effects of phenoxybenzamine to be advantageous, especially to provide adequate vasodilation during deep hypothermic CPB.[529–533]

Recently, an intraoral submucosal injectable formulation of phentolamine mesylate (OraVerse) was developed; it is used in pediatric dentistry to facilitate recovery from soft tissue local anesthesia.[534]

Angiotensin-Converting Enzyme Inhibitors

ACE inhibitors are administered to children with increasing frequency.[535-537] In the perioperative setting, they are given to control blood pressure after aortic coarctation repair or to relieve left ventricular outflow tract obstruction. In addition, ACE inhibitors are given on a more long-term basis to reduce afterload on the systemic ventricle and to improve ventricular performance in children with congestive heart failure or single ventricle physiology.[457,538,539] Among the growing number of ACE inhibitors, captopril, enalapril, and lisinopril are most often used in children, although data in children remain scant. A multicenter randomized controlled trial, investigating the efficacy of enalapril in infants with single ventricle physiology found it was associated with no weight gain, or improvement in ventricular function or heart failure symptoms.[540] Adverse effects common to all ACE inhibitors include angioedema, acute renal failure, and hyperkalemia; case reports of substantive complications have been published.[541-543] Cyanosis and coadministration of furosemide are independent risk factors for acute kidney injury in children undergoing cardiac surgery who were treated with ACE inhibitors.[539]

The contribution of ACE inhibitors to anesthetic-induced hypotension remains controversial.[544-548] Angiotensin receptor–blocking agents such as losartan and lisinopril can produce refractory hypotension with standard anesthetic induction techniques.[549] Because of this potential risk for substantive refractory hypotension that is usually unresponsive to volume expansion and requires substantial vasoconstrictor treatment, it is our practice to discontinue long-acting ACE inhibitors 1 day before surgery.

Captopril (Capoten)

Captopril has a relatively brief elimination half-life (<2 hours); clearance is by metabolism in the liver (captopril-cysteine disulfide and the disulfide dimer) and excretion by the kidney.[550] Oral dosing in neonates is 0.05 to 0.1 mg/kg every 8 to 24 hours, titrated up to 0.5 mg/kg every 6 to 24 hours. Infants initially receive 0.15 to 0.3 mg/kg every 6 to 8 hours. This can be titrated toward a maximum dose of 6 mg/kg per day in 4 divided doses. Oral dosing in older children is 0.3 to 0.5 mg/kg every 6 to 12 hours. The brief duration of effect, necessitating more frequent dosing, has led to increased use of the longer-acting ACE inhibitors (enalapril and lisinopril) in children.

Enalapril (Vasotec, Epaned) and Lisinopril (Prinivil, Qbrelis, Zestril)

Enalapril is metabolized in the liver to its active form, enalaprilat. Enalapril is the only ACE inhibitor currently available in the United States that has an IV formulation. It can also be given orally, once or twice daily, with daily doses ranging between 0.1 and 0.5 mg/kg. The IV dose is 0.005 to 0.01 mg/kg per dose, 1 to 3 times a day.[535] The initial oral dose for lisinopril is 0.07 mg/kg once daily, slowly titrated up to a maximal dose of 0.6 mg/kg.[551] Both enalapril and lisinopril are eliminated by the kidney. The duration of their hypotensive actions averages 24 hours but can extend to 30 hours.

Losartan (Cozaar)

Losartan blocks selectively angiotensin II type 1 (AT_1) receptors. It is used mainly to treat proteinuria and hypertension associated with renal disease in children and seems to be well tolerated.[552-556]

Losartan may also help to slow the rate of aortic root dilation in patients with Marfan syndrome.[557,558]

Hydralazine (Apresoline)

In the past, hydralazine was frequently used for long-term blood pressure control in children but has been largely replaced by ACE inhibitors. In contrast to its effect in adults, its ability to decrease pulmonary hypertension in children was disappointing.[559] Hydralazine directly relaxes smooth muscle without known effects on receptors. It reduces cardiac afterload but may cause reflex tachycardia. With long-term use, it may also cause fluid retention, requiring concurrent administration of a diuretic. Oral dosing is in the range of 0.75 to 1 mg/kg per day divided in 2 to 4 doses and is slowly increased over 3 to 4 weeks to a maximum dose of 5 mg/kg per day for infants and 7.5 mg/kg per day for children. In the perioperative setting, it is occasionally used by the IV route to control blood pressure and reduce afterload. IV doses are administered as a bolus of 0.1 to 0.2 mg/kg not to exceed 20 mg. The effects of IV hydralazine on PVR are variable.[559,560] Tachyphylaxis to the antihypertensive effects of IV hydralazine may occur. Important adverse effects include a drug-related fever, rash, pancytopenia, and lupus-like syndrome. The elimination half-life of the drug is approximately 4 hours, but the duration of its effective biologic half-life may be substantially greater because the drug binds to vascular smooth muscle.[561]

Prostaglandin E_1 (Alprostadil, Prostin)

The major indication for PGE_1 is to establish or maintain patency of the ductus arteriosus in neonates. It is best able to reopen a closing ductus in neonates up to 1 to 2 weeks of age but may occasionally be effective even in older infants.[21,562]

Ductal patency is important and often lifesaving for duct-dependent circulations—those in which either the lower body is supplied by right-to-left ductal flow (e.g., interrupted aortic arch, critical aortic stenosis, HLHS) or the PDA is the sole provider of pulmonary blood flow (e.g., pulmonary atresia, tricuspid atresia, severe TOF). Adverse effects of PGE_1 include systemic hypotension, apnea, increased risk of infection, leukocytosis, gastric outlet obstruction, and CNS irritability.[563-565] PGE_1 infusions usually start at 0.05 µg/kg per minute and may be increased to 0.1 µg/kg per minute or more; maintenance infusions range from 0.003 to 0.01 µg/kg per minute.[566,567] The risk of apnea may be related to the infusion rate. Tracheal intubation and ventilation are often required with infusion rates greater than 0.05 µg/kg per minute.[568,569] Prophylactic treatment with aminophylline was found to be effective in reducing the apnea risk.[570] Caffeine may also prove useful for those with apnea. PGE_1 has also been used to treat primary or acquired pulmonary hypertension with varying degrees of success.[571-576]

Inhaled Nitric Oxide (Inomax)

An important development in the treatment of pulmonary hypertension is inhaled NO gas, which can be delivered directly to the pulmonary circulation. NO is an endothelium-derived relaxing factor that acts on guanylate cyclase in vascular smooth muscle.[577] Endogenous NO is produced by endothelial cell NO synthase. NO synthases convert the amino acid l-arginine into NO and the by-product l-citrulline. NO then diffuses into the subjacent vascular smooth muscle. It produces relaxation by acting on smooth muscle guanylate cyclase to produce cGMP, which acts on a series of protein kinases and reduces intracellular calcium levels to inhibit muscle contraction (see Fig. 35.3A and B). Diffusion of NO in the other direction from the endothelial cell into the blood vessel lumen can decrease the adhesiveness of white blood cells and platelets. NO in the blood is rapidly bound by oxyhemoglobin, which is then oxidized to methemoglobin. From this reaction, NO is inactivated, and nitrite and nitrate are released in the blood. Red blood cell methemoglobin is subsequently reduced back to hemoglobin. The rapid binding and inactivation of NO in the blood means that inhaled NO has a minimal effect on the systemic circulation and functions as a very specific pulmonary vasodilator.

Reduction of PVR from inhaled NO has been demonstrated in adults with mitral stenosis, in neonates with persistent pulmonary hypertension of the neonate, in lung transplant recipients, and in children after surgical repair of a variety of CHDs.[578–582] Its potential antiinflammatory and neuroprotective role during deep hypothermic bypass is currently under investigation.[583] The efficacy of inhaled NO is in large part related to the ability to deliver it into the alveolus, which is in close proximity to the pulmonary vascular smooth muscle.

Inhaled NO has found several indications in children with CHD. In the cardiac catheterization laboratory, it is used to assess the reactivity of the pulmonary vasculature in children with pulmonary hypertension. This can help distinguish between children with fixed pulmonary vascular obstructive disease and those with a reversible component to pulmonary hypertension, thereby facilitating therapeutic management and operative planning.[584–587] Positive vascular reactivity is defined by a decrease in pulmonary artery pressures by at least 10 mm Hg with sustained cardiac output.[588]

In the postoperative period after the repair of CHD, NO can be used to reduce PVR and improve cardiopulmonary performance.[589–592] Experience thus far suggests that children with two ventricles who have increased LA pressure or its pathophysiologic equivalent (e.g., mitral stenosis, severe congestive heart failure, cardiomyopathy, large left-to-right shunt, TAPVR) are more likely to respond to NO in the postoperative period. Some children who do not respond to NO immediately after CPB in the operating room demonstrate reductions in PVR with NO several hours later. NO is administered in concentrations of 1 to 80 ppm in oxygen via a special delivery device attached to the ventilator or oxygen delivery system. Inspired gas is monitored for toxic nitrogen oxides; during long-term therapy with NO, blood methemoglobin concentrations should be assessed on a regular basis.[593]

Prostanoids
Members of the prostacyclin and prostaglandin families are often classified as *prostanoids*. All prostanoids are potent vasodilators and inhibitors of platelet aggregation. Since the 1980s, they have been used in the treatment of PA hypertension and are part of the official treatment guidelines (E-Fig. 16.4, E-Table 16.5),[594–599] even though they are not selective pulmonary vasodilators. Common adverse effects include flushing, hypotension, headache, jaw pain, skin rash, nausea and diarrhea, and nonspecific musculoskeletal pains. Tolerance can develop over time, requiring increasing doses.[600] Only three prostanoids are currently approved by the Food and Drug Administration (FDA): epoprostenol (Flolan), treprostinil (Remodulin), and iloprost (Ventavis). Beraprost is an oral prostacyclin analog licensed in several Asian countries and still being investigated.

Epoprostenol (Flolan, Veletri)
Continuous IV infusion of epoprostenol has been used for many years in children to treat PA hypertension of any cause. It improves hemodynamics by reducing PA pressure, increasing cardiac output, increasing oxygen transport, and improving symptoms such as exercise capacity and dyspnea.[601] It has been used with good results in the treatment of primary pulmonary hypertension and irreversible acquired pulmonary hypertension in CHD; in children awaiting heart, lung, or heart-lung transplantation; in children with primary pulmonary hypertension; in neonates with persistent pulmonary hypertension; and in pulmonary hypertensive crises.[602–610] The fact that children who were initially nonresponders may respond after prolonged use of NO suggests that its mechanism of action involves a degree of remodeling, although no absolute mechanism has been elucidated.

Unfortunately, epoprostenol is chemically unstable at room temperature and has a half-life of 6 minutes or less; it requires cooling for storage, continuous IV infusion via a central venous catheter, and a specific delivery system. Rapid and unintended decreases in the rate, dislodgments or occlusions of the central venous catheter, or pump malfunctions can lead to severe and life-threatening rebound pulmonary hypertension.[611,612] The infusion is usually started at 1 to 2 ng/kg per minute and gradually increased over several months to doses between 30 and 80 ng/kg per minute. In patients with pulmonary venous disease, IV epoprostenol can worsen the pulmonary edema; it can also increase the ventilation/perfusion mismatch in patients with pneumonia and thereby negatively affect oxygenation. In the acute setting, epoprostenol is increasingly used in the inhaled form to benefit from the selective pulmonary vasodilation and reduction of ventilation/perfusion mismatch.[600,613–615] Some centers have used inhaled epoprostenol as an alternative to the rather expensive NO, although the currently available delivery systems are far from ideal and may alter the delivered tidal volumes.[600]

Treprostinil (Remodulin)
Treprostinil was first introduced in 2002, initially only for continuous subcutaneous infusion, but later also for IV infusion in patients who could not tolerate the pain at the subcutaneous infusion site. The hemodynamic effects are similar to those of epoprostenol, with fewer adverse effects.[616–619] IV infusions of treprostinil are started at 1 to 2 ng/kg per minute and slowly increased over several weeks to 40 ng/kg per minute, occasionally even larger doses (80–120 ng/kg per minute) are used. One pediatric study confirmed the effectiveness of IV treprostinil in children.[620] Since 2009, inhaled treprostinil has been used for long-term outpatient management. Because of the relatively brief half-life, it must be administered every 6 hours.[621–624] A sustained-release oral form of treprostinil (Orenitram) has been investigated in adults; it showed some promising effects in treatment-naïve patients but failed to demonstrate significant long-term improvements in more advanced disease stages.[625–628] Side effects were common and included headaches, nausea, diarrhea, and flushing. The initial dose for adults is 0.25 mg every 12 hours or 0.125 mg every 8 hours. The pediatric experience with oral treprostinil is still limited. In a multicenter observational review, the authors described a high rate of adverse effects, especially nausea and headaches; on follow up, 50% of patients had discontinued the treatment.[629] Another small multicenter pharmacokinetic study in children transitioning from parenteral, inhaled or de novo additional treprostinil found the peak concentration at a median time of 3.8 hours with a wide variability. Optimal dosing guidelines are still unclear.[630] If more than two doses are missed (prolonged NPO status owing to gastrointestinal symptoms or surgical procedure), appropriate treatment with subcutaneous or IV treprostinil has to be initiated.

Iloprost (Ventavis)

Iloprost, approved by the FDA in 2004, is another prostaglandin I_2 analog that can be delivered by IV or via an ultrasonic nebulizer. It has a very brief elimination half-life of only 7 to 9 minutes, although its clinical efficacy is greater, with a half-life of 20 to 25 minutes. Frequent nebulized treatments (6 to 9 times each day) are required.[631] In adult studies, iloprost was shown to be beneficial in patients with PA hypertension of any cause, idiopathic PA hypertension, or chronic thromboembolic pulmonary hypertension. These patients demonstrated improvements in hemodynamics and in subjective parameters such as quality of life scores.[632–634] Studies in children are scarce and have involved only small numbers of patients, although numerous case reports are encouraging[600,635–643]; long-term effects and compliance are still under investigation.[644] When iloprost and NO were compared in children with CHD, the two agents produced similar effects.[645] In one study, combination therapy using both systemic and inhaled prostacyclin analog showed promise.[646] It has also been successfully used in the perioperative management of CHD patients with pulmonary hypertension[647] and for the postoperative transition from inhaled NO to an inhaled prostacyclin.[648] A study in lambs demonstrated an enhanced effect of prostacyclin and iloprost when combined with milrinone.[324]

Beraprost (Careload)

Beraprost sodium is an oral prostacyclin analog that is chemically more stable and has a prolonged elimination half-life but nevertheless requires dosing three to four times per day, reaching its peak blood concentration at 30 minutes. Two double-blind studies showed no long-term benefit, but there may still be a role for this drug in combination therapy because improvements have been observed in the exercise capacity of children with idiopathic PA hypertension.[649,650] Case reports of successful long-term treatment with beraprost and of combination therapy using oral beraprost and inhaled prostacyclin have been published.[646,651–653] Another case series described the use of beraprost for the treatment of persistent pulmonary hypertension in newborns.[654]

Endothelin-Receptor Antagonists

Endothelin-1 is a potent vasoconstrictor that is thought to be a key factor in the pathogenesis of PA hypertension. There are two known receptors on which it acts: endothelin A and endothelin B. Endothelin A receptors are present on smooth muscle cells, and agonist action causes vasoconstriction; endothelin B receptors are present on endothelial cells, and agonist action causes both relaxation and vasoconstriction through different pathways. In addition, endothelin B receptors are involved in the clearance of endothelin.

Bosentan (Tracleer)

Bosentan is an oral, nonselective endothelin-receptor antagonist. Adult studies have shown long-term benefit in patients with PA hypertension. It can also improve exercise capacity in adolescent and adult patients with a Fontan circulation.[655] Bosentan can cause abnormal liver function test results, although no severe liver dysfunction has been reported in adults.[656–660] Two studies in children showed both short-term reduction in PA pressure and PVR and longer-term improvement in symptoms and stabilization of the disease process.[601,661] In addition, three studies have suggested that the dose for children weighing more than 10 kg could largely follow adult guidelines, with the total daily dose not exceeding 125 mg. There is growing evidence, although few controlled studies, suggesting that bosentan is an effective and well-tolerated therapy in children.[662–664] Compared with the results in adult studies, hepatic dysfunction was less frequently reported but was still the most common adverse effect.[665–668]

Ambrisentan (Letairis)

Ambrisentan is a selective endothelial A receptor antagonist that has been extensively studied in the adult population.[669–671] It seems to be associated with an increased incidence of peripheral edema but a smaller risk for liver dysfunction.[672,673] The pediatric experience is limited but ambrisentan could be a safe and effective treatment alternative for some children with pulmonary arterial hypertension.[674]

Macitentan (Opsumit)

Macitentan is another oral, dual endothelin-receptor antagonist with promising results in adult studies[675]; however, there is only a limited pediatric experience.[676]

Selexipag (Uptravi)

Selexipag is an oral, selective prostacyclin agonist that was introduced as an additional component to various combination therapies[677] and is currently being investigated for the use in children.[678]

Phosphodiesterase Type 5 Inhibitors
Sildenafil (Viagra)

Sildenafil is a selective inhibitor of phosphodiesterase type 5, the isoform that is responsible for hydrolysis of cGMP in the pulmonary vasculature. By preventing the breakdown of cGMP, sildenafil increases cGMP concentrations and potentiates the pulmonary vasodilation caused by endogenous NO.[679–681] Sildenafil can also have positive effects on the ventricular contractility in patients with pulmonary hypertension because phosphodiesterase type 5 is highly expressed in the hypertrophied human right ventricle.[682] It has a long-standing track record in the adult population.[683–688] In the pediatric population, sildenafil is currently used as an adjunctive agent during weaning from NO, in the treatment of PA hypertension, for patients with congenital diaphragmatic hernia, for the perioperative management of patients after cardiac surgery, and also for persistent pulmonary hypertension of the newborn.[49,689–700] The benefit of combining oral sildenafil with inhaled iloprost for the treatment of severe pulmonary hypertension has also been demonstrated.[701] Most of the pharmacokinetic data for sildenafil are derived from adult studies with oral dosing. Sildenafil is rapidly absorbed; the bioavailability is 38% to 41% in the fasted state; and the maximum plasma concentration is achieved after 0.5 to 2.5 hours. It is highly metabolized in the liver into active metabolites. With a half-life of only 2 to 4 hours, sildenafil is relatively short-acting. Clearance decreases in patients with severe renal or hepatic dysfunction. Compared with healthy volunteers, patients with pulmonary hypertension have reduced clearance and greater bioavailability.[702–707] In adult patients, a 10 mg IV bolus and a 20 mg oral tablet have comparable effects.[708] According to in vitro studies, plasma concentrations of 50 to 400 ng/mL are necessary to provide a 50% to 90% inhibition of phosphodiesterase 5 activity.[709,710] Only a few pediatric pharmacokinetic studies are available. Children (1–17 years of age) with PA hypertension given oral sildenafil had a relatively high clearance (confounded by bioavailability).[711] Investigations in neonates demonstrated a larger volume of distribution, greater elimination half-life, and a rapidly increasing age-dependent metabolic clearance over the first month of postnatal life.[712,713] Oral therapy usually begins with 0.25 to 0.5 mg/kg every 4 to 6 hours with increasing doses as tolerated.[695,714,715] The IV use of sildenafil has been investigated in premature infants, neonates with persistent pulmonary hypertension, and children after congenital cardiac surgery[49,716–719]; sublingual administration of sildenafil has also been reported.[720] Sildenafil seems to be well tolerated; the most common adverse effects are headache, fever, respiratory infections, vomiting, and diarrhea,[711] but serious adverse events such as pulmonary hemorrhage, stridor, or hypotension have been occasionally observed.[665,711,721] In 2012, the results of a randomized, double-blind, placebo-controlled clinical trial (STARTS-1) investigating three different dose regiments of oral sildenafil for treatment-naïve children with pulmonary arterial hypertension were published. Body weight–adjusted groups were treated for 16 weeks with placebo, small- (10 mg tid), medium- (10–40 mg tid), or large-dose (20–80 mg tid) sildenafil. The effect was greater with the medium- and large-dose ranges.[711] A follow-up study (STARTS-2) after 2 years of treatment found an increased risk of mortality for the large-dose group,[722] which triggered the release of an FDA warning against the chronic use of sildenafil for children aged 1 to 17 years. The European Medicines Agency warned only against the use of large doses. The current controversy among pediatric cardiologists regarding the safety of sildenafil was fueled by several publications, which questioned the START-2 results.[721,723–725] In 2014, the FDA issued another statement clarifying that the risk-benefit profile of sildenafil might be acceptable for selected children in special situations. Oral phosphodiesterase 5 inhibitors are currently still part of the treatment guidelines for pulmonary hypertension in children.[588,595,596]

Tadalafil

Tadalafil is another selective phosphodiesterase 5 inhibitor. Compared with sildenafil, it has a longer duration of action, which permits once-daily dosing. Extrapolated data from adult studies suggest weight adjusted tadalafil doses of 1mg/kg per day. The initial experience in pediatric patients is promising.[726–729] A small multicenter pharmacokinetic study in pediatric patients >2years of age confirmed safety and established dosing guidelines for further research projects.[730]

ANTIARRHYTHMIC AGENTS

Antiarrhythmic agents have been traditionally categorized according to the Vaughan Williams classification, which is based on the presumed primary mechanism of action. For example, class I agents are sodium channel blockers. They are also called membrane-stabilizing agents because of their ability to decrease the excitability of the plasma membrane. Class I drugs can be subdivided into class IA, IB, or IC agents depending on their effects on the cardiac action potential (Table 16.10). Many antiarrhythmic drugs have multiple mechanisms of action and are therefore difficult to classify. Commonly used IV antiarrhythmic agents for children are described in Table 16.11.

Procainamide (Pronestyl)

Procainamide is one of the most commonly used class IA agents in children. It has sodium channel and moderate potassium channel blocking activities (class III effect). Its major effect is to delay repolarization; this effect is more pronounced at faster heart rates. IV procainamide is used to treat SVT associated with the Wolff-Parkinson-White syndrome, atrial flutter, and ventricular dysrhythmias unresponsive to lidocaine.[731–734] It may also be effective in postoperative junctional ectopic tachycardia.[735,736] In addition, electrophysiologists use it as a "procainamide challenge" to unmask the characteristic electrocardiographic changes of Brugada syndrome.[737,738]

TABLE 16.10	Vaughan Williams Classification of Antiarrhythmic Drugs	
Class	Mechanism	Examples
I	Sodium channel blockers	
IA	Increase length of action potential	Procainamide Quinidine Disopyramide
IB	Decrease length of action potential	Lidocaine Mexiletine Phenytoin
IC	No effect on length of action potential	Flecainide Propafenone
II	β-Blockers	Propranolol Atenolol Metoprolol Esmolol
III	Potassium channel blockers	Amiodarone Sotalol Bretylium Ibutilide Dofetilide Dronedarone
IV	Calcium channel blockers	Verapamil Diltiazem
V	Other or unknown mechanism	Adenosine Digoxin Magnesium sulfate

Data from Vaughan Williams EM. A classification of antiarrhythmic actions reassessed after a decade of new drugs. *Clin Pharmacol.* 1984;24:129-147; and Fuster V, Ryden LE, Cannom DS, et al. ACC/AHA/ESC 2006 guidelines for the management of patients with atrial fibrillation: a report of the American College of Cardiology/American Heart Association Task Force on Practice Guidelines and the European Society of Cardiology Committee for Practice Guidelines (Writing Committee to Revise the 2001 guidelines for the management of patients with atrial fibrillation). Developed in collaboration with the European Heart Rhythm Association and the Heart Rhythm Society. *Circulation* 2006;114:e257-e354.

Procainamide is the only class IA agent that is still clinically used in children, mainly for short-term IV therapy. A loading dose of 3 to 10 mg/kg is given over 30 to 60 minutes to infants younger than 1 year of age. Older children receive IV bolus doses of 5 to 15 mg/kg given over 30 to 60 minutes. After the bolus dose, an infusion is usually started at 20 to 80 µg/kg per minute. Infusion rates more than 100 µg/kg per minute are occasionally necessary, particularly in infants. Infusion rates are adjusted to achieve procainamide plasma concentrations of 4 to 10 µg/mL.[739] The first concentration should be measured 6 to 20 hours after initiation of the infusion. The infusion should be stopped if hypotension occurs or the QRS widens by more than 50%. Procainamide can have substantial negative inotropic effects, which may be more pronounced in the ischemic/reperfused or otherwise damaged myocardium.

The clearance of procainamide depends 50% on hepatic (phase II acetylation) metabolism and 50% on the renal clearance of the unchanged drug. Metabolism in the liver to N-acetyl procainamide (NAPA), which has class III antiarrhythmic effects,[740] depends on the individual's genetic polymorphism of N-acetyltransferase-2 as a slow or fast acetylator. In the past, procainamide and NAPA serum concentrations were added, with a therapeutic goal of 10 to 30 µg/mL. Currently, only

TABLE 16.11 | Intravenous Antiarrhythmic Agents

Agent (Vaughan Williams Class)	Dose	Comments
Procainamide (Class IA; sodium ± potassium channel blockade; antivagal effects)	Infant (<1 year): 3–10 mg/kg loading dose over 30–60 minutes Child (>1 year): 5–15 mg/kg loading dose over 30–60 minutes All ages, infusion rate: 20–80 µg/kg per minute	Used to treat SVT due to WPW, atrial flutter, junctional ectopic tachycardia (with patient hypothermia), lidocaine-resistant ventricular dysrhythmias; hypotension and negative inotropy; lupus-like syndrome.
Lidocaine (Class IB; sodium channel blockade; speeds repolarization)	1 mg/kg bolus; then 20–50 µg/kg per minute	Used for ventricular dysrhythmias; CNS toxicity (apnea, seizures, abnormal sensations).
Phenytoin (Class IB)	1–3 mg/kg q5 minutes up to 15 mg/kg loading dose, then 5–10 mg/kg divided q6 hours	Drug must be infused slowly (>30 minutes) due to potential hypotension; antidysrhythmic profile similar to that of lidocaine; may be useful to treat digoxin-induced dysrhythmias.
Propranolol (Class II; β-adrenergic blockade; sodium channel blockade also)	0.01–0.1 mg/kg slowly	Nonselective β-blockade; used mainly to treat SVT; bradycardia, hypotension, worsening of myocardial pump function; AV block; hypoglycemia; bronchospasm; depression; fatigue.
Esmolol (Class II; B-receptor blockade)	100–500 µg/kg loading dose (over 5 minutes); 50–250 µg/kg per minute infusion	Used to treat SVT; relatively selective β_1 blockade; short elimination half-life (7–10 minutes); hypotension, especially during bolus; if less than desired response after 5 minutes, can repeat or double bolus dose, followed by doubling infusion rate; non–organ-based metabolism by plasma and red blood cell esterases; infusion concentrations >10 mg/mL may predispose to venous sclerosis; dilute infusion at high rates increases risk of volume overload.
Amiodarone (Class III; prolongs repolarization; adrenergic and calcium blockade)	1–2.5 mg/kg bolus over 5–10 minutes (total loading dose up to 5–6 mg/kg); 5–15 mg/kg per 24-hour infusion	Used for resistant reentrant atrial and ventricular dysrhythmias; may be useful for postoperative junctional ectopic tachycardia; hypotension with bolus IV administration; bradycardia; AV block; rare proarrhythmia and torsades de pointes; pulmonary fibrosis; hypothyroidism; controversial association with acute perioperative lung injury.
Verapamil (Class IV; calcium channel blockade)	0.1–0.3 mg/kg bolus (maximum 5 mg)	Used for SVT in older children and adults; potential for hypotension and asystole contraindicates use in children <1 year of age; bradycardia; AV block; may increase ventricular response rate in some children with WPW.
Adenosine	0.05–0.1 mg/kg rapid bolus followed by flush; may repeat with doses increasing in increments of 0.05 mg/kg q2 minutes (maximum dose 0.25 mg/kg or 12 mg, whichever comes first)	Increases potassium channel flux and inhibits slow inward calcium current; causes transient sinus bradycardia and AV block; transient hypotension; rarely causes ventricular ectopy or atrial fibrillation; bronchospasm; used to terminate SVT; used diagnostically to transiently produce AV block. Reduce dose by 50% in heart transplant patients or if given through a central line.
Digoxin	Total digitalizing dose (TDD)[a]: Premature: 15–25 µg/kg Neonate (<1 month): 20–30 µg/kg Infant (<2 years): 30–50 µg/kg Child (2–5 years): 25–35 µg/kg Child (>5 years): 15–30 µg/kg Child (>10 years): 8–12 µg/kg	TDD given in divided doses: ½ TDD followed by ¼ TDD q8–12 hours × 2; slows sinus node and decreases AV node conduction; used to slow ventricular response in atrial flutter and fibrillation and may also treat junctional tachycardia or SVT; variable effect on accessory pathways; long half-life (24–48 hours) that is prolonged by renal dysfunction; numerous drug interactions; toxicity includes SVT, AV block, ventricular dysrhythmias; toxicity symptoms include drowsiness, nausea, vomiting; toxicity exacerbated by hypokalemia.
Magnesium sulfate	25–50 mg/kg bolus; maximum single dose 2 g; 30–60 mg/kg per 24-hour infusion	May be first-line therapy for torsades des pointes; also used for refractory ventricular tachycardia and ventricular fibrillation; hypotension and respiratory depression may accompany IV bolus dosing—IV calcium is an antidote.

[a]Daily maintenance dose varies by age; consult pharmacy or cardiologist.
AV, Atrioventricular; *CNS*, central nervous system; *IV*, intravenous; *SVT*, supraventricular tachycardia; *WPW*, Wolff-Parkinson-White syndrome.

procainamide plasma concentrations are monitored. Oral procainamide therapy is complicated by unreliable absorption, the need for frequent dosing, potential proarrhythmogenic effects, and a wide spectrum of adverse effects. Typical doses are 15 to 50 mg/kg per day, divided every 4 to 6 hours. A sustained-release form (administered every 8–12 hours) is available for older children.

The majority of procainamide-related adverse effects depend on the plasma concentration and the duration of therapy. A systemic lupus erythematosus–like syndrome is common, manifested as fevers, pleural effusions, pericarditis, arthralgias, myalgias, and rashes. A considerable number of children demonstrate positive antinuclear antibodies with chronic therapy, but they do not necessarily require discontinuation of the therapy.

Lidocaine (Lignocaine, Xylocaine)

Lidocaine is a member of the class IB antiarrhythmic agents, which include mexiletine and phenytoin. Proarrhythmogenia is less common with class IB agents. In addition to blocking fast sodium channels, they also reduce the duration of both the action potential and repolarization.[739] As with class IA agents, the effects of these agents may be greater at faster heart rates. Lidocaine primarily affects cells inferior to the AV node. It produces its greatest effects on cells with the action potentials with the greatest duration and thereby balances ventricular repolarization.

Because of its rapid hepatic metabolism, lidocaine is available only in an IV formulation. It is indicated for the emergency treatment of ventricular dysrhythmias.[741] Lidocaine is initially administered as an IV bolus of 1 mg/kg that can be repeated once within 5 to 10 minutes. Standard lidocaine infusion rates range from 20 to 50 µg/kg per minute.

The major adverse effects of lidocaine administration are well known to anesthesiologists. They primarily consist of CNS toxicity, which typically occurs at plasma concentrations in excess of 6 to 8 µg/mL. Mental status changes, abnormal taste or other sensations, apnea, and seizures may occur. Lidocaine doses should be reduced in children with decreased cardiac output because it has perfusion limited clearance. The administration of lidocaine to children with atrial tachydysrhythmias or a prolonged QT interval can increase the ventricular response rate.[742]

Phenytoin (Dilantin)

Phenytoin shares many similarities to lidocaine in terms of its antiarrhythmic effects, which are also restricted primarily to tissues inferior to the AV node and the bundle of His. Phenytoin primarily binds to sodium channels, maintaining them in the inactivated state. Very large concentrations may also affect calcium channels and automaticity. This drug is useful in treating refractory ventricular arrhythmias and especially digoxin-induced dysrhythmias.[743,744]

IV loading with phenytoin (fosphenytoin) is achieved by a bolus of 1 to 3 mg/kg. Larger loading doses (10–15 mg/kg) are used to treat status epilepticus. IV maintenance dosing is 5 mg/kg per day divided into two to three doses. IV phenytoin must be administered extremely slowly (>30 minutes) owing to its potential to cause hypotension. The oral dose in infants and older children is 5 mg/kg per day given every 12 hours, after a total loading dose of 15 mg/kg divided over 6 hours. Other typical adverse effects are well described from its use as an antiepileptic medication including gingival hyperplasia, aplastic anemia, ataxia, and nystagmus. Phenytoin should be avoided in patients who are pregnant or who may become pregnant because of its significant teratogenic profile (fetal hydantoin syndrome).

Genetic polymorphisms in the metabolism of phenytoin, especially via CYP2C9, can cause significant interpatient pharmacokinetic variability, potentially increasing plasma concentrations and the risk of toxicity.[745]

Flecainide (Tambocor) and Propafenone (Rythmol)

Flecainide and propafenone are class IC agents. As such, they have potent sodium channel blocking activity. In adults, flecainide is used to treat various tachyarrhythmias, and it has a special role in the pharmacologic cardioversion of recurrent atrial fibrillation in patients with normal hearts ("pill in a pocket").[746,747] Flecainide has also been extensively evaluated in children in whom it is frequently used in the treatment and prevention of supraventricular tachyarrhythmias.[748–756] It blocks activated slow sodium channels

but exerts less of an inhibitory effect on potassium channels. It appears to reduce the refractory time and decrease the automaticity in His-Purkinje cells. In contrast, the duration of the action potential and refractory period is prolonged in ventricular muscle, resulting in a greater duration of the QRS complex.

Clearance is achieved via renal excretion of the unchanged drug and by hepatic metabolism by CYP2D6; both are immature in neonates. Clearance in adults is slow, 4.6 to 12.1 mL/minute per kilogram. Clearance in neonates is immature but achieves adult rates by the first year of life, after which dose can be scaled using allometry. Relative bioavailability of the oral formulation is 90%. Neonatal dosing starts at 2 mg/kg per day orally, divided every 12 hours and titrated to clinical response; monitoring of serum concentration is advised. Infants over 1 month of age require 3 to 6 mg/kg per day. Typical dosages in infants are in the range of 80 to 90 mg/m² per day, given in two divided doses (40–45 mg/m² every 12 hours). Older children receive 100 to 110 mg/m² per day (50–55 mg/m² every 12 hours). Loading doses are not used. Serum elimination half-life is age dependent: approximately 1 day in neonates, 12 hours in infants younger than 6 months of age, and 8 to 12 hours in older children and adults. Therapeutic trough concentrations are believed to be in the range of 200 to 1000 ng/mL. IV flecainide is available outside the United States. A dose of 1 to 2 mg/kg given over 5 to 10 minutes has been used. Continuous infusions are avoided because of its prolonged elimination half-life.

Flecainide has mild to moderate negative inotropic effects. Substantial proarrhythmogenic effects have been observed in children with atrial tachydysrhythmias or significant abnormalities of myocardial anatomy and function. Proarrhythmia was considerably increased in adult patients who received flecainide after myocardial infarction.[757] In children and adults with paroxysmal SVT, a slow but incessant SVT may result on initiation of therapy; it is recommended to closely monitor these patients when initiating therapy. The efficiency and safety of class IC antiarrhythmic agents in children with an abnormal or damaged myocardium are unclear; many pediatric electrophysiologists would avoid these drugs in children with severe myocardial dysfunction, myocardial injury (e.g., immediately postoperatively), right- or left-sided hypertrophy (e.g., TOF), or aortic stenosis.[732,758] Nevertheless, a retrospective cohort study based on an administrative database from 43 pediatric tertiary care hospitals in the United States reported a trend toward increased use of flecainide in patients with CHD or cardiomyopathies (8.7% in 2011 compared with 4.6% in 2004) with a cardiac arrest rate comparable to other antiarrhythmic medications.[759] These findings were confirmed in another small retrospective multicenter study.[760]

The effects and risks of propafenone are similar to those for flecainide.[761] Propafenone can also control dysrhythmias that arise from automatic mechanisms and can be used to treat postoperative junctional ectopic tachycardia. Oral propafenone is administered at 200 to 600 mg/m² per day divided into three doses (for children under 15 kg, 10–20 mg/kg per day and for children over 15 kg, 7–15 mg/kg per day). IV propafenone is not available in the United States. An IV loading dose of 0.2 to 1.0 mg/kg should be given slowly over 10 minutes. The initial dose may be doubled to achieve a maximum 2-mg/kg total loading dose. Infusion rates of 4 to 7 µg/kg per minute have been reported.[762–767]

Hypotension, primarily attributed to its negative inotropic effects, can occur with a bolus of propafenone. Like flecainide, propafenone is probably contraindicated in children with significant structural or metabolic myocardial abnormalities, such as those related to severe pressure or volume overload, ischemia-reperfusion, or myocardial infarction. In addition, propafenone has the potential for proarrhythmogenic effects. Propafenone is extensively metabolized in the liver, with significant interindividual variability. Its reported elimination half-life ranges from 4 to 18 hours. Serum concentrations of propafenone do not correlate well with the clinical response.[768]

β-Blockers

β-Blockers are class II antiarrhythmic agents. Mechanism of action, relevance of subtype selectivity, metabolism, and other features are described in the section on vasoactive drugs. Here we focus on their indications as antiarrhythmic agents. In children, propranolol, atenolol, and esmolol are the most frequently used β-blockers.[432]

Propranolol (Inderal)

Propranolol is probably the most widely studied β-blocking agent in children.[769] Its primary indication is the treatment and prophylaxis of SVT.[770,771] Even infants seem to tolerate high-dose propranolol (up to 4 mg/kg per day) but require frequent weight-based dose adjustments to maintain effect.[772–774] In addition to nonselective β-blockade, propranolol has effects on the sodium channels and at high concentrations on calcium channels as well. It seems that conduction tissues of neonates are more sensitive to the drug than those of older children and adults.[744,775]

Atenolol (Tenormin)

Atenolol is a commonly used, longer-acting β-blocker.[748,776,777] It has more selective effects on β-adrenergic receptors, although the risk of bronchospasm may not be completely eliminated with this drug. Atenolol does not cross the blood-brain barrier, which may be a reason for its lower incidence of depression, fatigue, and malaise compared with propranolol.[439,778]

Esmolol (Brevibloc)

Esmolol is increasing in popularity for the control of perioperative tachydysrhythmias in children.[732] Esmolol acts predominantly on the sinus and AV nodes. It does not have important antiarrhythmic effects in the His-Purkinje or ventricular conducting tissues. Pharmacokinetics and the efficacy to terminate SVTs were found to be similar in children and adults.[443]

Class III Agents

The primary class III agents are amiodarone, sotalol, and ibutilide. They prolong depolarization and therefore increase refractoriness. All of these drugs have numerous other properties, including membrane-stabilizing effects, calcium channel blockade, and adrenergic blockade.

Amiodarone (Cordarone, Pacerone)

In addition to prolonging refractoriness, amiodarone has sodium channel blocking and noncompetitive α- and β-adrenergic receptor blocking properties. It may also interfere with potassium channels and inhibit the release of myocardial norepinephrine. Oral amiodarone is absorbed quite slowly and metabolized in the liver to an active metabolite, desethylamiodarone. Because of its high lipid solubility and large volume of distribution, tissue concentrations are maintained for 2 to 3 months after discontinuation of therapy. There are increasing data demonstrating the efficacy and safety of oral and IV amiodarone for the treatment of dysrhythmias in infants and children.[779–783] In addition to

resistant reentrant atrial and ventricular dysrhythmias, amiodarone may be effective in treating postoperative junctional ectopic tachycardia (target concentration 0.8–1.5 mg/L).[784–786] Amiodarone, in a dose of 5 mg/kg IV push, is also indicated for shock-resistant arrhythmias during cardiopulmonary resuscitation in infants and children.[741]

The loading dose for oral amiodarone is 10 to 15 mg/kg per day for 5 to 10 days. After the loading dose, long-term oral dosing is 2 to 5 mg/kg once daily. IV amiodarone is usually given in boluses of 1.0 to 2.5 mg/kg, reaching a total of 5 to 6 mg/kg, with each bolus administered over 5 to 10 minutes. In children with resistant dysrhythmias, the average loading dose was 6.3 mg/kg, with 50% of children requiring a continuous amiodarone infusion of 10 to 15 mg/kg per day.[781,787,788]

Hypotension is the major acute adverse effect of IV amiodarone therapy.[789] The effects of amiodarone may be synergistic with those of other agents that depress sinus node and AV node function. Important cardiac dysrhythmias include bradycardia and AV block. Proarrhythmogenic effects and torsades de pointes may occasionally occur. Long-term oral amiodarone therapy can lead to progressive and irreversible pulmonary fibrosis; all patients taking amiodarone chronically are usually monitored with pulmonary function tests at regular intervals.[790–792] The high iodine content of amiodarone can affect thyroid function, resulting in either hyperthyroidism or hypothyroidism; therefore, periodic thyroid function tests are indicated. Given the importance of thyroid hormone for brain development and growth, a rigorous surveillance regimen is recommended for infants and children.[793–795] Other effects include drug deposits in the cornea, skin photosensitivity, and chemical hepatitis with increased liver transaminases. Coadministration of amiodarone with other antiarrhythmic agents may result in increases in the plasma concentrations of the other drugs.[779,796]

The incidence of perioperative organ dysfunction in children who receive either acute or long-term amiodarone therapy is controversial. A syndrome with similarities to the adult respiratory distress syndrome has been described, particularly in children exposed to high inspired oxygen concentrations who are undergoing thoracic surgery or CPB.[797–800] This finding led to the recommendation that amiodarone be discontinued for several weeks before elective surgery.[801] Subsequent studies failed to demonstrate an increased incidence of injury to lungs or other organs in children undergoing surgery while receiving amiodarone. Because it is most frequently given to children with severe and life-threatening cardiac rhythm disturbances, the current recommendation is to continue amiodarone up to the time of surgery. However, it may be wise to attempt to limit the inspired oxygen concentration and other factors that may predispose the children receiving amiodarone to free radical and inflammatory injury.[802]

Dronedarone (Multaq)

Dronedarone is a noniodinated analog of amiodarone that was developed to reduce the iodine-associated adverse effects of chronic amiodarone therapy. Like amiodarone, it inhibits sodium, potassium, and calcium currents. It is mainly indicated for maintenance of sinus rhythm in patients with atrial fibrillation but is still undergoing investigations regarding its long-term safety profile.[746,803–805] After the initial drug approval, a high incidence of serious adverse events has been reported, including several cases of severe hepatocellular injury, which prompted the FDA to issue a warning in 2011.[806,807] There is also the concern about interactions with other drugs, especially new oral anticoagulants due to an increased risk for bleeding.[808] Pediatric data are not yet available.

Sotalol (Betapace, Sorine, Sotylize)

Sotalol is a class III antiarrhythmic that also acts as a nonselective β-blocker. At small doses, the β-adrenergic blocking effects predominate; at larger doses, the class III effects become more important. Sotalol is indicated for a number of refractory tachydysrhythmias, including fetal supraventricular tachyarrhythmias.[809] Current oral dosing recommendations for children start at target doses of 2 and 4 mg/kg in neonates, 3 and 6 mg/kg for children up to 6 years, and 2 and 4 mg/kg, divided into three doses, for children older than 6 years of age.[810] The major adverse effects of sotalol include mild cardiodepression associated with its β-blocking ability and prolongation of the QT interval and torsades de pointes due to its class III effects.[811] It should be avoided in children with asthma, heart failure, renal dysfunction, or QT interval prolongation. Sotalol may be used as an alternative to amiodarone in some children who are unable to tolerate the adverse effects associated with amiodarone. Adult studies have shown that sotalol is not as effective for pharmacologic conversion of atrial fibrillation compared with other strategies or medications, but it can be indicated for maintenance of sinus rhythm after an episode of atrial fibrillation, especially for patients with coronary artery disease.[747] It has also been recommended as an alternative to amiodarone for postoperative atrial fibrillation in cardiac patients, but for prophylaxis and rate control pure β-blockers are still preferred.[812–814] The pediatric experience with sotalol is steadily increasing, but most studies have been limited by relatively small numbers.[432,732,815–821]

Ibutilide (Corvert)

Ibutilide is one of the more recently released intravenous class III antiarrhythmic drugs. It prolongs repolarization by increasing the slow inward sodium current and by blocking the late rectifier current. It can be given intravenously and has a fast onset. Ibutilide is currently indicated for the rapid pharmacologic conversion of atrial fibrillation and atrial flutter, although it may be more efficacious for the latter. As with other class III drugs, ibutilide can prolong the QT interval and cause associated polymorphic ventricular tachycardia (torsades de pointes, which occur in 5%–8% of adults).[796,822] The elimination half-life of ibutilide is approximately 6 hours. It is recommended to observe children for several hours after an IV administration of this drug. A bolus dose of 10 to 25 µg/kg administered over 10 minutes has been used and this can be repeated once.[823] Ibutilide has been successfully used in neonates,[824] children with CHD,[825] and in children with accessory pathways.[826]

Dofetilide (Tikosyn)

Dofetilide is another oral class III antiarrhythmic drug that has been approved for treatment of atrial fibrillation and flutter.[747,827] It prolongs the effective refractory period by selectively blocking the rapid component of the delayed rectifier potassium current. The major adverse effect is the potential for torsade de pointes as a result of QT prolongation.[828,829] Compared with amiodarone, it has a shorter half-life (10 hours) but requires hospital admission for initiation of therapy. It has been successfully used in adult patients with CHD, but pediatric data are still lacking.[830]

Verapamil (Calan, Covera, Isoptin, Verelan)

Verapamil is a member of the class IV antiarrhythmic agents, the calcium channel blockers. Its primary action is depression of sinus node and AV node function.[831] Oral doses range from 4 to 8 mg/kg per day divided into three doses. A sustained-release preparation is available for older children. IV doses range from 0.1 to 0.3 mg/kg with a maximum dose of 5 mg. The most important side effect of verapamil occurs in children younger than 1 year of age, in whom IV administration can cause severe hypotension and asystole.[832] In fact, the drug is now contraindicated in infants (<1 year of age) because of this complication. Other side effects include bradycardia, AV block, and increased ventricular response in some children with Wolff-Parkinson-White syndrome.

Verapamil has been shown to be effective in terminating most SVTs in older children and adults.[732,833,834] Verapamil is also used to relieve outflow obstruction in hypertrophic cardiomyopathy[835] and as an antihypertensive in some children. The negative inotropic and AV conduction effects of verapamil are potentiated by β-blockers and anesthetic agents.[836,837] IV calcium and β-adrenergic drugs such as isoproterenol have been given to reverse the depressive effects of verapamil and other calcium channel antagonists.[838,839]

Adenosine (Adenocard, Adenoscan)

IV adenosine has markedly changed the therapy for SVTs. Its electrophysiologic effects are multiple and include increased potassium channel flux and decreased slow inward calcium current. These effects result in sinus bradycardia and transient AV block and are mediated primarily by stimulation of the A1-purinergic receptor subtype. Its onset of action is within 10 to 20 seconds. Bradycardia, AV block, and hypotension last an additional 10 to 30 seconds.

The best response to adenosine is achieved when it is rapidly administered into the central circulation. The initial central venous dose is 50 µg/kg and the initial peripherally administered dose is 100 to 150 µg/kg given as a rapid bolus, followed by a rapid fluid bolus given via a syringe to flush the medication into the circulation. If this is unsuccessful or the effect is not sustained, the procedure can be repeated doubling the dose (up to a maximum of 300 µg/kg). In adults, the starting dose is 6 to 12 mg.[840,841] Adenosine can also be used as a diagnostic tool to differentiate between SVT and other dysrhythmias. The slower HR caused by the transient AV conduction block often allows the recognition of specific electrocardiographic features, such as delta waves in Wolff-Parkinson-White syndrome.[842]

Other than the noted electrophysiologic changes, the major adverse effect from adenosine is transient hypotension. In children with an antegrade-conducting accessory pathway, adenosine can induce atrial fibrillation with a rapid ventricular response. Therefore it should be used only in an appropriate setting with electrocardiographic monitoring and available resuscitation equipment.[843] Dipyridamole and diazepam may inhibit the metabolism or cellular redistribution of adenosine. Either drug can significantly potentiate the effects of adenosine, resulting in more prolonged hypotension and AV node blockade.[844] Children with transplanted hearts can demonstrate prolonged bradycardia and asystole in response to adenosine. **The denervated heart is extremely sensitive to the AV node–blocking effects. It is recommended that the initial dose be reduced by 50% in these children.**[162,845] **This can be very important in the cardiac catheterization laboratory, where wire-induced supraventricular arrhythmias are common during surveillance biopsies.**[846] Adenosine has been reported to cause bronchospasm in children both with and without known reactive airway disease. It is usually mild and, if necessary, can be treated with IV aminophylline, which directly counteracts the receptor-mediated effects of adenosine.

Digoxin (Digitek, Digox, Lanoxicaps, Lanoxin)

Digoxin has antiarrhythmic as well as positive inotropic effects. Its basic pharmacology and therapeutic dosing were discussed earlier in the section on vasoactive drugs. As an antiarrhythmic agent, digoxin slows both atrial and AV node conduction. It slows the ventricular response in atrial flutter and fibrillation and may be used to treat children with junctional tachycardia and SVT.[432,732] Digoxin can have an unpredictable effect on the refractory period of accessory pathways[847,848] and is therefore relatively contraindicated in children with Wolff-Parkinson-White syndrome or other forms of SVT with accessory pathways. Digoxin easily crosses the placenta and remains the primary treatment for termination of fetal SVT.[846,849–852]

The dosing of digoxin in infants and children must be undertaken with care. Infants have greater myocellular concentrations of digoxin than adults.[328,853–855] The dosing schedule of digoxin, based on age, is shown in Tables 16.8 and 16.11. The onset of effect is more rapid with IV dosing (5–10 minutes) than with oral dosing (1–2 hours). The elimination half-life of digoxin is prolonged, approaching 1 to 2 days in young infants. Significant renal dysfunction and congestive heart failure can extend the elimination half-life. Cardiac injury (e.g., ischemia-reperfusion, myocarditis) may increase the sensitivity to digoxin.

Magnesium Sulfate

Magnesium plays an important role in many biologic processes. The catalytic actions of more than 300 enzymes, including those for ATP and DNA synthesis, depend on the presence of the Mg^{2+} ion, the physiologically active form. Myocardial conduction and contractility, transmembrane calcium flux, potassium transport, vascular smooth muscle tone, coronary reactivity, and NO synthesis are all regulated by magnesium. Only 1% of the total body magnesium is extracellular; 60% is found in bones and 39% is intracellular, especially in muscle cells. This distribution explains why serum concentrations of magnesium may be normal despite an underlying intracellular deficiency. Of the extracellular magnesium, 55% is in the active ionized form. Ionized magnesium is a better predictor of the intracellular magnesium status; age-specific reference values have been published.[856,857]

Magnesium sulfate is currently used for the correction of hypomagnesemia, for management of seizures and hypertension, for bronchodilation during status asthmaticus, and in the treatment of life-threatening arrhythmias. It is especially valuable in the treatment of long QT syndromes and torsades de pointes.[858,859] More recently, prophylactic magnesium supplementation during pediatric CPB has been advocated to reduce the incidence of postoperative junctional ectopic tachycardia.[860–862] The IV dose is usually 25 to 50 mg/kg over 10 minutes (0.2–0.4 mEq/kg), with a maximum single dose of 2 g. This dose can be repeated every 6 to 8 hours depending on renal function and serum concentrations. Because magnesium is excreted solely by the kidneys, renal

insufficiency requires increasing the intervals between doses to avoid toxicity. The normal serum concentration of magnesium is 1.5 to 2.5 mEq/L. Concentrations greater than 5 to 7 mEq/L can lead to increasing CNS and cardiac depression, initially manifested as loss of deep tendon reflexes and muscle weakness, potentially leading to respiratory depression and cardiac arrest (at levels >15–20 mEq/L). IV calcium directly antagonizes magnesium-induced toxicity.

ANNOTATED REFERENCES

Baum VC, Palmisano BW. The immature heart and anesthesia. *Anesthesiology.* 1997;87:1529-1548.

Review article describing the developmental changes in the immature heart and the implications for anesthesia on a physiologic, structural, and molecular level.

Cotts WG, Oren RM. Function of the transplanted heart: unique physiology and therapeutic implications. *Am J Med Sci.* 1997;314:164-172.

Classic article describing the physiologic changes in the denervated heart.

Hoffman JL, Kaplan S. The incidence of congenital heart disease. *J Am Coll Cardiol.* 2002;39:1890-1900.

Interesting literature review looking into the reasons for the wide range of incidence data on congenital heart disease.

Jolley M, Colan SD, Rhodes J, DiNardo J. Fontan physiology revisited. *Anesth Analg.* 2015;121(1):172-182.

Review article discussing the fundamental characteristics of the Fontan circulation.

Jone PN, Ivy DD, Hauck A, Karamlou T, Truong U, Coleman RD, Sandoval JP, Del Cerro Marín MJ, Eghtesady P, Tillman K, Krishnan US. Pulmonary Hypertension in Congenital Heart Disease: A Scientific Statement From the American Heart Association. *Circ Heart Fail.* 2023 Jul;16(7):e00080.

Scientific statement describing various subgroups of patients with CHD associated pulmonary hypertension, diagnostic modalities, and treatment options.

Kiserud T. Physiology of the fetal circulation. *Semin Fetal Neonatal Med.* 2005;10:493-503.

Review article with a thorough description of the fetal circulatory physiology and the implications of placental compromise.

Latus H, Delhaas T, Schranz D, Apitz C. Treatment of pulmonary arterial hypertension in children. *Nat Rev Cardiol.* 2015;12(4):244-254.

Review article summarizing the current treatment options for pediatric pulmonary hypertension.

Rhodes J, Tikkanen AU, Jenkins KJ. Exercise testing and training in children with congenital heart disease. *Circulation.* 2010;122:1957-1967.

Original article describing the exercise limitations in children with repaired congenital heart disease.

Wadia RS, Bernier ML, Diaz-Rodriguez NM, Goswami DK, Nyhan SM, Steppan J. Update on Perioperative Pediatric Pulmonary Hypertension Management. *J Cardiothorac Vasc Anesth.* 2022 Mar;36(3):667-676.

Review article summarizing the current diagnostic and therapeutic approach to pediatric pulmonary hypertension with a special emphasis on perioperative management.

Van Genuchten WJ, Helbing WA, Ten Harkel ADJ, Fejzic Z, Md IMK, Slieker MG, van der Ven JPG, Boersma E, Takken T, Bartelds B. Exercise capacity in a cohort of children with congenital heart disease. *Eur J Pediatr.* 2023 Jan;182(1):295-306.

Multicenter study demonstrating disease specific changes of exercise capacity during childhood in different subgroups of patients with congenital heart disease.

A complete reference list can be found online at Elsevier eBooks+.

17 Cardiopulmonary Bypass and Management

RALPH GERTLER, ERIN A. GOTTLIEB, AND DEAN B. ANDROPOULOS

Basic Aspects of Cardiopulmonary Bypass
The Circuit and Cannulas
Cardiopulmonary Bypass Pumps
Cardiopulmonary Bypass Prime
Special Coagulation and Hematologic Problems
Heparin-Induced Thrombocytopenia
Antithrombin III Deficiency
Recombinant Factor VIIa for Massive Hemorrhage
Fibrinogen Concentrate
Prothrombin Complex Concentrate
Desmopressin
Sickle Cell Disease
A Perspective on Blood Preservation: Cardiopulmonary Bypass in Jehovah's Witness Patients
Myocardial Protection
Phases of Cardiopulmonary Bypass
Prebypass Period
Heparin and Coagulation Management
Cannulation and Initiation of Bypass
Cooling Phase
Aortic Cross Clamping and Intracardiac Repair Phase
Deep Hypothermic Circulatory Arrest or Selective Cerebral Perfusion Phase
Removal of Aortic Cross Clamp and Rewarming Phase
Separation from Bypass
Postbypass Period

Particular Aspects of Management on Cardiopulmonary Bypass
pH-Stat Versus α-Stat Management
Hematocrit on Bypass
Flow Rates on Bypass
Conventional Ultrafiltration and Modified Ultrafiltration
Prebypass Anesthetic Management
Anesthesia on Cardiopulmonary Bypass
Changes in Pharmacokinetics
Changes in Pharmacodynamics
Special Techniques
Management of Deep Hypothermic Circulatory Arrest
Regional Cerebral Perfusion
Effects of Cardiopulmonary Bypass
Cardiac Effects
Systemic and Pulmonary Vasculature Effects
Pulmonary Effects
Neurologic Monitoring and Effects of Cardiopulmonary Bypass on the Brain
Systemic Inflammatory Response Syndrome
Coagulation Effects
Hepatic, Renal, and Gastrointestinal Effects
Immune System Effects
Endocrine System Effects
Transport to the Intensive Care Unit
Fast Tracking and Recovery

THIS CHAPTER REVIEWS THE equipment and strategies for cardiopulmonary bypass (CPB) in infants and children, focusing on how they differ compared with CPB in adults. We will review the effects of CPB on the key organ systems and discuss specific management issues that occur in daily practice.

Basic Aspects of Cardiopulmonary Bypass

The basic principles of cardiopulmonary bypass remain unchanged from when they were first introduced in the 1950s: the CPB machine assumes the functions of the heart and lungs during the time necessary to complete either an intracardiac or an extracardiac repair. A basic bypass circuit (Fig. 17.1) consists of an oxygenator, heat exchanger, and venous reservoir; pump heads for perfusion, cardiotomy suction, and cardioplegia; appropriate

tubing, cannulas, and monitoring and alarm devices.[1] Major differences exist between pediatric and adult CPB, stemming from anatomic, metabolic, and physiologic differences in these age groups (Table 17.1).

THE CIRCUIT AND CANNULAS

Circuit size cannot be reduced proportionately to the patient's size; this disproportion commonly leads to hemodilution and dilutional coagulopathies in children. Surgical procedures require extremes of temperature, hemodilution, and changes in flow rates. Because of the smaller vascular structures and greater flow rates (150 to 200 mL/kg per minute) in infants and children compared with flow rates of 2.2 to 2.4 L/minute per m² in adults, selection of appropriately sized cannulas is critical to maintain these flows. Shear stress is significant in small cannulas and several-fold greater

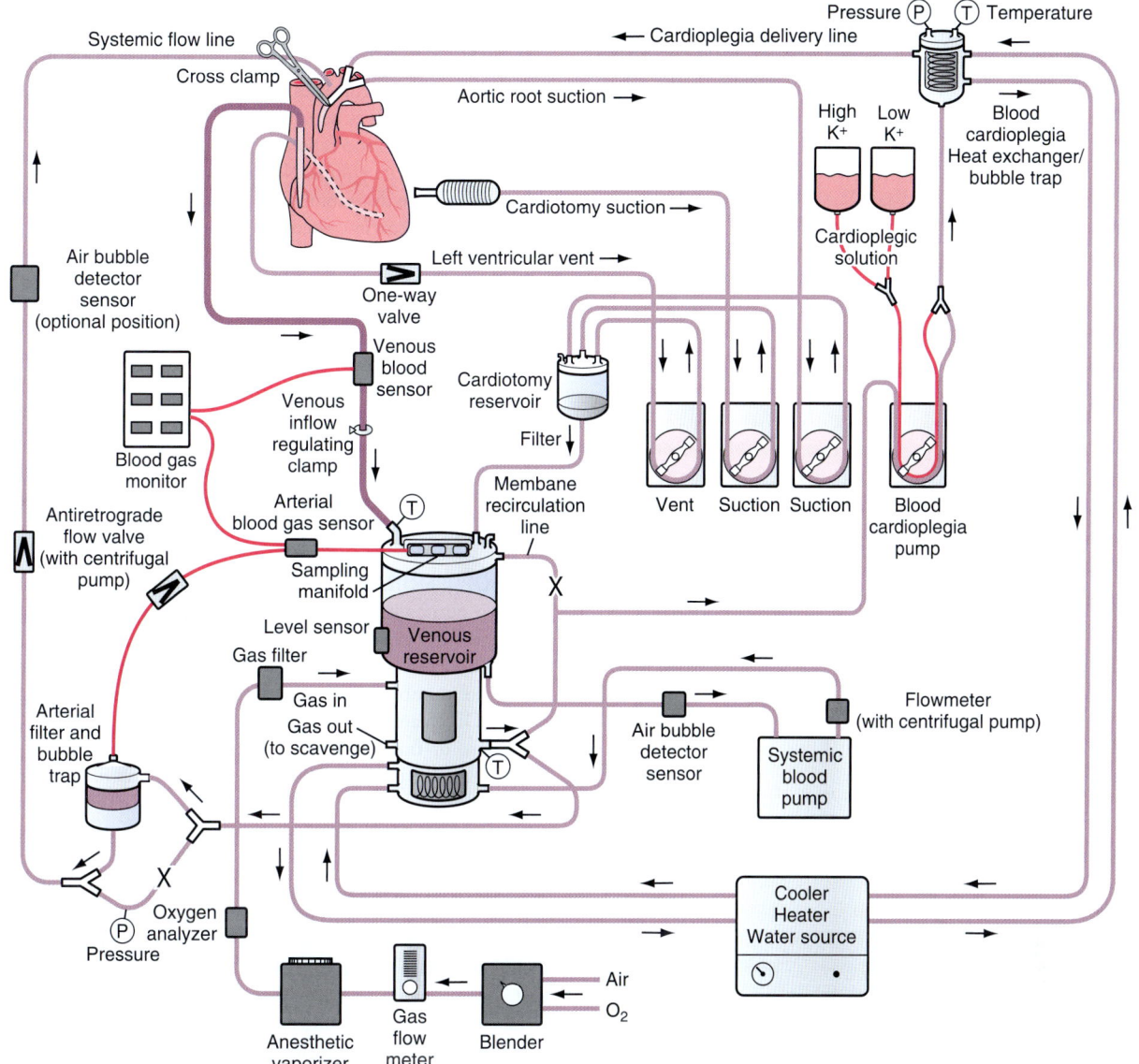

FIGURE 17.1 Schematic diagram of a cardiopulmonary bypass circuit. This scheme depicts a membrane oxygenator with integral hard-shell venous reservoir and external cardiotomy reservoir. Many circuits have the cardiotomy reservoir, venous reservoir, and oxygenator integrated into one single unit. The systemic blood pump may be either a roller or centrifugal pump. Most pediatric venous cannulations are bicaval with two separate venous cannulas instead of the single venous cannula depicted here. Carbon dioxide can also be added to the inspired gas to facilitate pH-stat blood gas management. *Arrows* indicate direction of flow; *P*, pressure sensor; *T*, temperature sensors; *X*, placement of tubing clamps. (From Hessel EA, Hill AG. Circuitry and cannulation techniques. In: Gravlee GP, Davis RF, Kurusz M, Utley JR, eds. *Cardiopulmonary Bypass: Principles and Practice.* 2nd ed. Philadelphia: Lippincott Williams & Wilkins; 2000:69-97.)

than needed for activation of blood cells and platelets, leading to an exaggerated systemic inflammatory response syndrome (SIRS).

Bypass Circuit
Currently, it is thought that more than 70% of infants weighing less than 5 kilograms and undergoing cardiac surgery could benefit from a bloodless circuit prime if miniaturized circuits were used.[2] Technical advances in the field of oxygenator construction and size, including the reduction of priming volumes to as small as 45 mL for neonatal oxygenators, have allowed marked reductions of circuit volumes over the past decade. Also, tubing sizes

can be reduced to ³⁄₁₆-inch diameters, which in combination with shorter length tubing, can allow the reduction of priming volumes to the range of 100 to 150 mL for neonates. The downside of very low volume CPB circuits is the common requirement for vacuum-assisted drainage, a technique that may entrain air through the venous line and result in red cell hemolysis. This can be avoided by the use of an effective negative pressure greater than 40 mm Hg, by tight purse-string sutures on the venous cannulas, and by monitoring the pressure in the venous reservoir. A summary of the Texas Children's Hospital sizing chart is shown in Table 17.2.

TABLE 17.1	Comparison of Pediatric Versus Adult Cardiopulmonary Bypass	
	Child	**Adult**
Hemodilution	3–15 × adult	Moderate
Perfusion pressure	30–40 mm Hg	Moderate (>50–80 mm Hg)
	Wide flow rates (0–200 mL/kg per minute)	Narrow range (CI 2.0–2.4 L/m² per minute)
Blood gas management	pH-stat (PCO₂ 20–80 mm Hg or greater)	α-stat (PCO₂ 30–45 mm Hg)
Cannulation techniques	Variable	Predictable
Aortopulmonary collaterals		Uncommon
Temperature ranges	Variable	DHCA occasionally
Glucose management		Predictable
Inotropic response	Negative	Positive
Perfusion circuit	Per kilogram weight	Standard
Parameters	Hematocrit often >55%–60%	
	PO₂ 40–80 mm Hg	±
	SaO₂ 75%–85%	
	Ultrafiltration (MUF/CUF)	±Ultrafiltration

CI, Cardiac index; *CUF*, conventional ultrafiltration; *DHCA*, deep hypothermic circulatory arrest; *MUF*, modified ultrafiltration.

TABLE 17.2	Cardiopulmonary Bypass Circuit Prime Volume and Constituents at Texas Children's Hospital	
Patient Weight	**Prime Volume**	**Prime Constituents**
<8 kg	350 mL	Whole blood or PRBC + FFP + crystalloid prime[a]
8–15 kg	650 mL	100 mL albumin 25% ± PRBC + crystalloid prime[a]
15–25 kg	900 mL	100 mL albumin 25% + crystalloid prime[a]
15–25 kg	1200 mL	Crystalloid prime[a]

[a]Crystalloid prime: 1/2 normal serum + PlasmaLyte + CaCl₂ + KCl.
FFP, Fresh frozen plasma; *PRBC*, packaged red blood cells.

Biocompatibility of Circuit Surfaces

Young children are more susceptible to the adverse effects of CPB than adults, and the inflammatory response to CPB may have serious consequences for neonatal and pediatric patients.[3,4] This is in part related to the surface area of the CPB circuit, which is large relative to the infant and child's blood volume. For example, a 3-kilogram neonate with a blood volume of 90 mL/kg has a total blood volume of approximately 270 mL, and with an average priming volume in many centers of 350 mL (120% of the neonate's estimated blood volume), the CPB circuit volume thus causes greater than 100% dilution. A 70-kilogram adult with 70 mL/kg blood volume has an approximately 5000-mL blood volume; with a CPB circuit prime of 1500 mL, this results in less than 33% dilution. Contact of blood with the surface of the circuit also plays an important role for activation of coagulation and fibrinolysis. Biocompatible coatings mimic properties of the endothelium. This is achieved using molecules such as heparin, poly2-methoxyethylacrylate, phosphorylcholine, siloxane/caprolactone, polyethylene oxide chains, and sulfate/sulfonate groups. No clear evidence was found that these materials decrease thrombin formation or confer any outcome benefit in adults.[5] Heparin-coated biocompatible bypass systems reduce this activation in children weighing less than 10 kilograms undergoing CPB.[6] They also reduce the activation of factor XII and the complement system.[7,8] This results in less kallikrein and bradykinin being produced, which in turn reduces the secretion of tissue plasminogen activator from endothelial cells. One study has documented more bleeding with a conventional, non–heparin-coated circuit compared with a heparin-coated circuit.[8] Overall, children who underwent surgery while supported with heparin-coated circuits have reduced inflammatory mediator release and fewer consequences thereof, such as prolonged postoperative ventilation and duration of stay in the intensive care unit (ICU).[9]

CARDIOPULMONARY BYPASS PUMPS

The two pumps used most commonly for CPB are roller pumps and centrifugal pumps. Roller pumps have the advantages of simplicity, low cost, ease, and reliability of flow calculation, and the ability to pump against increased resistance without reducing flow.[10] Disadvantages include the need to assess occlusiveness, spallation, or fragmentation of the inner tubing surface (potentially producing particulate arterial emboli), potential for pumping large volumes of air, and ability to create large positive and negative pressures. Compared with roller pumps, centrifugal pumps offer the advantages of less air pumping potential, less ability to create large positive and negative pressures, less blood trauma, and virtually no spallation. Disadvantages of centrifugal pumps include a greater cost, the lack of occlusiveness (creating the possibility of accidental patient exsanguination), and afterload-dependent flow that requires constant flow measurement. In the setting of short-term CPB for cardiac surgery, it remains uncertain whether the selection of a roller pump over a centrifugal pump, or of any specific centrifugal pump over another, has clinical importance. Pulsatile perfusion may prove to be beneficial in the future, but further outcome data and technical improvements are needed.[11]

CARDIOPULMONARY BYPASS PRIME

The optimal priming fluid in cardiac surgery is a topic of enduring debate. Crystalloid solutions, colloids, and mixtures of both are used. Children appear to benefit from a colloid prime.[12] Pure crystalloid prime can be routinely used in those with a weight greater than 7 kilograms, but has been used successfully even in neonatal cases.[13,14] If crystalloid is used for priming, it should not contain lactate or dextrose because CPB induces a metabolic acidosis[15] that is iatrogenic, not splanchnic, in origin.[16] The addition of lactate to the prime increases the serum concentration of lactate postoperatively and should be avoided.[17] Hyperchloremic metabolic acidosis is the second contributing component of a metabolic acidosis on CPB. This is often only detected by measuring the strong ion difference via the Stewart approach to the acid-base homeostasis.[18] Both acidifying events are attenuated by the dilutional hypoalbuminemia induced by the pump prime. Because a hyperchloremic acidosis of a mild degree seems to be well tolerated and not associated with a poor outcome, no intervention is necessary. Understanding the nature of CPB–associated acidosis, however, is likely to prevent unnecessary investigations or interventions.

Avoiding dextrose is particularly important during complex repairs using deep hypothermic cardiac arrest in which the risk of neurologic injury is substantive. The additives in banked blood, namely, glucose in citrate-phosphate-dextrose (CPD) storage solutions, also need to be considered as a source of glucose as well as potassium from the increased concentration in stored blood. We use a balanced electrolyte solution, such as PlasmaLyte, for the crystalloid component of our prime.

The proportionally large volume of the bypass circuit compared with the child's blood volume has impact on the coagulation factors and cellular components. Platelet count decreases and coagulation factors, including fibrinogen, are diluted after bypass thereby contributing to a coagulopathy. The fibrinogen concentration at the end of bypass correlates with the 24-hour chest drainage in children who weigh less than 10 kilograms.[19,20] This occurs more frequently in infants and neonates in whom the plasma concentrations of hemostatic proteins decrease postoperative by 56% immediately upon initiation of bypass[21]; younger age represents the single most important risk factor for coagulopathy and bleeding complications.[22]

One approach to offset this dilutional coagulopathy is the addition of whole blood to the circuit prime. Proponents cite two theoretical advantages: (1) improved hemostasis and (2) decreased SIRS with less edema formation and less organ dysfunction. However, the use of fresh whole blood has also been reported to increase perioperative fluid requirements, leading to a more prolonged duration of mechanical ventilation and ICU stay than in the single component group.[23] Also, platelet function is reduced secondary to the storage of the whole blood at 4°C and nonexistent after 24 hours of storage.[24] The only advantage of whole blood prime was fewer donor exposures, a problem we obviate by matching packed red blood cells (PRBCs) and fresh frozen plasma (FFP) from the same donor.[25] One retrospective analysis of donor exposures using fresh whole blood concluded that donor exposures were reduced in patients younger than 2 years of age compared with published reports using component therapy.[26] Unfortunately, fresh whole blood is frequently unavailable. However, when there is a commitment to use fresh whole blood for pediatric cardiovascular surgery, it is possible to build a sustainable operating protocol to provide this resource. An alternative approach is to use FFP in the prime.[27,28] Some investigators determined that the use of FFP led to greater fibrinogen concentrations at the end of surgery. On average, children in the FFP group needed 1.3 fewer donor exposures and tended to need fewer PRBCs. The reduced donor exposure was primarily the result of fewer transfusions of cryoprecipitate.[27] FFP may be safely substituted by 5% albumin in the prime, particularly above the neonatal age, and in children with less complex repairs and acyanotic lesions.[12,29] Whenever possible, we prefer fresh blood that is less than 5 days old. Fresh PRBCs are presumably more balanced metabolically than stored PRBCs; the former contain less potassium, greater concentrations of glucose, reduced concentrations of lactate, and a greater pH.[30] Also, postoperative morbidity increases with increasing age of red blood cells (RBCs).[31] Pulmonary complications, acute renal failure, and increased infection rates were among the main complications associated with increased red blood cell storage time. As far as potassium concentrations and acid-base balance are concerned, PRBC priming can be safely performed with stored PRBCs if the priming solution is circulated for 20 minutes before the initiation of CPB[32] or the red blood cells are processed with a cell saver.

Depending on the size and age of the child, and the complexity of the repair, a target hematocrit is chosen. Based on the child's blood volume and the prime volume, homologous blood is added using the calculation:

$$\begin{aligned} \text{Prime PRBC volume (mL)} = \ & (\text{Target hematocrit}) \\ & \times (\text{Patient blood volume [mL]} \\ & + \text{Prime volume [mL]}) \\ & - (\text{Patient PRBC volume [mL]}) \end{aligned}$$

The average prime volume of the circuits in use at Texas Children's Hospital is shown in Table 17.2. Other prime additives are heparin, antifibrinolytics, antiinflammatory agents (corticosteroids), antibiotics, vasodilators, and, sometimes, diuretics (mannitol, furosemide). At the end of the surgical repair and before separation from bypass, a blood gas sample should be analyzed to ensure the concentrations of electrolytes (including calcium and magnesium ions) and glucose, as well as the hematocrit are within a desired range. Acid-base changes and sodium concentration are corrected with sodium bicarbonate and wash solutions, and residual lactate is washed out with the help of the hemofiltration.

Antifibrinolytic Agents

Antifibrinolytic therapy is a pharmacologic cornerstone of a multimodal blood conservation program in cardiac surgery with or without CPB (see Chapter 18). The administration of antifibrinolytic agents during CPB reduces both perioperative blood loss and the requirements for transfusion of allogeneic blood products. It is a 1A recommendation for adult cardiac surgical procedures with CPB[33] and a 1B recommendation for pediatric cardiac surgery.[12] Since the withdrawal of aprotinin from the market in 2008 because of safety concerns, tranexamic acid (TXA) and ε-aminocaproic acid (EACA) have become the two most extensively used antifibrinolytic agents. All three agents are equally effective in pediatric cardiac surgery.[34]

Aprotinin

Inhibitors of serine proteases regulate and prevent uncontrolled activation of thrombin, coagulation factors, complement products, kallikrein, trypsin, elastase, and cathepsin among others of these potent enzymes. Of the serine protease inhibitors, the broad-spectrum agent aprotinin is the most widely studied in both experimental and clinical settings. Aprotinin is derived from bovine lung. It inhibits plasmin, kallikrein, trypsin, and other proteases, resulting in both antiinflammatory and antifibrinolytic effects and maintenance of glycoprotein homeostasis.

The first use of aprotinin in pediatric cardiac surgery was reported in 1990.[35] No reduction in blood loss or drainage was observed; there were no adverse effects, and the time to chest closure from the end of CPB was reduced. Despite the expense of aprotinin, follow-up studies reported more favorable results. Its use has reduced overall costs, because of a reduced number of blood products used, operative time, duration of postoperative ventilation, and hospitalization.[36,37] This was confirmed in a comparative analysis among antifibrinolytic medications.[38] However, this benefit was observed only in complex repairs and with the use of a high-dose regimen.[39] The lesser effect of a low-dose regimen may be attributable to the dilutional effects in pediatric surgery compared with the adult population.[40] In general, infants younger than 6 months of age and those with repeat sternotomies benefit from a high-dose aprotinin regimen[41] compared with reduced doses, despite greater drug costs. Economic studies have shown a cost-effective benefit of aprotinin in repeat cardiac procedures.[36,37]

Aprotinin influences the inflammatory response to CPB in children.[42] Postoperative lung function is improved[43,44] and pediatric studies have demonstrated decreases in the operative time for chest closure, in exposure to donor blood products, and in postoperative chest tube drainage.[43] Anaphylactic and anaphylactoid reactions may occur with aprotinin in 1% of first exposures, 1.3% of second exposures, and 2.9% of more frequent exposures.[45] A test dose should be given before administration of the loading dose or addition of aprotinin to the CPB circuit.

We used aprotinin for complex neonatal repairs, such as arterial switch operations or Norwood procedures, as well as for most repeat operative procedures and organ transplantations.[46,47] The drug is currently unavailable in the USA and Europe because of safety concerns in adults. Aprotinin has been shown to be safe and effective in the neonate.[48] Aprotinin continues to be used in Australia and New Zealand and has been reintroduced for adult coronary artery bypass graft surgery in Canada. The European Medicines Agency removed the suspension of use warning in 2012.[49] Our dosing regimen is based on a 60,000 KIU/kg loading dose IV and in the pump prime. The aprotinin infusion (7000 KIU/kg per hour) is started before skin incision and is discontinued just before leaving the operating room. Regimens based on body surface area are also used, along with a CPB prime dose that is based on the priming volume designed to achieve a plasma level above 200 KIU/mL.[36]

The Lysine Analogues: Epsilon-Aminocaproic Acid and Tranexamic Acid

Despite meticulous surgical technique, it is still frequently difficult to achieve adequate hemostasis after CPB, particularly in neonates. EACA and TXA are analogs of the amino acid lysine that exert their antifibrinolytic effect by interfering with the binding of plasminogen to fibrin, thereby preventing the activation of the active plasmin. TXA may also improve hemostasis by preventing plasmin-induced platelet activation. Both EACA and TXA exercise some antiinflammatory properties, but not to the same extent as aprotinin. In one study, EACA reduced bleeding postoperatively in 25 of 71 children undergoing cardiac surgery on CPB but only benefited children with cyanotic heart disease.[50] The empirical EACA loading dose was 75 mg/kg followed by an infusion of 15 mg/kg per hour, with an additional 75 mg/kg added to the CPB prime. A larger loading dose of 150 mg/kg that was followed by an infusion of 30 mg/kg per hour of EACA has also been studied. In the latter case, intraoperative blood loss was reduced, although postoperative blood loss did not differ between the treatments.[51] Blood coagulation measured with a thromboelastogram showed less fibrinolysis with EACA. The clearance of EACA is reduced in neonates compared with children and adults; dosing requirements in neonates are approximately half of those for children and adults. A regimen of 40 mg/kg as a loading dose, 30 mg/kg per hour infusion, and a pump prime concentration of 100 mg/L effectively maintained the plasma concentration more than 50 mg/L in 90% of neonates undergoing cardiac surgery utilizing CPB.[52] Dosing regimens for EACA at Texas Children's Hospital are displayed in Table 17.3. A recent meta-analysis established the efficacy of EACA in pediatric cardiac surgery.[53]

Tranexamic acid compares favorably with EACA but confers a particular benefit in children with cyanotic heart disease.[54] Those with acyanotic defects and those who required repeat sternotomies did not benefit from TXA, although that dosing regimen only included a single 50 mg/kg loading dose before incision. In children, the TXA plasma concentration between the peak of the loading

TABLE 17.3	Epsilon-Aminocaproic Acid Dosing (Texas Children's Hospital)		
Age (Weight)	Loading Dose to Patient	Infusion Dose	Loading Dose to Bypass Circuit
<30 days (3.5 kg)	40 mg/kg	30 mg/kg per hour	0.1 mg/mL of CPB prime volume
1 month–12 years (3.5–40 kg)	75 mg/kg	75 mg/kg per hour	75 mg/kg patient weight
>12 years (>40 kg)	5 grams	1 gram/hour	5 grams

Neonatal dose from Eaton MP, Alfieris GM, Sweeney DM, et al. Pharmacokinetics of epsilon-aminocaproic acid in neonates undergoing cardiac surgery with cardiopulmonary bypass. *Anesthesiology.* 2015;122(5):1002-1009.

Child dose from Ririe DG, James RL, O'Brien JJ, et al. The pharmacokinetics of epsilon-aminocaproic acid in children undergoing surgical repair of congenital heart defects. *Anesth Analg.* 2002;94(1):44-49.

dose and the end of CPB decreases ~80% when it is not followed by a continuous infusion.[55] For TXA, typical dosing regimens include a bolus of 10 to 30 mg/kg at the beginning of surgery followed by an infusion of 2 to 10 mg/kg per hour until weaning from CPB or sternal closure. Based on pharmacokinetics, we use 10 mg/kg TXA as a bolus followed by an infusion of 10 mg/kg per hour until the start of CPB, a 4 mg/kg bolus into the prime and a reduced infusion rate of 4 mg/kg per hour after the start of CPB to maintain TXA concentrations greater than 20 µg/mL,[56] which inhibits fibrinolysis about 80%.[57]

Although less efficient than aprotinin, EACA, and TXA are equally effective in reducing perioperative blood loss in pediatric cardiac surgery.[58] Given their safety profile, they may be even more appealing in the future. Pharmacokinetic simulation of EACA in neonates undergoing CPB suggests a loading dose of 40 mg/kg and infusion of 30 mg/kg per hour with pump prime concentration of 100 mg/L maintains plasma concentrations greater than 50 mg/L in most neonates.[52] We use EACA based on simulation results from a study in children and adults.[59] An initial loading dose of 75 mg/kg over 10 minutes followed by an infusion rate of 75 mg/kg per hour complemented a 75 mg/kg dose in the pump to maintain serum concentrations in excess of the therapeutic concentration (assumed to be 130 µg/mL) in more than 95% of children. In the future, point-of-care monitoring might allow for individualized dosing to suppress fibrinolysis optimally during the different stages of cardiac surgery.[60] Goal-directed therapy using point-of-care testing with coagulation factor concentrate-based algorithms has been used safely and effectively to treat coagulopathy and reduce transfusion in adult cardiac surgery patients, but there is a paucity of data in children.[61–63]

Special Coagulation and Hematologic Problems

HEPARIN-INDUCED THROMBOCYTOPENIA

The use of unfractionated heparin for anticoagulation for CPB in adults produces antiheparin antibodies in 25% to 50% of patients within 10 days postoperatively. In a small minority of these patients, high-titer IgG platelet-activating antibodies form and make immune complexes with heparin and platelet factor 4 (PF4).[64]

This results in activation of platelets (via their Fc receptors) and formation of procoagulant platelet micro particles, leading to thrombin generation and thrombosis. The major problem of this heparin-induced thrombocytopenia (HIT) is thrombocytopenia several days after heparin exposure accompanied by thrombosis, often in major vessels or structures. HIT appears to be less common, of milder course, and probably underrecognized in neonates and children. About 1% of children exposed to CPB have PF4 antibodies when tested before their second exposure to CPB, and actual HIT is much less common.[65] When HIT is suspected, either PF4 enzyme-linked immunosorbent assay or a functional assay for HIT can be used to make the diagnosis; if positive, no further heparin should be given. If CPB is necessary, alternatives to heparin, such as the direct thrombin inhibitors argatroban, lepirudin, and bivalirudin, may be used. None of these agents is approved for use in children for anticoagulation for CPB, but case reports and small series have documented their successful use when HIT is diagnosed.[66–68]

Bivalirudin effectively inhibits the coagulation cascade and has a short 25-minute half-life in patients with normal renal function. Monitoring of anticoagulation with bivalirudin is more challenging than with heparin. The ecarin clotting time correlates strongly with therapeutic bivalirudin concentrations but is not commonly available as a point-of-care test. Although not as accurate as the ecarin clotting time, the more commonly available celite activated clotting time (ACT) was found to have an acceptable correlation to ecarin clotting time determined bivalirudin concentration.[69] Bivalirudin has the broadest experience in pediatric patients undergoing cardiac surgery (with and without CPB) and in those with HIT and HIT thrombosis (HITT) requiring CPB. An age-corrected dosing schedule has been published.[70] Of note, a reversal agent is not yet available and restoring coagulation activity depends primarily on renal clearance and plasma proteolysis. Thus, treatment of post-CPB bleeding involves using ultrafiltration to increase clearance and the administration of blood products and coagulation factors.

ANTITHROMBIN III DEFICIENCY

Heparin produces anticoagulation by combining in a 1 : 1 ratio with antithrombin III (ATIII), which then binds to and causes a 2000- to 4000-fold increase in thrombin inhibition that enables systemic anticoagulation for CPB. Between 4% and 13% of adults exhibit resistance to normal doses of heparin for CPB; most instances occur because of a partial deficiency of ATIII, rendering heparin less effective at producing anticoagulation.[71] There is large between-subject variability in antithrombin concentrations and several isoforms exist in neonates, infants, and children that can be attributed to age, immaturity of the coagulation system, inflammation, and liver dysfunction.[72] Full-term neonates have plasma concentrations of antithrombin that are 50% to 75% of adult concentrations, whereas preterm neonates may have even lower concentrations. Adult concentrations are typically not attained until 6 to 12 months of age. Patients with low levels of antithrombin have lower heparin efficacy, and more heparin is required to maintain an adequate ACT. In children ATIII deficiency is often unknown, and the first suspicion of its deficiency may occur when the standard heparin dose of 300 to 400 units/kg fails to adequately anticoagulate before CPB; the ACT remains less than 300 seconds. The usual response is to administer another dose of heparin from a different vial and remeasure the ACT; if the ACT is still not adequately prolonged, a diagnosis of ATIII deficiency must be suspected. Infants less than 6 months of age

and children with congenital heart disease have decreased ATIII concentrations.[73] Therefore, heparin may not achieve adequate anticoagulation, and disorders in hemostasis and thrombosis and an exaggerated inflammatory response may occur. In this case, blood can be sent for ATIII concentration, but to proceed with CPB, the ATIII must be increased. This can be accomplished in two ways: (1) by supplementing ATIII with 75 units/kg of recombinant ATIII and ensuring that the ACT is adequately prolonged before proceeding with CPB, which is the current treatment of choice, or (2) by adding FFP to the CPB prime or administering it to the child prebypass.[71,74,75] In the presence of reduced baseline concentrations of ATIII, the total dose of heparin, the amount of thrombin that was generated during bypass, and the fibrinogen that was consumed and fibrinolysis that was produced increased in infants undergoing cardiac surgery with CPB. This can exacerbate coagulopathy and transfusion requirements after CPB.[76,77] Overall, routine preoperative measurement and supplementation to maintain values close to 100% of adult values was safe and protective in a blinded, randomized study, and no excessive bleeding was observed.[78,79]

RECOMBINANT FACTOR VIIA FOR MASSIVE HEMORRHAGE

Recombinant factor VIIa (rFVIIa) was originally approved for use in patients with hemophilia who possess inhibitors to factors VIII or IX, and was shown to effectively treat bleeding in these patients with doses of 45 to 90 µg/kg (see also Chapter 10).[80] Endogenous factor VII circulates in small concentrations in the plasma. At a site of tissue or blood vessel injury, tissue factor (TF) is exposed, and the extrinsic coagulation pathway is activated by the binding of factor VII to TF, resulting in the activation of factor X to factor Xa, leading to the generation of thrombin from prothrombin, with further activation of platelets and the coagulation cascade.[81] Large concentrations of rFVIIa activate the extrinsic pathway at the site of injury, theoretically without inducing systemic hypercoagulability. However, thrombotic complications are increased after its use. In the most recent study,163 pediatric patients with post-CPB bleeding who received rFVIIa were an estimated 3.9 times (95% confidence interval [CI] 2.6, 5.9) more likely to develop thrombotic complications when compared with propensity-matched controls.[82] Recombinant FVIIa also activates platelets, adding to the potential benefit of this agent during poorly controlled bleeding. Thus, this therapy seems appropriate for the treatment of surgical bleeding; a review of the off-label uses of rFVIIa in pediatric cardiac surgery patients found no evidence to support the routine or prophylactic use of rFVIIa. However, rFVIIa may be beneficial as a rescue therapy for severe life-threatening refractory bleeding; the authors caution against the use of rFVIIa in children at risk for thromboembolic complications.[83] A dose of 45 to 90 µg/kg, repeated every 2 hours, has been used. Recombinant FVIIa cannot produce hemostasis alone and should only be administered after the transfusion of sufficient amounts of platelets, plasma, and fibrinogen to form the substrate for hemostasis. The combination with other factor concentrates like 3-factor prothrombin complex concentrates is not advisable.

FIBRINOGEN CONCENTRATE

The relatively small concentration of fibrinogen in FFP of 2.5 to 3.0 g/L after thawing makes FFP unsuitable to replenish fibrinogen.[84] Therefore, both fibrinogen concentrate and cryoprecipitate are alternatives to replace fibrinogen after CPB. Cryoprecipitate not only contains concentrated fibrinogen but also von Willebrand factor, factor VIII, and factor XIII.[85] Compared with cryoprecipitate, fibrinogen concentrate, which is lyophilized and purified human plasma fibrinogen, has an improved safety profile because it has undergone viral inactivation and is devoid of microparticles that can cause vasoreactivity. In addition, fibrinogen concentrate contains a known amount of fibrinogen, and cryoprecipitate varies in the amount of fibrinogen per unit (range: 150 to 700 mg/unit). No difference in the safety and efficacy of fibrinogen concentrate compared with cryoprecipitate is reported when managing bleeding in children undergoing CPB.[86] The dose of fibrinogen concentrate required usually appears to be 50 to 60 mg/kg although larger doses (100 to120 mg/kg) have been used,[87–89] based on either empiric dosing, laboratory fibrinogen concentration, or thromboelastography (TEG). Using TEG or rotational thromboelastometry (ROTEM), a target of 9 to 14 mm of maximum clot firmness in the fibrin-based thromboelastometry assay is sought.[90]

PROTHROMBIN COMPLEX CONCENTRATE

FFP can be used to replenish coagulation factors; however, large volumes (up to 15 mL/kg) are required to increase coagulation factor levels by as little as 20%. Such a volume overload is often poorly tolerated immediately after CPB, particularly in small children. In addition, large volume FFP transfusion results in further hemodilution of hemoglobin and other coagulation proteins.

Factor concentrates like 3- or 4-factor prothrombin complex concentrates have been studied and introduced into clinical practice.[91,92] They do not require crossmatching, may be administered in a small volume, are readily available, and not associated with the same infectious and noninfectious risks as blood product transfusion. Despite the risk of excessive thrombin generation and excessive clotting with thrombosis, clinical studies are favorable and report a low rate of thrombotic events. We start at a low dose of 25 to 50 IU/kg and reevaluate the success by observing the surgical field and thrombelastography.[87] The goal is for judicious and targeted factor and platelet transfusions to manage bleeding.

DESMOPRESSIN

Desmopressin (DDAVP) is a vasopressin analog that increases circulating levels of coagulation factor VIII and von Willebrand factor by stimulating the release of stored von Willebrand factor from the Weibel Palade bodies in the endothelium. DDAVP is used mainly to improve hemostasis in patients with von Willebrand's disease, hemophilia A, and certain inherited disorders of platelet function at a dose of 0.3 μg/kg IV. The efficacy of DDAVP in reducing bleeding and transfusion in children undergoing cardiac surgery was not associated with a significant reduction in blood loss or blood product transfusion.[12]

SICKLE CELL DISEASE

Sickle cell disease (SCD), one of the most common hemoglobinopathies among patients of African American or West Indian origin (with a prevalence of 0.2% to 0.3% in that population), is the result of the substitution of valine for glutamic acid in position 6 of the β-hemoglobin chain. Normal adult hemoglobin is referred to as HbA, whereas hemoglobin containing the mutant β-hemoglobin chains is referred to as HbS. SCD is represented by a homozygous genotype (HbSS) with fractional concentrations of HbS in the range from 70% to 90%. Sickle cell trait, on the other hand, is a heterozygous manifestation (HbAS) with a prevalence of 8% to 10% in the same population. The definitive diagnosis of any sickle cell hemoglobinopathy is confirmed by hemoglobin electrophoresis (see Chapter 8).

Children with SCD are at particular risk for perioperative complications.[93,94] Sickling can be triggered by hypoxia, dehydration, acidosis,[95] hypothermia, stress, and infections. Hypoxia opens a Ca^{2+}-activated K^+ channel (Gardos channel) that causes intracellular dehydration.[96] Chain formation occurs that leads to increased blood viscosity with vasoocclusion. Opening of the Gardos channel depends on temperature, with greater potassium efflux at reduced temperatures.[97] Shrinkage of sickle erythrocytes may also result from activation of a K^+/Cl^- cotransport pathway under acidotic conditions.[98] Activation of this pathway can be blocked by increasing the abnormally low level of intracellular magnesium in sickled erythrocytes. The use of magnesium and hydroxyurea in the perioperative period therefore seems to be reasonable.[99]

Few data exist regarding sickle cell hemoglobinopathies other than sickle disease. In a recent retrospective, propensity-matched study of children from the Society of Thoracic surgeons congenital heart surgery database between 2014 and 2019 with sickle disease (n=75), sickle trait (n=411), and controls (n=36,500) undergoing CPB, the primary outcome, mortality, occurred significantly more frequently in children with sickle disease (5.5%) than in the matched controls (0%).[100] The remainder of the outcomes including postoperative complications did not differ among the three groups.

CPB, particularly for more complex surgical procedures, may involve periods of low flow or even circulatory arrest, as well as hypothermia with consequent local vasoconstriction, hypoxemia, and acidosis. There is some evidence that CPB can be safely undertaken in SCD.[101] Flow conditions are an important determinant of sickle erythrocyte adherence to endothelium. Under low-flow conditions, the adhesion of sickle cells to the endothelium increases with contact time in the absence of endothelium activation or adhesive proteins, whereas under low-flow conditions in venules, sickle cell adhesion occurs only after endothelial activation. During CPB, both low-flow conditions and endothelial activation may occur. Multiple triggers of sickling are likely to occur during CPB, and close attention should be paid to the conduct of all aspects of bypass.

In the past, routine exchange transfusion has been recommended to prevent these complications.[102] More recent experience provides evidence that not all children require an exchange transfusion.[103] The growing evidence of the harmful effects of blood transfusion adds to the need to carefully reconsider routine exchange transfusion.[104] For uncomplicated bypass surgery without periods of cardiac arrest, the omission of exchange transfusion has led to good outcomes.

Guidelines have been proposed for the perioperative management of children with sickle cell disorders.[103] It is essential to avoid hypothermia using tepid or warm CPB in its stead; blood transfusion only for a decrease in hematocrit to less than 20%; maintenance of intravascular volume and body temperature while on CPB; the avoidance of vasopressors; the use of postoperative multimodal pain therapy; and early incentive spirometry to prevent pulmonary complications.[105] In our practice, we use cerebral near-infrared spectroscopy (NIRS) to help determine an acceptable lower limit of hemoglobin for the individual child.

For children undergoing hypothermia, successful management with[106] and without[107] partial or complete exchange transfusion on bypass has been reported. Exchange transfusion can be performed preoperatively or on initiation of CPB.[108] For exchange transfusion during CPB, the extracorporeal circuit is primed with blood and the usual components. When CPB is commenced, the child's blood volume is drained into storage bags and separated. The platelet-rich plasma is reinfused at the end of CPB, and the concentrated sickle cells are discarded. Platelet and plasma sequestration in conjunction with exchange transfusion reduces the need for postoperative transfusion and protects the platelets from the negative effects of CPB.[109]

There is no consensus for a suitable target concentration of HbS. Reducing the absolute level of HbS may provide a greater benefit than targeting a particular ratio of HbA to HbS because the remaining sickle cells are still 100% at risk for sickling.[110] In SCD, exchange transfusion has been shown to favorably affect cerebral tissue oxygenation.[111] Exchange transfusion decreases both the proportion and absolute amount of HbS, but it does not remove every cell that may sickle. It may also improve hypoxic pulmonary vasoconstriction.[111] In this context, these children may benefit from continuous hemofiltration to reduce inflammatory mediators and improve pulmonary recovery.[112] Inhaled nitric oxide also has been recommended as an adjunct to prevent sickle cell crisis. It may improve the binding of oxygen, thereby reducing the formation of sickle cells, reduce pulmonary hypertension, and improve pulmonary function without adverse effects on normal hemoglobin.[113]

A Perspective on Blood Preservation: Cardiopulmonary Bypass in Jehovah's Witness Patients

Jehovah's Witnesses differ from other religious groups in their conscious objection to receive a therapeutic infusion of blood and blood components. They uniformly refuse the transfusion of red blood cells, and some individuals also refuse platelets and plasma, as well as predonated autologous blood. Individual choices that can be made are the acceptance of fractions of blood, such as albumin and globulins, dialysis, cell salvage, and acute isovolemic hemodilution.

Acute isovolumic reduction of hemoglobin to a concentration of 5 g/dL has been well tolerated in healthy children under anesthesia in one study and does not appear to reduce tissue oxygenation ominously.[114] Reduction of oxygen delivery to 7 to 8 mL/kg per minute under resting conditions does not increase the oxygen debt. This degree of anemia is compensated for in part, by an increased extraction, an increase in cardiac index, and a subsequent decrease in systemic vascular resistance.[115,116] In a retrospective study of the morbidity associated with reduced concentrations of hemoglobin in Jehovah's Witness patients, the hemoglobin concentration of those who died was less than 5 g/dL.[117] A safe limit of hemodilution in children has not been established. Hemodiluting acyanotic children up to 50% appears to be well tolerated and safe,[118] although in cyanotic children, hemodilution probably should not exceed 40%. If this level of hemodilution is exceeded, hemodynamic instability and inadequate oxygen delivery can occur. Hematocrit concentrations of 21.5% in infants on CPB is thought to increase adverse psychomotor developmental outcomes compared with concentrations of 27.8%.[119]

The most important and simplest strategy to avoid transfusion in the setting of cardiac surgery is to limit blood loss. Unnecessary and reduced amounts of blood removed for testing and sampling reduce the blood loss.[90] Pharmacologic agents, such as aprotinin, TXA, and EACA, reduce the risk of perioperative blood loss.[120] The administration of erythropoietin in the cardiac surgery setting has been shown to reduce the risk of exposure to allergenic blood.[121] Preoperative recombinant erythropoietin is an acceptable strategy to Jehovah's Witnesses to augment the red cell concentration. This strategy requires that oral iron (2–6 mg/kg of elemental iron in 2–3 divided doses) and vitamin C are started about 6 weeks before surgery followed by twice weekly erythropoietin (50–100 IU/kg) intramuscularly about 3 weeks before surgery. Hemoglobin concentrations should be tracked to ensure the concentration does not exceed 15 to 20 g/dL as venous thromboembolism may occur. Some Jehovah's Witnesses refuse albumin, a constituent in the preparation of erythropoietin that is supplied in glass ampoules. In the latter case, a lyophilized preparation of erythropoietin, which is albumin-free, may be used. The cost of erythropoietin can be substantial, and one cost analysis suggested that its use in cardiac surgery is not cost-effective.[122]

Intraoperative recovery of blood with a cell salvage device is also acceptable to many Jehovah's Witnesses. This involves the removal by suction of blood from the operative field followed by washing, filtering, and return of red blood cells to the patient. A randomized controlled trial of intraoperative cell salvage in cardiothoracic surgery has demonstrated a reduction in RBC transfusions and an increase in postoperative hemoglobin.[123]

Acute normovolemic hemodilution involves the preoperative removal of a volume of blood from the patient with the simultaneous administration of crystalloid or colloid to maintain circulating volume.[124] The collected blood is then reinfused during the operation. Some Jehovah's Witnesses find this process acceptable, especially if the blood remains in continuity with the patient throughout. Acute normovolemic hemodilution has other advantages, including lower costs, because the blood does not need compatibility testing; reduced possibility of administrative error; and a saving in patient time (see also Chapters 8 and 10). The development of artificial red cell substitutes could potentially obviate the need for compatibility testing, as well as vastly reduce infection risks, with none of the immunomodulatory side effects of allogeneic blood.[125] Some of these products would also be acceptable to Jehovah's Witness families. Substitutes include perfluorocarbons, hemoglobin solutions, intramolecular cross-linked hemoglobin, and liposome encapsulated hemoglobin. None of these has reached clinical practice. Lastly, autologous retrograde priming has been used in Jehovah's Witness patients and can further reduce the hemodilutional effects of the prime.[124,126] For this purpose, priming of the arterial line of the CPB circuit is accomplished with the patients' own blood.

Current bypass circuits reduce the priming volumes to less than 200 to 300 mL. Main components that are amenable to volume reduction on a regular circuit are the size and length of the lines, small oxygenators, and arterial filters, and priming the hemofilter for modified ultrafiltration with blood from the venous line after CPB. Line volumes, for example, may vary from 1.73 mL per 10 cm of a 3/16-inch tubing to 0.75 mL per 10 cm of a 1/8-inch tubing. The limiting factor, however, is the necessary flow. For a 3/16-inch arterial line, a maximum flow of 1.8 L/minute was established as the point at which the Reynolds number (reflective of flow patterns) reaches a value >2000, indicating a change to turbulent flow (https://www.britannica.com/science/Reynolds-number). Modified ultrafiltration at the end of CPB through a fluid warmer line to prevent heat loss or continuous ultrafiltration has been used. The venous line and the reservoir are emptied before discontinuation of bypass, the field is suctioned, and all blood is retransfused through the arterial line. Decannulation is achieved and protamine is given as usual. Crystalloid cardioplegia solution should be evacuated from the field by an external sucker to prevent dilution of the pump volume.

Postoperative care involves minimal blood sampling, and only on special indications. Noninvasive monitoring allows uncomplicated weaning from the ventilator.[127] The first report of successful outcomes in Jehovah's Witness children with congenital cardiac defects was in 1985[128]; 110 children older than 6 months of age successfully underwent operation, with a perioperative mortality rate of 5.3%. Only one death was attributed to blood loss. A weight <5 kilograms was considered by some as a contraindication for open-heart surgery and palliative procedures were advocated in the past.[129] For some lesions, however, no palliation is possible. The development of miniaturized circuits, preoperative optimization, use of antithrombolytic drugs, vacuum-assisted drainage to allow smaller tubing and cannula sizes, as well as the use of modified ultrafiltration, enabled the safe expansion of surgery into the neonatal population. Individualized heparin level–based anticoagulation management further results in a reduction of coagulation problems, blood loss, and transfusion requirements.[130] The addition of desmopressin, 0.3 μg/kg, may improve platelet activity and stimulate the release of von Willebrand factor after protamine infusion, although this belief is not evidence based.

In one study, when center-specific blood conservation strategies were employed, bloodless cardiac surgery was most successful in children greater than 18 kilograms in weight, followed by those 6, 10, and 18 kilograms in weight. All 73 patients less than 6 kilograms in weight were transfused during their hospitalization.[131]

All the aforementioned considerations are important in approaching the Jehovah's Witness patient; however, at Texas Children's Hospital, Jehovah's Witness children are not treated differently regarding blood transfusion practice than any other child. Cerebral NIRS is used to help determine the safe hemoglobin level for the individual child at all phases of surgery. Consent for blood transfusion in this situation is a complicated issue, because the legal status of children differs from that of an adult. Each institution must develop a legal informed consent process for blood transfusion for Jehovah's Witness children, in consultation with local legal authorities, social workers, ethnic group representatives, and representatives of the Jehovah's Witness faith. Currently, we have a release of liability form for the parents to sign that states that they request that no blood products be used, but acknowledges transfusions may be needed. The parent further agrees to release and hold harmless the physicians and hospital for any liability associated with blood transfusion. This form was developed in conjunction with the local Jehovah's Witness church representatives, and in our practice, this has been accepted by more than 95% of parents and has obviated the need for more extreme measures, such as temporary child protective services custody during the perioperative period, which was our former practice.

Myocardial Protection

Myocardial protection and the concept of chemical cardioplegia was introduced in 1955.[132] Before the popular use of chemical cardioplegia, topical cardiac hypothermia was used. In the late 1970s and early 1980s, the concept of cold hyperkalemic blood cardioplegia was introduced.[133] Potassium concentrations in cardioplegic solutions ranging from 12 to 30 mEq/L are typically used to achieve cardiac standstill within 1 to 2 minutes under hypothermic conditions, with greater concentrations for induction times required for normothermic conditions.

Myocardial edema after bypass and global ischemia can be reduced by a number of strategies that involve modifying the conditions of delivery and composition of cardioplegia solutions as they affect the movement of intracellular and interstitial fluid. In contrast to studies in adults, most studies conducted in neonates have shown little difference between blood and crystalloid cardioplegia.[134,135] Hypothermia also decreases myocardial oxygen consumption. The benefits of this approach appear to be optimal at myocardial temperatures between 24°C and 28°C. However, there is growing evidence that warm, intermittent blood cardioplegia may be advantageous compared with either cold crystalloid or cold blood cardioplegia.[136] The benefits of blood cardioplegia are more pronounced in younger, cyanotic children who require longer aortic cross-clamping. For acyanotic children, the cardioplegic technique is probably not as critical.[137] Avoidance or reduction of myocardial edema occurs by limiting the pressure of cardioplegia infusions and by providing moderately hyperosmolar cardioplegia solutions that contain blood. Buffering the acidosis that results from ischemia is achieved by including tromethamine, histidine-imidazole, or both in the cardioplegia solution. Close management of myocardial calcium balance to avoid extremes of intracellular hypercalcemia or hypocalcemia, especially during reperfusion, is very important.[138,139] The addition of magnesium may solve this dilemma by preventing damage from greater cardioplegic calcium concentrations by its action as a calcium antagonist.[139,140] This prevents mitochondrial calcium overload as a consequence of reperfusion injury. Magnesium also prevents the influx of sodium into the postischemic myocardium, which is exchanged for calcium during reperfusion. The addition of lidocaine for Na^+ channel blockade counteracts the negative effects of a hyperkalemic depolarized arrest by polarizing the cell membrane to some degree and preventing sodium and calcium accumulation within the cell.[141]

Every cardiac program has its own philosophy regarding cardioplegia and myocardial protection. At Texas Children's Hospital, plain crystalloid cardioplegia is used. The prime blood gas and electrolytes should physiologically mimic the child's arterial blood gas as closely as possible. If whole blood or packed cells are added to the prime, the target hemodilution range should be 28% to 30%; the prime should be recirculated continuously and warmed between 35.0°C and 36.5°C before initiation of bypass. In neonates and infants, albumin is added to the cardioplegic solution to maintain an appropriate colloid osmotic pressure. This may decrease edema formation of the arrested heart. In children undergoing circulatory arrest, long cross-clamp times, and large pump suction return cases, 20 mg/kg methylprednisolone is used, up to a maximum of 500 milligrams, to reduce the production of inflammatory mediators that result in myocardial dysfunction. Table 17.4 summarizes the Texas Children's Hospital protocols for cardioplegia and myocardial protection.

Phases of Cardiopulmonary Bypass

Surgery requiring CPB can be separated into several basic phases.

PREBYPASS PERIOD

This phase begins with surgical incision and lasts through initial dissection and preparation for cannulation. During this period, transesophageal echocardiography (TEE) is performed to confirm the diagnosis and establish a basis for postbypass comparison.

TABLE 17.4 | Cardioplegia Solution

CARDIOPLEGIA BASE SOLUTION (385 ML)			
Concentration		**Contents**	
Sodium chloride BP	3.54 grams/L	Sodium	23 mmol
Anhydrous glucose BP	6.65 grams/L	Potassium	15 mmol
Potassium chloride	2.92 grams/L	Calcium	0.35 mmol
Mannitol	6.54 grams/L	Chloride	39 mmol
Calcium chloride	135 mg/L	Glucose	2.52 grams
		Mannitol	2.48 grams
		Approximate pH 4.5	
		275 mOsm/L	

CARDIOPLEGIA BUFFER SOLUTION			
Concentration		**Contents**	
Sodium carbonate	9.37 grams/L	Sodium carbonate	0.28 grams
Sodium bicarbonate	27.0 grams/L	Sodium bicarbonate	0.81 grams

USES OF CARDIOPLEGIA SOLUTION DURING CARDIOPULMONARY BYPASS

Children weighing <10 kg

385 mL Cardioplegia base solution

26 mL Cardioplegia buffer solution

100 mL 25% Albumin

Note: This is usually delivered at a pressure of 30 mm Hg for newborns and 30–40 mm Hg for older infants.

Children weighing >10 kg

385 mL Cardioplegia base solution

100 mL 0.9% Sodium chloride

10 mL 25% Mannitol

5 mL 8.4% Sodium bicarbonate

Note: This is usually delivered at a pressure of 30–60 mm Hg. A good guide is to note the end-diastolic pressure of each child before bypass. This will be a guide to the normal filling pressure of the coronary arteries. When aortic incompetence is present, the CPS flow may need to be increased.

ADMINISTRATION OF CARDIOPLEGIA SOLUTION

For all patients:	
Temperature	8–12°C
Initial dose	110 mL/m^2 per minute for 4 minutes
Subsequent doses	110 mL/m^2 per minute for 2 minutes

Note: Following the initial dose, cardioplegia is to be delivered every 20 minutes during the cross-clamp period unless otherwise indicated by the surgeon. The perfusionist will remind the surgeon of the need for cardioplegia and keep track of the time. Because of the nature of the surgical procedure, it may be necessary to deliver cardioplegia directly into the coronary ostia via a hand-held delivery system. In this case the surgeon will direct the perfusionist. Close attention should be paid to the delivery line pressures.

EXAMPLES OF PRIMES	
Neonate: Whole Blood, If Available, Otherwise Reconstituted	
Whole blood	225 mL
PlasmaLyte A	50 mL
0.45% NaCl	125 mL
Heparin	2500 units
NaHCO$_3$	5 mEq
CaCl$_2$	250 mg
Pediatric: Packed Red Blood Cells	
PRBCs	250 mL
PlasmaLyte A	300 mL
0.45% NaCl	75 mL
25% Albumin	100 mL
Heparin	3500 units
NaHCO$_3$	20 mEq
CaCl$_2$	300 mg
Adult: Crystalloid Prime	
PlasmaLyte A	700 mL
0.45% NaCl	600 mL
25% Albumin	100–200 mL (volume varies depending on the size of the patient)
5% Dextrose	40 mL
Heparin	5000 units
NaHCO$_3$	40 mEq
CaCl$_2$	300 mg
KCl	2.4 mEq

BP, The material conforms to the specifications and procedures outlined in the British Pharmacopoeia; *CPS,* cardioplegia solution; *PRBCs,* packed red blood cells.

HEPARIN AND COAGULATION MANAGEMENT

After sternotomy and mediastinal dissection, the aorta is cannulated, along with either the right atrium, if single venous drainage is planned, or the superior and inferior venae cavae for bicaval venous drainage. After a large dose of heparin (300 to 400 units/kg) is administered intravenously, the adequacy of the anticoagulation is measured using the ACT *before initiating CPB.* Heparin requirements in children are much higher than in adults.[142] The target ACT is usually 480 seconds. High ACTs are maintained during CPB with the addition of heparin to the prime as needed, because larger doses of heparin lead to a reduced degree of consumptive coagulopathy, which translates into reduced blood product requirements.[130] Other methods of measuring anticoagulation include the Hepcon system (a plasma heparin concentration assay), which may allow for more accurate titration of heparin and protamine dosages since ACT is prolonged by hypothermia, hemodilution, platelet dysfunction, and low coagulation factor levels.[143,144] Although heparin management by concentration did not differ in the number of blood transfusions both in a meta-analysis in adults[145] and in a small study in children,[146] it is generally true that less coagulation activation occurs when using the heparin concentration system.[144,147,148]

Based on different volumes of distribution in children younger than 5 years and reduced circulating antithrombin activity, particularly in infants,[76] major differences in heparin and protamine doses are apparent. The extreme hemodilution in childhood is not adequately reflected by the ACT.[149] There is no correlation between the ACT and heparin level or anti-Xa activity after the initiation of the cardiac bypass or after protamine infusions.[150,151] Point-of-care diagnostics has decreased the need for blood transfusions.[152,153] Excessive protamine delivery contributes to platelet dysfunction and prolongation of ACT values.[154–156]

The thromboelastogram may also be used as a baseline measure of the coagulation system and then repeated during and after bypass, with heparinase added to more objectively assess each child's anticipated need for coagulation factors.[157,158] An improved preservation of the hemostatic system with subsequent reduction in blood loss and transfusion requirements has been demonstrated after maintenance of high heparin levels during CPB.[159] The additional maintenance of high ATIII concentrations may further contribute to a reduction of hemostatic activation.[160]

CANNULATION AND INITIATION OF BYPASS

Bicaval cannulation is used for all but the smallest children (less than 2 kg) to prevent venous return from interfering with the surgical field. A gradual transition to full CPB is then performed to minimize myocardial stress, using a prime that has essentially the same composition as the child's blood regarding temperature, pH, calcium, potassium, and hematocrit. CPB flows of 150 mL/kg per minute are used for infants weighing less than 10 kilograms, and 2.4 L/minute per m² is used for children weighing more than 10 kilograms. Flow rates may be reduced during periods of hypothermia, although many centers now prefer to maintain greater flows of up to 3.0 L/minute per m² throughout the bypass period. Misplaced cannulas can lead to significant morbidity. Obstruction of the inferior vena cava (IVC) by a misplaced IVC cannula can lead to increased venous pressure, which causes ascites and decreased perfusion pressure in mesenteric, hepatic, and renal vascular beds. Misplacement of the cannula in the superior vena cava can result in cerebral edema from inadequate venous drainage and a subsequent reduction in cerebral blood flow, potentially resulting in ischemia. Arterial cannula misplacement can also occur. If the cannula inadvertently slips beyond the takeoff of the right innominate artery, preferential perfusion to the left side of the brain can be observed. This can be detected on the NIRS monitor, which is proving a useful monitor during pediatric cardiac surgery.[161]

The presence of any anomalous systemic-to-pulmonary shunts can lead to shunting of blood away from the systemic circulation, through the pulmonary circuit, and then through the venous cannula to the CPB machine. Thus, the systemic perfusion is shunted away from the body in a futile circuit back to the CPB machine. Anatomic lesions where such shunting can occur include an unrecognized patent ductus arteriosus and large aortopulmonary collaterals, as found in pulmonary atresia. Bypass flow should be increased to compensate for these shunts until they can be controlled.

COOLING PHASE

Systemic cooling is used frequently in pediatric cardiac surgery, but normothermia is used with increasing frequency for selected cases.[162] Normothermia reduces time on bypass, improves serum lactate levels 2 to 4 hours after CPB and serum creatine 24 and 48 hours after CPB.[163] Hypothermia is classified as mild (30°C to 36°C), moderate (22°C to 30°C), or deep (17°C to 22°C). In general, the coldest temperatures are used for more complex operations that carry a greater potential for requiring periods of low-flow bypass or circulatory arrest. Cooling is primarily achieved extracorporeally through the heat exchanger in the bypass circuit; some surgeons may request that ice be applied to the head to prevent brain rewarming during circulatory arrest.

AORTIC CROSS-CLAMPING AND INTRACARDIAC REPAIR PHASE

The aorta is cross-clamped, with the heart then rendered asystolic after infusion of cardioplegia solution into the aortic root.

DEEP HYPOTHERMIC CIRCULATORY ARREST OR SELECTIVE CEREBRAL PERFUSION PHASE

If circulatory arrest is to be used, it is initiated after a slow cooling period of at least 20 minutes, and an attempt is made to limit the total duration of deep hypothermic circulatory arrest (DHCA) to less than 40 minutes. Special bypass techniques (see later in the chapter) have been developed to avoid the necessity of using DHCA and may also be performed during this time.

REMOVAL OF AORTIC CROSS-CLAMP AND REWARMING PHASE

After completion of the intracardiac repair and deairing of the heart, the aortic cross-clamp is removed, allowing reperfusion of the myocardium. Optimally, normal sinus rhythm and myocardial contractility are restored during this time, while the child is slowly rewarmed. During rewarming, surgery is completed, inotropic and vasoactive agents are started, the trachea is suctioned, and ventilation begins. Hemofiltration and blood transfusion are used to achieve the desired hematocrit. Left atrial and/or pulmonary artery monitoring lines, if indicated, are placed at this time, as are temporary atrial and ventricular pacing wires. If the child is incompletely rewarmed before separation from CPB, a precipitous postbypass reduction in core body temperature can occur. This can lead to vasoconstriction, shivering, increased oxygen consumption, and acidosis. However, postischemic hyperthermia can lead to delayed neuronal cell death.[164] Mild degrees of hypothermia and certainly the avoidance of hyperthermia are essential in the perioperative period.[165] In children, rectal temperature mostly reflects peripheral temperature. One study showed that the temperature of the foot was more sensitive than the temperature of the hand.[166] Another study revealed that for anatomic or physiologic reasons, temperature gradients in the toes develop more readily than those in the fingers.[167] Several endpoints have been proposed, such as nasopharyngeal temperatures greater than 35.0°C, bladder temperature greater than 36.2°C, or skin temperatures greater than 30°C[168,169]; we use an endpoint of 35.5°C rectal temperature.[170]

SEPARATION FROM BYPASS

The child's core body temperature, hematocrit, and metabolic variables should be optimized before attempting separation from CPB. Careful observation for air in the systemic ventricle, confirmation with the TEE, and concurrent inspection of electrocardiogram (ECG) changes should continue throughout the weaning process, with the child in the Trendelenburg position and the aortic root vented. While fluid volume is gradually added to the child by reducing the outflow to the venous reservoir until optimal filling pressures are achieved, CPB flow is then slowly reduced to zero. If inotropic support is anticipated to separate from CPB, infusions should be initiated before beginning separation.

POSTBYPASS PERIOD

This phase lasts until chest closure and transfer to the ICU have been accomplished. During this time, modified ultrafiltration (MUF) may be performed for 10 to 20 minutes after cessation of CPB. Cardiac function and the quality of the surgical repair are assessed using TEE, and if found to be satisfactory, protamine is administered to neutralize residual heparin. The usual dose of protamine is 0.6 to 1.0 mg/100 IU of heparin given at the onset of bypass.[171] Limiting protamine to this dose prevents an overdose with its associated effects on platelet function (reduction of the interaction of glycoprotein Ib receptor interaction with von Willebrand factor).[172] If the ACT remains increased or prime blood is given back to the child, an additional 10% of the initial dose of protamine is added and the ACT is rechecked, keeping in mind that high ACT values after bypass may be due to factors other than the presence of residual heparin.[150]

Early use of heparinase-assisted thrombelastography or protamine titration ACT will allow a diagnostic separation of residual heparin effect. However, particularly in infants, the administration of protamine and the persistent treatment of a suspected incomplete heparin reversal should not distract and delay the treatment of other commonly associated postbypass coagulopathies, such as thrombocytopenia, platelet dysfunction, hypofibrinogenemia, and other coagulation factor deficiencies. The child should be transferred to the ICU only after adequate hemostasis has been established since ongoing bleeding increases surgical mortality.[173]

Protamine reactions occur much less frequently in children younger than 16 years of age, approximately 1.8% to 2.9%.[174] Independent risk factors are a female gender, a larger protamine dose, and smaller heparin doses. Type I reactions (isolated hypotension) or effects during administration are rare and adding calcium does not change the hemodynamic consequences of injection.[175] Fortunately, severe anaphylactic reactions (type II) or catastrophic pulmonary vasoconstriction (type III) are rare but have been observed.[176] Administering the protamine over 5 minutes or longer reduces the severity and precipitous nature of any protamine reaction.

Unstable neonates and small infants may have their sternums temporarily left open, with surgical closure planned 24 to 72 hours later when cardiac function has improved, and myocardial edema has diminished.

Because CPB can have a multitude of adverse physiologic effects, attempts are made to minimize both the duration of CPB and ischemic (aortic cross-clamp) time; as much of the surgery as possible is performed outside of these phases. In general, physiologic responses to bypass are more extreme with decreasing age and size of the child. The neonate experiences a greater degree of hemodilution on bypass and colder temperatures on bypass and frequently requires longer aortic cross-clamp times, all of which can result in a greater inflammatory response. Table 17.5 summarizes clinical management issues during the major phases of CPB.

Particular Aspects of Management on Cardiopulmonary Bypass

pH-STAT VERSUS α-STAT MANAGEMENT

Some degree of hypothermia is used for nearly every cardiac operation to slow the metabolism and oxygen consumption of all organs, particularly the brain and heart.[177] During cooling, the

TABLE 17.5	Checklist for Bypass Management

Before CPB

1. Check temperature; maintain normothermia during induction and preparation
2. Supplement premedication
3. Ensure noninvasive monitoring: blood pressure, ECG, pulse oximetry, stethoscope
4. Perform inhalational induction after preoxygenation; intravenous induction if cannula is in place
5. Peripheral intravenous placement(s)
6. Neuromuscular blockade and ventilation
7. Intubation and mechanical ventilation according to shunt lesion (CO_2, O_2 control)
8. Monitoring:
   a. Arterial line and central venous line
   b. ECG electrodes
   c. Bladder catheter
   d. Temperature probes
   e. TEE probe (in infants >3 kg)
9. Positioning
10. Deepening of anesthetic level
11. Antifibrinolytics and corticosteroids, as indicated
12. Heparin, 300–400 U/kg, before arterial cannulation
13. Check activated clotting time >400 seconds
14. Supplement anesthetics on initiation of bypass

During CPB

1. Stop ventilation and drips when full flow is reached
2. Inspect head perfusion
3. Evaluate quality of perfusion (perfusion pressure, central venous pressure, diuresis, arterial blood gases, temperature gradient)
4. Prepare for separation
   a. Drips (inotropic drugs, calcium)
   b. Pacemaker
   c. Blood products
5. Set and control temperature and rewarming (heating blanket, room temperature)
6. Zero transducers
7. Check arterial blood gases in preparation for discontinuation of CPB; correct abnormalities
8. Suction and ventilate

After CPB

1. Separate when:
   a. Temperature >35.5°C
   b. Stable rhythm or pacing
   c. Heart contracting well
2. Fine-tune blood pressure; consider direct blood pressure measurement for hypotension at the aortic cannula; volume ± drips
3. Consider modified ultrafiltration
4. Check arterial blood gases
5. Evaluate with transesophageal echocardiography for residual defects
6. Give protamine, 1–1.3 mg/100 IU of initial heparin
7. Check activated clotting time and arterial blood gases
8. Chest closure and recheck arterial blood gases
9. Transport to the intensive care unit

CPB, Cardiopulmonary bypass; *ECG,* electrocardiogram; *TEE,* transesophageal echocardiography.

carbon dioxide contained in blood becomes more soluble and its partial pressure decreases. The $PaCO_2$ sensed by the body decreases as body temperature decreases, with the result that at a core temperature of 17°C to 18°C, if pH and $PaCO_2$ have not been corrected for temperature, the body experiences a pH of about 7.6 and $PaCO_2$ of 15 to 18 mm Hg (Fig. 17.2).[178] This very low $PaCO_2$ causes cerebral vasoconstriction, particularly during the cooling phase of bypass, which in turn leads to less cerebral blood flow, less efficient brain cooling, and less cerebral protection at a given temperature.[179] Because blood samples are normally heated to 37°C before measurement of pH, $PaCO_2$, and PaO_2, the use of pH-stat management indicates that blood gases are being corrected for the child's actual body temperature by increasing the $PaCO_2$ during bypass, as it is measured at 37°C, so that the body experiences a $PaCO_2$ of approximately 40 mm Hg and a pH of 7.4 at all temperatures. Conversely, α-stat management means not correcting the blood gases for temperature, as if the child's blood was always at 37°C, with the goal of pH 7.4 and $PaCO_2$ 40 mm Hg. In the early days of CPB, pH-stat was used to preserve cerebral blood flow at all ages.[178] Subsequently, in the 1970s and 1980s, randomized controlled studies in adults confirmed that acute, post-CPB neurologic problems were worse with pH-stat management.[180] α-Stat management was, therefore, adopted for both

adult and pediatric CPB. However, studies in a neonatal pig model have challenged this conclusion, proving that neurologic outcomes, both behavioral and neuropathologic, are significantly worse when α-stat management is used in infants.[179,181]

Advantages of pH-stat CPB have been shown to include:

- A decreased brain metabolic rate[182]
- An increased rate of brain cooling and reperfusion,[183] thereby providing better protection through more even and faster cooling and rewarming secondary to increased CBF[183,184]
- Molecular effects of altered PaO_2 and pH, including changes in cerebral oxygenation and brain enzyme activity, as well as decreased brain electrical activity[184–186]
- Decreased oxyhemoglobin affinity[187]
- Increased cortical oxygenation before arrest (through hypercapnic capillary vasodilation) and decreased oxygen metabolic rate, providing slower deoxygenation compared with α-stat management (~10 vs. ~7 minutes).[179,188] Cortical anoxia occurs at 36 minutes with pH-stat management compared with 24 minutes for α-stat management

In cyanotic infants with aortopulmonary collaterals, pH-stat management improves brain oxygenation when measured using NIRS oximetry.[189] A retrospective study of 16 infants revealed worse neurodevelopmental outcomes with α-stat management.[190]

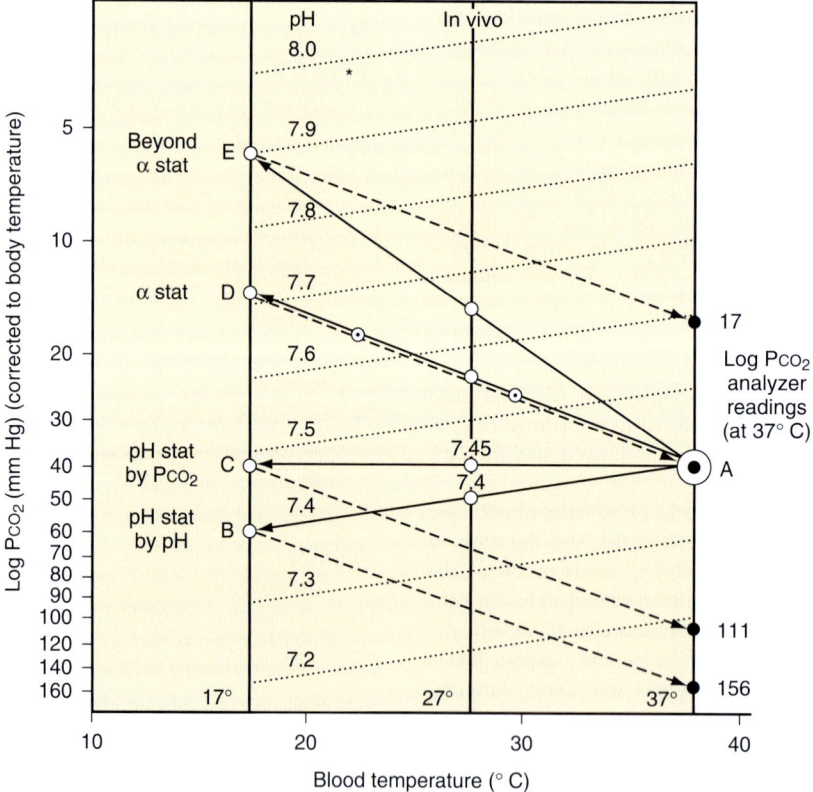

FIGURE 17.2 pH and PCO_2 changes when blood temperature is varied between 17°C and 37°C. Point A is the starting point, with pH 7.4 and PCO_2 40 mm Hg at 37°C. Points B, C, D, and E are the conditions the brain experiences at 17°C with various blood gas management strategies. pH-stat management (correcting the pH and PCO_2 for temperature) results in an acid-base environment that is neutral, whereas α-stat management (not correcting for temperature) results in a very alkalotic environment at 17°C. Warming the blood sample (as is done for blood gas measurement) results in very high PCO_2 values when pH-stat is used. The pH of blood becomes slightly more alkalotic with cooling, owing to the decreased dissociation of hydrogen ions. (From Jonas RA. Carbon dioxide, pH, and oxygen management. In: Jonas RA, DiNardo J, Lawson PC, et al., eds. *Comprehensive Surgical Management of Congenital Heart Disease.* London: Arnold Publishers; 2004:151-160.)

In a randomized prospective trial of pH- versus α-stat management in 182 infants younger than 9 months of age, there was moderate evidence for improved outcomes with pH-stat management, including earlier return of electroencephalographic activity, fewer seizures, and improved psychomotor development index.[191] Another study examined the effects of α-stat and pH-stat on developmental and neurologic outcomes after deep hypothermic CPB in infants.[192] Psychomotor development index scores of 110 patients did not differ significantly between the groups ($P = 0.97$). The results of the Mental Development Index scores were dependent on diagnosis. In all but the ventricular septal defect subgroup, the pH-stat group did not have statistically greater Mental Development Index scores. Abnormalities on the electroencephalogram ($P = 0.77$) and neurologic examination ($P = 0.70$) were similar with the two methods of blood gas management. The authors concluded that the use of α-stat or pH-stat strategy is not consistently associated with improved or impaired early neurodevelopmental outcomes in infants undergoing deep hypothermic CPB.[192] One reason for the differing results between pediatric and adult studies is that the increased cerebral blood flow produced by pH-stat management and the presence of atherosclerotic plaques in adults lead to microcerebral atherosclerotic plaque emboli. Emboli occur much less frequently in children and the primary cause of neurologic injury from CPB in children is hypoxic-ischemic,[193] thus, the increased cerebral blood flow observed on CPB with pH-stat management lessens this risk in children. Interestingly, this putative mechanism has been recently challenged by a study involving a controlled microembolic load and DHCA in pigs that revealed that pH-stat was still associated with improved outcomes when compared with α-stat.[194] pH-stat also improves oxygen delivery by counteracting the pH- and hypothermia-associated leftward shift in the oxyhemoglobin dissociation curve. Studies have also revealed a decrease in peak postoperative troponin levels, reduced ventilator dependence, and reduced ICU stays with pH-stat versus α-stat.[195] Most programs specializing in surgery for congenital heart defects currently use pH-stat management. This necessitates careful attention to $PaCO_2$ during all phases of bypass, and possibly reducing the sweep gas flow into the CPB oxygenator (to decrease the efficiency of CO_2 removal), and often adding inspired CO_2 to the sweep gas of the bypass circuit, particularly in small infants.

HEMATOCRIT ON BYPASS

The relatively small total blood volume in infants, along with the volume required to prime the CPB circuit, means that adding blood to the CPB prime is mandatory. However, this practice is institution specific with many centers adding either whole blood, PRBCs with FFP (for children less than 8 kg), or PRBCs alone (for children less than 12 to 15 kg) so as to ensure that the hematocrit on bypass is not <20%. As a result of increased transfusion-related concerns from bloodborne viral disease transmission during the 1980s and 1990s, and given that a low hematocrit is thought to be necessary to ensure adequate blood flow through capillary beds (because the blood viscosity increases at low temperatures), hematocrits of 20% or less on CPB with deep hypothermia were frequently tolerated.[196] There is increasing evidence that the practice of extreme hemodilution is detrimental to neurologic outcome in children. In a pig model, the incidence and degree of hypoxic-ischemic brain injury after a period of DHCA was greater with a hematocrit of 20% versus one of 30%, regardless of whether pH- or α-stat strategy was used.[197] In another pig model, using intravital microscopy of pial capillaries during deep

hypothermic CPB, a hematocrit of 30% did not impair cerebral microcirculation when compared with a hematocrit of 20%.[198] Finally, in a prospective randomized trial of CPB hematocrit of 20% versus 30% at the Boston Children's Hospital, children in the lower hematocrit group demonstrated reduced psychomotor development index scores 1 year after surgery.[119] In a follow-up study of hematocrit 25% vs. 35%, the same group did not observe a difference in neurodevelopmental outcomes.[199] However, when they combined all children from both hematocrit trials, they found that a hematocrit less than 24% was associated with poorer psychomotor index scores 1 year after surgery.[200] The hypoxic-ischemic damage possibly occurs during the cooling and rewarming phases of bypass, when cerebral oxygen metabolism is not suppressed, yet hematocrit and, thus, oxygen delivery, is reduced. Therefore, current guidelines now recommend maintaining hematocrits on CPB of at least 25%,[12] which either means using more donor blood products or using hemofiltration to raise the hematocrit during bypass.

The current quantifiable risk of viral transmission through blood product transmission in the United States is 1 in 1.9 million units for human immunodeficiency virus, 1 in 370,000 for hepatitis B virus, and 1 in 1.7 million units for hepatitis C virus.[201,202] The risk–benefit ratios therefore favor the greater hematocrit approach, a definitive change from previous practice patterns. Balanced against this practice of a greater hematocrit on CPB is the finding that greater transfusion of blood products in the intraoperative, and early postoperative periods, is associated with longer duration of mechanical ventilation in infants undergoing two-ventricle (biventricular) repairs.[203] Additional studies are required to optimize strategies for the use of blood products in infants and children undergoing CPB.

FLOW RATES ON BYPASS

The traditional practice in many institutions has been to decrease CPB flows, particularly during hypothermia, to reduce the volume of blood returning to the surgical field and allow more efficient completion of the surgery, particularly in small infants. This concept has been questioned in recent years owing to the inability to determine the safe low-flow bypass rate in the individual child. One report studied 28 neonates who underwent the arterial switch operation with α-stat blood gas management during CPB.[204] At 14°C to 15°C, bypass flow was sequentially reduced from 150 mL/kg per minute to 50 mL/kg per minute, and then further decreased in increments of 10 mL/kg per minute until circulatory arrest was begun (to 0 mL/kg per minute). All neonates had detectable cerebral blood flow by transcranial Doppler (TCD) at CPB flows above 20 mL/kg per minute, but 1 had no detectable perfusion at 20 mL/kg per minute, and 8 had none at 10 mL/kg per minute, leading the authors to conclude that 30 mL/kg per minute was the minimum acceptable flow in this population. A neonatal pig model determined that, at normothermia, bypass flows of at least 150 to 175 mL/kg per minute were necessary to ensure full oxygenation of all end organs and tissues.[205] Clinical studies of a high-flow bypass strategy, which included flows of 150 mL/kg per minute at all phases of bypass except during DHCA, minimal use of DHCA, and α-adrenergic receptor blockade with phenoxybenzamine to produce long-duration systemic vasodilation, demonstrated excellent short- and long-term clinical and neurodevelopmental outcomes, with no child scoring outside normal ranges for testing performed at a mean age of 9 years.[206] This strategy also has led to excellent early results for the Norwood operation, with an early perioperative survival of 83% for cases carried out from 1993 to 1999.[207] During the same era, one report documented that 26.7% of arterial switch children had neurologic abnormalities and 55% had at least one abnormal area on neurodevelopmental testing (performed at a mean of 10 years) when DHCA and low-flow bypass had been used.[207] However, it should be noted that abnormal brain development is common in children with congenital heart disease, particularly those with cyanotic disease, possibly leading to abnormal cognitive developmental outcomes even before any cardiac surgery.[208-210]

Vasoconstriction and increased vascular resistance, resulting in uneven regional organ perfusion, are among the adverse effects of CPB. Endogenous catecholamine production and the alkaline α-stat CPB technique, if used, are responsible for these effects. To be able to run full flow during hypothermic CPB without hypertension, vasodilators are often used. Agents currently used to provide systemic vasodilation and more even cooling and rewarming include phentolamine, milrinone, clonidine, nitroprusside, or nitroglycerin. Phenoxybenzamine, which is no longer available, was used as part of a treatment strategy after stage 1 palliation for hypoplastic left heart syndrome, and was associated with improved outcomes.[211,212] Phenoxybenzamine was more effective than sodium nitroprusside in improving peripheral circulation, as shown by temperature gradients intraoperatively.[213] Greater CPB flows are associated with an improved oxygen delivery, which can improve patient outcome.[214]

Phentolamine is a nonselective competitive α_1 and α_2 catecholamine receptor blocker. It has a half-life of 19 minutes and is eliminated mainly by the kidneys. Through postsynaptic α_1 and α_2 receptor inhibition it has a vasodilating and hypotensive effect that can improve cardiovascular variables and metabolic acidosis during CPB.[215] In children receiving phentolamine, increasing lactate concentrations at the end of the CPB period show a steady state toward the end of the surgery, whereas lactate continues to rise in patients who did not receive phentolamine.[215] These findings suggest that the use of phentolamine limits lactic acid production during the hypothermic period and aids the disposal of lactic acid from tissues. Seelye and associates called the physiologic state after hypothermia the "oxygen debt repayment" period in infants.[216] Although it has a beneficial effect on CPB management, the potential harmful effects of phentolamine, especially on the brain, have still not been fully elucidated. One study provided evidence that phentolamine increases S100B (a chemical marker of brain injury) protein and the pulsatility index in the middle cerebral artery (a measure indicative of altered cerebrovascular resistance) in infants given phentolamine during open-heart surgery.[217]

Nitroprusside has been used as an easily titratable agent with direct arterial smooth muscle relaxant properties through production of nitric oxide and enhancement of the cyclic guanosine monophosphate (GMP) pathway. In comparison to the prebypass values, a similar increase in the concentration of S100B protein was found 2 hours after the termination of CPB in the sodium nitroprusside-treated and nontreated neonates, which decreased over the subsequent 48 postoperative hours.[218] However, reduced postbypass serum levels of S100B protein were found in the sodium nitroprusside-treated group after 24 and 48 hours of treatment.[218]

Nitroglycerin has been used with the same success. The only proven benefit over other agents is its nitric oxide donation capacity.[219] In Japan, high-dose chlorpromazine has been used as part of a low-resistance strategy during CPB for the Norwood procedure.[220]

We routinely use phentolamine, 0.1 to 0.2 mg/kg, to provide normal CPB flow and mean arterial pressure in the range of the diastolic pressure. If hypotension develops during bypass, the flow should be increased up to 150% of predicted; also, one should examine the acid-base status in conjunction with cerebral oxygenation and mixed venous saturations. Often, severe hemodilution with oxygen debt is the cause and should be treated. After exclusion, we treat the hypotension carefully with vasoconstrictors, knowing that normal systemic pressures will not restore splanchnic hypoperfusion[221] and that vasoconstrictors will often lead to a greater base excess. Excessive α-adrenergic receptor blockade can be antagonized by vasopressin.[222] One study demonstrated that vasoconstrictor treatment results in the administration of more sodium bicarbonate to treat the acidosis and is associated with a later time to extubation and return of bowel function.[223] An α-adrenergic receptor blockade during bypass should be considered because of its benefits for tissue perfusion, but carefully executed and balanced against potential drawbacks afterwards.

CONVENTIONAL ULTRAFILTRATION AND MODIFIED ULTRAFILTRATION

Ultrafiltration involves placing a hemofilter in the CPB circuit and has become the standard of care for nearly all congenital heart programs.[224,225] Conventional ultrafiltration (CUF) is performed during CPB, with the filter placed between the arterial and venous sides of the CPB circuit. The hemofilter has thousands of fibers with pores, which allow water, electrolytes, and small molecules to be filtered out of the blood. Suction is applied to the hemofilter on CPB, and an ultrafiltrate of plasma is produced. Advantages of ultrafiltration include the ability to increase the hematocrit, fibrinogen, plasma proteins, and platelet count,[226,227] without necessitating further blood transfusion; the ability to remove excess free water and sodium (which contribute to excess intravascular volume, tissue edema, pulmonary and myocardial edema); the ability to correct acid-base and electrolyte imbalances; and to remove small molecules, such as interleukins and tumor necrosis factor-α (TNF-α) in particular,[228] which are involved in the postbypass inflammatory process.[229,230] This improves systolic and diastolic function of the myocardium and reduces endothelial dysfunction in the systemic and pulmonary vasculature.[230,231] Pulmonary function is better preserved, probably owing to a slight reduction in interleukin 6 (IL-6) and thromboxane B_2,[232] even though this is not a consistent finding.[233,234] Endothelin-1, another mediator of pulmonary damage and hypertension, is not reduced by any filtration method.[234] Clinically, however, any ultrafiltration method seems to benefit children, especially those undergoing complex repairs, neonates, and children with preexisting pulmonary hypertension.[233]

MUF is performed for 10 to 20 minutes immediately after the conclusion of CPB. It can be performed in an arteriovenous manner with a hemofilter placed between the aortic cannula and the IVC cannula, or in a venovenous fashion using bicaval cannulation or an internal jugular venous catheter.[235] MUF was developed in 1991[236] as an alternative method to reduce the adverse effects of CPB. CUF during bypass is often limited by the minimal venous reservoir levels and requires the addition of crystalloid or colloid to be able to continuously remove cytokines during ultrafiltration. During MUF, blood passes out of the aorta, through the hemofilter, and is returned through the IVC cannula. The theoretical advantage of MUF over CUF is that only the child's blood volume is filtered, yielding a more efficient system for achieving the goals outlined above. The disadvantages are that the child remains heparinized, and body temperature may decrease during the process (unless the circuit is modified to include the heat exchanger).[237] It also requires extra time; an aortic cannula is needed that can obstruct the aorta in small infants, and acute intravascular volume shifts may occur at a time when the child is prone to hemodynamic instability. Opposite to the expected effects of fluid removal, MUF actually increases arterial pressures despite decreasing filling pressures and improving myocardial performance.[238]

There is increasing evidence that the use of ultrafiltration reduces bypass-related postoperative morbidity; ultrafiltration improves myocardial and pulmonary function, lessens tissue edema, allows faster weaning from mechanical ventilation, and decreases the need for inotropic support.[239] Current guidelines recommend using hemofiltration or MUF for at least 10 minutes in all neonates and infants.[12] In that aspect it may be as efficient as the perioperative application of steroids.[240] Cytokines are created in tissues, have large volumes of distribution, and plasma concentrations restored to steady-state concentration after hemofiltration. The reduction of inflammatory transmitters is only temporary, because the concentrations of cytokines are restored after 24 hours.[241]

Although each method has its proponents, and some centers perform both techniques in the same children, controlled comparative studies revealed no difference in outcome between MUF and CUF.[239,242] We routinely use a balanced ultrafiltration technique for all cases on CPB because it removes fluids, cytokines, and reduces lactate, which can aggravate reperfusion injury.[243]

Prebypass Anesthetic Management

The objectives of the anesthetic management of children before bypass include maintenance of normal sinus rhythm and ventricular function and avoidance of extreme increases in heart rate, ventricular contractility, and pulmonary vascular resistance (PVR). Special attention should be given to maintaining adequate coronary perfusion. Methods for accomplishing these objectives are lesion-specific and may include the maintenance of PVR with controlled hypoventilation and delivery of a low fraction of inspired oxygen to avoid pulmonary overcirculation, diastolic runoff, and coronary hypoperfusion in patients with a large left-to-right shunt (truncus arteriosus, aortopulmonary window, large patent ductus arteriosus, central shunt). Vasoactive and inotropic infusions and temporary snaring of the pulmonary artery may be required to achieve these goals. The duration of the prebypass period varies greatly, particularly in children who have had previous surgery, and maintaining hemodynamic stability for prolonged periods of time can be challenging. Adequate anesthetic depth should be ensured to avoid increases in sympathetic stimulation and hypercyanotic spells, and temperature homeostasis should be maintained to avoid cardiac arrhythmias, especially when the duration of the pre-CPB surgical dissection is protracted. For children undergoing repeat sternotomy, blood products with an appropriate-capacity blood warmer should be readily at hand.

Neonates and children who have been receiving total parenteral nutrition preoperatively require frequent monitoring of glucose concentrations to avoid hypoglycemia or hyperglycemia; an infusion of 5% or 10% dextrose before CPB is common. Older children receive PlasmaLyte, a balanced electrolyte solution, at a reduced maintenance rate, allowing the administration of 5% albumin, if necessary, for volume augmentation.

The placement of purse-string sutures before cannulation, as well as the actual cannulation of the great vessels before CPB, can often precipitate arrhythmias, hypotension, and arterial desaturation, especially in small infants and children. It is common for volume replacement to be necessary during placement of the cannula; if the aortic cannula is already in place, it is our practice to coordinate the administration of fluid volume between the anesthesiologist and perfusionist while the surgeon completes cannulation. Calcium chloride (10 mg/kg) is also frequently useful to support hemodynamics at this time.

Anesthesia on Cardiopulmonary Bypass

CHANGES IN PHARMACOKINETICS

The initiation of CPB introduces additional volume to the intravascular space (hemodilution). Hemodilution and altered protein concentrations affect drug distribution and consequent plasma concentrations. Plasma protein binding,[244] hypotension, hypothermia,[245] pulsatility,[246] isolation of the lungs from the circulation, altered hepatic and renal function, ultrafiltration, and uptake of anesthetic drugs by the bypass circuit (adherence) are important factors that may affect pharmacologic responses.[247,248] Drugs in the blood exist in the free (unbound active form) or bound (inactive form bound to protein, e.g., albumin) forms and therefore may be subject to marked changes with alterations in plasma protein concentrations. CPB alters all these factors, which makes description of pharmacokinetic parameters during CPB problematic. The greatest changes occur within 5 minutes of initiation of CPB. The addition of the prime volume immediately reduces the protein concentration, and the ratio of bound-to-free drug in the circulation changes. Hemodilution occurs with marked dilution of drug concentrations, reducing the amount of drug available for interaction with the receptors. There is a transient (less than 5 minutes) reduction in drug concentration at initiation of CPB[249] and it would appear that the greatest risk for unwanted "lightening of anesthesia" is within this time frame. Additional doses of fentanyl, neuromuscular blocking drugs, and sedatives are generally administered just before or with the onset of CPB. The explanation for why unbound drug concentrations are sustained during CPB is that the volume of distribution for most anesthetic agents is large relative to the volume of the CPB prime and serves as a huge reservoir for drug after intravenous administration. A decrease in the plasma concentrations of medications as a result of hemodilution shifts drugs down their concentration gradient from tissue to plasma. Hypothermia contributes to the changes in plasma concentrations primarily by depressing enzyme function and slowing drug clearance by approximately half for every 10° reduction in temperature. When normothermia is reestablished, reperfusion of tissues might lead to washout of drug sequestered during the hypothermic CPB period. This may explain the secondary increases in plasma concentrations of opioids reported during the rewarming phase. The pH-stat management also affects the degree of ionization and protein binding of certain medications, leading to increased unbound drug. During CPB, the lungs are out of circuit and medications that are taken up by the lungs (e.g., opioids) are sequestered during CPB. These medications are released when systemic reperfusion is reestablished and concentrations transiently increase. The volume of distribution of many drugs is expanded because of the priming volume of the bypass circuit, especially with neonates and small infants, where the priming volume is often greater than the child's blood volume. Medications may be taken up by various components of the CPB circuit itself. Renal dysfunction associated with CPB reduces the clearance of drugs such as cephalosporin antibiotics, TXA, EACA, and milrinone.

CHANGES IN PHARMACODYNAMICS

The pharmacodynamic effects of anesthetic agents are affected primarily via the central nervous system, which undergoes major changes during CPB. For example, hypothermia reduces anesthetic requirements and causes a host of other effects, including decreases in receptor affinity (e.g., decreased opioid receptor affinity[250] and nicotinic acetylcholine receptor sensitivity),[251] enhanced effects of neuromuscular receptor blocking drugs at the neuromuscular junction,[252,253] and alterations in tissue blood flow that may affect the response to catecholamines.[254]

CPB also affects the degree of ionization and protein binding (hence free or unbound drug concentrations) of weak acids and bases, as well as the electrolyte balance achieved by the blood gas management strategy used during CPB. Plasma concentrations of calcium, magnesium, and potassium decrease during CPB,[255,256] and these changes may lead to muscle weakness, dysrhythmias, and digitalis toxicity. The number of receptors available for interaction with a ligand will determine the subsequent magnitude of a drug effect. A reduction in the number of cardiac receptors has been observed in congestive heart failure, and defects in receptor transduction, as well as impairment of synthesis and reuptake of norepinephrine occur.

Prolonged administration of β-adrenergic agonists has been associated with reductions of β-receptor numbers, with consequent diminished pharmacologic effect. Removal of β-adrenergic blockade may lead to β-adrenergic receptor upregulation and increased adrenergic responsiveness.[257] Changes in receptor density and function may occur very quickly and have been observed to occur during cardiac surgery. Many perfusionists, under the direction of the anesthesiologist, can also administer inhalation agents via a separate bypass mounted vaporizer. Alternatively, a propofol infusion can be administered during bypass to maintain anesthetic depth. Anesthetic requirements decrease with systemic hypothermia,[258] but as rewarming is initiated, additional anesthetic drugs, including a benzodiazepine, are added to the bypass circuit to ensure that amnesia is maintained. Further work is required to elucidate the mechanisms and clinical implications of these acute changes in receptor density and function.

Special Techniques

MANAGEMENT OF DEEP HYPOTHERMIC CIRCULATORY ARREST

In the early days of cardiac surgery and CPB, hypothermia was used to improve intracardiac surgical exposure. In 1950, Bigelow and colleagues were the first to show that hypothermia decreases the metabolic rate.[259] Since then, we have discovered other advantages of hypothermia, including decreases in the inflammatory response of CPB,[260] decreases in blood loss,[261] and myocardial[262] and neuroprotection.[263] The last effect relates primarily to the decrease in the metabolic rate (by approximately 64%) that is achieved by cooling from 37°C to 27°C. The disadvantages of DHCA include a prolongation of CPB duration and a greater tendency toward postoperative bleeding.[264] Postoperative recovery, however, is not prolonged by hypothermia.[265] The rate of wound infection is uninfluenced by hypothermic bypass.[266]

Hypothermia during cardiac surgery gained widespread acceptance only after the development of a heat exchanger that could be integrated into the CPB machine in 1959.[267] DHCA involves cooling the child's body temperature during CPB to 17°C to 18°C, stopping the bypass machine, draining the blood from the child into a venous reservoir, and removing the cannulas

from the heart. After the first reports of DHCA in the 1960s, this technique gained popularity in the 1970s and 1980s because the bloodless field it provided, thus facilitating complex intracardiac and aortic repairs in neonates and small infants,[268] as well as reducing myocardial edema. However, it soon became evident that DHCA was associated with neurologic morbidity. Choreoathetosis, seizures, coma, and hemiparesis were all noted, especially with prolonged (>60 minutes) DHCA. The incidence of these acute morbidities seemed to increase when α-stat management became the widely accepted standard. Long-term adverse neurodevelopmental outcomes have also been associated with long periods of DHCA, including abnormalities in mental development and in fine and gross motor skills.[269] The Boston Circulatory Arrest Study, in which 155 neonates undergoing the arterial switch operation from 1988 to 1992 were reviewed, was followed up to 8 years of age.[270] The CPB protocol in those years included α-stat management, routine hemodilution to a hematocrit of 20%, and the absence of an arterial filter on the CPB circuit. A DHCA time of greater than 40 minutes was associated with an increase in adverse long-term neurologic outcomes (Fig. 17.3). Although the 40-minute cutoff is now well-accepted, a number of changes have subsequently been made to bypass protocols. Results from animal

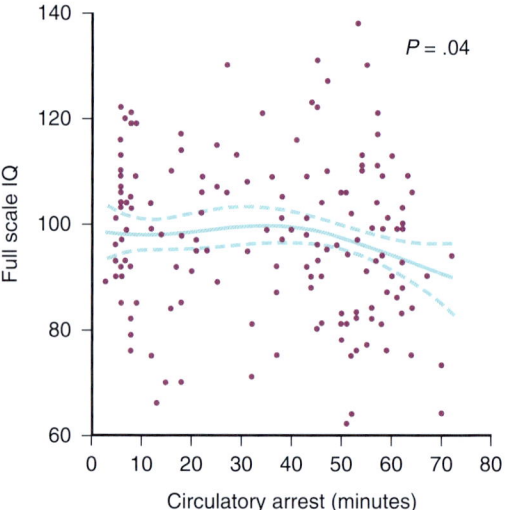

Variable	Cut-point estimate (minutes)	95% lower confidence limit (minutes)
Full-scale IQ	42	27
Verbal IQ	41	23
Performance IQ	47	31
Average achievement	43	4
Grooved pegboard	35	13
Mayo test for apraxia	40	29
Combined analysis (overall six outcomes)	41	32

FIGURE 17.3 Safe duration of circulatory arrest. From the Boston Circulatory Arrest Study, 155 8-year-olds underwent arterial switch operation for D-transposition of the great arteries as neonates. Bypass protocol used α-stat pH management, with hematocrit of 20% and temperature of 18°C. Above 40 minutes DHCA, both mental and physical performance test scores decreased significantly. (From Wypij D, Newburger JW, Rappaport LA, et al. The effect of duration of deep hypothermic circulatory arrest in infant heart surgery on late neurodevelopment: the Boston Circulatory Arrest Trial. *J Thorac Cardiovasc Surg.* 2003;126:1397-1403.)

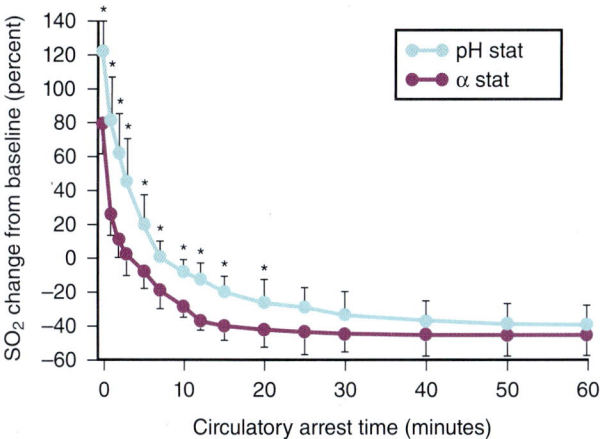

FIGURE 17.4 Cortical oxygen saturation *(SO₂)* during deep hypothermic circulatory arrest in pH-stat and α-stat groups. The cortical SO_2 half-life during arrest was significantly greater in the pH-stat than in the α-stat group. Mean ± SD, eight animals per group. *$P < 0.05$ between groups. (From Kurth CD, O'Rourke MM, O'Hara IB. Comparison of pH-stat and alpha-stat cardiopulmonary bypass on cerebral oxygenation and blood flow in relation to hypothermic circulatory arrest in piglets. *Anesthesiology.* 1998;89:110-118.)

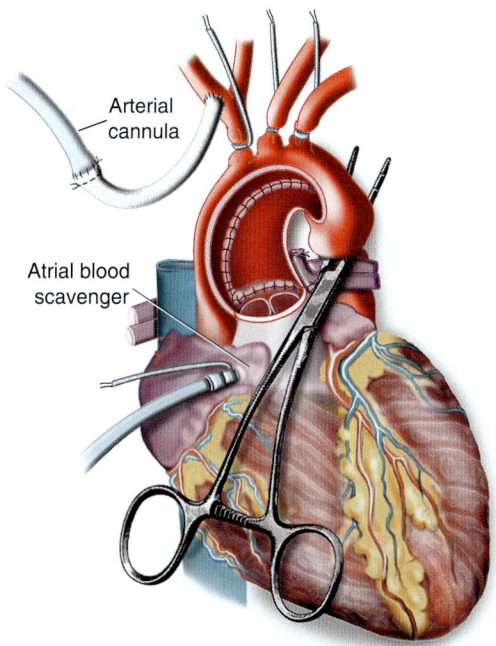

FIGURE 17.5 Selective cerebral perfusion for the Norwood stage I palliation for hypoplastic left heart syndrome. Arterial inflow for bypass is provided by a small polytetrafluoroethylene graft sewn to the right innominate artery. Instead of deep hypothermic circulatory arrest, flow is provided to the brain at low rates, while the brachiocephalic vessels and descending thoracic aorta are snared, providing a bloodless operating field. (From Pigula FA, Nemoto EM, Griffith BP, Siewers RD. Regional low-flow perfusion provides cerebral circulatory support during neonatal aortic arch reconstruction. *J Thorac Cardiovasc Surg.* 2000;119:331-339.)

experiments using a neonatal pig model of DHCA, as well as data from the Boston Circulatory Arrest Study, led to the following recommendations for increasing the child's safety margin when using DHCA:

- Hematocrit of 30% should be the target.[119]
- Systemic hypothermia should be achieved slowly, over no less than 20 minutes.[271]
- pH-stat blood gas management should be used, at least for cooling (Fig. 17.4).[179,181]
- Core body temperatures of 17°C to 18°C should be used, and ice bags should be applied to the head.[272]
- DHCA should be divided into periods of less than 20 minutes, allowing a reperfusion period of at least 2 minutes between each segment of DHCA, to improve neurologic outcome.[273]
- Low-flow CPB is better than DHCA. Selective regional cerebral perfusion may be better than full body low-flow CPB.[274]
- Normoxia should be maintained to decrease exacerbation of brain injury after DHCA.[275]

Neurologic monitoring (see discussion later in the chapter) may be useful in the individual child to aid in determining the safe duration of DHCA.[179,276]

Although there are situations in which DHCA must be used, many surgeons are avoiding it whenever possible, minimizing its duration and dividing the periods of its use, or using alternate methods, such as selective cerebral perfusion (see next section).

REGIONAL CEREBRAL PERFUSION

To avoid the use of DHCA, several novel CPB techniques have been developed. The purpose of these techniques is to allow perfusion of the brain during critical periods of surgery, such as aortic reconstruction during the Norwood operation.[277,278] These techniques are collectively referred to as selective cerebral perfusion. Regional cerebral perfusion (RCP) is one variation in which a small Gore-Tex graft of 3 to 4 mm is sewn onto the innominate artery before initiation of CPB and is then used as the aortic cannula during CPB (Fig. 17.5). During aortic reconstruction, snares are placed around the brachiocephalic vessels and CPB flow is

decreased, with only the brain receiving perfusion via the right carotid artery during this period. In this way, a bloodless operative field is achieved, just as if DHCA was being performed, yet the brain is still receiving blood flow and oxygen, theoretically increasing protection from hypoxic-ischemic brain injury. Another potential advantage of this technique occurs in neonates, who frequently have extensive arterial collaterals between the proximal branches of the aorta and the lower body via the internal mammary and long thoracic arteries. In this instance, the use of selective cerebral perfusion also provides some blood flow to the lower body, protecting renal, hepatic, and gastrointestinal systems from hypoxic damage as well.[279] This protection is, however, incomplete and RCP at 25°C is no more protective than DHCA.[280] Also, the ongoing perfusion prolongs the effective bypass time, leading to more cytokine release and capillary leakage, with worse pulmonary function, more weight gain, and decreased right ventricular function.[281]

A cohort of 57 neonates undergoing RCP for stage I palliation of hypoplastic left heart syndrome and other aortic arch reconstructions has been reported.[282] Mean RCP time was 71 ± 28 minutes and flow rate 57 ± 11 mL/kg per minute (38% of normal full CPB flow). Postoperative brain MRIs revealed no differences in patients undergoing RCP compared with standard CPB. Twelve-month neurodevelopmental outcomes assessed with the Bayley Scales of Infant Development-III revealed cognitive score of 100 ± 15, language score of 87 ± 15, and motor score of 88 ± 17. Increasing duration of RCP was not associated with adverse neurodevelopmental outcomes.

Neurologic monitoring, consisting of NIRS and transcranial Doppler measurements, was used to adjust the flow rate during RCP.[283,284] Radial arterial pressures of 30 to 40 mm Hg were maintained during RCP.[283]

Effects of Cardiopulmonary Bypass

CARDIAC EFFECTS

In addition to myocardial ischemic injury secondary to aortic cross-clamping, several other factors can contribute to perioperative myocardial dysfunction. The first is entrainment of air into the coronary arteries, which frequently occurs during weaning from bypass.[285] Despite meticulous deairing of the heart, air may enter the right coronary artery, producing ischemia that is heralded by a pale myocardium, poor contractility, and ST-segment elevation of the ECG. Should this occur, appropriate management involves remaining on CPB, increasing perfusion pressure, and "milking" the air through the coronary arteries, allowing time for recovery of the ECG and ventricular function before attempting to wean from bypass. Surgical factors, such as reimplantation of coronary arteries with possible resultant ischemia or residual surgical defects, can also occasionally contribute to myocardial dysfunction.

The inflammatory response to CPB has important implications for cardiac function.[286] This systemic response results in a capillary leak syndrome, which in turn leads to accumulation of edema fluid in interstitial and extravascular spaces, including the myocardium.[287] Myocardial edema can contribute to post-CPB myocardial dysfunction by impairing diastolic function and causing mechanical limitation of cardiac filling and outflow in small infants whose sternums have been closed. Additionally, myocardial edema has been implicated as a causative factor in the frequent decline in myocardial function that occurs 6 to 12 hours after conclusion of CPB. Inflammatory mediators also affect the responsiveness of the myocardium to catecholamines by interfering with their binding to the cell surface receptors,[288] rendering exogenously administered drugs, such as dopamine and epinephrine, as well as the child's endogenous catecholamines, less effective at augmenting cardiac function perioperatively.

Mechanisms for prevention and treatment of myocardial dysfunction include the use of ultrafiltration and antiinflammatory drugs, such as corticosteroids and aprotinin.[289,290] The prophylactic use of noncatecholamine inotropic agents, such as milrinone, has also been shown to prevent low cardiac output syndrome in infants, even if cardiac function is adequate in the immediate postoperative period.[291]

SYSTEMIC AND PULMONARY VASCULATURE EFFECTS

The inflammatory response to CPB often produces mediators that directly increase pulmonary and systemic vascular resistance. These include interleukins, leukotrienes, and endothelin.[292] Indeed, when pulmonary artery pressure is measured directly, it is often significantly increased immediately after bypass, even if surgical results are optimal. This increase can be extremely detrimental in children with large left-to-right shunts, those undergoing cardiac transplantation secondary to dilated cardiomyopathy, and those undergoing bidirectional cavopulmonary anastomosis, where right ventricular output depends on maintaining low PVR. Prevention and treatment of increases in PVR include maintaining an adequate depth of anesthesia, ventilating with 100% oxygen, and judicious use of hyperventilation. Milrinone will increase right-sided heart output via its actions as both an inotropic agent

and a pulmonary vasodilator. When PVR is increased, inhaled NO is often used to assist in the early postoperative period.[293] Although effective, its cost is not inconsequential, and because PVR almost always decreases with time, inhaled NO is generally reserved for selected cases of pulmonary hypertension. Other simpler, less expensive treatments include oral or intravenous sildenafil[294,295] and inhaled nebulized prostacyclin.[296]

PULMONARY EFFECTS

The lungs are not ventilated during CPB and are usually totally collapsed by intention, with the ventilator circuit disconnected, especially in small infants. This contributes to regional atelectasis; lung function can be improved by continuation of ventilation even on bypass.[297] The lungs are also at least partially ischemic during the bypass period, resulting in decreased production and reduced alveolar levels of surfactant.[298] In addition, reperfusion injury (pulmonary edema or hemorrhage after a sudden increase in pulmonary flow) can also occur after creation of a systemic-to-pulmonary artery shunt or pulmonary artery unifocalization. Inflammatory mediators liberated by the bypass run also predispose to increases in smooth muscle tone and resistance resulting in bronchospasm.[299]

In addition to complement, endotoxins and certain cytokines can also activate neutrophils and attract them toward sites of inflammation.[300] In animal studies, endotoxin-induced lung injury can lead to rapid (within 45 minutes) accumulation of neutrophils within lung capillaries. Activation of neutrophils, with up-regulation of adhesion molecules, neutrophil adhesion to the endothelium of lung vessels, and endothelial damage through proteases, appears to be the main step of the underlying pathophysiologic mechanism (Fig. 17.6). Macrophages play an important role in the evolution of the inflammatory acute lung injury through the secretion of cytokines, cytotoxic metabolites, and chemoattractants for leukocytes. Acute respiratory distress syndrome (ARDS) is often only one part of multiorgan failure, and lung injury should be seen as part of a more general state of systemic inflammation. The reported prevalence of ARDS after CPB in adults is 0.5% to 1.7%; the incidence in children is unknown. Interestingly, moderate hypothermia at 28°C failed to prevent the loss of adenosine triphosphate (ATP) and the accumulation of lactate in lungs.[301] Other methods that aim to protect the lungs during CPB, such as continuous lung perfusion, pneumoplegia, and inhaled NO ventilation at lung reperfusion prevent more severe hemodynamic deterioration and preserve reactivity of the pulmonary vasculature, but fail to prevent pulmonary dysfunction.

The severity of pulmonary dysfunction after CPB can be measured via changes in the alveolar-arterial oxygenation gradient, intrapulmonary shunt, degree of pulmonary edema, pulmonary compliance, and PVR. Treatment of pulmonary atelectasis includes careful reinflation of the lungs when weaning from bypass (by administering several vital capacity breaths), gentle but thorough suctioning of the tracheal tube, and prophylactic use of inhaled bronchodilators before separation from CPB. Using these measures, pulmonary function has been shown to improve immediately in most children with large left-to-right shunts, with the duration of CPB seemingly having little effect on pulmonary outcomes.[302] Thus, CPB itself has little effect on pulmonary function in most children. There is still an occasional child, however, who experiences classic "pump lung" ARDS, caused by the factors noted earlier. Treatment is supportive as for anyone with ARDS.

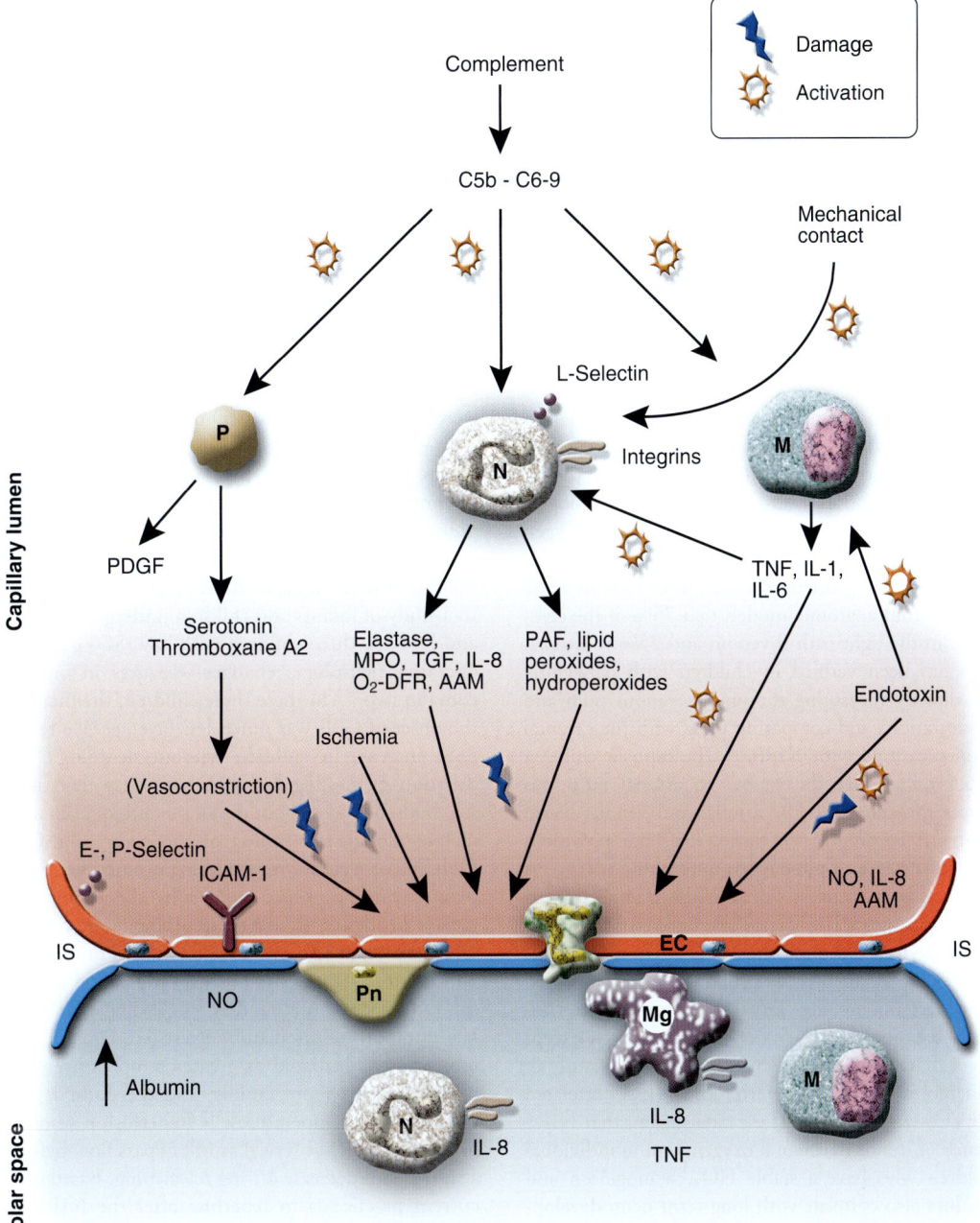

FIGURE 17.6 Leukocytes, endothelial cells *(EC)*, and humoral inflammatory mediators have been shown to play an important role in the cardiopulmonary bypass-induced lung injury. Complement *(C)* activation and complement-independent mechanical injury activates leukocytes, which, in their turn, secrete several inflammatory mediators, such as proteases and cytokines. Complement, cytokines, and ischemia-reperfusion also activate endothelial cells. Endotoxin, probably released from intestinal bacteria, exerts similar effects on leukocytes and endothelium. This process leads to disruption of endothelial and epithelial integrity and allows albumin, plasma, and activated leukocytes to enter the interstitial and alveolar space, causing tissue edema and reducing pulmonary compliance and blood oxygenation. *AAM,* Arachidonic acid metabolites; *ICAM-1,* intercellular adhesion molecule 1; *IL,* interleukin; *IS,* interstitial space; *M,* monocyte; *Mg,* macrophage; *MPO,* myeloperoxidase; *N,* neutrophil; *NO,* nitric oxide; *O_2-DFR,* oxygen-derived free radicals; *P,* platelet; *PAF,* platelet-activating factor; *PDGF,* platelet-derived growth factor; *Pn,* pneumocyte; *TGF,* tumor growth factor; *TNF,* tumor necrosis factor. (From Asimakopoulos G, Smith PL, Ratnatunga CP, Taylor KM. Lung injury and acute respiratory distress syndrome after cardiopulmonary bypass. *Ann Thorac Surg.* 1999;68(3):1107-1115.)

NEUROLOGIC MONITORING AND EFFECTS OF CARDIOPULMONARY BYPASS ON THE BRAIN

Cerebral monitoring can help to detect those children who are at risk for neurologic sequelae after bypass, promptly recognize and treat changes in cerebral blood flow/oxygenation, evaluate the effect of therapeutic interventions on cerebral physiology, optimize brain protection during the vulnerable periods of CPB, and potentially improve short- and long-term neurologic outcomes.[303] However, one must recognize that there is an increased frequency of congenital structural central nervous system (CNS) abnormalities in association with complex congenital heart disease that are present at birth in nearly half of these neonates and that cannot be reversed. Further damage can be prevented using specific management strategies during the perioperative period.[304]

The cerebral NIRS monitor measures brain tissue oxygenation (see Chapter 49). This device noninvasively measures the cerebral tissue oxygen saturation and displays a numerical value for the regional cerebral oxygen saturation (rSO_2), the ratio of oxyhemoglobin to total hemoglobin in the light path. Regional cerebral oxygen saturation is a measure of local microcirculatory oxygen supply-and-demand balance and is reported on a scale from 15% to 95%. It has been assumed from anatomic models that 75% of the cerebral blood volume in the light path is venous and 25% is arterial. This relationship has been verified in children with congenital heart disease by directly measuring the jugular venous bulb and arterial oxygen saturations and comparing these with the cerebral oxygen saturation measured with NIRS.[305] The ratio in children varied widely, but on average the venous to arterial ratio was 85:15. All devices measure both the arterial and venous blood oxygen saturations. Accordingly, this device does not provide a measure of the jugular venous bulb oxygen saturation ($SjVO_2$). A corollary of this is that maneuvers that increase arterial oxygen saturation (e.g., increasing FiO_2) increase cerebral oxygenation as measured by these devices, although the $SjVO_2$ may remain unchanged. In a study of 40 infants and children with congenital heart disease who were undergoing cardiac surgery or catheterization, NIRS correlated poorly with $SjVO_2$ measurements, except in infants younger than 1 year of age.[306] In contrast, in a study of 30 children undergoing cardiac catheterization, NIRS correlated very well with $SjVO_2$ ($r = 0.93$).[307] These data suggest that NIRS is a useful indicator of trends in cerebral oxygenation in individual infants and children who have a stable FiO_2, hemoglobin and $PaCO_2$. NIRS values also correlate with long-term neurodevelopmental outcomes in infant heart surgery. In a prospective study of 104 two-ventricle repairs, low rSO_2 in the intraoperative period did not correlate with death or major morbidity.[308] However, when these children underwent neurodevelopmental testing at 1 year of age, lower average and minimum rSO_2 in the 60-minute period immediately after CPB correlated with worse psychomotor development index scores. Low rSO_2 also correlated with remote ischemic changes on brain MRI at 1 year of age.[309]

Neurologic Monitoring for Low-Flow Hypothermic Bypass

Transcranial Doppler (TCD) ultrasonography has been used to determine the threshold of detectable cerebral perfusion during low-flow CPB. *TCD velocities reveal trends or changes in cerebral blood flow and not absolute values.* One report studied 28 neonates undergoing the arterial switch operation using α-stat blood gas management.[204] Their study suggested that NIRS and TCD may be useful to determine the minimum acceptable bypass flow rate for an individual neonate during low-flow hypothermic bypass.

Blood flow becomes insufficient at bypass flow rates less than 30 mL/kg per minute.[204,310] Inadequate blood flow to the brain during this technique could be undetected without such monitoring, and low-flow bypass may confer no advantage to the brain over DHCA in some children. Long-term outcome studies of this monitoring strategy are not available.

Neurologic Monitoring for Deep Hypothermic Circulatory Arrest

Despite clinical and experimental evidence that periods of DHCA that exceed approximately 40 minutes are associated with an increased risk of adverse long-term neurologic and developmental outcomes, this technique is still widely used in surgery to correct congenital heart defects. Recent recommendations for improving outcome after DHCA, based on both animal and clinical studies, were described previously. During DHCA, rSO_2 predictably decreases to a nadir 60% to 70% (relative change) below baseline values obtained before bypass. The nadir is reached at 10 to 20 minutes, after which there is no further decrease.[311] At this point, it appears that there is no additional oxygen uptake by the brain. Several studies suggest the potential for NIRS to determine the safe conduct and duration of DHCA in the individual child. In a study of infants and children undergoing surgery with bypass and DHCA, three children with low rSO_2 developed acute postoperative neurologic changes—seizures in one, and prolonged coma in two.[311] In these three children, the increase in rSO_2 after the onset of CPB was much less (average 3% relative increase vs. 33% increase in children without neurologic deficit) and the duration of cooling before DHCA less than in the remaining 23 children who did not develop neurologic changes. In a neonatal pig model, the timing of the nadir of rSO_2 values during DHCA correlated with neurologic outcome: a more prolonged period without oxygen uptake by the brain correlated with a greater incidence of adverse neurologic outcome. The maximum safe duration at 17°C without additional brain oxygen uptake was 30 minutes.[197] Interestingly, this time period correlates with clinical and experimental studies, suggesting that 40 minutes is the safe duration for circulatory arrest (see Fig. 17.3). When circulatory arrest is initiated at greater temperatures (e.g., 25°C), the rSO_2 decreases more rapidly, and the nadir is achieved sooner, than at lower temperatures.[312] Reperfusion results in an increase in rSO_2 to levels observed at full bypass flow before DHCA, with a subsequent decrease during rewarming. Based on these data, our current practice is to reperfuse after the NIRS nadir has been reached for a period of 20 to 25 minutes.

Neurologic Monitoring for Regional Cerebral Perfusion

Regional cerebral perfusion (RCP), also known as selective cerebral perfusion or antegrade cerebral perfusion, uses a polytetrafluoroethylene graft or a small aortic cannula as arterial inflow to the right innominate artery for neonatal aortic surgery, such as the Norwood stage 1 operation or aortic arch advancement. The other brachiocephalic vessels and descending thoracic aorta are snared, resulting in a bloodless operating field. The brain is perfused through the right innominate and right vertebral arteries only. This approach reduces or eliminates the use of DHCA for these operations and preserves brain perfusion, potentially improving neurologic outcome. Initial descriptions of this technique used the pressure in the radial artery or a predetermined bypass rate of 25 to 30 mL/kg per minute as an estimate for the bypass flow during RCP without neurologic monitoring. When flow rate was estimated on the basis of NIRS monitoring in individual children, it was determined that 20 to 25 mL/kg per minute was required.[277] However, NIRS was applied only to the right side of the skull (i.e., brain), the same side as the sole arterial inflow. Using a pH-stat blood gas strategy for RCP, we noted that the majority of our children had an rSO_2 of 95% (the maximum reading on the rSO_2 scale) when we used the left radial artery pressure of 20 to 25 mm Hg as the target for bypass flow. These children were theoretically at risk for excessive cerebral perfusion. Therefore, we performed a study using both NIRS and TCD of the right cerebral hemisphere, to determine if TCD could be used as a guide to RCP flow rate.[283] Bypass flow rate was adjusted to achieve a cerebral blood flow volume within 10% of baseline (e.g., TCD was used to determine necessary flow). The estimated flow rate, 63 mL/kg per minute (range, 24 to 94 mL/kg per minute), proved to be greater than that estimated in the earlier studies. This flow rate did not correlate with the pressure in the right or left radial artery. The rSO_2 was well maintained in all children, leading us to conclude that TCD was a useful monitor to ensure adequate but not excessive cerebral blood flow during RCP. Because RCP perfuses the brain through a single arterial inflow vessel, questions have arisen about the adequacy of cerebral blood flow and oxygenation to the left cerebral hemisphere. Although the circle of Willis is expected to be intact without stenoses in neonates, 10% of healthy full-term neonates exhibit deviations from normal flow patterns. Two studies concluded that although cerebral blood flow and oxygenation were adequate to both cerebral hemispheres in neonates during RCP, bilateral monitoring, at least of NIRS, may be warranted.[283,313]

SYSTEMIC INFLAMMATORY RESPONSE SYNDROME

The SIRS is thought to result from four main sources of injury: (1) contact of the blood components with the artificial surface of the bypass circuit, (2) ischemia-reperfusion injury, (3) endotoxemia, and (4) operative trauma. Inflammatory cytokines, together with endothelial activation and endothelial-leukocyte interactions, appear to play an important role in the induction of this systemic inflammatory response.

Exposure of blood to the artificial materials in the bypass circuit—plastics, polypropylene oxygenator fibers, and metal suction devices—initiates a cascade of inflammatory responses, including activation of the complement, kallikrein, and coagulation systems.[287] As a result, interleukins, tumor necrosis factor, endotoxin, heat shock protein, and many other inflammatory mediators are released into the circulation. Leukocyte activation also results in secretion of inflammatory mediators, such as proteases and cytokines (e.g., TNF-α and IL-1), which are secreted early in the evolution of the inflammatory process. This chemokine-mediated increased leukocyte activation constitutes an important link in the chain of the propagation of the inflammatory response (see Fig. 17.6).

This inflammatory response is counterbalanced by a complex system of inhibitors, such as IL-10 and soluble cytokine receptors.[314] Also, the inflammatory response of the neonate may be more exaggerated than that of the infant or older child,[315] justifying a more aggressive approach to its modulation in the neonate (see discussion later in chapter).

A number of novel treatments have been studied, including monoclonal antibodies for inflammatory products, such as complement, endotoxin, and tumor necrosis factor. Although theoretically attractive, no clinical difference has been noted with any of these treatments.

Effective treatments used every day in the operating room and ICU include: use of corticosteroids,[316] ultrafiltration,[289] aprotinin,[290]

leukocyte-depleted blood in prime and in-line arterial filter,[317] as well as initiation of bypass using normoxic management (FiO_2 of 21%) in severely cyanotic infants.

Corticosteroids interrupt the inflammatory response at several levels by entering cell nuclei and changing the rate of transcription of inflammatory molecules. Increasing evidence suggests that glucocorticoids act by regulating transcription or translation of antiinflammatory cytokines, such as IL-10, and altering expression of other proteins, such as endothelin-1 and inhibitor NF-κβ.[318,319] Because these processes take time to develop, the effects of corticosteroids are not immediate, taking up to several hours.[320] The common practice of adding corticosteroids to the CPB prime will not fully prevent the inflammatory response[321]; to be effective, corticosteroids may need to be administered 4 or more hours before the onset of CPB.[322]

Despite these theoretical advantages of using corticosteroids to modulate the inflammatory response the benefit is still unproven.[323] A large discharge database review of over 46,000 infants and children, in which 54% received corticosteroids, demonstrated no difference in mortality. Using propensity score matching, the authors concluded that corticosteroids were associated with greater length of hospital stay, greater rate of infection, and greater use of insulin. There was no difference in duration of ventilation. Steroids conferred no important benefit; conversely in the simpler surgery categories, there was increased morbidity with these drugs.[324] Although inflammatory activation from CPB definitely occurs, and it would seem intuitive that this would lead to worse outcomes in those patients with excessive inflammation, in contemporary practice, the correlation of the magnitude of this response and length of ICU stay and blood product administration, is statistically significant, but clinically modest, accounting for only 4% to 9% of the difference in these variables, in a large study of infants undergoing two-ventricle repairs.[325–327] Two randomized controlled trials of corticosteroid vs. placebo in neonates undergoing heart surgery will hopefully shed more light on the usefulness of corticosteroids in this setting. One study of 190 neonates found no difference in recovery following either 30 mg/kg methylprednisolone or placebo, but some benefit to those undergoing palliative procedures.[328] The STeroids to REduce Systematic Inflammation after Infant Heart Surgery (STRESS trial)[329] (clinicaltrials.gov/ct2/show/NCT03229538) concluded that prophylactic methylprednisolone did not reduce the likelihood of a worse outcome and was associated with postoperative hyperglycemia requiring insulin.

COAGULATION EFFECTS

Blood coagulation is frequently abnormal after CPB for several reasons. The risk factors identified can be summarized as follows: (1) hemodilution because of CPB, (prime, cardioplegia, and perioperative fluids), (2) activation of coagulation and fibrinolysis, (3) a consumptive coagulopathy, (4) anticoagulation using unfractionated heparin, and (5) other physiological disturbances (i.e., hypothermia, acidemia, hypocalcemia).[12] The inflammatory cascade activates the coagulation system, resulting in factor consumption and fibrinolysis, which, in turn, breaks down existing blood clots, leading to increased bleeding.[22] Treatment is adequate heparinization, reversal with protamine, and the use of an antifibrinolytic to inhibit fibrinolysis and improve platelet function.[43] In addition, the smaller the child, the greater the dilution of clotting factors by the bypass prime, and the greater the risk for low concentrations of clotting proteins and fibrinogen postoperatively. Platelets are also degranulated and consumed by the CPB circuit, leading both to low platelet counts and nonfunctioning platelets.[22]

The smaller the infant, the greater the duration of bypass, and the more complicated the surgery, the greater the incidence of coagulopathy after bypass. Efforts to minimize the postbypass coagulopathy in infants includes priming the CPB circuit with fresh whole blood for small infants, if available, or packed cells plus FFP if fresh whole blood cannot be obtained.[27,330] Treatment often involves administration of platelets to small infants as the first line of therapy, followed by the replacement of fibrinogen and FFP to replace clotting factors. If these factors are repleted and studies are normal, then surgical bleeding may be the cause and surgical reexploration may be warranted.[331] Coagulation can be monitored intraoperatively with thromboelastography (TEG), rotational thromboelastometry (ROTEM), or laboratory coagulation studies. Thromboelastography has been shown to be a cost effective monitor to decrease the amount of transfusions.[332] Factor rVIIa has also been used as a last resort in children who have significant postbypass bleeding unresponsive to standard measures.[81] Current interest exists in the use of factor concentrates

such as fibrinogen concentrate and 3- or 4-factor prothrombin complex concentrates for correction of coagulopathy in children undergoing cardiac surgery (see also Chapter 10). Fig. 17.7 presents the intraoperative coagulation monitoring and blood product and factor transfusion algorithm in use at Texas Children's Hospital.

HEPATIC, RENAL, AND GASTROINTESTINAL EFFECTS

The liver, kidneys, and gastrointestinal tract, like the brain and heart, may be rendered ischemic by prolonged CPB, DHCA, or low cardiac output syndrome. Renal function is compromised on CPB. This is manifested by the appearance of proteinuria and impaired tubular cellular function immediately after CPB. Renal dysfunction from ischemia is also common. Low urine output may occur secondary to secretion of antidiuretic hormone, a response to surgical stress. However, the latter appears to be transitory and usually resolves spontaneously.[333] The incidence of acute renal dysfunction after surgery with bypass to correct

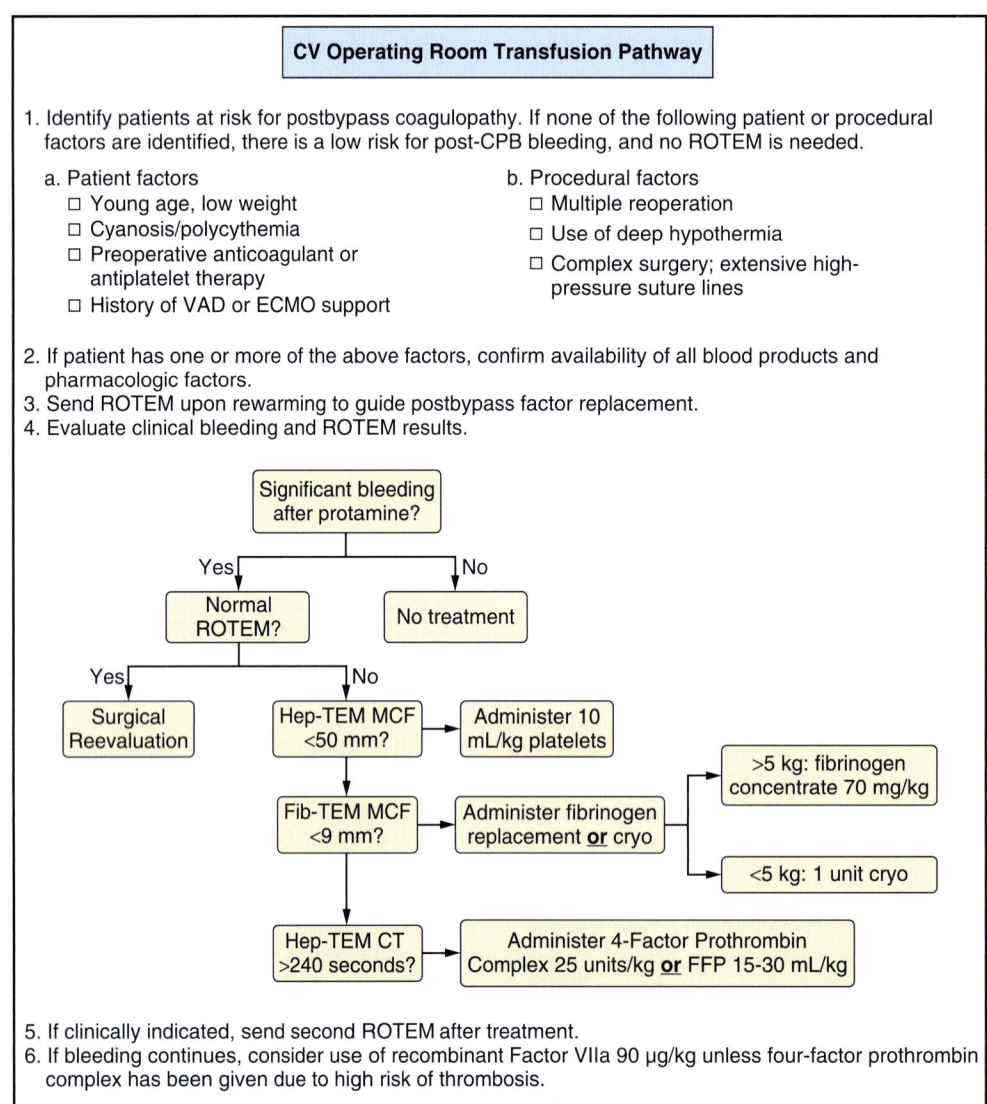

FIGURE 17.7 Texas Children's Hospital Coagulation Monitoring and Blood Product and Coagulation Factor Transfusion Algorithm. *CPB,* Cardiopulmonary bypass; *cryo,* cryoprecipitate; *ECMO,* extracorporeal membrane oxygenation; *FFP,* fresh frozen plasma; *Fib-TEM MCF,* fibrinogen-thromboelastometry maximum clot firmness; *Hep-TEM CT,* heparinase-thromboelastometry clotting time; *Hep-TEM MCF,* heparinase-thromboelastometry maximum clot firmness; *ROTEM,* rotational thromboelastometry; *VAD,* ventricular assist device.

congenital heart defects is on average 17%, ranging from 0.7% for atrial septal defect closure to 59% for arterial switch operations.[334] Deep hypothermic cardiac arrest subjects the kidney to additional ischemia-reperfusion injury.[335] Acute renal failure after CPB is uncommon in children, with fewer than 3% requiring dialysis perioperatively.[334,336] Infants who undergo cardiac surgery routinely receive diuretics or a peritoneal dialysis catheter, the latter prophylactically in some instances.[337,338] Although some have attributed the improved survival with early peritoneal dialysis to the prevention of fluid overload, others have attributed it to a more rapid clearance of CPB-induced proinflammatory cytokines.[339] Further study is required to clarify the mechanism of action of early peritoneal dialysis. In our center, neonates and children with a complex heart defect usually receive peritoneal dialysis immediately postoperatively to prevent fluid overload and decrease inflammatory cytokines. The use of aminophylline has been tested as an alternative renal rescue, but without success.[340,341]

Recovery of hepatic and gastrointestinal function follows hemodynamic recovery but may require several days. Therapy is mainly supportive. Splanchnic and renal perfusion can be monitored noninvasively using somatic oximetry. Somatic oxygenation may predict renal dysfunction and predict organ failure. Interventions based on the somatic NIRS may improve outcome.[342]

IMMUNE SYSTEM EFFECTS

Leukocytes are activated by the CPB circuit, although their numbers may be depleted by leukocyte filters, which are sometimes used to attenuate the inflammatory response. Despite the theoretical possibility that this may increase the risk of infection or neutrophil dysfunction, this has not been observed in published studies or clinical practice.[343]

ENDOCRINE SYSTEM EFFECTS

The magnitude of the inflammatory and endocrine responses after cardiac surgery depends in part on the duration of the surgical procedure and CPB.[344] In children undergoing brief operating times, postoperative blood concentrations of cortisol, adrenocorticotropic hormone, and β-endorphins are significantly greater than those in children undergoing prolonged operation times. In contrast, the serum concentrations of the proinflammatory cytokines IL-6, IL-1β, and TNF-α are similar in the two groups. Adrenocorticotropic hormone and cortisol concentrations correlated positively with the blood concentrations of IL-1β, IL-6, and TNF-α in the group of children with prolonged operation times.

The plasma concentrations of both epinephrine and cortisol increase after cardiac surgery.[345] In children, pre- and postbypass cortisol and norepinephrine increase during isoflurane anesthesia when 2 μg/kg of fentanyl is used rather than 25, 50, 100, or 150 μg/kg.[346] No noteworthy increase in the blood concentrations of these hormones occurred with any of the fentanyl doses of 25 μg/kg or greater. In addition to cardiovascular stability, continued use of larger doses of opioids during bypass minimizes the stress responses and stabilizes hemodynamics during and after bypass, but may delay recovery.[347] Also, growth hormone, glucose and insulin, lactate, glutamate, aspartate, and free fatty acid concentrations increase after cardiac surgery, whereas total triiodothyronine concentrations decrease.[348] Limiting the amount of opioids balances the negative effects of inflammation and stress with the opportunity to fast-track children's recovery after surgery for congenital heart disease.[349,350]

Transport to the Intensive Care Unit

Extreme vigilance is required during transfer of the child from the cardiac operating room to the ICU. Monitoring of ECG, arterial, venous, and atrial pressures, and end-tidal CO_2 and pulse oximetry must be maintained continuously; the battery charge of the monitor and the infusion pumps should be checked beforehand to prevent monitor failure and interruption of the infusions of vasoactive medications. Resuscitation drugs, airway equipment, and blood products should accompany the child to the ICU. Before leaving the operating room, a report should be given to the ICU staff. Children who are transported with tracheal tubes in situ are usually ventilated manually during transport with either 100% oxygen or, for those who require an FiO_2 less than 1.0, an oxygen-air blender. For children who require nitric oxide, a respiratory therapist should assist with transport to ensure that no interruptions in therapy occur and that a smooth transfer occurs in the ICU as well. On arrival in the ICU, vital signs are confirmed, all monitoring devices are transferred sequentially to the ICU monitors and rechecked to ensure they are in working order, and a detailed report is given to the ICU staff.

Fast Tracking and Recovery

Some institutions advocate continued ventilation, high-dose opioid sedation, and often paralysis during the initial postoperative care of the child with congenital heart disease. The aim is to improve outcome by minimizing the stress response to surgery and to prevent pulmonary artery hypertension. However, pulmonary hypertension can be triggered by events such as endotracheal suctioning. The potential adverse effects of prolonged mechanical ventilation also include laryngotracheal trauma, mucus plugging, accidental extubation, and ventilator-associated pneumonia. Positive pressure ventilation also reduces venous return, which can worsen hemodynamics, in particular in single ventricle physiology after stage 2 and 3 repairs,[351,352] increase PVR, and may lead to reduced pulmonary blood flow. Drugs used for sedation can also reduce myocardial function as well as prolong the time of exposure to potentially neurotoxic agents. On the other hand, early extubation reduces infusion requirements and the amount of vasopressors required to maintain adequate hemodynamics.[353,354] Extubation in the operating room after surgery was reported as early as 1980[355]; 61% of 197 patients younger than 3 years of age (including neonates) were successfully extubated in the operating room. Newer series report success rates for intraoperative extubation in 71.3% of cases and early extubation (<6 hours) in 89.4% of 613 children (including 97 neonates).[356] Norwood operations were the only procedure in which no patient was extubated within the first 24 hours. Early extubation (<24 hours) was associated with lower mortality and lower rates of reintubation compared to delayed extubation. Predictors of delayed extubation included the need for preoperative mechanical ventilation, weight <5 kilograms, longer procedure times, and the need for greater postoperative inotrope support. Immediate extubation in neonates was possible in 30% in another study.[357] Early extubation after cardiac surgery in children may result in a transient, mild to moderate respiratory acidosis that usually requires no intervention.[358] In summary, to quote from Kloth et al.,[359] *"successful early extubation of even young children is possible and easily accomplished in most children undergoing cardiopulmonary bypass, even with complex procedures, but advantages of extubation in the operating room vs. immediate ICU extubation remain unclear."*

ANNOTATED REFERENCES

Andropoulos DB, Easley RB, Brady K, et al. Neurodevelopmental outcomes after regional cerebral perfusion with neuromonitoring for neonatal aortic arch reconstruction. *Ann Thorac Surg.* 2013;95(2): 648-654; discussion 654-645.

This study reported MRI assessment and 12-month neurodevelopmental outcomes following RCP for neonatal aortic arch reconstruction. 57 infants were enrolled and RCP flows were determined by NIRS and transcranial Doppler monitoring. New postoperative MRI brain injury was observed in 40% of children. For 35 patients at 12-month follow-up, neurocognitive outcomes were at reference population normal values. Language and motor outcomes were lower than the reference population. The authors feel that this technique for monitoring RCP is effective in supporting the brain during neonatal aortic arch reconstruction.

Andropoulos DB, Fraser CD, Jr. Antithrombin levels during pediatric cardiopulmonary bypass: key to changing a decades-old paradigm for anticoagulation? *J Thorac Cardiovasc Surg.* 2016;151(2):305-306.

This was the accompanying editorial to the Manlhiot paper.

Dennhardt N, Sümpelmann R, Horke A, et al. Prevention of postoperative bleeding after complex pediatric cardiac surgery by early administration of fibrinogen, prothrombin complex and platelets: a prospective observational study. *BMC Anesthesiol.* 2020;20(1):302.

As a proof of concept, in 50 children at high risk for bleeding, coagulation factor management with thromboelastography was applied without either excessive bleeding complications or an increased risk of thrombosis.

du Plessis AJ, Jonas RA, Wypij D, et al. Perioperative effects of alpha-stat versus pH-stat strategies for deep hypothermic cardiopulmonary bypass in infants. *J Thorac Cardiovasc Surg.* 1997;114:991-1000.

In this study, 182 neonates and infants were randomized to pH-stat or α-stat CPB strategy. Important trends or statistically significant improved outcomes were seen with pH-stat management for deaths, EEG seizures, return of EEG activity, acidosis, hypotension, inotropic support, and length of mechanical ventilation. These improvements were most significant for arterial switch operation patients.

Gottlieb EA, Andropoulos DB. Current and future trends in coagulation management for congenital heart surgery. *J Thorac Cardiovasc Surg.* 2017;153(6):1511-1515.

Introduces the concept of goal-directed coagulation management in pediatric cardiac surgery. Besides thromboelastography, the combination of fibrinolysis inhibition, tight AT III monitoring and specific coagulation therapy enables the anesthesiologist to reduce bleeding complications.

Jonas RA, Wypij D, Roth SJ, et al. The influence of hemodilution on outcome after hypothermic cardiopulmonary bypass: results of a randomized trial in infants. *J Thorac Cardiovasc Surg.* 2003;126:1765-1774.

One hundred thirteen infants randomized to a target hematocrit of 20% (actual 21.5%) versus 30% (actual 28%) on CPB had lower neurodevelopmental outcome scores at 1 year of age: 82 on the Psychomotor Development Index of the Bayley Scales of Infant Development with lower hematocrit versus 90. The children with lower target hematocrit also had a greater incidence.

Manlhiot C, Gruenwald CE, Holtby HM, et al. Challenges with heparin-based anticoagulation during cardiopulmonary bypass in children: impact of low antithrombin activity. *J Thorac Cardiovasc Surg.* 2016;151(2):444-450.

The authors wished to study the impact of baseline antithrombin activity on response to heparin and thrombin generation during CPB. Detailed measurements revealed that low circulating antithrombin activity was associated with lower heparin efficacy, leading to lower ability to suppress thrombin generation during CPB. The authors suggested that determination of risk factors for heparin resistance may improve anticoagulation treatment.

Newburger JW, Jonas RA, Soul J, et al. Randomized trial of hematocrit 25% versus 35% during hypothermic cardiopulmonary bypass in infant heart surgery. *J Thorac Cardiovasc Surg.* 2008;135:347-54.

Perioperative hemodynamics during hypothermic CPB and developmental outcome and brain MRI at 1 year were evaluated. Hemodilution to hematocrit levels of 35% compared with those of 25% had no major benefits or risks overall among infants undergoing two-ventricle repair. Developmental outcomes at 1 year of age in both randomized groups were below those in the normative population.

Odegard KC, Zurakowski D, DiNardo JA, et al. Prospective longitudinal study of coagulation profiles in children with hypoplastic left heart syndrome from stage I through Fontan completion. *J Thorac Cardiovasc Surg.* 2009;137(4):934-941.

This prospective study examined coagulation profiles in patients with hypoplastic left heart syndrome from stage I palliation through completion of the Fontan. Healthy children were used as age-matched controls. Lower levels of procoagulation and anticoagulation factors were demonstrated until completion of the Fontan procedure. After the Fontan procedure there was a higher level of factor VIII. The cause of this acquired defect is unknown but the authors suggest that monitoring factor VIII levels could reveal a subset of patients at risk for thrombosis.

Pasquali SK, Li JS, He X, et al. Comparative analysis of antifibrinolytic medications in pediatric heart surgery. *J Thorac Cardiovasc Surg.* 2012;143(3):550-557.

This study examined outcomes data from 22,258 children from 25 centers and found no differences in outcome in children treated with aprotinin compared with aminocaproic acid. Tranexamic acid was associated with reduced mortality and bleeding requiring surgical intervention compared with aprotinin. The authors concluded that the use of aprotinin reduced bleeding and mortality in children undergoing heart surgery with no increase in dialysis.

Withington DE, Fontela PS, Harrington KP, Lands LC. Perioperative steroids in pediatric cardiopulmonary bypass: we still do not have all the answers. *Pediatr Crit Care Med.* 2016;17(5):475.

This editorial reviews the ongoing controversy regarding the pros and cons of prophylactic steroid administration for CPB.

Wolstencroft P, Arnold P, Anderson BJ. Dose estimation for bivalirudin during pediatric cardiopulmonary bypass. *Paediatr Anaesth.* 2021;31(6):637-643.

Anticoagulation on extracorporeal membrane oxygenation (ECMO) has shifted away from heparin-based anticoagulation to bivalirudin as an alternative. This study examines its use during pediatric CPB and provides dosing recommendations based on pharmacokinetics.

Wypij D, Jonas RA, Bellinger DC, et al. The effect of hematocrit during hypothermic cardiopulmonary bypass in infant heart surgery: results from the combined Boston hematocrit trials. *J Thorac Cardiovasc Surg.* 2008;135:355-60.

In this combined review of 271 infants, analysis was undertaken of the effects of hematocrit level at the onset of low-flow CPB. A hematocrit level at the onset of low-flow CPB of approximately 24% or higher was associated with higher psychomotor development index scores and reduced lactate concentrations.

Wypij D, Newburger JW, Rappaport LA, et al. The effect of duration of deep hypothermic circulatory arrest in infant heart surgery on late neurodevelopment: the Boston Circulatory Arrest Trial. *J Thorac Cardiovasc Surg.* 2003;126:1397-1403.

Neurodevelopmental outcomes were assessed with a battery of six tests in 155 8-year-olds who had a neonatal arterial switch operation using α-stat bypass management, hematocrit of 20% on bypass, and varying duration of DHCA at 18°C. Neurodevelopmental outcomes were not adversely affected for the group as a whole until the DHCA time exceeded 41 minutes (95% lower confidence limit 32 minutes).

Yamamoto T, Wolf HG, Sinzobahamvya N, Asfour B, Hraska V, Schindler E. Prolonged activated clotting time after protamine administration does not indicate residual heparinization after cardiopulmonary bypass in pediatric open-heart surgery. *Thorac Cardiovasc Surg.* Aug 2015;63(5):397-403.

This study examined the appropriate treatment for a prolonged ACT after protamine. The ACT and blood concentrations of heparin, coagulation factors, etc. were assessed and confirmed using rotational thromboelastometry. The authors concluded that prolonged ACT after heparin neutralization by 1:1 protamine administration does not necessarily indicate residual heparin effect but rather low blood concentrations of coagulation factors.

A complete reference list can be found online at Elsevier eBooks+.

Medications for Hemostasis

PHILIP ARNOLD AND NURIA MASIP

Physiology of Coagulation
Initiation
Amplification
Propagation
Clot Inhibition
Fibrinolysis
Developmental Coagulation
Genetics of Bleeding
Coagulopathy and Major Surgery
Coagulation Tests and Role in Management of Bleeding
Human Factors in Management and
Assessment of Surgical Bleeding
Alterations in Hemostasis During Pediatric Cardiac Surgery
Routine Anticoagulation

Failure Of Hemostasis Associated With Cardiac Surgery
Thrombosis and Heart Surgery
Medications Used for Hemostasis
Blood Products
Fractionated Human Blood Products
Desmopressin
Antifibrinolytic Drugs
Dosing Of Antifibrinolytic Medications
Which Antifibrinolytic Drug for Pediatric Cardiac Surgery?
Use of Antifibrinolytic Drugs in Other Types of Major Surgery
Antifibrinolytic Medication and Trauma
Authors' Recommendations for Use of Antifibrinolytics
New Drug Development

BLEEDING IS AN INEVITABLE CONSEQUENCE of surgery and trauma. Provided the coagulation processes are normal, a meticulous hemostatic surgical technique is usually adequate to achieve hemostasis for most surgical procedures. However, if the degree of injury is more extensive, major blood loss can occur, particularly if there is a coexistent deficiency of the normal coagulation process. Since the early part of the 20th century, it has been appreciated that transfusion of fluids and human (allogeneic) blood can prevent many of the adverse effects of blood loss. Despite this, it is important to appreciate the risks and limitations of transfusion: packed red blood cells (PRBCs) will fail to correct any existing coagulopathy, and immunologic and pathophysiologic adverse effects of exogenous stored blood products may occur.

This chapter examines the specific interventions to correct coagulopathy and strategies to reduce the requirement for transfusion of blood products by encouraging hemostasis. Although similar, these objectives are not synonymous. During many types of surgery, in vitro tests may demonstrate only mild coagulation defects, and yet the use of hemostatic medications may reduce blood loss and obviate the need to transfuse PRBCs.[1,2] In the absence of these medications, bleeding itself is often unlikely to be life-threatening. Benefit to the patient arises from avoidance of transfusion. In comparison, severe coagulopathic bleeding is immediately life-threatening. Transfusion of blood products cannot be avoided and the hemostatic "medications" used are often blood products themselves.

When considering the role of medicines in achieving hemostasis, some caution is required. Aprotinin, recombinant factor VIIa (rFVIIa), and fibrinogen concentrate have all been proposed as "magic bullets" able to restore hemostasis. As experience has grown, these agents have proved to have limitations. Their value is limited to specific indications and their use does not obviate the

need for attention to basic principles. In many respects, the management of severe bleeding has not greatly changed in recent years. Newer approaches continue to emerge, although at the time of writing, robust evidence of their risks and benefits for children is not available. Optimal management of severe bleeding requires:

- Good surgical hemostasis
- Adequate preparation, including availability of blood products and the means to administer them
- Targeting of coagulation defects that are either likely (given the clinical context) or have been identified by appropriate coagulation tests
- Avoidance (and recognition) of hypothermia, acidosis, and electrolyte disturbance

Patient blood management describes a package of measures aimed at reducing exposure to allogenic blood, in the belief that this will improve patient outcomes. The "three pillars" of patient blood management are: correction of anemia prior to surgery, minimizing perioperative blood loss, and defining thresholds for transfusion of red blood cells. It is sensible that when one measure is taken to reduce transfusion, other methods are also considered and employed. Use of medications to reduce blood loss, without considering preoperative treatment of anemia or defining thresholds for red cell transfusion, is likely to be less effective. Patient blood management in children has been recently reviewed.[3,4]

To justify these approaches, it is useful to consider why transfusion of allogenic blood may be undesirable. Many common ideas about the potential harm of transfusion are mistaken. An audit of the Serious Hazards of Transfusion (SHOT) organization in the United Kingdom reported 3239 adverse events over a 10-year period; this is only 0.013% of all blood transfusions.[5] These adverse events were more common in infants, but were reported in only 0.037% of infants who had transfusions. The true incidence of events is likely to be higher because of underreporting, although many of these "events" were procedural errors not associated with actual harm. The risk of immediate harm directly attributable to transfusion is exceptionally low. In localities with well-organized blood transfusion services and low incidence of blood borne disease, the risk of direct transmission of infection is particularly small. The risk of transmission of HIV from transfusion of blood in the United Kingdom is 1 in 5 million.[5] The greatest hazard of immediate harm is transfusion of incompatible blood and can be minimized with good attention to detail.[6] Subtle negative effects of transfusion on children's outcomes may be more important.[7]

Transfusion of blood may lead to deterioration in pulmonary function and immunologic effects that predispose children to infection. In addition, if the objective of transfused red cells is to boost tissue oxygenation by improving oxygen-carrying capacity, then transfused blood is less effective than the child's own blood for this purpose.[8] In adult patients there is a consensus that techniques of patient blood management are effective in reducing exposure to blood products; however, there are conflicting data on the effect on mortality or other important complications. A network meta-analysis of studies of adults undergoing major surgery demonstrated that although patient blood management interventions were effective at reducing exposure to transfusion, there was no associated reduction in 30-day mortality.[9] Additional considerations include the increasing costs of transfused blood products, the logistical difficulties of maintaining a secure blood supply (in both well-resourced and less well-developed health systems), substantially greater risks of transfusion in poorly developed health systems, and the possibility of new, unrecognized, infective agents entering the blood supply.

There are 2.3 million transfusions each year (37 per 1000 population) in the United Kingdom; 4.2% are given to children younger than 18 years of age (7.1 per 1000) and 1.7% to infants less than 1 year of age (52 per 1000). An audit of pediatric blood transfusion from Australia revealed 41% of blood transfused was given perioperatively,[10] and blood was transfused during 6.3% instances of anesthesia. Most units were used during heart surgery (58% of perioperative use), whereas a very small minority (4%) was used during major trauma surgery. Heart surgery (on and off cardiopulmonary bypass), craniosynostosis surgery, and liver transplantation were all commonly associated with blood transfusion. The epidemiology of major bleeding is less certain. Reports of blood use may be misleading: for example, neonates undergoing cardiac surgery may receive few blood units despite considerable bleeding; pump prime, blood scavenging, and hemofiltration may be adequate to maintain hemoglobin. Observational studies have reported very heavy blood loss associated with heart surgery in children, with increased (per kilogram) blood loss in smaller children and more complex procedures.[11,12] Cardiac surgery can probably be considered the main cause of major blood loss in children and accounts for most severe bleeding events in children younger than 1 year.

Physiology of Coagulation

The understanding of coagulation has shifted greatly in the last 2 decades.[13] The "traditional" model, which emphasizes the importance of a cascade of proteolytic enzymes, has given way to the "cell-based" model of coagulation that emphasizes the importance of cellular elements and presents coagulation as a complex web of interactions rather than a linear process.[13–15] Although this model has helped to explain a number of clinical aspects of coagulation, the complexity of the model can be confusing and

abstract compared with the decisions made in clinical care. Attempts have been made to apply this understanding more clearly to the management of bleeding[16]; this model can be used to generate useful hypotheses and explanations of the efficacy of different approaches. Evidence gained from experience and research in real patients can be added to such coagulation models to improve the model or investigate individual situations.[15,17–20] An understanding of the "modern" model of coagulation is useful and will be discussed in some detail below.

To achieve effective hemostasis, a platelet plug must form at the site of vessel injury. To prevent widespread thrombosis, this process needs to remain localized to the injured site. This is achieved through changes at the cell surface and localization of the procoagulant reactions on the surfaces of specific cells. Different cells possess different procoagulant and anticoagulant properties; these are incompletely understood, but platelets and cells bearing tissue factor (TF) are central to the process. Endothelium is vital to inhibition of coagulation, both by forming a physical barrier between components of the coagulation system (principally preventing activated factor VII and platelets from contacting collagen and tissue-factor–bearing cells) and by playing a more active role in the expression of inhibitory proteins such as thrombomodulin (TM). The phases of coagulation are often described as initiation, amplification, and propagation,[13] although in reality there is considerable overlap.

INITIATION

Coagulation is initiated by an interaction between circulating factor VIIa and TF (a membrane-bound lipoprotein expressed on subendothelial cells such as fibroblasts). A complex is formed between TF and factor VIIa (TF/VIIa, also known as "extrinsic tenase"), which activates factors IX and X. Factor Xa, in association with cofactor Va, also forms "prothrombinase" complexes on the surface of the TF-bearing cell, which activates a small amount of thrombin (factor IIa)[13] (Fig. 18.1), leading to activation of platelets and factors V and VIII.

This low level of thrombin production occurs constantly and is not sufficient to initiate widespread clot formation. Inhibitors, such as tissue factor pathway inhibitor (TFPI) and antithrombin (AT), provide a localizing function on factor Xa by inhibiting any factor Xa that becomes dissociated from the TF-bearing cell.

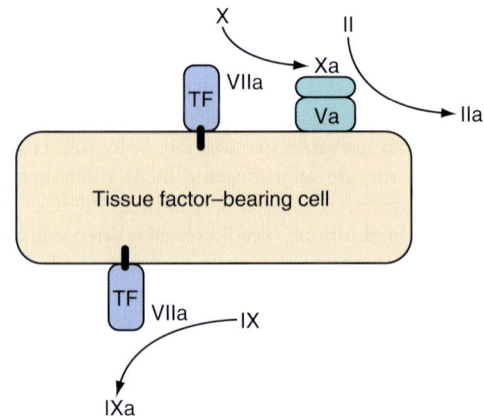

FIGURE 18.1 Initiation. The tissue factor (TF)/VIIa complex (also known as "extrinsic tenase") on the TF-bearing cell activates factors IX and X. The factor Xa/Va complex, known as the "prothrombinase" complex, forms small amounts of thrombin (factor IIa). (Reproduced from Hoffman M. Remodeling the blood coagulation cascade. *J Thromb Thrombolysis.* 2003;16:17-20.)

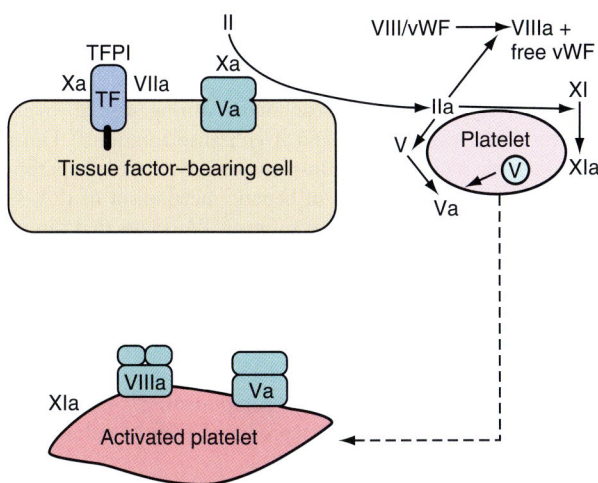

FIGURE 18.2 Amplification. Small amounts of thrombin (factor IIa) set the stage for large-scale generation of thrombin in the propagation phase. Platelets are activated along with other important coagulation enzymes and cofactors. *TF*, Tissue factor; *TFPI*, tissue factor pathway inhibitor; *vWF*, von Willebrand factor. (Reproduced from Hoffman M. Remodeling the blood coagulation cascade. *J Thromb Thrombolysis.* 2003;16:17-20.)

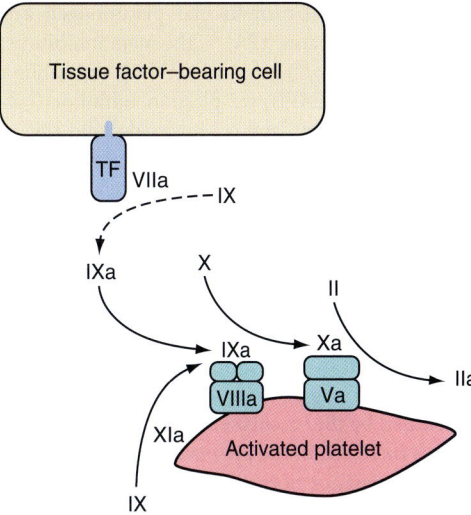

FIGURE 18.3 Propagation. Factor Xa is formed locally by the VIIIa/IXa complex (also known as "intrinsic tenase") on the surface of the activated platelet. A large amount of Xa/Va "prothrombinase" complexes will be formed, due to the large number of platelets recruited, causing a burst of thrombin (factor IIa) generation. *TF,* Tissue factor. (Reproduced from Hoffman M. Remodeling the blood coagulation cascade. *J Thromb Thrombolysis.* 2003;16-20.)

AMPLIFICATION

More extensive damage to the vasculature allows greater interaction between TF and factor VIIa and contact between platelets and extravascular components (including collagen and von Willebrand factor [vWF]).[14]

Small quantities of thrombin are generated on the TF-bearing cells. This sets up the subsequent propagation phase, during which thrombin is generated in larger quantities (Fig. 18.2). This thrombin has several functions:

- Activation of platelets, exposing receptors and binding sites for clotting factors
- Activation of cofactors V and VIII on the activated platelet surface, thereby releasing vWF to mediate additional adhesion and aggregation at the injury site
- Activation of factor XI to XIa[21]
- Activation of factor XIII (fibrin-stabilizing factor) and promotion of fibrin cross-linking
- Cleaving fibrinopeptides A and B from fibrinogen (forming fibrin)

The concept of platelet activation is important. Circulating platelets are discoid in shape. Upon activation, they change shape dramatically into spread and spiky cells to increase their surface area, increase expression of a variety of receptors and binding proteins, and release a series of chemicals (including clotting factors and platelet activators). These complex intracellular changes are central to normal coagulation and alterations in this process are central to the coagulopathy seen during surgery and major bleeding.[22,23] Once formed into a clot, the platelets will undergo a further change, fully spreading out to form a physical (platelet) plug.

PROPAGATION

Propagation occurs on the surface of activated platelets that are recruited to the site in large numbers. Activated factor IX (from both initiation phase and provided by factor XI on the surface of activated platelets) binds to factor VIIIa. The resultant VIIIa/IXa complex (also known as "intrinsic tenase") activates factor X on the platelet surface. Factor Xa then associates with factor Va and forms a large amount of "prothrombinase" complexes due to the large number of platelets recruited. These "prothrombinase" complexes cause a "burst" of thrombin generation to cause clotting via fibrinogen (Fig. 18.3).[14] An inability to form the VIIIa/IXa complex, and therefore this sustained burst in thrombin production, explains the bleeding tendency of children with hemophilia A (low levels of factor VIII).[14]

Traditional models of coagulation have also described an alternative pathway initiated by contact factors (XII, XI, prekallikrein, and high-molecular-weight kininogen [HMWK]). This pathway is of no physiologic importance in terms of coagulation activation; however, it provides important acceleration loops through feedback activation of factors VIII, IX, and XI[24] and is important in fibrinolytic and inflammatory pathways.[25]

CLOT INHIBITION

The clot is confined to the site of injury by direct and indirect thrombin inhibitory systems. The direct system consists of AT, α_2-macroglobulin, and heparin cofactor II (HCII). AT and HCII activities are accelerated greatly in the presence of heparin.

Several indirect systems inhibit thrombin, including the protein C/protein S/thrombomodulin system and tissue factor pathway inhibitor. Thrombin binds to thrombomodulin on the surface of intact endothelial cells and can no longer cleave fibrinogen to form fibrin. The thrombomodulin/thrombin complex is neither able to activate platelets nor activate factors V and VIII. Instead, this complex activates protein C, which binds to the cofactor protein S and inactivates factors Va (on the surface of endothelial cells and platelets) and VIIIa.[14,24]

FIBRINOLYSIS

Fibrinolysis, the breakdown of fibrin into soluble degradation products, is mediated by the proteolytic enzyme, plasmin. Plasmin is formed from an inactive zymogen, plasminogen, which is produced in the liver. This process is controlled by activators and inhibitors. The principal intravascular plasminogen activator is tissue plasminogen activator (tPA).[26] The main inhibitory proteins are plasminogen activator inhibitor 1 (PAI-1), thrombin-activated fibrinolysis inhibitor (TAFI), α2-plasmin inhibitor (α2-PI; also known as α2-antiplasmin), and α2-macroglobulin (Fig. 18.4).[27]

In addition to cleaving fibrin, plasmin metabolizes a number of other proteins, including the platelet receptor for fibrinogen (glycoprotein IIb/IIIa) and fibrinogen.[28] Furthermore, plasmin accelerates its own production by metabolizing the conversion of single-chain plasminogen activators to more active two-chain versions. The action of plasmin on fibrin produces a series of degradation products, some of which convey anticoagulant properties; this effect is achieved by preventing polymerization of fibrinogen and by inhibition of platelet function.

tPA is released by the vascular endothelium of small blood vessels. Release is increased in the presence of stimuli such as trauma, endotoxins, ischemia, or normal exercise. This effect is mediated via contact activation (through the kallikrein system) and by a series of other substances, including thrombin. Once released, tPA is rapidly metabolized by the liver with a half-life of approximately 5 minutes.[29] Fibrin binds both plasminogen and tPA and greatly accelerates the conversion of plasminogen to plasmin (facilitating its own degradation, but also localizing the process to areas of clot). An alternative mechanism for plasminogen activation exists by tPA binding to receptors expressed by certain cells (endothelium, white cells, and some tumor cells); the importance of this is unclear.

Primary hyperfibrinolysis can occur during cardiac bypass, massive blood loss, trauma, and liver transplantation.[29] During the an-hepatic stage of liver transplant surgery, there is hyperfibrinolysis because of the failure of hepatic metabolism of tPA. On reperfusion of the liver, a further surge of tPA occurs that can take several hours to return to normal. In coagulopathic patients, reduced thrombin formation may lead to reduced production of TAFI (important in inhibition of membrane-bound plasmin), whereas conversion of single- to two-strand tPA by plasmin may further sustain the process. Individual susceptibility is likely to be important and may have a genetic component.[30,31] Inhibition of fibrinolysis in these situations can produce beneficial reductions in blood loss.

Excessive fibrinolysis can also directly result from excess production of fibrin, as in disseminated intravascular coagulation. This is termed secondary hyperfibrinolysis and, in this context, the fibrinolysis is considered beneficial because it prevents widespread vascular occlusion. Therapy is directed at replacement of consumed clotting factors, inhibition of excessive coagulation, and treatment of the underlying cause. Inhibition of secondary fibrinolysis with antifibrinolytics is considered harmful.

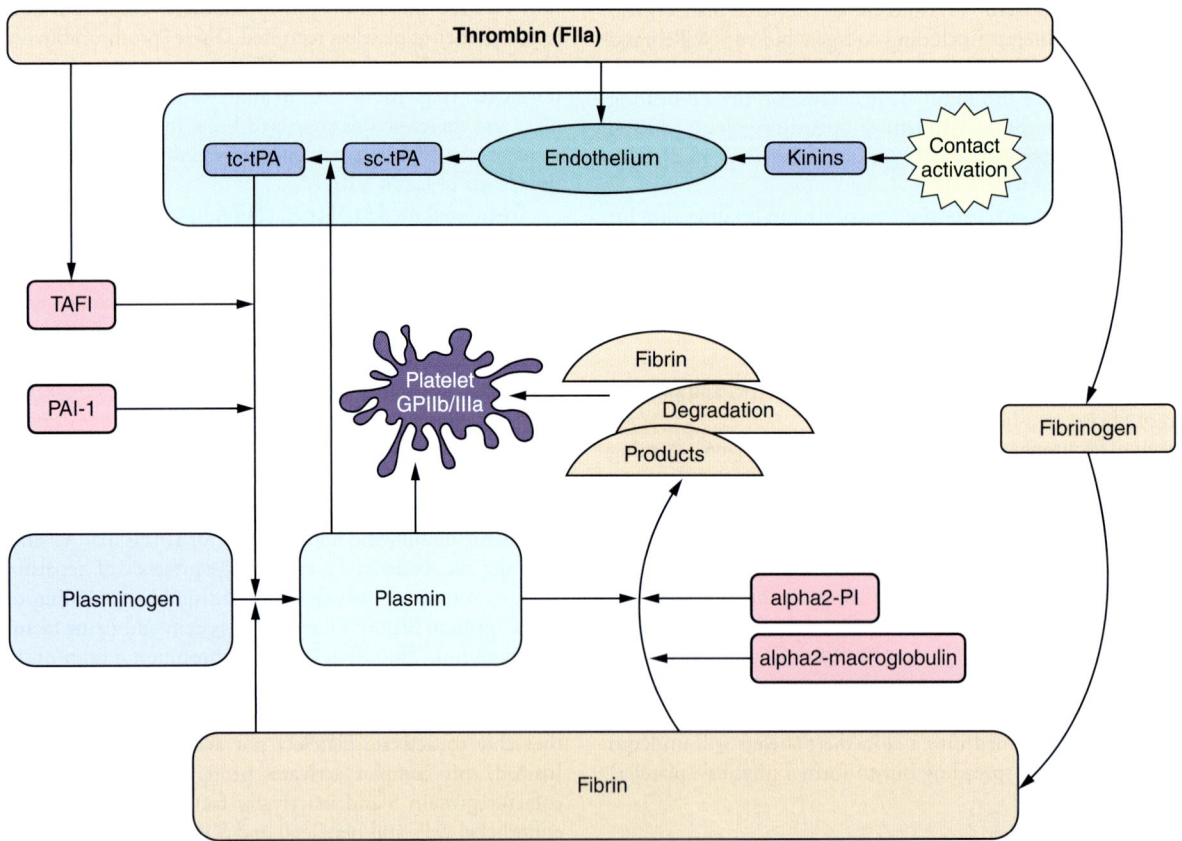

FIGURE 18.4 The main fibrinolytic pathway, leading to the breakdown of fibrin into fibrin degradation products (FDP). It is initiated by release of tissue plasminogen activator *(tPA)* from endothelial cells in response to contact activation and thrombin *(top of diagram)*. Plasminogen needs to be bound to fibrin to allow conversion to plasmin. *sc-tPA* and *tc-tPA* refer to single- and (more active) two-chain tPA, respectively. Endogenous fibrinolysis inhibitors are shown in *purple boxes*. α_2-*PI*, α_2-Plasmin inhibitor; *GP*, glycoprotein; *PAI-1*, plasminogen activator inhibitor; *TAFI*, thrombin-activated fibrinogen inhibitor.

Developmental Coagulation

The hemostatic system in neonates, infants, and children differs from that of the adult (see also Chapter 8). Although it is most pronounced in neonates, in whom development is rapid, differences persist throughout childhood.[32–34] Understanding these differences is necessary to correctly interpret coagulation tests and to select appropriate interventions to manipulate hemostasis in vivo.[35–37]

All fetal coagulation factors are produced independently of the mother; fibrinogen starts to be formed as early as 5.5 weeks gestation, and blood can clot at 11 weeks. The development of micro-assay techniques in the 1980s facilitated the determination of reference ranges for the coagulation factors beginning at 19 weeks gestational age.[24,32,33] A wider range of differences have now been noted.

The concentration of vitamin K–dependent factors II, VII, IX, and X in the neonate is only 50% of adult values; this leads to a slightly prolonged prothrombin time (PT) or international normalized ratio (INR).[24] Similarly, the concentrations of contact factors HMWK, prekallikrein, and factors XI and XII are approximately 50% of adult values.[24,38] The reduced contact factors account for a disproportionally prolonged activated partial thromboplastin time (aPTT). The reduced concentration of factors at birth is probably explained by the reduced synthesis by the liver; however, concentrations increase rapidly after birth, reaching approximately 80% of adult values by 6 months of age.[24,39] Although hemorrhagic disease due to vitamin K deficiency is rare, biochemical evidence of vitamin K deficiency occurs in 3% of healthy infants. Most infants will receive intramuscular vitamin K soon after birth; however, there is potential for error or for parental hesitancy in giving consent. Additionally, exclusively breastfed infants whose mother's diet is deficient in green vegetables or vitamin K, especially in low-income countries, may also develop a coagulopathy due to vitamin K deficiency.[40–42] Prior to surgery in neonates, efforts should be made to confirm that vitamin K has been given.[43,44]

In contrast, the plasma concentrations of fibrinogen and cofactors (factors V and VIII) at birth are similar to those in adults. A "fetal" form of fibrinogen predominates in term neonates and clots formed from either fetal, or a mixture of fetal and transfused adult fibrinogen, differs in structure from those formed with adult fibrinogen.[45,46] The physiological and clinical significance of this is not known. Concentrations of vWF in the first 2 months of life are greater than those in adults,[47] whereas platelet reactivity (to exogenous activators) is reduced in the first few days of life.

The inhibitor systems of coagulation also differ from adults. At birth, plasma proteins C and S are 35% of adult values and do not reach adult values until adolescence. Neonatal concentrations of AT and HCII are 50% of adult values; they reach adult concentrations by 6 months of age. The concentration of α_2-macroglobulin, however, is increased at birth and remains increased throughout childhood. It has been postulated that this may be one of the mechanisms that protects young children from thromboembolic complications.[48] Thrombin generation in vitro is reduced in children to approximately 75% of adult values.

Despite lower plasma concentrations of many procoagulant and anticoagulant proteins, healthy fetuses, neonates, and children do not suffer excessive hemorrhage in the presence of minor challenges, nor is spontaneous thrombosis common.[49] This is consistent with the thromboelastogram (TEG) studies of healthy children younger than 2 years of age; no defects in coagulation were noted using this test compared with adults, indicating an intact hemostatic system.[50] The general picture is of a coagulation system that is in balance. This is also true of children with stable cardiovascular disease.[51] In response to more severe disease or insult, this balance is lost, making sick infants and children susceptible to hemorrhage and thrombosis.

GENETICS OF BLEEDING

The hemophilias are a group of genetic diseases that cause excessive bleeding, often in response to minor trauma. Hemophilia A and von Willebrand disease are the most common variants (see also Chapters 8 and 10), associated with low levels of factor VIII and vWF respectively. A wide range of single-gene defects, resulting in deficiencies of single clotting proteins or regulatory proteins has now been described. A further group of single-gene disorders may result in thrombophilic disorders, associated with abnormalities of inhibitory proteins.

Unexplained variations have been observed in bleeding between apparently similar patients in the absence of specific factor deficiency. The causes of these variations are likely to be multifold, according to nuances of surgical technique and subtle difference in disease process and therapy. It might appear counterintuitive that genetic factors have any role in acquired bleeding resulting from surgery. However, the genetics of most clotting proteins has now been described, and common variations within populations have been revealed for some. As an example, a common polymorphism of PAI-1 has been well described. PAI-1 is an important endogenous inhibitor of fibrinolysis, and deficiency is associated with increased bleeding.[52] The $G5/G5$ polymorphism is common (about 20% in European populations) and is associated with reduced concentrations of PAI-1. It has been linked (though not consistently) to increased bleeding and to increased benefit from use of antifibrinolytics.[30,31] Should these findings be substantiated, then PAI-1 may still be an exceptional example. In general, the influence and consequences of genetic determinants of bleeding are likely to be more subtle. In infancy, an additional factor may be the relationship between developmental and genetic factors. Many clotting proteins are present in infants as isoforms distinct from those in adults; this implies a different gene expression in the young. It is possible that understanding genetically determined variations in bleeding will increase our understanding of bleeding and allow us to guide therapy for the individual child. The practical applications of such observations remain speculative.

Coagulopathy and Major Surgery

Bleeding is an inevitable consequence of invasive surgery. Severe bleeding can be associated with derangement of coagulation, which may increase the severity of bleeding or, alternatively, may put the child at risk for thrombosis. These two adverse events are not mutually exclusive: patients who bleed more and who demonstrate coagulopathic bleeding may also be at increased risk of thrombosis.

Coagulation changes during major surgery and bleeding are complex[53] and depend on the clinical context in which bleeding occurs. Coagulation changes that occur in surgical patients have some similarities to those who present after severe trauma. However, the balance of pathophysiologic factors is likely to be very different. The factors underlying these coagulation changes include:

- *Dilution.* Components of the coagulation system are lost in shed blood. The volume of blood lost is then replaced by crystalloid, colloid, or blood products that lack these components, leading to progressively lower concentrations of these coagulation components. To some degree such changes are balanced, as the concentration of coagulation inhibitors also decreases. In addition, coagulation components may be produced or released in response to trauma, which limits the reduction in concentration. To complicate this issue, a reduction in the concentration of one component of the coagulation system may not have the same clinical effect as the same reduction of another component. As an example of this important concept, substantial decreases in the concentration of many clotting proteins will not result in severe bleeding, whereas even modest decreases in the number of platelets or the fibrinogen concentration may cause clinically noteworthy bleeding (see also Chapters 8 and 10).

- *Effect of tissue damage.* Extensive interactions occur between inflammatory and coagulation pathways. Inflammation following trauma to tissues can be linked to excess activation of fibrinolytic pathways (resulting in excess bleeding) and to activation of procoagulant pathways (resulting in increased risk of thrombosis). Damage to endothelium or disruption in endothelial function is common in inflammation.
- *Physiologic derangement associated with blood loss.* Acidosis, hypothermia, and hypocalcemia are associated with excess bleeding.[54] Hypothermia slows proteolytic enzyme activity, reduces fibrin synthesis, and reduces platelet function. These effects are largely reversible on rewarming. Acidosis markedly reduces the activity of coagulation proteins.[55] These effects are not fully reversed by correcting acidosis. Dilution and the effect of citrate (contained in many blood products) causes plasma calcium concentration to decrease. During major bleeding, the concentration of calcium ions should be closely monitored and replaced as needed. Cryoprecipitate and fresh frozen plasma (FFP) contain high concentrations of citrate and rapid administration may cause a precipitous decrease in the plasma concentration of calcium (see Figs. 10.10 and 10.11).
- *Effects of treatment.* The use of some synthetic colloids may worsen bleeding to an extent greater than might be expected by dilution. Whether differences exist in coagulation effects of different starches is controversial.[56–58] Concerns about safety of starch solutions have limited their use in adults and children.
- *Use of specific techniques during surgery.* The important effects of cardiac bypass and anticoagulation are discussed later. Liver transplant surgery (see also Chapter 29) and major trauma (see also Chapter 37) are discussed in detail elsewhere in this book.

COAGULATION TESTS AND ROLE IN MANAGEMENT OF BLEEDING

Coagulation tests can also be useful to inform choices of different agents to treat coagulopathy during bleeding. They may be helpful when there is uncertainty as to whether the primary cause of bleeding is "medical" (due to coagulopathy) or "surgical" (due to physical disruption of the vasculature); however, these conditions can often coexist. No coagulation test can, with 100% accuracy, exclude an abnormality in coagulation, and abnormal tests do not exclude a hole in a blood vessel. All coagulation tests have limitations, and their role is generally secondary to clinical assessment of bleeding: in particular, the rate of ongoing blood loss. Abnormal coagulation tests should generally not lead to treatment in the absence of clinically problematic bleeding.

Coagulation tests primarily fall into two groups:
- Laboratory tests (such as prothrombin time or Clauss fibrinogen assay)

- Point-of-care tests: will usually refer to either crude tests of global coagulation such as activated clotting time (ACT), or to viscoelastic tests (rotational thromboelastometry [ROTEM] or thromboelastography [TEG]).

Other tests, such as various devices to analyze platelet function, are largely confined to research studies or to specific uses (such as monitoring medications). Most tests aim to simulate the activation of some part of the (in vivo) coagulation process, in vitro. Laboratory tests are usually conducted under highly standardized, reproducible, and quality controlled conditions, often on plasma. Most point-of-care tests will be conducted on whole blood under less rigorous conditions. Despite this lower level of standardization, point-of-care tests may provide more clinically relevant information by providing a more global picture of coagulation in a timely way. Compared to the in vitro coagulation process, the results will be modified by the artificial method of activation in vitro and by the absence of components of coagulation, especially the endothelium.

HUMAN FACTORS IN MANAGEMENT AND ASSESSMENT OF SURGICAL BLEEDING

Human factors (team behaviors rather than clotting proteins) are important in the clinical management of major bleeding and of children undergoing heart surgery.[59–61] Communication within teams and with more remote teams (such as transfusion laboratories), the logistics of transporting blood products and samples, and avoidance of error are vital. Simulation training has often focused on such events with the aim of improving team work and communication.

Human factors will also impact on the assessment of bleeding and on decision making. During cardiac surgery, bleeding will often occur toward the end of the case when teams are tired or experience time pressures. The surgeon and anesthesiologist may have a different, and poorly communicated, understanding of the cause and effect of the bleeding.[61,62] Handover of patients from the anesthetic to intensive care teams may lead to confusion. Professionals may be inappropriately attached to secondary objectives, such as reducing blood product usage. These factors may lead to either inappropriate treatment or inappropriate withholding of potentially useful treatment. Efforts should be made to maintain good communication; later discussion can improve management of subsequent cases.[61]

Alterations in Hemostasis During Pediatric Cardiac Surgery

ROUTINE ANTICOAGULATION

Without anticoagulation, blood will rapidly form thrombi on the artificial surface of the cardiopulmonary bypass (CPB) circuit. The major mechanism for activation of the coagulation cascade during CPB is via the "extrinsic" TF pathway, which is activated as a result of surgical trauma and inflammation.[63–66] Inflammatory mediators induce expression of TF on endothelial cells and monocytes. The "intrinsic" coagulation system is also activated when factor XII is absorbed onto the surface of the CPB circuit, causing activation of complement, neutrophils, and the fibrinolytic system via kallikrein.[63] Although the intrinsic system has little role in initiating coagulation, activations of kinins will lead to increased fibrinolysis and inflammation.[25]

Heparin
Heparin remains the most effective anticoagulant used to facilitate CPB.[67] The binding of heparin to lysine sites on AT (also termed

antithrombin III) causes a conformational change in AT. This results in an increase in AT potency; the inhibition of thrombin (factor IIa) and factors IXa, Xa, XIa, and XIIa is increased by a factor of 1000.[63,68] In infants, AT concentrations are low until 3 to 6 months of age and other heparin cofactors may have greater importance. However, neonates who require surgery for congenital heart disease have unusually reduced concentrations of all major heparin cofactors, and this may be one reason for the greater concentrations of thrombin produced in these patients.[69]

Heparin therapy is most frequently guided by the ACT. The ACT is an inexpensive and rapid on-site test, in which a small sample of blood is mixed with a coagulation activator such as celite, kaolin, or diatomaceous earth. The ACT is the time to produce a stable clot, with a normal value being between 80 and 140 seconds. A value greater than 400 seconds is required for CPB.

There are limitations to the use of the ACT. Firstly, the ACT is altered by hypothermia, hemodilution, platelet activation, activation of the hemostatic system, aprotinin therapy[70,71] and in children with cyanotic congenital heart disease (especially in those with secondary erythrocytosis).[72] Accordingly, it does not accurately reflect the heparin concentrations. One study reported that the heparin concentration decreased by 50% as soon as the children went on CPB, even though the ACT doubled.[73] The decrease in the heparin concentration was attributed to hemodilution. Secondly, in the bleeding child, the ACT is unable to differentiate bleeding because of excess heparin from that of other acquired hemostatic defects.[73]

The "gold standard" for measurement of heparin concentration is the antifactor Xa assay; however, this test remains too cumbersome for bedside use.

Protamine titration is an alternative point-of-care test (Medtronic Hepcon HMS Plus, Medtronic, Minneapolis, MN). In adult patients, use of this system reduces thrombin formation.[74] Reduced bleeding and reduced thrombin generation in children, as well as reduced thrombin formation in infants, have also been demonstrated with this system.[33,75] However, the accuracy of the device has been questioned,[76] and a trial in infants was terminated early when increased bleeding and increased length of stay were demonstrated in children in whom the Hepcon device was used.[77] In that trial, Hepcon underestimated heparin concentrations, leading to excess dosing of heparin and inadequate reversal with protamine. After modification of the protocol, use of the device demonstrated reduced bleeding, length of stay, and reduced thrombin formation compared with standard treatment.[77] Agreement between protamine titration, measures of heparin concentration, and laboratory measures has been demonstrated.[78]

A common feature of the pediatric studies using the Hepcon device is increased heparin use compared with regimens based on units-per-kilogram dosing or ACT. This is consistent with other studies of traditional dosing regimens. Using common pediatric heparin regimens (300 units/kg before CPB, then 100 units/kg to keep the ACT above 450 seconds), 50% of children on CPB had low levels of heparin (<2 units/mL).[73] It is suggested that reduced heparin concentrations during CPB is one factor responsible for activation of coagulation and fibrinolysis. It is likely that widely used regimens for dosing of heparin in children lead to inadequate dosing, and that units-per-kilogram dosing fails to allow for important pharmacokinetic (PK) and pharmacodynamic (PD) differences in children.

Even effective dosing of heparin does not completely abolish the production of thrombin. Low-grade thrombin production leads to activation of the coagulation cascade, platelets, fibrinolysis, and the endothelium. Thrombin generation and activity during CPB reflects the inability of the heparin/AT complex to inactivate fibrin-bound thrombin or to inhibit thrombin-induced platelet activation.[79] Theoretically, direct thrombin inhibition may be free of these limitations. Practically, the use of the current generation of thrombin inhibitors (such as hirudin and bivalirudin) is limited because of a lack of effective monitoring, agents for reversal, and dose uncertainty. Currently few reports exist of the use of thrombin inhibitors in children, although they would be indicated when heparin use is not possible.[80–85] Attempts using pharmacokinetic modeling to provide greater clarity for dosing of bivalirudin in children have not yet been clinically validated.[86]

Adverse effects of heparin are uncommon; hypotension can result from a reduction in calcium ions or, rarely, anaphylaxis. A benign transient decrease in the platelet count can occur. Heparin-induced thrombocytopenia is a rare but life-threatening prothrombotic condition.[83,87–92]

Reversal of Anticoagulation with Protamine

Protamine is a positively charged polypeptide derived from salmon sperm. It neutralizes heparin by forming an ionic bond with heparin. The resultant complex is removed by the reticuloendothelial system. The dose given should reflect the amount of heparin to be neutralized. Commonly used dosing schemes fail to take into account the range of concentrations of heparin that occur in infants and children after a similar dose.[67,75] The initial heparin dose is often used to guide the dose of protamine; however, it is unclear how this should be modified by various factors, such as additional doses of heparin administered (to prime or during bypass), duration of bypass, ultrafiltration, or developmental coagulation differences in children.[93]

Administration of protamine has been associated with catastrophic pulmonary hypertension and hemorrhagic pulmonary edema.[94,95] It is also known that protamine can be associated with coagulation abnormalities; an increasing ACT occurs at a protamine/heparin ratio of 2.6:1, and platelet aggregation occurs with a minimal excess in protamine.[96] Although some studies of regimens to titrate protamine in adults demonstrated encouraging results in terms of reduced bleeding,[97] others failed to demonstrate differences in transfusion requirements.[98]

The clearance of protamine is greater than that of heparin, and "heparin rebound" is described when tissue-bound heparin redistributes.[67] The diagnosis of residual heparin effect or heparin rebound is challenging. The ACT is not a specific measure of excessive heparin and is also poor at detecting heparin at low concentrations (<0.5 unit/mL).[99] The aPTT and PT are similarly nonspecific and may be increased after CPB in the absence of heparin.[100] An unmodified TEG does not reliably detect low concentrations of heparin.[101] The sensitivity of these tests may be improved by performing similar tests in parallel and comparing the results, such as a reptilase time (unaffected by heparin), or by eliminating residual heparin in vitro with heparinase or protamine. Protamine titration can be used to guide the protamine dose in children; however, in infants, protocols will require modification (50% greater than the calculated dose).[77] In practice, most anesthesiologists continue to give protamine empirically, at a protamine/heparin ratio of between 1 and 1.3 to 1. The authors' current practice is to give a standard dose of protamine (4 mg/kg) regardless of heparin dose, and to give a further 2 mg/kg in the presence of continued bleeding or unusually high ACT. In the presence of continued bleeding, a TEG or ROTEM may be run both with and without heparinase to exclude residual heparin.

FAILURE OF HEMOSTASIS ASSOCIATED WITH CARDIAC SURGERY

Complex abnormalities occur in the coagulation system during cardiac surgery owing to the profound surgical insult, hypothermia, acid-base disturbance, blood transfusion, anticoagulants, and use of cardiac bypass. In addition, children and infants with congenital heart disease may have preexisting coagulation defects or be taking medications that affect coagulation before surgery. The common preoperative and intraoperative risk factors for excessive bleeding are summarized in Table 18.1.

Antiplatelet drugs such as aspirin or clopidogrel may exacerbate bleeding. The clinician must balance the risk of perioperative bleeding against the risk of drug discontinuation when deciding if, and when, to withhold the drug before surgery. The authors' current practice is to discontinue aspirin for 5 days prior to major surgery in most children, but to continue until the day prior to surgery in children with polycythemia and circulation dependent on small arterial shunts or stents. Dehydration should be avoided during preoperative fasting in these patients. Prostaglandin E_1 can inhibit platelet aggregation at clinically relevant concentrations,[102] although this effect is too subtle to detect in vitro using the TEG.[51] For elective surgery in children receiving warfarin (or other vitamin K agonist) therapy, it is often possible to stop the drug before surgery, but "bridging" the patient with heparin may be necessary. An INR of less than 1.5 is usually considered acceptable for surgery. If urgent correction of anticoagulants is required, prothrombin complex concentrates, together with vitamin K, are more effective than FFP.[103] There is less experience with reversing the effects of newer, direct acting, oral anticoagulants. This group of drugs have much shorter durations of action than warfarin. Active reversal is likely to be needed only during bleeding or to allow emergency surgery. Dabigatran can be fully and rapidly reversed with idarucizumab (a monoclonal antibody). Similarly, andexanet alfa has been approved by the FDA for reversal of rivaroxaban, edoxaban, and apixaban in adults. It is a recombinant molecule, similar to Xa, which binds drugs which target factor Xa.[104] There are very limited data on use to reverse the effect of other drugs or concerning use in children. The high price of these drugs will also limit wider use in some health care systems. In the absence of specific antagonists, prothrombin complex concentrates could be used.[105]

In children with cyanotic congenital heart disease, hemostasis is impaired because of polycythemia; poor function and low numbers of platelets; reduced factors V, VII, and VIII; and increased fibrinolysis.[51,106] The degree of derangement is related to the degree of cyanosis.[107] Preexisting coagulopathy may also occur in children with severe underlying illness or poor nutritional status.[41,42]

Despite improvements in the design and materials of equipment, CPB and associated techniques still pose a considerable challenge to the coagulation system. Children are particularly vulnerable because of their small size (relative to the size of the circuit), the complexity of many surgeries, and a lack of reserve owing to developmental differences in the coagulation system.[108] As soon as CPB is established, there is a decrease in the concentration of all hemostatic proteins, with a commensurate decrease in platelet numbers as a result of dilution.[73,109] This effect is exacerbated owing to sequestration, mechanical disruption, and adhesion to the circuit.[110] Despite anticoagulation, there will be further platelet consumption resulting from activation of coagulation (and particularly platelets) on the surface of the bypass circuit and the contact of blood with the pericardium or air (and returned via pump suction). Further, it is likely that substances that interfere with coagulation accumulate during bypass (e.g., degradation products of fibrin and activators of fibrinolysis). The risk of greater coagulopathy (and of severe bleeding) is increased by more complex surgery, longer bypass, use of deep hypothermic circulatory arrest, and in smaller patients.[12,111,112]

A further feature of coagulopathy after heart surgery is platelet dysfunction.[22,23,73,113] As described previously, platelets exert many functions initiated by a range of different activators. Assessing this function in vitro can be difficult. Studies have used "multiplate platelet aggregometry" to access platelet function.[114–116] Platelet adhesion to an electrode is detected in response to specific agonists, with different agonists chosen to detect different pathways within the platelet. When assessing the effect of drugs used to inhibit individual pathways, the application of this is logical and relatively straightforward. It is less clear how this relates to a "global" measure of platelet function during coagulopathy. In a study conducted in children after heart surgery, three of these measures do appear to alter in tandem, suggesting a global change in platelet function. Recovery is observed at 24 hours, despite persistence of thrombocytopenia, with early signs of recovery seen by the time the patient is admitted to the intensive care unit.[23] The speed at which recovery to restore adequate hemostasis occurs, or whether this recovery will occur in patients during active bleeding, is unclear. More widely available testing using thromboelastography demonstrated an inconsistent relationship to "platelet function" measured in this way.[22] A further study demonstrated reduced platelet function, measured by exposure of P-selectin on platelet membranes in response to agonists rather than aggregometry.[117] This did not relate to the incidence of clinical bleeding. In the period soon after bypass, it should be assumed that platelet function is abnormal, especially in the patient with active bleeding.

Thrombosis and Heart Surgery

Bleeding is usually immediately apparent. Thrombosis is often more insidious in onset and many thrombi will go unnoticed unless symptomatic or specifically looked for. Despite this, thrombus can have life-threatening consequences due to occlusion of vascular shunts[118] or cerebral vessels. Venous thrombosis may lead to emboli or complicate subsequent treatment due to loss of central blood vessels. More speculatively, smaller multiple thrombi may be

TABLE 18.1	Common Predictive Factors for Bleeding
Preoperative	**Intraoperative**
Age <1 year or weight <8 kg	Individual surgeon
High hematocrit	Complex surgery
Congestive heart failure	Low platelet count during CPB
Repeat sternotomy	Prolonged CPB
Congenital and preoperative acquired coagulopathy	Duration of hypothermia on CPB
Cyanotic congenital heart disease	Deep hypothermic cardiac arrest

CPB, Cardiopulmonary bypass.
Data from Williams GD, Bratton SL, Ramamoorthy C. Factors associated with blood loss and blood product transfusions: a multivariate analysis in children after open-heart surgery. *Anesth Analg.* 1999;89:57-64.

an unsuspected cause for poor outcomes. A large opportunistic retrospective analysis demonstrated an incidence of thrombosis after heart surgery rising from 1.7% in 2004 to 4.4% in 2012.[119] Multiple possible explanations exist for this apparent rise. The authors and others have specifically identified increased use of rFVIIa perioperatively as a risk factor.[120,121] Other risk factors include age <28 days, more complex surgery, single ventricle anatomy, and infective complications.[119,122–124] Anatomical features, technical aspects, abnormalities in coagulation and genetic factors, including specific thrombophilia syndromes, will also influence the risk of thrombosis.[124–126] Mortality and hospital stay were substantially higher in patients who experience thrombosis. Causality for this association is likely to be mixed: sicker patients will develop more thromboses and thrombosis itself is likely to be a risk for mortality or slower recovery. Attempts at treatment of established thrombosis are often unsuccessful or associated with complications.[127,128] Strategies for avoiding thromboses are unclear. Good technique in placement of vascular shunts, reducing the time vascular lines are in position, and prophylaxis use of anticoagulants may be of benefit. The degree to which the use of agents to minimize bleeding may later increase the risk of thrombosis is uncertain. Although the use of rFVIIa is associated with a very high incidence of thrombosis, it is unknown whether this is also true for other agents. Enthusiasm for more aggressive treatment of bleeding or use of "novel" approaches should be tempered. The use of newer agents should be monitored for any increased risk.

Medications Used for Hemostasis

The pathophysiology of coagulopathies and bleeding in children during surgery is complex, with a multifactorial etiology (see Table 18.2). No single blood component or drug treatment can reverse the abnormal clotting profile. Initially, an attempt should be made to identify the causes of bleeding that may be remedied by surgical interventions. In the context of cardiac surgery, the anesthesiologist should attempt to ensure adequate reversal of heparin and restore normal physiologic variables, such as body temperature, serum calcium concentrations, and acid-base balance. In the postoperative period, platelets and other blood products, such as FFP and cryoprecipitate, remain the mainstays of treatment for excessive coagulopathic bleeding.[129] Medications and blood products (see also Chapter 10) are briefly discussed here, primarily within the context of pediatric heart surgery.

BLOOD PRODUCTS

It is frequently necessary to administer blood products on a largely empirical basis; laboratory tests describe only parts of the coagulation process[51] and it often takes too long to obtain results to guide the anesthesiologist in real time. Thromboelastography is frequently used to assess clot elasticity properties and more precisely delineate the bleeding and homeostasis profile. The role of thromboelastography and thromboelastometry during pediatric heart surgery has been reviewed.[130–133] The use of treatment algorithms based on viscoelastic testing (TEG/ROTEM) can limit transfusion of blood products in adults[134–138] and children.[139] In children, it may not be appropriate to use protocols originally designed for adults; alternative approaches have been proposed.[130]

Platelets

Platelet dysfunction and thrombocytopenia are common after cardiac bypass in infants. Hence, in the presence of bleeding, transfusion of platelets is logical. Coagulation variables that relate to platelet number and function (such as TEG maximum amplitude) are corrected by infusion of platelets, and clinical experience indicates that platelet transfusion reduces bleeding. This has been confirmed in a small study of children after cardiac surgery.[50] A platelet count of less than 108,000/mm^3 has been identified as a predictor of bleeding. Clot strength measured by TEG reduces steeply at platelet counts below 120,000/mm^3. It would appear sensible to follow the common current practice by targeting a platelet count of at least 100,000/mm^3 during bleeding after heart surgery,[140] whereas higher targets should be used in severe bleeding. In the absence of bleeding, platelet transfusion is generally not indicated unless thrombocytopenia is profound.[141] It would also appear reasonable to use platelets for the initial treatment of presumed coagulopathic bleeding (in the absence of specific clotting tests).

TABLE 18.2	Causes of Excessive Bleeding After Pediatric Cardiac Surgery
Preoperative Causes	
Liver immaturity	
Congenital coagulopathy	
Poor nutrition	
Cyanotic congenital heart disease	
Drugs: prostaglandin E$_1$, aspirin, clopidogrel	
Intraoperative Causes	
Surgical insult	
Inadequate surgical hemostasis before bypass	
Inflammatory cascade, fibrinolysis, and so on	
Cardiopulmonary bypass	
Inflammatory cascade	
Ongoing fibrinolysis	
Increased vascular permeability	
Capillary damage	
Hemodilution	
Platelet reduction	
Clotting factor reduction	
Fibrinogen reduction	
Complement activation	
Platelet abnormality	
Disseminated intravascular coagulation	
Postcardiopulmonary Bypass	
Inadequate surgical hemostasis	
Acidosis	
Hypothermia	
Hypocalcemia	
Excessive blood transfusion and clotting factor dilution	
Inadequate reversal of heparin with protamine	
Excess protamine	
Inadequate reversal of heparin in transfused pump blood	

Fresh Frozen Plasma

The case for the use of FFP, either as an empirical treatment of bleeding or guided by coagulation tests, is considerably weaker than for platelets. The use of FFP in cardiac surgery is based on the observation that the concentration of clotting factors is often reduced in bleeding patients, especially in the period after bypass. The PT (with its derived measure, INR) is the most common test used to detect the presence, and gauge the severity of, clotting factor deficiency. Unfortunately, observation studies have shown that PT correlates poorly with clinical bleeding and transfusion of plasma often achieves neither measurable change in the INR nor provides a clinical benefit (particularly if the INR was only marginally raised to <1.7).[142] Despite this, FFP is frequently transfused in the absence of either bleeding or increased PT.[143] Administration to patients with longer PT values is more effective in correcting clotting test results; however, large volumes may be required[142] even in the absence of ongoing loss of clotting factors. The situation is further complicated, in that initially normal coagulation test results deteriorate during severe bleeding.

Systematic reviews of the use of FFP to treat or prevent bleeding resulting from acquired coagulopathy failed to demonstrate benefit, although the trials examined were small, used a wide range of outcomes, and were conducted in heterogeneous populations.[144,145] In a small observational study of children undergoing heart surgery, a number of patients had coagulopathic bleeding after transfusion of platelets; if these patients were then given FFP, the bleeding increased, whereas if cryoprecipitate was given, bleeding decreased.[50]

It is possible that the lack of efficacy may be related to the dose of FFP used. The dose of FFP most frequently recommended (10 to 15 mL/kg)[143,146] may be inadequate to restore factor concentrations.[142] Modeling of FFP administration in major trauma suggests that larger doses (30 to 40 mL/kg) may be required to increase or maintain factor concentrations[147]; however, administration of such a large volume is often undesirable in the absence of severe ongoing bleeding. Addition of FFP to the bypass circuit or during modified ultrafiltration may allow administration of much larger doses, but benefit appears to be confined to small infants.[148,149]

Cryoprecipitate

Not all coagulation factors are of equal importance during bleeding. Fibrinogen is present in much greater concentrations than other clotting factors, and although other factors are mainly involved in initiating or amplifying thrombin formation, fibrinogen is the substrate for the production of fibrin. Deficiencies of fibrinogen are reflected in reduced strength of clot and increased bleeding.[150] Cryoprecipitate has a fibrinogen concentration four to eight times that of FFP. However, a unit of cryoprecipitate contains less fibrinogen than a unit of FFP, and multiple cryoprecipitate units are required in larger patients. One cryoprecipitate unit for each 10 kilograms should increase the fibrinogen concentration by 0.5 to 1.0 g/L. Cryoprecipitate is also a source of vWF and factors VIII and XIII, although the clinical significance of this to prevent bleeding is unclear. Cryoprecipitate has been effective in treating bleeding resistant to platelet concentrates alone during pediatric heart surgery.[50]

FRACTIONATED HUMAN BLOOD PRODUCTS

Products such as FFP or cryoprecipitate can be considered crudely purified blood products. It is possible to produce more refined products containing greater concentrations of a single clotting protein or relatively standardized concentrates of selected proteins. Examples of these are prothrombin complex concentrates and fibrinogen concentrate. These products are human blood products produced from pooled plasma; they are presented as a powder requiring reconstitution for use. They do not require freezing or cross-matching, which simplifies their supply, storage, and administration. Risk of viral transmission should be small[151] because of sourcing of plasma from low-risk populations, pooling of plasma from many individual donors (reducing viral load resulting from a single infected donor), and pasteurization. Although the effect of pasteurization on prion infection is less certain, the risk of transmission would be expected to be similarly low. Recombinant factor concentrates (as opposed to factor concentrates of human origin) are increasingly available and avoid cross infection. One such agent, rFVIIa, is discussed later in this chapter (see also Chapter 10). Although the agents discussed in this section are used in a manner similar to traditional factor supplementation to reestablish near-physiologic concentrations, rFVIIa is used very differently to produce factor concentrations greatly in excess of "normal."

Prothrombin Complex Concentrates

Prothrombin complex concentrates (PCCs) are mixtures of coagulation proteins and inhibitors whose production depends on vitamin K. Initially developed for treatment of hemophilia B (now superseded by the development of factor IX concentrates)[152] PCCs are now most commonly used for rapid reversal of oral anticoagulants,[153] although there is increasing interest in their use to treat other forms of abnormal coagulation.[154–159]

Factor concentrations in different preparations of PCC differ and the production of PCCs is variable.[160] All PCCs contain large concentrations of factors II (PT), IX, and X. They differ in the degree of activation of the factors, the addition of heparin and coagulation inhibitors (such as AT, proteins C and S) and the concentration of factor VII. Those with reduced concentrations of factor VII are referred to as three-factor PCCs, whereas those with greater concentrations, as four-factor PCCs. These differences affect both the risks of administration (largely thrombotic risk) and efficacy. Thrombotic risk is associated with low concentrations of inhibitors, high concentration of activated factors (principally VIIa), and possibly with greater activity of prothrombin (especially when given repeatedly).[161] Three-factor PCCs are considered less effective at reversing the effects of oral anticoagulants and would be expected to also be less effective in treating other causes of abnormal coagulation; indications are therefore limited.[160,162] A clear distinction should be made between inactive and active PCCs (containing activated factor VIIa). Activated PCCs, such as factor eight inhibitor bypassing activity (FEIBA), are discussed later, under activated products.

PCCs should be regarded as the agent of choice for reversal of warfarin[103]; they should be used only when rapid reversal is required (because of bleeding or the need for urgent surgery). In other cases, discontinuation of the anticoagulant is preferred. Vitamin K should be given simultaneously, as the duration of effect of the anticoagulant will exceed that of the PCC (and repeat administration may lead to increased risk of thrombosis). Oral anticoagulants are given to patients at risk of serious complications of thrombosis. When PCCs are given, there should be a clear plan about the timing of surgery and the need for continuing anticoagulation. Dosing depends on the PCC used, on the patient's INR, and on the target INR.

The use of PCCs in cases of severe coagulopathy (not associated with oral anticoagulants) has been described. These agents have been used in some European countries. The scientific rationale is that coagulopathy can result from low concentrations of clotting proteins leading to a failure of adequate thrombin production and failure to initiate and maintain coagulation. Agents such as FFP allow the administration of these clotting proteins, but only in a dilute form (reflecting normal adult population concentrations). PCCs may help to restore thrombin production by providing (as inactive zymogens) those clotting factors most critical to coagulation (i.e., principally in restoring prothrombin concentration). This is supported by experimental research[163] and observational studies.[154–158] One study, conducted ex vivo, used plasma from children after cardiac bypass in which a three-factor PCC was more effective than rFVIIa in restoring thrombin generation.[163] European Society of Anesthesiology (ESA) guidelines on management of massive bleeding, support the use of PCCs (at a dose of 20 to 30 IU/kg) in adults.[164,165] A meta-analysis comparing FFP to PCCs in adults undergoing heart surgery concluded that PCCs are more effective, while not increasing the risk of thrombosis.[159] A review of use in children undergoing heart surgery identified anecdotal reports only.[166] A systematic review of use in neonates, with medical causes for coagulopathy and bleeding, concluded that: *"there is insufficient evidence to allow a recommendation for use of PCC in neonates and infants."*[167] The current quality evidence is poor, and there are no randomized trials in adults or children. It would be wise to confine use to management of life-threatening bleeding when there is evidence of slow initiation of clotting (a long PT or latent period on TEG) and only after failure of more established therapies. Risk of thrombosis is unclear[168]; however, the risk benefit in this situation is likely to support measures that prove effective in reducing bleeding. Risk should also be compared with other therapeutic options in this situation. The dose in this situation (especially in children) is uncertain. The author has only rarely used these agents and would use a dose of 20 to 40 units/kg.

Fibrinogen Concentrate

The importance of fibrinogen depletion in coagulopathy and bleeding has been increasingly appreciated.[169,170] It has also been recognized that traditional cutoff values for supplementation of fibrinogen during bleeding (1.0 g/L) may be too low and that further advantage can be gained from greater targets, possibly as high as 2.0 g/L. This may be difficult to achieve with traditional blood products. FFP contains only physiologic concentrations of fibrinogen and only modest increases may be achieved, whereas cryoprecipitate requires administration of product from several donors to achieve meaningful increases in fibrinogen concentration (especially in larger patients). Fibrinogen concentrates contain a greater concentration of fibrinogen.

Initial reports on the use of fibrinogen concentrate to manage bleeding were largely positive.[171,172] This was supported by two systemic reviews[173,174]; however, the variable quality of early studies was noted. Three larger randomized trials reported a lack of efficacy in the management of postpartum hemorrhage,[175] prevention of bleeding after heart surgery,[176] and management of bleeding after adult cardiac surgery.[177] In all three studies the fibrinogen concentration was within the "normal" range (>1.5 g/L) in the majority of patients. The later study (randomized evaluation of fibrinogen versus PLACEbo [REPLACE] trial)[177] is of particular note. Patients were recruited if they demonstrated clinical evidence of substantial bleeding shortly after bypass. A low fibrinogen concentration was not required for recruitment, though dosing of the drug (or placebo) was based on the FIBTEM assay (Instrumentation Laboratory, Bedford, MA). The median fibrinogen concentration at recruitment was almost 2 g/L with a narrow interquartile range. Transfusion of allogenic blood products was increased in the group receiving fibrinogen. A later post hoc analysis by the original study authors identified a number of factors they felt responsible for this negative result.[178]

Several descriptions report individual children receiving fibrinogen concentrates with apparently good effect.[179,180] Siemens et al. reported reduced postoperative drain losses with use of fibrinogen concentrate versus placebo.[181] Two trials have compared fibrinogen concentrates with cryoprecipitate in children after heart surgery.[182,183] One described reduced intraoperative transfusion in infants, while the second described similar volumes of 48-hour blood loss. Neither of these small trials reported improvement in other outcomes. The role of this agent remains uncertain and initial enthusiasm should be tempered by more recent findings.[184] Further trials that may provide a clearer picture are under way in both adults and children.[185] Current use should be confined to the treatment of established bleeding in the presence of a low fibrinogen concentration. The decision to use fibrinogen concentrates in place of cryoprecipitate is likely to be dictated by their availability in different locations, costs, and logistical factors rather than presumed efficacy or safety.

Dosing and the optimal fibrinogen concentration in the presence of bleeding of different severities, and the means by which the fibrinogen concentration is measured, remain issues for further investigation.[186] A dose of 70 mg/kg is often used; however, the evidence to support this is poor. One study[181] described the use of ROTEM Delta to define dosing to be given prior to separation from bypass; a wide variation in dose was found (51 to 218 mg/kg). This was effective in increasing fibrinogen concentration into a target range of 1.5 to 2.5 g/L. Dosing recommendations used in the authors' hospital (note the reference range for the automated ROTEM Sigma device used differs from the ROTEM Delta[187]) are shown in Table 18.3. Fibrinogen concentrate is only given after administration of protamine and clinical assessment of bleeding. The assumption is that clinical response and further ROTEM measures will be assessed after administration and the possibility of further doses anticipated.

Other Factor Concentrates

Deficiency of factor XIII during and after CPB has been described, although the importance of this finding is uncertain.[188–191] Supplementation with human or recombinant factor XIII has been demonstrated to reduce bleeding after adult heart surgery, although possibly only in the presence of factor deficiency.[190,192,193] A study in children after heart surgery (in which FFP had been added to the prime) did not demonstrate clinically significant

Table 18.3	Fibrinogen Concentrate Dosing Suggestions		
Fibrinogen g/L	FIBTEM (ROTEM Sigma) MCF	Dose of Fibrinogen mg/kg	Maximum Dose
<0.5	<3	100 mg/kg	4 g
0.5–1	3–9	70 mg/kg	2 g
>1	>9	35 mg/kg	2 g

MCF, Maximum clot firmness.

deficiency or correlation between low concentrations of factor XIII and bleeding.[194] The action of factor XIII is to catalyze the formation of cross-bridges between fibrin molecules. High concentrations of factor XIII can be administered as cryoprecipitate, human factor XIII, and recombinant factor XIII. There is insufficient evidence to support its use in acquired bleeding.

It is possible that von Willebrand Syndrome may be acquired in infants undergoing heart surgery.[195,196] The hypothesis is that high sheer stresses related to areas of turbulent blood flow contribute to coagulation abnormalities. Factor VIII/ von Willebrand complex has been given to some of these infants with this acquired syndrome along with multiple other blood products. This approach cannot currently be recommended but may be an area for future research.

Activated Agents

The factor concentrates attempt to restore normal coagulation function by returning coagulation components to near normal levels. The philosophy of using 'activated agents' is different. The objective is to produce a sharp spike in thrombin production (usually for a short period of time) to allow hemostasis to occur. This bypasses, to a degree, the mechanisms that normally control coagulation, including those that localize clot formation and prevent widespread thrombosis. For this reason, these approaches are best confined to more extreme situations, in which the presumed greater risk is justified in the face of otherwise life-threatening blood loss.

Recombinant Factor VIIa

Recombinant activated factor VII (rFVIIa) is known to be safe and effective for treatment and prevention of hemorrhage in children with hemophilia who have circulating inhibitors to replacement factors (see also Chapters 8 and 10). It is also used in patients with Glanzmann thrombasthenia refractory to platelet transfusion and in patients with factor VII deficiency. Regulatory approval has been granted in Europe and the United States for these indications.

Off-label use of this drug grew steadily and by 2011 accounted for 97% of in-hospital use in the United States.[197] This has encompassed a number of indications involving treatment or prevention of acquired bleeding or coagulopathy of varying severity.[198–211] The most common off-label indications are treatment of bleeding related to cardiovascular surgery, trauma, and intracranial bleeds. Off-label use in children was also widespread. One retrospective study recorded 3655 off-label administrations (in 39 US pediatric hospitals over a 7-year period); 46% of uses were in children admitted to a surgical specialty or to a pediatric intensive care unit and more than 20% to cardiac surgery or cardiology. Administration was most common in children younger than 1 year of age.[212] Another report from a single US hospital reported use in 148 patients over 3 years. This was approximately 7% of cardiac surgeries in children performed at that hospital.[213]

The therapeutic effects of factor rFVIIa begin at doses up to 10 times greater than physiologic concentrations of the endogenous factor. To produce a "burst" of thrombin at the site of injury, two mechanisms likely work in synergy. The TF pathway is stimulated to augment generation of factor Xa and high concentrations of rFVIIa bind directly to the surface of activated platelets, again activating factor Xa (Fig. 18.5).[214] Sufficient concentrations of substrate are needed to produce a clot. Measures should be taken to ensure adequate fibrinogen concentration and platelet numbers before giving rFVIIa. In addition, factors such as acidosis and hypothermia reduce the efficiency of rFVIIa.[215] An adequate circulating concentration of prothrombin is also required and a

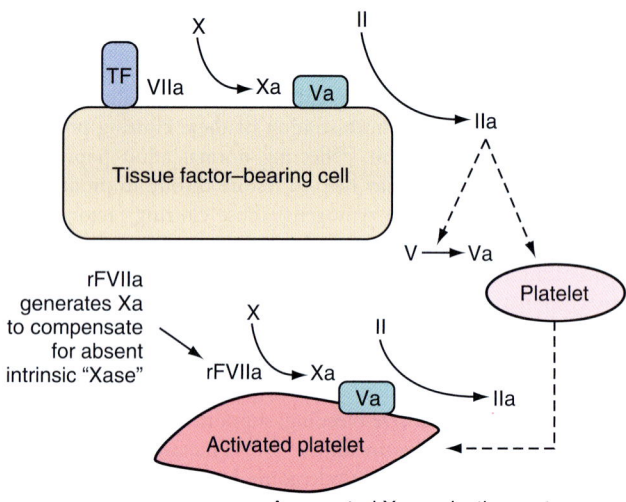

FIGURE 18.5 Schematic representation of the cell-based coagulation model and the proposed mechanism of how recombinant activated factor VII *(rFVIIa)* can potentially improve coagulation in hemophiliacs. At supraphysiologic concentrations, rFVIIa can bind to the phospholipid membranes of activated platelets, where it activates factor X independent of the tissue factor *(TF)* pathway, causing a large rise in thrombin at the platelet surface. It can therefore compensate for a lack of factor VIII or IX, a possible explanation for its effectiveness in platelet function disorders. (From Welsby IJ, Monroe DM, Lawson JH, Hoffmann M. Recombinant activated factor VIIa and the anaesthetist. *Anaesthesia.* 2005;60:1203-1212.)

synergy between administration of prothrombin concentrates and rFVIIa has been suggested. Given the expense of rFVIIa, in addition to doubts over its safety, it appears wise to use more established measures before administration.

Evidence that rFVIIa reduces bleeding comes mainly from case reports. Numerous anecdotes appear to demonstrate dramatic reductions in bleeding in apparently catastrophic situations. Demonstrations of even occasional success, in the face of an otherwise hopeless situation, might themselves be taken as a good reason to use the drug. However, rFVIIa is often used for patients at much lower risk of bleeding to death. Reported cases of off-label use in anesthesiology and surgical practice range from truly prophylactic use (in high-risk populations before evidence of severe bleeding), to use to control prolonged or severe (but not immediately life-threatening) bleeding, to compassionate use in immediately life-threatening bleeding after exhaustion of other treatments. The balance of risk and benefit will vary widely within these differing clinical scenarios.

Most controlled trials of rFVIIa have focused on prophylactic use, or use in less severe bleeding.[216–220] A meta-analysis of these trials demonstrated no reduction in mortality and only relatively modest reductions in bleeding and transfusion.[221] A study that examined adult patients with moderately severe bleeding (>200 mL/hour or >2 mL/kg for 2 consecutive hours) after heart surgery demonstrated a reduction in reexploration, bleeding, and in transfusion requirements.[218] The objective of the trial was to examine the safety of using rFVIIa. Unfortunately, the trial was terminated early, and any adverse effects result was inconclusive. The author of this study cautioned against wider use before further trials. A single randomized trial (*n* = 76) that examined prophylactic rFVIIa administration (40 µg/kg) in infants undergoing heart surgery[219] demonstrated neither efficacy nor toxicity in this group. A small trial of patients undergoing neurosurgical procedures appeared to demonstrate a dose-dependent reduction in bleeding.[222]

Risk of thrombotic complications is a concern with this drug. Propensity score-matched retrospective observational studies have been conducted in children undergoing cardiac surgery with mixed results. Downey et al. demonstrated an increased risk of thrombotic events.[223] Li and colleagues found no overall association between use of rFVIIa and thrombotic events; however, in a secondary analysis higher dose (>90 μg/kg) did increase this risk.[224] Zink et al. found no increased risk of thrombosis in neonates undergoing arterial switch operations[225]; whereas Christoff et al. concluded that in neonates who underwent surgery on bypass, the administration of rFVIIa was associated with an increased occurrence of thrombus formation.[121] In more mixed populations, two studies have systematically reviewed the data on toxicity.[226,227] In the first study, the rate of thrombosis was greater (10.2% vs. 8.7%) in those treated with rFVIIa. In the second study, data from observational trials reported that mortality was unaffected by treatment with rFVIIa, although the risk of thrombosis was increased in some groups (including adult cardiac patients). Both reviews combined data from studies on very different patient populations; caution is required in their interpretation. The risk of thrombosis in children is uncertain and data are inconclusive.[228] In a large multicenter registry, thrombotic complications occurred in 10.8% of children who received off-label rFVIIa and the overall mortality rate in those receiving rFVIIa was 34%.[212] In a further series of children receiving rFVIIa for severe bleeding, the reported rate of thrombosis was low; however, only events believed by the reporter to be directly related to use of rFVIIa or events with a fatal outcome were reported.[229] Neonates treated with either FFP or rFVIIa for similar indications had a similar incidence of thromboses (7%),[230] and administration of very large repeated doses in preterm infants did not produce thromboses.[231]

Both thrombotic complications and mortality are common in patients with bleeding serious enough to warrant use of this drug. Use of rFVIIa is likely to increase the risk of thrombosis, although the impact of this, and the benefit of the drug, vary in different clinical situations. The risk of thrombosis may be further increased in highly proinflammatory states resulting from damage to endothelium and expression of TF on circulating monocytes and platelets. For this reason, rFVIIa should be used very cautiously in patients supported by extracorporeal membrane oxygenation[228] and avoided when there is evidence of widespread activation of coagulation (disseminated intravascular coagulation). The importance of this to patients soon after separation from bypass is unknown.

A dosing regimen for off-label use of rFVIIa is not established. One of the difficulties is that there is no satisfactory laboratory test to monitor its effectiveness[232,233] and factor VII activity does not always predict efficacy.[234] Although it is known that the PT, aPTT, and TEG improve after rFVIIa during liver surgery,[235] they cannot reliably be used to determine a dosing regimen. If the main effect of rFVIIa is at the site of injury, clinical observation still remains the best indication of effect.[232] The dose used often closely relates to the dose indicated in hemophilia patients (90 μg/kg), although in practice doses are often rounded to the nearest vial.[235] Although a lower dose of 40 to 60 μg/kg has been proposed,[228] a dose of 40 μg/kg has been shown to have no effect.[219] Larger doses of 60 to 90 μg/kg may prove more effective. Differences in the pharmacokinetics may be a justification for use of larger dose in children (clearance is 67 mL/kg per hour in children vs. 37 mL/kg per hour in adults).[236,237] However, children managed with rFVIIa with hemophilia and those children undergoing heart surgery have different coagulation abnormalities. Lower

doses may retain efficacy while reducing the risk of thrombotic complications in surgical patients.

It is the authors' view that rFVIIa should be used only to treat life-threatening bleeding that has proved refractory to other treatments. Outside of properly conducted trials, it should not be used to prevent bleeding, for treatment of less severe bleeding, or as an alternative to blood products. Trials of use of rFVIIa to prevent bleeding can ethically only be justified in very high-risk populations. Its use should not delay surgical reexploration if indicated. Every attempt should be made to ensure an adequate hemoglobin concentration, platelet count, and fibrinogen concentration, as well as correction of acidosis, and near-normothermia before use.

Factor Eight Inhibitor Bypassing Activity

FEIBA is the only activated PCC generally available. Like rFVIIa, FEIBA was developed for the treatment of hemophilia in patients with inhibitory antibodies. It has been used for this indication for a considerable time.[238] It differs from rFVIIa in that it is a product of human origin, and it contains inactive prothrombin (factor II), factors IX and X, as well as factor VII, mainly its activated form. No randomized controlled trials (RCTs) have been conducted to examine the use of FEIBA during pediatric heart surgery. A very small feasibility study has been conducted in adult cardiac surgical patients and did not show a benefit.[239] There are case reports and small case series of use after heart surgery in children.[240] The presence of other factors may be attractive. As with rFVIIa, caution should be exercised in the use of this agent prior to evidence of efficacy, safety, and dosing.

Emicizumab

Emicizumab is a humanized asymmetric bispecific IgG4 antibody that mimics the function of factor VIIIa cofactor activity. It bridges activated factor IX and factor X to restore the function of missing activated factor VIII that is needed for effective hemostasis. Emicizumab has gained widespread use for prophylaxis to prevent bleeding and as a treatment option for severe bleeding in children with hemophilia.[241] Use to control severe bleeding during pediatric cardiac surgery has not yet been explored.

Reptilase

Reptilase (a batroxobin) is derived from the venom of pit vipers. It causes direct cleavage of fibrinogen leading to its polymerization. It therefore bypasses the normal coagulation pathway and is resistant to inhibitors. It is used in the laboratory test (the reptilase time). It has been used intravenously, as hemocoagulase, to promote hemostasis. A systematic review concluded that there was some evidence of efficacy but further well conducted trials were warranted.[242] Topical use to prevent pulmonary hemorrhage has been described, but use of reptilase has also been associated with serious anaphylaxis.[243] Given the nature of this agent, it would be prudent to avoid use in humans pending further evidence.

DESMOPRESSIN

Desmopressin acetate (1-desamino-8-D-arginine [DDAVP]) is a synthetic analog of vasopressin. The production of desmopressin involves alteration in the chemical structure of naturally occurring vasopressin. In the process, the antidiuretic effect is enhanced, and the vasopressor effect is virtually eliminated. Desmopressin is more resistant to enzymatic cleavage, and hence the duration of action is prolonged from 6 to 24 hours.[244] Desmopressin can cause endothelial release of factor complexes VIII/protein C and VIII/vWF. It has been used in mild hemophilia, von Willebrand disease, coagulopathy of uremia, liver failure, and in adults undergoing cardiac and spinal fusion surgery (see also Chapter 10). The maximum effect of desmopressin is observed at a dose of 0.3 µg/kg.

The most recent review in the use of desmopressin for minimizing perioperative blood transfusion, included 65 RCTs, of which 7 included only children.[245] Findings show small reductions in blood loss and in total volume of red cells transfused in cardiac surgery, but these are unlikely to be clinically important. No difference was found either in mortality or adverse events (such as thrombotic events), although event rates were very low. Subgroups of patients with platelet dysfunction or taking antiplatelet agents may gain benefit from perioperative use of desmopressin.

In children, desmopressin at 0.3 µg/kg failed to demonstrate any benefit during cardiac surgery.[246,247] Younger children are not as capable of releasing vWF from endothelial storage sites as older children, and the maximal release of vWF caused by the operative stimulus, cannot be enhanced by desmopressin.[248] Potential adverse sequelae from desmopressin include fluid retention, hyponatremia, tachyphylaxis, tachycardia, and mild hypotension.[249] Desmopressin is not currently recommended in pediatric cardiac surgery.[108,250]

ANTIFIBRINOLYTIC DRUGS

Two groups of drugs are used clinically to inhibit fibrinolysis:

1. Synthetic lysine analogs: tranexamic acid (TXA) and ε-aminocaproic acid (EACA)
2. Protease inhibitors: aprotinin

Synthetic lysine analogs are specific inhibitors of plasminogen activation, working by competitively binding to lysine-binding sites on the plasminogen molecule (Fig. 18.6). This blocks the

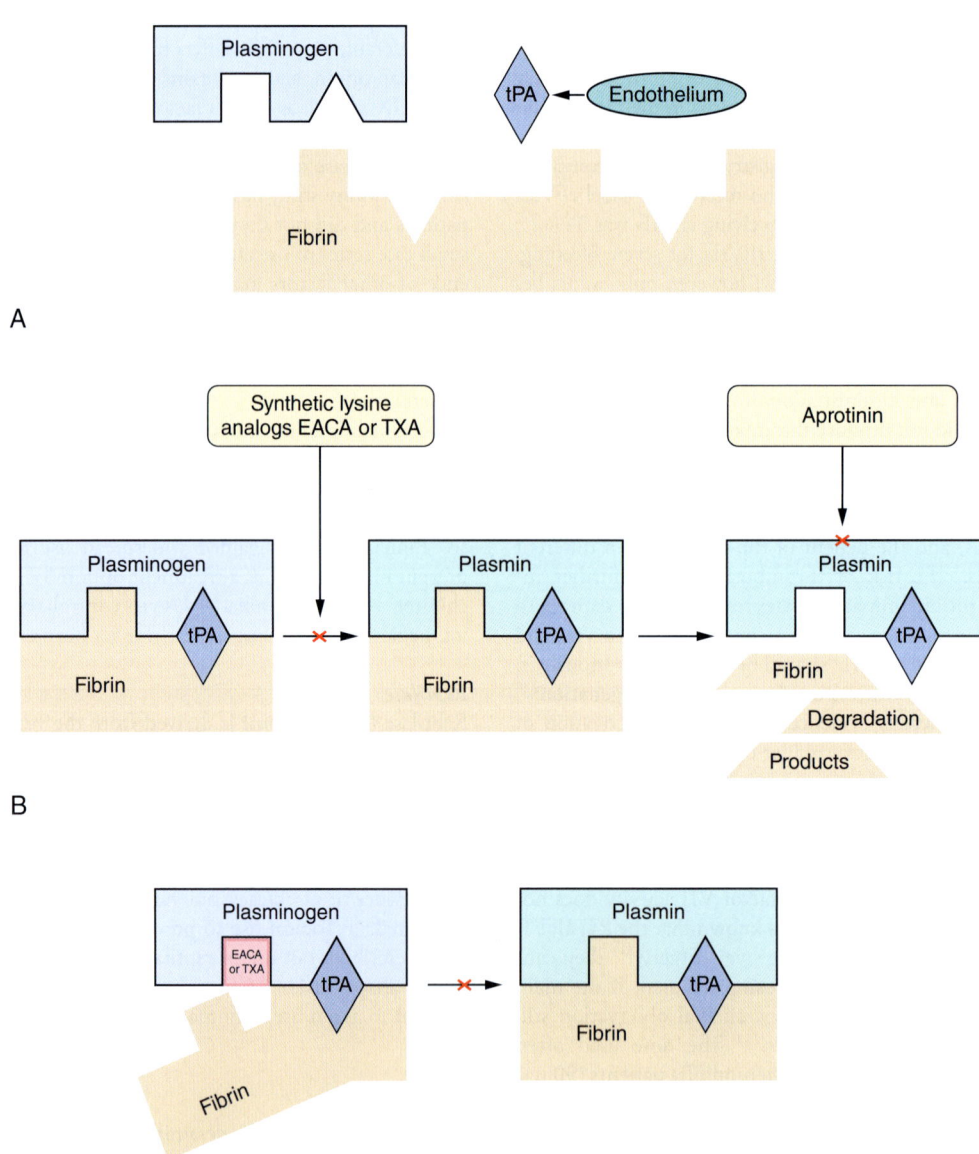

FIGURE 18.6 Activation of plasminogen and action of antifibrinolytics. **A,** Plasminogen is activated to form plasmin only after binding to fibrin. This binding requires an activator (typically t-PA[tissue plasminogen activator]). **B** and **C,** Synthetic antifibrinolytics prevent the binding of plasminogen to fibrin by blocking the binding site on the plasminogen molecule. This prevents activation of plasminogen and cleavage of fibrin. In contrast, aprotinin breaks down and inactivates plasmin.

binding of plasminogen to fibrin, a required step for the conversion of plasminogen to plasmin by plasminogen activators.[251] At larger doses, they may have additional effects through direct inhibition of plasmin; this includes inhibition of the plasmin-mediated effects on platelets.

Aprotinin (bovine-derived protein) is a less specific inhibitor of proteolytic enzymes; it has actions on the kallikrein-kinin (contact) system, as well as the enzymes involved in coagulation and fibrinolysis. In addition, aprotinin may be associated with greater preservation of platelet function, as well as an antiinflammatory effect. This wider spectrum of effects from aprotinin may have additional benefits over the antifibrinolytic lysine analogs.

Antifibrinolytic Drugs During Pediatric Heart Surgery

Fig. 18.7 summarizes the data currently available on the efficacy of antifibrinolytics during heart surgery in children to reduce postoperative blood loss.[248–267,354] Overall, almost 2000 children have been recruited into studies of these drugs. Some caution is required in the interpretation of these data. Most trials are small and trial methodology is of variable quality. The studies examine a diverse population, use variable dosages, and are statistically heterogeneous. Data from adult cardiac surgical patients are included in the figure for comparison.[252] Although these adult studies are also primarily small and of variable quality, they include almost 10,000 patients (in studies reporting postoperative blood loss) and seven trials with more than 200 participants. Given the available data on efficacy of antifibrinolytic drugs (e.g., TXA, EACA, and aprotinin) in children undergoing heart surgery and

the evidence of efficacy in different, but similar, patient populations, it is reasonable to conclude that these drugs are effective (compared with placebo) for reducing blood loss after heart surgery in children. In addition, the three drugs (TXA, EACA, and aprotinin) can all be shown to reduce blood loss individually. A recent updated meta-analysis reached similar conclusions.[253]

Efficacy is not the only consideration when choosing whether to use a drug. It should also be considered whether the reduction in blood loss is of a magnitude likely to produce a clinical benefit, whether any benefits are offset by adverse effects, how other outcomes are affected, if the drug also works in important subgroups of patients, and whether the benefits can be better realized by use of other medications. From the earlier analysis, a crude estimation of the expected reduction in bleeding in children can be made at 7.7 (3.9 to 11.6) mL/kg, whereas the mean blood loss across these studies is 28 mL/kg. This is a potentially useful reduction in blood loss. In a previous meta-analysis, the mean volume of red cell transfusion was also reduced, although only by relatively small volumes.[2] The use of these drugs has not been shown to increase the chance of avoiding transfusion completely or affect the risk of life-threatening bleeding, surgical reexploration, or mortality in children. In adults undergoing heart surgery, exposure to transfused blood and surgical reexploration is reduced, although the impact on mortality is unclear.

Children undergoing heart surgery are heterogeneous. Efficacy may be affected by the presence of chronic hypoxemia and polycythemia (owing to excessive fibrinolysis in cyanotic patients) or might differ in neonates as opposed to older children (owing to

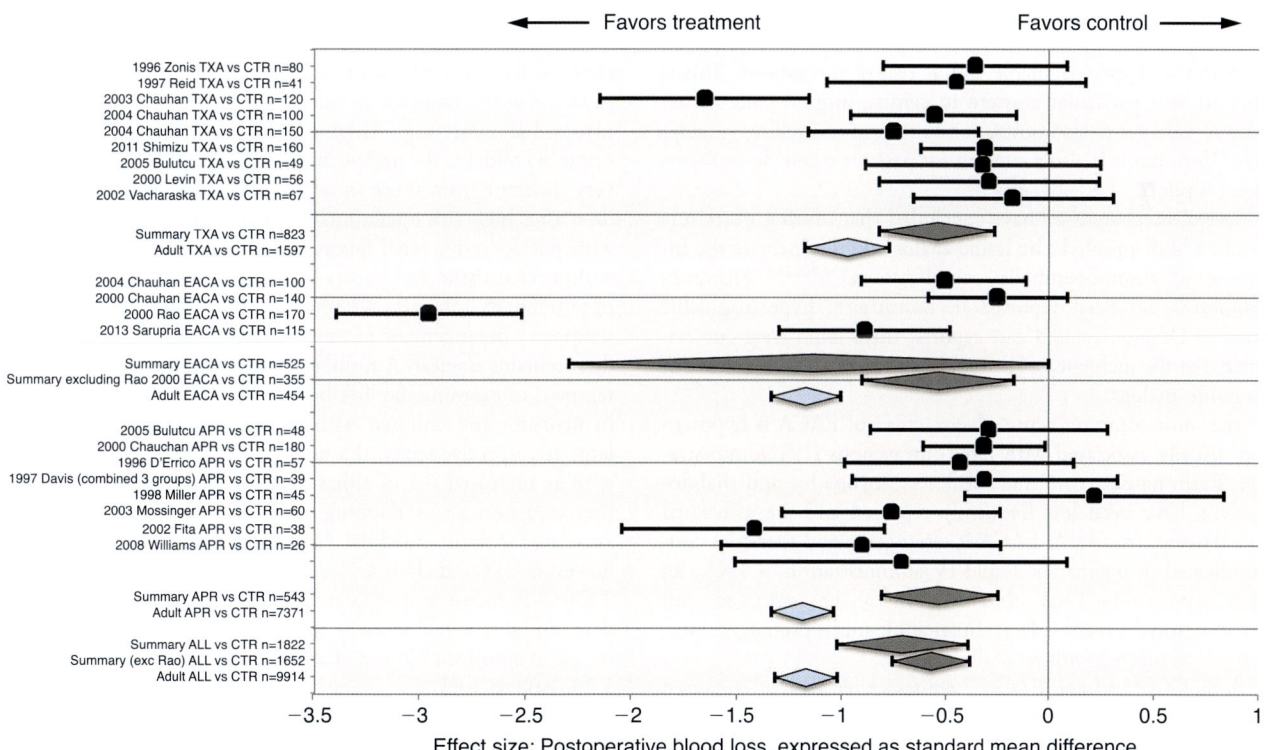

FIGURE 18.7 Efficacy of antifibrinolytic medications in reducing postoperative blood loss compared with control. Results of studies are shown as a standardized mean difference (the size of the treatment effect divided by the standard deviation of the outcome); the outcome used is expressed as milliliters per kilogram over the first 24 postoperative hours. Standardized mean difference is given to allow studies with similar but different outcome measures to be included and to allow a comparison with adult studies. The effect size expressed in this way is generally smaller than that seen in adults, indicating that other causes for variation in bleeding have a greater impact. All three drugs perform better than control.[252,254–260,262,263,300,319,348,349,352–358] *APR,* Aprotinin; *EACA,* ε-aminocaproic acid; *TXA,* tranexamic acid.

developmental differences in the coagulation system). Studies of synthetic antifibrinolytic drugs have been undertaken mainly in children with cyanotic heart disease and most studies originate from a single institution undertaking late correction of cyanotic heart disease.[254–258] From studies of TXA, data on 6-hour blood loss were available for 143 children who were not cyanotic, and a significant reduction in bleeding was not demonstrated (mean reduction 1.8 mL/kg, 95% confidence interval [CI] of −0.8 to 4.5 mL/kg).[259,260]

The fibrinolytic system of neonates differs from that of older children. Plasminogen concentrations are about 50% of adult values, and plasminogen activation occurs more slowly, whereas levels of inhibitor (PAI-1) are normal.[34] Reduced concentrations of TXA are required to inhibit fibrinolysis in cord blood.[261] Deficiency of substrate (fibrinogen and platelets) may be a greater risk factor for bleeding in neonatal patients than fibrinolysis,[150] implying that the relative benefits of antifibrinolytic medications may be less. Among studies of synthetic antifibrinolytics, only one recruited infants younger than 2 months of age[259] and it is not possible to identify any effect specific to this group of patients. In a study of the use of aprotinin in children undergoing arterial switch procedures, reduced blood loss, exposure to allogeneic blood products, and reexploration were demonstrated.[262] A further randomized trial of aprotinin in neonates was terminated early because of the concerns about reported toxicity in adults and did not show any advantage in indexes of bleeding or postoperative recovery.[263]

Adverse Effects of Synthetic Lysine Analogs

As with any drug used to promote hemostasis, there is concern as to the risk of thrombosis. After any major surgery or trauma, patients can be hypercoagulable and at risk of thrombosis. This is likely to be a particular concern in cardiac surgical patients because of vascular anastomoses, conduits, and indwelling vascular lines. Thrombosis is also a concern for patients receiving extracorporeal support.

Several meta-analyses have concluded that, during heart surgery in adults, prophylactic lysine analogs do not increase the incidence of thromboembolic complications.[252,264,265] However, thrombosis has been reported in nonsurgical hypercoagulable states.[266] Despite isolated case reports, there is no clear-cut evidence that the incidence of thrombosis is increased with either of the lysine analogs.

The most common acute adverse effect of EACA is hypotension, usually associated with rapid intravenous (IV) administration. Rash, nausea, vomiting, weakness, myopathy, and rhabdomyolysis have been less frequently reported and are associated with longer-term use.[244] EACA is teratogenic and therefore contraindicated in pregnancy. Rapid IV administration of TXA can cause hypotension. Oral administration can be associated with gastrointestinal adverse effects. In an adult study, prolonged infusion was associated with renal dysfunction.[267]

Both TXA[268–271] and EACA[272] are associated with an increased risk of seizures in a dose-dependent fashion. Possible mechanisms have been reviewed.[269,273] TXA crosses the blood-brain barrier[274] and causes seizures when applied directly to the brain of animals. The most probable mechanism is antagonism of inhibitory glycine receptors.[269] A similar effect can be observed with EACA at equivalent concentrations.[269] This effect is inhibited by general anesthetic agents including propofol and inhalational agents, but not by sedatives commonly used during intensive care. A recent large randomized trial in adults undergoing coronary surgery demonstrated an

increase in the incidence of seizures in those treated with TXA compared with placebo (0.7% vs. 0.1%).[275] This association has also been described in children undergoing heart surgery.[276] A national survey in Japan estimated an increased risk of seizures, from 0.2% to 1.6%.[277] Cerebral spinal fluid concentrations remain lower than plasma concentrations and peaks occur later. This may indicate slow equilibrium between these tissue compartments and may be a concern with more prolonged use.

Adverse Effects of Aprotinin

Adverse effects of aprotinin in adult cardiac patients include increased risk of renal failure, serious intravascular thrombosis (myocardial infarction and stroke), and death within 5 years of surgery.[278,279] In a large randomized trial, which was stopped early due concerns of a higher mortality in the aprotinin group, this effect was not seen with synthetic antifibrinolytics.[280] Excess deaths resulted from heart failure and myocardial infarction. The relative risk of death in adults treated with aprotinin compared with those treated with synthetic antifibrinolytics was 1.53 (95% CI 1.06 to 2.22). Data on bleeding in this study were inconclusive, although they suggested a small benefit for aprotinin in preventing severe bleeding. The conclusion of these papers was that aprotinin should not be used in the patient populations studied and led to the drug being effectively unavailable in several countries. Subsequently there has been a reevaluation of the evidence regarding adult patients, and aprotinin is again available with restrictions on its use. The European Society of Anaesthesiology has attempted to clarify current indications for use of aprotinin in adults.[281]

The implication of these studies for children and young adults with congenital heart disease is uncertain. The use of aprotinin in children has reduced within the United Kingdom.[282] The main cause of death reported in adult patients was from stroke and myocardial infarction. Although thrombotic complications do occur in children, the pathogenesis and underlying risk factors are very different from those in adults. Renal failure occurs in children after high-risk operations and may share pathogenic factors with postoperative renal failure in adults; aprotinin accumulates within renal tissue and affects local autoregulation of blood flow in response to ischemia. Whether aprotinin causes any more than temporary derangement of renal function tests in adults or children remains unclear. A number of retrospective studies have attempted to examine the link between aprotinin and renal failure in neonates and children with contradictory results.[283–289] In a large retrospective study, the use of aprotinin was not associated with an increased risk of either renal failure or death.[290] In a further study, on an overlapping data set, aprotinin was again not associated with increased risk (compared with no antifibrinolytic); however, risks of dialysis or death were lower in those treated with TXA.[291] A recent meta-analysis, pooling RCT and observational data, found that incidence of acute kidney injury was not altered by use of aprotinin but use of renal replacement therapy was (OR 1.29; 1.08 to 1.54).[292]

A further concern is the association between aprotinin and anaphylaxis.[293,294] The risk is small in children during primary exposure, but the risk increases with repeated exposure (estimated as 2.4%).[295] Therefore, administration of a test dose before the full dose is wise.

Secondary Benefits of Aprotinin

Although synthetic antifibrinolytics are selective inhibitors of fibrinolysis, aprotinin is a less specific inhibitor of proteolytic enzymes.[25] Proteolytic enzymes are important mediators of inflammation via contact activation and the complement system; it is postulated that aprotinin may exert a beneficial antiinflammatory effect. A number of studies have demonstrated a reduction in inflammatory markers, although other studies have failed to corroborate this effect.[296–298] One trial demonstrated that inflammatory markers were reduced postoperatively in infants treated with aprotinin compared with infants treated with TXA.[299] Another small study in older children undergoing mainly low-complexity surgery failed to demonstrate any effect of aprotinin on a series of inflammatory markers compared with control.[297] At the same time, it is important to appreciate that broad inhibition of inflammation may not always be beneficial: inflammation is, to some degree, a part of an appropriate physiologic response to tissue injury and contact activation may provide some protection against ischemic reperfusion injury.[25] There are no convincing clinical data to show any clinical benefit from an antiinflammatory action of aprotinin.[297] A trial designed to detect a reduction in ventilation days (as a marker of organ dysfunction) in neonates was terminated by the FDA before an adequate number of patients had been recruited to identify a significant effect.[263]

DOSING OF ANTIFIBRINOLYTIC MEDICATIONS

Both the beneficial and adverse effects of these drugs will depend on their doses. It is desirable that the dose is optimized to ensure a balance between these effects. This will require a knowledge of the pharmacokinetics of the drugs, and the relationship the plasma concentration has with effect and toxicity. Regimens based on a single dose have performed less well than those based on infusions or repeated intermittent dosing.[254,300] A reasonable approach is to aim to maintain effective concentrations of the drugs throughout surgery, and such regimens are best informed by pharmacokinetic studies.[301–307]

Experiments conducted in vitro can identify the concentration required to produce the intended biochemical effect (inhibition of fibrinolysis); however, these may not be identical to the concentration required to produce the intended clinical effect in vivo. The gold standard would be properly conducted dosing studies, using a pharmacokinetic-pharmacodynamic (PKPD) design based on clinically relevant outcomes. As yet, only limited dosing studies have been conducted in children.[254,300,308,309]

Dose of Tranexamic Acid

There has been considerable uncertainty regarding the dose of TXA.[282] Two studies have addressed the TXA pharmacokinetics (PK) in children undergoing heart surgery.[304,305] In children older than 1 year of age, there is good agreement between these studies and suitably scaled adult data.[302] In younger infants and neonates, the PK could not be extrapolated from data in adults or older children, and there were maturation changes in the PK during the first year of life. Table 18.4 lists three possible dosing schedules that target low, intermediate, and high plasma concentrations. Unfortunately, these studies could not link the drug concentration to a PD effect such as inhibition of fibrinolysis or a clinical effect on blood loss. In vitro, a concentration of 20 µg/mL is sufficient to inhibit fibrinolysis and the effect of plasmin on platelets.[261,310] Lower concentrations may be adequate to inhibit fibrinolysis in neonatal plasma. However, in adult cardiac patients, regimens that targeted larger concentrations may produce an improved clinical effect.[311] A "model based meta-analysis" attempted to define a dose in adult cardiac surgical patients, which balanced risks of seizure

TABLE 18.4	Three Possible Dosing Schedules Targeting Plasma Concentrations of Tranexamic Acid in Children		
		TARGET TXA CONCENTRATION	
		Low	Intermediate	High
Age		(20 µg/mL)	(60 µg/mL)	(150 µg/mL)
0–2 months	Loading dose (mg/kg)	15	50	120
	Infusion (mg/kg per hour)	2.5	7	17
	CPB prime dose (µg/mL prime)	20	60	150
2–12 months	Loading dose (mg/kg)	9 (6–12)[a]	26 (20–30)[a]	65 (45–85)[a]
	Infusion (mg/kg per hour)	2	6	14
	CPB prime dose (µg/mL prime)	20	60	150
>12 months ≤20 kg	Loading dose (mg/kg)	4	13	31
	Infusion (mg/kg per hour)	2	5.5	14
	CPB prime dose (µg/mL prime)	20	60	150
Adults[a,b]	Loading dose (mg/kg)	8	12.5	30
	Infusion (mg/kg per hour)	4	6.5	16
	CPB prime dose (mg/kg prime)	0.6	1	2

Suggested dosing regimen for tranexamic acid during heart surgery to achieve target concentrations of 20, 60, and 150 µg/mL. A dose is added to the circuit prime to prevent dilution on initiation of bypass. This is calculated according to the size of the circuit rather than the patient.

CPB, Cardiopulmonary bypass; TXA, tranexamic acid.

[a]The required loading dose in children aged 2 months to 1 year alters rapidly with age. The larger relative dose in the range is appropriate for infants close to 2 months whereas a smaller dose (relative to body size) is appropriate for children closer to 1 year.

[b]Adult low, intermediate, and high dosing would aim for target concentrations of 33 µg/mL, 52 µg/mL, and 126 µg/mL, respectively. The prime dose is in milligrams per kilogram rather than micrograms per milliliter.

Pediatric dosing estimations from Wesley MC, Pereira LM, Scharp LA, et al. Pharmacokinetics of tranexamic acid in neonates, infants, and children undergoing cardiac surgery with cardiopulmonary bypass. *Anesthesiology.* 2015;122(4):746-758. Adult dosing estimations from Dowd NP, Karski JM, Cheng DC, et al. Pharmacokinetics of tranexamic acid during cardiopulmonary bypass. *Anesthesiology.* 2002;97(2):390-399.

and reduction in blood loss. A "low" dose equivalent to 20 mg/kg in total was recommended.[312] A PK study of dosing during craniofacial surgery in infants and children recommended a loading dose of 10 mg/kg combined with an infusion of 5 mg/kg per hour,[313] and a similar low dose used in a trial reduced bleeding.[314] This regimen prevented large peaks associated with large loading doses and maintained a steady-state plasma concentration of 16 µg/mL. Factors such as bleeding and administration of large volumes of IV fluid may also affect the PK of the drug. The authors' practice is to routinely administer a dose similar to the intermediate concentration described (i.e., 60 µg/mL); although more drug is given during severe bleeding (see Table 18.4).

Dosing of ε-Aminocaproic Acid

Two small PK studies can be used to inform the dose of EACA in children and neonates.[301,315] A larger dose is required to maintain target concentrations assumed to be therapeutic in children older than 9 months compared with adults. A dose of 75 mg/kg at induction and repeated on bypass combined with an infusion of 75 mg/kg per hour was recommended.[301] This dose was more effective than two divided doses of 100 mg/kg in a study of patients undergoing late repair of tetralogy of Fallot.[300] A dose of 40 mg/kg, followed by 30 mg/kg per hour and 100 mg/mL added to the bypass prime, should be adequate to maintain a plasma concentration of 50 µg/mL in neonates.[315] This is, however, a lower concentration than targeted by the earlier study in children. As with TXA, the concentration required to produce an optimal clinical effect is uncertain. Generally, potency is around 10 times less than TXA and lower concentrations are effective in vitro using neonatal plasma.

Dosing of Aprotinin

Aprotinin rapidly redistributes into the extracellular space after IV administration. It is metabolized in the proximal renal tubules and eliminated in a biphasic pattern: in adults it has a distribution half-life of 40 minutes and an elimination half-life of 7 hours.[306,316] A PK study of aprotinin in children undergoing CPB examined aprotinin concentrations after administration of weight-based dosing (25,000 KIU/kg bolus before CPB, 35,000 KIU/kg in CPB prime, and 12,500 KIU/kg per hour infusion).[317] There was considerable variation in plasma concentration of aprotinin, with the lowest concentration seen in the smallest patients. This may explain inconsistent results from aprotinin trials in children. Concentrations less than 200 KIU/mL would be insufficient to inhibit contact activation on the CPB circuit. This is consistent with greater clearance (expressed as per kilogram) in children (see also Chapter 5, Fig. 5.5). A further PK study of aprotinin in neonates also demonstrated rapid clearance and suggested that considerably larger doses are required to maintain therapeutic concentrations: a 50,000-KIU/kg bolus, 40,000 KIU/kg for CPB priming, and continuous infusion of 54,000 KIU/kg per hour for 3.4 hours and 10,000 KIU/kg per hour for 3.4 hours. Calculation of the dose using nonlinear functions (e.g., body surface area or an allometric 3/4-exponent model; see Chapter 5), as opposed to the linear dose per kilogram, may provide more effective dosing. This would result in a 2.5 times greater dose in neonates than would otherwise be given.[307]

WHICH ANTIFIBRINOLYTIC DRUG FOR PEDIATRIC CARDIAC SURGERY?

A meta-analysis of trials in adult patients reviewed differences between EACA and TXA. Aprotinin was more effective than either TXA or EACA, and although that effect was marginal, only aprotinin reduced the risk of reoperation.[252] Direct comparisons between TXA and EACA demonstrated no differences in their effects in children.[256,318] Low-dose aprotinin (10,000 KIU/kg followed by 10,000 KIU/kg per hour) has been compared with EACA (100 mg/kg on induction, 100 mg/kg in the pump prime, and 100 mg/kg on weaning from CPB).[257] There was a reduction in postoperative blood loss and transfusion requirements in both groups compared with the control, but no significant difference between the two drugs. TXA (100 mg/kg before, during, and after CPB) was compared with a higher (but still low) dose of aprotinin (30,000 KIU after induction, 30,000 KIU in the pump, and 30,000 KIU after weaning off bypass). There was a reduction in the time to sternal closure, transfusion requirements, and blood loss compared with control, but there was no significant difference between the two drugs. When the two drugs were combined at the same doses, they showed no additional benefit.[319] A further small trial demonstrated no difference in outcomes between aprotinin and TXA.[320]

Retrospective studies have examined outcomes related to efficacy and adverse effects. Results have been contradictory; some studies reported greater benefit with aprotinin,[284,287,321] whereas others showed no differences.[322] One study reported reduced bleeding with aprotinin, but greater creatinine concentrations and more prolonged postoperative ventilation.[285] A large multicenter study (>22,000 patients) demonstrated a benefit with all these drugs; however, mortality and reexploration were least in those who received TXA.[291]

A meta-analysis has pooled RCT and observational studies in children. Not surprisingly, efficacy is shown compared with control. It is harder to extract a conclusion about adverse effects or to make a comparison with synthetic antifibrinolytics. The authors concluded that: "*comparative efficacy and safety of aprotinin versus lysine analogues remain controversial but our analysis seems to indicate the superiority of aprotinin over the two lysine analogues.*" Superiority was primarily in a reduction in red cell transfusion of 5.6 mL/kg. Other outcomes, including length of stay, were worse in the aprotinin group. The authors acknowledged the limitations of their approach and concluded that "*there is an urgent need for adequately powered RCTs.*"[292]

In the absence of convincing evidence of improved efficacy for any drug, the choice of antifibrinolytic depends on the adverse effects and cost. The incidence of important adverse effects is also uncertain. Both mechanistically and from the available data, the "safety" concerns about aprotinin in adults are not applicable to children. A more certain risk of aprotinin is anaphylaxis with repeated exposure. This is a concern because many pediatric cardiac patients undergo repeat surgery. In the absence of further studies, it is the authors' conclusion that if an antifibrinolytic is indicated, lysine analogs are preferred over aprotinin.

USE OF ANTIFIBRINOLYTIC DRUGS IN OTHER TYPES OF MAJOR SURGERY

There is a trend toward increased use of antifibrinolytic drugs (especially TXA) during noncardiac surgery; principally major orthopedic surgery (e.g., spinal instrumentation, see also Chapter 30) and craniofacial surgery (see also Chapter 33). Aprotinin is less commonly used because of reduced availability and its safety concerns.

Multiple trials have examined the use of TXA during orthopedic surgery in adults[252]; they report a 50% reduction in the relative risk of requiring a blood transfusion. In 20 of these trials, there was a reduction in the incidence of total blood loss of more than 400 mL. Almost all these studies were conducted in adults undergoing major joint replacement surgery. In one study of adults (n = 147) undergoing posterior spinal fusion, TXA appeared to reduce total blood loss but the reduction in blood products transfused was not statistically significant.[323] The popularity of antifibrinolytic use during scoliosis surgery in children and adolescents is reflected in two surveys, which show use in 70% to 80% of hospitals.[324,325] It is unclear whether this use is mostly confined to higher-risk cases; however, in the authors' institution, TXA is currently used during all scoliosis surgery as part of a program aimed at reducing the use of blood products.

Two meta-analyses and a further systematic review have examined this question (reviewing six and seven studies, respectively); no single prospective study included more than 45 patients.[2,326,327] These meta-analyses concluded that antifibrinolytic drugs reduce bleeding and the volume of red cells transfused. To date there has been no single prospective trial comparing different antifibrinolytics. A retrospective comparison of TXA and EACA appeared to show a superiority of TXA, but the doses used were not comparable.[328] The two meta-analyses failed to establish any difference between the drugs.[2,326] It is also not possible to determine whether reported benefits hold for all children undergoing scoliosis repair. Bleeding is greater in children with nonidiopathic scoliosis (including patients with Duchenne muscular dystrophy),[329] those with hemostatic disorders, and in those undergoing more extensive surgery; therefore, in these groups a greater advantage in terms of bleeding reduction might be expected. At least one study examined children with idiopathic scoliosis and demonstrated a reduction in blood loss with aprotinin (see also Chapter 30).[330] As with cardiac studies, there is a considerable range in the dose of drug used; in a survey of practice in the United Kingdom, the TXA dose ranged from 3-fold to 5-fold, whereas in published trials the dose varied 10-fold.[324]

Antifibrinolytics are also used widely in craniosynostosis surgery.[331–333] In a survey of North American practice, they were used in 20% of hospitals for strip craniotomy, increasing to 30% for more complex repairs.[334,335] Four small trials, three using TXA[314,336,337] and one using aprotinin,[338] (a total of 141 children) have addressed the use of these agents for this indication. All these trials demonstrated reductions in blood transfused and in bleeding. A further trial demonstrated a greater than 50% reduction in the volume of blood transfused and in the proportion of children transfused (70% vs. 37%).[314] Although all these studies were relatively small, it would appear likely that antifibrinolytics produce a useful reduction in blood loss during craniosynostosis surgery. An updated meta-analysis of use in children demonstrated benefit during heart surgery and craniofacial surgery, but not during scoliosis surgery.[253]

A further trend has been the use of antifibrinolytic drugs during surgery not commonly associated with transfusion.[339–342] The objectives are to prevent uncommon, but potentially life-threatening bleeding and to limit hematoma formation. It is likely that very large numbers of patients would require treatment to realize this benefit, and, in this context, even rare adverse effects may outweigh any advantage.

ANTIFIBRINOLYTIC MEDICATION AND TRAUMA

The Clinical Randomization of an Antifibrinolytic in Significant Hemorrhage 2 (CRASH-2) study (a blinded RCT of more than 20,000 patients) demonstrated a reduction in mortality with TXA in adult trauma patients with, or at risk of, significant hemorrhage; mortality was reduced from 16% to 14.5%.[343] Mortality related to bleeding was reduced from 5.7% to 4.9%. No difference was reported in the rates of vascular occlusive events. In a large follow-up trail of adults with traumatic brain injury (CRASH-3), TXA was safe but produced only small benefits in a subgroup with less severe injury treated early.[344] One nonrandomized study of 766 children younger than 18 years of age, who were victims of trauma in Afghanistan, evaluated 66 children who received TXA; the study found that TXA administration was independently associated with decreased mortality.[345] In the absence of prospective well-controlled studies in children and in the absence of definite evidence of toxicity, it would seem reasonable to use TXA as part of the treatment of severe bleeding from trauma or surgery. Some caution is required, and its use should be reserved for severe bleeding (e.g., bleeding requiring treatment with non–red cell blood products). A dose of 15 mg/kg followed by 2 mg/kg per hour has been recommended for use in trauma.[346] This represents a simple per-kilogram scaling of the dose used in the CRASH-2 study. A further caveat is that administration more than 3 hours after injury in adults appeared to increase mortality.[347] The significance of this is unclear; however, such late administration should be avoided.

AUTHORS' RECOMMENDATIONS FOR USE OF ANTIFIBRINOLYTICS

Many children and adults have been recruited for studies of antifibrinolytic drugs. Consequently, it is reasonable to use these drugs during cardiac surgery, during other surgery likely to require blood transfusion, and in the management of trauma associated with severe bleeding. Considerable uncertainty remains: the dose is uncertain, the incidence of important adverse effects is unclear, the choice of drug is open to question, and effectiveness in different patient subgroups and clinical situations is debatable. Any further studies should be designed very carefully to address these questions. In the absence of such studies, it is not possible to make solid recommendations. The authors' current practice is:

- Antifibrinolytics are used routinely during heart surgery in children with cyanotic heart disease, especially in the presence of polycythemia, or reduced saturations for a prolonged period.
- Antifibrinolytics are used during cardiac procedures in other children as part of a strategy to reduce transfusion. Greater benefit is likely, but not proven, in children with a greater tendency to bleeding, including smaller children, when bypass time is likely to be long, and during repeat surgery.[348,349]
- Antifibrinolytics are given during other major surgical procedures in children including scoliosis repair, multilevel joint surgery, and craniosynostosis repair, but only in combination with other, potentially more effective, measures to reduce bleeding and limit transfusion.
- Synthetic antifibrinolytics are used. Aprotinin is not.
- Dosing of TXA is as described in Table 18.4.
- These drugs are used together with other measures to reduce bleeding and transfusion. Concepts of patient blood management are followed.[3]

New Drug Development

Much of the previous discussion has concerned use of drugs and blood products that have been available for many years. Development of medications for treatment of bleeding is largely driven by a desire to improve long-term treatment of congenital hemophilias.[350] This has also led to new therapies for acute bleeding and acquired coagulopathy, and this may be the case in the future. A novel area of research that may be more directly applicable to management of surgical bleeding is development of novel inhibitors of fibrinolysis.[351]

Acknowledgment

I thank Andrew Wolf and Adam Skinner for their prior contributions to this chapter.

ANNOTATED REFERENCES

Faraoni D, Goobie SM. New insights about the use of tranexamic acid in children undergoing cardiac surgery: from pharmacokinetics to pharmacodynamics. *Anesth Analg.* 2013;117:760-762.

This editorial summarizes the challenges in optimizing the use of antifibrinolytic medications for use in children. It offers an insight into the problems of translating drugs widely used in adults to use in children and how pharmacokinetic, in vitro, and clinical studies can be used to make logical recommendations about dosing.

Faraoni D, Goobie SM. The efficacy of antifibrinolytic drugs in children undergoing noncardiac surgery: a systematic review of the literature. *Anesth Analg.* 2014;118(3):628-636.

A balanced review of the evidence regarding use of antifibrinolytic drugs in children during noncardiac surgery.

Goobie SM, Gallagher T, Gross I, Shander A. Society for the advancement of blood management administrative and clinical standards for patient blood management programs. 4th edition (pediatric version). *Paediatr Anaesth.* 2019;29(3):231-236.

Guidelines and a review of principles of patient blood management with respect to pediatric practice.

Guzzetta NA, Miller BE. Principles of hemostasis in children: models and maturation. *Paediatr Anaesth.* 2011;21:3-9.

An excellent review of the changes in coagulation with development, with a particular emphasis of the relevance of this to the use of rFVIIa in pediatric practice. This is part of an issue of Paediatric Anesthesia themed around topics related to coagulation.

Hoffman M. Remodeling the blood coagulation cascade. *J Thromb Thrombolysis.* 2003;16:17-20.

Hoffman explains the difficulties associated with the "old model" of coagulation cascade. The paper contains an excellent step-by-step discussion of the cellular-based model of coagulation.

New HV, Berryman J, Bolton-Maggs PH, et al. British Committee for Standards in Haematology. Guidelines on transfusion for fetuses, neonates and older children. *Br J Haematol.* 2016;175:784-828.

Extensive and informative guidelines produced in the United Kingdom covering aspects of transfusion in the child, infant, and fetus. Although written to reflect U.K. practice, the guidelines are informative for readers from other locations.

Rahe-Meyer N, Levy JH, Mazer CD, et al. Randomized evaluation of fibrinogen vs placebo in complex cardiovascular surgery (REPLACE): a double-blind phase III study of haemostatic therapy. *Br J Anaesth.* 2016;117:41-51.

The REPLACE trial is an important trial conducted in adult cardiac surgical patients. The findings cast doubt on the effectiveness of fibrinogen concentrates in the management of bleeding serving as a further warning that there is no "magic bullet" in the treatment of severe bleeding. Rather, there is a need for good surgical hemostasis and a methodical approach based on an understanding of the physiology and pathophysiology of coagulation.

Warren OJ, Rogers PL, Watret AL, et al. Defining the role of recombinant activated factor VII in pediatric cardiac surgery: where should we go from here? *Pediatr Crit Care Med.* 2009;10:572-582.

A thorough review of the use of rFVIIa in pediatric heart surgery.

Welsby IJ, Monroe DM, Lawson JH, Hoffmann M. Recombinant activated factor VIIa and the anaesthetist. *Anaesthesia.* 2005;60:1203-1212.

This is a very good overview of the mechanisms and use of rFVIIa.

A complete reference list can be found online at Elsevier eBooks+.

Mechanical Circulatory Support

ADAM C. ADLER, RANIA K. ABBASI, AND LAURA K. BERENSTAIN

Learning Systems and Databases
Indications for Mechanical Circulatory Support
Preoperative Stabilization
Failure to Wean From Cardiopulmonary Bypass
Cardiac Transplantation
Pulmonary Hypertension
Respiratory Failure
Cardiopulmonary Resuscitation
Other Indications
Contraindications
The Devices
Extracorporeal Membrane Oxygenation
ECMO Circuit Configurations
Ventricular Assist Devices

Short-Term Devices
Long-Term Devices
Perioperative Management of Mechanical Circulatory Support
Hemodynamics
Respiratory Considerations
Hematologic Considerations
Prevention of Infection
Anesthetic Considerations
Outcomes and Complications
Outcomes
Complications
Future Directions
Devices

THE NUMBER OF INFANTS and children who are hospitalized each year with cardiorespiratory collapse who require artificial support is substantive. Despite maximal medical therapy, failure of the cardiac and/or respiratory systems to provide adequate end-organ perfusion and oxygenation often results in the need for mechanical support of the circulation, either as an adjunct to cardiopulmonary resuscitation (CPR) or as a bridge to recovery or transplantation. The number of pediatric patients who require support has been increasing yearly and includes not only patients with primary cardiac dysfunction but also children and adolescents with primary respiratory failure.

The number of hospitalizations for pediatric heart failure (HF) along with the number of children awaiting cardiac transplantation in the United States continues to increase each year.[1] Improved recognition, medical management, and surgical and perioperative survival of patients with congenital heart disease (CHD) have significantly increased the number of both children and adults living with impaired ventricular function due to congenital heart disease. However, congenital heart disease remains the most common cause of heart failure in children.[2–4] Between 2004 and 2018 hospital admissions for pediatric heart failure in patients with congenital heart disease doubled.[5] Despite the increased number of hospitalizations, hospital mortality decreased in association with an increase in the use of ventricular assist devices (VAD) and extracorporeal membrane oxygenation (ECMO) as well as an increase in the number of heart transplantation procedures.[3,5] Due to earlier recognition and more aggressive medical management, more patients with cardiomyopathies are surviving the initial phase of their illness. Admissions for pediatric heart failure carry a mortality of approximately 10%, and 10% to 15% result in the institution of mechanical circulatory support (MCS).[6,7]

The prevalence of heart failure in adults has remained greater than in the pediatric population, and the development and use of MCS for adults with end-stage heart failure has correspondingly grown and matured at a faster pace than in children. First-generation VADs for adults came into routine use in the 1980s, and the use of MCS in adults has continued to rapidly evolve.[8] The use of VADs in children began with the application of adult devices in adolescents. Expansion of their use in children has proceeded more slowly as technologic challenges of effectively "miniaturizing" adult devices to accommodate pediatric weight ranges have resulted in fewer VAD options for children compared with the number and types of devices available for adults. Important considerations and differences between adult and pediatric patient populations include physiologic and anatomic variations, a dissimilar immunologic response to blood transfusions, the growth and development of pediatric patients, and greater thromboembolic risk owing to an immature coagulation cascade.[9,10] Finally, regulatory constraints of device evaluation in a small and heterogeneous patient population[11] have also made advances more challenging.

The number and type of MCS devices available for children remains comparatively limited, particularly for children weighing less than 20 kg in the United States. The use of extracorporeal life support (ECLS) in this population has also continued to grow. Initiatives by the National Heart, Lung, and Blood Institute (NHLBI) supporting the development of MCS devices for infants and children offer promising future alternatives.[12] Mechanical support can be provided either in the form of ECMO for cardiopulmonary support or in the form of VADs to support cardiac function and maintain perfusion.

Learning Systems and Databases

Although VAD support for children is becoming more common, the experience at most centers continues to be limited and low patient volume has been associated with suboptimal outcomes and decreased survival.[13] Recognizing this issue, a collaborative learning health care system, Advanced Cardiac Therapies Improving Outcomes Network (ACTION), was formed in April 2017.[14] ACTION's mission is to improve critical outcomes and the patient/family experience for children with heart failure by developing an international collaborative learning health network. The mission includes focusing on goals and outcomes that matter most to participants, using quality improvement methodology to assess impact and creating infrastructure that allows sharing and facilitates connection between institutions.[15] This learning health system was developed for the benefit of both inpatient and outpatient pediatric heart failure populations and thus differs from other inpatient registries and networks.[16] Although ACTION's mission encompasses all pediatric heart failure patients, the initial focus has been on the pediatric VAD population, with the goal of reducing the frequency and severity of stroke associated with VAD care.[16] The most recent Pediatric Interagency Registry for Mechanical Circulatory Support (Pedimacs) national registry report highlighted that pediatric patients predominantly suffer from ischemic stroke as opposed to hemorrhagic stroke, emphasizing the importance of the initial ACTION project to evaluate anticoagulation practices to reduce the incidence of stroke.[15]

Interagency Registry for Mechanically Assisted Circulatory Support (INTERMACS), an NHLBI-sponsored registry for FDA-approved durable MCS devices in the United States, began data entry on adult and pediatric durable device implants in June 2006. As part of this project, Pedimacs, a dedicated pediatric component, began registering patients on September 19, 2012. From September 2012 through December 2020, 47 institutions had enrolled 1229 devices in 1011 patients receiving temporary or long-term MCS devices.[17] This registry focuses on capturing data elements unique to pediatric patients, evaluating special issues in pediatric MCS, chronicling the variety of devices applied in the pediatric population, and identifying the particular cohort in whom therapy is most effective. Goals of this registry include delineating the best support strategies for VAD therapies, refining patient selection of VAD therapies, developing "best practices" by analyzing outcomes, and facilitating and guiding the development and clinical evaluation of pediatric devices.

Indications for Mechanical Circulatory Support

Decision making regarding the optimal timing for implementation of MCS is often challenging. It is generally agreed that MCS should be initiated earlier to avoid prolonged low cardiac output states and organ hypoperfusion with resultant end-organ damage.

Early institution of support better avoids end-organ dysfunction (e.g., renal or hepatic failure) and maximizes the opportunity for either recovery or bridge to transplantation. Indications for MCS in children can be divided primarily into cardiac and noncardiac indications (Table 19.1). The following criteria for implementation of MCS have been used in one institution: (1) cardiac index less than 2 L/minute per m² with inotropic dependence; (2) poor peripheral perfusion with metabolic acidosis and mixed venous oxygen saturation <40%; (3) signs of impending respiratory, renal, or hepatic failure; and (4) increased or rapidly increasing B-type natriuretic peptide (BNP) concentrations (Table 19.2).[18,19]

In general, with the exception of pulmonary hypertension and isolated respiratory failure, either ECMO or VAD can be used for all indications. Each device has pros and cons, with the optimal device depending on the acuity of the illness, patient comorbidities, potential for recovery, and anticipated duration of support.[20] Table 19.3 summarizes the numerous patient and device characteristics that must be considered when choosing a strategy for

TABLE 19.1	Indications for Mechanical Circulatory Support
Preoperative Stabilization	
Severe cyanosis/hypercyanotic spells	
Pulmonary hypertensive crises	
Myocardial dysfunction/cardiac arrest	
Malignant dysrhythmias	
Sepsis	
Postcardiotomy Patients	
Heart failure	
Early: inability to wean from cardiopulmonary bypass	
Late: prolonged low cardiac output syndrome	
Procedure related	
Stage I palliation for hypoplastic left heart syndrome	
After ALCAPA repair	
Persistent malignant dysrhythmias	
Bridge to Myocardial Recovery	
Acute myocarditis	
Cardiomyopathy	
Acute cardiac transplant rejection	
Bridge to Transplantation	
Direct bridge to transplantation	
Bridge to bridge (short- to long-term support)	
Noncardiac Indications	
Respiratory failure of oxygenation and/or ventilation	
Near-drowning	
Severe hypothermia	
Drug toxicity	
Critical airway (tracheal stenosis)	
Sepsis/shock	
Extracorporeal Cardiopulmonary Resuscitation	
Refractory Cardiopulmonary Arrest	

ALCAPA, Anomalous origin of the left coronary artery from the pulmonary artery.

TABLE 19.2	Suggested Clinical Criteria for Mechanical Cardiac Support Implementation

Rapid Circulatory Deterioration (CI <2 L/minute per m²)

Inotropic dependence

High or rapidly increasing B-type natriuretic peptide

Critical Peripheral Perfusion

Development of metabolic acidosis

Mixed venous oxygen saturation <40%

Signs of Renal, Hepatic, and Respiratory Failure

Ventilatory support with increasing FiO₂

CI, Cardiac index; *FiO₂*, fraction of inspired oxygen.
Modified from Hetzer R, Potapov EV, Alexi-Meskishvili V, et al. Single-center experience with treatment of cardiogenic shock in children by pediatric ventricular assist devices. *J Thorac Cardiovasc Surg.* 2011;141(3):616-623; and Potapov EV, Stiller B, Hetzer R. Ventricular assist devices in children: current achievements and future perspectives. *Pediatr Transplant.* 2007;11:241-255.

mechanical support. As pediatric VAD experience has grown, patients may now be considered not only for bridge to recovery or bridge to transplant but also bridge to decision or candidacy for transplantation, and destination therapy. In patients with cardiac failure, the primary goal is to allow the myocardium to rest and recover function (bridge to recovery). In the absence of myocardial recovery, heart transplantation is often considered. However, considering the paucity of available organs, the patient may be transitioned with long-term mechanical support (i.e., ECMO to a VAD) while awaiting a suitable organ (bridge to transplant). The use of MCS as destination therapy in the pediatric population continues to be rare, with no devices specifically approved for this indication in pediatric patients. A small but growing group of children and adolescents with Duchenne or Becker muscular dystrophy have undergone VAD placement as destination therapy, and a case report details a patient supported for more than 2100 days with a continuous flow VAD at the time of the report.[10,21,22] It is expected that this population will continue to grow because of strong advocacy by these patients and their families. An increasing number of patients with adult congenital heart disease who develop heart failure are eligible for MCS as either bridge to transplant, bridge to decision, or destination therapy if end-organ dysfunction or elevated pulmonary vascular resistance (PVR) precludes cardiac transplantation.[23] In the subgroup of failing Fontan patients with ventricular dysfunction who may not be transplant candidates, the potential role of destination therapy continues to be discussed.[24] Other pediatric patients who may ultimately benefit from destination therapy include children with chemotherapy-induced cardiomyopathy with ongoing malignancy and unlikely long-term remission, and children with cardiac dysfunction accompanied by multiple comorbidities or impairment that might preclude transplantation. The most recent Pedimacs registry data from 2012 to 2017 showed the primary VAD indication to be bridge to transplant 55%, bridge to decision 34%, and VAD implantation as destination therapy in 2% of patients.[25]

A critical early decision point in the deployment of VAD support in children is determining whether left ventricular (LV) support alone will suffice. For a left ventricular assist device (LVAD) to provide satisfactory support, adequate right ventricular (RV)

function is crucial to allow for adequate LV function and, ultimately, LVAD filling. Unlike heart failure in adults, pediatric heart failure is commonly associated with biventricular failure and/or increased PVR, both of which may limit left ventricular diastolic filling. Although early data showed that 29% to 35% of pediatric patients required biventricular VAD (BiVAD) support,[26,27] more recent data have shown a declining frequency in its use as decision making regarding implementation of MCS has improved. Adults requiring BiVAD support are now more likely to receive a SynCardia Total Artificial Heart (TAH), with better outcomes reported than with BiVAD HeartWare Ventricular Assist System (HVAD) support.[28] The use of BiVAD support has been associated with increased mortality in both adults and children, likely reflecting the severity of disease in patients requiring such intensive assistance.

PREOPERATIVE STABILIZATION

Preoperative cardiopulmonary stabilization may be required in children with profound hypoxemia and/or cardiovascular collapse resulting from hypercyanotic spells, pulmonary hypertensive crises, obstructed total anomalous pulmonary venous return, occlusion of systemic-pulmonary shunts, or cardiogenic shock (see Table 19.1).[19] Preoperative ECMO was used as a bridge to surgical repair or palliation in 26 children, with 62% surviving to discharge and no observed differences in outcome between single-ventricular and biventricular patients.[29] ECMO has also been successfully used to stabilize children with refractory dysrhythmias.[30–33] In a retrospective study, ECMO was used in nine infants with a variety of tachy- or brady-dysrhythmias, with all nine surviving to discharge.[34] ECMO has also been used to stabilize children in the cardiac catheterization laboratory, both preemptively before high-risk interventional procedures and as a rescue technique for catheter-induced complications, persistent low cardiac output, or hypoxemia.[35,36]

FAILURE TO WEAN FROM CARDIOPULMONARY BYPASS

Failure to wean from cardiopulmonary bypass (CPB) after congenital heart surgery is the most common cardiac indication for mechanical support.[37,38] In a review between 2000 and 2016 of children <18 years of age who required ECMO support for failure to wean from cardiopulmonary bypass, the number of children requiring support has continued to grow each year but in-hospital mortality has remained unchanged at approximately 55%.[39] Factors that contribute to lower survival rates included the presence of genetic syndromes, noncardiac abnormalities, comorbid conditions and cardiac arrest before surgery. Postcardiotomy myocardial dysfunction can manifest as either early (inability to wean from cardiopulmonary bypass) or late (sustained postoperative low cardiac output syndrome) failure with poor end-organ function, persistently increased plasma lactate concentrations, low mixed venous saturations (<40%), reduced cerebral saturation (>20% below baseline), and escalating inotropic support. It is essential to rule out the presence of residual surgical lesions, coronary insufficiency secondary to surgical manipulation, and mechanical problems (e.g., cardiac tamponade) before initiating MCS.[40] Early cardiac catheterization after institution of ECMO may be helpful to identify and treat residual lesions that can facilitate weaning from ECMO and promote increased survival.[41]

It is crucial to reiterate that early initiation of mechanical support leads to better outcomes. In a study of 81 children, those who had ECMO initiated in the operating room had a survival rate of 64% compared with 29% in those who had initiation of

TABLE 19.3   Characteristics of Commonly Used Pediatric Support Devices

Device	Patient Size Restrictions	Duration of Support	Type of Support	Pump Type	Flow	Advantages	Disadvantages	FDA Approval
Short-Term Support Devices								
ECMO	None	<3 weeks	Cardiac/Pulmonary	Continuous	Variable	• Central or peripheral cannulation • Extensive experience in all age groups • Rapid rescue capability • Can be placed at bedside • Less expensive • Easy decannulation	• Higher levels of anticoagulation needed • Increased neurologic complications • Increased bleeding/transfusions • No/limited patient mobility • Usually remain intubated • Need for trained personnel and continuous monitoring	Yes
Bio-Medicus BP-50 (Medtronic)	None	Days/weeks	Univentricular or biventricular	Continuous centrifugal		• Simpler setup than ECMO • Requires less anticoagulation than ECMO • Better ventricular unloading than ECMO	• No respiratory support • No/limited patient mobility • Generally remain intubated • Direct cannulation of the heart via sternotomy	Yes (6 hours)
CentriMag (Thoratec)	None		Univentricular or biventricular	Continuous centrifugal				
PediMag (Thoratec)	<20 kg, BSA <1.3 m²		Univentricular or biventricular	Continuous centrifugal	Up to 1.5 L/minute			
Jostra RotaFlow (Maquet)	None		Univentricular or biventricular	Continuous centrifugal	Up to 10 L/minute			
TandemHeart (CardiacAssist)	>40 kg, BSA >1.3 m²	Days	Univentricular or biventricular	Continuous centrifugal	Up to 5 L/minute	• Percutaneous placement possible • Extubation possible	• Transseptal puncture necessary • Risk of thromboembolism • Risk of pump dislodgment	
Impella (AbioMed)	BSA >0.93 m²	Days	Univentricular	Continuous axial	2.5–5 L/minute	• 3 pump sizes • Percutaneous placement possible • Improved unloading of ventricle • Extubation possible	• Pump migration may occur	
Long-Term Support Devices								
Berlin Heart EXCOR	>3 kg, BSA 0.2–1.3 m²	Months–years	Univentricular or biventricular	Pneumatic, pulsatile	Varies with pump size	• Extubation, ambulation possible • Less anticoagulation than ECMO	• Sternotomy required for implantation	Yes for BTT
HeartWare HVAD[a]	>15 kg or BSA >0.65 m²	Years	Univentricular or biventricular	Continuous centrifugal	Up to 10 L/minute	• Reduced anticoagulation requirements compared with older VADs	• Device exchange may be necessary	No, recalled in 2021[a]
HeartMate 3	>30 kg, BSA >1.5 m²	Years	Univentricular	Continuous axial	>2.5 L/minute	• Discharge home possible		Yes for BTT and DT
SynCardia TAH	BSA >1.2 m² (50 mL) BSA >1.7 m² (70 mL)	Years	Biventricular	Pneumatic, pulsatile	Up to 9.5 L/minute			Yes for BTT

BSA, Body surface area; BTT, bridge to transplantation; DT, destination therapy; ECMO, extracorporeal membrane oxygenation; FDA, US Food and Drug Administration; TAH, total artificial heart.
[a]The HeartWare device is on recall by the FDA at the time of updating this chapter. (UPDATE: Parameters of weight and BSA listed above are commonly recommended; however, anecdotal reports exist describing device usage outside these parameters.)

ECMO in the intensive care unit (ICU).[42] Risk factors for increased mortality for patients requiring ECMO support also include more complex cardiac surgery and CPB of greater duration.[41] Patients with single-ventricle physiology or cyanotic heart disease are more likely to require mechanical support after CPB. According to the 2015 Extracorporeal Life Support Organization (ELSO) registry,[43] hypoplastic left heart syndrome (HLHS) is the most frequent type of congenital heart disease requiring ECMO in neonates, and certain centers have advocated the routine use of mechanical support to optimize postoperative cardiac output following stage I Norwood procedures.[44] Both ECMO and LVADs have been used for postoperative ventricular support in infants with anomalous origin of the left coronary artery from the pulmonary artery trunk (ALPACA), either as a bridge to recovery or transplant.[45,46]

CARDIAC TRANSPLANTATION

In children without congenital heart disease, viral myocarditis is the most common cause of acute heart failure and ECMO has been successfully used as a bridge to either subsequent VAD therapy, transplantation, or recovery in this population.[47,48] Other cardiac pathophysiologic processes, such as coronary ischemia, graft rejection after cardiac transplantation, or end-stage heart failure owing to chronic cardiomyopathies, dysrhythmias, or congenital heart defects, may also warrant the use of mechanical support. ECMO has been used for patients with early and late ventricular dysfunction after cardiac transplantation. Acute graft failure is the most common reason for ECMO post transplantation.[49]

In a review of 2820 patients, 7.9% required ECMO after transplant, with risk factors including lower age (<1 year or 1–5 years), congenital heart disease, re-transplant, and ECMO or VAD support before transplant. Although in-hospital survival decreased with duration of ECMO support, long-term survival was no different compared with patients who did not require ECMO support.[50] ECMO is generally the initial modality of choice for support because of the speed of application, familiarity of use, and the ability to manage situations in which RV failure and/or high pulmonary artery vascular resistance are present.[51]

PULMONARY HYPERTENSION

Patients with pulmonary hypertension may be considered candidates for ECMO support. Both perioperative patients with reversible pulmonary hypertension (for example, patients with total anomalous pulmonary venous drainage with increased PVR that improve after surgical intervention) and those experiencing pulmonary hypertensive crises may benefit from ECMO support. Patients with severe medically refractory pulmonary hypertension may also require venoarterial (VA) ECMO as a bridge to lung or heart-lung transplant. Novalung (Novalung GmbH, Hechingen, Germany) has developed a paracorporeal pumpless interventional lung assist device using a low-resistance hollow fiber oxygenator that has been used in patients with cardiogenic shock secondary to pulmonary hypertension. Cannulas are placed in the pulmonary artery and left atrium and the high pulmonary pressures drive the blood through the oxygenator, removing carbon dioxide and improving oxygenation, without the need for a mechanical pump. This allows pulmonary pressures to decrease, off-loading the failing RV and thus facilitating recovery. Four infants and children, 23 days to 23 months of age, were bridged from ECMO to a pumpless paracorporeal lung assist device while awaiting lung transplantation for chronic lung disease and pulmonary hypertension. Three of the four were extubated while supported by the

device. One was bridged to recovery, one to transplant, and two died supported by the device while awaiting transplant.[52] One potential advantage of the device is its small size; it is much smaller than an ECMO circuit that may allow for easier patient transport when the device is used.

RESPIRATORY FAILURE

Multiple noncardiac indications exist for the use of ECMO, most importantly respiratory failure. Data from the 2020 ELSO Registry Annual Report showed that 41% of pediatric patients who received ECMO were neonates, the majority (55%) due to respiratory failure.[53] In neonates, the most common indications for ECMO were congenital diaphragmatic hernia, meconium aspiration syndrome, and persistent pulmonary hypertension of the newborn, with an overall survival rate following ECMO exceeding 70%.[38,54,55] Among the nonneonatal pediatric patients, 33% received support due to pulmonary compromise. With the H1N1 influenza pandemic, the number of pediatric patients supported by ECMO for respiratory failure increased dramatically.[38,56–58] Similarly, data are emerging on the use of ECMO in children for cardiopulmonary support after the height of the Coronavirus 2019 (COVID-19) pandemic.

Although adults comprised the vast the majority of patients requiring ECMO support during the COVID-19 pandemic, children and adolescents with COVID-induced pneumonia resulting in acute respiratory distress syndrome (ARDS) were also bridged with this therapy.[59–61]

CARDIOPULMONARY RESUSCITATION

Extracorporeal cardiopulmonary resuscitation (ECPR) was suggested by the American Heart Association Pediatric Advanced Life Support (AHA PALS) 2010 guidelines for use in refractory CPR during in-hospital cardiac arrests resulting from potentially reversible causes.[62] The AHA 2020 evidence summary continues to support the use of ECPR in pediatric patients, showing improved survival and more favorable neurologic outcomes compared with CPR alone.[63] Outcomes after ECPR for children with underlying cardiac disease have been better than for children without underlying heart disease. AHA 2020 guidelines recommend that ECPR be used for children with an underlying cardiac diagnosis who suffer in-hospital cardiac arrests in centers with ECMO protocols.[64] Data from the 2020 ELSO Registry Annual Report stated that approximately 10% of neonatal and 22% of pediatric ECMO is performed as ECPR with survival from ECMO being 68% and 57%, respectively.[65] Additionally, the survival to hospital discharge is 44% and 42% for neonatal and pediatric ECPR, respectively. In contrast, ECPR comprises approximately 15% of ECMO in adults with a survival from ECMO of 41% and survival to discharge of 29%. This improved survival in children is likely owing to the more reversible causes for pediatric cardiopulmonary arrest.[53]

OTHER INDICATIONS

ECMO can also provide short-term respiratory support for tracheobronchial reconstruction in infants and children with critical airways when conventional mechanical ventilation is either not feasible or has not been successful.[66] Other noncardiac indications for mechanical support include hypothermia, drug toxicity, and near-drowning. Septicemia was initially considered a contraindication to MCS; the necessity for greater flow requirements can make the use of ECMO challenging in this population. However, a recent review of the use of VA ECMO in children with sepsis showed high resource utilization but a 59% survival to discharge.[67] In fact, utilization of ECMO as a bridge to recovery in children with refractory ARDS or pneumonia has become widely accepted.[38] ECMO can provide a bridge to lung transplantation or re-transplantation. After transplantation it can be used in cases of severe primary graft dysfunction, although survival in these patient groups remains less overall than for other indications.[68–70]

Contraindications

Contraindications to implementation of MCS should be considered on a case-by-case basis but may include significant lethal chromosomal defects, neurologic compromise or intracranial hemorrhage, allogeneic bone marrow transplant recipients with pulmonary infiltrates, and incurable malignancy. High-risk candidates include those with advanced multisystem organ failure, active infection, and severe coagulopathy. Extreme prematurity, very low birth weight, and/or multiple congenital anomalies and preexisting chronic illness with poor long-term prognosis may also be considered relative contraindications.[71] Neonates with low birth weight, extreme prematurity, and preexisting intracranial hemorrhage pose a particular risk when considered for ECMO because of the risk of developing or worsening intracranial hemorrhage.[72] Most bleeds occur within the first 72 hours of birth so, in theory, the risk of hemorrhage or extension of existing hemorrhage may be less after 3 days of age. Most ECMO exclusion criteria include patients with grade 3 or 4 intracranial hemorrhage, and many consider a birth weight of less than 1.6 kg as a reasonable contraindication to ECMO, as a regression analysis suggested that a minimum weight of 1.6 kg was necessary to achieve a 40% survival in noncardiac ECLS.[73]

For children who require mechanical support secondary to a cardiac etiology, due consideration should be given to the likelihood of myocardial recovery before instituting support, and if recovery is unlikely, whether the child is a suitable candidate for cardiac transplantation. While there are no true contraindications, there are some common anatomic issues that should be considered before initiating MCS. These include the thickness of the ventricles, semilunar valve regurgitation, and presence of intracardiac shunts. Thick ventricles, such as in hypertrophic cardiomyopathy, can prevent proper device filling. In some patients with large atria, atrial cannulation may allow proper filling of the VAD. Aortic or pulmonary valve insufficiency may not permit adequate ventricular emptying. Instead, blood recirculates through the regurgitant valve, occasionally necessitating closure or repair of the valve at the time of VAD implantation.[74] Intracardiac defects will also need to be closed at the time of device placement to prevent embolization of thrombus, air, or right-to-left shunting.

The Devices

A variety of devices are available to provide mechanical support for the cardiopulmonary circulation in children. Devices are discussed sequentially based on the type and duration of support provided. Three types of continuous flow pumps have been proven in providing durable support: centrifugal, axial, and mixed flow pumps.[75]

Extracorporeal Membrane Oxygenation

Whereas adults generally have isolated LV failure, children more often require cardiopulmonary support because of hypoxemia,

pulmonary hypertension, or concurrent RV failure. For infants and children who require short-term or urgent cardiopulmonary support, ECMO remains the modality of choice. Initially reported for the treatment of cardiac failure in children in the 1970s, ECMO was subsequently used for mechanical support during interhospital transport.[76,77] Currently the most common cardiac indications for ECMO are failure to wean from CPB, emergent support after cardiac arrest with failure of conventional resuscitation, and early graft failure after cardiac transplantation. Since the ELSO registry began in 1989, ECMO has been the MCS modality with the most pediatric usage, with >7500 usages in neonates and children for cardiac indications and >26,000 usages in neonates for respiratory support.[38,78] Since 2015 alone, there have been 7500 reported uses of ECMO in neonates and 10,500 in children with continuously increasing survival.[53]

A typical ECMO circuit is composed of a pump (either a roller pump with a servo regulatory mechanism for controlling circuit flow or a centrifugal pump); a hollow fiber or membrane oxygenator; a heat exchanger; and cannulas (either venous, arterial, or both) (Fig. 19.1). A modified ECMO circuit composed of a heparin-coated circuit, Bio-Medicus centrifugal pump (Medtronic, Minneapolis, MN), hollow fiber membrane oxygenator, flow probe, and hematocrit/oxygen saturation monitor, allowing the circuit to be set up and primed in 5 minutes for rapid resuscitation, has been described.[79] Most hospitals supporting such a service have readily available trained personnel to assist with implementing and maintaining ECMO therapy. Versatility and suitability for rapid implementation are advantages of ECMO; venoarterial cannulation in postcardiotomy patients may be either transthoracic via the right atrial appendage and aorta, transcervical via the right internal jugular vein and common carotid artery, or femoral via the femoral artery and vein in larger patients. Heparin-bonded circuitry is often used to minimize surface-induced complement activation, platelet dysfunction, and anticoagulation requirements.[80] A dry circuit can be kept ready for rapid deployment, with crystalloid prime used during initiation of support and addition of blood products (packed red blood cells [PRBCs] and fresh frozen plasma [FFP]) as soon as they become available. Alternatively, use of non–cross-matched blood (O negative) can be used, especially in neonates, until type-specific blood becomes available. During resuscitative efforts, before institution of mechanical support, multiple doses of vasoconstrictors should be avoided. If possible, acidosis should be corrected, and the infant's head may be packed in ice in an effort to facilitate cerebral protection. Ultimately, the restoration of cardiac output, even with a low hematocrit, is the most important factor for successful resuscitation and long-term survival.[81,82]

Other advantages of ECMO include the ability to institute support in the intensive care unit, provide ultrafiltration or hemodialysis for children during mechanical support, and provide biventricular cardiopulmonary support even in very small neonates.

ECMO CIRCUIT CONFIGURATIONS

Three common configurations exist for ECMO circuits (see Fig. 19.1). The most commonly used configuration, VA ECMO, is similar to CPB. A venous cannula is placed centrally via the superior or inferior vena cava and an arterial cannula is placed in either the aorta (open chest), femoral, or carotid artery. Blood is drained from the venous cannula, bypassing the heart and lungs, and replaced into the patient via the arterial cannula. VA ECMO can provide gas exchange and hemodynamic support without assistance from the native heart. VA ECMO decreases

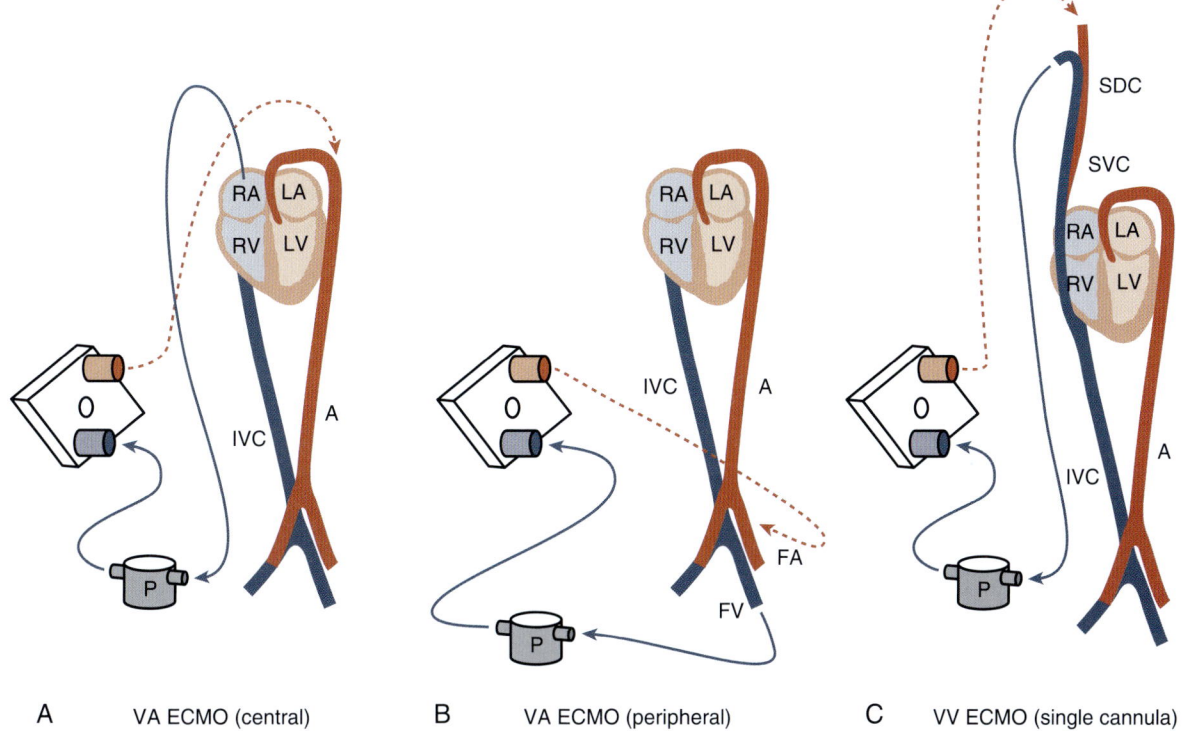

| A | VA ECMO (central) | B | VA ECMO (peripheral) | C | VV ECMO (single cannula) |

FIGURE 19.1 Schematic diagram of extracorporeal membrane oxygenation *(ECMO)* circuit configurations. *Dotted red arrow,* Oxygenated blood. The *solid blue arrow* designates deoxygenated blood. **A,** Venoarterial *(VA)* central ECMO. The dual venous cannula (right atrium *[RA]* and interior vena cava *[IVC]*) drain blood toward a pump *(P)* that pushes the blood through an oxygenator *(O)* with an integrated heat exchanger before returning via an aortic cannula placed in the ascending aorta *(A)*. **B,** VA peripheral ECMO. The venous drainage via a cannula in the femoral vein *(FV)* is pumped through the oxygenator and returned into the femoral artery *(FA)*. **C,** Venovenous *(VV)* ECMO: single dual-chamber *(SDC)* venous cannulation strategy. One chamber has the distal orifice in the inferior vena cava *(IVC)* and the proximal orifice in the superior vena cava *(SVC)*. Together they drain blood into the pump/oxygenator; blood returns through an outflow exit orifice into the RA. *LA,* Left atrium; *LV,* left ventricle; *RA,* right atrium; *RV,* right ventricle. Alternatively, this can be accomplished through cannulae in both femoral veins. (From Martinez G, Vuylsteke A. Extracorporeal membrane oxygenation in adults. *Continuing Education in Anaesthesia, Critical Care & Pain.* 2012;12(2):57-61.)

myocardial work and oxygen consumption and can be used to "rest" the native heart, especially in cases of myocarditis. If there is minimal ventricular ejection, care must be taken to avoid ventricular overdistention, which may necessitate placement of a left atrial vent.

Venovenous ECMO (VV ECMO) can be accomplished either with a double-lumen catheter or two venous cannulas placed in large veins (femoral, internal jugular). Blood is drained from the patient, gas and/or heat exchange occurs, and the blood is returned to the patient's venous circulation. VV ECMO can provide gas and/or temperature exchange and is mainly used for primary respiratory failure in patients with preserved cardiac function, because VV ECMO requires adequate function of the native heart. Although VV cannulation is technically more difficult and may be associated with a greater frequency of flow issues and cannulation site bleeding, neurologic injury is seen less frequently than with VA ECMO.[83]

In arterial-venous ECMO (AV ECMO), both arterial and venous cannulas are placed. The patient's own blood pressure and native heart function pump the blood through the ECMO circuit specifically for gas exchange. Basic ECMO configurations are described in Fig. 19.1. Cannulation strategies specific to ECPR are depicted in Fig. 19.2.

Cannulation in infants and small children is generally performed either directly through the chest (especially postoperatively) or via the neck (carotid and jugular) vessels, due to potentially inadequate flow from the femoral vessels in small patients. While they are supported by ECMO, patients generally remain continuously ventilated to allow for surfactant production and circulation and for mobilization and extrusion of secretions to avoid infection. "Lung rest" settings, with minimal inspiratory pressure and inspired oxygen and addition of positive end-expiratory pressure to prevent atelectasis, have been suggested.[54]

In a small series of 27 children who underwent VA ECMO for cardiac indications, both nonsurgical and postcardiotomy, the overall survival rate was 59%; of these, 56% required CPR at the time ECMO support was instituted, 73% survived.[84] Hemodynamic benefits of ECMO include decreased RV preload and pulmonary artery pressures. Owing to reentry of blood into the aorta, an increase in afterload often occurs and may require pharmacologic afterload reduction therapy such as milrinone.

Several management options exist for children with single-ventricle physiology and shunt-dependent pulmonary circulation who require ECMO support. The survival rate of 10 children who underwent single-ventricle palliation and subsequently required

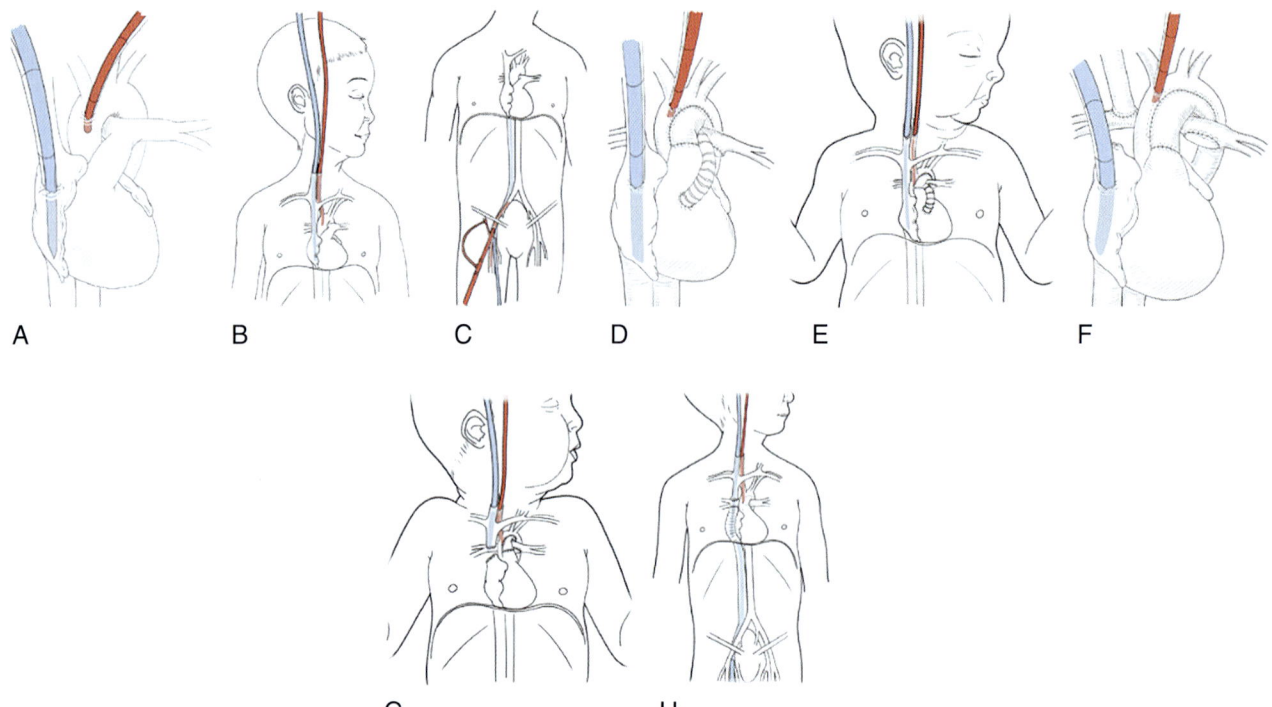

FIGURE 19.2 A–H, Cannulation strategies for rapid venous and arterial accesses for ECPR: **A, B,** and **C** show strategies for structurally normal hearts or biventricular circulation. **A,** Central cannulation with venous access in the right atrium and arterial access in the aorta. **B,** Peripheral cervical cannulation with venous access in the internal jugular vein and arterial access in the common carotid artery. **C,** Peripheral femoral cannulation with venous access in the femoral vein and arterial access in the femoral artery. Left atrial decompression may need to be considered as an additional intervention in all these approaches. For patients with single-ventricle physiology with a shunted or right ventricle to pulmonary artery conduit physiology (e.g., Norwood stage 1), strategies are shown in D and E. **D,** Stage 1 with central cannulation with venous access in the common atrium and arterial access in the aorta. **E,** Stage 1 with peripheral cannulation with venous access in the internal jugular vein and arterial access in the common carotid artery. Special care should be taken regarding cannula position in relation to the shunt as it may result in over circulation to the lungs or shunt. For patients with single-ventricle physiology with a superior cavopulmonary anastomosis (e.g., Norwood stage 2), strategies are shown in **F** and **G. F,** Stage 2 with central cannulation with venous access in superior vena cava or in common atrium and arterial access in aorta. **G,** Stage 2 with peripheral cannulation with venous access with internal jugular vein or femoral vein and arterial access with common carotid artery. If a femoral approach is only used for peripheral cannulation, one must remember that passive venous return must flow through the lungs and mechanical ventilation must be carefully optimized; added venous cannula may be required. For patients with single-ventricle physiology Stage 3 following a Fontan operation, a suggested strategy is shown in H and may be adapted to patient size. **H,** Peripheral cannulation with venous access in the internal jugular vein and or femoral vein with arterial access in the common carotid artery. Femoral venous cannula may be required depending on patient size and it is important to note that the femoral cannula should be long enough to reach the inferior vena cava drainage site into the Fontan baffle. (From Guerguerian AM, Sano M, Todd M, et al. Pediatric Extracorporeal Cardiopulmonary Resuscitation ELSO Guidelines. *ASAIO J.* 2021;67(3):229-237.)

ECMO support was greater in those in whom the aortopulmonary shunt was left open during ECMO.[85] Adequate alveolar ventilation must be provided, however, and greater ECMO flow rates are generally required to maintain adequate pulmonary and systemic circulations. In children with low PVR, pulmonary blood flow may prove to be excessive and limitation of shunt flow with surgical clips may become necessary. Although children with single-ventricle physiology have comparable overall survival rates after ECMO support compared with other cardiac patients,[84] in neonates who required ECMO after stage I palliation for HLHS, survival to hospital discharge ranged from 0% to 36%; reduced body weight, duration of support, and renal failure were associated with greater mortality.[86,87] ECMO has been successful in treating children with single-ventricle physiology who develop

acute shunt thrombosis or transient depression of ventricular function.[88] Of 44 children with single-ventricle physiology and shunts who required ECMO support, the indication for support was the strongest predictor of survival to discharge, with 81% of those cannulated for hypoxemia surviving, but only 29% of those cannulated for hypotension surviving to discharge.[89] Patients with Fontan physiology who require ECMO have a greater mortality rate (65%), possibly the result of long-standing ventricular dysfunction that is not easily reversible.[90]

ECMO for primary respiratory failure in larger pediatric patients and young adults was heavily used during the H1N1 pandemic as a number of children with respiratory failure and ARDS proved refractory to conventional and advanced modes of ventilation. According to the ELSO database, use of either VV ECMO or VA ECMO achieved a 60% survival rate in patients refractory to medical therapy.[38] Although ECMO has been used extensively during the COVID-19 pandemic in pediatric patients, currently published data regarding use and outcomes remain limited.

Disadvantages of ECMO include complex circuitry, reduced portability, the need for greater levels of systemic anticoagulation than required by VADs, the necessity for both blood prime and frequent transfusions, and decreased pulmonary blood flow. Compared with other support modalities, ECMO circuitry is complex and requires full-time supervision by trained personnel. Left atrial decompression may occasionally be inadequate, requiring either the placement of a left atrial vent or an atrial septostomy. Inadequate unloading of the left atrium can lead to mitral regurgitation and pulmonary edema or hemorrhage and can also minimize the chances of myocardial recovery when the left ventricle is not sufficiently unloaded. Most often moderate levels of ventilatory support must be maintained to ensure that well-oxygenated blood is provided to the coronary arteries, requiring tracheal intubation and sedation throughout the ECMO period.[91] However, there are recent case reports of awake or ambulatory ECMO (VV or VA) in children.[92]

Although effective for rapid rescue and short-term support, ECMO assist is most often maintained only for 1 to 3 weeks before complications limit its usefulness.[93] In children who require postcardiotomy ECMO assist, the need for prolonged support, renal failure, and low pH in the first 24 hours of support have been associated with a greater mortality.[94] Survivors of ECMO support also have greater risk of neurologic impairment than those supported with VADs, with poorer outcomes noted in younger children with more complex disease.[95]

Ventricular Assist Devices

VADs are used for cardiovascular support and are designed to reduce the work of the left ventricle, right ventricle, or both ventricles and to restore adequate cardiac output. They can be classified based on the duration of support, the mechanism by which they propel blood, and the indication for therapy (as discussed earlier). Commonly used devices in children are described in Table 19.3. The length of support is generally divided into short-term use (typically <2 weeks) and long-term

use (>2 weeks). Forward flow of blood can be achieved with a rotational device (e.g., centrifugal pumps), a pneumatic pusher plate (e.g., Berlin Heart [Berlin Heart GmbH, Berlin, Germany]), or axial flow (e.g., HeartMate 3 [Thoratec Corp., Pleasanton, CA]) (see Table 19.3).

Compared with ECMO circuits, VAD circuits have reduced priming volume owing to the lack of an oxygenator and shorter tubing and cause less trauma to blood cells. VAD circuits are composed of an inflow and outflow cannula, a pump (intracorporeal or paracorporeal), a power source with a driveline, and a system controller. Because they do not have an oxygenator or heat exchanger, they require reduced systemic anticoagulation compared with an ECMO circuit. For an LVAD, blood travels from the inflow cannula in the left atrium or the left ventricle, through the device, and into the aorta via the outflow cannula. For a right-sided VAD (RVAD), blood travels from the inflow cannula in the right atrium or the right ventricle, through the device, and into the pulmonary artery via the outflow cannula. In general, inflow cannulas in the ventricle achieve better unloading of the heart, thereby reducing wall stress, and allowing for better ventricular recovery and reduced incidence of thrombotic events.

SHORT-TERM DEVICES

The most commonly used short-term devices are centrifugal pumps providing continuous flow (Fig. 19.3). They include the Bio-Medicus Bio-Pump (Medtronic), CentriMag and PediMag (Thoratec), RotaFlow (Maquet Cardiovascular, Wayne, NJ), and TandemHeart (CardiacAssist, Pittsburgh, PA). The Impella (Abiomed, Danvers, MA) is a continuous flow axial device. The term *centrifugal pump* is not always synonymous with VAD because a centrifugal pump may also be used with an oxygenator to construct an ECMO circuit. Centrifugal pumps offer the advantage of excellent ventricular unloading and decreased wall stress, optimizing the chances of myocardial remodeling and recovery. Unloading the LV can also decrease its size and improve septal configuration, resulting in improved tricuspid valve function and RV inflow.[96] Decreased trauma to red blood cells and a less pronounced systemic inflammatory response are also observed compared with roller pumps.[97] A centrifugal pump spins, creating a vortex, with negative pressure at the inlet drawing blood into the cone and positive pressure at the outlet allowing nonpulsatile

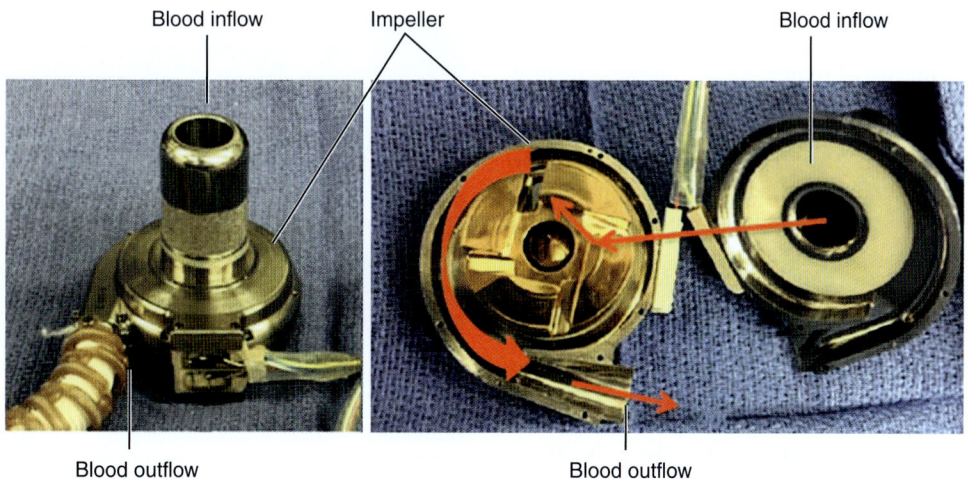

Blood inflow   Impeller   Blood inflow

Blood outflow   Blood outflow

FIGURE 19.3 In vitro example of an axial flow pump with inflow and outflow cannula *(left)*. The impeller spin provides suction to allow for propulsion *(right)*. (Courtesy of Adam C. Adler, MD.)

ejection at the base. Cardiac output from a centrifugal pump depends on preload, afterload, and the rotational speed of the pump. A flow probe is necessary because increases or decreases in preload and afterload can affect pump flow without changes in rotational speed. Excessive negative inlet pressures (hypovolemia) must be avoided because air can be entrained into the circuit. The main limitation of centrifugal pumps is the inability to provide long-term support related to issues with thrombosis, bleeding, and infection.

The RotaFlow pump is a paracorporeal, centrifugal, continuous flow device that has a rotating mechanism levitated in three magnetic fields with one point bearing, allowing laminar flow and reducing mechanical friction, heat production, and clotting potential compared with the Bio-Medicus pump (Table 19.3).[98] It can be used in patients of all sizes, irrespective of body surface area (BSA), and can flow up to 10 L/minute. It has a small priming volume (32 mL), surface area, and passage time, minimizing hemodilution and blood trauma, and can be used along with a membrane oxygenator as an ECMO circuit. It is approved by the US Food and Drug Administration (FDA) for up to 6 hours of use. However, one report described 2 months of support using the RotaFlow in an infant with a dilated cardiomyopathy.[99]

The PediMag is the pediatric version of the CentriMag. It is a paracorporeal, centrifugal, continuous flow device for children who weigh <20 kg (Table 19.3). The device does not contain bearings, instead relying on magnetically levitated technology to avoid any points of contact. This design may resist deterioration and thrombosis, contributing to its superior performance over ECMO.[100] It has a priming volume of only 14 mL and can provide up to 1.5 L/minute of flow. The PediMag is approved by the FDA for up to 6 hours of support and is also commonly used as part of an ECMO circuit.[101]

The TandemHeart is a paracorporeal, centrifugal, continuous flow device with a priming volume of 10 mL and is capable of flows up to 5 L/minute, with a hydrodynamic fluid bearing supporting the spinning rotor (Table 19.3; Fig. 19.4). Although size requirements (>40 kg) preclude its use in most children, it is advantageous because it can be placed percutaneously through the femoral vessels in either the operating room or the cardiac catheterization laboratory, with a transseptal extended-flow cannula allowing entry from the femoral vein into the left atrium. The arterial cannula can be placed directly into the femoral artery in larger patients, and in patients who weigh <80 kg, a vascular graft to the femoral artery may be cannulated to avoid lower extremity vascular compromise.[102] It is FDA approved for up to 6 hours of support.

The Impella is a microaxial continuous flow device contained in a single-pigtail catheter with three pump sizes: 2.5 L/minute (Impella 2.5 via 12 F), 3.3 L/minute (Impella CP via 14 F), and 5 L/minute (Impella 5.0 via 21 F), respectively (Fig. 19.5). The smaller pump is designed for use in adults requiring partial LV support during high-risk cardiac catheterizations and ablation procedures.[103] It can also provide full LV support in pediatric patients. In a recent multicenter study, a regression analysis was performed of cardiac MRI and echocardiography data to define minimum size requirements for placement of the smallest Impella.[104] A minimum LV apical length of 7.5 cm was required to accommodate the 7.5 cm catheter length, correlating to a height of 122 cm, weight of 23 kg, and BSA of 0.89 m².[104] The Impella is inserted retrograde through a femoral artery; with the device inlet zone resting in the LV cavity where blood is collected and propelled into the aorta, the deployment is performed under direct vision by fluoroscopy and transesophageal echocardiography

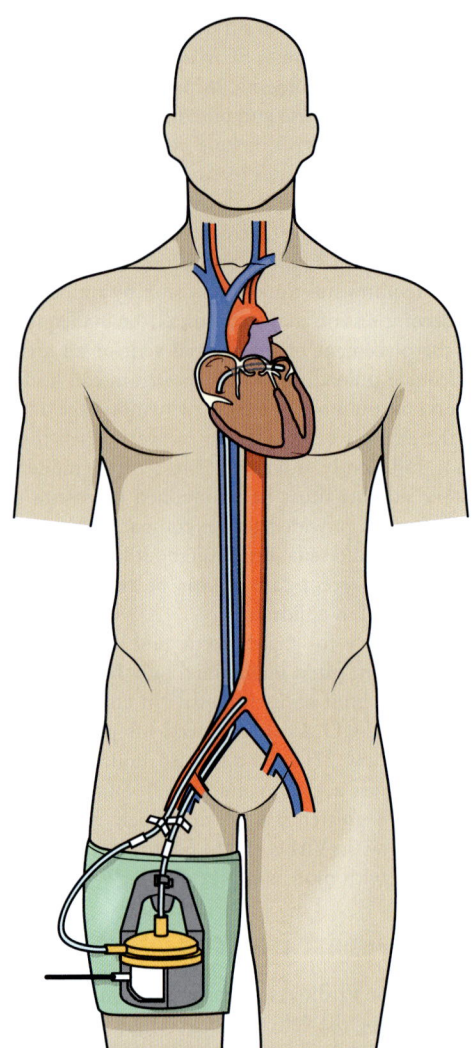

FIGURE 19.4 TandemHeart. A multistaged access cannula is inserted via the femoral vein, placed in the left atrium via a transseptal puncture. In the left atrium, left atrial blood is drained into the circuit, and returned to the systemic circulation via a single-staged return cannula in the femoral artery. (© LivaNova)

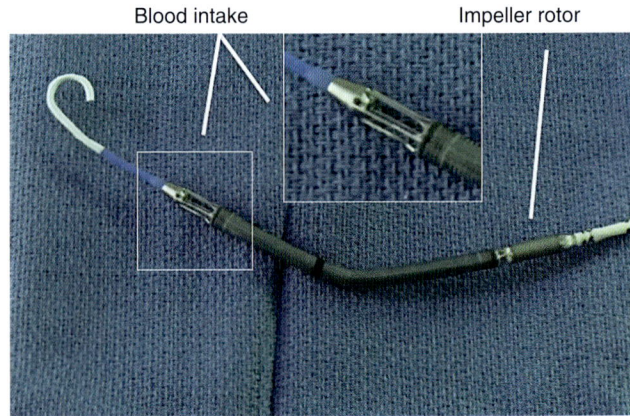

Blood intake   Impeller rotor

FIGURE 19.5 Impella microaxial continuous flow device pigtail catheter. The pigtail end with the blood intake is inserted into the left ventricle. The impeller rotor is positioned in the aortic root/ascending aorta and is electromagnetically powered, generating suction and driving blood through the outflow into the aorta. (Courtesy of Adam C. Adler, MD.)

(TEE). It has been placed into the ascending aorta in smaller patients via a sternotomy. Experience from 16 centers between 2009 and 2015 documented 39 Impella implantations, with a mean support duration of 45 hours with the primary indication cardiogenic shock.[105] This device can be placed either before or after induction of anesthesia for patients who are at high risk of developing arrhythmias or cardiac depression during the procedure.[103]

An analysis from the Organ Procurement and Transplantation Network of all children who received either ECMO or a temporary circulatory support device while awaiting transplantation between 2011 and 2015 showed an increasing trend in short-term temporary circulatory support device use. The most commonly used device, the CentriMag-PediMag (65%), had a median support duration of 24 days and demonstrated a significant survival advantage over ECMO.[100]

LONG-TERM DEVICES
Pulsatile Pumps

Pulsatile pumps are VADs that facilitate long-term support of the circulation while allowing tracheal extubation, enteral nutrition, and ambulation. They are paracorporeal and either pneumatically or electromechanically driven. Like centrifugal pumps, pulsatile VADs enjoy several advantages over ECMO. They are simpler in design, less expensive, require lower levels of anticoagulation, and may be used for left, right, or biventricular support of the circulation. Pulsatile pumps are suitable for long-term mechanical support, but until the advent of the Berlin Heart EXCOR (BHE), their use in infants and children was severely limited by patient size constraints.

The BHE ("Berlin heart") remains the most popular pediatric long-term support device. First used in adults in 1987, the BHE is a pulsatile, paracorporeal pump currently manufactured in several different pump sizes (10, 15, 25, 30, 50, and 60 mL) (Fig. 19.6).[106]

Smaller pumps are appropriate to support neonates and infants, while the 25- and 30-mL pumps will support children weighing 20 to 25 kg. The pediatric version was first used in 1992 and has since been successfully used in neonates and infants with a BSA as low as 0.2 m².[107,108] An investigational device exemption (IDE) trial was begun in the United States in 2007; before this, the BHE was used nearly 100 times in North America at 29 different institutions under compassionate use regulations. A review of 73 of these initial patients (weight 3–87.6 kg) revealed a 77% success rate in bridging to either transplant or recovery, with a median support time of 1.6 months. Younger age and the need for BiVAD support were risk factors for increased mortality.[109] The BHE received Humanitarian Device Exemption status in 2011 and postmarket approval in 2017 from the FDA. The FDA required postmarket surveillance of at least 60 patients, to be compared with patients from the previously reported BHE study. Utilizing data from the ACTION registry, the report found surveillance patients to be younger, smaller, more likely to have congenital heart disease, and supported for longer duration than those in the comparison group. Additionally, surveillance patients demonstrated greater success rates, reduced stroke rates, and reduced adverse events, suggesting improved care over time.[110]

The BHE consists of a pneumatically driven translucent polyurethane pump, trileaflet polyurethane inlet and outlet valves, and silicone inflow and outflow cannulas. The cannulas exit the skin to the paracorporeal location through the upper abdominal wall. One advantage to the external location is the ability to change the device if thrombus formation is identified. All blood-contacting surfaces, including the polyurethane valves, are heparin-coated (Carmeda AB, Upplands Väsby, Sweden). A flexible diaphragm in three layers divides the pump chamber into an air chamber and a blood chamber (Fig. 19.6), with the two diaphragm layers facing the air

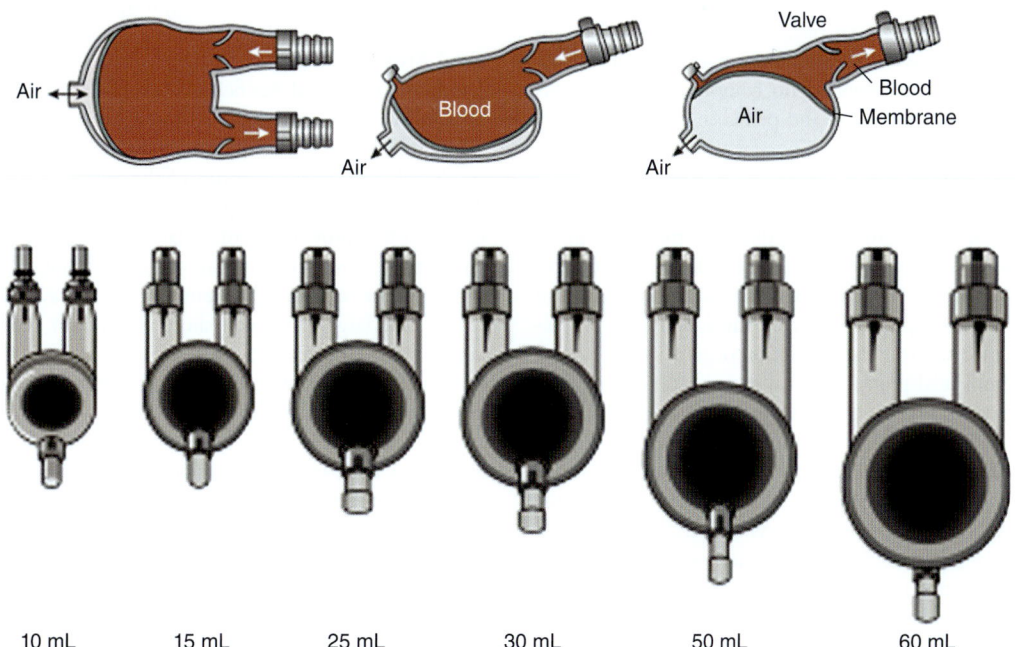

FIGURE 19.6 *Top panel,* Illustration of Berlin Heart EXCOR internal functionality. In the device, a flexible diaphragm in three layers divides the pump chamber into an air chamber and a blood chamber. (From Hetzer R, Potapov E, Stiller B, et al. Improvement in survival after mechanical circulatory support with pneumatic pulsatile ventricular assist devices in pediatric patients. *Ann Thorac Surg.* 2006;82:917-925.) *Bottom panel,* Berlin Heart EXCOR sizes 10, 15, 25, 30, 50, and 60 mL. (Reproduced with permission from Berlin Heart)

chamber serving as driving membranes and the third seamless blood membrane passively moved by the driving membranes.[111] During diastole, blood enters the pusher-plate polyurethane chamber through an inlet valve and negative pressure is generated to aid in pump filling. In systole, the blood-filled chamber is compressed from an air-filled chamber, creating pulsatile systolic flow ejected through the outlet valve into the aorta. Mechanical valves direct the flow, and there is no direct contact between the pumping mechanism and blood. The pump rate can be adjusted to between 30 and 150 beats/minute. The BHE has been successfully used to provide univentricular (left or right) or biventricular support, even in infants, and may be operated in a synchronous, asynchronous, or fill-to-empty mode. A rechargeable battery is available that can provide up to 5 hours of independent power supply for adult-sized pumps, but power requirements are greater for pediatric pump operation, owing to the greater flow resistance with small-diameter cannulas and greater pump rates.[112] A newer-generation pneumatic driver is under development that will permit discharge from the hospital for pediatric patients.[71]

Major benefits of BHE support include the ability to extubate the trachea, encourage enteral nutrition, and optimize patient mobility during long-term support. In addition, transfusions during mechanical support are less in children supported with the BHE compared with those supported with ECMO. In a study comparing 30 children receiving BHE support with 34 children supported by ECMO, transfusion requirements for platelets, packed RBCs, and FFP were significantly less in BHE patients. The overall mortality rate was also noted to be less in BHE patients.[113] Anticoagulation is currently initiated with unfractionated heparin, maintaining the activated thromboplastin time (aPTT) at 60 to 80 seconds. Thromboelastography (TEG) is also used, along with platelet aggregation tests, to monitor the use of aspirin and dipyridamole. Antithrombin III (ATIII) concentrations are closely monitored and substituted if the concentrations fall below 70%.[111] Low–molecular-weight heparin (LMWH), with monitoring of anti-factor Xa concentrations, has been used since 2007.[18] Pump exchange may be necessary if thrombus formation occurs in the valves, although one group reported no complications from this procedure during 15 years of adult and pediatric experience.[114]

Continuous Flow Pumps

The increased risk of thromboembolic events with the BHE and the current absence of an option for hospital discharge prompted interest in the pediatric application of adult continuous flow devices despite patient–device size mismatch. Continuous flow pumps can be either axial or centrifugal, depending on the design of the impeller, and are designed to limit the interaction of moving parts. Like a centrifugal pump, axial pump function depends on preload and afterload. Decreases in preload can cause emptying and collapse of the ventricle ("suction events"), whereas increases in afterload initially result in reductions in forward flow and ultimately can lead to regurgitant flow. Axial pumps offer several advantages over pulsatile pumps, including their small blood-to-device interface, the lack of a compliance chamber or artificial valves, and fewer moving parts. They are quieter than pulsatile pumps, which is a decided advantage for the child. Axial pumps can also allow some pulsatile flow to occur as the ventricle recovers, and cardiac output can increase in response to increased patient activity. The major disadvantages for children are the continuing size limitations for placement and the fact that the device provides only LV support.

The HeartMate 3 is an implantable, intracorporeal device that was FDA approved for use in adult heart failure in 2018, and

further approved with a pediatric device label in December 2020. This was based on ACTION Learning Network data from 35 pediatric patients.[115] The HeartMate 3 contains a rotor that relies on magnetic levitation rather than mechanical bearings, which reduces wear and thrombosis risk.[116] There is no minimum weight recommended by the FDA; however, according to the ACTION data, patients as small as 19 kg (BSA 0.78 m²) were implanted successfully.[116]

The HeartWare Ventricular Assist System (HeartWare Systems, Framingham, MA) (presently under recall at the time of writing this chapter) is a continuous flow device with a centrifugal pump directly attached to the inflow cannula.[117] It can provide up to 10 L/minute of flow. Although recommended for use in patients with a BSA >1.5 m², it is clear from the literature that multiple groups were using these devices off-label in smaller children[118–120]; use was reported in a toddler weighing 13 kg with a BSA of 0.65 m².[121] The HVAD is a small pump with a rotating impeller forcing blood through the device via hydrodynamic and centrifugal forces, that could be placed either adjacent to the heart in the pericardial space or in a small pocket created above the left hemidiaphragm.[122] In addition to its suitability for smaller patients, another advantage was that children could be discharged home and often return to school and pursue normal daily activities.[121] However, as of June 2021, Medtronic stopped the sale and distribution of the HeartWare due to increased risks of neurological events and mortality as well as potential for internal pump failure.[123] A retrospective analysis of 14 children implanted with the HeartWare device demonstrated increased blood trauma, as indicated by elevated lactate dehydrogenase and D-dimer values, at low pump speeds and flows.[124] In August 2021, the FDA issued a Class I recall of the device.[125] According to the Pedimacs registry, the HeartWare was implanted in 192 children between 2012 and 2017. Prophylactic explantation was not recommended. With the HeartWare withdrawal, the BHE remains the only long-term, approved device for children weighing <30 kg.[115]

Total Artificial Heart

The SynCardia Total Artificial Heart (TAH) (SynCardia Systems, Tucson, AZ) is an implantable biventricular device capable of providing to 9.5 L/minute of pulsatile flow (Fig. 19.7). Currently, there are 70-mL and 50-mL versions of the pump. It is a pneumatically driven pulsatile device designed with two prosthetic polyurethane ventricles that provide biventricular support. Each ventricle has two mechanical valves providing inflow and outflow. The TAH has the largest inflow and shortest distance of blood traveled of all available VADs. The large valves and short blood path provide little resistance, thereby decreasing stasis and thrombosis.[126,127] The 50-mL version allows application of the TAH in patients down to a BSA of 0.9 m² or in patients in whom virtual fit has determined that size is appropriate.[128,129] It is FDA approved for bridge to transplant and more than 1800 implants have occurred worldwide. Major advantages of the TAH include immediate elimination of concern regarding right heart failure, atrioventricular or aortic valve issues, dysrhythmias, LV clot, and intracardiac shunts.[71] Its use has also been described in patients with chronic graft dysfunction who are immunocompromised, as use of the TAH eliminates the need for immunosuppressive therapy.[130] A recent review of all pediatric patients under 18 years old in the SynCardia database showed 51 patients implanted with the TAH, 15 of which were supported with the newer 50-mL pump. Ten of these patients carried a diagnosis of congenital heart disease. Overall survival with the device or to transplantation was 71%.[129]

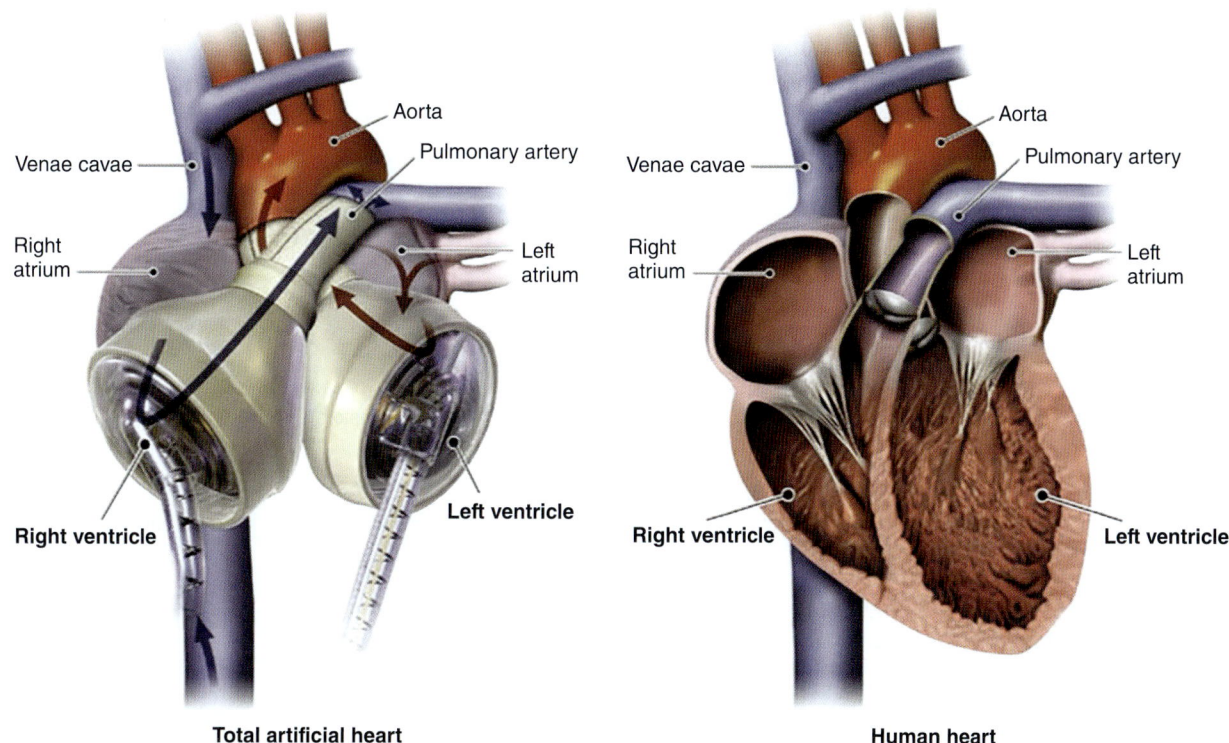

FIGURE 19.7 SynCardia Total Artificial Heart as compared with a native heart. (From Yaung J, Arabia FA, Nurok M. Perioperative care of the patient with the total artificial heart. *Anesth Analg.* 2017;124(5):1412-1422.)

Perioperative Management of Mechanical Circulatory Support

Successful management of critically ill children receiving mechanical support requires multidisciplinary expertise. The Hospital for Sick Children, Toronto, Ontario, developed an Interprofessional VAD Support Team involved in clinical care, education, and family support for patients receiving BHE support. In addition to physicians (cardiac surgeons, cardiac intensivists, heart failure and transplant cardiologists, hematologists, and psychiatrists) and nurses (cardiac and critical care), team members include pharmacists, respiratory therapists, dieticians, social workers, physiotherapists, biomedical engineers, and perfusionists.[131] Development of a team approach and use of interdisciplinary guidelines for care of these children can enhance communication, family support, and outcomes.[132–134]

HEMODYNAMICS

During ECMO support, central venous pressure (CVP) should remain low to ensure adequate venous drainage. Left atrial pressure should be closely monitored using echocardiographic evaluation of atrial septal position. An increase in left atrial pressure may indicate incomplete unloading of the left atrium and ventricle, potentially requiring a blade and/or balloon atrial septostomy or surgical placement of a left atrial vent.[135] Anatomic issues, such as the presence of aortopulmonary collateral vessels, aortic insufficiency, or a patent ductus arteriosus, can also result in a persistently increased left atrial pressure.

Increased arterial pressures and systemic vascular resistance (SVR) during ECMO can be due to large pump flows, but other causes, such as unrecognized seizure activity, inadequate pain or

sedation management, and hypothermia, should also be considered. High SVR during ECMO support can be pharmacologically managed. In general, mean arterial pressures should be maintained at a level appropriate to the child's size and body weight.

Unlike ECMO support, LVAD support requires maintenance of effective RV output to provide adequate LV preload. Right ventricular failure, pulmonary hypertension, and arrhythmias can all limit left ventricular filling and must, therefore, be aggressively treated.[136] Other potential causes of inadequate left ventricular filling include cannula malposition or low intravascular volume. CVP can be used to evaluate volume status. Serial echocardiograms are useful to assess RV function and estimate RV and pulmonary artery pressures. Clinical signs of right-sided heart failure include increased central venous or right atrial pressures, hepatomegaly, peripheral edema, and decreasing hemoglobin-oxygen saturations. Right ventricular function can be augmented pharmacologically with drugs such as milrinone or isoproterenol. Increased pulmonary artery pressures are best initially treated by ensuring adequate alveolar ventilation, and subsequently by using inhaled nitric oxide if necessary. Mechanical issues, such as cardiac tamponade, can also negatively affect hemodynamics. These can be diagnosed at the bedside using echocardiography. Inadequate LV decompression can increase left atrial and pulmonary artery pressures and may be treated by augmenting LVAD flow; if necessary, biventricular or ECMO support can be initiated.[137]

Children supported by VADs often require vasodilators to maintain the low SVR necessary for optimal pump function. Frequently used vasodilators include milrinone, hydralazine, β-blockers, angiotensin-converting enzyme (ACE) inhibitors, and clonidine. Left atrial pressure is optimally maintained at 3 to 4 mm Hg, while allowing some ventricular ejection to avoid stasis.

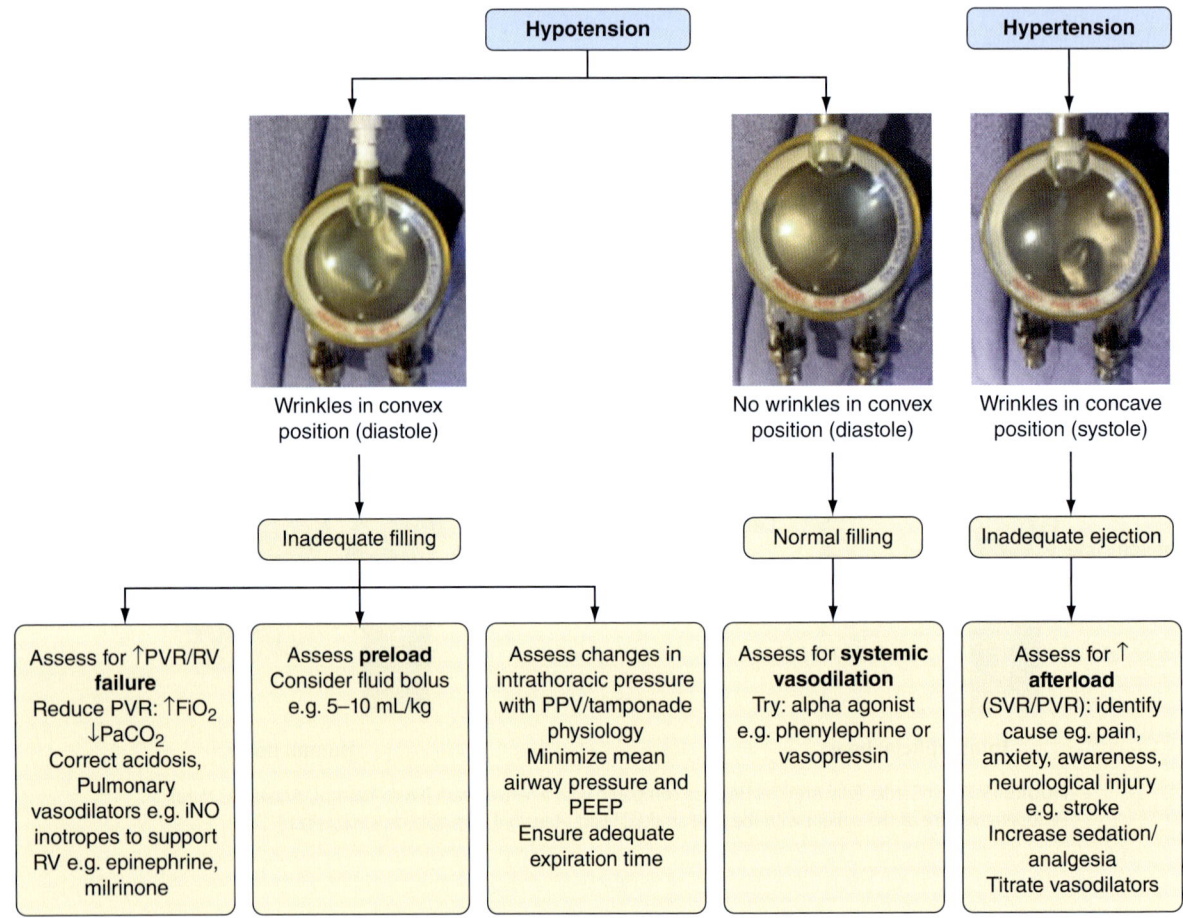

FIGURE 19.8 Berlin Heart EXCOR perioperative troubleshooting guide. Target MAPs and flows specific to the patient should be defined preoperatively. *iNO,* Inhaled nitric oxide; *PEEP,* positive end-expiratory pressure; *PPV,* positive pressure ventilation; *PVR,* pulmonary vascular resistance; *RV,* right ventricle; *SVR,* systemic vascular resistance. FiO_2, fraction of inspired oxygen; *MAP,* mean arterial pressure; $PaCO_2$, arterial partial pressure of carbon dioxide; *iNO,* inhaled nitric oxide; *MAP,* mean arterial pressure. (From Navaratnam M, Maeda K, Hollander SA. Pediatric ventricular assist devices: bridge to a new era of perioperative care. *Paediatr Anaesth.* 2019;29(5):506-518.)

Systemic mixed venous hemoglobin-oxygen saturation, either continuously via in-line monitoring with a centrifugal VAD, or intermittently with a paracorporeal pulsatile VAD, is a useful metric to monitor the adequacy of cardiac output. Strategies for maintaining hemodynamics with VAD support as well as treatment of hypotension are summarized in Figs. 19.8 and 19.9.

RESPIRATORY CONSIDERATIONS
Although ECMO can provide full cardiopulmonary support, tracheal intubation and mechanical ventilation help to avoid atelectasis and optimize oxygenation of blood returning to the left atrium that will provide coronary artery blood flow. Modest ventilator settings are generally recommended: (1) 6 to 8 mL/kg tidal volume, (2) 5 to 10 cm H_2O of positive end-expiratory pressure, (3) a rate of 10 to 12 breaths/minute, and (4) a fractional inspired oxygen value of 0.4 or less (to avoid oxygen toxicity). Recently "awake" VA ECMO has been reported in children, including allowing the tracheas to be extubated during support.[138] Maintenance of adequate ventilation is particularly important in children with single-ventricle physiology with an open systemic-pulmonary shunt. Because of the complexity of the ECMO circuit, mechanical issues such as oxygenator malfunction must be

considered when increasing hypoxemia occurs. After ruling out oxygenator failure, ECMO flow may be increased, or the membrane size may be increased to improve systemic oxygenation.

Children supported by VADs receive only cardiac support. With centrifugal VAD support, the trachea generally remains intubated, and the lungs mechanically ventilated. Paracorporeal pulsatile VADs and implantable VADs, on the other hand, allow children to be weaned to extubation. Anatomic issues, such as an atrial septal defect, should be recognized as potential causes of hypoxemia from right-to-left shunting.[139] Children who receive LV support via either a centrifugal or pulsatile VAD may also require inhaled nitric oxide to decrease PVR and augment RV function.

HEMATOLOGIC CONSIDERATIONS
Anticoagulation management continues to be one of the most challenging clinical issues in caring for children who require MCS, in part owing to age-based differences in the coagulation cascade (see Chapters 8 and 18).[140] Patients who require mechanical support are at risk for hemorrhage and/or thromboembolic complications.[141] Ongoing hemorrhage around cannulation sites is a frequent issue, particularly with ECMO support.

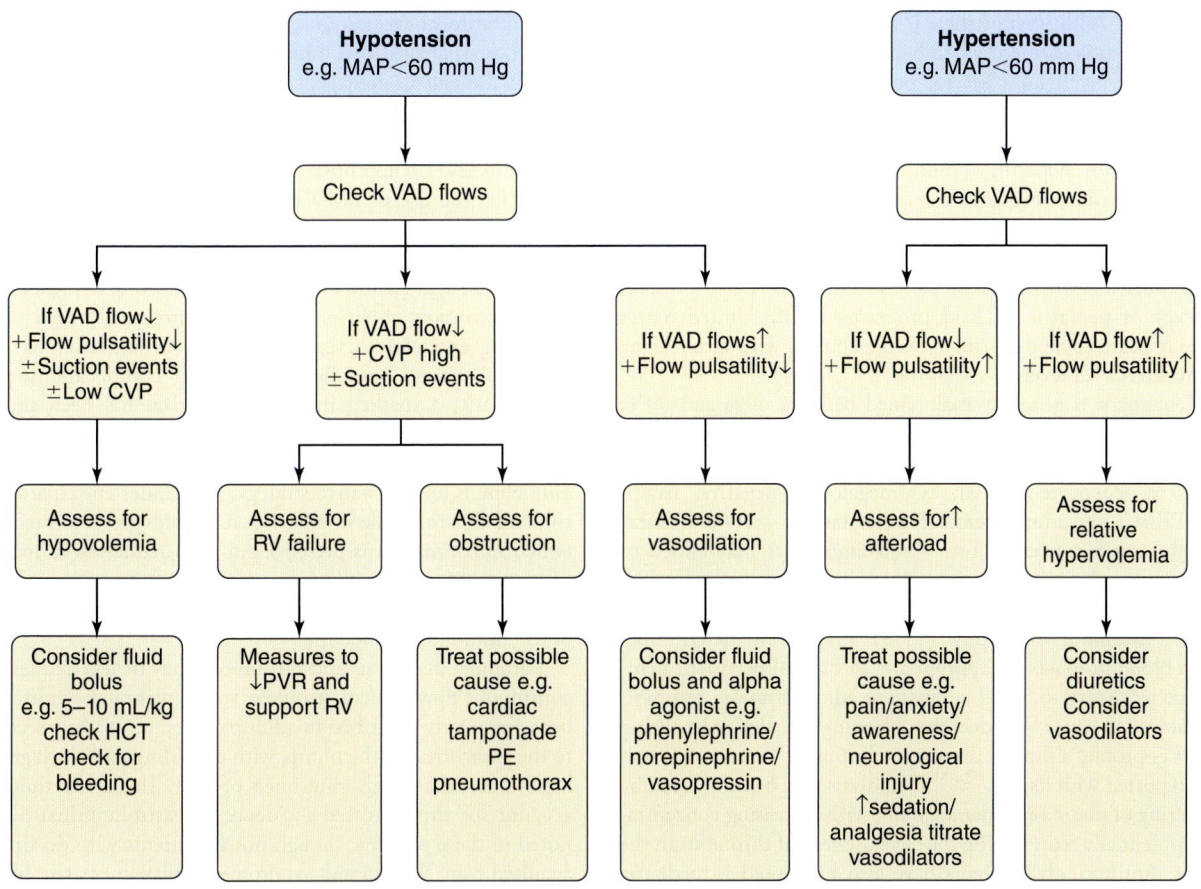

FIGURE 19.9 Continuous flow devices perioperative troubleshooting guide. Target MAPs and flows specific to the patient should be defined preoperatively. *CVP,* Central venous pressure; *LV,* left ventricle; *MAP,* mean arterial pressures; *PE,* pulmonary embolus; *PVR,* pulmonary vascular resistance; *RPM,* revolutions per minute (ventricular assist device speed); *RV,* right ventricle. (From Navaratnam M, Maeda K, Hollander SA. Pediatric ventricular assist devices: bridge to a new era of perioperative care. *Paediatr Anaesth.* 2019;29(5):506-518.)

Of greater concern are gastrointestinal (GI), pulmonary, or, more devastatingly, intracranial hemorrhage; infarctions or thromboembolic events may also occur. Serial ultrasonography of the head may be used to monitor for intracranial bleeding in infants and neonates, and, when possible, computed tomography may be used in older children.

Contact with the nonendothelial surfaces in an ECMO circuit can activate hemostatic agents, including platelets, factor XII, tissue factor, and von Willebrand factor (vWF). There is also a tendency toward fibrinolysis and release of proinflammatory cytokines. This leads to both a state of hypercoagulability and coagulopathy in ECMO patients. These effects are more pronounced in neonates and infants because of their lower blood volume relative to circuit size.[142] Destruction of platelets and coagulation factors and an increase in fibrinolysis can cause bleeding around cannula sites and, more detrimentally, in intracavitary spaces. Activation of tissue factor and the inflammatory system contribute to hypercoagulability, which can cause both internal and circuit thrombosis. It is the role of the ECMO team to balance this precarious state of coagulation.

Traditionally, unfractionated heparin has been the first-line drug for maintenance of anticoagulation during ECMO therapy. Heparin binds to ATIII, producing anticoagulation via inhibition of activated factors IXa, Xa, XIa, XIIa, and, to a lesser extent, IIA (thrombin). Infants tend to have reduced ATIII concentrations and can rapidly develop acquired ATIII deficiency during MCS, which is reflected by the need for increased supplementation of ATIII to provide adequate levels in this age group.[143,144] The anticoagulation effect of heparin is most commonly monitored with the activated clotting time (ACT), a real-time bedside test that measures whole blood clotting after exposing the blood to either kaolin or celite activators. Although ECMO protocols vary, ACTs are generally maintained between 180 and 220 seconds using heparin infused at 10 to 50 units/kg per hour. The use of heparin-bonded tubing can reduce the need for long ACTs. There are numerous concerns regarding the reliability of ACT monitoring and its correlation with heparin concentration in pediatric patients on ECMO. Many factors, including hemodilution, temperature, reduction in coagulation factors, and platelet dysfunction, may alter ACT results. Some centers rely on alternative monitoring tests including aPTT, anti-factor Xa concentration assays, anti-factor Xa range, TEG, and rotational TEG.[145,146] Recently, some centers have moved to using bivalirudin for systemic anticoagulation on ECMO.

Bivalirudin directly inhibits thrombin irrespective of ATIII and provides inhibition for both circulating and clot-bound thrombin.[147] Additionally, there is no requirement for monitoring of ACT as is required when heparin is used. A single-center reporting of bivalirudin use for pediatric anticoagulation during ECMO demonstrated shorter time to anticoagulation, reduced cost with no increase in adverse bleeding events when compared with heparin.[148] Additionally, bivalirudin has become more commonly used for neonatal ECMO, particularly in children with congenital diaphragmatic hernia requiring support.[149] Direct thrombin inhibitors may be well suited to this population with unpredictable levels of ATIII. At present, a survey of pediatric ECMO programs in the United States shows heparin to be the primary anticoagulant with monitoring of anti-factor Xa levels.[150]

Hematocrit is generally maintained between 40% and 50%, although efforts are made to limit transfusions because most children are potential candidates for cardiac transplantation. When necessary, leukocyte-reduced, cytomegalovirus-negative, irradiated PRBCs are administered. Platelet counts >100,000/mm³ and fibrinogen concentrations >100 mg/dL are maintained to minimize bleeding complications.[151] In the presence of continued bleeding, cryoprecipitate and/or FFP may be added to the circuit prime. Thromboelastography (TEG) may assist determining which blood products are appropriate. In cases of persistent hemorrhage refractory to blood component administration, recombinant activated factor VIIa decreases bleeding and aids normalizing the TEG profile, although disastrous clotting of circuitry has also been reported with its use.[152-155] Hemolysis may be monitored by measuring of plasma-free hemoglobin, with increasing concentrations potentially representing the development of thrombus in the circuit. Antifibrinolytic agents have also been used in pediatric patients receiving ECMO therapy, albeit with limited available data.[156] ε-aminocaproic acid has been associated with an increased frequency of thrombotic or cerebral events,[157] although recent evidence raises doubts about this concern.[158] Since 2011, the use of tranexamic acid during pediatric ECMO has increased, and is now used as frequently as ε-aminocaproic acid.[156,157]

Without an oxygenator in the circuit, anticoagulation requirements are not as stringent for children on VADs, and the ACT may be maintained between 140 and 180 seconds. A percutaneously placed VAD, such as the TandemHeart, requires a target ACT greater than 180 seconds. Most long-term VADs, such as the BHE, are placed while the patient is supported by CPB and under full anticoagulation. Once weaned from bypass, the heparin is fully reversed with protamine. In the first 24 hours after VAD placement, a reoperation to achieve hemostasis may be required. After the immediate postoperative period, the risk of bleeding decreases while the risk of thrombosis increases. Unfractionated heparin infusions are used with a target aPTT of 1.5 times normal. The ATIII concentrations are also monitored and maintained in excess of 70% to avoid thrombotic complications. The use of argatroban (a small molecule direct thrombin inhibitor) has been described in children with heparin-induced thrombocytopenia type II.[159] A recent multicenter study investigating the use of direct thrombin inhibitors for continuous flow devices demonstrated encouraging results.[24] There was an adverse event rate for major bleeding of 16% (2.6 events per 1,000 patient days) and a rate of stroke of 12% (1.7 events per 1000 patient days).[24]

There is a wide variability of in-hospital anticoagulation management for children with assist devices.[160] Most institutions follow the Edmonton antithrombotic protocol once the patient is discharged from the ICU. This protocol involves a three-drug regimen: aspirin, dipyridamole, and either warfarin (for patients ≥12 months of age) or enoxaparin (for patients <12 months of age). Enoxaparin is used more frequently in infants because warfarin is difficult to manage, as infants are more likely to use vitamin K–containing formulas and have changes in diet during their growth. There is also scant information about the dose of warfarin in infants and no appropriate formulations (i.e., suspensions) are available. The use of LMWH requires the use of anti-factor Xa activity monitoring.[161,162] After normalizing the platelet count and function, aspirin and dipyridamole are started, using TEG and platelet aggregation tests to monitor clotting tendency, with a target activation of 30%. Once an appropriately aged child is tolerating enteral feedings, a transition to warfarin may commence. Although embolic and bleeding complications remain problematic, a marked increase in survival has been noted in children undergoing BHE support with this management strategy compared with earlier regimens.[163] The Stanford Antithrombotic Guideline is an alternative strategy; it includes enoxaparin, aspirin, and dipyridamole in addition to clopidogrel and prednisone (when inflammation is present). An 84% reduction in incidence of stroke (0.8 vs. 4.9 events per 1000 days) was observed in patients using the Stanford Guideline when compared with the use of the Edmonton Guideline.[164]

Although hemolysis and thrombosis may be less frequent with continuous flow devices, acquired von Willebrand syndrome has been frequently described in adult patients, most likely secondary to the shear stress of the pump, with unfolding and cleavage of the high–molecular-weight multimers of vWF. This is also thought to account for the increased incidence of gastrointestinal bleeding noted in these patients, though not all patients with documented acquired von Willebrand syndrome display increased bleeding tendencies.[165,166]

PREVENTION OF INFECTION

Infection is a constant concern, particularly in children requiring intermediate- to long-term ECMO and VAD support. Devices with larger surface area and areas of turbulent flow are associated with greater infection rates owing to increased adherence of blood-borne pathogens. As a result, smaller, fully implantable devices and devices with improved flow dynamics may decrease the incidence of infection.[167,168] Devices such as the BHE allow for removal of tracheal tubes, indwelling catheters, and intravenous lines; minimize the need for blood transfusions; and offer a reduced risk of device-related infections.[113,169] Deep wound complications of inflow and outflow cannulas have been successfully treated with vacuum-assisted wound closure systems.[170] Children with the HeartMate 3 device can be discharged home and this may lessen hospital-acquired infection.

The use of MCS can result in immunologic dysfunction, further increasing infection risk.[171] Signs and symptoms of infection can be subtle, and a need for increasing inotropic support to maintain mean arterial pressure can often be a harbinger of infection. Endogenous reactions to infection can also result in activation of the coagulation cascade, increasing the difficulty of anticoagulation management.[172] Many children prophylactically receive antibiotics with Gram-positive coverage, as well as oral nystatin for fungal prophylaxis.

ANESTHETIC CONSIDERATIONS

In preparing for the anesthetic care of infants and children, either when ECMO or VAD support is being used or when implementation of MCS is imminent, initial planning centers on two main areas of concern: the child's current status and the location of the proposed procedure (Table 19.4). The need for emergency surgery, the child's condition at the time of surgery, the presence of preoperative multiorgan failure, and the need for CPB with cross-clamping of the aorta have all been shown to increase perioperative risk.[173]

A comprehensive preoperative evaluation is essential, encompassing knowledge of the underlying pathology necessitating MCS and the length of the child's illness, along with evaluation of other potential multiorgan dysfunction, including neurologic, hematologic, renal, hepatic, and pulmonary issues. Review of current drug therapy, particularly the duration and degree of current inotropic support, anticoagulation protocols, sedation regimens, cardiac function, intravascular volume status, and the presence and degree of preoperative hemorrhage, is also necessary. A detailed physical examination should include the airway and both current vascular access as well as potential sites for additional vascular access. In infants, ultrasonography of the head is useful before considering institution of MCS, as intraventricular hemorrhage is a relative contraindication to MCS. Similarly, infants on ECMO, especially those younger than 35 weeks gestation, are at high risk for cerebral bleeding and are often monitored with daily head ultrasounds.[174]

Preoperative laboratory evaluation should include a complete blood cell count (CBC) with platelet count, electrolytes, blood urea nitrogen and creatinine concentrations, prothrombin time and partial thromboplastin time, and liver function tests. Concentrations of BNP, produced in the myocardium, serve as a marker of ventricular overloading and have been shown in adults and children with congenital heart disease to correlate with the degree of ventricular dysfunction.[175,176] Serial BNP concentrations in

TABLE 19.4	Anesthetic Considerations
Preoperative Assessment *History*	**Intraoperative Management** *Availability of blood products* *Monitoring*

Etiology and duration of cardiac failure	Standard ASA monitors
	    Electrocardiogram
	    Noninvasive blood pressure
	    End-tidal CO$_2$
	    Temperature
	    Peripheral oxygen saturation

Review of system/end-organ dysfunction	
Pulmonary	
Renal	
Hepatic	
Neurologic	Assess need for invasive arterial or central venous monitoring
Medications Inotropic/vasoactive support	Urine output

Angiotensin-converting enzyme inhibitors
    Antiarrhythmic therapy
    Anticoagulation protocols
    Analgesic/sedative drugs
    Antibiotics
	Echocardiography

	Presence of septal defects
	Aortic insufficiency
	Mitral stenosis
Planned surgical procedure	Cardiac de-airing
Timing of procedure: elective/urgent/emergent	Ventricular function
Laboratory	*Management principles*

Hematology
    Complete blood cell count
    Platelet count
	Maintain adequate intravascular volume/preload for ventricular assist device
	    Avoid abrupt decreases in preload

Serum chemistries
    Electrolytes
    Liver function studies
    Blood urea nitrogen, creatinine
    B-type natriuretic peptide concentration
	Support right ventricular function, reduce pulmonary vascular resistance
	    Nitric oxide availability

	Maintain adequate ventilation
	Inotropic support: milrinone, prostaglandin E$_1$

Coagulation studies
    Prothrombin time/partial thromboplastin time
    Fibrinogen concentration
    Activated clotting time
    Thromboelastogram
	Hypotension can be treated with volume or α-adrenergic agonists

	Postoperative Issues
Physical examination	Transport to intensive care unit
Airway	Control of ongoing hemorrhage
Vascular access, both existing and available	Timing of extubation
Neurologic status	
Evidence of ongoing hemorrhage	
Assessment of intravascular volume status	

children supported with ECMO have also been used to predict clinical outcomes, with greater BNP concentrations noted after termination of ECMO support in nonsurvivors than in children who ultimately survived.[177]

Useful preoperative coagulation data includes recent TEG results, fibrinogen concentrations, and platelet function tests, if available. The most recent echocardiography data and chest radiograph should be reviewed. Blood products, including PRBCs, platelets, cryoprecipitate, and FFP, should be available at the bedside or in the OR, with provision for a continuing supply of products as needed. PRBCs should preferably be cytomegalovirus-negative, leukocyte-reduced, and irradiated, because all of these children should be considered potential transplant candidates (note that the potassium concentration of irradiated PRBCs may be greatly increased, resulting in acute hyperkalemia if administered rapidly). Appropriate antibiotic prophylaxis should be discussed with the surgeon.

Standard American Society of Anesthesiologists monitoring should be employed before induction of anesthesia. Depending on the child's condition and the type of surgery planned, the use of arterial and central venous lines should be considered if not already present. In children who have been in the ICU for a prolonged time or those undergoing current resuscitation, securing additional vascular access lines can be challenging and may occasionally require surgical assistance. In most centers, children undergo ultrasound assessment of vessels to assure their patency before implementation of a VAD. This is particularly important for children with congenital heart disease who have previously undergone cardiac surgeries and catheterizations. For children already receiving mechanical support, it is important to know that VAD ejection is usually asynchronous with the child's underlying heart rate, yielding a discrepancy between the observed electrocardiographic and the arterial line waveform. Multiple peripheral intravenous lines are useful for the administration of volume and blood products. If RVAD support is being used, special care must be taken not to entrain air if the great veins are accessed.

Anesthesia for the VAD Patient With Cardiac Disease

Etomidate is generally an advantageous drug for induction of anesthesia because it does not depress myocardial contractility at clinically relevant concentrations, even in children with severely compromised ventricular function.[178] Judicious and incremental doses of opioids and benzodiazepines may be used with consideration given to the patient's reduced cardiac output, slow circulation time, and limited ability to compensate for changes in preload or afterload. The choice of a neuromuscular blocking drug is usually based on the presence of hepatic or renal dysfunction or duration of block intended. Adequate depth of anesthesia should be ensured before tracheal intubation to avoid abrupt increases in PVR, particularly in children with marginal RV function. Children may be less responsive to β-adrenergic agonists owing to depletion of myocardial catecholamines and downregulation of β receptors.[179] This can also make them more susceptible to the myocardial depressant effects of ketamine.[179] Hypotension on induction of anesthesia and decreased responsiveness to catecholamines may also be observed in children receiving long-term ACE inhibitors for afterload reduction preoperatively.[55,180,181] Opioids, benzodiazepines, and neuromuscular blocking agents are generally used to maintain anesthesia before ECMO cannulation or initiation of CPB for VAD implementation, with the express goal of maintaining adequate cardiac output and resultant systemic perfusion to end organs. Serial serum lactate concentrations, mixed

venous hemoglobin-oxygen saturations, and the presence or absence of metabolic acidosis are useful indexes to evaluate the adequacy of cardiac output. Emergent institution of CPB may occasionally be necessary due to cardiac decompensation or ongoing hemorrhage in patients who have had previous sternotomies.

The effects of positive pressure ventilation should also be considered for patients whose lungs were not previously mechanically ventilated. Although patients with left heart failure might benefit from decreases in afterload reduction, high mean airway pressures and the use of positive end-expiratory pressure (PEEP) may prove detrimental for some patients, particularly those with single-ventricle physiology. In general, respiratory goals should aim to minimize mean airway pressures, and avoid prolonged inspiratory time or excessive PEEP.

Unless contraindicated, a TEE probe should be placed after the induction of anesthesia for use throughout the procedure. Initial TEE assessment is important to determine the presence of intracardiac shunts that would require closing before initiating mechanical support. Aortic valve competence should be evaluated because greater than trivial insufficiency can recirculate blood through an LVAD. The mitral valve should be examined for significant stenosis that could limit LV inflow. After device placement, TEE ensures that adequate cardiac de-airing has occurred, evaluates ventricular function, monitors the orientation of intracardiac cannulas, and evaluates whether the left atrium and ventricle have been decompressed after pump activation. In smaller patients, the potential impact of the TEE probe on respiratory dynamics should be noted. If the use of TEE is not possible, epicardial echocardiography may also be used.

For children undergoing LVAD placement, as the venous line from the CPB circuit is occluded, the pump speed is gradually increased. If LVAD flow (and rate when fill-to-empty mode is used) is less than desired, the major areas of concern center on hypovolemia or poor RV function. The RV should be monitored closely for signs of dysfunction or failure that can result in decreased LVAD output, high CVP, and RV distention on TEE. In children with preexisting RV dysfunction, pulmonary vasodilatory agents, such as milrinone, prostaglandin E_1, or inhaled nitric oxide, should be aggressively used to optimize right-sided heart function. In a recent single-center review of pediatric VAD implementation, inhaled nitric oxide was utilized on separation from CPB in 96% of patients.[182] Children with low pressures and signs of vasodilatory shock may require infusions of vasopressin, epinephrine, or norepinephrine to support the circulation; adequate volume loading and VAD output should be ensured. In patients with ongoing bleeding or a poorly contractile RV, the chest may be left open electively at the end of surgery.

Difficulty in predicting drug pharmacokinetics is another important consideration in patients undergoing VAD or ECMO placement.[183,184] These patients frequently have altered hepatorenal perfusion and function, drug interactions, reduced protein binding, and may additionally be receiving renal replacement therapy. ECMO, in particular, complicates drug pharmacokinetics related to the volume of the circuit, the polymer components, and altered perfusion and drug eliminations. At the time of commencing ECMO, the volume of fluid within the membrane oxygenator and tubing increases the circulating blood volume by 200 to 300 mL depending on the circuit. Drugs with large volumes of distribution such as fentanyl show little change in plasma concentration with the increases in circulating volume. However, drugs with smaller volumes of distribution such as nondepolarizing neuromuscular blocking agents and the antibiotics gentamycin and vancomycin, have larger changes in plasma concentration and may therefore have a prolonged elimination half-life. Hemodilution with ECMO may also be associated with reduced concentrations of plasma proteins, which in turn would increase the free fraction of highly protein-bound drugs. Drug adsorption can occur on the large surface area of the tubing or the membrane oxygenator of the circuit, further increasing the volume of distribution of drugs. The opposite may occur when a drug is discontinued; it is then released back into the circulation, adding further unpredictability to its disposition and potential prolongation of its effect.[185] The degree of this sequestration depends on both the materials used in the circuit and the nature of the drugs. In general, drugs that are lipophilic such as opioids, propofol, and benzodiazepines are more likely to adhere to the walls of the tubing.[186,187] Drug clearance may improve in children supported by ECMO, coincident with better organ function as oxygenated blood flow to those organs improves.[188] Multiple factors in this patient population make accurate prediction of drug doses extremely challenging and understanding of the variables involved is essential.

The timing of tracheal extubation depends on the child's preoperative condition, degree of preexisting pulmonary dysfunction, duration of the surgical procedure, extent of postoperative bleeding, and maintenance of appropriate hemodynamic parameters. Tracheal extubation at the conclusion of the procedure is not generally an option for those undergoing ECMO or centrifugal VAD support, but children receiving pulsatile VADs or axial pumps may potentially be candidates for tracheal extubation with minimal bleeding and appropriate hemodynamic parameters.

Anesthesia for the VAD Patient for Noncardiac Surgery

With the steadily increasing use of VAD support in infants and children, the need to provide anesthesia for noncardiac surgery during the period of support also continues to grow. Although these patients should generally be cared for in centers with personnel and resources accustomed to caring for children with VADs, the increasing number of children discharged to home while receiving mechanical support raises the possibility that these patients can require emergent care at other institutions. Care coordination is necessary, and it is prudent to conduct a preoperative discussion with all perioperative team members to discuss the specifics and concerns related to caring for a patient with a VAD. Whenever possible, consultation with an anesthesia provider who is experienced in caring for these patients should be sought.

Before surgery, the patient's baseline VAD flow parameters should be identified to readily identify any deviations from the new physiologic "normal." Whenever possible, assistance from the perfusion or device management team should be sought, and ideally a member of that team should be present throughout the procedure. The VAD should remain connected to wall power whenever possible and backup batteries should be fully charged. A mirror should be available for Berlin heart devices to assess chamber filling and emptying during the procedure, and for continuous flow devices the display screen or controller should remain visible throughout surgery.

Clear communication regarding ongoing therapies is essential. The need for temporary conversion from warfarin or LMWH to an unfractionated heparin infusion should be discussed with both the specific team managing the patient's anticoagulation strategies and the surgical team, and appropriate blood products ordered. Drugs such as ACE inhibitors, β-blockers, and diuretics, as well as infusions such as milrinone are often delivered. Preoperative

discussions should clearly delineate the desired perioperative management of these therapies. Specific considerations or vulnerabilities related to the patient's unique circumstances should also be considered, such as the presence of ongoing RV dysfunction or single-ventricle physiology.

Noninvasive blood pressure monitoring can be challenging in patients with VADs, and reliable noninvasive blood pressure monitoring may be difficult. Sampling errors and the ability to obtain reliable cuff pressures should be established before induction. Arterial access is often warranted to continuously measure mean arterial blood pressure. Intraoperative use of transthoracic or TEE may be helpful to continuously assess volume status, monitor inflow cannula patency, and to help diagnose any alterations in VAD output. Adequate venous access should be secured, particularly if significant blood loss or fluid shifts are anticipated.

VADs depend on adequate preload for filling and avoiding excessive afterload so as not to impede forward flow. For children receiving VAD support, appropriate pump function continues independently of the induction drugs used, provided adequate preload is maintained and no acute changes occur in SVR. With the BHE device, cardiac output is limited by the device chamber size and the programmed heart rate, making the patient sensitive to decreases in preload and SVR.[189,190] Continuous flow devices are preload-dependent and sensitive to increases in afterload. It is often prudent to administer a fluid bolus (5–10 mL/kg) before induction of anesthesia while monitoring chamber filling and emptying in the BHE and flow and pulsatility index for continuous flow devices.[191] When anesthesia is induced with ketamine, hypotension that requires support with a fluid bolus or α-adrenergic agonists is less likely to occur in children with BHE support.[189] In addition to inotropic medications, alpha-agonists such as phenylephrine or vasopressin should be available to treat vasodilation-induced hypotension. As continuing function of an LVAD relies on adequate right heart function, measures to maintain or increase right heart output may be required. Care should be taken to avoid conditions that can increases PVR, as right ventricular failure is the likeliest cause of decompensation in such patients. Nitric oxide and appropriate vasoactive drugs should be readily available if needed. When possible, spontaneous ventilation is preferred to enhance venous return and maintain hemodynamic stability.[103,190] Before induction of anesthesia, defibrillation pads should be applied as rhythms other than sinus may reduce VAD inflow.

For cases involving laparoscopic surgery, the use of minimal insufflation pressures should be discussed with the surgical team as excessive pressures can adversely affect VAD filling conditions. Additionally, extreme positioning maneuvers such as steep reverse Trendelenburg may decrease VAD preload resulting in hypotension and low cardiac output states.

Outcomes and Complications

OUTCOMES

According to data from the US Organ Procurement and Transplantation Network (OPTN), pediatric VAD implantation, particularly of the BHE and HeartMate 3, continues to rise.[192] Regardless of the type of mechanical support chosen, it has become increasingly apparent that the indication for and timing of initiation of support are major factors for determining outcome. Age can also affect outcomes, with patients under 1-year-old demonstrating a lower survival than older children.[17] Although the majority of children with cardiac disease have structural congenital defects, only 25% of children undergoing VAD implantation have structural disease.[17,193] Universally, survival has been greater in children who required support secondary to acute myocarditis or dilated cardiomyopathy compared with children who received support because of congenital heart defects or post cardiotomy failure.[17,194-196] Patients who present with a long-standing cardiomyopathy and who require VAD support as a result of gradual or acute decompensation represent a much different cohort than those who have congenital heart disease and require salvage VAD support postoperatively. Mortality in the latter group is greater, particularly if they also require ECMO to bridge them to VAD support.

When feasible, VAD support offers several major advantages over ECMO. The lack of an oxygenator simplifies the circuit and reduces the need for anticoagulation and trauma to blood elements. Neurologic deficits occur more commonly in patients supported by ECMO than in those supported with VADs, particularly in younger children with more complex heart disease,[95] although the frequency of neurologic complications with VV ECMO is less than with VA ECMO.[197,198] Additionally, evidence suggests that VAD support provides superior ventricular decompression and physiologic rest, promoting myocardial recovery in children with acute myocarditis or dilated cardiomyopathy by normalizing the ventricular geometry and reverse remodeling.[199-201] Children with chronic heart failure who are waiting for transplantation and who experience progressive multiorgan dysfunction benefit from the use of pulsatile VADs with recovery of pulmonary, renal, and hepatic function.[202]

In some children, transition to VAD support may follow initial ECMO support.[109,195] Patients supported with ECMO may require transition to a VAD if they do not achieve adequate myocardial recovery and cannot be weaned from ECMO. Most often these patients are supported with ECMO after congenital heart surgery or cardiopulmonary support. Rarely, children previously listed for transplantation deteriorate rapidly requiring emergent institution of MCS and thus are initially supported by ECMO. In evaluating VAD usage and outcomes, one review reported that 21% of 187 children with VADs had prior ECMO support.[195] Regardless of diagnosis, the use of ECMO to bridge patients to VAD is associated with significantly decreased survival; children in whom ECMO was initiated for cardiac failure after cardiac surgery and who required VAD support for continued cardiac dysfunction had particularly poor survival rates.

Single-center reports of the use of BHE in children in the United States increased in the early 2000s, with markedly improved transplant wait-list survival.[109,203] This resulted in the NHLBI-sponsored randomized, controlled trial of the BHE VAD in 2006, with results published in 2012.[27] This study, notable for being the first controlled trial of a VAD in children, led the FDA to issue IDE approval for the BHE. Using strict inclusion criteria, 48 patients were enrolled, 24 with BSA less than 0.7 m² and 24 with BSA 0.7 to 1.5 m². The prospectively enrolled patients were compared with a historical control group of patients who received ECMO support. Survival to transplantation occurred in a substantially greater proportion of patients supported with the BHE VAD compared with patients receiving ECMO, whereas the time for which support was provided without catastrophic neurologic events was significantly greater in the BHE VAD group.

The challenges involved in improving survival in the smallest patients with congenital heart disease are especially daunting because of their complex physiology and hemodynamics, immature coagulation systems, infection risk, and previous surgical correction.

Pump size in relation to BSA has been shown to have a major impact on the rate of thromboembolic events. Children supported with large pumps (>50 mL/m²) had significantly more thromboembolic events compared with those supported with small- or normal-for-BSA–sized pumps.[204] This was initially observed when adult VADs were implanted in older children who subsequently developed complications such as arterial hypertension and cerebral vascular accidents,[205] possibly attributable to pumping large stroke volumes into anatomically small sized aortas.[206] In 2013 a new 15-mL BHE designed specifically for children with a BSA of 0.3 to 0.5 m² was introduced, which could substantially reduce the risk of thromboembolic events in the subset of pediatric patients for whom the 10-mL device was too small and the 25-mL device was too large.[204] Postmarketing surveillance from 2018 to 2020 of young children on BHE (median BSA 0.4 m²) from the ACTION registry reported increased survival and decreased adverse events than those reported in the original BHE study 2007 to 2014, even though children in the surveillance study were deemed at greater risk for sequelae.[110] In a review of the BHE prospective registry, survival in the current era (2013–2017) improved in patients <5 kg (51% vs. 65%) and 5 to 10 kg (74% vs. 78%) compared with those from the previous era (2000–2012). In addition, congenital heart disease, preoperative ECMO, and biventricular support were no longer associated with increased mortality for the <5 kg group in the current era.[207]

Between September 19, 2012, and December 31, 2020, most devices were intracorporeal continuous flow (41%), followed by paracorporeal pulsatile (27%) and paracorporeal continuous flow (26%). The total artificial heart was least common (1%). According to the latest Pedimacs report, survival was affected by device type, with intracorporeal continuous flow devices and paracorporeal continuous flow devices demonstrating the greatest and least survival, respectively. However, patient populations varied widely between device types.[17]

The Effect of Mechanical Circulatory Support on Wait-List Survival

Of all patients wait-listed for organ transplantation in the United States, children listed for heart transplantation face one of the largest mortality rates on a waiting list, regardless of age.[208] Every year, approximately 500 additional pediatric candidates are added to the transplant waiting list, with approximately 17% dying each year while awaiting a donor heart.[209] The impact of MCS on cardiac transplantation is evident when considering the evolution of the proportion of patients supported by MCS devices at transplant. In 2000, fewer than 5% of patients were supported by durable devices at transplant, but by 2013 the frequency had increased to greater than 20%.[210] For critically ill children, the presence of a pediatric VAD program decreases the wait-list mortality by as much as 50%, despite the increased waiting time.[211] Importantly, the increased proportion of pediatric patients supported by MCS devices at the time of transplant has not adversely affected posttransplant survival.[212] Not only has the wait-list mortality decreased, many patients are actually stabilizing and rehabilitating, making the posttransplant period easier.

The UNOS database from 1999 to 2012 identified 5532 pediatric candidates (age ≤18 years) actively listed for pediatric heart transplant; 2191 were listed between 1999 and 2004 (Era 1) and 3341 were listed between 2005 and 2012 (Era 2). Wait-list mortality rates were less in Era 2 (8%) compared to Era 1 (16%). VAD therapy was used more frequently in Era 2 (16%) than in Era 1 (6%) and was associated with improved wait-list survival

($P < 0.001$). Independent predictors of wait-list mortality included weight less than 10 kg, congenital heart diagnosis, ECMO, mechanical ventilation, and renal dysfunction. Independent predictors of survival on the wait-list included VAD therapy, cardiomyopathy diagnosis, blood type A, and being listed in Era 2. Despite an increase in the number of children listed as status 1A, wait-list mortality decreased more than 50% during Era 2. Irrespective of other factors, those supported with a VAD were four times more likely to survive to transplant.[211] Patients awaiting transplantation requiring circulatory support care were managed with a device or by ECMO. Analysis of the Organ Procurement and Transplantation Network database identified device support, most commonly using CentriMag-PediMag, TandemHeart, Rota-Flow, or Impella as superior with respect to survival to transplantation when compared with support using ECMO (hazard ratio: 0.49; 95% CI: 0.30–0.79) including a reduced 90-day mortality from 45% with ECMO to 39% with VAD support.[100]

The first multiinstitution study to evaluate outcomes of VAD support in children revealed that 77% of children bridged to transplant survived.[213] Risk factors for mortality in the VAD cohort in this study included earlier era and congenital heart disease. There was no difference in 5-year survival after transplantation for patients with VADs at the time of transplant compared with those not requiring VAD support.[203] In addition, posttransplant survival was improved in VAD patients compared with patients supported with ECMO or those without mechanical support. VAD support is likely superior to ECMO for several reasons: increased need for sedation and mechanical ventilation with ECMO, the need for greater levels of anticoagulation, the persistent inflammatory response, and the possibly deleterious effects of nonpulsatile flow on renal perfusion in small children.[9,27,196] Although the use of ECMO as a bridge to transplant continues to be necessary in selected cases, especially for those whose congenital anatomy is not amenable to VAD support, every effort should be made to avoid its use when other methods of mechanical support are possible. Less favorable outcomes with the use of paracorporeal VADs were also observed, suggesting that conversion to other modes of support may improve posttransplant outcomes. Consistent with adult data,[214] researchers found that the poor survival with paracorporeal VADs extended to the posttransplant period. Although the use of paracorporeal devices to stabilize children may be necessary in some situations, there should be a timely conversion to an implantable device to improve outcomes. A retrospective study comparing children who received multimodality MCS before transplant with those who received single-modality MCS showed similar survival to transplant and discharge between groups, despite the greater duration of support required in patients with multimodality MCS.[215]

Of 259 children who were listed for isolated heart transplantation at Texas Children's Hospital between 1995 and 2013, the proportion of patients who received mechanical support while on the wait-list increased from 13% before 2005 (i.e., before BHE when only ECMO and centrifugal pumps were available for those <20 kg) to 37% after 2005 ($P = 0.0001$). Among the 70 patients who received MCS, a temporary device was used as an initial therapy in 27 (ECMO = 14 and short-term VAD = 13), whereas long-term VAD was the first device in 43 patients. Wait-list mortality before 2005 (25%), decreased after 2005 (11%) ($P = 0.0006$). Median MCS duration before 2005 (12 days) also increased compared with after 2005 (78 days) ($P = 0.004$). Kaplan-Meier estimates showed weak evidence ($P = 0.08$) for improved survival after bridge to transplant both at 1 year (70% before 2005 and 88% after 2005) and at 5 years (60% and 78%, respectively).[216] This reduction in wait-list mortality is likely attributable to both the increased use of MCS as well as improvements in medical management and the maturation and experience of their program.[129]

Mechanical Circulatory Support and Single-Ventricle Physiology

The most recent ELSO guidelines for pediatric cardiac failure include cannulation strategies for patients with single-ventricle physiology at each stage of repair.[19] Factors such as central cannulation and avoidance of thrombosis have been associated with increased survival in all stages.[217] Infants who require ECMO support after stage I palliation for HLHS experience considerable mortality. In a recent review of the ELSO database from 1998 to 2013, only 36% of children survive to hospital discharge for this population.[86] An analysis of ELSO data from 1999 to 2012 reported a 41% survival to hospital discharge in those who had undergone superior cavopulmonary anastomosis.[218] Of patients with single-ventricle physiology who required VV ECMO for oxygenation/ventilation, the majority of whom had stage I physiology, 48% survived.[219]

Not surprisingly, children with congenital heart disease who require VAD support are often anatomically more challenging to support and have a greater mortality rate compared with children with cardiomyopathy.[220–222] In multiple studies, congenital heart disease has been identified as a risk factor, with those with single-ventricle physiology at greatest risk.[223] Based on data from the Pediatric Heart Transplant Study (PHTS) and Cardiac Transplant Research Database, single-ventricle anatomy is the most common cardiac lesion necessitating heart transplantation from age 6 months to adulthood. Unfortunately, outcomes after VAD support have been disappointing in the growing population of patients with failed single-ventricle palliations, with only 50% survival compared with overall pediatric VAD survival rates of 70% to 86%.[17,109,222,224] Only 5% of children listed for heart transplant who underwent VAD placement from 2004 to 2019 had single-ventricle heart disease.[192,225] Of note, although patients on VAD support with congenital heart disease have worse survival than those with cardiomyopathy, patients with single-ventricle and biventricular congenital heart disease have similar outcomes.[17] Because most patients who have undergone palliative cavopulmonary connections ultimately develop heart failure, the Mechanical Support as Failure Intervention in Patients with Cavopulmonary Shunts (MFICS) registry has been developed to improve the quality of care in this population.[221]

Although MCS has been used after all stages of single-ventricle palliation, a multi-institutional analysis of BHE use in patients with functional single-ventricle physiology reported particularly poor outcomes in neonates who required support after stage I palliation for HLHS and successful bridge to transplant in only 40% of patients overall.[223] Only 11% of those who received an implant after stage I palliation survived, whereas 58% to 60% of patients after stage II or III palliation survived. A recent analysis of 14 single-ventricle VAD patients from a large-volume pediatric VAD center noted 57% of patients were successfully bridged to transplant. Of these, 100% of Fontan patients but only 20% of Glenn patients survived to transplant.[225] Difficulty in selecting the correct pump size for patients with parallel circulations, extra sources of collateral pulmonary blood flow, and difficulty in balancing systemic and pulmonary circulations may all contribute to the high mortality after stage I palliation.

Supporting the patient with failing Fontan circulation presents unique barriers for mechanical support. Two basic physiologic subsets exist, which importantly affect support options. When heart failure symptoms develop because of a failing systemic ventricle (primary ventricular dysfunction), either pulsatile or continuous mechanical support is quite feasible, typically including inflow from the systemic ventricle and pump outflow to the ascending aorta. If right-sided pressures have been markedly increased, fenestration can be added at the time of implant.[226] When increased PVR or increased cavopulmonary resistance exists (failing Fontan physiology), successful support is more difficult to achieve and may require the addition of a pump from the systemic venous to the pulmonary circulation, requiring revision of the Fontan pathway to separate systemic venous and pulmonary circulations. When ventricular function is preserved and PVR is the predominant issue, pump outflow can be directed toward the pulmonary artery, providing isolated right-sided MCS. In circumstances in which a patient has significant diastolic dysfunction or residual structural lesions, a SynCardia TAH may be the most viable option for support[227]; successful use has been described in a teenager with failing Fontan circulation.[228] A review using ACTION data from 2014 to 2019 counted 45 Fontan patients being supported with VAD. Although nearly 70% were transplanted 1 year after device implantation, 67% of patients experienced adverse events, most commonly neurologic, and 21.3% died.[229]

VAD implantation is also technically difficult after previous sternotomies. Cannulation of the systemic RV can be complicated secondary to dense trabeculations and septal positioning, predisposing to "suction" events in which the cannula is too closely opposed to the septum. After device implantation, Fontan patients generally have more bleeding and thrombotic complications related to inherent protein C and S deficiencies.

Predicting the Need for BiVAD Support

The pathology leading to left heart failure in children is also more likely to lead to RV failure than the typical adult ischemic cardiomyopathy.[230] As a consequence, BiVAD support is more often necessary in children, with reports of BiVAD use in 25% to 45% of patients.[109,231,232] Patients who receive BiVAD support have reduced rates of survival.[220,232–234] This may be related to the pathophysiology necessitating BiVAD support, or the fact that use of multiple devices can lead to an increased risk of adverse events including infection, bleeding, and clot formation. Outcomes are also worse in patients who have delayed RVAD placement.[235] RV dysfunction was assessed in 57 patients who underwent BHE implantation for bridge to transplant; 25% required BiVAD support and an additional 17% had RV dysfunction (defined as CVP >16 mm Hg with inotropic therapy and/or inhaled nitric oxide for >96 hours). Preoperative variables such as younger age; use of ECMO; and increased blood urea nitrogen (BUN), creatinine, and bilirubin were associated with RV dysfunction and increased blood urea nitrogen and need for ECMO were risk factors for BiVAD placement. Patients who developed RV dysfunction with LVAD support had complicated postoperative courses but excellent survival (100%) comparable with those with preserved RV function (91%). Survival of those patients who required BiVAD support was only 71%.[232] Another study demonstrated that patients who required biventricular support had a significantly greater postoperative mortality and that preoperative milrinone therapy decreased the risk of severe RV failure necessitating RVAD insertion and improved postimplantation survival.[26]

ECMO for Cardiac Arrest

Emergent use of ECMO for children during in-hospital cardiac arrest with failure of conventional resuscitation methods has increased over time, although overall survival has remained roughly 40%. According to combined data from ELSO and the AHA "Get with the Guidelines" (GWTG) registries of children under 18 years old requiring ECPR for in-hospital cardiac arrest, 40.5% died before decannulation and 59.4% died before hospital discharge. Factors increasing odds of death included noncardiac diagnosis, preexisting renal insufficiency, longer time to initiation of ECMO, and associated adverse events.[236] Previous analyses have demonstrated single-ventricle physiology and history of complex cardiac surgery to be negative predictors of survival in pediatric cardiac patients who received ECPR. Acceptable neurologic outcomes have been described in children after CPR of up to 3 hours in duration before institution of ECMO.[237] However, longer duration of cardiopulmonary resuscitation is associated with increased neurologic injury and mortality.[236]

COMPLICATIONS

VAD use is associated with neurologic, hematologic, GI, and immunologic complications, with the frequency and severity of many of these complications being device specific. The profiles of adverse events differ between pulsatile devices and currently used continuous flow pumps.

Stroke is the most feared complication related to MCS, occurring more commonly with pulsatile flow than continuous flow devices.[238,239] Strokes may be hemorrhagic or ischemic in nature owing to embolism from ventricular clot or device thrombus, the latter being more common. Of 3517 cardiac surgical patients who received ECMO support between the years 2002 and 2013, neonatal status, smaller weight for age, and greater duration of ECMO were associated with a greater stroke risk.[240] In the original BHE trial, stroke occurred in 29% of supported patients, with thromboembolic strokes occurring eight times more often than hemorrhagic strokes.[27] Temporally, neurologic events were more common during the first month of support and, overall, was the leading cause of death after pump implantation. Mortality was 42% among patients with at least one neurologic event versus 18% in the absence of this event ($P = 0.0006$). Patients weighing less than 10 kg have the greatest incidence of stroke.[213,241] Evidence suggests improvement over time. In the follow-up BHE postsurveillance study report, the incidence of stroke was reduced by 44% compared with the original study.[110] Similarly, analysis of the Pedimacs registry from 2012 to 2019 demonstrates a stroke rate of 10.7%.[239] Increased institutional experience and appointment of a single physician to manage a patient's anticoagulation therapy can decrease the risk of stroke.[242]

Bleeding is quite common after ECMO and VAD device placement and is usually most severe in the early postoperative period. One-third of patients in the Pediatric Heart Study assist device multiinstitutional study and up to 50% of those in the Berlin Heart Trial had bleeding requiring reoperation.[224] Major bleeding was also the most commonly encountered complication in patients enrolled in the randomized Berlin Heart Pediatric VAD study, occurring in 42% of the low-BSA and 50% of the high-BSA cohorts.[27] In the fifth annual Pedimacs report, bleeding was the most common adverse event (14%), particularly in those with paracorporeal continuous flow devices.[17]

Infection is a relatively common complication and occurs in 50% to 69% of patients,[27,243,244] with infection attributable to the prolonged hospitalizations and exposure to multiple invasive therapies. The potential also exists for VAD-specific (driveline, hardware, or pump pocket) or VAD-related (mediastinitis, endocarditic, or bloodstream) infections. Commonly implicated organisms include *Staphylococcus aureus*, coagulase-negative staphylococci, *Pseudomonas aeruginosa*, and *Candida* spp.[243] Aggressive antibiotic and/or antifungal therapy, in addition to source control, is crucial, particularly in the setting of antirejection medications at the time of transplantation. Patients with driveline infections are often maintained with suppressive oral antibiotic therapy until 2 weeks after cardiac transplantation. According to data from the Pedimacs registry, 17% of reported adverse events between 2012 and 2015 were attributed to infection.[244] For children requiring readmission after discharge on VAD support, 25.8% of those identified from ACTION centers via the Pediatric Health Information System database were due to infection.[245]

Immunologic complications related to VAD support involve the formation of antibodies against human leukocyte antigens (anti-HLA antibodies), a process that has been consistently observed. The mechanism of antibody formation is complex and likely involves factors specific to the device itself as well as clinical events occurring during VAD support, particularly blood product transfusion.[246] After taking into account the blood product usage, some studies still reported an increase in panel reactive antibodies.[247] The presence of HLA antibodies is of concern because their presence may limit the suitability of a donor organ should the donor have pre-formed anti-HLA antibodies against specific HLA antigens. Although the adult sensitization rates of patients supported with a VAD have been reported to be as great as 60% on modern devices,[248] the true incidence of anti-HLA antibody formation in children supported with VADs is difficult to ascertain. It is postulated that lower survival approximately 5 years after transplantation for patients who received VAD support could be related to increased graft failure, secondary to increased allosensitization in VAD patients.[213] The smaller surface area and materials used to make the newer continuous flow devices appear to decrease the incidence of anti-HLA antibody formation.

Increased rates of both aortic insufficiency and aortic valve leaflet fusion exist with continuous flow devices, thought to be explained by a larger gradient across the aortic valve and increased strain on valve leaflets.[249] An increased rate of pulmonary hypertension and GI bleeding in the adult population has also been reported with continuous flow devices.[250] GI bleeding occurs from a combination of factors, including anticoagulation, acquired vWF deficiency and decreased pulsatility, leading to the formation of arteriovenous malformations.[165] In the latest Pedimacs registry report, freedom from GI bleeding in pediatric patients was lowest in patients with paracorporeal continuous flow VADs, with only 79.6% free from GI bleeding at 3 to 12 months.[17]

VAD therapy is also associated with other GI complications, including the need for peritoneal disruption as part of implantation. It is estimated that 55% of adult patients experience abdominal complications with VAD support, with problems such as wound/pocket infection, *Clostridium difficile* infection, hepatic dysfunction, and pancreatitis.[251] The incidence of such complications in the pediatric population is unknown.

Future Directions

DEVICES

In the face of an increasing need for advanced circulatory support in children, the NHLBI developed a Pediatric Circulatory Support Program in 2004 that matured into the Pumps for Kids, Infants, and Neonates Program (PumpKIN) in 2010 with the goal of developing a pediatric continuous flow-VAD. The Jarvik 2015 VAD (Jarvik, Inc., New York, NY) is the first pediatric continuous flow VAD and the result of this program, with the first implantation reported in a 12 kg patient in 2019.[252] Although it is still being evaluated, the Jarvik 2015 has subsequently been used under the designation of "compassionate use" in two additional children.[253] Three children with dilated cardiomyopathy recently demonstrated successful implantation of the Infant Jarvik 2015, though additional studies are needed.[117]

Minimally invasive pulmonary replacement devices are also now in development; devices such as the Biolung[254] and others are being developed as an alternative to ECMO for gas exchange and may become available in the near future.

ANNOTATED REFERENCES

Adachi I, Fraser C. Mechanical circulatory support for infants and small children. *Semin Thorac Cardiovasc Surg Pediatr Card Surg Annu.* 2011; 14:38-44.
This review article summarizes currently available devices for support of children with acute heart failure.

Almond C, Singh T, Gauvreau K, et al. Extracorporeal membrane oxygenation for bridge to heart transplantation among children in the United States: analysis of data from the Organ Procurement and Transplant Network and Extracorporeal Life Support Organization Registry. *Circulation.* 2011;123:2975-2984.
The authors review data from two major databases, evaluating outcomes of children undergoing ECMO as a bridge to heart transplantation in the United States between 1994 and 2009.

Baldwin J, Borovetz H, Duncan B, et al. The National Heart, Lung, and Blood Institute Pediatric Circulatory Support Program: a summary of the 5-year experience. *Circulation.* 2011;123:1233-1240.
This paper presents a summary of the progress made and devices under development in the United States from the Pediatric Circulatory Support Program.

Barrett C, Bratton S, Salvin J, et al. Neurological injury after extracorporeal membrane oxygenation use to aid pediatric cardiopulmonary resuscitation. *Pediatr Crit Care Med.* 2009;10:445-451.
This is a retrospective cohort study of data from the Extracorporeal Life Support Organization registry, evaluating neurologic injury in children undergoing ECPR.

Blume E, Naftel D, Bastardi H, et al. Outcomes of children bridged to heart transplantation with ventricular assist devices: a multi-institutional study. *Circulation.* 2006;13:2313-2319.
This paper presents a multiinstitutional review of children undergoing heart transplantation, evaluating outcomes in those who required VAD support as bridge to transplantation.

Bhaskar P, Davilla S, Hoskote A, et al. Use of ECMO for Cardiogenic Shock in Pediatric Population. *J Clin Med.* 2021 Apr 8;10(8):1573.
This review highlights the use of ECMO for patients requiring cardiovascular support.

Hetzer R, Potapov E, Alexi-Meskishvili V, et al. Single-center experience with treatment of cardiogenic shock in children by pediatric ventricular assist devices. *J Thorac Cardiovasc Surg.* 2011;141:616-623.
The authors offer a review of management strategies and outcomes in 94 patients with Berlin Heart EXCOR support, between 1990 and 2009.

Jefferies J, Price J, Morales D. Mechanical support in childhood heart failure. *Heart Fail Clin.* 2010;6:559-573.
This is a comprehensive review of indications for MCS and currently available devices for children of all ages.

Lorts A, Smyth L, Gajarski RJ, et al. The creation of a pediatric health care learning network: the ACTION quality improvement collaborative. *ASAIO J.* 2020;66(4):441-446.

This article describes the creation of a learning network to improve the outcomes of children with congenital heart disease.

Maslach-Hubbard A, Bratton SL. Extracorporeal membrane oxygenation for pediatric respiratory failure: history, development and current status. *World J Crit Care Med.* 2013;2:29-39.

The authors provide a comprehensive review of the use of extracorporeal membrane oxygenation for respiratory failure in children.

Mossad E, Motta P, Rossano J, et al. Perioperative management of pediatric patients on mechanical cardiac support. *Paediatr Anaesth.* 2011; 21:585-593.

The authors review the demographics of children requiring MCS and perioperative management concepts for their care.

Navaratnam M, Maeda K, Hollander SA. Pediatric ventricular assist devices: bridge to a new era of perioperative care. *Paediatr Anaesth.* 2019;29(5):506-518.

This article reviews the anesthetics management for children with VAD support as well as suggests mechanisms to manage changing hemodynamic conditions.

Rais-Bahrami K, Van Meurs KP. Venoarterial versus venovenous ECMO for neonatal respiratory failure. *Semin Perinatol.* 2014;38(2):71-77.

The authors provide a good brief review of ECMO in neonates complete with cannulation pictorial.

Sani A, Spinella PC. Management of anticoagulation and hemostasis for pediatric extracorporeal membrane oxygenation. *Clin Lab Med.* 2014;34:655-673.

The authors provide a thorough review of various methods for anticoagulation and monitoring for patients on ECMO support.

A complete reference list can be found online at Elsevier eBooks+.

Interventional Cardiology

ELLEN RAWLINSON

Types of Procedures Performed
Diagnostic Catheterization
Interventional Catheterization
Hybrid Procedures
Electrophysiologic Catheterization
Choice of Vessel Access
Complications and Limitations of Procedures
Overall Mortality and Morbidity
Vascular Complications
Damage or Dysfunction of a Valve
Blood Loss
Dysrhythmias and the Catheterization Laboratory
Cardioversion
Desaturation
Embolization

Contrast Toxicity
Neurologic Events
Radiation
Hypothermia and Hyperthermia
Endocarditis
Overcoming Limitations
Anesthesia
Who and How?
Preprocedural Assessment and Management
Anatomy and Function
The Environment
The Cardiac Patient
Choice of Anesthesia
Future of Anesthesia in Interventional Cardiology

THE USE OF CATHETERIZATION in the care of children with congenital heart disease (CHD) was first described by Dexter and colleagues in 1947[1] with the first interventional procedure, balloon atrial septostomy, subsequently described by Rashkind and Miller in 1966.[2] Over the intervening decades the discipline of pediatric interventional cardiology has vastly expanded within the field of pediatric cardiovascular medicine.

Technologic advances have increased the scope of pediatric cardiac catheterization procedures. As echocardiography, computed tomography (CT), and magnetic resonance imaging (MRI) diagnostic capabilities have increased, the need for purely diagnostic cardiac catheterization has waned.[3] There has been a transition from diagnostics toward more therapeutic interventions, with interventional procedures now accounting for more than two-thirds of all pediatric cardiac catheterizations.[4] Interventional cardiology has afforded patients a wider range of nonsurgical options for the management of CHD, postponing or replacing the requirement for surgery. Hybrid procedures combining interventional cardiology with cardiac surgery have enabled the management of more complex cardiac lesions.[5] There has been a shift in patient demographics as more children with CHD survive into adulthood. Children presenting for interventional cardiology represent a diverse group from premature neonates to older adolescents, with simple to complex pathophysiology, and requiring procedures of varying complexity. Cardiac catheterization laboratories are often remote sites and can be challenging environments. Anesthesiologists providing care to children undergoing cardiac catheterizations must have a good understanding of the patient's pathophysiology and tailor anesthesia to the patient- and procedure-specific requirements. Adverse events are common during catheterization procedures.[6] The anesthesiologist must be able to anticipate, prevent, and treat complications that may arise in this high-risk population.

In this chapter, we outline the main procedures performed in interventional cardiology, describe the challenges and complications faced by anesthesiologists, and address the principles and details of anesthetic techniques.

Types of Procedures Performed

DIAGNOSTIC CATHETERIZATION

Diagnostic catheterization provides accurate measurement of pressure and oxygen content from different regions of the circulation, permitting quantification of intracardiac shunting and calculation of vascular resistances and cardiac output. This information will guide critical decisions, such as suitability for palliative or reparative surgery for congenital heart lesions and direction of medical therapy. Consistent and reproducible physiologic conditions are required during the procedure to allow correct interpretation and comparison of results.[7] Expected values for hemodynamic variables are listed in Table 20.1. There are no absolute values for these variables, which relate to the age of the child. The use of angiocardiography during catheterization to define complex cardiac anatomy is waning because of the increased use and capabilities of noninvasive imaging modalities such as echocardiography, CT, and MRI.[8]

INTERVENTIONAL CATHETERIZATION

Interventional procedures now account for approximately two-thirds of all cardiac catheterization cases in children of all ages.[9]

Procedures on Atrial and Ventricular Septa
Atrial Septostomy
An atrial communication may be required in conditions of inadequate mixing of blood (e.g., D-transposition of the great arteries

TABLE 20.1	Normal Values in Diagnostic Cardiac Catheterization
Structure	Value (mm Hg)
Right atrium	3–5 (mean)
Right ventricle	20–25/3–5 (systolic/end-diastolic)
Pulmonary artery	12–15 (mean)
Left atrium	7–10 (mean)
Left ventricle	65–110/3–5 (systolic/end-diastolic)
Aorta	65–110/35–65 (systolic/diastolic)

[D-TGA] with restrictive septum), or conditions with elevated left atrial pressures (e.g., patients receiving venoarterial extracorporeal membrane oxygenation [VA ECMO]).[10] Balloon atrial septostomy (the Rashkind procedure) involves passing a balloon-tipped catheter across the atrial septum: the balloon is then inflated and pulled back through the septum creating an intraatrial communication. The procedure can be performed in the catheterization suite under fluoroscopic guidance or at the bedside in the intensive care unit using echocardiographic guidance. Alternative techniques include using a Brokenbrough needle or radiofrequency catheter. Septal puncture may also be required during procedures accessing the left side of the heart (e.g., pulmonary vein access and anterograde aortic valvuloplasty).[11] The major risks associated with the procedure are vessel injury, paradoxical embolism, arrhythmia, and cardiac perforation; previous concerns of an association with increased brain injury do not seem to have been evidence-based.[12]

Atrial Septal Defect Closure

Atrial septal defect (ASD) closure is one of the most commonly performed endovascular procedures and is the treatment of choice for up to 90% of secundum ASDs. Surgical repair is still required in secundum ASDs where the septal rim is insufficient to support the device, sinus venosus ASDs, multiple defects, or an aneurysmal septum.[13] Closure is warranted where there is evidence of right heart volume loading and a defect that is unlikely to close spontaneously in the short to medium term. The size of the defect

may be measured by fluoroscopy or inflatable balloon, and deployment may be monitored in real-time by transesophageal ECHO. Devices are available in a wide variety of sizes and designs, but brand selection depends more on clinician preference than objective performance (Fig. 20.1).[14] Devices may be used to close surgically created fenestrations when no longer required (e.g., Fontan circulations), whereas some devices are designed to only partially occlude the ASD to facilitate shunting in the presence of high right-sided pressures. Daily aspirin in a dose of 3 to 5 mg/kg is recommended for a minimum of 6 months after the procedure. Specific perioperative complications include device embolization, which occurs in up to 1% of cases, usually within 24 hours. Devices are designed to allow percutaneous retrieval although surgery is occasionally required. Compression and edema of conducting systems can produce high level atrioventricular block, although this is usually self-limiting. In the long term, devices are well tolerated with atrial arrhythmias the most common problem, although life-threatening complications such as cardiac erosion have been reported.[15]

Ventricular Septal Defect Closure

Ventricular septal defect (VSD) closure presents a technically greater challenge than ASD closure and is associated with a greater incidence of complications. Muscular or apical VSDs are most suitable as poor visualization during surgery leads to a high risk of residual defects, although perimembraneous VSDs may also be closed percutaneously. To accommodate large delivery systems, the technique involves a snare in the right ventricle capturing a guidewire passed across the VSD from the left ventricle. The guidewire forms an arteriovenous rail along which the VSD device may be advanced across the defect from the right side of the heart (Fig. 20.2). A combined surgical and interventional approach may be required for certain cases, such as the small infant with an anterior apical VSD that is difficult to reach surgically.[16] The device is passed directly through the right ventricular free wall via a ministernotomy, with the ventriculotomy closed by purse-string suture once the sheath is withdrawn.[17] Perioperative hemodynamic instability is relatively common due to manipulation of large sheaths and device embolization occurs in 1% to 2% of cases, again

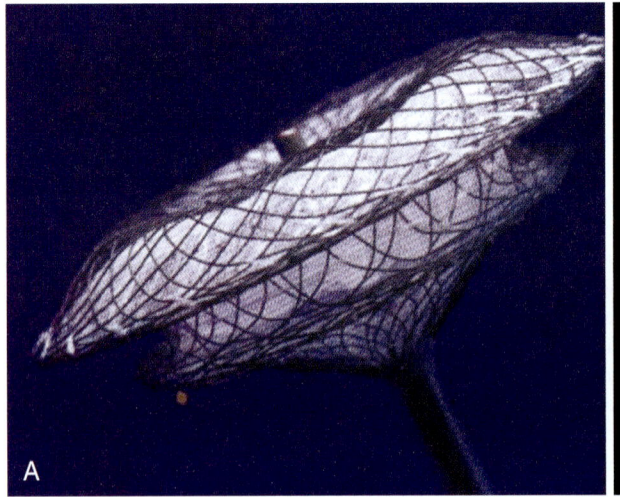
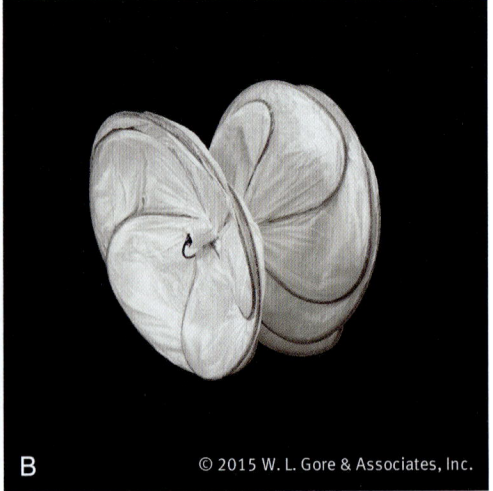

© 2015 W. L. Gore & Associates, Inc.

FIGURE 20.1 Devices for closure of an atrial septal defect. **A,** The Amplatzer (St. Jude Medical, St. Paul, MN) Septal Occluder. **B,** Gore Cardioform Septal Occluder. (**A,** Courtesy AGA Medical Corporation, Golden Valley, MN. **B,** Courtesy W.L. Gore & Associates, Flagstaff, AZ.)

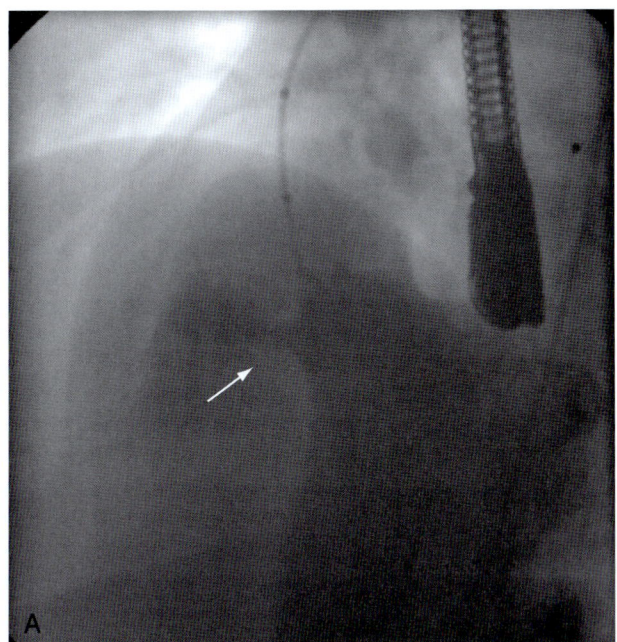

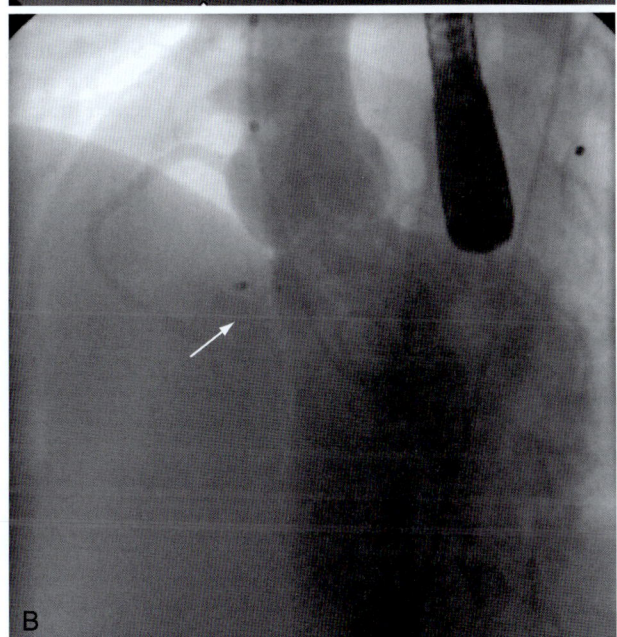

FIGURE 20.2 A, Angiography of a ventricular septal defect (VSD) device before deployment. Contrast agent passes through the perimembranous VSD *(arrow)*. **B,** Appearance of same region *(arrow)*, no contrast agent after deployment of the device.

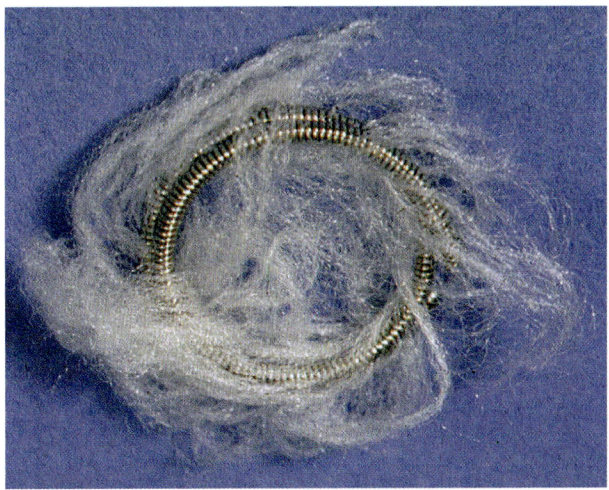

FIGURE 20.3 The coil is used for closure of a patent ductus arteriosus.

usually within 24 hours.[18,19] Early experience with VSD device closure was associated with a high incidence of complete heart block and aortic valve disruption owing to the close proximity of conduction pathways and the aortic valve apparatus. Many centers consider the risks unacceptable given good surgical outcomes, although more recent reports suggest that in selected subgroups of older children the risks may be broadly comparable.[20]

Procedures on Vessels and Valves
Ductus Arteriosus
Transcatheter closure of a patent ductus arteriosus (PDA) has a high success rate and the smallest incidence of adverse events of all

interventional procedures. It is indicated in any child with evidence of left ventricular overload. PDA morphology is very variable, so an aortogram is performed to define size and geometry. Persistent PDA in premature infants is linked to significant morbidity, such as chronic lung disease and necrotizing enterocolitis, but where medical management has failed, surgical intervention remains controversial.[21] However, technical advances now permit percutaneous closure in infants weighing less than 1 kg and there is some evidence to support reduced ventilator days and hospital stay in this population.[22] For closure of small and moderate PDAs, stainless steel coils (e.g., Gianturco, Cook Medical, Bloomington, IN) are most commonly used, whereas for larger PDAs, occluder devices (e.g., Amplatzer, St. Jude Medical, St. Paul, MN) are more appropriate.[23,24] Devices can be deployed with a retrograde or anterograde approach, and similar techniques may be employed to close other vascular connections such as major aortopulmonary collateral arteries (MAPCAs) and Blalock-Taussig (BT) shunts that are no longer required (Figs. 20.3 and 20.4). Complications include vascular injury, treatment failure, and device embolization, which can occur at the point of deployment or later: all are more common in lower-weight patients.[25]

In patients with duct-dependent circulations, stenting of the ductus arteriosus may be used as a bridge to palliative or definitive surgery. These are often high-risk procedures on small patients, whose complex anatomy is not immediately amenable to surgical repair. Perioperative ductal spasm, inadvertent occlusion, or vessel damage may require emergent open cardiac intervention.

Angioplasty and Stenting
Pulmonary artery angioplasty with or without stenting is a common intervention; improved pulmonary blood flow may assist with balancing of complex circulations and relief of right heart pressure. Complications are seen in 14% of interventions and include vessel rupture that can lead to life-threatening hemorrhage and may require surgical intervention.[4] Stent embolization is seen in up to 6% of cases.[26] Aortic coarctation may be treated with angioplasty and stenting, whether as a primary intervention or a response to postsurgical stenosis. The technique is increasingly being used in younger and smaller children but the elasticity of the aorta can limit the effectiveness of angioplasty alone.[27] Although rare, late aneurysm formation has been reported after stenting the aorta for coarctation.[28] Stents may be inserted within

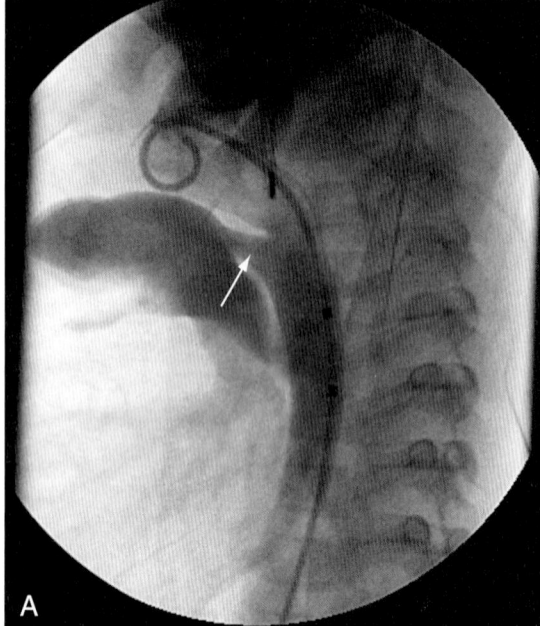

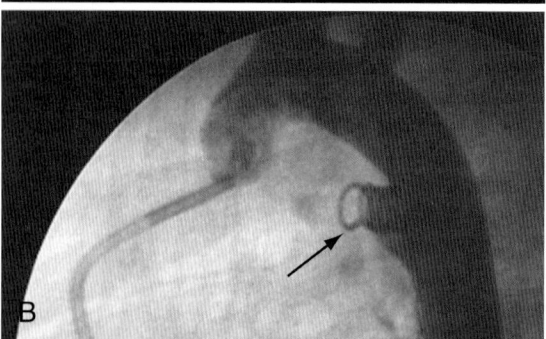

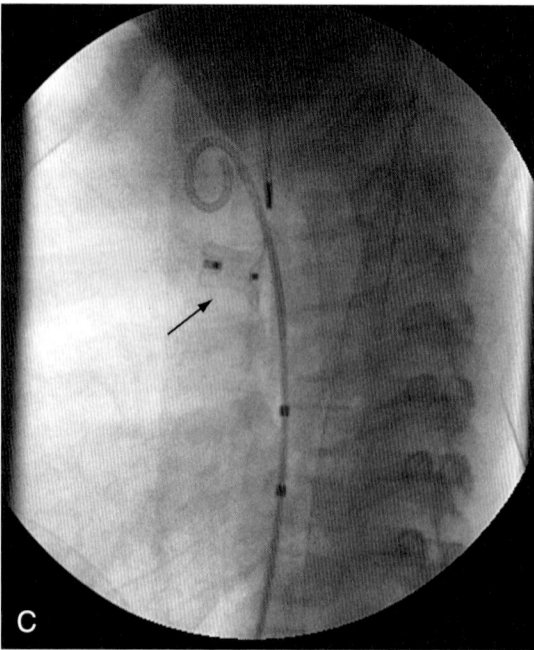

FIGURE 20.4 A, Lateral angiography demonstrates a patent ductus arteriosus (PDA) *(arrow)*. The PDA lies between aorta and pulmonary artery *(arrow)*. The angiography catheter is in the proximal aorta. **B,** Lateral angiography after closure of the PDA with a coil *(arrow)*. **C,** Lateral fluoroscopy after closure of the PDA with the Amplatzer Duct Occluder device. The device *(arrow)* is in the PDA.

surgically placed shunts as well as blood vessels, but in any situation when stenosis is due to external compression, the benefits may be short lived. The technique of implantation requires great precision with ever-present risks of malposition causing anatomical distortion and vessel obstruction.

Balloon Valvuloplasty

Stenotic valves may be dilated by inflating a balloon in the narrow orifice. For older infants and children with isolated lesions, pulmonary balloon valvuloplasty is often curative, whereas neonates with critical disease often require further interventions to supplement pulmonary blood flow.[29] Neonatal membranous pulmonary atresia may be similarly treated by perforating the membrane with the stiff end of a guidewire or with radiofrequency catheters.[30] There is increasing interest in stenting the right ventricular outflow tract (RVOT) as an initial palliative strategy in high-risk infants with tetralogy of Fallot.[31]

Inflation of a balloon or stent in the RVOT temporarily arrests right ventricular output and is often accompanied by transient hypotension, although this is generally well tolerated.[32] Paradoxically, those with tighter stenosis and little antegrade flow may maintain hemodynamic stability better, particularly if the duct is still open, as cardiac output is less disrupted.

Valvuloplasty for critical aortic stenosis remains controversial with concerns relating to longer-term outcomes and the rate of surgical intervention required in those treated initially with valvuloplasty. Moderate to severe aortic regurgitation is seen in up to 28% of cases at follow-up.[33] Neonatal aortic balloon valvuloplasty is a particularly high-risk procedure, often performed in patients with low–cardiac output requiring ventilation, inotropic support, and prostaglandin E_1 (PGE$_1$) infusion to maintain ductal patency. Catheterization can be complicated by arrhythmias (including asystole), the development of aortic regurgitation (which may require surgical intervention), and sudden death resulting from acute coronary ischemia.[34] The complication rate in older children is less than in younger children, yet transient hypotension, bradycardia, and left bundle branch block are commonly reported.[35]

Valve Replacement

Percutaneous pulmonary valve replacement (PPVR) offers an alternative to surgery in children with RVOT dysfunction, most commonly following tetralogy of Fallot repair. It may be used in both native RVOT and right ventricle to pulmonary artery (RV-PA) conduits.[36] Intervention is indicated when RV pressures exceed two-thirds systemic, or with symptomatic moderate to severe pulmonary regurgitation. High procedural success rates and satisfactory short- and medium-term valve function rely on careful patient selection; the procedure may be precluded by aneurysmal RVOT morphology.[37] The development of lower profile delivery systems and hybrid per-ventricular approaches are enabling the use of this technique in younger and smaller children.[38] Complications include RVOT tears, compression of aberrant coronary arteries, and the usual surgical risks of thrombus formation; infective endocarditis risks persist with percutaneous approaches.

Pulmonary valve systems have also been deployed percutaneously in the mitral valve position in children, with novel strategies being deployed to treat subsequent perivalvar regurgitation.[39]

HYBRID PROCEDURES

Hybrid procedures use both surgical and interventional techniques to provide treatment that is less invasive than surgery alone. As already described, per-ventricular access allows deployment of devices or valves where conventional catheter approaches would be limited by vessel size or hemodynamic instability from large sheaths in small hearts.

For children with hypoplastic left heart syndrome (HLHS), a hybrid strategy of ductal stenting and atrial septostomy combined with surgical pulmonary artery banding avoids the major physiological demands of the Norwood operation. Usually confined to particularly high-risk neonates (difficult to compare directly with primary surgical approaches), this strategy comes at the expense of more extensive stage II surgery at 4 to 6 months, and a high risk of further intervention being required for hypoplastic pulmonary arteries.[40] As well as avoiding the traditional Norwood operation, the stage III total cavopulmonary circulation can be set up during stage II surgery by forming the lateral tunnel but leaving an occluding patch that can be perforated percutaneously when required. This increases complexity of the stage II procedure but avoids the subsequent need for redo sternotomy.[41]

ELECTROPHYSIOLOGIC CATHETERIZATION

Endocardial catheters that record an electrocardiogram first became available in the early 1960s. Intracardiac electrograms, supplemented by external electrocardiogram leads, record electrical activity in the heart, and programmable stimulators aim to induce and terminate tachyarrhythmias. This allows arrhythmia mechanisms to be defined and arrhythmogenic foci to be mapped. Ablation catheters can then be guided to deliver local energy to the endocardium to destroy the source of the arrhythmia or interrupt aberrant conduction pathways. Ablation can be delivered as radiofrequency, cryoablation, laser therapy, or direct currents. Ablative procedures are indicated for both primary cardiac arrhythmias, particularly those of atrial origin, and those arising following surgery for CHD.[42]

The procedures are complex and often of longer duration than other catheterization procedures. They require multiple catheters to accurately measure electrical signals, and specially trained staff to interpret the data. Ablation of ectopic foci has a good success rate and small complication rate.[43,44] The main risks with this procedure are heart block, cardiac perforation, vessel injury, and stroke.

CHOICE OF VESSEL ACCESS

The most common approach for cardiac catheterization is the femoral route. Femoral venous catheterization avoids the risk of pneumothorax, and the vessel is often easier to access than the internal jugular vein in the unanesthetized child. The main alternative is internal jugular access, which may be specifically required for some VSD closures or investigation of cavopulmonary connections. Internal jugular approaches should be avoided whenever possible in children likely to require surgical cavopulmonary connection because of the risk of precipitating superior vena cava (SVC) thrombosis and occlusion. In neonates, the umbilical vein may be used, although difficulty can be encountered attempting to cross the ductus venosus to access the inferior vena cava. Patency of the ductus venosus can be assessed by ultrasound before the procedure to avoid unnecessary manipulation of the umbilical vein. An alternative route is transhepatic puncture, which has been used temporarily during catheterization and for long-term vascular access.[45]

Complications and Limitations of Procedures

The pediatric cardiac catheterization laboratory is a high-risk environment associated with major morbidity and mortality.[6] Of the

373 anesthesia-related cardiac arrests reported in the Pediatric Perioperative Cardiac Registry, 34% occurred in children with cardiac disease and 17% of these occurred in the catheterization laboratory.[46] Additionally, there are complications directly attributable to the procedures. Successful practice in this setting requires a thorough understanding of pathology, vigilance, excellent communication between team members, and appropriate backup from surgeons and other specialties. Standard procedures for predictable emergencies should be in place. An intensive care bed should be available for high-risk procedures. The facility for cardiopulmonary bypass or extracorporeal membrane oxygenation (ECMO) for high-risk patient groups or procedures may be beneficial,[19] although this type of therapy may not be available everywhere. Local policies on appropriate case mix should be based on experience and infrastructure; clear referral pathways for high-risk cases should be established.

OVERALL MORTALITY AND MORBIDITY

The **IM**proving **P**ediatric and **A**dult **C**ongenital **T**reatment (IMPACT) database of more than 16,000 pediatric catheterizations reports all-cause mortality for children undergoing catheterization during their admission as 2.1%, with the majority of deaths occurring within 14 days of the procedure.[4] Studies that focused on the immediate perioperative period (in the operating room or post anesthesia care unit) reported mortality rates between 0.05% and 0.28%.[23,36] Overall, despite the increasing complexity of both patients and procedures, it appears the mortality rate is decreasing.

Adverse events occur in 7.2% to 8.8% of catheterization procedures overall.[4,47,48] Morbidity may be classified as either major or minor. Major complications are life-threatening events requiring immediate medical or surgical intervention (e.g., cardiac arrest, removal of an embolized device) or which result in a permanent major lesion (e.g., embolic stroke, vessel aneurysm). The incidence of perioperative arrest in the cardiac catheterization laboratory from a multicenter cardiac arrest registry is between 0.8% and 1.6%, with bradycardia (with pulse) or pulseless electrical activity/asystole the most common presenting rhythm.[49] Minor complications are transient and resolve with specific treatment (e.g., tolerated dysrhythmias, transient arterial thrombosis). Complication rates have remained largely constant despite technologic advances, reflecting the changing nature of the patient population and interventions.

Certain patient and procedural characteristics confer increased risk of complications. Neonates are particularly vulnerable, with a 4.7% rate of major complications associated with interventional catheterization. This may be explained by reduced physiologic reserve, presence of uncorrected or partially palliated congenital heart defects, and an increased risk of obstruction to great vessels and cardiac chambers by wires and devices.[32] Age younger than 1 year and low body weight have been identified as independent risk factors for complications.[50] Specific cardiac lesions are also associated with greater risks of both morbidity and mortality, notably single-ventricle physiology, whether unrepaired or palliated, and significant left ventricular outflow tract obstruction (e.g., Williams-Beuren syndrome and hypertrophic cardiomyopathy).[51] The presence of pulmonary hypertension, particularly with an idiopathic etiology and suprasystemic pulmonary artery pressures, increases perioperative risk substantially.[52] With respect to procedural risk, interventional procedures have greater complication rates than diagnostic procedures for all age groups except neonates, in whom the complication rates are similar.[4,32,53] Specifically, high-risk procedures include VSD device closure; atrial septostomy where the septum is restrictive; balloon interventions for the mitral valve, pulmonary vein, pulmonary artery, and neonatal aortic valve; and stent placement in surgical shunts.[6,54] At the other end of the spectrum, PDA and ASD device closures have the least risk of complications.[32]

VASCULAR COMPLICATIONS

Vascular complications are the most common complication of pediatric catheterizations, accounting for almost one-third of the total.[53] They may be acute, leading to unexpected hemodynamic instability, or delayed, leading to longer-term morbidity. Many factors may contribute to unexpected hemodynamic instability, including blood loss, balloon- or catheter-induced interruptions in blood flow or coronary perfusion, arrhythmias, tamponade, vessel rupture, acute valve dysfunction, and device malposition.

Arterial Thrombosis and Occlusion

Arterial thrombosis is common after pediatric cardiac catheterization, with a reported incidence in two large studies of 4.3% and 11.4%.[55,56] Cannulation under ultrasound guidance does not reduce the incidence.[57] Young age, small size, larger sheath size, and repeated arterial catheter exchanges are independent risk factors for thrombosis; polycythemia and dehydration may further increase the risk.

Prophylactic heparin reduces but does not eliminate the risk of arterial thrombosis[58]; despite its widespread use, there is no consensus on the appropriate dose. Common schedules prescribe 50 to 100 IU/kg; larger doses do not appear to confer additional benefit. Most cases of reduced or absent pulse resolve either spontaneously or with additional heparin anticoagulation, and evidence of significant acute consequences is lacking.[59] Thrombolysis is a viable next step, but surgical intervention will be needed for thrombosis resistant to medical therapy, arterial tears or avulsion, and pseudoaneurysms. Percutaneous thrombectomy may be suitable in older children.[60,61] Occasionally, a pulse may be persistently reduced in a clinically well-perfused limb despite intervention. The long-term concern is delayed limb growth; cases have been reported but one small study failed to demonstrate limb-length discrepancy after median follow up of 3.5 years. Currently there are no means to identify those at risk.[60,62]

Venous Thrombosis and Occlusion

Isolated cases of femoral or iliofemoral venous occlusions with limb edema have been reported,[47] but two small prospective observational studies found very small incidences, 0% and 1.6%.[63,64] All affected children responded to heparin therapy without the need for further intervention. Using the smallest catheter necessary and heparin prophylaxis should limit the incidence.

Vessel Rupture, Perforation, and Dissection

Vessel rupture can occur at the site of vessel entry or at the site of intervention. This is a rare but potentially catastrophic event. One death caused by intraabdominal rupture of a femoral vein in a neonate was reported in a series of 4454 catheterizations.[32] Arterial or venous perforations were responsible for four major complications and six minor complications in a series of 4952 procedures, and groin hematoma occurred in 25 cases.[47]

Vessel rupture occurs most commonly during balloon dilation of branch pulmonary arteries and during RVOT valve implantation procedures, but also along the ascending aorta and arch after dilation of the aortic valve.[65] Occasionally, arterial dissection,

aneurysm, and pseudoaneurysm formation may occur. Rupture may cause hemopericardium or hemothorax, or both; pulmonary artery disruption after balloon dilation may manifest as hemoptysis.[60] If rupture and hemorrhage occur, hypertension should be avoided, the trachea should be intubated (if the airway is not already secured), and heparin should be reversed. In extremis, blood from pericardial or pleural drains may be returned directly to the patient via femoral cannulae until surgical intervention can be achieved.

Cardiac Perforation and Tamponade

Perforation of the myocardium during catheterization procedures is relatively common, with the atrial appendage and RVOT the most common sites. Procedures associated with a greater risk include atrial septostomy, balloon dilation of the mitral valve, and attempted radiofrequency perforation of membranous pulmonary atresia.[60] Signs suggesting perforation include wires appearing in unexpected places, atypical contrast appearance, lack of a return to baseline blood pressure after catheter-induced tachycardia, narrow pulse pressure, and hemodynamic instability. Echocardiography should always be immediately available to confirm a suspected perforation or tamponade. Perforation is often well tolerated and can frequently be managed conservatively, but the **C**ongenital **C**ardiac **C**atheterization **P**roject on **O**utcomes (C3PO) database of nearly 9000 cases recorded five neonatal deaths resulting from cardiac perforation during atrial septostomy.[66]

Cardiac tamponade is an uncommon complication of cardiac catheterization with an incidence reported at 0.1% to 0.2%.[4] In one series of 4952 patients, tamponade was responsible for two deaths: one neonate after a balloon atrial septostomy and one 4-year-old child after a recent Fontan procedure for stent insertion in a branch pulmonary artery.[47] Tamponade may be treated by needle pericardiocentesis, insertion of a pericardial drain, or occasionally, by the formation of a pericardial window by cardiac surgeons.

DAMAGE OR DYSFUNCTION OF A VALVE

Damage to a valve is uncommon but most often occurs with balloon valvuloplasty rather than with other procedures. The primary complication is creation of excessive regurgitation. The hemodynamic consequences of such a defect are more significant on the systemic side of the circulation than on the pulmonary side.[60] The mechanism of injury is most commonly leaflet avulsion during dilation, although the leaflet can be inadvertently perforated by the guidewire and then further damaged as the catheter wire is manipulated. Emergency repair is occasionally required.[60] Direct injuries to atrioventricular valves are rare, but placing wires and large sheaths across atrioventricular valves and septal defects can cause severe, albeit temporary, hemodynamic disturbance. This is particularly true during implantation of VSD occlusion devices.[18] ASD and PDA occlusions are less likely to produce significant hemodynamic disturbance.[67]

BLOOD LOSS

Blood loss may be sudden and massive after a vessel ruptures, but more often, it is slow and insidious owing to multiple blood samples and blood loss associated with catheter exchanges, exacerbated by systemic heparinization. Noteworthy blood loss is more likely to occur during procedures that involved placing a device because of the need for larger catheters and multiple catheter exchanges. A preoperative hematocrit and a current type and screen are advisable. For procedures with a greater risk of blood loss, a crossmatch should also be requested. Access to emergency blood and blood administration equipment should be readily available for unexpected hemorrhage.

DYSRHYTHMIAS AND THE CATHETERIZATION LABORATORY
Cardiac dysrhythmias are common during cardiac catheterization. Most are mechanically induced and repositioning the wire or catheter usually results in rapid resolution. Other causes of rhythm abnormality include coronary air embolism, electrolyte imbalance, and hypercarbia. Although most are minor and self-limiting, dysrhythmias can cause hemodynamic instability and are a common cause of major complications.[32,53] Young age and a prolonged duration of the procedure are both risk factors for developing dysrhythmias. Treatment may include defibrillation, pacing, or medical therapy and should be managed in collaboration with the cardiologist. The relevant equipment should always be available in the catheterization suite.

Types of Dysrhythmias
Dysrhythmias may originate from the atria, ventricle, or involve the conduction system with varying degrees of block. Atrial tachyarrhythmias are generally considered the most common but frequently resolve with adjustments to the catheterization technique or spontaneously. However, they may be poorly tolerated by children with single-ventricle physiology, mitral stenosis, or poor myocardial function; these children may need intervention earlier than others. Catheter-induced complete heart block is reported to be between 0.3% and 2.2% of cases; the latter study retrospectively searched specifically for catheter-induced heart block from a database of more than 6000 pediatric catheter cases.[53,68] In this series, 96% of catheter-induced heart block events resolved spontaneously shortly after the procedure, but six children required a pacemaker. First- or second-degree atrioventricular block is well tolerated at all ages. Device closure for VSD may cause severe junctional bradycardia or complete heart block in up to 10% of cases, and almost half of these children require pacing or isoproterenol.[18]

The overall incidence of ventricular tachycardia or fibrillation is ~0.3%, the most common rhythms causing major complications.[53] Children undergoing VSD device placement had ventricular arrhythmias that required lidocaine or cardioversion in 8.5% of cases.[18]

Children with obstruction to systemic flow (e.g., hypertrophic obstructive cardiomyopathy or aortic stenosis) are at a greater risk of developing ventricular fibrillation secondary to myocardial ischemia.

CARDIOVERSION
Histologic injury to the myocardium is rare when the starting power for cardioversion is set at 0.5 J/kg.[67] Systemic and pulmonary emboli are rare in children compared with adults, for whom the incidence is 1% to 2%. All forms of dysrhythmia may occur after cardioversion; factors that influence the incidence include the underlying pathology, electrolyte disturbance, residual drugs, and the strength of shock. Children with implantable pacemaker devices requiring cardioversion need special consideration. Electrode pads should be placed a distance from the generator and the pacemaker circuits, and pacemaker programming mode should be checked after the procedure.

DESATURATION
Arterial desaturation or cyanosis in the child undergoing cardiac catheterization may be respiratory or circulatory in origin. A systematic approach is required to diagnose and treat the underlying cause. A transesophageal echocardiographic (TEE) probe can cause desaturation by compressing the trachea, bronchi, or vessels, or precipitating bronchospasm. These events are more common in children weighing less than 10 kg.[67] Pneumothorax is rare but possible during cardiac catheterization. Hypercarbia, acidosis, excessive positive-pressure ventilation, contrast media, and hypoxia can increase pulmonary vascular resistance, which may lead to increased shunting and cyanosis. Hypercyanotic episodes are frequently observed,[47] particularly in infants with uncorrected tetralogy of Fallot. In one study, 12% of children with tetralogy of Fallot exhibited a hypercyanotic episode within 12 hours of catheterization despite adequate hydration, sedation, and the use of nonionic contrast media.

EMBOLIZATION
Introduced devices, native tissues, and air can all embolize. Children with aberrant connections between the right and left circulations are at risk to embolize material to the systemic circulation, with cerebral and coronary vessels at particular risk.

Device, Balloon, Thrombus, or Dislodged Material
All devices including coils, duct umbrellas, occlusion devices, and endovascular stents have embolized, although improvements in their design, particularly in retrieval techniques, have reduced these risks.[4,47] Similarly, the incidence of balloon rupture has decreased with technical improvements in materials and design. The use of an inflation device with an attached manometer is recommended to ensure that the inflation pressure does not exceed the burst pressure of the balloon. Thrombi may be dislodged from devices or catheters, and balloon dilation may dislodge calcium, intimal lining from conduits, and thrombus from surgical systemic-pulmonary shunts.

Air Embolism
Gas emboli may originate from sheaths, catheters, burst balloons, or anesthetic infusion lines. The many wire and catheter exchanges required during interventional procedures make air embolism an ever-present risk.[67] Balloons are dilated with a weak contrast mixture and, in view of the occasional balloon rupture, it is important to ensure all gas bubbles are eliminated from the contrast mix syringe and catheter before dilation is undertaken. All intravenous lines, injections, and infusions should also be free of air bubbles. Balloons used for flotation tip catheters should ideally be filled with carbon dioxide rather than air to minimize the potential embolic effect if the balloon bursts; carbon dioxide will be absorbed into the blood more rapidly than air. Nitrous oxide should be avoided because it expands air bubbles.

CONTRAST TOXICITY
Adverse reactions to intravascular media are relatively uncommon, but accurate recognition and management by the anesthesiologist is critical. Idiosyncratic reactions may be acute or delayed, but the pathophysiologic mechanisms underlying these responses are complex, varied, and remain to be fully elucidated.[69] Unless formal allergy testing has been undertaken, hypersensitivity is an appropriate term that does not misattribute a mechanism.[70] Both acute and delayed reactions can occur with first exposure to contrast media, and all grades of severity including anaphylaxis are possible.

Acute Reactions
Acute reactions to contrast agents can range from mild to severe; symptoms include tachycardia, bronchospasm, flushing, urticaria,

laryngeal edema, and cardiovascular collapse. Replacing high-osmolar (ionic) contrast solutions with isomolar or low-osmolar (nonionic) solutions has reduced the incidence substantively. In one series of more than 11,000 administrations of nonionic iodinated contrast media to children, acute reactions were noted in 20 (0.18%) cases; 16 were mild, 1 moderate, and 3 severe.[71] Reactions appear to be more common when contrast medium is given through an arterial access compared with venous access. Acute reactions should be managed in accordance with standard anaphylaxis protocols (i.e., oxygen, IV fluid, epinephrine, corticosteroids, and histamine 1- and histamine 2-antagonist therapy). If there is a history of an acute reaction to contrast agents, then prophylaxis with corticosteroids and antihistamines can be considered if further exposure is proposed. However, breakthrough reactions of all severity grades have been observed in up to 40% of all pretreated patients, so alternative agents or imaging modalities should be strongly considered.[70]

Delayed Reactions

Delayed reactions have a much broader spectrum of clinical symptoms including: headache, heat feeling, skin redness, fixed drug eruptions, **d**rug **r**eaction with **e**osinophilia and **s**ystemic **s**ymptoms (DRESS reaction), and Stevens-Johnson syndrome. With the increasing trend to day-case treatment, many such reactions occur once the child has been discharged. It is therefore important that a specific history is taken from children presenting for catheterization of any previous exposure and reactions to contrast media.

Renal Adverse Reactions and Prevention

The term contrast media nephrotoxicity refers to an increase in serum creatinine concentration by more than 25% or 0.5 mg/dL within 3 days of receiving IV contrast media in the absence of another cause.[72] The underlying mechanism of injury is unclear, although it is thought that contrast can reduce renal perfusion and is toxic to tubular cells. Contrast media nephrotoxicity occurs more frequently but not exclusively in children with preexisting renal damage; additional risk factors include dehydration, cardiac failure, and the subclinical renal insufficiency seen in cyanotic children. It has been suggested that infants and children who receive more than 5 mL/kg of nonionic contrast agent are at increased risk for contrast media nephrotoxicity.[73] Contrast for angiography does not increase the risk of post-bypass acute kidney injury[74] and most contrast media nephrotoxicity appears to resolve without intervention. However, a recent study of 233 heterogeneous children receiving contrast for CT scanning found an association between contrast media nephrotoxicity and unfavorable outcome, suggesting the process may not be as benign as previously hoped.[75] Many interventions have been given prophylactically to prevent contrast media nephrotoxicity; preliminary studies with N-acetylcysteine have been promising but no interventions have been more effective than normal saline hydration.[76] Currently, the only modifiable risk factors are hydration status and dose of contrast used. When possible, potentially nephrotoxic drugs should be stopped at least 24 hours before the procedure. Gadolinium-based contrast materials are considered nonnephrotoxic in the normal MRI dose of up to 0.3 mmol/kg. However, there is some evidence that the increased doses required for cardiac angiography may confer adverse renal effects.[77] Most radiologic contrast media have osmotic diuretic effects. During procedures requiring large volumes and/or repeated doses of contrast media, an impressive diuresis may occur, causing concealed fluid losses and potential hypovolemia. Additional IV fluid may be required to avoid dehydration. Occasionally, bladder distention and retention can also occur, which should be considered in a child with unexplained postoperative distress.

NEUROLOGIC EVENTS

Central and peripheral neurologic damage can occur as a complication of the catheterization procedure. In one prospective study, 0.38% of children suffered a neurologic complication, and the incidence was significantly greater after interventional than diagnostic procedures.[78]

Central Nervous System

Ischemic cerebrovascular events may occur because of embolization, damage to the carotid artery, or acute low–cardiac-output states causing hypoxic-ischemic encephalopathy. Thrombotic emboli may originate from any site in which there is endovascular or endocardial damage from the inner surface of the catheter or an implanted device. Factors that increase the risk during interventional procedures include large catheter size, more numerous vascular punctures, and procedures of increased duration. The most common complications after an embolic stroke are convulsions and hemiplegia, but children with this type of stroke often make a good recovery. The outcome is more guarded after hypoxic-ischemic encephalopathy occurring after a period of reduced cardiac output.[78]

Peripheral Nervous System

During catheterization procedures, the arms are frequently extended above the head to improve the lateral radiologic views of the heart; in these circumstances the brachial plexus may be injured.[79] Reduced cardiac output states associated with cardiac catheterization can augment this risk. To decrease the risk of injury, the elbows should be flexed with the hands up and the elbows then adducted a minimum of 15 cm above the table (many adduct the elbows until they are positioned directly above the shoulders and taped in position), while maintaining the head/neck in a neutral position.[79] At-risk positions should be adopted only when necessary, for the briefest time possible, and all precautions documented.[80]

RADIATION

Cardiac catheterization procedures deliver some of the largest radiation doses owing to the requirement for rapid-sequence screening and/or prolonged screening.[81] Complex interventional procedures require long fluoroscopy times with multiple angiographic or fluoroscopic acquisitions. This poses a risk to both the patient and staff. Radiation overexposure can lead to scarring and skin injury, cellular injury, gene mutation, cell death, radiation-induced cancers, and birth defects. The acronym ALARA (or ALARP), which stands for "**a**s **l**ow **a**s **r**easonably **a**chievable (or **p**ractical)," is a principle for radiation exposure that should be applied in the context of obtaining adequate diagnostic images.[82]

Radiation Exposure of Patients

Children are especially vulnerable to the oncogenic effects of radiation; their actively growing tissue and organs are more sensitive to radiation and a greater proportion of their bodies are irradiated during procedures. Many children with CHD will require more than one catheterization procedure and with improvements in long-term outcomes there are longer life spans to develop radiation-related problems.[83]

Oncogenic effects of radiation require a long latent time, often decades. The lifetime risk of cancer from radiation exposure may be estimated from age, weight, effective dose, and duration of radiation exposure. The risk for adult coronary angiography is 6% per sievert (Sv), and the average dose is about 10 mSv, which gives an increased risk of 0.06%. By contrast, an infant has a lifetime cancer risk of 11% to 15% per sievert (lower exposure but increased sensitivity). An exposure of 20 mSv (1 hour of fluoroscopy and 7 digital acquisition runs) gives a lifetime cancer risk of 0.03%.[84,85] Changes to imaging practices appear capable of reducing exposure without compromising clinical care and minimizing these risks further.[86]

Radiation Exposure of Staff

Most radiation exposure to staff comes from scatter from the beam entry point on the patient. Lesser amounts come from the x-ray tube and intensifier. The need for staff protection is well established and is accomplished by wearing lead aprons, thyroid shields, goggles, and suspended mobile glass lead screens for the head and neck. In addition, staff should aim to keep a maximal possible distance from the radiation source and minimize exposure time. All personnel working regularly in the catheterization suites should wear dosimeters to monitor cumulative radiation exposure.

HYPOTHERMIA AND HYPERTHERMIA

Catheterization procedures are often prolonged, increasing the need for close temperature monitoring. Hypothermia can exacerbate blood loss or dysrhythmias and hyperthermia may exacerbate any neurologic injury. External body and fluid warming devices should be used for all but the briefest procedures and central temperature should be measured.

ENDOCARDITIS

Under current recommendations, routine endocarditis prophylaxis is not indicated for cardiac catheterization procedures; however, the CHD patient population undergoing the procedures may warrant prophylaxis because of their increased risk of endocarditis.[87] Children with acquired valvular disease, hypertrophic cardiomyopathy, and previous infective endocarditis are at increased risk. Clinical practice varies between centers. Prophylactic antibiotics should be administered before any devices are implanted, and some centers continue to recommend endocarditis prophylaxis for a minimum of 6 months after implantation. Diagnostic or routine angioplasty procedures do not usually warrant antibiotic prophylaxis, but there is usually a residual flow disturbance after angioplasty procedures that some consider warrants preventive therapy.

OVERCOMING LIMITATIONS

The main limitation in the use of catheterization techniques in younger or smaller children has been the delay in development of equipment of appropriate size. To some degree this difficulty has been managed by the collaboration between surgeons and interventricular cardiologists in developing the hybrid approaches already discussed. Practical advances in this area continue to be made, as can be seen with the increased use of interventional techniques to close PDAs in very small premature infants. There are predictions that within 2 decades the primary treatment modality for tetralogy of Fallot will be percutaneous.[88]

The next major challenge is to develop equipment and techniques that are MRI compatible.[89] This would minimize radiation exposure to children and staff. However, there are significant technical obstacles that need to be overcome before this approach can fully replace catheterization laboratories using ionizing radiation.

Anesthesia

WHO AND HOW?

The aims of anesthesia care for pediatric interventional cardiology are to ensure the child is not distressed, to provide optimal conditions for accurate diagnostic measurements and successful interventions, and to manage any complications or alterations in the child's cardiovascular physiology during the procedure. These aims often require general anesthesia but occasionally may be met with deep sedation.

The choice of sedation or general anesthesia and the seniority of the anesthetic provider should match the complexity of the procedure and the child's cardiac pathology. Analysis of the IMPACT database suggests that operator-directed sedation is safe in selected patients in centers with an established program, and that clinical judgment was better at identifying suitable cases than preprocedural risk scores.[90] However, deep sedation can easily merge into general anesthesia so children undergoing sedation should be cared for by someone skilled at providing both and who possesses the ability to manage and resuscitate children with CHD.[91] Full standard patient monitoring should be available for all cases, and there must be adequate facilities for postprocedural recovery and emergency resuscitation.

Increasingly, there are fewer diagnostic procedures and more interventional procedures. This change is reflected in a shift from sedation to general anesthesia and the expanding role of specialized pediatric cardiac anesthesiologists.[92] Anesthesia providers for these children must have a high level of experience in pediatric anesthesia and a thorough understanding of pediatric cardiology and CHD. They must understand the physiology, the procedure, and the potential complications and have the ability to anticipate, diagnose, and respond to any hemodynamic changes or deteriorations.

PREPROCEDURAL ASSESSMENT AND MANAGEMENT

Children scheduled for elective interventional cardiology are often admitted to the hospital on the day of the procedure. Ideally, all children should have an anesthesia assessment at the same time as their preprocedural cardiologic workup. An efficient and complete anesthesia assessment requires good coordination and communication between cardiology and anesthesia units. The anesthesia preoperative assessment should establish the cardiac anatomy and details of any previous surgery, interventions, and investigations. Current functional status should be elicited, as should any signs of worsening function, cyanosis, or heart failure. Baseline observations for heart rate, blood pressure, and oxygen saturation should be recorded.[93]

Up to 25% of children with CHD have syndromes or other anomalies that may affect their anesthesia care. They are likely to have undergone previous procedures and anesthetics, and the family may be well informed about the child's condition, hospital process, and anesthesia. It is important that discussions include sedative premedication, parental presence, and the mode of induction of anesthesia (see Chapter 2). Sedative premedication may be particularly beneficial in children where anxiety and associated sympathetic activation and tachycardia are best avoided, such as those with left ventricular outflow tract obstruction or with sympathetically induced arrhythmias.

Interventional cardiology procedures may involve considerable physiologic trespass, and some children may have limited cardiac reserve. They should be in optimal health whenever possible. Intercurrent illness or infection may bias cardiorespiratory diagnostic values, increase the risk of endocarditis, and increase the risk of anesthesia-related complications. Respiratory illness in particular may lead to detrimental increases in pulmonary vascular resistance. The urgency and extent of the procedure must be carefully balanced against the cardiovascular status of the child before proceeding in a child with intercurrent illness.

ANATOMY AND FUNCTION

When assessing the anatomy and function, answers to four primary questions may affect anesthesia management:

- Where does the blood go?
- What is the ventricular function?
- How reactive is the pulmonary circulation?
- Is there a fixed or dynamic stenosis?

Answers to these and other questions can help the anesthesiologist determine the optimal approach to management:

- How well will hyperoxia or hypoxia be tolerated?
- What is the likely effect of increased sympathetic stimulation, vasodilation, or a reduction in myocardial contractility?
- What are the likely causes of cardiovascular collapse, and how should they be managed?

Most primary questions can be answered from the record, details of previous surgery, and recent echocardiographic results. However, an index of suspicion is always required: although very poor function may be readily detected, moderate levels of dysfunction may not be acknowledged or as easily detected clinically.

Preoperative blood tests may include hematocrit and a type and hold or crossmatch. Sedative premedication may consist of oral midazolam (0.5 mg/kg) or ketamine (up to 5 mg/kg). Larger doses of sedative premedication may be used to provide more reliable or greater sedation if required, but they may cause prolonged sedation and delayed recovery after the procedure. Topical anesthesia creams facilitate venous cannulation if an IV induction is planned. Care should be taken that these children do not become excessively dehydrated. In selected children, IV fluids should be considered (e.g., BT shunts) before the scheduled procedure.

THE ENVIRONMENT

The cardiac catheterization laboratory can be a challenging environment for the anesthesiologist. Ideally, the cardiac catheterization laboratory should be located near cardiac operating rooms to facilitate rapid availability of ECMO support for high-risk cases. In practice, they are often remotely located from the main operating room complex, limiting availability of immediate assistance and additional resources. Limited functional space may hinder access to the child during both procedures and emergency resuscitation. Blood gas analyzers should be readily available, and blood should be immediately accessible for urgent transfusion for procedures such as balloon dilation and device insertion.

Cardiac catheterization teams usually include many individuals from multiple disciplines so detailed briefing and communication are essential before proceeding. The use of a cardiac catheterization laboratory-specific checklist is associated with fewer complications, decreased radiation exposure, and faster turn-around times. They include planning for anticoagulation, vascular access, and any special equipment required.[51,94]

Lateral and anterior-posterior cameras used for imaging are in close proximity to the patient during procedures and, in combination

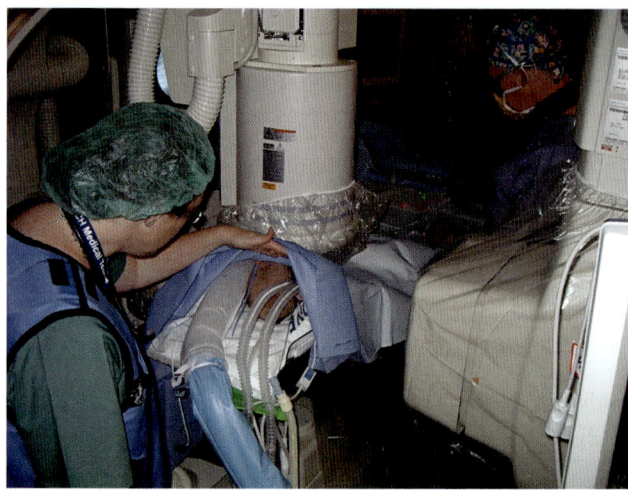

FIGURE 20.5 Typical setup of a catheterization laboratory showing limited access to a child.

with sterile drapes, limit access to the patient and the airway. Blind manipulation under the drapes can dislodge monitoring or the tracheal tube. X-ray cameras are liable to move during procedures to acquire different fields and magnifications, which risk dislodging airway devices, breathing circuits, and IV fluid lines. Meticulous care must be taken to ensure all equipment is well secured before draping and positioning of cameras. Intravenous line extensions are required to enable easy drug administration during the procedure. The catheterization laboratories are often cooled thus temperature should be monitored in all patients; small children will likely require active warming to maintain normothermia. Lighting is often subdued to enhance viewing of the radiographs (Fig. 20.5).

THE CARDIAC PATIENT

The management of anesthesia for children with CHD is discussed further in Chapters 14 to 16. Important considerations include the potential for myocardial dysfunction and identifying limited functional reserve. This may be a particular problem in children with hypertrophied right ventricles operating at near-systemic pressures or with volume-loaded dilated ventricles. Another important consideration is the status and reactivity of the pulmonary vasculature. Difficulties may be anticipated in the following circumstances:

- Increased reactivity of the pulmonary vasculature, such as neonates, or children with primary pulmonary hypertension
- Established pulmonary hypertension with irreversible, chronically increased pulmonary artery pressures and consequent right heart dysfunction
- Circulations that require balancing (e.g., BT shunts or duct-dependent situations), in which increases or decreases in pulmonary vascular resistance may lead to spiraling hypoxia or systemic ischemia and acidosis
- Circulations that rely on low pulmonary vascular resistance to function correctly (e.g., cavopulmonary shunts or after Fontan surgery)

CHOICE OF ANESTHESIA

Many anesthetic agents and techniques have been used safely in pediatric interventional cardiology; thus, the choice of technique should be guided by the patient's pathophysiology and procedural requirements. There is no specific anesthetic method that is appropriate for all children undergoing cardiac catheterization; what is important is that the provider understands the benefits and limitations of the choices they make.[51]

Sedation

The difference between deep sedation and general anesthesia is imprecise and controversial, especially for small children in whom consciousness and memory are harder to measure (see Chapters 43 and 44). When considering the suitability of sedation or general anesthesia, several issues are important:

- Does immobility need to be guaranteed?
- What level of stimulation is expected?
- Do oxygen and carbon dioxide tensions need to be controlled?
- What are the cardiovascular effects of the anesthetic agents?
- How likely is significant physiologic trespass?
- What is the anticipated duration of the procedure?

Sedation is often advocated to avoid the potential effects of general anesthesia on diagnostic measurements; spontaneous ventilation may maintain a more natural intrathoracic physiology promoting the acquisition of more accurate hemodynamic data. However, sedation can be associated with substantial respiratory changes and hypoxia or hypercarbia can have as much of an effect on the circulation as general anesthesia, altering hemodynamics and intracardiac shunts and thus limiting the theoretical advantages.[95–97] Diagnostic studies require controllable, reproducible physiologic conditions, such as consistent arterial carbon dioxide tension with manipulation of inspired oxygen concentrations. Such conditions may be difficult to achieve and/or reproduce in the sedated child. Many modern diagnostic and interventional techniques require the patient to be absolutely still for prolonged periods of time and may require breath-holds. Sedation can be associated with a degree of patient movement that makes procedures such as device placement or balloon dilation potentially difficult or dangerous. However, despite these concerns, sedation remains the technique of choice in some institutions, with evidence of a comparable safety record compared to general anesthesia. Reports from the C3PO database including more than 13,000 pediatric catheterizations reported 31% were performed using a spontaneous ventilation technique with a safety profile comparable to those managed with an artificial airway. In this series, 2% required conversion to general anesthesia with younger age and higher-risk procedures and pressor/inotrope requirements predictive of sedation failure. The eight institutions participating in C3PO had clearly established practice preferences, with two centers undertaking most cases under sedation and the remaining six using general anesthesia as their primary strategy.[98] If sedation is used, full standard monitoring should be undertaken, including monitoring of the airway and end-tidal carbon dioxide ($ETCO_2$), and provisions must be in place for rapid and expert transition to general anesthesia.

Sedation techniques have evolved over the past few decades, resulting in much more effective and titratable strategies. In the past, the classic lytic cocktail of intramuscular meperidine (pethidine), promethazine, and chlorpromazine was the standard for sedation. However, these cocktails had a high incidence of failure and oversedation, and intramuscular routes were associated with sterile abscess formation. Oral ketamine and midazolam provide more reliable sedation, but occasionally respiratory support is required.[95] In theory, IV ketamine is an excellent choice for sedation because it provides a stable or increased heart rate and blood pressure and has little or no effect on pulmonary vascular

resistance. However, prolonged recovery, vomiting, and dysphoric reactions may be problematic. Propofol is also widely used for sedation, but compared with ketamine, it causes a greater reduction in systemic blood pressure and systemic vascular resistance, with no effect on pulmonary vascular resistance. This may increase a right-to-left shunt, or in diagnostic procedures may attenuate the gradient across a stenosis, making the decision to dilate the stenosis more difficult.[99] The highly selective α-agonist dexmedetomidine produces sedation akin to natural sleep, anxiolysis, and sympatholysis without significant respiratory depression, but may not be sufficient in this environment as a sole agent.[100]

Multiple small studies have both described and investigated various combinations of the four major agents: midazolam, ketamine, propofol and dexmedetomidine. In general, the presence of two agents allows smaller doses of each and seems to effectively mitigate some unwanted adverse effects. For example, compared with propofol sedation, a combination of ketamine and propofol sedates similarly with less cardiovascular depression and the drug proportions can be tailored to the degree of stimulus anticipated.[101] However, with small data-sets, highly variable dosing schemes and overtly contradictory techniques, the optimal strategy remains impossible to identify.[102,103]

Local anesthetic infiltration at cannulation sites at the start of the procedure reduces the pain from catheter insertions and exchanges. Spinal anesthesia is an alternative to sedation or general anesthesia in high-risk infants younger than 6 months of age when the procedure is expected to take less than 90 minutes.[104]

General Anesthesia

In the pediatric population, more than 80% of catheterization procedures are performed with patients under general anesthesia.[4] General anesthesia with controlled ventilation has several advantages, including establishing a secure airway without the risk of obstruction and hypoventilation, controlling arterial carbon dioxide and inspired oxygen accurately, and ensuring immobility. In addition, many patients prefer general anesthesia for fear of being awake; as many children require repeat procedures, patient satisfaction with the whole process is important. However, there are also disadvantages. The increased intrathoracic pressure associated with positive-pressure ventilation may decrease preload to the pulmonary and systemic atria, increase afterload on the right ventricle, and decrease afterload on the left ventricle. These effects may be particularly pronounced in patients with right ventricular failure or those dependent on passive pulmonary blood flow (Fontan physiology). Spontaneous ventilation through a supraglottic airway device facilitates venous return and pulmonary blood flow, although the degree of hypoventilation often seen in this situation can result in respiratory acidosis and altered pulmonary vascular resistance. This may be particularly troublesome in patients with pulmonary hypertension. The decision to intubate the trachea or insert a supraglottic airway depends on several variables including patient factors, the duration of the procedure, the requirement for TEE, and whether the neck vessels will be accessed during the procedure.

A variety of general anesthetic agents have been used successfully for interventional cardiology, with no ideal agent identified. There are arguments for and against inhalational and intravenous anesthesia, but no outcome studies have provided strong evidence to recommend one technique over another. Great care should be taken to avoid myocardial depression or systemic vasodilation associated with excessive doses of either inhalational or intravenous anesthetic agents. Knowing that the level of stimulation during most catheterization procedures is minimal, a sufficient depth of anesthesia can often be maintained at a small minimum alveolar concentration (MAC) multiple or plasma concentration, particularly when supplemented with opioids and paralyzing agents, thereby mitigating some of the negative depressant effects of general anesthesia.

Inhalational agents are safe for both induction and maintenance of anesthesia for cardiac catheterization. Sevoflurane has a safe hemodynamic profile and isoflurane maintains cardiac output; both reduce hypoxic pulmonary vasoconstriction and increase ventilation-perfusion ($\dot{V}/\dot{Q}$) mismatch.[105] These changes may affect cardiac output calculations using the Fick principle (equations shown in Table 20.2).

Although nitrous oxide does not appear to affect the pulmonary vasculature in children (in contrast to its effects in adults), it can expand gas bubbles, which is an important consideration in children at risk of paradoxical air embolus. Accordingly, its use is usually limited to facilitating an inhalation induction rather than routine use for maintenance of anesthesia.[106]

Propofol has been safely and extensively used for maintenance of anesthesia in pediatric cardiac catheterization procedures. It has no effect on pulmonary vascular resistance, but dose-dependent reductions in cardiac contractility and systemic vascular resistance are well recognized. Care must be taken in patients with limited myocardial reserve, aortic stenosis, systemic-to-pulmonary shunts, or pulmonary hypertension. However in one study, neither the shunt fraction nor pulmonary-systemic flow (Qp/Qs) ratio changed with doses of 100 µg/kg per minute.[107] Propofol causes respiratory depression and loss of airway reflexes but has the ad-

vantage of reduced postoperative delirium and postoperative nausea and vomiting compared with inhaled agents.

Ketamine produces dissociative anesthesia while preserving airway reflexes and ventilation. It produces stable hemodynamics and, provided carbon dioxide is controlled, has no significant effect on pulmonary vascular resistance or pulmonary artery pressure in patients with pulmonary hypertension.[108] Disadvantages include dysphoria, nausea, prolonged recovery, and salivation. Furthermore, ketamine maintains cardiac output through stimulation of the sympathetic nervous system. A direct myocardial depressant effect may be seen when it is administered to children whose sympathomimetic responses are already maximally stimulated.[109]

Opioids are a useful anesthetic adjunct that reduces both the required dose of other anesthetic agents and the pulmonary vascular response to noxious stimuli. Appropriate dosing should avoid the adverse effects of respiratory depression and hypercarbia. In general, these are not painful procedures; longer-acting opioids, however, may confer postprocedure sedation in addition to analgesia, as the children must remain recumbent for several hours to preclude bleeding from the femoral access sites. Remifentanil may offer an advantage in long catheterization procedures compared with other opioids as the short, context-sensitive half-time allows for rapid clearance and awakening. Bradycardia may be prevented by prophylactic administration of glycopyrrolate.[110] Local anesthetic infiltration around vessel cannulation sites can significantly limit the degree of procedural stimulus and further reduce anesthetic requirements. Maximum safe doses should be calculated according to the child's weight and communicated to the interventionalist to reduce the risk of local anesthetic toxicity (see Table 40.2).

TABLE 20.2	Hemodynamic Calculations Using Cardiac Catheterization Data	
Hemodynamic Variable	**Equation**	**Normal Values**
Oxygen consumption	$\dot{V}O_2 = (CO \times CaO_2) - (CO \times CvO_2)$	Age-, heart rate-, gender-dependent[a]
Flow		
Pulmonary	$Q_P = \dfrac{\dot{V}O_2}{(S_{PV}O_2 - S_{PA}O_2) \times Hgb \times 1.36 \times 10}$	L/minute per m²: 3.5–5 3.5–5
Systemic	$Q_S = \dfrac{\dot{V}O_2}{(S_{AO}O_2 - S_{MV}O_2) \times Hgb \times 1.36 \times 10}$	
Shunt flow ratio	$\dfrac{Q_P}{Q_S} = \dfrac{S_{AO}O_2 - S_{MV}O_2}{S_{PV}O_2 - S_{PA}O_2}$	1:1
Resistance		Wood units:
Pulmonary	$PVR = \dfrac{PAP - LAP}{Q_P}$	Newborns: 8–10 Older children: 1–3 Newborns: 10–15 Older children: 15–30
Systemic	$SVR = \dfrac{AoP - RAP}{Q_S}$	

[a]LaFarge equation for $\dot{V}O_2$:
Boys $\dot{V}O_2 = 138.1 - [11.49 \times \log_e (\text{age in years})] + 0.378 (\text{heart rate})$
Girls $\dot{V}O_2 = 138.1 - [17.04 \times \log_e (\text{age in years})] + 0.378 (\text{heart rate})$
AO, Aorta; *AoP*, aortic pressure; *CaO₂*, arterial oxygen content; *CO*, cardiac output; *CvO₂*, venous oxygen content; *Hgb*, hemoglobin; *LAP*, left atrial pressure; *MV*, mixed venous; *Oₚ*, pulmonary flow; *Q_S* systemic flow; *PA*, pulmonary artery; *PAP*, pulmonary artery pressure; *PV*, pulmonary vein; *PVR*, pulmonary vascular resistance; *QP*, pulmonary blood flow; *QS*, systemic blood flow; *RAP*, right atrial pressure; *S_AoO₂*, aortic oxygen saturation; *S_MVO₂*, mixed venous oxygen saturation; *SO₂*, oxygen saturation; *S_PVO₂*, pulmonary venous saturation; *SVR*, systemic vascular resistance; *V̇o₂*, oxygen consumption.
Modified from Lam JE, Lin EP, Alexy R, Aronson LA. Anesthesia and the pediatric catheterization suite: a review. *Paediatr Anaesth*. 2015;25(2):127-134.

20

Radiofrequency ablation procedures may be protracted, require immobility, and precipitate arrhythmias requiring defibrillation. For these reasons, general anesthesia is usually preferred, but many anesthetic agents affect cardiac conduction and may prevent the generation of preexcitation and automatic tachycardia. Dexmedetomidine has useful sedative, anxiolytic, and analgesic properties without effects on respiratory drive. It depresses sinus and atrioventricular nodal function, and avoiding its use in electrophysiology settings has been recommended.[111] However, a study using the different techniques of anesthetists at one institution has recently challenged this. Induction and ablation of arrhythmias was not inhibited using dexmedetomidine, although slightly larger doses of isoproterenol were required in the higher-dose group.[112] Controversy has surrounded the use of inhalational agents for the maintenance of anesthesia during ablation procedures but sound clinical data are scant. It appears that for preexcitation, isoflurane and sevoflurane have little effect at less than 1 MAC, whereas propofol and opioids have no demonstrable effects at any dose. In contrast, automatic tachycardia may be suppressed by large doses of propofol and opioids. In a prospective, randomized trial, isoflurane- and propofol-based anesthesia resulted in a similar duration of anesthesia and effectiveness of ablation.[113] Reducing the dose of anesthesia may limit some of the unwanted effects on conduction.

Principles of Technique

The most important principle of anesthesia in this setting is that the anesthetic practitioner has a sound knowledge of CHD physiology, experience with the procedures, and sedation/anesthesia techniques that are reliable and with which they are familiar. Attention to detail is critical for the provision of safe anesthesia. Consideration of preprocedural anxiolysis, fluid management, full monitoring, expert assistance, and choice of anesthetic technique is critical, in addition to generating a functional interaction with the rest of the catheterization team.

Careful attention to volume status is very important. Prolonged preoperative fasting can cause dehydration, particularly in small infants, and should be actively avoided. Hypovolemia is poorly tolerated in most children with CHD, particularly those with shunt-dependent circulations and those who are preload dependent such as children with single-ventricle physiology. Prolonged procedures can be associated with gradual hypovolemia secondary to blood sampling, bleeding, and diuretic effects of contrast media. Volume overload is also a risk with liberal fluids and high-dose contrast, which may be poorly tolerated in children with congestive heart failure. Cyanotic patients or those with single ventricles are usually accustomed to or benefit from a larger hematocrit, which needs to be taken into consideration when replacing fluid losses. Large volume fluid replacement during diagnostic catheterization may affect filling pressures, gradient, and flow and should be communicated to the cardiologist.

Difficult IV access is prevalent in this patient population but reliable IV access is essential in case rapid resuscitation is required. Availability of ultrasound may facilitate access and intraosseous access should be available for emergency access (see Chapter 46). Intravenous access should ideally be placed in the upper extremities, as the femoral vessels are most commonly accessed for procedures in young children, and the presence of catheters may prevent reliable IV drug and fluid administration. Similarly, pulse oximetry and noninvasive blood pressure cuffs may be less reliable if placed on a limb used for cardiology access or with a BT shunt. Invasive central or arterial monitoring may be indicated for high-risk cases to monitor and treat any perioperative instability. During procedures to dilate the aortic arch or aortic valve, it may be prudent to have an arterial line (preferably a right radial line) to allow continuous blood pressure monitoring during the dilatation. If continuous arterial monitoring is not required from induction, arterial access obtained by the cardiologist for the procedure can sometimes be transduced for anesthetic monitoring using either a second stopcock or a slave monitor.

Problems associated with anesthesia-induced myocardial depression and hypotension are well recognized but inadequate anesthesia can create its own problems. Hemodynamic consequences of light anesthesia, such as hypoxia owing to laryngospasm, are poorly tolerated in children with pulmonary hypertension. Hypoxia or hypercapnia may lead to increasing pulmonary vascular resistance, which may increase cardiac shunts, further worsening hypoxia. Increased pulmonary artery pressures may also lead to significant decreases in pulmonary compliance, further increasing hypoxia and precipitating a downward spiral.

Catheterization procedures often involve long periods of very little painful stimulation with discrete periods of increased painful stimuli, such as during dilation of arterial and venous vessels, sheath changes, or balloon dilation. By maintaining good communication between the cardiologist and anesthesiologist, these periods can be anticipated, and the depth of anesthesia or sedation analgesia adjusted accordingly.

TEE is increasingly being used during diagnostic procedures and to guide intracardiac catheter placement. Insertion of a TEE probe can be very stimulating and often requires a deeper plane of anesthesia with the addition of opioids, neuromuscular blockade, or both. A tracheal tube is required to ensure a patent airway during TEE, and care must be taken to avoid dislodging the tracheal tube during manipulations of the TEE probe.

Procedures in the catheterization laboratory can often be lengthy with limited access to the patient. Extra care should be taken to ensure careful positioning of the patient to avoid pressure areas and potential nerve injury.

Coughing and straining on extubation may increase the risk of hematoma formation. For this reason, extubating the trachea during a deep level of anesthesia may be preferred. The advantages of deep extubation must be balanced against the risks of hypoxia, hypercapnia, and loss of airway control or laryngospasm that may ensue if the tracheal tube is removed before the child is fully awake.

Catheterization procedures are usually minimally invasive and are not associated with excessive postprocedural pain. Simple analgesics, such as paracetamol, combined with local anesthetic infiltration are usually adequate. Opioids are rarely required for postoperative analgesia and may contribute to postoperative nausea and vomiting. Emergence delirium and postoperative restlessness may increase the risk of bleeding at catheter puncture sites. Additional analgesia or sedatives may occasionally need to be administered by the anesthesiologist in recovery to gain control of an agitated patient and prevent such complications.

Effective teamwork is critical to the safe and effective pediatric cardiac catheterization procedure. This is particularly important for high-risk children and complex procedures that may involve many multidisciplinary professionals. Effective communication between the interventional cardiologist (and surgeon in hybrid procedures) and anesthesiologist should be maintained before and throughout the procedure to (1) plan and modify anesthesia and (2) anticipate any hemodynamic changes or adverse events. Often treatment of complications, such as bleeding or dysrhythmias, involves interventions using both cardiology and anesthesiology techniques. A good team approach is key to achieving the best possible patient outcomes.

FUTURE OF ANESTHESIA IN INTERVENTIONAL CARDIOLOGY

Anesthesia for interventional cardiac catheterizations will become more challenging as new interventions are developed for sicker children and more procedures are performed in combination with open surgery or MRI. As is often the case in pediatric practice, technologic advancements in cardiac catheterization have lagged behind those for the adult population. Focused development of smaller pediatric-appropriate devices will continue to expand the scope of pediatric interventional cardiology; promising potential for wider applications of transcatheter valve replacements is already on the horizon. More children are likely to require general anesthesia, and specialist pediatric cardiac anesthesiologists will be spending an increasing proportion of their time in interventional cardiology suites.

The ability to risk-stratify children and procedures prospectively to accurately predict and potentially prevent adverse events is key to improving patient safety in the catheterization laboratory.[51] Progress has been made in this area with the development of the **C**atheterization **RIS**k **S**core for **P**ediatrics (CRISP score; available online at https://www.evidencio.com/models/show/678), which uses patient demographics, current physiologic status, and procedural risk to predict the risk of adverse events for an individual child.[114] This ability to predict risk is potentially invaluable both for assessing the level of resources and expertise required and informing anesthetic strategies to minimize risk of harm to the children we seek to care for.

Acknowledgment

We thank Dr Natalie Forshaw for her previous contributions to this chapter.

ANNOTATED REFERENCES

Feltes TF, Bacha E, Beekman RH III, et al. Indications for cardiac catheterization and intervention in pediatric cardiac disease: a scientific statement from the American Heart Association. *Circulation.* 2011;123(22):2607-2652.

The American Heart Association has provided a comprehensive overview of the subject.

Odegard KC, Vincent R, Baijal RG, et al. SCAI/CCAS/SPA expert consensus statement for anesthesia and sedation practice: recommendations for patients undergoing diagnostic and therapeutic procedures in the pediatric and congenital cardiac catheterization laboratory. *Anesth Analg.* 2016;123(5):1201-1209.

A comprehensive review of anesthetic concerns in the pediatric catheterization laboratory.

Tierney N, Kenny D, Greaney D. Anaesthesia for the paediatric patient in the cardiac catheterisation laboratory. *BJA Education.* 2022;22(2): 60-66.

This is a good review of anesthesia for pediatric cardiac catheterization.

Twite MD, Friesen RH. The anaesthetic management of children with pulmonary hypertension in the cardiac catheterisation laboratory. *Anesthesiol Clin.* 2014;32(1):157-173.

An overview of managing the high-risk subgroup of patients with pulmonary hypertension.

Vincent RN, Moore J, Beekman RH, et al. Procedural characteristics and adverse events in diagnostic and interventional catheterisations in pediatric and adult CHD: initial report from the IMPACT Registry. *Cardiol Young.* 2016;26(1):70-78.

This paper describes complications in pediatric cardiac catheterization from the currently largest dataset.

A complete reference list can be found online at Elsevier eBooks+.

Anesthesia for Noncardiac Surgery in Children With Congenital Heart Disease

21

WANDA C. MILLER-HANCE

Selected Congenital Heart Defects
Atrial Septal Defects
Ventricular Septal Defects
Atrioventricular Septal Defects
Patent Ductus Arteriosus
Right Ventricular Outflow Tract Obstructions
Left Ventricular Outflow Tract Obstructions
Coarctation of the Aorta
Tetralogy of Fallot
D-Transposition of the Great Arteries
Congenitally Corrected Transposition of the Great Arteries
Truncus Arteriosus
Ebstein Anomaly
Interrupted Aortic Arch
Congenital Anomalies of the Coronary Arteries
Single Ventricle
Perioperative Considerations in Children With CHD during Noncardiac Surgery
Preoperative Assessment
Intraoperative Management
Perioperative Problems and Special Considerations
Hypotension

Cyanosis
Heart Failure
Ventricular Dysfunction
Ventricular Volume Overload
Ventricular Pressure Overload
Myocardial Ischemia
Altered Respiratory Mechanics
Endocarditis Prophylaxis
Pulmonary Hypertension
Eisenmenger Syndrome
Systemic Air Embolization
Anticoagulation
Conduction Disturbances and Arrhythmias
Pacemakers and Implantable Cardioverter-Defibrillators
Nerve Palsies
Mechanical Circulatory Support Devices
Cardiac Transplantation
Perioperative Stress Response
Types of Noncardiac Surgical Procedures in Children With CHD and Implications for Anesthesia Care
Outcomes of Noncardiac Surgery in Children With CHD and Risk Analysis

THE NATURAL HISTORY OF CONGENITAL HEART DISEASE (CHD) has been favorably impacted by remarkable advances in medical and surgical care over the past several decades. These refinements have resulted in decreased morbidity and improvement in long-term clinical outcomes in affected children. As survival rates further improve and life expectancy continues to increase,[1] an escalating number of children with CHD are presenting for noncardiac surgery or other procedures related or unrelated to their heart disease. The care of these children is becoming more common in all diagnostic and surgical venues, including in ambulatory standalone settings, free-standing hospital-based facilities, and quaternary-care institutions.[2,3]

A variety of extracardiac anomalies are well known to affect children with CHD[4–8] with a reported prevalence of associated malformations ranging between 10% and 33%.[9,10] The musculoskeletal, central nervous, renal-urinary, gastrointestinal, and respiratory organ systems are most often affected. Although many extracardiac malformations are relatively minor and have limited or no clinical implications, a considerable number of children with CHD have noncardiac comorbidities.[11,12] These pathologic and disease processes may necessitate diagnostic evaluation and/or surgical intervention under sedation or general anesthesia. This is also the case for other routine ailments that may affect these children. Chromosomal syndromes and genetic disorders, well known to be associated with CHD, may lead to conditions that necessitate anesthesia care.

As early palliation and corrective surgery has become the favored approach in most congenital cardiovascular malformations, children who have undergone these interventions represent the main patient group that an anesthesiologist is likely to encounter during elective, urgent, and emergent noncardiac surgery. In some cases, children may require noncardiac surgery before undergoing procedures to address their cardiovascular disease. In others, the cardiac condition may not necessitate or be amenable to surgical intervention.

The challenges of caring for children with CHD for noncardiac surgery are magnified by the wide range of defects, each with specific physiologic perturbations, hemodynamic consequences, and severity. This is further complicated by the variety of medical and surgical strategies available for the management of these conditions. Many children, but particularly those with more than mild disease, require an individualized approach to anesthesia care.[13–17]

Undoubtedly, optimal anesthesia care for children with CHD requires a thorough appreciation of the underlying cardiovascular anatomic abnormalities, pathophysiologic consequences of the defect, functional status, residua, sequelae, and expected long-term outcome, in addition to the planned procedure, implications regarding underlying cardiovascular disease, and potential complications. Given the importance of a general understanding of the cardiac defect during noncardiac surgery, this chapter presents an overview of malformations most likely to be encountered in the noncardiac perioperative setting. General principles of anesthesia practice pertaining to the care of children with CHD during noncardiac procedures are also reviewed. Unique perioperative considerations and issues applicable to high-risk patient groups are addressed. Finally, an overview is provided of current knowledge concerning outcomes and risk assessment in these children during noncardiac surgery. The American Heart Association has recently published a scientific statement addressing perioperative considerations for pediatric patients with CHD presenting for noncardiac procedures.[18] The reader is referred to this document as an additional resource on the subject discussed in this chapter.

Selected Congenital Heart Defects

Providing anesthesia care to children with CHD undergoing noncardiac surgery is influenced by the specific nature of the cardiovascular malformations, pathophysiology of the lesions, operative state (e.g., unoperated, prior palliative or definitive procedure), complications associated with the primary pathology or treatment, and other comorbidities. Accordingly, this section reviews selected cardiac defects most likely to be encountered during noncardiac surgery with an emphasis on anatomic features, hemodynamic consequences, and usual management strategies. Treatment, potential residua, sequelae (Table 21.1), and long-term outcomes of these lesions are also addressed, as well as considerations for anesthesia care.

ATRIAL SEPTAL DEFECTS
Anatomy and Pathophysiology
Defects in the interatrial septum, or atrial septal defects (ASDs) (see Fig. 15.1), are among the most common congenital cardiac anomalies in childhood (30% to 40% of CHD).[19,20] These occur in 1 of 1500 live births; several types of defects are identified based on their location within the atrium:

- *Ostium secundum or fossa ovalis defects* (75% of ASDs) result from a deficiency in the region of the fossa ovalis, representing a true defect in the atrial septum (see Fig. 15.1B). These anomalies can be associated with mitral valve prolapse and/or mitral regurgitation.
- *Ostium primum defects* (15% to 20% of ASDs) represent a form of atrioventricular (AV) septal (canal or endocardial cushion) defect (see Fig. 15.1A). The malformation is characterized by a deficiency in the inferior portion of the interatrial septum, separate AV valves (common junction), and is frequently associated with a commissure or cleft in the anterior leaflet of the mitral valve and various degrees of mitral regurgitation.
- *Sinus venosus defects* (5% to 10% of ASDs) typically are located at the superior aspect of the interatrial septum, at the junction of the superior vena cava and the right atrium (i.e., superior vena cava type-defect) (see Fig. 15.1C). An inferior-type defect (at the inferior vena cava) is less common. These defects are frequently associated with partial anomalous pulmonary venous drainage. It has been argued that this may not represent a defect in the true atrial septum but unroofing of venous structures in the right atrium and may be better considered a venovenous malformation.[21]

- *Coronary sinus defects* (<1% of ASDs) consists of a communication between the atria due to partial or complete unroofing of the tissue that normally separates the coronary sinus from the left atrium. The direction of shunting across the coronary sinus itself may be variable but left-to-right shunting usually occurs across the large coronary sinus orifice. This defect is often associated with a persistent left superior vena cava that drains directly into the left atrium (Raghib syndrome), resulting in a right-to-left shunt.

Other entities that may allow for interatrial shunting include a *patent foramen ovale* (PFO) at one end of the spectrum and a *common atrium* at the other. A PFO is a flap-like opening or channel between the two septa (septum primum and septum secundum) that divides the primordial single atrium into right and left atrial chambers. A PFO can be identified in approximately 25% of all individuals. The communication may have implications for perioperative care because of the potential for right-to-left shunting and paradoxical emboli.[22,23] In a common atrium, there is complete or near-total absence of the interatrial septum. This can be seen in complex congenital cardiac pathologies such as heterotaxy syndromes, a condition characterized by abnormal arrangements or sidedness of the abdominal viscera, heart, and lungs, and associated with a high likelihood of complex cardiovascular disease.

An atrial communication allows mixing of the pulmonary and systemic venous returns. A left-to-right shunt permits pulmonary venous blood to enter the right atrium. The magnitude of shunting correlates with the size of the defect, relative ventricular compliances, and pulmonary artery (PA) pressures. A clinically significant defect results in right-sided volume overload. A pulmonary-to-systemic blood flow ratio ($\dot{Q}_{pulm}/\dot{Q}_{sys}$) that exceeds 2:1 and the potential detrimental effects of chronic right-sided volume overload are indications for intervention.

Treatment Options, Residua, Sequelae, and Long-Term Outcomes
Surgical closure of secundum ASDs in childhood provides excellent results, almost normal long-term survival, and negligible mortality.[24–26] Normal ventricular function should be anticipated after repair of these defects. Rarely, children can demonstrate persistent right ventricular (RV) dilation and abnormal ventricular septal motion, but this may not result in a functional deficit. Atrial arrhythmias and ventricular dysfunction can occur after late repairs owing to chronic volume overload. Delayed defect closure can be a risk factor for the rare development of pulmonary hypertension later in life as the result the chronic abnormally increased pulmonary blood flow.[27,28]

Transcatheter device occlusion is an alternative approach to surgery for closure of secundum ASDs in selected children, with excellent success rates (see Chapter 20).[29,30] Complications are rare and can be associated with the catheter-based intervention or occur at a later time.

After surgical closure of ostium primum defects, morbidity manifests primarily as mitral valve dysfunction (e.g., mitral regurgitation or stenosis) or left ventricular outflow tract (LVOT) obstruction.[31,32] In most children, outcomes are favorable after repair at an early age. After closure of sinus venosus defects, potential problems include pulmonary venous obstruction and loss of sinus node function.[33–35] Repair of coronary sinus defects depends on the specific nature of the defect and associated anomalies. The surgical intervention usually consists of redirection of the coronary sinus blood and possibly the associated abnormal systemic venous return to the right atrium.[36] Patch closure of the

TABLE 21.1 | Potential Issues After Interventions for Selected Congenital Heart Defects

Atrial Septal Defects

Residual intracardiac shunt

Persistent right ventricular dilation and abnormal motion of interventricular septum

Atrial arrhythmias, ventricular dysfunction if late repair

Pulmonary venous obstruction (sinus venosus defect associated with anomalous pulmonary venous return)

Mitral valve problems, left ventricular outflow tract obstruction (ostium primum defect with cleft mitral valve)

Development of pulmonary vascular disease (rare)

Atrioventricular Septal Defects

Left atrioventricular valve problems (regurgitation, stenosis)

Left ventricular outflow tract obstruction

Residual intracardiac shunts

Atrioventricular block, conduction abnormalities

Prior palliation with pulmonary artery banding might have resulted in inadequate protection of pulmonary vasculature or distortion of pulmonary artery anatomy

Pulmonary hypertension may persist

Coarctation of the Aorta

Systemic hypertension

Residual or recurrent obstruction

Death from untreated pathology, related to heart failure, aortic rupture or dissection, infective endarteritis or endocarditis, premature coronary artery disease, or cerebral hemorrhage

Endocarditis risk with concomitant aortic valve disease

Congenitally Corrected Transposition of the Great Arteries

Residual defects (e.g., shunts, outflow tract obstruction)

Systemic (right) ventricular dilation, dysfunction, failure

Left-sided (tricuspid) valve regurgitation

Atrioventricular block or arrhythmias

Coronary artery anomalies

May go unsuspected for some time

Myocardial ischemia

Ventricular dysfunction

May present as syncope, or lead to sudden death

D-Transposition of the Great Arteries

Residual pathology (e.g., intracardiac shunts, outflow tract obstruction)

After atrial baffle procedure: baffle leak, obstruction of systemic or pulmonary venous pathways, progressive right ventricular dilation or failure, tricuspid regurgitation, sinus node dysfunction, or atrial arrhythmias

After arterial switch operation: aortic root dilation, aortic regurgitation, supravalvar stenosis (pulmonary or aortic), or coronary insufficiency

Ebstein Anomaly

Progressive tricuspid regurgitation and right-sided volume overload

Right/left ventricular dysfunction

Atrial tachyarrhythmias (particularly if Wolff-Parkinson-White syndrome)

Potential for paradoxical right-to-left shunting in the presence of an interatrial communication

Valve repair or replacement may be necessary

Interrupted Aortic Arch

Residual intracardiac defects

Subaortic obstruction

Residual or recurrent aortic arch obstruction

Left Ventricular Outflow Tract Obstructions

Residual or recurrent obstruction

Aortic regurgitation, aortic root dilation

Risk of endocarditis

Ventricular dysfunction

Potential subendocardial ischemia if ongoing ventricular pressure overload

Coronary ostial stenosis, diffuse arteriopathy (supravalvar aortic stenosis)

Need for reoperation in those with bioprosthetic or mechanical valves or conduits

After Ross procedure: autograft or right ventricular homograft failure, progressive aortic root dilation, or aortic regurgitation

Patent Ductus Arteriosus

Residual or recurrent shunting

Increased pulmonary vascular resistance (now rare)

Right Ventricular Outflow Tract Obstructions

Residual or recurrent obstruction resulting in ventricular pressure overload

Pulmonary regurgitation may require intervention

After right ventricle-to-pulmonary artery conduit: need for intervention or reoperation related to conduit failure

Single Ventricle

After aortopulmonary shunt: shunt stenosis or thrombosis with associated hypoxemia, ventricular volume overload, systemic ventricular dilation, distortion of pulmonary artery anatomy, or pulmonary hypertension

After bidirectional Glenn connection or hemi-Fontan procedure: progressive cyanosis owing to venous collaterals or other vascular communications, allowing venous pathways to bypass the pulmonary circuit, or owing to the development of pulmonary arteriovenous malformations (more likely with classic Glenn anastomosis)

After Fontan procedure: chronically increased systemic venous pressures, right atrial hypertension (with atriopulmonary connection), sinus node dysfunction, atrial rhythm disturbances, atrioventricular valve regurgitation, hepatic dysfunction, thrombotic complications, coagulation defects, protein-losing enteropathy, or progressive systemic ventricular dilation or dysfunction

Tetralogy of Fallot

Residual or recurrent pathology (e.g., intracardiac shunts, right ventricular outflow tract obstruction, distal pulmonary artery bed abnormalities)

Progressive pulmonary regurgitation with need for repeat intervention (e.g., right-sided heart dilation, dysfunction)

Arrhythmias associated with poor hemodynamics

Syncope or sudden death (arrhythmogenic cause)

Restrictive right ventricular physiology

Truncus Arteriosus

Residual intracardiac shunting

Revision of right ventricle-to-pulmonary artery reconstruction (for stenosis or regurgitation)

Truncal (aortic) valve stenosis or regurgitation

Ventricular Septal Defect

Potential residual defects

Risk of endocarditis (diminishes with time after repair)

Aortic regurgitation

Rarely, increased pulmonary vascular resistance that may not improve postoperatively atrial communication at the mouth of the coronary sinus may be all that is required in some cases, leaving a small right-to-left shunt as deoxygenated blood from the coronary sinus continues to drain directly into the left atrium. For most children with atrial communications, significant postoperative sequelae are unlikely, and outcomes are generally good. Transcatheter approaches for this defect have also been sporadically reported but these have been mostly beyond childhood.[37]

Considerations for Anesthesia Care
An important consideration in the child with an unrepaired interatrial communication is the avoidance of intravenous (IV) air in view of the potential for paradoxical gas embolism. In most cases, no major repercussion should be expected for future anesthesia care from a repaired defect.

VENTRICULAR SEPTAL DEFECTS
Anatomy and Pathophysiology
Ventricular septal defects (VSDs) are the most common of all congenital cardiac anomalies, occurring in 30% to 60% of CHD (excluding a bicuspid aortic valve), with an incidence of 2 to 6 cases per 1000 live births (see Fig. 15.2A).[38] VSDs can be found in isolation or within the context of other structural malformations. Large defects require early attention for symptoms related to pulmonary over circulation that result in congestive heart failure (CHF) or pulmonary hypertension. VSDs have a greater rate of spontaneous closure, reported anywhere between 60% to 75%, during childhood.[39]

Various classification schemes have been proposed for VSDs based on their anatomic location, size, restrictive versus nonrestrictive nature, and hemodynamic impact.[40,41] The following scheme categorizes defects as four major morphologic types *based on their anatomic location*. In some cases, the boundaries of a defect extend beyond the margin of a particular region of the ventricular septum into another and these are qualified as such.

- *Perimembranous defects* (most common types) are located in the membranous region, under the septal leaflet of the tricuspid valve and just below the aortic valve. They are frequently associated with redundant septal tricuspid valve tissue (e.g., aneurysmal tissue) that can limit shunting or eventually result in spontaneous complete defect closure.
- *Muscular defects* are located anywhere within the trabecular (muscle-bound) component of the ventricular septum. Multiple defects can give the appearance of a "Swiss cheese" septum, which complicates surgical closure.
- *Doubly committed, subarterial, conal, or supracristal defects* are found within the region of the subpulmonary infundibulum. They can be associated with aortic valve herniation or prolapse into the defect and aortic regurgitation.
- *Inlet defects* are located in the posterior aspect of the ventricular septum near the AV valves; associated valvar anomalies frequently coexist.

The characterization of VSDs *based on their size and likely hemodynamic importance* is extremely useful when caring for unoperated children:

- *Small defect:* The pulmonary-to-systemic systolic pressure ratio is less than 0.3 and the $\dot{Q}_{pulm}/\dot{Q}_{sys}$ is less than 1.4. The defect causes negligible to minimal hemodynamic effects. Normal RV systolic pressure, pulmonary vascular resistance, and LV size are typically found.
- *Moderate defect:* The systolic pressure ratio is greater than 0.3 and the $\dot{Q}_{pulm}/\dot{Q}_{sys}$ is 1.4 to 2.2. The defect can be associated with volume overload and congestive symptoms. Some degree of left atrial and LV dilation exists, as well as elevated PA pressures.
- *Large defect:* The systolic pressure ratio is greater than 0.3 and the $\dot{Q}_{pulm}/\dot{Q}_{sys}$ exceeds 2.2. The defect is associated with important symptoms (e.g., failure to thrive, CHF). Cardiomegaly and increased pulmonary vascularity are usual findings.

The physiologic effects of the communications that allow for ventricular-level shunting are determined by factors such as the size of the defect, amount of shunting, and relative pulmonary and systemic vascular resistances. Physiologically, isolated defects can be classified as pressure restrictive (i.e., RV pressure < LV pressure) or nonrestrictive defects (i.e., equal or near-equal ventricular pressures). Restrictive defects often imply limited flow through the communication. This is usually the case with small VSDs in which the pressure gradient determines the magnitude of shunting. If the defect is large and nonrestrictive, the amount of shunting depends on the ratio between the pulmonary and systemic vascular resistances. A low pulmonary vascular resistance in the context of a nonrestrictive VSD leads to a large left-to-right shunt, increased pulmonary blood flow, pulmonary hypertension, and increased myocardial work, as evidenced by a volume load to the left heart. Nonrestrictive left-to-right shunts result in pulmonary congestion and abnormal respiratory mechanics characterized by decreased lung compliance, increased airway resistance, and increased work of breathing. Increases in alveolar dead space and alveolar to arterial oxygen gradients are to be expected, as well as increases in minute ventilation and potential oxygen requirements.

Treatment Options, Residua, Sequelae, and Long-Term Outcomes
Surgical closure of VSDs early in childhood results in excellent outcomes, usually without sequelae.[42] Patient weight is considered a significant predictor of morbidity in these children.[43] Intervention in older children can lead to reduced LV function and increased LV mass. Small communications, although regarded as hemodynamically insignificant, may not be benign. This has led to ongoing controversy regarding the need for definitive intervention. Occasionally a young child with a defect of moderate size remains relatively asymptomatic until later life, when gradual decompensation may ensue related to increased end-diastolic volume and ventricular dilation. Defect closure in this setting is indicated if the magnitude of the increase in pulmonary vascular resistance is not prohibitive, which would be extremely rare. Severely increased pulmonary vascular resistance increases the perioperative risks, and it may not return to normal levels after the surgical intervention.[44] If postoperative pulmonary hypertension persists, the prognosis is unfavorable, with the potential for eventual RV failure. Development of Eisenmenger syndrome (i.e., pulmonary vascular obstructive disease and reversal in the direction of the ventricular-level shunt) has become rare owing to early recognition and management of children with these defects.

Postoperative sequelae after VSD closure include residual or, less commonly, recurrent defects, valvar regurgitation, subaortic obstruction, or arrhythmias or other conduction system disturbances. Although surgical closure is considered the gold standard, transcatheter closure by device placement is feasible for selected defects, typically muscular or postoperative residual defects. The experience to date demonstrates excellent closure rates with reduced rates of complications (see also Chapter 20).[45] Device occlusion of perimembranous defects has been successfully performed.[46–48] However, this approach has not been universally embraced due to potential serious complications such as the development of conduction system disturbances, including complete AV block.[49]

Considerations for Anesthesia Care

An important perioperative consideration for children with defects associated with increased pulmonary blood flow is the pulmonary steal phenomenon, which may result from decreases in pulmonary vascular resistance as left-to-right shunting increases at the expense of systemic blood flow.[50] This requires an appraisal of the factors that may influence pulmonary vascular tone to prevent compromises in systemic output. Children with a small defect or without residual pathology after undergoing VSD closure often have normal ventricular systolic function and should be expected to do well during future noncardiac procedures.

ATRIOVENTRICULAR SEPTAL DEFECTS

Anatomy and Pathophysiology

Atrioventricular septal defects (AVSDs), also referred to as AV canal defects or endocardial cushion defects, are characterized by deficiency of the AV septum and abnormal formation of the AV valves (see Fig. 15.2B). These defects represent only 4% of CHD cases, although they are prevalent in children with Down syndrome. Although the nomenclature of AVSDs has been the subject of confusion and even controversy, in general the lesions that represent the spectrum of pathologies can be classified as:

The *complete form* (i.e., common AV canal defect) consists of contiguous defects including an ostium primum defect and an interventricular communication at the superior aspect of the inlet or posterior muscular septum, and a large common AV valve. They are frequently associated with various degrees of AV valve regurgitation.

The *partial form* (i.e., incomplete form) is usually characterized by an ostium primum ASD accompanied by a cleft or commissure in the left-sided AV valve. Two functionally distinct AV valvar orifices are usually identified (refer to section on Atrial Septal Defects earlier in the chapter).

The *transitional or intermediate forms* represent variants of AVSDs. When considered as separate entities, a transitional defect is regarded as a partial form of the defect characterized by a primum ASD, a small inlet VSD (usually restrictive), and two distinct AV valve components. An intermediate defect refers to a variant of the complete form of the defect characterized by a primum ASD and a nonrestrictive VSD in the setting of a common AV valve annulus and two distinct AV valvar orifices separated by a tongue of tissue.

Complete defects are associated with nonrestrictive intracardiac shunting, excessive pulmonary blood flow, CHF, and systemic RV and PA systolic pressures. Without intervention, they can lead to early pulmonary vascular changes. The severity of AV valve regurgitation also influences the clinical presentation. Partial AVSDs are less likely to be associated with pulmonary over circulation of sufficient severity to cause significant heart failure.

Treatment Options, Residua, Sequelae, and Long-Term Outcomes

The surgical approach for complete defects is that of primary repair in infancy. The intervention consists of patch closure of the intracardiac communications, partition of the common AV valve, and closure of the left-sided valvar cleft (also known as zone of apposition). The long-term outlook after repair is generally good,

with a small likelihood of residual dysfunction.[51] Postoperative problems include left AV valve regurgitation or stenosis, residual intracardiac shunting, AV block, and subaortic obstruction.[31,52] Occasionally, pulmonary hypertension persists or develops postoperatively; it is more likely in children with Down syndrome. In the remote past, uncorrected defects associated with high pressure and high flow resulted in muscular development of the pulmonary vasculature and Eisenmenger physiology, accounting for major late morbidity and early death.[53] These patients are at high risk for anesthesia for any procedure (see Eisenmenger Syndrome later in the chapter).

Considerations for Anesthesia Care

Perioperative concerns like those previously described in children with nonrestrictive ventricular communications are applicable, but they also are magnified in those with unrepaired complete defects. In children with unrepaired defects with increased pulmonary vascular resistance and a reactive pulmonary bed, issues such as airway manipulation, light anesthesia, hypoxemia, or hypercarbia can lead to acute increases in PA pressures to suprasystemic levels and detrimental hemodynamic consequences. After surgical correction, important anesthesia considerations relate to degree of AV valve dysfunction, severity of LVOT obstruction when present, and potential pulmonary hypertension in some children.

PATENT DUCTUS ARTERIOSUS

Anatomy and Pathophysiology

The ductus arteriosus is an essential vascular structure in fetal life that connects the pulmonary trunk and thoracic aorta (see Figs. 15.4 and 16.1). It enables RV output into the descending aorta in the fetus, within the context of normally increased pulmonary vascular resistance. A patent ductus arteriosus (PDA) can be an isolated finding or can be associated with other forms of heart disease. Prematurity and CHD are important risk factors.

The magnitude and direction of great artery shunting depends on the size of the communication and the pulmonary vascular resistance. In children with moderate or large left-to-right shunts, the physiologic effects are those of increased pulmonary blood flow and LV volume overload.

Treatment Options, Residua, Sequelae, and Long-Term Outcomes

Children with a tiny or small PDA have a normal life expectancy. Those with hemodynamically important communications eventually develop symptoms related to LV volume overload that predispose them to pulmonary hypertension.[54] Although unlikely in the current era, in the past, the long-standing high-pressure and high-flow states associated with a moderate or large PDA resulted in Eisenmenger syndrome in some children.

Surgical ductal closure can be performed by ligation or division. This may be favored in the case of large communications or when catheter-based interventions may not be suitable. Percutaneous catheter occlusion can be accomplished with a good success rate in infants and children (see also Chapter 20).[55] Advances in occluder technology over the last several years now allow transcatheter closure even in preterm infants.[56] Interruption of this vascular structure is rarely associated with long-term issues.

Considerations for Anesthesia Care

In the preterm neonate with a hemodynamically significant PDA, the main concerns relate to prematurity (see Chapter 35), pulmonary over circulation, and the potential for a steal physiology similar to that described for intracardiac shunts. In general, children with a small to moderate size ductus or post transcatheter closure or ligation with normal cardiovascular reserve can be expected and should be managed using usual protocols during anesthesia care.

RIGHT VENTRICULAR OUTFLOW TRACT OBSTRUCTIONS

Anatomy and Pathophysiology

Pulmonary valve stenosis is the most common pathology among children with RV outflow tract (RVOT) obstruction. Other lesions that result in obstruction to pulmonary blood flow include infundibular (subpulmonary) stenosis, anomalous muscle bundles within the body of the RV, and structural alterations in the pulmonary arterial bed. These pathologies may be found in isolation or occur as part of more complex malformations. Such is the case in tetralogy of Fallot (discussed later in the chapter), in which multiple anatomic levels of RVOT obstruction are typically encountered (see Fig. 15.5).

Although isolated valvar pulmonary stenosis is congenital in most cases, the disease can be progressive. In the uncomplicated or pure variant, an interatrial communication in the form of a PFO or secundum ASD may be identified, and the ventricular septum is intact.

The magnitude of RVOT obstruction is directly related to the degree of valvar narrowing. This imposes an afterload burden on the RV, resulting in muscle hypertrophy and decreased diastolic compliance. Tricuspid regurgitation can be an associated finding. In severe cases, the RV systolic pressure may exceed that of the LV. Cyanosis in children with pulmonary stenosis usually reflects right-to-left interatrial shunting and reduced pulmonary blood flow. It can be associated with severe RV hypertrophy, myocardial fibrosis, and/or ventricular dysfunction.

Most children with mild to moderate valvar stenosis remain asymptomatic, and the pathology is relatively well tolerated chronically. Severe obstruction in older children is frequently associated with limited exercise tolerance.

Treatment Options, Residua, Sequelae, and Long-Term Outcomes

Percutaneous balloon valvuloplasty is very effective and currently is considered the treatment of choice for isolated valvar pulmonary stenosis, replacing surgical valvotomy in most cases. Outcomes are excellent, and long-term issues are rare.[57] Dysplastic valves have a less favorable response to catheter-based interventions, and affected children are more likely to require surgery. Indications for repeat intervention include residual outflow tract obstruction and progressive pulmonary regurgitation.

Considerations for Anesthesia Care

In children with RV hypertrophy undergoing noncardiac surgery, adequate ventricular preload and optimization of volume status are recommended. Preoperative fasting after clear liquids should be minimized and a judicious volume of balanced salt solution should be infused. Subendocardial ischemia is a potential risk in those with a hypertensive, hypertrophied RV. Management is directed at maintaining coronary perfusion and the inotropic state of the myocardium. Further increases in RV afterload should be avoided in those with residual or recurrent outflow tract obstruction.

LEFT VENTRICULAR OUTFLOW TRACT OBSTRUCTIONS

Anatomy and Pathophysiology

Left ventricular outflow tract obstruction can occur at the level of the aortic valve, supravalvar region, or subvalvar region. It may take place in isolation or as part of a complex malformation. A *bicuspid*

aortic valve is the most common of all congenital cardiac anomalies, occurring in approximately 2% of the general population.[58,59] Although it may not necessarily imply valvar stenosis, this abnormality can be associated with progressive obstruction or regurgitation as well as aortic root dilation. A bicuspid valve can be found in asymptomatic individuals or within the context of severe left heart obstruction. The prevalence of coexistent defects is relatively high and frequently includes PDA, VSD, aortic coarctation, and other abnormalities of the aorta and its branches.

Infants with *critical aortic stenosis* and those with severe obstruction require early intervention based on ductal dependency for systemic blood flow, heart failure symptoms, and the degree of ventricular dysfunction. *Hypoplastic left heart syndrome* (HLHS) represents an extreme form of LVOT obstruction (see Fig. 15.10).[60] It encompasses a constellation of malformations, affecting left-sided cardiac structures (e.g., mitral and aortic valves, aorta, aortic arch) (see Single Ventricle later in the chapter). It is usually characterized by aortic stenosis or atresia.

Older children with moderate to severe obstruction related to aortic stenosis can present with decreased exercise tolerance, syncopal episodes, or myocardial ischemia. Impedance to LV ejection results in elevation of LV systolic pressure and increased myocardial work. Ventricular hypertrophy is the compensatory response to the increased afterload. Contractile function is normal to increased, but diastolic impairment can occur.

In *supravalvar aortic stenosis,* the narrowing usually occurs at the sinotubular junction. The coronary arteries arise proximal to the area of obstruction and are subjected to increased systolic pressures equal to that of the LV. This pathology is seen most commonly in children with elastin arteriopathy, Williams syndrome (also known as Williams-Beuren syndrome).[61] A high incidence of cardiovascular abnormalities are known to occur in these children (80%) and most commonly include valvar and supravalvular aortic stenosis, and aortic coarctation.[62] Elfin facies, developmental delay, idiopathic hypercalcemia, and other features characterize Williams syndrome.[63] The arteriopathy can also result in obstruction to the pulmonary arteries, origins of the coronary arteries, or other vessels. Prolongation of the corrected QT interval has also been observed in 13% of affected children and is reported to be a risk factor for sudden death.[64]

Subvalvar aortic stenosis may take a variety of forms, including a discrete fibromuscular ridge or membrane, complex tunnel-like obstruction, or hypertrophy of the interventricular septum (i.e., hypertrophic cardiomyopathy). The association of LV pathology of an obstructive nature such as a bicuspid aortic valve, subaortic stenosis, aortic coarctation, and mitral valve inflow obstruction (e.g., parachute mitral valve, supravalvar mitral ring) is referred to as the *Shone complex.*

Common features of the anomalies that result in obstruction to LV output include a pressure gradient across the involved region, increased LV systolic pressure, altered myocardial force, and LV wall stress. With chronic obstruction, the hypertrophied myocardium is at risk for subendocardial ischemia because of an imbalance in the ratio between myocardial oxygen supply and demand. Factors such as increases in LV afterload, inadequate hypertrophic remodeling, and decreases in myocardial systolic or diastolic performance can compromise stroke volume and contribute to cardiac dysfunction and heart failure.[65]

Treatment Options, Residua, Sequelae, and Long-Term Outcomes

Individuals with a bicuspid aortic valve can remain asymptomatic for many years but are at risk for developing aortic stenosis and/

or regurgitation and concomitant hemodynamic alterations, as well as an aortopathy characterized by aortic root dilation. Some of those requiring surgical intervention during childhood undergo reoperation for recurrent stenosis or progressive regurgitation later in life.

Percutaneous balloon valvuloplasty may be a treatment option for critical or severe aortic valve disease.[66] Surgical alternatives include valvotomy, mechanical or bioprosthetic valve placement, and root replacement with homograft or autograft material. In the Ross operation, the native, diseased root is replaced by a pulmonary autograft, and an extracardiac conduit establishes continuity between the RV and main PA.[67] Repeat intervention for eventual failure of the RV conduit is anticipated in these patients. In addition to surveillance of the RVOT, monitoring for neoaortic root dilation and concomitant regurgitation are important components of follow-up. Ascending aorta aneurysm formation, dissection, and rupture also represent long-term concerns.

Myocardial fibrosis and ventricular dysfunction can be a feature of severe aortic outflow obstruction in infancy. Although adequate relief of the obstruction results in clinical improvement, abolition of CHF symptoms, and myocardial remodeling in most children, ventricular hypertrophy or dilation persists along with various degrees of systolic or diastolic impairment in many. Other problems include myocardial ischemia, ventricular failure, and risk of sudden death.

Management of discrete subaortic stenosis and the timing of surgery are controversial.[68] Postoperative issues include residual or recurrent obstruction and progressive aortic regurgitation. For severe supravalvar obstruction, surgical intervention is recommended resulting in adequate relief of the obstruction in most cases.[69]

Considerations for Anesthesia Care

The concern regarding anesthesia or sedation in children with Williams syndrome and supravalvar aortic stenosis is related to published reports of perioperative acute hemodynamic instability, cardiovascular collapse, and death likely related to the coronary artery abnormalities resulting in myocardial ischemia and severe biventricular outflow tract obstruction.[70-75] This syndrome represented one of the leading causes of cardiac arrest in the Pediatric Perioperative Cardiac Arrest (POCA) registry.[76]

In view of the increased risk in these children for cardiovascular decompensation and frequently unsuccessful resuscitative efforts, careful periprocedural risk stratification, perioperative/procedural planning, and strategies to mitigate untoward events are highly advisable.[77-81] Care should ideally be provided by pediatric anesthesiologists familiar with the syndrome and at facilities with the infrastructure capable of providing the necessary support for these children during an acute event. Affected children should be considered at increased risk for any procedure. The reader is referred to Chapter 14 for further discussion on the subject.

In children who have undergone either catheter-based intervention or surgery for valvar aortic stenosis, or relief of subvalvar or supravalvar stenosis, the main concerns during anesthesia and surgery revolve around residual obstructive pathology as well as aortic valve competency. Important are the potentially limited LV functional reserve and alterations of the fine balance between myocardial oxygen supply and demand. Maintenance of coronary perfusion and ventricular contractile function are keys in the care of these children. Pharmacologic agents with vasoactive and inotropic properties should be readily available during anesthesia care.

COARCTATION OF THE AORTA

Anatomy and Pathophysiology

Coarctation of the aorta is characterized by narrowing of the aortic lumen in the thoracic region.[82] The constriction can be discrete or diffuse. In infants, a long, narrowed aortic segment often is associated with hypoplasia of the transverse arch and aortic isthmus, in which case other structural cardiac malformations can also be present.[83] Associated defects include a bicuspid aortic valve, VSD, mitral valve abnormalities, and other types of left-sided obstructive lesions. In the neonate, if the aortic arch pathology is severe, it can represent a ductal-dependent lesion for systemic blood flow. Hemodynamic consequences result from obstruction to systemic blood flow and increased LV afterload. During infancy, ventricular dilation and heart failure predominate.

In older children, the presentation is usually that of arterial hypertension, with a gradient between the upper and lower extremities. There is typically an element of LV hypertrophy although ventricular function is well preserved. Collateral circulation develops when the pathology is long-standing.

Treatment Options, Residua, Sequelae, and Long-Term Outcomes

Symptoms associated with severe aortic arch obstruction or concomitant cardiovascular pathology lead the need for early intervention. In the neonate, alterations in ventricular systolic function usually resolve after relief of the obstruction. Various catheter-based and surgical approaches have been applied to the management of this lesion; each has advantages and disadvantages[84,85] (see also Chapter 20).

Repair at an early age is advocated in consideration of the reduced surgical risks for the younger age group and minimization of late morbidity with an early repair.[86] Long-term issues include systemic hypertension (independent of the hemodynamic result) and residual or recurrent aortic arch obstruction. LV hypertrophy may persist in some children after repair, particularly in those undergoing interventions later in childhood. Abnormalities in diastolic ventricular function have been reported after successful repair.[87] Catheter techniques (i.e., balloon angioplasty with and without stent implantation) have been effective in relieving the obstruction and normalizing blood pressure. This approach may be used either as primary therapy or to address residual or recurrent disease although there continues to be ongoing controversy regarding treatment.[88] Aortic aneurysms can occur around the area of coarctation or elsewhere in the aorta after surgical intervention or balloon angioplasty. Aortic coarctation has been associated with cerebral aneurysms.

Considerations for Anesthesia Care

Most children whose arch defects have been repaired have essentially normal cardiac function when presenting for noncardiac procedures. Hypertension may be a concern regardless of pre- or post-repair stage or type of prior intervention.[89] It might be wise in these children to record arterial blood pressures in the right upper extremity in the case of ongoing, residual, or recurrent obstruction.

TETRALOGY OF FALLOT

Anatomy and Pathophysiology

Tetralogy of Fallot (TOF) is the most common cyanotic cardiac lesion (see Fig. 15.5).[90] This malformation is characterized by RVOT obstruction/pulmonary stenosis, an interventricular communication, RV hypertrophy, and aortic override.[91] There is considerable variation in the severity of the disease, accounting for the wide clinical spectrum.[92] The subpulmonary obstruction is due to anterior deviation of the infundibular septum and typically has both dynamic and fixed components.[93] Pulmonary valve stenosis almost invariably exists, and the main PA and distal branches often demonstrate various degrees of hypoplasia. The limitation of pulmonary blood flow and magnitude of ventricular-level right-to-left shunting account for the degree of cyanosis.

Pressure overload results in hypertrophy of the RV myocardium. The large, nonrestrictive VSD and the outflow obstruction account for an RV pressure at systemic levels, whereas the PA systolic pressure in the classic form of TOF remains normal. Increases in the severity of the RVOT obstruction (infundibular spasm) or decreases in systemic vascular resistance exacerbate right-to-left intracardiac shunting and systemic arterial desaturation, increasing the level of cyanosis. These features characterize hypercyanotic episodes or "tet spells" in unoperated children.

Several TOF variants are recognized, including the "pink" or mild forms at one end of the spectrum, and complex defects, such as pulmonary atresia with diminutive or discontinuous distal PA branches, at the other. Associated cardiovascular anomalies in children with TOF include an atrial communication, right aortic arch, multiple VSDs, persistent left superior vena cava to the coronary sinus, complete AVSD, and abnormal origin or course of the coronary arteries.

Treatment Options, Residua, Sequelae, and Long-Term Outcomes

The surgical management of TOF has evolved from a strategy of a staged approach with initial palliation using a systemic-to-pulmonary shunt to a single-stage, definitive repair in infants. Ongoing controversy exists about the favored approach in the neonate or very young infant in need of an intervention.[94,95] In selected cases, percutaneous balloon pulmonary valvuloplasty has been performed as a palliative, temporizing measure.[96] The definitive repair of TOF, although a successful operation enabling most children to be free of symptoms, can be associated with postoperative residua. Volume loads arise from pulmonary regurgitation, residual shunts, and the presence of aortopulmonary collaterals. Ventricular pressure loads can result from residual or recurrent obstruction of the RVOT or the pulmonary arteries. This pathology is associated with RV hypertension, myocardial hypertrophy, and reduced ventricular compliance.

Conditions that can require repeat intervention in TOF include pulmonary regurgitation, residual or recurrent pulmonary outflow tract obstruction, and hemodynamically important residual intracardiac shunts. Catheter-based procedures can be effective in the management of obstruction of the pulmonary arteries and have been applied to rehabilitate the vascular tree in cases of significant underdevelopment. Children who have undergone RV-to-PA reconstruction by means of placement of an extracardiac conduit eventually develop conduit failure (i.e., stenosis or regurgitation) requiring catheter interventions or reoperation. Percutaneous valves that can be implanted in pulmonary position are now available, precluding the need for surgical valve replacement in some cases. Aortic root dilation can lead to increasing degrees of regurgitation and the need for surgery.

In the past, most children underwent definitive repair at an older age, consisting of an extensive right ventriculotomy to facilitate resection of the infundibular obstruction and closure of the VSD. Many were also subjected to procedures that included placement of a large patch that encompassed the subpulmonic region, valve annulus, and supravalvar region (i.e., transannular patch). Although effective in relieving the obstruction, this approach invariably resulted in pulmonary regurgitation, which was reasonably well tolerated over several years but progressed over time.

On late follow-up, pulmonary regurgitation has been identified as a major cause of morbidity, and it may result in progressive RV dysfunction owing to volume overload, ventricular arrhythmias with their associated disabilities, and even sudden death.[97] The LV systolic function can also be compromised in some cases. In recognition of the long-term morbidity linked to severe pulmonary regurgitation, the surgical strategy for this defect has undergone reappraisal and modification over the years. One such method uses a transatrial approach for closure of the VSD, minimizing the size of an infundibular incision (if one is required), and avoiding or limiting the size of the transannular patch in order for the RV to be able to potentially better cope in the long term.[98,99]

Although surgical refinements have led to overall improvements in postoperative outcomes, the preoperative evaluation of these children for noncardiac surgery should include inquiries regarding exercise tolerance as an indicator of functional status and an appraisal of RV and LV function, residual pathology, potential rhythm abnormalities, and conduction disturbances. Magnetic resonance imaging (MRI) is extremely useful in the evaluation of RV systolic function, quantitation of the severity of pulmonary regurgitation, and evaluation of the distal pulmonary vascular bed. If available, the results of these studies should be reviewed. Electrophysiologic testing and programmed ventricular stimulation may be indicated to refine antiarrhythmic drug therapy, for ablation of arrhythmia foci, or for implantation of a cardioverter-defibrillator system in adolescents or older patients.

After corrective surgery, a subset of children develops RV diastolic noncompliance, which is known as *restrictive RV physiology*. This may have acute and chronic consequences. In the late postoperative follow-up, it is associated with a reduced likelihood of progressive pulmonary regurgitation and RV dilation. The RV operates at a greater end-diastolic pressure in this setting, and affected individuals demonstrate superior exercise performance in addition to a reduced likelihood of developing ventricular rhythm abnormalities.[100]

Considerations for Anesthesia Care

Hypercyanotic episodes in children with TOF are usually the result of dynamic RVOT obstruction leading to exacerbation of ventricular-level right-to-left shunting and acute reductions in pulmonary blood flow.[101] These are triggered by catecholamine release owing to pain, stress, and light anesthesia. In infants, these may be due to emotional upset. Tet spells are rare during noncardiac surgery, probably because general anesthesia attenuates the triggers. Occasionally, however, increased cyanosis may occur without warning in response to obscure stimuli.

Factors that decrease systemic blood pressure and systemic vascular resistance, such as hypovolemia and extreme vasodilation, should be avoided. Treatment involves volume administration to augment RV preload and stroke volume, increasing the level of sedation or anesthesia, avoidance of exogenous catecholamines, and increasing systemic vascular resistance to enhance left-to-right shunting or minimize the amount of blood shunted in the right-to-left direction. Systemic vascular tone can be increased using either phenylephrine (bolus of 5 μg/kg IV initially and if needed, 0.1 to 2 μg/kg per minute by continuous infusion), norepinephrine (0.5 µg/kg IV initially, and then 0.05 to 2 µg/kg per minute by continuous infusion) or metaraminol (0.01 mg/kg IV initially and then 0.05 to 0.5 µg/kg per minute by continuous infusion). Vasopressin (infusion of 0.02 to 0.04 units/kg per hour) may be an alternative agent to increase systemic vascular resistance. Beta-blockade is also known to be helpful. Esmolol (starting dose 50 µg/kg per minute) has largely replaced propranolol in this setting (see also Chapters 14 and 15). Additional therapies include increasing the level of sedation or anesthetic depth. The administration of morphine (given IV, intramuscular [IM], or subcutaneous [SQ] has been one of the therapies traditionally advocated; however, in the intraoperative setting other sedatives are likely to be equally effective for tet spells.

Increasing the inspired oxygen concentration and reducing the inspiratory ventilatory pressures can also improve the clinical condition. Although the pulmonary vascular tone does not play a major role in this physiology, it is prudent to administer oxygen or increase the inspired oxygen concentration and limit factors that may increase pulmonary vascular tone and additional afterload stresses to the RV, which further impede pulmonary blood flow.

Perioperative goals for the child post tetralogy repair with pulmonary regurgitation and RV dysfunction include optimizing RV filling, maintaining or supporting RV function, and minimizing factors that may further increase RV work (e.g., increased pulmonary vascular resistance, increased peak inspiratory pressures). Review of data obtained by surveillance echocardiography and/or MRI is helpful in planning an anesthetic. Any detrimental factor that may affect the RV can also negatively affect the LV owing to the phenomenon of ventricular interdependence and should be kept in mind.

D-TRANSPOSITION OF THE GREAT ARTERIES
Anatomy and Pathophysiology
In D-transposition of the great arteries (D-TGA), the aorta arises from the anatomic RV, and the PA arises from the LV (see Fig. 15.6). This malformation accounts for the most common cause of cyanotic heart disease in the neonate. Associated defects include VSD(s), LVOT obstruction, aortic arch obstruction, and coronary artery variants.

In D-TGA, the systemic and pulmonary circulations operate in parallel rather than in series, resulting in cyanosis.[102] Mixing at the atrial, ventricular, or ductal level is essential for survival. Initial management depends on the degree of arterial desaturation. If significant, an infusion of prostaglandin E_1 may be initiated to maintain ductal patency and to enhance intercirculatory mixing. If restrictive, the interatrial communication may require enlargement by balloon atrial septostomy.

Because most neonates with D-TGA are otherwise healthy, the concerns before surgical correction of the cardiac defect(s) primarily are those associated with diagnostic procedures or interventions in the cardiac catheterization laboratory. Considerations for anesthetic management primarily are related to cyanosis. An inadequate communication for intercirculatory mixing results in hypoxemia, potentially progressing to metabolic acidosis caused by compromised tissue oxygenation. Less commonly, increased pulmonary vascular resistance may account for severe cyanosis despite prostaglandin E_1 therapy and an adequate interatrial communication.

Treatment Options, Residua, Sequelae, and Long-Term Outcomes
The arterial switch operation (i.e., Jatene procedure) is considered the standard surgical approach in neonates with D-TGA. The repair

establishes a normal, concordant relationship between the ventricles and their respective great arteries, achieving anatomic correction. The procedure involves transection of the arterial trunks above their respective semilunar valves, anastomotic connections to their appropriate outflows, translocation of the coronary arteries to the neoaortic root, and closure of existing intracardiac communications (see Fig. 15.7A–E). Associated defects are also addressed as needed. Normal physiology is restored, enabling the LV to function as the systemic chamber. This approach has excellent results, and is favorable long-term.[103] Potential postoperative problems include supravalvar pulmonary or aortic obstruction. Neoaortic root dilation and aortic regurgitation can be identified on follow-up in some children. Ventricular function is normal in most cases.

The approach to D-TGA many decades ago consisted of an atrial baffle (i.e., atrial switch) or redirection procedure (i.e., Mustard or Senning operations). Physiologic correction was accomplished by allowing systemic venous blood to enter the LV and PA while pulmonary venous blood was rerouted through the tricuspid valve into the RV and aorta. The RV remained as the systemic ventricle. These procedures, while relieving cyanosis and allowing reasonably good survival, led to long-term problems such as sinus node dysfunction and atrial rhythm disturbances.[104] Other issues included progressive obstruction of venous pathways and atrial baffle leaks with associated intracardiac shunting. Abnormal RV and LV responses to exercise have also been reported in these patients.[105] Progressive RV dilation, tricuspid (i.e., systemic AV valve) annular dilation, associated regurgitation, and eventual RV dysfunction or failure were causes of major morbidity.[106] In addition to the rhythm abnormalities and conduction defects, problems related to the RV were thought to account for sudden cardiac death in some individuals later in life.

Considerations for Anesthesia Care
Anesthetic management of children after the arterial switch operation in general should be the same as in those without structural or functional cardiovascular abnormalities. However, there is some degree of concern related to late coronary artery problems that may not be evident clinically or identified by routine surveillance methods. Investigations have demonstrated postoperative regional LV wall motion abnormalities, evidence of myocardial perfusion defects, and pathologic changes in the coronary vasculature following the arterial switch operation, suggesting a risk for coronary insufficiency in this cohort.[107,108] Thus, cognizance of these potential issues in this patient group is prudent.

CONGENITALLY CORRECTED TRANSPOSITION OF THE GREAT ARTERIES
Anatomy and Pathophysiology
Congenitally corrected transposition is characterized by AV and ventriculoarterial discordance, also referred to as "double discordance."[109] There is ventricular inversion and malposition of the great vessels. In this anomaly, the morphologic right atrium empties into an anatomic LV, which then contracts into the pulmonary trunk.[110] The morphologic left atrium opens into an anatomic RV, which ejects into the aorta. The aorta is usually oriented in a leftward and anterior position with respect to the PA, thus accounting for nomenclature of L-transposition of the great arteries (L-TGA) in most patients with this lesion.

Cyanosis is absent because the circulations are physiologically corrected. The anatomic RV functions as the systemic pump in this lesion. Associated defects are frequently present and include pulmonary outflow tract obstruction, an interventricular communication, and tricuspid valve (left-sided) abnormalities resulting in regurgitation. This pathology can remain undetected until the onset of cardiac rhythm disturbances or syncope owing to complete AV block or the effects of coexistent defects later in life.

Treatment Options, Residua, Sequelae, and Long-Term Outcomes

Without associated defects, children with corrected transposition may do well for many years. Development of complete AV block is common with increasing age. The surgical approaches for this lesion are variable. The "correction" consists of an anatomic or physiologic (also known as classical) repair. Young children with defects that maintain LV pressure at systemic levels might be suitable candidates for a surgical intervention that restores the LV as the systemic chamber.[110,111] This complex repair, known as the double-switch operation or a variation thereof, combines redirection of the systemic and pulmonary venous flows in an atrial baffle procedure with the arterial switch operation. This is referred to as an anatomic correction. A physiologic repair aims to address concomitant defects; however, the double discordance is maintained and the RV and tricuspid valve remain in the systemic circulation in the long-term.

Issues that require long-term surveillance in children with congenitally corrected transposition in addition to those related to the associated defects present in most cases include RV performance and tricuspid valve competency.

Considerations for Anesthesia Care

The primary issues in the care of children with congenitally corrected transposition relate to the presence of associated defects in the unoperated patient, ventricular function, valvar competence, and residual defects after repair. There may be additional considerations depending on the specifics of the repair.

TRUNCUS ARTERIOSUS
Anatomy and Pathophysiology

Truncus arteriosus is characterized by a single arterial trunk that gives rise to the aorta, pulmonary root, and coronary arteries (see Fig. 15.8). A ventricular communication is located underneath the single arterial root or truncal valve. Various anatomic types are recognized based on the origin of the pulmonary arteries from the arterial trunk.[112] Associated findings may include a right aortic arch, aortic arch interruption, abnormalities of the truncal valve (e.g., abnormal number of cusps, stenosis, regurgitation), and coronary artery anomalies. Approximately one-third of children with truncus arteriosus have DiGeorge syndrome (see Chapter 14).

Clinical features of the neonate with this defect largely depend on the status of the pulmonary vasculature. If the pulmonary vascular resistance is increased, the infant is well compensated. The normal decrease in pulmonary vascular resistance leads to symptoms related to pulmonary over circulation and CHF, accounting for the need for surgical intervention early in life. The physiology that characterizes a reduced pulmonary vascular resistance and a significant runoff setting is that of an increased arterial oxygen saturation, reduced diastolic arterial pressures (potentially leading to myocardial ischemia), systemic hypotension, impaired cardiac output, and hypoperfusion of distal beds.

Treatment Options, Residua, Sequelae, and Long-Term Outcomes

Surgery for truncus arteriosus consists of detaching the main PA from the truncal root, repairing the ensuing aortic wall defect, closing the VSD to allow LV output through the arterial root (neoaorta), and establishing continuity between the RV and the PA.

Neonates undergoing truncus arteriosus repair have excellent survival rates.[113,114] Late complications include RV-to-PA conduit failure, residual or recurrent PA obstruction, and truncal valve problems. Truncal valve dysfunction may require repair or replacement.

Considerations for Anesthesia Care

Truncus arteriosus is one of the structural malformations associated with major risk for adverse events during anesthesia before repair because balancing the pulmonary and vascular resistances can be challenging.[115,116] The main issues of concern in these children are those related to DiGeorge syndrome, when present, and the status of the RV-to-PA conduit (stenosis and/or regurgitation) and truncal root post-repair, consequences related to semilunar valve problems, and biventricular function.

EBSTEIN ANOMALY
Anatomy and Pathophysiology

The classic findings in Ebstein anomaly of the tricuspid valve include a large, sail-like anterior leaflet and apically displaced septal and posterior leaflets.[117,118] This configuration commonly results in an atrialized portion of the RV and tricuspid regurgitation. Some degree of RV dysplasia is common. An interatrial communication is a frequent finding, and it can produce right-to-left shunting and clinical cyanosis. The spectrum of disease ranges from minimal or no symptoms to intractable CHF. A neonatal presentation implies a major clinical problem and usually portends a poor prognosis. Symptoms in older children include cyanosis, palpitations, dyspnea, and exercise intolerance. The association of Wolf-Parkinson-White syndrome with Ebstein anomaly is well recognized. Initial presentation can be related to the development of supraventricular tachycardia (reported ~20% to 25% incidence of accessory pathways).

Treatment Options, Residua, Sequelae, and Long-Term Outcomes

The neonate with Ebstein anomaly and notable symptomatology is unlikely to tolerate noncardiac interventions; even diagnostic procedures can hold significant risk.[119,120] Children with this condition can be asymptomatic, requiring only conservative management and follow-up. Surgery is indicated for significant tricuspid valve regurgitation, closure of interatrial communications, or other associated problems.[121,122] In contrast to adults, children are less likely to require valve replacement. A cavopulmonary or Glenn connection is performed in some cases during the tricuspid valve repair as part of a so-called one-and-a-half ventricle strategy to limit the right-sided volume load associated with residual tricuspid regurgitation. Good functional outcomes and long-term survival have been reported after surgery.[123] Atrial arrhythmias in affected individuals are common before and after surgery. Electrophysiologic procedures to ablate arrhythmias may be performed during childhood or adolescence.

Considerations for Anesthesia Care

Given the variable disease spectrum, it is important to consider the severity of the underlying pathology and associated repercussions in the care of these children. In general, concerns depend on the presence of atrial level shunts, the degree of tricuspid valve dysfunction, and the functional state of both the RV and the LV.

The potential for perioperative rhythm disturbances should also be considered in children with accessory AV pathways.

INTERRUPTED AORTIC ARCH
Anatomy and Pathophysiology
Interrupted aortic arch is an uncommon malformation characterized by discontinuity between the ascending and descending thoracic aorta (see Fig. 15.14). Ductal patency is essential for systemic perfusion beyond the area of interruption. This anomaly is classified in terms of the site of interruption as follows: *type A* occurs distal to the left subclavian artery, *type B* between the left carotid and left subclavian arteries, and *type C* between the carotid arteries.[124] Type B interruption is the most common variant, followed in frequency by types A and C.

Interrupted aortic arch is typically associated with a posteriorly malaligned VSD, potentially resulting in subaortic obstruction. Other defects can include a right aortic arch, aberrant origin of a subclavian artery, and truncus arteriosus. Many children with this anomaly have DiGeorge syndrome.

Neonatal presentation of interrupted aortic arch may be related to ductal closure in the setting of aortic arch obstruction (e.g., CHF, poor perfusion, cardiovascular collapse, shock) and occasionally to differential cyanosis between the upper and lower extremities.[125] Stabilization of the infant and initiation of prostaglandin E_1 therapy is critical. An adequate response to prostaglandin E_1 therapy implies no significant gradient between the areas proximal and distal to the obstruction and an oxygen saturation differential (i.e., increased values in beds supplied proximal to the interruption, reduced values distally).

Treatment Options, Residua, Sequelae, and Long-Term Outcomes
Surgical intervention is necessary for interrupted aortic arch during the first few days of life. The goal is to establish aortic arch continuity and to address coexistent defects. The current approach favors a one-stage repair.[126,127] Survival in uncomplicated cases is excellent.[128] Problems after repair mainly are related to the LVOT.[129] Reoperation may be required and in some cases consist of LVOT enlargement (e.g., Konno procedure). Eventual aortic root or valve replacement or a Ross-Konno operation may be necessary. Aortic arch obstruction can occur in the long-term.

Considerations for Anesthesia Care
In the unoperated infant, the site of interruption and presence of coexistent anomalies can influence the selection of sites to monitor blood pressure and oxygen saturation.[124] This requires that the anesthesia provider be aware of the anatomic details and the severity of the pathology. This may also be important in the case of residual arch obstruction after surgery. Other relevant issues in the care of these children relate to DiGeorge syndrome, and the presence of intracardiac shunts or obstruction to the LVOT.

CONGENITAL ANOMALIES OF THE CORONARY ARTERIES
Anatomy and Pathophysiology
Congenital anomalies of the coronary arteries include an abnormal origin of one of the main branches, aberrant vascular course, or pathologic communications that involve the coronary circulation.[130] The most common anomalies detected during early childhood include anomalous origin of the left main coronary artery from the PA (ALCAPA), coronary artery-to-PA fistulas, and coronary cameral fistulas (i.e., connection between a coronary artery and cardiac chamber). Although rare, anomalous origin of a coronary artery from the incorrect (contralateral) sinus of Valsalva can occur in asymptomatic children and adolescents. In some instances, a major coronary artery courses between the great arteries. This situation can be associated with compromised coronary blood flow and myocardial ischemia during exercise, presumably related to dilation of the arterial roots to accommodate the increased stroke volume.

The clinical presentation varies depending on the nature of the anomaly. Infants and young children with ALCAPA typically exhibit severe ventricular dysfunction and mitral valve regurgitation, which are largely ischemic in nature. Children with fistulous coronary artery connections can present with a heart murmur or evidence of ventricular volume overload. Significant symptoms indicate CHF. Other coronary artery anomalies can manifest as myocardial ischemia, causing exertional syncope or chest pain, and in some cases, arrhythmias may lead to a near-sudden death event.

Treatment Options, Residua, Sequelae, and Long-Term Outcomes
After surgical intervention for ALCAPA, most children demonstrate reasonable recovery of myocardial function. Others continue to exhibit alterations in myocardial performance and can develop dilated cardiomyopathy; if the dysfunction is severe, they may require cardiac transplantation. A few children reach adulthood without symptoms or any intervention. Coronary artery fistulas resulting in congestive symptoms are usually referred for catheter-based interventions. Angina complaints, myocardial infarction, and sudden death are risks with certain types of anomalous aortic origin of the coronary arteries. The risk is greater when the left coronary artery originates from the right sinus of Valsalva and courses between the aorta and the RVOT.[131] Sudden death is most likely to occur during or immediately after strenuous exercise.

Considerations for Anesthesia Care
The implications of anesthesia for coronary artery anomalies primarily are related to the underlying potential for myocardial ischemia, effects of ventricular volume overload, and ventricular dysfunction.

SINGLE VENTRICLE
Anatomy and Pathophysiology
The single ventricle (i.e., univentricular heart) spectrum encompasses several congenital cardiac defects. They are characterized by abnormalities such as ventricular hypoplasia (e.g., HLHS), AV valve atresia (e.g., tricuspid atresia), or abnormal AV connections (e.g., double-inlet LV). Malformations with two distinct ventricles may also be considered in the functional single ventricle category because of associated defects that may preclude a biventricular circulation (i.e., unbalanced AVSD). Single ventricle lesions are commonly seen within the context of heterotaxy syndrome.

With single ventricle physiology, there is complete mixing of the systemic and pulmonary venous circulations at the atrial or ventricular levels. The output of the ventricle(s) supplies both the PA and the aorta. Aortic or pulmonary outflow tract obstruction is a common feature in affected children. An important management strategy early in the palliation pathway involves optimizing the balance between the pulmonary and systemic circulations, which in turn is influenced by the resistance to flow into the circulations.

Treatment Options, Residua, Sequelae, and Long-Term Outcomes

Surgical interventions available for children with a functional single ventricle include the following procedures.

Systemic-to-Pulmonary Artery Shunt

Infants with limited or ductal-dependent pulmonary blood flow require a reliable source of pulmonary blood flow. This can be accomplished by the percutaneous placement of a ductal stent in the cardiac catheterization laboratory or by the surgical creation of a connection between the systemic and pulmonary circulations. This most commonly takes the form of a Gore-Tex graft between the right subclavian and right pulmonary arteries (i.e., modified right Blalock-Taussig shunt). Potential problems include shunt malfunction associated with reductions in pulmonary blood flow and CHF related to excessive pulmonary blood flow. Several factors determine blood flow across an aortopulmonary shunt, with systemic arterial pressure playing a major role. In the case of a ductal stent, follow-up issues relate to occlusion or narrowing of the stented vessel. Distortion of the branched pulmonary arteries can occur with either catheter or surgical-based approaches.

Pulmonary Artery Banding

Pulmonary artery banding aims to limit pulmonary blood flow in children with minimal or no restriction. The intervention aims to protect the pulmonary vascular bed from increased flow and excessive pressure, an essential requirement for subsequent strategies in the child with a functional single ventricle.

Over or under tightening, as well as distortion of the proximal branch pulmonary arteries can result from band placement. The main considerations in these children are the usual presence of an intracardiac communication, associated shunting, ventricular volume load, the consequences of ventricular hypertrophy developed as a response to the mechanical limitation of pulmonary blood flow, and issues associated with coexistent defects. In a few children, PA banding can lead to ventricular dysfunction and the development of or an increase in the severity of AV valve regurgitation.

Norwood Procedure

In infants with HLHS, its variants, and other lesions with similar hemodynamic consequences, systemic blood flow largely depends on patency of the ductus arteriosus. Cerebral and coronary blood flow is usually provided in retrograde fashion across a typically hypoplastic transverse aortic arch.

The Norwood procedure is considered the first step along the three palliative stages for infants with HLHS or similar cardiac malformations.[132] The intervention, also referred to as stage I single ventricle palliation or reconstruction, is typically performed within the first few days of life. Surgery consists of aortic reconstruction or creation of a neoaorta, establishing continuity between the native main PA and aortic arch to provide for unobstructed systemic outflow from the RV; the creation of an unrestricted atrial communication by means of an atrial septectomy; and establishing a source of pulmonary blood flow (see Fig. 15.11). Pulmonary blood flow is allowed by the creation of a modified Blalock-Taussig shunt or placement of a RV-to-PA conduit (i.e., Sano modification and variations). Although the potential benefits of one approach over the other have been debated, additional studies, with long-term follow-up, are required to provide further information in this regard.[133,134] It should be emphasized that the single ventricle following stage I palliation handles both the systemic and pulmonary circulations and consequently it is a volume loaded ventricle.

This leads to changes in ventricular geometry that include progressive chamber dilatation and may be associated with problems such as the development of tricuspid regurgitation, systolic, and/or diastolic functional impairment.

Outcomes after the Norwood procedure vary; good results imply operative survival for 85% to 90% of infants. Immediate postoperative problems include inadequate or excessive pulmonary blood flow and decreased myocardial performance. Monitoring of mixed venous oxygen saturation and cerebral/somatic near-infrared spectroscopy (NIRS) are helpful in balancing the pulmonary and systemic circulations in this setting. Occasionally, aortic arch obstruction develops, and less commonly, the atrial septum becomes restrictive. Other problems include the development or progression of tricuspid regurgitation and/or RV dysfunction. Interstage mortality accounts for attrition among Norwood survivors.[135] In infants who have undergone placement of a RV-to-PA conduit, stenosis of the conduit associated with progressive cyanosis may require a catheter intervention or early second-stage palliation.

A hybrid stage I strategy has been used as an alternate approach to the Norwood procedure in the neonate.[136] The combined effort of an interventional cardiologist and surgeon aims at delivering a stent across the ductus arteriosus under fluoroscopic guidance and banding the branched pulmonary arteries via a median sternotomy. The interatrial communication is enlarged as needed at the same time or soon thereafter through balloon atrial septostomy.

Glenn Anastomosis or Hemi-Fontan Procedure

A cavopulmonary connection or Glenn procedure (i.e., stage II palliation) consists of the creation of a direct anastomosis between the superior vena cava and one of the pulmonary arteries (usually the right PA, see Fig. 15.12). This is considered an intermediary step in the sequential diversion of the systemic venous blood into the pulmonary vasculature in children with a functional single ventricle. The original or classic Glenn operation consisted of an end-to-end anastomosis of the transected superior vena cava onto a right PA, which had been disconnected from the main PA. Long-term issues included decreasing arterial saturation, attributed in many cases to the development of pulmonary arteriovenous fistulae. The current approach is to anastomose the superior vena cava to the right PA in end-to-side fashion, preserving PA continuity (i.e., bidirectional cavopulmonary anastomosis [BCPA] or bidirectional Glenn connection). Depending on the specific anatomic abnormalities, right, left, or bilateral BCPAs may be indicated.

An alternative approach in the second-stage of single ventricle palliation is the hemi-Fontan procedure. It directs superior vena cava blood to the pulmonary circulation while excluding entry of superior vena cava blood into the right atrium by placement of a patch (dam). This approach provides a step closer to lateral tunnel Fontan completion (see later in chapter). When present, a systemic-to-PA connection (shunt or conduit) is ligated and divided as part of stage II palliation, regardless of whether a BCPA or hemi-Fontan procedure is undertaken.

The second-stage intervention requires a low pulmonary vascular resistance because of the passive nature of the pulmonary blood flow. This approach provides adequate palliation to a significant number of infants at an early age while conferring favorable hemodynamic benefits. Diverting a portion of the systemic venous return directly into the pulmonary bed reduces the output requirements of the single ventricle while decreasing the ventricular volume load and myocardial work. As compared with the post-Norwood patient, the post-BCPA setting is generally considered less risky for noncardiac interventions.

Issues after stage II palliation include hypoxemia related to the development of collateral vessels that bypass the pulmonary circulation, AV valve regurgitation, and impaired ventricular function. Risk factors for interstage attrition between BCPA and the Fontan procedure in children with HLHS palliation are known to be tricuspid valve regurgitation and low body weight at the time of the BCPA.[137] These factors can also affect the anesthesia-related risks for noncardiac procedures required between these two stages of palliation.

Fontan Procedure

The Fontan procedure is the final step (i.e., stage III reconstruction) in the separation of the pulmonary and systemic circulations in children with a functional single ventricle. This intervention allows passive blood flow from the inferior vena cava into the pulmonary vascular bed while bypassing the heart, and achieves a circulation in series (see Fig. 15.13). The creation of a fenestration, or communication, between the systemic venous pathway and physiologic common atrium is favored in some cases as it allows for a pop off or right-to-left shunting, providing cardiac output that depends not only on pulmonary blood flow. It also alleviates potential problems associated with chronically increased systemic venous pressures. Common features of the various Fontan modifications are separation of the pulmonary and systemic circulations and relief of hypoxemia.[138] Pulmonary blood flow occurs without an intervening ventricular chamber, thus being critically dependent on the transpulmonary pressure gradient (or driving pressure across the pulmonary bed) and influenced by pulmonary vascular resistance. This blood flow determines cardiac output, emphasizing the importance of adequate hydration and maintenance of central venous pressure.

Several anatomic and hemodynamic variables influence Fontan physiology.[139,140] Critical factors include unobstructed systemic venous return, status of the pulmonary vasculature, reduced intrathoracic pressures, systemic AV valve competency, systemic ventricular function, unobstructed systemic outflow, and atrial contribution to ventricular filling. Long-term problems are related to sinus node dysfunction, loss of AV synchrony, atrial arrhythmias, AV valve regurgitation, ventricular dysfunction, venous pathway obstruction or thrombotic complications, and symptoms resulting from a chronic reduced cardiac output state.[141] Chronically elevated central venous pressures in children after the Fontan procedure can produce hepatic dysfunction (referred to as Fontan-associated liver disease), coagulation defects, protein-losing enteropathy, and plastic bronchitis, among other issues.[142–145] The quality of life after the Fontan operation can be compromised by a late decline in functional status, reoperations, arrhythmias, and thromboembolic events. Decreased exercise tolerance in most children represents limited cardiopulmonary reserve, which manifests as an inability to increase cardiac output to meet the metabolic demands associated with increased work. Children who develop problems such as intractable heart failure may need to undergo placement of mechanical circulatory support devices and/or cardiac transplantation.

Considerations for Anesthesia Care
Prior to and After Stage I Single Ventricle Palliation
A key strategy in the management of the neonate with single ventricle before cardiac surgery is to optimize systemic perfusion and the balance between the pulmonary and systemic circulations.[146–148] Alteration of this balance manifests with signs of inadequate systemic output (e.g., hypotension, lactic acidosis, decreased urine output) within the context of high systemic arterial oxygen saturation, reflecting the relatively excessive pulmonary blood flow. In this setting, maneuvers that increase pulmonary vascular resistance are indicated to improve hemodynamics, including limiting inspired oxygen concentrations, the administration of subambient gas mixtures, and increasing the partial pressure of carbon dioxide (PCO_2) by hypoventilation or the administration of inspired carbon dioxide. A comparison of hypoxia versus hypercarbia in infants with HLHS under conditions of anesthesia and muscle paralysis demonstrated that inspired CO_2 was more effective than hypoxic gas mixtures at increasing parameters associated with improved systemic output.[149] The administration of inspired carbon dioxide may be favored over hypoventilation as a means of judiciously increasing pulmonary vascular resistance and improving the overall clinical preoperative condition, although hypoventilation remains the more practical alternative in the intensive care unit.

The anticipated arterial oxygen saturation (SpO_2) after stage I surgery is expected to be in the range of 75% to 85%. During perioperative care and in the selection of monitoring sites in these infants, the presence of a Blalock-Taussig shunt can compromise ipsilateral subclavian artery flow and may prevent accurate blood pressure measurements. Although this is a more stable arrangement compared with the preoperative physiology, it remains a relatively fragile parallel circulation.[150] These infants display little tolerance to even the most common childhood conditions, and ailments such as dehydration, febrile illnesses, or other stresses can have catastrophic consequences. Despite these challenges, successful outcomes have been reported during noncardiac surgery for a variety of procedures, including those that may be associated with significant hemodynamic perturbations.[151,152]

After Stage II Single Ventricle Palliation
Considerations in children who have undergone BCPA palliation include the passive nature of the pulmonary blood flow, the importance of maintaining adequate intravascular volume (i.e., minimal fasting) to enhance pulmonary blood flow, and limiting significant increases in pulmonary vascular tone. Pulmonary blood flow and systemic arterial oxygenation are significantly influenced by the interplay between PA pressure (i.e., equal to the pressure in the superior vena cava), pulmonary venous pressure, and pulmonary vascular resistance. It should be noted that high peak inspiratory inflation pressures or positive-end expiratory pressure (PEEP) can reduce pulmonary blood flow. Targeting functional residual capacity should be the goal.[60] The expected systemic arterial oxygen saturation after BCPA ranges between 75% and 85%. Although factors that increase pulmonary vascular resistance can negatively influence pulmonary blood flow, the observation has been made that early after BCPA, moderate hypercapnia with respiratory acidosis improves arterial oxygenation and reduces oxygen consumption, enhancing overall oxygen transport in these children.[153] Hyperventilation can decrease cerebral oxygenation and should be avoided.[154] Near-infrared spectroscopy monitoring can be useful to guide ventilation strategy. The postoperative ventilatory goal in these children should be that of spontaneous ventilation.

After Stage III Single Ventricle Palliation
Several considerations are important in the perioperative care of children with Fontan circulation.[152,155,156] Even mild alterations in

factors that influence cardiac output, such as ventricular preload, AV synchrony, contractile function, afterload, and stress response, can adversely affect hemodynamics. Ensuring the adequacy of hydration, preserving sinus rhythm, and limiting the stress response are key goals. Maintenance of adequate ventricular function may require the administration of inotropic or vasoactive agents perioperatively. Because systemic venous pressures are typically increased, the potential for bleeding and its effects on ventricular filling should be considered. The likelihood of blood loss with ensuing hemodynamic instability is exacerbated by the coagulation defects in these children.[157] The potential for end-organ dysfunction related to chronically decreased organ perfusion, particularly in the renal and hepatic systems, should be considered, and problems may require interventions to minimize perioperative morbidity. Drugs or devices appropriate for cardiac rhythm or arrhythmia management should be readily accessible.

Important principles apply to airway and ventilation management after the Fontan operation. Although spontaneous ventilation favors phasic pulmonary flow patterns in these children, controlled ventilation is preferable in most cases. This approach minimizes the detrimental effects of factors, such as hypoventilation, atelectasis, hypoxemia, hypercarbia, and respiratory acidosis on pulmonary vascular resistance during spontaneous ventilation, limiting passive drainage of systemic venous blood into the pulmonary circulation. The pH and PCO_2 should be maintained within the normal range, and arterial oxygen saturation should remain close to baseline. The oxygen saturation may depend on the presence or absence of a fenestration in the Fontan pathway and the degree of right-to-left shunting. Mechanical ventilation with large lung volumes can impair pulmonary blood flow because high mean intrathoracic pressures transmitted to the pulmonary vascular bed increase PA pressures and decrease systemic venous return. Judicious use of mechanical ventilatory support is therefore warranted. Smaller than usual tidal volumes and reduced PEEP levels deliver the smallest mean airway pressure possible to optimize lung recruitment and normal to relatively small inspiratory times (i.e., normal to slightly prolonged inspiratory/expiratory ratios). Although adequate minute ventilation may require increases in the respiratory rate, the potential detrimental effects of very fast rates should also be considered. The goals are to maintain adequate lung volumes, functional residual capacity, and optimal gas exchange. Modes of assisted mechanical ventilation, such as pressure support ventilation with the ability to accurately control preset indexes, may also be suitable in this patient population. Laparoscopic procedures require special consideration since absorption of insufflated carbon dioxide may increase $PaCO_2$ and thus pulmonary vascular resistance, which together with the increased intraabdominal pressure from insufflation compromise venous return. Profound hypotension may ensue. To minimize the risk that these events occur, intraabdominal pressure should be minimized during laparoscopic surgery in children with HLHS (see Chapter 27). An open procedure might be preferable to avoid these risks.

Perioperative Considerations in Children With CHD during Noncardiac Surgery

PREOPERATIVE ASSESSMENT

A detailed preoperative evaluation is indispensable for identifying and anticipating factors that may place any patient with CHD at increased risk during anesthesia care (Table 21.2).[158–161] Thus, an

TABLE 21.2	Factors That May Increase Perioperative Risk in Children With Congenital Heart Disease During Noncardiac Surgery
Anticoagulation therapy	
Arrhythmias	
Cardiomyopathy	
Congestive heart failure	
Elastin arteriopathy	
Emergent surgery	
History of implanted device (pacemaker or defibrillator)	
Hypoxemia	
Long-standing cyanosis	
Major noncardiac surgery	
Older age at the time of cardiac intervention	
Older type of cardiac surgical procedure	
Pulmonary hypertension/pulmonary vascular disease	
Outflow tract obstruction	
Postoperative sequelae or residua	
Single-ventricle circulation or complex defects	
Syncope	
Unrepaired pathology	
Ventricular dysfunction	
Young age (infancy)	

important goal of the preoperative evaluation is to gather information regarding the specifics of the cardiovascular disease and prior therapeutic interventions. Determination of functional status is based primarily on clinical information. The history and physical examination, in addition to the laboratory data and ancillary tests, provide complementary information contributing to an overall risk assessment. Based on this clinical evaluation and consideration of the major pathophysiologic consequences of a particular condition, a systematic, detailed, organized plan is formulated for anesthesia and perioperative management. In some cases, the preoperative evaluation may establish the need to delay or defer elective noncardiac surgery, other interventions, or diagnostic procedures. If necessary, the child's pediatric cardiologist should facilitate information about the nature and severity of the cardiovascular disease, the child's overall clinical status, and prior problems/complications related to the underlying pathology. The perioperative care teams should be alerted to any concern that may affect the care of the child in order to identify those children who may be at increased risk and may benefit from preoperative optimization of their clinical condition. The anesthesiologist should have a detailed understanding of the child's cardiac defect, pathophysiologic consequences, nature of the medical and surgical therapies applied, functional status, and implications for perioperative management.

In patients at increased risk, pediatric anesthesia consultation is recommended before the procedure. In some cases, based on this assessment, an inpatient setting may be favored over an outpatient surgical facility. In addition, preparations for postoperative recovery, for example, in the critical care setting can be undertaken. Although the surgical team may not have an in-depth understanding of the child's cardiovascular disease, by discussing the details of the surgical plan and potential issues with the perioperative care providers, problems can be anticipated and proactively addressed. This is an important issue given that the overall risk assessment of the child also takes into account the type of noncardiac procedure, the urgency of the intervention, and likely impact on the underlying pathophysiology.

An additional important aspect of the preoperative visit is that it provides an opportunity to initiate psychological preparation of parents and children before the planned intervention. Issues regarding expectations on the day of surgery in terms of fasting, premedication, the potential need for preoperative IV access, plans for induction of anesthesia, the estimated duration of the procedure, postoperative recovery, and plan for pain management as appropriate, can be addressed at that time. In addition to the surgeon and anesthesia providers, other teams that may be part of this preoperative assessment may include the child's cardiologist, nursing, social work, child-life specialists, and other support services.

History and Physical Examination

As for all children undergoing anesthesia, the history and physical examination are essential components of a thorough preoperative evaluation. In addition to the details regarding the clinical symptoms related to the current illness and planned procedure, the history should focus on the overall health status, in particular as it relates to the cardiovascular system. Relevant information includes presenting symptoms, the type of cardiovascular disease and comorbid conditions, medications, allergies, prior hospitalizations, surgical procedures or other catheter-based interventions, anesthesia experiences, postoperative course, and complications. Symptoms, including tachypnea, dyspnea, tachycardia, fatigue, and those related to rhythm problems, should be sought. Feeding difficulties and diaphoresis can represent significant symptoms in infants, whereas decreased activity level or exercise intolerance may be a concern for older children. Palpitations, chest pain, and syncope should be characterized. The history should include an assessment of growth and development because these may be affected in children with CHD. Failure to thrive suggests ongoing cardiorespiratory compromise. Those with decompensated disease, complex pathologies, associated genetic defects or other syndromes, and coexistent noncardiac conditions may be particularly vulnerable. These along with underlying comorbidities are important considerations given their impact on perioperative risk. Recent illnesses such as intercurrent respiratory infections or pulmonary disease may increase the potential for perioperative complications and require careful appraisal of the risk/benefit ratio in elective cases.[162]

The physical examination should note the child's weight and height. Vital signs, including heart rate, respiratory rate, and blood pressure, should be documented, as well as the SpO_2. If the child is known or suspected to have or has been treated for any form of aortic arch obstructive pathology or has had any systemic-to-PA shunt, upper and lower extremity and the right and left upper extremity blood pressure recordings and palpation of the quality of pulses should be documented. This assessment provides information about the patency of arterial beds and helps in the selection of blood pressure monitoring sites. The examination should explore suitable sites for vascular access (venous and arterial) and identify potential difficulties. Emphasis should be given to the airway and cardiovascular system, with particular attention to any changes from previous examination findings.

General assessment includes the child's level of activity, breathing pattern, level of distress (if any), presence/degree of cyanosis, and hydration status. Respiratory evaluation focuses on the quality of the breath sounds and should indicate the presence or absence of labored breathing, intercostal retractions, wheezing, rales, or rhonchi. Abnormalities may suggest congestive symptoms or a pneumonic process. Cardiac auscultation should include assessment of heart sounds, pathologic murmurs, and gallop rhythms. The presence of a thrill, representing a palpable murmur, should be documented. The abdomen should be examined for the presence of hepatosplenomegaly. Assessment of the extremities should include examination of pulses, overall perfusion, capillary refill, cyanosis, clubbing, and edema. Noncardiac anomalies or pathology that may impact anesthesia care (e.g., specific syndrome complex, potentially difficult airway, gastroesophageal reflux) should be recorded.

An important objective of the preoperative evaluation is to identify children with functional cardiopulmonary limitations imposed by their cardiovascular disease. Symptoms and signs consistent with CHF, cyanosis, hypercyanotic episodes, and compromised functional status (i.e., significant exercise intolerance or syncopal episodes) should raise concerns about potential perioperative problems.

Ancillary Studies and Laboratory Data

The baseline systemic arterial saturation value should be determined by SpO_2 when the child is calm and, in most cases, while breathing room air. Acceptable values depend on many factors, including the specific cardiovascular defect(s), whether the child has a two- or a one-ventricle circulation, the preoperative versus postoperative status with respect to the cardiac disease, and the stage of palliation for those undergoing such a strategy. Children who have undergone definitive or corrective procedures should be expected to have a normal to near-normal SpO_2 value (at least 95%). As previously mentioned, depending on the particular palliative stage or intervention, acceptable SpO_2 values may range between 75% and 85%.

The value of routine preoperative testing in children has been questioned not only during minor ambulatory procedures but even prior to elective cardiothoracic surgery.[163,164] The extent of preoperative laboratory testing should largely depend on the status of the patient and the type, anticipated duration, and complexity of noncardiac surgery. It should also consider patient symptomatology and current medications. Analyses commonly obtained include hematocrit, hemoglobin, electrolyte concentrations, and coagulation tests. In cyanotic children, a complete blood cell count will identify the presence of polycythemia, anemia, and thrombocytopenia. Prothrombin time, partial thromboplastin time, and international normalized ratio (INR) provide an indication of clotting ability. Additional studies such as anti-factor Xa levels may be obtained in some cases. Cyanotic children usually have increased red blood cell mass and relatively small plasma volumes. The collection of specimens for coagulation testing may require sampling tubes that adjust the amount or concentration of citrate to prevent artifactually prolonged values. Children who may benefit from coagulation tests are those at risk for bleeding, such as those with cyanotic heart disease, receiving anticoagulation therapy, and post-Fontan palliation.[165] However, it should be noted than even elective and straightforward urologic surgery in children with complex heart disease has been associated with a greater risk of bleeding.[166] Conversely, various subgroups of children may be prone to thrombotic problems (thrombosis and thromboembolism) in the perioperative period.

These include those with: (1) single ventricle physiology palliated with systemic-to-PA Gore-Tex shunts, (2) cyanotic heart disease, and (3) implanted mechanical circulatory support devices.[167] Decisions regarding management of anticoagulation therapy should be discussed with the cardiology service and surgical team.

For those receiving diuretic therapy or digoxin, a basic metabolic panel can be useful. A comprehensive metabolic panel may be more appropriate in some to provide data including the electrolyte and acid-base balance, concentrations of blood glucose and blood proteins, and importantly, the status of the kidneys and liver. Blood typing and cross-matching should be performed if a blood transfusion may be required.

A recent electrocardiogram (ECG), if available, should be reviewed for any changes from prior studies (particularly regarding criteria consistent with chamber dilation or ventricular hypertrophy), the presence of rhythm abnormalities, and findings suggesting myocardial ischemia. If an arrhythmia is identified on the preoperative assessment, further evaluation is warranted because it may reflect an underlying hemodynamic abnormality that may impact the perioperative course. A continuous ECG recording (i.e., Holter monitor) and additional evaluations may be indicated in the child with a history of rhythm disturbance, palpitations, or syncope or with an ECG suggesting significant ectopy or arrhythmia. Additional cardiac testing may be indicated in some cases, guided by the recommendations of the child's cardiologist.

Review of a recent chest radiograph, including a lateral view, provides information regarding cardiac size, chamber enlargement, and pulmonary vascularity. Prior studies such as echocardiograms, cardiac catheterizations, electrophysiologic procedures, MRI, and computed tomography should be reviewed. Potential "red flag" indicators include the presence of significant ventricular systolic or diastolic dysfunction or pathology, either native, residual, or recurrent, of more than moderate severity. If there are symptoms that merit additional investigations or issues of concern it may be necessary to obtain further diagnostic information before proceeding with the planned procedure. These evaluations should be coordinated with the child's cardiologist. It is also important to consider whether the child may benefit from cardiac catheterization to undertake interventions addressing significant anatomic, functional, or hemodynamic abnormalities before the anticipated noncardiac procedure. In addition to further testing providing potentially helpful information, the clinical status of the child can be substantially improved in many cases by catheter-based interventions. This may be of significant benefit when the planned procedure is of an elective nature and considered to be major.

One of the goals of the preoperative evaluation is to obtain the most diagnostic information with the fewest tests and the least risk, discomfort for the child, and expense. The anesthesiologist is particularly suited to determine which tests are appropriate for optimal perioperative planning and whether additional data are needed.

Informed Consent

The physicians involved in the care of the child should meet with the patient and family to discuss the anesthetic plan and answer any questions. The preoperative consultation provides the opportunity to alleviate patient and parental anxiety. At the same time, the possible benefits and risks involved should be discussed. Although anesthesia and surgery in children with CHD, particularly in those with uncorrected defects, may carry an increased risk, it may not be possible to define the specific contribution of each factor to the overall risk.

Fasting Guidelines

The optimal period of fasting for children before surgery has been the subject of ongoing debate.[168–171] Most centers follow guidelines established by their national societies to reduce the risk of pulmonary aspiration.[172–174] Some institutions and other pediatric organizations have adopted more liberal fasting guidelines[175–177] expecting that the incidence of prolonged fasting in children is reduced although the most transparent evidence to address prolonged fasting is a simple text message to the parents the evening before surgery.[178]

The same fasting principles are generally applicable to children with CHD with a few additional concerns. Oral intake of clear fluids or the IV administration of balanced salt solutions should be considered in some children to ensure adequate hydration if the fasting period is anticipated to be prolonged. This is particularly important in small infants and in children with obstructive cardiovascular pathology, cyanotic heart disease, or single ventricle physiology. Adequate hydration and ventricular preload may minimize potential detrimental hemodynamic changes associated with anesthesia and surgery. When an IV is present, glucose-containing fluids, administered at maintenance rates, are appropriate for neonates and small infants.

Medications

Several medications are routinely used in the care of patients with CHD (Fig. 21.1). These include diuretics, angiotensin-converting enzyme inhibitors (ACEIs), β-blockers, and pulmonary vasodilators, among many others. A review of the medication list is thus essential in the preoperative evaluation because some drugs, along with factors such as a prolonged fasting period and anesthetic agents, can contribute to perioperative hemodynamic changes. In general practice, most medications are routinely administered with few exceptions until the time of surgery. In most centers, children are allowed to take scheduled oral medications with small sips of water preoperatively. In children receiving chronic pulmonary vasodilator therapy such as sildenafil, endothelin receptor antagonists, and prostacyclin analogs in particular, it is important for these drugs to be continued throughout the perioperative period.

Diuretics are usually held to avoid potential hypovolemia. The practice with respect to drugs such as ACEIs or angiotensin receptor blockers is variable. Although limited and conflicting data are available, mostly in adult patients, the concern relates to the vasodilatory properties of these drugs potentiating perioperative hypotension.[179–181] In children receiving antiplatelet drugs such as aspirin, anticoagulant agents such as warfarin, and any other drugs with a potential for intraoperative bleeding, a consideration of the risk-benefit ratio and other options should take place (see Anticoagulation later in the chapter).

Anesthesia Care Provider and Health Care Facility

Anesthesia care should be provided by individuals who are familiar and comfortable caring for children with CHD, the planned operative procedure, and the surgeon's usual approach. Although many specialized centers that care for these children have dedicated pediatric cardiac anesthesiologists, they may not be available at all facilities, nor at all times. Even if these providers are available, their number might be limited and they may not be able to support all noncardiac cases; in many instances, this type of advanced expertise may not be required.

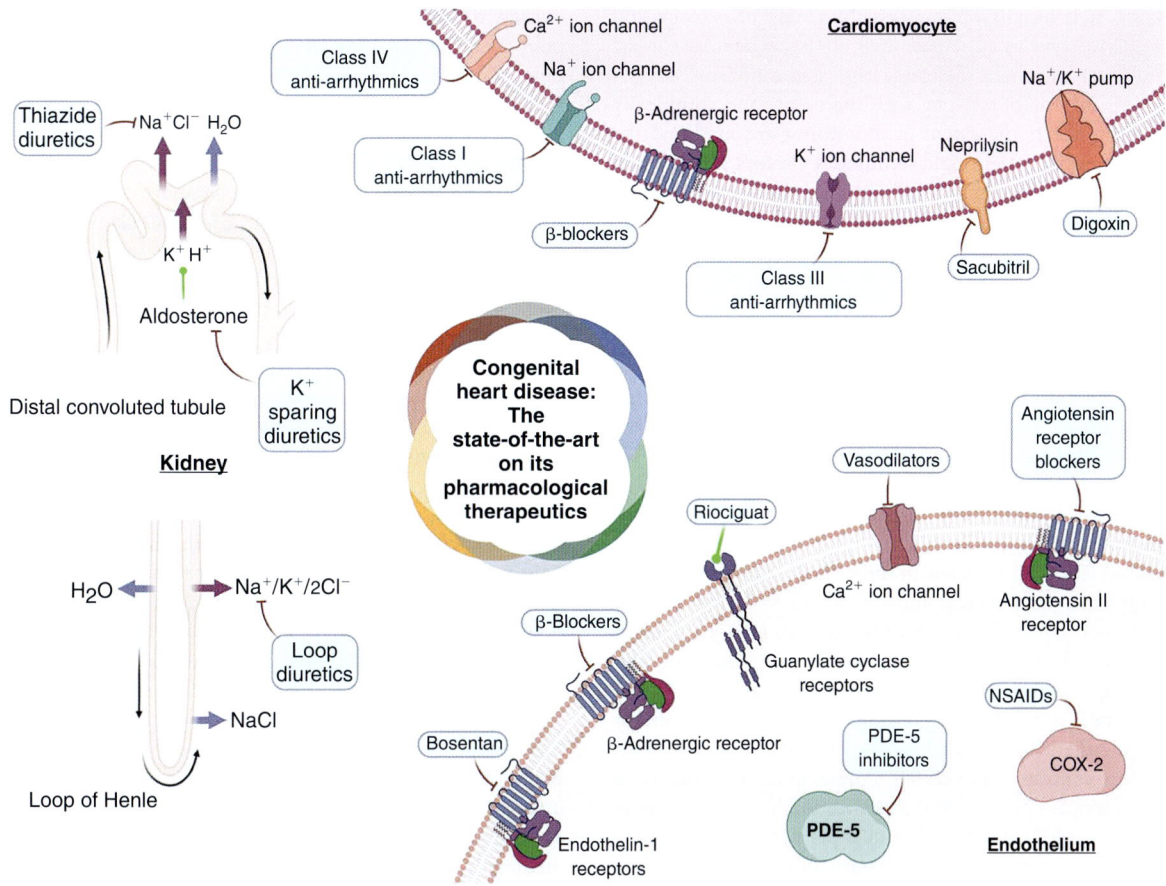

FIGURE 21.1 Medications in children with congenital heart disease. Drugs used for the treatment of children with congenital heart disease. The molecular targets on cardiomyocytes and endothelial cells are noted. (From Varela-Chinchilla CD, Sánchez-Mejía DE, Trinidad-Calderón PA. Congenital heart disease: the state-of-the-art on its pharmacological therapeutics. *J Cardiovasc Dev Dis.* 2022;9:201.)

An ongoing dilemma in CHD has been the optimal environment where care should be provided for affected children during noncardiac surgery.[182,183] Data regarding this specific issue and support for a strong recommendation are otherwise extremely limited. It has been suggested that high-risk children should be cared for at specialized centers. It is of interest that an outcome review from the United Kingdom concluded that procedures requiring general anesthesia could be performed safely in children from any of the three risk groups (low-, intermediate-, and high-risk) in a noncardiac center with the caveat that this requires close communication and careful planning among the various specialties.[184] Further data in this regard are necessary. A recent study addressing the type and location of hospitals where patients with CHD are cared for during noncardiac procedures reported that families are more likely to travel to a hospital setting with a structured cardiac program than otherwise.[3] This was particularly the case in those with single ventricle disease, other complex pathologies, or multiple chronic conditions.

Premedication

Premedication provides sedation and anxiolysis before most surgical procedures because some degree of fear or anxiety is expected. Sedation and anxiolysis facilitate parental separation, calm entry into the operating room, placement of monitors, and induction of anesthesia.

Commonly used premedications include oral or IV benzodiazepines, opioids, and small amounts of hypnotic agents. Alternative routes for premedication include IM, intranasal, and very rarely nowadays, rectal. Drugs such as barbiturates and ketamine are occasionally used. In recent years, the use of dexmedetomidine has increased, including for premedication, even in children with CHD.[185–188] One such example is the common practice of using intranasal dexmedetomidine for pediatric echocardiography sedation.[189–191]

The cardiorespiratory effects of premedication in children can be influenced by the underlying systemic disease.[192–197] Children with marginal clinical status or hemodynamic decompensation may require little or no premedication. Caution should also be exercised in children with a history of cardiovascular disease associated with pulmonary hypertension because hypoventilation and hypoxemia can be detrimental. Conversely, children susceptible to hypercyanotic episodes or those with catecholamine-induced arrhythmias can benefit from heavy premedication. In selected children, for example those affected by cyanotic conditions, SaO_2 after premedication should be considered and supplemental oxygen administered as needed.[193]

INTRAOPERATIVE MANAGEMENT

Anesthesia and surgery impose additional stresses on the cardiovascular system and provoke compensatory mechanisms to maintain homeostasis. It is important to assess the child's physiology and cardiovascular reserve to anticipate their ability to increase cardiac output to meet metabolic demands and assure optimal oxygen delivery. This information, along with the nature and complexity of the surgery, affects the extent of monitoring required and the selection of anesthetic agents and techniques. Prompt intervention is imperative if cardiopulmonary decompensation occurs. Good communication among the perioperative providers is essential in managing children with complex heart disease.

Induction of Anesthesia

Induction of anesthesia in children with CHD most commonly can be accomplished using the inhaled or IV route. The IM route (e.g., ketamine administration) may be preferable in rare cases, particularly in an uncooperative, developmentally delayed, or combative child. Less common induction techniques include intranasal, subcutaneous, and rectal administration of induction or sedative agents. These various approaches can also be used in combination (see Chapter 2).

An IV induction is preferable in some children given its potentially greater margin of safety, and the ability to titrate medications and rapidly correct hemodynamic alterations. Other benefits include the speed of effect, although this may be slowed in children with large left-to-right shunts owing to the recirculation of the drug in the lungs. Left-to-right shunting decreases the concentration of anesthetic agents reaching the brain and delays its onset of action. In contrast, right-to-left shunts speed IV inductions because a significant portion of the medication bypasses the lungs (where it is degraded) and directly enters the systemic circulation, reaching the brain more rapidly than with an intact circulation.

If IV access is not available, an inhalational induction is performed in most cases. A carefully titrated inhalational induction and early placement of an IV catheter usually is safe, even in children with moderate hemodynamic disturbances, particularly after premedication has been given. This produces loss of consciousness, with acceptable conditions for establishing IV access. Inhalational induction can be delayed in cyanotic children and those with right-to-left shunts, particularly for anesthetics with reduced blood solubility, because the decreased pulmonary blood flow limits the rate of increase in the concentration of the anesthetic in the systemic arterial blood. The rapidity of an inhalational induction is increased in the presence of a reduced cardiac output because the anesthetic partial pressure in the alveoli increases more rapidly as less anesthetic is removed by the smaller pulmonary blood flow (see Chapter 5). Left-to-right intracardiac shunts have limited effects on the speed of induction of inhaled anesthetics.

A single center investigation of induction techniques for children with CHD undergoing noncardiac procedures reported that etomidate, ketamine, or opioids tended to be used in those with greater American Society of Anesthesiologists (ASA) classes and CHD of more severity; sevoflurane or propofol were used less commonly. It was observed that the administration of intraoperative inotropes was more frequent when ketamine, etomidate, or opioids were used for induction; however, there was no difference in respiratory events among the various induction agents.[198]

Intravenous Access

Secure IV access is mandatory for administration of fluids and medications during anesthesia care in children with CHD. In most, IV access is established after an inhalational induction. In those considered at major risk, such as children with severe ventricular outflow tract obstruction, moderate to severe cardiac dysfunction, pulmonary hypertension, or potential for hemodynamic compromise, placing an IV should be considered before induction of anesthesia or very early in the process. The size of the IV catheter should be determined by the anticipated fluid/transfusion requirements and the age of the child. If peripheral access is poor and depending on the nature of the noncardiac intervention, central venous access may be necessary, particularly if large intravascular volume shifts are anticipated to allow central venous pressure to be monitored, and inotropic or vasoactive drugs to be administered. A central venous catheter should be placed with the assistance of point-of-care two-dimensional ultrasound imaging or less frequently today, by audio Doppler (see Chapter 46). In the small infant with single ventricle physiology, central venous cannulation with catheter placement in the superior vena cava may be undesirable given concerns of potential vascular complications (i.e., thrombus formation) that may affect pulmonary blood flow or subsequent surgical palliation. In these children, an alternative approach (e.g., femoral venous access) should be considered. In children with an existent or potential right-to-left shunt, all air must be removed from IV fluids and infusion tubing. Air filters can be difficult to use in the operating room because they potentially restrict the rate at which IV fluids or blood may be administered in emergency situations. They can be more useful in the preoperative and postoperative settings.

Emergency Drugs

Hemodynamic instability can occur in children with CHD under any circumstance and at any time. Therefore, drugs for emergency situations should be prepared in advance or be immediately available.

Monitoring

A fundamental principle of intraoperative monitoring is to use techniques or devices that provide useful information to facilitate clinical decision making and to avoid monitors that are distracting or redundant. Basic monitoring involves observation of the child, including skin color, capillary refill, respiration, pulse palpation, events on the surgical field, and color of shed blood. Standard noninvasive monitors used during most surgical interventions include oscillometric blood pressure assessment, electrocardiography, SpO_2, capnography, and temperature recordings. A precordial stethoscope, unfortunately rarely used today, can be extremely helpful for monitoring changes in heart tones that may suggest early hemodynamic compromise. In the child with CHD, relatively sophisticated and invasive monitoring may be needed.

Arterial Blood Pressure Assessment

Blood pressure monitoring begins with pulse palpation. Automated blood pressure measurements are used in most children. The selection of monitoring site is influenced by vascular anomalies (e.g., aortic arch pathology, aberrant origin and course of aortic arch vessels) or prior surgical interventions (e.g., Blalock-Taussig shunt, arterial cutdown). Direct blood pressure monitoring by an indwelling arterial catheter may be necessary for beat-to-beat assessment and for blood gas analysis. In most children, this is accomplished after induction of anesthesia. Percutaneous arterial cannulation can be achieved in most cases with a low risk of complications (see Chapter 46). The radial artery usually is preferred over the ulnar artery because avoiding the ulnar artery allows preservation of a larger contributor of blood supply to the hand. The ulnar artery often is the larger vessel and it can be cannulated if required. However, some centers have a policy that the ulnar artery should never be cannulated. This approach ensures that there is always at least one vessel (ulnar artery) available to perfuse the hand should the radial vessel be compromised. Ultrasound guidance with two-dimensional imaging or audio Doppler can facilitate cannulation. The need for invasive monitoring is largely based on the child's clinical condition and nature of the surgical procedure.

Electrocardiography

The ECG provides a surface recording of the electrical myocardial activity and is used to monitor heart rate, cardiac rhythm, and ST-segment analysis. One or multiple leads typically are displayed. Arrhythmias can occur because of hypoxia, electrolyte imbalances, acid-base abnormalities, intravascular or intracardiac catheters, and surgical manipulations near or around the thorax. Ischemia may be evident on direct examination of the ECG or ST-segment analysis. Although in adults such ST-segment changes may be associated with worsened outcome,[199,200] the implications for the pediatric population are unknown.

Pulse Oximetry

Placement of an oximeter probe is well tolerated, even by unco-operative children, and it is usually one of the earliest monitors applied during induction of anesthesia. Monitoring SaO_2 by SpO_2 is particularly useful in infants, cyanotic children, and those with complex anatomy or significant hemodynamic compromise. In addition to providing continuous assessment of oxygen-hemoglobin saturation and heart rate, the pulse oximeter waveform can indicate the adequacy of peripheral perfusion and cardiac output.[201,202] Other parameters that can be reflected by the SpO_2 include intracardiac or great artery-level shunting and to some extent, changes in the magnitude of pulmonary blood flow.

Capnography

Capnography confirms proper tracheal tube placement, helps to assess the adequacy of ventilation, and aids in the recognition of pathologic conditions such as bronchospasm, airway obstruction, and malignant hyperthermia. Capnography is also useful in spontaneously breathing, sedated children receiving supplemental oxygen through a nasal cannula; a prospective, observational study in children undergoing cardiac catheterization with sedation administered by nonanesthesiologists found that exhaled carbon dioxide values ($PetCO_2$) provided a reasonable estimate of arterial blood CO_2 values.[203] Although the absolute value for $PetCO_2$ may not be as reliable as in the presence of a tracheal tube, the capnograph waveform confirms the presence or absence of respirations and air exchange. End-tidal CO_2 monitoring also provides a gross index of pulmonary blood flow. In children with cyanotic heart disease, $PetCO_2$ values can underestimate arterial carbon dioxide tension ($PaCO_2$) measurements owing to altered pulmonary blood flow and ventilation-perfusion mismatch.[204,205]

Temperature Monitoring

Temperature should be routinely monitored during most procedures. Although temperature swings are usually not profound, some children, particularly small neonates, may become hypothermic because of the large body surface area/body weight ratio and decreased amount of subcutaneous tissue. This can influence oxygen delivery (i.e., increased oxygen consumption) and emergence from anesthesia, cause detrimental changes in hemodynamics, and

affect hemostasis. The neonate or small infant with CHD can be particularly vulnerable to the effects of hypothermia.

Urinary Output Measurements

The production of urine is a useful index of the adequacy of renal perfusion and cardiac output. Urine output is usually monitored during cases involving major fluid shifts or blood loss or when the surgical procedure is expected to be prolonged. No specific value for intraoperative urine output is predictive of good renal function in the postoperative period.

Echocardiography

Numerous publications have documented the utility of trans-esophageal echocardiography in general anesthesia practice,[206] as a rescue tool,[207] and as a monitoring device in high-risk adults undergoing noncardiac procedures.[208–222] Sporadic reports have demonstrated the utility of this imaging modality in children undergoing noncardiac surgery.[223–227] However, the application of transesophageal echocardiography in the pediatric age group or contributions in this particular setting has not been well defined and deserves further investigation.

Near-Infrared Spectroscopy

NIRS measures light absorbance utilizing various wavelengths of the electromagnetic spectrum to calculate the ratio of oxyhemoglobin to total hemoglobin. The technology has been used widely to monitor tissue oxygenation in the perioperative period and other clinical settings.[228,229] Applications have been reported in various pediatric populations including in neonates and children with CHD and those at high-risk of low perfusion.[230–236]

Regional cerebral oximetry monitoring using NIRS technology has been used as a surrogate of the adequacy of brain perfusion in children during cardiac and noncardiac surgery, and in those with CHD with a goal to reduce the potential for brain injury (Fig. 21.2).[237–239] Additional reported applications in the CHD population include abdominal sampling as an index of regional splanchnic tissue oxygenation in neonates at risk of gastrointestinal events such as necrotizing enterocolitis[240] and flank sampling for estimation of renal oxygenation.[241] In a pediatric cardiac intensive care setting, cerebral and somatic oximetry (Fig. 21.3) have been used to predict acute events such as cardiac arrest.[242] Algorithms are now being developed to apply combined cerebral and somatic NIRS during pediatric noncardiac surgery.[243] Although there are a number of limitations of NIRS monitoring, for example the potential inability to obtain a reading in children with cyanotic CHD and polycythemia,[244] the technology and applications will continue to evolve and likely expand to the fragile CHD population during noncardiac surgery.

Newer Technologies

Of significant interest over the last several years has been the growing use of point-of-care ultrasonography of the heart and lungs in various settings, including perioperatively.[245–247] The use of this technology in the qualitative determination of ventricular volume, systolic function, ventricular afterload, and the exclusion of physiologic causes of hemodynamic decompensation can be of significant benefit in the perioperative setting in children (Fig. 21.4). This is also an evolving field that is receiving increasing attention and may have significant applications in children with CHD during noncardiac surgery.[248,249]

Continuous noninvasive cardiac output assessment also represents an area of ongoing investigation in children using a variety

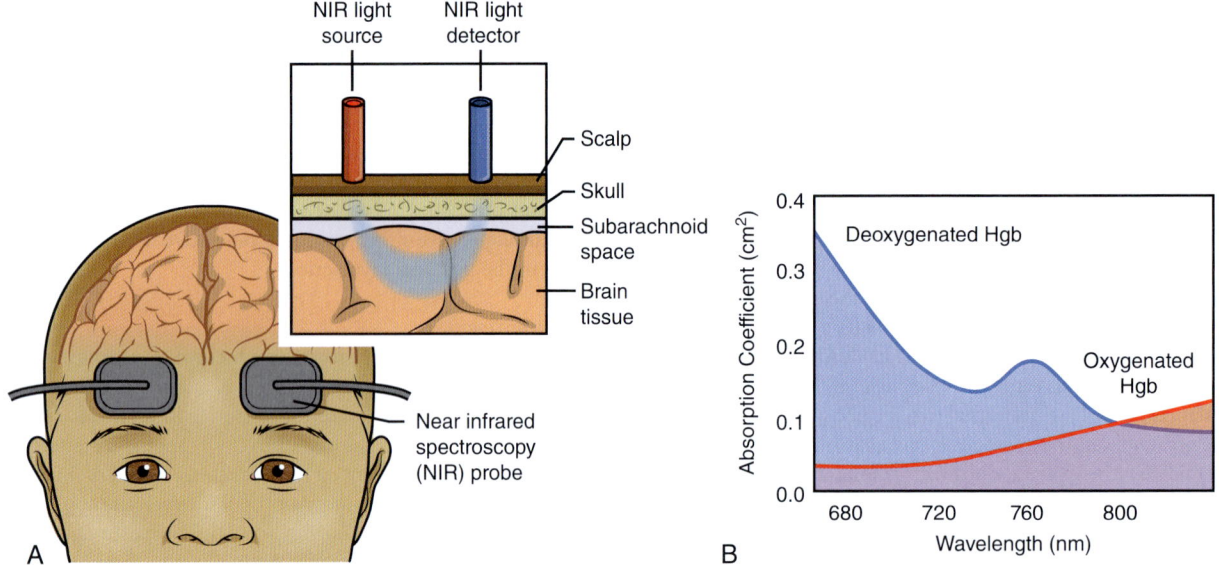

FIGURE 21.2 Regional cerebral near-infrared spectroscopy. **A,** Near-Infrared light source and detector. **B,** The different absorption wavelengths for oxy- and deoxy-hemoglobin are shown. *NIR, Near-infrared.* (From Rao A, Gourkanti B, Van Helmond N. Near-infrared spectroscopy monitoring in pediatric anesthesiology: a pro-con discussion. *Cureus.* 2021;13:e13875.)

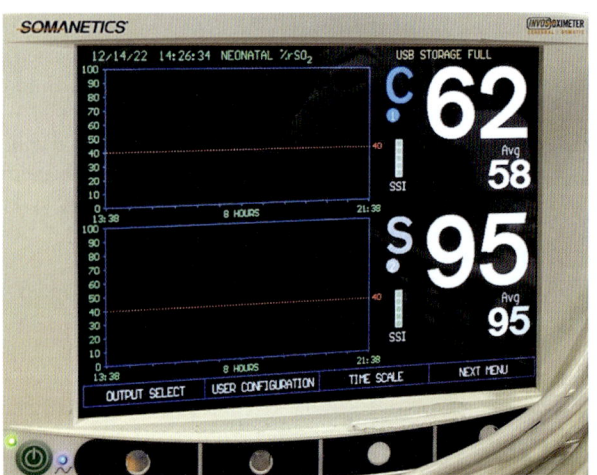

FIGURE 21.3 Cerebral and somatic near-infrared spectroscopy monitoring. The image displays monitoring of cerebral and somatic tissue oxygenation using near-infrared spectroscopy in the perioperative setting.

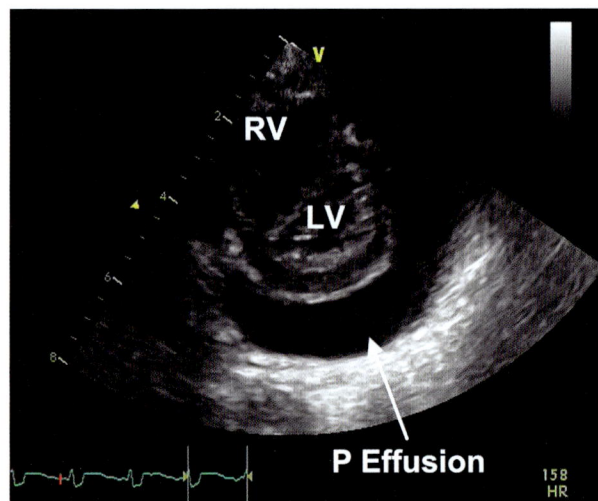

FIGURE 21.4 Point-of-care cardiac ultrasound. The image was obtained in a child with Down syndrome and post-repair of an atrioventricular septal defect undergoing Hickman line placement for treatment of newly diagnosed leukemia. There was acute hemodynamic deterioration during the procedure and cardiac perforation was suspected. A large pericardial (P) effusion is noted posteriorly on short-axis transthoracic cardiac imaging highlighting the utility of point-of care ultrasound in the acute setting. *LV,* Left ventricle; *RV,* right ventricle.

of techniques.[250–253] These monitoring modalities are likely to further enhance the practice of pediatric anesthesia in the future and especially benefit the CHD patient.

Maintenance of Anesthesia

After induction, anesthesia is usually maintained using an inhalational, IV, or combined inhalational and IV technique. In children with CHD, anesthesia can result in hemodynamic changes regardless of the technique, agents, or experience of the anesthesiologist. Some children may not tolerate even minor alterations in hemodynamics. Factors that may lead to cardiovascular decompensation in the marginally compensated child include hypovolemia, relative anesthetic overdose, increased vagal tone, positive-pressure ventilation, hypoxemia, airway obstruction, alterations in $PaCO_2$ or other factors that influence the balance between systemic and pulmonary

blood flow, myocardial ischemia, arrhythmias, and anaphylaxis. The anesthesiologist should be prepared to manage these rare but occasionally unavoidable occurrences at any time.

Selection of Techniques and Agents

Several anesthetic regimens have been used in children with CHD undergoing noncardiac surgery and during studies or procedures that require deep sedation or immobility. Although no single formula or protocol is recommended, the anesthetic techniques and agents used for a particular situation should be selected in consideration of the procedure, the child's disease and functional status, and the impact of the hemodynamic effects of the anesthetic and procedure on the pathophysiologic process.[254] Factors such as age, physical characteristics, and preferences of the anesthesiologist must be considered. The primary goals of anesthesia management with respect to the cardiovascular system are to optimize systemic oxygen delivery, maintain myocardial performance within expected parameters for the patient, and ensure the adequacy of cardiac output. A potentially limited cardiovascular reserve, reduced tolerance for perioperative stress, and detrimental alterations of the balance between pulmonary and systemic blood flow during anesthesia and surgery should be considered. A carefully titrated anesthetic, regardless of the specific agent or drug, should be the goal.

Anesthesia Technique

General anesthesia has the advantages of wide acceptance, ease of application, and certainty of effect. It is the appropriate choice for most children undergoing noncardiac surgery. Disadvantages include a greater potential for wide fluctuations in the hemodynamics and a prolonged recovery period. The IV route allows for rapid induction of anesthesia. If IV access is not available, inhalational induction can be performed. Inhalational anesthetics dilate vascular beds and reduce sympathetic responsiveness. These are desirable goals for most children, even those with heart disease, because adequate myocardial function and a reactive sympathetic nervous system are usual. However, sick children, and in particular those with ventricular dysfunction, may require an increased resting sympathetic tone to maintain systemic perfusion. Potent inhalational agents in this setting can further impair myocardial function, decrease sympathetic tone, and potentially lead to cardiovascular decompensation. These children and others with a relatively fixed cardiac output frequently require a balanced technique (combining several medications) to achieve anesthesia while minimizing the risk of hemodynamic compromise. A combined opioid, amnestic agent, and muscle relaxant technique minimizes myocardial depression and tends to leave sympathetic responsiveness intact while providing analgesia, amnesia, and immobility. Inhaled agents may also be added at low concentrations. The alpha-2 agonists (dexmedetomidine, clonidine) are options in the armamentarium of drugs that provide sedation and anxiolysis among several other benefits, and they reduce analgesic requirements intraoperatively and postoperatively.[185,186]

Regional anesthesia has been used safely and shown to be effective in children including those with CHD (see Chapter 40).[50,255–262] Advantages of regional anesthesia include an effect largely limited to the surgical site, decreased number of systemic medications, a potentially brief recovery period, and usually a more pleasant experience for the child. The administration of agents such as local anesthetics, opioids, or other adjuvants (e.g., alpha-2 agonists) into the caudal space can attenuate the sympathetic outflow associated with surgical manipulation and noxious stimuli and facilitate postoperative pain management.[263] Use of regional anesthesia, however, may not always be effective. Certain techniques retain the potential for hemodynamic alterations, particularly in hypovolemic children or those with a fixed cardiac output. It may also be contraindicated in those with coagulation defects.

The choice of technique affects the termination of anesthesia and emergence. Anesthesia performed with fewer agents is inherently simpler, usually easier, and more predictable to terminate. The use of ultra-short-acting opioids (e.g., remifentanil) and other

agents (e.g., dexmedetomidine) has avoided the need for postoperative ventilation solely related to residual effects of depressant drugs. Ventricular function and the presence of intracardiac shunts can affect uptake and distribution of inhalational anesthetics and the kinetics of IV medications (see Chapter 5).

Inhalational Agents

Inhalational anesthesia has been at the forefront of pediatric anesthesia practice for many decades.[264–266] Sevoflurane was introduced in the mid-1990s, replacing halothane for inhaled induction in many institutions. One of the known benefits of sevoflurane over halothane is its more pleasant and faster induction of anesthesia and very minimal risk of arrhythmias. When assessing the safety and efficacy of inhaled agents in infants and children with CHD during cardiac surgery, a study demonstrated twice as many episodes of hypotension, moderate bradycardia, and emergent drug use in those who received halothane compared with those given sevoflurane.[267] These data, combined with those from other studies that demonstrated the potential benefits of sevoflurane on hemodynamic stability and minimal impact on myocardial performance, led to sevoflurane becoming the preferred anesthetic agent for children, particularly those with heart disease.[268–272] Nonetheless, and although unusual today, in some jurisdictions and under some conditions, halothane may remain the primary anesthetic for children. After an inhalational induction with sevoflurane, this agent can be continued, or isoflurane may be used to maintain anesthesia.

Intravenous Agents

Propofol is one of the most frequently used medications for IV sedation and general anesthesia. It has been used in children with CHD in numerous settings.[273–276] The hemodynamic effects of propofol have been investigated in children with normal hearts and in those with cardiovascular disease. An echocardiographic study in infants with normal hearts undergoing elective surgery demonstrated that propofol did not alter heart rate, functional myocardial parameters such as shortening fraction or rate-corrected velocity of circumferential fiber shortening, nor cardiac index after IV induction.[277] However, propofol decreased arterial blood pressure to a greater extent than thiopental, an effect attributed to a reduction in afterload. A comparison of propofol and ketamine during cardiac catheterization found that propofol caused a transient decrease in mean arterial pressure and mild arterial oxygen desaturation in some children.[278] In view of the faster recovery, propofol infusion was identified as a practical alternative to ketamine for elective cardiac catheterization in children.

Another investigation in children with CHD undergoing cardiac catheterization demonstrated significant decreases in mean arterial blood pressure and systemic vascular resistance during propofol administration.[279] No changes in heart rate, mean PA pressure, or pulmonary vascular resistance were observed. In children with intracardiac shunts, the net result of propofol administration was a significant increase in the right-to-left shunt, a decrease in the left-to-right shunt, and a decreased pulmonary/systemic blood flow ratio, resulting in a statistically significant decrease in the PaO_2 and SaO_2, as well as reversal of the shunt direction from left-to-right to right-to-left in a small number of patients. Propofol could also cause further arterial desaturation in children with cyanotic heart disease. A study that examined the effects of propofol on cerebral oxygenation in children with CHD reported that propofol sedation increased cerebral tissue oxygenation despite a decrease in mean arterial pressure, stroke volume, cardiac output, and cardiac index.[280] The hemodynamic changes were not considered clinically relevant nor did they require intervention.

In children undergoing electrophysiologic testing and radiofrequency catheter ablation for tachyarrhythmias, propofol did not affect either sinoatrial or AV node function or accessory pathway conduction in Wolff-Parkinson-White syndrome.[281,282] However, ectopic atrial tachycardia can be suppressed.[283]

Collectively, these data support the judicious use of propofol in children with adequate cardiovascular reserve who can tolerate mild decreases in myocardial contractility and heart rate and mild to moderate decreases in systemic vascular resistance. Given the effects of propofol on the direction and magnitude of intracardiac shunts, this might be an important consideration in children with cyanotic heart disease and can influence the hemodynamic assessment of those undergoing evaluation of pulmonary/systemic blood flow ratios in the cardiac catheterization laboratory.

Ketamine is a dissociative anesthetic agent administered by the IV, IM, nasal, rectal, and oral routes. Its sympathomimetic effects increase heart rate, blood pressure, and cardiac output. This drug has been widely used in children with heart disease, particularly in young infants. The effects of this agent on systemic vascular resistance make it a suitable choice in children with right-to-left shunts because pulmonary blood flow is enhanced. This contrasts with inhalational agents, which by decreasing systemic vascular resistance, decrease pulmonary blood flow in the presence of an intracardiac communication and potentially worsen the severity of the cyanosis. In clinical use, however, SaO_2 typically increases with both agents. Additional favorable properties of ketamine include intense analgesia at subanesthetic doses and a lack of respiratory depressant effects.

Several investigations have addressed the concern of potential detrimental changes in pulmonary vascular tone resulting from ketamine, although no clinically important effects have been reported on pulmonary arterial pressures and pulmonary vascular resistance at the usual clinical doses.[284–288] Regarding its effect on myocardial performance, in vitro investigations have shown a direct myocardial depressant effect in animal species and the failing adult human heart.[289] This may be a consideration in the critically ill infant with a severely impaired cardiac reserve. Additional undesirable effects of ketamine include emergence reactions, excessive salivation, vomiting, and increased intracranial pressure.

Etomidate, a carboxylated imidazole derivative, has anesthetic and amnestic properties but is devoid of analgesic effects. This agent demonstrates favorable qualities over other IV drugs because it does not affect hemodynamics nor impair systemic and cerebral perfusion.[290–292] This, combined with laboratory and clinical data that support minimal effects on myocardial contractility, have made this drug a particularly desirable agent in critically ill children and in those with limited cardiovascular reserve.[293] Despite these benefits, several undesirable adverse effects are associated with etomidate, including pain on IV administration, myoclonic movements that may mimic seizure activity, and inhibition of adrenal steroid synthesis perioperatively.[294] Evaluation of this drug in a group of unrepaired children with TOF undergoing elective surgery demonstrated reduced clearance.[295] Although used primarily as an induction agent, etomidate has been administered for sedation of children during cardiac catheterization and in other settings in the past.[296–298]

Sodium thiopental, a rapid-onset short-acting barbiturate, was used for many years for induction of anesthesia until manufacturing of the drug was stopped in the United States approximately a decade ago. It was recognized that with administration of this drug in children with normal hearts, the cardiac index remained unchanged, although the shortening fraction decreased along with alterations in load-independent parameters of contractility.[277] The data regarding myocardial depressant properties of barbiturates and their effects on venodilation and peripheral blood pooling suggested that the administration of thiopental in a subset of children could cause hemodynamic instability. Thus, it was recommended that thiopental should be used with caution, particularly in those with limited reserve or increased sympathetic tone.

Dexmedetomidine is a selective α_2-adrenergic agonist agent increasingly used in the pediatric age group.[185] Compared with clonidine, the drug exhibits greater specificity for the α_2-adrenergic receptor over the α_1-adrenergic receptor. Favorable effects of the drug include sedation, anxiolysis, and analgesia. Other applications of dexmedetomidine include the reduction of emergence delirium, the treatment of symptoms associated with opioid withdrawal, and as an adjuvant agent in the operating room and postoperative settings.[299] In children with CHD, its benefits have been reported during monitored anesthesia care, diagnostic and interventional cardiac catheterization, intraoperative sedation, after cardiac and thoracic surgery, as a primary agent during invasive procedures, and in the treatment of perioperative atrial and junctional tachyarrhythmias.[300–307] The drug has also been used in children with pulmonary hypertension with good outcomes[308–310] and for deep tracheal extubation in children with CHD undergoing cardiac catheterization.[311]

The electrophysiologic effects of dexmedetomidine in children include substantial depression of sinus and AV nodal function.[312] Although dexmedetomidine has been described as an undesirable agent for electrophysiologic studies because it could be associated with adverse effects in patients at risk for bradycardia or AV block, another study reported that dexmedetomidine was not associated with any substantial or atypical ECG interval abnormalities, except for a trend toward a decrease in heart rate in children with CHD.[313] Until additional data are available, it may be prudent to be cautious when using dexmedetomidine in children with conduction abnormalities.

This medication provides hemodynamic stability, although adverse effects have been reported, including bradycardia, hypertension, and hypotension, all of which are dose dependent. A study of the hemodynamic effects in children undergoing dexmedetomidine sedation for radiologic imaging demonstrated modest decreases in heart rate and blood pressure. These changes in response to moderate doses were independent of age, required no pharmacologic interventions, and did not result in any adverse events; although, high-dose dexmedetomidine did cause bradycardia.[314,315] In those children with dexmedetomidine-induced bradycardia, administration of glycopyrrolate (5 µg/kg) has been proscribed as it precipitated severe persistent hypertension.[316] Although experience suggests an overall safety profile in children with CHD, fragile patients may not tolerate the heart rate and blood pressure fluctuations associated with dexmedetomidine; adverse effects include severe bradycardia progressing to asystole.[317]

The growing use of dexmedetomidine was reported in the Congenital Cardiac Anesthesia Society-Society of Thoracic Surgery Database in children with CHD even during cardiac surgery. In 2016, almost 30% of children received dexmedetomidine and it is likely that today, many more receive the drug.[318]

Opioids and *benzodiazepines* are widely used medications in pediatric anesthesia practice. Opioids attenuate the neuroendocrine stress response associated with anesthesia and surgery.[319,320] After repair of CHD, these medications blunt the stress response in the pulmonary circulation elicited by airway manipulations.[321] Morphine can release histamine and vasodilate, but this rarely has clinical importance when used in modest dose. Synthetic opioids can be administered in large doses without any "morphine-like" effects. These opioids maintain very stable hemodynamics with minimal perturbations in heart rate and blood pressure in children with CHD.[322] The primary concern about opioid administration is their central respiratory depressant effects because their primary cardiovascular effects are minimal. Benzodiazepines provide sedation and amnesia during the perioperative period. Midazolam may reduce the inspired concentration of inhalational anesthetic agents, which is a desirable feature in children with labile hemodynamics or in those considered at increased risk for the myocardial depressant properties of inhalational anesthetics. Studies of the effects of benzodiazepines in children with CHD are limited.[323]

Neuromuscular blocking drugs facilitate tracheal intubation and prevent reflex movement during surgery if the anesthetics alone are insufficient. All inhalational anesthetics potentiate the effects of nondepolarizing muscle relaxants. These medications have various onsets and durations of action and diverse hemodynamic effects. The cardiovascular and autonomic effects of muscle relaxants have been characterized mainly in adults with acquired cardiovascular disease (see also Chapter 5).[324-327] Drug selection is based on the need to facilitate tracheal intubation and surgical relaxation, hemodynamic adverse effects, and the anticipated duration of surgery. In children with cyanotic heart disease, the onset of action of rocuronium was more rapid than in children with acyanotic heart disease, likely due to bypassing the pulmonary circulation.[328]

Emergence From Anesthesia

Most children undergoing noncardiac surgical interventions are expected to awaken immediately at the completion of the procedure or shortly thereafter. This is achieved by reducing and then discontinuing IV or inhalational anesthetics, antagonizing neuromuscular blockade, and finally, extubating the trachea. Ensuring the return of protective reflexes and monitoring the adequacy of the airway and respirations are important considerations.

Postoperative Care

The postoperative management of the child with CHD involves many of the same physiologic principles applicable to intraoperative care. The extent of the postoperative care, optimal place for recovery (e.g., postanesthesia care unit, critical care unit), and need for monitoring and hospitalization depend in large part on the child's clinical condition and type and extent of the procedure. Immediately after surgery, most children awaken from anesthesia and recover from neuromuscular blockade, which may impose various stresses and hemodynamic changes. Adequate oxygenation and ventilation along with airway protection must be ensured and may need to be provided if the child cannot manage these functions on their own. Hypoventilation must be avoided during this time because it may negatively affect pulmonary vascular tone and overall hemodynamics in vulnerable children with CHD. Adequate pain control and, sometimes, sedation are very important postoperatively. This can be a challenging issue for the child who requires noncardiac surgery soon after a prolonged hospitalization in view of the increased likelihood for tolerance to analgesic and sedative drugs.

Observation and physical examination provide much information about the child's respiratory status, cardiac function, and

systemic perfusion during the postoperative period. Adequacy of oxygenation and ventilation can also be assessed with noninvasive monitoring and blood gas analysis as indicated. Monitoring urine output can be helpful.

Hemoglobin or hematocrit values are followed as a measure of oxygen-carrying capability in cases in which significant blood loss or the administration of fluids might have occurred. Serum electrolytes are screened if fluid shifts have taken place during the surgical and/or postoperative periods. Although digoxin is now used less frequently, attention should be given to the avoidance of hypokalemia in children receiving this drug. Serum glucose concentrations should be followed in neonates and small infants and dextrose-containing IV solutions administered as appropriate. Determination of ionized calcium (iCa^{++}) levels is indicated particularly for infants with DiGeorge syndrome because of a propensity toward hypocalcemia. Fluid replacement is dictated by the child's heart defect, type of surgery performed, and volume losses (see Chapters 7 and 10).

Perioperative Problems and Special Considerations

Several potential problems can be encountered during the perioperative period in children with CHD undergoing noncardiac interventions. This section highlights some of these issues to serve as a framework and outlines special considerations in this patient population.

HYPOTENSION

Hypotension can be related to hypovolemia owing to prolonged fasting, volume loss, arrhythmia, anesthetic agents, myocardial dysfunction, or mechanical influences associated with the operative procedure. A practical diagnostic approach to the hypotensive child is to consider factors that may affect ventricular preload, contractility, afterload, and the assessment of cardiac rhythm. Although the management of hypotension should be guided primarily by the causative factor, acutely increasing blood pressure by the administration of volume and/or an appropriate vasopressor, if indicated, often restores adequate perfusion while definitive therapy is instituted. Ensuring adequate intravascular volume with a fluid challenge often helps to restore perfusion and blood pressure, especially in the setting of hypovolemia. A pure α-adrenergic agent such as phenylephrine increases systolic blood pressure without increasing heart rate. Some children are unable to tolerate any degree of myocardial depression or reduction in sympathetic outflow and require continuous inotropic support or vasopressor infusions throughout and after the operative procedure. This is more likely to be needed in the child with a functional single ventricle after palliative strategies.

CYANOSIS

Cyanosis is a common finding in children with defects characterized by reduced pulmonary blood flow or intracardiac mixing. As surgical management strategies evolve to target the cardiac condition in the youngest of infants, the chronic effects of cyanosis may be limited. However, in those requiring delayed surgery, palliation, or staged correction of their defects, the effects of cyanosis can be long lasting. Chronic hypoxemia affects all major organ systems. Compensatory mechanisms that attempt to provide adequate systemic oxygen delivery in the presence of chronic hypoxemia include polycythemia (related to secondary erythrocytosis), increases in blood volume, alterations in oxygen uptake and delivery, and neovascularization. Despite the favorable effects of the adaptive responses, these alterations can be detrimental. Polycythemia, the most significant compensatory response, is associated with increases in blood viscosity and red cell sludging. The common occurrence of iron-deficiency anemia in cyanotic children further enhances hyperviscosity and the unfavorable consequences of this condition.[329] Several hemostatic abnormalities (e.g., thrombocytopenia, altered platelet function, and clotting factor abnormalities) have been described as a result of hypoxemia and erythrocytosis that may affect the coagulation system and increase perioperative risks.[165] This is compounded by increased tissue vascularity, with a larger number of blood vessels per unit of tissue. A concerning issue has been the identification of deranged vascular function as a sequel of chronic cyanosis and its implications in the pathogenesis of cyanosis-associated cardiovascular risk.[330]

The increased blood viscosity in children with cyanosis is associated with stasis and a risk for thrombotic events. If the hematocrit exceeds 65% preoperatively, some clinicians advocate phlebotomy to reduce the hematocrit to between 60% and 65%. This limits sludging of red blood cells and increases oxygen delivery to tissues. If blood is removed by preoperative phlebotomy, it may be saved for autologous transfusion in the perioperative period. Despite its potential benefits, phlebotomy in patients with secondary erythrocytosis has been controversial and is now reserved for those with significant symptoms related to hyperviscosity.

During the perioperative period, adequate hydration should be maintained in children with cyanotic CHD, and care should be taken to avoid prolonged venous stasis. Cyanotic children are at risk for paradoxical embolic events, mandating meticulous attention to IV lines during fluid or drug administration. This is a reasonable routine approach for all children with CHD, regardless of the nature of the anatomic abnormalities. The use of air filters in IV tubing or air removing devices should not replace vigilance.

HEART FAILURE

In infants, heart failure is most often due to ventricular volume overload resulting in congestive symptoms from ventricular or great artery-level communications.[331,332] Heart failure can also result from severe valvar regurgitation, obstructive disease, or intrinsic myocardial disease (e.g., cardiomyopathy).[333–335] Congenital defects can lead to heart failure due to poor myocardial contractility, compromising cardiac output and the ability of the cardiovascular system to meet systemic demands.

In children with significant pulmonary vascular congestion, issues such as poor airway control, hypoventilation, atelectasis, hypercarbia, and respiratory acidosis are detrimental and should be avoided. Positive-pressure mechanical ventilation may be necessary before and after surgery. In cases of elective noncardiac surgery in these children, it can be of benefit to optimize medical therapy and/or to address the cardiovascular defect(s) before the planned noncardiac procedure if not urgent or emergent.

In a retrospective review of 21 children with severe heart failure who underwent 28 general anesthetics, 10% had a cardiac arrest requiring unplanned postoperative admission to the intensive care unit, and 96% required perioperative inotropic support. The investigators concluded that general anesthesia for children with severe heart failure is associated with a noteworthy complication rate.[336] Given the potential for major morbidity and even mortality in children with acute decompensated heart failure it is vital to have careful multidisciplinary discussions and planning with all health

care teams involved (anesthesiology, cardiology, critical care, perfusion, nursing, cardiac surgery) before proceeding with anesthesia.[337,338] The nature of these discussions should address the risks and benefits, timing of the procedure, optimizing their clinical state, recovery/postoperative care, and options in the event that complications or acute deterioration occur.

VENTRICULAR DYSFUNCTION

Children with CHD can have ventricular dysfunction involving the right heart, left heart, both chambers, regional tissue, or global myocardium.[333,339] The impairment can be of a temporary or permanent nature. In systolic dysfunction, contractile function is primarily impaired. Diastolic dysfunction is associated with abnormal cardiac relaxation or impaired ventricular compliance.[340–342] Some children have both systolic and diastolic dysfunction. Ventricular dysfunction can result from factors such as age at the time of the operation and chronicity of the cardiac workload (pressure or volume); it can also be caused by the primary disease, myocardial hypertrophy, ischemia, or cyanosis, or can occur as a direct effect of surgery (e.g., ventriculotomy, cardiopulmonary bypass, ischemic time, circulatory arrest).[333–335] Diseases that affect cardiac muscle (e.g., myocarditis, dilated cardiomyopathy) can be associated with congestive symptoms due to impaired systolic or diastolic (e.g., restrictive cardiomyopathy) dysfunction.

In children with cardiomyopathy that was accompanied by severe ventricular dysfunction, general anesthesia for noncardiac procedures has been reported to be associated with more complications.[343] Children often required hospital support before and after the procedure that in many cases included intensive care management. Hospital stay was prolonged for children with severe ventricular dysfunction compared with those with a lesser degree of impairment. Based on these findings, perioperative intensive care support should be entertained early on to monitor and optimize cardiovascular therapy.

In any patient with ventricular dysfunction and/or heart failure the physiologic goals of the anesthesia care should include:

- maintaining/optimizing ventricular preload
- reducing ventricular afterload
- maintaining/optimizing the contractile state of the myocardium (this may imply, for example, supporting the ventricular function with inotropes, inodilators, pulmonary vasodilators, or other therapies as necessary)
- maintaining the atrial contribution to ventricular filling by ensuring sinus rhythm and AV synchrony, avoidance of the potentially detrimental effects of tachycardia or other rhythm disturbances that may shorten ventricular filling time
- preserving systemic cardiac output and oxygen delivery

VENTRICULAR VOLUME OVERLOAD

Ventricular volume overload, which manifests as increased left atrial pressure, LV end-diastolic pressure, and stroke volume, is a common feature in many children with unoperated CHD. Long-standing volume overload enlarges the atria, dilates the ventricles, and increases the heart size. In the postoperative child, residual valvar regurgitation can increase volume overload that, if significant, can result in congestive symptoms and ventricular dysfunction. Children with a palliated functional single ventricle are particularly vulnerable to conditions associated with ventricular volume overload such as systemic-to-PA shunts or valvar regurgitation. In these children, the volume of fluids infused must be carefully evaluated and titrated, guided by the cardiac filling pressures.

VENTRICULAR PRESSURE OVERLOAD

Pressure overload in the postoperative cardiac patient typically results from residual or recurrent muscular, valvar, or distal outflow obstruction or from increased PA pressure or vascular resistance. In children with abnormal distal pulmonary arterial beds, for example, the hypoplastic vessels may not be amenable to surgical repair or other intervention, although associated defects may be satisfactorily addressed. This results in increased proximal PA and RV pressures and compensatory myocardial hypertrophy. RV pressure can exceed systemic values and compromise LV function because septal shift can impair LV filling or result in obstruction to systemic outflow by the phenomenon of ventricular interdependence. Abnormal pressure loads to the RV can also result from progressive obstruction after procedures that involve outflow tract reconstructions. In children who have undergone outflow conduit placements, surgical interventions for successive conduit replacements are delayed as much as possible. This translates into long-standing pressure loads on the myocardium with associated wall hypertrophy and potentially some element of ischemia until the criteria for surgical intervention have been met. Another important cause of increased RV afterload in children with CHD is the presence of pulmonary hypertension (see section later in the chapter).

Whether the altered loading conditions affect the RV or LV primarily, the result is an increased myocardial demand because of the increased wall tension. This implies a susceptibility of the ventricular myocardium to the supply-and-demand relationship, a reduced tolerance for factors that may alter this fine balance, and an increased risk of ischemia.

MYOCARDIAL ISCHEMIA

Several factors can cause myocardial ischemia in children with CHD. They include chronic hypoxemia, increased systolic and diastolic wall stress, and decreased coronary perfusion owing to reduced diastolic pressures in the presence of large systemic-to-pulmonary shunts. The long-term effects of cardiopulmonary bypass, aortic cross-clamping, and surgery itself cannot be ignored. Other conditions with a propensity for myocardial ischemia include congenital coronary artery lesions, aortic stenosis, corrective procedures involving coronary transfer, and the increased blood viscosity associated with cyanosis. The deprivation of myocardial perfusion can lead to ventricular dysfunction and eventual development of myocardial fibrosis.

Detection of intraoperative myocardial ischemia during noncardiac surgery can be challenging in children. However, it is reasonable to assume that hypotensive episodes are likely to compromise myocardial perfusion and should be avoided and managed promptly.

ALTERED RESPIRATORY MECHANICS

Chronically increased blood flow and pressures in the pulmonary arteries result in progressive vascular changes, increased pulmonary vascular resistance, and alterations in lung mechanics. The primary effects on respiratory mechanics are related to increased airway resistance and decreased lung compliance. These alterations can have detrimental respiratory consequences in children with inadequate palliation or residual shunts. In some children, left atrial dilation can lead to respiratory compromise (e.g., air trapping, atelectasis) caused by bronchial compression. Although it is not possible to recommend a particular ventilatory strategy for these children, ventilatory parameters such as tidal volume, PEEP, I:E ratio, should be optimized and importantly, their influence on ventricular performance considered.

ENDOCARDITIS PROPHYLAXIS

The 2007 guidelines of the American Heart Association for infective endocarditis (IE) prevention[344] were updated in 2021 with minor changes.[345] The recommendation for prophylaxis was only for patients with cardiac conditions associated with the greatest risk of adverse outcome from infective endocarditis (see Chapter 14). In accordance with the guidelines, only a subset of children with CHD should be offered subacute bacterial endocarditis prophylaxis for specific surgical/procedural indications (see Table 14.2). Antibiotic prophylaxis is appropriate in the following cases:

- Patients with CHD
  - Unrepaired cyanotic CHD, including palliative shunts and conduits
  - Completely repaired congenital heart defect with prosthetic material or device, whether placed by surgery or by catheter intervention, during the first 6 months after the procedure
  - Repaired CHD with residual defects at the site or adjacent to the site of a prosthetic patch or prosthetic device
- Prosthetic cardiac valve or material
- Previous history of, relapse, or recurrent IE
- Cardiac transplant recipients who develop cardiac valvopathy

For patients with these underlying conditions, prophylaxis is recommended during all dental procedures that involve manipulation of gingival tissues or periapical region of teeth or perforation of oral mucosa. Although several respiratory tract procedures can result in transient bacteremia, no definitive data demonstrate a cause-and-effect relationship between these and IE. Caution may be warranted for children at high risk undergoing invasive procedures of the respiratory tract that involve incision or biopsy of the mucosa. Antibiotic prophylaxis solely for the prevention of IE is not recommended for genitourinary or gastrointestinal tract procedures, although it is advisable to verify the institutional practice with local surgeons and cardiologists.

Current recommendation for IE prophylaxis is to administer antibiotic prophylaxis 30 to 60 minutes before the procedure. In most cases, it is prudent to administer the antibiotics as soon as IV access is established to achieve adequate tissue levels before skin incision or other sources of bacteremia. If antibiotic prophylaxis is inadvertently not given, it may be given up to 2 hours after the procedure. The reader is referred to Table 14.3 for the AHA antibiotic guidelines. It should be highlighted that in the most recent recommendations, if the child is allergic to penicillin or ampicillin, and is unable to swallow oral medications, cefazolin or ceftriaxone should be used but not clindamycin. This change was made because of the potential for more frequent and severe reactions (e.g., *Clostridium difficile* infection) with clindamycin.

PULMONARY HYPERTENSION

Pulmonary hypertension had been traditionally arbitrarily defined as a mean PA pressure in the resting state equal to or greater than 25 mm Hg. However, the 6th World Symposium on Pulmonary Hypertension in 2018 proposed a revised definition to reduce this threshold to >20 mm Hg based on scientific evidence.[346,347] Pulmonary hypertension in children is mostly related to cardiac disease (Group 1 or pulmonary arterial hypertension in the World Symposium on Pulmonary Hypertension (WSPH) classification and pulmonary disease Group 3 or lung or hypoxia-related pulmonary hypertension).[348] Several factors can lead to increased PA pressures. These include increased pulmonary blood flow, pulmonary venous pressure, and pulmonary vascular resistance among many other causes.[349]

Unoperated CHD, a major cause of pulmonary arterial hypertension in children,[350] usually results from unrestricted pulmonary blood flow that arises from a communication between the intracardiac chambers or at the level of the great arteries. One of the benefits of correcting cardiac defects in early life is that the PA pressures and pulmonary vascular reactivity remain within normal limits or return to normal values. However, in some cases, pulmonary hypertension can persist or develop even after a corrective intervention.[351,352] Children with Down syndrome are particularly prone to developing pulmonary hypertension.[353,354] A less common entity known as increased pulmonary vascular resistance can occur, which can be reactive or fixed. Pulmonary hypertension and increased pulmonary vascular resistance pose significant risks for perioperative complications in patients, regardless of the underlying cause or the child's age.[287,355–361]

An acute increase in pulmonary vascular tone, also known as pulmonary hypertensive crisis, can result in cardiac arrest.[362,363] In the presence of an intracardiac communication that allows for shunting, acute increases in PA pressure can manifest as arterial desaturation, bradycardia, and systemic hypotension. In the absence of an intracardiac communication, the acute increase in RV afterload can encroach on the LV, caused by an unfavorable leftward shift of the interventricular septum, compromising LV filling and decreasing cardiac output. These events can be catastrophic.

Several factors can acutely affect pulmonary vascular tone (Table 21.3). An acute increase in pulmonary vascular resistance should be treated aggressively, reducing PA pressures using sedation, oxygen, hyperventilation to produce hypocapnia, and treating the acidosis.[357,364–366] The use of selective pulmonary vasodilators such as inhaled nitric oxide and inotropic support of the RV may be indicated. Manipulating the pulmonary hemodynamics is challenged by the difficulty of directly measuring the indices in children. Managing these critical situations requires a thorough understanding of the pathophysiologic process and experienced clinical judgment. The same principles apply in the postanesthetic care of affected children.[358] Because of the morbidity and potential periprocedural mortality for children with a history of severe pulmonary hypertension, the benefit of the planned procedure should outweigh the risk, and it must have an impact on the overall quality of life.

Children with pulmonary hypertensive vascular disease (PHVD) undergo initial cardiac catheterization to confirm diagnosis, assess disease severity, test for vasoreactivity, and gather data with prognostic implications.[366] Subsequent studies may be performed to determine the response to drug therapy.[367] Although a setting that may mimic an awake state might be desirable, it is useful to recognize that spontaneous ventilation during sedation raises the possibility of respiratory depression and hypercapnia, which may increase PA pressures and resistances. Thus, most children require general anesthesia for these procedures. The consensus statement of the Pulmonary Vascular Research Institute, Pediatric and Congenital Heart Disease Task Forces indicates: *"we recommend the presence of an anesthesiologist familiar with the management of neonatal and childhood PHVD when either sedation or general anesthesia is used."*[368] It is noted that general anesthesia and mechanical ventilation provide stable conditions for the cardiac catheterization procedure but require the availability of a trained pediatric anesthesiologist with experience in the management of children with cardiopulmonary disease.

EISENMENGER SYNDROME

Eisenmenger syndrome, rarely encountered in the current era, is characterized by progressive, irreversible pulmonary vascular disease in the patient with CHD usually owing to pathology associated with high-flow lesions and significant left-to-right shunting.[369,370] The PA pressure in such patients reaches systemic/suprasystemic values from increased pulmonary vascular resistance (usually exceeding 10 Wood units). Cyanosis is the result of reversal in the direction of an intracardiac or arterial level shunt (from the left-to-right to the right-to-left direction). Eisenmenger syndrome is most likely to occur in older children, adolescents, or adults with CHD. Morbidity relates to problems associated with chronic cyanosis and erythrocytosis. Other medical issues include hemoptysis, gout, cholelithiasis, hypertrophic osteoarthropathy, and decreased renal function. These comorbidities mandate careful appraisal of risk-benefits of the planned procedure and extensive preoperative preparation and testing whenever feasible. Laboratory studies of relevance include a hematologic profile, as well as assessment of renal and liver function. Other considerations include the possible need for preoperative therapeutic phlebotomy in selected patients, although this remains a controversial intervention. The blood removed should be saved for subsequent autologous transfusion as needed. It should be recognized that samples sent to the blood bank for typing and cross-matching may require additional processing time in these patients owing to the potential presence of antibodies from previous blood transfusions during prior surgeries.

The presence of a number of findings including syncope, increased RV end-diastolic pressure, and significant hypoxemia (i.e., SaO_2 <85%) have been associated with poor outcome in Eisenmenger syndrome. Life expectancy is reduced in affected individuals. Most succumb suddenly, probably from ventricular tachyarrhythmias. Surgical modalities that have been advocated in selected patients include combined heart and lung transplantation and lung transplantation alone. In the recent past, attention has focused on the ability of newer pharmacological agents to reduce pulmonary vascular resistance in these patients[371] and other surgical approaches.[372,373]

The considerable morbidity and mortality in patients with Eisenmenger syndrome during noncardiac surgery require not only expertise from the providers but also care at facilities capable of managing problems that may arise perioperatively. Despite the overall poor prognosis and the extremely high-risk of untoward events, several reports have documented good outcomes with a variety of anesthetic techniques and agents.[374–377] In a retrospective study of institutional outcomes in patients with Eisenmenger syndrome, arterial hypotension was reported in 26% and arterial desaturation in 17%.[378] These observations

TABLE 21.3	Factors Associated With Increased Pulmonary Vascular Tone
Acidemia	
Atelectasis	
Hypercarbia	
Hypothermia	
Hypoxemia	
Lung disease	
Stress response, stimulation, light anesthesia, pain	
Transmitted positive airway pressure	

led to the recommendation for blood pressure support with a vasopressor before or during induction to maintain systemic vascular tone and prevent worsening of the shunt flow. It is vital that the family and patient, if of appropriate age, understand these risks before undertaking any procedure that requires anesthesia or deep sedation.

SYSTEMIC AIR EMBOLIZATION

Intracardiac communications in children with CHD may cause right-to-left shunting and paradoxical embolization of systemic air. The increased right-heart pressures associated with many cardiac defects further increase this risk. It is well recognized that arterial gas embolism can lead to catastrophic consequences; thus, it is imperative to ascertain the presence of or likelihood for intracardiac or vascular shunting or to assume that this may potentially be the case in most children with CHD and consider appropriate precautions.

ANTICOAGULATION

Anticoagulants, antiplatelet drugs, and thrombolytic agents are increasingly used in children, particularly in those with CHD.[379–383] In most cases, anticoagulant treatment protocols in children are institution-based, representing a collaboration between cardiologists, surgeons, hematologists, and pharmacists.[384–386] This is due to the lack of guidelines supported by strong evidence specific to this age group and limited data regarding safety and efficacy of these drugs in pediatric practice.

Unlike detailed guidelines regarding perioperative management of antithrombotic therapy in adults,[387] management strategies in pediatrics are quite heterogeneous, and lack of consensus because of the paucity of studies in large cohorts of children. Decisions regarding the perioperative management of anticoagulation in children are primarily influenced by the nature of the procedure, urgency of the intervention, specific drug therapy, and expected effects or laboratory data. The risk of bleeding from the surgical intervention versus the risk of a thromboembolism from a reduced anticoagulant dose determines to what extent and for what duration the anticoagulant therapy should be modified.

Low-dose aspirin can be continued for most simple, superficial procedures, but if major surgery is planned, a preoperative discussion needs to take place to balance the risks and benefits of discontinuing the aspirin for 7 to 10 days before surgery. Recommendations to manage oral anticoagulation such as warfarin (Coumadin) and other antithrombotic therapy (e.g., direct oral anticoagulants; dabigatran, rivaroxaban) preoperatively in children vary widely.[388–391]

If the indications for the anticoagulation are for native valve disease or atrial arrhythmias, the risk of a major thromboembolic event is considered relatively small, and warfarin may be discontinued a week or two before the day of surgery. In those with mechanical prosthetic valves, the risk of thromboembolic events is greater. In some cases the oral anticoagulant is discontinued a few days before surgery allowing the prothrombin time to return to within 20% of normal.[392] Administration of parenteral vitamin K, factor concentrates, or fresh frozen plasma, may be required to restore the prothrombin time within an acceptable range, especially in those with liver disease and in emergency cases. The use of point-of-care studies (activated clotting time) and perioperative viscoelastic hemostatic testing such as thromboelastography (TEG) and thromboelastometry (ROTEM) should facilitate assessing the bleeding risk, in addition to guide reversing the anticoagulant and administering blood products.[393]

Elective preoperative admission is favored in some children, particularly those who are high risk, such as those with mitral or combined valve prostheses, in order to discontinue warfarin therapy and bridge with a heparin infusion, which is continued up until a few hours before surgery. Alternatively, low-molecular weight heparin may be considered the better option than unfractionated heparin because the perioperative conversion from warfarin therapy to the former heparin product can be accomplished without hospitalization.

Anticoagulation is usually reinitiated after 24 hours in children with valvular prostheses, and this may be achieved with a continuous heparin infusion or intermittent subcutaneous injections. The advantage of heparin is the ability to rapidly reverse the drug effect with protamine sulfate if bleeding complications occur. Oral anticoagulants are reinitiated 2 to 3 days after surgery if there are no bleeding concerns and oral medications can be taken. Although it has been suggested that anticoagulation therapy can be continued for minor procedures such as dental or ophthalmologic surgery in adults, the same is less clear in children.

CONDUCTION DISTURBANCES AND ARRHYTHMIAS

Acute rhythm disturbances can occur with the use of any anesthetic agent or technique and can be related to several factors. The administration of drugs with vagolytic or sympathomimetic properties requires consideration in patients with a prior history of arrhythmias or pathology associated with arrhythmias. Bradycardia can occur during induction of anesthesia, laryngoscopy, and tracheal intubation, particularly in infants and in children with Down syndrome.[394–396] In most cases, bradycardia is self-limited and requires no therapy, although if hypoxemia is the cause, it must be treated immediately.

Certain cardiac lesions can be associated with rhythm abnormalities and the potential for acute hemodynamic deterioration, increasing perioperative risks. Conduction system disorders and rhythm disturbances can occur after cardiac surgery as a direct result of the procedure or can develop owing to the inadequacy of the palliation or repair. Because cardiac arrhythmias are more prevalent among specific surgical subgroups, anticipation of their occurrence and planning for management are advocated. These cases may require prior consultation with a pediatric cardiologist or electrophysiologist, availability of specific medications, and the ability to electrically manage an acute rhythm disorder.

PACEMAKERS AND IMPLANTABLE CARDIOVERTER-DEFIBRILLATORS

An in-depth discussion of perioperative considerations related to implanted pacemakers or defibrillators can be found in Chapter 14. Consultation with a cardiologist or electrophysiologist is essential when caring for children with implanted units. Device interrogation and programming are required in most cases although the need for this recommendation has been recently challenged.[397,398] The main goal is to avoid problems with hardware malfunction related to electromagnetic interference (i.e., electrocautery). Chronotropic agents and backup pacing modalities (e.g., transvenous, epicardial, transcutaneous) should be readily available and carefully considered in the event of pacemaker malfunction associated with an inadequate underlying heart rate. A magnet should be accessible to enable asynchronous pacing if required. Perioperative ECG monitoring is essential, as is the use of monitoring modalities that can confirm pulse generation during pacing. Implanted devices should be interrogated and reprogrammed after the procedure.

NERVE PALSIES

Surgery for CHD can be associated with transient or permanent injury to the recurrent laryngeal and phrenic nerves. Recurrent laryngeal nerve injuries can result in abnormal phonation or airway difficulties and lead to aspiration, particularly in small infants. These injuries usually occur during or in association with aortic arch surgery (e.g., PDA ligation or aortic arch reconstruction) and may resolve. Diaphragmatic palsies resulting from phrenic nerve injuries are associated with abnormal lung mechanics and limited pulmonary reserve, both of which may account for perioperative morbidity.[399] These injuries can occur in association with a Blalock-Taussig shunt, arterial switch operation, Fontan procedure, and others.

MECHANICAL CIRCULATORY SUPPORT DEVICES

In recent years, an increasing number of mechanical circulatory support devices have been implanted in children, in most cases, as a bridge to cardiac transplantation.[400–408] These children may require sedation/general anesthesia for noncardiac procedures of a diagnostic or therapeutic nature, for placement of indwelling catheters used for long-term vascular access, and for other procedures. As the hardware is typically implanted at specialized cardiac centers, these children are usually well known to the anesthesia teams who are involved in multiple patient encounters during a usually relatively long hospital stay.

Several publications have highlighted the unique perioperative considerations in this patient group.[409–414] Key issues include familiarity with the various devices, their operation, control features, waveforms, and alarms.[415–417] In addition, it is important to understand factors that influence device output such as fluid status and systemic vascular tone. The functional status of the right heart influences device preload; thus, it is prudent to minimize any increases in RV afterload that can compromise device filling and stroke volume. Hypotension has been described as a common occurrence during anesthesia, necessitating the administration of IV fluid and α-adrenergic agents. This may be the result of vasodilation and a decrease in systemic afterload under conditions of a fixed cardiac output delivered by the device. Preparation and immediate access to drugs with vasoactive properties is key.

Patients with implanted devices, either temporary or durable hardware, are known to have underlying hematologic and coagulation system disturbances related to the devices. In addition, they require anticoagulation therapy to prevent clotting and major complications.[390,418] A carefully coordinated approach is key in these children and should be arranged with the input of anesthesiology, cardiology, surgical teams, and importantly hematologists who are familiar with these advanced circulatory support technologies. The common goal should be to balance the potential for bleeding and thrombotic complications.[419]

Although in adult patients a trend toward perioperative care by educated noncardiac anesthesiologists has been reported, the anesthesia care of these children has been primarily the responsibility of specialty providers.[420]

CARDIAC TRANSPLANTATION

In some cases of end-stage cardiac pathology because of congenital or acquired disease in children, cardiac transplantation may represent the best or only option for survival.[400,421–425] The preoperative assessment should note indications for transplant and specifically assess transplant organ function.

An important consideration is the lack of external nerve supply of the transplanted heart (i.e., no sensory, sympathetic, or parasympathetic innervations). The physiology of the denervated heart implies that the usual autonomic regulatory mechanisms are not operational, increasing the vulnerability of children receiving heart transplants to hemodynamic alterations.[426] Compensatory responses may be delayed, further increasing the potential for compromise.

In the child with a transplanted heart, the resting heart rate is greater than normal because of the loss of parasympathetic inhibition. Critical determinants of cardiac output are the systemic venous return (preload dependence) and maintenance of an adequate heart rate. During the early posttransplantation period, the heart rate may be supported by exogenous chronotropes or pacing. Subsequently, circulating catecholamines drive the heart rate. Regardless of the time interval from transplantation, while caring for these children the following are recommended: (1) availability of medications with chronotropic properties and drugs with direct action on the myocardium and vasculature, and (2) access to emergent cardiac pacing modalities (see also Chapter 16).[421,427,428]

Long-term immunosuppression in children who have undergone cardiac transplantation presents several issues during noncardiac surgery. First, administration of multiple medications, particularly immunosuppressant agents, throughout the perioperative period is a concern. In most cases, immunosuppressant medications are continued, if feasible, to maintain adequate blood concentrations and limit the potential to reject the transplanted organ. Children who receive long-term corticosteroid therapy can be at risk for adrenal crisis during an acute illness or other stress, such as may be encountered during surgery or other minor procedures. The perioperative administration of corticosteroids ("stress-dose") should be considered based on the procedure and severity of the illness (anticipated stress). Second, immunosuppressive therapy is associated with adverse effects that can impact various organ systems. Cyclosporine administration, for example, increases systemic arterial blood pressure, potentially influencing hemodynamics. The drug is also responsible for renal dysfunction. Anesthesia management must consider potential underlying alterations in hepatic and renal function. Third, strict aseptic technique is needed in managing a child with a compromised immune system in view of the infectious risk.

Immunosuppressant drugs such as cyclosporin, tacrolimus, and the mTOR inhibitors (sirolimus, everolimus) are cleared through the CYP 3A enzyme pathway. The use of ritonavir in those receiving treatment for HIV or COVID-19 increases concentrations of these drugs rapidly within 1 to 2 days. High concentrations of tacrolimus can speedily cause adverse effects including kidney injury, seizures, posterior reversible encephalopathy, and death. Ritonavir can also reduce the clearance of drugs commonly used in anesthesia (fentanyl, midazolam, rocuronium, ketamine). Therapeutic monitoring with subsequent dose reduction to maintain target concentration is imperative.[429]

An additional concern is the potential for cardiac allograft vasculopathy (i.e., small-vessel coronary artery disease).[430] Because older children or adolescents with ongoing myocardial ischemia may not experience angina symptoms, it is reasonable to assume that most of these children are at risk for ischemic events, particularly those who are several years after transplantation.

PERIOPERATIVE STRESS RESPONSE

The perioperative stress response is known to be characterized by endocrine and inflammatory effects. This is associated with an increase in the activity of the sympathetic nervous system and a surge in serum concentrations of catecholamines.[431,432] The typical physiologic response to painful stimuli in normal children consists of an increase in heart rate and blood pressure and a transient decrease in PaO_2. These normal patterns, however, can be detrimental to children with CHD. Tachycardia can shorten diastolic filling time and diminish cardiac output, whereas hypertension increases ventricular afterload. The reduced ability of the postoperative child with CHD to increase cardiac output in response to stimulation has been well described. Thus, in vulnerable children with limited cardiovascular reserve, it is essential to recognize the importance of modulating the perioperative stress response.

Several strategies have been employed to attenuate the associated sympathetic outflow and its negative impact in the cardiovascular system. These include the use of inhalational anesthetic agents, pharmacologic agents such as opioids and α_2-adrenergic agonists, regional anesthesia, and techniques such as minimally invasive surgical interventions.[432,433]

Types of Noncardiac Surgical Procedures in Children With CHD and Implications for Anesthesia Care

A study derived from a large multi-institutional administrative database from 2004 to 2014 reported outcomes on 8857 children with CHD, and stated that 41% who had cardiac surgery by 1 year of age also underwent noncardiac surgery by the age of 5 years.[2] More than half of these procedures involved either general (~32%) or otolaryngology surgery (~29%). Most cardiac procedures were performed in children with smaller Risk Adjustment for Congenital Heart Surgery (RACHS-1) scores. However, those with greater RACHS-1 scores had more surgical procedures compared with those in the lesser score groups. Significant variability was identified among institutions in the proportion of children undergoing noncardiac procedures. An analysis of 3010 children at a single, high-volume referral congenital center reported that otorhinolaryngology procedures were most common, followed by those performed in radiology and by general surgery. Approximately 40% of these were day cases.[434] At the same institution, the unplanned hospital admission in children with CHD undergoing ambulatory noncardiac surgical procedures was reported to be 2.7%.[435]

Infants with CHD may undergo procedures such as direct laryngoscopy and bronchoscopy, gastrostomy tube placement, at times with fundoplication, and diaphragm plication in the perioperative period usually after their initial cardiovascular intervention. A report in a very small number of infants with palliated HLHS undergoing laparoscopic Nissen fundoplication showed no intraoperative or postoperative complications with limited insufflation to 12 mm Hg.[151] A subsequent single institution series in a similar cohort also reported satisfactory outcomes in a variety of laparoscopic abdominal procedures.[436] A study that reviewed the open versus laparoscopic approach to Nissen fundoplication in infants with HLHS demonstrated frequent hemodynamic instability but no difference between the groups.[437] A large multi-center study in infants with HLHS (n=4287) examined hospital mortality related to two feeding modalities (gastrostomy versus no gastrostomy tube). Gastrostomy tube placement with or without fundoplication after stage I palliation did not place these infants at greater risk of mortality. Given the importance of optimal caloric intake for growth and survival of these infants, gastrostomy tube placement should be considered for persistent feeding difficulties.[438]

The potential physiologic implications of laparoscopic surgery in the patient with single ventricle circulation at the various stages of palliation have been highlighted in several publications.[439,440] Despite the benefits of a laparoscopic procedure, a concern in this setting is the potential for cardiorespiratory compromise owing to the physiologic effects of the pneumoperitoneum, patient positioning (Trendelenburg or reverse Trendelenburg), and increased carbon dioxide tensions. A study assessing cardiac function by transesophageal echocardiography in single ventricle patients reported a reversible decrease in shortening fraction during laparoscopic gastrostomy tube placement.[441] It is well recognized that in the single ventricle patient group there is also less tolerance for complications that might be associated with the procedure (e.g., gas embolism, pneumothorax, and pneumomediastinum), resulting in increased vulnerability for untoward events. During these procedures, communication between the anesthesia and surgical teams is imperative. Early consideration should be given to reducing the intraabdominal pressure by deflation of the pneumoperitoneum and possible conversion to an open procedure if hemodynamic, oxygenation, or ventilation difficulties are encountered (see Chapter 27).

Older children with CHD may undergo laparoscopic procedures, scoliosis surgery, or other types of interventions. A high prevalence of scoliosis has been reported in children with CHD, particularly those who undergo cardiovascular interventions early in life.[442] These spine deformities occur irrespective of cardiothoracic surgery or surgical approach (i.e., thoracotomy or sternotomy).[443] The orthopedic procedures for progressive spine deformities in older children generally aim to improve cardiorespiratory function. Particular issues of concern during these procedures relate to excessive blood loss, for example in children with Fontan circulation and high central venous pressures, and potential detrimental effects in vulnerable patients of techniques used during these types of orthopedic interventions to minimize bleeding such as a controlled hypotension.[444] A review of children with CHD who underwent spinal fusion between the years 1995 and 2015 identified an adverse event in 38.5% of patients, mostly related to perioperative fluid shifts.[445] An increased risk of major perioperative event was associated with more severe spine deformity and longer length of spinal fusion. Other factors that impacted risk included older age at time of surgery, single ventricle circulation, cyanosis, and patients taking cardiac medications at the time of surgery. A review of children with single ventricle palliation who underwent spine surgery over a 25-year span from 1995 until 2019 experienced a 52% incidence of postoperative complications, but no deaths or cerebrovascular events.[446] The frequency of complications in those who received tranexamic acid was less than in those who did not receive tranexamic acid (P=NS), although blood loss was less in those who received tranexamic acid ($P<0.016$).

Outcomes of Noncardiac Surgery in Children With CHD and Risk Analysis

Clinical outcomes for CHD depend on the nature of the structural abnormalities and the possibility of successful palliation or correction. The primary goal of palliative surgery is to favorably influence the natural history of the defect and decrease the likelihood of severe consequences of the disease. However, these children continue to have abnormal cardiovascular anatomy and physiology, and their abnormal circulation is associated with an increased risk of perioperative adverse events. Reparative, corrective, or definitive procedures are expected to improve hemodynamics and cardiac function while minimizing long-term ill effects of an abnormal circulation, improving the overall clinical outcome. Although the pathology might have been surgically treated, the cardiovascular system should not be considered normal. Therefore, repair of a congenital cardiac lesion should not be equated with a cure for many children.

Despite these considerations, for children with good hemodynamic results, the risks associated with noncardiac surgery may not be significantly different from those of others without CHD. These children are considered to be doing well clinically, have a good functional status, require few or no medications, have no exercise restrictions, and undergo routine surveillance. They require minimal or no adjustment in perioperative care compared with that provided to children without CHD. In others, however, residual abnormalities exist. In some who are less fortunate, pathology may remain or develop after cardiac surgery that is related to the primary disease or therapy. This may lead to severe cardiovascular or pulmonary impairment. These residua and sequelae may necessitate further medical, catheter, or surgical interventions and can increase perioperative morbidity during noncardiac surgery. Management of these children is guided by several factors, but to a significant extent by the residual problems of the disease and treatment and associated hemodynamic perturbations.

Many publications have examined the implications of anesthesia for children with CHD undergoing noncardiac surgery[13,15–17,150,182,259,434,447–460] Initial published data regarding this issue raised substantial concerns. An experience of 110 children with CHD over a 1-year period undergoing noncardiac outpatient surgery identified a 47% incidence of adverse events attributed to anesthesia, with more than 1 occurring in a significant number of children.[461] This study also noted an increased incidence for unplanned intensive care admissions. In another investigation involving 70 children with CHD, continuous monitoring of perioperative rhythm abnormalities and a history of ventricular arrhythmias documented a 35% and 87% incidence of intraoperative and postoperative ventricular arrhythmias, respectively.[462]

Among ongoing questions regarding risks in children with CHD undergoing noncardiac surgery, important ones include: which patients are specifically at risk, during which procedures, and what is the contemporary incidence of perioperative adverse events in this population. With respect to these questions the collected observations over the past several decades have been as follows:

- Cyanosis, treatment for CHF, poor health, and young age represent risk factors.[452]
- Perioperative risks involve major and minor interventions.[454]
- Children before stage II single ventricle palliation, those undergoing more invasive procedures, and those receiving inotropes, ACEIs, or digoxin are at risk for intraoperative hemodynamic instability.[463]
- An increased frequency of cardiac arrests is observed in children with CHD undergoing cardiac catheterization; the frequency of these events being greater compared with the incidence during pediatric noncardiac and cardiac surgery.[464]
- Children with major and severe CHD have an increased risk of mortality and a greater incidence of life-threatening postoperative outcomes compared with matched controls of children without CHD undergoing comparable procedures.[465]
- Single ventricle and complex CHD groups are at greater risk for adverse perioperative events.[17,435,452,454,463,465–474] It should

be noted, however, that risk in single ventricle patients may vary according to palliative stage, lesser risks generally being associated with more advanced palliative stages, although the exact risk for each stage has not been well defined.

- Children with Williams syndrome are at risk for perioperative morbidity and cardiac arrest.[79–81]
- In children with cardiomyopathy who require general anesthesia, especially those with severe systolic impairment, periprocedural complications are common (reported in 38% of procedures) and likely to be cardiovascular in nature.[343]
- Cardiovascular and respiratory events in patients with CHD undergoing noncardiac procedures are relatively common even at quaternary-care heart centers with large surgical volumes (11.5% and 4.7% respectively).[434]

There is extensive literature in adults with heart disease regarding perioperative cardiac complications and risks during noncardiac surgery, risk stratification schemes, and guidelines aimed at improving clinical outcomes. The lack of rigorous scientific data on this subject for children with CHD has made an equivalent effort challenging.[475] However, in recent years further information has become available.[78,183,434,465,472,474,476–479] The overall data suggest that younger age, higher ASA status, severe heart disease, and emergency procedures represent risk factors for poor outcomes during noncardiac surgery in patients with CHD. Predictors of in-hospital mortality have been reported to include: (1) preoperative markers of critical illness such as mechanical ventilation, inotropic support, preoperative cardiopulmonary resuscitation, and kidney injury; (2) type of cardiac disease (e.g., single ventricle physiology); and (3) functional severity of heart disease (e.g., severe CHD).[471] It is of interest that a related study on predictors found no correlation between the type and complexity of the noncardiac procedure and in-hospital mortality.[477]

Although patients with a functional single ventricle are widely known to be at risk for complications during noncardiac surgery regardless of their stage of palliation, it should also be recognized that it is feasible to deliver a safe anesthetic to these vulnerable patients provided one understands the pathophysiology present.[480–482] The fact that the escalating number of children with CHD presenting for noncardiac surgical procedures over time has been accompanied by an impressive decline in perioperative mortality rates (most recent reported incidence of 1.06% in 2019) is quite reassuring.[483] This is likely the result of careful perioperative planning, identification of patients at potentially increased risk for complications or poor outcomes, medical optimization, increased communication among health care providers, and the combined expertise of the perioperative team.

ANNOTATED REFERENCES

Faraoni D, Vo D, Nasr VG, DiNardo JA. Development and validation of a risk stratification score for children with congenital heart disease undergoing noncardiac surgery. *Anesth Analg.* 2016;123:824-830.

This study aimed to identify predictors for in-hospital mortality among children with CHD undergoing noncardiac surgery and to develop a risk stratification scoring system that could be applicable to clinical care. Data from large administrative databases (American College of Surgeons National Surgical Quality Improvement Program Databases) were used. The study reported that, in addition to preoperative markers of critical illness, the type of heart lesion (e.g., single-ventricle physiology) and the functional severity of the heart disease (e.g., severe CHD) are strong predictors of in-hospital mortality in children undergoing noncardiac surgery.

Faraoni D, Zurakowski D, Vo D, et al. Post-operative outcomes in children with and without congenital heart disease undergoing noncardiac surgery. *J Am Coll Cardiol.* 2016;67(7):793-801.

This study compares the incidence of mortality and major adverse postoperative outcomes following noncardiac surgery in children with and without CHD using a pediatric database of the American College of Surgeons National Surgical Quality Improvement Program. The review identified 4520 children with CHD who underwent noncardiac surgery. Children in each of three subgroups consisting of minor, major, and severe CHD were matched and compared with controls without CHD who underwent noncardiac surgery of comparable complexity. It was found that children with major or severe CHD who undergo noncardiac surgery have an increased risk of mortality with a higher incidence of life-threatening postoperative outcomes compared with children without CHD.

Latham GJ, Ross FJ, Eisses MJ, Richards MJ, Geiduschek JM, Joffe DC. Perioperative morbidity in children with elastin arteriopathy. *Paediatr Anaesth.* 2016;26(9):926-935.

The study presented a single institution rate of morbidity and mortality among children with confirmed elastin arteriopathy (most with Williams syndrome) who underwent anesthesia care to examine the patient characteristics that pose the greatest risk. Forty-eight patients underwent a total of 141 anesthetics. They reported seven cardiac arrests (15% of patients, 5% of anesthetics) and nine additional intraoperative cardiovascular complications (15% of patients, 6% of anesthetics) in this cohort. Risk factors for a cardiac arrest or complication were younger age (<3 years old) and biventricular outflow tract obstruction.

Patel A, Costello JM, Backer CL, Pasquali SK, Hill KD, Wallace AS, et al. Prevalence of noncardiac and genetic abnormalities in neonates undergoing cardiac operations: analysis of the Society of Thoracic Surgeons Congenital Heart Surgery Database. *Ann Thorac Surg.* 2016;102(5):1607-1614.

In this study the authors examined the contemporary prevalence and distribution of noncardiac congenital anatomic abnormalities (NC), genetic abnormalities (GA), and syndromes (S) in neonates undergoing cardiac operations using a large nationally representative clinical registry, The Society of Thoracic Surgeons Congenital Heart Surgery Database (STS-CHSD). Their study group included 15,376 index neonatal operations from 112 centers. They reported that 18.8% of operations were performed in neonates with NC/GA/S, with the highest prevalence in the entire cohort among those with atrioventricular septal defect (59.4%), interrupted aortic arch (43.7%), truncus arteriosus (36.8%), and tetralogy of Fallot (30.2%).

Ramamoorthy C, Haberkern CM, Bhananker SM, et al. Anesthesia-related cardiac arrest in children with heart disease: data from the Pediatric Perioperative Cardiac Arrest (POCA) registry. *Anesth Analg.* 2010;110:1376-1382.

This is a report from the Pediatric Perioperative Cardiac Arrest (POCA) registry on anesthesia-related cardiac arrests during the years 1994 to 2005, with a focus on children with heart disease. The data were provided by several North American institutions (average of 68 institutions enrolled each year). The study noted that children with heart disease who suffered a cardiac arrest were sicker than those without heart disease and more likely to suffer an arrest from cardiovascular causes. Mortality rates were greater for those with heart disease. The events were more likely to occur in the general operating room compared with the cardiac setting. The subset of children with a single ventricle was the most common category of heart disease to suffer cardiac arrest. Children with aortic stenosis (e.g., Williams Syndrome) and cardiomyopathy had the greatest cardiac arrest–related mortality rates.

Sebastian R, Ullah S, Motta P, Das B, Zabala L. Anesthetic considerations in pediatric patients with acute decompensated heart failure. *Semin Cardiothorac Vasc Anesth.* 2022;26:41-53.

This work reviews the etiology, pathophysiology, and clinical features of acute decompensated heart failure in children, in addition to perioperative care of these patients. Various aspects of perioperative care are addressed including preoperative risk assessment and planning, preoperative optimization, and intraoperative management.

Stein ML, Staffa SJ, O'Brien Charles A, et al. Anesthesia in children with pulmonary hypertension: clinically significant serious adverse events associated with cardiac catheterization and noncardiac procedures. *J Cardiothorac Vasc Anesth.* 2022;36:1606-1616.

The investigation aimed to describe the contemporary incidence of clinically significant adverse events in a large cohort of children with pulmonary hypertension undergoing anesthesia care during cardiac catheterization, noncardiac surgery, and diagnostic imaging. The study reported serious adverse events occurring in 26% of procedures. Variables associated with higher risk included younger age, procedure location in the cardiac catheterization laboratory, interventional catheterizations, and longer duration of the procedure.

Zabala LM, Guzzetta NA. Cyanotic congenital heart disease (CCHD): focus on hypoxemia, secondary erythrocytosis, and coagulation alterations. *Paediatr Anaesth.* 2015;25:981-989.

This is a comprehensive review that highlights several important clinical issues in patients with cyanotic congenital heart defects. The paper focuses on the systemic effects of long-standing hypoxemia, secondary erythrocytosis, and hemostasis.

A complete reference list can be found online at Elsevier eBooks+.

Essentials of Neurology and Neuromuscular Disorders

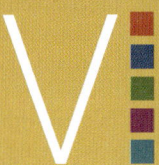

22

MARIE-AGNÈS DOCQUIER, MARIE-CÉCILE NASSOGNE, AND FRANCIS VEYCKEMANS

General Considerations
Static Neurologic Disorders
Cerebral Palsies
Malformations of the Nervous System
Disorders of Ventral Induction
Disorders of Cortical Development
Progressive Neurologic Disorders
Primary Brain Tumors
Inborn Errors Of Metabolism
Neuromuscular Disorders
Disorders of the Anterior Horn Cell

Axonal Disorders
Disorders of Muscle Fibers
Epilepsy
Antiepileptic Drugs
Ketogenic Diet
Vagal Nerve Stimulation
Surgical Treatment
Anesthesia Considerations
Refractory Seizures and Status Epilepticus

DISORDERS OF THE NERVOUS SYSTEM are common in childhood, and their diverse manifestations and complications may lead to diagnostic and surgical procedures that require anesthesia. Children with these disorders are also subject to the same acute illnesses, such as acute appendicitis, as other children. Moreover, many neurologic disorders exert profound effects on other body systems and medications taken for chronic conditions may interact with anesthetic agents, which in turn may have an impact on an underlying disorder. Anesthesiologists must have an understanding of the patient's neurologic or neuromuscular condition and its influence on anesthesia management to optimize perioperative outcomes.

General Considerations

The term *neurologic disorder* encompasses a wide variety of conditions that may have mild or serious effects. These disorders are likely to be associated with a degree of physical, cognitive, or combined disabilities. Many children with severe physical disabilities have normal intelligence and are competent to make decisions about treatment options. Those with mild cognitive impairment may wish to be consulted about treatment choices; adolescents in particular must be involved in decision making.[1] This approach is especially important for managing individuals with chronic disorders who are accustomed to thinking about health issues and who often have strong opinions about how they wish to be treated.[2]

When planning anesthesia for these individuals, physicians must be knowledgeable about these children and their conditions. Assumptions should not be made about their level of comprehension or about how they and their parents view the choices available.[3] It was formerly acceptable practice for children with chronic neurologic disorders to be excluded from the full range of therapeutic options, but it is now essential that all options are included in the discussion and review.[4]

Parents of children with chronic disorders of all types are usually accustomed to dealing with health care situations and often have thought carefully about the implications of treatments. They know their child best and are usually most qualified to make decisions by proxy. Many parents have become knowledgeable about their child's condition and about potential interventions through the widespread availability of the internet.[5] By becoming better informed about their child's disorder, parents can collaborate more effectively with physicians to determine the optimal management of their child although, the information may on occasion, be inaccurate or inappropriate for their child.[6] Misinformation can precipitate difficult situations for professionals, although one study reported that only 17% of parents used online information to influence the treatment decisions for their children.[7] In a survey of low-income families with special health care needs, more than 82% of families had internet access; however, only 50% felt confident to distinguish high quality from low quality information.[8] This may present challenges when there is a perceived disparity between the desires of the parents and the child and what the clinician considers to be in the child's best interest. The anesthesiologist must participate in the dialogue concerning procedural consent and the anesthetic prescription because anesthesia may be the part of a treatment that carries considerable risk.

Children with neurologic disorders usually have a regular physician overseeing their care, and this person should participate in preoperative decision-making. Cognitive, communication, and behavioral problems, coexisting diseases, and drug therapy that may influence anesthetic management should be evaluated at an early stage.

Verbal communication may be difficult for some children with neurologic disorders. Use of age-appropriate assisted communication devices may help to ensure open communication between physician and patient.[9] Parents' opinions and attempts to protect their children should be respected and understood as a consequence of previous experiences, stress, frustration, anger, and possible guilt. Each procedure must be assessed in terms of morbidity, mortality, and probability of improving quality of life. All aspects must be clearly and objectively discussed with parents or guardians and informed consent obtained.

Clinicians who are responsible for providing emergency care to children must have the knowledge and skills required to manage children with neurologic disorders. A preoperative assessment may be required on an urgent basis. A parent-held record of previous diagnoses and treatment is extremely helpful. Concurrent medications, previous reactions, and a history of complications such as respiratory insufficiency, electrolyte disturbance, or cardiac, renal, or hepatic dysfunction should be elicited before induction of anesthesia. A specific management plan for seizure medications is important for children who are likely to develop ileus postoperatively and thereby require a change from oral to intravenous (IV) medications.

Static Neurologic Disorders

CEREBRAL PALSIES

The definition of cerebral palsy has changed over the years. The current international definition is "*cerebral palsy describes a group of permanent disorders of the development of movement and posture, causing activity limitation, that are attributed to non-progressive disturbances that occurred in the developing fetal or infant brain. The motor disorders of cerebral palsy are often accompanied by disturbances of sensation, perception, cognition, communication, behavior, by epilepsy and by secondary musculoskeletal problems.*"[10,11] According to European data, the average incidence of cerebral palsy ranges from 1.5 to 3.0 per 1000 live births.[12] Registry data from 1999 to 2013 showed a decreasing frequency of cerebral palsy in Denmark attributed primarily to a decrease in children with bilateral spastic and dyskinetic cerebral palsy born fullterm[13]; similar reductions have occurred in other jurisdictions and throughout the world.[14]

The diagnosis of cerebral palsy is primarily clinical. Although the diagnosis can be suspected earlier in many cases, a minimum age of 4 to 5 years is recommended to confirm the diagnosis of cerebral palsy and establish its subtype. It is based on disorders of motor function and posture occurring in early childhood (excluding progressive disorders of motor function). The symptomatology is nonprogressive but can evolve with age. Once the diagnosis is made, it is imperative to investigate the etiology. Determining the cause of cerebral palsy, whether due to a malformation, a perinatal injury, or a genetic aberration, has consequences concerning risk assessment, family counseling, and the development of preventive and therapeutic strategies.

Causes of cerebral palsy are numerous and include a wide range of genetic or acquired disorders leading to brain dysgenesis or injury. Risk factors are classified according to the timing of the brain insult: prenatal, perinatal, and postnatal. Prenatal factors seem to be more often involved (~75% of cases) than perinatal risk factors (~10%–18% of cases).[15,16] One of the major associations is with prematurity and low birth weight. The incidence of cerebral palsy in premature infants with birthweights less than 1500 grams is 70 times greater than in infants with birth weight greater than 2500 grams.[17] Multifactorial prenatal and perinatal factors and the course of the pregnancy have been implicated: multiple pregnancy, placental abnormalities, intrauterine hypoxia (maternal smoking, diabetes, nutritional factors), intrauterine infections (cytomegalovirus, toxoplasmosis, Zika virus), maternal infection, hemorrhage, toxemia gravidis, trauma,[18] prolonged labor, birth asphyxia, meconium aspiration syndrome, instrumental/emergency cesarean delivery, neonatal seizures, respiratory distress syndrome, hypoglycemia, and neonatal infection.

During the neonatal and infancy period the main causes are infection (e.g., bacterial meningitis, viral encephalitis), intracranial hemorrhage, neonatal seizures, or metabolic disturbances (e.g., hypoglycemia, hypothyroidism, hyperbilirubinemia) and trauma (e.g., falls, child abuse).[15–21]

The clinical presentation of cerebral palsy is varied. A simple classification based on three major groups is currently used: spastic, dyskinetic, and ataxic. In mixed cerebral palsy forms (i.e., spasticity with ataxia and/or dyskinesia), the child is classified according to the dominant clinical features (Table 22.1).[22] Scales such as the Gross Motor Function Classification System[23] (Table 22.2) are helpful to categorize and assess the severity of the motor disorder. Initially designed to be used with children 2 to 12 years of age, the Gross Motor Function Classification System was revised in 2007 to include the ages 12 to 18 years by incorporating developmental milestones.[24]

TABLE 22.1	Clinical Classification of Cerebral Palsy. *Surveillance of Cerebral Palsy in Europe (SCPE)*
Spastic Type	Characterized by at least two of: • abnormal pattern of posture and/or movement • increased tone (not necessarily constant) • pathological reflexes (increased reflexes: hyperreflexia and/or pyramidal signs, e.g., Babinski response) May be either unilateral or bilateral
Dyskinetic Type	Characterized by both: • abnormal pattern of posture and/or movement • involuntary, uncontrolled, recurring, occasionally stereotyped movements May be either: • dystonic: hypokinesia (reduced activity, i.e., stiff movement) and hypertonia (tone usually increased) • choreoathetotic: hyperkinesia (increased activity, i.e., stormy movement) and hypotonia (tone usually decreased); so-called hypotonic-hyperkinetic
Ataxic Type	Characterized by both: • abnormal pattern of posture and/or movement • loss of orderly muscular coordination so that movements are performed with abnormal force, rhythm, and accuracy

From Christine C, Dolk H, Platt MJ, et al. Recommendations from the SCPE collaborative group for defining and classifying cerebral palsy. *Dev Med Child Neurol.* 2007;(109)(Supp):35-38.

TABLE 22.2	Classification of Child Autonomy Based on Five Levels of Functional Limitations (Motor Function). *Gross Motor Function Classification System for Cerebral Palsy (GMFCS)*
Level I	Walks without limitations
Level II	Walks with limitations (no mobility aid by 4 years of age)
Level III	Walks using a hand-held mobility device
Level IV	Self-mobility with limitations; may use powered mobility
Level V	Transported in a manual wheelchair

From Palisano R, Rosenbaum P, Walter S, Russell D, Wood E, Galuppi B. Development and reliability of a system to classify gross motor function in children with cerebral palsy. *Dev Med Child Neurol.* 1997;39(4):214-223.

22

Although neuroimaging is not a prerequisite to establish the diagnosis of cerebral palsy, it is essential in the evaluation of children with motor delay. Neuroimaging findings have strong correlations with clinical observations and are abnormal in more than 80% of children with cerebral palsy.[25] Neuroimaging can help parents and clinicians understand the structure-function relationship and assist with the child's future prognosis. The degree of disability in cerebral palsy depends on the area of the brain affected. The Surveillance of Cerebral Palsy in Europe (SCPE) network proposed an easy and reliable classification of MRI findings[26]; the "pathogenic patterns" described using MRI can also help characterize the stage of brain development at the time of insult.

Multisystem Comorbidities

Cerebral palsy is frequently associated with comorbidities such as epilepsy, feeding disorders, visual limitations, learning disorders, intellectual disability, attention-behavioral dysfunction, and secondary musculoskeletal problems with orthopedic deformities. Comorbidities affect the overall health and quality of life, including schooling. Children with cerebral palsy require multiple anesthetics throughout their lifetime: for imaging, common pediatric surgical conditions, or as a consequence of the associated comorbidities (including orthopedic or neurosurgical procedures, gastrostomy or tracheostomy, Nissen fundoplication, diagnostic endoscopy, dental surgeries, and more).[27,28] Many of these comorbid conditions can affect the anesthesia management. Understanding the pathophysiology and comorbidities of cerebral palsy allows anesthesiologists to anticipate and prevent perioperative complications. The major medical problems associated with cerebral palsy include[9,22,27–30]:

Gastrointestinal System
Most children with cerebral palsy have oromotor dysfunction. This is commonly associated with gastroesophageal reflux and may lead to recurrent aspiration, decreased respiratory reserve, esophageal stenosis, and malnutrition. Increased salivation and impaired swallowing due to impaired cranial nerve function may require the chronic administration of an antisialagogue (e.g., oral glycopyrrolate or scopolamine patch). Immobility, dehydration, and poor diet predispose patients to bowel stasis and constipation that can cause fecal impaction. Associated procedures include diagnostic upper endoscopy, fundoplication, percutaneous gastrostomy, and esophageal dilatation.

Malnutrition
Poor nutrition and laxative use for chronic constipation predispose the child to anemia, protein deficiency, and electrolyte imbalance; iron deficiency is common. The higher the Gross Motor Function

Classification System score, the greater the risk of iron and other nutrient deficiencies.[31,32] Malnutrition may compromise wound healing and depress immune responses. Preoperative assessment and correction of these parameters is essential.

Central Nervous System
Visual and hearing impairments are common, limiting our ability to communicate with these children. In children with more severe intellectual disability, anxiety and emotional lability can be challenging. Epilepsy occurs commonly, in up to 90% to 94% of children and adults with cerebral palsy.[21,33] Anticonvulsant therapy should be maintained until the day of surgery and restarted as soon as possible in the postoperative period. If oral ingestion may limited after surgery, the child's neurologist should be consulted to transition the child to intravenous antiseizure medications.

Respiratory System
Pulmonary complications are a common cause of death in children with cerebral palsy. Aspiration is exacerbated by excessive oral secretions, bulbar dysfunction with impaired swallowing, hypotonia of the respiratory muscles resulting in poor cough, inability to clear secretions, recurrent respiratory infection, and chronic lung disease. Concomitant scoliosis may restrict pulmonary function (see Chapter 30). Chronic respiratory failure can also lead to pulmonary hypertension, right ventricular hypertrophy, and cardiac failure.

Musculoskeletal Deformities
Spasticity leads to chronic contractures, spine deformities, and chronic pain. Orthopedic and neurosurgical operations are the most frequently performed procedures in children with moderate to severe cerebral palsy: they include tendon releases, femoral osteotomy, and hip adductor and iliopsoas releases. The current trend in orthopedic surgery is to perform multiple procedures involving tenotomies or osteotomies at different levels of all extremities during a single general anesthesia, rather than staging them during multiple operations. Scoliosis often requires surgery to prevent further deterioration in lung function and stabilization of the spine to facilitate ambulation and sitting. Spinal fusion is considered in all children with progressive curves greater than 40 to 50 degrees.[34]

Baclofen can be used to reduce pain associated with spasticity and may delay the development of contractures. It acts as an agonist at GABA$_B$ receptors in the dorsal horn of the spinal cord. Its intrathecal administration overcomes the problem of poor transfer across the blood-brain barrier. Intrathecal baclofen is considered the most effective treatment for severe spasticity and dystonia in children with cerebral palsy. The most common complications related to intrathecal administration are associated with pump and catheter delivery systems.[35]

Botulinum toxin is also used to reduce muscle spasticity in affected children.[36] It is commonly injected into motor points of spastic muscles during sedation or general anesthesia. Systemic effects are observed in 1% to 2% of children: it is recommended to limit the dose of injectate to 16 IU/kg, with a maximum of 400 IU in any one encounter.[37] Treatments are repeated every 3 to 6 months. Botulinum toxin causes a dose-dependent, reversible muscle denervation, and muscle atrophy if given long term. The toxin reduces spasticity and increases the range of motion, which is particularly useful in children with dynamic contractures; however, improvement in function has not been convincingly demonstrated.

Allergies
An increased incidence of latex allergy has been reported in children with cerebral palsy.[38] This may be the result of multiple

surgeries, or bladder catheterization with latex products. Prophylaxis against latex anaphylaxis has been unreliable; it is best to avoid latex in the perioperative period to prevent anaphylaxis.

Anesthesia Considerations for Cerebral Palsies

Table 22.3 summarizes the most important anesthetic considerations in children with cerebral palsy.[9,27–30] The management and assessment of perioperative pain in children with neurocognitive impairment is addressed in Chapter 42.

MALFORMATIONS OF THE NERVOUS SYSTEM

Central nervous system (CNS) malformations are common in pediatric neurologic practice and are a frequent cause of morbidity and mortality. The CNS develops very rapidly in the 2-week embryo and continues until several years after birth. The causes of CNS malformations are largely uncertain, but their timing appears to be more important than the nature of the insult in producing the specific type of malformation. Possible causative agents include maternal drugs such as sodium valproate, which is associated with neural tube defects; infections such as cytomegalovirus that can cause cerebral lesions, depending on the time during gestation of the infection; toxins such as alcohol; vitamin deficiency (e.g., folic acid), and genetic disorders. MRI can provide adequate images to enable an early and rather precise diagnosis in many instances (e.g., cortical dysplasia).[39]

Neural Tube Defects: Cranial and Spinal Dysraphism

The live birth incidence of neural tube defects is 5.7 to 6.7 per 10,000. Neural tube defects are a group of birth defects that result in failure of the neural tube to develop properly during the embryonic stage. Neural tube defects include anencephaly, encephaloceles, and spina bifida.

The cause of neural tube defects is multifactorial, with genetic and environmental factors the most important. Approximately 10% of the defects are caused by chromosomal abnormalities such as trisomies (i.e., 13, 18, and 21), triploidy, and 22q11 microdeletion. Some of the environmental causes include folate deficiency, maternal antiepileptic drugs (valproate, phenytoin, carbamazepine, and polytherapy), retinoids, and maternal diabetes.

Preconception folic acid supplementation has reduced the prevalence of neural tube defects ~30% to 50%.[40,41] Along with antenatal ultrasound examination, screening is done for increased maternal serum concentration of α-fetoprotein; termination of pregnancy in cases with positive test results has further reduced the prevalence of these defects.

Anencephaly is a lethal disorder resulting from the neural tube failing to close between the 23rd and 26th day following conception. This leads to disorganization of neural elements and the absence of skull formation.[42] Some deep cerebral structures may remain intact, and the brainstem may develop normally. Normal respiration and cardiovascular functions may develop, enabling the infant to survive for hours or days after birth. Other structures in the head and brain, including the eyes, face, and pituitary gland, may not develop normally. An infant with anencephaly is usually blind, deaf, and unable to feel pain. The anencephalic neonate has been used as an organ donor for neonates or small infants although this can be controversial.[43–45]

Encephalocele is a herniation of neural tissue and meninges out of the skull through deficient skin and bone either anteriorly or posteriorly (see Fig. 24.12A). Anterior encephaloceles are associated with underlying brain, orbital structures, or pituitary gland anomalies. Posterior encephaloceles are associated with

cerebral or cerebellar tissue that herniates through a bony defect in the posterior cranium. In both cases, care should be taken to avoid compressing the herniated structure during induction (e.g., from a face mask or the undersurface supporting the head) as well as during closure of the defect when cerebral tissue is reintegrated into the cranium (risk of acute intracranial hypertension).[46] Intranasal encephaloceles may be difficult to diagnose. Once diagnosed, they can be corrected either endoscopically or via a combined nasal and neurosurgical approach.[47] However, these defects carry a poor prognosis for long-term survival. The only treatment is reparative surgery; occasionally shunts are placed for hydrocephalus.[48]

Spina bifida refers to a group of conditions in which there is abnormal or incomplete formation of the midline structures over the neuraxis (see Fig. 24.12B).[42] Skin, bony, and neural elements may be involved singly or in combination. Congenital malformations of the spinal cord may exist in isolation or in association with brain anomalies. These defects may present at birth, as in the case of the more severe and open lesions (i.e., spina bifida aperta) or be identified later if the skin overlying the spinal defect is intact (e.g., spina bifida occulta). Those who develop a Chiari malformation may present with cervical cord or bulbar deficits, increasing their risk for respiratory difficulties (see Figs. 24.13 and 24.14). Children with spinal cord lesions are at increased risk for sensory deficits, making meticulous skin care and positioning essential to prevent pressure sores and damage to neuropathic joints.

In *spina bifida occulta* the overlying skin appears to be intact and normal. In many cases, a hairy patch or a dermal sinus (i.e., sacral dimple) may communicate with the meninges or attach to the spinal cord or a lipoma that causes a fatty swelling overlying the bony defect; these require further radiologic investigation.[49] The spinal cord may be tethered by internal connection to such structures, making it vulnerable to trauma at surgery and during growth, especially at puberty. The spinal cord may also be abnormally formed, with cartilaginous or bony spurs that damage or divide the cord during growth as the neural tissue grows at a slower rate than the surrounding bone (i.e., diastematomyelia). These infants may not be candidates for a caudal block because the spinal cord may end at an unusually low position.

Spina bifida cystica, the most common type of spinal dysraphism, manifests as an obvious lesion on the back (see Fig. 24.12B). The defect may be diagnosed antenatally. The abnormally developed spinal cord may be covered by a layer of meninges (i.e., myelomeningocele) or remain uncovered (i.e., open myelomeningocele). The spinal level of the lesion is the major determinant of morbidity. Myelomeningoceles need to be repaired within a few days of birth to prevent infection and further damage to the neural tissues. A cerebrospinal fluid (CSF) leak or frank dural rupture may develop, leading to intravascular volume and electrolyte abnormalities that should be treated preoperatively.

When the defect is identified at birth, it is optimally managed in a specialist center by a multidisciplinary team (i.e., pediatrician, neurologist, neurosurgeon, orthopedic surgeon, and others) who can anticipate, prevent, and treat complications and assist in the child's long-term care. Children with dysraphism often develop postoperative hydrocephalus because of disrupted CSF flow and require a ventriculoperitoneal shunt. Long-term complications, including paraparesis, neurogenic bladder and bowel, renal insufficiency, trophic limb changes, pressure sores, joint contractures, and scoliosis that may require surgical repair and future intervention.[50] Children with neural tube defects should

TABLE 22.3	Anesthesia Considerations for Children With Cerebral Palsy	
	Implications	**Management**
Preoperative concerns		
Clarify known cause of cerebral palsy:	Evaluate coexisting medical problems	
Clarify child autonomy: Gross Motor Function Classification System for Cerebral Palsy (GMFCS)	The more affected the child, the more likely they are to experience perioperative adverse events	
Assess frequently associated comorbidities:		
1. Malnutrition	Anemia, iron deficiency, hypoalbuminemia, electrolyte imbalance.[216]	Preoperative blood test + ferritin before major surgery
2. Gastroesophageal reflux	Antiacid medications Antireflux surgery	↑ risk of aspiration Continue antiacid and prokinetic medications
3. Hypersalivation	Antisialagogue treatment	To be continued
4. Recurrent respiratory infection	Hypotonia of the respiratory muscles with swallowing problems and inability to cough and clear secretions	↑ risk of aspiration Preoperative pulmonary physiotherapy Gentle suction the oropharynx before induction of anesthesia
5. Epilepsy	Antiepileptic drug therapy	To be continued and restarted as soon as possible
6. Evaluate spasticity and chronic pain	Oral or intrathecal baclofen	To be continued Should not be discontinued abruptly
7. Evaluate spine deformities	Scoliosis (restrictive pulmonary function, predisposing to chronic hypoxemia, pulmonary hypertension, and right ventricular hypertrophy)	Room air SpO_2 Preoperative pulmonary physiotherapy and bronchodilators Chest X-ray Cardiac echo Neuraxial block difficult
8. Evaluate abnormal dentition and temporomandibular joint dysfunction	Difficult airway examination: limited mouth opening, temporomandibular joint dysfunction, arched palate, teeth anomalies	Possible difficult airway
Check usual medications	Antiepileptic drugs, baclofen, antisialagogue, prokinetic, bronchodilator	To be continued
Check allergies	Increased risk of latex allergy	No latex protocol
Evaluate anxiety	Irritability or combativeness Spasticity may increase	Premedication may be indicated Presence of familiar caregiver or parent at induction of anesthesia EMLA cream if IV induction
Intraoperative Concerns		
Spasticity and contracture Spine deformity	Difficult positioning and IV access Possible difficult airway management	
Excessive salivation	Increased risk of aspiration	Postintubation endotracheal suction
Sensibility to hypothermia		Body and IV fluid warming devices from the start of anesthesia[217]
Risk of hypotension	Preemptive volume loading as soon as IV is secured[218] Careful titration of doses	Adjust anesthesia depth
Increased sensitivity to anesthetic agents[219–222]		Adjust anesthesia depth
Neuromuscular blockers[223–225]		Monitoring of anesthetic depth of neuromuscular-block
Monitoring of anesthetic depth [219–222]	Check baseline value of the cerebral function monitor (e.g. BIS) in the awake child	Use of a cerebral function monitor to avoid overdose
Emergence of anesthesia	Often slower	Check for hypothermia, seizures, hypoglycemia Extubation in fully awake child
Difficult positioning Osteoporosis	Prevent dislocations, fractures, and pressure sores	Careful positioning
Postoperative Concerns		
Difficult to identify the presence and location of pain Frequent resurgence of muscle spasms	Check for the presence, source, and intensity of pain with help of parents or familiar caregiver	Use multimodal opioid-sparing regimen[217,226] Provide regional anesthesia if possible Cautious use of low-dose muscle relaxants (e.g., diazepam or dantrolene)

be managed in a latex-free environment at all times, lest they develop latex allergy if repeatedly exposed to latex products.[51,52] The anesthesia considerations for neural tube defects are presented in Chapter 24.

Chiari Malformation

Chiari malformations[53] of the nervous system may coexist with other anomalies and manifest in the neonatal period or later in the early decades of life (Table 22.4). Surgical decompression at the foramen magnum and upper cervical spine is the treatment of choice for neuronal dysfunction.

Syringomyelia

Syringomyelia results from a glial cell–lined cavitation within the spinal cord. Diagnosis has been simplified by the use of MRI, which provides images of the spinal cord and the tubular fluid-filled space within.[42] Although the spectrum of Chiari I malformations is not usually associated with other cerebral abnormalities, syringomyelia is found in ~20% to 70% of patients, depending on the degree and extent of disruption of normal CSF flow between the spine and cranium. Syringomyelia manifests with dissociated sensory loss, usually in the upper limbs, causing loss or impairment of pain and temperature sensation, which may cause trophic changes in the fingers and neuropathic joints. It may progress to paralysis and hyporeflexia later in life. The lower limbs may exhibit pyramidal signs; some lesions may extend upward (i.e., syringobulbia) and produce lower brainstem signs, such as stridor and laryngospasm (i.e., vocal cord palsy).

Treatment of syringomyelia is controversial, especially if the lesion is asymptomatic. Management may focus on associated disorders as the size of the syrinx may remain static or slowly increase in size. Adequate surgical decompression at the foramen magnum and upper cervical spine is the treatment of choice for neuronal dysfunction, symptomatic syrinx, or hydrocephalus. Ventriculoperitoneal shunting may be required for hydrocephalus and syringostomy or syrinx shunting for cord drainage if the craniocervical decompression alone does not relieve the pressure in the syrinx.

Hydrocephalus

Hydrocephalus is defined as an increase in the volume of CSF in the brain, particularly the ventricles, associated with an increase in the intracranial pressure (ICP). It may be associated with syndromes such as craniosynostosis, tuberous sclerosis, achondroplasia, and others.[54] It results from either obstructed drainage or from overproduction of CSF within the brain. In practice, obstructed drainage of CSF is the most common cause of hydrocephalus. Obstruction results from intraventricular hemorrhage, Chiari malformation, brain tumor, and congenital aqueductal stenosis. In contrast, overproduction is an uncommon source of hydrocephalus most often resulting from tumors of the choroid plexus. Hydrocephalus may present with chronic or acute symptoms of ICP. Children typically present with a headache and irritability, but signs and symptoms can progress to lethargy, seizures, vomiting, and ophthalmoplegia as pressure within the brain increases. In infants, it presents as accelerated head growth, bulging fontanelle, poor feeding, sunsetting eyes sign, and developmental delay. If left untreated, it may lead to a reduced level of consciousness, oculomotor palsies, sluggish pupillary light reactions, bradycardia, and eventually respiratory arrest. Diagnosis of hydrocephalus is confirmed by neuroimaging, often with computed tomography (CT) in the acute situation, followed by MRI.

Surgery is the definitive treatment for hydrocephalus. It usually involves inserting a drainage system to shunt CSF from the brain to another site in the body (see Fig. 24.11). After insertion of a shunt, children should be closely monitored for shunt complications; these include infection, blockage or fracture of the shunt, and over drainage of CSF. The anesthetic considerations for treating hydrocephalus are discussed in Chapter 24. An endoscopic cerebral aqueductoplasty, choroid plexus cauterization, or third venticulostomy is often performed for obstructive hydrocephalus.[55]

DISORDERS OF VENTRAL INDUCTION

Holoprosencephaly (or frontonasal dysplasia) is a cephalic disorder in which the forebrain of the embryo fails to develop into discrete hemispheres with normal connections.[42,56]

There are four types on imaging:

1. Lobar: There is almost complete separation of the hemispheres, and the corpus callosum is almost absent.
2. Semilobar: The two hemispheres are divided posteriorly, with interhemispheric connections present anteriorly. The corpus callosum is absent anteriorly, and the thalami are fused in the midline.
3. Alobar: An undivided and small forebrain with a dorsal sac that may contain some cortex.
4. Syntelencephaly: The frontal, parietal, and occipital lobes are fused and the corpus callosum is absent but the hypothalamus is normal.

TABLE 22.4	**Chiari Malformations**		
Type	**Main Features**	**Associated Abnormalities**	**Neurologic Features**
Chiari I	Downward displacement of cerebellar tonsils >5 mm caudally through the foramen magnum	Syringomyelia (in 20%–70%); hydrocephalus	Later onset (>12 years of age), cervical cord signs: tetraparesis, sensory deficits of upper limbs
Chiari II	Downward displacement of cerebellar tonsils, vermis 4th ventricle and brainstem with obstruction of cerebrospinal fluid flow	Supratentorial and infratentorial abnormalities; myelomeningocele or meningocele in nearly all	Present in neonate, macrocephaly, increased intracranial pressure, cranial nerve palsies
Chiari III (rare)	Downward displacement of cerebellum into posterior encephalocele; elongation of 4th ventricle	Posterior defects: cervical spina bifida ± cranium bifidum	Present in neonate with signs of hydrocephalus ± brainstem and cervical cord signs
Chiari IV (extremely rare)	Cerebellar hypoplasia or primary cerebellar agenesis	Usually none	± Ataxia

Facial defects may be severe and include cyclopia (i.e., single orbit with fused globes), cebocephaly (i.e., single nostril), proboscis, and a midline cleft lip and palate. Associated malformations (e.g., congenital heart disease, scalp deficits, polydactyly) are common. Chromosomal anomalies (trisomy 13 or 18), a mutation of one of 13 different genes or a complex syndromic disorder (e.g., Pallister-Hall or Smith-Lemli-Opitz) may be associated with disorders of ventral induction. The diagnosis rests on a careful description of the external and internal morphology using MRI, followed by genetic assessment. Complications include hydrocephalus, endocrine pituitary defects, epilepsy, and severe complex disability, usually with a shortened life expectancy.

DISORDERS OF CORTICAL DEVELOPMENT

Malformations of the cerebral cortex are varied. Malformations of cortical development (MCD) are increasingly recognized as an important cause of epilepsy and developmental delay. It is estimated that up to 40% of children with refractory epilepsy have a cortical malformation. Malformations of the cerebral cortex encompass a wide spectrum of disorders with various underlying genetic etiologies and clinical manifestations. MRI has dramatically improved our recognition of these malformations, their identification, and their classification.[57] Disruptions at the various stages of development lead to characteristic malformations. Disorders of neurogenesis give rise to microcephaly (small brain) or macrocephaly (large brain). Disorders of early neuroblast migration give rise to periventricular heterotopia (neurons located along the ventricles), whereas abnormalities later in migration lead to lissencephaly (smooth brain) or subcortical band heterotopia (smooth brain with a band of heterotopic neurons under the cortex). Abnormal neuronal migration arrest leads to overmigration of neurons in cobblestone lissencephaly. Lastly, disorders of neuronal organization cause polymicrogyria (abnormally small gyri and sulci).

Environmental agents and genetic abnormalities have been identified for many of these malformations, and genetic derangements can produce a multisystem syndrome. Some of the genes involved are the *LIS1* gene, 4p− (Wolf-Hirschhorn), and 17p− (Miller-Dieker syndrome). Clinical effects vary, and the severity depends on the site and extent of the lesion. Children may have learning disabilities, epilepsy, focal neurologic deficits, motor dysfunction, and other system involvement.

Progressive Neurologic Disorders

PRIMARY BRAIN TUMORS

Children with primary brain or spinal cord tumors represent a major therapeutic challenge that requires the coordinated efforts of pediatric specialists in neurosurgery, anesthesiology, neuropathology, radiotherapy, pediatric oncology, neurology, rehabilitation, neuroradiology, endocrinology, and psychology, who have special expertise in the care of these patients.

Brain and other CNS tumors, both malignant and nonmalignant, comprise a constellation of over 100 histologically distinct subtypes with varying descriptive epidemiology, clinical characteristics, treatments, and outcomes. The classification of these tumors has changed in recent years in parallel with progress in molecular biology leading to a more accurate diagnosis.[58] Brain and other CNS tumors are broadly categorized as glial (e.g., astrocytomas, ependymomas), embryonal (e.g., medulloblastomas, atypical teratoid/rhabdoid tumors, and CNS primitive neuroectodermal tumors), germ cell (e.g., germinoma, teratoma), and others (e.g.,

choroid plexus tumors, craniopharyngiomas) (Table 22.5). The most common gliomas in children are astrocytomas, oligodendrogliomas, ependymomas, brainstem gliomas (including the diffuse midline glioma, previously referred to as diffuse intrinsic pontine glioma) and optic nerve gliomas. Pilocytic astrocytomas are more common in children and adolescents compared with adults (~25% of malignant tumors). Germ cell tumors and cystic tumors are also more common among children and adolescents than in adults.

Brain and other CNS tumors are the most common cause of cancer in children aged 0 to 14 years, with an average annual age-adjusted incidence rate of 5.85 per 100,000 (average annual age-adjusted incidence rate of malignant tumors of 3.87 vs. 1.97 for nonmalignant tumors).[58] Leukemia is the second most common neoplasm in the same population, with an average annual age-adjusted incidence rate of 5.09 per 100,000. Whereas the incidence of neurologic malignant tumors peaks in children aged 1 to 4 years and declines thereafter, the incidence of nonmalignant tumors decreases immediately after infancy but subsequently rises in adolescence. The male/female ratio is equal in these tumors except for a male preponderance in ependymal tumors, embryonal tumors, and germ cell tumors, and a female preponderance in pituitary tumors.[59] Brain tumors are most often supratentorial in infants and older children and infratentorial, located in the posterior fossa, (cerebellum and brainstem) in children aged 1 to 9 years.[58] During adolescence most tumors are located in the pituitary and craniopharyngeal duct.[59]

Some children are genetically predisposed to CNS tumors. These include neurofibromatosis (i.e., optic nerve gliomas, schwannomas of the spinal cord, peripheral nerve tumors, skeletal deformities) and tuberous sclerosis (i.e., subependymal glial cell astrocytoma, cardiac rhabdomyomas, renal angiomyolipomas) that require long-term follow-up. Some Mendelian syndromes are linked to an increased risk for CNS tumors such as familial adenomatous polyposis and Turcot syndrome type 1 and type 2 for medulloblastoma and gliomas. Children who received cranial radiation as a part of their treatment for acute lymphocytic leukemia are at particular risk for subsequent primary brain tumors.[60]

The clinical presentation depends on the child's age, the histology, growth rate, and location of the tumor. Some symptoms may not be easy to detect because they are similar to symptoms of other conditions.[61] Infants are typically irritable, with an increasing head circumference, failure to thrive, and developmental regression. Older children develop morning headaches, nausea and vomiting, seizures, gait disturbances, or visual deficits. Supratentorial tumors can present with seizures, focal neurological deficit, personality change, visual field defects (optic pathway gliomas), and endocrine dysfunction (craniopharyngiomas). Infratentorial tumors present with cerebellar ataxia, signs of increased ICP (morning headaches, nausea, and vomiting), cranial nerve, and pyramidal tract signs. If the lesion is rapidly expanding and is accompanied by cerebral edema or obstructive CSF drainage, ICP will increase. Occasionally, a hemorrhage occurs into the tumor, causing a dramatic increase in ICP with its associated signs and symptoms, necessitating emergency treatment. Ultimately, brainstem decompensation and death ensue if the lesion is left untreated.

Although many pediatric brain tumors are diagnosed by a CT scan of the head performed for indications such as vomiting, ataxia, or altered mental status, CT is insufficient to characterize a tumor. MRI is the gold standard for the diagnosis of CNS tumors and metastases[62]; a classic MRI is often associated with

TABLE 22.5 Central Nervous System Tumors in Children

Tumor Type	Percent of All Childhood CNS Tumors, Median Age at Diagnosis	Sites and Clinical Features	Treatment	Overall Survival
Medulloblastoma				
Three distinct clinical groups: • Average-risk medulloblastoma • High-risk medulloblastoma • Very young children medulloblastoma Four molecular subtypes	~20% 6 years	Location in posterior fossa: ↑ICP • early morning headache, vomiting and visual disturbances • progressive macrocephaly, in young children, lethargy and irritability • papilledema, signs of cerebellar dysfunction: slurred speech, ataxia, and nystagmus	Surgical excision ± radiotherapy ± chemotherapy and targeted therapies	70%–85% according to the molecular subtype
Ependymoma				
• Posterior fossa: 70% • Supratentorial compartment: 25% • Spinal canal: 5% (adolescent)	~12% 4–6 years	Location in posterior fossa (see above) Spinal cord: dorsal pain, sphincter disturbances, walking difficulties	Surgical excision: complete neurosurgical resection is still the most important prognostic factor ± Radiotherapy	40%–75% (lower <4 years of age) Excellent survival for spinal tumors
High-Grade (Malignant) Gliomas (HGG)				
• Anaplastic astrocytoma (WHO grade III) and glioblastoma (WHO grade IV). • Midline pediatric HGGs including diffuse intrinsic pontine glioma (DIPG)	~10% at any age	Cerebral white matter and deep midline structures: ↑ICP, focal neurological deficits, and/or seizures Classic triad on DIPG *Cerebellar signs* (e.g., ataxia, dysmetria, dysarthria) *Long tract signs* (e.g., increased tone, hyperreflexia, clonus, Babinski sign, hemiparesis), Unilateral or bilateral *cranial nerve palsies* (e.g., abducens and facial palsy) Obstructive hydrocephalus 10%	Surgery ± radiotherapy ± chemotherapy Stereotactic biopsy at diagnosis as part of "precision medicine" radiotherapy ± chemotherapy ± targeted therapy.	30%–60% 10% beyond 2 years and only 2%–3% long-term survivors
Low-Grade Gliomas				
Pilocytic astrocytoma Diffuse astrocytoma	39% 7.1 years	Posterior fossa: (15%–20%) (see above) Cerebral hemispheres, midline structures such as the ventricles, hypothalamus, thalamus, and brainstem (10%–15% for each subsite), Spinal cord: 3%–6% Focal neurologic deficits, including hemiparesis, monoparesis, aphasia, dysphasia, and other cranial nerve or long tract signs	Surgery ± radiotherapy ± chemotherapy Targeted molecular agents	> 85%
Optic pathway gliomas	4.3–8.8 years	Endocrine disturbances: precocious puberty, growth retardation, diabetes insipidus ↓ visual acuity, strabismus, proptosis, hemianopsia Associated disorders (e.g., nNF1)	Controversial and individualized	
Craniopharyngioma	4%	Midline location + association with the hypothalamic-pituitary axis, visual pathways Endocrine deficiencies, visual deficits, headaches, and, in more advanced cases, neurological deficits affecting cranial nerves and long-tracts	Surgery ± Radiotherapy Hormonal therapy	Survival variable: 60%–90%

CNS, Central nervous system; ICP, intracranial pressure; ±, with or without; ↓, decreased; ↑, increased.

functional MRI, perfusion imaging, or MR spectroscopy. Other imaging includes positron emission tomography. A biopsy may be done because tissue diagnosis is always desirable. If the tumor is hard to reach or in a sensitive area, a stereotactic needle biopsy can be used. Immunohistochemical analysis, cytogenetics, molecular genetics, and measures of proliferative activity are increasingly used in tumor diagnosis and classification. Targeted drug therapy can then be tailored to the individual's needs. MRI of the spine and CSF analysis (except in case of increased ICP) are necessary to exclude metastases and check for some specific tumor markers like beta-human chorionic gonadotropin (βhCG) and alpha-fetoprotein (AFP) in nongerminomatous germ cell tumors.

Treatment for a pediatric brain tumor depends on the type, size, and location of the tumor, as well as on the child's age and overall health status. Surgery is the mainstay of treatment and is usually combined with radiotherapy or chemotherapy, or both. Cerebral edema should be treated preoperatively with corticosteroids to reduce ICP, alleviate symptoms and signs, and enable correction of fluid and electrolyte abnormalities. Seizures require anticonvulsant therapy. Nutrition may be poor and necessitate aggressive management with enteral or parenteral feeding. Intervention for increased ICP may require CSF diversion by endoscopic third ventriculostomy or internal or external shunting. The timing of surgery depends on whether the tumor should first be treated with radiotherapy or chemotherapy. Aggressive surgery with the intent of completely resecting the tumor improves the prognosis for many tumor types but carries important risks of residual neurologic deficits. The anesthetic implications of tumoral neurosurgery are summarized in Table 22.6.

Irradiation has been shown to be associated not only with middle- and long-term neurologic toxicity but also with increased mortality in long-term survivors.[63] Proton beam therapy, which delivers greater targeted doses to brain tumors, and minimizes radiation exposure to nearby healthy tissue, is available for certain types of brain tumors (see also Chapter 9). Conventional adjuvant chemotherapy regimens are used for some tumors, and key molecular pathways have been identified and targeted drugs developed such as BRAF (the human gene that encodes a protein called B-Raf) inhibitors in tumors with the BRAF V600E mutant, mitogen-activated protein kinase (MEK) inhibitors (in tumors with the tandem duplication such as pediatric low-grade glioma) or member of the phosphatidylinositol 3-kinase-related kinase family (mTOR) inhibitors for subependymal giant cell astrocytoma.

Malignant brain and other CNS tumors among children aged 1 to 14 years have an average annual age-adjusted mortality rate of 0.7 per 100,000, are the fourth largest cause of mortality from the various causes referenced in this age group and are the most common cause of cancer death. Five-year survival is 80% overall for children and adolescents diagnosed with malignant tumors and 95% for nonmalignant tumors. Patients frequently have long-term physical and psychosocial sequelae related to the tumor and/or its treatment, with variation by type or location of the tumor, patient characteristics, environmental factors, and treatment received. Despite high survival rates, nonmalignant tumors may confer substantial long-term morbidity. Childhood and adolescent cancer survivors are at particular risk of long-term and late effects because of the insult to the developing brain during cranial irradiation, surgical treatment, and the toxicity of chemotherapeutic agents. Children who survive CNS tumors frequently have permanent neurologic deficits, including epilepsy, learning disabilities, visual or hearing impairment, and growth and endocrine disorders.[64] Short-term and long-term follow-up evaluations by

specialist teams are required, along with careful emotional and social support for children and their families.

Tumors of the spinal cord and cauda equina are rare in childhood and account for ~5.2% of all brain and other CNS tumors in childhood and adolescence, but they result in significant morbidity. The most common are ependymal tumors (~17.7%) followed by nerve sheath tumors (~17.4%). They may be benign or malignant, sited within the cord (intramedullary) or outside (extramedullary). Symptoms may initially be nonspecific, especially in young children. The diagnosis may thus be delayed with an increased risk of spinal cord compression. These may include dorsal pain, paresthesia, paresis, sphincter disturbance, spinal deformity, torticollis, and hydrocephalus (ependymoma). Delayed diagnosis and cord decompression can cause spinal cord vascular compromise, leading to total and irreversible paralysis and permanent disability. The diagnosis is best achieved by spinal MRI, which provides details of the lesion and adjacent structures. Treatment usually involves surgery to decompress the cord and excise or biopsy the lesion. Follow-up treatment with radiotherapy may be indicated. Children with established neurologic deficits require a rehabilitation program.[65]

INBORN ERRORS OF METABOLISM

Inborn errors of metabolism (IEM) are rare genetic disorders of the biosynthesis or breakdown of molecules within metabolic pathways. These approximately 1450 disorders are caused by partial or complete loss of function of a single enzyme, cofactor, or transporter and are mostly inherited as autosomal recessive or X-linked.[66] Protein, carbohydrate, and fatty acid metabolism or the mitochondrial energy metabolism can be involved (Table 22.7).

Symptoms fluctuate with changes in the metabolic state of the patient. Most of these disorders are diagnosed through biochemical investigations including blood gases, plasma glucose, lactate, ammonia and amino acids, urinary organic acids, and an acylcarnitine profile.

Disorders of Protein Metabolism

The aminoacidopathies result from abnormal breakdown of amino acids in the cytosol (e.g., phenylketonuria or homocystinuria) or in the mitochondria (maple syrup urine disease [MSUD]). Clinical symptoms are caused by the accumulation of toxic intermediates. The classical organic acidurias are deficiencies of enzymes in the mitochondrial metabolism of CoA-activated carboxylic acids, most of which are derived from amino acid breakdown.[67] Clinical features are caused by the accumulation of toxic intermediates but also by a disturbance of mitochondrial energy metabolism and carnitine homeostasis; they may include encephalopathy and metabolic acidosis. Organic acidurias are diagnosed through the analysis of urinary organic acids or acylcarnitines in the blood. The treatment of the aminoacidopathies and organic acidurias involves the restriction of the dietary protein intake, intake of the amino acid involved in the defective pathway, and the prevention or prompt treatment of catabolic states that lead to the breakdown of large quantities of proteins.

The breakdown of proteins produces large amounts of nitrogen in the form of ammonia that is highly neurotoxic but is normally converted to urea in the urea cycle and excreted in the urine.

Urea Cycle Defects

Urea cycle defects (UCD) can have acute, chronic, and intermittent clinical manifestations occurring at any age, having as

TABLE 22.6 | Perioperative Management of Intracranial Brain Tumor in Children

Preoperative Management	Implications
Clarify the (1) localization and (2) the nature of suspected brain tumor (1) Posterior fossa, brain stem, supratentorial tumor, craniopharyngiomas (2) Cystic or solid tumor	(1) Localization ⇨ surgical position (supine, prone, sitting) and surgical approach (craniotomy, endoscopic, transsphenoidal or transoral) (2) Anticipate red blood cell transfusions (3) Plan venous access and monitoring (large-bore IV access, central venous catheter, arterial blood pressure, TEE)
Check associated symptoms: hydrocephalus and increased ICP (lethargy, nausea, vomiting), seizures, cranial nerve palsies, focal muscle weakness, hypothalamic-pituitary axis hormonal deficiencies, SIADH	Adapt anesthesia to symptoms: Lethargy or nausea/vomiting at risk for aspiration of gastric content Substitute hypothalamic-pituitary dysfunction (diabetes insipidus, adrenal insufficiency)
Check medications: antiepileptic drugs, steroids, vasopressin	Given usual morning medication, provide hydrocortisone supplement
Check coexisting comorbidities associated with some syndromes (e.g., tuberous sclerosis)	Check cardiac or renal anomalies
Evaluate anxiety of the child and parents	Take time for explanations Consider caregiver presence during induction of anesthesia Premedication may be considered only if cerebral compliance allows it
Preoperative blood test: Hb, Hct, platelet, serum electrolytes and osmolality, urine-specific gravity, coagulation, blood group, and cross match	Correct electrolyte deficit Anticipate red blood cell transfusions

Intraoperative Management	Implications
Preserve neurological function and cerebral autoregulation and CPP	The most important factor in preserving CPP is an adequate MAP maintenance Keep in mind that: Hypercarbia and hypoxia may increase ICP (e.g., obstructed airway during induction) Lethargy or nausea/vomiting increase risk for gastric aspiration; consider rapid-sequence induction
Positioning requires meticulous care	Allow adequate access to the patient Excessive rotation of the head can impede cerebral venous return, impair cerebral perfusion, increase ICP and venous bleeding. Head elevation facilitates venous and CSF drainage from the surgical site but increases the risk of VAE Inadequate prone position leads to decreased lung compliance, venocaval compression, and bleeding (increased epidural venous pressure)
Normovolemia	Intraoperative maintenance with isotonic saline (mildly hyperosmolar, minimize cerebral edema); check for hyperchloremic acidosis Small infants require glucose-containing fluids: check blood glucose level
Massive blood loss	Aggressive treatment with crystalloid, blood, and vasopressors Caution to dilutional thrombocytopenia Consider early administration of fibrinogen, platelets, and FFP Consider prophylactic IV tranexamic acid
Intraoperative neurophysiologic monitors: facial nerve assessment, ECoG (resection of an epileptogenic focus)	Discuss with the surgical and neuromonitoring teams (e.g., neuromuscular-blocking agent) Adapt anesthesia depth
Intraoperative MRI	Prolongs anesthesia time Adapt monitoring to MRI environment
Surgical manipulations may have impact on BP and ECG	Trigeminocardiac reflex resulting in vagal stimulation Stimulation of brainstem centers
Early or delayed extubation	Discuss with surgical team

BP, Blood pressure; *CSF*, cerebrospinal fluid; *CPP*, cerebral perfusion pressure; *ECoG*, electrocorticogram; *FFP*, fresh-frozen plasma; *HT*, hypertension; *ICP*, intracranial pressure; *IV*, intravenous; *NM-blocking agent*, neuromuscular blocking agent; *SIADH*, syndrome of inappropriate antidiuretic hormone; *TEE*, transesophageal cardiac echography; *VAE*, venous air embolism.

clinical hallmark the hyperammonemic crisis (lethargy and anorexia, progressing to seizures, coma, and/or death). Hyperammonemia is triggered by catabolic events (e.g., change from intrauterine to neonatal life, fever), protein overload or intake of certain drugs.[68] A urea cycle defect should be suspected when unexplained encephalopathy occurs at any age, but particularly in neonates. Investigations include ammonia level, analysis of the amino acids in plasma and urine as well as urinary orotic acid. Treatment requires the reduction of protein intake (special diet), the avoidance of catabolic states, supplementation by arginine or citrulline, and the administration of ammonia scavengers such as benzoate and/or phenylacetate/ phenylbutyrate. Extracorporeal detoxification (hemo- or peritoneal dialysis) is sometimes required.

TABLE 22.7 | Inborn Errors of Metabolism

Disease	Defect (gene)
Disorders of Protein Metabolism	
Amino-Acidopathies	
Alkaptonuria	Homogentisate 1,2-dioxygenase (HGD)
Phenylketonuria	Phenylalanine hydroxylase (PAH)
Homocystinuria	Cystathionine β-synthase (CBS)
Hepatorenal tyrosinemia (Type I)	Fumarylacetoacetate hydrolase (FAH)
Maple syrup urine disease	Branched-chain 2-ketoacid dehydrogenase (BCKAD) complex (BCKDHA, BCKDHB, DBT)
Organic Acidurias	
Propionic acidemia	Propionyl-CoA carboxylase (PCCA, PCCB)
Methylmalonic acidemia	Methylmalonyl-CoA mutase (MMAA, MMAB, MMADHC, MUT)
Isovaleric acidemia	Isovaleryl-CoA dehydrogenase (IVD)
Glutaric aciduria (type I)	Glutaryl-CoA dehydrogenase (GCDH)
Disorders of the Urea Cycle	
Ornithine transcarbamylase deficiency	Ornithine transcarbamylase (OTC)
Carbamylphosphate synthetase 1 deficiency	Carbamylphosphate synthetase 1 (CPS1)
Citrullinemia type 1	Argininosuccinic acid synthetase (ASS1)
Argininosuccinic aciduria	Argininosuccinate lyase (ASL)
Argininemia	Arginase (ARG1)
Hyperornithinemia, hyperammonemia, homocitrullinemia (HHH) syndrome	Ornithine transporter 1 (SLC25A15)
Lysinic protein intolerance	Deficient transport of basic amino acids (SLC7A7)
Glutamine synthetase deficiency	Glutamine synthetase (GLUL)
Carbonic anhydrase VA deficiency	Carbonic anhydrase VA (CA5A)
Disorders of Carbohydrate Metabolism	
Galactosemia	Galactose-1-phosphate uridylyltransferase (GALT)
Hereditary fructose intolerance	Aldolase B (ALDOB)
Glycogen storage disease	
Type 0	Glycogen synthase (GYS2)
Type I (von Gierke)	Glucose-6-phosphatase (G6PC) or translocase (SLC37A4)
Type II (Pompe)	Acid alpha-glucosidase (GAA)
Type III (Cori or Forbes)	Glycogen debranching enzyme 0 (AGL)
Type IV (Andersen)	Glycogen branching enzyme (GBE1)
Type V (McArdle)	Muscle glycogen phosphorylase (PYGM)
Type VI (Hers)	Liver glycogen phosphorylase (PYGL)
Type VII (Tarui)	Muscle phosphofructokinase (PFKM)
Type IX	Phosphorylase kinase (PHKA2, PHKG2, PHKB, PHKA1)
Type XI (Fanconi Bickel)	Glucose transporter member 2 (SLC2A2)
Disorders of Fatty Acid Metabolism and Ketone Bodies	
Carnitine cycle defects	
Carnithine transporter deficiency	Carnitine transporter (SLC22A5)
Carnitine-acylcarnitine translocase deficiency	Carnitine-acylcarnitine translocase (SLC25A20)
Carnitine palmitoyl transferase I (CPTIA) deficiency	Carnitine palmitoyl transferase I (CPT1A)
Carnitine palmitoyl transferase II (CPTII) deficiency	Carnitine palmitoyl transferase II (CPT2)
β-oxidation defects	
Very long-chain acyl-CoA dehydrogenase deficiency	Very long-chain acyl-CoA dehydrogenase (ACADVL)
Medium chain acyl-CoA dehydrogenase deficiency	Medium chain acyl-CoA dehydrogenase (ACADM)
Short chain acyl-CoA dehydrogenase deficiency	Short chain acyl-CoA dehydrogenase (ACADS)
Long-chain 3-hydroxyacyl-CoA dehydrogenase deficiency	Long-chain 3-hydroxyacyl-CoA dehydrogenase (HADHA)
Mitochondrial trifunctional protein deficiencies	Mitochondrial trifunctional protein (HADHA, HADHB)
Electron transfer defects	
Multiple acyl-CoA dehydrogenase deficiency/glutaric aciduria type II	α-/β unit of ETF, ETF-coenzyme Q oxidoreductase (ETFA, ETFB, ETFDH)
Ketogenesis and ketolysis defects	
3-Hydroxy-3-methylglutaryl-CoA lyase deficiency (HMG CoA lyase deficiency)	3-Hydroxy-3-methylglutaryl-CoA lyase (HMGCL)
Succinyl-CoA 3-oxoacid CoA transferase deficiency	Succinyl-CoA 3-oxoacid CoA transferase (OXCT1)
Mitochondrial acetoacetyl-CoA thiolase deficiency	Mitochondrial acetoacetyl-CoA thiolase (ACAT1)

22

Continued

TABLE 22.7 | Inborn Errors of Metabolism—cont'd

Disease	Defect (*gene*)
Lysosomal Storage Diseases	
Mucopolysaccharidoses	
I-H (Hurler); I-S (Scheie);I-HS (Hurler-Scheie)	α-l-iduronidase *(IDUA)*
MPS II (Hunter)	Iduronate sulfatase *(IDS)*
Sanfilipo disease (MPS IIIA, MPS IIIB, MPS IIIC, MPS IIID)	Heparan sulfamidase *(MPS IIIA)*, N-acetylglucosaminidase *(MPS IIIB)*, Heparan-α-glucosaminide N-acetyltransferase *(MPS IIIC)*, N-acetylglucosamine 6-sulfatase *(MPS IIID)*
MPS IVA (Morquio A), MPS IVB (Morquio B)	Galactose-6-sulfate sulfatase *(GALNS)*; β-galactosidase *(GLB1)*
MPS VI (Maroteaux-Lamy)	N-acetylgalactosamine-4-sulfatase *(ARSB)*
MPS VII (Sly)	β-glucuronidase *(GUSB)*
Mucolipidosis II, III (I cell disease)	Uridine diphosphate-N-acetyl glucosamine (GNPTAB)
Sphingolipidoses	
Nieman-Pick disease A, B	Acid sphingomyelinase *(SMPD1)*
Fabry disease	α-galactosidase A *(GLA)*
Krabbe disease	Galactocerebrosidase *(GALC)*; saposin A *(PSAP)*
Gaucher disease	Glucocerebrosidase *(GBA)*; saposin C *(PSAP)*
Metachromatic leukodystrophy	Arylsulfatase A *(ARSA)*; saposin B *(PSAP)*
GM1-gangliosidosis	β-Galactosidase *(GLB1)*
GM2-gangliosidosis (Tay-Sachs disease /Sandhoff disease)	Hexosaminidase A and B *(HEXA, HEXB)*
Peroxisomal Disorders	
X-linked adrenoleukodystrophy	Adrenoleukodystrophy protein *(ABCD1)*
Classic/adult Refsum disease	Phytanoyl-CoA hydroxylase *(PHYH)*
Zellweger spectrum disorders	Peroxins *(PEX1, PEX10, PEX11B, PEX12, PEX13, PEX14, PEX16, PEX19, PEX2, PEX26, PEX3, ...)*
Inborn Errors of Cholesterol Synthesis	
Smith-Lemli-Opitz syndrome	3 beta-hydroxysterol-delta 7-reductase *(DHCR7)*

Disorders of Carbohydrate Metabolism

These disorders include diseases such as galactosemia, hereditary fructose intolerance, and glycogen storage diseases. Defects in the metabolism of galactose and fructose cause disease through accumulation of pathogenic metabolites. Children with galactosemia and fructosemia typically develop severe damage to the liver and/or kidney after dietary intake of lactose (milk, milk products) or fructose (fruit, sucrose), respectively. Treatment requires the elimination of the dietary intake of galactose or fructose. In hereditary fructose intolerance, special caution should be taken during any hospitalization.[69] All members of the team should be aware of the diagnosis of hereditary fructose intolerance (HFI) and the patient advised to wear a medically approved alert bracelet providing information about the diagnosis of hereditary fructose intolerance. "Red flags" should be placed in the patient's medical record to alert providers to the diagnosis and to the risks associated with exposures to foods and/or medications (oral or parenteral) containing fructose, sucrose, sorbitol, or sucralose. Many medications designed for pediatric use contain these substances: oral suspensions or chewable flavored tabs, injectable medications (e.g., trastuzumab, filgrastim, some intravenous immunoglobulins solutions), vaccines, and iron supplements, as well as enema solutions and rinsing aids. For many preparations, it may not be apparent that fructose or similar compounds are included.[69]

Disorders of gluconeogenesis and glycogen storage are revealed by hypoglycemia and lactic acidemia after short periods of fasting. Glycogen storage leads to hepatic enlargement and/or clinical myopathy in some subtypes. Treatment includes frequent meals, cornstarch supplementation, or continuous overnight tube feeding to avoid hypoglycemia.

Disorders of Fatty Acid Oxidation and Ketone Bodies

Mitochondrial fatty acid oxidation is required for the provision of energy during fasting, either through complete oxidation or through production of ketones in the liver that can serve as an alternative energy source for the brain. Disorders in this pathway present as hypoketotic hypoglycemia precipitated by fasting, leading to coma or epileptic seizures. In addition, some disorders cause severe liver disease and/or cardiomyopathy and/or rhabdomyolysis. The diagnosis is reached through the analysis of the acylcarnitine profile and urinary organic acids. Treatment consists of avoiding fasting and using medium chain fatty acid supplements in place of long-chain fatty acids.[70]

Lysosomal Storage Disease

Disorders of the biosynthesis and breakdown of complex molecules such as mucopolysaccharidoses and mucolipidosis II, show progressive clinical symptoms caused by their accumulation in several organs and are less likely to cause acute metabolic crises. Disorders in this group require specific investigations for their diagnosis. Lysosomal enzymes are involved in stepwise degradation of glycosaminoglycans (GAGs) and sphingolipids. Malfunction of an enzyme results in accumulation of the preceding metabolite: Clinical features of lysosomal storage disorders include dysmorphic features, organomegaly, and progressive neurological deterioration. Treatment approaches for most lysosomal storage disorders include enzyme replacement therapy and hematopoietic stem cell transplantation; gene therapy and substrate reduction therapy are currently being studied. Even if the child benefits from these treatments, the disease still progresses in some organs. Preoperative investigations should include echocardiography examining for involvement of the valves, a careful evaluation of the cervical vertebrae looking for instability, and an assessment of the upper airway (obstructive sleep apnea, involvement of the larynx and trachea, size and shape).[71]

Peroxisomal Disorders

Peroxisomes are organelles present in all cells except erythrocytes. They perform essential metabolic functions including β-oxidation of very long-chain fatty acids (VLCFAs) α-oxidation of phytanic acid, and biosynthesis of plasmalogen and bile acids. They include major subgroups: disorders of peroxisomal biogenesis and single peroxisomal enzyme/transporter defects. Peroxisome biogenesis defects, such as Zellweger spectrum syndrome (ZSS), are characterized by defective assembly of the entire organelle, whereas in single enzyme/transporter defects such as X-linked adrenoleukodystrophy, the organelle is intact, but one of its specific functions is disrupted. Peroxisomal biogenesis defects are clinically diverse and range in severity from neonatal lethal to later onset milder variants and cause a wide range of neurological symptoms as well as hepatointestinal dysfunction, skeletal abnormalities, dysmorphic features, and visual/hearing impairments. X-linked adrenoleukodystrophy (XALD) is the most common of the peroxisomal disorders, affecting 1 in 17,000 to 1 in 21,000 males with a wide range of phenotypic expressions: cerebral inflammatory (ALD), adrenomyeloneuropathy (AMN), Addison only, and asymptomatic. The first two phenotypes account for almost 80% of the patients. Treatment options are hormone replacement therapy, dietary intervention, or hematopoietic stem cell transplantation

Catabolism

The presence of an inborn error of metabolism has major implications in the perioperative period. The first step in successful management is being aware of the child's disease. As a rule, elective surgery should be carried out in centers experienced with the inborn error of metabolism, especially if the child is prone to acute metabolic decompensation. The main issues concerning the perioperative management of children with an inborn error of metabolism are detailed below.[72]

Conventional preoperative fasting, general anesthesia, and surgical stress are potential sources of catabolism and can be responsible for hypoglycemia, hyperammonemia, metabolic acidosis, or rhabdomyolysis in the presence of an inborn error of metabolism.

Prevention of hypoglycemia in disorders of fatty acid oxidation, glycogen storage diseases, and disorders of gluconeogenesis. The aim is to maintain glycemia greater than 4 mmol/L (70 mg/100 mL). The patient's history and tolerance of fasting should be documented before planning the anesthetic prescription. According to the recent fasting recommendations, children are now allowed to drink a clear glucose-containing solution up to 1 to 2 hours before induction of anesthesia.[73] However, in children who were fed overnight via a nasogastric tube, an intravenous infusion of glucose should be started before the nasogastric administration is discontinued. Intravenous 10% glucose with electrolytes (Na, K) administered at a rate of 2500 mL/m² for 24 hours adjusted based on regular measurements of glycemia can be started before hypoglycemia would be expected. The IV administration of glucose should be discontinued only after the child begins to drink and eat, and when the risk of vomiting has subsided.

Prevention of metabolic acidosis and ketosis in organic acidurias and maple syrup urine disease. This can be achieved first by avoiding hypoglycemia as described earlier. Intravenous lipid administration solution may be considered in case of prolonged postoperative fasting. One-third of the usual amino acid supplementation, or at least 0.25 g/kg, is recommended for children with maple syrup urine disease before anesthesia.

Prevention of hyperammonemia in disorders of the urea cycle and organic acidurias. Hyperammonemia is prevented by avoiding protein catabolism, which in turn is prevented by avoiding hypoglycemia (see earlier). Patients whose usual medication includes arginine or citrulline should be given intravenous arginine (the dose is the patient's usual dose diluted as 2.5 grams in 50 mL 10% glucose and piggybacked via a syringe pump to the glucose infusion). In children receiving sodium benzoate, phenylbutyrate, or both, an intravenous mixture of benzoate and phenylacetate is employed, again in a dilution of at least 2.5 grams of each per 50 mL and given via a piggyback pump. For brief procedures, these medications can be started postoperatively. For more prolonged procedures or situations likely to induce catabolism, and certainly in the presence of hyperammonemia, they can be given intraoperatively. It is also important to avoid any hidden intake of proteins such as blood swallowed during oropharyngeal surgery.

Prevention of rhabdomyolysis in disorders of fatty acid oxidation, especially in carnitine palmitoyl transferase II (CPT2), very long chain acyl-CoA dehydrogensase deficiency (VLCAD), and long chain 3-hydroxyacyl-CoA dehydrogenase deficiency / Mitochondrial trifunctional protein (LCHAD/MTP) deficiencies. This should be achieved by preventing hypoglycemia as described earlier, taking care that the child is not fasted for more than 6 hours. A propofol infusion should be avoided in these children for several reasons. Propofol inhibits the metabolism in mitochondrial myocytes by (1) inhibiting membrane-bound carnitine palmitoyltransferase I thus limiting the influx of lipids by active transport and (2) limiting electron transport in the respiratory chain via coenzyme Q, and cytochrome oxidases II and III, thus reducing available ATP.[74–76]

Positioning and Intubation

In children with lysosomal storage disorders, glycogenoses, and Smith-Lemli-Opitz syndrome, tracheal intubation may prove difficult because of small oropharyngeal space, necessitating a smaller than expected tracheal tube diameter. Instability of the atlantoaxial joint and severe kyphoscoliosis are also major problems in mucopolysaccharidosis (MPS), such as Morquio disease, but also in patients with MPS I, MPS II, and MPS VI; careful positioning is required, avoiding hyperextension or flexion of the neck. Glycosaminoglycans deposits may lead to macroglossia, adenotonsillar hypertrophy, upper/lower airway narrowing, and soft tissue thickening with a reduction in neck range of motion and mouth opening. A nasopharyngeal airway may be useful during induction and awakening. Furthermore, a video laryngoscope and supraglottic airway device have greatly improved the airway management for these children.

Aspiration pneumonia should be anticipated as these children can present with gastroesophageal reflux disease, esophageal dysmotility, and CNS disorders accompanied by oropharyngeal incompetence. Postoperative airway obstruction can occur. Postoperative pulmonary problems may result from failure to clear thick secretions. Recovery from anesthesia may be slow.

Concern exists regarding neurological complications from spinal abnormalities (kyphosis, narrow spinal canal) even when the surgery does not involve the spine. It is useful to employ evoked sensory and the motor potentials in the following clinical situations:

- kyphosis >60 degrees and an estimated surgical duration of >60 minutes
- kyphosis <60 degrees and an estimated surgical duration of >90 minutes

The basal values must be established with the child supine and then in the surgical position. In those in whom the spinal cord may be fragile (e.g., kyphosis, risk of intraoperative hypotension, long-lasting surgery, difficult surgical positioning), neurologic monitoring must be used during the entire anesthetic. The role of epidural anesthesia has been questioned because of difficulties inserting it and out of fear that it might mask spinal cord damage that occurred during the surgery.[77,78]

Coagulopathy

Abnormal liver function can affect the coagulation process. Thrombocytopenia can result from splenic sequestration in case of infiltrative disease or liver disease with subsequent portal hypertension, or in association with alterations in red and white blood cells in case of pancytopenia from bone marrow infiltration. Patients with cystathionine synthase deficiency (classical homocystinuria) are predisposed to the development of both arterial and venous thromboses. Automatic pneumatic compression stockings for deep vein thrombosis prophylaxis, adequate perioperative hydration, delivery of glucose-containing fluids, and low-molecular weight heparin thromboprophylaxis are sensible clinical strategies. The avoidance of nitrous oxide should be considered because it irreversibly oxidizes the cobalt of vitamin B_{12}, which in turn inhibits the cobalamin-dependent enzyme methionine synthase.

Seizures

Substrate deposits in the CNS interfere with neuronal functioning or affect the energy homeostasis of neurons and glia and can precipitate seizures. These patients are typically treated with anticonvulsants.

Neuromuscular Disorders

Neuromuscular disorders are caused by an abnormality of any component of the lower motor neuron system: anterior horn cell in the spinal cord, axon, neuromuscular junction, or muscle fiber (Fig. 22.1).[79] The cardinal features are weakness of skeletal muscles that is proximal, distal, or generalized in distribution, hypotonia, and reduced deep tendon reflexes. True fatigability suggests a defect of the neuromuscular junction. Neuropathy is characterized by distal weakness and sensory deficit. Joint contractures, scoliosis, respiratory, and cardiac involvement are common complications and some conditions are associated with cognitive deficits.

DISORDERS OF THE ANTERIOR HORN CELL

Spinal Muscular Atrophies

Spinal muscular atrophy (SMA) affects approximately 1 in 6000 live births, with a carrier frequency of approximately 1 in 50. Spinal muscular atrophies are a group of disorders in which there is progressive degeneration of the anterior horn cells of the spinal cord and brainstem nuclei, leading to death of motor neurons. The diagnosis of SMA is based on molecular genetic testing. Mutations in the *SMN1* (survival motor neuron 1) gene (5q13.2) account for the main causes of SMA, although an increase in the *SMN2* gene copy number can modify the clinical presentation.[80]

Classification of the SMN1-linked forms by age of onset and maximum function achieved is useful for prognosis and management.[81] Subtypes include:
- Type 0, SMA 0, with prenatal onset and severe joint contractures, facial diplegia, and respiratory failure. Some may have congenital bone fractures.

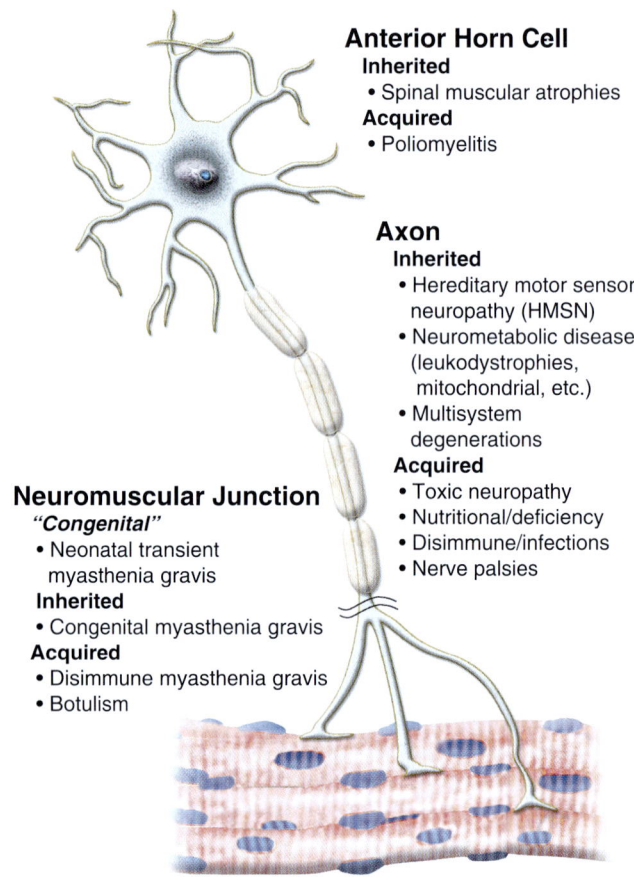

Anterior Horn Cell
Inherited
- Spinal muscular atrophies
Acquired
- Poliomyelitis

Axon
Inherited
- Hereditary motor sensory neuropathy (HMSN)
- Neurometabolic disease (leukodystrophies, mitochondrial, etc.)
- Multisystem degenerations
Acquired
- Toxic neuropathy
- Nutritional/deficiency
- Disimmune/infections
- Nerve palsies

Neuromuscular Junction
"Congenital"
- Neonatal transient myasthenia gravis
Inherited
- Congenital myasthenia gravis
Acquired
- Disimmune myasthenia gravis
- Botulism

Muscle Fiber
Inherited
- Congenital myopathies
- Muscular dystrophies
- Myotonias
- Metabolic myopathies
Acquired
- Disimmune myopathies (dermatomyositis)
- Endocrine myopathies
- Toxic (e.g., drug-induced [steroid])

FIGURE 22.1 Diagram of a lower motor neuron. (Modified from Dubowitz V. *Muscle Disorders in Childhood*. Philadelphia: WB Saunders; 1978. Courtesy A. Moosa, MD.)

- Type 1, SMA 1, with onset before age 6 months (Werdnig-Hoffmann disease). The infant appears neurologically normal at birth but demonstrates an abnormal breathing pattern as the intercostal muscles are affected, and respirations become increasingly diaphragmatic. The infant is usually very alert and interactive but severely weak and floppy. There is good facial expression and normal eye movements, but the tongue fasciculates, and the tendon reflexes are absent. The heart is not involved. Weakness, hypotonia, and bulbar involvement lead to progressive respiratory insufficiency and swallowing dysfunction, which are frequently complicated by episodes of aspiration.
- Type 2, SMA 2, with onset between age 6 and 12 months, is an intermediate form, but is the most prevalent. Because the weakness is milder, many children survive for years with meticulous multidisciplinary therapy, orthopedic and respiratory management, and care with nutrition. The clinical signs are

similar to those of type 1 SMA, and the children are bright, intelligent, and particularly verbal. Patients with type 2 SMA usually achieve independent sitting at some stage, but these children never walk. Respiratory infections are a particular problem, and noninvasive nocturnal respiratory support with a face mask and portable ventilator is well tolerated. This improves well-being and enables remarkably full activity despite weakness.[82,83] Joint contractures are almost inevitable, as is progressive scoliosis, which usually appears early, and are difficult to manage in the very young. Some children with type 2 SMA develop feeding difficulties because of weakness of bulbar musculature or as a complication of chronic nocturnal hypoventilation. Gastrostomy feeding may be required.

- Type 3, SMA 3 (Kugelberg-Welander disease) with onset after 18 months of age, is a mild variant with similar signs of flaccid and areflexic weakness of the lower limbs and with proximal predominance. These children often deteriorate around puberty, when the growth spurt causes the previously precariously balanced muscle groups to become dysfunctional. Obesity and joint contractures also may affect the situation. Aggressive measures to keep the child walking are often effective in delaying or preventing scoliosis and lower limb contractures.[84] Noninvasive respiratory support may be necessary for nocturnal hypoventilation. Prognosis for long-term survival is good.
- Type 4, SMA 4, with adult onset (>18 years) and mild course. This group includes those who can walk as adults, without respiratory and nutritional problems.

More than 20 forms of SMA not caused by SMN1 gene mutations have also been described: they are much rarer, and their distribution can be proximal, distal, or bulbospinal. Gene therapy including intrathecal nusinersen or gene-replacement therapy has stabilized the evolution of SMA 1 and 2 deterioration.[85] Collaborative interdisciplinary treatment improves the duration and quality of life.

Anesthesia Considerations for Spinal Muscular Atrophies

Children with SMA present for surgical and diagnostic procedures, including intrathecal drug administration, gastrostomy placement, tracheostomy, and spinal surgery.[86] In SMA 1 and 2, chronic denervation leads to changes in muscle metabolism with loss of glycogen, secondary carnitine deficiency, and alteration in β-oxidation of fatty acids: increased lipid catabolism should thus be avoided by providing adequate glucose supply.[87] Hypoplasia of the midface caused by chronic noninvasive ventilation with a facemask, temporomandibular joint ankylosis, or a stiff neck after scoliosis surgery can cause intubation difficulties.

Neuromuscular blockade may not be necessary for surgical anesthesia. If a nondepolarizing neuromuscular blocking drug is given, neuromuscular monitoring should be used. Sugammadex is effective antagonizing rocuronium and vecuronium.[88,89] Succinylcholine is contraindicated in these patients. Ultrasound-guided spinal and epidural anesthesia and postoperative epidural analgesia have been used without adverse effects. Postoperative respiratory support should be considered after assessing the child's preoperative respirator status. Repeated intrathecal administration of nusinersen in SMA 1 and 2 improves their evolution. This can be done under sedation or light general anesthesia without intubation, sometimes with CT or ultrasound guidance.

Poliomyelitis

Poliomyelitis is an infectious disease caused by poliovirus, a human enterovirus. Most poliovirus infections are asymptomatic.

If symptomatic, it occurs in two phases: an acute, nonspecific, febrile illness followed by aseptic meningitis and acute, flaccid, lower motor neuron paralysis. It typically manifests asymmetrically and may affect any muscle group. In children with respiratory involvement, lifelong ventilation may be needed. Immunization programs have made this a rare disease in many countries, but it can still be diagnosed in immigrants from economically poor and nonindustrialized countries, transmitted from patients who have received the oral polio vaccine, which contained attenuated live virus, and sporadically in vaccine-resistant enclaves even in industrialized communities[90,91](https://forward.com/opinion/511863/vaccine-hesitancy-haredi-jews-orthodox-hasidic-polio/). The post-poliomyelitis syndrome is not a relapse of the disease; it is caused by the late degeneration of the axonal fibers that proliferate to create giant motor units during the healing phase of acute poliomyelitis. It can present as progressive muscle weakness, dysphagia, chronic pain (both muscular and neuropathic), and sleep disordered breathing problems. The use of regional blockade remains controversial. If nondepolarizing neuromuscular blocking drugs are administered, neuromuscular monitoring should be used.[92]

AXONAL DISORDERS

Hereditary Neuropathies

The hereditary neuropathies are divided into two major subgroups: neuropathies in which the neuropathy is the sole or primary feature and neuropathies in which the neuropathy is part of a more generalized neurologic or multisystem disorder. There are five subgroups in the primary hereditary neuropathies[93]:

- ***Charcot-Marie-Tooth disease*** (CMT) or hereditary motor sensory neuropathy (HMSN): mutations of more than 40 genes result in variable decrease in nerve conduction velocity and myelinization, and peripheral nerves hypertrophy. Neuromuscular monitoring can be difficult.[94] Ultrasound-guided regional blockade is preferred to landmark techniques.
- ***Hereditary neuropathy*** with liability to pressure palsy (HNPP) (tomacular neuropathy): careful positioning is mandatory to avoid paralysis due to nerve compression.[95]
- ***Hereditary sensory and autonomic neuropathy*** (HSAN): this includes congenital insensitivity to pain with or without anhidrosis, and Riley-Day syndrome. The association of absent hemodynamic responses to pain and dysautonomia makes the anesthetic management challenging.[96]
- ***Distal hereditary motor neuropathy*** (dHMN), a distal form of spinal muscular atrophy (see earlier).
- ***Hereditary neuralgic amyotrophy*** (HNA) present with attacks of severe pain and muscle loss (mainly in the region of the brachial plexus) triggered by exercise, surgery, childbirth, or infection.

Neuropathies may also be part of a more widespread neurologic or multisystem disorder:

- ***Familial amyloid polyneuropathy*** (FAP) presents with muscle weakness with neuropathic pain; some patients also present with dysautonomia, a dilated cardiomyopathy and cardiac conduction defects.[97]
- ***Disturbances of lipid metabolism***. In the leukodystrophies (metachromatic and Krabbe disease),[98,99] demyelination affects central and peripheral axons, giving a clinical picture of combined upper and lower neuron feature. In case of adrenoleukodystrophy adrenal insufficiency is often present (see earlier: peroxisomal disorders).[100] Refsum disease is caused by the impaired α-oxidation of branched-chain fatty acids, resulting in buildup of phytanic acid and its derivatives in the plasma and tissues.[101]

Individuals with Refsum disease present with neurologic damage, cerebellar degeneration, and peripheral neuropathy.

Porphyria acute crisis.

Disorders with defective DNA (e.g., ataxia telangiectasia).

Neuropathies associated with hereditary ataxias: risk of aspiration due to bulbar involvement.

In children with mitochondrial diseases, peripheral neuropathy is often found, along with myriad other features (see later in the text).

Clinical presentation depends on the subtype and can occur at any age. Children usually present with disorders of gait or foot deformity, or may come to the attention of a neurologist or geneticist through an affected parent. Clinical signs are usually confined to the lower limbs in the early years and may lead to orthopedic intervention before diagnosis. When the neuropathy is associated with multisystem involvement (cardiac, autonomic, respiratory), a complete preoperative assessment is essential.

Acquired Disorders of the Peripheral Nerves

Acquired disorders of the peripheral nerves are rare in childhood. In clinical practice, neuropathies complicating metabolic or nutritional disorders and treatment for cancer are the most common forms. In underdeveloped parts of the world, nutritional deficiencies, especially of vitamins E, B_1, B_6, B_{12}, niacin, and thiamine, are important contributors. The neuropathic features may be overshadowed by the other characteristics of the disease.

Guillain-Barré Syndrome

Guillain-Barré syndrome (acute inflammatory demyelinating polyneuropathy) is an acute demyelinating disorder that causes progressive weakness.[102] It has an incidence of 1 to 2 per 100,000. The causal mechanism is an immunologic cross-reactivity process secondary to a prodromal illness within the previous 4 weeks, typically an upper respiratory tract infection or gastroenteritis. Implicated organisms include mycoplasma, cytomegalovirus, Epstein-Barr virus, *Campylobacter,* vesicular stomatitis virus, measles, mumps, hepatitis A and B, rubella, influenza A and B, coxsackievirus, and echovirus. Although the precise pathologic process has not been delineated, various antibodies, immune complexes, and complement components have been found, suggesting pathologic heterogeneity. Variants with a similar/related clinical picture include acute motor axonal neuropathy, acute motor and sensory axonal neuropathy with prominent sensory features (poor prognosis), and Miller Fisher syndrome (ophthalmoplegia, ataxia, and areflexia).

The disorder is rare in children younger than 3 years of age. Onset is usually sudden, although subacute presentations have been reported. The first sign is weakness in the lower limbs, which characteristically ascends the body, next affecting the trunk, the upper limbs, and occasionally the cranial nerves. It causes a flaccid paralysis, usually sparing sensory function but causing pain and areflexia at all levels. Autonomic neuropathy may develop, causing instability of blood pressure and cardiac arrhythmias. Involvement of respiratory muscles may produce acute respiratory failure or apnea that necessitates tracheal intubation.

Guillain-Barré syndrome is diagnosed clinically and confirmed by finding an increased protein concentration in the CSF (despite a normal cell count) and abnormalities on nerve conduction studies. MRI of the spine may show thickening and contrast enhancement of the nerve roots and cauda equina.[103]

Pediatric Guillain-Barré is usually a disease of shorter duration and more complete recovery than in adults. Patients with very mild symptoms that do not interfere with activities of daily living can be observed for deterioration without treatment. The natural course is improvement, generally in 2 weeks, but progressive weakness can be seen up to 4 weeks. It seems that the more rapid the onset of the disease, the more rapid its offset. Similarly, the slower the onset, the more prolonged the clinical findings and slower the recovery. One-third of children may have long-term sequelae, although these are usually mild. Supportive care in the intensive care unit may be needed for children with severe bulbar or respiratory weakness. In those children who are nonambulatory or with respiratory failure, IV immunoglobulin with or without plasmapheresis are the current treatment options.[102,104,105] Children with axonal neuropathies usually recover motor function more slowly than those with demyelination; it is believed that early treatment with IV immunoglobulin may speed recovery.[106,107] However, corticosteroids are ineffective and may delay recovery.

Chronic Inflammatory Demyelinating Polyneuropathy

Chronic inflammatory demyelinating polyneuropathy is extremely rare in childhood, and it is usually confined to older age groups. It manifests in a subacute, chronic progressive or relapsing and remitting pattern with prominent sensory involvement. Diagnostic investigations are similar to those for acute Guillain-Barré syndrome. Corticosteroids, IV immunoglobulin, and plasma exchange have been effective.[106] Although these treatments may be effective in the short term, recurrences may take place, and the usual pattern is that of a chronic, disabling, relapsing and remitting condition that does not threaten longevity, but interferes significantly with the quality of life.[107]

Nerve Palsies

Like neuropathies, nerve palsies are uncommon in childhood.[108] The most common palsy encountered in infants and children is neonatal brachial plexus palsy. Infants may present with reduced movement of an arm, reflecting the side of the brachial plexus injury after a difficult delivery involving traction of head and/or shoulders: Erb palsy (injury to C5,6), Klumpke paralysis (injury to C8, T1), or an injury to the whole brachial plexus with a limp arm and an associated clavicular fracture. The obstetric-related injuries may be categorized by the nerve roots involved using the Narakas classification and the severity of the nerve injury using the Seddon classification.[109] Radiologic investigations including MRI, ultrasound, and others are very useful in identifying the level of the injury (e.g., avulsion of the nerve root) and thus the potential role of surgical correction.[109,110] Cranial nerve palsies, especially those that involve the eye muscles, are usually related to intracranial disease such as increased ICP or cerebral tumor in children, but they may also be isolated findings that result from viral infections (e.g., Lyme disease for facial palsy); in the latter instances, recovery is the norm.

Peripheral nerve palsies such as carpal tunnel syndrome have been reported in childhood.[111] They may complicate severe juvenile arthritis[112] or storage disorders such as mucopolysaccharidoses. Because symptoms may be difficult to elicit from children, identifying palsies may be problematic in children with severe learning disabilities.

DISORDERS OF THE NEUROMUSCULAR JUNCTION
Myasthenia Gravis
Myasthenia gravis is a disorder of the neuromuscular junction that includes heterogeneous autoimmune diseases, with a postsynaptic

TABLE 22.8	Classification of Myasthenia Gravis

Based on serum antibody specificity:
1. Acetylcholine receptor (AChR) antibody–positive
2. Muscle-specific tyrosine kinase (MuSK) receptor antibody–positive
3. Low-density lipoprotein receptor–related protein 4 (LRP4) antibody–positive
4. Antibody-negative

Based on thymus histopathology:
1. Thymitis
2. Thymoma
3. Atrophy

Based on degree of involvement:
1. Only eyes: ocular myasthenia
2. Full body: generalized myasthenia
3. Mainly swallowing, speech: bulbar myasthenia

defect of neuromuscular transmission as the common feature. Weakness results from antibodies that block various receptors, inhibiting the excitatory effects of acetylcholine at the neuromuscular junction. This defective transmission at the junction results in a characteristic pattern of progressively reduced muscle strength with repeated use and recovery of muscle strength after a period of rest. Myasthenia gravis can be classified according to Table 22.8.

Juvenile myasthenia gravis is the pediatric form of the disease. It is also an autoimmune disease, with the production of antibodies against the acetylcholine receptor and sometimes other proteins as mentioned in Table 22.8. Management is similar to that for adult myasthenia gravis. Symptomatic treatment of myasthenia gravis with cholinesterase inhibition (e.g., pyridostigmine) is usually combined with immunosuppression. Azathioprine remains the first choice for immunosuppressive therapy, usually along with steroids.[113] Alternative immunosuppressive options include cyclosporin, cyclophosphamide, methotrexate, mycophenolate mofetil, and tacrolimus. Rituximab is a promising new drug for severe generalized myasthenia gravis. Emerging therapy options include monoclonal antibodies (e.g., belimumab, eculizumab)[114] and the granulocyte macrophage colony-stimulating factor. For decades, thymectomy has been performed in younger adults to improve nonparaneoplastic myasthenia gravis.[115] With optimal treatment, the prognosis is good in terms of daily functions, quality of life, and survival.[116]

Neonatal Transient Myasthenia Gravis

Neonatal myasthenia gravis is caused by placental transfer of antibodies to acetylcholine receptors from an affected or previously affected mother. The neonate may present with feeding difficulties or respiratory dysfunction. Treatment, which involves anticholinesterases, must be tailored to the severity of the weakness, and intensive support occasionally is required. Spontaneous recovery occurs 3 to 6 weeks following birth. It should be anticipated in the offspring of any woman who has active myasthenia gravis or a history of the disorder, because cases have been described even in neonates of mothers in remission.[117]

Congenital Myasthenic Syndromes

Congenital myasthenic syndromes (CMS) form a heterogeneous group of genetic diseases characterized by a dysfunction of neuromuscular transmission that usually becomes symptomatic during childhood; this causes muscle weakness that increases with exertion. The prevalence of congenital myasthenic syndromes is

estimated at 1 in 500,000 in Europe and is less common than autoimmune myasthenia. The classification of congenital myasthenic syndromes is based on where the defect occurs in the neuromuscular synapse: presynaptic, synaptic, and postsynaptic. Mutations of at least 34 genes can cause congenital myasthenic syndromes.[118] Clinical signs consist of ophthalmoplegia and ptosis, dysphonia and swallowing disturbance, facial paresis, muscle fatigability, and recurrent apneas. The occurrence of such clinical events, worsened by exertion, is characteristic of the disease. Acute respiratory failure may occur, triggered by infectious episodes, and is frequent in the first months of life. In the absence of respiratory assistance, the risk of death is high. The favorable effect of cholinesterase inhibitors is a significant argument in favor of a myasthenic syndrome. However, presynaptic mutations, slow channel syndrome, and acetylcholinesterase deficiency are actually worsened by cholinesterase inhibitors: ephedrine, salbutamol, or 3,4 diaminopyridine are used to treat these mutations.[118]

Although rare, congenital myasthenic syndromes should be considered in the differential diagnosis of any neonate or infant who presents with motor problems (e.g., weakness, hypotonia, fatigability), eye signs (e.g., ptosis, ophthalmoplegia, pupillary abnormalities), and respiratory insufficiency (e.g., recurrent apneas, ventilator dependence). Late-onset muscle weakness has been reported in adolescence or early adulthood. Diagnosis may be difficult because the classic features of myasthenia, including responses to anticholinesterase medications, may be absent. A Tensilon test, electromyography with repetitive nerve stimulation, a muscle biopsy, and molecular analysis in a specialist center should be sought to confirm the diagnosis.

Anesthesia Considerations for Myasthenia Gravis

The anesthesiologist may become involved in the management of children with myasthenia gravis for several reasons[119]:

- respiratory failure requiring tracheal intubation and mechanical ventilation
- need for central venous access to facilitate plasma exchange transfusion
- thymectomy
- elective or emergency surgery unrelated to myasthenia

The severity of the muscle weakness and the muscle groups affected by the disease should be documented, focusing on respiratory and bulbar function. Decreased density of acetylcholine receptors at the motor end plate means that children with myasthenia may require up to four times the calculated dose of succinylcholine to establish a depolarizing muscle block. Because succinylcholine is metabolized by acetylcholinesterase, its metabolism is reduced, and duration of action is prolonged in the setting of chronic acetylcholinesterase inhibition. For this reason, succinylcholine is best avoided. The activity and duration of effect of nondepolarizing neuromuscular blocking drugs is increased: their dosage should thus be titrated according to the patient's response as assessed by quantitative neuromuscular monitoring. If rocuronium or vecuronium have been administered, sugammadex can be used safely in myasthenic patients.[120]

Inhalational anesthetic agents decrease neuromuscular transmission, and these effects may be exaggerated in children with myasthenia gravis.[121] However, no clinically significant postoperative neuromuscular depression has been demonstrated with isoflurane, sevoflurane, or desflurane. These potential neuromuscular effects are not shared by propofol, making total intravenous anesthesia (TIVA) a useful option in these children. For all but the most minor surgery in the patient with stable myasthenia gravis without respiratory or bulbar compromise, a tracheal tube and intermittent positive-pressure ventilation are likely required. If possible, the trachea should be intubated without the use of neuromuscular blocking drugs. Tracheal intubation with inhalational anesthetics alone or propofol with a short-acting opioid has been described in these children.[122]

Myasthenia-Like Syndrome

The toxin of *Clostridium botulinum* produces a myasthenia-like syndrome that may occur through two mechanisms: ingestion of food contaminated by *C. botulinum* toxin (e.g., contaminated honey) and wound infection by *C. botulinum*. Features include blurring of vision with ptosis, dilated and unresponsive pupils, cranial nerve palsies, limb paralysis with areflexia, feeding difficulty, and respiratory insufficiency. Diagnosis depends on clinical suspicion, identification of the toxin in residual food, and electromyography. Treatment is supportive, and recovery may take weeks to months.[39] Succinylcholine is contraindicated in children with infections that affect the neuromuscular junction, including botulism and tetanus.[123,124]

DISORDERS OF MUSCLE FIBERS

Myopathies

Congenital Myopathies

Congenital myopathies (CM) are disorders that have many variations in the type and severity of features.[125] There can be clinical overlap between congenital myopathies and other neuromuscular disorders, including the congenital muscular dystrophies, myotonic dystrophy, congenital myasthenic syndromes, metabolic myopathies including Pompe disease, and spinal muscular atrophy. All these disorders can present in the neonate with marked weakness and/or hypotonia ("floppy infant"): prominent facial weakness ("carp-shaped mouth") with or without ptosis, generalized hypotonic ("frog-leg") posture with hyporeflexia, and weakness of the respiratory and bulbar muscles. The severity of weakness and disability varies widely, ranging from profound generalized weakness in neonates to patients with more subtle weakness.

Congenital myopathies may also present during childhood with signs of delayed motor milestones, or even later in life with symptoms of proximal weakness. Reduced muscle bulk is usually observed. Usually, the diagnosis is confirmed by characteristic findings on muscle biopsy (Table 22.9). Genetic diagnosis is

TABLE 22.9 | Congenital Myopathies

PATHOLOGIC FINDINGS AND GENOTYPES	
Disorder	**Genetics**
Core myopathies (including central core disease and multi-minicore disease)	*RYR1, SELENON, ACTA1, TTN, MYH7, KBTBD13, FXR1, CFL2, TNNT1*
Centronuclear myopathies	*MTM1, RYR1, DNM2, BIN1, SPEG, ZAK, CCDC78*
Nemaline myopathy (including cap disease, zebra body myopathy and core-rod myopathy since these appear to be pathologic variants of nemaline myopathy)	*ACTA1, NEB, TPM2, TPM3, TNNT1, CFL2, LMOD3, MYPN, KBTBD1, KLHL40, KLHL41*
Myosin storage myopathy (also known as hyaline body myopathy)	*MYH7*
Congenital fiber–type disproportion	*ACTA1, TPM3, RYR1, MYH7, MYL2, ZAK, SELENON*

now available for many of these as different mutations on the same gene can produce a different phenotype as illustrated in Table 22.9.[126] Support of respiration and nutrition may be necessary: for example, noninvasive nocturnal ventilation by face mask may help management at home. Regular passive movements and careful management of posture and positioning to prevent contractures, especially scoliosis, is essential. Meticulous care of skin, joints, bowels, and teeth help to avoid the need for more invasive management. A complete evaluation of cardiovascular and respiratory status is required before anesthesia and surgery.[127,128]

Malignant hyperthermia (MH) is a pharmacogenetic disorder of the skeletal muscle caused by mutations in the *RYR1, SCN4*, or *STAC3* gene that manifests in response to anesthetic triggering agents (succinylcholine, halogenated agents). This disorder is full reviewed in Chapter 39. Although most patients susceptible to malignant hyperthermia do not present with clinical signs of muscle involvement, core myopathies (central core disease and multi-minicore disease) caused by a *RYR1* mutation are associated with malignant hyperthermia.[129] Malignant hyperthermia and RYR1-associated myopathies are primarily disorders of calcium regulation in skeletal muscle.[130] The RYR1 gene encodes the channel that controls calcium release from the sarcoplasmic reticulum in the skeletal muscle. RYR1 abnormalities alter the channel kinetics for calcium inactivation, and calcium buildup causes excessive skeletal muscle contraction, leading to anaerobic metabolism and acidosis. Early manifestations of malignant hyperthermia include hypercarbia, tachypnea, and tachycardia. Late signs and symptoms include fever, sympathetic nervous system activation, hyperkalemia, muscle rigidity, disseminated intravascular coagulation, myoglobinuria, and multiorgan dysfunction and failure if not treated early with dantrolene and supportive measures.

The in vitro contracture test (IVCT) has been developed to confirm susceptibility to malignant hyperthermia by studying the contracture of muscle fibers in response to triggers such as caffeine and halothane. This is an invasive investigation because an open muscle biopsy is required, and only a few specialized centers perform this procedure; it is generally not performed in children younger than 10 years of age because of the size of the muscle biopsy required. However, DNA analysis can provide a fairly reliable test for susceptibility to malignant hyperthermia in family members of a patient with a positive contracture test.[129] The complexity of the situation is such that assessment and advice by a specialist is recommended so that the child and family may benefit from appropriate investigation and interpretation.[131,132] Any individual with core myopathy or any other myopathy possibly caused by a RYR1 mutation, and their family, should be informed about the clinical situation, diagnosis, and possible risks and complications, including malignant hyperthermia, and should be offered a specialized investigation. An individual who may be susceptible to malignant hyperthermia should carry information (e.g., a medical alert bracelet) to inform medical staff in an emergency.[133] Any elective operative procedure must be meticulously planned with the anesthesiologist. The clinical presentation of congenital myopathies varies and their genetic cause is often undetermined at the time of anesthesia; it is therefore safer to consider all these patients as at risk for malignant hyperthermia unless a RYR1 mutation has been excluded.[130]

Metabolic Myopathies

Metabolic myopathies (Table 22.10) are uncommon and complex. Most affected children have multisystem involvement that could mask the myopathic features. The most important concerns

TABLE 22.10 | Metabolic Myopathies

Disorders of purine nucleotide cycle: myoadenylate deaminase deficiency

Mitochondrial myopathies: see Table 22.11

Glycogen storage disorders:
- muscle phosphorylase deficiency (glycogen storage disease [GSD] type V: McArdle disease)
- lysosomal acid maltase disease (GSD type II: Pompe disease)

Disorders of fatty acid oxidation: carnitine palmitoyl transferase II or VCLAD deficiency

for the anesthesiologist are the risk of metabolic instability during surgery (see above: Catabolism section of inborn errors of metabolism): close liaison with the child's pediatrician is needed to plan fluid and electrolyte balance and nutritional management.[133,134]

Mitochondrial Disorders Underlying Myopathies

Mitochondrial disorders comprise the diseases that cause primary or secondary impairment of the production of adenosine triphosphate (ATP). The defective proteins are subunits of the respiratory chain complex, components of the final pathways of substrate breakdown such as the pyruvate dehydrogenase complex and the Krebs cycle, or various other components of mitochondrial homeostasis. They are a common cause of inherited neurologic disease in children, occurring in 1 of 5000 live births. They are caused by mutations in mitochondrial or nuclear DNA. The respiratory chain proteins are under bigenomic control: nuclear DNA codes for 85% and mitochondrial DNA for 15%. Nuclear DNA is inherited along Mendelian inheritance patterns, whereas mitochondrial DNA follows a maternal inheritance pattern. They manifest with symptoms of energy deficiency and a highly variable pattern of organ dysfunctions depending on the need for energy (concept of threshold) and the distribution of the mutated mitochondria (heteroplasmy) in the tissues. The brain, nerves, and muscles can be involved in isolation or in combination. In many cases, lactic acidemia and progressive neurodegenerative disease are present. Periods of metabolic stress such as an intercurrent infection or prolonged fasting may trigger a deterioration in the child's condition.

Neurologic symptoms and signs are varied and include myopathy, neuropathy, stroke-like episodes, ataxia, dementia, epilepsy, migraine, sensorineural deafness, and pigmentary retinopathy. The more common clinical scenarios in childhood are outlined in Table 22.11. Involvement of other organ systems,

such as diabetes mellitus, gastrointestinal disease, renal tubulopathy, and cardiomyopathy, may coexist or dominate the clinical picture.[135]

Assessment of the child with atypical and otherwise unexplained features should include a search for evidence of mitochondrial abnormalities. The diagnostic workup may be difficult. Recently, exome sequencing has emerged as the primary diagnostic approach.[136] The clinical details determine the investigative plan, which should include cerebral imaging with MRI and MR spectroscopy (to detect lactate peaks), blood biochemistry (i.e., creatine kinase, lactate, and glucose levels), tests of urinary amino and organic acids, cardiologic assessment (i.e., chest radiography, electrocardiogram, and echocardiogram), electroencephalography, and exercise testing and neurophysiology, leading to mitochondrial studies of muscle tissue.[135,137] Muscle biopsy investigations include histopathology (ragged red fibers), electron microscopy, respiratory chain enzymology, and molecular analysis of mitochondrial DNA. Further investigation with respiratory chain enzymes and molecular genetic analysis is indicated in some cases.

Treatment of mitochondrial disorders includes management of specific features such as antiepileptic therapy and efforts to maintain stability of metabolic pathways.[138] Vitamins and other supplements such as coenzyme Q_{10} (i.e., ubiquinone), riboflavin, thiamine, and carnitine are referred to as the *mitochondrial cocktail* used to treat most mitochondrial disorders,[139] based on the assumption that high doses of these agents may increase the energy output by mitochondria.[140]

Anesthesia Considerations for Mitochondrial Myopathies

The challenge for the anesthesiologist is to maintain metabolic stability. The main problems include respiratory failure (often associated with decreased sensitivity to hypoxemia and hypercarbia), cardiomyopathy, cardiac conduction defects, and dysphagia.[141] The preoperative fasting period should be kept to a minimum to avoid hypoglycemia and hypovolemia. Stresses that may provoke increased energy requirements, such as perioperative pain, hypothermia, or hyperthermia, must be minimized. The anesthetic implications of mitochondrial diseases are summarized in Table 22.12.

Inhalational and IV anesthesia have been used successfully in many children with mitochondrial disorders, although several cases of untoward perioperative complications have been reported.[142–145] However, the relationships between specific anesthetics and serious adverse effects remain tenuous. Retrospective

TABLE 22.11 | Mitochondrial Syndromes in Childhood

Syndrome	Features
Alpers-Huttenlocher, neuronal degeneration	Brisk onset of epilepsy, paralysis, ataxia, dementia, visual impairment, liver disease; death usually in months
Leigh encephalomyeloneuropathy	Brainstem signs predominant; relapsing/remitting or steadily progressive to death
Infantile myopathy and lactic acidosis	Hypotonia in infancy, feeding difficulties, respiratory problems, cardiomyopathy; fatal and nonfatal forms
Leber hereditary optic neuropathy (LHON)	Progressive visual loss in childhood, cardiac arrhythmias, dystonia
Kearns-Sayre (KSS)	Progressive external ophthalmoplegia, pigmentary retinopathy, deafness, heart block, choreoathetosis and ataxia, myopathy, endocrine disorders
NARP	Neuropathy, ataxia, retinitis pigmentosa
MELAS	Mitochondrial encephalomyopathy, lactic acidosis, stroke-like episodes, dementia
MERFF	Myoclonic epilepsy, myopathy with ragged red fibers, ataxia
MNGIE	Myoneurogenic gastrointestinal encephalopathy

TABLE 22.12	Perianesthetic Considerations in Patients With a Mitochondrial Disease
Preanesthetic Assessment	Neurologic: seizures?, spasticity?, amyotrophy?, contractures? Cardiac: ECG (conduction), echocardiography, pacemaker? Metabolic: liver enzymes, urea and creatinine, thyroid function Baseline blood lactates level Swallowing problems? gastroesophageal reflux? central or obstructive apnea? Current treatment: anticonvulsants, carnitine, ketogenic diet? Elective procedures should be best avoided in case of fever (risk of postoperative neurological deterioration?)
Anesthesia	Short fasting time or glucose 5% solution with electrolytes as soon as fasting starts (except in case of ketogenic diet) Usual dose of carnitine and anticonvulsants in the morning Induction: either IV (single bolus dose of propofol dose allowed except in case of current metabolic crisis) or inhalational (sevoflurane) using spectral EEG monitoring to avoid overdosing is recommended Total intravenous anesthesia with propofol is best avoided: possible increased risk of PRIS IV fluids: glucose 5% (or more according to glycemia) with electrolytes (avoid lactates) *except in case of ketogenic diet* Monitoring: glycemia and blood lactates Avoid hyper- and hypoventilation Avoid hyper- and hypothermia Avoid succinylcholine especially in the presence of any muscle involvement; if a nondepolarizing muscle relaxant is used, neuromuscular monitoring is mandatory Opiates: remifentanil could be a safe option Regional block: 1) neuraxial: Okay except in the presence of demyelination; could be difficult in case of scoliosis 2) peripheral: Okay except in the presence of axonal neuropathy
PACU and Postoperative Care	Risk of decreased response to hypoxemia and or hypercarbia Monitor: glycemia, blood lactates Central hyperthermia is possible (24–48 hours)

PACU, Postanesthesia care unit; *PRIS*, propofol infusion syndrome.

reviews of perioperative complications in children with known mitochondrial myopathies reported no complications after general anesthesia.[134,142,146] However, mitochondrial diseases represent a wide variety of molecular defects and thus a wide range of different diseases with similar phenotypes. It is likely that some types of defects, e.g., complex I deficiency, are more sensitive to inhibition by anesthetics than others, and therefore possibly more prone to untoward effects.[141,147] Moreover, although a mitochondrial disease is not associated per se with an increased risk of malignant hyperthermia, two cases of mitochondrial disease in malignant hyperthermia–susceptible patients have been reported.[148]

In vitro, all general anesthetics, except opioids, depress mitochondrial function at several levels.[141] Knowing that propofol interferes with the respiratory chain and fatty acid metabolism in mitochondria, it has been postulated that children who develop metabolic acidosis and myocardial failure after a propofol infusion for extended periods (>5 mg/kg per hour for more than 48 hours; known as propofol infusion syndrome [PRIS]) have a subclinical form of a mitochondrial disorder.[149] However, this is still speculative. The use of propofol for induction of anesthesia or for very brief procedures in children with mitochondrial myopathies is reasonable,[150] although children with mitochondrial myopathies who are treated with a ketogenic diet may be susceptible to lipid overload with propofol.[151] Sensitivity and resistance to nondepolarizing neuromuscular blocking drugs have been reported in children with these myopathies. To ensure appropriate dosing, neuromuscular blocking drugs should be titrated judiciously using neuromuscular monitoring. In addition to standard monitoring, blood glucose and lactates should be closely monitored in children with mitochondrial myopathies.

Muscular Dystrophies

These dystrophies represent a group of more than 30 inherited disorders of muscle that may appear in infancy, childhood, or adulthood (Table 22.13). The word *dystrophy* implies a destructive progressive process: one still distinguishes congenital muscular dystrophies (e.g., Ullrich muscular disease) and progressive muscular dystrophies (e.g., Duchenne muscular dystrophy [DMD]) according to their characteristic clinical course, although the classification could be adapted due to progress in genetics and molecular biology.[152]

The characteristic clinical features of muscular dystrophy include muscle weakness, the distribution of which varies from type to type, contractures, sluggish deep tendon reflexes, and involvement of respiratory muscles and the myocardium. Other features often coexist, including learning disabilities, deafness, and ophthalmologic disorders. The serum creatine kinase level may be normal or increased. Diagnosis rests on careful clinical assessment, creatine kinase level, molecular analysis, and muscle biopsy. Although there is no specific curative treatment for these disorders, advances in understanding the molecular genetic defect and the proteins responsible for the disease have focused the search for an effective pharmacologic treatment to reverse the clinical signs and symptoms.

Myotonic Dystrophy

Myotonic dystrophy is the most common inherited neuromuscular disorder in the general population, and many cases probably remain undiagnosed. The two forms of myotonic dystrophy are autosomal dominant.[153] DM1, the most common, is caused by the untranslated trinucleotide CTG that repeats in the *DMPK* gene (19q13). This CTG expansion varies from 80 to over 4000 repeats in DM1 patients, but there are usually no clinical signs in individuals with only 50 to 100 repeats of CTG. There is a mild correlation between repeat size and age of onset of DM1 when the number of repeats is <400. DM1 tends to become more severe in subsequent generations, a phenomenon called anticipation, which is commonly observed following maternal transmission. Three

TABLE 22.13 | Muscular Dystrophies

Disorder	Genetics
Myotonic dystrophy	
DM1 (98%), autosomal dominant (dystrophia myotonica, Steinert disease)	9q13.3, *DMPK* or *DM1*
DM2 (2%), autosomal dominant	3q21, *CNBP* (formerly *ZNF9*)
Other myotonic disorders	
Schwartz-Jampel (chondrodysplastic myotonia)	1p36.12, *HSPG2*, perlecan
Rippling muscle disease	3p25, *CAV3*, caveolin 3
Brody disease	16p12, *ATP2A1*
Isaacs syndrome (neuromyotonia)	12p13, *KCNA1*
Congenital Muscular Dystrophies	
Dystroglycanopathies	
Fukuyama type (also LGMDR13)	9q31.2, *FKTN*, fukutin
Muscle-Eye-Brain	1p34, *POMGNT1*; 19q13.32, *FKRP*; 14q24.3, *POMT2*; 3p27.31, *GMPPB*
Walker-Warburg (HARD[E], lissencephaly type 2) (also LGMDR11)	9q34.1, *POMT1*; 14q24.3, *POMT2*; 9p31.2, *FKTN*; 19q13.32, *FKRP*; 1p34.1, *POMGNT1*; 7p21.2, *ISPD*; 3p22.1, *POMGNT2*; 11q13.2, *B4GAT1*
Merosin-negative (MDC1A)	6q22-q23, *LAMA2*, laminin α2
Merosin-positive Collagen 6 related myopathies (Ullrich, Bethlem)	21q22.3, *COL6A1*, *COL6A2* 2q37, *COL6A3*
Progressive muscular dystrophies (Dystrophinopathies)	
Duchenne and Becker types	Xp21.2, *DMD*, dystrophin

Disorder	Genetics
Emery-Dreifuss muscular dystrophy	
X-linked recessive	Xq28, *EMD*, emerin; Xq27.2, *FHL1*
Autosomal recessive	1q21.2, *LMNA*, lamin A/C
Autosomal dominant	6q25.2, *SYNE1*, nesprine1; 14q23.2, *SYNE2*, nesprine 2; 3p25.1, *THEM43*, luma
Limb girdle muscular dystrophies	
Autosomal recessive (LGMDR) (90%)	>30 currently characterized. Most common: LGMDR1(25%): 15q15.1, *CAPN3*, calpain 3; LGMDR2: 2p13.2, *DYSF*, dysferlin; LGMDR 3-6: the sarcoglycanopathies
Autosomal dominant (LGMDD) (10%)	10 currently characterized
Facioscapulohumeral muscular dystrophy	
Autosomal dominant	FSHD1, *DUX4*, 4q35, FSHD2, *SMCHD1*, 18p11
Distal myopathies	5q31.2, *MATR3*, matrin 3
Oculopharyngeal	14q11.2, *PABPN1* (formerly *PABP2*)
Ion channel muscle diseases	
Na channel	17q23.3, *SCNA4*
Cl channel	7q35, *CLCN1*
K channel	1q23.2, *ATP1A2* 11p13.4, *KCNE3*
Ca channel	1q31-q32, *CACN1AS*

Data from Benarroch L, Bonne G, Rivier F, Hamroun D. The 2020 version of the gene table of neuromuscular disorders (nuclear genome). *Neuromuscul Disord.* 2019;29(12):980-1018. https://www.musclegenetable.fr.

distinct phenotypes are described according to age of onset, group of symptoms, and number of repeats:

- Congenital DM1: severely hypotonic and nearly immobile neonate; a clinical picture of *arthrogryposis congenital multiplex* caused by intrauterine immobility can be observed; equinovarus talipes; feeding difficulties and aspiration pneumonia; respiration failure.
- Childhood-onset DM1: normal or only moderately delayed motor development; weakness of facial and neck muscles; speech and learning difficulties because of some mental handicap; myotonia appears after 3 to 5 years of age[154]; cardiac problems (arrhythmias, cardiomyopathy) usually appear during the second decade.
- Adult-onset DM1: muscle weakness, difficulty walking, bilateral cataracts, arrhythmias, myotonia (difficulty in releasing handgrip), problems when swallowing or talking, bifacial weakness with mild ptosis and progressive wasting of the muscles of the temporal fossae and cheeks. Mild diabetes mellitus. Cardiac involvement is always present: progressive deterioration of atrioventricular and intraventricular conduction and/or dilated cardiomyopathy with cardiac failure. As there is an increased risk of sudden cardiac death, a pacemaker is sometimes inserted prophylactically.

- DM2: becomes symptomatic in adulthood; it is caused by an untranslated CCTG repeat in the *CNBP* gene (3q21) and results in the dysregulation of the expression of 530 genes (181 are identical to DM1). The muscular and systemic involvement in DM2 is usually less severe than in DM1.

Children with DM1 are at increased risk for respiratory complications of anesthesia.[155,156] Their preoperative evaluation should include ECG and echocardiography. They often present with central and obstructive sleep apnea and demonstrate a decreased response to hypercarbia as well as an increased sensitivity to opioids. The dose of sedative medications and neuromuscular blocking agents should be titrated judiciously. The administration of succinylcholine and contact with a cold surface should be avoided as they can induce a myotonic crisis. Sugammadex should be used instead of neostigmine to reverse a nondepolarizing muscular block.[157] Maximal use of regional nerve blocks or local infiltration with local anesthetic agents should be used whenever possible to minimize the need for opioids. Prolonged stay in postanesthesia care unit or high-dependency unit is recommended.

Rare conditions such as ion channel muscle diseases, Brody disease, Schwartz-Jampel syndrome, Isaacs syndrome, or Rippling muscles disease may present with features resembling myotonic dystrophy (see Table 22.13). Although they have different pathophysiology, it is safer to avoid succinylcholine and to monitor neuromuscular blockade after a nondepolarizing agent.[158,159]

Dystrophinopathies

The next most commonly encountered dystrophies are the dystrophinopathies. Duchenne muscular dystrophy (DMD) is the more severe phenotype, and Becker muscular dystrophy (BMD) is the milder phenotype with a later age of onset (adolescence). Both dystrophies are the result of mutations in the dystrophin gene (*DMD*, locus Xp21.2). They are inherited in an X-linked recessive pattern and affect boys almost exclusively, but among female carriers of a mutation, 2.5% present muscular signs and 70% show signs of cardiac involvement.[160] These disorders are caused by a deficiency of dystrophin (i.e., less than 3% of the normal content in DMD), a muscle membrane protein essential to the skeletal and cardiac muscle cytoskeleton and to neural tissue. Dystrophin reinforces the inner strength of the myocyte during lateral stretching and is involved in signal transduction (Fig. 22.2).

Affected children experience a progressive deterioration in muscle strength between the ages of 3 and 5 years that continues to progress until adolescence, at which time a wheelchair is usually required. Respiratory, orthopedic, and cardiac complications emerge with increasing age. From 10 years of age, however, primary focus shifts from deteriorating skeletal muscle to cardiac muscle. Aa a result, annual or biannual echocardiograms are recommended to assess cardiac function, specifically to diagnose a dilated cardiomyopathy. Respiratory surveillance includes sleep studies and early morning blood gas analysis to detect nocturnal hypoventilation early. As the lack of dystrophin also affects the integrity of neural tissue, progressive cognitive dysfunction may occur. Muscle damage is caused by tearing from normal stretching, increased intracellular calcium concentrations (secondary dysfunction of the ryanodine receptor) and an inflammatory reaction progressively replacing muscle with fatty tissue. Without intervention, Duchenne muscular dystrophy is usually fatal by a mean age of 20 years. With improvements in care, some patients are now surviving into the third decade. Death is usually the result of underlying respiratory or cardiac failure. Care is best provided in a multidisciplinary setting in which the individual and family can collaborate with specialists about the required multisystem management of Duchenne muscular dystrophy.

Glucocorticoids are used in the management of Duchenne muscular dystrophy; these agents slow the decline in muscle strength and function in the short term (up to 2 years), which reduces the risk of scoliosis and stabilizes pulmonary function.[161] Prednisone or deflazacort are commonly used. International guidelines outlined by the DMD Care Considerations Working Group[162,163] have established uniformity of care. Children who receive glucocorticoids should be monitored regularly to prevent secondary complications from the steroids: obesity, systemic hypertension, osteoporosis, mood changes, cataracts. Cardiac function may improve with the use of beta blockers and or angiotensin converting enzyme inhibitors. In case of nonsense mutations, oral ataluren may increase the synthesis of dystrophin. Gene therapy trials are underway.

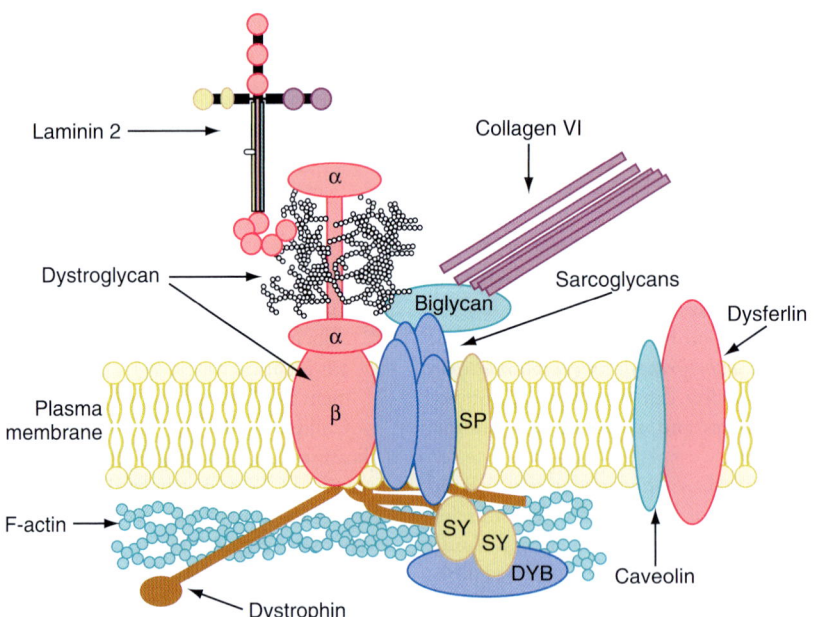

FIGURE 22.2 Schematic diagram of the proteins associated with dystrophin in skeletal muscle cells. The three key elements of the membrane skeleton and signal transduction path are laminin 2, which is the extracellular component; dystrophin-associated protein complex (DAPC) with its α- and β-dystroglycan, sarcoglycan, and cytoplasmic subunits, which is the transmembrane component; and dystrophin, which is the intracellular component. The cytoplasmic subunit of the DAPC consists of syntrophin *(SY)* and dystrobrevin *(DYB)*. Sarcospan *(SP)* has four transmembrane-spanning helixes, and its expression is lost in patients with Duchenne muscular dystrophy. Dystrophin is the pivotal element that reinforces the muscle cell cytoskeleton, and it mediates signal transduction across cell membranes through its interactions with syntrophin, dystrobrevin, and neuronal nitric oxide synthase. Notice that the noncontractile F-actin binds to the N terminus of dystrophin. (From Goodwin FC, Muntoni F. Cardiac involvement in muscular dystrophies: molecular mechanisms. *Muscle Nerve.* 2005;32:577-588.)

If lower limb contractures develop despite range-of-motion exercises and splinting, surgery can be considered to enable rehabilitation in long leg orthoses so that the ambulatory phase may be prolonged.[164] This is indicated for children between 8 and 12 years of age, and it is well tolerated and successful if supported by a specialist team.

Children who are not treated with glucocorticoids are at risk of developing progressive scoliosis.[165,166] Although glucocorticoids can reduce the risk of scoliosis, the risk of vertebral fracture is increased.[167,168] Spinal care should involve an experienced spinal surgeon and consists of scoliosis monitoring, support of spinal and pelvic symmetry, and spinal extension by the wheelchair seating system. Corrective spinal surgery improves posture and seating options, prevents pain from vertebral fracture (osteoporosis), and slows the rate of respiratory decline. The procedure is fraught with difficulty due to blood loss, postoperative respiratory weakness, and possible cardiac dysfunction. Careful multidisciplinary preparation is essential to reduce complications[169]; a plan for postoperative management, including the possibility of tracheostomy, should be made (see Chapter 30).[133]

Boys with undiagnosed Duchenne muscular dystrophy or Becker muscular dystrophy who are anesthetized with inhalational agents or given succinylcholine have developed acute rhabdomyolysis, hyperkalemia, and cardiac arrest.[170] To minimize the risk, clinicians should question family members during the preoperative evaluation about any history of muscle disease, mild signs of hypotonia (Gower sign), and motor weakness and delayed motor milestones. However, at least 30% of children present with de novo mutations. A brief developmental and neuromuscular history should be obtained, and if there is any question or suspicion, it is reasonable to measure a serum creatine kinase level preoperatively. It is for this reason that the routine use of succinylcholine is contraindicated and that its use in children should be reserved for those requiring emergency intubation, a full stomach, or to treat laryngospasm. Facioscapulohumeral dystrophy (FSHD) is less often encountered in childhood, and specific surgical and anesthesia issues are limited. There are several phenotypes in childhood, including a severe neonatal form and a variably progressive childhood type that may be associated with sensorineural deafness. These children may benefit from surgery to fix the scapulae, which improves functionality of the upper limbs.[171,172]

Limb girdle syndromes (LGMD) (no longer a single entity; see Table 22.13) occur infrequently. Some have cardiac and respiratory implications similar to Duchenne muscular dystrophy and require careful preoperative assessment. In Emery-Dreifuss muscular dystrophy (EDMD) cardiac conduction defects and dysrhythmias are very common, and syncope is usually the presenting complaint.[133] A preoperative cardiac workup is essential before general anesthesia; some patients may have a cardiac pacemaker or automated defibrillator.

Congenital Muscular Dystrophies

Congenital muscular dystrophy (CMD) comprises a group of muscular dystrophies that become apparent at an early age. They are slowly progressive or static, and can be associated with learning difficulties. The two most common forms of congenital muscular dystrophy are Ullrich congenital muscular dystrophy (owing to defective collagen VI) (50%) and merosin-deficient CMD (CMD 1A) (25%). These children have normal intellectual function. In contrast, congenital muscular dystrophies that are caused by a defect in the glycosylation of α-dystroglycan that produce an abnormal basal lamina formation in the brain and muscle can impair intellectual development. There is varying severity of disorganization of the cortical lamination, muscular dystrophy, and eye problems depending on the genetic defect. Examples of these are Fukuyama CMD (caused by fukutin defect), muscle-eye-brain disease (caused by a protein O-mannosyltransferase 1 [POMGnT1] defect), and Walker-Warburg syndrome (due to POMT1). Diagnosis is made from the clinical picture, creatinine kinase levels, muscle biopsy, presence or absence of cortical abnormalities, and finally, by genetic testing. Medical care for patients with CMD remains diverse and is outlined in a Consensus Statement on Standard of Care for Congenital Muscular Dystrophies.[173]

Anesthesia Considerations for Muscular Dystrophies

The anesthesia implications for muscular dystrophies are dictated by the age of the child and severity of the disease. All children with a known or suspected muscular dystrophy should have a preoperative ECG and echocardiogram to assess their cardiac function. They should also be evaluated for obstructive sleep apnea. Some are at risk for a difficult airway because of macroglossia (Duchenne muscular dystrophy), temporomandibular joint involvement (Ullrich), and or contracture of the neck muscles (extramedullary muscular dystrophy). These patients can present with severe rhabdomyolysis and hyperkalemia resulting in cardiac arrest when exposed to succinylcholine and/or inhalational anesthetics. This is known as Anesthesia Induced Rhabdomyolysis (AIR).[174-177]

Those most at risk for these complications are younger children who are undiagnosed until the perioperative rhabdomyolysis develops or in whom succinylcholine is given for emergency reasons.[170] Adolescents in whom muscle breakdown has waned and muscle mass has been lost and replaced by fatty infiltration have had uneventful perioperative courses when exposed to inhalational anesthetic agents and succinylcholine and could be at a lesser risk for rhabdomyolysis but are at a greater risk for cardiac failure. Even though anesthesia-induced rhabdomyolysis is rare and does not occur with every episode of using an inhaled agent or succinylcholine,[178] it seems prudent to avoid inhalational anesthetics and succinylcholine in patients with known or suspected Duchenne muscular dystrophy or Becker muscular dystrophy. By analogy, this caution is extended to children with a known or suspected progressive and congenital muscle dystrophy.

Total intravenous anesthesia (TIVA) (see Chapter 6) has emerged as the preferred alternative to inhalational anesthetics in these children. If the anesthesia workstation is used for a child with Duchenne muscular dystrophy, it should be prepared as it is for malignant hyperthermia. In some specific clinical situations such as the child with Duchenne muscular dystrophy for whom IV access cannot be established before induction of anesthesia, an inhalational anesthetic may be given to secure the airway followed by TIVA for maintenance. Case reports of rhabdomyolysis during and after inhalational anesthesia[170,174-176,179-181] warrant monitoring these children for signs of rhabdomyolysis (i.e., urine myoglobin, serum K+ level), even if the risk is small. If rhabdomyolysis occurs, the inhalational anesthetic should be discontinued and replaced with a TIVA anesthetic. The child should not be discharged home until the signs of rhabdomyolysis resolve; myoglobinuria should be managed with large volumes of IV balanced salt solutions.

The clinical presentation of anesthesia-induced rhabdomyolysis may mimic malignant hyperthermia but the risk of malignant hyperthermia in children with Duchenne muscular dystrophy is the same as in the general population.[170,181,182] Hyperkalemic arrhythmias or cardiac arrest are most effectively reversed by rapid IV administration of calcium (10–20 mg/kg of calcium chloride, 30–60 mg/kg of calcium gluconate),[183] which should be repeated until the arrhythmias abate. Other therapies, including hyperventilation, administration of bicarbonate, albuterol, insulin, and glucose, are also recommended. On rare occasions, the hyperkalemia associated with acute rhabdomyolysis may be refractory to the usual treatments and require a prolonged resuscitation or even ECMO[184] (see Chapters 7 and 38).

Ion Channel Muscle Diseases

Congenital dysfunction of some ion channels can result in muscle diseases and present as crisis of myotonia or paralysis (see Table 22.13).[185,186] Paramyotonia congenita results from a mutation of the *SCN4A* gene (17q23-25) resulting in gain of function of the α subunit of the Na$_v$1.4 of the muscle fiber. It is inherited in an autosomal dominant pattern. Myotonic episodes localized in the muscles of neck, face, and upper limbs appear during the first decade, they are usually triggered by exposure to cold or prolonged exercise. They are followed by a prolonged muscle weakness. Other mutations of the same gene can produce potassium-aggravated myotonias, sodium channelopathies presenting as myotonia fluctuans, myotonia permanens, or acetazolamide-responsive myotonia. Episodes of myotonia in the upper part of the body are triggered by ingestion of potassium, exposure to cold, or exercise.

A mutation of the *CLCN1* gene (7p35) results in a loss of function of the α subunit of the chloride channel of the muscle fiber, which is known as Thomsen or Becker disease, depending on the inheritance pattern, autosomal dominant or recessive, respectively. Cold environmental temperatures, hypothermia, succinylcholine, and anticholinesterases should be avoided. The serum potassium should be monitored in patients with this myotonic phenotype who present for anesthesia. These children are often treated with mexiletine. There is no increased risk of malignant hyperthermia.

Familial hypokalemic periodic paralysis is caused by a mutation of the *CACCN1AS* gene (Ca channel), the *SCNA4* gene (Na channel), or the *ATP1A2* or *KCNE3* genes (K channel). The episodes of flaccid often asymmetric paralysis are triggered by stress, cold, infection, or a carbohydrate-rich meal; paralysis may last for many hours. Typically, the oculomotor and swallowing muscles as well as the diaphragm are spared. Hypokalemia is severe and can be life-threatening. Thyrotoxic periodic paralysis is a rare form of hypokalemic paralysis associated with biological hyperthyroidism. It occurs mainly in boys of Asian origin and is probably the result of a genetic susceptibility.[187]

Familial hyperkalemic periodic paralysis is caused by a mutation of the *SCNA4* gene (Na channel); it presents as short-lasting episodes of localized paralysis following exercise, stress, exposure to cold, or hypoglycemia. Dysphagia and breathing difficulties may occur. Serum potassium increases rapidly during a crisis. In some cases, episodes of myotonia occur between paralytic crises. Familial normokalemic periodic paralysis is considered a variant of the hyperkalemic form. Stress, exposure to cold, hypothermia, and succinylcholine should be avoided, and serum potassium monitored. Intravenous glucose is best avoided in children with the hypokalemic form. In the hyperkalemic form, fasting should be avoided, and a glucose-containing balanced salt solution administered as soon as the preoperative fasting interval starts. A single case of malignant hyperthermia has been published in a patient with the hypokalemic form, but this may be a random coincidence or possibly a false positive contracture test.[188]

Undiagnosed Myopathy

The neonate or infant with a possible myopathy (e.g., floppy, hypotonic, motor developmental delay) but without a definitive diagnosis is a challenge for the anesthesiologist.[189] A careful, thorough history and physical examination should be completed preoperatively. Serum creatine kinase and lactate concentrations should be evaluated, and the child's pediatrician or pediatric neurologist contacted for advice. If a progressive muscular dystrophy cannot be excluded (e.g., in the presence of an increased creatine kinase concentration), it may be prudent to avoid inhalational anesthetics except for induction of anesthesia.

Epilepsy

Epilepsy is common in childhood, with a prevalence of 0.5% to 1% in school-age children.[190] Epilepsy is defined as "a chronic disorder of the brain characterized by an enduring disposition toward recurrent unprovoked seizures." Seizures are defined as a "transient symptoms and/or signs due to abnormal excessive or simultaneous neuronal activity of a population of neuronal cells in the brain." The diagnosis of epilepsy requires at least two seizures that occur more than 24 hours apart or one seizure with a relevant abnormal EEG pattern or brain imaging suggesting a high probability of a second seizure.[191]

The International League against Epilepsy has published a classification of seizures and the epilepsies.[192,193] This operational classification is based on three levels: (1) seizure type defined by their type of onset (focal; generalized; unknown), (2) epilepsy type, and (3) epilepsy syndrome. It emphasizes the importance of considering the etiology and comorbidities associated with epilepsy (Figs. 22.3 and 22.4).

In generalized seizures, the abnormal electrical activity (behavior or EEG) originates simultaneously on both sides of the brain and spreads rapidly via neuronal networks.

Generalized seizures include generalized tonic-clonic seizures (convulsive seizure), absences (loss of awareness for several seconds resulting in a vacant state that may be accompanied by more subtle signs, such as eyelids and mouth movements), and myoclonic jerks (sudden rapid contraction of a group of muscles). This group also includes atonic (loss of muscle tone) and tonic (more prolonged increase in muscle contractions) seizures which can result in falls or drop attacks and epileptic spasms.

In focal seizures, the abnormal electrical activity originates on one side of the brain. These can spread quickly to produce a "generalized tonic-clonic seizure" in some situations. Symptoms depend on the site of origin of the abnormal electrical discharges, the extent, and speed of their spread in the brain.

In some children, the seizure type may be unclear and reported as "unknown." The third level of diagnosis is the identification of the epilepsy syndrome. Seizure types, EEG changes, brain imaging abnormalities, and genetic analyses may help to narrow down the diagnosis. Some syndromes are generally associated with other signs or symptoms, such as intellectual and psychiatric problems. Knowing the possible causes of epilepsy may help to understand the problem and treatment choice. Six main etiologies are described (see Fig. 22.3).

Structural causes are related to anatomical abnormalities that are usually acquired (e.g., head injury, stroke, tumor, birth injury, brain infection, etc.) or may be part of a genetic disorder (e.g., cortical malformations). Genetic factors are probably the single

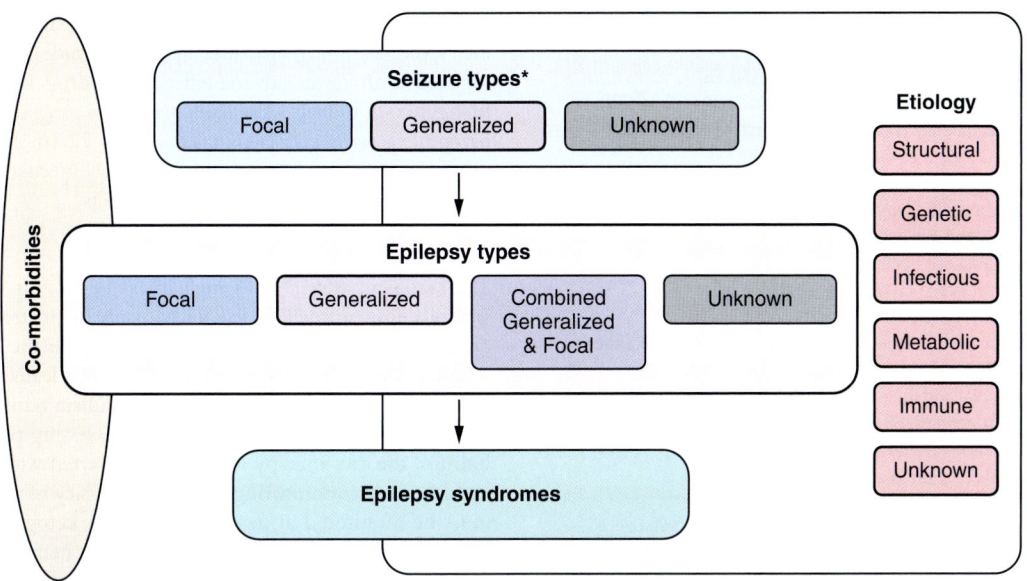

FIGURE 22.3 Framework for classification of the epilepsies with three levels of terminology involving (1) seizure type(s) defined by their type of onset (focal; generalized; unknown), (2) epilepsy type, and (3) epilepsy syndrome. In diagnostic stages, the search for a cause and identification of any associated disorders or comorbidities are primordial. (Scheffer IE, Berkovic S, Capovilla G, et al. ILAE classification of the epilepsies: position paper of the ILAE Commission for Classification and Terminology. *Epilepsia.* 2017;58(4):512-521. https://www.ilae.org/guidelines/definition-and-classification.)

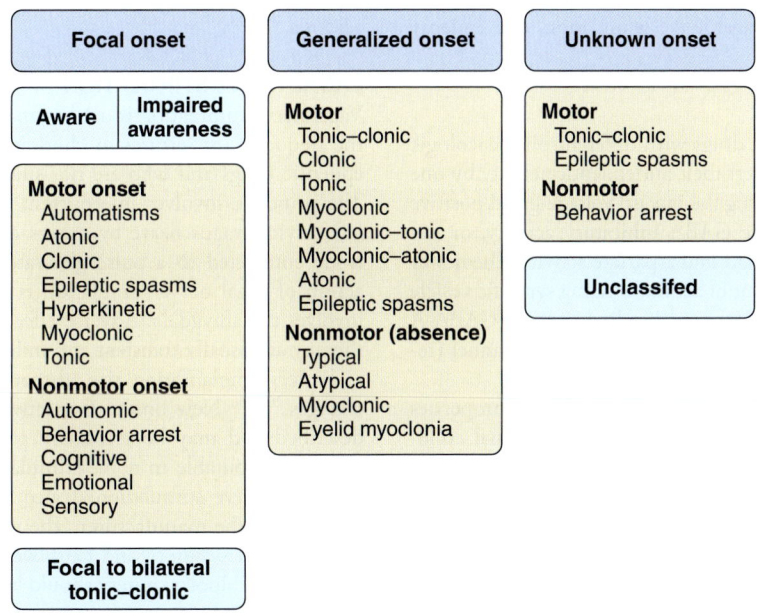

FIGURE 22.4 International league against epilepsy operational classification of seizure types. (Scheffer IE, Berkovic S, Capovilla G, et al. ILAE classification of the epilepsies: position paper of the ILAE Commission for Classification and Terminology. *Epilepsia.* 2017;58(4):512-521.https://www.ilae.org/guidelines/definition-and-classification.)

most important causative group. Infectious causes include tuberculosis, malaria, bacterial meningitis, and viral encephalitis. Metabolic and autoimmune causes are unusual but must be recognized to ensure that they are managed optimally. The International League against Epilepsy website (www.epilepsydiagnosis.org) provides the definition, classification, and descriptions of many seizure types along with epilepsy syndromes, and treatment guidelines. Table 22.14 describes epilepsy syndromes that begin in childhood (2–12 years).

Organization of forms of epilepsy is first by specificity: electroclinical syndromes, nonsyndromic epilepsies with structural-metabolic causes, and epilepsies of unknown cause.[193]

Management of epilepsy includes treatment of the underlying cause, if possible (e.g., tumors, infection, toxins, or metabolic disturbances), and the prevention of seizures using antiepileptic drugs. Selection of antiepileptic drugs is based on the seizure type and/or epilepsy syndrome, taking into account the child's age, associated disorders, and other medications.[190,194] The aim of the

TABLE 22.14 | Epilepsy Syndromes With Onset in Childhood

(1) **Self-Limited Focal Epilepsies of Childhood (SeLFE)**
   a) Self-Limited Epilepsy with Centrotemporal Spikes (SeLECTS)
   b) Self-Limited Epilepsy with Autonomic Seizures (SeLEAS)
   c) Childhood Occipital Visual Epilepsy (COVE)
   d) Photosensitive Occipital Lobe Epilepsy (POLE)
(2) **Genetic Generalized Epilepsies**
   a) Myoclonic-Atonic Epilepsy (MAE)
   b) Childhood absence epilepsy (AE)
   c) Epilepsy with Eyelid Myoclonia (E-EM)
   d) Epilepsy with Myoclonic Absences (E-MA)
(3) **Developmental and/or Epileptic Encephalopathies of Childhood**
   a) Lennox-Gastaut syndrome (LGS)
   b) Developmental and Epileptic Encephalopathy with spikewave activation in sleep (D/EE-SWAS)
   c) Febrile Infection-Related Epilepsy Syndrome (FIRES)
   d) Hemiconvulsion-Hemiplegia Epilepsy (HHE)

Childhood epilepsy syndromes from Scheffer IE, Berkovic S, Capovilla G, et al. ILAE classification of the epilepsies: position paper of the ILAE Commission for Classification and Terminology. *Epilepsia.* 2017;58(4):512-521.https://www.ilae.org/guidelines/definition-and-classification.

treatment is to eliminate all seizures with the smallest number of drugs in the smallest dose. When epilepsy fails to respond to antiepileptic drugs, nonpharmacological options may be considered including a ketogenic diet, vagal nerve stimulation, and epilepsy surgery.

ANTIEPILEPTIC DRUGS

A wide range of antiepileptic drugs with different pharmacologic profiles are available. They exert their antiepileptic activity by one of several mechanisms: reducing the inward voltage-gated positive Na^+ or Ca^{++}, increasing the GABA inhibitory activity, or decreasing the excitatory glutamate and aspartate activity. The newer drugs act via novel mechanisms of action: binding synaptic vesicle (SV2) protein (levetiracetam), steroid binding sites on GABA-A receptors (ganaxolone), and voltage-gated potassium channel (retigabine) (Table 22.15).

Optimal drug therapy seeks to maximize the desired properties while minimizing the undesired effects for the individual child. Every antiepileptic drug has potential adverse effects that range from behavioral problems (irritability, hyperactivity, depression, anxiety, sleep disruption, somnolence) to clinical disorders (mild to severe rashes and allergy, decreased bone density, hematologic or hepatic disorders). These drugs may have important pharmacokinetic interactions through enzyme induction or inhibition. Pharmacodynamic interactions may modify their therapeutic effects or the effects of the anesthetics.[195–197]

The *first-generation antiepileptic drugs* induce (phenobarbital, phenytoin, primidone, carbamazepine) or inhibit (valproate) cytochrome P450 hepatic isoenzymes resulting in a number of possible drug-drug interactions (see Table 22.15). Moreover, phenytoin, benzodiazepine, and valproic acid are highly protein bound. This may affect the free plasma concentrations of other drugs by competition for protein-binding sites. In the presence of hypoalbuminemia, malnutrition, nephrotic/uremic states, or liver disease or when a highly protein-bound antiepileptic drug is coadministered, a disproportionate increase in their free fraction increases the risk for adverse effects and toxicity.

The *second-generation antiepileptic drugs* (vigabatrin, lamotrigine, levetiracetam, pregabalin, and zonisamide) are generally associated with fewer adverse effects and drug interactions than first-generation drugs. The *third-generation drugs* comprise eslicarbazepine acetate and lacosamide. Table 22.16 shows the commonly used antiepileptic drugs with their mechanisms of action and their main possible adverse side effects.

KETOGENIC DIET

The ketogenic diet[198,199] is high in fat but low in carbohydrates and protein, compelling the body to use fat instead of carbohydrates to produce energy. The basic principle is the induction and maintenance of ketosis. This metabolic state leads to an effective reduction of seizures.[200] The exact mechanism remains unknown. After excluding contraindications and assessing possible comorbidities, the diet therapy is most often started with strict clinical and laboratory monitoring.[201,202] The efficacy of the diet therapy must be monitored at regular intervals. A ketogenic diet should be used for a minimum of 3 months and a maximum of 2 years. Although this diet is associated with adverse effects such as hyperlipidemia, hypoglycemia, metabolic acidosis, nephrolithiasis, pancreatitis, increased transaminases levels, constipation, abdominal pain, growth failure, and osteopenia, short- and long-term beneficial effects have been established for children with intractable epilepsy, even after discontinuation.[200,203] Metabolic changes associated with acute illness or surgery can precipitate loss of ketosis, thus worsening seizures, and induce metabolic acidosis.[151,198]

VAGAL NERVE STIMULATION

Vagal nerve stimulation is used as an adjunctive therapy to reduce the frequency of seizures in children who are refractory to antiepileptic drugs and who are not suitable for epileptic surgery.[204] The principle involves intermittent electrical stimulation of the left cervical vagus nerve by means of an implanted helical electrode connected to a pulse generator. The exact mechanism of action of vagal nerve stimulation is unknown but it most likely involves the amygdala. Adverse effects of vagal nerve stimulation therapy are usually transient and mild, including local discomfort at battery implantation site, throat pain, coughing, and voice changes.[205,206] New onset obstructive sleep apnea has also been described and may be secondary to changes in the respiratory pattern attributable to nerve stimulation activation.[207] Handling the vagal nerve stimulation device requires a magnet, which is supplied by the manufacturer. The pulse generator may be damaged by electrocautery and cardioversion/defibrillation. For surgery, either a bipolar cautery should be used, or the grounding pad of the monopolar electrocautery should be placed so that current flows away from the nerve stimulation generator. If defibrillation is required, the lowest setting should be used, and the pads placed as far away from the generator as possible. In case of cardiothoracic surgery or when a monopolar cautery is required, it is useful to stop the device and to keep the cautery pads as far away as possible from the device implantation site during surgery and to reprogram it as soon as possible after surgery.[204]

SURGICAL TREATMENT

Surgical treatment may be indicated for refractory epilepsy when the epileptogenic focus or interruption of a seizure pathway is possible. Surgical options include temporal lobectomy, amygdalo-hippocampectomy, lesionectomy, cortectomy, hemispherectomy,

TABLE 22.15 Commonly Used Antiepileptic Drugs (AEDs): Antiseizure Mechanism of Action, Possible Adverse Effects; not an Exhaustive List

AEDs	Mode of Action on	Adverse Effects	Interactions With AEDs and Non-AEDs		Effects of Non-AEDs or Disease
1st-Generation					
Clonazepam	GABA-A	Drowsiness, dizziness, depression, aggressiveness If sudden discontinuation, withdrawal seizures			
Carbamazepine (CBZ)	Na⁺	Hypersensitivity reactions, cardiac conduction abnormalities, hyponatremia, low platelet level	P-450 inductor	Enhances hepatic oxidation and conjugation of liposomal drugs	Erythromycin may ↑ its plasma concentration
Phenobarbital (PB)	GABA, GLU, Ca⁺⁺, CA	Cognitive and behavioral adverse effects, sedation, megaloblastic anemia, liver necrosis	P-450 inductor	Hepatic microsomal enzyme induction	
Phenytoin (PHT)	Na⁺	Rash and other hypersensitivity reactions, gingival hyperplasia, vestibular cerebellar dysfunction, megaloblastic anemia, Stevens-Johnson syndrome, hyperglycemia	P-450 inductor Highly protein bound	Induces oxidative metabolism of liposomal drugs ↓ serum concentrations of cortisol derivatives, dextropropoxyphene, calcium antagonists, fentanyl, statins, methadone, thyroxine	If hypoalbuminemia, ↑ in free fraction > ↑ risk for dose-dependent toxicity
Sodium Valproate (VPA)	Na⁺, Ca⁺⁺, GABA	Hepatotoxicity, platelet dysfunction, thrombocytopenia hyperammonemia (in case of mitochondrial cytopathy), pancreatitis, teratogenic, postnatal cognitive effects after fetal exposure	Hepatic microsomal enzyme inhibitor Highly protein bound	Enhances hepatic oxidation and conjugation of liposomal drugs Displaces diazepam from the binding site	If hypoalbuminemia, ↑ in free fraction > ↑ risk for dose-dependent toxicity
2nd-Generation					
Felbamate (FBM)	Na⁺, Ca⁺⁺, GLU, CA	Insomnia, anorexia, nausea, headache, irritability, aplastic anemia, leucopenia, and hepatotoxic effects	Enzyme inhibitor	The most toxic	
Lamotrigine (LTG)	Na⁺, Ca⁺⁺	Rash and other hypersensitivity reactions, bone demineralization Dizziness, diplopia, tremor Stevens-Johnson syndrome hyponatremia	P-450 induction	Hepatic microsomal enzyme induction	
Levetiracetam (LEV)	SV2 Binds to protein A2 (release of glutamate)	Irritability, mood changes anorexia, diarrhea, dyspepsia, skin changes, and pancytopenia			
Oxcarbazepine (OXC)	Na⁺				
Pregabalin (PGB)	Ca⁺⁺, Na⁺				
Rufinamide (RUF)	Na⁺				
Tiagabine (TGB)	GABA	Dizziness, asthenia, somnolence, anxiety, nausea, nervousness, tremor, abdominal pain, and cognitive disorders			
Topiramate (TPM)	Na⁺, Ca⁺⁺, GLU, CA	Metabolic and renal acidosis, cognitive effects, weight loss, paresthesia, nephrolithiasis, glaucoma			Interactions with carbonic anhydrase inhibitors, digoxin, hydrochlorothiazide, metformin, pioglitazone,
Vigabatrin (VGV)	GABA				
Zonisamide (ZNS)	GLU, Na⁺, Ca⁺⁺, CA	Sedation, asthenia, diplopia, hypohidrosis, skin changes, Stevens-Johnson syndrome, dizziness, headache, ataxia, anorexia, agitation, irritability, and nephrolithiasis, metabolic acidosis			
3rd-Generation					
Lacosamide (LCM)	Na⁺, collapsin	Dizziness, fatigue, nausea, and ataxia, prolonged PR interval			

CA, carbonic anhydrase; *Ca⁺⁺,* voltage-gated calcium channel; *GABA,* gamma-aminobutyric acid receptor; *GABA-A,* chloride associated gamma-aminobutyric acid receptor; *GLU,* glutamate receptor; *SV2,* synaptic vesicle 2 protein; *Na⁺⁺,* voltage-gated sodium channel.

TABLE 22.16 | Interactions Between Anti-Epileptic Drugs and Commonly Used Perioperative Drugs

Non-AEDs	Action/Interactions	Effects
Omeprazole	= inhibiting CYP2C19	Can ↑ PHT plasma concentrations resulting in toxicity
Corticosteroids	Metabolism ↑ by P-450 inducers such as PB, PHT, CBZ	Therapeutic efficacy ↓
Cyclosporine	Metabolism ↑ by P-450 inducers such as PB, PHT, CBZ	Therapeutic efficacy ↓
Amiodarone	Metabolism ↑ by P-450 inducers such as PB, PHT, CBZ	Therapeutic efficacy ↓
β-Blockers: propranolol, metoprolol	Metabolism ↑ by P-450 inducers such as PB, PHT, CBZ	Therapeutic efficacy ↓
Calcium channel Antagonists: nifedipine, felodipine, nimodipine, verapamil	Metabolism ↑ by P-450 inducers such as PB, PHT, CBZ	Therapeutic efficacy ↓
Antacids such as cimetidine	↓ absorption and excretion of gabapentin	Prolong half-life of gabapentin
Anesthetic Drugs: thiopentone, midazolam, opioids	Metabolism ↑ by P-450 inducers such as PB, PHT, CBZ	Duration of action is ↓
Propofol	Metabolism modified by AEDs (competitive inhibition of hepatic metabolism)	Propofol clearance ↓ (Lower required dose; longer time to emerge when compared with non-AEDs)
Nondepolarizing Blockers:		
Rocuronium, Pancuronium, Vecuronium Cisatracurium	Hepatic clearance ↑ by PHT, CBZ	Their duration of action is ↓ But acute administration of PHT potentiates the neuromuscular blockade of rocuronium
Atracurium Mivacurium	Not metabolized by hepatic enzymes	Duration of action not affected
Antibiotic		
Macrolides (particularly erythromycin)	= potent inhibitors of CYP3A4	Can ↑ CBZ toxicity
Carbapenem		Significant ↓ in serum VPA concentrations

The list is not exhaustive, only the most relevant effects are noted. *PB*, phenobarbital; *PHT*, phenytoin; *CBZ*, carbamazepine; *AEDs*, anti-epileptic drugs; *VPA*, sodium valproate.

corpus callosotomy, and multiple subpial transections.[208–210] Surgical excision of epileptogenic foci is generally performed under general anesthesia and combined with intraoperative brain surface electrocorticography (ECoG) to carefully delineate the epileptogenic foci. Preoperative diagnostic interventions include stereotactic electrode insertion, intracranial grid and strip electrodes to map the location of the seizure foci, or the Wada test to determine which is the dominant (speech) or seizure-triggering hemisphere using amobarbital or low-dose propofol injected into the carotid artery (see Chapter 24).

ANESTHESIA CONSIDERATIONS

A preoperative assessment should be conducted with special focus on epilepsy without overlooking coexisting medical problems. The anesthesiologist needs to confirm:

(1) the seizure history (nature of the seizure, frequency, allergy to antiepileptic drugs) and actual regular medication regimen;
(2) the factors that trigger seizures; and
(3) the pharmacological properties of the antiepileptic drugs and their possible interactions with anesthetics and other drugs used perioperatively (Tables 22.15–22.17).

Table 22.18 provides a checklist for the perioperative management of these children. Some disorders that cause epilepsy may be associated with other medical conditions, such as cardiorespiratory deficits, nutritional problems, craniofacial malformations, and other disabilities.

Many perioperative factors can provoke or increase the frequency of seizures (e.g., missed doses of antiepileptic drugs due to prolonged periods of fasting), sleep deprivation, exposure to proconvulsant drugs, hypoxia, hypocapnia (hyperventilation), electrolyte disturbance (e.g., hyponatremia), postoperative ileus resulting in poor drug absorption, changes in serum pH and albumin levels, drug interactions with antiepileptic drugs, loss of ketosis in a child using a ketogenic diet, direct effect of neurosurgery on the brain, cerebrovascular instability, or coincidental exacerbation of severe epilepsy.

To limit seizure activity, the perioperative fasting period should be kept to a minimum, and routine medications should be given pre- and postoperatively to minimize missed doses of antiepileptic drugs. In some instances, children will only take their antiepileptic drugs with solids or semisolids such as apple sauce or toast and peanut butter, which presents a problem preoperatively. Alternate arrangements may have to be made to continue the antiepileptic drugs preoperatively such as taking the drugs orally the night before the surgery or after the surgery or given perioperatively parenterally. Careful scheduling of the time of surgery may facilitate this because many children receive antiepileptic drugs on a twice-daily

TABLE 22.17 | Effects of Anesthetic Agents in Epileptic Patients

Anesthetic Agents	Action
Benzodiazepines	Used as first-line anticonvulsant drug
N_2O	Varying effects: excitatory and inhibitory effects Most of the time, described as suppressing epileptiform activity on ECoG monitoring for epilepsy surgery, continuing effect when N_2O administration is interrupted Can be safely used in epileptic patients provided hyperventilation is avoided
Sevoflurane	Normally safe <1.5 MAC Can provoke seizure-like activity, particularly in children at high concentrations (≥1.5 MAC) in conjunction with hypocapnia/hyperventilation The ususal anti-epileptic drugs should be given on the day of anesthesia
Isoflurane	Well-characterized anticonvulsant properties Can be used in refractory status epilepticus
Halothane	Anticonvulsant activity
Desflurane	No proconvulsant activity
Barbiturates (thiopental, methohexital, pentobarbital) Propofol	Anticonvulsant properties Methohexital = proconvulsant Propofol: at low dose reported to produce excitatory activity; abnormal movements as opisthotonus and myoclonia in normal as well as epileptic patients; at high doses, no seizure effect, can inhibit seizure. Barbiturates and propofol can be used for the treatment of refractory status epilepticus
Etomidate	Can be proconvulsant at clinical doses Anticonvulsant at high doses
Ketamine	Both pro- and anticonvulsant properties Low doses may facilitate seizures At sedative and anesthetic doses shows anticonvulsant properties Reported as beneficial in management of status epilepticus refractory to other agents
Alpha2-agonists clonidine dexmedetomidine	No pro- or anticonvulsant activity Sedation with dexmedetomidine shows EEG pattern similar to stage II sleep
Meperidine	Strongest association with myoclonus and tonic-clonic seizure activity (metabolite normeperidine)
Fentanyl, alfentanil, sufentanil, remifentanil, morphine	Generalized seizure reported after low-to-moderate dose, particularly after intrathecal use. Remifentanil and alfentanil can induce spike activity in localizing epileptogenic zones during epilepsy surgery; alfentanil appears to be the more potent activator
Neuromuscular blocking agents	No pro- or anticonvulsant effects Clinical evidence of seizures only in animals with laudanosine, the primary metabolite of atracurium
Anticholinergics	Can be used in epileptics Atropine and scopolamine can cross the blood-brain barrier and produce central anticholinergic syndrome (manifests as agitation with seizures, hallucinations, and restlessness or stupor, coma, and apnea) Glycopyrrolate does not cross the blood-brain barrier, does not produce these effects
Anticholinesterases	No reported proconvulsant activity
Local anesthetics	Subtoxic doses: anticonvulsants, sedative, and analgesic effects Higher concentrations can cause seizure activity
Droperidol	No proconvulsant activity
Antiemetics	Dopamine antagonists may cause extrapyramidal effects and dystonia that can be confused with epileptic activity

AED, Antiepileptic drug; *ECoG,* electrocorticographic monitoring.

regimen (8 AM and 8 PM). It is essential to restart the drugs in the postoperative period as soon as possible. When the fasting time exceeds 24 hours, parenteral replacement is necessary using an intravenous form (phosphenytoin, sodium valproate, levetiracetam) or suppository formulation (carbamazepine). If the patient's current antiepileptic medication is not available in a parenteral form or if the surgery is complex and expected to be prolonged, input from the child's neurologist should be sought regarding alternate antiepileptic drugs. If a sedative premedication is needed (anxious

or combative child), the interactions with actual antiepileptic drugs must be considered.

The choice of anesthetic agents can also affect the seizure threshold. Many anesthetic agents possess both proconvulsant and anticonvulsant properties. Their main effects are summarized in Table 22.17. Inhalation induction with sevoflurane may be associated with cortical epileptiform EEG signs especially at high concentration (MAC >2) and with hyperventilation.[211] This epileptiform EEG is usually asymptomatic and sevoflurane is not contraindicated

TABLE 22.18 | Perioperative Management of Children With Epilepsy

Preoperative Management

Clarify usual nature of the seizures, seizure types, frequency, and trigger factors

Review and document regular medication regimen

Check drug allergies and adverse reactions

Review rescue medication regimen

Check the eventual interactions and side effects of the medication (e.g., thrombocytopenia with valproate)

Check coexisting medical problems related to underlying pathology

Check with parents or familiar caregiver if epilepsy is stabilized, if not liaise with child's pediatrician or neurologist

If premedication is considered, check interactions with actual medication

Day of Surgery

Give usual morning medications

Avoid prolonged fasting

Aim for evening medication as usual

Keep in mind that factors such as hypoxia-hypercapnia, hypocapnia, hyponatremia, and hypoglycemia can precipitate seizures

If the child is treated with KD, ensure that all IV solutions and IV/oral medications are carbohydrate-free

Blood glucose, bicarbonate electrolytes and pH, and urine ketones (dipstick) should be monitored
Prolonged fasting must be avoided
Take advice from neurology team

If the child has a VNS therapy, place electrocautery grounding pad so that current does not flow through the device
Take advice from neurology team if the device must be stopped (e.g., before MRI)

If fasting exceeds 24 hours, parenteral replacement must be evaluated: IV levetiracetam, phenytoin, sodium valproate
Take advice from neurology team

If regular drug administration is not possible, consider:
Phenytoin: IV load of 15–20 mg/kg at a rate of 50 mg/minute and then twice-daily maintenance dose of 2.5–5.0 mg/kg
Levetiracetam: IV 20 mg/kg in 15 minutes following by 10 mg/kg twice daily. When switching from oral form, total daily IV dosage should be equivalent to dosage and frequency
Benzodiazepine: Give intravenously as rescue

IV, Intravenous; *KD,* ketogenic diet; *VNS,* vagal nerve stimulation.

provided the usual antiepileptic drug has been given and a high inspired concentration is not used for a long period of time.[211] Spontaneous movement and EEG changes are described with small doses of propofol; but in anesthetic doses, it suppresses EEG activity.[212] TIVA can be used in these children recognizing that there is a risk of propofol infusion syndrome in some cohorts.

Antiepileptic drugs interact with certain anesthetic agents. They reduce the required dose of propofol and prolong the time for emergence from anesthesia. Chronic treatment with phenytoin and carbamazepine increases the hepatic clearance of rocuronium, pancuronium, vecuronium, and cisatracurium, and decreases their duration of action.[213] However, acute administration of phenytoin potentiates the effect of rocuronium. These drugs also cause resistance to the analgesic effects of opioids.

Cytochrome P450 enzymes induced by chronic administration of phenobarbital speed the clearance of ketamine, thereby reducing its effect.[214] Intraoperative factors such as hypoxia-hypercapnia, hypocapnia, hyponatremia, and hypoglycemia can precipitate seizures and must be avoided. Hypercarbia and hypoxemia during emergence may increase the susceptibility for seizures or prolong the duration of the seizure.

It is mandatory to maintain ketogenesis in children using ketogenic diets during the perioperative period. All IV solutions and IV/oral medications should be carbohydrate-free.[215]

Intraoperatively, normal saline or a balanced solution without lactate is preferred. However, given in larger volume, normal saline might produce hyperchloremic acidosis, exacerbating preexisting metabolic acidosis. Throughout the perioperative period, blood glucose, pH, and electrolyte levels, and urinary ketones should be monitored (every 2–3 hours), especially in procedures lasting more than 3 hours. If a child develops metabolic acidosis, IV bicarbonate can be used. If blood glucose is less than 3 mmol/L (55 mg/dL), a glucose-containing IV fluid (glucose 2.5% or 5%) should be titrated to maintain blood glucose between 50 and 80 mg/dL.[202] Intravenous fluids should be continued postoperatively until oral fluids are tolerated. Finally, the ketogenic diet should be reintroduced as soon as possible after surgery. The transfusion of blood products might contain variable amounts of carbohydrate from the donor's plasma and preservative solutions. Drugs inducing hyperglycemia may also alter the ketotic state, but it is unlikely that a single low dose of dexamethasone will disturb that state (see https://www.gosh.nhs.uk/conditions-and-treatments/procedures-and-treatments/ketogenic-diet/). Discussion with the neurology team for children undergoing elective and long-lasting surgical procedures could lead to a temporary discontinuation of the diet before surgery, which would allow more therapeutic freedom for the anesthetic team, but may increase the risk of perioperative seizures.[204] Regional anesthesia is safe to use. It is possible that the threshold for seizures in cases of local anesthetic systemic toxicity (LAST) is lower than in nonepileptic children.

REFRACTORY SEIZURES AND STATUS EPILEPTICUS

Drug therapy is usually required for any seizures that last 2 minutes longer than the patient's habitual seizures. This treatment should be administered if the seizure continues beyond 5 minutes. Benzodiazepines are the first-line agents. Subsequent treatment with second line drugs (sodium valproate, phenobarbitone, levetiracetam, phenytoin/fosphenytoin, lacosamide, topiramate) depends on local drug availability, adverse effect profiles, the child's pathology, or the nature of the seizure activity. Guidelines for seizure and convulsive state management are available at: https://www.nice.org.uk/guidance/cg137/chapter/Appendix-F-Protocols-for-treating-convulsive-status-epilepticus-in-adults-and-children-adults-published-in-2004-and-children-published-in-2011.

ANNOTATED REFERENCES

Arzimanoglou A, O' Hare A, Johnston M, Ouvrier RA, (eds). *Aicardi's Diseases of the Nervous System in Childhood.* 4th ed. Wiley; 2018.
A comprehensive review of neurologic and neuromuscular conditions in children.
Bissonnette B, Luginbuehl I, Engelhardt T (eds). *Syndromes: Rapid Recognition and Perioperative Implications.* 2e. McGraw Hill; 2019.
Most neurologic and neuromuscular diseases are rare diseases: this textbook provides a short description and the anesthetic implications of most known rare diseases.

Nicolau S, Milone M, Liewluck T. Guidelines for genetic testing of muscle and neuromuscular syndromes. *Muscle & Nerve*. 2021;64:255-269.

A clear summary of the diagnostic approach in patients in whom a muscular or neuromuscular disorder is suspected accounting for the phenotypic overlap of many mutations.

Saudubray J-M, Baumgartner MR, Walter J (eds.) *Inborn Metabolic Diseases Diagnosis and Treatment*. 6th ed. Springer; 2016.

A comprehensive review of all inborn metabolic disease: mechanisms, diagnosis, and treatment.

Schieren M, Defosse J, Böhmer A, Wappler F, Gerbershagen MU. Anaesthetic management of patients with myopathies. *Eur J Anaesthesiol*. 2017;34:641-649.

A clear overview of the literature on anesthesia and neuromuscular diseases

Soriano SG, McClain CD (eds). *Essentials of Pediatric Neuroanesthesia*. Cambridge University Press; 2019.

All you need to know about anesthesia of a child with a neurologic pathology.

van den Bersselaar LR, Heytens L, Silva HCA, et al. The European Neuromuscular Centre Consensus Statement on Anaesthesia in Patients with Neuromuscular Disorders. *Eur J Neurol*. 2022;29(12):3486-3507.

A group of experts proposes evidence- or experience-based considerations on anesthesia for children and adults with a neuromuscular or muscular disease.

22

A complete reference list can be found online at Elsevier eBooks+.

23 Surgery, Anesthesia, and the Immature Brain

ANDREAS W. LOEPKE AND ANDREW J. DAVIDSON

Background
Normal Brain Development
Effects of Anesthetic Exposure on the Developing Brain
Apoptotic Cell Death
Long-Term Brain Cellular Viability, Neuro-
logic Function, and Behavior
Effects on Neurogenesis and Gliogenesis
Alterations in Dendritic Architecture
Decrease in Trophic Factors
Degeneration of Mitochondria
Abnormal Reentry Into Cell Cycle
Destabilization of the Cytoskeleton
Genomic, Proteomic, and Epigenetic Alterations
Effects on the Developing Spinal Cord
Putative Mechanisms for Neurotoxicity
Specific Anesthetic and Sedative Agents
Ketamine
Inhaled Anesthetics
Nitrous Oxide
Xenon
Benzodiazepines
Chloral Hydrate
Barbiturates
Propofol
Dexmedetomidine
Opioid Analgesics
Exposure Time, Dose, and Anesthetic Combinations

Deleterious Effects of Untreated Pain and Stress
Potential Alleviating Strategies
Anesthetic Neuroprotection
Critical Evaluation of Animal Studies and Interspecies
Comparisons
Duration of Exposure
Anesthetic Doses
Experimental Versus Clinical Conditions
Comparative Brain Development
Assessing Neurobehavioral or Cognitive Outcomes
Nonhuman Primate Studies
Long-Term Outcome in Children Exposed to Anesthesia and
Surgery
Major Surgery in the Neonatal Period
Study Design to Address Possible Anesthetic Neurotoxicity
The Data Linkage Studies
Longitudinal Cohort and Registry Datasets
Prospective Cohort Studies With Children
Randomized Trials
Combination Analysis the Gas, Mask, and Panda Studies
Prenatal Exposure
Outcome After Exposure to Anesthesia Outside of the
Operating Room
Limitations of the Available Clinical Studies
Future Research
Recommendations for Clinical Practice

MILLIONS OF CHILDREN UNDERGO SURGERY with anesthesia every year.[1] This powerful drug-induced coma has facilitated life-saving procedures in very young infants. During the perioperative period, these same infants are exposed to a multitude of stressors capable of interfering with normal brain development. Pain, stress, inflammation, hypoxia, and ischemia all adversely affect the immature central nervous system (CNS). However, evidence from studies in animals have indicated that sedatives and anesthetics—the very drugs used to shield patients from pain and stress—may themselves influence brain development undesirably, by triggering structural and functional abnormalities. In fact, this phenomenon has been one of the most intensely investigated laboratory research fields in anesthesiology and a passionately debated topic (Fig. 23.1). To date, close to 1000 animal studies have addressed the effects of anesthetics on the developing brain.[2] These laboratory studies in a variety of animal species have unequivocally found disruption of brain structural integrity immediately after prolonged exposure to a wide range of anesthetics and other perioperative medications. It is highly probable that several of these deleterious effects to some degree also occur in the developing human brain. Moreover, long-term cognitive and behavioral abnormalities have been found in several animal species, including nonhuman primates. However, laboratory findings cannot be directly extrapolated to humans in clinical settings and the long-term effects of the immediate brain structural abnormalities remain highly speculative.[3]

Importantly, primate and human epidemiological studies have found mixed evidence for an association between surgery with general anesthesia in childhood and subsequent neurobehavioral abnormalities. Some studies have identified learning disabilities or behavioral disorders in primates or children after general anesthesia early in life, whereas others have not. More recently, a randomized controlled human trial and several ambidirectional epidemiological studies have demonstrated zero or only limited long-term cognitive alterations after anesthesia and surgery early in life. This chapter explains the compelling laboratory data that demonstrate

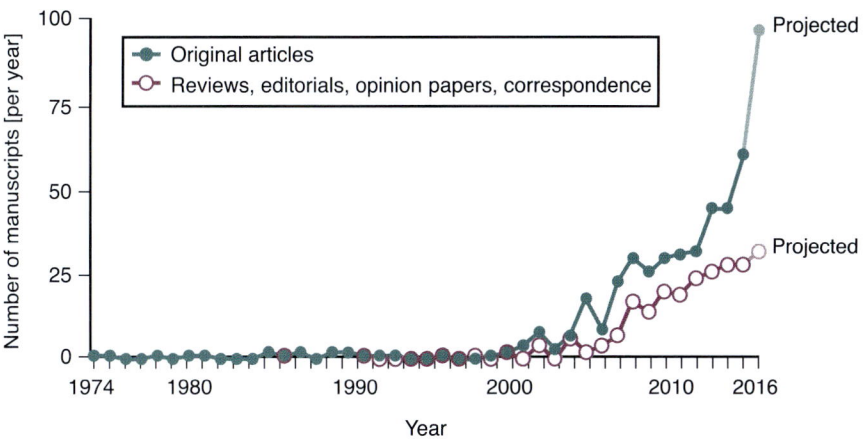

FIGURE 23.1 Research into the effects of anesthetic exposure in immature animals represents one of the most intensely investigated fields in anesthesiology and one of the most hotly debated topics. Graphical depiction of the annual publication of original articles *(solid circles)* and reviews, editorials, letters, commentaries, or opinion papers *(open circles)* spanning from 1974 to 2016, identified in a PubMed database search and screened for relevance using the terms "anesthesia or anesthetic or isoflurane or sevoflurane or desflurane or halothane or enflurane or ketamine or barbiturate or pentobarbital or benzodiazepine or midazolam or propofol or dexmedetomidine or xenon" and "neurotoxicity or apoptosis" and "neuron or brain." (From Lin EP, Lee J-R, Lee CS, et al. Do anesthetics harm the developing human brain? An integrative analysis of animal and human studies. *Neurotoxicol Teratol.* 2017;60:117-128.)

deleterious effects as well as protective effects of anesthetic exposure and discusses it in light of the limited discernable human phenotype.

Background

After the first public demonstration in the Western hemisphere of drug-induced, reversible coma by William T.G. Morton during a surgical procedure at the Massachusetts General Hospital in Boston more than 175 years ago, "anesthesia", derived from the Greek words *an-* (without) and *aisthēsis* (sensibility), has been a staple of modern medicine. According to estimates, worldwide more than 230 million patients of all ages benefit from general anesthesia during surgical procedures every year.[4] This positive impact has now been tempered by the possibility that anesthetics may adversely affect brain development. Combustibility of the anesthetic and substantial hemodynamic and respiratory adverse effects in the patient caused serious concerns during the first century of anesthetic use. General anesthesia was rarely used in critically ill neonates because of the fear of profound myocardial depression and hemodynamic instability. Perioperative drug regimens were often limited to neuromuscular blocking agents and nitrous oxide, which did not reliably provide loss of consciousness. With the realization that dramatic stress responses to painful stimulation are detectable even in preterm infants, that unopposed pain exerts deleterious effects on the developing brain, and that modern anesthetics and analgesics can abolish these responses without substantial hemodynamic compromise, modern pediatric anesthesia has afforded critically ill infants the benefits of amnesia, analgesia, stress-free conditions, and immobility during increasingly invasive procedures and surgeries. These stress-free interventions have saved countless lives and have preserved quality of life in this vulnerable population. All the while, the powerful coma induced by general anesthetics had been thought to be temporary and devoid of serious long-term adverse consequences after emergence. This notion of complete reversibility is now being seriously

questioned because of dramatic structural abnormalities, including dendritic, synaptic, cellular, and subcellular changes detected during and immediately after anesthetic exposure in neonatal animals and long-term cognitive abnormalities reported in animals and some human clinical studies after general anesthesia at a young age.

Normal Brain Development

Any brain structural abnormalities observed after exposure to anesthesia need to be put into the context of the natural changes experienced during normal brain development. The mammalian brain undergoes a complex and extended process of enormous growth in cell number, synapse formation, and connection forming during the perinatal period and into young childhood. Subsequent to this dramatic expansion in the number of cells and connections early in life, regressive processes occur all the way into adolescence. These expansive and regressive processes allow the human brain to fully mature to excel at complex tasks, such as talking, walking, reading, writing, calculating, acquiring social skills, perfecting fine motor dexterity, and accomplishing complex functions, including learning, abstract thinking, and planning and executing long-term objectives.

At birth, the size of the immature human brain is only one-third of the adult brain, doubling in weight within the first year of life, and reaching 90% of its adult size by 6 years of age.[5] This dramatic growth spurt coincides with a remarkable overabundance of neurons and neuronal connections. In fact, less than half the neurons generated during development survive into adulthood.[6,7] Superfluous neurons that lose in the competition for the limited amount of trophic factors are removed by an inborn cellular suicide program, also termed programmed cell death or apoptosis.[8]

After their rapid growth in number during early brain development, immature neurons subsequently form an excess of connections via synapses. Depending on the brain region, synaptic densities reach their maximum in infants and young toddlers between 3 to 15 months of age and undergo a progressive reduction by about half during adolescence and into adulthood.[9] According to Donald Hebb's adage "neurons that fire together, wire together," connections demonstrating continued electrical and chemical activity are sustained, whereas those with little or no activity are lost. Surviving axons are myelinated by oligodendrocytes, leading to progressive maturation of the CNS.

Brain architecture changes rapidly and dramatically throughout early life. Neuronal density is greatest during fetal life, and excess neurons are eliminated via apoptosis or programmed cell death, predominantly in utero, during the neonatal period and into infancy.[10] Rapid growth of dendrites and synaptic connections occur during infancy and early childhood, and underutilized dendrites and synapses regress, predominantly during later childhood and adolescence.[9,10]

Although these processes occur at slightly different stages of development for different regions of the brain, the first several years after birth represent a critical period for the entire developing CNS. Recent findings in animals suggest that exposure to anesthetics or sedatives during this period may interfere with proper neuronal development, brain architecture, and subsequent function. Although the exact molecular mechanisms by which anesthetics afford their therapeutic properties of amnesia, analgesia, and immobility are incompletely understood, their interaction with a wide variety of ion channels, such as sodium, calcium, and potassium channels, as well as several cell membrane proteins, including γ-aminobutyric acid (GABA), glycine, glutamate (N-methyl-D-aspartate [NMDA]), acetylcholine, and serotonin receptor systems, make it conceivable that anesthetics could interfere with important neurochemical processes during critical windows of brain development. In fact, both GABA and NMDA receptors, putative targets for many anesthetics, play pivotal roles in trophic signaling, regulation of neuronal maturation, and programmed cell death. During early brain development, GABA directs cell proliferation, neuroblast migration, and dendritic maturation.[11] In turn, developmental NMDA receptor stimulation directly fosters neuronal survival and maturation,[12,13] making it entirely plausible that anesthetics could interfere with these critical developmental processes.

Effects of Anesthetic Exposure on the Developing Brain

Concerns regarding protracted neurological effects in young children after exposure to general anesthetics were first raised more than half a century ago, when behavioral changes were observed following administration of vinyl ether, cyclopropane, or ethyl chloride for otolaryngologic surgery.[14] However, these abnormalities were regarded as psychological in nature because they were alleviated by the preoperative administration of sedatives.[14,15] Approximately 2 decades later the focus of research into the long-term effects of anesthetics shifted to occupational exposures of pregnant health care workers.[16–19] Delayed synaptogenesis and behavioral abnormalities were observed in neonatal rats born to rodent dams that were chronically exposed to subanesthetic doses of halothane during their entire pregnancy. Interest into the effects of anesthetics on brain development in children dramatically increased several decades later following a seminal study in neonatal rat pups, observing widespread neuronal degeneration after prolonged exposure to ketamine.[20] This initial discovery has now culminated in hundreds of animal and human studies into the

brain structural and/or functional effects of almost every sedative and anesthetic in current clinical use in a wide variety of immature animal species as well as numerous commentaries, editorials, and reviews (see Fig. 23.1).[21–68] The effects of opioid analgesics on the developing brain have also undergone scrutiny.[57,58] Accordingly, this chapter examines the specific cellular and structural effects that exposure to sedatives, anesthetics, and analgesics trigger in the immature brain.

APOPTOTIC CELL DEATH

The most widely studied deleterious structural consequence of exposure to sedatives or anesthetics on the immature mammalian brain is widespread apoptosis. Although neuronal apoptosis eliminates approximately 50% to 70% of neurons throughout the brain during the entire CNS developmental period, nerve cells eliminated by this natural process only represent a small fraction of all neurons at any particular time. Moreover, this natural process peaks at different time points in different regions of the brain. Exposure to anesthetics or sedatives briefly, but dramatically, increases the number of apoptotic neurons (Fig. 23.2). An up to 68-fold increase in the density of degenerating neurons has been observed after a combination of anesthetics in newborn rats compared with control animals.[69] A study in 7-day-old newborn mice found that a 6-hour exposure to a clinically relevant dose of isoflurane triggered apoptotic cell death in 2% of neurons in the superficial cortex, a region of the brain substantially affected at this age. In control animals, less than 0.1% of neurons underwent physiologic apoptosis in the same region, which represented a 20-fold increase in anesthesia-induced apoptosis.[70] The exact mechanism and selectivity of the cell death process remains under investigation, as dying neurons are located immediately adjacent to seemingly unaffected neighboring cells (Fig. 23.3). Increased neuroapoptosis has now been observed after in vitro and in vivo exposure to a wide variety of sedatives and anesthetics, including chloral hydrate, clonazepam, diazepam, midazolam, nitrous oxide, desflurane, enflurane, halothane, isoflurane, sevoflurane, ketamine, pentobarbital, phenobarbital, propofol, and xenon, as well as opioid receptor agonists in a wide variety of species, including fruit flies, nematodes, chicks, mice, rats, guinea pigs, piglets, and rhesus monkeys (E-Table 23.1).

Apoptosis represents an inherent, energy-consuming process using a cascade of enzymes called caspases. It is highly conserved among species and culminates in self-destruction and elimination of cells, even under physiologic conditions, when these cells are functionally redundant or potentially detrimental to the organism.[71] It involves an orderly breakdown of the cell by chromatin aggregation, nuclear and cytoplasmic condensation, and partitioning of cytoplasmic and nuclear material into apoptotic bodies for subsequent phagocytosis, without eliciting an extensive inflammatory response. This active process contrasts with features observed during another major form of cell death, necrosis, which is triggered during brain ischemia, and includes energy failure, cellular swelling, membrane rupture, and release of cytoplasmic content into the extracellular compartment, that triggers an inflammatory response.[71] However, cell death processes, such as apoptosis, necrosis, and autophagy, which were regarded as entirely separate processes in the past, are now appreciated to overlap and share pathways in common.[72] Apoptosis, which has also been termed cellular suicide or programmed cell death, is extensively used during tissue homeostasis, endocrine-dependent tissue atrophy, and normal embryogenesis (e.g., cardiac sculpting, ablation of tail tissue as part of tadpole metamorphosis in amphibians, or elimination of interdigital mesenchymal tissue of

23

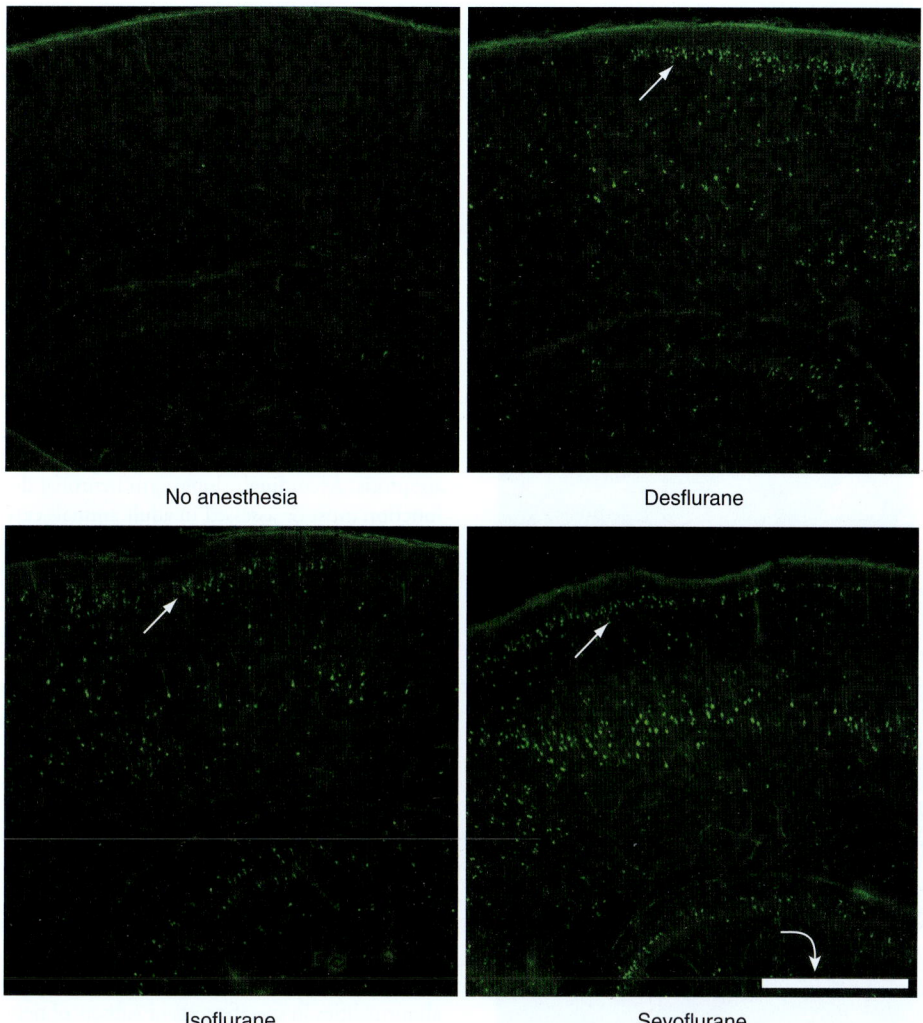

No anesthesia

Desflurane

Isoflurane

Sevoflurane

FIGURE 23.2 Prolonged exposure to anesthetics causes widespread apoptotic cell death in the developing animal brain. Representative photomicrographs of brain sections from 7- to 8-day-old mice exposed to 6 hours of equipotent doses of 7.4% *desflurane*, 1.5% *isoflurane*, 2.9% *sevoflurane* in 30% oxygen, respectively, or fasted, unanesthetized litter mates in room air *(no anesthesia)*. These doses were previously determined to represent 0.6 minimum alveolar concentration for the respective anesthetics. *Arrows* mark clusters of cells in layer II/III of the neocortex that are dying from programmed cell death and are therefore labeled for the apoptotic marker, activated caspase 3 *(bright green)*. Scale bar = 500 µm. (From Istaphanous GK, Howard J, Nan X, et al. Comparison of the neuroapoptotic properties of equipotent anesthetic concentrations of desflurane, isoflurane, or sevoflurane in neonatal mice. *Anesthesiology*. 2011;114:578-587.)

fingers and toes). Similarly, brain cells are produced in excess during normal brain development and are eliminated in large number during normal brain maturation in rodents, nonhuman primates, and humans.[6,7] This physiologic apoptotic cell death is critical to establish proper brain structure and function, and disruption of this physiological process can lead to considerable brain malformations and intrauterine demise.[73] In the developing brain, apoptotic cell death can also be triggered by pathologic extrinsic factors, such as hypoxia and ischemia.[74] It remains unclear whether anesthesia-induced neuroapoptosis accelerates physiologic programmed cell death or whether it eliminates cells not destined to die, as in pathologic apoptosis. Recent data suggest that a prolonged isoflurane exposure that eliminated up to 10% of immature dentate granule cells in neonatal mice may not lead to structural abnormalities in the surviving 90% of cells of this neuronal cohort 2 months following the exposure.[75,76]

Animal studies initially identified a narrow window of susceptibility to neuronal cell death induced by several anesthetic drugs, such as the NMDA antagonist ketamine, the GABA agonist isoflurane, or ethanol (a combined NMDA antagonist and GABA agonist). Ketamine-induced neuronal demise is most pronounced during exposure between 5 and 7 days of age in neonatal rodents or before 6 days of age in monkeys.[20,77,78] Similarly, a dramatic increase in neuronal apoptosis was detected in the cortex, thalamus, and amygdala of 3- to 10-day-old rodents after prolonged exposure to isoflurane, but minimal cell death was detected in 1-day-old animals or those older than 10 days of age.[79] However, data from one of these authors' laboratory has challenged the notion that anesthetic-induced neuroapoptosis is limited to a narrow age range. Similar to previous studies, neuronal apoptosis was observed in the cortex and hippocampus of 7-day-old mice after exposure to isoflurane; however, vulnerability extended to older

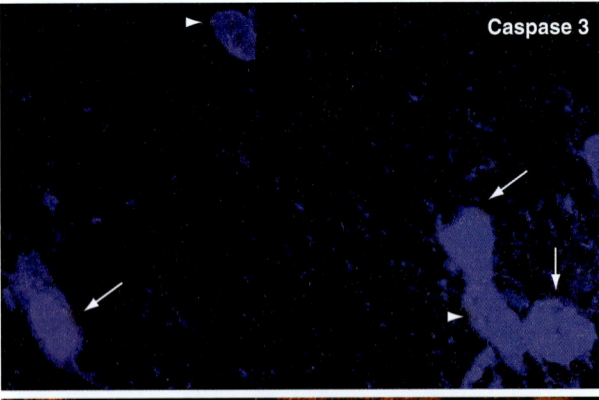

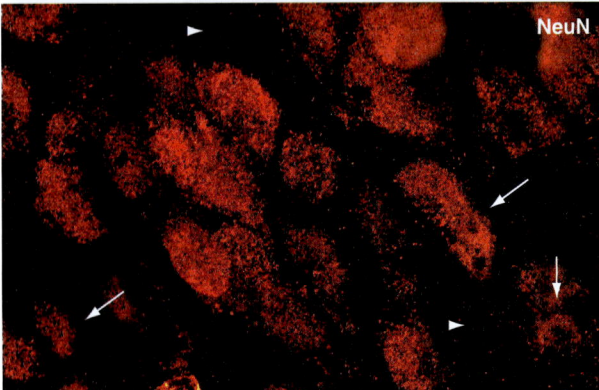

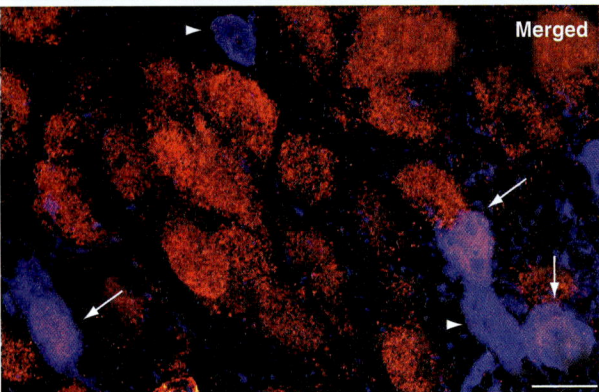

FIGURE 23.3 Neurons affected by apoptotic cell death following anesthetic exposure are surrounded by seemingly unaffected cells. Representative photomicrograph from a 7-day-old mouse following a 6-hour exposure to 1.5% isoflurane, showing neocortical cells stained for the apoptotic cell death marker activated caspase 3 *(blue, top)*, the neuronal marker NeuN *(red, middle)*, and a merged image of the two stains *(bottom)*. The majority of dying cells are identified as postmitotic neurons, as indicated by the purple cells coexpressing activated caspase 3 and NeuN in the bottom *(arrows)*, whereas some cells expressing caspase 3 are NeuN-negative *(arrowheads)*. Importantly, cells affected by anesthetic-induced neuroapoptosis are surrounded by numerous, seemingly unaffected neurons. Scale bar = 10 μm. (Image courtesy Loepke Laboratory.)

animals, even into adulthood, in brain regions experiencing ongoing neurogenesis, such as the dentate and olfactory bulb.[80] Importantly, neurons were found particularly vulnerable to isoflurane-induced apoptotic cell death under 14 days of cellular age and accordingly anesthesia-induced neurodegeneration would be expected to occur throughout life in neurogenic niches containing immature neurons.[81] Other studies suggest that intrauterine exposure to clinical doses of isoflurane in prenatal rats may actually

decrease physiologic apoptosis and improve subsequent memory retention,[82] whereas only supraclinical doses of isoflurane-induced neuroapoptosis in this setting.[83] Chronic opioid exposure in immature animal models can lead to long-term neurodegeneration[83–85]; however, no neuronal cell death was found immediately after a brief exposure to morphine in newborn rats.[86] Additional research is needed to further elucidate the timing of exposure and brain regional variability on cellular demise and the differential effects of anesthetics and analgesics on brain structural integrity.

LONG-TERM BRAIN CELLULAR VIABILITY, NEUROLOGIC FUNCTION, AND BEHAVIOR

To better understand the long-term effects of the dramatic escalation of the natural process of neuronal apoptotic cell death during anesthetic exposure, it is critical to appreciate whether anesthetics simply hasten natural apoptosis or whether they induce pathologic apoptosis. Accordingly, long-term neuronal density and neurologic function must be assessed in adult animals exposed to anesthesia as neonates. If exposure to anesthetics or analgesics only temporarily accelerated physiologic apoptosis, one would expect normal cellular density and function in adulthood. Conversely, permanent neuronal cell loss and long-term neurocognitive impairment after anesthetic exposure early in life would suggest that anesthesia-induced neuronal apoptosis may be pathologic in nature and that the organism was unable to compensate for the neonatal cell loss by postexposure neuronal plasticity and repair. To address these questions, several studies measured neurologic function, assessed behavior, and/or determined neuronal density in adult animals after anesthetic exposure in the neonatal period. Results from these studies, however, are conflicting. A number of studies reported long-term neurocognitive or behavioral abnormalities after neonatal exposure to enflurane, halothane, isoflurane, sevoflurane, propofol, or ketamine, or to a combination of isoflurane, nitrous oxide, and midazolam.[16,17,69,87–101] However, many of these studies only observed abnormalities in specific tests or subsets of neurocognitive batteries, whereas other neurobehavioral domains remained unaffected. For example, a 6-hour exposure to midazolam, isoflurane, and nitrous oxide in neonatal rats transiently impaired spatial learning in a water maze task in adulthood, whereas in the same animals, several other tests of behavior and learning, including acoustic startle response, sensorimotor tests, spontaneous behavior in an open field, and learning and memory in the radial arms maze, remained unimpaired.[69] After a 4-hour exposure to 1 minimum alveolar concentration (1 MAC) of isoflurane in 7-day-old rats, long-term memory retention was abnormal at two times, whereas performance at several other times, as well as in other tests of learning and memory, remained intact.[91] The relevance of these temporary and limited learning deficits remain unclear. Similar to humans, the performance of rodents and primates in learning tasks depends to a great extent on maternal behavior and rearing conditions, making them strong confounders of offspring cognitive performance.[102–105] Another obvious and important factor in neurocognitive testing is to verify that similar degrees of motivation were present when comparing separate groups of animals. For example, a 24-hour exposure to ketamine sedation early in life impaired subsequent performance of rhesus monkeys in learning and memory tests, in addition to decreasing their motivation to perform these tasks.[98]

Studies of prolonged opioid administration in immature animals have also yielded evidence of long-term impaired learning tasks,[106–111] and altered pain responses in adult animals after exposure to morphine, fentanyl, heroin, or methadone early in life.[83,112–116]

Conversely, several other investigations have observed no neurologic abnormalities after administration of midazolam, isoflurane, sevoflurane, or ketamine, even when using complex neurologic tests in neonatal animals.[82,90,99,102,117–123] It remains to be determined whether these differential findings are attributable to the anesthetic doses, exposure times, species, or are related to the specific testing conditions or the timing of the exposure or the assessment, relative to brain maturational state. Interestingly, escalating exposure times of isoflurane in neonatal rats caused neuronal apoptosis beginning at 2 hours of anesthesia, but no evidence of long-term neurologic abnormalities until 4 hours of anesthesia.[90] In another study, a 6-hour exposure to isoflurane caused significant apoptosis immediately after exposure in neonatal mice but no measurable long-term deficits in performance of complex neurologic tests as adult animals.[102] Moreover, brain neuronal density in adulthood was not diminished in regions significantly affected by anesthesia-induced neuroapoptosis compared with unanesthetized littermates.[102] Studies in mice exposed to 6 hours of isoflurane at 21 days of age did not observe subsequent diminution in dentate granule cells, despite considerable apoptotic cell death immediately after exposure.[124] These findings could either suggest that isoflurane may only accelerate physiologic apoptosis or that the developing brain's plasticity and capacity for repair can compensate for a pathologic insult early in life. Conversely, a study in similarly aged rats observed a permanent elimination of neurons, as well as neurologic abnormalities in adult animals, after exposure to isoflurane, nitrous oxide, and midazolam as neonates, suggesting that either the specific combination of anesthetic drugs (isoflurane alone vs. the combination exposure) or species differences (rats vs. mice) could affect relationships between neonatal neuroapoptosis and long-term function and neuronal density.[125] These conflicting results may be explained by the dissimilar testing environment because neurocognitive tests are not easily transferable among laboratories.[126] Another explanation posits that neonatal apoptosis may not be causally linked to adult neurocognitive performance at all, as evidenced by substantial apoptotic cell death observed immediately after carbon dioxide–induced hypercarbia in unanesthetized neonatal rats, which lacked long-term neurologic sequelae.[91]

EFFECTS ON NEUROGENESIS AND GLIOGENESIS

The generation of new neurons, or neurogenesis, as well as new astrocytes—gliogenesis—is most active in the immature brain in utero or soon after birth. Accordingly, several studies have investigated the effects of anesthetic exposure, primarily isoflurane, on progenitor viability and rates of neurogenesis. Although isoflurane did not kill neural progenitor cells in vitro, 3.4% isoflurane for 4 hours decreased the rate of neuronal proliferation and increased neuronal fate selection.[127] These findings have been confirmed as 2.8% isoflurane for 6 hours had no effect on neural stem cell viability, whereas larger doses inhibited cell proliferation.[128] In vivo studies in newborn mice failed to find significant cell death in radial glial-type progenitor cells in the dentate gyrus immediately after a 6-hour isoflurane exposure, although more mature neuroblasts made up a substantial number of cells affected by anesthesia-induced apoptotic cell death.[81] Morphine did not affect cell survival in a murine cerebellar neuronal precursor culture, although exposure decreased DNA synthesis.[129]

After a 24-hour administration of 3% isoflurane, the growth of cultured immature astrocytes was impaired and their maturation was delayed; however, even this extreme exposure showed no effect on cell viability.[130] Morphine increased apoptosis in neurons and microglia, but did not affect astrocytes in a study involving human fetal cell cultures.[131] A recent study in nonhuman primates found astrogliosis in several brain regions up to 2 years after exposing infant primates to isoflurane.[132]

ALTERATIONS IN DENDRITIC ARCHITECTURE

The immature brain accumulates an overabundance of neuronal connections in infancy, and the number of dendrites and synapses dramatically decreases after the first year of life. Several studies have examined the effects of a wide variety of anesthetics, such as propofol, isoflurane, sevoflurane, desflurane, midazolam, and ketamine on dendritic arborization and synaptic architecture.[133–142] A common theme in these studies is that anesthetics can affect dendritic arborization and synaptic density, and that the direction of any change, either an increase or a decrease in the number of dendritic spines, depends on the age at which the animals were exposed to anesthetics, and therefore, the developmental state of the brain. During the first 2 weeks of life, anesthetic exposure can lead to a decrease in synaptic and dendritic spine density in small rodents exposed to isoflurane, sevoflurane, or propofol-based anesthetics,[132,139,143,144] whereas exposure beyond this age can lead to an increase in the number of dendrites.[135,142] Other studies suggest that this differential effect may depend on the maturational switch of GABA from excitation to inhibition, which is related to the switch from the immature form of the potassium-chloride-cotransporter $Na^+-K^+-2Cl^-$ cotransporter 1 (NKCC1) to the mature K^+-Cl^- cotransporter 2 (KCC2). However, the permanence of these dendritic changes remains controversial because some studies have observed only a transient effect after ketamine, midazolam, or isoflurane anesthesia exposure early in life.[136,140]

DECREASE IN TROPHIC FACTORS

Isoflurane-, sevoflurane-, ketamine-, or propofol-based anesthesia in neonatal animals has been associated with a diminution in brain-derived neurotrophic factor (BDNF),[100,134,143,145–148] a protein integral to neuronal survival, growth, and differentiation. The cellular mechanism involves a reduction in tissue plasminogen activator and plasmin, which converts proBDNF to BDNF. As expected, isoflurane triggers proBDNF/p75[NTR] (p75 neurotrophin receptor) complex–mediated apoptosis in neonatal mice.[134] Similarly, prolonged exposure to opioid receptor agonists early in life alters nerve growth factors in the immature brain.[149,150]

DEGENERATION OF MITOCHONDRIA

Administration of inhaled anesthetics in neonatal rodents, such as repeated sevoflurane exposures, has been found to result in substantial homeostatic disruption of the cell's energy producing organelles, such as increased mitochondrial reactive oxygen species production and cytoplasmic calcium levels, opening of the mitochondrial permeability transition pore, and decrease in the mitochondrial membrane potential.[144] Ultrastructural morphologic abnormalities have been reported in mitochondria of pyramidal neurons in the subiculum of 7-day-old rats after 6 hours of isoflurane, nitrous oxide, and midazolam.[151] A morphometric analysis demonstrated mitochondrial enlargement, impaired structural integrity, and decreased mitochondrial density, indicating protracted mitochondrial injury after drug exposure.[152,153] Moreover, an ultrastructural examination with electron microscopy revealed increased autophagy, a form of cell death.[151] Exposure to several general anesthetics, such as isoflurane,[154] sevoflurane,[155] propofol,[156,157] and ketamine,[158,159] can lead to mitochondrial fission and apoptosis in immature animals and cell cultures.

ABNORMAL REENTRY INTO CELL CYCLE

Ketamine induces reentry of postmitotic neurons into the cell cycle in immature rats.[160] Similarly, cell cycle activation has been found to contribute to isoflurane-induced neurotoxicity in developing mice.[161] This could be one trigger for apoptotic cell death, since postmitotic neurons lose the ability of neuronal progenitor cells to enter the cell cycle during proliferation and are committing programmed cell death when forced to reenter the cell cycle.

DESTABILIZATION OF THE CYTOSKELETON

Structural integrity of the cellular cytoskeleton is critical for proper neuronal morphology and function. Actin is one of the major components of the cytoskeleton of all eukaryotic cells and participates in important cellular processes, including cell signaling, motility, and division. It is also essential for the formation of dendritic spines. Isoflurane has been found to depolymerize actin in neurons and astrocytes, initiating cytoskeletal destabilization, impairing astrocyte morphologic differentiation and maturation, and neuronal apoptosis.[130,162]

GENOMIC, PROTEOMIC, AND EPIGENETIC ALTERATIONS

Neonatal anesthesia leads to long-term alterations in gene and protein expression, as well as epigenetic modifications, heritable alterations in gene expression that are not a result of alterations of the DNA sequence. Neonatal rats exposed to 2 hours of sevoflurane on 3 consecutive days led to long-term cognitive impairment, hypermethylation of BDNF and Reelin genes, and subsequent downregulation of BDNF and Reelin genes, which decreased dendritic spines in the hippocampal pyramidal neurons in adolescence.[163] Repeated isoflurane or sevoflurane exposures in neonatal mice also led to disturbances in synaptogenesis, altered social interactions, and mRNA modifications that were associated with critical metabolic, developmental, and immune functions. The proteins altered by isoflurane were mainly associated with epilepsy, ataxia, and brain development, whereas sevoflurane altered proteins involved in social behavior.[164] Neonatal mice exposed to sevoflurane sustained impaired long-term memory that was associated with increased DNA (cytosine-5)-methyltransferase 1 (DNMT1), DNMT3a, and 5-methylcytosine levels and decreased ten-eleven translocation methylcytosine dioxygenase 1 (TET1) and 5-hydromethylcytosine levels. Sevoflurane subsequently induced hypermethylation of the hippocampal synaptic genes SHANK2, PSD95, SYN1, and SYP and downregulated the expression of synaptic proteins, which decreased synaptic density.[165] Sevoflurane-exposed rats also exhibited reduced hippocampal density of dendritic spines, levels of the BDNF, c-fos protein, microtubule-associated protein 2, synapsin1, postsynaptic density protein 95, pCREB/CREB, CREB binding protein, and acetylated histones H3 and H4, and increased levels of histone deacetylases 3 and 8.[166] Isoflurane, nitrous oxide, and midazolam caused epigenetic modulations manifested by histone-3 hypoacetylation and fragmentation of cAMP-responsive element-binding protein with decreased histone acetyltransferase activity that downregulated transcription of BDNF and the cellular Finkel-Biskis-Jinkins murine sarcoma virus osteosarcoma oncogene.[167] Unanesthetized male offspring of rat mothers who were anesthetized with sevoflurane as infants had transgenerational effects of decreased DNA methylation epigenetic modification of KCC2 expression.[168,169] Several hypermethylated genes, related to neurite growth and neuronal plasticity, were found in female macaques and twice as many in male macaques who were anesthetized as neonates and infants for three separate 4-hour sevoflurane

anesthetics.[170] Learning abnormalities observed after propofol anesthesia in neonatal rat pups were linked to downregulation of miR-132, noncoding microRNA molecules that regulate gene expression and play a critical role in hippocampal neuronal morphogenesis, mediating dendritic growth and spine formation.[171] A study observed miR-124 associated spatial learning abnormalities in neonatal mice anesthetized with ketamine.[172] This review provides additional discussion.[173]

EFFECTS ON THE DEVELOPING SPINAL CORD

Most animal studies have focused on the effects of general anesthetics and sedatives on the developing brain. However, it is important to also consider the developmental impact of anesthetics on the spinal cord. Neuroapoptosis is increased in the lumbar spinal cord of 7-day-old rats after 6 hours of 0.75% isoflurane with 75% nitrous oxide.[174] Increased neurodegeneration was also documented in the brain and spinal cord after 6 hours of 1% isoflurane in a similar model, but not after 1 hour of anesthesia or after spinal administration of bupivacaine.[175] Intrathecal ketamine can cause neuroapoptosis in the developing spinal cord of 3-day-old rats, but not of 7-day-old rats.[176] Preservative-free ketamine caused long-term alterations in spinal cord function and gait disturbances,[176] whereas in a separate study, even high-dose intrathecal morphine caused no evidence of spinal cord toxicity.[177]

Putative Mechanisms for Neurotoxicity

The exact mechanisms by which anesthetics and sedatives impact the immature brain and spinal cord remain unresolved. Elucidating these mechanisms will be critical in establishing the relevance of these findings for pediatric anesthesia and neonatal critical care medicine, as well as for developing mitigating interventions, if necessary. The current, overarching hypothesis is that anesthetics and sedatives interfere with normal GABA$_A$ and NMDA receptor mediated activity, which are the putative targets for unconsciousness, amnesia, and immobility,[178] and at the same time are essential for mammalian CNS development.[12,179] Administering GABA$_A$-receptor agonists and/or NMDA-receptor antagonists could potentially cause abnormal neuronal inhibition during a vulnerable period in neuronal development, triggering apoptosis in susceptible neurons, which in turn impairs neurocognitive development and decreases neuronal density into adulthood.[25,63,69,125] Other lines of evidence suggest that the NMDA receptor blocking properties of ketamine may upregulate NMDA receptors, rendering neurons more susceptible to excitotoxic injury caused by endogenous glutamate action on the increased number of receptors immediately after withdrawal of the anesthetic such as proposed for ketamine.[78,180] However, several observations partly contradict both hypotheses; neuronal cell death has been reported during exposure to anesthetics and not only after their discontinuation. Moreover, several anesthetics with minimal NMDA-receptor interaction, such as propofol and barbiturates, have demonstrated robust neurotoxic properties, whereas the neurotoxic potency of the NMDA antagonist xenon has been found to be limited, therefore casting doubt on receptor upregulation as the sole mechanism for anesthetic neurotoxicity. In terms of abnormal neuronal inhibition being the main trigger for apoptosis in developing neurons, GABA$_A$-receptor stimulation decreases neuronal activity in the mature brain; however, it also causes excitation in developing neurons,[181] thereby contradicting the inhibition hypothesis. In immature neurons, intracellular chloride (Cl$^-$) concentration is high; thus GABA-induced opening of Cl$^-$ channels allows this anion to exit the cell, leading to membrane depolarization. In mature neurons, the intracellular Cl⁻ concentration is low. When anesthetics open Cl⁻ channels in mature neurons, ions enter the cell, thereby hyperpolarizing the membrane. This reversal of the cellular Cl⁻ gradient occurs as a result of a switch from the immature potassium-chloride-cotransporter 1 to the mature brain form, potassium-chloride cotransporter 2.[182] Studies in neonatal rats demonstrated excitatory properties in the brain and episodes of epileptic seizures during sevoflurane anesthesia.[183] Isoflurane also triggers release of excessive amounts of Ca^{2+} from the endoplasmic reticulum via overactivation of inositol 1,4,5-trisphosphate receptors (InsP3Rs) in neonatal rats in vivo and in vitro.[184] A similar mechanism may be linked to the production of Alzheimer-associated increases in β-amyloid protein levels after anesthesia.[185] Although xenon and hypothermia inhibit neurons, they do not exacerbate isoflurane-induced neuronal cell death as expected by the cumulative inhibition of neurons, but rather significantly reduce it.[186–188] Isoflurane-induced diminution of aquaporin-4, a key protein in waste clearance pathways of the brain that is involved in synaptic plasticity and neurocognition, has been linked to more apoptotic cell death in neonatal rats.[189]

General anesthesia in developing animals triggers a neuroinflammatory response that can lead to oxidative damage, microglial activation, and production of interleukin-6 (IL-6), tumor necrosis factor alpha (TNF-α), and IL-1β.[190,191] Anesthesia-induced oxidative stress and neuroinflammation have been linked to immediate structural abnormalities and long-term cognitive impairment for several anesthetics, including propofol, ketamine,[145,192] isoflurane,[193] and sevoflurane.[144,194]

Evidence indicates that equianesthetic concentrations of the three contemporary inhaled anesthetics cause similar degrees of neuroapoptosis, suggesting that it is the anesthetic depth and not the specific doses or end-tidal concentrations of the anesthetics that determine cytotoxic potency.[195] However, other studies have failed to link the anesthetic and the apoptotic mechanisms. Specifically, although racemic ketamine and (S)-ketamine both elicit their anesthetic effects via NMDA-receptor blockade, (S)-ketamine induced up to 80% less cell death in vitro compared with equipotent doses of racemic ketamine.[196] Moreover, concomitant administration of the GABAₐ-receptor antagonist gabazine failed to attenuate neuroapoptosis induced by the GABA agonist isoflurane, in contrast to the α₂-agonist dexmedetomidine.[197] Decreases in anesthetic-induced neuronal activity may therefore be less important than the disruption of the neuronal balance of excitation and inhibition, as demonstrated by studies of changes in anesthesia-induced dendritic morphology in mice.[133,139] In a mechanistic study of brain development, simultaneous blockade of excitatory and inhibitory activity with tetrodotoxin did not cause structural changes during synaptogenesis that would have been expected from a causative relationship between neuronal inhibition and structural abnormalities; the administration of either GABAₐ-agonistic or NMDA-antagonistic compounds alone did alter synaptogenesis.[139]

It is not entirely clear at this time whether cytotoxicity is a direct effect of the anesthetic itself, of any anesthetic by-products, or if it is related to physiologic derangements observed during anesthesia, especially in small rodents.[91,102,198] Hypercarbia can trigger widespread neuroapoptosis,[91] even in unanesthetized neonatal rats exposed to increased partial pressures of carbon dioxide. Whereas apoptotic cell death was quantitatively indistinguishable from neurodegeneration in isoflurane-treated litter mates, which were also hypercarbic; neurocognitive impairment in adults was observed only in the isoflurane-treated animals.[91] However, widespread apoptotic neurodegeneration observed in anesthetized nonhuman primates, where carbon dioxide tensions were controlled by tracheal intubation and ventilation, suggests that metabolic derangements may not be sufficient to explain the structural abnormalities observed in immature animal species. Experimental models of neurodegeneration have also implicated reentry of postmitotic neurons into the cell cycle, leading to cell death. Ketamine exposure has been found to induce aberrant cell cycle reentry, leading to apoptotic cell death in the developing rat brain.[160] However, a causative link between neuronal degeneration immediately after exposure and subsequent cognitive abnormalities observed into adulthood have yet to be firmly established.

Specific Anesthetic and Sedative Agents

To provide a succinct overview of the available laboratory data, we briefly review the effects of each class of anesthetics separately. Although the effects of some anesthetics, such as ketamine and isoflurane, have been extensively studied in the developing brain, the effects of others, such as xenon and desflurane, have not been examined in depth. However, data suggest that all commonly used anesthetics exert deleterious effects to some degree (see E-Table 23.1 for a representative overview of animal studies). When examining the available animal literature, it is important to acknowledge that the potencies of inhaled anesthetics, as measured in MAC values (a concentration measure), are comparable across species, whereas doses for intravenous (IV) medications are not—that is, weight-based dosing rather than concentration varies substantively. Weight-based dosing of most IV medications to effect sedation or anesthesia in animals is approximately 6- to 10-fold greater than comparable doses in humans. The dosing is further complicated by the different routes used to administer these drugs in most neonatal animal models, frequently relying on the subcutaneous and intraperitoneal routes as opposed to the oral or IV routes used in humans. However, the possible importance of these interspecies pharmacodynamic differences on brain structural and functional outcomes has not yet been adequately addressed.

KETAMINE

The injectable anesthetic most frequently studied in this context is ketamine, an antagonist of the NMDA glutamate receptor that also interacts with other cell membrane proteins, such as muscarinic, nicotinic, and opioid receptors, and voltage-gated calcium channels. Ketamine's properties, which include potent analgesia, dissociative anesthesia, and relative hemodynamic stability, have made it a popular choice for procedural sedation and induction of anesthesia in children with concerns for hemodynamic stability, such as critical congenital heart disease or pulmonary hypertension.[199–201] However, a seminal study examining the effects of repeated intraperitoneal injections of ketamine on the brain of neonatal rats observed widespread apoptotic cell death.[20] Seven injections of 20 mg/kg of ketamine, administered to 7-day-old rat pups over a 9-hour period in evenly divided intervals, caused a 3- to 31-fold increase in degenerating neurons, depending on the brain region, compared with vehicle-injected control animals. This has led to speculation that these changes might contribute to subsequent neuropsychiatric disorders.[20] These initial findings for ketamine have been confirmed in several dozen rodent studies, as well as nonhuman primates, both in vitro and in vivo (see E-Table 23.1). Several of these studies have identified relationships between neurodegeneration and dose, number of injections, and animal species and age during exposure. Single doses up to 75 mg/kg or multiple intraperitoneal injections up to 17 mg/kg per hour for 6 hours were not neurotoxic to neonatal rats.[202] In contrast, single doses between 20 and 50 mg/kg subcutaneous in neonatal mice[95,203] or six or seven repeated injections of 20 to 25 mg/kg intraperitoneal consistently led to apoptosis in the neonatal rat brain.[20,202,204–206] Although these doses appear to be excessive compared with clinical practice, and plasma concentrations in these rodents were up to 7 times greater than those in humans,[204] these doses of ketamine were required for sedation owing to increased requirements for IV anesthetics in small animals based on body weight (refer to the later section Critical Evaluation of Animal Studies and Interspecies Comparisons). Moreover, coadministration of midazolam, diazepam, propofol, or thiopental can compound the neuronal injury caused by ketamine.[95,96,203] Studies in rats, mice, and nonhuman primates suggest that susceptibility to ketamine-induced neurotoxicity may be most pronounced during a brief period after birth, with a maximum impact between 3 and 7 days of age in small rodents and less than 35 days of age in monkeys.[20,78] In vitro electrophysiological studies suggest a compensatory enhancement of currents at NMDA receptors specific to the developing brain resulting in apoptotic cell death of immature neurons.[207] In addition to neuronal apoptosis, both small rodents and nonhuman primates that were anesthetized with ketamine also exhibited impaired learning tasks later in life.[87,94,98,164,208–212] Repeated neonatal ketamine exposure also interferes with the integration of adult-generated neurons into hippocampal dentate gyrus neural circuits and causes deficits in hippocampal-dependent spatial reference memory tasks.[213] Prolonged ketamine administration in pregnant mice led to attention-deficit/hyperactivity disorder (ADHD)-like behavior and depression in their offspring.[76] In murine neuronal cell culture, ketamine-induced neurotoxicity via endoplasmic reticulum stress-dependent apoptotic pathways,[214] as well as astrocyte-derived extracellular vesicles.[145] Ketamine also induces neural death, reactive oxygen species augmentation, neural apoptosis, and neurite degeneration in human embryonic stem cell-derived neurons.[215]

Ketamine is one of the earliest and most frequently studied anesthetics in terms of its neurotoxic effects, and has repeatedly been shown to cause widespread apoptosis (an effect that is exacerbated by the coadministration of other anesthetics). Moreover, during the brain developmental period, ketamine contributes to inflammation, autophagy, increases oxidative stress, and can lead to neurologic impairment in adult animals exposed early in life.[145,192,208] Ketamine impairs long-lasting learning and causes white-matter structural abnormalities in nonhuman primates, the closest animal model to humans.[98,164,212] It is unclear whether lack of motivation to complete learning tasks in this model may be linked to the observed learning abnormalities.[98]

INHALED ANESTHETICS

Another commonly studied class of drugs is the inhaled anesthetics (see E-Table 23.1). Desflurane, sevoflurane, isoflurane, enflurane, and halothane exert their anesthetic properties predominantly by their agonistic effects on the GABA$_A$ receptor, but also to differing degrees on glycine, NMDA, acetylcholine, serotonin (5-HT$_3$), α-amino-3-hydroxy-5-methyl-4-isoxazole-propionic acid (AMPA), and kainate receptors. Whereas GABA represents the main inhibitory neurotransmitter in the adult CNS, it has excitatory properties in the developing brain,[181] which may have implications for neurotoxicity, as discussed. Most studies of inhaled anesthetics examined either isoflurane by itself or in combination with midazolam and

nitrous oxide. This combination of GABA agonists and NMDA antagonists has been repeatedly found to cause widespread brain cell degeneration in neonatal animals.[69,79,148,216] In addition to the immediate deleterious effects on brain structure, long-term abnormalities in spatial learning tasks and decreased neuronal cell density in adult rats have also been observed after exposure to this anesthetic combination early in life.[69,125] One MAC of isoflurane administered to neonatal rats as the sole anesthetic for 4 hours led to neurocognitive deficits in rats when they matured to adults.[90,91] Up to 0.6 MAC for 6 hours in neonatal mice caused widespread neuronal degeneration immediately after exposure, although it failed to lead to neurocognitive deficits or decreases in neuronal density in adulthood.[102,118] These inconsistencies raise questions of whether neonatal neuronal apoptotic cell death during exposure is causatively linked to long-term behavioral and learning abnormalities observed in adult animals. In fact, similar degrees of neurodegeneration were observed in 7-day-old rats after a 4-hour exposure to either carbon dioxide or isoflurane; however, long-term neurocognitive deficits were observed only after the anesthetic exposure.[91] Widespread neuronal cell death has also been observed in neonatal rhesus monkeys after 5 hours of isoflurane in concentrations between 0.75% and 1.5%,[217] although long-term neurologic studies in this species have yet to be published.

Sevoflurane has also induced widespread neuroapoptosis in neonatal mice similar to isoflurane,[101,118,195] but the long-term effects on learning and behavior are conflicting.[101,117,118] Systemic inflammation exacerbated developmental neurotoxicity by worsening sevoflurane-induced neuronal damage and behavioral abnormalities in newborn mice.[218] Repeated sevoflurane anesthesia upregulated RNA N^6-methyladenosine (m6A) methylation in the prefrontal cortex of infant rhesus macaques, which may alter synaptic plasticity.[170] In a human neuroblastoma cell model, sevoflurane triggers both cell death processes, apoptosis and autophagy.[219] Few studies have examined desflurane in this context. Desflurane causes age- and species-dependent neuronal cell death in 7-day-old mice, but not 16-day-old rats.[133,195]

Several studies compared the neurotoxicity of contemporary inhaled anesthetics. Equianesthetic concentrations of 0.6 MAC of desflurane, isoflurane, or sevoflurane for 6 hours in neonatal mice caused a similar degree of neuronal degeneration in superficial neocortex, a brain region significantly affected in this model.[195] These results contrast with studies in which neonatal mice were exposed to much smaller concentrations of sevoflurane that resulted in less immediate neuronal loss compared with isoflurane, albeit no neurocognitive performance deficits were observed in adult animals with either regimen.[118] In another comparative study in mice, desflurane caused greater injury than isoflurane or sevoflurane, which demonstrated comparable degrees of neurodegeneration, and long-term neurologic impairment occurred only after exposure to desflurane.[117] In neonatal rats, 4 hours of 1 MAC of isoflurane or sevoflurane caused deficits in a spatial learning task evaluated 2 weeks after exposure, with slightly worse outcome after isoflurane.[220] The significance of these differential findings remains unclear but could be related to methodologic differences in the assessment of brain injury. However, these conflicting results prohibit any clinical recommendations for choosing one particular inhaled anesthetic over another.

Although largely phased out from clinical anesthesia practice, halothane and enflurane also induce brain abnormalities. These anesthetic vapors were initially studied in rat models of chronic occupational exposure during pregnancy, causing delayed synaptogenesis as well as behavioral and learning abnormalities.[16–19,88]

Inhaled anesthetics represent one of the most frequently used classes of anesthetics in pediatric anesthesia, and their neurotoxic properties have been extensively studied. Widespread apoptosis immediately after exposure in a large variety of animal models, including nonhuman primates, is a consistent finding. However, neurologic impairment in adult animals exposed to anesthesia early in life has not been consistently found, and in fact, some studies failed to observe any neurologic impairment at all. Accordingly, long-lasting impaired learning has not been convincingly linked to neonatal neuroapoptosis. Primate studies on long-term neurocognitive outcomes after inhaled anesthesia early in life have yet to be published.

NITROUS OXIDE

Nitrous oxide, an NMDA antagonist, is the oldest anesthetic still in clinical use, although its low potency (MAC of 115% in adult humans) necessitates the coadministration of other anesthetics to provide surgical anesthesia. Anesthetic combinations studied in this context have often included the GABA agonist midazolam, and the mixed GABA agonist/NMDA antagonist isoflurane.[69,79,125,148,216,221,222] In rats, nitrous oxide alone did not induce neuronal apoptosis,[69,79,186] whereas in an in vitro study, it caused neuronal cell death in hippocampal slices in mice.[186] When administered in combination with other anesthetics, however, nitrous oxide exacerbated neuronal cell death induced by isoflurane and also contributed to long-term neurologic abnormalities in rats when combined with isoflurane and midazolam.[69]

XENON

Because of the cost differential between other inhaled anesthetics and this rare, colorless, and odorless noble gas, xenon has not achieved widespread clinical use, despite its NMDA-antagonistic anesthetic properties.[223] Xenon has a relatively low anesthetic potency, with a MAC measuring between 65% and 70% in adults,[224,225] but a very low blood-gas solubility that facilitates a rapid onset and emergence from anesthesia.[226] Xenon's effects on neuronal apoptosis have been examined in two in vivo studies, with slightly differing results. Although 75% xenon for 6 hours did not cause neuronal apoptosis in 7-day-old rat pups,[186] 70% xenon for 4 hours increased neuroapoptosis in 7-day-old mice.[188] Both studies demonstrated that xenon decreased the neurodegeneration induced by isoflurane anesthesia,[186,188] which may have relevance to the phenomenon's putative mechanism (see later text). An investigation of xenon's effects on neuronal viability in hippocampal slice cultures observed neuronal cell death after exposure to more than 0.75 MAC of xenon for 6 hours.[227] In this setting, isoflurane pretreatment reduced neuronal cell death caused by 1 MAC of xenon,[227] again demonstrating the confusing finding that combinations of anesthetics can have both exacerbating and ameliorating effects related to their respective neurotoxic properties.

BENZODIAZEPINES

The effects of benzodiazepines, such as clonazepam, diazepam, and midazolam, on the immature brain, either alone or in combination with other drugs have been studied. These GABA agonists are most frequently used for anxiolysis in toddlers and older children in the perioperative setting, but they are also used in premature neonates in the critical care setting. Repeat exposure to benzodiazepines can increase neuronal degeneration in small-animal models, depending on the dose, region of the brain, species, and age of the animal studied. Repeat injections of midazolam for

6 hours increased neuronal cell death in neonatal rats,[228] whereas single doses of intraperitoneal 5 mg/kg of diazepam or 9 mg/kg of midazolam did not.[69,229] Although 5 mg/kg of subcutaneous diazepam caused neuronal cell death in some brain regions in mice, this was not associated with learning deficits in adulthood.[87] In these studies, the neuroapoptosis associated with diazepam was augmented by the coadministration of other sedatives, such as ketamine.[87] Similarly, the combination of midazolam and caffeine caused widespread neuroapoptosis in a premature mouse model.[230] The dose-dependence of neuroapoptosis observed in neonatal rats is highlighted by the fact that diazepam doses of 10 mg/kg or greater have been found to be injurious,[77,229] an effect that was prevented in one study by the coadministration of the benzodiazepine-antagonist flumazenil.[229] Two studies reported no neurocognitive learning disabilities in adult mice after they were sedated with diazepam or midazolam as neonates.[87,123] It is therefore unclear whether dose- or species-specific factors are responsible for the disparate findings.

CHLORAL HYDRATE

The sedative chloral hydrate, a chlorination product of ethanol that acts as a combined GABA agonist and NMDA antagonist, has been largely supplanted by barbiturates and benzodiazepines in pediatric clinical practice. However, it is still used in doses of up to 120 mg/kg for sedation for some imaging studies,[231] and its neurotoxic properties have been investigated in a single animal study. Preliminary results indicate that it causes neuroapoptosis in the cerebral cortex and the caudate-putamen complex in immature mouse pups in doses of 100 mg/kg or greater.[187] The neurofunctional outcome in adult mice, however, has not as yet been investigated.

BARBITURATES

Barbiturates act primarily via the $GABA_A$ receptor but also exert effects via nicotinic acetylcholine, AMPA, and kainate receptors. Thiopental in subcutaneous doses of 25 mg/kg does not induce apoptosis in neonatal mice, although when doses as small as 5 mg/kg are combined with 25 mg/kg of ketamine subcutaneously, neuronal degeneration and impaired long-term learning and memory are reported.[96] Pentobarbital and phenobarbital induce neurodegeneration in mouse and rat pups. Furthermore, after receiving these sedatives as neonates, long-term alterations in brain protein expression and abnormalities in learning and memory have been observed,[89,232,233] although in one study these long-term alterations may be attributable in part to hypoxia and hypercarbia during the neonatal sedation.[232] Interestingly, estradiol has been shown to attenuate phenobarbital-induced neuroapoptosis.[229,234]

PROPOFOL

Propofol predominantly acts via GABA and glycine receptor-agonistic properties, but also weakly on nicotinic, AMPA, and NMDA receptors. Its neurotoxic profile has been repeatedly studied both in vitro and in vivo. Propofol has consistently caused neuroapoptosis after single doses greater than 50 mg/kg (subcutaneous or intraperitoneal) or repeated doses greater than 20 mg/kg per hour for 4 to 5 hours in neonatal rodents.[96,99,235,236] Interestingly, lithium prevents propofol-induced neuroapoptosis in neonatal mice.[235] However, after 24 hours of IV anesthesia with propofol (6 mg/kg per hour) and fentanyl (10 μg/kg per hour), no evidence of apoptosis was found in a pig model.[237] Apart from overt neuronal cell death, propofol also decreased the effect of

GABAergic enzyme glutamic acid decarboxylase,[238] diminished nerve growth factors,[100,239] and caused neurite growth cone collapse in tissue culture.[240] In addition, propofol alters dendritic spine architecture in developing rats, depending on the age at the time of anesthetic exposure.[142] Specifically, dendritic spine density decreased during exposures in the first week of life, but increased if the exposure occurred during week 3 of life; the mechanism of these differing responses remains elusive.[142] Propofol has also been found to cause apoptotic degeneration of neurons and oligodendrocytes in fetal and neonatal rhesus monkeys after a 5-hour exposure.[241] Repeat doses of propofol in infant mice leads to impaired motor learning in adulthood.[242] In vitro, propofol induces neurotoxicity in murine cortical neuronal cell culture and dose-dependent apoptosis in human stem cell–derived neurons, respectively.[243,244] Accordingly, the overall consensus of this body of literature is that propofol, in a dose- and exposure time–dependent fashion, can dramatically affect the developing brain of animals and human stem cells.

DEXMEDETOMIDINE

Unlike other anesthetics and sedatives, dexmedetomidine is a sedative and analgesic that does not interact with GABA, NMDA, or opioid receptors, but rather interacts presynaptically with α_2-adrenergic receptors. Given this dissimilar mechanism of action and the fact that all anesthetics acting on GABA or NMDA receptors have been found deleterious to the developing brain, there has been substantial interest in the use of dexmedetomidine as an alternative sedative since it may not cause neurocognitive dysfunction. Several initial studies that examined the brain structure after dexmedetomidine administration in rodents and monkeys reported none to minimal neurodegeneration.[197,245–251] However, one study observed increased neuroapoptosis after a prolonged exposure to dexmedetomidine, albeit in brain regions distinct from those vulnerable to ketamine-induced apoptosis.[252] Additionally, dexmedetomidine reduces or even attenuates brain structural or long-term cognitive abnormalities caused by isoflurane, sevoflurane, ketamine, or propofol.[197,245,246,249,251,253,254] However, there is evidence that dexmedetomidine does not alleviate sevoflurane-induced neuroapoptosis in newborn rats.[255–257] Further laboratory studies in which dexmedetomidine is compared with standard anesthetic regimens at similar levels of sedation are warranted.

OPIOID ANALGESICS

Since all currently used general anesthetics can dramatically alter the structure of the developing brain, opioid analgesics represent a class of drugs that reduces anesthetic requirements and could therefore diminish the deleterious effects of anesthetics in the developing brain. To date, only one study has investigated neurotoxic properties of opioids compared with an inhaled anesthetic regimen. Mechanically ventilated, neonatal pigs, injected with an IV bolus of 30 µg/kg fentanyl followed by 15 µg/kg per hour for 4 hours, exhibited less neuroapoptosis in several regions of the brain compared with a balanced anesthetic of 1 mg/kg of midazolam, followed by 4 hours of 0.55% isoflurane and 75% nitrous oxide.[221] These initial findings are encouraging, although future neurotoxicity studies with opioid infusions need to also include adjuvants that produce amnesia as this is an expectation during clinical anesthesia. However, whether neonates and infants require the same level of amnesia as adults during surgery remains a hotly debated subject.[258,259] Finally, it is critical to confirm that equipotent anesthetic doses are used when comparing the effects of different regimens (e.g., IV vs. inhaled anesthetics) on neurotoxicity.

The long-term consequences of opioid administration to the immature brain need to be elucidated before recommending such a regimen as an alternative strategy for clinical practice. Similar to GABA and NMDA receptors, opioid receptors are also intimately involved in early brain development and synaptogenesis,[260,261] which would make it plausible that opioids could similarly affect brain development during the critical period of synaptogenesis. Moreover, repeated neonatal exposures could alter long-term opioid receptor composition. Increased neuronal cell death and decreased neuronal density after perinatal exposure to µ-receptor agonists, such as morphine and heroin, have been observed in developing animals after prolonged exposures.[83–85] Long-term buprenorphine and methadone treatment early in life diminished the concentrations of nerve growth factors in the immature brain.[149,150] Moreover, perinatal exposure to morphine has immediate and permanently reduced µ-opioid receptor density[262,263] that may be associated with long-term impaired memory and cognitive function in small animals,[106–111,264] as well as exaggerated nociceptive responses to a pain challenge later in life.[116,265] Stimulation of the κ-opioid receptor may amplify neuronal cell death induced by proapoptotic agents.[266] High-dose fentanyl exacerbates white-matter brain lesions induced by glutamatergic overstimulation in mice.[267] However, a single morphine injection of up to 10 mg/kg in 7- or 15-day-old rats does not affect either survival or dendritic differentiation of pyramidal neurons in the medial prefrontal cortex.[86] These animal data suggest that prolonged perinatal exposure to opioid analgesics could potentially cause structural and long-term functional alterations in the developing brain and may amplify proapoptotic stimuli, whereas a brief or single exposure may not. These data support the need for further studies into the interactions of opioid analgesics and anesthetics in the developing brain.

Exposure Time, Dose, and Anesthetic Combinations

As in the case of opioid analgesics, the impact of anesthesia during development seems to depend on the dose and/or duration of anesthesia for inhaled anesthetics, as well as the dose, route of administration, and number of doses (i.e., exposure time) for injectable anesthetics. Moreover, combinations of several anesthetics and sedatives have, in general, exacerbated the neuroapoptosis and long-term cognitive changes compared with single drugs. For example, combinations of midazolam, nitrous oxide, and isoflurane cause a much greater degree of neuroapoptosis in neonatal rats than isoflurane alone, even when the latter is administered at a greater inspired concentration.[69] In the case of ketamine, its neurodegenerative potency is amplified when coadministered with thiopental or propofol.[96] Anesthetic combinations of mixed GABA agonists and NMDA antagonists demonstrate exaggerated effects. This evidence supports the notion that a deeper level of anesthesia increases the neuroapoptotic injury. However, coadministration of two anesthetics, xenon and dexmedetomidine, as well as isoflurane before treatment (all of which attenuated the neurotoxic effects of isoflurane anesthesia),[186,188,197] seem to contradict this hypothesis.

The effects of neuromuscular blocking drugs on neurologic outcomes, although unlikely related to their insignificant permeation of the intact blood-brain barrier, have not yet been studied. Moreover, the study of local anesthetic toxicity has been limited to the developing spinal cord and has not yet been expanded to the developing brain. This line of investigation will require greater emphasis if the use of regional anesthetic techniques is expanded in infants and young children to reduce requirements for general anesthetics.

Deleterious Effects of Untreated Pain and Stress

Given the evidence for deleterious effects of anesthetics and analgesics on the developing brain and the paucity of complete anesthetics devoid of cytotoxicity, one approach would be to reduce or even withhold potentially toxic drugs at the expense of children experiencing pain and stress during surgery. Such practice would not only be unethical, but animal and clinical research actually suggest that these recurrent stressful and painful experiences also adversely affect the developing brain. Noxious stimulation in neonatal rodents has been associated with subsequent hyperalgesia as well as hypoalgesia, depending on the type and severity of injury.[268] In human neonates, repetitive painful skin lacerations for procedures as minor as blood draws lead to long-term, local sensory hyperinnervation.[269] In immature animals, in addition to these local responses, repetitive, inflammatory pain early in life results in hyperalgesia and lasting changes in nociceptive circuitry of the adult dorsal horn.[270] Repeated painful injections into the paws of rat pups induced a generalized thermal hypoalgesia.[268] In addition to altered pain processing and sensory perception, repetitive or persistent pain in the neonate alters behavior and cognitive function in adulthood, decreases pain thresholds, and increases vulnerability to stress and anxiety disorders or chronic pain syndromes later in life.[121,271–274]

In addition to painful stimulation, early adverse emotional experiences can also induce long-lasting abnormalities in animals such as imbalances of the inhibitory nervous system,[275] impaired normal development of the nociceptive system, long-term behavioral changes,[276] and impaired persistent learning.[109] Therefore, fetuses, neonates, and infants subjected to pain and stresses associated with invasive procedures without adequate anesthesia and analgesia may also be at risk for long-term adverse outcomes.

Preemptive administration of analgesics and sedatives such as morphine or ketamine attenuate the deleterious effects of pain in the neonate in some animal studies.[109,121,274] Either the presence of painful stimulation or 5 days of morphine administered to neonatal mice without pain independently impaired adult rewarded behavior, although the combination of pain and analgesia did not trigger behavioral abnormalities.[109]

Clinical reports have also demonstrated that human neonates and infants can mount a substantial metabolic and endocrine response to perioperative stress and painful stimulation, which include surges in catecholamine, cortisol, β-endorphin, insulin, glucagon, and growth hormone levels.[277–279] Some of these markers, such as cortisol, can remain increased for more than a year after the insult, possibly as a result of cumulative stress related to multiple painful procedures early in life.[280] Inhaled anesthetics, opioid analgesics, as well as regional anesthesia, inhibit intraoperative stress and improve postoperative outcomes.[278,281,282] Moreover, adequate perioperative anesthesia reduced the incidence of other complications, such as the incidence of sepsis and disseminated intravascular coagulation, leading to a decrease in overall mortality.[283] Even less invasive procedures, such as circumcisions performed without analgesia in young boys, can exaggerate responses to painful challenges (e.g., immunizations) later in life.[284]

Conversely, topical or regional anesthesia for circumcision not only mitigated the immediate humoral stress response during the procedure[285] but also blunted the pain-induced, long-term hyperalgesia.[284] In preterm neonates, painful stimulations early in life have also been associated with subsequent diminished cognition and motor function.[286] In a retrospective study of children older than 1 year of age who were born at less than 32 weeks' gestational age without significant neonatal brain injury or major sensorineural impairment, an increased number of skin-breaking procedures from birth to term (including heel sticks, intramuscular injections, chest tube placements, and central line insertions) predicted poorer subsequent cognitive and motor development (as assessed using the Bayley Scales of Infant Development II) when compared with term controls. Importantly, after controlling for severity of illness, the duration of morphine administration, and exposure to postnatal dexamethasone, gestational age at birth was not associated with poorer cognitive or motor outcomes. These findings suggest that repetitive pain-related stressful experiences and not prematurity per se were in part responsible for the altered neurodevelopmental outcome.[286] Although this study did not examine the effects of anesthetic or analgesic administration during painful stimulation on subsequent outcome, a small, retrospective report suggested an improvement in outcome after administering anesthesia during painful stimulation.[287] In this study, painful stimulation during reduction of herniated bowel without anesthesia in infants suffering from gastroschisis tended to more frequently lead to serious adverse events, such as bowel ischemia, the need for total parenteral nutrition, and unplanned reoperation, than in infants undergoing the same procedure with general anesthesia.[287]

Surprisingly, despite the persistently large numbers of painful and stressful procedures performed in vulnerable neonates, the majority of these procedures are still not accompanied by adequate analgesia or anesthesia.[288] In clinical practice, the relative effects of anesthetic exposure or inadequate anesthesia or analgesia during painful stimulation as the potential basis for cognitive abnormalities remain open to speculation.

Together, the data from animals and humans convincingly demonstrate that pain-related stress experienced early in life is deleterious to the developing nervous system, that pain in children remains undertreated, and that analgesics and/or anesthetics may alleviate many of the degenerative effects of unopposed pain and improve outcomes. However, if anesthetics protect from the deleterious effects of painful stimulation but at the same time confer their own cytotoxic effects, the quintessential question is whether other adjuvant compounds can alleviate these adverse effects.

Potential Alleviating Strategies

Whereas the translational relevance of anesthetic-induced neurotoxicity observed in neonatal animals to humans remains unresolved, several laboratory studies have investigated strategies to alleviate some of the deleterious effects of anesthetics and sedatives in animals, which may have relevance for clinical practice. These protective strategies have been directed at both the structural effects observed immediately after anesthesia, such as neuronal cell death, as well as the long-term abnormalities, such as neurocognitive impairment and learning abnormalities. Importantly, many animal studies administered adjuvants immediately before or during anesthesia, thereby maintaining an adequate level of anesthesia and analgesia to avoid the deleterious effects of unopposed pain.

The sedative dexmedetomidine and the anesthetic xenon possess limited neurotoxic potencies themselves but seem to significantly reduce isoflurane-induced neuroapoptosis.[186,188,197,245,246,249,251] The coadministration of dexmedetomidine also prevented long-term memory impairment after 6 hours of isoflurane in rats.[197] However, augmenting sevoflurane anesthesia with dexmedetomidine did not diminish neurotoxicity in newborn rats.[255–257] Preconditioning with a brief exposure of isoflurane conferred protection from the deleterious effects of a subsequent prolonged exposure to the same drug, both in vitro and in vivo.[289,290] In in vitro studies, the inositol triphosphate–receptor antagonist xestospongin C, tissue plasminogen activator, plasmin, inhibition of the neurotrophic receptor p75[NTR] or RhoA receptor, as well as prevention of cytoskeletal depolymerization with either jasplakinolide or TAT-Pep5 significantly attenuated isoflurane-mediated neuroapoptosis.[134,162,291] In addition, L-carnitine attenuated neuronal apoptosis after 6 hours of isoflurane and nitrous oxide in 7-day-old rat pups.[292] Supplementation with the naturally occurring hormones β-estradiol or melatonin prevented the deleterious effects on neuronal survival of a prolonged exposure to midazolam, isoflurane, and nitrous oxide.[79,148] Melatonin protected against isoflurane-induced endoplasmic reticulum stress, protein degradation, and chemotaxis behavioral abnormalities in the roundworm *Caenorhabditis elegans*,[293] and attenuated isoflurane's spatial learning and memory dysfunction in developing rats.[294] Coadministration of β-estradiol reduced phenobarbital-induced neuroapoptosis.[229,234] Prophylactic administration of progesterone prevented the adverse behavioral and neurocognitive effects of neonatal sevoflurane anesthesia exposure in rats.[295]

Blocking the GABA receptor with the antagonist gabazine does not attenuate isoflurane-induced neurodegeneration[197]; however, pilocarpine reduced neuroapoptosis induced by the GABA agonists isoflurane and midazolam, while augmenting the damage after administration of the NMDA antagonist phencyclidine, based on preliminary results from neonatal mice.[296] Preliminary data from the same laboratory also suggest that whole-body hypothermia with a targeted brain temperature of less than 30°C may protect from the neuroapoptotic ramifications of 4 hours of 0.75% isoflurane or 40 mg/kg of intraperitoneal ketamine in neonatal mice.[44,187] Supplementation of the brain developmental promotor monosialotetrahexosylganglioside (GM1) ameliorated the apoptotic and deleterious functional effects of ketamine exposure in neonatal rats.[210,297] Neuronal apoptosis immediately after ketamine in newborn rats and long-term spatial and memory abnormalities were attenuated by remote ischemic preconditioning with repeated ischemia/reperfusion cycles using an elastic rubber band tourniquet around the hind limb.[298] Another therapy that has been successfully tested in mouse pups as well as nonhuman primates that either received ketamine, propofol, or isoflurane was lithium, which abolished the anesthetic-induced neuroapoptosis in the cortex and the caudate-putamen complex.[235,299]

To further elucidate the mechanisms of developmental anesthetic neurotoxicity, several studies have used micro-RNAs to successfully modulate genes and cell signaling pathways at the posttranscriptional level to alleviate the deleterious effects of several anesthetics, including propofol,[171] ketamine,[172] and sevoflurane.[300]

Because the applicability and extent of anesthetic neurotoxicity has not been established in humans, it seems premature to recommend any of these protective strategies for children. Moreover, the safety of many of these drugs and interventions has yet to be determined in human neonates and infants. For example,

tissue plasminogen activator and plasmin promote fibrinolysis and may not be first-line treatments during invasive surgical procedures. The sex hormones β-estradiol and progesterone may not be a feasible adjuvant in prepubescent boys. The safety of pilocarpine in young children may be hampered by its proconvulsant activity observed in some animal studies.[301,302] Lithium has been labeled as harmful to the human fetus and may cause neurocognitive abnormalities in young children.[303–305] Whole-body hypothermia below 30°C is not a clinically feasible modality, because even mild perioperative hypothermia, at least in adults, has been causally linked to numerous complications, including increased blood loss and transfusion requirements, morbid myocardial outcomes, prolonged postanesthetic recovery and hospitalization, thermal discomfort, and an increased risk of surgical wound infections.[306] Therefore, pilocarpine, lithium, or hypothermia to treat or prevent anesthesia-induced neurotoxicity are unlikely to play a substantive role during routine pediatric anesthesia, but may have a role in infants undergoing hypothermic cardiopulmonary bypass for heart surgery. Unfortunately, the latter population often presents with neurocognitive abnormalities even before anesthetic exposure, which confounds the potential effects of anesthetics.[307] Xenon's scarcity renders it a very expensive adjuvant or anesthetic, although dexmedetomidine's more widespread availability and increasing familiarity among pediatric anesthesiologists makes it a more attractive option for further research into protective strategies.[308,309]

Anesthetic Neuroprotection

Although the adult brain represents 2% of the body weight, it accounts for approximately 20% of the body's energy and oxygen consumption. Neurons consume more than 50% of their produced adenosine triphosphate (ATP) for action potential generation and neurotransmission. Anesthetics reduce neuronal activity and concomitant energy consumption, increasing the limited tolerance of the brain to ischemia and attenuating neuronal injury and long-term neurologic impairment. Additionally, direct mitochondrial effects represent potential mechanisms for both neuroprotection as well as neurotoxicity.[152,153,310] Animal studies have repeatedly confirmed protective properties of anesthetics when administered before or during episodes of brain hypoxia-ischemia, albeit most of these studies have been conducted in adult animals and the longevity of the protective effects are controversial.[311] In immature animal models, anesthetics have also been found to reduce neurologic injury and improve functional outcome after brain ischemia.[68] Desflurane alleviates neuronal cell death and early neurologic dysfunction in a neonatal pig model during hypothermic cardiopulmonary bypass and deep hypothermic circulatory arrest.[312,313] Isoflurane treatment before hypoxia-ischemia protects the brain and improves survival in neonatal rats and mice.[314–316] Both xenon and sevoflurane protect the immature brain during simulated hypoxia-ischemia in vitro.[317] Furthermore, sevoflurane combines with mild hypothermia to protect brain structure and function in neonatal mice during hypoxia-ischemia.[318] These findings in immature animals suggest that critically ill human neonates could potentially benefit from these protective properties during clinical scenarios of greater risk for neurologic injury, such as cardiopulmonary bypass, neurologic surgery, or perioperative cardiocirculatory arrest; these potential benefits therefore should be weighed against the theoretical neurotoxic properties of current anesthetic regimens in young children.

Critical Evaluation of Animal Studies and Interspecies Comparisons

To determine whether findings from animal studies can inform clinical practice, it is critically important to evaluate how well animal studies represent the perioperative experience of young children.[5,26,69,90,91,98,102,190,319–323]

To date, no animal model exists that covers all aspects of human physiology and pathophysiology during surgical procedures. The task of modeling potential vulnerabilities of the developing human brain in animals is complicated by the fact that human CNS development is much more protracted than that of any of the model species. However, human neurocognitive performance is also much more complex compared with lower animals, and any potential neurologic injury might therefore have a greater or lesser impact on such an intricate system.

DURATION OF EXPOSURE

To elicit toxic effects, the designs of many animal studies include durations of anesthesia from 1 to 31.5 hours (Fig. 23.4). The majority of animal studies used exposure times of 6 hours—a duration extending far beyond the average time required for most routine pediatric anesthetics.[2] However, expressing the duration of anesthesia as a fraction of a subject's life span, thereby equating a 6-hour anesthetic in mice to a 2-week or greater anesthetic in humans, is probably an oversimplification. Life expectancy or even the relative duration of neurodevelopment may not be immediately relevant when considering the likelihood of injury at a cellular level. The extent of the injury and its functional implications may potentially be related to the duration of the entire brain developmental period, even though the mechanism of anesthetic-induced neurodegeneration is unknown. Because human brain development occurs at a much slower pace than in any of the other species, similar exposure times could potentially result in differential susceptibility and ability for postexposure repair among species. For example, the brain reaches adult size at 20 days of age in rats, 3 years of age in rhesus monkeys, 7 years of age in chimpanzees, and not until 15 years of age in humans.[5,324,325] Exposure to anesthesia during a larger proportion of the period of development could result in a greater impact on

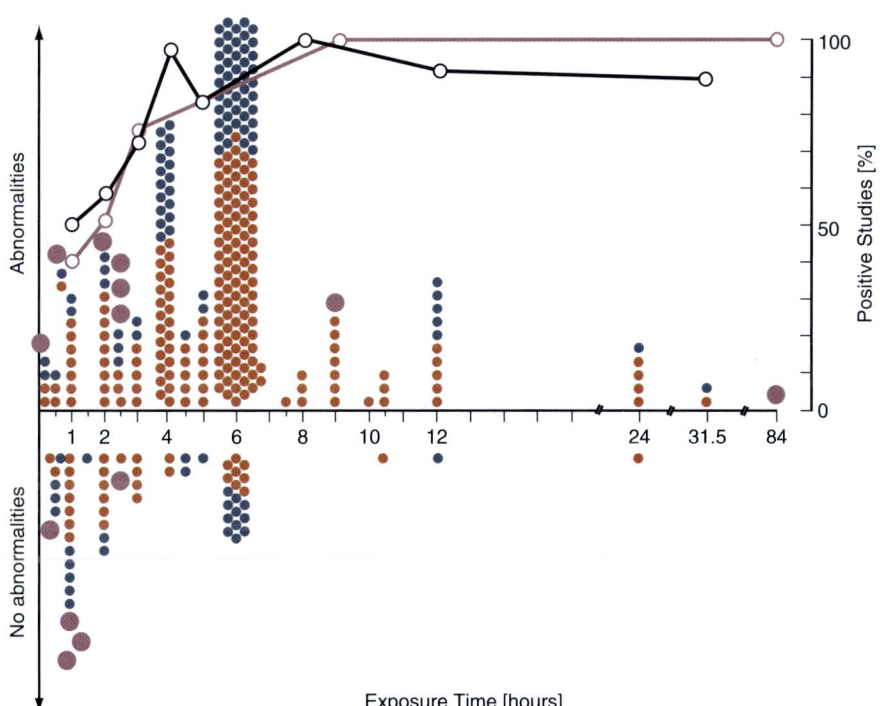

FIGURE 23.4 The majority of in vivo animal studies into the effects of anesthetic exposure on brain structure and function examine substantially longer exposure times than occurring in clinical practice. However, longer exposures trend toward more positive findings in both animal and human studies. Animal studies, inclusive of various anesthetic drugs and doses, reporting abnormal findings (above the horizontal line) or negative findings (below the horizontal line) for brain structural (*solid red circles*) or cognitive outcomes (*solid blue circles*), as a function of exposure time. *Solid purple circles* represent clinical studies of long-term cognitive outcomes in humans demonstrating abnormalities (above the horizontal line) or lack thereof (below the horizontal line). Exposure times denote all reported anesthetic durations, either single or cumulative, or estimated exposure times based on injection schedules, ranging from 10 minutes to 31.5 hours. For the purpose of analysis, results are reported separately for structural and functional outcomes, resulting in up to two circles, if both outcomes were reported, and may include opposing results, if structural and functional findings diverged. The graphs express the ratio of positive to negative studies in animals (*black*) or humans (*purple*); circles represent the percentage of positive studies for respective exposure epoch ranging from specific data point to next lower data point on the graph. Note that positive studies outnumber negative studies for all exposure times in both animals and humans, except for only 40% of human studies demonstrating cognitive abnormalities following anesthetic exposures of 1 hour or less. (From Lin EP, Lee J-R, Lee CS, et al. Do anesthetics harm the developing human brain? An integrative analysis of animal and human studies. *Neurotoxicol Teratol.* 2017;60:117-128.)

23

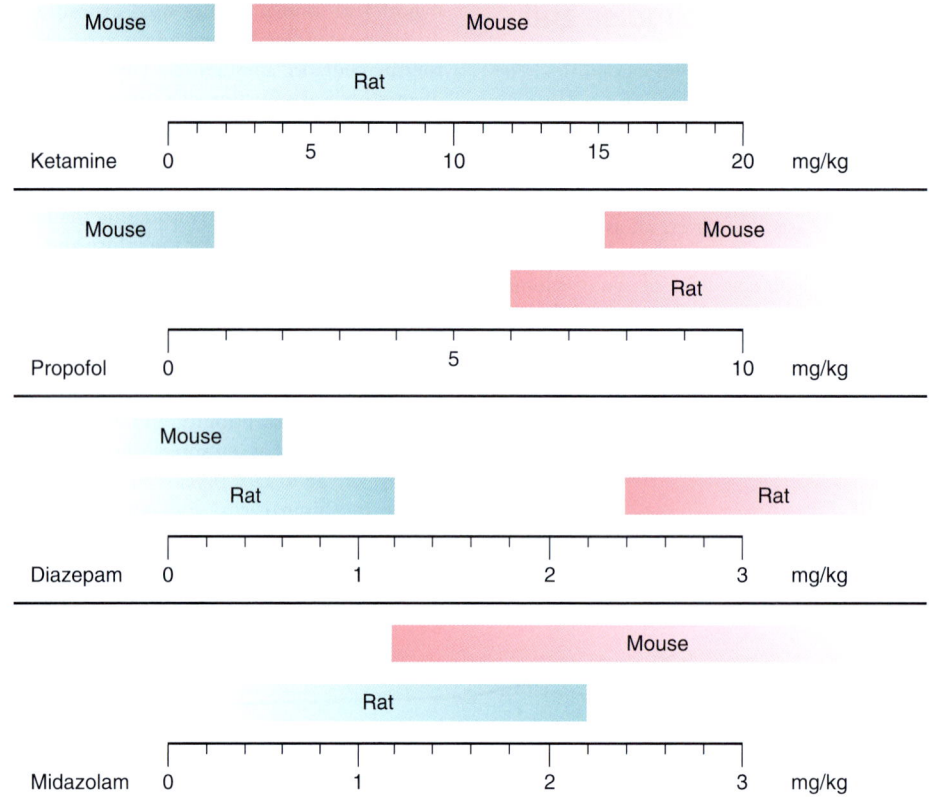

FIGURE 23.5 Neurodegenerative effects of injectable anesthetics in developing animals are dose-dependent. *Blue bars* represent doses of the respective anesthetics not causing neurodegeneration in rats and mice; *pink bars* represent doses causing neurodegeneration in animals. The figure includes only studies using single injections of anesthetics, and doses used in animals were scaled to doses for children by using an allometric scaling technique, based on calculations outlined in reference 329. Neurotoxic data are based on experiments described in references 20, 69, 77, 78, 87, 96, 202–204, 229, 239, and 341.

total development and maturation. Given the plasticity of the developing brain, it seems conceivable that brains with slower growth rates are afforded more time for repair.[326,327] Conversely, in complex organisms, such as humans, relatively minor injuries in crucial areas or at critical times during development could have profound effects on long-term cognitive and executive function. Accordingly, cognition may be altered by briefer periods of anesthetic exposure in children, compared with animals functioning on a simpler cognitive level.

ANESTHETIC DOSES

Animals are subjected to greater weight-based doses of injectable anesthetics, sometimes by orders of magnitude, compared with doses commonly used in human clinical practice. In the discussion of whether these doses have applicability to pediatric anesthesia practice, it is important to understand that small animals require larger weight-based doses of IV anesthetics to produce immobility than larger animals or humans. These differences can be explained, in large part, by the animals' smaller size, greater metabolic rate, and shorter physiologic time compared with humans.[328] Using a process called allometric scaling, which takes the differences among species into account, doses for injectable drugs in animals comparable with human doses have been estimated to be approximately 3-, 6-, or 12-fold greater for monkeys, rats, or mice, respectively (see also Chapter 5).[328,329] Whereas drug doses used in anesthetic neurotoxicity studies frequently still exceed

these comparable doses calculated using allometric scaling, they do not include a significant safety margin (Fig. 23.5). Using allometrically scaled doses, plasma concentrations for ketamine, for example, were approximately 3 to 10 times greater in monkeys and small rodents than those observed during clinical human practice.[78,204] This might suggest that the neurotoxic properties observed with large doses of injectable anesthetics, such as ketamine, could potentially have direct applicability to humans only if the anesthetic and the neurotoxic effects were based on the same molecular mechanism, which has yet to be verified. Otherwise, animal studies would expose subjects to much greater plasma concentrations of potential neurotoxicants than those used during anesthesia in humans, thereby possibly overestimating the neurotoxic effects of IV anesthetics in laboratory studies.

Doses for inhaled anesthetics generating immobility in animals, on the other hand, are much closer to human clinically used doses. Moreover, similar to human anesthesia, potency of inhaled anesthetics increases with subject age, necessitating larger doses in younger animals,[195,198,330] which could suggest closer clinical applicability of laboratory data using these compounds. The use of observed concentration or area under the curve might be a better measure of exposure than dose.

EXPERIMENTAL VERSUS CLINICAL CONDITIONS

An important distinction between laboratory studies in animals and clinical practice in humans is the presence of comorbidities and underlying disease, the genetic diversity in human populations, as well as the frequent occurrence of stress and pain associated with surgical procedures. Very few laboratory studies have examined the effects of surgical stress and pain on anesthesia-induced neurotoxicity. When tail clamping or injection of caustic substances were used to model surgical stress, results have varied; one study reported no influence of the painful stimulus on anesthesia-induced apoptosis,[331] whereas a second reported that painful stimulation increased anesthetic-induced neuroapoptosis.[332] Conversely, pain-induced neurodegeneration was attenuated by coadministration of small doses of analgesics or sedatives.[109,121] Neonatal surgery during sevoflurane anesthesia, but not sevoflurane alone, impaired learning and memory of juvenile mice.[333] The interactions between anesthetics and analgesics and the noxious stimuli encountered in the perioperative setting have not been thoroughly elucidated.

Studies that measured metabolic and respiratory variables during anesthetic exposure in small rodents reported abnormalities not routinely observed during pediatric anesthesia practice, such as extensive hypercarbia, metabolic acidosis, and hypoglycemia.[91,102,198] Tracheal intubation and mechanical ventilation do not necessarily completely obviate all of these abnormalities in rodents.[198] In stark contrast to anesthesia in children, administering clinical doses of anesthetics for periods greater than 4 hours can be lethal for up to 20% of small rodents,[102] even when intermittent painful stimuli are applied.[91] However, the growing evidence from nonhuman primate studies, in which animals were intubated, ventilated, had vital signs stringently monitored, and lacked mortality during anesthetic exposure, but still demonstrated comparable neuronal injury patterns observed in rodents,[241,334,335] suggests that the shortcomings in physiologic conditions in small-animal studies does not eliminate their potential biologic relevance to humans. Moreover, rearing conditions after anesthesia have a profound impact on the brain's repair mechanisms after injury. Environmental enrichment and exercise dramatically increase neurogenesis in rodents and therefore may facilitate plasticity and repair after anesthesia, compared with the customary bare cage housing environment of rodents.[336,337] Comparably, children face daily cognitive challenges in their normal "enriched" environment, substantially different from normal laboratory animal housing,[78,98,217,221] which could attenuate the postulated neurocognitive effects of anesthesia in humans. This is highlighted by recent animal studies in which environmental enrichment reversed the deleterious effects of prolonged or repeated anesthetic exposures on subsequent neurologic performance in rats.[331,338] These studies suggest that neurobehavioral outcomes depend on multiple factors, of which anesthesia represents only one of many other events important for the developing brain.

COMPARATIVE BRAIN DEVELOPMENT

A major challenge in translating any animal data to human clinical practice is properly matching brain maturational stages between model species and young children. The ongoing discussion regarding these comparisons is somewhat reminiscent of the cliché of 1 "dog year" being equivalent to 7 "human years." Because earlier animal studies have suggested that anesthesia-induced structural abnormalities may be most pronounced during very defined, early stages of development, such as neuroapoptosis in cortex and thalamus peaking between 3 and 10 days of age in small rodents[20,79] or between gestational day 120 and day 6 of life in rhesus monkeys, it becomes imperative to appropriately identify the equivalent period during human brain development to assess human applicability of the animal data and to adequately design clinical studies.

Brain architecture and rate of maturation, however, vary widely among mammalian species, both in magnitude and timing. Small rodents, such as mice and rats, have a smooth (lissencephalic) brain surface, whereas humans and monkeys exhibit the typical fissured, gyrencephalic brain surface of gyri and sulci. Overall brain size and the number of neurons differ by orders of magnitude between humans and animal species; the mature human brain contains approximately 86 billion neurons, compared with the rhesus macaque's 6 billion and the adult mouse brain's 70 million neurons.[339] Other important species differences exist in timing and duration of critical developmental events. Rodents are altricial species, meaning considerable brain development occurs postnatally during their first 2 to 3 weeks of life, whereas numerous critical developmental steps take place in utero in monkeys and especially humans.[319] Given these substantial differences, it is difficult to unequivocally associate specific ages in animals to humans. Older data, based on simple species comparisons of brain growth and still persistently quoted in the pertinent literature, equated the first week of life in small rodents, when the peak of vulnerability to anesthetic neuroapoptosis occurs for several cortical and subcortical brain regions, to an extended time span in humans from the third gestational trimester all the way to the third year of life.[5,25,320] However, more contemporary approaches using computational models have approximated the 7-day-old rat or mouse to be closer in brain maturity to human fetuses during the third trimester of pregnancy, whereas the immature rhesus monkey 5 to 6 days old is closer to the postnatal human brain in infancy, ~5 months of age (Fig. 23.6).[321–323,340] According to these models, stages of brain maturity equivalent to term human neonates are not reached in small rodents until after postnatal days 10 to 12 in rats or mice, respectively (an online calculator is available at https://www.translatingtime.org). In general, the majority of in vivo laboratory studies examine animals during developmental stages equivalent to the very immature human brain (Fig. 23.7) and the injury pattern of neuroapoptosis significantly changes in the subhuman animal models.[78,80] In aggregate, animal data do not clearly identify a "safe" age beyond which no deleterious anesthetic effects on brain development are observed.[2]

Limited human data seem to suggest that postnatal brain development may be most susceptible to anesthetic or sedative exposure, whereas animal data, including a recent nonhuman primate study,[334] demonstrated a greater degree of neuroapoptosis after exposure in the premature human brain. However, substantial differences in brain development still exist between humans and nonhuman primates. Development progresses at a much slower pace in humans compared with any other model species, including nonhuman primates, and developmental stages are up to 50% longer. Even on a cellular level, remarkable differences exist between humans and all other animals; cell cycle duration during cortical neurogenesis is approximately 17 hours in mice, 28 hours in macaque monkeys, and 36 hours in humans.[327] In aggregate, these differences undermine the notion of directly equating anesthetic effects in the developing brain of any animal species to clinical anesthesia practice in humans. The potential long-term effects of anesthetics have to be examined carefully in clinical studies before concluding that the results from animal studies portend similar outcomes in humans.

ASSESSING NEUROBEHAVIORAL OR COGNITIVE OUTCOMES

Translating neurodevelopmental outcomes from animals to humans is difficult. Human cognitive performance includes the vast capacity for learning, the ability for abstract thinking, the aptitude

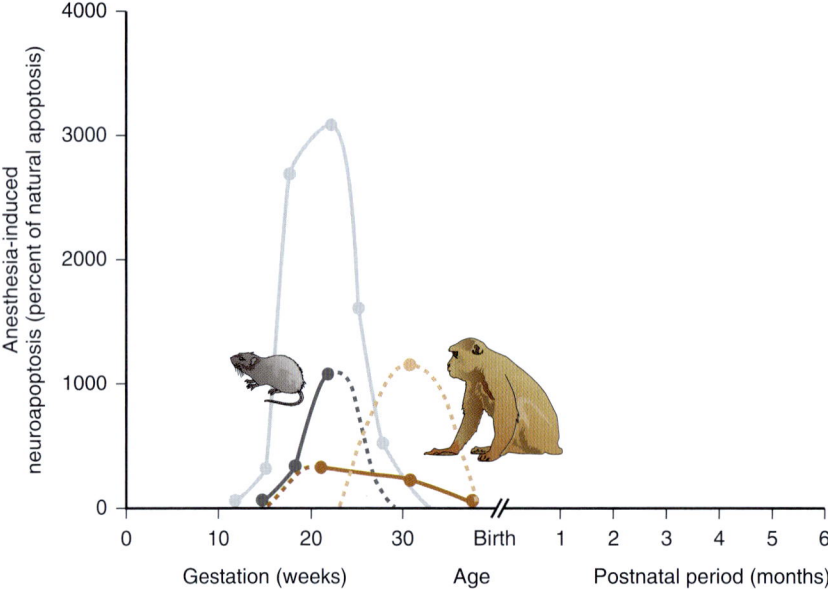

FIGURE 23.6 The degree of neuronal apoptotic cell death following anesthetic exposure is highly dependent on the age of the animal during exposure. Graphs demonstrate the percent increase of apoptotic cell death compared with natural apoptosis following an exposure to an isoflurane/nitrous oxide–based anesthetic in immature rats *(dark gray)* or very young macaque monkeys *(dark brown)* or prolonged exposure to ketamine in immature rats *(light gray)* or macaque monkeys *(tan). Solid lines* connect the available data points; *dashed lines* represent extrapolations of the available data. Neurotoxicity data were derived from references 20, 78, 148, and 217. To infer the potential age of anesthetic vulnerability in humans, respective brain maturity in the animal species during exposure was equated to the corresponding state of the developing human brain, and relative human ages for each data point were plotted accordingly, using a mathematical model outlined in references 322, 323, and 340, which is available in the online calculator at https://www.translatingtime.org.

for solving complex mathematical equations, and even the capability of inventing and operating complex machinery. Cognition is a complex process that includes such diverse processes as perception, attention, motivation, working memory, long-term memory, executive function, language, and social cognition. These brain functions are all difficult to model in animals.[190] It is therefore imperative to critically evaluate any animal model attempting to replicate human cognitive performance. Moreover, it is important to assess the validity of these models in the context of the critical period for human brain development that they are trying to represent. Current assessment of neurocognitive performance after developmental exposure largely depends on hippocampal-dependent tests, such as tests of spatial learning and memory, administered to adult animals after anesthetic exposure early in life.[69,90,91,98,102] However, it remains unclear whether these are the same functional domains that may potentially be targeted in children during anesthesia. Brain regions maximally affected by anesthesia may depend on their state of development and therefore change dependent on the age of the organism during exposure.[80,221,335] Accordingly, subsequent neurobehavioral abnormalities may vary, depending on the age at which anesthesia was administered.

This discussion does not entirely discredit the results from small-animal studies, but rather seriously limits their generalizability to clinical practice. Several large-animal models that more closely resemble clinical pediatric anesthesia practice have used tracheal intubation and mechanical ventilation.[217,221,334,335] However, these large-animal studies have only included minor stimulation, such as skin clamping, but not surgical stimulation during the anesthetic exposure.[78,98,217,221]

NONHUMAN PRIMATE STUDIES

Due to technical, economical, and ethical considerations, the great majority of preclinical studies into the effects of anesthetics on the developing brain have been conducted in small-animal or cell culture models. Studies in rodents and lower animals have been criticized for their inability to stringently monitor physiologic variables and the substantial anatomical, physiological, neurological, behavioral, biochemical, and pharmacological dissimilarities with humans. Accordingly, several large-animal and nonhuman primate studies have examined the immediate effects of anesthetic exposure on the immature brain and have attempted to elucidate the presence of a long-term behavioral or cognitive phenotype after exposure to anesthesia in infancy. Nonhuman primates are the closest living relatives to humans and share many similarities in anatomy and complex physiology, making them the most useful model for studying the effects of toxic substances on humans.

Studies in developmental anesthetic neurotoxicity in nonhuman primates have used the rhesus monkey *Macaca mulatta* or the cynomolgus monkey *Macaca fascicularis*. The specific anesthetics tested included exposures to ketamine,[78,98,180,212,335,341] propofol,[241] dexmedetomidine,[248] nitrous oxide,[342] isoflurane,[132,217,299,334,342–346] or sevoflurane,[347–355] as well as combinations of isoflurane and nitrous oxide.[342,356,357] The assessed outcomes included brain structural integrity immediately after the exposure in addition to long-term behavioral and neurocognitive evaluations. For ethical reasons and to guarantee translational relevance, nonhuman primate studies require the highest quality of experimental design, including randomization and blinding, adherence to clinical anesthesia monitoring and management standards, adequate sample size and

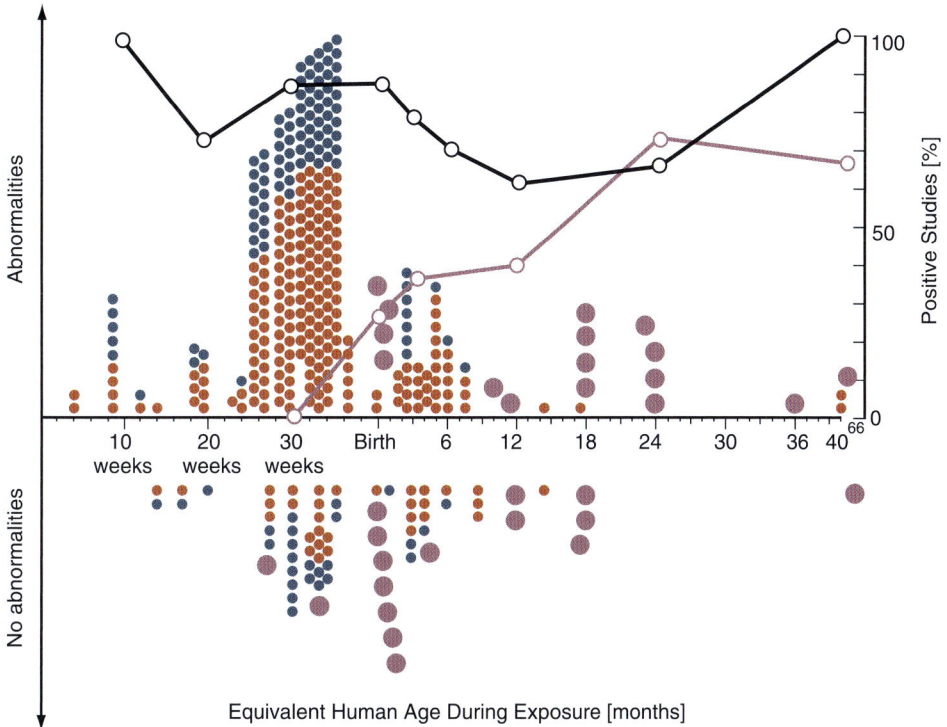

FIGURE 23.7 The majority of in vivo animal studies into the effects of anesthetic exposure on brain structure and function focus on brain developmental stages equivalent to premature neonates. Studies with negative results never outnumber those with positive results at any time point, suggesting that no age can be clearly identified at which anesthetics do not cause abnormalities. Animal studies, inclusive of various anesthetic drugs and doses, reporting abnormal findings (above the horizontal line) or negative findings (below the horizontal line) for brain structural (*solid red circles*) or cognitive outcomes (*solid blue circles*) are depicted as a function of maturational age of the animals' brain relative to the human brain during exposure. *Solid purple circles* represent clinical studies into long-term cognitive outcomes in humans. The animals' age during exposure was converted to the corresponding maturational stage of the human brain by using a computational neurodevelopmental model (https://www.translatingtime.org). For the purpose of analysis, reports with separate anesthetic protocols consisting of different anesthetic regimens or multiple exposure times of the same anesthetic were classified as separate studies. For repeated exposures at different ages, the equivalent mean age of the human brain is reported. The graphs express the ratio of studies with positive findings to those with negative findings in animals (*black*) or humans (*purple*); open circles represent the respective percentage of positive studies for age epochs ranging from specific data points to next lower data point on the graph. Note that animal studies with positive findings outnumber those studies with negative findings from conception until 40 months' equivalent age in humans, whereas this ratio does not turn positive for human studies until exposures between 12 and 24 months of age. (From Lin EP, Lee J-R, Lee CS, et al. Do anesthetics harm the developing human brain? An integrative analysis of animal and human studies. *Neurotoxicol Teratol.* 2017;60:117-128.)

statistical analysis, and reporting of all outcomes.[358] Although many studies did not meet the most stringent criteria for study design and reporting,[358] all found structural abnormalities in infant primates, most frequently neuronal apoptotic cell death after exposure to a variety of anesthetics. Importantly, the observed apoptotic neuronal cell death pattern in neonatal rhesus monkeys was strikingly similar for several anesthetics to those observed in immature rodents exposed at an early age, especially cortical layers II/III and V,[69,78,81,217] suggesting that a similar response of immature neurons to prolonged anesthetic exposure throughout the animal kingdom may exist.[81] Even if general anesthetics lead to the demise of developing neurons, primate studies have not been able to establish a direct link between the structural alterations observed in the developing brain and specific long-term behavioral abnormalities or learning deficits. Performance deficits in the Operant Test Battery (OTB) has been reported.[98] The OTB is a reward-based test of motivation, color and positional discrimination, learning and short-term memory function, and was investigated in rhesus monkeys (younger than 31 months of age) who were exposed to ketamine for 24 hours with spontaneous ventilation during their first week of life.[98] Subsequently, the same methodology demonstrated similar motivational impairment and abnormalities in motor function in older rhesus monkeys after exposure to isoflurane in neonates.[357] Importantly, the same test battery can also be administered in children and has been linked to intelligence quotient (IQ).[359] However, using a similar OTB task, no deficits were observed in school-age children and adolescents who required general anesthesia under 3 years of age compared with their unexposed peers.[360] In another study, novel object recognition was impaired 12 to 30 months after repeated 4-hour sevoflurane exposures in infant monkeys.[345] Characterizing adult behaviors in this cohort, the authors observed amplified hostility and anxiety at 6 months of age[348]; however, these abnormalities were not observed at the 1-year and 2-year follow-up, when increased stress behavior was detected.[355] Similarly, another group found anxiety-related behavior in 12-month-old monkeys who were triple-exposed to isoflurane in infancy, compared with single-exposed animals or unexposed controls.[344] In a 2-year follow-up, this was reversed; the single-exposure group now exhibited significant anxiety-related behavior, but the triple-exposed animals did not. However, the triple-exposed group now displayed social behavioral abnormalities.[346] None of the groups demonstrated impairments in any of the cognitive tests.[346]

Nonhuman primate studies have consistently demonstrated neuronal cell death after anesthetic exposures in infancy that is similar in pattern to some of the brain structural injury observed in neonatal rodents. However, long-term cognitive abnormalities have not consistently been found and behavioral abnormalities, such as social and anxiety-related behavioral deficits were not found at all ages and have not followed a dose-response relationship, rendering the current data derived from nonhuman primates inconclusive to advise clinical practice.

Long-Term Outcome in Children Exposed to Anesthesia and Surgery

The difficulties in translating animal data to clinical anesthesia in human infants raise the importance of identifying potential clinical evidence for or against a causal relationship between exposure to anesthesia in early life and later neurologic abnormalities. Several clinical studies have attempted to identify if such a relationship exists.

MAJOR SURGERY IN THE NEONATAL PERIOD

Several cohort studies have demonstrated an association between major surgery in the neonatal period and poor neurodevelopmental outcome.[361] Children born with esophageal atresia, for example, had a lower IQ and more frequently suffered from depression, emotional, and behavioral problems compared with the general population.[362,363] Children with congenital diaphragmatic hernia repair also have a greater rate of neurologic sequelae.[364] Extremely premature, low–birth-weight neonates who underwent laparotomy exhibited poorer neurodevelopmental outcomes compared with matched controls.[363] A cohort of infants who underwent major surgery did not perform as well in school as a matched control group of healthy infants or with infants who had major nonsurgical medical conditions.[365] In a randomized trial of indomethacin treatment in 426 infants who weighed less than 1000 grams at birth, neurologic impairment was present in more of the 110 children who had undergone surgery (53%) compared with that in the 316 children who had received medical therapy (34%).[366] In a study of extremely preterm infants, the IQ of those who had undergone surgery was lower at 5 years of age and exhibited more sensorineural disability than those who had not undergone surgery.[367]

An MRI study conducted soon after major surgery in neonates reported abnormalities in 75% of the brain studies in preterm infants and in 58% of term neonates.[368] Lastly, a systematic review of 23 studies that examined neurodevelopmental outcome after surgery for noncardiac congenital anomalies in neonates reported cognitive delay in 23% of children and motor delay in 25%, with children exposed to surgery performing one-half a standard deviation below normal, on average.[368]

Preoperative brain lesions and white-matter injury have also been observed in a substantial number of neonates suffering from major congenital heart disease.[369–373] These studies all included neonates and infants with major confounding factors, such as congenital malformations or very preterm birth, which might increase the risk of poor neurodevelopmental outcome independent of surgery and anesthesia. Surgery itself can lead to poor outcome from perioperative neurohumoral and inflammatory response, or the hemodynamic instability associated with major surgery. Severity of illness may also have been greater in surgical patients compared with their respective control groups. Selection bias may have resulted in the sicker children being treated with surgery, whereas less severely ill children received medical therapy. Although these studies suggest that some infants undergoing major surgery are at increased risk of poor neurodevelopmental outcome, none of the studies provide conclusive evidence that the anesthesia or even the surgical episode is the cause of the increased risk of poor neurodevelopmental outcome.

Neonates do have vulnerable brains. A recent and plausible theory is that rather than just considering anesthesia to be a direct neurotoxin, the combination of an immature vasculature and hence risk of altered perfusion distribution, the inflammation associated with major illness or major surgery, and a direct neurotoxicity from prolonged exposure to anesthetic agents may form "the perfect storm" and have a synergistic impact causing brain injury.[374]

STUDY DESIGN TO ADDRESS POSSIBLE ANESTHETIC NEUROTOXICITY

As well as the aforementioned studies, which focused on the impact of surgery, there are now numerous studies that have focused on determining the impact of anesthesia itself on neurodevelopmental outcomes. These studies can be broadly classified according to their designs and/or the outcomes assessed. Each strategy has both strengths and weaknesses inherent to the design.

1. *Data linkage population-based studies.* These use existing administrative datasets that can be linked to other datasets. Such datasets include school grades, readiness for school, prescription patterns, and diagnostic codes. These studies are retrospective, and the outcomes and exposure variables are limited to those collected for the original purpose of the dataset. The exposure data may be limited in detail and the outcome data may not be the most pertinent for neurobehavioral analysis. They do, however, have the advantage of increased power due to their size. They often include whole country or whole state datasets.

2. *Use of existing birth cohorts or longitudinal studies.* These studies extract subsets of data from existing longitudinal cohorts examining aspects of child development. They are often large and include access to more detailed outcome measures, including some psychometric outcomes, and may also include diagnoses of disability and school grades. Although often large, they are not as big as the population linkage studies. As for data linkage studies, details of exposure may be limited.

3. *Purpose built cohort studies.* These studies typically recruit children de novo or out of existing longitudinal cohorts, where children exposed to anesthesia are then matched to children who were not exposed. Both groups are then tested with a range of neuropsychometric tests. School grades, diagnoses of neurodevelopmental disorders, and parent-reported questionnaires

can also be used as outcomes. These studies enable deeper and broader psychometric testing, but are expense, and logistic constraints limit their size and hence power.

4. *Trials.* Trials form the strongest evidence when assessing causation. However, given that anesthesia is always provided in association with surgery or a diagnostic procedure, it is difficult to design a trial where the impact of surgery or anesthesia alone can be examined. One trial to date has endeavored to do this while a second is underway (see later). Trials are logistically difficult and the long period between randomization and outcome means the trials take many years to complete and loss to follow-up can be a problem.

When it comes to outcome measures used, the studies can be broadly divided into four domains, though some studies will measure outcomes across multiple domains.

1. *School grades or school readiness tests.* These are easy to obtain and often applied at a population level. However, they are an imperfect measure of neurodevelopment. Deficits in neurodevelopment may occur with no impact on school grades, and similarly school grades can be affected by many social and other determinants apart from neurodevelopment.[375]

2. *Diagnosis of a learning disorder or specific neurodevelopmental disorder.* These are also easily discovered in administrative datasets and have substantial importance for those affected; however, definitions of disorders vary between jurisdictions and over time.

3. *Psychometric testing.* These are the gold standard for assessing neurodevelopment. Many tests covering a wide range of neurodevelopmental domains are available. Apical tests, such as IQ, are composite scores that pool results from several domains. Apical tests have the best value as far as predicting future function but using apical tests may miss deficits in some subdomains.

4. *Imaging.* MRI can detect brain injury; however, these studies are usually small due to costs and logistic issues. Some injuries may not be easily detected with MRI and the link between MRI findings and functional outcome is not always clear.

THE DATA LINKAGE STUDIES

Several large studies have used data linkage to explore associations between exposure to anesthesia and surgery and later neurodevelopmental outcomes. Here some of the most pertinent studies are described.

In one of the first studies reported, a retrospective cohort analysis using the New York State Medicaid records matched 383 children who underwent hernia repair before 3 years of age with 5050 children who did not undergo inguinal hernia repair.[376] After adjusting for sex, age, and complicating birth conditions (such as low birth weight), children who had hernia repair were more than twice as likely to have a subsequent diagnosis of a developmental or behavioral disorder (hazard ratio [HR] 2.3; 95% confidence intervals 1.3–4.1). To reduce environmental confounding effects, the authors then proceeded to use the data from the New York State Medicaid program to construct a retrospective sibling birth cohort.[377] Once again, they assessed the association between exposure to anesthesia in children younger than 3 years of age and the subsequent risk of diagnosis of developmental or behavioral disorders. A total of 10,450 siblings were identified, 304 of whom underwent surgery before 3 years of age, with no history of behavioral or developmental disorders before the surgery, and 10,146 children who did not undergo surgery. The association of exposure to anesthesia with subsequent developmental or behavioral disorders was

assessed with both proportional hazards modeling and pair-matched analysis. As with their previous study, they found an association between surgery and poor neurodevelopmental outcome. The incidence of developmental or behavioral disorders was 128.2 diagnoses per 1000 person-years for those who had surgery and 56.3 diagnoses per 1000 person-years for those who did not. This association persisted when adjusted for sex, history of birth-related medical complications, and clustering by sibling status; the estimated hazard ratio (HR) of developmental or behavioral disorders associated with any exposure to anesthesia was 1.6 (95% confidence intervals 1.4–1.8). The risk increased from 1.1 (95% confidence intervals 0.8–1.4) for one operation to 2.9 (95% confidence intervals 2.5–3.1) for two operations and 4.0 (95% confidence intervals 3.5–4.5) for three or more operations. The number of siblings available for a matched analysis was relatively small; there were only 138 sibling pairs. In the pair-matched study, there was no evidence of an association between surgery and poor outcome, with a relative risk of 0.9 (95% confidence intervals 0.6–1.4); however, the small sample size may have limited the power of that analysis.

The same group used linked Medicaid claims in New York and Texas to explore the association between a number of types of surgery at various ages before 5 years of age and the subsequent diagnosis of any mental disorder, developmental delay, or ADHD. There were 38,493 children who had either pyloromyotomy, inguinal hernia repair, circumcision, or tonsillectomy and/or adenoidectomy who were matched to 192,465 controls. They found evidence for weak association; overall HR of mental disorder 1.26 (95% confidence intervals 1.22–1.30), developmental delay 1.26 (95% confidence intervals 1.20–1.32), and ADHD 1.31 (95% confidence intervals 1.25–1.37). Interestingly, the risk was not greatest in the youngest exposed and varied minimally among surgeries.[378] This study was criticized given that the diagnoses in Medicaid may be inaccurate, so they repeated the study looking at prescriptions of ADHD medications. Once again, they found an association between surgery and ADHD, as defined by having an ADHD medication prescribed, and once again the association was not greatest in the youngest. It did appear, however, that the risk was greater in tonsillectomy, but no definitive conclusions were drawn that one surgery had a greater risk. The investigators also sought to quantify any bias by looking at risk for receiving medication that were not plausibly linked to neurodevelopment such as antibiotics and diphenhydramine. They found that exposure to surgery increased the risk of having these medications prescribed, indicating that there was some bias; however, this increased rate of prescribing was consistent with the Medicaid population studied.[379]

Another US study used administrative datasets consisting of claims in a national insurance-based cohort. Children born between 2006 and 2012 were categorized as having one, multiple, or no exposures to anesthesia before the age of 5. The outcome of interest was the diagnosis of ADHD (those diagnosed with ADHD prior to an exposure were excluded). Among 185,002 children in the final cohort, 9179 were diagnosed with ADHD. Compared with unexposed children, a single exposure to anesthesia was associated with an increased risk of ADHD (HR 1.39, 95% confidence intervals, 1.32–1.47). Multiple exposures increased the risk further (HR 1.75, 95% confidence intervals 1.62–1.87). In the analyses evaluating potential moderators of the association between exposure and ADHD, only the interaction for race was statistically significant, with exposure increasing the risk of ADHD to a greater extent in non-White compared with White children.[380]

In contrast to the above, data from Taiwan reported no increased risk of ADHD in children who received general anesthesia.[381] In a matched cohort from a national insurance database of 16,465 children among whom 3293 were exposed to anesthesia before 3 years of age, the adjusted HR of developing ADHD was 1.06 (95% confidence intervals 0.86–1.31). The HRs for developing ADHD after a single anesthetic was 1.11 (95% confidence intervals 0.88–1.41) and for multiple exposures 0.96 (95% confidence intervals 0.71–1.31).[381] The same group examined a diagnosis of autism in children exposed to general anesthesia before 2 years of age and found no evidence for an association (HR 0.93, 95% confidence intervals 0.57–1.53).[382]

Hansen et al. used a very large Danish birth cohort of 2689 children who had inguinal hernia repair in infancy to compare academic performance with 14,575 children who were randomly selected as an age-matched sample from the general population.[383] Those who had hernia repair performed worse at school, although after adjusting for likely confounding variables, there was no evidence of any association between surgery and school performance. A similar but smaller study conducted in Iowa[384] in which investigators reviewed school test scores in 287 children who had surgery in infancy determined that scores in surgical infants were slightly lower than in the general population. However, the test scores from 12% of the children were in the lowest 5th centile in the general population. In a subset of 58 children with no risk factors for neurodevelopmental issues, the test scores were not below the average for the population, although 14% still scored in the lowest 5th percentile. These results suggest that a subset of the population may be particularly vulnerable to the neurocognitive effects of anesthetics.

Two similar population-based Canadian cohort studies examined the association between surgery in young children and their Early Development Index (EDI). The EDI is a test of readiness for school. The 103-item questionnaire is completed by teachers when children are 5 years of age. It has five domains: physical health and well-being, social knowledge and competence, emotional health and maturity, language and cognitive development, and communication skills and general knowledge. Both studies assessed the association between surgery and their EDI using data from the entire province of Ontario. The 28,366 children who had surgery before they performed the EDI[385] were compared with 55,910 controls who did not have surgery but were matched for gestational age at birth, mother's age at birth, rurality, gender, and year and quarter of birth, and excluded children with known physical disability health-related causes of impaired development, and those with a diagnosis of behavioral, learning, or developmental disorder. They also adjusted for aboriginal status, age, and household income. The primary outcome was defined as vulnerable (scoring in the lowest 10th centile in any domain). Vulnerability was increased slightly in those who had surgery: 7259/28,366 (25.6%) compared with 13,957/55,910 (25%) controls (odds ratio 1.05; 95% confidence intervals 1.01–1.08). Interestingly, the odds of vulnerability were greater in those younger than 2 years of age at the time of surgery (odds ratio 1.05; 95% confidence intervals 1.01–1.10), whereas the odds were not increased in those older than 2 years of age at the time of surgery (odds ratio 1.04; 95% confidence intervals 0.98–1.10). They also found no evidence of increased vulnerability in those who had multiple surgeries. In the second study, 4470 children who underwent surgery in Manitoba before the age of 4 years were matched with 13,586 controls for gestational age at birth, mother's age at birth, rurality, income quintile, gender, and year of birth.[386]

They excluded children with a diagnosis of any developmental disability. In their analysis, the authors adjusted for welfare status, gestational age, small or large for dates, mother's age at birth, child's age, and Johns Hopkins Resource User Band (which assesses medical resource utilization with a score of 0 to 5). As in the Ontario study, these investigators reported a small difference with children who had surgery performing worse than those who had not had surgery. However, the domains in which they performed poorly were not consistent with the Ontario study. Like the Ontario study, the Johns Hopkins study detected evidence for an association in children who had surgery at age greater than 2 years of age but no evidence for any association if surgery occurred at less than 2 years of age. They also found no evidence of a greater risk in those who had multiple surgeries compared with those who underwent only one surgery. Although the findings in these two studies may seem inconsistent with nonhuman studies that suggest a greater risk in younger animals, it is possible that the substantial differences in neurodevelopment between animals and humans means that exposures in the older children could affect more vulnerable neuronal networks. Alternatively, the association seen in these cohort studies could be due to factors other than the neurotoxicity observed in animal studies.

A large Swedish study examined the school grades of all children born in Sweden between January 1973 and December 1993. Of the 2,174,073 children, 33,514 had one anesthetic for a surgical procedure before the age of 4 years and no subsequent hospitalizations. These were matched to 159,619 children who had no exposure to anesthesia. 3640 children who had multiple anesthetics were also identified. The outcomes were mean school grades at 16 years of age and IQ test scores for those children who were conscripted into military service. The model that compared outcomes accounted for sex, month of birth, gestational age at delivery, Apgar score at 5 minutes, parental education, cohabiting parents, income, and sibling number. Exposure to 1 anesthetic was associated with a mean difference of 0.41% (95% confidence intervals 0.12–0.70) lower school grades. The effect size was similar between single and multiple anesthetic exposures. When subgroups based on age were examined, a statistically significant difference was only seen in the children exposed to anesthesia between 36 and 48 months of age.

The IQ test scores were obtained from 9198 exposed boys and 45,115 unexposed boys. The mean IQ test scores among boys with 1 exposure before the age of 4 years were 0.97% (95% confidence intervals, 0.15–1.78) lower than the scores among unexposed boys.

The investigators also studied the impact of sex, maternal educational level, or month of birth during the same year. Compared with exposure to anesthesia, these all substantially impacted school grades to a greater extent, leading the investigators to conclude that any impact related to surgery before 4 years of age was relatively small compared with other factors in development.[387]

A study from Australia also used data linkage to examine the association between surgery and school grades. Of 211,978 children born at term without major abnormalities or known neurodevelopmental disability, 82,156 had a school entry developmental assessment and 153,025 had grade 3 school test results, with 12,848 (15.7%) and 25,032 (16.4%) exposed to general anesthesia before 2 years of age, respectively. Children who underwent general anesthesia had 17%, 34%, and 23% increased odds of being developmentally high risk (adjusted odds ratio [aOR]: 1.17; 95% confidence intervals: 1.07–1.29); or scoring below the national minimum standard in numeracy (aOR: 1.34;

95% confidence intervals: 1.21–1.48) and reading (aOR: 1.23; 95% confidence intervals: 1.12–1.36), respectively.[388]

In summary, most, but not all data linkage studies have found evidence for a modest association between anesthesia and surgical exposure in early childhood and aspects of later school performance or school readiness. Some, but not all, have also found evidence for an association with learning difficulty and behavioral problems such as ADHD. These studies have not found that the association is greater in younger children. The association between exposure and behavioral problems does appear to be greater for children who have multiple exposures.

LONGITUDINAL COHORT AND REGISTRY DATASETS

In an established population-based, retrospective birth cohort, Wilder and colleagues studied the association between anesthetic exposure before 4 years of age and the subsequent development of learning disabilities.[389] Regression was used to calculate HRs for anesthetic exposure as a predictor of learning disability, with adjustment for gestational age at birth, sex, and birth weight. Of 5357 children in the cohort, 593 had been exposed to general anesthesia before 4 years of age. Compared with those not exposed to anesthesia, a single exposure was not associated with an increased risk of learning disability (HR 1.0; 95% confidence interval 0.79–1.27). However, children who underwent two separate episodes of anesthesia had an increased risk of a learning disability (HR 1.59; 95% confidence intervals 1.06–2.37) and those who underwent three or more separate anesthetics had an even greater risk (HR 2.60; 95% confidence intervals 1.60–4.24). The association between learning disability and multiple episodes of anesthesia remained after adjusting for the American Society of Anesthesiologists (ASA) physical status. The risk for a learning disability also increased according to the cumulative duration of anesthesia. However, this study suffered from several limitations. Because the study reported anesthetics administered between 1976 and 1982, the most common anesthetic treatment was halothane and nitrous oxide, and none of the children were monitored with pulse oximetry or capnography. It is not possible to determine how many of these children had excessive hyperventilation or unrecognized desaturation. Furthermore, the maternal birth histories were not described (e.g., magnesium may cause neuroapoptosis or be neuroprotective). Three different learning disabilities were considered with equipoise in the final analysis, and these disabilities were not tested in all children, but only when a teacher or parent requested testing. These questions limit the external validity of these data.

To reduce the impact of confounding factors, using the same population-based, retrospective birth cohort, the same group conducted further studies with a matched cohort design.[390] The researchers matched 350 children exposed to anesthesia before the age of 2 years to 700 children not exposed to anesthesia. The matching was based on several known risk factors for learning disabilities: sex, mother's education, birth weight, and gestational age at birth. Outcomes of interest included learning disability, need for individualized education program for an emotional or behavioral disorder, and group-administered achievement tests. In the analysis, an adjustment was also performed for burden of illness. The primary finding was that children exposed to two or more occurrences of anesthesia (but not a single occurrence) were at increased risk for having a learning disability (HR 2.12; 95% confidence intervals of 1.26–3.54), and an amplified need for individualized education programs for speech and language impairment. However, there was not an increased need for

a program for emotional or behavioral disorders. The authors also detected an association between multiple exposures to anesthesia and lower math testing scores. The same criticisms apply to this study as to the earlier study from this institution.[389]

Given that the above studies were conducted in a population who had potentially outdated anesthetic agents (e.g., halothane), they performed a similar set of studies in a cohort of children born between 1996 and 2000. Once again, the birth cohort from Olmstead County was used. Propensity was used to match children exposed and not exposed to general anesthesia before age 3 years. Outcomes included learning disabilities, ADHD, and group-administered ability and achievement tests. For the 116 multiply exposed, 457 singly exposed, and 463 unexposed children analyzed, multiple, but not single, exposures were associated with an increased frequency of both learning disabilities and ADHD (HR for learning disabilities = 2.17 [95% confidence intervals, 1.32–3.59]). Multiple exposures were associated with decreases in both cognitive ability and academic achievement. Single exposures were associated with modest decreases in reading and language achievement but not cognitive ability.[391]

The two Olmstead County cohort studies described earlier were combined in a subsequent analysis to provide a greater sample size with which to explore any association between exposure to anesthesia before 3 years of age and a subsequent diagnosis of a learning disability or ADHD. 5339 children were unexposed and 1054 had one exposure. In a weighted analysis, single exposure to anesthesia was not associated with either ADHD (HR 1.21, 95% confidence intervals 0.91–1.60) or a learning disability (HR 0.98, 95% confidence intervals 0.78–1.23).[392]

Studies involving identical twins are useful to reduce confounding environmental and genetic influences. A study from Denmark sought to identify a possible association between anesthesia exposure before 3 years of age and school performance in 1143 monozygotic twin pairs in The Netherlands Twin Registry.[393] In the identical twins who were discordant for exposure to anesthesia (one twin was exposed to anesthesia and the other was not), their school performance was identical. This would suggest that surgery with anesthesia may not be the cause of poor school performance. Interestingly, the school performance in both the discordant pairs and the pairs where both twins underwent surgery was poorer than that for concordant twin pairs in which neither twin was exposed to anesthesia. This finding could imply that there may exist an unknown genetic factor that increases the risk of both the need for surgery and poor school performance.

A number of investigations examined the association between surgery and neurodevelopmental outcome using the Western Australian Pregnancy Cohort (Raine). In one analysis they found an association between language and abstract reasoning deficits in 10-year-old children who were exposed to one or more anesthetics before age 3 years compared with unexposed children. After adjusting for confounders, any anesthetic before age 3 years increased the risk ratio of disability in receptive, expressive, or total language as measured by the Clinical Evaluation of Language Fundamentals (CELF-3) test, as well as abstract reasoning (Raven's Colored Progressive Matrices) to between 1.7 and 2.1 of unexposed controls, whereas other tests of vocabulary, behavior, and motor function were unaffected by exposure.[394]

The same authors performed a subsequent analysis, comparing the diverse outcome measures of neuropsychological testing, International Classification of Diseases, Ninth Revision (ICD-9)-coded diagnoses, and academic performance.[395] Of the 781 children who had all outcome measures, 211 had received an anesthetic before 3 years of age. Compared with the unexposed children, those who had received anesthesia demonstrated an increased risk of deficit in neuropsychological language assessment and an increased risk of an ICD-9-coded diagnosis of language or cognitive disorder. However, they did not demonstrate poorer academic performance. This finding highlights the limitations of using school performance as a measure of neurodevelopmental outcome. In the subset of children who were exposed at older ages (3- to 5-year-olds and 5- to 10-year-olds), there was no association between exposure and any deficit in any neuropsychological test except for children exposed between 3 and 5 years of age who demonstrated worse scores on motor function tests.[395]

In a British birth cohort, The Avon Longitudinal Study of Parents and Children Birth Cohort, the association between exposure to anesthesia before the age of 4 years and a range of subsequent neurodevelopmental outcomes was explored. 13,433 children born between 1991 and 1993 comprised the cohort; 8.3% were exposed to one anesthetic and 1.6% were exposed to multiple anesthetics. 46 neurodevelopmental outcomes were assessed between ages 7 years and 16 years in motor, cognitive, linguistic, educational, social, and behavioral domains using school examination results, parent and teacher questionnaires, and clinical assessments. Of these, the following reached predefined levels of statistical significance ($P<0.00652$): dynamic balance 0.3 standard deviations less in multiply exposed children (95% confidence intervals 0.1–0.5, $P<0.001$), manual dexterity performance was 0.1 standard deviation less in singly exposed children (95% confidence interval 0.0–0.2, $P=0.006$) and 0.3 standard deviations less in multiply exposed children (95% confidence interval 0.1–0.4, $P<0.001$), and social communication scores were 0.1 standard deviations less in singly exposed children (95% confidence interval 0.0–0.2, $P=0.001$) and 0.4 standard deviations less in multiply exposed children (95% confidence interval 0.3–0.5, $P<0.001$). Anesthesia and surgery did not impair the remaining neurodevelopmental measures; general cognitive ability; attention; working memory; reading, spelling, verbal comprehension, and expression; behavioral difficulties; or national English, mathematics, and science assessments.[396]

Another study used an established cohort of children 5 to 18 years of age who had MRI scans as part of a large language development study.[397] The cohort did not include children with any risk factors for poor neurodevelopmental outcome. Within this cohort, they found 53 children who had undergone surgery before the age of 4 years and matched these to 53 peers who had not, matching on age, gender, and socioeconomic status. All children underwent a battery of neuropsychological tests and brain MRI. Exposed children scored lower in listening comprehension and performance IQ but did not exhibit comparably decreased grey-matter density in the thalamus or retrosplenial cortex, as previously seen in rodent studies. Instead, they demonstrated diminished grey-matter volumes in the occipital cortex and cerebellum, associated with lower-performance IQ.

The studies that examined existing cohort data found an association between multiple exposures and subsequent learning disorder and ADHD, but not after a single exposure. Some of these studies also found an association between exposure and deficits in a variety of different neurodevelopmental domains on psychometric testing.

PROSPECTIVE COHORT STUDIES WITH CHILDREN

Studies in animals have also identified deficits in recognition memory tasks after general anesthesia. Recognition is based on recollection and familiarity. To test if humans had similar deficits in recollection, investigators studied 28 children aged 6 to 11 years who had undergone anesthesia in infancy compared with 28 age- and gender-matched controls.[398] They found that scores in tests of recollection in exposed children were less than in unexposed children, but scores in tests of IQ, behavior, and familiarity were similar.

Perhaps the most important cohort study was the Pediatric Anesthesia and Neurodevelopment Assessment (PANDA) study.[399] In this bidirectional cohort study, 105 children aged 8 to 15 years who had surgery for inguinal hernia repair before 3 years of age were compared with 105 matched siblings who were of similar age at testing but did not undergo surgery early in life. Children underwent a range of well-validated neuropsychological tests. The choice of tests was based on their psychometric properties and on their relevance to animal data and previous cohort study findings. The primary outcome was full-scale IQ. The median duration of anesthesia exposure was 80 minutes. There was no evidence for a difference in any of the IQ domains. In the exposed cohort, full-scale IQ was 111, performance IQ was 108, and verbal IQ was 111, whereas in the unexposed siblings, full-scale IQ was 111, performance IQ was 107, and verbal IQ was 111. Differences in mean IQ scores between exposed and unexposed siblings for full-scale IQ were 0.2 (95% confidence intervals, −2.6 to 2.9); performance IQ, 0.5 (95% confidence intervals, −2.7 to 3.7); and verbal IQ, −0.5 (95% confidence intervals, −3.2 to 2.2). There was also no evidence of differences in secondary outcomes that included memory and learning, motor and processing speed, visuospatial function, attention, executive function, or language. Exposed children did, however, have poorer scores in some aspects of behavior even when adjusted for gender. Subanalyses that addressed age at the time of exposure and duration of exposure reported no effects of either variable on outcome, although these analyses had limited power. This study is by far the most rigorous cohort study and provides strong evidence that approximately 1 hour of exposure to anesthesia in early childhood is unlikely to cause significant cognitive impairment at a later age.

Another important cohort study is the Mayo Anesthesia Safety in Kids (MASK) study.[400] Children unexposed to anesthesia, singly exposed, and multiply exposed who were born in Olmsted County, Minnesota, from 1994 to 2007 were sampled using a propensity-guided approach and underwent neuropsychological testing at 8 to 12 or 15 to 20 years of age. The primary outcome was the full-scale intelligence quotient standard score of the Wechsler Abbreviated Scale of Intelligence. Secondary outcomes covered several domains of neurodevelopment including both comprehensive neuropsychological assessment and parent reports. In the sample, 411 children were unexposed, 380 singly exposed, and 206 multiply exposed. The primary outcome of IQ did not differ significantly according to exposure status. The multiple-exposed and single-exposed children scored 1.3 points (95% confidence intervals, −3.8 to 1.2; $P=0.32$) and 0.5 points (95% confidence intervals, −2.8 to 1.9 $P=0.70$) less compared with unexposed children. Among the secondary outcomes, processing speed and fine motor abilities decreased in multiply but not singly exposed children and the parents of multiply exposed children reported increased problems related to executive function, behavior, and reading.

As a secondary analysis, the authors used factor and cluster analysis to investigate particular domains of outcomes. The factor analysis found the data fit well to a five-factor model. For subjects multiple (but not single) exposed to anesthesia, a factor reflecting motor skills, visual-motor integration, and processing speed was significantly less in exposed children (standardized difference of −0.35 [95% confidence interval −0.57 to −0.13]). No other factor was associated with exposure to anesthesia. The cluster analysis identified three groups with 106 children (10.6%) with the poorest performance in most tests, 557 (55.9%) with intermediate performance, and 334 (33.5%) with best performance in most tests. The odds of multiply exposed children belonging to the poorest performing cluster compared with the intermediate cluster was 2.83 (95% confidence intervals: 1.49–5.35; *P*=0.001) There were no other significant associations between exposure status and cluster group.[401]

As a part of the MASK study, children were also asked to perform the OTB. In one of the nonhuman primate studies, primates exposed to anesthesia performed more poorly in this test. The test has also been used previously in children, and applying the same test to children provided an avenue to compare nonhuman primate and human data directly. In the analyses however, none of the OTB test scores depended upon anesthesia exposure status when corrected for multiple comparisons.[360]

RANDOMIZED TRIALS

Cohort studies are inherently limited by the risk of confounding. Adjustments in the analyses can never completely remove the risk that the association is due to a factor apart from anesthesia. Only randomized trials can reliably reduce the risk of confounding. Randomized trials are difficult to perform as it is impossible to randomize for anesthesia versus no anesthesia in children undergoing surgery. It is, however, possible to randomize for two different anesthetic techniques. The general anesthesia compared with spinal anesthesia trial (GAS study) is the only randomized trial that has examined the effect of different anesthetic regimens in infancy on neurodevelopmental outcome.[402] In the GAS study, 722 infants younger than 60 weeks postmenstrual age were randomly assigned to awake-regional (nearly always spinal anesthesia) or sevoflurane general anesthesia for inguinal hernia repair. Children were then tested at 2 and 5 years of age. In this study, the median duration of sevoflurane exposure in the general anesthesia group was 54 minutes. The spinal failure rate was 19% and the loss to follow-up for the 2-year assessment was 14%. The trial was designed as an equivalence trial with predefined boundaries of equivalence being set at 5 IQ points in the primary outcome at 5 years of age. Five IQ points is one-third of a standard deviation and well within what would be regarded as a clinically insignificant effect size.

At 2 years of age, the cognitive score of the Bayley Scales of Infant and Toddler Development, Third Edition (Bayley-III) scale was a prespecified secondary outcome.[402] The Bayley-III has five domains: cognitive, language, motor, social emotional, and adaptive behavior. There was strong evidence of equivalence in all domains. In the as-per-protocol analysis using multiple imputation, the mean difference (awake-regional vs. general) in the cognitive composite score adjusted for gestational age at birth was 0.17 (95% confidence intervals −2.30 to 2.64). This was within the predefined equivalence margin of 5 points. The difference in language was 1.15 (95% confidence intervals −1.59 to 3.88), motor 0.60 (95% confidence intervals −1.77 to 2.97), social emotional 1.0 (95% confidence intervals −3.12 to 5.13) and adaptive behavior −0.89 (95% confidence intervals −3.52 to 1.73). The results were similar in intent-to-treat and complete case analyses, implying spinal failure and loss to follow-up did not bias the results.

At the five-year assessment point, the primary outcome was the Wechsler Preschool and Primary Scale of Intelligence, Third Edition (WPPSI-III) full-scale IQ.[403] A range of other neurodevelopmental domains were assessed with neuropsychometric testing and parent reporting. The full-scale IQ score was 99.8 in the awake-regional and 98.97 in the general anesthesia group, with a difference in means of 0.23 points (95% confidence intervals −2.59 to 3.06). This is strong evidence for equivalence, with the 95% bounds being well within predefined equivalence ranges. The intention-to-treat and as-per-protocol analyses gave similar results, as did complete case and multiple imputation analyses. There was evidence for equivalence in the verbal and performance subdomains of the IQ score. Among the secondary outcomes assessed with psychometric testing, the 95% confidence interval bounds of differences between groups were within half a standard deviation for all secondary outcomes exploring domains in verbal, language, perception, visuospatial, processing speed, attention, executive function, memory, learning, social perception, sensorimotor, and academic domains. These reinforced the premise that a single exposure of 1 hour of anesthesia has no impact on neurodevelopment as tested at 5 years of age. In the parent-reported outcomes examining executive function, adaptive behavior, and maladaptive behavior, the 95% confidence intervals around the differences in means between groups were also within half a standard deviation. In one test of executive function (the BRIEF), the 95% confidence intervals crossed 0 in favor of unexposed children performing worse; however, this result is difficult to interpret given the multiple outcomes measured and the likelihood that the bounds still fall within what would be regarded as clinically insignificant.

However, the trial does have three important limitations: first, the relatively brief anesthetic exposure (54 minutes); second, the lack of sensitivity to test higher executive function and memory even at 5 years of age; and third, only one anesthetic was administered.[404] Accordingly, future studies are needed to address these limitations.

COMBINATION ANALYSIS THE GAS, MASK, AND PANDA STUDIES

A meta-analysis was performed using data from the three prospective studies, the GAS, PANDA, and MASK studies. These studies were chosen assuming they were least likely to be biased. When combining the studies, outcome data were available across all three studies for the full-scale intelligence quotient (FSIQ); the parentally reported Child Behavior Checklist (CBCL) total, externalizing, and internalizing problems scores; and Behavior Rating Inventory of Executive Function (BRIEF). Of 1644 children identified, 841 who had a single exposure to general anesthesia were evaluated. Children exposed performed worse on the CBCL with a mean total score difference of 2.3 (95% confidence intervals 1–3.7, *P*=0.001). performance was also worse in the subscales; CBCL externalizing problems: 1.9 (95% confidence intervals 0.7–3.1, *P*=0.003); and CBCL internalizing problems: 2.2 (95% confidence intervals 0.9–3.5, *P*=0.001). Differences in the BRIEF were not significant after multiple comparison adjustment. Full-scale IQ was also not affected by general anesthesia exposure. The CBCL and BREIF scores are parent-reported scores and as such are open to bias if the parents are aware of the exposure status; in the GAS study some parents were unaware of exposure status. Interestingly a secondary analysis exploring the impact of being blinded or unblinded did not find that parents were more likely to score their children worse in the exposure groups if they were unblinded.[405]

PRENATAL EXPOSURE

Relatively few studies have examined the possible impact of prenatal exposure. To investigate a potential association between perinatal exposure to general anesthesia during cesarean delivery and subsequent diagnosis of learning disability,[406] the risk of a learning disability was compared in 193 children delivered via cesarean section with general anesthesia, 304 delivered via cesarean section with regional anesthesia, and 4823 delivered vaginally without any anesthesia. The association between mode of delivery and learning disability was adjusted for sex, birth weight, gestational age at birth, exposure to anesthesia before 4 years of age, and maternal education. The risk of disability was similar between children delivered vaginally with no anesthesia and cesarean delivery with general anesthesia, but risk of disability was less in children delivered via cesarean with regional anesthesia than vaginal delivery with no anesthesia (HR 0.64; 95% confidence intervals 0.44–0.92; $P=0.017$). The results implied that brief exposure to general anesthesia during delivery was not associated with subsequent learning disability, but the reason the risk was less with regional anesthesia compared with no anesthesia is unclear, although this may suggest the possibility of substantial confounding influences. To explore the possibility that the regional blockade was protective, the authors subsequently compared those born without general anesthesia by vaginal delivery with and without regional analgesia and found no difference in risk of learning disability.[407] Using the same epidemiologic cohort, the same research group detected an increased prevalence of ADHD in children who had undergone repeated surgical procedures with anesthesia, compared with none or only one exposure.[408]

Ing and colleagues used the Western Australian Raine cohort to evaluate any association between prenatal exposure to anesthesia for procedures during pregnancy and neuropsychological and behavioral outcomes at 10 years of age. Associations were assessed between exposure and six neuropsychological and behavioral tests using a multivariable linear regression model, adjusting for demographic and clinical covariates (sex, race, income, and maternal education, alcohol or tobacco use, and clinical diagnoses). Among 2024 children with available outcome scores, 22 (1.1%) were prenatally exposed to general anesthesia. Compared with unexposed children, the CBCL externalizing behavioral scores were greater in prenatally exposed children (score difference of 6.1 [99.17% confidence intervals, 0.2–12.0]; $P=0.006$). No significant differences were found in any other score.[409]

Outcome After Exposure to Anesthesia Outside of the Operating Room

The operating room is not the only area where anesthetic neurotoxicity may be relevant. Ketamine and benzodiazepines are frequently administered in the emergency room and in neonatal and pediatric intensive care units. These drugs may be administered for a prolonged period of time, in theory increasing the risks of neurotoxicity.[56,58]

Unfortunately, determining the clinical relevance of any neurotoxicity in intensive care patients is even more difficult than in the operating room. The total number of children who can be examined is smaller, the children tend to be a heterogeneous population, and most importantly, they often have multiple significant confounding comorbidities including exposure to anesthesia, which could significantly affect interpretation of adverse outcomes. To date, there is mixed evidence that exposure to anesthetic or sedative drugs is associated with poorer neurobehavioral outcome in this patient population. A Cochrane review found some evidence for worsened short-term outcome in neonates who had prolonged exposures to midazolam infusions.[410] In contrast, after correction for severity of illness, another study (using the Etude EPIdémiologique sur les Petits Ages GEstationnels [EPIPAGE] cohort) found no evidence of an association between prolonged sedation and adverse neurologic outcomes.[411] In that study, however, many children received opioids for sedation rather than benzodiazepines and the study was not powered to detect performance differences of less than 10%.

Limitations of the Available Clinical Studies

There are numerous reasons why clinical data on neurobehavioral outcomes after anesthesia are difficult to interpret. The response to a brain injury in a child varies according to the nature of the insult and the timing of the insult. The trajectory after injury is also substantially modified by the environment and genetic factors. Given the heterogeneity in surgical populations, ages of exposure, and ages when outcomes are assessed, and the wide variety of different outcome domains assessed, it is not surprising that the clinical studies often present somewhat conflicting results.

Confounding is a major limitation for all the observational studies. Confounding may be minimized by careful subject selection and matching or by adjusting for plausible known confounding factors in analyses such as multivariable regressions. However, these techniques are to some extent imperfect in reducing known confounding and cannot remove the impact of unknown confounding factors. Such confounding means that all observational studies can only at best identify associations and hence possible causation but cannot definitively prove causation. One important confounding factor is the impact of surgery and other perioperative factors. Observational studies are generally unable to separate the effects of surgery or the need for surgery from the potential anesthetic effects. Surgery may result in significant neurohumoral stress and/or inflammatory responses that may influence neurocognitive outcome in addition to metabolic, hemodynamic, and respiratory events that occur perioperatively. Data collection for some of these studies also occurred before continuous pulse oximetry and capnography monitoring were standard monitors and at a time when inhaled anesthetics with profound adverse cardiovascular effects such as halothane, were used.[389,390] Prospective studies of capnography and pulse oximetry have demonstrated that the very population considered to be at increased risk (those <2 years of age) had the greatest incidence of desaturation events, hypercarbia, and hypocarbia.[412–414]

Children undergoing surgery or diagnostic procedures early in life may suffer more frequently from concomitant chromosomal and genetic abnormalities or comorbidities such as prematurity, that have been linked to abnormal neurobehavioral outcomes. For example, children with cyanotic congenital heart disease often have abnormal neurocognitive development and some have smaller brain volumes before any surgical or anesthesia intervention.[307] The indication for surgery or for a diagnostic procedure requiring anesthesia, such as injury or infection, may artificially increase the incidence of neurodevelopmental abnormalities in the anesthetized cohort.[307] On the other hand, it has been argued that subjects suffering from underlying abnormalities adversely affecting neurodevelopment who do not receive the required surgery may be introduced into the pool of unanesthetized children, and therefore mask potentially toxic effects of anesthesia.[60]

Confounding cannot be mitigated by ever larger sample sizes. Replication also cannot rule out confounding. If multiple studies show similar results, this does not preclude confounding, as the confounding factor may be present across multiple populations. Similarly, associations seen in multiple domains can also be explained by the impact of a single confounding factor. Lastly, if there is confounding by indication, then the association between exposure and outcome will be greater if there are multiple exposures.

Further complicating the interpretation of data is the substantial gap in time between exposure and neurologic assessment. The advantage of performing neurologic assessments in school-age children includes the increased precision and greater predictive value of such assessments compared with neurobehavioral testing performed for children younger than 2 years of age and an ability to test wider domains of neurodevelopment, in particular higher executive function.[415] Some behavioral problems can only be diagnosed accurately in an older child. Also, if an injury occurs in early life the child may "grow into the injury" which means the impact becomes more obvious over time; alternatively, a child may recover. As mentioned above, the trajectory will vary with type and age of injury as well as the environmental and genetic make-up of the child.

Current animal studies do not provide sufficient guidance on the most vulnerable brain regions, the individual neurocognitive domains that may be affected, or the particular age at which the human brain may potentially be most susceptible to the neurotoxic effects of anesthetic exposure.

No consensus exists, even in the animal literature, concerning the duration of anesthesia exposure required to induce long-lasting injury. Although anesthetic exposure may represent a much larger fraction of an animal's life than a human's, at the cellular level apoptosis is likely triggered by a more similar duration of exposure. However, both cell cycle duration and the developmental period of the brain are considerably greater in humans than in rodents. It is therefore plausible, if an anesthesia-induced increase in apoptosis does occur in humans during a prolonged anesthetic exposure, that it may be functionally less important than the same increase in apoptosis over the same period of time in a rodent. Similarly, the plasticity and capacity for recovery may differ between species. It can be argued that the period of development in humans is greater than it is in animals, and hence there may be more time for recovery, but, as mentioned before, this may extend the potentially vulnerable period in humans into adolescence. Human development and subsequent cognitive performance are far more complex than in animal species and humans may therefore be more vulnerable, even following less severe neurodegeneration than that observed in laboratory studies. Injuries during critical periods of development may have an exaggerated effect compared with the same injury outside of these periods.[319,416] Accordingly, studies that find no evidence of association with shorter exposures may not be generalizable to all applications of anesthesia.

We currently lack adequate information from preclinical studies to know which specific domains to examine in humans following anesthetic exposure. Many of these studies use summary scores, such as IQ or average school grades. These outcome measures may miss subtle effects confined to specific neurobehavioral domains. Similarly, a diagnosis of developmental delay or behavioral problems may also miss more subtle changes in particular areas. However, broad batteries of detailed tests where analyses are not adjusted for multiplicity are likely to find at least one association purely by chance.

The vulnerable period in humans, if it exists, has not been clearly identified. Animal data seem to suggest that anesthetic exposure may be most relevant during pregnancy or in early infancy, but it could be possible that the period of vulnerability may extend beyond infancy and young age for some brain regions with ongoing neurogenesis. These critical uncertainties not only complicate the interpretation of published studies, but they also make the design of future prospective studies very difficult.

The possible neuroprotective effects of anesthesia complicate this conundrum even further. Infants undergoing surgery who experience major intraoperative adverse events, such as cardiopulmonary arrest, are generally expected to suffer from abnormal neurologic outcomes, irrespective of their anesthetic exposure. Neurologic abnormalities observed after an otherwise uneventful procedure are considered neurotoxic effects of anesthesia. However, because anesthetics may also, at least partially, protect from the harmful metabolic, immunologic, and humoral responses to surgery and pain,[278] an alternative explanation may be that inadequate levels of anesthesia, insufficient postoperative pain relief, or unabated inflammation may be the culprit for the neurodevelopmental abnormalities observed in epidemiologic studies. It is also possible that anesthetics may protect in major adverse settings but may be deleterious in the absence of toxic stimuli, causing injury during minor procedures but ameliorating injury during major surgery, such as complex heart surgery involving cardiopulmonary bypass.

For exposures of less than 1 hour in otherwise healthy infants, there is increasing evidence that there is no association between anesthetic exposure and poor cognitive outcome in human studies. This is consistent with animal studies not detecting brain structural abnormalities or functional deficits after exposures of 1 hour or less. It is pertinent, however, to note that more prolonged exposures (up to several hours) more consistently lead to deficits in preclinical studies. Since there are no data in humans reporting the neurobehavioral effects of several hours of exposure to anesthesia, this should be addressed in future studies. However, collection of more definitive data supporting a deleterious role for anesthetics during brain development will continue to be complicated by uncertainties regarding the toxic threshold dose for anesthetics, the lack of information about the age of maximum susceptibility, and ambiguity related to the most appropriate neurobehavioral domains to examine.

Future Research

Further animal data will continue to provide information on the mechanisms of and susceptibility to anesthetic neurotoxicity. Understanding the mechanisms will be critical in translating the animal findings to clinical settings. Future animal work may also assist in determining which domains of neurobehavioral outcome are most likely to be affected, and this would assist in the design of human clinical trials. If neurotoxicity is found to be clinically relevant, animal data will also guide in devising prevention strategies.

Further human clinical studies must also be performed. Cohort studies will better identify children most at risk and characterize the neurobehavioral changes that occur.[417] Future cohort studies should focus on those with multiple or prolonged exposures. Because of the multiple confounding factors, cohort studies will always have great difficulty determining if the outcomes are a result of the surgery, the comorbidities, or the anesthetic exposure.

Finding evidence for a lack of neurologic abnormalities in certain populations would provide some reassurance that laboratory studies in animal models lack immediate clinical relevance; however, it is important to note that such findings may not be automatically generalizable to all clinical settings.

To definitively answer this important health concern, clinical trials provide the strongest evidence. However, such trials are difficult to perform, as randomization to anesthesia or no anesthesia is impossible. It is, however, feasible to randomize for different types of anesthetic agents or approaches, such as regional versus general anesthesia. Finding a "nontoxic" anesthetic for longer procedures will be challenging. High-dose opioid with or without α_2-agonists might be a feasible nontoxic anesthetic for a trial. An international collaboration, the Trial of an alternative technique of Remifentanil and dEXmedetomidine (T-REX) study,[418,419] is designed to investigate an alternative anesthetic for infants consisting of dexmedetomidine, remifentanil, and caudal anesthesia with either ropivacaine or bupivacaine for lower abdominal/extremity surgery (https://clinicaltrials.gov/ct2/show/NCT02353182).

Even if anesthesia-induced neuroapoptosis is found to be clinically irrelevant, it is still important to recognize that there is a strong association between major surgery in neonates and abnormal neurobehavioral outcomes. Thus, the questions become which other factors may be causing the poor outcome and which perioperative interventions could be performed by anesthesiologists to improve outcomes in these children.

Recommendations for Clinical Practice

The currently available laboratory data are insufficient to make definitive recommendations for clinical pediatric anesthesia practice. As outlined previously, numerous laboratory studies have unequivocally documented deleterious effects of anesthetic exposure on the developing animal brain, including in nonhuman primates undergoing anesthetic management closely simulating clinical practice. Although these results should not be easily dismissed, the problems in translation from animal to human are substantial. Epidemiologic studies in children are somewhat contradictory; however, there is strong evidence suggesting that a single, short exposure does not have an impact on cognition. Epidemiologic studies have not ruled out an impact on behavior. Essentially no data exist about the neurobehavioral effects of prolonged exposure and the evidence pertaining to multiple exposures remains mixed and of poor quality.

SmartTots, a collaboration between the US Food and Drug Administration (FDA) and the International Anesthesia Research Society (IARS) has produced a consensus statement endorsed by many pediatric anesthesia societies. (http://smarttots.org/about/consensus-statement/). The statement indicates that:

The effect of exposure to anesthetic drugs in young children is unknown; however, some but not all studies have suggested that problems similar to those seen in animals could also occur in infants and toddlers. It is important to recognize that the studies in children suggest that similar deficits may occur. These studies in children have limitations that prevent experts from understanding whether the harmful effects were due to the anesthetic drugs or to other factors such as the surgery or related illness.... Because there is not enough information about the effects of anesthetic drugs on the brains of young children, it is not yet possible to know whether use of these medicines poses a risk, and if so, whether the risk is large enough to outweigh the benefit of the planned surgery, procedure, or test.

The statement goes on to advise health care providers to consider that:

Clearly, anesthetic drugs are a necessary part of the care of children needing any surgery, procedure, or test that cannot be delayed. Decisions regarding the timing of a procedure requiring anesthesia should be discussed with all members of the care team as well as the family or caregiver before proceeding. The benefits of an elective procedure should always be weighed against all of the risks associated with anesthesia and surgery.

Parents are advised to:

Discuss the timing of planned procedures with your child's primary care physician, surgeon/proceduralist and anesthesiologist. Concerns regarding the unknown risk of anesthetic exposure to your child's brain development must be weighed against the potential harm associated with cancelling or delaying a needed procedure.

Pediatric surgery is rarely entirely elective, and in neonates may be required to preserve life, such as for critical congenital heart disease, necrotizing enterocolitis, or congenital diaphragmatic hernia. Accordingly, calls to postpone infant surgery are not easy to accommodate. Delaying surgery is also problematic, as no vulnerable or safe period has been clearly identified in animal studies to guide this practice. It might be reasonable to delay purely elective surgeries; however, these represent only a very small fraction of surgeries performed in children.

It is well documented that neonates are at an increased risk for respiratory and cardiovascular complications during anesthesia, which influences the choice of anesthetic technique and drugs used in this population. It would be very unwise to change practice based on concerns over anesthetic neurotoxicity, while potentially increasing the risks of cardiovascular or respiratory complications. Similarly, it must be stressed that insufficient anesthesia and analgesia are definitely associated with poor neurologic outcomes.

When discussing the risks and benefits of anesthesia with parents, pediatricians, and surgeons, anesthesiologists need to be cautious not to cause undue alarm, while taking the matter of potential toxicity seriously and not hastily dismissing parental concerns.

ANNOTATED REFERENCES

Deng M, Hofacer RD, Jiang C, et al. Brain regional vulnerability to anaesthesia-induced neuronal cell death shifts with age during exposure and extends into adulthood for some regions. *Br J Anaesth.* 2014;113(3):443-451.

This animal study demonstrates that anesthesia-induced neuronal cell death pattern differs dramatically by brain region, dependent on the age during exposure, and extends into adulthood in some brain regions; suggesting that long-term effects from anesthetic exposure could also vary dependent on when the anesthetic exposure occurred in life.

Hofacer RD, Deng M, Ward CG, et al. Cell age-specific vulnerability of neurons to anesthetic toxicity. *Ann Neurol.* 2013;73(6):695-704.

This animal study supports an explanation for the differing neuronal cell death pattern by age of exposure, specifically that very immature, 2-week-old neurons are most vulnerable to anesthesia-induced neurodegeneration.

Ikonomidou C, Bosch F, Miksa M, et al. Blockade of NMDA receptors and apoptotic neurodegeneration in the developing brain. *Science.* 1999;283:70-74.

First animal study to examine the effects of anesthetic exposure early in life on brain structure, demonstrating widespread neuronal degeneration in newborn rats following a prolonged exposure to ketamine.

Ing C, Ma X, Sun M, et al. Exposure to surgery and anesthesia in early childhood and subsequent use of attention deficit hyperactivity disorder medications. *Anesth Analg.* 2020;131(3):723-733.

Utilizing a Medicaid database, this study found a single anesthetic exposure for a common surgical procedure under 5 years of age to be associated with a subsequent increased requirement for medications to treat ADHD, anxiety, depression, psychosis, or mood disorders.

Istaphanous GK, Howard J, Nan X, et al. Comparison of the neuroapoptotic properties of equipotent anesthetic concentrations of desflurane, isoflurane, or sevoflurane in neonatal mice. *Anesthesiology.* 2011;114:578-587.

First study in animals to compare the neurodegenerative properties of three contemporary inhaled anesthetics, finding no difference using equipotent doses and therefore no advantage of using one agent over another in regard to the degree of apoptotic neuronal cell death caused during exposure.

Jevtovic-Todorovic V, Hartman RE, Izumi Y, et al. Early exposure to common anesthetic agents causes widespread neurodegeneration in the developing rat brain and persistent learning deficits. *J Neurosci.* 2003;23:876-882.

Seminal study into the brain structural and long-term functional effects of a combined exposure to isoflurane, nitrous oxide, and midazolam in newborn rats, showing both increased neuroapoptosis immediately following exposure and long-term learning impairment.

McCann ME, de Graaff JC, Dorris L, et al. Neurodevelopmental outcome at 5 years of age after general anaesthesia or awake-regional anaesthesia in infancy (GAS): an international, multicentre, randomised, controlled equivalence trial. *Lancet.* 2019;393(10172):664-677.

The first human randomized trial to examine neurotoxicity comparing infants having awake-regional or sevoflurane anesthesia; the authors found no evidence of a difference in neurodevelopmental outcome measured at 5 years of age.

Paule MG, Li M, Allen RR, et al. Ketamine anesthesia during the first week of life can cause long-lasting cognitive deficits in rhesus monkeys. *Neurotoxicol Teratol.* 2011;33:220-230.

First study in nonhuman primates to link a prolonged exposure to ketamine very early in life to long-term neurobehavioral abnormalities as tested with OTB.

Sun LS, Li G, Miller TL, et al. Association between a single general anesthesia exposure before age 36 months and neurocognitive outcomes in later childhood. *JAMA.* 2016;315:2312-2320.

Most definitive cohort study, comparing children aged 5 to 8 years following hernia repair before the age of 3 years with their siblings, finding no evidence of a difference across a battery of neuropsychologic tests.

Warner DO, Chelonis JJ, Paule MG, et al. Performance on the Operant Test Battery in young children exposed to procedures requiring general anaesthesia: the MASK study. *Br J Anaesth.* 2019;122(4):470-479.

Study in children who required procedures with anesthesia before 3 years of age did not demonstrate any of the deficits that were observed in nonhuman primates in study by Paule et al., 2011, utilizing similar OTB tasks.

Wilder RT, Flick RP, Sprung J, et al. Early exposure to anesthesia and learning disabilities in a population-based birth cohort. *Anesthesiology.* 2009;110:796-804.

The authors provide one of the earliest epidemiologic studies to suggest an association between repeated exposure to surgery with anesthesia early in life to long-term neurobehavioral abnormalities in children.

A complete reference list can be found online at Elsevier eBooks+.

24 Pediatric Neurosurgical Anesthesia

CRAIG D. McCLAIN, JUE TERESA WANG, SULPICIO G. SORIANO,
AND CAROLYN G. BUTLER

Pathophysiology
Intracranial Compartments
Intracranial Pressure
Cerebral Blood Volume and Cerebral Blood Flow
Cerebral Perfusion Pressure
Cerebrovascular Autoregulation
Management of Anesthesia
Preoperative Evaluation
Premedication
Monitoring
Induction
Airway Management and Intubation
Neuromuscular Blocking Drugs
Positioning

Local Anesthesia
Maintenance of General Anesthesia
Apoptotic Neurodegeneration
Blood and Fluid Management
Temperature Control
Venous Air Emboli
Emergence
Special Situations
Trauma
Craniotomy
Hydrocephalus
Congenital Anomalies
Neuroradiologic Procedures

CHILDREN WHO REQUIRE NEUROSURGICAL PROCEDURES present unique challenges to pediatric anesthesiologists. In addition to addressing problems common to general pediatric anesthesia practice, anesthesiologists must consider the effects of anesthesia on the developing central nervous system (CNS) of children with neurologic disease. This chapter reviews the age-dependent physiology of the CNS of children undergoing neurosurgical procedures requiring anesthesia and addresses some of the unique situations that anesthesiologists face.

Pathophysiology

INTRACRANIAL COMPARTMENTS

The skull can be compared to a rigid container with almost incompressible contents. Under normal conditions, the intracranial space is occupied by the brain and its interstitial fluid (80%), cerebrospinal fluid (CSF, 10%), and blood (10%). In pathologic states, space-occupying lesions such as edema, tumors, hematomas, or abscesses alter these proportions. The Monro-Kellie hypothesis, elaborated in the 19th century, states that the sum of all intracranial volumes is constant. An increase in the volume of one compartment must be accompanied by an approximately equal decrease in the volume of the other compartments, except when the cranium can expand to accommodate a larger volume. Gradual increases in intracranial volumes, such as a slow-growing tumor or hydrocephalus, can be compensated by the compliant nature of open fontanelles and sutures in infants and young children; an increasing head circumference is the result.[1] However, herniation can occur even in children with open fontanelles if large increases in intracranial pressure (ICP) develop acutely. In the nonacute situation, the brain can compensate for pathologic increases in intracranial volume by intracellular dehydration and a reduction in the interstitial fluid.[2–4]

Under normal conditions, CSF exists in dynamic equilibrium, with the rate of absorption balancing the rate of production. The rate of CSF production in adults is approximately 0.35 mL/minute or 500 mL/day.[5] The average adult has 100 to 150 mL of CSF distributed throughout the brain and subarachnoid space. Children have correspondingly smaller volumes of CSF, but the rate of CSF production is similar to that in adults.[5,6]

Production of CSF is only slightly affected by alterations of ICP and is usually unchanged in children with hydrocephalus.[6] Some drugs, including acetazolamide, furosemide, and corticosteroids, are mildly effective in transiently decreasing CSF production.[1,7,8] There is an inverse relationship between the rate of CSF production and serum osmolality; an increase in serum osmolality decreases CSF production. Choroid plexus papillomas, which overproduce CSF, are rare but occur more commonly in childhood.

Absorption of CSF is not well understood, but the arachnoid villi appear to be important sites for reabsorption of CSF into the venous system. One-way valves between the subarachnoid space and the sagittal sinus appear to open at a gradient of about 5 mm Hg. Some resorption may occur from the spinal subarachnoid space and from the ependymal lining of the ventricles. Resorption increases with an increase in ICP. However, CSF absorption is decreased by pathologic processes that obstruct arachnoid villi or interfere with CSF flow, such as intracranial hemorrhage, infection, tumor, and congenital malformations.[9,10]

INTRACRANIAL PRESSURE

Increased ICP causes secondary brain injury by producing cerebral ischemia and ultimately causing herniation. Ischemia occurs when ICP increases and cerebral perfusion pressure (CPP) decreases. As cerebral blood flow (CBF) and the supply of nutrients wane, cell damage and death occur, leading to increased intracellular

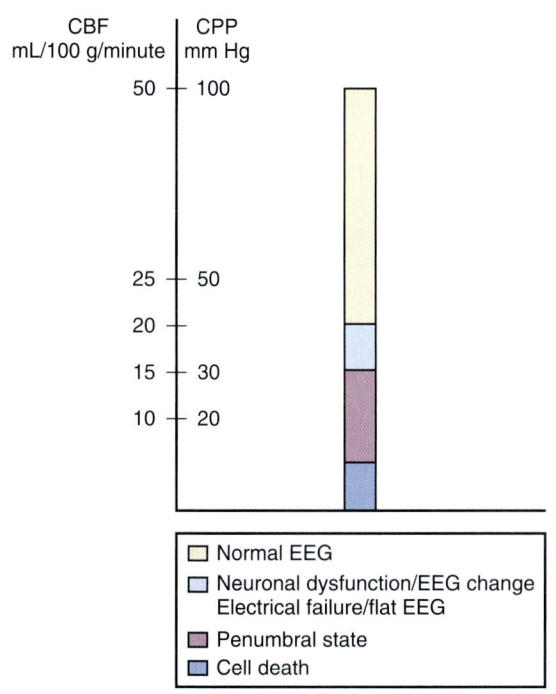

CBF
mL/100 g/minute

CPP
mm Hg

☐ Normal EEG
☐ Neuronal dysfunction/EEG change
    Electrical failure/flat EEG
☐ Penumbral state
☐ Cell death

FIGURE 24.1 Cerebral blood flow (CBF), cerebral perfusion pressure (CPP), and brain ischemia. Changes in CBF and CPP affect neuronal synaptic function and cellular integrity. When CBF decreases to 15 to 20 mL/100 grams per minute, there is distinct neuronal dysfunction on the electroencephalogram (EEG). At 15 mL/100 grams per minute, the EEG is essentially flat, and electrical activity ceases to function. At 6 to 15 mL/100 grams per minute, a penumbral state occurs in which there is energy for cellular integrity but insufficient energy for synaptic function. Neuronal survival is unlikely if this low CBF is allowed to persist for more than an ill-defined but critical period. At less than 6 mL/100 grams per minute, there is no energy for cellular membrane integrity. Infarction occurs at this stage unless reperfusion is accomplished immediately.

and extracellular water and further increases in ICP. When ICP increases, CPP decreases, the brain becomes ischemic, and cell death can ensue (Fig. 24.1).[11]

Herniation Syndromes
Several herniation syndromes exist. The most common is *transtentorial* herniation, in which the uncus of the temporal lobe is displaced from the supratentorial to the infratentorial space. Compression of the third cranial nerve and brainstem results in pathognomonic signs of pupillary dilatation, hemiparesis, and loss of consciousness. If this compression is not promptly relieved, apnea, bradycardia, and death occur.

In *cerebellar* herniation, the cerebellar tonsils herniate through the foramen magnum from the posterior fossa to the cervical spinal space. This can obstruct the circulation of CSF and lead to hydrocephalus. As the brainstem becomes compressed, cardiorespiratory failure and death ensue.

Signs of Increased Intracranial Pressure
The clinical signs of increased ICP in children vary. Papilledema, pupillary dilation, hypertension, and bradycardia may be absent despite intracranial hypertension, or these signs may occur with normal ICP.[9,12] When associated with increased ICP, they are usually late and dangerous signs.[13] Chronic increases in ICP are often manifested by complaints of headache, irritability, and vomiting, particularly in the morning. Papilledema may not be present even

in children dying as a result of intracranial hypertension.[14] A diminished level of consciousness and abnormal motor responses to painful stimuli are frequently associated with an increased ICP.[9] Computed tomography (CT) or magnetic resonance imaging (MRI) can reveal small or obliterated ventricles or basilar cisterns, hydrocephalus, intracranial masses, and midline shifts. Diffuse cerebral edema is a common finding when increased ICP is associated with closed-head injury, encephalopathy, or encephalitis.

Monitoring Intracranial Pressure
Techniques to monitor ICP in adults have been successfully used in children.[15–17] Noninvasive techniques seem to be less accurate than invasive methods.[18] Ventricular catheters are generally accepted as the most accurate and reliable means of measurement, permitting removal of CSF for diagnostic or therapeutic indications. The major risks of intraventricular catheters are infection and hemorrhage; although rare, they can lead to devastating complications. These catheters may be difficult to insert precisely when they are needed most, as in a child with severe cerebral edema and small ventricles. Compared with intraventricular catheters, subarachnoid bolts can be placed even when the ventricles are obliterated. This procedure minimizes trauma to brain tissue and poses less risk of serious infection and hemorrhage. The major disadvantages are that subarachnoid bolts may underestimate ICP, particularly in areas distant from their insertion site, and they are difficult to stabilize in infants with thin calvarias.

Epidural monitors that do not require a fluid interface can be implanted outside the dura, avoiding the risks of CSF contamination and the limitations of fluid-dependent systems.[19,20] Most epidural systems correlate well with intraventricular measurements, but they cannot be recalibrated after insertion. Epidural monitors have also been secured noninvasively to the open anterior fontanelle of infants and appear to reflect changes in ICP. Fiber optic catheters with self-contained transducers can also be used to measure ICP from intraventricular, subarachnoid, or intraparenchymal sites. These monitors avoid some of the problems of external fluid-filled transducers, but like epidural transducers, they cannot be recalibrated after insertion.

The normal ICP in children is less than 15 mm Hg. In term neonates, normal ICP is 2 to 6 mm Hg; it is probably even less in preterm infants. Children with intracranial pathology but normal ICP values occasionally exhibit pressure waves, which are considered abnormal.[9] In children with open fontanelles, the ICP may remain normal despite intracranial pathologic processes; increasing head circumference may be the first clinical sign. Bulging fontanelles may not develop, especially when the process evolves slowly.

Intracranial Compliance
The absolute value of ICP does not indicate how much compensation is possible. If the ICP increases considerably, compensatory mechanisms have failed. However, pathologic states may be present despite an ICP within the normal range. Intracranial compliance (i.e., the change in pressure relative to a change in volume) is a valuable concept. Fig. 24.2 is a schematic diagram of the relationship between the addition of volume to intracranial compartments and ICP. The shape of the curve depends on the time over which the volume increases and the relative size of the compartments. At normal intracranial volumes (point 1 in the figure), ICP is low, but compliance is high and remains so despite small increases in volume. If volume increases rapidly, compensatory

24

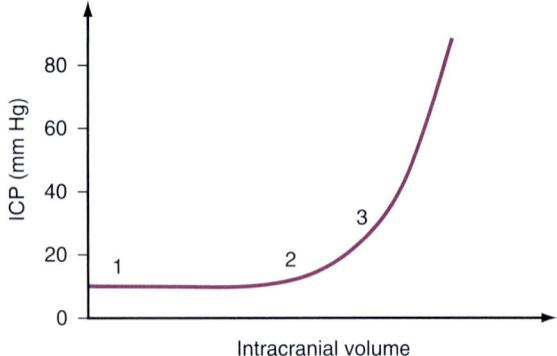

FIGURE 24.2 Idealized intracranial compliance curve for intracranial pressure *(ICP)* plotted against intracranial volume.

abilities are surpassed, and further increases in volume are reflected in increases in pressure. This can occur when the ICP is still within normal limits, but the compliance is low (point 2). If the ICP is already increased, further volume expansion causes a rapid increase in ICP (point 3). In clinical practice, compliance can be evaluated with a ventriculostomy catheter or by observing the response of ICP to external stimulation (e.g., tracheal suction, coughing, agitation).

Several physiologic and mechanical factors such as a greater percent of brain water, less CSF volume, and a greater percent of brain content to intracranial capacity decreased intracranial compliance in children compared with adults.[2] Children may be at increased risk for herniation compared with adults when similar relative increases in ICP have occurred. However, infants faced with a slowly increasing ICP may have a greater compliance because of their open fontanelles and sutures.

CEREBRAL BLOOD VOLUME AND CEREBRAL BLOOD FLOW

In addition to CSF, cerebral blood volume (CBV) represents another compartment in which compensatory mechanisms influence ICP. Although the CBV occupies only 10% of the intracranial space, changes related to dynamic blood volume occur, often initiated by anesthesia or intensive care procedures. As with other vascular beds, most intracranial blood is contained in the low-pressure, high-capacitance venous system. Increases in intracranial volume are initially offset by decreases in CBV. This response is apparent in hydrocephalic infants, in whom venous blood shifts from intracranial to extracranial vessels, producing distended scalp veins.[21]

In the healthy adult, CBF is approximately 55 mL/100 grams of brain tissue per minute.[22–24] This represents almost 15% of the cardiac output for an organ that accounts for only 2% of body weight. Estimates of CBF are less uniform for children. Normal CBF in healthy, awake children is approximately 100 mL/100 grams of brain tissue per minute, which represents up to 25% of cardiac output.[25,26] CBF in neonates and preterm infants (approximately 40 mL/100 grams of brain tissue per minute) is less than in children and adults.[27,28] In infants, CBF is modified by sleep states and feeding.[29]

Understanding CBF in neonates, infants, and other children is fundamental to being able to safely care for these most vulnerable patients during procedures requiring sedation and general anesthesia. CBF increases during the first 3 days of life then decreases slightly, followed by further increases during the first 3 years of life.[30] A number of factors contribute to adequate CBF in children undergoing general anesthesia. Classically,

teaching has focused on factors that underlie maintenance and autoregulation of CBF (e.g., mean arterial pressure [MAP], venous return, $PaCO_2$, and pH). Although these concepts remain critical underpinnings of neurophysiology, it is also incumbent upon anesthesia providers to have a broader understanding and approach to the idea of CBF.[31] Regulation of CBF is best understood as the nexus of different physiologic systems. These systems include the respiratory, cardiovascular, autonomic, nervous, and endocrine systems, metabolic processes, and the intracranial environment itself.[32] In light of this approach, CBF is regulated by integrative processes that involve respiratory gas exchange, hemodynamic parameters and their consequent effects on cerebrovascular resistance. In adults, the cerebral metabolic rate for oxygen consumption ($CMRO_2$) is 3.5 to 4.5 mL O_2/100 grams per minute; it is greater in children,[25] but less in preterm and term neonates. The $CMRO_2$ in preterm and term neonates is less than half adult values.[33] General anesthesia reduces $CMRO_2$ by as much as 50%.[34] Coupling of CBF and $CMRO_2$ is probably mediated by the effect of the local hydrogen ion concentration on cerebral vessels. Conditions that cause acidosis (e.g., hypoxemia, hypercarbia, ischemia) dilate the cerebral vasculature, which augments CBF and CBV. A reduction in brain metabolism (i.e., $CMRO_2$) similarly reduces CBF and CBV.[31] When autoregulation is impaired, CBF is determined by factors other than metabolic demand. If the CBF exceeds metabolic requirements, luxury perfusion or hyperemia exists. Many pharmacologic agents act directly on the cerebral vasculature to alter CBF and CBV.

CEREBRAL PERFUSION PRESSURE

CPP is a useful and practical estimate of the adequacy of the cerebral circulation, because CBF is neither easily nor widely measured. Defined as the pressure gradient across the brain, CPP is the difference between the systemic MAP at the entrance to the brain and the mean exit pressure (i.e., central venous pressure [CVP]). When ICP exceeds CVP, it replaces CVP in the calculation of CPP. In supine children, the mean CPP is the difference between the MAP and the mean ICP (CPP = MAP − ICP). If the brain and heart are positioned at different heights, all pressures should be referenced at the level of the head (e.g., external auditory meatus).

Fluctuations in cerebral perfusion during general anesthesia make anesthetizing neonates and infants a particularly challenging endeavor. Neonates already have an increased perioperative morbidity and mortality. Recent concerns for the risks of adverse neurocognitive outcomes from exposure to common anesthetic drugs have evolved into greater efforts in optimizing the physiologic management of neonates undergoing general anesthesia (see Chapter 23). An additional confounding factor is the underdeveloped cerebral vasculature in preterm infants that is unable to fully autoregulate, especially if perinatal ischemia occurred at birth.[35,36] It comes as no great surprise that part of this renewed effort to improve the care of neonates has focused on understanding the role of an adequate cerebral perfusion.[37–40] However, ensuring an adequate cerebral perfusion requires accurate blood pressure measurements,[41] knowledge of appropriate hemodynamic goals, and maintaining said normal hemodynamic ranges and hemodynamic goals while avoiding hypocapnia.[31,35,37,42]

CEREBROVASCULAR AUTOREGULATION
Effects of Blood Pressure

Classical teaching has maintained that in adults, CBF remains relatively constant over a MAP range of 50 to 150 mm Hg

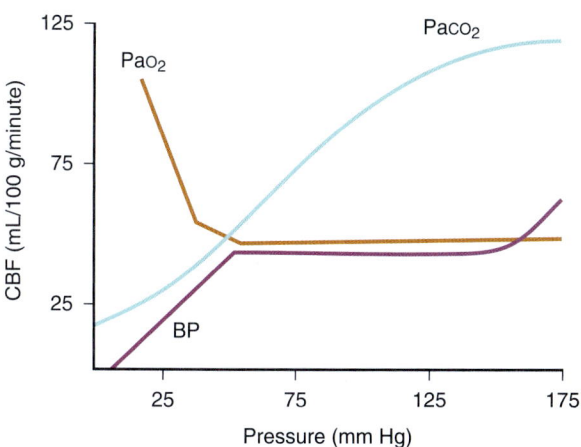

FIGURE 24.3 The effects of increasing mean blood pressure *(BP)*, arterial partial pressure of oxygen *(Pao₂)*, and arterial partial pressure of carbon dioxide *(Paco₂)* on cerebral blood flow *(CBF)* in the normal brain. (From Shapiro HM. Intracranial hypertension: therapeutic and anesthetic considerations. *Anesthesiology.* 1975;43:447.)

(Fig. 24.3), although this concept does not necessarily hold true in practice. Interpretation of a constant flow is the result of limitations to this research that include methods of measuring and the assumptions made by such methods (e.g., transcranial Doppler [TCD] and the assumption that the diameter of the measured vessel remains constant), the manipulation of CBF pharmacologically (the influence on cerebrovascular tone is not well understood and controversial), and the confounding effect of the arterial partial pressure of carbon dioxide ($PaCO_2$) alterations during pharmacologic manipulations of blood pressure.[32,42] Despite these limitations, as clinicians we still try to optimize the care using published interpretations.[31,35,36,38,41] It is useful to understand these new concepts but try to not simply disregard older, probably somewhat simple, ideas of maintenance of CBF in our patients under anesthesia.

We can view autoregulation as a mechanism that enables brain perfusion to remain relatively stable despite changes in MAP or ICP. The relationship between MAP and CBF is likely more pressure passive than originally thought. In fact, it seems as if stricter autoregulation occurs at greater values of MAP than smaller values.[33] Autoregulation is mediated by autonomic and myogenic control of vascular resistance, although there remains considerable debate regarding the exact mechanism and exact location of this modulation. When CPP decreases, cerebral vessels dilate to maintain CBF, thereby increasing CBV. When CPP increases, cerebral vasoconstriction occurs, maintaining the CBF with a reduced CBV. When ICP and CVP are low, MAP normally approximates CPP. Beyond the range of autoregulation, CBF becomes more pressure-dependent. In children with chronic hypertension, the upper and lower limits of autoregulation are increased. Cerebral autoregulation can be abolished by acidosis, medications, tumor, cerebral edema, and vascular malformations, even at sites far removed from a discrete lesion.[22]

The limits of autoregulation for normal infants and children are unknown, but autoregulation probably occurs at lower absolute values than in adults[43]; this is particularly true in preterm infants with immature cerebral autoregulation mechanisms.[36] Although the lower limit of autoregulation in adults is approximately 50 mm Hg MAP, this blood pressure may be beyond that

of the neonate. Intact autoregulatory mechanisms have been demonstrated within lower blood pressure ranges in newborn animals compared with mature animals.[36] In the past transcranial Doppler was used to assess CBF but more recently near-infrared spectroscopy (NIRS) has been used to interpret cerebral perfusion using regional oxyhemoglobin saturation as a surrogate measure of CBF.[44–46] In infants less than 6 months of age who were anesthetized with sevoflurane, CBF velocity decreased at a MAP of ≤~38 mm Hg (20% less than baseline).[41] In children undergoing craniofacial reconstruction (mean age 7.7 ± 1.9 months), cerebral perfusion during sevoflurane anesthesia was pressure passive, with limited autoregulation.[44] Cerebral autoregulation may even be abolished in critically ill humans, rendering CBF pressure passive.[47,48]

Effects of Oxygen

CBF is constant over a wide range of oxygen tensions. When the partial pressure of arterial O_2 (PaO_2) decreases to <50 mm Hg, CBF increases exponentially in adults; for example, at a PaO_2 of 15 mm Hg, CBF is double that at a normal PaO_2 (see Fig. 24.3).[47] The resulting increase in CBV increases ICP when intracranial compliance is low; the lower limit for PaO_2 is probably less in neonates. In a study of CBF in preterm infants during desaturation events and resaturation in the first 2 days of life, opposite responses that relate to gestation age were noted: in neonates <32 week's gestational age, CBF increased in the presence of hyperoxia, whereas in infants >32 week's gestational age, CBF increased in response to hypoxia.[49] The importance of these observations is amplified knowing that sick preterm infants lose cerebral autoregulation, rendering them even more susceptible to ischemic events.[47] Oxygen delivery is more important than the actual PaO_2 as hyperoxia decreases CBF in preterm neonates[50,51] and older adults.[37,52] Kety and Schmidt[38] demonstrated a 10% decrease in CBF in adults breathing 100% O_2, although Rahilly reported a 33% decrease in neonates breathing 100% O_2.[39] However, a decrease in MAP with sevoflurane anesthesia has also been reported to increase regional brain oxygenation as measured by NIRS.[53] This lends further credence to the complex interactions that modulate CBF; these factors are likely exacerbated in children with congenital heart disease.[54,55]

Effects of Carbon Dioxide

The relationship between the arterial partial pressure of carbon dioxide ($PaCO_2$) and CBF typically is linear (see Fig. 24.3). In adults, a 1-mm Hg increase in $PaCO_2$ increases CBF by approximately 2 mL/100 grams per minute.[38] The direct effect of changes in $PaCO_2$ on CBF and the consequent effect on CBV are the basis for the clinical practice of hyperventilating the lungs to reduce ICP. Likewise, increases in $PaCO_2$ increase the CBF, although the limits at which this occurs in neonates differ from those in adults. Neonatal studies using NIRS suggest that increases in CBF occur in preterm infants <29 week's gestational age when the $PaCO_2$ is greater than 55 mm Hg, particularly in the first days of life.[56] In lambs and monkeys, CBF does not change in response to a decreased $PaCO_2$.[40] The lower limits of $PaCO_2$ effect on CBF in human infants and children have not been defined. The $PaCO_2$ can vary considerably during surgical procedures. Blood gases from neonates (n = 112) obtained during noncardiac surgical procedures reported 13 neonates with a $PaCO_2$ <30 mm Hg and 2 with a $PaCO_2$ <25 mm Hg. Transient hypocarbia is common in this cohort, but the importance in terms of potential CBF is unknown.[57] Similarly, there is a paucity of information regarding the extent and duration of cerebrovascular responsiveness to hyperventilation in brain-injured and critically ill children. Moderate hyperventilation has been used to rapidly reduce ICP, but several reports have demonstrated worsening cerebral ischemia in children with compromised cerebral perfusion.[58–60]

Autoregulation of CBF is impaired in regions of damaged brain tissue.[61] Blood vessels in an ischemic zone are subject to hypoxemia, hypercarbia, and acidosis, which are potent stimuli for vasodilation. These vessels develop maximally reduced cerebrovascular tone or vasomotor paralysis. Small, localized lesions may impair autoregulation in areas far removed from the site of injury.[22] The extent of autoregulatory impairment varies in children with brain damage.

Management of Anesthesia

PREOPERATIVE EVALUATION

History

Preoperative evaluation of infants and children is discussed in Chapter 2. Children who are scheduled for neurosurgery might have been healthy until the onset of their symptoms, have been developmentally delayed from birth, or have impaired neuromuscular function. The anesthetic plan, including postoperative care, needs to consider the particular issues of each child and the disease state.

A history of food or drug allergies, eczema, or asthma may provide warning of an adverse reaction to contrast agents frequently used in neuroradiologic procedures. Special attention should be given to symptoms of allergy to latex products, such as lip swelling after blowing up a toy balloon or tongue swelling after insertion of a rubber dam into the mouth by a dentist, because latex anaphylaxis has been reported in some children who have undergone multiple operations, especially those with a meningomyelocele.[62–67] Children with latex allergy may also report allergies to fruits (e.g., kiwi, banana, avocado, strawberry, and others).[63,65]

Concurrent pediatric diseases and symptoms of neurologic lesions may influence the conduct of anesthesia. Protracted vomiting, enuresis, and anorexia related to intracranial lesions should prompt evaluation of hydration and electrolytes. Diabetes insipidus or inappropriate secretion of antidiuretic hormone are common. A history of the use of aspirin or aspirin-containing remedies for headaches or respiratory tract infections is information that is not usually forthcoming but may have important implications for operative and postoperative bleeding. Corticosteroids are often initiated at the time of diagnosis of intracranial tumors, and they should be continued with a pulse dose administered during the perioperative period. Therapeutic concentrations of anticonvulsants should be verified and maintained in the perioperative period. Children receiving long-term anticonvulsants may develop toxicity, especially if seizures are difficult to control; this is frequently manifested as abnormalities in hematologic or hepatic function, or both. Children receiving long-term anticonvulsant therapy may also require increased amounts of sedatives, nondepolarizing muscle relaxants, and opioids because of enhanced metabolism of these drugs (see also Chapters 5 and 22).[68–70]

Patients with drug resistant epilepsy may be prescribed cannabidiol or ketogenic diet therapy (e.g., developmental and epileptic encephalopathies).[71] The physiologic changes brought about by ketosis, glucose restriction, and increases in levels of polyunsaturated fatty acids increases the levels of inhibitory neurotransmitters such as γ-aminobutyric acid (GABA), resulting in decreasing seizure activity.[71,72] Another possible mechanism is caloric restriction leading to reduced cerebral glucose consumption inhibiting glycolysis, which inhibits neuronal excitation.[71] In addition, 2-deoxy-D-glucose has antiseizure properties relating to blocking seizure induced brain-derived neurotrophic factor and its receptor.[73] Multiple possible processes may be involved, although the exact mechanism of action remains unclear. These patients may need to avoid glucose in medications such as syrup used to mix oral medications as well as fluids containing lactate or dextrose. To prevent hypoglycemia due to prolonged fasting times during the perioperative period, patients should generally be scheduled as early in the day as possible.

Intraoperative glucose-containing solutions should be avoided; some medications contain large concentrations of glucose and should be used with caution (e.g., oral midazolam, oral acetaminophen, oral ibuprofen suspension).[73,74] It should also be noted that sugar concentrations vary greatly by the generic manufacturer. Both normal saline and lactated Ringer solution may be used safely in children on ketogenic diets.[73,75] Intraoperative glucose concentrations should be measured during prolonged procedures, and values <40 mg/dL should be treated.[73] Postoperatively, the serum glucose concentration and the pattern of the seizures should continue to be monitored; a review of the long-term complications of the ketogenic diet has been described.[76]

Physical Examination

The physical examination should encompass a brief neurologic evaluation, including level of consciousness, motor and sensory function, normal and pathologic reflexes, integrity of the cranial nerves, and signs and symptoms of intracranial hypertension. Examination of pupillary size and responsiveness can detect benign anisocoria. Preoperative respiratory assessment should include the effects of motor weakness, impaired gag and swallowing mechanisms, and evidence of active pulmonary disease, such as aspiration pneumonia. Muscle atrophy and weakness should be documented, because upregulation of acetylcholine receptors may precipitate sudden hyperkalemia after administration of succinylcholine and induce resistance to nondepolarizing muscle relaxants in the affected limbs.[77,78]

Laboratory and Radiologic Evaluation

In all but the most minor procedures, laboratory data should include a hematocrit determination. Blood typing and cross-matching should be performed for any major procedure. The need for additional studies, such as evaluation of coagulation parameters, serum electrolyte concentrations and osmolality, blood urea nitrogen and creatinine values, arterial blood gas analysis, chest radiography, or electrocardiography (ECG), is determined on an individual basis. Liver function tests and a hematologic profile should be obtained if not recently reviewed in children receiving long-term therapy with anticonvulsants. Specific neuroradiologic studies are usually obtained by the neurosurgeon and should be reviewed (e.g., the anesthesiologist should know which children with a ventriculoperitoneal shunt have "slit ventricles" because these children have special risks in the perioperative period)[79] (see the section on Hydrocephalus later in the chapter). Preoperative neurophysiologic studies, including electroencephalography (EEG) and evoked potentials, may provide a baseline for comparison of intraoperative and postoperative evaluations.

PREMEDICATION

Sedation is usually withheld from pediatric neurosurgical patients until they arrive in the preoperative area to allow titration of drug to desired effect while under direct supervision. Opioids are usually withheld because they may cause nausea or respiratory depression, especially in children with increased ICP; sedatives alone are usually adequate to relieve preoperative anxiety. Sedatives are administered in the parents' presence to facilitate a smooth separation and induction. Oral midazolam (~0.5 to 1.0 mg/kg) or incremental doses of intravenous midazolam (0.05 mg/kg) are commonly used.

MONITORING

Minimal monitoring for pediatric neuroanesthesia includes ECG, oxygen saturation, noninvasive blood pressure, expired carbon dioxide, and temperature. Neuromuscular blockade monitoring is also important as chronic anticonvulsant therapy may alter the clearance of neuromuscular blocking drugs. However, nerve stimulators may give misleading information about the extent of relaxation if applied to a denervated extremity.[80] If the child has paresis, the nerve stimulator should be sited where neurologic function is normal. Care should be taken to remove neuromuscular blockade monitors in those patients who are scheduled for an intraoperative MRI scan, as the electrodes could cause superficial burns.[81,82] Precordial Doppler ultrasound is recommended in children undergoing craniotomy, especially in the head-up position, because their risk for air emboli is increased on the basis of their relatively large head. Monitoring devices for ICP are used for the same indications as in adults. Intraoperative EEG and electrophysiologic monitoring require advanced coordination among the neurosurgeon, anesthesiologist, and neurophysiologist. Urinary output should be measured during prolonged procedures, in cases with anticipated large blood loss, and when diuretics or osmotic agents are administered.

An arterial catheter is placed for craniotomies in which there is a potential for sudden and severe hemodynamic changes; small patient size should not preclude the use of invasive monitoring and may actually be an indication for a more aggressive approach. An increase in the paradoxical arterial pressure waveform with positive-pressure ventilation may indicate intravascular volume deficiency and the need for fluid replacement (see Fig. 10.12). Intraarterial catheters can be placed percutaneously in the radial, dorsalis pedis, or posterior tibial arteries even in small infants, and it is rarely necessary to resort to femoral arterial catheter placement or surgical cutdown. The arterial transducer should be zeroed at the level of the head if the head and heart positions are different so that CPP can be accurately assessed. Both the lateral corner of the eye or the external auditory meatus are convenient landmarks as they approximate the level of the foramen of Monro. In the first days of life, the umbilical artery and the umbilical vein can be cannulated. These catheters should be discontinued as soon as alternative access is established because of the potential for serious complications.

Percutaneous central venous cannulation (i.e., external or internal jugular, femoral, or subclavian veins) using ultrasound and the Seldinger technique is possible even in the smallest infants (see Chapter 46). However, in children undergoing neurosurgical resections, consideration should be given to sites other than neck veins, such as the femoral vein, thereby avoiding the Trendelenburg position during catheter insertion and the risk of accidental carotid artery puncture and hematoma formation, which may compromise CBF and intracranial venous drainage. If there is no issue with ICP, the subclavian vein is a reasonable alternative.

Cannulation of antecubital veins may provide central venous access, but threading the catheter into the inlet of the right atrium may be technically difficult in small children. When rapid blood loss is a consideration in a small child in whom adequate peripheral venous access has proven difficult, a single-lumen, large-bore catheter inserted in a femoral vein will provide that access. Catheters inserted into the femoral veins usually are accessible to the anesthesiologist during most neurosurgical procedures. Multiple-lumen central venous catheters and peripherally inserted central venous catheters are inadequate for rapid blood transfusion. All central catheters should be removed as soon as possible after the procedure to minimize the risk of venous thrombosis.

Near-Infrared Spectroscopy Monitoring

Maintaining cerebral perfusion and oxygenation to prevent cerebral ischemia and brain injury is a critical goal for anesthetic management.[83] Although several of the standard monitors mentioned above such as arterial blood pressure provide a proxy for cerebral perfusion, none directly measure end organ perfusion.[45,84] Cerebral NIRS oximetry may provide a better measurement of cerebral perfusion and oxygenation.[84] Cerebral NIRS monitoring, interpreted together with continuously available contributing variables, may help avoid cerebral desaturation and its sequelae.[45]

NIRS oximetry applies light in the near-infrared range (760 to 1500 nm) to tissue 1 to 2 cm below the skin surface and compares the absorption of oxyhemoglobin and deoxyhemoglobin. This value expresses the percentage of tissue oxygenation, measured as regional cerebral oxygen saturation (rSO_2) or tissue oxygenation index. NIRS measurements are based on the high degree of transparency of brain tissue in the near-infrared range.[85] Light in the near-infrared range scatters less than light in other parts of the spectrum, thereby providing information from the inner body, and penetrating several centimeters through tissue and bone.[45] Although the hemoglobin saturation in all vessels located in the portion of the tissue scanned (arterioles, venules, and capillaries) is measured, the venous volume is the major compartment, contributing 75% to 85% of the total cerebral blood volume. Therefore, NIRS can be thought of as a surrogate for venous oxygen saturation.[45,85,86] There is a strong correlation between NIRS and the more invasive jugular venous oximetry in animal studies, with inconsistent replication in clinical studies.[87]

Pulse oximetry and NIRS can be distinguished by phase of flow and the type of tissue being sampled. Pulse oximetry provides information about pulmonary function, and the a-A gradient, while cerebral oximetry trends the ratio of regional oxygen delivery.[87] Pulse oximetry measures the fraction of oxygenated blood in arteries and depends on pulsatile blood flow, whereas NIRS measures the oxyhemoglobin/deoxyhemoglobin ratio in tissue, and does not depend on pulsatile blood flow. It can be thought of as a "nonpulsatile venous oximeter," providing real time information regarding rSO_2 and the oxygen uptake/consumption balance.[45,88] Consider the example of a child with cyanotic heart disease. For this child, the pulse oximeter could show an oxygen saturation of 85%, whereas the NIRS-derived cerebral rSO_2 value is around 70% (in the range of normal values in healthy children). Here, despite a decrease in peripheral saturation, the cerebral oxygenation is preserved through an increased level of hemoglobin.[45] NIRS values for this patient might better reflect cerebral desaturation events. Factors that interfere with the precision of rSO_2 levels include skull thickness, extracranial tissue saturation, CSF volume, head position, anesthesia status, $PaCO_2$, and device model.[83]

Multiple physiologic parameters contribute to cerebral oxygen delivery and the rate of oxygen consumption in the brain including cardiac output, CPP, oxygenation, temperature, and hemoglobin concentration. Most anesthetic agents decrease the metabolic rate of oxygen consumption with the exception of ketamine, which increases cerebral metabolic demand. NIRS is a "multidimensional monitor" that allows the interpretation of multiple variables influencing the balance of oxygen delivery and demand in the brain.[86] Perturbations in NIRS values can therefore be used to guide the management of other physiologic parameters and provide organ-specific goal-directed treatments.[88]

There is no consensus regarding the normal range and lower safety margin of cerebral rSO_2 in children. The rSO_2 values observed in full-term neonates revealed values of 43% at 1 minute of age, progressing to 52% at 5 minutes, and 57% at 10 minutes of age.[89] Studies in pigs show a functional neurological impairment at a threshold saturation of 33% to 44%.[55] Gomez-Pesquera et al. found that intraoperative cerebral rSO_2 values in children of less than 20% from awake baseline was associated with negative behavioral changes on postoperative day 7.[84] Other reports suggest that interventions should occur when the rSO_2 is 20% less than baseline or at an absolute value less than 55%.[88] Pediatric patients may be more sensitive to an intraoperative decrease in cerebral rSO_2 because of cerebral immaturity.[84] Some authors have advocated for an individualized approach to NIRS where a baseline rSO_2 measurement is obtained under awake conditions before the induction of anesthesia with the goal to maintain NIRS values greater than this baseline.[45] There is still much to be determined regarding the value of this monitor in noncardiac surgical procedures; some advocate simply using it as a trend monitor.[45]

Although NIRS has become a standard monitor in some pediatric cardiac surgery centers, with multiple studies demonstrating the benefits of regional cerebral oxygenation monitoring in cardiac and ICU patients, there is no firm evidence that NIRS improves patient outcomes in noncardiac surgery.[45,55,87,90] NIRS may be particularly helpful in patients at increased risk of anesthesia-associated hypoxic ischemic neurologic injury, or patients who may have impaired autoregulation either due to age or preexisting physiology. There are other potential applications for NIRS in the future. Some reports suggest that NIRS might serve to monitor perioperative analgesia; procedure-related transient increases in oxyhemoglobin and total hemoglobin concentrations are reported to accompany a concomitant behavioral pain response as assessed by the Neonatal Infant Pain Scale.[91] Changes in NIRS with nociception remain speculative.[92]

INDUCTION

For children with intracranial hypertension, the primary goals during induction are to minimize severe increases in ICP and decreases in blood pressure. Most IV induction agents decrease $CMRO_2$ and CBF, which consequently decreases ICP.[93] Historically, sodium thiopental (4 to 8 mg/kg) was the default induction agent for neurosurgical cases. However, sodium thiopental is no longer available in the United States, although it remains available in other countries. In the United States, propofol has become the IV induction agent of choice for most children. Propofol (2 to 4 mg/kg) appears to have similar cerebral properties and an antiemetic effect; however, its antiemetic effect is usually not relevant for lengthy procedures. Etomidate, a possible neuroprotective agent, can be used if hemodynamic stability is a concern.[94–96] In the past, ketamine was avoided because of its known ability to increase cerebral metabolism, CBF, and ICP, and sudden increases

in ICP have been reported after ketamine administration, especially in infants and children with hydrocephalus.[97,98] However, ketamine has been shown to reduce ICP on average by ~30% in ventilated children and prevented further increases in ICP during "distressing events."[99] The apparent differences in responses likely related to controlled ventilation rather than noncontrolled ventilation.[100,101] A systematic review of adult patients with traumatic brain injury concluded that ketamine may cause small but brief increases in ICP that were clinically unimportant and that its sedative properties offer advantages.[102]

Other measures to reduce ICP during induction include controlled hyperventilation and administration of opioids (e.g., fentanyl, remifentanil, or sufentanil) and supplemental hypnotics before laryngoscopy and intubation. Lidocaine (1.5 mg/kg) limits the increase in ICP when administered intravenously just before laryngoscopy.[103]

Sevoflurane has replaced halothane for inhaled inductions because of its more rapid onset, acceptability for pediatric patients, and hemodynamic stability. Similar to isoflurane in its cerebral physiologic effects, sevoflurane with hyperventilation appears to blunt the increase in ICP related to cerebral vasodilation from inhalational anesthetic agents alone.[104–106] Sevoflurane offers an additional advantage because it causes less myocardial depression compared with halothane.[107] As stated earlier, sevoflurane anesthesia can decrease MAP, but can also lead to an increase in regional cerebral oxygenation.[53] However, when sevoflurane is combined with hyperventilation, it may produce epileptiform-like activity on the EEG without clinical manifestations of motor seizures in children without a prior history of clinical seizures (see Chapter 5).[108] These epileptiform-like EEG recordings occur at small brain partial pressures of sevoflurane (e.g., in early phase of induction), but are less common in the presence of nitrous oxide or alfentanil.[109] Since epileptiform-like EEG activity is reported in as many as 20% of children,[110–112] its clinical relevance remains unclear (see Chapter 5 for a more complete discussion).

A common presentation is an uncooperative toddler who has an intracranial tumor and moderately decreased intracranial compliance and who is agitated and resistant to separation from parents. Some clinicians might argue that a crying, agitated child has demonstrated a tolerance to increased ICP and that an IV induction is safe. Fortunately, children who have severe intracranial hypertension typically have a decreased level of consciousness, and it becomes easier to insert an IV catheter in those situations when it is most necessary.

AIRWAY MANAGEMENT AND INTUBATION

Airway management must be effective and smooth to avoid the ICP-increasing effects of hypoxemia, hypercarbia, and coughing. Administering opioids and hypnotics before intubation improves cerebral compliance and minimizes increases in ICP caused by laryngoscopy and intubation.

Either oral or nasal intubation may be appropriate. Nasotracheal intubation offers the advantage of increased stability and increased comfort for children when postoperative intubation is necessary. Nasotracheal tubes are often used for children who will be in the prone position (e.g., for a posterior fossa craniotomy), children whose airway will be inaccessible during the surgical procedure, and for smaller children. Nasotracheal tubes also offer the advantage of a decreased risk of kinking intraoperatively, especially in prone positioning of small children for whom a smaller-sized tracheal tube is necessary. It is important that the nasotracheal tube selected is a straight non-premolded tube with the connector firmly inserted into the tube, because once in situ, the tube will have to pass over the lips toward the chin to connect to the anesthesia breathing circuit. In this position, it is essential that the direction of the tube is toward the chin to avoid excessive and prolonged pressure on the ala and ischemic necrosis of the ala. Before finalizing the position of the nasotracheal tube, it is critical to guarantee that the tip of the tube will not encroach on the carina when the neck is hyperflexed to expose the posterior fossa. To confirm this, we flex the neck so the chin rests on the chest while the child is still in the supine position. With the neck in the flexed position, we auscultate the lungs to confirm good air entry bilaterally and wheezing and bronchospasm are not present. If confirmed, the tracheal tube is taped and/or sutured in position.

Contraindications to nasal intubation include choanal stenosis, possible basilar skull fracture, transsphenoidal procedures, and sinusitis. If nasotracheal intubation is planned, it is advantageous to prepare the nares with topical vasoconstrictors, recognizing that systemic hypertension can occur in response to excessive nasally administered vasoconstrictors.[113] Placing a few drops of 0.25% phenylephrine (Neo-Synephrine) or oxymetazoline on cotton-tipped applicators and positioning them in the nares against the nasal mucosa can prevent overdosage and help to gauge the patency of the nasal passage when anesthesia has been induced. It may also be useful to use a red rubber catheter or a nonlatex nasal trumpet (the Robertazzi nasopharyngeal airway [Rusch Nasal Airway, Teleflex, Morrisville, NC]) to gently dilate the nares and minimize the risk of a nosebleed.[114] Directly spray of the nares with topical vasoconstrictors (e.g., 0.25% phenylephrine)[115,116] should be used with caution as there are reports of development of lethal cardiopulmonary compromise in children after such delivery.[117] Whichever route is chosen for intubation, it is important to secure the tracheal tube with care because loss of the airway intraoperatively in a child with head pins in the prone position or a child with limited airway access can result in disaster.

In prolonged, combined neurosurgical and craniofacial reconstructions, the tracheal tube may be sutured to the nasal septum or wired to the teeth. A nasogastric or orogastric tube is inserted after intubation to decompress the stomach and evacuate gastric contents; leaving it open to gravity drainage during the case can prevent positive pressure from building up in the stomach if air leaks around an uncuffed tracheal tube. The child's eyes should be closed, lubricated with eye ointment, and covered with a clear waterproof dressing.

NEUROMUSCULAR BLOCKING DRUGS

Because of its rapid onset and brief duration of action, succinylcholine (1 to 2 mg/kg given intravenously or 4 to 5 mg/kg given intramuscularly) was frequently used to facilitate intubation in children with a full stomach[118]; atropine (0.01 to 0.02 mg/kg) is often administered to prevent bradycardia, particularly if a second dose is used. Succinylcholine does not significantly increase ICP in humans.[119,120] Succinylcholine is contraindicated when it may induce life-threatening hyperkalemia in the presence of denervation injuries related to various causes, including severe head trauma, crush injury, burns, spinal cord dysfunction, encephalitis, multiple sclerosis, muscular dystrophies, stroke, or tetanus,[121] but not in children with cerebral palsy.[122]

In current practice, rocuronium (1.2 mg/kg) has an onset of action similar to that of succinylcholine, with equivalent intubating conditions achieved in approximately 30 seconds.[123] The advantage of rocuronium is that it avoids the undesirable side effects associated with succinylcholine, but still can be antagonized with

sugammadex to restore spontaneous respirations should intubation prove difficult or impossible.[124]

POSITIONING

Positioning is an especially important consideration in pediatric neuroanesthesia. Children with increased ICP should be transported to the preoperative holding area and operating room with the head elevated in the midline position to maximize cerebral venous drainage.

After securing the airway, both neurosurgeons and anesthesiologists must have adequate access to the child. In infants and small children, even slight movement of the tracheal tube may extubate the trachea or advance the tube endobronchially. During prolonged procedures, it is important for the anesthesiologist to be able to visually inspect the tracheal tube and circuit connections and to suction the tracheal tube when necessary. Using proper draping and a flashlight, the anesthesia provider can usually create a "tunnel" to ensure access to the airway. All but very small children are placed in pins using devices such as the Mayfield head holder (Integra, Plainsboro, NJ). Neonates and small infants have thin calvaria, so head-pining systems are often avoided. Instead, there are a variety of non–pin-based headrests available for these children. Adequate padding should be used in such situations (Figs. 24.4 and 24.5). Extreme head flexion can cause brainstem compression in children with posterior fossa pathology, such as a mass lesion or Arnold-Chiari malformation. Extreme flexion can also cause high cervical spinal cord ischemia and tracheal tube kinking and obstruction.[125]

Extremities should be well padded and secured in a neutral position (i.e., palm supinated or neutral to avoid ulnar nerve compression). It is important to avoid stretching peripheral nerves and to prevent skin and soft tissue pressure injury because of direct contact with surgical accessories such as instrument stands and grounding wires (see Fig. 24.5). It is also important to ensure that extremities that are not directly visible to the anesthesiologist (e.g., those on the opposite side of the operating room table) cannot fall off the table during surgery, even if the table is rotated. In older children and adolescents undergoing prolonged procedures, deep vein thrombosis prophylaxis should be considered using compression or pneumatic stockings.[126,127]

Prone Position

The prone position is commonly used for posterior fossa and spinal cord surgery. The torso should be supported to ensure free abdominal wall motion because increased intraabdominal pressure may impair ventilation, cause vena cava compression, and increase epidural venous pressure and bleeding. Proper positioning is achieved most easily by placing silicone rolls or rolled blankets laterally on each side of the child's chest running from the shoulders toward the pelvis. A separate silicone roll or rolled blanket under the pelvis may occasionally be necessary in larger children. These rolls must not press into the flexed hips or compress the femoral nerve or genitalia. Placing the rolls in this position should also allow a precordial Doppler monitor to be easily placed on the anterior chest without undue pressure.

The head position depends on the surgical procedure. If surgery is limited to the lower spine, the head may be rotated and supported by padding, with care taken to avoid direct pressure on the eyes and nose and to keep the ears flat. For posterior fossa surgery, the head usually is suspended in pins to maintain central alignment of the head and maximal flexion. For infants and toddlers, a cerebellar head frame is another alternative when the

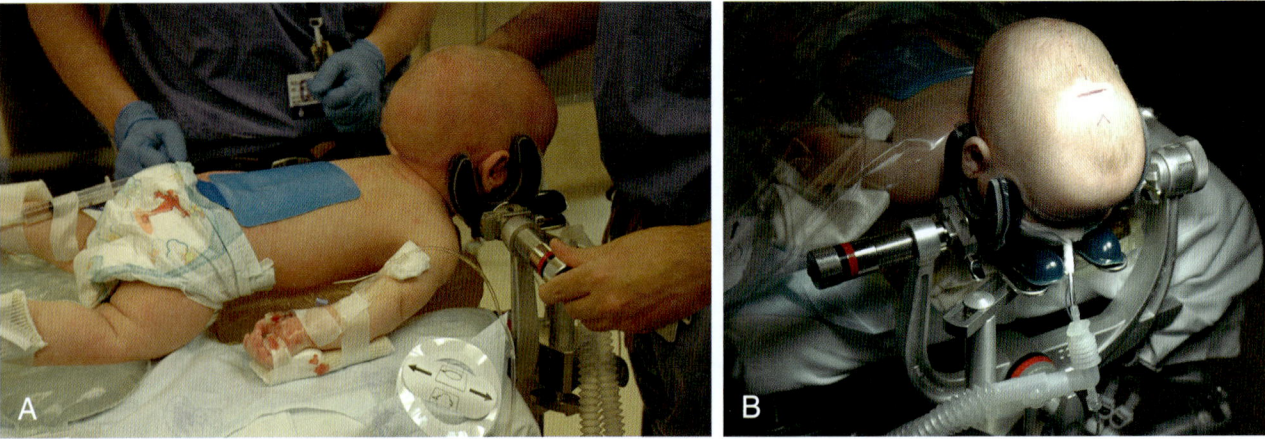

FIGURE 24.4 A, The child is positioned prone before surgery. Extreme head extension was needed for correction of craniosynostosis, but the equipment for securing the head was the same as that used for a prone craniotomy. **B,** This particular frame uses gel pads to support the chin, ears, and forehead.

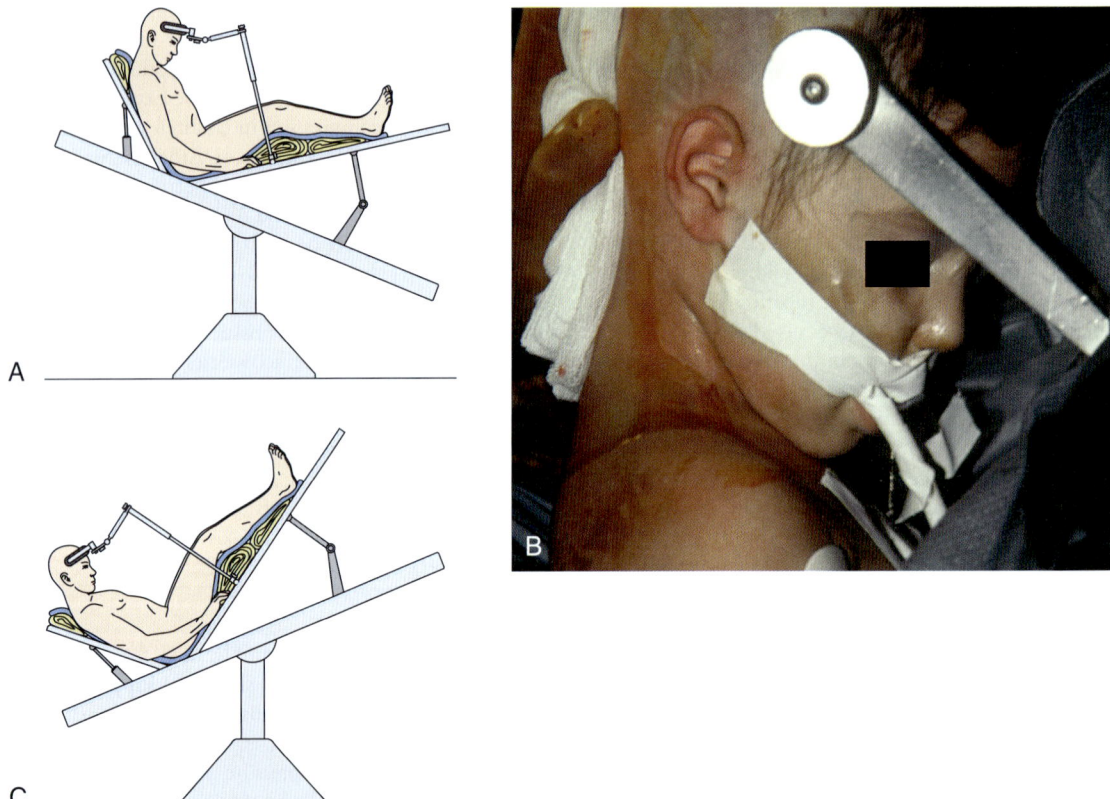

FIGURE 24.5 Resuscitation from the modified standard sitting position. The normal operative position **(A** and **B)** is compared with the resuscitation position **(C)**. The position can be expeditiously changed by one control of the operating table.

cranium is too thin for pins. In this situation, the child's forehead and cheeks rest on a well-padded head frame, and the eyes are free in the center of a horseshoe-shaped support (see Fig. 24.4). Ensure that the tracheal tube is properly positioned (after taping) and does not migrate to a main-stem position while repositioning the child prone. To avoid this, flexing the child's head maximally onto the chest and auscultating for equal air entry bilaterally will determine if there is risk for malposition before turning the child prone. Tape used to fix other tubes (e.g., gastric, esophageal) in

place should be separate from the tape used to secure the tracheal tube so that if these other tubes are accidentally dislodged, an extubation will not occur. For fixations where saliva and sterilizing solutions commonly soak the tape that stabilizes tubes, we use the 3M Multipore tape as it breathes fluids on its surface while remaining strongly adherent to the skin, unlike the pink waterproof polyethylene tape with zinc oxide adhesive that lifts off the skin when soaked with fluids. An emergency plan should be formulated to turn the child supine if it suddenly becomes necessary.[128]

Airway edema may develop in a child who is in the prone position for an extended period. Oral airways are best avoided because they can cause edema of the tongue by obstructing lymphatic and/or venous drainage. Alternatively, a folded roll of gauze is inserted between the lateral incisors to prevent the child from biting their tongue if cortical motor potentials are used for monitoring. Rarely, keeping the child intubated postoperatively may be necessary if facial swelling has developed during a prolonged surgery. Postoperative vision loss has been linked with prolonged spine surgery in the prone position and substantial blood loss.[129,130] Avoidance of direct pressure on the globe of the eyes,[131] staged procedures to decrease surgical time, and maintenance of stable hemodynamics with avoidance of excessive intraoperative fluid administration should be ensured in prone children.[129–132]

Modified Lateral Position

Insertion or revision of ventriculoperitoneal shunts may require the child to be rotated from the supine to the semilateral position. This is achieved by placing a roll under the child's dependent axilla (to prevent a brachial plexus injury). The knees should be supported in a slightly flexed position and the heels padded. This position is also used for some temporal and parietal craniotomies.

Sitting Position

The sitting position is now used less commonly in pediatric neurosurgical procedures and is rarely used in children younger than 3 years of age. However, this position may be used for morbidly obese children who cannot tolerate the prone position because of excessive intrathoracic and abdominal pressures. When the sitting position is used, precautions to prevent hypotension and air embolism must be followed. The lower extremities should be wrapped in elastic bandages. The head must be carefully flexed to avoid kinking the tracheal tube, advancing it into a bronchial position, or to avoid compressing the chin on the chest, which can block venous and lymphatic drainage of the tongue. Extreme flexion can also result in brainstem or cervical spinal cord ischemia, or both. As in the prone position, nasotracheal tubes are often used because they are more secure. The child's upper extremities are supported in the child's lap. Control levers to lower the head position should be easily accessible to the anesthesiologist and unencumbered by wires and drapes (see Fig. 24.5).

LOCAL ANESTHESIA

Local anesthetic should be injected subcutaneously before a skin incision to provide analgesia, and epinephrine is included in the local anesthetic to reduce cutaneous blood loss. If bupivacaine 0.25% with 1:200,000 epinephrine is used, the dose should be limited to 0.5 mL/kg (max 225 mg/dose and 400 mg/24 hours). When greater volumes are required, the solution can be diluted with normal saline. This dilute solution is still effective for vasoconstriction and provides a prolonged sensory block postoperatively. Specific blocks of supraorbital and supratrochlear nerves can provide analgesia from the frontal area to the midcoronal portion of the occiput and are particularly useful for awake craniotomies and ventriculoperitoneal shunt placement.[133] Blockade of the great occipital nerve provides analgesia from the posterior of the occiput to the midcoronal area of the occiput, whereas block of the supraorbital nerve provides analgesia to the front of the occiput (see Figs. 40.30 and 40.31).[134]

MAINTENANCE OF GENERAL ANESTHESIA

General anesthesia is required for most therapeutic and many diagnostic procedures in pediatric neurosurgery. Ventilation is controlled if intracranial hypertension is a concern. Although spontaneous ventilation provides another indication of brainstem function, its disadvantages (e.g., hypoventilation, increased potential for air embolism) are usually outweighed by the safety of controlled ventilation.

Maintenance of general anesthesia can be accomplished using inhalational anesthetics, IV infusions, or a combination. Anesthetics that decrease ICP and $CMRO_2$ and maintain CPP are most desirable (Table 24.1). The commonly used inhalational agents uncouple CBF and $CMRO_2$ such that CBF increases while $CMRO_2$ decreases. All potent inhalational agents are cerebral vasodilators, which increase both CBF and ICP. Low concentrations of isoflurane, sevoflurane, or desflurane, combined with ventilation to maintain normocarbia, minimally affect CBF and ICP.[104,105,135] Isoflurane is often the inhalational agent of choice for maintenance of neuroanesthesia. At two times the MAC, this dose of isoflurane induces a level of anesthesia that is associated with an isoelectric EEG while, unlike several other inhalational agents, maintaining hemodynamic stability. Other studies have demonstrated a similar effect with sevoflurane and hyperventilation.[136]

Practitioners debate the routine use of nitrous oxide for intracranial neurosurgical procedures. Opponents cite the increased risk of postoperative nausea and vomiting (PONV) with nitrous oxide in a surgical population already at greater risk for PONV.[137] Proponents cite studies that failed to demonstrate a substantive increased risk of PONV with nitrous oxide or appreciate that the risk is time-dependent, with a minimal effect for surgeries <2 hours.[138–140] Nitrous oxide can increase CBF in humans in a dose-dependent fashion through cerebral vasodilatation.[141,142] This increase in CBF can lead to an increase in ICP, which can be deleterious if the child already has reduced intracranial compliance.[143] Nitrous oxide can also suppress somatosensory and motor evoked potentials, especially if the inspired concentration exceeds 50%.[144–146] The more common use of intravenous anesthesia (e.g., propofol and remifentanil) obviates the need for nitrous oxide.

Proponents of the use of nitrous oxide for intracranial procedures cite its long track record of safety. Data from the two ENIGMA (**E**valuation of **NI**trous oxide in the **G**as mixture for **A**nesthesia) trials in 830 adults showed that nitrous oxide did not increase postoperative complications or prolong the hospital stay after neurosurgical procedures.[147] It is often of great clinical interest to obtain a neurologic assessment immediately after the conclusion of an intracranial procedure, and some practitioners prefer the use of nitrous oxide to aid in achieving this goal. Studies have demonstrated the safety of using nitrous oxide in a variety of combinations with other agents during intracranial procedures.[148,149] Nitrous oxide is relatively contraindicated, however, if the child has undergone a craniotomy within the past few weeks because air can remain in the head for prolonged periods after previous neurosurgery.[150]

Fentanyl is often administered as part of an opioid-based technique because it is easily titratable with minimal adverse effects. A common loading dose is 5 to 10 μg/kg, with a dose of 2 to 5 μg/kg per hour usually adequate for maintenance, recognizing that the context-sensitive half-life of fentanyl increases dramatically after 2 hours.[151,152] Adverse effects, including hypotension, can be avoided by giving the loading dose incrementally. Practitioners commonly use other opioids such as remifentanil and sufentanil.[151]

TABLE 24.1 | Neurophysiologic Effects of Common Anesthetic Agents

AGENT	MAP	CBF	CPP	ICP	CMRo₂	CSF Production	CSF Absorption	SSEP Amplitude	SSEP Latency
Nitrous oxide	0–↓	↑↑↑	↓	↑↑↑	↓↑	↑↓	↓↑	↓	↑-0
Inhalational Anesthetics									
Halothane	↓↓	↑↑↑	↑↑	↑↑	↓↓	↓↓	0–↓	↓	↑
Enflurane	↓↓	↑↑	↑↑	↑	↓↓	↑	↓	↓	↑
Isoflurane	↓↓	↑	↑↑	↑	↓↓↓	↓↑	↑	↓	↑
Sevoflurane	↓↓	↑	↑	↑	↓↓↓	↑	↓	↓	↑
Desflurane	↓↓	↑↑	↑	↑	↓	↑↓	↑	↓	↑
Hypnotics									
Thiopental	↓↓	↓↓↓	↑↑↑	↓↓↓	↑↑↑	↑↓	↑	↓	↑
Propofol	↓↓↓	↓↓↓	↓↓	↓↓↓	↑↓	↑	↑	↑	0–↑
Etomidate	0–↓	↓↓↓	↑	↓↓↓	↓↓↓	↑↓	↑	↑	↑
Ketamine	↓↓	↑↑↑	↓	↑↑↑	↑	↑↓	↓	↑	0
Benzodiazepine	0–↓	↓↓	↑	0–↓	↓↓	N/A	↑	↓	0–↑
Opioids	0–↓	↓	↑↓	0–↓	↓	↑↓	↑	↓	↑
Droperidol	↓↓	N/A	↑	↓	0–↓	N/A	N/A	N/A	N/A
Dexmedetomidine	↑↓	↑↓	↑	↓	0–↓	N/A	N/A	N/A	N/A

NOTE: The relative number of arrows refers to the degree of effect on the noted parameter. For example, CMRo₂ is decreased much more with isoflurane than opioids. In cells with up and down arrows, there are conflicting reports on the effect of the drug.
CBF, Cerebral blood flow; *CMRo₂*, cerebral metabolic rate for oxygen; *CPP*, cerebral perfusion pressure; *CSF*, cerebrospinal fluid; *ICP*, intracranial pressure; *MAP*, mean arterial pressure; *N/A*, not applicable; *SSEP*, somatosensory evoked potential; ↑, increased; ↓, decreased; *0*, no change.

Total intravenous anesthesia (TIVA) using propofol and remifentanil is popular when rapid emergence is required at the end of surgery (see Chapter 6). Note that the context-sensitive half-life for propofol increases with time but is particularly steep in infants[153–155]; in contrast, the context-sensitive half-life of remifentanil remains short in both children and neonates (see also Chapter 5). Dexmedetomidine, an α₂-agonist sedative, has also been used in children for neurophysiologic monitoring, for awake craniotomies,[156] to facilitate smooth wake-ups after neurosurgical procedures, and for neuroprotection.[157–160] The pharmacokinetic and pharmacodynamic limitations of IV infusion agents such as dexmedetomidine[161,162] must be appreciated if the surgeons expect a timely arousal to ensure that the CNS is intact.

APOPTOTIC NEURODEGENERATION

Several investigators have demonstrated that commonly used anesthesia drugs accelerate programmed cell death (i.e., apoptosis) in the CNS of immature rodents and rhesus monkeys.[163–165] This laboratory observation has provoked a heated debate about its relevance to anesthetizing neonates,[166–169] which has been extended to the lay press.[170] Although these experimental paradigms have yielded some surprising findings, extrapolating these data to the practice of anesthetizing human neonates is questionable (see Chapter 23 for a detailed discussion).[171]

BLOOD AND FLUID MANAGEMENT

Blood loss is difficult to estimate accurately during neurosurgery because most of the losses are absorbed by the operative drapes and the surgical field is difficult for the anesthesiologist to visualize.

Accuracy can be improved if all suctioned blood is collected in calibrated containers visible to the anesthesiologist and an overhead camera provides a view of the operative field at all times. Blood loss is usually greatest at the beginning of surgery, when the scalp is incised, and when a large bone flap is removed.

Fluid and blood product management are discussed in Chapters 7 and 10. Disruption of the blood-brain barrier by underlying pathologic processes, trauma, or surgery predisposes neurosurgical patients to cerebral edema, which may be exacerbated by excessive administration of IV fluids. Fluid management during neurosurgical anesthesia affects cerebral perfusion, cerebral edema, water and sodium homeostasis, and serum glucose concentrations.

In most cases, crystalloid solutions are commonly administered; blood transfusions are not planned and every effort is taken to avoid administering blood products with their associated risks. Lactated Ringer solution is not considered truly isotonic because its osmolality is 273 mOsm/L (normal: 285 to 290 mOsm/L). The resultant biochemical profile in adults undergoing elective craniotomy for supratentorial tumors includes hyponatremia and increased serum lactate concentrations.[172] Normal saline solution, which is slightly hypertonic (308 mOsm/L), is the fluid of choice because it maintains the serum osmolality. However, rapid infusion of large volumes of normal saline has been associated with a 24% incidence of hyperchloremic non-anion gap metabolic acidosis, hypocalcemia, and a 1.85-fold increase in the incidence or indices of acute kidney injury in adults.[172–178] The clinical significance of this acidosis is unclear. If large volumes of crystalloid solutions are required during surgery, bags of lactated Ringer solution should be alternated with normal saline solution to minimize the risks of hypernatremia, acidosis, hypoosmolality and acute kidney injury. Plasma-Lyte (Baxter Healthcare Corp., Deerfield, IL) is an acceptable crystalloid fluid as well, as it is only slightly hypotonic and yields fewer side effects than large volumes of normal saline.[178]

Inducing dehydration with osmotic and loop diuretics is a useful strategy to minimize cerebral edema and provide an optimal surgical field. However, hypotension and rebound effects may be associated with their use. Rapid administration of hypertonic solutions can cause profound but transient hypotension as the result of peripheral vasodilation.[179] Glucose-containing solutions are usually unnecessary during neurosurgical procedures because blood glucose concentrations are well maintained even in small children in the absence of IV glucose administration. However, glucose may be indicated when hypoglycemia is a risk, such as in diabetic children, children receiving hyperalimentation, preterm and full-term neonates, and malnourished or debilitated children. In these situations, glucose solutions should be administered at or slightly below maintenance rates (by constant infusion pump) and serum glucose concentrations monitored throughout surgery. The potential association of larger cerebral infarct size with hyperglycemia (i.e., blood glucose values >250 mg/dL) during ischemia is of particular concern.[180,181]

Meticulous management of fluids and blood products to minimize cerebral edema is a cornerstone of pediatric neuroanesthesia. Although cerebral hemorrhage is fortunately a rare event, when it does occur, it can be sudden and catastrophic. All children should have secure, large-bore IV access, and blood products should be available along with blood-warming devices.

TEMPERATURE CONTROL

Because the head accounts for a large proportion of an infant's body surface area, infants are particularly susceptible to heat loss during neurosurgical procedures. Attention should be focused on maintaining normal temperature from the time the child is brought into the operating room, although moderate hypothermia during neurosurgery may be salutary to decrease the $CMRO_2$. Ambient room temperature should be increased before the child enters the operating room. Infrared warming lights may be helpful for infants, and warming blankets may be useful for infants weighing less than 10 kilograms. Forced-air warming devices remain the most effective means to maintain body temperature in infants and children.[182–185]

VENOUS AIR EMBOLI

Venous air embolism (VAE) is a potential danger during intracranial procedures. The larger the pressure gradient between the operative site and the heart, the greater the potential for clinically meaningful entrainment of air into the central circulation.[186] For example, when the operative site is far above the heart (e.g., in a seated craniotomy) or when the CVP is low (e.g., acute blood loss during craniofacial procedures), it creates an environment for a VAE. Intracranial procedures are a particular concern because intracranial venous sinuses have dural attachments that impede their ability to collapse. Other potential air entry sites during neurosurgical procedures include bone, bridging veins, and spinal epidural veins. The sequence of events that should be followed when a VAE occurs is to identify the problem, stop further air entrainment, and support the circulation. Understanding the cause, prevention, and treatment of VAE is crucial because the consequences can be life-threatening.[187]

When air enters the central circulation, it can accumulate in the right atrium or the right ventricular outflow tract. Cardiac output may be reduced, depending on the size of the air lock. If enough air is entrained into the circulation, the preload to the right ventricle decreases, or the right-sided heart afterload increases acutely, which can lead to cor pulmonale, acutely decreasing left ventricular preload and ultimately causing cardiovascular collapse. In dogs, 1 mL/kg of air injected intravenously could increase pulmonary artery pressure 200% to 300%, mediated via vagal mechanisms.[188] Intracardiac shunts such as a patent foramen ovale, atrial or ventricular septal defects, and other congenital cardiac defects, may allow air to access the systemic circulation, including the coronaries and brain. The risk of VAE is even greater in infants and children because potential intracardiac shunts exist in many otherwise healthy infants and children. They may become clinically important if pulmonary hypertension develops acutely after a large air embolism. Some clinicians recommend preoperative echocardiographic screening for patent foramen ovale in any child being considered for a sitting craniotomy; others regard a patent foramen ovale to be an absolute contraindication to the sitting position.[189,190]

Although the incidence of VAE is greatest in the sitting position, the lateral, supine, and prone positions are not free of risk. VAE have also been observed during craniotomy for craniosynostosis, even when the operating room table was flat, and rarely when the surgery involved endoscopic strip craniectomy, although most occur without clinical sequelae.[191,192] The incidence of VAE in children undergoing suboccipital craniotomy in the sitting position is similar to that in adults, although children have a greater incidence of hypotension and a smaller likelihood of successful aspiration of central (intravascular) air.[193]

Several techniques may be used to detect VAE. Depending on the study design, the usual order of sensitivity of detecting air in the heart is transvenous intracardiac echocardiography (0.15 mL/kg) > transesophageal echocardiography (0.19 mL/kg) = precordial Doppler probe (0.24 mL/kg) > pulmonary artery pressure (0.61 mL/kg) = end-tidal CO_2 tension (0.63 mL/kg) = arterial O_2 tension > MAP (1.16 mL/kg) = arterial CO_2 tension.[194,195] Transvenous intracardiac echocardiography is commonly used to guide catheters in cardiac ablation procedures or insertion of foramen ovale occlusion devices, but it is invasive and infrequently used in pediatric anesthesia. A precordial Doppler probe has been traditionally placed over the fourth or fifth intercostal space at the right sternal border to best monitor right heart sounds, although evidence suggests that placing the Doppler probe at the left parasternal border may be at least as sensitive (Fig. 24.6).[196,197] Appropriate Doppler positioning can be confirmed by listening for the characteristic change in sounds after rapid administration of a few milliliters of saline solution into a venous catheter. The precordial Doppler probe is particularly valuable because it is inexpensive, easy to use, benign, and noninvasive. Although transthoracic or transesophageal echocardiography is the most specific method for detecting small air emboli, it is not easily used intraoperatively, especially in children during neurosurgical procedures.[189,198,199]

Monitoring end-tidal gas tensions is important during neurosurgical procedures. When VAE occur, there is a ventilation-perfusion mismatch caused by the air blocking passage of blood through the pulmonary circulation, increasing dead-space ventilation with a sudden decrease in end-tidal CO_2 partial pressure ($ETCO_2$) and activation of complement resulting in pulmonary interstitial edema, neutrophil infiltration, and lung injury (Fig. 24.7).[194] The $ETCO_2$ remains a useful and cost-effective strategy in diagnosing massive VAE, although its sensitivity has been surpassed by other approaches

AIR EMBOLISM
Relative sensitivity

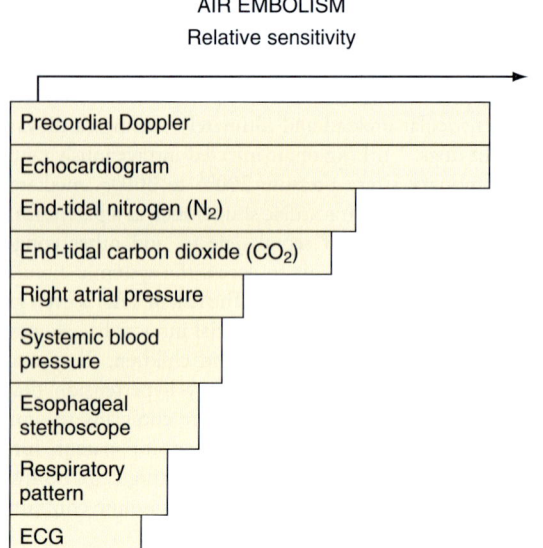

FIGURE 24.6 Relative sensitivities of air embolism–monitoring modalities. *ECG*, Electrocardiogram.

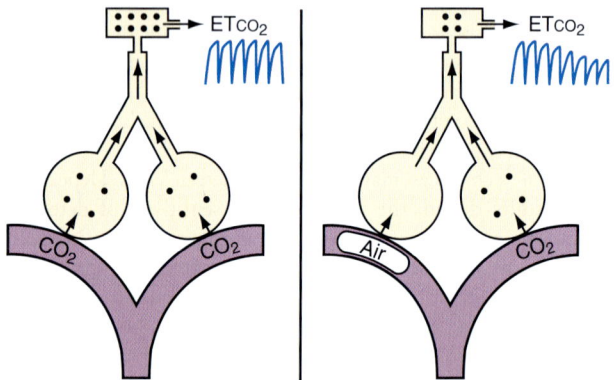

FIGURE 24.7 Mechanism of decreased end-tidal carbon dioxide *(ETCO₂)* after an air embolus. (Courtesy J. Drummond, MD.)

(see Fig. 24.6). An increase in end-tidal nitrogen partial pressure during continuous monitoring is a specific sign of air emboli. Although slightly more sensitive than a decrease in ETCO₂, an increase in end-tidal nitrogen is not detected by most infrared analyzers in practice and is usually of such small magnitude that it may be difficult to detect.

Less sensitive or more invasive methods to detect VAE include ECG changes, changes in heart rate, onset of a mill-wheel murmur (https://youtu.be/-jROC3RoaU0), decreases in systemic blood pressure, and increases in right atrial and pulmonary arterial pressures. Right atrial and pulmonary artery pressures increase quickly after the emboli develop (within 30 seconds). The magnitude of these increases correlates with the size of emboli, although these findings should not be relied on alone for monitoring and diagnosis.

On suspicion or diagnosis of VAE, immediate measures must be taken by the surgeons and anesthesiologists to prevent continued entrainment of air and consequent hemodynamic deterioration. The surgeon should immediately flood the field with saline solution and apply bone wax to exposed bone edges. The anesthesiologist should discontinue nitrous oxide and place the child in the Trendelenburg position, which has the effect of increasing cerebral venous pressure, stopping entrainment of air, augmenting the child's peripheral venous return, and increasing systemic blood pressure. Occlusion of the internal jugular veins in an attempt to increase cerebral venous pressure should be done with great care because occlusion of the carotid arteries can lead to cerebral ischemia. The application of positive end-expiratory pressure increases CVP but also decreases cardiac filling pressure, cardiac output, and blood pressure; extreme increases in positive end-expiratory pressure are usually unwarranted. Chest compressions, vasopressors, and aggressive fluid resuscitation may be required.

Aspiration of air from a central venous catheter is rarely successful unless massive amounts have been entrained. When central venous catheters are necessary, such as for a child in the sitting position or when massive blood loss is anticipated, an attempt should be made to place the tip at the junction of the superior vena cava and right atrium to provide the optimal location for aspiration of entrained air. More importantly, a central venous catheter is useful to estimate maintenance of circulating blood volume and to rapidly administer fluids and resuscitative medications when necessary. The position of a central venous catheter near the heart should be confirmed by radiograph, by transducing CVPs, or with the aid of ECG monitoring (i.e., biphasic P waves develop in a lead at the tip of the catheter). The threshold for aspirating air may be increased by properly positioning a multiple-orifice central venous catheter using a transvenous intracardiac echocardiography probe.[194] Because erosion of the catheter tip through the heart causing fatal pericardial tamponade has occurred after surgery in small children, soft silicone catheters are recommended.[200,201]

EMERGENCE

Protecting the brain is a major concern during neurosurgical procedures (Table 24.2). Emergence and extubation should be smooth and controlled to prevent fluctuations in ICP and in venous and arterial pressures.[202] To avoid vomiting during emergence, a multimodal antiemetic approach is advised.[203] Despite this approach, the incidence of PONV is high, which may be attributed to several factors: blood in the CSF is a potent emetic, opioids are often used to treat postoperative pain, and headache itself can precipitate emesis.

Intravenous lidocaine (1.0 to 1.5 mg/kg) or fentanyl (1 µg/kg) or propofol (0.5 to 1 mg/kg) given before extubation may help to suppress coughing and straining on the tracheal tube. An α- and β-adrenergic blocking agent, such as labetalol, can be administered incrementally to control blood pressure during the acute period of emergence; this is rarely necessary in children who have received adequate doses of opioids during surgery. For adolescents, IV labetalol (0.1 to 0.4 mg/kg given every 5 to 10 minutes until the desired effect is achieved) may be necessary, but does not generally have to be repeated after extubation. Esmolol is as effective as labetalol in controlling hypertension after intracranial surgery in adults.[204,205] However, esmolol should be used with caution in infants and smaller children because their cardiac output depends on a rapid heart rate. The role of esmolol in children for such an application has not been studied. Dexmedetomidine may be useful in facilitating a smooth emergence while still allowing the child's neurologic status to be evaluated.[206]

Neuromuscular blockade should be pharmacologically reversed because even the slightest residual weakness is poorly tolerated and may interfere with the neurologic examination.

TABLE 24.2 | Maneuvers of Neuroprotection

Goals	
	Avoid cerebral edema
	Avoid cerebral hypoxia
	Avoid cerebral hypoperfusion
	Avoid cerebral hypermetabolism
	Avoid neuronal membrane damage
Maneuvers	
Head of bed at 30 degrees in midline	Increases cerebral venous drainage while maintaining CPP
Corticosteroids	May improve outcome in spinal cord injury
	Decrease vasogenic cerebral edema in children with tumors
	Stabilize neuronal membranes
	Free-radical scavengers
Controlled ventilation	Maintain $Paco_2$ at normal to slightly low levels: prevents both cerebral vasodilation and increased ICP
Muscle paralysis	Avoids coughing, straining, child movement, and other causes of increased ICP
Ventricular drainage	Decreases ICP
Antihypertensives	Prevent further cerebral edema, ischemia, and cerebral hemorrhage
	Severe hypotension can significantly decrease CPP
Anticonvulsants	Prevent seizure activity and increased ICP
Hypothermia	Decreases $CMRo_2$ and CMRglu consumption
Barbiturate coma	Membrane-stabilizing effect
	Decreases CBF and $CMRo_2$

CBF, Cerebral blood flow; *CMRglu*, cerebral metabolic rate for glucose; *CMRo₂*, cerebral metabolic rate for oxygen; *CPP*, cerebral perfusion pressure; *ICP*, intracranial pressure; *Paco₂*, partial pressure of arterial carbon dioxide.

Adequate spontaneous ventilation and oxygenation and an awake mental status are required before extubation. If postoperative intracranial hypertension is possible or if the child does not meet respiratory or neurologic criteria for extubation, the tracheal tube should be left in place, sedation administered, and the child transported to an intensive care unit.

The child should be as fully alert as possible immediately after the operation to permit repeated neurologic examinations to assess recovery and to detect a deteriorating status. In unconscious children, ICP can be monitored invasively. CT scans can help to evaluate the cause of an increased ICP or deteriorating mental status.

Pain is usually not severe after a craniotomy, but it can be treated with incremental doses of opioids. Ketorolac is best avoided in the early postoperative period because of its effects on platelet function. Acetaminophen may be administered orally, rectally, or intravenously for mild pain.[207–209]

Diabetes insipidus or inappropriate secretion of antidiuretic hormone may complicate postoperative fluid and electrolyte management, particularly when surgery is in the region of the hypothalamus and pituitary gland (see Chapter 25). Careful observation of fluid status and repeated laboratory evaluation of blood and urine osmolality and sodium levels are important in this situation. When diabetes insipidus occurs, it can be managed with a continuous infusion of dilute aqueous vasopressin (0.001 to 0.01 U/kg per hour).[210] In such circumstances, large volumes of hypotonic IV solutions must be avoided because they may rapidly decrease the serum sodium concentration and osmolality. If normal saline solution is administered in strictly limited volumes, aqueous vasopressin can control the electrolyte and fluid balances of children with diabetes insipidus until they resume oral fluids. At that time, intranasal or oral desmopressin (DDAVP) can be substituted. When diabetes insipidus develops after surgery in the pituitary region (e.g., during resection of a craniopharyngioma), it may only be transient; it is important to repeatedly assess the need for vasopressin.

Portable EEGs and evoked auditory, somatosensory, and less commonly, visual potentials may be helpful in assessing children who are deeply sedated or paralyzed. Observation in an intensive care unit capable of managing children is essential for the prevention or early detection and treatment of postoperative complications. CT and/or MRI are often performed 1 or 2 days after a craniotomy or earlier if neurologic deterioration develops.

Special Situations

TRAUMA

Head Injury

Among children, trauma is the primary cause of death; head injuries from motor vehicle accidents produce most of this mortality ($\sim$1/100,000 in children 1 to 17 years of age) with homicide the next leading cause $\sim$0.9/100,000.[211] Approximately 3000 children die each year from traumatic brain injuries and $\sim$29,000 are hospitalized with a bimodal distribution of 0- to 4-year-olds and 15- to 19-year-olds suffering the greatest mortality.[212,213] Motor vehicle accidents continue to be the most frequent preventable cause of head injury, although sports-related head injury is also common in teenagers. Nonaccidental head trauma is more common in infants resulting in subdural hematomas and falls resulting in epidural hemorrhage (see Fig. 37.1 and 37.2).[212,213] Firearm-related injuries have now surpassed motor vehicle trauma as the leading cause of death in children and adolescents.[214]

Children with head trauma may have minimal neurologic abnormalities at the time of initial evaluation. However, increased ICP and neurologic deficits may progressively develop. They develop slowly because brain injuries occur in two stages. The primary insult that occurs at the time of impact results from the biomechanical forces that disrupt the cranium, neural tissue, and vasculature. The secondary traumatic brain injury is a consequence of parenchymal damage caused by the pathologic sequelae of the primary insult. These changes can result from hypotension, hypoxia, cerebral edema, or intracranial hypertension leading to altered regional CBF, metabolism, oxidative stress, neuroinflammation, increased excitatory transmitters, and disruption of the blood-brain barrier.[212,215–218] Whereas prevention of primary injuries must be addressed in a sociopolitical forum such as through seat-belt laws, sports injury prevention, and domestic violence legislation, anesthesiologists are instrumental in preventing or minimizing secondary insults (see Chapter 37).

There are major differences between children and adults in the pattern of CNS injuries. Although intracranial hematomas (i.e., epidural, subdural, or intraparenchymal) are common in adults, they are less common in children. In contrast, diffuse cerebral edema after blunt head trauma occurs more often in children than in adults.[218]

Scalp Injuries

One of the most common head injuries in children is scalp laceration. Most can be managed in the emergency department, but more serious injuries may require the operating room to provide immobility and comfort. Children can lose a considerable amount of blood from a scalp injury because a larger fraction of the cardiac output perfuses the head compared with adults. Infants younger than 1 year of age may become hemodynamically unstable from blood loss from a subgaleal hematoma alone, as in a closed scalp injury, and hypovolemia should always be considered and treated before induction of anesthesia. Coexisting intracranial or other injuries must be considered, and a preoperative CT scan may be warranted.

Skull Fractures

Skull fractures are a common manifestation of head trauma in children and these may be accidental or intentional. Fractures are divided into four types: (1) linear, usually temporal or parietal; (2) depressed, caused by direct hit to the head; (3) open; and (4) basal, involving the bones at the base of the skull.[219] Most are linear and do not require surgical treatment. These fractures are of concern primarily because the force required to produce them may damage the underlying brain and vasculature. A linear fracture over a major blood vessel (e.g., middle meningeal artery) or a large dural sinus may result in intracranial hemorrhage. Most children have an uneventful course after sustaining a simple isolated skull fracture.[220] A few develop a leptomeningeal cyst or growing fracture that eventually requires surgical treatment. Multiple skull fractures in the absence of documented major trauma should always raise the suspicion of child abuse (see Fig. 37.2), which is also referred to as *nonaccidental trauma*.

Depressed skull fractures often require surgical repair. They may occur even in the absence of a scalp laceration. However, displacement of the inner table of the skull requires greater force than that needed to produce a simple linear fracture and has greater potential to damage underlying tissues. Approximately one-third of all depressed fractures are uncomplicated, another third are associated with dural lacerations, and the remaining third are associated with cortical lacerations. The extent of cortical injury is the primary determinant of morbidity and mortality. Surgical debridement and elevation of the depressed bone are usually performed as soon as possible after the injury (Fig. 24.8A).

Basilar skull fractures are less common in children. Despite the force needed to produce these fractures, they typically have an excellent prognosis and rarely require surgical intervention. However, the possibility of a basilar skull fracture should be considered when caring for children with altered mental status, seizures, or associated trauma requiring surgery. Findings include periorbital ecchymoses ("raccoon eyes"), retroauricular ecchymosis (i.e., the Battle sign) (see Fig. 37.2B), hemotympanum, clear rhinorrhea, or otorrhea. Unless absolutely necessary (e.g., mandibular wiring), nasotracheal intubation or passage of a nasogastric tube is best avoided because these tubes have inadvertently traversed these skull fractures and entered the cranium.[221–223] Complications of basilar skull fracture include meningitis from a CSF leak, cranial nerve damage, and anosmia.

Epidural Hematoma

Epidural hematomas most commonly develop in the temporoparietal region because of arterial bleeding from a severed middle meningeal artery. They can also develop in the posterior fossa because of bleeding from a venous sinus. Approximately 85% of children will have an overlying laceration or skull fracture but the remainder do not.[224] The classic natural history in adults is a "lucid interval" between the initial loss of consciousness and subsequent

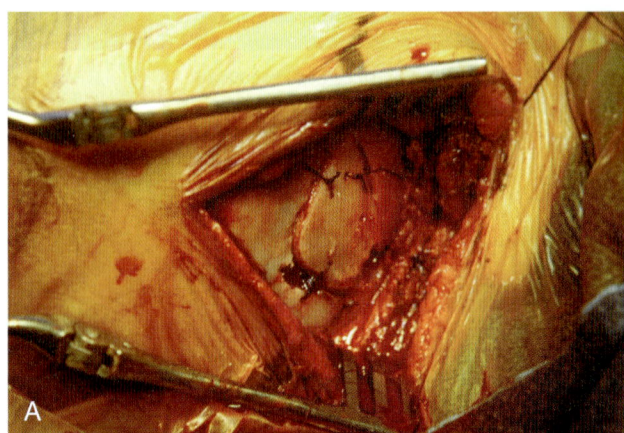

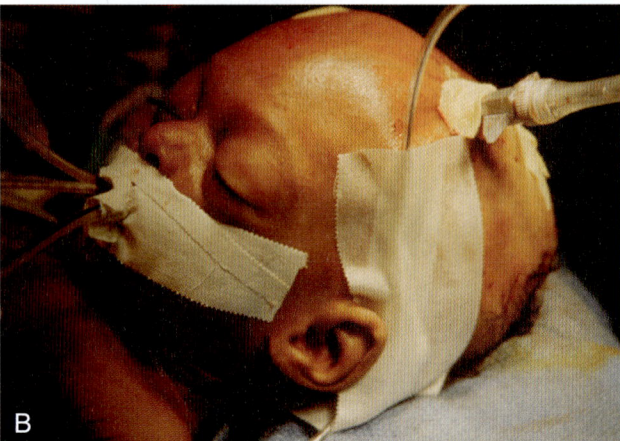

FIGURE 24.8 A, This depressed skull fracture required surgical intervention. **B,** Children with severe head trauma (in this case, a shaken baby) may present with marked increases in intracranial pressure.

neurologic deterioration. Infants and children may appear completely asymptomatic and not demonstrate an altered mental status in the early stages after the injury and present with a Glasgow Coma Scale of 15 (~40%).[224] However, as the hematoma expands, it can lead to a loss of consciousness, hemiparesis, and pupillary dilatation. This deterioration can be quite rapid once a mass effect occurs. Treatment is emergent surgical evacuation because delays are associated with increased morbidity. Medical therapy directed at decreasing ICP should be instituted as soon as a diagnosis is suspected but should not delay surgical repair (see Fig. 24.8B). Children recover well after these hemorrhages, although morbidity is usually a reflection of underlying brain injury or lengthy delay in treatment.

Subdural Hematoma

Subdural hematomas are usually associated with cortical damage resulting from direct parenchymal contusion or laceration of venous blood vessels. Acute subdural hematomas are almost always traumatic and are frequently a result of abuse, such as shaking of small children, particularly those younger than 1 year of age. Shaken baby syndrome (now called abusive head injury)[225] occurs when an infant is shaken so vigorously that neuronal disruption occurs and tears in the cortical bridging veins cause subdural hematomas.[226–228] These infants suffer brain damage complicated by episodes of apnea and further hypoxic insult. These babies present with the triad of subdural hematoma, retinal hemorrhages, and cerebral edema.[225,229]

Subdural hematomas occasionally result from birth trauma within the first hours of life. Vitamin K deficiency, congenital coagulopathies, and disseminated intravascular coagulation are considerations in these situations. Great force is required to produce a subdural hematoma, whether by direct impact, laceration of blood vessels, or traumatic separation of the brain and overlying dura. Cerebral edema, uncontrolled intracranial hypertension, and persistent neurologic deficits often characterize the postoperative course. Chronic subdural hematomas or effusions may also develop in infancy, although these children do not usually present with acute symptoms. Children are often diagnosed because they are irritable and vomiting or have an increased head circumference. Chronic subdural hematomas can increase in size, causing slow but significant increases in ICP. Although a craniotomy is sometimes performed, most children undergo some form of hematoma drainage or shunting procedure as definitive treatment.

Intracerebral Hematoma

Intracerebral hematomas fortunately are rare but have a poor prognosis. Deep parenchymal hematomas are most often extensions of cortical contusions in a child with severe neurologic injury. Rarely, a localized hematoma may be appropriate for surgical evacuation to decompress the brain. However, intraparenchymal hematomas are not evacuated for fear of damaging viable brain tissue. Anticonvulsants are usually administered prophylactically, and it is safest in the initial period after injury to avoid any medications that interfere with coagulation (e.g., ketorolac).

Spinal Injury

Although isolated cervical spine injuries are uncommon in children, those with severe head trauma should always be managed as if they also have a cervical spine injury.[230,231] Different causes of spinal injuries are associated with specific age groups. Motor vehicle accidents produce the largest number of injuries in older children and adolescents, whereas birth injuries and falls are the most common cause in infants and young children.[232] Spinal cord injury itself may be caused by a variety of forces, including hyperflexion, hyperextension, rotation, vertical compression, flexion rotation, and shearing. The injury may involve bony, ligamentous, cartilaginous, vascular, or neural components of the spine or adjacent structures. The biomechanics and functional anatomy of the pediatric spine depend on the age of the child. Older children and teenagers are more likely to sustain injuries in the thoracolumbar region or lower cervical spine (C5 to C6), whereas infants and younger children are more likely to suffer injuries in the high cervical region, particularly in the atlantoaxial region.[233] The cervical spine is at greater risk in the infant and younger child (C2 to C4) because of the relatively weak and flexible neck muscles, increased ligamentous laxity, incomplete vertebral ossification, that support a proportionally large and heavy head, with the atlantooccipital area acting as a pivot point.[233] Atlantooccipital dislocations are major neurologic injuries, leaving children neurologically devastated but not necessarily dead.

As with brain injury, spinal cord injury occurs in two phases. The primary insult results from biomechanical forces and bony fragments directly impacting the spinal cord. The secondary insult results from the pathologic sequelae of the primary insult: edema and ischemia owing to cortical compression, hypotension, or hypoxia. Inappropriate manipulation of a child with an unstable fracture can exacerbate primary and secondary injuries. Anesthesiologists who provide care for a child with a potential cervical spine injury should be aware that spinal cord injuries in children commonly occur without actual evidence of spinal bone fractures on plain cervical radiographs. These injuries are known as spinal cord injuries without radiologic abnormality (SCIWORA).[234] Injuries to the cervical spine in particular are often difficult to recognize but may be identified by odontoid displacement or prevertebral swelling on radiographs. As a result, a CT scan is frequently indicated when a spinal injury is initially suspected in a child with trauma.[233] A CT scan is more sensitive for bone injury but less for soft tissue or ligamentous injury where an MRI would be most useful.[235,236] After a child with a potential spinal injury is determined to be medically stable, these studies should be obtained as soon as possible. The child's airway and cardiorespiratory function must be continuously and closely monitored until a spinal cord injury can be ruled out. Sometimes, as with brain injury, there can be a delay in the onset of neurologic deficits with SCIWORA injuries.[233,237]

Respiratory failure is the most common cause of death after isolated cervical spine injury. The level of injury determines the degree of impairment. The phrenic nerve originates primarily from C4 but receives contributions of fibers from C3 and C5. Lesions at C5 leave partial diaphragmatic innervation but impair abdominal and intercostal accessory muscles. Lesions between C6 and T7 preserve diaphragmatic innervation but diminish accessory muscle function.

Children with a cervical spine injury may rapidly develop respiratory failure owing to decreased vital capacity, increased dead space, retention of secretions, and respiratory muscle fatigue. Resultant hypercarbia and hypoxia aggravate the secondary injury to the brain and spinal cord. Respiratory status may be further impaired by associated trauma to the chest, causing pulmonary contusion or pneumothorax, or by aspiration of gastric contents.

Prompt airway management is essential to avoid hypoxia, ensure adequate respiratory mechanics, preserve neural function, and prevent extension of spinal injury (see Figs. 37.4 and 37.5). The head and neck must be immediately immobilized; restraint of the extremities may also be required. Various tracheal tubes and laryngoscope blades should be available, as well as equipment and personnel for an emergency tracheostomy. Insertion of a laryngeal mask airway may be lifesaving until a more secure airway can be achieved with fiberoptic or other means.[238–243] Small fiberoptic bronchoscopes (2.2-mm diameter) can fit through infant-sized tracheal tubes (see Chapter 12). However, an unstable infant or child whose airway cannot be secured by conventional means is probably best managed by an emergency tracheostomy. As a temporizing measure, a cricothyroidotomy can be performed (see Figs. 12.27 to 12.29).[244] This permits oxygenation (although inadequate ventilation) until personnel and equipment for tracheostomy are assembled. An emergent surgical airway can be extremely difficult to perform on a small child or infant, even by experienced and skilled hands.

Hemodynamic instability may be a problem owing to hypovolemia from other injuries or severe head trauma. Other sites of bleeding such as long bone fractures, chest, and abdominal trauma should be ruled out. Children with spinal shock exhibit loss of vasomotor tone or loss of normal neurocardiac function with associated bradycardia and decreased myocardial contractility; IV fluids and vasopressors may be necessary.

The use of high-dose steroids as treatment of spinal cord injury remains controversial.[233] Although there are few data for adults and children, corticosteroids are still administered by some to patients with spinal injuries as soon as possible after the initial trauma in the hope of reducing the neurologic injury. The most commonly used drug is methylprednisolone; 30 mg/kg is administered over the first 15 minutes, followed by an infusion of 5.4 mg/kg per hour for the next 23 hours.[245,246] Such therapy is no longer recommended. A systematic review of five randomized controlled trials and seven observational studies evaluating methylprednisolone administration within 8 hours of injury found an increased risk for hyperglycemia and pneumonia; the authors concluded that these data failed to show a significant short- or long-term improvement in motor function or neurologic scores.[247]

If the spinal cord injury is more than 24 hours old, succinylcholine should be avoided because hyperkalemia may occur.[78,248] Physiologic changes may result from autonomic hyperreflexia, which frequently develops after cervical or high thoracic spinal lesions. Autonomic hyperreflexia can produce severe and life-threatening vasomotor instability with hypertension and arrhythmias.[249–251]

Concussion

Concussion is the mildest of traumatic brain injuries and is a clinical diagnosis defined by the American Association of Neurology as *"a clinical syndrome of biomechanically induced alteration of brain function, typically affecting memory and orientation, which may involve loss of consciousness."* [252] Loss of consciousness is not absolutely needed for the diagnosis. Diagnosing concussion can be difficult given the variety of symptoms. One easy diagnostic acronym utilizing clinical phenotypes of concussion was developed by Craton, et al is COACH CV: Cognitive dysfunction, Oculomotor dysfunction, Affective disturbance, Cervical spine disorders, Headaches, and Cardiovascular and Vestibular anomalies.[253] Clinical symptoms of concussion may include one or more of the following: memory impairment, attention impairment, visual changes such as blurred vision or abnormal extraocular movements, vestibular dysfunction, heart rate variability, headaches, mood changes, fatigue, and poor sleep. There are a variety of diagnostic assessment tools available, but it is generally advised to use one throughout disease evolution to allow for better tracking of symptom resolution or lack thereof. CT scans are not used for diagnosis and generally not recommended in order to avoid unnecessary exposure to ionizing radiation.

Once a diagnosis of concussion is made, a resting period of 24 to 48 hours followed by a plan for slow return to play or activity should be made with the guidance of a neurologist. Each plan is different and should be tailored to the patient's specific symptoms. Up to 10% to 15% of children will not make a full recovery after a resting period of 4 weeks and develop postconcussion syndrome, which has been renamed "major or mild neurocognitive disorder due to TBI" that warrants referral to a concussion specialist.[254] Another concern is the occurrence of a second concussion before resolution of symptoms from the first. Such injuries can result in catastrophic cerebral edema, failure of cerebral autoregulation, and activation of all the inflammatory and excitatory responses associated with acute brain injury.[255]

CRANIOTOMY

Tumors

Brain tumors are the most common solid tumors in children, exceeded only by the leukemias as the most common pediatric malignancy (~6/100,000).[256–258] Between 1500 and 2000 new brain tumors are diagnosed annually in children in the United States. Unlike those in adults, most brain tumors in children are infratentorial in the posterior fossa. They include medulloblastomas,

cerebellar astrocytomas, brainstem gliomas, and ependymomas of the fourth ventricle.[258,259] Because posterior fossa tumors usually obstruct CSF flow, increased ICP occurs early. Presenting signs and symptoms include early morning vomiting and irritability or lethargy. Cranial nerve palsies and ataxia are also common findings, with respiratory and cardiac irregularities usually occurring late. Sedation or general anesthesia may be required for radiologic evaluation or radiation therapy.

Surgical resection of a posterior fossa tumor presents a number of anesthetic challenges. Children are usually positioned prone, although the lateral or sitting positions are used by some neurosurgeons.[260] In either case, the head is flexed, and the position and patency of the tracheal tube must be meticulously ensured. In the event that the tracheal tube does become dislodged when the child is in a head holder and prone, successful emergent airway management has been described using a laryngeal mask airway.[261]

Arrhythmias and acute blood pressure changes may occur during surgical exploration, especially when the brainstem is manipulated or irrigated (Fig. 24.9). The electrocardiogram and arterial waveform should be closely monitored. Altered respiratory control may be masked by neuromuscular blocking drugs and mechanical ventilation. Even when ICP is only marginally increased, intracranial compliance is presumed to have decreased. This warrants precautions against further increases in ICP. If ICP is markedly increased or acutely worsens, a ventricular catheter may be inserted before the tumor is resected. Venous air embolism is a potentially serious complication that is not eliminated by the prone or lateral position because head-up gradients of 10 to 20 degrees are frequently used to improve cerebral venous drainage. In infants and toddlers, large head size relative to body size accentuates this problem.

Supratentorial tumors in the midbrain include craniopharyngiomas, optic gliomas, pituitary adenomas, and hypothalamic tumors and account for approximately 15% of intracranial tumors. Hypothalamic tumors (i.e., hamartomas, gliomas, and teratomas) frequently manifest with precocious puberty in children who are large for their chronologic age. Craniopharyngiomas are the most common parasellar tumors in children and adolescents and may be associated with hypothalamic and pituitary dysfunction. Symptoms often include growth failure, visual impairment, and endocrine abnormalities.[262]

Signs and symptoms of hypothyroidism should be sought, and thyroid function measured. Corticosteroid replacement (i.e., dexamethasone or hydrocortisone) usually is administered because the integrity of the hypothalamic-pituitary-adrenal axis may be uncertain. Diabetes insipidus can occur preoperatively and is a common postoperative problem. The history usually reveals this condition preoperatively, especially if attention is focused on nocturnal drinking and enuresis. Evaluation of serum electrolytes and osmolality, urine specific gravity, and urine output is helpful because hypernatremia and hyperosmolality, along with dilute urine, are typical findings. If diabetes insipidus does not exist preoperatively, it usually does not develop until the postoperative period because there is an adequate reserve of antidiuretic hormone in the posterior pituitary gland capable of functioning for many hours, even when the hypothalamic-pituitary stalk is damaged intraoperatively.

Postoperative diabetes insipidus is marked by a sudden large increase in dilute urine output associated with an increasing serum sodium concentration and osmolality. Protocols have been developed to guide intraoperative and postoperative management of diabetes insipidus (see Chapters 7 and 25).[210] Return of

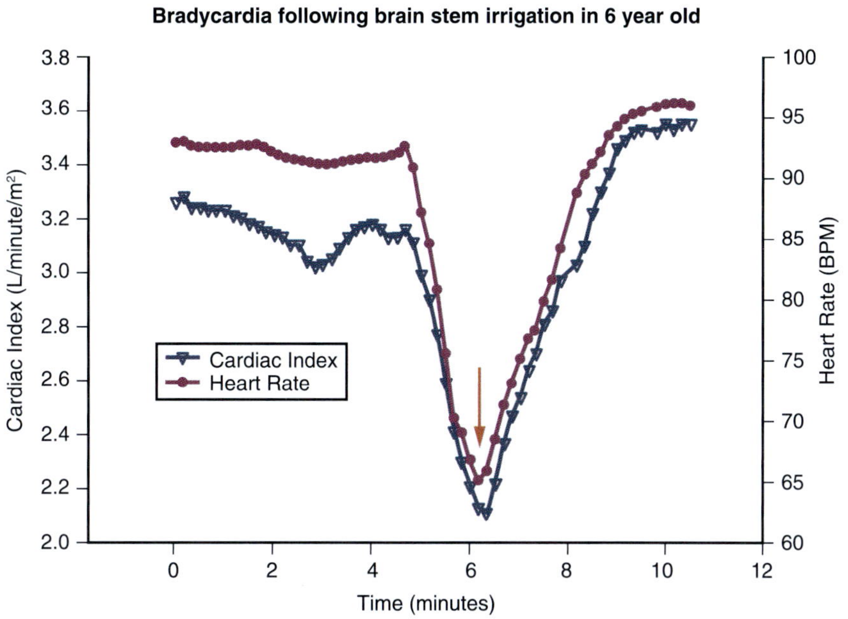

Bradycardia following brain stem irrigation in 6 year old

FIGURE 24.9 This graph illustrates the dramatic bradycardic response and accompanying decrease in cardiac index measured by a continuous noninvasive cardiac output monitor (Cardiotronic, Osypka Medical Inc., La Jolla, CA) in a 6-year-old child following brainstem irrigation. As soon as the surgeon stopped irrigation and atropine was administered (see down arrow), the heart rate and cardiac index were restored. (Courtesy Charles J Coté, MD.)

antidiuretic hormone activity a few days postoperatively may cause a marked decrease in urinary output, water intoxication, seizures, and cerebral edema if it is not recognized and fluid administration is not adjusted appropriately.

Transsphenoidal surgery typically is performed only in adolescents and older children with pituitary adenomas. However, it should be treated like other midbrain tumors in terms of monitoring and vascular access. Children are usually intubated orally to give the surgeon optimal access to the nasopharynx, and preparations for an emergent craniotomy should be anticipated in case unexpected massive bleeding develops. Because nasal packs are inserted at the end of surgery, the child should be fully awake before tracheal extubation.

Gliomas of the optic pathways occur with increased frequency in children with neurofibromatosis. Presenting symptoms include visual changes and proptosis; increased ICP and hypothalamic dysfunction are usually late findings.[263] Neurofibromas are of three types: Type 1, 2, and schwannomas.[264] Malignant neurofibromas tend to be highly vascular, and the anesthesiologist should be prepared for considerable blood loss.

Approximately 25% of intracranial tumors in children involve the cerebral hemispheres. They are primarily astrocytomas, oligodendrogliomas, ependymomas, and glioblastomas. Neurologic symptoms are more likely to include a seizure disorder or focal deficits. Succinylcholine should be avoided if motor weakness is present because it can cause sudden severe hyperkalemia. Nondepolarizing neuromuscular blocking drugs and opioids may be metabolized more rapidly than usual in children who are receiving chronic anticonvulsants. Choroid plexus papillomas are rare but occur most often in children younger than 3 years of age. They usually arise from the choroid plexus of the lateral ventricle and produce early hydrocephalus because of increased production of CSF and obstruction of CSF flow. Hydrocephalus usually resolves with surgical resection. When lesions lie near the motor or sensory strip, a special type of somatosensory evoked potential monitoring called

phase reversal may be used to delineate the locations.[265] If cortical stimulation is planned to help identify motor areas, neuromuscular blocking drugs must be permitted to wear off and the anesthetic technique adjusted to achieve immobilization without paralysis.

Stereotactic biopsies or craniotomies present special concerns regarding airway accessibility. Newer head frames have adjustable anterior positions so that the airway is readily accessible (E-Fig. 24.1). They are especially useful for stereotactic neurosurgery. It is more comfortable and less distressing for the child to be anesthetized before the head frame is applied, even though this means the anesthesiologist must induce anesthesia in the radiology suite and then transport the child from the CT scanner to the operating room. The wrench that is used to apply and remove the head frame should be taped to the frame at all times so that it is always readily available if emergent removal of the head frame becomes necessary (e.g., during transport).

Vascular Anomalies

Arteriovenous Malformations

Arteriovenous malformations consist of large arterial feeding vessels, dilated communicating vessels, and large draining veins carrying arterialized blood. Large malformations, especially those involving the posterior cerebral artery and vein of Galen, may manifest as congestive heart failure (i.e., high-output heart failure, often with pulmonary hypertension) in the neonate. Consumption of coagulation factors and platelet destruction may further complicate the clinical picture. The prognosis for these types of arteriovenous malformations is quite poor. Saccular dilation of the vein of Galen may manifest later in infancy or childhood as hydrocephalus owing to obstruction of the aqueduct of Sylvius. Malformations not large enough to produce congestive heart failure usually remain clinically silent unless they cause seizures or a stroke or until the acute rupture of a communicating vessel results in subarachnoid or intracerebral hemorrhage.[266] Intracranial hemorrhages are the most common presentation in this population, with an associated mortality rate of ~25%.

Treatment usually consists of embolization or irradiation of deep malformations, surgical excision (usually of the more superficial ones), or a combination of these modalities. The surgical technique may require coordination between multiple locations and a prolonged anesthetic. However, the extra time and transport is worth the generally good outcome and avoidance of subsequent craniotomies for further resection if there is a residual arteriovenous malformation. A postoperative obliteration rate of 100% using a protocol of immediate postcraniotomy cerebral angiography to confirm obliteration has been reported.[267]

Management for elective embolic procedures involves general anesthesia. Moderate hyperventilation may enhance visualization of abnormal blood vessels that do not respond with vasoconstriction. The anesthesiologist should be knowledgeable about the types of embolic agents that can be used and their potential complications. Anticonvulsant therapy is routine. Neonates in cardiac failure may be receiving inotropic agents. Bleeding, especially from the femoral arterial puncture site (which cannot always be visualized), should always be a consideration. Fluid overload may result from the large amount of contrast agents administered, especially in a young infant who may already be in high-output cardiac failure. The anesthesiologist should be prepared for the possibility of an emergency craniotomy if a vessel ruptures.

Aneurysms

Intracranial aneurysms most often result from a congenital malformation in an arterial wall with an estimated incidence of ~1 to 3/1,000,000.[268] Children with coarctation of the aorta or polycystic kidney disease have an increased incidence of these aneurysms.[268] They usually remain asymptomatic during childhood; most ruptures that occur in childhood are fatal. Symptoms of subarachnoid or intracerebral hemorrhage frequently appear suddenly in a previously healthy young adult. When technically feasible, the treatment of choice is surgical ligation or clipping of the aneurysm.[269]

Anesthesia for surgical resection of vascular malformations and aneurysms in children presents unique challenges, especially if the diagnosis has been preceded by an intracranial hemorrhage. Blood products should be in the operating room and verified before the start of the procedure. An adequate depth of anesthesia should be ensured before any invasive maneuver to prevent precipitous hypertension.[270] Adequate venous access to respond to sudden and massive blood loss is crucial but can wait until after induction of anesthesia. A blood-warming device, such as a rapid transfusion device, should be immediately available.

Controlled hypotension may be valuable in some situations for brief periods to reduce tension in the abnormal blood vessels and improve the safety of surgical manipulation.[271–273] It is not clear, however, whether the benefits of controlled hypotension are worth the risks, especially in small children (see Chapter 10). Controlled hypotension should not be used in children with increased ICP because of the risk of decreasing CPP, with resulting ischemia and further increased ICP. Although the absolute limits of acceptable hypotension are unknown, a mean blood pressure greater than 40 mm Hg for infants or 50 mm Hg for older children appears to be safe; teenagers should have a target MAP no less than 55 mm Hg. At the conclusion of the procedure, the blood pressure is returned to normal, but before closing the dura, the operative site should be inspected for bleeding.

Hemodynamic stability is important during emergence to avoid bucking, coughing, straining, and hypertension during extubation. Excessive hypertension can result in postoperative

bleeding, although in most cases of aneurysm clipping, a slightly increased blood pressure may be desirable postoperatively to minimize the risk of vasospasm. After resection of an arteriovenous malformation, there can be serious postoperative complications related to cerebral edema with increased ICP or hemorrhage. This *normal perfusion pressure breakthrough* is probably caused by hyperemia of the areas surrounding the previous arteriovenous malformation site, where vessels suffer from continued vasomotor paralysis and cannot vasoconstrict. Treatment is controversial but usually involves therapy for increased ICP (e.g., diuretics, moderate hyperventilation, head elevation) in addition to judicious use of moderate hypotension (while maintaining CPP) and moderate hypothermia. When surgery is completed, it is important that children can cooperate with a neurologic examination and that there is careful control of blood pressure in the intensive care unit.

Moyamoya Disease

Moyamoya disease is an anomaly that results in progressive and life-threatening occlusion of intracranial vessels, primarily the internal carotid arteries near the circle of Willis.[274] An abnormal vascular network of collaterals develops at the base of the brain, and the appearance of these many, small vessels on angiography was originally described by the Japanese name *moyamoya*, which roughly translates as "puff of smoke" (Fig. 24.10A). The congenital form of the disease can involve the systemic vasculature, including pulmonary, coronary, and renal vessels[275]; affected renal arteries are the most commonly identified angiographic lesion. The acquired variety (i.e., moyamoya syndrome) may be associated with meningitis, neurofibromatosis, chronic inflammation, connective tissue diseases, certain hematologic disorders, Down syndrome, or prior intracranial radiation.[276] Some children with neurologic symptoms from sickle cell disease may also have moyamoya.[277] Moyamoya disease appears to be more common among children of Japanese ancestry. Associated intracranial aneurysms are rare in children but may occur in more than 10% of affected adult patients. Abnormal ECG findings have been described with the syndrome in adults.

Moyamoya disease usually manifests as transient ischemic attacks progressing to strokes and fixed neurologic deficits in children.[275] These attacks may be precipitated by hyperventilation.[278] The morbidity and mortality rates are high if the condition is left untreated. Medical management consists of antiplatelet therapy, such as aspirin, or calcium channel blockers. The most common surgical operation for correction in children is pial synangiosis, which involves suturing a scalp artery (usually the superficial temporal artery) directly onto the pial surface of the brain to enhance angiogenesis (Fig. 24.10B).[275,279]

Careful and continuous monitoring of ETCO$_2$ is essential in anesthesia management.[280] Children with moyamoya disease have reduced hemispheric blood flow bilaterally, and hyperventilation may further reduce regional blood flow and cause EEG and neurologic changes.[281] *Normocapnia must be maintained throughout all phases of the procedure,* including induction of anesthesia.[275] Adequate hydration and maintenance of baseline blood pressure are indispensable. Most of these children have an IV catheter inserted the night before surgery and are given 1.5 times the amount of maintenance fluids to avoid dehydration during the perioperative period. EEG monitoring during these procedures can detect and help to treat ischemia that appears to be a result of cerebral vasoconstriction in response to direct surgical manipulation of the brain.[275,282] Normothermia is maintained, particularly at the end of the procedure, to avoid postoperative shivering and an

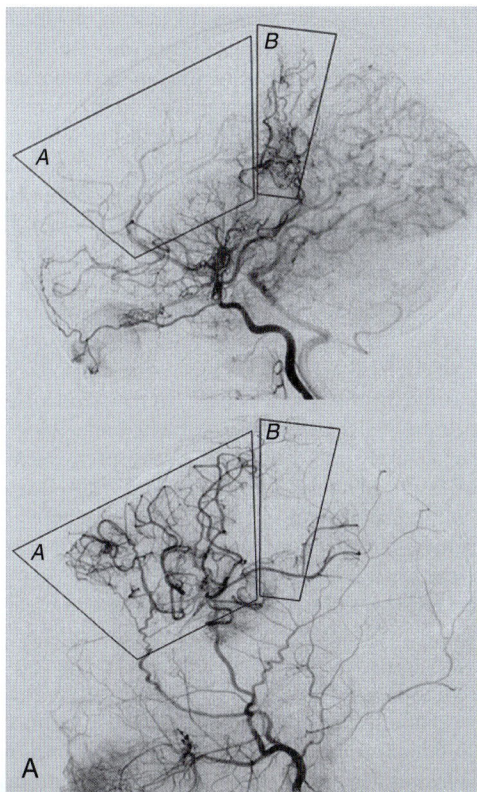

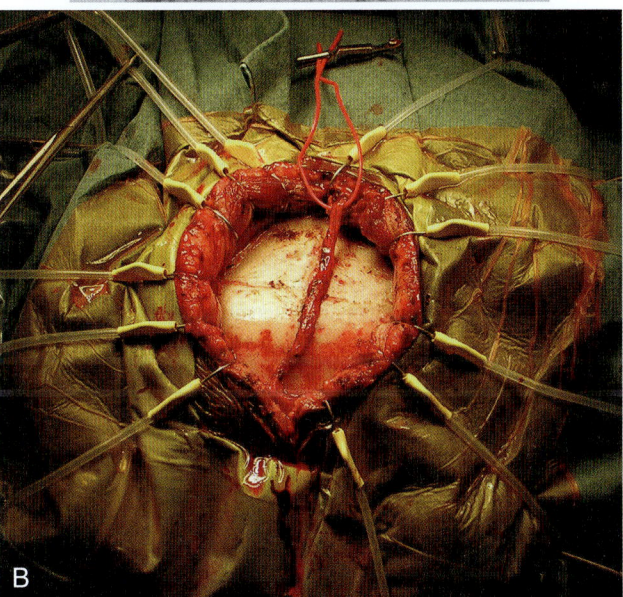

FIGURE 24.10 Moyamoya disease. **A,** The top angiogram shows the pattern of arterial filling after injection of the internal carotid artery in a child with moyamoya disease before pial synangiosis. *Area A* shows poor filling from the middle cerebral artery because of the disease process. *Area B* shows the characteristic hazy collaterals, or moyamoya vessels. The bottom angiogram is from the same child after pial synangiosis. The angiogram was obtained after injection of the superficial temporal artery, and it shows good filling in the middle cerebral artery distribution in *area A. Area B* does not fill from the middle cerebral artery. **B,** Pial synangiosis. The superficial temporal artery is prepared to be sutured to the pia of the cerebral cortex. After the craniotomy is completed, this artery can be sewn directly onto the underlying pia mater. The result of this procedure is improvement of blood flow to ischemic areas of the cerebral cortex.

exaggerated stress response. As with most neurosurgical procedures, a smooth extubation without hypertension or crying is desirable. Although scant literature exists regarding intraoperative and postoperative complications during moyamoya surgery, it appears that most complications (e.g., strokes) occur postoperatively and are associated with dehydration and crying (i.e., hyperventilation) episodes.[283] Those centers that regularly perform this surgery have better outcomes,[284] indicating that higher-volume centers are able to provide improved care and reduced mortality in children with moyamoya disease. Life-long antiplatelet treatment with aspirin is usually prescribed.[275] The most marked benefit displayed was for those patients who underwent surgical revascularization.

Seizure Surgery

Epilepsy is one of the most common neurologic disorders of childhood. Despite the development of new drugs and regimens, the prevalence of pharmacologically intractable seizures remains high. Advances in neuroimaging, functional MRI, and EEG monitoring provide epileptologists anatomic targets that mediate some medically intractable seizure disorders.[285,286] Advances in pediatric neurosurgery have exploited these technologies and dramatically improved the outcomes for infants and children.[287,288]

Children presenting for surgical management of seizures take anticonvulsant medications, which can have serious adverse effects, including abnormalities of hematologic function such as abnormal coagulation, depression of red or white blood cell production, and decreased platelet counts.[289] Other problems may arise from altered hepatic function. Specific anticonvulsant concentrations should be determined preoperatively to detect subtherapeutic or toxic concentrations. Many anticonvulsants enhance hepatic metabolism of nondepolarizing neuromuscular blocking drugs and opioids, increasing (up to 50%) the frequency of administration and total amounts of these drugs needed during a surgical procedure (see Tables 22.15 and 22.16 for interactions between seizure medications and commonly used anesthetic drugs).[290] The preoperative evaluation should detect underlying conditions that are causing the seizures and the disabilities that can result from progressive neurologic dysfunction.

A major concern during resection of seizure foci is avoiding harming brain tissue that controls vital functions, such as motion, sensation, speech, and memory (the so-called eloquent cortex), especially if a seizure focus is adjacent to cortical areas controlling these functions. Cooperative adolescents and adults can assist in determination of the limits of safe cortical resection if they can be continually assessed during the surgical procedure. The technique of awake craniotomy is often performed in carefully selected adolescents.[291] An awake craniotomy encompasses a wide variety of techniques whose common goal is to allow intraoperative assessment and feedback to determine if the eloquent cortex is at risk during resection.

Children are selected for this procedure on an individual basis. Most children younger than 12 years of age and many teenagers cannot tolerate an awake craniotomy. However, selected individuals may do well. The anesthesiologist should have detailed conversations with the child and parents to determine appropriateness before initiating such a procedure.

Some practitioners perform the entire procedure, including line placement, infiltration of local anesthetic, skull and dural opening, and resection, with the child completely awake or with minimal sedation. This particular approach requires an extremely motivated child. A variation on this technique uses short-acting sedatives and analgesics, such as propofol and fentanyl or remifentanil, titrated to induce unconsciousness but maintain spontaneous ventilation for instillation of local anesthetics, insertion of monitoring catheters, placement of head pins, and skull opening.[292] Subsequently, children can be allowed to awaken during surgical resection. They can then have sedatives and opioids reinstituted for the craniotomy closure.

Alternatively, some anesthesiologists use the asleep-awake-asleep technique.[291] It consists of inducing general anesthesia and maintaining airway control with a supraglottic device (i.e., laryngeal mask airway). General anesthesia is maintained for line placement, placement of head pins, and skull and dural opening. The child is then awakened, the supraglottic airway is removed, and the surgeons proceed with resection. At the conclusion of the resection, general anesthesia is again induced and the supraglottic airway is reinserted for closure of the dura, skull, and skin. There are several disadvantages to the asleep-awake-asleep approach. One of the major concerns with this approach is airway management during emergence and induction while the child is in head pins. If the child coughs or bucks while immobilized, cervical spine injuries or scalp lacerations can occur. Brain swelling is also a concern in a child who is breathing spontaneously under general anesthesia with an inhalational anesthetic and possibly with nitrous oxide.

Regardless of the technique chosen, the anesthesiologist must have an in-depth discussion with the child or adolescent about intraoperative needs and expectations.[293] The preoperative period is the time to decide whether the child is a candidate for an awake craniotomy. There are no randomized, controlled trials comparing the safety or effectiveness of the techniques described, particularly in adolescents.[291]

Younger children (<12 years of age) or uncooperative children of any age do not tolerate this approach and require general anesthesia throughout. In these circumstances, intraoperative electrophysiologic studies, such as somatosensory evoked potentials, EEG, and motor stimulation, may be used to help localize and determine the function of the site of planned resection. If EEG studies are to be performed, the anesthetic technique should be adjusted to maximize EEG signals. If direct cortical motor stimulation is planned, neuromuscular blocking drugs must be permitted to wear off. Occasionally, a seizure focus is difficult to identify intraoperatively. In these situations, hyperventilation may be helpful in lowering the seizure threshold and producing EEG seizure activity. Methohexital in small doses (0.25 to 0.5 mg/kg) has been used in the past to lower the seizure threshold.[294,295]

In some children, the site of origin of generalized seizures is difficult to determine. When this occurs, evaluation with intracranial EEG monitoring ("grids and strips") may be accomplished with direct electrocorticography (E-Fig. 24.2). The leads are placed on the surface of the cortex after a craniotomy performed with general anesthesia. Intraoperative EEG monitoring is limited during these procedures to ensuring that all leads are functional; monitoring for seizures takes place over the next several days to identify a focus that is amenable to resection. These children need to be observed carefully in the postoperative period because complications can develop from having intracranial electrodes in place. Because air frequently persists in the skull for up to 3 weeks after a craniotomy,[150] these children should not have nitrous oxide administered for a subsequent procedure (e.g., to resect a seizure focus, to remove the electrocorticography leads) until their dura has been opened to prevent the development of tension pneumocephalus.

The development of intraoperative MRI (iMRI) with laser-guided thermal therapy has aided in the surgical treatment of epilepsy. There continues to be great interest in the development of this technology to assist perioperatively with a variety of neurosurgical procedures and aid in facilitating optimal outcomes. This technology naturally lends itself to seizure surgery when a focal lesion can be identified. There is evidence in the adult literature supporting the use of iMRI in seizure surgery to facilitate higher resection volumes and consequently improved postoperative seizure outcomes.[296] A retrospective review of the role of iMRI in children undergoing resection for perieloquent cortical dysplasias and heterotopias has suggested that, in comparison with conventional surgical approaches in these patients, iMRI led to elevated rates of gross total resection and a seizure-free postoperative course. Further, the use of iMRI in these patients led to a decrease in postoperative neurologic deficits.[297] Similar results have been published using iMRI in pediatric patients undergoing surgical resection of focal cortical dysplasia.[298] A retrospective comparison of 185 MRI-guided thermal resection with 185 open surgical resections found that the open resection was superior to MRI-guided thermal resection but the latter resulted in shorter hospitalization and better safety profiles.[299]

When a focal resection is not possible, a lobectomy or corpus callosotomy may be attempted. However, children undergoing the latter procedure are often somnolent for the first few postoperative days, especially if a complete callosotomy is performed. This also occurs in children who have undergone insertion of multiple subdural grids and strips. Occasionally, small children undergo a hemispherectomy because their seizures are attributed to an abnormal hemisphere that is already severely dysfunctional, as when affected by hemiparesis. These can be challenging cases for the anesthesiologist because of high blood loss (from one-half to multiples of the estimated blood volume).[300] This procedure is usually performed when children are very young to permit the other hemisphere to take over the function of both sides. Large-bore IV access is necessary in these cases to facilitate rapid replacement of blood, crystalloid solutions, and medications. Arterial pressure monitoring is routine, and many practitioners also use CVP monitoring.

Recent advancements in minimally invasive surgical treatment of drug resistant epilepsy include stereotactic electroencephalography (SEEG) and laser interstitial thermal therapy (LITT). SEEG uses stereotactic guided intracranial electrodes to identify an epileptogenic zone with the goal of finding an anatomic location for the seizure onset zone that can be treated with either surgical resection or laser ablation.[301] SEEG is particularly useful when the underlying seizure focus is located deep within the brain such as in the hippocampus. Brain imaging via computed tomography (CT) and MRI are done prior to the electrode placement to provide a map for electrode insertion. Anesthetic management for SEEG placement should take the same precautions as with other seizure surgeries with special consideration being paid to patient positioning in relation to the head frame. Once a position is chosen, the patient must not move from that position as it will interfere with the accurate placement of the electrodes.[302] Postoperative recovery is faster than with large craniotomies and offers the benefit of avoiding a craniotomy if patients do not have surgically operable seizure foci. Although the potential risks with SEEG placement are low, they involve intracranial hemorrhage and infection.[303-305] Once seizure foci are identified for intervention, either surgical resection or thermal ablation are utilized for treatment. Thermal ablation (LITT) can be accomplished via a small burr hole through which a laser electrode is inserted. Benefits of LITT include the ability to reach deep lesions or lesions near sensitive areas of the brain.[305-308]

An advance in the treatment of epilepsy has been the development of the vagal nerve stimulator. Although its exact mechanism of action is not well understood, it appears to inhibit seizure activity at brainstem or cortical levels.[309,310] It is becoming a popular form of treatment because it has shown benefit with minimal side effects in many children who are disabled by intractable seizures.[311,312] A systematic review and meta-analysis of 101 pediatric trials supports the effectiveness of vagal nerve stimulators in the treatment of drug resistant seizures, although complete freedom from seizures is less common[313]; fewer antiseizure medications and older age at time of onset of seizures were associated with better outcomes.

The vagal nerve stimulator is a programmable device similar to a cardiac pacemaker and is placed subcutaneously under the left anterior chest wall. Bipolar platinum stimulating electrode coils, which are implanted around the left vagus nerve, are connected to the generator by subcutaneously tunneled wires. The device automatically activates for up to 30 seconds every 5 minutes. Although stimulation of the vagal nerve in this manner may affect vocal cord function, sudden bradycardia or other side effects are uncommon.[314] When children with vagal nerve stimulators return for subsequent operations, it may be appropriate to deactivate the stimulator while the child is receiving general anesthesia in order to prevent repetitive vocal cord motion.

HYDROCEPHALUS

Hydrocephalus is a condition involving a mismatch of CSF production and absorption, resulting in an increased intracranial CSF volume. It can be caused by a variety of pathologic processes, including arachnoid cysts (E-Fig. 24.3). Except for rare instances of excess CSF production, such as in choroid plexus papillomas, most cases of hydrocephalus result from some type of obstruction or an inability to absorb CSF appropriately. Commonly, this is a result of neonatal intraventricular or subarachnoid hemorrhage, congenital problems (e.g., aqueductal stenosis), trauma, infection, or tumors, especially those in the posterior fossa. Hydrocephalus can be classified as nonobstructive/communicating or obstructive/noncommunicating based on the ability of CSF to flow around the spinal cord in its usual manner.

Intracranial hypertension or decreased intracranial compliance typically accompanies untreated hydrocephalus in children. Intracranial compliance and acute development are both factors contributing to the severity of signs and symptoms of hydrocephalus. If hydrocephalus develops slowly in the young infant, the skull will expand, and the cerebral cortical mantle will stretch until massive craniomegaly (often with irreversible neurologic damage) occurs. However, if the cranial bones are fused or the cranium cannot expand fast enough, neurologic signs and symptoms rapidly become apparent. The child may become progressively more lethargic and develop vomiting, cranial nerve dysfunction (i.e., setting sun sign), bradycardia, brain herniation, and death.

Unless the cause of the hydrocephalus can be definitively corrected, treatment usually involves surgical placement of an extracranial shunt. Most shunts transport CSF from the lateral ventricles to the peritoneal cavity (i.e., ventriculoperitoneal [VP] shunts). The distal end of the shunt occasionally must be placed in the right atrium or pleural cavity, usually because of problems with the ability of the peritoneal cavity to absorb CSF. Newer shunt systems with programmable valves reduce the need for shunt revisions.[315]

The use of a percutaneous flexible neuroendoscope through a burr hole in the skull has provided an alternative to extracranial

shunt placement.[316,317] During these procedures, a ventriculostomy may be made to bypass an obstruction (e.g., aqueductal stenosis) by forming a communicating hole from one area of CSF flow to another using a blunt probe inserted through the neuroendoscope (Video 24.1). Common locations for a ventriculostomy are through the septum pellucidum (allowing lateral ventricles to communicate) or through the floor of the third ventricle into the adjacent CSF cisterns. Complications such as damage to the basilar artery or its branches or neural injuries can be life-threatening when they occur, and the anesthesiologist should be prepared for an emergency craniotomy during these procedures. Hemodynamic instability may occur intraoperatively if excessive cold irrigating solutions or large volumes are infused through the endoscope. As endoscopic techniques become more commonplace, it is important for anesthesiologists to understand the unique challenges endoscopic neurosurgical procedures present.[318]

The anesthetic plan for a child with hydrocephalus should be directed at controlling ICP and relieving the obstruction as soon as possible. Children with an increased ICP are at risk for vomiting and pulmonary aspiration. Rapid-sequence induction and tracheal intubation should be performed. The use of ketamine is now more acceptable[319]; in the past it was avoided because of its potential to cause sudden intracranial hypertension.[100] However, recent evidence indicates that ketamine may ameliorate the increased ICP in some children.[99,101] In infants, hydrocephalus often produces large, dilated scalp veins, and they can be used for induction of anesthesia if necessary. If IV access cannot be established, induction with sevoflurane and gentle cricoid pressure may be an alternative, although less desirable, method of induction.[320] This method results in venodilation and usually facilitates establishment of IV access. After an IV catheter is inserted, the child may be paralyzed, the lungs ventilated, the trachea intubated, and the inhalational agent decreased or discontinued. The possibility of venous air embolism during placement of the distal end of a ventriculoatrial shunt should always be considered. Postoperatively, children should be observed carefully because an altered mental status and recent peritoneal incision place them at increased risk for pulmonary aspiration after feeding begins. Analgesia may be provided with a variety of easily performed blocks of the head (see Figs. 40.31 and 40.32).

Anesthesiologists should be familiar with a few special situations involving shunts. Children who develop a shunt infection usually have the entire shunt system removed and external ventricular drainage established. They return to the operating room for insertion of a new shunt several days after the infection has been treated with antibiotics. While an external drain is in place, the operator must be careful not to dislodge the ventricular tubing. The height of the drainage bag should not be changed in relation to the child's head to avoid sudden alterations in ICP. For example, suddenly lowering an open drainage bag can siphon CSF rapidly from the head, resulting in collapse of the ventricles and rupture of cortical veins. When transporting children with CSF drainage or when moving them from a stretcher to an operating room table, it is best to close off the ventriculostomy tubing during these brief periods.

Anesthesiologists should be aware of the condition known as slit ventricle syndrome (Fig. 24.11). This situation develops in 5% to 10% of children with CSF shunts and is associated with overdrainage of CSF and small, slit-like, lateral ventricular spaces. Children with this condition do not have the usual amount of intracranial CSF to compensate for alterations in brain or intracranial blood volume. Special attention should be paid when CT

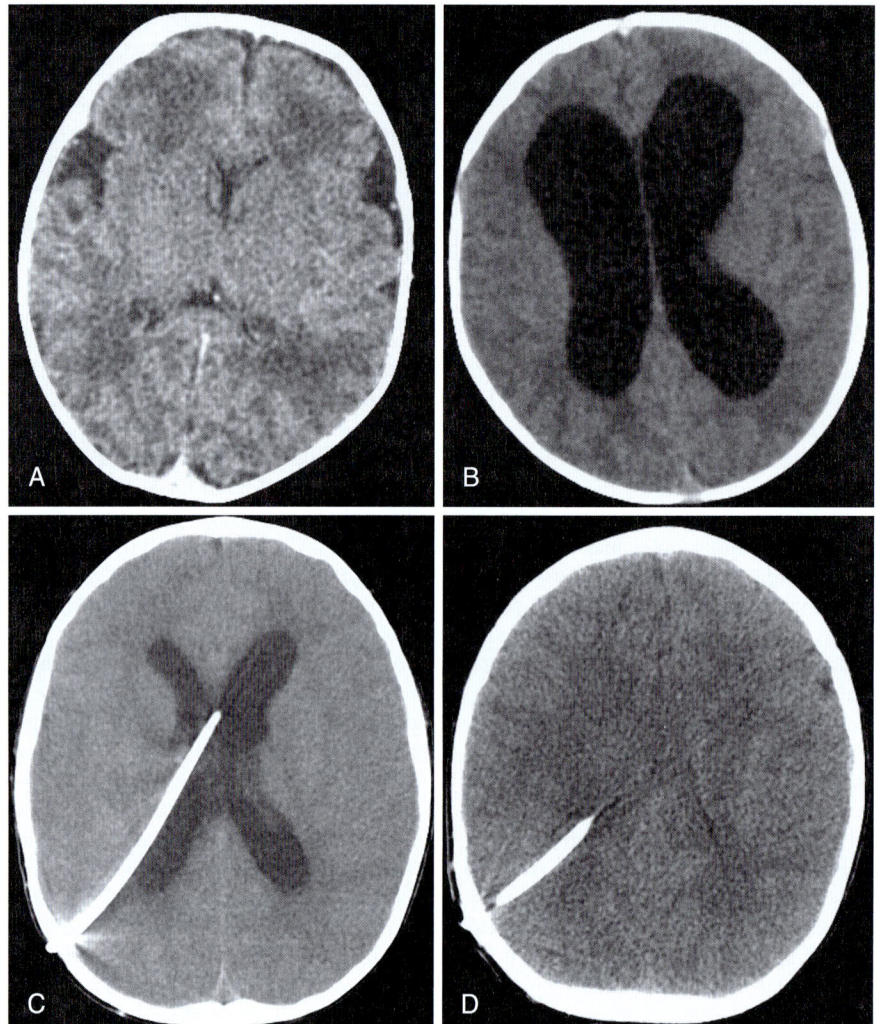

FIGURE 24.11 Computed tomographic scans of children with normal-sized ventricles **(A)**, untreated hydrocephalus **(B)**, hydrocephalus treated with a ventricular shunt **(C)**, and hydrocephalus treated with a ventricular shunt, resulting in slit ventricles **(D)**. (Courtesy Ellen Grant, MD.)

scans identify this condition. It is probably safest to avoid the administration of excess or hypotonic IV solutions in these situations in the intraoperative and postoperative periods to minimize the potential for brain swelling. Some of these children cannot accommodate to situations that otherwise healthy children can easily tolerate. Episodes of postoperative cerebral herniation have been reported after uneventful surgical procedures.[79]

CONGENITAL ANOMALIES

Congenital CNS anomalies typically occur as midline defects. This dysraphism may occur anywhere along the neural axis, involving the head (i.e., encephalocele) (Fig. 24.12A) or spine (i.e., meningomyelocele) (Fig. 24.12B). The defect may be relatively minor and affect only superficial bony and membranous structures, or it may include a large segment of malformed neural tissue.

Encephalocele

Encephaloceles can occur anywhere from the occiput to the frontal area. They can even appear to be nasal polyps if they protrude through the cribriform plate. They are rarely filled with so much

CSF that the defect can be almost as large as the head itself (see Fig. 24.12A). Large defects may present challenges to tracheal intubation. Blood loss can be severe, especially if venous sinuses are involved. Adequate IV access should be ensured and blood products readily available. If hemodynamic instability is anticipated, an arterial catheter is indicated.

Myelodysplasia

Defects in the spine are known as *spina bifida*. Meningoceles are lesions containing CSF without spinal tissue. When neural tissue is also present within the lesion, the defect is called a *meningomyelocele*. Open neural tissue is known as *rachischisis*. Hydrocephalus is usually present and is often associated with a type II Chiari malformation.

Most children with a meningomyelocele present for primary closure of the defect within the first 24 hours of life to minimize the risk of infection. Many are now scheduled electively before birth for repair because the defect is usually apparent on prenatal ultrasonography. Many neurosurgeons prefer to insert a ventriculoperitoneal shunt at the time of initial surgery. Alternatively, a shunt may be inserted a few days later or is occasionally deferred if there is no evidence of hydrocephalus at birth.

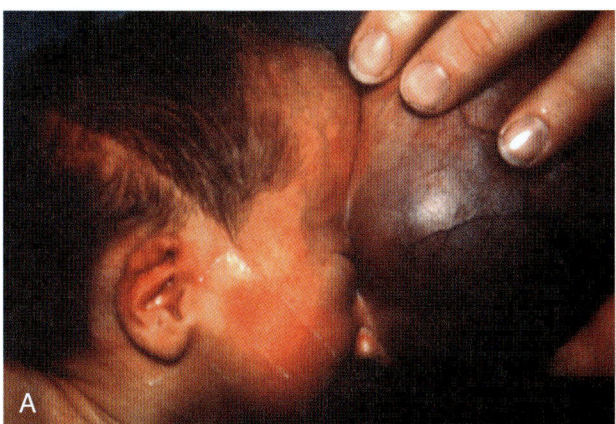

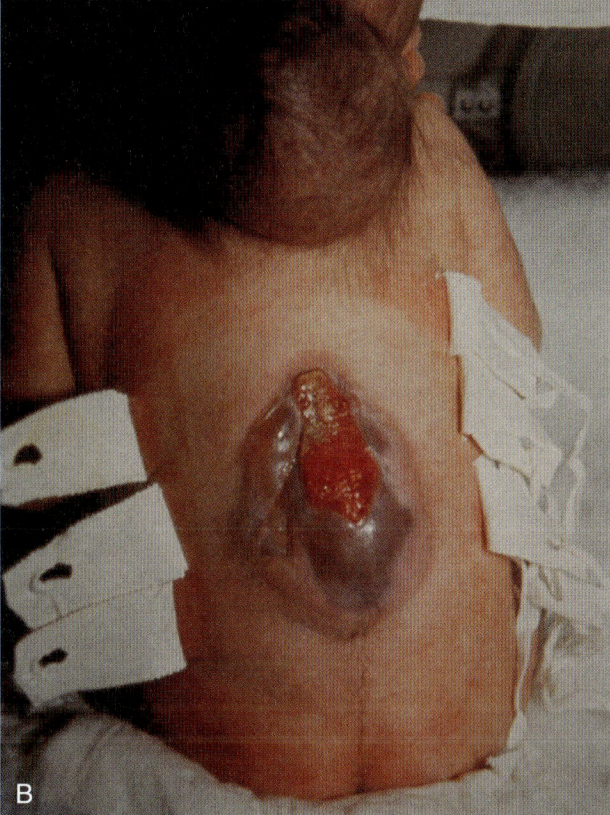

FIGURE 24.12 A, An infant with an anterior encephalocele. **B,** An infant with a posterior encephalocele and myelomeningocele defects. Notice the large exposed surface areas that make this child prone to dehydration. Difficulty may be encountered in positioning for induction of anesthesia and intubation; significant loss of blood and cerebrospinal fluid during surgical correction should be anticipated.

A major anesthesia consideration is positioning the neonate for induction at surgery. In most cases, tracheal intubation can be performed with the infant in the supine position and the uninvolved portion of the child's back supported with towels (or a donut ring) so there is no direct pressure on the meningomyelocele. For very large defects, it is occasionally necessary to place the infant in the left lateral decubitus position for induction and tracheal intubation. Succinylcholine is rarely needed for tracheal intubation, although it is not associated with hyperkalemia because the defect develops early in gestation and is not associated with muscle denervation.[321] Airway management,

mask fit, and intubation may be difficult in infants with massive hydrocephalus or very large defects. In such cases, a sedated "awake" intubation after preoxygenation and administration of atropine occasionally may be the safest alternative. Blood loss may be considerable during repair of a larger defect when skin is undermined to cover the defect.

Children with myelodysplasia are at high risk for latex sensitivity and possibly anaphylaxis.[62,64–66] This likely results from repeated exposure to latex products encountered during frequent bladder catheterizations and multiple (usually more than five) surgical procedures, during which latex gloves have been in contact with large mucosal surfaces. These children should be managed in a latex-free environment from birth to minimize the chances for sensitization.[64,65,67] Latex allergy should be suspected if signs and symptoms of anaphylaxis develop during surgery. Suspected anaphylaxis should be treated with IV epinephrine in a dose of 1 to 10 µg/kg, as required. Many hospitals have replaced most or all of their latex-containing supplies with nonlatex alternatives; this has resulted in complete elimination or marked reduction of latex anaphylactic reactions during anesthesia in some institutions.[66] Children who develop latex allergy exhibit cross-reactivity with some antibiotics[322,323] and foods, especially tropical fruits such as avocados, kiwi fruit, and bananas.[65]

Postoperatively, respiratory status should be carefully assessed. Pulse oximetry is valuable during recovery from anesthesia because breathing difficulties may occur after a tight skin closure and the ventilatory responses to hypoxia and hypercarbia may be diminished or absent when a Chiari malformation coexists.[324] Fetal surgery has been advocated as a way of diminishing the degree of damage caused by myelodysplasia.[325–327]

Chiari Malformations

There are several types of Chiari malformations (Table 24.3). The Arnold-Chiari malformation (type II) usually coexists in children with myelodysplasia. This defect consists of a bony abnormality in the posterior fossa and upper cervical spine with caudal displacement of the cerebellar vermis, fourth ventricle, and lower brainstem below the plane of the foramen magnum. Medullary cervical cord compression can occur (Figs. 24.13 and 24.14). Vocal cord paralysis with stridor and respiratory distress, apnea, abnormal swallowing and pulmonary aspiration, opisthotonos, and cranial nerve deficits may be associated with the Arnold-Chiari malformation and it usually manifests during infancy. Children with vocal cord paralysis or a diminished

TABLE 24.3	Types of Chiari Malformation
Type I	Caudal displacement of cerebellar tonsils below the plane of the foramen magnum
Type II (Arnold-Chiari; associated with myelomeningocele)	Caudal displacement of the cerebellar vermis, fourth ventricle, and lower brainstem below the plane of the foramen magnum Dysplastic brainstem with characteristic kink, elongation of the fourth ventricle, beaking of the quadrigeminal plate, hypoplastic tentorium with small posterior fossa, polymicrogyria, enlargement of the massa intermedia
Type III	Caudal displacement of the cerebellum and brainstem into a high cervical meningocele
Type IV	Cerebellar hypoplasia

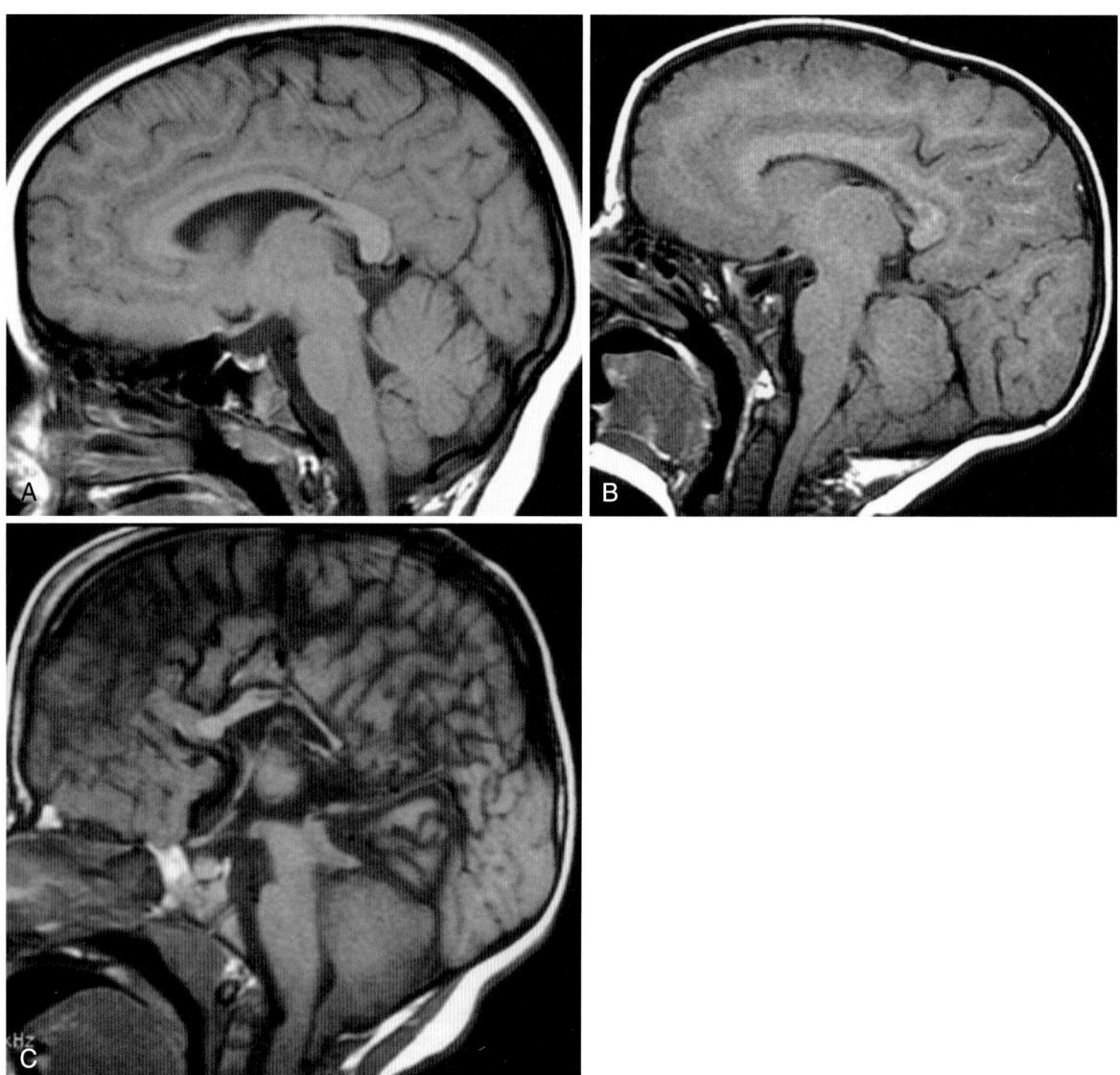

FIGURE 24.13 A, Sagittal, T1-weighted magnetic resonance imaging (MRI) of a normal child. **B,** Sagittal, T1-weighted MRI of a child with a Chiari I malformation, which consists of caudal displacement of the cerebellar tonsils at least 5 mm into the upper cervical spinal canal, often with no clinical symptoms. **C,** Sagittal, T1-weighted MRI of a child with a type II Chiari malformation, which is characterized by caudal displacement of the cerebellar tonsils, additional brain anomalies, and a meningomyelocele deformity. (Courtesy Ellen Grant, MD.)

gag reflex may require tracheostomy and gastrostomy to secure the airway and to minimize chronic aspiration. Children of any age may have abnormal responses to hypoxia and hypercarbia because of cranial nerve and brainstem dysfunction.[324,328] Extreme head flexion may cause brainstem compression in otherwise asymptomatic children.

Type I Chiari malformations can occur in healthy children without myelodysplasia. These defects also involve caudal displacement of the cerebellar tonsils below the foramen magnum, but children usually have much milder symptoms, sometimes manifesting only as headache or neck pain.[329] Surgical treatment usually involves a decompressive suboccipital craniectomy with cervical laminectomies.

Other Spinal Defects

Other spinal anomalies (e.g., lipomeningoceles, lipomyelomeningoceles, diastematomyelias, dermoid tracts) may manifest as tethered cords. Skin defects, typically over the lower lumbar region, may occur as dural sinus tracks or lipomeningoceles. Midline hair tufts, skin dimples, or fat pads may be associated with spinal defects. These anomalies sometimes manifest when toilet training or ambulation is observed to be abnormal or later in childhood when children complain of back pain. Children who have had a meningomyelocele repaired after birth may also develop an ascending neurologic deficit from a tethered spinal cord during growth. Early detection of a tethered cord is easily diagnosed with MRI. Prophylactic surgical untethering is common.

Anesthesia management for surgical release of a tethered cord usually entails monitoring the innervation of the lower extremities and bowel and bladder with nerve stimulators and rectal electromyelograms or manometry. Neuromuscular blocking drugs should be avoided or permitted to dissipate before intraoperative assessment.

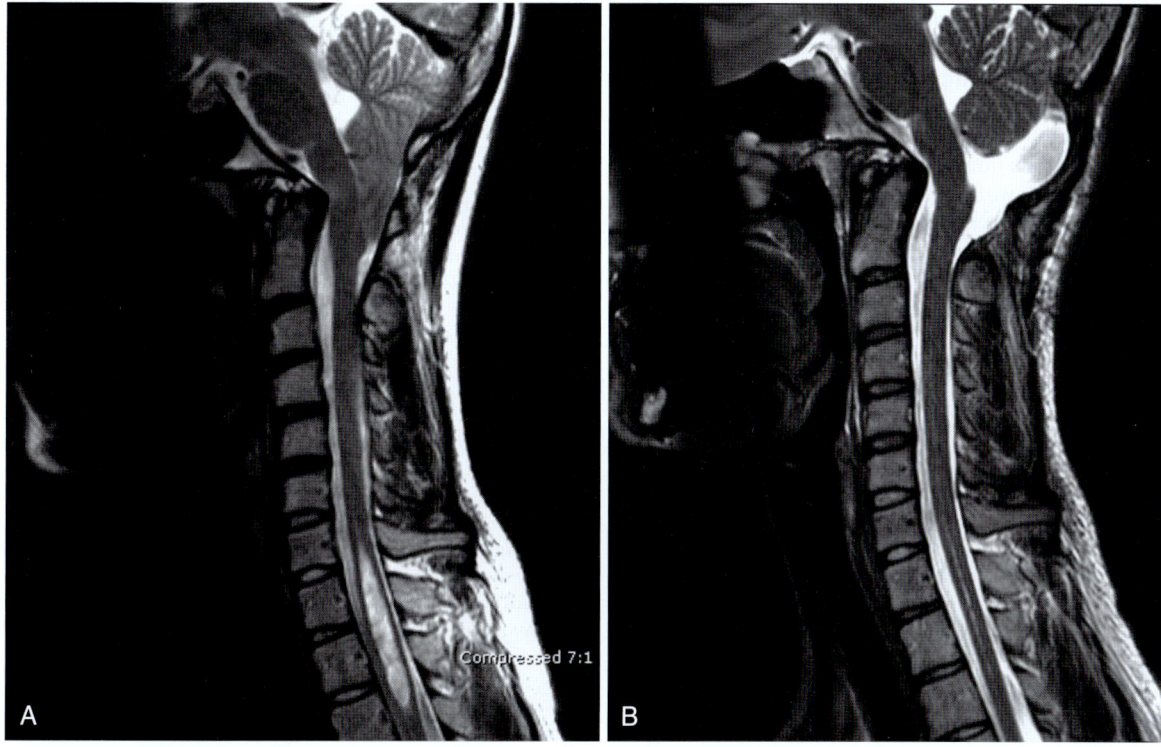

FIGURE 24.14 The images show the posterior fossa in a child with a Chiari II malformation before and after posterior fossa decompression. **A,** Notice the downward herniation of the cerebellar tonsils. **B,** Resolution of cerebellar tonsillar herniation after posterior fossa decompression.

NEURORADIOLOGIC PROCEDURES

Many neuroradiologic procedures are performed in children. Anesthetic considerations for neurodiagnostic procedures (e.g., CT, MRI) are discussed elsewhere (see Chapters 43 and 44), but certain therapeutic neuroradiologic procedures are addressed here.

iMRI was introduced in the mid-1990s to improve intraoperative navigation during intracranial procedures.[330] The combination of stereotactic imaging and iMRI allows neurosurgeons to better localize brain lesions and account for brain shift, the intraoperative movement of intracranial structures that occurs due to resection of tissue, surgical bleeding, CSF drainage, and hyperventilation.[293,330,331] iMRI has been shown to improve the extent of malignancy resection, increase the gross total resection, and more quickly identify intraoperative complications.[330] A variety of operating room suite designs encompass MRI machines (E-Fig. 24.4). The environment in these operating rooms presents special challenges for neurosurgeons and anesthesiologists, as the risks of a high powered magnet are combined with the management challenges inherent to neurosurgical procedures including blood loss, hemodynamic changes, and electrolyte disturbances.[332–336]

Anesthetic-specific considerations can be broken into several categories: risks from the physical forces of the MRI, equipment and monitoring issues, and risks related to poor access to the patient.[337] Complications related to iMRI include radiofrequency-induced burns, projectile, cryogen related, foreign metal object, and noise-related injury.[338]

Risks From MRI

Three physical forces from the MRI present a potential hazard to patients and operating room staff: the static magnetic field, the dynamic magnetic field, and the radiofrequency (RF) electromagnetic field. The static magnetic field generated by a 3-T iMRI scanner is 60,000 times stronger than that of the earth. This field can turn ferromagnetic objects into missiles.[330,339] The dynamic magnetic field is applied during image acquisition and generates a loud noise which may exceed 100 dB, which is dangerous to human hearing. Therefore, patients and personnel in the operating room should have ear protection. Finally, the radiofrequency field induces proton excitation, which generates heat and can cause burns, induce current in closed loops, and interfere with electrical equipment. To minimize the risks of burns, padding must be placed in skin creases to avoid skin-to-skin contact and no loops should be present in IV tubing or electrical wires.

Equipment and Monitoring Issues

As with anesthesia for diagnostic MRI scans, special monitors, infusion pumps, and an MRI-safe or MRI-conditional anesthesia machine are required. Some monitoring equipment found in conventional operating rooms (e.g., precordial Doppler ultrasonography, core temperature probes, fluid warmers) are not MRI-safe and must be accounted for and moved behind the 5-Gauss line or out of the room prior to scanning. In an airway emergency, conventional laryngoscope blades and emergency airway equipment such as fiberoptic and videoscopes are not MRI compatible and may pose a danger to the anesthetized patient and caregivers if the magnet is present. MRI compatible monitors have increased sensitivity to motion and artifact. ECG monitoring is particularly challenging as electrical interference creates difficulty with arrhythmia and ST analysis, and the short wires employed to minimize the risks of burns necessitate suboptimal lead placement.[330,339] Although patients may experience large fluctuations in temperature due to cooling in the operating environment and excessive heating when covered with plastic sterile drapes for an iMRI, most temperature monitoring systems are not MRI compatible.[293] Because of these monitoring difficulties, some institutions routinely exclude patients with severe coronary disease or small infants from iMRI.[82,339–341] However, a thorough risk-benefit discussion with the neurosurgery team, MR technologists, and nursing team is necessary for patients at high risk who might derive a strong benefit from iMRI.

Risks Related to Patient Positioning

Patients are positioned 180 degrees from the anesthesiologist, and often need to be located farther away from the anesthesia team for optimal placement inside the bore of the MRI. Extended circuits (often more than 1) and extensions on vascular lines are required. During the MRI scan the team is unable to have access to patients, so it is critical to perform a thorough pre-scanning positioning check (including an airway check), and ensure all necessary lines are accessible. Adjustments to standard circuits and ventilators may be necessary to overcome the increased dead space and compression volumes in these circuits; these issues may be a particular concern for smaller patients and those with poor lung compliance. In addition, airway access is limited and must be well secured (often a nasal intubation, particularly for prone patients.) Armored ETTs are not MRI compatible.

Despite these risks, numerous neurosurgical procedures have been safely performed in children in these MRI operating rooms, and the equipment for these procedures is rapidly evolving. Standardized protocols, checklists and close communication between neurosurgery, anesthesia, MRI technologists, and nursing teams can minimize errors and improve workflow, particularly when transitioning from a surgical field to a high-strength magnetic field.[293,342] Restricting access to iMRI suites to personnel with MRI-specific training as well as in situ, high fidelity simulation may allow for improved anticipation of and assignment of responsibilities in critical events.[341]

ANNOTATED REFERENCES

Coles JP, Fryer TD, Coleman MR, et al. Hyperventilation following head injury: effect on ischemic burden and cerebral oxidative metabolism. *Crit Care Med.* 2007;35:568-578.

Hyperventilation has a detrimental effect on brain tissue at risk after head injury. The authors refute the often-taught dogma regarding routine hyperventilation, especially after a traumatic brain injury. This article and several others on the same subject should give the anesthesiologist pause when hyperventilating children with intracranial pathology.

Ing C, Warner DO, Sun LS, et al. Anesthesia and developing brains: unanswered questions and proposed paths forward. *Anesthesiology.* 2022;136:500-512.

The authors review the current status of investigation into neuronal apoptosis. Although anesthetic agents disrupt neurodevelopment in animal models, evidence in humans is mixed. A brief or single early anesthetic exposure is not associated with deficits in a range of neurodevelopmental outcomes including broad measures of intelligence. The possibility that behavioral deficits are a phenotype, as well as the entire concept of anesthetic neurotoxicity in children, remains a source of intense debate. This report describes consensus and disagreement among experts, summarizes preclinical and clinical evidence, suggests pathways for future clinical research, and compares studies of anesthetic agents to other suspected neurotoxins.

Laochamroonvorapongse D, Theard MA, Yahanda AT, Chicoine MR. Intraoperative MRI for adult and pediatric neurosurgery. *Anesthesiol Clin.* 2021;39:211-225.

The authors review iMRI technology and its use in both adult and pediatric neurosurgery. They point out that the combination of risks from the MR environment with those of the operating room creates a challenging, zero-tolerance environment for the anesthesiologist. This article provides an overview of the currently available iMRI systems, the neurosurgical evidence supporting iMRI use, and the anesthetic and safety considerations for iMRI procedures.

Lassen NA, Christensen MS. Physiology of cerebral blood flow. *Br J Anaesth.* 1976;48:719-734.

This classic review article discusses the various physiologic mechanisms of control of CBF.

Pollack IF. Brain tumors in children. *N Engl J Med.* 1994;331:1500-1507.

Although this review is from the 1990s, it provides a comprehensive overview of the epidemiology of pediatric brain tumors and treatment approaches. Knowledge of various treatment approaches to different histologic types of tumors can inform the anesthesiologist about the extent of the process behind the procedure and how aggressive the surgery needs to be to achieve a desired outcome.

Reasoner DK, Todd MM, Scamman FL, Warner DS. The incidence of pneumocephalus after supratentorial craniotomy: observations on the disappearance of intracranial air. *Anesthesiology.* 1994;80:1008-1012.

This well-conceived study evaluates the length of time pneumocephalus persists after supratentorial craniotomy. The take-home message is that air persists in the head for several weeks after craniotomy, and care should be taken not to exacerbate the situation during subsequent administration of anesthetics. Nitrous oxide should be avoided in these children because tension pneumocephalus could develop.

Sultan I, Lamba N, Liew A, et al. The safety and efficacy of steroid treatment for acute spinal cord injury: a systematic review and meta-analysis. *Heliyon.* 2020;6:e03414.

A systematic review of five randomized controlled trials and seven observational studies evaluating methylprednisolone administration within 8 hours of spinal injury found an increased risk for hyperglycemia and pneumonia; the authors concluded that these data failed to show a significant short- or long-term improvement in motor function or neurologic function

Willie CK, Tzeng YC, Fisher JA, Ainslie PN. Integrative regulation of human brain blood flow. *J Physiol.* 2014;592(5):841-859.

This is a well-referenced review article that condenses current evidence on the regulation of CBF in humans. It makes a compelling argument that our current understanding is overly simplistic and argues that we really should be thinking about CBF regulation in terms of a multisystem approach. Finally, the authors make the point that we should rethink concepts of such tight control of CBF (autoregulation) over a variety of parameters including mean arterial pressure.

A complete reference list can be found online at Elsevier eBooks+.

Essentials of Endocrinology

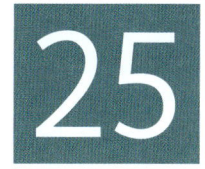

LIZABETH D. MARTIN, ERINN T. RHODES, CASEY A. QUINLAN,
ABHINASH SRIVATSA, ECHO ROWE, AND JOSEPH I. WOLFSDORF

Diabetes Mellitus
Classification and Epidemiology in Children
General Management Principles
Metabolic Response to Surgery
Metabolic Response to Anesthesia
Adverse Consequences of Hyperglycemia
Preoperative Consultation
Preoperative Management
Intraoperative Management
Perioperative Management of Type 2 Diabetes
Postoperative Management
Special Surgical Situations
Diabetes Insipidus
Diagnosis of Neurosurgical Diabetes
Insipidus: The Triple-Phase Response
Perioperative Management of Minor Procedures
Perioperative Management of Major Procedures
New Perioperative Diagnosis
Postoperative Management
Transient Medication-Induced Diabetes Insipidus
Syndrome of Inappropriate Antidiuretic Hormone Secretion
Perioperative Management

Thyroid Disorders
Hypothyroidism
Hyperthyroidism
Parathyroid and Calcium Disorders
Physiology of Calcium Homeostasis
Hypocalcemia
Hypercalcemia
Adrenal Disorders
Physiology
Causes of Adrenal Insufficiency
Testing for Adrenal Insufficiency
Perioperative Management of Adrenal Insufficiency
Hypercortisolism (Cushing Syndrome)
Pheochromocytoma
Etiology
Clinical Presentation
Diagnosis
Preoperative Management
Anesthetic Considerations

Diabetes Mellitus

Type 1 diabetes mellitus is a common chronic disease in children and adolescents and its incidence is increasing worldwide.[1–3] Crude estimates among the United States population for 2018 show that 210,000 children and adolescents younger than age 20 years (25 per 10,000) were diagnosed with diabetes, of whom 187,000 had type 1 diabetes.[4] Approximately 1:300 children in the United States have type 1 diabetes. Although type 2 diabetes in youth is considerably less prevalent than type 1 diabetes, its prevalence is also increasing.[2,3,5] In the United States, the incidence of type 2 diabetes among youths and adolescents increased more rapidly than that of type 1 diabetes, at 4.8% and 1.9% per year respectively,[2] in parallel with the increased prevalence of obesity.[2] Many children and adolescents require anesthesia for surgery, diagnostic procedures, or imaging studies. The use of various multicomponent insulin regimens that include novel insulin formulations, continuous subcutaneous insulin infusion systems (pumps), including hybrid closed-loop systems, and continuous glucose monitoring, has increased the complexity of perioperative management of children with diabetes. As the perioperative care coordinators for surgical patients with medical diseases, anesthesiologists must carefully plan for the specific

challenges in patients with diabetes mellitus. This includes consideration of the pathophysiology of the disease, as well as each child's specific treatment regimen, prior glycemic control, intended surgery, and anticipated postoperative course, when devising an appropriate perioperative management plan.[6] Standardized algorithms for perioperative diabetes management improve care[7–10] without markedly increasing costs.[9] Several guidelines and studies of perioperative management of children with diabetes are available in the literature and examples are discussed.[6,11–18]

CLASSIFICATION AND EPIDEMIOLOGY IN CHILDREN

Type 1 and type 2 are the most common, but not the only types of diabetes mellitus (Table 25.1).[19] Type 1 diabetes is characterized by an absolute deficiency of insulin, which usually results from immune-mediated destruction of pancreatic beta cells.[20] In contrast, type 2 diabetes is characterized by a combination of insulin resistance and relative insulin deficiency.[21,22] Children with type 2 diabetes typically are overweight or obese and frequently have a first- or second-degree relative with type 2 diabetes.[23] The high prevalence of obesity in children and adolescents in the general US pediatric population[24] has blurred the distinction between type 1 and type 2 diabetes, and children with phenotypic characteristics of type 2 diabetes may have pancreatic autoimmunity.[25–28]

TABLE 25.1	Classification of Less Common Forms of Diabetes Mellitus

Genetic Defects of Beta Cell Function

Monogenic diabetes (formerly referred to as maturity-onset diabetes of the young [MODY])

Neonatal diabetes

Mitochondrial disorders

Disease of the Exocrine Pancreas

Cystic fibrosis–related diabetes

Drug-Induced Diabetes

Steroids

Chemotherapeutic agents including post-transplantation diabetes

Genetic Syndromes

Prader-Willi syndrome

Down syndrome

Turner syndrome

Wolfram syndrome

Endocrinopathies

Autoimmune polyglandular syndrome

Cushing syndrome

Modified from Rhodes ET, Ferrari LR, Wolfsdorf JI. Perioperative management of pediatric surgical patients with diabetes mellitus. *Anesth Analg.* 2005;101(4): 986-999. Refer to American Diabetes Association. 2. Classification and Diagnosis of Diabetes: Standards of Medical Care in Diabetes–2021. *Diabetes Care.* 2021; 44(Suppl. 1):S15-S33,[31] for a comprehensive review of the diagnosis and classification of the causes of diabetes.

Moreover, up to 35% of children with a presumptive diagnosis of type 1 diabetes and who require exogenous insulin are overweight or obese at the time of diagnosis.[29,30]

Other forms of diabetes are considerably less common (see Table 25.1). Monogenic defects causing beta cell dysfunction, including maturity-onset diabetes of the young and neonatal diabetes, occur in less than 5% of the pediatric diabetes population. With improvements in care, patients with cystic fibrosis–related diabetes now account for a small but important fraction of the diabetic population at major pediatric medical centers.[31] Additional modifications to the perioperative treatment regimen may be necessary when diabetes is associated with genetic syndromes or other endocrinopathies, such as adrenal insufficiency (see later discussion).

Although the worldwide incidence of type 1 diabetes is quite variable, the incidence is increasing in almost all populations.[1] The SEARCH for Diabetes in Youth Study, which began in 2000, provides the most comprehensive estimates of the incidence and prevalence of type 1 and type 2 diabetes in US youth younger than 20 years of age.[2,3] Type 1 diabetes is the most common form of diabetes observed, with the greatest prevalence (2.79 per 1000) among non-Hispanic White youth.[3] The epidemic of obesity has contributed to a progressive increase in the incidence and prevalence of type 2 diabetes in US children[2,3] and recent data from the SEARCH study shows the prevalence of type 2 diabetes in 10- to 19-year-old youth ranged from 0.2 per 1000 among non-Hispanic White youth to 1.8 per 1000 among Black youth.[3]

During the period 2002 to 2015, the incidence of type 2 diabetes increased in youth aged 10 to 19 years in all age, sex, and race/ethnicity groups except White youth. During 2014–2015, the incidence differed by race/ethnicity, with the lowest rate among non-Hispanic White (4.5 per 100,000 person years) and highest rates among American Indians, Blacks, and Hispanics (32.8, 37.8, and 20.9 per 100,000 person years, respectively).[2] Increases in the incidence and prevalence of type 2 diabetes have also been noted in other parts of the world.[5,32–40]

GENERAL MANAGEMENT PRINCIPLES

Understanding both the pharmacokinetic and pharmacodynamic properties of insulin preparations and antihyperglycemic medications is essential to developing an appropriate perioperative plan.

Type 1 diabetes always requires treatment with insulin.[41] An increasing number of insulin preparations (Table 25.2),[42] multicomponent insulin regimens, and insulin delivery systems are now available.[43,44] The least complex regimens consist of two or three injections of insulin per day and incorporate a combination of an intermediate-acting insulin (neutral protamine Hagedorn [NPH]) or a long-acting insulin (e.g., insulin detemir [Levemir], insulin glargine [Lantus], or insulin degludec [Tresiba]) to provide basal coverage with a short-acting (regular) insulin or rapid-acting insulin (insulin aspart [NovoLog], insulin lispro [Humalog], or insulin glulisine [Apidra]) to provide prandial glycemic coverage. Intensive multicomponent insulin regimens have become the standard of care[45] and typically comprise a long-acting insulin (usually administered once daily) that provides a relatively constant 24-hour basal concentration of circulating insulin without a pronounced peak and simulates basal insulin secretion,[42] together with a rapid-acting insulin analog administered with food.

TABLE 25.2	Insulin Preparations Classified According to Their Pharmacokinetic Profiles			
Generic Name	**Brand Name**	**Time to Onset (h)**	**Time to Peak (h)**	**Duration (h)**
Rapid-Acting Insulin				
Lispro (U-100)	Humalog Admelog	Within 0.25	0.5–1.5	4–6
Aspart	Novolog Fiasp	Within 0.25	0.5–1.5	4–6
Glulisine	Apidra	Within 0.25	0.5–1.5	4–6
Short-Acting Insulin				
Regular Human Insulin (U-100)	Humulin R Novolin R	0.5	1.5–2.5	8
Intermediate- and Long-Acting Insulin				
NPH Insulin	Humulin N Novolin N	2–4	4–10	12–18
Detemir	Levemir	2–4	flat	14–24
Glargine (U-100)	Lantus Basaglar	2–4	flat	20–24
Degludec (U-100)	Tresiba	1	flat	>42

Reproduced with permission from the American Diabetes Association. Copyright 2019 by the American Diabetes Association.
Refers to subcutaneous dosing. Onset, peak, and duration of action may vary by individual. Duration is dose dependent (larger doses result in longer duration). NPH insulin 4–10 hour peak may predispose fasting patients to hypoglycemia.[6,42,350]

25

Increasing numbers of children with type 1 diabetes are managed with an insulin pump also referred to as continuous subcutaneous insulin infusion (CSII),[43,46–48] a device that administers a continuous infusion of insulin (typically a rapid-acting insulin, see Table 25.2) subcutaneously at a programmed basal rate that is supplemented by bolus doses of rapid-acting insulin given with meals and snacks. In addition, continuous glucose monitoring systems use has increased considerably in the pediatric diabetes mellitus population over the past decade.[48,49]

The continuous glucose monitor tracks the glucose concentration in the interstitial fluid through a sensor that is self-inserted subcutaneously and provides near real-time glucose measurements (with specific characteristics varying with the type of monitor).[50] In appropriately selected children, pump therapy has shown superiority over injection regimens including in a recent meta-analysis that compared the two treatment strategies.[51–57] Large observational studies have shown lower glycated hemoglobin (HbA1c) levels in children and adolescents who use either a pump or continuous glucose monitor or both.[48] Like HbA1c, continuous glucose monitoring provides a measure of long-term glycemic control but has the advantage of providing information about "time in range," time above or below specific thresholds, and glycemic variability. By consensus, time in range refers to the proportion of time spent in the individual's target glucose range (usually 70–180 mg/dL [3.9–10 mmol/L]) with a goal of at least 70%.[44,58] A recent randomized controlled trial in adolescents with type 1 diabetes also demonstrated a small but significant improvement in glycemic control with continuous glucose monitoring compared with standard blood glucose monitoring over 26 weeks (adjusted between-group difference, -0.37% [95% CI, -0.66% to -0.08%]; $P = 0.01$).[59]

In conjunction with the increasing use of continuous glucose monitoring, the use of sensor-augmented pump therapy, i.e., combining the use of insulin pump therapy and a continuous glucose monitor, has increased.[44,60] Depending on the format, these systems may be designed to suspend insulin administration to prevent hypoglycemia (low-glucose suspend) or have an algorithm designed to automate insulin delivery by changing the amount of insulin delivered in response to the sensor-derived glucose level.[60] Hybrid closed-loop systems refer to automated insulin delivery systems that require the additional input of information about food consumption and require the user to manually administer the appropriate prandial insulin coverage. The standard hybrid closed-loop system was the first introduced delivering microbursts of insulin to maintain a target concentration of 120 mg/dL. More recently, the advanced hybrid closed-loop system was introduced to permit the user to set their own target glucose concentration, with autocorrection of insulin boluses to maintain a target of 120 mg/dL. After a 6-month study of the two hybrid systems in 44 children and adolescents, HbA1c levels were 10% lower in the advanced loop system, which favored better glycemic control in younger children and those with more difficult glycemic control overall than the standard control.[61] In addition to FDA-approved automated systems, some patients may utilize "do-it-yourself" or DIY algorithms available on the internet.[60]

Providers should be familiar with the modality of insulin administration including the type of insulin pump that patients are using and the conditions under which insulin may be delivered, if applicable. Standard insulin preparations are U100, meaning that there are 100 units of insulin per milliliter. However, very young patients with type 1 diabetes may require diluted insulin

(e.g., U10, 10 units per mL) to enable accurate dosing of minute doses (less than 0.5 units) of insulin.[62–64] Parents of preschool-aged children, especially toddlers, with type 1 diabetes should be specifically educated and questioned about their use of diluted insulin.

Most children with type 2 diabetes are managed with oral metformin, which until recently, was the only antihyperglycemic agent approved for use in children with diabetes in the United States. It is often combined with insulin when monotherapy with metformin fails.[65–68] Metformin's primary action is to decrease hepatic glucose production and, secondarily to increase insulin sensitivity in peripheral tissues. Occasionally, other oral agents including sulfonylureas, which promote insulin secretion, and thiazolidinediones, which increase insulin sensitivity in muscle and adipose tissue, are used off-label in adolescents.[69,70] Nutritional therapy is always included in the management of children with type 2 diabetes.[67,68] The **T**reatment **O**ptions for Type 2 **D**iabetes in **A**dolescents and **Y**outh (TODAY) trial,[71,72] evaluated the optimal treatment for type 2 diabetes in children and adolescents, aged 10 to 17 years. In the TODAY trial, monotherapy with metformin was associated with durable glycemic control in approximately 50% of children and adolescents with type 2 diabetes. The addition of rosiglitazone, but not an intensive lifestyle intervention, was superior to metformin alone. Other medications used to manage adults with type 2 diabetes are now being evaluated for use in children. Incretins, including glucose-dependent insulinotropic polypeptide and glucagon-like peptide-1 (GLP-1), are gastrointestinal hormones released after eating that stimulate insulin secretion and are necessary for normal glucose tolerance.[73,74] GLP-1 acts through a G protein–coupled receptor to promote glucose-dependent insulin secretion, suppression of glucagon secretion, slowing of gastric emptying, and reduction in food intake.[74] To date, liraglutide, a GLP-1 analog that is injected daily and, more recently, extended-release exenatide, a once weekly injection, have been approved for use in patients with type 2 diabetes aged 10 years or older. GLP-1 agonists are associated with nausea, vomiting and delayed gastric emptying, which may increase the risk of aspiration of gastric contents under anesthesia. The American Society of Anesthesiologists Task Force recommends holding GLP-1 agonists on the day of surgery (daily dosing) or the week prior to surgery (weekly dosing), and considering the potentially increased aspiration risk in anesthetic planning.[74a] Liraglutide was evaluated in a randomized controlled trial in children and adolescents 10 to 17 years of age with type 2 diabetes; when liraglutide was added to metformin, with or without basal insulin, glycemic control improved over 52 weeks.[75] Extended-release exenatide was evaluated in a randomized placebo-controlled trial in suboptimally controlled children and adolescents with type 2 diabetes aged 10 to 17 years[76]; exenatide once per week lowered HbA1c levels. Inhibitors of dipeptidyl peptidase-intravenous,[77] the enzyme that degrades GLP-1, are also widely used to treat type 2 diabetes in adults, as are sodium-glucose cotransporter-2 (SGLT-2) inhibitors,[78] but have not yet been approved for use in children. The latter lower blood glucose concentrations by increasing urinary excretion of glucose. Pramlintide acetate (Symlin) is a synthetic amylin receptor agonist that is, occasionally, used as an adjunct to insulin therapy in adults with type 1 or type 2 diabetes.[79–82] Amylin, a 37-amino acid polypeptide islet hormone co-secreted with insulin from islet beta cells,[83] has three effects: delay of gastric emptying, inhibition of glucagon secretion, and modulation of satiety.[83]

METABOLIC RESPONSE TO SURGERY

Trauma of any kind, and surgery in particular, triggers a complex neuroendocrine stress response that includes suppression of insulin secretion and increased secretion of counterregulatory hormones (frequently referred to as "stress hormones"), particularly cortisol and catecholamines.[84,85] Insulin is the primary anabolic hormone that promotes glucose uptake in muscle and adipose tissue while suppressing hepatic glucose production (glycogenolysis and gluconeogenesis).[86] The counterregulatory or "stress" hormones, which include epinephrine, glucagon, cortisol, and growth hormone, exert the opposite effects, resulting in resistance to insulin action[87–89] and an increase in blood glucose concentration by (1) stimulating glycogenolysis and gluconeogenesis in the liver, (2) increasing lipolysis and ketogenesis, and (3) inhibiting glucose uptake and utilization in muscle and fat. Glucagon, secreted by alpha cells in the pancreatic islets, suppresses insulin secretion while stimulating hepatic glycogenolysis, gluconeogenesis, and ketogenesis.[86,87] Epinephrine, which acts via $\beta 2$- and $\alpha 2$-adrenergic receptors, stimulates glucagon production, increases glycogenolysis and gluconeogenesis, stimulates lipolysis, and decreases insulin secretion and glucose utilization in insulin-sensitive tissues.[86] Cortisol stimulates gluconeogenesis, proteolysis, and lipolysis and decreases glucose utilization.[87,90] Growth hormone augments glucose production, decreases glucose utilization, and accelerates lipolysis.[91] Proinflammatory cytokines may further stimulate secretion of counterregulatory hormones and alter insulin receptor signaling.[89] Collectively, these hormonal and metabolic changes increase catabolism, as evidenced by increased hepatic glucose production and breakdown of protein and fat. In the patient with diabetes with absolute or relative insulin deficiency, the enhanced catabolism resulting from surgical trauma can lead to marked hyperglycemia and even diabetic ketoacidosis.[92] A prolonged fast before surgery may exacerbate these metabolic effects.

METABOLIC RESPONSE TO ANESTHESIA

Although adequate analgesia is essential to minimize the neuroendocrine stress response to surgery, some anesthetics may also independently contribute to perioperative hyperglycemia.[11,93] Volatile anesthetics, such as isoflurane and sevoflurane, cause hyperglycemia by inhibiting insulin secretion[94–97]; the hyperglycemia results from both impaired glucose clearance and increased glucose production.[93] In contrast, epidural analgesia with local anesthetics prevents this hyperglycemic effect[98,99] by inhibiting endogenous glucose production.[93] Similarly, propofol and opioids attenuate the hyperglycemic response to surgery[93,100,101] through decreasing endogenous glucose production and whole-body glucose uptake.[93] Propofol may not impair glucose-stimulated insulin release the way that volatile anesthetics do.[102] Although these anesthetic agent differences are important to consider, the metabolic effects of anesthesia per se are relatively minor compared with the direct effects of surgery.[11]

Corticosteroids are routinely given during anesthesia to prevent postoperative nausea and vomiting or to decrease airway or brain edema. The risks and benefits in patients with diabetes must be carefully considered due to the catabolic effects and resulting hyperglycemia as detailed above. To date, one large trial and a systematic review indicate that blood glucose concentrations after a single dose of dexamethasone in both normal and diabetic adult patients are mildly increased during the first 12 hours postoperatively, particularly in those with greater HbA1c levels after 8 mg vs. 4 mg dexamethasone.[103,104]

ADVERSE CONSEQUENCES OF HYPERGLYCEMIA

Hyperglycemia can impair wound healing by hindering collagen production, which may decrease the tensile strength of the surgical wound.[105] Hyperglycemia may also have adverse effects on neutrophil function, including decreased chemotaxis, phagocytosis, and bactericidal killing.[106–109] Studies in adults with diabetes undergoing surgery have shown an association between postoperative hyperglycemia and infectious complications.[110,111] A meta-analysis showed that patients in surgical intensive care units (ICUs) benefit from intensive insulin therapy, whereas patients in other ICU settings do not.[112] These outcomes have obfuscated the specific glycemic targets and the means for achieving them in both critically and noncritically ill patients.

Several pediatric clinical trials in nondiabetic children have investigated whether a strategy of tight glycemic control with intravenous insulin should be used to normalize blood glucose concentrations after major surgery.[113–116] Unless combined with a continuous glucose monitor, this approach increases the risk of severe hypoglycemia.[115] The preponderance of published data indicates that tight glycemic control is not recommended as standard treatment for children who undergo cardiac surgery because it does not significantly change the infection rate, mortality, length of stay, or measures of organ failure compared with standard care.[117] Similarly, a randomized trial using a continuous glucose monitor in critically ill children (excluding postcardiac surgery patients) conducted at 35 centers, showed no benefit of tight glycemic control (target blood glucose 80–110 mg/dL [4.4–6.1 mmol/L]) compared with glycemic control targeting blood glucose in the range 150 to 180 mg/dL (8.3–10 mmol/L). No significant differences were observed in mortality, severity of organ dysfunction, or number of ventilator-free days; patients in the lower glucose target group had higher rates of infections and severe hypoglycemia.[116]

For pediatric patients with diabetes, the International Society for Pediatric and Adolescent Diabetes (ISPAD) Clinical Practice Consensus Guidelines for perioperative management suggest a target blood glucose concentration in the range 90 to 180 mg/dL (5–10 mmol/L) during all surgeries, and a target of 140 to 180 mg/dL (7.8–10 mmol/L) in the postsurgery ICU period.[18] The recommended practice for subspecialties, such as cardiac, neurosurgical, and solid organ transplant surgical patients, requires still more study, and it must be highlighted that few of the published investigations and meta-analyses have focused specifically on children.

PREOPERATIVE CONSULTATION

Preoperative consultation with the primary endocrinologist to assess the adequacy of metabolic control and coordinate a patient-specific perioperative plan is considered best practice (Fig. 25.1).[6,15,18] When feasible, children with diabetes should not undergo elective surgery until they are metabolically stable and glycemia is well controlled, that is, there is no ketosis, serum electrolytes are normal, and the HbA1c value approximates the recommended goal of <7% across all age groups,[118] similar to that for type 2 diabetes.[23]

If glycemic control is suboptimal, then one should consider delaying elective surgery. If that is not possible, hospital admission may be required to optimize glycemic control. There is no consensus regarding an HbA1c cutoff to define adequate glycemic control with regard to perioperative risk in children.[18] In adults with type 1 diabetes, an HbA1c value >8% warrants considering delaying surgery.[119] Both the endocrinology and anesthesiology services should participate in this assessment with the patient/family and surgeon. Whenever possible, surgery for children with

Preoperative medical assessment of diabetes control and planning

- Assess metabolic control with blood glucose, electrolytes, ketones (urine or blood), HbA1c
- Adjust diabetes treatment as needed to optimize glycemic control (ideally HbA1c<7%)
- Arrange additional investigations (ECG, chest radiograph, renal function) as needed
- Coordinate perioperative insulin and fasting plan with primary endocrinologist and patient/family
- If applicable, instruct patient to place insulin infusion set or Omnipod® and CGM in non-compressible locations distant from the surgical field prior to surgery
- Schedule surgery in the morning as FIRST case of the day

FIGURE 25.1 Preoperative assessment and planning for patients with diabetes mellitus. *CGM,* Continuous glucose monitor; *ECG,* electrocardiogram.

diabetes should be scheduled as the first case of the day to minimize fasting time and reduce the possibility of delays that may prolong the fasting time.[6,15,18,119–121]

Concern about slowed gastric emptying in those children prescribed GLP-1 medications has prompted guidance that recommends withholding these medications for at least a week prior to surgery and the morning following surgery (see also Chapter 27).[74a] Children who present for emergent surgery (e.g., trauma or acute surgical conditions) require a multidisciplinary preoperative assessment with collaborative involvement of both the endocrinology and anesthesiology services. Surgery often cannot be delayed even if metabolic control is poor, for example, a child requiring emergent surgery who presents with ketosis or in diabetic ketoacidosis. This has implications for the intraoperative management of such children; described later under "Special Surgical Situations."

PREOPERATIVE MANAGEMENT

General Principles

The regimen for managing diabetes before, during, and after a surgical or diagnostic procedure that requires the child to fast should aim to maintain near-normoglycemia, that is, a blood glucose concentration of approximately 100 to 200 mg/dL (5.6–11.1 mmol/L). Blood glucose concentrations in this range reduce the risks of osmotic diuresis, dehydration, electrolyte imbalance, metabolic acidosis, infection, and hypoglycemia in the sedated child who may be unable to communicate with staff.[122] Parents should receive explicit written instructions regarding appropriate modifications of their child's diabetes regimen before and on the day of surgery.

More detailed preoperative recommendations must be based on the individual child's usual treatment regimen. For most children with diabetes undergoing minor outpatient surgical procedures, insulin can be provided perioperatively with subcutaneous injections. For those undergoing more extensive procedures or for patients with poor glycemic control, transition to an intravenous infusion of insulin may be required.

Whatever the management strategy for the diabetes, it is most important that it is coordinated between the anesthesiology and endocrinology services, and that the modifications to the child's diabetes regimen at home be communicated clearly and in a timely manner to the family. Specific recommendations based on the usual treatment regimen and surgical context are provided here.

Day of Surgery

On the day of surgery, all patients should have an assessment of metabolic control, including a preoperative determination of the blood glucose concentration. The recommended perioperative blood glucose target is 90 to 180 mg/dL.[18] If the blood glucose is >250 mg/dL (14 mmol/L), check for ketones (urine or blood) to exclude ketosis or diabetic ketoacidosis. Positive urine ketones (≥small urine ketones) should be confirmed with a blood sample for β-hydroxybutyrate (BOHB).[18] If BOHB is ≥0.6 mmol/L, consult endocrinology to evaluate further. Delay nonemergent procedures until any problems with volume status and electrolytes have been corrected.[6]

On the morning of surgery, no rapid- or short-acting insulin should be administered *unless* the blood glucose concentration exceeds 250 mg/dL. If the blood glucose exceeds 250 mg/dL and BOHB is <0.6 mmol/L and no rapid-acting insulin has been given in the prior 3 hours, a conservative dose of rapid-acting insulin is administered to restore near-normoglycemia. The dose is determined using the child's usual insulin "correction factor," which refers to the decrease in blood glucose concentration expected after administering 1 unit of rapid-acting insulin. This can be calculated using the "1500 rule": divide 1500 by the child's usual total daily dose (TDD) of insulin. For example, if a child typically receives 30 units of insulin daily, this child's "correction factor" would be 1500 ÷ 30 = 50. In this example, 1 unit of rapid-acting insulin would be expected to decrease the child's blood glucose concentration by approximately 50 mg/dL over the ensuing 3 to 5 hours. Various correction factors have been described, including a "1500 rule" for short-acting insulin (regular) and an "1800 rule" for rapid-acting insulin, such as insulin lispro.[123,124] For simplicity and because insulin resistance typically occurs with surgical stress, the "1500 rule" is appropriate in this setting, even with the use of a rapid-acting insulin. To then calculate an appropriate corrective dose of insulin to restore near-normoglycemia, the anesthesiologist should aim for a target blood glucose concentration of 150 mg/dL.

A "correction factor" rather than a sliding scale is also used to manage a child with hyperglycemia and restore the blood glucose concentration to 150 mg/dL. For example, if the child has a correction factor of 1 unit of rapid-acting insulin to reduce the blood glucose concentration by 50 mg/dL, and the current blood glucose value is 300 mg/dL, to reduce the blood glucose concentration from 300 mg/dL to 150 mg/dL, a total dose of (300 − 150)/50 or 3 units of insulin would be required. At the start of the procedure, the "correction" dose may be administered subcutaneously (using rapid-acting insulin) or by intravenous infusion using regular insulin in those children who will be managed with an intravenous insulin infusion during the procedure. For children with type 2 diabetes who do *not* ordinarily require insulin (but who are, by definition, insulin resistant), an insulin dose of 0.1 unit/kg of rapid-acting insulin may be administered subcutaneously to correct a blood glucose concentration greater than 250 mg/dL.

If the blood glucose on presentation is <70 mg/dL, begin treatment for hypoglycemia. If intravenous access is established, administer 1 to 2 mL/kg of 10% dextrose intravenously and recheck blood glucose in 15 minutes. Basal insulin can be suspended, if necessary, for no more than 30 minutes, but should be restarted as soon as possible to prevent ketosis.[18] Sugar-containing clear fluids can also be given by mouth if time to surgery is more than 2 hours, or if no alternative is available.[6]

INTRAOPERATIVE MANAGEMENT

Intravenous Fluids

The insulin and fluid regimen during and after surgery depends on the duration of the procedure. If the procedure is likely to be brief (e.g., ≤2 hours) and one can reasonably anticipate that the child will be able to drink soon after the procedure, it may not be necessary to start a glucose-containing intravenous infusion for patients with normal preoperative blood glucose. If the duration of fasting is likely to be more prolonged, the patient is receiving an intravenous insulin infusion, or is otherwise at risk for hypoglycemia (e.g., receiving an insulin regimen that includes intermediate-acting insulin [NPH], or presenting with an abnormal blood glucose requiring intervention), dextrose-containing intravenous fluids should be started at a maintenance rate. Generally, fluids containing 5% dextrose administered at the patient's maintenance rate are sufficient, but 10% dextrose may be required if the patient is at greater risk for hypoglycemia such as in the setting of an initial blood glucose <100 mg/dL or continuous glucose monitor trend indicating rapidly decreasing glucose levels. Perioperative replacement of insensible losses and intravascular volume owing to blood or other body fluid losses should be with an isotonic solution.[125,126] Care should be taken to avoid potassium-containing resuscitation fluids in emergency surgery or metabolically unwell patients.

Glucose Monitoring

In all cases, blood glucose concentrations should be measured at least hourly and either insulin or dextrose adjusted, as necessary, to maintain blood glucose in the target range of 90 to 180 mg/dL. The frequency of monitoring should be increased to every 30 minutes if there is a change in therapy or to every 15 minutes if blood glucose is <80 mg/dL.[6] Either an increase in the rate of insulin infusion or subcutaneous administration of a rapid-acting insulin analog (not more often than every 3 hours to prevent "stacking") is used to correct intraoperative hyperglycemia as described earlier. An intraoperative intravenous bolus of regular insulin is not recommended because this causes a rapid supraphysiologic increase in serum insulin concentration, which, owing to insulin's short half-life (approximately 5 minutes), will have a short-lived effect on blood glucose concentration. In contrast, subcutaneously administered rapid-acting insulin analogs have a typical and reproducible pharmacologic profile. If the blood glucose exceeds 250 mg/dL, urine or blood ketones should also be measured.

The reliability of a continuous glucose monitor in the perioperative setting is uncertain and glucose values may not be accurate in the setting of hypoperfusion or hypothermia[50] or due to "compression artifact," which may falsely lower glucose readings if the sensor is located on a compressed body surface.[127,128] Interference caused by electrocautery in the operating room has also been observed.[129] The effects of anesthetic medications, per se, on continuous glucose monitors have not been thoroughly evaluated. Patients with a continuous glucose monitor device should be advised to place the device as far as possible from the anticipated surgical field and values from the continuous glucose monitor should only be used for trends in the perioperative setting; a blood glucose value must be obtained for treatment decisions.[18,130]

Some drugs (e.g., acetaminophen, hydroxyurea)[131] may also falsely increase the glucose concentration in continuous glucose monitoring systems. The degree of inaccuracy varies with time and between individuals. Acetaminophen's phenolic moiety is oxidized at the sensing electrode, particularly those amperometric glucose biosensors measuring hydrogen peroxide, producing an electrochemical signal not related to glucose. A mean difference from the true reading of 60 mg/dL (3.3 mmol/L) at 2 hours after acetaminophen ingestion has been described.[132] This problem has been overcome with recent sensors (e.g., Dexcom G7, San Diego, CA, USA), but physicians should be aware older sensors and monitoring systems may deviate and avoid overreacting and over-correcting the spurious readings.[50,133]

Methods of Insulin Administration

Subcutaneous Insulin Injection

Intermediate- and long-acting subcutaneous insulin may be continued for minor procedures (2 hours or less) according to the patient's usual regimen. For all patients on subcutaneous insulin, the usual regimen should be followed on the day before the procedure (Fig. 25.2). For the child using a basal-bolus regimen with long-acting insulin glargine or insulin degludec or once- or twice-daily with insulin detemir (plus rapid-acting insulin with meals at home), a dose of basal insulin is required to prevent hyperglycemia and ketosis. Less commonly, split-mixed insulin regimens may be used and involve two to three injections per day with a combination of intermediate-acting insulin (NPH) plus a rapid- or short-acting insulin. For children who use such a regimen, 50% of the usual morning dose of NPH should be administered on the morning of the procedure. Adjustments may be recommended by endocrinology if patterns of hypoglycemia have been observed or if the procedure cannot be scheduled for the morning.[18] Hyperglycemia (blood glucose >250 mg/dL) should be treated with subcutaneous rapid-acting insulin boluses as previously described.

Continuous Subcutaneous Insulin Infusion

Management of the child with an insulin pump depends on the duration of the surgery. Those undergoing minor procedures expected to last 2 hours or less can continue to receive their usual basal rate via their insulin pump. However, this approach requires the anesthesiologist to be familiar and comfortable with the use of an insulin pump in the operating room and have a diabetes care provider available to review pump functions with the anesthesia team.[15,18,121,134–136] If the patient is undergoing a major procedure, and someone experienced in managing these pumps is not available or the pump is not in an accessible location during the surgery, then the insulin pump should be discontinued and intravenous insulin administered.[18,121,137] Insulin pumps may also be contraindicated in some procedures involving radiology and electrocautery.[121,138]

If insulin is delivered via a pump perioperatively, the patient's usual basal rate should be continued. General day of procedure

---

Day of procedure

- Hold rapid- or short-acting insulin (regular, insulin lispro [Humalog], insulin aspart [NovoLog], insulin glulisine [Apidra])
- Omit breakfast
- Should be **FIRST** case of the day
- Obtain preoperative labs: blood glucose (BG) and ketones (urine or blood) if BG >250
- Consult with Endocrinology if moderate or large ketonuria or if blood β-hydroxybutyric acid is >0.6 mmol/L

FIGURE 25.2 General recommendations for the day of the procedure for children with diabetes mellitus.

guidelines as outlined in Fig. 25.2 should be followed. Hyperglycemia (blood glucose >250 mg/dL) should be treated with subcutaneous rapid-acting insulin boluses as previously described. Any unexplained hyper- or hypoglycemia or metabolic derangement in the immediate perioperative period warrants discontinuing the pump and commencing an intravenous insulin infusion. When a subcutaneous insulin pump is discontinued in a patient whose diabetes is well-controlled with near-normal glycemia, plasma insulin levels decline rapidly and plasma glucose and ketone concentrations increase within 60 minutes.[139] An intravenous insulin infusion should be started within 30 minutes[18,121] because even a brief period of interrupted insulin delivery can cause marked hyperglycemia.[139,140]

Other protocols include transitioning patients who use an insulin pump to an intravenous insulin infusion or subcutaneous long-acting insulin.[87] For procedures expected to last longer than 2 hours, children should be transitioned to an intravenous insulin infusion, as described later.

Children[11] and adults should be admitted to the hospital before *major* surgical procedures if their metabolic status needs to be optimized preoperatively.[87] If the surgery must be delayed for any reason, frequent blood glucose monitoring is mandatory to prevent perioperative hypoglycemia or hyperglycemia.

Intravenous Insulin Infusions

Children who require major surgery, especially procedures anticipated to last more than 2 hours, should have an intravenous infusion of regular insulin as the preferred perioperative diabetes management plan. Both children[13,141] and adults[7] have better glycemic control with intravenous insulin infusion compared with subcutaneous injections. Children should receive their usual regimen of insulin on the day before the procedure and general day of procedure guidelines as outlined in Fig. 25.2 should be followed. Insulin pumps should be physically removed before starting an insulin infusion.

A protocol for selecting the starting rate of intravenous regular insulin infusion (1 unit regular insulin per mL) via a syringe pump is shown in Fig. 25.3.[18] After starting the insulin infusion, titrate the dose by 0.01 to 0.03 units/kg per hour aiming to keep blood glucose within the target range of 90 to 180 mg/dL.[6] Intravenous insulin infusions should be administered with dextrose-containing maintenance fluids. Dextrose and insulin should be administered via a dedicated intravenous line, independently titrated, and physically separated from bolus fluids. The half-life of intravenous regular insulin is approximately 5 minutes.[142] Therefore, administration of a dose of subcutaneous insulin by injection or resumption of insulin pump therapy should be started at least 15 minutes before discontinuation of intravenous insulin infusion.

PERIOPERATIVE MANAGEMENT OF TYPE 2 DIABETES

Children with type 2 diabetes may require insulin and/or other antihyperglycemic agents. Metformin should be discontinued 24 hours before a major surgical procedure (e.g., expected to last more than 2 hours) because of its long duration of effect and the risk of lactic acidosis in the presence of dehydration, hypoxemia, or poor tissue perfusion.[143–146] For minor procedures, expected to last 2 hours or less, metformin may be discontinued on the day of the procedure.[17,147] Metformin may be restarted after 48 hours when oral intake resumes and provided that postoperative renal function is normal.[148] Patients using a sulfonylurea, thiazolidinedione, or alpha-glucosidase inhibitor should stop the medication on the day of surgery and can restart when oral intake resumes.[148] Given the risk of diabetic ketoacidosis with SGLT-2 inhibitors, these should be held for at least 24 hours before surgery and restarted when oral intake resumes and the patient has no nausea or vomiting.[149] While holding SGLT-2 inhibitors for at least 24 hours is the recommendation of the American Association of Clinical Endocrinologists and American College of Endocrinology,[150] the American Diabetes Association suggests considering holding SGLT-2 inhibitors for 3 to 4 days.[151] There are also varying recommendations regarding DPP-intravenous inhibitors and GLP-1 agonists. Given the low risk of hypoglycemia with these medications, some[152,153] but not all[151] guidelines suggest that these can be continued in the perioperative period. It should be noted that the risk of hypoglycemia increases if used in conjunction with other antihyperglycemic agents, and GLP-1 agonists can delay gastric emptying.[152] Recommendations about the management of antihyperglycemic agents in the perioperative period continue to evolve; specific pediatric information about management of these medications is not available. Clinical context, including the duration of the procedure and associated risks, should be considered.[74a] Children with type 2 diabetes who use a split-mixed or basal-bolus insulin regimen alone or in conjunction with an antihyperglycemic agent should also adjust their insulin regimen as outlined above.

POSTOPERATIVE MANAGEMENT

As soon as the child is able to resume drinking and eating normally, the usual diabetes regimen may be reinstituted, and the dextrose infusion discontinued. One exception to this approach is for children with type 2 diabetes who have discontinued metformin. In such cases, metformin should be withheld for 48 hours, and renal function must be within normal limits before its resumption. Intravenous dextrose and electrolyte solutions should be continued until oral intake resumes. An infusion of intravenous short-acting insulin (regular) or intermittent subcutaneous rapid-acting insulin should be administered, not more frequently than every 3 hours, to maintain blood glucose in the target range of 90 to 180 mg/dL as discussed earlier. Frequent blood glucose monitoring and monitoring blood or urine ketones is essential because of the variable effects of surgical trauma, inactivity, pain, anxiety, nausea and/or vomiting with poor oral intake, medications, and postoperative

---

Insulin infusion

- Use regular insulin 50 units in 50 mL NS via syringe pump
- Concurrently infuse 5% dextrose in Normal Saline at maintenance rate via the same venous access point
- Blood glucose (BG) checks at least hourly. Increase to every 30 minutes for change in therapy. Check BG every 15 minutes if BG <80 mg/dL
- Insulin Infusion starting rate
  - 0.025 units/kg/hour if BG <140 mg/dL
  - 0.05 units/kg/hour if BG 140–220 mg/dL
  - 0.075 units/kg/hour if BG 221–270 mg/dL
  - 0.1 units/kg/hour if >270 mg/dL
- Titrate infusion by 0.01–0.03 units/kg/hour to achieve target BG range of 90–180 mg/dL

FIGURE 25.3 Guideline for insulin infusion during surgery.[6,18]

infection. At the time of discharge from the hospital, children and their parents or care providers should be given appropriate guidelines regarding these issues. Those who are admitted to the hospital after surgery should be managed in consultation with the endocrinology service to coordinate appropriate scheduling and subsequent dosing of insulin.

SPECIAL SURGICAL SITUATIONS

Children with diabetes who need urgent surgery must have a full clinical and biochemical assessment (Fig. 25.4). If the emergent procedure is minor and the child is metabolically stable, subcutaneous insulin therapy may be continued for the procedure according to the guidelines outlined earlier. However, if the procedure is major, the child is metabolically unstable, or the patient's insulin status cannot be confirmed, then intravenous insulin should be administered. Patients who use an insulin pump should also be transitioned to an insulin infusion and the pump removed.[6,18] The problem necessitating surgery may have led to metabolic decompensation that must first be corrected and stabilized unless the need for surgery is immediate. These children are often dehydrated; therefore, in addition to administering insulin, rehydration and electrolyte replacement is critical to address their metabolic derangements and restore normovolemia to ensure adequate end-organ perfusion. Management of children with diabetic ketoacidosis is a high-risk situation that requires close collaboration between the anesthesiology and endocrinology services.

Diabetes Insipidus

Diabetes insipidus (DI) is caused by impaired secretion of or response to vasopressin (antidiuretic hormone), resulting in the production of large amounts of dilute urine. Central DI

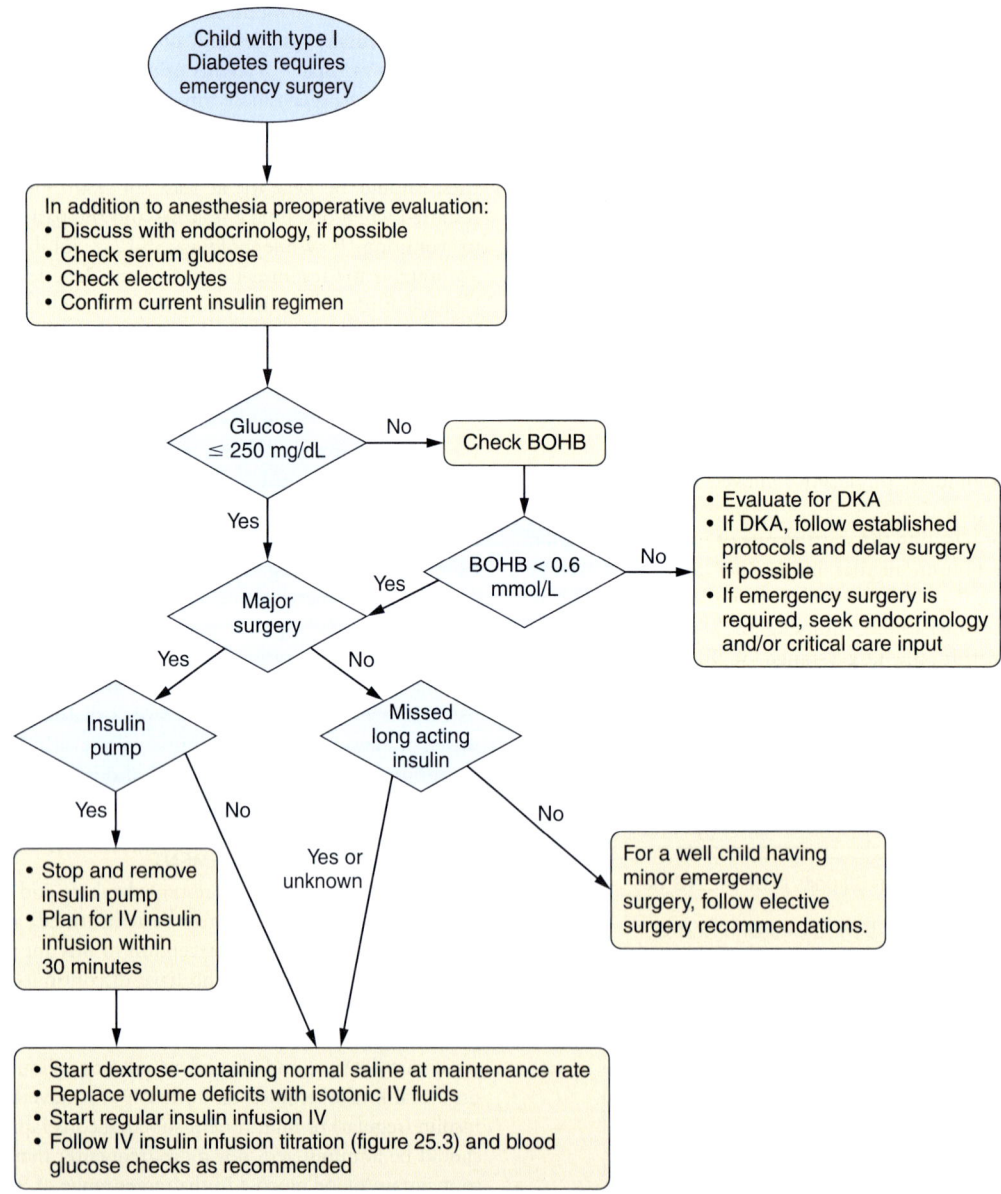

FIGURE 25.4 Emergency surgery algorithm.[6] *BOHB*, β-hydroxybutyrate; *DKA*, diabetic ketoacidosis. (Reproduced with permission from Martin, LD, Hoagland MA, Rhodes ET, Wolfsdorf JI, Hamrick JL. Perioperative management of pediatric patients with type 1 diabetes mellitus, updated recommendations for anesthesiologists. *Anesth Analg.* 2020;130(4):821-827.)

(also referred to as neurohypophyseal, neurogenic, or vasopressin-sensitive DI) is caused by a deficiency of the antidiuretic hormone, arginine vasopressin, which produces antidiuresis by stimulating V2 receptors on the principal cells of the kidney to promote reabsorption of water.[154] Central DI can be caused by disorders of vasopressin gene structure; accidental or surgical trauma to vasopressin neurons; congenital anatomic hypothalamic or pituitary defects; neoplasms; infiltrative, autoimmune, and infectious diseases affecting vasopressin neurons or fiber tracts; and increased metabolism of vasopressin. The etiology is unknown in approximately 50% of children with central DI. Nephrogenic DI occurs when there is renal resistance to the action of vasopressin, which may be hereditary or secondary to medications, urinary obstruction, or electrolyte abnormalities.

Children undergoing neurosurgical procedures for tumors in or near the pituitary gland, especially craniopharyngioma, often require management of DI, as do children with known DI who require anesthesia for surgical or radiologic procedures. The perioperative management of these children requires meticulous attention to fluid and electrolyte balance to prevent either overhydration or underhydration and electrolyte disturbances.

DIAGNOSIS OF NEUROSURGICAL DIABETES INSIPIDUS: THE TRIPLE-PHASE RESPONSE

It is important to distinguish polyuria (>2 L/m^2 per day) caused by the onset of acute postsurgical central DI from polyuria resulting from diuresis of salt and fluid given during surgery. In both cases, children may have a large volume (typically exceeding 200 mL/m^2 per hour or >4 mL/kg per hour) of urine. In DI, serum osmolality is increased whereas urine is inappropriately dilute (low osmolality). In comparison, a child with normal excretion of excess salt and water may have normal serum osmolality and concentrated urine (greater than 300 mOsmol/kg). A meticulous examination of the intraoperative and postoperative records and careful bedside assessment of volume status (jugular venous distention, capillary refill) help to distinguish between these two entities.

Of special interest is the triphasic pattern of vasopressin secretion often observed after neurosurgical procedures that interfere with the supraoptic-hypophyseal tract.[155] An initial phase of transient DI may be observed that lasts between 12 hours and 2 days after surgery. This may be explained by local edema that interferes with normal vasopressin secretion. If noteworthy vasopressin-secreting cell damage has occurred, release of stored vasopressin from damaged neurons leads to a second phase that involves water retention. The syndrome of inappropriate antidiuretic hormone secretion (SIADH) may last up to 10 days. Finally, a third phase, permanent neurogenic DI, may follow if more than 90% of vasopressin cells are destroyed. Prolonged SIADH in the second phase generally portends permanent DI in the final phase of the triple response. In children with vasopressin and cortisol deficiency (e.g., in combined anterior and posterior hypopituitarism after neurosurgical treatment of craniopharyngioma), symptoms of DI may be masked because cortisol deficiency impairs renal free water clearance. Institution of glucocorticoid therapy may precipitate polyuria, leading to the diagnosis of DI.

PERIOPERATIVE MANAGEMENT OF MINOR PROCEDURES

Children with preexisting DI who are scheduled for a minor procedure, that is, a procedure without substantial blood loss and not followed by a period of further fasting or fluid shifts (e.g., myringotomy, radiologic imaging, peripheral orthopedic procedures) are treated differently from those undergoing a more major procedure associated with blood loss or fluid shifts and delayed postoperative resumption of fluid intake (Fig. 25.5).

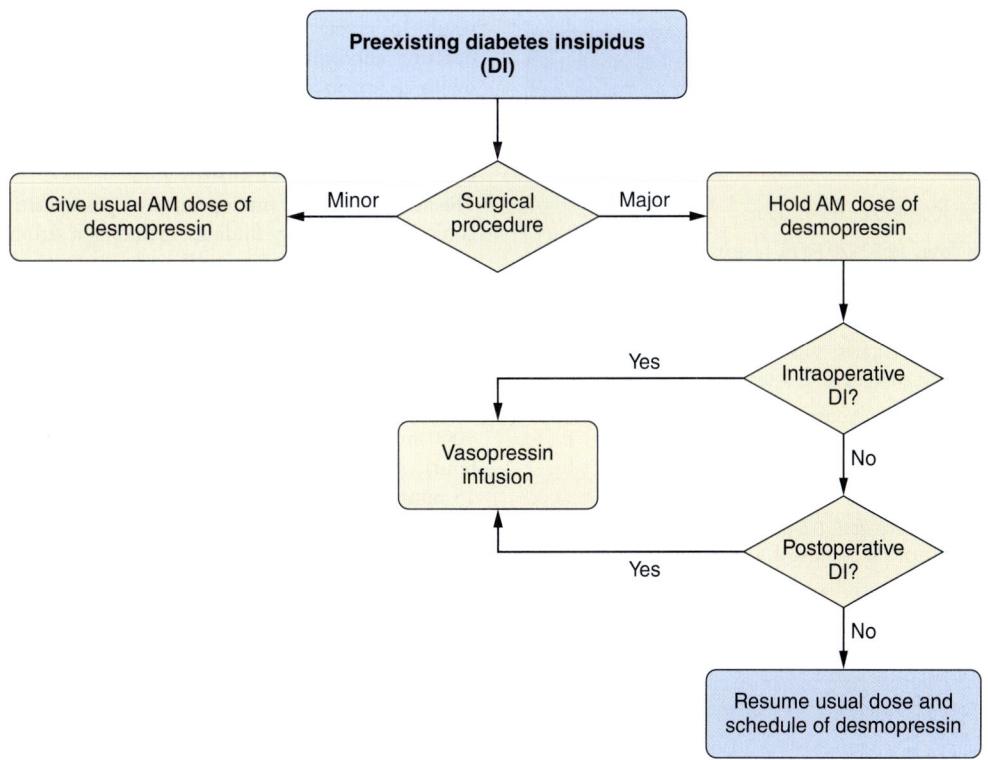

FIGURE 25.5 Perioperative management of diabetes insipidus.

The naturally occurring hormone, vasopressin, is a selective agonist of the vasopressin V2 receptors in the collecting ducts and distal convoluted tubules of the kidney. It has a short half-life, 5 to 15 minutes intravenously with powerful vasoconstricting properties.[156] Given its very brief half-life, it is suited as a continuous infusion during surgery to control DI. Current recommendations for vasopressin in shock is as a second-line treatment after norepinephrine or to reduce the dose of norepinephrine.[156] Except in the case of acute DI with shock where vasopressin infusion may be indicated, desmopressin is widely used for DI. Desmopressin, 1-deamino-8-D-argnine vasopressin, is a synthetic analog of vasopressin, that is formulated for oral, nasal, and parenteral routes (Table 25.3).[157] For the oral route, the dosing is greater, as this route has reduced bioavailability and a shorter half-life (6–8 hours). With an antidiuretic duration of action of 12 hours and limited vasoconstricting properties, desmopressin has become the formulation used widely to treat most forms of DI.

Children undergoing minor procedures with anesthesia should receive their usual morning dose of desmopressin (Table 25.3). The anesthetic technique should be tailored to the procedure. Arterial and urinary catheters are not required, and recovery may take place in the postanesthesia care unit (PACU). Once the morning dose of desmopressin has been administered, intraoperative and postoperative fluids should be restricted to the rate of 1 L/m² per 24 hours (approximately two-thirds of usual maintenance fluid requirement) to match insensible free water losses and obligatory urine output. Oral fluids may be offered once the child is awake. Although many patients may be discharged from the PACU without having successfully resumed oral fluids, discharge of the child with a history of DI should be delayed until the child tolerates oral fluids. Subsequent doses of desmopressin should be administered according to the child's usual preoperative schedule.

TABLE 25.3   Medications for Management of Central Diabetes Insipidus

Desmopressin acetate 100-, 200-µg tablets; nasal rhinal tube 10 µg/0.1 mL; nasal spray 10 µg/0.1 mL can only deliver fixed doses of 10 µg (0.1 mL) per spray	
Oral	Dose: 100–400 µg q8–12 hours
	Oral doses are 10–20 times intranasal doses of desmopressin
	Onset of action: ~1 hour
	Duration: 6–8 hours; dose dependent (0.4 µg has antidiuretic effect up to 12 hours)
Intranasal	Dose: ~10–20 µg/dose q12–24 hours
	Onset of action: within 1 hour
	Duration: 5–21 hours
Vasopressin (Pitressin) (20 units/mL); 0.5-mL, 1-mL, and 10-mL vials). Dilute in normal saline or 5% dextrose in water	
Intravenous	Dose: 0.5 mU/kg per hour; titrate upward in 0.5 mU/kg per hour increments to target urine output <2 mL/kg per hour
	Onset of action: rapid; maximum effect is achieved within 15 minutes of initiation of continuous infusion
	Duration: action ceases within 20 minutes of stopping intravenous infusion

PERIOPERATIVE MANAGEMENT OF MAJOR PROCEDURES

For a major surgical procedure, or any procedure followed by delayed resumption of unrestricted fluid intake, a child with DI should be scheduled as the first case of the day. On the day before the procedure, the child treated with either a twice-daily or once-daily morning dose of desmopressin should receive the usual doses. On the morning of the surgery, the morning dose of desmopressin should be withheld. In the case of the child who is treated with a single evening dose of desmopressin, the dose should be reduced by 50% on the evening before surgery (see Fig. 25.5). The child undergoing a major procedure should receive general anesthesia with conventional monitoring, as well as insertion of arterial and urinary catheters when appropriate, and after surgery should be admitted to an ICU for close fluid and electrolyte monitoring.

At the start of the procedure, an infusion of aqueous vasopressin (available as Pitressin 20 U/mL in a 1-mL vial, diluted to 20 U/1000 mL to yield a final concentration of 20 mU/mL) should be started at 0.5 mU/kg per hour (0.0005 U/kg per hour) and incrementally increased by 0.5 mU/kg per hour (0.0005 U/kg per hour) every 10 to 30 minutes until a urine output of less than 2 mL/kg per hour is achieved.[158] Normal saline with 5% dextrose intravenous fluids should be infused at a rate of 1 L/m² per 24 hours (two-thirds of the usual maintenance rate of fluid administration) during aqueous vasopressin therapy to approximate insensible losses and obligate urine output. Additional intravenous saline, isotonic fluids, or blood products may be given to replace blood and surgical fluid loss, to offset the third-space fluid losses, and to maintain hemodynamic stability. Fluid intake and output should be continuously monitored, and serum sodium concentration measured frequently to ensure water balance is maintained. Urine output should not routinely be replaced in the child receiving a vasopressin infusion. Accidental overdoses resulting from inadequate dilution of the highly concentrated stock vasopressin solution result in severe hypertension, and awake patients may also describe abdominal cramping, diarrhea, vomiting, and pallor owing to action at V1 receptors on smooth muscle in the gastrointestinal tract and blood vessels.

NEW PERIOPERATIVE DIAGNOSIS

The new diagnosis of intraoperative or postoperative DI is based on clinical and laboratory findings, including a serum sodium concentration greater than 145 mmol/L, polyuria (>4 mL/kg per hour) for 30 minutes or more, increased plasma osmolality (>300 mOsm/kg) in association with hypotonic urine (<300 mOsm/kg; specific gravity <1.005), and after excluding the presence of glycosuria and diuretic or mannitol administration as possible causes of polyuria.

When DI occurs, an infusion of aqueous vasopressin (20 U/1000 mL) is initiated at 0.5 mU/kg per hour (0.0015 U/kg per hour). Aqueous vasopressin has a brief plasma half-life of 5 to 15 minutes; the rate of infusion is increased every 30 minutes until urine output decreases to less than 2 mL/kg per hour, indicating that antidiuresis has been achieved. Once a urine output of less than 2 mL/kg per hour is achieved, the vasopressin infusion is maintained at a constant rate.[158] At a dose of 1.5 mU/kg per hour, aqueous vasopressin results in a supranormal blood vasopressin concentration of approximately 10 pg/mL, twice that needed for full antidiuretic activity.[159] The effect of vasopressin is maximal within 2 hours after starting an infusion.[159]

Intravenous desmopressin should *not* be used to manage postoperative central DI acutely. It offers no advantage over aqueous vasopressin and has a long half-life (8–12 hours) compared with that of vasopressin, which increases the risk of water intoxication and precludes dose titration. Furthermore, the synthetic analog is a weak vasoconstrictor, attenuating its effectiveness in hypotensive, shock patients. Once the diagnosis of DI is made, close monitoring of fluids, urine output, and serum sodium are essential, as severe and life-threatening complications including sodium imbalance, seizures, and brain injury, can rise from inadequate monitoring when hypotonic fluids and vasopressin are concomitantly administered.

POSTOPERATIVE MANAGEMENT

The child with DI should be cared for in an ICU after major surgery, as continued close monitoring (hourly if necessary) of fluid input and output, serum electrolytes, and osmolality are required. It is important to have a urinary catheter in place to distinguish postoperative urinary retention from oliguria and until stability is achieved. The vasopressin infusion initiated intraoperatively is continued in the ICU. Fluid administration is *not* adjusted according to urine output; however, fluid deficits are replaced, and blood pressure supported until antidiuresis (urine output <2 mL/kg per hour) is clearly established. In the patient with maximum antidiuresis, total (oral and intravenous) maintenance fluids should not exceed insensible plus obligatory urinary losses (i.e., approximately 1 L/m^2 per 24 hours or two-thirds of usual maintenance fluid requirement). In the postoperative period, appropriate maintenance fluid is generally 5% dextrose in half-normal saline (depending on the serum sodium concentration) solution with 0 to 40 mEq/L of potassium chloride (depending on the serum potassium concentration). Blood loss should be replaced with normal saline solution, 5% albumin, or blood products, as appropriate.

After hypothalamic, but not transsphenoidal surgery, greater initial concentrations of vasopressin are occasionally required to treat acute DI. This may be attributed to the release of a substance related to vasopressin from the damaged hypothalamo-neurohypophyseal system, which acts as an antagonist to normal vasopressin activity.[160] Much greater rates of vasopressin infusions, resulting in plasma concentrations greater than 1000 pg/mL, should be avoided because they may cause cutaneous necrosis,[161] rhabdomyolysis,[161,162] and cardiac rhythm disturbances.[162]

Children treated with vasopressin for post neurosurgical DI should be switched from intravenous to oral fluid intake at the earliest opportunity. With an intact thirst mechanism and access to free water, the patient will better regulate blood osmolality. Once oral intake has been resumed without nausea and vomiting (often by the morning of the day after surgery), the vasopressin infusion should be stopped. All intravenous infusions should also be stopped to avoid iatrogenic fluid overload, and oral fluids are permitted freely. Desmopressin is again reinstituted (nasally or orally) in the child with preexisting DI or begun in the child who has new-onset DI, in consultation with an endocrinologist (see Table 25.3).

TRANSIENT MEDICATION-INDUCED DIABETES INSIPIDUS

Although diabetes insipidus is typically classified as either central or nephrogenic, there has been a growing awareness of a phenomenon of transient, medication-induced diabetes insipidus that is particularly relevant for the anesthesiologist.[163] This diagnosis appears to be rare, but in cases of medication-induced DI, commonly implicated medications include dexmedetomidine, sevoflurane, ketamine, and propofol.[163] Patients typically present with profound polyuria in the setting of hypovolemia and rising serum sodium concentration. Untreated, this may lead to weakness, lethargy, myalgias, seizures, and in the most severe instances, coma or death.[163] Other symptoms of DI are typically impossible to appreciate under anesthesia, which may lead to delay in diagnosis. Furthermore, patients are unable to compensate with a thirst mechanism. A high index of suspicion is critical for prompt recognition and institution of therapy, which should ideally include removal of the suspected offending agent where possible, and management of hypovolemia and electrolyte abnormalities. Time to resolution of symptoms after withdrawal of the suspected medication is variable; in some instances, resolution is prompt, but in cases of prolonged exposure, resolution has taken 1 to 2 days or longer. Treatment with vasopressin may be necessary while awaiting resolution.

Syndrome of Inappropriate Antidiuretic Hormone Secretion

The SIADH is caused by the inability to excrete free water. Physiologically, it is characterized by hyponatremia, plasma hypoosmolality (<275 mOsm/kg), inappropriately concentrated urine (>100 mOsm/kg), natriuresis in the absence of edema and volume depletion, and normal renal and adrenal function.[164–166] Dilutional hyponatremia of SIADH develops secondary to inappropriately increased levels of plasma antidiuretic hormone (ADH, also known as arginine vasopressin) relative to plasma osmolality.[166] Antidiuretic hormone is produced in the hypothalamus and released from the posterior pituitary gland. In the renal collecting ducts, it binds to V2 receptors initiating an intracellular cascade that results in the insertion of aquaporin channels and water reabsorption in the collecting ducts and distal convoluted tubules.

The major causes of SIADH are neurologic and psychiatric diseases, pulmonary disorders and interventions, malignancies, surgery, and medications (Table 25.4).[165–168] Pain, stress, and nausea, which are common in the perioperative period, are also potential stimuli of ADH secretion.[168] Medications that cause SIADH can act by stimulating the release of ADH, by enhancing the effect of ADH, or by acting as an ADH analog.[165] Although ADH secretion impairs water excretion, the other mechanisms that regulate fluid volume and sodium balance (renin-angiotensin-aldosterone system and atrial natriuretic peptide) are intact. Volume expansion activates natriuretic mechanisms (decreased proximal sodium reabsorption and decreased aldosterone production), resulting in sodium and water excretion and the restoration of near euvolemia. With chronic SIADH, sodium loss is a more prominent feature than is water retention. Severe hyponatremia increases cell size because of entry of water into the cell along its osmotic gradient and may be associated with loss of intracellular potassium and other solutes to restore cell volume.

Hyponatremia caused by SIADH can lead to clinical symptoms. Inappropriate infusion of hypotonic fluids in the postoperative period can exacerbate the hyponatremia caused by SIADH.[169,170] The clinical manifestations of symptomatic hyponatremia are principally neurologic. Early symptoms include headache, nausea, vomiting, weakness, confusion, altered consciousness, and lethargy. Late symptoms include seizures, coma, decorticate posturing, and death.[171] The severity of symptoms is related to both the absolute serum sodium concentration (most patients with serum sodium levels >125 mEq/L are asymptomatic)

TABLE 25.4	Causes of Syndrome of Inappropriate Antidiuretic Hormone Secretion

Central Nervous System Disturbances

Head trauma

Brain tumor

Hydrocephalus

Subarachnoid hemorrhage

Stroke

Infection (meningitis, encephalitis, brain abscess, AIDS)

Acute psychosis

Drugs

Vasopressin, desmopressin

Carbamazepine, oxcarbamazepine

Cyclophosphamide

Vincristine or vinblastine

Cisplatin

Phenothiazines

Serotonin uptake inhibitors

Tricyclic antidepressants

Monoamine oxidase inhibitors

Methylenedioxymethamphetamine ("ecstasy")

Nicotine

Major Surgery

Major abdominal or thoracic surgery

Pituitary surgery

Pain

Severe nausea

Pulmonary Disease

Pneumonia, tuberculosis

Asthma

Atelectasis

Pneumothorax

Acute respiratory failure

Positive-pressure ventilation

Neoplasia

Carcinoma of lung, gastrointestinal tract, or genitourinary tract

Thymoma

Leukemia

Lymphoma

Sarcoma

Other tumors

Miscellaneous

Idiopathic

Hereditary SIADH

Gain-of-function mutation in the gene encoding vasopressin-2 receptor

and its rate of decrease, especially if greater than 0.5 mEq/L per hour. Children are at greater risk than adults for developing hyponatremic encephalopathy because of a larger brain/skull size ratio, which limits room for brain expansion.[171,172]

PERIOPERATIVE MANAGEMENT

Many of the causes of SIADH are transient and resolve spontaneously once the underlying condition is corrected. Treatment of SIADH consists mainly of water restriction (i.e., maintaining a daily water intake that is less than daily water losses). If dilutional hyponatremia is mild and asymptomatic, therapy may not be required. In adults, both moderate and severe hyponatremia (serum sodium ≤130 mEq/L) are associated with increased mortality.[173,174]

Hyponatremic encephalopathy should be treated immediately with hypertonic (3%) saline solution. For mild to moderate symptoms with a low risk of herniation, treatment consists of 3% saline at a rate of 0.5 to 2 mL/kg per hour.[175] For severe symptoms, treatment consists of a bolus of 2 mL/kg 3% saline (to a maximum of 100 mL) over 10 minutes.[171,172,175] This may be repeated once or twice until symptoms improve, with a goal of increasing serum sodium concentration of 5 to 6 mEq/L in the first 1 to 2 hours.[171,172,175] The greater the duration of hyponatremia and the lower the serum sodium concentration, the greater the concern for brain injury secondary to overcorrection of hyponatremia. Overcorrection of chronic hyponatremia can lead to serious, permanent, and even fatal neurologic complications from osmotic demyelination (central pontine myelinolysis).[171,172,176] Recommended safe limits for the rate of hyponatremia correction vary from 6 to 15 mEq/L per 24 hours.[172,175,177–179] The hypertonic saline infusion should stop when the absolute concentration of serum sodium reaches 120 to 125 mEq/L. Hypertonic saline solution is usually combined with furosemide to limit treatment-induced expansion of the extracellular fluid volume.[178] Thereafter, treatment should consist of fluid restriction.

Thyroid Disorders

Thyroid hormones play an important role in metabolic processes, growth, and development in children.[180] The thyroid gland develops from the embryonic pharyngeal floor and descends along the thyroglossal duct to its final position in the anterior neck. Thyroid hormone production is controlled by the hypothalamic-pituitary-thyroid axis. Two principal thyroid hormones are produced, thyroxine (T4) and triiodothyronine (T3). Although T4 is the predominant circulating thyroid hormone, T3, which is primarily formed by peripheral conversion from T4, is the major physiologically active thyroid hormone. Serum T4 and T3 concentrations in turn regulate hypothalamic thyrotropin-releasing hormone (TRH) and anterior pituitary thyroid-stimulating hormone (TSH) secretion via a negative feedback loop. Thyroid hormones are transported in the blood by carrier proteins, including thyroxine-binding globulin (80% of binding), prealbumin (10%–15% of binding), and albumin (5%–10% of binding). Protein-bound T4 and T3 are not biologically active. Only 0.03% of circulating T4 and 0.3% of T3 are unbound and active.[181]

HYPOTHYROIDISM

Classification and Epidemiology

Hypothyroidism is the most common thyroid disorder in children. Although iodine deficiency is the foremost cause of hypothyroidism worldwide,[182] as of 2020, 88% of the global population has iodized foods available for consumption.[183] The availability of iodized food has largely eradicated iodine deficiency in all but 21 noncompliant countries[183]; it is noteworthy that patients on long-term total parenteral nutrition remain at risk and this risk often goes unrecognized.[184] However, the most common causes of primary hypothyroidism where iodine intake is adequate are congenital hypothyroidism and Hashimoto thyroiditis.[180] The incidence of autoimmune hypothyroidism is increased in patients with trisomy 21, Turner syndrome, and other autoimmune diseases, including type 1 diabetes mellitus.[185,186] Other less frequent causes of primary hypothyroidism include sick euthyroid syndrome, hypothyroidism secondary to medications (thionamides, lithium, amiodarone), and radiation or surgery to the thyroid or neck.[180] Hypothyroidism can also be caused by disorders of the pituitary gland or the hypothalamus.

Subclinical hypothyroidism is characterized by a mildly increased TSH with normal concentrations of T4 and T3.[187] It is usually a self-limiting problem with a low rate of progression to overt hypothyroidism, although consensus on the treatment of subclinical hypothyroidism is still a matter of debate.[188–191]

Biochemical Tests of Thyroid Function

In general, measurement of serum TSH, T4, and unbound or free T4 is sufficient for initial assessment of thyroid function. Free T4 is preferable to total T4 since it eliminates the effects of variation in protein binding. Measurement of thyroid-stimulating hormone (TSH) is a sensitive test for diagnosing primary thyroid disorders and generally precedes noticeable changes in total T4 and T3 levels. In primary hypothyroidism, serum TSH is increased, whereas total T4 and free T4 are decreased. If the total T4 level is reduced but free T4 and TSH values are unchanged, thyroxine-binding globulin deficiency is the most likely diagnosis. No treatment is required for thyroxine-binding globulin deficiency since these individuals have normal concentrations of free T4 and are clinically euthyroid. If the hypothalamic-pituitary axis is not intact, such as in cases of secondary or tertiary (central) hypothyroidism, diagnosis and treatment is based on serum T4 levels and clinical signs and symptoms.

Clinical Manifestations

Since thyroid hormone affects all metabolically active cells, hormone deficiency leads to a wide array of systemic abnormalities. Classic signs and symptoms of hypothyroidism in children include short stature, fatigue, weight gain, dry skin, hair loss, coarse facial features, hoarse voice, and constipation. Myxedema coma is a rare, severe manifestation of hypothyroidism that can occur in profoundly hypothyroid individuals exposed to an external stress, such as infection, trauma, anesthesia, or cold temperature.[192] Myxedema coma can result in severe, life-threatening hypoxemia and hemodynamic instability and carries a high mortality even in the presence of prompt treatment.[192–195] Although myxedema coma is certainly rare, there have been increasingly frequent case reports of critically ill child presenting with this diagnosis.[195–198]

Neonatal Hypothyroidism

Congenital hypothyroidism remains the most frequent preventable cause of intellectual disability with an increased risk in neonates weighing less than 2 kg or more than 4.5 kg.[180,199] Thyroid dysgenesis or agenesis accounts for the majority of cases, whereas a smaller percentage results from thyroid dyshormonogenesis, secondary, or tertiary hypothyroidism.[180,200] Since most neonates do not exhibit the classic signs or symptoms of hypothyroidism during the perinatal period owing to the transplacental passage of maternal thyroid hormones, testing via the neonatal screen is necessary to diagnose congenital hypothyroidism.[180] Screening programs may measure T4, TSH, or both. Early detection and implementation of thyroid replacement are essential to avoid permanent neurologic sequelae. The classic syndrome of congenital hypothyroidism that develops in the first 3 months of life occurs in countries with no screening programs. The typical findings include macrosomia, enlarged fontanel, macroglossia, coarse facial features, bradycardia, hoarse cry, umbilical hernia, constipation, hypothermia, decreased activity, and neonatal jaundice (Fig. 25.6).[180] In general, affected children who receive adequate thyroid replacement starting early in the neonatal period lead normal lives.[201]

Treatment

The goal of thyroid replacement is to normalize T4 within 1 to 2 weeks and TSH within 4 weeks,[202] reversing the metabolic derangements caused by hypothyroidism. This is typically achieved with daily levothyroxine.[203] The appropriate starting levothyroxine dose varies with age and disease state. For neonates, the starting dose is 10 to 15 μg/kg per day,[180,202,204] which is much greater than the conventional replacement dose of 2 to 6 μg/kg per day in older children and adolescents.[180] Children with severe, chronic hypothyroidism are at risk for developing adverse effects, including headache, insomnia, hyperactivity, or pseudotumor cerebri when initiating treatment at replacement dose and may benefit from starting with smaller doses of levothyroxine and up titrating slowly.[180,205] After titration and stabilization of the dose, children and adolescents should continue to have regular clinical examinations and TSH monitoring owing to increased dose requirements during puberty or pregnancy.[206,207] Thyroid replacement can be given parenterally if needed. The intravenous dose of levothyroxine is approximately half of the oral dose, given once daily.

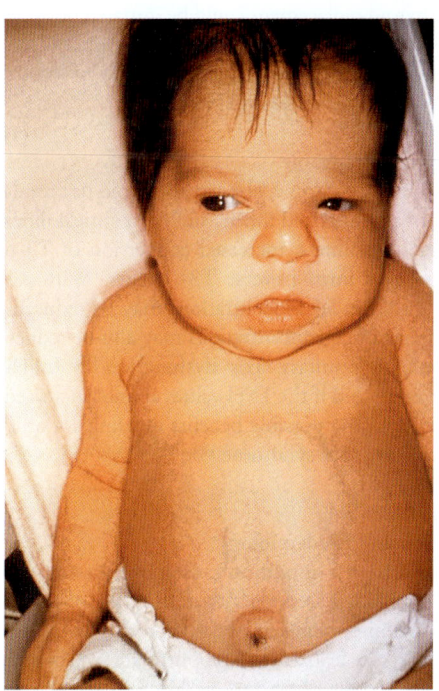

FIGURE 25.6 An infant with congenital hypothyroidism. ("Congenital hypothyroidism." Wikipedia: The Free Encyclopedia. Wikimedia Foundation, Inc., February 24, 2012, http://en.wikipedia.org/wiki/Congenital_hypothyroidism.)

Preoperative Management

Because thyroid hormones play a critical role in regulating metabolism, children should be clinically and biochemically euthyroid before undergoing elective surgery. Children with known hypothyroidism should have documented normal thyroid function tests before surgery. A detailed history should be obtained regarding previous thyroid disorders, head and neck radiation, radioiodine therapy, thyroid surgery, and family history of thyroid disease.[208] The majority of reported complications have occurred in patients with severe, unrecognized hypothyroidism.[209] Children at increased risk of primary hypothyroidism secondary to other autoimmune disorders or genetic syndromes should be screened preoperatively if symptomatic.[180,210–212]

In children with subclinical or mild hypothyroidism, review of limited available clinical data does not reveal an increase in perioperative risk.[178,213] However, for children with moderate to severe hypothyroidism, elective surgery should be postponed when possible, until thyroid hormone concentrations normalize on replacement therapy. Inadequate preoperative treatment increases the risk for impaired cardiac function, bradyarrhythmia, abnormal response to hypercapnia and hypoxia, delayed gastric emptying, hypothermia, and increased sensitivity to anesthetics.[209,214–217] Preoperative sedation should be minimized as these patients may be very sensitive to opioids and benzodiazepines.[214,215] When urgent surgery is required, perioperative treatment with intravenous levothyroxine should be given to minimize complications.[122,208,215] Since these children may also have adrenal insufficiency and because thyroid replacement may precipitate an adrenal crisis, glucocorticoids should also be administered.[209,215] An exception to this strategy applies to the child presenting for cardiovascular surgery or cardiac catheterization because of the concern that a rapid increase in thyroid function could increase myocardial oxygen demand, thereby precipitating or worsening unstable coronary syndromes. Several studies have reported no adverse outcomes in cardiac patients undergoing surgery without thyroid replacement.[122,208,213,218] Therefore thyroid replacement could be initiated postoperatively in children with cardiovascular disease; however, many endocrinologists recommend starting with a minimal dose of levothyroxine in consultation with the cardiologist.[215]

Sick Euthyroid Syndrome

In sick euthyroid syndrome, abnormal thyroid test results occur in the setting of a nonthyroid illness, such as a critical illness. During times of stress or illness, increased conversion of T3 to a metabolically inactive form (reverse T3) occurs. With more severe illness, T4 and free T4 concentrations may be reduced. Thyroid-stimulating hormone concentrations may also be reduced because of hypothalamic-pituitary axis dysfunction.[180] Individuals are considered euthyroid if the TSH values are not increased. Controversy exists regarding possible benefits of using T4 or T3 therapy to treat sick euthyroid syndrome.[180,219–221]

HYPERTHYROIDISM

Classification and Epidemiology

Hyperthyroidism is a condition caused by excess circulating thyroid hormones either secondary to destruction of thyroid follicles leading to inappropriate release of thyroid hormone or nondestructive processes leading to inappropriate synthesis of thyroid hormone. Excess thyroid hormone leads to increased metabolic activity in the peripheral tissues and hallmark clinical symptoms. Almost all children with hyperthyroidism have suppressed serum TSH concentrations resulting from negative feedback by the increased concentrations of T4 and T3. Overt hyperthyroidism is characterized by both biochemical and clinical manifestations of the disease. A child with subclinical hyperthyroidism has reduced TSH concentrations but is typically asymptomatic.[222,223]

In children, *hyper*thyroidism occurs less frequently than *hypo*thyroidism and is nearly always caused by Graves disease. Other causes of childhood thyrotoxicosis include autoimmune thyroiditis (Hashimoto thyroiditis), autonomously functioning thyroid nodules, infections of the thyroid gland, iodine-induced hyperthyroidism, TSH-secreting pituitary adenomas, thyroid hormone ingestion, and as a result of therapy for treatment of malignancy with checkpoint inhibitors or radiation therapy.[224–226] Hyperthyroidism can be associated with McCune-Albright syndrome, a triad of fibrous dysplasia of bone, café-au-lait skin spots, and precocious puberty.[226,227] A rare thyroid disorder that mimics the increased levels of T4 and T3 in hyperthyroidism is thyroid hormone resistance. However, unlike other causes of childhood thyrotoxicosis, thyroid hormone resistance should not be treated with antithyroid medications.[228,229]

Graves Disease

Graves disease is the most common cause of childhood hyperthyroidism. The pathogenesis of Graves disease is unclear but is believed to result from a complex interaction of genetic, immune, and environmental factors.[225,230] Graves disease occurs more frequently in children with other autoimmune diseases or with a condition associated with autoimmunity, as in Turner syndrome, trisomy 21, or DiGeorge syndrome.[231] In Graves disease, the immune system produces antibodies to the TSH receptor. These antibodies bind to and stimulate the TSH receptors found on the thyroid follicular cells, causing excessive synthesis and secretion of thyroid hormone. Most children with Graves disease have a smooth, diffusely enlarged goiter, ocular signs, as well as the systemic signs and symptoms associated with thyrotoxicosis.[225] Because few children with Graves disease enter spontaneous remission, treatment of hyperthyroidism is required.

Thyroiditis

The term *thyroiditis* is used to describe a heterogeneous group of disorders that result in inflammation of the thyroid gland with subsequent release of preformed thyroid hormone. Hashimoto thyroiditis is the most common form of thyroiditis in children.[226] Transient hyperthyroidism can result from the initial inflammatory process, and symptoms generally last up to about 8 weeks, until preformed stored thyroid hormone is depleted. The majority of children with Hashimoto thyroiditis present with a goiter but are asymptomatic.[180] In some children, antibodies that stimulate the TSH receptors on the thyroid follicular cells are present, prolonging the hyperthyroid phase.[232] In children who are symptomatic during the transient hyperthyroid phase, cardioselective β-blockers (e.g., metoprolol, atenolol) should be used to control symptoms. In children with stimulating TSH receptor antibodies, antithyroid drugs are needed to supplement the β-blockers since thyroid hormone is being produced.[232] Some children develop hypothyroidism after the recovery phase as a result of lymphocytic infiltration of the thyroid gland and destruction of thyroid tissue.

Thyroiditis can also manifest as painful inflammation of the gland and fever secondary to bacterial or viral infection. *Haemophilus influenzae*, group A streptococci, and *Staphylococcus spp.* are the most frequent causes of acute infectious thyroiditis, which can be complicated by thyroid gland cutaneous fistulae.[233] Viral infections of the thyroid gland are less severe. Owing to the

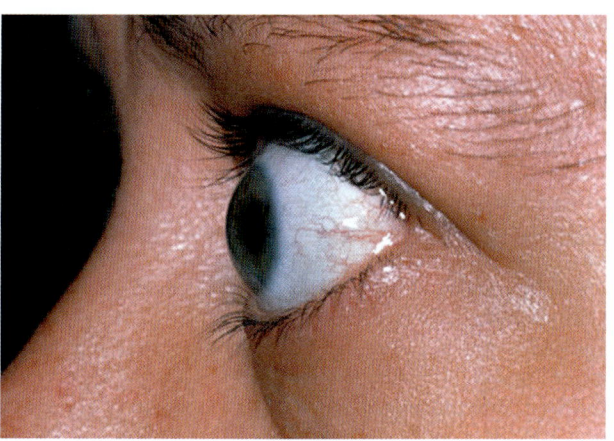

FIGURE 25.7 Proptosis of the eyes in a child with Graves disease.

difficulty in distinguishing bacterial from viral infections, all cases of infectious thyroiditis are treated with antibiotics. Treatment with antithyroid drugs is not indicated, but if the child is symptomatic, β-blockers should be used.

Clinical Manifestations

Most of the symptoms that children experience are ubiquitous regardless of the cause of hyperthyroidism. Classic signs and symptoms of hyperthyroidism include goiter, tachycardia, palpitations, dyspnea, fatigue, proximal muscle weakness, tremor, brisk reflexes, heat intolerance, insomnia, nervousness, increased frequency of bowel movements, and weight loss despite a normal or increased appetite.[225,230,234] Many children with hyperthyroidism have an inability to concentrate, resulting in poor school performance, and may be initially mistaken for attention deficit hyperactivity disorder. Other medical conditions associated with longstanding hyperthyroidism include growth acceleration and advancement in epiphyseal maturation, delay in onset of puberty, and irregular menses.[225,235]

Children with Graves disease may develop additional autoimmune manifestations. Pretibial myxedema and dermopathy are rare in children.[231,234] Ocular involvement in Graves disease is characterized by autoimmune inflammation and edema of the retroorbital tissue and extraocular muscles, resulting in proptosis and impaired ocular muscle function.[234] Children with Graves ophthalmopathy often complain of eye irritation or ocular dryness because of lid retraction, which is due to increased adrenergic tone of the ocular muscles resulting in a prominent stare (Fig. 25.7). If left untreated, corneal ulceration may develop and lead to irreversible eye damage, including blindness. Once hyperthyroidism is treated, the lid retraction and "adrenergic stare" resolve quickly, but proptosis from Graves ophthalmopathy usually persists or regresses only slightly.[225,236,237]

Treatment

Current treatment options include antithyroid medications, radioactive iodine therapy, or surgical removal of the thyroid gland.[225,230,236] Antithyroid medications are the least invasive treatment option and they remain the first line of treatment for children. Methimazole is the medication of choice for children with Graves disease. Minor adverse effects occur in 14% to 25% of children treated with thioamides and include nausea, skin rash, arthralgias, myalgias, gastrointestinal problems, and neutropenia.

Serious adverse effects occur in <2% of children and include agranulocytosis, hepatitis, liver failure, vasculitis with a lupus-like syndrome and Stevens-Johnson syndrome. Propylthiouracil is no longer recommended for treatment of Graves disease in children because of the unacceptable risk of hepatotoxicity and liver failure.[225,231] However, even after 2 years of therapy with antithyroid medication, the rate of sustained remission after withdrawal of the medication is low, approximately 25% to 40%.[225,231] Favorable predictors of remission in Graves disease after treatment include a small thyroid gland and milder disease at time of diagnosis, older age, postpubertal status, decrease in stimulating TSH receptor antibodies over time, presence of other autoimmune diseases, and duration of treatment longer than 2 years.[225,230] In those patients with relapsing disease after withdrawal of antithyroid medications, options for further treatment include continuing long-term therapy with methimazole, or consideration for radioactive iodine therapy or subtotal thyroidectomy.[238]

Definitive therapy with radioactive iodine is appealing to some patients as it carries less risk than surgery.[239] Radioactive iodine therapy is used for adolescents who fail initial therapy with antithyroid medications, either due to relapse after treatment noncompliance, or serious adverse reaction. It is also used for children older than 5 years of age who require immediate, definitive therapy. Although radioactive iodine therapy aims to induce hypothyroidism, it is notable that only 70% of patients achieve this result with initial treatment.[240] A subsequent dose may improve treatment success. Radioactive iodine has been considered a safe therapy for many years and longitudinal studies have shown that children are not at increased risk for developing thyroid cancer; however, a retrospective 24-year extension of the multicenter Cooperative Thyrotoxicosis Therapy Follow-up Study raised concern for a modest increase in death from solid cancer associated with radioactive iodine in adults.[225,231,241] In a small retrospective study that examined the applicability of adult guidelines for risk stratification after diagnosis and treatment of differentiated thyroid cancer to children, gender and pubertal status at the presentation of the disease influenced the clinical course and outcome.[242] Further studies are needed to assess longer-term risk in pediatric patients.[240]

Thyroidectomy is reserved for children and adolescents with a large thyroid gland, a history of failed drug therapy, severe ocular disease, or poor response to radioactive iodine therapy. Surgeons with expertise performing thyroidectomies in children should undertake the surgery because of the potential for serious complications, including hemorrhage, transient or permanent hypoparathyroidism, and vocal cord paralysis.[225,231]

Perioperative Management

Children should be euthyroid or slightly hypothyroid before surgery to minimize complications and avoid precipitation of thyroid storm, an endocrine emergency that can be difficult to diagnose and treat intraoperatively. The possibility of airway compromise related to a large goiter should be considered and carefully evaluated.

In children with uncontrolled hyperthyroidism, surgery should be postponed until thyroid hormone concentrations normalize with therapy. If presenting for emergency surgery, careful preparation of the patient is essential and may include administration of antithyroid drugs, iodine, β-blockers, and corticosteroids.[215,243] Uncontrolled hyperthyroidism can be ameliorated by administering oral iodine (Lugol solution or saturated solution of potassium iodine) to block further release of thyroid hormone from the thyroid gland.[215,244] Excess iodine transiently inhibits thyroid hormone release (the Wolff-Chaikoff effect).[244] Iodine should not be administered before methimazole treatment as it may paradoxically increase the amount of thyroid hormone released.[215,244]

Rarely, untreated or undertreated hyperthyroidism can lead to thyroid storm, which has a reported incidence of 0.1 to 3 per 100,000 hospitalized patients.[245] A systematic review of the risk of thyroid storm yielded no randomized studies and the remainder were of poor quality precluding an assessment of which patients were at increased risk for thyroid storm.[246] Based on case reports, the frequency of thyroid storm in hyperthyroid patients, whether treated or not, ranged from 0% to 14%.[246] In children without a history of thyroid disease, the incidence of storm is 1:1,000,000 children and 3:100,000 adolescents.[247] Thyroid storm is usually precipitated by a second superimposed insult, such as infection, trauma, surgery, or diabetic ketoacidosis.[244] The clinical signs of thyroid storm are nonspecific; however, laboratory tests are diagnostic: low to undetectable TSH levels and increased free T4 levels.[247] Thyroid storm may be difficult to differentiate from an acute malignant hyperthermia (MH) reaction.[248,249] However, in contrast to MH, thyroid storm has a more variable onset (usually an insidious onset 6–18 hours postoperatively, although it can develop precipitously during surgery), it induces a less severe metabolic acidosis than MH, and the serum creatine phosphokinase (CPK) remains unchanged. However, since the serum creatine phosphokinase peaks at 12 to 18 hours after an MH reaction, it is a late sign to differentiate thyrotoxicosis from MH. If the presentation proves difficult to distinguish from MH (both diseases may present with tachycardia, rigidity, and fever), it is prudent to administer dantrolene sodium 2.5 mg/kg intravenously.[250] However, if the hypermetabolic signs abate after dantrolene, one cannot conclude that the reaction was MH, since dantrolene attenuates the hypermetabolic signs of thyroid storm as well.[249] The differential diagnosis for such a presentation also includes neuroleptic malignant syndrome and pheochromocytoma.[215]

If thyroid storm is suspected, immediate, aggressive management is essential to avoid death.[193,224,248] The mortality rate from thyroid storm is 10% to 30%.[212,251,252] The recommended treatment for thyroid storm remains a multidrug approach to (1) block production and release of thyroid hormone, (2) prevent conversion of T4 to T3, (3) antagonize the peripheral (adrenergic) effects of thyroid hormone, and (4) control systemic disturbances with supportive therapy (Table 25.5).[194,236,244,253–257] Pharmacologic treatment includes administration of parenteral β-blockers, methimazole or propylthiouracil, glucocorticoids (which decrease conversion of T4 to T3 and prevents relative adrenal insufficiency), and antipyretics (acetaminophen).[215,243,248]

Parathyroid and Calcium Disorders

PHYSIOLOGY OF CALCIUM HOMEOSTASIS

The four parathyroid glands are usually present in two pairs on the posterior aspect of the superior and inferior poles of the thyroid gland, with the inferior pair occasionally ectopic elsewhere in the neck or chest. Parathyroid hormone (PTH) is released from

TABLE 25.5	Management of Hyperthyroid Crisis		
Drug Class	**Recommended Drug**	**Starting Dose**	**Mechanism of Action**
Iodine	Potassium iodide (SSKI)	3–5 drops by mouth q6 hours	Blocks release of thyroid hormone from gland
	Lugol solution	4–8 drops by mouth q6–8 hours	Blocks release of thyroid hormone from gland
β-Blockers	Propranolol	Infant: 2 mg/kg per day by mouth divided q8–12 hours	β-adrenergic blockade; decreased T₄ to T₃ conversion
		Child: 10–40 mg by mouth q6–8 hours	
	Esmolol	100–200 μg/kg per minute intravenous infusion	β-adrenergic blockade; decreased T₄ to T₃ conversion
Thioamide	Methimazole	0.4 mg/kg per day by mouth divided q8–12 hours	Inhibits new hormone synthesis
Supportive treatment	Intravenous fluid	20–40 mL/kg normal saline	Replacement of increased insensible losses resulting from fever, diaphoresis, vomiting, and diarrhea
	Cooling blankets, ice packs	Reduce fever	
	Acetaminophen	Children 2–12 years:	Reduce fever
		15 mg/kg q6 hours or 12.5 mg/kg q4 hours; maximum daily dose: 75 mg/kg per day (≤4 g/day)	
		Adolescents >12 years:	
		<50 kg: 15 mg/kg q6 hours or 12.5 mg/kg q4 hours; maximum single dose: 750 mg/dose; maximum daily dose: 75 mg/kg per day (≤4 g/day)	
		≥50 kg: 1000 mg q6 hours or 650 mg q4 hours; maximum single dose: 1000 mg/dose; maximum daily dose: 4 g/day	
	Hydrocortisone	2 mg/kg intravenous q8 hours (maximum single dose 100 mg)	Decreases T₄ to T₃ conversion; enhances vasomotor stability

SSKI, Saturated solution of potassium iodide.

secretory granules in response to a decrease in serum ionized calcium. Its secretion is inhibited by hyperphosphatemia, profound hypomagnesemia or hypermagnesemia, or increased 1,25-dihydroxyvitamin D (calcitriol). The calcium-sensing receptor in the parathyroid mediates PTH release. PTH has three primary modes of increasing serum calcium: (1) increased renal tubular reabsorption of calcium as well as decreased reabsorption of phosphate; (2) upregulation of osteoclast-mediated calcium and phosphate release from bone; and (3) renal conversion of 25-hydroxyvitamin D to the active metabolite, calcitriol. In turn, calcitriol increases absorption of calcium and phosphate from the gastrointestinal tract and has direct calcium-releasing effects on bone. Calcitonin is secreted by the thyroid C cells and has calcium-reducing properties via its own G protein–coupled receptor.

HYPOCALCEMIA

Neonatal Hypocalcemia

Although mild neonatal hypocalcemia is common and frequently asymptomatic, neonates with moderate to severe hypocalcemia typically present with tetany, seizures, apnea, or cardiac rhythm disturbances that can be life threatening.[258] Neonatal hypocalcemia owing to prematurity, perinatal stress/asphyxia, and maternal diabetes is common but typically transient.[259,260] Less common causes include maternal hyperparathyroidism, transient neonatal hypoparathyroidism, vitamin D deficiency, excessive diuretic use or phosphate load, and congenital hypoparathyroidism.[260] Maternal vitamin D deficiency remains a cause of infant hypocalcemia in the United States despite routine prenatal vitamin D supplementation and regardless of the infant's dietary intake.[258,261,262]

The most common cause of congenital hypoparathyroidism is DiGeorge syndrome (also known as velocardiofacial syndrome or 22q11.2 deletion).[259,260] The degree of parathyroid hypoplasia in DiGeorge syndrome is variable, so hypocalcemia may present during infancy, childhood, or only during periods of stress.[259] Other causes of congenital hypoparathyroidism include isolated hypoparathyroidism, hypercalciuric hypocalcemia, activating mutations in the calcium-sensing receptor, mitochondrial disorders (Kearns-Sayre syndrome, mitochondrial encephalopathy), and metabolic syndromes (Kenny-Caffey syndrome).[258–260,263] Reduced PTH or PTH resistance (pseudohypoparathyroidism) cause hyperphosphatemia beyond the already increased normal range in neonates, whereas vitamin D deficiency or resistance is associated with low to normal serum phosphate concentrations.

Childhood Hypocalcemia

Etiologies for hypocalcemia in children include hypoparathyroidism (congenital and acquired), insensitivity to PTH (pseudohypoparathyroidism), disorders of vitamin D supply or metabolism, and calcium/phosphorus/magnesium disorders.[259,264,265] Acquired hypoparathyroidism may be due to infiltrative disease of the parathyroid gland (hemochromatosis, Wilson disease, granulomatous disease, or metastatic cancer), autoimmune hypoparathyroidism (polyglandular autoimmune disease type1), or postsurgical complications of thyroid or parathyroid surgery.

Persistent hypocalcemia in infants and children can have many manifestations, including poor feeding, circumoral numbness, paresthesias, laryngospasm, tetany, seizures, myocardial dysfunction, and myopathy.[265] Initial evaluation of hypocalcemia includes measurement of serum calcium, phosphate, magnesium, alkaline phosphatase, creatinine, PTH, 25-hydroxyvitamin D, and 1,25-dihydroxyvitamin D, as well as assessment of urine calcium, phosphate, and creatinine. Therapy for acute hypocalcemia includes

parenteral calcium, followed by oral calcium supplementation and 25-hydroxyvitamin D if reduced,[262] and calcitriol. Notably, conventional long-term therapy for hypoparathyroidism with calcium and calcitriol can lead to treatment-related complications, including episodes of hypocalcemia from undertreatment or hypercalcemia from supratherapeutic dosing, sequelae of longstanding hypercalciuria, including nephrocalcinosis and ultimately chronic renal disease[266] and systemic calcific deposits, most notably in the basal ganglia, leading to potential for extrapyramidal symptoms and psychosis.[267,268] Although use of recombinant human PTH to treat hypoparathyroidism may be more physiologic and avoids many of these treatment-related adverse effects, widespread use in children and adults has been limited. Particularly in pediatric patients, there has been concern for potential risk of developing osteosarcoma based on animal models, which ultimately lead to a black box warning.[269] However, recombinant human PTH is used in the subset of patients who do not respond well to conventional therapy and available studies in adults and children have not shown an increased risk of malignancy.[264,269–272]

Perioperative Management

Hypocalcemia is usually managed by intravenous infusion of calcium in the form of calcium chloride or calcium gluconate, with frequent measurement of serum ionized calcium concentrations to guide therapy. Administration via a central venous catheter is recommended as inadvertent extravasation of hypertonic solutions of concentrated ionized calcium into the interstitial space causes intense local vasoconstriction that may lead to necrosis of the skin and subcutaneous tissues, and in some instances, gangrene of the affected limb. In the postoperative period after the child is tolerating oral intake, intravenous calcium supplementation may be converted to oral supplementation.

HYPERCALCEMIA

Hypercalcemia is an uncommon finding in children.[273,274] Parathyroid causes of hypercalcemia include neonatal hyperparathyroidism, primary hyperparathyroidism, parathyroid hyperplasia, familial hypocalciuric hypercalcemia (familial benign hypercalcemia), and rarely, parathyroid carcinoma.[275] In children and adolescents, 65% of cases of hyperparathyroidism may be attributed to a single parathyroid adenoma that is unresponsive to increases in serum calcium level.[273]

Parathyroid hyperplasia occurs in familial forms of hyperparathyroidism, including multiple endocrine neoplasia type 1 (MEN 1), in which hyperparathyroidism is the presenting manifestation the majority of the time.[273,276,277] MEN 1 is also associated with pancreatic and pituitary tumors.[276,277] Hyperparathyroidism is a less common manifestation of MEN 2A, in which medullary thyroid carcinoma and pheochromocytoma occur.[278] Some mutations in the calcium-sensing receptor gene result in a greater serum calcium set point in familial hypocalciuric hypercalcemia (familial benign hypercalcemia), an incidental diagnosis that is benign.[279,280] However, other mutations in the calcium-sensing receptor gene can also lead to a life-threatening form of neonatal severe hyperparathyroidism.[273] Secondary hyperparathyroidism with relatively normal calcium levels is a common pediatric phenomenon that accompanies renal failure, renal tubular acidosis, and hypophosphatemic rickets.[281]

When hypercalcemia is present, the differential diagnosis should also include Williams syndrome (associated with hypercalcemia in 15% cases), vitamin A intoxication, vitamin D intoxication, hypophosphatasia, granulomatous disorders, subcutaneous fat necrosis, immobility, and medications (thiazide diuretics, lithium, theophylline).[273,282] Solid tumors may secrete parathyroid hormone–related protein (PTHrP). Tumors, such as leukemias, lymphomas, and others, may release excess cytokines and osteoclast-activating factors. Not infrequently, hypercalcemia may be the presenting finding that leads to the diagnosis of a new malignancy.[283,284]

Signs and symptoms of hypercalcemia are usually nonspecific, such as nausea and vomiting, failure to thrive, irritability, polyuria, constipation, and fatigue. Initial laboratory evaluation of hypercalcemia is similar to that for hypocalcemia.[285] Moreover, evaluation of unexplained hypercalcemia may also warrant additional hormone or genetic testing for MEN syndromes, measurement of PTHrP for malignancy, blood for tumor markers, bone marrow biopsy, and relevant imaging. When hyperparathyroidism is found, ultrasonography is helpful to assess the parathyroid glands, but MRI or technetium-sestamibi scan is more precise, especially at locating ectopic tissue.[286]

Perioperative Management

Management of acute hypercalcemia begins with discontinuing or minimizing all sources of calcium (enteral/parenteral feeds, total parenteral nutrition). Children should be aggressively hydrated with isotonic fluids. The administration of a loop diuretic, such as furosemide, increases urinary calcium excretion and may be helpful once adequate hydration has been achieved.[287] Calcitonin, which inhibits bone resorption, helps to decrease the serum calcium concentration, although tachyphylaxis may occur within 1 or 2 days.[273] Bisphosphonates are potent inhibitors of bone resorption; a single dose can rapidly reduce the serum calcium concentration with an effect that lasts 2 to 4 weeks. Pamidronate is the preferred medication in children.[273,287] Glucocorticoids may also be useful as they inhibit synthesis of 1,25-dihydroxyvitamin D3.

Definitive therapy for primary hyperparathyroidism is parathyroidectomy.[273,286–288] Acute management after parathyroidectomy requires careful monitoring and replacement of calcium and possibly the use of calcitriol for persistent hypocalcemia, which is challenging to manage as described earlier. In isolated parathyroid hyperplasia, MEN, or secondary hyperparathyroidism, surgeons may elect to leave a portion of one gland in the forearm to avoid permanent hypoparathyroidism.

Adrenal Disorders

PHYSIOLOGY

Adrenal steroidogenesis begins with cholesterol as a precursor and results in three types of steroids: mineralocorticoids, glucocorticoids, and sex steroids (androgen precursors).[289] Most of the enzymes involved in adrenal (or gonadal) steroidogenesis are cytochrome P450 types. The adrenal cortex consists of three zones: the outer zona glomerulosa, which exclusively synthesizes mineralocorticoids owing to localized expression of *CYP11B2*, whereas the zona fasciculata and reticularis synthesize glucocorticoid and androgens owing to localized expression of *CYP17*.[290]

Cortisol, the end product of the glucocorticoid pathway, is the primary regulator of the hypothalamic-pituitary-adrenal axis (HPAA), providing a negative feedback loop regulating hypothalamic release of corticotropin-releasing hormone (CRH), pituitary secretion of adrenocorticotropic hormone (ACTH), and downstream adrenal production of steroids (Fig. 25.8). ACTH release follows a diurnal pattern with a peak between 0400 to 0800 hours. ACTH markedly increases in response to trauma, acute illness, high fever, and hypoglycemia.

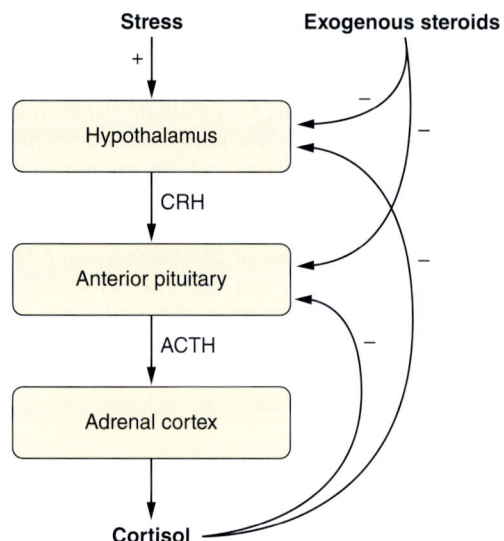

FIGURE 25.8 Hypothalamic-pituitary-adrenal axis. *ACTH*, Adrenocorticotropic hormone; *CRH*, corticotropin-releasing hormone; −, negative feedback; +, positive feedback. (Reproduced with permission from Liu MM, Reidy AB, Saatee S, Collard CD. Perioperative steroid management: approaches based on current evidence. *Anesthesiology*. 2017;127(1):166-172.))

Mineralocorticoid production is primarily controlled by the renin-angiotensin system, in which angiotensinogen is cleaved by renin to angiotensin I, which is then converted to angiotensin II.[291] The mineralocorticoid pathway is also responsive to ACTH; an increase in all mineralocorticoid precursors and the end product aldosterone occurs within minutes of exogenous ACTH stimulation. However, hypopituitarism does not lead to mineralocorticoid deficiency because an intact renin-angiotensin system can independently stimulate aldosterone synthesis.

Patients with ACTH deficiency may present with hyponatremia (because glucocorticoids are required for free water excretion) and hypotension. Cortisol enhances vascular responsiveness to catecholamines, maintains cardiac output, and stimulates inotropic activity.[292,293] Volume depletion from loss of salt and water together with absence of these hemodynamic effects are the most lethal potential consequence of adrenal insufficiency and requires the utmost caution on the part of pediatrician, endocrinologist, surgeon, or anesthesiologist. When any question regarding adequacy of the HPAA arises perioperatively, it is prudent to provide exogenous glucocorticoid.[294,295]

CAUSES OF ADRENAL INSUFFICIENCY

Primary adrenal insufficiency, also called Addison disease, is caused by the destruction of the adrenal gland, most commonly by autoimmunity, infection, or hemorrhage.[296] Affected patients may present with lack of energy, weight loss, nausea and vomiting, poor appetite, and, specifically, the characteristic skin hyperpigmentation that is secondary to melanocyte-stimulating hormone receptor cross-stimulation by ACTH. Treatment requires both glucocorticoid and mineralocorticoid replacement. Congenital disorders causing adrenal insufficiency include adrenoleukodystrophy,[297] congenital adrenal hypoplasia, X-linked adrenal hypoplasia congenita, ACTH receptor defects,[298] and congenital adrenal hyperplasia, which may or may not have associated mineralocorticoid loss.[299,300]

Secondary adrenal insufficiency occurs when congenital or acquired lesions of the hypothalamus or pituitary lead to ACTH deficiency. These conditions are typically associated with other pituitary deficiencies, particularly growth hormone or TSH deficiency. Central nervous system malformations associated with hypopituitarism including septo-optic dysplasia and associated midline defects are usually detectable by MRI.[301–303] Acquired lesions that lead to hypopituitarism include tumors such as craniopharyngioma, radiation, hydrocephalus, meningitis, infiltrative disorders,[304] and histiocytosis X.[305] Tumor resection, especially craniopharyngioma, cranial irradiation, and chemotherapy, can lead to multiple pituitary deficiencies, often evolving over years.[202] Secondary adrenal insufficiency usually requires glucocorticoid, but not mineralocorticoid replacement if the renin-angiotensin system is intact.

Iatrogenic adrenal insufficiency occurs when exogenous glucocorticoids are used in chronic treatment regiments such as autoimmune disorders, suppression of transplant rejection, and control of inflammatory processes. Exogenous glucocorticoids inhibit the HPAA, decreasing CRH and ACTH production (see Fig. 25.8). This leads to atrophy of the adrenal glands, which are unable to respond normally to stress caused by acute febrile illness, trauma, or surgical procedures. In awake patients, abdominal pain, nausea, hypotension, and weakness may be presenting symptoms. However, the typical presentation of adrenal insufficiency is hypotension during anesthesia that is poorly responsive to vasopressors and fluids. A high index of suspicion is required to make this diagnosis in anesthetized patients.

TESTING FOR ADRENAL INSUFFICIENCY

Physiologic serum cortisol concentrations follow a diurnal pattern, with concentrations peaking during an ACTH surge in the early morning and waning later in the day. A morning serum cortisol concentration of less than 5 μg/dL may be suggestive of adrenal insufficiency and should prompt further testing.[295] A reduced concentration at any other time of day is uninformative and should not be used to test for adrenal function.

Primary adrenal insufficiency is typically assessed with the ACTH stimulation test, where exogenous ACTH (cosyntropin [Cortrosyn]), is administered and cortisol subsequently measured. Measurement of morning cortisol and ACTH as a preliminary test may be used if ACTH stimulation is unavailable. More sophisticated strategies, including the nuances of high versus low dose ACTH stimulation, CRH stimulation, and in depth evaluation of the HPAA may be obtained in consultation with an endocrinologist.[295,306]

In contrast to glucocorticoid deficiency, primary mineralocorticoid deficiency can be diagnosed with a random serum sample that shows low aldosterone concentration despite markedly increased plasma renin activity.

Glucocorticoid Dosing

The adrenal gland normally secretes 8 to 10 mg/m² of cortisol daily, which may increase as much as 200 mg/day with illness or surgery. In general, the recommended starting replacement dose of hydrocortisone for primary adrenal insufficiency is 8 mg/m² per day.[295] Dosing is adjusted based on the child's growth rate, weight gain, appetite, and energy levels.[295] Fludrocortisone (Florinef) is added to the medication regimen if the child shows evidence of mineralocorticoid deficiency. The adequacy of mineralocorticoid therapy is determined by blood pressure monitoring and plasma renin activity. In congenital adrenal hyperplasia, where the primary goal of glucocorticoid therapy is not replacement but

TABLE 25.6	Steroid Equivalency Ratios and Doses[293,351]		
Steroid	Relative Antiinflammatory Potency	Relative Mineralocorticoid Potency	Equivalent Dose (mg)
Hydrocortisone (Cortisol)	1	1	20
Cortisone	0.8	0.8	25
Prednisone	4	0.8	5
Prednisolone	4	0.8	5
Methylprednisolone	5	0.5	4
Dexamethasone	25–50	0	0.5–0.75

suppression of ACTH secretion, the daily hydrocortisone dose is typically 10 to 15 mg/m², guided by laboratory monitoring of the serum concentrations of 17-hydroxyprogesterone, androstenedione, dehydroepiandrosterone sulfate, and testosterone.[300] Alternatives to hydrocortisone include prednisone, which is four to five times more potent than hydrocortisone. Dexamethasone is 30 to 40 times more potent than hydrocortisone, but carries more important risks of adverse effects with long-term replacement therapy such as growth impairment, osteopenia and aseptic necrosis of the femoral head.[300] In addition, dexamethasone does not have mineralocorticoid effects and is not the steroid of choice if both mineralocorticoid and glucocorticoid replacement is required (Table 25.6).

PERIOPERATIVE MANAGEMENT OF ADRENAL INSUFFICIENCY

For patients who have diagnosed HPAA suppression or who are at high risk for adrenal insufficiency, stress dose steroids are required for any procedures likely to cause physiologic stress, typically 50 mg/m² (up to 100 mg) of hydrocortisone at induction of anesthesia with redosing of 12.5 mg/m² every 6 hours during surgery.[295] A postoperative steroid taper should be planned depending on the patient and procedure for at least 24 hours after surgery. Stress dose steroids may not be required for minor low-stress procedures if the regular daily steroid replacement is continued through the perioperative period.[293,295,307]

Patients taking daily doses of prednisone less than 5 mg (in teenagers) or 10 mg/m² (in younger children) and with treatment periods of less than 3 to 4 weeks are unlikely to have HPAA suppression.[293,307] In these patients, it may be reasonable to continue their usual daily dose, monitor for signs of adrenal insufficiency, and only administer stress doses if signs of HPAA suppression are identified.[293,307]

Long-term high-dose treatment may require up to 6 to 9 months for complete return of normal HPAA function and necessitates a gradual taper. Perioperative steroid coverage should be administered if there is any concern about the integrity of the HPAA during an ongoing steroid taper.

For even the lowest risk patient where stress dosing is deferred, close monitoring and low threshold for stress dosing in the perioperative setting is recommended given the low risk of harm with short-term stress-dose steroid treatment compared with the life-threatening risk of perioperative adrenal crisis.[293,295,307]

HYPERCORTISOLISM (CUSHING SYNDROME)

Excess cortisol, whether exogenous or endogenous, results in muscle wasting, truncal obesity, moon facies, hypertension, hyperglycemia, osteopenia, and growth deceleration.[308,309] Iatrogenic hypercortisolism is common in pediatrics,[310] whereas Cushing disease or syndrome are rare.[311] Cushing disease refers to an ACTH-secreting pituitary adenoma. Cushing syndrome refers to other conditions of excess glucocorticoid, including ectopic ACTH-secreting tumors[312] and adrenal tumors that secrete cortisol.[313] An adrenal tumor (adenoma or carcinoma) is the most likely cause of hypercortisolism in a young child. These tumors can secrete any combination of steroids and commonly co-secrete androgens, resulting in virilization.[314] A unilateral glucocorticoid-secreting tumor typically causes HPAA suppression, requiring careful tapering of hydrocortisone replacement after resection to reestablish normal production of cortisol in the contralateral adrenal gland.[315]

Therapy for Cushing disease and Cushing syndrome is surgical.[316,317] Anesthetic considerations include the supportive management of secondary manifestations, such as obesity and its attendant airway concerns, hypertension, and skin and bone fragility.

Pheochromocytoma

Pheochromocytomas and paragangliomas are rare neuroendocrine tumors that arise from neural crest–derived cells. They can occur anywhere from the base of the skull to the pelvis where paraganglia are found.[318,319] Pheochromocytomas arise from the adrenal medulla whereas paragangliomas arise from extra-adrenal locations. The latter can be further subdivided into sympathetic and parasympathetic tumors. Functional tumors produce catecholamines and are known as chromaffin tumors. These tumors derive their name from the dark gray-brown immunostaining of chromogranin A by chromium salts.[320]

ETIOLOGY

Nearly 80% of functional paraganglial tumors occur in the adrenal medulla and are referred to as pheochromocytomas. The other 20% of cases arise from extra-adrenal paraganglionic tissue.[318,319] The overall incidence of pheochromocytoma is estimated in the general population at approximately 0.3 cases per million population per year.[320] About 10% to 20% of all pheochromocytomas are diagnosed in childhood, with an average age at the time of onset of 11 years.[318,320] In large registries of pediatric paraganglial tumors, there appears to be a male predominance in childhood, whereas during the reproductive years, this shifts to a greater female predominance with the net effect being an equal distribution in the sexes.[321] In contrast to adults, pheochromocytomas in children are more often benign, bilateral, multiple in number, and extra-adrenal.[320]

Although only 5% to 10% of pediatric paraganglial tumors are thought to be malignant, metastases can be widespread and have been found in the bones, lungs, lymph nodes, and liver.[318,319] The European-American Pheochromocytoma-Paraganglioma Registry reports that as many as 80% of patients diagnosed before 18 years of age had a germline mutation in one of the known susceptibility genes.[322] To date, mutations in at least 10 susceptibility genes have been linked with pheochromocytoma-associated cancer syndromes such as von Hippel-Lindau (*VHL*), multiple endocrine neoplasia (*MEN*) type 2, neurofibromatosis 1, paraganglionic syndromes types 1–4, and familial pheochromocytoma syndromes.[322,323] Germline succinate dehydrogenase gene mutations (SDHx) involving the mitochondrial enzyme complex are now a well described part of the familial paraganglioma and pheochromocytoma syndromes. Importantly the SDHB gene mutation

carries a high rate of malignancy.[324] Additionally, tuberous sclerosis and the Carney triad have also been associated with pheochromocytomas. Nearly one-half of patients with Carney triad syndrome will develop paraganglioma-pheochromocytomas, and tumors have decreased SDH enzymatic activity.[325]

CLINICAL PRESENTATION

The clinical presentation of paraganglial tumors in children can vary greatly and may be due to catecholamine secretion or from mass effect. Tumors may also be found as incidental radiologic findings or as part of screening for one of the hereditary syndromes.[320] Functional pheochromocytomas and paragangliomas can secrete different catecholamines, including epinephrine, norepinephrine, and dopamine. Norepinephrine is the most predominant hormone secreted, whereas only 10% to 20% of tumors secrete epinephrine and dopamine. However, there is no direct relationship between circulating catecholamine concentrations and overt symptoms.

Hypertension is the most typical presenting symptom in children, but it may be sustained rather than paroxysmal as is often the case in adults,[326] and is usually not associated with tumors that primarily secrete dopamine. Another common presentation in children is regular, intermittent headaches often associated with nausea and vomiting. Other reported findings include weight loss, polyuria, visual disturbances, and anxiety.[327] Although extremely rare, epinephrine-secreting tumors can actually present as circulatory shock owing to decreased intravascular volume and myocardial depression, the result of sustained high concentrations of catecholamines.

DIAGNOSIS

Because of the deleterious consequences of a missed pheochromocytoma diagnosis, testing should be performed for any child who presents with signs suggestive of pheochromocytoma or other paraganglial tumor.[328] Paragangliomas may be mistaken for the more common neuroblastomas because of their similar location and secretion of vanillylmandelic acid and homovanillic acid.[321] Initial screening should include biochemical testing for excess catecholamines,[328] followed by radiologic studies to find the anatomic location of a suspected catecholamine-secreting mass. Traditionally catecholamines and their metabolites are measured in a 24-hour urine collection; however, this is often difficult in children. Plasma free metanephrines (metanephrine and normetanephrine) are produced and secreted by tumors independent of catecholamine release caused by tumor or sympathetic responses.[329] Liquid chromatography mass spectrometry assays to detect plasma free metanephrine and normetanephrine are available with a 98% sensitivity.[330]

Once the biochemical diagnostic tests suggest the presence of a paraganglial tumor or pheochromocytoma, additional imaging to locate the mass is warranted. The most common location in children is in the abdomen, both within and outside the adrenal gland. Both CT and MRI can be used to locate these tumors[331]; considerations such as radiation exposure and possible need for general anesthesia may influence which technique is used, depending on the age of the child. The accuracy of locating a pheochromocytoma with these two techniques is similar,[331] although both have limitations in distinguishing a pheochromocytoma from other intraabdominal lesions less than 1 cm in diameter.[146] Pheochromocytomas often have a classic "lightbulb" appearance on T2-weighted images making MRI preferred.[332] Other imaging options include functional testing to assess metastatic disease, multifocal disease, or regional extension.[131] I-metaiodobenzylguanidine (MIBG) and ^{18}F-fluorodeoxyglucose PET can be helpful for identifying small tumors outside the adrenal gland as well as metastatic disease.[333] Ga-DOTATATE[68] has been shown to have even better sensitivity for both primary and metastatic pheochromocytomas and paragangliomas.[334]

A comprehensive preoperative workup should also include genetic screening and counseling. As many as 50% of patients will have germline mutations in one of the susceptibility genes: *RET, VHL, NF1, SDHAF2, SDHA, SDHB, SDHC, SDHC, SDHD, TMEM127,* and *MAX.*[335]

PREOPERATIVE MANAGEMENT

Once the diagnosis of a pheochromocytoma or paraganglioma has been established, additional workup is often needed as medical therapy is initiated before surgery. A few basic laboratory results can be helpful in detecting remote organ involvement. For example, hypokalemia may be present in the context of hyperaldosteronism, or an abnormal total and ionized calcium level may indicate parathyroid gland involvement, suggestive of MEN 2 syndrome. Excess catecholamines can also increase fasting glucose concentrations or cause an abnormal glucose tolerance test. Long-term exposure to increased circulating catecholamine concentrations causes vasoconstriction and relative hypovolemia and may lead to cardiomyopathy, congestive heart failure, and arrhythmias. Therefore, a preoperative electrocardiogram and echocardiogram should be obtained as part of the preoperative assessment.[331]

Surgical resection of pheochromocytoma should almost always be done on an elective basis after the child's medical status has been properly investigated, medical conditions stabilized, the location of the tumor(s) determined, and therapeutic α-adrenergic receptor blockade has been established. Preoperative α-adrenergic blockade is critical, and has been shown to reduce perioperative complications during pheochromocytoma resection from 60% to 3%.[336,337] Effective blockade is evidenced by normalization of blood pressures for age and resolution of other symptoms, such as palpitations and headache. It must be emphasized that β-adrenergic blockade should *never* be introduced until α-adrenergic blockade has been well established; otherwise, this could result in unopposed paroxysmal systemic hypertension, leading to acute congestive heart failure, an acute coronary event, stroke, and even death. β-Adrenergic blockade to control reflex tachycardia or arrhythmias should only be started once α-adrenergic receptor blockade has been well established.[320]

Preoperative preparation has traditionally been achieved with the noncompetitive α-adrenergic blocker, phenoxybenzamine. Phenoxybenzamine irreversibly alkylates α-adrenergic receptors, reducing the risk of an α-adrenergic–mediated increase in blood pressure during surgery. Phenoxybenzamine may be administered either orally or intravenously.[323] The effective oral dose usually ranges between 0.25 and 1.0 mg/kg per day and is given in divided doses. After the initial starting dose, increases should be titrated up every 2 to 3 days (owing to the drug's long half-life) until effective α-adrenergic blockade is achieved.[318] This may require doses as large as 2 mg/kg per day and take several weeks of titration to establish the desired effects.[320,323] Increased preoperative phenoxybenzamine dose has been shown to be a significant predictor of improved hemodynamic stability.[337]

Oral bioavailability of phenoxybenzamine is only 20% to 30% with a 24-hour onset of action.[323] Alternatively, intravenous phenoxybenzamine has been used to more rapidly and reliably block α1-receptors, although this requires close monitoring for peripheral vasodilatation and decreases in blood pressure, especially in the setting of relative hypovolemia. The disadvantage of irreversibly blocking α-adrenergic receptors, as conferred by phenoxybenzamine, is that reactive hypotension may follow removal of the tumor, with resistance to interventions that are intended to increase the peripheral vascular resistance. The action of phenoxybenzamine is terminated only by synthesizing new α-adrenergic receptors. Doxazosin is a competitive selective α-1 adrenergic receptor blocker, with a half-life of 20 hours and better availability worldwide, which has also been successfully used in preoperative management of hypertension in children. Since doxazosin does not block α-2 receptors, it is less likely to have associated reflex tachycardia.[338] The Pheochromocytoma Randomized Study Comparing Adrenoreceptor Inhibiting Agents for Preoperative Treatment (PRESCRIPT) trial compared phenoxybenzamine to doxazosin in 134 adults for pheochromocytoma resection; no difference in time in target hemodynamic range intraoperatively, postoperative hemodynamics, or adverse outcomes were observed. Phenoxybenzamine was associated with greater intraoperative stability and greater reflex tachycardia.[339] Calcium channel blockers may be used as second-line adjuncts to control blood pressure when blood pressures are not well controlled on alpha blockade or side effects preclude increased dosing.[338]

Ensuring adequate α-adrenergic receptor blockade, normalizing blood pressure, and expanding contracted intravascular volume are all essential before entering the operating room. Patients may develop nasal congestion and fatigue as alpha blocking medications are up titrated. The development of orthostatic hypotension may be used as an endpoint to access adequacy of alpha blockade and determine surgical timing, typically 1 to 2 weeks.[340,341] Careful follow-up to assess symptoms and blood pressure measurement is indicated during this titration phase, particularly in patients with longstanding hypertension. During this phase, salt and fluid loading may be prescribed to address the chronic underlying state of vasoconstriction and intravascular volume depletion, and to achieve the endpoint of intravascular volume loading with concurrent vasorelaxation.[340] Hemodilution may occur during this period and is another objective parameter that supports adequate preparation.

ANESTHETIC CONSIDERATIONS

Resection of a catecholamine-secreting tumor is one of the most challenging and rare cases in anesthetic practice. The surgical approach may be open or laparoscopic depending on the tumor location, size, and surgeon's preference. However, minimally invasive adrenalectomy has been associated with lower perioperative morbidity, less pain, and faster recovery.[342] The primary goal and challenge is maintaining stable hemodynamics both before tumor removal and immediately after. This requires careful planning preoperatively and anticipating intraoperative changes. Given the high-risk nature of these patients, surgical resection ideally should be done in a center with experience in such cases.[341]

Anxiolysis prior to placement of invasive monitors or induction is important to maintain circulatory homeostasis and mitigate any stressor that may trigger a catecholamine surge. If feasible, invasive monitors such as arterial catheters are placed before induction of general anesthesia. A central venous catheter is always indicated for fluid management monitoring and delivering vasoactive infusions, including both vasodilators and vasoconstrictors. In patients with evidence of myocardial dysfunction, noninvasive continuous cardiac output assessments, a pulmonary artery catheter, or transesophageal echocardiography are essential to tailor the intraoperative management.

The goal during general anesthesia induction and intubation is to limit hemodynamic stress. Depending on the age of the patient, this can be accomplished with either intravenous or inhalation agents. Use of medications that may cause histamine release, such as ketamine, morphine, curare alkaloids (NMBDs) should be considered carefully, and sympathomimetics such as ephedrine and meperidine titrated cautiously. Some have suggested that succinylcholine may trigger a sympathetic response via stimulation of the sympathetic ganglia or fasciculations and thus should also generally be avoided, although succinylcholine is now rarely administered in pediatric anesthesiology for other reasons. Airway instrumentation should be attempted only after adequate depth of anesthesia is established, and adjuncts such as opioids or intravenous lidocaine may be of benefit. Vecuronium or rocuronium are the preferred neuromuscular blockers owing to their lack of autonomic effects and histamine release.[343]

Hypertension can occur during the surgery, especially during manipulation of the tumor, despite α-adrenergic blockade. Measures to control the blood pressure include increasing the inspired concentration of inhalation anesthetic, sodium nitroprusside infusion, intravenous magnesium sulfate,[344] and, in refractory cases of hypertension, nicardipine and fenoldopam have been used successfully.[345] Use of intravenous magnesium may have additional benefit since it causes vasodilation of blood vessel walls, inhibits catecholamine release from the adrenal medulla, and directly blocks peripheral catecholamine receptors.[346] More recently clevidipine, a third generation dihydropyridine calcium channel antagonist, with a more rapid onset than nicardipine has been used successfully to manage intraoperative hypertension in pheochromocytoma resection.[347] Tachycardia may also occur intraoperatively, and esmolol would be the preferred β-adrenergic blocker to control heart rate due to its very brief duration of action.

Profound hypotension may occur as the tumor's blood supply is ligated because of the removal of the source of catecholamines and concomitant presence of irreversible α-adrenergic blockade. These factors, in conjunction with a contracted plasma volume, blood loss, and anesthetic agents, may lead to profound and persistent hypotension.[341] Hypotension may continue for several days postoperatively until new α-adrenergic receptors are synthesized. Supportive treatment with volume expansion and vasopressors such as epinephrine, norepinephrine, and vasopressin may be needed.[341,344] Alternative nonadrenergic agents such as methylene blue have also been used effectively in treating hypotension.[348] Angiotensin II infusion use in refractory shock following pheochromocytoma removal has also been described.[349] Postoperative management in an ICU should be expected as it may take several days for blood pressures to normalize.

Finally, reactive hypoglycemia may occur on removal of the source of catecholamines and the coexisting relative excess plasma insulin levels; thus, blood glucose concentrations should be measured frequently until stabilized. Consultation with an endocrinologist and steroid replacement should be initiated if bilateral adrenalectomy has been performed.[340,341]

ANNOTATED REFERENCES

Baylis PH. The syndrome of inappropriate antidiuretic hormone secretion. *Int J Biochem Cell Biol.* 2003;35:1495-1499.
The author reviews the cardinal diagnostic criteria, clinical features, and pathophysiology of SIADH, which develops because of persistent detectable or elevated plasma arginine vasopressin concentrations in the presence of continued fluid intake. Inappropriate infusion of hypotonic fluids in the postoperative state is a common cause. For symptomatic patients with chronic SIADH, the mainstay of therapy is fluid restriction.

Cameron FJ, Wherrett DK. Care of diabetes in children and adolescents: controversies, changes, and consensus. *Lancet.* 2015;385(9982):2096-2106.
A clinically focused, up-to-date review of epidemiology, pathophysiology, diagnosis, and management of diabetes in children and adolescents.

Chiang JL, Maahs DM, Garvey KC, et al. Type 1 diabetes in children and adolescents: a position statement by the American Diabetes Association. *Diabetes Care.* 2018;41(9):2026-2044.
This statement provides a comprehensive review of the diagnosis of diabetes, management of type 1 diabetes, and acute and chronic complications of type 1 diabetes.

Hanley P, Lord K, Bauer AJ. Thyroid disorders in children and adolescents: a review. *JAMA Pediatr.* 2016;170(10):1008-1019.
This review details the pathophysiology and epidemiology of disorders of the thyroid. It surveys the clinical presentation, diagnosis, and treatment of hypothyroidism, hyperthyroidism, and thyroid nodules.

Jefferies C, Rhodes E, Rachmiel M, et al. ISPAD Clinical Practice Consensus Guidelines 2018: management of children and adolescents with diabetes requiring surgery. *Pediatr Diabetes.* 2018;19 Suppl 27:227-236.
The authors review the perioperative management of type 1 and type 2 diabetes mellitus in children who require anesthesia both for minor and major procedures.

Lenders JW, Eisenhofer G, Mannelli M, Pacak K. Phaeochromocytoma. *Lancet.* 2005;366:665-675.
Pheochromocytoma is a rare and dangerous disorder with many hidden problems that may complicate anesthesia. This review provides a single but most thorough analysis of the basic science and practical clinical issues needed to safely anesthetize children with this disorder and to anticipate and minimize complications and risks.

Martin LD, Hoagland MA, Rhodes ET, et al. Perioperative management of pediatric patients with type 1 diabetes mellitus, updated recommendations for anesthesiologists. *Anesth Analg.* 2020;130(4):821-827.
This article provides recommendations for the perioperative management of pediatric patients with type 1 diabetes, including preoperative evaluation, insulin management and pumps, glucose monitoring including CGM, and postoperative monitoring. Algorithms are provided for both elective and emergency settings.

Nadeau KJ, Anderson BJ, Berg EG, et al. Youth-onset type 2 diabetes consensus report: current status, challenges, and priorities. *Diabetes Care.* 2016;39(9):1635-1642.
This report characterizes type 2 diabetes in children, describes differences between childhood and adult type 2 diabetes, describes treatment options, and describes challenges to and approaches for new therapies.

Oiso Y, Robertson GL, Nørgaard JP, Juul KV. Clinical review: treatment of neurohypophyseal diabetes insipidus. *J Clin Endocrinol Metab.* 2013;98:3958-3967.
This review summarizes information about the safety and efficacy of treatments for the types of diabetes insipidus caused by a primary deficiency of vasopressin.

Sarlis NJ, Gourgiotis L. Thyroid emergencies. *Rev Endocr Metab Disord.* 2003;4:129-136.
A concise review article on the presentation and management of extreme thyroid disorders, myxedema coma, and thyrotoxic storm.

Sherr JL, Tauschmann M, Battelino T, et al. ISPAD Clinical Practice Consensus Guidelines 2018: diabetes technologies. *Pediatr Diabetes.* 2018;19 Suppl 27:302-305.
An international group of experts comprehensively review technologies used in the management of diabetes including stand-alone pumps, hybrid closed-loop systems, continuous glucose monitoring systems that measure interstitial glucose concentrations, diabetes apps, automated decision support systems, bolus calculators, and telemedicine.

Sterns RH, Riggs JE, Schochet SS Jr. Osmotic demyelination syndrome following correction of hyponatremia. *N Engl J Med.* 1986;314:1535-1542.

This is a description of eight patients who developed a neurologic syndrome with clinical or pathologic findings typical of central pontine myelinolysis, which developed after they presented with severe hyponatremia. Each patient's condition worsened after relatively rapid correction of hyponatremia (>12 mmol of sodium per liter per day). The data suggest that the neurologic sequelae were associated with correction of hyponatremia by more than 12 mmol/L per day. When correction proceeded more slowly, patients had uneventful recoveries. Osmotic demyelination syndrome is a preventable complication of overly rapid correction of chronic hyponatremia.

TODAY Study Group, Zeitler P, Hirst K, et al. A clinical trial to maintain glycemic control in youth with type 2 diabetes. *N Engl J Med.* 2012; 366(24):2247-2256.

This is the primary report of the TODAY Study, a randomized trial of 699 adolescents with type 2 diabetes. The study found that monotherapy with metformin was associated with durable glycemic control in approximately half of children and adolescents with type 2 diabetes. The addition of rosiglitazone, but not an intensive lifestyle intervention, was superior to metformin alone.

Wise-Faberowski L, Soriano SG, Ferrari L, et al. Perioperative management of diabetes insipidus in children. *J Neurosurg Anesthesiol.* 2004; 16(1):220-225.

This clinically focused review of diabetes insipidus in children provides recommendations for management in the perioperative setting.

Zeitler P, Arsianian S, Fu J, et al. ISPAD Clinical Practice Consensus Guidelines 2018: type 2 diabetes mellitus in youth. *Pediatr Diabetes.* 2018;19 Suppl 27:28-46.

This consensus statement provides guidance on the diagnosis, management, and screening for complications of youth with type 2 diabetes and includes recommendations on population screening for type 2 diabetes in high-risk youths.

25

A complete reference list can be found online at Elsevier eBooks+.

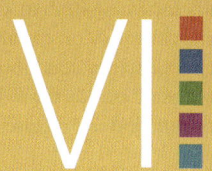

Essentials of Nephrology

26

REETI KUMAR, ANNABELLE N. CHUA, AND WARWICK A. AMES

Renal Physiology	Risk Factors
Fluids and Electrolytes	Prevention
Acid-Base Balance	Management of Acute Kidney Injury
Disease States	Anesthesia Concerns in Patients Presenting With Renal Failure
Acute Kidney Injury	Fluids and Blood Products
Chronic Kidney Disease	Anesthetic Agents
Intraoperative Management	Postoperative Concerns
Strategies for Renal Protection	

ANESTHESIOLOGISTS ARE OFTEN FACED with a child who has acute kidney injury or renal failure. Renal disease requires the practitioner to be vigilant about fluid homeostasis, acid-base balance, electrolyte management, choice of anesthetics, and potential complications. This requires a thorough understanding of the excretory and fluid homeostatic functions of the kidney, particularly in the neonate and younger child. If not managed assiduously, perioperative renal dysfunction can deteriorate into renal failure or multiorgan system failure resulting in considerable morbidity or mortality. The anesthesia provider must understand renal physiology, appropriate preoperative preparation, intraoperative management, and postoperative care of the child with renal disease.

Renal Physiology

The basic functions of the kidney are to maintain fluid and electrolyte homeostasis and metabolism. The first step in this tightly controlled process is the production of the glomerular filtrate from the renal plasma. The glomerular filtration rate depends on renal blood flow, which depends on the systolic blood pressure and circulating blood volume. The kidneys are the most highly perfused organs per gram of body weight. They receive 20% to 30% of the cardiac output maintained over a wide range of blood pressures through changes in renal vascular resistance. Numerous hormones play a role in this autoregulation including vasodilators (i.e., prostaglandins E and I_2, dopamine, and nitric oxide) and vasoconstrictors (i.e., angiotensin II, thromboxane, adrenergic stimulation, and endothelin). Congestive heart failure and volume contraction severely limit the ability of the kidney to maintain autoregulation.

When adjusted for body surface area or scaled using allometric theory (see Chapter 5), both renal blood flow and glomerular filtration rate double in the first 2 weeks of postnatal life and both continue to increase steadily, reaching adult values by 2 years of age (see Figs. 5.12 and 5.13).[1,2] The increases in renal blood flow over time parallel similar increases in cardiac output and decreases in renal vascular resistance. The initial glomerular filtration rate and the rate of increase during the first few years correlate with the neonate's postmenstrual age at birth. For example, the glomerular filtration rate (corrected using body surface area or allometry) of a neonate born at 28 weeks' gestation is one-half of that of a full-term infant (see Figs. 5.12 and 5.13).[3] Glomerular filtration rate may be estimated, in children ≥2 years of age, from the serum creatinine concentration and the height of the child according to the formula:[4–6]

$$\text{Glomerular filtration rate (mL/minute/1.73m}^2\text{)}$$
$$= \text{height (cm)} \times \text{k/serum creatinine}$$

In the equation, k is a constant 0.413 that applies to most children; the constant k is 0.33 in premature neonates and 0.7 in adolescents.[4,5,7]

The serum creatinine concentration reflects the maternal serum creatinine concentration and therefore cannot be used to predict neonatal renal function until at least 2 days after birth. Neonatal serum creatinine reaches a nadir by 1 to 2 weeks of life and then stabilizes for the first year of life.[8,9] Serum creatinine concentrations that are reported for age bands provide a rudimentary measure of renal function.[10]

Cystatin C (cysC) is another serum marker of kidney function that can be used independently or in conjunction with serum creatinine to estimate glomerular filtration rate. The advantage of cystatin C is that it is a low-molecular-weight protein produced by all nucleated human cells and is not affected by sex, age, race, muscle mass, or dietary protein intake as is serum creatinine.[11] One pediatric equation used to measure glomerular filtration rate is based on cystatin C and known as the creatinine-cystatin chronic kidney disease (C-based CKID) equation:

$$\text{estimated glomerular filtration rate} = 70.69 \times \text{cysC}^{-0.931}$$

Others acknowledge the change in serum creatinine with age reflects both creatinine production and maturation of renal elimination.[6,12]

FLUIDS AND ELECTROLYTES

The kidney regulates the total body sodium balance and maintains normal extracellular and circulating volumes.[13] The adult kidney filters 25,000 mEq of sodium per day, but it excretes less than 1% because of extremely efficient resorption mechanisms along the nephron. The proximal tubule resorbs 50% to 70%, the ascending limb of the loop of Henle resorbs about 25%, and the distal nephron accounts for 10% of the filtered sodium load. Several hormones, including renin, angiotensin II, aldosterone, and atrial natriuretic peptide, and changes in circulating blood volume, contribute to maintain the sodium balance.[14]

Serum osmolality is tightly regulated through changes in arginine vasopressin release and thirst.[15–17] Arginine vasopressin, also known as *antidiuretic hormone (ADH),* is synthesized in the hypothalamus and stored in the posterior pituitary, where it is released in response to an increase in plasma osmolality. Arginine vasopressin is also released in response to decreases in the circulating blood volume and hypotension, including responses to nausea, vomiting, opioids, inflammation, and surgery. Arginine vasopressin binds to receptors in the collecting duct, increasing the permeability of the tubules to water, which increases water resorption and concentrates urine. Neonates are much less able to conserve or excrete water compared with older children, rendering the fluid management and volume issues in this young age group important challenges for the anesthesiologist.[18]

The regulation of serum potassium is managed by the kidney and depends on the concentration of plasma aldosterone. Aldosterone binds to receptors on cells in the distal nephron, increasing the secretion of potassium in the urine. Neonates are much less efficient at excreting potassium loads compared with adults, and the normal range of serum potassium concentrations is therefore greater in neonates; Table 26.1 provides normal values.[19] Potassium regulation is affected by the acid-base status; excretion of potassium increases in the presence of alkalosis and decreases in the presence of acidosis. Causes of hyperkalemia and hypokalemia are presented in Tables 26.2 and 26.3, respectively.

ACID-BASE BALANCE

The kidney regulates acid-base balance and the response to the stress of illness. The kidney reclaims virtually all of the filtered bicarbonate in the proximal tubule and regenerates bicarbonate

TABLE 26.1	Normal Values of Serum Potassium
Age	**Serum Potassium Range (mEq/L)**
0–1 month	4.0–6.0
1 month–2 years	4.0–5.5
2–17 years	3.8–5.0
>18 years	3.2–4.8

TABLE 26.2	Causes of Hyperkalemia
Transcellular Shifts	
Acidosis	
β-Adrenergic blockers	
Insulin deficiency	
Burns	
Tumor lysis syndrome	
Rhabdomyolysis	
Succinylcholine	
Decreased Excretion	
Renal failure	
Potassium-sparing diuretics	
Cyclosporine	
Nonsteroidal antiinflammatory drugs	
Angiotensin-converting enzyme inhibitors	
Mineralocorticoid deficiency	
Adrenal insufficiency	
Congenital adrenal hyperplasia	
Hyporeninemic hypoaldosteronism	
Primary mineralocorticoid deficiency	
Mineralocorticoid resistance	
Prematurity	
Obstructive uropathy	
Pseudohypoaldosteronism	
Increased Intake	
Potassium supplements, oral or intravenous	
Blood transfusions	
Potassium-containing antibiotics	

TABLE 26.3	Causes of Hypokalemia
Transcellular Shift	
Insulin	
β-Adrenergic agonists	
Increased Excretion	
Vomiting	
Diarrhea	
Nasogastric suction	
Laxatives	
Diuretics	
Cisplatin	
Amphotericin B	
Renal tubular acidosis	
Bartter syndrome	
Corticosteroids	
Decreased Intake	
Malnutrition	
Anorexia nervosa	

(HCO_3^-) lost in the neutralization of acid generated by the normal combustion of food, especially protein, and the formation of bone. New bicarbonate is the product of cells in the distal nephron that decompose the carbonic acid (H_2CO_3) formed from water (H_2O) and carbon dioxide (CO_2) by carbonic anhydrase. The protons (H^+) that are generated from this process are pumped into the lumen of the collecting duct, where they combine with hydrogen phosphate (HPO_4^{2-}) or ammonia (NH_3) generated by the catabolism of amino acids, mainly glutamine, in the tubule cells.[20]

Infants, especially neonates, maintain a slightly acidotic blood (pH = 7.37) and decreased plasma bicarbonate concentration (22 mEq/L) compared with older children and adults (pH = 7.39; plasma bicarbonate = 24 to 28 mEq/L).[21] The reduced plasma concentration of HCO_3^- is the result of a reduced threshold or the plasma concentration at which HCO_3^- is incompletely resorbed by the kidney. Neonates maintain acid-base homeostasis but are limited in their ability to respond to an acid load[22]; this is especially true for preterm infants.

Disease States

The causes of and differences in renal diseases between children and adults are substantive. Depending on the cause of the renal disease, management may vary. Adult renal disease usually results from long-standing diabetes mellitus or hypertension with an associated compromise in cardiovascular function. Children may also have renal failure owing to diseases such as sickle cell disease or systemic lupus erythematosus, but cardiovascular function is far less commonly compromised.

ACUTE KIDNEY INJURY

Acute kidney injury is defined as an abrupt deterioration in the ability of the kidneys to clear nitrogenous wastes, such as urea and creatinine. Concomitantly, there is a loss of ability to excrete other solutes and maintain a normal water balance. This leads to the clinical presentation of edema, hypertension, hyperkalemia, and uremia in higher stages of acute kidney injury. However, even modest increases in serum creatinine or decline in urine output are associated with a dramatic increase in mortality. The Kidney Disease: Improving Global Outcomes (KDIGO) defines and stages acute kidney injury by serum creatinine and urine output (Table 26.4).[23]

The term acute kidney injury has often been incorrectly used interchangeably with *acute tubular necrosis (ATN),* which usually refers to a rapid deterioration in renal function occurring minutes to days after an ischemic or nephrotoxic event. Although acute tubular necrosis is an important cause of acute kidney injury, it is not the sole cause, and the terms are not synonymous.

Etiology and Pathophysiology

Acute kidney injury (AKI) is often multifactorial in origin or the result of several distinct insults; to treat acute kidney injury, it is important to understand its causes and pathophysiology. The etiologies of acute kidney injury are varied, but can be broadly classified as (Table 26.5)[24,25]:

- *Prerenal,* implying caused by insufficient renal perfusion
- *Intrinsic renal,* implying renal injury or inflammation within the renal parenchyma
- *Postrenal,* implying an obstruction to the excretion of urine

Prerenal insults comprise the majority (up to 70%) of cases of acute kidney injury. They usually result from massive losses of extracellular fluid, such as in gastroenteritis, burns, hemorrhage,

TABLE 26.4	Kidney Disease: Improving Global Outcomes (KDIGO) Staging of Acute Kidney Injury	
Stage	Serum Creatinine	Urine Output
1	1.5–1.9 times baseline or ≥0.3 mg/dL (≥26.6 μmol/L) increase	<0.5 mL/kg per hour for 6–12 hours
2	2.0–2.9 times baseline	<0.5 mL/kg per hour for ≥12 hours
3	3 times baseline or ≥4.0 mg/dL (≥353.6 μmol/L) increase or initiation of RRT or in patients <18 years a decrease in eGFR <35 mL/minute per 1.73 m²	<0.3 mL/kg per hour for ≥24 hours or anuria ≥12 hours

eGFR, Estimated glomerular filtration rate; *KDIGO,* Kidney Disease Improving Global Outcomes, *RRT,* renal replacement therapy.
From Khwaja A. KDIGO clinical practice guidelines for acute kidney injury. *Nephron Clin Pract.* 2012;120(4):c179-184.

or excessive diuresis, as well as from cardiac failure and sepsis. The common feature of this condition is diminished renal perfusion. In response to the reduction in renal blood flow, there is a compensatory increase in afferent tone, which decreases the glomerular filtration rate and increases the retention of salt and water. The net effect of these events is a drastic reduction in urine volume, often leading to oliguria and/or anuria.[24,25] If the underlying problem is recognized early and treated aggressively, progressive renal insufficiency may be averted. Nonsteroidal antiinflammatory drugs, angiotensin-converting enzyme (ACE) inhibitors, and angiotensin receptor blockers can aggravate prerenal azotemia by further reducing glomerular capillary pressure and the glomerular filtration rate.[24,26]

Parenchymal disease or injury accounts for 20% to 30% of the cases of abrupt onset of acute kidney injury. In infants, the common causes include birth asphyxia, sepsis, and cardiac surgery. In older children, the important causes of acute kidney injury include trauma, sepsis, and hemolytic uremic syndrome. Prolonged prerenal azotemia may result in overt renal injury. Similarly, intrarenal obstruction to blood flow from thrombi or vasculitis may cause renal failure. Drugs such as aminoglycosides, glycopeptides, amphotericin B,[27] and other nephrotoxins, including radiocontrast agents, may induce acute kidney injury through tubular or interstitial injury or as a result of allergic reactions, as has been described with penicillins.[28] Acute glomerulonephritis is another cause of acute kidney injury in children; rarely, pyelonephritis can lead to acute kidney injury.[24,25]

The remaining causes of acute kidney injury result from the obstruction to urine flow. These conditions account for less than 10% of all cases of acute kidney injury and may involve obstruction of both kidneys. Sudden anuria suggests a postrenal cause for the acute kidney injury. The obstruction can occur within the collecting system of the kidney (intrarenal), in the ureter, or in the urethra (extrarenal). Intrarenal obstruction may occur with the tumor lysis syndrome with the deposition of uric acid crystals, from myoglobinuria, hemoglobinuria, or from medications such as acyclovir and cidofovir. Acute tumor lysis has also resulted in fatalities after a single dose of steroids was given to a child with an

TABLE 26.5	Causes of Acute Kidney Injury	
Prerenal Failure	**Intrinsic Renal Failure**	**Postrenal Failure**

Hypovolemia
  Volume loss
  Gastrointestinal, renal losses
  Sequestration (burns, postoperative)
	Acute glomerulonephritis
	  Postinfectious
	  Membranoproliferative glomerulonephritis
	  Rapidly progressive glomerulonephritis
	  Glomerulonephritis due to systemic disease
	    (e.g., HUS, DIC, SLE)
		Obstruction
		  Intrinsic (papillary necrosis due to diabetes, sickle cell
		    disease, or analgesic nephropathy)
		  Intrarenal abnormalities, ureteral obstruction, obstruction
		    of the bladder or urethra
		  Extrinsic (tumor compression, lymphadenopathy)

Hypotension
  Shock
  Vasodilators
	Acute interstitial nephritis
	  Drug-induced hypersensitivity (penicillin)
	  Infections	

Decreased effective blood flow
  Low cardiac output
  Cirrhosis
  Nephrotic syndrome
	Tubular disease
	  ATN (ischemic, nephrotoxic)
	  Intratubular obstruction (uric acid, oxalate)	

Renal hypoperfusion
  Use of ACE inhibitors
  NSAIDs
  Hepatorenal syndrome
	Cortical necrosis
	  Gram-negative sepsis
	  Hemorrhage
	  Shock	

Vascular occlusion
  Thromboembolic phenomenon
  Aortic dissection
  Renal vein thrombosis (dehydration,
    hypercoagulable state, neoplasm)
	Acute Kidney Injury
	  Toxins
	  Organic solvents
	  Heavy metals
	  Insecticides
	  Hemoglobin
	  Myoglobin
	Chronic renal disease
	  Chronic interstitial nephritis
	  Chronic glomerulonephritis
	  Chronic glomerulosclerosis
	  Nephrocalcinosis
	  Obstructive uropathy
	  Hypertension	

ACE, Angiotensin-converting enzyme; *ATN*, acute tubular necrosis; *DIC*, disseminated intravascular coagulation; *HUS*, hemolytic uremic syndrome; *NSAIDs*, nonsteroidal antiinflammatory drugs; *SLE*, systemic lupus erythematosus.

untreated hematologic cancer in one case and to prevent postoperative nausea and vomiting in another.[29,30] The pathology in the latter reaction is a massive deposition of uric acid and calcium phosphate crystals in the kidney. Extrarenal obstruction can be caused by stones inspissated in the ureters or from external compression by lymph nodes or a tumor. As with other forms of acute kidney injury, prompt recognition and appropriate intervention to relieve the obstruction may facilitate full recovery of renal function and obviate a permanent reduction in renal function.[24,25]

The exact pathophysiology of acute kidney injury remains unclear, but several factors have been identified.[31] In the initial phase of acute kidney injury, profound renovascular vasoconstriction reduces glomerular filtration rate (Fig. 26.1). Factors known to increase renal vasoconstriction include increased activity of the renin-angiotensin and the adrenergic systems and endothelial dysfunction with increased endothelin release and decreased nitric oxide synthesis.[32] However, therapeutic interventions to vasodilate the intrarenal vasculature, such as prostaglandin and dopamine infusions, ACE inhibitors, calcium channel blockers, and endothelin receptor antagonists, have not reversed established acute kidney injury.[33]

Another factor in the pathogenesis of acute kidney injury is renal tubule cell injury, the direct result of a nephrotoxic agent or

from an ischemic insult (Fig. 26.2). Cellular injury leads to sloughing of the brush border, swelling, mitochondrial condensation, disruption of cellular architecture, and loss of adhesion to the basement membrane with shedding of cells into the tubular lumen.[32,34] These changes, which occur within minutes of an ischemic event, contribute to the decreased glomerular filtration rate by obstructing the lumen of the tubule.[32,35] These cellular changes allow the filtrate to leak back into the peritubular blood, reducing the excretion of solutes and the effective glomerular filtration rate.

Some of the cellular derangements in acute kidney injury, such as a reduction in ATP concentrations, cell membrane injury by reactive oxygen molecules, and increased intracellular calcium concentrations from changes in membrane phospholipid metabolism, lead to cell death. Reactive oxygen molecules also stimulate the production of cytokines and chemokines that play a role in cell injury and vasoconstriction.[32,35,36]

Neutrophils that are recruited during reperfusion injury after renal ischemia mediate parenchymal renal damage. Reperfusion injury increases intracellular adhesion molecule 1 (ICAM-1) on endothelial cells promoting the adhesion of circulating neutrophils and their eventual infiltration into the parenchyma. Neutrophils then release reactive oxygen molecules, elastases, proteases, and other enzymes that lead to further tissue injury.[32,37]

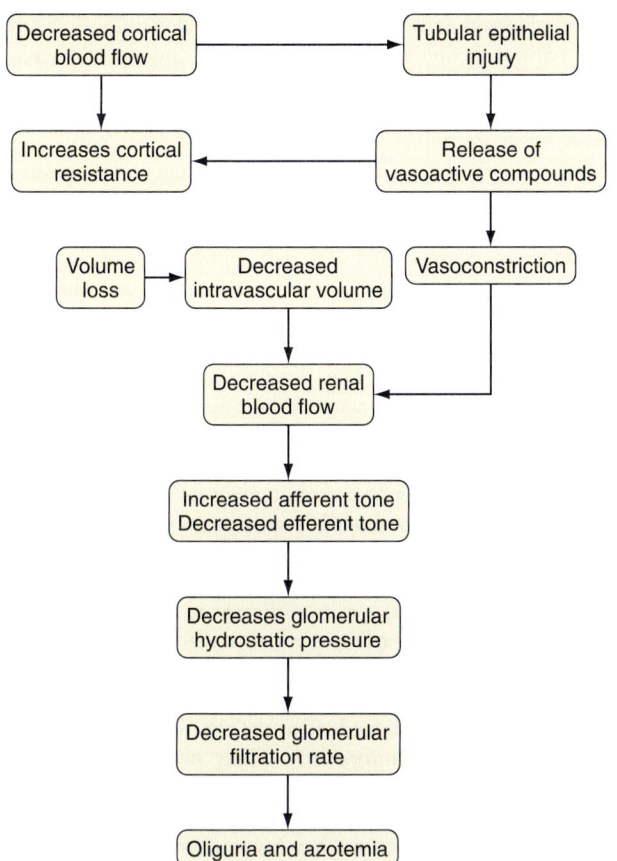

FIGURE 26.1 Hemodynamic factors in the pathogenesis of acute renal failure.

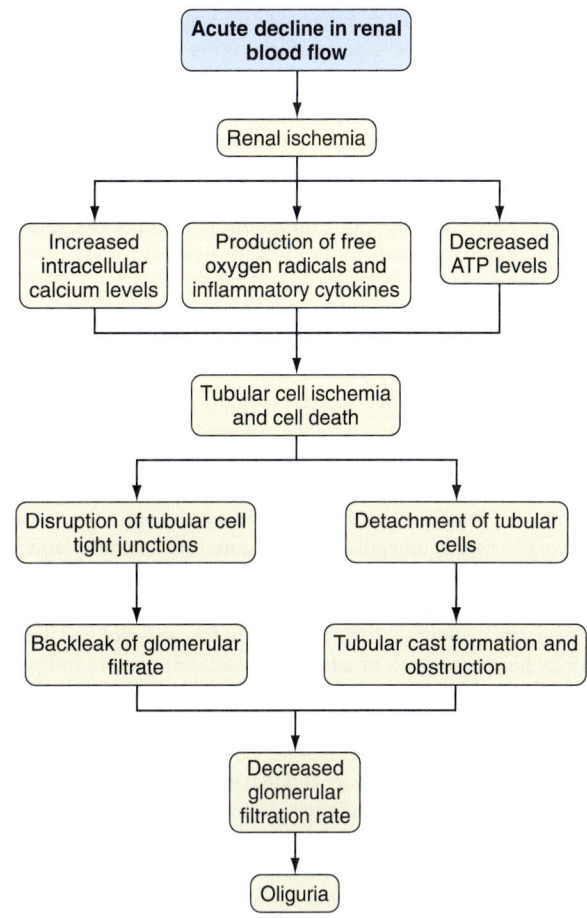

FIGURE 26.2 Influences of specific injuries on the nephron in the pathogenesis of acute renal failure. *ATP,* Adenosine triphosphate.

Diagnostic Procedures

A thorough history and physical examination can yield important insight into the likely causes of acute kidney injury. The initial laboratory assessment of a child with acute kidney injury should include the measurement of serum urea, creatinine, electrolytes, and a urinalysis. Prerenal azotemia is typically associated with a ratio of blood urea nitrogen (BUN) to creatinine that exceeds 20. In cases of renal parenchymal dysfunction, this ratio is closer to 10. Hematuria and proteinuria may be present in acute kidney injury, independent of the cause, although the presence of cellular casts, especially red blood cell casts, in the urinary sediment is suggestive of glomerulonephritis. Granular casts are associated with prerenal azotemia. Muddy brown casts and epithelial cell casts are associated with acute tubular necrosis.[38]

One test to distinguish prerenal azotemia from established renal failure from ischemia or nephrotoxins is the fractional excretion of sodium (FE$_{Na}$). The FE$_{Na}$ is calculated using the equation:

$$FE_{Na} = \frac{U_{Na} \times S_{Cr}}{S_{Na} \times U_{Cr}} \times 100\%$$

U$_{Na}$ and S$_{Na}$ are urine and serum sodium concentrations, and U$_{Cr}$ and S$_{Cr}$ are the urine and serum creatinine concentrations, respectively. In prerenal acute kidney injury, the FE$_{Na}$ is usually less than 1% for adults and children and less than 2.5% for infants. In established acute kidney injury from ischemia and nephrotoxins, but not acute glomerulonephritis, the FE$_{Na}$ usually exceeds 1%. Administration of diuretics and IV fluids may confound the interpretation of this test.[39]

In patients who have received diuretics, the fractional excretion of urea (FE$_{Urea}$) may be useful in distinguishing between prerenal and intrinsic renal injury. The FE$_{Urea}$ is calculated using the equation:

$$FE\,Urea, = \frac{U_{Urea} \times S_{Cr}}{BUN \times U_{Cr}} \times 100\%$$

U$_{Urea}$ and BUN are urine and serum urea concentrations. FE$_{Urea}$ <35% is indicative of prerenal acute kidney injury, whereas FE$_{Urea}$ >50% is indicative of acute tubular necrosis.[39]

The initial radiologic assessment of children with acute kidney injury is ultrasonography. Renal ultrasound does not depend on renal function and can define the renal anatomy, changes in parenchymal density, and possible outlet obstruction by demonstrating dilation of the urinary tract. Doppler interrogation of the renal vessels provides information on vascular flow. Further radiographic studies, such as voiding cystourethrography, nuclear renal flow scanning, dynamic functional MRI, and abdominal computed tomography (CT), may be indicated in select children and conditions.

Since the increase in the serum creatinine can be delayed in acute kidney injury, urinary biomarkers offer a promising area of research for the early detection, management, and prognosis of acute kidney injury. Markers of cell cycle arrest, tissue inhibitor of metalloproteinases-2 (TIMP-2), and insulin growth factor binding protein 7 (IGFBP7) are effective in risk stratifying critically ill adult patients with acute kidney injury stage 1. The combined urinary assay for TIMP-2 and IGFBP7 is the first clinical assay for acute kidney injury approved in the United States.[24,40,41] Unlike adults, adaptation of urinary acute kidney injury biomarkers requires the development of age-dependent reference ranges, which has delayed their adoption in pediatric clinical practice. In neonates, urine albumin, β-2 microglobulin, cystatin C, neutrophil gelatinase-associated lipocalin, uromodulin, osteopontin, and vascular endothelial growth factor (VEGF) have all shown promise for detection of acute kidney injury.[42]

Cystatin C, neutrophil gelatinase-associated lipocalin, interleukin-18 (IL-18), kidney injury molecular-1 (KIM-1), and liver fatty acid-binding protein are biomarkers that have been assessed for acute kidney injury prediction in pediatric patients undergoing cardiac surgery. Of these markers, neutrophil gelatinase-associated lipocalin has shown the most promise for the early detection of acute kidney injury in children undergoing cardiopulmonary bypass. Neutrophil gelatinase-associated lipocalin gene expression is upregulated after acute tubular injury and has been shown in several prospective studies to rise up to 10-fold within 2 to 6 hours after initiation of cardiopulmonary bypass in pediatric patients.[41,43–46] Further studies are required before urinary biomarkers can be adopted as useful diagnostic and prognostic tools in the management of pediatric acute kidney injury.

Therapeutic Interventions

Therapeutic interventions in children with acute kidney injury should be aimed at the underlying cause and at improving renal function and urine flow. Children with acute kidney injury caused by hypovolemia should be fluid resuscitated with at least 20 mL/kg over 30 to 60 minutes with normal saline or a balanced salt solution. For children with hypotension, an alternative choice is a colloid-containing solution. Children with oliguria caused by hypovolemia usually respond within 4 to 6 hours with increased urine output.

Diuretics have been commonly used to treat oliguric acute kidney injury. There are several theoretical reasons why mannitol, furosemide, and other loop diuretics may ameliorate acute kidney injury. First, diuretics may convert oliguric acute kidney injury into nonoliguric acute kidney injury. Second, loop diuretics decrease energy-driven transport in the loop of Henle, and this may protect cells in regions of hypoperfusion. However, neither mannitol nor loop diuretics can predictably convert an oliguric patient with acute kidney injury to a polyuric patient. Diuretics have not been shown in clinical studies to influence renal recovery, need for dialysis, or survival in patients with acute kidney injury. Diuretics should be used only after the circulating volume has been adequately restored and should be stopped if there is no early response.[47]

Dopamine has been widely used to prevent and manage acute kidney injury. In low doses (0.5–2.0 μg/kg per minute), dopamine increases renal plasma flow, glomerular filtration rate, and renal sodium excretion by activating dopaminergic receptors. Infusion rates in excess of 3 μg/kg per minute stimulate α-adrenergic receptors on systemic arterial resistance vasculature, causing vasoconstriction; cardiac β1-adrenergic receptors, increasing cardiac contractility, heart rate, and cardiac index; and β2-adrenergic receptors on systemic arterial resistance vasculature, causing vasodilatation. In three individual meta-analyses, dopamine did not prevent renal failure, alter the need for dialysis, or change the mortality rate.[48–50] From these data, the routine use of low-dose dopamine in patients with acute kidney injury cannot be supported.

Fenoldopam is a short-acting selective dopamine-1 agonist that reduces peripheral vascular resistance and promotes renal blood flow, natriuresis, and diuresis. In a meta-analysis of 16 studies and 1290 adult patients, fenoldopam reduced the incidence of acute kidney injury, the need for renal replacement therapy, length of intensive care unit (ICU) stay, and mortality in patients with acute kidney injury.[51] In a randomized trial of fenoldopam in 80 infants undergoing cardiopulmonary bypass, fenoldopam was associated with reduced incidence of postoperative acute kidney injury, use of diuretics, and vasodilators.[52] These initial studies show promise for its role in preventing acute kidney injury.

Renal replacement therapy through dialysis is life sustaining in patients with severe acute kidney injury. The indications for initiation of dialytic therapy are persistent hyperkalemia, volume overload refractory to diuretics, severe metabolic acidosis, overt signs and symptoms of uremia such as pericarditis and encephalopathy, removal of dialyzable toxins or drugs, and need to provide nutritional support in persistently oliguric patients. Ten percent fluid overload in patients with acute kidney injury unresponsive to diuretics is an indicator to initiate dialysis. In a multicenter study, pediatric patients who were initiated on continuous renal replacement therapy after they developed ≥20% fluid overload had higher mortality than patients who had 10% to 20% fluid overload at the time of continuous renal replacement therapy initiation.[53] Many nephrologists recommend dialysis if the BUN value approaches 100 mg/dL (35.7 mmol/L) or even earlier, especially in the oliguric patient, although subsequent outcome has not improved. An observation study of five medical centers compared low azotemia (BUN ≤76 mg/dL) vs. high azotemia (BUN >76 mg/dL) initiation of dialysis in adult patients suggested initiation of dialysis at lower BUN improved survival.[54] However, the timing of the initiation of dialysis remains an unresolved question.

Three strategies are available to replace renal function in critically ill children and adults: hemodialysis, peritoneal dialysis, and variations of continuous renal replacement therapy, such as continuous venovenous hemofiltration (CVVH), continuous venovenous hemodialysis (CVVHD), and continuous venovenous hemodiafiltration (CVVHDF). None of these strategies has been proven superior to the others. However, in the individual child, one strategy may be more practical than the others. Hemodialysis is technically more difficult than peritoneal dialysis in an infant and in hemodynamically unstable children. Continuous replacement therapies cause less hemodynamic instability compared with hemodialysis and offer more predictable solute and fluid removal than peritoneal dialysis. Hemodialysis and continuous replacement therapies require large-bore vascular access to achieve the large blood flows that are necessary to support these strategies. Peritoneal dialysis is often the modality of choice in neonates with acute kidney injury and infants who develop acute kidney injury following cardiac surgery.[55]

Although these three strategies differ technically, they share similar principles (Fig. 26.3). All three strategies remove nitrogenous wastes (i.e., urea), excess fluid, and excess solutes, especially potassium. This is achieved by circulating the child's blood over a semipermeable membrane that separates the blood from a salt solution (i.e., dialysate) on the contralateral surface. The movement of solutes across the membranes occurs by diffusion (i.e., solutes move across the membrane along their concentration gradients) and ultrafiltration (i.e., osmotic or hydrostatic pressures). The rate of removal of water and solute waste depends on the

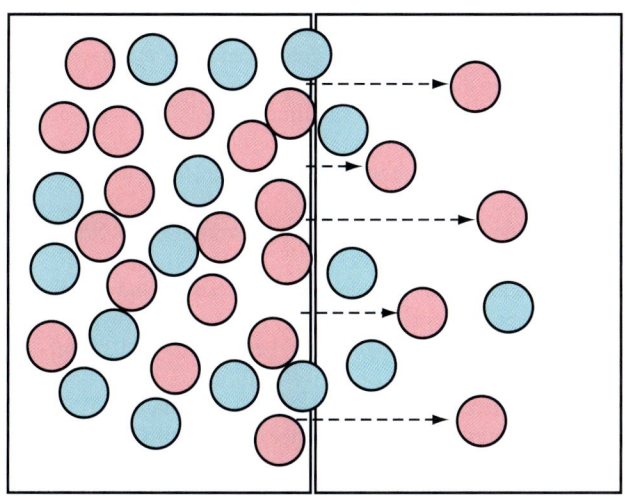

FIGURE 26.3 Principles of dialysis. Solute *(pink circles)* moves from the blood to the dialysate *(broken arrows)* in response to a concentration gradient (i.e., diffusion). The obligate passive movement of water *(blue circles)* attempts to maintain appropriate osmolarity. This flux of solute and water (i.e., ultrafiltration) may be enhanced by increased osmotic pressure (i.e., glucose in peritoneal dialysis fluid) or by increased hydrostatic pressure, which is created mechanically as transmembrane pressure in hemodialysis.

characteristics of the membrane (i.e., pore size and selectivity), diffusion, and ultrafiltration.[56]

The permeability characteristics and surface areas for the membranes are known for specific dialyzers used in hemodialysis and hemofiltration. The peritoneum serves as the dialysis membrane in peritoneal dialysis and remains physically unalterable, but changes in dialysate composition and length of time the dialysate is exposed to the peritoneal membrane changes the amount of solute and water removed. In all forms of renal replacement therapy, the therapeutic prescription is individualized for the child.[55]

Hemodialysis

Hemodialysis is very effective for acute kidney injury, being the best modality for the rapid removal of toxins, such as drug overdoses or other ingestions or metabolic toxins resulting from poisoning or inborn errors.[57,58] Hemodialysis is very efficient, reducing the BUN by 60% to 70%, normalizing the serum potassium concentration, and removing fluid equal to 5% to 10% of the body weight within 3 to 4 hours. Large-vessel venous access with a double-lumen catheter into the internal jugular, subclavian, or femoral vein is required to provide rapid blood flow rates (Qb) (5–8 mL/kg per minute). In small infants, two single-lumen catheters placed in different sites may be necessary to access and return the blood. Rarely, a single-lumen catheter may be used for both outflow and return of blood. For small infants and children whose total blood volume is <10% of the extracorporeal volume of the circuit (tubing volume + dialyzer volume), a blood prime using packed red blood cells diluted with saline to a hematocrit of 30% to 40% may be indicated.[59] Modern hemodialysis machines have microprocessors that can accurately measure the amount of fluid removed and this should be summarized for the anesthesiologist.

Hemodialysis usually requires systemic anticoagulation with unfractionated heparin, the effectiveness of which can be monitored by the activated clotting time (ACT). Alternatives to unfractionated heparin include low-molecular-weight-heparins (LMWHs), anticoagulant-free dialysis circuits using a rapid blood flow rate and frequently rinsing the blood circuit with saline (often used in children who are at considerable risk of bleeding) and regional anticoagulation with citrate that acts by binding ionized calcium.[60] However, clotting commonly forms within the circuit with subsequent loss of the extracorporeal blood.

In addition to the risk of bleeding, hemodialysis is associated with several other adverse effects, the most common of which is hypotension. This usually results from overly aggressive removal of fluid, although it can also result from sepsis or the release of cytokines and autokines from blood passing over the surface of the hemodialysis filter. Muscle cramps, headache, nausea, and vomiting are also commonly reported. A more serious complication of hemodialysis is the disequilibrium syndrome that is related to the rapid removal of solute from the bloodstream with slow equilibration with the tissues, particularly the brain. This can cause cerebral edema, manifested by headache, obtundation, seizures, or coma. The disequilibrium syndrome is usually reported in children undergoing dialysis for the first time.[61] This can be obviated by dialyzing for brief but frequent sessions initially and using less efficient dialyzers, especially if the BUN concentration is increased substantially and greater than 100 mg/dL, with goal urea reduction ratio of 30% for the first session. Infection of the dialysis catheter is another common problem that requires strict attention to sterile central line access techniques.

Peritoneal Dialysis

Peritoneal dialysis has a long history as renal replacement therapy in infants and children. It is relatively simple and easy to perform, does not require vascular access, and has less risk of hemodynamic instability. Although not as efficient as hemodialysis, optimal results are obtained if it is performed continuously to control solute and water balance. Peritoneal dialysis involves instilling dialysate fluid into the peritoneum for a set period and then draining the fluid and replacing it with fresh dialysate. This cycling removes waste products by diffusion and water by ultrafiltration as a consequence of a high glucose concentration in the dialysate. The efficacy of peritoneal dialysis depends on the volume of dialysate instilled per cycle and the number of cycles per day. Most children with acute renal failure are managed with 1- to 2-hour cycles of 10- to 30-mL/kg dwell volumes. Children with end-stage kidney disease are managed with greater cycle times and larger dwell volumes (1100–1400 mL/m^2). The amount of fluid removed can be controlled by changing the concentration of the glucose in the dialysate.[62] Short-term peritoneal dialysis can be accomplished with a nontunneled peritoneal dialysis catheter, but should dialysis be required beyond 3 to 5 days, a subcutaneously tunneled cuffed catheter is preferred to minimize the risk of peritonitis and leaks about the catheter insertion site.

The principal complications of peritoneal dialysis are infection (exit-site/tunnel infections and peritonitis), catheter-related problems, and mechanical problems related to the increased intraabdominal pressure. It is common to find poor drainage from the catheter, usually the result of fibrin occlusion of the catheter or from omentum or bowel covering the inlet holes.

Omentectomy at the time of peritoneal dialysis catheter placement may be necessary. The catheter may leak at its point of insertion, particularly if used within 2 weeks of catheter insertion.[63] Hernias, especially inguinal hernias in boys, may develop as a consequence of the increased intraabdominal pressure from the infused dialysate.[64] Mild hyponatremia may develop in infants because of the relatively low sodium concentration (130 mEq/L) in commercial dialysate. Less common but serious complications include bowel injury and intraabdominal hemorrhage from catheter insertion and sclerosing encapsulating peritonitis that can arise following prolonged peritoneal dialysis therapy.[65]

Continuous Renal Replacement Therapy

Continuous renal replacement therapy is commonly used in the management of acute kidney injury for the critically ill patient with hemodynamic instability due to its continuous nature allowing for gradual fluid removal and solute reequilibration. The solute clearance that continuous renal replacement therapy provides over 24 hours is comparable to the clearance obtained during a 4-hour hemodialysis session and is more efficient than peritoneal dialysis. In addition, the ability for precise continuous fluid removal allows for provision of necessary blood products and nutrition. Continuous renal replacement therapy can provide diffusive clearance through continuous venovenous hemodialysis, convective clearance through continuous venovenous hemofiltration, or both diffusive and convective clearance through continuous venovenous hemodiafiltration.[66] Indications for continuous renal replacement therapy include fluid overload, hyperkalemia, symptomatic uremia, hyperammonemia associated with inborn errors of metabolism, intoxication, or medication overdose.[67]

As with intermittent hemodialysis, vascular access is required, and blood priming is recommended if the extracorporeal circuit exceeds 10% of the circulating blood volume. Blood flow rates typically range from 3 to 5 mL/kg per minute in neonates and 5 to 10 mL/kg per minute in infants and 100 to 150 mL/minute in older children and adolescents. Additionally, anticoagulation using unfractionated heparin or regional citrate anticoagulation is essential to prevent the circuit from clotting, to preserve filter performance, and prevent blood loss. Whereas systemic anticoagulation with heparin can increase bleeding complications, regional citrate anticoagulation can predispose to metabolic alkalosis or citrate toxicity.[66] Challenges with continuous renal replacement therapy include need for specialized equipment, specialized nursing expertise, and greater nursing workload as compared to other dialysis modalities. Potential complications with continuous renal replacement therapy include catheter-associated complications and infections, hypothermia, and electrolyte abnormalities. In addition, continuous renal replacement therapy can have an important impact on drug dosing; therefore, when possible, drug concentration should be monitored.[55]

CHRONIC KIDNEY DISEASE

Based on clinical practice guidelines from KDIGO in 2012, pediatric chronic kidney disease is diagnosed by fulfilling one of the following clinical criteria:

- Glomerular filtration rate of less than 60 mL per minute per 1.73 m² for greater than 3 months with implications for health.
- Glomerular filtration rate greater than 60 mL per minute per 1.73 m² accompanied by evidence of structural damage or other markers of functional kidney abnormalities including proteinuria, albuminuria, renal tubular disorders, or pathologic abnormalities detected by histology or inferred by imaging.

The KDIGO chronic kidney disease staging for children older than 2 years of age stratifies the risk for progression of chronic

kidney disease and its complications based on glomerular filtration rate (GFR) and is used to guide management. The stages of chronic kidney disease are:

- G1 – Normal glomerular filtration rate is ≥90 mL per minute per 1.73 m²
- G2 – glomerular filtration rate between 60 and 89 mL per minute per 1.73 m²
- G3a – glomerular filtration rate between 45 and 59 mL per minute per 1.73 m²
- G3b – glomerular filtration rate between 30 and 44 mL per minute per 1.73 m²
- G4 – glomerular filtration rate between 15 and 29 mL per minute per 1.73 m²
- G5 – glomerular filtration rate <15 mL per minute per 1.73 m²; also referred to as end-stage kidney disease (ESKD)

Of note, children <2 years of age do not fit within this classification system as they normally have a low glomerular filtration rate even when corrected for body surface area. In these patients, calculated glomerular filtration rate based upon serum creatinine should be compared to normative age-appropriate values to detect kidney impairment.[68]

Managing a child with chronic kidney disease can be complex due to the variety of causes of chronic kidney disease and requires meticulous attention to electrolyte, fluid, and acid-base balance, metabolic bone disease, growth/nutrition, hematologic issues, and blood pressures/cardiovascular health. Attention should be focused on slowing the progression of renal disease and its complications to prevent end-stage renal disease, which in children, carries a 55-fold greater mortality than the general pediatric population.[69]

Electrolyte Balance

Despite losses of up to 90% of renal function, sodium homeostasis usually is well maintained in chronic kidney disease. With large decreases in the glomerular filtration rate, the kidney maintains normal serum sodium by increasing the FE_{Na} from less than 1% up to 25% to 30%, largely through decreases in distal tubular resorption. Some of the hormonal factors associated with this adaptation include aldosterone, atrial natriuretic peptide, and a poorly characterized natriuretic hormone that inhibits Na^+/K^+-ATPase. With worsening chronic kidney disease, the kidney loses its ability to handle a wide range of sodium intake, from 1 to 250 mEq/m² per day. Instead, the kidney may only be able to handle a narrow range of sodium intake of 50 to 100 mEq/m² per day. It may be possible to decrease this obligatory excretion of sodium to 5 to 20 mEq/m² per day, although it may occur only after weeks of decreasing the sodium intake slowly. Children with chronic kidney disease secondary to congenital anomalies of the kidney and urinary tract or tubulointerstitial disease may be unable to adjust to a decreased sodium intake and display a salt-losing nephropathy. These children are prone to dehydration with salt restriction and may need supplemental salt to ensure normal growth. On the other hand, children with chronic kidney disease due to acquired kidney diseases, such as glomerulonephritis, may develop sodium retention, volume overload, and hypertension with unrestricted sodium in their diet. As such, sodium intake must be individualized to fit the limitations of each child.

As in the case of sodium, the serum potassium concentrations usually remain normal until the glomerular filtration rate is less than 10% of normal. Potassium excretion normally occurs in the distal nephron. However, in response to an increase in potassium intake or loss of renal mass, Na^+/K^+-ATPase increases in the remaining collecting tubules; this is responsible, in part, for the augmented excretion of potassium per nephron. Approximately 13% of dietary potassium is excreted via the colon. This can increase to 50% by the activation of colonic Na^+/K^+-ATPase via aldosterone. An additional mechanism that plays an essential role in the adaptation to an acute potassium load is the redistribution of potassium from the extracellular to the intracellular compartment, which depends on insulin, β-adrenergic catecholamines, aldosterone, and pH. Despite the presence of total body potassium depletion in uremia, the uptake of potassium into the cells is impaired. This contributes to the intolerance to an acute potassium load in uremia despite the ability to excrete a potassium load.

Hyperkalemia is a major problem in chronic kidney disease.[70] Hyperkalemia can result from an extrinsic potassium load, but it may also be caused by fasting or acidosis, in which case the source of the potassium is the intracellular compartment. This can be a particular problem when a child has fasted before surgery and can be ameliorated by an infusion of glucose and insulin. Drugs that can cause hyperkalemia in renal failure include spironolactone, β-adrenergic blockers, and ACE inhibitors. When clinically significant hyperkalemia develops in a child with chronic kidney disease, the first-line therapy is to stabilize the myocardium with exogenous calcium and then to redistribute the potassium into the intracellular compartment with insulin and glucose. To deliver the same dose of ionized calcium, the dose of calcium gluconate (in milligrams per kilogram) should be three times that of calcium chloride.[71] All doses of calcium are optimally delivered through a central venous access line because calcium infusions are irritating to peripheral veins and can cause necrosis of the skin if extravasation occurs. At eight times the usual asthma dose, nebulized albuterol/salbutamol has been effective in redistributing potassium intracellularly, whereas sodium bicarbonate administration has not been effective (Table 26.6). More definitive correction of hyperkalemia is accomplished by removing potassium from the body using dialysis or medications such as sodium polystyrene sulfonate (Kayexalate), patiromer (Veltassa), or sodium zirconium cyclosilicate (Lokelma) (see also Figs. 7.7 and 7.8). In contrast, hypokalemia is unusual in the absence of potassium restriction, alkalosis, or diuretic therapy.

Fluid Balance

Water balance is also affected by chronic kidney disease. There is an obligatory total osmolar excretion that limits the ability of the kidney to excrete free water. The concentrating ability of the kidney is affected, limiting its ability to make a maximally concentrated or dilute urine. These limitations may result in water retention and hyponatremia or dehydration if water is administered in amounts exceeding the kidney's capabilities. These limitations must be considered when treating children with chronic renal failure, particularly before surgery when free access to water is restricted.

Metabolic Acidosis

Metabolic acidosis is common in those with chronic kidney disease.[72] In moderate chronic kidney disease, the type of metabolic acidosis is a non–anion gap acidosis, but in severe chronic kidney disease, the metabolic acidosis is an anion gap acidosis, because of the presence of excess phosphate, sulfate, and organic acids. The primary cause of metabolic acidosis in chronic kidney disease is the inability of the remaining proximal renal tubules to increase ammonium formation to keep pace with the loss of renal mass. The kidney becomes unable to generate the 1 to 3 mEq/kg per day of new bicarbonate that is necessary to compensate for the bicarbonate lost to buffering endogenous acids. The proximal renal tubule was thought to have a major role for the observed decreased resorption of bicarbonate in chronic kidney disease. Although this may occur in the presence of volume overload, severe secondary hyperparathyroidism, and disorders such as Fanconi syndrome, it is not a major cause of acidosis in chronic kidney disease. Except for severe phosphate depletion, decreased excretion of phosphate as a titratable acid normally does not contribute to metabolic acidosis.

Chronic Kidney Disease: Mineral Bone Disorder

As the mineral and endocrine functions of the kidney are critically important for regulation of bone formation and remodeling during growth, progression of chronic kidney disease leads to abnormalities in mineral metabolism and bone formation.[73] One of the earliest manifestations of chronic kidney disease is secondary hyperparathyroidism. Secondary hyperparathyroidism, which results from inadequate formation of 1,25-$(OH)_2$ vitamin D (i.e., 1,25-dihydroxyvitamin D_3 or calcitriol), develops in moderate chronic kidney disease in the presence of normal serum concentrations of calcium and phosphorus.[74] As chronic kidney disease progresses, overt hypocalcemia and hyperphosphatemia often develop. Hypocalcemia is caused by decreased calcium absorption from the gastrointestinal tract as a result of a true deficiency of 1,25-$(OH)_2$ vitamin D. Renal osteodystrophy, the term used to describe the impact of disordered mineral bone metabolism on the skeletal system, progresses with worsening chronic kidney disease and can result in skeletal deformities, fractures, muscle and bone pain, avascular necrosis, and growth failure.[75] Along with its effect on the skeletal system, disruption in mineral and bone metabolism also affects the cardiovascular system. Calcium and phosphate may be deposited in soft tissues as a consequence of hyperphosphatemia.

TABLE 26.6	Treatment of Hyperkalemia
Treatment	**Dosage**
Stabilization of Myocardium	
Calcium and bicarbonate	Calcium gluconate: 10% 30–100 mg/kg IV *or*
	Calcium chloride: 10% 10–33 mg/kg IV
	Sodium bicarbonate: 1 mEq/kg IV if acidotic
Shifting of Potassium to Intracellular Space	
Hyperventilation	
Insulin and glucose	Insulin: 0.10–0.3 unit/kg *or*
	0.1 U/kg per hour infusion
	Glucose: D_{50} 1–2 mL/kg *or*
	D_{25} 2–4 mL/kg IV *or*
	D_5 1–2 mL/kg per hour
Albuterol	Albuterol: 2.5–5 mg/mL nebulization
Decreasing Total Body Potassium	
Sodium polystyrene sulfonate (Kayexalate)	1 g/kg up to 40 grams every 4 hours PO or PR
Furosemide (diuretic)	0.5 mg/kg up to 40 mg

D, Dextrose; *IV*, intravenous; *PO*, per os (oral); *PR*, per rectum (suppository).

The kidney plays a key role in the maintenance of phosphate homeostasis by regulating its excretion. In the presence of a normal glomerular filtration rate, the kidney excretes 5% to 15% of the filtered load of phosphate. Fibroblast growth factor-23 (FGF-23) is a phosphaturic hormone secreted by the osteocytes that targets the kidney early in chronic kidney disease to increase phosphate excretion.[76] Through this adaptation, the kidneys are initially able to maintain a phosphate balance in chronic kidney disease, but they do so at an increased serum phosphate concentration. More importantly, the failing kidneys have no reserve with which to increase phosphate excretion in response to a phosphate load. In children with chronic kidney disease, a large phosphate load, such as with a phosphate-containing enema, can lead to life-threatening hyperphosphatemia and hypocalcemia.

Growth and Nutrition

Regular assessment of nutrition and growth is recommended for children with chronic kidney disease stage 2 or greater, as impaired growth increases as chronic kidney disease progresses.[77] Children with chronic kidney disease oftentimes experience anorexia, nausea, or vomiting as well as altered taste sensation, which leads to decreased caloric intake. The pathogenesis of short stature in children with chronic kidney disease is multifactorial, due to several possible causes that include malnutrition, metabolic bone disease, abnormalities in growth hormone–insulin like growth factor-1 (IGF-1) axis, fluid and electrolyte disturbances, metabolic acidosis, inadequate dialysis, and medications.[78] Management of these potential contributors to growth failure is essential to optimize growth. As the impact of nutrition on growth in infants is especially important, many infants and young children with chronic kidney disease or end-stage kidney disease need a gastrostomy tube to provide sufficient caloric intake for growth.[79] Even with optimization of the nutrition, acid-base balance, electrolyte disorders, chronic kidney disease, and metabolic bone disease, patients may require recombinant human growth hormone (rhGH) for improved growth.[80]

Uremia

The term *uremia* refers to the symptoms of anorexia, nausea, lethargy, and somnolence that results from chronic renal failure. Uremia ultimately leads to death unless dialysis therapy or renal transplantation is performed. Initiating dialysis or transplanting a kidney is referred to as end-stage renal disease care.

Hematologic Problems

One of the most common manifestations of chronic kidney disease is anemia. The anemia of chronic kidney disease is the result of impaired erythropoiesis, hemolysis, and bleeding. Of these, impaired erythropoiesis is most important and usually results from a deficiency of erythropoietin production. Erythropoietin is synthesized and secreted by the peritubular cells in the renal cortex in response to decreased tissue oxygenation. It acts on receptors on the erythroid burst-forming units and erythroid colony-forming units. With loss of renal mass, erythropoietin secretion does not respond adequately to hypoxia, and anemia ensues. Anemia is present in 95% of children with end-stage renal disease, although the incidence is less in those with chronic kidney disease.[81] In one study, 30% of those with chronic kidney disease stages 1 and 2 were anemic, 66% in stage 3, and 93% in stages 4 and 5.[81] Correction of the anemia reduces mortality. In a study of children undergoing peritoneal dialysis over a >3 year period, mortality was 62% greater in those with a hemoglobin <11 gm% compared with those >11 gm%.[82] Hence, treatment regimens

strive for Hb values >11 gm%, although erythropoietin was associated with a hazard ratio of 1.33 for death if the dose exceeded 6000 IU/m^2 per week compared with less than 6000 IU/m^2 per week.[82] 94% of children with chronic kidney disease are treated with erythropoietin stimulating agents (ESAs) when their hematocrit decreases to less than 30%.[83]

Recombinant human erythropoietin has a short half-life necessitating thrice weekly administration. The introduction of darbepoetin alpha extended the half-life to permit twice weekly treatment in the 1990s and a continuous erythropoietin receptor activator was introduced in 2007 to permit dosing one to two times per month.[84] All formulations of erythropoietin appear equally effective and equally safe.[85] Although erythropoietin therapy has been associated with several serious complications in adults (hypertension, stroke, and death), the association is less clear in children. Dose escalation of erythropoietin in adults to Hb values >12.5 gm% has resulted in a greater incidence of complications including mortality, which although unproven in children, resulted in the acceptance of moderate increases in Hb to 11.0 to 12.0 gm%.[84] The independent association of large erythropoietin doses with mortality has limited the dose of erythropoietin in children.

Children who are scheduled for erythropoietin therapy should begin oral iron, vitamin C (a cofactor for iron absorption from the gastrointestinal tract), and folic acid 2 to 3 weeks in advance of erythropoietin to ensure adequate iron and folic acid stores to facilitate erythropoiesis. The most common cause for failure of erythropoietin, and therefore erythropoiesis, is concurrent iron deficiency. Current recommendations recommend maintaining serum ferritin concentrations in excess of 250 ng/mL and a transferrin saturation greater than 20%. Other causes for the failure of erythropoietin to increase or maintain the hematocrit are occult infections, hemolysis, aluminum overload, severe hyperparathyroidism, and occult bleeding. Complications of erythropoietin therapy include worsening of hypertension, a possible increased incidence of thrombosis of polytetrafluoroethylene vascular grafts, and polycythemia.

The other major hematologic problem in chronic kidney disease is bleeding. This classic and lethal complication in children with terminal uremia results from platelet dysfunction in the presence of a normal coagulation profile and normal platelet counts.[86] The best indicator of platelet dysfunction in children with chronic kidney disease is a prolonged bleeding time. The platelet dysfunction is the result of poorly described abnormalities attributed to the uremic environment, rendering platelet transfusions ineffective. Dialysis improves platelet dysfunction, as does improvement in the hematocrit with transfusions or erythropoietin therapy.[87] Preoperative IV desmopressin acetate (1-deamino-8-d-arginine vasopressin, DDAVP) (0.3 μg/kg) improves the bleeding time in children with uremia.[88]

Cardiovascular Complications

Hypertension is one of the most common complications of chronic kidney disease and contributes significantly to the morbidity and mortality of these children. Approximately 4% of children and adolescents have hypertension and up to 14% have pre-hypertension.[89] The cause is multifactorial and includes volume overload and hormonal abnormalities, such as increased secretion of renin, which result from the underlying renal disorder as well as genetic factors, obesity, and ethnicity.[89] In children undergoing dialysis, volume overload is the result of inadequate removal of volume during dialysis. The goal of ultrafiltration is to remove sufficient salt and water to achieve the dry weight that is appropriate for each child. The *dry weight* is the weight at which the child has no signs of volume overload but below which the child has hypotension. The initial response to volume overload is to increase the cardiac output. Later, the cardiac output returns to normal, but the peripheral resistance increases because of peripheral vasoconstriction, resulting in hypertension. These children may have no other signs of volume overload, such as edema, but with a reduction in total body salt and water content, the blood pressure can be controlled with little or no antihypertensive medication.[62]

In other children, intrinsic renal abnormalities play a primary role in hypertension. Oral antihypertensive agents are often effective in controlling the severe refractory hypertension, although in some, bilateral nephrectomies may be required to control the hypertension. In an interesting "n-of-1" study to compare the efficacy of three antihypertensives to control their blood pressure without unacceptable side effects in 42 children, a Bayesian analysis concluded 49% preferred lisinopril, 24% amlodipine, and 12% hydrochlorothiazide.[90] Of the mechanisms that cause hypertension in these children, increased renin secretion is the best understood. Renin activates the formation of angiotensin I, which is then converted to angiotensin II, a powerful vasoconstrictor. Children with renin-dependent hypertension respond poorly to control of blood pressure by salt and water removal alone but respond well to ACE inhibitors such as captopril.

Cardiovascular disease is the most common cause of death in patients undergoing long-term dialysis, including children.[91] Females fare worse than males with advanced chronic kidney disease as they appear more susceptible to vascular stiffening.[92] Children with chronic kidney disease or end-stage kidney disease can have abnormalities of the pericardium, myocardium, cardiac valves, and coronary arteries. Pericarditis was once considered a sign of the terminal phase of uremia, but it occurs in 15% of children who are undergoing dialysis and can be either symptomatic or clinically silent. Intensive dialysis often results in its resolution within ~2 weeks in uremic patients with pericarditis who are not undergoing dialysis. Some children require surgical procedures such as pericardiocentesis, pericardial drainage with a catheter or through a pericardial window, or pericardiectomy.

Left ventricular failure is also a common complication of chronic kidney disease.[93] In older patients, coronary artery disease may lead to myocardial dysfunction, severely limiting cardiac output. Volume overload and hypertension, which increase preload and afterload, respectively, are important causes of heart failure. With proper fluid management and antihypertensive medication, these abnormalities can be controlled. Anemia is another contributing factor that can be controlled with the use of erythropoietin. An array of metabolic abnormalities associated with chronic kidney disease, such as secondary hyperparathyroidism, electrolyte and acid-base imbalances, and the accumulation of nonspecific uremic toxins, contribute to abnormal myocardial function.[94]

Causes of Chronic Kidney Disease

The causes of chronic kidney disease and end-stage kidney disease can be correlated with age (Table 26.7). The chronic kidney disease that is commonly encountered in early infancy results largely from congenital anomalies or perinatal asphyxia. Later in childhood, chronic kidney disease may result from dysplasia, or acquired lesions, whereas those affected in adolescence may have deterioration of function related to acquired disease, manifestation

TABLE 26.7	Causes of Chronic Renal Failure and Associated Syndromes	
Infancy (Congenital Anomalies)	**Childhood**	**Adolescence**
Prune-belly syndrome	Dysplasia	Focal segmental glomerulosclerosis
Congenital obstruction	Agenesis	Membranoproliferative glomerulonephritis
Posterior urethral valves	Autosomal dominant PKD	Secondary glomerulonephritis
Multicystic dysplasia	Reflux nephropathy	Systemic lupus erythematosus
Agenesis	Obstruction	Sickle cell disease
Autosomal recessive PKD	Focal segmental glomerulosclerosis	HIV-associated nephropathy
Reflux nephropathy	Membranoproliferative glomerulonephritis	Diabetes mellitus Vasculitis Hemolytic uremic syndrome Henoch-Schönlein purpura Interstitial nephritis Malignancy

HIV, Human immunodeficiency virus; *PKD,* polycystic kidney disease.

of inherited disease, or secondary lesions resulting from other illnesses (e.g., systemic lupus erythematosus, sickle cell disease) or their treatments.

Intraoperative Management

Anesthesia is a unique physiological challenge to a patient's normal homeostasis. Given the morbidity and mortality associated with acute kidney injury,[95] the anesthesiologist must be cognizant of the potential for causing acute kidney injury. This might occur in a child with preexisting chronic renal failure or end-stage renal disease, in whom further renal damage would be catastrophic or a patient who is at risk of acute kidney injury based on their degree of risk or the specific surgical encounter (e.g., cardiopulmonary bypass is the most widely reported).[96] There are suggested strategies for renal protection in both scenarios and clearly some considerable overlap. The most important tenant of anesthesia in regard to acute kidney injury is that prevention is vital because treatment options are limited.

STRATEGIES FOR RENAL PROTECTION

Described as an underrecognized problem, the incidence of perioperative acute kidney injury is variously reported but occurs in ~27% of critically ill children.[97–99] Despite the standardization of what constitutes acute kidney injury in children,[100] it remains underdiagnosed, leading to increased morbidity and mortality.

RISK FACTORS

To begin to understand the risk for acute kidney injury, the anesthesiologist should identify vulnerable patients and the associated risk factors. Although creatinine concentration and urine output are actually poor indicators of acute kidney injury in children, an increased creatinine at baseline is an important predictor of postoperative acute kidney injury.[101,102] Risk factors for neonates include low birth weight (and early gestational age), low APGAR score (and hypoxic ischemic encephalopathy), nephrotoxic medications, use of mechanical ventilation and extracorporeal life support, and antenatal corticosteroids.[103,104] In a recent meta-analysis of available data, binary risk factors included pulmonary hypertension, cyanotic heart disease, single ventricle anatomy, a Risk Adjustment for Congenital Heart Surgery (RACHS-1) score ≥ 3, use of nephrotoxic or vasopressors drugs, cardiopulmonary bypass, and sepsis. Continuous risk factors were younger age, lower body weight, surgery of greater duration, aortic cross-clamp time, bypass time, and greater volume of red blood cells transfused.[105]

Any child undergoing cardiopulmonary bypass is susceptible to acute kidney injury, with age and consequent kidney maturation important risk factors. Children under the age of 2 to 3 years may have difficulty accommodating the inflammatory and ischemic insults associated with surgery; diabetic children with poor glycemic control are also at increased risk.[106] In noncritically ill children exposed to three or more nephrotoxic medications or at least 3 days of aminoglycoside therapy, the incidence of acute kidney injury is 30%.[95,107] Identifying risk factors can lead to appropriate risk stratification and timely implementation of preventive and therapeutic strategies for acute kidney injury.

PREVENTION

Historically, measures that prevent acute kidney injury in adults were limited to "renal dose dopamine" and large doses of furosemide, although both may be injurious.[108] Pharmacological study is now aimed at antiinflammatory, antiapoptotic, and antioxidative agents to prevent acute kidney injury, although few drugs have shown clinical efficacy. Novel drug therapies aimed at reducing further damage through alterations in microcirculations and reduction of inflammatory mediators, are being proposed. For example, exogenous angiotensin II, which raises intraglomerular pressure and thus glomerular filtration rate, may potentially help to mitigate ischemic events, but this remains experimental.[109] Remote ischemic preconditioning seems to periodically carry favor in organ preservation strategies. Brief periods of ischemia and reperfusion of remote organs or tissues can result in protective adaptive responses in other organs, such as the kidneys. Although promising data have been reported in adults undergoing cardiac surgery,[110] there is no evidence as to its efficacy in the pediatric population. It is also unlikely to be well tolerated. In truth very few preemptive measures have proven effective in preventing acute kidney injury.[98,111]

Despite this scarcity of high-quality evidence, KDIGO recommendations include a "bundle" of measures to minimize the risk of acute kidney injury (https://kdigo.org/guidelines/acute-kidney-injury/). Optimization of volume status and hemodynamics, functional hemodynamic monitoring, avoidance of nephrotoxic drugs, and prevention of hyperglycemia in at-risk patients are all measures that, when clinically embraced and adopted in the perioperative management, could reduce acute kidney injury.

Fluid management and the correction to intravascular euvolemia *is* a key component of the prevention and management of acute kidney injury. Excessive fluid resuscitation should be avoided as it has been associated with the development of acute kidney injury.[112] There is clear evidence that more than 10% to 15% fluid overload by body weight is associated with adverse outcomes.[113] The most popular crystalloid historically has been 0.9% sodium chloride but a recent retrospective study indicates that the resulting hyperchloremia and hyperchloremic non–anion gap acidosis may increase adverse outcomes such as acute kidney injury.[114] Ideally, a physiologically composed balanced isotonic electrolyte solution such as Lactated Ringer solution is preferred for fluid resuscitation.[115] In adult studies some colloids, such as the hydroxyethyl starches, have been found to be nephrotoxic and therefore avoided in critically ill patients.[116] Controversy remains in pediatric practice.[117,118]

A recent perioperative quality initiative in adults concluded that intraoperative mean arterial pressure less than 60 to 70 mm Hg was associated with increased risk of acute kidney injury and death.[119] The hypotensive episodes could be of brief duration and may even occur between induction of anesthesia and surgical incision. It is unknown if this observation translates to children, but it is possible. Individualized blood pressure control is probably protective against acute kidney injury. Optimal fluid management along with selective vasopressor use are the tenants of perioperative care.

Avoidance of nephrotoxic drugs in the perioperative period will attenuate the risk of acute kidney injury. Medications associated with acute kidney injury include amphotericin B, chemotherapy, contrast media, acyclovir, and nonsteroidal antiinflammatory drugs. Glycemic control is a modifiable independent predictor of negative outcomes in critically ill children. While avoiding hypoglycemia, attempts at reasonable glycemic control are important. In children, wider intraoperative glycemic fluctuation, and not necessarily hyperglycemia alone, is associated with an increased incidence of postoperative acute kidney injury.[120]

Preoperative anemia has been linked with acute kidney injury for cardiac and noncardiac surgery in adults. Decreased oxygen delivery to vulnerable tissues such as the kidney inevitably leads to a greater oxidative stress. However perioperative blood transfusion has been identified as an independent risk factor for acute kidney injury. Both anemia and transfusion are associated with acute kidney injury giving rise to difficult decisions as to how to manage anemia.[121]

There are specific anesthesia-based preventive measures that are initiated with the avoidance of acute kidney injury in mind. The long-established fasting guidelines adopted by the global anesthesia community are currently being challenged.[122] Theoretically, shorter fasting times may decrease the risk of perioperative acute kidney injury, by reducing metabolic stress and attenuating insulin resistance.[123] Rather than adopt a 1-hour preoperative fast after clear fluids, strategies that reduce the risk of prolonged preoperative fasts after clear fluids include quality improvement and texting parents on the evening before surgery.[124,125] Nephrotoxic medications should be stopped as should angiotensin-converting enzyme inhibitors (ACE-1) to prevent intraoperative hypotension.[126]

As for anesthesia medications, inhalational agents may have reno-protective properties,[127] specifically sevoflurane and enflurane. However, the use of propofol or dexmedetomidine may be more so. Propofol is associated with increased kidney protection when compared with sevoflurane, possibly through an antioxidant mechanism,[128] but this may not be clinically important. Dexmedetomidine, an α_2-adrenoceptor agonist, has diuretic properties through its suppression of vasopressin secretion. Glomerular filtration rate and renal blood flow are enhanced, thereby increasing urine output. Some advocate its use in protecting against contrast-induced nephropathy, and it has an antiinflammatory effect.[129] Reduction in levels of harmful inflammatory molecules such as tumor necrosis factor-α (TNF-α) and increase of proteins such as bone morphogenetic protein-7 (BMP-7) are thought to protect against sepsis-induced acute kidney injury.[130] The clinical efficacy of this also has yet to be established, as the broader metrics of postoperative mortality, length of ICU stay or duration of mechanical ventilation have failed to show any benefit[131] but dexmedetomidine has been associated with improved short-term mortality in adult patients with sepsis and children after surgery for congenital heart disease.

New evidence suggests that acetaminophen may be one pharmacological intervention that preemptively reduces the risk of acute kidney injury. Although a modest influence, children undergoing cardiopulmonary bypass for congenital heart disease had a reduction in acute kidney injury in the first 48 hours following surgery.[132]

Regional anesthesia has a theoretical advantage of increased vasodilatation and therefore visceral perfusion, thus preserving renal blood flow. There are adult data describing an association with fewer dialysis requirements with combined general and regional anesthesia[133] but there are no pediatric data to support this theory.

Mechanical factors in the perioperative period should be considered. Compression of renal parenchyma with high insufflation pressures associated laparoscopic surgery results in oliguria, but whether this leads to acute kidney injury is unclear. Mechanical lung ventilation has multifactorial detrimental associated effects on renal function, with as much as a 3-fold increase in the odds of developing acute kidney injury compared with spontaneous ventilation.[134] A reasonable approach to high-risk surgical patients would be low tidal volume ventilation with optimal positive end-expiratory pressure (PEEP) to avoid hypoxia and hypercarbia.[126,135] Finally, poor patient positioning, and prolonged immobilization or use of a tourniquet can lead to compartment syndrome and rhabdomyolysis. The breakdown products of myocyte necrosis have long been associated with acute kidney injury, with prompt detection, volume resuscitation, and early renal replacement therapy, key tenants can reverse any renal damage.

MANAGEMENT OF ACUTE KIDNEY INJURY

After making the diagnosis of acute kidney injury, management of acute kidney injury should begin with treating the underlying cause and preserving tissue perfusion. Avoidance of nephrotoxic drugs is key. Renal replacement therapy, whether it be continuous renal replacement therapy and hemodialysis vs. peritoneal dialysis, has improved survival outcomes among pediatric acute kidney injury patients.[99] Nondialytic management via fluid therapy is effective in pediatric acute kidney injury, specifically with isotonic crystalloids.[136]

ANESTHESIA CONCERNS IN PATIENTS PRESENTING WITH RENAL FAILURE

It is also important to consider how anesthesia may be impacted by a child with chronic renal failure. This child will present with other unique issues that further complicate anesthesia management such as strategies for preserving renal function, optimization of hemodynamics and intravascular volume, and the avoidance or cautious use of drugs that are nephrotoxic. Considerations regarding the complications of chronic renal failure, such as anemia, and differences in the pharmacokinetics of anesthetic agents in children with renal failure are also important.

Preoperative Assessment

Specific information pertaining to the renal impairment is desired: the cause, duration, and severity, the last dialysis (if requiring renal replacement therapy), and mode of dialysis. What is a normal blood pressure for each patient and what disease-specific medications are prescribed. If hypertension is an issue, an echocardiogram and electrocardiograph may be required as part of the preoperative assessment. The decisions to stop ACE inhibitors remains with the anesthesiologist with the knowledge that any hypotension under anesthesia will need to be treated with vasopressors and intravenous fluids.

Hemodynamic Control

Intraoperative measures at maintaining hemodynamic stability are key. Both hypertension and hypotension can adversely affect the renal microvasculature in kidneys with impaired autoregulation. Advanced hemodynamic monitoring may be required. As mentioned earlier, dopamine has long been considered renally protective but conventional wisdom would now suggest that its efficacy is variable and unpredictable. Fenoldopam, a selective dopamine 1–receptor agonist, increases glomerular filtration rate without the hypertension associated with the use of dopamine. It significantly reduces creatinine more than dopamine and may have a role in renoprotection. Although several empirical measures have been recommended for renal protection in the perioperative period, a Cochrane review concluded that no interventions, whether pharmacologic or otherwise, protected the kidney in the perioperative period.[137]

FLUIDS AND BLOOD PRODUCTS

In the child with renal insufficiency, fluid management requires a balanced approach. The child must receive adequate hydration to prevent further renal deterioration in an otherwise injured kidney. Children with renal failure and a history of hypertension are at risk for both hypotension and hypertension and require some degree of fluid resuscitation for stability. However, they also may have hypoalbuminemia with low oncotic pressure that predisposes to pulmonary edema. Ideally, if the child is euvolemic, standard fluid therapy based on typical surgical fluid management is preferred. Fluid overload must be avoided in all anuric children and in outpatients. As discussed earlier, the type of fluid is also important. Normal saline solutions should be eschewed as they cause hyperchloremic acidosis and worsen renal failure; buffered isotonic solutions are preferred.

Children with renal failure are at a greater risk for bleeding in the perioperative period. This is a classic and lethal complication in children with terminal uremia that results from platelet dysfunction in the presence of a normal coagulation profile and normal platelet counts. As a consequence, the hemoglobin concentration should be monitored closely. Blood and component therapy may be used in accordance with surgical losses and to maintain the hemoglobin concentration but as mentioned above, blood transfusion itself is associated with increased risk of acute kidney injury and should not be undertaken lightly.

ANESTHETIC AGENTS

The pharmacokinetics and pharmacodynamics of anesthetic agents and perioperative medications may be altered in children with renal failure. The medications most likely to be affected are those that depend on renal excretion, such as the hydrophilic, highly ionized agents.

Induction of anesthesia may be carried out safely as long as the child is euvolemic and the pharmacokinetics and pharmacodynamics of the induction agent are understood and accounted for. Anesthetic agents may be affected by the presence of anemia, acidosis, and altered drug binding owing to hypoproteinemia in children with renal disease.

The dose of propofol to induce anesthesia (loading dose is principally volume related) using the bispectral index and clinical signs to indicate the state of hypnosis in adult patients with renal failure were greater than in those without renal disease.[138] When propofol is delivered as an infusion, no differences in pharmacokinetic (principally clearance) or pharmacodynamic parameters have been observed.[139] There is also some evidence to suggest that propofol, when compared with sevoflurane, may be reno-protective as a result of its ability to attenuate the perioperative increase in proinflammatory mediators.[140]

There are insufficient data regarding the use of inhalational anesthetics for induction in children with renal impairment. For maintenance of anesthesia in adults, desflurane and isoflurane do not further impair renal function in those with preexisting renal disease.[141] Sevoflurane at low flows is associated with increased circuit concentrations of compound A, which is nephrotoxic in rats but not in humans.[142] Overall, sevoflurane is considered safe in patients with renal disease, but low flows are best avoided.

Neuromuscular blocking drugs have evolved over the years to provide a choice of relaxants for use in children with renal disease. Children with chronic renal failure may have existing autonomic neuropathy and associated delayed gastric emptying that puts them at risk for aspiration. Along with renal implications, aspiration should be anticipated when choosing a neuromuscular blocking drug for airway management. Succinylcholine is often avoided in children with renal failure because of its well-known propensity for increasing serum potassium. However, succinylcholine does not increase the plasma potassium concentration in patients with chronic renal failure any more than in patients with normal renal function (0.5–0.8 mEq/L of potassium) unless a peripheral neuropathy is present.[143] The plasma concentration of potassium is chronically increased in renal failure, which implies that the intracellular and extracellular potassium concentrations are in equilibrium. As a result, the usual 0.5- to 1-mEq/L increase in serum potassium after succinylcholine causes no clinical manifestations, despite the large absolute concentration of potassium. This contrasts with patients with acute hyperkalemia in whom the intracellular and extracellular potassium concentrations are in disequilibrium, which predisposes these children to ventricular arrhythmias after succinylcholine. In the latter case, succinylcholine is relatively contraindicated, whereas in the former case, it is not contraindicated.

The pharmacodynamics of neuromuscular blocking drugs in children with renal insufficiency merit consideration. The onset time of rocuronium in children with renal failure is greater than in children with normal renal function.[144,145] This difference was attributed to a greater volume of distribution, decreased serum albumin concentrations, and possibly to a reduced cardiac output in children with renal failure who were taking antihypertensives. The slower onset time of rocuronium in children with renal failure must be considered when a rapid-sequence intubation is required, and succinylcholine is contraindicated. The durations of action of rocuronium in children with normal renal function and end-stage renal disease are similar.[146] This is not surprising because the elimination of rocuronium is predominantly via the biliary system and not the kidneys.

Neuromuscular blocking drugs such as atracurium and cisatracurium are ideal choices for children with renal insufficiency because their elimination is completely independent of the kidney. Despite the fact that both agents undergo spontaneous degradation by plasma esterase and Hofmann elimination, neuromuscular blockade should still be monitored.[147] Therefore, with appropriate monitoring and dosing, atracurium, cisatracurium, vecuronium, and rocuronium are all acceptable neuromuscular blocking drugs in children with renal disease and provide reliable durations of action after a single bolus dose.[147] Prolonged infusions of atracurium and cisatracurium may lead to moderate accumulation of laudanosine, possibly resulting in hypotension, bradycardia, and seizures.[148,149]

If a prolonged neuromuscular blockade occurs, hypermagnesemia should be ruled out. In this case, calcium may be administered to help antagonize the blockade. The elimination of neostigmine may be delayed beyond elimination of atropine or glycopyrrolate, and muscarinic effects such as bradycardia, increased secretions, or bronchospasm may theoretically occur postoperatively after antagonism.

Sugammadex is a binding agent selective for aminosteroidal neuromuscular blocking drugs such as rocuronium and vecuronium. It is entirely renally excreted with an elimination half-life of approximately 100 minutes. As discussed elsewhere, rocuronium is metabolized almost entirely in the liver but when it is bound to sugammadex, it is both inactivated and effectively removed from the circulation; the rocuronium-sugammadex complex is eliminated by the kidney. Special consideration should therefore be given to patients with renal failure.[150] Sugammadex dosing in mild to moderate renal dysfunction is the same as in patients with normal renal function; it is not recommended for those with severe renal failure.[151] In a patient with normal renal function, rocuronium can be redosed in about 25 minutes after sugammadex administration. Because there are currently no redosing data for patients with renal failure, the use of sugammadex should be carefully considered.

Opioids do not have any direct toxic effects on the kidney but there is potential for alteration of pharmacokinetics of the parent drug and the metabolites. Morphine for example has an active metabolite, morphine-6-glucuronide whose metabolism is dependent in part on the kidneys. Morphine should be used with caution in children with end-stage renal disease.[141]

Doses of other opioids should be reduced by 30% to 50% to avoid respiratory depression in children with chronic renal failure. Active metabolites of hydromorphone and meperidine (no longer recommended for children other than to treat shivering) can likewise accumulate in patients with renal failure, whereas those of fentanyl and sufentanil do not. Dialysis may be required to eliminate these active metabolites.[152]

Remifentanil may be a preferred choice for a maintenance opioid in the intraoperative period in children with renal insufficiency because of its rapid metabolism by nonspecific blood and tissue esterases. The pharmacokinetics and pharmacodynamics of remifentanil are not altered in patients with renal disease, but the principal metabolite of remifentanil has reduced elimination, which is not clinically relevant.[153]

Although dexmedetomidine is metabolized in the liver, none of the renally excreted metabolites are active. The reno-protective effect of dexmedetomidine therefore may make it a logical sedation and anesthetic choice in children who are vulnerable to acute kidney injury, further increasing its appeal for use in children with renal disease.[154,155] There is concern that with the reduced plasma protein binding in end-stage renal disease, sedation may increase; this should be considered.[141]

Delayed emergence, vomiting and aspiration, hypertension, respiratory depression, and pulmonary edema are potential problems that should be anticipated during emergence from anesthesia. Hyperkalemia as a consequence of tissue injury, catabolism, blood transfusion, and acidosis may occur. Children with chronic renal failure usually have chronic metabolic acidosis with limited buffer reserve. Modest hypercapnia with emergence may lead to significant acidosis and hyperkalemia. Careful attention should be given to the fluid needs of the child postoperatively to minimize volume overload and potential pulmonary edema.

Regional anesthesia is a viable alternative to general anesthesia or an adjunct in many cases. The anesthesia team must pay particular attention to coagulation studies and signs of coagulopathy before embarking on any central block because abnormal platelet function puts the renal failure patient at risk for an epidural hematoma.

POSTOPERATIVE CONCERNS

The postoperative care of the child with renal disease must consider the level of renal function, anemia, and preexistence of hypertension. In the child with limited ability to excrete a salt and water load, care must be given to the rate and volume of postoperative fluids administered, with consideration of the volume given during the procedure and operative losses. In children with renal insufficiency, nephrotic syndrome, or tubular disorders (especially those with concentration impairments), it is common to administer fluid volumes that approximate anticipated output and insensible needs. This volume needs to be adjusted for third spacing, ongoing losses, and the administration of blood and blood products.

For children with known renal disease, care must be taken to identify medications that need to be resumed in the immediate postoperative period. Children who have been on chronic antihypertensive medications may be able to resume oral medications when awake. It may be necessary to treat isolated hypertensive episodes with intravenous medications during the immediate postoperative period. It is important to assess the contribution of pain and anxiety to increased blood pressures to avoid overtreatment of hypertension.

Because of ischemic tissue injury, it is possible that preexisting metabolic acidosis and hyperkalemia may worsen in the postoperative period. In children who have renal failure, careful monitoring of electrolytes during and after the procedure may prevent untoward emergencies. When clinically significant hyperkalemia develops in a child with chronic renal failure, treatment is imperative.

Acute hypertension can be treated with a variety of intravenous and oral medications. The therapy for acute symptomatic hypertension should be directed toward rapid normalization of blood pressure. Prompt and effective therapy must be initiated, often before the cause has been discerned. The rate of change of blood pressure can be just as important as its absolute level in the pathogenesis of hypertensive emergencies. Blood pressure itself may be a poor determinant of the severity of the clinical situation and the need for aggressive parenteral therapy. The decision to use aggressive parenteral therapy should be based on an absolute number and on clinical findings that define the situation as emergent (Table 26.8).

Hemodialysis or peritoneal dialysis can be safely resumed on the first postoperative day, except for children who have operative placement of a dialysis access port for more emergent therapy. In these children, the timing of renal replacement therapy must be individualized in consultation with the child's nephrologist.

Uremic encephalopathy may occur and should be considered in any child who exhibits confusion or prolonged sedation in the postanesthesia care unit. These children should be transferred to

an intensive care setting for monitoring, stabilization, and airway management during further evaluation.

With a careful preoperative assessment and review of preexisting disease, many postoperative complications can be anticipated and avoided. Hypervigilance during the entire perioperative period allows children with renal disease to be managed in a safe manner.

TABLE 26.8	Management of Acute Malignant Hypertension	
Drug	Dose	Side Effects
Sodium nitroprusside	1–10 μg/kg per minute IV	Possible cyanide and thiocyanate toxicity, acute hypotension
Enalaprilat[a]	0.01–0.06 mg/kg IV 6 hourly	Onset 15 minutes in neonates; hypotension, angioedema, anaphylactoid reaction, and increase serum creatinine; avoid with increased plasma renin levels, acute kidney injury, and CKD
Labetalol	0.1–0.4 mg/kg per hour *or* 0.2–1 mg/kg IV every 10 minutes (maximum 40 mg)	Bradycardia; caution in children with head injuries at risk for hypotension
Nicardipine	0.5–5 μg/kg per minute IV (maximum 20 mg/hour)	Acute hypotension; possible superficial thrombophlebitis if administered through a peripheral IV
Hydralazine	0.1–0.5 mg/kg IV or IM, not to exceed 2 mg IV 6 hourly	
Esmolol	100–500 μg/kg IV over 2 minutes LOAD 50–100 up to 300 μg/kg per minute IV infusion	Bradycardia, acute hypotension

[a]Intravenous angiotensin-converting enzyme inhibitor.
AKI, Acute kidney injury; *CKD,* chronic kidney disease; *IV,* intravenous.

ANNOTATED REFERENCES

Cavalcante CTdMB, Cavalcante MB, Castello Branco KMP, et al. Biomarkers of acute kidney injury in pediatric cardiac surgery. *Pediatric Nephrology* 2022;37(1):61-78.
This article provides an up-to-date and comprehensive review of biomarkers that may be useful in predicting AKI in pediatric cardiac surgery.
de Galasso L, Picca S, Guzzo I. Dialysis modalities for the management of pediatric acute kidney injury. *Pediatr Nephrol.* 2020;35(5):753-765.
This article provides a comprehensive review of the available renal replacement therapy modalities available for treatment of children with AKI requiring dialysis, with a focus on indications, prescription considerations, advantages, disadvantages, and limitations of each modality.
Ricci Z, Luciano R, Favia I, et al. High-dose fenoldopam reduces postoperative neutrophil gelatinase-associated lipocaline and cystatin C levels in pediatric cardiac surgery. *Critical Care.* 2011;15(3):R160.
This article reviews the potential benefits of fenoldopam in preventing AKI in infants with congenital heart disease undergoing pediatric cardiac surgery.

Ronco C, Bellomo R, Kellum JA. Acute kidney injury. *Lancet.* 2019; 394(10212):1949-1964.

This article provides a comprehensive review of the definition, etiology, pathophysiology, prognosis, prevention, and management of AKI.

Van den Eynde J, Cloet N, Van Lerberghe R, et al. Strategies to prevent acute kidney injury after pediatric cardiac surgery: a network meta-analysis. *Clin J Am Soc Nephrol.* 2021;16(10):1480-1490.

This article recognizes the risk of AKI in a vulnerable population and comprehensively reviews the strategies to minimize this risk.

Zaccharias M, Gilmore ICS, Herbison GP, et al. Interventions for protecting renal function in the perioperative period. *Cochrane Database Syst Rev.* 2008;(4):CD003590.

This work reports the evidence for interventions that are successful for protecting the kidney in the perioperative period.

A complete reference list can be found online at Elsevier eBooks+.

General Abdominal and Urologic Surgery

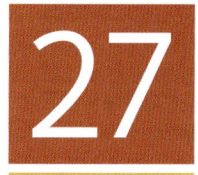

TOM G. HANSEN AND JERROLD LERMAN

General Principles of Abdominal Surgery
"The Full Stomach": The Risk for Pulmonary Aspiration of Gastric Contents
Rapid-Sequence Induction
Indications for Preoperative Nasogastric Tube Placement
Fluid Balance
Potential for Strangulated or Ischemic Bowel and Sepsis
Presence of Abdominal Compartment Syndrome
Preoperative Laboratory Testing and Investigations
Monitoring Requirements
Choice of Anesthetic
General Principles of Urologic Surgery
Reduced Renal Function
Systemic Arterial Hypertension
Corticosteroid Medications
Infection or Sepsis
Monitoring Requirements
Laparoscopic Surgery
Pneumoperitoneum
Respiratory Effects
Cardiovascular Effects
Central Nervous System Effects

Renal Effects and Fluid Requirements
Pain Management
Robot-Assisted Surgery
Specific General Surgical and Urologic Conditions
Nissen Fundoplication
Pectus Excavatum
Circumcision
Hypospadias and Chordee
Cryptorchidism and Hernias: Inguinal and Umbilical
Torsion of the Testis
Posterior Urethral Valves
Prune-Belly Syndrome
Ureteral Reimplantation
Pyeloplasty
Nephrectomy
Neuroblastoma
Wilms Tumor
Bladder and Cloacal Exstrophy
Bariatric Surgery in Children
Multidisciplinary Approach to Bariatric Surgery in Adolescents
Anesthetic Implications of Obesity in Adolescents

ABDOMINAL SURGERY AND UROLOGIC interventions make up a large fraction of anesthetic practice for the pediatric anesthesiologist. The field is rapidly evolving, with the increased use of laparoscopic surgery, including robot-assisted procedures.[1] This chapter focuses on the specific issues related to abdominal and urologic surgery, particularly in young children. The management of infants for pyloromyotomy and other neonatal abdominal procedures is discussed in Chapter 35.

General Principles of Abdominal Surgery

"THE FULL STOMACH": THE RISK FOR PULMONARY ASPIRATION OF GASTRIC CONTENTS

Most abdominal surgery is emergent and requires a rapid induction of anesthesia and protection of the airway to prevent regurgitation and pulmonary aspiration. Adhering to fasting guidelines for elective surgery does not ensure that the stomach of a child with an acute abdomen is empty of liquids and solids. The only metric that has been associated with gastric emptying after an acute emergency in children is the time interval between the last food ingested and the occurrence of the pathologic event or trauma.[2] However, there is no firm fasting interval after a trauma that predicts a zero risk of regurgitation and aspiration. The presence or absence of bowel sounds is also not predictive of gastric emptying or the risk of regurgitation.

Preoperatively, some children who present with an acute abdomen are administered an oral contrast agent before abdominal ultrasonography and/or computed tomography (CT) to visualize the stomach contents and estimate their volumes. These radiologic tools may not provide reliable estimates of the volume of gastric contents; however, the increased use of ultrasound assessments can provide further guidance.[3–8] Indeed, the absence of gastric contents in these assessments does not eliminate the risk of vomiting and regurgitation. Consequently, there is no evidence to delay a surgical procedure to empty the stomach of foods or reduce the risk of regurgitation; postponing may increase the risk of complications by delaying the urgently needed surgical attention to the acute abdomen.

RAPID-SEQUENCE INDUCTION

Rapid-sequence induction (RSI) is recommended for children with a full stomach to quickly secure the airway. This approach is intended to minimize the risk of aspiration, although it is not evidence-based. The strategy is to predetermine the drug doses for the child and have all the required airway equipment (age and size appropriate) ready to use. The predetermined drug doses are administered in a rapid sequence and when muscle relaxation has been achieved, the trachea is intubated and the tracheal tube cuff (if used) inflated. Many clinicians apply cricoid pressure to occlude the esophageal lumen during RSI, although not a single randomized trial has compared the frequency of regurgitation and aspiration with cricoid pressure during RSI with an inhalational or slow IV induction in children.[9] In the only published randomized, controlled trial of 3472 adults, the frequency of aspiration with and without cricoid pressure, 0.6% and 0.5%, were similar, but not noninferior, primarily because the *a priori* assumptions were too liberal.[10] In another study, the presence of microaspirates in the tracheas of 95 adults at risk for regurgitation (obese, those with diabetes, and those with gastroesophageal reflux) was compared with and without cricoid pressure during induction of elective surgery. The frequency of microaspirates in the two groups were similar.[11] This lack of evidence, combined with both theoretical and actual complications associated with RSI and cricoid pressure in children, has led to great skepticism regarding their roles in preventing pulmonary aspiration in children who are at risk, even though large population-based studies are lacking.[12] Only 74% of anesthesiologists in Northern Ireland perform RSI for children scheduled for appendectomy, 78% in the United States use it for pyloromyotomy, and 83% in England use it for forearm fractures within 2 hours of eating and after recent opioid administration.[13–15] In several surveys of pediatric anesthesiologists from the UK, India, and South Africa over the past 20 years, fewer than half of the practitioners used cricoid pressure in children during RSI and fewer than 20% used it in neonates and infants younger than 1 year of age.[16–18] In two surveys, 16% and 28% of anesthesiologists in the United States and the United Kingdom, respectively, reported that many children with full stomachs had experienced gastric regurgitation despite using RSI with cricoid pressure; several of them progressed to serious harm and even death.[14,19]

Despite the lack of evidence that cricoid pressure during RSI in children with full stomachs prevents regurgitation and thus aspiration,[20] some continue to cautiously recommend this approach for the majority of children at risk, recognizing that cricoid pressure is imperfect. Whether cricoid pressure during RSI effectively reduces the risk of regurgitation remains unclear. Evidence from nonrandomized controlled studies (RCTs) in a Cochrane review concluded that cricoid pressure may not be necessary to secure the airway during a RSI.[9] The authors called for well-designed and properly conducted RCTs to assess the safety and effectiveness of cricoid pressure in infants and children. However, these RCTs would require enrolling thousands of children to prove that without cricoid pressure, the risk of harm (e.g., aspiration) was significantly greater than using it and that investigators may find resistance when seeking approval from institutional review boards.[9] The National Emergency Airway Registry for Children, which is a large multinational database of airway management in critically ill children, determined the frequency of regurgitation to be 1.4% and aspiration to be 0.7% during 7825 tracheal intubations in children in 35 pediatric intensive care units.[21] When the contribution of cricoid pressure was evaluated as a factor in the frequency of regurgitation, regurgitation occurred in 1.9% of the intubations with cricoid pressure and in 1.2% without ($P = 0.018$). A sensitivity analysis of propensity score-matched cohorts showed that cricoid pressure was associated with a **greater** frequency of regurgitation ($P = 0.036$, odds ratio [OR] 1.01). Complications from RSI for the most part, relate to improperly performed RSI (e.g., excessive cricoid pressure distorting the anatomy of the airway[22] causing difficulty to pass a tracheal tube), force improperly applied to the thyroid cartilage or trachea rather than the cricoid ring or

applied askew, insufficient force to occlude the esophagus, or poor selection of patients (those with a known difficult airway, where a more measured approach must take precedence over concerns for possible aspiration).[23,24]

A RSI in infants and children requires more planning than in older children and adults because in the former, medications must be flushed into the vein to ensure they are delivered rapidly and they desaturate rapidly due to their greater oxygen consumption and reduced oxygen reserve. Succinylcholine remains useful for rapid-sequence tracheal intubation for brief procedures; however, concerns about the risk of hyperkalemia after succinylcholine in children with undiagnosed neuromuscular diseases (especially in males younger than 8 years of age). As a result, its use has dramatically decreased. With the shift from succinylcholine to nondepolarizing neuromuscular blocking drugs for rapid paralysis in young children, the inability to intubate and prolonged paralysis may present serious, possibly life-threatening dilemmas. However, with the availability of sugammadex, rocuronium in a dose of 1.2 mg/kg has become a safe alternative to succinylcholine to secure the airway[25] as it can be rapidly reversed should a "cannot intubate, cannot ventilate" scenario occur.[26–30] Since preoxygenation can occasionally be difficult in infants and children because they commonly resist the tight application of the face mask needed to fully denitrogenate the lungs, failure to adequately ventilate the lungs after induction of anesthesia but before tracheal intubation may result in desaturation. This occurs more rapidly in young infants and children than in older children and in those with respiratory tract infections or other causes of a limited oxygen reserve.[31–34] Therefore, some advocate a modified RSI during which the lungs are gently ventilated with a facemask and 100% oxygen before undertaking laryngoscopy and intubation to attenuate the nadir in oxygen saturation.[33,35] Another concern is that the force needed to occlude the esophagus when applying cricoid pressure to infants and children is poorly taught, often poorly applied, can distort the view of the larynx during laryngoscopy, may not occlude the lumen of the esophagus, and may deform the lumen of the trachea if excessive force is applied.[12,22,36] For example, as little as 10-Newtons of force will distort the shape of the subglottic airway and reduce the lumen by 50% or more in children younger than 5 years of age.[22] Effective cricoid pressure that occludes the esophagus in children and permits bag-and-mask ventilation with up to 40 cm H_2O peak inspiratory pressure without gastric insufflation[37] is known as a modified RSI. Thus, if the first attempt at tracheal intubation fails or the child desaturates during laryngoscopy, properly maintained cricoid pressure allows bag-and-mask ventilation to restore oxygenation, without increasing the risk of regurgitation. Another approach is to use low peak inflation pressures, known as the controlled or modified RSI technique.[35,38]

INDICATIONS FOR PREOPERATIVE NASOGASTRIC TUBE PLACEMENT

Although there are no published guidelines for placing nasogastric tubes preoperatively, it is reasonable to insert a tube preoperatively to allow drainage of gastrointestinal fluids in cases of documented bowel obstruction (e.g., ileus, strangulated bowel, pyloric obstruction) or in other situations in which the risk of aspiration is judged to be substantial. The child may experience discomfort when a nasogastric tube is inserted preoperatively, but this must be balanced against the need to decompress the stomach and reduce the risk of regurgitation during induction of anesthesia. For every other indication, the nasogastric tube may be placed after tracheal intubation. It should be noted that the presence of a nasogastric tube may decrease the tone of the lower esophageal sphincter, increase the risk for reflux, and reduce the ability to clear refluxed gastric contents from the distal esophagus.[39,40] Thus, the anesthesiologist is faced with the dilemma of whether or not to remove the nasogastric tube that was placed before induction of anesthesia. It may be reasonable to apply suction to the nasogastric tube, evacuate all of the gastric contents, and then remove the nasogastric tube before inducing anesthesia because it is unclear whether cricoid pressure, even if properly applied, prevents the wicking of gastric contents along the path created by the nasogastric tube. Although one can never guarantee that the stomach has been completely emptied with a well-placed nasogastric tube, suctioning the stomach contents in the supine, right, and left lateral decubitus positions has been reported to remove 97% of the residual fluid volume.[41]

FLUID BALANCE

Many children with acute abdominal emergencies have associated and pronounced abnormalities in their circulating blood volume, mainly in the form of dehydration, electrolyte losses, and third-space fluid shifts, resulting in hypovolemia. In most instances, correction of these derangements is mandatory before proceeding with anesthesia and surgery. However, when a large fraction of the bowel becomes strangulated and ischemic, surgical intervention is emergent despite large volumes of fluid sequestered in the bowel. In these cases, hypovolemic volume resuscitation is initiated as anesthesia is rapidly induced. In some elective cases (e.g., a bowel resection because of inflammatory bowel disease), fluid and electrolyte resuscitation should also be considered because the child may not be fully compensated at the time of surgery.

To date, published studies have suggested that resuscitation with crystalloid fluids and colloids has equipoise.[42] In children, initial resuscitation is usually undertaken with balanced salt solutions; a Cochrane review concluded that the use of isotonic intravenous (IV) fluids with sodium concentrations similar to that of the plasma reduces the risk of hyponatremia.[43] Although colloids may result in less tissue edema and less volume infused, the expense may not justify their routine use. Some have even questioned the use of colloids in patients with sepsis.[44]

POTENTIAL FOR STRANGULATED OR ISCHEMIC BOWEL AND SEPSIS

The need for anesthesia and surgery becomes more urgent when the bowel is potentially ischemic and/or necrotic. For example, if a volvulus is suspected, immediate action is necessary; otherwise, the child is at risk for massive bowel necrosis, necessitating resection of the dead bowel with subsequent short bowel syndrome, a condition associated with serious lifelong medical problems or even death. Even if the child is far from optimally resuscitated, anesthesia must be induced and maintained, preferably with anesthetics that maintain circulatory homeostasis, while simultaneously correcting the dehydration (or hypovolemia) and electrolyte imbalance. The situation is somewhat less critical in the child with an incarcerated inguinal hernia, although the delay of even this surgery should be minimized.

Ischemic bowel may release a host of mediators that can cause severe hemodynamic instability.[45] Children with an acute intraabdominal disease should always be regarded as being at risk for bacterial translocation and possible septicemia.[46] Those with overt sepsis are usually easy to identify and may have already been admitted to the pediatric intensive care unit. However, children

with incipient or early sepsis may not exhibit overt signs. Accordingly, the signs of sepsis should be actively sought. If septicemia is present or suspected, appropriate IV antibiotics should be administered without delay, preferably before anesthesia and surgery. Children with sepsis or presepsis can be extremely unstable and may require inotropic and/or vasoactive drugs. Immediately after induction of anesthesia, vascular sympathetic tone may be attenuated, leading to sudden hemodynamic instability. Thus, when a substantial segment of the bowel becomes ischemic, the anesthesiologist must maintain anesthesia without depressing the circulation excessively, acutely resuscitate the child with appropriate fluids, correct electrolyte imbalances, particularly potential hyperkalemia, and administer inotropic and/or vasoactive medications as indicated. It should be noted that hemodynamic instability might acutely worsen when the ischemic bowel is manipulated, suddenly reperfused, or immediately after the abdominal cavity is opened. In such cases, close communication with the surgeon is paramount. Furthermore, the presence of sepsis, complicated by an acute abdomen, cardiovascular compromise and acute lung injury may further reduce pulmonary compliance. The anesthesiologist needs to prepare for placing invasive monitoring lines (arterial and central venous pressures) and to have available an intraoperative ventilator that is capable of delivering positive end-expiratory pressure (PEEP).

PRESENCE OF ABDOMINAL COMPARTMENT SYNDROME

Acute intraabdominal processes may lead to critically increased intraabdominal pressure (IAP)[47] if the IAP exceeds the capillary perfusion pressure of the intraabdominal organs. Organ perfusion will become compromised and ischemia and/or necrosis may develop. The most commonly affected organs in this situation are the bowels, kidneys, and liver. Abdominal compartment syndrome occurs less frequently in children than in adults.[48] Causes of abdominal compartment syndrome include burns, extracorporeal membrane oxygenation,[49] closure of gastroschisis or omphalocele (see Chapter 35),[50] abdominal trauma,[51,52] abdominal surgery,[53] and a host of other intraabdominal pathologies,[54] including necrotizing enterocolitis, Hirschsprung enterocolitis, perforated bowel, diaphragmatic hernia, and Wilms tumor.[49,55,56] Insufficient perfusion of the bowel may cause an ileus, translocation of bacteria, lactate accumulation, and production of mediators that cause hemodynamic instability.[57] Increased IAP can reduce liver blood flow, which will in turn reduce hepatic function,[58] mainly manifested as an inability to metabolize lactate; impaired drug metabolism;[58,59] and, in severe cases, impaired synthesis of coagulation factors. Because the pressure is also transmitted to the retroperitoneal space, renal function may become impaired, resulting in oliguria or anuria and reduced excretion of drugs.[55] In addition, cranial displacement of the abdominal contents and splinting of the diaphragm may seriously compromise ventilation.[60]

If acute intraabdominal compartment syndrome is suspected, then the IAP should be monitored to prevent the pressures from exceeding the critical threshold of 20 to 25 mm Hg. IAP can be measured indirectly by transducing a nasogastric tube or bladder catheter.[61,62] Some define compartment syndrome as when the vesicular (bladder) pressure exceeds 10 to 12 mm Hg.[63,64] The diagnosis of intraabdominal compartment syndrome should be suspected when the triad of (1) massive abdominal distention, (2) increased bladder pressures and increased peak inspiratory airway pressures, and (3) evidence of hepatic, renal, and/or cardiac dysfunction are present.[56,65–67]

Children with acute intraabdominal compartment syndrome are often hemodynamically unstable. Although decompression of the abdomen by a laparotomy will immediately normalize the IAP, reperfusion of the ischemic tissues almost always releases a host of biologically active substances that cause profound hypotension.[57] These substances may also precipitate acute renal failure and lead to disseminated intravascular coagulopathy. As in the case of sepsis, the anesthesiologist must be fully prepared to address these challenges by ensuring that blood products are present in the operating room and vasopressors are drawn up and available before induction of anesthesia. Some children will require a patch abdominoplasty as a temporizing measure to protect abdominal organs that require delayed primary closure of the anterior abdominal wall.[56,65]

PREOPERATIVE LABORATORY TESTING AND INVESTIGATIONS

Most minor elective cases (e.g., umbilical or inguinal hernia repair) do not require any preoperative workup beyond a basic history and physical examination. Many centers require a preoperative urine (or hemoglobin) screen for pregnancy in females who have reached menarche (see Chapter 2).[68,69] More complex elective cases may warrant additional laboratory testing, including basic hematology screening and electrolyte profile.

Preoperative laboratory testing is strongly advised in more critically ill children. Liver and renal function tests, coagulation profile, and serum albumin concentration should be assessed and blood typed and crossmatched. In children with sepsis or who have an acute intraabdominal compartment syndrome, a preoperative chest radiograph may indicate the severity of pulmonary involvement. An echocardiogram may be needed to assess myocardial contractility and volume status if cardiac dysfunction is suspected.

MONITORING REQUIREMENTS

Routine elective cases rarely require more than standard monitoring equipment. In children undergoing major intraabdominal procedures, invasive arterial and central venous blood pressure monitoring may be indicated (see Chapter 46). A multiple-lumen central venous line inserted at the beginning of the procedure will facilitate the administration of inotropic and/or vasoactive drugs, in addition to measuring central venous pressure; ultrasound-guided insertion is strongly recommended.[70] These lines are of great value in the immediate postoperative period for blood sampling, drug administration, ongoing assessment of intravascular volume status, and parenteral nutrition; they will not, however, be adequate for rapid volume blood or fluid administration. Large-bore peripheral access is preferred. Transesophageal echocardiographic, transesophageal Doppler, or continuous noninvasive cardiac output (CO)[71–73] evaluation may provide valuable intraoperative and postoperative information regarding the child's volume status, as well as cardiac contractility (see also Chapter 49).[74–84]

A urinary catheter with a pediatric urometer (i.e., a graduated collection receptacle), which provides an accurate measure of urine output, is a useful monitor for most intraabdominal procedures. Maintaining a stable hourly urine output may safeguard against the development of hypovolemia and possibly prerenal azotemia (see the section "Laparoscopic Surgery" for a discussion of changes in urine output with increased IAP).

Monitoring IAP is important during laparoscopic surgery, although it is of minimal value in omphalocele and gastroschisis surgeries, as long as the abdomen remains open. Once the abdomen is closed, however, IAP provides useful prognostic information regarding intraabdominal organ (e.g., renal) blood flow, circulatory stability, and respiratory embarrassment (see Chapter 35).[60]

CHOICE OF ANESTHETIC

The anesthesiologist may use their personal preference for anesthetic technique for the management of both elective and emergency intraabdominal surgery in children. It is expected that the use of inhalational anesthetic agents will decline in the future given their effects (i.e., desflurane in particular) on the environment.[85] However, in a simulation of the environmental impact and carbon footprint of intravenous (e.g., total intravenous anesthesia [TIVA]) or inhalational anesthetics in infants and children, the carbon footprint for TIVA was unsurprisingly less than that after induction of anesthesia with an inhalational agent followed by either TIVA or inhalational anesthesia for maintenance.[86] In the case of an inhalational induction followed by TIVA for maintenance, however, the carbon footprint was only less than an inhalational induction and maintenance in children <20 kilograms if the anesthetic lasted >77 minutes and in children 30 to 50 kilograms if the anesthetic lasted >105 minutes. Hence, the addition of TIVA in this simulation only reduced the carbon footprint in children anesthetized with an inhalational anesthetic for procedures of prolonged duration. Surgical procedures in children that have prolonged durations, that is >80 minutes, comprise a minority of children (≤25% of those to 12 years of age).[87]

Airway management associated with intraabdominal surgery requires careful consideration. Even when the child is not at increased risk for regurgitation and aspiration, the risk of regurgitation can be increased if the surgeon positions the child in the Trendelenburg position and/or insufflates the peritoneal cavity with carbon dioxide (CO_2) during laparoscopic surgery. A particular concern arises when the surgeon decides to decompress the distended bowel by creating an enterotomy and directly draining the fluid, or by "milking" or "stripping" the bowel in a retrograde direction until the contents can be vented with a nasogastric tube. This can cause a massive regurgitation that can exceed the capacity of the nasogastric tube to decompress the stomach resulting in pulmonary aspiration.[88] It is for this reason that a laryngeal mask airway (LMA) should not be used during intraabdominal surgery; we strongly recommend that the trachea should be intubated with a cuffed tube as standard practice in these cases. A tracheal tube serves a dual purpose in these surgeries: it reduces the risk of aspiration and ensures that adequate peak inspiratory pressures can be delivered if the lung compliance decreases.

Regional anesthetic techniques may be useful adjuncts in children undergoing both minor and major abdominal surgery. Those who have had open abdominal procedures will require IV opioids or the use of a continuous epidural infusion of local anesthetics with or without additives (e.g., opioids or α2-agonists) for perioperative pain management (see Chapters 40 and 41). Analgesia is commonly supplemented with parenteral nonsteroidal antiinflammatory drugs (NSAIDs) and/or acetaminophen. In most children who have had laparoscopic surgery, adequate postoperative analgesia may be achieved by infiltrating local anesthetics at the port insertion sites. However, referred shoulder pain, the result of accumulated air under the diaphragm, may require IV opioids.[89] In critically unstable children or those with sepsis, the use of neuraxial anesthesia is not recommended because sympathetic blockade may further exacerbate the hemodynamic instability and the catheter could provide a nidus for infection.

General Principles of Urologic Surgery

Except for acute drainage of urinary obstruction (i.e., ultrasound-guided nephrostomy or cystostomy procedures) and torsion of the testis, most pediatric urologic surgeries are elective. In the vast majority of cases, these children are otherwise healthy or have stable medical conditions that do not require more than a careful history, physical examination, and review of the child's medical record. Children who undergo urologic procedures may be suffering from emotional disturbance because of repeated interventions and the sensitivity of the surgical site. This mandates special psychological attention before and after anesthesia.

Worldwide, the prevalence of latex allergy has been estimated to be 9.7%, 7.2%, and 4.3% among health care workers, susceptible patients, and the general population, respectively.[90] In the 1990s, the prevalence of latex allergy in children with spinal dysraphism exceeded 70%. Two decades later, the prevalence had decreased to <17%, and the most recent evidence suggests that the prevalence may be only 3% to 4.5% in those with dysraphism when cared for in a nonlatex environment.[91,92] Latex anaphylaxis is of particular concern in children with chronic urologic disorders;[93–96] in the past, children with spina bifida developed latex allergy more frequently than those without spina bifida[97–100] because the former were repeatedly catheterized with latex urinary catheters beginning early after birth. All children with congenital malformations of the urinary tract who were repeatedly exposed to latex via their mucous membranes beginning in the neonatal period were at increased risk for developing latex hypersensitivity.[101,102] However, a widespread shift in practice to avoid exposure to all latex products in these children has been extremely (but not 100%) effective in attenuating the prevalence of this allergy.[92,103] The exceptions usually occur when someone unfamiliar with the child's latex allergy introduces a latex product and sensitizes the child or triggers a reaction. Thus latex-free management is highly recommended in this population.[92,103–105]

REDUCED RENAL FUNCTION

Children with chronic renal disease have impaired renal function, which may affect drug dosing and disposition, as well as cause secondary effects on the cardiovascular system. In the most severe cases, the child may require dialysis to balance fluids and electrolytes. In children with renal disease, it is essential to consult the child's nephrologist to determine the degree of renal impairment and review current blood work such as the serum creatinine, blood urea nitrogen, sodium, and potassium concentrations (see also Chapter 26). Because renal impairment may also affect clotting, a coagulation profile, including platelet count, should be reviewed preoperatively if substantial blood loss is anticipated. These children are prone to fluid overload, particularly those who are anuric and dialysis dependent. Apart from clinical signs associated with fluid overload, measuring the child's weight and comparing it with their normal weight is a simple means to assess the child's current volume status. If the cardiac function or volume status remains in doubt, an echocardiogram should be obtained. Children with chronic renal insufficiency often have impaired left ventricular function even before they require dialysis, so a preoperative echocardiogram may be indicated[106–110]; pericardial effusion is also a concern.[107,111,112]

For children undergoing dialysis, the most recent date of dialysis should be documented. Overhydration and/or hypervolemia and hyperkalemia should be corrected preoperatively with dialysis. Although dialysis corrects these abnormalities, and may transiently improve platelet function (peritoneal dialysis yielding more consistent improvement than hemodialysis), it is best to avoid dialysis within 12 hours of anesthesia to preclude relative hypovolemia and to allow sufficient time for body fluids and electrolytes to reequilibrate (see Chapter 26).[113,114] Postdialysis laboratory indexes of serum electrolytes (particularly potassium), hemoglobin or hematocrit, renal function (creatinine and blood urea nitrogen), and the child's weight loss should be assessed. For children who undergo hemodialysis, IV access and blood pressure measurements should not be obtained in the extremity ipsilateral to the arteriovenous fistula.

SYSTEMIC ARTERIAL HYPERTENSION

Systemic hypertension is common in renal insufficiency in adults but is far less common in children. Nonetheless, some children with urologic disorders develop systemic hypertension associated with disturbances in the renin-angiotensin system.[115–118] As in adults, it is important to control systemic hypertension before induction to avoid wide swings in blood pressure. In contrast to adults, however, hypervolemia is an important cause of hypertension in children with renal insufficiency that should be considered and treated preoperatively. Children and adults are often treated with the same antihypertensive medications, in weight-adjusted doses (see Chapter 26).[117,118] All medications should be continued up to and including the morning of surgery to maintain intraoperative and postoperative hemodynamic stability except for angiotensin-converting enzyme inhibitors (ACE) and angiotensin II receptor blocking drugs (AIIRB). Some recommend stopping these medications on the day of surgery to avoid intraoperative hypotension although this recommendation remains debated.[119–122] Withholding these medications may lead to rebound hypertension in the perioperative period requiring intervention; however, if these medications are not withheld, vasopressors may be required to treat intraoperative hypotension.[123] The results of an ongoing multicentered trial to examine the perioperative consequences of withholding or not withholding these medications preoperatively in noncardiac adult surgery have not been published.[124] However, a consensus statement from the Society of Perioperative Assessment and Quality Improvement[125] recommended holding ACE inhibitors and AIIRBs preoperatively (except for low-risk minimally invasive surgery with minimal sedation or local anesthesia) but continuing β-adrenergic blocking agents, calcium channel blockers, digoxin, and direct-acting vasodilators on the morning of surgery. These recommendations continue to evolve as more evidence is published. Because therapy-resistant renal hypertension is an indication for nephrectomy, one should anticipate and be prepared to treat wide fluctuations in blood pressure, including severe hypertension during the first stage of the operation and profound hypotension when the responsible kidney is removed. Therefore, long-acting antihypertensive agents are best avoided during the early stages of nephrectomy in a child.

CORTICOSTEROID MEDICATIONS

Children with renal disease may be chronically treated with corticosteroids as part of their medical management (e.g., children with proteinuria or who have undergone previous renal transplant surgery). In such cases, a stress dose of parenteral corticosteroids during surgery is indicated, with continued supplementation until the child resumes their normal corticosteroid medication by the enteral route. In more complex situations, consultation with a pediatric nephrologist or endocrinologist is warranted to optimize corticosteroid supplementation, although in more straightforward cases, a dose of 2.5 mg/kg of IV hydrocortisone 2 to 3 times each day is usually adequate (see Chapter 25).

INFECTION OR SEPSIS

Obstructive urinary tract disease or chronic renal insufficiency increase the risk of urinary tract infections. If treated properly, the infection should not interfere with anesthesia. However, in children with overt signs of systemic illness or septicemia, the anesthetic, and postoperative courses may be difficult.

MONITORING REQUIREMENTS

Standard noninvasive monitoring is adequate for the vast majority of urologic procedures, as they are of minor or moderate magnitude (e.g., circumcision, orchiopexy, pyeloplasty, and uretero-reimplantation). The anesthetic care required for infants and children undergoing penile surgery is routine, including a forced-air heating mattress to prevent hypothermia for surgery lasting longer than 1 hour. However, recognizing the minimal amount of skin that is exposed during this type of surgery, the child's temperature often increases, necessitating close monitoring of the child's temperature to avoid overheating.

Invasive monitors (i.e., arterial and central venous access for pressure monitoring and administration of vasoactive drugs) may be indicated in major surgical interventions, and when major co-morbidities are present (e.g., decreased renal function, significant hypertension, associated cardiac dysfunction, sepsis). If central venous access is deemed necessary, the coagulation status of the child should be evaluated because platelet function may be substantially compromised. Ultrasound guidance improves safety while securing central venous access in cases in which a coagulopathy is present or suspected on clinical grounds (see Chapter 46). In the unstable child, even more complex monitoring (e.g., esophageal Doppler monitoring, transesophageal echocardiography, or continuous noninvasive cardiac output monitoring)[71] should be considered (see Chapter 49). Despite very limited evidence, the use of near-infrared spectroscopy (NIRS) in neonates and infants is increasing.[31] It is important to monitor urine output, although the volume of urine may not reflect renal function, especially in the presence of renal disease. During surgery that involves the bladder or in children who are anuric, urine output will not be available for part or all of the surgery. Hence, other indices of fluid status and perfusion must be used. Heart rate and systolic blood pressure are reliable indices of volume status and perfusion in most children, although central venous pressure and invasive arterial pressure measurement may be indicated in special cases. Surgeons may be heartened to observe urine flowing into the bladder after reimplantation of ureters and kidney transplantation in place of measuring it. Preloading with a balanced salt solution may be useful in such circumstances; occasionally a loop diuretic is requested.

Laparoscopic Surgery

Laparoscopic surgery was introduced more than 100 years ago, although its role in pediatric surgery only became pervasive in the past 15 to 20 years as technical challenges in the quality of the optics and miniaturization of the instruments were overcome. An increasing number of general and urologic surgical procedures (including appendectomy, cholecystectomy, and splenectomy, as well as those to treat inguinal hernia and undescended testicles) are performed either laparoscopically or with robotic techniques

in children of all ages (Figs. 27.1 to 27.4).[126–134] More sophisticated laparoscopic techniques have enabled the performance of

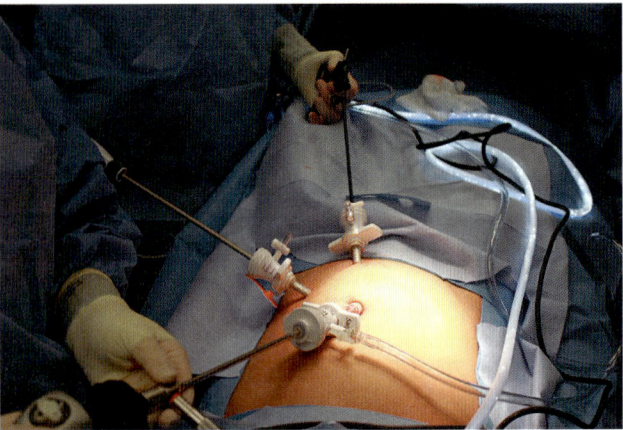

FIGURE 27.1 A child undergoing laparoscopic appendectomy, presented as a paradigm for the surgical setup for any multiple-trocar laparoscopic surgery. Three incisions were made, two in the anterior abdominal wall and the third in the umbilicus. The first two trocars carry instruments to manipulate the appendix, whereas the third holds the camera for viewing by all personnel in the operating room. All cables swing widely off the surgical field.

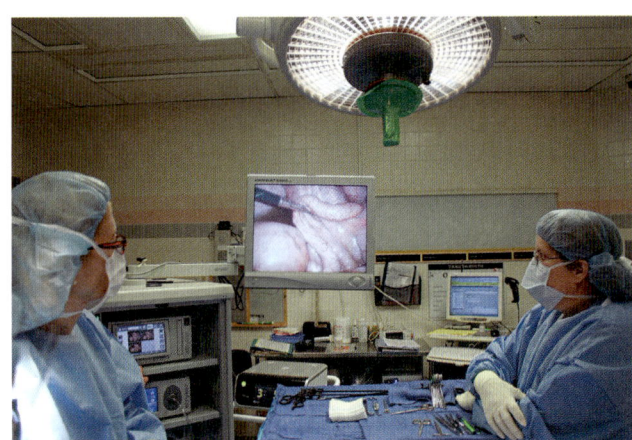

FIGURE 27.2 Wide-angle view of the operating room with surgeon and scrub nurse viewing the appendix being held by the grasper, shown on the overhead monitor.

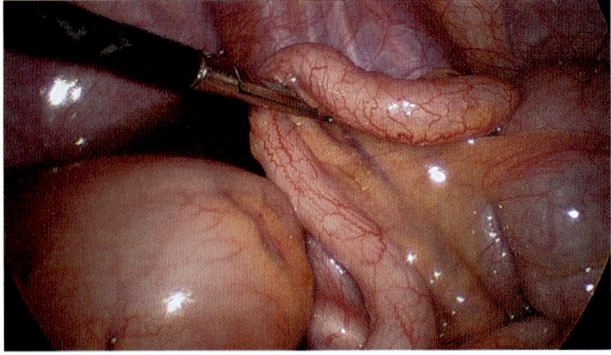

FIGURE 27.3 Inside the abdominal cavity with a view of the inflamed appendix that has been mobilized. The peritoneal attachments must be peeled off the appendix before it is ligated and removed.

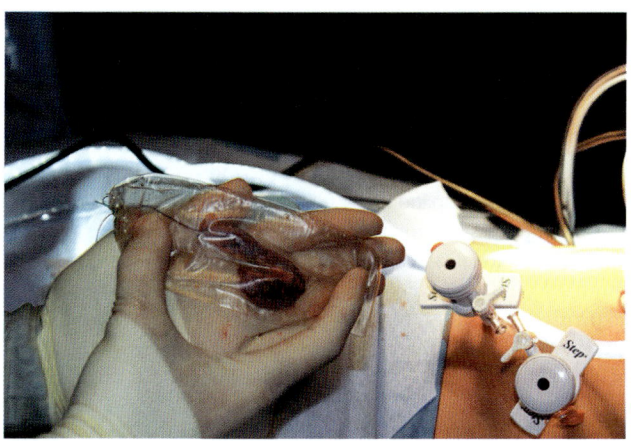

FIGURE 27.4 The appendix is ligated, inserted into a plastic container, and withdrawn, usually through the trocar or incision site without contaminating adjacent tissues. The appendix is shown in the surgeon's hand after removal.

complex surgical procedures,[135] including Nissen fundoplication, colectomy, pyeloplasty, bowel pull-through, and removal of large organs, including the kidney and spleen.[132,136–139] Technological advances now permit laparoscopic surgery in neonates and small infants, including those with hypoplastic left heart syndrome after stage 1 or 2 repairs.[134,140–142] It must be noted, however, that laparoscopic surgery in children with cyanotic heart disease carries with it a substantial risk that exceeds most other populations having this form of surgery. Although several reports suggest that infants and children of all ages, at all stages of palliative repair of their cyanotic heart disease, tolerate laparoscopic surgery,[142–144] the risk for those with Fontan physiology undergoing laparoscopic surgery is substantial. It is essential to understand that in Fontan physiology, pulmonary blood flow is passive, and decreases in venous return (whether from increases in intrathoracic pressure or head-up positioning) or increases in pulmonary vascular resistance (because of increased CO_2 partial pressures or decreased minute ventilation) could severely reduce cardiac output.[145] Creating a pneumoperitoneum for laparoscopic surgery and extreme positions increase IAP and arterial CO_2 tensions (increasing pulmonary artery pressure) thereby reducing venous return and increasing the risk of a diminished cardiac output in children with Fontan physiology (see later discussion). Successful management of these children during laparoscopic surgery requires a multidisciplinary team that functions in concert to enhance the child's outcome by (1) optimizing the child's condition preoperatively including fluid homeostasis and identifying any cardiac issues; (2) recruiting surgeons who can complete the surgery quickly and efficiently; (3) maintaining the children in the supine position throughout the surgery; (4) maintaining normocapnia; (5) monitoring the child with a transesophageal echo probe as needed, as well as with an arterial invasive pressure monitor for blood gas analysis; and (6) insufflating the abdomen to the minimal (<8 mm Hg) IAP that is surgically feasible. Larger studies are required before children with cyanotic heart disease, particularly those with Fontan physiology, should be candidates to undergo laparoscopic surgery in any center routinely, except those with specialized teams.

Laparoscopic surgery offers several advantages over open surgery, including more rapid emergence from anesthesia, faster ambulation, earlier discharge from the hospital, and reduced perioperative complications.[146–151] Because laparoscopic surgery involves the insufflation of gas into the abdominal cavity to visualize the intra-abdominal organs, the stomach should be decompressed using a nasogastric or orogastric tube for upper abdominal surgery, whereas the bladder should be emptied using a urinary catheter for lower abdominal surgery. Surgical access to the peritoneal cavity is achieved with trocars introduced through one to three small (3- to 10-millimeter in diameter) incisions; the laparoscopic instruments and a camera are then passed through the trocars. There are several laparoscopy procedures: laparoendoscopic single-site (LESS); single-port, single-incision laparoscopic surgery (SILS); and single-incision multiport laparoscopy (SIMPL), or "belly button" surgery, in which all instruments pass through a single incision and a single large trocar (often in the umbilicus) (E-Figs. 27.1 to 27.3).[152–156]

PNEUMOPERITONEUM

Pneumoperitoneal pressure is a major concern for all laparoscopic approaches. Experimental evidence in adult and newborn pigs demonstrated that the risks of cardiorespiratory consequences and potentially fatal emboli were directly related to the peak pneumoperitoneal pressure.[157,158] In infants and children, the optimal pneumoperitoneal pressure is the least pressure that enables adequate surgical access. CO_2 should be insufflated through one of the trocars until the IAP reaches 6 to 15 mm Hg; most surgeons currently limit the IAP in neonates and young infants to 6 to 8 mm Hg and in children to 10 to 12 mm Hg.[159] The IAP is maintained throughout the surgery by intermittently insufflating additional CO_2. Although CO_2 is most commonly used, many gases have been investigated (see later discussion).[160] CO_2 is the preferred gas because it does not support combustion, is rapidly cleared from the peritoneal cavity at the end of the surgery, and does not expand into bubbles or spaces.[137,161,162]

The increased IAP during laparoscopic surgery may cause many physiochemical side effects, including cardiorespiratory depression, hypothermia as the result of dry gas leakage, pneumothorax or subcutaneous emphysema, endobronchial intubation resulting from the upward shift of tracheal bifurcation, or injury resulting from paracentesis.

Carbon Dioxide

The major disadvantage of using CO_2 to insufflate the peritoneal cavity stems from its rapid absorption, which increases the peak end-tidal partial pressure of CO_2 ($PETCO_2$) if ventilation is not increased, an effect that is greater in infants than in older children.[163,164] The inverse relationship between age and the rate of CO_2 absorption from the abdomen has been attributed to the smaller absorptive surface, thinner peritoneal tissues, and the reduced peritoneal fat deposits in the abdomen of infants compared with older children.[164,165] Because CO_2 is so readily absorbed, particularly in infants, both the $PETCO_2$ and $PACO_2$ may increase 20% to 50% above baseline.[138,159,161,163,166] The resultant hypercapnia, which occurs more commonly in surgery lasting longer than 1 hour, particularly in neonates,[167] necessitates an increase in minute ventilation (from 50% to 100% above the baseline) to maintain a physiologic pH.[137,168] The difference between the partial pressures of arterial and end-tidal CO_2 ($PACO_2 - PETCO_2$) often increases during insufflation of CO_2.[166,168] In one report, the $PACO_2 - PETCO_2$ gradient before and after a carbon dioxide pneumoperitoneum increased from a mean of 5.7 to 13.4 mm Hg.[169] It should be noted that in neonates and in children with cyanotic congenital heart disease, the $PETCO_2$ may not reliably track the $PACO_2$ during

CO_2 insufflation, leading some to recommend arterial blood gas monitoring to validate the PETCO2 measurements.[166,169,170]

Increased $PACO_2$ may also trigger spontaneous respiratory efforts that could interfere with surgery. In addition, it may initiate a sympathetic response, including increases in the heart rate, blood pressure, and cerebral blood flow, as well as precipitate ventricular arrhythmias, although this occurs rarely with sevoflurane. A sudden increase in PETCO2 may also suggest a diagnosis of malignant hyperthermia if accompanied by sudden onset of tachycardia.[171–173] If this diagnosis proves to be difficult to confirm or reject (in malignant hyperthermia expect venous PVO_2 <40 mm Hg; see Chapter 39), it may be necessary to desufflate the abdomen and determine if the clinical and laboratory findings suggestive of malignant hyperthermia resolve.[165,174]

Gas Emboli

Gas emboli have been reported in several laparoscopic studies, most of which were interesting curiosities of no clinical consequence, although, in several, profound cardiovascular collapse ensued.[175–177] The frequency of CO_2 embolism is rare, estimated to be between 59:10,000 to 1:100,000, but associated with a mortality that may reach 28%.[178] Most consider the emboli to be intravascular CO_2 bubbles, although there is evidence to suggest that some emboli contain nitrogen or air.[179] Intravascular embolization of CO_2 may occur when the insufflation pressure exceeds the venous pressure, forcing CO_2 bubbles into the venous circulation, and resulting in sudden cardiovascular collapse.[176] Continuous precordial Doppler or expired CO_2 partial pressure is effective in detecting a gas embolus, although the Doppler may be overly sensitive, with numerous false-positive results. It has been suggested that many episodes of subclinical gas embolism are unrecognized because the symptoms are mild and nonspecific.[180] However, children with right-to-left shunts or potential right-to-left shunts, such as a patent foramen ovale, are vulnerable to the systemic effects of these emboli. Although CO_2 is soluble in blood and rapidly buffered, CO_2 emboli dissolve slowly in blood, taking 2 to 3 minutes to disappear.[181] Hence, large emboli may block blood flow in the heart for several minutes or more before they dissolve. The minimum rate of infusion of CO_2 into the blood that triggers cardiovascular collapse in pigs is 1.2 mL/kg per minute[181]; comparable data in humans are lacking. Anesthesiologists should be aware of the high-risk conditions that predispose to CO_2 emboli (e.g., increased abdominal insufflation pressure, hypovolemia and reduced venous pressure, spontaneous respirations, and resection of vessel-rich parenchymatous organs) and communicate closely with the surgeons at all times.

Some investigators suggest that clinically important gas emboli are comprised of nitrogen, not CO_2,[176] whereas transient emboli are thought to be comprised of CO_2.[176] Nitrogen is insoluble in the blood (blood/gas partition coefficient of 0.014), which explains its persistence as an embolus. These emboli may arise from the air, either present in or entrained by the trocar during insufflation of the peritoneum, which is forced into a transected blood vessel while the carboperitoneum is pressurized.[176] This mechanism is a rare source of gas in the circulation, which may explain, in part, why the emboli that occur during laparoscopy very rarely result in cardiovascular instability and arrest.

In contrast to CO_2, insufflation with oxygen, air, and nitrous oxide for laparoscopic surgery has been eschewed because they all support combustion. However, repeat desufflations of the pneumoperitoneal gas during laparoscopy in pigs whose lungs were ventilated with 66% nitrous oxide in oxygen prevented the concentration

of nitrous oxide from exceeding 10% in the pneumoperitoneal cavity.[182] Nitrous oxide is still avoided for both insufflation and as an adjunctive anesthetic gas during laparoscopy because it also expands into gas-filled cavities should gas emboli appear in the circulation.[161] Its use during laparoscopic surgery may distend the bowel in the case of bowel obstruction and obscure the surgeon's view; it may also expand any CO_2 emboli that develop.

The inert gases argon and helium were also candidate gases for insufflation to create a pneumoperitoneum as they cannot be oxidized (and therefore ignited), although they are much more expensive than CO_2. When argon was used to create a pneumoperitoneum in pigs, embolization occurred more frequently than with CO_2.[183] In theory, both argon and helium can cause serious sequelae if embolized into the vascular system because they are insoluble in blood (blood/gas solubility of helium is 0.007 and argon is 0.029) and therefore likely to persist.[137,161,162,183]

RESPIRATORY EFFECTS

As the pressure within the peritoneal cavity increases, the frequency of adverse respiratory effects also increases, particularly at IAP greater than 15 cm H_2O. The respiratory manifestations of increased IAP include cephalad displacement of the diaphragm, decreased excursion of the diaphragm, and decreases in pulmonary and thoracic compliance, vital capacity, functional residual capacity, and closing volume.[184] Cephalad displacement of the diaphragm shifts ventilation to the nondependent parts of the lungs, creating a ventilation-perfusion mismatch. With a small functional residual capacity in children, cephalad displacement of the diaphragm further compresses the lungs, causing a collapse of the small airways, ventilation-perfusion mismatch, and possibly hypoxemia. Other adverse pulmonary mechanics after insufflation include increased peak inspiratory pressures of up to 27% and decreased compliance by as much as 39%.[185] These physiologic changes are compounded by the extreme body tilting (i.e., extreme head-up or head-down positions) often requested by surgeons.[161,186] Positioning the child head down (i.e., Trendelenburg position) first decreases compliance by 17%, and second, adding a pneumoperitoneum decreases compliance by an additional 27%, requiring increases in peak inflation pressures of 19% and 32%, respectively.[187] In a study in which the pneumoperitoneum was created before Trendelenburg positioning in children whose lungs were ventilated using pressure control and 5 cm H_2O PEEP, a pneumoperitoneum of 12 cm H_2O decreased both dynamic compliance and tidal volume by 42%.[188] The addition of 20 degrees of Trendelenburg positioning only decreased these values by an additional 10%. All of these changes in pulmonary function can be offset by increasing minute ventilation (rate and peak inflation pressure) by as much as 50% to 100%. Pulmonary function appears to be restored more readily after laparoscopic than open surgery.[137]

In addition, a pneumoperitoneum when combined with the extreme Trendelenburg position can shift the tracheal tube in a rostral direction, as far as 1.2 to 2.7 centimeters. The tip of the tube may then impact the carina or pass into a bronchus and lead to bronchospasm and difficulty ventilating the lungs.[189] With these changes, inspired oxygen concentrations greater than 30% may be required, in combination with PEEP and alveolar recruitment to restore adequate oxygenation. A persistent 5% decrease in oxygen saturation has been associated with partial or intermittent endobronchial intubation.[190]

Securing the airway for laparoscopic surgery requires particular attention. Cuffed tracheal tubes are preferred over uncuffed tubes to ensure effective alveolar ventilation despite the conditions described earlier,[170] although LMAs and ProSeal supraglottic airways (Teleflex Medical Inc.; Research Triangle Park, NC) have been used for brief procedures during laparoscopic surgery without complications.[162,191] If the child has a mature tracheotomy, the air leak around the tracheotomy must be assessed before surgery and if the leak is excessive, the tracheotomy tube should be replaced with a cuffed tube, or an armored (cuffed) tracheal tube. If the air leak around the tracheotomy is insignificant, then ventilation should be adequate even in the presence of increased IAP during laparoscopic surgery.

Excessive IAP may cause gas to track across the diaphragm, causing a pneumomediastinum or pneumothorax.[162] This is more common in hiatus hernia surgery and Nissen fundoplication, during which dissection of the esophagus may create passages for gas to traverse the diaphragm. Pneumomediastinum should be suspected if subcutaneous emphysema appears. If surgery creates a transdiaphragmatic passage for CO_2 to accumulate in the pleural space, the resulting pneumothorax may produce cardiorespiratory manifestations. A chest radiograph should be obtained if subcutaneous emphysema appears during or after surgery, or if there is a high index of suspicion that a pneumothorax has formed. Both pressure- and volume-controlled ventilation have been used during laparoscopic abdominal surgery in infants and children. In a single randomized study, both ventilation strategies with 5 mm Hg PEEP maintained effective ventilation and gas exchange.[192]

To avoid the cardiorespiratory compromise of a pneumoperitoneum, a gasless laparoscopic approach has been described.[193] This requires lifting the anterior abdominal wall to create an intra-abdominal tent.[162,194] Implementation of the gasless approach in pediatric medicine has been rather slow,[195] presumably because of technical difficulties and the scarcity of instruments for infants and children.

CARDIOVASCULAR EFFECTS

Three major factors may contribute to adverse cardiovascular responses during pneumoperitoneum: (1) IAP, (2) position (i.e., steep head-up or reverse Trendelenburg), and (3) release of neurohumoral vasoactive substances.[162,184,194] Increased IAP exerts a biphasic effect on venous return and cardiac output. In neonatal pigs, the cardiac index decreased by 55% when IAP exceeded 20 mm Hg.[162] In the animal model, the magnitude of the increase in IAP determined the degree to which the circulation was depressed.[170,196] For example, at IAPs 15 mm Hg or less, blood is compressed out of the splanchnic circulation, increasing venous return, which either increases or results in no change in cardiac output. In contrast, at IAPs greater than 15 mm Hg, the inferior vena cava is compressed, reducing venous return and therefore cardiac output. Studies in children yielded similar results; when the IAP exceeded 12 mm Hg, myocardial contractility[197] and venous return[161] decreased. In both infants and children, CO_2 insufflation to IAP 10 to 13 mm Hg decreased cardiac index by approximately 13%.[198–200] In studies in infants and children in which the cardiac index decreased during increased IAP (10 to 12 mm Hg), the cardiac index returned to preinsufflation values when the abdomen was desufflated.[197–199] Left ventricular systolic function was diminished, and septal wall motion abnormalities have been reported with an IAP of 10 to 12 mm Hg in children with a CO_2 pneumoperitoneum.[197,198] No significant changes in echocardiographic indexes of left ventricular work, preload or afterload, have been noted if the IAP is 10 mm Hg or lower during

the pneumoperitoneum.[159] When standard indexes of hemodynamics were measured in infants and young children during laparoscopic Nissen fundoplication, IAP of 10 mm Hg or less yielded no significant changes in heart rate and blood pressure but a slight increase in cardiac index.[201,202] If IAP is maintained at 10 mm Hg or less, then the impact on hemodynamics (particularly cardiac output) should be clinically insignificant, because venous return may be enhanced as a result of displacement of blood from the splanchnic bed, and afterload is not increased.[161,170,201] Most importantly, if the IAP is less than 5 mm Hg, cardiac index is maintained in infants during a CO_2 pneumoperitoneum[201]; these low insufflation pressures are those often used to examine the contralateral side of a hernia defect during surgery.

Body position during laparoscopic surgery may exaggerate cardiovascular changes. For Nissen fundoplication, a steep head-up position (>20-degree incline) has been used, which reduces venous return.[186] In adult pigs, laparoscopic surgery for Nissen fundoplication increased pleural and mediastinal pressures that, in turn, reduced cardiac output episodically at an IAP of 15 mm Hg.[203] These decreases in cardiac output were manifested by episodes of hypotension and hypoxia. When children were positioned in the steep head-up position, they developed transient hypotension and bradycardia that were reversed immediately with fluid loading and atropine.[204]

It is imperative to continuously monitor IAP to minimize the cardiorespiratory effects of laparoscopic surgery and to avoid excessive insufflation pressures. In adults, induction of anesthesia, insufflating the IAP to 14 mm Hg, and a 10-degree head-up tilt decrease the cardiac index by more than 50%.[205] Some clinicians recommend a maximum IAP during laparoscopy in children of 6 to 8 mm Hg to limit the cardiorespiratory effects,[206] although most studies favor pressures of 10 to 12 mm Hg.[188,196,198,207] In neonates and infants, the maximum IAP should not exceed 6 to 8 mm Hg to minimize cardiorespiratory effects. Based on the current literature, the net cardiovascular effects of insufflating the abdomen to pressures of 12 mm Hg or less, combined with the head-up position, are likely to be well tolerated if adequate hydration is maintained and bradycardia is avoided.[204]

CENTRAL NERVOUS SYSTEM EFFECTS

Laparoscopic surgery must be carefully evaluated if planned for a child with increased intracranial pressure (ICP) or in the presence of a ventriculoperitoneal shunt. The combination of increased IAP, increased systemic vascular resistance, increased $PACO_2$ tension, and Trendelenburg position (as in lower abdominal surgery) may dramatically increase ICP. In adults during extreme head-down position (40 degrees) for prolonged periods, such as in robot-assisted surgery in the pelvis, cerebral tissue oxygen saturation is well maintained, as evidenced by near-infrared spectroscopy.[208] Under similar surgical conditions, intraocular pressure increased by up to 100%, and there was risk that scleral edema and blurred vision may develop.[209] In anesthetized children during laparoscopic surgery, intraocular pressure increased 30% after insufflation (<15 mm Hg IAP) compared with open laparotomy surgery.[210]

The patency of a ventriculoperitoneal (VP) shunt should be evaluated before the procedure to prevent sudden increases in ICP during the procedure. Children with reduced brain ventricular system compliance may sustain dramatic increases in ICP if the IAP is sufficient to attenuate the drainage of cerebrospinal fluid into the abdominal cavity. In these children, laparoscopic surgery may be relatively contraindicated.[186] The risks should be thoroughly explored and discussed with the neurosurgeon, general surgeon, anesthesiologist, and the family. Children with VP shunts have shown a range of responses to laparoscopy from dramatic increases in ICP to no change at all.[184,211,212] Accordingly, a variety of approaches have been suggested. Some advocate externalizing the shunt and clamping the distal (intraabdominal) end of the shunt before surgery to prevent CO_2 from passing retrograde up the shunt or from the laparoscopic pressure disrupting the shunt valve, although these valves are stable with an IAP up to 80 mm Hg.[213] Another approach has been to temporarily isolate the tip of the VP shunt in an Endopouch bag (Ethicon, Somerville, NJ) while insufflating pressures to 12 mm Hg and then removing the bag at the end of the procedure.[214] Others discourage externalizing the shunt as sequelae have been reported and instead recommend monitoring the ICP to prevent and detect increases in ICP and further recommend retraction of abdominal tissue during the laparoscopic surgery.[213] For the surgeon, using a single-incision laparoscopic approach in these children reduces the risk of both traumatizing and infecting the VP shunt.[215] One retrospective review reported that laparoscopy in children with VP shunts was not associated with an increased risk of shunt infection compared with open procedures.[213] No single strategy can provide optimal management for every child with a VP shunt undergoing laparoscopic surgery.

RENAL EFFECTS AND FLUID REQUIREMENTS

Increased IAP decreases renal blood flow, renal function (creatinine clearance and glomerular filtration rate), and urine output, although the mechanisms for each are incompletely understood.[170,184,216] Renal oxygenation, as reflected by near-infrared spectroscopy, did not produce renal hypoxemia when age-appropriate IAPs were used (<6 mm Hg in neonates, <8 mm Hg in 2- to 12-month-old infants, <10 mm Hg 1 to 2 years of age, <12 mm Hg 2 to 8 years of age). These same authors also reported increased cerebral oxygen saturation, heart rate, and mean arterial pressure likely attributable to the increased cerebral blood flow from the increased arterial CO_2.[217] Decreases in urine output during laparoscopic surgery in children vary, in part, with the age of the child: oliguria occurs in older children and anuria in infants younger than 1 year of age.[184,186,218] The etiology of renal dysfunction and oliguria is multifactorial but includes direct and indirect effects of IAP on renal perfusion, antidiuretic hormone (ADH), endothelin, and nitric oxide.[184,219] ADH concentrations increase because renal blood flow decreases, which causes resorption of water, and decreased urine output. IAP increases renal endothelin (endothelin-1), resulting in renal venoconstriction, which further reduces renal blood flow and urine output.[184,219] Inhibiting endogenous nitric oxide exacerbates renal dysfunction during pneumoperitoneum through several mechanisms including reduced renal perfusion and increased salt and water resorption (e.g., oliguria).[219] In theory, pretreating patients with a nitric oxide donor (such as L-arginine or nondepressor doses of nitroglycerin) may attenuate the detrimental effects of a carbon dioxide pneumoperitoneum on renal function.[219] Renal tubular injury does not contribute to the renal dysfunction associated with increased IAP.[220] In adult donor nephrectomy patients, an overnight infusion of fluids followed by a colloid bolus immediately before the pneumoperitoneum attenuated the adverse hemodynamic effects and reduced the magnitude of changes in creatinine clearance associated with increased IAP.[221] Comparable data in children have not been forthcoming.

Fluid administration during laparoscopic surgery should be carefully monitored. Open abdominal surgery may require 10 to 15 mL/kg per hour of balanced salt solution to offset third-space fluid losses from extensive bowel manipulation. Although the existence of and manipulation of a real "third space" are debated, the conceptual fluid shift is real. During laparoscopic surgery, however, these fluid requirements are reduced because little fluid is lost and the bowels are minimally manipulated. Care must be taken to avoid fluid overload. Urine output is often used as an index of preload in children undergoing abdominal surgery, but 88% of infants and 33% of children develop anuria or oliguria during laparoscopic surgery. Because these issues are completely resolved within several hours of desufflation, a fluid challenge is not necessary for these children as fluid overload is a real possibility.[218] Transient oliguria in children after laparoscopic surgery should not be viewed as an early indicator of impending renal dysfunction.

PAIN MANAGEMENT

Postoperative pain after open general and urologic surgery primarily results from skin and muscle incisions. With the small incisions used during laparoscopic surgery, perioperative pain is less than with open surgery.[222–224] Pain after laparoscopic antireflux surgery in children has not been reported in depth; between 0% and 50% are reported to require postoperative opioids.[225,226] Intraperitoneal administration of local anesthetic has also been evaluated as a strategy to attenuate pain after laparoscopic surgery such as appendectomy in children.[227–229] This technique demonstrated some benefit, although the dose of local anesthetic is limited by the child's weight. Intraperitoneal implants that deliver a lidocaine infusion have also shown promise.[230] Additional studies are needed to fully assess the effectiveness of these approaches.[231] Most recently, a national study of ERAS (Enhanced Recovery After Surgery) for elective gastrointestinal surgery in adolescents is underway to evaluate the benefits of preoperative NSAIDs, reduced opioids, limited fluids, and early ambulation to enhance recovery (reduce pain) and discharge from hospital.[232] ERAS studies have shown benefits in children undergoing laparoscopic appendectomy and other surgeries.[233–236] To date, there has been a dearth of studies investigating pain after laparoscopic surgery in children.

Pain after laparoscopic surgery arises from several sources, including the incision sites, residual gas in the abdomen, referred pain from the diaphragm, and stretch on nerves from peculiar patient positions. A long-acting local anesthetic should be infiltrated around the incision sites at the end of laparoscopic surgery to prevent postoperative incisional pain. Some children develop pain after laparoscopic surgery, including back and shoulder pain. In these instances, multimodal pain therapy including acetaminophen, NSAIDs, and (less commonly) opioids are effective.[138,139,162] Recent evidence suggests that single-incision multiport laparoscopy for appendectomy may cause less pain than surgery with a multiport system.[237]

Robot-Assisted Surgery

Robot-assisted surgery is relatively new to pediatric surgery and urology, with only limited published experience, although it has been used extensively in adults since the late 1990s to facilitate minimally invasive endoscopic surgery. Enhanced with three-dimensional magnifying views and feedback-controlled enhanced motions of human hands, robot-assisted surgery enables very fine manipulation of surgical instruments while eliminating natural human tremors. It has great potential as the future direction for pediatric surgery and urology.[1,208,238–243]

Robotic surgery was initially introduced as a tool for remote battlefield surgery. It is now available to assist pediatric surgeons in performing complex surgery, with less tissue and organ damage on extremely small surgical targets. Most of the information currently available is limited to one product (da Vinci Surgical System; Intuitive Surgical, Sunnyvale, CA) and adult urologic procedures. However, rapid innovation and miniaturization of equipment have resulted in several pediatric centers undertaking robot-assisted laparoscopic surgery, with excellent outcomes (Video 27.1 and 27.2).[244–246] Concerns from the anesthesiologist's perspective regarding this relatively new approach are summarized in Table 27.1. Most of the perceived problems relate to the extended duration of procedures and the steep Trendelenburg position used, although numerous surgeries have been performed without this position.[208,238] Published evidence with robot-assisted surgery has yielded outcomes comparable to laparoscopic surgery in children,

prompting many to question whether this new and expensive surgical venture is justified.[247–249] However, rapidly advancing technology offers enormous opportunities for robot-assisted surgery in children, for very fine and technical dissection in small and constrained spaces.[250–253]

Specific General Surgical and Urologic Conditions

NISSEN FUNDOPLICATION

This surgery is indicated for children with documented gastric fluid reflux for whom medical management has failed. It involves mobilizing the muscles around the esophagus and suturing them tightly around the esophagus at the level of the lower esophageal sphincter. This surgery requires general anesthesia and tracheal intubation and is usually performed laparoscopically, with the increasing application of robot-assisted technology.[254,255]

Children who require a Nissen fundoplication often have a neurologic injury (i.e., cerebral palsy) that causes esophageal dysmotility. This dysmotility heralds esophageal reflux that, if severe, may result in recurrent aspiration pneumonia. If medical and gastric tube therapies fail, a Nissen fundoplication may be considered. The anesthetic considerations are few because surgery is not associated with postoperative pain, large fluid shifts, or large blood loss. Positioning a bougie within the esophagus during surgery allows the surgeons to gauge how tight to tie the muscles around the esophagus; without a bougie, the muscles around the esophagus may be overtightened, causing an esophageal obstruction. Care must be taken to avoid dislodging the tracheal tube while manipulating the bougie. At the end of the procedure, it is common for the surgeon to request that 50 to 60 milliliters of air be insufflated into the stomach via the gastric tube to ensure there are no anastomotic leaks. In general, surgery is completed in less than 1 hour in experienced hands, with a complication rate of about 10% and an average hospital stay of about 1.6 days. Postoperative pain is usually easily managed; however, open procedures may require continuous analgesia for 2 to 3 days.[256,257] Five-year outcomes in young children (including those less than 2 years of age at the time of surgery) after laparoscopic Nissen fundoplication prove the benefit in resolving gastroesophageal reflux disease (GERD) with few complications.[258,259]

PECTUS EXCAVATUM

Pectus excavatum is a deformity of the anterior chest wall in which the sternum and the ribs that insert into it are depressed. If severe, this deformity can compromise cardiorespiratory function, as well as lead to psychological issues and delayed cognitive development.[260] By correcting this deformity surgically, evidence is now clear that many of the sequelae from pectus excavatum can be attenuated and even reversed.[260,261]

Although this is a deformity of the chest wall, pediatric surgeons most often carry out the corrective procedure. The classic approach to correcting a pectus excavatum involves an open procedure with fracture of the sternum, removal of multiple costal cartilages, and elevating the sternum with fixation, using one or two stainless steel bars. The Nuss procedure is a less invasive technique,[262,263] whereby a U-shaped bar is blindly passed through the thorax hugging the undersurface of the sternum. Once across the chest, the bar is flipped, through which process the sternum is pushed anteriorly without fracturing it, thus avoiding the creation of a flail chest by the removal of the costal cartilage. A systematic review of 1432 pediatric and adult patients found no difference in outcomes or

TABLE 27.1	Issues Regarding Current Robotic-Assisted Procedures From the Anesthetist's Perspective

Dependence on Extreme Body Position, Such as Extreme Trendelenburg Position (Because of Absence of Adequate Surgical Assistance for Surgical Field Exposure), May Lead to:

Increased intracranial pressure, ocular pressure, and impairment of cerebral perfusion

Optic nerve or retinal morbidity

Cerebrofacial congestion, airway edema, vocal cord palsy, delayed awakening

Possible overstretching of nerves passing through the axilla and nerve plexus damage

Extended lithotomy leading to compartment syndrome in the lower legs

Tendency to apply greater intraabdominal pressure

Circulatory depression and respiratory depression

Carbon dioxide insufflation related complications

Absence of Touch, Traction, and Compression Sensations of Holding Instruments or Tissues:

All the manipulations are dependent exclusively on the visual sense

Inability to know the events occurring in an invisible place, overt tissue damage

Possibility of overlooking overt bleeding or tissue damage

Absence of Robot Legs and Easy Movability:

Once fixed, it is hard to change the position of the robot or the child's position

Difficulty in checking IV access sites and the airway

Unlimited and unexpected surgical approaches

Exploration of new surgical approaches and complex tasks at awkward angles

Greater surgical and setup times, hypothermia, and pressure sores

Unpredictable movement of robot and camera arms

Hitting or compressing the child's face

Organization of all tubing and cables, including intravenous tubing and breathing hoses

Need for Emergency Undocking of the Robot in Case of Mechanical Failure or Critical Events

complications between techniques in children but a greater incidence of complications in adults with the Nuss approach.[264]

The Nuss procedure has since been modified, whereby the bar is passed through the thorax under direct vision, using thoracoscopy to reduce possible perforation of major structures (e.g., the heart or lungs).[265–267] Although the risks associated with the Nuss procedure under direct vision are infrequent, complications may still occur even during minimally invasive surgery.[268–271]

Both blind and thoracoscopic approaches cause severe postoperative pain, which may be treated with a variety of approaches including patient-controlled analgesia, a thoracic epidural catheter, a lumbar epidural catheter and epidural morphine (see Chapters 40 and 41), cryoablation,[272] or erector spinae plane blocks.[273–277] Because these procedures are generally performed in teenagers, the thoracic epidural is preferably placed with the teenager awake but sedated. Two instances of transient paraplegia, bowel and bladder dysfunction have been reported after thoracic epidurals for Nuss procedures in children who recovered after a protracted course. This resulted in some centers abandoning thoracic epidurals for these procedures although no deficiency or specific causes for the complications were identified.[271] Compliance with inserting the epidural catheter while awake may be difficult in less mature teenagers. The analgesic efficacy and limited side effects of thoracic epidural analgesia warrants consideration for this procedure, a combination of bupivacaine and clonidine was associated with fewer adverse effects than bupivacaine and fentanyl or bupivacaine, fentanyl, and clonidine.[278] A retrospective review of 78 adolescents who received either an erector spinae block, thoracic epidural, or patient-controlled analgesia for analgesia after a Nuss procedure suggested the impact of analgesic modality; the opioid consumption and length of stay with the erector spinae block were less than with a thoracic epidural or patient-controlled analgesia.[279] In a prospective comparative study of multimodal postoperative pain management after the Nuss procedure, bilateral paravertebral blocks with a continuous infusion, bilateral paravertebral blocks with a continuous infusion and a right-sided intercostal nerve (T3–T7) cryoablation, or a bilateral single-shot paravertebral blocks with cryoablation were evaluated.[280] Of the 17 children who had bilateral block and cryoablation, 11 were discharged the same day and 3 more the day after surgery. Compared with those who had bilateral paravertebral blocks and infusion alone, the length of stay (4.4 vs. 0.7 days) and opioid use (0.92 vs. 0.47 mg/kg morphine equivalents) were less for those with bilateral single-shot block and intercostal nerve cryoablation.

Children return after several years to have the pectus bar removed. Complications during removal are rare,[281,282] although the bar may become adherent to the pericardium or lung resulting in a severe, sudden, and catastrophic rupture of a major vessel or chamber in the heart when the pectus bar is removed.[283] It would be prudent to establish ample IV access to provide the means to rapidly transfuse fluids and blood should a catastrophic blood loss occur and to be prepared for possible emergent thoracotomy or sternotomy.[284] A single institution retrospective review of 1628 Nuss bar removals revealed seven patients to have blood loss of more than 150 milliliters and two children had a blood loss of more than 2000 milliliters.[284]

CIRCUMCISION

Globally, the prevalence of circumcised males is 40%, with half of these surgical procedures performed for religious or cultural reasons.[285] Circumcision is performed in neonates, infants, children, and adults with local, regional, or general anesthesia. The indications for circumcision include phimosis, recurrent balanitis, religious beliefs, and parental preference. Inhalational anesthesia supplemented by a regional block is preferred. Classic circumcision involves cutting the foreskin and cauterizing and suturing the skin edges. The duration of surgery is usually less than 1 hour. The type of anesthetic and airway management does not affect perioperative outcomes. The most common complication arising from circumcision is bleeding.

In infants and children, circumcision is performed with the patient under general anesthesia. Multimodal pain therapy includes acetaminophen (e.g., 10 to 15 mg/kg orally or 30 to 40 mg/kg rectally before starting surgery) or 10 to 15 mg/kg IV, parenteral opioids (i.e., morphine 0.05 to 0.1 mg/kg), and/or local anesthetic without epinephrine (dorsal penile block, caudal block, subcutaneous ring block, and topical lidocaine-prilocaine [eutectic mixture of local anesthetics (EMLA)]) (see Chapter 40).[286,287] In a comparative study, the suprapubic penile block provided better analgesia than the subcutaneous ring block of the penis.[288] When a caudal block was compared with penile blocks and parenteral analgesics, a Cochrane review concluded that both rescue analgesia and nausea and vomiting were comparable with all three techniques, although the analysis was limited because of small numbers and poor methodology.[289,290] Oral sucrose and swaddling or music have been effective in supplementing other methods of pain management.[287]

HYPOSPADIAS AND CHORDEE

This congenital malformation occurs in 1 of 250 liveborn males. It often occurs in isolation, without other congenital anomalies. *Hypospadias* refers to a malposition of the meatus of the urethra: rather than opening at the distal tip of the penis, the urethra opens along the undersurface of the penis anywhere from just proximal to the glans to the scrotum (Fig. 27.5). The majority of hypospadias defects are distal, occurring near or at the glans of the penis. Between 15% and 50% of instances of hypospadias have an associated chordee, whereas 8% have an undescended testis. A small number of children with hypospadias have urethral openings remote from the glans of the penis, including the scrotum (Fig. 27.6; E-Figs. 27.4 and 27.5).

Surgery is undertaken with an expected duration of between 1 and 4 hours depending on the severity of the hypospadias. It is important to establish an understanding with the urologist of the type of regional block that will suit the extent of surgery: those requiring a minor hypospadias repair, (i.e., a single-stage procedure with meatal advancement and glanuloplasty technique or Mathieu repair), may be managed with a face mask, LMA, or tracheal tube. The anesthetic prescription is at the discretion of the anesthesiologist; the children are outpatients and receive either a penile block or a single-shot caudal block. Those in need of more extensive hypospadias repair and requiring longer surgery may be managed with either an LMA or a tracheal tube. They may be admitted to a hospital for 1 to 2 nights and need a strategy for continuous postoperative analgesia. For the latter, either a caudal or a lumbar epidural catheter may be inserted after induction to reduce the anesthetic requirements and provide postoperative analgesia. If opioids are avoided, a caudal-epidural block consisting of only local anesthetic (e.g., bupivacaine 0.125% to 0.175% plain) does not delay micturition after the urinary catheter has been removed.[291]

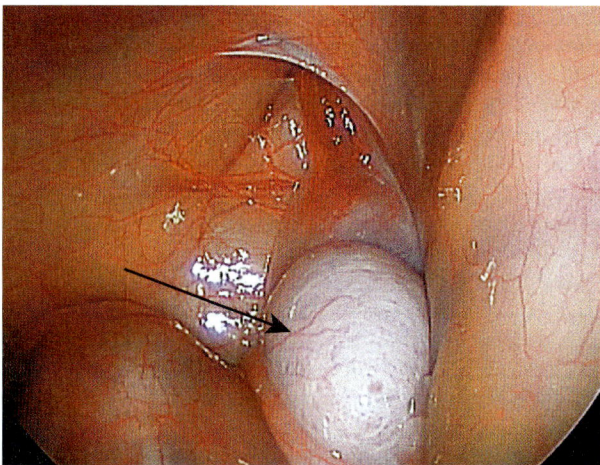

FIGURE 27.7 Intraabdominal testis *(arrow)* in the hernia ring, discovered during laparoscopy for an undescended testicle. (Courtesy Dr. P. Williot, Pediatric Urology, Women and Children's Hospital of Buffalo, Buffalo, NY.)

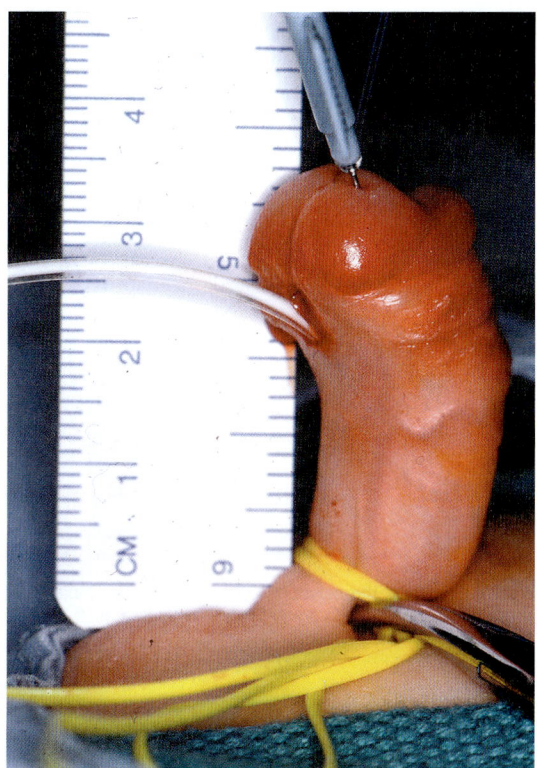

FIGURE 27.5 Classic hypospadias. Saline solution is injected to perform an erection test before surgical correction. (Courtesy Dr. P. Williot, Pediatric Urology, Women and Children's Hospital of Buffalo, Buffalo, NY.)

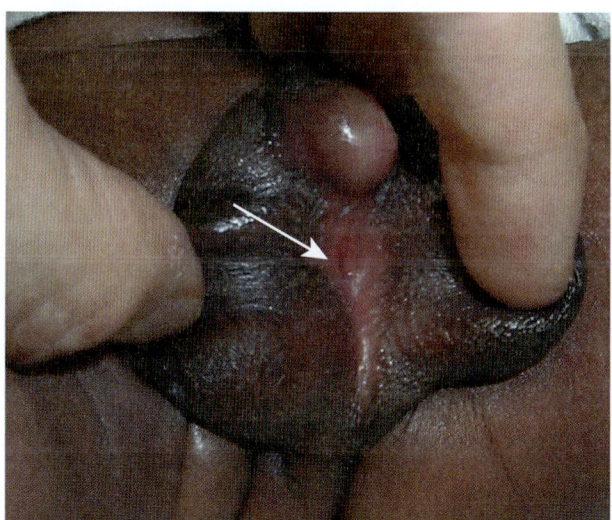

FIGURE 27.6 Scrotal hypospadias with the urethra opening in the midline of the scrotum. (Courtesy Dr. P. Williot, Pediatric Urology, Women and Children's Hospital of Buffalo, Buffalo, NY.)

CRYPTORCHIDISM AND HERNIAS: INGUINAL AND UMBILICAL

These surgeries, together with hydrocele repair, are common outpatient procedures. *Orchiopexy* refers to mobilizing the undescended testis that is either in the inguinal canal or, less commonly, within the abdominal cavity (Fig. 27.7), and securing it firmly in the scrotum. Approximately 33% of preterm infant males are born with one undescended testis, whereas only 3% of full-term males

are similarly affected. Although the incidence of undescended testis decreases to 1% by 3 months of age, the incidence remains at 1% thereafter. Cryptorchidism usually occurs in isolation, although it is associated with many conditions, including Prader-Willi syndrome, Noonan syndrome, and cloacal exstrophy.[292]

Undescended testes are categorized, based on physical examination, to include truly undescended testes, those that are ectopic, and those that are retracted. Retracted testes are not truly undescended because they can be massaged into the scrotum and require no further treatment. In the case of true undescended testes, the testes must be located, mobilized, and then fixed within the scrotal sac to ensure viability. Failure to mobilize the testes out of the inguinal canal or abdomen may result in atrophy, torsion, testicular cancer, or hernias.

An *inguinal hernia* in a child is a congenital failure of the processus vaginalis to obliterate. In this case, a loop of the bowel protrudes beyond the internal ring, causing a bulge in the inguinal region or scrotum. These protuberances may appear periodically, with complete resolution in the interim. On occasion, a small sac of fluid is present in the scrotum, known as a *hydrocele*, and is confused for a loop of bowel in the scrotum (E-Fig. 27.6). Hydroceles are removed electively with the same approach as for an inguinal hernia. On occasion, the loop of the bowel does not reduce spontaneously from the hernia and remains trapped in the canal, necessitating a visit to the emergency department. A surgeon is often required to manually reduce the trapped bowel. In these cases, the hernia repair is then scheduled as an urgent or elective surgery, depending on whether there is suspicion of persistent or potential recurrent ischemia to the bowel. In some cases, the entrapped bowel cannot be reduced and an incarcerated hernia or obstructed bowel is diagnosed. Incarcerated hernias and bowel obstructions are surgical emergencies that require general anesthesia and neuromuscular blockade to reduce the strangulated bowel. The emergency nature of the surgery requires careful questioning regarding the time interval between the last meal and the onset of abdominal pain and strangulated bowel. It is usually assumed that these children have full stomachs. At the time of an open reduction, if the bowel does not appear to have adequate perfusion, a segment of the ischemic or necrotic bowel may have to be resected.

Management of cryptorchidism and inguinal hernia requires general anesthesia (face mask, LMA, or tracheal tube) and a pain management strategy. When the surgeon pulls on the foreskin, hernia sac, or testis during surgery, laryngospasm may occur if the depth of anesthesia is inadequate. Anesthesia can be deepened most rapidly by an IV bolus of propofol; increasing the inspired concentration of inhalational anesthetic may also deepen the anesthetic. Multimodal pain therapy, as described earlier, may be used together with a regional block. Regional blocks (ilioinguinal, iliohypogastric, scrotal block; caudal-epidural block; or transversus abdominis plane block) are used for both orchiopexy and inguinal hernia surgery, using either a landmark-based or ultrasound-guided method (see Chapters 40 and 41).[293]

An *umbilical hernia* is a 1- to 5-centimeter defect in the anterior abdominal wall (usually halfway between the umbilicus and the xiphisternal junction), with an intermittent protuberance of the bowel through the defect. This defect occurs in 15% of children, more commonly in children of African rather than European descent, and equally in both sexes. It also occurs frequently in preterm and low-birth-weight infants. Many resolve spontaneously in the first year of life, but those that persist require surgical closure. If the defect is small, then an LMA may be sufficient, provided a deep level of anesthesia is maintained when the suture needles pass through each side of the rectus muscle. If the defect is large, tracheal intubation and, depending on the surgeon, neuromuscular blockade may be required. When closing the defect, a deep level of anesthesia should be established, muscle relaxation or an IV bolus of propofol (1 to 2 mg/kg) to reduce the risk that a suture perforates the serosa of the bowel or bowel wall itself. A periumbilical or rectus sheath block can be used to supplement postoperative analgesia.[294–297] A continuous infusion of bupivacaine into the rectus sheath has been used for more prolonged postoperative analgesia.

TORSION OF THE TESTIS

When a male presents with a history of sudden onset of acute scrotal pain in the absence of trauma, immediate investigation (and possible surgery) is required to preserve a potentially viable testis.[298] The differential diagnosis of acute onset of torsion of the testis (Fig. 27.8) includes torsion of the testicular appendix, torsion of the spermatic cord, epididymitis, and incarcerated hernia. The majority of testes can be saved if surgery is performed within 6 hours of the onset of pain if the diagnosis is confirmed by Doppler ultrasonography or suspected on clinical grounds.[299] The salvage rate for the testis decreases to 50% if surgery is undertaken 6 to 12 hours after the onset of pain. Children with suspected acute testicular torsion should be considered "an acute abdomen" and assumed to have a full stomach and require RSI and tracheal intubation. Although pain at the time of induction of anesthesia may be intense, when the torsion is relieved, the pain abates. Hence, after surgery, many of these children no longer have substantive pain that warrants aggressive treatment.

POSTERIOR URETHRAL VALVES

Posterior urethral valves are a spectrum of urethral obstruction that varies from mild to severe. The diagnosis is often made antenatally (preferably by 24 weeks gestation) by ultrasound identification of bladder distention, megaureters, and hydronephrosis. When posterior urethral valves is diagnosed antenatally, the severity of the disease tends to be greater.[300] Decompression of the urogenital system may be achieved by a vesicoamniotic shunt in utero. Although some recommend that an intervention should be undertaken as quickly as possible to minimize the impact on renal

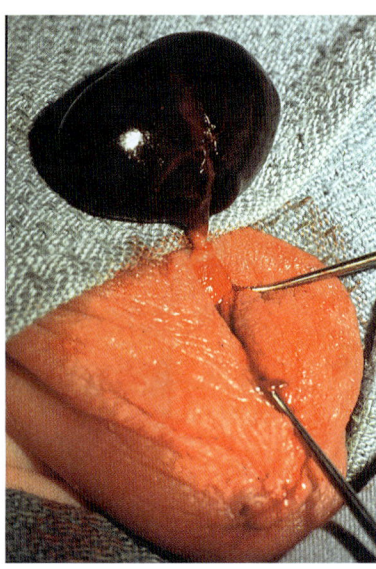

FIGURE 27.8 Torsion of the newborn testis. (Courtesy Dr. Daniel P. Doody, MD, Pediatric Surgery, MassGeneral Hospital for Children, Boston.)

function, evidence suggests that early intervention does not affect the outcome, because renal damage may have already occurred in utero.[24,301,302]

Postnatally, a lack of or decrease in urine output, urinary retention, or a poor urine stream may be the only indications of the presence of these valves.[303] Affected children can have associated renal insufficiency resulting from congenital renal dysplasia and urethral valve obstruction.[302] Because the renal concentrating mechanism is often impaired, these infants commonly present with greater than normal urine output. Consequently, careful monitoring of urine output and balanced salt solution infusion rate is necessary. Primary valve ablation is required to decompress the urogenital system.

Several indexes have been postulated as predictors of poor long-term renal function in infants with posterior urethral valves, including a creatinine value of 0.8 mg/dL (70 µmol/L) or greater at birth, antenatal diagnosis, proteinuria, moderate or severe hydronephrosis, and renal dysplasia.[300,304] One study indicated that a nadir creatinine greater than 1 mg/dL (88 µmol/L) and bladder dysfunction were the only independent predictors of long-term renal dysfunction.[305] Children with posterior urethral valves are scheduled for elective surgery. A general anesthetic is required, with the specific management left to the discretion of the anesthesiologist; there are few special considerations needed.

PRUNE-BELLY SYNDROME

Prune-belly syndrome is a disorder that occurs predominantly (97% of the time) in males, with an incidence of 3.8 in 100,000 births.[306] Affected infants present with a range of findings, from stillborn to a full-term neonate, with a host of possible organ and chromosomal abnormalities.[304,307] Affected systems include: orthopedic in 50% (congenital hip dislocation and scoliosis), gastrointestinal in 30% (malrotation and volvulus), congenital heart disease in 10% (tetralogy of Fallot and ventricular septal defect), and chromosomal defects (trisomy 18 and trisomy 21).[304]

In utero, the child's abdomen often swells with fluid (in the presence of oligohydramnios) that is resorbed by birth, leaving the

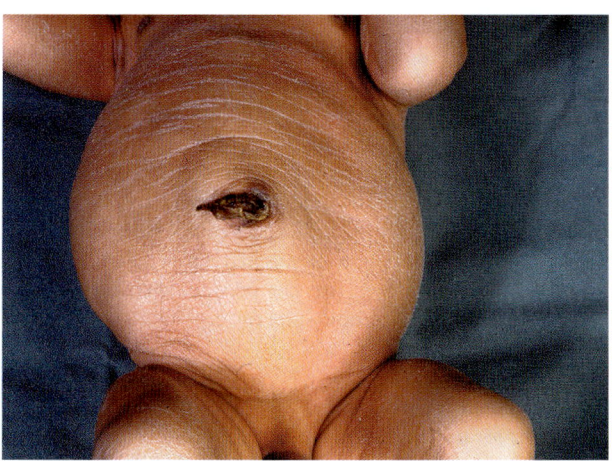

FIGURE 27.9 Prune-belly syndrome. View of the distended, weak-muscled abdomen; the muscle wall is so thin that the abdominal surface is bulging in front of the bowels. (Courtesy Dr. P. Williot, Pediatric Urology, Women and Children's Hospital of Buffalo, Buffalo, NY.)

characteristic wrinkled redundant abdominal wall (Fig. 27.9 and E-Fig. 27.7). The pathophysiology of this syndrome is unclear, but it has been suggested that a urethral obstruction in utero leads to dilatation of the urethra (megaurethra is a common finding), which, combined with bladder distention and ascites, causes distention of the abdomen in utero. This ultimately leads to vesicoureteral reflux and ureteral dilatation in 80% of affected children.

Abdominal overdistention in utero causes weak rectus abdominis muscles that undermine the child's ability to exhale forcefully and generate a strong cough to clear secretions. As a result, chronic aspiration pneumonia may contribute to an early demise. Some have suggested that aggressive intervention to correct the weak rectus muscles by plication and muscle transfer may improve respiratory function,[306,308–310] reduce back strain and pain, decrease bladder volume, and arrest scoliosis. However, this view is not shared by others who prefer to observe the child for signs of regurgitation and aspiration before intervening.[311] Controlling the type of feeds, preventing gastrointestinal reflux disease and constipation, and using antibiotics to treat pneumonia permit the child to grow. Pneumonia must be aggressively treated and completely resolved before entertaining surgery. Percutaneous endoscopic gastroscopy tubes are generally eschewed in these children when feeding is a problem, as abdominal wall surgery is difficult. These children often require urologic surgery to correct vesicoureteral reflux and orchiopexy.[306] Urethral obstruction may be due to the angulation of the urethra within the prostate.

Trisomy 18, the second most common autosomal trisomy, occurs in 1 in approximately 7000 live births and is associated with the prune-belly syndrome. In contrast to the simple prune-belly syndrome, 60% to 80% of these infants are female. Trisomy 18 is characterized by severe neurologic developmental problems (including microcephaly), micrognathia and/or retrognathia, microstomia, auricular abnormalities, and others. In fact, 95% die in utero, with only 5% to 10% surviving 1 year and only 1% reaching 10 years of age. Mortality results from cardiac anomalies (90% of affected children have a ventricular septal defect, valvular heart defect, atrial septal defect, hypoplastic left heart syndrome, tetralogy of Fallot, or other cardiac defects), renal anomalies, failure to thrive, and apnea.[312,313] Additional findings include pulmonary

hypoplasia and gastrointestinal anomalies (including omphalocele, ileal atresia, and esophageal atresia).

General anesthesia with tracheal intubation is required for most surgeries in children with prune-belly syndrome. Controlled ventilation is recommended because of the variability in the strength of the abdominal muscles. It is prudent to suction the lungs once the trachea has been intubated to assess the severity of the secretions. As little muscle relaxant as possible should be used during the surgery, with preferably no neuromuscular blocking drugs administered during the last hour, to ensure the child's muscles have had time to recover to maintain an adequate tidal volume after extubation. Opioids should be used cautiously to limit respiratory depression; regional anesthesia may be preferred because of the child's difficulty with clearing secretions from the tracheobronchial tree.[314]

URETERAL REIMPLANTATION

Vesicoureteral reflux, in which urine passes retrograde up the ureter, is a congenital disorder affecting 0.5% to 2% of children.[315] It occurs 10 times more commonly in White than Black children, is more common in male neonates but 5 to 6 times more common in females younger than 1 year of age, and more commonly occurs in red-haired children.[315] There is a genetic component to this disorder, with 34% of siblings affected, although the pattern of inheritance is unknown.[316] Recurrent episodes of pyelonephritis may occur, leading to renal scarring and reduced renal function, depending on the severity of the reflux.[317] The pathology is thought to be an anatomically abnormal insertion of the ureter into the bladder that fails to close tight when the bladder fills and contracts. A voiding cystourethrogram is a definitive test to diagnose reflux and assess its severity. Mild forms of vesicoureteral reflux are managed with daily antibiotics until the child outgrows the reflux.[317] This conservative approach has made ureteric reimplantation surgery less common.[318] However, more severe forms, or those who develop kidney infections despite antibiotic therapy require surgical correction. The classic surgical approach for vesicoureteral reflux is an open procedure in which the affected ureters are reimplanted into the bladder wall, recreating a normal muscle flap valve.[319] This involves a lower abdominal incision and 2 to 4 hours of surgery. Postoperatively, the pain is often intense, necessitating 2 to 3 days of continuous infusion of local anesthetic via an indwelling caudal or epidural catheter.

More recently, laparoscopic techniques have been developed, with and without robotic control, for reimplantation of the ureters.[317,319] Preliminary evidence suggests an excellent success rate (>90%) for this approach,[320] although the time for the surgery is more than twice that with the open technique, and more complications were identified in children with small bladders.

In the past 20 years, the search for alternatives to surgery has spawned several compounds to inject into the terminal submucosal tract of the ureter to prevent reflux. Initially, polytetrafluoroethylene (Teflon; Chemours, Wilmington, DE) was used but more recently a safer, more durable polymer comprised of dextranomer and hyaluronic acid (Deflux; Valeant Pharmaceuticals International, Bridgewater, NJ) supplanted Teflon. In this way, surgeons create a swelling just inferior to the opening of the ureter into the bladder that prevents urine from refluxing (Fig. 27.10, before and after injection of polymer). The technique is successful in 80% to 100% of cases of grade 1 to 2 reflux after one injection and in 85% of cases of grade 3 to 4 reflux after two injections (where the grade of reflux was related to the ureterorenal involvement).[321] Although

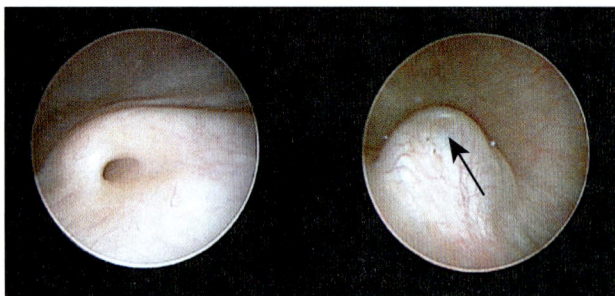

FIGURE 27.10 A child with ureteral reflux. Preinjection *(at left)* with the bladder orifice wide open with no valve to prevent the backwash of urine up the ureter. Polymer was injected into the submucosa of the bladder, raising a mound to seal off the orifice of that ureter. Postinjection *(at right)* with the orifice now appearing as a dimple on the peak of the mound *(arrow)*. (Courtesy Dr. P. Williot, Pediatric Urology, Women and Children's Hospital of Buffalo, Buffalo, NY.)

this procedure still requires general anesthesia, its advantages far outweigh its disadvantages in that the duration of the procedure is very brief (usually 15 to 30 minutes), avoids an abdominal incision, causes no postoperative pain, and may be performed as ambulatory surgery. However, the results of this injection technique continue to be monitored because long-term outcomes and sequelae have not been determined.[322]

PYELOPLASTY

Ureteropelvic junction obstruction occurs in 0.1% to 0.2% of neonates, approximately twice as frequently in males as females. Pyeloplasty is performed to decompress the renal pelvis either because of intrinsic (congenital) or extrinsic (major vessel) compression of the ureter. A distended renal pelvis is often diagnosed antenatally and, in some instances, decompressed in utero by percutaneous nephrostomy. The ureteric narrowing often occurs at the ureteropelvic junction, where the ureter exits the renal pelvis. Surgery involves disconnecting the ureter at the renal pelvis, reshaping it, and then reinserting it into the kidney. Such surgery is often performed with the patient in the lateral or prone position, with the table jackknifed. The duration of this surgery is approximately 2 hours and has a success rate of approximately 95%. Dissection is often retroperitoneal, but the incision is placed immediately below the rib cage. This procedure has been performed laparoscopically and with the use of robotics.[149,323,324]

Anesthetic considerations include the prone or lateral decubitus position (complicated by placing the table in the jackknife position), postoperative pain, and adequate fluid resuscitation. IV access should be established in an upper extremity to maintain adequate cardiac filling pressures. If the table is placed in the jackknife position, it is very important to measure the child's blood pressure before and after the table is jackknifed, because venous return may become compromised, necessitating reducing the extent of the jackknife and resuscitating the child with fluid. For postoperative pain management, an indwelling high lumbar or low thoracic epidural catheter is placed. We administer lidocaine 2% with 1:200,00 epinephrine immediately after inserting the catheter to set the block before the table is jackknifed. Thereafter a bupivacaine or ropivacaine epidural infusion may be used.

The laparoscopic[325] approach to pyeloplasty may be used; CO_2 is insufflated in the retroperitoneal space to provide surgical access.[326] Because of the anatomic differences between the retroperitoneal and intraperitoneal spaces, greater pressures may be required to provide adequate surgical visibility. A mean retroperitoneal pressure of 12 mm Hg increases $PETCO_2$ and peak inspiratory pressures, and decreases blood pressure.[327] Early evidence indicates that laparoscopic surgery yields outcomes similar to the open approach, although the duration of surgery is approximately one-third greater.[328,329] In part, this has been attributed to the learning curve of this technique. Evidence suggests that the laparoscopic and robotic-assisted approaches combined with an ERAS protocol decrease the length of hospital stay and may decrease postoperative pain[149,329–331] (see the previous discussion of pain management after laparoscopic surgery).

NEPHRECTOMY

Indications for nephrectomy and partial nephrectomy in children include nonfunctioning kidney, dysplastic kidney, urolithiasis, Wilms or other tumors, end-stage renal failure (pretransplantation or to control hypertension), hemolytic uremic syndrome, and polycystic disease. Children who need a nephrectomy require a thorough preoperative assessment in terms of history, physical examination, and laboratory testing, depending on their underlying pathology. These children are often anemic because of chronic disease and possibly decreased erythropoietin concentrations. If the child is being staged for a kidney transplant, the nephrologists may prefer to avoid blood transfusions at this time. If time is available and the patient is anemic, oral ferrous sulfate and vitamin C should be commenced 3 to 6 weeks before surgery (vitamin C increases gut absorption of ferrous sulfate) to increase the hemoglobin concentration, particularly if erythropoietin supplementation is planned.[332,333] These children are often small in size and this should be considered when preparing the anesthetic equipment.

Nephrectomies are commonly performed using a retroperitoneal approach with the child in the lateral decubitus position and the table jackknifed. The incision is usually large and located just subcostal to the twelfth rib. If an open approach is planned, an epidural catheter may be placed (see "Pyeloplasty" earlier). If, however, a laparoscopic or robotic-assisted approach is planned,[132] then a neuraxial block is not necessary but the same surgical approach occurs. Outcomes after laparoscopic nephrectomy in children are similar to those after an open procedure, according to the experience from one center,[334] although evidence points to less pain and earlier discharge from the hospital.[132]

NEUROBLASTOMA

The adrenal glands are located in the retroperitoneal space, adjacent to the superior pole of the kidneys. Masses that arise in the adrenal gland may be tumors, hemorrhages, infections, or cysts. The tumors in the adrenal glands may arise from the cortex (as in adenoma) or medulla (including the sympathetic chain, as in neuroblastoma or ganglioneuroma) and may be either hyperfunctioning or nonfunctioning.

Neuroblastoma is the most common extracranial solid tumor that presents in childhood, representing 10% of all tumors and 15% of all deaths from tumors.[335,336] It is the second most common abdominal tumor after Wilms tumor.[337] Its incidence is approximately 1 in 100,000 children in the United States.[338,339] Neuroblastomas arise in the abdomen in 75% of cases and along the sympathetic chain anywhere from the neck to the pelvis in 25%. Only one-third of those that arise in the abdomen arise in the adrenal glands. The median age at presentation is 2 years, with up to 90% occurring in children younger than 5 years with equal sex prevalence. In some series, up to 50% of cases appear in the first month of life, with some diagnosed antenatally; reports of familial neuroblastoma are rare.[335] However, these tumors may be associated with other disorders, including Beckwith-Wiedemann syndrome, neurofibromatosis, Hirschsprung disease, and central hypoventilation syndrome.[335]

Most neuroblastomas are first detected as palpable masses in the abdomen. The symptomatic presentation may present as local pressure on adjacent organs or structures (liver, kidney, or spine), as metastases (lymph nodes, bone marrow, liver, and skin), or with manifestations of excess neurohumoral production (that is, from catecholamines [e.g., systemic hypertension] or vasoactive intestine polypeptides [e.g., diarrhea]).[335] Urinary catecholamines are increased in greater than 90% of children (>1 year of age) with neuroblastoma. In a minority of instances, the diagnosis is made through incidental examination, either by radiography or ultrasonography.

The staging of these tumors follows two protocols.[338] The International Neuroblastoma Staging System depends on tumor resectability, lymph node involvement, and metastases. However, if patients are not surgical candidates, the staging score holds little relevance. To further stage these tumors, a second scoring system was developed, the International Neuroblastoma Risk Group classification system,[340] which is based on the preoperative radiologic findings only. Survival likelihood depends on a low score, extraabdominal (as opposed to intraabdominal) primary tumor, and younger age. Therapeutic intervention is tailored to the staging of the tumor at presentation and the size of the tumor. Those with favorable tumor biology, no distant metastases, and age younger than 18 months are often curable with surgical resection alone.[341] Those with less favorable tumor biology, metastases, and a large tumor size that may present a challenge surgically, are ideally treated with a combination of chemotherapy, radiation, and/or bone marrow transplantation to reduce the tumor size first and then with surgical resection. Patients with less favorable biology present a challenge for surgical resection because of local infiltration, large tumor size, and vascular extension. The most promising treatments for neuroblastomas with poor prognoses include molecular profiling of the tumor.[338] The long-term survival after treating these tumors is 88% for infants and children younger than 18 months, 49% for children 18 months to 12 years of age, and 10% for those 12 years of age and older.[342]

Preoperative assessment requires a general systems review, with a particular focus on the organ systems involved with the tumor. These tumors may present as a large intraabdominal mass that compromises respiration, most commonly manifested as tachypnea. Those with catecholamine-secreting tumors may also present with chronic hypertension. This is mitigated to a large extent if the tumor is shrunk preoperatively, but intraoperative hypertensive episodes still occur in 25% of the children (with elevated urinary catecholamines). Children with catecholamine-secreting neuroblastomas should have both α-adrenergic and β-adrenergic blockades established preoperatively (see Chapter 25) to avoid swings in blood pressure during manipulation of the tumor.[343] Less frequently, chronic diarrhea from vasoactive intestine polypeptides may cause chronic dehydration and electrolyte derangements that require correction.

The anesthetic plan depends on the nature and extent of the surgery. A general anesthetic with tracheal intubation and controlled ventilation, as well as standard anesthetic monitors, is required. These should be supplemented with invasive monitoring, including arterial and central venous access for catecholamine-secreting tumors, large tumors, and those that are expected to bleed excessively.[336] Anticipation of massive blood loss will

necessitate using large-bore upper extremity IV access, blood warmers, and possibly a rapid transfusion device. No specific anesthetic regimen has been recommended for these surgeries.

Although the blood pressure may be controlled with an established α-adrenergic blockade, manipulation and squeezing of the tumor during its removal may cause a surge in catecholamine release, necessitating the use of antihypertensive medications intraoperatively (see Chapter 25).[343] Labetalol may be effective in children with hypertension during resection of neuroblastomas[343]; however, it may cause paroxysmal hypertension and heart failure in children who have only β-adrenergic blockade established because of the predominant β-adrenergic blocking action of labetalol.

WILMS TUMOR

Renal tumors represent 2.5% to 7% of tumors in children. Wilms tumor is the most common abdominal tumor, with an incidence of 1 in 100,000 children younger than 15 years of age, and the most common solid renal tumor beyond the first year of life.[339,344] These tumors arise from persistent immature parenchymal renal tissue (referred to as Wilms tumorlet cells), often in the periphery of the kidney (as opposed to the collecting ducts), enclosed by a pseudocapsule. They may achieve a large size before detection, often compressing adjacent renal parenchyma (Fig. 27.11). Histologically, the tumor often includes up to three distinct tissue cell lines: epithelial, blastemal, and stromal cells.[344] The presence of anaplastic cells (in 4% of Wilms tumors) and, more specifically, whether the cells are focal or diffuse in the tumor, and older age at the time of presentation suggest a less favorable response to chemotherapy and less favorable long-term prognosis.[344] With tailored multimodal therapy, the survival from Wilms tumor in the past several decades has increased dramatically, from ~30% to ~90%.[345,346]

Eighty percent of the children with Wilms tumor present between 1 and 5 years of age (peaking at 3–4 years of age) with no gender or racial predominance.[339,344] The presentation of Wilms tumor is similar to that of other intraabdominal tumors in the form of an incidental mass on physical examination; approximately 6% are bilateral. Congenital anomalies coexist with Wilms

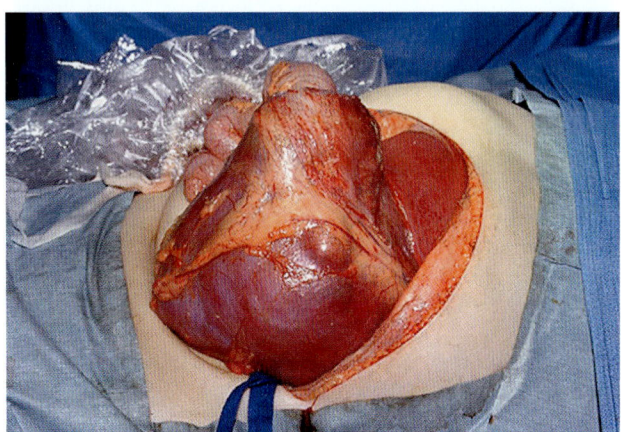

FIGURE 27.11 A Wilms tumor was mobilized and exteriorized from the abdomen. Note that it is encapsulated and contiguous with the left kidney. (Courtesy Daniel P. Doody, MD, Pediatric Surgery, MassGeneral Hospital for Children, Boston.)

tumors in 12% of children, notably genitourinary anomalies (5%), hemihypertrophy (2.5%), and aniridia (1%).[344] Several genetic syndromes are associated with Wilms tumors (e.g., Beckwith-Wiedemann, Fanconi syndrome, and Trisomy 18).[339,346] Wilms tumors occur twice as frequently in children with horseshoe kidneys than in those with normal kidneys and are also more frequent in those with multicystic dysplastic kidneys.

Preoperatively, most children with Wilms tumors appear well, presenting with constitutional findings including weight loss, loss of appetite, and malaise; a palpable abdominal mass is present in 75% to 90%. Laboratory investigations before nephrectomy include routine complete blood cell count, electrolytes, renal function, as well as coagulation indexes. Polycythemia may be present from tumor-induced excess erythropoietin production; acquired von Willebrand disease is present in less than 10%.[339] Microscopic hematuria occurs in 25%, whereas overt hematuria is rare,[344] suggesting tumor invasion of the collecting ducts. Systemic hypertension is present in 25%, presumably as a result of hyperreninemia. Preoperative investigations should include radiography and ultrasonography, the latter highlighting hyperechogenic structures within the kidney. Tumor extension into the ipsilateral renal vein and inferior vena cava must be examined before embarking on surgery, as chemotherapy may lead to the involution of these tumors (Fig. 27.12).[339] Magnetic resonance imaging (MRI) and CT are valuable tools for delimiting the tumor borders within the kidney, as well as metastases in the lungs or other organs.[339] Radiologic investigations may require additional interventions, including echocardiogram and lung scan, to determine the presence of tumors in the heart and lungs, respectively. An echocardiogram may be specifically required to

evaluate myocardial function if doxorubicin and other anthracycline chemotherapeutic agents have been administered.[339]

Anesthetic management of children with Wilms tumor is similar to that with neuroblastoma. No specific anesthetic regimen is preferred. The potential for massive and rapid blood loss must be anticipated and appropriate blood products should be immediately available. Invasive monitoring and large-bore IV access (upper extremities should the tumor extend into or compress the inferior vena cava) with adequate blood warming capability is mandatory; a rapid infusion device should be close at hand. Hypertension (precipitated by tumor handling), coagulopathy (acquired von Willebrand disease), the extension of the tumor into the proximal inferior vena cava or right atrium, pulmonary tumor emboli, acute right heart failure, and considerations concerning preoperative or previous treatment with chemotherapeutic drugs are anticipated potential complications during anesthesia.[339] These drugs may impair hepatic or hematopoietic function (actinomycin D), cause inappropriate antidiuretic hormone release (vincristine), or myocardial damage (anthracyclines) (see also Chapter 9).[339] Postoperative pain may be controlled using either IV opioids or regional anesthesia, though the risk of coagulopathy must be ruled out before placing an epidural block.

BLADDER AND CLOACAL EXSTROPHY

Bladder exstrophy is a rare congenital anomaly of the genitourinary tract occurring in 3.3 per 1,000,000 births[347] with a 2:1 male/female ratio, more common in White than non-White.[348,349] It occurs as a failure of the abdominal wall to close during fetal development and results in defects of the anterior wall of the bladder and overlying midline abdominal wall. Bladder exstrophy may present with a spectrum of anomalies, including widening of the symphysis pubis, and genital anomalies, such as epispadias, bifid clitoris, and undescended testes (Fig. 27.13). Some regard bladder and cloacal exstrophies as distinct entities, whereas others consider them both extremes in a continuum of antenatal defects.[350] Cloacal exstrophy includes features of bladder exstrophy, plus an omphalocele and spinal defects, and always includes an imperforate anus. Because the antenatal diagnosis of bladder exstrophy using ultrasound may be technically difficult, and thus dependent on indirect signs (absence of bladder filling, a low-set umbilicus, widening of the pubic ramus, small external genitalia, or a lower abdominal mass), the diagnosis is usually

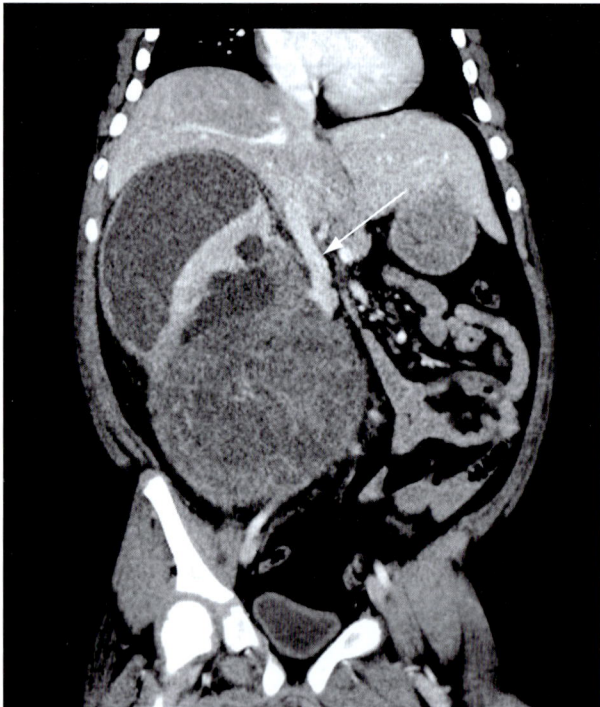

FIGURE 27.12 Coronal view of the CT scan of a Wilms tumor. Note the massive tumor enveloping the inferior vena cava, as the vena cava is only visible where it enters the liver in the upper midportion of the radiograph (*arrow*). (Radiograph courtesy Daniel P. Doody, MD, Pediatric Surgery, MassGeneral Hospital for Children, Boston.)

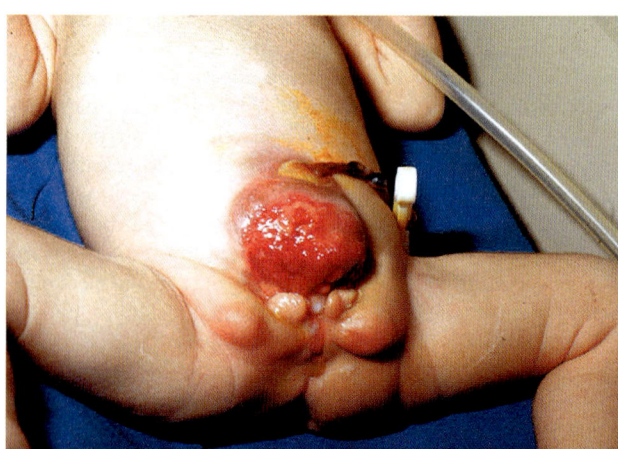

FIGURE 27.13 Bladder exstrophy in a neonate. Note the open anterior abdominal wall, protuberant bladder, distorted genitalia, and splayed hips.

confirmed at birth when the anterior abdominal wall defect with the exposed bladder mucosa is evident (Fig. 27.13).

Therapy is aimed at the surgical reconstruction of the bladder with preservation of renal function while achieving urinary continence and satisfactory appearance of the external genitalia.[347,351,352] In a select group of infants, surgical management may be carried out as a single-stage procedure[353]; however, the majority require a staged surgical repair directed at the closure of the bladder, posterior urethra, and abdominal wall.[354] In addition, a bilateral iliac osteotomy may be performed to facilitate surgical closure, decrease the stress on the midline soft tissues, and reduce the risk of postoperative wound dehiscence.

Wound dehiscence, bladder prolapse, and multiple attempts at bladder closure are among the risk factors for decreased bladder growth and the inability for the later development of continence.[355] In addition to the immediate postoperative complications, children who have undergone surgical repair of bladder exstrophy carry an increased risk for the development of renal, bladder, and colon adenocarcinoma.[356] Children who require frequent bladder catheterizations or repeat surgeries are at risk of developing latex allergy if latex products are used[96]; however, today bladder catheters are manufactured latex-free.

Surgical management of the epispadias is usually performed at 6 to 12 months of age, and reconstruction of the bladder neck by 5 years, the latter to allow for bladder training.[354] After the initial surgical repair, children are immobilized for 4 to 6 weeks,[357] with a successful outcome likely when a modified Buck traction with an external fixator or a modified Bryant traction[358] and adequate postoperative analgesia is used.[359]

The preoperative assessment should evaluate the presence and severity of all congenital anomalies, particularly cardiac abnormalities. Signs or symptoms of renal insufficiency and electrolyte imbalance may be present. If the child has renal insufficiency, the dose and frequency of administration of potentially nephrotoxic drugs, as well as the commonly used anesthetic drugs, must be carefully evaluated. Typically, surgery is performed with the child in the supine and lithotomy positions. The duration of surgery is often prolonged, requiring alternating urologic and orthopedic teams for their respective segment of the surgery, and repositioning the child depending on the stage of the surgery, thus requiring judicious management of fluids, blood loss, and temperature control. It is essential to communicate with the surgical teams to ensure an optimal perioperative strategy for balanced salt solutions, colloids, and blood products; a preoperative plan for multimodal perioperative pain management and anticipation of possible postoperative ventilatory support is essential.[354] After applying the standard monitors, anesthesia may be induced either by inhalation or IV; after induction, at least one large-bore peripheral IV line should be placed. A second IV line may be placed, or a central venous catheter and possibly an arterial catheter. In general, if blood loss occurs, it is slow and steady, but if posterior iliac osteotomies are performed, the blood loss may become brisk, requiring aggressive fluid resuscitation and administration of blood products. Beat-to-beat variability of arterial blood pressure and serial laboratory evaluations are valuable during goal-directed resuscitation. Appropriate padding, a fluid warmer, and a forced-air heating system should be standard. The anesthetic prescription varies with the age of the child and whether the surgery is completed in a single or staged repair. Postoperatively, children are transferred directly to the pediatric intensive care unit for recovery.

A general anesthetic in combination with an epidural or caudal continuous infusion technique is often used if there are no associated spine abnormalities, and if the catheter can be positioned out of the surgical field.[360] Maintenance of anesthesia may be achieved using either an inhalation or TIVA anesthetic combined with a caudal/lumbar epidural using intermittent boluses (0.5 to 1 mL/kg) or continuous infusions of bupivacaine (0.125% to 0.25%) or ropivacaine (0.2%). A protocol using regional anesthesia with sedation (dexmedetomidine and remifentanil) has been advocated to address concerns about apoptosis after inhalational anesthesia by some clinicians, although whether such an approach is superior to sevoflurane anesthesia remains unclear.[361,362] Caudal or epidural analgesia may be provided by advancing the catheter to the appropriate surgical dermatomal level after induction of anesthesia. In neonates, epidural infusions of bupivacaine (0.2 mg/kg per hour) provide excellent analgesia although total blood concentrations of bupivacaine steadily increase by 2 days (see later text). The catheter is either secured directly to the skin or tunneled using the epidural insertion needle[363]; a continuous infusion of a local anesthetic may be maintained for several days to provide analgesia and a mild motor blockade that favors immobility. However, care must be taken to avoid systemic toxicity. Neonates are at increased risk for developing local anesthetic toxicity because of their low serum protein concentration and immature metabolism. Albumin and α1-acid glycoprotein are reduced in this age group,[364] which may increase unbound bupivacaine and ropivacaine concentrations. However, the situation is confusing because AAG is a reactive protein that increases after surgery.[365–367] Further, it is unbound drug that is cleared, not bound and the two forms are in equilibrium. While total concentration increase after surgery as a result of AAG increases, unbound concentrations may increase because of immature clearance, increasing the risk of cardiac and neurologic toxicity.[368,369] It is for this reason that the upper limit of infusion of bupivacaine or ropivacaine is limited to 0.2 mg/kg per hour (for 48 hours), which is half that used in children older than 6 months, to minimize the risk of local anesthetic toxicity.[370–372] Unfortunately, (free, unbound) serum bupivacaine concentrations are rarely monitored and so that concentration in neonates with immature clearance remains poorly described. Lidocaine 0.1% (0.8 mg/kg per hour) is another option, but that drug is also bound to AAG. Chloroprocaine may be preferable (see also Chapters 40 and 41) because it is cleared by plasma esterases that are mature at birth.

The outcome of this complex surgery is determined primarily by surgical expertise. Urologic incontinence, bladder prolapse, and epispadias revisions require additional urologic surgery. Renal function is usually well maintained throughout; complications of complete repair are reported to be similar to those of the staged repair but usually involve additional soft tissue defects.[373]

Bariatric Surgery in Children

Obesity has become a major threat to public health worldwide.[374] The prevalence of pediatric obesity has increased exponentially, affecting every country over the past few decades. In the United States, the incidence of obesity in children 2 to 19 years old has increased from ~7% in 1980 to ~20% in 2020[375]; one-third of US children are either obese (BMI ≥95th percentile) or overweight (BMI between the 85th and 95th percentiles).[376,377] The causes of obesity are multifactorial: excess caloric intake, poor nutritional choices, and lack of exercise. However, evidence suggests that obese children are obese before the age of 5 years and that the underlying causes may have their provenance in early infancy and childhood.[378] Furthermore, the serious complications from obesity, for example, arterial hypertension, cardiovascular disease, fatty liver, diabetes, asthma, and obstructive sleep apnea (OSA), are recognized earlier in childhood,[379] often serving as precursors for gross and intractable obesity in adulthood.[380] A systematic review has reported an increase in medical/surgical complications in hospitalized obese children.[381] Thus, the societal burden of obesity is enormous (estimated at $147 billion dollars in yearly health care costs)[382] and is mainly driven by several associated comorbidities (e.g., diabetes, hypertension, sleep apnea, and depression). If left untreated, obesity may result in earlier mortality.[383,384]

The degree of obesity can be quantified using several metrics, the most common being the body mass index (BMI), defined as the weight (in kilograms) divided by the height squared (in meters squared). In adults, the degree of obesity can be defined by single BMI values (Table 27.2). However, in children, the degree of obesity is more difficult to quantify because BMI and other indexes of growth increase nonlinearly with age and gender. As a result, clinicians now define the degree of obesity in children based on growth charts for weight-dependent age and gender (Table 27.2).

To address these worrying statistics, bariatric surgery has emerged as one means to help the most extreme cases of adolescent obesity, especially those who are motivated toward weight loss and are psychologically prepared.[382,385,386] Bariatric surgery is designed to either bypass part of the small bowel to reduce caloric absorption (Roux-en-Y procedure) or to minimize the size of the stomach (laparoscopic vertical sleeve gastrectomy). The latter approach has replaced the more complex Roux-en-Y gastric bypass surgery as the most commonly performed surgical procedure for obesity in the United States.[387] These surgeries have proven to be safe, cost-effective means of achieving permanent weight loss and providing partial resolution of comorbidities, especially diabetes in adolescents.[388–391]

MULTIDISCIPLINARY APPROACH TO BARIATRIC SURGERY IN ADOLESCENTS

Developing a successful approach to bariatric surgery in children requires a multidisciplinary team with collaboration from many pediatric subspecialists, including bariatric surgeons, anesthesiologists, endocrinologists, gastroenterologists, cardiologists, pulmonologists, psychologists, dietitians, and others.[385,392,393] Only children who are motivated to lose weight and who exhibit a positive psychological approach to this intensive process should be admitted to these programs.

TABLE 27.2	Obesity Indexes in Adults and Children	
Classification of Obesity	Adult (BMI)	Children (Percentile on BMI Growth Chart)
Normal weight	18.5–24.9	5–85
Overweight	25–29.9	85–95
Obesity	30–39.9	>95
Severe obesity	≥40	>120% of the 95th percentile

Based on https://www.cdc.gov/obesity/basics/index.html and Pan L, Blanck HM, Sherry B, Dalenius K, Grummer-Strawn LM. Trends in the prevalence of extreme obesity among US preschool-aged children living in low-income families, 1998–2010. *JAMA.* 2012:308(24);2563-2565.[468]

ANESTHETIC IMPLICATIONS OF OBESITY IN ADOLESCENTS

Organ Dysfunction

Obesity is associated with several organ disorders including cardiovascular disease (hypertension, dyslipidemias),[394] respiratory (asthma and OSA),[395,396] renal dysfunction,[397] endocrinopathies (diabetes, metabolic syndrome), liver dysfunction (nonalcoholic fatty liver disease and nonalcoholic steatohepatitis).[398,399] Childhood obesity is associated with early pathologic cardiovascular changes. Hypertension, previously seen most frequently in children with renal disease, is increasingly identified in obese children. The risk of hypertension in obese children is 3-fold greater than non-obese children and increases as BMI increases. Cardiac risk factors in obese children as young as 5 years of age have been described, including hypercholesterolemia, hypertension, and hyperinsulinemia. Left ventricular hypertrophy has been identified in obese children as young as 10 years of age and is common in adolescents presenting for bariatric surgery. Research is underway to determine if changes in cardiac architecture and function are reversible with weight loss.

Preoperative Preparation

Preoperative preparation for bariatric surgery is an involved and prolonged process. A thorough preoperative review and investigation of multiple organ systems are warranted before proceeding with anesthesia. Once screening is complete, the children must be educated about appropriate nutritional and attitudinal principles for achieving and maintaining weight loss. The recent approval of glucagon-like peptides (GLP-1) agonists, originally approved for the treatment of type II diabetes, for weight loss in adolescents in the United States are associated with gastrointestinal adverse effects including nausea, vomiting, and delayed gastric emptying.[400] This raises the specter of an increased risk of regurgitation and aspiration at induction of anesthesia: a 10-fold greater risk of residual food in the stomach after a 12-hour fast in adult diabetics taking GLP-1 medications compared with matched diabetics not taking GLP-1 medications (5.4 vs. 0.49%, respectively).[400,401] These drugs were originally designed as a second line treatment for type II diabetes mellitus after metformin and other oral hypoglycemics, acting as incretins to stimulate beta cells to release circulating insulin and to antagonize glucagon secretion to limit hepatic gluconeogenesis. There are several groups of GLP-1 drugs available: exenatide (subcutaneous administration, $T_{1/2}$ 3 hours), semaglutide (subcutaneous or oral, $T_{1/2}$ 7 days), liraglutide (subcutaneous $T_{1/2}$ 12.5 hours), and dulaglutide (subcutaneous, $T_{1/2}$ 4.5 hours).[402] Currently, these drugs are in great demand because in addition to their effectiveness in controlling diabetes, they can cause rapid weight loss.[403–405] The semaglutides may be administered subcutaneously, either daily or weekly, with those given less frequently preferred by most patients. Oral formulations are also available. The mechanism of action of these drugs to reduce weight is incompletely understood; it is likely that weight loss occurs via mechanisms other than just delayed gastric emptying.[406,407] Consequently, this effect may critically impact how we manage the airway during general anesthesia as several cases of gastric regurgitation and aspiration have been reported at induction of anesthesia in patients taking this class of medications.[408–410] Currently, there is no evidence of the onset and severity of the delayed gastric emptying in patients taking a GLP-1 nor has evidence been forthcoming about when normal gastric emptying resumes after the GLP-1 drug has been stopped. It is possible that gastric ultrasound may be used to determine whether residual solid food is present in the stomach preoperatively. Delayed gastric emptying occurs in obese patients especially those with GERD, those with diabetes and those who are critically ill, which may be further exacerbated by GLP-1 medications.[411] Without an ultrasound assessment, patients who take a GLP-1 medication and who fast overnight and longer, even in the absence of GERD or diabetes, may present with residual food in the stomach at induction of anesthesia and an increase in the risk of regurgitation and aspiration.[408–410] As a result, an increasing number of anesthesiologists intubate the trachea with an RSI when general anesthesia is planned in patients taking GLP-1 medications.[411a]

After evaluating the major organ systems and optimizing organ dysfunction, a preoperative anesthetic interview should be completed. During this evaluation, the anesthesiologist should review the investigations and laboratory results, ensure compliance with all medications and interventions (e.g., continuous positive airway pressure [CPAP] device), and then describe the anesthetic process with the patient and family in detail. Although these children appear large, many are psychologically immature and very anxious. Anxiolytic premedication should be offered on the day of surgery. During the interview, the airway should be assessed (see later text) and if a difficult airway is identified, supplementary airway equipment should be immediately available. Children with CPAP devices should be advised to bring them on the day of surgery for possible use postoperatively. Routine fasting instructions and urine pregnancy testing for females who have reached menarche should be ordered or if complete, the results documented. If the child is unable to walk to the operating room, a wheelchair or stretcher rated for the child's weight should be used. The upper extremities should be examined for IV access as this may be difficult in obese patients[412]; ultrasound may be useful to establish venous access. In advance of undertaking bariatric surgery, appropriately sized operating room tables should be present. Operating room tables are rated for the patient's weight; for normal size patients, they may be rated for a maximum of 500 (227 kg) or 600 pounds (272 kg), and obese patients, 1000 (454 kg) or 1200 pounds (544 kg). In all cases, the children should be strapped to the table to prevent the child from rolling off the table. Unlocking the bed and shifting the tabletop while the patient is on the table may cause the table to tip, even if the child's weight is within the table rating. This is more likely to occur if the tabletop is shifted off-center, if the child is placed in reverse orientation, or if a strong force is applied in one direction to the table.[413]

Drug Dosing

Designing appropriate drug dosing in obese children requires an understanding of the scalars that may be used to estimate the correct dose.[414] Total body weight (TBW) consists of two compartments: fat-free mass and fat mass.[415] Loading dose is determined by volume of distribution. It is often assumed, but not proven, that the fat-free mass is the volume into which hydrophilic drugs tend to be distributed, whereas fat mass is the volume into which lipophilic drugs are distributed. Because most drugs have different lipophilic and hydrophilic properties, the distribution of each drug must be considered to define its dose. Unfortunately, few of the drugs used for anesthesia in obese children have been studied, thus limiting the evidence on which to base drug doses. Alternatively, dose may be limited by toxicity fears so that we grossly underdose drugs such as acetaminophen to the extent where therapeutic analgesic concentrations can never be achieved. This, despite an understanding that it is concentration, not dose that causes toxicity.[416,417]

The primary parameter that determines maintenance dose is clearance. The relationship between clearance and weight is curvilinear with a flattening of the curve as weight increases. Dose follows that trend with a decrease in dose (expressed as per kilogram) as weight increases. Most size scalers exemplify this pattern.[418] Recommendations for any size scaler are tempered by expert opinion that presumes dose in the obese child will be determined by better pharmacokinetic understanding[419–421] The best size scaler is possibly normal fat mass (NFM),[414] a scaler that is applicable to both lean and obese, useful for all ages, applicable to both loading and maintenance dose, accommodates each individual drug and differing fat mass proportions and is increasingly used in target controlled infusion pumps.[418]

Total body weight (TBW) is a poor size scaler and ideal body weight (IBW), which has a nonlinear relationship to clearance (i.e., rate of clearance increase slows as size increases), is currently the only alternative body weight scaler to total body weight[422] mentioned in the British National Formulary for Children.[423] Fat-free mass,[424] a measure similar to lean body mass,[425] may be considered the sum of the ideal body mass plus the additional mass required to support the physical and metabolic demands of the fat mass. The latter is derived primarily from an increased muscle mass as well as minor contributions from increased vessel-rich organ mass (heart, liver) and the fluid compartments. As the total body weight increases, the fat mass increases in proportion; fat-free mass increases up to a BMI of 40 kg/m^2 with a plateau thereafter.[426,427]

The ideal body weight of a child can be obtained from tables, graphs, or simple equations.[428] Sample equations include

$$IBW = 2 \times Age\,(years) + 9\ for\ children \leq 8\ years\ and$$
$$3 \times Age\,(years)\ for > 8\ years$$

The lean body weight may be estimated using a nomogram[428] or from a simple equation:

$$LBW = IBW + 0.3 \times (TBW - IBW)$$

Drugs used to induce anesthesia are distributed into the central compartment and throughout the vessel-rich group of organs (e.g., the brain). Even though these drugs are lipophilic, the induction dose is ideally based on the acute volume of distribution (V$_d$), which is more appropriately based on ideal body weight or lean body weight than total body weight.[429] Drugs used in anesthesia invariably conform to multicompartment models with drug movement between compartments and dose is further tempered by toxicity concerns.[430] Lean body weight might be a reasonable sized metric for the dose of propofol for induction of anesthesia,[431] but total body weight (with allometry) is better for maintenance/infusion (see also Chapter 5).[432] Current dosing recommendations remain, for the most part, based on empiric estimation.[433]

Other considerations in obesity include changes in plasma proteins, liver and renal functions, cytochrome enzyme activities,[434] cardiac output, and regional blood flow.[435] Obesity may compromise organ function (e.g., dexmedetomidine clearance is reduced in obese adults).[432] The pharmacokinetics of drugs in obesity depends on the physicochemical characteristics of the drugs. For the loading dose of drugs, if the Vd/TBW ratio is reduced in obesity, then the drug is not distributed to the fat mass and should be based on the lean body weight or ideal body weight.[426] In contrast, if the Vd/TBW ratio is unchanged or increased in obesity, then the drug is predominantly lipophilic and the dose should be based on total body weight.[436,437] For drugs administered for maintenance, the dose should be based on its clearance. All size scalers flatten in terms of the clearance-size relationship as weight increases.[415] Even total body weight, when used with allometry, demonstrates the same pattern. Recent target controlled pumps incorporate normal fat mass with allometry into their programs.[438-440] The use of cerebral function monitors (e.g., bispectral index in teenagers) greatly simplifies propofol infusion dosing by allowing titration of dose to a target effect.

Studies reporting the pharmacokinetics/dynamics of specific anesthetic drugs in obese children are limited.[433,441] Based on the best "available" data, a summary of the doses for induction or maintenance of anesthesia is presented in Table 27.3[442]; as more detailed evidence emerges, the basis for the dose of the drugs continues to evolve.

Inhalational anesthetic agents with low blood gas solubility are ideal in this setting although some advocate TIVA with a depth of anesthesia monitor.[443,444] Rapid induction and emergence from anesthesia can be achieved and facilitated in this population with agents of low solubility such as desflurane although that drug may be removed from the market for environmental reasons. Although that course is not imminent,[85,445] some individual institutions have already made the decision to no longer use the drug. The context-sensitive half-life of desflurane is superior to sevoflurane owing to lower solubility in blood and tissues; thus the former facilitates a more rapid recovery than the latter, particularly for surgeries longer than 2 hours when inhalation anesthetics accumulate in fat.[446] However, desflurane induces more bronchoconstriction than sevoflurane; thus in children with asthma or who smoke cigarettes, sevoflurane's bronchodilatory properties make it preferable to desflurane.

Airway management should take into consideration several basic principles. The presence of increased abdominal girth, shallow tidal volumes, and supine position predispose to rapid desaturation once anesthesia is induced. To preclude desaturation, patients should be preoxygenated in a reverse-Trendelenburg position of more than 25 degrees.[447] This provides an adequate reserve of oxygen during laryngoscopy and tracheal intubation, mitigating the risk of desaturation and attenuating atelectasis. To view the glottis aperture, the elevation of the head in the sniffing position should be doubled

(from a normal distance of ~7 cm) to ~14 centimeters. This may be achieved by combining the ramped position with the usual head elevation (7 cm).[448] The quintessential alignment that must be ensured to successfully visualize the larynx in obese children is that the tragus of the ear is at or above the level of the sternal notch in the sniffing position.[449] If the tragus is not elevated above the sternal notch, then the head must be propped up further. An RSI is not usually required in most obese children; those who have gastroesophageal reflux are controlled medically. Gastric fluid volume is increased in obesity, but the fluid pH is not decreased.[450] Therefore, the risk of pneumonitis should aspiration occur is no greater than in a nonobese patient.

Ventilation may be a challenge in obese children, particularly during laparoscopic surgery. The pulmonary challenges from laparoscopic surgery are compounded by the large abdominal girth compressing the basal lungs. Increased inspired oxygen concentration may prevent hemoglobin desaturation but may lead to absorption atelectasis. Optimal strategies for ventilation while avoiding barotrauma include low tidal volumes (6 to 8 mL/kg based on lean body weight, not total body weight), periodic alveolar recruitment maneuvers, PEEP (8 to 15 mm Hg), a respiratory rate to maintain normocapnia or permissive hypercapnia, particularly during pneumoperitoneum), and a sufficient inspired oxygen concentration to maintain an adequate saturation.[451-453] The ventilation mode has little bearing on the outcomes after anesthesia. At the end of surgery and after extubation, the child should be positioned in the semirecumbent position, administered oxygen by face mask, and monitored en route to the recovery room. Postoperative pain may be managed with either intermittent IV opioids or patient-controlled analgesia.

OSA is common in children who are morbidly obese, a more common finding in males and non-Hispanic Black and Hispanic populations.[454,455] Many use nightly CPAP devices, although obese adolescents exhibit poor compliance with these devices.[456] Given the known risks of OSA causing opioid sensitivity, opioids should be administered in reduced doses (one-third to one-half the usual doses).[457-459] Intermittent hypoxia commonly complicates the postoperative period. Hence, patients should bring their own CPAP or nasal CPAP devices to the hospital for postoperative use. Children may be discharged home after uncomplicated surgery on postoperative day 3.[460-462]

Drug dosing after gastric bypass surgery is poorly understood.[463,464] After gastric bypass surgery, whether Roux-en-Y or the more popular laparoscopic vertical sleeve gastrectomy surgery, rapid weight loss occurs. This often results in the resolution of many comorbidities associated with morbid obesity such as systemic hypertension, diabetes, and so on. However, failure to adjust drug dosing in parallel with the weight loss, reduced gastric residence time, reduced exposure to intestinal cytochrome enzymes (e.g., CYP3A4, increasing atorvastatin blood concentrations), and the resolution of the severity of the associated diseases may lead to relative drug overdoses and the associated consequences.[464] For example, after Roux-en-Y gastric surgery, approximately 50% of drugs taken orally have reduced area under the concentration-time curve, whereas 25% have unchanged and 25% have increased area under the concentration-time curves.[465] Oral morphine kinetics after Roux-en-Y showed dramatically increased blood concentrations within the first 2 weeks after surgery that persisted for at least 6 months.[466] The risks of an opioid overdose from the changes in pharmacokinetics not accounting for the effects of comorbidities may be substantial. In one meta-analysis, the range of postoperative to preoperative drug exposure

TABLE 27.3	Dosage of Intravenous Anesthetics in Obese Children	
Drug	**Induction Dose Based on**	**Maintenance Dose Based on**
Thiopenthal	LBW	
Propofol	LBW	TBW
Synthetic opioids (fentanyl, alfentanil, and sufentanil)	TBW	LBW
Morphine	IBW	IBW
Remifentanil	LBW	LBW
Nondepolarizing neuromuscular blockers	IBW	IBW
Succinylcholine	TBW	
Sugammadex	TBW	

IBW, Ideal body weight; *LBW*, lean body weight; *TBW*, total body weight.
Reproduced with permission. Mortensen A, Lenz K, Abildstrøm H, Lauritsen TL. Anesthetizing the obese child. *Paediatr. Anaesth.* 2011;21(6):623-629.[442]

ratio extended from a 10-fold greater ratio for penicillin to a 33% lower ratio for phenytoin and ampicillin.[464] The pharmacokinetics of midazolam after gastric bypass surgery in adults yielded similar bioavailability after oral dosing but greater clearance one year after bypass surgery.[467]

Currently, laparoscopic vertical sleeve gastrectomy surgery has eclipsed Roux-en-Y surgery in the United States in popularity, including in the adolescent age group. Laparoscopic vertical sleeve gastrectomy surgery is not associated with the same extent of gastric dumping as Roux-en-Y surgery, but gastric residence time and absorption with laparoscopic vertical sleeve gastrectomy are reduced. Until practice recommendations are forthcoming, it seems prudent to titrate all parenteral drugs to effect during the period of rapid weight loss in particular and to adjust the doses of all oral drugs using therapeutic drug monitoring and individual clinical responses.

Acknowledgments

The authors thank Steen W. Henneberg for his prior contributions to this chapter.

ANNOTATED REFERENCES

Alqahtani A, Elahmedi M, Al Qahtani AR. Laparoscopic sleeve gastrectomy in children younger than 14 years: refuting the concerns. *Ann Surg.* 2016;263(2):312-319.

This retrospective study compared the outcomes after laparoscopic sleeve gastrectomy in children younger than 14 years at the time of surgery with adolescents older than 14 years. The authors concluded that sleeve gastrectomy in children younger than 14 years is both safe and effective.

Kim PH, Patil MB, Kim SS, et al. Early comparison of nephrectomy options in children (open, transperitoneal laparoscopic, laparo-endoscopic single site [LESS], and robotic surgery). *BJU Int.* 2012;109:910-915.

This review provides comparative results of both laparoscopic techniques and robotic surgery in children.

Kobori T, Onishi Y, Yoshida Y, et al. Association of glucagon-like peptide-1 receptor agonist treatment with gastric residue in an esophagogastroduodenoscopy. *J Diabetes Invest.* 2023;14(6):767-773.

This case-controlled study of the residual gastric fluid measured via direct observation after a 12-hour fast in 205 diabetic adults taking a GLP-1 agonist matched with a cohort of the same size who were not taking a GLP-1 medication. The results demonstrated a 10-fold greater frequency of food in those taking GLP-1 medications (5.4%) than in those who were not taking GLP-1 medications (0.49%). This introduces an increased risk of regurgitation and aspiration at induction of anesthesia.

Mortensen A, Lenz K, Abildstrøm H, Lauritsen TLB. Anesthetizing the obese child. *Paediatr Anaesth.* 2011;21(6):623-629.

This review presents the epidemiology, pathophysiology, and pharmacology of drugs used in obese children who require anesthesia.

Morse J, Cortinez LI, Anderson BJ. Considerations for intravenous anaesthesia dose in obese children: understanding PKPD. *J Clin Med.* 2023;12(4):1642.

The authors explore size models used for drug dosing in children with obesity. The influence of fat mass on both volume (determining loading dose) and clearance (determining maintenance dose is discussed). The size scaler, normal fat mass, a versatile scaler that can be used in both obese and lean children is now increasingly programmed into intravenous anesthesia pumps. An understanding of how this size scaler is determined improves dosing prediction in obese children.

Narayanan H, Raistrick C, Pierce JMT, Shelton C. Carbon footprint of inhalational and total intravenous anaesthesia for paediatric anaesthesia: a modelling study. *Br J Anaesth.* 2022:129(2):231-243.

These authors assessed the carbon footprint of inhaled and TIVA anesthesia in infants and children using inhaled inductions with clinically relevant fresh gas flows and TIVA dosing based on age groups. The models revealed a reduced carbon footprint for pure TIVA compared with pure inhaled anesthetics up to 6 hours in duration. However, when TIVA is compared with an inhaled induction followed by a TIVA technique, the carbon footprint for the two techniques up to 4 to 6 hours was indistinguishable.

Neira VM, Kovesi T, Guerra L, et al. The impact of pneumoperitoneum and Trendelenburg positioning on respiratory system mechanics during laparoscopic pelvic surgery in children: a prospective observational study. *Can J Anaesth.* 2015;62(7):798-806.

The authors investigated the physiologic impact of 12 mm Hg pneumoperitoneum followed by 20-degree Trendelenburg positioning. They found that both dynamic compliance and tidal volume (normalized to weight) decreased after insufflation of the pneurmoperitoneum (by 42%) but decreased only 10% further after 20-degree Trendelenburg positioning. These changes could be offset by increasing the peak inspiratory pressures during pressure-controlled ventilation with PEEP in children undergoing laparoscopic surgery.

Phillip-Hohne C. Anaesthesia in the obese child. *Best Pract Res Clin Anaesthesiol.* 2011;25(1):53-60.

This review highlights the epidemiology of obesity in children, physiologic changes, and anesthetic considerations.

Walker RW, Ravi R, Haylett K. Effect of cricoid force on airway calibre in children: a bronchoscopic assessment. *Br J Anaesth.* 2010;104(1):71-74.

This investigation documents the magnitude of the external force required to distort the cricoid ring from infants until adolescents. In infants, force as little as 5 Newtons distorts the cricoid rings. The force required to distort the ring increases with age, reaching 15 to 25 N in adolescents.

A complete reference list can be found online at Elsevier eBooks+.

28

Essentials of Hepatology

JAMES E. SQUIRES, CAROL VETTERLY, AND DANIELA DAMIAN

Anatomy
Principles of Hepatic Drug Metabolism
Phase I Reactions
Cytochrome P-450 Activity
Phase II Reactions
Anesthetic Agents
Inhalation Anesthetic Metabolism
Neuromuscular Blocking Drugs
Sedatives, Opioids, and Liver Disease

Anesthetic Effects on Hepatic Cellular Functions
Carbohydrates
Protein Synthesis
Bilirubin Metabolism
Hepatotoxicity
Perioperative Considerations in Liver Disease

Anatomy

THE LIVER AND BILIARY TREE are derived from the endoderm of the dorsal foregut during the late third to the early fourth week of gestation. By the sixth week, the fetal liver primarily serves as a hematopoietic organ, and critical biologic functions such as glycolysis, bile acid synthesis, and metabolic waste processing are managed by the maternal liver through the fetoplacental circulation. Oxygenated blood is shunted from the placenta to the right atrium through the ductus venosus. Functional closure of the ductus begins immediately after birth, with complete functional closure occurring by 2 weeks of age in up to 95% of infants. Anatomic closure occurs shortly thereafter.

The functional development of the liver is reflected in the complex changes in hepatic enzyme efficiency and metabolic performance throughout gestation. In early gestation, the liver is the primary site of hematopoiesis. Hepatic hematopoiesis develops in utero at 5 to 6 weeks' gestation, followed closely by protein synthesis.[1] The ability to metabolize carbohydrates and lipids begins by 10 weeks' gestation, followed by the development of drug-metabolizing systems. Several patterns of hepatic enzyme development have been described that correlate with the needs of the developing fetus.[2]

The term neonate has a liver that weighs between 120 and 160 grams although it remains structurally and physiologically immature. Peripheral branches of the intrahepatic biliary system require an additional 4 to 8 weeks before they can be identified histologically. The liver is composed of eight structurally independent segments, each with a feeding hepatic artery, portal vein, draining hepatic vein, and bile duct. Segment 1 is the caudate lobe. Segments 2 and 3 form the left lateral segment, and with segment 4, the left lobe of the liver is defined. Segments 5, 6, 7, and 8 constitute the right lobe of the liver.

The liver receives blood from two sources: the portal vein that drains the spleen and intestine, and the hepatic artery that provides systemic oxygenated blood directly to biliary epithelium and to the hepatic sinusoids. The portal vein accounts for approximately 70% of the blood flow to the liver. In the hepatic sinusoids, the hepatic arterial and portal venous blood mix and intercalate among hepatocytes, fenestrated sinusoidal cells, and a host of resident immune cells (e.g., Kupffer cells). Sinusoids drain into terminal hepatic venules, which eventually coalesce to form the left and right hepatic veins. The veins merge into the inferior vena cava immediately before entering the right atrium. At any given time, the liver contains approximately 13% of the circulating blood volume.

During the neonatal period, liver function is immature and its ability to metabolize and clear most xenobiotics is poor. Factors that affect the clearance of medications include both hepatic blood flow and the developmental status of hepatic transport and enzyme systems. Size alone does not account for this observed degree of immaturity, because the fetal and neonatal liver account for a greater percentage of body weight than the adult counterpart (3.6% of body weight vs. 2.4% in adults).[3] The neonatal liver contains approximately 20% fewer hepatocytes than the adult liver, and the cells are almost one-half the size of adult hepatocytes. These structural features may play some role in the functional deficiencies exhibited by infant livers. Cellular growth and hypertrophy of the liver continue at a rapid pace into young adulthood.

The structural unit of the liver parenchyma is the lobule, a hub-and-spoke structure with the central vein serving as the hub that is bordered by portal tracts, which contain a bile duct and tributaries of the portal vein and hepatic artery. The mixed venous and arterial blood flows from the portal triad to the central vein; bile flows in the opposite direction through a canalicular matrix that then enters the bile ductule in the portal tract. The functional unit of the liver is the hepatic acinus, which is centered on the portal track and extends in three concentric zones (i.e., zones of Rappaport) outward to the central vein (Fig. 28.1). The more central zones (zones 1 and 2) are most active in oxidative processes, whereas the distal zone 3, which is closer to the central vein, depends on glycolysis and is more susceptible to ischemic and toxic injury.

The liver has the greatest regenerative capacity of any organ in the body. Only half of the original liver mass is required for the organ to regenerate back to full size. Although an acutely damaged liver can regenerate to an equivalent size and weight to that before the injury, chronic disease with loss of hepatocytes often

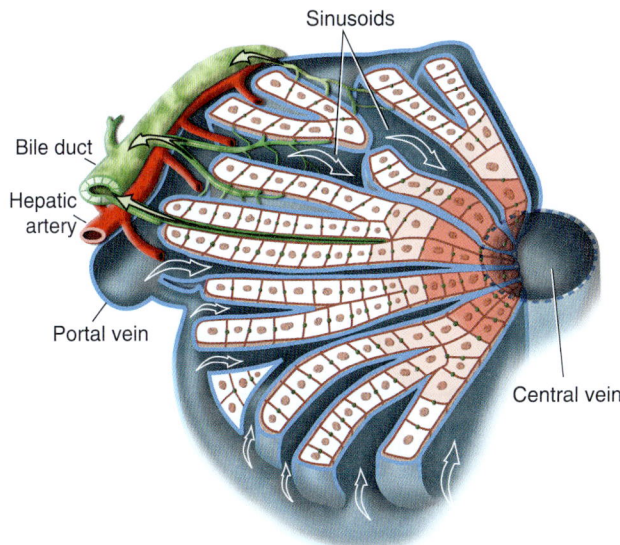

FIGURE 28.1 Blood flows from the hepatic arteries and portal vein along sinusoids toward the central vein. The hepatic triad consists of the bile duct, a branch of the portal vein, and the hepatic artery, with zone 1 *(white)* surrounding the triad, followed by zone 2 *(pink)*, and zone 3 *(red)*. Cytochrome P-450 expression is higher in zone 3 with more extensive drug metabolism. (From Oinonen T, Lindros KO. Zonation of hepatic cytochrome P-450 expression and regulation. *Biochem J.* 1998;329:17-35.)

has adverse consequences, including fibrosis, cirrhosis, and liver neoplasia.[4] This regenerative capacity after acute injury is recognized in Greek mythology. Prometheus angered the Gods by stealing fire and giving it to humans. Punishment involved having his liver eaten by birds of prey (eagles) by day and hepatic regeneration by night.

Principles of Hepatic Drug Metabolism

Lipid solubility, an important and desired feature of many anesthesia drugs, facilitates passive diffusion across cellular membranes. Lipophilic drugs are also difficult to excrete. They have a propensity to accumulate in the body's fat stores and then slowly recirculate from deep compartments back into plasma. Renal and biliary excretion of lipid-soluble compounds can be resorbed across their respective membranes. A major role of the liver is to transform lipid-soluble drugs into water-soluble compounds that become easily excreted metabolites. An interesting example of the need for this biotransformation is the anesthetic compound thiopental, which if it were not transformed into its less lipophilic counterpart, would have a plasma half-life of approximately 25 years.[1]

The primary family of liver enzymes assigned the task of metabolizing these exogenous substances is the cytochrome P-450 (CYP) family. *P* designates a red *pigment*, which is related to a heme molecule and absorbs light at a wavelength of 450 nm.[5] The primary reactions involved in the drug biotransformation and metabolism are hydroxylation and conjugation. Hydroxylation (i.e., a phase I reaction) prepares the metabolite for conjugation (i.e., phase II reaction). The CYP family of enzymes is responsible for most phase I reactions, and the members were first thought to be chemically similar to mitochondrial cytochromes (see Chapters 4 and 5).

PHASE I REACTIONS

The CYP enzymes likely evolved as a mechanism by which the host was able to protect itself from toxins ingested from the environment. Most enzymes involved in hepatic drug metabolism are categorized in three distinct families: CYP1, CYP2, and CYP3. Each family is further divided into subfamilies that are designated with capital letters and numbered in the order in which they were discovered. The CYP enzymes are generally conserved across species, but their regulation and catalytic activity vary among species, which highlights the challenges associated with laboratory analysis of drug metabolism.[5]

Genetic and nongenetic factors contribute to the variability in the enzymatic activity across all CYP enzymes.[6,7] Genetic factors that impact the variability include specific polymorphisms, gene expression regulation, and sex (see Chapter 4).[8,9] For example, approximately 5% of White populations lack CYP2D6 activity, which is associated with altered metabolism of ~15% of drugs.[10] A deficiency of CYP2D6 activity enhances the effect of some drugs such as haloperidol and metoprolol that require the enzyme for efficient metabolism, and decreases the effect of others such as codeine, which depends on CYP2D6 activity to convert it to morphine, the active analgesic metabolite of codeine.[11-13] Conversely a duplication of CYP2D6 enzymes or a polymorphism with increased 2D6 activity may cause a relative overdose of morphine from converting a greater fraction of codeine to morphine.[14,15] Furthermore, ethnicity has emerged as another important factor that contributes to the variability in CYP pharmacokinetics with differences appreciated between cohorts comprised of different races (see Chapter 4).[8,11-13]

Nongenetic factors that influence CYP activity include concomitant disease states, malnutrition,[16] and exposure to a host of pharmacologic and naturally occurring compounds.[9] Many drugs can inhibit or stimulate the enzyme system (Table 28.1).[17,18] There are several mechanisms of inhibition of the CYP enzyme system. One type occurs when drugs compete for the same enzyme and can be competitive or noncompetitive and may be reversible. Others can be mechanism-based inhibition, which may be irreversible.[19] The degree to which this competition becomes clinically important depends on five factors: (1) the relative amount of the specific CYP enzyme, (2) the concentrations of each drug, (3) the degree of pharmacologically active metabolite generated through this system, (4) the importance of the enzyme in elimination of the drugs, and (5) the therapeutic index of the drug.[5]

An example of strong inhibition of CYP3A is that of the protease inhibitor, ritonavir. The drug is used to manage the human immunovirus and is currently part of an oral antiviral drug combination (nirmatrelvir-ritonavir) treatment for the early treatment of COVID-19–positive patients aged 12 years and over who have recognized comorbidities. The CYP3A enzyme system is responsible for clearance of numerous drugs used in anesthesia (e.g., alfentanil, fentanyl, methadone, rocuronium, bupivacaine, midazolam, ketamine). Ritonavir impacts drug clearances that are influenced by the ritonavir plasma concentration, anesthesia drug intrinsic hepatic clearance, metabolic pathways, concentration-response relationship, and route of administration. Drugs with a steep concentration-response relationship (ketamine, midazolam, rocuronium) are mostly affected because small changes in concentration have major changes in the effect response. An increase in midazolam concentration is observed after oral administration because CYP3A

TABLE 28.1	Major Human Liver Cytochrome P-450s		
P-450	**Substrate**	**Inhibitors**	**Inducers**
CYP1A2	Caffeine	Ciprofloxacin	Carbamazepine
	Clozapine	Fluvoxamine	Rifampin
	Olanzapine		Tobacco smoke
	Theophylline		
	Propofol (minor)		
CYP2A6	Nicotine		Phenobarbital
	Propofol (minor)		(weak)
CYP2C8	Rosiglitazone	Clopidogrel	Rifampin
	Paclitaxel		
CYP2B6	Methadone		
CYP2C9	Diclofenac	Fluconazole	Carbamazepine
	Ibuprofen		(weak)
	Warfarin		Secobarbital
	Fosphenytoin		(weak)
			Rifampin
CYP2C19	Omeprazole	Fluvoxamine	Rifampin
	Propofol (minor)	Ketoconazole	
	Fosphenytoin	Fluconazole	
CYP2D6	Codeine	Fluoxetine	
	Chlorpromazine	Quinidine	
	(minor)	Methadone	
	Dextromethorphan	(weak)	
	Haloperidol		
	Metoprolol		
	Propofol (minor)		
CYP2E1	Acetaminophen	Isoniazid	Ethanol (weak)
	Halothane		Isoniazid (weak)
CYP3A4	Ketamine	Diltiazem	Carbamazepine
	Midazolam	Erythromycin	Phenobarbital
	Indinavir	Grapefruit juice	Phenytoin
	Lovastatin	Ketoconazole	Rifampin
	Methadone	Ritonavir	
	Nifedipine	Voriconazole	
	Tacrolimus	Propofol (weak)	

Adapted from Watkins PB. The role of cytochrome P450s in drug-induced liver disease. In: Kaplowitz N, Deleve LD, eds. *Drug-Induced Liver Disease*. New York: Marcel Dekker; 2003:15-33.

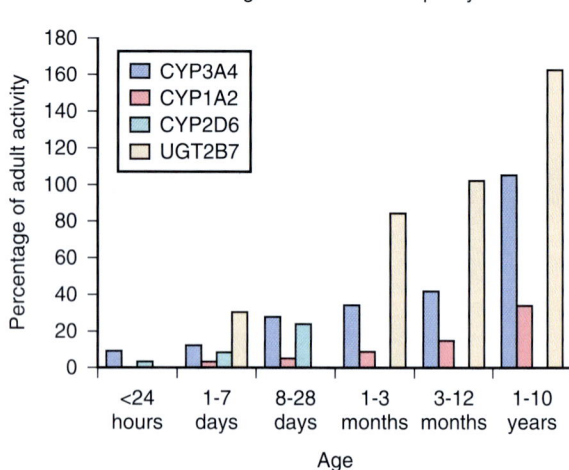

Changes in Metabolic Capacity

FIGURE 28.2 Changes in metabolic capacity versus percentage of adult activity. (Modified from Kearns G, Abdel-Rahman SM, Alander SW, et al. Developmental pharmacology—drug disposition, action, and therapy in infants and children. *N Engl J Med.* 2003;349:1157-1167.)

metabolism of xenobiotics. The three identified isoforms are CYP3A4, CYP3A5, and CYP3A7. CYP3A4 is the most abundant single enzyme in the human liver, accounting for the metabolism of approximately 50% of clinically used pharmaceuticals.[23] CYP3A5 is more commonly found in the kidneys and lungs and to a lesser degree in the liver. CYP3A7 is the predominant isoform in the neonatal liver but is replaced after birth by CYP3A4. Given its critical involvement in hepatic biotransformation of xenobiotics, the CYP3A4 family of enzymes is used to study estimated hepatic drug clearance in various age and gender groups.

Changes in the distribution and activity of the CYP enzyme systems occur with hepatic growth and maturation (Fig. 28.2). The CYP3A family is homogeneously distributed across the liver parenchyma in the fetal liver and shortly after birth. However, during postnatal growth, expression of the CYP3A protein shifts toward the periportal region of the acinus (i.e., Rappaport zone 1). By adulthood, expression of CYP2A becomes increasingly limited to the zone 1 and zone 2 hepatocytes, with sparse expression occurring in zone 3.[24] Other examples of developmental changes in the CYP system include the CYP2C and CYP3A3/4 subfamilies, which have negligible expression in the first few weeks of life.[25,26] CYP2D6 reaches adult activity levels within 1 month chronological age; variability thereafter is determined primarily by genetic polymorphisms.[27] Additionally, patterns of CYP enzyme expression can be altered in disease states such as cancer.[28]

Changes in activity of CYP enzyme families and subfamilies have correlated with drug clearance. For example, midazolam clearance correlates with changes in CYP3A4 activity, with decreased clearance in fetal neonatal livers, and adult clearance rates achieved by 3 months of age.[29,30] In contrast, CYP3A7 activity peaks at about 1 week postpartum and steadily diminishes during the first year of life, reaching approximately 10% of fetal liver activity by adulthood. Clearance of methadone (a drug metabolized by the CYP3A system) in neonates is similar to that in adults as a consequence of these changing CYP3A4/CYP3A7 ratios with age.[31] Advances in our understanding of CYP ontogeny have improved the integration of physiologic, developmental, and physiochemical knowledge to

in the gastrointestinal wall is inhibited, causing a large increase in relative bioavailability.[20]

Enhanced CYP expression occurs after amplified transcription of the specific gene that is induced by a variety of compounds. For example, rifampin and phenytoin induce CYP3A4 by binding the cytosolic human pregnenolone-X-receptor (hPXR) or the steroid and xenobiotic receptor (SXR).[21] The activated receptor translocates into the nucleus, where it binds the regulator elements of the CYP3A4 gene and promotes increased transcription of CYP3A4, which can lead to toxic concentrations of intermediate compounds, as is the case with erythromycin, or to subtherapeutic concentrations of cyclosporine in transplant recipients.[22]

CYTOCHROME P-450 ACTIVITY

The superfamily of CYP enzymes is divided into subfamilies based on sequence homology and on demonstration of broad substrate specificities. An important example is the CYP3A subfamily, which is the most abundant group of cytochromes involved in the design more accurate pharmacokinetic modeling systems and guide optimal dosing regimens for children.[14,32]

PHASE II REACTIONS

Conjugation of lipophilic compounds increases their water solubility to facilitate renal excretion.[33] Conjugation reactions (i.e., glucuronidation, sulfation, glutathione conjugation, acetylation, and methylation) in infants are generally decreased compared with those in adults.[34]

Glucuronidation is catalyzed by uridine 5′-diphosphate (UDP)–glucuronosyltransferase (UGT) family of enzymes, which are derived from assimilation of proteins from separate genes or alternate splicing from single-gene transcripts.[35] UGT enzymes are responsible for the metabolism of several drugs, including phenols, estrogens, and opioids (see Chapters 4 and 5).[36] As with the CYP enzymes, individual UGT enzymes demonstrate substrate specificity and can act in concert to metabolize single compounds. Glucuronidation is not fully active in neonates because of decreased mRNA transcript production.[37] As such, this population is at risk for toxic drug accumulation (e.g., chloramphenicol causing gray baby syndrome).[38] Hepatic UGT enzyme concentrations are reduced during fetal and early postnatal development. At 3 months of age, the levels of many UGTs are 25% of those in adults.[39]

UGT1A enzyme activity, which is involved in the conjugation of bilirubin and ethinylestradiol, is decreased in the fetus, but it increases to adult rates within 3 to 6 months after a term delivery.[40] UGT1A6, which conjugates acetaminophen and naproxen, has 10% of adult activity in the fetus and neonate, and it achieves only 50% of adult activity by 6 months of age.[34] UGT2B7 is active in the metabolism of the nonsteroidal antiinflammatory drugs (NSAIDs), naloxone, morphine, and lorazepam. Fetal activity of this enzyme approaches 10% to 20% of adult levels, with a rapid increase to adult activity levels by 2 months of age.[41]

Sulfation is accomplished by sulfotransferases, a family of cytosolic enzymes that are divided into two categories: catechol and phenol sulfotransferase. These enzymes conjugate inorganic sulfate from 3′-phosphoadenosine-5′-sulfophosphate (PAPS) with compounds containing functional hydroxyl groups. The catechol transferases develop earlier in fetal life than the phenol counterparts and appear to exhibit decreased activity in the developing neonate. Although specific sulfotransferase substrates require identification, the activity of these enzymes is increased in fetuses and neonates compared with that in adults and is considered to be an efficient conjugation pathway in this age group. Interestingly, with the obesity epidemic, UDP-UGT and sulfotransferase expression and function are altered in patients with nonalcoholic fatty liver disease.[42]

Glutathione S-transferases (GST) conjugate glutathione with a broad spectrum of lipophilic and electrophilic compounds. The GST family is composed of up to five different groups in various classes designated μ, α, θ, σ, and π, which are derived from at least three genetic loci.[43] Tissue-specific expression of these enzymes has been demonstrated, with the liver expressing the greatest amount of protein. Variable time-dependent expression has also been shown, with α- and π-class GSTs having enhanced expression between 16 and 24 weeks gestation, whereas only the α-class enzymes predominate in the neonate and adult liver.[44] The hepatic π-class enzymes disappear from their hepatocellular location by 6 months of age and can be found only in the epithelial cells of the biliary canaliculi. Variations in the

developmental expression of this class of enzymes have made it challenging to fully appreciate what is likely a multitude of clinical interactions.[44]

Acetylation reactions are catalyzed by N-acetyltransferases (NAT) that transfer an acetyl group from acetyl coenzyme A to a variety of substrates (e.g., p-aminobenzoic acid, p-aminosalicylic acid, procainamide). Two genes, NAT1 and NAT2, are responsible for yielding two specific enzymes with different allelic forms. Despite having 87% sequence homology, these enzymes exhibit different substrate specificities.[45] Both are cytosolic enzymes involved in the biotransformation of several drugs and the bioactivation of several human carcinogens. NAT1 is present in multiple fetal and postnatal tissues and accounts for the most N-acetyltransferase substrate metabolism in children younger than 1 year of age. NAT2 is located primarily in the liver and becomes the dominant acetylator after 1 year of age. NAT2 has polymorphisms with enzyme kinetics that differentiate patients with slow or rapid acetylation capabilities. Infants younger than 1 year of age usually are slow acetylators; subsequent age-dependent alterations lead an individual's targeted acetylator status.[46] Individuals who are genetically destined for rapid acetylation manifest this feature by 2 to 4 years of age.

Anesthetic Agents

INHALATION ANESTHETIC METABOLISM

Inhalational anesthetics are poorly metabolized, with 15% to 20% of halothane undergoing biotransformation. Although both oxidative and reductive pathways are involved, the primary pathway of metabolism of halothane is through oxidation to a reactive intermediate, trifluoroacetyl chloride,[47] which then undergoes glutathione conjugation.[48]

Isoflurane is metabolized by CYP2E1 to a limited extent (0.2%).[49] Isoflurane is excreted as inorganic fluoride and trifluoroacetic acid after oxidative metabolism in the liver.[50] Desflurane is the least metabolized (0.02%) of the volatile anesthetics, which is approximately 10% of the rate of isoflurane.[51] Both are metabolized in the liver along similar paths because the urinary metabolite for desflurane, trifluoroacetic acid, is the same as for isoflurane.

Only 2% to 5% of inhaled sevoflurane is metabolized in humans by means of the hepatic CYP2E1 enzyme, as occurs for the other ether anesthetics.[52] Oxidation of sevoflurane generates the intermediate formyl fluoride, a highly reactive species thought to generate liver protein adducts. Carbon dioxide and inorganic fluoride are released through this oxidative mechanism, and the final product is hexafluoroisopropanol, which undergoes glucuronide conjugation and is further excreted in the urine (see Chapter 5).[53]

NEUROMUSCULAR BLOCKING DRUGS

Neuromuscular blockade is achieved by depolarizing or nondepolarizing neuromuscular blocking drugs (NMBDs) (see Chapter 5). The only depolarizing agent still in use is short-acting suxamethonium (i.e., succinylcholine).[54] Succinylcholine is hydrolyzed completely by plasma cholinesterases, which are synthesized by the liver.[55] Enzyme activity varies with age and single nucleotide polymorphisms, but it is decreased in liver disease and has been used as a metric of liver prognosis.[56,57]

Nondepolarizing NMBDs are divided into aminosteroids (i.e., pancuronium, vecuronium, and rocuronium) and benzylisoquinolinium diesters (i.e., doxacurium, mivacurium, atracurium, and cisatracurium besylate). Renal and hepatic diseases affect their safety and efficacy.[58] Hepatic elimination depends on protein binding, hepatic blood flow, and drug extraction. The volume of drug distribution is increased in hepatic disease, leading to lower concentrations. In children with cholestatic liver disease, such as biliary atresia, uptake of these compounds by the liver is decreased, which reduces plasma elimination and prolongs their effects.[59,60] Approximately 75% of the administered dose is bound to plasma proteins, with most bound to albumin. Despite these problems, children with liver disease and a correspondingly low albumin concentration are at minimal risk for the adverse effects from this group of drugs.[61]

Rocuronium is an analog of vecuronium with a more rapid onset of action. Only 12% to 22% of rocuronium is cleared through the kidney.[62] In patients with hepatic disease, the volume of distribution of rocuronium increased by 33% compared with that in healthy controls,[63] and patients with cholestasis exhibit prolonged duration and a longer recovery index after repeated doses.[64] In patients undergoing liver transplantation, the clearance of rocuronium was only slightly reduced by the diseased native liver compared with the functioning allograft and healthy individuals.[65] Reduced infusion requirements of rocuronium during liver transplantation may indicate graft dysfunction.[66]

Although aminosteroid NMBDs may not possess drug-drug interactions directly related to the CYP-450 enzymes, clinically enhanced neuromuscular blocking effects may occur in combination with aminoglycosides, vancomycin, calcium channel blockers, ketorolac, protease inhibitors, and corticosteroids. Decreased neuromuscular blocking effects may result when combined with inducers, including carbamazepine and fosphenytoin; opioid interactions in combination with aminosteroid NMBDs are not reported.

Hepatic elimination of the benzyl isoquinolinium agents is poorly understood, but hepatic dysfunction does impact their effectiveness. Despite increased concentrations in biliary secretions, the pharmacokinetics of doxacurium are unchanged in the presence of hepatocellular injury, but recovery indexes are prolonged.[67] Although no longer available in the United States, mivacurium is a mixture of three stereoisomers. Clearance of the *trans-trans* and *cis-trans* isomers is reduced in patients with liver disease,[68] whereas clearance of the *cis-cis* isomer is unchanged. Prolonged recovery occurs as a result of a decrease in plasma cholinesterases in significant liver disease.[68] Clearance of cisatracurium is decreased, although patients with liver disease experience no delay in recovery and minimal delay in onset of action. Children with liver disease, regardless of cause, usually tolerate this class of compounds, and there is no observed toxicity.[69]

SEDATIVES, OPIOIDS, AND LIVER DISEASE

The commonly used sedatives midazolam, propofol, and ketamine undergo hepatic metabolism through oxidation and conjugation. These compounds are all lipid soluble, and their effects are altered by liver disease.[70] Midazolam has an extraction ratio of 0.3 to 0.5 and depends on both hepatic blood flow and intrinsic clearance. Midazolam may have an increased clearance rate if hepatic blood flow is increased. In children with cirrhosis, the clearance of midazolam is halved with a corresponding doubling of the half-life compared with that in healthy controls.[71,72] With 95% to 97% of midazolam bound to albumin, diseases that decrease the concentration of albumin dramatically increase

the free fraction of drug, which leads to a greater effect from the unbound drug.[38,73,74] Propofol has high intrinsic clearance and blood flow changes determine clearance. Although clearance is through a combination of both UGT and CYP enzymes (CYP2B6, 2C9, 2A6), hepatocellular injury does not alter its pharmacokinetics.[75] Ketamine is also highly lipophilic and undergoes metabolism in the liver. However, unlike the other drugs described, it does so through methylation, and its clearance is minimally affected by liver dysfunction.[76]

Clinical effects from opioids result from their binding to opioid receptors. A greater plasma concentration of opioid binds a greater number of receptors, resulting in a correspondingly greater opioid effect. Hepatic clearance and protein binding govern the serum concentration of an opioid.[77] Most opioids are oxidized in the liver. However, morphine and buprenorphine undergo glucuronidation, and remifentanil is metabolized by plasma and tissue esterases that are mature in term neonates. The ability of the diseased liver to oxidize opioids is diminished, leading to increased oral bioavailability owing to decreased first-pass metabolism and decreased drug clearance. The clearance of morphine, despite being metabolized by glucuronidation, is also negatively affected by the presence of cirrhosis.[78]

The clearance of drugs that are highly extracted by the liver, such as meperidine and morphine, depends on hepatic blood flow (i.e., perfusion limited clearance).[79] Hepatic clearance (CL_H) is a function of hepatic blood flow (Q_H) and the extraction ratio (ER), describing the ability of the liver to efficiently remove the drug from the circulation:

$$CL_H = Q_H \times ER$$

When the extraction ratio exceeds 0.7, as is the case with meperidine, lidocaine, and pentazocine, hepatic clearance (CL_H) approaches hepatic blood flow (Q_H). Conditions that alter hepatic blood flow, such as cirrhosis, portal vein thrombosis, congenital heart disease patients needing vasoactive support,[80] and portacaval shunting, significantly impact the clearance of opioids. Drugs with a low extraction ratio, such as diazepam, methadone, and naproxen, do not depend on hepatic blood flow. The metabolic activity of the liver and the plasma protein-binding fraction affect the clearance to a greater degree. The hepatic clearance of these drugs is described by the equation:

$$CL_H = CL_{INT} \times f_u$$

In the formula, f_u is the fraction of unbound drug and CL_{INT} describes the metabolic activity. When f_u is small, as with methadone (<0.1), clearance is mainly affected by reduced enzyme capacity.[77]

The pharmacology of the opioids is variably affected by liver disease. The analgesic effect of codeine, obtained after its demethylation to morphine, is reduced in the presence of liver disease. Liver disease can affect glucuronidation, thereby decreasing the clearance of morphine and increasing its half-life.[81] The protein binding and clearance of alfentanil are reduced in the presence of hepatic dysfunction,[82,83] whereas the half-life and volume of distribution of methadone are increased.[84] The pharmacokinetics of fentanyl, remifentanil, and sufentanil are unchanged in the presence of significant hepatic dysfunction.[85–87] Because the degree of hepatic dysfunction exhibits interindividual variability, adverse events of these medications also varies. Careful dosing or opioids and monitoring of children with liver disease is required when administering opioids.

Anesthetic Effects on Hepatic Cellular Functions

CARBOHYDRATES

Glucose metabolism is influenced by the availability of the substrate, the rate of entry into cells, and the ability of the target organ to convert glucose into energy, or to use it to synthesize fats. In healthy individuals, hepatic glucose production accounts for most whole-body glucose production and is narrowly regulated directly and indirectly by insulin.[88] Insulin directly inhibits gluconeogenesis and glycogenolysis by binding to insulin receptors in the liver, thereby diminishing hepatic glucose production. Of the glucose available to the liver, about 50% undergoes glycolysis and is converted to energy. Between 30% and 40% is converted to fat for storage, and 10% to 20% is shunted to glycogen.[89] Anesthetics inhibit glucose uptake by hepatocytes, an action referred to as the *antiinsulin effect of anesthesia*.[90] Although all inhalational anesthetics exhibit this tendency, halothane had the greatest impact on serum glucose, with isoflurane and sevoflurane having lesser effects.[91] Inhalational anesthetics at 1 to 2 minimum alveolar concentrations inhibit glucose uptake by up to 50%. The combined effects of anesthetics and the stress from surgery or trauma (as well as steroids that may be used as antiemetics) increase the serum glucose concentration, which is one reason why glucose-containing intravenous fluids are no longer recommended for most healthy children undergoing elective surgery.

PROTEIN SYNTHESIS

The impact of anesthesia and surgery on protein synthesis and metabolism is poorly understood. Albumin, a large, soluble, single-polypeptide protein with a molecular weight of 66 kD, is an important protein synthesized by the liver. Between 6 and 12 grams of albumin are produced each day, and production can increase 2-fold to 3-fold according to the individual's needs. Albumin functions as a binding and transport protein and maintains colloid oncotic pressure. Hepatic dysfunction may result in decreased synthesis of albumin and other proteins. Anesthetics may also inhibit protein synthesis. Diethyl ether causes reversible inhibition of protein synthesis in rat hepatocytes,[92] whereas halothane and enflurane block protein synthesis in a dose-dependent manner.[93] Halothane, sevoflurane, and enflurane inhibit protein synthesis and secretion, which may be an early indicator of hepatic cytotoxic injury (see also Chapter 5).

BILIRUBIN METABOLISM

Bilirubin, the final product of heme metabolism, is converted to unconjugated bilirubin by macrophages in the spleen and bone marrow and transported to the liver bound to plasma albumin. Unconjugated bilirubin is transported into the hepatocyte by bile acids and bacterial endotoxins. In the hepatocyte, bilirubin is conjugated with glucuronate, taurine, and, to a lesser extent, glucose by glucuronyl transferase. Deficiencies of glucuronyl transferase manifest clinically in Gilbert syndrome, with more severe forms in Crigler-Najjar syndrome types I and II. Gilbert syndrome affects 4% to 16% of individuals, who have increases in the unconjugated fraction of bilirubin associated with stress or fasting.[94] Although postoperative jaundice has been described, Gilbert syndrome has not been associated with serious adverse effects in the perioperative period.[95] Patients with Crigler-Najjar syndrome can be managed safely by minimizing their exposure to drugs that may displace bilirubin from albumin and by using anesthetics that are minimally metabolized by the liver.[96–98]

HEPATOTOXICITY

Increases in serum aminotransferase concentrations and bilirubin up to two times the upper limit of normal occur commonly in the postoperative period.[99,100] These increases are typically self-limited and inconsequential. However, serious liver injury can be caused by anesthetics.[101,102] The Drug-Induced Liver Injury Network (DILIN), established by the National Institutes of Health in 2003, has and continues to standardize the nomenclature and causality assessment of drug-induced liver injury (DILI).[103–105] Diagnosis of DILI is entertained when increases in alanine aminotransferase (ALT), aspartate aminotransferase (AST), alkaline phosphatase, γ-glutamyl transferase (GGT), and bilirubin occur coincident with xenobiotic exposure. Patterns of injury are classified as (1) hepatocellular, with predominantly increased ALT and AST levels; (2) cholestatic, with increases in alkaline phosphatase, GGT, and bilirubin; (3) and mixed pattern, with features of both hepatocellular and cholestatic injury. Although not specific to anesthetic medications, DILIN analyses concluded that mortality from DILI in individuals with preexisting liver disease or concomitant severe skin reactions is significantly greater than in patients without liver disease.[104] In April of 2012 the website LiverTox (https://www.ncbi.nlm.nih.gov/books/NBK547852/) was launched as a joint effort of the Liver Disease Research Branch of the National Institute of Diabetes and Digestive and Kidney Diseases (NIDDK) and the Division of Specialized Information Services of the National Library of Medicine (NLM), National Institutes of Health. The purpose of LiverTox is to provide up-to-date, accurate, and easily accessed information on the diagnosis, cause, frequency, patterns, and management of liver injury attributable to medications, herbals, and dietary supplements.

It is important to note that even though increases in liver-specific enzymes may reflect drug-induced injury, they are poor markers of liver function. In the absence of a unique test to assess liver function, surrogate markers for liver dysfunction include a prolonged prothrombin time (PT) >15 seconds or an international normalized ratio (INR) greater than 1.5, or both. Other clinical and biochemical markers, such as hypoalbuminemia, hypoglycemia, and an altered mental status, should be included in the assessment of hepatic dysfunction, but they can also result from conditions unrelated to liver function, such as malnutrition, protein-losing enteropathy or nephropathy, or medications for sedation or pain management (see also Chapters 8 and 10). It is critical that in the setting of suspected drug-induced liver injury that liver function is also determined.

An additional confounder relating to the incidence of anesthesia-induced liver injury is the obesity epidemic in children. The growing disease burden associated with nonalcoholic fatty liver disease and nonalcoholic steatohepatitis have raised concerns that these children may be at increased risk for DILI.[106,107] Obesity and hypercholesterolemia can induce CYP2E1, which may facilitate liver injury.[108] Few data are available to guide the best practice of anesthesia for the obese child; adequately powered prospective studies are warranted.

Perioperative Considerations in Liver Disease

Patients with known or suspected liver disease should be assessed for hepatocellular and bile duct injury, coagulopathy, ascites, and encephalopathy. Hepatopulmonary syndrome and portopulmonary hypertension are rare but important complications in children with known chronic liver disease, and they may serve as relative contraindications to elective surgery.[109,110] Perioperative mortality is greatest among those who have acute hepatitis compared with those with chronic liver disease.[109,111,112] The physiologic stress associated with surgical procedures decreases portal blood flow. Liver disease may decrease the degree to which hepatic artery blood flow can compensate for reduced portal blood flow, which can increase the risk of developing ischemic injury.

Parenteral nutrition–associated liver disease (PNALD) occurs in children requiring parenteral nutrition for longer than 60 days. Children with short bowel syndrome are at greatest risk for PNALD. Aside from the disturbances to hepatic and portal blood flows in children with liver disease, those exposed to total parenteral nutrition (TPN) are at increased risk for perioperative glucose derangements.[113–115] Frequent perioperative glucose monitoring with adjustment of dextrose infusion appears to be the standard of care, which is associated with various rates of tapering TPN. A survey administered to members of the Study Group on Pediatric Anesthesia found that approximately 50% of respondents checked glucose levels as often as every 1 to 2 hours. They also found that 19% discontinued TPN and administered a glucose-containing solution, whereas 35% decreased the fluids to one-half of maintenance rates and 33% continued maintenance rates unchanged.[116]

ANNOTATED REFERENCES

Bjorkman S. Prediction of drug disposition in infants and children by means of physiologically based pharmacokinetic (PBPK) modeling: theophylline and midazolam as model drugs. *Br J Clin Pharmacol.* 2004;59:691-704.

This paper attempts to generate data for an age group that provides significant challenges to study and examines two very different drugs. The predicted pharmacokinetics are then thoroughly compared with the adult literature, with very reassuring results.

Chalasani N, Bonkovsky HL, Fontana R, et al. Features and outcomes of 899 patients with drug-induced liver injury: the DILIN prospective study. *Gastroenterology.* 2015;148(7):1340-1352.e7.

Chalasani reports the first patients enrolled in this prospective observational longitudinal study. Mortality from DILI was higher in individuals with preexisting liver disease or concomitant severe skin reactions compared with patients without. Further results from ongoing enrollment are awaited.

Kharasch ED, Hankins D, Mautz D, Thummel KE. Identification of the enzyme responsible for oxidative halothane metabolism: implication for prevention of halothane hepatitis. *Lancet.* 1996;347:1367-1371.

This paper outlines a rare but serious complication of the inhaled anesthetic and provides a mechanism for its toxicity. These researchers also tested the hypothesis that the involved cytochrome enzyme was cytochrome P-450 2E1 (CYP2E1).

Real M, Barnhill MS, Higley C, Rosenberg J, Lewis JH. Drug-induced liver injury: highlights of the recent literature. *Drug Saf.* 2019;42(3):365-387.

This paper reviewed publications relating to liver injury from medications, herbal products, and dietary supplements in 2017 and 2018. The US DILIN prospective study highlighted several areas of ongoing interest, including the potential utility of human leukocyte antigens and microRNAs as DILI risk factors and new data on racial differences, the role of alcohol consumption, factors associated with prognosis, and updates on the clinical signatures of autoimmune DILI, thiopurines, and herbal and dietary supplements.

Svedmyr A, Hack H, Anderson BJ. Interactions of the protease inhibitor, ritonavir, with common anesthesia drugs. *Pediatr Anesth.* 2022;32:1091-1099.

The protease inhibitor, ritonavir, is a strong inhibitor of CYP3A. Use for the early treatment of patients with COVID-19 highlights the ubiquitous nature of this enzyme and its role in the clearance of numerous drugs used in pediatric anesthesia (e.g., alfentanil, fentanyl, methadone, rocuronium, bupivacaine, midazolam, ketamine). Ritonavir is classified as mechanism-based irreversible inhibitor and its perioperative use has consequences for clearance and relative bioavailability of anesthesia drugs.

A complete reference list can be found online at Elsevier eBooks+.

Organ Transplantation

JULIANNE MENDOZA AND KAITLIN M. FLANNERY

Liver Transplantation
Epidemiology and Demographics
Pathophysiology of Liver Disease
Preoperative Evaluation
Intraoperative Care
Surgical Technique
Outcomes
Immediate Postoperative Care
Long-Term Issues
Renal Transplantation
Pathophysiology
Surgical Technique
Anesthetic Management
Long-Term Issues
Cardiac Transplantation
Demographics and Epidemiology
Pathophysiology of The Disease
Congenital Heart Disease
Dilated Cardiomyopathy
Hypertrophic Cardiomyopathy
Restrictive Cardiomyopathy
Repeat Transplantation

Contraindications
Waitlist and Donor Selection
Preoperative Evaluation
Surgical Technique
Intraoperative Problems and Management
Immediate Postoperative Management
Survival and Quality of Life
Anesthesia and the Transplanted Heart
Pediatric Lung and Heart-Lung Transplantation
Demographics and Epidemiology
Pathophysiology of the Disease
Cystic Fibrosis
Pulmonary Hypertension
Contraindications
Waitlist and Donor Selection
Preoperative Evaluation
Surgical Technique
Intraoperative Problems and Management
Immediate Postoperative Management
Long-Term Concerns
Survival and Quality of Life

Liver Transplantation

The first successful pediatric liver transplant was performed by Tom Starzl and colleagues in 1967, but the history of liver transplantation began in 1955 with Stuart Welch in Albany, NY and Jack Cannon at the University of California, Los Angeles (UCLA). Welch was the first to describe auxiliary liver transplantation in the dog and Cannon was the first to attempt orthotopic liver transplantation (OLT) in dogs. Unfortunately, none of the dogs survived the operation.[1] Francis Moore and Tom Starzl continued research with the dog model. From 1958 to 1959, they each successfully transplanted the liver, but all the dogs died from rejection within 4 to 20 days. These deaths highlighted the barriers that prevented the first OLT application in humans.

In the early stages of animal experimentation, the main barriers to success involved surgical technique, organ preservation, and immunosuppression. Livers were initially preserved with chilled electrolyte solutions such as lactated Ringer and normal saline; preservation time was only 5 to 6 hours. In 1987, the University of Wisconsin developed a solution that increased the preservation of livers for 18 to 24 hours. The third barrier, immunosuppression, was most important and likely explained most of the canine deaths. Medawar[2] reported the role of the immune system in organ rejection. Several subsequent attempts to deliberately weaken the immune system and control rejection failed. It was not until an animal model demonstrated that the combination of azathioprine and prednisone were synergistic and ameliorated rejection. This combination was first used in human kidney transplants and then expanded to liver transplantation.

The first human liver transplantation was performed in 1963 in a 3-year-old boy with biliary atresia. This attempt ended in failure caused by fatal intraoperative hemorrhage from venous collaterals. Six more attempts at three different institutions (Denver, Boston, and Paris) produced the same result. Attempts to control the intraoperative hemorrhage with coagulation factor replacement and ϵ-aminocaproic acid resulted in clots and fatal pulmonary emboli in the venovenous bypass system. Inadequate immunosuppression also played a major contributing role in these fatalities. At that time a self-imposed moratorium was established. In 1967, antilymphocyte globulin was introduced, providing lymphoid depletion while supplemental azathioprine and prednisone provided better immunosuppression,[3] allowing Starzl to successfully transplant a liver into a 1-year-old with hepatoblastoma who survived for 13 months.

Despite the initial success of the first pediatric liver transplant, the 1-year survival rate remained no greater than 50%. With the introduction of cyclosporine in 1979, this survival rate increased to 70%.[4,5] In 1989, tacrolimus replaced cyclosporine[6] and the 1-year patient survival further increased to approximately 80%.

EPIDEMIOLOGY AND DEMOGRAPHICS

There has been a steady increase in the number of liver transplants performed yearly in the United States (from 2690 per year in 1990 to 8906 per year in 2020). Most of this increase is attributed to adult transplants; since 1993 the number of pediatric liver transplants doubled whereas during the same period the number of adult transplants has increased 6-fold.[7] The total number of pediatric liver transplants in 1990 was 512; and the pediatric liver transplant volume nationally has remained between 500 and 600 per year over the past 30 years (Fig. 29.1) (https://www.unos.org/data/).

Indications for liver transplantation in children include the presence of an underlying primary liver pathology with acute or chronic liver failure caused by cholestatic liver disease, fulminant hepatic failure, metabolic disorders, tumors, and other derangements (e.g., Budd-Chiari syndrome) (Table 29.1).[8] The most common cause for liver transplantation in children is cholestatic liver disease secondary to biliary atresia across all ages.[9,10] This is especially true in patients younger than 1 year of age, in whom it accounts for more than 50% of liver transplants. Biliary atresia continues to be the most common overall cause for liver transplantation and the most common cholestatic cause.[11] Cholestatic liver disease secondary to total parenteral nutrition (TPN) has become more prominent over the past 10 years, accounting for ~6% of all pediatric liver transplants in the Society of Pediatric Liver Transplantation (SPLIT) registry data between 2011 and 2018.[11] After cholestatic liver disease, metabolic disorders are the next most common causes for pediatric liver transplantation. Historically, the most common metabolic disorders in decreasing frequency were α_1-antitrypsin deficiency, tyrosinemia, Wilson disease, oxalosis, and glycogen storage diseases. Tumors and fulminant

hepatic failures are the third and fourth most common reasons for pediatric liver transplantation, accounting for ~11% each of the SPLIT registry data.[11] The etiology of fulminant hepatic failure was not identified in more than 50% of pediatric patients. A viral cause (e.g., hepatitis A, B, or C) may account for almost half of the acute hepatic failures in infants and children. Acetaminophen is the most common overall cause of drug- or toxin-induced liver failure.[12]

There are few absolute contraindications to pediatric liver transplantation. Children with neoplastic processes such as hepatocellular carcinoma and infections with human immunodeficiency virus (HIV) have received transplants. However, patients with acute infections from bacterial or fungal agents, metastatic neoplasm, or disease processes that are considered an immediate threat to life (severe cardiopulmonary disease, sepsis/septic shock) generally do not undergo transplantation.

Allocation of available livers to appropriate recipients has been a challenge. Initially liver transplant candidates were prioritized based on geographic location and medical condition defined by the Child-Turcotte-Pugh (CTP) score. Patients were ranked as status 1, 2a, 2b, or 3. Status 1 patients received the highest priority and were defined by the presence of acute liver failure of less than 6 weeks or a failed liver transplant within 1 week. Status 2a, 2b, and 3 were defined by their CTP score and time on the waitlist.[13] Efforts by the United Network for Organ Sharing/Organ Procurement and Transplantation Network (UNOS/OPTN) Liver Disease Severity Scale (LDSS) committee to identify predictors of mortality in children with chronic liver disease resulted in the implementation of the **M**odel for **E**nd-Stage **L**iver **D**isease (MELD) and the **P**ediatric **E**nd-Stage **L**iver **D**isease (PELD) severity score in 2002.[14] The PELD and MELD scoring systems assign a score to reflect probability of mortality within the next 3 months. The PELD score incorporates variables for age, growth failure, serum albumin, bilirubin, and international normalized ratio (INR). PELD was initially applied to children younger than 18-years-old until 2005, but now only pertains to children younger than

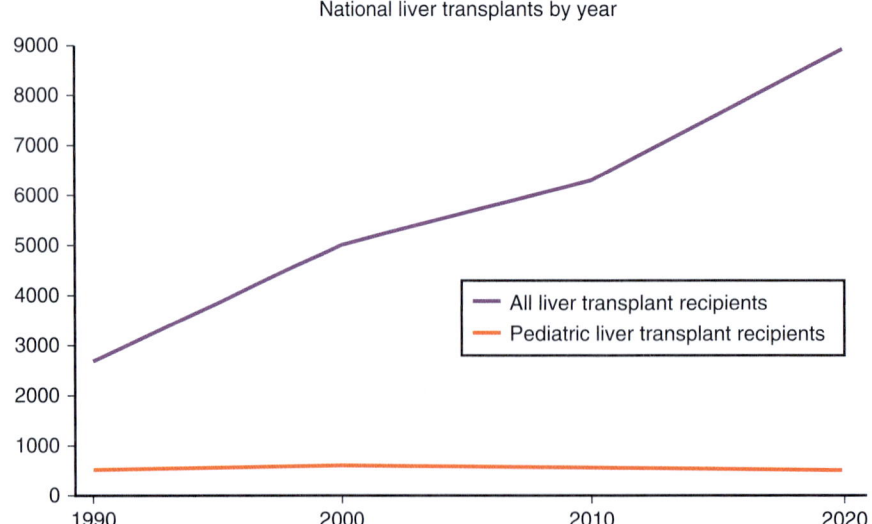

FIGURE 29.1 Graph of national liver transplant volume by year from 1990 to 2020. The *orange line* represents the pediatric liver transplant recipients defined as age <18 years at time of transplant. The *blue line* represents all liver transplant recipients in the United States. (United Network for Organ Sharing [UNOS] Scientific Registry, 2021; https://www.unos.org/data/)

TABLE 29.1	Primary Diagnosis of Liver Disease in Pediatric Patients: 1988–2015
Primary Diagnosis	
Total	13,340
Cholestatic	52.0%
Biliary atresia	
TPN-induced cholestasis	
Alagille syndrome	
Primary sclerosing cholangitis	
Secondary biliary cirrhosis	
Familiar cholestasis (Byler, others)	
Biliary hypoplasia	
Primary biliary cirrhosis	
Neonatal cholestatic disease	
Other causes of cholestasis	
Acute hepatic necrosis	13.3%
Neonatal hepatitis	
Drug-induced	
Hepatitis A	
Hepatitis B	
Hepatitis C	
Unknown	
Other causes of hepatic necrosis	
Metabolic disorder	12.9%
α_1-Antitrypsin	
Cystic fibrosis	
Wilson disease	
Tyrosinemia	
Oxalosis	
Glycogen storage disease	
Maple syrup urine disease	
Hemochromatosis	
Other metabolic disorders	
Cirrhosis	8.0%
Idiopathic	
Autoimmune	
Hepatitis C	
Chronic active hepatitis	
Hepatitis B	
Drug/toxin	
Hepatitis A	
Combined exposure (alcohol, hepatitis A, B, C)	
Alcoholic	
Other causes of cirrhosis	
Hepatic tumors	4.8%
Hepatoblastoma	
Hepatocellular carcinoma	
Hemangioendothelioma	
Benign tumor	
Other tumors	
Other	9%
Congenital hepatic fibrosis	
Budd-Chiari syndrome	
Graft-versus-host secondary to nonliver toxicity	
Trauma	
Other miscellaneous diagnoses	

12 years. The MELD score is now used for children 12 years of age and older. The MELD score, which incorporates creatinine, bilirubin, and prothrombin international normalized ratio has a maximum score of 40. Serum creatinine (SeCr) was incorporated into the MELD score because it predicts mortality for adult patients awaiting liver transplantation. Although serum creatinine may predict survival after liver transplantation, it does not predict mortality in the child awaiting liver transplantation.[15]

Children younger than 18 years of age at the time of listing for transplantation may be assigned one of the following scores: pediatric status 1A, pediatric status 1B, calculated PELD or MELD score, exception PELD or MELD score, or inactive status. Liver candidates who are younger than 18 years of age at the time of listing and who remain on the waiting list after turning 18-years-old are classified as 12 to 17 years for the purposes of allocation. A transplant program may apply to the National Liver Review Board for exception points to the calculated MELD or PELD score if the program believes that the patient's current score does not reflect the medical urgency for transplant or for specific diagnoses. Exception PELD/MELD scores may adjust for the underestimation of 90-day pretransplant mortality predicted by the calculated PELD/MELD score. Analysis of 4298 pediatric liver transplant recipients from 2002 to 2010, comparing calculated PELD scores to actual 90-day pretransplant mortality, found that 1413 patients received exception PELD points, and that the calculated PELD score underestimated pretransplant mortality.[16] Status 1A applies to a patient with one of the following 4 diagnoses: fulminant liver failure, primary nonfunction of transplanted liver (within 7 days of transplant), hepatic artery thrombosis in transplanted liver (within 14 days of transplant), or acute decompensated Wilson disease. Status 1B applies to a patient with one of the following diagnoses: biopsy-proven hepatoblastoma without metastatic disease, organic acidemia or urea cycle defect and an approved MELD or PELD exception for metabolic disease for at least 30 days, chronic liver disease with a calculated MELD or PELD greater than 25 and one of the following: on a mechanical ventilator, gastrointestinal bleed requiring at least 30 mL/kg of red blood cell transfusions within 24 hours, on hemodialysis (continuous or intermittent) or on continuous venovenous hemofiltration (CVVH), or Glasgow coma score (GCS) less than 10 within 48 hours.[17] Once a patient is listed for transplantation, they begin to accrue waiting time that is converted to points; points from waiting time and blood type are used with the PELD/MELD scores to create a rank list for organ allocation.

The allocation of deceased liver donors has changed with the new MELD/PELD policy. Prior to this policy, organs from donors younger than 18 years of age were distributed only to pediatric recipients. With the current policy, status 1A adults may receive a liver from a pediatric donor aged less than 17 years, however, since 2009, fewer liver pediatric donors were being used for adult recipients (11.7% in 2009 to 7.7% in 2019).[18] The introduction of the MELD/PELD score has decreased the waitlist mortality and increased posttransplant survival.[19] Analysis of pre- and post-MELD/PELD data for recipients of all ages indicates that the median time to transplant, defined as the number of days for half of the new registrants to receive organs, decreased from 981 days in 2002 to 361 days in 2007.[20] For pediatric recipients from 2010 to 2015, the median time on the waitlist was 39 days.[21]

Survival after deceased donor transplants is age-dependent. SPLIT registry data from 2011 to 2018 for all transplant recipients aged <18 years demonstrated a 1-year patient survival of 97.3% and 1-year graft survival of 96.6%.[11] Analysis of data from the SPLIT registry from 2011 to 2018, on 1033 patients less than 3 years of age at time of liver transplant, demonstrated similar overall 1-year patient survival of 97% and 1-year graft survival of 95%.[22] Of note in that study, 30 patients <3 months of age at transplantation had a 1-year patient survival of 93% and 1-year graft survival of 93%.[22] Data from outcomes before the implementation of the PELD scoring system showed the 10-year survival was 77% for infants <1 year of age, 79% for children 1 to 5 years of age, and 81% for children 6 to 11 years of age.[20]

There also appears to be a difference in recipient survival between living-donor and deceased-donor grafts. Children receiving a living-donor organ had 10-year survival rates >90%, whereas recipients of deceased donor organ had a 10-year survival rate <90%.[23] In addition to survival, other outcomes still need to be evaluated in children (e.g., growth and cognitive function).[12]

Split liver transplantation was introduced to increase available donor livers of appropriate size to infants and children who require transplantation. Recent evidence suggests that this approach is underutilized; fewer than 5% of livers that could be split for transplantation are actually split. Moreover, children who were transplanted with these split livers would have led to earlier transplantation and possibly reduced risk of death while on the transplant waitlist.[24,25]

PATHOPHYSIOLOGY OF LIVER DISEASE

The liver is the only organ that can regenerate itself when damaged. The stigmata and multiorgan involvement from end-stage liver disease occurs because of loss of hepatocytes and the resulting fibrosis. The hepatic injury and loss of hepatocytes leads to decreased synthetic function. This cellular dysfunction results in coagulopathy, hypocholesterolemia, hypoalbuminemia, and encephalopathy. Attempts at regeneration result in fibrosis and destruction of the portal triad with increased resistance to blood flow through the liver. Portal hypertension is the final consequence of this increased resistance. Many of the characteristic features of liver disease occur because of portal hypertension, specifically varices (esophageal, bowel), hemorrhoids, ascites, spontaneous bacterial peritonitis, splenomegaly with thrombocytopenia, and hepatic encephalopathy.

Cardiac Considerations

Cardiac disturbances occur because of altered physiology, congenital heart defects, and toxic medication-induced adverse effects. A hyperdynamic circulation with a compensatory increase in cardiac output secondary to vasodilation characterizes the altered cardiac physiology from liver disease. Vasodilation is central to the hyperdynamic circulation that accompanies portal hypertension. It likely is the result of the presence of vasoactive mediators. These mediators or gut-derived "humoral factors" (nitric oxide [NO], tumor necrosis factor [TNF]-α, endocannabinoids) enter the systemic circulation through portosystemic collaterals and bypass the hepatic detoxification that usually occurs.[26] Shunting also occurs in the skin and lungs. Mixed venous saturation is increased in patients with liver disease. Poor oxygen extraction and increased cardiac output likely explain the increased mixed venous saturation. The arterial-venous oxygen difference is reduced because of decreased oxygen consumption and arterial-venous shunting.

Cardiomyopathy associated with portal hypertension in adults is well described, but in children with liver disease, information is lacking. However, children with liver disease can have a cardiomyopathy for other reasons. Inborn errors of metabolism including Wilson disease, oxalosis, glycogen storage disease type III,

tyrosinemia, and Gaucher disease,[27] and other syndromes are associated with cardiomyopathies and cardiac anomalies. Tacrolimus and cyclosporine A have also been associated with hypertrophic cardiomyopathy in animal studies and in pediatric liver transplant recipients.[28–31] Although cardiac function is generally well preserved in children undergoing liver transplant who receive tacrolimus, there may be subtle cardiovascular changes that predispose a small percentage to develop hypertrophic cardiomyopathy.[32,33] Alagille disease is commonly associated with congenital heart disease (CHD) such as pulmonary stenosis, coarctation, tetralogy of Fallot, and atrial and ventricular septal defects. Diastolic dysfunction has been described and is associated with increased mortality after transplantation.[34]

Prolongation of QT interval (ECG; see Chapter 14) has been described in adult patients with alcoholic liver disease and may be associated with sudden cardiac death.[35] A decrease in K^+ currents in cardiomyocytes in rats with cirrhosis may provide a possible mechanism for the QT prolongation. Children with liver failure may have an increase in QTc interval; a QTc greater than 450 msec has been reported in 18% of children with liver disease.[36] These findings may increase the risk of ventricular arrhythmias; however, there are conflicting data regarding resolution after liver transplantation.[36,37] Nonselective β-blockade has also been shown to reduce the QT prolongation, but it is unclear if this reduces the risk of arrhythmias or improves survival.[38,39] The presence of prolonged QT has been associated with a greater PELD score and portal hypertension.[40,41] Children with chronic liver disease and prolonged QT may be at increased risk of mortality while waiting for a transplant.[42]

Pulmonary Considerations

Pulmonary hallmarks of liver disease are hypoxia and pulmonary hypertension. Hypoxia can occur for several reasons including hepatopulmonary syndrome and $\dot{V}/\dot{Q}$ mismatch from atelectasis owing to ascites, hepatosplenomegaly, or pleural effusions. Hepatopulmonary syndrome is characterized by hypoxia from intrapulmonary arteriovenous shunting (caused by increased angiogenesis)[43] and intrapulmonary vascular dilatation.[44] The diagnosis is based on either arterial hypoxia (PaO_2 <70 mm Hg) or an increased alveolar-arterial gradient greater than 20 mm Hg in the setting of pulmonary vascular dilatation. Intrapulmonary vascular dilatation is best demonstrated using echocardiography or a lung perfusion scan with macroaggregated albumin.[45] Hepatopulmonary syndrome, which occurs in at least 15% to 20% of adults with cirrhosis,[46] is described in 0.5% to 20% of all children with liver disease. It has been reported in infants as young as 6 months of age. It appears to be more prevalent in children with biliary atresia and polysplenia syndrome.[47,48] When adjusted for the severity of hepatic disease, hepatopulmonary syndrome does not affect mortality.[49] Normal oxygen saturation in children with cirrhosis does not necessarily rule out hepatopulmonary syndrome. Children with normal oxygen saturation may exhibit other criteria for the diagnosis (intrapulmonary vasodilatation and alveolar-arterial gradient greater than 15 mm Hg) and may be at increased risk for morbidity and mortality.[50]

Treatment for hypoxia is long-term supplemental oxygen. Definitive treatment may occur with liver transplantation; children with hepatopulmonary syndrome who had successful transplants have recovered from their hepatopulmonary syndrome post transplantation. The average time required to correct hypoxia after transplantation was ~24 weeks.[51]

29

Portopulmonary hypertension (PPH) is defined by the World Health Organization (WHO) as pulmonary artery hypertension (pressure >25 mm Hg) in the setting of normal pulmonary capillary wedge pressure and portal hypertension.[52] The incidence of PPH is 0.2% to 0.7% in adults with cirrhosis but increases to 2% to 6% in adults presenting for liver transplantation.[53,54] Case series and autopsy data suggest that the incidence of PPH is 0.5% to 5% in children with portal hypertension.[55,56] Signs and symptoms at the time of presentation included new heart murmurs, dyspnea, and syncope. Echocardiography can successfully identify pulmonary hypertension in children and adult patients with PPH.[57] The severity of PPH predicts mortality. The mortality in adult patients with mild PPH during orthoptic liver transplantation was unchanged compared with those without PPH; however, the mortality in those with moderate PPH (pulmonary artery pressure [PAP] = 35–45 mm Hg) and severe PPH (PAP >50 mm Hg) was 50% and 100% respectively.[58,59] With a pretransplant mortality of 29% in patients with PPH, aggressive targeted therapies to reduce pulmonary artery hypertension should be initiated as soon as a diagnosis of hypertension is made.[54] 3-year survival in adults undergoing liver transplantation with PPH that was aggressively treated before and after transplantation is steady at 77%.[54]

There are no definitive guidelines for the management of children with PPH. Early identification is essential, and all children who present for liver transplantation should be evaluated for the presence of PPH with echocardiography.[55,60] If present, cardiac catheterization is indicated to confirm the diagnosis, measure PAPs, and assess the response to pulmonary vasodilators (e.g., NO, epoprostenol). Children who respond to medical management may be candidates for liver transplantation.[61] In a review of six children with PPH, all were aggressively treated with pulmonary hypertension specific treatments (e.g., phosphodiesterase type 5 inhibitors and/or endothelin receptor antagonists and/or prostacyclin analogues).[62] Three benefited from shunt closure alone and three from liver transplantation as well. Pulmonary artery hypertension was stabilized or improved in five of the six patients, and all had survived to the 39-month follow-up.[62] Severe PPH is generally a contraindication for liver transplantation because of the increased mortality.

Neurologic Considerations

Hepatic encephalopathy is a neurologic complication of liver disease classified as either acute (seen in fulminant hepatic failure) or chronic (seen in chronic cirrhosis or chronic portal hypertension). Severity of hepatic encephalopathy is graded using West Haven criteria.[63] Diagnosis of hepatic encephalopathy in children especially those younger than age 4 years may be difficult but should include assessment of mental status, reflexes, neurologic signs, and EEG changes.[64] Minimal encephalopathy, diagnosed with neuropsychological testing, may be present in as many as 50% of children with chronic liver disease.[65] The pathophysiology is not entirely known but cerebral edema is a feature of both acute and chronic hepatic encephalopathy. The cerebral edema is more severe in acute hepatic encephalopathy and can result in increased intracranial pressure (ICP) and risk of brainstem herniation. Ammonia is repeatedly implicated in the pathogenesis of hepatic encephalopathy and may participate in the process by causing astrocytes to swell, resulting in low-grade cerebral edema.[66,67] Ammonia crosses the blood-brain barrier where it is converted with glutamate to glutamine.

Glutamine acts as an osmolyte and increases cerebral volume.[63] The two major sources of ammonia in humans are catabolism of endogenous protein and gastrointestinal absorption of exogenous protein. Bacterial breakdown of nitrogen-containing products in the gut results in ammonia formation, which is then absorbed in the portal circulation. Factors that can increase blood ammonia concentrations in combination with decreased clearance of ammonia by the failing liver can exacerbate the signs and symptoms of hepatic encephalopathy. These typically include increased catabolism from infection, catabolism of protein load from blood products, or increased gut absorption from high-protein diets, constipation, and gastrointestinal bleeding. Other factors that have been implicated in the exacerbation of hepatic encephalopathy include benzodiazepines, hyponatremia, and inflammatory cytokines, which may all share a final common pathway to increase cerebral edema.

Management of hepatic encephalopathy should begin with assessing the child's ability to manage their airway. Children with grade 3 and 4 hepatic encephalopathy may require tracheal intubation to protect the airway to ensure adequate oxygenation and ventilation. Otherwise, management typically focuses on reducing gastrointestinal production and absorption of ammonia. Lactulose is often prescribed to create an osmotic diarrhea and to acidify the lumen of the gut to trap ammonia and minimize absorption. Antibiotics such as neomycin and metronidazole have been used to kill the gastrointestinal bacteria involved in metabolizing nitrogen products to ammonia. Other medications include sodium benzoate, which combines in the liver with ammonia-genic amino acids, such as glycine, to facilitate their excretion.[68] Ornithine aspartate may also provide a substrate to the liver for enhancing the urea cycle and glutamine synthesis and to reduce ammonia concentrations. Flumazenil has been postulated to reduce the symptoms of hepatic encephalopathy by inhibiting endogenous benzodiazepines and γ-aminobutyric acid. However, this benefit was not demonstrated in children who received 0.01 mg/kg flumazenil for hepatic encephalopathy in the setting of fulminant hepatic failure.[69]

Patients with fulminant hepatic failure can have increased ICP, which is the major cause of mortality and may be a contraindication for liver transplantation. Intracranial hypertension occurs in 38% to 81% of patients with fulminant hepatic failure.[70] Invasive ICP monitoring may be considered in patients with fulminant hepatic failure with grade 3 to 4 hepatic encephalopathy although there is a risk of intracranial hemorrhage secondary to coagulopathy. This risk can be reduced by replacing clotting factors and platelets and by placing an extradural rather than a subdural ICP monitor.[71] Noninvasive methods to monitor ICP and cerebral perfusion may be preferred because there is limited evidence of a positive impact of invasive cranial pressure monitoring on patient outcome.[72] Near-infrared spectroscopy (NIRS) and transcranial Doppler (TCD) ultrasound are two noninvasive techniques that can allow for continuous monitoring of cerebral blood flow, though the challenge remains to correlate such data to the increased ICP, cerebral perfusion pressure, and most importantly patient outcomes.[72]

Management strategies for patients with increased ICP should focus on maintaining a cerebral perfusion pressure greater than 60 mm Hg and an ICP less than 20 mm Hg. Often this includes tracheal intubation and ventilation. Patients should be positioned with their heads midline and slightly elevated to 30 degrees to facilitate venous drainage. Ventilation should focus on achieving a

PaCO$_2$ of 30 to 35 mm Hg with minimal positive end-expiratory pressure (PEEP). Medical management to reduce ICP includes administering barbiturates or propofol to minimize stimulation and to reduce ICP.[73] Hyperosmolar therapy with mannitol or hypertonic saline can be administered if ICP remains increased though serum osmolality and serum sodium should be closely monitored. Hypothermia has also been described in a small trial with 14 patients with fulminant hepatic failure; maintaining core body temperature at 32°C to 33°C reduced ICP, but the impact on outcome is less certain.[74] Patients with increased ICP may demonstrate signs of Cushing triad with bradycardia, systolic hypertension, and irregular respirations. Orthotopic liver transplantation is the definitive treatment for patients with acute or chronic hepatic encephalopathy.

Hematologic Considerations

Anemia is common and occurs because of a combination of gastrointestinal bleeding, poor nutritional state, and decreased erythropoietin production from renal failure. Portal hypertension can result in splenomegaly, which causes platelet sequestration, thrombocytopenia, and leukopenia. The liver synthesizes procoagulants, anticoagulants, and fibrinolytic factors, all of which are diminished as synthetic function declines, resulting in a "rebalanced hemostasis."[75] Although the rebalanced hemostasis may explain the lack of spontaneous hemorrhage in liver failure patients, despite abnormal traditional coagulation tests such as prothrombin time (PT) and activated prothrombin time (APTT), it is easily unbalanced in favor of hemorrhage or thrombosis. More comprehensive evaluations of a patient's coagulation status such as with viscoelastic tests may provide guidance in addition to traditional coagulation tests to make informed decisions about the risk for hemorrhage or thrombosis.

Renal Manifestations

Multifactorial renal failure is common in patients with acute and chronic liver disease. Renal failure can be classified as prerenal azotemia, acute tubular necrosis (ATN), or hepatorenal syndrome. Prerenal azotemia from hypovolemia occurs secondary to diuretic therapy, gastrointestinal bleeding, splanchnic pooling, and sepsis. Acute tubular necrosis occurs because of decreased central blood volume secondary to central splanchnic pooling and decreased prostaglandin synthesis. The hepatorenal syndrome is characterized by renal failure in the setting of liver failure and portal hypertension. The incidence in adults with chronic liver disease is ~10% to 15%. The lower incidence in children (5%) possibly reflects the lack of criteria for the diagnosis of hepatorenal syndrome in children.[76] It occurs secondary to intense renal vasoconstriction from activation of the renin-angiotensin, arginine vasopressin, and sympathetic nervous systems. This activation is a homeostatic response to the profound splanchnic vasodilation that occurs in patients with portal hypertension.[77] Hepatorenal syndrome appears similar to prerenal azotemia (increased serum creatinine, decreased urine Na (U$_{Na}$) <10 mM, fractional excretion of sodium [FE$_{Na}$] <1%]) but it is differentiated by its lack of response to a fluid challenge (see Chapter 26). Hepatorenal syndrome is classified into two types distinguished by the rate of progression of renal failure. Type 1, which has a worse prognosis, is characterized by a rapid progression of renal failure with a 100% increase in serum creatinine in less than 2 weeks. It usually occurs in acute liver failure. Type 2 progresses over weeks to months and usually occurs in children with chronic liver disease. Regardless of the type, prognosis is

poor in patients with hepatorenal syndrome with a mortality rate of 80% to 95%.[76] The definitive treatment for hepatorenal syndrome is liver transplantation because the renal failure is reversible if the liver is replaced.[78]

The primary goal in the management of patients with liver disease and renal failure is to exclude treatable and reversible causes of renal failure such as nephrotoxins (e.g., nonsteroidal antiinflammatory drugs), hypovolemia (e.g., diuretics, gastrointestinal bleeding), and sepsis (e.g., spontaneous bacterial peritonitis [SBP]). All nephrotoxins should be stopped and patients should be given a fluid challenge, ideally with a colloid solution. If sepsis is suspected, extensive cultures should be obtained and antibiotics that are not nephrotoxic started.

Pretransplant renal function predicts mortality in adults undergoing transjugular intrahepatic shunt and liver transplantation. This underscores the importance of renal function and explains why serum creatinine is used in the MELD score. Preexisting renal failure is also a major determinant of survival after liver transplantation in adults. Efforts to improve renal function pretransplant may improve post transplantation outcome.[79] It is not clear whether serum creatinine is a predictor of mortality in children with liver disease.[15] Type 1 hepatorenal syndrome can be managed by treating reversible causes such as providing antibiotic treatment for spontaneous bacterial peritonitis before transplantation. Critically ill children may require continuous renal replacement therapy (continuous venovenous hemofiltration, continuous venovenous hemodiafiltration) and vasopressors as a bridge to transplantation.[80]

Metabolic Considerations

Metabolic derangements include glucose, ammonia, electrolyte, and acid-base disturbances. Electrolyte abnormalities include hyponatremia, hypokalemia, hyperkalemia, hypocalcemia, and hypomagnesemia. Hypoglycemia often occurs in patients with fulminant hepatic failure or abrupt discontinuation of total parenteral nutrition and should be closely monitored for and promptly treated. Hyperglycemia is more common in the intraoperative and postoperative period. Patients with chronic liver failure may present with chronic hyponatremia that puts them at risk for developing central pontine myelinolysis upon rapid correction of serum sodium. Central pontine myelinolysis is more commonly seen in adult liver failure patients after transplant and can present as encephalopathy, seizures, hemiparesis, or ataxia.[81,82] The diagnosis is confirmed by MRI of the brain. Risk factors for developing central pontine myelinolysis include serum sodium <120 mmol/L and correction of chronic hyponatremia greater than 8 mEq/L per day.[81] Care should be taken when using sodium bicarbonate and albumin for resuscitation during transplantation as these both contribute to increasing serum sodium. In patients with metabolic disorders, metabolic acidosis pretransplant may be an early sign of metabolic crisis. Identification and treatment of the underlying cause for the metabolic crisis must occur in addition to correction of the acidosis prior to proceeding to liver transplant.

PREOPERATIVE EVALUATION

The preoperative evaluation begins with a history and physical examination to identify the primary cause of liver failure and to identify liver and nonliver-related alterations in physiology that may affect the anesthetic and surgical plan. A complete review of systems identifies most of the perioperative concerns (Table 29.2).

TABLE 29.2	Preoperative Evaluation of Liver Transplant Candidates

History and Physical Examination

Cause for liver failure

Identifiable syndrome or metabolic disorder

Past medical history: non–liver-related medical problems (e.g., asthma)

Past surgical history: portoenterostomy (Kasai), previous anesthetic concerns

Medications: diuretics, lactulose

Allergies

Family history of anesthesia-related problems

NPO history

Cardiovascular

Echocardiography: to identify cardiomyopathy, pulmonary HTN, congenital cardiac defects, and intrapulmonary vasodilation

Electrocardiogram: to identify arrhythmias and QT prolongation

Pulmonary

Oxygen saturation (possible arterial blood gas): to assess hypoxia, A-a gradient (HPS)

Chest x-ray: to identify pleural effusions and central line position

Hematology

Complete blood cell count: to assess anemia, leukocytosis/leukopenia (sepsis)

Prothrombin time and partial thromboplastin times

Platelet count

Thromboelastography

Renal

Blood urea nitrogen

Creatinine

Bicarbonate: to assess degree of metabolic acidosis

Neurologic

Assessment of increased intracranial pressure in acute/fulminant hepatic failure

Hepatic encephalopathy: ammonia level

Electrolytes

Na^+ and K^+: hyponatremia and hypokalemia secondary to diuretics

Calcium

Albumin

Magnesium

Glucose

A-a gradient, Alveolar-arterial gradient; *HPS*, hepatopulmonary syndrome; *HTN*, hypertension; *NPO*, nothing by mouth.

The primary cardiovascular concerns include acquired cardiomyopathies from liver disease and inborn errors of metabolism, congenital cardiac defects, and QT prolongation. Aside from a cardiovascular physical examination, the preoperative cardiac evaluation should include an echocardiogram and 12-lead ECG.

The pulmonary manifestations of concern include hypoxia and PPH. Oxygen saturation on room air and with oxygen identifies hypoxic patients and their response to oxygen. Children with noteworthy intrapulmonary shunts from hepatopulmonary syndrome will not increase their oxygen saturation. Hepatopulmonary syndrome, with a varied incidence from 4% to 47% of adults with cirrhosis,[83] can be diagnosed by demonstrating intrapulmonary vascular dilatation on echocardiography with macroaggregated albumin[45] and by the severity of the hypoxemia.[83]

Screening for PPH can usually be accomplished using echocardiography (if tricuspid regurgitation jet is present) but the gold standard for diagnosis remains a right heart catheterization.[58] Catheterization will define the severity of the PPH and its responsiveness to pulmonary vasodilators. Children with severe pulmonary hypertension (PAP >50 mm Hg) are at increased risk of perioperative mortality and liver transplantation may be contraindicated.[59]

Anemia and thrombocytopenia are common in children with liver disease and a complete blood cell count should be obtained. In addition, because of decreased synthetic function and because of reduced vitamin K absorption, concentrations of clotting factors II, VII, IX, and X may be low. Prothrombin and partial thromboplastin times and platelet counts should be assessed. A viscoelastic test if available, such as ROTEM (rotational thromboelastometry) or TEG (thromboelastography), should be considered before surgery to assess the coagulation status.

In adults, renal failure is a common finding in liver failure and predicts decreased survival during the posttransplant period.[84] Blood urea nitrogen (BUN) and serum creatinine measurements should be obtained preoperatively. Children who require hemodialysis or continuous venovenous hemofiltration in the preoperative setting warrant special consideration for intraoperative planning.

Baseline laboratory values should be obtained for liver function tests, sodium, potassium, calcium, glucose, and albumin. Hyponatremia and hypokalemia are common with diuretic therapy. Hypocalcemia may be present due to vitamin D deficiency, low albumen, and possible hypoparathyroidism; ionized calcium would be further acutely reduced during rapid infusion of citrated blood products, which chelate calcium. Hypoglycemia occurs secondary to depleted glycogen stores in the failed liver and/or removal of long-term total parenteral nutrition.

Children should be evaluated for evidence of altered mental status, particularly those with acute hepatic failure. There are no studies that define the optimal monitoring of intracranial pressure in children with hepatic encephalopathy; both noninvasive and invasive monitoring have been used.[72] Noninvasive monitoring includes transcranial Doppler ultrasound, tympanic membrane displacement, optic nerve sheath diameter, near-infrared spectroscopy, and jugular venous oxygen saturation. Each modality has its limitations. Invasive monitoring involves an intracranial bolt associated with a 7% incidence of bleeding.[72] Increased intracranial pressure is a common cause of mortality in those with fulminant hepatic failure. Altered mental status may also be caused by hepatic encephalopathy. An ammonia concentration should be obtained as part of their evaluation. Children with advanced hepatic encephalopathy (grade 3 and 4) may require orotracheal intubation to protect their airway and mechanical ventilation to control $PaCO_2$.

A key portion of the preoperative evaluation is the preparation of the patient and family for the anticipated risks, benefits, and clinical course. Specifically, a critically ill child will likely remain intubated and mechanically ventilated in the immediate postoperative period and may have significant facial and extremity edema. Infants and children with less severe disease or disease that does not result in portal hypertension (e.g., maple syrup urine disease) may be extubated at the end of surgery. Similarly, informing the family about the potential number and location of the intravascular catheters and their associated risks can be helpful in preparing them to see their child after surgery. Informed consent should also include a discussion regarding the need for blood products, risks associated with prolonged positioning (peripheral nerve injury, occipital alopecia), and the possibility of intraoperative death.

INTRAOPERATIVE CARE

Appropriate intraoperative care of the pediatric liver transplant patient requires an understanding of the surgical and anesthetic issues. Several factors affect the patient's physiology, including the underlying pathophysiology of liver disease, surgical technique, and response to anesthetic drugs. The surgical approach for OLT in children is similar to that for adults. The major difference is the smaller size of the recipient. The obstacles imposed by the size of the patient include a smaller blood volume, more challenging vascular access, size restriction of donor graft, less frequent use of venovenous bypass (VVBP), and thus transient decrease in preload, and surgical complications such as hepatic artery thrombosis.

Anesthetic management begins with a thorough preoperative evaluation. Children older than 1 year of age will likely be anxious during the preoperative period. They can be premedicated with an anxiolytic like midazolam, which may be administered intravenously, orally, nasally, or rectally. Patients with hepatic encephalopathy should not receive sedative premedication.

Most children are considered to have full stomachs because of delayed gastric emptying from ascites, gastrointestinal bleeding, hepatic encephalopathy, and the nonelective nature of most transplants. The exception may be those presenting for an "elective" transplant without any stigmata of portal hypertension (e.g., Crigler-Najjar syndrome or maple syrup urine disease). Venous access should be sited in the lower extremities preoperatively because lower extremity veins cannot be used intraoperatively as the vena cava (VC) will be cross clamped during the transplant. Furthermore, this preserves the veins in the upper extremities to establish large-bore access for blood transfusion during transplantation. Patients who are considered to have a full stomach should receive a rapid-sequence induction. Induction agents should be tailored to meet the needs of the patient, but etomidate (0.2–0.3 mg/kg), propofol (2–4 mg/kg), or ketamine (2 mg/kg) are suitable options. Appropriate neuromuscular blocking drugs for rapid-sequence induction include succinylcholine and high-dose rocuronium.[85] Some children may require greater inspiratory pressures to achieve adequate ventilation in the intraoperative and postoperative period compared with unaffected children because of atelectasis from pleural effusions and ascites, surgical retractors placed on the abdominal and chest wall, and a tight abdominal closure; a cuffed tracheal tube is appropriate for these children. PEEP is recommended for all patients; PEEP (10–15 cm H_2O) has no negative effects on liver function in donors[86] or recipients.[87]

An inhalation induction with sevoflurane and nitrous oxide is appropriate for children who are not at risk for aspiration. Nitrous oxide is not recommended after induction of anesthesia because it may distend the bowel and expand gas emboli. Anesthesia is typically maintained with an inhalational agent, an opioid, and a neuromuscular blocking drug. Isoflurane and sevoflurane are commonly used because they are readily available, undergo minimal hepatic metabolism, and have minimal adverse effects on the liver.[88,89] Desflurane also undergoes minimal hepatic metabolism and appears to be quite safe, although there are reports of hepatotoxicity after desflurane exposure.[90] Sevoflurane provided more stable hemodynamics than desflurane in one study.[91] Hepatotoxicity has been reported after all inhalational agents; it follows the order halothane>enflurane>isoflurane>desflurane>sevoflurane.[92] Although hepatotoxicity has been reported after sevoflurane anesthesia, it is rare. Serum glutathione S-transferase alpha (α-GST) concentration has been measured as a metric of hepatocellular injury in anesthetized patients after inhalational anesthesia. A 24-hour increase in α-GST after sevoflurane anesthesia has been attributed to a polymorphism in glutathione S-transferase gene, GSTA1, which is distinctly different from the transient and mild increase in α-GST 1-hour after sevoflurane.[93] Propofol (with or without remifentanil, total intravenous anesthesia [TIVA], see Chapter 6) is also an option to maintain anesthesia during liver transplantation. Although the primary metabolic pathway is hepatic, extrahepatic metabolism occurs in the lung, kidney, and intestine,[94,95] and dosing can be titrated using modified EEG monitoring. Neuromuscular blockade can be maintained with a variety of agents. Rocuronium, vecuronium, pancuronium, atracurium, and cisatracurium have all been described. Pancuronium has the added advantage of increased heart rate, long duration, and reduced cost. The disadvantage of pancuronium, rocuronium, and vecuronium is their partial hepatic metabolism (see Chapter 5), but this can be overcome with appropriate monitoring and dose adjustments. Dose requirements of continuous infusions of rocuronium, vecuronium, and pancuronium are reduced during the anhepatic phase of liver transplantation but return to initial infusion rates after reperfusion.[96] There is no change in the dose requirements of atracurium during the anhepatic phase.[97] Atracurium or cisatracurium may be ideal in patients with combined hepatic and renal insufficiency because they do not rely on hepatic or renal function for elimination.

The liver metabolizes all opioids, except for remifentanil, which is metabolized by plasma and tissue esterases. The metabolic pathway for most opioids is oxidation, although morphine undergoes glucuronidation.[98] There is evidence that the elimination half-life and clearance of alfentanil and fentanyl are not dramatically altered in patients with cholestatic and cirrhotic liver disease.[99,100] Fentanyl, sufentanil, alfentanil, and morphine have all been described and used in children undergoing liver transplantation. Fentanyl is commonly selected and is usually administered as a bolus during induction (2–10 μg/kg) and maintained as an infusion throughout the anesthetic and the immediate postoperative period (2–5 μg/kg per hour). The use of a fentanyl infusion intraoperatively does not preclude extubation at the end of the procedure if it is stopped early (usually during the biliary reconstruction) and total intraoperative fentanyl dose is 10 to 20 μg/kg.

Vascular access is important for resuscitation and monitoring. At least two large-bore peripheral IV catheters should be placed in the upper extremities along with a multilumen central venous line (CVL) for administration of drug infusions, vasopressors, and assessment of volume status. The CVL can also be used to monitor trends in central venous pressure (CVP) and measure superior vena cava oxygen saturation (a surrogate marker for SvO_2). Rapid infusion catheters are recommended for larger patients. Venous access must be secured above the diaphragm because of the risk that the inferior vena cava (IVC) will be cross clamped intraoperatively. Blood loss can be large during liver transplantation with estimates ranging from 0.5 and 25 blood volumes (mean = 3.95 blood volumes).[101] Fluid warmers and infusion devices (Level 1 Fast Flow Fluid Warmer, Smiths Medical, Rockland, MA; Belmont Rapid Infuser, Belmont Instrument Corporation, Billerica, MA) need to be available to facilitate volume resuscitation if massive hemorrhage occurs (see Chapters 10 and 49). The early version of the Level 1 Fast Flow Fluid Warmer was associated with massive air emboli, but the newer models are equipped with air detectors. Nevertheless, all infusion bags must be deaired before starting the device.[102] The choice of resuscitation fluids should be limited to 0.9% normal saline solution and PlasmaLyte. Lactated Ringer solution is not recommended because the lactate will remain unmetabolized during the anhepatic stage. Many patients with liver disease are hypoalbuminemic, so the use of 5% albumin is appropriate. However, 5% albumin is hypertonic, and care must be taken when administering this to children with hyponatremia because rapid hyponatremia correction can cause adverse cerebral pressure changes.

Standard monitoring should include five-lead ECG, pulse oximetry (upper and lower extremities), noninvasive blood pressure, invasive arterial blood pressure, CVP, and temperature. Other high-technology monitoring commonly used in adult liver transplantation includes transesophageal echocardiography (TEE), continuous cardiac output (CCO) catheter, bispectral index (BIS), venoveno bypass, and more than one arterial catheter. There are limitations to the use of these monitors in children because of patient size. Continuous noninvasive or minimally invasive cardiac output (CO) monitors such as the Cardiotronic ICON (Osypka Medical, La Jolla, CA), which simply requires four ECG pads to assess changes in bioimpedance or small esophageal Doppler monitors (Deltex Medical, Chichester, West Sussex, England) may prove to be of great value in the future (see Chapter 49).[103,104]

Hematologic and electrolyte changes are common during liver transplantation, and measurements of arterial blood gases, sodium, potassium, calcium, magnesium, hemoglobin platelets, and coagulation parameters (PT, PTT, fibrinogen and D-dimers, TEG or ROTEM) need to be performed frequently throughout the procedure. Point-of-care testing with TEG (E-Fig. 29.1) may reduce transfusion requirements in patients having liver transplants.[105,106] However, only 28% of US pediatric transplant centers used TEG.[107]

Acid-base disturbances commonly occur during liver transplantation. Children with renal disease may have a preexisting metabolic acidosis from increased bicarbonate elimination. A metabolic acidosis is typically present during the dissection and anhepatic phase of surgery, but it is usually most pronounced immediately after reperfusion. Lactic acid and citrate (from blood products) are not metabolized during the anhepatic phase and contribute to the acidosis. Cross clamping of the IVC and aorta alters blood flow to gut and lower extremity tissue beds and may also contribute to the development of a lactic acidosis. Once the liver graft begins to function, a metabolic alkalosis can develop as the lactate and citrate are metabolized.[101]

During the dissection and anhepatic phase there are several causes of hyperglycemia. Serum glucose will increase if there is an exogenous source or if there is altered glucose metabolism. Exogenous sources of glucose include glucose from blood products,[101] dextrose-containing IV fluids, and damaged hepatocytes from the liver graft.[108] Typically, glucose concentrations will increase immediately after reperfusion. Glucose uptake is altered from the administration of methylprednisolone because of steroid-induced insulin resistance. Hepatic denervation likely results in alterations in insulin and glucose clearance during the postoperative period and may explain the frequent occurrence of impaired glucose tolerance and diabetes in liver transplant recipients.[109,110] Lack of hyperglycemia after reperfusion may be an early sign of delayed graft function or primary graft nonfunction.

Positioning is critical to prevent soft tissue and peripheral nerve injuries. All extremities should be padded, and all cables and wires need to be wrapped and protected from the skin. The head should be rotated and repositioned periodically, or a gel ring used to support the head to prevent pressure sores and/or alopecia from developing. To minimize the risk of peripheral neuropathy, the upper extremities should not be abducted more than 90 degrees, the hands pronated, and the wrists should not be hyperextended for the arterial catheter.

Temperature changes may be drastic during the procedure especially in infants and small children. The patient should be actively warmed using a forced-air warming blanket; consider wrapping an infant's head and extremities to prevent heat loss.

SURGICAL TECHNIQUE

The surgical approach can be divided into four stages: hepatectomy, anhepatic, reperfusion, and biliary reconstruction.

Hepatectomy (Stage 1)

The initial description of OLT is referred to as the "classic" technique. In the classic approach, the liver is dissected to its vascular supply and the suprahepatic and infrahepatic vena cava (VC) are clamped along with the portal vein and hepatic artery. The liver is removed en bloc (Fig. 29.2). The disadvantage of this approach is the VC cross clamp and the associated reduction in preload as well as impaired venous drainage of the kidneys and splanchnics during the anhepatic phase. The piggyback technique was described in 1989 and is the preferred approach for pediatric transplants because there is more flexibility with the organ size and it requires only partial clamping of the vena cava.[111,112] The piggyback technique is used for all living-donor liver transplants since the donor allograft does not contain an intrahepatic vena cava (Fig. 29.3). The liver is dissected away from the IVC, the short hepatic veins, left, right, and middle hepatic veins at the hepatic vein confluence, and the portal vein and hepatic artery. This approach requires careful dissection to leave the intrahepatic vena cava intact since breaches may cause venous air emboli. During this dissection phase for piggyback techniques the liver may be twisted around the axis of the hepatic vein confluence causing sudden changes in preload. The donor infrahepatic vena cava is oversewn, and the donor suprahepatic vena cava is anastomosed to the recipient hepatic vein confluence (see Figs. 29.2 and 29.3). This requires only partial clamping of the IVC. A temporary portocaval shunt can be established for patients who do not tolerate clamping of the portal vein (Fig. 29.4). Typically, these are patients who have not developed collateral flow secondary to portal hypertension (e.g., maple syrup urine disease).

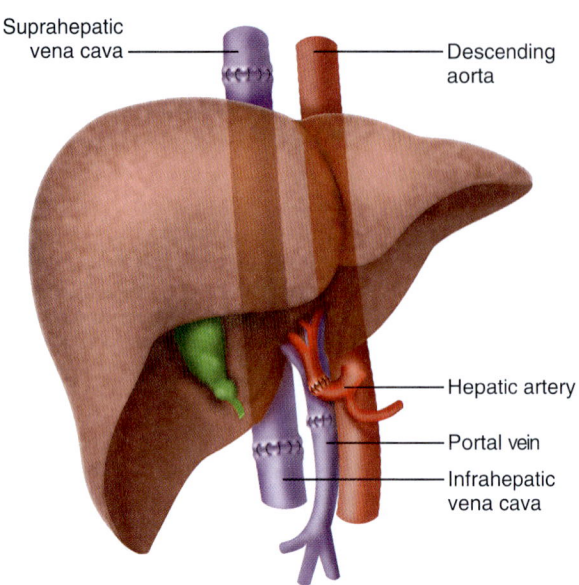

Suprahepatic
vena cava

Descending
aorta

Hepatic artery

Portal vein

Infrahepatic
vena cava

FIGURE 29.2 The classic approach for orthotopic liver transplantation. The suture lines are visible at the suprahepatic and infrahepatic anastomoses. (From Starzl TE, Iwatsuki S, Van Theil DH, et al. Evolution of liver transplantation. *Hepatology.* 1982;2[5]:614-636.)

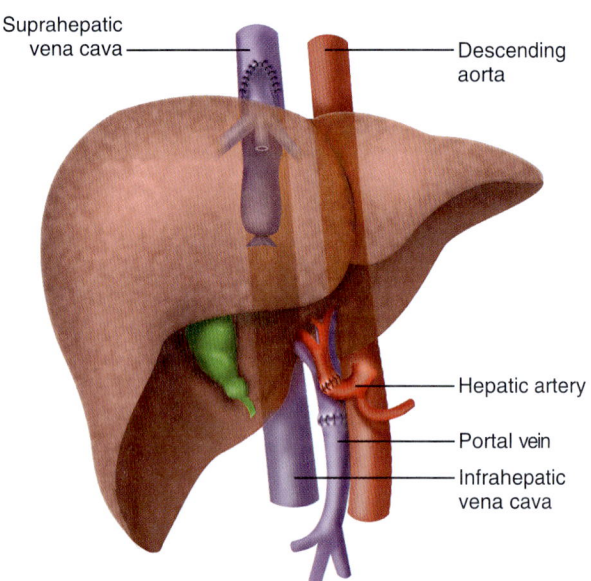

Suprahepatic
vena cava

Descending
aorta

Hepatic artery

Portal vein

Infrahepatic
vena cava

FIGURE 29.3 The piggyback technique preserves the inferior vena cava (IVC). This is the view of the liver graft after the recipient's hepatic confluence is anastomosed to the donor's IVC (the infrahepatic IVC of the donor is ligated). (From Tzakis A, Todo S, Starzl TE. Orthotopic liver transplantation with preservation of the inferior vena cava. *Ann Surg.* 1989;210[5]:649-652.)

Several physiologic considerations that take place during the hepatic dissection affect the anesthetic management. Hypotension is common and can occur from surgical manipulation, and changes to the cardiovascular, hematologic, and metabolic systems. The most common cause of hypotension includes hypovolemia secondary to hemorrhage and third-space volume losses. Resuscitation with citrated blood products can result in hypocalcemia (see Fig. 10.11) and surgical manipulation can cause mechanical

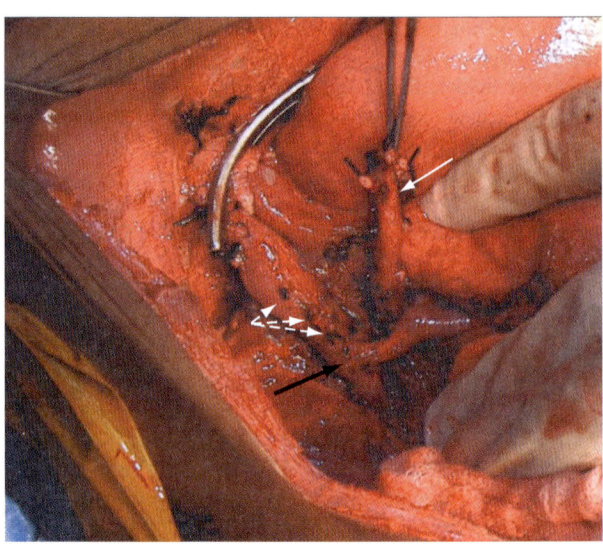

FIGURE 29.4 The native liver has been removed. There is a clamp across the right, middle, and left hepatic veins. The *black arrow* shows the portacaval shunt. The *solid white arrow* shows the hepatic artery. The *dashed white arrows* show the short hepatic veins. (From Kuo PC, Davis RD. *Comprehensive Atlas of Transplantation*. Philadelphia: Lippincott Williams & Wilkins; 2005:132.)

compression of the IVC or right ventricle. Bleeding occurs from fragile collaterals, adhesions from prior surgery (e.g., Kasai procedure), and coagulopathy.[113] Blood conservation with a reduction in allogeneic blood exposure may have a benefit on perioperative morbidity including infections, intensive care unit (ICU) length of stay, and hospital length of stay.[114] One technique to reduce blood loss is the maintenance of a low CVP (decrease of 30% from baseline) as has been described in adults.[115] The reported benefit of a low CVP is less bleeding with subsequent decrease in allogeneic blood requirements and decreased morbidity.[112] Some studies have also suggested an overall reduction in morbidity and 1-year mortality.[116,117] The technique is controversial and the potential risks include end-organ injury, such as renal or graft failure.[118] This technique has not been described in the pediatric liver transplant population. Close monitoring of end-organ perfusion with frequent arterial blood gas analysis and serum lactate should be monitored when maintaining a low CVP to decrease blood loss.

Hematologic abnormalities include anemia, thrombocytopenia, coagulation factor deficiency, and low fibrinogen.[75] A progressive coagulopathy can develop during this stage. Metabolic derangements including hyperkalemia, hypocalcemia, hypomagnesemia, and acidosis may occur from volume resuscitation with blood products.

Anhepatic Stage (Stage 2)

The anhepatic phase begins once the hepatic veins, hepatic artery, and portal vein are cross clamped and dissection of the recipient's liver is completed and removed. This phase ends when the hepatic and portal vein cross clamps are removed, and the graft is reperfused.

Cardiovascular changes that occur during this stage can result in hypotension. This occurs from the IVC cross clamp, which decreases the preload. Hemodynamically, CO, CVP, and PAP decrease while systemic vascular resistance increases.[113] Preload should be gently augmented to maintain mean arterial pressure (MAP) with the minimum filling pressures possible since hypervolemia may cause hepatic congestion during reperfusion. Inotropic agents may be needed to maintain mean arterial blood pressure. A temporary portocaval shunt may attenuate these hemodynamic changes by preserving preload from the portal vein. In adult-sized patients, venovenous bypass may be instituted at this point to preserve preload from below the diaphragm. Unmetabolized citrate causes hypocalcemia and hypomagnesemia since it chelates both cations. Acidosis occurs from the unmetabolized citrate, lactate, and other acids. Bicarbonate may be administered if there is severe metabolic acidosis, although there is no evidence outcomes are improved.[119] In fact, a mild metabolic acidosis during reperfusion may not be detrimental since it will be later offset by the metabolism of citrate, which produces bicarbonate.

Once the liver allograft is out of the ice and on the field, then warming starts and ischemia time begins. The time to reperfusion will be brief and the patient must be readied. The potassium level should be low-normal, and the calcium level should be high-normal, hemoglobin should be maintained between 9 and 10 g/dL. If the potassium is greater than 5 mEq/L, steps need to be taken to reduce it. This includes increasing the serum pH with hyperventilation and the administration of sodium bicarbonate (1–3 mEq/kg), β_2-agonists, and glucose and insulin infusion (see Chapters 7 and 25). Potassium-wasting diuretics such as furosemide (0.5–1 mg/kg) can also be used. Administering fresh blood or washed red blood cells minimizes the increase in potassium during transfusion therapy. Calcium and epinephrine should be immediately available for reperfusion.

Reperfusion (Stage 3)

The liver graft can be reperfused once the caval or hepatic and portal vein anastomoses are complete. Before reestablishing hepatic blood flow, the graft is flushed to remove the high potassium preservation solution to minimize reperfusion syndrome.

Many changes can occur acutely during the reperfusion period secondary to cardiovascular, hematologic, and metabolic derangements. Reperfusion syndrome is characterized by a decrease in mean arterial pressure of greater than 30%.[120] Factors participating in this event include myocardial dysfunction, arrhythmias, and bleeding. The myocardial dysfunction is attributed to the release of NO and TNF-α.[121] Cardiovascular collapse can occur and patients may require epinephrine to correct the hemodynamic effects of reperfusion.[120] Hyperkalemia arising from acute metabolic acidosis, transfusion of blood products, and flushing the vessels of the donor liver occurs commonly immediately after reperfusion and may lead to ventricular arrhythmias.[122,123] Hyperkalemia should be treated with calcium chloride (10–30 mg/kg) initially to stabilize the cardiac membrane and then with insulin and dextrose, hyperventilation, furosemide, β_2-agonists, and sodium bicarbonate to decrease the serum potassium concentration as needed (see previous section). The increased potassium content of the preservation solution is the primary cause of the hyperkalemia. The commonly used University of Wisconsin solution contains large amounts of potassium (120 mmol/L). Histidine-tryptophan-ketoglutarate solution was introduced in 1980 as a cardioplegic solution and contains less potassium (10 mmol/L) than the University of Wisconsin solution.[124] Viscosity is reduced with histidine-tryptophan-ketoglutarate solution compared with the Wisconsin solution and may introduce itself more easily into the vascular spaces in the donor liver.[125] Although hyperkalemia is the hallmark electrolyte disturbance in the immediate reperfusion period, hypokalemia is more common in children throughout the intraoperative period and may require correction.[126]

Fibrinolysis can occur after reperfusion and in one study it occurred in 60% of children and 80% of adults.[127] Viscoelastic tests will demonstrate fibrinolysis if present (see E-Fig. 29.1 and Chapter 10). Fibrinolysis occurs from increased tissue plasminogen activator activity and decreased synthesis of fibrinolysis inhibitors. Heparin effect occurs from endogenous heparinoids from the graft and residual heparin from the preservation solution and the release of tissue plasminogen activator from endothelial cells of the revascularized graft. Antifibrinolytic medications blunt this process, but there is concern that there may be an association with antifibrinolytics and intraoperative thrombotic events (hepatic artery and portal vein thrombosis) in pediatric patients receiving liver transplants. Children can have a mixed coagulation picture after transplantation and may be hypercoagulable because of a decrease in protein C and antithrombin III.[128] This may result in hepatic artery thrombosis.[129–131] Tranexamic acid, ϵ-aminocaproic acid, and other methods to reduce transfusion needs in adult liver transplants have been advocated, but there are no pediatric transplant data to support or refute the use of tranexamic acid or ϵ-aminocaproic acid and the adult series have small sample sizes.[132–134]

Biliary and Hepatic Artery Reconstruction (Stage 4)

The final step is reestablishing hepatic artery blood flow and reconstructing the biliary system. The hepatic artery may require an anastomosis via a conduit to the infrarenal aorta in infants. This requires temporary cross clamping of the aorta. Biliary reconstruction is established by either directly connecting the graft and the recipient's common bile ducts or by connecting the common duct of the graft to a Roux-en-Y limb of the recipient's jejunum.

During biliary reconstruction, metabolic and hematologic alterations are addressed. As the liver graft begins to function, the citrate administered during the previous three phases is metabolized and the patient can develop a metabolic alkalosis. One of the hemodynamic goals includes maintaining a normal CVP. If the CVP is increased (>8–10 mm Hg), there is concern that the liver graft can become congested and not function properly. The risk of hepatic artery thrombosis ranges from 0% to 25% and is greater in infants and children.[130,131] This risk may be increased if the PT and PTT are corrected to normal values. Also, the viscosity from a greater hematocrit may increase the risk of hepatic artery or portal vein thrombosis. The hematocrit does not need to be corrected to normal values; maintaining the hemoglobin at 8 to 9 g/dL is safe and reasonable. Surgical techniques to reduce the risk of hepatic artery thrombosis include anticoagulation with heparin, dextran, aspirin, and alprostadil.

Split Liver Techniques and Living-Donor Liver Transplants

Advances in surgical technique, tissue preservation, and immunosuppression have improved the survival in patients undergoing liver transplantation. The result is more patients awaiting liver transplantation without an increase in available organs. Children are at a disadvantage because of the size limitations. Two techniques have attempted to address these issues. In 1984, Bismuth and Houssin split an adult liver and transplanted it into a child.[135] The reduced liver technique does not increase the number of available grafts and efforts were made to perform split liver techniques to make two grafts from one adult donor. The initial results were poor, with an increase in complications and mortality.[136,137] The technique has evolved and today the graft is split while still in vivo (in the heart-beating donor) compared with ex vivo (splitting performed after the graft is removed from the donor). This decreases cold ischemia time and facilitates hemostasis of the liver edge. The result is improved patient and graft survival.[138] Patient survival has increased from 60% to 70% in the 1990s to 80% to 90% in 2003. In one series, 218 split liver technique grafts were transplanted between 1995 and 2002; overall patient survival at 1 year was 81.7% and overall graft survival was 75.8%. Surgical complications that caused a return to the operating room were bleeding (9.2%), bowel perforation (8.3%), and biliary problems (7.5%). Hepatic artery complications occurred in 6.7%.[138]

Living-donor liver transplantation was first described in 1989.[139] The result has been a reduction in mortality among children awaiting liver transplantation. The benefit of a living donor (especially if related) is improved posttransplant results because of better graft quality, shorter ischemic times, and better immune compatibility. One- and five-year patient survival rates were 94% and 92%, respectively.[140] The left hepatic segment is removed for pediatric recipients, whereas the right hepatic lobe is removed for adult recipients. The regenerative capacity of the liver allows the donor to regenerate the liver without hepatic insufficiency. Despite the success of this technique for the recipients, there is considerable risk to the donor. Complications include exposure to blood products, short- and long-term peripheral nerve injuries, biliary leakage, abdominal wall defects, pleural effusions, pneumonia, pulmonary emboli, and death.[140,141]

OUTCOMES

The SPLIT registry was initiated in 1995 and consists of 50 centers in the United States and Canada. In the past, patient age younger than 1 year was considered an increased risk factor for mortality, but over the past 20 years little difference is seen between patients younger than 2 years and those older than 2 years of age. Analysis of data from the SPLIT registry from 2011 to 2018 patients less than 3 years of age at the time of liver transplant demonstrated an overall 1-year patient survival of 97% and 1-year graft survival of 95%.[22] Of note, in that study, 30 patients less than 3 months of age at the time of transplant demonstrated a slightly lower 1-year patient survival of 93% and 1-year graft survival of 93%.[22] There was also no difference between male and female sex.[139]

Review of the MELD/PELD data indicates that survival also depends on the preoperative MELD/PELD score. Patients stratified to status 1 had a lower 1-year survival rate compared with other transplant recipients (76% vs. 87%). Adults with greater MELD scores (scores >35) demonstrated decreased 1-year patient and graft survival. Pediatric patients with greater PELD scores showed a trend toward decreased 1-year patient and graft survival but the association was not statistically significant. The overall 1-year survival rate remained excellent at >85%.[142] Children who are liver transplant recipients are at risk for cognitive deficits; long-term cognitive and academic deficits persist with verbal comprehension, working memory, mathematical computation, and executive function deficits.[143,144] Factors that predicted cognitive deficits included operative complications and intraoperative transfusion volume.[144] Conversely, liver transplantation improved global functioning in some children.[145] In a small cohort of children, medical complications pre- and posttransplant but not intraoperative were predictive of cognitive impairment.[146] In another study, cognitive deficits and behavioral problems were identified in a minority of children after transplant, particularly in those with single parents and parents with lower education levels.[147]

IMMEDIATE POSTOPERATIVE CARE

At the completion of surgery, the child is transported to the ICU. Even though the old liver has been removed, much of the preoperative pathology persists into the postoperative period. Patients with underlying cardiac, pulmonary, and renal dysfunction will be more difficult to manage.

Patients continue to lose intravascular volume after liver transplantation because of ongoing bleeding and third-space losses. These losses need to be replaced to maintain a normal CVP and adequate urine output (0.5–1 mL/kg per hour). Replacement with a lactate-free isotonic solution (0.9% normal saline solution or PlasmaLyte) and albumin is appropriate. Particular attention should be paid to children with underlying ventricular dysfunction or persistent PPH because they will not tolerate fluid overload. In adults, there is some evidence that fluid overload was responsible for ICU readmission in liver transplant patients.[148] This, however, must be balanced against the risks of hypovolemia, which could cause renal failure and may increase the risk of hepatic artery and portal vein thrombosis. Preexisting pulmonary hypertension does not dissipate immediately after transplantation and children who previously took prostaglandins need to continue these infusions in the operating room and into the postoperative period. Systemic hypertension is common after liver transplantation and has been described in as many as one-third of patients.[149] It is typically related to cyclosporine therapy or chronic kidney disease.[150,151]

Almost all children require tracheal intubation and mechanical ventilation in the immediate postoperative period; however, some centers extubate those who are stable immediately after surgery. Early extubation may be associated with decreased morbidity and improved graft and recipient survival.[152] It is unclear if postoperative intubation is just an association or a cause of adverse outcomes. Children who may be appropriate candidates for early extubation (extubation in the operating room) include those with reduced blood loss, hemodynamic stability, alveolar-arterial gradient less than 150 mm Hg, and absence of hepatic encephalopathy.[153] Children with important comorbidities such as respiratory insufficiency and reoperation are more likely to require continued intubation or reintubation.[154]

Postoperative ventilation may be more appropriate for smaller children who have received a relatively large graft and in children with underlying lung disease (hepatopulmonary syndrome). Ascites, pulmonary edema, and pleural effusions have been described after transplantation (possibly associated with the degree and duration of preoperative portal hypertension) and may necessitate prolonged mechanical ventilation.[155] Efforts to minimize atelectasis include positive-pressure ventilation with PEEP.[87] Diuretics may be needed on the second or third postoperative day to treat edema and effusions. There is speculation that prolonged mechanical ventilation may have a negative effect on the hemodynamics of transplant patients and may contribute to overall morbidity and mortality.[156] Increased levels of PEEP may contribute to this morbidity. Some have advocated for early extubation to decrease the incidence of pulmonary complications and to facilitate discharge from the ICU.[149]

Renal failure secondary to hepatorenal syndrome usually resolves after successful liver transplantation. The goal in the immediate postoperative period is to maintain normovolemia and to avoid nephrotoxic agents. These include aminoglycoside antibiotics and immunosuppressant agents such as cyclosporine and tacrolimus. The immunosuppressant agents may need to be delayed until renal function begins to improve.

Neurologic complications after liver transplantation are also common. In the adult population these complications occur in 10% to 30% of patients.[157] Pediatric information is lacking. In adults, the complications present as encephalopathy, seizures, or coma. The causes of encephalopathy and coma include drugs (immunosuppressive agents such as tacrolimus and OKT3), infection (meningitis and brain abscess), strokes (bleeding), and hyponatremia with central pontine myelinolysis. The most common cause of seizures is an adverse drug reaction associated with immunosuppressant drugs.[158] Hyponatremia can contribute to neurologic complications. If the correction proceeds faster than the recommended rate, there is weak evidence from an animal model that dexamethasone administered within 6 hours of the correction may minimize the risk of central pontine myelinolysis.[159]

Surgical complications that occur after transplant include vascular complications, acute rejection, and infections; frequent monitoring for their occurrence is important to ensure prompt management. Vascular complications include hepatic artery thrombosis, portal vein thrombosis, bleeding, and bowel perforation.[149,160] Hepatic artery thrombosis is identified with frequent hepatic Doppler flow imaging. Patients may undergo anticoagulation with aspirin, heparin, dextran, and alprostadil to reduce the risk of thrombosis.[160] Infections are common in immunosuppressed transplant patients and contribute to significant morbidity. The primary source for infections appears to be central venous access lines, percutaneous catheter drainage, and mechanical ventilation. Acute rejection should be suspected in patients with fever and increased liver enzymes. The diagnosis is made by histologic examination.[149]

Rejection is an immune response and efforts to understand and control this immune response lie at the heart of transplant medicine. Initial efforts to control the response involved suppressing the recipient's immune system. There has been a move away from immunosuppression to immunotolerance. Immunotolerance describes the concept of immune cells from both the recipient and the donor coexisting without attacking each other.[161] The goal of immunosuppression medication is to reach this state of tolerance. In this state of immunotolerance, minimal immunosuppression can be used. The benefits of decreasing immunosuppression include a reduced risk of infection, hypercholesterolemia, malignancy, hypertension, and diabetes mellitus. Protocols to induce tolerance include exposing patients to lymphoid-depleting agents (antilymphoid antibody) such as antithymocyte globulin before liver engraftment to reduce the antidonor response to a more controllable range and allow maintenance therapy (tacrolimus) to begin with one agent. Other agents are added if there is evidence of rejection.[162] The immunosuppressant agents currently used include calcineurin phosphatase inhibitors, such as tacrolimus and cyclosporine, that provide the mainstay of therapy. Other options include azathioprine or mycophenolate mofetil for patients who cannot tolerate the calcineurin phosphatase inhibitors because of toxicity. Adverse effects of the calcineurin phosphatase inhibitors include hypertension, tremor, and renal failure. Newer agents such as mammalian target of rapamycin inhibitors (e.g., everolimus IL-2; sirolimus, IL-5) and monoclonal antibodies against interleukins (e.g., basiliximab) are also being used.[163]

LONG-TERM ISSUES

Recipients of liver transplants return to the operating room for a variety of reasons (central line placement, wound irrigation, dental rehabilitation, bowel obstruction, cholangiogram, biliary dilation, esophagogastroduodenoscopy). A primary concern in the posttransplant patient is the adverse effects of immunosuppressant agents. Most organ systems become involved, and a thorough review of systems is important.

The cardiovascular effects of immunosuppressant agents include hypertension from cyclosporine and cardiomyopathy (rare) from tacrolimus.[30,164] Renal insufficiency can occur secondary to cyclosporine, diuretics, or hypertension. Baseline BUN and creatinine should be obtained preoperatively in patients with a history of renal insufficiency, and medications or their active metabolites (e.g., morphine 6-glucuronide, aminoglycosides) that are renally cleared must be adjusted or avoided. Hyperkalemia may accompany renal failure and should be evaluated before induction of anesthesia.

Pediatric liver transplant recipients can develop multiple hematologic abnormalities. Azathioprine can cause anemia, leucopenia, and thrombocytopenia. Another cause of anemia includes unrecognized gastrointestinal bleeding from steroid-induced ulcers. Patients who have been taking azathioprine should have a complete blood cell count before surgery, particularly if they are having a procedure that may involve blood loss.

The endocrine effects of chronic steroid exposure include diabetes, growth retardation, and adrenal insufficiency. Patients who are taking long-term steroid therapy need stress-dose steroids during the perioperative period (see Chapter 25). Those receiving insulin for diabetes need intraoperative blood glucose monitoring and dextrose-containing IV fluids if they are hypoglycemic or are at risk of developing hypoglycemia.

Most recipients of a liver transplant have been exposed to multiple procedures and may have significant anxiety in the preoperative period. These patients should receive an anxiolytic to reduce anxiety and the risk of postoperative behavioral changes.[165] Midazolam is an appropriate and safe medication, provided there is no evidence of residual hepatic encephalopathy. Anesthesia can be induced with an inhalational technique, provided oral intake guidelines have been followed and the liver graft is functioning normally. Children who are hospitalized, with sepsis, bleeding, encephalopathic, or rejection should have an IV induction and their airway secured with a tracheal tube. Isoflurane, sevoflurane, and desflurane may be used for maintenance of anesthesia.

Renal Transplantation

The causes of end-stage renal disease in children differ from those in adults. The main causes in adults are diabetes, hypertension, glomerulonephritis, and cystic kidney disease,[166] whereas the main causes in children are congenital anomalies of the kidneys or urinary tract, and acquired lesions such as glomerulonephritis, and focal segmental glomerulosclerosis (FSGS).[167] There are approximately 700 to 800 pediatric renal transplants performed in the United States yearly.[168] The number of children on the waitlist for kidney transplantation increased from 2000 in 2009 to a stable number of 2500 per year between 2014 and 2019.[167] From 2009 to 2019, the pediatric waitlist by age has also been stable with ~20% age <6 years, ~20% 6 to 11 years, and ~60% between 12 and 17 years of age.[167]

OPTN implemented changes to the allocation system for deceased donor kidneys, the kidney allocation system, to increase donor organs to highly sensitized patients, decrease regional variability in access, and increase donor organ longevity.[169] Before 2014, pediatric recipients received priority for all deceased donor kidneys less than age 35 years. However, since 2014, highly sensitized adults and former living donors are prioritized before pediatric patients, who then receive priority for the top 35% Kidney Donor Profile Index (KDPI).[169] KDPI is a scoring system derived from adult patient data that is applied to kidney donors to predict graft survival; however, this scoring system does not accurately predict pediatric graft survival.[170] Although 10% to 12% of deceased donor kidneys come from pediatric donors each year, if they are not within the top 35% KDPI, then they are not prioritized for pediatric recipients.[169,170] Since the kidney allocation system was implemented, young pediatric patients received fewer deceased donor kidneys from pediatric donors overall and instead received more kidneys from donors over age 35 years.[169] The importance of this change in donor allocation to pediatric recipients is reflected in the increased incidence of delayed graft function, a risk factor for decreased donor organ longevity, in the post-kidney allocation system era.[169]

Both graft and patient survival have improved dramatically over the past 4 decades.[166,168,171,172] Improvements in immune-suppression therapies, advancements in surgical technique, improved donor selection, and a greater understanding of pediatric pharmacokinetics have all contributed substantively to improving patient survival and quality of life. Patient survival is >80% at 10 years postrenal transplant.[173] Age-related changes in survival continue to exist and differ slightly from the earliest years of transplantation. Children <5 years of age have better graft survival, whereas adolescents have the worst outcome (Fig. 29.5).[166] Graft survival from living-related donors (LDs) appears slightly better than from deceased donors (DDs). Recipients who received a kidney transplant in 2012 to 2014, had 1- and 5-year graft survival of 95.7% and 83.2% for DD recipients and 96.9% and 91.4% for LD recipients.[167] Multivariate analysis of risk factors for graft loss include Black race, history of prior transplantation, more than five transfusions, and HLA-B mismatch (Table 29.3).[171]

PATHOPHYSIOLOGY

The pathophysiology of renal disease in children involves cardiovascular, hematologic, and metabolic abnormalities. Cardiovascular changes include hypertension, coronary artery disease, dyslipidemia, left ventricular hypertrophy, and diastolic dysfunction.[174–187] Anemia occurs with a loss of renal function and as a consequence of decreased erythropoietin production.[188–190] Growth retardation is common, thought to be due to a combination of protein and calorie malnutrition, growth hormone resistance, anemia, renal bone disease, and chronic metabolic acidosis. In some instances, steroids used to treat an underlying pathology can further exacerbate growth retardation. Metabolic abnormalities and fluid and electrolyte disturbances are common in renal failure and are a consequence of the kidney's inability to eliminate waste products and regulate fluids and electrolytes. Hyperkalemia is a potential life-threatening complication of end-stage renal disease. Metabolic acidosis is a consequence of the failing kidney to excrete an acid load and can exacerbate hyperkalemia. Renal osteodystrophy occurs secondary to an increased concentration of parathyroid hormone and to decreased concentrations of active vitamin D. Because growth retardation and nutritional insufficiency are common in children with end-stage renal disease, cognitive function[191–196] and development can also be impaired.[191–194]

SURGICAL TECHNIQUE

The surgical techniques used in the pediatric recipient differ from those in adults and depend on the child's size and underlying pre-existing abnormalities. The surgical approach may be either intra-peritoneal or extraperitoneal. The extraperitoneal approach may be more technically difficult than the intraperitoneal approach in younger recipients. Native kidneys are removed either concurrently or (ideally) in advance. Native nephrectomy may be required for polycystic kidney disease, uncontrollable hypertension, urinary tract infection, or nephrotic syndrome with its associated hypoal-buminemia, malnutrition, and hypercoagulability.[197–200] The risks associated with concurrent native nephrectomy include increases in surgical time and cadaveric graft ischemic time. This approach is also a risk factor for ATN in the grafted organ.

In children >20 kg in weight, the surgical approach is similar to that in adult recipients. A lower-right quadrant incision is used, the kidney is placed in the iliac fossa, and the vascular anastomoses are to the common iliac vein and artery.[198,199] This extraperitoneal approach has the advantage of increased ease of future graft biopsy and offers the ability to resume peritoneal dialysis in cases of delayed graft failure.[166] In the past, the donor organs for renal transplantation in children <20 kilograms in weight were restricted to those that were size-compatible. These small cadaveric donor organs presented technical challenges, sometimes resulting in a vascular thrombosis, acute rejection, and graft loss.[166,201,202] Adult-sized donor kidneys are now used in infants and young children. The surgical approach may use a midline incision with mobilization of the cecum and right colon or an alternate approach involving a right-lower quadrant incision and an extraperitoneal dissection. The donor organ may be anastomosed to either the common iliac artery and vein, or directly to the aorta and vena cava.[198,199,203–207]

ANESTHETIC MANAGEMENT
Preoperative Evaluation
Immediately before transplantation, the child should be hemodynamically stable and fluid/electrolyte imbalances corrected before transplantation; blood should be typed and crossed. It is important to assess urine output (anuric, polyuric) so that appropriate intraoperative fluid replacement can be administered before unclamping of the donor organ during surgery. Active infection is a contraindication to transplantation; any concurrent systemic disorders should be optimized. The unpredictable availability of cadaveric organs means that many patients who present for cadaveric transplantation present with full stomachs and appropriate precautions must be undertaken. The need for premedication should be assessed on an individual basis and either an oral or IV anxiolytic (midazolam) administered. If time permits, patients may receive immunotherapy perioperatively to assist developing immunotolerance[208] of the implanted graft and, potentially, delaying the administration of the nephrotoxic calcineurin phosphatase inhibitors. Infusion of these induction antilymphocyte antibody agents (alemtuzumab [Campath], antilymphocyte globulin [equine] [Atgam], and anti-thymocyte globulin [Thymoglobulin]) cause a cytokine release. This cytokine response, which includes fever, chills, rigors, and malaise, can be attenuated by pretreatment with acetaminophen, corticosteroids, and diphenhydramine.[208,209]

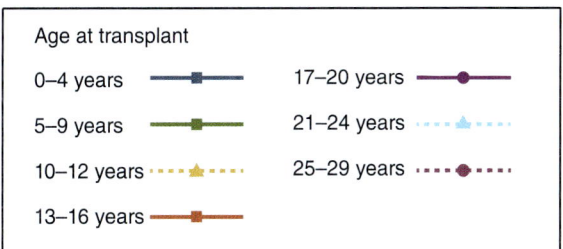

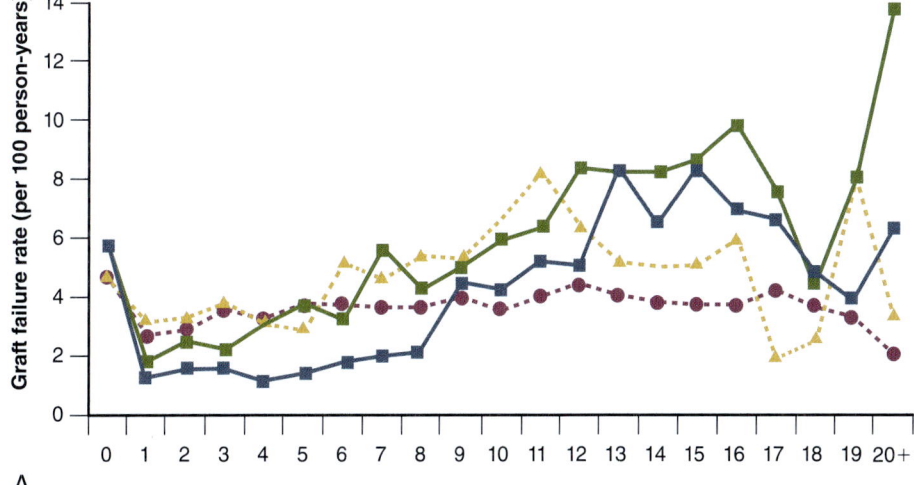

A

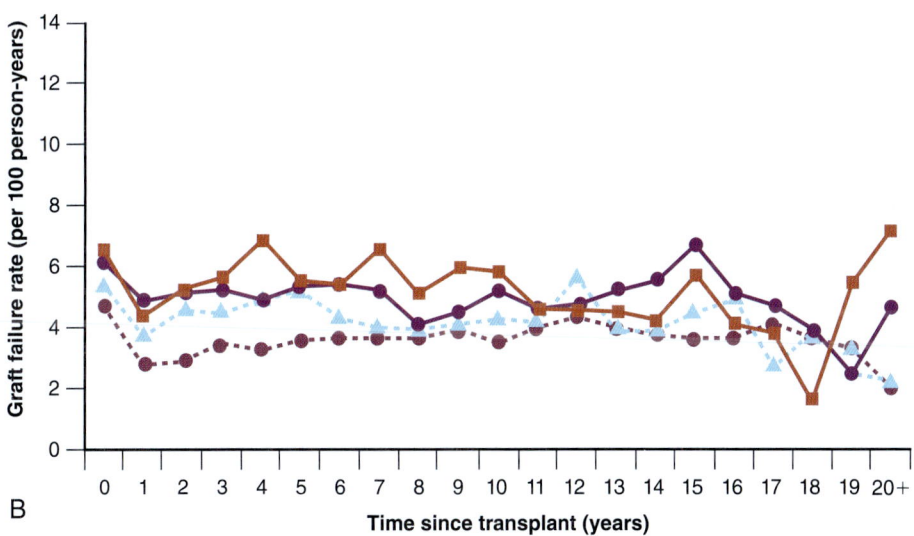

B

FIGURE 29.5 Age at transplant stratified crude death-censored graft failure rates (failures per 100 person-years) in each 1-year interval after transplant are shown for recipients0-4, 5 to 9 and 10-12 years at transplant in **A**, and 13 to 16, 17 to 20, and 21 to 24 years at transplant in **B**: recipients 25 to 29 years at transplant are shown as a reference in **A** and **B**. Timing of peak failure rates depended on age at transplant. Colored horizontal bars provide a guide as to the interval during which individuals of different ages at transplant would have reached the high-risk interval provide of 17 to 24 years of age identified with adjusted analysis. For example, individuals who were between 10 and 12 years at transplant would reach 17 years of age a minimum of 5 years posttransplant (12 plus 5) and would reach 24 years of age a maximum of 14 years posttransplant (10 plus 14). The youngest recipients showed peak failure rates 13 to 17 years posttransplant (when they had reached 17-22 years of age), whereas those who received transplants during adolescence were at highest risk in the years immediately after the transplant. The rates presented here are crude rates; the timing of peak failure rates for any age at transplant group depends on the mix of ages at transplant within each group. For example, in the 5-9 years at transplant group, the majority of patients were at the upper end of this age interval at transplant. Therefore, most would have reached 24 years of age by 15-16 years posttransplant; this may explain the decline in failure rates observed before the end of the identified high-risk interfal. Foster BJ. Association between age and graft failure rates in young kidney transplant recipients. *Transplantation.* 2011:92(11):1237-1243.

TABLE 29.3	Multivariate Model of Renal Graft Survival						
			LIVING DONOR		**DECEASED DONOR**	
Characteristic	Comparison Group	Reference Group	Rh	P Value	Rh	P Value
Recipient age	≥24 months	<24 months	1.23	0.0698	0.67	0.0036
Transplant history	Prior transplants	No prior transplants	1.50	<0.0001	1.45	<0.0001
Induction therapy	Induction	No induction	0.84	0.0051	0.92	0.1405
Transfusion history	>5	≤5	1.22	0.0164	1.25	0.0006
HLA-B mismatch	0 mismatches	1–2 mismatches	1.32	0.0183	1.15	0.017
HLA-DR mismatch	0 mismatches	1–2 mismatches	0.82	0.0532	1.13	0.0333
Recipient race	Black	Non-black	1.94	<0.0001	1.58	<0.0001
Dialysis history	Prior dialysis	No prior dialysis	1.16	0.0375	1.23	0.0326
Cold storage time	>24 hours	≤24 hours	—	—	1.15	0.0201
Native nephrectomy	Not removed	Tissue removed	0.86	0.0264	0.92	0.2335
Gender	Male	Female	0.88	0.0382	0.85	0.0039
Transplant year	Per year 1987–2010		0.95	<0.0001	0.94	<0.0001

Rh, Relative hazard, the ratio of two hazard rates.
From Smith JM, Martz K, Blydt-Hansen TD. Pediatric kidney transplant practice patterns and outcome benchmarks, 1987–2010: a report of the North American Pediatric Renal Trials and Collaborative Studies. *Pediatr Transplant*. 2013;17(2):149-157.

Anesthetic Induction

Anesthesia may be induced either intravenously or by inhalation. Succinylcholine may be used in the absence of contraindications such as hyperkalemia, although chronic hyperkalemia is not a contraindication to succinylcholine (see Chapter 5). Because renal failure affects both protein binding and the volume of distribution of drugs, anesthetic agents and adjuncts should be titrated to effect. One should not assume the new graft will function fully immediately after decannulation of the vessels. Drugs that undergo organ-independent elimination (cisatracurium, remifentanil), do not depend on renal elimination (morphine-6-glucuronide), do not rely exclusively on the kidney for metabolism (propofol), and have metabolites that are inactive (midazolam, fentanyl) are preferred. Drug metabolites that are eliminated through the kidney and are toxic (i.e., meperidine) should be avoided entirely. Although rocuronium is eliminated by both the kidney and the liver, children in renal failure are no more sensitive to the drug nor do they demonstrate an increased duration of action for a given dose compared with children with normal renal function.[210] However, the onset of action of rocuronium may be delayed in renal insufficiency and failure.

Monitors and Vascular Access

Standard monitors, including invasive arterial and central venous catheters if indicated, should be placed after induction of anesthesia. The need for vascular access reflects third-spacing requirements and the potential for brisk blood loss inherent in a prolonged intraabdominal procedure in which large arteries and veins must be accessed directly. Central venous access should be considered, depending on the type and preparation of intravenous immunosuppression the patient will require in the perioperative setting. Urine output may not reflect the child's intravascular volume status during the surgery as the native kidney may be dysfunctional, the grafted kidney may be discontinuous from the urinary catheter, the grafted kidney may not begin to function immediately, or the reperfused graft may develop polyuria.[197,198]

Smaller-sized children will have the most severe fluid shifts and will be the most vulnerable to graft hypoperfusion. In addition, the use of adult donors in small infants sequesters a disproportionate amount of the infant's blood volume and CO,[197,198,211,212] necessitating large amounts of fluids or blood transfusion to adequately perfuse the donor kidney. To prevent this possibility, the CVP should be maintained near the upper limit of normal immediately before declamping the vessels. Accordingly, central venous and arterial pressures should be monitored intraoperatively and postoperatively, although the need for invasive arterial monitoring must be balanced against the rare possibility of the need for an atrioventricular fistula in the future.[197,198,212]

Maintenance of Anesthesia

Virtually all combinations of anesthetic agents and anesthetic techniques have been used. Combined general-regional techniques have been employed, but they have been associated with larger intraoperative fluid requirements and the need for IV opioid supplementation in half the patients.[213] A hypnotic drug supplemented with an opioid to minimize the inhalational anesthetic requirements is common. Avoiding nitrous oxide in a long intraabdominal case is prudent. One nonrandomized, single-center study of 240 patients reported similar creatinine values in patients anesthetized with sevoflurane and isoflurane with slightly greater blood urea values and reduced urine volumes in the sevoflurane patients.[214] However, the use of sevoflurane in renal transplant recipients has not resulted in any negative outcomes.[214,215]

The anesthetic prescription should account for the hemodynamic conditions needed to maintain adequate perfusion of the donor kidney. Optimal hemodynamic conditions for reperfusion are more important when the size of the native organ is discrepant from the graft. At the extreme, aggressive fluid management would be required in an infant who is scheduled to receive an adult graft. In children, the CVP should be maintained at 8 to 12 cm H_2O and 16 to 20 cm H_2O immediately before declamping the renal vessels,[205,212] with most centers recommending pressures in the middle range.[198] Some authors suggest a systolic blood pressure in excess of 120 mm Hg[198] and mean arterial pressure exceeding 65 to 70 mm Hg.[197,198] Surgeons and anesthesiologists should confer before and during the transplant to ensure that the CVP and blood pressure target values are achieved and maintained once the donor kidney has been reperfused and is making urine. In the smaller child, especially those receiving disproportionately large donor kidneys, a large percent of the child's blood volume will be sequestered in the graft, volume that will have to be rapidly replaced to prevent hypotension and hypoperfusion of the newly grafted kidney.[197,198,212] The arterial anastomosis may have to be partially clamped during this period, until the hemodynamics are stabilized or the vessels repeatedly clamped and unclamped while the preload is increased to maintain stable hemodynamics with the clamps completely removed. Low dose heparin (10 units/kg) may be requested by the surgeon before incising the aorta for anastomosis. Both preload supplementation with blood, crystalloid, and colloid, and possible dopamine infusion to optimize CO may be necessary.[197,198] Furosemide and mannitol are administered at the completion of the vascular anastomoses to promote a diuresis that will continue postoperatively and necessitates continued large-volume resuscitation to maintain adequate perfusion to the donor kidney. Sodium bicarbonate may be administered after aortic unclamping to attenuate the underlying acidosis,[197–200] which worsens during the procedure. Frequent monitoring of the patient's arterial blood gas and electrolytes is essential to detect the possibility of hyperkalemia. Hyperkalemia can be treated with hyperventilation, calcium and bicarbonate, glucose and insulin, and β-adrenergic agents (see also Chapter 7). Avoidance of blood products is desirable, as patients with more than five lifetime transfusions are at increased risk of ATN, but transfusion may be necessary in an infant receiving an adult kidney. Although anemia should be avoided in the chronic management of the renal transplant patient, an optimal hematocrit in the immediate postoperative period has not been identified.

Immediate Postoperative Management

In the immediate postoperative period, maintenance of the child's blood volume remains important. Most patients can be extubated in the operating room. In small children, volume resuscitation required to adequately perfuse the graft may preclude early extubation.[199,205,212,213] Maintenance of an adequate blood volume continues into the postoperative period, where usually copious urine output is replaced milliliter for milliliter.[197–199,206,212] Prevention of graft hypoperfusion and subsequent ATN potentially prevents acute rejection,[202] as ATN in the early postoperative period is a major risk factor for graft loss.[216,217] Maintenance of the circulating blood volume continues to be important even in the late postoperative period. Preservation of perfusion pressure and circulating blood volume to the donor kidney should be considered during subsequent general anesthetics in renal transplant recipients (e.g., ureteral stent removal under anesthesia).

LONG-TERM ISSUES

Much has been accomplished in preservation of graft function for kidney transplant patients. Unfortunately, cardiovascular morbidity, infection, and malignancy are the major long-term concerns. Almost half of renal transplant recipients die with a functioning graft.

Infection

Success with immunotolerance for transplant recipients places the patient at risk for opportunistic infections. Fungal and bacterial infections are most common in the first 30 days after renal transplant with activation of latent pathogens such as Epstein-Barr virus (EBV) or cytomegalovirus (CMV) occurring after the first 30 days.[173] After the first 5 months, infection is a greater cause of hospitalization in the transplanted patient than acute rejection; in particular, fungal infection is a major risk for graft loss.[217,218] EBV–related adenotonsillar hypertrophy is common in the transplant population, occurring in 11 of 16 patients in one series.[219] Risk factors for EBV–related adenotonsillar hypertrophy include young age and seronegativity at time of transplant.[220,221] Posttransplant lymphoproliferative disorder (PTLD), a result of EBV infection, is common and occurs earlier in the renal transplant population (1%–2% within the first 5 years after transplant) but is not a contraindication to later retransplantation.[222–225] Human BK polyomavirus (BKPyV) is common in the general population as a latent infection of the urinary tract, but in pediatric postrenal transplant patients, BKPyV can cause nephropathy associated with acute rejection and graft failure.[173]

Malignancy

Malignancy is a major concern after renal transplantation in children, estimated to be 10 times greater than that of the general pediatric population. The crude estimate is about 2.5%, with greater than 82% lymphoproliferative in nature.[172]

Summary

Anesthetic management of the pediatric renal transplant patient may be complicated by many factors. Impaired renal function may be present before and after transplant. Comorbidities because of impaired renal function are numerous and may require altered anesthetic management. Although the renal transplant patient has a lifetime of medical issues, the continued function of the transplanted kidney allows for near-normal function, growth, and development. Therefore the ultimate goals of management are the preservation of the graft, thereby improving the quality of life.[226]

Cardiac Transplantation

Adrian Kantrowitz performed the first heart transplant in an infant in 1967.[227] Since that time, pediatric heart transplantation has matured considerably and is now an established treatment for children with CHD and heart failure unresponsive to other therapy.[228] The indications for pediatric cardiac transplantation continue to evolve; however, donor organ availability remains the major limiting factor.[229,230] Improved graft and child survival, fewer side effects, and an improved quality of life are the result of advancements in immunosuppression coupled with a better understanding of rejection. Unfortunately, infection, rejection, and posttransplant neoplasia continue to be the major causes of death.

DEMOGRAPHICS AND EPIDEMIOLOGY

Cardiac transplantation is a valuable treatment option for a broad range of causes of pediatric heart failure. The distribution of pediatric heart transplant recipients by age has remained stable for over 20 years with ~24% of the pediatric recipients younger than 1 year of age, ~23% between 1 and 5 years, ~15% between 6 and 10 years, and ~38% between 11 and 17 years (Fig. 29.6).[231] The major indications for pediatric heart transplant are congenital heart disease (CHD), cardiomyopathy, and retransplant. The frequency of these indications for transplantation varies by age

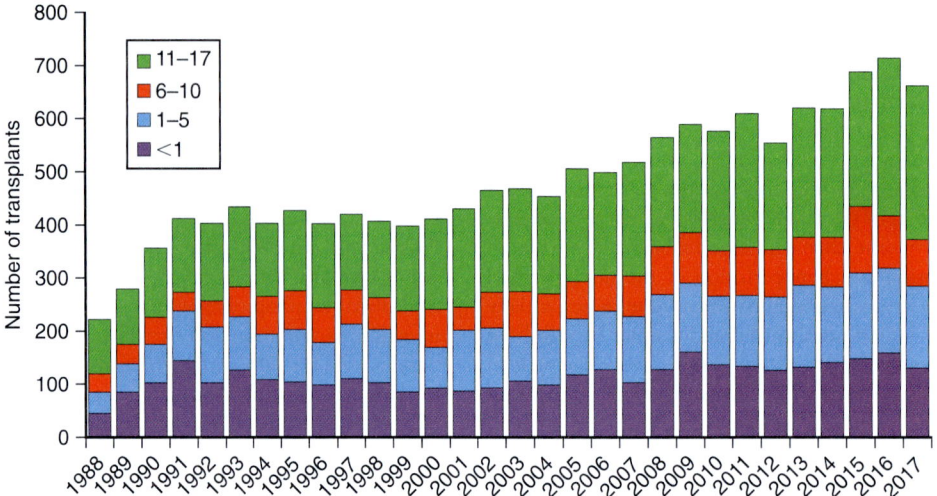

FIGURE 29.6 Age distribution of pediatric heart recipients by year of transplant. (From Rossano JW, Tajinder PS, Cherikh WS. The Registry of the International Society for Heart and Lung Transplantation: Twenty-second Pediatric Heart Transplantation Report—2019; focus theme: donor and recipient size match. *J Heart Lung Transplant.* 2019;38(10):1015-1066.)

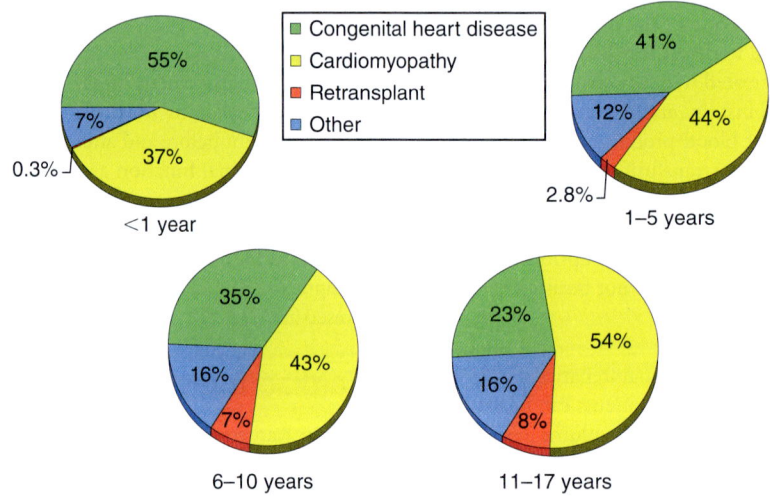

FIGURE 29.7 Diagnosis in pediatric heart transplant recipients by age group. (From Rossano JW, Wida SC, Chambers DC. The Registry of the International Society for Heart and Lung Transplantation: Twentieth Pediatric Heart Transplantation Report—2017; focus theme: allograft ischemic time. *J Heart Lung Transplant.* 2017;36[10]:1060-1069.)

group. In infants younger than 1 year of age, the primary indication for cardiac transplantation is a severe structural congenital cardiac defect, and the secondary indication is cardiomyopathy.[231] Cardiomyopathies represent the most common indication for heart transplant in children between 1 and 17 years of age, whereas CHD represents a decreasing proportion with increasing age (Fig. 29.7).[231]

PATHOPHYSIOLOGY OF THE DISEASE

The key to safe perioperative management of children presenting for heart transplantation requires an understanding of the basic cardiac anatomy and pathophysiology. Many transplant recipients with CHD have underlying lesions that alter the balance between systemic and pulmonary blood flow. The hemodynamic effects that accompany normal anesthetic management can radically alter

this balance and thereby result in the recipient's deterioration. Other recipients have marginal cardiac output secondary to their underlying myopathies or structural defects that hinder normal myocardial function.

CONGENITAL HEART DISEASE

This group of children includes those with complex lesions for which no option for palliation exists, children with end-stage heart failure after surgical repair of congenital heart defects, children with failed palliation for single-ventricle physiology (Fontan type), and neonates with hypoplastic left heart syndrome (HLHS). This population of patients is growing in incidence at US centers that perform large-volume heart transplants, which are defined as those performing greater than 10 pediatric heart transplants per year.[231] Children with CHD who undergo transplantation may have undergone surgical palliation with successful early results. They present later in life with dilated cardiomyopathies secondary to long-standing valvular regurgitation, ventricular outflow tract obstruction, or dysrhythmias. The majority of these children have single-ventricle physiology and are referred to as "failing the Fontan" procedure.[232–236] Although the right ventricle has been shown to be capable of adapting to work as the "systemic" ventricle in cases of HLHS or in children who have undergone an "atrial-type" switch operation for transposition of the great vessels, systemic right ventricles fail with time and develop both systolic and diastolic dysfunction. Transplantation is indicated in these children when they have acute decompensated heart failure refractory to medical therapy and not amenable to other reparative surgery or palliation.

DILATED CARDIOMYOPATHY

Dilated cardiomyopathy is the most common cardiomyopathy and reason for heart transplantation in children. The etiology is often unknown, but causes include infectious, drug-induced, ischemic, metabolic (disorders of fatty acid, amino acid, glycogen and mucopolysaccharide metabolism), or neuromuscular/genetic/mitochondrial disorders.[237,238] Dilated cardiomyopathy is characterized by systolic dysfunction and ventricular dilation with signs and symptoms of congestive heart failure. Predictors of poor outcome include a family history of cardiomyopathy, syncope, ventricular arrhythmia, left ventricular end-diastolic pressure greater than 25 mm Hg, and left ventricular ejection fraction less than 30%.

HYPERTROPHIC CARDIOMYOPATHY

Hypertrophic cardiomyopathy is a concentric thickening of the left ventricular wall not caused by a downstream obstruction that can lead to both a fixed and a dynamic obstruction to left ventricular outflow (see Chapter 14). A large septal muscular prominence can lead to mitral regurgitation secondary to abnormal systolic anterior motion of the mitral valve leaflets. The majority of hypertrophic cardiomyopathy is idiopathic (>70%), whereas inborn errors of metabolism (e.g., Pompe disease), malformation syndromes (e.g., Noonan, Beckwith-Wiedemann syndromes), and children with neuromuscular disorders account for the remainder.[239] Those who present as infants with hypertrophic cardiomyopathy have the worst outcome. If there is evidence of obstruction, more than 25% of infants will manifest congestive heart failure with symptoms of failure to thrive and feeding intolerance. Risk factors for sudden death include a family history of sudden death,[240,241] marked concentric left ventricular wall thickness, age at presentation, and a smaller fractional shortening z score.[242] The indication for transplantation is a progression to dilated or restrictive cardiomyopathy.

RESTRICTIVE CARDIOMYOPATHY

Restrictive cardiomyopathies are uncommon disorders with generally poor prognoses that are associated with infiltration of the myocardium, such as glycogen storage disease, amyloidosis, mucopolysaccharidosis, hemochromatosis, sickle cell disease,[243] and sarcoidosis. Myocardial infiltration results in diastolic dysfunction and diminished stroke volume. Endocardial fibroelastosis also causes a restrictive cardiomyopathy and an increased pulmonary vascular resistance (PVR).[244,245] The increased PVR is secondary to an increased left ventricular end-diastolic pressure with associated increases in pulmonary arterial pressure. The poor survival rates after diagnosis of restrictive cardiomyopathy prompt early consideration for transplantation.[246]

REPEAT TRANSPLANTATION

Repeat transplantation is uncommon in children, representing only 2.7% of all transplants in 2017.[247] Over the last decade, retransplant has accounted for between 2.7% and 7% of all pediatric cardiac transplants. Most cases of retransplantation occur at least 5 years after initial transplant and the indication is moderate graft vasculopathy with or without abnormal ventricular function.[229] Overall survival is lower compared with primary transplantation, irrespective of the cause for the primary transplant, whether it was dilated cardiomyopathy or congenital heart disease.[248,249]

CONTRAINDICATIONS

Contraindications to pediatric cardiac transplantation include multiple severe congenital anomalies, prematurity (<36 weeks), low birth weight (<2 kg), ectopia cordis, diffuse pulmonary artery hypoplasia, pulmonary venous hypoplasia, active malignancy, active infection, severe metabolic disease, and irreversible noncardiac end-organ damage. These contraindications are considered by some to be relative, rather than absolute, contraindications to cardiac transplantation. For instance, combined heart/liver, heart/lung, heart/kidney transplants are performed,[250,251] whereas advances in HIV treatment have led to the consideration of transplantation in HIV-positive patients.[229,252] PVR, and the potential reversibility of an elevated PVR, is usually assessed during cardiac catheterization. Although the upper limit of PVR associated with successful cardiac transplantation has not been established in children, most centers generally limit transplantation to those with a PVR less than 6 Wood units/m^2 or a transpulmonary pressure gradient of 15 mm Hg or less.[253] Some centers accept an increased PVR; however, it is understood that there is a greater risk of early mortality from right ventricular failure.[254,255] Finally, severe psychosocial problems, the lack of reliable caretakers, and an unstable family structure are critical factors in the decision to offer transplantation as a treatment option.

WAITLIST AND DONOR SELECTION

The waitlist mortality rate for pediatric heart transplant recipients was ~16% in the United States between 1999 and 2004.[256] The mean time from listing for transplant to actual surgery is about 3 months but varies with the child's age, blood group, and list status. With increasing use of ventricular assist devices (VADs), the waitlist mortality rate in the United States from 2005 to 2012 decreased to 8% despite an increase in mean waiting time.[257] Waitlist mortality remained high in high-risk VAD candidates, specifically patients less than 10 kg and those with CHD.[257] Infants experience the greatest waitlist mortality with risk factors that include weight less than 3 kg, high level of invasive support, and children with CHD requiring prostaglandin infusion.[258]

In July 2016, changes were made by UNOS and OPTN in an attempt to decrease waitlist mortality and reduce the disparities in outcomes that exists between patients listed for transplant with CHD compared to dilated cardiomyopathy (Table 29.4).[259] The changes included redefining the criteria for pediatric heart status 1A and 1B, as well as criteria and allocation priority for ABO-incompatible (ABOi) heart transplants.[260] The immaturity of the infant immune system and the lack of production of ABO

TABLE 29.4	OPTN/UNOS Heart Allocation Policy

Pediatric Status 1A Requirements

1. Continuous mechanical ventilation and admitted to the hospital where the candidate is registered

2. Assistance of an intraaortic balloon pump and admitted to the hospital where the candidate is registered

3. Ductal dependent pulmonary or systemic circulation, with ductal patency maintained by stent or prostaglandin infusion and admitted to the hospital where the candidate is registered

4. Congenital heart disease diagnosis, requiring infusion of multiple intravenous inotropes or a high dose of a single intravenous inotrope, and admitted to the transplant hospital where the candidate is registered

5. Assistance of a mechanical circulatory support device

Pediatric Status 1B Requirements

1. Infusion of one or more inotropic agents but does not qualify for pediatric status 1A

2. Less than 1 year old at the time of the candidate's initial registration and has a diagnosis of hypertrophic or restrictive cardiomyopathy

antibodies during the first 3 to 6 months of life provide a unique opportunity for ABOi heart transplantation. Multiple studies have documented similar survival and freedom from rejection similar to ABO-compatible donors[261,262]; ABOi heart transplantation has succeeded in reducing waitlist time mortality in Canada,[263] with similar results from the Pediatric Heart Transplant Registry that includes infant heart transplants from Canada, the United States, and the United Kingdom.[258,264,265] In an effort to increase infant donor heart utilization, UNOS/OPTN changed the isohemagglutinin titer to 1:16 from 1:4 or less for status 1A/1B candidates who are 1 year of age or older but registered before their second birthday. Initial evaluation of the effects of the 2016 changes shows an increase in the proportion the status 1A patients with CHD, but no improvement in waitlist mortality for patients with CHD. Waitlist mortality did not change for patients with dilated cardiomyopathy and waitlist mortality worsened for those with restrictive and hypertrophic cardiomyopathy.[259]

Donor selection for pediatric heart transplantation is often complicated by difficult social settings associated with the death of the donor. The increasing frequency of donation after circulatory determination of death also creates a potentially controversial mechanism to increase the donor pool (see also Chapter 3).[266,267] Donor size is also an important factor to consider in pediatric cardiac transplantation. Donor-to-recipient weight ratios up to 3.0 have been used successfully. In a comparison with more equally matched donor/recipient weight ratios, children who received hearts from oversized donors had no differences in ICU ventilator days, fractional shortening as assessed by echocardiography, ability to close the chest, or duration of inotropic support.[268] In contrast to the use of oversized donor organs, undersized donor organs were associated with an increased rate of donor organ failure. Recipient PVR is a major determinant for appropriate donor selection, and larger donor hearts should be considered for those with increased PVR to permit the right ventricle to compensate for the increased afterload.[269] Myocardial preservation of the donor organ is aimed at minimizing the ischemia time. Greater than 4 hours of ischemia time is independently associated with increased 1-year and 5-year mortality.[270]

PREOPERATIVE EVALUATION

A comprehensive, multidisciplinary evaluation of a potential cardiac allograft recipient is required to determine the recipient's suitability for transplantation. This evaluation includes an assessment of the child's underlying cardiopulmonary, hepatic, renal, neurologic, infectious disease, and immune system status, as well as socioeconomic and psychosocial function (Table 29.5).

Assessment of cardiopulmonary function usually begins with a thorough history with attention to exercise tolerance, oxygen requirements, and need for diuretics and inotropic support. Examination of the ECG, chest radiographs, echocardiograms, and Holter monitors may be helpful in the discovery of pleural or pericardial effusions, conduction disturbances, cardiac function, and arrhythmias. Radionuclide angiography may be useful in defining systemic ventricular dysfunction in children with complex cardiac morphology. The pretransplant assessment ultimately includes cardiac catheterization with angiography. The anatomy and hemodynamics of the recipient must be carefully delineated because these factors influence anesthetic management, surgical donor harvesting, and recipient transplant technique. For instance, in children with unrepaired HLHS, the donor harvest team must harvest a large segment of donor aorta to facilitate reconstruction of the recipient aorta. Determination of the pulmonary vascular resistance index (PVRI), transpulmonary gradient (TPG), and reactivity of the pulmonary vascular bed to pharmacologic manipulation is crucial to the assessment of suitability for cardiac transplant:

$$PVRI \ (units/m^2) = PAP \ (mm\ Hg) - PAWP \ (mm\ Hg)/CI \ (L/min/m^2)$$
$$TPG \ (mm\ Hg) = PAP \ (mm\ Hg) - PAWP \ (mm\ Hg),$$

where PAP is the mean pulmonary artery pressure, PAWP is the mean pulmonary artery wedge pressure, and CI is the cardiac index.

An endomyocardial biopsy can identify acute myocarditis and myocardial infiltrates. Pulmonary function studies may be useful in older children with chronic lung disease.

Laboratory evaluation should include serum electrolytes, complete blood cell count with differential, coagulation profile, viral titers for possible latent viral infections such as coronavirus, CMV, and EBV, and metabolic or genetic workups. Donor matching is based on ABO typing, although transplantation of ABOi hearts is an increasingly used option in infants.[264,271,272] and is also being offered to older children.[273,274] The use of triple-volume exchange transfusions also minimizes the potential reaction to maternally transmitted preformed ABO antibodies.[275]

Another important laboratory assessment is a panel reactive antibody (PRA) screen. Panel reactive antibodies are pre-formed circulating human leukocyte antigen (HLA) alloantibodies that, in high titers, are associated with diminished graft survival.[276-278] HLA matching with a donor is not possible due to time constraints. Therefore, listed patients undergo PRA screens for "virtual crossmatching." HLA antibodies arise from blood transfusions and the use of homograft material.[279] A patient with a PRA screen >10% is considered sensitized. From 1992 to 2000, ~7% of recipients had a PRA screen >20%. In recent years, 2010 to 2018, perhaps driven by the increased use of mechanical circulatory support and resultant exposure to multiple blood transfusion, 24% of recipients had a PRA screen >20% with 6% of recipients with a PRA screen >80%.[280] Treatments to reduce PRAs are institution specific, rapidly evolving, and have included IV immunoglobulin, cyclophosphamide, and plasmapheresis.[281]

TABLE 29.5 | Routine Precardiac Transplant Evaluation

History and Physical Examination

Age, height, weight, body surface area

Diagnoses

Medical history

Medications

Allergies

Immunization record

Laboratory Data

Liver and kidney function studies

Urinalysis

Glomerular filtration rate

Prothrombin time/partial thromboplastin time/INR, platelet count

Complete blood cell count with differential

PPD skin test

Serologies for HIV, hepatitis, cytomegalovirus, Epstein-Barr virus, toxoplasmosis, syphilis

ABO type

Panel reactive antibody

Cardiomyopathy Workup

Thyroid function studies

Blood lactate, pyruvate, ammonia, acyl carnitine

Urine organic acids, acyl carnitine

Skeletal muscle biopsy

Karyotype

Cardiopulmonary Data

Electrocardiogram

Chest radiograph

Echocardiogram

Radionuclide angiography

Cardiac catheterization

Endomyocardial biopsy

Pulmonary function studies

Oxygen consumption

Psychosocial Evaluation

History of abuse or neglect

Parental substance abuse

Long-term supportive care and reliability of caregivers

Possible relocation

Consultations as Needed

Dental services

Social services

Other

INR, International normalized ratio; *PPD*, purified protein derivative.
Adapted from Boucek MM, Shaddy RE: Pediatric heart transplantation. In: Allen HD, Gutgesell HP, Clark EB, et al., eds. *Moss and Adams' Heart Disease in Infants, Children, and Adolescents Including the Fetus and Young Adult.* 6th ed. Philadelphia: Lippincott Williams & Wilkins; 2001:295-407.

Rituximab, an anti-CD20 antibody that targets B cells, and bortezomib, a proteasome inhibitor directed against plasma cells, can be used to reduce circulating antibodies.[282,283]

Medical stabilization of patients listed for heart transplant frequently includes the use of diuretics, inotropic agents, afterload reduction, arrhythmia therapy, and respiratory support including mechanical ventilation. β-Blockade therapy is also used in the management of children with dilated cardiomyopathy and chronic heart failure.[284,285] Those with severe chamber enlargement, arrhythmias, and low CO may require systemic anticoagulation to prevent thrombus formation and systemic embolization. Implantable defibrillators have been effective in children large enough for these devices, and biventricular pacing is showing promise as well.[286,287]

Children with end-stage myocardial failure will require mechanical circulatory support as a bridge to transplantation (see Chapter 19). The proportion of children bridged to transplant from mechanical circulatory support has steadily increased from ~22% in 2005 to ~36% in 2017.[247] Extracorporeal membrane oxygenation (ECMO) remains a time-limited bridge to transplant, whereas pulsatile VADs such as the Berlin Heart EXCOR (Berlin Heart GmbH, Berlin, Germany) in infants allows for more prolonged support with fewer complications. The Berlin EXCOR regulatory database shows a median duration of support of 40 days, with 75% survival at 12 months.[288] Intracorporeal continuous flow devices such as the HeartMate 3 (HM3, Abbott, Chicago, IL) and HeartWare HVAD (Medtronic, Minneapolis, MN) are used for adolescents and larger children. The use of these mechanical circulatory support devices has improved waitlist survival; however, sepsis, neurologic injury, bleeding, and thromboembolic events are serious complications.[289,290] Transplantation from ECMO continues to be associated with perioperative and early posttransplant mortality; however, children with transplantation from mechanical circulatory support devices such as a VAD have survival similar to those undergoing transplantation without mechanical circulatory support.[231,291]

CHD is the primary indication for cardiac transplantation in infants younger than 1 year of age. In many patients, the patency of the ductus arteriosus must be maintained with prostaglandin E_1 initially as a continuous infusion and perhaps by stenting the ductus in the catheterization laboratory later if a suitable donor organ is not found. Alteration of flow across the atrial septal defect can be addressed as well by the interventional cardiologist (see Chapter 20). If the balance between systemic and pulmonary blood flow cannot be managed medically, pulmonary artery banding may be necessary to reduce pulmonary over circulation while waiting for a donor organ.

SURGICAL TECHNIQUE

The original orthotopic technique devised by Lower and Shumway in adults was popular for many years in pediatric cases when the anatomy was straightforward.[292] This technique avoided individual systemic and pulmonary venous anastomoses by leaving a large cuff of right and left atrial recipient tissue behind and anastomosing the donor right and left atria to these cuffs. The resulting atrial chambers were a combination of donor and recipient atria that contracted asynchronously. Because the atrial contribution to cardiac output may be augmented with total cardiac transplantation, most centers have converted to the "bicaval" technique with a modification to use the standard left atrial anastomosis.[293–295] This technique improves sinus node function, causes less tricuspid regurgitation, and improves exercise tolerance.[296,297]

Cardiac transplantation in children with CHD may require surgery of greater complexity involving reconstruction of the great vessels or alterations in venous anastomoses. It is important that the donor-harvesting team understand the recipient's anatomy and the potential harvest needs that may require large portions of aorta, pulmonary arteries, and venae cavae. In children with HLHS who require aortic arch reconstruction, deep hypothermic circulatory arrest may be necessary.[298–300]

The recipient is placed on cardiopulmonary bypass (CPB) after median sternotomy with aortic and bicaval cannulation. Cannulation may be modified depending on the cardiac anatomy encountered. The aorta is cross clamped, and both the aorta and the pulmonary artery are divided at the level of their semilunar valves. The superior and inferior vena cavae are transected, preserving a cuff of atrial tissue on each to facilitate the anastomoses. The interatrial groove is prepared, and an encircling left atriotomy is performed and the recipient heart is removed from the field. The donor organ is prepared and brought to the field. The left atrial anastomosis is completed first, followed by the aortic anastomosis. A vent is placed in the left ventricular cavity for decompression and evacuation of air as the caval anastomoses are completed while the child is rewarming. The cross clamp is removed, and the donor heart is reperfused while the pulmonary arterial anastomosis is completed. Ventilation is resumed, and the child is separated from CPB after return of cardiac function is documented by TEE. Epicardial pacing wires are placed, mediastinal drainage tubes are positioned, and the chest is closed.

INTRAOPERATIVE PROBLEMS AND MANAGEMENT

Close coordination of operating room time with the donor team is needed to ensure the briefest possible ischemic time for the donor organ. The team should consider if anesthesia induction, line placement, or sternotomy may require additional time given the child's history. Crossmatched blood products should be available since this process can be prolonged in highly sensitized patients. Communication with the medical transplant team is needed to understand the immunosuppression induction plan as these medications may need to be administered by the anesthesia team.

Children listed for cardiac transplantation may be hemodynamically stable and living at home. Others may be on low dose vasoactive infusions or stable with mechanical circulatory support and extubated in an inpatient unit. In these children, preoperative fasting and NPO status may be an issue when a donor organ becomes available. The anesthesiologist must carefully assess the relative risks of a full stomach compared with the potential complications associated with hemodynamic changes and an unexpected difficult airway in a child undergoing a rapid-sequence induction. It is equally likely that the pediatric recipient is admitted to the ICU and requires a host of treatments designed to promote hemodynamic stability while a donor organ is sought. These children have minimal cardiovascular reserve. Anesthetic agents, positive-pressure ventilation, and surgical stress frequently result in hemodynamic instability. Anesthetic preparation should include the immediate availability of a variety of medications for the perioperative manipulation of myocardial function and hemodynamics.[301] For children with underlying CHD, the anesthesiologist needs to understand the child's underlying pathophysiology. The anesthetic management before CPB is similar to nontransplant cardiac surgery. For children with end-stage myocardial dysfunction, the sympathetic nervous system is chronically activated with downregulation of the cardiac β_1-receptors and an impaired response to β-agonists.[302] Reduced renal perfusion stimulates the renin-angiotensin system, leading to increases in vasoconstriction, venoconstriction, and increased intravascular volume. These compensatory changes further aggravate the congestive heart failure by increasing preload and afterload. A dysfunctional, dilated myocardium is very sensitive to changes in preload, afterload, heart rate, and contractility. Both systolic and diastolic myocardial function are impaired, and a high mean atrial pressure is needed to ensure adequate ventricular filling volume. Increasing heart rate results in a decreased diastolic filling time and, therefore, a diminution in stroke volume because of the poor systolic and diastolic ventricular function, atrial pressure increase, and atrial enlargement. There is a loss of preload reserve, resulting in cardiac output depending more on the heart rate. Finally, small increases in afterload increase end-systolic volume, decrease stroke output, and further decrease cardiac output. Dysrhythmias are poorly tolerated in these children.

More frequently, patients who present for heart transplant have been bridged with mechanical circulatory support. The level of circulatory support depends on the device. For patients with LVADs, right ventricular dysfunction should be assessed. Patients with mechanical circulatory support will often tolerate the hemodynamic changes of anesthesia induction better as their circulation is supported. Due to anticoagulation used during mechanical circulatory support, the primary concern pre-bypass is bleeding with sternotomy and dissection.

Premedication is best administered under monitored conditions. If the child was receiving supplemental oxygen, it should be continued during the preinduction period. Before induction, monitoring devices such as ECG, noninvasive blood pressure cuff, and pulse oximeter are applied. Meticulous airway management is critical because hypoxemia and hypercarbia may increase PVR and further decrease the cardiac output. A wide variety of anesthetic agents have been used depending on the nature of the cardiac disease and the risk of pulmonary aspiration. After induction, invasive monitoring does not differ from that used during routine pediatric cardiac open-heart surgery. Some centers avoid right internal jugular vein cannulation because that vessel may be repeatedly accessed for posttransplant endomyocardial biopsy. TEE is useful to assess graft function, mechanical issues, and pulmonary hypertension. Many experienced centers do not use pulmonary artery catheters routinely because the value of the information gained does not warrant the additional risk. In children who have undergone multiple cardiac operations, the potential risks of reoperation should be addressed and include the need for adequately sized vascular catheters, the availability of blood products and a rapid transfusion device in the operating room, the preparation for alternate cannulation sites, and the use of antifibrinolytics. Anesthesia is generally maintained with opioids, benzodiazepines, isoflurane, and a nondepolarizing neuromuscular blocking drug.[301]

The principles of CPB management are reviewed in Chapter 17 and are not different in a patient undergoing heart transplantation. One alteration is the use of exchange transfusion with the initiation of CPB in children with high PRA screens or in children receiving an ABOi transplant to reduce antibody concentration.[303] The use of ultrafiltration during CPB may be beneficial by removing free water, hemoconcentrating red blood cells and coagulation factors, and modulating the inflammatory response.[301,304–310]

In the preparation for termination of CPB, it is critical that the hemodynamics are optimized. A stable cardiac rhythm and acceptable heart rate are desirable. Chronotropic support using IV therapy with β-adrenergic agents or the use of epicardial pacing may be needed to maintain an appropriate heart rate between 120 and 150 beats/minute. The denervated transplanted heart does not respond in the normal fashion to hypotension. Medications with indirect cardiac effects such as atropine, glycopyrrolate, and ephedrine will likewise be ineffective. Direct-acting medications such as dopamine, dobutamine, epinephrine, and isoproterenol are required if inotropic or chronotropic support is needed (Table 29.6).[311] Some children benefit from vasodilator infusions to improve left ventricular stroke volume and cardiac output.[312] The use of inotropic agents to separate from CPB and provide early postoperative stability is common; the selection of drugs is based largely on the perceived balances between pulmonary and systemic vascular resistance, and myocardial dysfunction to blood pressure and cardiac output.[301] Ventilation should be managed to ensure mild respiratory alkalosis and adequate oxygenation. Factors that increase PVR such as hypothermia, acidosis, hypercarbia, hypoxemia, increased adrenergic tone secondary to light anesthesia, and polycythemia should be avoided. Children with increased PAP before bypass show a greater response to ventilatory changes than those without increased PAP. In addition, children with CHD and associated pulmonary hypertension may develop severe pulmonary hypertension in response to hypoxemia.[313–315] The narrow range of afterload that the donor right ventricle is capable of handling is critical; if success in managing the pulmonary hypertension with conservative methods fails, more aggressive pharmacotherapy is warranted. The use of prostaglandin, prostacyclin, nitroglycerin, high-dose milrinone, calcium channel blockers, sildenafil, and inhaled NO (iNO) have all been effective in treating pulmonary hypertension in children (see Chapter 16).[316–328] In extreme cases, mechanical assist devices or ECMO have been used (see Chapter 19).[329,330]

Dysrhythmias are common in the post-bypass period and, depending on the technique of implantation, there may be two independent P waves on the ECG, one from the recipient sinoatrial node and the other from the donor sinoatrial node. It is only the donor sinoatrial node that transmits impulses to the atrioventricular node and thus to the ventricle. The most common dysrhythmias are junctional rhythms, underscoring the utility of direct-acting β-agonists and epicardial atrioventricular sequential pacing. This denervated state results in the loss of the baroreceptor reflex, forcing cardiac output to depend primarily on venous return and circulating catecholamines; the denervated heart is unable to respond acutely to changes in the circulating blood volume and blood pressure.[331,332]

After separating from CPB, stabilizing hemodynamics, and controlling surgical bleeding, protamine sulfate is administered slowly to reverse anticoagulation. Risk factors for hypotension in children after protamine include female sex, larger protamine doses, and smaller heparin doses.[333] Transfusion of blood products should be guided by the balance of the need weighed against the associated risks of administration. Acid-base and electrolyte disturbances may be associated with large-volume transfusions. These disturbances may be lessened by washing the cells before transfusion.[334–336] Donor blood should be screened for CMV and, ideally, CMV-negative recipients should receive blood screened negative for CMV.[337] Leukocyte reduction by filtration may be associated with a diminished risk of exposure to CMV through transfusion.[338,339] Another concern associated with transfusion in cardiac transplant recipients is the risk of transfusion-associated graft-versus-host disease (TA-GVHD). This results from active T lymphocytes in the transfused blood of a recipient who is unable to reject them, such as a neonate, those undergoing chemotherapy, and the otherwise immunocompromised child.[340,341] To limit the risk of TA-GVHD in cardiac transplant recipients, some centers routinely gamma irradiate cellular blood products before administration. At recommended doses, gamma irradiation has an insignificant effect on platelet, red blood cell, or granulocyte function but it may increase the potassium concentrations (see Chapter 10).[342]

Transport of the child from the operating room proceeds as in any other open-heart procedure. In selected recipients with excellent allograft function and hemodynamics, the trachea may be extubated in the operating room or within a few hours of arrival in the ICU. It is important that these children are pain-free and ventilating adequately to prevent atelectasis, hypoxemia, or hypercarbia that may increase PAP and thus strain the donor right ventricle. Sedative agents such as dexmedetomidine may facilitate early extubation in these children.[343] Other children may require sedation and mechanical ventilation because of hemodynamic instability or delayed sternal closure, particularly if a large donor-to-recipient size mismatch is present.

IMMEDIATE POSTOPERATIVE MANAGEMENT

Early postoperative management consists primarily of maintaining hemodynamic stability. Infusions and fluid volume needs are adjusted to optimize the preload, afterload, cardiac output, and peripheral perfusion. Attention should be directed toward maintaining

TABLE 29.6	Properties of Vasoactive Drugs After Heart Transplantation				
Drug	Peripheral Vasoconstriction	Cardiac Contractility	Peripheral Vasodilation	Chronotropic Effect	Arrhythmia Risk
Isoproterenol	0	++++	+++	++++	++++
Dobutamine	0	+++	++	+	+
Dopamine	++	+++	+	+	+
Epinephrine	+++	++++	+	++	+++
Milrinone	0	+++	+	++	++
Norepinephrine	++++	+++	0	+	+
Phenylephrine	++++	0	0	0	0
Vasopressin	++++	0	0	0	0

Modified from Costanzo MR, Dipchand A, Starling R, et al. The International Society of Heart and Lung Transplantation guidelines for the care of heart transplant recipients. *J Heart Lung Transplant*. 2010;29(8):914-956.

normal acid-base and electrolyte balance. In some children, pulmonary hypertension remains a serious concern and management of sedation, ventilation, inotrope infusions, and pulmonary vasodilator administration is required to optimize right ventricular function. Ventilation modes may need to be adjusted to reduce the mean intrathoracic (airway) pressure. Additional approaches to manage right ventricular function are illustrated in Fig. 29.8. Renal dysfunction continues to be a major source of morbidity and mortality after cardiac transplantation; the UNOS database showed ~7% incidence of perioperative renal failure after pediatric heart transplantation.[344] Posttransplant survival is decreased in children with posttransplant renal failure. Risk factors for developing posttransplant renal failure include the use of ECMO, the need for mechanical ventilation, and inotropic support at the time of transplant listing. A peritoneal dialysis catheter placed during transplantation can be used to reduce ascites and improve ventilatory mechanics in those with right-sided heart dysfunction and to treat renal insufficiency. Arrhythmias in the postoperative period may herald rejection.

Induction of immunosuppression can begin with corticosteroids, antithymocyte immunoglobulin, or IL-2 receptor antagonists. Induction therapy has increased from ~59% of pediatric transplant patients during 2004 to 2009 to ~74% from 2010 to 2018, although there is no evidence that graft survival improves in primary pediatric heart transplantation with induction.[231,247] However, transplant recipients with panel reactive antibodies >50% or with congenital heart disease, benefit from induction immunosuppression as reflected by improved survival.[345] Maintenance therapy is guided largely by institutional experience and the recipient's clinical profile. The goal of maintenance therapy is to prevent acute and chronic rejection while minimizing the adverse effects of immunosuppression. All maintenance regimens involve a calcineurin phosphatase inhibitor (tacrolimus more commonly than cyclosporine) along with antiproliferative agents such as azathioprine or mycophenolate mofetil (CellCept). Corticosteroids may also be used, although most centers limit or avoid their long-term use. Sirolimus (rapamycin) is a macrolide antibiotic that acts synergistically with the calcineurin phosphatase inhibitors and can be used to reduce the dose of cyclosporine or tacrolimus. Sirolimus may also inhibit the process of coronary arteriopathy.[346]

First-line therapy to treat acute rejection is high-dose corticosteroids. Other agents, including monoclonal and polyclonal anti–T-lymphocyte antibodies, are reserved for refractory or recurrent severe acute rejection or rejection with severe hemodynamic compromise.

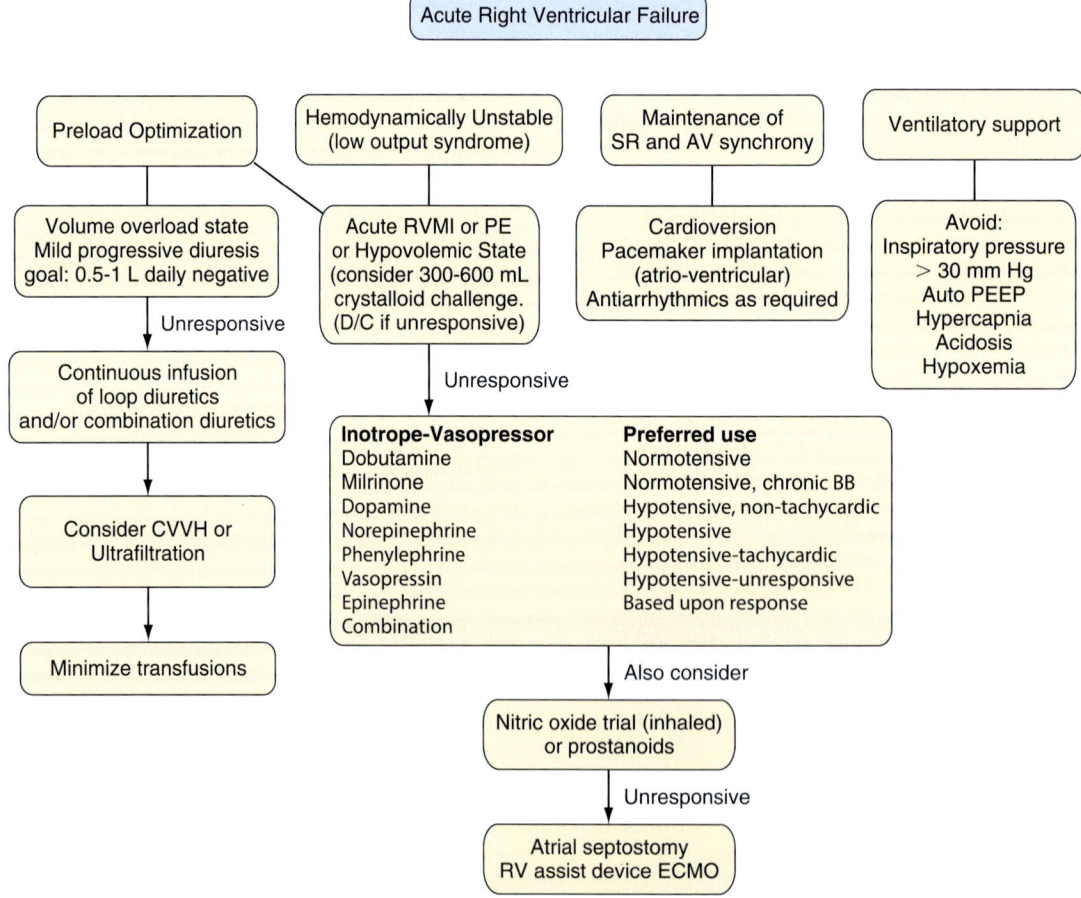

FIGURE 29.8 Management of right ventricular dysfunction. *AV,* Atrioventricular; *BB,* beta blocker therapy; *CVVH,* continuous venovenous hemofiltration; *D/C,* discontinue; *ECMO,* extracorporeal membrane oxygenation; *MI,* myocardial infarction; *PE,* pulmonary embolism; *PEEP,* positive end-expiratory pressure; *RV,* right ventricular; *RVMI,* right ventricular myocardial infarction; *SR,* sinus rhythm. (Modified from Haddad F, Hunt SA, Rosenthal DN, Murphy DJ. Right ventricular function in cardiovascular disease, part II: pathophysiology, clinical importance, and management of right ventricular failure. *Circulation.* 2008;117:1717-1731.)

Recurrent moderate rejection is usually controlled with modulation of the maintenance therapy dosing.[347]

Graft failure continues to remain the major cause of death after transplantation, with the greatest mortality in the first year post-transplant.[231] Experiencing an episode of rejection requiring treatment in the first year following transplant worsens the child's survival prospects. Fortunately, there has been a decline in treated rejection from hospital discharge to 1-year posttransplant. From 2004 to 2009, ~24% of recipients had an episode of treated rejection; this is down to ~13% from 2010 to 2018.[247,348] Some studies suggest that transplantation before 1 year of age offers protection from episodes of acute rejection and greater freedom from rejection and time to first rejection.[349] Monitoring and diagnosis of allograft rejection remain a challenge. The clinical assessment includes nursing and parental accounts of changes in the child's activity and appetite, nausea, emesis, malaise, resting heart rate 15 to 20 beats/minute above normal, and the presence of ectopy. Echocardiography plays a very important role in the postoperative follow-up, especially in neonates. These studies are performed frequently, especially in the first months after transplant. Acute changes in left ventricular end-diastolic dimension, posterior wall thickness, and shortening fraction are potential signs of acute rejection.[350] Endomyocardial biopsy remains the gold standard in the diagnosis of acute cardiac allograft rejection. The initial biopsy is performed 1 to 2 weeks following transplant. The biopsy schedule moving forward is institution specific and dependent on symptoms and prior episodes of rejection. In the first year, biopsies often occur every 3 months and then decrease to every 6 months or annually. A biopsy provides tissue for both precise documentation of the presence or absence of rejection and allows more accurate titration of immunosuppression to avoid the adverse effects of increased use of immunosuppression based on clinical and noninvasive examinations only. Biopsy specimens are analyzed for signs of humoral rejection, vascular rejection, and for evidence of lymphocytic accumulations in the graft interstitium and perivascular tissue; in severe cellular rejection, myocardial necrosis and polymorphonuclear cell infiltrates are evident. Over time, it is also possible to develop chronic rejection, which is primarily a vasculopathy.[351] This produces a diffuse and concentric stenosis affecting the mid and distal coronary arteries and is often asymptomatic. Although annual coronary angiography is recommended, accelerated graft arteriosclerosis is underestimated angiographically.

SURVIVAL AND QUALITY OF LIFE

The survival of pediatric heart transplant recipients continues to improve. The overall median survival for pediatric heart transplant recipients is grouped by age at the time of transplantation, with a median of 24.5 years for infants, 20.2 years for children with transplants at 1 to 5 years of age, 15.9 years for children with transplants at 6 to 10 years of age, and 14.3 years for adolescents with transplants at 11 to 17 years of age (Fig. 29.9).[247] Mortality in the first year after the transplant is the greatest, so the median conditional survival after 1 year is even better (Fig. 29.10). The most common causes of death in the first year after transplant include graft failure (~28%), multisystem organ failure (~17%), acute rejection (~12%), cerebrovascular event (~9%), and non–CMV infection (~8%) (see Table 29.7). By 10 years after transplant, graft failure and coronary artery vasculopathy account for most mortality. Patients who had transplants for the diagnosis of CHD have a greater risk for mortality after transplantation compared with those with a diagnosis of cardiomyopathy (Fig. 29.11). Other risk factors for mortality in the first year after transplant include retransplant, pretransplant ECMO support, and pretransplant dialysis.[231]

ANESTHESIA AND THE TRANSPLANTED HEART

Pediatric cardiac recipients often return to the operating room for noncardiac procedures. Preoperative evaluation requires an understanding of the unique features associated with the transplanted heart, such as its denervation, risk of vasculopathy (coronary artery disease), and arrhythmias.[301] The interaction of the immunosuppressive regimens with anesthetic agents and their association with hypertension and renal dysfunction are additional considerations. Interruption in the administration of immunosuppressive

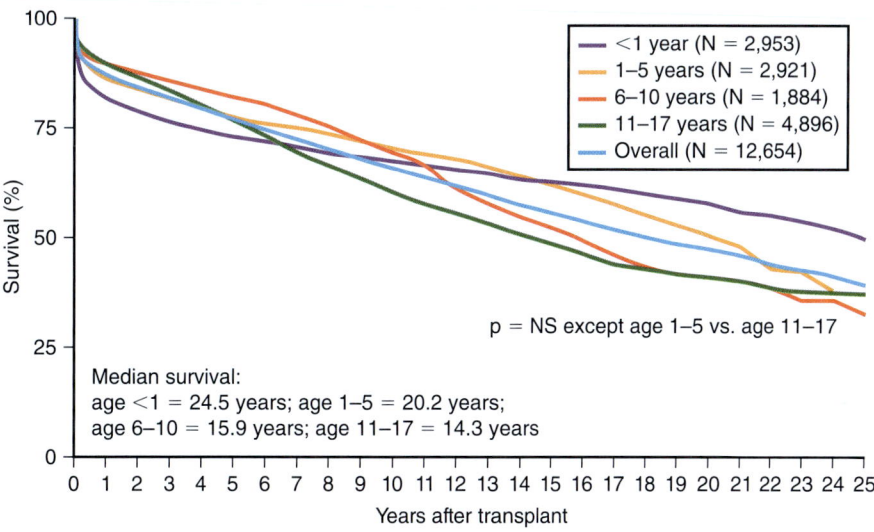

FIGURE 29.9 Survival curve for pediatric heart transplant recipients (Kaplan-Meier). (From Rossano JW, Tajinder PS, Cherikh WS. The Registry of the International Society for Heart and Lung Transplantation: Twenty-second Pediatric Heart Transplantation Report—2019; focus theme: donor and recipient size match. *J Heart Lung Transplant.* 2019;38[10]:1028-1041.)

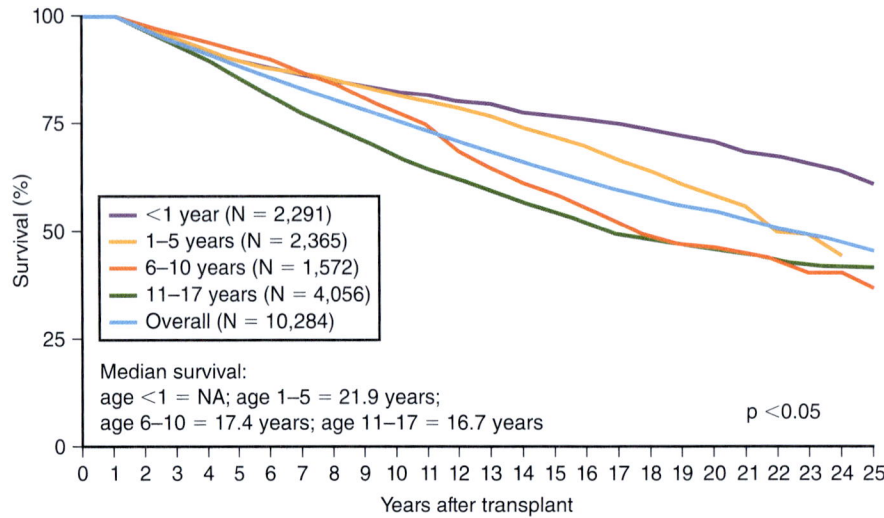

FIGURE 29.10 Conditional survival curve for pediatric heart transplant recipients (Kaplan-Meier). (From Rossano JW, Tajinder PS, Cherikh WS. The Registry of the International Society for Heart and Lung Transplantation: Twenty-second Pediatric Heart Transplantation Report—2019; focus theme: donor and recipient size match. *J Heart Lung Transplant.* 2019;38[10]:1028-1041.)

TABLE 29.7	Risk Factors for 1-Year Mortality: Pediatric Heart Transplants (January 2002–December 2015)	
Cause of Death	**N (493)**	**Percent**
Graft failure	138	28
Multisystem organ failure	82	16.6
Acute rejection	60	12.2
Cerebrovascular event	45	9.1
Infection, non–CMV	42	8.5
Technical	20	8.5

CMV, Cytomegalovirus.
Adapted from Dipchand AI, Rossano JW, Edwards LB. The Registry of the International Society for Heart and Lung Transplantation: Eighteenth Official Pediatric Heart Transplantation Report—2015; focus theme: early graft failure. *J Heart Lung Transplant.* 2015;34(10):1233-1243.)

medications in the perioperative period should be minimized. Medication and monitoring choice should be tailored to the individual needs of the child to minimize anesthetic morbidity. Most medically stable cardiac transplant patients can undergo routine noncardiac surgical procedures in a similar fashion to children without transplants (see Chapter 21). It is important to remember that reflex mechanisms are impaired in the denervated heart and circulatory changes that may result from light anesthesia, hypovolemia, or contractility will be delayed until circulating catecholamines can influence the cardiac β-receptors directly.[352,353] As cardiac transplant patients live longer, the risks of coronary vasculopathy increase, with coronary ischemia becoming a major concern. Attention to the maintenance of coronary perfusion is paramount. As in all immunocompromised patients, these children are vulnerable to infection, and strict adherence to aseptic and sterile technique is mandatory. In transplanted patients with valvular disease, endocarditis prophylaxis is warranted in high-risk procedures.[354]

Pediatric Lung and Heart-Lung Transplantation

Pediatric lung and heart-lung transplant patients are similar and share many underlying disease management processes. These children, with end-stage pulmonary and cardiopulmonary disease, undergo a variety of pretransplant and posttransplant interventions and require special considerations in all phases of their anesthetic care.

DEMOGRAPHICS AND EPIDEMIOLOGY

The first lung transplant was performed in 1963 on an adult with carcinoma occluding the left mainstem bronchus. A single lung transplant was performed and was successful from a technical aspect with adequate oxygenation and ventilation postoperatively. Azathioprine and radiation were administered for immunosuppression. The patient had renal failure before the transplant and ultimately died as a result of renal failure in the first month after transplant.[355] It was another 2 decades before the first pediatric lung and heart-lung transplantation occurred. Advances in surgical technique and immunosuppressive therapy ushered in the modern era of lung transplantation in the early 1980s.[356] The first successful pediatric heart-lung transplant was performed at the Children's Hospital of Pittsburgh in 1985 and the first successful pediatric lung transplant followed in Toronto 2 years later.[357]

Thirty-seven hospitals performed a total of 101 pediatric lung transplants in 2017. For the past decade, between 97 and 136 pediatric lung transplants have been reported to the International Society for Heart and Lung Transplantation (ISHLT) registry. In 2017, only three infant lung transplants were reported. Most centers performing pediatric lung transplants perform one to four transplants annually with only one center reporting performing more than 10 in 2017. The frequency of pediatric heart-lung transplants peaked in the early 1990s. Many of these combination transplants were performed in small patients who required lung transplantation before surgical techniques improved for lung transplantation in small patients. Transplanting the heart and lungs

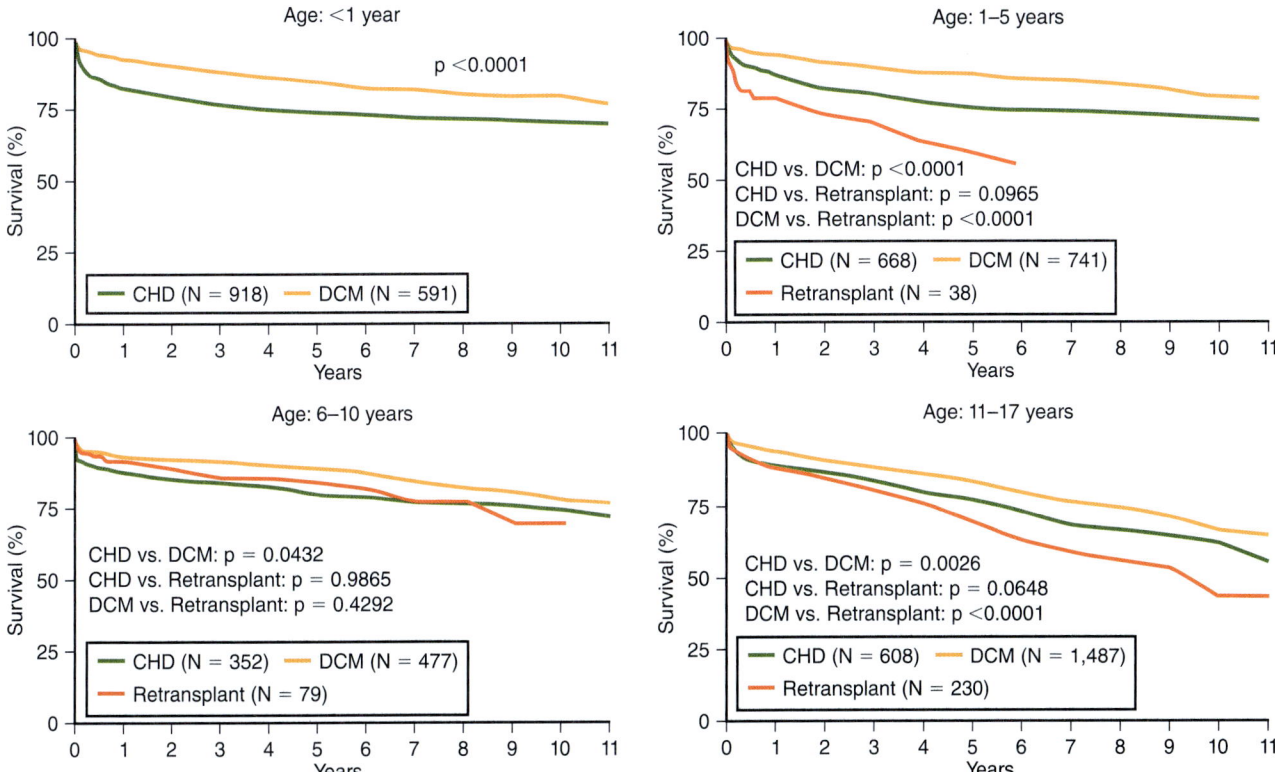

FIGURE 29.11 Survival by diagnosis for pediatric heart transplant recipients (Kaplan-Meier). (From Rossano JW, Tajinder PS, Cherikh WS. The Registry of the International Society for Heart and Lung Transplantation: Twenty-second Pediatric Heart Transplantation Report—2019; focus theme: donor and recipient size match. *J Heart Lung Transplant.* 2019;38[10]:1028-1041.)

"en bloc" was technically less demanding. Outcomes of combined heart-lung transplants are generally worse, and the frequency has decreased. In 2017 only three heart-lung transplants were reported to the ISHLT registry.[358]

PATHOPHYSIOLOGY OF THE DISEASE

The indication for lung transplantation is severe end-stage pulmonary disease for which there is no other medical treatment, with a life expectancy of <2 years. Additional considerations when deciding to list include functional status, quality of life, hemodynamic parameters, and the natural history of the underlying disease. Most pediatric lung transplants (~75% annually) are performed in patients 11 to 17 years old. The most common diagnoses in this age group are cystic fibrosis (65%) and idiopathic pulmonary arterial hypertension (IPAH, 8.9%).[358] In patients aged 1 to 5 years undergoing lung transplantation, the most common causes are idiopathic pulmonary arterial hypertension (~26%) and pulmonary hypertension from other causes (~21%). Infants who require lung transplantation have a variety of relatively rare diseases, such as surfactant B deficiency, primary alveolar proteinosis, or pulmonary vascular disease causing pulmonary hypertension.[359] These infants are often severely ill at the time of their transplants and are frequently intubated and ventilated or on ECMO support (Table 29.8).[360,361]

CYSTIC FIBROSIS

Cystic fibrosis (CF) accounts for nearly half of all pediatric lung transplants. It is an autosomal recessive disease caused by mutation in the cystic fibrosis transmembrane conductance regulator (CFTR) protein, a chloride channel (see also Chapter 11). Altered ion movement due to the mutation produces viscous mucous that leads to multiorgan dysfunction, most prominently in the lung and pancreas. Ninety-five percent of patients with CF will eventually die from pulmonary causes. Clinical markers of advanced disease include a forced expiratory volume in 1 second (FEV$_1$) <40%, PaO$_2$ <55 mm Hg, or a PaCO$_2$ >50 mm Hg.[362] In a study of children less than 18 years of age with CF from 1994 to 2005, independent risk factors for mortality included digital clubbing, ability to auscultate abnormalities on examination, pseudomonas infection, unknown CFTR mutation, and weight below the 50th percentile.[363]

Over the past several decades, diagnosis of CF with newborn screening and improved systems of care have increased life expectancy. CFTR modulators that appear to improve respiratory function and quality of life in the 90% of CF patients with Phe508del CFTR mutation have been developed. Elexacaftor-tezacaftor-ivacaftor is FDA approved for patients aged 12 years and older with at least one Phe508del CFTR mutation. Initiation of this medication has allowed some patients with CF listed for lung transplantation to be removed for the list due to improvement in lung function.[364,365]

PULMONARY HYPERTENSION

Pulmonary hypertension is the second most common cause of pediatric lung transplantation. It is the leading indication in infants and children aged 1 to 5 years. It is also the primary indication for

TABLE 29.8 | Indications for Pediatric Lung Transplants by Age Group (Transplants January 2002–June 2018)

Diagnosis	<1 year N (%)	1–5 years N (%)	6–10 years N (%)	11–17 years N (%)
Cystic fibrosis	0 (0)	4 (3.4)	116 (48.1)	823 (65.4)
IPAH	7 (11.3)	31 (26.7)	24 (10)	112 (8.9)
Obliterative bronchiolitis				
Retransplant	0 (0)	4 (3.4)	7 (2.9)	35 (2.8)
No transplant	0 (0)	10 (8.6)	32 (13.3)	60 (4.8)
Pulmonary fibrosis				
Idiopathic	5 (8.1)	6 (5.2)	5 (2.1)	39 (3.1)
Other	6 (9.7)	10 (8.6)	21 (8.7)	51 (4.1)
Retransplant, not obliterative bronchiolitis	0 (0)	5 (4.3)	7 (2.9)	43 (3.4)
Pulmonary hypertension not IPAH	16 (25.8)	25 (21.6)	7 (2.9)	27 (2.1)
Surfactant deficiency	20 (32.3)	11 (9.5)	3 (1.2)	3 (0.3)
COPD/emphysema	2 (3.2)	1 (0.9)	3 (1.2)	11 (0.9)
Bronchopulmonary dysplasia	3 (4.8)	4 (3.4)	3 (1.2)	3 (0.2)
Bronchiectasis	0 (0)	0 (0)	2 (0.8)	25 (2)
Other	3 (4.8)	5 (4.3)	11 (4.6)	26 (2.1)

COPD, Chronic obstructive pulmonary disease; *IPAH*, idiopathic pulmonary arterial hypertension.
Adapted from: Hayes DJ, Cherikh WS, Chambers DC, et al. The International Thoracic Organ Transplant Registry of the International Society for Heart and Lung Transplantation: Twenty-second Pediatric Lung and Heart-Lung Transplantation Report—2019; focus theme: donor and recipient size match. *J Heart Lung Transplant*. 2019;38(10):1015-1027.

the few annual heart-lung transplants. Pulmonary hypertension is defined as mPAP >20 mm Hg with PVRi >3 Wood units. Pediatric patients with idiopathic pulmonary artery hypertension progress rapidly and often die within 3 years of initial diagnosis. Early referral for transplantation should be considered, especially in patients with suprasystemic right heart pressure and episodes of hemoptysis despite maximal medical therapy.[357,366]

CONTRAINDICATIONS

Primary contraindications for lung transplantation are (1) active malignant disease within the prior 2 years, (2) significant active infectious processes (including HIV and hepatitis B and C), (3) significant coexisting cardiac disease, (4) hepatic or renal disease (although these patients may be candidates for multiple-organ transplants), (5) collagen vascular disease, (6) major irreversible neurologic injury, and (7) patient or family history of poor medical compliance or severe psychiatric illness that would preclude the patient from effective posttransplant care. Relative contraindications include (1) significant musculoskeletal disease, (2) invasive ventilation, (3) colonization with atypical mycobacterium or fungi, (4) poor nutritional status (body mass index [BMI] at either extreme), and (5) inability to reduce dependency on corticosteroids.[367]

WAITLIST AND DONOR SELECTION

As many as one-third of children listed die before receiving lung transplantation due to the scarcity of organs for transplantation. Only about 15% of cadaveric lungs are acceptable for donation. Patients aged 12 to 17 years have the greatest mortality of ~19.7 per 100 transplant waitlist years.[368–370] The average waiting time for cadaveric lungs is 20 months for adolescents and 6 to 12 months for children younger than 2 years of age.

UNOS has separate allocation systems for pediatric patients under age 12 years and patients aged 12 to 17 years. Children younger than 12 years of age are categorized by priority levels, with the most gravely ill children given a priority 1 ranking. Priority 1 candidates have respiratory failure requiring continuous mechanical ventilation, a fractional inspired oxygen (FiO_2) greater than 0.5 to maintain arterial oxygen saturation levels of more than 90%, an arterial or capillary $PaCO_2$ >50 mm Hg, or a $PvCO_2$ >56 mm Hg and/or pulmonary hypertension despite medical therapy. Children not meeting the above conditions are listed as priority 2. Donor lungs are first allocated to the priority 1 candidate with the longest waiting time who matches the donor's blood type and size. If there is no suitable priority 1 candidate, the lungs are then offered to the priority 2 candidate with the longest waiting time. For patients aged 12 to 17 years, a lung allocation score is calculated. The score is based on the individual patient's age, underlying illness, forced vital capacity, functional status, and need for supplemental oxygen.[371] The score ranges from 0 to 100 with higher scores indicating more severe disease. Patients with the highest lung allocation score are offered compatible organs first. Waiting time on the list is not a factor for patients aged 12 to 17 years.[372]

Standard criteria for donor lungs include: donor age <55 years, a clear chest x-ray, PaO_2 >300 mm Hg on 100% oxygen with PEEP of 5 mm Hg, nonsmoker, no chest trauma, no malignancy, no pulmonary infection, and no pulmonary aspiration. One study showed no difference in hospital length of stay, pulmonary function tests, graft function at 1 and 5 years, and 5-year survival in pediatric patients who received lungs from extended criteria donors (ECD). ECDs do not meet one of the standard criteria listed previously. By expanding the pool of donors, waitlist mortality may be improved.[373]

Donation after circulatory death (DCD) donors are another potential source for suitable organs for lung transplantation.[374,375] DCD donors are typically younger than traditional donors and therefore could expand the pool of organs for patients on the pediatric lung transplant waitlist. One report detailed a single center's experience with pediatric lung transplantation from DCD donors. From 2012 to 2017 the center performed 22 pediatric lung transplants of which 9 had DCD donors. The results showed no difference in median ICU stay, graft function or 5-year survival in patients who received organs from DCD donors versus from brain-dead donors.[376]

Living-related donation of adult lobes for transplantation into the child offers an additional organ donor source as well as elective transplant scheduling.[377,378] Inherent size mismatch limits use of this technique to children 5 years of age and older. Typically, the left lower lobe is harvested from one donor with the right-lower lobe harvested from another donor. The harvest technique is similar to a lobectomy; however, the harvested lobes require an appropriate length of bronchus as well as adequate vascular pedicles. Donor morbidity is high and as a result none have been reported to the IHLTS registry since 2013.[379]

Once harvested, lungs are perfused with a preservative solution and prostaglandins. The lungs are inflated, and the trachea stapled closed to maintain an inflated position. The organs are then transported to the recipient at a temperature of 4°C. Ischemic times <8 hours are desired, whereas <3 to 4 hours is ideal.[380]

PREOPERATIVE EVALUATION

Children listed for lung transplantation undergo an extensive workup that includes chest radiographs, pulmonary function tests, arterial blood gases, complete metabolic panel, ECG, and echocardiogram. Those with pulmonary hypertension and/or associated cardiac defects will also require cardiac catheterization to better define the anatomy and hemodynamic profile, specifically, PVR.

SURGICAL TECHNIQUE

Children most commonly receive bilateral lung transplants with the use of CPB[381-383] through a bilateral anterolateral transsternal "clamshell" incision. As much dissection as possible is carried out before instituting CPB. Bilateral bronchial anastomosis has been found to produce better results without the concern for tracheal stenosis. The most popular technique is the telescoping anastomosis in which the larger bronchus is telescoped several centimeters over the smaller bronchus portion with peribronchial tissue wrapped around the anastomosis to ensure blood supply, as bronchial blood supply is not reestablished. If the older end-to-end anastomosis technique is used, an omental wrap is placed around the suture line. The pulmonary artery is reanastomosed after the bronchus is reanastomosed. The pulmonary venous component of the donor lung includes an atrial cuff, which is sutured directly to the left atrium of the recipient. This avoids the complication of pulmonary vein stenosis. Although donor lungs are selected for size match, occasionally lungs are too large and cannot be used in total without exposing the recipient to significant areas of atelectasis. In this instance, volume reduction of the donated lung is performed to remove areas prone to atelectasis.[384-387]

Single lung transplants are uncommon in children and are specifically avoided in CF patients to avoid soiling from the remaining diseased lung. If single lung transplantation is performed for a non–CF patient, the most diseased lung is transplanted. Additionally, if emphysematous changes are present, the most emphysematous lung is removed to decrease the risk of compression of the donor lung. Single lung transplants are most often performed without cardiopulmonary bypass. After anesthesia is induced, single lung ventilation is achieved, a thoracotomy is performed, and the bronchus and vessels are exposed. A test occlusion of the pulmonary artery to the proposed explant lung is then performed by the surgeon to evaluate the ability of the patient to hemodynamically tolerate the procedure without CPB. Presuming the patient tolerates the test clamp, the surgery proceeds with the removal of the native diseased lung. The donor lung is anastomosed by first connecting the pulmonary vein atrial flap to the native left atrium followed by reanastomosing the pulmonary artery, and then the smaller of the two bronchial ends is telescoped into the other with an overlap of one cartilage ring. The lung is then gently inflated. Air within the lung vasculature is vented via the pulmonary artery or the atrial cuff with the left atrium partially occluded. Once de-airing is accomplished, ventilation and perfusion of the donor lung are both established.

INTRAOPERATIVE PROBLEMS AND MANAGEMENT

Patients arriving for lung and heart-lung transplant are often critically ill. The anesthesiologist commonly has limited time to collate all data and perform the preoperative evaluation. Although preoperative anxiolysis may be beneficial, it is important to not significantly decrease respiratory drive and worsen hypoxemia, hypercarbia, and right heart failure.

Due to the short interval between notification of impending transplantation and operating room time, the patient may not be appropriately fasted. In such circumstances, a rapid sequence or modified rapid sequence should be used to facilitate induction of anesthesia. A one-size-fits-all anesthetic technique is not appropriate for heart-lung and lung transplants. The choice of induction agents is broad and must consider comorbid illnesses, such as significant right heart dysfunction, or other congenital anomalies in addition to the end-stage pulmonary disease.

Once standard monitors have been applied, propofol, etomidate, ketamine, or volatile anesthetics may be considered as primary induction agents either alone or in combination with narcotics or benzodiazepines. Ketamine does not appear to significantly alter PVR in infants[388] and may be considered as a first-choice drug.[388-391] Given the desire to rapidly intubate and control the airway, a relatively rapid onset neuromuscular blocking agent, such as high-dose rocuronium, is most commonly used.[89] Much of the peritransplant anesthetic considerations focus on the optimization of PVR, particularly with heart-lung transplant patients, and those with pulmonary hypertension and right heart dysfunction. Increases in PVR may cause acute right ventricular failure, resulting in reduced cardiac output. Right-sided pressures may increase such that major right-to-left shunting occurs through intracardiac defects and results in desaturation.

Initial ventilator settings must consider the underlying disease process. Fibrotic lungs may be better served by smaller tidal volumes with a faster respiratory rate that allows for a decreased peak inspiratory and plateau pressures while preserving minute ventilation. Conversely, severe obstructive disease may be best served by a slower respiratory rate, and a prolonged expiratory time to limit or prevent auto-PEEP. PEEP may be beneficial to improve oxygenation and ventilation and decrease atelectasis. Should hemodynamic collapse occur with the institution of positive-pressure ventilation in a patient with severe obstructive lung disease, dynamic hyperinflation should be immediately considered among the possible etiologies. Both dynamic hyperinflation and PEEP, by increasing intrathoracic pressure, may decrease venous return and cause hemodynamic compromise, particularly in relatively hypovolemic patients. Rapid treatment is provided by just disconnecting the patient from the ventilator circuit and allowing the patient to exhale. When ventilation is reinstituted, care must be taken to allow for adequate expiratory time. Attention should be paid to the patient's preoperative $PaCO_2$. This is often increased in patients with end-stage pulmonary disease. If mechanical ventilation targets a normal $PaCO_2$, respiratory alkalosis will result, and cause decreased cerebral perfusion.

Maintenance anesthesia is most commonly a balanced anesthetic using a combination of opioids and volatile anesthetic with the possible addition of ketamine, benzodiazepines, and dexmedetomidine. Regional anesthesia may also be considered for intraoperative and postoperative care. Because of the typical use of CPB and its need for systemic heparinization, epidural thoracic catheters used for postoperative pain control are generally placed postoperatively when the patient's coagulation profile has normalized. The anesthesiologist must communicate closely with the medical transplant team to ensure all necessary perioperative antibiotics and immunosuppressive medications are administered at the correct time during the transplantation.

Most pediatric lung transplants are performed with the assistance of CPB, in contrast to the non–CPB technique most commonly used for adults. There are several reasons for this distinction, particularly when considering the two most common indications for pediatric lung transplantation. CF patients have a significant risk of cross-contamination of the donor lung during a bilateral sequential lung transplant. This risk of soiling is minimized by the simultaneous removal of both lungs. Pediatric patients with pulmonary hypertension are frequently too unstable to tolerate single lung ventilation. Additionally, many children are too small to accommodate a double-lumen tube and single lung ventilation may be difficult. CPB alleviates these issues and allows the surgeon a quiet field with good exposure and predictable hemodynamics, thus speeding the time for anastomosis and decreasing the overall ischemic time.

If the patient undergoes either single lung transplant or off-pump sequential bilateral lung transplant, continual vigilance and reassessment of the patient's condition is required. Single lung ventilation often precipitates hypoxemia and hypercarbia. The combination of increased afterload on the right heart by clamping of the pulmonary artery along with hypercarbia and hypoxemic-induced pulmonary hypertension on the other lung may precipitate right heart failure. Pulmonary vascular dilators and inotropes, such as milrinone, prostaglandins, and NO, along with maintaining adequate right-sided filling pressures may be used to diminish pulmonary hypertension. Nonetheless, continued right heart failure may necessitate CPB. If the patient tolerates pulmonary artery clamping, the gas exchange typically improves as the shunting through the nonventilated lung is stopped and the perfusion-ventilation mismatch is diminished.

Bilateral sequential lung transplants performed on CPB do not offer these problems. Nonetheless, CPB comes with a cost. During CPB the patient is typically cooled to 32°C, which introduces the concerns associated with moderate hypothermia. Gas exchange may worsen because of reperfusion injury, pulmonary edema, and decreased lung compliance. CPB also results in inflammatory mediator release that contributes to the reperfusion injury in the transplanted lungs. The systemic heparinization required for CPB increases the risk for perioperative bleeding and the need for transfusion of blood products. Packed red blood cells, platelets, and clotting factors are typically required. Fibrinolytics may somewhat mitigate bleeding.

When the procedure is performed with CPB, airway management is performed with a single-lumen tracheal tube. Cuffed tracheal tubes are typically chosen for the ability to provide a better tracheal fit and allow for the potential ventilation of the lungs with relatively high pressures. In the rare circumstances that the operation of pediatric lung transplantation is performed without CPB, single lung ventilation will be required. Double-lumen tubes may be used in older patients (see Chapter 13). If a double-lumen tube is used, it is exchanged for a single-lumen tube at the conclusion of the operation unless there is a desire to continue with differential lung ventilation or there is a concern about lung soiling. In small children, either a bronchial blocker or selective intubation of a single bronchus may be considered. These options, however, preclude the ability to suction the nonventilated lung.

Once the patient has been intubated, additional invasive monitoring is placed, typically an arterial catheter and a central venous catheter, along with large-bore peripheral intravenous catheters. Some centers place a pulmonary artery catheter in addition to or in place of the percutaneous central venous catheter. Occasionally, the surgeon will place a right atrial catheter. If a pulmonary artery catheter is placed, it must be withdrawn into the main pulmonary artery before the pneumonectomy. A TEE probe is frequently placed to assist in evaluation of residual cardiac abnormalities and cardiac performance, particularly right ventricular performance.[392]

Perioperative bleeding is common, both in the operating room after coming off CPB and in the immediate postoperative period. Extensive pulmonary to systemic collaterals, coagulopathies caused by hepatic dysfunction, and adhesions from prior surgery or CF may make the surgical dissection difficult and precipitate blood loss. Fibrinolytics have been demonstrated to reduce bleeding in patients with prior thoracic surgery.[393]

Lungs with CF are uniformly colonized with bacteria. After the native lungs are removed; their tracheal stump is irrigated with antibiotic solution to reduce contamination of the transplanted lungs. Despite best efforts, these patients occasionally develop sepsis owing to liberation of bacteria and toxic mediators during the removal of the native lungs. These patients require intensive therapy and most often do poorly.

After the first lung has been implanted, a small amount of blood is allowed to eject into the pulmonary artery while the second lung is anastomosed, thereby reducing the ischemic time for the first lung. After the second lung is implanted, the lungs are ventilated to remove areas of atelectasis. Posttransplant ventilation strategy limits tidal volumes to maintain peak inspiratory pressures <25 cm H_2O and PEEP in the range of 5 to 10 cm H_2O. Supplemental oxygen should be reduced as tolerated and limited to 40% to 50% or less. It is typical to augment myocardial performance with inotropic support before termination of CPB. Occasionally, a combination of inotropes, dilators, or vasopressors may be required. Some centers routinely use inhaled NO and/or prostaglandin E_1 (PGE_1) to reduce PVR, whereas others reserve their use only for those in whom pulmonary hypertension is problematic. Fiberoptic bronchoscopy may be performed to assess the bronchial anastomotic sites in the operating room along with a lung perfusion scan performed within the first 24 hours postoperatively.

In the heart-lung transplant patient, weaning from CPB is analogous to that for cardiac transplantation as described earlier. There remains the need to support the denervated heart with adequate fluids and inotropy. Maintaining adequate fluid status in these patients may require a bit more effort because of increased bleeding compared with heart transplant patients. Blood products are uniformly required in these patients. Bleeding is further exacerbated in these patients owing to extensive collaterals and bronchial circulation, which have often developed.

The onset of acute graft dysfunction may present with persistent hypoxemia after weaning from CPB. Although this may be attributable to relatively reversible causes, such as inadequate ventilation, atelectasis, or right ventricular dysfunction with right-to-left shunting, a more ominous problem may be reperfusion injury. Free radicals and inflammatory mediators are readily produced by the lung during both the ischemic time as well as during reperfusion. Reperfusion injury is correlated with longer ischemic times and presents as hypoxemia in the face of adequate ventilation and no other clear etiology of the hypoxemia. Pink frothy secretions noted in the tracheal tube may indicate reperfusion injury. PGE_1 may reduce reperfusion injury risk and symptoms. The optimal ventilation strategy aims to maintain oxygenation and ventilation with adequate PEEP and as low a peak inspiratory pressure as possible. FiO_2 is targeted to keep the PaO_2 less than 120 mm Hg to avoid oxygen toxicity. Inhaled NO has not been shown to prevent reperfusion injury when administered prophylactically. However, inhaled NO in the dose range of 20 to 60 ppm has been demonstrated to be effective in patients with increased pulmonary artery and right heart pressures coupled with hypoxemia.[394–399] Inhaled prostacyclin has also been demonstrated to be safe and effective in the treatment of pulmonary hypertension and reperfusion injury.[400] Occasionally, all these measures are inadequate and ECMO is instituted to allow the donor lungs to recover.[401–404]

IMMEDIATE POSTOPERATIVE MANAGEMENT

Immediate postoperative care is individualized based on the child's age, pretransplant diagnosis, and pretransplant comorbidities. Older patients with CF require mechanical ventilation for several days with their time to discharge from the critical care unit averaging less than 1 week.[405] Non–CF infants and children, typically more acutely ill before transplant, require an average of more than 3 weeks of mechanical ventilation and average nearly 2 months of critical care stay.[406] These younger transplant patients are smaller, have an increased incidence of airway complications, and may suffer from associated congenital cardiac defects. Patients with significant pretransplant pulmonary hypertension often manifest significant hemodynamic instability postoperatively. As such, these patients remain intubated, sedated, and frequently paralyzed for the first 2 postoperative days.

The cough reflex is absent and mucociliary transport is disrupted across the bronchial suture line in posttransplant patients, necessitating aggressive chest physiotherapy to avoid lung congestion that could lead to infection and respiratory failure. Frequent tracheal suctioning is mandatory; therapeutic bronchoscopy for pulmonary toilet may also be required. In addition to the risk for infections owing to pulmonary considerations, surgical sites, catheters, and drains add to the risk of infection. Prophylactic antibiotics are given perioperatively, including antivirals and antifungals, particularly if underlying fungal infection or viral infection (such as CMV) are present in either the donor or recipient.[407] Transplanted lungs do not have lymphatics reanastomosed. This loss of lymphatic drainage increases the risk for pulmonary edema postoperatively. After initial postoperative bleeding has been controlled, additional intravenous fluid should be administered judiciously and diuresis should be initiated to target a CVP of 4 to 6 mm Hg if hemodynamically tolerated.[408]

Postoperative pain control with judicious use of opioids is critical to ensure effective pulmonary toilet. Patient-controlled analgesia may be considered in patients capable of using such a device. Regional anesthesia may also be used, but because of the systemic heparinization in CPB, many are reluctant to place a catheter before bypass. If regional anesthesia is desired, a thoracic epidural or paravertebral catheters may be placed postoperatively when the coagulation status of the patient has normalized. Dexmedetomidine may also be used for adjunct pain management by providing arousable sedation with minimal effect on respiratory drive with the additional benefit of opioid sparing.

LONG-TERM CONCERNS

A variety of perioperative complications may occur (Table 29.9).[409] More than one-third of patients who receive chronic immunosuppression develop hypertension during the first posttransplant year.

TABLE 29.9	Cumulative Morbidity Rates in Pediatric Lung Transplant Survivors Within 1, 5, and 7 Years After Transplant (Follow-Ups April 1994–June 2014)					
Outcome	Total With Known Response (N)	Within 1 Year (%)	Total With Known Response (N)	Within 5 Years (%)	Total With Known Response (N)	Within 7 Years (%)
Hypertension[a]	765	41.4	229	67.7	—	—
Renal dysfunction	795	9.4	247	29.6	138	42.8
Creatinine (≤2.5 mg/dL)		6.5		23.1		32.6
(abnormal) >2.5 mg/dL		1.9		4.0		6.5
Chronic dialysis		0.8		1.6		0.7
Renal transplant		0.3		0.8		2.9
Hyperlipidemia[a]	781	5.1	231	17.7	—	—
Diabetes[a]	797	21.3	250	35.2	—	—
BOS	739	12.2	192	35.9	93	41.9

[a]Data are not available 7 years after transplant.
BOS, Bronchiolitis obliterans syndrome.
Goldfarb SB, Benden C, Edwards LB, et al. The Registry of the International Society for Heart and Lung Transplantation: Eighteenth Official Pediatric Lung and Heart-Lung Transplantation Report—2015; focus theme: early graft failure. *J Heart Lung Transplant.* 2015;34(1):1255-1263.

By 5 years, that number has reached almost three-quarters of all survivors. Additionally, a number of these children, particularly those receiving tacrolimus, develop chronic renal insufficiency marked by a lower creatinine clearance. Chronic kidney disease is a major comorbidity in pediatric lung transplant recipients.[410,411] More than one-third of patients have a degree of renal dysfunction within 7 years of transplantation. Occasionally, renal insufficiency progresses such that the child requires dialysis and renal transplantation.[412] Renal dysfunction is associated with increased mortality.

The large endothelial surface in the lungs and the resulting large number of immunologically active cells cause an extreme lymphocyte-directed host response. Due to this, immunosuppressive drugs are used in larger doses in lung transplant and heartlung transplant patients than in other organ transplants. Induction immunosuppression was used in 86% of pediatric lung transplants in 2017 though survival data do not yet demonstrate improvement with induction immunosuppression.[358,413] Most transplant centers use triple therapy for maintenance immunosuppression. Most patients are on long-term systemic corticosteroids with the goal of titrating to the lowest dose.[414] The International Pediatric Lung Transplant Collaborative has recommended that tacrolimus, mycophenolate mofetil, and prednisone constitute the mainstay of immunosuppressive therapy. The most widely used regimens rely on a calcineurin phosphatase inhibitor coupled with a cell cycle inhibitor and a corticosteroid. The most commonly used calcineurin phosphatase inhibitors are cyclosporine and tacrolimus. Neither appear to offer a benefit over the other in preventing bronchiolitis obliterans from occurring. The major adverse effects of tacrolimus include hyperglycemia, alopecia, possibly worsening renal function, and possibly increased risk of posttransplant lymphoproliferative disorder. Cyclosporine's major adverse effects include hypercholesterolemia, hirsutism, gingival hyperplasia, and hypertension. Cyclosporine may prolong the neuromuscular blockade of atracurium and vecuronium.[415] Cyclosporine blood concentrations must be monitored closely, particularly in CF patients who are prone to variable absorption. Increased concentrations of cyclosporine have been implicated in central nervous system adverse effects such as seizures, headaches, and even strokes.[416,417] Steroids are included in nearly all lung transplant programs. Over time, the steroid dose is weaned to prevent complications such as hyperglycemia and osteoporosis, yet at 1 and 5 years after transplant, nearly all lung transplant patients continue to take prednisone. Cell cycle inhibitors are used in addition to the calcineurin phosphatase inhibitors and corticosteroids. Mycophenolate use is increasing but has not yet demonstrated benefit over azathioprine. Azathioprine may prolong the neuromuscular blockade of succinylcholine.[415] Sirolimus acts by blocking IL-2–induced T-cell proliferation. Its role as a primary medication is limited by its inhibition of wound healing, potentially contributing to a dehiscence. It may be used as rescue therapy in patients with bronchiolitis obliterans with mature suture lines.

Posttransplant patients are followed closely for signs of rejection, infection, and/or bronchiolitis obliterans. Surveillance requires flexible fiberoptic bronchoscopies with bronchoalveolar lavage and transbronchial biopsies. This is the most common indication for general anesthesia in posttransplant patients, as they are performed at regular intervals, typically every 3 months. The choice of anesthetic for posttransplant patients must be individualized, accounting for comorbidities such as continued right heart dysfunction, decreased ability to handle secretions,

current graft function, and particular caution regarding any potential to cross the bronchial suture line.[418] A laryngeal mask airway is the preferred manner of airway management. The laryngeal mask airway lumen is significantly larger than that of the corresponding tracheal tube and allows the bronchoscopist to use a larger fiberoptic bronchoscope, facilitating improved view, improved suctioning, and easier bronchoalveolar lavage along with enhancing the ability to obtain adequate transbronchial biopsies.[419]

Acute rejection is common in the first several weeks to months after transplant. Acute rejection is often asymptomatic and presents as a >10% decrease in FEV_1. It may also present similar to a common upper respiratory tract infection. Radiographic findings may include infiltrates and pleural effusions. Diagnosis is confirmed by bronchoscopy, bronchoalveolar lavage, and transtracheal biopsy. Acute rejection is graded on a scale of A0 to A4. Grade A2 scores and above are treated with increased immunosuppression. The major manifestation of chronic rejection, bronchiolitis obliterans,[420] occurs in up to 50% of all post–lung transplant patients within 5 years of transplant. Bronchiolitis obliterans is the leading cause of death after the first posttransplant year. It presents as progressive deterioration of exercise tolerance and deterioration in airflow. Bronchiolitis obliterans is characterized by fibrosis of small airways and thickening of blood vessels. Diagnosis is defined by a decrease in FEV_1 compared with the immediately previous FEV_1.[421] Known risk factors for bronchiolitis obliterans include prolonged ischemic time of the donor lung, more than two rejection episodes, and age >3 years.[359] Unfortunately, there is no effective treatment for bronchiolitis obliterans. A variety of immunosuppressive medications have been used with variable results. The primary treatment is immunosuppressive prevention of acute rejection and prompt CMV treatment. In severe instances of bronchiolitis obliterans, retransplantation is the only treatment option, though survival following retransplantation is poor.[422]

Posttransplant airway complications may be devastating.[423] Although life-threatening bronchial dehiscence is uncommon, bronchial stenosis and tracheomalacia remain problematic.[424,425] Bronchial stenosis may be related to relative ischemia at the anastomotic site, recurrent infections, and possibly high-dose corticosteroids. Initial treatment of stenosis is balloon dilation; however, up to half of the patients with bronchial stenosis will require placement of bronchial stents. In younger patients, dynamic obstruction may be a complication that makes extubation difficult. This dynamic airway obstruction usually is self-limited, improves over time, and does not require intervention.

Posttransplant vascular complications are uncommon, but important. Most are caused by mechanical obstruction of blood flow secondary to redundant tissue in either the pulmonary artery or at the cuff of the atrial tissue, impeding venous return. Vascular complications may be difficult to distinguish from reperfusion injury, as both present with increased right atrial and pulmonary pressures and pink frothy secretions. Pulmonary arterial or venous stenosis may be diagnosed in the operating room or at bedside with an echocardiogram; in some cases, cardiac catheterization may be required. Depending on the findings, the patient may be treated with a stent placed during cardiac catheterization or reoperation to alleviate the stenosis.

Phrenic, recurrent laryngeal, and vagus nerve injuries are common after lung transplant.[426] Although phrenic nerve injury is typically transient, the resulting diaphragmatic paralysis may cause prolonged need for mechanical ventilation or even consideration of placement of a diaphragmatic pacer. Recurrent laryngeal nerve injury may occur in up to 1 of every 10 pediatric lung transplant patients; left recurrent laryngeal nerve–induced vocal cord paralysis is the most common, although most children will recover.[426] Gastroesophageal reflux disease and gastroparesis may be precipitated by vagal nerve injury. Gastroesophageal reflux disease is a major post–lung transplant problem, which increases the risk for bronchiolitis obliterans and aspiration pneumonia, both of which contribute to graft failure.[427,428] Delayed gastric emptying results in unreliable absorption of immunosuppressive drugs. A number of patients with GERD require a Nissen fundoplication.[429] Additionally, children with CF have a high incidence (10%) of intestinal obstruction after lung transplantation.[430]

Infection is a leading cause of morbidity and mortality following lung transplantation. Viral infections are associated with decreased 1-year survival. Of particular concern is CMV infection. CMV infections may present with mild symptoms, but they may progress to pneumonitis, gastrointestinal symptoms, or even a sepsis syndrome with multiorgan failure. CMV has been associated with both acute cellular rejection and chronic rejection.[431,432] Antiviral medications have decreased the severity of this infection.[433] Prophylactic treatment is often considered if either the donor or the recipient were CMV positive. Children with CF remain at a greater risk for infection postoperatively with *Pseudomonas aeruginosa* or fungal organisms.

Posttransplant lymphoproliferative disorder is another cause of morbidity in pediatric lung transplant patients. From 1995 to 2007, the IHLST registry found the rate of malignancy to be 4.8% in patients 1 year following transplant and 9.3% in patients 5 years out. The majority of these malignancies are lymphoma.[358] Posttransplant lymphoproliferative disorder has a greater incidence in lung and heart-lung transplant patients than in other solid organ transplants, perhaps owing to the greater level of immunosuppression required. Additionally, the CF subgroup has an increased incidence of posttransplant lymphoproliferative disorder. Posttransplant lymphoproliferative disorder includes a group of tumors, ranging from B-cell hyperplasia to immunoblastic lymphoma. Mortality from posttransplant lymphoproliferative disorder has been reported to be up to 60%; a number of these deaths have been attributed to graft failure as a result of treating the posttransplant lymphoproliferative disorder by decreasing immunosuppressive therapy.[434] Posttransplant lymphoproliferative disorder is, in most cases, associated with EBV infection, either as a reactivation of the virus with immunosuppression or with new infection acquired from the donor lung. EBV is uncommon in patients who are seropositive for EBV before transplant. For those who are seronegative before transplant, EBV-associated disease occurs in one in five patients. The diagnosis of posttransplant lymphoproliferative disorder is made by the symptoms, biopsy, and the presence of EBV DNA or RNA in the biopsied tissue. Posttransplant lymphoproliferative disorder presents with a variety of nonspecific symptoms including a mononucleosis-type syndrome. The most common symptoms include fever, lymphadenopathy, and gastrointestinal symptoms. EBV infection results in both a humoral and cellular immune reaction. In immunodeficient patients, the normal immune responses are blunted. The natural regulation by T cells and natural killer cells is impaired. The immunosuppression required to prevent graft rejection impairs T-cell immunity and allows for

unchecked proliferation of EBV-infected B cells. The treatment of posttransplant lymphoproliferative disorder is reduction or withdrawal of immunosuppressive therapy.[435,436] Unfortunately, reduction or withdrawal of immunosuppressive therapy places these children at risk for graft failure. Additional effective treatments include localized excision of the lesion, antiviral therapy,[437] monoclonal antibodies,[438] interferon,[439,440] immunoglobulin, and cytotoxic T lymphocytes.[434] Chemotherapy does not appear to offer an advantage and may worsen survival.[436]

Dysrhythmias, although possible, are relatively uncommon (<5%) after transplant and typically do not require treatment. Atrial dysrhythmias associated with extensive left atrial suture lines were among the first dysrhythmias to be described.[441,442] However, the types of dysrhythmias after lung transplant surgery includes nonsustained ventricular tachycardia, accelerated junctional rhythm, sinus bradycardia, nonsustained supraventricular tachycardia, ectopic atrial tachycardia, and second-degree heart block; treatment is not generally required.[443]

Postoperative lung transplant patients fall behind their contemporaries in height and weight, and their growth curves lie between the 5 and 10 percentiles for age, with the overall growth rate only two-thirds of the predicted value. It appears, based on pulmonary function tests, radiographic studies, and histologic examination, that the growth of the transplanted lung(s) in the recipient is appropriate for the recipient's height and weight. Functional reserve capacity,[444] airway size,[445] and absolute number of alveoli grow as height and weight increase in a manner comparable to their normal counterparts. Furthermore, recipients of mature living-related lobar lungs are also noted to grow. Transplanted mature lung lobes expand and fill the entire chest. In these mature lung lobes, however, although the airways appear to grow in size, the alveoli appear to become distended rather than increasing in absolute number.

SURVIVAL AND QUALITY OF LIFE

The survival of pediatric transplant patients has improved in the recent era defined as 2002 to 2017 compared with 1992 to 2001. (Fig. 29.12) Median survival for children is ~5.7 years. If patients who die in the first year after transplant are excluded, the median survival for pediatric patients is ~9 years. Survival was similar between pediatric recipients of different age groups and diagnostic indication for transplantation.[358]

Risk factors for mortality after lung transplant include renal dysfunction, older donors, female recipients, and patients undergoing retransplantation. Infants have a substantive early death rate of 25%. Early deaths within the first month are caused by primary graft failure, technical issues, and cardiovascular failure. The leading cause of death from 1 month through 1 year posttransplant is non–CMV infections. After 3 years, bronchiolitis obliterans is the leading cause of death, accounting for nearly half of all deaths. In those patients who do survive, functional status is good with over 80% having no or minimal activity limitations. Additionally, ~57% of survivors did not need to be hospitalized for any reason in posttransplant years 4 to 5.[358]

Acknowledgements

We wish to thank Franklyn P. Cladis, Brian Blasiole, Martin B. Anixter, James Gordon Cain, and Peter J. Davis for their prior contributions to this chapter.

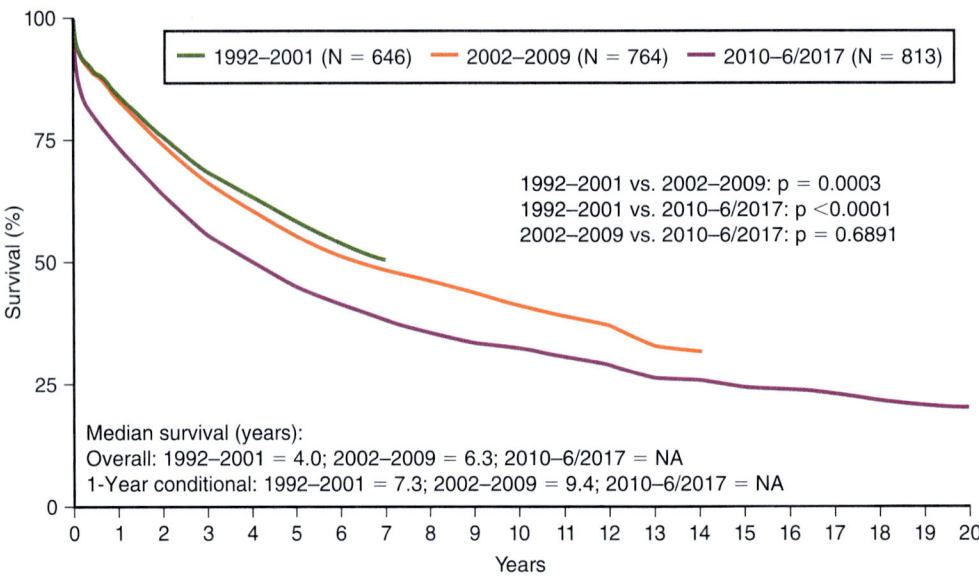

FIGURE 29.12 Pediatric lung transplants. Kaplan-Meier survival by era. (From Hayes DJ, Cherikh WS, Chambers DC, et al. The International Thoracic Organ Transplant Registry of the International Society for Heart and Lung Transplantation: Twenty-second Pediatric Lung and Heart-Lung Transplantation Report – 2019; focus theme: donor and recipient size match. *J Heart Lung Transplant.* 2019;38(10):1015-1027.)

ANNOTATED REFERENCES

Zafar F, Castleberry C, Khan MS, et al. Pediatric heart transplant waiting list mortality in the era of ventricular assist devices. *J Heart Lung Transplant.* 2015;34(1):82-88.

The authors of this paper utilize information from the UNOS database to evaluate pediatric heart transplant waitlist mortality before and after the wide use of pediatric VADs. From 1999 to 2004, VADs were utilized in 6% of patients, and waitlist mortality was 16%. From 2005 to 2012, VADs were utilized in 16% of patients, and waitlist mortality was 8%. During this time, changes were made to organ prioritization and there was continued improvement in the management of patients pretransplant. However, these data show the large impact of VAD support in pediatric patients, a 50% decrease in waitlist mortality.

Dharnidharka VR, Fiorina P, Harmon WE. Kidney transplantation in children. *N Engl J Med.* 2014;371(6):549-558.

This review paper summarizes the latest surgical and immunologic advances in pediatric kidney transplantation. The paper includes outcome data of graft and patient survival broken down by patient age and era of time that the transplant was performed.

Lancaster TS, Miller JR, Epstein DJ. et al. Improved waitlist and transplant outcomes for pediatric lung transplantation after implementation of the lung allocation score. *J Heart Lung Transplant.* 2017; 36(5):520-528.

In 2005, the lung allocation score (LAS) was implemented to determine prioritization of lung recipients 12 years of age and up. With this change, the severity of illness instead of time on the waitlist determined prioritization. The LAS was not utilized for younger patients on the transplant list except in special circumstances. At the time of LAS implementation, geographical sharing of child donors to child recipients was expanded. The authors of this paper evaluated time on the waitlist, waitlist mortality, and median survival following transplantation in patients before and after implementation of LAS. They found a decrease in wait time for all age groups, a decrease in waitlist mortality in all age groups, and an increase in median survival following transplant for adults and children.

Lee J, Yoo YJ, Lee JM, et al. Sevoflurane versus desflurane on the incidence of postreperfusion syndrome during living donor liver transplantation: a randomized controlled trial. *Transplantation.* 2016; 100(3):600-606.

This prospective, randomized, controlled trial investigated postreperfusion syndrome and use of vasoactive agents in 62 adult liver transplant recipients receiving either sevoflurane or desflurane. There was significantly less postreperfusion syndrome (38% vs. 77%) and vasoactive agent (19% vs. 45%) use in adults receiving sevoflurane. There does not appear to be an advantage to using desflurane over sevoflurane during reperfusion.

Sorensen LG, Neighbors K, Martz K, et al. Longitudinal study of cognitive and academic outcomes after pediatric liver transplantation. *J Pediatr.* 2014;165(1):65-72.e2.

This is a prospective multicenter longitudinal study investigating intellect, academic performance, and executive function over time. Pediatric liver transplant recipients 2 or more years after liver transplant were evaluated at 5 to 6 years and 7 to 9 years, after liver transplant. A pattern of cognitive and academic deficits was detected in patients that persisted over time. Factors that seemed to predict cognitive deficits included operative complications and intraoperative transfusion volume.

A complete reference list can be found online at Elsevier eBooks+.

Orthopedic and Spine Surgery

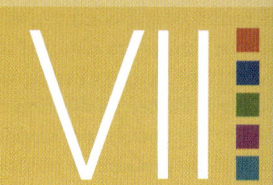

NIALL C. WILTON AND BRIAN J. ANDERSON

Scoliosis Surgery
Terminology, History, and Surgical Development
Classification
Pathophysiology and Natural History
Risk Minimization and Improving Outcome from Surgical Intervention
Respiratory Function and Other Complications in the Early Postoperative Period
Long-Term Changes
Spinal Cord Injury During Surgery
Etiology
Risk of Spinal Cord Injury and Spinal Cord Monitoring
Methods of Monitoring Spinal Cord Function
The Patient Journey: Preparation, Planning, and Pathways
Preoperative Assessment and Postoperative Planning
Respiratory Assessment and Planning for Postoperative Ventilatory Support
Cardiovascular Assessment
Postoperative Care
Anesthetic and Intraoperative Management
Positioning and Related Issues
Temperature Regulation
Patient Monitoring

Minimizing Blood Loss and Decreasing Transfusion Requirements
Managing Blood Loss
Effects of Anesthetics on Somatosensory Evoked and Motor Evoked Potentials
Choosing Anesthetic Drugs and Techniques
Tourniquets
Indications and Design
Physiology
Complications
Recommended Cuff Pressures
Acute Bone and Joint Infections
Pathophysiology
Clinical Presentation
Treatment Options
Anesthesia Considerations
Pain Management
Common Syndromes
Cerebral Palsy
Spina Bifida
Osteogenesis Imperfecta
Duchenne Muscular Dystrophy
Arthrogryposis Multiplex Congenita

ANESTHESIA FOR ORTHOPEDIC AND SPINAL SURGERY provides a multitude of challenges. Children often present with concomitant diseases that affect cardiovascular and respiratory function. The ability to maintain a clear airway during anesthesia is not straightforward for some children, such as those with arthrogryposis multiplex congenita.[1] Operating times can be protracted. Considerable blood loss can occur that requires strategies for blood product management and transfusion reduction (see Chapter 8). Major trauma causing orthopedic injuries invariably involves other organ systems that may adversely interact with or compromise anesthesia management (see Chapter 37). The risks of pulmonary aspiration of gastric contents and the requisite fasting times, after even minor trauma involving an isolated

forearm fracture, continue to be debated. Fat embolus is uncommon in children with long-bone fractures but should be considered in any child with hypoxia and altered consciousness in the perioperative period.[2] Tumor surgery may be complicated by chemotherapy, altered drug disposition, or bone grafting considerations akin to those for plastic and reconstructive surgery (see Chapter 33), and complex postoperative pain management may be required (e.g., phantom pain, reflex sympathetic dystrophy) (see Chapters 41 and 42).

Children with chronic illnesses present repeatedly for surgical or diagnostic procedures. A single bad experience can blight attitudes about anesthesia for a long time. Positioning children on the operating table involves care, especially for those with limb deformities and contractures (Video 30.1). Padding, pillows, and special frames are required to protect against damage from inadvertent pressure ischemia while achieving the best posture for surgery. Plaster application, particularly around the hip, should allow for bowel and bladder function, avoid skin breakdown caused by pressure or friction, and allow access to epidural catheters. Postoperative management of casts on peripheral limbs must account for the possibility of compartment syndromes attributable to restrictive casts or compartment pathology. Major plexus blocks may mask pressure effects under plaster casts or compartment syndrome, but epidural blocks using low-dose amide anesthetics do not mask the discomfort of pressure.[3,4] Intraoperative temperature regulation may be affected by tourniquet application or disease (e.g., osteogenesis imperfecta, arthrogryposis multiplex congenita). The use of radiology is common during orthopedic surgery; anesthesiologists should take precautions against excessive radiation exposure.

Regional anesthesia (see Chapter 40) reduces anesthesia requirements intraoperatively and provides analgesia postoperatively. The use of ultrasound techniques to locate neural tissue improves the rate of successful blocks and reduces local anesthetic doses (see Chapter 40).[5,6] This has heralded increasing use of peripheral nerve blockade rather than central blockade for unilateral lower limb surgery. Acetaminophen (paracetamol) and nonsteroidal antiinflammatory drugs (NSAIDs) are the most common analgesics prescribed for moderate pain. Regular administration of acetaminophen and NSAIDs decreases the amount of systemic opioids administered,[7] but NSAIDs decrease osteogenic activity and may increase the incidence of nonunion after spinal fusion in adults.[8,9] Intravenous acetaminophen improves the early effectiveness of this drug before the child is able to tolerate oral intake.[10] Long-term pain associated with limb-lengthening techniques may require oral opioids after hospital discharge but these must be limited and closely monitored to minimize abuse potential.

Scoliosis Surgery

Children presenting for scoliosis surgery represent a spectrum, ranging from uncomplicated adolescents to severely compromised patients with neuromuscular disease, respiratory failure, and cardiac problems. The age range at presentation varies from infancy to young adulthood. Anesthesia techniques for scoliosis surgery vary with individual patient requirements.[11,12] Approaches aimed at minimizing blood loss and transfusion requirements have progressed from extremes of hypotension and hemodilution to a more balanced approach involving moderate degrees of both, use of antifibrinolytic agents, predonation programs, and intraoperative cell salvage. The impact of anesthetic agents on complex physiologic signals has become increasingly important as more sophisticated measurements of neural transmission using somatosensory evoked potentials (SSEPs) and motor evoked potentials (MEPs) have become the standard of care.

TERMINOLOGY, HISTORY, AND SURGICAL DEVELOPMENT

The terms scoliosis (i.e., crooked), kyphosis (i.e., humpbacked), and lordosis (i.e., bent backward) originated with the Greek physician Galen. *Scoliosis* is a lateral deviation of the normal vertical line of the spine, greater than 10 degrees when measured by radiographs. Scoliosis consists of a lateral curvature of the spine with rotation of the vertebrae within the curve. *Lordosis* refers to an anterior angulation of the spine in the sagittal plane, and *kyphosis* refers to a posterior angulation of the spine as evaluated

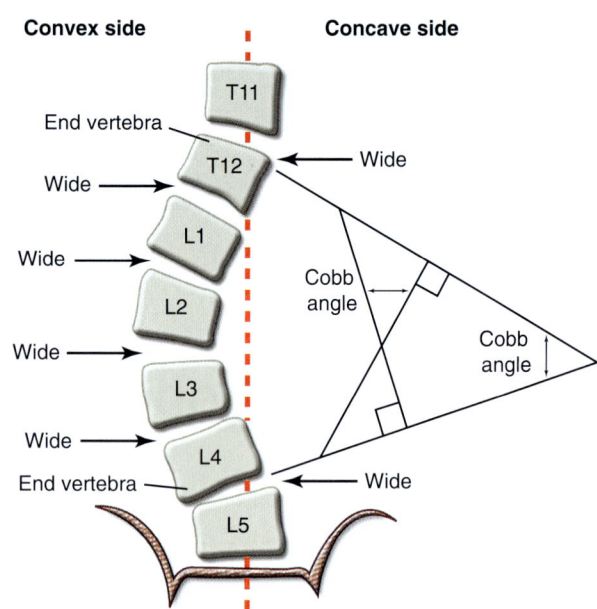

FIGURE 30.1 Diagram of an anteroposterior spinal radiograph shows the Cobb method of scoliosis curve measurement.

on a side view of the spine. Curves may be simple or complex, flexible or rigid, and structural or nonstructural. Primary curves are the earliest to appear and occur most frequently in the thoracic and lumbar regions. Secondary (or compensatory) curves can develop above or below the primary curve and evolve to maintain normal body alignment. Various combinations of curve types have different pathophysiologic consequences.

The magnitude of the scoliosis curve is most commonly measured using the Cobb method.[13] Measurement is made from an anteroposterior radiograph and requires accurate identification of the upper and lower end vertebrae involved with the curve. These vertebrae tilt most severely toward the concavity of the curve. The Cobb method of angle measurement is shown in Fig. 30.1.

Spinal deformities were managed nonsurgically until 1839, when a surgical treatment in the form of a subcutaneous tenotomy and myotomy was described by a French surgeon, Jules Guerin.[14] Posterior spinal fusion was first described for tuberculous spinal deformity.[15] The original spinal instrumentation system was the Harrington rod system.[16] Modification of this technique that allowed segmental fixation of the rods and early mobilization followed.[17] These systems treated the lateral curve but did not allow for correction of the axial rotation. Subsequent developments allowed both corrections by cantilever maneuvers using Cotrel-Dubousset instrumentation.[18]

Pedicle screws rather than hooks were the next advance and were found to enhance correction and stabilization, even when used with hooks for the more proximal curves (i.e., hybrid constructs).[19] Pedicle screw instrumentation techniques for total curve correction offer better correction than hook techniques[20] or the hybrid pedicle screw and hook technique.[21] Sublaminar polyester bands are also used in children with dysmorphic or osteoporotic spines because of concerns about pedicle screw placement,[22] although bands may be associated with more neurologic complications.[23] Posterior column (Ponte) osteotomies may be performed with kyphotic or complex deformity corrections.[24] The relevance for anesthesiologists is that the procedure includes excision of the posterior ligaments (supraspinous, infraspinous, and ligamentum flavum) exposing the epidural space, thus rendering epidural pain management less effective. They are also associated with a greater incidence of critical intraoperative neuromonitoring changes.[25]

CLASSIFICATION

Classification of scoliosis deformities is imperfect because the systems used are clinically rather than etiologically based. Most classifications are surgically based and used for surgical decision making. Curves can be described on the basis of age at onset, associated pathology, and anatomic configurations of the curve, such as single, double, or triple curves; amount of pelvic tilt; curve flexibility; and three-dimensional (3D) analysis of the curve.[26] Children younger than 5 years of age with early-onset scoliosis or with independent cardiac or pulmonary disease appear to be at increased risk for respiratory failure, whereas those with idiopathic scoliosis in whom the curve develops at adolescence appear to have minimal risk.[27] A classification adapted from that proposed by the Scoliosis Research Society in 1973 remains relevant for anesthesiologists (Table 30.1).[28]

The Lenke classification system, developed in 2001 for idiopathic scoliosis, provides a means to categorize curves and guide surgical treatment.[29] The system has three components: curve type (1–6), a lumbar spine modifier (A, B, or C), and a sagittal thoracic modifier (−, N, or +). The six curve types have specific characteristics, on coronal and sagittal radiographs, which differentiate structural and nonstructural curves in the proximal thoracic, main thoracic, and thoracolumbar/lumbar regions. The lumbar spine modifier is based on the relationship of the center sacral vertical line to the apex of the lumbar curve and measures the degree of lateral shift away from the midline caused by the curve. The sagittal thoracic modifier measures the degree of thoracic kyphosis with 10% to 40% being considered normal (N) [29]; these are summarized in E-Fig. 30.1.

PATHOPHYSIOLOGY AND NATURAL HISTORY

Vertebral rotation and rib cage deformity usually accompany any lateral curvature. With progression of the curve, the vertebral bodies in the area of the primary curve rotate the convex aspect of the curve and the spinous process to the concave side. This vertebral rotation can be determined by measuring the position of the pedicles from the midline (i.e., Moe method).[30] The vertebral bodies and the disks develop a wedge-shaped appearance, with the apex of the wedge toward the concave side. On the convex side of the curve, the ribs are pushed posteriorly, which narrows the thoracic cavity and causes the characteristic hump. On the concave side, the same rotation forces the ribs laterally, with consequent crowding toward their lateral margins (Fig. 30.2). These changes result in an increasingly restrictive lung defect. Exactly when this becomes a clinical problem depends on the accompanying pathology. The thoracic and lumbar regions are the most common sites of the primary curve. In children in whom the primary curve is in the lumbar region, the rotation of the vertebral bodies and spinous processes should be taken into consideration when attempting to place a spinal or epidural block because the spinal canal is relatively displaced toward the convex aspect of the curve.

The physical distortion in the thorax results in restriction of lung volumes and function. Ventilation depends on the mobility of the thoracic cage, the volume of each hemithorax, and the muscle power and elastic forces required to move the thorax.

Children with idiopathic scoliosis with a mild decrease in vital capacity also have reduced forced expired volume at 1 second (FEV_1), gas transfer factor, and maximal static expiratory airway pressures (PE_{max}). The predominant deformity of lateral flexion and vertebral rotation results in the lung on the concave side being able to achieve a near-normal end-expiratory position but not end-inspiratory position, whereas the lung on the convex side achieves a normal end-inspiratory position but cannot reach a normal end-expiratory position. The concave side contributes less than normal at total lung capacity, resulting in a decrease in PE_{max}. Similarly, because the convex side does not reach a normal end-expiratory position, the intercostal muscles and hemidiaphragm will be less efficient, resulting in a reduced maximum static inspiratory airway pressure (PI_{max}), although this reduction may not be quite so marked.[31] The main effect of scoliosis on respiratory function is mechanical, and the anatomic changes in the chest wall cause impaired movement and reduced compliance. Potential long-term respiratory problems when these defects are left untreated include hypoxemia, hypercarbia, recurrent lung infections, and pulmonary hypertension.

Congenital, Infantile, and Juvenile Scoliosis: Early-Onset Scoliosis

Congenital spinal anomalies are caused by failures of formation and segmentation that result in scoliosis and kyphosis. Hemivertebra, caused by failure of formation, is the most common anomaly. Fully segmented hemivertebrae contribute to progressive deformity during periods of rapid spinal growth (e.g., the first 5 years of life). The most severe deformities are seen in the thoracolumbar spine. Congenital spinal anomalies may be associated with malformations of the ribs, chest wall, and hemifacial microsomia.[32] Children with congenital scoliosis have an increased risk of cardiac and urological abnormalities. Bracing or casting techniques are not effective for this form of scoliosis. These children may have obstructive lung disease in addition to their restrictive disease, possibly owing to mainstem bronchial compression from spine rotation.[33] Surgical options for these children include fusion in situ, convex hemiepiphysiodesis, hemivertebra excision, growing rods, and vertical expandable prosthetic titanium rib (VEPTR) treatment.[34] Although short-term correction is easily achievable, a short thoracic spine or even thoracic insufficiency syndrome (inability of the thorax to support normal breathing and lung growth) can result.[35] Approximately one-half of the children who have extensive thoracic fusions and those whose fusions involve the proximal thoracic spine develop restrictive pulmonary disease (FEV_1 <50%).[36] Expansion thoracoplasty and stabilization using a VEPTR may be used.[37]

Infantile and juvenile scoliosis are part of the spectrum of idiopathic scoliosis but are considered here because they manifest and require treatment at an early age. Infantile scoliosis accounts for less than 1% of idiopathic scoliosis and is defined as scoliosis appearing between birth and 3 years of age.[34] It usually occurs in the thoracic spine, and the curve is usually convex to the left. Bracing and serial casting techniques are used for infantile scoliosis; improvement and resolution in some cases have been achieved at 9-year follow-up.[38]

Treatment of infantile scoliosis may begin as early as 4 to 5 months of age or as soon as the diagnosis of scoliosis has been made. Body casting appears useful in selected children, such as those with smaller, flexible spinal curves, but curve progression and the need for secondary treatments affect a significant proportion.[39] Bracing is considered when the curve reaches 30 degrees.[34]

TABLE 30.1	Classification of Scoliosis With Associated Key Anesthetic Risk Factors			
Classification	**Issues Associated With Scoliosis Surgery**	**Increased K⁺ With Succinylcholine**	**Expected High Blood Loss**	**Respiratory Complications and Ventilatory Support**
Idiopathic				
Infantile <3 years of age	Repeat operations, small size	✓		✓
Juvenile 3–9 years of age				
Adolescent 9–18 years of age	Regarded as cosmetic by patient; perfect result expected			
Congenital				
Bony abnormalities	Acute angle deformity; high risk of spinal cord injury, genitourinary malformations			
Neural tube defects				
Meningomyelocele, spina bifida, syringomyelia	Latex allergy, pressure sores, hydrocephalus, Arnold-Chiari and Chiari malformations (avoid neck extension)			
Neuromuscular				
Neuropathic				
Upper motor neuron				
Cerebral palsy, cerebral hypoxia	Upper airway obstruction, recurrent pneumonia, postoperative pain management		✓✓	✓✓
Lower motor neuron				
Poliomyelitis				
Myopathic				
Progressive				
Duchenne muscular dystrophy	Cardiomyopathy, mitral valve prolapse, conduction abnormalities	✓	✓✓	✓✓
Spinal muscular atrophy	Electrocardiographic abnormalities	✓	✓	✓
Facioscapulohumeral muscular dystrophy	Hypertrophic cardiomyopathy, cardiac failure	✓		
Other				
Friedrich ataxia		✓		
Neurofibromatosis	Hypertension, other neurofibromas			
Mesenchymal				
Marfan syndrome	Mitral and aortic regurgitation			
Mucopolysaccharidoses (e.g., Morquio syndrome)	Atlantoaxial subluxation, difficult intubation			
Arthrogryposis	Difficult intubation, severe contractures		✓	
Osteogenesis imperfecta	Small size			
Trauma				
Tumor				

✓, Anesthetic risk is likely; ✓✓, anesthetic risk is very likely.
Modified from Goldstein LA, Waugh TR. Classification and terminology of scoliosis. *Clin Orthop Relat Res.* 1973;93:10-22.

Success has also been reported for more severe curves (60 degrees) when casting was started before 20 months.[40] After induction of anesthesia, the child is positioned on the frame (first described by Cotrel and Morel[41]), securing the pelvis to the caudal end of the frame and tethering the head by a chin strap to the rostral end. The spine is mildly distracted, but the main maneuver derotates the spine through the ribs (Fig. 30.3A,B). General anesthesia with tracheal intubation is required to facilitate positioning the child, stretching the spine, and molding the body cast. Hemoglobin desaturation frequently occurs when the cast is molded to correct the spinal deformity; hypoxemia or breathlessness may occur following its application. Peak inspiratory pressure (PIP) may double if using positive-pressure ventilation intraoperatively; this can be partially improved by cutting a window in the cast.[42]

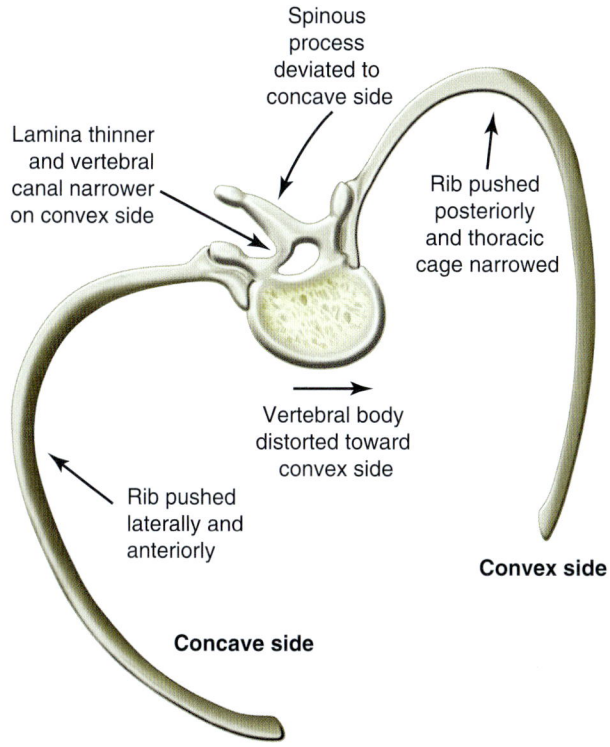

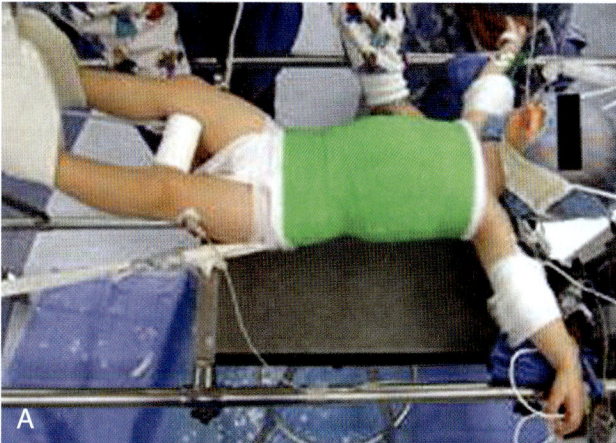

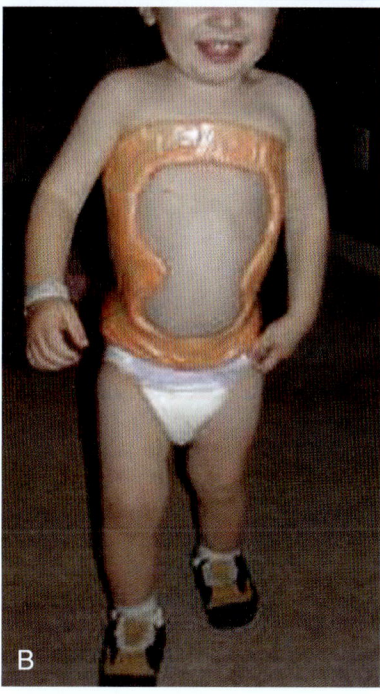

FIGURE 30.2 Characteristic distortion of the vertebra and ribs in thoracic scoliosis. (Modified from Kleim HA. Scoliosis. In: *Ciba Foundation Symposium*. Vol. 1. Summit, NJ: Ciba; 1978:609; Anesthesia for orthopedic surgery. In: Gregory GA, ed. *Pediatric Anesthesia*. 3rd ed. Edinburgh: Churchill Livingstone; 1994.)

FIGURE 30.3 A, Nonoperative correction of scoliosis in infants and toddlers may be achieved with repeated casting. **B,** Cutting and trimming of the cast allows correction of the spine while facilitating daily living.

An oral airway is also needed to prevent compression of the tracheal tube after the chin strap is applied and tightened (Fig. 30.3A). After the cast has hardened, it is cut back and trimmed to maintain the correction to the spine while facilitating breathing, gastrointestinal function, and day-to-day living (see Fig. 30.3B). Halo traction may be used to stretch and improve the curves but infections occur in ~50%.[43]

Juvenile idiopathic scoliosis represents 10% to 15% of idiopathic scoliosis and is defined as scoliosis that is first diagnosed between the ages of 4 and 10 years of age. Approximately 20% of these children and those with infantile scoliosis with a curve greater than 20% have an underlying spinal condition, most commonly Arnold-Chiari malformation and syringomyelia.[44] Although bracing is used to manage these curves, almost all children in this group with curves greater than 30% require surgical intervention.[45]

Growing rods may be used for congenital, infantile, or juvenile scoliosis to maintain the correction obtained at initial surgery while allowing spinal growth to continue. Several procedures are required before a definitive fusion.[46] All the systems (i.e., growing rods and VEPTR) have a moderate complication rate (i.e., rod breakage and hook displacement).VEPTR systems are being used to correct large-magnitude curves in this group of children when conservative treatment is inadequate.[47]

Idiopathic Scoliosis

Although adolescent idiopathic scoliosis is relatively common, severe morbidity develops only in children with early-onset (infantile or juvenile) idiopathic scoliosis.[48] Respiratory deterioration alone is seldom the reason for surgery in those who develop

scoliosis after the age of 5 years.[27] This is explained by the fact that the respiratory alveoli are mature by this age.[49,50]

Scoliosis evolves during growth spurts. The earlier the age of onset and the more immature the bone growth at the time the process begins, the more severe the outcome. The relentless progression of infantile-onset idiopathic scoliosis with rapidly deteriorating curves and lung function is often not amenable to surgery. Treatment involving spinal instrumentation and anterior epiphysiodesis does not prevent the reappearance of the deformity or the decrease in pulmonary function.[51]

Impaired lung function correlates directly with the magnitude of the thoracic curve. Severity of the scoliosis is the most accurate predictor of impaired lung function.[52] The morphology of the thoracic curve, the number of vertebrae in the major curve, and the rigidity of the curve also are associated with deteriorating pulmonary function.[53] Conventional wisdom has held that there is minimal impact on the vital capacity until the curve exceeds 60 degrees, with clinically relevant decreases in respiratory function occurring only after the thoracic scoliosis has progressed beyond 100 degrees.[36] Forced vital capacity (FVC) may decrease below normal (<80% of predicted) after the magnitude of the thoracic curve exceeds 70 degrees; FEV_1 decreases below normal after the main thoracic curve exceeds 60 degrees.[37] Twenty percent of children with a thoracic curve of 50 to 70 degrees have moderate or severe pulmonary impairment (i.e., FEV_1 <65% of predicted) (Fig. 30.4A).[54] Those with thoracic hypokyphosis are more likely to have moderate or severe impaired lung function; complex curves have a greater prevalence of moderate or severe pulmonary impairment, and the number of vertebrae in the thoracic curve is the most significant predictor of impaired lung function (see Fig. 30.4).[55] Children with a structural cephalad thoracic curve, a major thoracic curve spanning eight or more vertebral levels, or thoracic hypokyphosis are at increased risk for moderate to severe pulmonary impairment. Bracing patients with adolescent idiopathic scoliosis decreases the progression of high-risk curves[56] but is associated with worse pulmonary function test (PFT) results at the time of surgery.[57]

Neuromuscular Scoliosis

Children with neuromuscular scoliosis have the burden of deteriorating muscle function in addition to mechanical distortion. Crowding of the ribs on the concave side of the curve limits chest wall expansion, and the sitting posture restricts diaphragmatic excursion. This inevitably leads to more rapid deterioration in the curve and respiratory function. These children also have the potential for rapid and unpredictable deterioration of the curve.[38] It is important to consider the natural history of the specific neuromuscular disease when trying to balance the risks of surgery against conservative management.

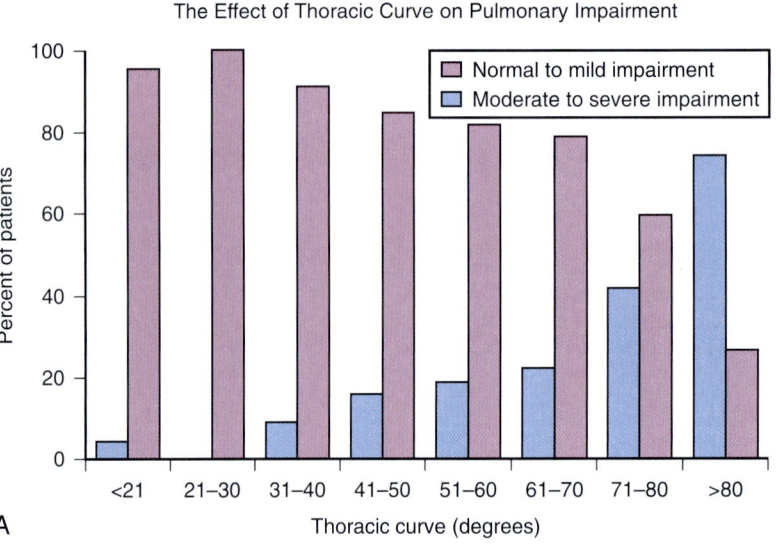

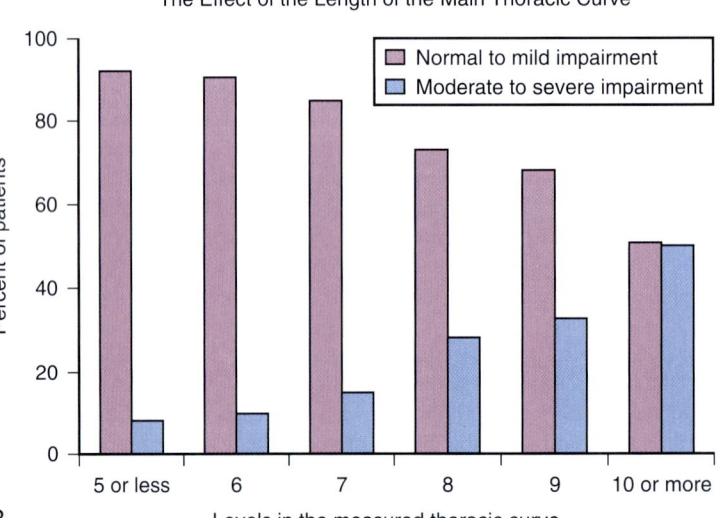

FIGURE 30.4 A, The bar graph demonstrates increasing pulmonary impairment with increasing curve severity as measured by degrees. **B,** Pulmonary impairment increases with increasing length of the thoracic curve. (From Newton PO, Faro FD, Gollogly S, et al. Results of preoperative pulmonary function testing of adolescents with idiopathic scoliosis. A study of six hundred and thirty-one patients. *J Bone Joint Surg Am.* 2005; 87:1937-1946.)

Children with Duchenne muscular dystrophy (DMD) suffer from progressive muscular weakness and increasing disability until death occurs, usually by the beginning of the third decade.[58] These children tend to become wheelchair-bound by 8 to 10 years of age because of increasing motor muscle weakness. Scoliosis then progresses with an acute deterioration during the growth spurt between the ages of 13 and 15 years, such that it becomes difficult or impossible to sit unaided. After the lumbar curve exceeds 35 degrees, further progression becomes inevitable.[59] A normal cough requires an inspiratory effort of more than 60% of total lung capacity and effective glottic closure to produce an effective peak flow (more than 160 L/minute in adults). Forced expiratory flows are typically reduced in proportion to the decrease in lung volume. As muscle weakness progresses, patients hypoventilate, initially at night. If nocturnal ventilatory support is not provided at this stage, diurnal hypercapnia will result.[60]

There have been two important changes in the overall management of children with DMD: the use of steroids and the earlier use of nocturnal noninvasive positive-pressure ventilation (NPPV). Steroid treatment in the early phase of the disease appears to slow disease progression for a few years; treatment with prednisone can stabilize strength and function for 6 months to 2 years.[61] This may delay the presentation of children for corrective surgery. Earlier adoption of nocturnal NPPV for nocturnal hypoventilation improves survival and quality of life. Clinically unsuspected nocturnal hypoventilation occurs in about 15% of patients with DMD and can be predicted by moderate impairment according to PFT results (FVC <70% and FEV$_1$ <65% of predicted) and scoliosis. Those with nocturnal hypoventilation have increased gas trapping, decline of muscle strength, and worse perception of health status despite NPPV.[62]

A 2007 multidisciplinary "Consensus Statement on the Respiratory and Related Management of Patients with Duchenne Muscular Dystrophy undergoing Anesthesia or Sedation" provided recommendations to standardize the approach to these patients[63] and others with flaccid neuromuscular diseases undergoing anesthesia. The most important of these recommendations are: an FVC <50% of predicted indicates an increase in postoperative respiratory complications; an FVC <30% suggests a further increase in risk. PFTs should be part of the preoperative evaluation when possible and should include FVC, P$_{I}$max, P$_{E}$max, peak cough flow, oxygen saturation by pulse oximetry (SpO$_2$) on room air, and partial pressure of carbon dioxide (PaCO$_2$) if the SpO$_2$ value is less than 95%. Consider preoperative training and postoperative use of NPPV if FVC is less than 50% of predicted, and strongly consider NPPV if FVC is less than 30%. Consider preoperative training and postoperative use of manual and mechanically assisted cough in those with impaired cough. In older children, this can be predicted by a peak cough flow less than 270 L/minute or maximal expiratory pressure less than 60 cm H$_2$O. Strongly consider planning to extubate the trachea directly to NPPV when the FVC is less than 30%.

Dilated cardiomyopathy occurs in up to 90% of DMD individuals older than 18 years of age; the severity of their physical disability often masks the clinical symptoms of cardiac failure. Cardiomyopathy is responsible for 20% of deaths, but this proportion may increase in the future for individuals in whom NPPV prevents respiratory-related mortality[61] (see also Chapter 21).

Risk Minimization and Improving Outcome From Surgical Intervention

RESPIRATORY FUNCTION AND OTHER COMPLICATIONS IN THE EARLY POSTOPERATIVE PERIOD

Lung volumes and flow rates decrease after scoliosis surgery as they do after thoracic and upper abdominal surgery. The FVC and FEV$_1$ decrease with a nadir at 3 days and are about 60% of preoperative values 7 to 10 days after surgery (Fig. 30.5). It is not until 1 to 2 months after surgery that PFTs return to baseline values. The magnitude of these decreases is unaffected by the type of surgery or whether the scoliosis is idiopathic or has an underlying neuromuscular cause.[64] Surveys from the British Scoliosis Society and Scoliosis Research Society report mortality rates before 2014 of 1.5 to 1.9 per 1000 cases[65,66]; but rates have decreased to 1.1 to 1.2 per 1000 cases in 2019 and 2020.[67] Before 2014, mortality rate was less in adolescents with idiopathic scoliosis (0.4 per 1000) and greater in those with neuromuscular disease (3.6 per 1000)[66]; by 2019 and 2020, rates for neuromuscular disease were 3.0 and 2.5 per 1000.[67] Overall, deep infections occurred in 2.8% and a permanent neurologic defect in 0.45% of

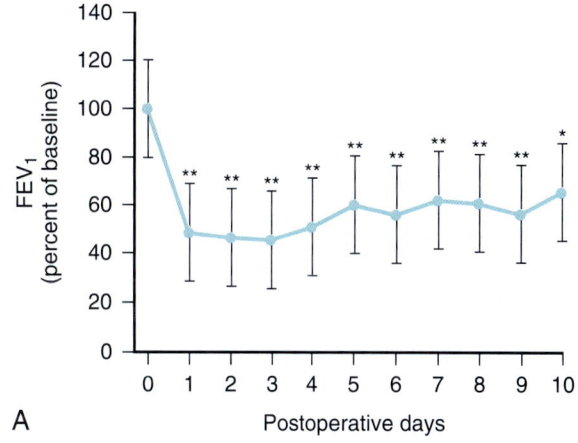

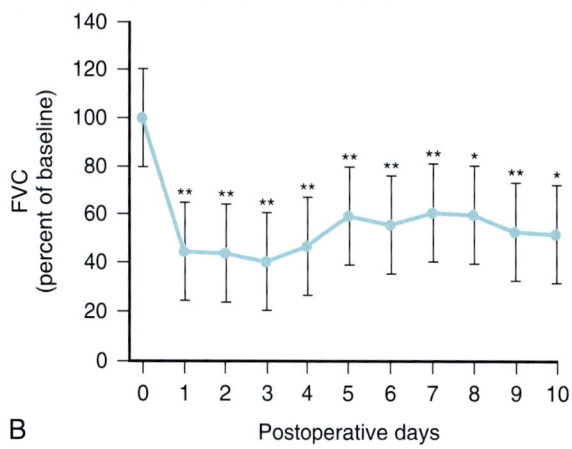

FIGURE 30.5 A, Changes in forced expiratory volume in 1 second (FEV$_1$) during the 10 days after scoliosis surgery. **B,** Changes in forced vital capacity (FVC) during the 10 days after scoliosis surgery. (From Yuan N, Fraire JA, Margetis MM, et al. The effect of scoliosis surgery on lung function in the immediate postoperative period. *Spine* 2005; 30:2182-2185.)

children in reports up to 2014[65]; deep infections decreased to 0.95% and permanent neurologic deficits were 0.71%.[67]

Early-Onset Scoliosis

Early-onset scoliosis has a dismal prognosis when untreated, and repeated spinal lengthening procedures are associated with a complication rate of 80% and a mortality rate of 18%.[68] Magnetic growing rods, by reducing the number of operative interventions, may be associated with fewer complications and improved pulmonary function.[69]

Idiopathic Scoliosis

Complications in children with adolescent idiopathic scoliosis are uncommon. A small body mass index (BMI <10%) is an independent predictor of increased blood loss, pneumonia, and readmission.[70] An increased body mass index is associated with a 3-fold increase in postoperative adverse events. Instrumentation of more than 13 segments and operating times greater than 6 hours are associated with an increased length of stay. Any complication during the hospital stay is associated with readmission; the most common cause is surgical site infection (SSI).[71] Scheuermann kyphosis is associated with an 8- to 10-fold increase in major complications, SSI, and reoperations compared with adolescent idiopathic scoliosis.[72] The Nationwide Inpatient Database of operations from 2002, involving 36,335 patients with adolescent idiopathic scoliosis reported that 7.6% of patients developed at least one in-hospital complication. The three most common complications were respiratory failure (3.5%), reintubation (1.3%), and implant related (1.1%). Major complications such as death, pancreatitis, disseminated intravascular coagulation, visual loss, spinal cord injury, cardiac arrest, sepsis, nerve root injury, deep vein thrombosis, pulmonary embolism, shock, myocardial infarction, and iatrogenic stroke each had an incidence of ≤0.2%. Combined anterior-posterior procedures were 3 times more likely to experience a complication (19.8%) than posterior fusion alone (6.7%).[73] Surgeon-reported complications from the British Scoliosis Research Society Morbidity and Mortality database of operations from 2004 to 2016 involving 84,320 patients found an overall complication rate of 1.5%; respiratory complications were not reported. Death occurred in 12 patients (0.014%). The three most reported complications were SSI 0.52%, new neurological deficit 0.35%, and implant-related complications 0.20%. The overall complication rate decreased from 4.95% during 2004 to 2007 to 0.98% during 2013 to 2016.[74]

Neuromuscular Scoliosis

Children with neuromuscular disease are more likely to require prolonged mechanical ventilation after spinal surgery because of more severe preoperative respiratory impairment.[75] The marked decrease in vital capacity and peak flows is undoubtedly related to the risk of postoperative complications, but determining when it is no longer safe to anesthetize those with a restrictive lung defect remains an imperfect science.

Postoperative management of children with impaired respiratory function is the routine use of NPPV and cough augmentation therapy that should be planned if the preoperative FVC is less than 30%. Cough augmentation can be provided manually by hyperinflation and forced expiration, alone or together, and by mechanical insufflation-exsufflation (MIE) therapy.[76] The effectiveness of mechanical insufflation-exsufflation may be limited in children with a weak or enlarged tongue if it blocks exsufflation flow.

Less extensive surgery with the newer pedicle screw systems decreases the need for pelvic fixation to correct pelvic obliquity. The procedures require less extensive surgery and shorter operating times, which may benefit children with impaired respiratory function.[77–80]

Respiratory complications after surgery for adolescent idiopathic scoliosis are relatively uncommon; however, they are 5-fold more common in children with neuromuscular scoliosis.[81,82] Anterior spinal procedures are associated with a greater incidence of complications than posterior spinal fusion; some consider this to be the main risk factor for postoperative respiratory complications.[82] Current pedicle screw systems may decrease the need for anterior procedures, thereby decreasing the complication rate.[83]

Atelectasis, infiltrates, hemothoraces, pneumothoraces, pleural effusions, and prolonged intubation have the greatest incidence, whereas pneumonia, pulmonary edema, and upper airway obstruction occur less frequently. These problems are more common when the scoliosis is associated with developmental delay; the greatest complication rate is in those with cerebral palsy and flaccid neuromuscular scoliosis.[81–84] Respiratory complications increase as the severity of scoliosis and degree of respiratory impairment increase but complication rates vary considerably. Children with neuromuscular scoliosis have a respiratory complication rate of 15% to 30%[84–88] and minimal mortality. One study, which separated three groups according to respiratory impairment (FVC <30%, FVC = 30% to 50%, FVC >50%), reported an overall complication rate of 31% independent of the degree of respiratory impairment,[84] possibly reflecting improved modern management techniques (Table 30.2).

A systematic review and meta-analysis of neuromuscular scoliosis patients (n = 15,218) demonstrated a large incidence of complications: pulmonary (22.7 %), followed by implant complications(12.5%), infections (10.9%), neurological complications (3.0%), and pseudoarthrosis (1.88%)[89]; these were all greater than those observed in patients with adolescent idiopathic scoliosis. A national database interrogation of short-term outcomes in patients with cerebral palsy showed that the most common nonsurgical complications were acute respiratory failure requiring mechanical ventilation (11.4%), paralytic ileus (8.2%), wound complications (4.9%), and urinary tract infections (4.6%), with a

TABLE 30.2	Incidence of Pulmonary Complications[84]					
Forced Vital Capacity	Total Number of Patients	Patients With Pulmonary Complications	Pneumonia	Atelectasis	Pneumothorax	Ventilator Care (>3 days)
<30%	18	6	3	0	1	2
30%–50%	18	7	3	1	0	4
>50%	38	10	2	1	0	7

90 day readmission rate of 17.6%, due in almost equal part to wound dehiscence, surgical site infection, other infection, dehydration, feeding issues, or acute respiratory failure.[90]

Surgical Site Infection

SSI results in high morbidity and cost. Rates are much greater after nonidiopathic scoliosis repair, increasing from 2.6% with adolescent idiopathic scoliosis to 9.2% with neuromuscular scoliosis. The most common pathogens are *Staphylococcus aureus,* coagulase-negative staphylococci, and *Pseudomonas aeruginosa.*[91] Almost half of the infections in children with neuromuscular scoliosis contain at least one Gram-negative organism and half are polymicrobial. SSI was more common in children with spina bifida than in those with other diagnoses (OR = 3.0).[92] Increased body mass index for age ≥95th percentile is associated with increase rate of SSI (relative risk [RR] = 2.8) and hospital readmission (RR = 1.8).[93] More severe curves, nonambulatory status, and increased length of stay increase the risk of infection.[94] A systematic review was unable to find evidence for many measures used to minimize SSIs; chlorhexidine skin wash the night before surgery, preoperative nasal swabs for *S. aureus,* chlorhexidine skin disinfection, perioperative prophylaxis with intravenous vancomycin, or gentamicin powder in the surgical site or graft.[95] Application of structured protocols by two institutions using many of these measures as a "bundle of care" has resulted in markedly decreased infection rates from 8.6% and 10% to 2.2% and 1%.[96,97]

Gastrointestinal

Children with neuromuscular scoliosis suffer gastrointestinal tract complications in up to 13% of cases.[98] Paralytic ileus, gastroparesis, and dysphagia are among the most common postoperative adverse events. Important risk factors are preoperative main curve >90 degrees (RR = 5.5) and adverse intraoperative neuromonitoring changes (RR = 6.0). Hospital stay was 6 days longer in those with gastrointestinal problems.[99] Children with cerebral palsy have additional problems associated with their lack of muscular control (e.g., swallowing incoordination, excessive salivation, gastroesophageal reflux) and may have developmental delay that contributes to a postoperative complication rate of 30%.[85,86,98] Nonambulatory children and those with curves greater than 60 degrees are at increased risk for major complications; nonambulatory patients are almost four times more likely to have a major complication.[86] Gastrointestinal dysmotility in cerebral palsy patients can be exacerbated after scoliosis surgery and cause persistent vomiting and bloating.[100] Pancreatitis may occur in up to 30% of cerebral palsy patients after surgery, with a greater incidence among those with documented gastroesophageal reflux and reactive airway disease.[101]

LONG-TERM CHANGES

Idiopathic Scoliosis

Improvements in pulmonary function are not impressive after correction of idiopathic scoliosis. Early studies suggested that spinal fusion stabilized the respiratory dysfunction that existed preoperatively but failed to offer any improvement.[102] Improvements are possible in some subgroups of patients with some surgical techniques. For example, children undergoing a posterior procedure for a preoperative curve less than 90 degrees experienced an increase in vital capacity of slightly greater than 10%, improved maximum voluntary ventilation, and improved maximum respiratory mid-flow rate after 2 years. In contrast, those who underwent anterior surgery did not improve similarly.[103] Harrington rod instrumentation in children with idiopathic scoliosis resulted in only a small improvement in vital capacity.[104]

Pulmonary function returns to preoperative values within 3 months after the posterior approach using the newer instrumentation systems, with additional improvements occurring and sustained for 2 years.[105] Pedicle screws provide greater curve correction in adolescent idiopathic scoliosis, with some slight improvement of pulmonary function after 2 years compared with other instrumentation techniques.[21] Lung volumes measured by 3D computed tomographic scans do not change even with an increase in patient height, suggesting a dynamic rather than static improvement from hemithoracic symmetry.[106,107] A 10-year follow-up analysis demonstrated an absolute increase in the FVC (3.25 L to 3.66 L) and FEV_1 (2.77 L to 3.10 L) but no changes in percent of predicted values in children who underwent a posterior fusion only. In the same analysis, those with chest wall disruption experienced no change in FVC and FEV_1 over 10 years, but a significant decrease in predicted FVC (79% vs. 85%,) and FEV_1 values (76% vs. 80%).[108]

Chest cage disruption (i.e., thoracoplasty or anterior thoracotomy) is associated with reduced pulmonary function at 3 months and a 10% to 20% decrease in total lung capacity (TLC) and FVC. These values do not return to baseline until 1 to 2 years after surgery. Improvements in lung function with this approach rarely occur.[48,49] Video-assisted thoracoscopic surgery (VATS) for anterior release and instrumentation incur less pulmonary morbidity and a smaller decrease in pulmonary function at 3 months. One year after surgery, values for children treated thoracoscopically return to baseline, but not for those undergoing open thoracotomy (Fig. 30.6).[109,110] Two- and 5-year follow-up evaluations of those after VATS showed no significant changes with regard to the correction of the major Cobb angle (56% ± 11% and 52% ± 14%, respectively) or average predicted TLC (95% ± 14% and 91% ± 10%).[111]

Improving surgical techniques may challenge these findings in the future. A 2-year postoperative study concluded that VATS for thoracic curves and open anterior procedures for thoracolumbar curves resulted in minimal to no permanent pulmonary impairment 6 months after the procedure compared with posterior spinal fusion, despite a short-term decrease observed after VATS.[112]

Posterior spinal fusion with pedicle screws improved back pain and health-related quality of life compared with patients with

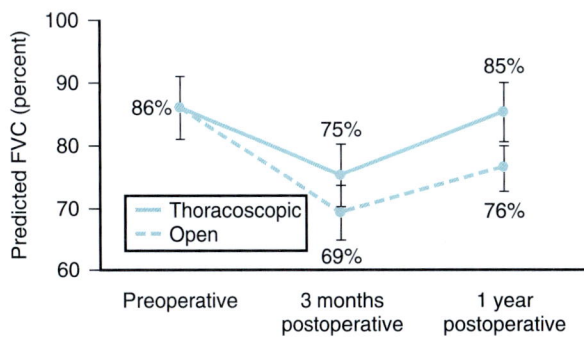

FIGURE 30.6 Changes in percent of forced vital capacity (FVC) for thoracoscopic versus open anterior instrumentation during the first year after surgery. (From Faro FD, Marks MC, Newton PO, Blanke K, Lenke LG. Perioperative changes in pulmonary function after anterior scoliosis instrumentation: thoracoscopic versus open approaches. *Spine.* 2005; 30:1058-1063.)

untreated adolescent idiopathic scoliosis at 5 years post-surgery. These patients had similar health-related quality of life to that of the healthy control group without adolescent idiopathic scoliosis, except for reduced function.[113]

The most exciting possible advance in scoliosis surgery for idiopathic surgery is minimally invasive spine surgery that involves three 2-inch incisions or the "coin-hole" technique.[114,115] Early studies with minimally invasive scoliosis surgery were of longer duration than conventional surgery and with smaller correction of the curve, but with more experience, the times for surgery decreased. In meta-analysis and systematic reviews of minimally invasive surgery versus conventional surgery, minimally invasive surgery yielded smaller scars, less blood loss, less pain, and shorter length of stay, with similar rates of complications, and prolonged duration of surgery.[116–118] As the instruments for scoliosis surgery continue to improve, surgeons adapted minimally invasive robotic-assisted surgery to scoliosis as a means to improve the accuracy of the surgery, specifically pedicle screw placement.[119] As newer surgical techniques are introduced into scoliosis surgery, it is conceivable that perioperative problems after scoliosis surgery will wane and become clinically inconsequential.

Neuromuscular Scoliosis

Improvements in the scoliosis angle and the degree of pelvic obliquity are achieved after spinal instrumentation in children with neuromuscular disease. Although there is consensus for the start of the proximal fusion (T1 or T2) to prevent a kyphosis from developing, debate rages whether the distal fusion should terminate at L4/L5 or L5/pelvis, particularly since fusing of the L5/pelvis for pelvic obliquity is a major source of postoperative surgical complications.[120,121] Recent evidence from 47 children with neuromuscular scoliosis showed similar degrees of L5 and pelvic tilt by terminating the fusion at L4/L5 and L5/pelvis, but a 2-fold greater incidence of complications terminating the fusion at L5/pelvis versus L4/L5.[120] Improvement in the quality of life was perceived by the child or caregiver and in the ability to sit unaided, particularly if children are unable to do so beforehand.[80,122–127]

Improvement in respiratory function is less certain. A review of the long-term survival of children with DMD after spinal surgery and nocturnal ventilation demonstrated that those having spinal surgery and ventilation had a median survival of 30 years, whereas those receiving nocturnal ventilation only survived to 22.2 years. This result occurred despite a decrease in mean vital capacity from 1.4 L to 1.13 L in the first postoperative year.[128] Posterior spinal fusion for scoliosis in DMD was associated with a slowing in the rate of decrease in respiratory function; the rate of 4% per year before surgery decreased to 1.75% per year (over 8 years) after surgery.[129] The mean rate of decrease in percent of FVC after surgery was 3.6% per year in those with an FVC of less than 30%.

However, there is little evidence for any improvement in respiratory function in this group of children, although there may be a period of delay or even stabilization of the inevitable deterioration in respiratory function.[58,123,130] No difference in respiratory function 5 years after surgery was noted when compared with patients managed conservatively.[125,131] There is progressive loss of vital capacity after surgery with a decrease of 25% over 4 years, with 66% of children requiring mechanical respiratory assistance by that time.[124] A Cochrane review failed to identify any randomized clinical trials to evaluate the effectiveness of scoliosis surgery in patients with DMD, leaving authors to suggest: "*Patients with*

scoliosis should be informed as to the uncertainty of benefits and potential risks of surgery for scoliosis. Randomized controlled trials are needed to investigate the effectiveness of scoliosis surgery, in terms of quality of life, functional status, respiratory function, and life expectancy."[132,133]

Less outcome information is available for children with cerebral palsy. Surgery is perceived to have a positive impact on patients' quality of life, overall function, and ease of care by parents and other caregivers,[134] despite the high complication rates. A 3-year follow-up after a pedicle screw construct for scoliosis in 52 children with cerebral palsy demonstrated an improved functional ability in 42% of children.[83] Most children had improved sitting balance with a reduced pelvic obliquity from 9.2 degrees to 5.2 degrees and less nursing care requirements. A 32% complication rate occurred; most were pulmonary in origin but ultimately reversible. Two perioperative deaths and one transient neurologic deficit caused by screws that impinged in the spinal canal, which resolved when they were removed.[83]

Less morbidity has been claimed for the same-day (one-stage) surgery compared with the two-staged approach in children with neuromuscular disease requiring anterior and posterior spinal surgery.[135,136] However, it seems reasonable to avoid anterior thoracotomy in neuromuscular patients in view of the poor respiratory function after chest cage disruption.[105,109] Currently, pedicle screw systems in children with neuromuscular scoliosis produce outcomes similar to those of earlier systems but with shorter operating times and less blood loss.[78]

Spinal Cord Injury During Surgery

ETIOLOGY

Spinal cord injury can occur by four main mechanisms: direct contusion of the cord during surgical exposure; contusion by hooks, wires, or pedicle screws; distraction by rods or halo traction; and reduction in spinal cord blood flow.[137] Epidural hematoma should be included in the differential diagnosis of deficits occurring postoperatively. The areas of the spinal cord most vulnerable to ischemic injury are the motor pathways, which are supplied by a single narrow anterior spinal artery. This is fed in a segmental manner by the radicular arteries that arise from the vertebral, cervical, intercostals, lumbar, and iliolumbar arteries. The largest radicular artery is the artery of Adamkiewicz, which arises between T8 and L4. A watershed area between T4 and T9 is prone to ischemia because the blood supply in this region of the cord is poorest (Fig. 30.7).[138,139] Paraplegia is the most feared neurologic complication, but partial spinal cord injury resulting in areas of localized weakness and numbness as well as bladder and bowel disturbances have also been reported.

The increasing use of pedicle screws in spinal surgery raises the possibility of increased risk to individual nerve roots. A systematic review of pedicle screw complications that involved a total of 4570 pedicle screws in 1666 patients reported an overall 4% malposition rate that increased to 16% in studies that systematically examined their patients postoperatively.[140] Eleven patients required revision surgery for the malpositioned screws, and there was one temporary neurologic complication (i.e., epidural hematoma). No vascular injuries were reported, although six cases of aortic abutment were described. Robotic-assisted minimally invasive scoliosis surgery has been shown to improve the accuracy of pedicle screw placement during minimally invasive surgery.[119]

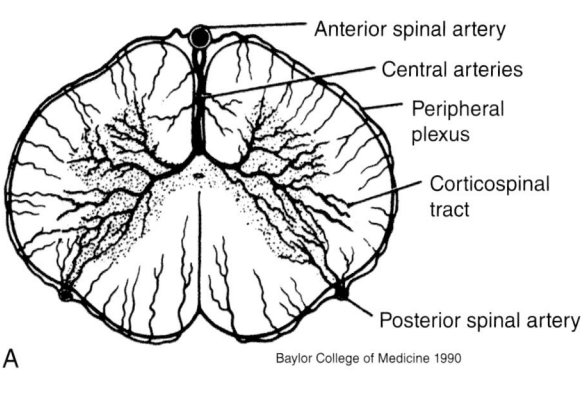

A

Baylor College of Medicine 1990

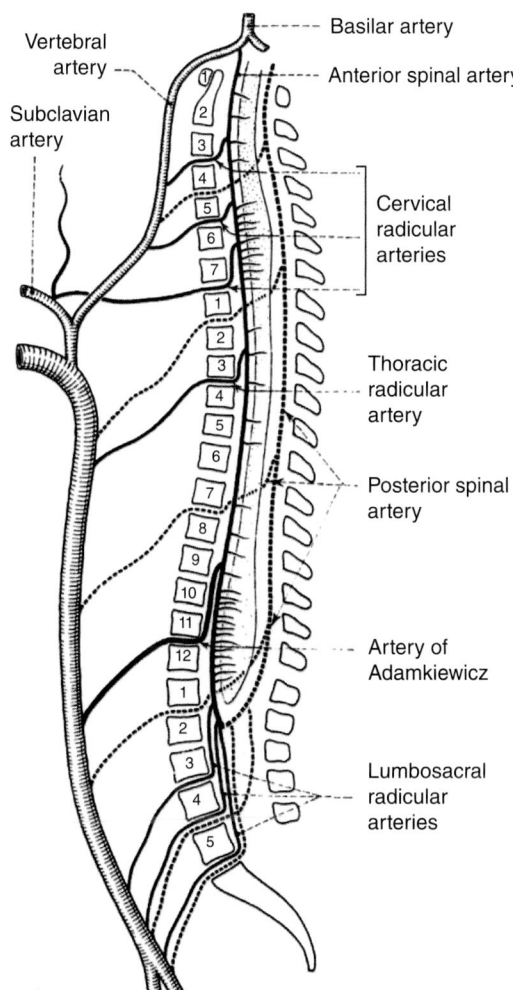

B

FIGURE 30.7 Spinal cord blood supply. **A,** Axial view. **B,** Longitudinal view. (From Macdonald DB, Skinner S, Shils J, Yingling C, American Society of Neurophysiological M. Intraoperative motor evoked potential monitoring – a position statement by the American Society of Neurophysiological Monitoring. *Clin Neurophysiol.* 2013;124:2291-2316, with permission.)

RISK OF SPINAL CORD INJURY AND SPINAL CORD MONITORING

Surveys undertaken by the Scoliosis Research Society investigating idiopathic scoliosis reported in 1975 an incidence of neurologic impairment of 0.72%,[141] which in 2000 had decreased to 0.3%. All of the deficits were partial cord lesions.[137] Patients with curves greater than 100 degrees, congenital scoliosis, kyphosis, and post-irradiation deformity appear to be at greatest risk for complications. The use of pedicle screws may have increased the immediate neurologic complication rate. In 2007, nine neural complications were reported among 1301 patients, for an incidence of 0.69%. Three thecal penetrations occurred, two because of pedicle screws, all without sequelae. There were two nerve root injuries and four spinal cord injuries, all of which resolved within 3 months.[142]

A retrospective review of 19,360 cases of pediatric scoliosis showed different overall complication rates among idiopathic (6.3%), congenital (10.6%), and neuromuscular (17.9%) scoliosis. Neurologic deficits had a different distribution, with the greatest rate among congenital cases (2%), and smaller rates with neuromuscular (1.1%), and idiopathic scoliosis (0.8%).[143] Mortality rates of 0.3% were observed for neuromuscular and congenital scoliosis, with an idiopathic scoliosis rate of 0.02%. Rates of new neurologic deficits were greater with anterior screw–only constructs (2%) or wire constructs (1.7%) than with pedicle screw constructs (0.7%). Surgery for high-grade spondylolisthesis appears to be associated with a particularly high risk of neurologic deficit with a rate of 11.5%.[144]

Spinal cord function is monitored to ensure that the complication rate is as small as possible. The Scoliosis Research Society issued an information statement in 2019, which stated that intraoperative neuromonitoring (IONM) was "*... a standard modality that is a nearly universally used adjunct to improve safety of surgical deformity correction procedures when the spinal cord is at risk. It has been conclusively demonstrated that intraoperative spinal cord monitoring facilitates detection of impending spinal cord deficit and facilitates early interventions that are likely to preserve spinal cord function.*"[145] For any monitoring technique to be effective, it needs to have a sensitivity and specificity that allows true changes to be immediately recognized with very low false-negative and false-positive results to allow the problem to be reversed or prevented. Older tests, such as the wake-up test and ankle clonus test, have largely been superseded by monitoring of SSEPs, MEPs, and triggered electromyographic (EMG) techniques. The importance of using a multimodal approach is increasingly recognized[146–149]; the capabilities and limitations of the various techniques are summarized in E-Table 30.1.

METHODS OF MONITORING SPINAL CORD FUNCTION
Wake-Up Test
The wake-up test measures gross motor function of the upper and lower extremities.[150] The test requires limiting or antagonizing muscle relaxation and reducing the depth of anesthesia sufficiently to enable the patient to follow commands during the surgery; failure to move the feet and toes while being able to squeeze a hand suggests a problem with the spinal cord. When the test was initially described, 3 of 124 patients were identified as having no movement and were saved from paraplegia.[150] A major limitation is that the test is conducted after maximal spinal correction when any neurologic insult has already occurred; however, subsequent removal or modification of the spinal instrumentation within 3 hours of the onset of the neurologic deficit has been reported to prevent permanent neurologic sequelae.[151] The wake-up test is unlikely to detect isolated nerve root injury or sensory changes and is limited to patients with an appropriate developmental age who can follow instructions.

With the clinical application of SSEP and MEP monitoring (Fig. 30.8) well established and in the absence of intraoperative

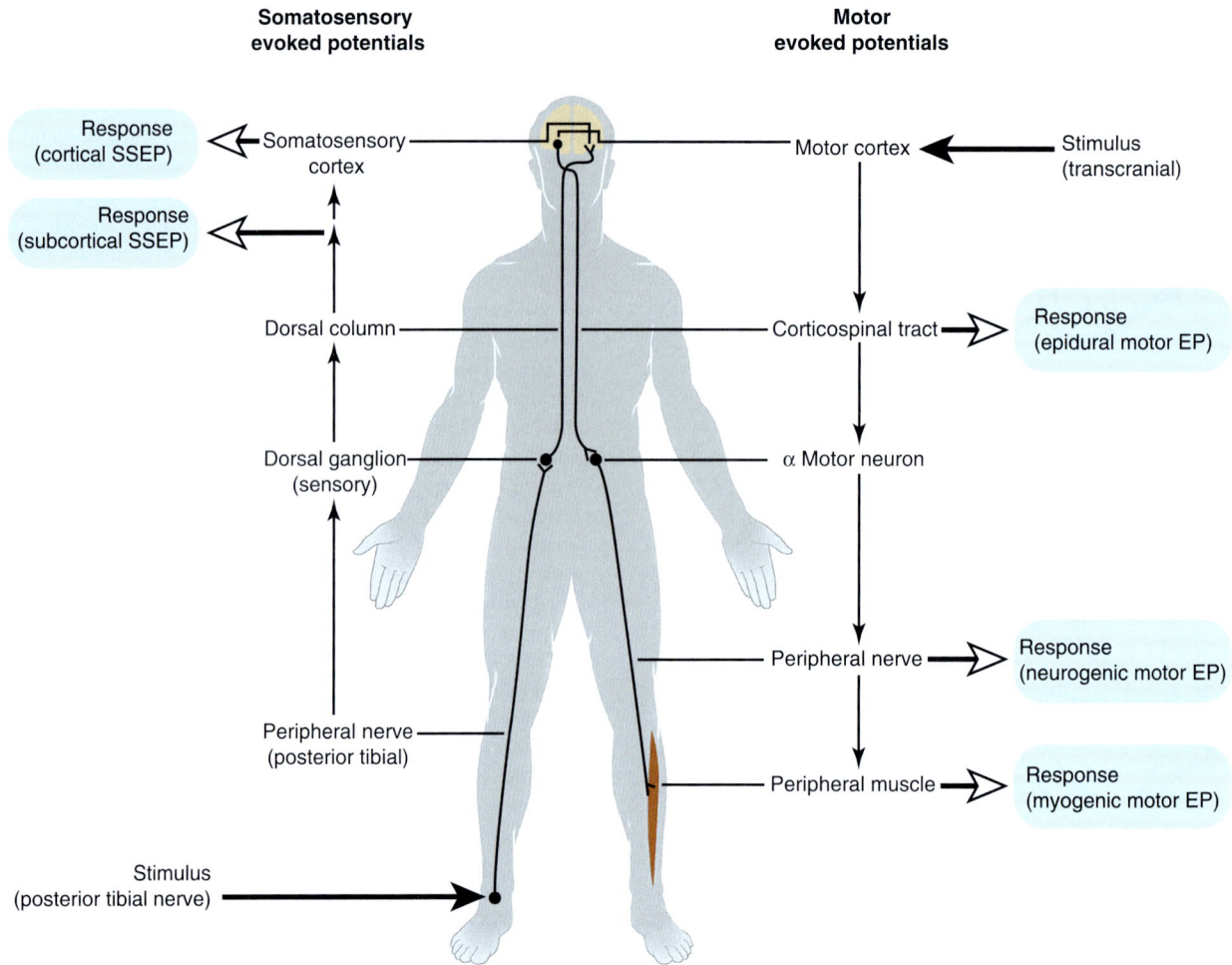

FIGURE 30.8 Comparison of pathways involved in somatosensory evoked potential *(SSEP)* and motor evoked potential *(motor EP)* monitoring. (Modified from de Haan P, Kalkman CJ. Spinal cord monitoring: somatosensory- and motor-evoked potentials. *Anesthesiol Clin North Am.* 2001;19:923-945.)

changes, there is no justification to routinely perform the wake-up test.[152] Nonetheless, some surgeons still regard the wake-up test to be the gold standard, and it may be used to confirm changes demonstrated by SSEP or MEP monitoring.[153,154] Risks associated with the wake-up test include lack of nerve root and sensory information, accidental extubation, dislodgment of the instrumentation, intraoperative recall with subsequent psychological trauma, air embolism, and cardiac ischemia. If a wake-up test is planned, it is prudent to warn the patient at the preoperative visit that they will be awakened during the surgery (but reassure them that they should not feel pain) and to instruct the surgeon to fill the wound with saline to reduce the risk of an air embolism.

Ankle Clonus Test

The ankle clonus test uses the clonus that occurs just before consciousness is regained during wakening from anesthesia. Rhythmic muscle contractions are thought to result from spinal reflexes returning while the higher neurologic centers remain inhibited by anesthesia, and the oscillations demonstrate an intact spinal cord. Inability to demonstrate clonus suggests spinal cord injury.[155] Like the wake-up test, it is a post hoc test rather than real-time monitoring. However, in a review of more than 1000 patients undergoing spinal procedures in which six postoperative neurologic deficits occurred, this test identified all the deficits but

produced three false-positive findings, giving a sensitivity of 100% and a specificity of 99.7%. In comparison, the wake-up test produced false-negative results for four of the five patients who developed deficits.[155]

Somatosensory Evoked Potentials

SSEPs involve stimulating a peripheral nerve and measuring the response to that stimulation using scalp electrodes (i.e., cortical SSEPs).[156,157] Alternatively, the response can be measured subcortically near the spinal cord by electrodes placed in the epidural space, interspinous ligament, or spinous processes of the vertebrae.[158] The advantage of the subcortical evoked potential is that the responses are more stable, reproducible, and resistant to the effects of anesthetic agents.

The signal produced with SSEP monitoring travels from the peripheral nerve through the nerve root and up the ipsilateral dorsal column. The impulses then cross over at the level of the brainstem and progress rostrally through the thalamus to the primary sensory cortex. Up to 30% of patients with adolescent idiopathic scoliosis may have abnormal SSEP signals preoperatively.[159]

The rationale for using SSEP to monitor motor deficits is because the sensory tracts are in proximity to the motor tracts of the spinal cord. Injury to the motor tracts indirectly affects the sensory tracts and causes changes in the SSEP. When spinal cord function is impaired, there is usually an increase in latency and a decrease in amplitude in the SSEP, with eventual loss of signal. A 10% increase in latency of the first cortical peak (P1) or 50% decreases in the peak-to-peak amplitude (P1N1) suggest a need for intervention.[160,161] Although SSEP signals primarily monitor transmission through the sensory dorsal columns, they are effective,[161] and SSEP monitoring is associated with a 50% decrease in the incidence of neurologic deficits.

It is unusual for motor tract injury to occur when SSEPs remain unchanged, but false-positive and false-negative results have been reported.[161,162] Seventy percent of the postoperative complications were detected by the monitor, but 30% (false negatives) were not detected. Pedicle screw misplacement leading to radiculopathy may not be detected by SSEP monitoring.[163] Several case reports of paraparesis also attest to the limitations of SSEP monitoring. Further evaluation of the technique demonstrated that SSEPs alone have an unacceptably low level of sensitivity (i.e., spinal cord injuries can be missed).[164] These concerns encouraged development of methods to monitor the motor tracts of the spinal cord. SSEP monitoring is possible in patients with cerebral palsy, whereas MEP monitoring may not be.[165]

Motor Evoked Potentials

The motor pathways can be activated by transcranial stimulation of the motor cortex or by spinal cord stimulation. Transcranial stimulation in spinal surgery is usually achieved using electrical or magnetic stimulation applied to the scalp by applying high-voltage pulses to the scalp using corkscrew, needle, or surface electrodes. The stimulation pulses can be applied as single stimuli or brief pulse trains with intervals between the pulse trains. Multiple stimuli result in a stronger signal with less variability owing to temporal summation of the excitatory postsynaptic potential.[166] Epilepsy and proconvulsant medicines are considered relative contraindications to MEP monitoring because of concerns about brain injury from prolonged seizure activity caused by the electrical current required for stimulation.[167,168] Not surprisingly, MEPs may be difficult to record and interpret in patients with cerebral palsy and should not be attempted if the child has seizures.

MEP monitoring may be a problem in younger children, particularly those younger than 6 or 7 years of age.[167,169] Younger children require a greater stimulating voltage and pulse train frequency for MEP monitoring, probably because of immaturity of the central nervous system, specifically the descending corticospinal tracts.[170] Use of spatial summation in addition to temporal summation in children younger than 6 years of age enabled reliable MEPs to be documented in 86% (18 of 21).[169] Improving techniques allow satisfactory recordings in children under age 4 years, but true-positive findings are rare, whereas low MEP amplitude and poor waveforms are common.[171]

Spinal cord stimulation can be applied using electrodes placed outside or inside the spinal cord rostral to the area of interest. Single stimuli rather than brief pulse trains typically are used for spinal cord stimulation.[172] This approach is not commonly used in scoliosis surgery.

Responses can be recorded anywhere distal to the area of interest. They have included the lower lumbar epidural space (i.e., epidural MEP), peripheral nerve (i.e., neurogenic MEP), and peripheral muscles using compound muscle action potential (CMAP) (see Fig. 30.8).[173] Each recording site has its limitations regarding the accuracy of the information displayed and the susceptibility to anesthetic drug interference. Epidural MEPs are the least affected by neuromuscular blocking drugs

(NMBDs), but they monitor only conduction in the corticospinal tract and provide no information about the anterior horn gray matter.[174] They have a much slower response to acute spinal cord ischemia compared with myogenic responses (i.e., CMAPs).[175] Neurogenic MEPs are also resistant to anesthetic interference but appear to not accurately measure motor conduction. Most of the spinally elicited peripheral nerve responses seen with neurogenic MEPs occur through the dorsal columns in a retrograde fashion and are sensory rather than motor.[176] Anterior spinal cord injury has been demonstrated with normal neurogenic MEPs.[177] CMAPs after transcranial stimulation are thought to be exclusively generated by motor tract conduction, and unlike epidural MEPs, they include the ischemia-sensitive anterior horn alpha motor neurons.[173] These responses are very sensitive to anesthetic agents. The responses obtained with CMAPs after spinal cord stimulation also appear to contain signals that include transmission through the dorsal columns and may represent a mixed response.[178]

An ongoing problem with MEP monitoring is deciding what degree of signal change is indicative of spinal cord injury.[179] A negative predictive value of 100% is important and a feature of all reports but there is variability in the positive predictive value. Some centers use the same criteria they adopted for SSEP monitoring (i.e., 50%),[180] whereas others use a greater degree of change. A decrease in amplitude of 80% had a sensitivity of 1.0 and a specificity of 0.91 when used as the sole monitor during spinal surgery.[181] A 65% decrease in amplitude identified all postoperative motor deficits (SSEP changes identified only 43%) in children with idiopathic scoliosis.[164] An alarm threshold using a decrease in amplitude of >70% and delay in onset latency of >10% from baseline has high specificity that reduced false-positive results while retaining a negative predictive value of 100% (false negative of 0%).[182] Using an amplitude decrease of >80% for MEPs and 50% for SSEPs, a sensitivity of 100%, specificity of 99.3%, positive predictive value of 55.6%, and negative predictive value of 100% was observed. Sensitivity was 100% for MEPs compared with 20% for cortical or cervical SSEPs.[183]

The dorsal columns may be injured without involvement of the motor tract.[184] Occasionally, adverse changes in SSEPs occur without changes in MEPs.[172,185] Because of these reports, MEP monitoring should be used in addition to SSEP monitoring rather than as a replacement.[146–149,186] SSEP monitoring alone is no longer considered an acceptable standard of care,[145] despite some institutions reporting sensitivity of 95%, specificity of 99.8%, a positive predictable value of 95%, and a negative predictive value of 99.8%.[187] However, multimodal intraoperative monitoring (combination of SSEP and MEP) demonstrated improved sensitivity when compared with either modality alone.[154,183] Examples of IONM monitoring are shown in E-Figure 30.2.

The relationship between neuromonitoring alerts and new neurological defects (NNDs) was explored in a detailed study of 275 patients undergoing scoliosis surgery with SEP and MEP monitoring. Alerts occurred in 51 patients (18.5%) and following intervention, signals improved in 42: one patient developed an NND (false negative), but the others did not. In the nine patients without signal improvement, six developed NND (true positive) and three did not (false positive). Among the remaining 224, 221 had no NND (true negative) but three had a NND (false negative). All patients made complete long-term recoveries.[188] Of particular interest is the breakdown of anesthetic and surgical related factors and the interventions performed (Fig. 30.9). Hypotension was a factor in >50% of alerts. Although volatile

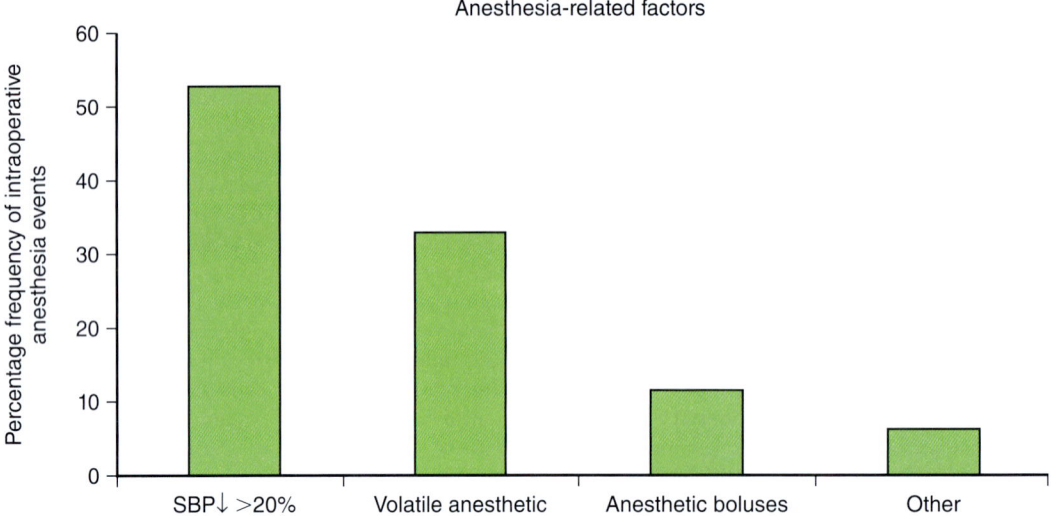

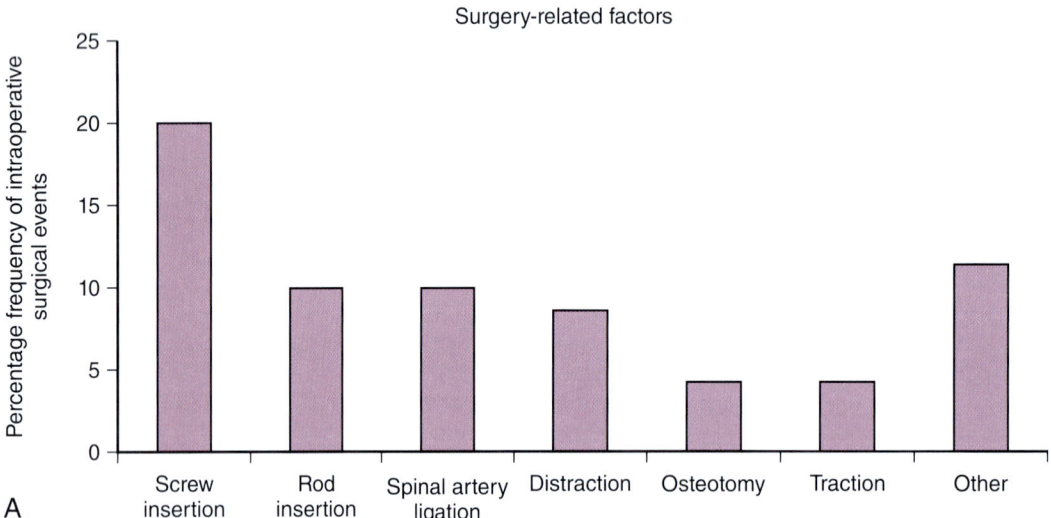

FIGURE 30.9 A, Frequency of anesthesia and surgery related factors at the times of alerts. Note the higher percentages in the anesthesia related factors. *SBP <20%*, Decrease in systolic blood pressure of more than 20% from the baseline.

anesthetics were used in 30% of cases, they were not specifically related to the alerts, but bolus anesthetic doses were used 10% of the time. Vasopressors, fluid bolus, and/or transfusion were the most common anesthetic interventions and on the surgical side, modification of surgery, release of halo traction, and decreased distraction were most common.

Triggered Electromyographic Techniques

The increasing use of pedicle screws allows greater curve and rotational correction than earlier techniques but has an additional risk of direct nerve root trauma. Triggered EMGs using a monopolar needle or bipolar handheld stimulator have been described, with a threshold stimulation level of more than 8 mA considered to be normal, 5 to 8 mA to be critical, and less than 5 mA to be pathologic, indicating that there is insufficient distance between the screws and the neural tissue.[186,189] This technique requires monitoring rectus abdominis or intercostal muscles when used for thoracic curves.[190,191]

The Patient Journey: Preparation, Planning, and Pathways

A more comprehensive approach to managing these complex patients has developed in recent years, key components being, increased patient involvement in decision making through education and explanation, improved communication between team members and outside specialist consultants, and better discharge planning. Although the delivery of care is institutional, many guidelines endorsed by national societies have been promulgated and given identifying names such as Perioperative Surgical Home (PSH) and Perioperative medicine–the pathway to better surgical care.[22,192] These models of care also encompass aspects of Enhanced Recovery After Surgery (ERAS) protocols[193] to deliver planned and standardized approaches to care, yet tailored to individual patient needs.[194–197] Component parts include preoperative teaching of parents and patients, setting expectations, standardized

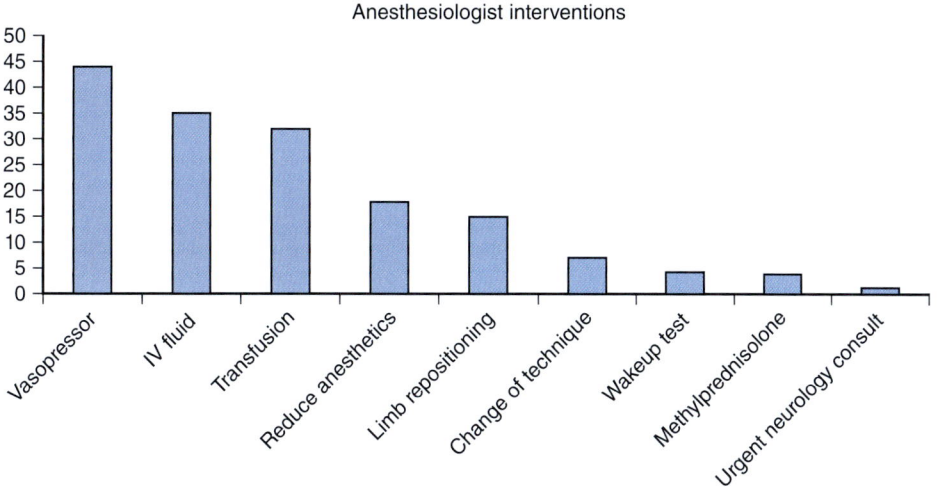

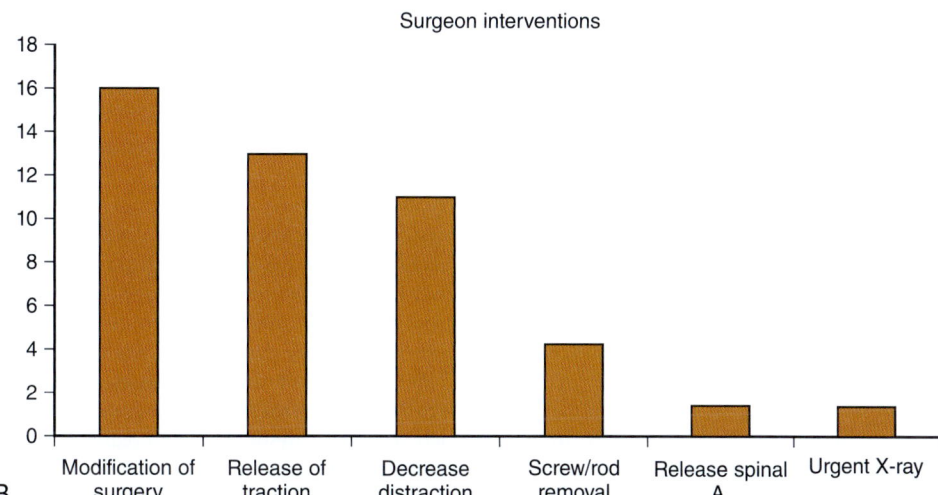

FIGURE 30.9, cont'd B, Frequency of interventions performed by the anesthesiologists and surgeons according to the guidelines when alerts occurred. Note higher percentages of interventions performed by the anesthesiologists. *A.,* Artery; *IV,* intravenous. (From Neira VM et al. Diagnostic accuracy of neuromonitoring for identification of new neurological deficits in pediatric spinal fusion surgery. *Anesth Analg.* 2016; 123: 1556-66, with permission.)

approach to intraoperative anesthetic and surgical management, and immediate to long-term postoperative medical management over and above pain management. This involves shortening time to first solid food intake, and time to ambulation plus minimizing adverse effects of medication such as postoperative nausea and vomiting (PONV), sedation, and constipation. An accelerated discharge pathway emphasizing early transition to oral pain medications, mobilization with physical therapy 2 to 3 times/day, and discharge regardless of return of bowel function resulted in a 50% decrease in hospital stay with no difference in readmissions or wound complications. Expectations were set with the family before surgery for early discharge.[198] Such approaches have resulted in most or all of the following: earlier urinary catheter removal, earlier discontinuation of patient-controlled analgesia (PCA) pumps, decreased postoperative pain scores and opioid use, reduction in postoperative complications, earlier feeding and ambulation, and shortened length of hospital stay, in children undergoing corrective surgery for adolescent idiopathic scoliosis.[194–197]

A meta-analysis and systematic review of ERAS–like protocols reinforces the earlier statements but makes the point that the literature is restricted largely to retrospective studies with nonrandomized data and initial cohort studies, lacking formal control groups.[193]

PREOPERATIVE ASSESSMENT AND POSTOPERATIVE PLANNING

This is an important opportunity to build rapport with the patient and family. The most common concerns raised by patients and their parents are regarding pain, ability to return to activities after surgery, and the possibility of surgical complications, particularly neurological injury.[199,200] Using a structured questionnaire, Patient Generated Index (PGI), the three most common patient-reported concerns before surgery were sports, general function, and general fitness, whereas the three most common parent-reported concerns were general function, sports, and appearance.[201] The preoperative interview is the time to discuss such issues, premedication, and what to expect in the early postoperative period. Neuromuscular patients have the burden of coexisting disease that may be a concern to the patient and parents. All benefit from a comprehensive explanation of the anticipated process and a realistic discussion regarding postoperative comfort and outcome.

RESPIRATORY ASSESSMENT AND PLANNING FOR POSTOPERATIVE VENTILATORY SUPPORT

The preoperative pulmonary assessment should identify patients at increased risk for postoperative respiratory compromise. Since patients with idiopathic scoliosis generally have less compromised pulmonary function, most studies have focused on nonidiopathic patients.[81] For planning purposes, patients with idiopathic scoliosis and preexisting respiratory disease, such as asthma or bronchopulmonary dysplasia, maybe expected to spend a day longer in hospital than those without.[202]

The rate of postoperative pulmonary complications correlates broadly with the decrease in vital capacity.[75,203,204] Vital capacity less than 30% to 35% of predicted values indicates marginal respiratory reserve and a level at which complications and a need for postoperative respiratory support are likely. Many patients with low vital capacity are unable to cough effectively, rendering them prone to postoperative atelectasis, pneumonia, and respiratory failure.

Studies of a mixed population of disorders with a vital capacity less than 40% reported that despite the occurrence of short-term and middle-term pulmonary complications, these patients can be successfully discharged home, although some require prolonged postoperative ventilation.[205–207] Modest numbers with a vital capacity less than 25% of the predicted value are included in these studies and do not have greater complication rates than those with greater vital capacities. Anterior or combined approaches increase the likelihood of respiratory complications, particularly owing to pleural effusion.[205,206]

Children with neuromuscular scoliosis are likely to need postoperative ventilation that may be prolonged.[75,204] These patients may also have abnormalities in the central control of breathing and impaired airway defense mechanisms. Impaired coordination of laryngeal and pharyngeal muscles may result in impaired swallowing and inadequate cough with increased risk of aspiration. A vital capacity of <35% of predicted, is often associated with the need for a brief period of postoperative ventilation.[110] The earlier use of nocturnal NPPV and use of NPPV in the postoperative period may alter our perception of this risk by decreasing the impact or severity of postoperative respiratory complications while allowing children with increasingly severe respiratory impairment to be considered for surgery. Scoliosis surgery can be successfully undertaken in patients with a vital capacity less than 35% of predicted, often with no more than 24 hours of planned ventilation followed by a period of noninvasive ventilation (e.g., bilevel positive airway pressure [BiPAP]).[75,84,208,209] The overall complication rate was similar whether the FVC was greater than or less than 30%, and the average hospital stay was approximately 3 weeks (see Table 30.2) in one small study (n = 30). Tracheostomy was required in two children, and the overall pulmonary complication rate was 30%[209]; similar results are reported by others.[84] It seems reasonable to anticipate using noninvasive ventilator support for several days after spine stabilization surgery in children with a vital capacity less than 25% of predicted values. Even children with a mean FVC of 20% of predicted have been successfully managed with a brief period of postoperative ventilation and transition to

BiPAP within 48 hours.[210] Whether a child should be denied surgery requires consideration of individual patient factors. The successful management of children with a vital capacity of 15% to 20% of predicted has been reported, although the sample size is small.[205,206,208,209] Although the risk of an unsuccessful outcome can increase at this level of pulmonary dysfunction, individual circumstances may justify the risk. The successful introduction of perioperative NPPV will likely lead to children who were previously considered unsuitable for surgery now being offered surgery, challenging the established limitations.[211]

CARDIOVASCULAR ASSESSMENT

Many children with complex cardiac comorbidities can successfully undergo scoliosis surgery because of improvements in understanding, monitoring, anesthesia, and surgical techniques. A greater need for blood transfusion should be expected. A preoperative curve greater than 80 degrees is a risk factor for major complications in children who have had congenital cardiac defects corrected.[212] Children with residual cardiac abnormalities will require prolonged stays in the intensive care unit and hospital. Those with single ventricle or Fontan physiology have increased morbidity and mortality.[213] Increased bleeding is almost always a problem because of high venous pressures; the need for inotropic support and the occurrence of arrhythmias and pleural effusions are common.[213]

Muscle disorders may affect the myocardium and the skeletal system. Children with DMD develop a cardiomyopathy in the second decade that may be difficult to evaluate because the child is wheelchair bound by that age. Sinus tachycardia is an early manifestation. Cardiac function deteriorates during early adolescence[214] as more than 90% of adolescents with DMD have subclinical or clinical cardiac involvement.[215,216] Most patients will be receiving angiotensin-converting enzyme inhibitors which delay left ventricular dysfunction and reduce mortality.[217] Echocardiography is an essential aspect of the preoperative evaluation of any wheelchair-bound patient presenting for scoliosis surgery (see also Chapters 16 and 21). Cardiac magnetic resonance imaging may be better than echocardiography to assess cardiac function in children with DMD, particularly those with poor acoustic windows. Furthermore, cardiac magnetic resonance imaging also assesses myocardial fibrosis.[218] A dobutamine stress echocardiogram is rarely needed to provide additional information.

POSTOPERATIVE CARE

Pain Management

Scoliosis surgery is associated with severe pain that lasts for at least 3 days.[219] Effective analgesia minimizes postoperative respiratory complications by allowing deep breathing, chest physiotherapy, early ambulation, and rehabilitation. Pain may begin preoperatively, perioperatively, or postoperatively and may be managed with systemic or epidural analgesia. A multimodal approach is likely to be most effective. The wide variety of treatment options described suggests no single optimal pain management plan.

Intraoperative Intrathecal and Intravenous Opioids

Intraoperative intrathecal morphine (2–5 µg/kg) provides effective analgesia during the first 24 hours after spinal fusion.[220,221] Intrathecal morphine also decreases the amount of remifentanil required intraoperatively, contributing to less pain when remifentanil is discontinued.[222,223] This benefit does not occur when IV morphine is used intraoperatively.[224] A meta-analysis of intrathecal morphine in pediatric scoliosis surgery confirms its analgesic effect, decreased opioid consumption in the initial 48 hours after surgery without an increase in complications such as respiratory depression, nausea, vomiting, or pruritus.[225]

Methadone (0.2 mg/kg) decreases pain scores and opioid requirements for 36 hours.[226,227] This drug is used in adult spinal surgery and reports of its use in children are increasing.[228,229] A prescription proposed to maintain adequate plasma concentrations for 24 hours would include an IV bolus (0.25 mg/kg) of methadone followed by an infusion (0.1–0.15 mg/kg per hour) for 4 hours during spinal surgery.[229] In a single center retrospective study of methadone to reduce perioperative hydromorphone use after posterior spinal instrumentation, supplemental hydromorphone was least required in those who received the following regimen: methadone 0.2 mg/kg IV before incision, 0.1 mg/kg IV for pain in postanesthesia care unit (PACU) and then 0.1 mg/kg IV 6 hours after postanesthesia care unit compared with children who received zero methadone and those who received a single preoperative dose of methadone and a hydromorphone PCA.[226]

Nonsteroidal Antiinflammatory Drugs

Acetaminophen is commonly used together with NSAIDs; both act on different parts of the Prostaglandin H2 synthetase enzyme with additive effect.[230–232] NSAIDs, but not acetaminophen, impair fracture healing in animal models.[233] Cyclooxygenase-2 (COX-2) activity plays an important role in bone healing, and the use of NSAIDs decreases osteogenic activity that may increase the incidence of nonunion after spinal fusion.[8,9] The effect on osteogenic activity is dose dependent and reversible.[234] Similar effects have not been demonstrated in humans and the use of these drugs after scoliosis surgery varies in different parts of the world.[235] NSAID use is generally in consultation with the surgeon during the first 3 to 5 days after scoliosis surgery.[236]

Systemic Analgesics

Morphine remains the mainstay of systemic analgesic regimens. Morphine infusions of 10 to 40 µg/kg per hour are required during the first 48 hours after surgery. Achieving a balance of effective analgesia while avoiding sedation can be difficult in children with developmental delay. Frequent assessment of these children is important to minimize complications. PCA is appropriate for children older than 6 to 7 years of age. It can be used with a typical bolus dose of 20 µg/kg and a lockout interval of 5 to 10 minutes. The use of a background morphine infusion may be effective in some patients.[237,238] Our preference is to use a nighttime background infusion at 5 to 10 µg/kg per hour but to use PCA alone during the day (see also Chapter 41). The addition of acetaminophen improves analgesia but does not decrease opioid requirements.[239] Nurse- and parent-controlled analgesia are effective if the child is too young or unable to use PCA.[240] Intrathecal morphine plus PCA appears to offer the optimal combination of effective analgesia and minimal adverse effects in patients with idiopathic scoliosis compared with PCA morphine alone or epidural morphine.[241] The demands/deliveries ratio of PCA is predictive of increased opioid requirements, with a ratio greater than 1.5 associated with greater pain scores, opioid-related adverse effects, and duration of hospitalization; a ratio greater than 2.5 suggests a possible benefit from switching opioids.[242]

Low-dose ketamine infusion (0.05–0.2 mg/kg per hour) has been used as an adjunct to morphine infusions or PCA, with mixed effects. Ketamine has not been effective to reduce opioid requirements after lower abdominal surgery in children,[243,244] although it has been effective in reducing post-scoliosis pain in patients who were opioid tolerant.[245] The effective ketamine dose was 0.2 mg/kg IV in the postanesthesia care unit followed by 0.12 mg/kg per hour for 24 hours. A postoperative 72-hour ketamine infusion did not decrease morphine consumption or pain scores in children or adults undergoing scoliosis surgery.[246–248] Ketamine is effective; however, if used to treat pain resistant to morphine or in heroin-addicted patients.[249,250] Ketamine added to morphine PCA has produced mixed results, with no clear beneficial effect in orthopedic surgery, despite such evidence being apparent for thoracic surgery.[251] If added to PCA, the optimal combination of morphine/ketamine in adults (spine and hip surgery) was found to be a 1:1 ratio with an 8 minute lockout.[252] Although scoliosis is a very painful surgery, it is probably best to reserve the use of ketamine for those with major preoperative pain or morphine-resistant pain.[245]

Gabapentin and pregabalin may provide some benefit with an opioid-sparing effect,[253] although postoperative nausea and vomiting benefits are limited.[254] Gabapentin (15 mg/kg followed by 5 mg/kg three times daily for 3 days) after scoliosis surgery in adolescents reduced morphine consumption by about 30% during the study period but without any improvement in morphine's adverse effects. Improved pain relief was observed only until the morning after surgery.[255] A systematic review of gabapentin for postoperative pain demonstrated a very small reduction (1–2/10 score) in pain and preoperative anxiety and mildly increased patient satisfaction.[256] Further studies involving patients with adolescent idiopathic scoliosis, neither gabapentin nor pregabalin had any effect on postoperative pain or chronic pain after surgery.[257–259] Although gabapentin has only a modest effect on analgesia at best, it has been associated with a decrease in time to completing physical therapy goals.[260] However, a multimodal analgesic pathway based on preoperative acetaminophen and gabapentin, combined with intraoperative infusions of lidocaine and ketamine, did not improve recovery in patients who had multilevel spine surgery.[257,258,261]

Other Drugs

Other drugs or drug combinations used perioperatively or early postoperatively may have a positive effect on postoperative pain management. Dexamethasone continued for 3 days postoperatively (8 mg/day) after posterior spinal fusion in adults was associated with a 40% decrease in opioid use, with no increase in wound complications.[262] Patients were also more likely to walk at the time of the initial physical therapy evaluation.[262] A single dose of dexamethasone, 0.15 mg/kg IV, at induction of anesthesia reduced nausea and vomiting for 48 hours after surgery.[263]

The role of lidocaine infusions remains uncertain. Intravenous lidocaine may have a role in postoperative pain management after spine surgery. An intraoperative infusion at 2 mg/kg per hour IV improved pain scores and decreased opioid consumption for 48 hours postoperatively, and improved quality of life at 1 and 3 months assessed using the acute short-form (SF-12) health scores.[264] Lidocaine reduced postoperative pain and long-term postoperative back pain intensity measured at 3 months.[265] However, others report that lidocaine had no effect on pain scores, morphine consumption, or quality of life during the first postoperative day 1 using SF-12 physical and mental composite scores.[145] In children with adolescent idiopathic scoliosis, lidocaine infusions at 1 mg/kg per hour continued for 6 postoperative hours was associated with decreased pain scores for the first

9 hours, a 30% decrease in morphine consumption over the first 48 hours, and earlier oral intake and ambulation.[266]

Dexmedetomidine infused at 0.4 µg/kg per hour for 24 hours after idiopathic scoliosis surgery provided the equivalent analgesia to a morphine infusion (10 µg/kg per hour) with less PONV and the times to oral intake, ambulation, and first bowel movement were also less.[267]

Epidural Analgesia

Continuous epidural analgesia using single- and double-catheter techniques may provide effective analgesia after spinal surgery.[268] The single-catheter technique using bupivacaine-fentanyl and sited at T6–7 for patients undergoing a mean 12-level scoliosis surgery yielded similar analgesia as PCA but with more PONV and pruritus. Bowel sounds returned earlier in the epidural group, but liquid intake and hospitalization time were similar.[269] Similar results were reported with a bupivacaine-morphine combination in patients undergoing 10-level spinal fusions. Full diet and discharge from hospital were achieved one-half day earlier with the epidural technique than with PCA.[270] A retrospective review of more than 600 patients treated with an epidural or PCA for analgesia after scoliosis surgery that involved an average 8.5 fused segments confirmed the effectiveness of epidural analgesia.[271] In that study, a bupivacaine-hydromorphone epidural combination effectively controlled the pain, although it was associated with more complications. Respiratory depression and transient neurologic changes were the most common complications observed.[271] Effective analgesia and a large incidence of PONV and pruritus have been features of studies that combined bupivacaine and morphine.[272,273]

Patient-controlled epidural analgesia (PCEA) has been successfully used in children older than 5 years of age for orthopedic surgery and thoracotomies.[274] In scoliosis surgery, the pain score with PCEA with bupivacaine and hydromorphone was slightly superior to that with PCA.[275] PCEA with a single- or double-catheter technique, depending on the number of spinal segments involved, with a combined bupivacaine-fentanyl-clonidine solution effectively controlled pain with a relatively small incidence of complications.[276]

Improved pain control and bowel function, and decreased adverse effects may be possible by using a double-epidural technique using moderate amounts of fentanyl and clonidine with local anesthetics.[277] Double-epidural techniques, position one catheter in the upper to middle thoracic segments and a second catheter in the upper to middle lumbar level.[278,279] This technique improved pain control and was associated with fewer gastrointestinal adverse effects when compared with a single epidural catheter and morphine PCA.[268] Failure rates due either to inadequate analgesia or technical problems with epidurals at reported rates of 13% to 38%.[271,275]

A Cochrane review in 2019 that sought to compare the postoperative efficacy of epidural analgesia with systemic analgesia after thoracolumbar spine surgery, reported that epidural analgesia reduced pain at rest at all times, although the reduction in pain was not clinically meaningful. At 6 to 8 hours after surgery, the mean pain score with systemic analgesia was 3.1 (VAS 0–10) and with epidural analgesia was 1.32 points less; by 72 hours the difference was 0.8. A similar margin of improvement was observed with pain on movement.[280] There was no difference in PONV and only weak evidence to support earlier return of bowel function, earlier ingestion of liquid or solid food, with epidural local anesthetics alone. The difference in time to ambulation was minimal, (mean difference 0.08 days, 95% CI 0.24–0.39).

Optimizing Postoperative Pain Management to Facilitate Early Ambulation and Discharge

The variety of alternative analgesic options attests to the fact that a superior single analgesic regimen does not exist. Although opioids remain an integral part of postoperative pain relief, there is increasing interest in the use of other drugs to minimize reliance on opioids. This includes coadministration of gabapentin or pregabalin, tramadol or tapentadol, ketamine, lidocaine, dexamethasone, dexmedetomidine, and clonidine, alone or in combination plus the use of epidural analgesia.

Anesthetic and Intraoperative Management

POSITIONING AND RELATED ISSUES

The patient must be positioned so that extreme pressure points are avoided, the limb positions are adjusted to prevent nerve injury, and the abdomen is free to minimize venous congestion. This is usually achieved by the use of the Relton-Hall frame or a variant.[281] The frame consists of four well-padded supports arranged into V-shaped pairs, with the upper pads supporting the thoracic cage and the lower pair supporting the anterolateral aspects of the pelvic girdle at the anterior iliac crests. The arms must not be abducted or extended more than 90 degrees from their natural position. The weight of the arms is evenly distributed across the forearm to avoid pressure on the ulnar nerve at the elbow. The range of motion of the shoulders should be assessed preoperatively for optimal positioning during anesthesia. This can present quite a challenge in children with severe deformities, and creative positioning may be required. Some cover the nipples with Tegaderm (3M, St. Paul, MN, USA) and position them free of direct pressure. It is also essential that the head is maintained in a neutral position and that pressure is evenly distributed between the forehead and face, avoiding direct pressure on the eyeballs. The use of a DuoDERM extra thin dressing to cover the face and allow all taping to be applied to the dressing, helps minimize eye swelling and minor skin tears that can occur with prolonged periods in the prone position (E-Fig. 30.3A,B). Care must be taken to avoid any direct pressure on the knees, and the patient's weight should be distributed throughout the lower limb (Fig. 30.10). Reston self-adhering foam (3M, St. Paul, MN, USA) may be used to pad the pelvic brim, elbows, and knees.

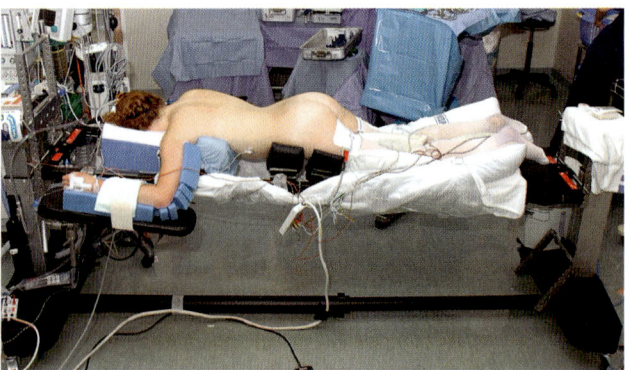

FIGURE 30.10 Positioning on the Orthopedic Systems Incorporated (OSI) Jackson frame (Mizuho OSI, CA, USA), showing protected pressure points and an underframe forced-air warming blanket.

Not all spinal tables and frames affect cardiac function in the same way. The Jackson spine table (Mizuho OSI, CA, USA) or longitudinal bolsters have fewer effects on cardiac function, whereas Wilson and Andrews frames may negatively impact cardiac function.[282] However, an average decrease in cardiac index of 18.5% (0.5 L, 95% CI 0.3–0.7 L) was observed after placing patients prone on the Jackson table, without a notable change in blood pressure.[283] The use of two chest pads rather than a single pad with the Jackson frame results in smaller average and maximum chest pressures at the expense of increasing the pelvic pressures.[284]

Postoperative visual loss is an uncommon, unpredictable, and devastating complication associated with spinal surgery in the prone position. The reported incidence is up to 0.2% of cases, although the incidence has been decreasing over the past decade. Most reports of blindness after spine surgery involve adult patients, but it has involved older children as well.[285,286] The most common outcome is posterior ischemic optic neuropathy and it occurs bilaterally in 50% of cases.[287] Its cause has remained obscure. Prolonged operating time (>6 hours), large blood loss, blood transfusions, male sex, obesity, and increased age are features.[287–291] The phenomenon is unrelated to pressure on the globe and is usually an isolated ischemia event.[291] Evidence is conflicting regarding an association between blindness and hypotension, controlled hypotension, anemia, hemodilution, blood loss, rotational positioning of the head, diabetes, and others.[288,291–293] A practice advisory for perioperative visual loss associated with spine surgery 2019 from the American Society of Anesthesiologists cautioned clinicians to use controlled hypotension *"only when the anesthesiologist and surgeon agree that its use is essential and to treat prolonged significant decreases in blood pressure."* They further stated that *"staged spine procedures may be used on a case-by-case basis for high-risk patients."* Regarding blood loss and anemia they state that *"a transfusion threshold that would eliminate the risk of perioperative visual loss related to anemia cannot be established at this time."*[294]

TEMPERATURE REGULATION

The long preparation time and exposure of undraped patients on a spinal frame render them susceptible to hypothermia. Hypothermia is associated with hemodynamic instability and increased blood loss.[295] A 3-fold increase in surgical wound infection occurs with a 2°C-decrease in core temperature.[296] Preoperative warming reduces the amount of time that the patient is hypothermic during surgery by almost 2 hours without affecting the temperature at the end of surgery.[297] Efforts should be made to increase the ambient temperature in the operating room while the patient is prepared for surgery. Subsequent hypothermia can be minimized if the room temperature is maintained at 24°C during this period rather than at 18°C to 21°C.[298] After the patient has cooled during preparation and positioning, it may take several hours before the core temperature begins to return to normal. Even with forced-air warming systems, it is often difficult to restore normothermia because only a small amount of the patient's body is exposed to these devices. It may be possible to position a warming blanket underneath the frame to improve warming (see Fig. 30.10 and Video 30.1). In addition to less bleeding and shorter operating times, aggressive maintenance of normothermia throughout the perioperative period in patients with adolescent idiopathic scoliosis also resulted in a shorter hospital stay.[299]

PATIENT MONITORING

Patient monitoring needs to be tailored to the individual case, but at minimum, arterial oxygen saturation, end-tidal carbon dioxide ($ETCO_2$), electrocardiographic (ECG) patterns, core temperature, and urine output should be recorded. In most cases, invasive arterial and central venous pressures are monitored because of large blood losses, fluid shifts, and the risk of cardiovascular instability. Externally applied pressure by the surgeon during dissection or curve correction may compromise cardiac function or filling. Central venous pressure is an accurate and valid measurement in the prone position, providing the zero is adjusted for the patient's position on the spinal frame. Patients with a kyphotic component are at increased risk for venous air embolism and should be monitored for this possibility. Depth of anesthesia monitoring should be used when MEP monitoring limits the concentrations of anesthetic drugs and total IV anesthesia (TIVA) is used. Care should be taken when positioning the head because pressure on the forehead by the sensor while the patient is in the prone position for many hours may cause erythema, localized swelling, and tissue necrosis; contact dermatitis from the adhesive has been reported.[300] Mixed venous oxygen tension trends may be helpful for children with myocardial compromise. Transesophageal echocardiography can be useful for determining ventricular filling and function when hemodynamic compromise is identified or suspected preoperatively. Dynamic indices, such as pulse pressure variation (PPV) may assist in managing fluid responsiveness when managing the circulation. PPV is based on the heart-lung interaction and reflects cyclical changes in stroke volume (and thus pulse pressure) induced by mechanical ventilation that occur in cases of biventricular preload responsiveness. Systematic reviews identified that PPV >12.5% was accurate in predicting volume responsiveness.[301,302] In the prone position a similar degree of PPV (14%) indicated fluid responsiveness.[303] PPV may not be as reliable in children as in adolescents.[304] Although utility of PPV in cardiac surgery has been demonstrated,[305] this is less so in neurosurgery.[306] Other less invasive methods assessing noninvasive continuous cardiac output such as bioimpedance- and bioreactance-based devices may be of value as well.[307,308]

MINIMIZING BLOOD LOSS AND DECREASING TRANSFUSION REQUIREMENTS

Scoliosis surgery involves exposure of a large wound over a considerable period. Positioning the patient with the abdomen free to avoid venous compression is important to control and minimize blood loss. Increased intraabdominal pressure attributable to positioning can double intraoperative blood loss.[309]

More blood is lost in posterior spinal fusion procedures than in anterior procedures. Blood loss increases as the number of vertebrae included in the fusion increases. The estimated blood loss (EBL) is approximately 750 to 1500 mL in patients with idiopathic scoliosis, or 60 to 150 mL per vertebral segment fused. The blood loss of 1300 to 2200 mL (100–190 mL per vertebral segment) is greater in patients with cerebral palsy. Children with DMD experience the largest EBL: 2500 to 4000 mL (200–280 mL per vertebral level).[310]

Children with neuromuscular scoliosis demonstrate a prolonged prothrombin time and a decrease in factor VII activity intraoperatively, suggesting that consumption of clotting factors and dilution of clotting factors enhance the blood loss.[311] It has been postulated that children with DMD lack dystrophin in all muscle types and that the poor vascular smooth muscle vasoconstrictor response may be a factor in the increased blood loss.[312] Hypothermia exacerbates blood loss by decreasing platelet function, decreasing coagulation factor activity, and slowing vasoconstriction.[295]

Adverse reactions to blood appear to be more common in children than adults, with human error as the most common cause.[313] Several techniques have been used to decrease blood loss and minimize exposure to blood products (see also Chapter 10).

Hypotensive Techniques

Controlled hypotension has been used to minimize blood loss during scoliosis surgery since it was first described more than 30 years ago. Spinal cord blood flow is considered to mirror cerebral autoregulation, where stable blood flow is maintained when mean arterial pressure (MAP) is above 50 mm Hg. It is still unclear what blood pressure is sufficient to ensure spinal cord perfusion. In adults a consensus statement suggests maintaining mean BP no lower than 60 to 70 mm Hg to avoid harm[314] but no data exist for children. In contemporary practice more moderate degrees of hypotension are being employed due to concerns of impaired neuromonitoring associated with decreases in blood pressure, particularly at the time of rod insertion and spinal distraction.[315,316] A target mean arterial pressure of 50 to 65 mm Hg has been widely used.[12] Concerns that the margin of safety for optic, cerebral, and spinal cord ischemia has reduced the use of controlled hypotension, particularly for operations of prolonged duration.[294] Additionally, there is the potential that periods of unexpected hypovolemic hypotension may exacerbate and complicate drug-induced (controlled) hypotension.[317,318] The incidence of these feared complications is fortunately very small with or without hypotension. Renal function appears well preserved even when hypotensive anesthesia is used during scoliosis surgery.[319,320] Because of these concerns and the concomitant use of hemodilution, less extreme degrees of hypotension are suggested (see also Chapter 10).

Moderate hypotension with good control of the heart rate can often be achieved without the use of specific vasoactive drugs by using a remifentanil infusion titrated to the desired blood pressure.[321,322] Although not considered a hypotensive agent, intrathecal morphine decreases blood loss and may facilitate blood pressure control, particularly when combined with a remifentanil infusion. At an analgesic dose of 5 μg/kg, a decrease in EBL from 41 to 14 mL/kg has been reported.[221] Using this technique, blood pressure control can frequently be achieved without any additional agents. Dexmedetomidine may be used as part of a technique for controlling blood pressure.[323,324] Its use resulted in a mean blood pressure of 66 mm Hg (a 20% decrease compared with nonuse), with reduced blood loss (782 vs. 465 mL) and fewer children requiring transfusion.[325]

Short-acting calcium channel blockers have been used to control hypotension in patients undergoing scoliosis surgery, and although these agents are effective, experience is limited. The blood loss during nicardipine for hypotension was less at the same mean arterial pressure compared with sodium nitroprusside, although blood pressure returned to baseline more slowly (27 vs. 7 minutes) with the former.[326,327] Clevidipine has been used without evidence of clear benefit, but it may be associated with an increase in heart rate.[328] If a hypotensive technique is to be used, invasive arterial monitoring is essential, and central venous pressure catheters are useful for the safe conduct of anesthesia (see also Chapter 10).

Hemodilution

Decreasing the hemoglobin concentration by removing red blood cells and replacing the volume with a combination of crystalloid and colloid means that for a given volume loss, fewer red blood cells are lost (see also Chapter 10). The decreased metabolic rate during anesthesia suggests that oxygen delivery can be maintained with a reduced hemoglobin concentration if normovolemia is maintained.

It has been estimated that more than 2 to 3 units of blood must be removed during hemodilution to reduce transfusion requirements. Hemodilution modeling in adult patients has suggested that as many as 5 units of blood must be removed before there is a decrease in transfusion requirements.[329] Deciding on the degree of hemodilution and establishing a threshold for transfusion may be difficult. In scoliosis surgery, reduction to an initial hematocrit of 30% has been effective for reducing and minimizing transfusion requirements.[330] Some posit that only modest benefits are gained from this technique.[331] Hypotensive anesthesia, hemodilution, and a cell saver used as part of a "bloodless surgery" program with erythropoietin and supplemental iron resulted in an average estimated blood loss of 855 mL (blood returned by the cell saver averaged 341 mL), with an average decrease in hemoglobin after surgery of 3.1 grams/dL.[332]

Tachycardia and hemodynamic instability are common at hemoglobin concentrations less than 7 grams/dL. Myocardial ischemia becomes a risk at hemoglobin concentrations less than 5 grams/dL.[333] At this level of anemia, cyanosis cannot develop because 5 grams/dL of desaturated hemoglobin is required for cyanosis to be detected. Extreme hemodilution techniques such as these are reserved for patients who oppose blood transfusion. We generally advocate maintaining the hemoglobin in the 8 to 10 grams/dL range. Information regarding critical hemoglobin concentrations is lacking but combining hemodilution with controlled hypotension is not recommended.[294]

Autologous Predonation

Preoperative strategies, including predonation of blood and preoperative red cell augmentation, may be used alone or in addition to intraoperative techniques to minimize exposure to blood (see also Chapter 10). In idiopathic scoliosis surgery, preautologous blood donation plus intraoperative red cell salvage and controlled hypotension resulted in an average EBL of 1055 mL, avoided transfusion, and decreased the hematocrit by only ~10% (35.6% preoperatively to 32.4% at discharge)[334]; again, because of the overall improved safety of blood products, and the potential for visual loss, we no longer recommend the combined techniques of hemodilution and controlled hypotension. The advantages of preoperative erythropoietin in addition to preautologous blood donation include a greater preoperative hemoglobin concentration and fewer donated units. Its effect on blood use depends on the total blood loss.[335,336] In children with neuromuscular scoliosis, erythropoietin alone did not affect the amount of blood transfused, although the preoperative and discharge hematocrits were greater in treated patients.[337]

Antifibrinolytic Agents

The use of synthetic antifibrinolytic agents to decrease perioperative blood loss during scoliosis surgery has become almost routine. A meta-analysis of aprotinin, tranexamic acid, and ε-aminocaproic acid on blood loss and use of blood products in children undergoing scoliosis surgery showed that all antifibrinolytic drugs decreased the amount of blood transfused and that aprotinin, tranexamic acid, and ε-aminocaproic acid were equally effective.[338] In patients with adolescent idiopathic scoliosis, however, tranexamic acid was more effective in reducing perioperative blood loss and allogenic transfusion requirement compared to ε-aminocaproic acid.[339] Tranexamic acid has emerged as the preferred agent due to the withdrawal of aprotinin in many countries. ε-Aminocaproic acid (Amicar) may be as effective but variable results are reported and its use has decreased. To be most effective, an effective plasma concentration of the antifibrinolytics should be established before skin incision (see also Chapter 18).

There is evidence of antifibrinolytic activity during posterior spinal fusion for adolescent idiopathic scoliosis that is attenuated by tranexamic acid.[340] Systematic reviews specifically addressing tranexamic acid administration in adolescent idiopathic scoliosis confirmed that patients treated with tranexamic acid showed lower blood loss intraoperatively and in total[341,342]; lower rates of allogenic blood transfusion than the control groups have also been reported.[343,344] The correct dose of tranexamic acid remains undetermined. Low dose (10 mg/kg bolus plus infusion 1 mg/kg per hour) appears inferior to higher dosing regimens.[341,345] Many recent high-dose studies used infusion rates of 10 mg/kg per hour although there is evidence that 5 mg/kg per hour, following a bolus dose of 10 to 50 mg/kg is effective in reducing both blood loss and transfusion requirements.[341,342,345–347] Patients with greater intraoperative blood loss spent a longer time in the hospital.[348] Continuing tranexamic acid postoperatively using three doses at 6 hourly intervals, either IV (0.5 g) or orally (1 g) resulted in decreased postoperative bleeding and transfusion.[349]

Systemic reviews of adults undergoing spinal deformity surgery have also demonstrated decreased blood loss and transfusion requirements with tranexamic acid use.[342,350,351] Anaphylaxis to tranexamic acid is extremely rare but is reported.[352,353]

Patients with neuromuscular scoliosis probably benefit more from tranexamic acid.[354] ε-aminocaproic acid in patients with neuromuscular scoliosis also reduced mean intraoperative blood loss, total perioperative blood loss, and transfusion requirements compared with placebo.[339,355]

Reduced blood loss has cost savings from decreased operating room time and blood product use.[356] Desmopressin is ineffective for decreasing blood loss associated with spinal surgery. Initial beneficial results with desmopressin[357] have not been reproduced in patients with idiopathic scoliosis[358,359] or in those with neuromuscular scoliosis.[360,361]

Intraoperative Salvage of Shed Blood

Decisions concerning the use of intraoperative salvage of shed blood (e.g., cell saver) depend on the anticipated blood loss, size of the child, and use of other methods to minimize blood transfusion, such as predonation and hemodilution (see also Chapter 10). Cell salvage is most useful in procedures with the potential for a large blood loss, e.g., neuromuscular scoliosis. In patients with adolescent idiopathic scoliosis where blood loss is quite small or none, institutional knowledge should assist in guiding cell salvage use. A retrospective study from one institution that compared several blood conservation strategies reported that the cell saver garnered a mean transfusion volume of 230 mL from 23 of 43 subjects and prevented transfusion in only 5%.[330] At the other extreme, cell saver reduced allogeneic transfusion rates from 55% to 18%.[362] The allogeneic transfusion relative risk was 2.04 for patients undergoing surgery lasting more than 6 hours and 5.87 for patients not receiving cell saver blood.[362] Cost may also be a factor. Charges for cell salvage set-up and processing of one bowl was much higher than for one allogeneic unit ($1200 vs. $462) in the United States, so transfusing small volumes of autologous cell saver blood may not be cost effective. The use of cell

saver resulted in the return of more than 250 mL (similar volume to one allogeneic unit) in only 6.5% of cases, although 41% of patients received a cell saver return mean volume of 167 mL.[363] Donor transfusion reduction is most effective when intraoperative cell salvage is combined with either preoperative autologous blood donation or postoperative collection and retransfusion.[364]

Pediatric systems are available with small spinning bowls (55–75 mL). These systems benefit children with smaller body weights and greater than anticipated blood loss such as patients with neuromuscular scoliosis undergoing extensive spinal fusion.[311,365] Among children undergoing anterior instrumentation for thoracolumbar curves, cell saver use decreased the number requiring allogenic blood transfusion from 39.4% to 6.7% and with similar mean postoperative hemoglobin values (10.2 vs. 9.6 grams/dL).[366]

MANAGING BLOOD LOSS

Autologous blood donation before surgery requires an organized schedule of donation with or without the administration of erythropoietin.[367,368] This may be the safest and most effective method of avoiding or minimizing the use of allogenic blood products.[369] A predonation program was effective in minimizing blood exposure in adolescent idiopathic scoliosis patients undergoing surgical correction for their scoliosis. A mean of 3.7 units of blood was donated by each patient before surgery, and 97% of adolescents avoided the use of allogeneic blood during and after surgery.[367] Similar results have been reported without predonation. Ninety-five percent of adolescent idiopathic scoliosis patients avoided transfusion just by using a cell saver with a transfusion trigger of 7 grams/dL. The average drop in Hb was 4.1 grams/dL with nadir on postoperative day 2.[370] However, preoperative blood typing for crossmatch is always warranted.

Measurement of blood loss during scoliosis surgery is difficult. Accuracy is lost as measurements embrace blood suctioned from the operative field that includes irrigation fluid, weighing or estimating blood collected on swabs and sponges, approximations of blood on drapes and gowns, and estimations of evaporation from the wound.

The decision about when to administer blood component therapy (i.e., non–red cell blood components) is often based on clinical judgment. Dilutional thrombocytopenia is expected only after several blood volumes have been lost and depends on the preoperative platelet count (see also Chapter 10). Platelet concentrations should be measured after loss of one blood volume and at periodic intervals after this. Dilution of coagulation factors may also lead to surgical bleeding when only packed red blood cells are used to replace blood loss. Prolongation of prothrombin time and activated partial thromboplastin time may occur when the blood loss exceeds one blood volume, and these coagulation times should be checked. These coagulation tests are not usually associated with increased bleeding until values are greater than 1.5 times mean control values, at which time increased surgical bleeding can be effectively treated with fresh frozen plasma.[371] Platelet counts after one blood volume loss, whether associated with normal or abnormal clotting, were within the normal range.[371] Blood component therapy should probably be based on abnormal clotting test results, uncontrolled bleeding, or the absence of normal clotting in the surgical field. It is preferable to intervene with blood component therapy before uncontrolled bleeding develops. If pooled blood in a dependent part of the operative field fails to show evidence of clotting, it is time to transfuse with blood components, starting with fresh frozen plasma and administering platelets only if this approach is not effective.[371]

Massive transfusion protocols, in which predefined ratios of red blood cells, plasma factors, and platelets (usually in a 1 : 1 : 1 ratio) are administered early in the resuscitation phase of massive trauma, are being increasingly used in all situations of uncontrolled blood loss (see Chapter 10).[372,373] Evidence that these protocols decrease morbidity and mortality in the trauma setting has resulted in their implementation for blood loss during surgery.[374,375] By adopting these protocols, proportionally greater quantities of factors and platelets are transfused compared with conventional approaches in severe hemorrhage, but it is associated with increased survival.[376] An evidence-based multidisciplinary developed pathway with ongoing quality improvement addressing blood loss management is likely to produce the greatest reward. One institution reduced the proportion of patients transfused from almost 90% to less than 20% over a 15-year period; when scoliosis patients required transfusion, the units administered per patient decreased from an average of nine to just two.[377]

The thromboelastogram is useful in refining blood product administration if multiple blood volumes are required for resuscitation.[374,376] Scoliosis surgery in patients with neuromuscular scoliosis or cerebral palsy, particularly in those with severe complex curves in whom pelvic stabilization and iliac crest grafts are considered, fulfill these criteria. In this group of patients, early administration of blood and factors using a massive transfusion protocol may be beneficial.[378] Recombinant factor VII (rFVIIa) may be a useful therapy for patients with a dilutional coagulopathy who are unresponsive to blood component replacement therapy. Successful use with doses as small as 20 µg/kg has been described in spinal surgery.[379–382]

EFFECTS OF ANESTHETICS ON SOMATOSENSORY EVOKED AND MOTOR EVOKED POTENTIALS

Anesthetic agents act by directly inhibiting synaptic pathways or by indirectly changing the balance of inhibitory and excitatory influences.[383] The greater the number of synapses and the more complex the neuronal pathway being monitored, the greater the potential impact of anesthetic agents on the evoked potentials. Most anesthetic agents depress the amplitude and increase the latency of SSEPs and MEPs. For this reason, cortical SSEPs are more sensitive than spinal cord- or brainstem-measured SSEPs. MEPs are susceptible to anesthetic agents at three sites: the motor cortex, the anterior horn cell, and the neuromuscular junction. Consequently, transcranial stimulation with peripheral muscle detection (using CMAPs) is most susceptible to anesthetic interference. Although inhalational anesthetics and most IV anesthetics markedly depress SSEPs and MEPs, ketamine and etomidate appear to enhance the amplitudes of both, possibly by attenuating inhibition.[384]

Inhalational Anesthetics

Inhalational anesthetics cause a dose-dependent depression of both SSEP and myogenic MEP, although at equipotent concentrations, the MEP is affected to a greater degree than the SSEP. This means that although inhalation agents can be used during SSEP monitoring, they often need to be administered in subanesthetic doses during MEP monitoring. Adequate cortical SSEPs and subcortical SSEPs can be measured with up to one minimum alveolar concentration (MAC) of isoflurane, sevoflurane, and desflurane, although some increase in latency and decrease in amplitude may be detected.[385,386] It is important to maintain constant end-tidal concentrations throughout anesthesia after baseline measurements have been established.

Myogenic MEPs (i.e., CMAPs) are recordable only at low concentrations of inhalational anesthetics. The exact concentration depends on the system being used and is greatly influenced by the number of pulses in the stimulus. Single-pulse transcranial stimuli may be inhibited by end-tidal concentrations as small as 0.2 MAC and abolished by end-tidal concentrations as small as 0.5 MAC.[387–389] This suppression can be partially overcome by using greater intensity stimuli with multi-pulse stimulation of up to 6 pulses per stimulus. An increasing number of patients lose recordable myogenic MEPs, even when multi-pulse stimuli are used, as the concentration of inhalational anesthetic exceeds 0.5 MAC. At end-tidal concentrations in excess of 0.75% isoflurane, monitoring conditions become unacceptable.[390–394] Stimulus intensity and pulse train frequency probably are factors in determining successful myogenic MEPs with inhalational anesthetics. Using direct stimulation of the cortex during craniotomy, CMAP was easily recordable at 1 MAC of isoflurane and sevoflurane.[395] Similar results have been demonstrated with sevoflurane using transcranial stimulation.[396] Information regarding desflurane is limited, and although it causes a dose-dependent depression, myogenic MEPs have been successfully recorded at 0.5 MAC.[394,397] Using a multi-pulse stimulation technique, intraoperative recording of MEPs was equally successful during desflurane or propofol anesthesia.[398] Desflurane anesthesia allowed MEP monitoring when used to provide a depth of anesthesia that maintained the bispectral index (BIS) at 40 to 60 or at a concentration of 0.6 to 0.8 MAC.[399,400] There was no difference in the amplitude or latency of SSEPs compared with propofol (150–300 µg/kg per minute) titrated to a similar BIS.[400] Low-dose desflurane is a viable alternative to propofol infusion and may be associated with a shorter wake-up time.[400] Concerns about the environmental impact of desflurane have limited its use in recent years.[401,402]

Nitrous oxide reduces the amplitude of the cortical SSEP, but comparisons with other inhalational anesthetics are limited. Nitrous oxide (0.5 MAC) depresses SSEPs to a greater extent than isoflurane at a similar MAC.[403] Similarly, 66% nitrous oxide depressed SSEPs to a greater extent than propofol (6 mg/kg per hour; 100 µg/kg per minute).[404] Nitrous oxide depresses myogenic MEPs.[386] The effect relative to other inhalational anesthetics is difficult to determine. Nitrous oxide appears to affect CMAP amplitude to a lesser extent than isoflurane.[405] Multi-pulse stimulus techniques can partially reverse nitrous oxide–induced depression of amplitude. Compared with a propofol infusion designed to maintain a target concentration of 3 µg/mL, 50% nitrous oxide decreases CMAPs with single or paired stimuli to a lesser extent.[406] When 60% nitrous oxide was added to low-dose propofol infusion, at a target concentration of 1 µg/mL, adequate CMAPs were obtained using multi-pulse transcranial stimulation.[407] Conversely, the addition of nitrous oxide to a variety of different total IV techniques significantly depressed the CMAP such that some were not recordable.[408] With the widespread availability of remifentanil and the variable but mostly negative effects of nitrous oxide on SSEP and MEP signals, the latter is best avoided when monitoring spinal cord potentials.

Propofol

Propofol decreases the amplitude of the cortical SSEP, but adequate signals can be recorded, even in the presence of nitrous oxide, at doses used for anesthesia (6 mg/kg per hour; 100 µg/kg per minute).[409] Propofol better preserves cortical SSEP amplitude and provides a deeper level of hypnosis as measured by processed electroencephalographic values than combinations of low-dose isoflurane and nitrous oxide or low-dose isoflurane or sevoflurane alone.[410–412] Compared with propofol/remifentanil, cortical but not cervical SSEP signals were more suppressed with a desflurane/remifentanil anesthetic.[413,414]

Propofol depresses the amplitude of myogenic MEPs. In addition to its cortical effect, it suppresses activation of the alpha motor neuron at the level of the spinal gray matter.[415,416] Low-dose propofol infusions have become popular as part of the anesthetic technique used with MEP monitoring owing to the rapid improvement of signals when the drug is terminated and because multi-pulse stimulation techniques can improve the response amplitude.[391,417] Propofol, even in combination with nitrous oxide, depresses multi-pulse transcranial CMAPs less than isoflurane.[391] Propofol (5 mg/kg per hour; 83 µg/kg per minute) combined with 66% nitrous oxide produced satisfactory CMAP recordings in 75% of patients when a four-pulse stimulation sequence was used. In contrast, no recordings were possible with 1 MAC of isoflurane.[392] The infusion rates or target concentrations that allow acceptable myogenic MEP recordings vary considerably and reflect different adjuvants (e.g., opioids, ketamine, nitrous oxide), degrees of neuromuscular blockade, and transcranial pulse rates. Propofol at a target of 4 µg/mL or at an infusion rate of 6 mg/kg per hour (100 µg/kg per minute) produces acceptable signals with multi-pulse stimuli.[417–419] Current target-controlled infusion pumps underpredict propofol concentration in early teenagers (see Chapter 6).[420] MEPs appear particularly sensitive to depth of anesthesia, but processed EEG monitors are agent specific and so their role to assess anesthesia depth when using multiple agents in teenagers remains uncertain.

α₂-Adrenoreceptor Agonists: Clonidine and Dexmedetomidine

The cerebral effects of the α_2-agonists act primarily at the locus coeruleus, rather than by the more generalized inhibition of synaptic pathways, as is the case with general anesthetics.[421] Clonidine at 2 to 5 µg/kg IV had minimal effects on cortical SSEPs when combined with isoflurane[422–424] and exhibits anesthetic-sparing properties with inhalational agents and propofol.[424–426] Its effects on MEPs, however, are more dramatic, decreasing the amplitude 60% to 80% after a bolus of 1 to 2 µg/kg during a low-dose propofol infusion (2–3 mg/kg per hour); these decreases persisted for at least 30 minutes.[427]

Dexmedetomidine minimally impacts SSEPs at the usual clinical doses.[428–430] The reported effects on MEPs are variable. Initial studies using either dexmedetomidine target-controlled infusion (TCI) of 0.3 or 0.6 ng/mL added to a constant propofol infusion or an infusion at 0.5 µg/kg per hour with propofol adjusted to maintain BIS at 45 to 60 showed no notable effect on MEP.[431–434] A dose-dependent effect was demonstrated with target-controlled infusion of 0.4 ng/mL dexmedetomidine and 2.5 µg/mL propofol having a minimal effect on the amplitude of the transcranial-MEP (tcMEP) signal but larger infusion rates (TCI 0.6 or 0.8 ng/mL) significantly decrease tcMEP amplitude.[85] Dexmedetomidine infusions at 0.6 µg/kg per hour added to a propofol infusion titrated to maintain a BIS of 30 to 55 yielded no adverse effects on the SSEP and MEP signals.[430] Similarly a dexmedetomidine infusion of 0.5 µg/kg per hour with propofol titrated to a BIS of 45 to 60 maintained MEPs

unchanged.[435] In contrast, dexmedetomidine infusions of 0.3 and 0.5 µg/kg per hour reduced MEP by greater than 50% in 4 of 6 muscle groups measured, with anesthetic depth maintained constant using referenced-EEG.[436] Collectively these data suggest that if dexmedetomidine is used as part of the anesthetic technique, the drug should be introduced slowly, infused at no more than 0.5 µg/kg per hour, and depth of anesthesia, as well as MEPs monitored early during administration. Propofol infusion should be reduced during dexmedetomidine infusions.

Opioids

Alfentanil, fentanyl, sufentanil, and remifentanil minimally depress SSEP and MEP signals.[437,438] Dose-dependent depression of the CMAP occurs at doses of opioids that far exceed those used in clinical anesthesia.[439,440] When alfentanil, fentanyl, and sufentanil at doses sufficient to suppress noxious stimuli were compared for their effects on evoked potentials, sufentanil suppressed the potentials the least of the three.[439] A similar study that included remifentanil showed that it depressed the signals the least, with CMAPs measurable at infusion rates of 0.6 µg/kg per minute.[440] It is likely that greater doses can be used if clinically indicated.

Ketamine and Etomidate

Ketamine enhances the cortical SSEP amplitude and has a minimal effect on subcortical and peripheral SSEP responses.[441] It also produces minimal effects on the myogenic MEP responses as a bolus of 0.5 mg/kg[442] or when used as a low dose infusion (1 mg/kg per hour) to supplement a nitrous oxide–opioid anesthesia.[442,443] Experimental evidence suggests S(+)-ketamine modulates the CMAP by a peripheral mechanism at or distal to the spinal alpha motor neuron.[444] Ketamine at a low dose (0.5 µg/kg per minute) may improve and augment MEPs.[435] When added to propofol in a 1:4 ratio, and infused to maintain BIS 40 to 60, ketamine administration resulted in a 40% increase in MEP amplitude and was associated with more stable hemodynamics (see also ketofol, Chapter 6).[445] Higher doses (4 µg/kg per minute) have been successfully used with MEP monitoring during propofol-remifentanil anesthesia for scoliosis correction.[169,446]

Etomidate behaves more like ketamine in its effects on evoked potentials. It improves the quality of SSEPs and increases the amplitude of MEPs.[447] It produces minimal changes in MEPs compared with barbiturates or propofol.[415] Etomidate infusions (10–35 µg/kg per minute) produce adequate MEP monitoring signals.[442,448] Concerns regarding adrenocortical depression with etomidate infusions remain and limit its widespread use.[449] Bolus doses of etomidate, however, can transiently depress MEPs.[442] New etomidate analogs are under investigation that will have a half-life of minutes with no associated adrenocortical depression and no active metabolites[450,451]; when commercially available, this drug may provide an alternative to propofol (see Chapter 5).

Midazolam

Midazolam 0.2 mg/kg IV decreases the SSEP amplitude by 60%.[452] This does not occur with subcortical SSEPs, for which a slight increase in latency but no change in amplitude has been demonstrated.[453] Although midazolam (0.5 mg/kg) markedly depresses MEPs in nonhuman primates that persisted during awakening,[454] this finding does not hold true in human studies. MEP amplitude was unaffected by a midazolam-ketamine infusion technique compared with propofol-ketamine or propofol-alfentanil techniques.[408] Midazolam did not suppress myogenic

TABLE 30.3	Effect of Anesthetic Drugs on Somatosensory Evoked Potentials and Motor Evoked Potentials		
Drug	SSEP Amplitude	MEP Amplitude	Additional Information
Propofol	1–2	2	
Volatile anesthetics <0.5 MAC	1–2	2	
Volatile anesthetics >0.5 MAC–1 MAC	2	3	*Exception: 0.8% desflurane= propofol at same BIS
Nitrous oxide	2	2	Additive effect with other agents
Oral midazolam	?	?	No studies
IV midazolam	1–2	0–1	Limited studies
Clonidine	1	2	Limited studies: following bolus
Dexmedetomidine	1	1–2	Variability in studies: infusion <0.5 µg/kg per hour BIS adjusted to 40–60
Opioids	0	0	Includes remifentanil up to 0.6 µg/kg per minute
Ketamine	0+1	+1	May increase MEP amplitude 40%
Gabapentin/pregabalin	0	0	

CODE: +1 augmentation; 0 no change; 1 mild decrease in amplitude–monitoring likely; 2 moderate decrease in amplitude–monitoring possible; 3 marked decrease in amplitude–monitoring unlikely.
MEP, Motor evoked potentials; *SSEP*, somatosensory evoked potentials.

MEPs, even at doses sufficient to produce anesthesia.[440] Effects were similar to those with etomidate.[440]

Neuromuscular Blockade

NMBDs exert little or no effect on the SSEP. They prevent or limit recording of CMAPs during myogenic MEP recording because of their effects on the neuromuscular junction. Partial neuromuscular blockade may be used during MEP monitoring because it improves conditions for surgery by providing adequate muscle relaxation when retraction of the tissues is required and limits any patient movement during the stimulus generation. Partial muscle relaxation may also reduce noise caused by spontaneous muscle movement. Constant neuromuscular blockade must be maintained during the procedure and should be evaluated in the specific muscle groups that are used for electrophysiologic monitoring because different muscle groups have different sensitivities to the NMBDs. Many centers avoid neuromuscular blockade after intubation, the initial incision, and muscle dissection.

Patients with preoperative neuromuscular dysfunction demonstrate a greater effect after partial neuromuscular blockade than those with normal preoperative motor function. It is appropriate to avoid neuromuscular blockade in most of these patients.[448]

Other Medications

Preoperative pregabalin and gabapentin do not impact spinal cord monitoring.[455] Droperidol, at low dose used for antiemesis (20 µg/kg), is associated with a notable decrease in MEPs, so if indicated, should not be given until the end of surgery.[456] Lidocaine infusions have been used in spine and scoliosis surgery. At infusion rates of 1 to 1.5 mg/kg per hour, lidocaine decreased sevoflurane or propofol requirements, without an effect on SSEPs or MEPs.[457,458]

CHOOSING ANESTHETIC DRUGS AND TECHNIQUES

The choice of anesthesia depends on the patient's pathology and the type of electrophysiologic monitoring for the operation. Increased use of MEPs and advances in MEP techniques have

occurred worldwide. CMAPs appear to provide the most useful data for minimizing the risk of spinal cord injury.

The key to success is to use a technique that allows a stable concentration of the hypnotic component of anesthesia. Whatever technique is applied, minimal amounts of anesthetic agent and/or adjuncts should be used. This is facilitated by processed EEG monitoring with most studies keeping BIS values between 40 to 60. Although concentrations of inhalational anesthetics approaching 1 MAC may be compatible with multi-pulse MEP monitoring systems, propofol infusions have become the most widespread anesthetic technique.[459]

Remifentanil is a rapidly titratable analgesic that minimally affects spinal cord monitoring. Clonidine or dexmedetomidine, ketamine, and lidocaine all decrease the concentration of hypnotic drugs needed during SSEP and MEP monitoring. Even at low doses, ketamine facilitates MEP monitoring. Clonidine and dexmedetomidine exert variable effects so the depth of anesthesia should also be monitored. If processed electroencephalographic monitoring is used to determine anesthetic depth, the addition of ketamine may confound the reading by increasing it.[460,461] This occurs despite a deepening level of hypnosis.[460] A NMBD improves the SSEP monitoring and may be used in conjunction with MEP monitoring within the confines described earlier. However, even in patients with idiopathic scoliosis, adequate operating conditions after the initial muscle dissection can be produced in the absence of neuromuscular blockade. In the absence of muscle relaxation, muscle contractions, including those of the masseter muscles, occur during stimulation. In this situation, it is prudent to insert a soft bite block to prevent obstructing the tracheal tube or biting the tongue, or simply to intubate nasally. The effects of anesthetic drugs on SSEPs and MEPs are summarized in Table 30.3.

Tourniquets

INDICATIONS AND DESIGN

The tourniquet was used by the Romans to control bleeding during amputation.[462] The arterial tourniquet is used during orthopedic procedures to reduce blood loss and provide good operating conditions, for IV regional blockade and sympathectomy, and for isolated limb perfusion in the management of localized malignancy.[463]

The word *tourniquet* is derived from the French verb *tourner,* meaning "to turn," referring to the twisting or screwing action applied to the constricting bandage to tighten it. In 1873, von Esmarch introduced the use of a flat rubber bandage wrapped repeatedly around a limb.[462] Although this rubber bandage is still used to render a limb bloodless, the pneumatic tourniquet, introduced by Cushing in 1904, has replaced the rubber bandage to maintain ischemia. Compressed nitrogen or air is used for inflation. The target pressure is preset, and compensatory feedback mechanisms maintain that pressure during inflation. Curved and wider tourniquet cuffs, which are designed to fit conical limbs, are associated with lower arterial occlusion pressures than standard cuffs.[464] A soft dressing applied to the limb before tourniquet application prevents wrinkles and blisters that may occur when the skin is pinched.[465] Adequate exsanguination can also be achieved by raising the arm at 90 degrees or the leg at 45 degrees for several minutes before inflating the tourniquet.[466,467]

PHYSIOLOGY

Ischemia

Ischemia leads to tissue hypoxia and acidosis. The severity and consequences of the associated changes (e.g., increased capillary permeability, coagulation alteration, cell membrane sodium pump activity) depend on the tissue type, duration of ischemia, and collateral circulation. Muscle is more susceptible to ischemic damage than nerves. Histologic changes are more pronounced in muscle beneath the tourniquet compared with muscle distal to the tourniquet.

Reperfusion

Reperfusion removes toxic metabolites and restores energy supplies. There is a sudden release of lactic acid, creatinine phosphokinase (i.e., creatine kinase), potassium (peak increase of 0.32 mEq/L), and CO_2 (peak increase of 0.8–18 mm Hg) when the cuff is deflated suddenly. Metabolic changes increase after prolonged periods of ischemia but return to baseline within 30 minutes. Muscle damage may release myoglobin, which can collect in the collecting tubules of the kidney, precipitating renal insufficiency or failure.

Systemic effects after deflation of the tourniquet include a shift of blood volume back into the limb with a transient decrease in blood pressure that is exacerbated by a postischemic reactive hyperemia in the limb. CO_2 release transiently increases the minute volume. The rapid increase in CO_2 is also associated with a transient (8–10 minutes) increase in cerebral blood volume that may affect patients with raised intracranial pressure.[463]

Increased microvascular permeability of muscle and nerve tissue occurs with tourniquet release after 2 to 4 hours of ischemia. Interstitial and intracellular edema and capillary occlusion owing to endothelial edema and leukocyte aggregation may take months to resolve.

Ischemic Conditioning

Short periods of ischemia followed by reperfusion render muscle more resistant to subsequent ischemia. Ischemic preconditioning improves skeletal muscle force, contractility, and performance and decreases fatigue of skeletal muscle. This preconditioning may enable prolongation of orthopedic and reconstructive procedures.[468]

COMPLICATIONS

Local Complications

Muscle Damage

Histologic changes in the muscle beneath the tourniquet occur after 2 hours of tourniquet time (at 200 mm Hg [26.7 kPa]), but similar changes can occur in the distal ischemic muscle after 4 hours of tourniquet use. Direct pressure and mechanical deformation contribute to increased severity of muscle damage under the cuff.[463] These changes include an increase in the number of inflammatory cells in the perivascular space, focal fiber necrosis, and signs of hyaline degeneration.

The combination of muscle ischemia, edema, and microvascular congestion contributes to post-tourniquet syndrome: edema, stiffness, pallor, weakness without paralysis, and subjective numbness of the extremity without objective anesthesia. The common use of postoperative casts may conceal the true incidence of this syndrome. Recovery usually occurs over 7 days.[469]

Nerve Damage

The cause of nerve injuries after use of a tourniquet is likely from direct compression under the cuff rather than ischemia. Sheer forces that are maximal at the upper and lower edges of the tourniquet cause the most damage. These forces are greater with the Esmarch bandage than with the pneumatic tourniquet. The incidence of nerve injuries in the upper limb (1 case per 5,000 patients) is greater than in the lower limb (1 case per 13,000 patients); in the upper extremity, the order of nerves from most to least vulnerable to tourniquet-associated injury is radial > ulnar > median and in the lower extremity, the sciatic nerve is most vulnerable.[470,471] Tourniquet application of 1 hour or less produces minimal ischemic cell injury.[472] One study of 505 adults found no tourniquet-related events up to 2 hours of tourniquet inflation pressures of 250 mm Hg or less.[473] Complete recovery of tourniquet-related nerve injury occurred in 90% of instances in both the upper and lower extremities in 1 study.[470]

Vascular Damage

Arterial injury is uncommon in children. It is an injury of adults with atheromatous vessels, and the tourniquet should be avoided in patients with absent distal pulses, poor capillary return, a calcified femoropopliteal system, or a history of vascular surgery on the involved limb.[474]

Skin Safety

Pressure necrosis and friction burns may occur with poorly applied tourniquets, and some form of skin protection should be used routinely.[475] A "limb protection sleeve" may help reduce wrinkling, shearing, and pinching of soft tissues. Chemical burns may result from antiseptic skin preparations that seep beneath the tourniquet and are then retained and compressed against the skin. Chemical burn under pneumatic tourniquet caused by povidone-iodine is an iatrogenic injury rarely reported. Special attention should be paid to children, whose skins are more delicate and vulnerable.[476]

Tourniquet Pain

The tourniquet causes a vague, dull ache that becomes intolerable after approximately 30 minutes.[477] This pain is associated with an increase in heart rate and blood pressure that is not ameliorated by general anesthesia and neuraxial blockade.[477] The pain is transmitted by unmyelinated C fibers, which are normally inhibited by fast pain impulses transmitted by myelinated A-delta fibers, but in this case, mechanical compression reduces transmission through the larger A-delta fibers.[478] Narrow silicon ring tourniquets may be associated with less pain than wide tourniquets.[479]

Systemic Complications
Temperature Regulation
The combination of decreased heat loss from the ischemic limb and reduced heat transfer from the central to ischemic peripheral compartment increases core body temperature.[480,481] Bilateral tourniquets increase the temperature more than unilateral tourniquets.[481] Children who require intraoperative tourniquets should not be aggressively warmed during surgery.[481] Redistribution of body heat and the efflux of hypothermic venous blood from the ischemic area into the systemic circulation after deflation of the tourniquet decreases the core body temperature, which may switch off thermoregulatory vasodilation and decrease the skin-surface temperature.[482]

Deep Vein Thrombosis and Emboli
The incidence of emboli after release of the tourniquet in children is unclear. The tourniquet appears to have no influence on deep vein thrombosis, but release of the tourniquet may be associated with an increased risk of embolism in adults. Some clinicians have suggested that heparin be used during total joint arthroplasty in adults to prevent emboli formation,[483] although this practice is not routine in children. Some surgeons use such therapy in adolescents.

Sickle Cell Disease
Hypoxia, acidosis, and circulatory stasis contribute to the sickling of sickle cells in susceptible individuals. However, several institutions routinely use tourniquets in children with sickle cell disease while maintaining acid-base status, hydration, and oxygenation throughout the procedure.[484,485] The use of tourniquets for patients with sickle cell disease has been poorly studied. Several papers suggest that vasoocclusive crisis is rare and that tourniquets can be used with relative safety with proper care (thorough exsanguination, limited ischemia time, minimizing tourniquet inflations pressures).[486–488] Each case must be assessed individually for the balance between the advantages of a bloodless field and the risks of precipitating sickling crises (see Chapter 8).

Drug Effects
Antibiotics given after the tourniquet is inflated do not produce effective concentrations in the interstitium of the ischemic limb. Inflation of the tourniquet should be delayed at least 5 minutes after administration of the antibiotics.[489,490] Medications administered before inflation of the tourniquet may be sequestered in the ischemic limb and then re-released into the systemic circulation when the tourniquet is deflated. The antibiotic effect depends on the amount of antibiotic sequestered, the tissue binding, and the concentration-response relationship for the antibiotic, although the impact is minimal for most medications used in anesthesia. Volume of distribution may be reduced if the drug is administered after the tourniquet is inflated, but the plasma clearance remains unaffected.

RECOMMENDED CUFF PRESSURES
Most clinicians limit the duration of tourniquet inflation to a maximum of 1.5 to 2 hours. Techniques such as hourly release of the tourniquet for 10 minutes, cooling of the affected limb,

and alternating dual cuffs may reduce the risk of injury.[491] Nerve and muscle injuries that occur beneath the tourniquet cuff are related to the pneumatic pressure. Consequently, the minimum pressure that maintains ischemic conditions should be sought. Hypotensive anesthetic techniques have been used in adults to reduce the need for high cuff inflation pressures,[492] but there seems to be little need for this in children. It has been suggested that the arterial occlusion pressure in each child should be measured by Doppler and the tourniquet pressure set to 50 mm Hg in excess of this value.[493] Alternatively, the tourniquet pressure may be set to 20 mm Hg in excess of the arterial occlusion pressure.[494] However, these empiric formulas ignore the typical fluctuations in blood pressure that occur during surgery. The optimal tourniquet pressure may be one that fluctuates with the systemic blood pressure.[495] Pediatric maximum mean cuff pressures recommended for the upper and lower extremities are 173.4 ± 11.6 mm Hg (range, 155–190 mm Hg) and 176.7 ± 28.7 mm Hg (range, 140–250 mm Hg), respectively.[493] Wider cuffs exert less force per unit area and reduce the risk of local sequelae. Recommendations for adults suggest that the cuff should exceed the circumference of the extremity by 7 to 15 cm. This is difficult to achieve in infants, in whom the proximal limb length is proportionally shorter than in adults and the wide cuffs impinge on the surgical field. New disposable narrow elastic ring tourniquets may improve access for short-duration adult surgery, but concerns about injury risk limit their use in children.[496]

Acute Bone and Joint Infections

The mainstays of management for osteomyelitis and septic arthritis are antibiotics and surgical drainage. The incidence of these infections is increasing, particularly in immunocompromised children with HIV infection. Tuberculosis remains a scourge in many developing countries. Mortality rates for hospital-acquired staphylococcal disease in compromised children[497] and community-acquired disease in healthy children[498–500] range from 8% to 47% for those presenting with severe sepsis.[501] *Mycobacterium* and *Staphylococcus* species resistant to conventional antibiotics increase morbidity and mortality rates.

PATHOPHYSIOLOGY
Staphylococcus aureus is the most common pathogen. Osteomyelitis develops after bacteremia and occurs mostly in prepubertal children. Normal bone is highly resistant to infection, but *S. aureus* adheres to bone by expressing receptors for components of bone matrix, and the expression of collagen-binding adhesin permits the attachment to cartilage.[502] After the microorganisms adhere to bone, they express phenotypic resistance to antimicrobial treatment.[502]

The metaphyseal region around the growth plate is the predominant area of infection. Sluggish blood flow in the metaphysis predisposes children to bacterial infection, and endothelial gaps in developing vessels allow bacteria to escape into the metaphysis. Subsequent abscesses may decompress into the joint or subperiosteally. Infection may involve adjacent tissue planes, and hematogenous spread causes multiple pathologic processes beyond the primary site of infection.

Septic arthritis is more common in neonates because transphyseal vessels link the metaphysis and epiphysis. Growth plate and epiphyseal destruction may occur in this age group. Articular cartilage damage is attributable to the release of proteolytic enzymes by the pathogen and activated neutrophils.

CLINICAL PRESENTATION

Most children with staphylococcal disease present with musculoskeletal symptoms and fever, but those with disseminated disease may be critically ill (4%–10%) with severe sepsis, lung disease, and extracutaneous foci.[498,499,503,504] One report found that one-half of extracutaneous foci of staphylococcal infection were not detected on hospital admission, and one-third of these lesions were observed for the first time at autopsy.[497] There is often a history of trauma.[498,499] An absolute polymorphonuclear cell count of greater than $10,000/mm^3$ or an absolute band-form count of greater than $500/mm^3$, or both, correlates with the presence of one or more inadequately treated sites of staphylococcal infection.[497] Tuberculosis is the great mimic and must always be suspected in endemic areas.

Diagnosis is confirmed by blood, bone, or joint aspirate culture. Radiologic procedures (e.g., plain radiographs, computed tomography, magnetic resonance imaging, radionuclide scans) are often required to identify foci, and the anesthesiologist is often requested to provide sedation.[505]

TREATMENT OPTIONS

Antibiotic therapy is the mainstay of treatment. Initial antibiotic choice is dictated by age and by local pathogen and sensitivity profiles. Antibiotic treatment should be extended to cover Gram-negative enterococci in neonates and *Streptococcus* in older children. *Haemophilus influenzae* remains a pathogen in unvaccinated regions. Surgical decompression of acute osteomyelitis that responds poorly to antimicrobial therapy may release intramedullary or subperiosteal pus that leads to clinical improvement. Pus within fascial planes also requires release. Venous thrombosis attributable to pus in soft tissue planes around major joints is associated with a high mortality rate.[498] Determining and eradicating the primary focus improves the mortality and reduces recurrence rates.[506] An aggressive search for foci and surgical drainage of infective foci is required.

Highly active antiretroviral therapy (HAART) has positively altered the mortality rates for HIV-infected children. However, acute bone and joint infections still occur,[507] and these drugs can cause significant morbidity resulting from changes in fat distribution, lipid profiles, glucose concentrations, homeostasis, and bone turnover.[508] Infarction may replace infection as the major cause of morbidity and mortality from HIV.[508] Malnutrition, advanced stage of HIV infection, lower CD4 count at the time of evaluation, and longer duration of disease are associated with increased frequency of musculoskeletal manifestations.[509] It remains uncertain whether HAART should be continued during acute osteomyelitis. Worsening cell-mediated immune function may occur during tuberculosis treatment if HAART is continued.[510] The combination of HIV infection and tuberculosis can be lethal in children; antituberculosis treatment should be continued for 12 to 18 months.

ANESTHESIA CONSIDERATIONS

Anesthesiology services are commonly required for sedation during diagnostic investigation, anesthesia for surgical exploration and release of pus or fixation of pathologic fractures, management of pulmonary complications (e.g., intercostal chest drain insertion, pleurodesis), central venous cannulation for long-term antibiotic treatment, and analgesic modalities.

Children with disseminated staphylococcal disease may be critically ill with multisystem disease and require fluid volume augmentation, inotropic support, positive-pressure ventilation, extracorporeal renal support, and coagulation factor replacement. Others may appear clinically stable before induction of anesthesia; the assessment of hypovolemia in children is subject to moderate to poor interrater agreement.[511] IV access and rehydration are required before beginning anesthesia to avoid a precipitous blood pressure drop immediately after induction. Bacteremic showering during manipulation and drainage of pus causes further decompensation necessitating initiation of vasoactive support. Excessive bleeding owing to altered coagulation status should also be anticipated.

The presence of a septic arthritis in the shoulder or neck may cause cervical ligamentous laxity predisposing to C1–2 subluxation during intubation.[512] Pneumatoceles from staphylococcal pneumonia can rupture during positive-pressure ventilation. A spontaneous breathing mode, however, may be difficult to achieve because of laryngospasm, breath-holding, increased secretions, and bronchospasm. The use of NMBDs and positive-pressure ventilation in these patients with a low threshold for introducing inotropes to support the cardiovascular system is an easier option. Vigilance is required for acute pneumothorax.

Myocarditis, pericarditis, and pericardial effusions compromise myocardial function. A 12% prevalence of infective endocarditis among children with hospital-acquired *S. aureus* bacteremia has been reported.[513] This prevalence of infective endocarditis is frequently associated with congenital heart disease and the necessity for multiple blood cultures.[513] The incidence of infective endocarditis among children with community-acquired disease without preexisting cardiac abnormalities is low,[498] suggesting that echocardiography could be reserved for children with preexisting cardiac disease, those with suspicious clinical findings, those whose temperature fails to stabilize, or those who have prolonged bacteremia without an obvious source of infection.

PAIN MANAGEMENT

Morphine and acetaminophen are the analgesics commonly used for postoperative pain management. NSAIDs are relatively contraindicated in the presence of coagulation disorders, altered renal function, and COX-2–mediated osteogenesis.

The performance of regional blockade in children with acute bone or joint infection is controversial. There are no studies addressing the risk/benefit ratios of regional techniques in this population. It seems reasonable to use these techniques only after 24 hours of appropriate antibiotic therapy in apyrexial children who show no signs of a coagulopathy.

Common Syndromes

Children with some specific conditions present repeatedly for orthopedic procedures (see Chapter 22). It is worthwhile maintaining a database that details their anesthetic management. There should be 24-hour access to standard texts or electronic information concerning anesthesia and uncommon pediatric diseases.

CEREBRAL PALSY

Clinical Features

Cerebral palsy is an umbrella term that describes a group of nonprogressive, motor impairment syndromes caused by lesions or anomalies in the brain that occur during the early stages of its development.[514] It is the leading cause of motor disability during childhood, with a prevalence of approximately 2 per 1000 live births in developed countries.[515]

Disorders include cognitive impairment, sensory loss (i.e., vision and hearing), seizures, and communication and behavioral disturbances. Systemic disorders resulting from cerebral palsy affect the gastrointestinal, respiratory, urinary tract, and orthopedic systems. Cerebral palsy is divided into three broad categories: spastic (70%), dyskinetic (10%), and ataxic (10%). Children with spastic cerebral palsy commonly present for orthopedic procedures because of contractures at major peripheral joints.[516,517] Functional improvement after surgery in children with spastic diplegia and spastic hemiplegia is better than in those suffering spastic quadriplegia.[516]

Orthopedic Considerations

Orthopedic manipulations form only part of the treatments designed to improve performance or improve the ease of care.[518] Management, including orthopedic surgery, physical and occupational therapy, recreational therapy, orthotics, and assistive devices, improves functional outcomes. Medical modalities such as intramuscular injections of botulinum toxin and intrathecal administration of baclofen by means of an implanted pump may also be of benefit.[519] Selective dorsal rhizotomy has been used to control spasticity.[520,521]

The indications for and timing of surgical interventions vary. Gait analysis increases the age of the patient at the first orthopedic surgical procedure, and botulinum toxin type A treatment delays and reduces the frequency of surgical procedures on the lower extremities.[522,523] Bone and soft tissue surgical procedures are designed to lengthen or weaken spastic muscles to give opposing muscles a chance to attain muscle balance.

Anesthetic Considerations

Children with cerebral palsy who present for orthopedic surgery often have previous experience with operating rooms. They should be handled with sensitivity because communication disorders and sensory deficits may mask mildly impaired or normal intellect. They may be accompanied by a parent or caregiver and/or premedicated before induction of anesthesia. If there is a communication problem, the parent or caregiver should be present before and after anesthesia[516,524] as this cohort benefit from their caregiver or parents in recovery. These children have an increased risk of postoperative complications, which correlates with the severity of the child's preoperative condition.[525] Preoperative risk factors associated with increased risk for perioperative hypotension, hypothermia, seizures, delayed emergence, and upper airway obstruction, included an American Society of Anesthesiologists physical status score >2, history of seizures, upper airway hypotonia, and those undergoing general surgery procedures.[525] Children with cerebral palsy with or without epilepsy are at increased risk for obstructive sleep apnea.[526]

Medical conditions (e.g., seizure control, respiratory function, gastroesophageal reflux) should be optimized preoperatively.[527] Contracture deformities, spinal deformities, decubitus ulceration, and skin infection must be considered when positioning the child for anesthesia and surgery. Poor nutritional status affects postoperative wound healing and the risk of infection. Concurrent medications may influence anesthesia; sodium valproate can cause platelet dysfunction and affect drug metabolism, and anticonvulsants increase the resistance to NMBDs (See also Table 22.16).[528] A history of latex allergy should be sought because of exposure to latex allergens from an early age.[529]

IV access may be difficult. Drooling, a decreased ability to swallow secretions, and gastroesophageal reflux may dissuade some from performing inhalational inductions in these children, although there is no evidence that a rapid-sequence induction is safer. Succinylcholine may be used because it does not cause hyperkalemia in these children, whose muscles have never become denervated. Noncommunicative or nonverbal children with cerebral palsy require less propofol to obtain the same BIS values (i.e., 35–45) than do otherwise healthy children.[530] The MAC of halothane is 20% less in children with cerebral palsy regardless of whether they took anticonvulsant drugs (MAC of 0.62 and 0.71, respectively).[531] A similar study suggested lower BIS values at similar MAC concentrations in children with cerebral palsy compared with unaffected children.[532]

Intraoperative hypothermia is common in children with disordered temperature regulation caused by hypothalamic dysfunction, reduced muscle bulk, and fat deposits. Thermal homeostasis should be managed aggressively from the moment the child enters the operating room.

Extensive plaster casting is an important component of bone and soft tissue surgical procedures. These casts may conceal blood loss, and limb swelling within the cast may contribute to compartment syndromes. Plaster jackets and hip spicas have been associated with mesenteric occlusion and acute gastric dilatation.[533,534]

Pain and spasm are regular features postoperatively. Epidural analgesia is particularly valuable when major orthopedic procedures are performed. Occasionally, two epidurals at different spinal sites may be required for multilevel surgery. The addition of either fentanyl or clonidine to bupivacaine in an epidural reduced the incidence of muscle spasm, although the incidence of vomiting was greater in the fentanyl group.[535] Systemic benzodiazepines, baclofen, dantrolene, and clonidine have been used to reduce muscle spasms. Selective dorsal rhizotomy is associated with severe pain, muscle spasms, and dysesthesia. Epidural and intrathecal forms of morphine as well as IV morphine and midazolam have been used to control this pain.[536] Oral benzodiazepines may be required to reduce the incidence and severity of muscle spasms but should be used with caution if combined with opioid analgesia.

Chronic pain is very prevalent (77%) in children and adolescents with predominant dyskinetic and mixed (dyskinetic/spastic) motor types.[527] Pain occurs across multiple body locations and less commonly recognized locations of pain include the face, jaw, and temple.[527] Pain can be difficult to assess in children with cerebral palsy, but several scoring systems are available (see also Chapter 42).[537,538] The opinions of parents and caregivers are extremely valuable in assessing pain in these children and in discriminating pain from other factors, such as irritability on emergence from anesthesia, poor positioning, a full bladder, or nausea.

SPINA BIFIDA

Spina bifida is characterized by developmental abnormalities of the vertebrae and spinal cord that may be associated with changes in the cerebrum, brainstem, and peripheral nerves. The failure of fusion of the vertebral arches is commonly known as *spina bifida*. *Spina bifida occulta* refers to spina bifida that occurs when skin and soft tissues cover the defect. *Spina bifida aperta* is used to describe lesions that communicate with the outside as a meningocele or a myelomeningocele (incidence of 1 per 1000 live births). The myelomeningocele sac contains nerve roots that do not function below the level of the lesion (see Chapters 22 and 24).

Clinical Features

Nerve root dysfunction results in muscle paralysis and a neurogenic bowel and bladder. Eighty percent of children develop hydrocephalus because of aqueductal stenosis (Arnold-Chiari [type II] malformation). Skeletal abnormalities such as clubfoot and congenital dislocation of the hip are common. Scoliosis may result from congenital vertebral abnormalities or, more commonly, abnormal neuromuscular control. Epilepsy and learning disorders can also occur, but most children have normal intelligence.

Orthopedic Considerations

Denervation causes muscle imbalance that results in abnormalities at the hip, knee, and foot. The aims of surgery are to reduce flexor posture at the hip and knee and plantigrade feet. Children with clubfeet, hip subluxation, or scoliosis commonly present for orthopedic correction.

Anesthetic Considerations

The potential for infection of the central nervous system dictates closure of the sac within the first few days of life. Subsequent surgical procedures and urinary catheterizations set the stage for sensitivity to latex.[539] Primary prophylaxis (i.e., avoiding all latex materials and using a latex-free operating room) is recommended for prevention of latex allergy and anaphylaxis.[540]

Preoperative assessment should include motor and sensory deficits, respiratory and renal function, and functioning of a ventriculoperitoneal shunt. Positioning on the operating table may require additional pillows for support of limbs with contractures. As a result of hypesthesia in the lower extremities, IV cannulae can be inserted painlessly. However, venous access is usually poor in the lower extremities because of limited limb use. The risk of endobronchial intubation is increased because of a short trachea (36% of children).[541] Kyphoscoliosis may distort tracheal anatomy. Renal dysfunction may dictate the choice of NMBD as well as the avoidance of NSAIDs. Succinylcholine may be used because it does not cause hyperkalemia in these children.[542] A reduced hypercapnic ventilation response means that these children should be closely observed in the recovery period.

OSTEOGENESIS IMPERFECTA

Osteogenesis imperfecta (OI) is thought to have afflicted Ivar the Boneless (Ivar Ragnarsson), a Viking chieftain who led a successful invasion of the East Anglia region of England in AD 865. Because he "had legs as soft as cartilage," he was unable to walk and had to be carried on a shield. Ivar's name is also associated with an early form of thoracoplasty. When King Ælla of Northumbria was captured, Ivar subjected him to the horrific "Blood Eagle" ordeal. His ribs were torn out and folded back to form the shape of an eagle's wings, and his lungs were removed.

Clinical Features

OI is a genetically determined disorder of connective tissue that is characterized by bone fragility. The disease state encompasses a phenotypically and genotypically heterogeneous group of inherited disorders that result from mutations in the genes that code for type I collagen.[543] The disorder manifests in tissues in which the principal matrix protein is type I collagen—mainly bone, dentin, sclerae, and ligaments. Musculoskeletal manifestations vary in severity along a continuum ranging from perinatal lethal forms with crumpled bones to moderate forms with deformity and propensity for fracture to clinically silent forms with subtle osteopenia and no deformity.[543]

Classification (types I through IV) is based on the timing of fractures or on multiple clinical, genetic, and radiologic features. Type I is the most common (1 case per 30,000 live births), and types I and IV have autosomal dominant inheritance patterns. These children have the classic triad of blue sclera, multiple fractures, and conductive hearing loss in adolescence. Bowing of the lower limbs, genu valgum, flat feet, and scoliosis develop with age. Type IV is characterized by osteoporosis, leading to bone fragility without many of the other features of type I. Type II, the most severe, is also known as perinatal lethal OI. Types II and III are more severe forms of OI and have autosomal recessive inheritance patterns. Molecular genetic studies have identified more than 150 mutations of the COL1A1 and COL1A2 genes, which encode for type I procollagen.[543] Ongoing studies in OI have been instrumental in the development of new and targeted therapeutic approaches, such as sclerostin inhibition and transforming growth factor-β inhibition.[544,545]

Orthopedic Considerations

The goals of treatment of OI are to maximize function, minimize deformity and disability, maintain comfort, achieve relative independence in activities of daily living, and enhance social integration. Physiotherapy, rehabilitation, and orthopedic surgery[546] are the mainstays of treatment for moderate and severe forms of OI.[547] Medical treatment with the antiresorptive bisphosphonates (e.g., pamidronate, alendronate) can decrease pain, lower the fracture incidence, and improve mobility.[548] Initial investigations have demonstrated an acceptable safety profile for bisphosphonates and long-term follow-up suggests a reduction in fractures, improved pain profiles, and improved physical activity with no major safety concerns.[549-554] Long-term IV bisphosphonate therapy was associated with higher z scores for lumbar spine, bone mineral density, and vertebral reshaping, but long-bone fracture rates were still common and the majority of patients developed scoliosis.[555] Medical therapies other than bisphosphonates, such as growth hormone and parathyroid hormone, have only minor roles; gene-based therapy remains in the early stages of preclinical research.[556,557]

Operative intervention is indicated for recurrent fractures or deformity that impair function.[543] Fractures in mild to moderately severe cases of OI type I are treated using the same methods as for patients without OI. Deformed bones that are fracturing are realigned, frequently followed by providing external or internal support. In selecting various modes of treatment, it is important to consider the natural history of the particular type of OI and to set realistic goals.[558-562]

Anesthetic Considerations

In common with other children suffering chronic disabilities, children with OI are veterans of the operating room. Chronic pain from frequent fractures complicates handling; deafness may hinder communication. Preoperative assessment centers on the chest wall deformity because it determines the severity of restrictive lung disease and subsequent cardiovascular compromise. Neck mobility, mouth opening, and dentition should also be assessed.

There is a risk of causing further fractures with positioning, tourniquet application, airway handing, and use of a blood pressure cuff. Invasive pressure monitoring may be less traumatic than a blood pressure cuff for some patients. Blood loss can be substantial in the more severe forms of the disease.[563] In a review of 252 children with cerebral palsy, massive blood loss occurred in 18% of children that was primarily related to the duration of surgery and the number of bone segments involved, but not to the classification of the OI.[564] If noninvasive blood pressure monitoring is used, less frequent monitoring of the blood pressure is recommended if possible. A laryngeal mask airway may avoid pressure from face masks. An individual history may help determine the risk/benefit ratio for each child. Succinylcholine has the potential to cause fasciculation-induced fractures. Regional, neuraxial and spinal techniques have been used successfully in these children.[565,566]

Abnormal temperature homeostasis may result in intraoperative hyperthermia that may be severe and accompanied by tachycardia and metabolic acidosis. This response is different from that of malignant hyperthermia in that there is an absence of respiratory acidosis and muscle rigidity.[567] Surface cooling is usually effective in restoring thermal homeostasis.

DUCHENNE MUSCULAR DYSTROPHY

Clinical Features

DMD is the most common of the progressive muscular dystrophies. It is an X-linked recessive disorder with an incidence of 3 per 10,000 births (see also Chapter 22). The *DMD* gene (located at Xp21.2) codes for a large sarcolemmal membrane protein, dystrophin, which is associated with muscle cell membrane integrity and signal transduction. Dystrophin is missing or nonfunctional in DMD patients; both sexes can carry the *DMD* mutation, but girls rarely exhibit signs of the disease.

Children usually present before school age with a waddling gait and later develop a lumbar lordosis and difficulty climbing stairs. Children use their arms to assist standing up (i.e., Gowers sign) because of proximal weakness of the hip girdle. Distal muscles, such as the calves, appear hypertrophied. The disease process is progressive, with increasing muscle weakness occurring with age. These boys often become wheelchair-bound by 10 to 11 years of age. Respiratory weakness, often exacerbated by scoliosis and by difficulty swallowing secretions related to pharyngeal involvement, can progress to a terminal pneumonia in the late teenage years.[568] By late adolescence, most children with DMD have cardiac disease, whether it is an abnormal electrocardiogram, arrhythmias, or a cardiomyopathy. Death from cardiorespiratory failure usually occurs before age 30, although respiratory support is extending life expectancy. Corticosteroids are the only treatment documented to improve strength and function in boys with DMD.[569] Gene editing offers hope for the future.[570]

Duchenne muscular dystrophy is not a static disease but evolves in end-organ implications with age.[571,572] In early childhood, skeletal muscle is constantly catabolized and becomes unstable. The use of membrane-destabilizing medications such as succinylcholine and potent inhalational anesthetics (halothane in particular) in these young children can result in hyperkalemia, rhabdomyolysis, and cardiac arrest.[573] However, after the children reach adolescence, the bulk of the skeletal muscle catabolism has arrested, and membrane-destabilizing medications are left with less substrate. Succinylcholine and potent inhalational anesthetics may be used with caution in the majority of cases without sequelae in adolescents with DMD who are undergoing scoliosis surgery and instrumentation,[574] although other anesthetic techniques are generally recommended (see also Chapters 6 and 22).

In contrast to its very limited effect on cardiac and smooth muscles in childhood, in adolescence DMD may cause substantive and life-threatening cardiac complications including arrhythmias. The anesthesiologist must appreciate the developmental changes of DMD with age and recognize the varying risks that may be associated with the use of succinylcholine and inhalational anesthetics in children and adolescents with this disease.

Duchenne muscular dystrophy can affect cardiac smooth muscle. Left ventricular hypertrophy is the most common cardiac finding followed by right ventricular hypertrophy.[215] Sophisticated cardiac imaging indicates that diastolic dysfunction may precede systolic dysfunction and may begin as early as 6 years of age, which has led to the recommendation for biannual echocardiograms until age 10 and annual evaluations thereafter. Right ventricular function may be compromised by nocturnal oxygen desaturation and sleep apnea contributing to pulmonary hypertension. Sinus tachycardia and arrhythmias may occur at an early age, but clinically apparent cardiomyopathy usually does not develop before 10 years of age. One-third of children have some degree of intellectual impairment.

DMD should be suspected in male preschool children with delayed walking ability; measurement of high serum creatinine phosphokinase concentrations provides a screening tool. Steroids are increasingly used for the management of DMD because they appear to increase muscle mass by decreasing protein breakdown.[575]

Becker muscular dystrophy (BMD) is a milder form of DMD with an onset at puberty or later in adolescence. Clinical expression varies, but even adolescents presenting with mild or subclinical weakness can develop cardiomyopathy with age progression. Death from cardiac or respiratory failure does not usually occur until the fourth or fifth decade. Because of improvements in respiratory care, dilated cardiomyopathy has become the major cause of death.[576]

Becker muscular dystrophy is an autosomal recessive myopathy that also results from mutations of dystrophin caused by a deletion of the exons 11 to 13 in the *DMD* gene (located at Xp21.2).[577] Dystrophin exerts its effect at the voltage-gated chloride channel 1 (CLCN1). Genetic analysis is an essential step in confirming the diagnosis. Additional EMG procedures may be of diagnostic value even when muscle biopsy may reveal no evidence of dystrophy.

Of importance to anesthesiologists, two-thirds of patients with mild or subclinical BMD have evidence of right ventricular dilation, and one-third have evidence of left ventricular dysfunction.[578] A thorough cardiac evaluation (similar to that for DMD) is recommended before scoliosis surgery.[576] Hyperthermia and heart failure, mimicking malignant hyperthermia and hyperkalemia with rhabdomyolysis after inhalational agents, have been reported in patients with BMD.[579,580] Therefore, inhalation agents and succinylcholine should be avoided. Despite these reports, neither DMD nor BMD has been associated with malignant hyperthermia.[581]

Orthopedic Considerations

Orthopedic surgery is indicated to improve or maintain ambulation and standing. Early treatment of contractures of the hips and the lower limbs prevents severe contractures and delays the progression of scoliosis.[571,582] Techniques designed to improve deformities and permit early postoperative mobilization include subcutaneous release of contracted tendons and percutaneous removal of cancellous bone with corrective manipulation of the feet.

Maintenance of upright posture extends the ability of patients to attend to the tasks of daily living.[583] Spinal deformities attributable to muscle imbalance or a collapsing spine are corrected to improve or maintain sitting posture. Spinal fusion may also decrease the rate of deterioration of respiratory function, although this has been questioned.[584]

Anesthetic Considerations

Respiratory and cardiovascular compromise dominates preoperative assessment.[585] Preoperative cardiac assessment should include an electrocardiogram and an echocardiogram. Chronic steroid use must be considered and perioperative use reviewed.[586,587] Deformities and contractures of limb joints hinder vascular access, regional anesthetic techniques, and positioning on the operating table. Hypertrophy of the tongue[588] may cause difficulty during intubation. Gastric motility is delayed, and gastric emptying times are prolonged.[589] Tracheobronchial tree compression has been described in a child positioned prone for spinal instrumentation.[590] These children often have greater blood loss during surgery. The precise cause remains unclear, but it may be because fat and connective tissue have replaced muscle or because of abnormalities in the blood vessels.[312]

Nondepolarizing NMBDs, at standard doses, have a slow onset and prolonged duration of action.[591–593] All NMBDs should be monitored with a peripheral nerve stimulator.[594] *Succinylcholine is contraindicated in these children because of the risk of hyperkalemia, muscle rigidity, rhabdomyolysis, myoglobinuria, arrhythmias, and cardiac arrest.* If a rapid-sequence intubation is indicated, then a large dose of rocuronium ($>3x$ ED$_{95}$) with later reversal with sugammadex is reasonable.[595,596] There is no known link between DMD and malignant hyperthermia.[597,598] The predominant candidate gene (*RYR1*) for malignant hyperthermia is located on the long arm of chromosome 19, whereas the *DMD* gene is located on the short arm of the X chromosome.[599] Although inhalational anesthetic agents continue to be used in young children with DMD, rhabdomyolysis and hyperkalemia have been reported in the recovery room after halothane, isoflurane, desflurane, and sevoflurane anesthesia.[600–604] Potent inhalational anesthetics are best avoided in young children with DMD; instead, alternative anesthetics that do not trigger rhabdomyolysis and hyperkalemia, such as propofol, remifentanil, ketamine, opioids, α$_2$-agonists, and benzodiazepines (remimazolam[605]), are preferred (see Chapters 5 and 6).[606] Total intravenous anesthetic techniques such as propofol and remifentanil[607] or even ketamine supplemented with dexmedetomidine or propofol has proven useful for brief procedures such as muscle biopsy.[608,609]

Regional techniques such as epidurals may be technically more difficult because of kyphoscoliosis and obesity. The use of ultrasound-guided peripheral nerve blockade can improve the quality and reduce complications of neuronal blockade.[6] Opioids are not contraindicated in the postoperative period but should be used with caution in children with respiratory compromise. Noninvasive ventilation support using BiPAP or continuous positive airway pressure is sometimes required after major surgery or in those already receiving this treatment overnight.

ARTHROGRYPOSIS MULTIPLEX CONGENITA
Clinical Features

Arthrogryposis multiplex congenita is a spectrum syndrome of multiple, persistent limb contractures often accompanied by associated anomalies, including cleft palate, genitourinary defects, gastroschisis, and cardiac defects.[610] The incidence is 1 case per 3000 births. Joint contractures are present at birth and are a result of immobility in utero, commonly related to a neurogenic abnormality or myopathy.[611] These children have been likened to a "thin, wooden doll," because muscles connected to affected joints are atrophic and replaced by fibrous tissue and fat.[612] The temporomandibular joint may also be involved, causing restricted mouth opening (microstomia) and micrognathia. Scoliosis commonly develops. Restrictive lung disease, rib cage deformities, and pulmonary hypoplasia predispose to recurrent chest infections.

Orthopedic Considerations

The aim of surgery is to improve function. Most operations involve the soft tissues, tendons, and osteotomies of the lower limbs and hips.[613] Upper limb surgery is less common. Extension contracture of the elbow joint may make it difficult or impossible to reach the mouth or to perform hygienic necessities. Improvement in passive elbow flexion by capsulotomy or in active flexion by triceps transfer can increase independence and personal hygiene. When both arms are involved, consideration may be given to maintaining one arm in flexion for reaching the head and mouth passively or even actively and one arm in extension for basic hygiene cares.[614]

Anesthetic Considerations

Arthrogryposis multiplex congenita is commonly associated with other syndromes that may complicate anesthesia.[610,615–617] Venous cannulation is difficult because veins tend to be small and fragile. The concavity of joints is difficult to access. Regional blockade can also be difficult, although use of ultrasound improves success rates for the femoral and sciatic nerve block.[618] Care must be taken in positioning the patient on the operating table and protecting skin overlying bony joints to prevent pathologic fractures.

These children should be evaluated for a difficult airway because of temporomandibular joint dysfunction, mandibular hypoplasia, and micrognathia.[619–622] Fusion or underdevelopment of the first and second cervical vertebrae may further complicate laryngoscopy and tracheal intubation with a severe reduction in neck mobility. Tracheal intubation may become progressively more difficult with age. During infancy, however, evaluating mouth opening may be difficult; it may be necessary to insert a tongue blade to determine whether the mandible can be distracted from the maxilla.

Succinylcholine has been used without incident in these children, although teleologically, the use of a depolarizing muscle relaxant in the presence of anterior horn cell disease is contentious. The response to nondepolarizing NMBDs should be monitored.

Hyperthermia and persistent tachycardia have been reported during general anesthesia.[610,623–625] Although intraoperative cardiovascular instability is reported, intraoperative hyperthermia or hypermetabolic responses are less certain to occur.[626] Hyperthermia, if present, responds to simple cooling techniques.

Pulmonary dysfunction and an increased sensitivity to opioids dictate suitable monitoring postoperatively. Regional techniques may be difficult in the presence of contractures, but if successful, they offer intraoperative and postoperative analgesia.[612] Success can be improved by using ultrasound-guided techniques.

ANNOTATED REFERENCES

Birnkrant DJ, Bushby K, Bann CM, et al. Diagnosis and management of Duchenne muscular dystrophy, part 1: diagnosis, and neuromuscular, rehabilitation, endocrine, and gastrointestinal and nutritional management. *Lancet Neurol.* 2018;17:251-267.

Birnkrant DJ, Bushby K, Bann CM, et al. Diagnosis and management of Duchenne muscular dystrophy, part 2: respiratory, cardiac, bone health, and orthopaedic management. *Lancet Neurol.* 2018;17: 347-361.

These two papers present a comprehensive review of current treatment and management of Duchenne muscular dystrophy.

Harper CM, Ambler G, Edge G. The prognostic value of preoperative predicted forced vital capacity in corrective spinal surgery for Duchenne's muscular dystrophy. *Anaesthesia.* 2004;59:1160-1162.

Performing scoliosis surgery on children with Duchenne muscular dystrophy who have a forced vital capacity (FVC) of 30% has been questioned because of the high incidence of postoperative pulmonary complications. This clinical paper demonstrated that with careful attention to detail, children with an FVC less than 30% can undergo scoliosis surgery with results similar to those with an FVC greater than 30%. Early extubation followed by the use of noninvasive ventilation was identified as key to reducing respiratory complications.

Holdefer RN, Furman M, Sangare Y, Slimp JC. A comparison of the effects of desflurane versus propofol on transcranial motor-evoked potentials in pediatric patients. *Childs Nerv Syst.* 2014;30:2103-2108.

Martin DP, Bhalla T, Thung A, et al. A preliminary study of volatile agents or total intravenous anesthesia for neurophysiological monitoring during posterior spinal fusion in adolescents with idiopathic scoliosis. *Spine.* 2014;39:E1318-E1324.

These two studies demonstrate that adequate neurophysiologic status using SSEPs and MEPs during scoliosis surgery can be obtained with either a desflurane- or propofol-based anesthetic technique. Current opinion favors a total IV anesthetic (propofol) technique, but desflurane is an acceptable alternative. Both studies used modest doses of either agent (0.6–0.8 MAC desflurane, propofol 150–300 µg/kg per minute). Adequate SSEPs and MEPs were obtained in all patients, but a higher stimulating voltage was required in both papers when desflurane was used. A potential benefit of desflurane is a shorter wake-up time, which may be advantageous if signal changes are observed.

Julien-Marsollier F, Michelet D, Assaker R, et al. Enhanced recovery after surgical correction of adolescent idiopathic scoliosis. *Paediatr Anaesth.* 2020;30(10):1068-1076.

Pennington Z, Cottrill E, Lubelski D, et al. Clinical utility of enhanced recovery after surgery pathways in pediatric spinal deformity surgery: systematic review of the literature. *J Neurosurg Pediatr.* 2020;27(2): 225-238.

Both of these studies show that ERAS protocols as a standardized pathway, reduced length of stay and improved postoperative care. These studies emphasize that standardizing the approach to these patients prior to and throughout their hospitalization produces benefits to patients and institutions.

Karimi S, Lu VM, Nambiar M, et al. Antifibrinolytic agents for paediatric scoliosis surgery: a systematic review and meta-analysis. *Eur Spine J.* 2019;28(5):1023-1034.

This systemic review and meta-analysis concludes that antifibrinolytics lead to reductions in perioperative blood loss, intraoperative blood loss, reduced fresh frozen plasma requirements and reduced postoperative blood loss.

Neira VM, Ghaffari K, Bulusu S, et al. Diagnostic accuracy of neuromonitoring for identification of new neurologic deficits in pediatric spinal fusion surgery. *Anesth Analg.* 2016;123(6):1556-1566.

Tsirikos AI, Duckworth AD, Henderson LE, Michaelson C. Multimodal intraoperative spinal cord monitoring during spinal deformity surgery: efficacy, diagnostic characteristics, and algorithm development. *Med Princ Pract.* 2020;29(1):6-17.

These two studies investigated the incidence of new neurologic deficits (NNDs) and estimated sensitivity and specificity of intraoperative neuromonitoring modalities (IONM). Both sensitivity and specificity are impacted substantially by assumptions of the impact of interventions on alerts and NND. Properly designed, controlled, multicenter studies are required to establish diagnostic accuracy of IONM in scoliosis surgery. Anesthesia and surgery related factors at the time of the alert and the interventions undertaken to improve or reverse those alerts are described. The second study confirmed that multimodal IONM is highly sensitive and specific for spinal cord injury. An algorithm of intraoperative action to allow close cooperation between the surgical, anesthetic, and neurophysiology teams to prevent neurological deficits is described.

Solla F, Lefebvre R, Clement JL, et al. Prevention of surgical site infections in pediatric spines: a single-center experience. *Childs Nerv Syst.* 2021;37(7):2299-2304.

Tipper GA, Chiwera L, Lucas J. Reducing surgical site infection in pediatric scoliosis surgery: a multidisciplinary improvement program and prospective 4-year audit. *Global Spine J.* 2020;10(5):633-639.

Standardized pathways determined by examining the impact of multidisciplinary led multimodal improvements reduced surgical site infections. Pathways were similar in both papers. Common to both studies were standardized antibiotic prophylaxis, including vancomycin powder into the wound and pulsed lavage wound irrigation.

Yuan N, Fraire JA, Margetis MM, et al. The effect of scoliosis surgery on lung function in the immediate postoperative period. *Spine.* 2005;30: 2182-2185.

The decrease in pulmonary function in the days after scoliosis surgery are described, explaining why children are at risk for pulmonary complications during this period. Pulmonary function tests decreased by up to 60% after surgery, with a nadir at 3 days. The FEV1 and FVC values were still only at 60% of the preoperative values on the 10th postoperative day.

A complete reference list can be found online at Elsevier eBooks+.

Otorhinolaryngologic Procedures

KIMMO MURTO, MICHELE M. CARR, AND JERROLD LERMAN

Anesthesia for Otologic Procedures
Myringotomy and Tube Insertion
Middle Ear and Mastoid Surgery
Cochlear Implants and Bone-Anchored Hearing Aids
Anesthesia for Rhinologic Procedures
Adenotonsillectomy
Indications
Surgical Approach
Obstructive Sleep Apnea
Preoperative Evaluation of the Child with OSA
Indications for Adenotonsillectomy
Risk Stratification for Perioperative Adverse
Events and Disposition Planning
Anesthetic Considerations
Perioperative Considerations
Postoperative Considerations
Admission Policies
Opioids and Risk for Postoperative Respiratory
Depression in Children With OSA
Adenotonsillectomy Complications
Emergence and Recovery
Posttonsillectomy Hemorrhage

Peritonsillar Abscess
Anesthesia for Endoscopy
Direct Laryngoscopy and Bronchoscopy
Esophagoscopy for Foreign Bodies
Upper Airway Obstruction
Laryngomalacia
Acute Epiglottitis
Laryngotracheobronchitis (Croup)
Laryngeal Papillomatosis
Congenital and Acquired Upper Airway Obstruction
Tracheotomy
Management of the Child With a Tracheostomy In Situ
Tracheocutaneous Fistula
Airway Trauma and Inhalational Injury
Laryngotracheal Injury
Surgical Repair
Upper Airway Inhalational Injury
Laryngeal Clefts
Laryngotracheal Reconstruction
Surgical Approach
Anesthetic Considerations

ELECTIVE OTORHINOLARYNGOLOGIC SURGERY is commonly performed in infants, children, and adolescents. Anesthetic management is provided by both pediatric and general anesthesiologists in ambulatory surgery centers, hospitals, and office practices.[1] In addition, anesthesiologists are often consulted to help manage potentially life-threatening airway emergencies caused by croup, foreign body aspiration, airway trauma, bacterial tracheitis, posttonsillectomy bleeding and, rarely, acute epiglottitis.[2] In both the elective and emergent scenarios, the pathophysiology is critical to designing the optimal anesthetic plan, which should be discussed in advance with the surgeon with whom the airway will be shared so as to ensure safe anesthetic management and ideal surgical conditions.

Anesthesia for Otologic Procedures

MYRINGOTOMY AND TUBE INSERTION

A myringotomy is a surgical procedure to create an opening in the tympanic membrane that allows the pressure within the middle ear to equalize with ambient pressure and serves as a route for middle ear fluid to drain. It is indicated for children with recurrent otitis media or persisting middle ear effusions; often a small plastic tube (tympanostomy tube or gromet) is placed to ensure myringotomy incision patency. The tube facilitates continuous ventilation of the middle ear and is naturally extruded by 6- to

12-months after placement, or it can be surgically removed at a later date.[3] Coincidentally, a film, paper patch or fat graft may be placed over the myringotomy incision to stimulate healing of the tympanic membrane. Most young children require general anesthesia to place a tympanostomy tube, although occasionally adolescents may tolerate the procedure using only topical anesthesia.

Myringotomy with tube insertion is a very brief ambulatory procedure (usually 5–10 minutes), commonly performed under general anesthesia with an inhalational agent (e.g., sevoflurane). Since head movement is amplified through the surgeon's microscope, such movements while the knife is in the ear canal may cause inadvertent injury to important structures including the facial nerve and carotid artery (within the petrous temporal bone behind the middle ear). Head movement can be minimized by ensuring a patent upper airway using a jaw thrust (subluxing the temporomandibular joint) or an oropharyngeal airway and gently assisting ventilation while the anesthesiologist stabilizes their own forearm using the table for support. For children with trisomy 21 or achondroplasia, the table may be tilted laterally (i.e., airplaned) rather than rotating the head if there are concerns of atlantoaxial subluxation.[4–10] Occasionally, a laryngeal mask airway is used when the procedure is expected to be prolonged due to narrow ear canals, a difficult airway is anticipated, or a second procedure will occur.

Most children undergoing myringotomy can be managed safely without intravenous (IV) access[11,12] although IV equipment should be immediately available. In those with severe underlying medical or surgical conditions or who are at risk for an adverse respiratory event or who require a supraglottic airway (SGA), IV access may be prudent despite the anticipated brief duration of the procedure. Premedication is infrequently used since the duration of action of the medication will likely outlast the expected duration of surgery and may prolong recovery; children with behavior disorders may benefit from premedication and/or the assistance of parents at induction.

There is a divergence of opinion regarding the severity of the pain and its management after myringotomy and tube surgery. A large retrospective study determined that more than 50% of children experienced pain despite receiving ketorolac.[13] Factors that were more likely to lead to postoperative pain included younger age, surgery of greater duration, normal appearing middle ears, and the individual surgeon. Normal/unilateral infected ears at the time of pediatric myringotomy are associated with a greater incidence of moderate-to-severe postoperative pain following intraoperative fentanyl/ketorolac administration, but the predictive value of the ear condition on pain is limited.[14]

Discomfort after myringotomy and tube insertion is usually addressed with acetaminophen and nonsteroidal antiinflammatory drugs (NSAIDs) such as ibuprofen or ketorolac,[15] but many other analgesics have successfully provided analgesia, such as, dexmedetomidine, fentanyl (oral [PO], intramuscular [IM], or intranasal [IN]), codeine, and butorphanol.[16] Acetaminophen (10–20 mg/kg PO or 30–40 mg/kg rectally), has been shown to be as effective as ketorolac and fentanyl in providing pain relief.[17–19] The analgesic effect for acetaminophen and NSAIDs is concentration dependent. Larger oral doses or IV administration achieve greater blood concentrations and are more effective for immediate postoperative analgesia (Fig. 31.1).[18,20–23]

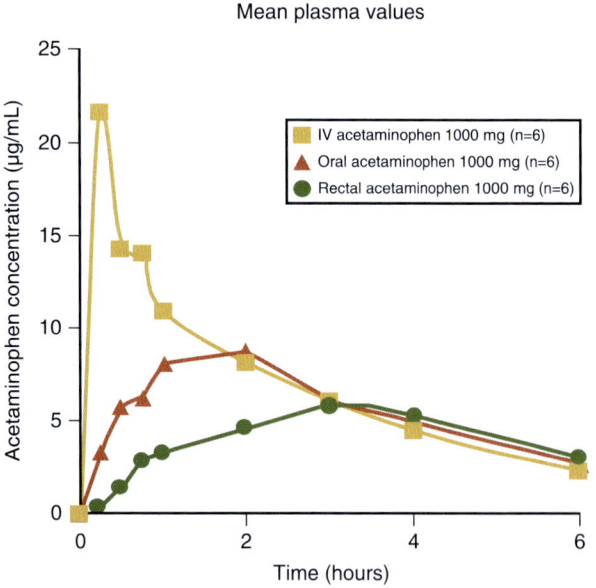

FIGURE 31.1 Plasma time-concentration profile for 1000 mg acetaminophen via three routes: intravenous, oral, and rectal (IV, PO, and PR, respectively). PR acetaminophen reflects standardization of 1300 mg dose to 1000 mg (linear kinetics). (Adapted from Singla NK, Parulan C, Samson R, et al. Plasma and cerebrospinal fluid pharmacokinetic parameters after single-dose administration of intravenous, oral, or rectal acetaminophen. *Pain Pract.* 2012;12[7]:523-532.)

Intranasal medications may be instilled as liquid drops or by an atomizer.[24] Dexmedetomidine (2 mg/kg IN) provides analgesia,[25] but sedation is associated with a prolonged stay in the postanesthesia care unit (PACU).[26,27] Intranasal fentanyl (1–2 µg/kg) has been used to reduce pain and emergence agitation,[28,29] particularly in preschool-aged children after sevoflurane anesthesia (see Chapter 2).[28,29] Combination analgesia is usually superior to single agent therapy, but most combinations have a maximum effect similar to single agent therapy in a larger dose.[20–22] For example, the combination of IM fentanyl (≥1.5 µg/kg) and ketorolac (≥0.75 mg/kg) was superior to either analgesic.[30] If powerful opioids such as fentanyl are used intraoperatively, preoperative oral acetaminophen or ibuprofen conferred no additional analgesia.[31] In a retrospective single center review of IV or IN fentanyl, IV or IM ketorolac, or the combination of fentanyl and ketorolac reported similar pain scores in the children (mean age 1.7 years).[32] Equivalent analgesia following a nerve of Arnold block (0.2 mL 0.25% bupivacaine) or IN fentanyl (2 µg/kg) is reported with no difference in the need for pain rescue, vomiting, or time to discharge (see Chapter 40). The analgesic approaches to pain after myringotomy are many.[33]

Children should be offered clear fluids, but not forced to drink in PACU to reduce postoperative nausea and vomiting (PONV).[34] When this strategy was applied to children whose faces, legs, activity, cry, and consolability (FLACC) pain scores were ≥4, the incidence of PONV and the need for analgesics in those who accepted fluids was one-half those who were restricted clear fluids.[35] However, children in that study were also offered opioids, and opioid use influences the incidence of nausea and vomiting. Avoidance of opioids for a simple 10-minute sevoflurane anesthetic in healthy children is associated with little nausea and vomiting.

Chronic otitis media is often accompanied by adenoidal hypertrophy or allergies with persistent rhinorrhea or recurrent upper respiratory tract infections (URI) (see Chapter 11). If a child presents with copious, clear rhinorrhea with or without recurrent mild upper respiratory symptoms, a nasal decongestant (e.g., oxymetazoline) may be instilled to reduce secretions and the risk of perioperative airway events. This practice is tempered by concerns that vasoconstrictors are systemically absorbed from the nose and can have adverse effects such as hypertension if administered in excessive doses.[36]

Children with chronic otitis media often also suffer from recurrent URIs. Generally, there are four reasons to cancel a child with an active URI: (1) copious, green, mucopurulent nasal discharge; (2) lower respiratory tract signs (wheezing that does not clear with a cough), (3) fever >38.5°C; and (4) a change in sensorium (not eating or behaving normally).[37] However, tympanostomy surgery may still be required in these children to break the cycle of recurrent ear infections, prevent hearing loss, and/or mastoiditis.

MIDDLE EAR AND MASTOID SURGERY

Tympanoplasty and mastoidectomy are two common major pediatric ear operations. Typically, these are performed as day-surgery cases with general anesthesia that consists of either an inhalational agent or total intravenous anesthetic (TIVA). Neuromuscular blockade with an intermediate acting neuromuscular blocking agent will facilitate tracheal intubation, but this effect should be allowed to wear off to permit facial nerve monitoring.

To gain access to the surgical site, the child's neck will be laterally rotated; to avoid extreme rotation, the table can be airplaned. The anesthesiologist and surgeon must be especially vigilant to ensure that nerves, muscles, and bony structures are not injured because of this unusual positioning; the sternocleidomastoid muscles generally limit the safe degree of lateral head rotation. Caution should be exercised when rotating the neck of children with trisomy 21 or achondroplasia.

Positioning of the operating table to allow access to the middle ear and to accommodate the additional surgical equipment can be challenging. Depending on the room configuration, the table is rotated 90 or 180 degrees away from the anesthesia workstation, necessitating the use of extension tubing on the anesthesia breathing circuit (E-Fig. 31.1). Draping must allow immediate access to the airway if required and drape adhesives should not be placed directly on the tracheal tube or breathing circuit.

Bleeding may be reduced by using a mild degree of hypotension (i.e., mean arterial pressure 10%–20% less than baseline) and the topical application of concentrated epinephrine (1:10,000) applied to the mucosa of the middle ear. The dose of epinephrine used must be limited to prevent arrhythmias and wide swings in blood pressure, (e.g., epinephrine 10 μg/kg) repeated after 30 minutes. Alternatively, topical oxymetazoline (0.05%) may be used to induce vasoconstriction.

The middle ear and sinuses are air-filled, nondistensible cavities; an increase in the volume of gas within these cavities increases the pressure therein. Nitrous oxide diffuses along a concentration gradient into air-filled middle ear spaces. Given that the solubility of nitrous oxide in blood is 33 times greater than that of nitrogen, 33 molecules of nitrous oxide enter the space for every molecule of nitrogen that leaves. This exchange of gases may increase the pressure within the middle ear, possibly exceeding the ability of the eustachian tube to vent the middle ear, particularly if the eustachian tube function is compromised due to infection or the surgical procedure.[38] The increase in middle ear pressure from nitrous oxide may increase the incidence of PONV, an effect attributable to labyrinthine, vestibular, and/or central nervous system dysfunction mechanisms.[39] In addition, the resulting intermittent venting of the middle ear causes fluctuations in middle ear pressure and movement of the tympanic membrane.[40] It seems prudent to discontinue nitrous oxide before procedures in which the tympanic membrane is replaced or a perforation is patched, to reduce the potential for pressure-related displacement of the graft.[41] To offset the absence of nitrous oxide, the concentration of sevoflurane should be increased by ~25% in children.[42] It should be noted that after nitrous oxide is discontinued, it is quickly resorbed, creating a void in the middle ear, that could generate a negative pressure. This negative pressure may lead to a serous otitis, disarticulation of the ossicles in the middle ear (especially the stapes), and impaired hearing, which may last up to 6 weeks postoperatively.[40,43]

PONV after middle ear surgery occurs in 62% to 80% of patients.[44] The etiology of PONV remains unclear but depends on a multitude of factors including the general anesthetic (inhaled versus TIVA), the prolonged use of nitrous oxide, opioids and their effects on the vestibular system, and low-frequency sounds generated by drilling near the middle ear apparatus (known as the Tullio phenomenon whereby sound triggers vertigo or nystagmus).[39,45] The negative pressure created by the reabsorption of nitrous oxide stimulates the vestibular system by producing traction on the round window. The risk of PONV after inhaled agents is greater than that after TIVA, but the difference is attenuated in the presence of antiemetics.[46,47] Children anesthetized with sevoflurane for less than 1 hour showed that the addition of nitrous oxide did not increase the incidence of PONV.[48] Age also affects

the risk of PONV: infants younger than 1 year exhibit a low risk, whereas those older than 6 years exhibit the greatest risk of PONV.[49] Strategies to minimize PONV after middle ear surgery include prophylactic administration of antiemetics (e.g., dexamethasone and ondansetron), IV fluids (30 mL/kg per hour),[50] replacing long-acting opioids with regional anesthesia, avoiding nitrous oxide for long cases, and either substituting sugammadex for an anticholinesterase to reverse long-acting neuromuscular blocking drugs (NMBDs) or avoiding them altogether.[51,52] TIVA is finding increasing popularity.[53,54] A preoperative block of the great auricular nerve provides comparable pain relief as that of 0.1 mg/kg IV morphine and reduced the incidence of PONV during hospital stay and at home. (see Chapter 40).[55]

A smooth, quiet emergence after tympanoplasty and/or mastoidectomy is desirable. Deep tracheal extubation or replacement of the tracheal tube with a laryngeal mask airway (LMA) before the application of the head bandage dressing may be considered. Alternately, a smooth emergence with minimal coughing at the time of extubation can be achieved by gently suctioning the oropharynx and IV administration of a short-acting opioid, dexmedetomidine (0.5–1.0 μg/kg) or lidocaine (0.5–2.0 mg/kg).[56,57] Efforts should be made to reduce the potential for a tumultuous emergence with emergence delirium; strategies should be incorporated to minimize its possibility (see Chapters 2 and 5).[58]

COCHLEAR IMPLANTS AND BONE-ANCHORED HEARING AIDS

Cochlear implants are indicated in children with profound sensorineural hearing loss. The surgery involves opening the cochlea and attaching an electrode to a receiver-stimulator device placed on the outside of the skull in the postauricular region.[59] Forty percent of children who present for cochlear implantation have syndromic comorbidities associated with deafness, as well as those associated with premature birth, neurologic development, and congenital heart disease.[60,61] An endoscopic-assisted technique reduces intraoperative bleeding, requires less muscle dissection, and reduces postoperative pain.[62]

Many children with conductive hearing loss are not candidates for traditional hearing aids due to chronic ear drainage, microtia, or aural atresia. These children may be candidates for a bone-anchored hearing aid device.[59,63] The bone-anchoring hearing aid surgical approach involves placing a titanium implant in the bone of the skull behind the ear; sound vibrates the implant and the bone to transmit sound directly to the inner ear.

For both cochlear implants and bone-anchored hearing aids, the surgical technique requires meticulous care with hemostasis, soft-tissue dissection, and bone drilling, as bleeding from bone can be difficult to control and can complicate the surgical outcome. A great auricular nerve block reduces the incidence of PONV both in hospital and after discharge.[55] Table 31.1 (the "5 Ps"; Patient, Preoperative, Position, Procedure, and Postoperative) summarizes the anesthetic considerations for middle ear, mastoid, and cochlear implant surgery.

Anesthesia for Rhinologic Procedures

Chronic sinusitis in children is often caused by antibiotic-resistant bacteria and usually treated with broad-spectrum antibiotics. In some children with obstructive adenoid hypertrophy, adenoidectomy improves the signs and symptoms of sinusitis, but the primary method of surgical treatment for chronic sinusitis is functional endoscopic sinus surgery (FESS). The surgeon visualizes the

TABLE 31.1 Anesthetic Considerations for Middle Ear, Mastoid, and Cochlear Implant Surgery

Patient
- Prone to recurrent URIs
- Communication (↓ hearing/speech delay) and cooperation challenges

Preoperative

Optimize
- Sedation vs. PPIA/retain hearing aid for induction.

Disposition Planning
- Ambulatory or inpatient surgery

Position
- Supine with lateral neck rotation/extension
  - Caution with atlantoaxial instability
- Lateral rotation of the child's neck/airplane the OR table
  - Safety straps
- OR table rotated 90–180 degrees.
  - Extra-long or extensions for the breathing circuit
  - Limited access to the airway
- Protective padding:
  - Dependent eye and ear and other vulnerable pressure points
- Reverse Trendelenburg
  - Venous air embolism risk

Procedure

Goals
- Provide bloodless surgical field
- Plan for smooth emergence/deep extubation
- Mitigate postoperative pain & PONV risk
- Avoid pressure injury
- Maintain normothermia

Anesthetic Approach
- Anesthetic technique:
  - GA with inhalational agents and/or TIVA
  - Avoid neuromuscular blockade during facial nerve monitoring
  - Avoid N₂O during prolonged middle ear surgery
  - Deep vs. awake extubation
- Medications:
  - Analgesia:
    - Opioid-sparing or minimize the dose of opioids
    - NSAIDs (to be discussed with surgeon)
    - Supplemental regional blockade/LA infiltration
  - Antiemetic drugs and adjuvant techniques
- Complications include:
  - Accidental extubation
  - Arrhythmias/hemodynamic instability due to:
    - Local anesthetic infiltration or topical vasoconstrictor
  - Bleeding
  - CSF leak, facial nerve injury, or VAE with sigmoid sinus injury

Postoperative
- Replace hearing aid
- Discharge criteria
- Risk for:
  - Emergence delirium, pain, and PONV
- Facial nerve paralysis (injury vs. local anesthesia) or vertigo

CSF, Cerebral spinal fluid; *GA,* general anesthesia; *N₂O,* nitrous oxide; *NSAID,* nonsteroidal antiinflammatory drug; *OR,* operating room; *PONV,* postoperative nausea and vomiting; *PPIA,* parental presence at induction of anethesia; *TIVA,* total intravenous anesthesia; *URI,* upper respiratory tract infection; *VAE,* venous air embolism.

sinonasal cavity directly and cleans out sinus tissue (using sharp dissection instruments and/or a microdebrider).[64] Many children who require functional endoscopic sinus surgery have coexisting medical problems, such as asthma and/or cystic fibrosis, which must be optimized before surgery. An alternative to functional endoscopic sinus surgery in select cases is balloon sinuplasty to dilate the natural maxillary, frontal, or sphenoidal ostia without bone or soft-tissue removal, thus reducing bleeding.[64,65]

Most rhinologic procedures require tracheal intubation with a preformed cuffed orotracheal tube that permits unobstructed access to the maxilla and sinuses; it should be noted that the distance from the bend-to-tip distance varies among manufacturers, especially for nasotracheal tubes.[66] A cuffed tracheal tube eliminates gas leaks that could fog the endoscopic instruments and trigger a fire if cautery is used. A throat pack may be required to absorb blood draining from the surgical site. It is critically important that the throat pack is removed before the trachea is extubated.

To reduce bleeding from the nasal and sinus mucosa, the nasal cavity is often packed with gauze soaked with a vasoconstrictor such as oxymetazoline (0.025%–0.05%), phenylephrine (0.25%–1%), epinephrine (0.05%) (1:2000), and less frequently, cocaine (4%–10%).[67] In a comparison of the three vasoconstrictors, oxymetazoline (0.05%), phenylephrine (0.25%), and cocaine (4%) applied to the nasal mucosa in children undergoing functional endoscopic sinus surgery, bleeding was less severe after oxymetazoline compared with the other two vasoconstrictors, and the increase in blood pressure 10 minutes after phenylephrine was greater than after the other vasoconstrictors.[68] Knowing that systemic absorption of vasoconstrictors can cause severe hypertension, reflex bradycardia, and cardiac arrest,[69–71] the anesthesiologist and the surgeon should discuss the type and dose of the vasoconstrictor to ensure that a subtoxic dose is used.[72,73] Additional measures to prevent toxicity include removing (e.g., suction) excess drug from the pharynx to prevent additional mucosal absorption.

Topical oxymetazoline is FDA-approved only for children older than 6 years of age and is usually dosed as two to three sprays per nostril (30 μL/spray) for a total of 180 microliters administered from an upright spray bottle. If oxymetazoline is delivered from a metered dose device, the orientation of the device during actuation markedly affects the dose delivered; the dose delivered in the inverted position, 606 microliters, is 10-fold greater than in the upright position, 62 microliters.[74] Importantly, administering oxymetazoline via a spray bottle inverted or using prolonged placement of oxymetazoline-soaked cotton nasal pledgets may deliver up to 16- to 50-fold greater volumes, respectively.[72] In children, the initial topical dose of phenylephrine should not exceed 20 micrograms per kilogram to a maximum of 0.5 milligrams (equivalent to 4 drops of a 0.25% solution), greater doses may lead to hypertension, pulmonary edema, and even intraoperative death.[69,75] The practice of wringing out pledgets after being soaked in a vasoconstrictor reduces the risk of administering a toxic dose.[76] Local injection of vasoconstrictors in functional endoscopic sinus surgery in adults is controversial and is not recommended for children.[77]

Paroxysmal hypertension induced by topically applied vasoconstrictors generally resolves spontaneously, but if extreme in magnitude or prolonged in duration, may require aggressive treatment using alpha₁-antagonist drugs such as hydralazine (administer 80–150 μg/kg IV, onset 5–15 minutes, and peak effect 10–80 minutes).[78] β-adrenergic blockers are not recommended to control blood pressure in these circumstances as they can increase peripheral vascular resistance and depress cardiac output, resulting in pulmonary edema and cardiac arrest.[69] Similarly calcium channel blockers are not recommended as cardiac depression is additive to that produced by inhalation agents commonly used to treat the hypertension in this circumstance.[69]

An anesthetic technique that ensures adequate analgesia, minimizes bleeding, and promotes a rapid return of consciousness at the end of surgery is desirable. Both TIVA and inhalational techniques are used, often augmented with opioids, alpha-2 agonists, and a regional block; there is no consensus on the preferred anesthetic technique for this surgery.[79] Placing the bed at a 15 to 20 degree reverse Trendelenburg position is a simple approach to reduce blood in the surgical field.[77] Unilateral or bilateral infraorbital nerve block, performed via the intraoral or extraoral route can provide supplemental analgesia (see Chapter 40).[80] The combination of topical lidocaine 1% and epinephrine 1:200,000 reduces bleeding and prolongs analgesia.[79]

A Cochrane review of 14 studies that involved 942 patients (12 studies) and children (2 studies) demonstrated with moderate certainty that tranexamic acid reduces the surgical field bleeding and the overall surgical blood loss during functional endoscopic sinus surgery.[81] In adults, tranexamic acid as a 15 mg/kg bolus (± an infusion) or administered topically as a 5% solution combined with phenylephrine reduces the operative time and intraoperative blood loss, and improves surgical satisfaction.[67] This has been attributed in part to its antiinflammatory as well as antifibrinolytic activity.[81,82] In children, a randomized study reported that a single dose of tranexamic acid (25 mg/kg) improved surgical field visibility, reduced intraoperative bleeding, and shortened the duration of surgery.[83]

After the procedure, the surgeon usually leaves an absorbable stenting material in the nasal cavities, which may interfere with nasal breathing. Non-selective cyclooxygenase (COX) 1 and 2 NSAIDs should be avoided in children with asthma and sinusitis secondary to nasal polyps (Samter triad)[84,85]; selective COX-2 NSAIDs may be a safer alternative.[86]

Adenotonsillectomy

Adenotonsillectomy is one of the most performed pediatric procedures worldwide. One in eight American children will undergo adenotonsillectomy[87,88]; most adenotonsillectomies in children older than 3 years of age are performed as outpatient procedures.[89]

INDICATIONS

Sleep-disordered breathing and its extreme form, obstructive sleep apnea (OSA), are the most common indications for adenotonsillectomy, followed by recurrent tonsillitis (Table 31.2).[90]

Sleep-Disordered Breathing (SDB)

A polysomnogram is the gold standard to diagnose sleep-disordered breathing and OSA, although there is a lack of consensus on the criteria and severity of disease in children to warrant surgery, which may explain the widespread variability in undertaking adenotonsillectomy for OSA. However, when polysomnography is not readily available, other metrics have been investigated to diagnose OSA. Questions around clinical characteristics of children with potential OSA that can be asked of parents are included in Table 31.3.

Overnight pulse oximetry (e.g., McGill oximetry score) has been used to assess severity but not to diagnose sleep-disordered breathing in children, particularly in resource-limited centers.[91–93] In an observational study of 162 children with polysomnogram-confirmed OSA, the Nonin 3150 WRISTOX$_2$ confirmed OSA

TABLE 31.2	Indications for Adenotonsillectomy

Indication

Obstruction

Nasal airway (adenoids)
Pharyngeal airway (tonsils)
Obstructive sleep-disordered breathing/sleep apnea
Failure to thrive with large tonsils
Cor pulmonale due to airway obstruction

Infection/Inflammation

Acute tonsillitis or adenoiditis
Recurrent tonsillitis or adenoiditis
Chronic tonsillitis or adenoiditis
Complicated tonsillitis (streptococcal complications)
Peritonsillar abscess
PFAPA (periodic fever, aphthous stomatitis, pharyngitis, adenitis)
PANDAS (pediatric autoimmune neuropsychiatric disorders associated with streptococcal infections)
Posttransplant lymphoproliferative disease
Halitosis
Tonsilloliths

Mass Lesion

Tonsillar/adenoidal (benign/malignant)
Unilateral tonsil hypertrophy (asymmetrical tonsils)

TABLE 31.3	Common Signs and Symptoms of Children with Obstructive Sleep Apnea

1. **Predisposing physical characteristics:**
   Body mass index greater than 95th percentile for age and sex
   Craniofacial abnormalities affecting the airway
   Anatomic nasal obstruction
   Tonsils nearly touching or touching in the midline
2. **History of apparent airway obstruction during sleep** *(two or more of the following)*:
   Loud snoring (loud enough to be heard through a closed door)
   Frequent snoring
   Observed pauses in breathing during sleep
   Frequent arousal from sleep
   Intermittent vocalization during sleep
   Parental report of restless sleep, difficulty breathing, or struggling respiratory efforts during sleep
   Child with night terrors
   Child sleeps in unusual positions
   New-onset nocturnal enuresis
3. **Somnolence (one or more of the following):**
   Parent or teacher comments that the child appears sleepy during the day, is easily distracted, is overly aggressive, or has difficulty concentrating
   Child often is difficult to arouse at the usual awakening time

Note: If signs and symptoms in at least two categories are present, there is a significant probability of moderate obstructive sleep apnea (OSA). If severe abnormalities are present, children should be treated as having severe OSA.
Modified from Gross JB, Bachenberg KL, Benumof JL, et al. Practice guidelines for the perioperative management of patients with obstructive sleep apnea: a report by the American Society of Anesthesiologists Task Force on Perioperative Management of patients with obstructive sleep apnea. *Anesthesiology.* 2006;104:1081-1093.

with a 92% positive predictive value and a 53% negative predictive value.[94] The indications for adenotonsillectomy, surgical approaches and techniques, screening for OSA, airway management, planning for postoperative disposition, and perioperative analgesic regimens, as well as posttonsillectomy bleeding and peritonsillar abscess management in this patient population provide a number of anesthetic challenges.[95,96]

Obstructive sleep-disordered breathing describes abnormal breathing patterns during sleep caused by increased upper airway resistance and pharyngeal collapse that leads to hypercarbia, transient oxygen desaturations, and microarousals. Phenotypically, this disordered breathing is characterized by snoring, paradoxical chest wall motion, and/or increased respiratory effort.[97] The spectrum in increasing order of severity ranges from (1) primary "benign" snoring (estimated prevalence 7.45%) occurring more than three nights per week, (2) upper airway resistance syndrome, clinically indistinguishable from the former and comprised of snoring, increased work of breathing, and frequent arousal episodes, (3) obstructive hypoventilation unique to children and characterized by snoring and increased end-expiratory carbon dioxide partial pressure during >25% of sleep time and no obstructive events, and (4) recurrent events of partial or complete upper airway obstruction (obstructive or mixed apneas or hypopneas) with oxygen desaturation, and disruption of ventilation and sleep patterns.[96,98]

An apnea is defined as a decrease in airflow of ≥90% with a duration that is at least the duration specified for the type of apnea: (1) obstructive apnea = two breaths, (2) central apnea = 20 seconds or greater for at least two breaths associated with arousal or ≥3% desaturation, (3) mixed apnea = if apnea criteria are met for at least two breaths during baseline breathing and associated with absent respiratory effort during one portion of the event.[96] A hypopnea event is defined as a decrease in airflow of ≥30% with a reduced respiratory effort for two or more breaths coupled with a ≥3% decrease in oxygen saturation or electroencephalographic evidence of an arousal. OSA also implies associated end-organ dysfunction including possible cardiopulmonary disease, metabolic perturbations, and neurocognitive and behavioral disorders. If left untreated, OSA can change the patient's health trajectory and cause premature death.[99]

Recurrent Tonsillitis

Recurrent acute tonsillitis refers to repeated episodes of streptococcal tonsillitis. Positive and negative group A, C, or G type of β-hemolytic streptococcus infections are distinguished by their associated morbidity. Associated group A β-hemolytic streptococcus infection accounts for approximately 5% of related medical consultations.[100]

The evidence to justify adenotonsillectomy in children with recurrent tonsillitis is modest at best. The current indication is based on an annual frequency of infections and includes one or more of the following: temperature >38.3°C, cervical lymphadenopathy, tonsillar exudate, and positive test for group A β-hemolytic streptococci.[100] Surgery is generally not indicated if there have been fewer than seven episodes of tonsillitis in the previous year, fewer than five episodes per year in the past 2 years, or fewer than three episodes per year in the past 3 years.[95,101,102]

SURGICAL APPROACH

Surgical techniques for adenotonsillectomy are generally divided into "cold" and "hot" techniques.[103] A "cold steel" technique uses sharp and blunt instruments to excise tissue followed by measures to control bleeding. A "hot" technique uses thermal instruments for incision, excision, and simultaneous control of bleeding using various technologies such as unipolar or bipolar electrocautery, bipolar radio frequency ablation (coblation), and laser. Overall, there is no evidence that one surgical technique is consistently superior to the others in terms of postoperative pain, bleeding, or

wound healing,[104,105] although one prospective study reported less pain and a smaller frequency of posttonsillectomy hemorrhage after intracapsular tonsillectomy using coblation compared with bipolar and cold steel approaches.[106] Tonsillotomy (intracapsular tonsillectomy, subtotal tonsillectomy) is becoming more common because postoperative pain, pharyngeal swelling, and the risk of bleeding is less than more invasive approaches[107,108]; long-term data are lacking.[109,110]

Adenoidectomy is often performed in conjunction with tonsillectomy, although it can be performed as a separate procedure. Indications for adenoidectomy alone include nasal obstruction with adenoid hypertrophy, chronic or recurrent adenoiditis, recurrent otitis media, and chronic sinusitis.[111] In children, adenoid enlargement may lead to nasal obstruction, mouth breathing, poor feeding resulting in failure to thrive, speech disorders, recurrent otitis media, and sleep-disordered breathing or OSA.

The surgical approach to tonsillectomy may result in variable pain responses. Extracapsular tonsillectomy (traditional tonsillectomy) consists of complete removal of the palatine tonsils and its surrounding capsule, whereas intracapsular tonsillectomy (tonsillotomy) involves debulking the tonsil preserving a thin layer of the capsule with a variable amount of tonsil tissue. This latter technique preserves the nerve supply and blood vessels to the region as well as potentially reducing postoperative pain, bleeding, and readmission rates and more rapid return to normal diet.[112,113] Despite its advantages, intracapsular tonsillectomy is performed in only a minority of surgeries in North America. A 2007 survey revealed that 73% of pediatric otolaryngologists routinely use extracapsular tonsillectomy for sleep-disordered breathing and 97% use it for recurrent tonsillitis.[112–114]

There are alternate surgical procedures that may be helpful in treating OSA in children not amenable to adenotonsillectomy including midfacial maxillary advancement, palatal expansion, inferior turbinate reduction, uvulopalatopharyngoplasty, supraglottoplasty, and tongue base procedures.[115,116] Tracheostomy is reserved for children with severe OSA who fail to respond to noninvasive ventilation or to other treatment approaches. Although most of these surgeries improve symptoms, they are not uniformly curative.[117]

OBSTRUCTIVE SLEEP APNEA

Incidence

Between 10 and 50 million children worldwide (prevalence 1%–5% and >50% in syndromic children) have OSA.[118–120] In children, OSA is associated with environmental stressors that include exposure to second-/third-hand smoke, early childhood respiratory infections, neighborhood disadvantage (e.g., lower socioeconomic status) and a positive history in first-degree relatives.[96,121–123] OSA is found equally in prepubertal boys and girls, although boys are at greater risk after puberty.[124] The prevalence of OSA is greatest in children 1 to 8 years of age, Black and Hispanic children,[125–127] in obese children (body mass index [BMI] >95th percentile), those with a history of prematurity, and syndromic (trisomy 21) children.[128–130] Children with OSA may present with body habitus: underweight, normal weight, or obese. The risk of obese children developing OSA is 2- to 5-fold greater than in nonobese children. Severe OSA is 12.5 times greater in African Americans than Caucasians, with the greatest incidence in children under 2 years of age.[130] The peak incidence of pediatric OSA (3–8 years of age) coincides with augmented adenotonsillar growth, which exceeds the increase in airway diameter.[129]

Children with OSA are frequent users of health care resources including excessive use of antibiotics for respiratory tract infections and asthma. They are reported to have an increased frequency of head injuries, early onset of atheromatous cardiovascular disease, a low quality of life, and possibly premature death.[99,131]

Mechanisms

The pharynx is a collapsible muscular tube contained within a rigid bony structure surrounded by tissue; the proximal and distal ends extend from the inferior nasal turbinates to the glottic opening (see Chapter 12). In children, the smaller diameter muscular tube affords greater muscle tone to prevent collapse, resulting in fewer obstructive apneas compared with adults.[132] Augmented adenotonsillar growth at 3 to 8 years of age exceeds the increase in airway diameter.[129] This leads to areas of narrowing in the upper airway, with the most severe narrowing found in the retropalatal region, reflecting an increase in adenotonsillar volume in children with OSA.[133] Increased proximal or distal airway resistance exacerbates the severity of the underlying OSA. The apnea hypopnea index (AHI), which is the number of apneas and hypopneas per hour, is a common metric to diagnose the severity of OSA.

Endotypes

Upper airway anatomical features in OSA include infant, child, and preteen/teen phenotypes, and their associated anatomical endotypes (Table 31.4). Adenotonsillar hyperplasia is the prototypical endotype responsible for increased upper airway resistance in children and is the result of an interaction between environmental stressors (e.g., passive smoking, a viral infection in the

airway) and an underlying genetic predisposition of the child. In addition, abnormal orofacial features from premature birth (<34 weeks) can also result in abnormal nasal airway resistance and associated oral facial hypotonia, mouth breathing, and changes in maxillary-mandibular growth, possibly as a consequence of prolonged invasive or noninvasive airway ventilation.[134,135] In infants, collapse of aryepiglottic folds into the glottic opening causes upper airway obstruction known as laryngomalacia. Whereas adenotonsillar hypertrophy contributes to prominent narrowing at the juncture of the nasal and oropharyngeal airway and contributes to a smaller retroglossal airway which is exacerbated by excessive soft tissue (e.g. obesity), a smaller boney enclosure of the airway (e.g. craniofacial syndromes); these factors create a relative tissue excess referred to as an anatomical soft tissue-bone imbalance.[136] Anatomic endotypes and airway phenotypes may underlie the pathogenesis of OSA including common medical conditions and syndromes listed in Table 31.4. Neuromuscular and genetic-syndrome–related OSA airway endotypes can span all ages (e.g., trisomy 21).[137]

Pathophysiology

The pathophysiology of OSA in children is characterized by a narrowed upper airway that is vulnerable to muscular collapse with negative inspiratory airway pressure during sleep. Upper airway neuromotor dysfunction is implied by the presence of residual airway obstruction after adenotonsillectomy and the absence of daytime obstructive symptoms.[137,138] It is unclear if neuromotor dysfunction is inherent or acquired due to recurrent nocturnal hypoxemia-related reactive oxygen species and/or inflammation altering neuromotor plasticity. Collapse of the pharyngeal airway has been attributed to relaxation of the genioglossus muscle and other pharyngeal dilator and tensor muscles. Two mechanisms may explain the airway collapse as described in Figs. 31.2 and 31.3.[136,139,140] Negative pressure generated by the diaphragm and intercostal muscles with inspiration against an obstruction, extralumen compression due to excessive fat and tissue deposition and/or a relatively small boney enclosure (e.g., small mandible) may each contribute to airway collapse.

Airway obstruction during induction of anesthesia in patients with moderate-to-severe OSA leads to diminished neural input to pharyngeal muscle tone with consequent greater collapse. This anesthetic-induced obstruction augments an underlying soft tissue-bone imbalance with further narrowing and obstruction of the pharyngeal airway; this collapse may in part be offset with positive end-expiratory pressure. In the absence of anesthesia medications the usual course of events would be reliant on a negative-pressure reflex, increased ventilatory drive from hypoxemia/hypercarbia, and finally, "airway self-rescue" through arousal to maintain airway patency.[139,141] The negative pressure and airway self-rescue reflexes are blunted in children with OSA, whereas in adults, the ventilatory drive is maintained (E-Table 31.1).[132] All anesthetic agents, with the possible exception of alpha-2 agonists and ketamine, which are considered "pharyngeal sparing", further compromise the interaction between anatomic and neuromotor mechanisms to maintain patency of the airway.[142] In addition, the decrease in lung volume during an inhalational anesthetic induction reduces thoracic tension on the upper airway structures, which, when combined with vigorous initial inspiratory efforts due to OSA-related ventilatory control instability (i.e., "high loop gain"), worsening negative upper airway pressure occurs and airway collapse is further exacerbated (see also Fig. 12.11). OSA is associated with neuromotor (e.g., cerebral palsy) and muscular

TABLE 31.4	Pediatric Obstructive Sleep Apnea Upper Airway Phenotypes by Age and Anatomical Endotypes		
	OSA AIRWAY PHENOTYPES		
OSA Anatomical Airway Endotypes	Infant (0–1 year)	Child (2–8 years)	Preteen/Teen (9–21 years)
Lymphoid hyperplasia (adenoids +/− tonsils)	+/−	++++	++
Soft tissue			
Obesity	+/−	++	+++
"Genetic" (e.g., mucopolysaccharidosis, Prader Willi)	++	+++	++
Craniofacial syndromes			
Vault and mandible (e.g., craniosynostosis, Pierre Robin)	+++	++	+/−
Foramen magnum (e.g., Arnold-Chiari, achondroplasia)	++	++	+/−
Neuromuscular (e.g., cerebral palsy and trisomy 21)	++	+++	+++
Prematurity (<32–34 weeks)	+++	++	−
Inflammatory (e.g., asthma, sickle cell disease)	+/−	+++	++

Modified from Murto KT, Zalan J, Vaccani JP. Paediatric adenotonsillectomy, part 1: surgical perspectives relevant to the anesthesiologist. *Br J Anaesth Educ.* 2020;20(6):184-192.[154]

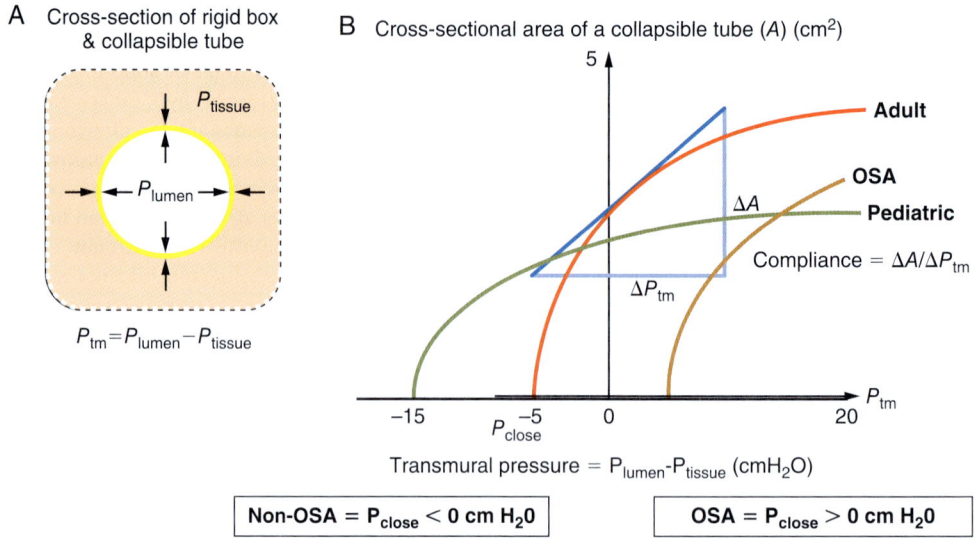

FIGURE 31.2 Pathophysiology of pediatric OSA. Airway collapse occurs via two mechanisms. **A,** Depicts a decreased pharyngeal transmural pressure (P_{tm}) due to negative pressure on inspiration (P_{lumen}) and/or extralumen positive pressure from tissue and/or bony encroachment (P_{tissue}); **B,** Depicts reduced longitudinal pharyngeal traction by the trachea due to gravity or small lung volumes. The critical "closing" pressure (P_{close}) is a measure of upper airway collapsibility in which airflow ceases and is greater (less negative) in people with OSA. (From Isono S. Physiology and dynamics of the pharyngeal airway. In: Kushida CA, ed. *Encyclopedia of Sleep*, vol. 1. Waltham, MA: Elsevier; 2013:533-44.)

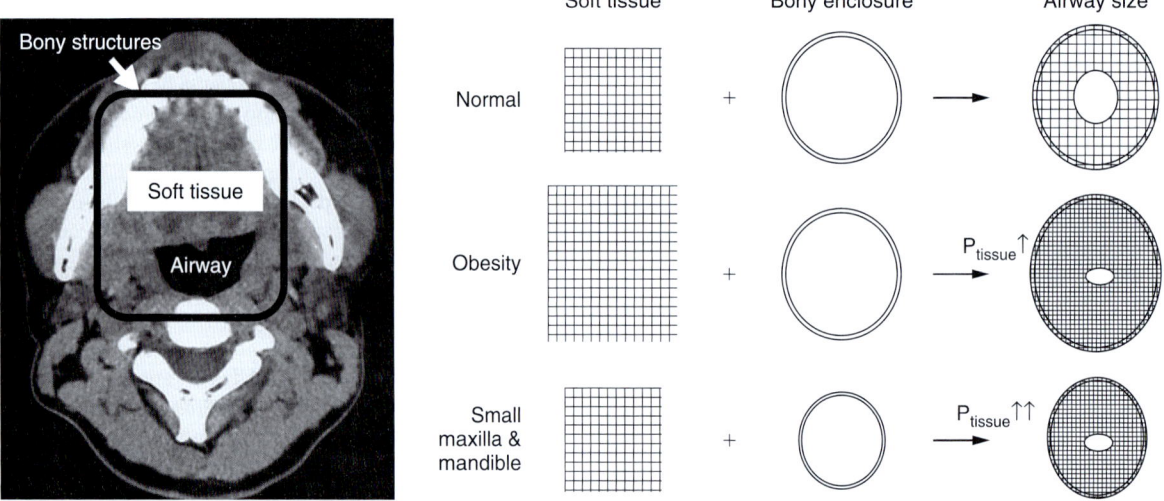

FIGURE 31.3 The left image represents the collapsible upper airway, a muscular tube, within a bony enclosure consisting of vertebral bodies, the mandible, and the maxilla. The image on the right represents the interaction between soft tissue and the upper airway bony enclosure and their combined effect on airway size. P_{tissue} is the pressure exerted by soft tissue on the collapsible airway and it is determined by the balance between the amount of soft tissue inside the bony enclosure and the size of the surrounding rigid box. Obesity and other medical diseases associated with excessive soft tissue (e.g., mucopolysaccharidosis) and/or a small bony enclosure led to a relative excess of soft tissue inside the rigid bony box leading to increased P_{tissue} and a predisposition to pharyngeal airway collapse. (Modified from Watanabe T, Isono S, Tanaka A, Tanzawa H, Nishino T. Contribution of body habitus and craniofacial characteristics to segmental closing pressures of the passive pharynx in patients with sleep-disordered breathing. *Am J Respir Crit Care Med.* 2002;165(2):260-265, modified with permission.)

disorders (e.g., Duchenne muscular dystrophy) that may further decrease pharyngeal tone. In addition to enhanced airway collapsibility, other neuromotor endotypes are also associated with OSA (see E-Table 31.1).[132,143,144]

The obstructive events that characterize OSA result in recurrent episodes of hypoxia, hypercarbia, and sleep disruption, a trilogy that has been linked to the development of multiple medical sequelae (Fig. 31.4). OSA has a spectrum of severity based on the frequency and severity of the obstructive respiratory events during sleep which occur most often during rapid eye movement (REM) sleep and are worse after midnight.[145–147]

Both obesity and OSA share similar inflammatory mechanisms, suggesting they may reciprocally contribute to their adverse consequences (Fig. 31.5).[148,149] Furthermore, obesity and

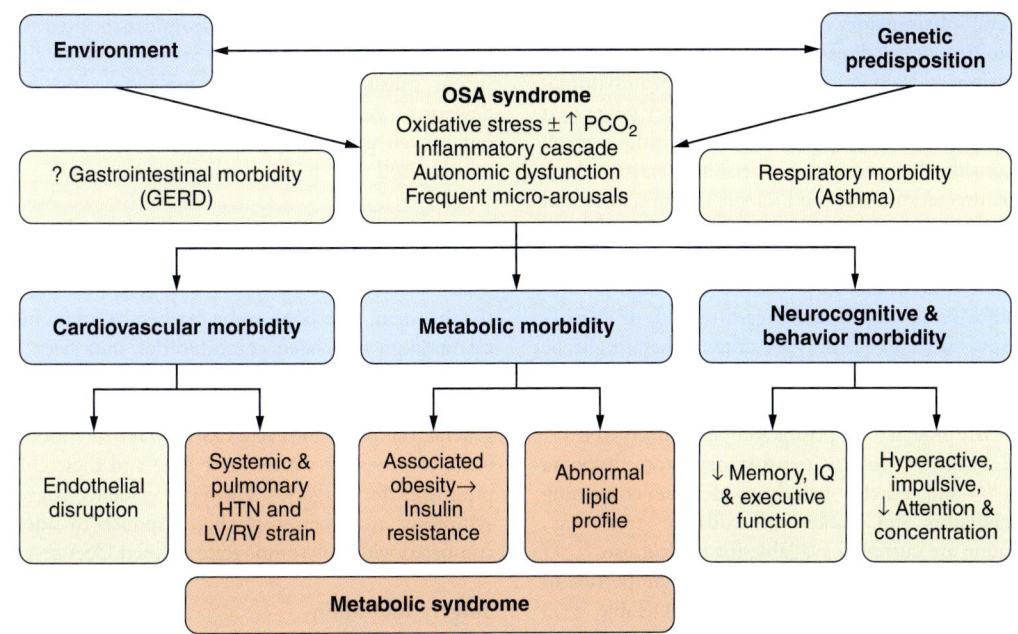

FIGURE 31.4 Pathophysiology of obstructive sleep apnea *(OSA)* syndrome and end-organ dysfunction. *GERD,* Gastroesophageal reflux; *HTN,* hypertension; *IQ,* intelligence quotient; *LV,* left ventricle; *RV,* right ventricle. Classifying tonsil size may be helpful in evaluating the degree of airway obstruction. (Adapted from Tan HL, Gozal D, Kheirandish-Gozal L. Obstructive sleep apnea in children: a critical update. *Nat Sci Sleep.* 2013;5:109-123.)

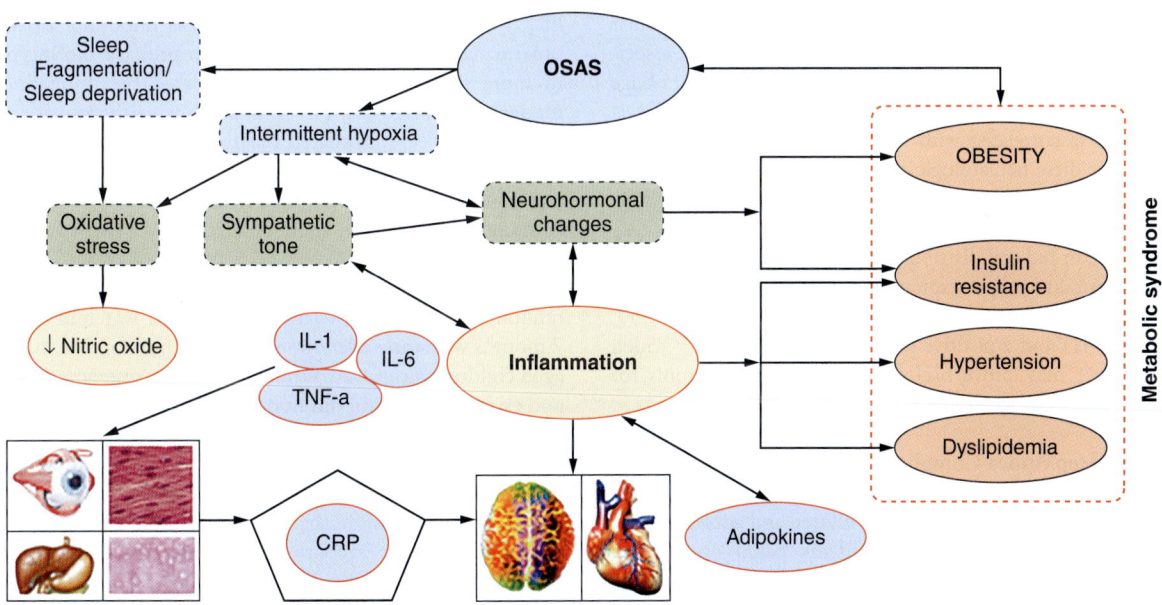

FIGURE 31.5 Schematic diagram outlining potential inflammatory pathways linking obesity and obstructive sleep apnea syndrome *(OSAS)* in children. *CRP,* C-reactive protein; *IL-I,* interleukin-1; *IL-6,* interleukin-6; *TNF-a,* tumor necrosis factor alpha. (Adapted from Gozal D, Kheirandish-Gozal L, Bhattacharjee R, Kim J. C-reactive protein and obstructive sleep apnea syndrome in children. *Front Biosci (Elite Ed).* 2012;4(7):2410-2422.)

OSA might also be linked via an imbalance between leptin and ghrelin, two hormones crucial in regulating satiety and hunger. OSA has been shown to be associated with leptin resistance and increased ghrelin levels that favor the development of obesity.[150]

There is considerable phenotypic variability of OSA on end-organ disease, possibly mediated by different compensatory mechanisms, genetic and environmental factors, and individual variability (E-Table 31.2).[98] Evidence of the phenotypic variability is apparent as the AHI does not correlate with neurocognitive or behavioral

dysfunction. In the genetically predisposed child, the oxidative stress from recurrent hypoxemia increases the concentrations of endorphins and reactive oxygen species. This upregulates brainstem mu-opioid receptors and causes systemic inflammation-prone epigenetic alterations that lead to variably increased sensitivity to the respiratory effects of opioids, reduced perception of pain, and decreased opioid requirements after adenotonsillectomy in groups with a greater prevalence of OSA (e.g., those of African-American descent).

There are several inflammatory cascades that are central to the initiation and progression of disease morbidity related to OSA, including local airway and systemic proliferation of proinflammatory cytokines and DNA methylation of inflammatory genes that impact systemic inflammatory expression.[151,152] Within a given level of OSA, considerable phenotypic variability exists, which suggests complex interactions between biologic inflammatory and oxidative stress pathways activated by environmental factors (e.g., diet, physical activity, pollution) in genetically susceptible populations.[153–156] To that end, studies have focused on potential biomarkers from saliva, serum, urine, and breath-related, to identify preclinical, noninvasive, and phenotypic criteria that might be used to predict treatment success and resolution of symptoms.[157–160] Biomarkers under investigation include: tumor necrosis factor,[161] interleukins, C-reactive protein,[148,162] plasma adropin,[163] microRNA,[164] salivary cortisol levels,[165] urinary neurotransmitters, hypoxia inducible factor,[166] and exhaled breath condensate containing inflammatory mediators and markers of oxidative stress (e.g., 8-isoprostane); none are currently available for clinical use.[167–169] A number of urinary proteins showed promising properties to noninvasively identify children with OSA.[170,171] E-Table 31.3 provides a summary of the various approaches to the preoperative assessment of OSA in the child scheduled for adenotonsillectomy. Another biomarker is red cell distribution width (RDW), a measure of heterogeneity of red cell size, which is considered a biomarker for OSA severity in adults; an increase is thought to be secondary to increased oxidative stress, red cell turnover, and inflammation. Both red cell distribution width (RDW >13.1%) and mean corpuscular hemoglobin concentration (MCHC >34.9 grams/dL) were associated with moderate-to-severe OSA in children, independent of age and BMI.[172] Furthermore, an oxygen-desaturation index (ODI) >3% and >4% correlated with red cell distribution width. The mechanism for these hematologic changes may be explained by repeated hypoxic events that upregulate erythropoietin or other hormones that respond to chronic hypoxia.

An increase in red cell distribution width >14.7% in children predicted minor and major respiratory complications after adenotonsillectomy with an odds ratio (OR) of 7.8 (95% CI, 4.30, 13.28; $P<0.001$) and a positive predictive value of 91.2.[173] Such indices as these may prove useful as future screening tools for moderate-severe OSA in children.

Obstructive Sleep Apnea Complications

The American Heart Association has formally recognized the risk of OSA on the cardiovascular health of children and adolescents.[174] A classification of congenital heart disease based on residual disease burden and functional status is found in E-Table 31.4. Cardiovascular, metabolic sequelae, behavior disorders, impaired neurocognition, and end-organ dysfunction in children with OSA are illustrated in Fig. 31.4.[98,148,149,157,175–202]

With adenotonsillar hyperplasia, some children develop swallowing disorders, speech abnormalities, (i.e., oral-motor dysfunction) and gastroesophageal reflux disease (GERD), particularly younger children, that may contribute to upper airway inflammation.[203–205] Adenotonsillar hypertrophy may result from recurrent infections in the upper airway that are manifest by periodic fever, aphthous stomatitis, pharyngitis, or adenitis. Recurrent streptococcal bacteremia secondary to infected tonsils increases the risk of endocarditis.

While polysomnography-confirmed OSA resolves spontaneously within 7 months in children with mild-to-moderate disease, this is less likely to occur in children with moderate-to-severe disease and those with syndromic-associated OSA.[206] Factors associated with persistent or worsening OSA include obesity, persistent tonsillar hypertrophy, male sex, and African-American descent.[207] Acute tonsillitis/tonsillitis-pharyngitis (with or without proven group A β-hemolytic streptococcus) is usually self-limiting and only requires symptom support.

Treatment Thresholds

Approximately two-thirds of pediatric adenotonsillectomy patients have OSA as their indication for surgery.[88,90,208–211] A consensus on the treatment thresholds to be reached based on history and physical findings, associated comorbidities, and sleep laboratory measurements, however, is lacking and the surgical "window of opportunity" to halt or reverse end-organ dysfunction remains unclear. In general, moderate-to-severe OSA (AHI >5 episodes/hour) is more likely to persist or worsen over time and these children should be prioritized for surgery.[95] However, evidence suggests that patient symptoms may better predict response to adenotonsillectomy compared with polysomnogram defined OSA severity.[191,192,212,213]

Surgery Indication

In general, the decision to remove the tonsils and subject the child to a potentially risky and painful airway procedure must be undertaken with care.[100] In appropriately selected children, tonsillectomy can decrease upper airway resistance, improve or resolve the OSA and sleep-disordered breathing, decrease the incidence of recurrent tonsillitis, and improve the child's health and quality of life.[206] Identification of these children is important because approximately one-third of children with primary snoring progress to more severe forms of sleep-disordered breathing, including moderate-to-severe OSA[137,177] and many with primary snoring (mild or no sleep-disordered breathing) show impaired behavior (e.g., hyperactivity), physical symptoms (e.g., difficulty swallowing food), mild neurocognitive defects, and reduced quality of life. Although controversial, these children may benefit from adenotonsillectomy.[201,202]

The Childhood Adenotonsillectomy Trial (CHAT) was a randomized controlled trial that compared watchful waiting for 7 months with early adenotonsillectomy in more than 400 school-aged children with OSA. While the primary outcome of attention and executive function did not differ between the two groups, the secondary outcomes for polysomnographic, behavioral, and quality-of-life metrics normalized in 79% of the children after adenotonsillectomy compared with 46% in the watchful-waiting group.[87,207] Follow-up studies more than 6 months after adenotonsillectomy in children with OSA reported that symptoms completely resolved in those with mild OSA (AHI <10) but are persistent in up to 35% of those with severe OSA (AHI >20).[214–216] Comorbid conditions that improve with adenotonsillectomy include quality of life, uncontrolled asthma, poor school performance, behavioral problems, metabolic syndrome, oral-motor dysfunction (e.g., articulation), and recurrent otitis media among others.[95,217] Central sleep apnea also improves after adenotonsillectomy.[218,219] Excessive weight gain is not associated with adenotonsillectomy for OSA.[220]

In North America, undertaking adenotonsillectomy to treat sleep-disordered breathing is largely driven by its potential to improve behavior, cognition, and quality of life, independent of the underlying OSA.[116,221,222] A Cochrane review concluded that there is moderate evidence that adenotonsillectomy in nonsyndromic children 5 to 9 years of age with mild-to-moderate OSA have improved quality of life, symptoms, and behavior, and high quality evidence that the polysomnogram improves compared with no surgery.[206] The results of an ongoing trial (Pediatric Adenotonsillectomy Trial for Snoring [PATS]) will prospectively examine the benefits of adenotonsillectomy versus watchful waiting.[223]

PREOPERATIVE EVALUATION OF THE CHILD WITH OSA

The preoperative evaluation of the child for adenotonsillectomy must distinguish the child with OSA from the child with primary snoring or chronic infectious tonsillitis. Obstructive sleep-disordered breathing is an independent risk factor for a 2-fold increased risk of severe critical respiratory events[211]; children with OSA are five times more likely to develop severe perioperative respiratory adverse events (PRAE)[224] including apnea, hypoxemia, laryngospasm, bronchospasm, airway obstruction, and rarely, the need for reintubation.[9,224–231] Deaths after adenotonsillectomy from presumed sleep apnea have occurred in the PACU, on the ward, and at home or in an automobile after discharge from a monitored setting,[127,232] likely related to associated OSA and use of opioids.[127,233]

Identification of At-Risk Children

Identification of children at risk for OSA is based on history, physical, and laboratory assessments; history alone has only a 65% positive predictive value.[96] The initial assessment of children with sleep-disordered breathing is a medical history and physical examination (see Table 31.3 and E-Table 31.3). Although clinical features obtained from demography, parental report, and physical findings do not differentiate primary habitual snoring (with a prevalence of ~10% in children) from snoring associated with OSA or its severity,[234–241] parents should be asked about nocturnal and daytime symptoms and associated OSA risk factors. Parents should be questioned whether their child snores loudly (and can be heard through a closed door), snores more than three nights per week, if there are observed gasps or pauses in respirations, and if the child's breathing at night is of serious concern to the parent/caregiver.[242–246] New onset of OSA-associated nocturnal enuresis may be secondary to blunted arousal reflexes or related to increased brain natriuretic peptide levels.[247–250]

Daytime symptoms of OSA include attention-deficit disorder-like behavior or poor school performance, whereas daytime somnolence is more commonly associated with obesity complicating OSA and severe disease (see Table 31.3).[243,251] The prevalence of OSA is increased in infants who have suffered an acute life-threatening event (sudden infant death syndrome); they also have a greater incidence of OSA in childhood and adolescence.[229–231] Prematurity (born <34 weeks), failure to thrive, GERD, asthma, a family history of OSA, and exposure to passive smoking are also factors that portend OSA.[242] As the number of these risk factors increases, so does the risk that OSA will develop.

A home audiovisual recording during sleep may provide additional nocturnal history, but it may miss late night airway obstruction during rapid eye movement (REM) sleep. Smartphone audiovisual applications to screen for OSA are being developed.[252–254]

Questionnaires

In contrast to the Snoring, Tired, Observed, Pressure, Body mass index, Age, Neck size, Gender (STOP-BANG) questionnaire for OSA in adults,[255] the questionnaires developed to diagnose OSA in children lack diagnostic accuracy, a reliable positive predictable value, and have insufficient validation to justify their widespread adoption to diagnose OSA in at-risk children.[227,228,246,256–261] The

STOP-BANG questionnaire in adults performed as well as the GOAL (Gender, Obesity, Age, and Loud snoring) and NoSAS (Neck circumference, obesity, Snoring, Age, and Sex) questionnaires as screening tools with any level of OSA, and all performed better than the ESS (Epworth Sleepiness Scale).[262–264] In one study in adolescents (10–18 years of age), a STOP-BANG score of <3 indicated a small risk for OSA, whereas a score >4 indicated a greater risk for OSA.[257] Furthermore, omitting neck circumference in a STOP-BAG score yielded similar predictive values in adolescents.

Abbreviated OSA questionnaires for children have been developed to assess snoring, sleepiness, and inattention/hyperactive behavior, and are typically derived from the 22-item Pediatric Sleep Questionnaire-Sleep-related Breathing Disorder subscale (PSQ-SRBD), which encompasses three domains: snoring, sleepiness with OSA-related symptoms, and inattentive/hyperactive behavior, that has an overall sensitivity and specificity of 0.85.[265] The PSQ-SRBD predicts moderate-to-severe OSA in children[266]; however, in children with craniofacial anomalies, the correlation between PSQ-SRBD score and AHI severity was less sensitive for those with syndrome or chromosomal anomalies.[267] In terms of predicting OSA in children, the sleep-related breathing disorder (SRBD) scale is the most validated of the screening tools with a sensitivity and specificity of 78% and 72%, respectively.[265] This scale is reliable, inexpensive, easily administered/scored in a preoperative setting, and can predict posttonsillectomy outcomes, including resolution of neurobehavioral outcomes and the risk of residual OSA.[268] Both the PSQ-SRBD and the more involved sleep clinical record (SCR) have been recommended for use by the European Respiratory Society Task Force.

The ASA 2006 OSA questionnaire correlated poorly with a severe OSA diagnosis,[269] compared with polysomnogram, and the associated risk score did not predict respiratory complications in children after tonsillectomy[270]; the ASA 2014 questionnaire has not been evaluated in children.[246] Other scales that remain research tools are the "I'M SLEEPY" brief questionnaire[260] and a daytime sleepiness and hyperactivity questionnaire.[271] The OSA-18 questionnaire, which was originally developed to assess quality of life, has been repurposed to screen for the severity of OSA in children.[272] Despite attempts to focus the factors in the most meaningful domains, this questionnaire did not reliably predict the severity of OSA. Subsequently, an abbreviated version of the OSA-18 questionnaire narrowed to five questions (OSA-5 questionnaire) to screen for those at risk for OSA: snoring, breath holding, choking, mouth breathing, and parental concern.[273] This brief questionnaire yielded a sensitivity for OSA of 82% and a negative predictive value of 81% for moderate/severe OSA. To further simplify the questionnaire, a revision that required only dichotomous responses (yes or no) to "selected features" from previous questionnaires included four questions: (1) During the past month has your child breath held or paused in breathing at night? (2) Does your child breathe through the mouth in the daytime? (3) Has your child's growth rate since birth stopped? (4) Is your child overweight? This questionnaire eliminated redundancy and yielded slightly greater accuracy than PSQ-SRBD for AHI >10 (0.73 vs. 0.65, P=0.04).[274] The external validity of this questionnaire remains to be established.

To assess whether a questionnaire can predict if adenotonsillectomy will improve the quality of life of a child with sleep-disordered breathing, the OSA-18 and PSQ questionnaires were prospectively compared.[275] The OSA-18 was a better predictor of improved quality of life than the PSQ. A systematic review and meta-analysis of questionnaires to diagnose OSA in children with AHI >1 also focused on the PSQ-SRBD and the OSA-18.[276] The PSQ-SRBD more accurately diagnosed OSA in children at an AHI >1 than the OSA-18, but the evidence was insufficient to supplant the polysomnogram as the gold standard.

Physical Assessment

The physical assessment of the child includes determining evidence for age and sex adjusted hypertension. One may appreciate swollen nasal mucosa or "adenoidal facies". Hyponasal speech and nasal congestion may be evident.[277] Although tonsillar hypertrophy may be present in the absence of OSA, the combined adenotonsillar volume correlates with the severity of OSA.[133] However, upper airway obstruction can occur even in the absence of adenotonsillar hypertrophy including obesity, craniofacial disorders, laryngomalacia, and neuromuscular disorders.[278] It is unclear if anthropomorphic measures (e.g., neck circumference) improve the diagnostic performance of OSA questionnaires, but they indicate increased risk of OSA in older children and adolescents.[235,243,279] Both flexible nasal endoscopy and a lateral-view x-ray can be used to assess adenoid size, but they depend on the patient's cooperation and/or specialist expertise. Low radiation 3-D cone beam computed tomography can identify smaller airway volume and cross-sectional area in children with moderate-severe OSA.[280]

The Polysomnogram

The polysomnogram is the gold standard diagnostic test for evaluation of OSA, which in children should ideally be carried out in dedicated pediatric centers. An attended polysomnogram provides an audiovisual record of the patient and simultaneously records the electroencephalogram (EEG), electrocardiogram (ECG), bilateral electrooculogram (EOG), electromyogram (EMG), and pulse oximetry and other various measures of ventilation (e.g., oronasal airflow and end-tidal carbon dioxide) (E-Fig. 31.2).

The AHI component is used to quantify the severity of sleep-disordered breathing. It is comprised of the number of mixed, obstructive, and central apneas and hypopneas per hour of sleep and is equivalent to the respiratory disturbance index (RDI). Normal infants and children may have a considerable number of short central pauses in respirations not associated with desaturation or arousal[281] and their number is inversely proportional to postmenstrual age.[96] In children younger than 18 years of age, OSA is defined using the number of mixed and obstructive apneas and hypopneas per hour of sleep, but excludes central apnea. Most sleep centers consider a normal obstructive AHI ≤1 event per hour total sleep time, mild OSA obstructive AHI >1 to 5 events per hour, moderate OSA obstructive AHI 6 to 10 events per hour, and severe OSA obstructive AHI >10 events per hour of sleep. A central AHI of ≥5 events per hour is considered pathological central sleep apnea.[282] Children with trisomy 21 exhibit more frequent episodes of central apnea that can markedly increase the AHI and RDI, but not the obstructive AHI. The polysomnogram also records oxygen-desaturation indexes; an oxygen-saturation nadir <92% is considered abnormal.[283]

Although a polysomnogram provides a detailed evaluation of both sleep quality (the amount and distribution of the various sleep stages, sleep disturbance, arousal, and awakening) and sleep-related breathing events (quantification of abnormal respiratory and gas-exchange events against time spent asleep),[234] the procedure is costly and access is limited, with only ~13% of North American children undergoing a polysomnogram before adenotonsillectomy.[209,284]

Current surgical guidelines recommend that symptomatic children younger than 2 years of age, those with complex high-risk medical conditions (e.g., neuromuscular disorders) who are at greater risk for general anesthesia, children in whom the indication for tonsillectomy is uncertain, or children where there is discordance between the physical examination and reported severity of symptoms should undergo a polysomnogram.[95,96,212,285] Some sleep specialists score children who are 13 years of age or older for OSA risk using adult criteria. As a result, a survey of the American Society of Pediatric Otolaryngology reported that the polysomnogram was underused in children with sleep-disordered breathing, obesity, younger than 2 years of age, and trisomy 21 before adenotonsillectomy, with only 29% to 55% of these children completing a preoperative polysomnogram (E-Fig. 31.3).[286] Ultimately, the final diagnosis of the severity of OSA is determined by a sleep medicine specialist and is based on a constellation of patient symptoms, associated comorbidities including evidence for end-organ disease, and polysomnogram parameters that include measures of gas exchange.

Overnight Pulse Oximetry

Home respiratory polygraphy studies (polysomnograms without EEG, EMG, and electrooculogram studies), represent an alternative to a complete polysomnogram and are being used with increased frequency due to the ease of set-up, scoring, and cost.[287,288] Some centers have reported good agreement with in-lab polysomnograms; however the AHI may be underestimated due to missed hypopnea resulting in arousal but not desaturation.[289,290] Oximetry-based pulse-transit-time has been associated with subcortical arousal and may help to minimize AHI underestimation in home respiratory polygraphy.[291,292] Overnight oximetry is equivalent to home respiratory polygraphy in unattended settings for children with a high pretest probability,[293] and both compare favorably with a formal polysomnogram.

Metrics obtained from overnight pulse oximetry may be used to estimate the severity of OSA, although they fall short of being diagnostic for OSA.[91,92,294–296] A low intercluster SpO_2 is reported in children with diseases of the lower airways, such as bronchiolitis, and abnormalities of ventilatory control.[297–299] Examples of oximetry metrics used to diagnose OSA include the McGill oximetry score, oxygen-desaturation nadir (nSAT; the minimum SpO_2 recorded during sleep), (ODI; specifically the number of decreases in $SpO_2 \geq 3\%$ [ODI_3] or 4% from baseline [ODI_4]) and proportion of total sleep time spent with $SpO_2 < 90\%$, which all attempt to quantify the cumulative nocturnal hypoxemic burden. The McGill oximetry score system (Fig. 31.6) further classifies the severity of nocturnal hypoxemia;[300] the severity of the desaturation nadir determines the score. McGill oximetry scores of 2, 3, and 4 correspond to oxygen-desaturation nadirs less than 90%, 85%, and 80%, respectively.[91] However, it may miss obstructive events without desaturation or capture desaturations related to central apnea reflected by a relatively low sensitivity of 43%.[96,301] In resource-limited settings or in uncooperative children, nocturnal oximetry may be the preferred first test as it is readily available, cheap, and easily performed at home,[302] although monitoring for only one night may be insufficient in some children.[303]

The nadir saturation (nSAT), which is the lowest SpO_2 recorded during sleep, correlates inversely with the AHI.[304] An nSAT of 92% is the minimum normal SpO_2 in children.[295,305–307] In children, the ODI_3 (oxygen desaturation ≥3%) measured using unattended home oximetry offers future possibilities to

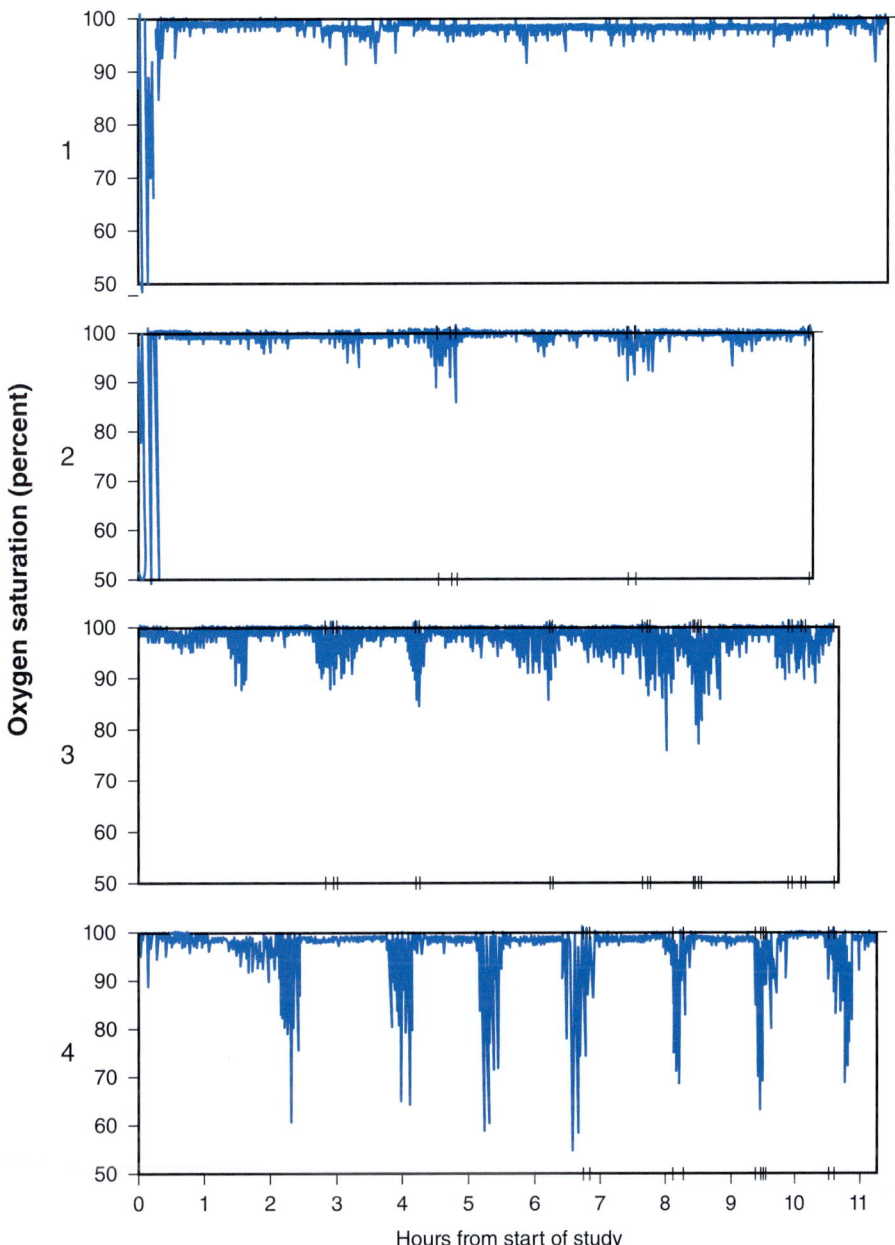

FIGURE 31.6 Representative figures for McGill oximetry scores 1 to 4. McGill oximetry scores 2 to 4 are abnormal in that they all show at least three clusters of desaturation. The severity of the SpO_2 nadir determines the score such that McGill oximetry scores 2, 3, and 4 correspond to SpO_2 nadirs of less than 90%, less than 85%, and less than 80%, respectively. (From Nixon GM, Kermack AS, Davis GM, et al. Planning adenotonsillectomy in children with obstructive sleep apnea: the role of overnight oximetry. *Pediatrics.* 2004;113[1 Pt 1]:e19-e25.)

reliably differentiate children with and without OSA.[293] The 95th percentile for the ODI_4 (oxygen desaturation $\geq$4%) is 2.2 episodes per hour,[295] which correlates closely (r=0.94) with the AHI,[94,308] although there is currently no consensus on the cutoff value of ODI_4 in pediatric OSA.[234] The ODI has been incorporated into an algorithm to treat obstructive sleep-disordered breathing in that an ODI_3 >3.5 episodes per hour and/or ODI_4 >1.5 episodes per hour predicts improvement in nocturnal desaturations after adenotonsillectomy in more than 95% of children.[137,309] Data from children that evaluated the relationship between the proportion of time spent with oxygen saturation less than 90% and the AHI are limited, but preliminary evidence indicates that

it correlates (r=0.85; *P*<0.001) with the McGill oximetry score in medically complex patients.[300] Overall, the combination of the McGill oximetry score and the nSAT and ODI may represent a simple yet pragmatic composite metric to objectively screen for OSA in children.[234,310]

An ODI greater than 3% from baseline for at least 10 seconds (ODI_3) independently predicted more than 29 postadenotonsillectomy respiratory events,[311] and an index of more than 15 predicted events in children with severe OSA.[312] In the absence of opioids during adenotonsillectomy for sleep-disordered breathing, ODI_4 more than eight episodes per hour predict respiratory complications (OR=1.07).[313] Mild hypercarbia in the polysomnogram[312,314–322] did not predict adverse respiratory events, unplanned admission, or increased length of stay after adenotonsillectomy as well as peak $ETCO_2$ >60 mm Hg or $ETCO_2$ >50 mm Hg for ≥25% total sleep time.[315]

Drug-Induced Sleep Endoscopy

Drug-induced sleep endoscopy is a diagnostic tool to characterize the severity and location of upper airway obstruction in children who snore and have OSA under conditions similar to that which occurs during natural sleep. The results help determine the correct surgical procedure needed to mitigate the OSA. Several consensus statements describe the indications for and the optimal anesthetic techniques that yield the greatest diagnostic value.[323,324] Although adenotonsillar hypertrophy is the primary cause of OSA in children, those with comorbidities such as obesity, trisomy 21, and craniofacial abnormalities may experience airway obstruction at multiple levels within the upper airway (e.g., tongue base or aryepiglottic folds) unrelated to the tonsils and adenoids.[325] Diagnostic anatomical evaluation of airways using drug-induced sleep endoscopy or cine MRI is indicated for: (1) persistent OSA after adenotonsillectomy or presurgery with small-sized adenoids and tonsils; (2) a discrepancy between clinical findings and OSA severity; (3) suspicion of multilevel airway obstruction (e.g., trisomy 21 or craniofacial syndromes); (4) inability to tolerate noninvasive positive airway therapy; (5) treatment planning before airway surgery or initiation of appliances.[117,325–329]

During drug-induced sleep endoscopy, the airway is directly visualized for obstruction during spontaneous breathing. Anesthetic induction usually begins with an inhaled agent to establish IV access. It is then converted to a TIVA technique while maintaining spontaneous ventilation and stable vital signs.[142] The two

most commonly used anesthetics preferred by otolaryngologists are dexmedetomidine (50%) and propofol (58%), the former providing greater respiratory stability and the latter providing more reliable sedation.[324] Propofol decreases the anteroposterior airway diameter as the dose increases but has a rapid onset and offset of action.[330] In contrast, dexmedetomidine minimally alters the dimensions of the upper airway and does not depress respirations,[27] but has a slower onset of action and more prolonged recovery.[142] It is unknown to what degree if any, dexmedetomidine mimics REM sleep, when obstructive events are most likely to occur.[142,146] Oxygen desaturations to <85% during drug-induced sleep endoscopy with dexmedetomidine and ketamine are less than with either propofol alone or a combination of propofol and sevoflurane.[331]

The endoscopy is performed with the smallest flexible scope possible to avoid distorting the airway. Topical administration of lidocaine and oxymetazoline to the nasal mucosa may be useful to ensure smooth passage of the scope into the hypopharynx. Endoscopy may commence once a good view is obtained and either airway turbulence is palpated or snoring is heard.

INDICATIONS FOR ADENOTONSILLECTOMY

The indications for adenotonsillectomy should be clearly delineated in the surgical care plan including a diagnosis of OSA or the results of laboratory tests distinguishing between viral and bacterial infection, in the case of recurrent tonsillitis.[100] Beyond a complete history, review of comorbidities, a physical examination, and a focused airway examination (Fig. 31.7) is required.[332] Additional preoperative investigations are unnecessary before adenotonsillectomy in healthy children. Concurrent medical treatment (e.g., airway devices, nasal antiinflammatory agents) for OSA,

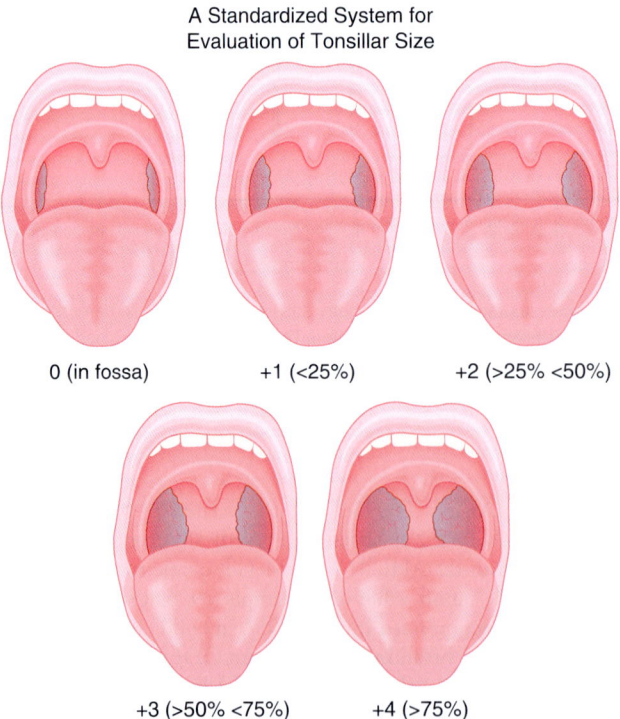

A Standardized System for Evaluation of Tonsillar Size

0 (in fossa)   +1 (<25%)   +2 (>25% <50%)

+3 (>50% <75%)   +4 (>75%)

FIGURE 31.7 Classifying tonsil size may be helpful in evaluating the degree of airway obstruction. Children classified as +3 or greater (i.e., having more than 50% of the pharyngeal area occupied by hypertrophied tonsils) are at an increased risk of developing airway obstruction during anesthetic induction. (Modified from Brodsky L. Modern assessment of tonsils and adenoids. *Pediatr Clin North Am.* 1989;36[5]:1551-1569; illustration by Jon S. Krasner.)

summarized elsewhere, should be reviewed prior to adenotonsillectomy.[117] URIs are frequent in these children and can interfere with the timing of adenotonsillectomy and increase the risk of respiratory compromise and hemorrhage.[333-336] Asthma is commonly associated with obstructive sleep-disordered breathing, and OSA is an independent risk factor for in-hospital asthma exacerbation severity[337]; however, routine chest x-rays and pulmonary function tests are generally not indicated.[338]

Coagulation studies are not warranted for adenotonsillectomy although a history of bleeding warrants investigation.[339,340] A history of medications that interfere with coagulation should be sought, including aspirin, NSAIDs, valproic acid, and nutraceuticals, particularly garlic, ginkgo, ginseng, green tea, saw palmetto, St John's wort, and fish oil.[341,342] Preoperative discontinuation of some medications is sometimes problematic, and a preoperative consultation may be indicated.

Tests in adolescents with obesity, for insulin resistance, abnormal liver structure and function, and evidence of dyslipidemia are recommended to exclude a metabolic syndrome. Although routine preoperative echocardiography is not necessary in the child with obesity due to low yield for positive findings,[343] it is recommended in patients with signs of right ventricular dysfunction, systemic hypertension, or severe desaturation (hemoglobin oxygen saturation $[SaO_2] < 70\%$) during a polysomnogram.

Full cardiac evaluations are only warranted in children at greater risk for secondary cardiopulmonary complications including those with Prader Willi, the mucopolysaccharidoses syndromes, and trisomy 21.[143,314] A preoperative electrocardiogram or echocardiogram may show evidence of right or left ventricular hypertrophy, diastolic dysfunction, and/or pulmonary hypertension.[179,184] A blood gas may reveal an increased concentration of bicarbonate or evidence for polycythemia, consistent with a chronic respiratory acidosis or recurrent nocturnal hypoxemia.[344]

RISK STRATIFICATION FOR PERIOPERATIVE ADVERSE EVENTS AND DISPOSITION PLANNING

Children undergoing adenotonsillectomy, particularly those who have OSA with extreme obesity, are at increased risk for perioperative complications that can result in anoxic neurologic injury associated with a difficult airway, pulmonary aspiration of gastric contents including blood, and apnea that is not associated with opioid sensitivity. These events may occur in the operating room, PACU, in hospital, during transport home, and at home.[127,232,233] This may be explained in part by evidence for worsening airway obstruction on the first night of surgery (E-Fig. 31.4), OSA being associated with a heightened analgesic and respiratory sensitivity to opioids, and in some patients, an increased pain experience.[345] Most studies that evaluated perioperative respiratory events during adenotonsillectomy were observational, small in size, and heterogeneous. Although pediatric otolaryngologic surgery is an independent risk factor for major respiratory events,[211,346] North American surgical databases surprisingly do not consider adenotonsillectomy a high-risk surgical procedure.[347,348] Given the complexity of risk factors influencing postoperative disposition planning (including intra- and postoperative course), site-specific information should be taken into consideration in the final decision-making process.[349]

Clinical factors such as age younger than 3 years, ASA physical status >I, an associated syndrome, morbid obesity (BMI>99th percentile for age and sex) and a preexisting pulmonary disease are independent risk factors for developing critical perioperative respiratory events after adenotonsillectomy, with the latter two factors having an odds ratio (OR)>2.5.[350] The 'Kids Inpatient Database', a retrospective review of adverse events associated with adenotonsillectomy, demonstrated that complications were more common in obese than in nonobese children, males, those with concomitant asthma, and those of low socioeconomic status, independent of race or insurance status.[351] The risk of respiratory complications after adenotonsillectomy overall is small, but the underlying etiology is usually multifactorial, influenced by demographic, clinical factors, surgical/provider factors, medications, polysomnogram parameters, and other laboratory results. Although severe OSA may be associated with perioperative respiratory events, OSA does not influence the risk of major respiratory complications such as laryngospasm, pulmonary edema, pneumonia, or the need for postoperative reintubation.[352] Factors associated with adverse respiratory events after adenotonsillectomy in children are summarized in Table 31.5.[353]

TABLE 31.5	Summary of Preoperative Factors Associated with Perioperative Adverse Respiratory Events and Adenotonsillectomy in Children
Factors Related to History/Physical Exam Ination	**Factors Related to Tools or Laboratory Investigations**
Demographic Factors: Age <3 years, prematurity (<34 weeks GA), male sex, African descent, low socioeconomic status; ASA PS classification ≥II; "comorbidities"	**Prediction Tools:** STBUR Questionnaire; COLDS inventory; ambulatory perioperative respiratory adverse events tool
Clinical Factors: Craniofacial disorders including foramen magnum stenosis and mucopolysaccharidosis Seizures Asthma, upper airway infections and airway hyperresponsiveness; Congenital heart disease and pulmonary hypertension Obesity Failure to thrive Gastroesophageal reflux disease Neuromuscular disease including trisomy 21, cerebral palsy, and muscular dystrophy Sickle cell disease Adenoid size	**OSA Metrics and Nocturnal Sleep Investigations:** Polysomnography oAHI >10 AHI>20–24 Oxygen-saturation nadir (nSAT) <80% 25% TST $ETCO_2$>50 mm Hg or peak $ETCO_2$>60 mm Hg 4% TST SpO_2<90% Nocturnal Oximetry: McGill Oximetry Score (MOS) 2–4 ODI_3>29 (>15 with severe OSA) and ODI_4>8
Medications: Benzodiazepines, opioids, and bronchodilator/antireflux medication	**Lab:** Red cell distribution width >14.6%
Surgical/Provider Factors: Surgical timing later in day; surgical indication for obstructive SDB/OSA; anesthesia provider experience	**Experimental:** Genetic variants of OCT1 and ABCC3

ABCC3, ATP-binding cassette subfamily C member 3; *AHI*, apnea hypopnea index; *ASA PS*, American Society of Anesthesiologists' physical classification; *oAHI*, obstructive apnea hypopnea index; *OCT1*, Organic Cation Transporter 1; *ODI*, oxygen-desaturation index; *OSA*, obstructive sleep apnea; *oSDB*, obstructive sleep-disordered breathing; *GA*, gestational age; *RDW*, red cell distribution width; *STBUR*, Snoring, Trouble Breathing, UnRefreshed; *TST ETCO2*, total sleep time end-tidal carbon dioxide.
Data abstracted in part from:[127,130,173,211,224,232,247,311,314–318,343,346,348–407,410–416,418,419]

Patients younger than 3 years of age have a 2-fold increase in respiratory events after adenotonsillectomy compared with a similar cohort aged 3 to 5 years.[354] Children younger than 2 years of age have a greater occurrence of OSA, although correlation with major respiratory events is weak.[135] Children with OSA commonly have a history of prematurity (<34 weeks gestational age),[135] are underweight, of African American or Hispanic descent, are obese, and have an associated syndrome.[130,355] A history of prematurity doubles the risk of serious adverse respiratory events, the etiology of which is multifactorial, including residual upper airway neuromotor dysfunction, deficits in the respiratory center in the pons and medulla, persisting alveolar-capillary gas-exchange impairments, and bronchopulmonary dysplasia/bronchial hyperreactivity or subglottic stenosis from prolonged intubation at birth.[135,211,356-358] Adenotonsillectomy is an uncommon procedure in infants aged younger than 12 months; adenoidectomy in this age group carries a high risk (28%) for postoperative adverse events requiring pediatric intensive care unit (PICU) admission, usually related to increased perioperative oxygen requirements.[359]

Ethnicity is a risk factor. African American children are known to be at greater risk for major perioperative respiratory events (adjusted OR=1.82; 95% CI, 1.05–3.14])[315,360] and other post-adenotonsillectomy adverse events including bleeding, pain, or fever/dehydration (OR=1.36; 95% CI, 1.10–1.67) than others.[361,362] In part, these adverse events may be due to a reduced socioeconomic status (e.g., reduced access to health care,[351] presenting with advanced OSA), a greater incidence of sickle cell disease and associated OSA, and single nucleotide polymorphisms in the CYP2D6 isoform metabolizing codeine rapidly into its active metabolite.[361,363-365] Insurance payer status is not associated with perioperative respiratory complications.[351,366,367] Hydroxyurea, an antiinflammatory agent, effectively reduces episodes of pain and other complications in patients with sickle cell disease[368]; it has also shown promise to reduce OSA in patients with sickle cell disease.[369-372]

Comorbidities are associated with both major and minor perioperative adverse respiratory events, prolonged PACU stay, and unexpected admissions after adenotonsillectomy.[232,314-316,360,366,373-383] ASA physical status score ≥2 is independently associated with adverse respiratory events.[350,384] The absence of comorbidities protects against these adverse respiratory events, whether major or minor.[385-388]

Upper and lower respiratory tract infections and asthma are associated with an almost 3-fold increase in adverse respiratory events (relative risk=3.15) including bronchospasm, desaturation (OR=1.6; 95%C, 1.1–2.4) compared with unaffected children,[346,373,389] as well as an increased incidence of unplanned admissions and hospital revisits (OR=1.38).[351,361,374,390] It is unclear how long procedures should be postponed after the last URI before proceeding with adenotonsillectomy, provided other comorbidities are well controlled and risk reduction strategies are employed. In a multivariate analysis of the risk factors that contributed to perioperative adverse respiratory events in children undergoing ambulatory surgery, five factors were identified: surgery as opposed to radiology (OR=2.71), morbid obesity (OR=3.05), preexisting pulmonary disease (OR=3.95), ASA P/S ≥III (OR=2.37) and age ≤3 years (OR=1.73).[350] Children who are exposed to passive smoking are at increased risk for events and those with a positive respiratory history[211] (nocturnal dry cough, wheezing during exercise, wheezing more than three times in the past 12 months, history of past or current eczema) are also at risk

for bronchospasm, laryngospasm, perioperative cough, and hypoxemia.[127,232,346]

Children with major and severe congenital heart disease (CHD) (see E-Table 31.4) undergoing noncardiac surgery are at greater risk for cardiac arrest, reintubation, and death compared with children with minor or no CHD.[391] The risk of adverse respiratory events in children with CHD undergoing adenotonsillectomy has not been well defined,[374-376,382,392,393] nor has the risk stratification score been validated for less severe postoperative complications.[391,394] Pulmonary hypertension is associated with a greater frequency of adverse respiratory events in children undergoing adenotonsillectomy[376,395] and should be factored into the anesthetic plan for children with severe OSA (nSAT<70%) or with predisposing conditions including Prader Willi, the mucopolysaccharidoses syndromes, and trisomy 21.[396] Systemic hypertension and echocardiographic findings of valvular dysfunction and ventricular dilation do not increase the risk of adverse respiratory events.[314,316,317,343] Children with major or severe CHD or pulmonary hypertension that is poorly compensated undergoing elective, urgent, or emergent adenotonsillectomy, regardless of their OSA severity, are at greater risk for untoward events and may require specific anesthetic considerations, including overnight admission for monitoring and observation.[348,397] After discharge from the hospital, neither major nor minor CHD was associated with a spike in 30-day return visits.[398]

Obesity is a very common comorbidity in children who present for adenotonsillectomy. Morbid obesity increases the risk of perioperative respiratory events and unplanned hospital admission independent of other systemic or respiratory disorders.[399] Children who are obese with mild OSA and no associated comorbidities (e.g., hypertension, asthma, and diabetes) may be suitable to undergo ambulatory surgery,[232,311,315,318,360,384,393,400,401] although the presence of comorbidities increases the risk for both adverse respiratory events and/or unplanned admissions.[247,395,402,403] Residual polysomnogram-measured OSA and sleep architecture abnormalities are reported in obese children immediately after surgery.[404] Drug doses must be adjusted in these children to minimize adverse respiratory events from the use of opioids.[350,358,405] Size scalars based upon theoretical pharmacokinetic modeling and allometry (see Chapter 5) may prove helpful for dose determination.[406-409]

Weight less than 14 to 20 kilograms is independently associated with increased risk for perioperative adverse respiratory events after adenotonsillectomy[373,374,382]; however, it is unclear if this association reflects the younger age of the patient or a weight indexed scalar for failure to thrive.[173,315,360,410] Large adenoids are associated with increased risk for postoperative adverse respiratory events, especially in younger children, those with GERD, nasal obstruction, and prematurity.[311,392,411]

In children undergoing adenotonsillectomy, GERD is associated with increased frequency of adverse respiratory events including bronchospasm, prolonged length of stay, prolonged PICU intubation, and unplanned admission after adenotonsillectomy.[316,389,390,392,412,413]

The frequency of major adverse respiratory events after adenotonsillectomy in children with trisomy 21 (17%–25%),[320,394,404,414-417] is more than double the frequency in unaffected healthy children (9.4%).[224] Severe OSA (obstructive AHI >10 events/hour and minimum oxygen saturation <80%), ASA physical status classification >II, preoperative PICU admission, and aerodigestive comorbidities in children with trisomy 21 are additional risk factors for respiratory complications particularly on the first night or first postoperative day.[394,415]

A systematic review identified cerebral palsy to be an independent risk factor for respiratory complications after adenotonsillectomy such as requiring supplemental oxygen (OR=3.4–6.8), PICU admission (OR=8.08), or a prolonged PACU length of stay compared with healthier children with OSA undergoing adenotonsillectomy.[418] Close monitoring of these children in PACU for up to 5 hours without incident may permit them to be safely discharged to the ward overnight.[419]

ANESTHETIC CONSIDERATIONS

The anesthetic goals for adenotonsillectomy are to (1) induce anesthesia smoothly; (2) provide optimal operating conditions; (3) anticipate potential intraoperative complications; (4) optimize analgesia and IV fluids, and prevent PONV; and (5) provide rapid emergence without adverse respiratory events. The anesthetic techniques for adenotonsillectomy are varied and include the choice of an inhalational or TIVA technique, the choice of a tracheal tube or LMA, and the choice of spontaneous or controlled ventilation. Anesthetic considerations for pediatric adenoidectomy are summarized in Table 31.6.

PERIOPERATIVE CONSIDERATIONS

The use of premedication varies widely. Many children require no premedication. Family and patient preparation involving a child life specialist using distraction techniques during parental presence can be helpful for the anxious child.[420–422] If premedication is required, then the most commonly used drug is midazolam. It is not consistently associated with either an increased risk or no risk of severe perioperative adverse respiratory events in patients with OSA.[211,345,390,423–425] However, when adverse events occur they are usually dose specific[426] or attributed to concurrent opioid use.[427] Midazolam premedication does not increase emergence or discharge times in children with OSA.[428–430] Reduced doses of midazolam premedication and the dose of hydromorphone resulted in similar emergence times and frequency of perioperative adverse events in all patients.[431] The intranasal midazolam (0.1 mg/kg) preparation was considered inferior to IN dexmedetomidine premedication (2 µg/kg).[432]

Most clinicians modify opioid dosing in children perioperatively based on the severity of the OSA and nocturnal desaturation nadir; the evidence to reduce the dose of benzodiazepines to avoid adverse events in children remains ambiguous, although in adults with OSA, evidence suggests that benzodiazepines increase the risk of adverse events.[431,433–437] Current evidence indicates that oral midazolam is a safe premedication for children with OSA, although the dose should be adjusted to reflect comorbidities and ancillary medications.[143,246,433,438,439]

The etiology of associated adverse respiratory events after adenotonsillectomy is multifactorial including increased upper airway collapse, synergy with other anesthetic agents and opioids, central apnea, and impairment of respiratory drive through decreased arousal responses to hypoxemia and hypercapnia.[142,440]

In children with severe OSA, desaturation in PACU is less likely to occur if the surgery was performed in the morning compared with the afternoon.[441] The reasons behind this observation remain elusive. Urgent surgery in children appears to be a predictor of increased morbidity and mortality,[211,319,346,442] and urgent adenotonsillectomy for severe OSA is associated with postoperative adverse respiratory events.[319,443,444]

Clinical education and experience of the anesthesia provider is inversely associated with perioperative adverse respiratory events, with approximately a 1% decrease per year of experience.[211,346,445]

TABLE 31.6 | Anesthetic Considerations for Pediatric Adenotonsillectomy

Pediatric Patient
- Indication for surgery: OSA vs. recurrent tonsillitis or other diagnosis
- Specific airway anatomy/physiology/associated medical diagnosis (e.g., asthma or recent URI)
- Drug dosing considerations: i.e., opioids and sedatives

Preoperative

Optimization
- Preoperative investigations (e.g., polysomnogram/nocturnal oximetry)
- Age-related psychosocial issues-sedation/proton-pump inhibitor/distraction techniques
- Analgesic (acetaminophen and/or NSAID)
- Upper/lower airway reactivity-bronchodilators

Disposition Planning
- Diagnosis/suspicion of OSA severity
  - Ambulatory or admission postoperatively
  - Potential need for postoperative intensive care/monitoring

Position
- Supine with neck extension
  - Caution with atlantoaxial instability
- OR table rotated 90 degrees.
  - Shared/limited access to airway

Procedure

Goals
- Mitigate risk of adverse respiratory events
- Mitigate postoperative pain, PONV, and bleeding risk
- Fire precautions

Anesthetic Approach
- Anesthetic technique:
  - GA with inhalational agents and/or TIVA
  - Oral RAE tube or reinforced LMA
  - Aim FiO_2 <30%
  - Prepare for difficult bag/mask ventilation ± airway visualization/intubation
  - Deep vs. awake extubation
- Medications:
  - Analgesia:
    - Titrate opioids based on nocturnal oxygen saturation nadir and other comorbidities
    - Parenteral NSAIDs based on institutional practice
  - Antiemetic drugs and adjuvant techniques (e.g., superhydration, dexamethasone)
- Complications:
  - Accidental extubation or tracheal tube/LMA compression
  - Laryngospasm, bronchospasm, and apnea; continuously monitor oxygen saturation
  - Airway fire
  - Bleeding

Postoperative
- Discharge criteria vs. overnight admission
- Risk for:
  - Perioperative adverse respiratory events
  - Bleeding, emergence delirium, pain, PONV

LMA, Laryngeal mask airway; *NSAID*, nonsteroidal antiinflammatory drug; *OR*, operating room; *OSA*, obstructive sleep apnea; *TIVA*, total intravenous anesthesia; *PONV*, postoperative nausea and vomiting; *URI*=upper respiratory tract infection.

Complex patients or those recognized to be at increased risk for complications should be cared for by the most experienced pediatric anesthesiologist or referred to a tertiary-care center. Despite the provider's level of experience, opioid administration and the postoperative monitoring environment can contribute to the risk of adverse events[349]; implementation of institutional OSA guidelines with locally developed interventions specific to adenotonsillectomy reduces unanticipated admissions and the rate of adverse respiratory events.[247,384,446,447]

Three tools have been validated to predict perioperative respiratory events: The STBUR (snoring, trouble breathing, unrefreshed) questionnaire,[256] the COLDS inventory,[448] and the Ambulatory Perioperative Respiratory Adverse Events Assessment Tool.[350] The STBUR noted that the presence of three symptoms predicted a 3-fold increase in the risk of perioperative adverse respiratory events, and the presence of five symptoms, predicted a 10-fold increase in events.[449] The questionnaire's large negative predictive value and specificity may be used as an effective screening tool to predict those children who are at low risk for a prolonged early phase recovery stay and supplemental support.[450]

The COLDS scoring tool is an acronym for **C**urrent signs/symptoms of a URI, **O**nset, presence of **L**ung disease, the airway **D**evice used, and type of **S**urgery where each is subdivided into three outcomes assigned 1, 2, or 5 points, yielding a maximum score of 25. This score demonstrated good predictive ability for perioperative respiratory events[448]; children whose COLDS score was >16 had a 55% risk of developing a perioperative adverse event.[448] Other screening tools have been reviewed elsewhere.[356]

Aggregate outcomes may be useful to predict perioperative respiratory adverse events.[451] The acronym PRAE has been adopted to describe five variables: laryngospasm, airway obstruction, bronchospasm, desaturation (<95%), and recurrent coughing.[452] Most such events were easily managed, were less prevalent if the airway was intubated, and decreased by ~8% with each year of increasing patient year of age. However, the variables have not been clearly defined in terms of their severity (except for a desaturation threshold), the level of intervention (laryngospasm treated with continuous positive airway pressure [CPAP] or succinylcholine), or duration.[452] Moreover, each of the variables carries equal weight in terms of outcome although most practitioners would not equate the sequelae from laryngospasm with recurrent coughing, and the significance of one, two, or more variables in the perioperative respiratory adverse events aggregate has neither been defined nor validated.[453] Many questions remain about the validity of the PRAE score.

Routine polysomnogram is not warranted in healthy children or those with controlled comorbidities, as clinical factors alone can predict those at risk for adverse respiratory events after adenotonsillectomy (see earlier discussion).[95,353,454] An AHI >20 events per hour has been associated with breath holding during induction, postoperative complications, and unplanned admissions[315,403]; a respiratory disturbance index (RDI), which is equivalent to an AHI >30, has been associated with laryngospasm and desaturation during emergence; and an RDI >40 associated with comorbidities or age <24 months may require ICU admission.[95,375] Only a few studies have assessed the utility of both the AHI (RDI) and obstructive AHI to predict adverse respiratory events after adenotonsillectomy, but a difference in associated nocturnal hypoxemia was not assessed and neither scoring system was found to be better at predicting adverse events after adenotonsillectomy.[300,316,404] Criteria for elective PICU admission after adenotonsillectomy for children with severe OSA are institution and surgeon specific.[375] The American Academy of Pediatrics 2012 guideline recommends that an AHI >24 requires a preemptive admission due to the increased risk of perioperative adverse events.[96] Perhaps the threshold for a postoperative admission warrants a greater threshold, AHI (>20) compared with obstructive AHI (>10) because gas-exchange abnormalities only become apparent at these levels of OSA, regardless if the pathogenesis is obstructive or central.[455,456] A multivariable analysis of 278 children with severe OSA (polysomnogram AHI >10) after adenotonsillectomy yielded three variables that predicted an escalation of airway management or prolonged PICU stay: intraoperative respiratory complications, polysomnogram $ETCO_2$ >60 mm Hg, and the presence of neuromuscular disease.[457]

Cumulative nocturnal hypoxemic burden or nadir SpO_2 desaturation is associated with perioperative adverse respiratory events,[300,455] and may better predict these events when compared with standard polysomnogram variables such as AHI.[207,300,311,312,315,455] A polysomnogram-derived nadir saturation <80% is a robust predictor for perioperative adverse events, prolonged PACU length of stay, unplanned admission, and sensitivity to opioids after adenotonsillectomy.[196,300,312,315,352,389,393] Current guidelines recommend preemptive admission postadenotonsillectomy for children who have a nadir saturation <80%.[95,96,212] The McGill oximetry score correlates well with the polysomnogram and was discussed above.[91,300,301,458,459]

The severity of OSA depends on the AHI, patient symptoms, comorbidities (including end-organ disease), and other polysomnogram variables including abnormal gas exchange, which are then interpreted by a sleep medicine specialist. A sleep medicine specialist diagnosis of OSA severity is preferred over an AHI, although the obstructive AHI, AHI (RDI), and nadir SAT should be sought for risk stratification.[246]

Pharmacogenomic variability may lead to opioid-related adverse respiratory events after adenotonsillectomy (see Chapters 4 and 5).[460] Polymorphisms affect both pharmacokinetics and pharmacodynamics at multiple sites.[461] For example, genetic variants of the ATP-binding cassette gene ABCC3, which facilitates hepatic morphine glucuronide metabolite (M3G and M6G) efflux, is associated with respiratory depression after adenotonsillectomy.[462]

POSTOPERATIVE CONSIDERATIONS

Adverse Respiratory Events

Children who are scheduled for adenotonsillectomy have a greater incidence of difficult bag-and-mask ventilation and critical adverse respiratory events including coughing, oxygen desaturation, airway obstruction, laryngospasm, stridor, and bronchospasm.[211,346] The majority (25.6%) of these events occur in the PACU, followed by 18.5% during emergence, 16% during induction, and 2.1% during maintenance anesthesia.[463] As part of the real-time assessment of community transmission (REACT) trial, pretreatment with 100 micrograms salbutamol (albuterol) administered twice within 20 minutes of surgery reduced the potential for these events in children at risk for airway reactivity, including those with obstructive sleep-disordered breathing/OSA, by 50% with the number needed to treat of 5[464]; children with asthma should be administered salbutamol (albuterol) before induction.[465] However, the external validity of the results from the REACT study in children may be limited, as 25% to 30% of the children reported a URI in the 2 weeks preceding adenotonsillectomy, fewer than 18% had a history of asthma, 8% reported wheezing with exercise, and 40% of the children were exposed to passive smoking. The role of albuterol (salbutamol) to attenuate

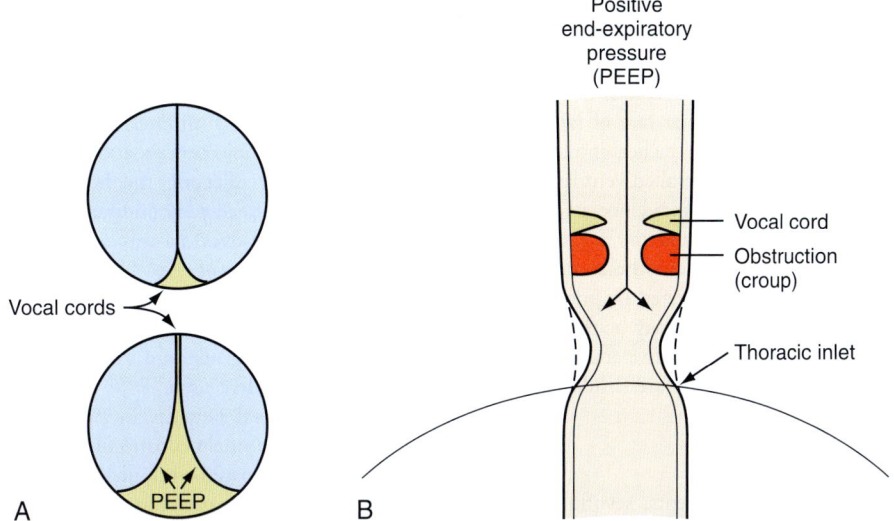

Positive
end-expiratory
pressure
(PEEP)

Vocal cord
Obstruction
(croup)

Thoracic inlet

Vocal cords

A   PEEP   B

FIGURE 31.8 When a child has upper airway obstruction caused by laryngospasm **(A)** or mechanical obstruction, application of approximately 10 cm H_2O of positive end-expiratory pressure *(PEEP)* during spontaneous breathing often relieves obstruction. PEEP helps to hold the vocal cords apart **(A)** and the airway open *(dashed lines* in **B)**. (From Coté CJ. Pediatric anesthesia. In Miller RD, ed. *Miller's Anesthesia.* 8th ed. New York: Churchill Livingstone; 2012.)

perioperative respiratory events in children undergoing adenotonsillectomy who are not diagnosed with asthma and routinely treated with salbutamol (albuterol) is inconsistent with other studies. Two puffs of salbutamol (albuterol) preoperatively did not reduce the incidence of respiratory adverse events in children undergoing surgery (adenotonsillectomy comprising only 5%–6%) with at least two risk factors for perioperative respiratory adverse events.[466]

Induction of anesthesia either intravenously or with inhalational anesthetics must recognize the increased risk of airway collapsibility and decrease in genioglossus muscle activity particularly in children with severe OSA.[138,467] Intravenous induction permits the use of transnasal humidified rapid-insufflation ventilatory exchange or nasal cannula to provide oxygen before and during tracheal intubation.[468,469] In children with severe OSA, securing IV access before induction of anesthesia will expedite drug administration should pharyngeal obstruction or laryngospasm occur. An inhalational induction with rapid intravenous placement may be associated with a 2- to 3-fold increased risk of critical adverse respiratory events in children who present with a recent upper respiratory tract infection or wheezing, or if the care provider is inexperienced, compared with an intravenous induction.[211,346,396,470] However, many clinicians would defer anesthesia in children who present with a recent infection (<2 weeks) or wheezing.[476]

Airway patency can be maintained after induction by offsetting the reduction in pharyngeal muscle tone, genioglossus muscle activity, and impaired ventilatory drive using the jaw thrust maneuver,[471] manual neck extension, head-up elevation, and CPAP with moderate lateral head tilt, which acts as a pneumatic splint, taking advantage of tethering forces in the mediastinum and thorax through increased lung volumes to reduce upper airway collapsibility (see Fig. 12.11 and Fig. 31.8A,B)).[127,139,472–477] Small increments of CPAP between 5 and 10 mm H_2O increase the dimension of the pharyngeal airway dramatically (Fig. 31.9). A slowing of the heart rate, after the peak sevoflurane-induced tachycardia, is a sign of sufficient depth of anesthesia to avoid

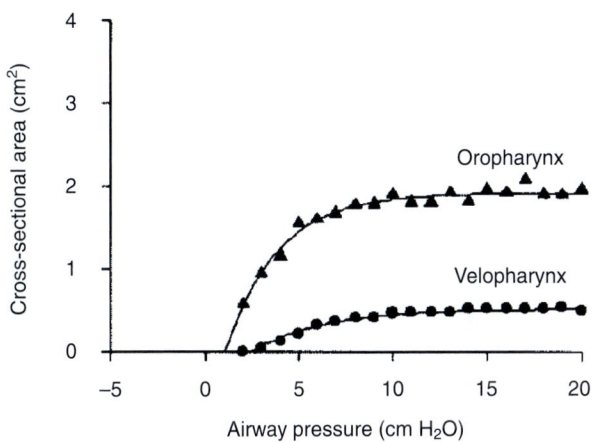

FIGURE 31.9 The relationship between airway pressure and the cross-sectional area of the pharynx. Maximal airway dimension is achieved between 15 and 20 cm H_2O. At reduced airway pressures, around 5 cm H_2O, small increments in airway pressure make a large difference in airway caliber. (From Isono S, Tanaka A, Nishino T. Dynamic interaction between the tongue and soft palate during obstructive apnea in anesthetized patients with sleep-disordered breathing. *J Appl Physiol.* 2003;95[6]:2257-2264.)

placing an oral airway prematurely and triggering laryngospasm during an inhalational induction.

Airway Control

Cuffed tracheal tubes (TT) are increasingly used in children of all age groups because of the reduced risk of an air leak and the bubbling of secretions and blood that can interfere with surgery, minimized anesthetic gas pollution, and decreased risk of an airway fire when electrocautery is used.[478] However, a cuffed TT has been associated with more adverse respiratory events in children compared with SGA (relative risk 3.31 vs. 1.67).[211] Although the TT remains the airway of choice, some prefer a flexible spiral, metal reinforced LMA for adenotonsillectomy.[479,480] SGAs offer several advantages over the TT including a reduced incidence of postoperative stridor, bronchospasm, and possibly laryngospasm,[481,482] as well as less coughing and gagging. Even though the SGA reduces the time in the operating room and favors successful deep extubation, this must be balanced against a greater rate of failure (obstruction by the Boyle-Davis gag and rescue tracheal intubation) of 15%, which is related to younger age, controlled ventilation, and surgeon experience.[482–485] Although the incidence of laryngospasm during emergence with the LMA and the TT is similar, removal of the SGA during a deep level of anesthesia may reduce the risk of postoperative laryngospasm triggered by pooled secretions,[424] particularly after a recent URI and may be the preferred technique in the child with asthma. Perioperative adverse respiratory complications after adenotonsillectomy are similar for both deep and awake extubation.[373,486]

Anesthetic Choice

Of the currently available inhalational agents, sevoflurane provides a smooth induction of anesthesia. An algorithm for the anesthetic management of the child with a recent URI is provided in Fig. 31.10, highlighting the value of preoperative inhaled salbutamol (albuterol) for children with moderate to severe asthma, avoiding desflurane, and the benefits of airway management using

an SGA in this population.[384,385] The benefits of sevoflurane as a bronchodilator and propofol to blunt reflex bronchoconstriction as well as other drugs are detailed in E-Table 31.5.[424,487] These drugs can be combined with an IV infusion of dexmedetomidine (1–2 µg/kg over 5–10 minutes) or a single IV dose of clonidine (1 µg/kg),[488] to supplement sedation and analgesia intraoperatively without adversely affecting the hemodynamics. Some advocate a bolus dose of dexmedetomidine (0.5 µg/kg over 5 seconds), although severe bradycardia was reported in this small cohort of children 5 to 10 years of age.[489] Rapid IV boluses or large doses of dexmedetomidine are best avoided.[490]

There is no single preferred anesthetic technique to manage children undergoing adenotonsillectomy, and both inhalational and TIVA are widely used.[491–493] A propofol-based TIVA technique offers several benefits in preserving upper airway tone, blunting reflex bronchoconstriction and reducing the risk of laryngospasm compared with inhalational anesthetics. These characteristics of TIVA are particularly relevant for the child with OSA and asthma or an URI.[424,465] Propofol is also an antiemetic,[494] does not trigger emergence delirium,[495] and does not pollute the operating room.[496] In contrast, an inhalational anesthetic technique with sevoflurane is simple to deliver, rapidly titratable with measurable concentrations, does not require awake IV access, and

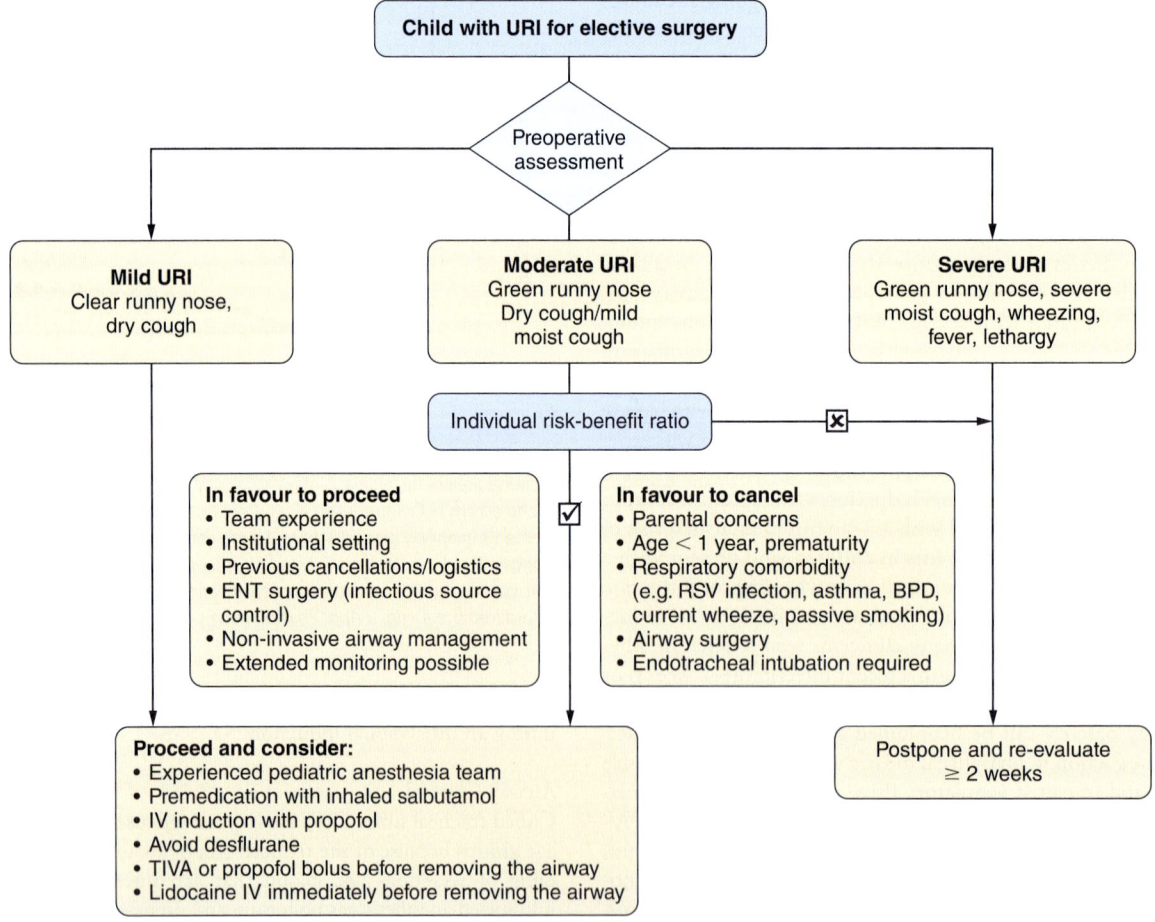

FIGURE 31.10 Algorithm to guide perioperative management in children with URI scheduled for elective surgery. *BPD*, Bronchopulmonary dysplasia; *ENT*, ear, nose, and throat; *IV*, intravenous; *RSV*, respiratory syncytial virus; *TIVA*, total intravenous anesthesia; *URI*, upper respiratory infection. (Modified from Regli A, Becke K, von Ungern-Sternberg BS. An update on the perioperative management of children with upper respiratory tract infections. *Curr Opin Anaesthesiol.* 2017;30(3):362-367.)

the recovery time may be more predictable. Maintenance of anesthesia with desflurane may provide a rapid emergence and recovery but is relatively contraindicated in children with airway reactivity secondary to asthma or URI.[487,497]

Postoperative Nausea and Vomiting

Adenotonsillectomy is an independent risk factor for postoperative vomiting (POV) and/or PONV.[51,494] Emesis and poor oral intake are common comorbid conditions after adenotonsillectomy. Risk factors for POV and PONV in children undergoing adenotonsillectomy include patient factors (age older than 3 years, personal or family history of POV/PONV or motion sickness, and postpubertal females), duration of surgery (>2 hours), surgical factors (ear surgery and others) and anesthetic factors (opioids, inhalational anesthetics, anticholinesterase drugs, limited intraoperative fluids, and forcing oral fluids before discharge).[51,494] Opioids, especially long-acting agents used in the postoperative period, increase the incidence of PONV, highlighting the benefits of nonopioid analgesics including NSAIDs and acetaminophen.[498–502] Hydration (20–30 mL/kg IV balanced salt solution) administered during adenotonsillectomy reduces the incidence of POV by 25% in children who did not receive intraoperative antiemetic prophylaxis compared with normal fluid volumes (10 mL/kg IV).[503] Most cases of adenotonsillectomy do not require neuromuscular blocking drugs, particularly if OSA is present, as spontaneous respiration is used to test the effect of small doses of opioids on the respiratory rate in children who severely desaturate at night. Nonetheless, if a neuromuscular blocking drug has been administered, atropine and neostigmine are preferred to glycopyrrolate and neostigmine because the former is associated with less PONV.[504] The introduction of sugammadex into clinical practice has reduced concerns regarding the emetic effects of anticholinesterase agents.

Intraoperative IV ondansetron (0.15 mg/kg)[505–509] combined with dexamethasone (single intraoperative dose 0.15 mg/kg)[510–512] are recommended to reduce the incidence of emesis after adenotonsillectomy. The use of TIVA may be considered in high-risk patients (≥3 risk factors).[494,513,514] It should be noted that a randomized dose-escalation study of dexamethasone for tonsillectomy found no difference in the incidence of PONV, pain, or time to first liquid intake following 0.0625 to 1.0 milligrams per kilogram (Fig. 31.11).[510] There is a small but acceptable risk for an absolute increase in bleeding rates with dexamethasone.[515] Dexamethasone also reduces perioperative adverse respiratory events.[51,381,516] If dexamethasone is contraindicated (e.g., risk of tumor lysis syndrome),[517,518] droperidol 0.025 milligrams per kilogram may serve as an alternative. Intravenous tropisetron 0.1 milligram per kilogram (max 2 mg) may substitute for ondansetron (see Chapter 5).[519,520]

Emptying the stomach with an orogastric tube does not reduce nausea and vomiting in children.[510,521] It remains unclear how PC6 (Nei-Kuwan) stimulation using needle acupuncture, acupressure,

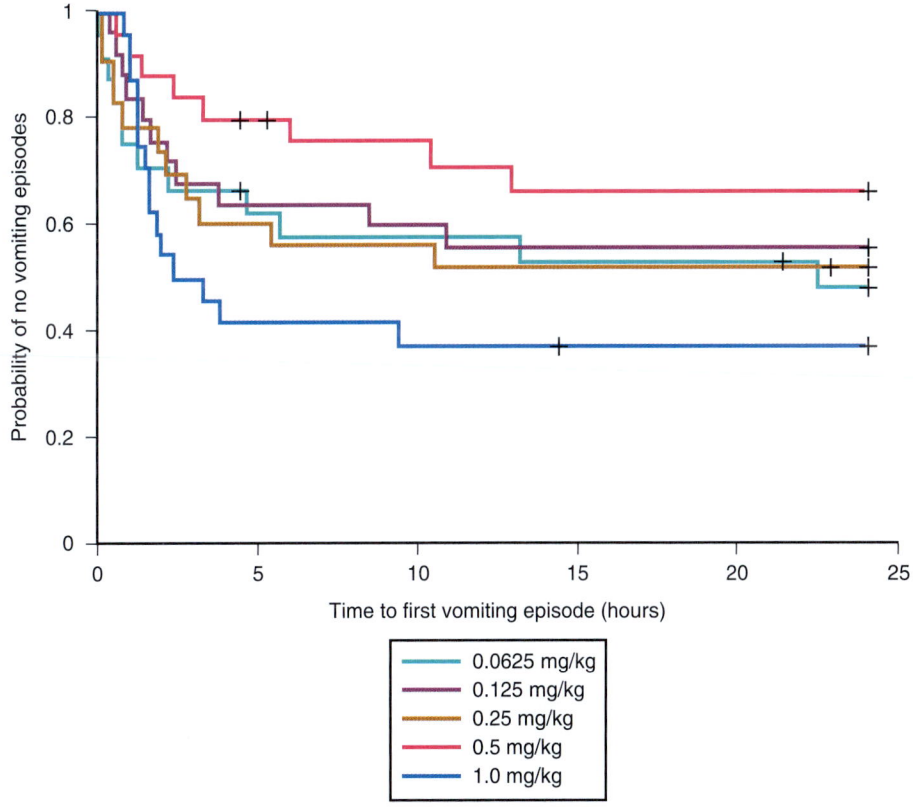

FIGURE 31.11 Effect of dexamethasone to prevent vomiting in children undergoing tonsillectomy was independent of the dose administered. Time-to-event analysis for first vomiting episode was performed; *plus signs* indicate time of censoring for patients who did not have complete follow-up (*N*=13). No significant difference was found between dose levels, *P*=0.28 (Cox proportional hazard likelihood ratio test). (Redrawn with permission from Kim MS, Coté CJ, Cristoloveanu C, et al. There is no dose-escalation response to dexamethasone [0.0625–1.0 mg/kg] in pediatric tonsillectomy or adenotonsillectomy patients for preventing vomiting, reducing pain, shortening time to first liquid intake, or the incidence of voice change. *Anesth Analg.* 2007. 104[5]:1052-1058.)

needle, or transcutaneous electrical stimulation can be used as part of a perioperative multimodal treatment to reduce the risk of PONV in children.[522–526]

Perioperative Pain

Children experience pain and severe functional limitations for up to 7 days after adenotonsillectomy,[527–529] unlike with adenoidectomy where recovery is considerably faster and the severity of the pain is less.[528] Barriers to optimal analgesia after adenotonsillectomy may be attributed to either inadequate analgesia (child and parent factors) or prescription issues (medication or system factors).[530] Child factors include anxiety and previous acute pain experience,[531–533] culture and ethnicity,[534] certain obstructive sleep-disordered breathing/OSA phenotypes,[535,536] obesity,[537,538] genetic predisposition to altered pain perception, polymorphisms (drug pharmacokinetics) or altered pharmacodynamics (opioid sensitivity with repeated hypoxemia events),[461,539–543] and reluctance/inability to swallow the analgesic preparations. Parental factors include attitudes, misconceptions (e.g., fear of addiction), and knowledge deficits[544,545] compounded by poor pain assessment and an anxiety pain-catastrophizing overlap.[546]

Although child and parent factors may partly explain the growing evidence for two distinct "early" and "late" postoperative pain recovery populations,[547–549] inadequate or inappropriate perioperative analgesic administration/prescription[550] and poor provider communication and/or lack of discharge information are leading causes of insufficient pain management in children undergoing adenotonsillectomy. Reduced system access to opioids due to drug shortages and opioid epidemic-related concerns over opioid abuse, misuse, and diversion has further worsened the pain experience.[551–553] Concerns have also been raised over ethnic and racial disparities in pain assessment, treatment, and outcomes in children.[541,554–556]

There is growing interest in opioid-free enhanced recovery protocols after adenotonsillectomy.[557–559] A systematic multimodal analgesic approach is recommended.[560,561] Medication choices should be individualized as there is no one ideal class of medication, dose, or dosing frequency that is optimal to manage pain in all children undergoing adenotonsillectomy; however, there is increasing interest in an opioid-free multimodal analgesic approach.[557–559] Perioperative pharmacologic analgesic approaches to pain management are multiple.[95,561–565]

Acetaminophen is insufficient to provide complete analgesia on its own and is frequently used in combination with other medications.[566] An IV formulation may provide greater analgesic predictability than the oral and rectal routes (see Fig. 31.1), but the oral route provides consistent serum drug concentrations at lower cost.[567]

NSAIDs are effective analgesic agents that are opioid-sparing and associated with less PONV. They are particularly effective as a preemptive analgesic, and they can reduce dynamic pain (e.g., with swallowing). NSAIDs are also considered first-line treatment after adenotonsillectomy in several guidelines,[562,563,565] including the current American Academy of Head and Neck Surgery (AAO-HNS) tonsillectomy guideline, which recommends ibuprofen (5–10 mg/kg) every 6 to 8 hours for postadenotonsillectomy pain.[95] The intensity and duration of the effect of ibuprofen to reversibly inhibit platelet function (via inhibiting platelet aggregation and thromboxane A_2 synthesis) is dose dependent. For example, in adults a single dose of 5 to 10 milligrams per kilogram inhibited platelet dysfunction within 2 hours of administration, a duration that lasted 6 to 11 hours respectively, and an offset within 12 to 24 hours.[568]

Adverse effects after NSAIDS were traditionally associated with ketorolac in large doses; a reduced dose decreased bleeding rates.[569–571] Some practitioners advocate deferring ketorolac until intraoperative hemostasis has been achieved[569,572–574]; but this is not common pediatric practice for other NSAIDs.[558,575] Meta-analyses on NSAIDs and postoperative bleeding provide conflicting results and are limited by variable treatment indications, surgical approaches/techniques, and posttonsillectomy hemorrhage definitions and heterogeneity in NSAID type, doses, dosing intervals, and perioperative timing.[576–581] Despite concerns regarding the effect of ibuprofen to increase the intensity of posttonsillectomy hemorrhage related to reversible COX-1 inhibition (responsible for platelet aggregation), ibuprofen continues to be widely used clinically.[582,583] Large retrospective observational studies demonstrated that routine postoperative use of ibuprofen after adenotonsillectomy is not associated with an increased risk of bleeding.[583–586] A noninferiority randomized controlled trial did not reveal a greater rate of severe bleeding with ibuprofen (10 mg/kg 6 hourly) compared with acetaminophen (15 mg/kg 6 hourly).[582]

Combination therapy (e.g., acetaminophen and ketorolac or ibuprofen or celecoxib) reduces the dose of each drug required to achieve an analgesic effect and prolongs the duration of that effect.[20,22] High dose single drug therapy can achieve the same effect.[20,22,587] Consequently drug combinations vary from region to region and may involve different NSAIDS (e.g., celecoxib,[588] diclofenac, and others[21,498]). In a prospective quality improvement study of 353 children after adenotonsillectomy, increasing the dosing interval of ibuprofen (10 mg/kg) alternating with acetaminophen (15 mg/kg) from 3 to 4 hours reduced the postadenotonsillectomy bleeding rate from a median of 5% to 0%.[589] Aspirin is not commonly used in children. However, the aspirin antiplatelet effect is not reversible and caution should be exercised if NSAIDs are prescribed after adenotonsillectomy in children who have been taking aspirin.[590]

Although COX-2 specific analgesics (e.g., celecoxib or parecoxib) cause no platelet dysfunction,[591] they remain off-label in children in North America, despite evidence that they are effective analgesics[547,588,592–594]; an editorial and recent systematic review suggest that this class of analgesic drugs warrants further attention in adenotonsillectomy patients.[595,596] Selective COX-2 inhibitors may be better suited to those with NSAID allergy, mild-to-moderate asthma, and known aspirin- or NSAID-exacerbated respiratory disease.[86] Although the AAO-HNS has endorsed selective COX-2 inhibition to reliably circumvent antiplatelet effects and risk for bleeding in adult otolaryngologic surgery,[597] and a large adult trial has established celecoxib as noninferior for cardiac risk and having fewer gastrointestinal and renal adverse events compared with ibuprofen,[598] more evidence is needed before COX-2 agents can be routinely recommended for children after adenotonsillectomy.[599]

Intraoperative IV dexamethasone may reduce postadenotonsillectomy pain and edema when administered alone or in combination with other analgesics.[512,562] Dexamethasone is recommended by the AAO-HNS[600–606]; a dose response for analgesia is as yet undefined.[607] Dexamethasone (0.3–1 mg/kg) has been associated with reduced parental- and physician-rated pain scores after adenotonsillectomy (E-Table 31.6)[608,609]; however a dose-escalation study found no difference in time to first analgesic with single doses ranging from 0.0625 milligrams per kilogram to 1.0 milligram per kilogram.[510] Children with obstructive sleep-disordered breathing/OSA undergoing adenotonsillectomy are commonly given IV dexamethasone (0.25–0.3 mg/kg, some advocating up to

1 mg/kg); the larger dosing is compatible with the reduced risk of adverse respiratory events.[381,562,607] The optimal dose for dexamethasone for its antiemetic effect and possible analgesia is as yet to be defined. No reports of aseptic necrosis of the hip or infections has been reported after a single dose of dexamethasone; however, it has precipitated acute tumor lysis syndrome.[518,610,611]

Several studies suggest that a preoperative course of oral steroids improves the severity of documented OSA and reduces perioperative respiratory adverse events,[612,613] whereas a short postoperative course after adenotonsillectomy may decrease the risk of postoperative tonsillectomy hemorrhage and pain-related phone calls from families. However, rates of hospital revisits remain unchanged when compared with a nonsteroid cohort.[614,615] The benefits of dexamethasone beyond a single intraoperative dose remain unproven.

ADMISSION POLICIES

Guidelines recommend that children with severe OSA should be treated in an inpatient setting; however, no validated pediatric-specific risk assessment scoring system exists to identify children with OSA who are inappropriate for daycare surgery.[127] The AAO-HNS 2019 tonsillectomy guideline recommends that suspected "severe OSA" (i.e., obstructive AHI >10 events per hour and/or nSAT <80%) and/or the presence of other comorbidities (e.g., trisomy 21, cardiac complications of OSA, neuromuscular disorders, or obesity) increase the risk for perioperative adverse respiratory events that warrants a preemptive overnight admission, especially in younger children (<3 years of age).

It is recommended that children younger than 3 years of age are admitted overnight preemptively (92% of surveyed otolaryngologists).[616] However, the threshold of 3 years of age should be considered a "starting point" to discuss postoperative disposition planning given that adenotonsillectomy is a high-risk surgical category,[211,346] and this age independently predicts critical respiratory events in pediatric perioperative data in Europe, Australasia, and North America.[211,346,350]

For children who are otherwise healthy or those with well-controlled comorbidities, disposition decisions based on the diagnosis of OSA can be challenging. Polysomnogram data are often lacking, and symptomatology or clinically based assessment methods have not been fully validated. Furthermore, predicting the risk of a serious adverse event postoperatively must be balanced with the cost of a preemptive overnight admission.[617] Unsurprisingly, rates of preemptive inpatient admissions after adenotonsillectomy vary widely (3%–100% of all adenotonsillectomies), with no apparent difference in 7- and 30-day revisit rates for any cause.[618,619]

Site-specific preemptive admission guidelines have reduced adverse respiratory events and postoperative readmission rates.[247,384] Children with severe OSA can be observed for a severe adverse respiratory event in a PACU-like setting for 2 hours after adenotonsillectomy; if a severe event occurs (reported in 8% of children), a PICU admission can be evaluated. If an event did not occur, the child may follow the usual postoperative course (Fig. 31.12).[320,620] This criterion resulted in a negative predictive value of 98% for no worse than a mild adverse event after an uncomplicated 2 hour PACU stay.[320] A combination of a high suspicion for OSA based upon nocturnal symptoms, an increasing number of risk factors for OSA, and adverse respiratory events, and when available, objective measures of sleep parameters (e.g., overnight oximetry) combined with complications that developed during/after surgery should reduce the threshold to consider an overnight admission after adenotonsillectomy.

Some children may be treated at home with CPAP or bilevel positive airway pressure therapy to improve airway patency and

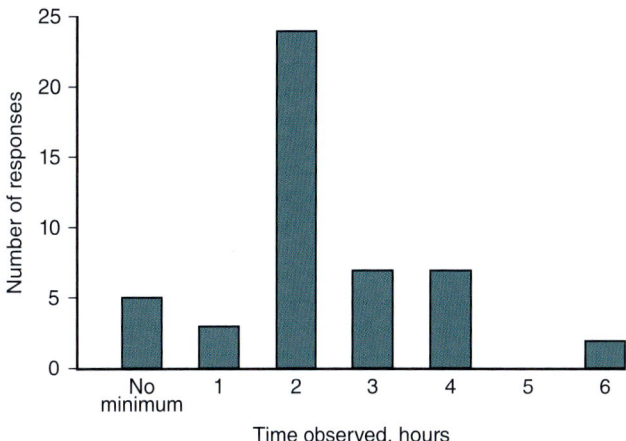

FIGURE 31.12 A survey of observation time from pediatric otolaryngologists from 72 pediatric otolaryngology divisions at tertiary-care children's hospitals after outpatient adenotonsillectomy regarding the minimum time that a patient was observed before discharge home. (Modified from Nardone HC, McKee-Cole KM, Friedman NR. Current pediatric tertiary-care admission practices following adenotonsillectomy. *JAMA Otolaryngol Head Neck Surg.* 2016;142[5]:452-456.)

reduce pulmonary hypertension.[396] Noninvasive ventilation devices, especially for children who are compliant with their use, should be brought to the hospital for adjunct use to improve oxygenation and ventilation postoperatively. In some hospitals, documentation of PACU noninvasive ventilation device compliance may forego the need for an ICU admission. Fig. 31.13 depicts a suggested decision-making algorithm for risk stratification and discharge planning for a child scheduled for adenotonsillectomy.[463] Factors that should be considered for an ICU admission after adenotonsillectomy include young age (<2 years), ASA P/S ≥III, difficult airway, prolonged PACU stay due to repeated or major adverse respiratory events in the PACU, urgent/emergent surgery, or severe OSA.[315,378,621] Young children with profound oxygen desaturation during sleep, severe obstructive desaturation index/nadir, and severe carbon dioxide (CO_2) retention should be admitted to the PICU to be optimized before and/or after adenotonsillectomy.[622,623] Interventions such as electively inserting a nasopharyngeal airway after surgery in children with severe OSA may reduce postoperative obstructive events.[378,624] Additional extrinsic factors including syndromic facies, the family living more than 1 hour from a hospital, children with behavioral factors, or those with an uncertain social setting, should also be considered for preemptive admission. Alternative care options include transfer to a tertiary-care center with specialist pediatric services, or delay to further optimize the child's health status can also be explored. It should be noted that despite these recommendations, deaths related to apnea have occurred even in the protected environment of the PACU[127]; the bottom line is one of great caution in this cohort.

OPIOIDS AND RISK FOR POSTOPERATIVE RESPIRATORY DEPRESSION IN CHILDREN WITH OSA

Children with oxygen nadir of <85% may be at greater risk for opioid-induced respiratory depression, possibly due to an increased density of μ-opioid receptors in the respiratory-related areas of the brainstem related to intermittent desaturation events and hypoxia.[625–628] This opioid-induced respiratory depression may be especially exaggerated in younger children (Figs. 31.14 and 31.15).[434,436,629] Perioperative opioid doses in children with severe

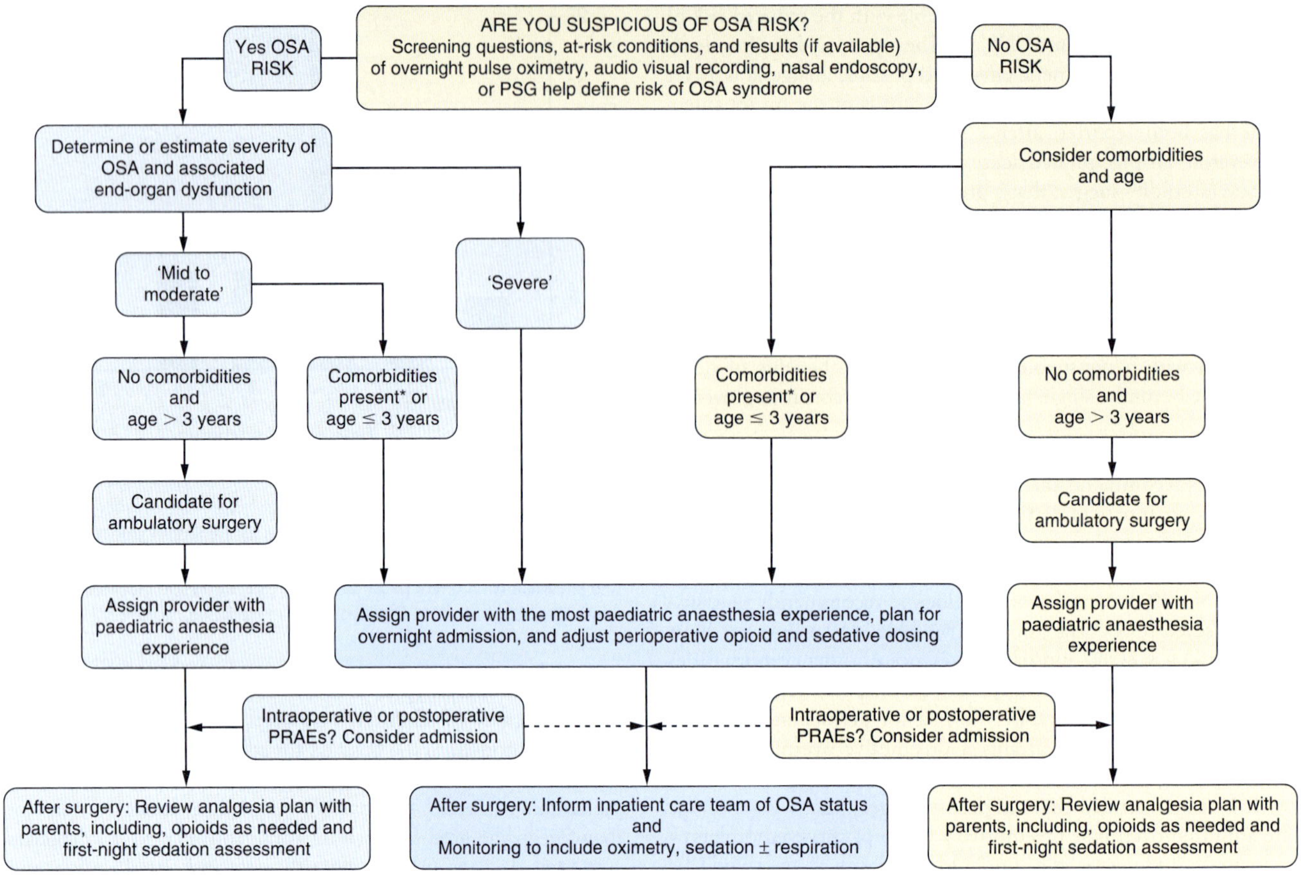

ARE YOU SUSPICIOUS OF OSA RISK?
Screening questions, at-risk conditions, and results (if available) of overnight pulse oximetry, audio visual recording, nasal endoscopy, or PSG help define risk of OSA syndrome
Yes OSA RISK
No OSA RISK
Determine or estimate severity of OSA and associated end-organ dysfunction
Consider comorbidities and age
'Mid to moderate'
'Severe'
No comorbidities and age > 3 years
Comorbidities present* or age ≤ 3 years
Comorbidities present* or age ≤ 3 years
No comorbidities and age > 3 years
Candidate for ambulatory surgery
Candidate for ambulatory surgery
Assign provider with paediatric anaesthesia experience
Assign provider with the most paediatric anaesthesia experience, plan for overnight admission, and adjust perioperative opioid and sedative dosing
Assign provider with paediatric anaesthesia experience
Intraoperative or postoperative PRAEs? Consider admission
Intraoperative or postoperative PRAEs? Consider admission
After surgery: Review analgesia plan with parents, including, opioids as needed and first-night sedation assessment
After surgery: Inform inpatient care team of OSA status and Monitoring to include oximetry, sedation ± respiration
After surgery: Review analgesia plan with parents, including, opioids as needed and first-night sedation assessment

FIGURE 31.13 Decision-making algorithm for risk stratification and discharge planning for children with OSA after adenotonsillectomy. *Comorbidities include obesity; failure to thrive; craniofacial and genetic syndromes; neuromuscular, respiratory and hematological disorders; congenital heart disease; and diabetes mellitus. PRAE is perioperative respiratory adverse event. (From Zalan J, Vaccani JP, Murto KT. Paediatric adenotonsillectomy, part 2: considerations for anaesthesia. *BJA Educ.* 2020;20[6]:193-200.)

Morphine (mg/kg)
0.20
0.16
0.12
0.08
0.04
0.00
80
60
40
20
0
Age (months)
50
60
70
80
90
100
SaO2 nadir (percent)

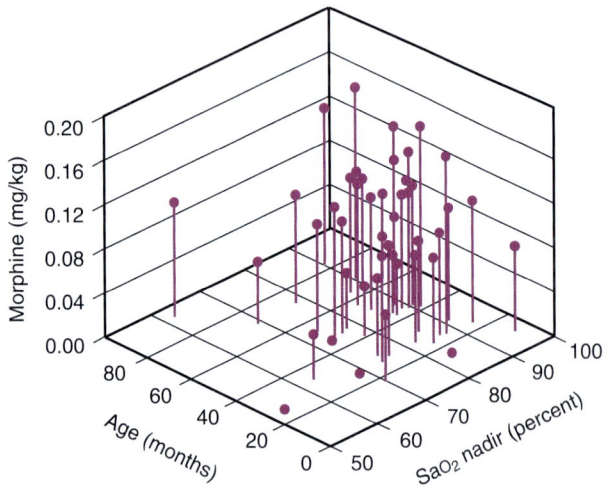

FIGURE 31.14 Relationship between morphine requirement, age, and the preoperative arterial oxygen-saturation nadir in 46 children who were otherwise well. The lengths of the stems supporting the 46 dots are proportional to the morphine equivalent dose. The stems in the foreground are shorter than those in the background, indicating a significant correlation between the three variables. Sao_2, Arterial oxygen saturation. (From Brown KA, Laferrière A, Moss IR. Recurrent hypoxemia in young children with obstructive sleep apnea is associated with reduced opioid requirements for analgesia. *Anesthesiology.* 2004;100[4]:806-810.)

Total analgesic dose (mg/kg)
0.25
0.20
0.15
0.10
0.05
0.00
*
*
<85%
≥85%
Oxygen saturation nadir
Calculated
Standard

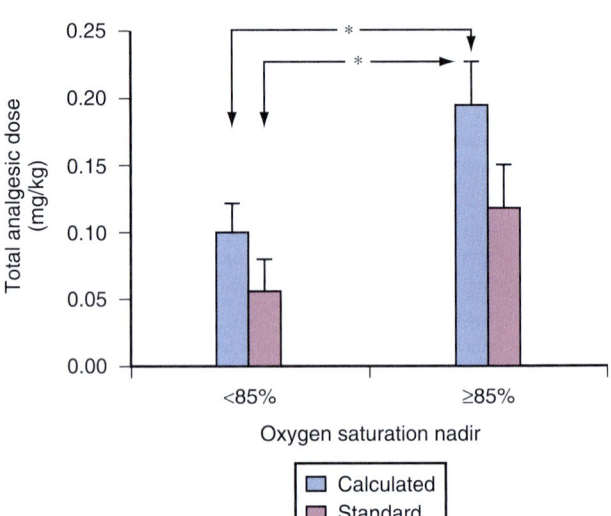

FIGURE 31.15 The total analgesic dose of morphine equivalents required to achieve a uniform analgesic endpoint in children with obstructive sleep apnea (OSA). Children were grouped by severity of OSA into those who had a preoperative SpO_2 nadir of <85% or ≥85%. The *asterisks* indicate post hoc differences between groups, $P<0.05$. (From Brown KA, Laferrière A, Lakheeram I, Moss IR. Recurrent hypoxemia in children is associated with increased analgesic sensitivity to opiates. *Anesthesiology.* 2006;105[4]:665-669.)

OSA may exaggerate the respiratory depression.[373,437,630] Therefore, opioid dosing must be adjusted for the child's weight, severity of nocturnal desaturation and pharmacogenomic differences, and observed individual analgesic responses; for obese children the ideal or lean body-weight is commonly used to avoid such overdosing.[406,461,631]

Dose Titration

In children at risk for opioid-induced respiratory depression from chronic nocturnal desaturations, one technique involves the use of spontaneous respirations during maintenance of anesthesia with sevoflurane and observation of response to incremental opioid doses (e.g., fentanyl 0.5 µg/kg or morphine 10 µg/kg IV).[434,632] To test whether individualized opioid dosing responses reduced the frequency of perioperative respiratory adverse events, 280 children undergoing adenotonsillectomy with a parental history of snoring and pharyngeal obstruction from tonsils were randomized to either an individualized opioid dosing regimen or a standard dosing regimen.[633] All children received fentanyl 1 µg/kg IV before extubation. For those in the individualized dosing group, if their respiratory rate decreased ≥50% after the dose of fentanyl, they received small, serial doses of morphine (10 µg/kg IV) for pain in the PACU, whereas if their respiratory rate decreased <50%, they received morphine increments of 50 µg/kg IV. In the control group, every child received 25 µg/kg IV morphine to treat pain. The frequency of perioperative respiratory adverse events in the individualized group (~12%), was about half that in the standard dosing regimen (~22%) ($P=0.025$).

The Society of Pediatric Anesthesia recommends that in patients with OSA, opioid doses should be reduced by ~50%, with extended monitoring (level B evidence).[553] In children who desaturate to <85% at night or who are clinically diagnosed as having severe OSA, a trial of a dose of opioid before emergence to assess the child's sensitivity to opioids is warranted (as described above), with a plan to reduce the postoperative opioid administration if the response to the trial shows an increased sensitivity.

Codeine and CYP2D6

There is no preferred oral opioid to treat perioperative pain after adenotonsillectomy; however, codeine should be avoided,[634-636] as it may increase the risk of critical opioid-induced respiratory depression due to CYP2D6-genotype dependent liver metabolism leading to unpredictable plasma levels of more potent active metabolites.[635-639] Tramadol has also come under criticism, despite a lack of any evidence that the metabolite might cause harm.[640] Both codeine and tramadol are currently contraindicated in children <18 years of age undergoing tonsillectomy based on revised FDA guidance.[435,635,637-639] It is noteworthy that some CYP2D6 metabolism also occurs with oxycodone and hydrocodone, producing the more potent metabolites noroxymorphone and hydromorphone, respectively. Children undergoing adenotonsillectomy managed with oxycodone and hydrocodone postoperatively may therefore be subject to some metabolic heterogeneity and increased risk of opioid-induced respiratory depression,[641,642] particularly with concomitant use or discontinuation of CYP3A4 inhibitors (e.g., clarithromycin) that increase hydrocodone and oxycodone plasma concentrations that could result in fatal respiratory depression.[643,644] As with tramadol, this remains unproven.

Oral morphine, which undergoes glucuronidation to produce less potent glucuronide metabolites,[645] has been prescribed at a dose of 100 to 200 micrograms per kilogram[646] every 3 to 4 hours as needed in children 2 to 12 years old.[646,647] However, all opioids are associated with considerable pharmacokinetic and pharmacodynamic variability; a smaller oral dose of 100 micrograms per kilogram is prudent. The continued use of opioids in children with severe OSA postoperatively may further impair arousal mechanisms,[648-652] which may have been a contributing factor in the reports of deaths from apparent apnea after hospital discharge.[127,225,653] Concerns have been raised regarding opioid-associated hyperalgesia with short-acting agents (e.g., remifentanil)[654]; however, it is unclear if this occurs in the pediatric adenotonsillectomy population.[655,656] Finally, an opioid stewardship program should be implemented to oversee opioid use within and outside of the hospital to address the potential for abuse, diversion, addiction, or accidental ingestion (especially by young children) by the patient or other household members.[552,657]

Avoidance of Opioids

Preliminary evidence suggests that implementing an enhanced recovery after surgery (ERAS) protocol improves pain, anxiety, and diet in the first week after surgery.[658] Measures to reduce anxiety including parental presence in the PACU,[659] preoperative and postoperative parental and child pain education,[660] improved written discharge instructions, and follow-up instructions, have only modestly improved postoperative pain[661]; relaxation, simple distraction, and guided imagery have a negligible impact.[662]

Complete avoidance of opioids is an alternative approach. Ketamine can be administered intravenously, orally, infiltrated locally, or applied topically; a systematic review and two meta-analyses have examined the advantages and disadvantages of these analgesic techniques.[562,663,664] A single dose of IV ketamine (0.25-0.5 mg/kg) improves short-term (<8 hours) and long-term (up to 24 hours) pain, reduces morphine consumption, and alone,[665] or at a reduced dose (0.15 mg/kg) combined with dexmedetomidine (0.3 µg/kg), reduces the incidence of emergence delirium.[666] Ketamine has been associated with increased sedation,[667,668] although, hallucinations, nightmares, and dissociative symptoms are uncommon and the need for prophylactic antisialogues is not usually required at doses <0.5 milligrams per kilogram.[556] Low-dose IV ketamine (0.25-0.5 mg/kg) alone or when combined with IV dexamethasone is associated with a reduced rate of PONV because of effective pain control and reduced analgesic requirements, including opioids.[664,667,668]

Infiltration of the tonsillar bed with ketamine (0.5 mg/kg) compared with placebo is reported to provide short-term analgesia (<5 hours)[663,664] and may reduce analgesic requirements up to 24 hours either alone[667,669] or when combined with bupivacaine (0.25%).[670] While IV or infiltrated ketamine provide similar pain relief, infiltration is associated with less dynamic pain with swallowing and analgesic consumption for the first 24 hours; when combined with local anesthetic this approach may delay the time to first analgesia by an additional 8 hours.[667,670,671] Preliminary evidence also suggests that even topically applied ketamine (20 mg) may prolong postoperative analgesia and reduce the need for acetaminophen compared with placebo in the first 24 hours,[672,673] whereas oral ketamine (5 mg/kg) is less effective than an equivalent dose injected locally.[674] Other routes of ketamine administration (intranasal, nebulized, and rectal) require further investigation.[609,675,676] In patients where acetaminophen and/or NSAIDs are contraindicated, a single intraoperative dose of IV ketamine (0.2-0.5 mg/kg) is recommended as part of an opioid-free and opioid-sparing multimodal analgesic protocol.[562,677,678] The benefit of combining ketamine with a basic analgesic regimen (including opioids) beyond 24 hours is unclear.

Clonidine[679] is described as an oral preoperative (2–4 µg/kg)[680] or postoperative (1–2 µg/kg) analgesic in some guidelines for tonsillectomy[563]; however, studies have failed to demonstrate any incremental analgesic benefit from oral,[681] intramuscular,[682] or locally infiltrated clonidine.[683] Administering clonidine 60 to 90 minutes preoperatively presents additional challenges to consider, including a delayed recovery; although this delay is dose dependent,[488] it can be a major consideration for a busy list of brief surgical procedures.

Dexmedetomidine has also been advocated for postoperative analgesia.[562,684–686] The oral bioavailability of dexmedetomidine is poor, but when administered intranasally (2–3 µg/kg), it is well tolerated, easily administered, and has an 83% success rate, but has a delayed time to peak blood concentration (37 minutes) and sedation (20–40 minutes) compared with oral midazolam.[687–689] The half-life of IV dexmedetomidine is brief (1.8 hours) in children[690] and 1 microgram per kilogram has analgesic equivalence with IV morphine (100 µg/kg).[27] An infusion of dexmedetomidine (2 µg/kg IV over 5–10 minutes followed by 0.7 µg/kg per hour) may reduce postoperative opioid requirements,[691] with greater doses of dexmedetomidine (2 and 4 µg/kg) increasing the opioid-free interval and decreasing postoperative opioid requirements but prolonging PACU stay.[692] The opioid-sparing quality of intraoperative IV dexmedetomidine (0.3–1.0 µg/kg) has appeal in patients with severe obstructive sleep-disordered breathing/OSA,[558,684,691] as it has minimal effect on the tone of the upper airway muscles and ventilatory drive while providing effective, but short-lived (30 minutes) postoperative analgesia and better analgesia when compared with fentanyl.[562,685] In addition, IV dexmedetomidine reduces anesthetic requirements[693] and risk for emergence delirium (95% effective dose 0.38 µg/kg)[694] but it does not delay discharge from PACU, although more sedation in the early recovery phase has been reported.[685] The reduced incidence in emergence agitation and PONV did not impact discharge from PACU.[695,696] Dexmedetomidine may protect against respiratory adverse events associated with benzodiazepines in the presence of OSA.[155,429,678] The benefit of adding dexmedetomidine to a basic analgesic (including opioids) regimen beyond 24 hours still requires clarification.

Blockade of neural input to the upper airway dilator musculature in children with OSA is problematic. Serious life-threatening complications including severe upper airway obstruction, loss of protective reflexes, and pulmonary edema[697] may occur. In children with OSA, the larynx is smaller in size,[477,698] more collapsible,[140,330,699] and susceptible to compromised airway patency with the application of topical anesthesia.[700]

Topical lidocaine spray may provide short-term (20 minutes) postoperative analgesia,[701] and a meta-analysis was equivocal about its use after adenotonsillectomy although the reporting quality of the included trials was poor.[702] A systematic review found that local anesthetic infiltration reduced pain after adenotonsillectomy in only half of the published pediatric studies.[562] Although local anesthetic infiltration into the tonsillar fossa during tonsillectomy can provide brief postoperative pain relief (E-Fig. 31.5),[703] it is associated with life-threatening complications such as inadvertent intraarterial injection and at best provides only a modest reduction in pain after adenotonsillectomy[704,705] such that injection of local anesthesia in the tonsillar fossa does not have a favorable risk-benefit ratio.[697,706] The benefit of adding local anesthetic infiltration to a basic analgesic regimen (including opioids) beyond 24 hours is unclear.

Glossopharyngeal nerve blocks reduce postoperative pain (including pain with swallowing), analgesic requirements, and time to first analgesia for up to 12 hours after adenotonsillectomy[707–709]; an obtunded gag reflex correlates with clinical analgesia. Although 5 milliliters of 0.25% bupivacaine plain is considered safe and efficacious,[709] it can also cause life-threatening upper airway obstruction by producing unintended block of adjacent nerves that adduct the vocal cords (recurrent laryngeal nerves) and loss of motor function of the tongue and upper pharyngeal muscles (hypoglossal nerves); hypertension and tachyarrhythmias (concurrent glossopharyngeal and vagal neural blockade), and subsequent postobstructive upper airway pulmonary edema may occur.[697,710] The impact of the block on upper airway function in children with obstructive sleep-disordered breathing/OSA is unclear. The suprazygomatic maxillary nerve block, which limits glossopharyngeal nerve involvement, has been proposed as a safe alternative block[711]; however, evidence for its effectiveness in children undergoing adenotonsillectomy remains anecdotal (see Chapter 40).[712]

A preoperative oral dose of gabapentin (10–20 mg/kg) reduced pain scores and analgesic requirements in children undergoing adenotonsillectomy up to 18 hours after surgery compared with placebo, acetaminophen, or when combined with acetaminophen.[713,714] However, no clinically significant analgesic effect for the perioperative use of gabapentinoids has been observed in adult patients.[715] The usefulness of this drug for acute pain management is doubtful. It is suggested that single-dose preoperative gabapentin is only indicated when acetaminophen and/or an NSAID are contraindicated, opioids cannot be tolerated, or the child exhibits opioid tolerance.[562] It is possible that gabapentin may reduce the opioid dose requirement, and limit respiratory depression, excessive sedation, dizziness, and prolonged PACU stay[715–717]; however, this is unproven.

Several meta-analyses suggest that magnesium sulfate may provide a small analgesic benefit when administered locally (not systemically) and may reduce the incidence of laryngospasm and emergence delirium.[718–720] Repeat topical applications of sucralfate as an oral rinse may have a weak adjunct analgesic benefit, in the first postoperative week, particularly after a "cold" surgical technique.[721–723] Several Cochrane reviews demonstrated that prophylactic antibiotics neither reduce pain nor the need for analgesics after adenotonsillectomy.[724]

Other treatment modalities have been reported.[725] Acupuncture can reduce pain and analgesic requirements after adenotonsillectomy.[562] Honey reduced pain scores and postoperative analgesia requirements, although benefits were small.[726–729] Active preoperative nutrition counseling and a standardized liberal oral fluid intake up to 2 hours before surgery may improve patient well-being and reduce analgesic requirements after adenotonsillectomy.[730–732] However postoperatively, restricting resumption of eating and activity had no impact on the severity of pain.[733]

The surgical technique can impact the severity and duration of postoperative pain. "Hot" techniques cause greater postoperative pain than "cold" techniques, possibly the result of increased thermal tissue injury,[608,734–736] whereas an intracapsular tonsillotomy is associated with less pain and morbidity than the conventional extracapsular approaches (see earlier).[653,737,738]

ADENOTONSILLECTOMY COMPLICATIONS

Complications from adenotonsillectomy are organized by their timing relative to the surgery (Table 31.7). Operative complications are uncommon but include trauma to the teeth and other

TABLE 31.7	Complications Associated with Adenotonsillectomy in Children
Onset	**Description**
Immediate	• Trauma or burn (secondary to surgical technique or airway device ignition) to eyes, lips, teeth, mandible, temporomandibular joint, cervical vertebra, tongue, uvula, soft palate, pharynx, carotid artery, and larynx • Compression or dislodgement of airway device • Bleeding at surgical site
Intermediate **(in PACU or** **within the** **first 24 postop** **hours)**	• Emergence delirium • Pain including referred otalgia • Major respiratory event including postobstructive pulmonary edema and aspiration • Nausea and/or vomiting • Primary bleeding (due to surgical technique) including need for blood transfusion • Death secondary to respiratory adverse event and/or bleeding
Delayed **(after the first** **24 postop** **hours)**	• Pain including referred otalgia • Nausea and/or vomiting • Dehydration, delayed feeding, or fever • Secondary bleeding (due to wound healing) including need for blood transfusion up to 2 weeks • Speech disorders (e.g., velopharyngeal incompetence) • Injury to hypoglossal, glossopharyngeal, or vagal nerve causing transient/permanent dysphagia or altered taste • Persistent or recurrent obstructive SDB/OSA • Tonsil regrowth or recurrent tonsillitis • Nasopharyngeal stenosis • Neck infection • Internal jugular vein thrombosis • Death secondary to respiratory adverse event and/or bleeding

OSA, Obstructive sleep apnea; *PACU*, postanesthesia care unit; *SDB*, sleep-disordered breathing.
Modified from Murto KT, Zalan J, Vaccani JP. Paediatric adenotonsillectomy, part 1: surgical perspectives relevant to the anesthesiologist. *Brit J Anaesth Educ.* 2020; 20(6):184-192.

airway anatomy structures, carotid artery injury causing bleeding or accidental intraarterial injection of local anesthetic causing arrhythmia, eye injury, mandibular subluxation, condylar fracture, perioral cautery burns, and ignition of the TT.[95] Adopting a hot surgical technique has reduced intraoperative bleeding, although burns, airway fires, and increased postoperative pain may occur.[739] Decreasing the risk of injury associated with an airway fire includes reducing the inspired oxygen concentration to ≤30% before using cautery, being prepared to extinguish a fire should one occur, and removing an ignited TT immediately. Compression or accidental dislodgement of the airway device due to placement or removal of the Boyle-Davis gag should not be confused with bronchospasm. Complications after local anesthetic infiltration in the tonsillar fossa including intracranial hemorrhage, bulbar paralysis, deep cervical abscess, cervical osteomyelitis, medullopontine infarct, and cardiac arrest have been reported; these complications may outweigh the potential benefits especially since the duration of analgesia is brief.[697,706]

Emergence and Recovery

Extubation

Blood, secretions, and/or irrigation fluids in the oropharynx after surgery should be suctioned before emergence from anesthesia to prevent aspiration and laryngospasm. Historically extubation was preferred when the child was fully awake[740] but a careful deep extubation is increasingly being advocated; major respiratory complications requiring positive airway pressure, administration of drugs, airway manipulation, or instrumentation are similar after deep or awake extubation (~11%).[373] Inserting an oropharyngeal airway (or nasopharyngeal airway placed by the surgeon) before extubation is useful.[396] To increase both the cross-sectional area and total volume of the upper airway compared with the supine position,[741] the child should be positioned in the lateral "recovery" or "tonsil" position with the head slightly down to avoid blood and secretions from pooling in the laryngeal inlet during emergence. This position is maintained during their transport to and stay in the PACU until the child is fully awake (Fig. 31.16).

Neuromuscular Compromise

Residual neuromuscular blockade will selectively depress the integrity of the upper airway dilators compared with the diaphragm, promoting collapse of the pharyngeal airway.[742] Therefore, quantitative neuromuscular blockade monitoring is recommended if paralysis was used and the neuromuscular blockade should be antagonized before emergence and extubation.[358,743,744] Atropine administered after induction of anesthesia has been reported to decrease the risk of postoperative adenotonsillectomy respiratory complications,[443] possibly enhancing the activity of the genioglossus muscle,[745] whereas neostigmine has been shown to selectively depress the activity of the pharyngeal dilator muscles[746] and in adults, excessive dosing is associated with increased postoperative respiratory complications.[747] Sugammadex, is considered a "pharyngeal muscle sparing drug" compared with neostigmine and may be a better choice of reversal agent in children with severe OSA.[748–751] Avoiding nondepolarizing muscle relaxants in patients with severe OSA may be prudent as relaxants blunt the carotid body sensitivity to hypoxemia in healthy adult volunteers, which is not reversed by antagonists[752]; similar evidence in children is lacking. In addition, opioids depress activity in the pharyngeal dilator muscles, including the genioglossus muscle.[626,753–755] Given the increased sensitivity to both analgesic and respiratory effects of opioids in children with severe OSA, small doses of naloxone may alleviate upper airway obstruction after adenotonsillectomy if a relative "overdose" of opioids has been administered.

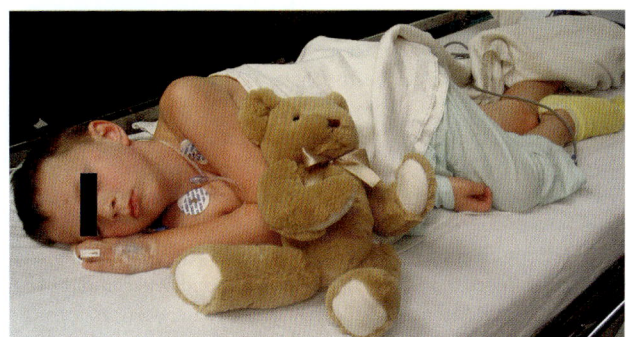

FIGURE 31.16 Child in the recovery position, lateral decubitus, for transfer from the operating room to the recovery room.

Respiratory Events

Children are at an increased postoperative risk for major adverse respiratory events (laryngospasm and bronchospasm, apnea, obstruction, and oxygen dependence), transient desaturation, PONV, pain including referred otalgia, emergence delirium, and bleeding,[95] with an overall frequency of postoperative complications of 19% immediately after adenotonsillectomy.[224] Depressed respirations, hemorrhage, pain, fever, nausea and vomiting, and dehydration are the most frequent early postoperative complications. The rate for a major adverse respiratory event after adenotonsillectomy in children is ~5.8% (95% CI, 4.2%–7.4%),[353] which may be as much as five times greater in children with OSA.[224] Children younger than 3 years of age are particularly prone to respiratory complications such as obstructed breathing after adenotonsillectomy.[756,757]

As described earlier, opioids should be carefully titrated in small incremental doses while observing respiratory responses intraoperatively in those with moderate-to-severe OSA.[381] Such a systematic approach to opioid administration has been associated with a reduced incidence of adverse respiratory events, abbreviated recovery time, and a 3-fold reduction in hospital admission.[338,381,498,633] In PACU, children with SDB after a number of painful surgeries were found to experience increased pain as well as increased sensitivity to the analgesic and respiratory effects of opioids.[439,535,536,758]

Measures to maintain postextubation airway patency include insertion of a nasal airway, administration of bronchodilators, and racemic epinephrine; reintubation is rarely required. The application of noninvasive ventilatory support (e.g., CPAP or BiPAP, high-flow nasal oxygen), particularly in children with preexisting neurologic disorders, may also be useful.[759,760] Children with complex medical diseases, who depend upon upper airway musculature function may benefit from delayed extubation. Noncardiogenic pulmonary edema may result from the acute relief of chronic upper airway obstruction and may present perioperatively and require supportive measures.[761–763]

Postoperative Nausea and Vomiting

PONV is common after adenotonsillectomy (~21%; range: 13%–32%), where the incidence of at least one episode of vomiting ranges from 89% without PONV prophylaxis to 11% in the absence of opioids, a confounder in many of these studies and with prophylactic medications.[501,764–766] PONV is associated with aspiration, bleeding, and prolonged length of stay and is one of the most common reasons for unplanned admission.[767] Rescue treatment for PONV in the PACU should include an antiemetic from a different class than the prophylactic drugs already used, such as droperidol (0.025 mg/kg), promethazine, dimenhydrinate (0.5 mg/kg), or metoclopramide (0.15–0.25 mg/kg).[51,494] However, this recommendation discounts the possible poor effect of the 5-HT$_3$ antiemetics due to single nucleotide polymorphisms (see Chapter 4).[768–771] Redosing the 5-HT$_3$ antiemetic should be considered in the absence of genetic identification of polymorphisms. Droperidol is contraindicated in patients with long QT syndrome and may occasionally cause extrapyramidal effects; these adverse effects are more common with promethazine and metoclopramide and these antiemetics are not recommended for children younger than 1 year of age.[51] Oral ondansetron has been approved for children as young as 4 years of age whereas intravenous ondansetron is approved as young as 1 month of age. Ondansetron tablets can prevent emesis at home in the first 3 days after adenotonsillectomy provided the child can swallow ondansetron in a pill form.[772,773] Children may be offered oral fluids before discharge after adenotonsillectomy, although forcing them to ingest oral fluids increases the frequency of vomitng.[51]

Postoperative Admission Guidelines

Obstructive apnea and worsening of desaturation events during sleep should be anticipated in children with severe OSA on the first night after adenotonsillectomy (E-Fig. 31.6),[345,774] underscoring the need to admit these children for continuous overnight monitoring. In addition to pulse oximetry, common monitors in the postoperative setting include photoplethysmography, transthoracic impedance, and capnography. Respiratory events are multifactorial, usually occurring within the first 24 hours of surgery but potentially preventable with improvements in care-team awareness of the OSA diagnosis with related adjustments in sedative and opioid dosing and bedside assessment of sedation level, monitoring of oxygenation, and ventilation.[433,775] Excessive sedation predicts impending respiratory arrest, whereas supplemental oxygen can provide a false sense of security by maintaining adequate oxygen-saturation levels in the face of increasing carbon dioxide tensions.

A limitation of transthoracic impedance is that obstructive respiratory efforts may be falsely interpreted as respirations with a patent airway.[776,777] Postadenotonsillectomy nasal capnography in the setting of nasal secretions may be poorly tolerated and inaccurate. Transcutaneous CO_2 monitors may be useful in somnolent children, but they do not provide second-to-second data. Without a consensus for factors that warrant an ICU admission, local guidelines determine this decision, which incorporates preoperative risk stratification and factors related to the patient's intraoperative and postoperative course.

Although children without apnea can undergo ambulatory surgery, *adenotonsillectomy for obstructive breathing in children with severe OSA should be undertaken as an inpatient.* Obese children, children younger than 3 years of age, those with comorbid conditions affecting the airway (e.g., trisomy 21), and those with severe polysomnogram documented OSA should be admitted and closely observed due to the increased risk of perioperative respiratory adverse events.[95,96,127,212,246,247,399,616] The implementation of posttonsillectomy admission guidelines decrease the overall rate of unplanned admission to the hospital after adenotonsillectomy[247]; the current pediatric tertiary-care admission practices after adenotonsillectomy show considerable variability among institutions. (Fig. 31.17).[616,778] Oxygen-desaturation nadir and peak ETCO$_2$ may be more important than AHI in predicting respiratory adverse events in children undergoing adenotonsillectomy.[315,318,779] As fewer than 12% of children are evaluated with a polysomnogram before surgery, overnight pulse oximetry, a metric of the cumulative nocturnal oxygen debt, is a useful alternative screening tool for OSA as described above when a polysomnogram is unavailable.[91,96,295,780]

In children with suspicion or diagnosis of OSA, different algorithms are available to guide the disposition planning and indications for postoperative admission.[246,396,463,777] Because the onset of respiratory complications in children with severe OSA may be delayed,[345,441,454] practice guidelines from the AAO-NHS, the American Academy of Pediatrics (AAP), and the American Society of Anesthesiologists all recommend that discharge criteria from a monitored setting should include observation with SpO$_2$ monitoring during sleep[95,190,246] and should extend beyond the commonly used minimum 2-hour observation period,[616] so as not to miss the delayed onset of sleep-related respiratory compromise and deaths from apparent apnea after adenotonsillectomy.[127,232]

Criteria for admission

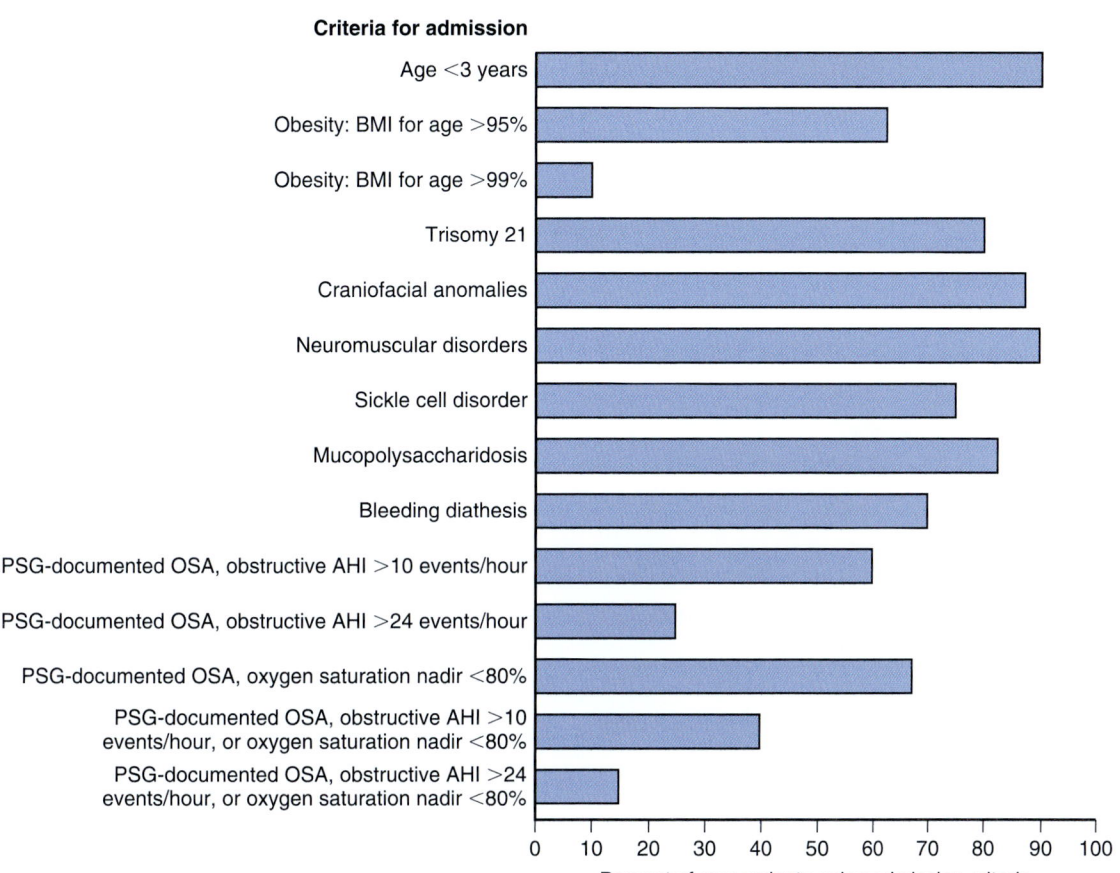

FIGURE 31.17 Admission criteria after adenotonsillectomy. Percentage of respondents from 72 pediatric otolaryngology divisions at tertiary-care children's hospitals using the criteria shown as an indication for admission. It is surprising and counterintuitive that the children with documented obstructive sleep apnea *(OSA)* and the highest apnea hypopnea index *(AHI)* or desaturation (<80%) criteria had the lowest use by otolaryngologists. *BMI,* Body mass index; *PSG,* polysomnography. (From Nardone HC, McKee-Cole KM, Friedman NR. Current pediatric tertiary-care admission practices following adenotonsillectomy. *JAMA Otolaryngol Head Neck Surg.* 2016;142[5]:452-456.)

Not requiring oxygen beyond 3 hours and maintaining oxygen saturations ≥90% on room air for >20 minutes while asleep is one approach to establish the child's fitness for discharge.[779] Table 31.8 presents common admission criteria post-tonsillectomy; criteria vary widely amongst otolaryngologists.

Postoperative Adenotonsillectomy Adverse Events

Postoperative adenotonsillectomy pain, PONV, dehydration, and bleeding may result in an unplanned hospital revisit or postsurgical admission and can occur up to 3 weeks after surgery.[781,782] Pain including otalgia, fever, bleeding, emesis, poor oral intake, and dehydration are the most common reasons for a return to the emergency department after hospital discharge, occurring most commonly in adolescents (11–18 years of age) followed by the very young (0–3 years old). Pain is among the most likely reason for hospital revisit/admission across all age groups.[782,783] Children older than 10 years of age are most prone to secondary tonsillectomy hemorrhage (defined as a hemorrhage 24 hours after surgery), whereas younger children are most prone to poor oral intake, dehydration, and respiratory complications.[784] Posttonsillectomy hemorrhage in children with OSA is less likely than that in children without OSA (OR=0.4).[224]

Long-term complications after adenotonsillectomy are infrequent, but include atlantoaxial subluxation manifesting as neck pain and torticollis, altered taste, cervical adenitis, cervical osteomyelitis, velopharyngeal insufficiency, nasopharyngeal stenosis, and death.[95,333,785] The mortality rate associated with adenotonsillectomy ranges from 0.6 to 4 per 10,000 for outpatient and inpatient procedures, respectively, in the United States.[782,783,786–788] Children with complex chronic conditions undergoing adenotonsillectomy are particularly vulnerable with a reported mortality rate triple of that reported for otherwise healthy children: 11.7 per 10,000 procedures.[789]

Residual obstructive sleep-disordered breathing is more likely to persist after adenotonsillectomy in older (>7 years of age) and obese children, those with severe OSA, those with trisomy 21 or other craniofacial syndromes, those with nocturnal enuresis, African-American children, and those having a history of asthma or allergic rhinitis. Children with these conditions should undergo follow-up assessments that may include polysomnogram and/or drug-induced sleep endoscopy.[128,207,606,790–792] Since OSA affects cardiac autonomic regulation including heart rate variability in children, serial assessments of cardiac autonomic function may hold promise as a biomarker of the presence of OSA.[793] Although controversial, it has been proposed that tonsillotomy may be a risk factor for the recurrence of OSA and may require surveillance compared with tonsillectomy.[109] The reader is directed to excellent reviews concerning the management of residual or recurrent OSA in children.[791,794]

TABLE 31.8	Criteria for Overnight Admission After Adenotonsillectomy

Patient/family demographics

Age <3 years

Live >1 hour away (precludes adequate time to address bleeding/breathing issues at a hospital)

Unstable home environment (precludes adequate supervision or analgesic management)

Patient comorbidities

Craniofacial abnormalities (e.g., trisomy 21, Treacher Collins syndrome)

Morbid obesity

Possible or documented coagulopathy

Sleep disturbance (moderate to severe OSA)

Indication for surgery

Moderate-to-severe OSA

Postoperative problems

Examples include fever, not tolerating oral fluids, or persistent postoperative nausea/vomiting, hypoxemia, or pain

OSA, Obstructive sleep apnea.
From Zalzal G: Personal communications, survey of major pediatric hospitals, 2006.

POSTTONSILLECTOMY HEMORRHAGE

Posttonsillectomy hemorrhage is a surgical emergency that can occur within the first 24 hours of surgery (primary bleeding) or from 2 to 14 days after surgery (secondary bleeding). Primary bleeding is due to failure to establish surgical hemostasis, and is more common in obese and older children,[127,795] whereas secondary bleeding, due to eschar sloughing, is attributed to nonsurgical complications, including specific medications, a bleeding diathesis, or infection. Posttonsillectomy hemorrhage is less likely to occur in children undergoing adenotonsillectomy for obstructive sleep-disordered breathing/OSA than for recurrent infections.[224] In terms of bleeding risks, OSA is not associated with abnormal indices of traditional measures (nonviscoelastic) of coagulopathy in children.[796] Primary bleeding occurs in 0.2% to 2.2% of patients, whereas secondary bleeding requiring surgery occurs in ~3% of children, the latter associated with a 1.6% hospital admission rate.[95,208] Posttonsillectomy hemorrhage originates from the tonsillar fossa (67%), nasopharynx (27%), or both (7%).[797] Commonly used periods of observation for primary hemorrhage depends in part on the surgical techniques: 6 hours for blunt (cold) and 4 hours for hot dissection,[498,797,798] although, observation periods of lesser duration have been advocated.[208]

The anesthetic management of children with posttonsillectomy hemorrhage can be stressful because the parents are anxious and the child is frightened, anemic, hypovolemic, and likely has a stomach full of blood.[799] In one retrospective study of adults and children, nebulized or IV tranexamic acid reduced bleeding and the need for proceeding to surgery to cauterize the tonsillar fossa, but did not affect the hospital stay or rate of blood transfusion.[800] In another similar study, nebulized tranexamic acid reduced the need for operative intervention from 60% to 36% and repeat bleeding from 14% to 5%.[801] The effectiveness of tranexamic acid in posttonsillectomy hemorrhage remains controversial.

The anesthetic record of the original surgery should be reviewed for information about the surgical indication, comorbidities, medications, airway management and any airway difficulties encountered, intraoperative blood loss, and fluid replacement. The duration of bleeding, the estimated volume of blood the child has vomited, current vital signs, IV fluids administered, and physical examination of the child provide information about child's current volume status. Aggressive fluid resuscitation and blood grouping before induction may be required if there is a history of dizziness with orthostatic hypotension (suggesting a blood volume loss >20%).[802] Even without evidence of hypotension, these children may be hypovolemic and have a decreased cardiac output due to peripheral vasoconstriction and reduced intravascular volume.[803]

Acute blood loss precipitates an outpouring of catecholamines resulting in peripheral vasoconstriction, which can be offset once general anesthesia is induced resulting in profound hypotension. To restore the cardiac output and achieve hemodynamic stability before induction of anesthesia, vigorous fluid resuscitation with crystalloids (repeated boluses of 10–20 mL/kg of balanced salt solution) and/or O-negative blood is required. A preoperative hemoglobin or hematocrit should be interpreted based on the child's volume status and the volume of IV fluids administered. For severe hypovolemia, one or more units of red blood cells should be typed and grouped before the child reaches the operating room. *The child must be adequately volume resuscitated before proceeding to the operating room with the goal of achieving an age-appropriate heart rate and blood pressure.*

A child who presents with a tonsillar hemorrhage should be considered to have a stomach that contains swallowed blood. Pulmonary aspiration of blood does not generally induce the same severity of inflammatory injury as acid aspiration, but if a sufficiently large volume of blood is aspirated, it may prove difficult to oxygenate the child due to small airway obstruction. Bleeding arises from two sources in posttonsillectomy hemorrhage: venous (slow bleeding, most common) or arterial (rapid bleeding). However, if bright red blood is observed, the child may quickly exsanguinate if it is not controlled. In this case, bleeding may be temporarily controlled by compressing the carotid artery on the ipsilateral side to the bleeding source and the airway secured as quickly as possible followed by rapid intervention to stop the bleeding. Visualizing the larynx may be difficult if bleeding cannot be controlled by external pressure and if blood clots fill the pharynx.

Before induction of anesthesia, styletted and cuffed TTs, one the same size as that used in the original adenotonsillectomy and one a half-size smaller should be prepared along with two sets of well-illuminated laryngoscope blades and handles, and two large-bore Yankauer-type suction devices (see also Chapters 2 and 12). After routine monitors are applied and the child has been preoxygenated, a rapid-sequence induction (with or without cricoid pressure) should be undertaken.[804,805] Preoxygenation may prove difficult in the very anxious child, especially if the child is actively bleeding. In this situation the child will likely prefer the left lateral position to the supine position, and slight Trendelenburg to drain blood away from the larynx (Fig. 31.18). The left rather than right lateral decubitus position is preferred to insert a right-handed laryngoscope blade at the right commissure to expose the larynx. If the bleeding has subsided, the child may remain supine in the preoperative period for preoxygenation and induction of anesthesia. Anesthesia may be induced with propofol (1–2 mg/kg), ketamine (1–2 mg/kg) or etomidate (0.2 mg/kg), adjusting the dose according to the child's hemodynamic status. Induction should be followed immediately by atropine (0.02 mg/kg) combined with succinylcholine (1.5–2 mg/kg) or rocuronium (1.2 mg/kg) to facilitate a rapid

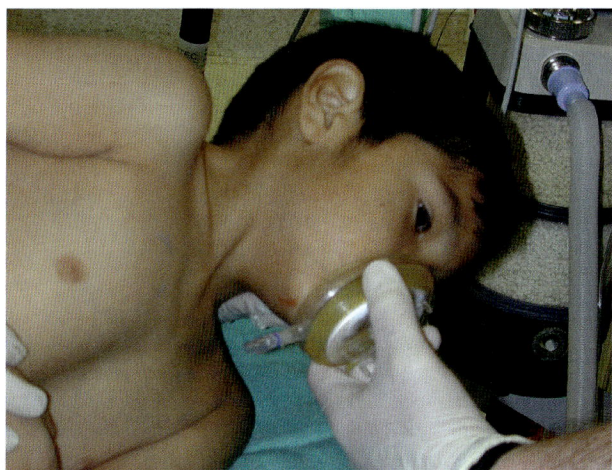

FIGURE 31.18 Preoxygenation with the patient in the lateral position to control posttonsillectomy bleeding before induction of anesthesia.

tracheal intubation. Either rocuronium or succinylcholine can be used in these cases, recognizing that an unexpected difficult intubation combined with arterial bleeding in the oropharynx could rapidly lead to an hypoxic injury if the airway cannot be rapidly secured.[445,806] In the event that brisk bleeding starts once anesthesia is induced and the glottic opening cannot be visualized, the child should be turned to the left lateral decubitus position if they were not already in that position, placed in Trendelenburg, and the oropharynx suctioned using two suctions. The use of a video laryngoscope in an actively bleeding airway may be problematic as blood that soils the camera lens cannot be wiped clean. If securing the airway proves impossible, an emergency surgical airway may be required, recognizing that this requires the child to be supine.

After intubation the concentration of inhalational agent is titrated with nitrous oxide or air in a balance of oxygen.[487] In the majority of tonsil rebleeds, opioids are not required as the mucosal surface and nerve endings therein have already been cauterized during the first surgery.[807] Prophylactic antiemetics such as ondansetron and dexamethasone are commonly readministered.

Children should be extubated when they have regained control of their upper airway reflexes, ideally in the lateral (recovery) position (see Fig. 31.16) to minimize the risk of aspiration should they regurgitate during emergence. If rocuronium 1.2 mg/kg had been used and the duration of surgery was brief, then the train of four should be evaluated and relaxation antagonized with sugammadex as needed.[808–811] A postoperative hemoglobin concentration determination may be indicated to assess whether blood is warranted. When a source of bleeding has not been clearly identified, blood should be sent for fibrinogen, and coagulation indices (prothrombin time, partial thromboplastin time, and platelet count) to rule out a bleeding diathesis (Table 31.9).

PERITONSILLAR ABSCESS

Peritonsillar abscess (quinsy tonsil) is a common deep neck infection. Pus is located between the tonsillar capsule and the superior pharyngeal constrictor muscle, often extending into the soft palate near the superior pole of the tonsil. The most commonly cultured organisms are aerobes, such as *Streptococcus pyogenes, S. milleri, S. viridans,* β-hemolytic streptococci, *Haemophilus influenzae,* as well as anaerobes, such as *Fusobacterium* and *Prevotella* species.[812] The antibiotic of choice is commonly penicillin or a penicillin derivative as most of these organisms are sensitive to this class of antibiotics.[812]

TABLE 31. 9	Anesthetic Considerations for Pediatric Posttonsillectomy Bleed

General
- Emergency surgery versus observe
- Primary vs. secondary bleeding/arterial vs. venous
- Surgical vs. medical bleeding
- Hemodynamic instability
- Aspiration risk
- Bleeding airway

Preoperative
Optimization
- Fluid resuscitation-achieve adequate age-dependent HR/BP
- Type and cross packed red blood cells
- Rule out bleeding diathesis, review blood work

Disposition Planning
- Inpatient surgery
  - Potential need for intensive care

Position
- Supine with neck extension or left lateral decubitus if bleeding is too brisk to remain supine
  - Caution with atlantoaxial instability in trisomy 21
- OR table rotated 90 degrees after airway has been secured
  - Shared/limited access to airway

Procedure
Goals
- Mitigate aspiration
- Maintain hemodynamic stability
- Prepare for a challenging airway

Anesthetic Approach
- Anesthetic technique:
  - Experienced anesthesiologist
  - Preoxygenate
  - Advanced airway equipment available
    - Styletted tracheal tube & two sets of direct laryngoscopy blades/handles
    - Two large-bore suctions
    - Surgeon in OR: rigid bronchoscope and rapid tracheotomy kit ready for use
- IV induction with rapid-sequence induction
  - *If unable to visualize the larynx despite two large-bore suctions, adopt Trendelenburg position, then add left lateral decubitus position. Consider pressure on the right carotid artery if the bleeding is arterial from the right hypopharynx*
- Suction stomach before extubation
- Extubate awake
- Medications:
  - Analgesia:
    - Opioid-sparing or avoid opioids
  - Antiemetic drugs and adjuvant techniques (e.g., superhydration)
  - Other: consider tranexamic acid
- Complications (in addition to those for adenotonsillectomy):
  - Hypoxemia from aspiration
  - Hemodynamic instability/hypovolemia

Postoperative
- Admit overnight
- Risk for (adenotonsillectomy plus):
  - Aspiration
  - Anemia & ongoing bleeding/ hemodynamic instability

BP, Blood pressure; *HR,* heart rate; *IV,* intravenous; *OR,* operating room.

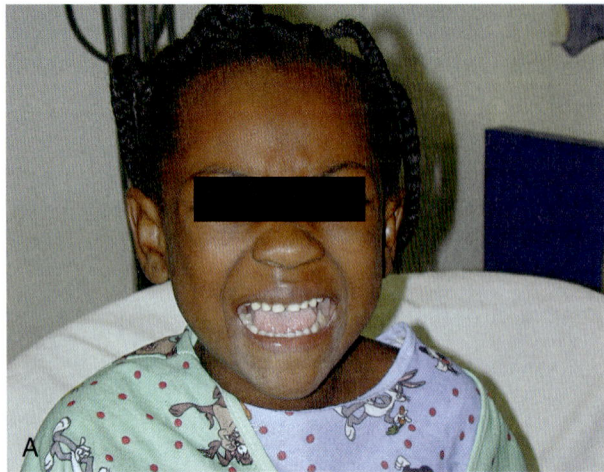

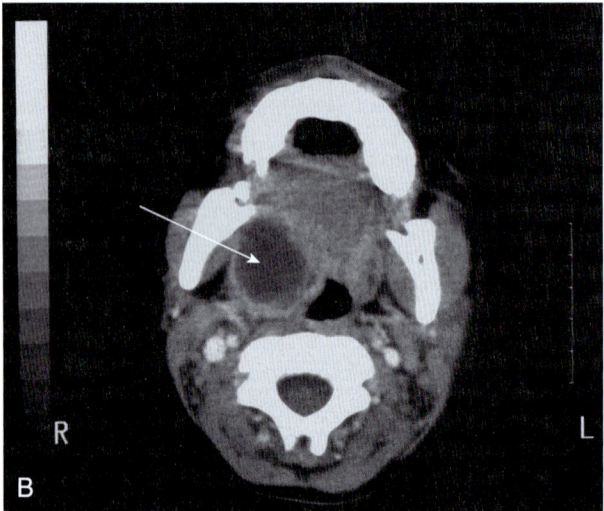

FIGURE 31.19 A, Peritonsillar abscess with trismus. **B,** Axial enhanced computed tomography scan through the oropharynx showing a 3-cm ring-shaped, enhancing, low-density mass *(arrow)* replacing the left tonsil, typical of a tonsillar abscess.

Clinically, children with peritonsillar abscess present with fever, pharyngeal swelling, sore throat, dysphagia, odynophagia, torticollis, and often trismus, which in aggregate can lead to dehydration. Trismus primarily results from pain when the child opens their mouth and is not a structural limitation that would prevent mouth opening for tracheal intubation once the child is anesthetized. Computed tomography of the tonsillar area will identify evidence of any deviation in or compression of the airway and the extent of the abscess in the neck (Fig. 31.19A,B); transcutaneous ultrasound has been increasingly used to confirm the diagnosis.[813] A left-sided abscess is less likely to impact visualizing the glottic opening than a right-sided abscess, although if large enough, an abscess on either side could render the glottis difficult to vizualize. However, such a circumstance could occur and should be anticipated with a backup plan to secure the airway in such an eventuality.

While awaiting the results of the blood cultures, treatment begins with establishing IV access, hydration, and appropriate antibiotic coverage. Nonoperative approaches (antibiotics and analgesics including NSAIDs) have been used with limited success. Early surgical intervention enhances recovery from deep neck infections and reduces the postoperative length of stay,[814] especially for infants and younger children, those with a compromised airway, and those whose abscess exceeds 2 cm in diameter.

Procedures used to drain a peritonsillar abscess include needle aspiration, incision and drainage, and abscess tonsillectomy.[815] Surgical outcomes are similar for incision and drainage versus quinsy tonsillectomy interventions.[816] While most children undergo general anesthesia for treatment by incision and drainage, moderate to deep sedation has been used successfully, although it requires very careful monitoring of the airway for patency and avoidance of spilling pus into the larynx and lungs.[817] If the abscess does not respond to aspiration or incision and drainage, a quinsy tonsillectomy is performed.

The anesthetic management of children with a peritonsillar abscess can be challenging. Most peritonsillar abscesses are in a fixed location in the lateral pharynx and do not interfere with mask ventilation or visualization of the vocal cords. Laryngoscopy should be undertaken avoiding excessive manipulation of the larynx and impinging on the abscess, which may be more difficult because of pharyngeal swelling and distortion of normal anatomy, particularly if the abscess is in the right side of the neck.

The operating room should be prepared as for a difficult airway including different sizes of TTs, stylets, two sets of well-illuminated laryngoscopes, a video laryngoscope, and two working tonsil-tip suctions. The surgeon must be present in the operating room during induction of anesthesia with cricothyrotomy or tracheotomy equipment immediately available to intervene emergently should the airway become obstructed.

Preoperative sedation before induction of anesthesia is generally not required in older children but may be helpful in toddlers. If trismus is present, an inhalational induction should be performed using sevoflurane and oxygen while assessing temporomandibular joint mobility and avoiding an oropharyngeal airway to reduce puncturing the abscess. A neuromuscular blocking drug or propofol may be given to facilitate tracheal intubation once a deep level of anesthesia has been achieved and any trismus resolves. Alternately, a rapid-sequence IV induction may be undertaken after adequate preoxygenation if airway distortion is minimal and to avoid traumatizing the abscess.[2] A cuffed TT is recommended with the child placed in the Trendelenburg position to avoid aspiration of purulent material during intubation and drainage. The trachea should be extubated after antagonism of neuromuscular blockade with the child awake, in the lateral decubitus (recovery) position as in Fig. 31.16.[2]

Anesthesia for Endoscopy

Direct Laryngoscopy and Bronchoscopy

Diagnostic Laryngoscopy and Bronchoscopy

Although diagnostic suspension laryngoscopy and bronchoscopy are generally brief procedures, the anesthetic management can be challenging, especially in small infants and those with comorbidities. In this population, inspiratory and/or expiratory stridor (see Chapters 12 and 13), or noisy breathing caused by obstructed airflow from laryngomalacia is a common indication for a diagnostic laryngoscopy and bronchoscopy (Table 31.10). The evaluation of a child with stridor begins with taking a thorough history including age of symptom onset, which may suggest the etiology (e.g., laryngotracheomalacia and vocal cord paralysis usually present at or shortly after birth, whereas cysts or mass lesions may develop later). Positions that make the stridor better or worse should be determined before induction of anesthesia to reduce the severity of the obstruction. Listening to the child during quiet breathing and crying

TABLE 31.10	Causes of Stridor

Supraglottic Airway

Choanal atresia
Cyst
Mass
Large tonsils
Infection (tonsillitis, peritonsillar abscess)
Large adenoids
Craniofacial abnormalities
Foreign body

Larynx

Laryngomalacia
Vocal cord paralysis
Hemangiomas
Cysts
Laryngocele
Laryngeal web
Infection (epiglotittis)
Foreign body

Subglottic Airway

Subglottic stenosis
Tracheomalacia
Tracheal web
Vascular ring
Foreign body
Infection (croup)
Hemangiomas

provides an indication of whether the airway problem is dynamic or fixed. Suprasternal and supraclavicular retractions, particularly when the child cries, suggest an extrathoracic obstruction. A chest radiograph and barium swallow are infrequently beneficial in diagnosing the airway problem. Similarly, computed tomography and magnetic resonance imaging are not routinely indicated because many airway problems are dynamic, and these radiological assessments are static. Nonetheless, if these investigations are available, they can help to understand the nature of the child's airway problems.

The percentage of airway obstruction and grade may be estimated by comparing the outer diameter of the appropriate TT with the inner diameter of the child's larynx and trachea with a TT that is passed with minimal resistance. Grade I obstruction involves up to 50% of the airway, whereas grade III is greater than 70% (Fig. 31.20A,B).[818] If ventilation is adequate and the anesthetic depth is not excessive after evaluating the severity of the obstruction, the trachea can be extubated and the child transferred breathing 100% oxygen by a face mask.

Laryngomalacia is the most common congenital cause of stridor in infants younger than 1 year of age and most often results from an epiglottis that prolapses posteriorly, redundant arytenoid mucosa that collapses anteriorly, and shortened aryepiglottic folds that collapse medially.[819] The definitive diagnosis is made by flexible laryngoscopy during spontaneous respirations. To rule out a second airway lesion in the trachea or main bronchi, a rigid or fiberoptic bronchoscopy may follow the laryngoscopy. To investigate tracheobronchomalacia, a dynamic 3-phase flexible bronchoscopy approach has also been described that includes static and dynamic assessments of the airway during an induced cough and with the airways distended.[820]

Preliminary examination is usually carried out in the surgeon's office or in the operating room in a lightly anesthetized child during spontaneous respirations with topicalization of the nasal mucosa, whereby a flexible fiberoptic laryngoscope is inserted through the nose into the oropharynx to view the movement of the vocal cords and pharyngeal structures. After movement of the vocal cords is observed and recorded, the anesthetic depth can be increased as appropriate to evaluate the subglottic airway, the trachea, and bronchi using a rigid bronchoscope (or just the telescope in small infants).

Rigid bronchoscopy is useful for the diagnosis and treatment of a variety of airway disorders from the larynx to the proximal bronchi. Rigid bronchoscopy permits dilation of stenosis or scar tissue, marsupialization or debulking of cysts or tumors, biopsy of lesions, and brushing for cytology/bronchoalveolar lavage specimen acquisition.[821] Rigid bronchoscopy has distinct advantages in certain clinical scenarios such as stenting an obstructed airway, retrieval of an obstructing foreign body or assessment during airway hemorrhage. The fiberoptic component of the rigid scope, the Hopkins telescope, may be removed and used to perform tracheal intubation via the Seldinger technique, although a flexible bronchoscope remains the preferred technique.[822] The Hopkins telescope, however, has no suction and does not have any means to ventilate the lungs. Its main advantage is its small diameter to reach narrower airway structures or visualize difficult airways.

Rigid bronchoscopy is the preferred tool to examine the bronchial tree beyond the carina and main-stem bronchi. It is increasingly preferred to assess laryngeal and glottic function with minimal distortion of the airway during spontaneous respirations.[821] In contrast, the flexible scope may be used with local anesthesia and sedation in older children to assess laryngeal and glottic function. Applications of fiberoptic bronchoscopy are evolving and may include electromagnetic, cryo-, and laser technologies, foreign body removal, and the use of airway balloons for dilation, among others.[823–826] Newer endoscopic approaches and techniques include the "triple endoscopy," which allows an interdisciplinary team of an otolaryngologist, pulmonologist, and gastroenterologist to perform their respective endoscopies during a single anesthetic to reduce the number of anesthetics.[820,827,828]

Indications for Endoscopy

The indications for endoscopic evaluation and therapeutic intervention are listed in Table 31.11. The benefits of flexible and rigid endoscopy for various diagnostic assessments and therapeutic interventions in children are compared in E-Table 31.7.[821] Although both endoscopic airway approaches may have roles in managing the difficult airway, particularly in infants, other technologies such as video laryngoscopy are equally effective for intubation as measured by similar success rates of first attempt at intubation.[445,829–831]

Airway endoscopy in children carries with it a greater risk for a compromised airway, and in the setting of a foreign body aspiration, it necessitates close communication between the anesthesiologist and surgeon. The perioperative pediatric mortality reported for foreign body aspirations is approximately 100 deaths per year.[832,833] Children undergoing rigid or flexible bronchoscopy may have associated comorbidities related to feeding, swallowing, breathing, and airway integrity, some arising from underlying neurologic deficits that require careful coordination of anesthetic/surgical plans between the procedural team and the anesthesiologist to minimize risks to the child.[820]

In general, endoscopic airway intervention in children can be broadly categorized into three clinical scenarios: (1) diagnostic laryngoscopy and bronchoscopy; (2) relief of acute airway obstruction;

Percent Subglottic Stenosis by Tracheal Tube Size (mm ID)

A Age	ETT	2	2.5	3	3.5	4	4.5	5	5.5	6
Preterm (<1500 grams)		40								
Preterm (>1500 grams)			30							
0-3 months			48	26						
3-9 months	No detectable lumen	75		41	22					
9 months to 2 years		80			38	20				
2 years		84	74		50	35	19			
4 years		86	78			45	32	17		
6 years		89	81	73			43	30	16	
	Grade IV	Grade III			Grade II		Grade I			

No obstruction

B Obstruction classification	From	To
Grade I	No obstruction	50% obstruction
Grade II	51% obstruction	70% obstruction
Grade III	71% obstruction	99% obstruction
Grade IV	No detectable lumen	

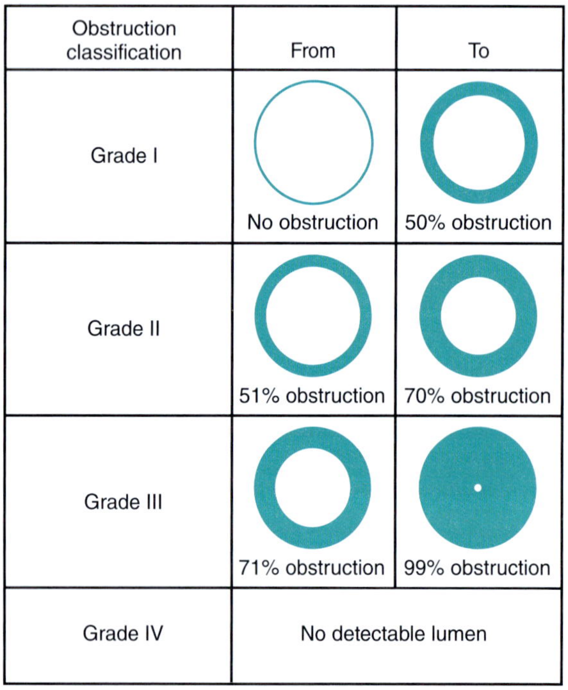

FIGURE 31.20 **A,** Method for estimating the percentage of airway obstruction. After easy passage of an uncuffed tracheal tube (TT), a manometer is placed at the connection of the elbow of the anesthesia circuit and the TT. A stethoscope is placed over the larynx and the circuit is slowly pressurized. The pressure at which a leak is auscultated (10–25 cm H_2O) is matched with the age of the child and the size of the TT to estimate the percent of laryngeal narrowing shown in numbers in teal boxes. Clear boxes indicate the usual size TT for child's age. Grade I, *light teal*; Grade II, *medium teal*; and Grade III, *dark teal*. **B,** Schematic representation of subglottic stenosis classification system. This chart is based on one institution's experience, and the manufacturer of the TTs was not described, thus the actual external diameter of the TTs used is unknown. *ID,* Internal diameter. (Reproduced and modified with permission from Myer CM III, O'Connor DM, Cotton RT. Proposed grading system for subglottic stenosis based on endotracheal tube sizes. *Ann Otol Rhinol Laryngol.* 1994;103[4]:319-323.)

and (3) shared airway surgery. The goals of anesthesia for these three endoscopic indications are similar and include adequate oxygenation, ventilation, circulation, and effective analgesia while acquiring the anatomic and/or physiologic information for diagnostic purposes or to safely and effectively perform a procedure.[834]

The Anesthetic Plan

Anesthetic considerations for airway endoscopy are outlined in Table 31.12. Before induction of anesthesia, a detailed anesthetic and operative plan should be discussed with the surgeon and case-specific drugs and airway equipment checked and organized.

TABLE 31.11 Diagnostic and Therapeutic Indications for Airway Endoscopy in Children

Diagnostic	Therapeutic
Bronchoalveolar lavage (e.g., for cystic fibrosis diagnosis)[a]	Removal of aspirated foreign body or particulate matter[a]
Bronchomalacia, tracheomalacia, or laryngomalacia	Atelectasis unresponsive to treatment
Caustic or smoke inhalation injury	Bronchial blocker placement
Congenital airway anomaly suspected (e.g., laryngeal cleft)	Difficult pediatric airway management[a]
Cough (chronic)	Double-lumen tube placement
Croup (recurrent)	Mucus plugging
Hemoptysis or pulmonary hemorrhage[a]	Pneumonia unresolving/ recurring or requiring toilette[a]
Stenosis or scar[a]	Tracheal esophageal fistula identification and management[a]
Stridor	Tracheostomy evaluation and management[a]
Trauma[a]	Tumors or other airway/ mediastinal lesions[a]

[a]May be both diagnostic and therapeutic.
Modified from Londino AV III, Jagannathan N. Anesthesia in diagnostic and therapeutic pediatric bronchoscopy. *Otolaryngol Clin North Am.* 2019;52(6): 1037-1048.

Some clinicians use a topical lidocaine nebulizer (1%–4%) or a spray (2–4 mg/kg),[835] IV atropine or glycopyrrolate (antisialagogue), aerosolized albuterol (salbutamol), and aerosolized epinephrine to reduce distal bronchial airway edema in the presence of an aspirated foreign body. The vocal cords and subglottic airway are topicalized to decrease the incidence of coughing or straining during instrumentation.

Premedication should be individualized. For these procedures, an inhalational induction with sevoflurane is commonly performed. Nitrous oxide may be used for induction of anesthesia but should then be discontinued to attenuate the risk of oxygen desaturation during the bronchoscopy. Although many embark on anesthesia using sevoflurane as the sole anesthetic, if V/Q mismatch is present because of either a pulmonary or cardiac shunt, if ventilation is intermittently interrupted during the bronchoscopy, or if ventilation becomes very difficult when the telescope is present in the 2.5 to 3.5 millimeter rigid bronchoscope, then supplemental IV agents such as propofol (1–2 mg/kg IV boluses or a 50- to 100-µg/kg per minute infusion), ketamine (0.25–1 mg/kg IV boluses) or changing to a TIVA technique may become necessary to maintain an adequate depth of anesthesia and to prevent coughing and bucking when the bronchoscope is in the airway (E-Table 31.8).

Some practitioners use an insufflation technique by inserting a nasopharyngeal airway with a TT connector attached to deliver anesthetic gases. However, the reliability of this technique is quite variable as the presence of the bronchoscope in the glottic opening dramatically increases the resistance to gas flow across the vocal cords and most surgeons prefer not to be exposed to inhalation agents. Low-dose, short-acting opioids such as fentanyl (0.5 µg/kg bolus) or a remifentanil infusion (0.05–0.2 µg/kg per minute) may smooth the anesthetic, although bolus doses of remifentanil

are generally avoided as they may cause apnea or chest wall rigidity.[53] Dexmedetomidine as a single IV bolus (0.5 µg/kg) or low-dose infusion can also be used to minimize the need for opioids. As TIVA is used increasingly for bronchoscopy, both a hybrid technique using sevoflurane and TIVA or a gas-free TIVA approach are acceptable.[836–838] By ventilating the lungs through the side port on the rigid bronchoscope, anesthesia may be maintained with sevoflurane in oxygen and air. However, when the Hopkins telescope is in the bronchoscope, the lumen of the bronchoscope is occluded with the telescope and attempts at ventilation are met with very high resistance, limiting gas exchange. To offset this resistance, manual ventilation requires greater than usual respiratory rates with 8% sevoflurane in 100% oxygen. This is not the time to reduce the inspired concentration of sevoflurane, but it is the time to administer supplemental IV anesthesia and discuss with the surgeon the need for a pause in the procedure to remove the optical scope, occlude the bronchoscope with a thumb, and allow unimpeded ventilation of the lungs as needed.

During laryngoscopy, additional oxygen may be delivered to the lungs by connecting an oxygen source to the side port of the Parson or suspension laryngoscope, or using the anesthesia circuit by connecting it to a standard 22 millimeter ventilating side port of the rigid bronchoscope. Placing a shortened oral preformed TT at the corner of the mouth or a 3- to 5-centimeter long cut TT within the lateral commissure of the mouth to deliver oxygen is another option. Oxygenation and ventilation in the absence of a TT can be accomplished safely using low and/or high-frequency jet ventilation, typically provided by a Sanders injector via a supraglottic, transglottic, or a transtracheal approach.[839]

In addition to the standard ASA monitors, a precordial stethoscope confirms pulmonary ventilation; without a precordial stethoscope, ventilation may be confirmed by observing the chest rise and fall with ventilation. Continuous monitoring of ventilation by capnography during bronchoscopy is usually not possible because exhaled gases pass through the vocal cords rather than through the bronchoscope.

The main anesthetic considerations for elective airway endoscopy in children include an inhalational induction, IV placement, and then strategies to maintain oxygenation and ventilation depending on the indication for the endoscopy.[833] A deep plane of anesthesia is required to prevent airway reflex responses and oxygen desaturation as well as to prevent movement, which could result in a bronchial or tracheal laceration or perforation with subsequent pneumothorax or pneumomediastinum.

Before finalizing the anesthetic prescription, it is important to confirm the purpose(s) of the bronchoscopy, in terms of whether dynamic or static events will be assessed. If movement of the vocal cords or trachea will be the focus, then the anesthetic should maintain spontaneous respirations, whereas if a mass is sought, then the anesthetic could also include controlled ventilation possibly with muscle paralysis. Oxygenation during the procedure depends on whether the airway is secured or not; apneic oxygenation via low-flow nasal cannula may be considered as an inexpensive adjuvant for most bronchoscopies, regardless of anesthetic technique.[840] Ventilation also varies depending on the procedure to be undertaken and whether spontaneous ventilation is preferred. The choices include using the side port of the rigid bronchoscope or an SGA in the case of flexible bronchoscopy, a continuous or intermittent placement of a TT or low- or high-frequency jet ventilation or apneic oxygenation using transnasal humidified rapid-insufflation ventilatory exchange.

TABLE 31.12	Anesthetic Considerations for Airway Endoscopy

Patient
- Prone to adverse respiratory events
- Potential challenging airway
- Aspiration risk
- Diagnostic vs. therapeutic (e.g., relief of airway obstruction)
- Emergent/urgent vs. elective/repeat procedure

Preoperative
Optimize
- Sedation ± proton-pump inhibitor
- Antisialogue
- Bronchodilator
- Review imaging

Disposition Planning
- Ambulatory or inpatient surgery
  - Potential need for intensive care/extra monitoring

Position
- Supine with neck extension
  - ± shoulder roll
  - Caution with atlantoaxial instability
- Rotate OR bed 90 degrees
  - Limited airway access
- Shared/unprotected airway

Procedure
Goals
- Ensure adequate oxygenation/ventilation
- Minimize patient movement
- Laser precautions
- Rigid vs. flexible bronchoscopy
- Spontaneous vs. controlled ventilation determined by team
- Closed-loop communication with team

Anesthetic Considerations
- GA with inhalation agent and/or TIVA
- Advanced airway equipment available
- Additional monitors include precordial stethoscope and ECG derived respiratory rate

- Surgeon present at induction
- Topical lidocaine to vocal cords
- Multiple methods of oxygenation/ventilation
  - ± Jet ventilation

Medications
- Airway edema: steroids and nebulized epinephrine
- Nebulized bronchodilators
- Airway reflex blunting drug(s)
- Neuromuscular blocking drugs available

Complications
- Failed intubation requiring emergent cricothyrotomy
- Bronchospasm/laryngospasm
- Complete airway obstruction due to a foreign body
- Hypoxemia/hypercarbia
  - ECMO if in extremis
- Hypotension
- Cardiac arrythmias
- Airway trauma
- Pneumothorax/pneumo mediastinum
- Cardiac arrest
- Airway fire with laser
- Aspiration
- Dental damage
- Unretrievable foreign body requiring thoracotomy

Postoperative
- Risk for:
  - Airway edema and obstruction
  - Respiratory adverse events
  - Pneumothorax/pneumo mediastinum
- PACU instructions
  - CXR after removal of a foreign body
  - Delay oral intake after topicalizing the upper airway with local anesthesia

CXR, Chest x-ray; *ECG*, electrocardiogram; *ECMO*, extracorporeal membrane oxygenation; *GA*, general anesthesia; *OR*, operating room; *TIVA*, total intravenous anesthesia.

At the conclusion of bronchoscopy, one of several approaches is undertaken depending on the child's anesthetic state. If the child is breathing spontaneously, an oxygen facemask may be applied, and the child transferred to the PACU. However, if the child remains deeply anesthetized or paralyzed and apneic, a TT may be inserted, and ventilation controlled until the child recovers sufficiently to support their own airway. Intraoperative dexamethasone is commonly administered for its antiemetic effects, although there is no evidence that it is salutary for postbronchoscopy laryngeal edema.[841] If croup develops postbronchoscopy, nebulized racemic epinephrine may be administered. Children who undergo a diagnostic bronchoscopy may be discharged home the same day, but children in whom airway surgery was performed are best observed either in an ICU or a monitored setting overnight.[842] Children in whom a foreign body was removed from the lower airways are usually observed for 12 hours and then discharged if their lungs remain clear.

Jet Ventilation

The principle of jet ventilation involves intermittent pulses of 100% oxygen, that entrains room air into the trachea or bronchoscope via a venturi effect. It is delivered at various driving pressures (10–15 psi if age ≤1 year, 15–35 psi if age > 1 year, and 35–59 psi for adolescents/adults to a maximum of 60 psi), through the tip of a 16-gauge catheter attached to a suspension laryngoscope or a rigid bronchoscope where the pressure is adjusted by a regulator sited near the hand-set.[839,843] In the case of a supraglottic technique, this pulse of oxygen and room air mixture, typically achieving an FiO_2 of 0.8 to 0.9, directly inflates the lungs. Common starting pressures of 10 to 15 psi are incrementally increased until the desired chest movement is detected visually, delivering 8 to 10 breaths per minute to allow adequate time for exhalation via passive recoil of the lungs and chest wall.[844] Although this technique is usually effective for both oxygenation and ventilation in experienced hands, a number of potential problems exist and are listed in E-Table 31.9.[844–846] It is possible to perform supraglottic high-frequency jet ventilation either alone or in combination with low-frequency ventilation for upper airway endoscopy, foreign body retrieval, and laryngotracheal surgery.[846–848] Major concerns remain for obstruction to expiratory flow and other complications including barotrauma, pneumothorax, pneumopericardium, CO_2 retention, necrotizing tracheobronchitis, and gastric rupture.[849,850]

Subglottic jet ventilation can be achieved either by a transglottic or transtracheal approach. A transglottic approach to jet ventilation may be achieved by either placing a specialized catheter below the glottic opening[851] or administering it through the rigid bronchoscope. Transglottic high- or low-frequency jet ventilation utilizes a specialized catheter made of nonflammable, laser-resistant material that has the advantages of creating a favorable pressure gradient for egress of exhaust gases. The FiO_2 is titratable and a second lumen is used to measure the airway pressure and $ETCO_2$ at the expense of having a catheter in the surgical field.[852] Transtracheal jet ventilation is rarely used in children because it is fraught with complications due to the small caliber of the patient airways and anatomical landmarks, making it difficult to place a transtracheal catheter in an awake child for elective surgery. Jet ventilation may be preferred in an emergency using a percutaneous needle cricothyrotomy approach.[839,853] Patency of the upper airway or a transtracheal orifice that is at least twice the diameter of the catheter are needed to allow for egress of gas and avoid barotrauma. Newer devices for transtracheal ventilation are being evaluated that enable active expiration based on the venturi principle.[854]

High-Flow Nasal Oxygenation

Transnasal humidified rapid-insufflation ventilatory exchange (nasal prongs, which can administer a high-flow ($\geq$2 L/kg per minute) heated and humidified air/oxygen mixture via a nasal cannula may provide adequate oxygenation during airway interventions in small spontaneously breathing infants with abnormal airways who are sedated or receiving TIVA; however, ventilation may be difficult to sustain and monitor in older children.[468,855–858]

Complications from Airway Endoscopy

Complications from airway endoscopy depend upon the approach, underlying airway pathology, technique of diagnostic or therapeutic intervention, experience of the surgeon, and the child's age and comorbidities. The most common complications are related hypoxemia, which can lead to bradycardia and, potentially, cardiac arrest; mortality from foreign body aspiration is approximately 4%.[832] Most morbidity data are reported during bronchoscopy for removal of tracheobronchial foreign bodies; common complications and their rate per 10,000 are provided in Table 31.13.

The laryngoscope, Hopkins telescope, and rigid bronchoscope can damage the lips, teeth, gingiva, or surrounding soft tissue. A tooth guard or saline-soaked gauze and adequate hand positioning minimize this risk. When placing tooth guards or gauze in the airway, it is critical to communicate this to operating personnel to ensure they are removed before emergence, to avoid aspirating these devices or obstructing the airway. Laceration and/or laryngeal fracture and damage to the arytenoids or vocal folds have been reported during bronchoscopy. The bronchoscope itself or a therapeutic intervention could cause a pneumothorax or pneumomediastinum that presents as subcutaneous emphysema. If a laser is used, appropriate laser-protective precautions should be utilized including covering the child's eyes with a saline-soaked gauze eye pad. To mitigate the risk of a fire during laser surgery in the airway, saline should be immediately available on the bronchoscopy set; the FiO_2 should be minimized to reduce the fire risk.

Aspirated Foreign Bodies

Objects within the nose or ear of children are usually benign in nature and simple to remove; however, small button-sized battery foreign bodies require urgent removal because of their potential to cause extensive local tissue inflammation and damage.[859] Impacted or displaced objects present greater challenges for the

TABLE 31.13	Morbidity Associated with Bronchoscopy for the Removal of Tracheobronchial Foreign Body in Children	
Complication		**Rate per 10,000**
Major nonfatal complications		96
Tracheal or bronchial tear requiring surgery		5
Nonfatal cardiac arrest		12
Pneumothorax or pneumomediastinum		29
Failed bronchoscopy requiring:		39
Thoracotomy		29
Tracheotomy		11
Laryngeal edema or bronchospasm requiring tracheotomy or reintubation		45
Death		42
Due to bronchial rupture		2
Cardiac/respiratory arrest:		11
During bronchoscopy		3
Postoperative		3

Abstracted from Fidkowski CW, Zheng H, Firth PG. The anesthetic considerations of tracheobronchial foreign bodies in children: a literature review of 12,979 cases. Anesth Analg. 2010;111(4):1016-1025.

anesthesiologist and airway endoscopist as there is a danger of misplacement within the respiratory tract.[860]

Tracheobronchial foreign body aspiration is most common in toddlers 1 to 3 years of age. Incomplete dentition and immature swallowing coordination coupled with a tendency to be easily distracted while eating, or challenges associated with parental supervision contribute to a greater risk of aspiration.[861,862] Although food products are most commonly aspirated in young children, aspiration of inorganic products (e.g., Legos, pen caps, coins, etc.) are more common in older children.[863,864] A history of a choking or gagging event followed by a cough and/or cyanosis while eating or playing is highly suspicious for a foreign body aspiration; however, a persistent cough, or wheezing that does not respond to medical treatment may be the only manifestation, delaying the diagnosis for weeks to months. The majority (95%) of foreign bodies lodge in the right main-stem bronchus.[865] A foreign body that impacts at or near the glottis or in the trachea may present as acute airway emergency, hoarseness, and stridor with a 45% mortality rate[866] from asphyxiation or as chronically hoarse "funny voice" and cough.[855] Foreign bodies too large to pass the carina may lodge in the trachea (<5% of airway foreign bodies),[867] signs of which may include a brassy cough with or without abnormal voice, biphasic stridor, or complete airway obstruction. Although cylindrical-shaped batteries are ingested mostly by adults, button batteries that are disk shaped are mostly ingested by infants or children; in some instances, impacting the supraglottic mucosa or actually aspirated into the airway, resulting in potentially catastrophic consequences if not addressed promptly.[868] Battery diameters may be less than 7 millimeters, but those more than 20 millimeters cause the most serious complications. For comparison, a pencil eraser is 7 millimeters in diameter, a dime 18 millimeters in diameter, and a quarter 24 millimeters in diameter.[868] Some lithium batteries have been inserted into the external auditory canal causing tympanic membrane perforation and in the nose, but the vast majority are swallowed into the esophagus.[869] In 2013, approximately

10.5 patients per million ingested button batteries with a fatality rate of 0.5%. Even after retrieving an ingested lithium battery from the esophagus, bronchoscopic examination of the tracheobronchial tree is warranted to ensure that damage to the tracheobronchial wall has not occurred in cases in which removal of the battery was delayed, if the negative pole impacted the posterior esophageal wall, or the child failed to improve after the battery was removed.[870–872] Aspiration of these batteries constitutes a surgical emergency as damage begins within 2 hours of aspiration, particularly if the negative pole is in contact with mucosa and has a charge >1.5 volts.[871] Any sharp object, or any object that causes acute upper airway obstruction with cyanosis and an inability to maintain ventilation, requires emergent removal.

Similarly, the child who presents with a history of cyanosis after aspiration of a nut very likely has aspirated material into the trachea or into the lungs bilaterally as cyanosis is not a common finding with unilateral bronchial aspiration. Such findings warrant an immediate assessment. Differentiating a coin in the trachea from one in the esophagus is determined with anterior-posterior and lateral radiographs: a coin in the esophagus appears as a flat radio-opaque solid white circle because the esophagus is a flattened tube in the anteroposterior view whereas a coin in the trachea/bronchi may appear end-on because the trachea is oval (anteroposterior axis is greater than the left-to-right axis) (Fig. 31.21A,B).

The type of object aspirated may influence the degree of a local inflammatory response. Unroasted peanuts (with unsaturated double bonds in the oils) should be removed promptly because the oil can induce an inflammatory response in the lungs, resulting in pneumonitis and swelling, rendering later removal of the peanut fragments very, very difficult (Fig. 31.22).[873] In contrast, roasted peanuts (with saturated double bonds in the oils) can remain in the lungs for greater periods (than unroasted nuts) without triggering as severe an inflammatory response. In addition, peanuts tend to swell, fragment, and crumble over time, making "en bloc" removal challenging. Types of bronchial obstruction secondary to the foreign body aspirated and their manifestations on chest x-ray are provided in Table 31.14 and (Fig. 31.23A–C).[855] The more distal the object is lodged in the airway, the more atelectatic changes are noted in the lung segment. A normal chest examination should not exclude the suspicion of an aspirated foreign body as 14% to 45% of children with abnormal bronchoscopic findings have a normal preoperative physical examination.[874–876] High-resolution spiral CT of the chest may be required to diagnose a foreign body when consolidation is present on x-ray.[877] Retrieval of a foreign body is essential due to the risk of atelectasis, bronchiectasis, chronic pneumonias, and granulation tissue formation.[878]

The anesthetic management for bronchoscopy to remove a foreign body depends on the level, degree, and duration of obstruction. Most pulmonologists use flexible fiberoptic bronchoscopy, whereas surgeons use rigid bronchoscopy to remove foreign bodies, with rigid bronchoscopy being the more common approach. However, improved equipment retrieval rates with fiberoptic bronchoscopy approach that of rigid bronchoscopy (99%).[879–881] An additional advantage is that the smaller flexible bronchoscope can reach foreign bodies in more distal airways.

There is no consensus on the optimal anesthetic technique for foreign body removal.[254,882] Most children who present with a foreign body also have a full stomach. In general, removal of the foreign body takes precedence over the full stomach as the child could cough the foreign body into the trachea at any time, totally obstructing their airway and succumb. Nonetheless, if

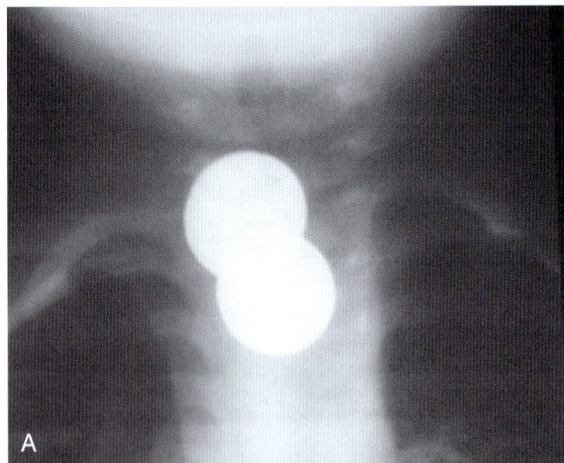

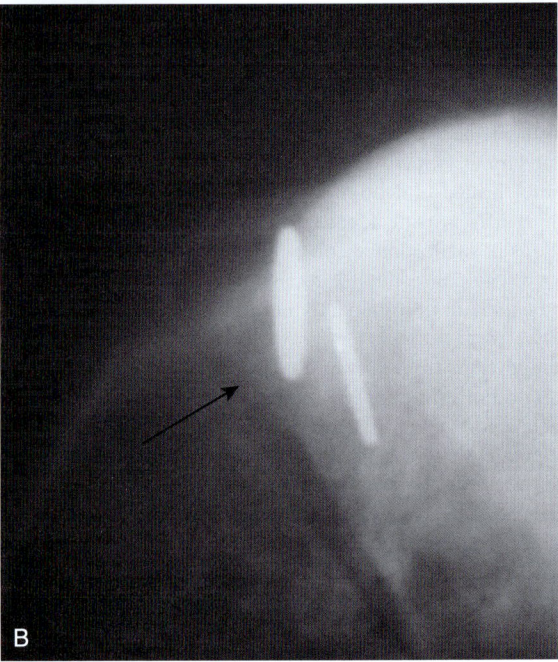

FIGURE 31.21 Anteroposterior **(A)** and lateral **(B)** neck radiographs of a child who swallowed two coins wedged at the cricopharyngeus muscle (upper esophagus). The coins are in the esophagus because in the anteroposterior (A) view, they appear as round solid circles lying in the flat esophagus. Note: these solid foreign bodies in the esophagus are compressing the tracheal lumen (*arrow*).

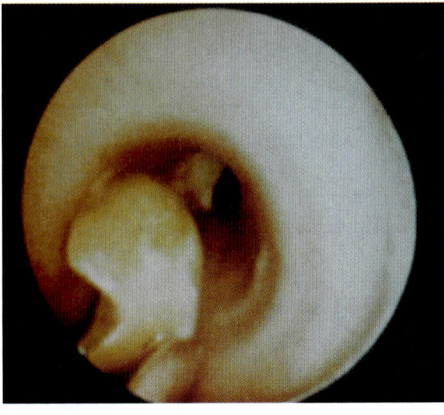

FIGURE 31.22 Classic view of a fractured peanut in the bronchus. Note the irritation as reddened mucosa caused by the oil of the peanut.

TABLE 31.14	Types of Bronchial Obstruction and Their Manifestation on Chest X-Ray	
Type of Bronchial Obstruction	**Explanation**	**Chest X-Ray Manifestations**
Ball-valve	Partial intermittent obstruction of the affected bronchus due to prolapse of foreign body, distal hyperinflation from air trapping may occur	Hyperinflated lung during the expiratory phase may be the only indication of an aspirated foreign body
Bypass-valve	Partial obstruction on both phases of respiration	Normal
Check-valve	Air is inhaled but cannot be expelled during expiration	Hyperinflation of the ipsilateral affected lung with inspiratory/expiratory films
Stop-valve	Air passage is impeded in both phases of respiration	Consolidation of the involved bronchopulmonary segment with subsequent collapse

From Zur KB, Litman RS. Pediatric airway foreign body retrieval: surgical and anesthetic perspectives. *Paediatr Anaesth.* 2009;19 Suppl 1:109-117.

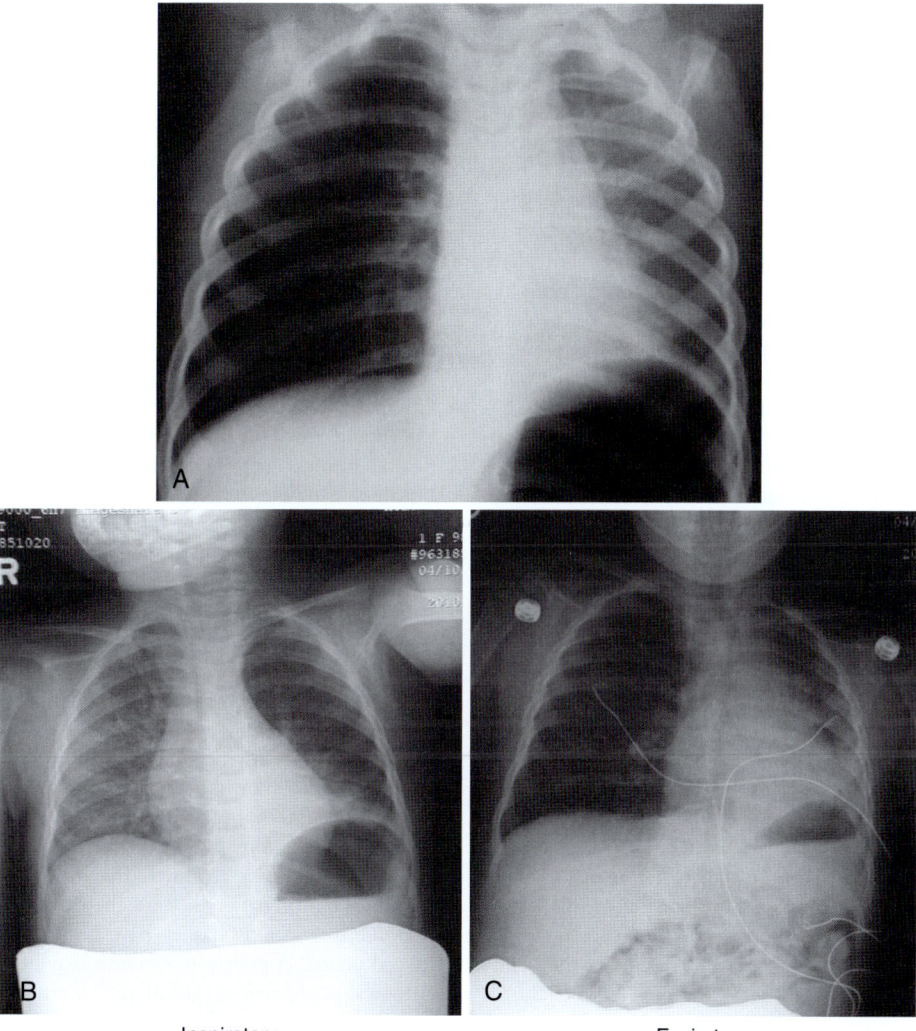

Inspiratory   Expiratory

FIGURE 31.23 A, Expiratory radiograph of the chest demonstrates marked right-sided hyperinflation because of air trapping by the ball-valve effect of the foreign body. The chest radiograph may appear normal during inspiration after foreign body aspiration. **B,** A hyperinflated right lung and **C,** a leftward mediastinal shift during expiration suggests a foreign body in the right main-stem bronchus. (Radiographs courtesy Sjirk J. Westra, MD, Division of Pediatric Radiology, Massachusetts General Hospital.)

there is no evidence of respiratory compromise, some endoscopists delay the bronchoscopy for at least 6 hours to allow gastric emptying or use gastric ultrasound to determine whether food is present in the stomach before proceeding.[882] The decision on which anesthetic technique to use to induce general anesthesia is usually left to the discretion of the anesthesiologist.[833,882] Furthermore, if the child aspirated several pieces of peanut, some pieces may be coughed up and then aspirated into the contralateral lung, contaminating both lungs and increasing the child's morbidity and mortality risks. If surgery is delayed, there is no guarantee that the stomach has emptied even if that involves several hours. If an IV has not been sited, an inhalational induction is performed with the child in the decubitus position in case vomiting occurs during induction. The left lateral decubitus position is preferred as the trachea can be more readily intubated in this position but not in the right decubitus as standard laryngoscope blades are designed to be inserted into the right commissure of the mouth. If an IV is in situ, metoclopramide (0.15 mg/kg) may be given to hasten gastric emptying but it neither guarantees that the stomach will be completely empty of food nor is it widely used in children due to reports of dystonic reactions.[883,884] In the past, an anticholinergic agent was administered to reduce secretions and prevent vagally-induced bradycardia from inserting a rigid bronchoscope, but these are infrequently used today.[855] Anesthetic agents used to blunt reflex bronchoconstriction and promote bronchodilation are detailed in E-Table 31.5.[465,885]

The intraoperative management of an aspirated tracheobronchial foreign body consists of a laryngoscopy followed by a formal bronchoscopy. The anesthetic management is the same as described above for elective diagnostic bronchoscopy with a few notable exceptions. Extraction forceps or extraction baskets for the fiberoptic or rigid bronchoscope should be immediately available. An inhalational induction in 80% oxygen and 20% or more air (as tolerated to prevent atelectasis) will require extra time, particularly for an insoluble anesthetic such as sevoflurane, as shunts delay the wash-in of insoluble agents to a much greater extent than soluble agents (such as halothane) (see Chapter 5). Patience is required to achieve an adequate depth of anesthesia when such an induction is performed.[2,886,887] Alternately, the depth of anesthesia can be increased rapidly with an opioid,[888] propofol, or a combined approach of inhalational agent (sevoflurane in oxygen) with TIVA drugs such as propofol, remifentanil, or dexmedetomidine. An adequate depth of anesthesia is achieved when there is no patient response to stimulation and spontaneous ventilation is maintained during laryngoscopy, appreciating that children younger than 3 years old tolerate greater doses of remifentanil that maintain spontaneous respirations compared with older children; the airway is topicalized with an appropriate dose of lidocaine.[889]

Once the child is at the desired depth of anesthesia, the airway is passed to the endoscopist who places either a protective wet gauze (edentulous infants) or a plastic dentition guard before inserting a rigid scope. The endoscopist performs laryngoscopy and may apply additional topical local anesthetic to the vocal cords and supraglottic structures.

One of the major controversies in the anesthetic management of foreign body aspiration is whether to control ventilation or allow spontaneous respirations during the bronchoscopy.[833,890] Often the choice is determined by a combination of the child's condition, location of the foreign body, and preference of the attending endoscopist or anesthesiologist. Although rigid bronchoscopy is the most commonly used approach, flexible bronchoscopy inserted through an SGA during spontaneous ventilation is increasingly being used. The foreign body is retrieved with the flexible scope using a basket or cryo retrieval through the bronchoscope's suction.[881,882,891,892] An SGA sized from 1.5 to 2.5 can accommodate flexible bronchoscopes with 2.8- and 4.0-millimeter external diameters, respectively with foreign body baskets (1.2 and 2.0 mm) inserted through their respective suction ports. Theoretical concerns of controlled ventilation further impacting or dislodging the foreign body to worsen gas exchange or creating a ball-valve effect have not been born out in retrospective analyses and a large meta-analysis.[34,833,893] Advantages of a spontaneously breathing child include improved ventilation/perfusion matching, especially for some obstructive lesions and decreased risk of barotrauma. However, disadvantages include oxygen desaturation and respiratory acidosis, as well as hemodynamic instability if the anesthetic depth needs to be adjusted. Neuromuscular blocking drugs ensure immobility during the most stimulating parts of the procedure. Positive-pressure ventilation offers better oxygenation and ventilation, but at the expense of intermittent apnea during extraction of the foreign body.[34,821,855] Conversely, positive-pressure ventilation may advance the foreign body distally. Dexamethasone may be given IV to limit the edema from airway manipulation although this is not evidence based. Nebulized epinephrine may be administered through the bronchoscope to reduce proximal inflamed and edematous mucosa to help reveal an impacted foreign body.

The equipment required to extract a foreign body using rigid bronchoscopy (E-Fig. 31.6) includes a Hopkins telescope with various sizes of laryngeal forceps (upper photo), suspension laryngoscopes with rigid bronchoscopes of different diameters, defogging agent, and a soaked gauze/plastic guard to protect the gums/teeth (lower photo).[821] The size of the rigid bronchoscope is determined by its external diameter, and a bronchoscope of the largest external diameter that can pass the child's subglottic region and not damage the laryngeal structures should be selected (E-Table. 31.10).[821] Fiberoptic bronchoscopy is performed using an endoscopy mask or an SGA and a swivel elbow adapter with a bronchoscopy access port. In smaller children, flexible bronchoscopy through a TT is limited to small-diameter bronchoscopes that may not have a suction port to extract a foreign body. Compared with a TT, an SGA allows the endoscopist to visualize the supraglottic and laryngeal structures and use larger diameter flexible bronchoscopes with a suction port to nebulize topical lidocaine, insufflate oxygen, or blow away secretions.

Intraoperative and immediate postoperative complications for bronchoscopic retrieval of aspirated foreign bodies include hypoxemia, hypercarbia, laryngeal laceration or fracture, and hemodynamic instability. Intraoperative desaturation may range from worsening ventilation/perfusion mismatch and pneumothorax requiring chest decompression to simply informing the surgeon to withdraw the rigid bronchoscope proximally until the distal side ventilating port is able to ventilate the unaffected lung. Anesthesia should be sufficiently deep or the child paralyzed to minimize the risk of a bronchial or tracheal laceration or perforation leading to a possible pneumothorax or pneumomediastinum.[833] In a minority of instances, the foreign body cannot be dislodged endoscopically and a thoracotomy is required. This may occur with an unroasted peanut or button battery because these often elicit an inflammatory response, particularly if they have been in the airway for a prolonged period. A patient in extremis may be a candidate for extracorporeal membrane oxygenation.[894] Complete airway obstruction can result if the object being removed is dropped in the larynx or trachea, or if the object crumbles (as in a peanut) and becomes lodged in the large airways, necessitating urgent maneuvers such as pushing the object distally into smaller airways. To facilitate removal and reduce the risk of accidentally dropping the object, the clinician can relax the vocal cords with IV propofol or a muscle relaxant. If hypotension occurs, its etiology can be multifactorial, including excessive anesthetic, a pneumothorax, acid-base disturbances, or anesthetic agent-related arrhythmias (e.g., halothane).

After removing the foreign body, a repeat bronchoscopy is performed to rule out the presence of residual matter (5% of the time) within the same or contralateral airway or an airway injury, which may need further evaluation postoperatively.[895] The child can emerge from anesthesia with or without a TT in place depending on the degree and duration of difficulty of the procedure, evidence of airway swelling, hypoxia, or hypercapnia, or complications and medical complexity of the patient. In rare cases, the airway may remain intubated and transferred to the PICU until the airway edema has resolved. Prolonged stays in the PACU due to mild hypoxemia should be anticipated. A detailed handover should occur with the PACU staff and include the specific time the airway was topicalized to avoid aspiration when oral intake (which should be delayed for ~60 minutes after topicalization) is resumed. If the child has postoperative croup in the PACU, nebulized racemic adrenaline (epinephrine) 1 to 5 milligrams should be given and the surgeon informed. If two or more doses are required, the child may benefit from an overnight admission for PICU observation; reintubation is rarely required.[886]

ESOPHAGOSCOPY FOR FOREIGN BODIES

Removal of foreign bodies from the esophagus may fall under the purview of the otorhinolaryngologist, general surgeon or gastroenterologist. Rigid esophagoscopy is commonly used by surgeons, and flexible esophagoscopy by gastroenterologists using an anesthetic technique similar to that used to examine the esophagus for elective procedures. However, in these cases the children usually have a full stomach and require a rapid-sequence induction to secure the airway; contraindications to cricoid pressure are discussed elsewhere (see Chapter 2 and Table 2.10). There are no specific anesthetic issues for these procedures except that the child should remain still during the esophagoscopy; analgesics are not generally required as there is usually minimal pain following the procedure.

Swallowed Objects

Millions of small objects have been swallowed by young children from peas to chunks of food to coins, razors, safety pins, and more.[896] Larger objects cannot pass through the superior constrictor muscle, whereas smaller objects pass through this muscle but often fail to pass through the esophagus into the stomach. Most children who swallow a foreign body present with an anterior-posterior and lateral chest x-ray. Radio-opaque foreign bodies such as metal objects in the esophagus will appear on the radiograph, with coins for example appearing flat and wide on the x-ray because the esophagus is wide and soft,[897] a finding that contrasts with the disk-like appearance of a coin aspirated in the airways, which appears end-on as a narrow line because anterior-posterior dimension of the trachea exceeds its width (see Fig. 31.21). In contrast, nonradio-opaque foreign bodies such as plastic objects will not be visible on a chest x-ray.

Sharp foreign bodies in the esophagus are dangerous and present a daunting task for removal. A sharp object that pierces the wall of the esophagus may enter the aorta or other mediastinal structures, causing mediastinitis and possibly death. To remove the sharp foreign object, the tip is grasped by the forceps to prevent it from piercing any tissues as it is dragged out of the airway. In contrast, a piece of broken glass has several sharp sides, each of which can tear through the mucosa. To remove a piece of glass, trapping the glass in a bag used to withdraw tissue biopsies may protect against mucosal tears as the object is removed. A very difficult esophageal foreign body is the open safety pin. If the open end faces cephalad, the spring is pushed into the stomach, the pin turned around and then pulled up through the esophagus. If the open end faces rostral, the spring can be grasped and pulled cephalad slowly, although the risk of trauma may persist. To preclude damage from the tip of the open safety pin, a Clerf-Arrowsmith safety pin closer or grasper is passed, grabs the two sides of the open pin, and closes it before withdrawing the safety pin.[862]

Lithium (Button) Batteries

Batteries are common objects that are swallowed with ~1:10,000 pediatric emergency department visits annually for battery-related reasons with the highest rate among 1 year olds. Battery ingestion is the fourth leading cause of calls to poison control centers in children <5 years of age; ~85% of these result from swallowing button batteries.[898] The ingestion of button batteries has been increasing steadily in the past 20 years.[899]

All batteries are visible on chest x-ray. Button batteries appear as a double halo on the anterior-posterior view and with a step off appearance on the lateral view.[900] Battery ingestion of alkaline batteries confers less damage than other batteries, in part because the anode and cathode are at opposite ends of a cylindrical battery. However, if the acid/alkali gel leaks out, it can corrode adjacent mucosal tissue. Rechargeable batteries contain nickel, cadmium, lithium, or mercury, which themselves are poisonous.[901]

In the case of button batteries, the positive and negative charges are millimeters apart, giving the opportunity to induce isothermic hydrolysis at the edge of the battery, which can lead to an alkaline caustic injury.[902] In addition, button batteries can cause pressure necrosis along with heavy metal toxicity, and caustic damage from leakage.[900] The severity of the esophageal injury depends on the size of the button battery (injuries are greatest in those >20 mm in diameter), the orientation of the negative pole, the duration of contact, and the presence of symptoms.[903] In animal models, button batteries cause mucosal burn injury within 30 minutes of contact and that burn increases over the subsequent 2 to 6 hours, resulting in stricture.[902] The extent of the injury may include a mucosal burn, through and through perforation of the esophageal mucosa, tracheo-esophageal fistula, esophageal stricture, erosion into the aorta resulting in a massive hemorrhage, recurrent laryngeal nerve injury, and death.[900,904,905] Hence, there is a multifaceted approach to limiting the severity of the injury, to neutralize the risk of hydrolysis, and extract the battery as soon as possible. A national battery ingestion hotline has been set up (800-498-8666) for advice on identifying the battery and treatment.[897] The national capital poison center button battery ingestion triage and treatment guideline recommends: (1) establishing that a button battery is in the esophagus, (2) determining if the orientation of the battery's negative pole is contacting mucosa (the narrower side of the battery on the lateral view of the x-ray is adherent to the mucosa), (3) determining the size of the battery (urgency increases if the battery is >20 mm diameter), (4) assuring administration of sucralfate or honey (in children older than 1 year of age) to neutralize the alkalinity and minimize the injury until the battery can be extracted,[906] and then (5) extracting the battery as soon as possible (Fig. 31.24).[897] Once the battery has been extracted, it is imperative to examine the esophagus to determine if an injury is present, put the esophagus to rest by maintaining NPO status, and admit the child for the first 24 to 48 hours after removal to observe for sequelae (mediastinitis, abscess, hemorrhage). If mucosal injury has occurred, antibiotics should be commenced, and an esophagogram performed 1 to 7 days after removal to exclude an esophageal perforation before allowing the child to commence an oral diet. A second esophagogram, rather than upper endoscopy, should be repeated 1 to 2 weeks afterwards to rule out an esophageal stricture.[897]

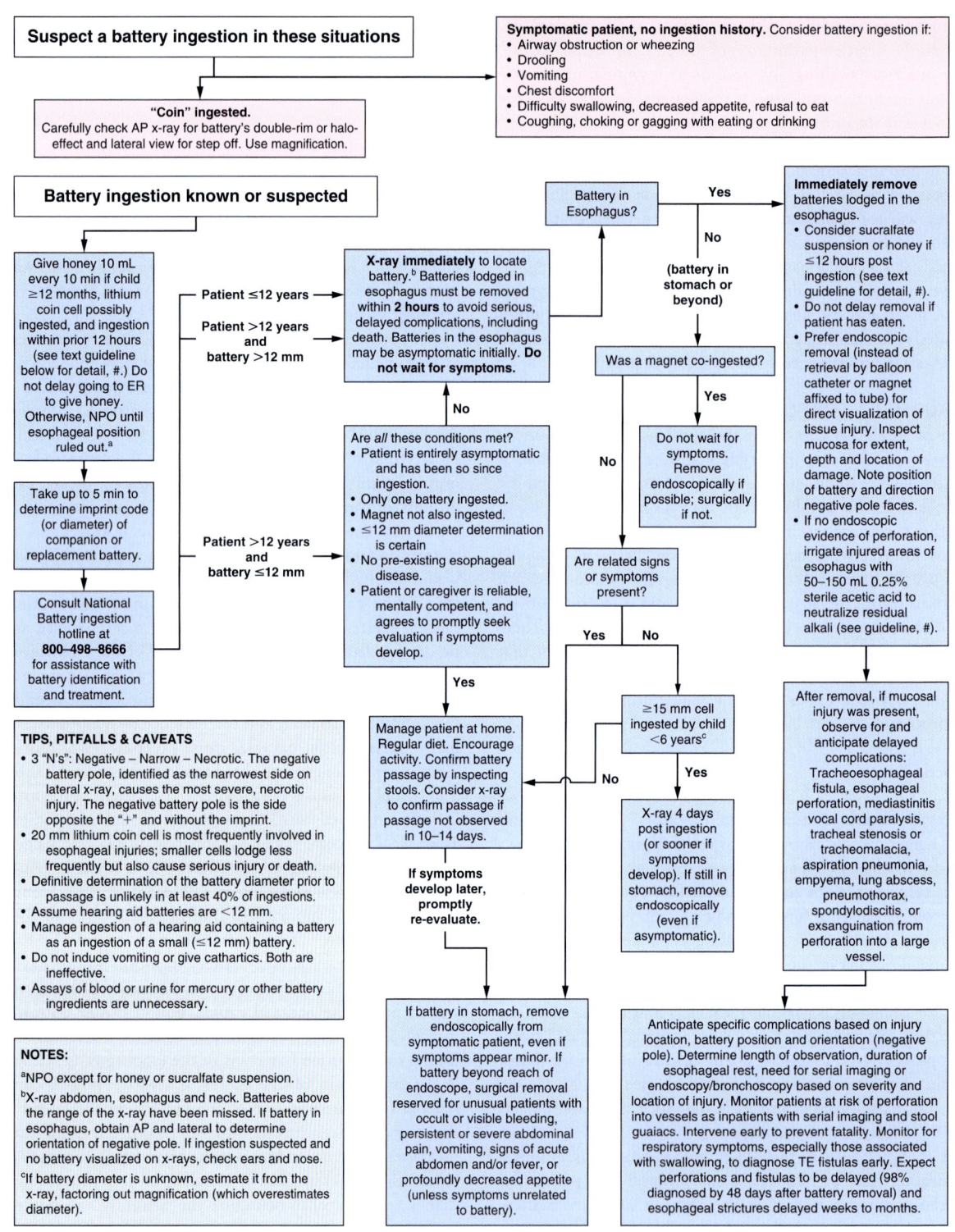

FIGURE 31.24 Button battery decision-making algorithm. *TE,* Transesophageal. (From Holtestaul T, Franko J, Escobar MA Jr, Barlow M. Pediatric ingestions. *Surg Clin North Am.* 2022;102(5):779-795.) (National Capital Poison Center 2024) (# Note that this guideline has 18 recommendations and the reader is referred to their web site https://www.poison.org/battery/guideline)

Prevention and deterrence measures are likely most effective to preclude injury from ingestion of button batteries. Some manufacturers have begun to double package the batteries to make them more difficult to access.[899] In addition, one company has added a deterrent directly onto the battery so the child will be less likely to swallow it if it reaches their mouth;[899] a nontoxic bitter coating is applied to 2032, 2025, and 2016 lithium button batteries. The coating, comprised of denatonium benzoate, is applied to one side of the battery so that when the child puts the battery on their tongue, contacting the bitter coating prompts a physical response and hopefully the child spits it out. The combination of these two strategies should be extended to all sizes of button batteries and to all manufacturers to deter children from accessing and swallowing these dangerous objects.

Upper Airway Obstruction

LARYNGOMALACIA

Congenital laryngomalacia is the most common cause of inspiratory stridor in infants.[907] Supraglottic structures including a combination of the arytenoids cartilages, aryepiglottic folds, and/or the epiglottis collapse into the laryngeal inlet during inspiration, causing upper airway obstruction. The stridor typically worsens with feeding, crying, supine positioning, agitation, and exercise. Usually, symptoms are not present at birth, but develop within the first 4 months of life and peak at 4 to 8 months of age. The natural course is that the symptoms usually resolve by 2 to 5 years of age. As laryngomalacia is considered to be a self-limiting disease, typical treatment consists of either a wait-and-see approach or for children with severe disease (<10%), an endoscopic supraglottoplasty, with ~95% success rate.[908,909] Some children may present with OSA later in life. Comorbidities are present in approximately one-half of patients and include neurologic and cardiac disease, genetic syndromes, GERD, and associated airway lesions (e.g., tracheal or pharyngomalacia). All are associated with increased risk of surgical failure that require revision surgeries or the insertion of a feeding tube.[908,910] Tracheotomy may be required in those patients with multiple comorbidities.[387]

Supraglottoplasty is the most common surgical approach with division of the aryepiglottic folds and/or trimming of the arytenoid mucosa using either a cold steel, coblation, or a CO_2 laser performed endoscopically, utilizing a small indwelling endotracheal tube or with intermittent intubation and an apneic oxygenation technique. Complications include airway edema, aspiration, airway fires, and granuloma formation, the last necessitating repeat surgeries to remove scarring.[911] Hence, these children must be closely monitored after surgery with continuous pulse oximetry[842]; overnight intubation may be indicated when a laser has been used because swelling often occurs

ACUTE EPIGLOTTITIS

Although rare in children today, acute epiglottitis is a potentially fatal infection that can lead to sudden and complete upper airway obstruction. It is a clinical and pathologic condition that results in generalized toxemia characterized by inflammatory edema of the supraglottic structures including the arytenoids, the aryepiglottic folds, and lingual surface of the epiglottis. Infectious epiglottitis commonly occurs between the ages of 3 and 5 years; however, as many as 41% of pediatric cases reported in 2006 occurred in infants younger than 1 year of age.[912] With widespread *H. influenzae* B vaccination, the incidence of epiglottitis in children has decreased dramatically[2,913–917] with a concomitant decrease in mortality from 0.064 to 0.001 per 100,000.[918] Nonetheless, *H. influenzae* epiglottitis may still occur because of a vaccine failure or a failure or refusal to immunize.[919,920] Although rare, pediatric cases of epiglottitis caused by group A β-hemolytic streptococcus,[921] staphylococcus,[922] candida,[923] and other fungal pathogens[924] have been reported.[925] Currently, infectious epiglottitis is more common in adults than children with an incidence of 1 to 4 per 100,000 in the United States.[926,927] Noninfectious causes of epiglottis such as direct laryngeal trauma, chemical or thermal burns, fungal infection, acute leukemia, or reactions to chemotherapy present similarly with the same anesthetic considerations for upper airway obstruction.[928–930]

The onset of infectious epiglottitis in children is usually abrupt with a brief history of a high fever, severe sore throat, dysphagia, and inspiratory stridor or expiratory snore, with little or no hoarseness (because this is a supraglottic disease). The mnemonic SNORED is useful: **S**eptic, **NO** cough, **R**apid onset, **E**xpiratory snore, **D**rooling. The child presents in a sitting (tripod) position, leaning forward to improve airflow past the swollen epiglottis, and breathing slowly. These children appear toxic, exhausted, tachycardic, with a flushed face, and drooling because dysphagia and odynophagia prevents them from swallowing (E-Fig. 31.7).

Although bacterial tracheitis has overtaken acute epiglottis as an infectious cause of life-threatening airway obstruction,[931,932] acute epiglottitis is a clinical diagnosis that should remain prominent in the differential diagnosis of a child presenting with signs and symptoms of upper airway obstruction. When the clinical presentation of acute epiglottitis is inconclusive, a lateral radiograph of the neck often demonstrates a swollen epiglottis and aryepiglottic folds (Fig. 31.25 and E-Fig. 31.8), but a radiograph should never be undertaken unless a physician who can establish an airway accompanies the child throughout the radiologic examination and the child should not be placed supine. Otherwise, lateral neck radiographs are avoided. A bedside ultrasound is an alternate approach being used increasingly to assess airway structures and to diagnose epiglottitis, although this approach depends on a degree of patient cooperation, end-user expertise, and is most useful in adults.[933]

In children with epiglottitis, examination of the pharynx and larynx should only be attempted in an area with adequate equipment and staff prepared to establish an airway should complete airway obstruction suddenly develop; ideally, this would take place in the operating room. No attempts to examine the larynx should be undertaken in the emergency room.[2] Given the rarity of epiglottitis in children, most clinicians today have never experienced the sudden and catastrophic deterioration that accompanies complete airway obstruction without the ability to ventilate or intubate the glottic opening. To preserve a patent airway, the child should remain in the sitting position at all times and never be forced into the supine position.

Premedication is neither recommended nor needed for children with acute epiglottitis because they are septic and usually exhausted from labored breathing. If anxiolysis is indicated, parental presence may be the preferred approach. The child should be brought to the operating room where standard monitors are applied and standard difficult airway equipment for tracheal intubation including a video laryngoscope, rigid bronchoscope, and needle cricothyrotomy set are available. Personnel who are very experienced with a rigid bronchoscope should be present before anesthesia is induced. General anesthesia is induced with sevoflurane in oxygen with the child in the sitting position and spontaneous respirations maintained as the child is gently allowed to recline. CPAP may be required as the child reclines to prevent airway obstruction. In the moribund child, preoxygenation with gentle CPAP and an awake intubation may be considered.

Once a surgical stage of anesthesia has been achieved, IV access should be established. A fluid bolus of 20 to 40 mL/kg of a balanced salt solution should be infused because these children are severely dehydrated and may become hypotensive as the anesthetic plane deepens. Epiglottitis is marked by progressive swelling of the lingual surface of the epiglottis with obliteration of the vallecula (Fig. 31.26A,B). Viewing the glottic opening without traumatizing the epiglottis is difficult but can be accomplished with a slightly different laryngoscopic approach: the tip of the

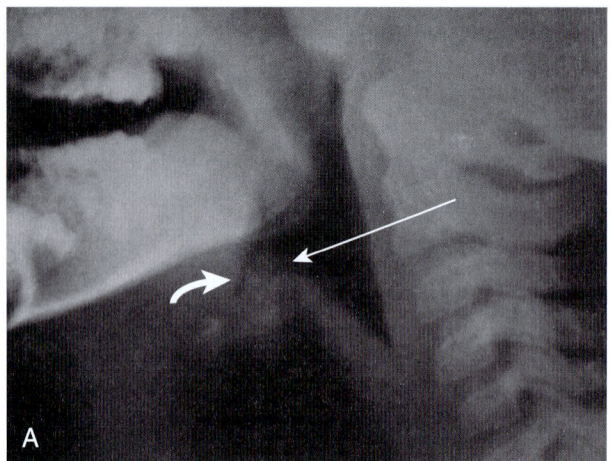

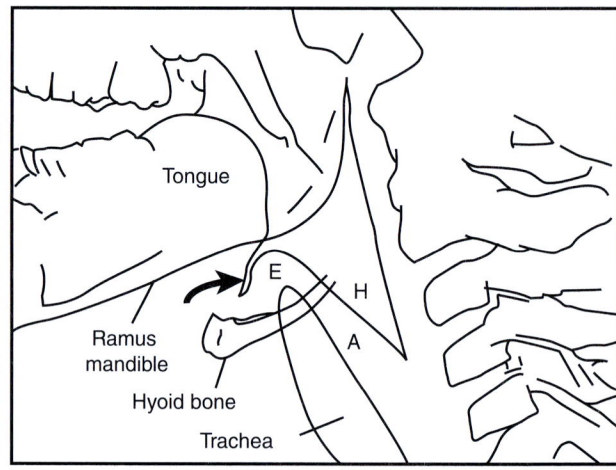

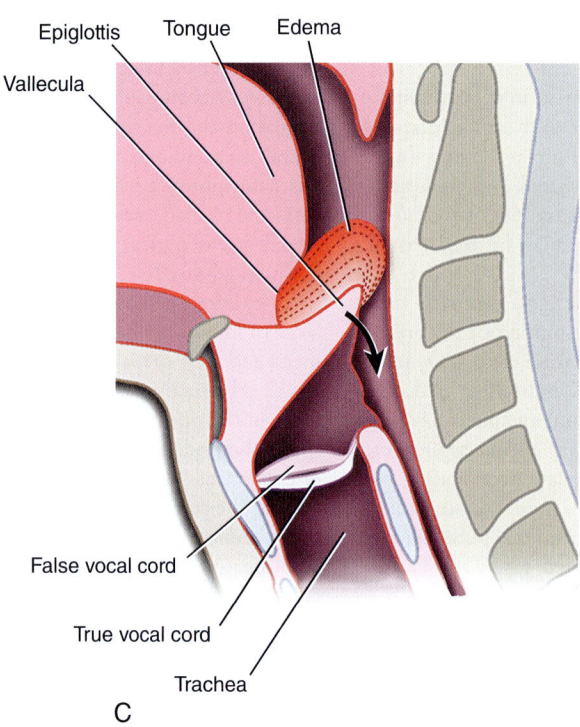

FIGURE 31.25 A, Lateral neck radiograph of child with epiglottitis. Note the marked thickening of the aryepiglottic folds *(straight arrow)*. **B,** Schematic representation of **A**. Note the marked thickening of the aryepiglottic folds *(A)*, loss ("amputation") of the vallecula *(curved arrow)*, swelling of the epiglottis *(E)*, and distention of the hypopharynx *(H)*. **C,** Schematic representation of epiglottitis demonstrating progressive swelling of the lingual surface of the epiglottis, resulting in "amputation" of the vallecula. Progressive swelling leads to trapdoor-like occlusion of the glottic opening *(curved arrow)*. For additional views, see E-Fig. 31.8.

laryngoscope blade is inserted following along the center of the base of the tongue into the vallecula while advancing the tip of the blade to pin the base of the tongue. This allows exposure of the glottis by lifting the base of the tongue, without directly touching the epiglottis. A stylet within the TT provides increased rigidity to facilitate passage of the tube through a partially obstructed glottic aperture. It is suggested that the internal diameter of the cuffed TT should be one-half–size smaller than estimated for patient age to reduce the risk of pressure necrosis on the mucosa; however, this is usually unnecessary since the laryngeal inlet and subglottic regions are normal sized. An inspiratory air leak at 20 centimeters of H_2O with the cuff deflated is usual because swelling is supraglottic. If the epiglottis is very swollen and the glottic aperture not

visible, the chest may be gently compressed to illicit bubbles in the saliva that should be followed to the glottic opening. After orotracheal intubation, the tube may be replaced by a nasotracheal tube of appropriate size, but only if the glottic opening is easy to visualize after oral intubation; if the laryngoscopy was difficult, then the TT should be left in an oral position. If one is unable to intubate the trachea, then a rigid bronchoscope should be used. If both of those maneuvers fail, then a tracheotomy or cricothyrotomy should be urgently performed (see Figs. 12.28 and 12.29).[934,935] Intraoperative complications include bronchospasm, laryngospasm, airway obstruction/loss, or hemodynamic instability with associated arrhythmias due to concurrent hypoxemia and/or hypercarbia.

the human parainfluenza virus, or other causative viruses such as influenza A and B viruses, respiratory syncytial virus, rhinovirus, coronavirus, human metapneumovirus, and adenovirus.[941] Laryngotracheitis affects boys more than girls (1.4 : 1) and is more common in children younger than 3 years of age.[942] Compared with the acute onset of epiglottis, croup has a gradual onset, and most commonly occurs in the fall or winter. Laryngotracheitis is common after a URI in a young child; the child is able to lie flat, presents with a low-grade fever, and has an acute onset of a barky cough, without dysphagia or drooling (Table 31.15). Children requiring more than one hospitalization for croup should be

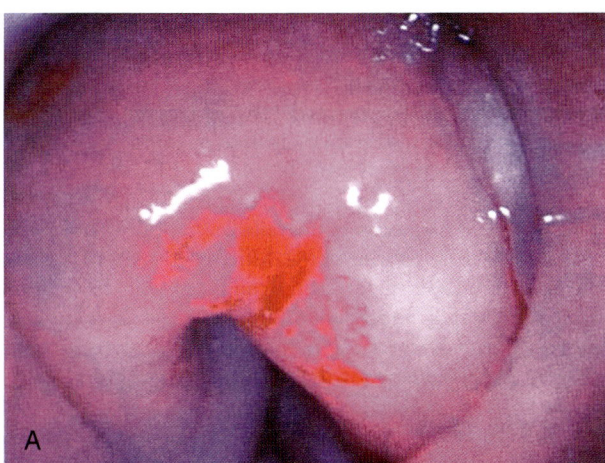

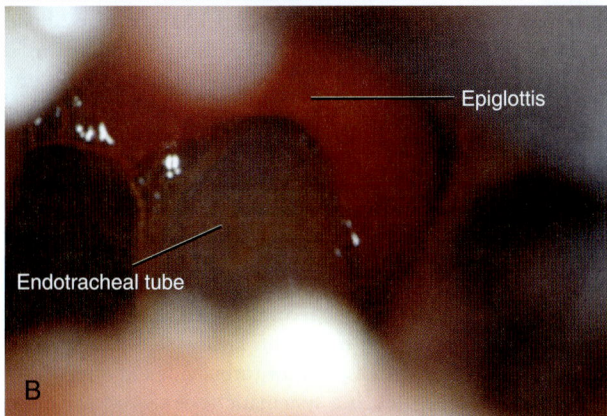

Epiglottis

Endotracheal tube

FIGURE 31.26 Acute epiglottitis. **A,** The entire upper airway is inflamed and there is marked swelling of the epiglottis. **B,** Photograph taken after securing the airway with an endotracheal tube.

Once the airway has been secured, a swab of the pharynx and a blood culture should be obtained. Antibiotics in the form of a cephalosporin (e.g., ceftriaxone 50 mg/kg per day)[912,936,937] can then be initiated.[2] Prophylactic antibiotics may be recommended for other family members or contacts.[938,939]

The duration of treatment in the intensive care unit is controversial, although a 3- to 5-day regimen of IV antibiotics followed by oral therapy is usually the minimum. Supportive measures include IV hydration, airway care, sedation as necessary, and acetaminophen for fever. Administration of steroids are usually not required.[940] Negative-pressure pulmonary edema can develop after tracheal intubation in children with severe epiglottitis.[761] Medically complex patients may develop an epiglottic abscess or descending necrotizing mediastinitis.[925] Extubation should be considered at 24 to 48 hours after initiation of therapy provided the child is afebrile and able to swallow. In some cases direct laryngoscopy under deep sedation is indicated to evaluate the extent of the edema and appropriateness for extubation.[925]

LARYNGOTRACHEOBRONCHITIS (CROUP)

Croup is characterized by inspiratory stridor; suprasternal, intercostal, and substernal retractions; barking cough; and hoarseness. Croup is caused by swelling of the mucosa in the subglottic area of the larynx, which narrows that portion of the upper airway and results in stridor.[2]

Viral laryngotracheitis is by far the most common form of infectious croup, and is caused by many viruses, most commonly

TABLE 31.15	Differential Diagnosis of Croup and Epiglottitis	
	Croup[a]	**Epiglottitis**
Incidence	More common	Less common
Obstruction	Subglottic	Supraglottic
Age	Younger (<3 years)	Older (3–6 years)
Etiology	Viral	Bacterial
Recurrence	Possible (5%)	Rare
Clinical features		
Onset	Gradual (days)	Sudden (hours)
Fever	Low grade	High
Dysphagia	None	Marked
Drooling	None	Present
Posture	Recumbent	Sitting
Toxemia	None	Present
Cough	Barking	Usually none
Voice	Hoarse	Clear to muffled
Respiratory rate	Rapid	Normal/slow
Larynx palpation	Not tender	Tender
Leukocytosis	+ (Lymphocytic)	+++ (Polymorphonuclear cells)
Neck radiographs	Anteroposterior: steeple sign	Lateral: thumb-like mass
Clinical course	Longer	Shorter
Treatment		
Primary therapy	Medical and supportive	Secure airway first
O$_2$ and humidity	Essential	Usually desirable
Hydration	Oral or intravenous	Intravenous
Racemic epinephrine	Usually effective	No value
Corticosteroids	Controversial, commonly used	Not indicated
Antibiotics	Not indicated	Effective
Airway support	Occasionally needed (<3%)	Always indicated (100%)
Preferred airway	Nasotracheal Tracheostomy (rarely)	Nasotracheal
Extubation	4–7 days	1–3 days

[a]Foreign bodies in the airway should also be considered.
From Hannallah R. Epiglottitis. In: Stehling L, ed. *Common Problems in Pediatric Anesthesia.* 2nd ed. St. Louis: Mosby–Year Book; 1992:277-281.

evaluated for subglottic narrowing from stenosis or cysts. Clinical scoring systems are helpful to follow the progress of the disease and to judge the effectiveness of therapy (E-Table 31.10).[943] In the case of stridor failing to improve with therapy, the differential diagnosis includes bacterial tracheitis, epiglottitis, upper airway abscess, and foreign body aspiration.[941]

Recurrent croup also has several noninfectious causes including allergies, gastroesophageal reflux, asthma, and structural problems (e.g., subglottic stenosis). It has been considered an allergic reaction to viral antigens and not a viral infection per se, but this remains controversial.[944] In general, management of noninfectious recurrent croup is supportive.

Radiographic studies are only indicated in children with atypical symptoms and an unclear diagnosis or if they fail to respond to treatment.[941] In such cases, anteroposterior radiographs of the neck will identify a foreign body in the airway, whereas a lateral neck x-ray can rule out epiglottitis.[945] The viral nature of laryngotracheitis causes edema in the subglottic region of the larynx such that blurring of the tracheal air shadow and symmetric narrowing of the subglottic air shadow (i.e. "steeple", sharpened pencil sign, or wine bottle sign) present on anteroposterior films, (Fig. 31.27 and E-Fig. 33.9).

Most cases of laryngotracheitis resolve quickly with conservative measures that include breathing humidified air or oxygen and hydration. Although humidification of inspired gases is not evidence-based practice,[946] oxygen is essential to prevent or to treat hypoxemia due to secretions that cause ventilation-perfusion mismatch, and hydration prevents thickening of tracheal secretions. Less than 6% of cases require hospitalization for respiratory difficulty, and of those, fewer than 3% require an artificial airway.[819,941,947] Tracheal intubation is required in ~1% to 3% of children with croup, with death occurring very rarely (1:7000 to 1:30,000 children whose airways were intubated).[941,948] The child should be kept calm and comfortable during treatment as agitation can worsen the symptoms.

Both corticosteroids and nebulized epinephrine are beneficial to treat croup. Corticosteroid therapy for laryngotracheobronchitis has become the standard of care.[941,949,950] Single-dose oral dexamethasone therapy is indicated for mild to severe croup.[941,951] In cases of moderate-to-severe laryngotracheobronchitis, IV dexamethasone (0.5–1 mg/kg) may be indicated.[952] Intramuscular dexamethasone (0.6 mg/kg) is an acceptable alternative route of administration if IV access is unavailable.[953,954] In a child with severe croup who is vomiting or too distressed to take oral medication, nebulized budesonide (2 mg) combined with epinephrine may be used. Rapid clinical improvement 12 and 24 hours after steroid treatment is associated with a decrease in admission rates by 50%, a 5-fold reduction in the need for intubation, and a 33% decrease in length of stay.[955–959]

Nebulized racemic epinephrine or L-epinephrine (1 mg/mL; i.e., 1/1000 or 1% solution) are both effective drug therapies to treat croup in children with peak benefit within the first 2 hours and reduced length of stay for admitted patients[960]; the latter may have a more prolonged effect.[956,960] Racemic epinephrine is provided as a 2.25% solution which is then diluted in 2 mL of water or saline solution based on the patient's weight (i.e., 0.25 mL of diluted racemic epinephrine for children 0–20 kg, 0.5 mL for children 20–40 kg, and 0.75 mL for children >40 kg).[961,962] The dose of a 1% solution is 0.5 milliliters per kilogram (maximum 5 mL). Because the duration of action of racemic epinephrine is brief, treatments are required every 1 to 2 hours and rebound edema may occur. ECG monitoring is recommended along with at least 2 hours of observation after treatment. Heliox, (a mixture of oxygen and helium) may decrease airflow turbulence and improve the work of breathing, although a systematic review of small studies suggests that it does not benefit those with moderate or severe croup.[963] Antibiotics are generally not indicated in the treatment of uncomplicated viral croup.

If treatment with steroids and nebulized epinephrine is unsuccessful, obstruction may be caused by thick, inspissated secretions

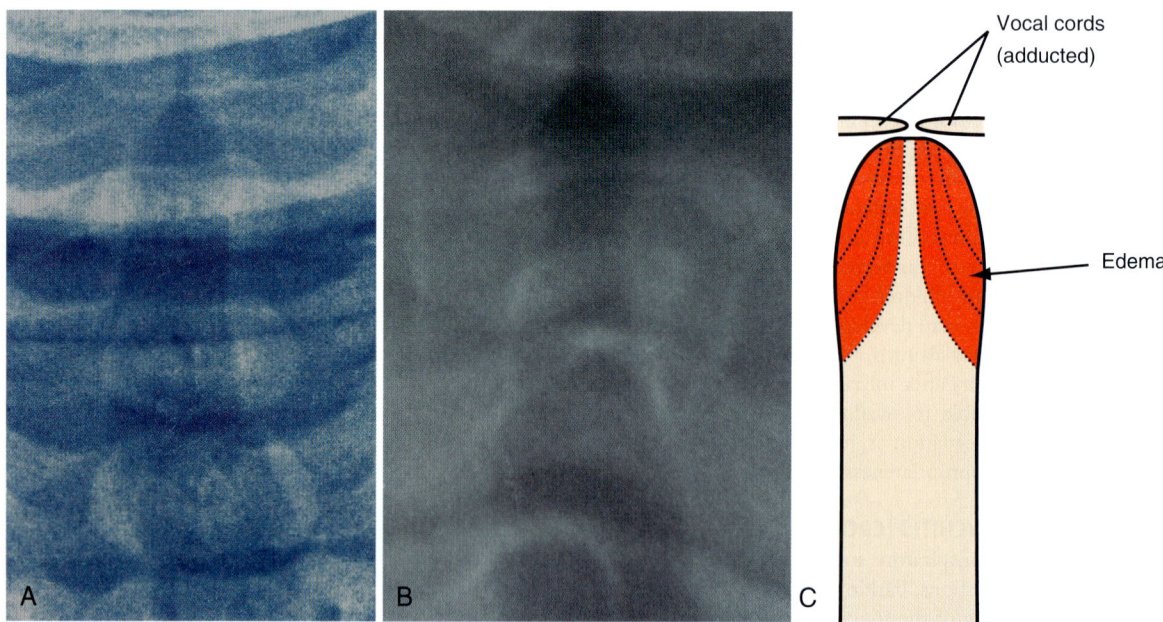

FIGURE 31.27 A, Xerogram radiograph of the normal upper airway (anteroposterior view). Note that the subglottic area is rounded. **B,** Laryngotracheobronchitis (croup) produces swelling (edema and inflammation), which obliterates the normal rounded subglottic area, producing the so-called sharpened pencil or steeple sign. **C,** Schematic representation showing progressive swelling of the subglottic area. For an additional view, see E-Fig. 31.09.

related to bacterial superinfection (e.g., bacterial tracheitis).[964,965] The symptoms and signs of bacterial tracheitis are intermediate between epiglottitis and croup. Onset at any age, an antecedent viral infection followed by rapid severe illness with a high fever, respiratory distress, and cough associated with copious secretions and retrosternal chest pain are presenting symptoms. Dysphagia and drooling are absent, and the child can lie flat. When the child appears exhausted from the increased work of breathing (i.e., SpO_2 <90% on room air, decreasing level of consciousness, or slowing ventilatory frequency),[966] tracheal intubation, followed by pulmonary suctioning, is required to relieve the obstruction. If possible, rigid bronchoscopy before intubation to remove purulent debris from the trachea may avoid blockade of the TT with inspissated pus.[966] Finally, tracheal intubation and suctioning may also be required in the case of laryngotracheobronchitis, where an inability to clear secretions from the lower airways contributes to atelectasis and arterial oxygen desaturation.

Approximately 6% of children with sternal and chest retractions on admission who fail to respond to conventional medical therapy require tracheal intubation,[967] which should be performed in the operating room under controlled anesthetic conditions. To avoid aggravating the subglottic edema and possibly causing subglottic stenosis,[968–970] the TT should be at least one-half–size smaller (0.5-mm internal diameter [ID]) and an air leak is commonly absent. After nasotracheal intubation (preferred for pulmonary toilet and child comfort), children are admitted to the ICU, and special care is provided for suctioning of inspissated secretions. TTs are usually placed for 2 to 4 days but may be required for up to 10 days. Extubation criteria include diminished or thinner tracheal secretions, and an audible air leak that develops around the TT as the edema subsides.[971]

LARYNGEAL PAPILLOMATOSIS

Recurrent respiratory papillomatosis, also known as juvenile laryngeal papillomatosis, is the most common pediatric upper airway/laryngeal tumor and is usually found in the larynx on the vocal cord margins, epiglottis, pharynx, or trachea (Fig. 31.28). The papillomata are caused by the human papilloma virus (HPV) 6 and 11 and used to occur in approximately 1 in 400 births. While in the past 10% to 25% of pregnant women presented with an active or a latent viral infection,[972] disease incidence is markedly decreasing following the introduction of HPV vaccines.[973–976] If left untreated, symptoms of aphonia, respiratory distress, hoarseness, stridor, right ventricular hypertrophy, and cor pulmonale may occur. It has been known to mimic other diseases including recurrent croup, asthma, laryngeal hemangioma, and tracheomalacia.[977]

The main goal of the treatment for papillomatosis is to reduce the bulk of the lesions without scarring or permanently damaging the underlying mucosa. Surgically, papillomatous tissue can be removed using the CO_2 laser under microscopic or telescopic visualization,[978] although some advocate the KTP (potassium titanyl phosphate) and pulse-dyed lasers as these cause less thermal damage without disrupting the basement membrane.[979,980] A laser is useful for endoscopic procedures because the beam may be directed down open-tube endoscopes and is invisible, thereby affording the surgeon an unobstructed view of the lesion during resection. However, modern CO_2 laser beams are carried on fibers that can be directed to the lesion through the bronchoscope or with a laryngeal handpiece. This improves access and reduces the risk of collateral burns of the mouth or face. The thermal energy produced by the laser beam cauterizes capillaries as it vaporizes tissues, thereby reducing the risk of bleeding and postoperative edema. Wet towels should be applied to the skin of the face and neck and moist eye pads applied over the eyelids during the procedure to prevent inadvertent damage from the laser.[981] Flammable objects such as TTs (see later) and surgical drapes must be kept remote from the path of the laser beam to prevent a fire or explosion. Syringes and a bag (500 or 1000 mL) of normal saline solution should be immediately available to douse ignited tissues in the event of an airway fire. Papillomas can also be surgically debulked using an ultrasonic microdebrider or cup forceps. This can be followed by laser treatment and topical application of mitomycin C.[982] Nonsurgical options in children include treatment with interferon alfa-N1.[983]

Given the recurrent nature of papillomas in the airway, frequent debulking treatments are required and many children return to the operating room monthly or bimonthly to prevent airway obstruction from developing, while avoiding emergent endoscopic resection. During each visit, the child and/or parents should be queried about changes in voice or increased difficulty breathing, as this may indicate progressive airway obstruction.

Airway management is challenging and depends on the degree of airway obstruction and the type and location of the papillomas.[984–987] Although these children can become psychologically sensitized to frequent hospital visits, premedication is usually avoided if the degree of airway obstruction is significant and there are concerns about compromising spontaneous respirations. In the extremely anxious child, distraction techniques (e.g., a video game) may be supplemented with parental presence at induction of anesthesia to attenuate the anxiety. As pedunculated papillomas can produce complete ball-valve obstruction of the upper airway, monitors should be placed before induction and spontaneous respirations maintained until the anesthesiologist confirms that assisted or controlled ventilation is possible, and the airway has been examined. During induction, the surgeon must be present in the operating room with an array of rigid bronchoscopes and a tracheostomy-cricothyrotomy set to intervene should complete airway obstruction occur.

Depending upon the surgical approach, debulking of airway papillomas can be achieved with or without a TT. If a TT is preferred, it is important to know that polyvinylchloride (PVC) TTs are flammable and can be ignited and vaporized by a laser. The

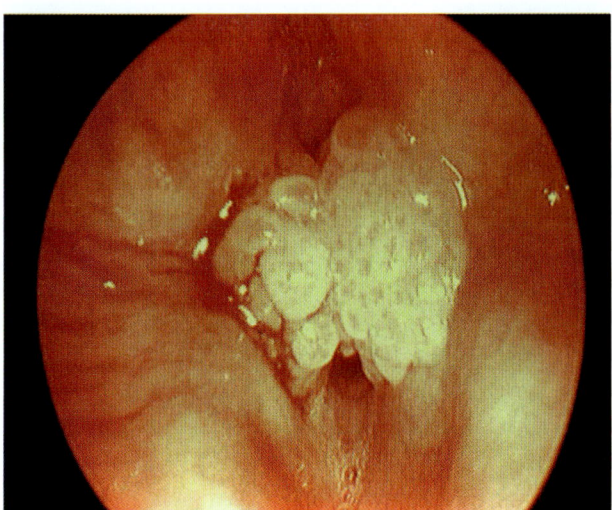

FIGURE 31.28 Large pedunculated papillomas obstructing the laryngeal inlet.

risk of ignition is reduced if the cuff is filled with water, FiO_2 is maintained at <40%, the laser power is limited to <8 watts, and the intermittent stimulation mode on the laser is used.[988] Red rubber TTs wrapped with metallic tape resist ignition and enjoyed a vogue,[989] but are rarely available.

The ASA recommends using laser-resistant TTs in the airway to minimize the risk of fires along with methylene blue colored saline in the cuff to detect a disrupted cuff during lasering.[990] If the tube is wrapped with metallic tape, the tape is applied along the stem as far down as the cuff, which increases the risk of laser damage to the tube below the vocal cords.[991] To address these issues, laser-resistant tubes have been designed specifically for use during laser surgery and may include: (1) a double cuff to protect the airway in the event the outer cuff is damaged; (2) a matte finish that can deflect the laser beam along its entire length; (3) nonreflective flexible stainless steel TTs; and (4) specifically wrapped TTs (E-Fig. 31.10). Because the outer diameters of these laser tubes are larger than their polyvinylchloride counterpart, their use may be limited in very small infants or children with severely narrowed airways (Table 31.16).

Anesthesia is typically induced with sevoflurane in an air/oxygen fresh gas mixture while the anesthesiologist gradually assists respirations as the depth of anesthesia increases. An antisialagogue and dexamethasone (0.5 mg/kg, maximum dose 10–20 mg) may be given once intravenous access is established to reduce secretions and mucosal swelling. Once a deep level of anesthesia is achieved, the larynx may be topicalized with lidocaine (3–4 mg/kg). The airway is then evaluated for a TT. If intubation is preferred, a smaller than usual size TT is inserted as the larynx may be scarred from previous resections and to maximize the surgeon's view or access to the lesions. When a nonlaser approach is planned, spontaneous ventilation is maintained while the FiO_2 is reduced to 30%. Sevoflurane is continued via a very small TT or by using a large double-lumen central venous catheter whereby one port is used to deliver low-flow 8% sevoflurane in air/oxygen and the other port used to sample carbon dioxide.[992] Supplemental propofol may be required to maintain an adequate depth of anesthesia.

Although the goal for laryngoscopy is to secure the airway with the child still spontaneously breathing, partial airway obstruction is frequently encountered before achieving an adequate depth of anesthesia. In such cases, upper airway obstruction is relieved by applying a jaw thrust and continuous positive airway pressure of 10 to 20 centimeters H_2O using the adjustable pressure limit valve (APL) valve (see Chapter 12). If complete obstruction is encountered, then a single IV bolus of propofol (2–3 mg/kg) or a short-acting neuromuscular blocking drug may be necessary to reestablish an airway by tracheal intubation or rigid bronchoscopy.

Once anesthesia has been induced and an intubation technique is planned, a neuromuscular blocking drug can be administered and a TIVA technique with propofol (200–300 µg/kg per minute) and fentanyl (2–3 µg/kg) or remifentanil infusion (0.1–0.25 µg/kg per minute or more) is commenced once the TT is positioned.

If a nonintubation technique is preferred, the choice for ventilation is either intermittent intubation with apnea or jet ventilation.[845] An apneic anesthetic technique with intermittent placement of a TT offers the best unobstructed view of the larynx and avoids the presence of flammable material in the path of the laser beam. The child is positioned for suspension laryngoscopy and the microscope and CO_2 laser equipment are aligned. The TT is then removed, and surgical resection is carried out during repeated periods of apnea. The need to reintubate the trachea, which is readily performed by the surgeon, is guided by the adequacy of oxygenation. After each reintubation, the lungs are manually reinflated to restore both the SpO_2 and $ETCO_2$ to baseline values, at which point the trachea is extubated and the process repeated as needed until the surgery is complete.[2]

Supraglottic jet ventilation is a modification of the apneic technique that avoids tracheal intubation. In this case, the lungs are inflated by intermittently delivering pressurized O_2 through a catheter mounted on the suspension laryngoscope. The pressure is preset to deliver <15 pounds per square inch pressure to preclude damaging the airway. The rapid delivery of oxygen entrains ambient air, thereby reducing the oxygen concentration. Although this technique eliminates large excursions of the diaphragm and provides a quiet surgical field and uninterrupted ventilation, it carries a greater risk of pneumothorax in infants and children than the transglottic approach (see Laryngoscopy and Bronchoscopy earlier).[845] Tension pneumothorax and pneumomediastinum have been reported because of excessive peak inspiratory pressures during jet ventilation disrupting the mucosa.[849] This risk has been sharply reduced by including a pressure-reducing valve on the wall

TABLE 31.16	External Diameter of Standard Plastic Versus TTs Used for Laser Surgery						
	EXTERNAL DIAMETER (MM)						
ID (mm)	Standard TT (Uncuffed)[a]	Standard TT (Cuffed)[a]	Laser-Shield (Cuffed)[b]	Laser-Flex (Uncuffed)[a]	Laser-Flex (Cuffed)[a]	Lasertubus (Double Cuffed)[c]	Red Rubber (Cuffed Without Copper Wrap)
3.0	4.2	4.2		5.2			4.7
3.5	4.9	4.9		5.7			5.3
4.0	5.5	5.5	6.6	6.1		6.0	6.0
4.5	6.2	6.2	7.3		7.0		6.7
5.0	6.8	6.8	8.0		7.5	7.3	7.3
5.5	7.5	7.5	8.6		7.9		8.0
6.0	8.2	8.2	9.0		8.5	8.7	8.7

[a]Mallinckrodt Inc., St. Louis, Missouri.
[b]Medtronic Inc., Minneapolis, Minnesota.
[c]Willy Rüsch GmbH.
TT, Tracheal tube; ID, internal diameter.

source of oxygen; this is especially important for neonates and infants. Another disadvantage is the theoretical risk that jet ventilation may distribute papilloma virus throughout the tracheobronchial tree, thus spreading the disease. A technique other than jet ventilation should be considered in morbidly obese children and in those with small airways where effective ventilation may be difficult.[993] Once surgery is complete, a TT may be inserted and secured until the child has awakened. It should be noted, however, that jet ventilation in pediatric patients is rarely used. Postoperative measures to minimize laryngeal edema such as racemic epinephrine inhalation and/or the use of dexamethasone are usually indicated.

CONGENITAL AND ACQUIRED UPPER AIRWAY OBSTRUCTION

Congenital or acquired anomalies of the upper airway arise from the larynx, subglottis, and trachea. These anomalies often present in infancy, with stridorous or noisy breathing, chest wall retractions, apnea, and possibly feeding difficulties or repeated aspiration.[994] The presentation, which is often airway obstruction, varies according to the age of the child and underlying etiologies.[909]

Laryngeal Atresia and Congenital Laryngeal Webs

Laryngeal atresia and congenital laryngeal webs result from a failure to recannulate the laryngeal lumen after epithelial obliteration. These anomalies may be incompatible with life if they are not recognized and dealt with emergently with a tracheostomy performed at birth. When diagnosed antenatally, such an intervention is undertaken before placental separation, described as an operation on placental support, or the ex-utero intrapartum treatment (EXIT) procedure (see Chapter 36). If severe, an unrecognized tracheal or laryngeal web or stenosis may be fatal after delivery if an alternate airway is not secured immediately via bronchoscopy, tracheal intubation, or tracheotomy. Laryngeal atresia is the most common cause of congenital high airway obstruction syndrome (known by the acronym as CHAOS) in which the neonate is unable to clear alveolar fluid and inflate the alveoli to begin ex-utero breathing.[994–996] Less severe cases may present as incidental findings later in life when the anesthesiologist finds the TT for the child's age/size will not pass the subglottic region. Laryngeal webs occur in 1:10,000 births and congenital webs account for ~5% of all congenital laryngeal lesions. The majority of these webs (~75%) occur at the level of the glottis with the remaining 25% supra- or subglottic. Up to 10% are accompanied by subglottic stenosis. They can occur in isolation or in association with pulmonary and neurologic sequelae of prematurity or other comorbidities including congenital heart disease and genetic syndromes, especially musculoskeletal and digital anomalies.[996,997] As many as 65% of anterior laryngeal webs are associated with DiGeorge syndrome (22q11.2 chromosome defect). Given the frequency of this association, all children with anterior webs should be investigated for congenital cardiac defects before undergoing elective surgery.[994] Laryngeal webs generally require treatment if >50% of the lumen of the glottis is obstructed by the web.[998] The treatment approach involves endolaryngeal techniques including dilatation, lysis with a laser, and stenting.

The treatment of glottic stenosis depends on the severity of laryngeal obstruction. Severe defects may require immediate tracheal intubation or tracheostomy (see E-Fig. 31.11), although most membranous defects can be broken by passing a rigid bronchoscope through the lumen, incising the defect with a surgical knife or scissors, or using a laser to destroy the tissue.

The anesthetic management of glottic stenosis is similar to that for children undergoing laser excision of laryngeal papillomatosis.

Acquired Laryngeal and Subglottic Stenosis

Acquired laryngeal and subglottic stenosis may result from endolaryngeal surgery, trauma, caustic ingestion, infection, or prolonged intubation.[999,1000] The grading system for subglottic stenosis is the Myer-Cotton scale (see Fig. 31.20); the grade is determined by the ratio of the outer diameter of the largest uncuffed TT that passes through the stenosis with a normal pressure leak to standardized subglottic dimensions for children of the same age.[818,1001] Treatment for subglottic stenosis may require laryngotracheal reconstruction (discussed later).

Tracheotomy

Tracheotomy in infants and children is usually performed electively after a TT has been present for a prolonged period and the child requires ongoing airway support, although a small number of children require tracheotomy on an emergent basis because of an acute obstruction.[1002] Currently, common indications for a planned tracheotomy include the need for long-term ventilation, treatment for fixed upper airway obstruction, or pulmonary toilet to help clear secretions (E-Table 31.12)[1003–1005]; approximately 0.2% of inpatient pediatric patients require this procedure.[1005] Children with complicated cardiopulmonary, craniofacial, or upper airway conditions may undergo tracheotomy between the ages of 4 to 6 months, unlike those with neurological disorders or trauma who usually undergo this procedure at 2 to 3 years of age.[1005] Advances in the management of critically ill children and improved airway management techniques and equipment (e.g., video laryngoscopes) have reduced the number of emergency tracheotomies performed in children.[1003] Contraindications to tracheotomy are rare. They have even been performed in children on extracorporeal membrane oxygenation (ECMO).[1006] The length of time a child's trachea should remain intubated before a tracheotomy is performed is debated, as children tolerate tracheal intubation (particularly with a nasal tube) for longer periods than adults without sequelae.[1007] In general, a child with a TT in place for 1 to 2 weeks should be evaluated for possible tracheotomy provided the child is in a stable medical condition.[1007,1008]

A tracheotomy may be temporary such as in cases of upper airway obstruction (~2 years) or permanent in children requiring long-term ventilation.[1007] Tracheostomy tubes come in a range of sizes and materials, including metal, polyvinyl chloride, or silicone, the last being more pliable.[1003] Pediatric tracheostomy tube components are shown in E-Table 31.13. Pediatric tracheostomy tubes are designed with variable lengths according to the age of the child and classified by their internal diameter, where 4 + patient's age/4 corresponds to the appropriate internal diameter in millimeters (uncuffed). Tracheostomy tube sizing is important as internal/external diameters and length vary among manufacturers.[1009] The optimal protocol to decannulate a tracheostomy in a child is unclear but is usually determined on a case-by-case basis, with rates of successful decannulation ranging from 0% to 45%.[1007,1010] Failing to decannulate successfully may be expected in children with a history of prematurity, bronchopulmonary dysplasia, gastrostomy tube placement, craniofacial or genetic syndromes, hydrocephalus, moderate-to-severe sleep-study defined OSA, and parental insistence.[1011–1013] Once the tracheostomy tube has been removed, most stomas heal spontaneously. Up to one-third of patients require surgical closure of a trachea-cutaneous fistula.[1014]

The comorbidities and small body habitus of children presenting for an open tracheotomy are an anesthetic challenge. Unlike in adults, percutaneous tracheotomy is rarely performed because of the greater technical difficulty and risk of lethal perioperative complications, especially in young children and infants.[1007] Most children scheduled for elective tracheotomy have major medical comorbidities (e.g., neuromuscular disease) with one-quarter presenting with a difficult airway.[1015,1016] Approximately one-third of tracheotomies are performed in children under 1 year of age and two-thirds in children under 4 years of age.[1003,1017] Surgical access is complicated by a shorter, fatter neck, and a larynx that is more superiorly located, rendering palpation of anatomic landmarks difficult. The tracheas in these children are small, short, mobile, and pliable with a tendency to collapse and are predisposed to accidental endobronchial migration of the tracheostomy tube or TT. The airway mucosa is lax and more prone to edema. The extension of the pleura into the neck and the close proximity of the common innominate artery increases the risk for pneumothorax and bleeding, respectively. The incidence of intraoperative complications during tracheotomy is generally small (<3%), but is more likely in emergency tracheotomy or in severely ill young children (Table 31.17).[1014]

When a child is scheduled for tracheotomy, the anesthesiologist should be prepared to intubate the trachea orally. If the child has a known difficult airway, appropriately sized rigid and flexible bronchoscopes, video laryngoscopes, needle cricoidectomy kit, and SGAs should be prepared in advance of inducing anesthesia (see also Chapter 12).[1015] The anesthesiology, otolaryngology, and nursing teams should discuss airway management plans and assign roles to all team members in case of an emergency. The surgeon will often want to perform a thorough examination of the airway (i.e., diagnostic laryngoscopy and bronchoscopy) before proceeding with the tracheotomy to help determine the size of the tracheostomy tube. Although intubation of the trachea is preferred during tracheotomy, an SGA or facemask can provide a temporary and effective airway where intubation is not possible. The TT may remain present throughout the tracheotomy, although if a bronchoscopy is planned it will have to be removed and reinserted. For a rigid bronchoscopy, the child should be positioned supine, a shoulder roll placed, and the head extended and taped to the end of the bed. A separate clean anesthesia circuit is generally recommended to hand to the surgeon to connect to the freshly inserted tracheostomy tube. Clear surgical drapes enable visualization of the child and facilitate manipulation of the upper airway and withdrawing the TT when appropriate.

Anesthesia should be undertaken with an inhalational agent in an air/oxygen mixture or TIVA with spontaneous respirations. If the trachea is intubated, the tape or apparatus that holds the TT should be partially released before drapes are applied to the head and neck. The minimum oxygen concentration in air should be provided throughout the procedure to reduce the risk of fire but maintain an acceptable minimum oxygen saturation. In addition, ventilation should be spontaneous instead of controlled or supported once the lumen of the trachea has been exposed. At this point, the TT is withdrawn until its tip passes above the tracheostomy stoma where it is stabilized while the tracheotomy is fitted and secured. This is the interval during which serious complications such as fire and hypoxia may occur. If the tracheostomy tube cannot be positioned and an airway must be established urgently, a sterile TT may be inserted by the surgeon into the stoma or the

TABLE 31.17	**Complications Associated with Pediatric Tracheotomy**	
Immediate (During procedure to first hours after)	**Early** (≤10 days)	**Late** (>10 days)
A/W obstruction: • A/W loss/creation of a false passage • Hemorrhage/secretions • Endobronchial placement	**A/W obstruction:** • Accidental decannulation • Creation of a false passage • Mucus plugging/blood clot	**A/W obstruction:** • Accidental decannulation • Mucus plugging/secretions • Tracheal granuloma
Air leak: • Subcutaneous emphysema • Pneumothorax/pneumo mediastinum	**Air leak:** • Subcutaneous emphysema	**Tracheal lesions:** • Granulomas-suprastomal/distal • Tracheocutaneous fistula • Tracheitis • Tracheoeosophageal fistula (rare) • Suprastomal-stenosis/malacia (rare)
Cardiopulmonary: • Cardiac arrest/death • Pulmonary edema (sudden relief A/W obstruction)	**Cardiopulmonary:** • Cardiac arrest/death	**Cardiopulmonary:** • Cardiac arrest/death • Pneumonia (aspiration/infectious)
Hemorrhage: • Thyroid gland • Aberrant vessel • Innominate artery	**Hemorrhage:** • Stomal • Tracheal mucosa	**Hemorrhage:** • Stomal and/or granuloma • Tracheal mucosa and/or granuloma • Tracheoinnominate fistula (rare)
Injury to surrounding structures: • Cricoid cartilage • Esophagus • Recurrent laryngeal nerve • Tracheal tear/fistula • Fire	**Stoma:** • Infection	**Stoma:** • Granulation tissue • Infection • Skin breakdown **Other:** • Swallowing difficulties

A/W, Airway.
Information from: [1007,1014,1020,1022,1023]

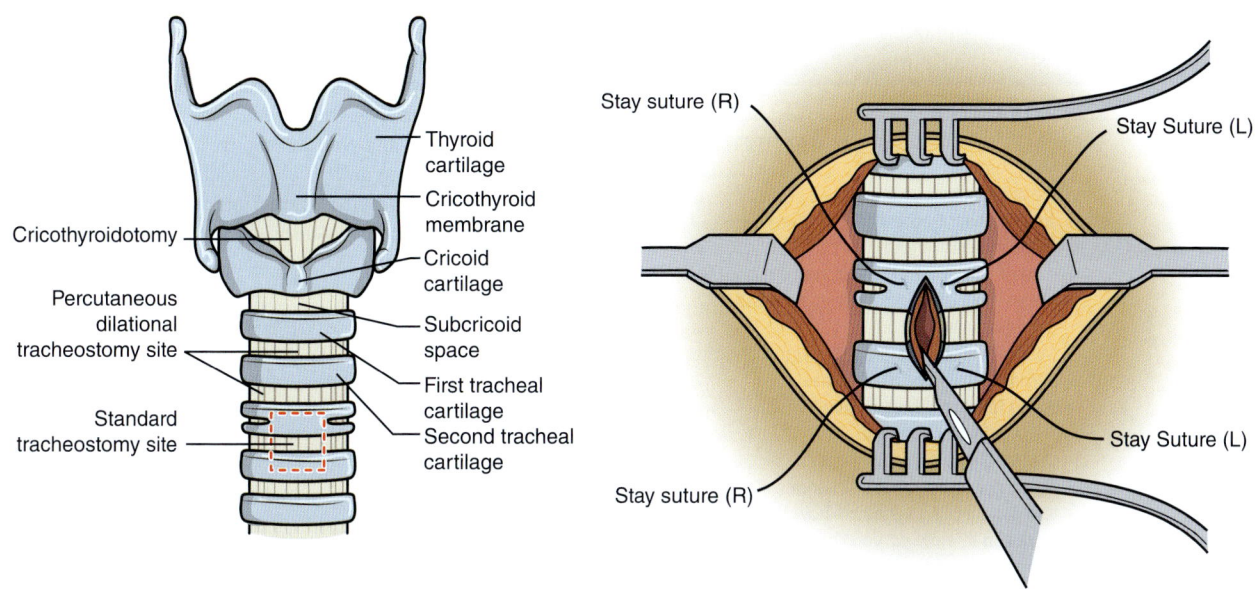

FIGURE 31.29 Tracheostomy anatomy in a child with stay sutures.

TT that was secured above the stoma advanced under direct vision in the trachea and beyond the incision. Once vital signs have been reestablished and ventilation restored, the tube can be again withdrawn, and the tracheotomy tube inserted into the stoma. Once the tracheotomy tube is properly positioned a clean anesthesia circuit is attached and the lungs ventilated; at this point the TT may be completely withdrawn and discarded. Two paramedian tracheal nonabsorbable "rescue" or "stay" sutures are placed to secure the tracheostomy tube (Fig. 31.29 and E-Fig. 31.11).

In the event that the tracheostomy tube is accidentally dislodged, pulling up on the external ends of these sutures will identify the tracheotomy and allow the tracheostomy tube to be reinserted. The child should not leave the operating room without these potentially lifesaving sutures in place and their laterality (right vs. left) properly identified. Importantly, reinsertion of a dislodged or removed tracheotomy tube may cause bleeding, creation of a false passage, or trauma to the tracheal wall.

Children whose airways preclude intubation may undergo an "awake" tracheotomy with sedation using ketamine and/or a dexmedetomidine infusion while maintaining spontaneous respirations.[1018]

A chest-x-ray should be performed immediately after the procedure to confirm correct tracheotomy tube placement and to rule out a pneumothorax. Guidelines for the prevention and management of life-threatening pediatric tracheotomy emergencies recommend that: (1) postoperative care staff should be trained on managing a fresh tracheotomy; (2) signs at the bedside identifying a new tracheotomy including the size, type of tracheotomy tube, and appropriate suction catheter size to use, as well as any upper airway abnormality; (3) an emergency tracheostomy box with itemized contents to accompany the patient; and (4) care is guided utilizing a published algorithm for associated life-threatening emergencies.[1019]

To prevent a thrashing, agitated, and crying child during emergence after the new tracheotomy has been inserted, sedation, opioids, and local anesthetic infiltration should be used to keep the child calm and comfortable during the recovery period.

Children with a tracheotomy have a greater risk of adverse events and mortality, which are largely secondary to their comorbidities

rather than the tracheotomy.[1007] A systematic review of 49 pediatric reports involving 14,270 patients 0 to 18 years of age reported an average complication rate of ~40%; these complications were associated with age, birth weight, prematurity, comorbidities, and emergency procedures.[1020] Skin lesions and granuloma formation accounted for ~44% of complications but more life-threatening complications such as tracheocutaneous fistula (9.5%), accidental decannulation (8.3%), cannula obstruction (8%), pneumothorax (4.2%), pneumomediastinum (3.4%), and others were reported. Leading up to the first tube change 5 to 7 days after surgery, approximately 10% of patients will experience tube occlusions, stoma breakdown, accidental decannulations, and ventilator issues.[1014] Overall, 15% to 19% of children experience a tracheotomy-related complication,[1021] but this can be as great as 77% in the first 2 years after a tracheotomy if minor complications (e.g., lower respiratory tract infections) are included.[1007,1014,1022,1023] Less than 3.5% of deaths are directly attributable to the tracheotomy and are most commonly related to accidental decannulation or obstruction.[1005,1014,1021,1024] The risk of death is, however, increased for tracheotomies performed in emergency situations, severely ill patients, and especially in children compared with adults.[1007] Children with a pulmonary indication for tracheotomy have a shorter time to death, whereas those who have a seizure disorder, underlying neoplasm, or congenital cardiac anomalies have a greater time to risk of death.[1005,1025] Quality improvement initiatives to reduce the mostly preventable adverse events promote a multidisciplinary coordinated approach to tracheotomy tube insertion, care, and decannulation and require appropriate tracheotomy training and intense support for parents and caregivers.[1005,1026]

MANAGEMENT OF THE CHILD WITH A TRACHEOSTOMY IN SITU

It is possible for a child to come to the operating room with a tracheotomy in situ scheduled for either a related (e.g., laryngeal reconstruction) or unrelated (e.g., dental extractions and restorations) procedure. In such cases, the preoperative history and physical should identify: (1) the indication for the tracheotomy; (2) evidence for respiratory compromise (e.g., history of tracheostomy tube obstruction, O_2 dependency, or diagnosis of pulmonary

TABLE 31.18	Preoperative Assessment of a Child with a Tracheostomy Tube In Situ
System	**Relevant Questions**
Airway	Able to intubate orally/how was airway managed for last surgery Tracheostomy tube: • Indication for tracheotomy • Type/size and length • Size of suction catheter, appropriate insertion depth, how often, and recent change in secretions • When last changed/difficulty with change • Stroma erosion or granulomas • Need for supplemental oxygen Requires ventilatory support: • 24 hours/day or just at night • Ventilator settings/recent changes • Did patient bring ventilator/how do you start and stop it? How do you charge the battery? • Most responsible physician and when was last visit • Size of leak around tracheostomy tube when ventilated
Cardiorespiratory	• Recent infections/increased secretions or bleeding • Requires bronchodilators • History of pulmonary hypertension • History of obstructive sleep apnea/recent sleep study • History of arrhythmias (e.g., associated with congenital central hypoventilation)
Other	Relevant comorbidities including prematurity, cardiac, neuromuscular, genetic, oncologic, etc.

From Ross P. Anesthesia for the pediatric patient with a tracheostomy. *Sem Anesth, Periop Med Pain.* 2007;26:153-157.

hypertension); and (3) associated comorbidities (Table 31.18). A focused airway-specific evaluation includes documentation of the type, size, and length of the tracheotomy tube and as well as the appropriate suction catheter size and acceptable insertion depth. Plans for postoperative disposition (day surgery, hospital short stay unit, or ICU) should be in place before going to the operating room. Appropriate tracheotomy "bed signs" should be available and consultation with the child's pulmonologist is recommended.

Specific considerations for a child with a tracheostomy tube in situ include the child's assigned pediatric tracheostomy box, which should include the same and half-size smaller regular, and cuffed tracheostomy tubes with obturators, an appropriately sized suction catheter, and similar sized internal diameter TTs. If a nasogastric tube or gastrostomy tube is in place, it should be vented before beginning the procedure. An otolaryngologist should be consulted before induction if the tracheotomy is fresh (less than 7 days old) or unreliable. If the leak around an uncuffed tracheotomy is too large to permit adequate ventilation, an inhalation induction may be delayed (due to entraining ambient air) or impossible.[1003] In such a case, an IV induction may be undertaken and a cuffed TT inserted into the tracheotomy stoma to maintain the airway. A corrugated connector placed between the tracheotomy tube's 15-millimeter connector and the breathing circuit facilitates access and reduces torque and accidental dislodging of the tracheotomy. A finger should fit under the tracheal tie to ensure that it is not too snug, which could lead to venous obstruction.

Before commencing anesthesia, the size of the leak around the uncuffed tracheostomy tube must be determined. If there is too large a leak around a tracheostomy tube before anesthesia begins, then large fresh gas flows may be required during the anesthetic induction and ventilating the lungs could become challenging should lung and/or chest wall compliance decrease. This can be anticipated before induction of anesthesia by asking the child to vocalize and listening to how loud their voice is around the tracheotomy. A large leak or loud audible voice speaks to the need to change the tracheostomy tube to a cuffed tracheostomy or TT to be completely safe. How one proceeds will also depend on the surgery type, context (emergent or elective) and duration, the comfort-level of the anesthesiologist, need for positive-pressure ventilation, and associated patient comorbidities (e.g., risk of aspiration).

There are four techniques to manage the airway during maintenance (E-Table 31.14). The first includes leaving the tracheostomy tube in situ with ventilation settings adjusted to account for a leak around the tracheotomy tube and/or upper airway.[1027] The second involves replacing the existing uncuffed tracheostomy tube with a cuffed one, a half-size smaller and inflating the cuff carefully to just occlude the leak. The third involves replacing the tracheostomy tube with either a half-size smaller internal diameter cuffed TT or a reinforced TT with padding placed beneath and secured to the chest wall with a surgical adhesive, tape, or a suture. The fourth technique is to remove the tracheostomy tube and orally intubate the airway with a TT from above and inflating the cuff after it passes the stoma. Do not inflate the cuff if any resistance is encountered. Techniques to manage placing a difficult tracheotomy are presented in E-Table 31.14 and E-Table 31.15.[1027] Increased muscle tone associated with emergence from anesthesia at the end of the procedure will decrease the leak around the tracheotomy. In many cases, the child can be brought to the recovery room and placed on their home ventilator and sent home if the duration of surgery was brief and/or noninvasive, adjusting the dose of analgesia and sedation accordingly.

TRACHEOCUTANEOUS FISTULA

Tracheocutaneous fistula is a complication after tracheostomy decannulation that occurs in 12% to 32% of children.[1014,1028] Closure of the tract can be achieved by excision and closure in layers with or without drain insertion or by allowing healing by secondary intention without primary closure.[1029] Success rates are the same with both techniques.[1029] Usually, a preliminary endoscopic assessment of the stoma site and removal of residual granuloma is performed to make sure the airway is clear so that closure is safe.[1030,1031] Failure to ensure a clear airway before attempting to close a tracheocutaneous fistula can result in postoperative airway obstruction.[1031] With layered sutured tracheocutaneous fistula closure, there is a rare risk of life-threatening pneumothorax or pneumomediastinum within the first week[1030]; conditions that require emergent removal of sutures include: reestablishment of a tracheostoma, and rarely thoracostomy and/or pericardial drainage.[1032] These risks do not occur with a secondary intention healing approach.

The anesthetic technique generally includes maintaining spontaneous respirations while sedating sufficiently to minimize coughing or straining at the time of extubation, which may result in residual air leak and the development of subcutaneous emphysema.[1033–1037] After surgery, some children require postoperative ventilation, but most are extubated and admitted for observation. Recovery is uneventful thereafter.

Airway Trauma and Inhalational Injury

Nasal fractures are frequently seen in older children and adolescents, usually as a result of a direct hit (fight) or an accident.[1038] Because the nasal mucosa is very vascular, a lot of blood may have been swallowed and retained in the stomach for the first 24 to 48 hours after injury. A rapid-sequence intubation is the safest approach during that period; however, once gastroparesis has resolved, a SGA may be considered. During these brief operations, a topical vasoconstrictor may be applied intranasally with a pledget before the fracture is reduced. The dose of vasoconstrictor should be confirmed by the anesthesiologist to prevent local anesthetic toxicity and arrhythmias (see Anesthesia for Rhinologic Procedures). Frequently, the surgeon will leave a nasal pack in situ and apply an external splint over the nose. If a throat pack was not inserted, then the pharynx and stomach should be suctioned to remove any remaining blood. The TT or SGA should be removed only when the child is awake, cooperative, and understands the need for mouth breathing.

Closed or open injuries to the larynx and trachea in children are rare but can result from bicycle accidents, falls, direct trauma from sharp objects, or a "clothesline" injury. Blunt (vs. penetrating) trauma accounts for most injuries, most commonly in boys older than 2 years of age.[1039] The cephalad location (C3–4 vs. C6) of the pediatric larynx behind the mandibular arch and the pliability of the cricothyroid structures usually limit the extent of injury[1038]; however, early diagnosis and treatment is critical due to the small size of the laryngotracheal airway and the potential for soft tissue swelling from the loose attachment of the submucosal tissue to the perichondrium.[1040,1041] Injuries can range from minor laryngeal hematoma to a severe form of laryngotracheal separation, an often fatal condition that can occur after a clothesline injury and is associated with bilateral vocal cord paralysis.[1040] Laryngotracheal injury presentation may be deceptive, initially appearing asymptomatic, followed by rapid onset of stridor and subsequent respiratory decompensation.[1039] Although hoarseness, cough, hemoptysis, dysphagia, and dysphonia suggest laryngeal damage, respiratory distress is reported to be the only factor to correlate with the severity of laryngeal injury.[1039]

LARYNGOTRACHEAL INJURY

Laryngotracheal injury is characterized by anterior neck ecchymoses or edema, loss of laryngeal topical landmarks and palpable cartilage fractures or hyoid bone elevation, whereas signs of air leak (e.g., subcutaneous emphysema or pneumothorax) suggest disruption of the laryngotracheal complex. Up to half of patients with this injury will have an associated cervical spine fracture, so precautions are recommended.[1042] Once the patient is stable and the airway has been evaluated, a computed tomography may be indicated to determine the extent of laryngeal injury and the correct course of action (observation vs. surgery).[1043,1044] False negative reports for laryngeal injury have occurred, diagnosed only by subsequent laryngoscopy.[1045]

Positive-pressure ventilation by mask, excessive coughing, or struggling can worsen the subcutaneous emphysema and cause the airway to further deteriorate. Nitrous oxide, cricoid pressure, multiple laryngoscopies to attempt intubation, and passage of blind nasotracheal/nasogastric tubes may create a false passage through a mucosal tear and should be avoided. Initial assessment to secure the airway ranges from observation to placement of a TT, cricothyrotomy, or tracheotomy. If the child is stable, a flexible fiberoptic bronchoscope can visualize the airway for tracheal intubation. The airway of the spontaneously breathing child should ideally be secured in the operating room by an experienced physician using supra- and infraglottic airway visualization and a smaller that normal size TT inserted after induction of general anesthesia with an inhalational agent.[1044] However, this approach has raised concerns that it may cause further injury (e.g., create a false passage), leading to rapid airway destabilization. An alternative approach is a tracheostomy below the level of the injury, under local anesthesia or over a rigid bronchoscope under general anesthesia, should major reconstruction be required.

SURGICAL REPAIR

Surgical repair of the airway may involve an open, endoscopic, or combined open and endoscopic repair,[1041,1046] performed after panendoscopy of the upper and lower airway and esophagus. The success of endoscopic management and the postoperative morbidity and recovery time after the procedure depend on both the characteristics of the laryngeal injury and the skill of the surgeon.[1047] Treatment algorithms for blunt laryngotracheal trauma in children have been published elsewhere.[1040,1044] Table 31.19 classifies and recommends management for laryngeal injuries.[1039,1040,1044,1048–1050] Stents are considered short-term adjuncts to primary surgical care. Typically, injuries ≥ grade 3 require surgical intervention, with early surgical repair yielding better results.[1041] The resolution of other complications such as subcutaneous emphysema, pneumothorax, or pneumomediastinum will determine the length of PICU stay. Postoperative analgesia is titrated to balance the need for analgesia with the adequacy of ventilation. Asymptomatic patients without evidence of injury progression 24 to 48 hours after the initial event may be safely discharged.[1040]

TABLE 31.19	Schaefer-Fuhrman Laryngeal Injury Classification and Treatment Recommendations	
Grade	Description	Treatment Recommendations
1	Minor endolaryngeal hematoma or laceration, no detectable fracture	Conservative (humidified oxygen, observation)
2	Edema, hematoma, minor mucosal injury without exposed cartilage, nondisplaced fracture on CT	Conservative treatment vs. tracheostomy, panendoscopy
3	Massive edema or hematoma, mucosal tears with exposed cartilage, vocal cord immobility, displaced fractures	Tracheostomy, panendoscopy, exploration, and repair
4	As with Grade 3, but with severe mucosal disruption, multiple fractures, disruption of anterior commissure, unstable laryngeal framework	Tracheostomy, panendoscopy, exploration, and repair with possible stent placement
5	Complete laryngotracheal separation	Emergent tracheostomy, exploration, and repair

CT, Computed tomography
Abstracted in part from:[1039,1040,1044,1048,1050]

UPPER AIRWAY INHALATIONAL INJURY

Inhalation injury of the upper and lower airway is the result of heat exposure (fire or steam) and/or smoke. Up to one-third of children hospitalized for a burn injury have a concomitant inhalation injury,[1051] which increases the risk of mortality 2-fold.[1052] Although the definition of what constitutes an inhalation injury remains undefined, it is generally considered a combination of direct thermal damage to the upper airway, local chemical irritation of the upper and lower respiratory tract, and systemic toxicity due to inhalation of toxic substances (e.g., carbon monoxide and cyanide). Evidence-based treatment of an inhalation injury including airway management and lung ventilation strategies are lacking.[1051] Direct thermal injury is thought to be confined to airway structures above the carina due to efficient upper airway heat dissipation, reflex closure of the larynx, and low heat capacity of air.[1053] Airway swelling from thermal injury may take time to manifest (accelerating at 4–8 hours and peaking from 12–36 hours), such that an initial evaluation for airway edema may be misleading. The airway is more likely to be compromised in those who were exposed to heat in an enclosed space (house, car, or boat cabin) and those who develop hoarseness, stridor, cough, and inability to swallow secretions.[1054] Diagnostic findings that point to an airway burn include singed nares, eyebrows and eyelashes, soot or char around the mouth, and soot in the oropharynx. In these victims, time is of the essence and the airway should be intubated prophylactically before it becomes unrecognizable from rapid swelling during ongoing volume resuscitation, which may make later intubation impossible.[1055] Excessive crystalloid administration, and dislodging or blocking the TT are potential issues.[1056] Tracheotomy is often not an option because the front of the neck is swollen and stiff from the burn injury and fluid accumulation (see also Chapter 34).[1057]

Laryngeal Clefts

Laryngotracheal clefts occur in 1:10,000 to 1:20,000 children and result from failure of fusion of the tracheoesophageal septum. These infants present with chronic aspiration and difficulty feeding, likely from spillage of food from the esophagus into the trachea. Embryologically, this septum forms from caudad to rostral so that the defect is classified in severity from rostral to caudad using the Benjamin-Inglis grading system[994]: a type I cleft extends caudad from the larynx to the vocal cords, type II extends caudad past the vocal cords into the posterior cricoid cartilage, type III extends caudad to the cervical trachea, and type IV extends to the thoracic trachea as far as the carina (Fig. 31.30). Types I, III, and

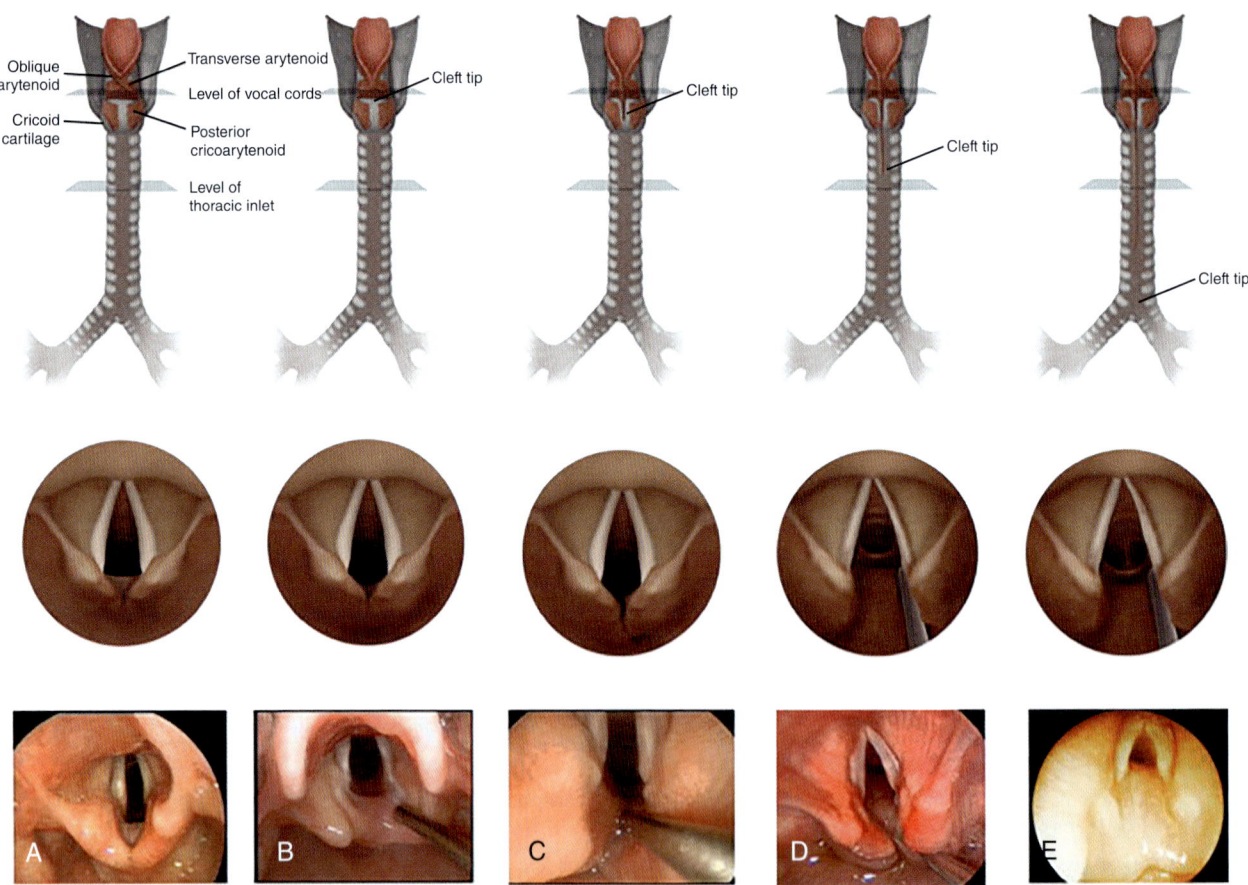

FIGURE 31.30 Laryngeal cleft anatomical classification. (Types I to IV). Posterior view (top row), superior view (middle row) and endoscopic view (bottom row) of Benjamin and Inglis classification of laryngeal and laryngoesophageal clefts: column **A,** normal larynx; column **B,** type I extends to the level of the vocal cords; column **C,** type II extends below the vocal cords into cricoid cartilage; column **D,** type III extends through cricoid cartilage to cervical tracheal esophagus; column **E,** type IV extends to level of thoracic tracheal esophagus. It is difficult in endoscopy view to show depth of type IV cleft as there is frequently redundant mucosa. (Modified from Johnston DR, Watters K, Ferrari LR, Rahbar R. Laryngeal cleft: evaluation and management. *Int J Pediatr Otorhinolaryngol.* 2014;78(6):905-911.)

IV primarily present with swallowing difficulties, whereas type II tend to present with stridor and aspiration.[1058] About 60% to 70% of these clefts have associated gastrointestinal anomalies such as tracheoesophageal fistula as well as cardiac, urological, and craniofacial anomalies.[1059] Laryngeal clefts also appear in several syndromes such as CHARGE, VACTERL, Pallister-Hall, and Opitz-Frias or G Syndrome.[1060] Types II, III, and IV require surgical treatment whereas type I is often managed conservatively.[1058,1060] Investigations including chest x-ray, swallowing studies, and flexible fiberoptic laryngoscopy/endoscopy identify the presence and nature of the defect.[1060] As described for other airway defects, general anesthesia with rigid bronchoscopy and esophagoscopy is required. Surgery for laryngeal cleft requires general anesthesia as described earlier for other airway anomalies using suspension laryngoscopy and a two-layer closure. Types III and IV defects require more involved approaches that may require ECMO or cardiac bypass to fully expose the defect and close it primarily or by using tissue flaps. Surgical correction depends on the defect. Type I clefts that do not extend beyond the vocal cords may be managed conservatively by observing if the defect resolves naturally or proceeding with injection laryngoplasty or endoscopic repair. In one review, less than 20% of type I clefts resolved with conservative care.[1058,1060]

Laryngotracheal Reconstruction

Congenital subglottic stenosis is the second most common congenital laryngeal anomaly after laryngomalacia.[1061] Acquired subglottic stenosis results from prolonged tracheal intubation in infants born prematurely or develops 2 to 4 weeks after laryngeal or other trauma in older children. The frequency of subglottic stenosis in neonates after intubation is unclear, but is reported to be up to 9% with an incidence in neonates from prolonged intubation of ~1%.[1062]

Laryngotracheal stenosis presents with respiratory insufficiency, similar to subglottic stenosis but is extremely rare.[1063] Congenital tracheal stenosis is reported to comprise <0.5% of laryngotracheal stenoses with the most common cause being complete tracheal rings (e.g., agenesis of the trachealis muscle).[1064] In this case, the pathogenesis is complete tracheal rings that develop in the first trimester of pregnancy extending from just below the larynx to the bronchi. These rings are associated with several syndromes including trisomy 21, VACTERL, tracheal bronchus, and cardiac anomalies including pulmonary artery sling in 30% of these patients, and tetralogy of Fallot.[1064,1065] Tracheal stenosis may be acquired after prolonged inflammation or airway manipulation. The mortality associated with surgical repair of congenital tracheal stenosis has decreased in the past three decades from 50% to <10% with improvements in cardiopulmonary bypass (in infants) and the introduction of the slide tracheoplasty. Surgery is almost always indicated as the diameter of the lumen precludes adequate oxygenation and ventilation and only becomes more laborious with age/growth. Only those with very short segments of complete tracheal rings live beyond infancy.

Symptoms usually relate to changes in the airway, voice, and/or feeding. Progressive respiratory difficulty with biphasic stridor, dyspnea, air hunger, and retractions are typical with a tendency toward prolonged courses of URIs. In children with subglottic and complete tracheal rings, a full evaluation for congenital anomalies or comorbidities (e.g., neurologic, cardiac, and pulmonary) is required, and assessment for gastroesophageal reflux is recommended as it may contribute to the development and exacerbation of the stenosis.

SURGICAL APPROACH

The dimensions of the lesions are obtained primarily from rigid and flexible endoscopy of the airway and esophagus in the operating room as laryngeal cartilages show poorly on soft-tissue radiographs and computed tomography scans.[1066] Because of the small diameter of the airways, a Hopkins rod and/or a flexible bronchoscope are used to visualize the larynx and trachea beyond the obstruction. To differentiate neurogenic vocal cord paralysis from posterior glottic stenosis, suspension microlaryngoscopy is needed. The arytenoids can be passively moved if the vocal folds are paralyzed. After tracheal intubation, the degree of air leak around the TT establishes the degree of subglottic stenosis (Fig. 31.20) and predicts the success rate of laryngotracheal reconstruction, which can be negatively impacted by glottic involvement and associated patient comorbidities.[818,1067] The McCaffrey system classifies laryngotracheal stenosis on the basis of the subsites involved and the length of the stenosis: stage I lesions involve the subglottis or trachea and are <1 cm in length; stage II lesions involve only the subglottis and are >1 cm in length; stage III lesions involve the subglottis/trachea, but not the glottis; and stage IV only involve the glottis.[1068] Computed tomography, magnetic resonance, and three-dimensional (3D)[1069] reconstructions are useful for assessing intrathoracic airway narrowing due to congenital cardiovascular anomalies or tumors.

The surgical management of infants with subglottic stenosis must be individualized according to the degree of obstruction and the condition of the child.[1070] Most cases of moderate or severe subglottic stenosis (grades II to IV)[818] require a tracheotomy with sufficient length of well-vascularized, normal trachea between the subglottic stenosis and the tracheostomy to facilitate future airway management. For less severe cases, initial endoscopic balloon dilation or endoscopic CO_2-laser scar excision may be sufficient; however, this approach may increase the risk of unplanned urgent intervention compared with laryngotracheoplasty.[1071]

The most severe cases of laryngeal stenosis require external reconstruction. Airway stenting is transient to keep a cartilage graft in place and lend support to the reconstructed area during healing.[1066] Surgical options include simple anterior cricoid split, single- or double-staged laryngotracheal reconstruction, or the more extensive partial/extended cricotracheal resection.[1062] The simple anterior cricoid split (Fig. 31.31A,B) avoids a tracheotomy and is used in children with early subglottic stenosis who fail extubation and have no baseline oxygen requirement.[1061] A partial/extended cricotracheal resection involves segmental excision of the stenotic segment and is used to treat isolated subglottic stenosis grades III to IV in healthy infants where there is an adequate margin of tissue between the stenosis and the vocal cords. The more common single-stage laryngotracheal reconstruction involves splitting the cricoid cartilage and expanding the framework with an anterior or posterior costal cartilage graft for grades I to III (and some grade IV) stenosis (including posterior glottic stenosis).[1061,1072] A two-stage procedure is reserved for children with a history of difficult intubation or reconstruction failure and multiple levels of obstruction or comorbidities.[1073]

Open laryngotracheal reconstruction surgical techniques such as cricoid and laryngeal splits, tracheal resection, cartilage grafts, and stenting are done at the youngest age possible to help with speech and language development. The anterior cricoid split operation is performed with the infant positioned with a shoulder roll in place to extend the head and the largest possible TT is inserted through the nose. An incision is made through the cricoid, allowing the cartilage to spring open; the TT should be readily

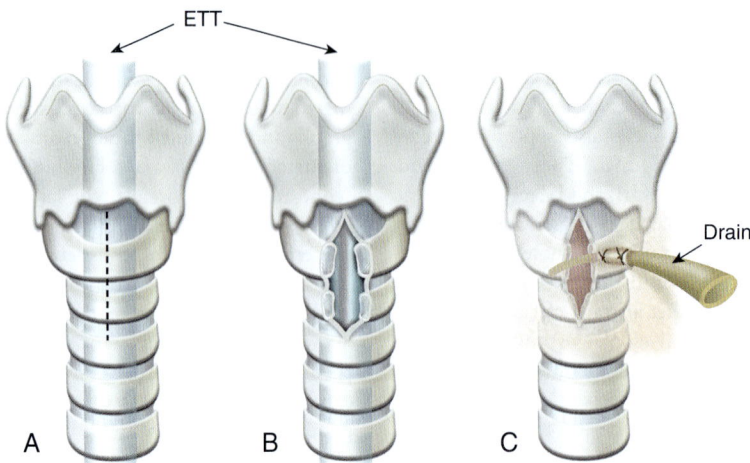

FIGURE 31.31 Anterior cricoid split. After a midline laryngeal incision through cartilage and mucosa **(A)**, the cricoid cartilage is decompressed, and the large endotracheal tube *(ETT)* is properly positioned with the tip distal to the incision **(B)**. The skin is loosely closed with a *drain* **(C)**. (From Zalzal GH, Cotton RT. Glottic and subglottic stenosis. In: Cummings CE, ed. *Cummings Otolaryngology Head & Neck Surgery.* 5th ed. St. Louis: Mosby; 2010:2912-2934.)

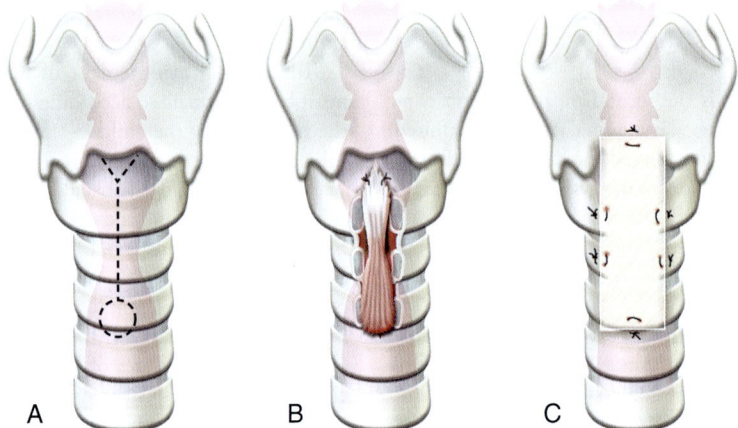

FIGURE 31.32 A, Laryngotracheal resection with anterior cartilage graft. **B,** After a midline incision into the thyroid cartilage, the intraluminal scar and lining mucosa are incised along the length of the stenotic segment. **C,** A piece of costal cartilage is shaped into a modified "boat" and placed in position with the lining of the perichondrium facing internally. (From Zalzal GH, Cotton RT. Glottic and subglottic stenosis. In: Cummings CE, ed. *Cummings Otolaryngology Head & Neck Surgery.* 5th ed. St. Louis: Mosby; 2010:2912-2934.)

visible in the lumen. Frequently, the incision is extended to include the proximal two tracheal rings and even the distal third of the thyroid cartilage. Stay sutures are placed on each side of the incised cricoid, and the skin is loosely approximated. The TT is left in place for about 7 days to act as a splint while the mucosal swelling subsides and the split cricoid heals. Endoscopy is not usually required, but corticosteroids are administered before extubation. A single-stage laryngotracheal reconstruction is sometimes used in children without noteworthy obstruction and in some cases a nasotracheal tube is used to support the cartilage graft for 3 to 7 days. Immediate decannulation may allow a tracheostomy to be avoided altogether, making this approach appealing in appropriate candidates (Fig. 31.32). The more common two-staged laryngotracheal reconstruction has the tracheostomy cannula replaced with a TT through the stoma to afford airway access. A sterile, shortened, preformed oral tube when sutured to the neck is ideal to allow secure fixation and avoid bronchial intubation. A costal cartilage graft is harvested and fashioned to fit the intended

site of transplantation (anterior or posterior). A stent is sutured into place and will counteract scar contracture and provide a scaffold for epithelium to cover the lumen of the airway; it is eventually removed endoscopically.[1074] Patient-specific 3D printed models designed with high-resolution imaging (e.g., computed tomography) are likely to revolutionize this approach through the use of 3D designed external stents (Fig. 31.33) and allow for a more precise understanding of anatomical relationships.[1075–1079] Prognosis for success after laryngotracheal reconstruction depends upon several factors as determined from a multiinstitutional retrospective analysis of more than 500 children. These include the stage and level of the stenosis as well as pulmonary and gastrointestinal comorbidities.[1080] The success rate for laryngotracheal reconstruction is ~69% after one procedure and ~86% after subsequent procedures.

Complete tracheal rings are often corrected on cardiopulmonary bypass using a slide tracheoplasty Fig. 31.34 after endoscopy to determine the diameter and length of the stenotic rings; the

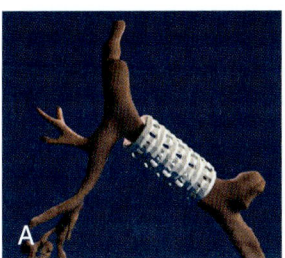
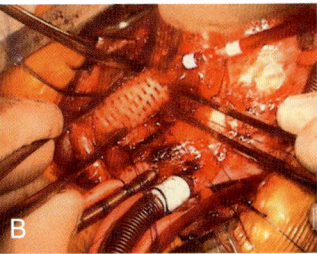

FIGURE 31.33 **A,** Three-dimensionally printed airway anatomic model defining the airway anatomy with a 3D-rendering of an airway splint individually designed to fit over the left main-stem bronchus. **B,** Intraoperative photograph of splint being placed along the patient's left main-stem bronchus. (From Van Koevering KK, Hollister SJ, Green, GE. Advances in 3-dimensional printing in otolaryngology: a review. *JAMA Otolaryngol Head Neck Surg.* 2017;143[2]:178-183 [with permission].)

median age for reconstruction is ~6 months. Intubation should be performed with a small TT (possibly 3.0-mm ID). To reduce resistance and add length, both a 3.0- and 3.5-millimeter internal diameter uncuffed TTs are transected and the upper half of the larger TT telescoped over the lower half of the smaller tube.[1064]

ANESTHETIC CONSIDERATIONS

Anesthetic considerations for pediatric airway surgery are outlined in Table 31.20. Both the preoperative endoscopic evaluation and the planned surgical intervention for glottic and subglottic stenosis present anesthetic challenges. The presence of associated congenital anomalies and comorbidities including gastroesophageal reflux and the sequelae of prematurity need to be evaluated and optimized when possible. A difficult airway should be anticipated, and appropriate preparations made, including a plan for tracheotomy. Preoperative team planning includes management of intraoperative complications and in the operating room concise closed-loop communication is critical. A quiet surgical field is essential. In the shared airway the TT will need to be intermittently removed for surgical access and to place a stent. A pneumothorax during the harvesting of the cartilage

graft is a possible complication that should be kept in mind. Timely administration of antibiotics and maintaining normal blood pressures attenuate the risk of dehiscence of the anastomosis postoperatively.[1066] The choice of the anesthetic technique, either a TIVA or combined TIVA and inhalational agent technique, is left to the discretion of the anesthesiologist.[1081] An adequate air leak at 20 centimeters H_2O around the TT should be the objective. In the ICU, a combination of sedative and analgesic drugs with/without neuromuscular relaxation is commonly used. Dexmedetomidine is a favored postoperative sedative.[1082,1083] It is critical to ensure that the stent, or the nasotracheal tube, is not dislodged in the ICU; accidental extubation must be prohibited.

Postoperative anastomotic dehiscence can result from anastomotic tension, inappropriate anastomotic technique, infection, or tracheal devascularization.[1066] The smaller size of the subglottis in infants and children compared with adults makes preventing extubation challenging and is dependent on perfect mucosal approximation at the anastomotic site to avoid granulation tissue formation and restenosis.[1066] Nonetheless, experience suggests that single-stage laryngotracheal reconstruction with an anterior costal cartilage graft is an effective treatment for subglottic stenosis grades I to III with immediate extubation after the surgery possible.[1084] The diagnosis and treatment of congenital tracheal stenosis, laryngotracheal clefts, and tracheomalacia is covered elsewhere.[1073,1085]

For complete tracheal stenosis, slide tracheoplasty has resulted in an overall success of 87% in one retrospective review, although recovery may be protracted, requiring repeat reinterventions including balloon dilatations and stenting.[1086,1087] Mortality is greatest in those who require preoperative ventilation and in those who present with single lung tracheal anatomy (~30%).

Acknowledgments

The authors thank Drs. Jarmila Kim and Sarah Leir for reviewing the content of the current chapter, and for helping to design the "5Ps" anesthesia flowcharts. The authors also thank RS Hannallah, KA Brown, and ST Verghese for contributions to this chapter in previous editions.

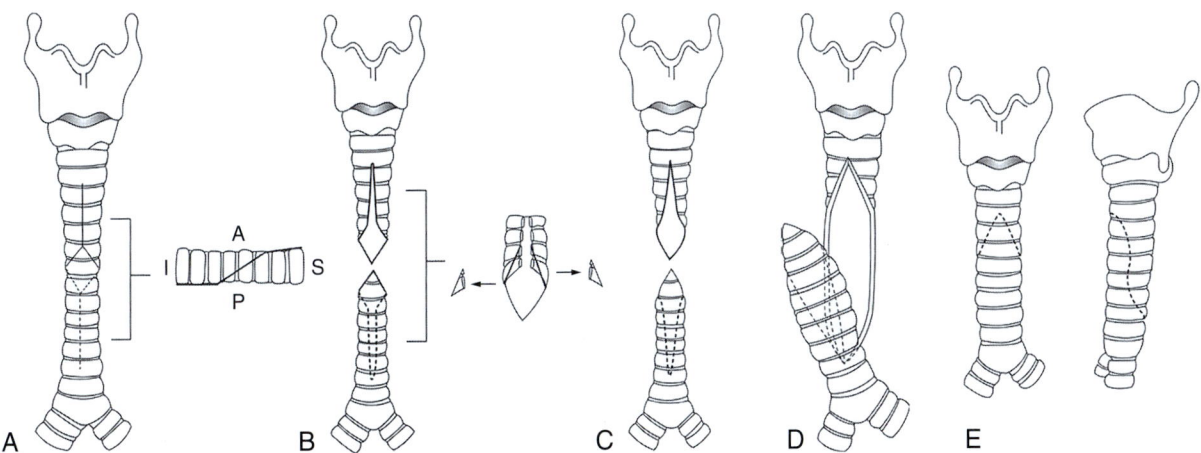

FIGURE 31.34 **A,** Tracheal transection is made at midpoint of stenosis with bevel. **B,** Opposing longitudinal incisions made in proximal and distal segments. **C,** Small triangles of cartilage are removed from the corners of the proximal and distal tracheal segments to round the edges. **D, E,** Anastomosis is performed in a running fashion. (From Richardson CM, Hart CK, Johnson KE, Gerber ME. Slide tracheoplasty complete tracheal rings and beyond. *Otolaryngol Clin N Am.* 2022;55;1253-1270.)

TABLE 31.20 | **Anesthetic Considerations for Pediatric Airway Surgery**

Patient
- See airway endoscopy considerations
- Syndromic and medically complex patients
- Potential for placement/in situ tracheostomy tube

Preoperative
Optimize
- See airway endoscopy considerations

Disposition Planning
- See airway endoscopy considerations

Position
- Supine with neck extension
  - ± Shoulder roll
  - Caution with atlantoaxial instability/c-spine injury
- OR table rotated 90–180 degrees.
  - Extra-long breathing circuit
  - Limited airway access
- Shared/unprotected airway

Procedure
Goals
- Ensure adequate oxygenation/ventilation
- Minimize patient movement
- Laser precautions
- Tracheostomy tube precautions
- Rigid vs. flexible bronchoscopy
- Spontaneous vs. controlled ventilation determined by team
- Closed-loop communication with team

Anesthetic Approach
Anesthetic technique:
- GA with inhalational agents and/or TIVA
- Intubation vs. nonintubation techniques
- May require smaller tracheal tube
- Advanced airway equipment available
- Additional monitors include precordial stethoscope and ECG-derived respiratory rate
- Surgeon present at induction
- Multiple methods of oxygenation/ventilation
  - ± Jet ventilation
  - Placement/in situ tracheostomy tube

Medications:
- Airway edema: steroids and nebulized epinephrine
- Nebulized bronchodilators
- Airway reflex blunting drug(s)
- Neuromuscular blocking drugs available
- Timely antibiotics

Complications:
- Failed intubation requiring emergent cricothyrotomy
- Associated with tracheostomy tube placement (see text)
- Airway trauma
- Pneumothorax/mediastinum
- Bleeding
- Bronchospasm/laryngospasm
- Accidental extubation/loss of airway
- Hypoxemia/hypercarbia
  - ECMO if in extremis
- Hypotension
- Cardiac arrythmias
- Cardiac arrest
- Airway fire with laser
- Dental damage

Postoperative
Risk for:
- Airway edema and obstruction
- Respiratory adverse events
- Pneumothorax/mediastinum
- Bleeding
- Pain
- PONV
- Prolonged intubation
- Tracheostomy tube complications (see text)

PACU instructions
- CXR
- Delay oral intake post topicalizing the upper airway with local anesthesia
- Appropriate tracheotomy care/signage/equipment

CXR, Chest x-ray; *GA*, general anesthesia; *ECMO*, extracorporeal membrane oxygenation; *OR*, operating room; *PONV*, postoperative nausea and vomiting; *TIVA*, total intravenous anesthesia.

ANNOTATED REFERENCES

Aldamluji N, Burgess A, Pogatzki-Zahn E, et al. PROSPECT guideline for tonsillectomy: systematic review and procedure-specific postoperative pain management recommendations. *Anaesthesia.* 2021;76(7):947-961.

A systematic review with recommendations for various analgesic drug classes and other modalities for children undergoing tonsillectomy.

Anderson BJ, Cortinez LI. Perioperative acetaminophen dosing in obese children. *Children (Basel).* 2023;10(4):625.

The concentration-response for analgesia from acetaminophen is explained. The target concentration concept uses pharmacokinetic information to determine dose for different routes of administration. Size models for fat mass account for obesity. Current dosing schedules do not achieve the target concentration because size is unaccounted. A more rational approach is required for acetaminophen dose to achieve concentrations that provide effective analgesia after otolaryngological surgery.

Brown KA, Laferrière A, Lakheeram I, Moss IR. Recurrent hypoxemia in children is associated with increased analgesic sensitivity to opiates. *Anesthesiology.* 2006;105(4):665-669.

This study makes a clear case that younger children with OSA syndrome are at increased risk from opioid-induced respiratory depression; equal analgesia can be achieved with one-third to one-half the usual opioid dose.

Combs D, Goodwin JL, Quan SF, Morgan WJ, Parthasarathy S. Modified STOP-BANG tool for stratifying obstructive sleep apnea risk in adolescent children. *pLoS One.* 2015;10(11):1-11.

Validation of the adult STOP-BANG tool to predict OSA in adolescents.

De Luca Canto G, Pacheco-Pereira C, Aydinoz S, et al. Adenotonsillectomy complications: a meta-analysis. *Pediatrics.* 2015;136(4):702-718.

OSA was identified as an independent predictor of increased respiratory complications (OR 4.90), but less postoperative bleeding (OR 0.41) compared with non-OSA children undergoing tonsillectomy.

Doherty C, Neal R, English C, et al. Multidisciplinary guidelines for the management of paediatric tracheostomy emergencies. *Anaesthesia.* 2018;73(11):1400-1417.

An excellent guideline for the management of pediatric in situ tracheostomy emergencies that includes appropriate patient signage, management algorithms, and methods to provide effective oxygenation and ventilation.

Mitchell RB, Archer SM, Ishman SL, et al. Clinical Practice Guideline: tonsillectomy in children (update). *Otolaryngol Neck Surg.* 2019; 160(1_suppl):S1-S42.

A practical guideline from the American Academy of Otolaryngology Head and Neck Surgery Foundation that addresses all perioperative aspects of the pediatric patient undergoing tonsillectomy including indications for

31

preoperative polysomnography, need for inpatient monitoring, and pain management.

Ohn M, Eastwood P, Ungern-Sternberg BS. Preoperative identification of children at high risk of obstructive sleep apnea. *Pediatr Anesth.* 2020;30(3):221-231.

An excellent review of various approaches to preoperative OSA assessment in children.

Schaefer SD. Management of acute blunt and penetrating external laryngeal trauma. *Laryngoscope.* 2014;124(1):233-244.

A contemporary review and associated treatment algorithm for blunt and penetrating external laryngeal trauma that highlights optimal treatment, including early identification through a directed history and physical.

Wang JT, Peyton J, Hernandez MR. Anesthesia for pediatric rigid bronchoscopy and related airway surgery: tips and tricks. *Paediatr Anaesth.* 2022;32(2):302-311.

A resource for perioperative anesthetic management for children undergoing rigid bronchoscopy or upper airway surgery.

A complete reference list can be found online at Elsevier eBooks+.

32 Ophthalmologic Surgery

SAMUEL A. HUNTER, WILLIAM ANNINGER, AND PHILIP D. BAILEY, JR.

Preoperative Evaluation
Common Ophthalmologic Diagnoses Requiring Surgery
Comorbidities Encountered in Ophthalmologic Surgery
Prematurity
Down Syndrome
Alport Syndrome
Marfan Syndrome, Homocystinuria, and Ehlers-Danlos Syndrome
Mucopolysaccharidoses
Craniofacial Syndromes
Phakomatoses
Ophthalmologic Physiology
Intraocular Pressure
Oculocardiac Reflex
Ophthalmologic Pharmacotherapeutics and Systemic Implications
Emergent, Urgent, and Elective Procedures

Induction and Maintenance of Anesthesia
Specific Ophthalmologic Procedures
Strabismus Surgery
Cataract Surgery
Anterior Chamber Paracentesis and Washout
Probing And Irrigation of Nasolacrimal Duct, or Dacryocystorhinostomy
Ptosis Repair
Retinoblastoma
Enucleation
Vitrectomy
Retinopathy of Prematurity Treatment

THE INFANT OR CHILD who presents for elective ophthalmic surgery requires careful preanesthesia assessment. In addition to ophthalmologic issues, the infant or child may have associated or unassociated systemic disorders. In this chapter, we review the essential issues that should be addressed preoperatively and difficulties that may be anticipated in the perioperative period.

There are a variety of reasons a pediatric ophthalmology patient will require anesthesia. Most ophthalmologic diagnoses can only be made by examining a cooperative infant or child. An examination under anesthesia (EUA) can be essential for an accurate evaluation of children, because these children are often too young or cognitively impaired to cooperate for a detailed clinical examination when awake. Common diagnoses for which EUAs are necessary include autism, developmental delay, refractive error, glaucoma, trauma, tumors such as retinoblastoma, infiltrative diseases, coloboma and anterior segment issues, and diseases of the retina. As a result, the anesthesiologist assumes an integral role as a member of the team, to provide optimal conditions for ophthalmologic diagnostic and therapeutic techniques.

Ophthalmologic procedures that require an immobile child for maximum safety include strabismus or eye muscle surgery, lacrimal and oculoplastic procedures, retinal lasers, intraocular injections, and surgeries in which the globe is open, such as repair of an open globe injury, cataract removal, vitrectomy, retinal detachment repair, and anterior chamber paracentesis.

The child in need of ophthalmologic surgery typically requires general anesthesia or deep sedation rather than exclusive use of local or regional anesthesia. Although small movements may be tolerable during an EUA, large head or eye globe movement during an ophthalmologic procedure should be prevented. Regional blocks (e.g., sub-Tenon, retrobulbar, peribulbar) are infrequently performed in pediatric patients,[1] but the complications associated with these blocks in adults are equally likely to occur in children.[2,3]

Preoperative Evaluation

The perioperative environment should be welcoming to the child and family.[4,5] All team members should be comfortable with anesthetic considerations for infants and children having ophthalmologic procedures.[5] Concerns over postoperative nausea and vomiting (PONV) and the severity of the pain afterward are essential as these are common sources of anxiety.[6,7] It is helpful to explain to both the child and parents that the pain afterwards is mild and that we will provide pain medications before the child awakens. Letting the child and parent know that the pain afterwards feels like "sand in the eye", a grainy discomfort that is mildly painful may help to assuage fears of excessive pain.

Before an elective ophthalmologic procedure, the child should undergo a thorough physical examination to determine whether the ophthalmologic condition or other underlying systemic conditions might impact the choice of airway management or affect the ability to obtain an appropriate mask fit. This evaluation must also include a review of all systems, a complete medical, surgical, and anesthesia history, a list of current medications, known allergies, and family history.[8] Some conditions have important cardiorespiratory and/or central nervous system (CNS) implications for perioperative management and should be fully evaluated before anesthesia (see Chapter 2). Many procedures are performed on preterm infants or formerly preterm infants, and appropriate monitoring for apnea after anesthesia is essential.[9,10]

For children who are old enough to understand the nature of their surgery, it is helpful to discuss how the surgery is performed and how they will feel afterwards. Even parents often benefit from a frank discussion. For example, both children and parents recognize the impact of strabismus on self-esteem and appearance.[11] Reinforcing the positive aspects of the outcome is important for both the child and the parent.

Common Ophthalmologic Diagnoses Requiring Surgery

Common pediatric diagnoses and surgical procedures are listed in Table 32.1. A diagnosis may exist in isolation or be one aspect of a more complex group of diagnoses. Many involve systemic illnesses, and the anesthesiologist should be familiar with the implications of ophthalmologic disease in these settings.[12]

Some procedures and examinations can be performed without insertion of an artificial airway; however, communication with the ophthalmologist about position and possible immobility requirements is essential when planning the anesthetic. Other procedures may be performed very quickly and require only induction of anesthesia (often by mask in children) and then removal of the face mask from the nasal bridge to give the ophthalmologist full access to both orbits, eyelids, and nasolacrimal ducts. The EUA may be brief or intermediate in length, and as information is generated, surgical correction may be contemplated during the same anesthetic, possibly requiring insertion of an artificial airway.

Communication and flexibility are essential since anesthesia may start with a plan for a brief EUA using an inhalational anesthetic with a face mask and no intravenous (IV) catheter; however, if corrective surgery becomes necessary, then airway control may require placement of a supraglottic airway (SGA) or tracheal tube. IV access is usually required to administer medications, including those to prevent or treat the oculocardiac reflex (OCR), nausea and vomiting, and postoperative pain.[13]

For procedures of brief or intermediate duration, the use of an SGA generally allows excellent access to all periorbital structures. Compared with mask anesthesia, the SGA has the advantage of decreasing environmental contamination by inhalational anesthetics and may reduce head movement during spontaneous respiration. These are relatively easy to insert and remain secure, while eliminating the need to hold a face mask near the eyes.

TABLE 32.1	Common Ophthalmologic Procedures in Children
Examination under anesthesia	
Strabismus repair	
Canalicular system probing and stenting	
Retinopathy of prematurity: laser or intraocular injection	
Ptosis repair	
Cataract extraction with or without intraocular lens placement	
Evaluation and repair of eyelid and facial lacerations, as well as penetrating eye injuries	
Dacryocystorhinostomy and dacryocystocele repair	
Enucleation	
Retroorbital cellulitis decompression	
Vitrectomy	

An SGA does not increase the heart rate, blood pressure, and intraocular pressure (IOP) to the same degree as a tracheal tube.[14] In our experience, an SGA with a flexible neck that can be angled over the child's chin is less intrusive on the surgical field but these devices may be challenging to insert. A stylet is usually needed in the SGA stem to advance the airway to its optimal location within the mouth.

Comorbidities Encountered in Ophthalmologic Surgery

PREMATURITY

The preterm infant may present for many surgical procedures early in life. Retinopathy of prematurity (ROP), congenital cataracts, and glaucoma may require EUAs and surgery even in infants who weigh less than 1000 grams. The preterm infant may have systemic illnesses that include acute and chronic pulmonary disease,[15] respiratory failure and pulmonary hypertension, congenital heart disease (CHD; unrepaired or with a limited palliative repair), and intraventricular hemorrhage,[16] with or without obstructive hydrocephalus.

Acutely ill preterm infants and those younger than 1 year of age are at greater risk than older children and adults for perioperative complications.[17] Careful attention to airway management, assisted ventilation, and titration of oxygen therapy with specified goals are essential for success.[18] In preterm infants, whose airways are already intubated and whose lungs are ventilated mechanically, the anesthesiologist should confirm the position of the tracheal tube, transport the infant safely to the operating room, and limit the concentration of oxygen to the minimum needed to maintain an acceptable oxygen saturation. Although institutional goals are not uniform regarding supplemental oxygen therapy,[19] communication with the neonatal team is often helpful in gauging the infant's previous oxygen requirement and current targeted goals (e.g., hemoglobin-oxygen saturation of 91%–95%).[20–22] Because most inhalational anesthetics impair hypoxic pulmonary vasoconstriction, a greater fraction of inspired oxygen (FiO_2) may be necessary to maintain the targeted hemoglobin saturation.

Hypercarbia and hypoxia may increase choroidal blood volume and increase IOP. Partial pressures of carbon dioxide (PCO_2) and oxygen (PO_2) should be controlled and monitored continuously. Infants are at greater risk for the OCR than older children and adults. Hence, IV access should be obtained before the surgical procedure or any examination or manipulation that may involve traction on the extraocular muscles or pressure on the globe.

Extremely low-birth-weight infants require many weeks to grow and develop to a weight of approximately 1800 grams and maintain their body temperature without special environmental control. Screening for ROP is widely practiced; serial preliminary examinations for ROP requires analgesia, which may involve any one of several strategies.[23,24] These infants commonly have a history of short-term or intermediate-term assisted ventilation and may or may not require supplemental oxygen before an EUA or planned operative procedure for ROP.[25] Many of these infants undergo ophthalmologic examinations while their lungs are ventilated in the neonatal intensive care unit,[26] although for those whose airways are extubated, sedation has been used to avoid reintubating the airway and the cycle of weaning again, particularly in those born extremely premature.[27,28] During surgical therapy (i.e., laser or intraocular injection) for ROP, these infants may require anesthesia to provide optimal conditions[29] (Fig. 32.1).

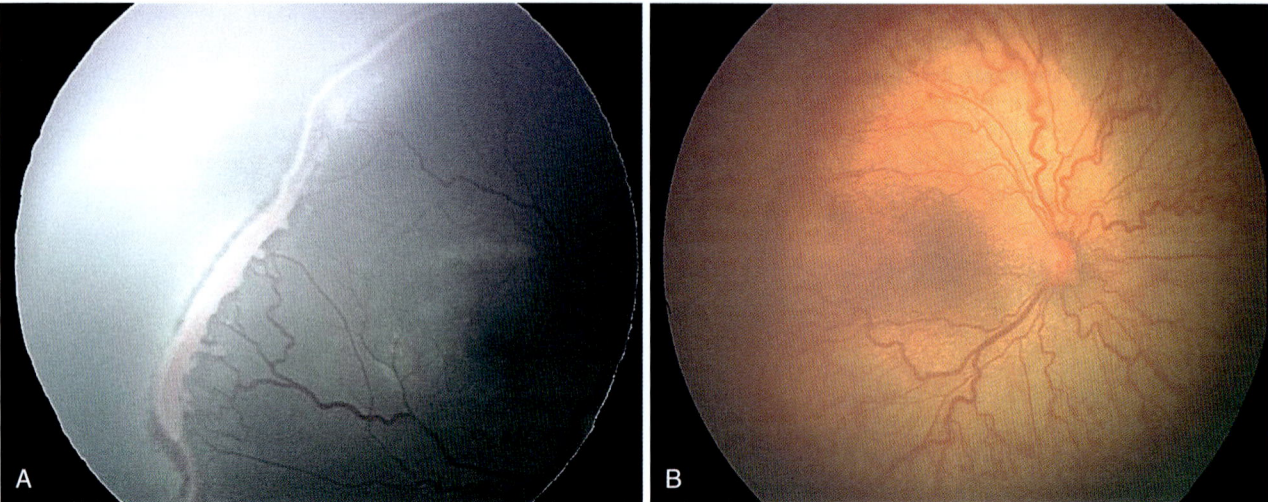

FIGURE 32.1 **A,** Stage 3 retinopathy of prematurity (ROP), the retinal vasculature ends abruptly in a large neovascular ridge **B,** Plus disease, is a severe stage of ROP characterized by venous dilation and arterial tortuosity venous dilation and arterial tortuosity. Stage 3 ROP with Plus disease are the standard criteria for the surgical treatment of ROP.

Perioperative apnea may preclude tracheal extubation or require close postoperative monitoring after anesthesia.[9,10,29]

Perioperative apnea in the preterm infant is widely described.[9,10,30] Whether the child is still hospitalized or presenting for elective surgery as an outpatient, the preoperative assessment should determine the pattern and frequency of apnea before the planned surgical procedure and anesthesia. The current use of respiratory stimulants (i.e., caffeine or theophylline) and oxygen should be determined. Is an apnea monitor being used, or has it been discontinued? Guidelines have not been developed to manage some of the scenarios, but infants who continue to require supplemental oxygen, who are younger than 60 weeks postmenstrual age, or who are monitored for apnea or bradycardia should have continuous cardiorespiratory and oxygen saturation monitoring postoperatively for at least 12 hours or until they are apnea free after both sedation and general anesthesia (see Chapter 2). The risk of apnea after general anesthesia and sedation decreases with advancing gestational age at birth and with advancing postmenstrual age. The risk of apnea is independent of opioid use; its multifactorial origins include the presence of general and neuraxial anesthetics and the immature CNS and respiratory centers in the preterm infant. Flexible planning for possible postoperative ventilatory support is essential, and families should be informed of this possibility preoperatively.

The airway of the preterm infant who is younger than 52 to 60 weeks postmenstrual age is usually intubated for ophthalmologic surgery owing to the immature respiratory drive, unpredictable respiratory response to anesthetic agents, and possible lag before recovery of respiratory drive after completion of the procedure and discontinuation of anesthetic agents.[29] If the infant does not appear to have a stable respiratory drive and strength after anesthesia, postoperative assisted ventilation should be continued as indicated; planning for this contingency is vital. *Ophthalmologic procedures may be brief and have a low risk of blood loss, but the risks of general anesthesia mandate full postoperative support.* Intensive care resources for assisted ventilation in preterm and formerly preterm infants should be available before embarking on anesthesia.

Although chronic lung disease related to prematurity is prevalent, its intensity has been reduced with the routine use of surfactant, steroids, and advances in ventilation management

strategies. Long-lasting respiratory effects from prematurity may include reactive airway disease, subglottic stenosis from prolonged intubation, and alveolar or interstitial disease with an oxygen requirement lasting weeks to years.[15] Because many anesthetics impair hypoxic pulmonary vasoconstriction, an increased oxygen requirement in the perioperative period should be anticipated. Tracheal intubation, a light level of anesthesia, or topical use of β-adrenergic antagonists may exacerbate reactive airway disease, requiring further treatment to reduce air trapping and hypercarbia.

In addition to assessing for airway and alveolar diseases, the anesthesiologist should determine whether pulmonary hypertension or right ventricular dysfunction is or was present.[31] Infants with pulmonary hypertension and episodes of hypoxemia when they cried or slept may be treated with continuous oxygen therapy and concomitant therapy (e.g., surfactant, sildenafil). If pulmonary hypertension was diagnosed previously, an updated evaluation is warranted. Because pulmonary hypertension is exacerbated by hypoxia and hypercarbia, tracheal intubation is indicated to ensure control of ventilation and oxygenation. At emergence, pulmonary hypertension may be exacerbated as hypercapnia develops, causing physiologic or anatomic shunting with systemic hemoglobin-oxygen desaturation. Immediate and continued evaluation of the airway is imperative to rule out an independent respiratory contribution to the systemic hypoxia.

Congenital cardiac disease may be diagnosed in the preterm neonate, infant, or child who presents for ophthalmologic procedures. Congenital cardiac anomalies require assessment before elective surgery. The various complex congenital cardiac lesions have a wide spectrum of interactions with anesthetic agents and vary in their risk for noncardiac surgery.[32,33] Many cardiac conditions require surgery or palliation (e.g., systemic-to-pulmonary shunts) before elective ophthalmologic procedures. There may be an urgent need for ophthalmologic evaluation (e.g., congenital tumor, cataract, glaucoma) before repair of the congenital cardiac condition. A ductus arteriosus may remain patent even after administering cyclooxygenase inhibitors. This may lead to persistent congestive failure, reduced pulmonary compliance, and complications of fluid management. Preoperative consultation with the infant's pediatric cardiologist can provide useful information on the infant's current cardiac status and the risk of dysrhythmias associated with cardiac defects.

Intraventricular hemorrhage is a major source of morbidity and mortality in preterm infants.[16,34] Obstructive hydrocephalus may occur and require cerebrospinal fluid diversion procedures to decompress the obstructed ventricular system and treat the associated increased intracranial pressure. Many of these infants require ophthalmologic surgery for repair of strabismus caused by a neurologic insult. If a ventriculoperitoneal shunt is in place, its proper function should be determined by direct evaluation. The anesthesiologist should assess whether there is inappropriate macrocephaly or a bulging or tense fontanelle. Obstructive hydrocephalus may occur after the infant's discharge from hospital, even though a ventriculoperitoneal shunt was not required previously. The preoperative assessment should include the child's developmental and neurologic status at the time of surgery. Because intraventricular hemorrhage is associated with long-term morbidity, any history of seizures should be elicited, and the antiepileptic drugs being used should be documented.

Preterm and small infants rapidly lose heat when anesthetized. Prevention of hypothermia is essential in the perioperative environment. Hypothermia decreases the metabolism of most drugs, depresses respiratory drive in preterm infants and if severe, interferes with coagulation (see Chapter 35).

DOWN SYNDROME

Children with Down syndrome (trisomy 21) frequently present for ophthalmologic surgery or EUA because of associated pathologic processes such as neonatal cataracts, refractive errors (e.g., hypermetropia, astigmatism), strabismus, glaucoma, keratoconus, nasolacrimal duct obstruction, and nystagmus.[35-37] Infants with trisomy 21 should have an ophthalmologic evaluation in the neonatal period. If this requires an EUA, the anesthesiologist should be prepared for the extensive medical implications associated with trisomy 21.[38,39] Almost half of these infants are born with CHD, including septal defects, complete or partial atrioventricular canal, tetralogy of Fallot, transposition of the great arteries, and valvular insufficiency or stenosis. Any child with a left-to-right shunt may develop pulmonary hypertension, and children with trisomy 21 can develop irreversible pulmonary hypertension at an earlier age. Bradycardia (25%–60%) and hypotension (12%–73%) have been reported during sevoflurane anesthesia in these children.[40,41] The child's cardiac defects should be clearly defined before planning the anesthetic prescription (see Chapters 14 and 16).

Airway abnormalities such as narrowed nasopharyngeal passages, macroglossia, pharyngeal hypotonia, and subglottic stenosis, as well as obstructive sleep apnea, are frequently observed in children with trisomy 21. These abnormalities may contribute to development of chronic intermittent hypoxia, further exacerbating pulmonary hypertension, and airway obstruction and hypoxia after general anesthesia.[42]

Children with trisomy 21 have a wide spectrum of developmental delays. Cervical spine instability occurs, and occiput-C1 and C1-C2 instabilities have been described.[43,44] Subluxation of the cervical spine has rarely been reported in these children during anesthesia. Nonetheless, the anesthesiologist and the surgeon should avoid extremes of neck flexion, extension, or lateral rotation during head positioning for laryngoscopy and surgery. Before the child is anesthetized, the parents should be questioned about a history of clumsy hand grip, wide based gait, or stumbling while walking. If cooperative, the child should be asked to flex and extend their neck to elicit neck pain and the presence of numbness

or tingling in the hands or feet in a particular position. Previous spine and neck investigations or operations should be reviewed. No consensus exists for the need to radiologically investigate a child with trisomy 21 who has an asymptomatic cervical spine, although many children undergo radiological evaluation before 5 years of age.[45]

Children with trisomy 21 may have congenital or acquired hypothyroidism. If the child is found to have a goiter on examination or has symptoms consistent with hypothyroidism (i.e., prolonged jaundice, hypothermia, constipation, dry skin, macroglossia, or relative bradycardia), thyroid function studies should be obtained before scheduling anesthesia. Children with trisomy 21 may develop junctional bradycardia during sevoflurane anesthesia,[46] which may be associated with or result from occult hypothyroidism.

ALPORT SYNDROME

Alport syndrome (i.e., progressive hereditary nephritis) is a disorder in a group of familial oculorenal syndromes that includes Lowe (oculocerebral) syndrome and familial renal-retinal dystrophy. Alport syndrome involves sensorineural hearing loss, progressive renal disease, and multiple ophthalmologic disorders, including cataracts, retinal detachment, and keratoconus.[47,48] Development of a myopathy and renal failure constitutes the major anesthesia concerns. If the patient has a myopathy, it is prudent to avoid succinylcholine and the risk of a hyperkalemic response and rhabdomyolysis. Renal insufficiency may impact on the choice of pharmacologic agents during anesthesia.

MARFAN SYNDROME, HOMOCYSTINURIA, AND EHLERS-DANLOS SYNDROME

Marfan syndrome, homocystinuria, and Ehlers-Danlos syndrome are considered together only from the perspective of a general body phenotype. The metabolic and molecular causes of these syndromes are well described.[49,50] They share problems with connective tissue development, possible joint laxity, and cardiovascular disorders.

Marfan syndrome is caused by a defect in the fibrillin 1 gene (FBN1), which affects elastic and nonelastic connective tissues. These children have an increased risk of lens dislocation, glaucoma, and retinal detachment (E-Fig. 32.1).[51] They may have pulmonary (scoliosis) and cardiovascular problems,[52] which includes aortic, mitral, or pulmonic valve insufficiency. Preoperative cardiovascular evaluation is indicated to determine the progression of cardiovascular abnormalities that inevitably occur. Acute and chronic blood pressure control is essential to prevent aortic dissection.

Homocystinuria has at least three forms and different inborn errors.[53] Enzymatic deficiency of the metabolism of sulfur-containing amino acids causes the intermediate metabolite, homocysteine, to accumulate. These children suffer from cataracts, retinal degeneration, optic atrophy, glaucoma, and lens dislocation. The cardiovascular pathology includes coronary artery disease at a young age. Thromboembolic phenomena occur more frequently because they may be hypercoagulable.[54] Nitrous oxide should be avoided because it inhibits methionine synthase, further limiting the conversion of homocysteine to methionine, which may lead to seizures and apneas.

Thirteen subtypes of Ehlers-Danlos syndrome have been described.[55] Not all forms express ocular pathology. From the anesthesiologist's perspective, positioning is important to avoid trauma to the skin because these children develop hemorrhages with minor trauma and experience delayed wound healing. A thorough preoperative assessment should be performed for cardiac lesions. Hypertension should be avoided to reduce the risk of rupturing an aneurysm. The duration of effect of local anesthetics in patients with type III Ehlers-Danlos syndrome may be less than that in unaffected patients, and contingency plans should be in place to address this possibility.[56]

MUCOPOLYSACCHARIDOSES

The mucopolysaccharidoses are a group of disorders with enzyme defects that result in incomplete degradation of glycosaminoglycans.[57] Affected children have various degrees of cognitive dysfunction, macroglossia, airway obstruction, cervical spine instability, and systemic involvement with deposition of mucopolysaccharide material. This leads to cardiac and respiratory dysfunction, airway obstruction, corneal opacities, and glaucoma.

The systemic complications of these disorders are sufficiently severe that even well-planned anesthesia management for ophthalmologic procedures may cause death.[58,59] Airway management can be extremely difficult with poor mask fit, dynamic airway obstruction with narrowed passages, a floppy epiglottis, and difficulty visualizing the larynx.[60] Infiltrative material may be deposited in the laryngeal inlet and pretracheal tissues; an SGA is particularly useful in maintaining a patent airway. Tracheal intubation may require the use of advanced airway visualization and management techniques, and the anesthesiologist should have several plans for airway management (see Chapter 12). Cardiac evaluation should be considered before an elective procedure to assess ventricular function and arrhythmias. IV access may be difficult due to subcutaneous deposition of mucopolysaccharides.

CRANIOFACIAL SYNDROMES

Craniofacial syndromes may manifest as craniosynostosis or have only middle and lower facial structure involvement.[61] Apert and Crouzon syndromes are both disorders of craniofacial development caused by a mutation in the fibroblast growth factor receptor 2 gene *(FGFR2)*. Apert syndrome manifests a more severe phenotype than Crouzon and is distinguished by the presence of syndactyly in fingers or toes (E-Fig. 32.2). They share the potential for many ocular disorders, including severe proptosis, making mask airway management difficult.[62] Other mutations of the *FGFR2* cause Antley-Bixler and Pfeiffer syndromes. These children may develop chronic airway obstruction, and some have complete tracheal rings (also known as tracheal cartilaginous sleeves); tracheal narrowing should be anticipated, and smaller tracheal tube sizes should be used.[63,64]

Children with asymmetry of facial and mandibular bone growth may present with limited mouth opening. Children with Goldenhar syndrome (i.e., hemifacial microsomia), Treacher Collins syndrome, and Pierre Robin sequence can be expected to present a challenge to airway management that differ developmentally: the airway in Goldenhar syndrome is either very difficult or easy with a 50:50 split in incidence that does not change with age; the airway in Treacher Collins syndrome becomes increasingly difficult with age, and the airway in Pierre Robin sequence infrequently presents a challenging tracheal intubation beyond 2 to 3 years of age as the size of the mandible grows to ultimately catch up to the maxilla (see Chapters 12 and 33).[65] Children with craniosynostosis have an increased risk of CHD and a cardiac evaluation should be performed before anesthesia.[66] Neurologic morbidity and seizure disorders occur more frequently in this group of patients.

PHAKOMATOSES

The phakomatoses are neurocutaneous syndromes with multiple ocular pathologic processes. These syndromes include neurofibromatosis,[67,68] encephalotrigeminal angiomatosis (i.e., Sturge-Weber syndrome),[69] tuberous sclerosis,[70,71] incontinentia pigmenti, and ataxia telangiectasia. CNS involvement varies with each of these diseases. Patients may have developmental delay, seizures, and neurologic morbidity. Anticonvulsant drug history and effectiveness should be reviewed; continue these medications in the perioperative period.

OPHTHALMOLOGIC PHYSIOLOGY

Two major considerations of ophthalmologic physiology are of great interest to the anesthesiologist. The first is the dynamics of aqueous humor production and transport, and their effects on IOP. The second is the OCR that may occur during any surgery around the orbit. Anesthetic agents affect the IOP. In a patient with a penetrating eye injury that is a laceration, any increase of IOP may be associated with extravasation of elements of the globe and irretrievable loss of vision.

INTRAOCULAR PRESSURE

IOP is pressure exerted by the internal components of the globe on the covering (i.e., sclera and conjunctiva). The normal IOP is 12 to 21 mm Hg; an IOP greater than 21 mm Hg is considered abnormal. IOP in children is unaffected by sex, but has a diurnal variation and is greater in obese compared with asthenic children.[72] Aqueous humor is a clear fluid that is secreted by the ciliary body into the anterior chamber of the globe where it bathes the iris. It then drains through the canal of Schlemm into the episcleral and then systemic veins (Fig. 32.2).[73–75] The posterior chamber, which is larger than the anterior chamber, is composed

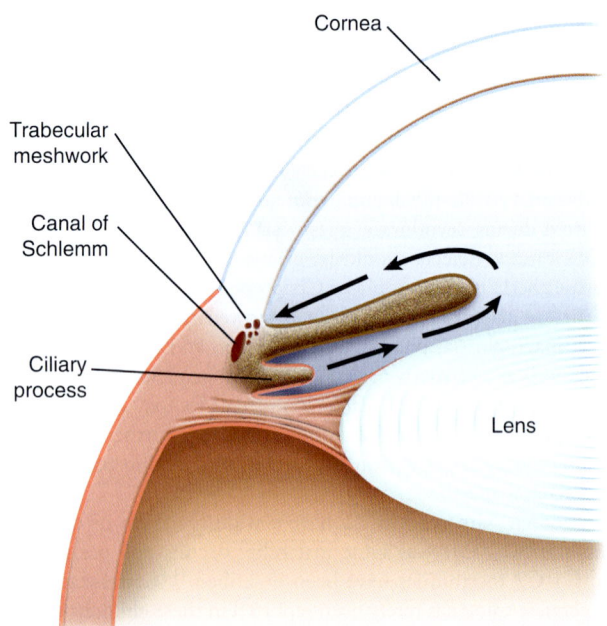

FIGURE 32.2 Aqueous humor is synthesized in the ciliary process and then circulates around the iris *(arrows)*, and into the anterior chamber. After flowing through the trabecular meshwork, aqueous humor enters the canal of Schlemm, which drains into the episcleral venous system. Pathologic conditions that increase venous pressure, obstruct the canal of Schlemm, or increase aqueous humor production may increase intraocular pressure.

of a gelatinous mix known as vitreous humor. The sclera and cornea that encase the intraocular constituents are relatively noncompliant and are protected by the bony orbit. However, intraorbital masses may impinge on the globe and increase the IOP or obstruct the drainage of aqueous humor from the anterior chamber and increase the IOP. If the drainage of aqueous humor into the episcleral veins is obstructed, fluid accumulates within the anterior chamber and the IOP increases.[74,76,77] Any increase in the central venous pressure (e.g., Trendelenburg position, coughing, Valsalva maneuver, straining, increased intrathoracic pressure) attenuates the drainage of aqueous humor from the anterior chamber and increases the IOP. Arterial pressure changes within the normal range indirectly affect the IOP: as arterial blood pressure increases beyond the normal range, approximately 30% of the increase in systolic blood pressure is reflected in IOP increases.

The formation of aqueous humor is described in the equation:

$$IOP = K[(OP_{aq} - OP_{pl}) + P_c],$$

where K is the coefficient of outflow, OP_{aq} is the osmotic pressure of aqueous humor, OP_{pl} is the osmotic pressure of plasma, and P_c is the capillary pressure. Accordingly, the IOP may be reduced by acutely increasing the plasma osmolality with mannitol. This increases the osmolality gradient and draws water out of the aqueous humor, thereby reducing the IOP.

In the relatively noncompliant globe, any pharmacologic or metabolic process that increases choroidal blood volume (e.g., hypercapnia, coughing, increased central venous pressure) produces choroidal congestion and an increased IOP. Although well tolerated in the healthy eye, this congestion may lead to extrusion of contents if the globe is open. The anesthesiologist should carefully control the child's physiology during the induction and maintenance of anesthesia to minimize increases in IOP, regardless of whether there is a preoperative concern about increased IOP.

Congenital or trauma-induced glaucoma requires therapy to reduce the IOP. If the IOP remains increased for a prolonged period, vision may be lost, primarily from damage to the optic nerve. Unfortunately, there are many causes of glaucoma in childhood. Hypercarbia, hypoxia, and drugs known or suspected to increase IOP (e.g., succinylcholine, ketamine) should be avoided or used with care. Reducing a child's apprehension and crying and avoiding increases in central venous pressure are also important considerations.

External pressure on the globe by a facemask or a finger increases the IOP.[78]

The effect of succinylcholine on IOP is well documented.[79–81] Succinylcholine increases IOP 6 to 10 mm Hg, an effect that begins within 1 minute after administration and continues for up to 10 minutes, at which time the IOP returns to normal. This effect has been attributed to four possible mechanisms:

- Cycloplegia induced by succinylcholine, which obstructs the outflow of aqueous humor.
- Tonic contraction of extraocular muscles.
- Increased choroidal blood volume.
- Relaxation of orbital muscles, which increases external pressure on the globe.

Specific muscles develop a sustained tonic tension after succinylcholine that in the presence of an open globe may cause extrusion of intraocular contents.[82] Extrusion in response to increased IOP depends on the diameter of the orifice; a smaller laceration/pinhole (<2 mm) is less likely to extrude intraocular contents than a larger laceration/incision (>4 mm). Alternatively, rocuronium (1.2 mg/kg IV) provides optimal intubating conditions within 30 seconds for the child with an open globe injury while minimizing the risk for aspiration or succinylcholine-associated increases in IOP. Rocuronium increases the IOP to a smaller extent than succinylcholine as part of a rapid-sequence induction of anesthesia.[83] Concerns associated with prolonged paralysis after large doses of rocuronium for a brief procedure or a failed intubation have been resolved with the widespread availability of sugammadex.[84]

Most general anesthetics decrease IOP,[78] although ketamine IV or intramuscular (IM) has been reported to exert a variable albeit minimal effect on IOP; an effect that may be attributed to ventilation control and consequent $PaCO_2$ rather than the drug.[85–88] Oral ketamine does not increase IOP. When IV access is unavailable or the cardiovascular status of the patient warrants the use of ketamine, the child's overall safety takes precedence over the possible ramifications of ketamine on IOP. IOP is measured by tonometry on the external surface of the globe and takes several seconds to complete. Tonometry is often performed early in the EUA during general anesthesia. Many ophthalmologists prefer to measure the IOP as soon as consciousness is lost to limit the effects of the anesthetic on the IOP.

OCULOCARDIAC REFLEX

First described in 1908, the OCR, also known as the trigeminovagal reflex or Aschner-Dagnini reflex, describes a reflex decrease in heart rate that is triggered by stretching or traction on the extraocular and levator (eyelid elevator) muscles or pressure applied to the globe. Although the criteria for diagnosing the OCR varies among centers, it is observed in roughly 10% of children undergoing strabismus surgery if anticholinergic prophylaxis is not administered. Routine prophylaxis is often not given due to widespread understanding of its pathogenesis and how to avoid a severe incidence of the OCR.[89] Sudden strenuous versus slow, gentle traction on the extraocular muscle evokes a more profound bradycardic OCR.[89] In addition, stretching the inferior oblique muscle is reported to evoke a greater OCR response than stretching the lateral rectus muscle.[90] The pathway for the reflex involves an afferent signal conducted through the ophthalmic (V1) branch of the trigeminal nerve via the ciliary ganglion that activates parasympathetic output through the vagus nerve, resulting primarily in sinus or junctional bradycardia or atrioventricular block[89] (Fig. 32.3A), although other dysrhythmias including ventricular ectopy and asystole may occur, usually in adults undergoing strabismus surgery (Fig. 32.3B). In the early days, some recommended a retrobulbar block with local anesthetic to attenuate the OCR, whereas others found that the block may precipitate the OCR by applying external pressure on the globe.[89] A sub-Tenon block before pulling on the eye muscle may effectively block this reflex.[12]

If the OCR occurs frequently with a surgeon or in practice, an anticholinergic medication, such as atropine (20 μg/kg) or glycopyrrolate (10–20 μg/kg), may be given IV prophylactically, at induction of anesthesia or earlier.[89] Although these medications do not absolutely prevent bradycardia, both decrease its severity and duration. Because anticholinergics cause pupillary dilatation, they do not present a problem for the ophthalmologist, but they may increase the IOP slightly.

If a clinically concerning decrease in heart rate occurs based on the child's age and clinical status, then the surgeon should be asked to immediately release the traction on the extraocular muscle or stimulation in the surgical field. Heart rate will spontaneously return to its "pretraction" value within a very brief period. An IV dose of atropine (5–20 μg/kg) will interrupt the reflex and restore the heart rate, although the correction may be evanescent

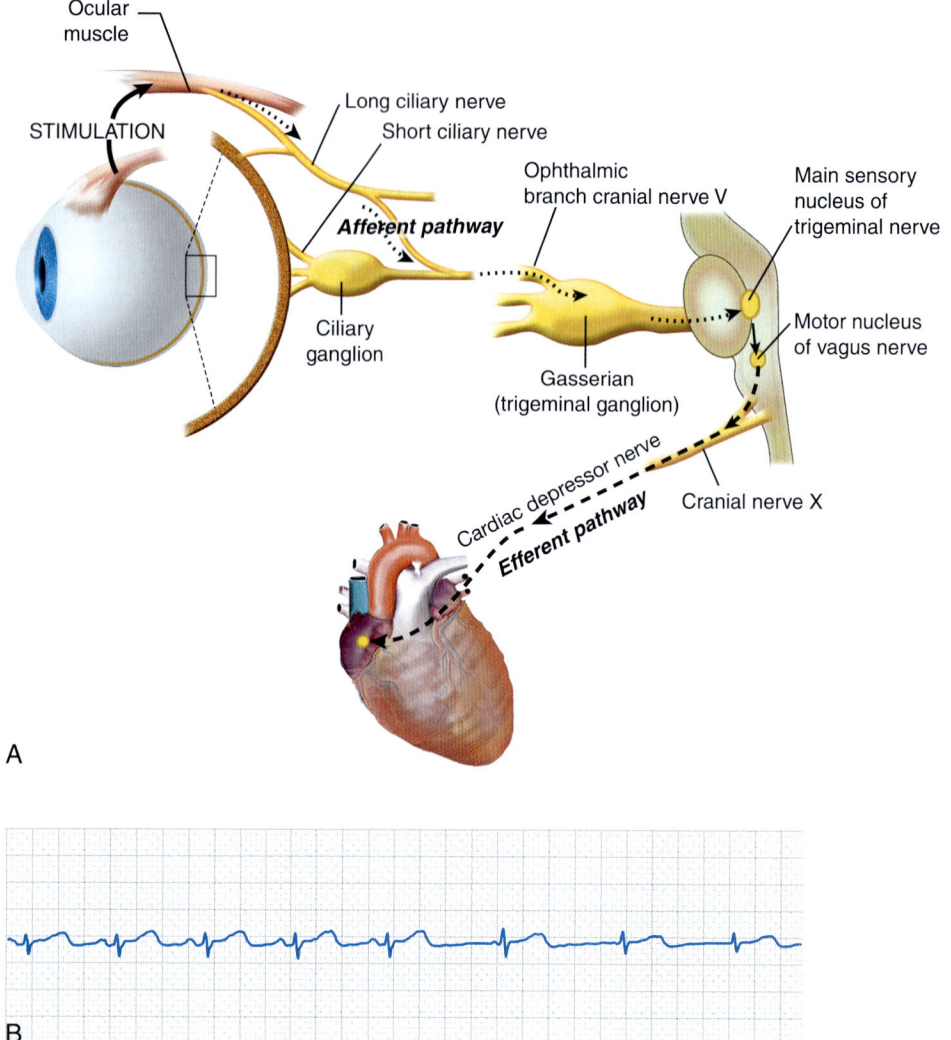

FIGURE 32.3 Traction on the extraocular muscles elicits the oculocardiac reflex (curved arrow). **A,** The afferent limb consists of the long and short ciliary nerves, which synapse in the ciliary ganglion *(dotted arrows)*. The ophthalmic division of the trigeminal nerve (cranial nerve V) carries the impulse to the gasserian ganglion, and the arc continues to the sensory nucleus of cranial nerve V in the brainstem. Fibers in the reticular formation synapse with the nucleus of the vagus nerve (cranial nerve X). Efferent fibers from the vagus nerve terminate in the heart *(dashed arrow)*. The neurotransmitter from the vagus nerve to the sinoatrial node is acetylcholine, and the reflex is blocked by antimuscarinic pharmacologic agents (i.e., atropine and glycopyrrolate). **B,** Electrocardiogram shows conversion from normal sinus rhythm to a nodal rhythm.

and dysrhythmias may recur. IV epinephrine (1–10 μg/kg) is rarely necessary but should always be available. The anesthesiologist should provide adequate oxygenation and ventilation because hypercarbia or hypoxia may compound or intensify the reflex activity.

The incidence of the OCR varies with the anesthetic: the incidence during sevoflurane and desflurane anesthesia is similar and less than that during total intravenous anesthesia with propofol.[91,92] When the incidence of OCR was compared among inhalational anesthetics, propofol and ketamine, the smallest incidence of OCR occurred during ketamine anesthesia.[93] Other strategies to attenuate the OCR include topically applied lidocaine[94] or IV ketamine.[95] Deeper levels of anesthesia during pediatric strabismus surgery when measured by EEG attenuate the OCR, although this has not been consistently demonstrated.[91,96,97]

OPHTHALMOLOGIC PHARMACOTHERAPEUTICS AND SYSTEMIC IMPLICATIONS

Topical ophthalmologic medications are usually placed directly on the cornea or in the inferior cul-de-sac. Most of these agents need several minutes up to 1 hour for maximal effectiveness and thus must be administered before entering the operating room, or soon after induction of anesthesia. Medications delivered topically to the eye are absorbed through the conjunctiva and nasal mucosa into the systemic circulation; their pharmacologic mechanisms of action predict the systemic consequences. Therefore, some medications are diluted for use in children to reduce the risk of systemic toxicity.[98,99] Anticholinergics, sympathomimetics, and antihistamines can cause pupillary dilation and decrease the movement of aqueous humor, thus increasing the IOP. Table 32.2 lists the more commonly used pediatric topical agents.

TABLE 32.2	Commonly Used Ophthalmologic Agents	
Drug	**Indication**	**Side Effect Profile**
Cholinergic Agents		
Acetylcholine	Induce miosis	Bradycardia
Carbachol	Induce miosis	Corneal edema, retinal detachment
Pilocarpine	Glaucoma	Corneal edema, retinal detachment
Cholinesterase Inhibitors		
Physostigmine	Glaucoma	Retinal detachment, miosis
Echothiophate	Glaucoma	Retinal detachment, miosis
Muscarinic Antagonists		
Atropine	Cycloplegic retinoscopy, mydriasis	Photosensitivity, blurred vision, increased heart rate, dry mouth
Scopolamine	Antiemetic, mydriasis	Photosensitivity, blurred vision, increased heart rate, dry mouth
Homatropine	Cycloplegic retinoscopy, mydriasis	Photosensitivity, blurred vision, increased heart rate, dry mouth
Cyclopentolate	Cycloplegic retinoscopy, mydriasis	Photosensitivity, blurred vision, increased heart rate, dry mouth
Tropicamide	Cycloplegic retinoscopy, mydriasis	Photosensitivity, blurred vision, increased heart rate, dry mouth
Sympathomimetic Agents		
Dipivefrin	Glaucoma	Photosensitivity, hypersensitivity
Epinephrine	Glaucoma	Photosensitivity, hypersensitivity
Phenylephrine	Mydriasis	Photosensitivity, hypersensitivity
Apraclonidine	Glaucoma	Photosensitivity, hypersensitivity
Brimonidine	Glaucoma	Photosensitivity, hypersensitivity
Cocaine	Local anesthetic	Anisocoria, corneal injury, photosensitivity, hypersensitivity
Hydroxyamphetamine	Glaucoma	Anisocoria, photosensitivity, hypersensitivity
Naphazoline	Decongestant	Photosensitivity, hypersensitivity
Tetrahydrozoline	Decongestant	Photosensitivity, hypersensitivity
α- and β-Adrenergic Antagonists		
Dapiprazole (α)	Reverse mydriasis	Conjunctival hyperemia
Betaxolol (β₁-selective)	Glaucoma	Bradycardia, hypotension
Carteolol (β)	Glaucoma	Decreased heart rate, blood pressure, bronchospasm
Levobunolol (β)	Glaucoma	Decreased heart rate, blood pressure, bronchospasm
Metipranolol (β)	Glaucoma	Decreased heart rate, blood pressure, bronchospasm
Timolol (β)	Glaucoma	Decreased heart rate, blood pressure, bronchospasm
Recombinant Monoclonal Antibodies		
Bevacizumab	ROP, retinoblastoma, retinal venous thrombosis, diabetic retinopathy	Drug introduced directly into eye; systemic effects minimal

ROP, Retinopathy of prematurity.
Modified from Brunton LL, Lazo JS, Parker KL, eds. *Goodman and Gilman's The Pharmacological Basis of Therapeutics.* 11th ed. New York: McGraw-Hill; 2006.

Topical mydriatic agents dilate the pupil. The most common mydriatic is phenylephrine (2.5% solution), an α_1-adrenergic agonist that is rapidly absorbed but may cause hypertension in small infants. If severe hypertension occurs, reflex bradycardia and asystole may ensue.

Topical cycloplegic agents also dilate the pupil, as well as eliminate lens accommodation by paralyzing the ciliary muscle. This aids in retinal evaluation with the indirect ophthalmoscope and in evaluating refractive errors because accommodation of the lens is paralyzed. These agents are muscarinic cholinergic antagonists (i.e., antimuscarinic agents). One such agent is cyclopentolate hydrochloride (0.5%), which can cause CNS toxicity with disorientation, seizures, and blurred vision. It is also marketed in

a combination with phenylephrine, which has caused a cardiac arrest in young infants.[98] Atropine (0.5%–2.0%) and scopolamine (0.25%) solutions are also cycloplegics that dilate the pupil. Tropicamide (0.5% and 1.0%) is another commonly used topical cycloplegic. When systemically absorbed, these agents may cause antimuscarinic, anticholinergic toxicity, including tachycardia, dry mouth, pupillary dilation, flushing of the skin, heat intolerance or fever, and disorientation (E-Fig. 32.3).

β-Adrenergic blockers (e.g., timolol, betaxolol) also decrease the IOP in patients with glaucoma.[100] However, when absorbed systemically from the eye, they bypass first-pass metabolism and in the case of timolol and its analogues are subject to CYP450 2D6 single nucleotide polymorphisms for metabolism.[101] As a consequence, when patients already treated with beta-blocker or at risk to develop complications from sympathetic nervous system blockade receive topical beta-blockade, bradycardia, asystole, and cardiovascular collapse, and bronchospasm may ensue, although this is supported only by anecdotal evidence, not randomized controlled trials.[102] Some advocate preoperative genotyping for CYP2D6 and continuous ECG monitoring when applying topical beta-blockers to the globe.[101] If β-adrenergic intoxication is suspected, direct-acting cardiovascular stimulants (epinephrine) should be used to antagonize the β-adrenergic blockade rather than indirect-acting stimulants such as ephedrine.

Topical local anesthetics are infrequently used in children except for the very cooperative child for tonometry or removal of sutures. Proparacaine and tetracaine (ester local anesthetics) may be used topically, whereas lidocaine and bupivacaine (or levobupivacaine, ropivacaine, which are amide local anesthetics) are used for ophthalmic blocks. Ester local anesthetics confer a small risk for systemic toxicity because they are extensively metabolized by plasma cholinesterases. Ophthalmic amide agents, however, may cause systemic toxicity (i.e., cardiac dysrhythmias and seizures), but these agents are infrequently used in children. Topical cocaine is very rarely used in pediatric ophthalmology except to test for Horner syndrome and as a vasoconstrictor to reduce nasal bleeding during nasal and nasolacrimal duct surgery.

Nonsteroidal antiinflammatory drugs (NSAIDs) are used for certain inflammatory conditions of the eye, but perioperative use in a child is uncommon. Some NSAIDs (i.e., ketorolac and ibuprofen) pose a concern for ophthalmology because their anticoagulant profiles may increase local perioperative bleeding. However, several NSAIDs are approved for ocular use, and systemic NSAIDs are used postoperatively for their antiinflammatory effects.

Echothiophate (i.e., phospholine iodide) is a cholinesterase inhibitor used to induce miosis in the treatment of glaucoma. When absorbed systemically, it impairs plasma cholinesterase, reducing the metabolism of some drugs (e.g., succinylcholine) and prolonging their duration of action. Decreased metabolism of acetylcholine may result in increased relative cholinergic tone, inducing bradycardia and bronchiolar muscle activity resulting in bronchospasm. Toxicity from echothiophate may be antagonized by administration of pralidoxime (2-pyridine aldoxime methyl chloride [2-PAM]) (25 mg/kg IV). Otherwise, its action to reduce effective systemic cholinesterases lasts 4 to 6 weeks.

Pilocarpine, a direct-acting cholinergic agonist that is used to treat glaucoma, has replaced echothiophate iodide. Through multiple actions, it improves the flow of aqueous humor; if absorbed, it may acutely cause bradycardia.

Many vitreal substitutes are used in ophthalmologic procedures. They include nonexpansile and expansile gases (e.g., sulfur hexafluoride), perfluorocarbon liquids, and silicone oils. The anesthesia team should be informed when the ophthalmologist plans intraocular use of one of these substances. If a gas pocket is anticipated, nitrous oxide should be discontinued or avoided completely. The patient and parent should be informed of any intraocular gas use, and the patient should wear an alert bracelet for the expected duration of absorption, usually no longer than 6 to 12 weeks, so that inadvertent use of nitrous oxide does not occur during that interval. When a perforated globe is closed, any residual environmental air pocket can be expanded by nitrous oxide; increased ocular pressure and reduced retinal blood flow may result.

Novel antivascular endothelial growth factor agents are being used in the treatment of retinal angiogenic diseases (e.g., macular degeneration, ROP, retinoblastoma) which inhibit the formation of new blood vessels.[103–105] The most commonly used are recombinant monoclonal antibodies (e.g., bevacizumab), which in the doses prescribed should not raise concerns for anesthesia.

EMERGENT, URGENT, AND ELECTIVE PROCEDURES

One of the greatest controversies in pediatric anesthesia is defining the optimal technique to induce anesthesia in a child with an open globe injury and a full stomach.[81,82] The issue of aspiration while securing the airway versus the possible extravasation of intraocular contents caused by an increase in IOP is a difficult risk/benefit assessment. In 2006, a postal survey of UK anesthesiologists revealed that 21% had never anesthetized and 55% had anesthetized fewer than 5 children with an open eye injury.[106] Interestingly, succinylcholine was used by 43% of anesthesiologists who had anesthetized >10 cases of open eye injuries compared with 10% of those who had managed <5 cases. The debate is likely to continue because the risks are real and the incidence of either phenomenon is rare and difficult to study.

The ophthalmologist should be intimately involved in the entire process. Ideally the patient should have a metal or plastic shield secured over the injured eye as soon as possible, as an agitated patient could easily harm the injured eye in the preoperative area or during induction.

Among adults, aspiration is an uncommon event with a small mortality rate. The incidence of aspiration in children is ~1/10,000 elective cases but is greater in emergent cases; mortality secondary to aspiration is <1/200,000 children.[107–110] The use of succinylcholine for rapid-sequence induction in the treatment of a perforated globe has been challenged because of its known propensity to increase the IOP. Rocuronium (1.2 mg/kg) has an onset equivalent to that of succinylcholine, provides excellent intubating conditions,[111] and increases IOP less than succinylcholine as part of a rapid-sequence induction.[83] However, if the child is not adequately anesthetized and fully paralyzed during instrumentation of the airway, coughing, retching, and increased systolic blood pressure may increase IOP. Lidocaine (1–2 mg/kg IV) usually attenuates the hemodynamic responses to laryngoscopy and tracheal intubation, but this is not a consistent experience.[112,113] Opioids blunt the IOP response to intubation, but may also induce vomiting, indirectly increasing the IOP transiently. Regardless of how it is achieved, adequate depth of anesthesia and akinesia before airway instrumentation is important to prevent the increase in IOP that accompanies sympathetic activation and patient movement.

IV access is essential for a rapid induction of anesthesia. In most instances, children with ruptured globes present with IV access because IV antibiotics are started as soon as possible (i.e., within 6 hours of the rupture) to prevent endophthalmitis. If antibiotics are not given early after the injury, complete loss of vision is more likely to be a long-term consequence. In some instances, however, IV access has not been established or the IV access has been lost. In this case, other options may include:

- Ultrasound-guided IV catheter placement with topical anesthesia.
- Gaseous induction with sevoflurane with the child in the lateral decubitus position.
- IM ketamine (and succinylcholine or rocuronium).
- Placement of a central line (e.g., femoral vein) or intraosseous needle.

The increase in IOP after IM succinylcholine is less than that after IV administration[114]; however, absorption of agents given IM varies widely. Although IM succinylcholine (4–5 mg/kg) will paralyze a child in 2 to 8 minutes depending on the dose, the child may cry from pain, develop hypertension, or vomit during the induction, all of which may increase IOP. Knowing that the airway reflexes are gradually lost after an IM injection in the child with a full stomach is a clinically important risk that must be considered when selecting a method to secure the airway.

Some clinicians recommend placing an intraosseous needle for induction when IV access has not already been established. Even when local anesthesia has been used to establish IV access, placing an intraosseous needle may be poorly tolerated in awake children.

Despite the presence of a full stomach, induction of anesthesia with sevoflurane may be used with caution, but a deep plane of anesthesia is required before attempting to establish IV access or manipulating the airway because coughing and vomiting may occur with a light plane of anesthesia. IV access should then be established. If this is unsuccessful, an IM dose of a neuromuscular blocking drug may be administered.[115-117] In this circumstance, IOP may increase and regurgitation remains a possibility.

A moderate approach to the child who needs emergent or urgent ophthalmologic surgery is to secure IV access as quickly and painlessly as possible (ultrasound with topical analgesia). Oral premedication with midazolam or a combination of midazolam and ketamine may be used to facilitate IV or intraosseous access if the patient will accept oral medication administration. An attempt is made to preoxygenate the child without causing distress. If a tight mask fit is not easily achieved, forcing the tight fit to the child's face is not desirable because of the likelihood of increasing the IOP as the child resists. Anesthesia may be induced via IV access with lidocaine, propofol, and rocuronium. After 30 to 60 seconds timed by the clock or with train-of-four monitoring, tracheal intubation is expeditiously performed, and gastric contents evacuated.

Other urgent procedures may include treatment of retinopathy or decompression of orbital cellulitis. These procedures may be urgent but still allow several hours of *nil per os* (NPO) status. Concern about aspiration may not be as great. Nonetheless, the surgeon will wish to proceed as expeditiously as is safe. Options for induction and maintenance may or may not include succinylcholine.

Most ophthalmologic procedures are performed on a scheduled basis, allowing routine preoperative evaluation and planning. This includes establishing all relevant medical information about the child, implementing NPO status, and placing an IV catheter if desired.

INDUCTION AND MAINTENANCE OF ANESTHESIA

Infants do not generally require a premedicant for anxiolysis, and the use of premedication after the first year of life is usually discussed with the parents and child. Separation anxiety or struggling during induction usually does not affect most ophthalmologic diagnoses, except for a penetrating eye injury, which may become worse if the child struggles. IV propofol, etomidate, or ketamine produce a smooth induction, as does an inhalational induction with oxygen, nitrous oxide, and sevoflurane. If laryngospasm develops during induction, an IV bolus of propofol (1–2 mg/kg IV) should be promptly administered. Atropine (20 μg/kg) may be given IV or IM before bradycardia occurs. IM succinylcholine or rocuronium may also break laryngospasm if an IV catheter has not been placed.[109-113,115-120] For elective tracheal intubation, an IV nondepolarizing muscle relaxant is preferred because succinylcholine may increase the IOP.

Alternative induction methods include IM ketamine (4–10 mg/kg) and, in infants, rectal methohexital (25–30 mg/kg). Ketamine may

increase IOP, but it has been successfully used in ophthalmologic procedures in children.[95]

For most ophthalmologic surgery, an anesthetized child is sufficient as most eye surgery is extraocular; however, for intraocular surgery such as a vitrectomy, the surgeon may request tracheal intubation and paralysis to ensure the child does not cough or buck when the eye is open. In the latter instances, we prefer to use a cuffed oral Ring-Adair-Elwyn (RAE) preformed tracheal tube (Mallinckrodt, Inc. St. Louis, MO) although a straight tracheal tube is equally safe. The tracheal tube is secured so that the sterile surgical field is maintained during the procedure. Access to the tracheal tube and anesthesia circuit by the anesthesia care team without trespass of the surgical field is imperative. Extensions to the individual limbs of the anesthetic circle circuit have no bearing on the dead space of the breathing circuit, whereas extensions between the Y connector in the circuit and the patient (i.e., adjacent to the tracheal tube) add dead space that may increase $PaCO_2$. For extraocular surgery, an SGA provides a patent airway, has less effect on the IOP than tracheal intubation, and requires a lighter plane of anesthesia to maintain.[78]

Anesthesia can be maintained with a variety of techniques. Inhalational sevoflurane, isoflurane, or desflurane provide excellent conditions for maintenance of anesthesia[121] and rapid emergence. Total IV anesthesia is also gaining popularity (see Chapter 6) and reduces PONV. When neuromuscular blockade is necessary to reduce the potential for movement, we routinely use nondepolarizing neuromuscular blocking drugs and train-of-four monitoring to ensure the adequacy of neuromuscular blockade. Since most ophthalmologic surgery results in minimal pain, an enhanced recovery after surgery (ERAS) protocol is used in many centers, which includes preoperative oral acetaminophen combined with intraoperative ketorolac and possibly dexmedetomidine.[122,123] Small doses of opioids may be titrated postoperatively as needed but are often not required.

Eye surgery is among the most common surgeries associated with PONV in children. Strabismus surgery in children is associated with the greatest incidence (45%–85%) of PONV, especially in the absence of antiemetic prophylaxis.[124,125] The type of ventilation does not attenuate the incidence of PONV.[126] However, several strategies have been shown to reduce the incidence of PONV including infusing 30 mL/kg balanced salt solution IV during surgery (Table 32.3).[127] Avoiding opioids[128,129] and replacing them with nonopioid analgesics such as acetaminophen,[130] diclofenac,[131] and ketorolac[128,129] lessen the risk of PONV. If opioids are needed, short-acting medications such as remifentanil, alfentanil, or fentanyl are preferred.

A host of medications are reported to affect the risk of PONV.[132] Preoperative use of benzodiazepines,[133] avoidance of nitrous oxide,[134] and superhydration with balanced salt solutions[127]; use of propofol,[134,135] clonidine,[136] dexmedetomidine,[137] 5-HT$_3$ receptor antagonists,[138-140] dimenhydrinate,[141,142] metoclopramide,[143] or dexamethasone[144-148]; all attenuate the incidence of PONV. Dose-response relationships with PONV have been described for some of these drugs (clonidine and 5-HT$_3$ receptor blockers, dexamethasone).[136,138,144] Older antiemetics such as droperidol that effectively attenuate the incidence of PONV[130,149-151] have fallen into disfavor because of their sedative side effects and risk of prolonging the QT interval,[152] although the latter has not been a common problem in children.[153] Anesthesiologists have adopted a multimodal approach to PONV in the case of strabismus surgery.[153] A commonly used regimen includes premedication with oral midazolam, choice of anesthesia,

TABLE 32.3	Antiemetic Strategies for Prophylaxis and Treatment of Postoperative Nausea and Vomiting
Strategy	**Drug and Dose**
Butyrophenone (dopamine antagonist)	Droperidol (10–70 µg/kg)
Serotonin (5HT$_3$ receptor antagonists)	Ondansetron (0.1 mg/kg)
	Granisetron (10–40 µg/kg)
	Dolasetron (0.35 mg/kg)
Propofol-based total IV anesthesia	Propofol (100–175 µg/kg per minute)
Local anesthetic	Lidocaine local-topical and systemic (1–1.5 mg/kg)
Opioid-sparing analgesics or anesthetics	Retrobulbar block with bupivacaine
Other pharmacology	Dexamethasone (10–500 µg/kg); maximum, 8 mg
	Dimenhydrinate (0.5–1 mg/kg)
	Metoclopramide (0.15–0.25 mg/kg)
	Benzodiazepines (e.g., lorazepam, midazolam) (10–100 µg/kg)
	Avoid nitrous oxide (N$_2$O)
	Avoid opioids
	Use ketorolac (Toradol) (0.5 mg/kg PO, IV, IM), acetaminophen (30–40 mg/kg PR or 15 mg/kg IV), or diclofenac (1 mg/kg PR), or short-acting opioids (e.g., remifentanil, alfentanil, fentanyl)
Nonpharmacologic adjuvants	IV hydration
	Gastric decompression
	Acupressure, specifically PC6 acupoint stimulation

IM, Intramuscular; *IV*, intravenous; *PO*, per os (oral); *PR*, per rectum (suppository).

liberal hydration with IV fluid, and the combination of 5-HT$_3$ receptor antagonists and dexamethasone. There is no evidence in children undergoing strabismus surgery that dosing of 5-HT$_3$ receptor antagonists at the end of surgery provides better protection against PONV than earlier in the surgery, probably because this surgery is brief, less than 1 hour.[154] However, dosing of 5-HT$_3$ receptor antagonists during emergence in children with congenital prolonged QT interval increases the risk of adverse events.[155] There is a dichotomy of practice with respect to the use of nitrous oxide for maintenance of anesthesia during strabismus surgery. Some avoid nitrous oxide, maintaining anesthesia by propofol infusion and including the previously mentioned adjunct medications. Others use nitrous oxide and an inhalational anesthetic for maintenance but also include the remainder of the preoperative and intraoperative adjunct medications. Use of at least dual-agent prophylaxis (5-HT$_3$ receptor antagonist and dexamethasone) for prevention of PONV after strabismus surgery seems prudent, is supported by evidence (from adults) that the effect of nitrous oxide is markedly diminished if two antiemetics are given prophylactically,[156] exerts a limited effect in surgeries that last less than 1 hour,[157] and is in accordance with consensus guidelines for the management of pediatric PONV.[158]

IV fluid replacement can reduce PONV.[158,159] Children who present for elective surgery may drink clear fluids up to 2 hours before surgery, reducing the fasting period. However, it is important to identify those who have fasted for a prolonged period and to administer sufficient IV fluids (10–20 mL/kg per hour of a balanced salt solution) depending on the severity of dehydration to reestablish euvolemia. Antidiuretic hormone release dictates reduced postoperative fluid requirements (e.g., infusion rate at one-half of the previously considered rate, using 2 mL/kg per hour for the first 10 kg, 1 mL/kg per hour for the next 10 kg, and 0.5 mL/kg per hour for every kilogram greater than 20 kg until the child takes fluids by mouth).[160-162] When the surgical procedure is not likely to involve an increased IOP, we routinely replace almost 100% of the calculated deficit. We have not observed children to experience urinary retention or hypertension from this strategy, most likely because children can redistribute the excess fluid more efficiently than adults.[163] However, if the duration of surgery exceeds 3 hours, we catheterize the bladder to reduce the risk of urinary retention and overdistention of the bladder.

At the completion of surgery, neuromuscular blockade is antagonized, maintenance agents are discontinued, and the child is allowed to awaken. Deep extubation is preferred by some to reduce coughing and increases in IOP at the time of extubation.[164] Others prefer extubating the trachea when the child is fully awake with intact airway reflexes, although coughing and increases in IOP may occur. For most procedures in children, a short interval of increased IOP does not damage a surgical correction, such as strabismus, ptosis, or ROP treatment. Appropriate postoperative analgesics may include local anesthetics, acetaminophen, and opioids. Nonsteroidal agents are effective, but their use should be discussed with the surgeon in case there is concern regarding postoperative bleeding.[128] In our experience, IV ketorolac is acceptable for use during strabismus surgery, but not for intraocular procedures. Benzodiazepines (e.g., lorazepam) may also have some utility.[133]

Specific Ophthalmologic Procedures

STRABISMUS SURGERY
Corrective strabismus surgery realigns the divergent visual axes of the eyes by detaching and reattaching extraocular muscles to the globes (Fig. 32.4). The procedures are brief if only one or two muscles are involved. In infants, inhalational or IV induction is performed, and neuromuscular blockade is provided with nondepolarizing neuromuscular blocking drugs. Strabismus may be an isolated finding in a child or a manifestation of other systemic diseases or syndromes. The anesthesiologist should carefully review the birth history, history of prematurity, CNS disorders, syndrome identification, possible coexistent myopathy, and cardiovascular and respiratory history. If OCR is anticipated, prophylactic prevention with IV atropine or glycopyrrolate may be considered.

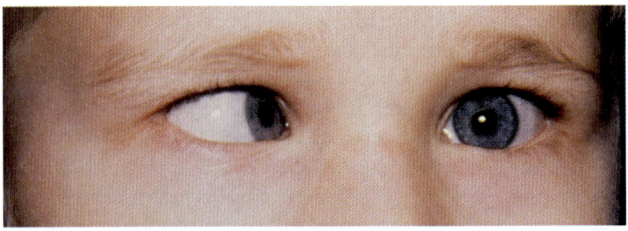

FIGURE 32.4 Strabismus repair is a common pediatric ophthalmologic procedure. The child demonstrates significant right esotropia that requires surgical correction.

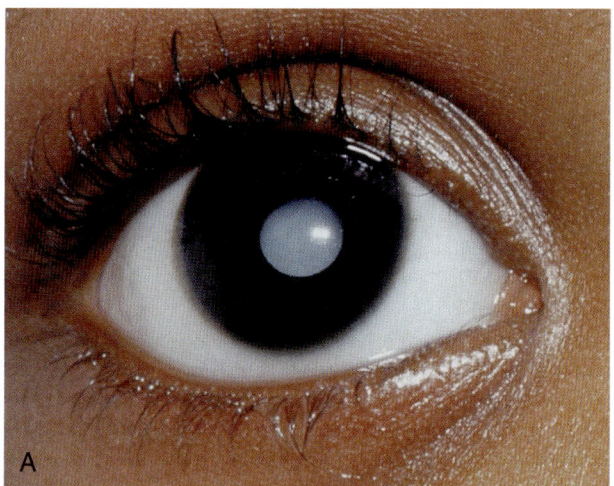

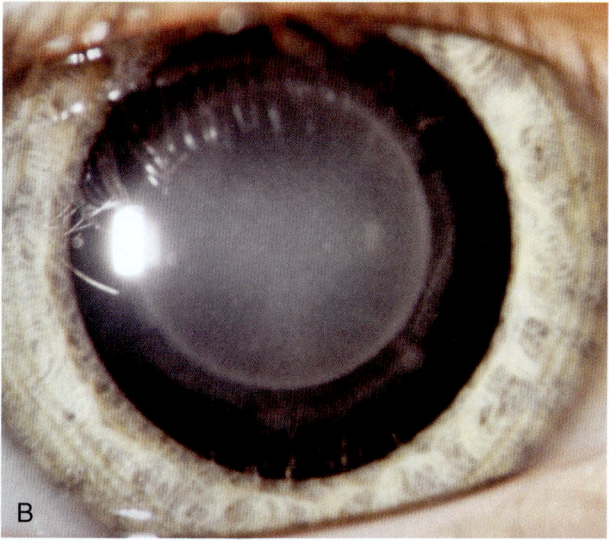

FIGURE 32.5 A, The red reflex is absent in the child with this cataract; this requires surgical removal. **B,** The close-up photograph shows a lamellar/nuclear cataract, which can be associated with inborn errors of metabolism in childhood.

infant may require monitoring for postoperative anesthetic-induced respiratory depression or apnea. In infants, bilateral cataracts may be corrected simultaneously, during the same anesthesia episode, or during staged procedures separated by days or weeks. There is no documented increased incidence of surgical or anesthetic complications when both cataracts are corrected simultaneously.[170] Pediatric cataracts can be associated with some systemic diseases or genetic abnormalities. Intraocular lens implants are often done in pediatric cataract surgery, although typically not in newborn congenital cataracts.[171] The child should be examined carefully for dysmorphology, with close attention to issues of airway management and the cardiorespiratory system.

ANTERIOR CHAMBER PARACENTESIS AND WASHOUT

An anterior chamber paracentesis may be performed in children to wash out blood products to lower IOP in a nonclearing hyphema, or for pathologic sampling in cases of uveitis, infection,[172] or presumed leukemia.[173] Because the field needs to be sterile and the needle must enter a small target area of the anterior chamber, the child should undergo general anesthesia to make the field immobile for the surgeon. As in the scenario of an open globe emergency, these procedures are intraocular and so an anesthetic approach must take control of IOP into consideration.

PROBING AND IRRIGATION OF NASOLACRIMAL DUCT, OR DACRYOCYSTORHINOSTOMY

Infants may be born with nasolacrimal duct stenosis (i.e., congenital dacryostenosis) (Fig. 32.6 and E-Fig. 32.4). If conservative measures do not improve the drainage of tears, the ophthalmologist may need to pass a metal probe through the duct to break the adhesion or pierce a hole in an intact membrane.[174,175] To perform either maneuver in infants and children, general anesthesia is required. Anesthesia is induced by inhalation and maintained with a facemask for the few minutes needed to complete the surgery. The smallest size facemask is preferred to permit the surgeon to work around the cushion of the mask and probe the ducts in the upper and lower lids. To confirm that the duct is patent, the ophthalmologist should establish metal-metal contact using one probe within the duct and a second probe within the nostril,[176] or

We usually avoid succinylcholine in children; however, if succinylcholine is used, the surgeon should be informed because it may alter their surgical approach.[165] After induction of anesthesia and airway management, the operating room table is rotated to permit complete access to the orbits. It is common to use a preformed airway device, such as an oral RAE or flexible SGA, that lies flat against the mandible.[166,167] The airway device is then positioned away from the surgical field. Ventilation may be spontaneous or controlled according to the anesthesiologist's preference. If the surgery is intraocular or medical conditions dictate, controlled ventilation should be considered. Two antiemetics are routinely given to children undergoing strabismus surgery. Although a regional block is performed in some adults, general anesthesia is preferred in children.

CATARACT SURGERY

Cataracts are opacifications of the lens of the eye (Fig. 32.5). Cataracts in children may be congenital, posttraumatic, or metabolic in origin.[168] Congenital cataracts require surgery very early in life to allow for normal visual development.[169] Although the surgery can be performed as an outpatient, the formerly premature and young

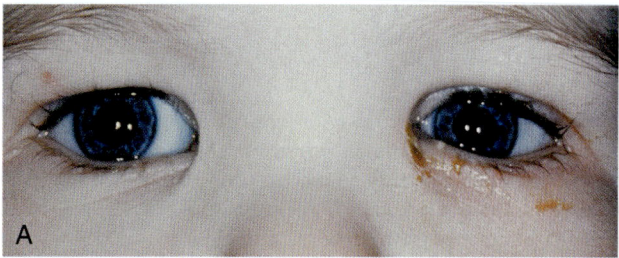

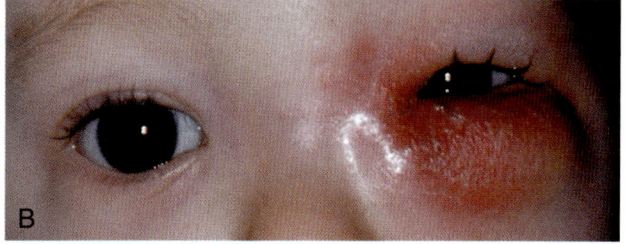

FIGURE 32.6 Nasolacrimal duct obstruction manifests with different degrees of infraorbital inflammation, from mild obstruction with mucoid material accumulation **(A)** to severe obstruction with dacryocystitis and periorbital or preseptal cellulitis **(B)**.

inject fluorescein into the nasolacrimal duct and detect the fluorescein with suction or on a pipe cleaner in the nasal airway. The surgeon may choose to place a small silicone stent in the nasolacrimal duct (monocanalicular tube) if they have concern the duct may restenose. Frequently the ophthalmologist will irrigate the nasal cavity with oxymetazoline to stop nasal bleeding. Oxymetazoline, saline, fluorescein, or blood may reach the larynx and trigger breath-holding or laryngospasm. To prevent this, it is prudent to tilt the operating table to a 5- to 10-degree Trendelenburg position and place a small roll under the child's shoulders to pool the fluids away from the larynx. These secretions are suctioned out of the oropharynx and nasopharynx before the roll is removed and emergence commences. Anesthesia may be maintained by face mask inhalation, laryngeal mask airway, or with IV agents. The infant is awakened preferably in the left lateral decubitus position (the recovery position to permit residual blood or fluorescein to drain from the mouth), and postoperative analgesia may be offered with acetaminophen or opioids, or both, as necessary.

For complicated or recurrent nasolacrimal duct obstructions, or when a dacryocele or dacryocystitis is present, an endoscopic nasal approach may be used to assist the procedure.[177,178] Endoscopic-assisted probing increases the duration of the procedure and requires airway control to facilitate the surgeon's approach and to protect the child from aspirating blood during the procedure. In older children with bilateral obstruction, endoscope-assisted probing increased the long-term success rate.[179,180] If a patent duct cannot be established, a new passageway can be created in a more involved procedure called a dacryocystorhinostomy.

PTOSIS REPAIR

Ptosis (i.e., blepharoptosis) means "drooping of the eyelid." This condition can be congenital or acquired, and it may cause amblyopia by depriving the eye of vision or by inducing astigmatism. If eyelid closure is complete in infancy, severe occlusion amblyopia will occur without correction, and this will require urgent attention. If mild, surgery for ptosis is often performed electively later in childhood. These children should be investigated for an underlying cause (e.g., chromosomal deletion, genetic syndrome, neuromuscular disease such as myasthenia gravis, and malignant hyperthermia).[181] The surgical approaches require a quiet surgical field, and the surgeon makes a great effort to produce a symmetric repair.

RETINOBLASTOMA

Mutations in specific genes are believed to cause retinoblastomas, which are the most common primary malignant tumors in children.[182,183] The pathognomonic defect is a mutation in the *RB1* gene on chromosome 13. These tumors have a strong familial and hereditary component with sporadic mutations and may be unilateral or bilateral.[184] They are most commonly recognized by a lack of the typical red light reflex in the infant's pupil.[185] Treatments include systemic chemotherapy,[186] injection of monoclonal antibodies (e.g., bevacizumab),[187,188] intraarterial chemotherapy, proton beam radiation, and occasionally surgical removal of the eye.[189,190]

Infants as young as 2 months of age may present for intraarterial chemotherapy.[191] Intraoperative complications of intraarterial chemotherapy include bronchospasm (29% of patients), bradycardia, and hypotension, which typically occur upon catheter placement into the internal carotid artery or ophthalmic artery, and all of which respond promptly to administration of epinephrine.[192]

Many children retain useful vision with proton beam treatments and there does not seem to be an increased incidence of associated secondary malignancy.[193] These children require multiple anesthetics for the initial evaluation, CT planning, EUAs for monitoring, and construction of a fiberglass mask for immobilization during treatments. This is then followed by placement of central venous access, which allows all 25 to 30 subsequent treatments to be performed under deep propofol sedation with maintenance of a natural airway with spontaneous respirations (see also Chapter 43). Children with extraocular disease are treated with larger doses of chemotherapy followed by delayed enucleation.[194]

ENUCLEATION

Enucleation of the eye may be necessary when a child has an intraocular tumor (e.g., retinoblastoma threatening extraocular involvement) (Fig. 32.7),[195] a ruptured globe or ocular trauma beyond repair,[196] or a blind, painful eye. The OCR may occur during this procedure and may be attenuated by infiltration with a local anesthetic. Prophylactic antiemetics are often administered because PONV is common.

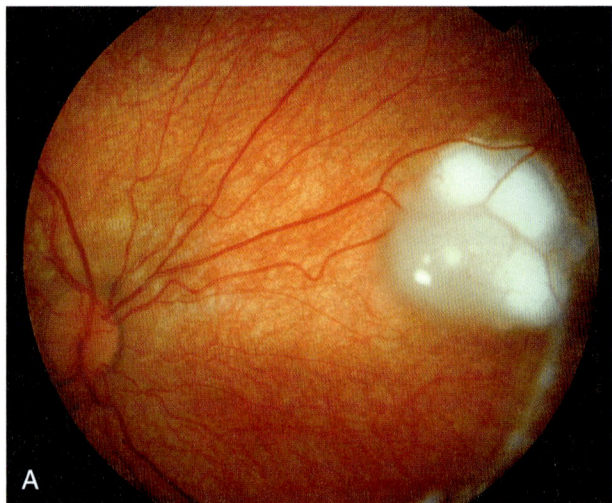

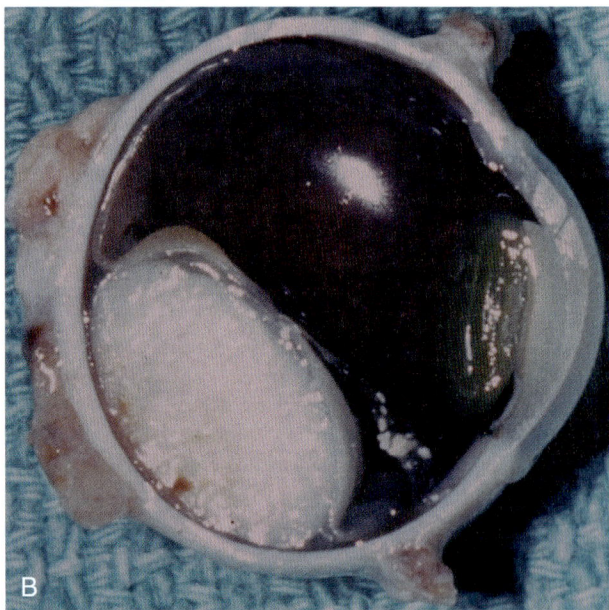

FIGURE 32.7 Retinoblastoma is one of many intraocular tumors that may require enucleation. **A,** Retinoblastoma seen by direct ophthalmoscopy. **B,** Pathologic specimen of a retinoblastoma in the globe after enucleation.

VITRECTOMY

Vitrectomy may be necessary for nonclearing intraocular hemorrhage, retinal injury, or detachment. These are most commonly caused by high myopia, trauma, or ROP.[197]

RETINOPATHY OF PREMATURITY TREATMENT

Preterm infants may present with multiple ocular pathologic conditions, but none is more common than ROP. It has been extensively studied,[25] and multiple collaborative trials have reported their results and recommendations for medical and surgical interventions, including retinal laser and intravitreal bevacizumab injection.[198–207] The cause is not fully understood, but oxygen-related theories and loss of maternal growth factors have been described as contributory. Because of this concern, targeting an oxygen saturation range between 91% to 95% has become common[208–210] to balance the risks of systemic hypoxemia with oxidative stress[211] on the infant.

Laser and intraocular medication injections are common treatments for this condition.[198,199] These treatments are frequently completed at the bedside in the neonatal intensive care unit. Because of the delicacy and exacting accuracy required in laser procedures, we routinely intubate the trachea and use neuromuscular blocking drugs. This facilitates the immobile field necessary for the surgeon and provides better perioperative physiologic stability for the infant.[212] The complications of prematurity determine whether extubation is possible, and many infants require postoperative ventilation, if only for a brief period or overnight.[213] The operative environment should be kept warm to reduce thermal stress on the infant.

Acknowledgment

We wish to acknowledge the prior contributions to this chapter from, Joseph R. Tobin, and R. Grey Weaver.

ANNOTATED REFERENCES

Arnold RW. The oculocardiac reflex: a review. *Clin Ophthalmol.* 2021;15:2693-2725.
This is a very nice summary of current knowledge regarding etiology, prevention, and treatment of the oculocardiac reflex.
Cunningham AJ, Barry P. Intraocular pressure—physiology and implications for anaesthetic management. *Can Anaesth Soc J.* 1986;33:195-208.
This review elegantly details the physiology of intraocular pressure and conditions that may increase it. Structural, physiologic, and pharmacologic considerations are reviewed in detail.
Donahue SP. Clinical practice. Pediatric strabismus. *N Engl J Med.* 2007;356:1040-1047.
Strabismus is a common presenting condition requiring surgical therapy in children. Significant improvements in the detection and treatment of strabismus are reviewed. Surgical approaches and recent advances are presented.

Lewanda AF, Matisoff A, Revenis M, et al. Preoperative evaluation and comprehensive risk assessment for children with Down syndrome. *Pediatr Anesth.* 2016; 26:356-362.
Children with Down syndrome have multiple systemic conditions of importance to the anesthesiologist. They are not exclusively of interest owing to CHD. Anesthesia-related complications occur more frequently in children with Down syndrome than other children presenting for noncardiac surgery, and prevention of complications is essential by means of thorough evaluation and planning, particularly appropriate consultation with cardiologists regarding residual or current CHD and the possibility of cervical spine instability.
Lewis H, James I. Update on anaesthesia for paediatric ophthalmic surgery. *BJA Educ.* 2021;21(1):32-38.
This paper provides a nice discussion of anesthetic management for both common and less common ophthalmic conditions requiring surgery in children; considerations for emergency procedures requiring anesthesia are also presented.
Murgatroyd H, Bembridg J. Intraocular pressure. *Contin Educ Anaesth Crit Care Pain.* 2008;8:100-103.
This paper presents a very succinct summary of the physiology of intraocular pressure and vitreous fluid dynamics.
Sanatkar M, Dastjani Farahani A, Bazvand F. Ketamine analgesia as an alternative to general anesthesia during laser treatment for retinopathy of prematurity. *J Pediatr Ophthalmol Strabismus.* 2022;59(6):416-421.
Although this paper represents a small series of patients, it describes the use of ketamine as a possible means of avoiding the need for general anesthesia with intubation in this vulnerable population; three minor complications were observed, which resolved without incidence.
Saugstad OD, Aune D. In search of the optimal oxygen saturation for extremely low birth weight infants: a systematic review and meta-analysis. *Neonatology.* 2011;100:1-8.
Advances in neonatology continue to reduce morbidity and mortality for these fragile children. Oxygen-saturation targeting is becoming a mainstream technique. This has implications for the management and oxygen support strategies for infants coming to the operating room for ocular and other surgical procedures. Because volatile anesthetics impair hypoxic pulmonary vasoconstriction, a supplemental oxygen requirement should be anticipated, but oxygen-saturation targets should be considered for optimal care.
Shen YD, Chen CY, Wu CH, et al. Dexamethasone, ondansetron, and their combination and postoperative nausea and vomiting in children undergoing strabismus surgery: a meta-analysis of randomized controlled trials. *Paediatr Anaesth.* 2014;24(5):490-498.
This meta-analysis examined 13 randomized controlled trials and found that PONV occurred in 68% of placebo-treated children compared with 34% of dexamethasone-treated children and 37% of ondansetron-treated children. The combination was significantly more effective at reducing PONV than either drug alone.
Stephen E, Dickson J, Kindley AD, et al. Surveillance of vision and ocular disorders in children with Down syndrome. *Dev Med Child Neurol.* 2007;49:513-515.
Children with Down syndrome have many different ocular disorders. In addition to the multiple systemic issues of concern for the anesthesiologist described in the chapter, this reference provides insight into the ocular diseases that may require surgical therapy.

A complete reference list can be found online at Elsevier eBooks+.

33 Plastic and Reconstructive Surgery

OLIVIA NELSON, PAUL A. STRICKER, JOHN E. FIADJOE, AND JERROLD LERMAN

Cleft Lip and Palate
Anesthetic Considerations
Craniosynostosis
Airway Management
Blood Loss, Coagulopathy, and Hyponatremia
Intracranial Pressure
Venous Air Embolism
Prolonged Surgery
Orbital Hypertelorism
Midface Procedures
**Hemifacial Microsomia, Treacher Collins Syndrome,
and Goldenhar Syndrome**
Airway Management

Orthognathic Surgery
Lymphatic Malformations and Hemangiomas
Möbius Sequence
Brachial Plexus Surgery
Otoplasty
Congenital Hand Anomalies
Tissue Expanders
Hairy Pigmented Nevi
Cosmetic Procedures
Trauma

PEDIATRIC PLASTIC SURGERY is performed in children of all ages, even in utero.[1] However, the majority of children who undergo plastic surgical and reconstructive procedures are between 2 and 9 years of age, with a median age of 5 years. A wide spectrum of associated craniofacial abnormalities, underlying medical conditions, and surgical procedures characterize this pediatric population. Consequently, a thorough preoperative assessment, consultation with medical and surgical teams, and anticipation and preparation for potential complications are of paramount importance to ensure a successful perioperative outcome. Many procedures are performed on the head and neck and require thoughtful coordination between the anesthesiologist and surgeon. A thorough understanding of the procedure allows for selection of the optimal anesthetic plan. The incidence of major morbidity and mortality has been reduced over the past 30 years from 16.5% and 1.6% to less than 0.1% and 0.1%, respectively, in children undergoing major craniofacial surgeries.[2]

Cleft Lip and Palate

Cleft lip and palate are among the more common congenital malformations, occurring in approximately 1 in 600 births worldwide.[3,4] This malformation is more common in males and people of Asian and Latin American descent, and is least common in African Americans. It likely results from both environmental and genetic causes. Paternal farming increases the risk of cleft lip or palate in the offspring, whereas the maternal occupation presents no additional risk.[5] Folate metabolism disturbances and increased maternal homocysteine concentrations also may be contributory.[6] Cleft lip with or without cleft palate has been linked to several loci on chromosomes 1, 2, 4, 6, 14, 17, 19, and 22, suggesting a genetic basis for some of these anomalies.[7–10] Three genes have been associated with syndromic cleft lip and palate: T-box transcription factor-22, poliovirus receptor–like-1, and interferon regulatory factor-6 *(IRF6)*. Gene mutations have been identified in only a small fraction of nonsyndromic cleft lip and palate.

These disorders are associated with more than 400 syndromes; the more common of which are presented in Table 33.1. Cleft lip and palate begin as a defect in palatal growth in the first trimester of pregnancy. Fetal magnetic resonance imaging (MRI) provides a greater degree of resolution of defects in the posterior palate and of the lateral extent of clefts with greater diagnostic accuracy than ultrasound. MRI also enables early detection of potential syndromic conditions by providing a complete study of the fetal head and biometric development of the facial bones.[11]

Primary cleft lip repair is usually undertaken at approximately 2 to 3 months of postnatal age, whereas primary cleft palate repair occurs at 6 to 10 months. Surgery for lip or nose revision usually takes place in early childhood, and palatal revision and alveolar bone grafts occur at approximately 10 years of age. Rhinoplasty and maxillary osteotomy complete the repair at 17 to 20 years of age. Pharyngoplasty may be required for velopharyngeal incompetence secondary to anatomic or neurologic dysfunction to improve speech development and prevent nasal regurgitation during eating.

ANESTHETIC CONSIDERATIONS

Surgical correction of a cleft lip defect is usually performed at 2 to 3 months of age to allow sufficient time for maturation and associated abnormalities to become apparent. Preoperative assessment may reveal abnormalities such as mandibular hypoplasia in Pierre Robin sequence (Fig. 33.1 and E-Fig. 33.1) or restricted neck movement as in Klippel-Feil syndrome (E-Fig. 33.2).[3] Pierre Robin sequence is defined as the triad of micrognathia, glossoptosis (caudally displaced insertion of the tongue), and respiratory distress in the first 24 to 48 hours after birth. The presence of

TABLE 33.1	Syndromes Commonly Associated With Cleft Lip and Palate
Pierre Robin sequence	
Down syndrome	
Klippel-Feil syndrome	
Treacher Collins syndrome	
Velocardiofacial syndrome	
Fetal alcohol syndrome	
Nager syndrome	
Goldenhar syndrome	

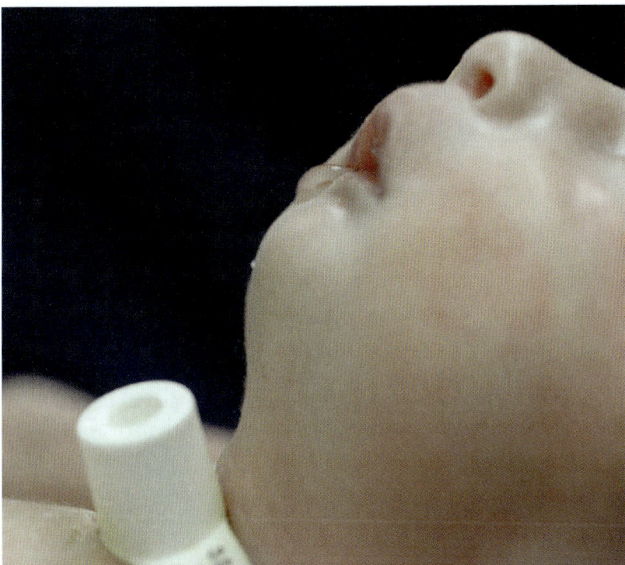

FIGURE 33.1 Child with Pierre Robin sequence who required a tracheostomy because of respiratory distress in the first 24 hours postnatally. The retrognathia is often associated with glossoptosis, which makes visualization of the glottic aperture more difficult.

other anomalies might warrant additional clinical or laboratory investigations. Cleft lip repair usually involves minimal blood loss, so for children with a hematocrit greater than 30%, additional preoperative laboratory testing is unnecessary. A sample for type and screen is usually sufficient for infants with a hematocrit value less than 30%.[12]

Upper respiratory tract infections are common in this age group. If an upper respiratory infection is present, then strong consideration should be given to delay surgery until it has resolved.

Airway Difficulties

The frequency of difficult airways in children with cleft lip and palate varies from 2.9% to 23%.[13–17] The incidence of difficult laryngoscopy in children with bilateral cleft lip and palate (16.5%) is 3-fold greater than that with unilateral cleft lip (5.1%) and the incidence decreases with increasing age.[15] The incidence of difficult direct laryngoscopy is approximately 50% in children with micrognathia but only about 4% in those without. Furthermore, micrognathia is an independent predictor of a difficult intubation.[15] In neonates and infants, micrognathia may be subtle and not always easily detected by physical examination. Micrognathia

is more apparent when examining the lateral profile of the child's head, as the mandible may appear receded relative to the maxilla. Recent MRI evidence has shed light on the effect of micrognathia. In children with Pierre Robin sequence, those with an airway cross-sectional area >37 mm^2 predicted a difficult airway with a positive predictive value of 79% and negative predictive value of 100%.[18] In children with mandibular hypoplasia, difficult intubation was predicted using a regression analysis of the airway dimensions from 3-D CT scans of the face. After accounting for age and sex, a diminished anterior distance of the hyoid bone (distance from the hyoid bone to the mentum [odds ratio 0.79, $P <0.03$], estimated by the thyromental distance) and increased inferior pogonial angle (angle formed by the intersection of the two rami of the mandible at the mentum (odds ratio 1.10, $P <0.04$) predicted a difficult intubation.[19] The presence of microtia predicts a difficult intubation, with an incidence of 42% with bilateral microtia compared with an incidence of 2% with a unilateral defect. The presence of mandibular hypoplasia should also raise the possibility of a hemifacial microsomia or Treacher Collins syndrome.[20] The incidence of a difficult intubation by direct laryngoscopy in an isolated micrognathia decreases with increasing age, with the greatest difficulty presenting in infants younger than 6 months. This has been attributed to rapid postnatal growth of the mandible, which catches up to the maxilla by 2 years of age in most cases. A careful review of previous anesthetic records may forewarn of a difficult airway. In a second study that reported the frequency of difficult intubations in young infants with cleft lip, cleft palate without Pierre Robin sequence, cleft-lip-palate and cleft palate, and cleft palate with Pierre Robin sequence was 0%, 2.7%, 10%, and 23%, respectively.[17] Difficult airways increased with early airway and feeding problems ($P <0.0001$); in the isolated cleft palate, a wider cleft was associated with a significantly more difficult laryngoscopy.

Induction of anesthesia via face mask is usually uncomplicated in infants with cleft lip and palate. Laryngoscopy may be performed using a straight blade via a right paraglossal approach (blade inserted into the pharyngeal gutter with tongue displaced to the left),[21] taking care to avoid dropping the blade into the cleft (see also Fig. 12.31A–C). In the presence of a hypoplastic mandible, external laryngeal manipulation is usually required to visualize the larynx. In some centers, the tongue is sutured to either the mandible or lower lip (glossopexy) to preclude airway obstruction in infants with Pierre Robin sequence in the postnatal period. In such instances, the tongue cannot be displaced to the left to expose the larynx, rendering laryngoscopy more difficult. To facilitate laryngoscopy in such cases, the tongue is first released from the lower lip using ketamine sedation followed by direct laryngoscopy. Alternatively, selection of a primary airway management strategy other than direct laryngoscopy (e.g., video laryngoscopy, fiberoptic intubation through a supraglottic airway) circumvents this problem and may be a preferable approach with a greater success rate on the first attempt (see Chapter 12).[22]

A variety of tracheal tubes can be used to secure the airway for cleft lip and palate surgery, although the ideal tracheal tube is perhaps the oral Ring-Adair-Elwyn (RAE) tube, which can be fixed centrally to the chin to facilitate optimal surgical access. It should be noted that preformed uncuffed and cuffed tracheal tubes vary in length from the bend to the tip.[23] Seven brands of preformed tracheal tubes were compared for the same size inner diameter tubes; the distance from the bend to the tip varied by 0 to 1 cm for oral cuffed tubes but from 0 to 4 cm for uncuffed oral tubes. Variability in the same bend-to-tip distance with preformed nasal tubes was even greater; cuffed nasal tubes varied by 0 to 5.5 cm and uncuffed varied from 2 to 9 cm. The risk of an endobronchial intubation when a cuffed oral preformed tube replaced an uncuffed tube of the same diameter was 0% to 27%, whereas when a cuffed nasal preformed tube replaced an uncuffed tube of the same size, the risk increased to 50% to 100%. The risk for endobronchial intubation varies among manufacturers and may be greater with nasal than oral preformed tracheal tubes.

Intraoperative Considerations

Throat packs usually impinge on the surgical field and are not normally required for cleft palate repair. Ventilation is usually controlled for the duration of the procedure (~1 to 2 hours). Inhalational or intravenous (IV) anesthetics combined with a short-acting opioid such as fentanyl (1–2 μg/kg) are used to maintain anesthesia. Bilateral infraorbital nerve blocks may be used to provide postoperative analgesia for cleft lip repairs (see Fig. 40.32 and Chapter 40 videos). Correct identification of the infraorbital foramen is essential. The infraorbital foramen is located within 2 mm of the midpoint between the nasospinale and jugale based on an anatomic study of dry crania from infants, children, and adolescents.[24] Such blocks reduce the need for opioids and antiemetics, improve the ability to feed postoperatively,[25,26] and increase parental satisfaction.[27] Additional evidence suggests that the incidence of emergence agitation is reduced with the use of infraorbital nerve blocks, although this most likely reflected less pain that was conflated with emergence agitation.[28] A combination of infraorbital and external nasal nerve blocks for pain control after cleft lip repair is an effective alternative approach.[29]

Postoperative Care

During cleft palate surgery, the pharyngeal space is reduced dramatically, and postoperative nasopharyngeal airways (usually placed by the surgeon intraoperatively) may be required to maintain a patent airway postoperatively and permit suctioning without damaging the palatal repair (Fig. 33.2 and E-Fig. 33.3A,B). At the end of surgery, the trachea is extubated after the upper airway reflexes have returned and the child is completely awake. These children are at particular risk for acute upper airway obstruction in the immediate postextubation period as a result of upper airway narrowing, edema, blood, and residual anesthetic effects.[30–35] Accordingly, the key elements to ensure a completely successful emergence is to site and secure a nasopharyngeal airway before emergence begins and to extubate the trachea only when the child is completely awake. Intraoperative dexamethasone (0.5 mg/kg) may be administered to attenuate postoperative airway edema. Late postoperative edema[36] and severe subcutaneous emphysema are additional complications. Upper respiratory tract infections, usually viral in origin, are common in this age group. Antibiotics may be indicated if the infection is bacterial in origin.[37] Adverse airway events, including postoperative airway obstruction, oxyhemoglobin desaturation, bronchospasm, laryngospasm, reintubation, and unplanned postoperative intensive care unit (ICU) admission have been identified in as many as 23% of children undergoing cleft palate repair (e.g., palatoplasty).[38,39] Modifiable independent risk factors that in aggregate, yielded a 37-fold greater risk of adverse perioperative events, included multiple intubation attempts (difficult intubation), duration of surgery greater than 160 minutes, opioid dose (e.g., morphine dose >0.32 mg/kg), both surgeon and anesthesiologist experience <5 years, and lack of neuromuscular blockade reversal; however, weight 9 to 13 kilograms reduced the risk for adverse events.[39]

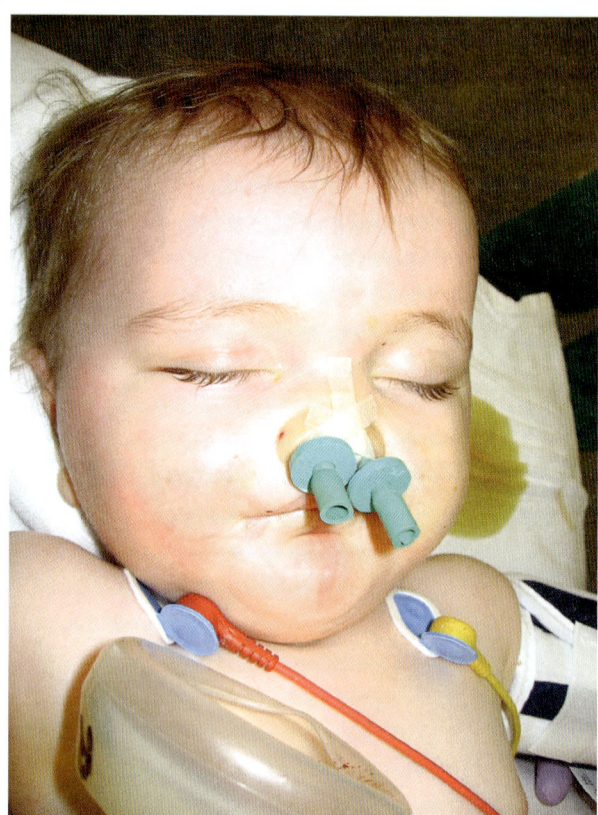

FIGURE 33.2 Nasal airways are often placed at the end of cleft palate or pharyngoplasty surgery to ensure that a patent airway is maintained.

Arm restraints are used in many centers to prevent the infant from disrupting the sutures and pulling out the nasopharyngeal airway. These children are monitored for signs of upper airway obstruction during the recovery period for approximately 48 hours.[30] As soon as the child is awake, feeding with clear fluids is allowed. Postoperative pain is managed with a combination of simple analgesics (e.g., acetaminophen and NSAIDs). Opioid or tramadol is infrequently required. Rectal acetaminophen administered before surgery does not reduce postoperative opioid requirements in children undergoing cleft palate repair.[40] In part, this may be attributed to local infiltration at the surgical site and the slow and variable absorption of acetaminophen by the rectal route.[40] However, IV acetaminophen has opioid-sparing effects that may be useful in certain scenarios.[40,41]

Peripheral nerve blocks including sphenopalatine and infraorbital nerve blocks (see Chapter 40, Fig. 40.32) with a long-acting local anesthetic at the end of the procedure prevent pain after cleft lip and palate repair.[25] Palatal nerve block (nasopalatine, greater and lesser palatine)[42] or a bilateral suprazygomatic maxillary nerve block also reduce postoperative pain (and opioid requirements) and favor early feeding.[43–46]

Complete cleft palate defects cross the alveolar ridge. In such cases, a residual defect is often present after the primary repair. Secondary alveolar bone grafting occurs during the period of mixed deciduous and permanent dentition to provide support for the incoming permanent teeth. The bone graft is harvested from the iliac crest and this donor site can cause more discomfort than the oral incisions, although packing the iliac crest site with bupivacaine-soaked gauze attenuates the postoperative pain and facilitates early activity.[47,48]

Pharyngoplasty Surgery

Children who are scheduled for elective pharyngoplasty are usually school age, having undergone cleft palate repair at an earlier age. The primary objective of this procedure is to restore velopharyngeal competence for speech development, which can be achieved by a pharyngeal flap, sphincter pharyngoplasty, or palatal lengthening (Furlow double-opposing Z-plasty palatoplasty). The anesthetic goals and management are similar to those discussed for cleft palate repair.

Craniosynostosis

Craniosynostosis, a congenital anomaly in which one or more cranial sutures close prematurely, occurs in approximately 1 in 2000 to 3000 births, affecting males more frequently than females.[49–51] Embryologically, the cranial vault starts to ossify 8 weeks postconception; fusion of the parietal and frontal bones is usually complete by 7 months postconception. Postnatally, the anterolateral fontanelle closes by 3 months, the posterior fontanelle by 3 to 6 months, the anterior fontanelle by 9 to 18 months, and the posterolateral fontanelle by 2 years. Premature osseous obliteration of a bony suture might result from the absence of osteoinhibitory signals from the suture. Craniosynostosis may be categorized as simple (or nonsyndromic) (60%–80% of cases), involving closure of one suture, or syndromic (complex) (20%–30%), involving closure of two or more sutures and is often associated with a variety of clinical features and metabolic diseases (Table 33.2).[50,52,53]

In the child with craniosynostosis, fusion of a cranial suture restricts normal bone growth perpendicular to the affected suture. Compensatory growth and expansion of the cranial vault occurs parallel to the affected suture, and there is a characteristic skull deformity associated with the different sutures involved (Fig. 33.3 and E-Fig. 33.4).[50] The frequency of single-suture closures varies with the specific suture: sagittal (50%), coronal (20%), and metopic (10%).[52] The coronal suture (especially bicoronal synostosis) is more commonly associated with syndromic craniosynostosis. Although approximately 80% of premature suture closures are isolated defects, the remaining 20% involve multiple suture closures associated with more than 400 syndromes that present with a myriad of clinical features (see Table 33.2); the more common syndromes that require craniofacial reconstruction are described later.[50,52] Syndromic craniosynostoses are commonly associated with gene defects including the fibroblast growth factor receptor (FGFR), which is involved in bone and cartilage development.[54,55]

Apert syndrome occurs in less than 1 in 100,000 live births, usually as a sporadic mutation, although autosomal dominant inheritance patterns can occur with the *FGFR2* gene on chromosome 10. This syndrome phenotypically manifests as cloverleaf skull (craniosynostosis), hypertelorism, proptosis, midface hypoplasia, and syndactyly (upper or lower extremity). Development is often complicated by increased intracranial pressure (ICP) and obstructive sleep apnea (OSA).[56,57] Whether children with Apert syndrome develop a normal intelligence quotient (IQ) is unclear; one study reported that 32% had an IQ greater than 70.[58] The timing of cranial surgery may affect the child's IQ; surgery in the first year of life was associated with an IQ greater than 70 in more than 50% of children in one study, whereas surgery after the first

TABLE 33.2	Classification of Craniosynostosis
Nonsyndromic (primary) ~80%: Single-suture closed, isolated finding	
Syndromic ~20%: Two or more sutures closed, often with associated clinical findings. More than 150 syndromes have been described; the more common syndromes are:	
Crouzon	
Apert	
Pfeiffer	
Saethre-Chotzen	
Carpenter (acrocephalopolysyndactyly type II)	
Muenke	
Crouzonodermoskeletal	
Shprintzen-Goldberg	
Loeys-Dietz	
Jackson-Weiss	
Beare-Stevenson	
Cole-Carpenter	
Kleeblattschädel	
Fibroblast growth factor receptor mutations 1 and 2	
Metabolic and other causes	
Rickets	
Bone metabolic disorders (hypophosphatasia)	
Achondroplasia	
Prematurity	

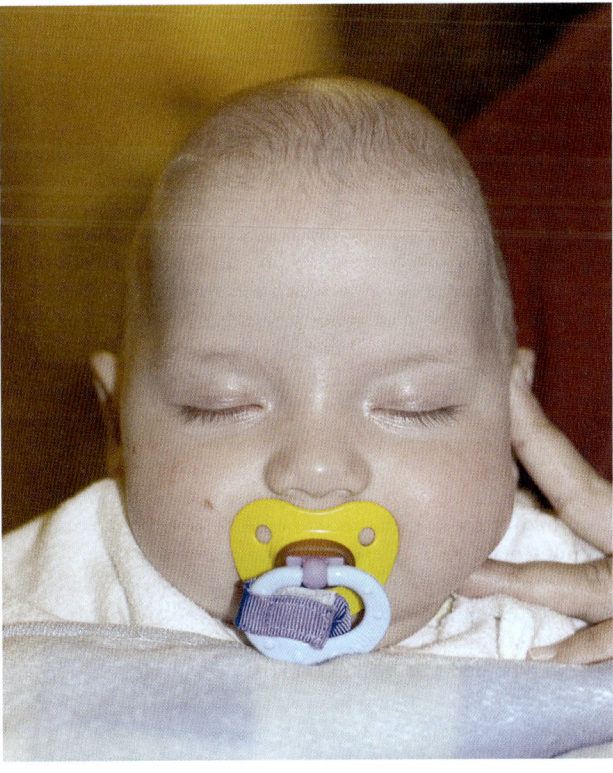

FIGURE 33.3 Infant with classic craniosynostosis. The shape of the child's head may not reflect the severity of the defect. The defect is best appreciated by three-dimensional magnetic resonance imaging reconstruction.

year of life was associated with an IQ greater than 70 in only 7%.[58] Two other factors predicted improved IQ: absence of a defect in the septum pellucidum and noninstitutional residence (i.e., family home residence). In contrast, more recent evidence failed to substantiate a salutary effect of early surgery on cognitive development. Indeed, cognitive development was related to the quality of the family environment and parental education and unrelated to brain malformation and the age of surgery.[59]

Crouzon syndrome is phenotypically similar to Apert syndrome but has different ophthalmologic defects, specifically, optic atrophy occurring in up to 20% of cases, and the absence of hand and foot defects (e.g., syndactyly).[50,60] 50% of Crouzon syndrome defects are sporadic mutations, and the remainder are familial with the same gene defect as Apert; FGFR2 on chromosome 10.

Pfeiffer syndrome occurs in approximately 1 in 25,000 live births. Most cases are familial with an autosomal dominant inheritance pattern that has its origin in defects in the FGFR1 and FGFR2 genes on chromosome 10, although many remain sporadic. The phenotype of Pfeiffer syndrome is similar to that of Apert syndrome but includes broad thumb, large first toe, polydactyly, and may be associated with a cartilaginous sleeve trachea. Children with Pfeiffer syndrome have normal intelligence.

Carpenter syndrome is associated with craniosynostosis, syndactyly, cardiac defects, and obesity.[61] Cognitive impairment is common.[61] Muenke syndrome is more common, occurring in 1 in 30,000 births. It results from a mutation in the FGFR3 gene. Affected patients have midface hypoplasia, ocular hypertelorism, strabismus, developmental delay, and intellectual disabilities.[50] A relatively new but rare syndrome, Shprintzen-Goldberg, is characterized by craniosynostosis and a phenotype that resembles that of Marfan syndrome.

Indications for cranial vault reconstruction include increased ICP, severe exophthalmos, OSA, craniofacial deformity, and psychosocial reasons. If uncorrected, the deformed cranium may cause severe neurologic sequelae including visual loss and developmental delay.[62–74] Because rapid brain growth during infancy determines skull shape, surgical correction is undertaken within the first months of life to achieve the best cosmetic results.

Cranial vault reconstruction may involve the anterior or posterior aspect of the skull or both (total cranial vault reconstruction).[51] Less invasive approaches to correct craniosynostosis are available and may reduce morbidity. Surgical correction may involve an open approach in which the synostotic suture is excised followed by barrel-stave osteotomies to release the adjacent cranium and allow the skull shape to normalize with subsequent brain growth (Fig. 33.4 and E-Fig. 33.5). This technique is used in children younger than 6 months of age and is believed to be less invasive than total cranial vault reconstruction.[75,76] Endoscopic strip craniectomy is increasingly used in early infancy because it reduces the transfusion requirements and hospital stay compared with the open procedures. A multicenter comparison of endoscopic versus open craniosynostosis repair reported decreases in the transfused volume of red blood cell–containing products, blood donor exposures, surgical and anesthesia times, and the number of days spent in the ICU and hospital in patients who underwent endoscopic compared with open repair. Complications including venous air embolism (VAE), hypothermia, and hypotension requiring vasopressor support were similar with the two surgical approaches.[77] The principal disadvantage of the endoscopic approach is the need for the child to wear a helmet for 4 to 6 months postoperatively to promote a normal shaped skull.[51]

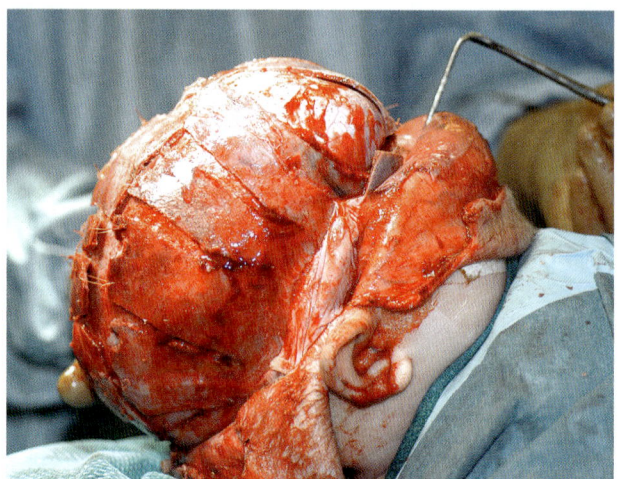

FIGURE 33.4 Child immediately before surgical closure after total cranial vault reshaping using strip craniectomy for sagittal craniosynostosis.

Spring-assisted cranioplasty, a technique preferentially used in infants younger than 6 months, involves performing a midline osteotomy along the fused sagittal suture and placing springs across the osteotomy to increase the biparietal dimension.[51] Spring-assisted cranioplasty may result in reduced blood loss and transfusion requirement, and a shorter duration of hospital stay.[78] The primary disadvantage of this approach is the need for a second surgery to remove the springs. A meta-analysis of the outcomes from calvarial remodeling, strip craniectomy, and spring-mediated cranioplasty in nonsyndromic sagittal synostosis demonstrated that the cephalic index (which is the ratio of the width of the outermost tables of the vault to the length of the outermost tables)[79] with calvarial vault remodeling was superior to strip craniectomy and that the former approach required more surgical time, involved more blood loss, a prolonged hospital stay, and greater costs than the other two approaches (P <0.0001).[80] In infants undergoing either endoscopic strip craniectomy or spring-assisted cranioplasty for sagittal synostosis, transfusion rates were similar although those undergoing spring-mediated cranioplasty had prolonged intensive care and hospital stays compared with those undergoing strip craniectomy.[81] In a systematic review of strip versus spring-assisted cranioplasty for nonsyndromic sagittal craniosynostosis, neither technique was superior with outcomes similar for both.[82]

Cranial vault distractors to achieve distraction osteogenesis is a technique that is used increasingly in children with syndromic forms of craniosynostosis.[83–85] This technique involves a craniotomy (usually without reconstruction of the cut bone flap) combined with placement of distractors that are subsequently incrementally lengthened by turning an externalized screw beginning a few days postoperatively and continuing until the targeted cranial vault expansion is achieved. This technique has the advantage of shorter surgery and allows for greater expansion of the cranial vault than can be achieved with a traditional cranial vault reconstruction. These children also return to the operating room for removal of the distraction hardware. A systematic review reported that standard or spring-mediated distraction osteogenesis treated the primary condition, which was deformity or increased ICP, in 98% of patients. Results likely to require surgical revision occurred in 1.3%.[86]

Preoperative assessment of children with craniosynostosis should focus on airway management, eye protection, and ICP. An important consideration in children with syndromic midfacial hypoplasia is its common association with OSA (50%–70% incidence) owing to associated narrowing of the nasopharyngeal space.[57,87,88] Although some recommend preoperative adenotonsillectomy to treat OSA in children with syndromic craniosynostosis, neither airway dimensions nor propensity toward airway collapse are improved. Midfacial advancement may be required to resolve OSA, and even then, residual airway obstruction may persist.[57,87] Preoperative endoscopy has been recommended to assess the severity of midfacial hypoplasia and whether OSA is likely to persist after midface advancement. Careful titration of opioids in the perioperative period is indicated if the child exhibits severe nocturnal desaturation (i.e., if the SaO_2 nadir is <85%) (see Chapter 31, Fig. 31.6). Children with OSA who have severe nocturnal desaturation require half the dose of opioids that children without nocturnal desaturation require; a normal dose of opioid may be a relative overdose in this population (see Chapter 31, Fig. 31.14).[89] Upper airway obstruction may also occur postoperatively in children who received opioids as a direct effect of opioids on the hypoglossal nucleus.[90] Preoperative laboratory assessment should include a complete blood cell count and a specimen for blood type, antibody screening, and crossmatching of blood. Many centers also routinely screen for coagulation abnormalities with a preoperative prothrombin time and the activated partial thromboplastin time.

Postoperative pain is generally not severe and is managed effectively with a combination of acetaminophen, nonsteroidal antiinflammatory drugs (NSAIDs), and IV opioids. Opioids remain the mainstay of pain management, but careful titration is indicated if OSA is present. Given the small incidence of craniosynostosis and the large variability in the management of these patients, there remains a need to determine the optimal management strategy for these children.[91]

AIRWAY MANAGEMENT

Meticulous preoperative planning and evaluation of the airway are essential, particularly for children with known or possible OSA.[87] Upper airway obstruction during induction of anesthesia in children with midface hypoplasia should be anticipated. This is usually readily managed with a jaw-thrust/subluxation technique or insertion of an oral airway.[92] Occasionally, however, face mask ventilation may prove challenging owing to difficulty in obtaining a good mask seal.[93] External fixator devices on the face may also present challenges in managing the airway (E-Fig. 33.6), and it is essential to craft the optimal plan and make necessary preparations should problems arise (e.g., emergent hardware removal, wire cutting). A laryngeal mask is a valuable rescue tool in these scenarios and should be readily available before anesthetic induction.

In most children with craniosynostosis, the anatomy of the mandible and the temporomandibular joint is normal, as are upper airway dimensions, resulting in an easy direct laryngoscopy and tracheal intubation. Rarely, mandibular hypoplasia and limited neck mobility may complicate an otherwise straightforward laryngoscopy and tracheal intubation. Apert, Crouzon, and Pfeiffer syndromes are associated with fusion of cervical vertebrae in a minority of children, occasionally involving fusion of C2/C3 but more commonly involving lower cervical levels.[94–97] Because fusion does not involve the skull/atlas or atlas/axis joints, neck extension during laryngoscopy is rarely limited.[98] Syndromic craniosynostoses are also associated with tracheobronchial anomalies including the tracheal cartilaginous sleeve in which tracheal rings are replaced by a continuous cartilaginous segments.[99] A retrospective study of airway management in patients with Crouzon or Pfeiffer syndrome reported that about one-third of patients experienced upper airway obstruction during induction and bag mask ventilation, with the obstruction almost always relieved when a laryngeal mask airway was placed. The Cormack-Lehane grade was I or II in 85% of children during direct laryngoscopy.[100]

BLOOD LOSS, COAGULOPATHY, AND HYPONATREMIA

Crystalloid solutions are commonly administered for minimal to moderate surgical blood loss and fluid shifts during craniosynostosis surgery. Isotonic balanced solutions may be the best choice for crystalloid management; lactated Ringer solution (Hartmann solution) is most commonly used in North America. Normal saline solutions are more likely to induce nonanion gap metabolic acidosis than lactated Ringer solution in infants undergoing craniosynostosis.[101] If present, hyponatremia is usually mild, self-limited, and asymptomatic. An association between hyperchloremic metabolic acidosis attributed to normal saline and morbidity, mortality, and increased resource use has been reported in adults,[102,103] but consequences in adults[104,105] have been questioned[90,91] and in children remain very uncertain.

Surgery for craniosynostosis is associated with the potential for cardiac arrest as a result of sudden massive blood loss or underestimated blood loss.[2,52,106,107] Although these procedures are extradural, major bleeding from the scalp and cranium can occur, especially after inadvertent tears of dural venous sinuses. The risks of massive blood loss and the need for invasive monitoring are primarily determined by the type of surgery.[107] In children undergoing endoscopic strip craniectomy, weight less than 5 kilograms, those undergoing sagittal endoscopic craniectomy, those with syndromic craniosynostosis, and earlier date of surgery are associated with the need for blood transfusion.[108] Some centers advocate commencing blood transfusions at the time of skin incision (particularly in infants) to prevent hemodynamic instability and the need for a rapid transfusion in patients undergoing complex cranial vault reconstruction. At a minimum, blood products should be immediately available. Patients undergoing endoscopic procedures require fewer transfusions but continue to face the risk of sudden massive surgical bleeding (see later discussion).

To manage the large volume and rapidity of the blood loss, it is essential to establish adequate peripheral venous access. Central venous access (see also Figs. 46.5 to 46.7), usually via the internal jugular vein, is commonly reserved for children in whom obtaining adequate peripheral venous access proves difficult.[109] Strategies that are important to avoid hyperkalemic cardiac arrest include transfusion through peripheral rather than small bore central access,[51] infusing blood stored less than 7 days, minimizing the time between red blood cell irradiation and transfusion, washing red blood cells that are older or have been irradiated, (see Wake Up Safe; http://wakeupsafe.org/wp-content/uploads/2018/10/Hyperkalemia_statement.pdf) and (most importantly) avoiding hypovolemia to preclude the need to rapidly infuse large volumes of blood.[51,110,111] Estimation of ongoing blood loss can be difficult because large volumes of irrigation fluid are frequently used and there is difficulty quantifying blood loss onto surgical drapes and gowns.[112] The Pediatric Craniofacial Collaborative Group collected data for 1223 cases of whom 935 were younger than 2 years of age; 95% of these 935 received at least one blood transfusion.[109] Invasive arterial blood pressure monitoring and serial blood gas sampling are indicated in this type of surgery (see Chapter 46). A urinary catheter should be inserted to monitor urine output.

Several blood conservation strategies have been proposed for this type of surgery, including preoperative recombinant human erythropoietin, acute normovolemic hemodilution, antifibrinolytics, induced hypotension (see Chapter 12 for a more detailed discussion), and use of intraoperative blood salvage with use of cell-saver devices.[113,114] Bleeding from the scalp incision may be reduced by infiltration with a dilute (1:400,000) epinephrine-containing solution. The use of the reverse Trendelenburg position may help to decrease venous pressure and blood loss from osteotomy sites but may increase the risk of venous air embolism (with a reported frequency of 5%–80%; see later discussion). For this reason, the horizontal position is preferred.

Blood-conserving dual therapy with recombinant human erythropoietin (to optimize preoperative hematocrit) and use of a cell saver has reduced transfusion in children undergoing craniosynostosis repair.[113–115] Administration of preoperative recombinant human erythropoietin, in combination with elemental iron (4 mg/kg per day, given in divided doses, orally to a maximum of 200 mg/day for 6 weeks) increases the preoperative hematocrit value and may decrease the need for autologous blood transfusion.[116–119] If iron stores are at all compromised, iron therapy combined with oral vitamin C (to increase gastrointestinal absorption) should begin 3 weeks before erythropoietin therapy.[120]

Little evidence exists to suggest that autologous blood donation decreases perioperative morbidity in craniosynostosis surgery.[121,122] Although infants as young as 3 months of age have predonated, this technique is of questionable value and should not be pursued in this population. Instead, simpler and more cost-effective techniques should be used such as meticulous surgical attention to hemostasis and administration of antifibrinolytics.[123]

Acute normovolemic hemodilution is a labor-intensive technique in which blood is collected from the child after induction of anesthesia but immediately before surgery and replaced with an appropriate volume of crystalloid or colloid, such as 5% albumin. This technique has been used in combination with other techniques such as preoperative erythropoietin to reduce transfusions in craniosynostosis surgery.[124,125] The maximum potential blood savings with this technique is modest at best.[126] Despite some reports of efficacy, owing to the labor-intensive nature of the technique and modest blood savings, this technique is rarely used in craniofacial surgery.

The coagulation profile and clotting factors after fresh frozen plasma (FFP) or 5% albumin during craniofacial surgery have been compared in a nonrandomized study in infants less than 1 year of age.[127] The increases in activated partial thromboplastin time and decreases in the plasma concentration of factors XI and XIII and antithrombin III were less after intraoperative FFP than after 5% albumin. Fibrinogen concentrations remained stable in the FFP-treated group but decreased in the albumin-treated group. A hemostatic resuscitation strategy, like that used in massive hemorrhage from trauma, has been applied in pediatric craniofacial surgery. With this approach, blood loss is replaced using red blood cells and FFP in a 1:1 ratio. The central tenet of this approach is to prevent dilutional coagulopathy (see also Chapter 10). At one center where blood loss frequently exceeds blood volume, FFP and packed red blood cells from the same blood donors were used to replace blood loss; this technique essentially eliminated coagulopathy, and resulted in fewer perioperative blood donor exposures.[128] Another transfusion strategy to decrease blood donor exposures and avoid dilutional coagulopathy is the use of whole blood.[129] Recombinant factor VIIa has been used successfully for intractable hemorrhage during cranial vault reconstruction in an infant, although this was an extreme circumstance in an isolated case[130]; its use should not be routine (see Chapter 18).

Antifibrinolytic therapy is recommended to reduce blood loss during craniofacial surgery in children. Tranexamic acid has been shown to reduce surgical blood loss and decrease transfusion volumes intraoperatively and postoperatively in complex cranial vault remodeling.[131–133] The recommended dosing regimen is a loading dose of 10 mg/kg followed by a continuous infusion of 5 mg/kg per hour.[134] The incidence of adverse events, including seizures and thromboembolic events, in children treated with or without antifibrinolytics during craniofacial reconstructive surgery was similar.[135]

Another antifibrinolytic, ε-aminocaproic acid (EACA), has been effective in reducing bleeding in cardiac and spinal procedures. In observational studies, ε-aminocaproic acid has been associated with reduced blood loss and transfusion in craniosynostosis surgery although these findings have not been confirmed in a controlled study.[136,137] The dosing for infants undergoing craniofacial surgery is a loading dose of 100 mg/kg followed by 40 mg/kg per hour.[138,139] An observational study failed to find a difference in calculated blood loss or transfusion volumes in patients who received either ε-aminocaproic acid or when compared to tranexamic acid.[140]

A single-center prospective study of 120 infants undergoing craniosynostosis repair used thromboelastography and the platelet-fibrinogen product to guide the administration of blood products.[141] Using multivariate analysis and receiver operating curves to assess four parameters: K-time >2:1, MA <55 mm, α-angle <62 degrees, and the platelet-fibrinogen product <343; infants with all four predictors had a 92% probability of a blood loss of 60 mL/kg or more, whereas those with none of these parameters had an approximately 10% probability.

Induced hypotension, defined as a 10% to 20% reduction in the mean arterial blood pressure, may decrease intraoperative surgical blood loss and operating time,[142] although its effectiveness and safety during craniosynostosis surgery is unknown. The lower limits of safe blood pressure reduction in infants are unknown. A variety of pharmacologic agents have been used to induce hypotension, including inhalational agents, vasodilators, β-blockers, and remifentanil.[142,143] Invasive arterial pressure monitoring is essential whenever hypotensive anesthesia is used. Induced hypotension should be used with great caution in the presence of increased ICP because of the risk of compromising cerebral perfusion pressure (i.e., the difference between mean arterial pressure and either ICP or central venous pressure, whichever is greater). The risks of inadequate cerebral and end-organ oxygen delivery during hypotension are magnified if anemia is also present. It is considered prudent to maintain normovolemia and normocapnia when induced hypotension is used (see Chapter 10). Many practitioners have determined that the potential benefits (reduction of blood loss, shorter surgery) of this technique are outweighed by the risks (cerebral ischemia and irreversible brain injury, blindness, end-organ damage). Some advocate a strategy of deliberate normotension where the anesthetic is tailored to avoid blood pressures greater than baseline rather than an approach of induced hypotension.

Even if employing some or all of the aforementioned techniques, the clinician caring for patients undergoing craniofacial surgery should be prepared for the possibility of rapid transfusion, particularly in children less than 24 months of age.[109] In addition to age less than 24 months, a study of risk factors for red blood cell–containing transfusion products found it was associated with American Society of Anesthesiologists (ASA) status of II or greater, preoperative anemia, and the lack of use of an antifibrinolytic, intraoperative cell saver, and transfusion protocol.[144] A machine learning model to predict the need for transfusion in craniosynostosis surgery reported that the most important variables associated with need for blood transfusion were the child's platelet count, preoperative hematocrit/hemoglobin, and age or weight, in addition to the institutional surgical case volume.[145] In a retrospective review of 60 children who underwent craniofacial surgery at a single institution, half of the children required fewer transfusions and had a reduced length of stay that were attributed to the preoperative use of iron and erythropoietin, the use of a blood-recycling device intraoperatively, and a reduced minimum hemoglobin concentration for transfusion (<7 mg/dL) compared with a placebo group.[146] Given the potential for acute large-volume blood loss, IV access with large-bore catheters remains essential and at least two units of packed red blood cells (PRBCs) should be crossmatched and available in the operating room at all times. Intravenous fluids should be administered via a fluid warmer to maintain normothermia. Maintaining normothermia preserves coagulation function and theoretically reduces bleeding and transfusion-related complications.[147] Based on adult data, coagulopathy from dilution of soluble clotting factors on average develops when 142% of the circulating blood volume has been lost and replaced with PRBCs and crystalloid, and with thrombocytopenia developing after an average of 2 to 3 blood volumes are lost (see also Figs. 10.6 and 10.7 and Table 10.10).[148] Useful empiric and clinical indicators for the need for hemostatic blood product administration include estimation of the blood loss based on the number of blood volumes of blood products administered, physical estimates of blood loss, and an assessment of hemostasis in the surgical field. Serial determinations of the international normalized ratio prothrombin time (INR), partial thromboplastin time (PTT), platelet count, and fibrinogen concentration and the use of thromboelastography help to identify coagulopathy and guide hemostatic blood product administration.[141,149] Avoidance of hypofibrinogenemia is important to maintain hemostasis[141,149,150]; however, prophylactic fibrinogen concentrate during open cranial vault remodeling did not reduce the transfusion volume required.[151]

Endoscopic repair of craniosynostosis has become an accepted surgical approach to reduce bleeding and decrease morbidity.[77,152,153] Independent risk factors for bleeding during endoscopic strip craniectomy include body weight <5 kilograms, sagittal suture surgery (related to proximity to the sagittal venous sinus), syndromic craniosynostosis, and earlier date of surgery.[108]

Hyponatremia and cerebral salt-wasting syndrome are associated with craniosynostosis repair.[154–158] Both intraoperative and postoperative hyponatremia have been described, with the latter occurring in approximately 30% of children. Postoperative hyponatremia has been associated with preoperative increased ICP, blood loss, and female sex with normal preoperative ICP.[158] The average reduction in sodium concentration was more pronounced in children who received hyponatremic (hypotonic) (5% dextrose and 0.2% or 0.5% NaCl) compared with normonatremic (isotonic) postoperative IV fluids.[158] The perioperative use of balanced salt solutions is recommended to prevent hyponatremia (see also Chapter 7).

INTRACRANIAL PRESSURE

Early surgery for craniosynostosis is often indicated to prevent increases in ICP.[53,56] One-third of children with craniofacial dysostosis syndrome and 15% to 20% of children with single-suture craniosynostosis have increased ICP (>15 mm Hg).[159] Approximately 40% to 50% of children with syndromic craniosynostosis have hydrocephalus, although differentiation from nonprogressive ventriculomegaly may be difficult.[159–161] Timing of surgery may affect neurocognitive development and intelligence because these are adversely affected by sustained increased ICP. Associated OSA resulting in hypoxemia and hypercapnia may lead to an increase in cerebral blood volume that exacerbates intracranial hypertension.[162] Untreated intracranial hypertension may lead to optic atrophy and visual impairment.[60,163] As a consequence, when increased ICP has been identified either preoperatively or postoperatively, placing a ventriculoperitoneal shunt should be considered[161]; this occurs more commonly in Crouzon and Pfeiffer syndromes.[161]

Basic principles of neuroanesthesia to prevent further increases in ICP and decreases in cerebral perfusion pressure should be followed in children with increased ICP (see also Chapter 24). It may be prudent to use protective measures to attenuate the hypertensive response to laryngoscopy and intubation, including the administration of a short-acting opioid, a β-blocker, or topical local anesthesia to the upper airway. Intraoperatively, the anesthesiologist faces numerous challenges to control ICP. Strategies to control ICP include mild to moderate hyperventilation (end-tidal carbon dioxide [$ETCO_2$] of 30 to 35 mm Hg), especially when signs of herniation are evident; avoidance of hypervolemia; and, where indicated, appropriate use of hypertonic (3%) saline solution, mannitol, furosemide, and dexamethasone to reduce ICP, reduce brain volume, and facilitate brain retraction. Although cranial vault reconstruction increases intracranial volume and reduces ICP,[164] children remain at risk of increased ICP after surgery and require close ophthalmologic and clinical follow-up, even after a cosmetically successful cranial expansion.[165,166]

VENOUS AIR EMBOLISM

Venous air embolism may occur during any operative procedure in which the operative site is above the level of the heart and noncollapsible veins are exposed to atmospheric pressure.[167–174] The incidence of venous air embolism in children undergoing craniectomy for craniosynostosis repair has been reported to be as great as 83%,[174] although hemodynamically significant venous air embolism is rare. The incidence of embolism associated with endoscopic craniectomy is reported to be between 2% and 8%,[108,173] similar to that during open repair.[71] Hypovolemia resulting from surgical blood loss can lead to a decrease in both systemic and central venous pressures and the development of a pressure gradient between the right atrium and the surgical site. This gradient increases the potential to entrain air via open dural sinuses or bony venous sinusoids.[174,175] If the volume of air that is entrained is sufficiently large, right ventricular outflow obstruction may ensue, causing acute right-sided heart failure and cardiovascular collapse. Smaller volumes of air may reduce cardiac output, and cause hypotension, and myocardial or cerebral ischemia.[172] Transesophageal echocardiography (documenting the presence of air in the right ventricular outflow tract), precordial Doppler ultrasonography (continuous windmill murmur), end-tidal carbon dioxide (precipitous decrease in carbon dioxide tension), and nitrogen monitoring (sudden increase in nitrogen concentration in the exhaled breath) have been used to identify venous air embolism with varying sensitivity, well before cardiovascular collapse occurs (see Figs. 24.6 and 24.7).[172,176–179] Applying bone wax to the open edges of cut bone, reducing the degree of or avoiding the reverse Trendelenburg position, maintaining positive-pressure ventilation with 5 cm of positive end-expiratory pressure (PEEP), and ensuring normovolemia help to prevent venous air embolism. Fluid resuscitation, vasopressors, and aspiration of air from the right side of the heart may prevent progression to cardiovascular collapse.[168,174,179]

PROLONGED SURGERY

As with all surgeries that last several hours, preventing the complications associated with prolonged anesthesia is paramount.[180] Nerve palsies, pressure ulcers of the skin, ophthalmic complications, hypothermia, and acidosis may occur. Careful positioning of the extremities, use of an egg-crate–type mattress or foam padding, and avoiding pressure to the eyes, particularly when the surgical procedure requires the prone position, will prevent most of these adverse outcomes. In children with proptosis, such as Crouzon syndrome, it may be necessary to suture the eyelids closed (temporary tarsorrhaphy) after applying lubrication to keep the corneas moist and prevent corneal abrasions. Anterior ischemic optic neuropathy, which can cause transient or permanent postoperative blindness, is a rare complication that occurs in the absence of external pressure to the eyes.[181,182]

Hypothermia, another major concern, is largely preventable. Factors that predispose to hypothermia include the large surface area exposed during surgery and the potential infusion of large volumes of relatively cold IV fluids. Effective measures to prevent hypothermia include warming the operating room, using forced-air warmers and radiant warming lamps, insulating the child, and using warming devices for blood and IV fluids. Attention to preventing hypothermia during induction of anesthesia and placing IV and arterial lines is paramount. Preventing hypothermia and limiting blood loss and transfusion requirements are key factors in preventing the development of perioperative metabolic disturbance[183]; even mild hypothermia has been associated with increased blood loss and transfusion.[184]

Orbital Hypertelorism

The term *orbital hypertelorism* describes abnormally widely separated orbits. This deformity may occur in isolation or in association with other congenital abnormalities, such as facial clefts and Apert syndrome (Fig. 33.5). Surgical repair involves mobilizing and repositioning the orbits through either a subcranial approach, which leaves the roof of the orbit intact, or an intracranial approach via a frontal craniectomy. This procedure is performed in children older than 5 years of age who may have already undergone extensive surgical reconstruction. Surgical manipulation of the globe may elicit the oculocardiac reflex, resulting in bradyarrhythmias or asystole. Oculocardiac reflex may also occur during frontoorbital advancement, midface, and orthognathic procedures (see also Fig. 32.3A,B).[185] These arrhythmias are generally without hemodynamic consequence and extinguish over time. Usually release of any orbital/periorbital pressure or tension being applied by the surgeon facilitates return of the heart rate to normal values. Hemodynamically important bradycardia can be treated, and further episodes prevented by administering an anticholinergic such as atropine (10–20 μg/kg) or glycopyrrolate (5–10 μg/kg).

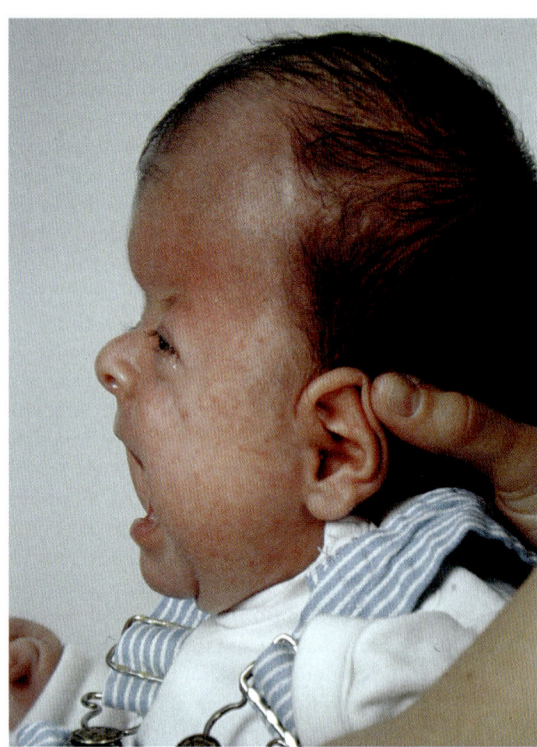

FIGURE 33.5 Child with Apert syndrome. Notable features include proptosis, cloverleaf skull, maxillary hypoplasia, and syndactyly (syndactyly is present in Apert syndrome but not in Crouzon syndrome).

After establishing IV access, the airway should be secured using an orotracheal tube; confirmation of bilateral breath sounds is essential after positioning.[23] Blood loss from multiple osteotomies may be substantial, and, as in the case of craniosynostosis surgery, methods to reduce the use of homologous blood should be considered. Intraoperative management follows the principles outlined for craniosynostosis surgery. At the conclusion of surgery, the trachea is extubated, and the child is monitored overnight in a high-dependency setting with the capability of managing acute airway obstruction and monitoring of neurologic status.

Midface Procedures

Midface advancement to improve facial appearance is commonly required for children with maxillary hypoplasia, such as those with Crouzon, Apert (see Fig. 33.5), and Pfeiffer syndromes (E-Fig. 33.7).[186–188] This procedure is typically performed in children age 5 to 7 years, although complications such as proptosis, corneal ulceration, ocular dislocations, and airway obstruction may necessitate intervention at a younger age.[188–191] A LeFort II procedure is similar to a LeFort III, with the difference being that the osteotomy is oriented vertically through the infraorbital rim. Thus, the nasal pyramid and the maxilla move forward as a single unit. Le Fort III osteotomy and monobloc procedures (Fig. 33.6) have the potential for significant complications, including massive blood loss, airway difficulties, blindness, cerebrospinal fluid leak, and infection.[180,182,192–194]

Anesthetic concerns are similar to those for orbital hypertelorism and craniosynostosis surgeries. Children with Apert and Crouzon syndromes often present with incomplete or complete nasal obstruction that results from choanal atresia or midface intraoperative change from the oral to the nasal tracheal position after completing the midfacial osteotomies.[195] To perform the latter maneuver, the anesthesiologist wears a sterile surgical gown and gloves and uses sterile equipment, including laryngoscope, Magill forceps, and tube exchange catheter (see E-Fig. 34.6A–G). Visualizing the glottis during surgery may be difficult because of the presence of airway edema and blood in the hypopharynx. A tube exchange catheter is passed through a naris and into the trachea alongside the orotracheal tube. The nasal tube is then passed over the exchange catheter, and its tip is positioned at the glottic opening. The oral tube is then withdrawn while the nasal tube is advanced (rotating the bevel 90 degrees clockwise or counterclockwise as needed to pass the vocal cords and arytenoids)[196,197] and visualized as it passes through the glottic aperture. Once the tube position is confirmed, the catheter is removed and the nasal tube is secured, possibly suturing it to the nasal septum.[23] Given the proximity of the tracheal tube to the surgical site, damage to the tracheal tube can occur during surgery.[198–200] Vigilance is required to detect an accidental disconnection or damage to the tracheal tube. The anesthesiologist must be prepared to respond immediately to an unexpected interruption in ventilation and replace the tracheal tube.

A nasogastric tube is placed after surgery to prevent gastric distention and reduce the likelihood of postoperative vomiting. A wire cutter must be available at the bedside at all times if intermaxillary fixation is used to stabilize the facial bones and mandible. In the ICU, the presence of an audible leak around the tracheal tube, whether uncuffed or cuffed and deflated, is one criterion to determine absence of laryngeal or periglottic edema and therefore readiness for tracheal extubation.[198] Intraoperative blood loss with LeFort III and monobloc procedures can be extensive.[201] Moderate hypotensive anesthesia may reduce or prevent the need for blood transfusions during maxillary orthognathic surgery and can improve visualization of the surgical field during the period of downfracture and osteotomy creation.[202]

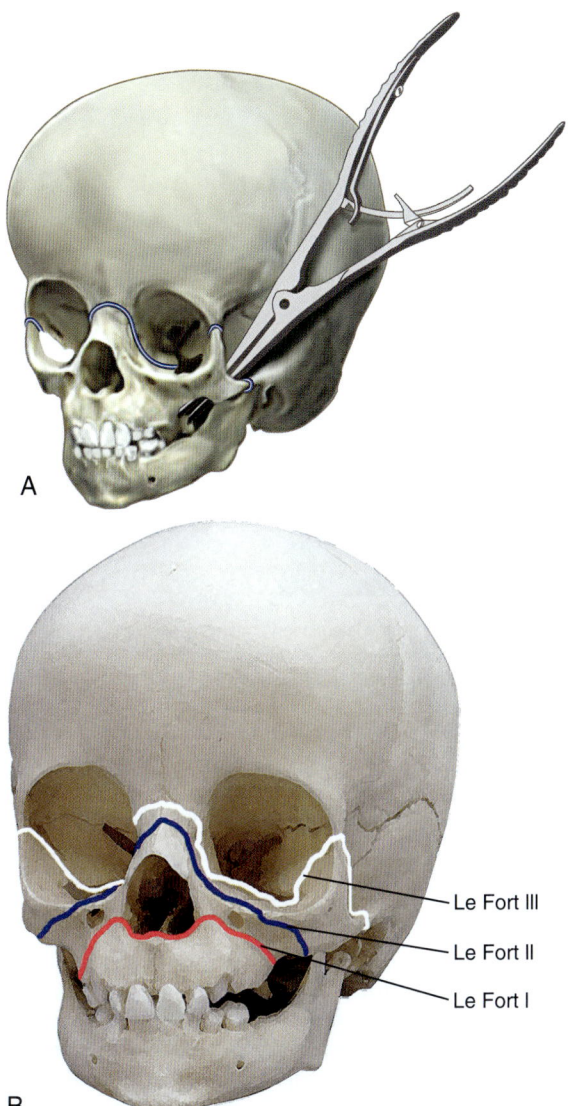

FIGURE 33.6 Le Fort III and monobloc procedures for correction of midface hypoplasia. **A,** The osteotomies in the Le Fort III procedure pass through the nasofrontal junction, across the medial orbital wall and floor, and into the inferior orbital fissure. A cut through the frontozygomatic suture, pterygomaxillary junction, and zygomatic arch allows separation of the midface. **B,** The monobloc procedures are similar, but the nasofrontal junction and frontozygomatic suture are not mobilized. This technique allows simultaneous correction of supraorbital and midface deformities at the expense of an increased incidence of postoperative complications.

Hemifacial Microsomia, Treacher Collins Syndrome, and Goldenhar Syndrome

Hemifacial microsomias, also known as otomandibular dysostosis (Fig. 33.7), result from a malformation of the first and second branchial (or pharyngeal) arches. This is the second most common facial defect after clefts. These disorders are organized according to the clinical classification system **O**rbital distortion, **M**andibular hypoplasia, **E**ar anomaly, **N**erve involvement, and **S**oft tissue deficiency (OMENS).[3,203–207]

Piezosurgery is a technique used to perform osteotomies using ultrasonic frequencies during mandibular distraction in children with hemifacial microsomia.[208] Airway difficulty increases with the complexity of the defect from unilateral to bilateral mandibular or temporomandibular involvement. The disorder may include mandibular hypoplasia, temporomandibular joint dysostosis, cleft palate, and auricular, ophthalmologic, and facial nerve defects. Goldenhar syndrome (Fig. 33.8 and E-Fig. 33.8) is the most common form of this disorder; vertebral anomalies are present in 40% and congenital heart defects occur in 35%. Airway management is complicated by midfacial hypoplasia, asymmetry, and limited size of the mouth opening, and mandibular retrognathia. The airway anomalies associated with this syndrome predispose to OSA. Overall, tracheal intubation in children with unilateral hemifacial microsomia is easy in 70% and very difficult in 9%.[203]

hypoplasia. Consequently, mask anesthesia can be difficult, even with an oral airway in situ (see discussion of syndromic craniosynostosis). However, a supraglottic airway often relieves upper airway obstruction and laryngoscopy and tracheal intubation in these children is usually uncomplicated. The diameter of the tracheal tube requires careful consideration because these children may require prolonged postoperative ventilation until postoperative facial and laryngeal edema have resolved. Although a tracheotomy is sometimes performed, orotracheal intubation is generally preferred and is the most straightforward method. In the latter case, the tube is wired to a nondeciduous tooth or secured with a circum-mandibular wire. A nasotracheal tube can also be used throughout the procedure, or the surgeon may request an

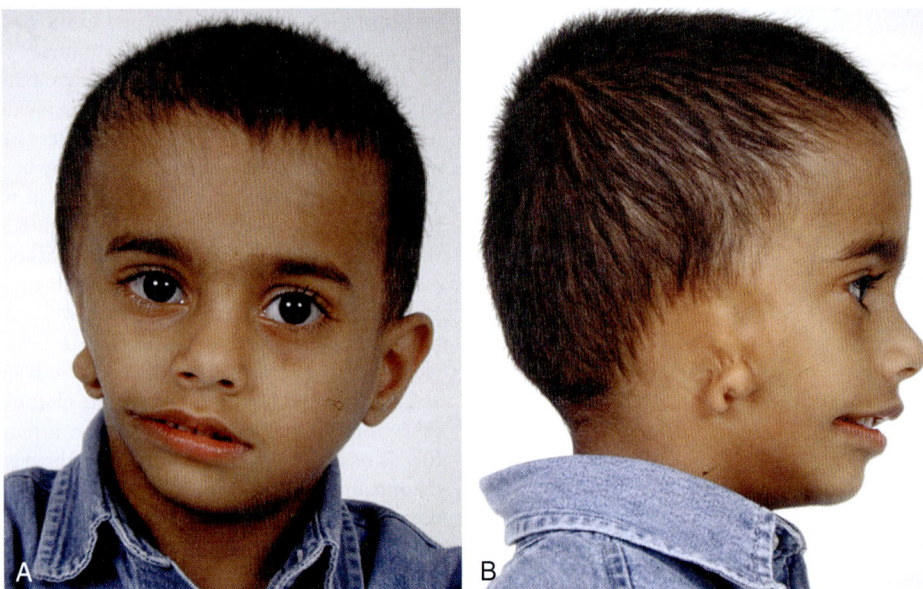

FIGURE 33.7 Frontal **(A)** and lateral **(B)** views of unilateral hemifacial microsomia. In the lateral view, microstomia and mandibular and ocular deformities are evident. These children may present with either unilateral or bilateral hemifacial microsomia, a hypoplastic mandible and maxilla, and ear deformities.

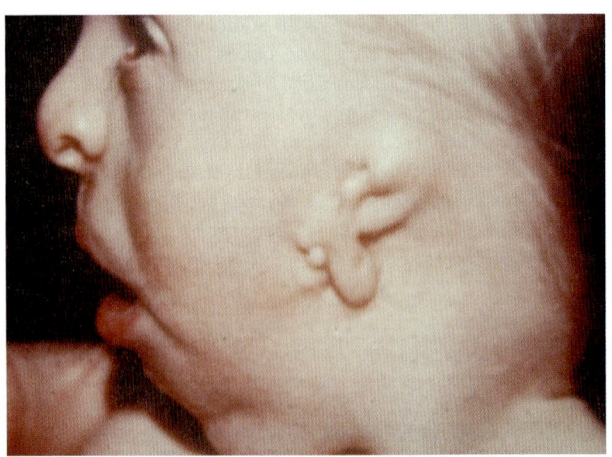

FIGURE 33.8 Goldenhar syndrome in an infant. This is one of the most common forms of hemifacial microsomia. With unilateral hemifacial microsomia, the airway is usually managed and instrumented without difficulty, but with bilateral mandibular hypoplasia, the airway may be very difficult to manage in one-third of afflicted children.

In contrast, tracheal intubation in children with bilateral mandibular hypoplasia is evenly distributed among easy, difficult, and very difficult.[203]

The craniofacial abnormalities of mandibular hypoplasia, macrostomia, and cleft palate in Treacher Collins syndrome (E-Fig. 33.9) often present difficulties for airway management that increase with age.[3,203] Other clinical features of the syndrome include hypoplastic zygomatic arches, ophthalmic features (including sloping palpebral fissures, coloboma of the eyes, and notched lower eyelids), microtia, choanal atresia, cardiovascular defects, and renal anomalies. Mandibular distraction osteogenesis is a surgical option considered when upper airway obstruction is due to mandibular deficiency. This avoids

tracheostomy or other surgical intervention and allows for future growth of the mandible. Children with hemifacial microsomia have a poor psychosocial outcome.[209]

AIRWAY MANAGEMENT

Airway management of children with hemifacial dysostoses is difficult. It is essential that all equipment for management of the difficult airway be present in the operating room before induction of anesthesia (or administration of sedatives/local anesthetic in cases where a sedated/awake approach is used) (see Table 12.9). For infants and children with difficult airways, an inhalational induction is the most commonly used technique. In a case series of 136 children with hemifacial microsomia who underwent 311 anesthetics, bag mask ventilation with or without oral airways was possible except for one child who required two practitioners for bag mask ventilation.[210] In older children and adolescents, either an inhalational induction or IV sedation (using dexmedetomidine and/or propofol) with topical local anesthesia applied to the upper airway may be used to facilitate tracheal intubation. In all cases, primary and backup plans to manage the airway should be prepared together with the equipment and personnel required to execute them.

A variety of techniques may be used to control the difficult airway, including a flexible fiberoptic bronchoscope, GlideScope (Verathon Inc., Bothell, WA), the C-MAC (Karl Storz S.E. & Co., Tuttlingen, Germany), the Airtraq optic laryngoscope (Prodol Meditec S.A., Vizcaya, Spain), and supraglottic airway devices,[211] (see Chapter 12). We have used the two-person intubation technique, in which the first anesthesiologist applies external posterior laryngeal pressure while performing laryngoscopy to optimize the view of the glottis, while the second anesthesiologist inserts the tracheal tube into the trachea when the view is adequate (Fig. 33.9).[212] The second anesthesiologist also may assist with more advanced airway management both in terms of helping to observe the child and assisting with the use of advanced airway

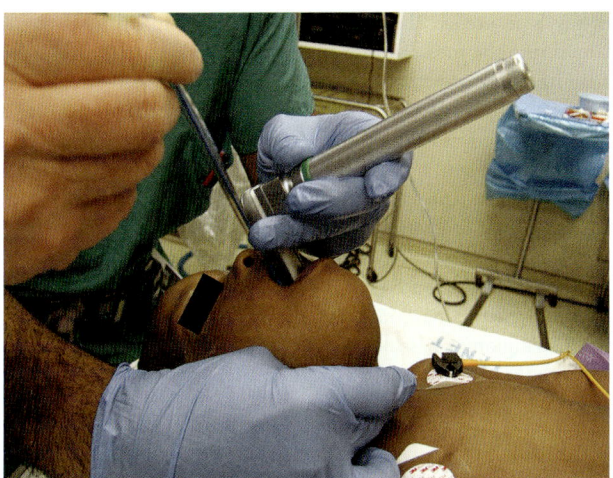

FIGURE 33.9 Two-person intubation technique. The intubator (first person) performs laryngoscopy and manipulates the larynx with external laryngeal manipulation (gloved hands). With the larynx in view, the intubator cocks their head to the left while holding position and the assistant (second person, nongloved hand), who is standing on the intubator's right, then passes the tracheal tube through the larynx.[212]

devices. Videolaryngoscopy can be used to stabilize mandibular structures and expose the glottis to facilitate intubation with a fiberoptic bronchoscope.

Preformed tracheal tubes are generally used via the oral or nasal route, depending on the site of surgery. When a nasotracheal tube is used, it can be secured by suturing it to the membranous nasal septum or taping it after the skin has been prepared with benzoin. An oral tube may be wired to the mandible or to a nondeciduous tooth. Care must be taken to ensure that the tip of the preformed tube is mid-tracheal, as the length of preformed nasotracheal and, to a lesser extent orotracheal tubes, exceeds that of the uncuffed version of the same diameter tube.[23] A supraglottic airway can be very effective in maintaining airway patency during induction of anesthesia or as a guide to facilitate a fiberoptic intubation.

For children with a history of upper airway obstruction or midfacial hypoplasia who present with a tracheostomy, the tracheostomy tube can be replaced with a cuffed tracheostomy tube or an armored tube that is sutured in place for the duration of the surgery. The use of a cuffed tracheostomy tube separates the aerodigestive tracts, facilitates controlled ventilation and the delivery of adequate positive end-expiratory pressure, and prevents atelectasis during prolonged procedures. Changes in the position of the head and neck can displace the tracheal tube, so care should be taken to confirm the position of the tracheal tube after the child is positioned for surgery.[23,213] This is especially important for cranial vault procedures that involve extremes of neck extension, such as might occur during reconstruction of the supraorbital bar. Airway equipment and additional tracheal tubes must be available in the operating room at all times. It is essential to document an audible leak around the tracheal tube at the time of tracheal intubation (with the cuff on the tracheal tube deflated), because the presence of a leak is often used postoperatively to determine suitability for extubation when significant airway edema has developed. OSA associated with midfacial anomalies may result in upper airway obstruction during induction and emergence.[87,93]

Orthognathic Surgery

Malocclusion secondary to maxillary or mandibular hypoplasia (such as occurs in hemifacial microsomia and Treacher Collins syndrome), tumors, trauma, as well as temporomandibular joint dysfunction are generally accepted indications for orthognathic surgery. LeFort I procedures for maxillary hypoplasia involve a transverse incision through the maxilla to advance the upper teeth into normal occlusion with the mandible. These procedures are usually performed in adolescents because surgery is performed once maxillary and mandibular growth is complete. Because this age group usually exhibits increased perioperative anxiety, preoperative assurance and education, as well as an adequate premedication based on the operator's preference are often necessary.

Airway management is a major concern, particularly in children with a hypoplastic mandible or temporomandibular dysfunction.[3] A high index of suspicion for atlantoaxial instability is required if the underlying disease process is juvenile rheumatoid arthritis. The anticipated difficult airway can be managed using fiberoptic intubation, with sedation or topical local anesthesia or an inhalation induction and maintenance of spontaneous ventilation until the trachea is intubated, as discussed earlier. Tracheal intubation in children with adequate mouth opening can be managed with a video/indirect laryngoscope or using a laryngeal mask as a conduit for fiberoptic intubation; these techniques are best suited for orotracheal intubations. However, for orthognathic surgery, nasotracheal intubation (using a preformed tracheal tube) is often preferred with transseptal suturing.[23] Excessive pressure on the ala nasi (causing ischemia) can be avoided by fixing the preformed nasal tube to the forehead with the nasal curve positioned away from the ala. LeFort I advancements require close communication between the surgery and anesthesia teams because the nasotracheal tube can be dislodged once the maxilla is fully mobilized or cut when the maxillary osteotomies are performed. If intermaxillary fixation is used postoperatively, wire cutters must be immediately available at all times while the child is monitored in an intensive care setting.

To reduce intraoperative blood loss, moderate controlled hypotension is commonly used by means of any of a range of pharmacologic agents, including inhalational anesthetic agents, β-blockers, and remifentanil. The literature is extensive on the salutary effect of induced hypotension in reducing intraoperative blood loss and improving the quality of the surgical field during orthognathic surgery.[202,214–223] However, many practitioners have moved away from controlled hypotension because of concerns regarding complications, particularly blindness. Regardless of anesthesia technique, invasive arterial monitoring facilitates intraoperative monitoring and evaluation of blood gases and hematocrit. In many cases, mild hypotension provides optimal surgical conditions (systolic blood pressure 85 to 90 mm Hg). Dexamethasone (0.5 mg/kg) may reduce postoperative airway edema.[224] After awakening the child, the trachea is extubated once protective airway reflexes have returned. The child is monitored overnight in a high-dependency setting with the ability to establish an airway should acute airway obstruction develop. In some cases, at the conclusion of surgery, mandibulomaxillary fixation may be used with either metal wires or elastic bands. Emergency wire cutters should be immediately available in the postoperative period in the event of the need for emergency airway management.

Lymphatic Malformations and Hemangiomas

Lymphatic malformations are rare congenital malformations of the lymphatic system occurring with an incidence of 1 in 20,000 births, most frequently involving the axilla and neck (Fig. 33.10 and E-Fig. 33.10). The pathology consists of multiple loculated cysts that contain lymph fluid or blood (see Fig. 33.10B). Historically, macrocystic lymphatic malformations (cysts >1–2 cm) were called cystic hygromas and microcystic lymphatic malformations (cysts <1–2 cm) referred to as lymphangiomas. Approximately 50% of lymphatic malformations are present at birth, with most developing within the first 2 years of life. They can often be identified prenatally with fetal ultrasound or fetal MRI.[225] Most require treatment which can include repeated aspirations, sclerotherapy, or surgical excision to debulk the mass (see E-Fig. 33.10B).[226–228] Lymphatic malformations can be associated with other chromosomal abnormalities such as Noonan and Turner syndromes, in which case the anesthetic management is guided by the underlying syndrome. Large lymphatic malformations that are diagnosed prenatally may require delivery with an ex-utero intrapartum treatment to allow time for airway management; others are managed expectantly after birth with close monitoring for the need for urgent intubation or tracheostomy to relieve an obstructed airway. Aspiration of cysts at the time of delivery may help temporarily relieve the obstruction (see Chapter 36).[225,229] During the preoperative assessment, the airway should be examined and evaluated by radiographs for involvement of supraglottic and infraglottic structures. Acute airway obstruction can occur during induction if lymphatic malformations are present in the upper airway. Fiberoptic intubation may be required if the larynx is distorted, in which case spontaneous ventilation should be maintained until the airway is secured.[230] Lower cervical lymphatic malformations can extend into the mediastinum and should be evaluated with further imaging.[225] Postoperative complications of surgical excision include laryngeal edema, airway obstruction, pneumonia, facial palsy, and infection.[226,227,231] Sclerotherapy with doxycycline, bleomycin, or other sclerosing agents can cause edema after the procedure that can lead to airway obstruction, depending on the location of the lymphatic malformations (see Chapter 36). For either surgical resection or sclerotherapy of lesions adjacent to the airway, postoperative intubation may be prudent by securing the airway with a nasotracheal tube.[225]

Hemangiomas, also known as juvenile or infantile hemangiomas, are the most common benign tumors in infancy, affecting up to 4.5% of infants.[232] The natural course begins with a proliferation phase during the first few months postnatally with 80% reaching their final size by 3 months of age, followed by an involution phase. Ninety percent of cases have completely involuted by the age of 4 years.[232] Deeper lesions can be slower growing and slower to involute. Most hemangiomas are uncomplicated and require no treatment. Complications requiring treatment occur in 10% to 15%.[232] Hemangiomas can affect all organs, and intervention is required when the lesion affects the function of vital organs such as the eyes, airway, or liver.[233] Hemangiomas that occur in the subglottic region must be considered in the differential diagnosis of a noninfectious cause of croup in infants younger than 3 months of age. When present on the face, particularly around the eyes or in the chin region (Fig. 33.11), hemangiomas are often associated with lesions in the airway.[232,234,235] They can occur in any part of the airway and can cause airway and feeding difficulties. Airway procedures to resect or remove hemangiomas are generally undertaken between 1 and 11 months of age.[236] Limb hemangiomas generally present with cosmetic concerns and bleeding. Rarely, children with large hemangiomas develop high-output heart failure. Up to 30% of

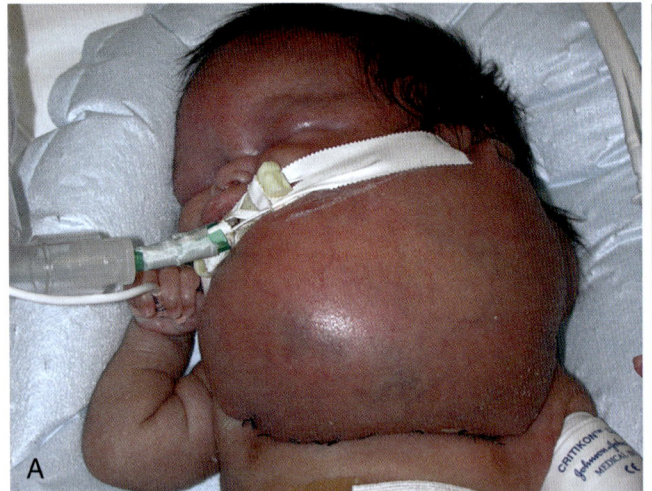
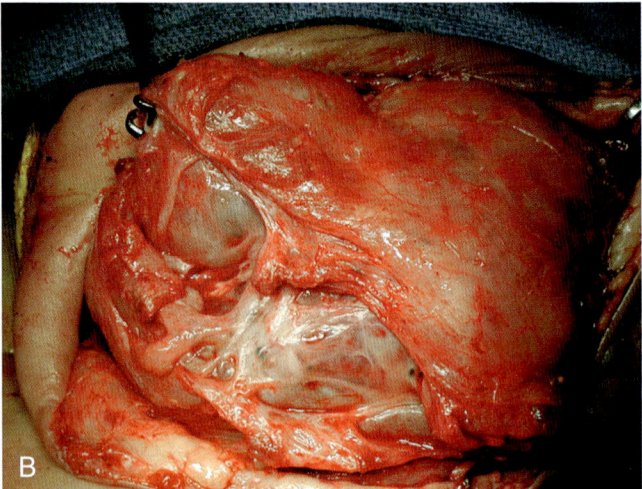

FIGURE 33.10 A, Lymphatic malformation. Note that the bulk of the tumor is extraoral and extralaryngeal, although extension into the tongue and supraglottic region may complicate direct laryngoscopy. The tumor on the surface of the neck may rapidly expand owing to bleeding into the cysts or accumulation of fluid in the lymphatics. Such large tumors may put the overlying skin under great tension. They may also be situated such that they preclude tracheostomy. **B,** Gross pathologic examination consists of a combination of multiloculated cysts that may contain a combination of lymph fluid and blood. Debulking may result in substantial blood loss. Sequential debulking of the hygroma may be required as the residual cysts expand with fluid and blood and re-expand the malformation.

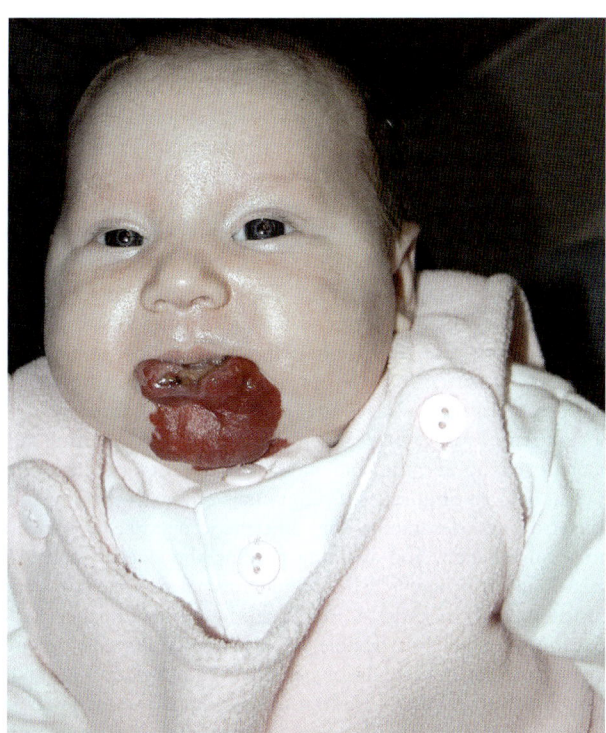

FIGURE 33.11 Facial hemangioma on the lip and chin of a child. The hemangioma involves the skin overlying the mandible centrally from the lower lip to the tip of the mandible. Hemangiomas vary widely in size but can enlarge precipitously as a result of bleeding into the tumor.

large facial hemangiomas are associated with anomalies in the PHACE syndrome (**P**osterior fossa malformations; **H**emangiomas; **A**rterial, **C**ardiac, and **E**ye abnormalities; and sternal or umbilical raphe). If present, cerebral artery anomalies can predispose these patients to ischemic stroke, and they may also have aortic arch abnormalities such as coarctation of the aorta.[232]

Since many hemangiomas spontaneously involute, continued monitoring is appropriate for uncomplicated hemangiomas. Oral propranolol is first line treatment for complicated hemangiomas.[232,237] In addition to propranolol, other treatment options include systemic corticosteroid treatment, corticosteroid injection, surgical excision, and laser ablation.[238–241] Propranolol reduces the need for surgical intervention but requires 6 months to 1 year of therapy.[242] Rare side effects relevant to the anesthesiologist include bronchospasm, bradycardia, hypotension, hypoglycemia, and unmasking of a previously undiagnosed atrioventricular conduction block.[232] Surgical treatment is reserved for superficial hemangiomas in locations that are surgically accessible.[233] Laser treatment for superficial lesions is commonly performed as an outpatient procedure,[243] and routine anesthetic precautions including fire precautions for facial hemangiomas, should be taken. Children with hemangiomas who had airway procedures received more steroids and had increased admissions and mortality compared with those without airway procedures.[236] Facial lesions with concern for PHACE syndrome or large lesions with the potential for increased cardiac output may warrant preoperative evaluation with echocardiography. Multifocal intrahepatic infantile hemangiomas are associated with disseminated intravascular coagulation.[232] Hemangiomas can trap platelets, leading to a consumptive thrombocytopenia with depletion of clotting factors and coagulopathy, known as Kasabach-Merritt syndrome.[244] Children

who undergo excision of hemangiomas often require blood products during surgery, but platelets should be transfused with care because an accumulation within the malformation may increase its size.[245] NSAIDs should be avoided because of their effects on platelet function.

Arteriovenous malformations are present at birth but can go unrecognized for years, especially when they are intracranial. Large arteriovenous malformations may cause high-output cardiac failure, necessitating therapeutic intervention. Treatment options may include chemotherapy, corticosteroid therapy, embolization, and surgical excision (see also Chapter 24).[246–248]

Möbius Sequence

Möbius sequence is a rare neurologic disorder (2–20 in 1,000,000 births) characterized by congenital palsy of the facial (VII) and abducens (VI) cranial nerves, resulting in unilateral or bilateral facial weakness and defective extraocular eye movement (E-Fig. 33.11). It is thought to arise from abnormal rhombencephalic development and is therefore primarily a disorder of the caudal brainstem.[249,250] These classic features may be associated with other cranial nerve palsies, ophthalmic abnormalities, developmental delay, and various craniofacial, limb, and musculoskeletal malformations, resulting in a variable pattern of clinical expression.[251–255] Involvement of cranial nerves IX and X is associated with pharyngeal dysfunction, dysphagia, feeding difficulties, retention of oral secretions, and recurrent aspiration pneumonia. Associated micrognathia, microstomia, limited mouth opening, and other orofacial abnormalities may make tracheal intubation difficult.[256,257] Other associations include gastroesophageal reflux, hypotonia of skeletal muscles, congenital cardiac abnormalities, spinal abnormalities, and peripheral neuropathies. Central alveolar hypoventilation syndrome has been described in association with Möbius sequence and may be secondary to hypoplasia of midbrain respiratory centers.[258] Central alveolar hypoventilation, compounded by upper airway hypotonia and the effects of sedatives, opioids, and anesthetic agents, can predispose to postoperative respiratory compromise. The absence of facial expression secondary to paresis of the facial nerve may complicate the assessment of postoperative pain.[259] The anesthetic plan for the child with Möbius sequence must be tailored to the individual based on the clinical expression of the syndrome. There is a single, isolated report of fatal malignant hyperthermia in a 7-month-old. The absence of other reported cases renders a connection between malignant hyperthermia and Möbius sequence exceedingly unlikely.[260]

The most common surgical procedure performed in children with Möbius sequence is segmental gracilis muscle transplantation, in which the muscle is transplanted to the face and revascularized to the facial artery and vein.[261] Motor innervation of the gracilis requires a functioning cranial nerve such as the masseter branch of the trigeminal nerve. The aim of this facial reanimation is to facilitate facial expression and provide lower lip support to reduce drooling and improve speech.[261] Anesthetic considerations include those for prolonged surgery, avoidance of neuromuscular block to facilitate intraoperative nerve stimulation, and avoidance of hypocapnia, hypothermia, and hypotension to ensure graft perfusion. The latter considerations are also applicable to the postoperative period. Other surgical procedures commonly performed in children with Möbius sequence include strabismus surgery and orthopedic procedures to improve limb function.

Brachial Plexus Surgery

Brachial plexus injury occurs in 0.5 to 5 infants per 1000 live births as a result of birth trauma.[262,263] Erb palsy involves damage to nerve roots C5, C6, and C7, whereas Klumpke palsy involves roots C8 and T1.[263] Complete plexus palsies are the most devastating injuries, resulting in a flail and insensate arm.[263,264] Although 75% of brachial plexus injuries resolve spontaneously and completely within the first month after birth, 25% result in permanent disability and impairment.[263,265–267] Surgical intervention is indicated if the motor function does not improve after 3 months of age.[265,266] Clinically significant diaphragmatic palsy is associated with 2.4% of neonates with brachial plexus injury. In the very young, diaphragmatic palsy requires aggressive intervention before brachial plexus repair. For brachial plexus surgery to be successful, the nerve root cannot be completely avulsed from the spinal cord. Therefore, detailed imaging is required to characterize the nature of the injury: avulsion of the nerve root from the spinal cord, disruption of the nerve within the nerve sheath, or disruption of the nerve and the nerve sheath. Because irreversible loss of the neuromotor end plate may occur, surgery is often undertaken before 12 months of age.[262,265,266,268–270] Microsurgical intervention is performed in infants with global lesions and Horner syndrome by 3 months of age. The aim is to improve function with no expectation of complete recovery; without intervention these children have severe functional deficits. Conversely, if recovery of the biceps occurs by 3 months, treatment is performed without microsurgical intervention.[271] The treatment of choice includes resection of neuromas with interpositional nerve grafting.[272] Nerve grafting is being increasingly performed for treating neonatal brachial plexus injury. Donor nerves include motor branches of C4, intercostal nerves, inferior branches of cranial nerve XI, pectoral nerves, and sural nerves.[273] Synthetic collagen nerve conduits have been approved as nerve guidance channels in microsurgery and may be an option for the future.[274]

A preoperative MRI to assess bone and joint deformities may require administration of general anesthesia. Repair of the brachial plexus may be challenging because the only extremity for IV access and monitoring (blood pressure and pulse oximetry) is the contralateral upper extremity. Both lower extremities are usually prepped and draped for harvesting the sural nerves or other donor nerves for the repair. This surgery often takes up to 12 hours, so the considerations for prolonged anesthesia must be invoked, such as protecting pressure points during positioning. Neuromuscular blocking drugs are avoided to facilitate intraoperative electrophysiologic testing.[275] An indwelling urinary catheter decompresses the bladder. Analgesic requirement is minimal except during brief periods of surgical stimulation. Remifentanil provides excellent intraoperative analgesia and permits rapid adjustment of the depth of anesthesia. Maintenance of normothermia and prevention of fluid overload are important during this prolonged surgery. Blood loss is minimal, and maintenance fluids usually suffice.[262] Propofol infusion is an option, but is often not used because of unsubstantiated and theoretical fears of propofol infusion syndrome or delayed emergence from prolonged propofol anesthesia. In its stead, remifentanil combined with inhalation agent or dexmedetomidine has been used. Postoperative analgesia requirements are minimal, and acetaminophen and NSAIDs usually provide adequate pain relief. Shoulder spica casts may be applied to avoid sudden neck movements postoperatively if the lower branches of the accessory nerve are used for reconstruction.[275]

Otoplasty

Protruding ears (commonly known as "bat ears") are common in the Caucasian population, occurring with an incidence of up to 5% (E-Fig. 33.12).[276] Children with protruding ears are generally healthy, with about two-thirds undergoing surgical correction before the age of 8 years or as soon as the child expresses concern about the deformity.[277] Younger children are more likely to require general anesthesia, whereas those older than age 8 years may tolerate the procedure using local anesthetic infiltration or nerve blocks.[278] Laser techniques are now used increasingly to perform cartilage reshaping.[279] The main complication of general anesthesia is postoperative nausea and vomiting, which can last up to 2 days after surgery in approximately 80% of children.[280] However, postoperative nausea and vomiting may be reduced by surgical and anesthetic techniques, including multimodal techniques with combined pharmacotherapy (ondansetron and dexamethasone), anesthetic maintenance with a propofol infusion, and avoiding packing the external auditory meatus and concha.[280,281] To provide optimal surgical access and positioning of the child, a preformed, low-profile tracheal tube may be required, but flexible laryngeal mask airways provide equally satisfactory conditions in the ventilated or spontaneously breathing child.[282] Infiltration with local anesthetic attenuates the surgical stimulus and reduces intraoperative opioid requirements. The use of a long-acting local anesthetic combined with acetaminophen and NSAIDs provides adequate postoperative analgesia in most children. This multimodal approach may obviate the need for opioids and reduce the incidence of postoperative nausea and vomiting.[283]

Congenital Hand Anomalies

Congenital limb malformations exhibit a wide spectrum of phenotypic manifestations. Syndactyly may occur as an isolated malformation (Fig. 33.12 and E-Fig. 33.13) or part of a syndrome. The most commonly associated syndrome is Apert syndrome. In Poland syndrome, congenital unilateral absence or hypoplasia of the pectoralis major muscle occurs in association with brachydactyly or syndactyly. These patients may also have other skeletal abnormalities as well as renal and cardiac malformations.[284] Limb malformations are more frequent in males than females, and they affect both upper and lower limbs in approximately 50% of children with a deformity. Early separation of digits is favored if the ring and little fingers or index finger and thumb are involved, because the differing longitudinal growth rates will lead to greater deformities.[285] Surgery is usually performed between 6 and 18 months of age.[286,287] An association has been reported between syndactyly and prolonged QT interval, with life-threatening arrhythmias reported in one child during anesthesia.[288] Timothy syndrome is a multisystem disorder with cardiac, facial, limb, and neurodevelopmental features.[289]

Duplicated thumb can be present as an isolated anomaly and is present in approximately 1 in 3000 births. Hypoplastic thumbs are associated with systemic syndromes such as Holt-Oram syndrome; Vertebral, Anal, Cardiac, Tracheal, Esophageal, Renal, Limb (VACTERL) anomalies; Fanconi anemia; Nager syndrome; and thrombocytopenia-absent radius.[290] A complete evaluation of the child is generally warranted because abnormalities can occur in the cardiovascular, neurologic, and hematopoietic systems.[290] Genetic testing is not generally needed in isolated thumb duplications.

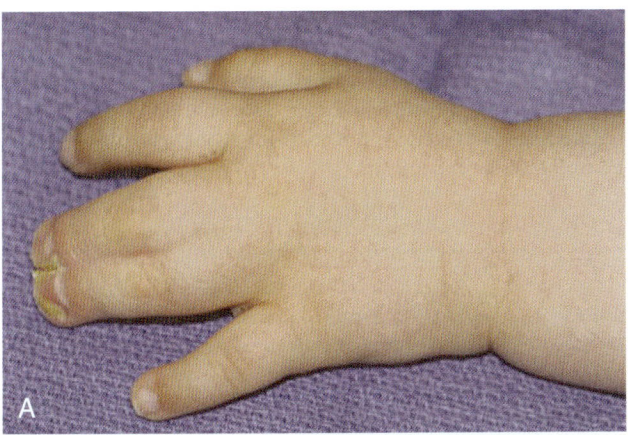
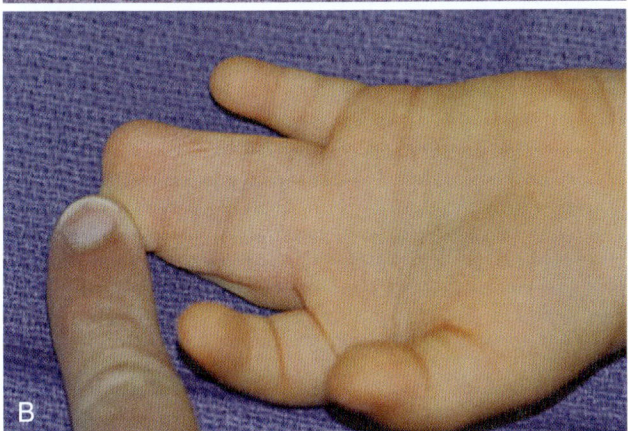

FIGURE 33.12 Syndactyly of the first and second digit of an infant: dorsal aspect **(A)** and volar aspect **(B)**.

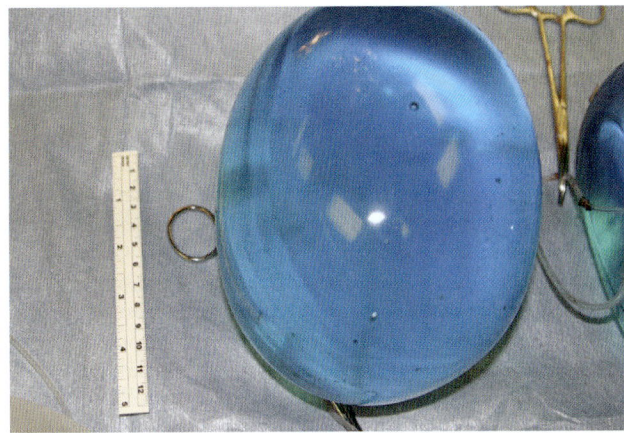

FIGURE 33.13 Tissue expander that is approximately 18 cm long. These expanders are inserted in a partially deflated state and then expanded by sequentially injecting saline solution over a period of weeks.

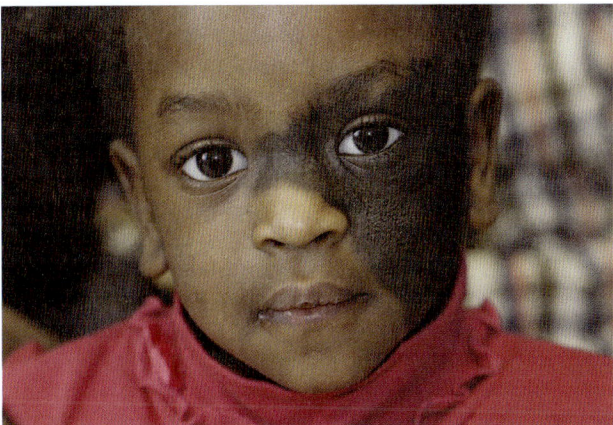

FIGURE 33.14 A heavily pigmented nevus covers the lateral aspect of the face from the eyebrow, over the bridge of the nose, and down to the skin covering the mandible. These large and disfiguring pigmented nevi must be resected in staged events.

Tissue Expanders

Tissue expansion has become a major treatment modality in the management of giant congenital hairy pigmented nevi (E-Fig. 33.14), hemangiomas, meningomyelocele, abdominal wall defects, and secondary reconstruction of extensive burn scars.[291–299] Tissue expanders effectively allow removal of the affected area and preserve sensation in a durable flap with minimal donor site morbidity.[300] These devices consist of a silicone shell that stretches to accommodate serial injections of saline solution when placed subcutaneously or, in the case of the scalp, under the galea, through an incision made in normal tissue adjacent to the lesion or defect (Fig. 33.13).[295,301] Osmotic tissue expanders have been used in burn scars, congenital nevi, alopecia, or foot deformities with reduced infection rates and low cost. Tissue expansion requires at least two surgical procedures: one to insert the expander and a second to remove it when expansion is complete; some children may require serial insertions or multiple expanders.[295] Reconstruction of areas of the head and neck constitute a particular challenge because expansion without oral, visual, or airway compromise is required.[302] Complications of tissue expansion include infection, skin erosion, leakage, migration, and flap necrosis.[298,303–306] Perioperative antibiotics are given at insertion and removal, although their effectiveness in preventing infection has not been established.[293,298,300,304,305]

Hairy Pigmented Nevi

Congenital melanocytic nevi characteristically vary in size, shape, surface texture, and hairiness. They are frequently excised because they are disfiguring and have the potential to become malignant. Serial surgical excision is common, but skin grafting and tissue expanders are also used (see E-Fig. 33.14).[300] The position and size determine the frequency of excision and anesthetic technique. If the face, head, or neck is involved, airway management should be discussed between the anesthesiologist and surgeon to ensure a secure airway while maximizing surgical access (Fig. 33.14).

In general, these children are healthy. In the cooperative and motivated child, subcutaneous infusion of a very dilute long-acting local anesthetic mixed with epinephrine can be used to provide painless tumescent anesthesia.[307] The local anesthetic is infused through a 30-gauge needle at an initial rate of 120 mL/hour. Blanching of skin identifies the area that is anesthetized. This method has been used successfully in children 6 years of age and older.[308] To avoid toxicity, local anesthetic volume and dosing guidelines should be followed (see Chapter 40). Repeated reconstructive procedures are often required, and attention should be paid to providing appropriate premedication where necessary (see Chapter 2).

Cosmetic Procedures

According to the American Society of Plastic Surgeons, the most common cosmetic surgery performed in adolescents is nose reshaping, male breast reduction, ear surgery, laser hair removal, laser treatment of leg veins, and laser skin resurfacing.[309] Breast implants and liposuction are the most controversial cosmetic procedures performed, although combined they represent only ~5% of cosmetic surgery in this age group. In 2011, 73% of male breast reduction and 28% of otoplasty occurred in this age group.[309] The breast augmentation procedures were performed on an outpatient basis.[310] These patients are generally healthy. Routine anesthetic induction with endotracheal intubation with no additional invasive monitoring is generally all that is required. This group of patients may be at increased risk of postoperative nausea and vomiting and will benefit from multimodal prophylaxis. Postoperative discomfort is common, requiring administration of systemic opioids or nerve blocks.

Liposuction is usually scheduled as outpatient surgery, although extensive liposuction may require an overnight admission to the hospital. This latter procedure is associated with acute complications, including itching, bruising, and swelling; damage to nerves or vital organs; blood loss; and embolization of fat or blood. Lidocaine toxicity and fluid accumulation at the surgical site are directly proportional to the volume of aspirated fat and number of treated sites.[311] Based on a study in healthy adult volunteers, the maximum safe dose of lidocaine is 28 mg/kg without liposuction and 45 mg/kg with liposuction; the difference is likely attributable to the delayed absorption during liposuction.[312] However, surgeons are increasingly using bupivacaine without adequate clinical study to determine the appropriate dose, the maximum dose, and safety recommendations.[313]

Trauma

Plastic surgical procedures in children are commonly performed for trauma and emergency surgery. Procedures include treatment of simple lacerations, animal bites, tendon, nerve, and vascular repair, reimplantation of digits and limbs, and treatment of burns (see Chapter 34). The cooperative and fasted child with minor trauma can often undergo minor surgical procedures using local anesthesia, commonly administered by the plastic surgeon in the emergency department. This can be supplemented with inhalation of a 50:50 mixture of nitrous oxide and oxygen (Entonox),[314] IV administration of small doses of a benzodiazepine and opioid (e.g., midazolam 50 μg/kg, and fentanyl 0.5 μg/kg) or ketamine according to locally established sedation protocols (see Chapter 44). Alternatively, a single-injection digital nerve block is safe and effective for minor surgical procedures.[315]

Surgery for extensive injuries to digits and limbs usually requires general anesthesia because children do not tolerate prolonged application of a tourniquet. The severity and urgency of the injury dictate the timing of the surgery. The general principles of care for the child with trauma should be followed (see Chapter 37), with particular attention directed to identifying more life-threatening injuries. For urgent surgery in the presence of a full stomach, precautions against aspiration of gastric contents should be considered. For postoperative pain control, a combination of regional anesthesia or systemic analgesia is usually adequate. Continuous brachial plexus or other nerve blocks may improve tissue perfusion[316] and facilitate cooperation during postoperative physiotherapy for procedures such as digital reimplantation. Continuous nerve block may attenuate the signs associated with compartment syndrome, and frequent and meticulous attention must be paid to perfusion of the extremity.

ANNOTATED REFERENCES

Antony AK, Sloan GM. Airway obstruction following palatoplasty: analysis of 247 consecutive operations. *Cleft Palate Craniofac J.* 2002; 39(2):145-148.

Two hundred forty-seven children underwent palatoplasty, yielding a 6% incidence of perioperative airway obstruction. The airway obstruction occurred as late as 48 hours postoperatively. Of the 14 children with severe airway compromise, 12 required continued tracheal intubation, reintubation, and tracheostomy. Of these 14 children (93%), 13 had coexisting craniofacial abnormalities, with 7 having Pierre Robin sequence.

Chiono J, Raux O, Bringuier, et al. Bilateral suprazygomatic maxillary nerve block for cleft palate repair in children: a prospective, randomized, double-blind study versus placebo. *Anesthesiology.* 2014;120(6): 1362-1369.

This randomized trial of bilateral suprazygomatic maxillary nerve blocks found less morphine use during the first 48 hours and fewer patients who required a continuous morphine infusion in the treatment group.

Faberowski LW, Black S, Mickle JP. Incidence of venous air embolism during craniectomy for craniosynostosis repair. *Anesthesiology.* 2000; 92(1):20-23.

This case series of 23 children undergoing craniosynostosis reported an 83% incidence of venous air embolism using precordial Doppler monitoring. Although cardiovascular collapse did not occur, 32% developed hypotension. Detection and early intervention are important strategies to prevent cardiovascular collapse associated with this type of surgery.

Gallant SC, Chewning RH, Orbach DB, et al. Contemporary management of vascular anomalies of the head and neck-part 1: vascular malformations: a review. *JAMA Otolaryngol Head Neck Surg.* 2021; 147(2):197-206.

This review details the etiology and treatment of lymphatic malformations, venous malformations, and arteriovenous malformations. Recommendations regarding preoperative assessment and postoperative airway management of patients with lymphatic malformations are provided.

Garcia-Marcinkiewicz AG, Stricker PA. Craniofacial surgery and specific airway problems. *Paediatr Anaesth.* 2020;30(3):296-303.

This review describes airway anomalies associated with types of syndromic craniosynostosis. The authors provide a detailed description of the approach for intubation in an awake sedated patient.

Goobie SM, Haas T. Bleeding management for pediatric craniotomies and craniofacial surgery. *Paediatr Anaesth.* 2014;24(7):678-689.

This review summarizes patient blood conservation techniques and their application in pediatric craniofacial surgery and in children undergoing craniotomies. The management of massive blood loss and North American and European guidelines for transfusion management are discussed.

Goobie SM, Staffa SJ, Meara JG, et al. High-dose versus low-dose tranexamic acid for paediatric craniosynostosis surgery: a double-blind randomised controlled non-inferiority trial. *Br J Anaesth.* 2020; 125(3):336-345.

This trial randomized patients undergoing open cranial remodeling for craniosynostosis to receive a low (10mg/kg bolus followed by infusion at 5mg/kg per hour) versus high dose (50mg/kg bolus followed by 5mg/kg per hour) of tranexamic acid. Low-dose tranexamic acid was noninferior for the primary outcome of intraoperative blood loss. Transfusion volumes of red blood cell and coagulation products were not statistically different between the two groups.

Jackson O, Basta M, Sonnad S, et al. Perioperative risk factors for adverse airway events in patients undergoing cleft palate repair. *Cleft Palate Craniofac J.* 2013;50(3):330-336.

33

Three hundred children younger than 2 years of age undergoing primary cleft palate repair using the modified Furlow technique were reviewed for the occurrence of perioperative adverse airway events. Adverse airway events occurred in 23% of patients overall. Airway complications were more likely in children with a craniofacial syndrome, preoperative airway problems, and with less experienced providers.

Léauté-Labrèze C, Harper JI, Hoeger PH. Infantile haemangioma. *Lancet*. 2017;390(10089):85-94.

This review article details the natural history, syndromic associations, and treatment options for pediatric hemangiomas.

Nargozian C. The airway in patients with craniofacial abnormalities. *Paediatr Anaesth*. 2004;14(12):53-59.

This review summarizes the salient features and airway implications of the major craniofacial disorders that affect children, including Pierre Robin sequence, Treacher Collins syndrome, Goldenhar syndrome, and Klippel-Feil syndrome. The anatomic pathology is very well described, and the clinical implications of the pathologic condition are thoroughly discussed.

Thompson DR, Zurakowski D, Haberkern CM, et al. Endoscopic versus open repair for craniosynostosis in infants using propensity score matching to compare outcomes: a multicenter study from the Pediatric Craniofacial Collaborative Group. *Anesth Analg*. 2018;126(3): 968-975.

This prospective observational multicenter data registry study assessed differences in blood and ICU use, length of hospitalization and perioperative complications in endoscopic strip craniectomy versus open repair in infants with craniosynostosis with propensity score matching of patients. There were 311 patients who underwent endoscopic repair and 1071 patients had open reconstruction surgery. Fewer patients who underwent endoscopic strip craniectomy received red blood cell and coagulation product transfusions. Complications such as hypotension requiring vasopressors, hypothermia, and suspected venous air embolism were not significantly different between the two groups.

A complete reference list can be found online at Elsevier eBooks+.

34 Burn Injuries

JOHN H. NICHOLS, CHARLES J. COTÉ, AND J.A. JEEVENDRA MARTYN

Pathophysiology
Cardiac
Pulmonary
Renal
Hepatic
Central Nervous System
Hematologic
Gastrointestinal
Endocrine
Skin
Metabolic
Calcium Homeostasis
Neuropsychiatric
Pharmacology

Resuscitation and Initial Evaluation
Airway and Oxygenation
Carbon Monoxide and Cyanide Poisoning
Volume Resuscitation
Associated Injury
Circumferential Burns
Electrical Burns
Abdominal Compartment Syndrome
Guidelines to Anesthetic Management
Special Considerations
Ultrasound-Guided Vascular Access, Regional
Analgesia, and Cardiovascular Assessment
Pain Management and Postoperative Care

MILLIONS OF PEOPLE ARE TREATED FOR BURNS every year throughout the world with a mortality that is associated with the severity of burn and considerable long-term morbidity in the recovered burned patients.[1–4] The Global Burn Registry, still in development, compared burns from low-income and low-resource countries with those from high-income, high-resource countries, and found a similar age distribution, but burns were more severe and there was an approximate 4-fold greater mortality in low-income, low-resource countries.[5] The US National Burn Repository Report (125 burn centers, not only US hospitals) for 2014 reviewed its 10-year experience (2003–2013) finding 175,099 burns reported,[6] of which 19% or 35,198 were children less than 5 years of age. Approximately 72% of adults and children were burned in their homes. The racial distribution for all burns, adults and children, was ~59% White, ~20% Black, 14% Hispanic, 2.4% Asian, and ~4% other. Most pediatric injuries in children less than 5 years of age were caused by scalds or contact with hot objects with a greater predominance in non-White (60%) vs White children (40%). Isolated inhalation injury accounted for only 1.4% of cases. Child abuse was suspected as the cause in 1718 cases.[7] The United States National Burn Repository Report for 2014 also reported that the overall mortality was reduced ~1% in both males and females compared with the previous epoch. Mortality varied from 0.6% in those with less than 10% body surface area (BSA) burns to ~86% for those with greater than 90% body surface area burns. Concomitant inhalation injury increased mortality.[8]

In the United states, approximately 486,000 burn injuries (adult and pediatric) are treated in the emergency department each year; ~300/day are pediatric[9] with the majority less than 6 years of age suffering from scald burns.[6,9,10] Firepit-related burns in 10,951 children younger than 19 years of age were reported from 2006 to 2017, with the majority occurring in children less than 5 years of age having fallen into or onto a firepit.[11] Children with burn injuries are well managed only when their care providers thoroughly understand the pathophysiologic and pharmacologic abnormalities associated with burn injury.[12,13] These abnormalities include metabolic derangements, neurohumoral responses, massive fluid shifts, sepsis, and the systemic effects of massive tissue destruction. An often overlooked yet overarching issue that must also be considered by the team managing the care of the child is the psychological impact of the child's mental well-being and the family members' guilt for the injury and failure to protect their child when a burn occurs. In this chapter we address the pathophysiology, the initial evaluation and resuscitation, and the anesthetic and pain management of children with burn injuries.

The mortality rate from burn injuries has declined steadily over the past decades, owing to the advent of dedicated burn centers,[14,15] improved surgical techniques, intensive care management and safer anesthetic management. The publication of expert guidelines for adults and children will likely further improve outcomes.[16] Safety prevention efforts such as smoke detectors have not reduced pediatric flame injuries because many flame injuries are related to children playing with matches or candles.[17–19]

Pathophysiology

Thermal injury to the skin disrupts the vital barrier responsible for temperature regulation, bacterial defenses, and fluid and electrolyte balance.[20] Even minor, localized burn injuries may be associated with diffuse and dramatic systemic responses that can have an impact on all systems of the body.[12] Mediators released from the burned areas (complement, arachidonic acid metabolites, cytokines, oxygen radicals, and damage-associated molecular patterns [DAMPs])[21–24] activate local and systemic inflammatory

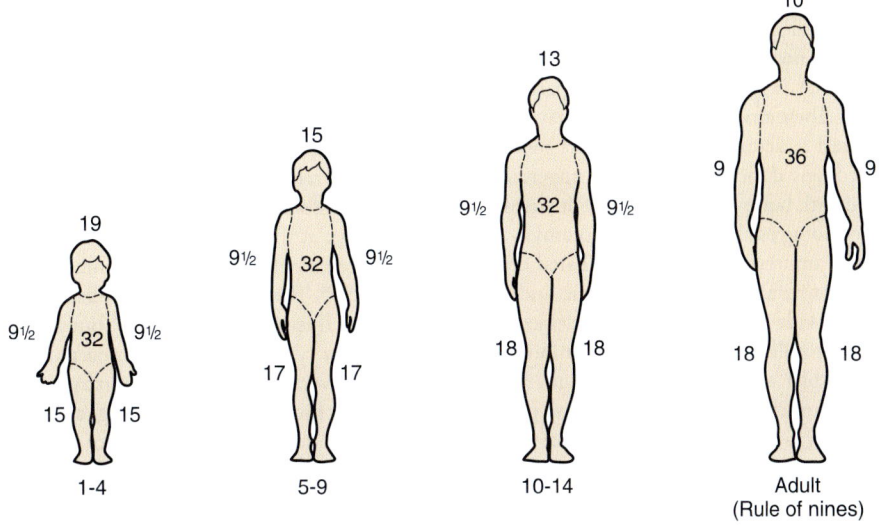

FIGURE 34.1 The different proportions of body surface area are illustrated for the calculation of percentage of burn according to a patient's age. Note the large proportion of body surface area that the head and face account for in an infant. (From Carvajal HF, Goldman AS. Burns. In: Vaughan VC III, McKay RJ, Nelson WE, eds. *Nelson's Textbook of Pediatrics.* Philadelphia: WB Saunders; 1975:281.)

responses.[13,25] Abnormal cytokine values reflect the severity of injury, and these abnormalities may persist for years after injury.[26–30] Endotoxins, which are frequently detected immediately after the burn, correlate with the size of the burn and can predict multiorgan failure and mortality.[31] The clinical symptoms and pathologic changes are relatively more severe in children, and unfortunately the gravity of the injury is often underestimated because of their greater body surface area/weight ratio (Fig. 34.1).[32,33]

Within the first few hours after a burn, massive fluid volumes (plasma and crystalloid loss in the absence of red blood cells) shift from the vascular compartment to burned tissues and nonburned areas of the body resulting in hemoconcentration.[12,34] Despite this massive fluid redistribution, systemic blood pressure is usually maintained by vasoconstriction through an outpouring of catecholamines and antidiuretic hormone (ADH).[35] In the first 4 days after a moderate- or large- (~40% body surface area) sized burn, an amount of albumin equal to approximately twice the total body plasma content is lost through the wounds. In addition to the direct effects of the burn (thrombosis, increased capillary permeability), changes in vascular integrity occur in areas remote from the injury, resulting in widespread edema,[36] including life-threatening pulmonary edema. A review of the outcomes of 821 children noted a very high mortality rate when three or more organs failed; respiratory failure occurred primarily in the first 5 days, cardiac and renal failure in the first 3 weeks, and hepatic failure with increasing duration of hospital stay.[37]

CARDIAC

Immediately after an injury, cardiac output is dramatically reduced.[38,39] This is related to the rapid reduction in circulating blood volume, the vascular effects of catecholamines and ADH causing increased systemic vascular resistance, impaired mitochondrial capacity,[40,41] and the severe compressive effects of circumferential burns on the abdomen and chest that may impair cardiac output and venous return.[42] Despite volume replacement and adequate cardiac filling pressures, cardiac output often remains reduced because circulating myocardial depressant factors

such as interleukins, tumor necrosis factors, altered β-adrenergic receptor modulation,[43] and oxygen free radicals in victims with extensive third-degree burns directly depress the myocardium.[44–47] Transesophageal echocardiography or noninvasive continuous cardiac output monitors may guide supportive care in the early phase.[48–52] Our experience is that acutely burned children frequently require early inotropic support for multiple reasons (e.g., depressed cardiac function, ongoing hypovolemia, or resuscitation volume overload).

Children develop a hypermetabolic state 3 to 5 days after a burn injury. This state is associated with a twofold to threefold increase in cardiac output that persists for weeks to months, depending on the extent of the injury and the time needed for wound closure. Heart rate, cardiac output and cardiac index are increased until complete healing of burn wounds in patients with burns involving more than 40% body surface area.[53] Some children develop a reversible cardiomyopathy.[54] In children with severe burn injuries (59% ± 19%), cardiac dysfunction may persist into adulthood[55,56] with continued systolic and diastolic dysfunction; an ~18% incidence of myocardial fibrosis has been reported.[57] Intermittent or continuous hypertension also occurs during this hypermetabolic period, which may be related to inadequate pain control as well as mediators such as increased catecholamines, atrial natriuretic factor, renin-angiotensin, endothelin-1, vasopressin (ADH), and others.[58–62] Closure of the burn wound usually decreases metabolic demand, resulting in a concomitant reduction in cardiac output.[63,64]

Some children may benefit from treatment with propranolol,[65] which reduces cardiac work and decreases the systemic inflammatory responses but does not appear to impact mortality.[66–68] Despite the widespread use of propranolol in both adults and children to attenuate this hypermetabolic response,[69] neither randomized studies nor a consensus regarding dosing has been forthcoming.[69,70]

PULMONARY

Pulmonary function may be adversely affected from the upper airway to terminal alveoli.[71–73] The upper airway is an excellent heat exchanger; just as it warms cold air, it effectively cools hot air. The air in a closed space (e.g., house or automobile fire) may reach 538°C (1000°F) 2 feet above floor level; cooling of hot inspired air causes a severe thermal injury to laryngeal structures, particularly those above the glottis.[74,75] These airway burns cause massive edema of all laryngeal and tracheal structures above the carina rendering tracheal intubation exceedingly difficult.[71] Moreover, upper airway burns are often associated with burns and/or edema of the tissues in the front of the neck precluding establishing a tracheotomy.

The thermal insult also injures or destroys the ciliated epithelium and mucosa in the proximal bronchi. Phosgene and toxic fumes, such as nitrogen dioxide and sulfur dioxide released from burning plastic are small aerosolized molecules that combine with water in the tracheobronchial tree to form nitric and sulfuric acids, damaging the distal bronchi, alveoli, and surfactant production.[76] Upper airway injury is usually a thermal insult, whereas lower airway injury is a chemical or toxic insult. Wool and cotton combustion forms aldehydes, which in concentrations as small as 10 ppm may cause coughing and "respiratory braking" that reduce the rate and depth of breathing and cause pulmonary edema.[77,78] Combustion of synthetic materials (insulation, wall paneling), particularly in enclosed-space fires, releases hydrogen cyanide[79] leading to histotoxic hypoxia and death,[80] while mimicking carbon monoxide poisoning.[81,82]

Inhalation of carbon monoxide can further compromise both hemoglobin's oxygen-carrying capacity (altered shape) and its ability to release oxygen to tissues (left shift of the oxygen-hemoglobin dissociation curve).[83] Carbon monoxide also impairs oxygen usage at the cellular level (cellular respiration).[84] Inhalation of hydrogen cyanide is an often unrecognized cause of immediate death.[85–87] The role of hydroxocobalamin and hyperbaric oxygenation in this setting is unclear[88] but recommended by some centers when cyanide toxicity is suspected.[88–93]

The overall effect of a pulmonary inhalation injury is necrotizing bronchitis, bronchial swelling, alveolar destruction, exudation of protein, loss of surfactant, loss of the protective bronchial lining, loss of cilial function, and bronchospasm, all of which contribute to bronchopneumonia (Figs. 34.2 and 34.3).[71,94,95] Inhalation of particulate matter (smoke, soot) and lower airway edema also obstruct the airway mechanically.[71] Edema of the bronchi,

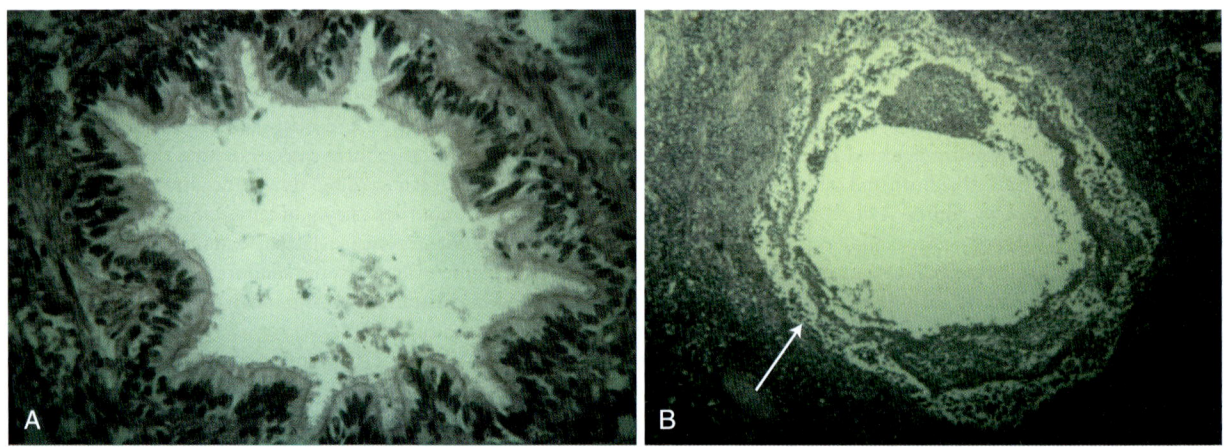

FIGURE 34.2 A, Cross section of a normal bronchiole. Note the ciliated epithelial layer. **B**, Compare with a cross section of a distal bronchiole from a child who died of an inhalation injury. Note the marked thickening of the bronchial wall, the massive inflammatory cell infiltrate, the sloughing of the mucosa *(arrow)*, and the total destruction of the ciliated columnar epithelium.

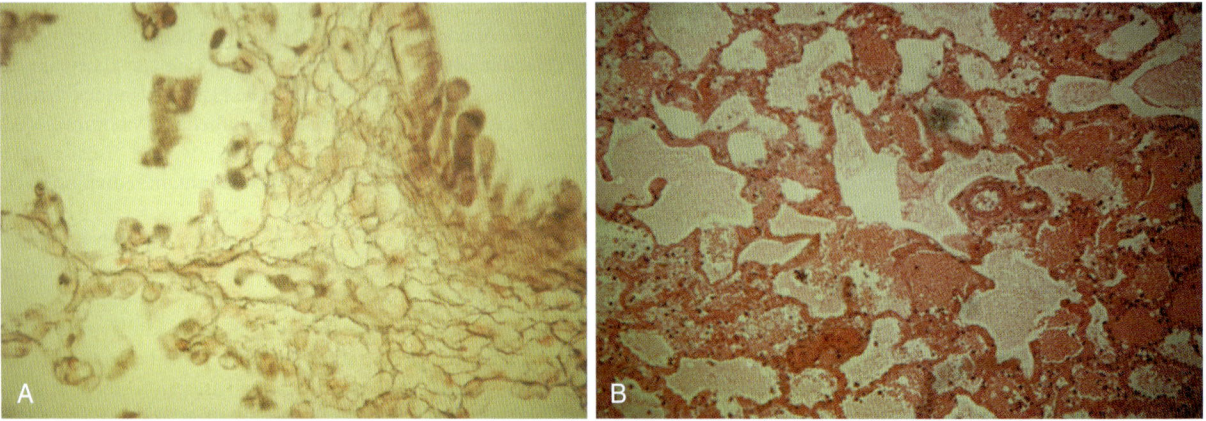

FIGURE 34.3 A, Normal alveoli. **B**, Inhalation alveolar injury is generally related to noxious fumes such as nitrogen dioxide and sulfur dioxide that are carried far down the tracheobronchial tree, combine with exhaled water, and form nitric acid and sulfuric acid, resulting in pulmonary congestion, alveolar injury, and hyaline membrane formation.

combined with loss of integrity of the pulmonary capillary endothelium, decreases pulmonary compliance. Circumferential chest burns may have a tourniquet-like effect that decreases chest wall compliance; escharotomy even in the prehospital setting may be lifesaving.[42,96] All of these injuries lead to ventilation-perfusion abnormalities and right-to-left intrapulmonary shunting, with hypoxemia and hypercarbia. In adults, the arterial partial pressure of oxygen/fraction of inspired oxygen (PaO_2/FiO_2) ratio and baseline carboxyhemoglobin concentrations are predictive of mortality.[97] The use of high-frequency oscillatory ventilation,[98] prone positioning,[99] and extracorporeal membrane oxygenation have had mixed results.[100–103] Inhaled heparin and acetylcysteine to assist clearing of mucus plugging[104] have been utilized with mixed results.[95,105–110] Severe smoke inhalation alone may occur without externally visible injuries.[85,86,111,112] One clue that smoke inhalation has occurred is the presence of singed nasal hairs or nasal passages. Steam inhalation can also cause supraglottic edema that presents with symptoms similar to epiglottitis related to edema rather than infection.[113]

Reduction in cardiac output in the presence of significant shunt can also contribute to hypoxemia.[114] Thus, correction of arterial oxygen desaturation requires evaluation of both extrapulmonary and intrapulmonary factors,[36,114] including cardiac output, mixed venous oxygen content or saturation, and shunt fraction.[38,115] Additionally, after a burn injury, obese children are at significant risk for obstructive sleep apnea.[116]

RENAL

Renal function immediately after injury may be adversely affected primarily as a result of myoglobinuria and hemoglobinuria but also from hypoxemia, hypotension, or inhaled toxins leading to acute tubular necrosis.[117] Myoglobinemia and rhabdomyolysis most commonly occurs after electrical injury,[118–120] whereas hemoglobinemia is common after severe cutaneous burns covering 40% or more of body surface area. Catecholamines, angiotensin, and vasopressin production increase, and release of vasoactive peptides such as endothelin-1 cause systemic vasoconstriction, compounding the renal dysfunction.[121–124] Fluid retention is common during the first 3 to 5 days after a burn injury and is followed thereafter by a diuresis. Glomerular filtration rate decreases soon after the injury, although 3 to 7 days after the burn injury, it actually increases *pari passu* with an increased cardiac output and metabolic rate, thus affecting the clearance of many antibiotics and other medications that are renally excreted.[125–130] Children who sustain a burn affecting 40% or more of body surface area demonstrate renal tubular dysfunction with an inability to concentrate urine.[35] Even during hyperosmolar states, antidiuresis is not observed, suggesting an inadequate renal response to antidiuretic hormone and aldosterone; an adequate urine output may be observed even in the presence of hypovolemia.[131] The estimation of the blood urea nitrogen to creatinine ratio (>20) is a reasonable indicator of the intravascular volume status.

A Cochrane review of 8200 adult patients from 33 studies reported an equal distribution of mild, moderate, and severe acute kidney injury after burns, but a greater incidence of acute kidney injury in several subgroups: the elderly, those with a greater percent burn (likely resulting in rhabdomyolysis), those with associated inhalation injury, sepsis, and assisted ventilation.[132] A meta-analysis and systematic review confirmed these observations.[133] Episodic or persistent hypertension is frequent in children after burns, in part mediated by an increase in circulating renin, ADH, and catecholamines.[134,135] Treatment of hypertension with propranolol may be indicated in some children.[66,136]

HEPATIC

Hepatic injury caused by hypoxemia, hypoperfusion caused by inhaled or absorbed chemical toxins, hypovolemia, or hypotension can occur during the early postburn phase.[137,138] Reperfusion injury may harm the liver when an adequate circulation is reestablished. Hepatic dysfunction may also result from drug toxicity, sepsis, the hypermetabolic response to burns, or blood transfusions.[30] Increased hepatic blood flow, increased protein synthesis and breakdown, and increased hepatic gluconeogenesis during the hypermetabolic phase of burn injury have been reported.[139]

Sustained increases in hepatic blood flow deliver more drug to the liver; this effect, combined with drug-induced enzyme induction, may increase the clearance of some drugs.[140] However, reports of the capacity of the liver to metabolize drugs are conflicting; this is possibly related to clearance differences in the hypodynamic (early) and hyperdynamic (late phases) of injury.[141–146] Coadministered drug interactions, alterations in protein binding, and volume of distribution changes also contribute to the conflicting reports of changes in drug half-lives.[147]

With the onset of sepsis, hepatic glucose output and alanine uptake may decrease sharply although hepatic blood flow and oxygen usage can remain increased.[137,148] Fatty infiltration of the liver secondarily associated with total enteral nutrition has also been reported.[149]

CENTRAL NERVOUS SYSTEM

The central nervous system (CNS) may be adversely affected by inhalation of neurotoxic chemicals or by hypoxic encephalopathy; other contributing factors include sepsis, hyponatremia, and hypovolemia.[150] CNS dysfunction includes hallucinations, personality changes, delirium, seizures, abnormal neurologic symptoms, and coma,[151] which may be due to the burn injury or to the drugs necessary for sedation, anxiolysis, and analgesia[152]; these effects usually clear after several weeks. Abnormalities of CNS neurotransmitters have been postulated to mediate the anorexia associated with extensive burn injury.[153]

Cerebral edema, increased intracranial pressure, and an altered blood-brain barrier may occur during the initial phases of burn injury.[154] Strategies to manage intracranial pressure should be instituted (see Chapter 24). Rapid overcorrection of hyponatremia may be associated with cerebral injury.[155] Microglia are activated even with a small burn injury with release of inflammatory cytokines causing neuroinflammation.[156]

HEMATOLOGIC

Blood viscosity may increase with hemoconcentration secondary to fluid shifts and alterations in plasma protein content in the acute phase after injury.[157] Ongoing microangiopathic hemolytic anemia is common.[158] An inhibitor of erythroid stem cells may contribute to the anemia of burns, even though the erythropoietin response to anemia is appropriate.[159] The half-life of red blood cells is diminished and multiple diagnostic blood sampling further contributes to the development of anemia.[160,161] The possible role of recombinant erythropoietin in the care of burn patients is unclear,[162–167] but evolving evidence suggests that recombinant erythropoietin may promote skin and burn wound healing.[168–172]

In the early stages, thrombocytopenia secondary to increased platelet aggregation particularly within the lungs, with a nadir at approximately 3 days after the burn, is followed by an increase in platelet count on days 10 to 14 days after the burn. The aggregation of platelets within the lungs contributes to the pulmonary insult. A prolonged period of thrombocytopenia and low nadir platelet count are both associated with sepsis and increased mortality.[173,174] In some patients, thrombocytopenia may persist for several months.[161,173] An increase in fibrin split products (disseminated intravascular coagulopathy), which lasts for 3 to 5 days, may also occur.[128] Factors V, VII, VIII, and fibrinogen are increased several-fold over baseline for the first 3 months after severe injury uncomplicated by sepsis.[175,176] Children with increased platelet counts (thrombocytosis >1 million/mm^3) who then developed sepsis in our unit experienced a marked decrease in the platelet count; the sudden onset of thrombocytopenia should prompt an evaluation for sepsis.[173,174,177] Likewise, large swings in the fibrinogen concentration can occur (up to 2 g/dL),[178] although these do not appear to herald an increase in the incidence of thrombotic events.

GASTROINTESTINAL

Gastric stasis and intestinal ileus occur immediately after thermal injury.[179] At 48 to 72 hours after a burn injury, when generalized edema is resolving, gastrointestinal function usually resumes but gastroparesis may continue with ongoing opioid administration.[180] Opioid-induced gastric stasis can be ameliorated with the peripheral opioid antagonist, methylnaltrexone.[181] Early postpyloric enteral feeding with close monitoring of gastric residuals is the norm and should be established at this time to provide calories, to blunt the hypermetabolic response, and to attenuate gluconeogenesis and stress ulceration.[157,182–185] Early enteral feeding has the added advantages of diminishing muscle catabolism, reducing bacterial translocation through the intestinal mucosa, and reduced mortality.[186–189] In children who do not tolerate enteral feeding, parenteral nutrition must be initiated.[182,185,190,191]

Stress ulcers (Curling ulcers) are associated with any burn injury and may be life-threatening. Antacid therapy may not adequately protect from increases in gastric acidity.[126,127] Frequent feedings when tolerated and the liberal use of antacids, combined with larger or more frequent doses of H$_2$-receptor antagonists (or proton pump inhibitors) may be required to prevent stress ulcers.[126,157,179,192] The current management of systemic hypoperfusion, early gut feeding, and improved pharmacologic control of gastric acidity has reduced the development of stress ulcers.[193] There is weak evidence that mechanical ventilation and coagulopathy are independent risk factors for stress ulcers.[194] Overt gastric bleeding in burned patients is now uncommon; routine guaiac fecal occult blood testing is no longer performed.

ENDOCRINE

Stimuli that trigger endocrine responses include the thermal injury itself, type of burn (scald vs. flame) and subsequent fluid shifts, as well as the stress responses associated with critical illness.[195,196] These may include reduced circulating hormone concentrations of triiodothyronine, dehydroepiandrosterone, and testosterone, as well as increased concentrations of other hormones such as antidiuretic hormone, catecholamines, renin, angiotensin II, and cortisol.[197]

Replacement therapy with synthetic androgenic steroids (e.g., oxandrolone) modulates the systemic inflammatory responses,[198] promotes wound healing,[199] reduces acute hospital stay, reduces scarring,[200] and improves body composition (lean body mass), muscle protein deposition,[201,202] and hepatic protein synthesis.[203,204] A 5-year follow-up study found that oxandrolone-treated children had increased height percentile, bone mineral content,

and improved cardiac function and muscle strength; no adverse effects from long-term administration were noted.[205]

Glucose control may be poor owing to the increased levels of cortisol and insulin resistance. This may persist for up to 36 months after the burn injury.[206–209] Tight control of hyperglycemia may improve mitochondrial oxidative capacity,[209] reduce protein turnover,[210] and decrease the incidence of urinary tract infection. The effect of tight glucose control on survival of critically ill burn patients is conflicting.[211–213] A systematic review reported increased mortality in children with loose glycemic control but recommended further study.[214] Tight glycemic control needs to be balanced against the increased risk of hypoglycemic events that, in turn, may be associated with increased mortality.[210,212,215] Avoiding hyperglycemia may attenuate the risk of cerebral injury from hypoperfusion states (see Chapters 24 and 37) and a target blood glucose concentration of 130 to 150 mg/dL has been suggested.[214] Blocking the renin-angiotensin system may improve the insulin response after burn injury.[66–68,216]

SKIN

Extensive skin destruction results in the inability to regulate body heat, conserve fluids and electrolytes, and protect against bacterial invasion and infection.[217] Because children have a much greater body surface area/weight ratio compared with adults, they are more likely to become hypothermic (see Fig. 34.1). Thus, it is important to keep children covered as much as possible to increase the environmental temperature, and to use radiant warmers, plastic wrap around extremities, reflective insulated blankets, artificial "noses" (in-line moisture and heat exchangers), and hot-air heating blankets.

Topical antibiotic and parenteral antibacterial therapy are necessary to prevent burn wound sepsis.[218–223] There is mixed evidence regarding the role of stem cell therapy to improve burn wound healing and reduce scar formation.[224–232] Late complications relate to progressive scar formation in any part of the body including the face and neck, resulting in movement-restricting contractures.[42,233]

METABOLIC

The metabolic changes after extensive burn injury are greater than after any other trauma.[234,235] Catabolism of glucose, fat, and protein (particularly muscle protein breakdown)[236,237] after burn injuries increases oxygen demand and carbon dioxide production.[2,137,157,190,219,238–244] These metabolic changes are mediated by interleukin-1, tumor necrosis factor, catecholamines, prostanoids, and other stress hormones.[2,245] Centrally mediated or sepsis-induced hyperthermia also increases oxygen consumption and carbon dioxide production. Some of these abnormalities may persist even after the burn wounds are completely covered with scar tissue.[26,28,30,64,67,246] Intravenous (IV) alimentation, particularly with increased glucose concentrations, may also increase carbon dioxide production and ventilatory requirements.[190] The increase in oxygen demand[247] and carbon dioxide production must be compensated for during controlled mechanical ventilation; treatment of fever reduces metabolic demand.[248] The exaggerated metabolism is one of the many reasons why burned patients desaturate quite rapidly.

CALCIUM HOMEOSTASIS

Ionized calcium concentrations in acutely burned patients decrease dramatically. Marked abnormalities of calcium and magnesium metabolism, including hypoparathyroidism in both acute and recovery phases, may persist for weeks after the injury (E-Fig. 34.1) and differ in children in whom the parathormone response is reduced compared with that in adults.[249–251] Increased bone resorption with failure of bone calcium uptake, resorption due to raised IL-1 and IL-6 concentrations, as well as decreased concentrations of vitamin D and a markedly reduced conversion in burned skin of dehydrocholesterol to previtamin D, reduce bone density.[252–255] Supplemental vitamin D and treatment with pamidronate, a drug that inhibits bone resorption, conserves bone mass and reduces muscle protein turnover after burn injury,[256,257] but the use of vitamin D and pamidronate is not routine in burn care.[255,256,258–262] Hypophosphatemia and hypermagnesemia revert toward normal values during the latter phase of recovery. The usual reciprocal relationship between calcium and inorganic phosphate is not evident in those with major burns. Supplemental calcium therapy is required.

Ionized hypocalcemia, evident during rapid infusions of colloid or fresh frozen plasma,[263] impairs myocardial contraction.[264] Frequent small boluses of calcium are safer and more effective than intermittent large boluses (see also Figs. 10.10 and 10.11).[265] Doses of 5 mg/kg calcium chloride or 15 mg/kg calcium gluconate ionize at equivalent rates and produce equivalent increases in ionized calcium concentrations.[265]

NEUROPSYCHIATRIC

Psychological trauma and its associated long-term sequelae are common after burn injury.[266,267] Many acutely burned children and their parents suffer acute stress or develop posttraumatic stress disorders.[266–272] Risk factors for developing these disorders include the size of the burn, the degree of pain, the pulse rate, ethnicity, and parental issues.[270,273] Long-term consequences spawned by parental guilt, self-conscious emotions regarding their child's scarring, depression, the child's adjustment to a new self-image, and other stressors are quite common.[274–278] Targeted preventive psychologic interventions reduce the duration and extent of the posttraumatic stress.[279] Treatment with antidepressants has proven useful.[280–282]

Delirium is common in children with burn injuries while in the intensive care unit. Its frequency is greater in children <2 years of age, those who are critically ill, those whose lungs are ventilated, and those with poor nutritional status.[283] Pharmacological management can be difficult because some medications have altered pharmacokinetics in burn patients that dictate formulation or dose changes.[284] The use of haloperidol or ziprasidone to treat hypoactive or hyperactive delirium in the intensive care unit did not significantly alter the duration of delirium.[285]

Pharmacology

Burn injuries induce many physiologic changes that affect drug pharmacokinetics and pharmacodynamics.[286] The pharmacologic perturbations that occur after a moderate or severe burn injury are unique to the two phases of metabolic regulation that occur after a burn: the early or "ebb" phase and the late or "flow" phase. During the ebb phase, large volumes of fluid shift from the vascular and extracellular compartments into the burned tissues, resulting in hypovolemia, decreased cardiac output state, and decreased metabolic rate.[287] This period usually lasts up to 48 hours. During the subsequent 5 days, the late or hypermetabolic phase emerges with a steadily increasing metabolic rate that is characterized by a hyperdynamic circulation and insulin resistance, with increased stress mediators and impaired glucose metabolism. This phase

lasts for 12 or more months, although it does not resolve when the wounds are completely healed. The hypermetabolic phase may persist for up to 3 years after the burn.

During the early hypovolemic phase, the uptake of drugs is usually reduced because gastrointestinal function and/or muscular and cutaneous perfusion are reduced.[2,141–143,288,289] Drugs administered via the oral, subcutaneous, and intramuscular routes may be poorly absorbed. During the hypermetabolic phase, the activity of organs that clear drugs from the circulation (e.g., the liver and kidneys) may be enhanced because of enzyme induction, increased blood flow, and an increased metabolic rate.[125,126,129,137,146,288–297] An adequate target plasma concentration of antibiotics, for example, may not be achieved.[297–300] Edema can increase the volume of distribution, loss of drugs through burn wounds might increase apparent clearance, and other drugs compete for elimination pathways.[301] As a general rule, children with burn injuries require larger than normal doses of almost all IV medications, including antibiotics.[2,108,125–127,140,144–146,198,289,293,294,296,298,299,301–312]

Children with burns typically clear drugs more readily than children without burns.[142–144,301–303,312] The enhanced elimination kinetics contribute to increased dose requirements for neuromuscular blocking drugs, opioids, and benzodiazepines.[145,146] Curiously, the clearance of oral ketamine is unaffected in children with small burns, although gastric absorption of the oral formulation is delayed.[313]

Pharmacodynamic changes related to cellular responses induced by the injury also contribute to a greater dose requirement.[314–317] A burn injury may affect the number or sensitivity of receptors in tissues.[140,145,153,288,294,318–324] The cardiovascular responses to catecholamines may be attenuated because of a reduced affinity of β-adrenergic receptors for ligands and diminished second messenger responses,[324] resulting in larger drug doses than usual to achieve the desired clinical response. Thermal injuries greater than 30% body surface area cause an upregulation of acetylcholine receptors and consequent resistance to neuromuscular blocking drugs.[140,319,320,322–326] Other aberrant responses include altered sensitivity to succinylcholine at the neuromuscular junction, increased sensitivity to dopamine in the pulmonary circulation, and decreased sensitivity to nondepolarizing neuromuscular blocking drugs.[140,289,318,320,321,325,327,328] The pharmacodynamics responses to dexmedetomidine (see later discussion) may also be altered in the burned child because of α_{2a}-adrenoceptor-induced hypotension. Attention must be paid to ensure euvolemia before administering the dose to preclude hypotensive and bradycardic responses.[329]

Many drugs are highly bound by plasma proteins, rendering only a small unbound fraction that determines the drug activity. The two major binding proteins, α_1-acid glycoprotein and albumin, increase and decrease, respectively, after a burn injury. These changes may exert substantive effects on the free fractions of the drugs depending on the initial fraction of protein binding.[289,294,330]

Due to the decreased albumin concentrations the free unbound fraction of diazepam was higher; the clearance, however, was decreased in burned patients, probably due to enzyme inhibition possibly by the co-administered cimetidine.[145] An increased tolerance to diazepam despite a greater fraction of the pharmacologically active compounds combined with a decreased clearance suggests resistance at tissue receptors similar to that observed for neuromuscular blocking drugs at the neuromuscular junction.[145] A similar tolerance has been observed with opioids due to drug and injury-induced changes in neuronal and nonneuronal microglia cells.[156,314] The persistence of such pharmacodynamic changes for both neuromuscular blocking and anesthetic drugs long after they have recovered from the burn render the clinical response to medications somewhat unpredictable and point to the need to titrate drugs to the patient's respon ses.[289,304,331,332] Therefore, clinical effects should always be closely monitored and plasma concentrations, protein binding, and clearance evaluated where possible.[126,129,289,304–307,333]

Resuscitation and Initial Evaluation

Resuscitation of children with a burn injury requires a clear and secure airway, as well as maintenance of adequate oxygenation, perfusion, and circulating blood volume; evaluation for associated injuries is essential.

AIRWAY AND OXYGENATION

Every burn patient, especially those with inhalation injuries, must be considered hypoxemic and exposed to carbon monoxide. During transport to the hospital and on admission, administration of high inspired concentrations of oxygen is mandatory, pending evaluation of the severity of carbon monoxide poisoning and pulmonary injury (see later discussion).[333] Direct injury to the airway and alveoli occurs in children with inhalation of smoke, flames, superheated air, noxious gases, or steam.[77,111,115,233,245,334–361] When a child is burned in an enclosed space (house, automobile) or if thermal burns or carbonaceous materials are evident in the vicinity of the mouth and nares, an inhalational injury is quite likely.[344,362] Upper airway obstruction caused by edema of the lips, nose, tongue, pharynx, glottis, and subglottis is very common.[75] The resultant airway obstruction can be compared with the combined effects of acute macroglossia, epiglottitis, macro uvula, and laryngotracheobronchitis. Deterioration of the airway after a burn

injury occurs very rapidly because the columnar epithelium of the upper airway swells precipitously in the first hours after the injury. A delay in instrumenting the airway early on may render the airway impossible to intubate even a few hours later. (Fig. 34.4).[95]

This airway edema may persist for several days. Prophylactic intubation should be performed in all cases in which severe facial burns or pulmonary burn and upper airway inhalation injury are suspected. Mortality is related to the presence or absence of inhalation injury.[111,115,351–361,363]

General anesthesia may be required to secure the airway in children. Early tracheostomy (usually after 10 days) minimizes laryngotracheal damage from prolonged tracheal tube intubation,[364,365] which contrasts with an old report[366] that found that tracheostomy in thermally injured children was associated with substantial mortality rates. Early tracheostomy may also reduce the risk of subglottic stenosis[367,368]; the duration of tracheostomy is related to body surface area burn and not age.[369] Tracheostomy for children expected to require long-term ventilation is increasingly common.[370,371] Although there is no consensus from the American Burn Association, the current trend based on views of otolaryngologists and pediatric surgeons at Shriners Hospital for Children, Boston, is that tracheostomy is performed within 10 to 14 days, provided there is no contraindication (e.g., excessive bleeding) at that time.[75] When early airway instrumentation is indicated, a cuffed tracheal tube is preferred to ensure that increased peak inspiratory pressures can be delivered should lung compliance decrease (from the burn), thus avoiding the need to change the tracheal tube.[372] We routinely use cuffed tracheal tubes, appreciating the added flexibility they offer as airway edema recedes, and it is common to allow permissive hypercarbia to

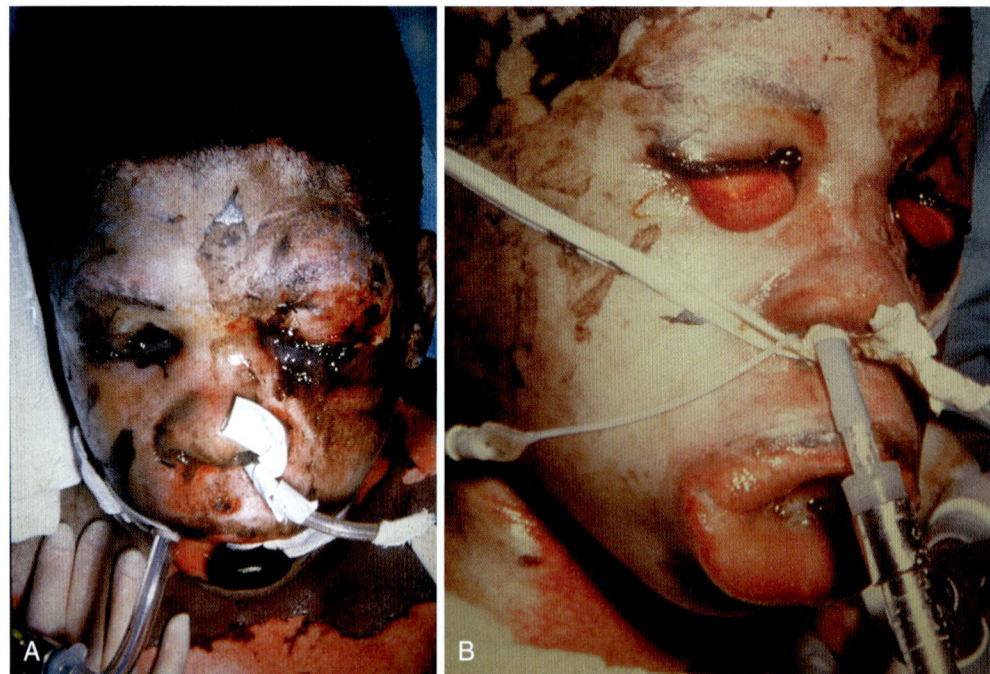

FIGURE 34.4 A, A young child who had just sustained a facial burn in a closed space. Note the early onset of facial edema. **B**, Several hours later there is massive edema that extends into the oropharynx, larynx, and trachea (similar to the combined effects of macroglossia, epiglottitis, and laryngotracheobronchitis). Early prophylactic intubation is mandatory in any facial burn or in any child when there is potential for inhalation injury. Note that the cuffed endotracheal tube was changed from an oral to a nasal position and that it is secured with cloth tape rather than adhesive tape.

34

reduce barotrauma.[373] Tracheal tubes with a more distally placed cuff and a cuff composed of thinner material may reduce the potential for airway injury (see also Figs. 12.18 and 12.20), but in the hot environment of a burn unit, they have a greater tendency toward kinking.[374–380]

CARBON MONOXIDE AND CYANIDE POISONING

Most smoke inhalation victims have carbon monoxide poisoning[71,94,112]; direct measurement of carboxyhemoglobin is important to guide treatment. Estimates of carboxyhemoglobin concentrations are best determined by measuring (not calculating) oxygen saturation or arterial oxygen content. The half-life of carboxyhemoglobin is approximately 5 hours when the patient is breathing room air but decreases to less than 90 minutes when 100% oxygen is administered.[381–384] One hundred percent oxygen should be administered to the child immediately upon arrival of first responders and continued in the hospital to achieve the maximum possible PaO_2. Positive-pressure ventilation[385–387] and hyperbaric oxygen remain possible options in some centers.

Standard pulse oximeters cannot accurately monitor the arterial saturation of oxygen (SaO_2) in patients with carbon monoxide poisoning because carboxyhemoglobin overestimates the true oxygen saturation; the photodetector interprets both carboxyhemoglobin and oxyhemoglobin as oxyhemoglobin.[388–391] An eight-wavelength pulse oximeter is capable of distinguishing carboxyhemoglobin and methemoglobin from oxyhemoglobin.[392–398] The SaO_2 in neonates and young infants also falsely overestimates the oxyhemoglobin saturation in the presence of carboxyhemoglobin because of the effect of fetal hemoglobin.[398,399]

Carboxyhemoglobin is produced by the combination of carbon monoxide with the iron of the heme radical at the oxygen-binding site. Carbon monoxide combines more slowly with hemoglobin than oxygen but is bound 200 times more firmly.[83,400] Inhalation of 1% carbon monoxide for just 2 minutes yields a carboxyhemoglobin concentration of 30% (E-Fig. 34.2).[401] The toxic effects of carbon monoxide poisoning are due to tissue, organ, and cellular hypoxia from decreased oxygen delivery because carbon monoxide reduces oxygen-binding capacity to the hemoglobin molecule at the tissue level and to cytochromes in the respiratory chain at the cellular level. Carboxyhemoglobin shifts the oxygen dissociation curve to the left (E-Fig. 34.3), reducing release of oxygen from hemoglobin.[77,83,333,385,401–404] For example, if an individual had 40% carboxyhemoglobin, this would reduce the oxygen-carrying capacity from 20 mL/100 grams of hemoglobin to 12 mL/100 grams with the leftward shift, further compromising oxygen delivery.

Evidence supporting the use of hyperbaric oxygen therapy as an adjunct therapy for burns remains controversial.[157,405–410] A Cochrane review concluded that the current data are insufficient to demonstrate that hyperbaric oxygenation therapy reduced adverse neurologic outcomes and that additional research is needed to *"better define the role, if any, of hyperbaric oxygenation in the treatment of patients with carbon monoxide poisoning."*[411] The most common indication for hyperbaric therapy in burned children is concomitant carbon monoxide poisoning.[77,412–416] Children with carbon monoxide exposure are at risk of developing both acute and delayed neurologic sequelae. The pathophysiology of neurologic sequelae is unknown, although imaging studies suggest a potentially reversible demyelinating process.[417,418] The important practical question is whether hyperbaric treatment will decrease the frequency and severity of delayed neurologic sequelae in children with carbon monoxide poisoning. This is a difficult question

because the incidence of delayed sequelae is unknown and determining the severity of the carbon monoxide poisoning is difficult because there is a poor correlation between serum carboxyhemoglobin and degree of carbon monoxide exposure.[419,420] Prolonged loss of consciousness, a reduced Glasgow Coma Score, increased troponin T and blood lactate concentration, and rescue by ventilation are major indicators for late neurologic sequelae.[421–423]

The severity of delayed neuropsychological sequela is not related to the carboxyhemoglobin concentration at the time of presentation.[424] Delayed sequelae include headaches, irritability, personality changes, confusion, memory loss, and gross motor deficits; a symptom-free interval of several days is commonly reported. Hyperbaric treatment may relieve symptoms, and spontaneous resolution of delayed sequelae may be expected in up to 75% of patients within one year.[425–431] Evidence in support of using hyperbaric oxygen to prevent and treat these complications is weak,[432–439] although the seriousness of sequelae encourages its use in institutions with ready access.[407,408,440,441] Some clinicians believe that a history of unconsciousness suggests a severe exposure that warrants treatment.[421,423,425,442–444] However, the few randomized prospective studies of hyperbaric oxygen to prevent sequelae have returned conflicting results.[438,439] Hyperbaric oxygen treatment is not without expense, inconvenience, and risk; the indications for treatment of burned children with concomitant carbon monoxide poisoning are unsettled.[416,445] Complications during treatment include emesis (6%), seizures (5%), agitation requiring restraints or sedation (2%), cardiac dysrhythmias or cardiac arrests (2%), arterial hypotension (2%), and tension pneumothorax (1%).[416] Complications may be expected more frequently in the critically ill.[446] Hyperbaric oxygen treatment is possibly appropriate in burned children with documented or strongly suspected serious carbon monoxide poisoning who are hemodynamically stable, not requiring ongoing burn resuscitation, and not wheezing or showing evidence of air trapping and in whom such treatment does not require interfacility transport.

Cyanide toxicity is associated with inhalational burn injuries due to hydrogen cyanide inhalation.[71,86,94,112,447] Fires that burn plastics and some furniture upholstery are the most common sources of cyanide poisoning.[82,448] If cyanide poisoning is confirmed, administration of hydroxocobalamin or sodium thiosulfate, alone or in combination, are indicated (see Chapter 10).[81,449] Hyperbaric oxygenation therapy facilitates movement of cyanide out of tissues and into blood, and should be considered for combined smoke and carbon monoxide inhalation. However, the logistics for caring for a patient with concomitant burns is logistically difficult.[88,447,450]

VOLUME RESUSCITATION

The formulas for determining fluid replacement are estimates and often need modification that depend on clinical and laboratory findings.[2,12,31,157,242,245,451–462] The most widely accepted fluid protocols in current use for fluid resuscitation in burn patients are the Parkland (Baxter) and Brooke formulas (Table 34.1). Both formulas not only estimate the fluid volume required for resuscitation, but also include normal maintenance fluid requirement for each day. *These formulas are of great value in guiding the fluid resuscitation of older children; however, serious underestimation of the fluid volume may occur if applied to infants weighing less than 10 kilograms. In such infants, it is reasonable to estimate the normal hourly maintenance fluid requirements and then add to this the fluid volume of the Parkland or Brooke formula.*[2,463] Alternatively, the crystalloid fluid regimen for resuscitation can

TABLE 34.1	Parkland and Brooke Formulas		
	FLUID THERAPY		
Formula	Crystalloid (mL/kg)	Colloid (mL/kg)	
Parkland	4.0	+0	× Percent burn × weight (kg)
Brooke	0.45	+1.5	× Percent burn × weight (kg)

NOTE: Half this volume is administered during the first 8 hours and the remainder during the next 16 hours. **Infants who weigh less than 10 kg may have even greater fluid requirements (see text).**

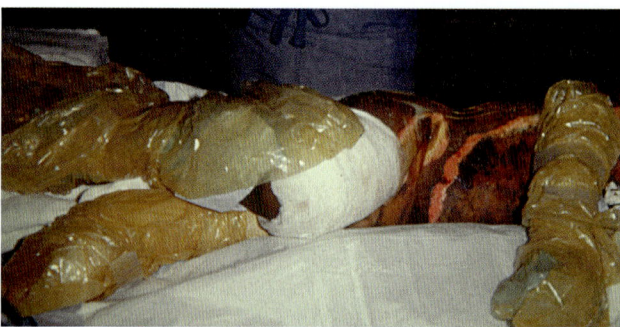

FIGURE 34.5 Children with extensive burn injury can be kept warm by having the extremities wrapped with sterile plastic bags. Covering the head is also an important method of heat preservation.

be increased to 6 mL/kg × the percent surface area burn per 24 hours.[464,465] All formulas and guidelines for fluid therapy require modification according to the individual child's response[13]; the most important metric of fluid homeostasis remains a good urine output (0.5 to 1 mL/kg per hour).

Goal-directed fluid therapy, using a noninvasive or a minimally invasive cardiac output monitor, may be beneficial for tailoring fluid administration.[466] The development of continuous noninvasive cardiac output monitors may soon be routinely used in the fluid and inotropic management of burn victims (see Chapter 49). These devices include Fick calculation using expired carbon dioxide rebreathing, esophageal Doppler, pulse contour analysis, thoracic impedance, and bioreactance (E-Fig. 34.4).[52,467–474]

The degree of edema depends on the volume and composition of the resuscitation fluid administered. Consequently, colloids or hypertonic saline solution (with or without albumin) are used in some burn centers during early burn wound resuscitation; these modified regimens are purported to be particularly effective in the very young and the elderly, resulting in less tissue edema.[2,157,245,456,457,462,464,465,475,476] A Cochrane review of 15 studies using hypertonic saline solution found that less IV fluid was needed for resuscitation and greater sodium concentrations occurred, although the overall morbidity and mortality were unchanged.[477] Further work is required before routinely advocating hypertonic fluid regimens in burned children.[478] A growing practice in burn centers has been to resuscitate children with colloid, usually 5% albumin, instead of crystalloid in the early phase after a burn injury.[479–482] Length of stay, number of graft and debridement procedures, and infection rates are less in those who were randomized to receive albumin early in the fluid resuscitation period (6–12 hours after burn) compared with those who received albumin later in the resuscitation period (24 hours after burn).[482] We begin with 5% albumin at a maintenance rate immediately upon admission. We administer an amount equal to that of their calculated crystalloid requirements, tapering the crystalloid first and continuing the albumin infusion for 48 hours.

The syndrome of hyperosmolar hyperglycemic nonketotic coma (severe dehydration, marked hyperglycemia, serum hyperosmolality, and coma in the absence of ketoacidosis) may be associated with burns and is a cause for concern as the associated mortality rate is substantial.[451] Glucose-containing solutions should be restricted, particularly during the initial volume resuscitation. Serum glucose concentrations should be measured frequently during this period; we recommend administering insulin as indicated to maintain a target blood glucose of approximately 130 to 150 mg/dL.[213]

The general appearance of the child and their sensorium provide important guides to the effectiveness of the resuscitative therapy. Urine output is a useful metric to determine the need for additional fluid administration, recognizing that antidiuretic hormone secretion may be increased, and renal tubular dysfunction may be present.[35,290] Every effort must be made to protect kidney function by providing adequate perfusion and fluid replacement.[2,478] Renal failure in the presence of a major burn is usually fatal.[37] However, overly aggressive fluid administration may induce pulmonary and tissue edema. Commonly used endpoints of satisfactory volume resuscitation include heart rate, systemic arterial blood pressure, urinary output, central venous pressure (CVP), arterial oxygenation, and pH. Noninvasive assessment of cardiac output may provide better guidance than clinical assessments alone regarding the decision to use a vasopressor or provide additional volume loading.[52]

The evaporative fluid losses in a child exceed 4000 mL/m² of burn surface each day, compared with only 2500 mL/m² in an adult.[456] Concomitantly, for each square meter of burn surface, 2500 to 4000 kcal of heat are lost each day. Minimizing caloric expenditure and providing caloric supplementation simultaneously are the only ways to minimize catabolism of body tissues. The tendency for children to be poikilothermic, particularly in the absence of protective skin as a result of the burn injury, causes profound temperature derangements. Efforts to maintain a normal body temperature are essential in both the operating room and the intensive care unit, especially during the initial volume resuscitation and in the operating room when dressings are removed (Fig. 34.5).

ASSOCIATED INJURY

Associated injuries such as a tension pneumothorax, a ruptured spleen or liver, long-bone fractures, or head injury may be missed, especially during the initial assessment and early phase of burn wound fluid resuscitation. Taking a detailed history, especially from the emergency medical personnel and family, combined with a careful physical examination, is mandatory because such injuries may compound or be hidden by the need for an increased volume of resuscitation fluids. The type of burn injury (e.g., explosion, electrical) may also trigger concerns for associated injuries (e.g., shrapnel, exit wounds, traumatic brain injury).[483]

CIRCUMFERENTIAL BURNS

Adverse cardiovascular and respiratory responses are immediate consequences to circumferential burns of the chest, abdomen, and extremities.[2,42,233,348] Circumferential burns of the thorax can restrict respiratory effort, resulting in respiratory failure from

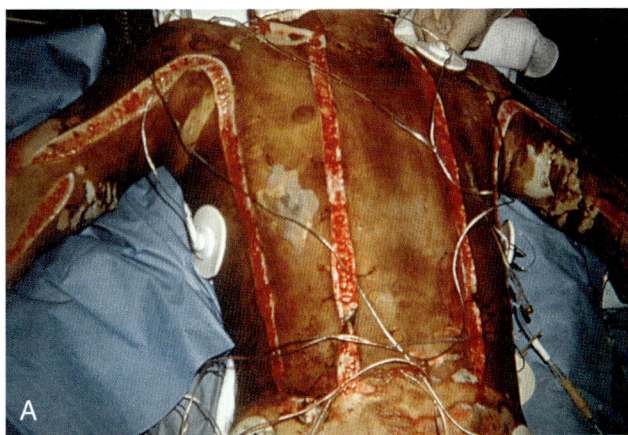

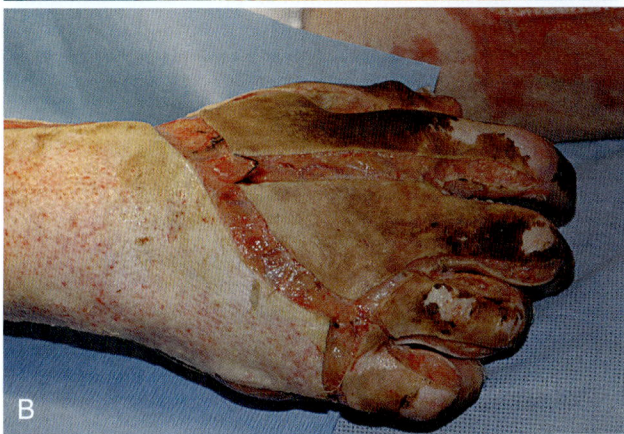

FIGURE 34.6 A, Circumferential chest burns result in severe impairment of respirations secondary to the tourniquet effect of the shrinking eschar and subcutaneous edema. The widely separated escharotomy lines indicate the severity of the constriction. **B,** Similar effects occur in circumferentially burned extremities. Early escharotomy may help to preserve blood flow and obviate amputation.

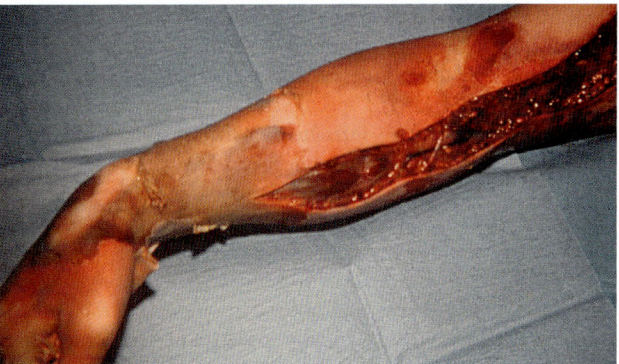

FIGURE 34.7 Electrical injuries tend to follow neurovascular structures and have an entry as well as an exit wound. The skin might appear normal, but the underlying structures may have had extensive injury. These children require a fasciotomy rather than just a simple escharotomy to preserve blood flow to the deep structures. In general, this is required on the first day of injury for best results in tissue preservation.

decreased chest wall compliance; reduced functional residual capacity with airway closure and atelectasis can lead to profound hypoxemia.[77,233,335–339,342–349,484] Deep circumferential burns of the chest and abdomen may generate excessive intrathoracic and intraabdominal pressures, which, in addition to restricting movement of the thorax and diaphragm, may further reduce the already decreased cardiac output by impairing venous return (Fig. 34.6).[42,233,348] When this occurs, both extrapulmonary and intrapulmonary factors contribute to the arterial desaturation.[114] The edema of damaged tissue generates severe compressive forces, restricting or occluding the blood flow to burned extremities. The net result may be ischemia of the limb and/or digits, which if left untreated, may lead to partial or total amputation. Escharotomies of circumferential burns of the chest, abdomen, and extremities must be performed urgently because impaired hemodynamics and respiratory mechanics can cause irreversible damage within hours of the burn injury (Fig. 34.7). Escharotomy is often undertaken without the need for general anesthesia because a full-thickness burn usually destroys skin innervation.

ELECTRICAL BURNS

Electrical burns occur with household (low-voltage, e.g., electric cords and sockets)[485] and nonhousehold high-voltage current (power line or lightning). Children often disconnect extension cords by stabilizing one end in their mouths and pulling the other end with a hand, resulting in circumoral and lingual burns.[10,118,486,487] High-voltage injuries are often associated with loss of limbs and other injuries that are not immediately obvious.[488–492] The extent of this injury is unpredictable. The surface injury is often small, but the extent of underlying tissue damage and necrosis can be massive. Such an injury is a combination of electrical and thermal damage.[491,493] Victims often have concurrent injuries such as fractures of vertebrae or long bones, ruptured organs, myocardial injury, or numerous contusions. Even children with low-voltage injuries may have abnormalities of cardiac conduction.[489] Children with electrical burns may be unconscious or have persistent seizures at the time of admission to the hospital. Muscle tissue adjacent to bone is usually more damaged than superficial muscles because bone is a poor conductor of electrical current, and therefore heats up when high currents pass through it, resulting in damage to the surrounding muscles. Early fasciotomy may be needed to preserve the blood flow to extremities (Fig. 34.7). Myonecrosis necessitates general anesthesia during the first day of injury at the time when fluid shifts, hyperkalemia, and myoglobinuria are maximal. Massive myonecrosis and hemolysis may cause hyperkalemia, as well as myoglobinuria and hemoglobinuria. In the presence of hemoglobinuria or myoglobinuria, increased fluid administration will stimulate a diuresis (>1 mL/kg per hour) that helps to preserve renal function.[494,495] Mannitol or alkalization of the urine reduces the risk that these proteins precipitate in the renal tubules, but evidence in support of this notion is weak.[496] Follow-up of patients with electrical injuries often reveals unpredictable sequelae, which may manifest months to years later. These injuries may occur in organs or areas that do not appear abnormal during the acute course of illness. These late complications most frequently include neurologic dysfunction, ocular damage, damage to the gastrointestinal tract, circumoral strictures, changes in the electrocardiogram, and delayed hemorrhage from rupture of large vessels.[493,495]

ABDOMINAL COMPARTMENT SYNDROME

Abdominal compartment syndrome may develop in children who require large-volume resuscitation, as tissue edema and free fluid (ascites) accumulate, and the abdomen reaches its maximal compliance. Abdominal compartment syndrome occurs when increased intraabdominal pressure (>20 mm Hg in adults, >10 mm Hg in infants/children) is accompanied by end-organ failure. Intraabdominal pressure should be maintained below these thresholds, but it remains unclear if a specific abdominal perfusion pressure (mean arterial pressure – intraabdominal pressure) is salutary.[497] Abdominal compartment syndrome is considered to be a "two-hit" process. The first hit occurs during the early phase of a severe burn, where an ischemia-reperfusion process occurs, followed by a systemic inflammatory response, increased mesenteric capillary permeability, and extravasation of fluid into the bowel wall. The ensuing bowel wall edema is the second hit, increasing the intraabdominal pressures, reducing fluid drainage, and decreasing bowel wall perfusion, all of which combine to cause increasing bowel injury and edema, further raising the intraabdominal pressures. This vicious cycle can be exacerbated with the administration of large fluid volumes.[498]

Abdominal compartment syndrome affects multiple organ systems outside of the gastrointestinal tract (Fig. 34.8). Increased intraabdominal pressures transmit pressure to the thoracic cavity, decreasing pulmonary compliance and lung volumes, and increasing airway pressures, the work of breathing, atelectasis, hypoxia, and hypercapnia. Increased intraabdominal pressure has detrimental effects on preload, afterload, and contractility of the heart, all of which may result in a low cardiac output state. This low cardiac output state can lead to renal hypoperfusion which will lead to further fluid retention and increase intraabdominal pressures.[497]

The incidence of abdominal compartment syndrome in burn patients with total body surface area burns more than 40% may exceed 30%. Mortality in pediatric abdominal compartment syndrome has been reported between 40% and 60%, and remains high despite abdominal decompression, illustrating the critical importance of early detection and avoidance of progression from increased intraabdominal pressures to abdominal compartment syndrome. Detection of evolving compartment syndrome is most effectively achieved by routine monitoring of bladder pressure.[484,497,499]

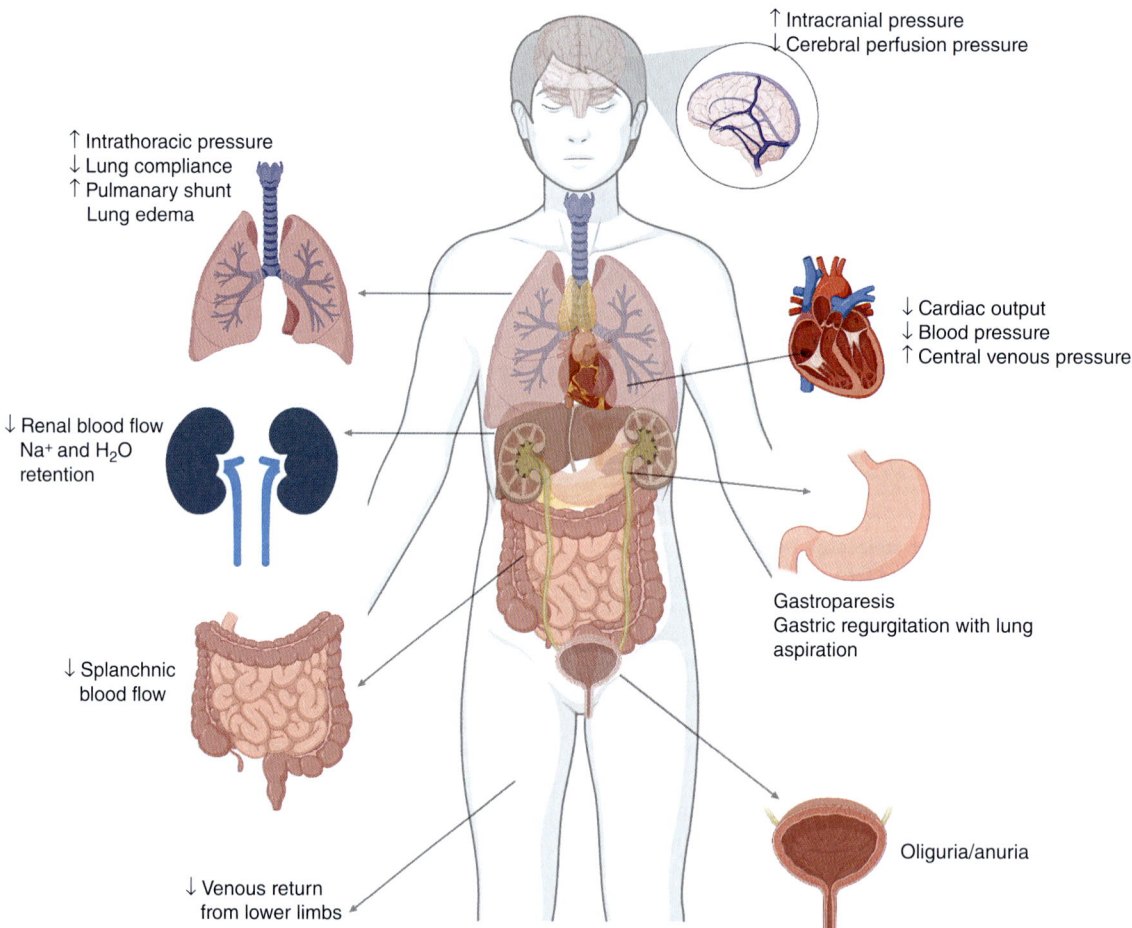

↑ Intracranial pressure
↓ Cerebral perfusion pressure

↑ Intrathoracic pressure
↓ Lung compliance
↑ Pulmanary shunt
Lung edema

↓ Cardiac output
↓ Blood pressure
↑ Central venous pressure

↓ Renal blood flow
Na⁺ and H₂O retention

Gastroparesis
Gastric regurgitation with lung aspiration

↓ Splanchnic blood flow

Oliguria/anuria

↓ Venous return from lower limbs

FIGURE 34.8 Abdominal compartment syndrome (ACS) occurs when intraabdominal pressure is increased beyond 20 mm Hg (infants) and 10 mm Hg (children). Failure to recognize and manage ACS can lead to high mortality and morbidity. It is usually seen in mechanically ventilated patients receiving over-enthusiastic fluid resuscitation after major burns or during sepsis. The cardiac sequelae include decreased cardiac output and blood pressure due to decreased venous return from splanchnic circulation and lower limbs and increased ACS-induced systemic vascular resistance. The central venous pressure artificially elevated. The pulmonary effects encompass decreased lung compliance and increased pulmonary shunt together with increased peak airway pressures. Central nervous system effects can include increased intracranial pressure and decreased cerebral perfusion pressure with encephalopathy. Renal effects consist of decreased glomerular filtration rate with oliguria or anuria. Gastroparesis and increased gastric pressure can lead to regurgitation and aspiration of gastric contents.

Guidelines to Anesthetic Management

Anesthetic management of children with severe thermal injury begins with the initial resuscitation and continues for many years through reconstructive surgery.[500] Knowledge and understanding of the pathophysiology of burn injury enable planning of appropriate anesthetic management and recognition and treatment of complications arising as a result of burn injury or its therapy (Table 34.2).[2,20,34,501]

Children who require surgery for burn wound excision and grafting require physiological and psychological preparation. Children who have not had surgical debridement and have had the burn for a week or longer should be considered septic. Such children often demonstrate severe cardiovascular instability during burn wound excision, likely because of acute bacteremia. In such cases, it is advantageous to have an inotrope infusion prepared for administration before induction of anesthesia.

Psychological support must be provided to parents, nurses, and physicians, by trained psychologists. Families of children who have sustained a severe burn injury feel a great deal of psychological stress and guilt. This stress may be manifested as anger toward the physicians, nurses, and other members of the burn care team. The parents are angry that their child has sustained a devastating injury and occasionally vent their anger and frustration.

The entire burn care team should understand this response, listen to the parents' concerns, and emphasize all that is being done to ensure the very best care for their child. Specific nurses and physicians should be designated to communicate with the family to avoid any misunderstandings and confusion about issues of patient care that result if disparate information comes from multiple sources. The anesthesia care team must emphasize the extensive monitoring and the central role that anesthesiologists have in ensuring the well-being of their child as well as explaining the risks of anesthesia. Special emphasis is on methods for minimizing physical and psychological pain during transport to the operating room, in the operating room, and postoperatively.

Keeping children with severe burn injuries starved (NPO) for 8 hours or longer before sedation for a dressing change or anesthesia for a surgical procedure severely compromises caloric intake; therefore, we advocate the use of continuous orojejunal or nasojejunal (postpyloric) alimentation. In general, children who receive oral calories up to about 4 hours before sedation or induction are unlikely to present with large gastric residual fluid volumes. Because children with moderate to severe burns are in a negative energy balance, it is preferable to minimize interruptions in feeds. Some continue jejunal feeds throughout the perioperative period but insert a nasogastric tube to monitor whether feeds are actually present in the stomach due to the jejunal tube migrating retrograde or feeds

TABLE 34.2	Systemic Effects of Burn Injury	
System	**Early Effects**	**Late Effects**
Cardiovascular	↓ CO as a result of decreased circulating blood volume, myocardial depressant factor	↑ CO as a result of sepsis ↑ CO 2 to 3 times > baseline for months (hypermetabolism) Hypertension secondary to vasoactive substances such as renin
Pulmonary	Upper airway obstruction as a result of edema Lower airway obstruction as a result of edema, bronchospasm, particulate matter, sloughing of airway mucosa ↓ FRC ↓ Pulmonary compliance ↓ Chest wall compliance	Bronchopneumonia Tracheal stenosis, vocal cord granuloma ↓ Chest wall compliance
Renal	↓ GFR secondary to ↓ circulating blood volume Myoglobinuria Hemoglobinuria Tubular dysfunction	↑ GFR secondary to ↑ CO Tubular dysfunction
Hepatic	↓ Function as a result of ↓ circulating blood volume, hypoxia, hepatotoxins	Hepatitis ↑ Function as a result of hypermetabolism, enzyme induction, ↑ CO ↓ Function as a result of sepsis, drug interactions
Hematopoietic	↓ Platelets ↑ Fibrin split products, consumptive coagulopathy, anemia	↑ Platelets ↑ Clotting factors
Neurologic	Encephalopathy Seizures ↑ ICP	Encephalopathy Seizures ICU psychosis
Skin	↑ Heat, fluid, electrolyte loss	Contractures, scar formation, difficult IV access, difficult intubation
Metabolic	↓ Ionized calcium	↑ Oxygen consumption ↑ Carbon dioxide production ↓ Ionized calcium
Pharmacokinetics and Pharmaco-dynamics	Altered volume of distribution Altered protein binding Altered pharmacokinetics Altered pharmacodynamics	Tolerance to opioids, sedatives Enzyme induction, altered receptors Drug interaction

↓, Decrease in; ↑, increase in; *CO*, cardiac output; *FRC*, functional residual capacity; *GFR*, glomerular filtration rate; *ICP*, intracranial pressure; *ICU*, intensive care unit.

refluxing into the stomach. If feeds are detected in the stomach, then jejunal feeds should be interrupted and resumed almost immediately after the procedure. In children with large injuries who will quickly develop a negative nitrogen balance with cessation of enteral feedings, short-term use of parenteral protein-sparing support is justified and safe.[502]

Adequate sedation and pain control are necessary before moving children to the operating room; IV fentanyl and midazolam are particularly helpful to provide analgesia and amnesia. The drug dose required to achieve a satisfactory clinical response may increase over time.[503,504] The dose of sedative or opioid should be titrated to effect while the child is carefully observed and monitored. It is not unusual for children with burns in excess of 25% of the body surface area to require 1 to 3 mg/kg per hour of both morphine and midazolam to provide adequate analgesia and sedation. However, we believe that opioid-sparing techniques including regional anesthesia and adjunct medications (e.g., dexmedetomidine or ketamine) are useful to reduce opioid and benzodiazepine use.

Correction of intravascular volume before induction of anesthesia may require fluid boluses during and after sedation and before transport. Establishing adequate IV access preoperatively may be especially difficult in children with large burns. We use both topical anesthetic creams and needle-free subcutaneous local anesthetics to help make this process painless and stress free.

Strategies should be implemented to attenuate heat loss during both transport and in the operating room. Multiple blankets or thermal reflective covers are effective. Open wounds should be covered to minimize heat loss due to evaporation. To minimize radiation and convective heat loss, the temperature in the operating rooms should be set to 37°C to 38°C during extensive excisions.[245] Equipment that is effective in maintaining the body temperature should be used including a warming blanket, radiant warmer, blood warmer, heat/moisture exchangers and forced hot-air warmers. Wrapping the extremities in sterile plastic bags and covering the head with plastic or thermal insulation material markedly reduces heat and fluid losses (see Fig. 34.5). Although a hot operating room is uncomfortable for staff, maintaining the child's temperature is essential to attenuate heat loss and avoid coagulopathies and loss of calories from thermogenesis should hypothermia develop. Each calorie saved is one more that can be used for tissue healing.

Adequate monitoring for major blood loss and fluid shifts includes standard American Society of Anesthesiologists (ASA) monitors as well as arterial and central venous cannulas, an esophageal stethoscope/temperature probe, and a urinary catheter. Continuous noninvasive cardiac output monitoring can be useful to assess cardiac output in children who may be septic or develop a cardiomyopathy.[52] A secure IV route for volume infusion is essential. If the potential for rapid blood loss exists, multilumen catheters may not be adequate because of their small calibers and resistance to rapid infusions. In such cases, a rapid infusion device may be needed (see Chapter 49).[505–507] Large venous access may be provided by cannulating the femoral, internal jugular, or subclavian veins (see Chapter 46). Invasive arterial and CVP monitoring can be established after induction of anesthesia in most children.

Propofol, thiopental (if available), or ketamine in incremental doses are usually well tolerated, provided the children are not hypovolemic (see Video 5.1). Ketamine can cause hypotension during the hyperdynamic phase. Studies in children long recovered from acute burn injury reported a 40% increase in the thiopental dose needed to eliminate the lid reflex compared with

children without burn injuries (E-Fig. 34.5).[331] Our clinical experience with propofol in children with burn injuries suggests that the clinical response is similar to that of thiopental, although studies are lacking. Ketamine may be preferred if hypovolemia is present or invasive monitoring lines must be inserted before induction. Tolerance to ketamine is rare[508]; one child is reported to have received a 37-day infusion with no evidence of tolerance.[509] High-dose fentanyl or morphine combined with nitrous oxide for children who will undergo ventilation postoperatively is commonly used with an inhalation agent titrated to clinical effect to supplement the opioid-based anesthetic.

In the absence of intravenous access, a slow inhalation induction is preferable for children with a compromised airway, bearing in mind the potential for aspiration if a full stomach is present, and cardiovascular depression if hypovolemia is present.[510] A difficult airway cart with appropriate advanced airway adjuncts should be in the operating room.

Succinylcholine is contraindicated in burned children 24 hours after the burn insult because of a potentially lethal efflux of potassium from muscle.[140,318,323] The hyperkalemia after succinylcholine is more related to the immature (fetal) receptors,[323] and the resistance to neuromuscular blocking drugs is more because of de novo expression of α7 acetylcholine receptors in the junctional and extrajunctional areas.[511,512] The massive efflux of potassium in response to IV succinylcholine after certain injuries including burns is attributed to the upregulation of acetylcholine receptors over the entire muscle membrane after the injury, compared with the limited acetylcholine receptor numbers located just at the myoneural junction in the normal state.[323] This peak release of potassium response after a dose of succinylcholine in a burn patient peaks in 2 to 5 minutes and usually lasts less than 15 minutes, although it can persist for a prolonged period.[323] The endpoint for succinylcholine-induced hyperkalemia is unknown. We recommend avoiding succinylcholine in children with large burns (≥40% body surface area) for at least 1.5 to 2 years after the burn. However, there is no definite time interval following a burn or after it is completely scarred after which succinylcholine will not trigger a hyperkalemic response. The smallest burn reported to trigger a hyperkalemic response was a 9% body surface area burn.

Since the muscle tissue of burn victims demonstrates resistance to nondepolarizing muscle relaxants (Fig. 34.9),[140,513] the hyperkalemic response likely persists long after the acute injury phase of the burn. A case report demonstrating marked resistance to nondepolarizing relaxant 463 days after burn injury indirectly supports the notion that a hyperkalemic response to succinylcholine may last long after the acute injury phase.[332] Studies of all neuromuscular blocking drugs have demonstrated that both the total dose and the serum concentration necessary to attain a given degree of muscle twitch depression in children with burns in excess of 25% of their body surface area are three to five times greater than in children without burn injury.[140,288,289,293,306,307,514] An increase in the number of acetylcholine receptors at junctional and extrajunctional areas and an altered affinity for the neuromuscular blocking drugs by those receptors both contribute to the increased demand for nondepolarizing neuromuscular blocking drugs.[320,325,513] With the availability of sugammadex, we now recommend rocuronium (1.5 mg/kg, 5 × ED$_{95}$)[515] if rapid control of the airway is needed (see Fig. 34.10).[516] Even with this dose of rocuronium (1.5 mg/kg), the onset time is prolonged compared with that in nonburned children (Fig. 34.10).[517]

Pharmacologic reversal of neuromuscular blockade, however, poses no special problem in burned children. Protein binding

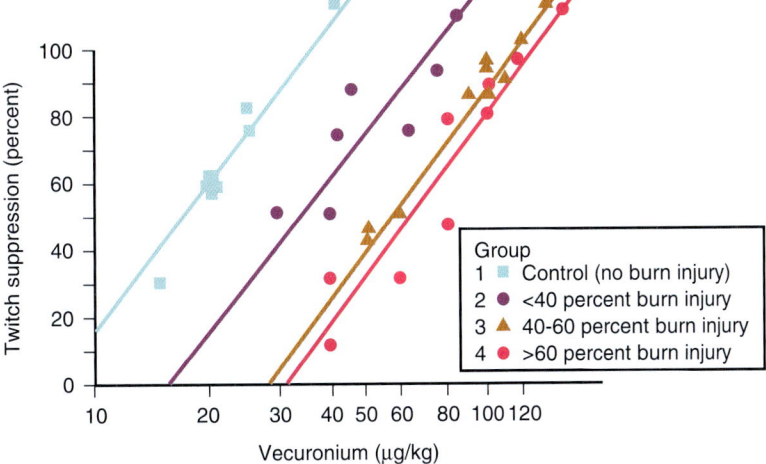

FIGURE 34.9 Logarithm of dose versus twitch suppression for vecuronium in control subjects and burned children. In the presence of acute injury, the vecuronium effective dose values increased with increasing burn size. The slopes of the curves were not different, but the intercepts were significantly different ($P<0.01$). *Solid squares,* children without burn injury; *purple circles,* children with less than 40% burn injury; *triangles,* children with 40% to 60% burn injury; *pink circles,* children with greater than 60% burn injury. (From Mills AK, Martyn JA. Neuromuscular blockade with vecuronium in paediatric patients with burn injury. *Br J Clin Pharm.* 1989;28[2]:155-159.)

and pharmacokinetic studies indicate that these two factors contribute little to the enhanced requirements.[140,288,289,293] Recovery from neuromuscular blockade has been observed at serum concentrations that would cause 100% twitch depression in children without burn injury.[316] Neuromuscular blocking drug hyposensitivity correlates well with the magnitude of burn ($r = 0.88$) (see Fig. 34.9).[306–310]

Maintenance of anesthesia is usually accomplished with nitrous oxide, oxygen, neuromuscular blocking drugs, and an opioid or inhalation agent; all potent anesthetic agents can be safely administered to burned children. Sevoflurane offers an advantage of smooth inhalation induction; any inhalation agent can be used for maintenance, but all cause a concentration-dependent decrease in cardiac output. In very ill children, anesthetic doses, but not neuromuscular blocking drug requirements, are drastically reduced. In this circumstance, high-dose fentanyl-oxygen-nitrous oxide/air anesthesia is well tolerated. Ketamine may be the anesthetic agent of choice in specific circumstances, including those in which we wish to avoid airway manipulation after application of fresh facial grafts, for very brief procedures, or for children who are unable to open their mouth for a standard laryngoscopy (Video 5.1). Ketamine may also be used along with midazolam for sedation before a trial of extubation. E-Fig. 34.6 illustrates extubation of a child with a severe facial burn with the use of an airway exchange catheter to provide a ready means for possible reintubation should the trial fail. Some burn centers use ketamine as the sole anesthetic and find it quite satisfactory.[518] The postoperative analgesia and somnolence for prolonged periods produced by high-dose ketamine may be considered an advantage in some instances in which postoperative agitation might dislodge fresh skin grafts.[509] However, prolonged somnolence will delay reinstitution of critical enteral nutrition. Low-dose ketamine may be used postoperatively for its opioid-sparing effects.[519,520] An emerging experience with dexmedetomidine appears to demonstrate safety and efficacy in reducing otherwise common opioid tolerance and dose escalation.[521] Ketamine, either alone or with propofol or midazolam, is commonly used for burn dressing changes[518,522,523]; rectal ketamine (6 mg/kg)

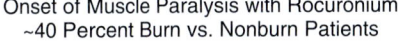

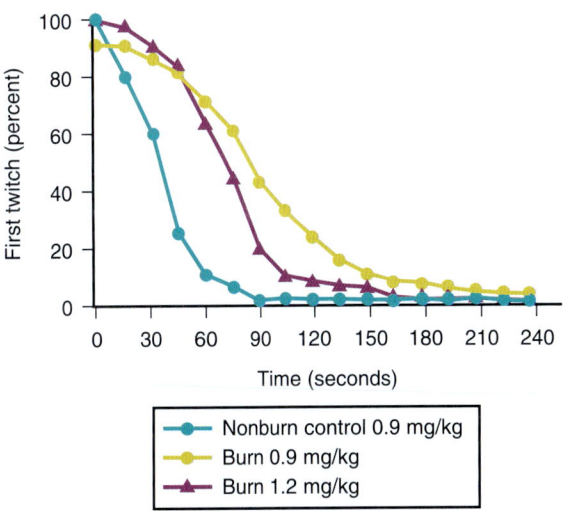

FIGURE 34.10 This dose escalation study of rocuronium in burned adults (approximately 40% body surface area) demonstrated severe resistance to the onset of neuromuscular blockade (percent of train-of-four first twitch). The time of onset could be reduced with higher doses; however, a dose of 1.2 mg/kg did not achieve complete paralysis until longer than 2 minutes had elapsed. These data suggest that if a rapid sequence induction were needed in patients with severe burns, an even greater as yet undefined dose would be required to shorten the time to complete relaxation. (Modified from Han TH, Kim HS, Bae JY, et al. Neuromuscular pharmacodynamics of rocuronium in patients with major burns. *Anesth Analg.* 2004;99[2]:386-392.)

has been combined with midazolam (0.5 mg/kg) as an alternative route for burn dressing change sedation.[524]

The inspired oxygen concentration is regulated according to the arterial blood gases and oxygen saturation. A pulse oximeter may not function properly on tissue discolored with silver nitrate; scraping the fingernail and cleaning the skin allow proper transmission and reception of the pulse oximeter light.[525,526] A pulse oximeter probe generally can function even on burned digits; however, if a child's digits are swollen, or in the presence of severe vasoconstriction, alternative sites such as the earlobe, nasal septum, or tongue must be sought. We have found the tongue to be useful for oximetry measurements when digital detection is poor[527]; a sealed oximeter probe that prevents electrical current leakage can be easily modified (E-Fig. 34.7).[527,528] Reflectance oximeters may also be valuable in the care of burned children.[529,530]

The combination of increased metabolic rate-induced carbon dioxide production and inhalation injury often necessitates an increase in alveolar ventilation compared with healthy children. Blood gas analysis assessed early and frequently throughout the anesthetic procedure does have merit. Continuous end-tidal carbon dioxide monitoring is essential, although shunting and dead-space ventilation in children with severe pulmonary injury after a burn may cause arterial to expired carbon dioxide gradients. *For these reasons, capnometry may be particularly effective for trending and as a disconnect alarm but should not be relied upon to adjust and assess ventilation until the end-tidal and arterial blood gas carbon dioxide tensions have been shown to correlate.* The tracheal tube must be secured with tracheostomy tape because standard adhesive tape does not stick to burned tissue and wet dressings. Electrocardiographic pads also do not adhere to the skin. These pads should be placed under dependent portions of the body or sutured or stapled onto the skin after the child is anesthetized. The standard measures for protecting the cornea from drying (including ophthalmic ointment and closing the eyelids when possible) and for positioning the limbs to prevent nerve compression must be observed.

The most important consideration of the intraoperative course is monitoring and correcting a child's blood losses. For this reason, invasive intravascular monitoring is essential. Children may lose as much as one to three blood volumes during each burn excision (surgeon dependent).[531] It is therefore necessary to be familiar with the surgical approach to burn excision. During a tangential excision (Fig. 34.11; Videos 34.1 and 34.2), a child might lose three to five times more blood than during excisions down to fascia (Video 34.3). The liberal use of very dilute concentrations of epinephrine (500 μg/L in normal saline) injected subcutaneously in both donor and excision sites markedly reduces surgical blood loss (Fig. 34.12 and Video 34.4)[532]; our institution uses a 1:2,000,000 epinephrine-containing solution (0.5 μg/mL). Large doses of epinephrine are well tolerated and

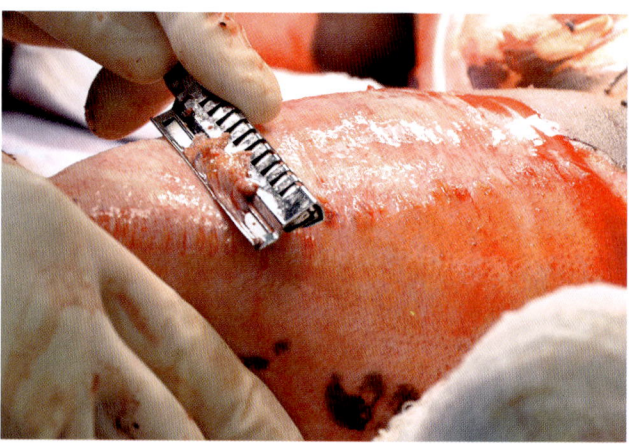

FIGURE 34.11 Tangential skin excision in which multiple thin areas of burn tissue are excised until a viable vascular bed is achieved. This is indicated by brisk bleeding. This type of excision results in less scarring because the majority of fat tissue remains intact. However, this also results in significantly greater blood loss.

markedly diminish bleeding. In a series of 25 consecutive children undergoing extensive layered excision, we used a total dose of epinephrine averaging 25 ± 3 μg/kg without complication[532]; as much as 10 μg/kg epinephrine may be injected every 20 minutes. One center reported their experience using a phenylephrine based tumescent solution in children with burns and found a 69.8% incidence of hypertension with some children requiring treatment.[533] It is unclear if epinephrine offers advantage due to its combined alpha and beta effects compared with the pure alpha effects of phenylephrine but it is clear that phenylephrine should be used with caution. Another concern is that some centers use electric infusion pumps to inject dilute epinephrine-containing saline solution; such devices have been associated with complications such as acute pulmonary edema and carpal tunnel syndrome, suggesting that hand injection may be safer.[534] Fluid overload may not become evident until several hours after surgery if excessive clysis or tumescent fluid is injected to facilitate harvesting of skin (Video 34.4). We have observed a number of infants (≤10 kg) who later developed pulmonary edema; therefore, the amount of fluid injected must be taken into consideration with the amount administered intravenously. Since it

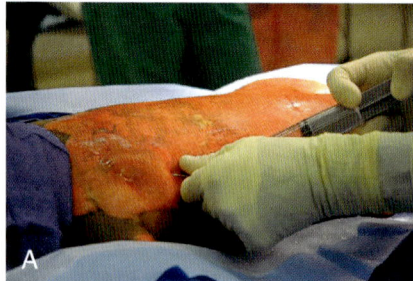
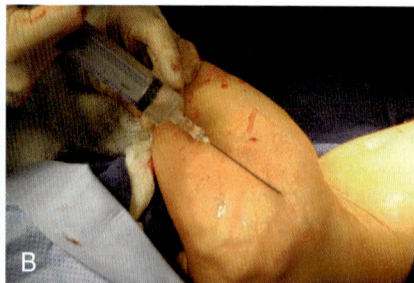
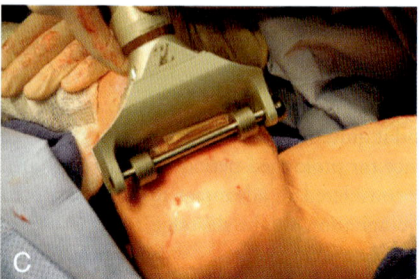

FIGURE 34.12 **A**, Subcutaneous injection of normal saline with a dilute concentration of epinephrine (0.5 μg/mL) from an area to be excised. **B**, Note the blanching of the donor skin secondary to the epinephrine. This helps to greatly reduce the amount of blood loss from both the donor sites and burn wound excision. It should be noted, however, that in the case of a large quantity administered to a small patient, late absorption can result in fluid overload. **C**, Skin is now harvested with minimal blood loss owing to the vasoconstriction of the tumescence solution.

is difficult to estimate blood and fluid loss, other indicators of circulating blood volume, such as urine output, central venous pressure, arterial pressure, and shape of the arterial waveform (see Fig. 10.12), should be closely monitored.

Early excision of full-thickness burns has improved survival and shortened hospital stays.[535–537] In the past, we routinely observed that 5% of the blood volume was lost for every 1% body surface area excised and grafted.[538,539] This extensive blood loss was a major source of morbidity and expense.[540,541] More recently, effective blood-conserving techniques for excision have drastically reduced intraoperative blood loss. These techniques include (1) clearly planning the excision to be performed before its initiation; (2) performing all extremity excisions under pneumatic tourniquet, exsanguinating the extremity before tourniquet inflation, and wrapping the extremity in a hemostatic dressing (epinephrine/saline soaked dressings) before tourniquet deflation; (3) conducting all fascial excisions with coagulating electrocautery; (4) performing major layered excisions as soon as possible after injury, before significant wound hyperemia develops; (5) executing all layered torso excisions after subeschar epinephrine clysis; (6) maintaining normothermia, primarily through maintaining a hot operating room (near 98.6°F [37°C]); (7) using multiple electrocautery devices simultaneously; and (8) subcutaneous injection of saline diluted epinephrine (with and without dilute bupivacaine) in donor areas.[311] Based on preoperative and postoperative hematocrit and known volume of transfusion, the percent of the total blood volume lost per percent of total wound excised generated an average 0.98% ± 0.19% of the blood volume per percent of the body surface excised. This was about one-fifth of our earlier experience with this type of excision.[542,543]

Chronic ionized hypocalcemia is commonly observed with major thermal injury.[249] Prophylactic intermittent administration of calcium chloride or calcium gluconate is strongly recommended during the rapid infusion of citrated blood products.[263,544–546] Some children have experienced electromechanical dissociation or cardiac arrest during the rapid administration of fresh frozen plasma. This observation prompted a controlled prospective study in which a highly significant decrease in the serum ionized calcium concentration occurred when fresh frozen plasma was administered at a rate of 1 mL/kg per minute or greater (see Figs. 10.10 and 10.11).[263] Interestingly, there was no correlation between adverse cardiovascular responses, the rate of fresh frozen plasma infusion, and the serum ionized calcium concentration. A careful review of the previous cases of cardiac arrest/electrical mechanical dissociation revealed that all children were anesthetized with halothane, whereas in our prospective study, most were anesthetized with "balanced" techniques. Because all inhalation agents depress cardiac function, in part through their calcium channel-blocking activity, a sudden citrate-induced decrease in ionized calcium would be expected to exacerbate the cardiac dysfunction of standard dose inhalation anesthesia. Studies in our laboratory have documented this interaction.[263,264] Additional exogenous calcium is administered during rapid infusion of fresh frozen plasma or citrated whole blood, especially in infants (see Chapter 10).[264] It is our clinical impression that the rapid administration of fresh frozen plasma or citrated whole blood through a central line, without additional exogenous calcium, may be more likely to induce severe hypotension, bradycardia, and electrical mechanical dissociation. Our experience has been that rapid administration of citrated blood products, particularly fresh frozen plasma or whole blood, is safer through

peripheral lines; rapid administration of packed red blood cells does not cause ionized hypocalemia. However, calcium administered simultaneously in the same IV line with fresh frozen plasma or citrated blood products may precipitate clot formation; we recommend giving exogenous calcium through a separate rapidly running IV line or preferably slowly through a central line.

SPECIAL CONSIDERATIONS

Methemoglobinemia

A less common but important source of intraoperative cyanosis and hypoxemia is methemoglobinemia. When silver nitrate dressings are used on the burn sites, some strains of Gram-negative bacteria reduce nitrates to nitrites, which diffuse into the bloodstream and convert hemoglobin into methemoglobin.[218,219,451] Methemoglobin decreases the available oxygen-carrying capacity of hemoglobin and increases the affinity of the unaltered hemoglobin for oxygen, thereby further impairing oxygen delivery. Consequently, the oxygen-hemoglobin P50 curve is shifted to the left.

Methemoglobinemia should be considered in the differential diagnosis of cyanosis. Approximately 5 grams of deoxyhemoglobin for each deciliter of blood is necessary to produce visible cyanosis, but a comparable skin color is produced by 1.5 to 2 grams of methemoglobin for each deciliter of blood. Blood that contains more than approximately 10% methemoglobin usually appears dark red or even brown, despite the presence of a high measured PaO_2, and does not change color even with vigorous agitation in room air. Measured oxygen saturation is low; however, the decrease in saturation provides a falsely increased value.[389,390] Treatment consists of removing the toxic agent and administering methylene blue (2 mg/kg) and high inspired oxygen concentrations. Other possible sources of methemoglobinemia include the absorption of excessive doses of eutectic mixture of local anesthetics cream (EMLA) or benzocaine cream applied to reduce pruritus from a burn wound.[547,548]

Tracheal Tube Size

Because burned children frequently undergo multiple anesthetic procedures, special considerations must be given to the tracheal tube type and size. Cuffed tracheal tubes are preferable to uncuffed tubes to minimize the number of reintubations. The size of the tracheal tube, the volume of air inflated into the cuff, and the pressure at which an audible air leak occurs should be recorded on each anesthetic record. It is common to note that the diameter of the tracheal tube decreases as weeks go by after the burn injury suggesting the development of a subglottic lesion (stenosis, granuloma), which should be investigated with bronchoscopy. When nitrous oxide is used, the intraoperative cuff pressure should be checked to avoid excessive pressure on the tracheal mucosa. Microcuff (Halyard Health, Inc., Alpharetta, GA) tubes may provide a greater margin of safety than conventional tracheal tubes (see Chapter 12) but they are more prone to kinking in a hot operating room. We generally inflate the cuff to the minimum pressure that allows controlled ventilation and check the cuff pressure regularly.

Airway Control

The child with a burn may present an especially difficult airway challenge (Fig. 34.13). This may be due to external airway factors, such as temporomandibular joint limitation, macroglossia from thermal injury, and neck contractures.[20,510] It also may be due to direct thermal or inhalational injuries to the glottis and respiratory tree. A detailed history and physical examination focusing on

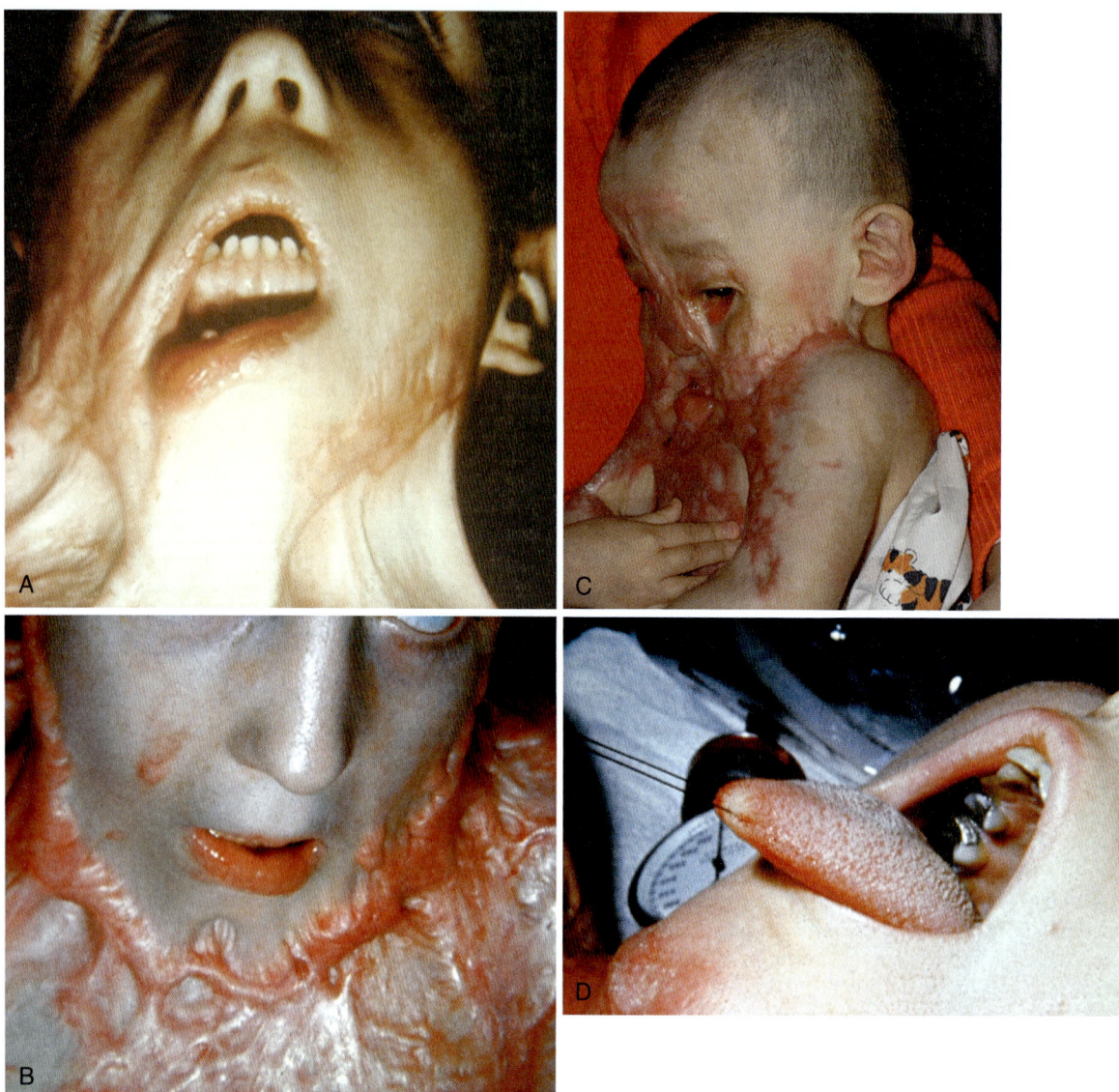

FIGURE 34.13 A, Child with inadequately treated facial burn. Note that skin contracture has resulted in complete distortion of the face with inability to close the right eye. **B**, Child with another example of an inadequately treated neck burn; note that her chin is fused with the sternum, resulting in very difficult airway management. **C**, An acute burn injury with an even more extreme example of inability to access the airway. To manage this child safely for the initial neck release, extracorporeal membrane oxygenation was used. This child is also unable to close her eyes. **D**, Some children with severe neck burns may have their airway visualized only by pulling back on the tongue (0 silk suture, suction applied to the tip of the tongue, or grasping forceps may be used [see also Fig. 12.32]) so as to pull the tongue and larynx cephalad.

airway injury is vital. History details such as a victim of fire in a closed space (e.g., house or automobile fire [very commonly associated with inhalational injuries]), vocal changes, stridor, singed nares, and hoarseness may be important predictors of difficulty in establishing an airway.

Fiberoptic intubation is frequently used after induction when we are confident that we can maintain a mask airway. We have used dexmedetomidine or high-dose ketamine as our sole sedative (combined with topical anesthesia) while performing fiberoptic intubations with spontaneously breathing children. A dexmedetomidine infusion (without a loading dose) may provide a relatively stable, hemodynamic environment, without respiratory depression or excessive secretions.

Fiberoptic intubation is often aided with manual distraction of the tongue (especially if macroglossia is present); a stitch through the tongue, and a jaw lift. If the tongue is difficult to grasp, moderately high suction applied to the tip of the tongue or a gauze wrapped around the tongue and then gently pulling the tongue forward facilitates visualization of glottic structures (Fig. 34.13D; see also Fig. 12.32).[549] Fiberoptic intubation sometimes is more easily performed if the bronchoscope is guided through a supraglottic airway (SGA) that has already been seated and used to ventilate the lungs. This can be especially advantageous if there is a great deal of perioral edema from inhalational burn injury.

In addition to direct laryngoscopy, fiberoptic intubations, and supraglottic airway–assisted intubations, the GlideScope

(Verathon, Bothell, WA) has proven particularly helpful; other techniques including retrograde wires and light-wand intubations may be difficult to use in a child with a severely burned neck and contractures. In these children, the surgeon may release the contracture during ketamine sedation and spontaneous ventilation to facilitate access to the airway (Video 5.1). The airway may then be instrumented either directly or indirectly (see Chapter 12). A useful review of airway management in pediatric head and neck burns that details successful strategies we use for securing the airway is available elsewhere.[550]

Hyperalimentation

Hyperalimentation fluids are frequently administered to burned children.[182,551] These fluids should be continued intraoperatively; however, we generally reduce the rate of infusion to one-half to two-thirds of the initial infusion rate because the metabolic rate is usually decreased during anesthesia. These fluids should be administered with a constant-infusion pump to avoid accidental over infusion or under infusion. If the hyperalimentation fluids must be terminated (e.g., to permit blood transfusion), monitoring of blood glucose concentration is recommended. Dangerous rebound hypoglycemia may occur if infusions are abruptly interrupted, and no compensation is made with other glucose-containing solutions. Compatibility of hyperalimentation solutions with drugs, blood, and other infusions must be addressed.

Awakening

In the immediate postoperative period, oxygen consumption increases even in the absence of shivering.[63] If oxygen debt develops (metabolic acidosis), appropriate measures must be taken to correct it. Special consideration also must be given to the likelihood of severe pain. Analgesic drugs should be administered in increasingly liberal doses because of increased drug tolerance. Adequacy of air exchange and patency of the airway, however, must be given priority. It is important to assess the leak pressure at the end of the surgical procedure. Airway patency in the burned child is dynamic; the child whose airway had minimal edema at the beginning of a procedure may have become very edematous at the end and be a poor candidate for extubation.

ULTRASOUND-GUIDED VASCULAR ACCESS, REGIONAL ANALGESIA, AND CARDIOVASCULAR ASSESSMENT

Ultrasound can serve as an adjunct for vascular access, regional anesthesia, and cardiopulmonary diagnosis. Placing CVP and arterial catheters in the operating room under carefully controlled conditions is associated with a low rate of acute mechanical complications and deep vein thrombosis (~1%), even in children with multiple prior cannulations, a hypercoagulable state from the burn, and long periods of being bedbound.[552] Ultrasound is useful to rapidly access arteries and veins but also to diagnose clotted vessels, reducing futile attempts at obtaining vascular access.[553] Ultrasound also helps establish the location of cannulas. We use ultrasound to assist in placing peripherally inserted central catheters (PICCs), then place the probe over the internal jugular to verify that the PICC is not traveling cephalad, and then scan the subclavian vein to verify correct placement.

Ultrasound-guided regional anesthesia is also a valuable tool in children undergoing reconstructive surgery. Typically, the complaints children have after reconstructive procedures most often involve the pain of the graft donor site. Postoperative experience can be improved by placing ultrasound-guided blocks of donor

sites, sometimes with catheters for more prolonged postoperative analgesia. These blocks include transversus abdominal plane blocks for truncal analgesia where both single-shot blocks and catheters are used (E-Fig. 34.8). Other specific blocks we have found very useful include the lateral femoral cutaneous nerve and fascia iliaca (Fig. 34.14) to cover the most common donor site, the lateral thigh or lower abdomen. Ultrasound has greatly improved success and reliability over typical blind techniques.[554,555] Our experience is that lateral femoral cutaneous nerve or fascia iliaca blocks provide better pain control for the donor site than infiltrating the donor site with local anesthetics; more prolonged analgesia is provided by leaving a catheter in place. We usually place fascia iliaca catheters since these are easier to place with a shorter learning curve than for placement of lateral femoral cutaneous nerve catheters.[556] Intraoperative single-shot regional blocks that cover both graft and donor sites in children (age 7 months to 14 years) undergoing reconstructive surgery had Face, Legs, Activity, Cry, Consolability scale (FLACC) scores of 0/10 in 93% of patients by the time of postanesthesia care unit (PACU) discharge (average discharge time of 70 minutes) and mean PACU morphine

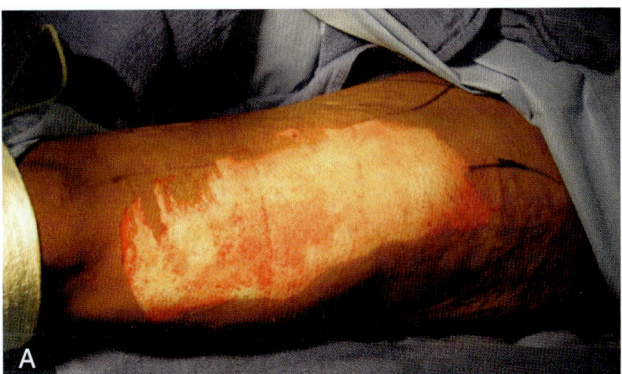
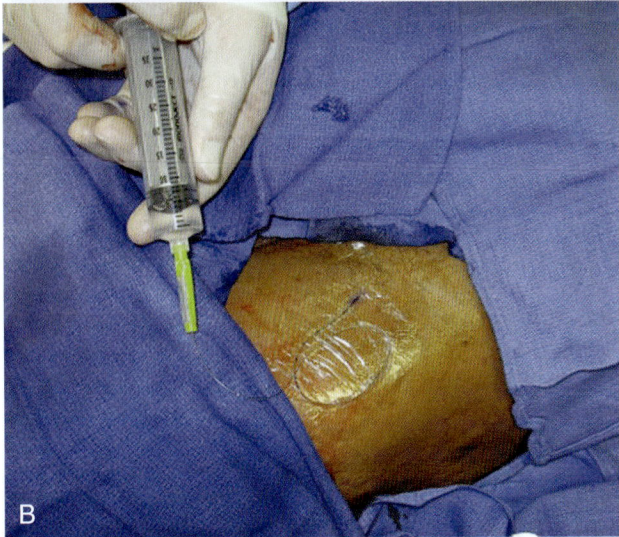

FIGURE 34.14 **A**, It is common for the thigh to be a donor site. In this case, a single-shot lateral femoral cutaneous nerve block is placed for postoperative analgesia. **B**, The fascia iliaca block will cover the distribution of the lateral femoral cutaneous nerve (lateral thigh) but also covers anterior and medial sensation (femoral and obturator nerves). In this case, the patient's legs are on the left and the lower abdomen to the right. A catheter was placed at the level just above the femoral crease allowing an infusion of low-dose local anesthetic for 2 to 4 days. Note that the catheter is secured with a coil to provide more stable placement.

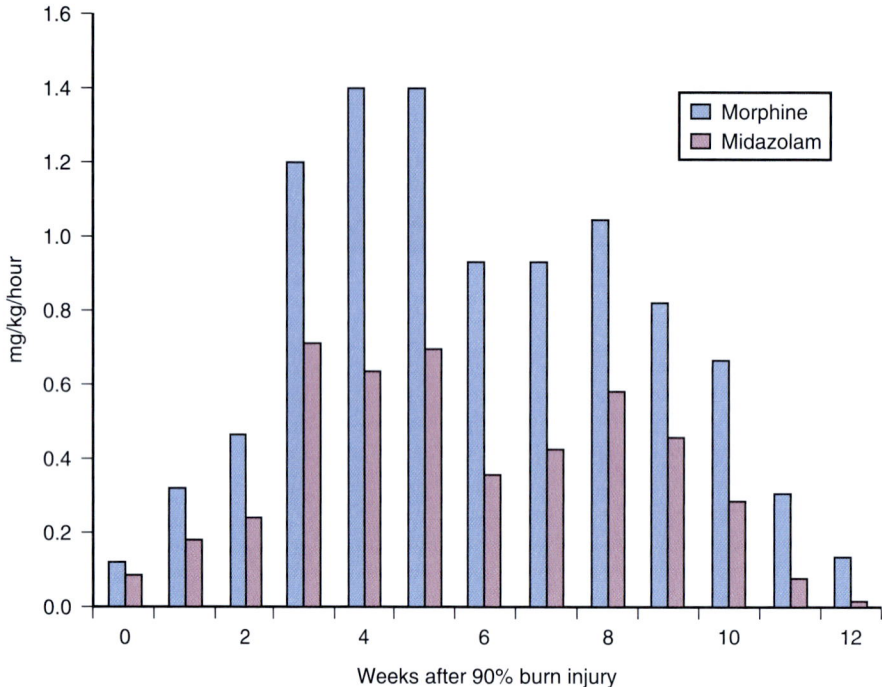

FIGURE 34.15 Morphine and midazolam requirements of a 16-year-old boy who had suffered an approximately 90% body surface area burn injury. Note the marked rapid rise in analgesia and sedation requirements during the first 4 to 5 weeks after injury and then the rapid decline in requirements as his wounds were successfully grafted.

requirement equivalents of 0.06 mg/kg.[557] Regional anesthesia is a valuable tool in children suffering burns, and can be used to better control postoperative pain and minimize opioid use.

Ultrasound is also one of several strategies during burn surgery. Hemodynamic measurements can be used to rapidly assess intraoperative cardiac function and the Bedside Assessment for Trauma/Critical Care (BEAT) examination used to assess volume status.[558,559] Ultrasound during decompression of a pneumothorax in a burn patient indicates the lung has reexpanded by the return of the pleural "sliding" sign.[560–562] Bladder scans avoid the need for a bladder catheter in some instances.[563,564]

PAIN MANAGEMENT AND POSTOPERATIVE CARE

Treatment of burn pain, both perioperatively and in the intensive care unit, remains a major challenge. Nearly every maneuver involving the care of these children, including dressing changes, excision and grafting, physical therapy, weighing, and line placements, is associated with pain.

Opioid administration for pain control has been an evolving science; 25 years ago, there was fear that treatment of pain with opioids would create addictions. However, no reports of children developing opioid addiction after therapeutic uses of opioids have been published and studies in adults revealed a very low addiction rate.[565–569] This has led to liberalization of opioid dosing in children with burns; it is not unusual for children to receive more than 1 to 3 mg/kg per hour of IV morphine and similar doses of midazolam while recovering from burn injuries. Once the thermal wounds are closed, opioid requirements rapidly decrease, and a weaning protocol introduced (Fig. 34.15).

Part of the challenge in managing burn pain is due to the overlay of physiologic and psychosocial responses to thermal injury. Besides physical stimulation of nociceptors and other direct pain mechanisms, there is also the very real anticipation, anxiety,

and fear associated with these procedures. Evidence suggests that skillful communication and explanations for specific treatments are necessary, despite the pain caused, and that such communications decrease analgesic requirements.[503,570–572] Hand and foot burns, elevated baseline pain preoperatively, deep partial thickness burns, burn size, and multiple areas of burn in particular are associated with increased pain.[573]

Animal data suggest that thermal injury causes a hyperalgesic state with both reduced effectiveness of morphine (presumably from downregulation of spinal μ receptors) and increases in N-methyl-D-aspartate (NMDA) receptors. The increases in NMDA receptors induced by burns provide the rationale for the widespread use of ketamine to treat pain in these children. Opioids may also increase the sensitivity to pain. In a mouse model, morphine downregulates μ-opioid receptors within the spinal cord and causes injury to spinal inhibitory interneurons.[568,569] In the same model, opioids cause postburn immunosuppression.[574] Additionally, opioid tolerance and opioid-induced hyperactive behaviors have, in a rat pup model, been exacerbated when midazolam has been concomitantly administered. This may be important as midazolam is frequently used as a clinical adjunct.[317] These potential opioid disadvantages have led to a search for alternative analgesics. Among these are potentially dexmedetomidine,[575–581] gabapentin,[582] and, until their withdrawal from the market, cyclooxygenase-2 inhibitors.[583–585]

Dexmedetomidine is an α_2-adrenoceptor agonist with good sedative and anxiolytic properties. In adults, it decreases opioid requirements postoperatively.[576–580,586] In children with burns, it has been used successfully for sedation,[521,575] although larger doses of dexmedetomidine may be needed than those required in nonburned adults or nonburned children.[575] Dexmedetomidine is not analgesic for children with burns.[587] In a prospective study of dexmedetomidine in acutely burned children,[588,587] a

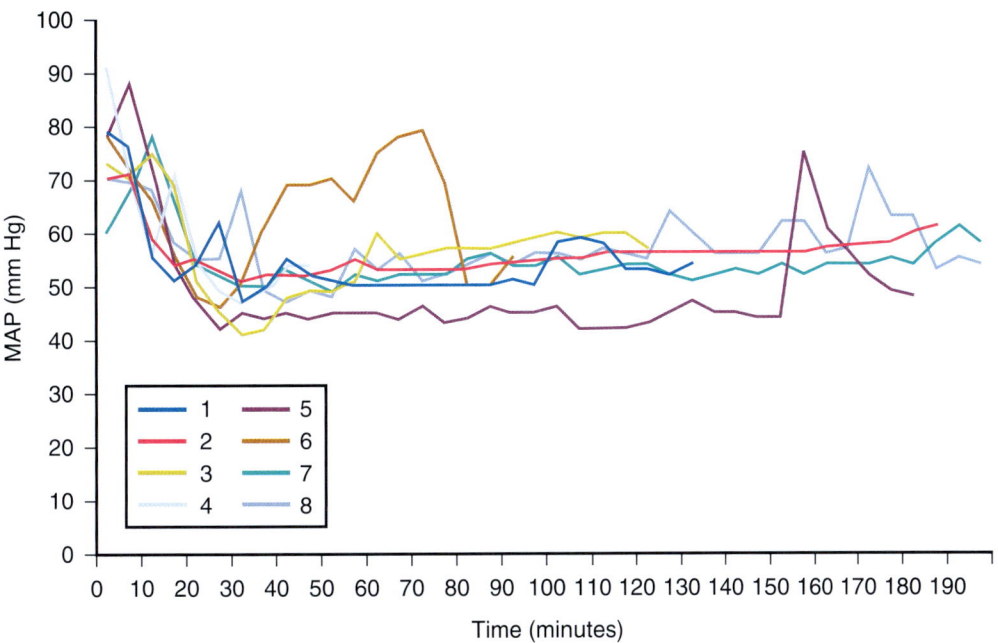

FIGURE 34.16 Change in mean arterial pressure (MAP) after bolus dose of dexmedetomidine in eight consecutive acute pediatric burn patients. *Note:* Given these observations, we now avoid a bolus dose; however, should a bolus dose be considered necessary, we suggest that the need for volume resuscitation (≥10 mL/kg of balanced salt solution) or mild pressor support must be anticipated. (From Shank ES, Sheridan RL, Ryan CM, Keaney TJ, Martyn JA. Hemodynamic responses to dexmedetomidine in critically injured intubated pediatric burned patients: a preliminary study. *J Burn Care Res.* 2013;34[3]:311-317.)

bolus dose of dexmedetomidine (1 µg/kg over 10 minutes) was followed by an ascending infusion protocol (0.7 µg/kg per hour to 2.2 µg/kg per hour).[575] A bolus dose of dexmedetomidine causes vasodilation,[589] which decreases the mean arterial blood pressure (Fig. 34.16).[588] This occurs in children of all ages studied (2–18 years), although the decrease in the mean arterial pressure does not correlate with size of burn, time since the burn, or central venous pressure. Volume loading using a balanced salt solution (10 mL/kg) or mild pressor support before commencing the dexmedetomidine may ameliorate hypotensive effect. In the absence of a loading dose, blood pressure was maintained with dexmedetomidine infusion.[521] Dexmedetomidine pharmacokinetics in nonburned children appear similar to those in adults.[590–592] It is anticipated that children with burn injuries are likely to have increased clearance compared with unaffected children.

When dexmedetomidine and ketamine were co-administered for sedation and analgesia during burn dressing changes, they provided better sedation with less hemodynamic instability than midazolam.[593] Dexmedetomidine has also been used as an intranasal premedication in anxious children with burns.[594] Intranasally, dexmedetomidine (2 µg/kg) induced sedation more rapidly and was equally effective to oral midazolam (0.5 mg/kg) for induction conditions and rapidity of emergence. However, children prefer oral midazolam despite its bitter aftertaste. Pharmacodynamic responses after a slow intravenous (15 minutes) and intranasal administration of dexmedetomidine were similar in both adults[594] and children.[595] Intranasal bioavailability was 40.6% (95% confidence interval [CI] 34.7%–54.4%) in children without burns. Sedation score, modeled using a sigmoidal Emax model had an equilibration half time of 3.3 (95% CI 1.8–4.7) minutes and an EC_{50} of 0.903 (95% CI 0.445–2.344) µg/L.

Dressing changes sometimes present one of the greatest analgesic challenges.[523,596,597] This is because they are very painful. Dressing changes cause a rapid increase above baseline pain, children develop opioid tolerance, and the child associates them with anticipation of impending pain. Strategies to manage this pain include additional opioids and benzodiazepines, ketamine,[518,524,596] intranasal fentanyl,[598] remifentanil,[599] immersive virtual reality,[600,601] and music therapy.[602] Management of the child's pain depends on physiologic and pharmacologic factors, as well as the psychological state of the child. Unfortunately, some children become so tolerant that one author observed that doses of IV fentanyl as large as 100 µg/kg administered as a bolus to a teenager did not cause respiratory depression nor did it control the pain (CJC).

When poorly controlled, pain and anxiety have adverse psychological[270,603,604] and physiologic effects.[30,31] Posttraumatic stress disorder occurs in up to 30% of those with serious burns[269,270,272,273,604,605] and may be related to both the accident and the treatment, particularly in the setting of inadequate control of pain and anxiety.[269,273,275,279] An inconsistent approach to pain and anxiety will be associated with inappropriate degrees of child discomfort, nonuniform drug selection with inconsistent dosing of unfamiliar drugs, varying tolerance of child discomfort among staff members, and bedside disagreements over management of the child's distress.

To address this issue, a pain and anxiety guideline should be developed by all facilities that routinely treat burned children.[604–609] We developed one such guideline that we have followed for several years (Table 34.3).[504] The ideal characteristics of such a guideline include (1) safety and efficacy over the broad range of ages and injury acuities seen in the particular unit; (2) explicit recommendations for drug selection, dosing, and escalation of dosing; (3) a limited formulary that generates staff familiarity with agents used; and (4) regular assessment of pain and anxiety levels and guidance

TABLE 34.3	Pain Treatment Plan				
Clinical State	Background Anxiety	Background Pain	Procedural Anxiety	Procedural Pain	Transition to Next Clinical State
Mechanically ventilated acute burn	Midazolam infusion	Morphine infusion	Midazolam intravenous titration	Morphine intravenous titration	Wean infusions 10%–20% per day and substitute "nonmechanically ventilated acute burn guideline"
Nonmechanically ventilated acute burn	Scheduled enteral lorazepam	Scheduled enteral morphine	Lorazepam intravenous titration or enteral dose	Morphine enteral or intravenous titration	Wean scheduled drugs 10%–20% per day and substitute "chronic acute burn guideline"
Chronic acute burn	Scheduled enteral lorazepam	Scheduled enteral morphine	Lorazepam enteral dose	Morphine enteral dose	Wean scheduled and bolus drugs 10%–20% per day to outpatient requirements and pruritus medications
Reconstructive surgical patient	Scheduled enteral lorazepam	Scheduled enteral morphine sulfate	Lorazepam enteral dose	Morphine enteral dose	Wean scheduled drugs and bolus drugs to outpatient requirement

for intervention as needed through dose ranging. We have found this structured approach to be effective over the broad range of injury severity and child ages. Substantial escalation of drug doses, particularly in children with large injuries, is commonly required; doses should be titrated to the child's needs.

When the child is being weaned toward extubation, background medications should be tapered to yield a sensorium consistent with airway protection; many tracheas are safely extubated while the children are still receiving opioid and benzodiazepine infusions. Following this, they are transitioned to oral medications, usually methadone. Finally, it is essential to emphasize that the most effective of all analgesics and anxiolytics is prompt, definitive wound closure.

Tolerance to opioids occurs over time and must be considered so that adequate analgesia is provided throughout the recovery period. It is common to observe children who receive 1 mg/kg of morphine at the beginning of a 2-hour operative procedure not only to be ready for extubation but also to require additional opioids for continued pain relief postoperatively. Similar trends have been observed for fentanyl[301]; scenarios are well described in children with long-term opioid use.[610] As the child recovers, the painful stimuli diminish, and the opioid requirements are gradually reduced. This is generally such a prolonged process that withdrawal is not an issue. Anesthesiologists can have a key role in the treatment of thermal injury pain and, with an understanding of pharmacology, pharmacokinetics, and pharmacodynamics, are a vital resource for the care of these children (see also Chapters 41 and 42).

Acknowledgment

We wish to thank Erik S. Shank for his previous contributions to this chapter.

ANNOTATED REFERENCES

Caruso TJ, Janik LS, Fuzaylov G. Airway management of recovered pediatric patients with severe head and neck burns: a review. *Paediatr Anaesth.* 2012;22(5):462-468.

Pediatric airways in burned children may present some of the greatest airway challenges for the anesthesiologist. This is a useful review of some of these challenges and the techniques used to meet them.

Haag AC, Landolt MA, Kenardy JA, Schiestl CM, Kimble RM, De Young AC. Preventive intervention for trauma reactions in young injured children: results of a multi-site randomised controlled trial. *J Child Psychol Psychiatry.* 2020;61(9):988-997.

This randomized controlled trial presents the importance of targeted preventive intervention measures to accelerate recovery from posttraumatic stress disorder (PTSD) for both children and their family in these unique one-time traumatic family events.

Han T, Kim H, Bae J, et al. Neuromuscular pharmacodynamics of rocuronium in patients with major burns. *Anesth Analg.* 2004;99(2):386-392.

Currently, rocuronium is the fastest-acting nondepolarizing muscle relaxant available. This paper discusses its pharmacodynamics in burn patients and describes both delayed onset and resistance in burned adults with doses as great as 1.2 mg/kg.

Holbert MD, Kimble RM, Jones LV, Ahmed SH, Griffin BR. Risk factors associated with higher pain levels among pediatric burn patients: a retrospective cohort study. *Reg Anesth Pain Med.* Mar 2021;46(3):222-227.

This retrospective cohort study examined particular risk factors for postoperative pain in pediatric patients with burn injuries. They observed that four factors were associated with increased postoperative pain: hand burns, foot burns, increased burn size, and four or more body areas of involvement. Other factors seemed to be initial treatment at a nonburn specialty center and time to hospital presentation.

Shank ES, Martyn JA, Donelan MB, et al. Ultrasound-guided regional anesthesia for pediatric burn reconstructive surgery: a prospective study. *J Burn Care Res.* 2016;37(3):e213-e237.

This is the first randomized, prospective study in pediatric burn patients demonstrating the efficacy of peripheral regional nerve blocks—especially in patients with continuous indwelling catheters—in the postoperative analgesic management of reconstructive surgery. This study suggests that regional anesthesia should be used for most reconstructive surgeries to minimize narcotics and optimize analgesia.

Song L, Wang S, Zuo Y, et al. Midazolam exacerbates morphine tolerance and morphine-induced hyperactive behaviors in young rats with burn injury. *Brain Res.* 2014;1564:52-61.

This animal study demonstrated that the coadministration of midazolam and morphine did exacerbate morphine tolerance and hyperactive behavior. It appears the morphine tolerance is mediated through a spinal NMDA/protein kinase C mechanism. Since it is very common to sedate pediatric burn-injured patients in the intensive care unit with both midazolam and morphine, this study may have important implications for this population.

Weaver LK. Carbon monoxide poisoning. *Undersea Hyperb Med.* 2020;47(1):151-169.

This paper reviews three randomized clinical trials as well as animal data and presents an up-to-date review of the pros and cons for hyperbaric treatment of patients with carbon monoxide and cyanide poisoning.

A complete reference list can be found online at Elsevier eBooks+.

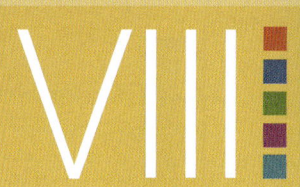

The Extremely Premature Infant (Micropremie) and Common Neonatal Emergencies

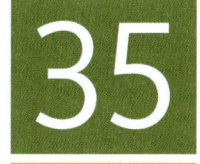

35

JAMES P. SPAETH AND JENNIFER E. LAM

Physiology of Prematurity Related to Anesthesia
Respiratory System
Cardiovascular System
Neurologic Development
Temperature Regulation
Renal and Metabolic Function
Gastrointestinal and Hepatic Function
Hematologic Function
Anesthetics and the Neonate/Premature Infant
Anesthetics and the Immature Brain
Inhalational Anesthetics
Intravenous Anesthetics
Regional Anesthetics

Neonatal Surgical Emergencies
Preparation for Surgery
The Operating Room
Monitors
The Family
Emergency Surgery
Respiratory Pathology
Abnormalities of the Airway
Gastrointestinal Pathology
Ligation of Patent Ductus Arteriosus
Retinopathy of Prematurity

THE PREMATURE INFANT IS DEFINED as birth before 37 weeks gestation. Premature births can be classified as low–birth-weight (LBW) infants (<2500 grams), very low–birth-weight (VLBW) infants (<1500 grams), and extremely low–birth-weight (ELBW) infants (<1000 grams). Alternatively, they may be classified as moderate to late prematurity (32 to <37 weeks), very premature (28 to <32 weeks), and extremely premature (<28 weeks). A neonate is an infant in the first 28 days after birth. "Premies" are commonly referred to as infants rather than neonates as a group because gestation may be very short (e.g., 24 weeks) and thus even at 37 weeks postmenstrual age (PMA), they are truly infants with a postnatal age of 13 weeks (24 + 13 = 37). Documentation for these infants should refer to both gestational age (i.e., at birth) and postnatal age (i.e., age after birth). The use of current post-conception age (PCA) or PMA (approximately 10 days older) helps define the maturation of physiologic processes.

Morbidity and mortality in this population has decreased considerably compared with 30 years ago, especially in ELBW infants.[1–4] This decrease is the result of influences such as the development of specialized maternal-fetal medicine and neonatal care units, antenatal corticosteroid administration, surfactant use shortly after birth, increased cesarean deliveries, and implementation of strategies to reduce lung injury; these include decreased delivery room intubations and increased use of continuous positive-airway pressure (CPAP).[1,2] Although survival and morbidity-free survival rates continue to increase, the trend over the past 20 years has plateaued. The last 5 years have shown a decrease in chronic lung disease, perhaps due to early initiation of noninvasive ventilator measures aimed at prevention rather than treatment of sequelae during extrauterine growth.[5] The cost of care is escalating, as are the number of surgical procedures and the need for specialized care these high-risk infants require.[6] The first part of this chapter will focus on the VLB and ELBW infant, or "micropremie," and discuss developmental physiology and its impact on anesthetic care.

Physiology of Prematurity Related to Anesthesia

RESPIRATORY SYSTEM

Airway

Anatomic Differences and Work of Breathing

The anatomic differences of the pediatric airway are detailed in Chapter 12; however, there are specific challenges unique to the airway of the premature infant. The small airways predispose the

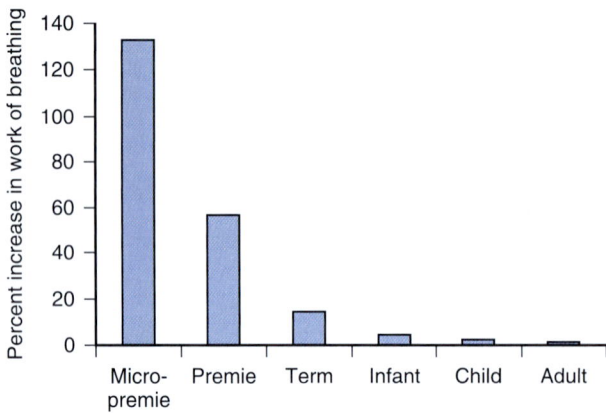

FIGURE 35.1 Change in work of breathing after placement of an appropriately sized endotracheal tube in extremely low–birth-weight infants (<1000 g), premature infants (1500 g), full-term infants, children, and adults (see text for details). (Redrawn with permission from Spaeth JP, O'Hara IB, Kurth CD. Anesthesia for the micropremie. *Semin Perinatol.* 1998;22(5):390-401.)

TABLE 35.1 Lung Function in Infants and Adults

Variable	Infants	Adults	Infant/Adult Ratio
Oxygen consumption (mL/kg per minute)	5–8	2–3	2
Respiratory rate (breaths/minute)	40–60	12	3–5
Tidal volume (mL/kg per minute)	6–8	7	1.0
Total lung capacity (mL/kg)	53	85	0.6
Airway diameter (mm)			
Trachea	5	14–16	0.3
Bronchus	4	11–14	0.3
Bronchiole	0.1	0.2	0.5

Data from Polgar G, Weng TR. The functional development of the respiratory system: from the period of gestation to adulthood. *Am Rev Respir Dis.* 1979;120(3): 625-695.

micropremie to obstruction and difficulty with ventilation. Resistance to airflow is inversely proportional to the fifth power of the radius in the upper airway and to the fourth power of the radius beyond the fifth bronchial division (see also Fig. 12.8). As a result, insertion of a tracheal tube (TT) increases resistance and the work of breathing far more for the micropremie (2.5- or 3-mm inside diameter [ID]) than for a larger infant (4-mm ID), child (5-mm ID), or adult (7-mm ID) (Fig. 35.1). Similarly, partial occlusion of the TT by secretions, blood, or kinking increases the work of breathing to a much greater extent in the micropremie. Partial occlusion of the natural airway from loss of muscle tone during anesthesia and sedation also increases the work of breathing more in the micropremie. Consequently, general anesthesia often requires placement of a TT to ensure airway patency and provide assisted ventilation to overcome the increased work of breathing.

Diseases that narrow the airway, such as subglottic stenosis, tracheal stenosis, and tracheobronchomalacia, occur commonly in the micropremie, and the associated reduction in airway diameter further increases both resistance to airflow and work of breathing. Subglottic stenosis necessitates the placement of a smaller TT than would otherwise be placed, further increasing airflow resistance. Although tracheal stenosis near the carina may not necessitate a smaller TT, it still increases airway resistance from the stenosis distal to the endotracheal tube (ETT). With tracheobronchomalacia, the intrathoracic airways collapse during exhalation, again increasing resistance and the work of breathing (see also Fig. 12.11 and Fig. 31.8). Positive end-expiratory pressure (PEEP) or CPAP helps stent open the airway. Mechanical ventilation, rather than spontaneous ventilation during anesthesia, prevents fatigue from increased work of breathing, and maintains ventilation and oxygenation. During anesthesia, the use of smaller inspiratory-to-expiratory ratios prevents air trapping and hyperinflation of lung segments.

The cardiopulmonary system of the neonate is driven by the need to deliver sufficient oxygen (O_2) to maintain a high metabolic rate. The O_2 consumption of an average neonate is 5 to 8 mL/kg per minute, whereas that of an adult is 2 to 3 mL/kg per minute (Table 35.1); the O_2 consumption rate in the premature infant is nearly 3 times that in the adult, consistent with allometric theory (see Chapter 5).[7,8] It is this enormous O_2 consumption rate that explains the rapid decrease in blood O_2 partial pressures in the

neonate during periods of hypoventilation. Although ventilatory gas exchange volume is nearly 10-fold greater in adults than in neonates, the tidal volume relative to body weight for both is approximately equal (6 mL/kg). In neonates, increasing the respiratory rate facilitates the elimination of carbon dioxide (CO_2) generated by their relatively high metabolic processes; alveolar ventilation is approximately 130 mL/kg per minute in the perinatal period, compared with 60 mL/kg per minute in adulthood.

Lungs

Pulmonary Gas Exchange

The structure and function of the immature lung predisposes to alveolar collapse and hypoxia. The premature alveoli are primarily composed of thick-walled, fluid-filled saccular spaces that are surfactant deficient and require greater pressures to initially expand. Production of surfactant by type II alveolar pneumocytes begins between 23 and 24 weeks gestation, although surfactant concentrations often remain inadequate until 36 weeks gestation. These factors lead to the development of respiratory distress syndrome (RDS), which causes reduced lung volumes and lung compliance, increased intrapulmonary shunting, and ventilation-perfusion mismatch. It is clinically characterized by grunting respirations, nasal flaring, and chest retractions that develop shortly after birth. Decreased lung volumes and ventilation-perfusion mismatch may also occur as a consequence of anesthesia. The effects of immature structures, disease, and anesthesia on lung function all increase the risk of hypoxia during surgery and anesthesia.

In neonates, atelectasis might also be caused by anatomic forces that decrease lung volume. For example, the relatively large abdomen in a neonate displaces the diaphragm cephalad, placing the closing capacity within the expiratory reserve volume (see also Fig. 1.8). Moreover, increases in intraabdominal pressure from gastric distention associated with overzealous assisted ventilation with a face mask; replacement of bowel in the abdomen during repair of gastroschisis or omphalocele; or surgical retraction or manipulation of the abdominal contents also might shift the closing capacity to within the infant's expiratory reserve volume. The resulting atelectasis and intrapulmonary shunting may require controlled ventilation with PEEP to recruit closed lung units and improve oxygenation, emptying of the stomach, or changes in surgical maneuvers.

Micropremie lungs are particularly susceptible to volutrauma. Mechanical lung injury is no longer thought to be caused by the use of high peak-inspiratory pressures, but rather related to increased end-inspiratory lung volumes and frequent collapse and reopening of alveoli. A ventilation strategy using small tidal volumes (4–6 mL/kg), greater respiratory rates, PEEP sufficient to avoid alveolar collapse, and permissive hypercapnia reduces lung injury in the premature lung.[9] Permissive hypercapnia (arterial partial pressure of CO_2 [$PaCO_2$] 45–55 mm Hg) results in smaller periods of assisted ventilation and a reduced incidence of bronchopulmonary dysplasia (BPD), without an increase in adverse neurodevelopmental outcomes.[10] A systematic review,[11] however, found contradictory results, with delayed development of BPD with no further benefit from higher $PaCO_2$ values; there was a suggestion of greater risk for intraventricular hemorrhage. It appears that the role of permissive hypercapnia remains unclear. Conversely hypocapnia may result in cerebral ischemia.

Bronchopulmonary Dysplasia

BPD is a chronic lung disease of prematurity, defined as the need for supplemental oxygen for 28 postnatal days.[12–15] Traditionally, BPD has been associated with premature infants subjected to high levels of O_2 and ventilation therapy that causes a lung injury-induced increase in cytokine activation. Other factors that increase the risk for developing BPD include chorioamnionitis and the persistence of a large patent ductus arteriosus (PDA).[16]

Alveolarization begins around 36 weeks gestation. Therefore, lung injury in the premature infant interrupts pulmonary maturation, resulting in larger but fewer alveoli than normal lungs. Decreased lung development in infants with BPD diminishes the surface area for pulmonary gas exchange, which increases O_2 requirements. Moreover, some infants with BPD have reduced lung compliance and increased airway resistance and hence have prolonged pulmonary time constants. Some infants with severe BPD have abnormal muscularization of the vessels in the periphery of their lungs, leading to pulmonary hypertension and right ventricular hypertrophy.

Several strategies may be implemented to prevent the development of BPD. Modalities include antenatal corticosteroid administration to the mother and early postnatal administration to the infant, exogenous surfactant therapy, and specific ventilatory strategies, such as early and aggressive use of CPAP instead of intubation with positive-pressure ventilation, and high-frequency oscillatory ventilation.[17,18] A systematic review of 15 studies, including 2038 neonates, found no difference in the risk for developing BPD between CPAP and high-flow nasal cannula.[19] Treatment of existing BPD often requires ventilatory and medical therapies.[20,21] Ventilation goals should be aimed at the avoidance of intubation if possible, and the use of permissive hypercapnia and smaller tidal volumes in those whose lungs are intubated. Infants with BPD are often treated with diuretics to decrease pulmonary alveolar and interstitial edema. As a result of chronic furosemide treatment, metabolic abnormalities may exist. Hypercalciuria from furosemide may lead to secondary hyperparathyroidism and nephrocalcinosis in some infants. Hydrochlorothiazide and spironolactone produce less severe metabolic abnormalities. Bronchodilators such as aminophylline, albuterol, or ipratropium may be beneficial for reducing airway resistance in some infants with BPD, although data are conflicting.[13,21] Finally, large doses of steroids, especially dexamethasone after the first week of life,[22] provide relief for infants with severe BPD that is refractory to other medical and ventilator therapies.[23,24] However, dexamethasone may cause systemic

TABLE 35.2	Severity-Based Diagnostic Criteria for Bronchopulmonary Dysplasia (BPD)
Gestational age	<32 weeks
Time point of assessment	Postmenstrual age 36 weeks or discharge home, whichever comes first
	Therapy with oxygen >21% for at least 28 days
Mild BPD	Breathing room air
Moderate BPD	Need for <30% oxygen
Severe BPD	Therapy with oxygen >21% for at least 28 days, continued need for ≥30% oxygen and/or positive-pressure ventilation or nasal continuous airway pressure

From Ehrenkranz RA, Walsh MC, Vohr BR, et al. Validation of the National Institutes of Health consensus definition of bronchopulmonary dysplasia. *Pediatrics.* 2005; 116(6):1353-1360.

hypertension, hyperglycemia, hypertrophic cardiomyopathy, and alteration of neurologic and pulmonary development in some children.[25,26] Emerging therapies include the use of sildenafil to improve alveolarization and preserve vascular development, high-frequency oscillatory ventilation with lower tidal volumes, and stem cell therapy.[17,18,27–30]

A severity index for BPD based on the need for supplemental oxygen and/or positive-pressure ventilation or nasal CPAP has been developed and shown to identify a spectrum of risk for adverse pulmonary and neurodevelopmental outcomes in preterm infants (Table 35.2).[31] Although this severity index has not been studied in the context of anesthetic risk, experience suggests that such infants requiring supplemental oxygen, positive pressure, or medications for reactive airways are at greater risk for perioperative pulmonary complications. Anesthetic goals include minimizing the inspired oxygen concentration and tidal volumes while maintaining adequate arterial oxygen saturation (SaO_2 90%–94%) and ventilation ($PaCO_2$ 50–55 mm Hg). The use of smaller tidal volumes decreases the risk of pneumothorax and interstitial emphysema. Preoperative evaluation of infants with BPD requires a very careful history and physical examination, particularly focused on the pulmonary and cardiovascular systems.

Hyperoxia

Some prematurity-related diseases, such as retinopathy of prematurity (ROP) and BPD, have been associated with neonatal exposure to supplemental oxygen (hyperoxia). Oxygen toxicity from hyperoxia leads to the formation of reactive oxygen intermediaries that impair intracellular macromolecules, leading to cell death. The formation of oxygen free radicals also promotes an extensive inflammatory response, leading to secondary tissue damage and cell death. Oxygen-induced vascular endothelial growth factor signals disturbances associated with abnormal angiogenesis; it may be detected in both ROP and BPD.[14]

Controversy exists over the optimal oxygen saturation to target in the premature infant.[32–36] Two studies, the SUPPORT trial (**S**urfactant, **P**ositive **P**ressure, and Pulse **O**ximetry **R**andomized **T**rial) from the United States and the BOOST II trial (**B**enefits **O**f **O**xygen **S**aturation **T**argeting) from the United Kingdom, Australia, and New Zealand reported that a reduced oxygen saturation target range of 85% to 89% had a lower incidence of ROP but an increased mortality compared with a target range of 91%

to 95%.[37–39] However, the COT (**C**anadian **O**xygen **T**rial) and BOOST-NZ (BOOST New Zealand) trials found no differences in either death or disabilities among the two target ranges.[40,41]

A more graded approach according to gestational age uses increasing oxygen saturation targets with increasing age, rather than a generalized approach that aims to target a single goal, has been suggested.[36] For example, an infant younger than 33 weeks (gestational age) should have an oxygen saturation target between 83% and 89%, whereas an infant between 33 and 36 weeks should have a goal between 90% and 94%.[36] However, the optimal range for the graded approach remains controversial. The timing and duration of oxygen therapy may be more important than a targeted oxygen concentration.[42–44] Because of the possible increase in mortality, most practitioners use the 91% to 95% target range for oxygen saturation.

Respiratory Control

Micropremies possess a biphasic ventilatory response to hypoxia. Initially, ventilation increases in response to hypoxia, but after several minutes, ventilation decreases and apnea may ensue.[45] The ventilatory response to CO_2 is decreased in the micropremie, and hypoxia further blunts this response.[46,47] Anesthetic drugs depress the ventilatory responses to both hypoxia and hypercapnia. Hypoxia and hypercapnia occur commonly because of apnea and hypoventilation during emergence and recovery from anesthesia. Thus the combination of anesthetic effects and an immature respiratory control system (see also Fig. 12.12), as well as immature intercostal and diaphragmatic muscles, increases the risk of hypoxia, hypercapnia, and apnea in the postoperative period (see also Figs. 2.13 and 2.14).[48,49]

Apneic episodes occur commonly in the micropremie but decrease with advancing PCA.[50] PCA is defined as the sum of the conception age and the postnatal age. These apneic episodes usually involve both a failure to breathe (central apnea) and/or a failure to maintain a patent airway (obstructive apnea). Central apnea results from decreased respiratory center output, although it may be precipitated by abrupt changes in oxygenation, pulmonary mechanics, brain hemorrhage, hypothermia, or airway stimulation. Apnea may also occur without a precipitating event (i.e., idiopathic). Premature infants with apnea do not increase ventilation in response to hypercapnia, compared with those without apnea, thereby delaying resumption of breathing and prolonging the apneic episode.[51] During obstructive apnea, the airway becomes obstructed in the hypopharynx and larynx as a result of pharyngeal muscle incoordination. Anesthetic drugs may further decrease pharyngeal muscle tone, precipitating airway obstruction during recovery from anesthesia. The combination of anesthetic effects and immature respiratory control places the micropremie at risk for central and obstructive apnea for a prolonged period during recovery from anesthesia.

Not surprisingly, apnea occurs commonly after anesthesia and surgery in premature infants.[52,53] Like apnea of prematurity, postoperative apnea may be central, obstructive, or mixed in origin.[54] The term *postoperative apnea* usually means prolonged apnea (≥15 seconds) or brief apnea accompanied by bradycardia (heart rate ≤80 beats/minute). Postoperative apnea typically occurs as a cluster of episodes over several minutes, with minutes of normal breathing in between the clusters. Bradycardia may occur with apnea, usually beginning at the onset of apnea and is not a response to hypoxia but likely a vagal-mediated response.[55] Arterial oxygen desaturation usually follows the apnea, although many apneic episodes may not have any associated desaturation. Arterial

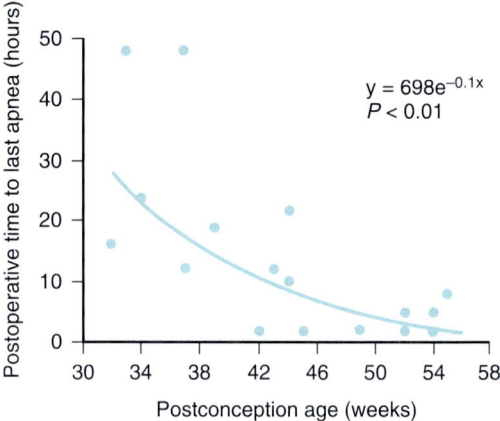

FIGURE 35.2 Time from the end of anesthesia to the last episode of postoperative apnea in prematurely born infants ($r^2 = 0.49$.) (Redrawn with permission from Kurth CD, Spitzer AR, Broennle AM, et al. Postoperative apnea in preterm infants. *Anesthesiology*. 1987;66(4):483-488.)

desaturation is worse with obstructive apnea than with central apnea.[54]

The incidence of postoperative apnea depends on PCA, hematocrit, and the type of surgical procedure (Figure 35.2; see also Fig. 2.12 and E-Fig. 2.7).[52–54,56] The most significant risk factor is the PCA; the lower the PCA, the greater the risk, with the incidence of postoperative apnea in the micropremie greater than 50%.[52,53] Postoperative apnea can occur in the micropremie even without a history of apnea of prematurity.[52] The initial decrease in postoperative apneic events in premature infants occurs at ~44 weeks PCA, but episodes similar to those in full-term infants may occur up to ~60 weeks PCA.[52] Therefore, most centers have adopted a policy where premature infants need to be monitored for 12 continuous hours of apnea-free events after anesthesia when younger than 60 weeks PCA. Many admit these infants for overnight monitoring. Anemia (hematocrit <30%) and younger gestation increase the risk of apnea for a given PCA.[53,56] Postoperative apnea usually begins within an hour of emergence from anesthesia.[52] In the micropremie, it can continue to occur up to 48 hours postoperatively, despite the elimination of anesthetic agents (see Fig. 35.2). In fact, postoperative apnea can occur after surgery with desflurane- or sevoflurane-based anesthetics, or even after surgery for which a regional anesthetic was administered and no general anesthetic drugs were used.[57–60] Although spinal anesthesia may reduce the incidence of apnea within the first 30 minutes in the postanesthesia care unit (PACU), the incidence of late apnea is the same as that after general anesthesia. Postoperative apnea is more common after major procedures, such as a laparotomy, compared with peripheral surgical procedures, such as inguinal hernia repair. These observations indicate that the neurohormonal response to surgery and postoperative pain may play an important role in the origins of postoperative apnea.

Management of postoperative apnea includes close observation with a cardiorespiratory monitor and pulse oximeter, administration of intravenous (IV) methylxanthines, such as caffeine or theophylline (Table 35.3), and prevention/treatment of anemia or hypovolemia. However, we would not recommend routine transfusion unless the neonatology team supported this management preoperatively. There is weak evidence that treatment with caffeine reduces the incidence of BPD, ROP, intraventricular hemorrhage, and the need to treat PDA, but shows no effect on necrotizing

TABLE 35.3 Primary Categories of Apnea in Infants

Cause	Treatment

Central	Increase O$_2$ delivery
	Increase fraction of inspired O$_2$
	Increase hematocrit (?)
	Xanthine derivatives:
	    Theophylline
	    Caffeine

Obstructive	Neck extension Prone or lateral position Oral airway Nasal continuous positive-airway pressure

TABLE 35.4 Circulating Blood Volume in Micropremies, Premies, Full-Term Neonates, Infants, and Children

	Blood Volume (mL/kg)	Weight (kg)	Total Blood Volume (mL)	25-mL Blood Loss Proportion of Total Blood Volume (%)
Micropremie	110	1	110	23
Premie	100	1.75	175	14
Full-term neonate	90	3	270	9
Infant	80	10	800	3
Child	70	20	1400	2

enterocolitis (NEC).[61] Caffeine has a very favorable risk/benefit ratio[61] and is generally preferred over theophylline because it has a longer half-life ($\sim$100 hours)[62–64] and needs less frequent dosing (see also E-Fig. 2.8). Another advantage is that its enteral absorption is more reliable, it has fewer adverse effects (tachycardia and feeding intolerance), and generally does not require serum drug monitoring. A loading dose of 10 mg/kg (IV or oral) is followed by a maintenance dose of 2.5 to 5 mg/kg daily.[65] Aminophylline 5 to 10 mg/kg, a prodrug of theophylline, can also be used intravenously but it is associated with greater irritability than caffeine.[66] Apnea can be exacerbated by opioids in the premature neonate, so their avoidance, if at all possible, is recommended. Obstructive apnea often responds to changes in head position, insertion of an oral or nasal airway, or placing the infant in a prone position. Nasal CPAP, high-flow nasal prongs (HFNP), or tracheal intubation and mechanical ventilation may be required for several days postoperatively if these measures fail.[52]

CARDIOVASCULAR SYSTEM
Immature Versus Adult Heart
The micropremie remains at greater risk of cardiovascular collapse during anesthesia and surgery than does the full-term infant for several reasons. The fetal heart differs from the infant heart in that it has more connective tissue, less organized contractile elements, and increased dependence on extracellular calcium concentration. In addition, the less compliant fetal heart has a flatter Frank-Starling curve (Figs. 16.3 and 16.4) and is less sensitive to catecholamines because of near-maximal baseline β-adrenergic stimulation (see also Chapter 16).[67,68] Consequently, cardiac output in the micropremie depends more on heart rate than it does in the term neonate. The increased resting heart rate in the micropremie also does not permit cardiac output to increase to the same extent as in an infant or child. Additionally, the vagotonic response caused by succinylcholine or its metabolites (succinylmonocholine) and synthetic opioids may lead to bradycardia. These cardiac reflexes can be offset by the vagolytic effects of pancuronium or atropine.[69,70]

The micropremie has a greater blood volume per kilogram, but it has a smaller absolute blood volume (Table 35.4). Therefore, relatively little blood loss during surgery can cause hypovolemia, hypotension, and shock. Because autoregulation is not well developed in the micropremie, the heart rate may not increase with hypovolemia, and blood flow and oxygen delivery to the brain and heart may decrease with relatively little blood loss.[71] Anesthesia blunts baroreceptor reflexes in the micropremie, further limiting the ability to compensate for hypovolemia.[72] The combination

of limited ventricular stroke volume reserve, an increased heart rate, small blood volume, and limited autoregulation predispose the micropremie to cardiovascular collapse during major surgery.

Transition From Fetal to Neonatal Circulation
The lungs are not required for gas exchange in utero because the placenta performs this function. The fetal circulatory pattern consists of atria and ventricles working as units in parallel (see Figs. 16.1 and 16.2). As little as 10% of the fetal right ventricular output may circulate through the lungs.[73] Most of the blood returned from the lower extremities and a portion of the umbilical venous blood supply passes into the pulmonary arteries and subsequently through the ductus arteriosus into the systemic circulation (see Chapters 14 and 16; Fig. 16.1). The superior vena caval blood supply circulates through the foramen ovale (FO) into the left atria and subsequently into the systemic circulation. With expansion of the lungs and increase in oxygen tension during the first breath, pulmonary vascular resistance decreases and blood flow to the lungs increases, matching perfusion with new ventilation; the increased systemic vascular resistance causes a rise in left atrial pressure to close the flap valve of the foramen ovale.[73,74] The increased oxygen tension and loss of prostaglandin E$_2$-based relaxation are thought to result in closure of the ductus arteriosus.[75] Any factor that increases pulmonary vascular resistance (e.g., hypoxia, hypercarbia, acidosis, and hypothermia) may cause the circulation to revert to a fetal circulatory pattern with shunting of deoxygenated blood from the right to the left side of the heart via a patent foramen ovale or PDA (flip-flop circulation).[76–78] This right-to-left shunting of blood explains in part why some infants remain hypoxemic despite ventilation with 100% O$_2$ after a severe desaturation event.

Patent Ductus Arteriosus
In addition to aeration of the lungs, the removal of prostaglandins from the placenta and release of vasoactive substances at birth cause the ductus arteriosus to constrict and functionally close around 12 to 24 hours after birth, with anatomic closure in 2 to 3 weeks. Failure of the ductus arteriosus to close at birth occurs in $\sim$1/2000 full-term births, but affects up to 80% of ELBW infants with the incidence increasing with decreasing gestational age.[79,80] It is thought to be due to immaturity and failure of smooth muscle cells within the ductus to constrict, as well as immaturity of the lungs, which are responsible for metabolizing prostaglandins.[75]

With the increase in systemic vascular resistance and decrease in pulmonary vascular resistance at birth, a PDA often results in considerable left-to-right shunting of blood, causing excess pulmonary blood flow, congestive heart failure, and respiratory failure. Diastolic runoff of blood into the pulmonary artery leads to a widened pulse pressure (owing to low diastolic blood pressure) and risk of coronary ischemia. In a neonate with respiratory distress syndrome or persistent pulmonary hypertension, right-to-left shunting across the PDA may occur, producing cyanosis. Paradoxical embolism is another concern with a PDA, as well as a patent foramen ovale.[78] Fluid restriction and diuretic therapy, often used to treat congestive heart failure from left-to-right shunting through a PDA, further increase the risk of hypotension during surgery. The use of nonsteroidal antiinflammatory drugs to close the PDA can cause renal compromise.[81–83]

Persistent Pulmonary Hypertension and Inhaled Nitric Oxide
Persistent pulmonary hypertension of the newborn (PPHN) and refractory hypoxemia in neonates occurs in approximately 2/1000 live births.[84,85] PPHN is diagnosed when right-to-left shunting of blood occurs through a PDA and/or patent foramen ovale in the absence of other congenital heart disease. Right-to-left shunting results from the failure of the pulmonary vascular resistance (PVR) to decrease at birth, thus preventing the conversion from fetal to neonatal pulmonary blood flow. The exact etiology of PPHN is not understood, but has been attributed to a variety of factors, including increased muscularization of pulmonary arterial vessels, impaired endothelial release of nitric oxide (NO), increased production of vasoconstrictors (e.g., endothelin-1), and impaired vascular endothelial growth factor.[86] It can be associated with circumstances leading to perinatal distress (meconium aspiration, sepsis, asphyxia), be idiopathic, and rarely, genetic.[87]

PPHN is suspected in severely hypoxic neonates who do not have an increase in postductal O_2 saturation despite mechanical ventilation with an increased fraction of inspired oxygen (FiO_2). A greater preductal versus postductal O_2 saturation supports the diagnosis because it reflects the extrapulmonary right-to-left shunting of deoxygenated blood via the PDA. An echocardiogram excludes the presence of a congenital heart defect as the cause of or a contributing factor of pulmonary hypertension and/or right-to-left shunt. It is imperative to diagnose and treat PPHN in a timely fashion as the morbidity, including neurodevelopmental delay, cerebral palsy, deafness, blindness, and mortality are substantive.[88–91] Premature infants tend to have worse outcomes and have more severe PPHN, requiring extracorporeal membrane oxygenation (ECMO) support earlier and more frequently than full-term neonates.[92]

The American Heart Association and American Thoracic Society have published guidelines for the diagnosis and treatment of PPHN. Treatment strategies aim to maintain adequate systemic blood pressure, maximize oxygen delivery, and optimize ventilator management to protect lung volume and function.[89,92] Normal lung expansion should be the goal of mechanical ventilation. Caution must be taken to avoid overdistending the lung, which can increase PVR. In cases of severe parenchymal lung disease, such as meconium aspiration, in which airway disease can lead to atelectasis and intrapulmonary shunt, PEEP and exogenous surfactant may be used to recruit alveoli. Although inspired O_2 is a potent vasodilator, maximum dilation of the pulmonary vasculature is achieved by relatively low levels of oxygen tension, and hyperoxia can potentiate lung injury. For these reasons, increasing the FiO_2 often does not improve gas exchange in PPHN. Acidosis causes pulmonary vasoconstriction and should be avoided; this led to the practice in the past of inducing alkalosis by hyperventilation of the lungs or by infusing sodium bicarbonate. However, there is no evidence of any long-term benefit with this approach, and such

management has been shown to worsen pulmonary vascular tone and lead to worse neurodevelopmental outcomes.[92,93] ECMO should be considered in those infants with severe sustained hypoxemia or compromised hemodynamic function.

Inhaled nitric oxide (iNO) is a selective pulmonary vasodilator used to treat PPHN.[94–96] NO is normally produced by the endothelium and diffuses into subjacent smooth muscle cells, where it increases cyclic guanosine monophosphate (cGMP) levels that play a role in intracellular calcium levels and vasomotor protein function, leading to vascular relaxation (Fig. 35.3). iNO decreases PVR, limiting right-to-left shunting of blood, increases systemic O_2 partial pressures, and reduces the need for ECMO support in neonates with pulmonary hypertension.[92,93,97,98] However, not all infants respond to iNO,[99] and the use of iNO may not reduce mortality, length of stay in the hospital, or risk of neurodevelopmental impairment.[92,93,100] In contrast to full-term neonates, the success of iNO in the micropremie with hypoxic respiratory failure and pulmonary hypertension remains unclear.[92,93,97] Even among full-term neonates, some conditions such as congenital diaphragmatic hernia (CDH) do not respond well to iNO.[93,101]

When iNO is administered, the optimal initial dose is 20 ppm (Fig. 35.4). There is no advantage in terms of improvement in oxygen requirements to starting iNO at doses greater than 20 ppm. Moreover, doses greater than 20 ppm for extended periods may produce methemoglobinemia and/or nitrogen dioxide.[102] Methemoglobin concentration should be monitored if large concentrations of iNO are used. Fig. 35.4 delineates both treatment and weaning algorithms for iNO. Care must be taken to slowly wean the iNO to avoid rebound pulmonary hypertension. Weaning should cease if the oxygen requirements increase at any stage during the weaning process and be resumed once the oxygen requirements stabilize. Some who encounter hypoxemia during weaning may benefit from phosphodiesterase inhibitors such as sildenafil or milrinone that prolong the duration of action of endogenous NO. Sildenafil (Revatio) is a phosphodiesterase-5 inhibitor that selectively reduces PVR. It has been recommended for PPHN that is refractory to iNO, although the US Food and Drug Administration (FDA) issued a black box warning in 2012 against chronic use of sildenafil in children. It may be administered orally or intravenously. Milrinone may also be added to treat infants with PPHN when left ventricular dysfunction is present. Prostacyclin-I_2 (e.g., epoprostenol IV or treprostinil oral, IV or subcutaneous) has been used to treat PPHN (as well as iNO-resistant PPHN); however, it has a very brief half-life (5 minutes) and requires permanent vascular access for continuous administration.[84,85] Any interruption in therapy will rapidly result in profound rebound pulmonary hypertension with many untoward adverse effects. Inhaled prostaglandin-I_2 analogs (e.g., iloprost) and endothelin receptor antagonists (e.g., bosentan) may also be used in iNO refractory PPHN.[103]

NEUROLOGIC DEVELOPMENT
Immature Brain
The central nervous system (CNS) is incompletely developed at birth. Regions of the CNS develop at different times during gestation; consequently, the impact of premature birth depends on gestational age at birth and the severity of cardiovascular, respiratory, and other postnatal stressors. The area of the brain most susceptible to injury in the micropremie is the periventricular white matter.[98,104] The white matter consists of preoligodendrocytes,

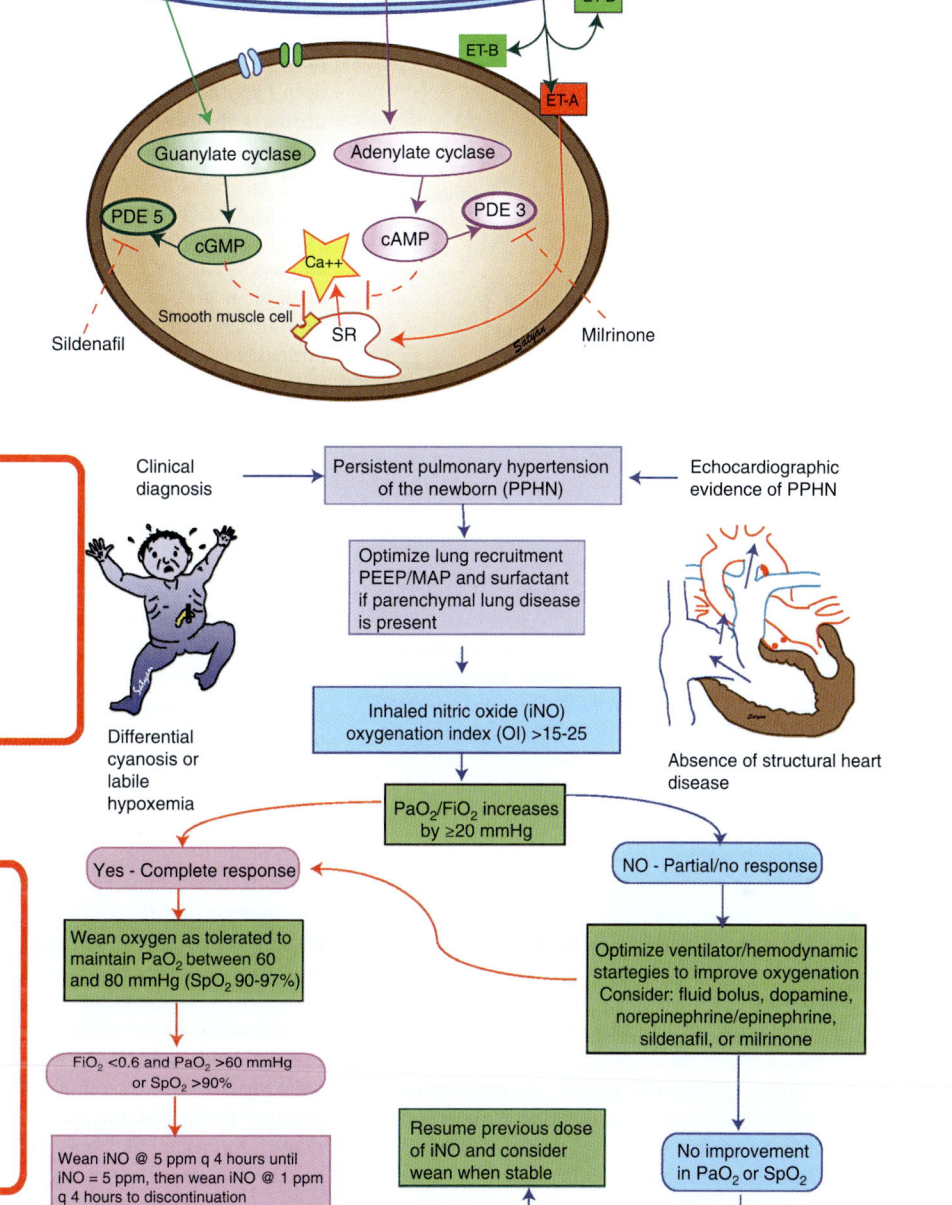

FIGURE 35.3 A, Nitric oxide *(NO)* produced by nitric oxide synthase in endothelial cells diffuses into subjacent smooth muscle cells, interacts with soluble guanylate cyclase, and increases the concentration of cyclic guanosine monophosphate *(cGMP)* to cause vascular relaxation. The effect of NO is decreased by metabolism of cGMP by specific phosphodiesterases *(PDE)*. **B,** Treatment algorithm for persistent pulmonary hypertension of the newborn *(PPHN)*. *ECMO,* Extracorporeal membrane oxygenation; *ET-A,* endothelin type A; *ET-B,* endothelin type B; *FiO2,* fraction of inspired oxygen; *L-arg,* L-arginine; *MAP,* mean arterial pressure; *OI,* oxygenation index; *P/F,* Pao2/ Fraction of inspired oxygen; *Pao2,* arterial oxygenation; *PEEP,* positive end-expiratory pressure; *Spo2,* oxygen saturation as measured by pulse oximetry; *SR,* sarcoplasmic reticulum.

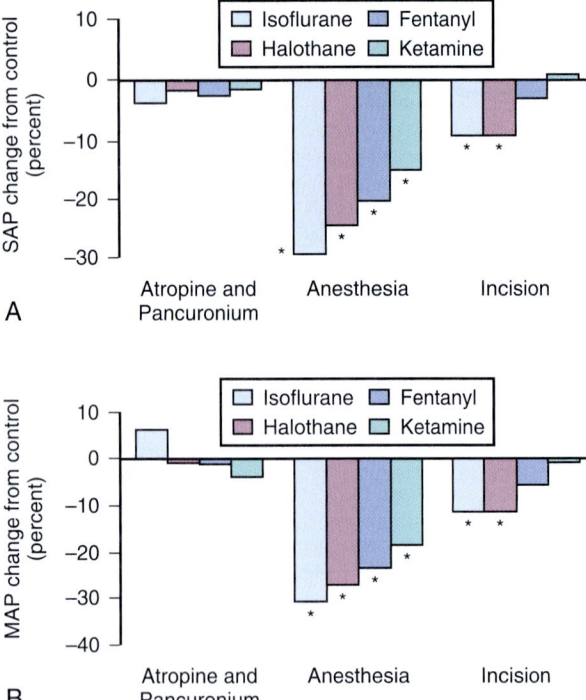

FIGURE 35.4 A, Changes in systolic arterial pressure *(SAP)* in preterm infants after anesthesia with either isoflurane, halothane, fentanyl, or ketamine, and after surgical incision. **B,** Changes in mean arterial pressure *(MAP)* in premature infants after anesthesia with either isoflurane, halothane, fentanyl, or ketamine, and after surgical incision. (Reprinted with permission from Friesen RH, Henry DB. Cardiovascular changes in preterm neonates receiving isoflurane, halothane, fentanyl, and ketamine. *Anesthesiology.* 1986;64(2):238-242.)

astrocytes, and neuronal axons. Late in the second trimester (24 to 27 weeks gestation), preoligodendrocytes and astrocytes multiply tremendously and most cortical and subcortical structures begin to develop.[98] The periventricular white matter is perfused by arteries penetrating from the cortical surface and by lenticulostriate arteries from the circle of Willis. During this period, the periventricular white matter is particularly susceptible to neurologic injury as it is a "watershed region," susceptible to poor perfusion and hypoxic-ischemic injury during hypotension, reduced cardiac output, hypoxemia, and hypocarbia.[105,104]

Neural pathways responsible for the perception of pain develop during the first, second, and third trimesters (see also Chapters 1, 41, and 42).[100] During the first trimester, peripheral sensory receptors and spinal reflex arcs mature, yielding the "withdrawal reflex" to non-noxious stimuli. Neurons that transmit nociception appear in the dorsal root ganglia at 19 weeks gestation, and afferent neurons from the thalamus reach the cortical subplate and cortical plate between 20 and 24 weeks gestation. However, it is not until early in the third trimester (29 weeks gestation) that pathways between the thalamus and somatosensory cortex are functional. Controversy exists regarding the exact gestational age at which perception and memory of pain occur,[106,107] particularly before 24 weeks gestational age.[108] The hormonal responses to pain and stress may be exaggerated in neonates, although the clinical significance of this has not been defined.[109,110] Nevertheless, current practice in the micropremie is to administer anesthesia during surgery and provide pain management postoperatively.

Glucose and the Brain

The neonatal brain requires a larger percentage of glucose production because of the greater brain weight in proportion to body weight. Hyperglycemia has been implicated as detrimental to the adult brain during global and focal ischemia, such as with a cerebral or hypoxemic ischemic event and during cardiac surgery with deep hypothermic cardiac arrest.[111] In contrast, hyperglycemia in neonates appears to protect the brain from ischemic damage or at the very least be less harmful than hypoglycemia.[112,113] Both neonatal rat and pig hypoxia-ischemia models observed less brain damage with greater glucose concentrations. Many mechanisms exist for this strikingly different outcome between neonates and adults.[114] Relatively mild hypoglycemia is known to cause brain damage in preterm infants.[115,116] Micropremies with critical illness are especially prone to hypoglycemia because they contain limited stores of glucose and consume glucose anaerobically. Thus the administration of dextrose-containing fluids (carefully controlled with an infusion pump to minimize wide serum glucose fluctuations) and close monitoring of blood glucose concentrations are vital during anesthesia.[104] Mild or moderate hyperglycemia during surgery is best managed by reducing the rate of infusion of dextrose-containing solutions and not administering insulin, with its attendant risk of hypoglycemia.

Complications of Prematurity

Despite decreases in mortality in the micropremie, long-term neurologic and developmental disabilities remain common in this group and include cerebral palsy, cognitive deficits, behavioral abnormalities, and hearing and visual impairment.[98,117] In a study of ELBW infants, only 25% were classified as "normally developed" at 5 years of age; 20% exhibited major disabilities.[117] Brain magnetic resonance imaging (MRI) has identified a spectrum of abnormalities in these infants. The most common abnormality is diffuse high signal intensity on T2-weighted imaging in the periventricular cerebral white matter. Diffusion-weighted imaging shows increased apparent diffusion coefficient values, indicative of increased water content and delayed white matter maturation, suggesting ischemia-reperfusion injury in periventricular white matter, which has activated microglia and damaged preoligodendrocytes.[98,118] Damage to preoligodendrocytes impairs myelination of cerebral white matter axons and accounts for many of the fine motor, speech, and cognitive deficits. On MRI, tissue volumes in the basal ganglia, corpus callosum, amygdala, and hippocampus are reduced and correlate with smaller full-scale, verbal, and performance IQ scores.[119] Collectively, these MRI findings indicate that different regions of the brain vary in their susceptibility to injury during development and that such injuries lead to specific long-term disturbances in neurocognitive function.[120]

Intraventricular Hemorrhage

Intraventricular hemorrhage (IVH) occurs in as many as one-third of micropremie infants. Although an association has been noted between the incidence of IVH and fluctuations in blood pressure, it is difficult to confirm any causal relationship. The severity of IVH, as defined by head ultrasound, is graded as:

- Grade 1: hemorrhage limited to the germinal matrix
- Grade 2: hemorrhage extending into the ventricular system
- Grade 3: hemorrhage into the ventricular system and with ventricular dilatation
- Grade 4: hemorrhage extending into brain parenchyma

Although micropremie infants with grade 3 or 4 IVH are more likely to exhibit severe long-term neurocognitive sequelae, even micropremie infants with grade 1 and 2 IVH display poorer neurodevelopmental outcomes compared with those without IVH.[119,121,122] Early onset of IVH appears during the first day of life. Risk factors include fetal distress, vaginal delivery, reduced Apgar scores, metabolic acidosis, severe hypercapnia, and the need for mechanical ventilation.[123–125] Late onset of IVH appears days to weeks after birth with contributing factors including respiratory distress syndrome, seizures, pneumothoraxes, hypoxemia, acidosis, severe hypercarbia, and the use of vasopressor infusions.[123,126] Lack of autoregulation leading to rapid fluctuations in cerebral blood flow, cerebral blood volume, and cerebral venous pressure, as well as fragile cerebral blood vessels, appear to play a role in the development of IVH.[71,126,127] Factors that may decrease the incidence and severity of IVH include administration of antenatal glucocorticoids or indomethacin.[128] Indomethacin helps to blunt the hyperemic response to hypoxia, improve cerebral autoregulation, and promote microvessel maturation of the germinal matrix. Although indomethacin decreases the incidence and severity of IVH, there is no evidence that long-term outcomes are improved.[128,129] Corticosteroids produce vasoconstrictive effects on fetal cerebral blood flow, protecting the fetus against IVH at rest and when challenged by conditions causing vasodilatation such as hypercapnia, leading to a significant reduction in IVH.[130]

TEMPERATURE REGULATION

The micropremie is very susceptible to hypothermia. Heat loss occurs by four possible routes: radiation (39%), convection (34%), evaporation (24%), and conduction (3%). In the micropremie, evaporative heat loss and insensible fluid loss are increased because the epidermis has less keratin.[131] Conductive and convective heat losses are also increased because the micropremie has little subcutaneous fat for insulation and a large surface area/mass ratio. Thermal regulation is not well developed in the micropremie. Even full-term neonates do not have the capability to shiver or sweat, relying instead on nonshivering thermogenesis. Nonshivering thermogenesis, which depends on brown fat stores (that do not develop until 26- to 30 weeks gestation), is decreased in the micropremie and regulation of skin blood flow is less efficient.[132–134] During anesthesia, measures should be undertaken to minimize radiation and convective heat loss by warming the operating room (OR) to 80°F to 85°F (26.7°C–29.4°C) before the neonate arrives, and minimizing convective heat loss during transport (i.e., use a thermoneutral incubator or a warming mattress, and keep them covered). The most effective means to maintain normothermia and to warm the micropremie is a forced-air warmer. Other strategies that may be useful to maintain normothermia include using a warming pad on the operating table to reduce conductive heat loss, overhead heat lamps to reduce radiant heat loss, and keeping the skin dry to reduce evaporative heat loss. Additional strategies to reduce heat loss include using humidified gases in the ventilator circuit, covering the head, and warming IV and irrigation fluids before they are used.[135] Temperature should be carefully monitored as overheating of the infant may readily occur.

RENAL AND METABOLIC FUNCTION
Renal Function
The kidneys are not fully developed at birth.[136] Full-term neonates have a glomerular filtration rate (GFR) that is only 30% of

normal adult rates owing to fewer nephrons and smaller glomerular size.[137–140] In fact, the GFR does not reach normal adult values until approximately 1 year of age (see Fig. 5.13).[138] Maternal transplacental transfer of creatinine in utero increases the creatinine level in the neonate for the first few days of life.[141] The baseline plasma concentrations of creatinine increase with increasing prematurity and remain increased until approximately 3 weeks of age because of immature renal function and the consequent lower creatinine clearance compared with full-term infants.[142] These factors affect the metabolism and elimination rate of many drugs in the neonate. The renal excretion of medications such as penicillin, gentamicin, and some neuromuscular blocking drugs such as pancuronium may be prolonged, resulting in increased duration of action or the development of high blood concentrations. This effect is particularly important when administering medications to an extremely premature infant. Thus, the use of neuromuscular blocking drugs that do not require renal function are advantageous (e.g., cisatracurium). Alternatively, if neuromuscular blocking drugs such as rocuronium or vecuronium are used, it is advised to reverse with sugammadex.[143] The neuromuscular blocking drug-sugammadex complex is also renally excreted; however, evidence has shown rapid and optimal reversal of neuromuscular blockade without recurarization in patients with renal disease.[144–148]

Very premature infants easily become hyponatremic because of reduced proximal tubular reabsorption of sodium and water and reduced receptors for hormones that influence tubular sodium transport. As many as one-third of ELBW neonates develop hyponatremia.[139] Frequent assessments of the serum concentration of sodium and free water requirements are important during critical illness. Increased serum concentrations of potassium occur in premature infants during the first few days after birth. The increase results from a shift in potassium from the intracellular to extracellular spaces.[140] These increases are greater as gestational age and birth weight decrease.[149] Reduced cardiac output and urine production may further increase serum concentrations of potassium and predispose to cardiac arrhythmias.[150]

The total body water content in neonates is greater than in infants, children, and adults. In a term infant, 70% of the body weight is water (see also Figs. 5.9 and 5.10).[151] By 6 to 12 months of age, 50% to 60% of the body weight is water. In the premature infant, 75% to 85% of the body weight is water. In general, the smaller the PCA of the neonate, the greater the percent of water present. Differences among the total body water, renal maturity, and serum protein concentrations in a neonate affect the volume of distribution and protein binding of many medications. Because the volume of distribution of drugs confined to the extracellular fluid is increased, the initial doses of some medications (e.g., neuromuscular blocking drugs, aminoglycosides) may be greater on a weight basis in neonates than adults to achieve the desired blood concentration. In contrast, because of immaturity of renal function, the interval between doses of these drugs must be increased.

Fluid Management
The basic principles of fluid maintenance in neonates are similar to those in older children and adults. The highly variable body fluid composition, degree of renal maturity, neuroendocrine control of intravascular fluid status, and insensible fluid loss with age make precise estimates of fluid requirements in neonates challenging.[152–154] Urine volume and concentration may be difficult to determine intraoperatively and may not always correlate with volume status. Moreover, blood pressure and heart rate may not

correlate with intravascular volume status in premature infants, and anesthetics may mask subtle cardiovascular changes that occur with changes in intravascular volume. Increased insensible fluid loss, which often occurs in the OR environment, requires judicious titration of IV fluids. Congenital abnormalities (e.g., gastroschisis, omphalocele) may markedly increase insensible fluid loss through exposure of large mucosal surfaces. The use of humidified gas mixtures reduces insensible fluid loss through the respiratory tract. However, overzealous intraoperative administration of fluids can result in pulmonary complications and worsened third spacing of fluids, particularly in preterm infants.[155–157] It is recommended to use volume-controlled devices for fluid management, such as an infusion device that holds limited quantities of IV fluids or medications or an IV infusion pump, to ensure accurate fluid administration.

Calcium Homeostasis

During the third trimester, calcium is delivered to the fetus from the mother via placental transfer, resulting in fetal hypercalcemia. At birth, serum calcium concentrations decrease with the abrupt loss of maternal calcium and reach a nadir at 2 days.[158,159] By the third day of life, the combination of parathyroid hormone (PTH) secretion, dietary calcium intake, renal calcium reabsorption, skeletal calcium stores, and vitamin D allow the serum calcium concentrations in the full-term neonate to return to normal.[160]

Infants who are born prematurely do not benefit from the transfer of maternal calcium and are at greater risk for hypocalcemia after birth.[161] In addition, premature infants experience hypocalcemia owing to hypoalbuminemia (reduces serum but not ionized calcium), limited oral intake, impaired secretion and response to PTH, increased calcitonin levels, and increased urinary losses as a result of increased renal excretion of sodium. Hypocalcemia has been observed in nearly 40% of critically ill neonates.[162–164] Causes of hypocalcemia in the latter population include PTH insufficiency and peripheral resistance to PTH, inadequate calcium supplementation, and altered calcium metabolism caused by transfusion with citrated blood products, bicarbonate administration, or diuretics (e.g., furosemide).

Calcium exists in the serum in three fractions: protein bound; chelated to bicarbonate, phosphate, and citrate; and free or ionized calcium (iCa^{2+}). The ionized fraction is the physiologically active component; however, there is not always a clear relationship between total serum calcium and iCa^{2+}. The correlation is poor with hypoalbuminemia or acid-base disturbances, as seen in premature and critically ill neonates. Hypocalcemia is defined as a total serum calcium concentration less than 8 mg/dL (2 mmol/L) in full-term infants and less than 7 mg/dL (1.75 mmol/L) in premature infants. An iCa^{2+} less than 4 mg/dL (1 mmol/L) defines hypocalcemia in both populations.

Hypocalcemia may be asymptomatic or accompanied by nonspecific symptoms such as neuromuscular irritability (myoclonic jerks, exaggerated startle, or seizures), tachycardia, prolonged QT interval, and decreased cardiac contractility. Diagnosis rests on the determination of total and iCa^{2+} levels. Neonatal hypocalcemia is a feature of DiGeorge syndrome (chromosome 22q11.2 deletion),[165] also known as velocardiofacial syndrome, secondary to underdeveloped or absent parathyroid glands. The syndrome also involves abnormal facial characteristics, cardiac defects, thymic hypoplasia, and cleft palate.

Symptomatic hypocalcemia may be treated with 90 mg/kg calcium gluconate or 30 mg/kg calcium chloride[166] by slow IV infusion over 5 to 10 minutes while monitoring the electrocardiogram, as bradyarrhythmias may develop in response to rapid increases in the serum concentration of calcium.[160] The IV site must also be closely monitored for extravasation as exogenous calcium supplementation may cause tissue necrosis and subcutaneous calcification deposits. Alternatively, if calcium chloride is administered, it should ideally be infused through a central IV line.[160] If using an umbilical venous catheter (UVC), caution must be taken to ensure the tip of the catheter is in the inferior vena cava (IVC) because direct infusion into the portal system can cause hepatic necrosis. Maintenance calcium gluconate dosing is administered at 80 mg/kg per day for the first 48 hours, followed by 40 mg/kg per day for the next 24 hours, and then discontinued. The clinical response and serum iCa^{2+} concentrations should be monitored. Treatment of hypocalcemia is not effective in the presence of hypomagnesemia. In such a situation, parenteral administration of supplemental magnesium and calcium and treatment of the underlying cause of hypocalcemia are necessary.[162] Persistent hypocalcemia necessitates determination of magnesium, phosphorus, PTH, and vitamin D concentrations.

Glucose Homeostasis

Early in gestation, the fetal liver begins to store glycogen while a continuous supply of glucose is delivered by transplacental transfer from the mother. In the third trimester, glycogen stores begin to develop in fetal skeletal and cardiac muscle, as well as in the kidneys, intestines, and brain. At birth neonatal glucose concentrations decrease rapidly to 30 mg/dL within the first 1 to 2 hours, stimulating glycogenolysis and gluconeogenesis.[167,168] The glucose flux usually stabilizes at values greater than 45 mg/dL (2.5 mmol/L) by 12 hours.[167,168] The premature infant is prone to hypoglycemia owing to immature glucoregulatory mechanisms, reduced levels of glycogen storage, increased energy demands, and limited adipose stores (reduced free fatty acids and ketones available as alternative sources of energy).[167] Full-term infants who have been excessively fasted, small-for-gestational-age (SGA) infants, and infants of diabetic mothers are also prone to develop hypoglycemia.[169]

The definition of hypoglycemia varies in the literature and among institutions. In full-term neonates, hypoglycemia is defined as a glucose concentration less than 40 mg/dL (2.2 mmol/L) during the first 24 hours after birth and less than 60 mg/dL (3.3 mmol/L) at 36 hours. In premature infants or those at risk for hypoglycemia,[170] the threshold for hypoglycemia at 24 hours is less than 45 mg/dL and at greater than 24 hours is less than 50 mg/dL (2.8 mmol/L).[167,171] Signs and symptoms of hypoglycemia tend to be nonspecific and many are masked under anesthesia.[167,172] Hypoglycemia may manifest as respiratory distress, apnea, cyanosis, seizures, tremors, high-pitched cry, irritability, limpness, lethargy, eye-rolling, poor feeding, temperature instability, and sweating.[172,173]

A bolus of 0.25 to 0.5 grams/kg (1–2 mL/kg of dextrose 25% in water [$D_{25}W$] or 2.5–5 mL/kg of $D_{10}W$) and an increase in the basal glucose infusion are prudent measures to treat hypoglycemia. Full-term infants require a glucose infusion rate of 5 to 8 mg/kg per minute to prevent hypoglycemia. However, premature and SGA infants have greater glucose requirements, and thus require infusion rates of 8 to 10 mg/kg per minute. It is extremely important to reassess the blood glucose concentration after these treatments to determine the effectiveness of the therapy. A single bolus of glucose without subsequent infusion can stimulate insulin production with consequent return to the hypoglycemic state.

Infants undergoing surgical procedures often require less glucose supplementation.[174,175] This reduced need may be attributed to hormonal responses that decrease glucose uptake as a result of catecholamine release in excess of insulin activity, as well as a decrease in metabolic demand from the effects of the anesthetic agents.[109,110,176] Nonetheless, it is important to administer glucose-containing solutions using a constant-infusion device to avoid large fluctuations in blood glucose concentrations and to monitor blood glucose concentrations in critically ill neonates.[177] All other fluids (e.g., to replace third-space losses, blood loss, and fluid deficits) should be glucose-free to avoid hyperglycemia.[174,175] Infants treated with glucose via total parental nutrition (TPN) may develop severe hypoglycemia if the infusion rate is abruptly lowered; thus, it is important to continue these infusions (possibly at a slightly reduced rate) during surgery and to check the serum glucose concentrations.

GASTROINTESTINAL AND HEPATIC FUNCTION

The anatomic structures of the fetal gastrointestinal (GI) tract are formed in the second trimester; however, the functional maturation does not occur until later in gestation and continues after birth.[178] For example, compared with adults, gastric emptying in neonates is prolonged and lower esophageal sphincters are incompetent, making reflux of stomach contents common, even in the full-term neonate.[178]

Premature infants, however, are susceptible to a multitude of complications because of the immaturity of the GI system at birth. Intestinal motility increases between 29 and 32 weeks gestation and is stimulated by enteral feeds. A full-term infant usually passes meconium within the first 48 hours; however, less than 50% of micropremies pass meconium in that time frame, and it may be delayed by days to weeks. Intestinal motility is also important to decrease the time allowed for colonization of harmful bacteria in the GI tract.[179] Increased time for bacterial growth, coupled with decreased bactericidal gastric and pancreatic secretions and immature GI immune defenses, renders the micropremie at risk for infections and the development of NEC. Enteric feeds increase intestinal motility in premature infants. However, controversy exists over the optimal time to start enteral feeds and which type of nutrition is best (mother's milk, donated human milk, or various types of formulas).[180–182] Early feeding of premature infants with hypertonic or trophic feeds (<10–20 mL/kg per day) is well tolerated, although the volume and frequency should be increased very gradually in premature infants to limit the risk of feeding intolerance.[180,183] A Cochrane review failed to associate early trophic feeding with the development of NEC or other bowel difficulties in extremely premature infants compared with prolonged enteral fasting.[181,182,184]

Hepatic metabolism is immature in neonates, particularly in premature infants. Drug metabolism may be slow because of immaturity of enzymatic processes, reduction of hepatic proteins, and relatively low hepatic perfusion (less drug delivered to the liver)(see also Chapters 4 and 5). Any factor that further compromises hepatic blood flow (e.g., increased intraabdominal pressure) may have profound adverse effects on drugs with perfusion-limited hepatic clearance.[185] Therefore, careful titration of these drugs (e.g., opioids, propofol) is required to optimize therapeutic effects and prevent toxicity. Just as consideration is given to immature renal function, the use of neuromuscular blocking drugs that do not require hepatic metabolism is advantageous (e.g., cisatracurium). The use of remifentanil (a drug cleared by plasma esterases that mature at birth) during the procedure, followed by a small dose of longer-acting opioid or regional block at the end of the procedure might facilitate early extubation.

In addition, reduced albumin synthesis decreases albumin concentrations compared with term neonates, enhancing the free (unbound) concentration of anesthetic drugs that are highly bound to albumin (see E-Fig. 5.2 and Figs. 5.8 and 5.10). Increased concentrations of unbound serum bilirubin introduces the risk of kernicterus, particularly in infants who are premature, hypoxemic, and acidotic and have low serum protein concentrations.[186,187] Highly protein-bound agents such as furosemide, sulfonamides, ceftriaxone, and benzyl alcohol (found as a preservative in many drugs such as diazepam) may displace bilirubin and increase the possibility of kernicterus.[186] The micropremie is also at particular risk for spontaneous liver hemorrhage.[188,189] This occurs most commonly during laparotomy for NEC, is associated with large IV fluid resuscitation, and is difficult to control surgically. Vitamin K–dependent coagulation factors may be less; one case report described the apparent successful use of recombinant factor VIIa to stop liver hemorrhage when administration of other blood products had failed.[190]

HEMATOLOGIC FUNCTION

Full-term newborns are born with an average hemoglobin (Hgb) concentration of 16.8 g/dL. This increase in Hgb is the result of increased production of fetal Hgb (Hgb-F) during the second and third trimesters, as well as an increase in the production of adult Hgb (Hgb-A) between 34 and 36 weeks gestation. This prepares the infant for the physiologic anemia of the newborn that develops between 8 and 12 weeks of life as the result of the fall in Hgb-F at birth and slow rise in erythropoietin (EPO) levels. The kidneys start transcribing EPO at 17 weeks gestation; however, production is not noteworthy until around 30 weeks. At birth EPO production is initially decreased because of greater oxygen tensions and is subsequently stimulated by the anemia of the neonate. Therefore, the premature infant has several reasons for being more susceptible to anemia at birth (average Hgb of 9.4 g/dL),[191] which is more pronounced than the full-term neonate (average Hgb of 11.0 g/dL).[192] The leftward shift of the oxygen-Hgb dissociation curve resulting from the decreased affinity of Hgb-F for 2,3-diphosphoglycerate is also more pronounced in the premature infant, further contributing to reduced effective oxygen carrying capacity.

The ideal hematocrit for the micropremie remains controversial. In the micropremie with reduced oxygen saturations and cardiac output, tissue oxygen delivery is maximized by maintaining the hematocrit between 44% and 48%. In a randomized study of liberal versus restrictive transfusion in neonates weighing between 500 and 1300 grams, intraparenchymal brain hemorrhage, periventricular leukomalacia, and episodes of apnea occurred more frequently in the restrictive transfusion group.[193,194] However, another more recent retrospective study favored restrictive transfusion using the same outcome measures[195]; a meta-analysis found no increase in short- or long-term mortality.[196] The risks of blood transfusion in the micropremie must be balanced against the benefits of improved oxygen delivery and fewer medical complications.

Thrombocytopenia (platelet count <150,000/mm³) occurs in as many as 70% of micropremies and neonatal platelets have relative hypoactive function compared with older children and adults.[197–199] Although the etiology of thrombocytopenia is often unknown, pathophysiologic processes such as sepsis, disseminated intravascular coagulation, and NEC are common causes. Platelet transfusions in general should be guided by clinical bleeding as there is an increased mortality with liberal rather than restrictive indications.[198,200] In addition to thrombocytopenia, premature infants are at increased risk for bleeding as the result of increased capillary fragility and decreased concentration of vitamin K–dependent coagulation factors. Preoperative evaluation should include a recent platelet count and coagulation studies; the availability of platelets and fresh frozen plasma and/or cryoprecipitate for major procedures should be assured.

Anesthetics and the Neonate/Premature Infant

ANESTHETICS AND THE IMMATURE BRAIN

Research in immature animals indicates that anesthetics are both neuroprotective and neurotoxic. Inhalational anesthetics protect against hypoxic-ischemic injury in neonatal pigs and rats.[201–203] The anesthetic must be administered before and during the ischemic event at a concentration of 1 minimal alveolar concentration (MAC) to be effective. Thus, for surgery in which there is a risk of brain ischemia, use of an inhalational anesthetic may afford some advantage over IV agents. Cardiac surgery, ventricular shunt insertion, and vein of Galen embolization represent examples of procedures performed in preterm infants that carry a significant risk of brain ischemia. The MAC for sevoflurane has not been established in premature infants, and unfortunately many sick preterm infants cannot tolerate even modest concentrations of potent anesthetic agents.

Of particular concern are the reports in immature rats and other animals, including primates, that prolonged exposure to commonly used anesthetics, such as isoflurane, ketamine, and midazolam, induces apoptosis in many regions of the brain (see Chapter 23).[204,205] If this phenomenon applies to humans, the premature infant could potentially be more susceptible to anesthetic neurotoxicity than is the full-term infant.

A confounding factor is that neurodegeneration and apoptosis is a normal developmental phenomenon in the maturing fetal brain. Furthermore, anesthesia-induced neuronal cell death in neonatal animals may not directly translate into long-term neurologic abnormalities. Indeed, evidence suggests that sevoflurane-induced cognitive impairment, in the form of short-term memory deficiency in neonatal rodents, is offset by delayed exercise.[206] Moreover, immature animals that undergo painful procedures without anesthesia experience neuronal degeneration.[207,208] Premature infants who receive anesthesia and sedation for painful procedures experience less morbidity and mortality than those who do not.[209,210] Curiously, the combination of surgery and anesthesia in neonatal rats produces more apoptosis than either intervention alone, suggesting that in this model, anesthetics are neither neuroprotective themselves nor do they offset the apoptotic effects of surgery.[211] In summary, the neurodegeneration precipitated by inhaled anesthetics, ketamine, and benzodiazepines depends on developmental age, brain region, and duration of exposure. Based on the animal models, the micropremie exposed to several hours of inhaled agents with nitrous oxide (N_2O) and midazolam is potentially at risk, as is the micropremie who is insufficiently anesthetized during surgery. One anesthetic approach is to use opioids (e.g., fentanyl, remifentanil), neuromuscular blocking drugs, minimal or no inhaled agent, and regional anesthesia whenever possible.

Of even greater concern may be the sedatives that are administered for prolonged periods of time in the intensive care unit (ICU), although one study found "no evidence of an association between dose and duration of sedation and/or analgesia drugs given during the preoperative, intraoperative, and postoperative period and major adverse developmental outcomes" in children undergoing repair of congenital heart disease in the first 6 weeks of life.[212]

INHALATIONAL ANESTHETICS

The MAC defines the minimum alveolar concentration for inhaled agents at which 50% of patients respond to a painful skin incision with withdrawal. This measure allows comparison of the effects of inhaled anesthetics at equipotent doses. The MAC of isoflurane in the micropremie (<32 weeks PCA) is approximately 20% less than that in full-term neonates (see also Fig. 5.18), and at equipotent doses of isoflurane (1 MAC), systolic arterial pressure decreased similarly in all age groups, 20% to 30%.[213] Sevoflurane affords a rapid induction and emergence from general anesthesia. Desflurane is contraindicated for induction of anesthesia but is widely used for maintenance of anesthesia administered through a tracheal tube. However, desflurane causes more airway irritability than isoflurane or sevoflurane, and as a result, it is not recommended for infants with severe BPD. Desflurane, sevoflurane, and isoflurane decrease arterial blood pressure in a dose-dependent manner, possibly through decreasing the systemic vascular resistance or by myocardial depression. One possible mechanism to explain the myocardial depression is that the baseline ionized calcium concentrations in premature infants, especially critically ill neonates, are less.[163,164] Premature infants may be more susceptible to the cardiodepressant effects of inhalational anesthetics because inhalational anesthetics block the calcium channels,[214] and the neonatal heart depends on the plasma ionized calcium for contractility to a greater extent than do the hearts of older children[215] (see also Chapters 5 and 16).

N_2O is not routinely used in the micropremie for several reasons. First, N_2O must be delivered in inspired concentrations ranging from 50% to 75% to reduce the MAC of other agents; its role in micropremies, a group often requiring supplemental oxygen, is limited. Second, even if supplemental oxygen were not required, 60% N_2O only decreases the MAC of sevoflurane and desflurane in children by ~25%.[216,217] Third, because of its blood gas solubility, N_2O rapidly enters air-filled cavities; therefore, it is not recommended for use in infants with bowel obstruction, NEC, pulmonary interstitial emphysema, or pneumothoraxes, pathologies that are common disorders in micropremies.[218] Fourth, in neonatal and young rats, N_2O demonstrates no antinociceptive effects, which contrasts with its antinociceptive effect in adolescent and adult rats.[219] This observation requires validation in humans.

INTRAVENOUS ANESTHETICS

Intravenous agents include opioids, benzodiazepines, barbiturates, propofol, ketamine, and dexmedetomidine. Fentanyl possesses analgesic and sedative properties; however, it does not reliably produce unconsciousness or amnesia and, by itself, is not considered an anesthetic in children or adults. Nonetheless, the use of fentanyl as an anesthetic has been justified in preterm infants because they were deemed to be inherently amnestic by virtue of their age, although the age at which consciousness and memory occurs is unknown.[210] Premature infants (<1500 grams) who receive IV fentanyl (30–50 μg/kg) and pancuronium for ligation of a PDA exhibit remarkable hemodynamic stability, with only a 5% decrease in blood pressure.[220] A dose of 10 to 12.5 μg/kg of fentanyl administered together with an neuromuscular blocking drug maintained hemodynamic stability for 75 minutes in neonates undergoing a variety of thoracic and abdominal procedures.[221] Hypertension and tachycardia did not occur with skin incision, suggesting that analgesic concentrations necessary for surgery are achieved with this dose of fentanyl.

The pharmacokinetics of fentanyl (30 μg/kg) in premature infants yielded plasma concentrations that remained constant for up to 120 minutes, indicating a reduced clearance.[222] The elimination half-life of fentanyl ranged from 6 to 32 hours in premature infants, greater than the 2- to 3-hour half-life observed in children and adults.[222] The clearance of fentanyl increases with gestational age from 7 mL/minute per kilogram at 25 weeks, to 10 mL/minute per kilogram at 30 weeks, and 12 mL/minute per kilogram at 35 weeks PCA.[223] These studies demonstrated that the half-life and volume of distribution of fentanyl are increased and the clearance is reduced in premature infants compared with adults.[185] These changes may be explained by immature CYP450 3A4, the major enzyme responsible for clearance (see also Chapters 4 and 5). In a subset of infants with increased intraabdominal pressure (after repair of a gastroschisis or omphalocele), the elimination half-life of fentanyl is 1.5- to 3-fold greater than that in other infants of the same age, possibly due to decreased hepatic blood flow.[185] Thus for some drugs, including fentanyl, clearance may be impaired consequent to reduced hepatic blood flow as the result of increased intraabdominal pressure (although maldistribution of blood away from regions of concentrated CYP450 3A4 activity and reduced hepatic function may play a greater role), and decreased cardiac output.[185,224] The increased volume of distribution decreases the initial plasma concentration of fentanyl compared with that in adults.[185] These pharmacokinetic differences, combined with an increased propensity to apnea, serve to prolong analgesia and respiratory depression, increase the risk of postoperative apnea, and slow recovery of consciousness. In the micropremie, mechanical ventilation may be required for several days after large doses of fentanyl.

Similarly, the elimination half-life of morphine is markedly prolonged in premature infants compared with that in children and adults.[225–228] The elimination half-life of morphine ranges from 6 to 16 hours in the micropremie, compared with 2 to 4 hours in the adult. The clearance (normalized to a 70-kg person) of morphine increased with PMA between 23 and 35 weeks, reaching 50% of the mature clearance by 50 weeks PMA, and mature values by 80 weeks PMA.[226] The active water soluble metabolite, morphine-6-glucuronide, also has reduced elimination because of immature renal function.[229] Fentanyl is preferred to large-dose morphine for anesthesia because the former has fewer hemodynamic adverse effects.[223,228]

Remifentanil is rapidly inactivated by plasma and tissue esterases and, because of its short half-life, is administered by continuous infusion. The half-life of remifentanil in adults is 3 to 4 minutes, independent of the duration of infusion, and similar to that in infants or children.[230] A multicenter study that compared halothane and remifentanil for maintenance of anesthesia in infants undergoing pyloromyotomy showed similar intraoperative hemodynamic stability with the two techniques, but fewer "new-onset apneas" with remifentanil compared with halothane.[231,232] Clearance of remifentanil is greatest in infants and children younger than 2 years of age, thus allowing an intense opioid effect

intraoperatively that rapidly dissipates upon terminating the infusion.[233] Remifentanil has been used to provide anesthesia in infants weighing 400 to 580 grams with apparent good hemodynamic stability.[234,235] A study examining cord blood from premature infants found high nonspecific esterase activity, comparable with that of term infants, thus suggesting that preterm infants rapidly metabolize remifentanil.[236] If a remifentanil infusion is indicated, it is best to use a dilute concentration (5 μg/mL) piggybacked as close to the IV as possible with a continuous carrier to achieve a constant rate of administration (see Chapters 5 and 6).

Ketamine, a phencyclidine derivative, affords several advantages compared with inhaled and other IV agents. It provides analgesia, amnesia, and unconsciousness yet minimally depresses cardiovascular function (Fig. 35.4).[237] However, ketamine anesthesia depresses ventilation and airway reflexes, which predisposes to airway obstruction, apnea, and gastric aspiration. The use of an airway device when ketamine is used for surgical procedures in the micropremie is recommended. In the setting of brief painful procedures, IV ketamine can be used as an anesthetic without a tracheal tube.[238]

Dexmedetomidine is an alpha-2 agonist that produces sedation while maintaining spontaneous respirations. The drug has antiinflammatory properties, possesses neuroprotective effects, may improve gut motility, and mitigate ventilator-induced lung injury. Although limited, data suggest that dexmedetomidine shortens the duration of mechanical ventilation and oxygen supplementation, as well as decreasing opioid and benzodiazepine requirements in neonates. Bradycardia and hypotension can be seen with dexmedetomidine; however, studies show a stable hemodynamic profile when it is administered in slow, small boluses and used with lower infusion rates, related to lower clearance in this cohort.[239–243]

Other IV agents include thiopental, propofol, and benzodiazepines. These agents induce loss of consciousness but possess less analgesia than ketamine. The micropremie requires less thiopental for induction than does the infant (2–3 mg/kg vs. 5–6 mg/kg, respectively), a relationship similar to the MAC of isoflurane.[244] In the past, we used only thiopental for neurosurgical procedures involving increased intracranial pressure in these infants. However, thiopental is no longer available in the United States; propofol has largely replaced thiopental for this purpose. A word of caution is needed regarding the use of propofol for induction of anesthesia in neonates. Several reports highlight episodes in otherwise stable infants of protracted hypotension and low cardiac output that appear to be dose dependent,[245,246] and that were associated with hypoxia after propofol boluses (1–3 mg/kg IV). The mechanism underlying these responses remains unclear, although systemic vasodilation and acute pulmonary hypertension with reversion to persistent fetal circulation remains a strong possibility.[247,248] In our experience, a propofol infusion (50–200 μg/kg per minute) supplemented with fentanyl as needed for analgesia can anesthetize the micropremie (see Chapters 5 and 6).[249,250] Recovery from propofol anesthesia is delayed in micropremies compared with term infants, because micropremies have both less fat and muscle tissue to redistribute the drug, and reduced clearance.[251] In the pediatric ICU, propofol infusions have been implicated in unexpected deaths (propofol infusion syndrome).[252] Use of propofol infusion in neonates remains limited because of these concerns.

Benzodiazepines, such as midazolam and diazepam, have been used in the neonatal intensive care unit (NICU) for sedation. As with thiopental and propofol, these drugs do not provide analgesia and are not recommended as the sole anesthetic for surgery.

However, the combination of a benzodiazepine and opioid provides satisfactory anesthesia for surgery. Midazolam clearance is markedly decreased in the micropremie compared with the term neonate or infant, and will be further prolonged in the setting of immature liver function.[253,254] Midazolam can cause systemic hypotension, depress ventilation, and impair airway reflexes in premature infants. The hypotension caused by midazolam is greater in the presence of fentanyl; both drugs must be titrated in small doses when administered concomitantly.[255] One study noted an 8% to 23% decrease in arterial pressure after a bolus of 0.1 mg/kg of midazolam in premature infants.[256]

REGIONAL ANESTHETICS

Regional anesthesia (see Chapter 40) is possible in premature infants and offers the advantage of the avoidance of sedative, volatile, and opioid medications that may lead to apnea, bradycardia, and hypotension. However, there is conflicting evidence of the superiority and reduction of adverse events of regional anesthesia compared with general anesthesia in this population.[59,60,257] In neonates the conus medullaris extends to a lower segment of the spine than adults; however, there does not appear to be a difference in location between term and premature neonates (see Fig. 40.18), thus it is generally recommended that lumbar punctures are made at L4–L5 or L5–S1 interspaces in this age group.[258] Larger doses of local anesthetics per kilogram are required in infants because of their larger volume of distribution of cerebrospinal fluid (see E-Fig. 40.3), relatively increased surface area of the spinal cord and nerve roots, and increased cardiac output with proportionally greater blood flow to the spinal cord. However, faster drug distribution, uptake, and elimination of local anesthetics from the CSF also abbreviate their duration of action. Adjuncts to local anesthetics, such as clonidine, may increase the duration of the block but also increase the risk of sedation, bradycardia, apnea, and hypotension. The optimal dose, timing and, side effects of these adjuncts in this age group are controversial.[259]

Neonatal Surgical Emergencies

Neonatal emergencies can present at any time, occurring immediately at birth or within weeks after delivery. Advances in perinatology have improved the morbidity and mortality of critically ill newborns. Nonetheless, whether acquired or congenital in nature, these emergencies can be truly life-threatening and require the skill and expertise of an anesthesiologist who is knowledgeable about the nuances of neonatal anatomy and physiology. The goal of this section is to describe common neonatal surgical emergencies and the considerations important to the anesthesiologist caring for this very special population.

PREPARATION FOR SURGERY
The "Urgent" Emergency
In the past, many conditions classified as neonatal emergencies were expeditiously taken to the OR, often within hours of diagnosis. However, with newer technology and medical advances, along with better outcome data, immediate surgical intervention is not always necessary or preferable. In most circumstances, there is time to medically optimize the neonate and correct any hemodynamic instability and/or metabolic derangement, although the optimal timing for surgical correction is not always straightforward and must be determined on a case-by-case basis.[260–263]

THE OPERATING ROOM
Environment
Owing to the immature and inefficient measures neonates use to regulate body temperature, precautions must be made to prevent heat loss. Warming the OR to 80°F to 85°F (26.7°C–29.4°C), using radiant warming units, using forced-air heating pads, and adding humidity to the inspired gases in the circuit help maintain the neonate's temperature in the neutral thermal range (see Chapter 49).[264–266] Other methods used to prevent heat loss include using a head cover and warming IV and irrigation fluids before they are used.[267,268] Precautions should also be used during transport, such as the use of an incubator/radiant warmer or a portable heated mattress as this has been identified as a critical period during which premature infants can become hypothermic.[135,269,270]

MONITORS
Routine standard monitoring equipment includes an electrocardiograph, chest or esophageal stethoscope, blood pressure monitor, temperature probe, pulse oximeter, and an end-tidal carbon dioxide (ETCO$_2$) and agent analyzer. Cerebral near-infrared spectroscopy (NIRS) is used increasingly in neonates (see Chapter 49) with cardiac pathology, neonatal intensive care, and the OR. Non-invasive continuous cardiac output monitors may become routine in these infants in the future (see Chapter 49).[271,272]

Oxygen Saturation
It is recommended to limit the use of oxygen in neonates to maintain an oxygen saturation as measured by pulse oximetry (SpO$_2$) of anywhere between 83% and 95% in order to decrease oxidative stress.[32–35] However, an increased inspired fraction of oxygen (FiO$_2$) may be required during anesthesia and surgery owing to their deleterious effects on oxygenation, such as reduced functional residual capacity (FRC), ventilation-perfusion mismatch, and hypoventilation. Perhaps more importantly, many neonatal emergency surgeries are intrathoracic or intraabdominal in nature, further exacerbating difficulties in oxygenation with limited recruitment maneuvers available. If the ductus arteriosus is still patent, a preductal pulse oximeter should be placed on the right hand, and a postductal oximeter placed on the left hand or foot to determine the severity of any extrapulmonary shunting of deoxygenated blood via the PDA. If the infant has a right-sided arch, the pulse oximeter should be placed on the left hand instead of the right for preductal monitoring.

End-Tidal Carbon Dioxide
ETCO$_2$ measurements have been shown to correlate generally well with PaCO$_2$, even in neonates.[271,273–275] However, most of these studies have taken place in ICUs, not in the OR, where the anesthesia circuits tend to carry more dead space (VD). The increase in dead space, along with the small neonatal tidal volumes (Tv) in neonates exacerbates the PaCO$_2$–ETCO$_2$ gradient, as evidenced by the Enghoff modification of the Bohr equation:

$$V_D/V_T = (PaCO_2 - ETCO_2) / PaCO_2$$

In addition, it has been noted that the correlation of PaCO$_2$ to ETCO$_2$ in neonates with severe lung disease who demonstrate an arterial oxygen saturation (SaO$_2$) to FiO$_2$ ratio of less than 200 is not as strong.[271,276] Neonates presenting for emergency surgery may harbor some degree of lung disease, and most will be subject to a large dead space, making it important to recognize that the $ETCO_2$ may significantly underestimate true $PaCO_2$. A more accurate estimate of $ETCO_2$ concentration may be obtained by using a special tracheal tube with a sample port located at its tip (mainstream monitoring) or by inserting a narrow catheter through the CO_2 sampling port in the elbow and into the lumen of the tracheal tube.[275,277,278] Measures to limit dead space include eliminating the elbow from the anesthesia circuit and shortening the ventilation circuit as much as possible.

Invasive Monitors

In neonates, changes in blood pressure, heart rate, and the intensity of heart sounds are excellent indicators of cardiac function, intravascular volume status, and depth of anesthesia. Invasive monitors may not be indicated in all cases. They can be difficult to place, lead to adverse events, and contribute to a significant decrease in hematocrit owing to multiple blood draws from a very small circulating volume. However, in cases in which major blood or fluid losses are expected, or the physiology is complicated by the presence of cardiac disease, a central venous catheter is warranted. Likewise, any neonate with significant underlying cardiovascular instability should have an arterial catheter placed for continuous monitoring of blood pressure and to provide means to obtain arterial blood samples for determination of blood pH, serum glucose, and electrolyte concentrations. Some neonates arrive in the OR with umbilical venous and/or arterial catheters (UAC) in place. Umbilical catheters can be used during the first 5 to 7 postnatal days of life, but are rarely used beyond 7 to 10 days. High-lying UACs (above the diaphragm) are associated with fewer complications, such as ischemia, thrombosis, and hypoglycemia, than low-lying catheters (above the aortic bifurcation).[279] UVCs should lie in the IVC at its junction to the right atrium (see Fig. 46.12). A UVC that lies within the portal system or wedged within the liver will not accurately reflect central venous pressure (CVP) and can lead to hepatic necrosis with infusions of hypertonic solutions.[280] Care must be taken to verify where the tips of each of these catheters lie before using them.

Ventilator

There is often a large amount of dead space from anesthesia circuits to a neonate who requires a very small tidal volume. In addition, these infants may have intrinsic lung pathology, which when coupled with intrathoracic or intraabdominal surgery that compresses the lungs, can render it extremely difficult to ventilate with a conventional anesthesia machine. It may be necessary to manually ventilate the lungs in these infants during parts of the surgery, particularly if a primitive ventilator is used. In certain circumstances it may be beneficial to have the ICU bring one of their ventilators to the OR for use during surgery, but this will preclude the ability to administer volatile agents.

Equipment Setup

Anesthesiologists need to be well prepared for these surgical cases. A sick neonate can have extremely labile hemodynamics even before the induction of anesthesia or surgical incision. Table 35.5 lists basic equipment for conducting emergency anesthesia in a neonate (see Figs. 35.5 and 35.6).

Fluids and Medication

Particular attention must be paid to ensuring the accurate delivery of medications and fluids. These infants require only small fractions of the medications in most vials and ampoules. As a

TABLE 35.5	Suggested Equipment for Emergency Neonatal Anesthesia		
Airway Equipment	**Environment**	**Agents**	**Intravenous Fluids[a]**
Suction catheters	Room temperature (80°–85°F; 26.6°–29.5°C)	Gases	Lactated Ringer's solution
Oral airways		Air/O_2/iNO	
Face masks		Volatile anesthetics	$D_{10}W$
Breathing circuit	Forced warm air delivery device	Drugs	Normal saline solution
Miller 0, 1, blades and handle		IV anesthetics	
		Propofol	5% albumin
Uncuffed tracheal tubes (ID 2.5, 3.0, 3.5, 4.0 mm)	Underbody warming blanket	Ketamine	PlasmaLyte
		NMBDs	
	Circuit humidifier	Succinylcholine	
	IV fluid warmer	Cisatracurium	
	Infusion pumps for both maintenance fluid and for opioid or vasoactive drugs	Vecuronium	
		Pancuronium	
Stylet		Rocuronium	
Cuffed tracheal tubes (ID 3.0, 3.5 mm)		Opioids	
		Fentanyl	
		Morphine	
		Remifentanil	
		Local Anesthetics	
		Tetracaine 1.0%	
		Bupivacaine 0.25%	
		Ropivacaine	
		Emergency Drugs	
		Atropine	
		Epinephrine (1:10,000)	
		Norepinephrine	
		Dopamine	
		Calcium	
		Bicarbonate	

ID, Inner diameter; *IV*, intravenous; *NMBDs*, neuromuscular blocking drugs; *NO*, nitric oxide; *O_2*, oxygen.
[a]Some guidelines suggest 1% glucose should be added to an isotonic fluid for maintenance during anesthesia.[459]

result, either tuberculin syringes should be used to carefully measure the very small aliquots of medications or the medication in the vial should be diluted so that a measurable and accurate fraction of the content of the vial can be given. Tuberculin syringes present several challenges, including difficulty in removing air bubbles from the syringe, and the very small volume that will be administered. The volume of medication may be so small that it is no larger than the volume of the stem of the clave or stopcock, resulting in less drug than intended being administered to the infant. To ensure the drug is not lost in the dead space of the IV set, each clave or stopcock should be flushed with saline solution after the medication has been given. Diluting medications introduces the risk of a drug dose error that could lead to an overdose or underdose of the medication. In all instances, it is prudent to verify the dose and dilution of the medication with a colleague and carefully label the contents. All medications should be administered into the IV set as close to the patient as possible to minimize the volume of fluids needed to flush the medication into the child (see Fig. 49.2).

Fluid overload is always a concern in these small infants.[154] To minimize the fluids administered, all IV infusions are best delivered through a pump. Free-flowing IVs are dangerous sources for fluid overload, which may open a ductus arteriosus

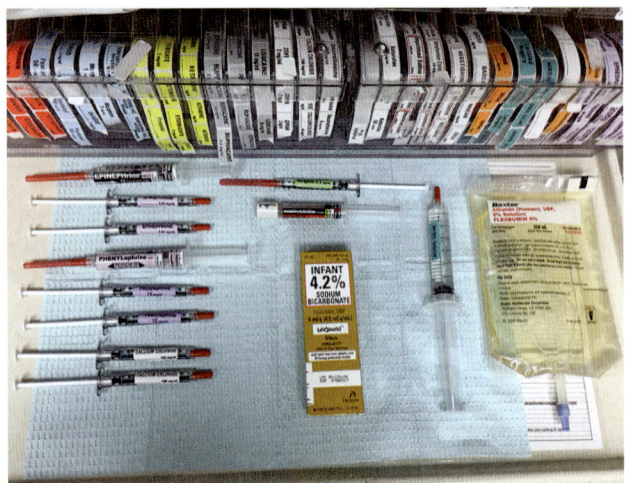

FIGURE 35.5 Example of emergency drug setup on anesthesia cart.

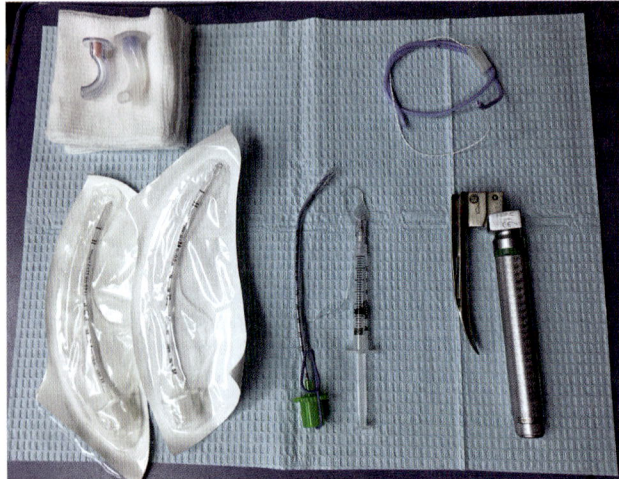

FIGURE 35.6 Example of neonatal airway setup on anesthesia machine.

and cause congestive heart failure. Finally, meticulous care must be taken to remove air bubbles from all IV administration systems, solutions, and medications that are administered. See Chapter 49 for further discussion on infusion pumps and the implications of IV administration VD on drug delivery (see also Figs. 49.2 and 49.3).[281,282,283]

Intraoperative fluid management in micropremies should begin with continuing the solution that arrives with the infant from the NICU; usually this is a calcium- and/or glucose-containing solution. Alternatively, some infants may arrive with a hyperosmolar glucose or dextrose (10%) parenteral nutrition solution. In both cases, these solutions should not be discontinued. The standard practice has been to maintain the infusion at the same rate (by pump) throughout the surgery to avoid reactive hypoglycemia from increased circulating insulin concentrations; however, recent evidence, albeit from a retrospective review of laparotomies in neonates, suggests the contrary. Halving the infusion rate greatly reduced the frequency of postoperative glucose concentrations exceeding 200 mg% (200 mg/dL, 11 mmol/L) which is severe hyperglycemia, (from 19% to 8%, ~50%) and did not increase the incidence of hypoglycemia postoperatively.[175] These results undermine

the two arguments for maintaining constant preoperative glucose infusions perioperatively: to prevent hypoglycemia from increased circulating levels of insulin in the blood and that hyperglycemia is unlikely to occur; neither of these concerns are supported by these data. Hyperglycemia will occur with unchanged maintenance infusion rates when combined with stressful surgery. Additionally, several studies have demonstrated that morbidity and mortality rates, as well as ICU and hospital lengths of stay, are increased in critically ill children who are hyperglycemic.[104,284] In another cohort of 178 surgical procedures in neonates, 33 weeks gestation and 1790 to 2140 grams in weight, with postoperative hyperglycemia defined as a glucose exceeding 150 mg% (8.3 mmol/L), 54% of the neonates experienced hyperglycemia postoperatively with the intraoperative glucose infusion rate the only modifiable risk factor for hyperglycemia.[177] The relationship between gestational age and postoperative glucose concentrations was nonlinear. If no solution is being infused, a balanced salt solution (e.g., lactated Ringer's solution or PlasmaLyte) could be initiated at 4 mL/kg per hour, supplemented with the same solution for third-space loss (at least 10 mL/kg per hour), and replacement of blood loss. If a glucose solution is not being infused, then a balanced salt solution containing glucose may be administered through a pump. The importance of including glucose as an infusion in these very small infants cannot be overstated as glycogen stores in VLBW neonates are minimal. Wherever possible, serum glucose concentrations should be monitored regularly to avoid hypoglycemia. Third-space losses including evaporation and vascular leak are replaced with a balanced salt solution.

Bedside Procedures in the ICU
Occasionally, neonates may be so critically ill that simply transporting the infant to the OR may be life-threatening. To decrease the risk, many institutions now perform surgical procedures at the infant's bedside or in a specialized surgical suite within the NICU, minimizing the period of transport and providing optimal surgical conditions.[285] Providing surgical and anesthetic care at the bedside has its challenges. There is reduced access to the child, suboptimal lighting, reduced sterility, limited monitors (usually capnography is absent), unfamiliar ventilators and an inability to control room temperature, although NICU incubators commonly include a built-in overhead radiant heater.

Adapting to the working environment requires planning and organization in concert with communication with the surgeons, neonatologists, and nurses in the NICU.[285] If bedside anesthesia is to be provided, then appropriate IV equipment for transfusion, pumps, and monitors compatible with electrocautery and expired CO_2 monitoring should be available, just as in the OR.

THE FAMILY
Close interaction between the parents and the anesthesia, medical, surgical, and nursing staff promotes effective communication of medical concerns and continued emotional support for parents. The birth of a premature neonate or illness in a full-term infant often does not allow time for emotional preparation for or acceptance of the situation by the family. With the institution of aggressive medical and surgical interventions, parents sometimes feel excluded from the care of their infant and develop feelings of isolation and lack of control. The development of rapport between the parents of critically ill infants and hospital staff is essential to ensure adequate psychological support during this intensely anxiety-provoking event.

Emergency Surgery

RESPIRATORY PATHOLOGY

Lesions of the respiratory system can be categorized into those that involve the large and small airways and those that involve the lung parenchyma.

ABNORMALITIES OF THE AIRWAY

Airway surgery presents unique operative challenges. The airway must be shared between the anesthesiologist and surgeon, while the operating table is rotated 90 degrees, hindering immediate access to the child's airway. Bronchoscopy with a rigid scope is very stimulating and may require a deep level of anesthesia, which may lead to cardiac and respiratory depression. There is intermittent and often inadequate ventilation because of leakage around the scope or during periods where the insufflation port is removed or just the telescope is used. These factors make it difficult to maintain an adequate level of anesthesia when inhalational agents are used. It may be more prudent to provide local anesthesia (topical lignocaine) with IV medications, such as propofol or ketamine, with intermittent boluses or with the use of a constant infusion for longer cases together with opioids (see also Chapters 5 and 6).

Choanal Atresia

Choanal atresia is a developmental failure of the nasal cavity to communicate with the nasopharynx owing to the persistence of the nasobuccal membrane. It occurs in approximately 1/7000 live births with a female predominance.[286] Choanal atresia is often associated with other congenital anomalies, such as CHARGE syndrome (**C**oloboma, **H**eart disease, **A**tresia choanae, **R**etarded growth, **G**enital anomalies, **E**ar anomalies), Treacher Collins, Pfeiffer, and VATER (**V**ertebral defects, **A**nal atresia, **T**racheoesophageal fistula with **E**sophageal atresia, and **R**adial and renal anomalies).[287,288] Unilateral choanal stenosis is usually diagnosed later in childhood or adulthood and is characterized by unilateral nasal discharge and persistent nasal obstruction. Bilateral stenosis, however, is considered a surgical emergency owing to the obligatory nasal breathing pattern in neonates. They often present within the first days of life with respiratory distress and cyanosis, usually while feeding, which is relieved by crying. Other diagnostic criteria include noisy breathing, difficulty feeding, and the inability to pass a 5 Fr or 6 Fr catheter into the nasopharynx. Definitive treatment involves perforation of the persistent membrane via an endoscopic transnasal approach (most common) or via a transseptal approach (usually reserved for patients with other significant craniofacial abnormalities).[287,289,290] Nasal stenting is often performed at the end of the procedure with stents left in place for about 4 weeks. Serial balloon dilations may replace nasal stenting in order to prevent relapse.[291] These neonates may develop airway obstruction during anesthetic induction, therefore early placement of an oral airway may aid in airway management.

Laryngeal and Upper Tracheal Obstruction

Because of the narrow diameter of neonatal airways, even a small obstruction can lead to significant resistance to airflow, leading to life-threatening respiratory distress. Therefore, timely recognition and treatment of laryngeal and upper tracheal abnormalities, such as webs, congenital subglottic stenosis, and hemangiomas is essential in reducing morbidity/mortality. (Figs. 35.7 and 35.8 and Video 35.1; see also Videos 12.1, 12.5, and 12.18).

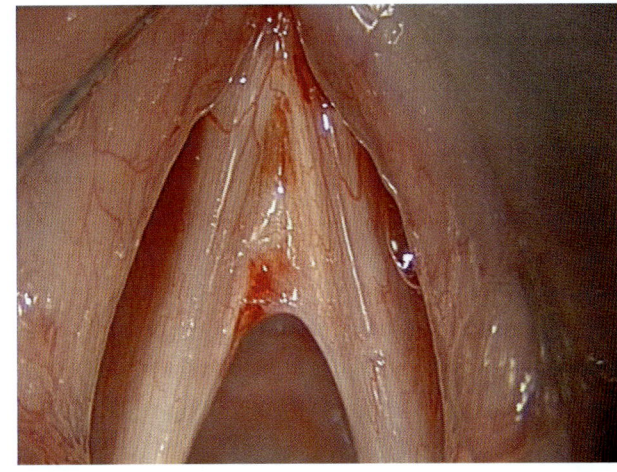

FIGURE 35.7 Laryngeal web in a neonate. (Courtesy Dr. Christopher Hartnick.)

As resistance increases inversely with the airway radius to the fifth power, ventilatory assistance is required to overcome this substantial increase in the work of breathing. The greater time constants that result from the increased airway resistance require a greater time for expiration to avoid gas trapping. In the most severe cases of obstruction, tracheal intubation may not be possible or is unable to provide adequate ventilation past the stenosis, and a tracheostomy may have to be placed before treatment.

WEBS. Laryngeal and tracheal webs are fibrous membranes that develop as the result of incomplete recanalization of the larynx during early gestation, resulting in variable degrees of airway obstruction and acute respiratory distress or stridor shortly after birth (see Fig. 35.7).[292,293] Some infants may succumb at birth because of a complete or near-complete tracheal web if this airway defect has not been identified antenatally. If a tracheal web has been identified in utero, an ex utero intrapartum treatment (EXIT) procedure may be a lifesaving maneuver (see Chapter 36). Anterior glottic webs are associated with velocardiofacial syndrome (also known as 22q11.2 deletion or DiGeorge syndrome) in 65% of cases, and many also include concurrent subglottic stenosis.[293] Endoscopic web excision is the preferred treatment via microlaryngoscopy. Many surgeons will elect to keep the airway intubated for 24 hours after surgery to allow the raw edges to remucosalize.

CONGENITAL SUBGLOTTIC STENOSIS. Subglottic stenosis is the most common indication for neonatal tracheostomy placement.[294] It is thought to be the result of malformed cricoid cartilage in utero, or, in rare cases, owing to severe gastroesophageal reflux, eosinophilic esophagitis, or infection.[293] The degree of symptomatology and treatment options vary with the degree of narrowing. Lower-grade stenoses can be treated with endoscopic interventions such as balloon dilation and steroid injection. However, the more severe stenoses require more extensive surgical repair. In the past, these neonates received long-term tracheostomy placement with the expectation that they would outgrow the stenosis. Currently the surgical options include cricotracheal resection and laryngotracheoplasty, involving an anterior with or without a posterior cricoid split and the placement of a cartilage graft, usually from the thyroid or costal cartilage, to enlarge the subglottic lumen. This may or may not include the temporary placement of a tracheostomy or tracheal tube while the incision heals (see also Chapters 13 and 31).[294] A small case series reports use of a CO_2

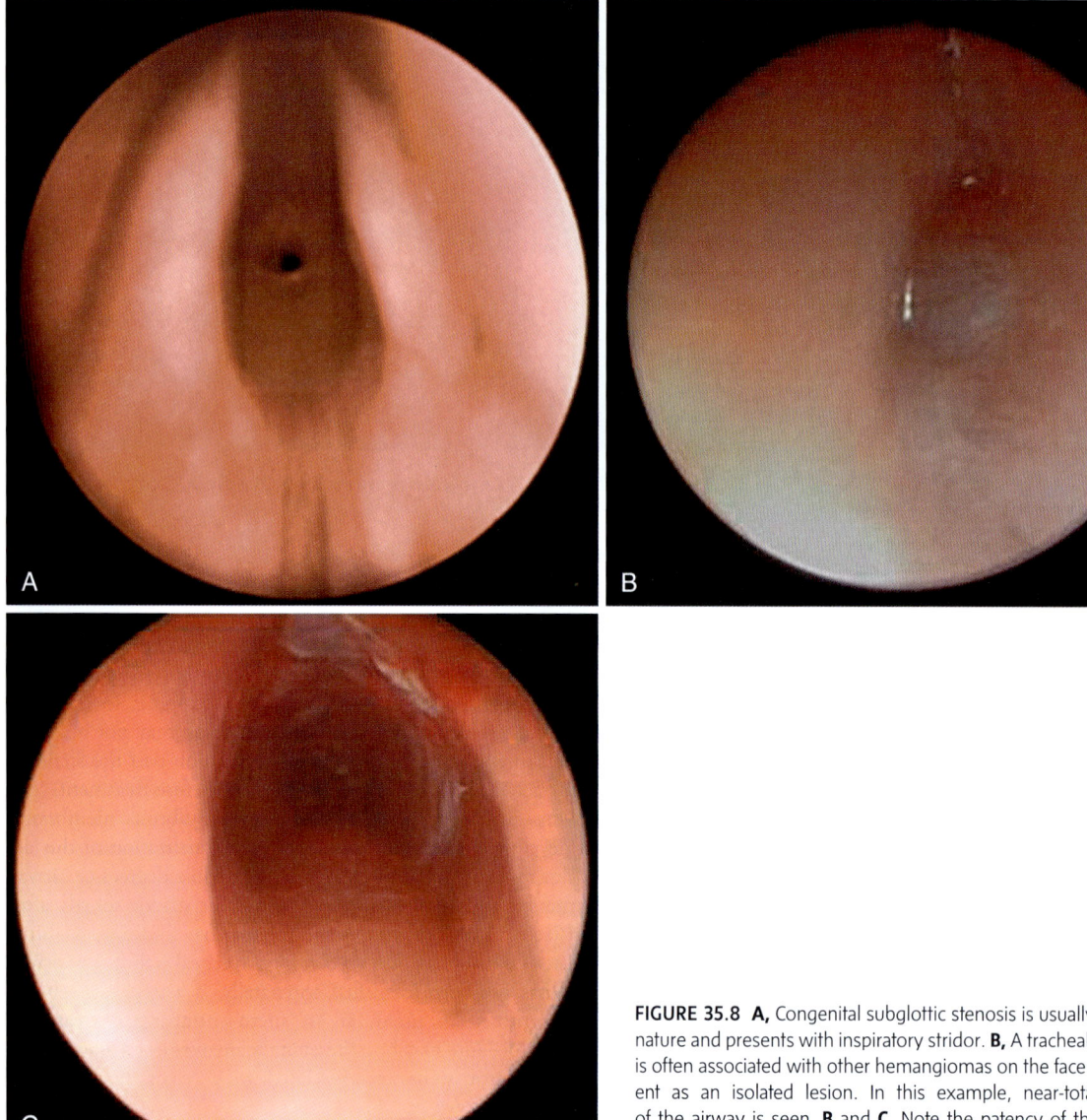

FIGURE 35.8 **A,** Congenital subglottic stenosis is usually concentric in nature and presents with inspiratory stridor. **B,** A tracheal hemangioma is often associated with other hemangiomas on the face but may present as an isolated lesion. In this example, near-total obstruction of the airway is seen. **B** and **C,** Note the patency of the airway after resection. (Courtesy Dr. Christopher Hartnick.)

laser to resect the stenosis without any mechanical dilation and may be the future of treatment.[295,296]

SUBGLOTTIC HEMANGIOMA. Infantile hemangiomas are the most common type of vascular tumor, affecting 4% to 10% of infants, and the most common tumor to involve the pediatric airway (see Fig. 35.8).[297,298] Its cause is not well understood. Any child with a cutaneous hemangioma, especially if in the V3 "beard" distribution on the face, should be evaluated for a concomitant subglottic hemangioma (20%–30% coincidence), although they can occur anywhere in the airway.[297,299] Airway hemangiomas can also be associated with PHACES syndrome (**P**osterior fossa malformation, **H**emangioma, **A**rterial lesions of the head and neck, **C**ardiac abnormalities, **E**ye abnormalities, **S**ternal cleft or **S**upraumbilical hernia). Symptoms, which include respiratory distress and stridor, are generally absent immediately after birth but can develop quickly as the hemangioma rapidly grows between 6 and 12 weeks of life. This proliferation continues until approximately 12 to 18 months of age, and the hemangioma then gradually begins to shrink. First-line medical therapy includes oral propranolol, followed by systemic and intralesional injection of steroids. Propranolol can cause bradycardia, hypotension, hypoglycemia, and hyperkalemia. Surgical options include laser therapy or open excision and are generally offered to those in whom medical therapy with persistent airway obstruction fails. Laser therapy achieves focal tissue ablation with the use of either the yttrium-aluminum-garnet (YAG) laser or a diode laser via an endoscopic approach through direct laryngoscopy. This therapy is reserved for smaller, focal lesions. Open excision is performed via an anterior airway incision around the cricoid cartilage, which may require a rib or thyroid cartilage graft to avoid subglottic stenosis. These children will remain intubated for several days after the procedure.[293,297] Subglottic hemangiomas are easily compressed when a tracheal tube is passed to intubate the airway, although bleeding is always a possibility and should be anticipated. However, when the practitioner is unaware of the presence of a hemangioma, the first recognition of the lesion may be the absence of an air leak around an appropriately sized tracheal tube.

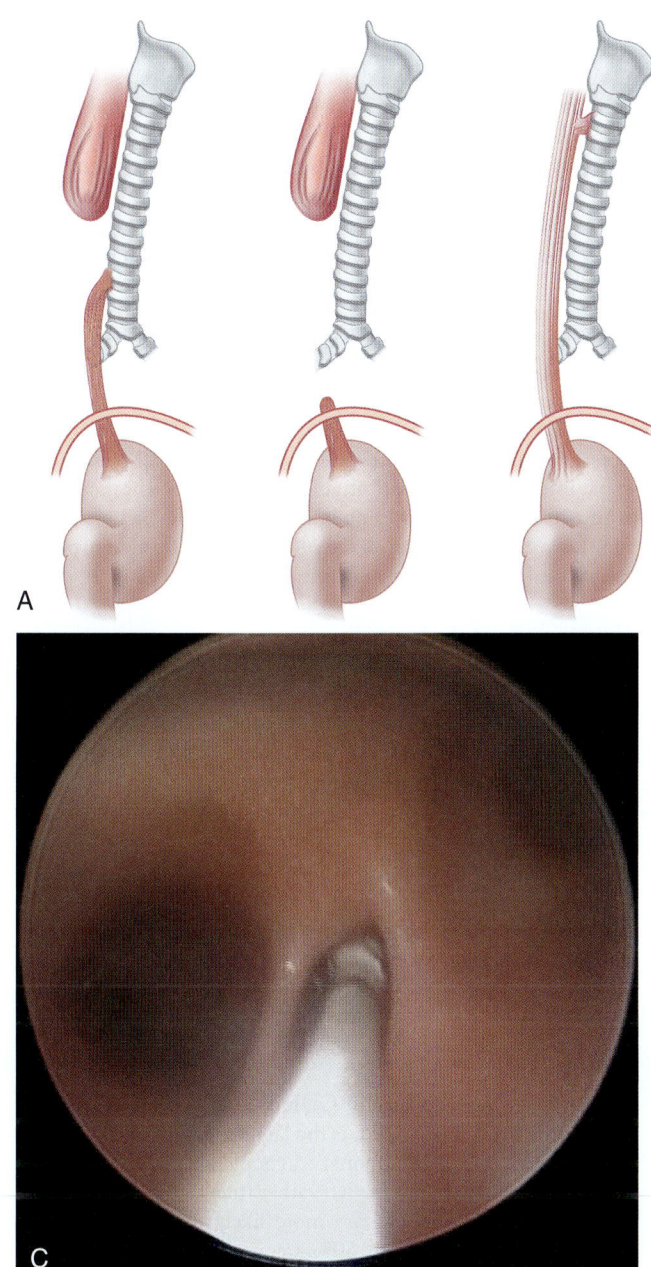

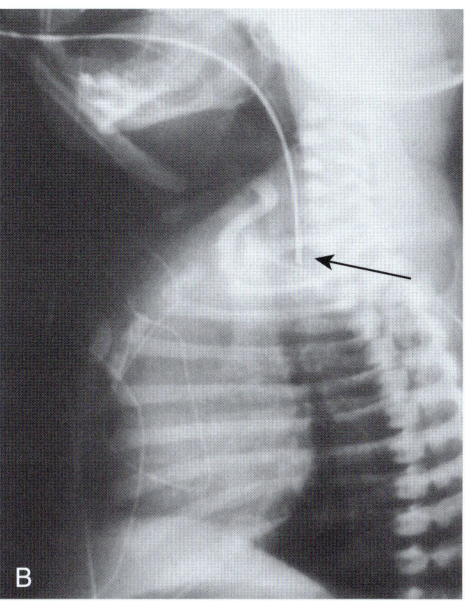

FIGURE 35.9 **A,** The three most common forms of esophageal atresia are presented. The most common form (~85%) consists of a dilated proximal esophageal pouch and a fistula between the distal trachea and distal esophagus *(left)*. The second most common form consists of esophageal atresia alone *(middle)*. Neonates with tracheoesophageal fistula alone *(right)* often present with pneumonia as the initial manifestation. **B,** The classic presentation is of a newborn with excessive secretions who spits up during the initial feeding; inability to pass a nasogastric tube *(arrow)* is pathognomonic. **C,** A catheter is placed inside the tracheoesophageal fistula, located near the carina. (**A,** From Coran AG, Behrendt DM, Weintraub WH, Lee DC: *Surgery of the Neonate.* Boston: Little, Brown; 1978:46. **B** and **C,** Courtesy Dr. Daniel P. Doody.)

Tracheoesophageal Fistula/Esophageal Atresia

Tracheoesophageal fistulas (TEFs) occur in 1/3000 live births in a mostly sporadic, nonsyndromic manner with no preference for sex or race. They are due to an error in separation of the trachea from the floor of the foregut around the fourth to fifth week of gestation. They are often associated with other congenital anomalies, in particular the VACTERL association (**V**ertebral anomalies, imperforate **A**nus, **C**ongenital heart disease, **T**racheoesophageal fistula, **R**enal abnormalities, **L**imb abnormalities).[300,301] There are two main systems of classifications of TEF (Gross and Vogt) that describe the lesions in terms of whether or not esophageal atresia (EA) is present and where the tracheoesophageal connection occurs in relation to the trachea (Fig. 35.9A) (see also Fig. 13.13).

The most common type (Gross classification C) consists of a blind proximal esophageal pouch with a distal TEF just above the carina (80%–90% of cases).

TEF can be diagnosed prenatally with signs of polyhydramnios (the fetus cannot swallow), small or absent fetal stomach bubble, and/or blind-ending upper pouch in the fetal neck. Early postnatal signs and symptoms include excessive salivation, choking/coughing/regurgitation at the first feed leading to cyanosis and/or respiratory distress, and a distended abdomen owing to the stomach filling with air every time the baby cries, which may compress the lung and embarrass respirations. Diagnosis of TEF/EA can be confirmed by the inability to pass a nasogastric (NG) tube into the stomach, a dilated proximal esophagus with air in conjunction with air in the distal stomach on x-ray, computed tomography scan, or direct visualization via bronchoscopy/esophagoscopy (Fig. 35.9B,C; E-Fig. 35.1 and Video 35.2) (see also Fig. 13.13).

Several classification systems (Waterston and Okamoto,[302] Spitz[303]) use weight, congenital anomalies, and comorbidities such as congenital heart disease to determine surgical risk and guide planning. This helps determine whether the child should undergo more immediate surgical correction, should undergo more extensive stabilization before correction, or requires a more drawn-out staged repair. Generally, there is enough time to stabilize and optimize the infant before surgery. This involves establishing IV access, correcting anemia and electrolyte imbalances, typing and crossmatching blood, evaluating for other anomalies (especially cardiac echocardiography), and possible placement of a gastrostomy tube, which can be completed using local anesthesia to vent the stomach.

Surgical repair has traditionally been performed with an open thoracotomy and manual lung retraction. However, in the past 2 decades, thoracoscopic repair has become increasingly popular even in infants <2000 grams.[304–306] A systematic review of 382 neonates (830–3960 grams) reported that 1/10 procedures had to be converted to open with 1 tracheal rupture and 16 other deaths due to cardiopulmonary failure or sepsis.[307]

Single-lung ventilation is not required, as low-flow, low-pressure intrathoracic CO_2 is used instead to collapse the right lung to improve surgical exposure. The patient is placed in the left lateral decubitus position for a right thoracotomy to avoid the aortic arch. The anesthesiologist will place a nasoesophageal tube to aid the surgeon in identifying the proximal esophageal pouch. The fistula is ligated first to avoid further entrapping air into the stomach, followed by a primary end-to-end anastomosis of the esophagus. Endoscopic TEF repair is feasible with good overall success and lower morbidity, albeit at the expense of repeated procedures.[308]

Several approaches may be used to secure the airway in these infants. One option is to keep the infant spontaneously breathing. Avoiding positive-pressure ventilation reduces the amount of gas entering the stomach, which can impede the ability to ventilate. This can be achieved by means of an awake intubation with topicalization and/or sedation, or with an inhalational induction. However, the awake approach can be traumatic and difficult, and a crying infant will only put more air into the stomach. Inhalational inductions in neonates can (but rarely does) cause major cardiovascular instability. An IV induction is quicker (less crying) and may be more stable, allowing for the use of neuromuscular blocking drugs to optimize intubating conditions. Positive-pressure ventilation is usually successful because the compliance of the lungs is greater than that of the distended stomach. Gentle mask ventilation with low peak pressure ventilation will decrease the amount of air that enters the stomach. If a gastrostomy has been performed, a Fogarty catheter can be passed retrograde through the gastrostomy to occlude the fistula from below.[309]

Although one-lung ventilation is usually not required, the tip of the tracheal tube must be placed above the carina but distal to the fistula. This can be achieved by purposefully placing the tracheal tube into the right main stem bronchus (with the bevel facing anterior to block the aperture of the fistula) and then very slowly withdrawing the tracheal tube while auscultating the left thorax until breath sounds are first heard. A fiberoptic scope can also be used to guide the TT into position and to confirm correct placement. The tracheal tube must be carefully secured to prevent accidental movement above the fistula. Frequent suctioning of the

tracheal tube may be required because of the accumulation of blood and secretions.

After correction of the defect, absorptive atelectasis may require ventilation with long inspiratory times to reexpand alveoli. Early extubation is desirable because it prevents prolonged pressure of the tracheal tube on the suture line. However, many surgeons request that the airway remains intubated postoperatively for several days because the tip of the tracheal tube may perforate the sutured trachea at the level of the fistula during an emergency reintubation or to prevent pneumonia and atelectasis. The tracheal tube provides a means to suction and expand the lungs during the first 24 hours of greatest risk. It is important to maintain the head in a neutral position so as not to pull on the esophageal anastomosis.[310] An epidural catheter threaded from the caudal to the thoracic space may provide a postoperative analgesia and aid in successful extubation (E-Fig. 35.2). Local anesthetic infusion through an intrapleural catheter is another means of providing analgesia after open surgery, but this may risk local anesthetic toxicity owing to rapid absorption from the pleural cavity combined with a lower clearance in neonates.

Abnormalities of the Lung
Congenital Diaphragmatic Hernia
CDH has an incidence of 1 to 2/5000 live births. It occurs around the eighth week of gestation owing to the failure of complete closure of the pleural and peritoneal canal, resulting in herniation of the abdominal organs into the thorax, inhibiting normal lung growth. This affects not only the division of the airways, but also the formation of pulmonary vasculature, leading to a decreased number of bronchi and alveoli (diminished surface area for gas exchange), as well as decreased cross-sectional area and numbers of pulmonary artery branches. This, in turn, increases the PVR and degree of primary pulmonary hypertension. The degree of abnormality depends on the timing of the herniation in utero and the amount of abdominal contents in the thorax. The ipsilateral lung is usually the one affected, but the contralateral lung may be involved as well.

The most common type of CDH occurs at the posterolateral foramen of Bochdalek (90%), is the largest, and is associated with the greatest degree of pulmonary hypoplasia; CDH occurs five times more frequently on the left rather than right side. Neonates with the Bochdalek hernia are more likely to have other birth defects including a 20% to 40% frequency of congenital heart defects and a 5% to 15% frequency of chromosomal abnormalities.[311] A Morgagni type of defect is reported in about 2% of CDHs with the remaining occurring through the esophageal hiatus. CDH is associated with genitourinary and GI malformations, as well as chromosomal anomalies, including trisomy 13, trisomy 18, tetrasomy, and 12p mosaicism.

Prenatal diagnosis can be made via ultrasound findings of polyhydramnios, an intrathoracic gastric bubble (stomach above the diaphragm), and mediastinal shift away from the herniation site (E-Fig. 35.3) (see also Fig. 13.11).[312] Antenatal predictors of poor outcome rely on the observed/expected lung/head ratio and the presence or absence of a thoracic liver in left-sided lesions. Lung/head ratios of <25% are associated with 25% survival, whereas those with ratios greater than 45% are associated with 100% survival.[312,313] An abdominal chest x-ray displaying intestinal loops and/or abdominal organs in the thorax and ipsilateral lung compression aids in postnatal diagnosis. Signs and symptoms are related to the degree of lung hypoplasia and pulmonary hypertension and associated defects that might be present. Owing to the increase in PVR, right-to-left shunting via the patent foramen ovale and ductus arteriosus may occur with hypoxemia. Infants most often present with respiratory distress, and tachycardia, tachypnea, and cyanosis can be observed shortly after delivery. A scaphoid (concave) abdomen and barrel chest may also occur from displacement of the viscera into the thorax. Bowel sounds in the chest are fairly uncommon.

Emergent surgical closure of the defect used to be the standard of care because of the prevalent belief that reduction of the herniated viscera would facilitate lung growth and a return toward normal lung size and function. However, this was untrue. A thorough understanding of the specific pathophysiology of the defect prompted the application of new medical therapies and changed the timing of open surgical repair.[314] Now the focus is to stabilize these neonates medically, optimize the infant's condition before surgery, and adopt measures to improve pulmonary hypertension and reduce PVR. Respiratory support is given, as needed, which may include tracheal intubation with gentle mechanical ventilation to avoid pneumothorax or barotrauma (especially in the normal [contralateral] lung), as in the use of an oscillator or ECMO. ECMO and/or iNO are used to bridge ventilation and oxygenation during the early postnatal life if the child is persistently hypoxic and/or acidotic despite conventional ventilation strategies.[315] Care is provided to avoid introducing air into the GI tract via the use of an NG tube and to avoid CPAP and prolonged mask ventilation, which will only further impinge on the lungs. These infants may also need pharmacologic cardiovascular support. Timing of the procedure is uniquely variable but should be based on the individual condition of the infant and institutional experience.[316–319]

Open surgical correction is achieved with a transabdominal approach, and primary closure is usually possible. If the defect is too large, artificial tissue may be used for closure. In most instances, the abdomen is too small to accommodate the bowels when they are returned to the abdominal cavity. The net effect is a dramatic decrease in pulmonary compliance (in the good lung), desaturation, and hypercapnia. Alternately, the viscera are placed in a Silo pouch (Bentec Medical, Woodland, CA) outside the body until growth allows their return to the abdominal cavity. A chest tube may be placed on the contralateral side before surgery in the event of a pneumothorax. In the past 2 decades, thoracoscopic repair has been used with excellent success in infants who are medically stable.[314,316]

This approach can be performed without single-lung ventilation by use of low-flow, low-pressure CO_2 insufflation, which collapses the lung and gently allows the return of the herniated viscera back into the abdomen. The infant is positioned in the lateral decubitus, with the upper arm supported without interfering with surgical instruments. Both of these techniques can also be performed if the child requires ECMO, but in the latter case these surgeries are usually undertaken in the NICU.[314,316] The surgical timing for neonates who require ECMO remains contentious. Some believe that surgery should be either performed early, before ECMO, whereas others believe that later surgery is preferred.[320] These arguments arise because bleeding during surgery in anticoagulated infants during ECMO can be excessive. In addition, some centers offer advanced treatment options such as fetal-based corrective surgical procedures.[317,321] Temporary fetoscopic tracheal plugging, performed between 25 and 28 weeks gestation, prevents the normal outflow of surfactant-rich fetal lung fluid.[322] The retained volume subsequently enlarges the fetal

lungs, accelerates growth, and reduces the mass effect of herniated viscera. A prospective randomized trial (**T**racheal **O**cclusion to **A**ccelerate **L**ung **G**rowth [TOTAL]) is currently enrolling patients to better define outcomes and advantages or disadvantages compared with standard surgical approaches.[323] A reanalysis of two trials at 14 centers concluded that "fetoscopic endoluminal tracheal occlusion increases survival for both moderate and severe lung hypoplasia"[324]; they also felt that separate analyses were confounded by small sample sizes.

Anesthetic management is aimed at avoiding the harmful effects of volutrauma (by maintaining frequent small tidal volumes and limited peak-inspiratory pressures) and those conditions known to increase PVR (hypoxemia, acidosis, hypothermia, hypercarbia). A nasogastric tube should be passed before induction of anesthesia to empty the stomach while the airway is ventilated at low peak-inspiratory pressures by face mask before the tracheal tube is placed. N_2O should be avoided because it will expand air-filled cavities (bowel) and limit the inspired oxygen concentration. Postoperatively, the trachea remains intubated. The use of an epidural catheter or intercostal nerve block (thoracoscopic approach) aids in postoperative comfort.

Congenital Lung Malformations

CONGENITAL BRONCHOGENIC AND PULMONARY CYSTS. Congenital bronchogenic and pulmonary cysts result from the abnormal development of the ventral foregut and lung budding during the first trimester.[325] These cysts may be centrally located within the mediastinum and produce obstruction by a mass effect.[326] They may also be located at the carina and cause obstruction or distal gas trapping by a ball-valve effect. Those located in the hilum, in the paratracheal region, or in the lung parenchyma may lead to chronic respiratory illness from infection and abscess formation.[327,328] Congenital cysts are occasionally diagnosed only after rupture of the cyst produces hemorrhage or bronchopulmonary fistula formation.[325,328] Urgent surgical resection via thoracotomy or thoracoscopically is recommended for symptomatic cysts, and at 3 to 6 months of age for asymptomatic cysts to promote lung growth and prevent malignant transformation.[329–332]

The anesthetic should be designed to prevent further enlargement of the cyst because a communication may exist with the airway. Awake (sedated) intubation or intubation after an inhalation induction, followed by maintenance of spontaneous ventilation, if possible, until the thorax is opened may reduce the potential risk of a sudden expansion of the cyst. If assisted ventilation is required, low peak-inspiratory pressures should be used. Should the cyst be fluid filled or infected, selective bronchial blocking may be helpful to protect the unaffected lung (see Chapter 13).[333,334] N_2O and positive-pressure ventilation without adequate expiratory time should be avoided to decrease the possibility of enlarging the cyst. If these attempts are unsuccessful and the cyst enlarges to the point of occluding the airway or compromising the circulation, needle aspiration may be required to reduce the size of the cyst and facilitate oxygenation and ventilation. If this approach is unsuccessful, emergency thoracostomy may be lifesaving.

CONGENITAL LOBAR EMPHYSEMA. Congenital lobar emphysema, also known as congenital lobar overinflation or infantile lobar emphysema, is the hyperinflation of one or more pulmonary lobes (Fig. 35.10) (see also Fig. 13.10). The incidence is approximately 1/20,000 with a 3:1 preference for males. The left upper lobe is most frequently involved (43%), followed by the right middle lobe (32%), and right upper lobe (20%), with bilateral

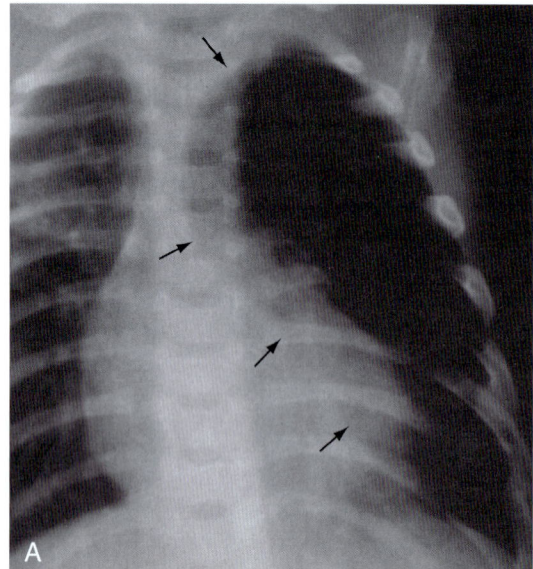

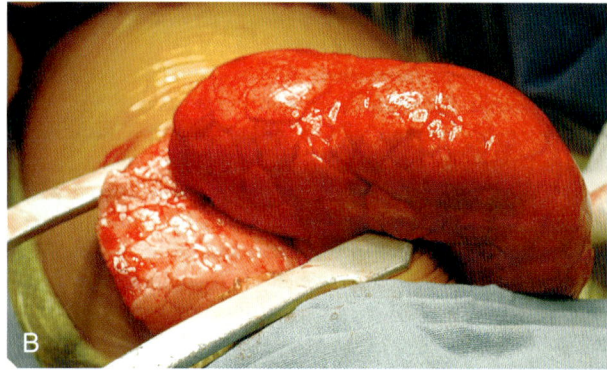

FIGURE 35.10 A, Radiograph from an infant with congenital lobar emphysema demonstrates hyperinflation of the left lung with herniation across the midline *(arrows)* and mediastinal shift. **B,** Intraoperative photograph shows the emphysematous lobe bulging through the thoracotomy incision. (From Coté CJ. The anesthetic management of congenital lobar emphysema. *Anesthesiology.* 1978;49(4):296-298.)

involvement in 20%. In 12% to 14% of cases there is associated congenital heart disease or vascular anomaly.[335] The exact etiology is unknown; however, it is thought to result from a disruption in the development of the bronchial cartilage that causes bronchial collapse.[336,337] This lack of cartilaginous support leads to a ball-valve effect with consequent overinflation. The hyperinflated lung causes an increase in intrathoracic pressure and compression atelectasis on the ipsilateral or contralateral lung, resulting in mediastinal shift and ventilation-perfusion (V/Q) mismatch.[335] Typically, a V/Q scan highlights the degree of hyperinflation; however, single-photon emission computed tomography with computed tomography has been used more recently, which allows for better delineation of function to determine which patients might benefit from surgical intervention.[338]

Surgical lobectomy of the affected segments via an open thoracotomy or thoracoscopically is the definitive treatment.[339] In infants with asymptomatic lobar emphysema, thoracoscopic lobectomy has become the most common approach with recent evidence demonstrating that thoracoscopic lobectomy is noninferior to open lobectomy.[340] Avoiding N_2O and positive-pressure ventilation prevents the expansion of the emphysematous lobe,

which could compress normal lung tissue.[341,342] If positive pressure is required, low peak pressures and tidal volumes should be used. There have been reports of using single-lung ventilation while the affected lobe is resected. Frequent tracheal tube suctioning is suggested; an epidural catheter threaded from the caudal to the thoracic space may provide pain control.[335,337]

GASTROINTESTINAL PATHOLOGY

Emergency surgical conditions of the GI tract are most frequently due to obstructive lesions, lesions that compromise intestinal blood supply, or both. Infants with obstructive lesions should be considered to have a full stomach, as the retention of gastric fluid increases the risk of aspiration during induction. A rapid-sequence induction (RSI) should follow suctioning of gastric contents (usually with a vented catheter in supine, right, and left positions),[343] and N_2O should be avoided to minimize intestinal distention. Desaturation after a brief period of apnea during an RSI occurs more rapidly in neonates than in older infants,[344] emphasizing the importance of preoxygenation and the rapid establishment of an airway. Some providers advocate the use of a modified RSI technique, with gentle mask ventilation before tracheal intubation.[345] Unless life-threatening compromise of organ blood flow occurs, these lesions do not require immediate surgical correction, and the priority is to correct any metabolic derangements and establish euvolemia before undergoing corrective surgery.

Infants with lesions that compromise intestinal blood supply and cause ischemia are extremely ill. They may present with hypotension, metabolic abnormalities, particularly hyperkalemia, anemia, and thrombocytopenia. Emergency surgery is required in these circumstances and is directed at removing the necrotic tissue, closing perforations, and reestablishing normal perfusion to the intestine. Blood products and emergency drugs should be readily available. Good IV access is required, and a centrally located catheter may be necessary for the administration of vasoactive drugs, as well as an arterial line for close blood pressure monitoring. Infants with compromised intestinal blood supply are usually considered to have full stomachs and N_2O is avoided, as well.

Obstructed Lesions
Hypertrophic Pyloric Stenosis
Hypertrophic pyloric stenosis is the result of hypertrophy and hyperplasia of the muscularis layer of the pylorus, causing a functional gastric outlet obstruction (Fig. 35.11). It occurs in 1/500 live births and more frequently in first-born males.[346,347] In a systematic review of publications on possible factors that were associated with developing pyloric stenosis, first-born males, bottle feeding, maternal smoking, and African ethnicity were significant.[348] Infants usually present between 2 and 8 weeks of age with protracted nonbilious projectile vomiting. Diagnosis of a thickened pylorus may be confirmed by palpation of a small olive-sized mass in the upper right quadrant, although a recent systematic review demonstrated that ultrasound (>3 mm pyloric muscle thickness) has a 98% sensitivity and 99% specificity for the diagnosis.[349] Persistent vomiting will result in hypokalemic, hypochloremic metabolic alkalosis; severe cases may progress to dehydration and a metabolic acidosis.[350] The kidneys attempt to maintain a normal blood pH by excreting bicarbonate. To maintain euvolemia and retain sodium cations, the kidneys excrete hydrogen and then potassium cations to maintain charge neutrality. Paradoxical aciduria occurs in hypovolemic infants (after prolonged

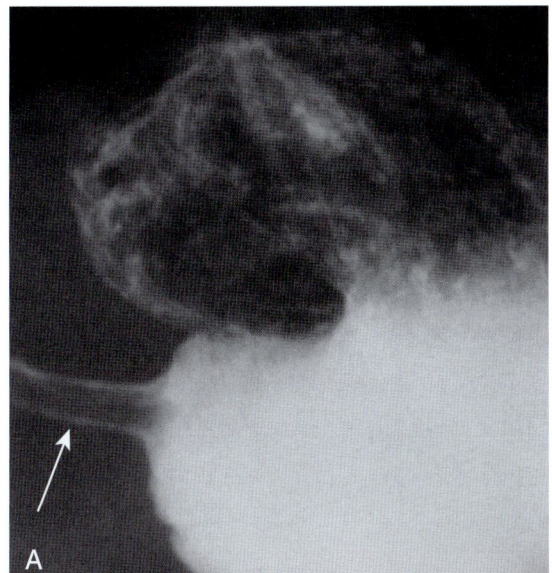

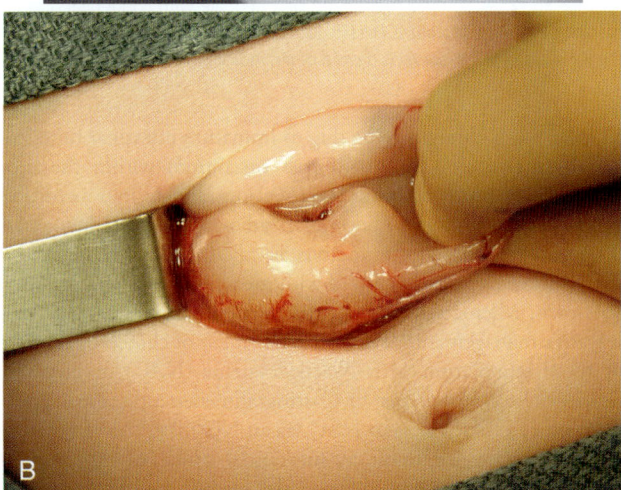

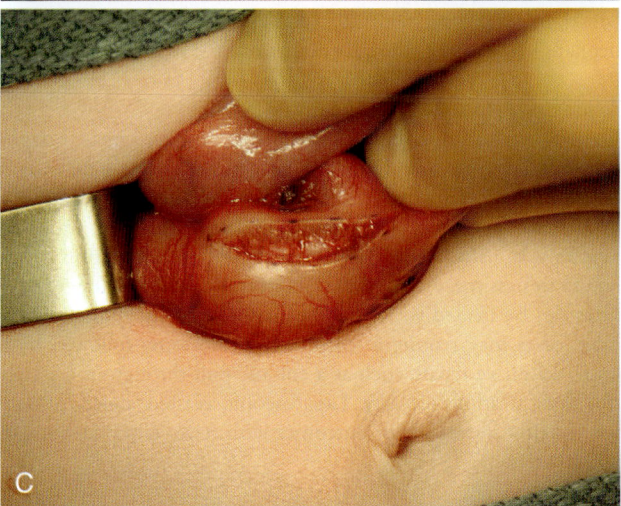

FIGURE 35.11 A, Barium swallow and abdominal radiograph of an infant with pyloric stenosis demonstrates a high degree of obstruction of the gastric outflow tract with a "wisp" of barium escaping through the pylorus *(arrow).* **B,** The hypertrophied pylorus. **C,** Surgical myotomy relieved the obstruction. (Courtesy Dr. Daniel P. Doody.)

vomiting) when the urine appears acidic, whereas the pH in the blood is alkaline. Since this disorder is not a life-threatening emergency, time should be taken to correct the metabolic derangements and ensure proper rehydration; this may take 24 to 48 hours although investigators reported that by adopting an institutional fluid management strategy for infants with abnormal electrolyte concentrations (Cl^- ≤85 or 97 mmol/L and $HCO3^-$ ≥33 or 40 mmol/L), the time to correcting the electrolyte concentrations, number of blood draws, and postoperative length of stay were all significantly reduced.[351] Before considering an anesthetic in these infants, the skin turgor and the urine output (1–2 mL/kg per hour) should be restored, a serum sodium greater than 130 mEq/L, potassium greater than 3.0 mEq/L, and a chloride concentration greater than 85 mEq/L. A Delphi Analysis resulted in recommendations that these children should have a pH ≤7.45, base excess ≤3.5, bicarbonate <26 mmol/L, sodium ≥132 mmol/L, potassium ≥3.5 mmol/L, chloride ≥100 mmol/L, and glucose ≥4.0 mmol/L, and that isotonic crystalloid with 5% glucose and 10 to 20 mEq/L potassium should be used for volume resuscitation.[352] Diagnosis is commonly made via ultrasonography or rarely with a barium swallow and radiographic examination.[353,354] Most infants are quickly diagnosed with pyloric stenosis, resulting in only a minority who now present with severe fluid and electrolyte imbalances.[355]

Treatment is surgical pyloromyotomy by means of an open periumbilical incision or laparoscopic approach (E-Fig. 35.4 and Video 35.3).[356] The laparoscopic approach speeds time to return to oral feeds, reduces hospital stay, and provides better cosmesis.[357–359] Some assert that the laparoscopic approach may have a greater rate of perforation and incomplete relief of gastric obstruction, although there is a lack of substantial evidence.[360–362] Endoscopic pyloric balloon dilation and endoscopic pyloromyotomy are novel techniques that are starting to gain popularity as an alternative to surgery.[363–365]

Three techniques have been used to secure the airway in infants with pyloric stenosis: an RSI, a modified RSI, or an inhalational induction. An RSI is generally recommended because of the gastric outlet obstruction and the risk of aspiration, although some have performed inhalational inductions successfully.[366] The risk of hypoxemia developing during an RSI in infants during induction of anesthesia is based on a retrospective review of 296 infants' data from Boston Children's Hospital between 2012 and 2018. Standard RSI had an odds ratio for hypoxemia of 6.5 compared with a modified RSI (which includes mask ventilation after induction of anesthesia but before tracheal intubation).[367] The odds ratio was increased to 18 for developing hypoxemia during multiple attempts at intubation compared with a single intubation attempt. Interestingly, cricoid pressure was used during induction whether using an RSI or modified RSI in 70% to 76% of infants. However, many practitioners have abandoned cricoid pressure during laryngoscopy in these infants in part because of its lack of proven benefit and in part because of the increased difficulty it poses during laryngoscopy when adult's fingers press on the infant's short neck. In two postal surveys from the UK in 1994 and 2007, 45% to 50% of consultants used cricoid pressure during induction of anesthesia in infants undergoing pyloromyotomy.[368,369] In a more recent survey from South Africa, 10% of respondents used cricoid pressure in neonates compared with 56% in children and 21% in infants undergoing RSI.[370] In fact, only 15% used cricoid pressure during laryngoscopy in infants undergoing pyloromyotomy, which likely reflects current practice. Difficult intubation was diagnosed in 7.5% to 8% of infants with pyloric stenosis, which is out of proportion to that otherwise expected in infants at this age according to the NECTARINE study.[371] The explanation for this finding was unclear: true difficult intubations, increased difficulty due to cricoid pressure, or lack of expertise by operators. The duration of surgery whether open or laparoscopic is brief (30 minutes), although neuromuscular blockade is usually required to maintain optimal surgical conditions. Sugammadex may be a good option for reversal if rocuronium is used as the paralytic often outlasts the short duration procedure; atracurium or cisatracurium are alternatives because of their metabolism through Hoffman elimination. Another study examined the effects of preoperative volume resuscitation with anesthetic emergence in 529 laparoscopic pyloromyotomies.[372] The times to emergence correlated positively with a serum bicarbonate concentration ≥24 mEq/L, increasing with each further 1 mEq/L rise in bicarbonate; also a preoperative bicarbonate <30 mEq/L predicted a 5.4 minute more rapid emergence from anesthesia than a bicarbonate value ≥30 mEq/L.[372]

Pain following pyloromyotomy is usually managed by the infiltration of local anesthetic into the trochar sites or incision site and a nonopioid agent such as acetaminophen or a nonsteroidal antiinflammatory agent. With postoperative pain of minimal intensity, opioids are generally not required for this surgery. Specific perioperative anesthetic management is as detailed earlier for obstructed lesions.[357,358]

Complications have been reported infrequently in association with anesthesia for pyloromyotomy. A recent report suggested that >1 episode of hypoxemia occurred in the perioperative period after pyloromyotomy in >50% of infants, primarily at induction or emergence[373]; 3/539 had at least one episode of postoperative apnea and 2 of these were former preterm infants. An analysis of data from 9752 pyloromyotomies reported to the National Surgical Quality Improvement Project between 2016 and 2020 revealed that the laparoscopic approach, which has been steadily increasing in utilization, has led to a reduced complication rate (2%) and shorter length of stay compared with the open approach.[374]

Duodenal Atresia and Meconium Ileus

The exact etiology of **duodenal atresia** is unknown; however, with its close association with multiple other congenital anomalies (50%–70%), it is believed to occur early in gestation. It is one of the more common causes of intestinal abnormalities, occurring in 1/6000 live births. Approximately 20% to 30% of these neonates also have trisomy 21, and up to 25% of these infants will have a cardiac anomaly. Diagnosis can be made with high reliability prenatally with ultrasound[375] or postnatally with an abdominal radiograph demonstrating the "double-bubble" sign, formed by fluid/air seen in the dilated stomach and proximal duodenum, with the remaining bowel devoid of fluid/air (Fig. 35.12).[376] Neonates born with duodenal atresia usually present with bilious vomiting beginning within the first 24 to 48 hours after birth, leading to dehydration and electrolyte imbalances. After medical stabilization, open or laparoscopic surgical correction is required. A peripherally inserted central catheter (PICC) may be placed in the event of continued obstruction and the need for long-term total parenteral nutrition.

Meconium ileus is an intestinal obstruction of the newborn caused by inspissated meconium in the terminal ileum. Most cases are associated with cystic fibrosis (10%–15% of neonates with cystic fibrosis will have meconium ileus).[377] Other cases have been reported in premature infants, especially those with VLBW and

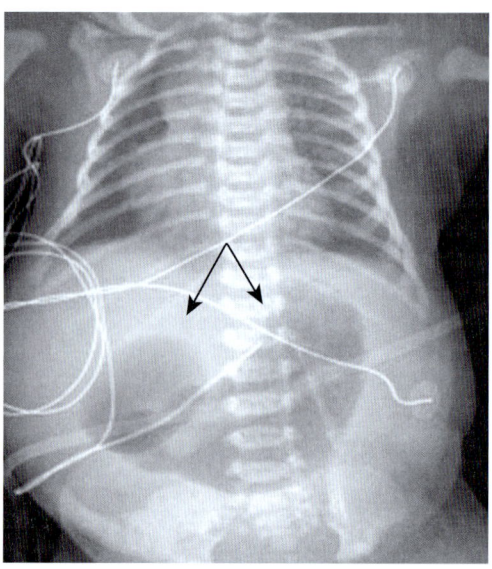

FIGURE 35.12 Abdominal radiograph of a neonate with congenital duodenal atresia demonstrating a classic double-bubble sign *(arrows)*. Note that the remainder of the bowel is devoid of air, indicating complete obstruction.

ELBW, and is thought to be due to immature intestinal function and dysmotility.[378] Failure to pass meconium within the first 24 hours of birth, abdominal distention, and bilious vomiting support this diagnosis. Abdominal radiographs reveal low small bowel obstruction with numerous air-filled loops of bowel and a soap-bubble effect of gas mixed with meconium in the right lower abdomen. Microcolon is often seen with a barium enema. Conservative management is the initial treatment of choice, consisting of rectal stimulation with *N*-acetylcysteine (NAC) or glycerin, simple enemas,[379] contrast or Gastrografin enemas, or the administration of Gastrografin or NAC via an NG tube.[376,378] Hyperosmolar enemas may result in substantial shifts in intravascular volume, leading to hypovolemia and electrolyte imbalances. If conservative management fails and persistent ileus ensues, the neonate may require surgical evacuation.

Imperforate Anus

The etiology of imperforate anus remains unclear but is thought to occur between 5 and 7 weeks of gestation. The incidence is 1/5000 births and is more prevalent in males. It is a part of the VACTERL association (see earlier).[301] The diagnosis of imperforate anus is usually made by initial physical examination or by failure to pass meconium within the first 48 hours of life. Milder cases can be treated with a perineal anoplasty, but more complicated cases may require a temporizing colostomy followed by a more definitive repair, such as a colonic pull-through or a posterior sagittal anorectoplasty. Laparoscopic-assisted anorectoplasty has recently shown better outcomes with fewer complications in select patients.[380,381]

Compromised Intestinal Blood Supply
Inguinal Hernia

Failure of the process vaginalis to close during the last few weeks of gestation can result in the protrusion of abdominal cavity and gonadal structures through the inguinal canal. Most inguinal hernias manifest within the first 6 months of life, affecting 1% to 5% of full-term infants and children, and up to 30% of premature infants. The prevalence is greater in males. In 60% of infants, the hernia occurs on the right, in 30% it occurs on the left, and in 10% there is bilateral involvement. Clinical manifestations include the visualization and/or palpation of a bulge in the inguinal or scrotal region that is more prominent when crying or straining and generally reduces while at rest.

Hernias that do not spontaneously resolve need to be surgically corrected because of the risk of incarceration; however, surgery can be performed on a semi-elective basis as an outpatient.[382] Both open and laparoscopic approaches are employed.[383] When the contents of the hernia become incarcerated or strangulated, they are at risk for ischemia and necrosis, and emergency surgical correction is indicated. Elective repair can be performed with the infant under either general or regional anesthesia (caudal or spinal block). In fact, regional anesthesia has been associated with lower risk of prolonged postsurgical intubation, early apnea, and desaturation.[384,385] Premature infants less than 60 weeks PCA should be observed for at least 12 apnea-free hours for signs of apnea, whether anesthetized with general or spinal anesthesia before discharge.[53,59,60] Anesthetic management for incarcerated or strangulated hernias should proceed as mentioned earlier for ischemic lesions.

Necrotizing Enterocolitis

NEC is a multifactorial disease that can lead to bowel necrosis and is a leading cause of neonatal mortality.[386] It affects 5% to 11% of premature and LBW infants and has a mortality rate of 10% to 50%.[387–389] The pathogenesis is not completely understood, but is thought to be due to unbalanced inflammatory responses of bowel mucosa; alterations in normal intestinal flora by antibiotics and feeds[386]; lack of a fully developed intestinal mucosal barrier, which leads to the breakdown of the intestinal wall and bowel necrosis; and prenatal factors such as intrauterine inflammation and infection.[387,388,390,391] Increasing evidence suggests that modulation of gut flora with probiotics and prebiotics may be indicated for prevention in preterm infants.[392] In addition to prematurity, NEC has also been associated with low systemic cardiac output, hypoxia, PDA, infection, red blood cell transfusion, and enteral feedings (especially formula-fed neonates).[393,394] In fact, human breast milk is now touted as the preferred strategy to prevent NEC in preterm infants.[395] Oxygen saturations in the lower range of 85% to 89% have been associated with an increased risk of surgical NEC, compared with oxygen saturations in the higher 91% to 95% range.[396]

NEC can be insidious in onset or rapidly progress to multisystem organ failure or death. Early signs tend to be nonspecific and include temperature instability, poor feeding with residual volumes or vomiting, lethargy, apnea, bradycardia, mild abdominal distention, and bloody stools, although evidence points to specific biomarkers to facilitate early diagnosis (fecal calprotectin and S100A12, serum fatty acid–binding protein, and urine biomarkers).[397,398] Tachycardia, poor perfusion/hypotension, metabolic acidosis, thrombocytopenia, abdominal tenderness, and peritonitis are findings in later, more severe cases.[387,393] An abdominal x-ray may initially suggest an ileus with thickened bowel walls and dilated bowel loops and later demonstrate gas in the intestinal wall (pneumatosis intestinalis) and in the hepatobiliary tract or portal venous system (Fig. 35.13). The finding of free air in the abdominal cavity (pneumoperitoneum) warrants prompt surgical intervention (Fig. 35.14).

Historically, initial therapy has been conservative and included making the neonate *nil per os* (NPO), initiating broad-spectrum antibiotics, and decompressing the bowel with low continuous

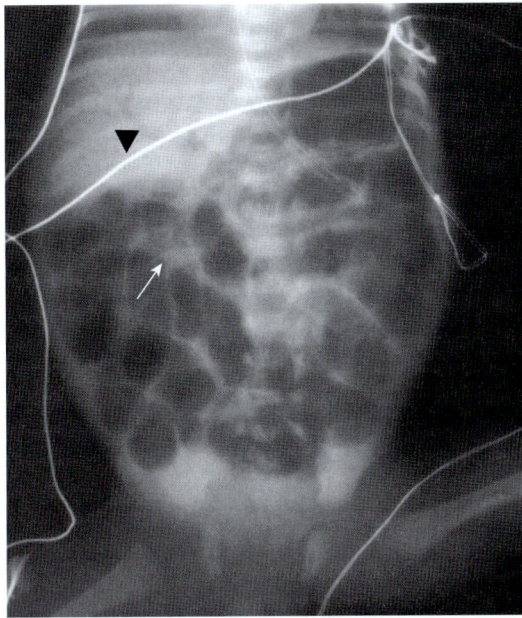

FIGURE 35.13 Abdominal radiograph of a neonate with necrotizing enterocolitis demonstrates generalized bowel distention (ileus), a small amount of pneumatosis intestinalis in the left upper quadrant *(arrow)*, and gas outlining the intrahepatic portal vein *(arrowhead)*. (Courtesy Dr. Sjirk J. Westra.)

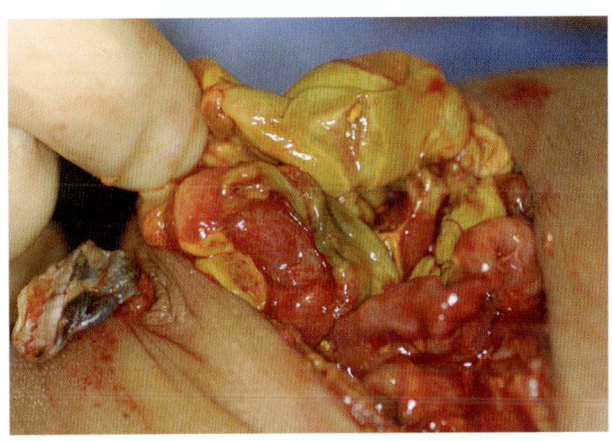

FIGURE 35.14 Early necrotizing enterocolitis with bowel perforation. Note that the perforation was diagnosed early and that there is soiling of the peritoneum but there does not appear to be any dead bowel. This type of perforation is generally associated with a positive outcome.

gastric suction. Recent data support standardized feeding protocols with human milk[395] (probiotic supplements when human milk is not available)[392,396] and warns against the use of empirical antibiotics, which have not been shown to reduce NEC and may even contribute to it.[386,399] Supportive measures to correct metabolic and hematologic abnormalities, as well as fluid resuscitation, are also involved. If conservative management fails or signs of necrosis or viscus perforation appear, an exploratory laparotomy is indicated for resection of necrotic bowel (Fig. 35.15). These infants are critically ill. Preoperative preparation in a timely fashion is vital. NEC predisposes to hypovolemia, cardiovascular and respiratory failure, capillary leak syndrome, disseminated intravascular coagulation, and hypoglycemia. These infants may be septic and volume depleted with very large fluid requirements as the

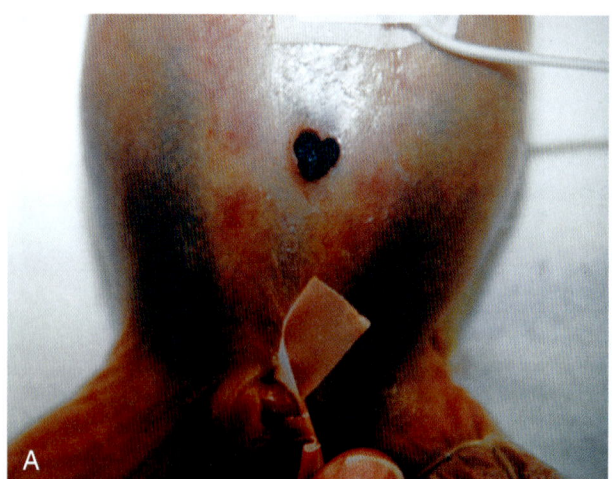
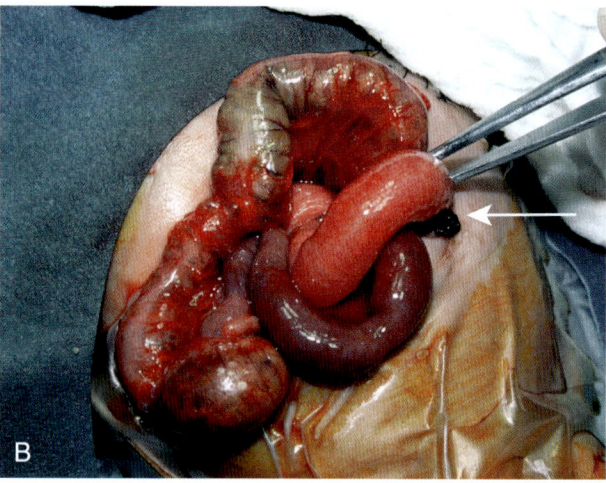

FIGURE 35.15 A preterm neonate with severe necrotizing enterocolitis and intestinal necrosis. **A,** Abdominal discoloration consistent with dead bowel. **B,** Necrotizing enterocolitis with a segment of dead bowel *(top)* and evidence of free stool in the abdomen *(arrow)*. These infants often have bowel perforation and hemorrhage from the bowel or liver. They can have severe hypotension requiring vasopressor support and enormous volume requirements. Moreover, because of hemorrhage and disseminated intravascular coagulopathy, these infants will generally require transfusions of blood, platelets, and fresh frozen plasma. Some practitioners also advocate administration of vitamin K. (Courtesy Dr. Daniel P. Doody.)

TABLE 35.6	Comparison of Omphalocele and Gastroschisis	
Comparison Factors	**Omphalocele**	**Gastroschisis**
Cause	Failure of gut migration from yolk sac into abdomen	Occlusion of omphalomesenteric artery
Location	Within umbilical cord	Periumbilical
Associated lesions	Beckwith-Wiedemann syndrome (macroglossia, gigantism, hypoglycemia, hyperviscosity) Congenital heart disease Exstrophy of bladder	Exposed gut inflammation, edema, dilation, and foreshortened

result of massive third-space losses. Often there is an enormous need for 5% albumin just to maintain intravascular volume (up to 1 blood volume or more) because of third spacing. There is nearly always a need for transfusion of platelets and fresh frozen plasma. Terminal, irreversible, hyperkalemia with renal failure is common; central venous access is usually required for inotropic support (e.g., dopamine, epinephrine).

Omphalocele and Gastroschisis

Defects in the abdominal wall can lead to herniated organs with impaired blood supply, intestinal obstruction, and major intravascular fluid defects in neonates with omphalocele and gastroschisis. The differences between omphalocele and gastroschisis are summarized in Table 35.6.

Omphalocele represents a failure of the gut to migrate from the yolk sac into the abdomen during gestation (Fig. 35.16A).[400,401] It occurs in ~1 to 2/10,000 births.[402,403] Infants with omphalocele may have associated genetic, cardiac, urologic (exstrophy of the bladder; Fig. 35.16B), and metabolic abnormalities (e.g., Beckwith-Wiedemann syndrome with visceromegaly, macroglossia, hypoglycemia, and polycythemia).[404] The herniated viscera

emerge from the umbilicus and are covered with a membranous sac. The bowel is morphologically and usually functionally normal. Nearly all omphaloceles are associated with reduced chest capacity and pulmonary hypoplasia, making them prone to respiratory disorders.[405]

Gastroschisis is defined as visceral herniation through the abdominal wall not covered by a membrane. Evidence suggests that there is a defect of the umbilical ring rather than the abdominal wall due to a vascular-thrombotic event of the umbilical vein.[406] It occurs in ~4.5/10,000 births and is usually not associated with other congenital anomalies.[402,406] The herniated viscera and intestines are periumbilical, usually on the right, and are exposed to amniotic fluid in utero and to air after delivery, resulting in inflammation, edema, and dilated, foreshortened, functionally abnormal bowel (Fig. 35.16C).[407–409]

Management of these neonates until surgical repair is directed at maintaining perfusion to the herniated viscera and reduction of fluid loss from exposed visceral surfaces by covering the mucosal surfaces with sterile, saline-soaked dressings. A plastic wrap aids in decreasing evaporative volume losses and the tendency to develop hypothermia, which is more pronounced with gastroschisis. These defects represent a wide spectrum of pathology and require individualized assessment of associated anomalies, intravascular volume status, and fluid replacement.[410] If complete reduction is not possible, a staged reduction is carried out.[411,412] The abdominal contents are covered with a Silastic pouch, and the size of the pouch is subsequently reduced in stages, thus allowing the abdominal cavity to gradually accommodate the increased mass without severely compromising ventilation or organ perfusion.[413,414] Tissue expanders and skin grafting may also be necessary for closure.

Anesthetic management is directed at continued volume resuscitation and measures to prevent hypothermia. Primary abdominal closure may be associated with markedly increased intraabdominal pressure (E-Fig. 35.5). Intraabdominal pressure may be monitored by transducing either an intragastric or urinary catheter.[415]

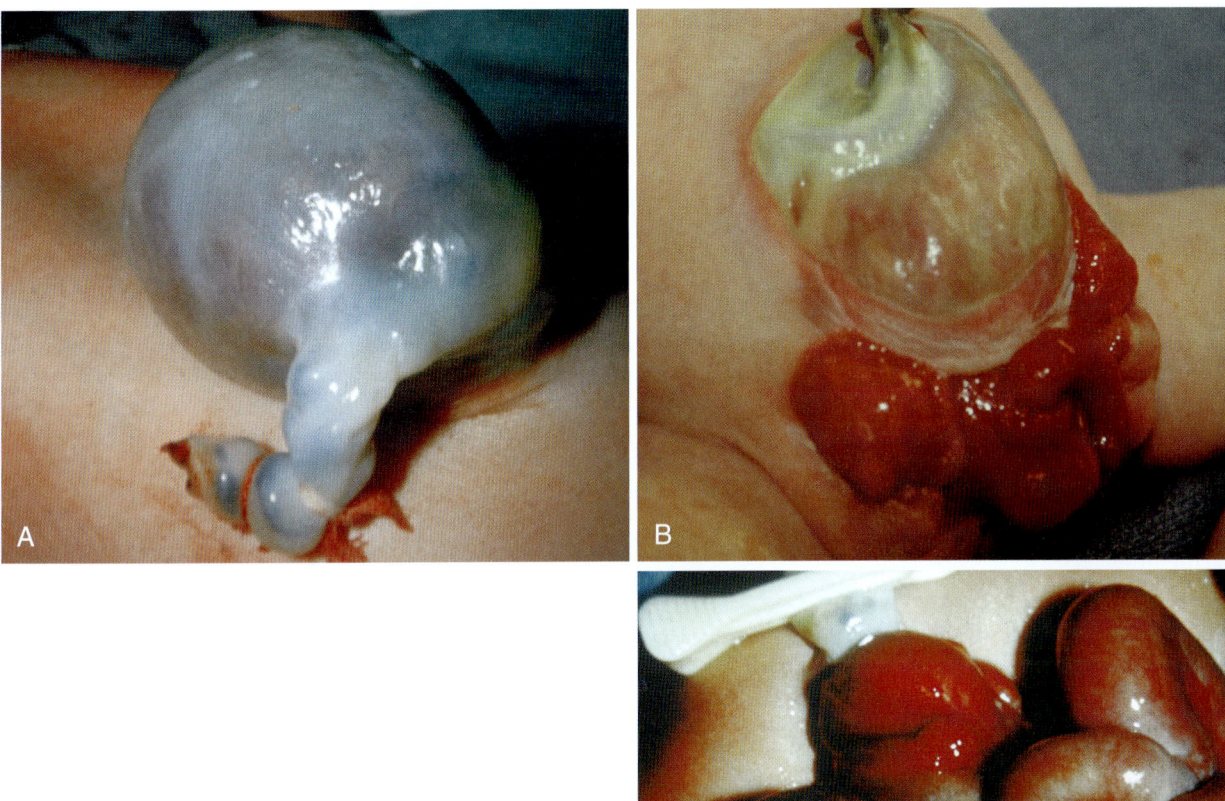

FIGURE 35.16 A, Omphalocele covered with a membranous sac; the defect arises at the umbilicus. **B,** Omphalocele with associated exstrophy of the bladder. **C,** Gastroschisis; note the absence of a membranous sac. In contrast to omphalocele, the gastroschisis anomaly is periumbilical.

Increased intraabdominal pressure can decrease organ perfusion and ventilatory reserve, including perfusion of the intestines, kidney, and liver as well as secondarily impaired organ function. This may lead to markedly altered drug metabolism and prolonged drug effects.[185] A bladder pressure that exceeds 20 mm Hg after primary closure is likely to cause abdominal ischemia and necessitate an urgent reoperation.[416] The bowel may become edematous, and urine output may be reduced as a result of poor renal perfusion. Venous return from the lower body also may be reduced, resulting in lower extremity congestion and cyanosis. Blood pressure and pulse oximetry determinations from a lower extremity may be different from those in the upper extremity. Decreased diaphragmatic function and bilateral lower lobe atelectasis may occur, contributing to respiratory failure.[417]

Malrotation and Midgut Volvulus

Malrotation and midgut volvulus result from abnormal migration or incomplete rotation of the intestines from the yolk sac back into the abdomen.[418] It occurs in ~1/500 births and 30% to 60% of affected patients have associated congenital anomalies. Rotation of the intestine around the mesentery may produce the abnormal location of the ileocecal valve in the right upper quadrant and kinking or compression of its vascular supply. This kinking can be seen on an abdominal CT scan or ultrasound as a

"whirlpool sign"; the twisting of the mesentery and superior mesenteric artery and vein.[419] If the malrotation occurs during development, atretic segments of bowel are formed. If the kinking or compression occurs after the bowel is normally developed, bowel necrosis may result.

These infants present with bilious emesis, a tender and distended abdomen, and increasing abdominal girth. Bloody stools are an ominous sign. They may have hypotension, hypovolemia, and electrolyte abnormalities. Neonatal diagnosis of a volvulus can be difficult due to fluctuating signs/symptoms.[420] Because delay in surgery may result in necrosis of the entire small intestine, fluid and electrolyte resuscitation with stabilization should not delay surgical correction. This is a true neonatal emergency, and surgery should proceed as expeditiously as possible with ongoing perioperative resuscitation. Surgery involves either an open Ladd's procedure or a laparoscopic Ladd's (lap-Ladd) procedure to correct the volvulus.[421]

Hirschsprung Disease

Hirschsprung disease is the absence of parasympathetic ganglion cells (Auerbach and Meissner plexuses) in the large intestine.[422,423] This deficiency creates a nonperistaltic segment of variable length, a tonically contracted anorectal sphincter, and delayed passage of meconium. Functional obstruction occurs at the level of the affected segment. Its incidence is ~1/6000 with a male predominance and is relatively rare in premature infants. Approximately 60% of patients will have an associated anomaly. Diagnosis is confirmed by the absence of ganglionic cells on rectal biopsy.

Infants with Hirschsprung disease present with symptoms consistent with bowel obstruction, such as bilious vomiting and abdominal distention. However, the bowel may occasionally become distended to the point that its blood supply is compromised, leading to perforation. If left untreated, enteric bacteria may invade the bowel wall and enter the bloodstream, leading to toxic megacolon (Fig. 35.17). These infants are critically ill and may require massive volume replacement and vasopressor support. Surgical repair depends on the extent of intestinal involvement and includes anorectal myomectomy, mucosal resections, diverting colostomies, and transanal pull-throughs. Future prospects include human-derived enteric cell transplants through stem cell research and tissue engineering.[424]

LIGATION OF PATENT DUCTUS ARTERIOSUS

Controversy exists regarding whether a PDA should be treated at all, the timing of therapy if treated, and merits of medical versus surgical therapy.[425–427] This controversy is the result of trials that have failed to show that early PDA closure leads to any benefit in premature neonatal outcomes.[427,428] It is possible that although a PDA is associated with morbidity in the neonate, it is not a causative factor, although delayed closure has been linked with bronchopulmonary dysplasia, NEC, intraventricular hemorrhage, and pulmonary hypertension. Medical therapy involves the administration of a cyclooxygenase inhibitor, such as indomethacin or ibuprofen.[428–430] Indomethacin therapy is less likely to close the PDA in micropremies compared with premature infants, and is more likely to produce complications, including thrombocytopenia, renal failure, hyponatremia, and intestinal perforation.[431] Ibuprofen is equally effective for PDA closure in the micropremie, with a reduced frequency of renal failure.[432] Both the probability of PDA closure and the probability of adverse effects relate to plasma nonsteroidal antiinflammatory drug concentration. The concentration achieved after a standard dose changes with PMA

because clearance increases with PMA; failure to account for a changing clearance with age contributes to confusion in the literature.[433,434] More recently, paracetamol (acetaminophen) has been used with equal effectiveness in those infants in whom cyclooxygenase inhibitor therapy has failed or in whom those drugs are contraindicated, although further efficacy evidence is required.[427,433,435–437] Surgical ligation of the PDA has a low incidence of major intraoperative complications when performed by an experienced team.[438] However, as many as one-third of premature infants develop severe cardiovascular instability following PDA ligation, termed postligation cardiac syndrome, which is due to an abrupt increase in left ventricular afterload with decreased preload, leading to low cardiac output, hypotension, and myocardial dysfunction.[426,427,439] In addition, some studies show an increased risk of chronic lung disease, ROP, and neurosensory impairment after surgical ligation.[426,440]

Surgical ligation of the PDA can be performed in the OR or in the NICU (usually reserved for micropremies and ELBW neonates). It is achieved via left thoracotomy with manual retraction of the lung. The aorta and pulmonary artery lie in proximity to the PDA; thus severe bleeding may occur abruptly and unexpectedly during the procedure. Blood should be immediately available for transfusion. In addition, it can be difficult to distinguish the PDA from the aorta, as the diameter of the PDA may be the same or even greater than that of the aorta. Monitoring blood pressure and pulse oximetry on the right arm (preductal) and oximetry on the foot (postductal) will assist the surgeon to identify the correct vessel to be ligated. The surgeon will place a temporary clamp on what is believed to be the PDA. A loss in postductal oximetry indicates clamping of the aorta, whereas a decrease in both oximeters and $ETCO_2$ suggests clamping of the pulmonary artery, most frequently the left. A successful PDA ligation results in a "step up" in mean arterial pressure owing to an increase in diastolic blood pressure with no decrease in either of the pulse oximeters

Transcatheter occlusion of the PDA can be accomplished using either coils or an occluder device in the catheterization laboratory as an alternative to surgical ligation with similar efficacy (see Chapter 20). Like the surgical option, device occlusion is performed only after failed conservative and medical attempts. In the past, the small vessel size of the extremely premature infant prevented the use of a large enough sheath to implant the device. However, advances over the past 5 to 10 years produced devices capable of transcatheter occlusion in smaller infants. In 2019, the first device for infants weighing less than 700 grams was approved with excellent results.[441,442] The extremely small size of the femoral artery in the micropremie predisposes it to injury, and is best avoided. Instead the PDA is accessed via the femoral vein and its precise location directed with the assistance of a transthoracic echocardiogram and placement of an esophageal catheter.[443,444] In some instances, they are even being deployed at the bedside using only echocardiographic guidance. In addition to avoiding the complications of a surgical repair, the transcatheter approach has shown a more rapid recovery of respiratory function. The most common complications include femoral artery thrombosis, left pulmonary artery stenosis, and aortic coarctation.[80,445–448]

RETINOPATHY OF PREMATURITY

Retinopathy of prematurity (ROP) can lead to blindness if left uncorrected. The exact cause of ROP is unknown; however, it is associated with prematurity, low birth weight, supplemental oxygen therapy, postnatal hypotension, use of surfactant or inotrope,

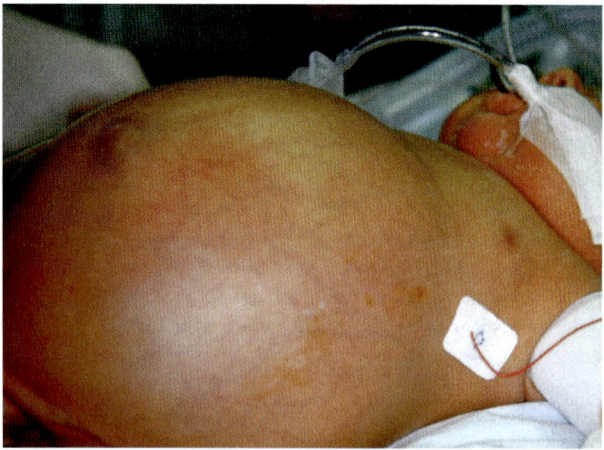

FIGURE 35.17 Toxic megacolon results in massive abdominal distention, fluid requirements, and sepsis. These infants require special consideration in airway management because of the high risk for aspiration and increased abdominal pressure.

and need for mechanical ventilation.[449,450] It is thought to be initiated by oxygen-induced retinal vasoconstriction and endothelial cell death, followed by unchecked neovascularization from angiogenic factors, such as vascular endothelial growth factor, that do not respond to normal regulation because of immaturity.[451–453] Its incidence increases with decreasing gestational age. ROP may be treated with cryotherapy, laser photocoagulation, scleral buckling surgery, and/or vitrectomy (see Chapter 32).

Cryotherapy involves applying a freezing probe under direct visualization to the avascular retina anterior to the fibrovascular ridge. It requires general anesthesia and is usually performed in the OR. Diode laser photocoagulation, currently the gold standard of care, is typically performed at the bedside in the NICU.[454] It has been shown to be as effective as cryotherapy for moderate ROP, and is most commonly used because the systemic adverse effects are fewer, the ocular tissues are less traumatized, and it has a smaller incidence of late complications than cryotherapy. Laser photocoagulation may be performed using topical anesthesia alone, with IV sedation, or with the patient under general anesthesia. However, the incidence of cardiorespiratory complications is greater with topical anesthesia alone than with topical anesthesia with sedation or general anesthesia.[449] The procedure takes 10 to 30 minutes to perform and often involves a series of treatments every few weeks. Anesthetic goals are to provide optic analgesia and to prevent eye and head movement. Many premature infants younger than 32 weeks PCA are naturally inactive and may remain motionless with topical anesthesia alone.

Scleral buckle surgery and vitrectomy, performed for more severe ROP with retinal detachment, are less frequently used because early detection and treatment with laser photocoagulation prevents ROP progression to severe disease. It is usually performed in older infants between 6 months and 1 year of age and requires general anesthesia in the OR.

The latest form of therapy includes intravitreal injection of bevacizumab, a recombinant humanized monoclonal antibody aimed at reducing vascular endothelial growth factor. Results are encouraging; however, more data are needed to establish safety and efficacy.[452,455,456] Ranibizumab has recently been approved by the European Medicines Agency for the treatment of ROP with fewer adverse effects and better outcomes compared with laser therapy.[457] As discussed previously, the optimal oxygen saturation target is controversial. Hyperoxia should be avoided, if at all possible, with a suggested target range of 91% to 95%.

It should be noted, however, that ROP has been reported in infants with cyanotic heart disease and infants never exposed to oxygen; thus hyperoxia is but one factor associated with ROP (see also Chapter 32).[455,458]

ANNOTATED REFERENCES

Bischoff AR, Jasani B, Sathanandam SK, et al. Percutaneous closure of PDA in infants 1.5 kg or less: a meta-analysis. *J Peds.* 2021;230:84-92.

Extremely premature, low birth weight neonates with patent ductus arteriosus had few options other than surgery in the past for closure when pharmacologic treatment failed. Today, with better technology, neonates <1.5 kg can have their PDA closed percutaneously with very few major adverse effects.

Kaemf J, Morris M, Steffen E, et al. Continued improvement in morbidity and reduction in extremely premature infants. *Arch Dis Child Fetal Neonatal Ed.* 2021;106:F2265-F2270.

This report from 10 English-language NICUs comprising nearly 6000 infants demonstrates that with current collaboration and better practice toolkits, premature infants born between 23 to 27 weeks are sustaining improved morbidity rates. Understanding these collaborations is fundamental in furthering the care of extremely premature infants.

Kamata M, Cartabuke RS, Tobias JD. Perioperative care of infants with pyloric stenosis. *Paediatr Anaesth.* 2015;25(12):1193-1206.

This article reviewed the current techniques in use for the perioperative management of infants with pyloric stenosis. They conclude that the optimal approach to airway management is not known, and several different techniques may be used, such as rapid-sequence induction or modified rapid sequence with gentle mask ventilation.

Sola A, Golombek SG, Montes Bueno MT, et al. Safe oxygen saturation targeting and monitoring in preterm infants: can we avoid hypoxia and hyperoxia? *Acta Paediatr.* 2014;103(10):1009-1018.

This study sought to define a more targeted range of oxygen saturations in premature infants to reduce morbidity and mortality. They concluded that there was an increase in mortality with reduced oxygen saturations, yet a greater morbidity with hyperoxia in the higher ranges, leading them to recommend a broader range of intermediate targets.

Stoll BJ, Hansen NI, Bell E, et al. Trends in care practices, morbidity, and mortality of extremely preterm neonates, 1993–2012. *JAMA.* 2015;314(10):1039-1051.

This prospective study of more than 34,000 premature infants born at the Neonatal Research Network centers looked at maternal and neonatal care, morbidities, and survival. They concluded that over the past 20 years there have been several advances in maternal and neonatal care that have contributed to improved outcomes.

A complete reference list can be found online at Elsevier eBooks+.

36

Fetal Intervention and the EXIT Procedure

MARLA B. FERSCHL AND MARK D. ROLLINS

Indications For Fetal Intervention
Twin-Twin Transfusion Syndrome
Twin-Reversed Arterial Perfusion Sequence
Lower Urinary Tract Obstruction
Congenital Heart Defects
Congenital Diaphragmatic Hernia
Congenital Pulmonary Lesions
Sacrococcygeal Teratoma
Myelomeningocele
Maternal Physiology
Respiratory and Airway Considerations
Cardiovascular Considerations
Pharmacologic Consequences of Pregnancy
Fetal Physiology and Monitoring
Fetal Cardiovascular Physiology
Fetal Oxygenation

Fetal Central and Peripheral Nervous
System Physiology and Pain Perception
Fetal Monitoring
Anesthetic Considerations
Preoperative Considerations
Intraoperative Management
Postoperative Considerations
The EXIT Procedure
Fetal Diseases Eligible for the EXIT-to-Airway Procedure
EXIT to Extracorporeal Membrane Oxygenation
EXIT to Resection
EXIT to Separation
Preoperative Considerations
Intraoperative Considerations
Postoperative Considerations
Future Directions

FETAL INTERVENTION ALLOWS SURGICAL correction or amelioration of known congenital defects in utero. With improvements in prenatal imaging and surgical techniques, fetal therapies have grown to include diagnoses associated with intrauterine demise, as well as diseases associated with substantial postnatal morbidity. The goal of fetal intervention is to improve the chances of normal fetal development and minimize ongoing irreversible harm to the fetus. Increasingly, surgical and imaging advances have changed some procedures from open in utero interventions, which are associated with considerable maternal risk, to percutaneous or fetoscopic techniques that improve the maternal-risk to fetal-benefit ratio. Fetal surgery often requires the anesthesiologist to care for two or more patients at once, all with distinctive and, at times, conflicting requirements. The first is the mother who can express her level of discomfort, who can be monitored directly, and to whom drugs can be easily administered. The second is the fetus. For the latter, detecting physiologic stress depends solely on indirect evidence, monitoring is limited at best, administering drugs is more complicated, and there is the possibility of long-term effects from procedures and drugs administered during early development. The anesthesiologist is required to provide maternal and fetal anesthesia and analgesia while ensuring both maternal and fetal hemodynamic stability. In addition, a plan must be prepared to resuscitate the fetus if problems occur during the intervention.

Guidelines for performing fetal interventions have been established by the International Fetal Medicine and Surgery Society.[1,2] Current criteria include (1) the fetal lesion is accurately diagnosed; (2) the progression and severity of the anomaly is predictable and well understood; (3) other severe anomalies that would

contraindicate fetal intervention are excluded; (4) the fetal abnormality would lead to fetal demise, irreversible organ damage, or severe postnatal morbidity if left untreated before birth, and intervening before birth would potentially benefit the neonate's outcome; (5) the maternal risk is acceptably low; (6) animal models have demonstrated feasibility of the surgical technique; (7) fetal interventions are performed at specialized institutions using protocols approved by the institution's ethics committee and with maternal informed consent; and (8) the patient has access to multidisciplinary specialists, including bioethical and psychological counseling.[3,4] Critical to successful fetal interventions is a multidisciplinary, team-based approach with open and collaborative planning and communication before, during, and after the procedure. Risks, benefits, and alternatives of the proposed fetal intervention should be carefully deliberated, and the family should receive extensive counseling, including the option of continuing the pregnancy without intervention and the option of elective pregnancy termination.

The success of modern fetal therapy is largely attributable to advances in imaging techniques. Both ultrasound and magnetic resonance imaging (MRI) quality have substantially improved and allowed for more accurate prenatal diagnosis and a more thorough understanding of the progression of the pathophysiology. Modern ultrasound transducer hardware and digital signal processing improvements have resulted in better resolution and the ability to perform real-time interventions with safety and accuracy. In addition, ultrasound is used for assessment of fetal well-being during interventions and can guide surgical and anesthetic techniques to optimize fetal stability.[5,6]

TABLE 36.1 | Fetal Conditions Currently Considered for Intervention

Fetal Condition	Therapy Rationale	Type	Intervention
Fetal anemia or thrombocytopenia	Prevention of heart failure and fetal hydrops	FIGS-IT	Intrauterine transfusion
Aortic stenosis, intact atrial septum, or pulmonary atresia	Prevention of fetal hydrops, myocardial dysfunction, and hypoplastic left (and right) heart	FIGS-IT	Percutaneous fetal valvuloplasty or septoplasty
Lower urinary tract obstruction	Bladder decompression with reduction in renal dysfunction, pulmonary hypoplasia, oligohydramnios, and limb malformation	FIGS-IT or fetoscopy	Percutaneous vesicoamniotic shunting or fetoscopic posterior urethral valve laser ablation
Twin-reversed arterial perfusion	Prevention of high-output cardiac failure in the normal twin by stopping flow to acardiac twin	FIGS-IT or fetoscopy	Image-guided radiofrequency ablation or fetoscopic coagulation of acardiac twin umbilical cord Percutaneous coiling or ligation of umbilical cord is also used
Twin-twin transfusion syndrome	Reduction of twin-twin blood flow and prevention of cardiac failure	Fetoscopy	Fetoscopic laser photocoagulation of placental vessels and amnioreduction
Amniotic band syndrome	Prevention of limb loss	Fetoscopy	Fetoscopic band ablation
Congenital diaphragmatic hernia	Prevention of pulmonary hypoplasia	Fetoscopy	Fetoscopic tracheal occlusion
Myelomeningocele	Reduction in hydrocephalus and hindbrain herniation, with reduced spinal cord damage and improved neurologic function	Open or fetoscopy	Closure of fetal defect through hysterotomy
Sacrococcygeal teratoma	Prevention of high-output cardiac failure, hydrops, and polyhydramnios	FIGS-IT or open	Ablation of tumor vasculature or open fetal tumor debulking
Congenital cystic adenomatoid malformation	Reversal of pulmonary hypoplasia and cardiac failure	FIGS-IT or open	Thoracoamniotic shunting or open surgical resection
Fetal airway compression	Secured open airway and/or circulatory support to prevent respiratory compromise at birth	Open intrapartum	Ex-utero intrapartum therapy (EXIT) that allows fetal stabilization while on uteroplacental circulation

FIGS-IT, Fetal image-guided surgery for interventional therapy.
Modified from Partridge EA, Flake AW. Maternal-fetal surgery for structural malformations, *Best Pract Res Clin Obstet Gynaecol.* 2012;26:669-682; and Hoagland MA, Chatterjee D. Anesthesia for fetal surgery. *Pediatr Anasth.* 2017;27:346-357.

Surgical interventions have also been refined, with advances in surgical equipment and innovative research in animal models. The first fetal intervention occurred in the 1960s when Sir (Albert) William Liley treated erythroblastosis fetalis with an intraperitoneal blood transfusion.[7] Fetal surgery began in the 1980s when, after many years of animal research, a successful fetal vesicostomy was performed in a fetus with congenital lower urinary tract obstruction.[8] Anesthetic techniques for open fetal procedures that promote uterine relaxation while promoting optimal maternal and fetal outcomes were initially investigated by Mark Rosen,[9] and continue to be refined today.

Three categories of fetal interventions are in current practice: minimally invasive procedures, open fetal procedures, and intrapartum procedures. Conditions amenable to fetal intervention, their rationale, and the typical therapeutic interventions are listed in Table 36.1. The following sections provide a review of the pathophysiology of the more common lesions and the perioperative anesthetic considerations for minimally invasive, open, and intrapartum fetal interventions.

Indications for Fetal Intervention

TWIN-TWIN TRANSFUSION SYNDROME

Twin-twin transfusion syndrome (TTTS) is a serious complication that occurs in 10% to 15% of monozygotic monochorionic twin pregnancies. Although all monochorionic twin pregnancies demonstrate one or more placental vascular anastomoses, TTTS represents a pathologic form of circulatory imbalance between the monochorionic twin fetuses.[10] As a result of this imbalance, a net feto-fetal transfusion occurs, from one twin (the donor) to the other (the recipient) (Fig. 36.1). Donor twin symptoms include hypovolemia, oliguria, oligohydramnios, and growth retardation. In turn, the recipient twin develops hypervolemia, polyuria, polyhydramnios, and signs of circulatory volume overload, resulting in congestive heart failure.[11] In severe cases, untreated TTTS may result in intrauterine fetal death and miscarriage. Even if twins with TTTS survive, there remains a high incidence of secondary neurologic and pulmonary morbidities.

The diagnosis of TTTS requires: (1) a monochorionic, diamniotic pregnancy and (2) discordant amniotic fluid volumes with

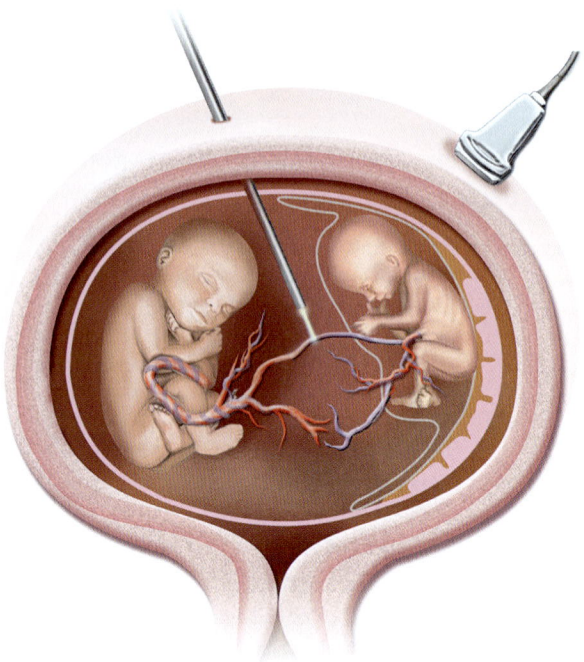

FIGURE 36.1 Schematic representation of umbilical cord ligation in twin-reversed arterial perfusion sequence. (Courtesy T.M. Crombleholme, MD.)

TABLE 36.2	Stages of Twin-Twin Transfusion Syndrome
Stage	**Ultrasound Findings**
I	**Amniotic Fluid:** Oligohydramnios in donor twin sac with MVP <2 cm and polyhydramnios in recipient twin sac with MVP >8 cm
II	**Fetal Bladder:** Stage I criteria AND no visualization of donor twin bladder with over 1 hour of ultrasound observation
III	**Doppler Flow:** Stage II criteria AND (1) absent or reversed umbilical artery end-diastolic flow, (2) reversed ductus venosus a-wave flow, OR (3) pulsatile flow in the umbilical vein
IV	**Fetal Hydrops:** Either stage I or stage II criteria AND fetal hydrops in either twin
V	**Fetal Demise**: Fetal demise in either or both twins as assessed by absent fetal cardiac activity

MVP, Maximal vertical pocket.
Staging data based on criteria from Quintero RA, Morales WJ, Allen MH, et al. Staging of twin-twin transfusion syndrome. *J Perinatol.* 1999;19:550-555.

an ultrasound measurement of the maximal vertical pocket of amniotic fluid less than 2 cm in the oligohydramniotic twin and more than 8 cm in the polyhydramniotic twin. Severity is measured using the Quintero staging system (Table 36.2).[12,13] Severity can be further quantified by using fetal echocardiography, assessing for progression of fetal hypertrophic cardiomyopathy in the recipient twin.[14,15] A greater mortality rate is associated with more

advanced disease stages; stage 1 has an 85% survival rate, whereas stage 4 can have an 80% mortality if left untreated.[16,17]

Several treatment options exist for TTTS. Historically, serial amnioreduction was performed to reduce polyhydramnios, thereby improving placental perfusion and reducing the potential for preterm delivery.[18] Perinatal survival rates among patients treated with amnioreduction alone range from 55% to 65%.[19,20] The best option for treatment of TTTS between 18 to 26 weeks gestation is selective fetoscopic laser photocoagulation (SFLP) of the vascular anastomosis between the twins. Selective fetoscopic laser photocoagulation is based on three fundamental assumptions: (1) the syndrome occurs in the presence of vascular communications between fetuses in a monochorionic gestation, (2) obliteration of these vessels can halt the pathophysiologic process, and (3) both deep and superficial communications can be interrupted at the surface of the placenta.[21] To perform fetoscopic laser photocoagulation, a 3-mm trocar is inserted into the recipient's amniotic sac under ultrasound guidance. Vessels that cross the membrane dividing the amniotic sac are visually identified and selectively coagulated using Doppler imaging, with an effort to spare normal vascular cotyledons. Some centers prefer the use of a sequential coagulation technique, whereby an effort is made to create a net flux of blood from the recipient to the donor. Although this technique may be associated with better outcomes, it is technically more challenging and results in longer procedural times.[22] An additional modification is the Solomon technique, which involves coagulation of the entire vascular equator at the end of the procedure.[23] Though this technique may result in a lower incidence of recurrence of TTTS, it may also carry an increased risk of placental abruption.[24]

A randomized multicenter trial that compared fetoscopic laser photocoagulation to serial amnioreduction in patients with severe TTTS at 15 to 26 weeks gestion[25] found that laser treatment increased survival of at least one twin at 28 days and 6 months of life. Additionally, laser-treated fetuses had improved neurological outcomes compared with the amnioreduction group. A more recent systematic review evaluated 25 years of fetoscopic laser coagulation in TTTS.[26] Among the 3868 treated patients, mean survival of both twins and at least one twin increased from 35% to 65% and 70% to 88%, respectively. The mean gestational age at birth from all series was 32.4 ± 1.3 weeks.

The most common complication of fetoscopic laser photocoagulation is premature rupture of the membranes (PROM), leading to preterm labor and delivery. Other potential complications include placental abruption, hemorrhage, and chorioamnionitis. Overall, the benefits of fetoscopic laser photocoagulation favor intervention in stage 2 or greater TTTS; further investigation is needed to determine optimal timing and long-term neurologic outcomes for these patients.

TWIN-REVERSED ARTERIAL PERFUSION SEQUENCE

Twin-reversed arterial perfusion sequence (TRAP) sequence is an abnormality that occurs in 1 per 100 monozygotic twin pregnancies.[27] With TRAP, one twin is not connected to the placenta and has an absent or nonfunctioning heart; blood flow is supplied in a retrograde fashion, primarily through the umbilical artery. This results in inadequate perfusion, leading to acardia and acephalus in the recipient twin. As the normal twin is generating flow for itself and the acardiac twin, it is prone to high-output cardiac failure, hydrops fetalis, and preterm birth. Left untreated, this condition results in a 35% to 55% demise rate and a mean gestation age of 29 weeks at birth.[28–31]

Treatment of TRAP involves disrupting the vascular communication between the twins, resulting in the death of the nonviable fetus and improvement of the high-output cardiac failure of the donor fetus. Several approaches can be used; however, the most effective is radiofrequency or laser ablation of the acardiac twin's umbilical cord base. A multicenter review of 98 cases of TRAP treated with radiofrequency ablation of the umbilical cord base found a survival rate of 80% for the donor twin and a mean gestational age of 37 weeks at delivery.[32] Although optimal timing is not definitively established, intervention before 16 weeks is likely warranted to reduce progression to cardiac failure and death.[33] Complications of the procedure include PROM, preterm delivery, and intrauterine fetal demise.

LOWER URINARY TRACT OBSTRUCTION

LUTO can occur at the level of the ureteropelvic junction, ureterovesical junction, or at the urethra; severity depends upon location. Bilateral or urethral obstruction is associated with up to a 90% perinatal mortality rate, and half of the survivors have long-term renal impairment.[34] Furthermore, inadequate urine production results in oligohydramnios, which in turn causes fetal pulmonary hypoplasia and neonatal respiratory failure. Posterior urethral valves are the most common cause of LUTO in male fetuses, whereas urethral obstruction is the most common cause in females. Severity has been graded based on several classifications systems, which use amniotic fluid index, ultrasonographic appearance of the kidney and bladder, and fetal urine chemistry to predict long-term morbidity.[35,36]

Two primary fetal interventions are performed to correct fetal LUTO: vesicoamniotic shunts (VAS) and fetal cystoscopy. Vesicoamniotic shunts are valveless double-coiled shunts that are inserted using a minimally invasive percutaneous approach with the use of local anesthesia. One end of the shunt is deployed in the fetal bladder, and the other in the amniotic cavity, with the shunt providing bladder decompression to improve renal and bladder development and increasing amniotic fluid levels to improve lung development.[37] A common complication of shunt placement is shunt malfunction or migration, necessitating a repeat procedure. Other complications include preterm PROM, fetal trauma, and infection.[38] Fetal cystoscopy can differentiate the causes of LUTO as well as treat posterior urethral valves with laser ablation. Fetal cystoscopy can be technically challenging and is not therapeutic for other causes of LUTO.[39]

A randomized controlled trial, the percutaneous vesicoamniotic shunt trial (PLUTO), was designed to evaluate the effectiveness of vesicoamniotic shunts compared with conservative management of fetal LUTO.[40] The study was prematurely concluded in 2010 because of insufficient recruitment. However, among the 31 patients recruited, it demonstrated improved survival at 28 days, 1 year, and 2 years in fetuses treated with vesicoamniotic shunts compared with those with conservative management. There was an overall poor postnatal renal prognosis in both treated and untreated fetuses.

A 2020 systematic review and meta-analysis examined survival and renal outcomes of antenatal intervention for LUTO. Of the 355 included fetuses, perinatal survival was greater in the vesicoamniotic shunts treated group (57%) versus control (39%) (odds ratio [OR]: 2.54, 95% confidence interval [CI]: 1.14–5.67).[41] Five studies reported improved postnatal renal function in the VAS group compared with the conservative group. Two studies examined 45 fetuses who underwent fetal cystoscopy. Survival and normal renal function were greater in the cystoscopy group compared with the conservative management group.[41]

More recent work has centered on serial amnioinfusion for fetuses with LUTO to prevent pulmonary hypoplasia in the setting of diminished renal function and oligohydramnios. With improved lung function, it is hypothesized that these fetuses could be more likely to survive the neonatal period and begin peritoneal dialysis. The Renal Anhydramnios Fetal Therapy (RAFT) trial (NCT03723564) is an ongoing prospective study that is examining this intervention.[42]

CONGENITAL HEART DEFECTS

A variety of congenital heart defects (CHDs) may be considered for fetal intervention, including critical aortic stenosis with evolving hypoplastic left heart syndrome (HLHS), hypoplastic left heart syndrome with highly restrictive or intact atrial septum, pulmonary atresia with intact intraventricular septum and hypoplastic right heart, and congenital cardiac tumors.[43–46] The most commonly performed is aortic balloon valvuloplasty for severe aortic stenosis with evolving hypoplastic left heart syndrome. This lesion is associated with high neonatal mortality and poor long-term outcome.[47] Severe aortic stenosis reduces blood flow through the left ventricle in this lesion, preventing normal ventricular growth and development (see Chapter 14). Without prenatal intervention, severe aortic stenosis leads to marked left ventricular dysfunction, arrest of left ventricular growth, and ventricular fibroelastosis. It has been hypothesized that relief of valvular stenosis in utero could reverse the progression toward ventricular hypoplasia and that there may be a window of opportunity when ventricular growth can be salvaged. Because most routine prenatal ultrasonographic screening is performed between 16 and 24 weeks gestation, the window of opportunity for prenatal intervention is likely between 20 and 26 weeks gestation.

Aortic valve dilation may be performed percutaneously with ultrasound guidance. Optimal fetal positioning, placental location, or maternal habitus may require exposure of the uterus through a maternal abdominal incision. A maternal laparotomy is performed in certain cases to optimize fetal positioning and improve access to the fetal thorax; in this case maternal general anesthesia is usually employed. These procedures have been performed with both maternal regional and general anesthesia.[48] After ultrasonographic confirmation of placental location, the maternal abdomen and uterus are accessed with a 22-gauge spinal needle. An intramuscular (IM) injection of fentanyl and a neuromuscular blocking drug (with or without atropine) is administered to the fetus. A 19-gauge needle is subsequently directed into the fetal thorax, and access to the fetal heart is obtained. A small diameter coronary balloon-tipped catheter is threaded over a guidewire through the needle and passed through the stenotic valve or closed septum. The catheter balloon is then expanded, and blood flow is confirmed using Doppler imaging (Fig. 36.2). An ultrasonographer continually monitors the fetal heart during placement of the intracardiac needle and during catheter balloon inflation. A continuous echocardiogram is also useful for measuring fetal heart rate, contractility, and volume status. Fetal resuscitation medications should be prepared and immediately available to the procedural team.

Technical success for this procedure is defined as an ~75% increase in flow through the aortic valve.[49] Improved valvular function leads to improved left ventricular function, valvular development, and delivery of a live fetus in 90% of cases.[50,51] Complications include fetal bradycardia, pericardial effusion, ventricular thrombosis, fetal and neonatal death, and preterm delivery.[52–55] Biventricular circulation is present at birth in approximately half

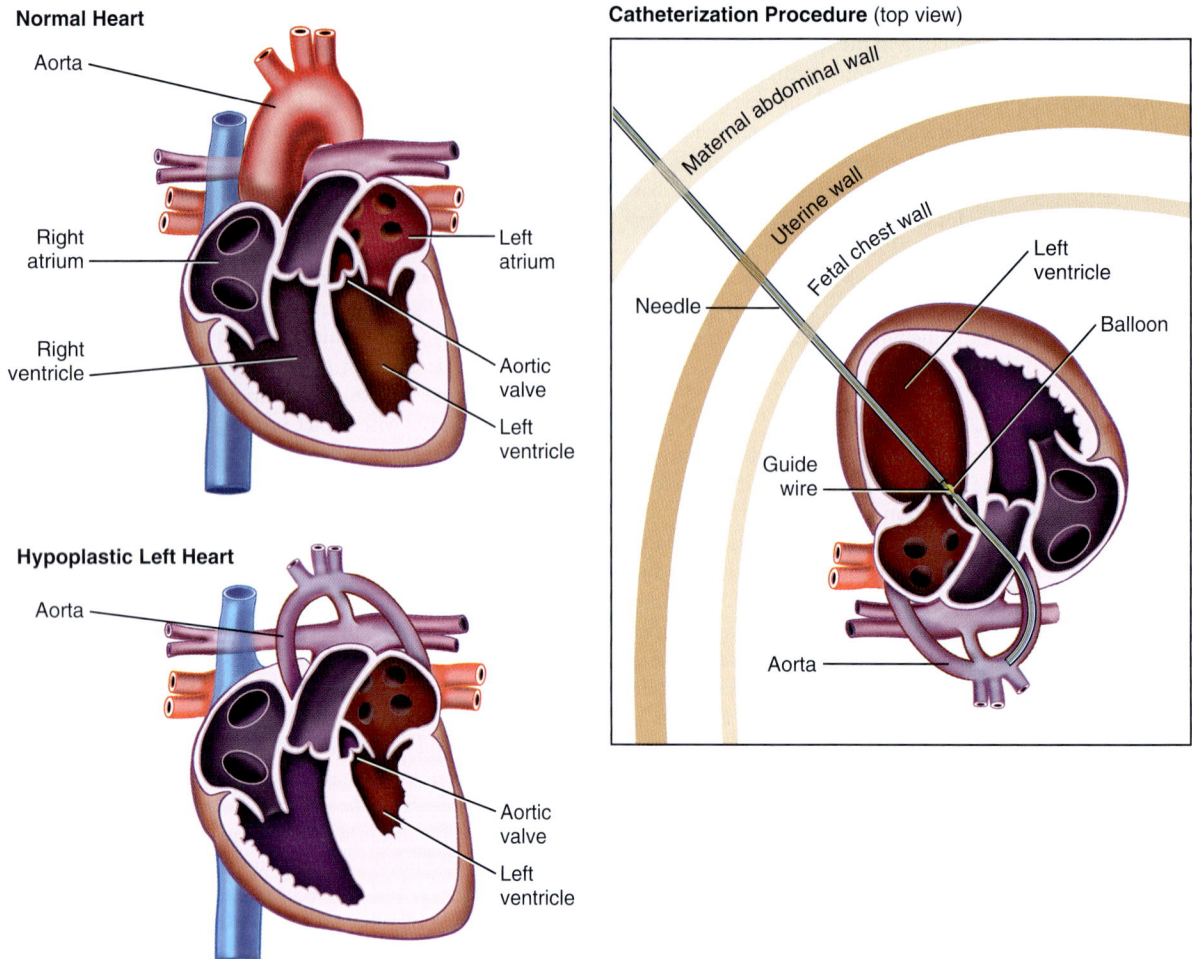

FIGURE 36.2 Technique for balloon dilation of a stenotic aortic valve in a fetus with hypoplastic left heart syndrome. (Reproduced with permission from *Dream Magazine*, Spring/Summer 2002. Boston: Children's Hospital Boston; 2002:20.)

of successful cases. In the future, larger, prospective investigations are warranted to determine the efficacy of these procedures.

CONGENITAL DIAPHRAGMATIC HERNIA

An incomplete closure of the diaphragm in the first trimester of pregnancy results in the development of a congenital diaphragmatic hernia (CDH). Abdominal contents herniate though the defect, compromising lung growth and development. This results in significant neonatal morbidity and mortality from both lung hypoplasia and pulmonary hypertension.[56] Prenatal intervention for CDH is focused on promoting pulmonary development to reduce these morbidities.

Initial investigations involved open fetal surgical repair of the CDH, but outcomes were poor and a prospective clinical trial did not demonstrate improved survival compared with the standard of care.[57] Subsequently, tracheal occlusion was promoted as a strategy to enhance fetal lung development. The fetal lungs secrete 100 mL/kg per day of fluid; by preventing the egress of this fluid via the trachea, the goal is to promote an increase in lung volume and reduce the growth restriction caused by the abdominal viscera.[58–60] Initial attempts were performed with an open fetal procedure, using foam tracheal plugs or surgical clips; however, neither device improved outcomes. Subsequently, minimally invasive

endoscopic techniques were attempted.[61] Ultimately, the use of a small detachable balloon after endoscopic tracheal intubation proved to be a reliable and reversible method of fetal tracheal occlusion. A neuromuscular blocking drug and fentanyl were administered IM to the fetus to ensure fetal immobility during the procedure. Initially, balloons were removed at delivery via an ex-utero intrapartum therapy (EXIT) procedure (see section on EXIT procedures later), although it was determined that removing the balloon before birth could improve surfactant production and allow for a vaginal delivery.[62] Typically, these balloons are placed at 27 to 29 weeks and removed at 34 weeks gestational age. Fetoscopic endoluminal tracheal occlusion (FETO) is frequently performed with maternal local or neuraxial anesthesia.

Not all patients with CDH have a degree of CDH that will benefit from fetal intervention; some neonates do well with a postnatal surgical repair. The ratio of the fetal lung area to the fetal head circumference (LHR) and the presence of an intrathoracic liver are often used as predictors of fetal outcome; fetuses with a lung-to-head ratio of <0.7 and an intrathoracic liver are unlikely to survive.[63] Fetal lung-to-head ratios change with gestational age, and are frequently corrected by creating an observed to expected (o/e) lung-to-head ratio.[64] With this ratio, fetuses can be classified as having severe (15%–25%), moderate (26%–35%), or mild (36%–45%) disease, with an expected survival of 20%, 55%, and 85%, respectively. More recently, fetal MRI has been used to quantitate lung volume and predict survival.[65,66]

The benefit of fetoscopic endoluminal tracheal occlusion for those with severe CDH was recently established with a multi-institutional randomized controlled trial, the **T**racheal **O**cclusion **To A**ccelerate **L**ung Growth (**TOTAL**) trial.[67] Fetuses with severe CDH treated with fetoscopic endoluminal tracheal occlusion at 27 to 28 weeks gestation were more likely to survive to discharge compared with fetuses who did not undergo fetal intervention (40% vs. 15%). The benefit of this intervention persisted until 6 months of age.[67] However, this effect was not present when the CDH was less severe.[68] Fetuses with moderate CDH who underwent fetoscopic endoluminal tracheal occlusion at 30 to 32 weeks of gestation did not have better survival to neonatal intensive care unit discharge or a reduction in the need for oxygen supplementation at 6 months of age.[68] In addition, the risk of preterm PROM was 4.5 times greater in the severe CDH cohort and 3.8 times greater in the moderate CDH cohort than the expectant group, and the rate of preterm birth was 2.6 times greater in the severe CDH cohort and 2.9 times greater in the moderate CDH cohort compared with the nontreated patient group.[67,68]

CONGENITAL PULMONARY LESIONS

Congenital pulmonary airway malformations (CPAM) of the lung consist of cystic masses of pulmonary tissue and bronchial structures, neither of which participate in gas exchange.[69] There are five subtypes of CPAM that arise from differing lung tissue; these lesions can be cystic or solid.[70] Large CPAM can compress surrounding lung tissue and impede normal lung development, resulting in pulmonary hypoplasia, cardiac compression, and mediastinal shift, leading to hydrops fetalis. Lesion size and growth characteristics are most predictive of prognosis.[71] Ultrasound measurement of CPAM lesion volume to fetal head circumference ratio (CVR) is used to predict outcome; with a CVR >0.56 predictive of a poor postnatal outcome and a CVR >1.4 to 1.6 associated with hydrops fetalis.[71–74] Untreated, fetuses with CPAM and hydrops fetalis have a survival rate of less than 5% without intervention.[75]

Fetal treatment for CPAM can be performed either fetoscopically or with an open procedure. Lesions with large cystic components or a large pleural effusion can undergo fetoscopic placement of a thoracoamniotic shunt. Like vesicoamniotic shunts, these devices are valveless double-coiled stents that allow for passive drainage of fluid from the cystic lesion to the amniotic cavity. Also, these shunts often migrate (8.5%) or malfunction, resulting in the need for multiple procedures.[76] However, proper shunt placement can reverse hydrops. One retrospective analysis of 75 fetuses demonstrated a decrease in cyst size by 55% ± 21%, and a resolution of hydrops in 83% of fetuses. The overall neonatal survival in this group was 68% and correlated with gestational age at birth and resolution of symptoms.[77]

Open fetal procedures are reserved for lesions with largely solid components, not amenable to percutaneous intervention. These procedures, which involve an open fetal thoracotomy and lobectomy, carry significant risk, including the possibility of fetal hemorrhage and the need for fetal resuscitation. Open resections in fetuses with hydrops fetalis carry a survival rate of 50% to 60%, and when successful, allow for lung growth and resolution of hydrops fetalis.[78] However, even when successful, patients are at risk for PROM, chorioamnionitis, and placental abruption.

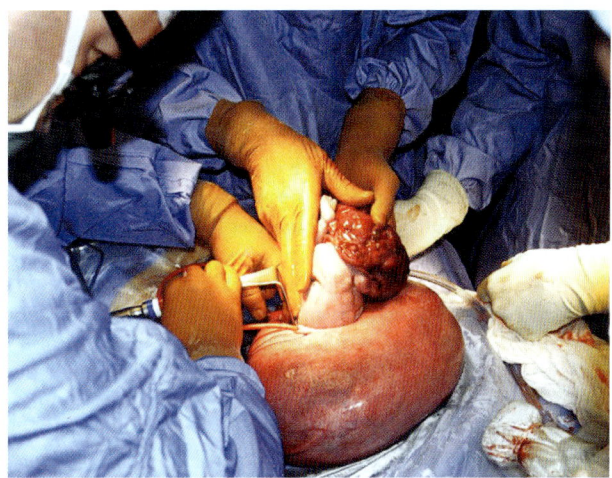

FIGURE 36.3 Fetal sacrococcygeal teratoma before in utero resection in a fetus at 22 weeks gestation. (Courtesy N. Scott Adzick, MD, Children's Hospital of Philadelphia.)

SACROCOCCYGEAL TERATOMA

Sacrococcygeal teratomas (SCTs) (Fig. 36.3) are one of the most common congenital neonatal tumors (1 per 15,000–40,000 live births).[79] A variety of tissues from the three primary germ layers are usually found, and the size of the tumor is quite variable.[80,81] The majority include both solid and cystic components, with the tumor composition and location determined by fetal MRI.[82] Although usually benign, sacrococcygeal teratomas can cause secondary morbidity in select cases because of its mass effect and vast blood supply. High-output cardiac failure can occur in the fetus.

With smaller tumors, complete surgical resection usually occurs after delivery under elective, controlled conditions. In more extreme cases, large tumor size can cause fetal congestive heart failure (usually high-output failure), and even fetal demise if no treatment is provided.[83] Death is usually secondary to an enlarged tumor mass and associated polyhydramnios, resulting in preterm labor and delivery, with survival ultimately depending on fetal lung maturity. Massive hemorrhage into the tumor with fetal exsanguination may occur spontaneously in utero or be precipitated by preterm labor and delivery. Additionally, maternal mirror syndrome, in which maternal physiology mimics the abnormal hydropic fetal physiology, can occur. The pregnant patient develops hypertension, pulmonary and peripheral edema, and a high cardiac output. Mirror syndrome can lead to severe maternal complications that include anemia, hypertension, proteinuria, and pulmonary edema.[84–86]

The diagnosis of a sacrococcygeal teratoma before 30 weeks gestation carries a poor prognosis and fetal intervention may be considered.[87] Options include minimally invasive intervention of the tumor blood supply, cyst drainage, or open fetal resection. Minimally invasive techniques include radiofrequency ablation, embolization, and thermocoagulation of the tumor or its blood supply.[88] Larger, prospective studies of these minimally invasive techniques are needed to determine their efficacy. Open fetal resections of sacrococcygeal teratomas are limited to case reports and case series. Like all open fetal procedures, these carry an increased risk for the fetus and the mother. Fetal intravenous access is necessary to provide adequate resuscitation and fetal medications and blood products should be readily available for transfusion. The optimal timing and criteria for open fetal sacro-coccygeal teratoma resection is unclear.[89,90]

MYELOMENINGOCELE

Myelomeningoceles (MMC) are congenital neural tube defects that arise from incomplete closure of the vertebra and overlying tissues, resulting in herniation of the meninges and spinal cord. As a result, patients with myelomeningoceles have sensory and motor defects below the level of the lesion, as well as bowel and bladder dysfunction, sexual dysfunction, and impaired cognition. In addition, these patients often have an Arnold Chiari II malformation and hydrocephalus that require ventriculoperitoneal shunting. Though these deficits are caused by the herniation of the neural tissue, it is hypothesized that the severity of the defect is exacerbated by exposure of these elements to amniotic fluid, which is neurotoxic, and by direct trauma. The goal of fetal repair of a myelomeningocele is to reduce the exposure of the neural tissue in order to improve overall outcomes for these patients.

The efficacy of fetal intervention for myelomeningocele repair was demonstrated in a prospective randomized clinical trial (the Management of Myelomeningocele Study [MOMS]) of 183 patients that compared prenatal intervention (at 19–26 weeks) with standard postnatal repair.[91] Prenatally treated patients had improved motor outcomes, less need for ventriculoperitoneal shunting and decreased hindbrain herniation at 30 months of age. Long-term study analysis continues, but ongoing results suggest that motor function improvements persist over time.[92] Unfortunately, those who underwent a fetal intervention were at greater risk for preterm labor and delivery as well as maternal uterine dehiscence compared with the postnatal intervention group. In addition, infants treated prenatally were more likely to have respiratory distress syndrome.

Fetoscopic myelomeningocele repair has been pursued to reduce complications from open hysterotomy. These procedures can be performed either with a maternal laparotomy followed by a fetoscopic intervention through the uterus or entirely fetoscopically through ports in the maternal abdominal wall. A systematic review and metanalysis of open and fetoscopic myelomeningocele repair suggests that a maternal laparotomy followed by a fetoscopic repair results in a reduced risk for maternal uterine dehiscence, allowing for the possibility of labor and vaginal delivery.[93] Several disadvantages of fetoscopic interventions include a greater operative time, a greater rate of myelomeningocele wound dehiscence and the need to reoperate after delivery. Shunt rates are similar to open fetal procedures.[93] A more recent study, from the International Fetoscopic Neural Tube Defect Repair Consortium, performed a retrospective registry review of 300 fetoscopic repairs at 14 centers worldwide. Mean gestational age at delivery in fetoscopically treated patients was similar to those who had prenatal open surgical repair in the MOMS trial at 34 weeks.[91] None of the fetoscopic patients had uterine dehiscence, and ventriculoperitoneal shunting rates were similar to those who had prenatal open surgical repair.[91] Long-term motor and neurocognitive outcomes were not assessed in this study.[94] More prospective studies are needed to elucidate the efficacy of the fetoscopic technique compared with open surgical repair.

Maternal Physiology

RESPIRATORY AND AIRWAY CONSIDERATIONS

Anatomic and hormonal influences, coupled with the increase in metabolic demand of both the mother and the fetus, account for

TABLE 36.3	Anesthetic Considerations of Respiratory Changes of Pregnancy
Decreased functional residual capacity	
Faster denitrogenation	
Rapidly prone to hypoxia during apnea	
Faster induction and emergence of anesthesia with inhaled agents	
Increased oxygen consumption	
Rapidly prone to hypoxia during apnea	
Capillary engorgement of the respiratory mucosa	
Predisposes upper airway to trauma, bleeding, and obstruction	
Laryngeal edema increases the frequency of difficult intubation	
Decreased $PaCO_2$ and no $PETCO_2$-$PaCO_2$ gradient	
Capnograph reading similar to $PaCO_2$	
Hyperventilation may lead to a reduction in uterine blood flow	

$PaCO_2$, Arterial partial pressure of carbon dioxide; $PETCO_2$, End-tidal carbon dioxide partial pressure.

changes in maternal pulmonary physiology (Table 36.3). Pregnancy results in progressive increases in maternal oxygen consumption and minute ventilation, along with a decreased pulmonary residual volume and functional residual capacity.[95] The increased metabolic demands and functional changes can make adequate oxygenation and perfusion of the mother and the fetoplacental unit a challenge during maternal general anesthesia. During periods of apnea or hypoventilation, the pregnant patient is prone to rapidly developing hypoxia and hypercapnia. The arterial oxygen partial pressure (PaO_2) in an apneic, anesthetized pregnant patient decreases more rapidly compared with the nonpregnant woman.[96] Acidosis rapidly develops from hypoxia during difficult airway situations because of a decreased buffering capacity during pregnancy. The decreased pulmonary oxygen stores and increased oxygen consumption make pregnant patients more susceptible than nonpregnant patients to the consequences of airway mismanagement.

Not all physiologic changes of pregnancy are deleterious to the performance of anesthesia. For example, both the induction of and emergence from anesthesia with inhalational anesthetics occur more rapidly in pregnant patients than in nonpregnant patients. The combination of increased alveolar ventilation and decreased functional residual capacity speed the rate at which denitrogenation occurs and at which inspired and alveolar concentrations of inhalational anesthetics equilibrate.[97]

CARDIOVASCULAR CONSIDERATIONS

Cardiovascular function is appropriately increased during pregnancy to meet the increased metabolic demands and oxygen requirements of the mother (Table 36.4). Cardiac output increases by 35% to 40% by the end of the first trimester and continues to increase steadily throughout the second trimester until it reaches a level 50% greater than that in nonpregnant women.[98] Heart rate increases 15% to 25% and stroke volume increases 25% to 30% compared with prepregnancy values by the end of the second trimester, after which they both remain stable until term.[99,100] Aortocaval compression by the gravid uterus can decrease cardiac output; lesser decreases occur in the sitting or semirecumbent positions. Maternal position is a major factor contributing to hypotension and fetal well-being.[101]

TABLE 36.4	Anesthetic Considerations of Cardiovascular Changes of Pregnancy

Aortocaval compression

   Supine position leads to a decline in cardiac output

   May lead to supine hypotensive syndrome

   Mostly prevented by left or right uterine displacement

Decreased colloid oncotic pressure

   Parturient is at greater risk for developing pulmonary edema

Increased maternal blood volume

   Parturient tolerates more blood loss than nonparturients

   Hypotension and acidosis may develop with significant blood loss

TABLE 36.5	Placental Transfer of Common Anesthetic Drugs[a]	
Drugs That DO NOT transfer	**Drugs That DO transfer**
Glycopyrrolate	Atropine
All neuromuscular blocking drugs	Ephedrine
Insulin	Esmolol, labetalol
Heparin	Benzodiazepines
	Propofol
	Ketamine
	Opioids[b]
	Inhalational anesthetics
	Local anesthetics[c]

[a]The major mechanism of transfer is passive diffusion of largely lipid-soluble, nonionized substances with low molecular weight (<500 D). Bulk flow, pinocytosis, and passage through the intervillous spaces are negligible sources of reliable transfer.
[b]Epidural or intrathecal opioids, to a lesser extent, generally produce minimal neonatal effects.
[c]Fetal acidosis produces higher fetal/maternal local anesthetic drug ratios because binding of hydrogen ions to the nonionized form causes trapping of the local anesthetic in the fetal circulation.

Maternal blood flow and pressure are directly linked to fetal perfusion via the placenta, and uterine blood flow represents about 10% of maternal cardiac output. It is imperative to prevent aortocaval compression by uterine displacement. Because large doses of inhalational anesthetics are often necessary to relax the uterus during fetal interventions, prompt treatment of hypotension is critical. A decrease in maternal blood pressure decreases placental blood flow and, therefore, blood flow to the fetus because uteroplacental blood flow is not autoregulated. Intravenous ephedrine or phenylephrine effectively treats maternal hypotension; often times a phenylephrine infusion is necessary to maintain normotension in the setting of large concentrations of inhalational anesthetic agents.[102,103]

Careful attention to the volume status of the parturient is imperative; aggressive volume hydration, the normal decrease in colloid oncotic pressure that occurs during pregnancy, and the use of tocolytic agents (e.g., magnesium or β-adrenoceptor agonists) may all predispose the parturient to pulmonary edema.

PHARMACOLOGIC CONSEQUENCES OF PREGNANCY

Physiologic changes of pregnancy alter the pharmacokinetics and pharmacodynamics of many anesthetic drugs. An increase in total body water and adipose tissue, and a decrease in plasma protein concentrations alter the volume of distribution of drugs. Increased renal blood flow and glomerular filtration rate enhance the elimination of renally excreted drugs. Hepatic metabolism of some drugs may be inhibited by competition with steroid hormones during pregnancy, whereas others may have a greater clearance associated with the increased basal metabolic rate and hepatic blood flow. Therefore, drug administration must consider the pharmacokinetics within the maternal-placental-fetal unit. Most maternally administered medications, including inhalational anesthetics and opioids, cross the placenta. Lipid solubility, the pH of both maternal and fetal blood, the degree of ionization, protein binding, perfusion, placental area and thickness, and drug concentration are factors that influence the extent of transplacental drug diffusion (Table 36.5).[104] The fetus has reduced plasma protein binding, producing relatively greater concentrations of free drug (i.e., unbound and available to cross biologic membranes).[105] Despite detection of oxidation and reduction reactions in the fetal liver from as early as 16 weeks, enzyme concentrations and reaction rates are reduced, exposing the fetus to more prolonged drug effects than occur in the mother.[106] Early in gestation, the primary mode of drug excretion is via blood flow to the placenta, but later, as the fetal kidneys mature, they become a route of drug excretion into the amniotic fluid for water-soluble drugs and metabolites. Amniotic fluid, however, can also act as a reservoir for drugs, from which they can be reabsorbed.[105]

Fetal Physiology and Monitoring

FETAL CARDIOVASCULAR PHYSIOLOGY

The differences between the fetal and postnatal circulations are complex (Fig. 36.4). In the fetal circulation, oxygenated blood returns from the placenta via the umbilical veins and ductus venosus (bypassing the liver) into the right atrium. At 20 weeks, 30% of the umbilical venous return (40–60 mL/kg per minute) is shunted through the ductus venosus.[107] This flow decreases over the second half of gestation as hepatic blood flow increases so that by term only 20% of umbilical venous return (<20 mL/kg per minute) is shunted through the ductus venosus.[107] Hypoxia and hemorrhage increase the resistance in the liver, shunting a greater proportion of blood toward the brain and heart through the ductus venosus.[108] The proportion of blood that perfuses the liver, which exits with an oxygen saturation 15% less than when it went in, rejoins the ductus venosus blood in the inferior vena cava. However, this deoxygenated blood flows more slowly into the right atrium toward the right ventricle.[108] The greater-velocity oxygenated blood from the ductus venosus is preferentially directed through the foramen ovale into the left side of the heart and out through the aortic arch to the developing head and upper body. The integrity of the foramen ovale is thus imperative. Blood returning from the placenta along the umbilical vein is 80% to 85% saturated. Despite this streaming within the right atrium, some mixing does occur, resulting in blood that is 65% saturated in the ascending aorta. The blood in the left ventricle, however, has an oxygen saturation that is 15% to 20% greater than the blood in the right ventricle. Most of the deoxygenated blood in the right ventricle bypasses the high-resistance pulmonary vasculature to enter the ductus arteriosus, and from there the descending aorta to supply the lower body or pass through the umbilical arteries for reoxygenation in the placenta. In contrast to extrauterine life, when the two ventricles have equal outputs, before

FETAL CIRCULATION

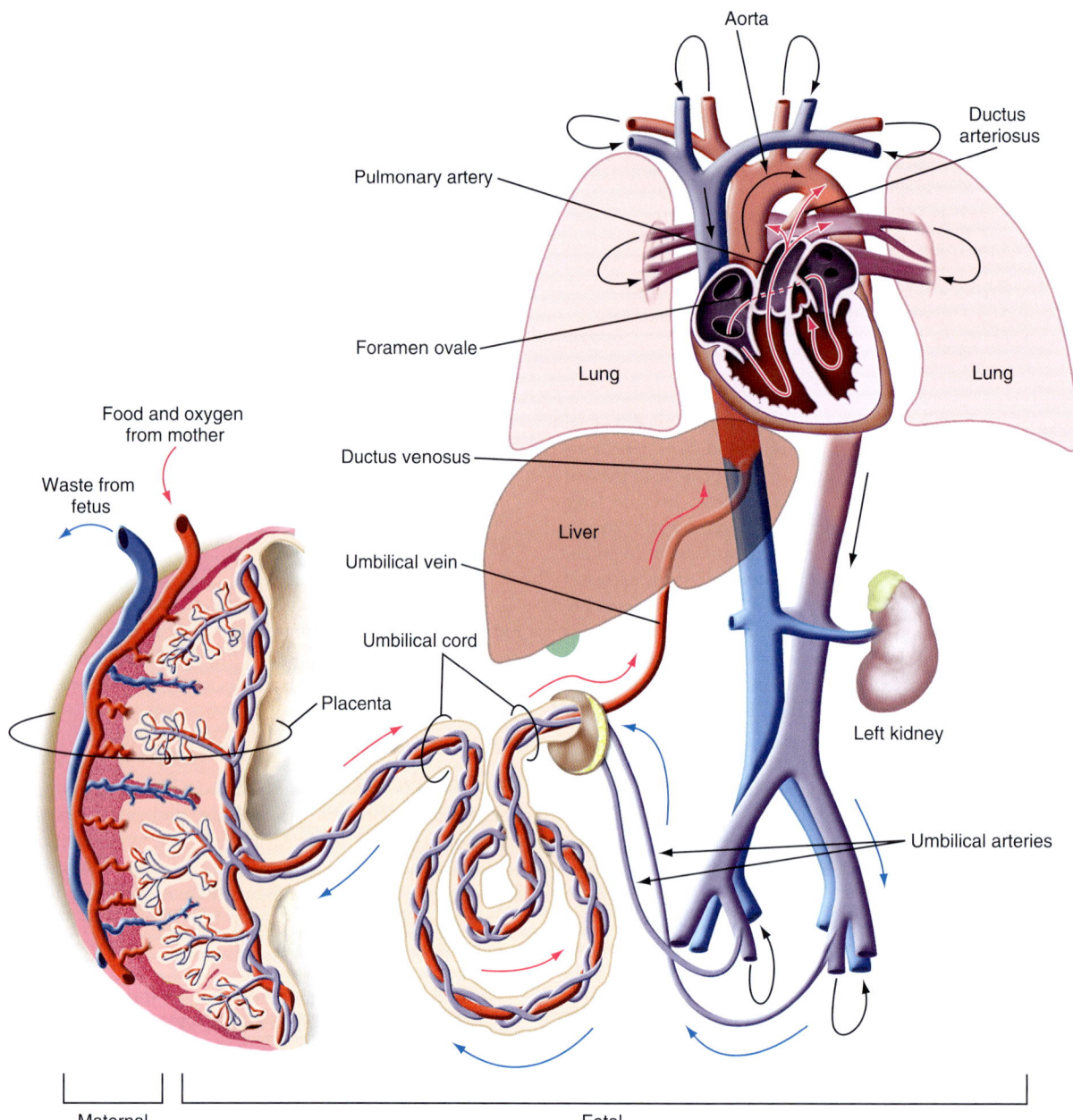

FIGURE 36.4 Fetal circulation. *Red arrows* represent flow of oxygenated blood and *blue arrows* represent flow of deoxygenated blood. *Black arrows* indicate direction of blood flow and represent travel of blood from the central circulation through capillary membranes and return to central circulation. *Shading (from red to purple to blue)* represents the corresponding relative oxygenation of the blood at that site, from oxygenated to deoxygenated. Note the mixing of blood as the ductus venosus delivers oxygenated blood from the placenta to the central fetal circulation and the progressive desaturation of blood in the fetal aorta secondary to shunts, consumption, and the return of deoxygenated blood from the fetal pulmonary circulation.

birth they have dissimilar outputs. In the third trimester, the cardiac output from the right side of the heart is greater than the left side, as determined by Doppler ultrasonography studies, and evidenced by a 28% greater stroke volume in the right versus the left side.[107]

The fetal heart rate (FHR) exceeds the intrinsic rate of the sino-atrial node by a combination of vagal and sympathetic inputs, and circulating catecholamines.[109–111] However, the fetal heart rate decreases throughout gestation,[112,113] accompanied by an increase in

stroke volume as the heart grows. Hypoxic stress in late gestation produces a reflex bradycardia, with a normal heart rate or tachycardia developing a few minutes later. The later tachycardia is a result of an increase in plasma catecholamines causing β-adrenergic stimulation.[114] Fetal hemorrhage can also produce increases in fetal heart rate, probably via a baroreceptor reflex.

Cardiac output in the fetus is determined to a large extent by the heart rate.[115] The combined ventricular output of the left and right ventricles in the human fetus is 450 mL/kg per minute.[115] During development, the ability of the fetus to increase stroke volume is limited by a reduced proportion of functioning contractile tissue and a limited ability to increase the heart rate because of a relatively reduced β-adrenergic receptor density and immature sympathetic drive. If the blood volume is reduced by hemorrhage, the heart cannot compensate by increasing stroke volume, or conversely, if volume is increased, the walls are less able to distend, and cardiac efficiency is reduced (although this second effect is reduced substantially by the huge, relatively compliant placental circulation). Thus, the only mechanism by which the fetus can increase its cardiac output is to increase its heart rate. The development of acidemia indicates that the fetus is unable to compensate. Acidosis shifts the oxygen dissociation curve to the right, thereby decreasing fetal hemoglobin oxygen saturation but improving release of oxygen from hemoglobin.

Neonatal blood volume increases throughout gestation. By mid-gestation, the fetoplacental blood volume is estimated to be 100 to 160 mL/kg. Approximately one-third of this blood is contained in the fetus and two-thirds is contained in the placenta.[116,117] The hemoglobin concentration increases in a linear fashion throughout gestation from 11 g/dL in a 17-week fetus to 18 g/dL in a term fetus.[118]

FETAL OXYGENATION

The fetus exists in an environment of low oxygen tension, with the PaO_2 approximately one-fourth that in the adult. The maximum PaO_2 of umbilical venous blood is approximately 30 mm Hg. The affinity of fetal hemoglobin (hemoglobin F) for oxygen is modulated in utero by two principal factors: fetal hemoglobin structure and 2,3-diphosphoglycerate (2,3-DPG). The hemoglobin oxygen dissociation curve is shifted to the left because of fetal hemoglobin, thereby increasing the affinity for oxygen. In addition, 2,3-DPG is present and might be expected to shift the oxyhemoglobin dissociation curve to the right, decreasing the affinity of the fetal hemoglobin for oxygen and favoring oxygen unloading. However, 2,3-DPG appears to only exert approximately 40% of the effect on fetal hemoglobin as it does on adult hemoglobin, thereby preserving a net leftward shift on the oxyhemoglobin dissociation curve. Thus, for any given PaO_2, the fetus has a greater affinity for oxygen than the mother. The P50 (the PaO_2 at which hemoglobin is 50% desaturated) is approximately 27 mm Hg for the nonpregnant adult, 30 for the pregnant mother, and 20 mm Hg for the fetus. The concentration of 2,3-DPG increases with gestation, as does the concentration of hemoglobin A[119]; the greater hemoglobin concentration (18 g/dL) results in a greater total oxygen-carrying capacity.

Oxygen supply to fetal tissues depends on several factors (Table 36.6). First, the mother must be adequately oxygenated. Second, there must be adequate flow of well-oxygenated blood to the uteroplacental circulation. This blood flow may be reduced from maternal hemorrhage (reduced maternal blood volume) or compression of the inferior vena cava (reduced venous return), which increases uterine venous pressure, thus reducing uterine perfusion. Additionally, aortic compression reduces uterine arterial blood flow.[120] Care must be taken to position the mother in such a way as to prevent aortocaval compression.[121,122] The surgical incision of a hysterotomy itself reduces uteroplacental blood flow in sheep studies, whereas fetoscopic procedures with uterine entry have no measurable effect.[123]

TABLE 36.6	Causes of Impaired Blood Flow and Oxygenation to Fetal Tissues
Causes of Impaired Uteroplacental Blood Flow/Oxygenation	**Causes of Impaired Umbilical Blood Flow/Fetal Circulatory Redistribution**
Reduced maternal oxygenation/hemoglobin concentration	Umbilical vessel spasm
Maternal hemorrhage	Reduced fetal cardiac output
Aortocaval compression	Fetal hemorrhage/reduced hemoglobin concentration
Drugs reducing uterine blood flow	Fetal hypothermia
Uterine trauma	Impaired uteroplacental blood flow/oxygenation
Uterine contractions	Umbilical cord kinking
Placental insufficiency (PET, IUGR)	
Polyhydramnios: pressure effect	
Maternal catecholamine production increasing uteroplacental vascular resistance	Fetal catecholamine production increasing fetoplacental vascular resistance

IUGR, Intrauterine growth restriction; *PET*, preeclamptic toxemia.

Even if the uterine circulation is adequate, the fetus still depends on uteroplacental blood flow and umbilical venous blood flow for tissue oxygenation. Care must be taken not to interrupt umbilical vessel blood flow by manipulation or kinking the cord, which can cause vasospasm. Umbilical vasoconstriction can also occur as part of a fetal stress reaction resulting from a release of fetal stress hormones (Fig. 36.5). Increases in amniotic fluid volume increase amniotic pressure and can impair uteroplacental perfusion.[124,125] Placental vascular resistance may increase, thereby increasing fetal cardiac afterload via a surge in fetal catecholamine production stimulated by surgical stress.[126] Fortunately, animal studies suggest that adverse effects on the arterial blood gas in the fetus do not occur acutely until uteroplacental perfusion has been reduced by 50% or more.[127]

FETAL CENTRAL AND PERIPHERAL NERVOUS SYSTEM PHYSIOLOGY AND PAIN PERCEPTION

Development of the brain and spinal cord begins as early as postconceptual week 3 with neural crest cells migrating laterally to form peripheral nerves from about 4 weeks, and the first synapses between them forming a week later.[128] Synapses within the spinal cord develop from about 8 weeks gestation, suggesting that the first spinal reflexes may be present at this time. Neuronal development is maximum between 8 and 18 weeks gestation. The first neurons and glial cells develop in the ventricular zone (an epithelial layer), along which the newly formed neurons migrate out in waves to form the neocortex. Synaptogenesis occurs after neural proliferation, first in peripheral structures and, second, more centrally from approximately 20 weeks; this process depends in part on sensory stimulation.[129] For all intents and purposes, the spinal cord is completely formed by the beginning of the second trimester.

The development of the nociceptive apparatus proceeds in parallel with the development of the basic central nervous system. The first essential requirement for nociception is the presence of sensory receptors, which develop first in the perioral area at around 7 weeks gestation. From here, they develop in the rest of

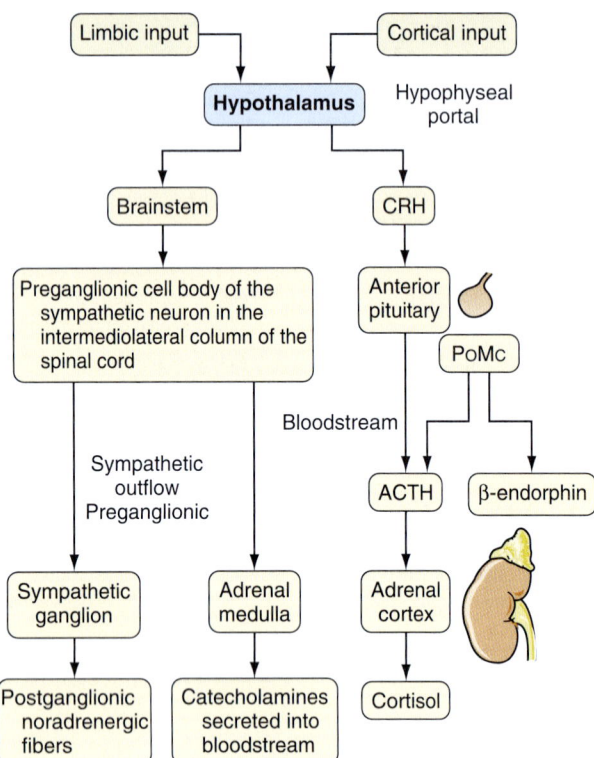

FIGURE 36.5 Human fetal endocrine responses to stress. *ACTH*, Adrenocorticotropic hormone; *CRH*, corticotropin-releasing hormone; *PoMc*, proopiomelanocortin.

the face and in the palmar surfaces of the hands and soles of the feet from about 11 weeks gestation. By 20 weeks, they are present throughout all of the skin and mucosal surfaces.[130] The nociceptive apparatus is initially involved in local reflex movements at the spinal cord level without higher cortical integration. As these reflex responses become more complex, they in turn involve the brainstem, through which other responses, such as increases in heart rate and blood pressure, are mediated. However, such reflexes to noxious stimuli have not been shown to involve the cortex and, thus, are not available to conscious perception.[131,132] The nature of fetal consciousness itself is complicated, both physiologically and philosophically, and a discussion of such is beyond the scope of this chapter. However, there is a working consensus that there must be electrical activity in the cerebral cortex for consciousness to be present.[133] It appears that, far from being "switched on" at any one moment, consciousness evolves in a gradual process that has been likened to a "dimmer switch," making attribution of fetal consciousness to any particular developmental moment a difficult undertaking.

When considering the effects of noxious stimuli on the developing fetus and the rationale for fetal anesthesia and analgesia, one must consider not just the need to alleviate the possible distress of a sensation eliciting a stress response, but also whether being subjected to surgical stress during early development might cause permanent alterations in physiology. This concept is known as *programming*, defined as *"the process whereby a stimulus or insult at a critical, sensitive period of development has permanent effects on structure, physiology, and metabolism."*[133,134] Studies in rats and nonhuman primates have shown that the numbers of hippocampal and hypothalamic glucocorticoid receptors in the offspring of antenatally stressed animals were permanently reduced. This

attenuates the negative feedback response, resulting in increased basal and stress-induced cortisol concentrations in the offspring that persist into adulthood. Behavioral changes, such as poor coping behaviors, have also been observed.[134]

Consequently, though it is unlikely that the fetus can perceive pain at the gestational age most in utero procedures are performed, it is recommended by both the American Society of Anesthesiologists and the Society of Maternal-Fetal Medicine that opioid analgesia should be administered to the fetus during invasive fetal procedures to attenuate the fetal stress response and its deleterious consequences.[135,136] Typically, IM opioid (e.g. fentanyl 10–20 µg/kg) is administered along with a neuromuscular blocking drug (e.g., rocuronium 2–3 mg/kg), with or without an anticholinergic (atropine 20 µg/kg) to reduce the possibility of bradycardia associated with opioid administration. For open maternal-fetal procedures using general anesthesia, inhalational anesthetics do not reliably blunt the fetal stress response necessitating supplementation with opioids. Maternal administration of remifentanil has been shown to transfer opioids to the fetus.[137] The umbilical cord and placenta do not have pain receptors, so procedures only involving these tissues (e.g., laser ablation for twin-twin transfusion syndrome) do not require administration of opioid analgesics.

The impact of anesthetic agents on the development of the brain should be considered when providing anesthesia for fetal procedures. Histologic changes in the brain as well as learning and memory deficits have been shown in animals with prolonged exposure to anesthetic agents in the fetal and neonatal period.[138,139] Human studies are less convincing, including two prospective trials that did not demonstrate neurocognitive deficits after a single brief exposure to anesthesia in the early postnatal period.[140,141] Nonetheless, a US Food and Drug Administration advisory committee issued a warning in 2016 that *"repeated or lengthy use of general anesthetic and sedation drugs during surgeries or procedures in children younger than 3 years or in pregnant women during their third trimester may affect the development of children's brains."*[142] To date, no studies have examined the impact of mid-gestion fetal surgery on cognitive development in humans,[143] though an international registry has been established to better assess this outcome (https://clinicaltrials.gov/ct2/show/NCT02591745).

FETAL MONITORING

The goal during any fetal intervention is to optimize fetal well-being by avoiding fetal hypoxia and hypothermia while optimizing fetal hemodynamics. It is essential that the physiologic response of the fetus to anesthetic and surgical stresses be understood and addressed to avoid the known detrimental effects of stress on an already compromised fetus. Direct ultrasound monitoring of fetal heart rate, umbilical blood flow, and fetal echocardiography are the most commonly employed methods of assessing fetal well-being.

Fetal heart rate monitoring with Doppler ultrasonography is the standard for the intrapartum assessment of fetal well-being. Fetal heart rate monitoring is also used perioperatively during fetal interventions. The fetal heart rate is documented before the mother is anesthetized to (1) serve as a baseline for comparison and (2) reassure the perinatologist, surgeon, and anesthesiologist that the fetus is stable before starting the procedure. The fetal heart rate may be continuously or periodically monitored intraoperatively; this requires the presence of a skilled ultrasonographer working in the operative field. When technically feasible, looping fetal echocardiography should be available to assess fetal myocardial contractility and function, heart rate, intravascular volume status, and amniotic fluid volume. The serial examination of flow in the ductus arteriosus and/or the umbilical artery can also be followed to assess for fetal distress.[5,144] If intraoperative monitoring detects fetal distress, immediate corrective actions should occur to improve uteroplacental perfusion. This can include increasing maternal blood pressure and/or cardiac output, altering maternal or fetal positioning, and promoting additional uterine relaxation. If these maneuvers do not improve fetal well-being, administration of fetal resuscitation medications should be considered, or if the fetus is of viable age, delivery can be considered.

Temperature monitoring is also critical for open fetal procedures. The fetus is unable to thermoregulate in utero and relies on maternal body temperature for euthermia. In the setting of maternal general anesthesia, which can decrease the maternal core temperature, and/or an open hysterotomy, the fetus can become hypothermic, leading to fetal bradycardia.[145,146] Important measures to consider include the use of maternal forced air warming blankets, a warm operating room temperature, and the use of warmed fluid for intrauterine irrigation. During open procedures, both maternal and amniotic cavity temperatures should be monitored continuously.

Anesthetic Considerations

PREOPERATIVE CONSIDERATIONS

Maternal safety should be the cornerstone consideration for fetal interventions. A multidisciplinary team approach to planning for an intervention should occur, with input from fetal surgeons, perinatologists, ultrasonographers, anesthesiologists, genetic counselors, nurses, and social workers. Anesthesiologists in particular are well-suited to determine if maternal risk is acceptably low for the potential fetal benefit. Pregnant patients should be well counseled regarding the procedure risks and benefits as well as outcome and complications data. Experimental investigative procedures should be distinguished from evidence-based procedures in the consent process. Alternatives, such as nonintervention and pregnancy termination must also be discussed. The pregnant patient should understand how the intervention will affect the current and future pregnancies, as well as the delivery plan. In the case of a viable fetus, additional discussion should occur before the procedure regarding a plan for emergent delivery and resuscitation.

INTRAOPERATIVE MANAGEMENT

Minimally Invasive Procedures

The intraoperative management of fetal procedures should follow considerations for nonobstetric surgery during pregnancy. Patients should be fasted preoperatively given a nonparticulate antacid before entering the operating room. Often tocolysis is provided as a rectal indomethacin suppository before the procedure. The majority of fetoscopic procedures can be performed under monitored anesthesia care with local infiltration at the trocar entry site. Supplemental maternal anesthetic medications, including midazolam, fentanyl, and/or remifentanil can be added to provide maternal anesthesia or anxiolysis. The use of remifentanil (0.1 µg/kg per minute) may reduce fetal movement and improve operating conditions.[137] Mild to moderate sedation should be sufficient, with a level of consciousness maintained so the patient can be directed as needed to facilitate a successful procedure.[147] Deep sedation should be avoided in pregnant patients with an unprotected airway. Excessive maternal intravenous fluid administration should also be avoided during minimally invasive fetal procedures as pressurized uterine crystalloid into the amniotic cavity may lead to pulmonary edema.[148]

In some fetoscopic cases, such as when maternal immobility is desired (fetal cardiac procedures), or multiple trocar insertion sites are anticipated, a neuraxial technique is preferred. Most of the time, general anesthesia is not necessary for percutaneous procedures; an exception is fetoscopic myelomeningocele repair, which tends to be a prolonged procedure that requires maternal and fetal immobility.

Many interventions require fetal immobility. This can be achieved with an IM neuromuscular blocking drug administered directly to the fetus (rocuronium 2 to 3 mg/kg IM, vecuronium 0.25 mg/kg IM), with or without atropine (20 µg/kg). Additionally, direct fetal analgesia (fentanyl 10 to 20 µg/kg) should be administered IM if noxious stimulation is involved (e.g., shunt placement, fetal cardiac interventions). Fetal resuscitation medications including atropine (20 µg/kg) and epinephrine (10 µg/kg) should be prepared in sterile syringes for surgical team to administer if fetal distress develops. Ongoing distress in the setting of a viable fetus may require a cesarean delivery and neonatal recusation. The anesthesiologist should be prepared for both scenarios.

Open Fetal Procedures

Open fetal procedures involve a maternal hysterotomy and require profound uterine relaxation. These procedures carry a greater maternal risk, due to alternations in hemodynamics and the potential for blood loss. The anesthesia team should be prepared for maternal and fetal resuscitation, maternal and fetal blood replacement, and emergent delivery. Ongoing fetal monitoring is essential for fetal well-being, and direct administration of fetal medications is necessary. A thorough preoperative evaluation and surgical planning meeting should occur before the day of surgery.

Neuraxial anesthesia is often used for postoperative pain control after open fetal surgery. Most often, an epidural catheter is placed before induction, but local anesthetic is not instilled to avoid intraoperative hypotension. Typed and cross-matched blood should be prepared for the fetus; the fetal blood should be O-negative, cytomegalovirus-negative, irradiated, leukocyte-depleted, and maternally cross-matched with the mother. Weight-based fetal resuscitation medications (atropine 20 µg/kg and epinephrine 10 µg/kg) should be sterilely prepared in unit doses and transferred to the scrub nurse. A maternal nonparticulate antacid should be given preoperatively, and an indomethacin suppository is often placed for tocolysis.

Sequential compression devices should be placed on the maternal lower extremities and the patient should be positioned with left uterine displacement. Before induction of general anesthesia, fetal well-being should be assessed via ultrasound. A rapid-sequence induction with propofol and a neuromuscular blocking drug is usually performed. After induction, care should be taken to maintain both maternal blood pressure and heart rate within 10% of preinduction values to ensure adequate uterine perfusion. Maternal ventilation should target an $EtCO_2$ of 28 to 32 mm Hg to match the typical minute ventilation of pregnancy. Additional large-bore intravenous access should be established, and an arterial line considered for more direct hemodynamic monitoring.

After induction of anesthesia and throughout the operative procedure, the fetus should be monitored to assess for fetal distress. Maternal anesthetic administration, positioning, and hemodynamic changes can significantly affect the fetus. An early sign of fetal distress is absent or reversed umbilical arterial blood flow.[5] Additionally, assessments of blood flow across the ductus arteriosus and fetal cardiac function are important ways to evaluate fetal well-being.[6,144,149] Nonreassuring assessments should trigger immediate measures to improve the fetal well-being, including alterations in maternal or fetal position, and increasing maternal blood pressure and/or cardiac output. A vasoconstrictor such as phenylephrine is typically used to maintain maternal mean arterial blood pressure within 10% of baseline, as this medication has been shown to have little effect on fetal acid-base status.[150] Additionally, ephedrine or glycopyrrolate can increase maternal heart rate and cardiac output.[151]

Uterine relaxation to prevent uterine contractions is of utmost importance during open fetal surgery. During open fetal surgery, uterine contractions can reduce uteroplacental blood flow and gas exchange, leading to fetal hypoxia and distress. Inhalational anesthetics are potent smooth muscle relaxants and are commonly used to provide tocolysis during open fetal procedures. This effect is dose dependent; in the absence of other tocolytic medications, 1.5 to 2.0 minimum alveolar concentration (MAC) is necessary for adequate relaxation.[152] Unfortunately, most inhalational anesthetics have several disadvantages that limit their effectiveness. Once discontinued, their effect disappears, so they are not adequate for postoperative tocolysis. At large doses, they cause both maternal and fetal physiologic derangements, including cardiovascular depression and hypotension, as they readily cross the placenta. Over 60% of fetuses develop progressive cardiac dysfunction during open fetal surgery,[149] although the etiology of this dysfunction is not always entirely attributable to inhalational anesthetics.[5]

Several strategies have been investigated to reduce the total dose of inhalational anesthetic agents used and mitigate the consequences of larger dose volatile anesthetic agents. Initially, supplemental intravenous anesthesia with propofol and remifentanil infusions before the uterine incision reduces the maximum concentration of desflurane needed for uterine relaxation, as well as a decrease in the fetal left ventricular dysfunction and fetal distress.[6] More recently, remifentanil alone has been used throughout open fetal surgeries to reduce the desflurane dose to relax the uterus.[153] An additional technique involves administering magnesium sulfate for tocolysis at the beginning of the surgical procedure. Patients administered 6 grams of magnesium sulfate over 20 minutes followed by 2 grams/hour intraoperatively received less inhalational anesthetic than those who did not get magnesium sulfate at the beginning of the procedure.[154]

In rare instances in which inhalational anesthetics are contraindicated (e.g., patient history of malignant hyperthermia), uterine relaxation can be achieved with intravenous nitroglycerine at doses up to 20 µg/kg per minute in combination with a neuraxial anesthetic technique.[155] Both prolonged nitroglycerin infusions and the use of magnesium sulfate can be associated with maternal pulmonary edema, so caution should be taken to limit the volume of intravenous fluids administered.[156]

Before uterine incision, the surgical team should manually assess uterine tone. The uterus should be flaccid and the placement of initial sutures into the uterine wall should not cause uterine contractions. Should uterine contractions be noted, the concentration of inhalational anesthetics can be increased, or 200 to 400 µg boluses of nitroglycerine given intravenously to relax the uterus. The absence of adequate uterine relaxation despite

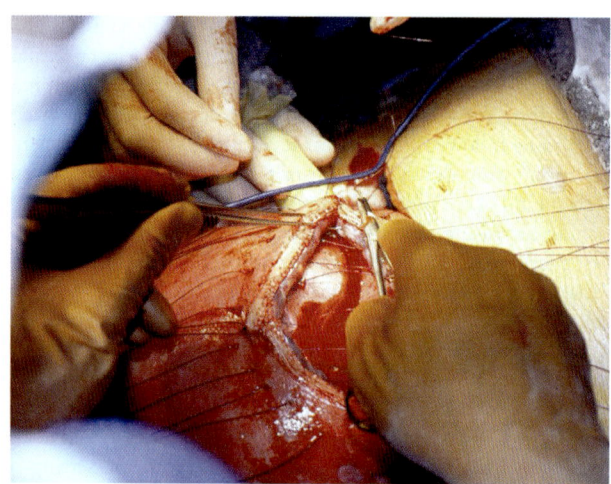

FIGURE 36.6 Hysterotomy closure. (Courtesy N. Scott Adzick, MD, Children's Hospital of Philadelphia.)

these interventions should prompt serious consideration to aborting the fetal intervention in order to avoid premature birth or fetal demise.

After assessing uterine tone, the placenta is mapped and a small hysterotomy is made away from the placenta. The excision is extended with a special lactomer stapling device that seals the amniotic membrane to the endometrium and tamponades the cut uterine wall (Fig. 36.6). During the hysterotomy, blood loss can be rapid and difficult to quantify, so vigilance of the surgical site and communication with the surgical team is essential. The fetus should be given an IM dose of neuromuscular blocking drug and opioid either just before or immediately after uterine incision. As uterine incision usually results in the egress of amniotic fluid, the surgical team must replace it with a warmed crystalloid solution to ensure proper fetal positioning and avoid umbilical cord kinking. An intrauterine temperature probe should be placed for continuous intrauterine temperature monitoring.

If a fetal mass resuscitation is planned (e.g., sacrococcygeal teratoma, congenital pulmonary airway malformation), fetal intravenous access should be established, so that the anesthesiologist can provide the fetus fluid, blood, and medications for resuscitation. It is essential that all fluids delivered to the fetus are adequately warmed. If fetal volume is required urgently and intravenous access has not yet been established, fluid can also be administered directly into the umbilical vein.

In case of maternal cardiac arrest, aggressive resuscitation should be initiated. If, after 4 minutes of resuscitation, maternal hemodynamics have not been restored, the fetus should be delivered to reduce aortocaval compression and improve the chance for maternal survival.[157] A neonatology team should be readily available for the care of the neonate, and depending on gestational age, neonatal resuscitation should occur following established neonatal resuscitation guidelines.[158]

At the conclusion of a fetal repair, magnesium sulfate should be administered for tocolysis if not yet given. Inhalational anesthetics can be weaned after magnesium has been administered, and the epidural activated for postoperative pain control after a test dose. When the incision is completely closed, neuromuscular blockade has been antagonized, and hemodynamic stability achieved, the tracheal tube may be removed once the mother is awake and breathing spontaneously.

POSTOPERATIVE CONSIDERATIONS

Postoperative care of patients undergoing fetal procedures center on fetal tocolysis and fetal monitoring. Though minimally invasive procedures usually do not require postoperative tocolysis, additional tocolytic agents in the postoperative period are important to prevent premature labor after more invasive fetoscopic or open fetal procedures. Options for tocolysis include indomethacin, magnesium sulfate, terbutaline, and calcium-channel blockers.

Indomethacin is a nonsteroidal antiinflammatory drug that blocks the action of cyclooxygenase, preventing the formation of prostaglandins (see Chapter 5). In vitro studies of indomethacin have found consistent inhibition or complete arrest of overall myometrial activity. Fetal echocardiography should be regularly performed when indomethacin is used, as it can cause premature closure of the ductus arteriosus. Indomethacin may also lead to fetal oliguria. These fetal effects limit the duration of indomethacin therapy.[159] However, after short-term use, these adverse effects are fully reversible within 72 hours from cessation of treatment.[159] Longer-term use of indomethacin has been associated with renal dysfunction and increased rates of necrotizing enterocolitis, intracranial hemorrhage, and patent ductus arteriosus in infants delivered at less than 30 weeks gestation.[160]

Magnesium sulfate competes with calcium for transmembrane channel entry into cells.[161] Because the myometrium depends on stores of calcium for adequate contraction, a decrease in intracellular transport prevents the activation of the actin and myosin complex, resulting in uterine relaxation. After a loading dose of 4 to 6 grams intraoperatively, it is maintained at an infusion of 1 to 2 grams/hour. Magnesium sulfate can cause maternal weakness and malaise. It also reduces fetal heart rate variability[162] and depresses fetal right ventricular function.[163] Because this drug rapidly crosses the placenta but is excreted more slowly by the fetal kidneys than by the maternal kidneys, there are concerns about fetal toxicity, resulting in respiratory and central nervous system depression.[164]

Calcium-channel blockers are generally well tolerated and are useful in postponing delivery, especially in those women with intact membranes.[165] Neonates born to women treated with calcium-channel blockers have a reduced frequency of respiratory distress, necrotizing enterocolitis, and intraventricular hemorrhage.[166] The most serious adverse effect of nifedipine is maternal hypotension. Hence, maternal blood pressure should be closely monitored when nifedipine is used.

In addition, robust maternal pain control is essential after a fetal intervention. Inadequate pain control can increase plasma oxytocin levels and precipitate preterm labor.[167] After open fetal procedures, an epidural infusion of a dilute local anesthetic solution and opioid is usually continued for a minimum of 48 hours postoperatively for analgesia. If an epidural is not placed, intravenous opioid medications can be used as an alternative, though this may decrease fetal heart rate variability.[168] For minimally invasive fetal procedures, analgesia is typically sufficient with a combination of oral opioids and acetaminophen.

Open fetal procedures increase the risk for infection, premature rupture of the membranes, premature labor, and uterine rupture.[169] These risks, combined with the need for ongoing assessment of fetal well-being, require the pregnant patient to remain close to the fetal intervention center in the initial weeks following intervention. If there is concern for premature delivery, a course of steroids should be administered to improve fetal lung maturity. Cesarean deliveries are planned for 37 weeks gestion, though preterm labor may hasten delivery. Due to the recent hysterotomy, uterine rupture is a real concern.[170] Furthermore, all subsequent pregnancies must be delivered via cesarean after an open fetal procedure.

The EXIT Procedure

EX-utero **I**ntrapartum **T**reatment, or the EXIT procedure, was initially described as a method for reversal of tracheal occlusion in fetuses with prenatally diagnosed severe congenital diaphragmatic hernia that had undergone in utero tracheal clip application.[171] Although these infants demonstrated no reduced morbidity compared with those who underwent conventional treatment, this novel technique provided a new therapeutic option for fetuses with a variety of potentially fatal diseases. Improvements in prenatal imaging and widespread use of prenatal ultrasonography have increased the identification of potentially lethal fetal structural malformations, which has had a direct impact on perinatal management and outcomes.

The EXIT procedure allows for a controlled delivery and intrapartum assessment strategy to treat fetuses with certain life-threatening diseases. By maintaining uteroplacental circulation with only partial delivery of the infant, crucial time is provided to perform procedures critical to infant survival. These procedures include direct laryngoscopy, bronchoscopy, intubation, tracheostomy, tumor decompression and resection, and extracorporeal membrane oxygenation (ECMO) cannulation before exteriorizing the entire infant and clamping the umbilical cord (Fig. 36.7). In this way, continuous oxygenation is maintained to the threatened neonate at all times, thereby improving the chances of overall survival. The EXIT procedure is now used for neonates in whom prenatal imaging suggests a very low probability of survival with conventional treatment methods. This group includes fetuses with known tracheal obstruction and other life-threatening airway abnormalities, as well as those who will likely require ECMO support (i.e., congenital cardiac disease and diaphragmatic hernia).[172]

Unlike many other fetal interventions, however, a planned delivery of the neonate is the end result of these interventions. This unique difference creates significant increases in maternal

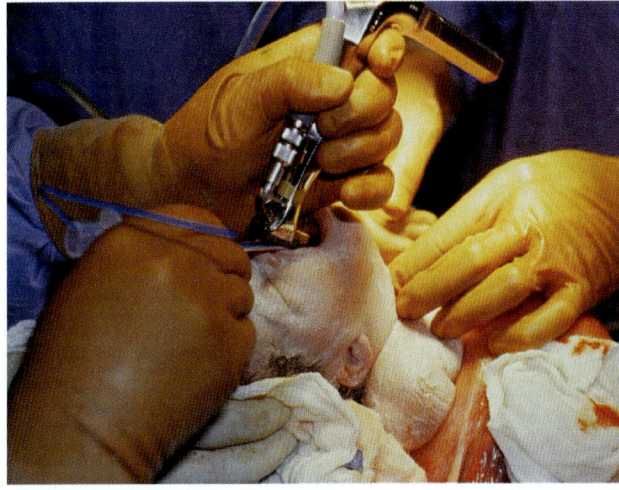

FIGURE 36.7 Fetal rigid bronchoscopy during an ex utero intrapartum treatment (EXIT) procedure. (Courtesy N. Scott Adzick, MD, Children's Hospital of Philadelphia.)

morbidity because these procedures require complete uterine relaxation before delivery and serious maternal hemorrhage can occur if the relaxation is not adequately reversed following delivery.[173] An intimate understanding of the EXIT procedure, the fetal pathophysiology involved, and pregnancy-induced alterations directly affecting anesthesia care (see Table 36.4) is required to minimize maternal and fetal morbidity and mortality.

FETAL DISEASES ELIGIBLE FOR THE EXIT-TO-AIRWAY PROCEDURE

Cervical Teratoma

Cervical teratomas are rare (1 per 20,000–40,000 live births) and can extend from the mastoid process to the sternal notch inferiorly and to the trapezius muscle posteriorly. They can also invade the oral floor and extend into the anterior mediastinum. Many of the larger teratomas diagnosed prenatally cause maternal polyhydramnios, which is secondary to esophageal compression by the tumor and impaired fetal swallowing. Most of these tumors are benign but are associated with substantial mortality caused by airway compression and difficulty in establishing an adequate airway after delivery (Fig. 36.8).[94,174] Of neonates with cervical teratomas, 30% die of airway obstruction shortly after delivery[175,176]; for neonates whose tumors are not diagnosed prenatally, mortality rates are even greater.[177,178] In addition, some larger tumors may interfere with normal delivery methods and necessitate emergent alterations in maternal care, placing the mother at increased risk.[174,179]

With the introduction of the EXIT procedure, precious time is provided to locate the trachea and provide a definitive airway in a controlled manner before clamping the umbilical cord, thereby maintaining continuous fetal oxygenation, and decreasing morbidity and mortality.

Cystic Hygroma

Cystic hygromas arise from the failure of the jugular lymph sacs to join the lymphatic system early in fetal development, resulting in the development of endothelium-lined cystic spaces that eventually compress normal surrounding structures. This compression may result in fetal hydrops, including skin edema, ascites, and pleural or pericardial effusions (Fig. 36.9).[177,178] In infants with isolated cervical cystic hygroma and no evidence of hydrops, airway compromise at birth or shortly thereafter is the main therapeutic concern. These infants are candidates for EXIT procedures.

Congenital High Airway Obstruction Syndrome

Congenital high airway obstruction syndrome (CHAOS) is a clinical syndrome consisting of extremely large echogenic lungs, flattened or inverted diaphragms, a dilated tracheobronchial tree, ascites, and evidence of nonimmune hydrops, including fetal ascites, placentomegaly, and pleural or pericardial effusions.[180–182] Airway obstruction may be because of laryngeal atresia, laryngeal cyst, or tracheal atresia. Diagnosis of prenatal CHAOS is confirmed by ultrasonographic evidence of complete or near-complete upper airway obstruction. Most diagnostic findings result from increased intratracheal pressure and distention of the tracheobronchial tree secondary to the accumulation of fluid in the lungs. Cardiac changes include the appearance of an elongated heart, septal shift, and small, compressed heart chambers.[178]

Management guidelines for fetuses with CHAOS are not definitive. In third-trimester fetuses with a diagnosis of CHAOS and no evidence of hydrops, there is most probably incomplete airway obstruction, and management is aimed at establishing an airway before complete delivery. This subset of fetuses would likely benefit from an EXIT procedure.[178,183] Those fetuses with a diagnosis of CHAOS made in the second trimester and those with evidence of complete airway obstruction and/or nonimmune hydrops present a dilemma, because insufficient data exist to determine their best treatment options. Several centers are performing fetoscopic ultrasound-guided decompression of the laryngeal atresia by inserting a wire across the atretic region and performing balloon dilation for these patients, and when successful, proceeding with an EXIT procedure in the third trimester.[184]

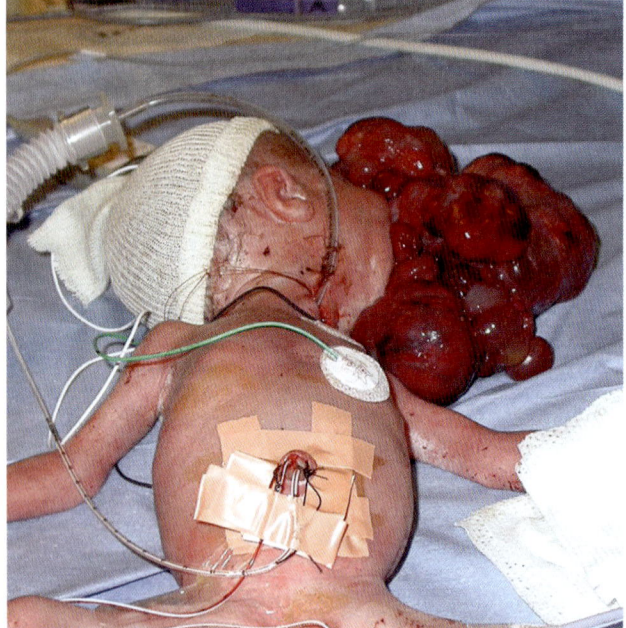

FIGURE 36.8 Newborn with a massive oropharyngeal cervical teratoma immediately after ex-utero intrapartum treatment was performed to secure the airway. Immediate resection of the teratoma followed in an adjacent operating room.

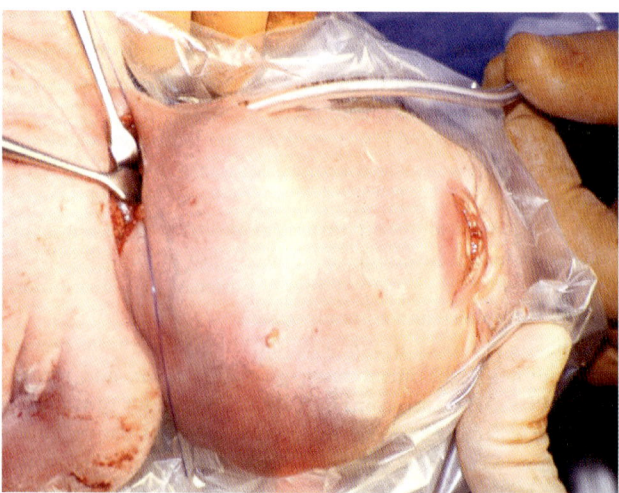

FIGURE 36.9 Fetus (with a cystic hygroma) that underwent ex-utero intrapartum treatment to establish a surgical airway before delivery. (Courtesy N. Scott Adzick, MD, Children's Hospital of Philadelphia.)

Congenital Goiter

Congenital goiter is associated with fetal hypothyroidism, euthyroidism, or hyperthyroidism. Goiter associated with fetal hypothyroidism is almost always associated with the transplacental passage of a thyroid-stimulating immunoglobulin G antibody from the mother. Such antibodies are present in 90% of women with Graves disease. These antibody levels may not reflect maternal thyroid status, making the fetus of any woman with Graves disease at increased risk for fetal goiter. Less common causes include iodine deficiency, iodine intoxication, congenital metabolic disorders of thyroid hormone synthesis, or hypothalamic-pituitary hypothyroidism.

Ultrasonographic findings of fetal hyperthyroidism include cardiac hypertrophy, tachycardia, or nonimmune hydrops fetalis. Fetal hypothyroidism may be associated with fetal cardiomegaly and heart block. Fetal blood sampling is required to determine the fetal thyroid status.[178,185,186] The possibility of significant airway compression immediately after delivery is similar for all fetuses with goiter. In severe cases, even the presence of experienced personnel in the delivery room may not ensure prompt ability to secure the airway. These infants may benefit from the EXIT procedure; it can provide time to identify and secure the compromised airway.

Microretrognathia

The EXIT procedure has also been used in those fetuses with severe micro or retrognathia who may develop severe airway obstruction at birth with inadequate ability to ventilate and oxygenate.[187] This is due to glossoptosis, (a posteriorly displaced base of the tongue due to a hypoplastic mandible) that reduces the already narrow hypopharynx. The severity of mandibular hypoplasia can be assessed in prenatal ultrasound, though care must be taken to view the mandible in the true sagittal plane to ensure accurate measurement.[188]

EXIT TO ECMO

In addition to airway management, the EXIT procedure may be considered for other instances in which separation from uteroplacental support is expected to cause critical cardiac or pulmonary compromise. Fetuses with congenital heart disease who are expected to need emergent ECMO at birth and fetuses with poor-prognosis congenital diaphragmatic hernias may benefit from the "EXIT to ECMO" strategy.[173,189] Neonates undergoing this procedure are partially delivered via the EXIT procedure, and arterial and venous cannulas are inserted while uteroplacental perfusion is maintained. Although congenital diaphragmatic hernia remains the most common disease entity considered for potential EXIT to ECMO therapy, this technique has been used for neonates with other disease processes associated with almost certain chance of immediate cardiorespiratory collapse after conventional delivery.

EXIT TO RESECTION

For fetuses with large intrathoracic lesions causing mediastinal compression or airway compromise, an EXIT to resection strategy can be considered. In these instances, the fetal lesion is resected on placental support. These cases require careful fetal monitoring and often volume resuscitation and blood transfusion. Conditions where EXIT to resection are considered include bronchogenic cysts, congenital pulmonary airway malformations, mediastinal masses, and intrathoracic tumors.[190]

EXIT TO SEPARATION

EXIT to separation can be used in the setting of conjoined twins. Typically, this strategy is reserved for fetuses where one twin is not viable. By performing an EXIT procedure, the viable twin can survive.[191]

PREOPERATIVE CONSIDERATIONS

A multidisciplinary team consisting of an obstetrician, pediatric surgeon, ultrasonographer, anesthesiologist, neonatologist, scrub nurses, and technicians provides the expertise in each respective field to aid in the overall success of the procedure. In cases in which immediate surgical intervention is planned after delivery (e.g., resection of a neck mass), a prepared adjacent operating room with separate personnel should be available. A meeting of the entire team is held before the start of the case to clearly identify individual roles and to discuss any concerns or questions. This is also a good opportunity to address any clinical changes, either in radiographic findings or in fetal position, or other factors that may alter the surgical plan.

INTRAOPERATIVE CONSIDERATIONS

General anesthesia is typically used for EXIT procedures, though neuraxial anesthesia with nitroglycerine for uterine relaxation has been described.[155] After a rapid-sequence induction, the maternal airway is secured and additional intravenous access is obtained. Arterial access should be considered. Maternal blood pressure is maintained within 10% of baseline, and large doses of inhalational anesthetics are used to relax the uterus as described in the open fetal surgery section.

To preserve maternal-fetal gas exchange at the placental interface and ensure fetal oxygenation, it is of primary importance to ensure complete uterine relaxation throughout the duration of fetal uteroplacental support. Factors affecting uterine blood flow include, but are not limited to, anesthetic induction agents, maternal hyperventilation, maternal hypotension, maternal catecholamine release, and other causes of increased noradrenergic activity and uterine tone. Any increase in uterine vascular resistance decreases uterine perfusion, in the same way as uterine contractions do. Of all factors ensuring the overall success of the EXIT procedure, minimal uterine vascular resistance and maintenance of uterine atony are the most important because decreases in uterine blood flow or early disruption of the placental interface will cause fetal hypoxemia, acidosis, and, potentially, fetal demise.[192]

After the hysterotomy site has been created and hemostasis achieved, the fetal head, neck, and shoulders are delivered. Because many of these procedures involve large neck masses, a generous hysterotomy incision is needed to partially deliver the fetus without injury to the mass or fetus. Furthermore, if a uterine contraction occurs at this time, inadvertent expulsion of the fetus could occur, interrupting the fetoplacental unit and thus critically jeopardizing the viability of the fetus. In some cases, a fetal extremity may be delivered to apply a pulse oximetry probe and to obtain IV access.[193,194] Although the fetus is anesthetized via placental transfer of maternally administered inhalational anesthetics in most cases, additional analgesia and paralytics are administered (e.g., fentanyl, atropine, neuromuscular blocking drug). The analgesics are critical to blunting the fetal stress response despite use of inhalational agents. The additional medications may be given as a single IM dose in an upper extremity or can alternatively be delivered under ultrasound guidance before hysterotomy. An advantage to earlier administration is increased time for fetal absorption via the IM route. If peripheral IV access is obtained, additional medications can be given through this route.

Most EXIT procedures are currently performed to access a compromised fetal airway before delivery; successful access depends on meticulous preoperative evaluation and careful preparation.[195,196] Portions of the trachea can be completely compressed and distorted such that even successful intubation may result in an inability to achieve adequate ventilation. For this reason, most surgeons perform a direct laryngoscopy and bronchoscopy to examine the status of the fetal airway. In one series, successful tracheal intubation by conventional means was reported in 77% of cases.[173] In those cases in which tracheal intubation is impossible, a surgical tracheostomy can be performed as soon as the trachea is identified.

Regardless of the method used to secure the trachea, the anesthesiologist must be prepared to control ventilation in the fetus. In some institutions, an anesthesiologist may be scrubbed at the operative field to assume this responsibility. In other institutions, one of the surgeons or neonatologists assumes this role. Ventilation should result in increases in fetal oxygen saturation to greater than 85%. If this does not occur, the position of the tracheal tube should be rechecked, and the lungs should be auscultated with a sterile stethoscope. Ultrasound examination for the presence of air bronchograms may also be used to confirm tracheal intubation. Ventilation occurs most commonly with the aid of a sterile Jackson-Rees circuit. When adequate ventilation has been established, the fetus can be delivered.

Before umbilical cord clamping and delivery, coordination between the surgery and anesthesia teams is crucial to prevent uterine atony and excessive maternal hemorrhage. Because a decrease in the tocolytic agent, whether it is an inhalational or an IV agent, would increase uterine vascular resistance and decrease fetal oxygenation, reversal of the tocolysis must not occur before the umbilical cord is clamped. However, at clamping, a near-total reversal of tocolysis is required to limit uterine bleeding. This is best achieved with an inhalational anesthetic with a low solubility (e.g., desflurane). As the cord is clamped, the anesthetic is immediately discontinued, and oxytocin is administered as a bolus followed by a continuous infusion and titrated to uterine response. Additional uterotonic medications may be necessary and must be immediately available should uncontrolled maternal hemorrhage occur.[197] These medications include methylergonovine, carboprost, and misoprostol. Use of a total intravenous anesthetic (TIVA) with propofol (see Chapter 6) and no inhalational agent may also be beneficial to maximize uterine tone. Anticipation of massive and rapid maternal hemorrhage is essential. Appropriate IV access (e.g., rapid infusion catheters, introducer sheaths) with a rapid infusion device in place for blood product administration may be lifesaving, should uncontrolled and persistent bleeding occur. In cases of uncontrolled hemorrhage despite maximal drug therapy, a hysterectomy may be necessary.

A separate team of neonatologists, anesthesiologists, and nurses should be available for the neonate because additional medications, blood products, and vascular access may be needed. A brief physical examination, confirmation of bilateral breath sounds, and hemodynamic stability must be ensured soon after delivery. In some instances, immediate surgical intervention is planned, necessitating entirely separate anesthetic, surgical, and nursing teams in an adjacent operating room as the maternal abdomen is closed.

POSTOPERATIVE CONSIDERATIONS

Mothers recovering from an EXIT procedure differ from those who undergo standard cesarean deliveries. Potential postoperative complications include wound dehiscence, infection, bleeding, and urinary retention.[173] Often, fetal anatomy necessitates an extended hysterotomy, or a hysterotomy location that is not a low-transverse incision. As a result, these patients are at increased risk of uterine rupture in any subsequent pregnancy. In most cases, neuraxial anesthesia is performed and mothers either have neuraxial opioids administered or epidural catheters placed to provide postoperative analgesia. Practitioners should also consider the fact that, unlike with a standard cesarean section, the parents cannot immediately interact with or even view their neonates after delivery. Because many of these neonates undergo immediate surgical intervention, the parents' first glimpse of their child will be of an intubated, sedated child with monitors, invasive catheters, and swollen, distorted facies. Continued emotional support, social services, and education will help ease this transition.

Future Directions

The indications for fetal intervention will continue to expand with the advances in surgical and anesthetic techniques as well as imaging technologies. It is anticipated they will move from treatment of only life-threatening fetal pathologic processes toward preemptive management of fetal disorders that are not necessarily life-threatening but certainly have disabling postpartum morbidities. However, these benefits must be balanced with maternal and neonatal risks. Improvements in the management of preterm labor, as well as the prevention of premature delivery are both important areas for future advancement, as both lead to better morbidity and limit the current scope of fetal practice.

Novel fetal therapeutics require thorough preclinical investigation in animal models to establish their utility and benefit. This must be followed with rigorous translational research investigation, followed by multicenter clinical trials. Ongoing research is needed to determine the optimal timing for fetal intervention as well as appropriate maternal and fetal patient selection.

Several interesting future research directions are evolving in fetal therapy. In utero stem cell and gene therapies hold promise to correct otherwise severe or lethal genetic disorders.[198,199] Artificial placental units hold promise for the support of preterm neonates. These systems provide extracorporeal support vial the umbilical cord as well as a warm, continuous fluid exchange, and have been shown to be successful in animal models.[199,200]

Within anesthesia, alternative anesthetic techniques that optimize maternal and fetal stability require examination. Additional investigation into the neurocognitive effects of anesthetic exposure in utero is also of great interest. Strategies to optimize placental perfusion and reduce uterine tone, both intraoperatively and postoperatively, are needed. Advances in fetal monitoring, including assessment of the fetal stress response, will help improve anesthetic techniques. Clinically, the development of standard guidelines[201] as well as formalized training in fetal anesthesia will continue to advance this unique subspecialty.

Acknowledgment

The authors would like to thank the previous author of this chapter, Dr. Roland Brusseau for his contributions.

ANNOTATED REFERENCES

Adzick NS, Thom EA, Spong CY, et al. A randomized trial of prenatal versus postnatal repair of myelomeningocele. *N Engl J Med.* 2011;364(11):993-1004.

This prospective, multicentered, randomized controlled trial established the efficacy of open fetal intervention for myelomeningocele repair. Neonates who underwent fetal intervention were less likely to need a ventriculoperitoneal shunt and had improved cognitive and motor outcomes at 30 months of age. Fetal intervention patients were also more likely to have preterm delivery and had a high rate of uterine dehiscence.

Boat A, Mahmoud M, Michelfelder EC, et al. Supplementing desflurane with intravenous anesthesia reduces fetal cardiac dysfunction during open fetal surgery. *Paediatr Anaesth.* 2010;20(5):748-756.

In a retrospective study, Boat and colleagues found that early institution of high concentrations of volatile agents for extended periods before hysterotomy resulted in the development of intraoperative fetal bradycardia, most notably when desflurane was used as the maintenance agent. They suggest supplemental IV anesthesia with propofol and remifentanil until just before the hysterotomy incision is made, at which point high volatile anesthetic concentrations may be used to achieve the desired uterine relaxation.

Chatterjee D, Arendt KW, Moldenhauer JS, et al. Anesthesia for Maternal-Fetal Interventions: A Consensus Statement from the American Society of Anesthesiologists Committees on Obstetric and Pediatric Anesthesiology and the North American Fetal Therapy Network. *Anesth Analg.* 2021;132(4):1164-1173.

This consensus statement from the American Society of Anesthesiologists (ASA) summarizes important recommendations for fetal intervention. Input from representatives from the ASA Committees of Obstetric and Pediatric Anesthesia and the Board of Directors of the North American Fetal Therapy Network was used to craft these recommendations, which include important preoperative, intraoperative, and postoperative considerations for the care of these patients.

Deprest JA, Nicolaides KH, Benachi A, et al. Randomized trial of fetal surgery for severe left diaphragmatic hernia. *N Engl J Med.* 2021;385(2):107-118.

This prospective, multiinstitutional study randomly assigned 27- to 29-week fetuses with severe congenital diaphragmatic hernia to fetoscopic endoluminal tracheal occlusion or standardized postnatal care. The authors found that fetal intervention resulted in a higher rate of survival to discharge compared with standard postnatal care, despite the fact that intervention increased the risk of preterm, prelabor rupture of membranes and preterm birth.

Donepudi R, Huynh M, Moise Jr KJ, et al. Early administration of magnesium sulfate during open fetal myelomeningocele repair reduces the dose of inhalational anesthesia. *Fetal Diagn Ther.* 2019;45(3):192-196.

This prospective observational study of fetuses going open mid-gestational fetal myelomeningocele repair compared the administration of magnesium sulfate for tocolysis at the end of the procedure to its administration at the beginning of the surgical procedure. The authors found that early administration of magnesium sulfate allowed for reduced volatile anesthetic agent use for these cases. Overall difference in maternal vasopressor administration was unchanged.

Ferschl MB, Rollins MD, Chatterjee D. Error traps in anesthesia for fetal interventions. *Paediatr Anaesth.* 2021;31(3):275-281.

The authors discuss five common pitfalls in fetal anesthesia. The challenges include failure to preserve uteroplacental perfusion, failure to maintain uterine relaxation, failure to adequately monitor the fetus, failure to prepare for maternal hemorrhage, and failure to treat uterine hemorrhage. Each error trap is outlined, and guidelines presented to practitioners to prevent these problems during fetal procedures.

Ferschl MB, Feiner J, Vu L, Smith D, Rollins MD. A comparison of spinal anesthesia versus monitored anesthesia care with local anesthesia in minimally invasive fetal surgery. *Anesth Analg.* 2020;130(2):409-415.

In this retrospective study, the authors compare the use of neuraxial anesthesia to local anesthesia with monitored anesthesia care in patients undergoing minimally invasive fetal procedures for twin-twin transfusion syndrome and twin-reversed arterial perfusion sequence. Patients treated with local were no more likely to require conversion to general anesthesia compared with those treated with a neuraxial technique. Furthermore, the patients treated with local anesthesia required less vasopressor, less intravenous fluid, and had a reduced total operating room time, without adversely affecting the surgical procedure length.

Lin EE, Moldenhauer JS, Tran KM, Cohen DE, Adzick NS. Anesthetic management of 65 cases of ex utero intrapartum therapy: a 13-year single-center experience. *Anesth Analg.* 2016;123(2):411-417.

This article describes the indications and anesthetic techniques for the EXIT procedure. Data on 65 cases at a single institution are reviewed, including data on anesthetic agent administration, blood loss, transfusion requirements, vasopressor use, and fetal resuscitation measures.

Marsh BJ, Sinskey J, Whitlock EL, Ferschl MB, Rollins MD. Use of remifentanil for open in utero fetal myelomeningocele repair maintains uterine relaxation with reduced volatile anesthetic concentration. *Fetal Diagn Ther.* 2020;47(11):810-816.

The authors report the use of remifentanil to as a supplemental intravenous anesthetic agent. In this retrospective study, they found that a continuous remifentanil infusion reduced volatile anesthetic agent use as well as maternal vasopressor administration without adversely affecting fetal outcome.

Ngamprasertwong P, Michelfelder EC, Arbabi S, et al. Anesthetic techniques for fetal surgery: effects of maternal anesthesia on intraoperative fetal outcomes in the sheep model. *Anesthesiology.* 2013;118(4):796-808.

Using an instrumented mid-gestational ewe model, the authors compared maternal and fetal hemodynamics, acid-base status, and left ventricular function in the setting of both high-dose desflurane anesthesia and lower-dose desflurane anesthesia with supplemental infusions of propofol and remifentanil. In this crossover design study, high-dose desflurane resulted in more maternal hypotension, reduced uterine blood flow, and greater fetal acidosis when compared with the lower-dose desflurane/intravenous agent technique.

Ngan Kee WD, Khaw KS, Tan PE, et al. Placental transfer and fetal metabolic effects of phenylephrine and ephedrine during spinal anesthesia for cesarean delivery. *Anesthesiology.* 2009;111(3):506-512.

The authors randomly assigned 104 healthy parturient undergoing elective cesarean section under spinal anesthesia to receive infusions of either phenylephrine or ephedrine, titrated to maintain approximate baseline systolic blood pressure. The authors found that, although ephedrine crosses the placenta to a greater extent and undergoes less early metabolism (or redistribution) in the fetus compared with phenylephrine, its associated increased fetal concentrations of lactate, glucose, and catecholamines may favor phenylephrine as the preferred vasopressor for such indications, despite historical evidence suggesting uteroplacental blood flow may be better maintained with ephedrine.

A complete reference list can be found online at Elsevier eBooks+.

37 Trauma and Mass Casualties

DANIEL STOCKI, DANIEL BRAUNOLD, YITZHAK BRZEZINSKI SINAI,
NADAV SHEFFY, ELIAHU SIMHI, AND AMIT LEHAVI

Epidemiology of Pediatric Trauma
Nonaccidental Trauma
Prehospital Care of the Pediatric Trauma Patient
Trauma Systems
Prehospital Airway Management
Emergency Department Evaluation and Management of the Pediatric Trauma Patient
In-Hospital Triage
Initial Management
Airway Management
Head Trauma
Chest Trauma

Abdominal Trauma
Blood Resuscitation
Intraoperative Management of the Pediatric Trauma Patient
Preoperative Evaluation
Intraoperative Management of Brain Injury
Intraoperative Management of Chest Trauma
Intraoperative Management of Abdominal Injury
Intraoperative Management of Orthopedic Trauma
Mass Casualty Events
Cricoid Pressure
Pain Management
Future Directions in Pediatric Trauma

ANESTHESIOLOGISTS COMMONLY PROVIDE CARE TO CHILDREN who have suffered traumatic injuries of varying complexity. They range from the healthy, older child with an isolated elbow fracture to the infant with a life-threatening epidural hematoma. The anesthesiologist should view the management of children with traumatic injuries as a continuum of care that may originate in the prehospital setting with emergency medical services (EMS), progression to the emergency department (ED) that continues to the operating room, the postanesthesia care unit (PACU), and the intensive care unit (ICU). Anesthesiologists have a role in all phases of care of the injured child. The care required to properly manage the injured child may be complex but can be effectively accomplished in a collaborative environment incorporating a standardized process for initial evaluation and management.[1] Anesthesiologists should be familiar with these processes to effectively continue this care into the perioperative setting.

Operative interventions demand the full involvement of the anesthesiologist. In many institutions, anesthesiologists also provide emergency airway and critical care management. In addition, anesthesiologists are highly skilled in airway management, ventilation, hemodynamic resuscitation, metabolic management, and control of pain, all of which can be important in the care of the injured child.

This chapter reviews the key principles of anesthesia management for children with traumatic injuries. Discussion is intended to augment the principles established in the widely accepted advanced trauma life support (ATLS) program, which is produced by the American College of Surgeons Committee on Trauma.[2] Additional resources for the management of the pediatric trauma patient include the advanced pediatric life support (APLS) and pediatric advanced life support (PALS) courses administered by the American Academy of Pediatrics and the American College of Emergency Physicians.[3,4]

Epidemiology of Pediatric Trauma

Injuries are the most common cause of death within the United States for children older than 1 year of age[5]; traffic accidents have consistently remained the leading cause of disability-adjusted life

year (DALY) rates among adolescents aged 10 to 24 years globally, despite a 33.6% decrease in age standardized DALY from 1990 to 2019, with self-harm ranked third and interpersonal violence fifth.[6] Approximately 10,000 children aged 1 to 19 years die annually in the United States as a result of trauma.[7] In 2019, motor vehicle accidents accounted for 91,000 injuries in children younger than 12 years of age with 608 deaths.[8] The epidemiology of trauma reflects its continued growth as an important health risk for children of the world. Table 37.1 lists the death rates for traumatic causes of childhood death within the United States in 2014.[7] Unintentional injuries consistently rank as the leading causes of death among pediatric patients for ages greater than 1 year, but child abuse is one of the leading causes of death in children younger than 1 year of age.[9]

Pediatric injury patterns differ by age groups, with falls being the major mode of injury for children aged 0 to 9 years[10] and motor vehicle collisions for those aged 10 to 18 years.[11] Injury patterns also differ between higher and lower income countries, with motor vehicle collisions constituting an even greater percentage of injury compared with falls in lower income countries.[12]

Traumatic brain injuries are the leading cause of death among children and there has been an increase in traumatic brain injuries diagnosed in children presenting to emergency departments in the United States; there was a 22.2% increase in traumatic brain injury diagnoses between 2006 and 2012.[13] The incidence of head injury globally varies widely with rates reported from 47 up to 280 per 100,000 children.[14] An important factor that contributes to the greater rate of head injury in children compared with adults is the child's proportionately larger (and heavier) head. Airborne children invariably land on their heads. Cervical injuries are prominent in infants restrained in forward-facing car seats

Thoracic injuries are the second leading cause of death for pediatric trauma patients. With their increased rib cage pliability from a lack of bony calcification and the presence of a flexible cartilaginous component, severe internal thoracic and upper

TABLE 37.1	Total Deaths and Death Rates[a] for Traumatic Causes of Childhood Death Within the United States[b]				
		AGE (YEARS)			
Cause of Death	Total	1–4	5–9	10–14	15–19
Unintentional	4335	831 (10.2)[a]	450 (4.3)[a]	500 (4.7)[a]	2554 (23.5)[a]
Assault	1590	184 (2.3)[a]	73 (0.7)[a]	95 (0.9)[a]	1238 (11.4)[a]
Self-Harm	1595	0	245 (2.3)[a]	1350 (12.4)[a]	

[a]Death rate is per 100,000 population.
[b]Abstracted from National Vital Statistics Reports, Vol. 65, No. 2, February 16, 2016
https://www.cdc.gov/nchs/data/nvsr/nvsr65/nvsr65_02.pdf.

abdominal injuries can occur in children without obvious external signs such as rib fractures.

Nonaccidental Trauma

Nonaccidental trauma, or injuries after child abuse, is an epidemic that continues to grow in virtually every part of the world. The COVID-19 pandemic that began in 2020 brought about global forced quarantines and enhanced psychosocial stressors, and is feared to have increased the size and implications of nonaccidental trauma/child abuse.[15-17] Almost 3 million cases of child maltreatment were filed in the United States in 2020; about half of those were further investigated, and of the confirmed 618,000 cases of neglect and abuse, 16.5% were physically abused and 9.4% sexually abused.[18]

The youngest children, particularly infants, are the most vulnerable to abuse (Fig. 37.1).[19–21] Every state has stringent laws for reporting nonaccidental trauma. These laws are designed to assist the health care provider who suspects abuse and to punish health care providers who do not appropriately report potential abuse and neglect. It is the responsibility of every physician who is involved in a child's care, including the anesthesiologist, to be aware of the potential for nonaccidental trauma in all infants and children and to report all suspicious observations to the appropriate authorities.[21,22]

Features of nonaccidental trauma include a history inconsistent with the characteristics and extent of the injuries and a delay in obtaining medical care.[23,24] Children experiencing nonaccidental trauma have a greater level of injury severity on average when compared with children sustaining injuries from accidental trauma; they also suffer worse outcomes and greater mortality even for similar injury severity scores in accidental trauma.[20,25–27] Nonaccidental trauma should be considered when the history appears suspicious.[28] Funduscopic examination may disclose retinal hemorrhages or papilledema, which suggests forceful shaking of the head or increased intracranial pressure (ICP), respectively. Examination of the skin may show bruises (especially in unusual locations, e.g., neck and perineum), burns, or other injuries in several stages of healing (Fig. 37.2). A skeletal survey, with added bone scintigraphy in equivocal cases, may reveal multiple fractures of various ages occurring typically at the metaphysis of long bones.[29] Occasionally, a child who has previously been silent in the company of the parents or caregiver reveals details to operating room or recovery room personnel about the events surrounding their injuries. These reports should be carefully documented and conveyed to the appropriate personnel.[30] Anesthesiologists have a key role in recognizing, reporting, and responding to child abuse.[31–34] Abused children are often terrified of painful procedures and the need for sensitivity as well as reassurance in these settings cannot be overemphasized.

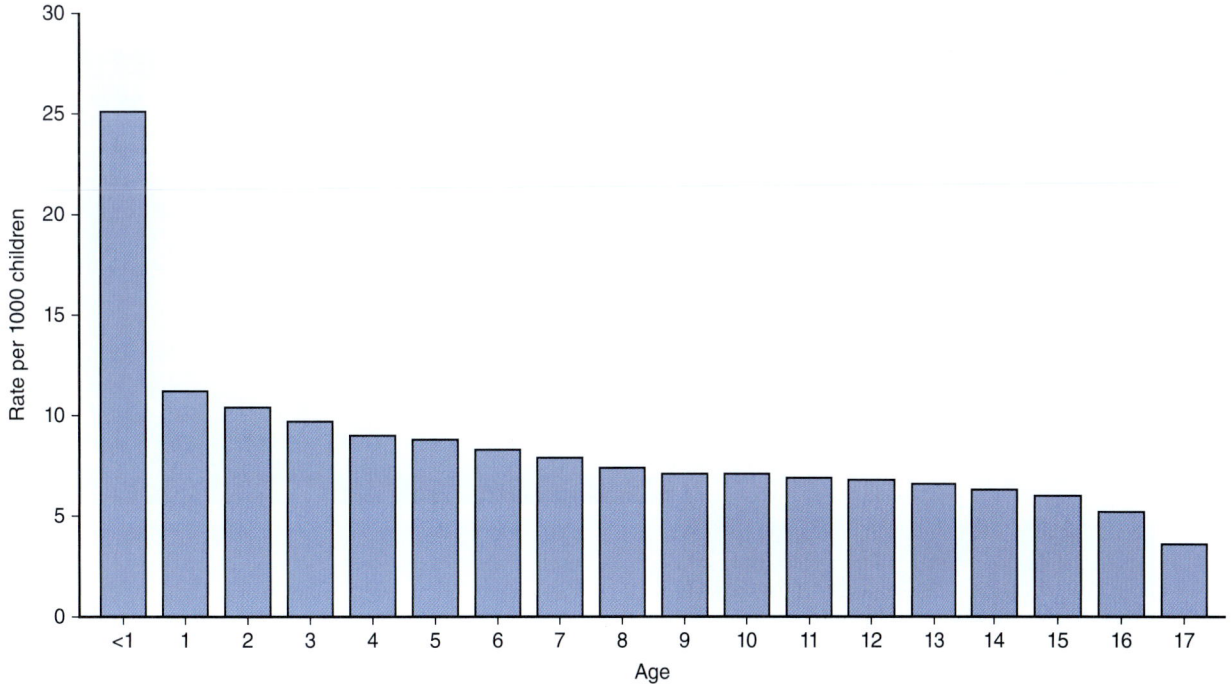

FIGURE 37.1 The rate of maltreatment per 1000 children by age group in years. The youngest children, particularly infants, were the most vulnerable to maltreatment. (Data from the US Department of Health and Human Services, Administration for Children and Families, Administration on Children, Youth, and Families, Children's Bureau; Child Maltreatment 2020. https://www.acf.hhs.gov/sites/default/files/documents/cb/cm2020.pdf.)

Although the role of the anesthesia team encountering a potential victim of nonaccidental trauma as part of the perioperative team is often not emphasized, the anesthesiologist may be in a unique position to provide the first impartial assessment of the child's status.[35–37] Historical data associated with the event may be inaccurate or fictitious at the time of initial presentation. A careful evaluation by the anesthesiologist in preparation for operative intervention may reveal the first objective evidence of nonaccidental trauma. Indications of mistreatment may be subtle, ranging from lack of parental availability for perioperative evaluation to the irrational refusal of consent for a necessary intervention.[36]

Prehospital Care of the Pediatric Trauma Patient

TRAUMA SYSTEMS

The evolution of pediatric trauma systems has improved outcomes and quality of life for trauma victims.[38,39] Countries such as the United States have a trauma system philosophy more in line with the military approach in which prehospital personnel such as paramedics are the first team summoned to make rapid assessments, initiate efforts at stabilization, establish radio contact with the medical facility, and transport the child to the trauma center

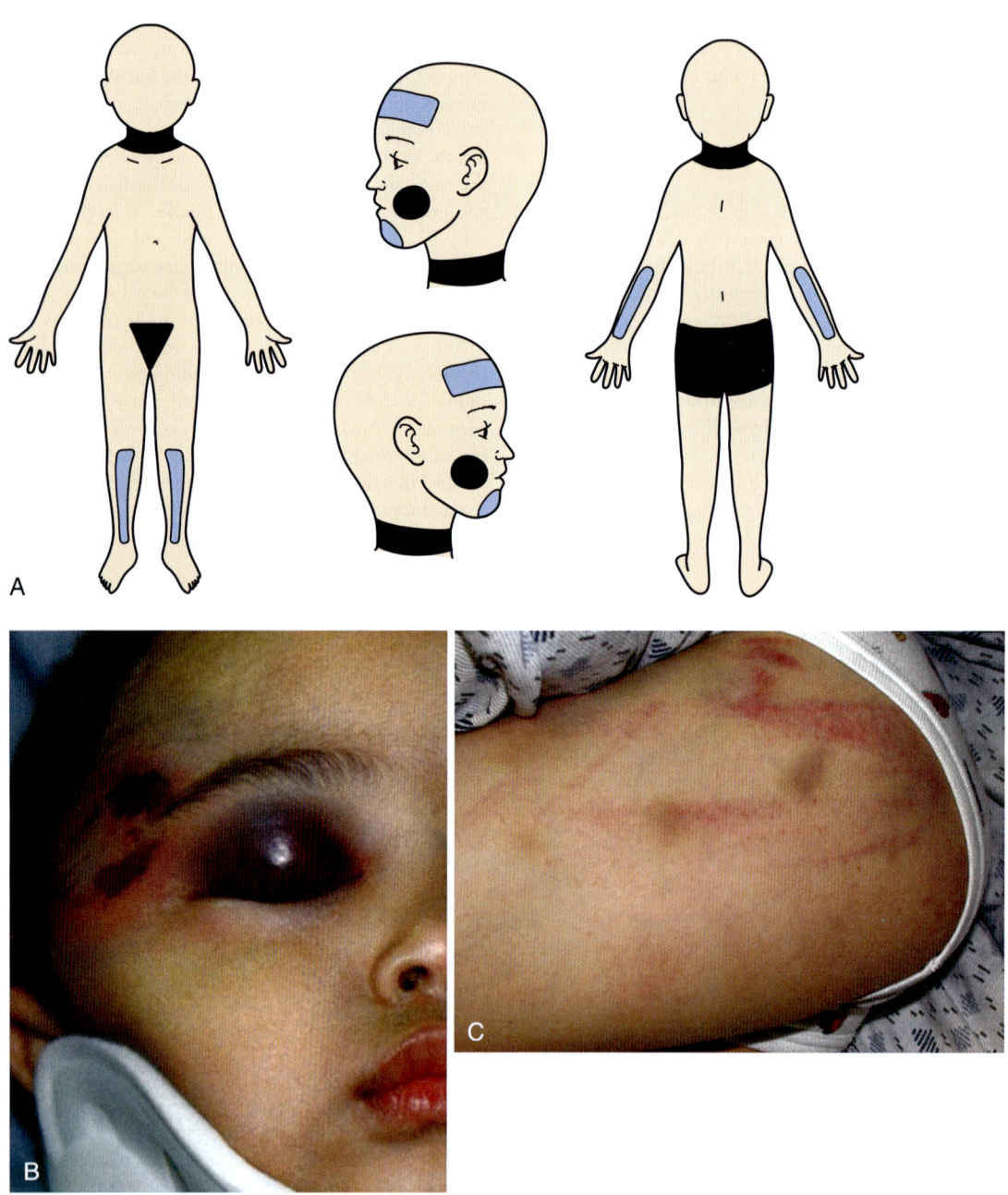

FIGURE 37.2 Common examples of child abuse, also referred to as nonaccidental trauma, are shown. **A**, Typical areas on children where bruising can be detected. The *blue areas* indicate regions where normal bruising may occur. The *black areas* are regions of unusual bruising. Any bruise in the black areas must be considered for possible nonaccidental trauma. **B**, A child with obvious facial trauma. **C**, A whipping injury from a belt plus additional bruises.

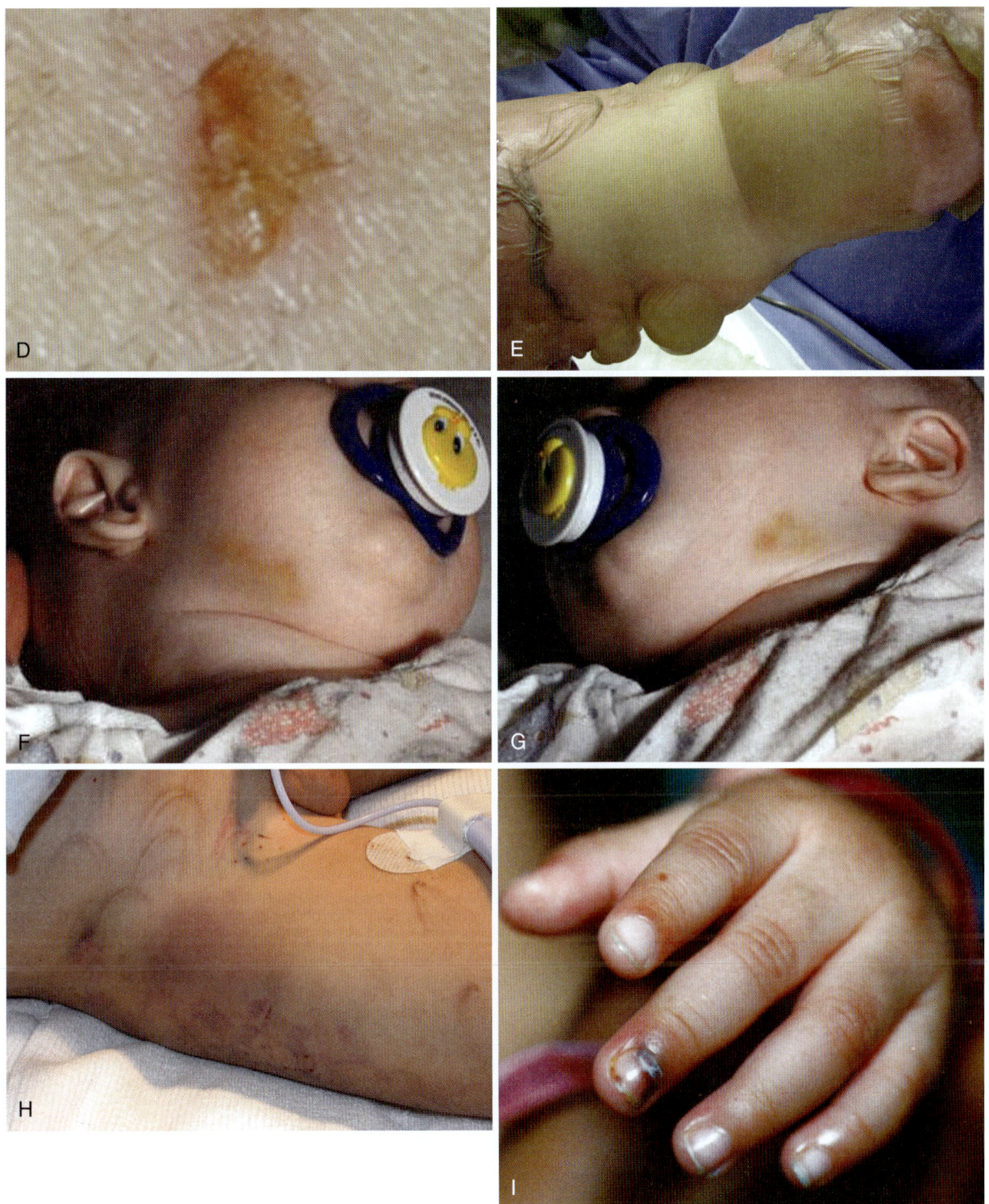

FIGURE 37.2, cont'd D, A cigarette burn. **E**, An immersion burn; notice sparing of the popliteal fossa, which is typical of this type of injury. **F** and **G**, Facial bruises. **H**, Whipping injury from an electrical cord. **I**, Unusual finger injuries in an infant. (Photographs courtesy several child advocates from several institutions who asked to remain anonymous.)

as rapidly as possible.[40] This philosophy of minimizing the time on the scene and emphasizing prompt transport to the closest trauma center is termed *scoop and run*.

In parts of Canada and several European countries, initial resuscitation of injured children is commonly performed by physicians who are charged with evaluating the child at the scene, securing the airway, initiating resuscitative measures to maintain hemodynamic stability, and transporting the child to an appropriate trauma center. Instituting these management procedures may result in additional time on the scene. This approach has been termed *stay and play*. Many aspects of this system are being integrated into existing American trauma systems as part of mass casualty disaster management plans.[41,42] The ideal approach is to minimize time on the scene and initiate resuscitation while enroute to the hospital.[43]

The Israel Air Force was for many years the only actor operating a medical airborne evacuation program for mass casualty events in both civilian and military scenarios. The airborne medical personnel consisted of medical doctors, often anesthesiologists and surgeons, with expertise in trauma and emergency care, as well as paramedics. The need for airborne rescue and evacuation in Israel arose out of the prolonged transport time from the site of injury to the hospital or because the terrain made it difficult to reach and rescue patients by any other route. Often the airborne rescue team arrives at the same time as the second treating team, thus focusing on minimizing interventions on the ground in favor of the scoop and run technique. A search of the Israeli trauma database from 2006 to 2021 identified 146 cases of airborne evacuation of pediatric trauma patients, which fell into three categories: motor vehicle accidents (MVA) 41%, falls 32%, and combat injuries, 10%. Of these evacuations, three died, all from motor vehicle accidents.

Developing a systematic approach to the care of the pediatric trauma patient is crucial. This includes acquiring age- and size-appropriate equipment. Luten and Broselow developed a system that identifies appropriate sized equipment and drug doses based on the child's length.[44–47] This system assigns a specific color based on the child's body length (E-Figs. 37.1A,B). A corresponding color-coded, length-based wristband that designates drug doses, and devices that match the assigned color are placed next to the child; these items can then be obtained from a color-coded compatible supply cart (E-Figs. 37.2A,B and 37.3). This system is designed to minimize delays, medication errors, and equipment errors.

Over the past 2 decades, there have been dramatic advances in the capability of prehospital providers to initiate resuscitation of pediatric trauma patients. Part of this progression has been attributed to developing trauma systems and committed trauma centers to provide more effective medical direction to prehospital providers. Effective management for the continuum of care in trauma patients is optimized if the prehospital personnel communicate the details regarding the child's injuries directly to the responsible hospital-based personnel. This information may include details about the mechanism of injury, traumatic forces involved, time elapsed from the event, loss of consciousness, estimated blood loss, treatment given (e.g., IV access, airway management), and a summary of suspected injuries.

As trauma systems have evolved and emergency departments have become overwhelmed by larger patient volumes, effective triage for the pediatric trauma patient has become increasingly important. Care of traumatically injured children requires the use of personnel and resources from many services, including the operating room and ancillary services such as diagnostic imaging and transfusion medicine.[48] Inappropriate triage may waste precious time and resources and limit access to patients most in need if every patient with traumatic injuries, regardless of their severity, is sent to a trauma center. Conversely, failure to recognize a child who needs the resources of a trauma center may increase morbidity and result in preventable deaths.[49–51]

The Glasgow Coma Scale (GCS) and the modified GCS for children (Table 37.2) are the most common scales used to estimate the severity of neurologic injury. The GCS assigns a total score with a range of 3 to 15 that quantifies eye opening, verbal response, and motor function; a GCS score of 8 or less implies severe neurologic injury and the need for placement of an advanced airway. The pediatric trauma score was developed to facilitate the initial assessment and triage of injured children by categorizing the overall severity of their injuries (Table 37.3). As trauma systems have matured and prehospital providers have become more experienced with assessment and field management, the GCS and pediatric trauma score have emerged as effective tools for determination of the need for direct transfer to a trauma

TABLE 37.2 | Modification of the Glasgow Coma Scale (GCS) for Pediatric Patients

Type of Response	Score*	AGE-RELATED RESPONSES		
		>1 Year	<1 Year	
Eye-opening response	4	Spontaneous	Spontaneous	
	3	To verbal command	To shout	
	2	To pain	To pain	
	1	None	None	
		>1 Year	<1 Year	
Motor response	6	Obeys commands	Spontaneous	
	5	Localizes pain	Localizes pain	
	4	Withdraws to pain	Withdraws to pain	
	3	Abnormal flexion to pain (decorticate)	Abnormal flexion to pain (decorticate)	
	2	Abnormal extension to pain (decorticate)	Abnormal extension to pain (decorticate)	
	1	None	None	
		>5 Years	2–5 Years	0–2 Years
Verbal response	5	Oriented and converses	Appropriate words, phrases	Babbles, coos appropriately
	4	Confused conversation	Inappropriate words	Cries but is consolable
	3	Inappropriate words	Persistent crying or screaming to pain	Persistent crying or screaming to pain
	2	Incomprehensive sounds	Grunts or moans to pain	Grunts or moans to pain
	1	None	None	None

*Total GCS is determined from adding scores for each of the 3 sections together to predict the extent of neurologic injury: severe <9; moderate 9–12; mild 13–15.
Modified from James HE, Trauner DA. The Glasgow Coma Scale. In: James HE, Anas NG, Perkin RM, eds. *Brain Insults in Infants and Children.* Orlando: Grune & Stratton; 1985:179-182.

TABLE 37.3 | The Pediatric Trauma Score (PTS)

Factor	SCORE +2	+1	−1	Totals*
Size (weight)	>20 kg	10–20 kg	<10 kg	
Airway	Patent	Maintainable	Not maintainable	
Systolic blood pressure	>90 mm Hg	50–90 mm Hg	<50 mm Hg	
Central nervous system	Awake	Obtunded or loss of consciousness	Unresponsive	
Open wound	None	Minor	Major or penetrating	
Skeletal trauma	None	Closed fracture	Open or multiple fractures	

*The Pediatric Trauma Score (PTS) is the sum of all 6 categories. Scoring: minor injury, 12 (maximum); severe injury, <7; uniformly fatal, −6 (minimum).

center.[52,53] The Israeli airborne evacuation and rescue team database shows that 61% of pediatric trauma patients were alert (GCS≥13), whereas 21% were severely injured (GCS=3). Almost half (44%) of children with a GCS=3 were 0 to 3 years of age.

PREHOSPITAL AIRWAY MANAGEMENT

Providing effective airway management within the prehospital environment has many challenges including poor access to the child, unavailability of pharmacologic agents, inclement weather, trauma to the face, and demanding environments such as within an ambulance or helicopter. Several studies of adult patients undergoing tracheal intubation in the prehospital setting have reported an increased incidence of difficult tracheal intubation,[54] need for multiple attempts before success,[55] and undiagnosed esophageal intubation. These events have been reported by all levels of providers, including anesthesiologists,[56] although anesthesiologists have more success and fewer complications when performing tracheal intubation compared with other providers.[57–59]

Unsuccessful prehospital airway management in children may be due to a combination of training, experience, equipment, and environmental issues. Unsuccessful prehospital tracheal intubations often result from ineffective operator training and lack of professional experience. Most prehospital providers such as paramedics, receive minimal dedicated training in pediatric airway management, insertion of supraglottic airway devices (SGAs), and tracheal intubation.[60] These providers may not have had an opportunity to either acquire or sufficiently maintain the necessary skills and in the face of an emergency, are unable to successfully intubate. Over time, psychomotor skills for all interventions decay, which likely contributes to the increased complication and failure rates associated with tracheal intubation in children in the prehospital setting.[61]

Guidelines that recommend that instrumentation of the airway be avoided in the prehospital setting yield similar outcomes to those that recommend intubating the trachea for pediatric trauma patients.[62] For example, the American Heart Association PALS guidelines state, "Bag-mask ventilation can be as effective as ventilation through an endotracheal tube for short periods and may be safer."[63] The 2010 PALS guidelines state, *"In the prehospital setting, ventilate and oxygenate infants and children with a bag-mask device, especially if transport time is short."*[63] Furthermore, the 2015 PALS guidelines state, *"The likelihood of successful endotracheal tube placement with minimal complications is related to the length of training and supervised experience in the operating room and in the field."* [64] However, if tracheal intubation is performed, we strongly recommend that a carbon dioxide detector is used to confirm tracheal placement. The current PALS guidelines state, *"When available,*

exhaled CO$_2$ detection (capnography or colorimetry) is recommended as confirmation of tracheal tube position" (E-Fig. 37.4) (It should be noted that if a colorimetric device is used it must be of appropriate size as too large a device may not detect CO$_2$ even when the tracheal tube is correctly positioned, e.g., pediatric for 1–15 kg and adult for >15 kg.) As a result, many emergency medical services agencies have developed policies based on a scoop and run philosophy for pediatric trauma patients that avoid definitive airway management if the transport time is brief and bag-mask ventilation is effective. Several investigators have also questioned whether prehospital tracheal intubation is the best approach in children who require positive-pressure ventilation. The infrequent need for tracheal intubation in pediatric trauma patients has created obstacles for members of the emergency medical teams to maintain their skills. Mortality rates are greater and neurologic outcomes worse for adult patients who received prehospital tracheal intubation compared with those who received standard bag-mask ventilation.[65,66] Several studies that focused on children also reported increased complication rates associated with prehospital tracheal intubation,[67–70] particularly in infants.[62] A meta-analysis of 17 studies involving 8772 pediatric patients reported a failed intubation rate that ranged from 0.4% to 52.6%, which overall was 3.5 times more likely than in adults; esophageal intubation ranged from 0.9% to 8%.[71] An analysis of the Cardiac Arrest Registry to Enhance Survival (CARES) examined 1724 out-of-hospital cardiac arrests and found that bag-valve-mask ventilation was associated with greater survival to discharge compared with either tracheal intubation or placement of a supraglottic device[72]; a systematic review reported similar statistics.[73]

Despite these reports, there is a trend toward using alternative airway devices in the field in both adult and pediatric trauma patients. Among the devices that have found support, SGAs have proved the easiest to use with high reliability in the field. Although these devices do not protect the airway from gastric regurgitation and pulmonary aspiration, they may provide adequate oxygenation and ventilation during transport particularly if traditional bag-mask ventilation is inadequate. One meta-analysis of prehospital alternative airway devices in adults and children indicated that SGAs were very successful in the hands of anesthesiologists and nonphysician flight crews (success rate of 96%) and slightly less successful in the hands of nonphysician clinicians (83%).[74] However, there is no evidence for an SGA in pediatric trauma unless it is used as a rescue device. There are many variations of SGAs available, but the ProSeal (Teleflex Medical Inc., Research Triangle Park, NC) offers the added advantage of greater sealing pressure while providing access to suction the stomach over other devices.[75]

The Israeli airborne evacuation and rescue team database showed that two-thirds of pediatric trauma patients required some sort of airway or breathing intervention to maintain SpO_2 above 90%, mostly supplemental oxygen by an oxygen mask during transport. However, nearly a quarter (23%) required ventilation; a minority were managed by bag-mask ventilation with 20% requiring tracheal intubation. Rarely was there a clinical need to treat pneumothorax during transport by placing a chest tube with drainage (5%). Needle placement for immediate release of a tension pneumothorax before placing a chest drain was performed in half of the patients needing such interventions.

Emergency Department Evaluation and Management of the Pediatric Trauma Patient

IN-HOSPITAL TRIAGE

In an ideal scenario, before a trauma patient arrives at the emergency department, their imminent arrival is announced and basic information such as the mechanism of injury, age and weight of the child, and current status are provided. This allows time for suitable staff to gather and for age- and size- appropriate equipment to be organized. In addition, the doses of resuscitation medications, analgesics, and fluids can be calculated and prepared in a calm environment to minimize the risk of errors.

The number of staff that attends a pediatric trauma call depends on the hospital and the availability of staff. As a minimum, a physician from the emergency department, an anesthesiologist, a pediatric or trauma surgeon, a pediatrician, and pediatric nurses from the emergency department should meet the patient. Other members of the team may be required depending upon the mechanism or severity of trauma (e.g., neurosurgery, cardiac surgery, and intensive care).[76] Roles for each member of staff should be assigned and one member should be designated team leader to provide oversight and coordinate the treatment plan.

Once the child arrives, they should be taken to the trauma bay and a primary survey completed (Table 37.4). Depending on the status of the child, severity of the injury and age of the child, having the parent accompany the child during the initial assessment may be challenging. Obviously in a severe head trauma that requires immediate ventilation, the appropriate place for the parent is not holding or physically comforting their child. But in the case of less serious traumas, the initial assessment can include the parent to keep their child calm in such a stressful environment and provide a history of medical conditions and the trauma event.

According to advanced trauma life support algorithms, the primary survey starts with an assessment of airway, breathing, and circulation with immediate interventions taken if required.[77]

TABLE 37.4	The Advanced Trauma Life Support Primary Survey Management Priorities
Priority Level	**Management**
Highest	Airway and cervical spine immobilization
	Breathing and ventilation
	Circulation and hemorrhage control
	Disability and neurologic status
Lowest	Exposure and environmental

With a large team to treat the child, initial monitoring and assessment can be conducted simultaneously. For example, the airway can be assessed while the anesthesiologist provides oxygen and a nurse applies monitors: an oximeter probe, ECG electrodes, and a blood pressure cuff. Two large-bore IV lines should be sited that are appropriate for the child's age. After two failed attempts including femoral access, intraosseous access should be established (see also Chapter 49).[78] When a cannula is placed, blood should be drawn for laboratory testing and cross matching. Concurrently, a surgeon conducts a formal primary survey to assess injuries.

One must remember to ensure the child has adequate analgesia while assessing the injuries. This will aid in smoother ventilation and in assessment of their injuries.[79] After completion of the primary survey (**A**irway, **B**reathing, **C**irculation), interventions and initial resuscitation can then be performed and appropriate imaging organized.

INITIAL MANAGEMENT

After the primary survey, key information is obtained to facilitate appropriate treatment strategies. Initial management of trauma depends on the severity of the injuries and which vital organs have been involved. Is the child in shock? What type and degree of shock? What is the mechanism of the injury and what structures are suspected of being injured? What imaging needs to be performed? Fig. 37.3 presents an algorithm for prioritizing management goals.

AIRWAY MANAGEMENT

Emergency management of a child's airway is challenging on many levels. Distressed children who are experiencing pain or anxiety from unusual surroundings, or separation from their parents can make pre-oxygenation very difficult. In addition, the injury may compromise ventilation and gas exchange causing hypoxia; trauma increases the metabolic rate above an already increased oxygen demand compared with adults, leading to rapid arterial oxygen desaturation.[80]

To adequately provide oxygen to combative children, some advocate a "delayed sequence induction" technique be used. This permits a dose of IV ketamine (0.5–1 mg/kg) to be given before a rapid sequence intubation (RSI), allowing adequate oxygenation with a tight-fitting oxygen mask.[81] Smaller children might not be able to tolerate the 45 seconds of apnea that is required for a neuromuscular blocking drug to work,[82–84] so gentle assisted ventilation may be needed in these children to maintain low peak inspiratory pressures until intubation to avoid desaturation, while remaining cognizant of the potential risk of aspiration.[85] Oral cuffed tracheal tubes as opposed to noncuffed tubes are preferred as they provide protection from aspiration and a better seal to optimize ventilation (Table 37.5).

Intubation in the setting of trauma requires manual in-line stabilization of the head and cervical spine, which can make the procedure much more difficult (Figs. 37.4 and 37.5).[86] This usually requires four individuals: (1) one to stabilize the neck, (2) one to perform cricoid pressure if indicated, (3) one to administer medications, and (4) one to perform tracheal intubation. Although video laryngoscopy can be valuable in some circumstances, blood or debris in the mouth might obscure the camera (importantly, if blood or other liquid soils the camera lens, it cannot be cleaned without autoclaving it). In these circumstances, intubation may be more challenging.[87] A backup plan including an SGA and an alternative plan to secure the airway should be delineated before beginning to secure the airway.

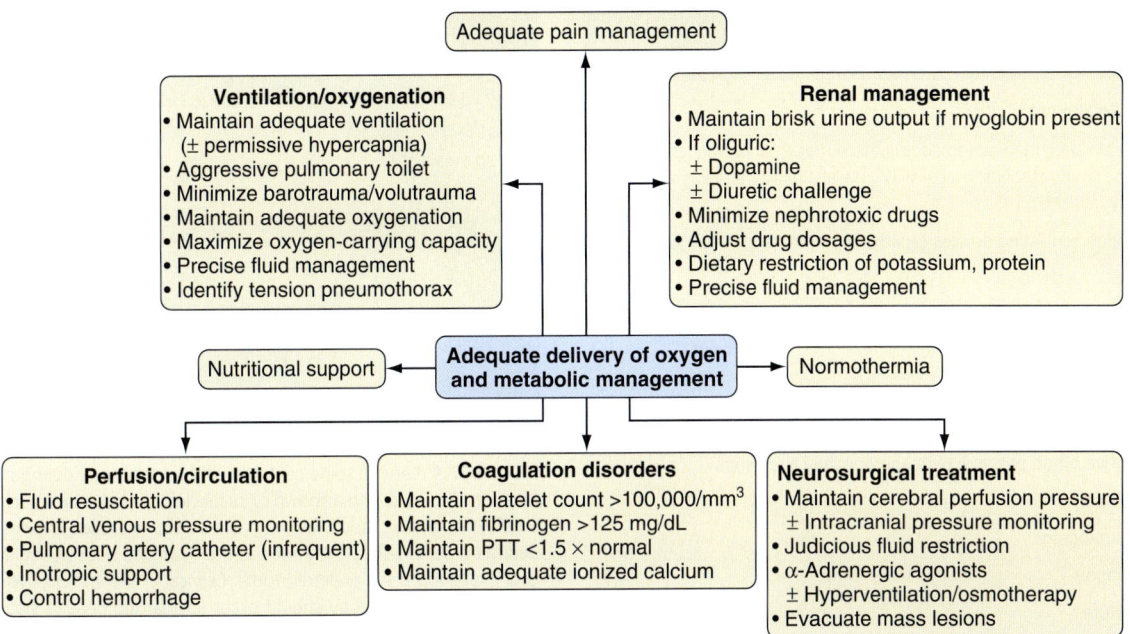

FIGURE 37.3 Diagram of the management priorities for pediatric trauma patients. The primary goals are delivery of oxygen, appropriate ventilation, perfusion to vital organs, maintenance of normothermia to mild hypothermia, stability of renal and neurologic function, correction of coagulopathies, avoidance of overhydration, and meticulous management of metabolic demands. *PPT,* Partial thromboplastin time. (Modified from Todres ID, Fugate JH, eds. *Critical Care of Infants and Children.* Boston: Little, Brown; 1996:17.)

A fluid bolus should be administered before inducing anesthesia to prevent hypotension. If the patient is actively bleeding, then depending on the extent of the blood loss, one should consider blood products instead of crystalloids to prevent a dilutional coagulopathy.

The selection of induction agents varies among practitioners, but the choices are generally based on hemodynamic indices and cardiac stability. Provided a sensible regimen is selected, and the whole clinical picture of the child's organ functions are considered, then most induction agents are acceptable. Regimens such as of fentanyl 1 µg/kg, ketamine 1 to 2 mg/kg and rocuronium 1.2 mg/kg are usually appropriate.[88] Table 37.6 illustrates a list of potential drugs and doses commonly used when performing a rapid sequence induction to control the airway. An algorithm for airway management of children without traumatic brain injury is presented in Fig. 37.6.

After tracheal intubation, an appropriate C-spine collar can be placed. It is no longer advised to place a hard neck brace (e.g., Philadelphia collar) on a child when they are awake/distressed after being injured and before the airway is secured. A distressed child could wriggle and thrash about in an ill-fitting collar and it could do more harm than good by placing one.[89,90]

HEAD TRAUMA

Head injury is the most common cause of traumatic death in children.[91] Although the principles of managing head injuries in children with polytrauma are, for the most part, similar to those in adults, there are several noteworthy differences. In contrast to adults, intracranial bleeding can lead to hypovolemic shock in neonates and infants because the head is proportionally larger and comprises a greater fraction of the total body weight. Furthermore,

the vessel-rich organs receive a substantially greater fraction of the cardiac output. The open fontanelles in neonates and infants may provide a potential space for a proportionately larger amount of blood to accumulate that can be monitored by palpation. However, the open fontanelles provide minimal additional protection against increases in ICP because the dura mater is relatively noncompliant.

The main target when managing neurological trauma is the prevention of a secondary brain insult and patients often require intubation for control of ventilation and rapid CT imaging. One must have strict physiological control to prevent hypoxia, hypercarbia, hyperthermia, and hypoglycemia. Sedation reduces cerebral metabolism and therefore its metabolic demand. Patients should have their heads elevated ~30 degrees to help promote cerebral venous drainage. Mannitol or 3% hypertonic saline should be given to patients with severe head injury to reduce ICP and prevent brain herniation. The challenge in complex multitrauma patients is to find the balance between appropriate permissive hypotension to limit ongoing abdominal hemorrhage and blood pressure support to maintain sufficient cerebral perfusion pressure.[92] If a child has sustained both head and significant abdominal injuries that require a laparotomy, then ICP monitoring can help guide hemodynamics. Fig. 37.7 presents a proposed algorithm to manage the airway in this subpopulation of trauma patients.

CHEST TRAUMA

There are a large number of structures potentially injured after thoracic trauma, and their management ranges from treating them immediately to conservative management in intensive care.[93] Table 37.7 illustrates the types of potential injuries, what needs to be treated, and the urgencies to treat.

TABLE 37.5	Recommended Equipment for Resuscitation of a Pediatric Trauma Patient

Airway Equipment

Appropriate sizes (neonate to adult) of face masks, endotracheal tubes, stylets, laryngoscopes, oral airways, nasal airways, and supraglottic airway devices

Self-inflating ventilating devices capable of administering >90% oxygen

Anesthesia machine

Difficult airway equipment in appropriate sizes including fiberoptic bronchoscopes, video laryngoscopes, and cricothyrotomy kits

Suction

Monitoring Equipment

Noninvasive blood pressure with appropriately sized cuffs

Pulse oximetry

Electrocardiogram

Capnography

Temperature

Transducers and monitors for direct arterial and central venous pressures

Surgical Instruments

Tracheostomy tray

Thoracotomy, laparotomy, craniotomy trays

Vascular tray

Resuscitation (Code) Cart Immediately Available

Vascular Access Equipment

Intravenous catheters and tubing prepared to administer crystalloids and blood products

Bedside ultrasound device

Intraosseous devices

Medications

Anesthetic drugs

Vasoactive drugs

Other Equipment and Adjuncts

Universal precautions equipment (e.g., gloves, masks, eye protection)

Infusion pumps and pressure bags

External warming devices

Blood-warming devices

Cognitive aids and treatment algorithms

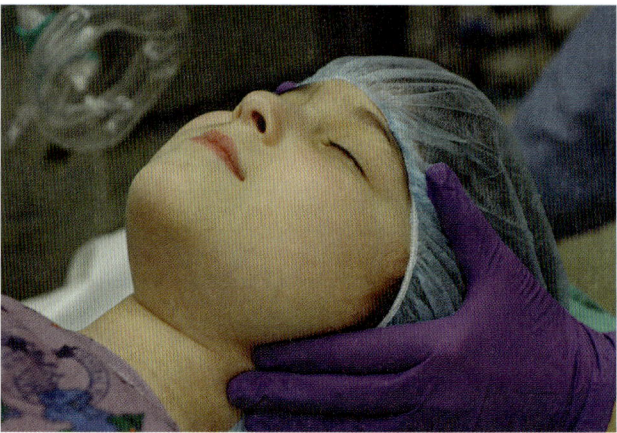

FIGURE 37.4 Cervical spine control must be maintained during tracheal intubation. The child with a known or suspected cervical spine injury requiring a definitive airway should be intubated under controlled circumstances. A dedicated person should immobilize the head and neck during intubation. Oral intubation is the preferred route. Cervical in-line immobilization before attempts at laryngoscopy should occur so that the head is stabilized and prevented from rotating side to side and into flexion or extension.

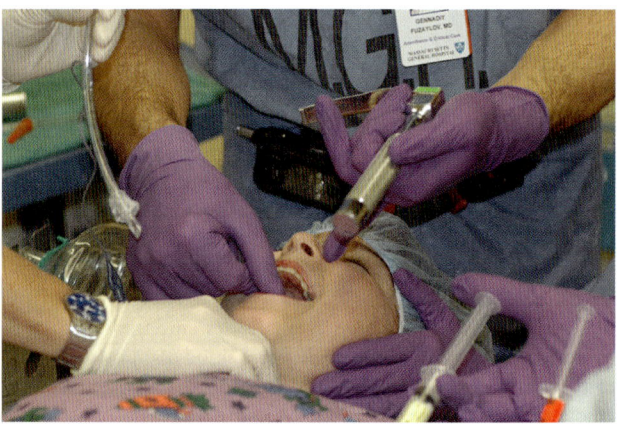

FIGURE 37.5 Intubation of a child with a cervical fracture may require up to four individuals: one person to provide in-line immobilization, a second person to perform tracheal intubation, a third person to perform cricoid pressure, hold the endotracheal tube, and perhaps retract the cheek, and a fourth person to administer the medications.

Lung contusions are very common in children who undergo thoracic trauma, estimated at 35% to 100%. Most, if not all, will need some ventilatory support in the form of supplemental oxygen, continuous positive airway pressure (CPAP), or invasive ventilation; ~30% of pediatric chest trauma patients require mechanical ventilation.[94]

Ventilation strategies for children with acute lung injury are similar to adults with an analogous injury. Commonly, peak inspiratory pressure is limited to ~28 cm H_2O, tidal volume 5 to 8 mL/kg, and positive end-expiratory pressure (PEEP) 10 to 15 cm H_2O titrated according to oxygenation and hemodynamic responses. Severity of lung injury tends to be measured against the maximum oxygen saturation achievable.[95,96]

Pneumothoraces and hemothoraces identified on chest radiograph should be drained if seen, or after a bedside focused abdominal sonography for trauma (**FAST**) scan.[97,98] An output of 25% of the total blood volume via chest drain warrants urgent thoracotomy.[99] If there is a large air leak despite adequate chest drains, then one should suspect tracheobronchial injury. In cases such as these, the tracheal tube can be advanced past the lesion emergently to allow ventilation while occluding the tear.[100] In cases of bronchial avulsion, a chest drain is urgently required along with immediate surgery, possibly with extracorporeal membrane oxygenation (ECMO) support. If a bronchial or tracheal

TABLE 37.6 Medications, Dosages, Advantages, and Disadvantages of Common Medications Used to Perform a Rapid Sequence Induction (RSI) in Pediatric Trauma Patients

Medication	Intravenous Dose (mg/kg)	Advantages	Disadvantages
Atropine	0.01–0.02	Attenuates vagal response	Flushed skin, tachycardia, mild hyperpyrexia; possible sedation/agitation
Glycopyrrolate	0.01	Attenuates vagal response and antisialagogue; lacks sedation/agitation	Longer acting than atropine
Lidocaine	1–1.5	Attenuates hemodynamic and intracranial responses to airway management	Can cause toxicity in large doses (e.g., >5 mg/kg)
Fentanyl	0.001–0.003	Analgesic and attenuates hemodynamic and intracranial responses to airway management	Can cause bradycardia, glottic and chest wall rigidity
Midazolam	0.05–0.2	Sedation, amnesia, anxiolysis, increases seizure threshold, minimal respiratory depression	May cause hypotension when combined with opioids in hypovolemic patients; rarely may cause paradoxical agitation
Ketamine	1–2	Sympathomimetic, used when hypovolemia is suspected, bronchodilation	Increases oral secretions (administer with atropine or glycopyrrolate to reduce secretions), may increase intracranial pressure if $PaCO_2$ is uncontrolled, hypotension possible if catecholamine depleted, causes nystagmus
Propofol	1–3	Sedative-hypnotic, some neuroprotective properties, antiemetic, lower ICP	May cause hypotension especially if hypovolemia present, painful on injection
Etomidate	0.2.–0.3	Hemodynamic stability; useful in patients with hypovolemia or cardiac instability	Possible adrenal suppression; painful on injection
Rocuronium	0.6–1.2	Rapid onset/long duration (with high doses), vagolytic properties; is an acceptable substitute for succinylcholine	Intermediate to long duration depending on dose
Succinylcholine	1–2 (precede with atropine or glyco-pyrrolate)	Rapid onset and ultra-short duration	May rarely cause bradycardia; may cause hyperkalemia, malignant hyperthermia, and rhabdomyolysis in susceptible children (muscular dystrophy, crush injury, prolonged immobilization, burns, intraabdominal sepsis, and upper and lower motor neuron lesions); may increase intracranial, intraocular, intragastric pressures
Sugammadex	2–16 2 4 16	Dosing for reversal of rocuronium or vecuronium: At least 2 twitches present with train of four (TOF) At least 1–2 posttetanic counts (PTC) but no twitches to TOF No twitches including posttetanic are present; reversal of neuromuscular blockade quickly, (approximately 3 minutes) after administration of 1.2 mg/kg of rocuronium	Most commonly reported adverse reactions include nausea, vomiting, headache; bradycardia, anaphylaxis, and increases in coagulopathy parameters have all been reported; not indicated for use in patients with severe renal failure

tear is suspected, the presence of subcutaneous air (crepitus) or a pneumothorax or pneumomediastinum, paralytics should be avoided until the airway is secured as positive-pressure ventilation could precipitate a tension pneumothorax or pneumomediastinum. Spontaneous ventilation should be maintained until a chest tube has been confirmed.

Hemodynamic collapse in the emergency department requires tracheal intubation, bilateral thoracostomies, blood resuscitation, and a FAST scan to rule out cardiac tamponade. Performing an emergency department thoracotomy carries a very high mortality rate. Penetrating cardiac injuries in children carry >70% mortality and survival of an emergency department thoracotomy ranges from 0% to 26%.[101] Blunt thoracic injury patients who arrive in the emergency department with no signs of life have almost zero chance of surviving a thoracotomy and it should probably be avoided. Although children do have a better chance of surviving an emergency department thoracotomy due to thoracic injury compared with adults, this does not always translate to better neurological outcomes.[102]

ABDOMINAL TRAUMA

About 25% of pediatric major trauma patients have an abdominal injury; it is the most common cause of unrecognized fatal injury in children. Abdominal trauma is the third leading cause of death in this population, after head and thoracic injuries. Pediatric abdominal trauma is typically blunt in nature with the spleen being the most common organ injured; nonoperative management is employed in over 95% of patients.[103–105] Advances in interventional radiology and the ability to catheterize small vessels warrants its consideration in pediatric trauma. In cases of liver, splenic, and renal injury, with a contrast blush on the CT indicating active bleeding,[106–108] embolization may avoid the need for surgery in cases of a falling hemoglobin, ongoing vasopressor support, and persistent tachycardia.

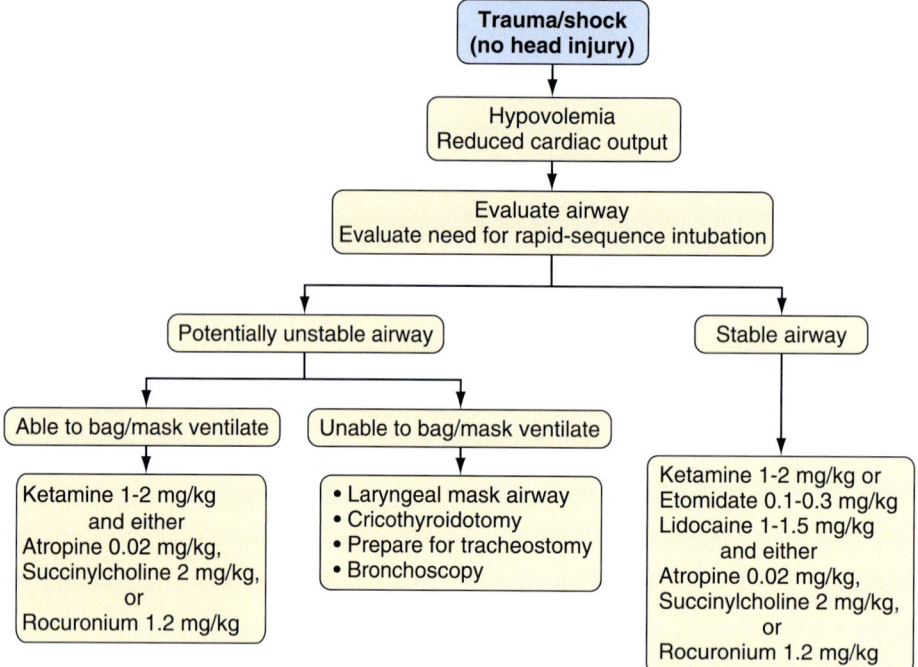

FIGURE 37.6 A proposed algorithm for airway management in children with traumatic injuries but without traumatic brain injury. The selection of medications and airway management techniques should be individualized to each patient. (Modified from Todres ID, Fugate JH, eds. *Critical Care of Infants and Children.* Boston: Little, Brown; 1996:36.)

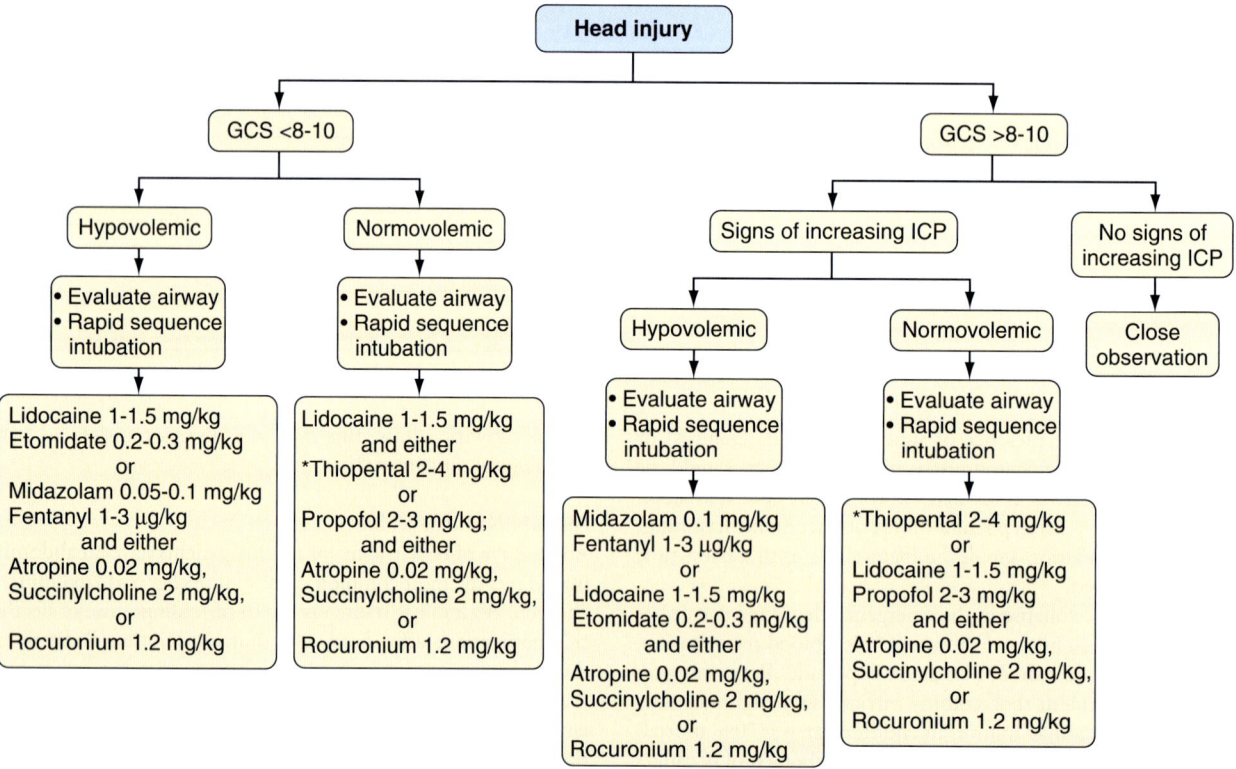

FIGURE 37.7 A proposed algorithm for airway management in children with traumatic injuries including known or suspected traumatic brain injury (TBI). The selection of medications and airway management techniques should be individualized to each patient. *GCS,* Glasgow Coma Scale score; *ICP,* intracranial pressure. *Thiopental is no longer available in the United States. (Modified from Todres ID, Fugate JH, eds. *Critical Care of Infants and Children.* Boston: Little, Brown; 1996:36.)

TABLE 37.7	Chest Trauma[93]	
Life-threatening Events	Potentially Life-threating Events	Non–life-threatening Events
Tension pneumothorax	Pulmonary contusion	Rib fractures
Open pneumothorax	Diaphragmatic hernia	Simple pneumothorax
Massive hemothorax	Myocardial contusion	Simple hemothorax
Flail chest	Esophageal rupture	Chest wall contusion
Cardiac tamponade	Trachea-bronchial injuries	

TABLE 37.8	Abdominal Trauma: Indications for Emergency Laparotomy in Children
Evisceration of intraperitoneal contents
Hemodynamic instability despite maximal resuscitative efforts (transfusion of greater than 50% of total blood volume)
Gunshot wound to the abdomen or other penetrating traumas
Free intraperitoneal air
Development of peritonitis post injury

Splenectomy should be avoided if possible, and splenic preservation (at least partial) should be attempted. Full splenectomy introduces the risk of postsplenectomy sepsis, which carries a high mortality rate. These patients should receive immunization against *Streptococcus pneumoniae*, *Haemophilus influenzae*, and *Neisseria meningitidis*, and may require ongoing antibiotic prophylaxis.[109]

Liver injuries are one of the most frequent life-threatening injuries in trauma patients. Nonetheless, as with other intraabdominal solid organ injuries, nonoperative management is considered optimal in most pediatric patients with liver injuries[110,111]; however, duodenal perforation and abdominal vascular injuries are treated operatively.[112] Despite advances in both diagnostic and therapeutic technologies, because of their devastating nature, abdominal vascular injuries remain a major source of morbidity and mortality among trauma patients.[105]

The biggest risk of nonoperative management in penetrating trauma is a missed abdominal injury, especially a hollow viscus perforation. However, mortality rates with missed hollow viscus perforation have not increased in patients without peritonitis on admission.[111]

Patients with moderate to severe traumatic brain injuries and spinal cord injuries combined with abdominal injuries are managed differently, requiring greater perfusion pressures than is otherwise advisable in trauma management. This is necessary to maintain adequate cerebral perfusion pressure to reduce the subsequent burden of disability and mortality. For example, penetrating liver injuries will hemorrhage more with an increased perfusion pressure; it is generally considered safer to manage this injury surgically in the setting of an associated traumatic brain injury.[111] The indications for emergency laparotomy are listed in Table 37.8.[103]

In pediatric patients, hemodynamic stability is considered a systolic blood pressure of 70 mm Hg plus twice the child's age in years (70 + [2 × age in years]). An acceptable hemodynamic status in children is considered a positive response to fluid resuscitation after 2 boluses of 20 mL/kg of crystalloid replacement before initiating blood replacement. The response should be a decrease in heart rate, cleared sensorium, return of peripheral pulses, normal skin color, increase in blood pressure and urinary output, and an increase in warmth of the skin in the extremities.[109–111] If there is a negative response, urgent blood transfusion is indicated.

BLOOD RESUSCITATION

When simultaneously stabilizing a child's airway and establishing adequate ventilation, the patient might require immediate blood resuscitation if there has been extensive bleeding. Based on their physiology, children often do not become hypotensive until ~40% or more of their total blood volume has been lost. Subtle signs such as increased respiratory rate, tachycardia, and delayed capillary refill are useful metrics of impending hypovolemia during the initial assessment.[113]

Blood volume also varies greatly by age and/or weight in childhood, as do physiological baseline values for heart rate, respiratory rate, and blood pressure. For example, 150-mL blood loss in a 6-month-old weighing 8 kilograms is >20% of their circulating blood volume, whereas the same volume blood loss in a 20-kilogram 4-year-old is approximately 10% of their blood volume.

If blood is required immediately (before cross matching) because of massive rapid hemorrhage, then O negative should be given at a dose of 10 to 20 mL/kg. If there is time, then blood should be cross matched. Blood replacement therapy largely follows adult massive transfusion protocols with a 1:1:1 ratio of packed red blood cells, fresh frozen plasma, and platelets. If there is a need for ongoing transfusion after the initial first round of blood products, then viscoelastic hemostatic assays and concurrent clinical judgment guide further blood product management.[114] It is vital to ensure normothermia, prevent acidosis, and treat hypocalcemia that may develop from citrate in fresh frozen plasma to ensure a coagulable state and maintain blood pressure.[115,116] Calcium chloride 10% (20 mg/kg) or calcium gluconate 10% (60 mg/kg) to treat an ionized calcium <1.0 mmol/L is appropriate. Antifibrinolytics such as tranexamic acid or epsilon aminocaproic acid are also useful and safe to be given to trauma patients to help achieve hemostasis (see Chapter 18) It is possible in the near future that noninvasive continuous cardiac output assessments will provide immediate feedback regarding the adequacy of volume resuscitation and/or the need to supplement with inotropic agents.[117]

Intraoperative Management of The Pediatric Trauma Patient

PREOPERATIVE EVALUATION

Advances in health care have produced an increased patient population with preinjury comorbid conditions. For example, children with repaired congenital heart disease may be victims of a traumatic injury. It is common for an acutely injured child to have a preexisting diagnosis of a medical condition such as asthma, developmental delay, seizure disorder, obesity, or psychosocial issues exacerbated by an unstable home environment. Each of these issues must be carefully considered when planning appropriate anesthesia management.

Emergency surgery can be a large source of fear and anxiety for children and their parents.[118] The suddenness of the event provides little time for the child and family to adjust to the crisis and

TABLE 37.9	Suggested Focus Items During the Preoperative Evaluation of the Pediatric Trauma Patient
Vital signs	
Airway/cervical spine evaluation	
Planned surgical procedure(s)	
List of known injuries	
Management since arrival	
Relevant laboratory/imaging results	
Past medical/surgical history/family history	
Allergies/current medications	
Fasting time	

often limits the time the anesthesiologist has to develop rapport with the child and parents. A calm and reassuring anesthesiologist is of great benefit to all parties.

If the child's condition permits, the preoperative evaluation should include a complete assessment. Vital signs should be stable and appropriate for age. Sensorium, urine output, capillary refill, and vital signs can be used to evaluate and estimate the child's preoperative volume status. A comprehensive airway examination should be completed, including assessment of the cervical spine. Past medical and surgical histories, medications, and allergies are recorded when feasible. A list of known injuries and interventions taken should be acquired before entering the operating room. Special attention to fluid management helps to estimate preoperative volume status and assist with intraoperative fluid administration. Assessment should include review of available laboratory reports such as hemoglobin, electrolytes, coagulation studies, and arterial blood gas results. Results from diagnostic imaging studies, including plain radiographs and CT scans, should also be obtained. The suggested items for emphasis during the preoperative evaluation of the pediatric trauma patient appear in Table 37.9.

Evidence suggests that the gastric residual volume in children undergoing emergency surgery is greater than in those undergoing elective surgery.[119,120] There is also evidence to suggest that in emergency cases, the size of the gastric residual volume (measured in milliliters per kilograms) depends in part, on the time interval between the last food ingestion and the injury, (i.e., the longer the time from ingestion to injury, the less the gastric residual volume).[120] The probability that gastric emptying is further delayed and the risk that residual solids are present in the stomach is exacerbated if opioid analgesics are administered to treat pain. There is some reassurance in these numbers, but the anesthesiologist should consider acutely injured children to have full stomachs and take appropriate measures to reduce the risk of pulmonary aspiration of gastric contents.[121–124] In those who likely have food in their stomach and are old enough, a regional block is an alternative. Otherwise, an RSI is mandatory and a laryngeal mask airway (LMA) is contraindicated.

Premedication before emergency procedures is administered when indicated by the intravenous route. Benzodiazepines, such as midazolam, may help to reduce preoperative anxiety. If pain is present, opioids may be beneficial for children who are hemodynamically stable and have no airway compromise. Other than ketamine, anesthetics rarely cause profuse secretions, and the use of an antisialogogue before induction should be reserved for specific indications.

INTRAOPERATIVE MANAGEMENT OF BRAIN INJURY

The anesthesiologist who manages the patient with head trauma must be familiar with the patient history, the mechanism of injury, and the indication for surgery. Intraoperatively, the anesthesiologist must maintain and adjust the care of the patient to optimize cerebral perfusion pressure (CPP).[125]

Care must be provided with the head in the neutral position, so as not to obstruct venous return. If there is a neck collar, it is usually removed before induction of anesthesia. Before surgery (but usually after induction) the anesthesiologist must secure adequate vascular access: two to three large-bore peripheral IVs, an arterial line, and possibly, a central line. Many anesthesiologists prefer a femoral line to use as a central line since the patient might require a neck collar. In addition, a central venous catheter to the internal jugular vein could limit cerebral venous drainage and a complication such as hematoma could compound this problem.

The anesthesiologist should be ready to treat acute increases in ICP.[92,126] Mannitol or hypertonic saline 3% should be administered as indicated to reduce ICP. In cases where there is an external ventricular device, cerebrospinal fluid (CSF) can be drained to reduce the ICP, and the patient should be placed with 30 degrees head up position.[127] A brief period of hyperventilation (to 30–35 mm Hg) to reduce cerebral blood flow will temporarily decrease ICP before the surgical intervention has begun, although cerebral perfusion may be compromised by concomitant vasoconstriction. Hypotension must be diligently avoided, and adequate fluid volume, but rarely vasopressors, should be administered to allow an appropriate cerebral perfusion pressure (see Chapter 24). Adrenergic and dopaminergic receptors are present in the cerebral vasculature, leading clinicians to consider vasopressors such as phenylephrine, dopamine, or ephedrine to treat hypotension. In the only study of the effects of phenylephrine, dopamine, or norepinephrine (3-hour infusions) in children after moderate to severe traumatic brain injuries, norepinephrine infusion increased cerebral perfusion pressure and reduced ICP compared with the other two pressors.[128] In a cross-over study in adults anesthetized with total intravenous anesthesia (TIVA), both phenylephrine and ephedrine increased blood pressure, although only phenylephrine decreased cardiac output and cerebral tissue oxygen saturation.[129] Ephedrine maintained both indices unchanged. The authors concluded that in adults without traumatic brain injury, phenylephrine is inferior to ephedrine to correct hypotensive adults. Comparable studies in children have not been forthcoming.

The operating room must be kept warm, and the anesthesiologist should use warming devices to prevent hypothermia, which would worsen possible coagulopathy. Hyperthermia must also be avoided as it increases cerebral metabolic demand.

Surgery to treat traumatic brain injuries, such as decompressive craniotomy or evacuation of hematomas, might be complicated with venous air emboli, especially if the patient is in reverse Trendelenburg position. Early recognition and treatment of venous air emboli is crucial. With the opening of the skull and dura, the tamponade effect might be lost. Often, bleeding occurs with an associated decrease in blood pressure. In preparation, blood should be readily available, as should vasoactive drugs. In the case of massive bleeding, blood products should be given early to prevent and treat coagulopathy. There should be frequent monitoring of the patient including urine output and assessments of glucose, hematocrit, electrolytes, and blood gas as indicated. If bleeding persists, then thromboelastogram (TEG)/ rotational thromboestastometry (ROTEM) can help guide management.

INTRAOPERATIVE MANAGEMENT OF CHEST TRAUMA

Intraoperative management of chest trauma can often be challenging, with the anesthesiologist having to balance sedation and analgesia against hemodynamic collapse from the patient's injuries. In extreme situations, management starts in the emergency room or even prehospital, but the same principles still apply. All major chest trauma patients invariably need large-bore IV access, an arterial line, central venous access, a urinary catheter, a temperature probe, an oral/nasal gastric tube, and a tracheal tube.

One of the key points in treating chest trauma is timing; a delay in placing invasive lines in a hemodynamically compromised patient is not warranted. Compromised children make cannulation difficult and arterial lines can be even more challenging. Each case must be evaluated individually, with decisions made before induction of anesthesia:

- What vascular access and monitoring should be placed before induction?
- What vascular access should be placed after induction but before surgery?
- What vascular access can be placed once surgery has started?

It should be remembered that these situations are dynamic, and these patients can often destabilize after induction. Surgery might need to commence immediately. Central access might be necessary but should not delay surgery and it should be remembered that resuscitation fluids can be given more rapidly through large-bore peripheral IVs than through standard central vein access catheters.

Most chest traumas will need blood and blood products in large quantities during their surgery so the operating room should be equipped with appropriate fluid warmers and rapid infusion devices. It is advisable to warm the operating room and immediately initiate actively warming the patient. Hypothermia is a common comorbidity in trauma, especially emergency procedures; hypothermia may exacerbate a patient's coagulopathy.

Pneumothorax/hemothorax, cardiac tamponade and tracheobronchial injuries must all be considered and assessed. A pneumothorax will need to be drained, but it is unnecessary to drain it before securing the airway, unless the child is showing hemodynamic compromise due to a tension pneumothorax. One should be prepared for a needle thoracostomy after induction in case the pneumothorax has evolved into a tension pneumothorax.[79]

Known cardiac tamponade seen on a focused abdominal sonography for trauma scan will require an emergency sternotomy/thoracotomy to repair. If the patient is not in severe shock when assessed in the emergency room, then it is best to induce anesthesia in the operating room. Typically, these patients are very easily compromised and can collapse after induction due to the increase in intrathoracic pressure from positive-pressure ventilation, which will decrease venous return. This in turn further decreases cardiac output and can lead to cardiac arrest. It is suggested that such patients should be prepared and draped while awake on the operating table before induction of anesthesia begins; this will shorten the time to open the chest and drain the tamponade to allow resumption of efficient cardiac output. While this is possible in the adolescent, this technique is near impossible for younger children with penetrating chest injuries. Ketamine is the preferred induction and maintenance agent for these procedures to prevent hypotension from occurring. In a tamponade state, the child cannot increase cardiac output in response to hypotension. Communication between the surgical and anesthesia teams

is critical to develop a plan and make decisions about where and what should happen and in which order.

Patients with tracheobronchial injuries can be very difficult to ventilate. Suspicion for such injuries should arise when there remains a significant pneumothorax despite adequate drainage with suction. The treatment for such an injury in children depends on the specific level of injury to the tracheobronchial tree. Tracheal injuries require the tracheal tube to be advanced past the level of the injury and can often be treated conservatively, whereas more extreme injuries such as an avulsion of the bronchus will require a surgical intervention to restore the integrity of the airway. One should try to advance the tracheal tube past the lesion with use of a fiberoptic scope, to avoid ventilating the pleural chest cavity/chest drains.[130,131]

INTRAOPERATIVE MANAGEMENT OF ABDOMINAL INJURY

In pediatric patients, nonoperative management should be considered the optimal management approach. The decision to proceed with surgery should be made by a multidisciplinary team and be based on the physiology of the patient, the anatomy of the injury, and the associated lesions. Operative management remains the gold standard in unstable patients, after failure of nonoperative management, and in many injuries caused by penetrating mechanisms.[109–111]

However, diagnostic laparoscopy is being used in lieu of exploratory laparotomy in hemodynamically stable children to evaluate and repair many types of abdominal injuries.[132]

Assessment of hemorrhage and immediate volume resuscitation should be carried out with blood products. Ideally, two large-bore IVs (in the upper extremities in case there is caval disruption) should be placed; this can be challenging in the very young or those patients between 9 months to 2 years of age where identifying veins for cannulation can be tricky. Ultrasound can be useful and the threshold for central venous cannulation should be low. Arterial line placement is an extremely useful hemodynamic monitor and port for point of care testing, but emergency surgery should not be delayed in favor of its placement.

Hypothermia is a major comorbidity that worsens a hypercoagulable state and should be aggressively treated and prevented. Children are very prone to hypothermia due to their large ratio of weight to body surface area. The operating room should be warmed, a forced hot air warming device (e.g., Bair Hugger) and other warming mechanisms placed, and a temperature probe inserted. Urinary catheterization is necessary for monitoring fluid input/output.

In order to control the source of the bleeding, surgeons might use different maneuvers such as the Pringle maneuver (compression of the hepatoduodenal ligament to stop blood flow to the liver) for liver injury,[133] the use of resuscitative endovascular balloon occlusion of the aorta (REBOA), and even resuscitative endovascular balloon occlusion of the vena cava (REBOVC) at the level of the retrohepatic vena cava to allow damage control procedures. The anesthesiologist should be familiar with the different maneuvers and devices and be prepared for hemodynamic shifts.

INTRAOPERATIVE MANAGEMENT OF ORTHOPEDIC TRAUMA

Orthopedic injuries are common in pediatric multitrauma and although skeletal trauma is rarely life threatening, it can lead to major morbidity[134–137] and should be aggressively managed even in the presence of severe brain injury because there is excellent recovery potential in children.[137] Historically, open fractures required wound debridement within 6 hours of injury. However, this recommendation was not evidence-based and delaying surgical irrigation and debridement for up to 24 hours does not increase infectious complications for open fractures.[138]

Children who require immediate surgical intervention due to brain, chest, or abdominal injury often have accompanying orthopedic injuries. Aggressive treatment is required to prevent the lethal triad of hypothermia, acidosis, and coagulopathy as a direct result of trauma and secondary injury from the systemic response to trauma with resulting postinjury multiorgan failure. However, postinjury multiorgan failure is rare in children, and when compared with adults with equivalent injuries, it is less severe when it occurs.[139] Thus, it appears to be safe to continue surgery and allow orthopedic interventions as long as the child is not hypothermic (<35°C), acidotic (pH <7.15 or increasing lactate), or coagulopathic.[140] Inadequately resuscitated children should only undergo damage control, covering all wounds, aligning deformed limbs, and documenting neurovascular status of the limb. Initial treatment includes splints or external fixators while avoiding skeletal and skin traction. Sufficient room should be left for venous access. Always reassess circulation in the injured limb after reducing the deformity. Unlike adults, pelvic fractures in children are not a cause for mortality, although it is evidence of high energy trauma and should raise suspicion for associated head and visceral injuries, which may be fatal.[141] Assessment for possible fat embolism syndrome (respiratory and neurologic symptoms and skin/scleral petechiae) should be performed as well.[142]

When positioning the child on the operating table, keep in mind their relatively large head to chest size and ensure adequate chest elevation to avoid cervical spine flexion or hyperextension that could displace an unstable cervical spine injury. Children under 2 years of age rarely have a bony cervical spine injury visible on x-ray. The hypermobility of their cervical spine can normally withstand most injuries but in extremes can result in neurovascular tearing. This spinal cord injury is missed on radiographs (and CTs) and is referred to as spinal cord injury without radiological abnormality (SCIWORA).[143,144] Initial treatment is directed at nonsurgical immobilization and evaluation with an MRI.[145–147]

Mass Casualty Events

A mass casualty event is an incident where the number of affected persons or the rate of their arrival to a health care facility overwhelms the available resources and the capability to provide care promptly.[141,148] Mass casualty events involving numbers of children are rare but unfortunately increasing in the United States with the easy availability of guns and drug-related gang activity. In 2019, there were 187 shooting events involving at least five individuals in the United States; 54 such events involved one or more pediatric patients <18 years of age.[149] Unfortunately, in 71% of such events the nearest hospital was not a trauma center and for more than half of these events the nearest pediatric trauma center was at least 10 miles distant. These data emphasize that all hospitals must have systems in place to manage and triage mass casualty events. Examples of events that involved large numbers of children worldwide include leak of toxic gases, plane crashes, earthquakes, bombings, terrorist (both homegrown and foreign) attacks (as in school shootings), hurricanes, tornadoes, and drug overdoses.[150]

When examining the world experience of mass casualties involving children, we encounter mostly gunshot scenarios that involve teenagers. In the Israeli database, we found events with up to 15 pediatric patients involved in a bus accident (age 7–15 years) requiring evacuation to hospital, with the only injury being mild hypothermia. Mass casualties involving large numbers of small children and infants are rare. Some of the difficulties reported in the literature are the relative clinical inexperience and skills among prehospital medical personnel of managing children, and sometimes lack of age- and size-appropriate equipment.[150] When considering triage involving pediatric mass casualties, there are unique physiological differences in children, including their ability to mask blood loss, vulnerability to develop hypothermia, and greater respiratory demands that justify considering pediatric trauma patients for emergent evacuation and where possible, in the company of a caregiver.[151] The younger and more severely injured children are preferentially evacuated to pediatric trauma centers. Teenagers and less severely injured children may be evacuated to adult trauma centers to minimize the impact on limited resources and personnel in the pediatric centers.[152]

Cricoid Pressure

Cricoid pressure, popularized for RSI by Sellick in his seminal report in 1961,[153] has come into question (see Chapter 27). A Cochrane review from 2015 suggested that cricoid pressure may not be necessary to undertake an RSI safely.[154] A multicenter study that examined cricoid pressure during induction and mask ventilation before tracheal intubation in critically ill children in pediatric intensive care units found that it did not reduce the regurgitation rate.[155] A multicenter, randomized controlled study in adults that compared cricoid pressure to sham procedures found no difference between the two groups for pulmonary aspiration. However, cricoid pressure resulted in prolonged intubation times, worse intubating views, and increased difficulty during intubation with more patients requiring more than two intubation attempts.[155,156] Radiologic evidence suggests that cricoid pressure may not completely occlude the lumen of the esophagus because the contours of the vertebral bodies are asymmetric and the esophagus is not aligned directly over the vertebral bodies.[157] The application of cricoid pressure in children may result in further lateral displacement of the esophagus than in adults.[158] Moreover, as little as 5 N force can deform the shape of the cricoid ring in infants, reducing the diameter of the cross-sectional area by 50%.[159] Cricoid pressure is usually applied by operating room nurses or anesthesia assistants whose level of knowledge of and expertise in performing cricoid pressure have not been confirmed, possibly applying cricoid pressure in the incorrect part of the neck and with insufficient or too much force, contraindications to cricoid pressure are presented in Table 2.10.[160–162] In the current medicolegal climate, many providers have perceived an obligation on their part to continue performing cricoid pressure for RSI as seen by the results of a survey documenting that even though 71% of practitioners do not believe cricoid pressure occludes the esophagus, 90% use it when there is an increased risk for pulmonary aspiration.[163] Even though we do not use cricoid pressure in children for RSI for the reasons given earlier, it is controversial and currently may be left up to the discretion of the intubating anesthesiologist. Consideration should be given to other verifiable factors associated with regurgitation and pulmonary aspiration, including inserting a nasogastric tube preoperatively, pharmacologic prophylaxis to decrease gastric fluid volume and acidity, optimizing the patient's position before induction of anesthesia, and rapid induction of a deep level of anesthesia and muscle relaxation to decrease the risks of coughing, straining, and retching, and routine tracheal extubation after return of airway reflexes.[164]

Pain Management

Some practitioners fear that if they treat pain after a traumatic injury, they may mask the symptoms of injury. Historically, adults have received more analgesia after injuries than children.[165] This unfortunate practice, leading to unnecessary suffering, must be avoided. Successfully treated pain associated with trauma improves outcome, early mobilization, recovery, and discharge from hospital. Inadequate treatment increases the risk for delayed recovery and chronic pain. Titration of opioids to the desired effect, along with appropriate monitoring ensure their safe administration. Children have unique age and developmental factors that must be taken into consideration during assessment and management of posttraumatic pain, using an appropriate pain assessment tool (Table 37.10).

A multimodal approach is recommended to managing pain in trauma, including pharmacology, nonpharmacological tools, and regional or nerve block techniques. Nonpharmacological tools include immobilizing fractures, comfort, heat or cold packs, positive reinforcement, distractions, relaxation exercises, and psychological support. The pharmacological treatment should be based on maximizing the use of nonopioid drugs. Often this means scheduling doses of acetaminophen and/or nonsteroidal antiinflammatory drugs (NSAIDs) around the clock. There is often a benefit to combining two nonopioids to achieve improved analgesia by additivity while decreasing adverse effects.[166,167] Opioids are added either as needed for breakthrough pain or in a scheduled manner with the option for additional doses for breakthrough pain.

Peripheral nerve blocks are easy and safe to perform using ultrasound-guided techniques, preferable in the sedated or anesthetized child, providing effective analgesia for limb injuries. Regional, epidural analgesia, is easy and safe to perform in the anesthetized child, providing excellent quality of analgesia for lower limbs, abdominal, and thoracic injuries. Precise transfer of relevant information with the surgical team is advised so that there are no miscommunications about the ability to perform sensory and motor examinations as well as coordination for the administration of additional analgesic medications.

An alternate route to deliver medications, especially when venous or intraosseous access is not initially present, includes the nares. This route can be used until other routes for drug administration are established or in lieu of intravenous catheters placed solely for minor procedures (i.e., fracture reductions in the emergency department). Nasal diamorphine,[168,169] sufentanil,[167] ketamine,[170,171] and fentanyl[172] are commonly used. Improved nasal delivery systems provide accurate dosing and broaden the drug choices (e.g., ketorolac).[173]

Compartment syndrome is a concern and should be suspected in high-velocity limb trauma and burns (see Chapter 34). An open fracture, or the presence of an open wound, does not prevent the occurrence of compartment syndrome. Careful and frequent assessment, preferably by the same physician, is essential in identifying compartment syndrome. As opposed to adults, the 5 "Ps" (**p**ain, **p**allor, **p**aresthesia, **p**aralysis, and **p**ulselessness) are not always reliable and one should instead look for 3 "A's" (increasing **a**nalgesia requirement, **a**nxiety, and **a**gitation). Breakthrough pain and inadequacy of a previously well-functioning epidural or nerve block should raise the suspicion that the child is developing a compartment syndrome. The treatment is urgent fasciotomy of all affected compartments. The risk for developing compartment syndrome does not preclude the use of adequate analgesia, either opioid based or using regional or peripheral blocks.

Future Directions in Pediatric Trauma

Further advances in interventional radiology and the ability to catheterize small vessels warrant its consideration in pediatric trauma. In cases of liver, splenic, and renal injury, with a contrast blush on the CT, embolization may avoid the need for expansive open surgery when appropriate.

The use of resuscitative endovascular balloon occlusion of the aorta in adult patients is gaining evidence as a temporizing measure for severe abdominal and pelvic trauma in various settings. A small number of reports in pediatric trauma patients[174] suggest that including resuscitative endovascular balloon occlusion of the aorta in pediatric acute trauma care may benefit a significant segment of the major pediatric trauma population.[175]

Acknowledgment

We thank David A. Young, MD, David E. Wesson, MD for their prior contributions to this chapter.

ANNOTATED REFERENCES

DeRoss AL, Vane DW. Early evaluation and resuscitation of the pediatric trauma patient. *Semin Pediatr Surg.* 2004;13(2):74-79.
This review article focuses on the initial management of the pediatric trauma patient.
Heydinger G, Tobias J, Veneziano G. Fundamentals and innovations in regional anaesthesia for infants and children. *Anaesthesia.* 2021;76 suppl 1:74-88.
Regional anesthesia in children incorporates both central regional analgesia and peripheral nerve blocks, allowing additional avenues for providing opioid-sparing analgesia while optimizing analgesia.
Kochanek PM, Tasker RC, Carney N, et al. Guidelines for the Management of Pediatric Severe Traumatic Brain Injury, 3rd ed.: Update of the Brain Trauma Foundation Guidelines, Executive Summary. *Neurosurgery.* 2019;84(6):1169-1178.
These guidelines provide up to date evidence-based recommendations for the treatment of severe traumatic brain injury in pediatric patients.
Lynch T, Kilgar J, Al Shibli A. Pediatric abdominal trauma. *Curr Pediatr Rev.* 2018;14(1):59-63.
This article reviews diagnostic tools and management of pediatric abdominal trauma.

A complete reference list can be found online at Elsevier eBooks+.

TABLE 37.10	Age-Appropriate Pain Assessment Tools
Tool	**Age Group**
FLACC – Face Legs Activity Cry Consolability	2 months to 7 years; nonverbal older and/or cognitively impaired
Pain Word Scale – (none, a little, medium, a lot)	3 to 7 years; older children unable to use 0–10 NRS
FPS-R – Faces Pain Scale	5 to 12 years
NCCPC-PV – Non-communicating Children's Pain Checklist-Postoperative Version	3 to 18 years; postoperative/ procedural pain assessment in hospital, in children unable to speak due to cognitive impairments and disabilities.
NRS – Numerical Rating Scale 0–10	7 years and older

38 Cardiopulmonary Resuscitation

POOJA NAWATHE, IRIS MANDELL, AND CHARLES L. SCHLEIEN

Historical Background
Epidemiology, Prevention, and Outcome of In-Hospital Cardiopulmonary Arrest
Diagnosis of Cardiac Arrest
Mechanics of Cardiopulmonary Resuscitation
Airway
Breathing
Circulation
Defibrillation and Cardioversion
Electric Countershock
Practical Aspects of Defibrillation in Children
Open-Chest Defibrillation
Automated External Defibrillation
Transcutaneous Cardiac Pacing
Vascular Access and Monitoring During Cardiopulmonary Resuscitation
Vascular Access and Fluid Administration
Endotracheal Medication Administration
Monitoring During Cardiopulmonary Resuscitation
Medications Used During Cardiopulmonary Resuscitation
Adrenergic Agonists

Epinephrine
Vasopressin
Atropine
Sodium Bicarbonate
Calcium
Glucose
Amiodarone
Lidocaine
Special Cardiac Arrest Situations
Perioperative Cardiac Arrest
Hyperkalemia
Anaphylaxis
Supraventricular Tachycardia
Pulseless Electrical Activity
Adjunctive Cardiopulmonary Resuscitation Techniques
Open-Chest Cardiopulmonary Resuscitation
Extracorporeal Membrane Oxygenation
Active Compression-Decompression
Post-resuscitation Stabilization (Post–Cardiac Arrest Care)
The 2020 AHA Pediatric Advanced Life Support Guidelines Update

THE PEDIATRIC ANESTHESIOLOGIST must be prepared to resuscitate a child who suffers a cardiac arrest in the course of a routine elective anesthetic, during a high-risk surgery, or outside the operating room during the delivery of an anesthetic or, as a vital part of the "code team." This chapter aims to provide pediatric anesthesiologists with an in-depth understanding of cardiopulmonary-cerebral resuscitation physiology and current evidence for cardiopulmonary resuscitation.

Historical Background

A description in poetic form of the Rules of the Humane Society (c. 1814) for recovering drowned persons included the following description of mouth-to-mouth resuscitation[1]:
Let one the mouth, and either nostril close
While through the other the bellows gently blows.
Thus the pure air with steady force convey,
To put the flaccid lungs again in play.
Should bellows not be found, or found too late,
Let some kind soul with willing mouth inflate;
Then downward, though but lightly, press the chest.
And let the inflated air be upward prest.

External cardiac massage was successfully performed more than 100 years ago in two children aged 8 and 13 years after circulatory arrest precipitated by chloroform anesthesia during a surgical procedure[2] In 1904, Crile described the effectiveness of external cardiac compressions in maintaining the circulation of dogs[3]

After multiple reports that attested to the effectiveness of mouth-to-mouth resuscitation[4–6] in 1958 the National Academy of Sciences National Research Council recommended mouth-to-mouth resuscitation with maximum backward tilt of the head as the preferred technique for all individuals requiring emergency artificial ventilation. In 1960, external cardiac compression was revived as a resuscitation technique when its effectiveness[7] was demonstrated when combined with artificial respirations. Many of the patients had sustained cardiac arrest during anesthesia. Before this study, internal cardiac compression was the accepted technique, demonstrated by experience in cardiac bypass surgery. The first successful internal defibrillation of a human heart was performed in 1947,[8] and in 1956, the first successful external defibrillation was performed[9]

Epidemiology, Prevention, and Outcome of In-Hospital Cardiopulmonary Arrest

A 2009 review of cardiac arrest events submitted to the National Registry of Cardiopulmonary Circulation included 3342 pediatric events, excluding events in a delivery room or neonatal intensive care unit (NICU).[10] Seventy-three percent of the inpatient cardiac arrests had occurred in an ICU, 7% in a general inpatient area, 11% in an emergency department, and 3% in an operating room or postanesthesia care unit (PACU). Return of spontaneous circulation was achieved in 65%, 24-hour survival occurred in 47%, and 30% of children survived until hospital discharge. Other large series of in-hospital pediatric cardiac arrest reported that between 14% and 44% survived until hospital discharge[11–14] with a 44% survival rate from cardiac arrests that had occurred in a pediatric cardiac ICU. In another multicenter cohort study of in-hospital pediatric cardiac arrests,[15] 48.7% of the 353 children survived until hospital discharge. Survivors had greater body temperatures, greater pH values, and reduced serum lactate concentrations compared with nonsurvivors. Nonsurvivors were more likely to have had a tracheal tube before the arrest and to have received sodium bicarbonate, calcium, and vasopressin during the arrest. In this study, postoperative cardiopulmonary resuscitation (CPR) was associated with decreased mortality. A retrospective review of more than 29,000 discharges with in-hospital cardiac arrest between 1997 and 2012 revealed a discharge survival of 54% overall, increasing from 49% in 1997 to 60% in 2012.[16] The incidence of in-hospital cardiac arrest was greater for males, neonates and infants, Black children, and children from metropolitan regions and from families with lower median incomes. Survival rates were lower for teenagers, Black and Hispanic children, and children from metropolitan regions. More than 15,000 children annually experience in-hospital CPR during their stay, with 80% to 90% surviving the event but most do not survive until discharge.[17] Confirming our current understanding, most cardiac arrests occurred in intensive care units and other monitored settings and were associated with respiratory failure or shock. The initial rhythm in half of the arrests was bradycardia with only 10% of the arrests presenting with a shockable rhythm.

Inpatient quality improvement and patient safety-focused programs have identified interventions and recognized risks to prevent cardiac arrest events. Rapid response teams and early warning screening scores have become mainstays that reduce the prevalence of cardiac arrest.[18–21] Perioperative physicians have spearheaded the development of risk-stratification instruments for assessing patient's risk of morbidity and mortality such as the American Society of Anesthesiology Classification physical status and airway visualization scoring methods.[22] These screening and stratification instruments identify necessary resources and help to develop plans for high-risk patients.[23–28] The perioperative physician should also identify potential risks to the patient and consult closely with surgical and subspecialty colleagues. The increased survival of children with uncommon chronic morbidities, syndromes, and metabolic illness requires consultation from a host of specialists as the breadth of knowledge and experience necessary for their safe, effective care is extensive and complex. In complicated cases, broad consultation may be necessary before an anesthesia plan is formulated. The operative and anesthesia plan and potential risks should be conveyed to the patient as well as a management plan for their chronic conditions.

Diagnosis of Cardiac Arrest

Electronic monitoring usually alerts the anesthesiologist to an actual or impending cardiac arrest in the operating room. The electrocardiogram (ECG) may indicate nonperfusing rhythms such as ventricular fibrillation, pulseless electrical activity (PEA), and asystole; end-tidal carbon dioxide (ETCO$_2$) may decrease precipitously, reflecting a decrease in cardiac output due to reduced delivery of carbon dioxide (CO$_2$) to the lungs. A pulse oximeter may lose its regular waveform in the absence of pulsatile blood flow. Despite the importance of these monitors, the diagnosis of cardiopulmonary arrest still rests on the absence of a pulse in a major artery (e.g., carotid, femoral, or brachial artery) determined by palpation in the presence of unconsciousness and apnea.

In the early minutes of CPR, the reason for the cardiac arrest should be sought. A blood gas analysis and serum electrolyte concentrations (ideally as point-of-care testing) may prove helpful in determining the cause of the arrest. In many instances, resuscitation will not be successful without the identification and correction of the underlying cause. A focused physical examination should be conducted, and a brief history should be elicited if it is not already known. If not present, a cardiorespiratory monitor should be placed, and the ECG analyzed. In an intraoperative arrest, the surgeon may be able to provide clues to the diagnosis, such as excessive blood loss, compression of major blood vessels, decreasing venous return to the heart, manipulation of anatomic structures (e.g., manipulation of the peritoneum resulting in severe vagal bradycardia or asystole), or air embolism. Equipment malfunction must always be considered as a potential cause of arrest.

Mechanics of Cardiopulmonary Resuscitation

Basic life support (BLS) and pediatric advanced life support (PALS) guidelines recommend that CPR should follow the airway, breathing, circulation (ABC) algorithm. However, there has been discussion regarding transition to circulation, airway, and breathing (CAB) algorithm with the goal to minimize delay in return of circulation, as findings confirm that the shorter time elapsed between cardiovascular collapse and the first chest compression is a reliable predictor of sustained return of spontaneous circulation.[29,30] The 2015 Consensus Guidelines[31] opted to continue the recommendation of the ABC algorithm as the majority of pediatric arrests are asphyxial in nature. The ABC algorithm applies to all children except for the child with ventricular fibrillation or pulseless ventricular tachycardia who should receive electrical defibrillation without delay. The ABC algorithm has been reaffirmed in the 2020 Consensus Guidelines for health care providers, with the exception of adult and children drowning victims, in whom CAB should be considered for laypersons performing resuscitation.[32] Airway access in children with ventricular fibrillation or pulseless ventricular tachycardia should be performed secondarily and CPR should continue without interruption until a shock can be delivered. There is no evidence that any one airway device is superior to the other in terms of survival or neurological outcome.[33]

AIRWAY

Before tracheal intubation, the child's airway can be managed effectively with bag-valve-mask (BVM) ventilation with proper head positioning and jaw thrust. Although tracheal intubation ensures optimal control of the airway for adequate ventilation, multiple attempts at tracheal intubation by an inexperienced operator may seriously compromise the airway and increase the cumulative duration of "no flow" (i.e., no CPR).

In the child without an artificial airway and proper jaw thrust application, bag-valve-mask devices can inflate the stomach and

TABLE 38.1	Ventilation and Chest Compressions During Pediatric Cardiopulmonary Pulmonary Resuscitation (all ages)		
	Respirations	**Chest Compressions**	**Notes**
Bag-mask ventilation	2 respirations after each 15 chest compressions (if one rescuer only, 2 respirations after each 30 compressions)	100–120/minute	Aspirate (vent) the stomach if gastric inflation interferes with ventilation
Endotracheal intubation	1 breath every 2–3 seconds (20–30 breaths per minute)	100–120/minute	Do not pause compressions during ventilation; After each compression, rescuers should allow the chest to recoil completely

cause regurgitation and pulmonary aspiration of gastric contents.[34] Abdominal distention (gastric and bowel) can compromise oxygenation; therefore, the stomach should be vented when excessive gastric inflation occurs. The incidence of pulmonary aspiration in a series of failed resuscitations is reported to be as great as 28%.[35] For this reason, as well as the risk of barotrauma and volutrauma, excessive inflation pressures should be avoided. Visualizing bilateral chest excursions and listening to the quality of the breath sounds rather than setting a preset maximal inflation pressure best judges effective bilateral ventilation. Placement of a supraglottic device such as a laryngeal mask airway (LMA) may serve as a bridge to establishing a more definitive airway in the hands of those inexperienced in airway management.

Tracheal intubation should be performed as soon as appropriate personnel and equipment are available. Some centers advocate placing a supraglottic airway device due to the delay and technical challenge of direct laryngoscopy and endotracheal tube placement. However, this is not a universally reported practice in the care of pediatric cardiac arrest.[36,37] The $ETCO_2$ is a valuable method of confirming the correct placement of the tracheal tube. In the absence of capnography, a disposable colorimetric $ETCO_2$ device may be substituted (E-Fig. 37.4). However, it is important to appreciate that $ETCO_2$ measurements are meaningful only in the presence of effective pulmonary circulation, such that a lack of color change may reflect either improper placement of the tube or a lack of pulmonary blood flow resulting from ineffective chest compressions or a massive pulmonary embolism. It is also essential to use the proper size colorimetric device for the child's weight because the adult size may not detect CO_2 and may lead the user to misdiagnose a successful intubation as unsuccessful. Selection of a cuffed endotracheal tube should be considered in infants and children to improve capnography as well as ventilation.[38–40]

BREATHING

Equipment to artificially ventilate the lungs should be readily available for all inpatients. The anesthesiologist needs to be familiar with the available equipment in different locations within the hospital because equipment for emergency ventilatory support may differ from standard equipment in the operating room. Anesthesiologists are skilled providers of ventilatory support, but in the context of a cardiac arrest, they must return to the basics and remember that *if there is no chest movement, there is no ventilation or oxygenation.* If no chest movement occurs during bag-valve-mask ventilation despite an apparently good seal between the mask and the child's face, the underlying cause must be investigated.

Overventilation is common during CPR, resulting in greater mean intrathoracic pressures than required, which decreases venous return and reduces cardiac output.[41] In cardiopulmonary arrest, less than usual minute ventilation may be appropriate, because cardiac output and delivery of CO_2 to the lungs are

diminished. If an artificial airway is not in place for *single-person rescue*, two breaths should be given for every 30 chest compressions. If an artificial airway is not in place for *two-person rescue*, two breaths should be given after every 15 chest compressions. Once an artificial airway is in place, updated recommendations suggest a target of 1 breath every 2 to 3 seconds, with goal of 20 to 30 breaths per minute (Table 38.1).[42]

CIRCULATION

During cardiac arrest, chest compressions provide the sole pump to perfuse a child's vital organs; therefore, optimal performance of CPR is critical. Key elements to providing quality chest compressions include (1) ensuring an adequate rate (100 compressions per minute),[43] (2) ensuring adequate chest wall depression (one-third to one-half of the anteroposterior chest diameter), (3) releasing completely between compressions to allow full chest wall recoil, (4) minimizing interruptions in chest compressions,[44] and (5) ensuring that the child is on a sufficiently hard surface to allow effective chest compressions.[45] The strategy for successful CPR is to push hard and push fast, release completely, and do not interrupt compressions unnecessarily. A recent systematic review of adult and pediatric studies of the effects of the back surface on chest compressions during CPR suggested that at best, a hard surface increased the depth of compressions by only 3 mm.[46]

Be mindful that incomplete recoil during CPR is associated with greater intrathoracic pressures and decreased venous return, coronary, and cerebral perfusion.[47]

If the child is younger than 6 months of age, the person performing chest compressions can comfortably encircle the chest with their hands. Chest compressions should be performed using the circumferential technique, with thumbs depressing the sternum and the fingers supporting the infant's back and circumferentially squeezing the thorax (Fig. 38.1). In larger infants, the sternum can be compressed using two fingers, and in the child, either one or two hands can be used, depending on the size of the child and of the rescuer.[47,48] Whichever method is used, attention should be focused on delivering effective compressions with *minimal interruptions.*[44,49] In all cases other than circumferential CPR, a backboard should be used. Properly delivered chest compressions will quickly fatigue the provider. To maintain effective CPR, providers should rotate approximately every 2 minutes to prevent fatigue and deterioration in the quality and rate of chest compressions.[47]

Mechanisms of Blood Flow

External chest compressions generate cardiac output via two mechanisms: the cardiac pump and the thoracic pump. The cardiac pump mechanism generates cardiac output by squeezing blood out of the heart when compressed between the sternum and the vertebral column. Blood exits the heart in an anterograde direction because the atrioventricular valves close during ventricular

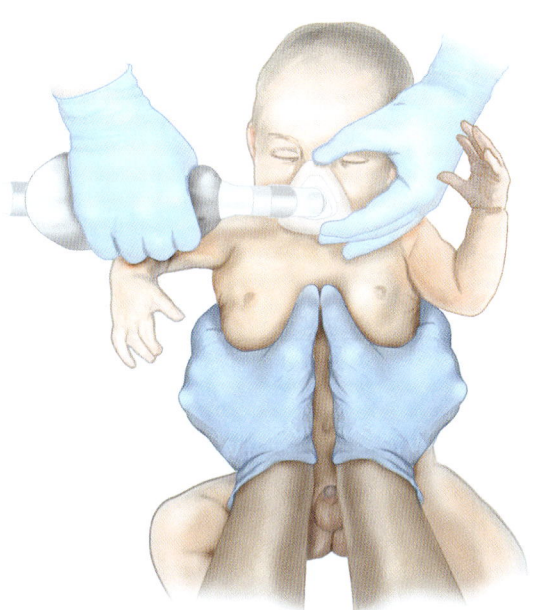

FIGURE 38.1 Chest-encircling method for cardiac compressions in a neonate: thumbs are placed one finger's breadth below the nipple line. (Modified from Todres ID, Rogers MC. Methods of external cardiac massage in the newborn infant. *J Pediatr.* 1975;86:781-782.)

Cardiac Pump

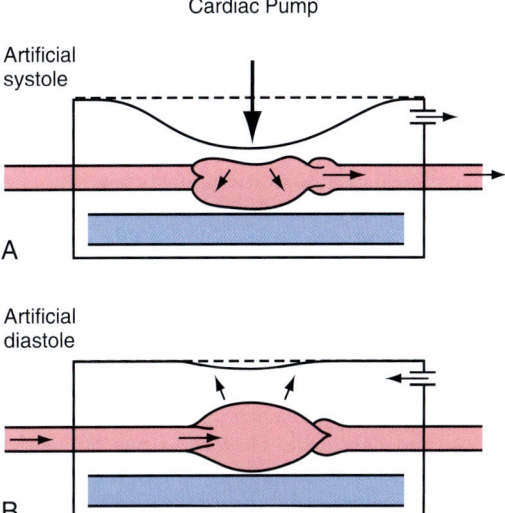

FIGURE 38.2 **A,** Cardiac pump mechanism by which the heart is directly squeezed between the sternum and vertebral column, representing artificial systole. **B,** Artificial diastole occurs with relaxation of the compressions. (From Babbs CF. New versus old theories of blood flow during CPR. *Crit Care Med.* 1980;8:191-195 with permission from Williams & Wilkins.)

Thoracic Pump

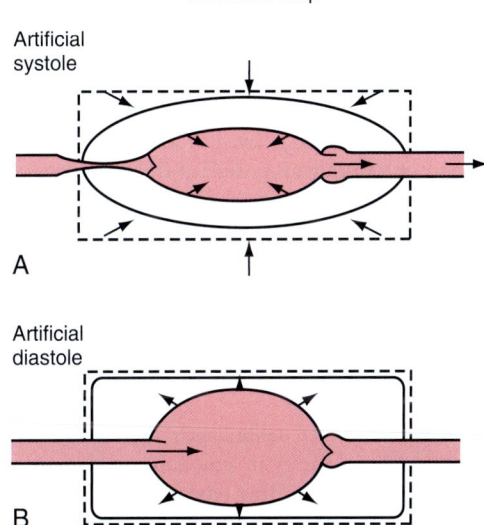

FIGURE 38.3 **A,** Thoracic pump mechanism by which blood flow occurs through a general increase in intrathoracic pressure with external compressions (i.e., the heart is a passive conduit). **B,** Artificial diastole occurs with release of external compressions. (From Babbs CF. New versus old theories of blood flow during CPR. *Crit Care Med.* 1980;8:191-195 with permission from Williams & Wilkins.)

compression. Between compressions, ventricular pressure decreases below atrial pressure, allowing the atrioventricular valves to open and fill the ventricles. This sequence of events resembles the normal cardiac cycle. Although the cardiac pump is likely not the dominant mechanism that generates cardiac output during most closed-chest CPR, specific clinical situations have been identified in which the cardiac pump mechanism is more prominent. For example, a smaller, more compliant chest may allow for more direct cardiac compression (Fig. 38.2). Increasing the applied force during chest compressions also increases direct cardiac compression and emptying of the ventricles.

The cardiac pump is not the primary mechanism generating cardiac output during CPR. Angiographic studies show that blood passes from the vena cava through the right heart into the pulmonary artery and the pulmonary veins through the left heart into the aorta during a single chest compression.[50,51] Echocardiographic studies show that the atrioventricular valves are open during blood ejection.[50,52,53] Without closure of atrioventricular valves during chest compression, the cardiac pump mechanisms cannot account for anterograde movement of blood during CPR.

The thoracic pump mechanism is the second mechanism by which cardiac output is generated during CPR. In 1976, several patients who developed ventricular fibrillation during cardiac catheterization were noted to produce enough blood flow to maintain consciousness by repetitive coughing.[54] The increase in thoracic pressure with coughing produced anterograde blood flow without direct cardiac compression. This describes the thoracic pump mechanism, in which the heart acts as a passive conduit for blood flow. The intrathoracic pressure is greater than the extrathoracic pressure during the compression phase of CPR. At this time, blood flows out of the thorax, with venous valves preventing excessive retrograde blood flow (Fig. 38.3). Experimental and

clinical data support both mechanisms of blood flow during CPR in human infants.

Rate and Duty Cycle

The recommended rate of chest compressions for all children is 100 per minute, with great care taken to minimize interruptions in chest compressions and to ensure adequate compression depth.[44,49] This rate represents a compromise that attempts to maximize contributions from both the thoracic pump and cardiac pump mechanism of blood flow.

The duty cycle is defined as the percent of the compression-relaxation cycle devoted to compression. If blood flow is generated by direct cardiac compression, then the force of compression determines the stroke volume. Prolonging the compression (increasing the duty cycle) beyond the time necessary for full ventricular ejection should not affect the stroke volume. Increasing the rate of compressions should increase cardiac output because a fixed volume of blood is ejected with each cardiac compression. In contrast, if the thoracic pump mechanism produces blood flow, the volume of ejected blood comes from a large blood reservoir contained within the chest's capacitance vessels. With the thoracic pump mechanism, flow is enhanced by increasing either the force of compression or the duty cycle, but is not affected by changes in the compression rate over a wide range of rates, given a set duty cycle.[55]

Animal models yield conflicting results as to the optimal compression rate and duty cycle. However, a rate of compressions during conventional CPR of 100 per minute satisfies both those who prefer the faster rates and those who support a longer duty cycle. This is true because it is easier to produce a longer duty cycle when compressions are administered at a faster rate.[56,57]

Defibrillation and Cardioversion

In children with ventricular fibrillation or pulseless ventricular tachycardia, the immediate management should be defibrillation, without delay to secure an airway.

ELECTRIC COUNTERSHOCK

Electric countershock, or defibrillation, is the treatment of choice for ventricular fibrillation and pulseless ventricular tachycardia. Defibrillation should not be delayed to secure an airway, because the likelihood of restoring an organized rhythm decreases as the duration of fibrillation increases. Ventricular fibrillation is terminated by simultaneous depolarization and sustained contraction of a critical mass of myocardium,[58] allowing the return of spontaneous, coordinated cardiac contractions, assuming the myocardium is well oxygenated and the acid-base status is relatively normal. Drug treatment may be required as an adjunct to defibrillation, but by itself cannot be relied on to terminate ventricular fibrillation.

An older generation of defibrillators that is still present in many hospitals delivers energy in a monophasic damped sinusoidal waveform (Fig. 38.4A). This type of instrument delivers a single, unidirectional current with a gradual decrease to zero current. By contrast, the newer generation of biphasic defibrillators delivers a current in a positive direction for a set period, followed by a reversal in current (Fig. 38.4B). Biphasic defibrillators are more effective than monophasic defibrillators for terminating ventricular fibrillation in adults; therefore, their use is recommended where possible. Pediatric attenuator pads or a pediatric mode on the automated external defibrillator should be used in children 1 to 8 years of age if it is available, but if it is not (and a standard defibrillator is similarly unavailable), an unmodified automated external defibrillator can be used.

In most of adult cases, energy levels of 100 to 200 J are successful when shocks are delivered with minimal delay.[59,60] The goal of defibrillation is to deliver a minimum amount of electrical energy to a critical mass of ventricular muscle while avoiding excessive current that could further damage the heart. The most reliable predictor for the success of defibrillation is the duration of fibrillation before the first countershock[61]; acidosis and hypoxemia decrease the success of defibrillation.[61]

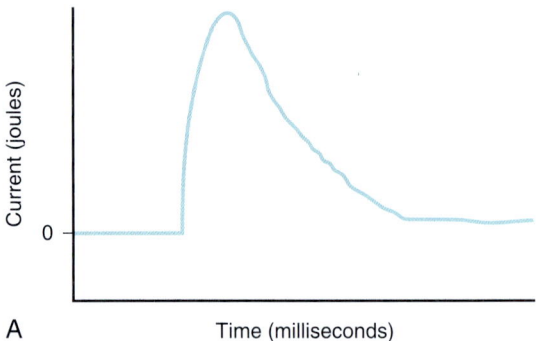

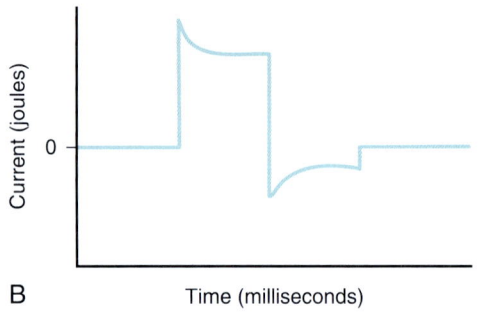

FIGURE 38.4 Energy delivery during conventional monophasic **(A)** and biphasic truncated exponential **(B)** defibrillation.

PRACTICAL ASPECTS OF DEFIBRILLATION IN CHILDREN

Correct paddle size and position are critical to the success of defibrillation. The largest paddle size appropriate for the child should be used because a bigger size reduces the density of current flow, thereby reducing myocardial damage. In general, adult paddles should be used in children weighing more than 10 kilograms and infant paddles should be used in infants weighing less than 10 kilograms. Paddle force is important as well. If the entire paddle does not rest *firmly* on the chest wall, a current of increased density will be delivered to a small contact point. Therefore, paddles should be positioned on the chest wall so that the bulk of myocardium lies directly between them. One paddle is placed to the right of the upper sternum below the clavicle; the other is positioned just caudad and to the left of the left nipple. For children with dextrocardia, the position of the paddles should be a mirror image. An alternative approach is to place one paddle anteriorly over the left precordium and the other paddle posteriorly between the scapulae.

The paddle and chest wall interface can be gel pads, electrode cream, or electrode paste. The electrode cream produces less impedance than the paste. *Electric current follows the path of least resistance, so care should be taken that the interface material from one paddle does not touch that of the other paddle. This is especially important in infants, in whom the distance between paddles is small.* If the gel is continuous between paddles, a short circuit is created and an insufficient amount of current will traverse the heart. Use of bare metal paddles increases the risk of arcing and worsens cutaneous burns from defibrillation. The use of self-adhesive pads is preferable when feasible.

In the past, sparking from poorly applied defibrillator paddles was a fire risk. As a result, all sources of free-flowing oxygen were maintained at a distance of at least 1 meter from the child. However, the use of pads rather than paddles has reduced the risk of fire, allowing the nasal oxygen or mask oxygen supply to remain in place during defibrillation. It is unnecessary to disconnect the ventilator from the child's tracheal tube, but if the ventilator is disconnected, the fresh gas flow should be turned off.

For children with in-hospital ventricular fibrillation or pulseless ventricular tachycardia, defibrillation should be attempted as soon as possible, with optimal CPR until the defibrillator is ready to deliver a shock. For the first defibrillation, 2 J/kg of delivered energy should be administered (Fig. 38.5). After delivering the shock, CPR should resume immediately with chest compressions for five duty cycles (2 minutes). If the first shock fails to restore normal sinus rhythm, the incremental benefit of a second immediate shock is small. Resumption of CPR is likely to confer a greater benefit than a second shock. CPR may restore coronary perfusion, increasing the likelihood of defibrillation with a

subsequent shock. It is crucial to minimize the time interval between chest compressions and delivery of the shock and between delivery of the shock and resumption of CPR.[49] Approximately 2 minutes of CPR should be delivered before a second shock is delivered at twice the original energy level (4 J/kg).[49]

If ventricular fibrillation or pulseless ventricular tachycardia persists beyond the second defibrillation, standard doses of epinephrine should be administered (with subsequent doses every 3 to 5 minutes during persistent cardiac arrest). Another defibrillation should be attempted after 2 minutes of CPR, further defibrillation attempts should be followed by intravenous amiodarone (5 mg/kg) or lidocaine (1 mg/kg). It is not necessary to increase the energy level on each successive shock after the second attempt. However, successful defibrillation has been reported with currents above 4 J/kg, up to a maximum dose not exceeding 10 J/kg or the adult level, whichever is less, without adverse sequelae.[49] This sometimes occurs when a fixed energy level, adult automated external defibrillator is used in a small child.

OPEN-CHEST DEFIBRILLATION

If the chest is already open in the operating room or easily opened as in a postoperative cardiac patient, ventricular fibrillation should be treated with open-chest defibrillation, using internal paddles applied directly to the heart. These should have a diameter of 6 cm for adults, 4 cm for children, and 2 cm for infants. Handles should be insulated. One electrode is placed behind the left ventricle and the other over the right ventricle on the anterior surface of the heart. The energy level used should begin at 5 J in infants and 20 J in adults.

AUTOMATED EXTERNAL DEFIBRILLATION

The use of automated external defibrillators is now standard therapy in out-of-hospital resuscitation of adults.[47,59] Automated external defibrillators are now deemed appropriate for use in children older than 1 year of age. If available, pediatric attenuator pads or a pediatric mode on the automated external defibrillator should be used in children 1 to 8 years of age, but if unavailable (and a standard defibrillator is similarly unavailable), an unmodified automated external defibrillator should be used.

TRANSCUTANEOUS CARDIAC PACING

In the absence of in situ pacing wires or an indwelling transvenous or esophageal pacing catheter, transcutaneous cardiac pacing is the preferred method for temporary electrical cardiac pacing in children with asystole or severe bradycardia. Transcutaneous cardiac pacing is indicated for children whose primary problem is impulse formation or conduction, with preserved myocardial function. It is most effective in sinus bradycardia or high-grade atrioventricular block, with slow ventricular response but adequate stroke volume. Transcutaneous cardiac pacing is not indicated for children during prolonged arrest, because in this situation it usually results in electrical but not mechanical cardiac capture and its use may delay or interfere with other resuscitative efforts.

One electrode is placed anteriorly at the left sternal border and the other posteriorly just below the left scapula to set up pacing. Smaller electrodes are available for infants and children, but adult-sized electrodes can be used in children weighing more than 15 kilograms. ECG leads should be connected to the pacemaker, the demand or asynchronous mode selected, and an age-appropriate heart rate should be used. The stimulus output should be set at zero when the pacemaker is turned on and then increased

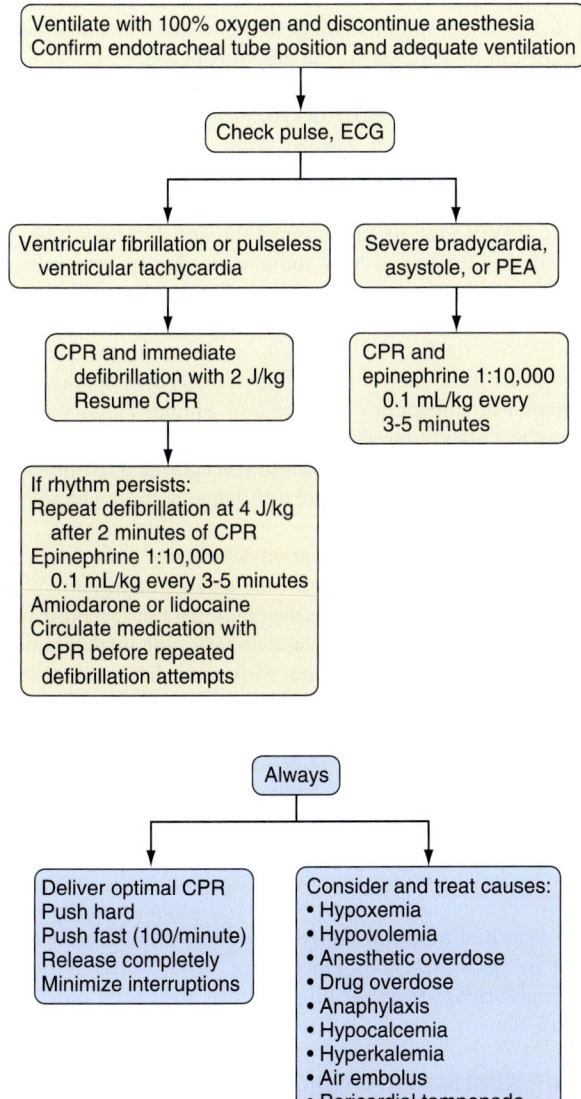

FIGURE 38.5 Algorithm for diagnosis and treatment of acute cardiac dysfunction in the operating room. *CPR,* Cardiopulmonary resuscitation; *ECG,* electrocardiogram; *PEA,* pulseless electrical activity.

gradually until electrical capture is identified on the monitor. After electrical capture is achieved, it must be determined if an effective arterial pulse is generated. If not, additional resuscitative efforts should be initiated.

The most serious complication of transcutaneous cardiac pacing is the induction of ventricular arrhythmias. Fortunately, this is rare and may be prevented by pacing only in the demand mode. Mild transient erythema beneath the electrodes is common. Skeletal muscle contraction can be minimized using large electrodes, 40-millisecond pulse duration, and the smallest stimulus required for capture. If defibrillation or cardioversion is necessary, 2 to 3 cm must be allowed between the electrode and paddles to prevent arcing of the current.

Vascular Access and Monitoring During Cardiopulmonary Resuscitation

VASCULAR ACCESS AND FLUID ADMINISTRATION

One of the critical aspects of successful CPR is establishing a route to administer fluids and medications. If intravenous access cannot be established rapidly, the intraosseous (see Chapter 46 and Figs. 46.3 and 46.4) or tracheal route should be used.

Intravenous Access

Many children who suffer an in-hospital cardiac arrest will already have established vascular access. For children with impending cardiac arrest and no vascular access, a brief attempt should be made to secure peripheral intravenous access. If access is not achieved quickly, an intraosseous needle should be placed. For young children in cardiac arrest without vascular access, an intraosseous needle should be placed immediately to avoid any delay from repeated attempts to establish intravenous access.

Intraosseous Access

The intraosseous route provides access to the systemic venous circulation via the marrow cavity, which establishes a noncollapsible entry point into the central circulation for emergency infusions.

Current applications of intraosseous access primarily include the emergent resuscitation of infants and children when intravenous access cannot be readily obtained. Intraosseous access has been used for the administration of fluids, vasoactive medications, isotonic crystalloids, and blood products (fresh frozen plasma, whole blood, and packed red blood cells). In children, the preferred site of access is the anteromedial surface of the tibia, approximately 1 to 2 cm below the tibial tuberosity, where the cortex is thinnest.[62,63] Other reported sites for intraosseous access have included the distal femur, lateral or medial malleoli, iliac crest, and sternum. Placing an intraosseous needle in an older child (older than 10 years of age) and adult, although possible, is more difficult because of the thicker bony cortex. Nonetheless, the success rate of establishing intraosseous access in these age groups is 50% to 60%.[62,64] However, in the case of intraosseous insertion in infants <6 months of age, the success rate was 47%; inserting a 15 mm intraosseous needle was successful in 83% but with a 25 mm intraosseous needle, it was 0%.[62]

The technique of establishing intraosseous access is straightforward.[65] An intraosseous needle or, if unavailable, a standard 16- or 18-gauge needle, a spinal needle with stylet, or bone marrow needle may be inserted into the anterior surface of the tibia 1 to 2 cm below and 1 cm medial to the tibial tuberosity (avoiding the epiphyseal plate). The needle is directed at 90 degrees to the anteromedial surface of the tibia, just distal to the tuberosity (see Figs. 46.3 and 46.4). A sudden loss of resistance is sensed when the needle passes through the cortex and into the marrow cavity. If the needle has reached the marrow cavity, it will remain upright without support. If, however, the needle is in the subcutaneous tissue, it will not remain upright without support. Correct placement of the intraosseous needle is confirmed by aspirating blood or bone marrow and by easily infusing (free flow by gravity) crystalloid without evidence of extravasation. Intraosseous access has a low complication rate,[66] although the complications could include osteomyelitis, fat and bone marrow embolism, and compartment syndrome. To avoid these complications, intravenous access should replace intraosseous access as soon as possible. The onset of action and concentration of most drugs after intraosseous administration are comparable with venous administration.[67] The EZ-IO system (Vidacare, Shavano Park, TX) provides a rapid means to establish intraosseous access (see Fig. 46.4). Although the rate of gravity-driven fluid flow with intravenous administration is generally faster than an intraosseous infusion, flow rates up to 10 mL per minute with gravity and over twice that under pressure can be achieved via the intraosseous route.[68,69]

ENDOTRACHEAL MEDICATION ADMINISTRATION

In the absence of other vascular access, medications including lidocaine, atropine, naloxone, and epinephrine (mnemonic LANE or LEAN; vasopressin is occasionally used in adults with the mnemonic NAVEL) can be administered through a tracheal tube.[70,71] Ionized medications such as sodium bicarbonate and calcium chloride should not be administered through the tracheal tube. The peak concentration of epinephrine or lidocaine administered through the tracheal tube, at similar doses, maybe less than through the intravenous route.[72] For example, the peak drug concentration of epinephrine after tracheal administration was only 10% of that after intravenous administration in anesthetized dogs. The recommended dose for tracheal epinephrine is 10 times the intravenous or intraosseous dose or 0.1 mg/kg for bradycardia or pulseless arrest.

The volume and the diluent in which the medications are administered through a tracheal tube may be important. When large volumes of fluid are used, the pulmonary surfactant may be altered or destroyed, resulting in atelectasis. The total volume of fluid delivered into the trachea with each drug administered should not exceed 10 mL in children and 5 mL in infants and neonates.[73] However, administering an adequate volume of a drug is important to reach a large surface area beyond the tip of the tracheal tube to achieve rapid absorption. Absorption into the systemic circulation may be further enhanced by deep intrapulmonary administration by passing a catheter beyond the tip of the tracheal tube deep into the bronchial tree. The duration of the effect of lidocaine, epinephrine, and atropine administered via the tracheal tube is prolonged compared with the same drugs given by the intravenous route. This "depot" effect is due to slower absorption from the lung and the larger drug doses used via this route.[72]

MONITORING DURING CARDIOPULMONARY RESUSCITATION

A basic clinical examination is vital during cardiac arrest. The chest is carefully observed for adequacy of bilateral chest expansion with artificial ventilation and equal and normal breath sounds. In addition, the depth of compression and the position of the rescuer's hands should be constantly reevaluated while performing chest compressions by palpation of a major artery. Palpation of an artery is essential for both confirming the absence of a pulse and for assessing the adequacy of blood flow during chest compressions. Palpating the peripheral pulses may be inaccurate, especially during intense vasoconstriction associated with the use of epinephrine, so it is prudent to palpate only large arteries such as the brachial, femoral, or carotid artery.

An indwelling arterial catheter is a valuable monitor to assess the arterial blood pressure. Specific attention should be paid to diastolic blood pressure as it relates directly to the adequacy of coronary perfusion during CPR. In addition, arterial access allows for frequent blood sampling, particularly for the measurement of arterial pH and blood gases. Pulse oximetry can be used during CPR to determine the oxygen saturation and may be of value in assessing the adequacy of cardiac output, as reflected in the plethysmograph. The ECG can suggest metabolic imbalances and diagnose electrical disturbances.

The $ETCO_2$ monitor provides essential information during resuscitation. Capnography confirms correct placement of the tracheal tube, monitors the quality of CPR, and provides an early indicator of return of spontaneous circulation.[74] Because the generation of exhaled CO_2 depends on pulmonary blood flow, $ETCO_2$ can provide a useful indicator of the adequacy of cardiac output generated by chest compressions. As the cardiac output increases, the $ETCO_2$ increases and the difference between end-tidal and arterial CO_2 diminishes.[75] In animal models, $ETCO_2$ during CPR correlates with coronary perfusion pressure and with return of spontaneous circulation.[76,77] A reduced $ETCO_2$ may occur transiently in the presence of adequate chest compressions after administration of epinephrine owing to an increase in intrapulmonary shunting. The International Liaison Committee on Resuscitation acknowledges that small values of $ETCO_2$ are associated with small probability of survival. The committee believes, however, that there are insufficient data to support or refute a specific cutoff value of $ETCO_2$ as a prognostic indicator of outcome during adult cardiac arrest.[78] $ETCO_2$ monitoring may be considered to evaluate quality of chest compressions, but there is no pediatric evidence that it improves or predicts outcomes after cardiac arrest.[31,79,80] However, we strongly advocate the use of $ETCO_2$ monitoring as a surrogate to monitor effective chest compressions.

Temperature should be monitored during and after CPR. The resuscitation of the child with hypothermia as the cause of cardiac arrest must be continued until the child's core temperature exceeds 95°F (35°C). A glass bulb thermometer measures the temperature to very low values. Repeated measurements of core body temperature should be made at several sites (rectal, bladder, esophageal, axillary, or tympanic membrane) where possible to avoid misleading temperature readings from a single site, because local body temperature may vary with changes in regional blood flow during CPR. Hyperthermia should be aggressively treated in the periarrest period, because postarrest hyperthermia is associated with worse outcomes in children.[81] Although early data suggested a benefit to induced hypothermia after resuscitation from cardiac arrest in adults[82,83] and after perinatal hypoxic or ischemic injury,[84] current evidence supports a temperature of 36°C rather than 33°C. The Therapeutic Hypothermia After Pediatric Cardiac Arrest study concluded that therapeutic hypothermia did not confer a benefit over therapeutic normothermia for survival with good functional outcome at 1 year.[85]

Medications Used During Cardiopulmonary Resuscitation

ADRENERGIC AGONISTS

In 1963, only 3 years after the original description of closed-chest CPR, early administration of epinephrine in a canine model of cardiac arrest was shown to improve the success rate of CPR.[86] In addition, the administration of α-adrenergic agonists increased the aortic diastolic pressure, which improved the success of resuscitation. The evidence suggested that vasopressors such as epinephrine were valuable during resuscitation because they increased peripheral vascular tone and, hence, coronary perfusion pressure. The relative importance of α- and β-adrenergic agonist actions during resuscitation has been widely investigated. In a canine model of cardiac arrest, only 27% of dogs that received a pure β-adrenergic receptor agonist along with an α-adrenergic antagonist were resuscitated successfully, compared with 100% of dogs that received a pure α-adrenergic agonist and a β-adrenergic antagonist. Others demonstrated that the α-adrenergic effects of epinephrine resulted in intense vasoconstriction of the resistance vessels of all organs of the body, except those supplying the heart and brain.[87] Because of the widespread vasoconstriction in nonvital organs, adequate perfusion pressure and thus blood flow to the heart and brain could be achieved despite the fact that cardiac output was poor during CPR.[87–89]

The increase in aortic diastolic pressure associated with epinephrine administration during CPR is critical for maintaining coronary blood flow and enhancing the success of resuscitation.[90,91] Even though the contractile state of the myocardium is increased in the presence of β-adrenergic agonists in the spontaneously beating heart, β-adrenergic agonists may actually decrease myocardial blood flow by increasing intramyocardial wall pressure and vascular resistance during CPR.[92] By its inotropic and chronotropic effects, β-adrenergic stimulation increases myocardial oxygen demand, which, when superimposed on low coronary blood flow, increases the risk of ischemic injury.

Any medication that causes systemic arterial vasoconstriction can be used to increase aortic diastolic pressure and resuscitate the heart. For example, pure α-adrenergic agonists can be used in place of epinephrine during CPR. Phenylephrine and methoxamine, two α-adrenergic agonists, have been used in animal models of CPR with success equal to that of epinephrine.[93] Their use results in a greater oxygen supply to demand ratio in the ischemic heart and at least a theoretical advantage over the combined α- and β-adrenergic agonist effects of epinephrine. These agonists, as well as other classes of vasopressors such as vasopressin, have been used successfully for resuscitation.

The merits of using a pure α-adrenergic agonist during CPR have been questioned by some investigators. Although the inotropic and chronotropic effects of β-adrenergic agonists may have deleterious hemodynamic effects during CPR for ventricular fibrillation, increases in both heart rate and contractility will increase cardiac output when spontaneous coordinated ventricular contractions are achieved.[94]

EPINEPHRINE

Epinephrine (adrenaline) is an endogenous catecholamine with potent α- and β-adrenergic stimulating properties. The β-adrenergic property increases systemic (both systolic and diastolic blood pressures) and pulmonary vascular resistance. The increase in diastolic blood pressure directly increases coronary perfusion pressure, thereby increasing coronary blood flow and increasing the likelihood of return of spontaneous circulation.[90,91] The β-adrenergic effect increases myocardial contractility and heart rate and relaxes smooth muscle in the skeletal muscle vascular bed and bronchi. Epinephrine also increases the vigor and intensity of ventricular fibrillation, increasing the likelihood of successful defibrillation.[95]

Epinephrine has been an integral part of CPR for more than a century. Although standard doses during CPR are associated with an early return of spontaneous circulation, the total dose does not improve neurologic outcomes up to 3 months after cardiac arrest.[96,97] Larger than necessary doses of epinephrine may be deleterious. Epinephrine may worsen myocardial ischemic injury secondary to increased oxygen demand and may result in post-resuscitative tachyarrhythmias, hypertension, and pulmonary edema. Epinephrine causes hypoxemia and an increase in alveolar dead space ventilation by redistributing pulmonary blood flow.[75,98] Prolonged peripheral vasoconstriction by excessive doses of epinephrine may delay or impair reperfusion of systemic organs, particularly the kidneys and gastrointestinal tract.

Routine use of large-dose epinephrine for in-hospital pediatric cardiac arrest should be *avoided*. The use of high-dose epinephrine in children with in-hospital cardiac arrest refractory to initial standard-dose epinephrine has not been encouraging. Survival was reduced at 24 hours compared with those given standard-dose epinephrine, with weak evidence of decreased survival to hospital discharge in the children who received large doses of epinephrine.[99] Despite these data, large doses of epinephrine may be considered in special cases (e.g., β-blocker overdose), particularly when diastolic blood pressure remains low despite excellent chest compression and several standard doses of epinephrine. No prospective pediatric trial has established the efficacy of epinephrine for improving survival outcomes, but delays in epinephrine administration are associated with worse outcomes in children. For patients with nonshockable rhythms, the earlier epinephrine is administered after CPR initiation, the more likely the patient is to survive. There is still inadequate research and consensus on the frequency of epinephrine administration. In a retrospective review of 1630 in-hospital pediatric cardiac arrests, longer average dosing intervals (5–8 minutes and 8–10 minutes) than currently recommended for epinephrine administration during pediatric in-hospital cardiac arrests were associated with improved survival to hospital discharge.[100] Contrast to that in an adult out-of-hospital cardiac arrest study, a shorter average epinephrine dosing interval was associated with improved survival with favorable neurologic status.[101]

VASOPRESSIN

Vasopressin is a long-acting endogenous hormone that causes vasoconstriction (V1 receptor) and reabsorption of water in the renal tubule (V2 receptor). In experimental models of cardiac arrest, vasopressin increases blood flow to the heart and brain and improves long-term survival compared with epinephrine.[102,103] In a randomized trial of epinephrine and vasopressin in shock-resistant out-of-hospital ventricular fibrillation in adults, vasopressin produced a greater rate of return of spontaneous circulation.[104] In a study of in-hospital adult cardiac arrest, epinephrine and vasopressin produced similar rates of survival to hospital discharge.[105] A recent meta-analysis of vasopressin for cardiac arrest did not demonstrate any overall benefit or harm.[106] The National Registry of Cardiopulmonary Resuscitation 2009 review concluded that vasopressin was associated with reduced return of spontaneous circulation and weak evidence for reduced 24-hour and discharge survival.[107]

However, the increases in coronary perfusion pressure and importantly, cerebral blood flow were consistently greater after vasopressin rescue than after rescue with a second dose of epinephrine in a recent animal model study.[108] Given that vasopressin induces vasoconstriction through the activation of V1a receptors rather than as an adrenergic agonist, vasopressin could hypothetically be advantageous in specific scenarios.[109] For example, in patients with pulmonary hypertension, the potentially harmful increase in pulmonary vascular resistance with epinephrine may be mitigated by vasopressin that largely spares the pulmonary vasculature from its effects.[17]

ATROPINE

Atropine, a parasympatholytic agent, blocks cholinergic stimulation of the muscarinic receptors in the heart, increasing the sinus rate and shortening atrioventricular node conduction time. Atropine may activate latent ectopic pacemakers. Atropine has little effect on systemic vascular resistance, myocardial perfusion pressure, or contractility.[110]

Atropine is indicated for the treatment of bradycardia associated with hypotension, second- and third-degree heart block, and slow idioventricular rhythms. Atropine is no longer recommended for asystole or pulseless electrical activity.[111] Atropine is particularly effective in clinical conditions associated with excessive parasympathetic tone. *However, for children with asystole or symptomatic bradycardia associated with severe hypotension, epinephrine is the medication of choice and atropine should be regarded as a second-line drug.*

A dose of 0.02 mg/kg with no minimum dose may be considered when atropine is recommended as a premedication for emergency intubation.[31] Although a minimum dose of 0.1 mg of atropine has been entrenched in the pediatric literature because of paradoxical bradycardia, this dose was not evidence-based.[112,113] There is no minimum dose of atropine in young infants and children.[114] Atropine may be given by any route, including intravenous, intraosseous, endotracheal, intramuscular, or subcutaneous. After intravenous administration, its onset of action is within 30 seconds and its peak effect occurs in 1 to 2 minutes. The recommended adult dose is 0.5 mg every 3 to 5 minutes until the desired heart rate is obtained, up to a maximum of 3 mg.

SODIUM BICARBONATE

Acidosis may depress myocardial function, prolong diastolic depolarization, depress spontaneous cardiac activity, decrease the electrical threshold for ventricular fibrillation, and reduce the cardiac response to catecholamines.[115–117] Acidosis also vasodilates systemic vessels and attenuates the vasoconstrictive response of peripheral vessels to catecholamines,[118] which is the opposite of the desired vascular effect during CPR. In children with a reactive pulmonary vascular bed, acidosis causes pulmonary hypertension. Therefore, correction of even mild acidosis may help to resuscitate children with increased pulmonary vascular resistance. In addition, the presence of severe acidosis may increase the threshold for myocardial stimulation in a child with an artificial cardiac pacemaker.[119]

The routine use of sodium bicarbonate during CPR is not supported by current data.[120,121] Routine administration of sodium bicarbonate is not recommended in pediatric cardiac arrest in the absence of hyperkalemia or sodium channel blocker (e.g., tricyclic antidepressant) toxicity.[122]

Potentially deleterious effects of bicarbonate administration include metabolic alkalosis, hypercapnia, hypernatremia, and hyperosmolality. The use of sodium bicarbonate was associated with increased mortality in a multicenter cohort study of in-hospital pediatric cardiac arrest.[15] Alkalosis causes a leftward shift of the oxyhemoglobin dissociation curve and thus impairs release of oxygen from hemoglobin to tissues at a time when oxygen delivery may already be reduced.[123] Alkalosis also can result in hypokalemia by enhancing potassium influx into cells and in ionic hypocalcemia by increasing protein binding of ionized calcium. The marked hypercapnic acidosis that occurs during CPR in the venous circulation, including the coronary sinus, may be exacerbated by the administration of bicarbonate.[124] Myocardial acidosis during cardiac arrest is associated with decreased myocardial contractility.[117] Hypernatremia and hyperosmolality may decrease tissue perfusion by increasing interstitial edema in microvascular beds.

Paradoxical intracellular acidosis after bicarbonate administration can occur with the rapid entry of carbon dioxide into cells with a slow egress of hydrogen ions out of cells; however, in neonatal rabbits recovering from hypoxic acidosis, the administration of bicarbonate increased both arterial pH and intracellular brain pH as measured by nuclear magnetic resonance spectroscopy.[125,126] Likewise, in rats, intracellular brain adenosine triphosphate concentration did not change during severe intracellular acidosis in the brain produced by extreme hypercapnia.[126] In a separate animal study, bicarbonate slowed the rate of decrease of both arterial and cerebral pH during prolonged CPR, suggesting that the blood-brain pH gradient is maintained during CPR.[127] Given the potentially deleterious effects of bicarbonate administration, its use should be *limited to cases in which there is a specific indication*.

CALCIUM

Calcium administration during CPR should be restricted to those with a specific indication for calcium (e.g., hypocalcemia, hyperkalemia, hypermagnesemia, and calcium channel blocker overdose).[128] These restrictions are based on the possibility that exogenously administered calcium may worsen ischemia-reperfusion injury. Intracellular calcium overload occurs during cerebral ischemia by the influx of calcium through voltage-dependent and agonist-dependent (e.g., N-methyl-D-aspartate [NMDA]) calcium channels. Calcium plays an important role in the process of cell death in many organs, possibly by activation of intracellular enzymes such as nitric oxide synthase, phospholipase A and C, and others.[129]

The calcium ion is essential in myocardial excitation-contraction coupling, in increasing ventricular contractility, and in enhancing ventricular automaticity during asystole. Ionized hypocalcemia is associated with decreased ventricular performance and the peripheral blunting of the hemodynamic response to catecholamines.[130,131] Severe ionized hypocalcemia has been documented in adults suffering from out-of-hospital cardiac arrest[131] and in animals during prolonged CPR.[132] Children at risk for ionized hypocalcemia should be identified and treated as expeditiously as possible. Both total and ionized hypocalcemia may occur in children with either chronic or acute disease. Ionized hypocalcemia also occurs during massive or rapid transfusion of blood products (particularly whole blood and fresh frozen plasma, see Fig. 10.11) because citrate and other preservatives in stored blood products rapidly bind calcium. Because of this effect, ionized hypocalcemia is a known cause of cardiac arrest in the operating room and should be treated immediately with calcium chloride or calcium gluconate (see Chapter 10 and Figs. 10.10 and 10.11). The magnitude of hypocalcemia in this setting depends on the rate and volume of blood products administered and the hepatic and renal function of the child.

Administration of fresh frozen plasma at a rate ≥ 1 mL/kg per minute decreases the ionized calcium concentration in anesthetized children.[133]

The pediatric dose for resuscitation is of calcium chloride 20 mg/kg and or calcium gluconate 60 mg/kg with a maximum dose for both of 2 grams. Calcium gluconate is as effective as calcium chloride in increasing the ionized calcium concentration (see Fig. 10.10).[134,135] Calcium should be given slowly through a large-bore, free-flowing intravenous cannula, or preferably a central venous line. When administered too rapidly, calcium may cause bradycardia, heart block, or ventricular standstill. Severe tissue necrosis occurs when calcium infiltrates into subcutaneous tissue.

Observational studies examining the administration of calcium during cardiac arrest demonstrated worse survival and reduced return of spontaneous circulation with calcium administration.[136,137] Calcium administration is not recommended for pediatric cardiopulmonary arrest in the absence of documented hypocalcemia, calcium channel blocker overdose, hypermagnesemia, or hyperkalemia (class III, level of evidence B). Routine calcium administration in cardiac arrest provides no benefit and may be harmful.[119,137,138]

GLUCOSE

The administration of glucose during CPR should be restricted to children with documented hypoglycemia because of the possible detrimental effects of hyperglycemia on the brain during or after ischemia. The mechanism by which hyperglycemia exacerbates ischemic neurologic injury may be an increased production of lactic acid in the brain by anaerobic metabolism. During ischemia under normoglycemic conditions, brain lactate concentration reaches a plateau. In a hyperglycemic milieu, however, brain lactate concentration continues to increase for the duration of the ischemic period.[139]

Clinical studies have shown a direct correlation between the initial serum glucose concentration after cardiac arrest and poor neurologic outcome,[140–143] although the greater glucose concentration may be a marker rather than a cause of more severe brain injury.[141] However, given the likelihood of additional ischemic and hypoxic events in the post-resuscitation period, it seems prudent to maintain serum glucose concentrations within the normal range. The benefit from tight control of serum glucose after cardiac arrest over risk of iatrogenic hypoglycemia is uncertain. Some groups of children, including preterm infants and debilitated children with small endogenous glycogen stores, are more prone to developing hypoglycemia during and after a physiologic stress such as surgery. Bedside monitoring of the serum glucose concentration is critical during and after a cardiac arrest and allows for the opportunity to administer glucose before the critical point of small substrate delivery has been reached. The dose of glucose generally needed to correct hypoglycemia is 0.5 g/kg given as 5 mL/kg of 10% dextrose in infants or 1 mL/kg of 50% dextrose in an older child. The osmolarity of 50% dextrose is approximately 2700 mOsm/L and has been associated with intraventricular hemorrhage in neonates and infants; a more dilute concentration is recommended in infants.

AMIODARONE

Early reports on the use of oral amiodarone in children were favorable.[144–146] However, recent data on amiodarone have been limited to case reports and descriptive case series. Nevertheless, it is now used widely for serious pediatric arrhythmias in the nonresuscitation environment. It appears to be effective, with an acceptable short-term safety profile.

The pharmacology of amiodarone is complex and may explain its wide range of usefulness. It is primarily classified as a Vaughn-Williams class III agent that blocks the adenosine triphosphate–sensitive outward potassium channels, causing prolongation of the action potential and refractory period; however, this effect requires intracellular accumulation. After intravenous loading, the antiarrhythmic effects of amiodarone are primarily due to noncompetitive α- and β-adrenergic receptor blockade, calcium channel blockade, and effects on inward sodium current, causing a decrease in anterograde conduction across the atrioventricular node and an increase in the effective atrioventricular refractory period. The α-adrenergic blockade leads to vasodilation, which may increase coronary blood flow. It is poorly absorbed orally, requiring intravenous loading in urgent situations. The full antiarrhythmic impact requires a loading period of up to 1 to 3 weeks to achieve intracellular concentrations and full potassium channel–blocking effects.

Hypotension is commonly reported with intravenous bolus administration and may limit the rate at which the drug can be given. However, the development of hypotension is less common with the aqueous formulation.[147] The overall hemodynamic impact of intravenous administration will depend on the balance of its effect on rate control, myocardial performance, and vasodilation. Dosage recommendations for children are based on limited clinical studies. The dose is extrapolated from data on adults; 5 mg/kg intravenously is used for life-threatening arrhythmias. This dose can be repeated if necessary to control the arrhythmia. Intravenous loading doses are followed by a continuous infusion of 10 to 20 mg/kg per day if there is a risk that the arrhythmia will recur. The ideal rate of a bolus administration is unclear; once it has been diluted, it is given as an intravenous push in adults. Amiodarone is best administered over 20 to 60 minutes to avoid profound vasodilation. We recommend a slow intravenous push (2 to 3 minutes) for pulseless ventricular tachycardia or ventricular fibrillation until the arrhythmia is controlled and then a slower bolus (up to 10 minutes) for the remainder of the dose. An alternative dosing regimen for children is a 1 mg/kg by intravenous push every 5 minutes up to 5 mg/kg. The use of the small aliquot bolus technique may be particularly appropriate for infants younger than 12 months of age.

Amiodarone-induced torsades de pointes has been described.[148] The use of amiodarone should be avoided in combination with other drugs that prolong the QT interval, as well as in the setting of hypomagnesemia and other electrolyte abnormalities that predispose to torsades de pointes. Severe bradycardia and heart block have also been described, especially in the postoperative period, and ventricular pacing wires are recommended in this setting. Both amiodarone and inhalation anesthetic agents prolong the QT interval; however, no specific data exist to evaluate the use of amiodarone for ventricular arrhythmias in children receiving inhalation anesthetics. It would seem prudent to be especially vigilant for this adverse effect in this circumstance.

Noncardiac adverse effects are often seen, especially with chronic dosing.[149] The most serious of these is interstitial pneumonitis seen most commonly in patients with preexisting lung disease.[150] The incidence in children is unknown. Rarely, an acute illness similar to acute respiratory distress syndrome has been reported in both infants and adults at the initiation of treatment.[151] The lung disease may remit with early discontinuation of the drug. Hypothyroidism, hepatotoxicity, photosensitivity, and corneal opacities are also reported with chronic use.[149]

The 2005 and 2010 pediatric advanced life support guidelines recommend administering amiodarone in place of lidocaine to manage ventricular fibrillation and pulseless ventricular tachycardia. Paradoxically, an observational study demonstrated that the return of spontaneous circulation after lidocaine was superior to that after amiodarone.[152] A recent study concluded that there was no significant difference in clinical outcomes between those receiving lidocaine compared with those receiving amiodarone.[153] There was no association between lidocaine or amiodarone use and the odds of survival to hospital discharge. Consequently, the 2015 and 2020 pediatric cardiac arrest algorithm[31,154] reflects the change in recommendation that either lidocaine or amiodarone can be used for refractory ventricular fibrillation or pulseless ventricular tachycardia.

LIDOCAINE

Lidocaine is a class IB antiarrhythmic that decreases automaticity of pacemaker tissue that prevents or terminates ventricular arrhythmias because of accelerated ectopic foci. Lidocaine abolishes reentrant ventricular arrhythmias by decreasing the action potential duration and the conduction time of Purkinje fibers and increases the effective refractory period of Purkinje fibers, reducing the nonuniformity of contraction. Lidocaine has no effect on atrioventricular nodal conduction time, so it is ineffective in the treatment of atrial or atrioventricular junctional arrhythmias. In healthy adults, no change in heart rate or blood pressure occurs with lidocaine administration. In patients with cardiac disease there may be a slight decrease in ventricular function when a lidocaine bolus is administered intravenously.

In children with normal cardiac and hepatic function, an initial intravenous bolus of 1 mg/kg of lidocaine is given, followed by a continuous intravenous infusion at a rate of 20 to 50 μg/kg per minute. If the arrhythmia recurs, a second intravenous bolus at the same dose can be given. In children with severely decreased cardiac output, a bolus of no greater than 0.75 mg/kg may be administered followed by an infusion at the rate of 10 to 20 μg/kg per minute. In children with severe hepatic disease and reduced hepatic blood flow, dosages should be decreased by 50%. Children with renal insufficiency have normal lidocaine pharmacokinetics; however, the active toxic metabolite (monoethylglycinexylidide) may accumulate in children receiving infusions over a long period and affect sodium channels. In children with hypoproteinemia, the dose of lidocaine also should be reduced because of the increase in free fraction of the drug.

Toxic effects of lidocaine may occur when the serum concentration exceeds 7 to 8 μg/mL. These effects include seizures, psychosis, drowsiness, paresthesias, disorientation, agitation, tinnitus, muscle spasms, and respiratory arrest. The treatment of choice for lidocaine-induced seizures is a benzodiazepine (midazolam or lorazepam) or a barbiturate (e.g., phenobarbital); chronic therapy also increases the hepatic metabolism of lidocaine.[155] Conversion of second-degree heart block to complete heart block has been described,[156] as has severe sinus bradycardia. Either lidocaine or amiodarone may be used in ventricular fibrillation or pulseless ventricular tachycardia.[152,153]

Special Cardiac Arrest Situations

PERIOPERATIVE CARDIAC ARREST

The incidence, causes, and risk factors associated with anesthesia- and operative-related cardiac arrest have been evaluated by the Pediatric Perioperative Cardiac Arrest registry.[157,158] Cardiovascular causes of cardiac arrest were the most common (41% of all arrests), with hypovolemia from blood loss and hyperkalemia from transfusion of stored blood the most common identifiable cardiovascular causes. Among respiratory causes of arrest (27%), airway obstruction from laryngospasm and bronchospasm was the most common cause.[159] Vascular injury incurred during placement of central venous catheters was the most common equipment-related cause of arrest. The cause of arrest varied by phase of anesthesia care.

Cardiac arrest in the operating room should have the greatest potential for a successful outcome, because it is a witnessed arrest with virtually instantaneous availability of skilled personnel, monitoring equipment, resuscitative equipment, and medications. Whenever a cardiac arrest occurs in the operating room, the circumstances causing the arrest should be rapidly determined. The circumstances of the arrest may provide a clue as to the cause, such as hyperkalemia after succinylcholine administration or rapid blood transfusion; hypocalcemia during a rapid infusion of fresh frozen plasma or large blood transfusion; or a sudden fall in $ETCO_2$ indicating air, blood clot, or tumor embolism. The most important causes of bradyarrhythmia are first, hypoxemia, second, an anesthetic overdose (real or relative), and third, a vagal reflex caused by surgical or airway manipulation. Administering 100% oxygen and establishing adequate ventilation should be the first maneuvers to implement, regardless of the cause of the bradycardia. In reflex-induced bradycardia, atropine may be the first drug of choice, but in extreme cases of bradycardia, whatever the mechanism, epinephrine is preferred in place of atropine. Hypotension and a low cardiac output state must be rapidly corrected by administration of intravenous fluids, vasopressors, and adequate chest compressions to circulate drugs to have the desired clinical effect. Once chest compressions are required, the standard American Heart Association recommendations for CPR apply and these include the frequent administration of epinephrine, with the goal to administer the first dose within 5 minutes of cardiac arrest.[154] Fig. 38.5 presents an algorithm for the differential diagnosis and treatment of the more common causes of acute operating room–associated cardiac dysfunction.

HYPERKALEMIA

A child with a hyperkalemic cardiac arrest may be identified by history, by the progression of ECG changes leading up to the arrest (Fig. 7.7), or by initial laboratory results. A high index of suspicion must be maintained for hyperkalemia as a cause of cardiac arrest because it requires specific therapy. Along with the usual resuscitation algorithms, immediate therapy to antagonize the acute effects of the increased serum potassium concentration on the myocardial cells is necessary to reestablish sinus rhythm. Calcium gluconate or calcium chloride antagonizes the effects of hyperkalemia on the myocardial cell membrane by increasing the threshold potential so that the gap between the threshold potential and the resting membrane potential is reestablished, curtailing the depolarization of random myocardial cells. Sodium bicarbonate and hyperventilation increase the serum pH and shift potassium from the extracellular to the intracellular compartments, and insulin (with concomitant dextrose) shifts potassium intracellularly (0.1 U/kg of insulin with 0.5 grams/kg of dextrose; 2 mL/kg of dextrose 25%). The serum potassium concentration must be monitored frequently during this treatment, preferably by point-of-care testing. Because these therapies simply shift potassium intracellularly, therapy to remove potassium from the body (furosemide, hemodialysis, sodium polystyrene sulfonate) should be instituted (see Chapter 26, Table 26.6).

ANAPHYLAXIS

Anaphylaxis is a rare, but usually reversible, cause of cardiac arrest. Classic anaphylaxis is defined by the triad of dermatologic (usually flushing, pallor, or urticaria), respiratory (airway edema and possible obstruction and bronchospasm), and cardiovascular signs. Anaphylaxis may be particularly severe in situations of decreased endogenous catecholamines, such as in a child taking β-blockers or in children receiving spinal or epidural anesthesia.

Resuscitation of the child with anaphylaxis rests on reversing airway obstruction and restoring intravascular volume and vascular tone. In the child with mild anaphylaxis (as manifested by mild bronchospasm and hypotension), epinephrine 1 to 2 μg/kg intravenous in repeated doses should be given until signs abate. In the child in cardiac arrest from anaphylaxis, the dose of epinephrine should be 10 μg/kg or 0.01 mL/kg of intravenous or subcutaneous epinephrine (1:1000 concentration). Some may require a continuous infusion of both epinephrine and neo-synephrine to maintain a stable blood pressure. Children with anaphylactic shock have profound intravascular depletion requiring rapidly administered, large-volume fluid resuscitation (20-mL/kg boluses of balanced salt solutions). In addition to the usual resuscitation medications, treatment should include an antihistamine and corticosteroid, such as diphenhydramine 1 mg/kg, and methylprednisolone 2 mg/kg. Intravenous and, to a lesser extent, inhaled bronchodilators such as albuterol/salbutamol may help relieve the bronchospasm. If severe airway obstruction occurs, tracheal intubation or even cricothyroidotomy may become difficult or impossible. Therefore, the airway should be secured by a skilled practitioner early in the course of the reaction.

SUPRAVENTRICULAR TACHYCARDIA

Supraventricular tachycardia, despite being a common arrhythmia in infants and children, is uncommon during the intraoperative period in children without cardiac disease.[160] Supraventricular tachycardia may be associated with severe circulatory compromise or even cardiac arrest. Therapy for this arrhythmia should be based on the child's hemodynamic status. Supraventricular tachycardia associated with inadequate circulation should be treated immediately with synchronized cardioversion beginning at a dose of 0.5 J/kg. If intravenous access is available, adenosine can be administered while cardioversion is being prepared; however, cardioversion should not be delayed to establish intravenous access.

Adenosine is the medical treatment of choice for supraventricular tachycardia. The underlying mechanism in children is usually a reentry circuit involving the atrioventricular node. Adenosine causes a temporary block in the atrioventricular node and interrupts this reentry circuit. The initial dose is 0.1 mg/kg given as a rapid intravenous bolus. Central venous administration is preferable because the drug is rapidly metabolized by red blood cell adenosine deaminase and therefore has a half-life of only 10 seconds. When the drug is given peripherally, the intravenous line should be immediately and rapidly flushed with 10 mL of saline. If there is no interruption in the reentry circuit, successive doses of 0.2 and 0.4 mg/kg should be given. In neonates, a smaller initial dose of 0.05 mg/kg is given and increased by 0.05 mg/kg per dose until termination of the arrhythmia up to a maximum dose of 0.3 mg/kg.[161] When supraventricular tachycardia appears without any circulatory compromise, conversion of the arrhythmia may first be attempted with a vagal maneuver such as ice to the face. If this is ineffective, then adenosine should be used. *Note that the denervated transplanted heart is extremely sensitive to the atrioventricular blockade and that half the normal starting dose is recommended.*

Other medications used to treat supraventricular tachycardia have a greater incidence of adverse effects than adenosine. Digoxin is often ineffective and causes frequent arrhythmias. Verapamil should be avoided in infants because of its association with congestive heart failure and cardiac arrest because of its negative inotropic effects.[162] Flecainide is effective in treating supraventricular tachycardia but has many cardiac and noncardiac adverse effects[163]; its role for hemodynamically unstable supraventricular tachycardia remains to be established. Other therapies include β-adrenergic blockers, edrophonium, and α-agonists. If supraventricular tachycardia persists despite medical therapy and the child progresses to circulatory instability, electrical cardioversion should proceed immediately.

PULSELESS ELECTRICAL ACTIVITY

Pulseless electrical activity is defined as organized ECG activity, excluding ventricular tachycardia and fibrillation, without clinical evidence of a palpable pulse or myocardial contractions. It may occur spontaneously after cardiac arrest or as an intervening rhythm associated with treatment for cardiac arrest. The causes of pulseless electrical activity are divided into primary (cardiac) and secondary (noncardiac) causes. Primary pulseless electrical activity, associated with cardiac arrest, is due to depletion of myocardial energy stores and responds poorly to therapy. Drugs used to treat primary pulseless electrical activity include epinephrine, atropine, calcium, and sodium bicarbonate.

The causes of secondary pulseless electrical activity are often remembered using the 4 Hs and 4 Ts mnemonic: **H**ypovolemia, **H**ypoxia, **H**ypothermia, and **H**ypo- or **H**yper-electrolytemia (e.g., hyperkalemia, hypocalcemia), **T**ension pneumothorax, pericardial **T**amponade, **T**hromboembolism, and **T**oxins (anesthetic overdose). In secondary pulseless electrical activity, intervention is directed at the underlying disorder and usually results in a successful resuscitation. When the cause of pulseless electrical activity is unknown and the child does not respond to medications, giving a fluid bolus and inserting needles into the pleural space to rule out pneumothorax and into the pericardial space to rule out cardiac tamponade are recommended.

Adjunctive Cardiopulmonary Resuscitation Techniques

OPEN-CHEST CARDIOPULMONARY RESUSCITATION

The use of open-chest cardiac massage, although generally replaced by closed-chest CPR, still has an active role in the operating room and ICU, especially during and after thoracic surgery. Compared with closed-chest CPR, open-chest CPR generates greater cardiac output and vital organ blood flow. During open-chest CPR, the intrathoracic, right atrial, and intracranial pressures increase to a lesser extent, resulting in greater coronary and cerebral perfusion pressure and greater myocardial and cerebral blood flow compared with closed-chest CPR.[164–166]

Typically, in the operating room and ICU, open-chest CPR is preferable to closed-chest CPR in the child who has had a recent sternotomy. Open-chest CPR is also indicated for selected children when closed-chest CPR has failed, although exactly which children should receive this method of resuscitation under this condition is controversial. When initiated early after failure of closed-chest CPR, open-chest CPR may improve outcome.[167–169]

When performed after 15 minutes of closed-chest CPR, open-chest CPR significantly improves coronary perfusion pressure and the rate of successful resuscitation.[170] It has been reported that 50% of patients who received open-chest CPR during resuscitation for an in-hospital cardiac arrest had a favorable neurologic outcome when evaluated one year after the event.[171]

EXTRACORPOREAL MEMBRANE OXYGENATION

Extracorporeal cardiopulmonary bypass may be considered for refractory pediatric cardiac arrest when the condition leading to arrest is reversible and when the period of no flow (cardiac arrest without CPR) was brief. This intervention depends on the institution's ability to rapidly mobilize an extracorporeal circuit. Survival with a good neurologic outcome is possible after more than 50 minutes of CPR in selected children by using extracorporeal cardiopulmonary bypass.[172,173] Emergency extracorporeal membrane oxygenation in children with in-hospital CPR 10 minutes or longer in duration has been associated with improved survival to hospital discharge and survival with favorable neurologic outcome compared with failed conventional CPR (see Chapter 19).[174] It has also been reported that there is a 58% survival rate for pediatric cardiac patients requiring extracorporeal membrane oxygenation support, with an even greater survival rate (89%) in pediatric patients with cardiomyopathy.[175] Cardiopulmonary bypass techniques such as extracorporeal membrane oxygenation require major technical support and sophistication but can be rapidly implemented in hospitals set up to do so. However, absence of a formal rapid deployment extracorporeal membrane oxygenation team does not preclude resuscitation with extracorporeal membrane oxygenation in pediatric cardiac patients with good results.[176]

ACTIVE COMPRESSION-DECOMPRESSION

Active compression-decompression CPR uses a negative-pressure "pull" on the thorax during the release phase of chest compression using a handheld suction device. This technique improves vascular pressures and minute ventilation during CPR in animals and humans.[177–181] The hemodynamic benefit of this technique is attributed to increased venous return by the negative intrathoracic pressure generated during the decompression phase. When this technique was used with a device adding impedance to inspiration, vascular pressures and flow increased further.[182] Its effectiveness in adults shows promise, with increased survival and weak evidence for neurologic improvement in prehospital victims.[183–185] However, larger trials did not demonstrate improved survival in in-hospital or prehospital victims of cardiac arrest, nor did any subgroup demonstrate benefit from active compression-decompression CPR.[186–188] The complication rate, including fatal rib and sternal fractures, may be greater with this technique.[189]

Post-Resuscitation Stabilization (Post–Cardiac Arrest Care)

Negovsky and Gurvitch in 1995 first proposed the term "post resuscitation disease" to refer to central nervous system and systemic pathological processes resulting from hypoxia-ischemia and occurring during recovery.[190] Neumar et al. described the cellular and pathophysiological inflammatory response in post–cardiac arrest syndrome.[191] Brain injury, myocardial dysfunction, systemic ischemia and reperfusion response, and persistent inciting pathology are the elements of the post–cardiac arrest syndrome.[191,192]

The goals of post-resuscitation care are to prevent secondary organ injury, preserve neurologic function, diagnose and treat the cause of the illness, and prevent a recurrence of the arrest. Respiratory support should be tailored to minimize the risk of oxidative damage while maintaining adequate oxygen delivery. FiO_2 should be limited to the minimum necessary to maintain an adequate saturation. Ventilation should be closely monitored because both hypercarbia and hypocarbia may confer deleterious effects.

Blood pressure and telemetry monitoring along with specific hemodynamic goals to maintain systolic blood pressures greater than fifth percentile for age and sex should be maintained using fluid resuscitation with or without vasopressor or inotropes.[192] Temperature monitoring along with preventing and treating fever promptly after arrest is vital and related to improved outcomes. Mitigation of neurologic injury after cardiac arrest has been a goal of many investigator groups. In adult patients with out-of-hospital ventricular fibrillation and in asphyxiated newborns,[84] therapeutic hypothermia was believed to offer some benefit. However, the effectiveness of hypothermia therapy was neither supported nor refuted in a retrospective study.[193] A target temperature of 36°C proved better than 33°C in adults.[194] Similar results have been reported in children. Therapeutic hypothermia in children did not confer a significant benefit in survival with a good functional outcome at 1 year.[85] Hyperthermia should be avoided.

The 2020 AHA Pediatric Advanced Life Support Guidelines Update

Current guidelines suggest that focus should be placed on providing 1 breath every 2 to 3 seconds during pediatric CPR, which is 20 to 30 breaths per minute.[31] Placement of a cuffed tracheal tube is thought to be more advantageous than an uncuffed tracheal tube. Routine use of cricoid pressure when placing a tracheal tube has been shown to decrease the rate of success and is no longer recommended. Early administration of epinephrine (described as within 5 minutes of initiation of CPR) is recommended. Using diastolic blood pressure as a guide to effective CPR is recommended, noting that diastolic blood pressure is the driver for coronary blood flow.[31]

Cardiopulmonary resuscitation of children with a nonnative airway should use $ETCO_2$ carbon-dioxide monitoring as a surrogate for effective compressions. This is of relevance for the perioperative physician as patients should have $ETCO_2$ monitoring as part of their routine anesthetic care. Attention should focus on an adequate depth and frequency of compressions with sufficient recoil. The compressor should be monitored for fatigue and rapid change of practitioners (~every 2 minutes) should be instituted if compressions are judged to be inadequate because of poor technique. Examination of patients for successful return of spontaneous circulation should not occur within the 2-minute epochs of compression as the quality of compressions could be compromised. Compressions should be extended 2 minutes after the confirmation of the return of spontaneous circulation.

ANNOTATED REFERENCES

Topjian AA, Raymond TT, Atkins D, et al. Part 4: Pediatric Basic and Advanced Life Support: 2020 American Heart Association Guidelines for Cardiopulmonary Resuscitation and Emergency Cardiovascular Care. *Circulation.* 2020;142(16 suppl 2):S469-S523.

This publication provides comprehensive guidelines for pediatric and adult advanced life support with comprehensive references.

Morgan RW, Kirschen MP, Kilbaugh TJ, Sutton RM, Topjian AA. Pediatric in-hospital cardiac arrest and cardiopulmonary resuscitation in the United States: a review. *JAMA Pediatr.* 2021;175:293-302.

Pediatric IHCA occurs frequently and has a high mortality rate. Early identification of risk, prevention, delivery of high-quality CPR, and post–cardiac arrest care can maximize the chances of achieving favorable outcomes.

Lasa JJ, Alali A, Minard CG, et al. Cardiopulmonary resuscitation in the pediatric cardiac catheterization laboratory: a report from the American Heart Association's Get with the Guidelines-Resuscitation Registry. *Pediatr Crit Care Med.* 2019;20:1040-1047.

The majority of children experiencing cardiac arrest in the cardiac catheterization laboratory analysis survived to hospital discharge, with no observable difference in outcomes between surgical and medical cardiac patients. Future investigations that focus on stratifying medical complexity in addition to procedural characteristics at the time of catheterization are needed to better identify risks for mortality after cardiac arrest in the cardiac catheterization laboratory.

A complete reference list can be found online at Elsevier eBooks+.

39

Malignant Hyperthermia

JERROLD LERMAN

Clinical Presentation

Patient Evaluation and Preparation

Monitoring

Pathophysiology and Laboratory Testing

Management of Malignant Hyperthermia

Immediate Management

Dantrolene

Postreaction Follow-Up

Stress-Triggered Malignant Hyperthermia

Genetics

Physiology

Normal Skeletal Muscle: Excitation-Contraction Coupling

Pathophysiology of Malignant Hyperthermia

Molecular Mechanisms and Physiologic Effects of Dantrolene

Laboratory Diagnosis

Contracture Testing

Genetic Testing

Noninvasive Testing

Other Disorders and Malignant Hyperthermia

Myopathic Syndromes

Malignant Hyperthermia Mimics

Neuroleptic Malignant Syndrome

MALIGNANT HYPERTHERMIA IS A PHARMACOGENETIC disease of skeletal muscle that may precipitate a potentially fatal sequence of metabolic responses in the presence of triggering anesthetics. The primary triggers for malignant hyperthermia (MH)—inhalational anesthetics and succinylcholine—induce an uncontrollable release of intramyoplasmic calcium (Ca^{2+}) that results in sustained muscle contractures, which in turn produce a hypermetabolic response. The hypermetabolic response is manifest by hypercarbia, hyperpnea, tachycardia, and if not treated early, a mixed metabolic and respiratory acidosis. An acute reaction is usually accompanied by muscle rigidity either as isolated muscle rigidity (e.g., masseter muscle tetany in the temporomandibular joint) or total body muscle rigidity (e.g., sustained contraction of major peripheral muscle groups) that may be followed by a progressively increasing core body temperature, that if untreated, may exceed 41°C (106°F), resulting in multiorgan failure, brain damage, and death.

MH was first described by Denborough and Lovell in 1960, who reported a 21-year-old man who was hesitant to undergo general anesthesia to repair his fractured leg because family members had died under anesthesia.[1] After 10 minutes of halothane, he became hemodynamically unstable with hypotension, tachycardia, and mottled skin that was hot to the touch. The soda lime canister was found to be hot and was changed because it appeared to be exhausted. The anesthetic was discontinued, the patient was packed in ice, and he recovered without sequelae. Subsequent physical examination and laboratory investigations failed to reveal a medical condition to explain the acute findings. A careful family history, however, disclosed that 10 blood relatives had died after ether anesthesia, suggesting an autosomal dominant inheritance pattern. For a subsequent surgery, this patient received a spinal anesthetic without incident.[2] Consequent reports from around the world established this disorder as a familial disorder that was potentially fatal.[3,4] The term *malignant hyperpyrexia*, which was subsequently changed to *malignant hyperthermia*, was coined in 1967 at the first international meeting on malignant hyperthermia in Toronto, Canada.

The incidence of MH based on the frequency of MH reactions is reported between 1:50,000 and 1:100,000 adults and between 1:3000 and 1:15,000 children.[5,6] Regional differences in the prevalence of MH may account for an even greater frequency of reactions (of all levels of severity) in some jurisdictions—for example, 1:16,000 anesthetics in adults in Denmark and 1:4200 adults when an inhaled anesthetic and succinylcholine were combined.[7] The "best" recent estimate of the incidence of MH in the United Kingdom is 1:250,000 anesthetics.[8] A review of discharge diagnoses from New York state ambulatory centers reported a prevalence of MH of 1:500,000,[9] and a review of almost 10 million inpatient discharges in 4 states found a prevalence of MH of 1.7:100,000 inpatient discharges and 2.4:100,000 surgical inpatient discharges.[10] A survey in a pediatric hospital in the United States during the halothane era revealed an MH incidence of 1:20,000 to 1:40,000 children, almost one-half of that reported previously.[11] The incidence of fulminant MH (defined as a rapid increase in temperature accompanied by life-threatening metabolic changes, arrhythmias, and increased serum creatine kinase level) is estimated to be 1.4:100,000 in the United States (based on 700 MH reactions/year and 50 million anesthetics administered)[12,13] and 0.6:100,000 in the United Kingdom.[8] A survey from Denmark in 1985 reported the incidence of masseter muscle spasm (considered a forme fruste of MH) to be 1:12,000 anesthetics among children who received succinylcholine, whether in combination with inhalational or intravenous (IV) anesthetics.[7] Clinically, the demographic data suggested that the incidence or suspicion of MH was greater among children and young adults than older adults and the elderly, greater in males than females, even greater among children in whom succinylcholine was used, and similar across racial groups.[10,14]

Genetic testing has become sufficiently pervasive to permit estimates of the prevalence of MH in the population based on genetic mutations to be between 1:3000 and 1:8500.[15] One report suggested a prevalence as great as 1:200 to 1:400 individuals in the Manawatu region of New Zealand.[15,16] This high prevalence was possibly contributed by a Danish sailor who carried the genetic mutation and was stationed on a whale station in that region in the early 1800s. The frequency of MH reactions is greatest in childhood (up to 52% of acute MH reactions), with a peak age of 3 years, with the youngest confirmed cases with acute reactions and genetic testing reported in early infancy.[17–20] In one case, a known genetic mutation (G2434R) consistent with the diagnosis of MH was identified in the cord blood of a neonate born to an MH-susceptible parturient with the same mutation, although a reaction did not occur during the birth.[21]

Many believe that the incidence of acute MH reactions has decreased in the past 2 decades because (1) families with a genetic predisposition to MH have been identified and patients bring it to the attention of their surgical and anesthetic care providers preoperatively and (2) the routine use of succinylcholine has decreased dramatically as a result of concerns of rare complications, such as hyperkalemic cardiac arrest. The latter resulted in a black box warning from the FDA admonishing against the routine use of succinylcholine in children during elective surgery, particularly male children younger than 8 years of age who may have unrecognized muscular dystrophy or other myopathy.[22,23] Whether true or not, some have challenged the notion that the frequency of MH reactions is decreasing.[24]

All inhalational anesthetics (except xenon) and succinylcholine trigger MH reactions in susceptible patients[25–31]; no other drugs used for IV or regional anesthesia trigger MH reactions. A comprehensive list of triggering and nontriggering drugs is available from the Malignant Hyperthermia Association of the United States (MHAUS; https://www.mhaus.org/).

The mortality rate from MH reactions in patients of all ages has decreased dramatically from more than 80% in the 1960s to ~5% or less more recently (Fig. 39.1)[24,32–35]; the mortality rate in children is only 0.7%, (20-fold <adults), but 11% to 14% based on an inpatient database.[10,24] A report of the National Inpatient Sample and the Kid's Inpatient Database between 1988 and 2010 yielded a 2.9% mortality rate in children <18 years of age, a rate between the two previous mortality rates for MH in children (0.7% and 4.6%).[36,37] The overall mortality rate in children from MH reactions in Japan between 1960 and 2020 was 15.5%, whereas the mortality between 2000 and 2020 was lower (8.8%), despite using dantrolene in 78% of reactions.[38] This lower mortality rate over the later epoch has been attributed to several factors: better identification of MH-susceptible individuals; the routine use of perioperative capnography and pulse oximetry to identify an evolving MH reaction[39,40]; a better understanding of the pathogenesis of MH; and the widespread availability and use of dantrolene early in the reaction.[41]

Clinical Presentation

The most common presentation of MH is a hypermetabolic response to an inhalational anesthetic, with or without concomitant succinylcholine (Table 39.1). Among the earliest and most frequent clinical signs of MH is a steadily increasing end-tidal carbon dioxide (ETCO$_2$) that occurred in 92% of MH reactions in the MHAUS summary of clinical events.[14] Hypercarbia persists despite attempts to control and reduce it by increasing ventilation either mechanically or intrinsically during spontaneous respiration by increasing the respiratory rate and tidal volume.[34,42] Tachycardia is another early sign of MH that occurred in 73% of

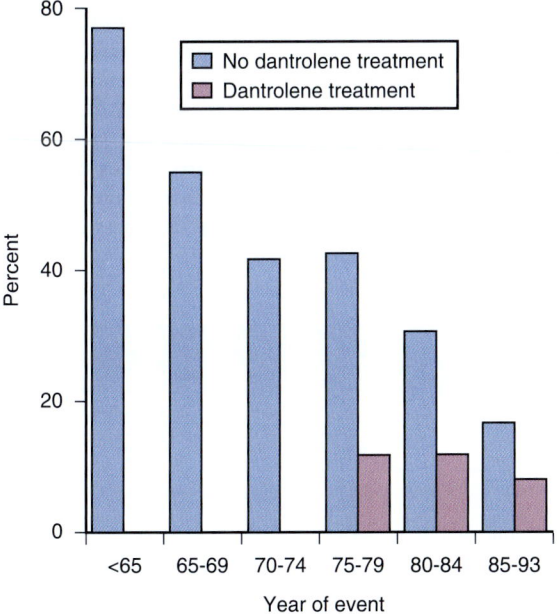

FIGURE 39.1 The trend in fatality rates from malignant hyperthermia is shown over time. The *blue bars* represent data from 361 patients, and the *magenta bars* represent data from 142 patients. Notice the marked decrease in mortality with dantrolene treatment. (Modified from Strazis KP, Fox AW. Malignant hyperthermia: a review of published cases. *Anesth Analg.* 1993;77[2]:297-304.)

TABLE 39.1	Clinical and Laboratory Findings in an Acute Malignant Hyperthermia Reaction
Clinical Findings	**Laboratory Findings**
Temperature, tachycardia, tachypnea, and hypertension	Increasing heart rate, respiratory rate, and blood pressure; increased temperature is a late finding
Hypercarbia (ETCO$_2$)	Increasing PaCO$_2$
Greatly increased minute ventilation	Acidosis (mixed respiratory and metabolic)
Hemoglobin desaturation	Relative hypoxia, increased alveolar to arterial partial pressure gradient for oxygen
Generalized muscle rigidity (unresponsive to nondepolarizing muscle relaxants)	Hyperkalemia Increased CK level (usually a late sign) Increased plasma lactate concentration
Skin mottling	
Hyperthermia (late sign)	
Cardiac arrhythmias (hyperkalemia-induced: PVC, VT, VF)	
Cola-colored urine (late sign)	Myoglobinuria, myoglobinemia
Disseminated intravascular coagulation (late)	Abnormal coagulation studies (late sign)

CK, Creatine kinase; *ETCO$_2$,* end-tidal carbon dioxide; *PaCO$_2$,* arterial partial pressure of carbon dioxide; *PVC,* premature ventricular contraction; *VF,* ventricular fibrillation; *VT,* ventricular tachycardia.
Data from Malignant Hyperthermia Association of the United States. https://www.mhaus.org.

patients in the MHAUS database.[14] Severe masseter muscle spasm (i.e., masseter muscle rigidity), a very early sign that occurs immediately after administration of succinylcholine, is the **inability** to insert a laryngoscope blade into the mouth—the so-called "jaws of steel"—despite a zero twitch response on the train-of-four monitor. Masseter muscle rigidity only occurred in 27% of cases of MH in the MHAUS database although it was likely the reason the time from induction of anesthesia to diagnosis of the MH reaction was 0 minutes in 5/6 cases.[14] Although many clinicians regard this finding as strongly suggestive of MH susceptibility (Fig. 39.2), an attempt to correlate DNA with patients who had had in vitro contracture testing found no link between the severity of masseter muscle rigidity and MH susceptibility.[43] The differential diagnosis of severe masseter spasm should include the possible presence of the ultrarapid polymorphism of pseudocholinesterase, the C5 (E Cynthiana or Neitlich) variant (see Chapter 5), which terminates the action of succinylcholine more rapidly than usual.[44] In vitro live muscle biopsy testing revealed a 28% to 50% incidence of MH susceptibility among children with jaws of steel, with an extensive differential diagnosis (Table 39.2).[45–47] Generalized skeletal muscle rigidity develops as a result of the excessive accumulation of myoplasmic Ca^{2+} concentrations in MH-susceptible skeletal muscle exposed to the triggers, resulting in sustained muscle contractures; this was reported in only 41% of MH reactions in the MHAUS database.[42] This small incidence of skeletal rigidity may have resulted from the early diagnosis and intervention with dantrolene. Nonetheless, skeletal muscle rigidity will occur even in the presence of neuromuscular blockade with nondepolarizing neuromuscular blocking drugs.

Hyperthermia, often reported as a late sign of an MH reaction, results from the greatly increased aerobic and anaerobic metabolic activity of contracted skeletal muscle; core temperature rapidly and steadily increases as the reaction progresses unabated, a finding in 65% of MH cases in the MHAUS database. The overlying skin and carbon dioxide absorbent soon become hot to the touch. In many instances, the large muscle groups such as calf or thigh muscles feel tight or knotted.

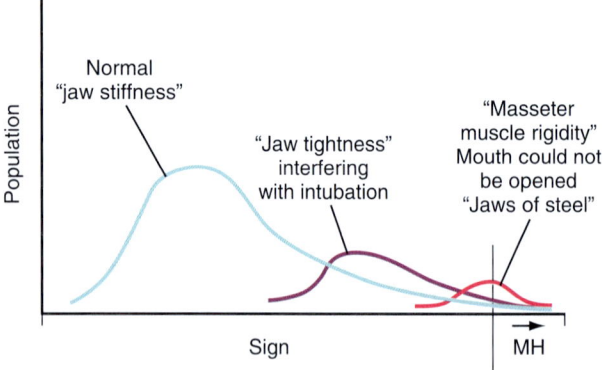

FIGURE 39.2 The spectrum of masseter muscle responses to succinylcholine varies from a slight jaw stiffness that does not interfere with endotracheal intubation to the extreme "jaws of steel," which is masseter muscle tetany that does not allow the mouth to be opened. The latter response is likely highly associated with malignant hyperthermia *(MH)*. Even with the inability to open the mouth, the child's lungs should still be able to be ventilated by bag and mask because all other muscles are relaxed. (From Kaplan RF. Malignant hyperthermia. Annual refresher course lectures. Washington, DC: American Society of Anesthesiologists; 1993.)

TABLE 39.2	Limited Excursion of the Mandible: Differential Diagnosis

Temporomandibular joint dysfunction: congenital, inflammatory/infectious, trauma, neoplasm, collagen vascular disease (rheumatoid arthritis)

Muscle disease: malignant hyperthermia, Duchenne or Becker muscular dystrophy, myotonia congenita

Integumentary disease: inflammatory or infectious disease, neoplasm, radiation effects, collagen vascular disease (scleroderma)

Neurologic injury

Ultrarapid metabolizer of succinylcholine (Neitlich or E Cynthiana [C5 enzyme] variant of pseudocholinesterase) (see Chapter 5)

Ineffective or expired succinylcholine

Serum lactate concentrations also increase rapidly, fueled by the widespread increase in glycogenolysis and glycolysis (i.e., mixed respiratory and metabolic acidosis).[48,49] If an acute MH reaction is diagnosed and treated early before the body becomes unable to sustain this exaggerated aerobic metabolism, arterial blood gases may show an almost pure respiratory acidosis (Table 39.3). A mixed venous or peripheral venous blood gas analysis will demonstrate an increased partial pressure of CO_2, but more importantly there will be significant oxygen desaturation (mixed venous O_2 saturation <40 mm Hg, despite administering supplemental oxygen for which the expected mixed venous O_2 saturation should be >60%), consistent with increased metabolism and oxygen consumption.

In fulminant, untreated cases, the rate of increase of the core temperature may be as rapid as 1°C every 10 minutes.[42] In one case, the temperature reached 43.8°C (110.8°F) within 18 minutes of the onset of the reaction.[50] In addition to the profound hypercarbia and tachycardia, if not rapidly treated with dantrolene, severe hypoxia, skin mottling, exuberant metabolic acidosis, rhabdomyolysis, coagulopathy, and hyperkalemia may follow, progressing to cardiovascular instability, ventricular arrhythmias, pulmonary edema, disseminated intravascular coagulation, cerebral hypoxia or edema, and renal failure; the latter is caused by the deposition of myoglobin in the renal tubules which is often associated with fatal outcomes.

TABLE 39.3	Arterial Blood Gas Data From a Child in Early Malignant Hyperthermia

	TIME AT MEASUREMENT			
Data	08:52	08:59	09:05	09:27
pH[a]	7.34	7.03	7.29	7.39
$PaCO_2$ (mm Hg)	46.3	109.4	47.9	42.7
PaO_2 (mm Hg)	236	159	589	635
Base excess	−1	−2	−3	1
HCO_3 (mmol/L)	25.1	29	23.1	25.6

[a]Notice the pure respiratory acidosis in this patient from Fig. 39.3 and the rapid decrease in $PaCO_2$ after dantrolene administration between 08:59 hours and 09:05 hours. (Corresponds to ~60 minutes in Fig. 39.3.)
$PaCO_2$, Arterial partial pressure of carbon dioxide; PaO_2, partial pressure of oxygen.

Before dantrolene was available to stop acute MH reactions, and even today in locations where dantrolene is unavailable, early, aggressive, symptomatic treatment is the mainstay of therapy. A review of cases from China where medications specific for MH are not available found 92 cases between 1985 and 2020; the vast majority had received succinylcholine (76 of 92).[51] Interestingly the majority of cases (78%) were male, presenting symptoms were increased expired CO_2 ($\sim$34%), increased heart rate ($\sim$25%), rapidly increasing temperature ($\sim$20%) and masseter spasm ($\sim$11%); the incidence of desaturation, reduced or elevated blood pressure, muscle rigidity, and many others was <5%. Arterial CO_2 values as great as 152 mm Hg, heart rates as great as 190 beats per minute, creatine kinase (CK) levels reaching 440,000 U/L, and temperature to 43.1°C were recorded with a mortality rate of 42%. Interventions to treat were not detailed in this report but likely included the classic treatment of the acidosis and hyperkalemia with bicarbonate, using insulin with glucose and active cooling with iced saline solution gastric lavage and infusion of cold IV saline solutions. In the past, infusions of procainamide were advocated but subsequently have been shown to be ineffective. These interventions reduce the mortality rate from more than 80% in the past to 36% to 42% more recently.[51] With MH-specific treatment, mortality is dramatically decreased to less than 5%.[36,52,53]

The natural course of acute MH reactions is variable, ranging from an immediate onset of muscle rigidity with induction of anesthesia to an insidious, and slow onset of symptoms commencing postoperatively; a course that has become less severe and more insidious as the use of succinylcholine has dwindled and sevoflurane replaced halothane in clinical practice.[54,55] In the MHAUS database of reactions reported between 1987 and 2006, 33% of the 268 reactions reported the first sign suggesting an MH reaction within 30 minutes of induction of anesthesia.[14] Six cases reported the first sign 0 minutes after induction, with five likely from masseter muscle rigidity. In a more recent summary of MH reactions, the (median) time interval from induction of anesthesia to the first presenting signs of an acute MH reaction (see also Table 39.1) was 1.3 hours (range of 0 to 18 hours),[51] although not all features of a classic MH reaction were immediately evident. Reports now attest to these reactions also occurring in awake patients as well as postoperatively, although the latter occurs in only $\sim$2%.[42,56,57] A review of postoperative MH reactions from the MHAUS reported an average onset time of less than 40 minutes after the end of anesthesia.[56,58] The greatest interval between the conclusion of anesthesia and the onset of an MH reaction was >10 hours.[51,58] The likelihood that an MH-susceptible patient will develop MH in the presence of inhalational anesthetics is exasperatingly unpredictable, with some positing that preoperative exercise and/or the presence of a fever account in part for the variability in susceptible MH patients developing acute reactions.[59] In one study, 50% of susceptible individuals reported two or more uneventful general anesthetics before an MH reaction was triggered.[14,34] Only 6.5% of probands in a retrospective review reported a family or personal history of MH.[14] A negative personal or family history is insufficient to conclude that a child is not susceptible to MH. One patient was reported not to trigger until 30 exposures to anesthesia.[60] Other disease states that may be confused with MH (Table 39.4) must be distinguished from it to provide correct therapy.

In a retrospective review of the MH database from Japan between 1960 and 2020, the clinical presentation of MH in 187 children younger than 18 years of age were grouped by age,

TABLE 39.4	Differential Diagnosis of Malignant Hyperthermia
Diagnosis	**Distinguishing Traits**
Hyperthyroidism	Patients often present with similar symptoms and physical findings; blood gas abnormalities gradually evolve; creatine kinase value does not increase substantively
	Unresponsive to dantrolene
Sepsis	Usually, blood gases are normal early, and metabolic acidosis occurs late; creatine kinase remains normal
Pheochromocytoma	Similar to malignant hyperthermia (MH), except for marked blood pressure swings, hypercarbia, and venous desaturation
Metastatic carcinoid	Flushing, diarrhea, hypotension
Cocaine intoxication	Fever, rigidity, rhabdomyolysis similar to NMS
Heat stroke	Similar to MH, except that the patient is outside the operating room, often exercising in a hot environment
Masseter muscle rigidity	May progress to MH; total body spasm more likely than isolated masseter muscle rigidity
Neuroleptic malignant syndrome (NMS)	Similar to MH but evolves over weeks; usually associated with the use of antipsychotics
Serotonergic toxicity	Similar to MH and NMS; associated with the administration of mood-elevating drugs (e.g., selective serotonin reuptake inhibitors)
Non-malignant hyperthermia syndrome	Reported only once; severe hyperthermia seemingly associated with fentanyl

0 to 2 years (n=15), 2 to 12 years (123) and 13 to 18 years (n=49).[38] Three clinical findings of MH occurred in all three age groups: hyperthermia, sinus tachycardia, and respiratory acidosis. The most frequent initial findings in the youngest age group were hyperthermia (47%) and generalized muscle rigidity (27%), in the middle age group were masseter spasm (35%) and generalized muscle rigidity (20%), and in the eldest age group were hypercarbia (26%) and tachycardia (22%).[38] Masseter spasm, generalized muscle rigidity, and dark urine (myoglobinuria) occurred significantly more commonly after succinylcholine.[38] These observations contrast with previous reports that the early warning signs of an MH event were tachycardia and hypercarbia and that hyperthermia was a late sign of an MH reaction.

Given the variability of the clinical presentation of MH and the dearth of pathognomonic signs for this syndrome, establishing the diagnosis can oftentimes be challenging. In response to the need for an objective measure to verify a clinical episode of MH, a retrospective, multivariable clinical grading scale was developed.[61] This grading scale was devised to clarify the cutoff value for a positive muscle caffeine-halothane contracture test (CHCT) result. Although the scale was not intended to be used as a guide to treatment in the operating room and knowing that it is more conservative in its application, Tables 39.5A and 39.5B are provided to assist clinicians identify true MH reactions. Although these clinical grading scales are somewhat cumbersome and have not been prospectively validated in clinical settings for use by nonexperts, they do serve as educational tools for the clinician.

TABLE 39.5A Clinical Indicators for Determining the Malignant Hyperthermia Raw Score

Process	Indicator	Points
Rigidity	Generalized muscular rigidity	15
	Masseter spasm	15
Muscle breakdown	CK >20,000 IU/L after succinylcholine	15
	CK >10,000 IU/L with no succinylcholine	15
	Cola-colored urine in perioperative period	10
	Myoglobin in urine >60 µg/L	5
	Myoglobin in serum >170 µg/L	5
	Blood, plasma, or serum K^+ >6 mEq/L, no renal illness	3
Respiratory acidosis	$PETCO_2$ >55 mm Hg with controlled ventilation	15
	Arterial $PaCO_2$ >60 mm Hg with controlled ventilation	15
	$PETCO_2$ >60 mm Hg with spontaneous ventilation	15
	Arterial $PaCO_2$ >65 mm Hg with spontaneous ventilation	15
	Inappropriate hypercarbia, anesthesiologist's call	15
	Inappropriate tachypnea	10
Temperature increase	Inappropriately rapid increase	15
	Inappropriately increased temperature >38.8°C (101.8°F)	10
Cardiac involvement	Inappropriate sinus tachycardia	3
	Ventricular tachycardia or fibrillation	3
Family history	Positive family history for first-degree relative	15
	Positive family history for more distant relative	5
Others	Arterial base excess more negative than −8 mEq/L	10
	Arterial pH <7.25	10
	Rapid reversal of malignant hyperthermia (MH) signs after intravenous administration of dantrolene	5
	Positive MH family history with another indicator from the patient's anesthesia experience other than increased CK level	10
	Increased CK level and a family history of MH	10

CK, Creatine kinase; *PaCO₂*, arterial partial pressure of carbon dioxide; *PETCO₂*, end-tidal pressure of carbon dioxide.
From Larach MG, Localio AR, Allen GC, et al. A clinical grading scale to predict malignant hyperthermia susceptibility. *Anesthesiology.* 1994;80:771-779.

TABLE 39.5B Malignant Hyperthermia Clinical Grading Scale

Raw Score Range	Rank	Likelihood
0	1	Almost never
3–9	2	Unlikely
10–19	3	Somewhat less than likely
20–34	4	Somewhat greater than likely
35–49	5	Very likely
≥50	6	Almost certain

Modified from Larach MG, Localio AR, Allen GC, et al. A clinical grading scale to predict malignant hyperthermia susceptibility. *Anesthesiology.* 1994;80:771-779.

anesthesia should signal to the surgeon and anesthesiologist to consider MH or another anesthesia-related life-threatening event. These questions assume that the patient is part of a classic nuclear family, but with increasing levels of adoption, artificial insemination, surrogate motherhood, and egg donations, standard probing may not elicit clear family histories. The anesthesiologist must be sensitive but decisive in determining the true genetic relationship between the guardians and the child. Despite attempts to obtain an accurate history, misinterpretation of the questions may occur. In one case, an adopted child died of succinylcholine-induced hyperkalemic cardiac arrest, even though the parents denied that anyone in the family had anesthesia problems or muscle disease during the preoperative assessment. Only immediately after the event did the parents reveal that the child had been adopted and that the child's birth uncle had muscular dystrophy.

If the anesthesiologist is informed that the child has a blood relative who had an MH reaction or who has a myopathy with high concordance with MH, the most prudent course of action is to schedule the case for the first of the day to minimize exposing the children to inhalational anesthetics in the operating or recovery room.[62–65] With the abundance of evidence that stress alone can trigger an MH reaction, preoperative anxiolytics such as midazolam are warranted, except possibly for the most minor procedures (e.g., myringotomy and tubes). Prophylactic dantrolene is not recommended for MH patients who receive a trigger-free anesthetic as the frequency of MH reactions is very small.[66–68] The anesthetic prescription must include nontriggering agents such as total IV or regional anesthetics, or both. In the rare circumstance in which triggers must be used such as during an inhalational induction for a child with epiglottitis, extreme vigilance and anticipation to treat an acute MH reaction are of the utmost importance, although the airway was secured in a 7-year-old child with acute epiglottitis recently using total intravenous anesthesia (TIVA) rather than inhalational anesthesia.[66,67,69]

When a child with a known susceptibility to MH is scheduled for general anesthesia, the anesthesia workstation (AWS) must be prepared to prevent the delivery of triggering agents. First, succinylcholine should be removed from the local vicinity to avoid inadvertent administration (refer to Laryngospasm algorithm, see E-Fig. 12.1. NB. substitute rocuronium for succinylcholine). Second, all vaporizers should be physically disengaged from the AWS, to preclude leakage of trace concentrations of inhalational anesthetics, even in the off state; if they cannot be physically removed from the AWS, they should be covered with tape while in the off position to warn unsuspecting individuals against turning them on.[70] Third, to accelerate the washout of anesthetics, the removable sections of the AWS should be replaced with new

Patient Evaluation and Preparation

Optimal treatment begins with prevention and preparation. Obtaining an accurate family history of suspicious or unusual life-threatening reactions during general anesthesia in blood relatives, unexpected admissions to intensive care after surgery, or unexplained sudden death during or immediately after general sections (i.e., a new CO_2 canister should be installed together with a new anesthetic breathing circuit).[70-72] Fourth, to eliminate trace inhalational anesthetics from the AWS, many clinicians follow a standardized protocol of flushing the workstation with 10 to 20 liters per minute of oxygen for 10 to 20 minutes based on published recommendations and age of the machine.[73] However, the flushing protocols and times to purge the AWS to below the purported threshold of 1 to 10 parts per million is wildly variable, with times exceeding 2 hours in some AWSs and requiring replacement of internal components. During this purging period, the ventilator should be operating to clear anesthetic from the internal circuit. The objective in purging inhalational anesthetics from the AWS is to reduce the anesthetic concentration to 1 to 10 parts per million, which is the purported threshold below which an MH reaction is not triggered,[8,74,75] although the minimum concentration of inhalational anesthetic that triggers an MH reaction has never been confirmed in humans.[73] Moreover, clinical analyzers are incapable of detecting such small concentrations of inhalational anesthetics precluding verification that the target concentration, <10 parts per million, was achieved. This is particularly an issue with the newer AWS, which are more complex in construction and more likely to contain internal working parts made of plastic that can act as reservoirs for inhalational anesthetics.[76] To address the various types of AWS, the duration of flushing with large fresh gas flows and the need to exchange contaminated internal components with clean versions must be determined for each. For some types of AWS, more than 1 to 2 hours may be required to reach anesthetic concentrations (<10 ppm).[73,76-78] To achieve an anesthetic concentration <10 parts per million in the Dräger Primus, Fabius, and Zeus machines (Drägerwerk AG & Co. KGaA, Lübeck, Germany) in a timely manner, the ventilator diaphragm and integrated breathing system should be replaced with autoclaved components and then flushed for 20 minutes at a fresh gas flow of 10 liters per minute.[77,78] Table 39.6 lists the published times required to achieve an anesthetic concentration of <10 parts per million.[73,74,76,78,79] These data support the notion that the previously held protocols to wash out inhalational anesthetics from older AWSs may not hold true for some of the newer AWSs and may be time consuming and complicated to achieve on the morning of surgery.

After the AWS has been flushed with 10 liters per minute of an air and oxygen mixture, most anesthesiologists reduce the fresh gas flow (to 2 to 5 L/minute) during anesthesia. However, evidence has shown that when the fresh gas flow is reduced, the concentration of inhalational anesthetic rebounds (≥50 ppm), and the magnitude of that rebound directly depends, in part, on the new fresh gas flow rate.[75,79] Those who reduce the fresh gas flow after purging the AWS may theoretically expose their patients to concentrations of inhalational anesthetics that may trigger an MH reaction, although no instances of this have been published.[73] To avoid confusion, a single, consistent, effective, and reliable intervention is required to prevent MH reactions in patients exposed to trace gases from a previously contaminated AWS; placing charcoal absorbers in the inspiratory and expiratory limbs of the anesthesia breathing circuit in part, address this issue.

A commercially available charcoal filter (Vapor-Clean, Dynasthetics, LLC, Salt Lake City, UT) fitted to the expiratory and inspiratory limbs of the AWS reduces the concentration of inhalational anesthetics to <5 parts per million within several minutes.[80] These filters are sold in pairs. The manufacturer recommends inserting a filter into both the inspiratory and expiratory limbs of the anesthesia breathing circuit just distal to the valves.

TABLE 39.6 Time to Wash Out Inhalational Anesthetics to Less Than 10 ppm AWSs

Datex-Ohmeda-GE AWSs	Time (minutes)	Other AWSs	Time (minutes)
Modulus I[a]	5–15	Narkomed[a] (Dräger)	20
Excel 210	7	Dräger Primus[a,b]	39–70
AS/3[c]	30	Dräger Fabius GS[a]	104
Aestiva (sevoflurane)[d]	22	Dräger Zeus[b,e]	35–85
Aisys (sevoflurane)[d]	25	Kion[f] (Siemens)	>25
Avance[b]	39	Perseus[b] (Dräger)	15
		Felix AInOC[b] (Taema, Air Liquide)	135
		Flow-i[b] (Maquet)	46
		Leon[b] (Heinen + Löwenstein GmBH)	106

AWSs, Anesthesia workstations
Data are from:
[a]Kim TW, Nemergut ME. Preparation of modern anesthesia workstations for malignant hyperthermia-susceptible patients; a review of past and present practice. *Anesthesiology.* 2011;114:205-212.
[b]Cottron N, Larcher C, Sommet A, et al. The sevoflurane washout profile of seven recent anesthesia workstations for malignant hyperthermia-susceptible adults and infants: a bench test study. *Anesth Analg.* 2014:119;67-75.
[c]Schonell LHB, Sims C, Bulsara M. Preparing a new generation anaesthetic machine for patients susceptible to malignant hyperthermia. *Anaesth Intens Care.* 2003:31;58-62.
[d]Sabouri AS, Lerman J, Heard C. Effects of fresh gas flow, tidal volume, and charcoal filters on the washout of sevoflurane from the Datex Ohmeda (GE) Aisys, Aestiva/5 and Excel 210 SE anesthesia workstations. *Can J Anesth.* 2014:61;935-942.
[e]Shanahan H, O'Donoghue R, O'Kelly P, Synnott A, O'Rourke J. Preparation of the Dräger Fabius CE and Dräger Zeus anaesthetic machines for patients susceptible to malignant hyperthermia. *Eur J Anaesthesiol.* 2012;29:229-234.
[f]Petroz GC, Lerman J. Preparation of the Siemens KION anesthetic machine for patients susceptible to malignant hyperthermia. *Anesthesiology.* 2002;96(4):941-946.

The manufacturer cautions against using just a single charcoal filter in elective cases involving MH patients citing two reasons:

1. Clinicians may fail to correctly identify the inspiratory limb of the anesthesia breathing circuit (with an arrow pointing toward the patient end) and
2. If the one-way valve in the expiratory limb becomes incompetent, exhaled (and contaminated) gases may be rebreathed thereby triggering an MH reaction.[81]

Most pediatric surgery is ambulatory. Naturally, clinicians questioned whether it was safe to discharge MH-susceptible children on the day of surgery after an uneventful, elective anesthetic. Evidence from several studies suggest that the risk of developing an MH reaction after such an anesthetic was exceedingly small, but not zero.[66-68] Ambulatory surgery centers should have protocols in place and regular drills for staff to maintain familiarity with acute MH reactions, IV dantrolene on site if succinylcholine or inhalational anesthetics are used, and a protocol to transfer patients who develop MH reactions to a specialized hospital.[82] Postoperative monitoring for an MH reaction has gradually been reduced from 6 hours to 2 hours or the standard interval in the surgical center before discharge.[83-85] In such cases, parents should be provided with a written description of the signs and symptoms of an MH reaction, advised to treat all fevers with oral acetaminophen and sponge baths, and to contact the on-call anesthesiologist for further advice and consultation. This advice is particularly important if fever is accompanied by tachycardia and tachypnea. In this circumstance, the parents should notify the on-call anesthesiologist and immediately return the child to the hospital. Families should contact an anesthesiologist directly rather than return to the emergency department for evaluation because the anesthesiologist is the doctor who is most familiar with the signs of MH, particularly in children.

Monitoring

The routine use of capnography, ECG, core temperature, and pulse oximetry should provide the earliest warning signs of an evolving MH event.[14,86] The site where the body temperature is measured may also reflect the sensitivity of this measure to detect an MH reaction and prevent death.[52] Some suggest that the core body temperature may be a late sign of MH but that temperature measurements in the axilla (opposite the extremity with the IV line) may yield an earlier sign of MH because venous blood passes through the large pectoral muscle girdle in the axilla. Moreover, data from a retrospective review of MH deaths suggested that the relative risk of mortality from an MH reaction when temperature was not measured was 14-fold greater, and if skin temperature was measured, 9.7 fold greater than when the core temperature was measured,[52] with the relative risk of any complication increasing 2.9-fold for every 2°C increase in body temperature.[14,52] Evidence also confirmed that crystalline skin temperature tapes did not reliably track core temperature changes during MH reactions.[14]

Pathophysiology and Laboratory Testing

With the underlying disorder in MH a hypermetabolic reaction that arises from persistent skeletal muscle contractures (i.e., increased CO_2 production and oxygen consumption),[32,87] massive volumes of CO_2 are released into the circulation, which rapidly increase the partial pressure of CO_2 ($PaCO_2$) and respiratory rate in the unparalyzed child (E-Fig. 39.1). This respiratory acidosis triggers tachypnea and an increased minute ventilation. The cardiovascular response is an increased cardiac output, heart rate, and in some cases, blood pressure. The first clinical signs and symptoms of this hypermetabolic reaction in a spontaneously breathing patient are hypercarbia, sinus tachycardia, and tachypnea (see Table 39.1).[14] **A steady and relentless increase in the end-tidal CO_2 ($PETCO_2$) is the earliest sign of a reaction** and is usually evident regardless of whether respirations are spontaneous or controlled. In some instances, the increase in $PETCO_2$ and heart rate occur contemporaneously, alerting the clinician to consider an evolving MH reaction (Fig. 39.3). In a retrospective review of 264 children in the North American MH Registry, the most common signs of an MH reaction were sinus tachycardia in 73% and hypercarbia in 69%, which were most common in adolescents.[53] Hyperthermia appeared in fewer than half (48%) of the children.[53] Greater temperatures and peak potassium concentrations were more common in adolescents, whereas greater peak lactic acid concentrations and reduced peak CK concentrations were present in the younger children.

The presenting signs of an acute MH reaction are nonspecific and may suggest several possible disease states or equipment problems. The differential diagnosis of an increase in $PETCO_2$,

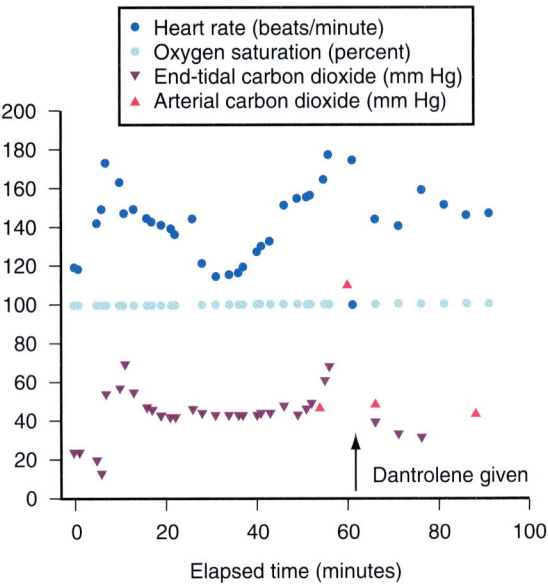

FIGURE 39.3 Response of physiologic parameters to dantrolene during an apparent intraoperative episode of malignant hyperthermia. Notice the rapid decrease in arterial and end-tidal carbon dioxide pressures after dantrolene (2.5 mg/kg) administration *(arrow)*. (Courtesy Steven C. Hall, MD.)

the earliest sign of an MH reaction, may result from one or more of three factors that define the CO_2 mass balance equation:

$$PETCO_2 = \frac{\dot{V}CO_2}{\dot{V}A} + FiCO_2$$

The circulating $PaCO_2$ depends on the production of CO_2 ($\dot{V}CO_2$), the elimination of CO_2 (i.e., alveolar ventilation [$\dot{V}A$]), and the fraction of inspired concentration of CO_2 ($FiCO_2$).

The differential diagnosis of an increased PCO_2 can be analyzed by considering the causes for each of these three factors: $\dot{V}CO_2$, $\dot{V}A$, and $FiCO_2$. An increased $\dot{V}CO_2$ can result from fever, MH, thyroid storm, and sepsis. This may pose a particular challenge to diagnose during laparoscopic surgery.[88,89] A decreased $\dot{V}A$ can result from a deep level of anesthesia (during spontaneous respiration), endobronchial intubation, bronchospasm, and a kinked tracheal tube or airway breathing circuit. An increased $FiCO_2$ can result from an incompetent expiratory valve, exogenous source of CO_2, low fresh gas flows with a partial or nonrebreathing circuit, and an expired CO_2 absorbent. The initial evaluation should include a rapid assessment of the integrity of the breathing circuit, the presence of bilateral breath sounds and absence of wheezing, and examination of the CO_2 absorbent.

During airway obstruction or hypermetabolic states such as thyrotoxicosis and sepsis, an increased $PETCO_2$ can be readily corrected by increasing the minute ventilation, whereas during an MH reaction this may prove very difficult, even with very vigorous hyperventilation.[40] The CO_2 production is sometimes so great that the CO_2 absorbent rapidly becomes exhausted in an exothermic reaction, and the absorbent container becomes hot to touch. Thyrotoxicosis can also be distinguished from an acute MH reaction by the absence of general muscle rigidity, less severe metabolic acidosis, near normal peak CK levels, and the absence of an effect by dantrolene on the clinical findings.

A child's response to surgery during light anesthesia often includes tachycardia and may sometimes include bronchoconstriction. However, a dramatic and unexpected increase in heart rate from 120 to 180 beats per minute in a healthy, 7-year-old child (or an increase from 70 to 120 beats per minute in an adult) strongly suggests a pathologic process, and a differential diagnosis beyond light anesthesia should be seriously considered. Before intervening, it is important to quickly scan all the monitors to determine whether the aggregate indexes point to a specific diagnosis. If tachycardia is associated with an increase in body temperature, a differential diagnosis of fever and tachycardia under anesthesia should be considered. Fever related to sepsis or viral infection usually has a slow onset, whereas fever from an MH reaction typically has a rapid onset. The differential diagnoses include iatrogenic external overheating and an MH reaction (see Table 39.4). A rapid increase in the inspired concentration of desflurane and isoflurane, but not sevoflurane, may cause a sympathetic-based tachycardia that in isolation should not suggest a diagnosis of MH because the $PETCO_2$ remains unchanged.[90,91] Of the inhalational anesthetics, halothane appears to be the most likely to trigger an MH reaction and the best discriminator for the CHCT; sevoflurane and isoflurane are intermediate, and preliminary data suggest that xenon does not trigger MH reactions.[31,55,92–94] If none of these factors appears to be causative and a deeper level of anesthesia (achieved with propofol with or without an opioid) fails to abate the signs, arterial and/or venous blood gases should be analyzed to determine whether the patient has or is developing a hypermetabolic state.

Peak serum CK concentrations that exceed 18,000 U/L correlate with MH susceptibility based on contracture and DNA testing.[43] However, the CK values increase slowly not precipitously, after muscle injury including an acute MH reaction, reaching peak median CK values at 12 to 18 hours after an acute MH reaction.[95] A level of >20,000 U/L is listed as a major determinant of an MH reaction after succinylcholine in a clinical grading score.[61] With muscle injuries, the CK concentration does not peak until 24 to 48 hours after the initial insult and return to normal values by 3 to 5 days after injury.[96] Measuring carbonic anhydrase III and aldolase concentrations specifically reflect skeletal muscle injury that when combined with increased CK concentration are highly suggestive of muscle injury.[97] In contrast to the slow elimination half-life of CK (1.5 days), serum myoglobin is rapidly and massively released after a muscle insult with an elimination half-life of 2 to 4 hours, returning to normal values 6 to 8 hours after the injury.[96] Evidence holds that the peak serum/plasma myoglobin concentration is a stronger predictor of acute kidney injury after a nontraumatic muscle injury than the CK value.[96]

Rhabdomyolysis may appear as part of the spectrum of an acute MH reaction, but it usually occurs later in the course of an incompletely treated or untreated MH reaction compared with anesthesia-induced rhabdomyolysis, which is the presenting finding after the administration of succinylcholine with or without an inhaled

TABLE 39.7	Differences Between Malignant Hyperthermia and Anesthesia-Induced Rhabdomyolysis		
		Anesthesia-Induced Rhabdomyolysis	**Malignant Hyperthermia**
Early Signs	Clinical	History of muscle injury, drug-induced, and others[96]	Skeletal muscle rigidity, Masseter spasm
	ECG	Peaked T waves (from hyperkalemia); Bradycardia, dysrhythmia, ± cardiac arrest	Tachycardia
	Oxygen saturation	Normal until cardiac arrest	Hemoglobin desaturation
	Airway gas monitoring		Hypercarbia; ↑ Oxygen consumption[a]
	Laboratory results	Marked hyperkalemia; Increased CK	Hyperkalemia
Late Signs		Acidosis, Hypercarbia, ± Hyperthermia (rare) Myoglobinemia & myoglobinurea; CK >1000 U/L (may exceed 40,000)	Mixed respiratory and metabolic acidoses, Hyperthermia, Increased CK (>20,000); Myoglobinemia & myoglobinurea; Ventricular arrhythmia, Cardiac arrest; Coagulopathy
Timing (unless succinylcholine has been given)[b]		May occur at any time, particularly later in the anesthetic or in recovery room	Any time
Treatment Priority		CPR; Stop halogenated agent, switch to TIVA; Antagonize and reduce hyperkalemia; "Clean" source of oxygen	Stop halogenated agent, switch to TIVA; Insert charcoal filters; Hyperventilate; Dantrolene; Antagonize and reduce hyperkalemia

CK, Creatine kinase; *CPR*, cardiopulmonary resuscitation; *ECG*, electrocardiogram.
[a]Represented by widening inspired to expired oxygen concentration in the face of unchanged fresh gas flows.
[b]If succinylcholine has been given, malignant hyperthermia or anesthesia-induced rhabdomyolysis may occur precipitously.
Table modified by the author; reproduced with permission; from Gray RM. Anesthesia-induced rhabdomyolysis or malignant hyperthermia: is defining the crisis important? *Paediatr Anaesth.* 2017;27(5):490-493.

anesthetic to a young child with an undiagnosed myopathy (e.g., Duchenne muscular dystrophy).[98] The presenting features of MH and anesthesia-induced rhabdomyolysis are contrasted in Table 39.7. Note that MH rarely presents with isolated rhabdomyolysis and in contrast to anesthesia-induced rhabdomyolysis, it is responsive to dantrolene. Nonetheless, the potential for hyperkalemia developing after muscle breakdown and acute renal failure from myoglobin deposition in the renal tubules exists as a late complication.

A moderate but gradual increase in body temperature may occur in children excessively draped, those heated with forced-air warming devices for prolonged periods, those with bilateral limb tourniquets, children with arthrogryposis, and those covered with plastic occlusive wrap. However, the sudden onset of a high fever must be more thoroughly investigated because it may result from several potentially fatal causes (see Table 39.4).[99–102]

Management of Malignant Hyperthermia

Management of an acute MH reaction is the model for which anesthetic crisis resource management (ACRM) was developed. The decision-making process for every aspect of managing the MH reaction (from differential diagnosis to counseling for MedicAlert bracelets [MedicAlert Foundation, Salida, CA] https://www.medicalert.org) together with excellent communication and human resource management ensure an optimal outcome after the reaction.[103] Given the rarity of these reactions, ACRM can be built into the simulation scenario for MH to teach leadership and decision making in the time of crisis (see Chapter 50).

IMMEDIATE MANAGEMENT

If the anesthesiologist suspects that a child is experiencing an MH reaction, the inhalational anesthetic should be immediately discontinued, 100% oxygen administered at a large fresh gas flow rate ($\geq$10 L/minute), and the surgeon informed; if surgery cannot be aborted, it must be completed expeditiously while administering TIVA to sedate the child until surgery is complete. Today, forced-air heating devices are commonly used in children of all ages. These devices should NOT be turned off when a reaction is suspected, but rather continued at a low temperature (32°C or less), to replace the hot air under the surgical drapes with cooler air to offset the patient's increasing temperature.

As soon as the anesthesiologist declares an MH reaction in the operating room, the MH cart (as described in Table 39.8) should be retrieved and additional personnel summoned to assist to deliver dantrolene, obtain and send blood specimens to the laboratory, and ensure timely charting. Minute ventilation should be increased to restore normocapnia. It is suggested that charcoal filters be inserted into both limbs of a new anesthesia breathing circuit (E-Fig. 39.2). The MH-treatment algorithm available on the MHAUS website or the locally available MH website, can be accessed to ensure compliance with optimal care. We recommend attaching an updated MH-treatment algorithm to every MH cart and anesthesia machine and that operating room personnel hold practice drills for the treatment of an MH crisis (see "Emergency Therapy for Malignant Hyperthermia" on the inside back cover of this text and at Elsevier eBooks+). If the patient experiences what is believed to be an MH reaction, the care provider should call the MH emergency response line (1-800-644-9737 or 001-1-315-464-7079 if calling from outside the United States) for consultation with experienced anesthesiologists who are available 24 hours every day.

By placing a charcoal filter in both the inspiratory and expiratory limbs of the breathing circuit, the child is protected from residual anesthetic in the AWS and the AWS is protected from anesthetic expelled from the patient.[80] The manufacturer recommends that the filters can maintain the concentration of inhalational anesthetic <5 parts per million for 60 minutes if the AWS was purged first. However, experimental evidence from an Ohmeda Aisys AWS indicated that the charcoal filters have a finite capacity to absorb inhalational anesthetics, particularly when the AWS has not been purged of inhalational agent *a priori*.[104] After contaminating an AWS with desflurane in a simulation scenario, the desflurane concentration decreased to <5 parts per million within 3 minutes of inserting two charcoal filters into the breathing circuit. However after 30 minutes, the desflurane concentration rebounded to >5 parts per million.[104]

TABLE 39.8	Contents of a Pediatric Malignant Hyperthermia Emergency Cart		
FLUIDS			
3 L COLD NORMAL SALINE, LACTATED RINGER SOLUTION OR PLASMALYTE			
Number of Containers	**Drug**	**Concentration**	**Container**
	Dantrolene IV[a]		
36	Dantrium or Revonto (see Table 39.9)	20 mg in 60 mL of sterile water (0.33 mg/mL)	1 vial
3	Ryanodex	250 mg in 5 mL of sterile water (50 mg/mL)	1 vial
25	Sterile injectable water		100 mL
4	Sodium bicarbonate	1 mEq/mL	50 mL vial
2	50% dextrose, to treat hyperkalemia	500 mg/mL	50 mL vial
1	Regular insulin, to treat hyperkalemia	100 units/mL	10 mL vial
4	Calcium gluconate or chloride (10%)		10 mL
3	Lidocaine (2%)[a]	20 mg/mL	5 mL
10	20- and 22-gauge IV catheters		
10	18- and 20-gauge needles		

IV, Intravenous; *TB*, tuberculin.
[a]Avoid lidocaine if wide QRS complex is present.
Charcoal filters should be immediately available if they are not present on the malignant hyperthermia cart.

The results of this one study strongly suggest that charcoal filters can become saturated with inhalational anesthetic after a brief use if the AWS has not already been flushed or purged of anesthetic. Until further evidence is forthcoming, we recommend replacing the charcoal filters in a contaminated AWS after 30 minutes.

If the anesthetic continues beyond 30 minutes, the charcoal filters should be replaced but an attempt to purge the AWS of anesthetic should be considered. To accomplish this, an external self-inflating or anesthesia-type bag with an exogenous source of oxygen should be used to hyperventilate the lungs while sedation/ anesthesia is maintained with TIVA. In the interim, the AWS should be purged of anesthetic and the disposable components replaced in anticipation of returning the AWS to use. If the airway was not intubated, the trachea should be intubated and ventilation controlled to restore a normal PETCO$_2$. Once purged of inhaled anesthetics, new charcoal filters should be inserted into the breathing circuit to deliver anesthetic-free gases to the child during the final stages of surgical closure.

Moderate external cooling measures may be instituted to control a rapidly increasing temperature, although ice should never be applied directly to the skin because it may cause tissue injury and intense cutaneous vasoconstriction. The latter may decrease heat loss further by accelerating acidosis and pyrexia. It is important to avoid overshooting with cooling measures (i.e., stop aggressive cooling at a temperature of about 38.5°C), because hypothermia may ensue, particularly if dantrolene has been administered. A urinary catheter should always be inserted during an MH reaction to identify myoglobinuria and to facilitate bladder emptying.

Initial laboratory assessments should be obtained before the bolus dose of dantrolene, and in addition to arterial and venous blood gases, determinations should include electrolyte, glucose, blood urea nitrogen, and creatinine levels; a complete blood cell count with platelets; prothrombin and partial thromboplastin times; serial CK concentrations; and serial serum and urine myoglobin levels. Because the CK concentration does not increase within the first couple of hours of an MH reaction, it is prudent to obtain a baseline blood CK value as soon as an MH reaction is suspected and collect serial blood samples every 6 hours for at least 24 hours or until the CK values abate. Blood and urine samples for myoglobin should be collected immediately after the bladder is catheterized and then hourly for the subsequent 12 hours to document the time course of the serum myoglobin concentration and myoglobinuria. Placing an arterial catheter facilitates continuous monitoring of blood pressure and for serial determinations of arterial blood gases, electrolytes, and CK.

The potential for life-threatening acidosis—an observed respiratory acidosis attributable to CO$_2$ production in muscles that occurs early in the syndrome and is poorly responsive to increases in minute ventilation,[105] followed by a mixed metabolic/respiratory acidosis—always exists. The excess PaCO$_2$ associated with MH results from aerobic muscle catabolism. When the intracellular oxygen and ATP become depleted in the muscle fibers, metabolic acidosis begins resulting in a mixed respiratory and metabolic acidosis as evident in the blood/gas results. *To preclude this dangerous deterioration in the child's condition, early dosing of IV dantrolene (see later) is critical.* Metabolic changes (acidosis, hyperkalemia) are often initially managed with sodium bicarbonate (e.g., 1 to 2 mEq/kg IV) before the dantrolene is available. If hypercarbia persists despite aggressive hyperventilation and dantrolene administration, further administration of sodium bicarbonate should be withheld so as not to further exacerbate the respiratory acidosis. An acute MH episode is also associated with

catecholamine stress, hemodynamic instability including tachycardia and dysrhythmias that may be related to hyperkalemia; intervention should proceed according to advanced cardiac life support protocols.

Acute hyperkalemia is common in patients with MH complicated by rhabdomyolysis and acidosis. Glucose and insulin should be immediately available and combined with the judicious use of exogenous IV calcium (see also Chapters 7 and 26). There is no evidence that the use of calcium in this setting exacerbates an MH reaction but it would oppose the cardiac effects of hyperkalemia and restore the cardiac output.[106,107] Dihydropyridine calcium channel blockers such as nifedipine, amlodipine and nicardipine do not trigger, exacerbate, or treat acute MH reactions, although other calcium channel blockers such as diltiazem and verapamil when co-administered with dantrolene, have been reported to cause hyperkalemia, myocardial depression and bradycardia in anecdotal reports and animals.[108–110] Although the dihydropyridine calcium channel blockers may increase intracellular calcium concentrations in in vitro models even in the presence of dantrolene, they do not modulate the flux of calcium out of the sarcoplasmic reticulum as occurs in MH reactions.[111] On balance, it remains prudent to avoid this class of drugs during MH crises.

DANTROLENE

Dantrolene, a nitrofurantoin derivative that was developed in 1967, was initially targeted to treat muscle spasticity in children. In South Africa around the same time, Gaisford Harrison was confronted with a series of pigs (subsequently identified as Landrace pigs that carry the MH gene) that died when they were anesthetized for liver transplantation.[112] Upon advice, he prepared a slurry of oral dantrolene that was passed through a nasogastric tube during an acute MH reaction, saving the pigs. Subsequently, he managed to dissolve dantrolene and saved seven of eight pigs that developed MH reactions during halothane anesthesia. The one pig that died survived the initial reaction but experienced a recrudescence that proved fatal.

The original dantrolene formulation (Dantrium, Par Pharmaceutical, Par Sterile Products, Chestnut Ridge, NY) for human use was packaged as a lyophilized yellow powder (E-Fig. 39.3) with constituents that contain mannitol and an alkaline pH to speed its dissolution in water (Table 39.9). This formulation of dantrolene that required 60 mL of sterile water in each vial containing 20 mg dantrolene took ~2 minutes to fully dissolve. Several strategies to speed the dissolution were identified: shaking the vial and warming the sterile water are very effective. Warming the sterile water to 40°C sped up dissolution by 6.7-fold.[113] Although heating the water to 40°C dramatically sped up the dissolution of dantrolene in one study, heating the water to 45°C in a second study only increased the rate of dissolution by ~20%.[114] Once the solution is clear of crystals, it should be withdrawn immediately from the vial and administered intravenously as rapidly as possible to stop the MH reaction; the earlier the administration of dantrolene, the greater the reduction in the fatality rate.[115] Given the extreme alkaline pH of the dantrolene solution, it should be infused into a large vein to reduce the risk of phlebitis. Extravasation of dantrolene into interstitial tissues must be avoided as it can cause tissue necrosis. Additionally, a prolonged continuous infusion of dantrolene may cause thrombophlebitis or thrombosis of large and small veins.[60,116,117] Some have recommended continuous infusions of small doses of dantrolene in adults after the initial bolus, although the risk/benefit ratio of this practice remains unproved in adults and untested in children.[118]

TABLE 39.9	Characteristics of Three Formulations of Dantrolene IV		
	Dantrium[a]	Revonto[b]	Ryanodex[c]
Dose (mg)/vial	20	20	250
Volume of diluent (mL)	60	60	5
Mannitol content (mg)	3000	3000	125
Time to dilute	129 seconds or "until solution is clear"[a]	20 seconds or "until solution is clear"[a]	<10 seconds
	"Shake the vial to ensure an orange-colored uniform suspension. Visually inspect the vial for particulate matter and discoloration prior to administration."		
pH of reconstituted solution	9.5	9.5	10.3
Number of vials recommended by MHAUS (for a 70-kg patient)	36	36	3 (equivalent to ~720 mg dantrolene)
Shelf-life from date of manufacturing (months)	36a	36	33
Acquisition cost/vial (USD wholesale)	$95	$82	$3320
Cost to treat a 70-kg adult (USD)	$3420	$3000	$9960

[a]Dantrium (Par Pharmaceutical Companies Inc., Spring Valley, NY).
[b]Revonto (dantrolene sodium; DSM Pharmaceuticals Inc., Greenville, NC); package insert revised November 2016. Prices accessed Aug 15, 2023
[c]Ryanodex (dantrolene sodium; Eagle Pharmaceuticals, Inc., Woodcliff Lake, NJ); package insert revised July 2014. Prices accessed Aug 15, 2023
Data were summarized in part from *Cleveland Clinic Clinical Rx Forum*, 2016:4(5);4-5.

In 2010, the Revonto formulation was introduced using the same formulation as the original Dantrium, but with a manufacturing process that abbreviated the time to dissolution to 20 seconds or until the solution was clear. The change in the manufacturing process has been attributed to the use of tert-butyl alcohol.[119]

In 2014, a novel formulation of lyophilized dantrolene (Ryanodex, Eagle Pharmaceuticals, Woodcliff Lake, NJ) was introduced in the United States that further streamlined the dissolution of dantrolene resulting in a rapid reconstitution with only 5 mL of sterile water in <10 seconds (Table 39.9) (https://www.ryanodex.com).[120,121] This preparation contains more dantrolene (250 mg) than the standard vial (20 mg), a greater concentration of dantrolene (250 mg/5 mL vs. 20 mg/60 mL), less mannitol (125 mg vs. 3000 mg per vial), and only 5 milliliters instead of 60 milliliters of bacteriostatic water per vial (see Table 39.9).[121] Preliminary evidence suggests that the clearance and elimination half-lives of Dantrium and Ryanodex are similar.[118,119,122,123] The shelf life of Dantrium, 36 months, is now indistinguishable from Ryanodex, 33 months. Table 39.9 compares and contrasts the characteristics of the three formulations of dantrolene; the marked

advantages of Ryanodex (the rapidity of dissolution, small volume of water required, ease and rapidity of preparation time) are offset by the cost, which is ~3-fold greater than Dantrium and Revonto.

The pharmacokinetics of IV dantrolene have been studied in MH-susceptible children 2 to 7 years of age.[122] A loading dose of 2.5 milligrams per kilogram produced predictable blood concentrations (≥3 µg/mL) for about 6 hours (Fig. 39.4).[122] Based on these pharmacokinetic data, if half of the loading dose of dantrolene that stopped the reaction were repeated at 6 hours after the loading dose, therapeutic blood concentrations of dantrolene would be maintained for a total of 15 hours and possibly prevent a recrudescence.[122]

An initial bolus dose of 2.5 milligram per kilogram controls most MH reactions if the dantrolene is administered as soon after the onset of the reaction as possible (see Fig. 39.3).[124] Delay in instituting dantrolene increases the probability of a failed or incomplete arrest of the MH episode and increased risk of death.[14,115] For a 70-kilogram patient, the initial dose is nine vials of Dantrium or one vial of Ryanodex.

Given the morbidity and mortality risks of an MH reaction, particularly if not treated early, intravenous dantrolene should be administered as soon as the diagnosis is suspected, even before it is confirmed, provided all the necessary blood work and laboratory tests have been collected (see Fig. 39.1).[14] The probability of developing complications from an acute MH reaction increases almost 3-fold for every 2°C increase in body temperature and 1.6-fold for every 30-minute delay in administering IV dantrolene during a reaction.[14] Cardiac arrest and death during an MH reaction correlate with a muscular physique and a greater interval between induction of anesthesia and the maximal value of $PETCO_2$.[35] Other possible diagnoses should continue to be considered while the treatment for the suspected MH reaction is organized (see Table 39.4). It should be emphasized that a positive response to dantrolene is not diagnostic of MH because other conditions may respond with resolution of their signs similarly.

The response to dantrolene should be evident within minutes, with a marked reduction in $PETCO_2$, heart rate, and respiratory rate (see Fig. 39.3). If a response is not observed within 3 to 5 minutes, the initial dose should be repeated at 3-to 5-minute intervals until signs that the event is abating, as evidenced by

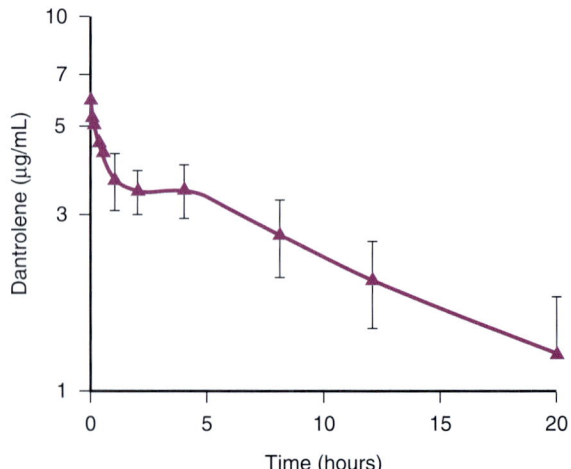

FIGURE 39.4 Pharmacokinetics of dantrolene in children. (From Lerman J, McLeod ME, Strong HA. Pharmacokinetics of intravenous dantrolene in children. *Anesthesiology.* 1989;70[4]:625-629.)

changes in the physiologic variables. The clinical endpoints include resolution of the hypercarbia, tachypnea, hyperthermia, and tachycardia; resolution of muscle rigidity; restoration of clear urine output; return of normal consciousness when sedation is discontinued; self-correction of blood gas abnormalities; and resolution of electrolyte disturbances. If these do not occur or are incomplete, additional doses of dantrolene should be administered rapidly until all signs and symptoms of the MH reaction have abated or the diagnosis is reevaluated.[124] There is no upper limit to the amount of dantrolene that can or should be given acutely to stop an MH reaction. In rare instances of persistent MH or recrudescence, a cumulative dose of up to 40 milligrams per kilogram has been required.[125] As dantrolene is a fairly potent muscle relaxant, it may cause the child to feel weak and develop labored breathing if the airway has not been secured. In such cases, induction of sedation/anesthesia and tracheal intubation should be undertaken.

Although dantrolene is effective in terminating acute MH reactions, this effect may wane as the blood concentration of dantrolene decreases and a recrudescence may occur. The prevalence of recrudescence may be as great as 20% and associated with several predictive factors, including muscular body type and a greater time interval between induction of anesthesia and the development of the initial reaction.[126] However, the first episode of recrudescence may occur any time after the initial reaction was successfully treated, up to and as late as 36 hours.[127] The possibility of recrudescence must always be considered during the first 2 to 3 days after an MH reaction has occurred. Because recrudescence cannot be predicted, all children who experience an MH reaction must be admitted to the pediatric intensive care unit or a monitored bed until the reaction resolves and the child's metabolic indices return to and remain normal for 2 to 3 days. MHAUS recommends that 1 milligram per kilogram of dantrolene be administered intravenously every 6 hours for 24 to 48 hours after an MH reaction to prevent recrudescence. This recommendation remains empirical because there are no data to support the effectiveness of dantrolene in preventing recrudescence, although these dosages are consistent with pharmacokinetic data in children.[122] We recommend continued vigilance, frequent physical examinations for muscle tightness (every 30 minutes), repeated laboratory tests (e.g., blood gas analyses), and monitoring of vital signs, particularly heart rate, respiratory rate, and expired CO_2 tension for evidence of a recrudescence during the first 48 hours after an MH episode. If recrudescence does occur, additional IV dantrolene should be administered until the reaction again abates.

There have been no reports of acute dantrolene toxicity, although acute administration of dantrolene may result in side effects that include skeletal muscle weakness (15%), phlebitis (9%), and gastrointestinal upset (4.3%).[60] Respiratory failure was reported in 3.8% of patients who received dantrolene, although distinguishing the cause of the failure to the underlying MH or the dantrolene has proven difficult.[60] Extravasation of dantrolene into subcutaneous tissue may cause tissue necrosis.[121] Not surprisingly, neostigmine is ineffective in reversing the effects of dantrolene because the latter acts intracellularly, not at the neuromuscular junction (see the section on molecular mechanisms of dantrolene). **It may be advisable to maintain control of the airway (combined with IV sedation) until the need for dantrolene has subsided**.

Preoperative oral dantrolene, initially recommended in MH-susceptible children 3 decades ago, caused much consternation as

the children developed muscle weakness, dysarthria, sialorrhea, and diplopia. Moreover, it did not prevent MH reactions.[66] As a result, this practice was discontinued.[66]

Chronic long-term use of oral dantrolene to treat skeletal muscle spasticity caused liver dysfunction and fatal hepatitis in about 1% and 0.1% of patients, respectively.[128] In a retrospective review of 476 adults who were MH-susceptible on the basis of muscle biopsies between 1994 and 2018, 193 complained of muscle symptoms and 164 took oral dantrolene for relief over a 25-year period.[129] No serious adverse events were reported although 28% experienced mild to moderate adverse effects. More than 40% complained of chronic muscle pain. Of the 164, 13% discontinued treatment due to adverse events or no improvement and the remaining 87% reported clinical improvement in their myalgias, fatigue, and hyper-creatine-kinaseemia at a median dose of 50 milligrams per day (25 to 400 mg per day range). Those with confirmed ryanodine receptor 1 gene (RyR1) variants were more likely to respond positively to the dantrolene (odds ratio 6.4).[129]

POSTREACTION FOLLOW-UP

Late Complications

After the acute crisis has abated, late complications including severe rhabdomyolysis may develop. It is important to follow both serial serum and urine myoglobin concentrations, urine for color as well as seral serum concentrations of CK as described earlier. Close review of the myoglobin concentration in the first 6 to 8 hours should prompt alkalinizing of the urine, avoid potassium and lactate-containing solutions, and induce a diuresis.[130] The precipitation of myoglobin in the renal tubules is inversely related to the urine pH: if the pH <5, 73% of the myoglobin precipitates, whereas if the pH is 6.5, only 4% precipitates.[96] Similarly, if the peak CK concentration exceeds 10,000 international units, the urine should be alkalinized and a forced diuresis (>2 mL/kg per hour) induced with mannitol should be induced. The enormous fluid requirements and edema associated with rhabdomyolysis may produce a compartment syndrome, which requires immediate surgical treatment.

Other organ systems may be affected after an acute episode of MH. It is common for markers of liver function to increase 12 to 36 hours after the crisis; some liver enzymes, including lactate dehydrogenase, aspartate aminotransferase, and alanine aminotransferase, can also originate from muscle. Accompanying increases in γ-glutamyltransferase and bilirubin suggest liver involvement. Disseminated intravascular coagulation as part of multisystem organ failure is an ominous late complication.[131] Coagulation profiles should be followed serially to guide treatment appropriate to the case.

Diagnostic Muscle Biopsy

Ideally, after treating a child for MH, the anesthesiologist should arrange for referral of the child and first-degree relatives to an MH-diagnostic biopsy center. It is only at such centers that the CHCT can be performed in adults. The CHCT is the only test that can produce a true negative diagnosis (i.e., not MH-susceptible),[132] but the sensitivity and specificity of this test are less than 100%. False-negative test results may occur, albeit rarely.[133] When the anesthetic management of a small number of MH biopsy-negative patients was reviewed, more than one-half were given inhalational anesthetics, although the biopsy results for the remainder may not have been known at the time of anesthesia because they were given trigger-free anesthetics.[134]

Because control muscle biopsy data for prepubescent children are not available, contracture testing is not usually performed in this age group. Instead, children are more often fitted with MedicAlert bracelets, and the parents are counseled regarding their own need for biopsies. The children may be reconsidered for muscle biopsy upon reaching puberty.

Many persons suspected of having MH have normal muscle responses on the CHCT. In the event that an adult who experienced an MH reaction has a normal CHCT result, they should be referred to a neurologist with an interest in muscle diseases to determine whether an occult myopathy is responsible for the clinical events. Alternatively, the diagnosis may be incorrect, and other diagnoses should be considered (see Table 39.4). Individuals suspected of being MH-susceptible should undergo CHCT; the family should also be evaluated and counseled accordingly.

Genetic Investigation

Patients with strongly positive CHCT results should undergo screening for the ryanodine receptor 1 gene (RyR1), because mutations in this gene have been found in about 60% of family members who had an MH episode (conversely, this means that ~40% test negative genetically but are clinically MH positive). However, if neither an MH reaction nor a positive CHCT result has occurred, DNA testing for RyR1 gene mutations based on a vague history offers such a poor yield of positive results that it cannot be justified at the present time.[135] If an MH-associated mutation (discussed later) is found in RyR1, first-degree relatives have a 50% probability of having a similar defect.[15] Diagnostic testing for RyR1 is performed on DNA obtained from a blood specimen, obviating the need to travel to an MH-diagnostic biopsy center or undergo muscle biopsy for the genetic test. Genetic testing of relatives can be undertaken through the office of the primary care physician or by the anesthesiologist, a process that will simplify evaluation of the family. Failure to identify an MH-causative RyR1 mutation (E-Fig. 39.4) does not confirm a negative diagnosis (i.e., not MH-susceptible) because more than one gene is associated with MH susceptibility, and not all are known.

Genetic testing and counseling can be arranged by the anesthesiologist or primary care physician by scheduling an appointment; one such center is located at the Center for Medical Genetics & Genomics at the University of Pittsburgh. The genetic counselors have extensive experience in counseling patients on the utility of the RyR gene test for evaluation of MH susceptibility. The center currently screens 12 exons of genomic RyR1 that commonly contain MH mutations (exons 6, 9, 11, 14, 17, 39, 40, 44, 45, 46, 101, and 102). A private commercial laboratory that also offers RyR1 testing is Prevention Genetics (https://www.preventiongenetics.com), which screens for MH mutations. It has adopted a two-tiered approach: tier 1 involves bidirectional sequencing of exons 2, 6, 8, 9, 11, 12, 14, 15, 17, 39, 40, 41, 44–47, 95, and 100–104. These 22 exons contain most of the conclusively documented MH and central core disease causative mutations in the RyR1 gene (European Malignant Hypothermia Group https://www.emhg.org/genetics/). If the first tier is uninformative, their second-tier screen covers the remaining 84 exons of the 106 making up the human RyR1 gene. The Prevention Genetics company corresponds only with physicians and does not provide patient or family counseling.

As DNA sequencing has become more automated and the cost has drastically declined, many private companies have arisen that purport to diagnose the entire panoply of human genetic diseases and resultant predispositions, including MH. We have no information about the reliability of their screening, or the recommendations based on their findings. If no causative RyR1 mutations are found, nothing more can be determined from genetic testing about susceptibility, because more than one mutated gene is linked to MH.

Notification

We strongly encourage completion of an adverse metabolic reaction to anesthesia (AMRA) report by members of the team who provided anesthesia and postoperative care to the child. These forms can be downloaded (https://www.mhreg.org), sent by the hotline consultant, or obtained from the MHAUS office through regular mail. The data contained in the completed AMRA forms allow the North American Malignant Hyperthermia Registry (NAMHR) and MHAUS to produce better data regarding the variability of MH crises and the effectiveness of treatment. Because anesthesiologists should take a leading role in managing these patients, the families should be strongly encouraged to register the proband before leaving the hospital for MedicAlert identification that provides critical health information, such as "malignant hyperthermia susceptible, avoid inhaled anesthetics and succinylcholine."

Stress-Triggered Malignant Hyperthermia

In 1974, Wingard described an MH-susceptible family with a history of exercise- and emotion-induced fevers and sudden death not associated with anesthesia or surgery; he considered the possibility that MH was part of a spectrum of human stress syndromes.[136] Likewise, the porcine model of MH, also known as porcine stress syndrome, was first described as an awake, stress-induced syndrome brought about by tightly packing pigs in a train, car, or truck for shipment.[137] Dantrolene-responsive cases of awake and heat stroke–induced MH have been reported.[138,139] Heat stress–induced MH also seems to be characteristic of susceptible animal models.[140–142] A fatal case of exercise-induced MH in a 12-year-old boy who had previously survived a suspected episode of MH during general anesthesia to set a fractured humerus has been reported.[143] Eight months after surgery, while playing a game of football, the child became hyperthermic, collapsed, and died. Postmortem DNA testing revealed an MH-associated RyR1 mutation in the child and his surviving father.[143] More cases of stress-induced MH have been reported, substantiated by genetic testing and in vitro contracture testing (IVCT).[144,145]

Screening for MH susceptibility in heat stroke patients and those suffering postexercise cramps or rhabdomyolysis using the in vitro CHCT has led to the laboratory diagnosis of MH susceptibility in some patients.[63,146–152] Although there is laboratory evidence of similarities in skeletal muscle metabolism in exertional heat stroke and MH,[153] and one of the mouse MH knock-in models exhibits environmental heat triggering,[154] there is as yet little evidence that these are anything more than clinically similar presentations.[63,155,156] For this reason, dantrolene has rarely been recommended to treat heat stroke.[157] Nonetheless, some subsets of MH-susceptible patients may be more sensitive to exertional heat stroke and thus should be tested for MH susceptibility.[158]

Heat stroke may occur from passive heat exposure, known as classic heat stroke or from physical exertion that leads to exertional heat stroke.[159] The former is more common at the extremes of ages, when vulnerable individuals are left in closed vehicles or houses overheat to temperatures that are dangerously high. The latter, exertional heat stroke, is a major cause of death in athletes and young military recruits during intense physical exertion that may lead to critical physiological and pathological events up to and including death.[156,159] The pathophysiology in exertional heat stroke differs from MH, although in a small number of cases heat stroke victims have been found with RyR1 mutations and positive CHCT.[146,151,160] Currently, a relationship between exertional heat stroke and the RyR1 mutation is speculative.

The prevailing opinion to date is that dantrolene is a second line treatment for severe heat stroke reserved for the patient whose condition does not respond to active cooling,[161,162] although a small preliminary study suggested that when dantrolene was combined with total body cooling, twice as many participants achieved a Glasgow coma scale ≥13 within the first 90 minutes after randomization.[163] Until further evidence is forthcoming, dantrolene remains a second line treatment for exertional heat stroke.

MH reactions have been reported infrequently in susceptible patients who received a nontriggering anesthetic.[67,164,165] Of 2214 patients who presented for muscle biopsy for MH susceptibility, 5 (0.46%) of 1082 who had MH-positive biopsy results developed MH reactions in the recovery room. None of the patients with negative biopsy results developed MH reactions. There is a small incidence of MH reactions among susceptible individuals that may occur despite a safe anesthetic regimen. Whether this is caused by stress or trace anesthetic concentrations that were inhaled is unclear. Massive rhabdomyolysis has been reported on rewarming from cardiopulmonary bypass despite the patient having received a nontriggering anesthetic.[164,165] The mechanism of these responses may be stress, but evidence is lacking.

Genetics

MH in humans follows an autosomal dominant inheritance pattern with incomplete penetrance and variable expressivity.[42,166,167] In the context of MH, incomplete penetrance means that there are fewer patients with MH susceptibility than would be predicted by simple autosomal dominant inheritance. Variable expressivity means that the presence of a genetic mutation defining susceptibility is documented, but it does not mean that a patient will have an MH reaction when exposed to triggering agents. Several explanations for the variable phenotypic responses of MH-susceptible patients to known triggers have been posited including differences among the RyR1 mutations[168] and the need for an antecedent infection (evidenced by a fever >37.5°C) or severe exercise to prime the muscle to respond to inhalational triggers.[59] One patient in the NAMHR received 30 anesthetics before an MH reaction was triggered.[14] Another was discovered to be MH-susceptible by IVCT during screening of a proband's family and later was inadvertently anesthetized with succinylcholine and isoflurane, but these drugs did not trigger a reaction.[169] However, it seems that once an MH reaction has been triggered, a reaction will always occur when the patient is exposed to the trigger agents.

The molecular and cellular bases of these phenomena remain unknown. Naturally occurring susceptibility to MH seems to follow autosomal dominant inheritance patterns in dogs[170] and horses[171] but follows a recessive inheritance pattern in pigs.[172] This suggests that other genetic and epigenetic factors may play a role in determining the degree and timing of MH susceptibility.

The first breakthrough in finding a gene that predisposed to MH was the serendipitous finding of a similar syndrome in pigs.[87,173] When anesthetized with halothane and succinylcholine or with halothane alone, the pigs developed full-blown MH

reactions (E-Fig. 39.5). The pig model has been a primary pathophysiologic, genetic, and pharmacologic model for the study of MH over the past 5 decades. A second serendipitous event introduced a South African anesthesiologist, G.G. Harrison, to dantrolene, and he successfully tested it in his pig model of MH.[112,174] This observation was quickly followed by the successful treatment of a patient with dantrolene.[175] An interview about Harrison's discovery of dantrolene is available from the Wood Library-Museum of the American Society of Anesthesiologists (https://www.woodlibrarymuseum.org/library/media).

One of the most surprising findings was that six separate breeds of pigs at different locations worldwide shared this MH susceptibility to inhalational anesthetics and succinylcholine. All reactions were treated successfully with dantrolene, and all were determined to have an autosomal recessive inheritance pattern. It was established that MH was associated with an uncontrolled increase in intramyoplasmic Ca^{2+}, presumably the result of an exaggerated release of Ca^{2+} from the sarcoplasmic reticulum (SR).[176,177] Much effort has been expended in understanding the physiologic basis of excitation–Ca^{2+}-release coupling (ECRC) as part of the general mechanism of skeletal muscle excitation-contraction coupling.

By the mid-1980s, an allosteric ion channel located on the sarcoplasmic reticulum (and endoplasmic reticulum) membrane was identified by its ability to bind the insecticidal toxin, ryanodine, which was extracted from the South American plant, *Ryania speciosa*.[178] It was named the ryanodine receptor, RyR, and subsequently noted to have properties consistent with a Ca^{2+} channel.[179–181] This ion channel proved to be the largest channel in mammals, exceeding 2 mega Daltons and was comprised of a homotetramer, each containing 5000 amino acids. Since then, more than 700 mutations in the RyR gene have been identified and several of which have associated with potentially fatal diseases including MH, ventricular tachycardia, sudden death, and several neurodegenerative disorders.[182] These receptors are present throughout the body in tissues including neurons, lymphocytes, epithelial and exocrine cells, and muscle. In 1988, this presumed primary Ca^{2+}-release channel of the sarcoplasmic reticulum was found to have gap junction–like channel properties.[183] It was hypothesized that this receptor might be the site of mutations that caused MH. Within a year, the complementary DNA (cDNA) for the skeletal muscle ryanodine receptor was cloned.[184] In 1990, both porcine and human MH were linked to the same region on chromosome 19q12-13.2 at the glucose phosphate isomerase locus, suggesting that MH in both species was due to point mutations in homologous genes.[185] Concurrently, a linkage study in eight families demonstrated that RyR markers cosegregated with MH phenotypes, providing compelling evidence that mutations of RyR determine MH susceptibility.[186] Two years after the initial cloning of RyR1, the identical single amino acid mutation (Arg615Cys) was discovered in this channel in all six breeds of MH-susceptible pigs.[187]

Detailed genetic evaluations have linked MH susceptibility to chromosome 19q12-13.2, the location of the human RyR1 gene (19q13.1), in MH-susceptible families. This is the locus for MH-susceptibility type 1, symbolized by RyR1 (formerly designated MHS1) (Table 39.10).[166,188,189] Of the more than 400 mutations identified in RyR1 (ClinVar-National Center for Biotechnology Information; https://www.ncbi.nlm.nih.gov/clinvar/), only about 30 have been shown to cause MH (https://www.emhg.org provides a comprehensive list of known causative mutations in RyR1). RyR1 mutations account for 50% to 70% of MH-susceptible individuals. Not all MH-susceptible families have disorders linked

TABLE 39.10	Malignant Hyperthermia Loci	
Designation	**Chromosome Locus**	**Gene**
Ryanodine receptor 1 (skeletal) (formerly malignant hyperthermia susceptibility 1 [MHS1])	19q13.1	RyR1
Malignant hyperthermia susceptibility 2	17q11.2-q24	MHS2
Malignant hyperthermia susceptibility 4	3q13.2	MHS4
Calcium channel, voltage-dependent, L-type, α-1S subunit (formerly malignant hyperthermia susceptibility 5 [MHS5])	1q32	CACNA1S
Malignant hyperthermia susceptibility 6	5p	MHS6

to this chromosome, however (see Table 39.10), indicating that this syndrome is genetically heterogeneous.

Three isoforms of the RyR receptor have been described in mammalian tissues: RyR1, RyR2, and RyR3. Each is expressed by a separate gene although they share 70% of the same sequencing; RyR1 is located on chromosome 19q13.2, RyR2 on chromosome 1q43 and RyR3 on 15q13.3-14.[190] The RyR1 and RyR3 isoforms are expressed primarily in skeletal muscle, and are inhibited by dantrolene.[191,192] Although present in striated muscle, smooth muscle, and neural tissue, the RyR3 isoform is expressed in much smaller concentrations than the RyR1 isoform.[191,193] In contrast, the RyR2 isoform, expressed primarily in heart muscle, has been associated with 320 point mutations that may lead to polymorphic ventricular tachycardia and right ventricular cardiomyopathy.[168,194] The RyR2 isoform is relatively resistant to inhibition by dantrolene although the extent of the resistance depends on the mutation. All three RyR isoforms are also expressed in mammalian neural tissue; RyR1 and RyR2 are limited to the cerebellum whereas RyR3 is located pervasively throughout the brain and in neural tissue in humans.[191,195]

The second gene mutation associated with MH-susceptible, MHS5, codes for the α1 subunit of skeletal muscle dihydropyridine receptor L-type calcium channel. This gene, CACNA1S, codes for only 1% of MH-susceptible subjects.

Several additional loci have been mapped to MH susceptibility, although the genes have not been identified. These include MHS2, linked to chromosome 17q11.2-q24 in North Americans; MHS3 locus, located on 3q13; MHS3 located on 7q21-q22; and MHS6 located on 5p.[15]

Complicating the potential of genetic testing for MH even further is the phenomenon of gene silencing. This phenomenon mimics a recessive mutation in heterozygous individuals by allowing expression of only the affected allele while silencing the other, normal, allele.[196] Because MH is an autosomal dominant susceptibility, it is conceivable that a mechanism underlying the variability in MH triggering seen in patients with identical, monoallelic RyR1 mutations results from skeletal muscle–specific silencing of the affected gene. It follows that inhalational anesthetics or succinylcholine, after multiple exposures, may release a gene from the silenced state, allowing triggering to occur. This may be an explanation for discordance among genetics, linkage analysis, and trait expressivity.

Although the inheritance of human MH is described as autosomal dominant, there are a few individuals who are allelically homozygous for an RyR1 mutation,[197,198] intra-allelically heterozygous for two different RyR1 mutations, or compound heterozygotes containing one mutation in RyR1 and a second mutation at another locus for MH susceptibility.[199] Surprisingly, no overt myopathies have been reported in these affected individuals.

Physiology

NORMAL SKELETAL MUSCLE: EXCITATION-CONTRACTION COUPLING

The neurochemical signal that triggers excitation-contraction coupling begins with the release of acetylcholine from the motor nerve terminal at the skeletal muscle nicotinic synapse, resulting in depolarization of the surface membrane, the sarcolemma. Sarcolemmal membrane depolarization travels along the muscle cell and penetrates the interior of the muscle cell via specialized invaginations in the surface membrane known as transverse tubules, which occur at regular intervals along the muscle cell (Fig. 39.5). The T-tubule membrane is studded with the skeletal muscle isoform of the voltage-dependent L-type Ca^{2+} channel known as the dihydropyridine receptor (DHPR). Thus, opening the RyR1 Ca^{2+} channel in skeletal muscle is a depolarization, rather than Ca^{2+}-induced calcium release as is the case in RyR2 (cardiac muscle).[200] In skeletal muscle, DHPR does not transmit Ca^{2+} in response to sarcolemmal depolarization, rather, it functions as a sarcolemmal voltage sensor.

In response to depolarization, the intrachannel charge moves across the T-tubule membrane inducing a conformational change in the DHPR. The T-tubule is surrounded by specialized portions of the cellular organelle (i.e., sarcoplasmic reticulum) responsible for maintaining the cellular Ca^{2+} store, and the sarcoplasmic reticulum contains a high-capacity Ca^{2+} storage protein called calsequestrin, which regulates the ability of the RyR1 channel to open.[201] The face of the sarcoplasmic reticulum R junctional membrane apposing the T-tubule contains a packed, regular array of RyR1 proteins in close apposition to the DHPR. Physically, the DHPR and RyR1 receptor proteins overlie each other in a unique arrangement of four DHPRs (tetrad) per one RyR1, with every other RyR1 lacking a tetrad (Fig. 39.6).[202] Physical interaction of the DHPR with RyR1 after depolarization causes the RyR1 channel to open, and sarcoplasmic reticulum-stored Ca^{2+} is released into the myoplasm. Orthograde and anterograde communication between the DHPR and RyR1 results in reciprocal regulation of both entities.[203,204]

In the myoplasm, the troponin C subunit of the troponin complex is bound to tropomyosin, which in the resting state inhibits myosin interaction with actin and maintains a relaxed muscle. Ca^{2+} binding to troponin C causes a conformational change in troponin and allows the complex to move away from tropomyosin, which rotates along the actin filament in a way that permits myosin head interaction with this fibrous protein. Fiber shortening and muscle contraction then occur in a myosin-ATPase–driven ratcheting reaction. The muscle relaxes when the sarcoplasmic reticulum membrane–bound Ca^{2+}-ATPase transports free myoplasmic Ca^{2+} back into the sarcoplasmic reticulum against its concentration gradient in an energy-dependent reaction, thereby driving myoplasmic Ca^{2+} concentrations down to resting levels. Troponin I, with its bound Ca^{2+} removed, moves back to block the myosin interaction with actin, thereby preventing muscle contraction and inducing its relaxation. Although a

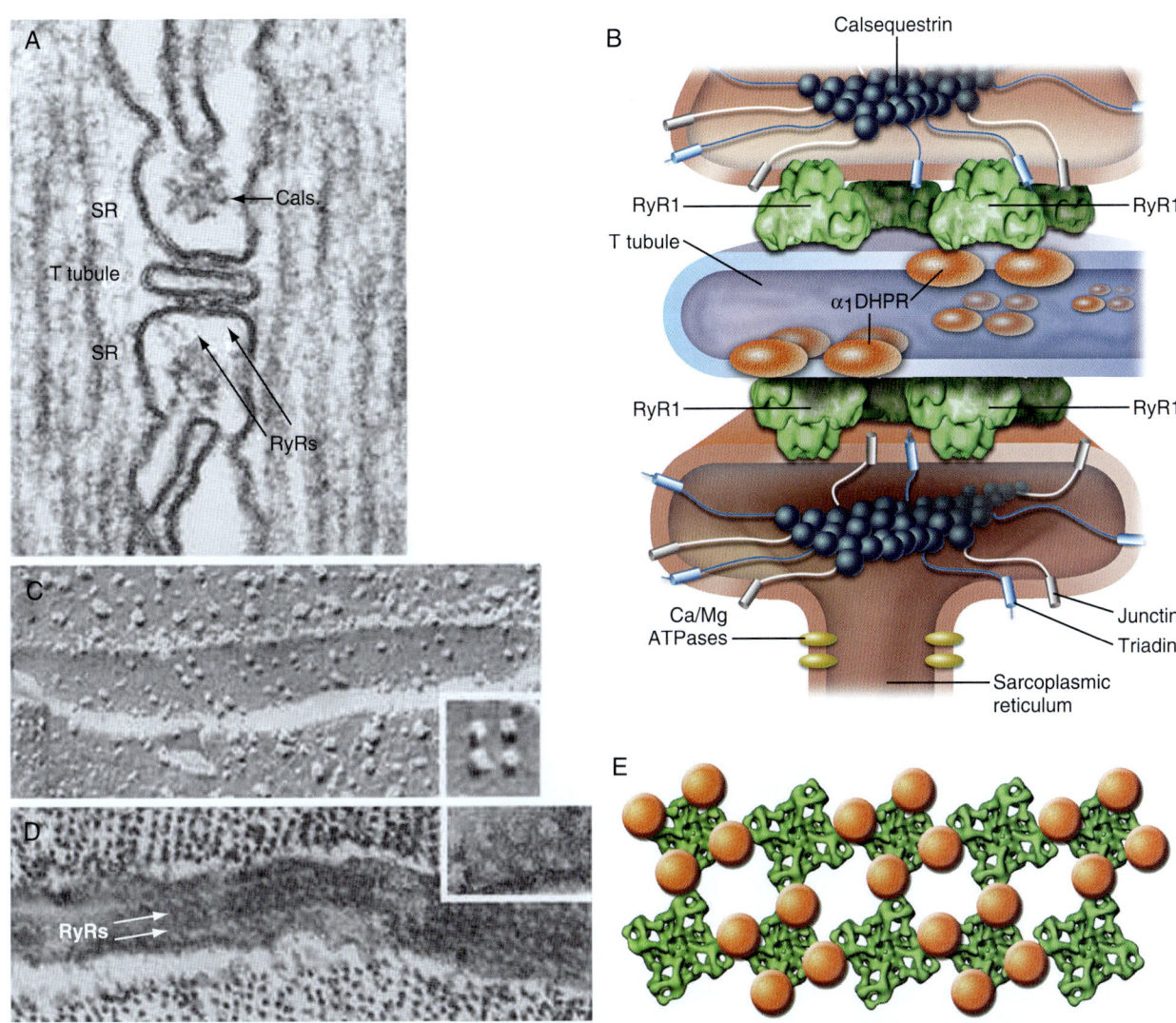

FIGURE 39.5 Structure of calcium release units in adult skeletal muscle fibers. In adult skeletal muscle, junctions are mostly triads: two sarcoplasmic reticulum *(SR)* elements coupled to a central transverse tubule *(T-tubule)*. **A,** A triad from the toadfish swimbladder muscle in thin-section electron microscopy shows the cytoplasmic domains of the SR Ca^{2+} release channel (RyR1), or feet, and calsequestrin *(Cals.)*, the SR Ca^{2+} storage protein. **B,** A tridimensional reconstruction of a skeletal muscle triad shows the ultrastructural localization of ryanodine receptors *(RyRs)*, dihydropyridine receptors *(DHPR)*, calsequestrin, triadin, junctin, and Ca^{2+}/Mg^{2+}-ATPases. Notice the localization of DHPR in the T-tubule membrane; DHPRs are intramembrane proteins that are not visible in thin-section electron microscopy but can be visualized by freeze-fracture replicas of T-tubules (in C). **C,** DHPRs in skeletal muscle form tetrads, a group of four receptors *(inset)*, that are linked to subunit of alternate RyRs (in **B** and **E**). **D,** In sections parallel to the junctional plane, RyR feet arrays *(white arrows)* are clearly visible in toadfish swimbladder muscle; the feet touch each other close to the corner of the molecule *(inset)*. **E,** The model summarizes the findings of **C** and **D**: RyRs *(green)* form two (rarely three) rows, and DHPRs *(orange)* form tetrads that are associated with alternate RyRs. The T-tubule is shown in *blue* in **B,** and sandwiched between two portions of the SR in **A.** (**A,** Courtesy Clara Franzini-Armstrong; **B,** courtesy T. Wagenknecht; from Protasi F. Structural interaction between RyRs and DHPRs in calcium release units of cardiac and skeletal muscle cells. *Front Biosci.* 2002;7:d650-d658.)

detailed description of the complexity of this process is beyond the scope of this chapter, reviews of excitation-contraction coupling are available.[205,206]

PATHOPHYSIOLOGY OF MALIGNANT HYPERTHERMIA

Advances in the pathophysiology of MH have been reviewed in great detail elsewhere.[207210] In brief, at the cellular level, MH is characterized by an inhalational anesthetic–induced, uncontrolled increase in intramyoplasmic Ca^{2+} levels,[211,212] which precedes the metabolic and clinical signs of this syndrome[213] (see Fig. 39.6). Increased intramyoplasmic Ca^{2+} has been demonstrated by directly measuring intracellular Ca^{2+} in anesthetic-triggered pigs[211] and by substantiating the sensitivity of stored Ca^{2+} release by isolated sarcoplasmic reticulum from MH-susceptible pigs.[176,177,214,215] There is also a significant loss in the ability of magnesium (Mg^{2+}), the natural inhibitory divalent cation that competes with Ca^{2+} for binding sites on RyR1, to inhibit Ca^{2+} release in MH-susceptible skeletal muscle.[216218]

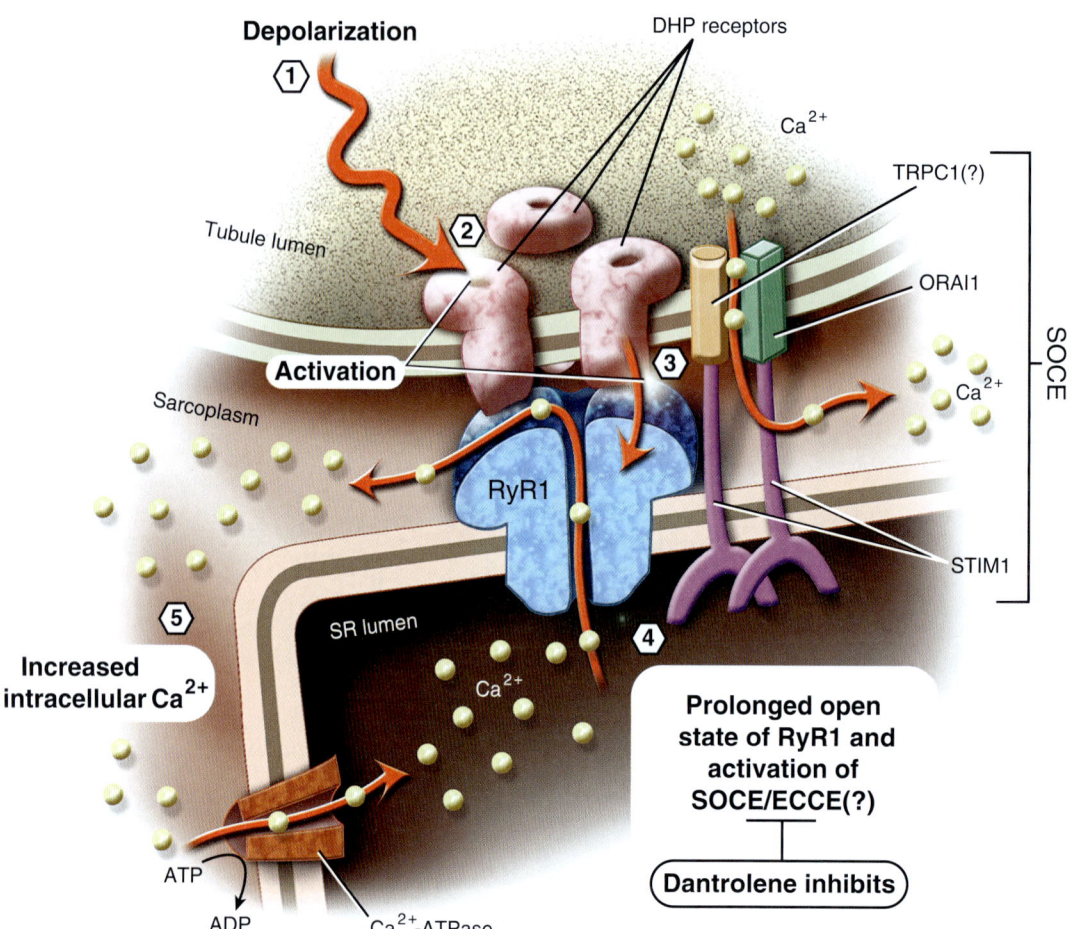

FIGURE 39.6 Schematic of the known pathophysiology of malignant hyperthermia (MH). Exposure of an individual who has a genetic susceptibility because of a ryanodine receptor (RyR1) or dihydropyridine *(DHP)* receptor mutation to an anesthetic triggering agent may result in MH. Normally, muscle cell depolarization **(1)** is sensed by the DHP receptor **(2)**, which signals RyR1 opening by a direct physical connection **(3)**. The conventional view of the genesis of MH is that RyR1 opening is easier and more sustained in the presence of volatile anesthetics **(4)**, allowing a sustained rise in the Ca^{2+} concentration in the myoplasm **(5)** that surpasses the sarcoplasmic reticulum Ca^{2+} reuptake activity of the Ca^{2+}/Mg^{2+}-ATPase. This results in unrelenting muscle contraction and uncontrolled anaerobic and aerobic metabolism, which translate into the clinical manifestations of respiratory and metabolic acidosis, muscle rigidity, and hyperthermia. If the process continues unabated, adenosine triphosphate *(ATP)* depletion eventually causes widespread muscle fiber hypoxia with resultant cell death and rhabdomyolysis. Rhabdomyolysis manifests clinically as hyperkalemia and myoglobinuria and an increase in the serum creatine kinase level. Dantrolene sodium binds to RyR1, presumably causing it to favor the closed state and stemming the uninhibited flow of calcium into the myoplasm. The contributions of store-operated Ca^{2+} entry *(SOCE)* to myoplasmic Ca^{2+} fluxes and its inhibition by dantrolene suggest that MH may have a significant component from SOCE or excitation-coupled Ca^{2+} entry *(ECCE)*, or both, and dantrolene may inhibit the RyR1-dependent activation of SOCE or ECCE. TRPC1, ORAI1, and STIM1 are proteins involved in calcium transport. *ADP*, Adenine diphosphate; *SR*, sarcoplasmic reticulum. (Modified from Litman RS, Rosenberg H. Malignant hyperthermia: update on susceptibility testing. *JAMA.* 2005;293[23]:2918-2924.)

RyR1 isolated from MH-susceptible pigs demonstrate greater open probabilities, greater sensitivity to Ca^{2+} activation, less sensitivity to Ca^{2+} inactivation, and reduced inhibition by Mg^{2+}. As a result, the affected RyR1 channels spend more time in the open state and less time in the closed state than normal channels.[219-223] Although not formally confirmed, this mechanism presumably underlies the sensitivity of RyR1 channels to volatile anesthetics and to the increase in intramyoplasmic Ca^{2+} seen in MH-susceptible skeletal muscle.

Similar single-channel studies of the Ca^{2+} responsiveness of human MH-susceptible RyR1 channels have yielded more equivocal results,[224] presumably because of the genetic heterogeneity of the human MH-susceptible population. Even within a single individual, heterozygosity for an MH mutation permits a given RyR1 channel that is supposed to be made up of four identical subunits to contain any combination of zero to four MH-susceptible subunits in combination with wild-type, normal RyR1 subunits. When examining single channels from a population of channels isolated from a heterozygous, MH-susceptible patient, the clinician can expect a wider range of channel responses than in the homozygous, inbred, porcine population used for MH models.

Several laboratories have created knock-in mice containing one of two known MH-related RyR1 mutations: Tyr522Ser and Arg163Cys.[141,142] In contradistinction to the pig model, but consistent with their MH-susceptible human counterparts, these knock-in MH mice are heterozygous. Their homozygous littermates die in utero on day 17. These heterozygous mice become rigid, hyperthermic, and hypermetabolic when exposed to inhalational anesthetics. These mice die after exposure to inhalational anesthetics or heat stress, and respond therapeutically to dantrolene. They display exaggerated responses to the RyR1 agonists caffeine and 4-chloro-m-cresol and to potassium depolarization. As with MH-susceptible humans and pigs, their muscle is less sensitive to inhibitory Mg^{2+} and possesses greater resting Ca^{2+} concentrations than wild-type animals. These experimental animals display a physiologic MH phenotype remarkably similar, if not identical, to the human syndrome and should prove extraordinarily useful in working out the details of MH pathophysiology.

Development of MH seems to require some form of neural input to muscle, because epidural anesthesia in the porcine MH model completely inhibits expression of MH.[225] However, complete inhibition of neural input to skeletal muscle in this model using competitive, nondepolarizing, nicotinic cholinergic receptor antagonists such as D-tubocurarine, pancuronium, and vecuronium before a halothane challenge does not prevent triggering an acute MH reaction.[226,227] Together, these results suggest that a neurologically significant contribution to MH arises from the central nervous system by means of sympathetic outflow or the neuroendocrine axis, rather than direct skeletal muscle stimulation. This theory is consistent with the awake or stress-related episodes of MH described earlier.

MOLECULAR MECHANISMS AND PHYSIOLOGIC EFFECTS OF DANTROLENE

Dantrolene (Fig. 39.7) is a hydantoin derivative originally synthesized as part of an effort to examine the muscle relaxant properties of a series of substituted furan derivatives.[228] Thinking that they might have discovered a new neuromuscular blocking drug, scientists investigated its mechanism of action but found that it differed from the known skeletal muscle relaxants. Dantrolene affected the intrinsic properties of skeletal muscle without affecting the central nervous system, neuromuscular transmission, electrical properties of the sarcolemma or the T-tubule, electromyogram, or train-of-four method for testing neuromuscular blockade. Its action was intracellular (Fig. 39.8).[229] Indirect evidence pointed to dantrolene interfering with Ca^{2+} fluxes that were intrinsic to skeletal muscle contraction.[230–232] Direct observations[233,234] demonstrated that dantrolene suppressed the rate and amount of Ca^{2+} released from the sarcoplasmic reticulum without completely abolishing it. Subsequently, it was demonstrated that dantrolene inhibited halothane-induced Ca^{2+} release from the isolated sarcoplasmic reticulum of MH-susceptible pigs,[214,235,236] but was devoid of any effect on calcium reuptake into the sarcoplasmic reticulum.[108,237]

After sarcoplasmic reticulum Ca^{2+} release was identified as the likely target of dantrolene's activity, several attempts to identify a dantrolene binding partner in the sarcoplasmic reticulum proved unsuccessful, primarily because of the difficulties of conducting detailed pharmacologic receptor analyses with a drug as hydrophobic as dantrolene.[238,239] In 1995, an assay for radioactively

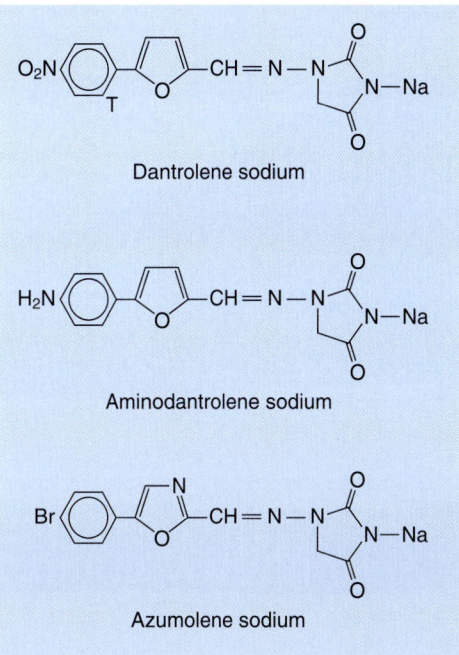

FIGURE 39.7 Dantrolene and its congeners. Dantrolene and azumolene are equipotent drugs, but azumolene is far more water soluble. Only dantrolene is approved by the US Food and Drug Administration for treatment of malignant hyperthermia. Aminodantrolene is a poorly active congener, demonstrating how small changes in drug structure can result in large changes in activity. (Modified from Parness J, Palnitkar SS. Identification of dantrolene binding sites in porcine skeletal muscle sarcoplasmic reticulum. *J Biol Chem.* 1995;270[31]:18465-18472.)

labeled dantrolene helped to elucidate specific binding sites in porcine skeletal muscle sarcoplasmic reticulum.[240] Dantrolene inhibits RyR1-dependent cellular Ca^{2+} fluxes in skeletal muscle, albeit incompletely, but it does not seem to affect RyR1 channel activity or its ability to transport Ca^{2+}.[241] Curiously, dantrolene proved to be ineffective in attenuating Ca^{2+} release through single RyRs inserted into lipid bilayers in most in vitro studies.[242] This inconsistency between the in vitro and in vivo studies has been attributed to dantrolene's codependency on adequate concentrations of both calmodulin,[243] which binds to RyR, ATP and Mg^{2+}, which accumulates from the hydrolysis of magnesium adenosine triphosphate (MgATP) during an MH reaction.[194,244]

A second physiologic process, called store-operated Ca^{2+} entry (SOCE), contributes to the increase in intracellular Ca^{2+} as a result of the RyR1 channel opening in skeletal muscle.[245–247] SOCE is a process by which the sarcoplasmic reticulum store of Ca^{2+} is replenished from the extracellular milieu after significant loss of Ca^{2+} from the sarcoplasmic reticulum.[248] Experiments with azumolene, a more water-soluble congener of dantrolene (Fig. 39.7), have demonstrated inhibition of skeletal muscle RyR1-dependent SOCE, not sarcoplasmic reticulum Ca^{2+} release.[249] Clinically, azumolene blocked skeletal muscle contractures in mouse and mammalian muscles in response to caffeine stimulation, and reversed an acute MH reaction in MH-susceptible swine in a dose equipotent with dantrolene.[250,251] These results raise profound questions. Do the induced Ca^{2+} fluxes during excitation-contraction coupling, experimental manipulation, and MH that result in an increase in intracellular Ca^{2+} all result from RyR1-dependent Ca^{2+} release or RyR1-dependent Ca^{2+} entry, or both?

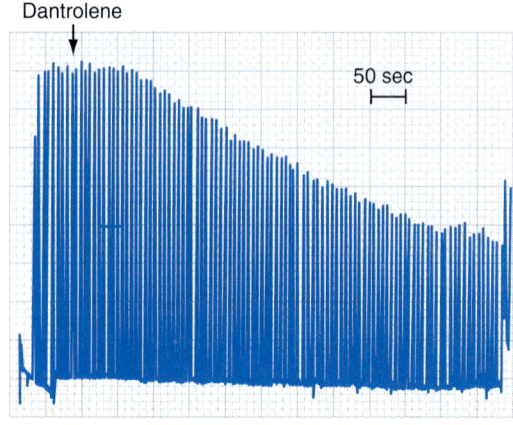

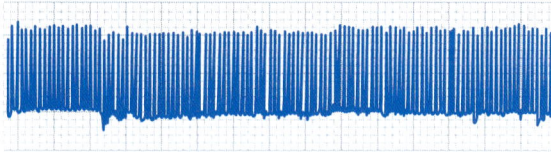

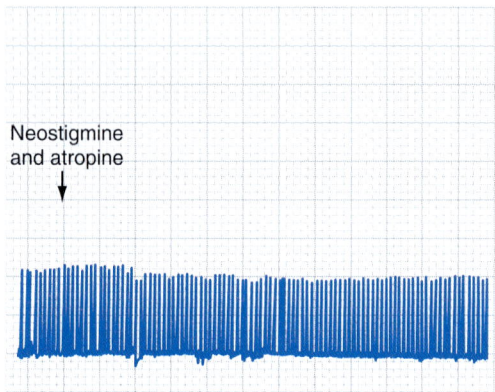

FIGURE 39.8 Intraoperative electromyogram of a child given intravenous dantrolene (2.4 mg/kg). The twitch tension decreased about 75% after dantrolene but was not reversed by administration of neostigmine, demonstrating the lack of involvement of the neuromuscular junction in the action of dantrolene.

Evidence of a dantrolene-sensitive, excitation-coupled Ca^{2+} entry mechanism of skeletal muscle (ECCE) that is more easily activated in MH skeletal muscle has been described, as well.[252–255] ECCE is different from SOCE in that it does not require depletion of the sarcoplasmic reticulum Ca^{2+} store and is activated by high-frequency electrical stimulation of the skeletal muscle membrane. ECCE and SOCE present new physiologic targets of investigation into the pathophysiology of MH that involve Ca^{2+} entry rather than Ca^{2+} release (see Fig. 39.6).

Elucidation of the pathophysiology of MH and the mechanism of action of dantrolene has radically transformed our understanding of muscle physiology and pathophysiology. As our understanding continues to evolve, the future for advances in therapy and testing capabilities hold great promise.

Laboratory Diagnosis

CONTRACTURE TESTING

The standard for testing susceptibility to MH in the human population is an in vitro contracture test that assesses live human muscle fibers from the vastus lateralis in a physiologic bath. With one end of the muscle tissue attached to a strain gauge, the degree of tension developed at baseline and on electrical stimulation is measured as a function of the concentrations of halothane or caffeine. The test is based on the observation that fresh muscle isolated from MH-susceptible patients behaved abnormally when exposed to halothane or caffeine in vitro (Fig. 39.9).[256–259] Two variations of this test have been developed and adopted: the CHCT by the North American Malignant Hyperthermia Group (NAMHG) and the IVCT by the European Malignant Hyperthermia Group (EMHG). The NAMHG test measures the response in separate muscle fascicles to a bolus of 3% halothane or incremental increases in the caffeine concentration,[33,260,261] and it requires a positive response to one of the challenges for a diagnosis of MH susceptibility. Those not responding are considered normal. The EMHG test measures the response to graded increases in the halothane concentration up to 2% and incremental increases in the caffeine concentration in different fascicles. The diagnosis of MH susceptibility by the IVCT requires a positive response to both challenges, whereas a positive response to one of the challenging agents results in equivocal diagnostic categorization (i.e., MH equivocal).[262–264]

Even though the EMHG protocol may prevent excess false-positive and false-negative results compared with the NAMHG protocol, overall results are comparable.[265] The EMHG reports that the sensitivity and specificity of its protocol are 99% and 94%, respectively,[263] whereas the NAMHG reports that its sensitivity and specificity are 97% and 78%, respectively.[266] Because the North American protocol is less specific and tends to over diagnose MH susceptibility, it has a very small likelihood of failing to diagnose an MH-susceptible individual. The fact that there are some false-positive findings in the contracture testing demonstrates that other myopathic conditions that are not necessarily concordant with MH have muscle tissue that is also capable of giving an abnormal response to halothane and caffeine exposures. Discordance between the results of an IVCT and the presence of MH mutations in RyR1 can occur in MH families such that 3.1% to 19.4% of family members who do not carry an MH mutation respond positively to an IVCT challenge.[263,267] This presumably indicates that there are other factors (e.g., a second MH susceptibility mutation in RyR1, another MH sensitivity locus, a sensitivity to caffeine and halothane that does not reflect MH susceptibility) in these individuals that give a positive IVCT result, but it does not necessarily mean that they are MH-susceptible.

GENETIC TESTING

Limited examination of the RyR1 gene is available for the purpose of diagnosing MH susceptibility at two Clinical Laboratory Improvement Amendments–approved laboratories in North America, as discussed earlier. Any physician can write a prescription for the ryanodine receptor gene test for MH susceptibility or fill out the requisition form and send blood for genetic testing. However, the probability of a positive outcome with genetic testing depends in part on the results of the in vitro CHCT, as the clinical signs of MH are nonspecific. Current genetic testing indicates that about 60% of those who have positive CHCT results also have positive genetic results, whereas only 20% of those without a positive CHCT result yield positive genetic results.[267] Thus, a negative gene screening test does not eliminate MH susceptibility, but a positive gene screen can be used to trace a family pedigree.

"Next-generation sequencing" is a more rapid, more accurate, and less expensive technique that has become increasingly available worldwide to assist in the genetic analysis of neuromuscular

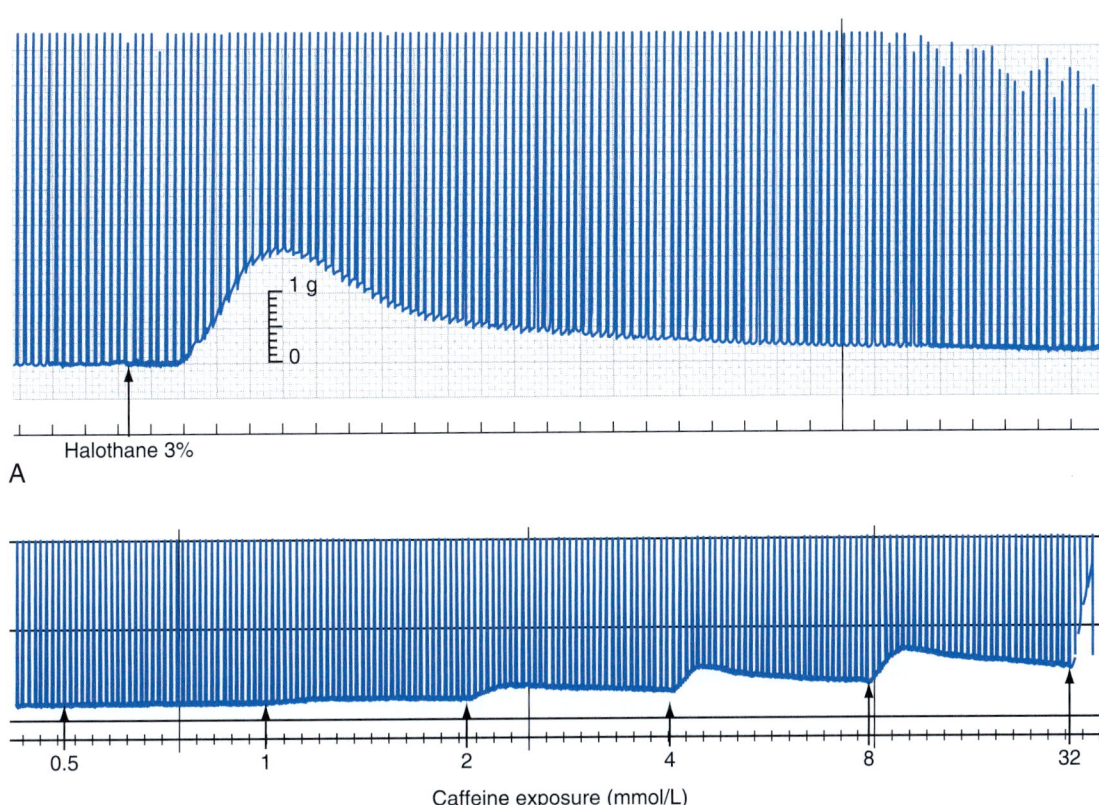

FIGURE 39.9 Caffeine-halothane contracture test. **A,** Abnormal (positive) response to 3% halothane. Each small box represents 0.1 grams of tension. The contracture response in this case is 1.6 grams. A normal response to 3% halothane is a contracture up to 0.7 grams. After exposure to halothane, 32 mmol/L of caffeine is added to the bath to determine maximal response. **B,** Abnormal (positive) response to caffeine. Caffeine exposure is increased to 0.5, 1.0, 2.0, 4.0, 8.0, and 32 mmol/L for 4 minutes. A contracture of greater than 0.3 g to 2 mmol/L of caffeine or less indicates susceptibility. (Modified from Rosenberg H, Antognini JF, Muldoon S. Testing for malignant hyperthermia. *Anesthesiology.* 2002;96[1]:232-237.)

disorders, including patients who are MH-susceptible (with a possible RyR1 variant) and those who have never experienced an MH event but present with an undiagnosed muscle disorder or heat-related event (heat stroke). It is for these reasons and its noninvasive nature compared with a muscle biopsy, that this sequencing technique is emerging as the first-line diagnostic criterion for MH and a host of possible-RyR1 variant causes of muscle disorders. In the case of genetic variants for MH, an expert panel was convened to recommend criteria to classify the pathogenicity of the 335 genetic variants of RyR1 that have been associated with MH.[268] If the criteria to diagnose MH were not met, a caffeine-halothane contracture test was recommended. In a retrospective, multi-institutional review of referrals to the MH units in four countries between 2010 and 2019, a personal history of an adverse anesthetic event was present in 41%, a family history in 22%, and exertional or recurrent rhabdomyolysis in 9%.[269] Over the decade reviewed, the proportion of referrals without an anesthesia-related history increased from 28% to 44% to diagnose muscle disorders and possible RyR1 variants. Of those with a personal or family history of an anesthesia-related event, 60% were more likely to be diagnosed as MH-susceptible than those without a history, with 39% based on the expert panel criteria for pathogenetic RyR1 variants. Interestingly, in 28% of the MH-susceptible patients, RyR1, CACNA1S, or STAC3 variants were not found, underscoring the need for further research to identify additional genes that harbor MH-susceptible variants. As this "next-generation sequencing"

expands, further studies on the CACNA1S and STAC3 variants and their pathogenicity will need to be added to fully characterize those at risk for developing MH reactions.

NONINVASIVE TESTING

Muscle ultrasound is an emerging diagnostic tool to noninvasively assess neuromuscular disorders. Currently, qualitative analysis yields ~70% sensitivity to diagnose disorders although quantitative analysis yields sensitivities up to 92%. An analysis of 40 MH-susceptible patients confirmed with RyR1 variants, yielded 38% with an abnormal ultrasound result that included muscle hypertrophy and increased echogenicity, the latter particularly prominent in the gastrocnemius, proximal vastus lateralis, and paraspinal muscles.[269] These findings occurred in patients both with and without muscular symptomatology.

Other Disorders and Malignant Hyperthermia

MYOPATHIC SYNDROMES

An incriminatory association between various myopathies and MH susceptibility, now known to be far more restricted than originally thought, was described in the 1970s and 1980s with much debate over the biochemical and pathophysiologic character of the clinical episodes that resulted from exposure to MH-triggering agents.[270,271]

Did the clinical episodes represent true MH; did the episodes relate to the instability of myopathic muscle membrane with attendant destruction of muscle cells and release of intracellular proteins; and was there sometimes an associated hyperthermic reaction with these exposures? Although both types of episodes may result in increased CK levels, hyperkalemia, myoglobinemia, and myoglobinuria, one results from exaggerated ramping of cellular energy and heat production, and the other results from cellular destruction that does not involve abnormal cellular metabolism as a primary cause. Of the congenital myopathies, central core disease, the related multi-minicore disease, and the myopathy of King-Denborough syndrome are the only myopathies known to have a definite relationship with true MH (see Chapter 22).[272,273]

MALIGNANT HYPERTHERMIA MIMICS

Malignant Hyperthermia–Like Syndrome in Pediatric Diabetes Mellitus

Diabetes mellitus has two well-characterized, life-threatening childhood presentations: diabetic ketoacidosis (DKA) and hyperglycemic hyperosmotic nonketotic syndrome (HHNS).[274–277] DKA, which is associated with type 1 diabetes, usually manifests as nausea, vomiting, dehydration, and weakness, but shock and coma are uncommon (1% to 2%) in the absence of cerebral edema. Fever is rarely a symptom and usually spurs a search for an underlying infection. HHNS is usually associated with type 2 diabetes and classically manifests with symptoms of increasing polyuria, polydipsia, and lethargy that develop over a few days. The estimated mortality rate is between 12% and 46%, somewhat more dramatic than that seen for DKA (2% to 10%), presumably because most cases of HHNS occur in adults with many other medical problems. The greatest rates of mortality with HHNS occur in adults older than 75 years of age or those with osmolarity values greater than 350 mOsm per liter. The incidence of HHNS among US children has been rapidly increasing and appears to be associated with the increase in childhood obesity. Despite this increase, pediatric HHNS is rare, and the presence of fever, as in DKA, usually prompts the search for an underlying infection.

A novel malignant hyperthermia–like syndrome (MHLS) against the background of pediatric diabetes mellitus was described in six adolescent boys between 14 and 18 years of age; the cases were culled from three tertiary care facilities in the United States.[278] The features of the syndrome included HHNS with coma, fever, rhabdomyolysis, and severe cardiovascular instability. Among the six adolescents with MHLS, five were obese, five had acanthosis nigricans, four were African American, and four died. Two more cases were later described; one patient died 14 hours after admission as a result of too rapid a correction of serum osmolarity and resultant cerebral edema and cardiovascular collapse, and a second patient was treated with dantrolene and completely recovered despite developing compartment syndrome in her left upper extremity as the result of rhabdomyolysis.[279] The survivor was tested for metabolic abnormalities, and a deficiency in short-chain acyl-coenzyme A (acyl-CoA) dehydrogenase was found.

Investigators recommend that anyone presenting with symptoms of HHNS and MHLS should be treated with dantrolene as soon as the syndrome is recognized, and that fluid and insulin therapy be used for an appropriate rate of correction of serum osmolarity. A search of the literature reveals a similar case described 10 years earlier as fulminant MH associated with DKA in a patient who survived with the addition of dantrolene to his treatment regimen.[280] Although it is difficult to ascertain the efficacy of dantrolene in abrogating the deleterious effects on skeletal muscle and in saving critically ill patients with MHLS during HHNS with such a small number of successfully treated patients, it seems prudent to initiate immediate treatment with dantrolene in these cases until the data can inform us about the true efficacy of this drug in MHLS.

Disorders of Fatty Acid Metabolism

Growing numbers of reports have documented cases of rhabdomyolysis in patients with disorders of fatty acid metabolism that in some ways mimic awake MH. These disorders arise from mutations in the enzymes responsible for the metabolism of various fatty acids and for ensuring adequate energy substrate for the mitochondria during periods of reduced glucose availability, such as during stress. Although these disorders have profound effects on energy metabolism, they should not be confused with mitochondrial myopathies, which result from completely different molecular defects and have mutations in the proteins of the mitochondrial respiratory chain (see Chapter 22). In neither case has a real association with MH been established, but there have been case reports of rhabdomyolysis and cardiac arrest in patients with carnitine palmitoyl transferase II deficiency.[281–283]

Various forms of acyl-CoA dehydrogenase deficiencies (i.e., very-long-chain, long-chain, medium-chain, and short-chain forms) lead to different types of myopathy that can have severe clinical consequences, including hypoglycemia and rhabdomyolysis with attendant multiple-organ dysfunction, which in some deficiencies are brought about by stress, particularly heat and severe exercise.[284,285] These diseases can manifest early in childhood or late in adolescence or young adulthood, and they can be a particular problem for individuals in the military or those who participate in intense sports.[285] Patients with the very-long-chain acyl-CoA dehydrogenase deficiency can present with acute hypercapnic respiratory failure.[286] Dantrolene has been used successfully to treat one case of recurrent rhabdomyolysis in a patient with very-long-chain acyl-CoA dehydrogenase deficiency,[287] and it may be useful to treat acute intraoperative rhabdomyolysis in these patients, although there is a dearth of evidence in this regard.

Children may present for surgery without a diagnosis of an inborn error of fatty acid metabolism and develop intraoperative rhabdomyolysis, mimicking aspects of a fulminant MH reaction. This may be the first manifestation of the child's fatty acid metabolism disorder. Preoperative increases in serum CK and uric acid levels, presumably owing to subclinical rhabdomyolysis, suggest an inborn error of metabolism or myopathy,[288] but these tests are not part of the usual preoperative panel of blood tests in normal pediatric anesthesia practice. Perioperative stress that may result from fasting, fear, disease states, and other causes can induce metabolic decompensation and hypoglycemia. As a consequence, an IV glucose-electrolyte solution is recommended for affected children.[289] Because of a few reports of rhabdomyolysis when these children are anesthetized with inhalational anesthetics, there has been some reluctance to use inhalational anesthetics.[289,290] It is, however, likely that the number of patients with inborn errors of fatty acid metabolism who undergo surgery is far greater than the paucity of reports of adverse outcomes with inhalational anesthetics. Because these patients vary considerably in their responses to stress, it is not surprising that most do well with any well-managed anesthetic. The available evidence suggests that the perioperative risk is no greater with any anesthetic in these children.

If the clinician elects to avoid inhalational anesthetics, two alternatives remain: regional anesthesia and TIVA. In children, peripheral limb surgery often allows for the use of IV sedation and regional anesthesia that may be suitable depending on the age of the child,[263] but most children do not tolerate this technique. However, a propofol based TIVA (see Chapter 6) is often used in children.[291]

Propofol infusion syndrome, a rare, usually lethal complication of prolonged infusions of propofol, is diagnosed by cardiovascular collapse associated with lipemic plasma, enlarged fatty liver, severe metabolic acidosis, and rhabdomyolysis or myoglobinuria.[292–294] In this syndrome, a large increase in particular fatty acids (i.e., malonylcarnitine and C5-acylcarnitine) that points to impaired entry of long-chain fatty acids into mitochondria and to resultant failure of mitochondrial respiration at complex II has been identified.[295] Others suggest that propofol infusion syndrome may uncover medium-chain acyl-CoA dehydrogenase deficiencies, although this remains unproved.[292] The notion that propofol can impair fatty acid uptake and subsequent oxidation raises the possibility that the acute administration of propofol to a patient with a defect in fatty acid metabolism can precipitate a metabolic crisis, although this has never been reported. It has also been suggested that the lipid load from a propofol infusion in the absence of adequate carbohydrate intake can expose a carnitine deficiency as a model for propofol infusion syndrome.[296] Moreover, propofol itself has been shown to inhibit mitochondrial respiration, possibly compounding the effects of fatty acid oxidation deficiencies.[292] In these children, the use of propofol may be associated with an unclear risk of inducing a metabolic crisis. If their metabolic abnormalities are subclinical, there is no easy, inexpensive preoperative screening tool to establish a diagnosis for a rare abnormality. Even if the child is diagnosed with one of the subsets of fatty acid oxidation deficiencies, it is impossible to predict preoperatively which children will be sensitive to propofol and, if they are, how sensitive they are.

Other TIVA regimens that may be considered include ketamine, dexmedetomidine, benzodiazepines, and opioids. In these instances, the preoperative discussion with the parents, children, and surgeons must address the perioperative risks, including the lack of evidence that any particular anesthetic is more likely to precipitate rhabdomyolysis and an MH-like reaction than others.

NEUROLEPTIC MALIGNANT SYNDROME

Neuroleptic malignant syndrome (NMS) is a rare, potentially lethal reaction to neuroleptics (0.1% to 2.5% of patients), which is characterized clinically by the slow onset of fever, muscle rigidity, altered consciousness, and autonomic instability over a protracted period of time.[297] Laboratory findings include increased CK levels, leukocytosis, increased liver enzyme values, and reduced serum iron or potassium concentrations.[297] Neuroleptic malignant syndrome is similar to MH, and the distinction between the two is often difficult to make,[298] except by medication history; neuroleptics are associated with NMS, and inhalational anesthetics and succinylcholine are associated with MH.

NMS has developed in children taking neuroleptics that block all dopamine D_2 receptors (i.e., high-potency neuroleptics, such as haloperidol; atypical neuroleptics, such as thiothixene; low-potency D_2-receptor antagonists, such as metoclopramide; and tricyclic antidepressants) and in those with the withdrawal of

antiparkinsonian medications. Although this syndrome has been attributed to a deficiency of central dopamine, other pathophysiologic mechanisms have also been proposed to explain the many clinical findings that cannot be explained by the lack of dopamine.

Successful therapy for NMS depends on early recognition, cessation of the offending medications, and intensive medical and nursing care geared toward hydration and restoration of electrolyte balance.[297] Specific pharmacologic therapy with dopamine agonists such as bromocriptine or with dantrolene has been advocated, although the use of dantrolene is controversial. Despite the fact that dantrolene is listed in psychiatric textbooks as a first-line pharmacologic treatment for NMS, there is no evidence that it is effective in treating NMS, except for the occasional case report declaring dantrolene to be effective.[297,299,300]

Children with psychiatric diagnoses who require treatment with neuroleptics make up a significant percentage of these pediatric patients. NMS in this pediatric population continues to be a problem, even with the newest drugs. The perioperative period for the pediatric patient taking neuroleptics is one fraught with potential diagnostic dilemmas. For example, one report described postoperative NMS in a child with severe cerebral palsy and seizure disorder who was not taking any neuroleptics and who was successfully treated three times with dantrolene.[301] Was this NMS or a mild form of MH? The answer remains unclear.

Many clinical scenarios in pediatric anesthesia can mimic MH and challenge our diagnostic acumen and our ability to deliver anesthesia safely. Not all metabolic syndromes that reveal themselves under inhalational anesthesia are MH, and not all metabolic syndromes that respond to dantrolene are MH. The examples given here underscore the need for expert advice during a case of suspected MH. Providers are urged to make use of the Malignant Hyperthermia Hotline when the need arises.

Acknowledgment

The author thanks Jerry Parness for his thoughtful prior contributions.

ANNOTATED REFERENCES

Hopkins PM, Girard T, Dalay S, et al. Malignant hyperthermia 2020. Guideline from the Association of Anaesthetists. *Anaesthesia.* 2021;76(5):655-664.
Excellent review of diagnostic criteria for MH and crisis management of an acute reaction.

Lanner JT, Georgiou DK, Joshi AD, Hamilton SL. Ryanodine receptors: structure, expression, molecular details, and function in calcium release. *Cold Spring Harb Perspect Biol.* 2010;2:a003996.
This review explores the chemistry, genetics, and physiology of ryanodine receptors in mammals as they affect skeletal and cardiac muscles.

Lerman J, McLeod ME, Strong HA. Pharmacokinetics of intravenous dantrolene in children. *Anesthesiology.* 1989;70(4):625-629.
This paper describes the pharmacokinetics of a single IV dose of dantrolene in children and the effect of a second bolus after 6 hours on serum concentration.

Litman RS, Rosenberg H. Malignant hyperthermia: update on susceptibility testing. *JAMA.* 2005;293(23):2918-2924.
The authors offer an excellent, understandable review of the clinical pathophysiology and testing strategies for malignant hyperthermia.

Riazi S, Kraeva N, Hopkins PM. Updated guide for the management of malignant hyperthermia. *Can J Anaesth.* 2018;65(6):709-721.
This publication summarizes the latest epidemiology of MH, the triggers of MH reactions, diagnostic criteria for MH including the clinical grading scale and

genetic mutations that predispose to MH. Intraoperative monitoring and treatment as well as postoperative management complete this in-depth review.

Rosenberg H, Pollock N, Schiemann A, Bulger T, Stowell K. Malignant hyperthermia: a review. *Orphanet J Rare Dis.* 2015;10:93.

This article is a comprehensive review of all aspects of MH, including the clinical diagnosis and management, as well as the preparations of dantrolene, genetics, and ongoing controversies related to associated medical disorders.

Rossi AE, Dirksen RT. Sarcoplasmic reticulum: the dynamic calcium governor of muscle. *Muscle Nerve.* 2006;33:715-731.

The article reviews the molecular pathophysiology of malignant hyperthermia and central core disease.

Ruffert H, Bastian B, Bendixen D, et al. Consensus guidelines on perioperative management of malignant hyperthermia suspected or susceptible patients from the European Malignant Hyperthermia Group. *Br J Anaesth.* 2021;126;120-130.

This detailed review provides an updated compilation of the perioperative preparation and management of MH-susceptible patients scheduled for elective and ambulatory surgery, monitoring, postoperative management, and follow-up from the European Malignant Hyperthermia Group.

van den Bersselaar LR, Hellblom A, Gashi M, et al. Malignant hyperthermia susceptibility diagnostics in patients without adverse anesthetic events in the era of next-generation sequencing. *Anesthesiology.* 2022;136:940-953.

A retrospective review of 520 patients referred to MH clinics over a 10-year period in three countries concluded an increasing fraction of referrals had no personal or family history of an MH reaction; patients with a personal/family history of a reaction were more likely to be diagnosed MH-susceptible.

A complete reference list can be found online at Elsevier eBooks+.

Regional Anesthesia

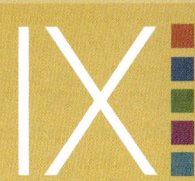

DAVID M. POLANER, MANOJ KUMAR KARMAKAR, RANI SUNDER, SANTHANAM SURESH, AND CHARLES J. COTÉ

Pharmacology and Pharmacokinetics of Local Anesthetics
Amides
Esters
Toxicity of Local Anesthetics
Prevention of Toxicity
Treatment of Local Anesthetic Systemic Toxicity
Hypersensitivity to Local Anesthetics
Ultrasound Equipment
Use of Ultrasound
Principles of Ultrasound
Modes of Ultrasound
The Ultrasound Machine
Essentials of Musculoskeletal Ultrasound Imaging
Axis of Scan
Probe and Image Orientation
Echogenicity
Axis of Intervention
Needle Visibility
Anisotropy
Identification of Structures
Nerves
Tendons
Muscle
Fat
Bone

Fascia
Blood Vessels
Pleura
Special Ultrasound Techniques
Tissue Harmonic Imaging
Compound Imaging
Panoramic Imaging
Artifacts
Scanning Routine
Use of a Nerve Stimulator
Specific Procedures
Central Neuraxial Blockade
Peripheral Nerve Blocks
Head and Neck Blocks
Truncal Blocks
Upper Extremity Blocks
Selective Peripheral Nerve Blocks of the Upper Extremity
Lower Extremity Blocks
Intravenous Regional Anesthesia
Technique
Selection of Drugs
Complications

THE USE OF REGIONAL anesthetic techniques in children has become a standard part of anesthesia practice.[1–11] Although regional anesthesia is most commonly used in conjunction with general anesthesia in children, in certain circumstances regional anesthesia may be the sole technique. In addition to central neuraxial blocks, peripheral nerve blocks are used with increasing frequency; the introduction of high-resolution portable ultrasound imaging has opened new vistas to ensure that these blocks are safe and effective. Ultrasound-guided visualization of anatomic structures permits both greater precision of needle or catheter placement, confirmation that the drug has been deposited at the site of choice, reduces the volume of drug needed to achieve successful blockade, and reduces local anesthetic toxicity.[11,12] Ultrasound guidance has also facilitated the performance of numerous blocks, including truncal blocks, approaches to the brachial plexus (supraclavicular and infraclavicular blocks), and several lower extremity blocks (midthigh saphenous and adductor canal blocks) that could not be otherwise performed accurately or safely in children using landmark or nerve-stimulation techniques.[13,14] Evidence from several large-scale collaborative studies of regional blockade in children supports the trend that peripheral nerve blockade is assuming greater prominence in pediatric anesthesia, and data from the Pediatric Regional Anesthesia Network (PRAN; a large prospective multicenter study) suggests that the increased use of ultrasound guidance may, at least in part, be driving this trend.[14–16] Supplementing a general anesthetic with a nerve block can result in a pain-free awakening and postoperative analgesia without the potentially deleterious adverse side effects associated with parenteral opioids.[17] This benefit may be of particular importance to neonates, former preterm infants, children with cystic fibrosis, and children with other conditions that render them vulnerable to adverse opioid effects.[4] There is also evidence that suggests that regional anesthesia may improve pulmonary function in children who have undergone thoracic or upper abdominal surgery.[18–21] The predominance of "same day surgery" in recent years has made the advantages of regional anesthesia, such as rapid awakening, enhanced postoperative analgesia with no sedation or altered sensorium, and lack of opioid-induced nausea or vomiting, even more apparent. Adjunctive agents that prolong effective blockade and devices such as elastomeric pumps permit continuation of analgesic blockade well into the post-operative recovery period.[22,23] The safe and effective use of these techniques in children, however, requires an understanding of the anatomy of the region in which the block is placed, developmental pharmacology of local anesthetic drugs, and an appreciation of the potential cognitive and performance errors that can occur.[24] Although there is strong evidence and consensus that ultrasound guidance affords numerous advantages in safety and precision over landmark techniques for most peripheral nerve blocks,[11,25,26] this chapter will continue to describe both traditional landmark-guided and ultrasound techniques for situations in which ultrasound technology may not be available. It should be noted that guidelines for managing patients taking anticoagulants are available elsewhere.[27]

Pharmacology and Pharmacokinetics of Local Anesthetics

There are two classes of clinically useful local anesthetics, the amino amides (amides) and the amino esters (esters) (Table 40.1). The amides are degraded in the liver by cytochrome P450 enzymes, whereas the esters are hydrolyzed primarily by plasma cholinesterases.[28] These degradation pathways account for some of the metabolic maturation differences of local anesthetics, particularly in neonates when compared with adults.[29] For example, the clearance of bupivacaine at 1 month of age is approximately one-third of adult values and at 6 months of age is approximately two-thirds of adult values.[30] Another contributing factor leading

to potential toxicity is that infants have lower concentrations of alpha-1-acid glycoprotein, the major protein binding local anesthetics, resulting in more unbound drug than in older children.[30–33] Anatomic factors may also affect drug absorption. For example, the nature of the epidural space in infants differs from that in adults due to increased vascularity and less fat, which may alter absorption. Anatomic studies have shown that the epidural fat is spongy and gelatinous in appearance, with distinct spaces between individual fat globules.[34,35] With increasing age, epidural fat becomes more tightly packed and fibrous.

AMIDES

Amide local anesthetics commonly used in children include lidocaine, bupivacaine, and its isomers levobupivacaine and ropivacaine. The choice of agent often depends on the desired speed of onset and duration of action of the block, but in small infants and children, issues related to potential toxicity are also important. The neonate's and infant's ability to oxidize and reduce drugs, in particular, is immature.[36–43] Neonates do not metabolize mepivacaine, with most of it excreted unchanged in the urine.[44–50] Some cytochrome families are mature at birth, whereas others do not achieve adult function until 6 to 12 months of age (see Chapters 4 and 5).[36,39–41,46]

The absorption half-time of epidural levobupivacaine decreases from 0.36 hours at 1-month postnatal age (PNA) to 0.14 hours at 6-months PNA (E-Fig. 40.1). This, combined with reduced clearance (by the cytochrome P450, CYP3A4), decreases the time to maximum plasma concentration (T_{max}) from 2.2 hours at 1-month PNA to 0.75 hours (80% of the mature value) by 6-months PNA.[51] Older children also differ from adults with respect to the pharmacokinetics of local anesthetics. The steady-state volume of distribution (Vdss) of amides in children is greater than that in adults, whereas their clearances (Cl) are similar.[52–54] Because the elimination half-life ($T_{1/2}$) is related to the volume of distribution and clearance,

$$T_{1/2} = (0.693 \times Vdss)/Cl,$$

a larger Vdss prolongs the elimination half-life. However, it is clearance that determines steady-state concentrations with continuous amide infusions; reduced clearance in neonates implies that repeated doses and continuous infusions of local anesthetics will accumulate (see E-Fig. 40.1).[55–57] Infusion rates and local anesthetic concentrations must be reduced in this vulnerable age group when amide local anesthetics are administered for prolonged periods for postoperative analgesia.[29]

Pharmacokinetic differences between adults and children may be further amplified by the location and type of block. It is critical to realize that the concept of a single toxic threshold dose of a local anesthetic is overly simplistic because systemic absorption rates and blood concentrations that result from drug deposition vary among different locations. That said, there remains a range within which safe dosing can be generalized. Children achieve peak plasma concentrations of amide local anesthetics after intercostal nerve blocks more rapidly than adults, but at similar times (~30 minutes with lidocaine and bupivacaine) after caudal epidural administration.[52,58,59] Ilioinguinal nerve blocks in children who weigh less than 15 kilograms may yield plasma concentrations of bupivacaine in the toxic range at doses exceeding 1.25 mg/kg.[60]

Bupivacaine

Bupivacaine may still be the most commonly used amide local anesthetic agent for regional blockade in infants and children at some institutions, although ropivacaine and levobupivacaine are

TABLE 40.1	Commonly Used Local Anesthetics	
Esters	**Amides**
Procaine	Lidocaine
Tetracaine	Mepivacaine
2-Chloroprocaine	Bupivacaine
	Levobupivacaine
	Ropivacaine
	Etidocaine

increasingly used. Bupivacaine's duration of action varies greatly with the site of blockade, but is generally several hours, although somewhat less in infants and considerably less for subarachnoid block. The concentration used depends on the site of injection, the desired density of blockade, the toxic threshold of the drug, and dose limitations imposed by the concomitant administration of other local anesthetics, such as local infiltration by the surgeon or intravenous (IV) or topical laryngotracheal administration of lidocaine. The most commonly used concentration for peripheral nerve blocks is 0.25%, with reduced concentrations of 0.0625% to 0.125% used for continuous epidural administration. The 0.5% concentration is infrequently used in children, although it may be used for peripheral nerve blocks where subsequent doses and drug accumulation are of limited concern and where the volume of administered drug is sufficiently small to permit that concentration to be used without toxicity. Greater concentrations also increase the density of the motor block, an effect that may be desirable depending on the clinical situation.

Bupivacaine is highly bound to plasma proteins, particularly to α_1-acid glycoprotein.[30] It is a racemic mixture of the levorotary and dextrorotary enantiomers; the *l*-isoform is bioactive with regard to clinical effect, and the *d*-isoform contributes more to toxicity. Hence, the *l*-enantiomer of bupivacaine, levobupivacaine, retains the efficacy and duration of blockade as the racemic formulation, yet carries up to a 30% reduced risk for cardiac and central nervous system (CNS) toxicities.[61,62] Although the safer toxicity profile of levobupivacaine has led to its widespread use, it is currently unavailable in the United States and Switzerland.[63]

Several experimental preparations of local anesthetics have the prospect to prolong analgesia with a reduced potential for toxicity.[64–66] Bioerodible encapsulated microspheres of bupivacaine administered for peripheral neural blockade[67] release local anesthetic over many hours to several days, depending on the formulation of the microsphere, yielding very prolonged analgesia.[68] The addition of dexamethasone to the microspheres prolongs the block up to 13-fold, and plasma bupivacaine concentrations in animal studies were far below the toxic threshold, yielding no adverse local reactions.[69] Several different preparations have been developed and studied, including synthetic bioerodible microspheres, protein-lipid-sugar spheres, and liposheres.[70–72] The first such commercially available preparation (Exparel, Pacira Pharmaceuticals, Inc., Parsippany, NJ) looked promising in initial studies, but a meta-analysis of nine trials in 619 patients cast doubts on its utility, finding clinically unimportant improvement in postoperative pain scores compared with plain local anesthetic.[73–76] New drugs appear to be on the horizon with novel mechanisms of action that may offer more promise. Site 1 sodium channel blockers such as neosaxitoxin have low toxicity and high efficacy and are currently undergoing early clinical trials (see Chapter 41).[77–82] Potential applications include intercostal blockade for rib fractures, postoperative analgesia for ambulatory surgery, and children in whom an indwelling epidural catheter poses an excessive risk of infection.

Ropivacaine

Ropivacaine, like levobupivacaine, is an *l*-enantiomer that in animal models has reduced risks of cardiac and neurologic toxicities compared with bupivacaine.[83,84] Ropivacaine is also reputed to produce a less dense motor block at equianalgesic potency to other local anesthetics, although data are conflicting in this regard, especially in infants and children.[84,85] Ropivacaine produces a denser blockade of the Aδ and C fibers than bupivacaine

when low concentrations are used, lending mechanistic credence to the idea of differential blockade.[86] Several studies in infants and children report a prolonged duration of analgesia with ropivacaine, despite using a solution of reduced potency.[85,87,88] This may be due to its intrinsic vasoconstrictive properties; it is thus not available as an epinephrine-containing solution.[89,90] Most clinical studies have used a 0.2% solution (2 mg/mL); the volume of drug injected is similar to that of bupivacaine. Concentrations of 0.1% for infusions with opioid or clonidine for continuous lumbar epidural postoperative analgesia are often used, whereas concentrations up to 0.2% may be used for thoracic epidural infusions and peripheral and plexus blocks.

Lidocaine

Lidocaine has a relatively short duration of action compared with bupivacaine and ropivacaine; it is rarely used for single-injection blocks in pediatric regional anesthesia, where a prolonged effect for postoperative analgesia is usually a priority. It is very effective for analgesia for IV placement, especially when applied via a transcutaneous jet (J-Tip); it is frequently used by spray or atomization for topical anesthesia of the upper and lower airway.

ESTERS

Chloroprocaine

The pharmacokinetics of the ester local anesthetics are also affected by the quantitative and qualitative difference in plasma proteins. Although data suggested that plasma pseudocholinesterase activity in neonatal umbilical blood was decreased compared with adults,[91] this was inconsistent with the increased clearance of ester anesthetics in neonates. Clearance maturation is mature at birth; a situation similar to that noted for remifentanil and succinylcholine (see Chapter 5). The metabolic capacity of plasma esterases in neonates and young infants permits larger local anesthetic infusion rates of chloroprocaine without drug accumulation[92–94] compared with amides. 2,3-chloroprocaine has been recommended for continuous regional techniques in neonates,[95–97] particularly for epidural, paravertebral, and plexus blockade.[98,99] Limited data suggest that 2,3-chloroprocaine is safe in this setting and that toxic accumulation does not occur after many hours of infusion of a 1.5% concentration.

Prilocaine

Another enzymatic system with decreased activity in neonates is methemoglobin reductase, which is responsible for maintaining hemoglobin in a reduced valence state where it is capable of binding and transporting oxygen. Hepatic metabolism of prilocaine yields *o*-toluidine, which can produce methemoglobinemia, thereby rendering red blood cells less capable of carrying oxygen.[100] The decreased activity of methemoglobin reductase and the increased susceptibility of fetal hemoglobin to oxidization make prilocaine an unsuitable local anesthetic for use in neonates. Although prilocaine is no longer available for use in the United States as an injected local anesthetic, it is one of the components of EMLA cream (eutectic mixture of local anesthetics, prilocaine and lidocaine as well as polyoxyethylene fatty acid esters, carboxypolymethylene, and sodium hydroxide buffered to a pH of 9, AstraZeneca, Wilmington, DE), a commonly used transdermal local anesthetic.[101] The total dose and surface area for EMLA application must therefore be limited in neonates, infants, and toddlers because methemoglobinemia has been reported after excessive and repeat doses (see Chapter 5).[102–104] EMLA should only be applied to normal intact skin in appropriate doses (0–3 months or weight <5 kilograms, 1 gram applied to a maximum of approximately 10 square centimeters surface area; 3–12 months and >5 kilograms, 2 grams to a maximum of 20 square centimeters; 1–6 years and >10 kilograms, 10 grams applied to a maximum of approximately 100 square centimeters surface area; 7–12 years and >20 kilograms, 20 grams applied to a maximum of approximately 200 square centimeters surface area). The dose must be reduced if EMLA is applied to mucosal surfaces (such as the glans of the penis) or oropharyngeal mucosa. The duration of action persists for 1 to 2 hours after the cream is removed. Adverse reactions include skin blanching, erythema, itching, rash, and methemoglobinemia. Infants who are taking drugs that may induce methemoglobinemia, such as phenytoin, phenobarbital, and sulfonamides, may be at increased risk, and caution is warranted. It is contraindicated in children with congenital or idiopathic methemoglobinemia.

Topical amethocaine or tetracaine 4% (Ametop, Smith & Nephew Healthcare, Mississauga, Ontario, Canada) has a more rapid onset of analgesia and increased depth of penetration through the skin and produces minimal vasoconstriction of the skin compared with EMLA.[105,106] However, amethocaine is only available in Canada, Europe, and the United Kingdom, but not in the United States. Other local anesthetics, particularly topical agents, such as benzocaine, are potentially dangerous in infants because of the risk of methemoglobinemia by this same mechanism.[107]

TOXICITY OF LOCAL ANESTHETICS

Except for uncommon effects, such as producing methemoglobinemia, the major toxic effects of local anesthetics are on the cardiovascular system and the CNS. A consistent sequence of symptoms can be observed as plasma local anesthetic concentrations progressively increase, although this may not be readily apparent in infants and small children or those under general anesthesia. Because of the smaller threshold for cardiac toxicity with bupivacaine, cardiac and CNS toxicity may occur virtually simultaneously in infants and children; cardiac toxicity may even precede CNS toxicity.[108] Local anesthetics readily cross the blood-brain barrier to effect alterations in CNS function. One review found 11/47 reports of local anesthetic toxicity (LAST) were associated with

penile blocks[108]; however, data from PRAN found only 7 cases among 112,000 pediatric regional anesthetics, the majority of which occurred after caudal blocks.[109] Under general anesthesia the early recognition of CNS toxicity may not be apparent until devastating cardiovascular effects occur.[110]

In awake patients, the earliest sign of local anesthetic toxicity is circumoral paresthesia, which is the result of the high tissue concentrations of local anesthetic rather than CNS effects. The development of circumoral paresthesia is followed by prodromal CNS symptoms of lightheadedness and dizziness, which progress to both visual and auditory disturbances, such as difficulty in focusing and tinnitus. Objective signs of CNS toxicity are shivering, slurred speech, and muscle twitching. As the plasma concentration of local anesthetic increases, CNS excitation occurs, resulting in generalized seizures followed by respiratory depression and respiratory arrest. Cardiovascular toxicity manifested by systemic blood pressure decreases due to peripheral vasodilation and direct myocardial depression, which leads to progressive bradycardia and ultimately cardiac arrest. In large doses, bupivacaine produces ventricular dysrhythmias, including ventricular tachycardia, peaked T waves, and ST-segment elevation that suggest myocardial ischemia, especially when epinephrine-containing solutions are used. Bupivacaine has a particularly strong affinity for the fast sodium channels, as well as the calcium and slow potassium channels in the myocardium. These effects explain why it is so difficult to resuscitate children from a toxic dose of bupivacaine.[111–113] Stereoselectivity of the sodium channel in the open state, however, has not been demonstrated. There is also evidence that the slow or "flicker" potassium channels may play a major role in bupivacaine toxicity.[114]

With an intravascular injection of bupivacaine with epinephrine, characteristic changes on the electrocardiogram (ECG) may be observed in the absence of symptoms of CNS toxicity, depending on the background anesthetic. Fig. 40.1 shows an ECG tracing obtained during an unintended intravenous injection of bupivacaine with and without epinephrine (positive test dose) under halothane anesthesia. Even a small IV dose of 1 to 2 µg/kg of epinephrine in a 1:200,000 solution with 0.25% bupivacaine produces peaked T waves with elevated ST segments, particularly in the lateral chest leads.[115–117] When the ECG effects of bupivacaine, with and without epinephrine, and epinephrine alone were compared in children anesthetized with sevoflurane, the most reliable ECG

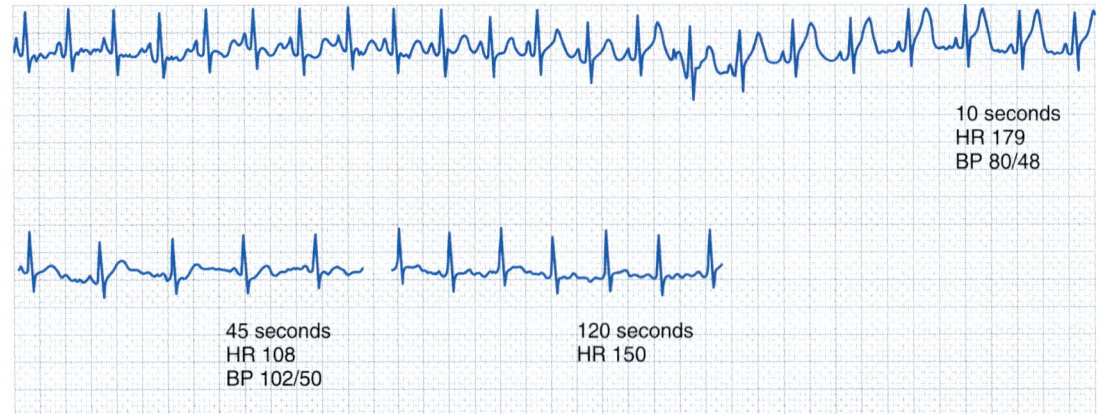

FIGURE 40.1 Electrocardiographic changes associated with the intravenous injection of bupivacaine and epinephrine 1:200,000. Note the marked increase in the height of the T waves at 10 seconds. *BP*, Blood pressure; *HR*, heart rate. (From Freid EB, Bailey AG, Valley RD. Electrocardiographic and hemodynamic changes associated with unintentional intravascular injection of bupivacaine with epinephrine in children. *Anesthesiology.* 1993;79[2]:394-398.)

changes, [peaked T waves (>25%) at 1 minute, and an increase in arterial pressure (≥15 mm Hg) and heart rate (≥10 bpm)], required at least 0.25 µg/kg epinephrine.[118,119] It should be noted, however, that these changes in the T waves depended on age, with diminished responsiveness in children beyond 8 years of age. These data suggest that careful observation of the ECG during test dose administration may be a sensitive indicator of unintended intravascular injection of bupivacaine (see Technique of Administration later) during inhalational anesthetics.[120,121] In contrast, T-wave morphology on the ECG is an unreliable metric to diagnose local anesthetic toxicity during total IV anesthesia (propofol/remifentanil).[122] Increases in systolic blood pressure >10% was found to be the optimal metric to detect local anesthetic toxicity (see later).

Plasma protein binding is an important pharmacologic factor that determines the toxicity of local anesthetics, particularly for amides, because it is the free (unbound) fraction of the drug that produces toxicity. Reduced plasma protein concentrations cause more drug to remain in the unbound active form with greater potential for toxicity (see Chapter 5). Concentrations of α_1-acid glycoprotein in neonates are less than in older infants and children, producing greater concentrations of free lidocaine and bupivacaine compared with older children and adults.[30,31,33,55,123–126] Current data suggest that the plasma concentration of unbound drug is increased in infants younger than 6 months of age and even greater in preterm infants than in adolescents.[32] The unbound fraction of lidocaine, bupivacaine, and ropivacaine in neonates is approximately 60%, 20%, and 20%, respectively, and gradually decreases during the first year of life.[30,127] The unbound fraction in children aged >1 year is similar to that in adults, approximately 35% for lidocaine and 5% for bupivacaine, levobupivacaine, and ropivacaine. α_1-Acid glycoprotein is an acute-phase reactant whose concentration increases after surgery or stress. Concentrations of α_1-acid glycoprotein in infants are less in those undergoing elective rather than emergency surgery.[128] It is not known whether these increased α_1-acid glycoprotein concentrations are sufficient to afford protection from the toxicity of bupivacaine accumulation in the perioperative period. Lower rates of infusions are therefore indicated in neonates and infants younger than 1 year of age, as reduced clearance contributes to drug accumulation and consequent high concentrations of unbound drug (see later).[129,130]

Plasma concentrations of lidocaine that depress the cardiovascular and respiratory systems in neonates are about half those that cause similar toxicity in adults.[131] Animal studies may yield different results, limiting extrapolation of those data to humans; 2-day-old guinea pigs were less susceptible to the toxic effects of bupivacaine than 2-week or 2-month-old guinea pigs, even though the blood concentrations in the 2-day-olds were greater.[110] Data regarding toxicity in infant versus adolescent versus adult rats for both bupivacaine and ropivacaine are similar.[84] Young dogs, however, have a decreased threshold to both seizure and cardiac toxicity caused by excessive doses of bupivacaine.[132] Because species differences are important in toxicity studies, it is difficult to predict which study represents the human neonate.[133] No human data exist regarding age-dependent differences in the toxic threshold of bupivacaine at a given blood concentration. Seizures and cardiovascular collapse have been reported in human infants at the same blood concentrations of bupivacaine as in adults. Whereas data from some animal studies suggest that the greater volume of distribution of amides in younger children may protect against bupivacaine toxicity because initial concentrations are reduced. Retrospective analyses of large databases of infants who have received epidural infusions indicate that continuous infusions or repeated dosing can cause toxicity because the

clearance of the local anesthetics is reduced and the blood concentrations are increased in neonates. Several reports document that infants and children may develop systemic toxicity, including dysrhythmias, seizures, and cardiovascular depression from the accumulation of epidural infusions of bupivacaine.[55,129,134–136] Meticulous attention must be paid to the total dose of local anesthetic administered, the rate of administration, the site of injection, and the use of vasoconstrictors to diminish the rate of uptake of the local anesthetic as well as improving recognition of an intravascular injection.[33,121] This is particularly important when a continuous regional anesthetic technique is used postoperatively or during prolonged surgery when repeated doses of local anesthetic are administered.

We recommend that both the bolus (less α_1-acid glycoprotein) and infusion dose (decreased clearance) of amide local anesthetics be reduced by approximately 30% for infants younger than 6 months of age to decrease the risk of toxicity. This would limit the maximum infusion rate of bupivacaine to ≤0.3 mg/kg per hour.[56] Whereas these recommendations are particularly applicable to continuous infusions of bupivacaine for postoperative analgesia, the same caveats apply to large single injections, repeated injections, and continuous infusions of local anesthetics during long surgical procedures.

The d-stereoisomer (or enantiomer) of racemic mixtures of local anesthetics may also be a primary factor in the risk for both cardiac and CNS toxicity.[113] As described earlier, both ropivacaine and levobupivacaine, which are l-enantiomers, have decreased toxicity compared with bupivacaine, a racemic mixture, as demonstrated in adults and experimental animals.[114] This may be due in part to the reduced affinity of cardiac and CNS tissues for the l-enantiomer.[83] It remains uncertain if the inclusion of levobupivacaine and ropivacaine into the clinical armamentarium has proven beneficial in decreasing local anesthetic toxicity because the dose of bupivacaine was reduced due to a better understanding of its pharmacokinetics, its use has decreased, and the use of intralipid to treat toxic concentrations of local anesthetics all occurred almost simultaneously. Certainly, current practice has moved toward isomer use, especially in younger children.[127]

PREVENTION OF TOXICITY

Few data have correlated the anesthetic block, blood concentration (total or unbound) of local anesthetic, and dose in infants and children. Most dosing guidelines have been extrapolated from studies in adults. Table 40.2 lists the maximum recommended doses of local anesthetics, as well as their approximate durations of action. To avoid overdose and the possibility of toxic effects, it is prudent to remain within these guidelines until studies in children clarify the pharmacokinetics and pharmacodynamics of local anesthetics for specific nerve blocks. As discussed earlier, all of these doses should be reduced by ~30% in infants younger than 6 months of age.

Toxic reactions from local anesthetics are a function of (1) the total dose administered; (2) the site of administration; (3) the rate of uptake; (4) pharmacologic alterations in toxic threshold; (5) the technique of administration; (6) the rate of degradation, metabolism, and excretion of local anesthetic; and (7) the acid-base status of the child.[137–142] Thus recommendations (including those of the authors) of a specific dose limit for a given drug are both overly simplistic and potentially misleading.[122] Because of the multiplicity of factors that drive the final concentration of unbound local anesthetic, and in the absence of definitive and comprehensive data, conservative dosing remains the most prudent course.

TABLE 40.2	Maximum Recommended Doses and Duration of Action of Commonly Used Local Anesthetics	
Local Anesthetic	Maximum Dose (mg/kg)[a]	Duration of Action (minutes)[b]
Procaine	10	60–90
2-Chloroprocaine	20	30–60
Tetracaine	1.5	180–600
Lidocaine	7	90–200
Mepivacaine	7	120–240
Bupivacaine	2.5	180–600
Ropivacaine	3	120–240

[a]These are maximum doses of local anesthetics. Doses of amides should be decreased by 30% in infants younger than 6 months of age. When lidocaine is being administered intravascularly (e.g., during intravenous regional anesthesia), the dose should be decreased to 3 to 5 mg/kg; there is no need to administer long-acting local anesthetic agents for intravenous regional anesthesia, and such a practice is potentially dangerous.
[b]Duration of action depends on the concentration, total dose, site of administration, and the child's age.

Total Drug Dose

The dose of local anesthetic should be determined by a child's age, physical status, the area to be anesthetized, and body mass. A severely ill child who is in congestive heart failure, for example, has a reduced capacity to metabolize amide local anesthetics because of a reduced cardiac output and hepatic blood flow that impact metabolic clearance. Similarly, a markedly obese child must not be given a larger dose (expressed as per kilogram total body weight) simply based on the increased body weight. If a large volume of local anesthetic is required for a particular procedure, a dilute concentration should be used to avoid exceeding the maximum recommended safe dose. Doses can be calculated based on an alternative body mass index (e.g., the lean body weight of the child). For example, a 20-kilogram child could receive up to 50 milligrams of bupivacaine. An easy approximation for bupivacaine is 1 mL/kg of 0.25% bupivacaine, reduced by approximately one-third for infants younger than 6 months of age.

Studies of large pediatric populations using the PRAN database have revealed highly variable doses of local anesthetics for all the commonly performed blocks.[143,144] This variability, which even exceeded the median dose for the block itself, was evident whether analyzed by volume or milligram per kilogram. It was primarily related to the institution performing the block, but there was large variability within centers as well. Eliminating unindicated dose variability is a priority strategy for reducing toxicity risk (particularly at larger doses), but we do not yet have either adequate evidence or a method to determine the optimal dose for a given block. Ultrasound guidance for peripheral blocks can reduce the volume and concentration of local anesthetic needed to achieve a successful block[145–148]; a potential method for determining the best volume/dose might be to visualize the deposition of local anesthetic around the target area with ultrasound.

Site of Injection

Injection of local anesthetics into vascular areas leads to greater blood concentrations than the same dose injected into less vascular areas. The order of uptake (i.e., maximum blood concentration) of local anesthetics (in order from greatest to least) from regional blocks in adults is (1) intercostal nerve blocks, (2) caudal

blocks, (3) epidural blocks, and (4) brachial plexus and femoral-sciatic nerve blocks.[149] An easy way to remember this is by the mnemonic ICE Block:

I = intercostal
C = caudal
E = epidural
Block = peripheral nerve blocks

Blood concentrations of bupivacaine twice those measured in older children have been reported in children weighing less than 15 kilograms after ilioinguinal nerve block for herniorrhaphy using only 1.25 mg/kg of 0.5% bupivacaine without epinephrine, which is half the usual recommended maximal dose.[60] Greater concentrations have also been reported when ultrasound localization is used, most likely due to more precise deposition of drug near the target.[147] This can be offset by the smaller local anesthetic volume required to achieve successful blockade.

However, the fascia iliaca block in older children produced blood concentrations of bupivacaine that were within the acceptable safe range.[150] Neonates who received a transversus abdominis plane block of 0.125% bupivacaine for a total volume of 1 mL/kg had the greatest plasma concentration (0.38 µg/mL) at 30 minutes after the block; this is one-quarter to one-fifth the reported toxic threshold of 1.5 to 2.0 µg/L.[151] Local infiltration of the wound in herniorrhaphy has not been associated with large blood concentrations of local anesthetics,[152] but scalp infiltration during neurosurgery may produce relatively greater blood concentrations.[153] As would be expected, spinal anesthesia results in very small blood concentrations, even in neonates.[126]

Rate of Uptake

The rate of uptake of a local anesthetic depends on the vascularity of the site of injection. Increased perfusion increases uptake, whereas decreased perfusion decreases uptake.[154] The rate of uptake in children is usually more rapid than in adults. In general, the addition of a vasoconstrictor to the local anesthetic reduces the rate of uptake and prolongs the duration of the block.[155] We have used as much as 10 µg/kg of epinephrine in children, with a maximum dose of 250 micrograms during halothane anesthesia without evidence of ventricular irritability[156–158]; these doses are likely safer with the ether inhalational anesthetics, which do not sensitize the myocardium to the arrhythmogenic effects of epinephrine. An epinephrine concentration of 1:100,000 should not be exceeded, and 1:200,000 or less is generally used. A quick reference for converting local anesthetic concentrations and the amount of epinephrine in various dilutions is presented in Tables 40.3 and 40.4. Use of greater concentrations of epinephrine has possibly contributed to ischemia of tissue supplied by end-arteries. *Epinephrine is contraindicated in blocks in which vasoconstriction of an end artery could lead to tissue necrosis, such as for digital and penile blocks, although this historical practice appears to have little scientific evidence and has been challenged, setting the stage for prospective studies.*[159–162]

TABLE 40.3	Epinephrine Dilution and Conversion to µg/mL
Epinephrine Dilution	µg/mL
1:100,000	10
1:200,000	5
1:400,000	2.5
1:800,000	1.25

TABLE 40.4	Local Anesthetic Concentration and Its Conversion to mg/mL
Concentration (percent)	**mg/mL**
3	30
2.5	25
2	20
1	10
0.5	5
0.25	2.5
0.125	1.25

Alteration in Toxic Threshold

Benzodiazepines increase the seizure threshold (i.e., the threshold for CNS toxicity) and can be valuable adjuncts to regional anesthesia.[163,164] In mice, the concomitant use of diazepam and bupivacaine decreased the elimination of bupivacaine from serum and cardiac tissue[165]; this effect was not a result of changes in protein binding,[166] but probably from competition for CY3A4, the major clearance pathway. Although premedication with a benzodiazepine prevents manifestations of CNS toxicity, the threshold for cardiovascular toxicity is unchanged.[167] Thus, cardiovascular collapse can occur without warning because the symptoms of CNS toxicity may be blunted.[167]

Technique of Administration

Whenever regional anesthesia is performed, the operator must be prepared for an adverse reaction, and resuscitation supplies, including drugs, suction, and airway equipment, must be immediately available. The needle or catheter must always be inspected for blood as soon as it is positioned and before injecting the local anesthetic, to determine if the tip is within an artery or a vein. It is preferable to observe the needle or catheter for passive blood flow rather than to actively aspirate for blood because the blood vessels, such as the epidural venous plexus, are thin walled and collapse readily when negative pressure is applied. As a result, the inability to aspirate blood is not absolute proof that the needle or catheter is not in a blood vessel, and even the absence of passive flow is a not a completely reliable indicator. For this reason, a small volume of local anesthetic with a marker for intravascular injection, such as epinephrine in a concentration of 1:200,000, is administered first, while the ECG is observed for 30 to 60 seconds and thereafter during subsequent incremental injections.[121] Data from awake adults indicate that the heart rate will increase within 1 minute of intravascular administration.[168] When the drugs are administered during general anesthesia, however, the efficacy of the test dose to detect an intravascular injection may be greatly reduced if one relies solely on the heart rate as an indicator. Heart rate increases in only 73% of children after an IV injection of 0.5 μg/kg of epinephrine during halothane anesthesia, suggesting that this marker of an intravascular injection is not very reliable.[169] Administration of atropine several minutes before the test dose increased the rate of positive responders to 92%, suggesting that vagal tone and the anesthetic's blunting of the sympathetic reflexes are responsible for the reduced sensitivity to the test dose. Test doses during isoflurane anesthesia appear to have the same limitations.[170] With sevoflurane, positive results were obtained in 100% of children if the threshold for a positive response was an increase in heart rate of 10 beats per minute and a dose in excess of 0.5 μg/kg of epinephrine was used; positive results were obtained in 85% if 0.25 μg/kg of

epinephrine was used.[119] In all children, a change in the T-wave amplitude was a reliable indicator of intravascular injection with both doses of epinephrine (see Fig. 40.1). All children in that study were pretreated with atropine (10 μg/kg). It is not known if increasing the dose of epinephrine to 1.0 μg/kg or increasing the concentration of epinephrine in the test dose solution to 1:100,000 during general anesthesia would increase the sensitivity of the heart rate response test without atropine. Systolic blood pressure increased by more than 10% within 60 seconds of the test dose injection, suggesting that an increase in blood pressure may be a more sensitive indicator of intravascular injection than heart rate during inhalation anesthesia. ST-segment and T-wave changes are important indicators of intravascular injection of bupivacaine with epinephrine (97% positive)[116]; these investigators did not confirm the efficacy of pretreatment with atropine on the heart rate. During total IV anesthesia with propofol and remifentanil, however, quite different results have been reported; T-wave changes in children who received an IV injection of bupivacaine with epinephrine as a simulated positive test dose were inconsistent and could not be relied upon to diagnose that an intravascular injection had occurred.[122] The only consistent and reliable indicator of an intravascular injection was an increase in blood pressure (particularly diastolic) that exceeded 10% in all subjects.

Knowing that every test dose regimen is fallible, and that interpreting a negative test dose may be challenging, the European Society of Regional Anaesthesia and Pain Therapy (ESRA)/American Society of Regional Anesthesia and Pain Medicine (ASRA) practice advisory have deemed their use discretionary.[171] Nonetheless, some clinicians continue to use an epinephrine-containing test dose before administering the therapeutic dose of local anesthetic for neuraxial blocks.[119] In particular, blood aspiration, positive test doses, and local anesthetic systemic toxicity are most common with caudal blocks.[109] The test dose should be repeated before subsequent bolus injections are administered through a catheter. If the drug injection is visualized in real time using ultrasound, test dosing may be less critical, as the actual drug deposition can be visualized during the injection, although this, too, may be fallible. Data from the PRAN registry detected no intravascular injections during ultrasound-guided (USG) peripheral nerve blocks, and test dosing during these blocks has become uncommon. If the child is receiving a general inhalation anesthetic, blood pressure and the ST-segment configuration, in addition to the heart rate, should be carefully and frequently observed after injection of the test dose.[120] Pretreatment with atropine (10 μg/kg) may increase the rate of detecting an unintended intravascular injection. Slow, incremental injection of the therapeutic dose of local anesthetic otherwise referred to as giving the entire dose as a series of multiple test doses is always recommended (over several minutes) as this may further increase the safety of regional blockade; a partial or even completely intravascular, but slow injection may not exceed the toxic threshold.

TREATMENT OF LOCAL ANESTHETIC SYSTEMIC TOXICITY

Treatment of toxic reactions to local anesthetic overdose requires knowledge of the signs and symptoms previously described and has changed dramatically with the introduction of lipid rescue therapy.[108,172–174] The signs of local anesthetic systemic toxicity (LAST), with the exception of the catastrophic cardiovascular events, are all masked by general anesthesia. Indeed, inhaled anesthetics may raise the threshold for seizures and thereby delay the detection of toxicity until cardiovascular collapse occurs. Even in the unanesthetized child, the progression from prodromal signs to cardiovascular collapse may be very rapid and the initial resuscitative therapy needs to be directed at maintaining oxygenation while reestablishing circulation and normal cardiac rhythm, including the timely institution of standard pediatric advanced life support (PALS) (but not epinephrine, see later), until definitive treatments are instituted. The timely administration of a CNS depressant that alters the seizure threshold may prevent seizures. Administration of midazolam (0.05–0.2 mg/kg IV) or propofol (1–3 mg/kg IV) effectively prevents or terminates seizure activity; however, propofol is also a potent myocardial depressant and should be used with great caution. If seizure activity is present and the airway has not been secured, succinylcholine or a nondepolarizing muscle relaxant may facilitate tracheal intubation to ensure adequate ventilation and prevent aspiration. It is important to recognize that muscle paralysis does not prevent seizures.[175] Securing the airway to prevent hypoxia takes precedence over controlling seizure activity. CNS excitability is exacerbated in the presence of hypercarbia; thus, mild hyperventilation should be employed to attenuate seizure activity. None of these interventions should supplant or delay the administration of lipid emulsion to simultaneously treat the toxic plasma concentrations of local anesthetic. A lipid emulsion (but not propofol) may reverse the CNS symptoms of LAST in the absence of cardiovascular collapse and is now accepted as the first-line therapy of LAST (see also End Matter for the AAGBI safety guideline).[175–179]

Advances in the treatment of LAST have completely altered the therapeutic interventions that should be initiated in the event of cardiovascular collapse or suspicion of LAST after a large intravascular injection of an amide local anesthetic. IV lipid emulsion (20% intralipid) has been shown in animal models and human reports to be effective to resuscitate a cardiac arrest caused by both bupivacaine and ropivacaine.[180] A clear relationship between the tissue concentration and the response has also been established.[181] Lipid emulsion was superior to epinephrine, which fared no better than the control in restoring metabolic and hemodynamic indexes in a rat model of bupivacaine toxicity.[182] These animal studies have been corroborated by anecdotal reports of rescue from cardiac arrest in humans.[183–186] The mechanism of action of lipid emulsions to treat bupivacaine toxicity is not entirely understood, but studies in isolated rat heart preparations suggest that the lipid treatment elutes bupivacaine from the myocardium and accelerates the recovery from bupivacaine-induced asystole.[187] This "lipid sink" hypothesis suggests a novel mechanism of action compared with more conventional antidysrhythmic drugs,[188] and the treatment appears to be more effective. An inverse relationship between the concentration of lipid emulsion and the myocardial bupivacaine concentration (greater lipid concentrations were more effective at decreasing the bupivacaine concentration in the myocardium) suggests that this lipid sink hypothesis is correct.[181] A study in infant pigs suggested that administering epinephrine in the initial arrest phase may actually impair resuscitation with lipid emulsion, preventing a sustained response to treatment, and that treatment with lipid alone was superior to both treatment with epinephrine and treatment with lipid plus epinephrine.[189]

The most recent practice advisory from the American Society of Regional Anesthesia (ASRA)[175] recommends 100 mL of 20% lipid emulsion for patients >70 kilograms and 1.5 mL/kg for patients <70 kilograms over 2 to 3 minutes followed by an infusion of 200 to 250 milliliters over 15 to 20 minutes for patients >70 kilograms and 0.25 mL/kg over 15 to 20 minutes for patients <70 kilograms. If the patient has not stabilized, consider another bolus dose or increasing the rate of infusion by 0.5 mL/kg per minute. The infusions should be continued for an additional 10 minutes after circulatory stability. Several pediatric events report success with this intervention, with a range

of doses similar to those reported in adults.[184,190–193] However, excess intralipid emulsion has been administered to a child, emphasizing the importance of administering weight-based infusion rates in children[194,195]; the FDA has recommended a limit of 12 mL/kg.[175] There is a consensus that 20% lipid emulsions should be immediately available in any location where regional anesthesia is performed[175,196] to permit rapid treatment of cardiac toxicity. Our practice is to include a bag of lipid emulsion and a dosing guide in the local anesthetic drug kit dispensed by the pharmacy for regional blockade. Although propofol is compounded in a lipid emulsion, it **_must not_** be substituted for lipid emulsion to resuscitate patients with LAST because propofol is a myocardial depressant that may impair recovery.

Because the initial stage of cardiovascular toxicity consists of peripheral vasodilation, supportive treatment should include IV fluid loading (10–20 mL/kg of isotonic crystalloid) and, if necessary, titration of a peripheral vasoconstrictor, such as phenylephrine (initial rate of 0.1 µg/kg per minute) or low-dose epinephrine. In the presence of cardiovascular collapse, the most important factor is effective CPR to circulate the intralipid so that it can remove the local anesthetic from cardiac tissue. Large doses of epinephrine and vasopressin are not recommended.[175,197] If necessary cardiac bypass could be instituted.[198]

HYPERSENSITIVITY TO LOCAL ANESTHETICS

Hypersensitivity reactions to local anesthetics are rare.[199–201] Ester local anesthetics are metabolized to *p*-aminobenzoic acid, which is usually responsible for allergic reactions in this group. However, these agents may cause allergic phenomena in children who are sensitive to sulfonamides, sulfites, or thiazide diuretics.[202,203] True allergies among the amide local anesthetics are rare.[204] These drugs may contain the preservative, methylparaben, which can produce allergic reactions in those sensitive to *p*-aminobenzoic acid.[203,205] When in doubt, local anesthetic allergy must be ruled out.[206] Detailed protocols are described elsewhere.[204,207]

Placement of Blocks in Patients Under General Anesthesia

Although concerns about the risks of neural injury in the unconscious patient have been raised in the adult literature, this is based entirely on anecdotal case reports with questionable practices, and the standard of care in pediatric anesthesia has long been to administer most regional blocks to children who are anesthetized.[208] The safety of this practice has now been confirmed by a large prospective study from the PRAN registry in an unselected cohort of more than 51,000 consecutive regional blocks in children.[209] Block placement in children under general anesthesia was determined to be as or more safe as placement in the awake or sedated child, with postoperative neurologic symptoms occurring at a rate of 0.93/1000 (95% confidence interval [CI] 0.7–1.2) compared with 6.82/1000 (95% CI 4.2–10.5) in sedated and awake patients. The authors concluded that administering regional blocks to children under general anesthesia is safe, remains the standard of care, and that prohibitive recommendations based on anecdote or case reports were unsupported. These conclusions are further supported in a joint consensus statement by the ASRA and the European Society of Regional Anesthesia (ESRA) with level B2 evidence.[171]

Ultrasound Equipment

USE OF ULTRASOUND

The availability of high-resolution portable ultrasound (US) machines has revolutionized regional anesthesia in children.[26,210] Evidence suggests that ultrasound guidance, by providing direct visualization of the anatomy, the needle and the injectate, increases success rates, reduces pain scores, prolongs block duration, reduces total dose of local anesthetic, reduces the time of block performance and reduces the number of needle passes, particularly in younger children.[26] Indeed, the most recent ASRA practice advisory regarding LAST suggests changing demographics is likely due to increased use of ultrasound and that nearly half the more recent cases of LAST were not associated with anesthesiologists.[175] Although this practice requires expensive equipment and the acquisition of new skills, it now has an essential role in pediatric regional blockade. The cost-effectiveness of acquiring these devices is justified because they serve multiple purposes (e.g., for placing invasive central lines, peripheral and arterial catheters, assessing tracheal tube position and identifying residual gastric volume).[13] Small point-of-care handheld devices are becoming available as well.[211–214] Because ultrasound might still not be available to every practitioner, particularly in limited resource environments, we present both landmark- and ultrasound-guided approaches, but it should be noted that the use of landmark techniques are especially limited for fascial plane blocks, as these require ultrasound guidance for visualizing the fascial compartments to be injected.

Peripheral nerve blocks provide anesthesia and analgesia during the perioperative period.[26,146,148,215–217] Success depends on the ability to accurately place the needle—and thereby the local anesthetic—close to the target nerve without causing injury to the nerve or adjacent structures. In the past, clinicians relied on anatomic landmarks,[215–217] fascial clicks,[218] loss of resistance,[219] or nerve stimulation[220] to position the needle in the vicinity of the nerve. Anatomic landmarks provide valuable clues to the position of the nerve, but they are markers that lack precision,[221] vary among children of different ages, and may be difficult to locate in obese children. Even nerve stimulation may not always elicit a motor response,[222] and its use does not guarantee success or preclude complications.[223] Moreover, the accuracy of needle placement cannot be predicted with any of these methods, which may lead to multiple attempts to place the needle and may result in an incomplete or failed nerve block.

Various imaging modalities, such as fluoroscopy,[224] computed tomography (CT),[225] and magnetic resonance imaging (MRI),[221] improve the accuracy of block placement in adults. However, these adjuncts are rarely used except for chronic pain blocks, and are impractical in the operating room. The use of ultrasound to guide peripheral and central neuraxial blocks has improved both accuracy and safety in both adults and children.[226–235]

PRINCIPLES OF ULTRASOUND

The use of ultrasound for regional anesthesia dates back to 1978, when la Grange et al. used a Doppler flow detector to locate the subclavian artery and guide supraclavicular brachial plexus blocks.[236] In 1994, Kapral and colleagues published the first report on direct sonographic visualization in regional anesthesia.[237] They used ultrasound to directly visualize the brachial plexus and observe the spread of the local anesthetic in real time during supraclavicular brachial plexus block. Today, ultrasound is commonly used to guide regional anesthesia techniques in both adults and children. Improvements in ultrasound technology and the availability of portable ultrasound machines with high-resolution imaging capabilities allow direct visualization of the peripheral nerves and central neuraxial structures in children; this can be compared to removing a blindfold from the anesthesiologist performing regional anesthesia. Currently, outcome data that prove ultrasound increases the safety and efficacy of regional anesthesia in children are rapidly accumulating.[16,143,144,238]

Sound is a form of mechanical energy that propagates through a medium as a wave of alternating pressure, causing local regions of compression and rarefaction (Fig. 40.2). The frequency (f) of sound is the number of cycles of oscillations per second made by the sound source and the particles in the medium through which it moves. It is expressed in hertz (Hz, cycles per second). Sound waves propagate symmetrically away from the source at a constant velocity (v), which is the speed of sound in the medium. Distance between the wavefronts is the wavelength (λ) of the sound. The speed of sound through a medium can thus be represented as:

$$v = f \times \lambda$$

Amplitude is the strength of a sound wave, and the unit used to describe it is decibels (dB). The velocity of transmission of sound through a medium depends on its acoustic impedance and is determined by factors such as the stiffness, elasticity, and density of the medium. This accounts for the varying velocity of sound transmission through different tissues in the human body (Table 40.5). The average velocity of sound transmission through biologic tissue is 1540 meters per second. If the time taken by the ultrasound signal to return to the transducer is known, the distance of the target from the transducer (depth) can be computed.

The human ear can detect sound between 20 and 20,000 Hz. Ultrasound has a frequency beyond 20,000 Hz (20 kHz). For medical imaging, ultrasound typically uses a frequency between 1 million and 15 million Hz (megahertz [MHz]) produced by a

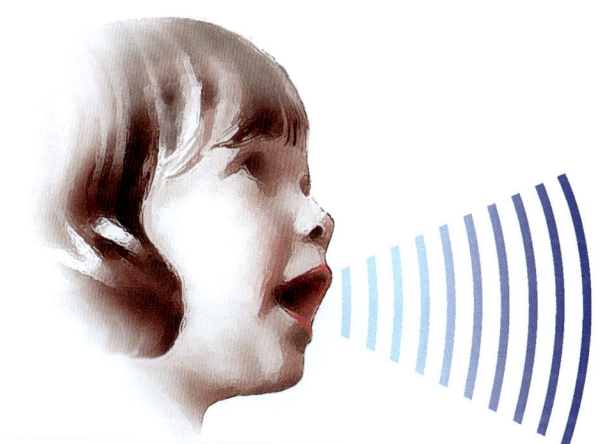

FIGURE 40.2 Sound wave.

TABLE 40.5	Propagation Velocity of Sound in Body Tissues
Tissue	**Propagation Velocity of Sound (m/second)[a]**
Bone	4080
Muscle	1580
Blood	1570
Kidney	1560
Liver	1550
Soft tissue (average)	1540
Water	1480
Fat	1450
Lung	600
Air	330

[a]Medical ultrasound device measurements are based on an assumed average propagation velocity of 1540 m/second.

piezoelectric crystal (element) within the transducer. When an electrical field is applied to the surface of an element in a transducer, it undergoes dimensional changes that cause it to vibrate and produce sound. The element is typically driven by a pulsed alternating voltage. This results in the generation of short pulses of ultrasound that are emitted into body tissues. Between successive short pulses of ultrasound generation, the transducer does not transmit but rather functions as a receiver of the reflected ultrasound energy (i.e., the echoes). The percent of time that a transducer is transmitting is termed the *duty factor* and is typically less than 1%. The ultrasound transducer thus has a dual function—it functions as both a transmitter and a receiver.

The emitted ultrasound signal travels through the tissue medium, and when it encounters a tissue interface, it is reflected back. The degree of reflection of ultrasound from tissues is related to the changes in acoustic impedance (Z) between two tissue interfaces. The reflected echoes are detected by the transducer and converted into electrical energy; they are then processed by the ultrasound machine according to their strength and displayed as dots on the monitor. The brightness of each dot corresponds to the strength of the echo signal. Strong echoes produce bright white dots, weak echoes produce gray dots, and anatomic structures that do not reflect ultrasound appear as black dots. The vertical position of the dot on the monitor represents the depth from which the echo is received. When all of these dots are combined, they produce a complete image of the area scanned.[239–241]

MODES OF ULTRASOUND

B-Mode (Brightness) or Two-Dimension Mode

B-mode (brightness) or two-dimensional (2D) mode, is the most commonly used ultrasound mode. In this mode, the echo is converted to a dot and the brightness of the dot represents the amplitude of the returning signal.[239–241] The vertical position of the dot on the display represents the depth from which the signal is returning and depends on the round-trip time of the ultrasound signal. Multiple scan lines across a plane are combined to produce a single 2D grayscale image. A series of frames are then displayed in rapid succession to give the impression of constant motion, the quality of which depends on the number of images displayed per second, that is, the *frame rate*.

M-Mode (Motion)

Motion, or M-mode, ultrasound is directed along a single scan line (sample line) and reflected signals along this scan line are converted to a brightness scale and displayed against a time axis. Because M-mode is produced from ultrasound signals along a single scan line, the 2D anatomy of the underlying body tissues should be studied first using the 2D mode. M-mode is of particular interest when time resolution is necessary, such as when examining a target with rapid movement (e.g., the mitral valve during echocardiography).[242]

Doppler Ultrasound

Doppler ultrasound (based on the Doppler principle) detects a shift in frequency between the emitted ultrasound waves and their echoes. It is used to detect and measure blood flow, and the major reflector for this purpose is red blood cells.[243–246] Several modes are available:

Color Doppler measures and color codes the direction and magnitude of the mean Doppler frequency shifts that occur in moving red blood cells and superimposes a color depiction of these data on the grayscale image (Fig. 40.3A).

Power color Doppler depicts the amplitude, or power, of the Doppler signals (Fig. 40.3B). This allows better sensitivity for visualization of small vessels, but at the expense of directional information.

Pulsed Doppler allows a sampling volume (or gate) to be positioned in a vessel visualized on the grayscale image and displays

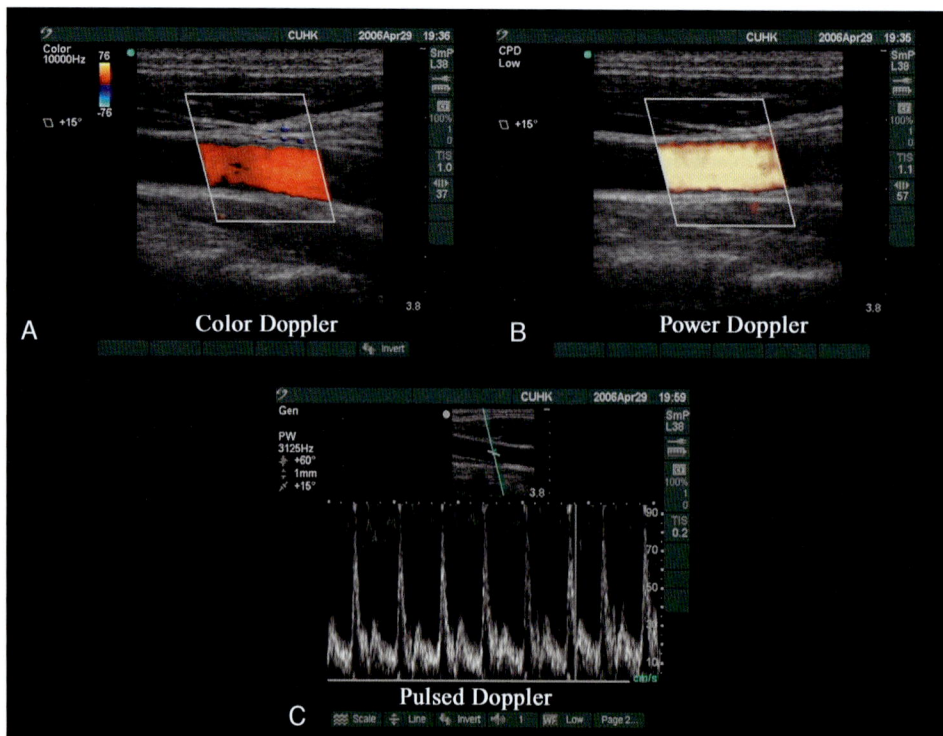

FIGURE 40.3 Doppler ultrasound. **A,** Color Doppler. **B,** Power Doppler. **C,** Pulsed Doppler.

a spectrum of the full range of blood velocities within the gate plotted as a function of time (Fig. 40.3C).

THE ULTRASOUND MACHINE

Ultrasound machines are comprised of the following components: a *monitor* (where the clinical images are displayed), the *ultrasound unit* (where the signals are processed), the *control panel* (with the knobs and controls), one or more *transducers*, and a *data storage device*.[247–249] For an anesthesiologist's first encounter with an ultrasound machine the wide array of knobs and controls available may be confusing. However, several controls are common in most ultrasound machines, and a clear understanding of their function—colloquially termed *knobology*—is essential for optimal imaging.

Presets

Most ultrasound machines have several presets, which are factory defined, to allow optimal ultrasound imaging of a specific area of the body or type of examination. Some of the categories of presets that are available include small part, vascular, breast, nerve, musculoskeletal, abdominal, and so on. For example, if a small part preset is chosen, the ultrasound machine assumes that the operator is scanning for small, relatively superficial structures and automatically adjusts the depth, power, focus, gain, and time-gain compensation (TGC) to allow optimal imaging of superficial structures. Some ultrasound machines also allow customized presets according to clinical requirements. Power output is the amount of energy transmitted from the ultrasound transducer. In most machines, the power cannot be adjusted by the operator but is automatically set when a particular preset is chosen.

Frequency

This control is used to select the desired frequency, within certain limits, of a broadband transducer—that is, a transducer that serves a range of frequencies. In some ultrasound systems (Edge, SonoSite Inc., Bothell, WA), this is available as an image optimization control. In the "Res" (resolution) setting the greatest frequency of the broadband transducer is selected; in the "Pen" (penetration) setting the lowest frequency is selected; and in the "Gen" (general) setting an intermediate frequency is selected.

Gain

The gain control adjusts the amplification of the returning acoustic signals and is used to optimize the image. Reduced gain produces a dark image (Fig. 40.4A) and detail is masked. In contrast, too much gain produces a white image and detail is saturated (Fig. 40.4B). Some ultrasound machines have separate controls for overall gain and gain for the near and far fields. "Autogain," by which the ultrasound machine automatically adjusts the gain to optimize the image, is also available in some machines (Fig. 40.4C).

Time-Gain Compensation

Ultrasound energy is progressively attenuated as it travels through tissue. Therefore, signals returning from reflectors at a depth are weaker in strength. By selectively amplifying the echoes from greater depths, using the TGC method or depth-gain compensation (DGC), equal reflectors at unequal depths are displayed as structures of equal brightness on the monitor. TGC is preset to a large degree, and the operator can make fine adjustments if necessary. The TGC control is presented as a series of sliders arranged in a vertical fashion on the control panel. Each of the sliders adjusts the amplification of the returning ultrasound signals at a specific image depth.

Depth

Adjustment in the displayed depth may be necessary, depending on the location of the target, the patient's body size, or other anatomic

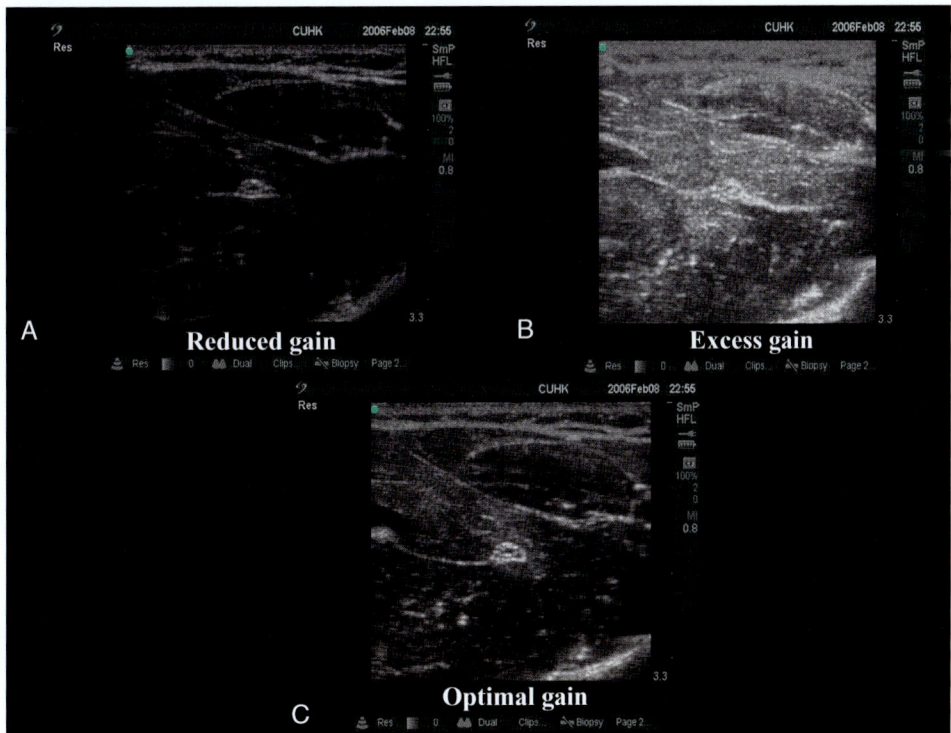

FIGURE 40.4 Transverse sonogram of the forearm demonstrating **A,** reduced gain, **B,** excess gain, and **C,** optimal gain.

factors. A depth greater than necessary should not be chosen because this reduces the frame rate and resolution of the image.

Focus (Focal Zone)

The focus of the ultrasound signal occurs at a point at which the beam is at its narrowest width. It is also the region where lateral resolution is the best. The focus point should therefore be positioned at the depth at which the relevant anatomic structures are located. In some ultrasound machines, the operator can select multiple focal zones, but this markedly reduces the frame rate and thus should not be routinely used.

Freeze and Unfreeze

The "freeze" function allows the operator to lock a static image on the monitor. A number of frames (usually 20 or more) are also simultaneously stored in a memory bank. These stored frames can be scrolled back and forth. The selected still image can then be used for annotation, documentation, storage, review, or teaching. Pressing the freeze button once again will unfreeze the image.

Ultrasound Transducers

The transducer functions both as a transmitter and a receiver of the ultrasound signal.[247–249] Three types of transducers are currently used (Fig. 40.5): (1) in a linear-array transducer, the piezoelectric crystals are arranged in a linear fashion and sequentially fired to produce parallel beams of ultrasound in sequence, creating a field of view that is rectangular and as wide as the footprint of the transducer (see Fig. 40.5A); (2) a curved linear-array transducer has a curved surface, creating a field of view that is wider than the footprint of the probe (see Fig. 40.5B), but at the cost of reduced lateral resolution in the far field as the scan lines diverge; (3) a phased-array transducer has a small footprint, but the ultrasound beam is steered electronically to produce a sufficiently wide far field of view. The ultrasound beam diverges from virtually the same point in the transducer (see Fig. 40.5C). Phased-array transducers are routinely used for transthoracic echocardiography.[248] The footprints of these transducers are small enough to fit between the ribs and still produce a wide far field of view to image the heart. Ultrasound transducers are typically broadband and can serve a range of frequencies. For example, a transducer with the notation HFL38/13-6 indicates that it is a high-frequency broadband (13-6 MHz) linear transducer with a 38-millimeter footprint. Note that the nomenclature used for transducers varies among manufacturers of ultrasound devices.

Ultrasound Transducer Selection

Resolution is the ability to distinguish two objects that are close together. *Axial resolution* is the ability to distinguish two objects that are along the axis of the ultrasound beam, and *lateral resolution* is the ability to distinguish two objects that are side by side. High-frequency ultrasound (13-6 MHz) has a higher axial and lateral resolution compared with low-frequency ultrasound but cannot penetrate as deeply into body tissue. Therefore high-frequency ultrasound is used to image superficial structures such as the brachial plexus in the interscalene groove or supraclavicular fossa. A lower-frequency ultrasound transducer (10-5 MHz) is suited for slightly deeper structures, such as the brachial plexus in the infraclavicular fossa, whereas a low-frequency ultrasound transducer (5-2 MHz) is used to image deep structures, such as the lumbar plexus or the sciatic nerve. Broadband transducers allow a single transducer to be used for scanning over a wide range of depths. Because regional blocks are performed at relatively shallow depths in neonates, infants, and young children, high-frequency linear transducers are used for most procedures. High-frequency linear transducers with a small footprint (13-6 MHz, 25 mm), in either a hockey stick or linear configuration, are particularly suited for young children.

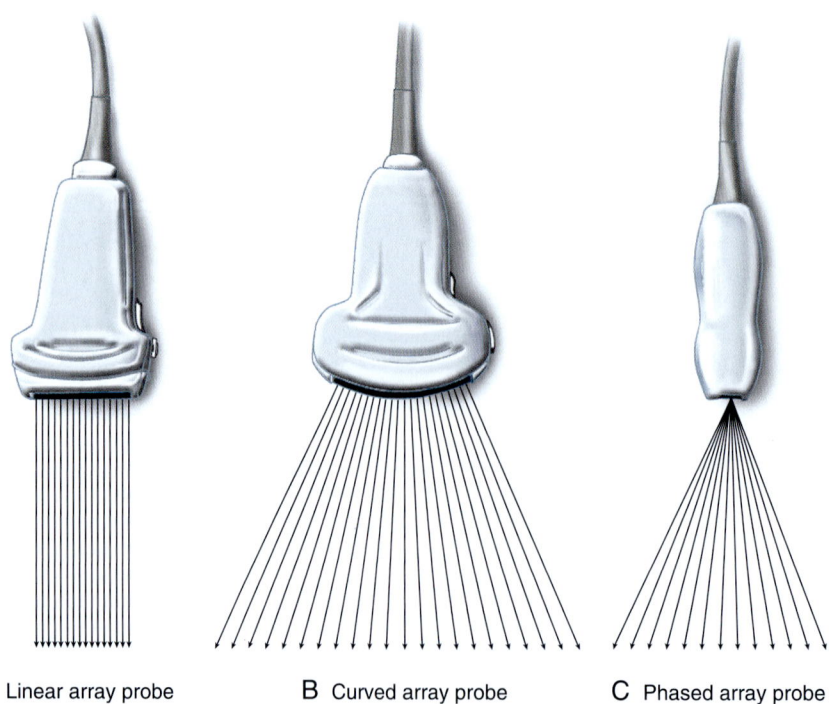

A Linear array probe   **B** Curved array probe   **C** Phased array probe

FIGURE 40.5 Schematic diagram illustrating the different types of ultrasound transducers. Note how the ultrasound beam is emitted from each of these transducers.

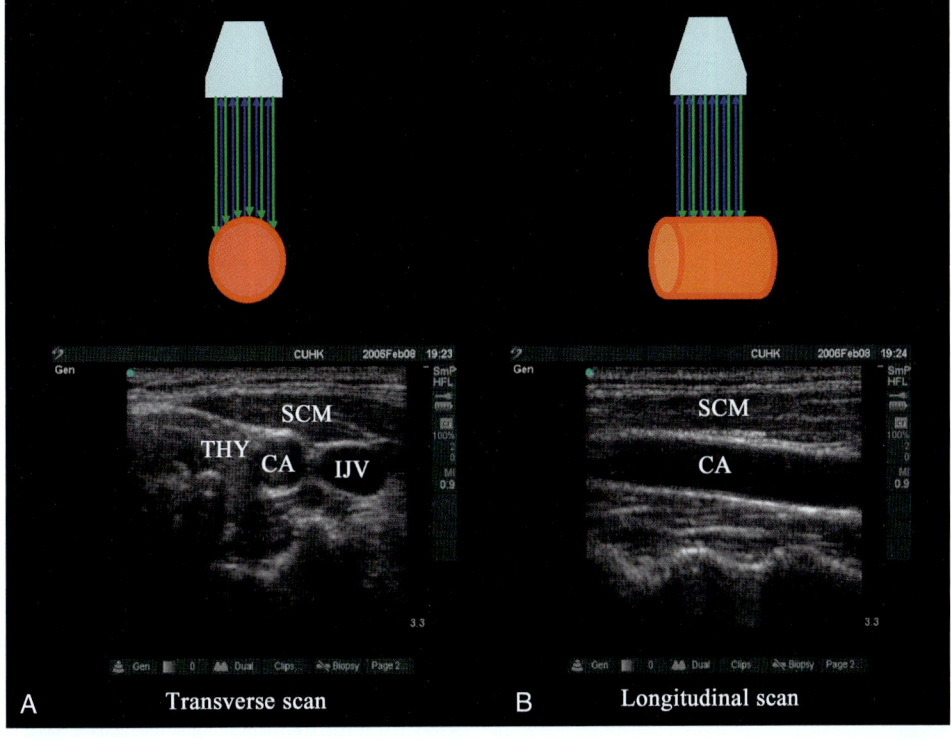

FIGURE 40.6 Axis of scan. **A,** Transverse scan. **B,** Longitudinal scan. *CA,* Carotid artery; *IJV,* internal jugular vein; *SCM,* sternocleidomastoid muscle; *THY,* thyroid.

Essentials of Musculoskeletal Ultrasound Imaging

AXIS OF SCAN

In diagnostic ultrasonography, scans are performed in the transverse, longitudinal (sagittal), oblique, or coronal axis. During a transverse (axial) scan the transducer is oriented at right angles to the target, producing a cross-sectional display of the structures (Fig. 40.6A). During a longitudinal scan, the transducer is oriented parallel to and along the long axis of the target (e.g., a blood vessel or nerve) (Fig. 40.6B). During ultrasound-guided regional anesthesia procedures, ultrasound scans are most commonly performed in the transverse axis. In this axis, the nerves, the adjoining structures, and the circumferential spread of the local anesthetic are easily visualized.

PROBE AND IMAGE ORIENTATION

The ultrasound image must be properly oriented to accurately identify the anatomic relations of the various structures on the monitor. To facilitate this, all ultrasound probes have an orientation marker, which is usually represented by a groove or a ridge on one side of the transducer and corresponds to a green dot (or a logo) on the monitor. By convention, the orientation marker on the transducer is directed cephalad when performing a longitudinal scan and directed toward the right side of the patient when performing a transverse scan. This way the orientation marker on the left upper corner of the monitor always represents the cephalad end during a longitudinal scan or the right side of the patient during a transverse scan. The top of the display monitor therefore represents superficial structures and the bottom of the monitor the deep structures.

ECHOGENICITY

Certain terms are frequently used to describe the sonographic appearance of musculoskeletal structures (Fig. 40.7):

Echogenic: A bright white structure against a dark background
Reflective: Synonymous with an echogenic structure
Isoechoic: A shade of gray that is of the same brightness or echogenicity as the surrounding tissues
Hyperechoic: A shade of gray that is bright white or brighter than the surrounding tissues
Hypoechoic: A shade of gray that is dark or less bright than the surrounding tissues
Anechoic: An absence of echoes, hence blackness

AXIS OF INTERVENTION

The plane of ultrasound imaging is approximately 1 millimeter thick (Fig. 40.8); for a needle to be visible during ultrasound imaging it must lie within this narrow plane of imaging. During ultrasound-guided regional anesthesia procedures, the block needle is inserted either outside of the plane (out-of-plane approach) (Fig. 40.9) or within the plane of the ultrasound beam (in-plane approach) (see Fig. 40.9B). In the out-of-plane approach, the needle is inserted in the short axis and is initially outside the plane of imaging and therefore not visible. It becomes visible only when the needle crosses the plane of imaging and is seen as an echogenic dot on the monitor (see Fig. 40.9A). It is important to note that this echogenic dot may be just the cross-sectional image of the shaft of the needle as it passes through the plane of the ultrasound beam and thus may not represent the tip of the needle. In the in-plane approach, the needle is inserted along the long axis of the transducer in the plane of imaging and therefore both the shaft and tip of the needle are visible.

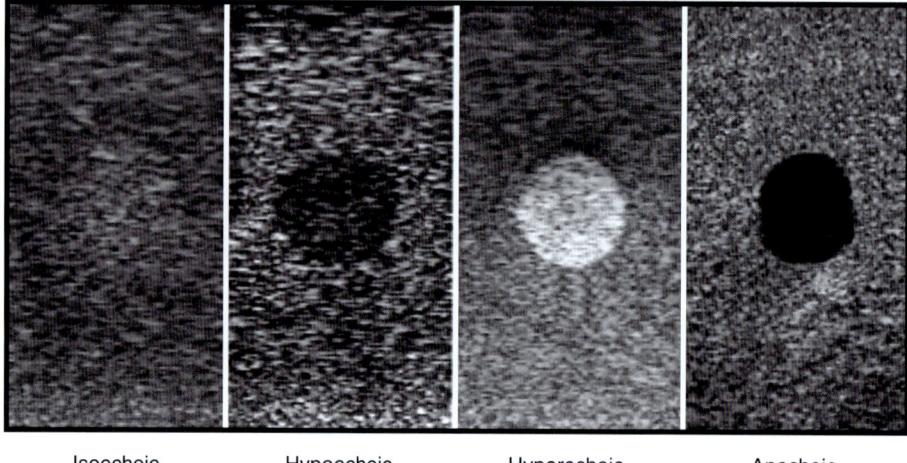

| Isoechoic | Hypoechoic | Hyperechoic | Anechoic |

FIGURE 40.7 Schematic diagram to demonstrate the relative echogenicity of various tissues.

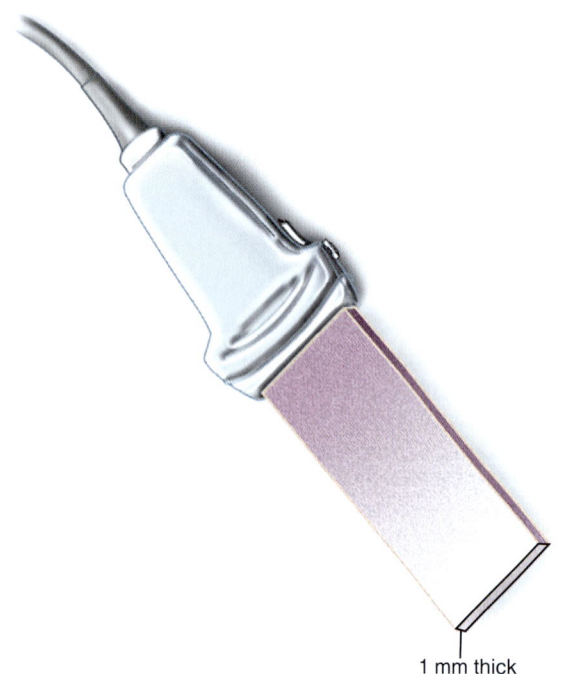

1 mm thick

FIGURE 40.8 The plane of ultrasound imaging. Note that the ultrasound beam is only 1 mm thick and for a needle to be visible during an ultrasound-guided intervention it must lie within this plane of imaging.

Both approaches are commonly used and complement each other. Proponents of the out-of-plane approach[227,228,250] have had great success with this method and claim that it causes less needle-related trauma and pain because the needle is advanced through a shorter distance to the target. However, critics express concerns that the inability to reliably visualize the needle and to use tissue movement as a surrogate marker to locate the needle tip during a procedure can lead to complications. The needle is better visualized in the in-plane approach,[251,252] but this requires good hand–eye coordination. Moreover, there are claims that the in-plane approach also causes more discomfort in awake patients because longer needle insertion paths are required.[227,228,250]

NEEDLE VISIBILITY

The ability to visualize the needle during an ultrasound-guided procedure is critical for precision, safety, and success. However, this is often limited by the dispersion of the reflected ultrasound signals away from the transducer. Several factors have been identified that can influence needle visibility.[253–255] The shaft of the needle is better visualized in the long axis than in the short axis, and its visibility decreases linearly with steep angles of insertion and smaller needle diameters. The needle tip is better visualized when it is inserted in the long axis for a shallow angle of insertion (<30 degrees) and in the short axis when the angle of insertion is steep (>60 degrees). To overcome the effect of angle on needle visibility, some machines allow the operator to steer the ultrasound beam toward the needle ("beam steering") during steep needle insertions.[256] However, this requires experience and decreases in needle visibility can still occur. Manufacturers have incorporated microscopic glass beads or reflectors onto the surfaces of block needles or have laser-etched the tips of block needles to improve their visibility (echogenic needle) on the ultrasound image.[257–259]

The anesthesiologist's skill in aligning the needle along the plane of imaging is by far the most important factor influencing needle visibility because minor deviations of even a few millimeters from this plane will result in inability to visualize the needle. Even with experience, needle tip visibility is a problem when performing blocks at a depth in areas that are rich in fatty tissue. Under such circumstances, gently jiggling (rapid in-and-out movement) the needle and observing tissue movement or performing a test injection of saline solution or 5% dextrose (0.5–1 mL) and observing tissue distention can help locate the position of the needle tip. 5% dextrose is the preferred solution for the latter when nerve stimulation is used because it does not increase the electric current required to elicit a motor response.[260]

ANISOTROPY

Anisotropy, or angular dependence, is a term used to describe the change in echogenicity of a structure with a change in the angle of insonation, or the angular orientation relative to the target structures, of the incident ultrasound beam (Fig. 40.10).[261] It is frequently observed during scanning of nerves, muscles, and tendons. This occurs because the amplitude of the echoes returning to the transducer varies with the angle of insonation. Nerves are best visualized when the

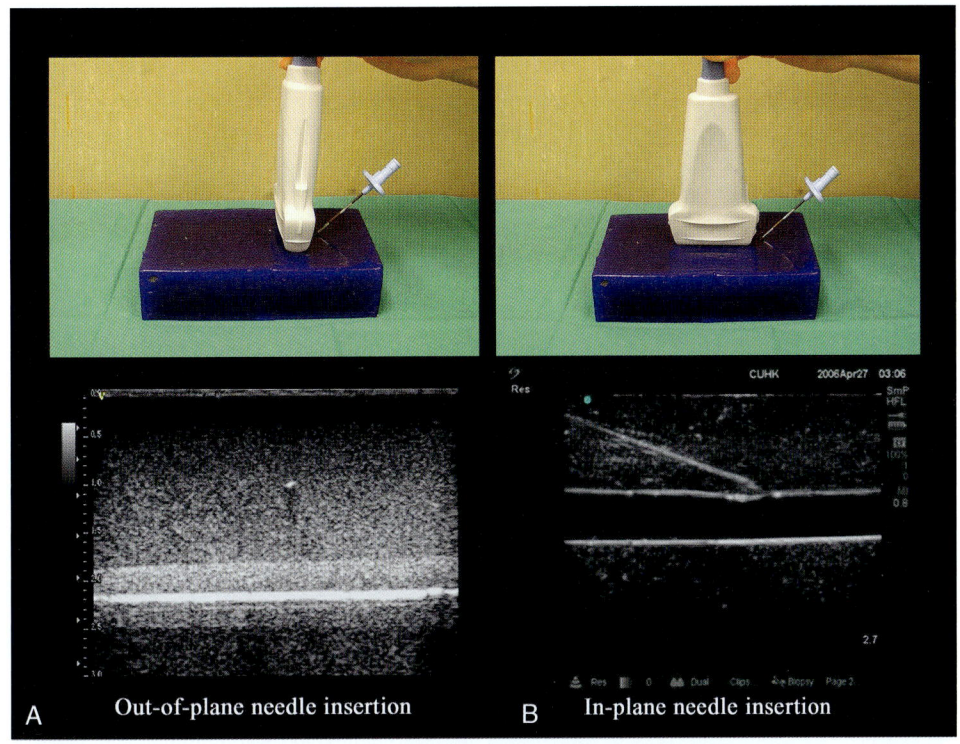

FIGURE 40.9 Axis of intervention. **A,** Out-of-plane and **B,** in-plane techniques.

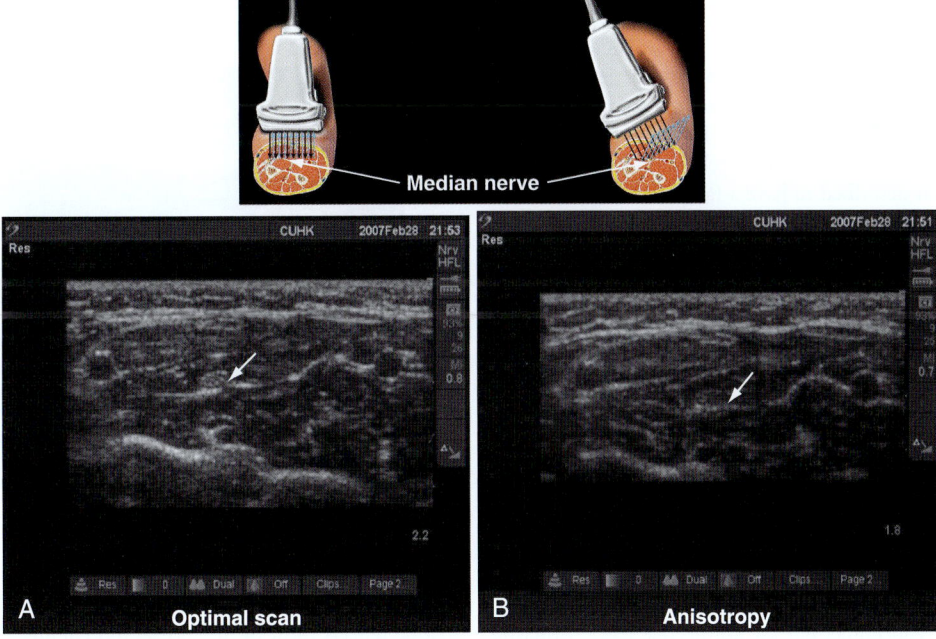

FIGURE 40.10 Anisotropy. Note how a small change in the angle of the ultrasound beam from the neutral position (**A**) has affected the visibility of the median nerve *(white arrow,* **B**) in the forearm.

incident beam is at right angles (see Fig. 40.10A); small changes in the angle away from the perpendicular can significantly reduce their echogenicity (see Fig. 40.10B). Therefore, during ultrasound-guided regional anesthesia procedures, the transducer should be tilted, from side to side, to minimize anisotropy and optimize visualization of the nerve.[262]

Identification of Structures

NERVES

On a transverse scan, nerves appear round, oval, triangular, lip-shaped, or even flat.[263] Nerves also assume different shapes along their course, depending on the surrounding structures. The

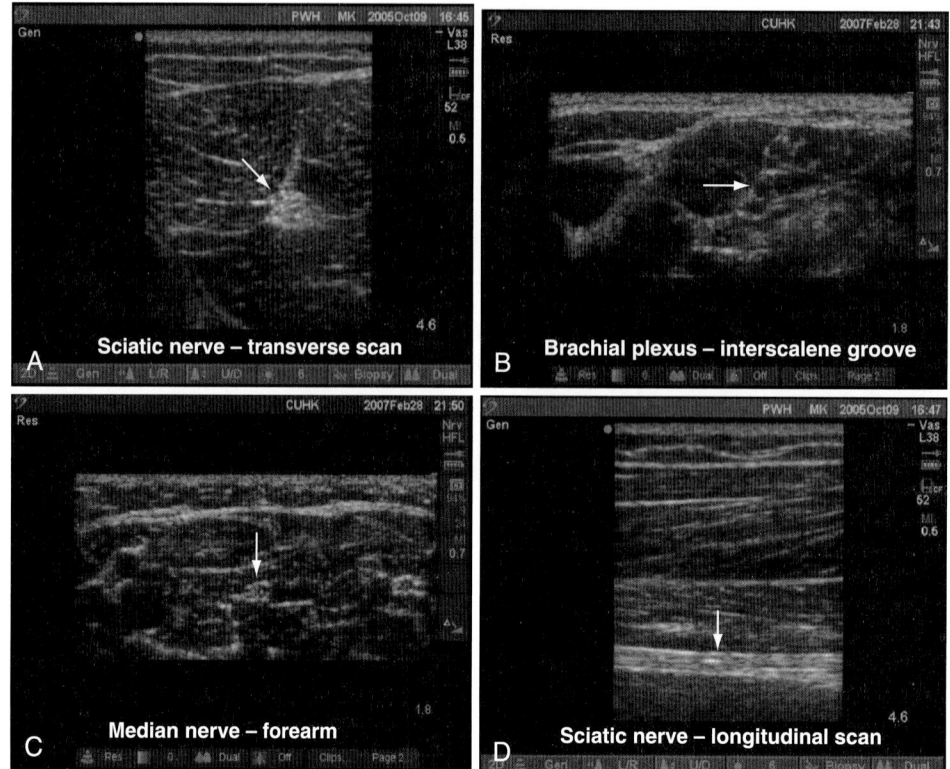

FIGURE 40.11 Ultrasound appearance of peripheral nerves. **A,** Transverse sonogram of the sciatic nerve in the thigh. **B,** Transverse sonogram of the brachial plexus in the interscalene groove. **C,** Transverse sonogram of the median nerve in the forearm. **D,** Longitudinal sonogram of the sciatic nerve in the thigh.

echogenicity of nerves also varies and depends on the nerve and area scanned. They are generally hyperechoic and stand out in the background of the hypoechoic muscles (Fig. 40.11A), but they can also appear hypoechoic with a hyperechoic rim (Fig. 40.11B). They also have been described to have a fascicular or honeycomb appearance (i.e., echogenic structures with internal punctate, echo-poor spaces) (Fig. 40.11C). On longitudinal scan, the appearance of peripheral nerves has been likened to a "tram track"; that is, parallel hyperechoic lines are seen against a background of echo-poor space (Fig. 40.11D).

TENDONS
Tendons appear to have numerous fine, parallel hyperechoic lines separated by fine hypoechoic lines (fibrillar pattern) on long-axis scans.[264] Compared with nerves, tendons have more hyperechoic lines and move more than adjacent nerves when the corresponding muscle is contracted or passively stretched.

MUSCLE
Muscle fibers are hypoechoic, but the connective tissue structure enveloping the entire muscle (epimysium) is hyperechoic.[265,266] The perimysium that envelops individual muscle fascicles is also hyperechoic. Muscle fibers converge to become tendons or aponeurosis.

FAT
Fat lobules appear as round to oval hypoechoic nodules separated by fine hyperechoic septa. Fat tends to be superficially distributed (subcutaneous fat), slightly compressible, and similar on transverse and longitudinal scans.

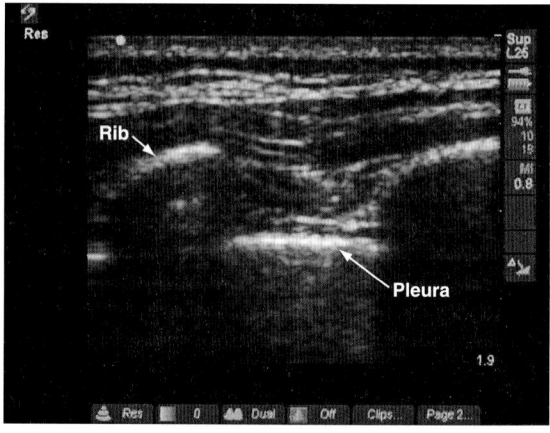

FIGURE 40.12 Longitudinal sonogram of the intercostal space demonstrating the ultrasound appearances of bone and pleura.

BONE
Bone reflects most of the ultrasound energy. Therefore, it appears bright and has a hyperechoic edge on ultrasound imaging, with a large anechoic shadow (acoustic shadow) distal to it (Fig. 40.12).

FASCIA
Fascia, peritoneum, and aponeurosis appear as thin hyperechoic layers on ultrasound imaging.

BLOOD VESSELS
Arteries are identified by their pulsatility, are not easily compressible, and have anechoic lumens. Veins are not pulsatile, are easily

compressible, and have anechoic lumens.[13] Color Doppler or power Doppler modes can also be used to demonstrate blood flow pattern and differentiate arteries from veins (see Fig. 40.3).

PLEURA

The pleura appear as a hyperechoic line on ultrasound imaging (see Fig. 40.12).[267–270] During scanning of the intercostal space, the pleural line is located slightly below the hyperechoic ribs. "Comet-tail" artifacts may be present as a series of vertical lines arising from the pleura. On real-time imaging, lung sliding movement between the parietal and visceral pleura can be discerned from movement of the comet-tail artifacts ("lung sliding sign").

Special Ultrasound Techniques

TISSUE HARMONIC IMAGING

The term *harmonic* refers to frequencies that are integral multiples of the frequency of the transmitted pulse (which is also called the fundamental frequency or first harmonic). The second harmonic has a frequency of twice the fundamental frequency. Harmonics are generated in the tissues by the nonlinear propagation of sound.[271–273] Tissue harmonic imaging (THI) is a technique in which the harmonic signals reflected from tissue interfaces are selectively displayed.[228] This results in reduced image artifacts, haze, and clutter, and improved contrast resolution (Fig. 40.13).

COMPOUND IMAGING

Ultrasound imaging depends on the reflection of the ultrasound from tissue interfaces. Not all tissues are good reflectors,

and certain structures also cause scattering of the ultrasound signals. Unlike reflected signals, scattered signals radiate in all directions. As a result, only a small amount of energy is reflected back to the transducer. The scattering of the ultrasound signal results in speckle artifacts, also described as noise, which reduces image resolution and makes the ultrasound image appear grainy or noisy. Compound imaging is a technique used to improve resolution by reducing the contrast-to-noise ratio.[274] The ultrasound beam from the transducer is electronically steered, and the same structure is imaged from several different angles. The returning echoes are then processed with simultaneous filtering of the artifacts in real time, producing a composite image that has reduced noise or speckle and improved definition (Fig. 40.14).

PANORAMIC IMAGING

B-mode (2D) ultrasonography has a limited field of view and allows visualization of only a small portion of any large structure. Panoramic imaging, as the name implies, is a technique used to extend the field of view so that larger structures and their surrounding tissues can be visualized together.[275] During a panoramic scan, the operator slowly slides the ultrasound transducer across the area of interest. During this motion, multiple images are acquired from many different transducer positions across the area of interest. The registered image data are accumulated in a large buffer and then combined to form the composite panoramic image (Fig. 40.15). Although useful for annotation, documentation, teaching, and research, it is rarely used in children during ultrasound-guided regional anesthesia procedures.

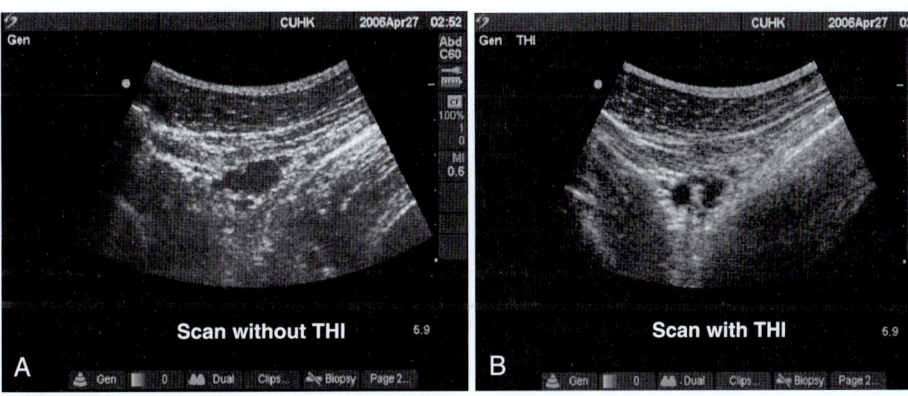

FIGURE 40.13 Tissue harmonic imaging *(THI)*. Sagittal sonogram of the infraclavicular fossa. **A,** Conventional scan. **B,** Conventional scan with THI.

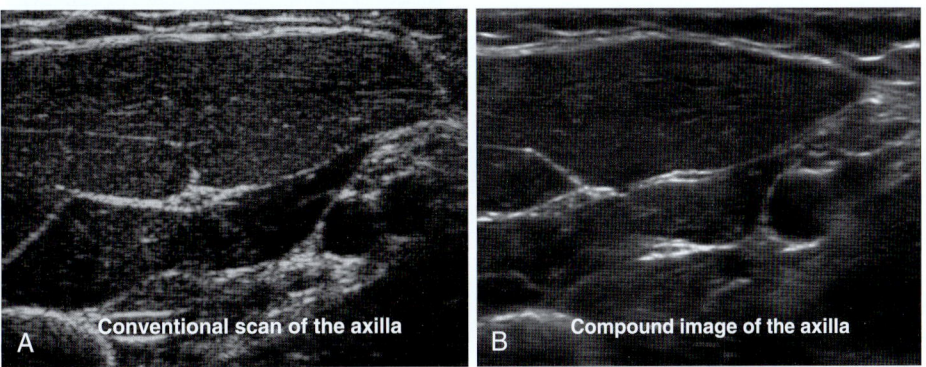

FIGURE 40.14 Compound imaging. Transverse sonogram of the axilla. **A,** Conventional scan. **B,** Conventional scan with compound imaging.

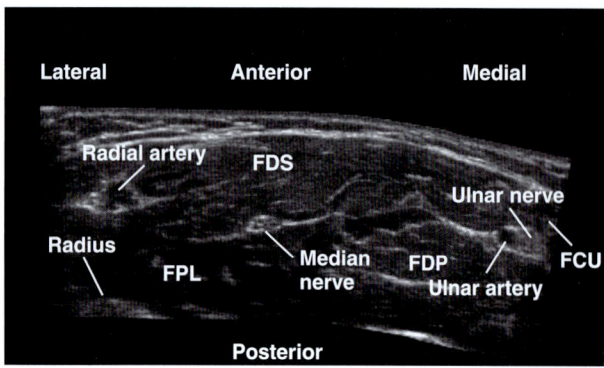

FIGURE 40.15 Panoramic imaging. Transverse panoramic scan of the forearm. *FCU,* Flexor carpi ulnaris; *FDP,* flexor digitorum profundus; *FDS,* flexor digitorum superficialis; *FPL,* flexor pollicis longus.

ARTIFACTS

Ultrasound artifacts are structures that are visible in the ultrasound image that do not correlate with any anatomic structure.[276] The ultrasound machine makes the following assumptions when generating an image:

1. The ultrasound beam is considered to travel only in a straight line, with a constant rate of attenuation.
2. The average speed of sound through body tissue is considered to be 1540 meters per second.
3. The ultrasound beam is assumed to be infinitely thin, with all echoes originating from its central axis.
4. The depth of a reflector is calculated by determining the round-trip time of the ultrasound signal.

When a deviation from any of these assumptions occurs, the ultrasound machine is unable to determine it. This results in the display of an echo that has no relation with the interface that actually produced the echo; that is, an artifact is produced. Some artifacts are undesirable and interfere with interpretation, whereas others help identify certain structures. It is essential to recognize them to avoid misinterpretation. Therefore, when a structure appears abnormal on ultrasonography, it must be examined in two planes to avoid making a wrong interpretation. Real anatomic structures are visible in both planes of imaging, whereas artifacts are visible in only one plane.

Contact Artifact

The contact artifact is the most common artifact produced when loss of acoustic coupling occurs between the skin and the transducer. This could occur because the transducer is not touching the skin, but more frequently it is due to air bubbles that are trapped between the skin and the transducer. Therefore, it is prudent to apply liberal amounts of gel to exclude air from the skin and transducer interface.

Reverberation Artifact

Reverberation artifacts, also known as repetitive echoes, occur when repeated reflection of ultrasound occurs between two highly reflective surfaces.[277] Some of the ultrasound signals returning to the transducer are reflected back, then strike the original interface, and are reflected back toward the transducer a second time. As a result, the first reverberation artifact is twice as far from the skin surface as the original interface. A second or third reverberation artifact also may be seen. Because of attenuation, the intensity of the artifacts decreases with increasing distance from the transducer.

Reverberation artifacts are frequently seen during ultrasound-guided axillary brachial plexus block, particularly when the needle is inserted in the long axis.

Mirror Image Artifact

Mirror image artifact is a type of reverberation artifact that occurs at highly reflective interfaces.[278] The first image is displayed in the correct position, and a false image is produced on the other side of the reflector because of its mirrorlike effect.

Propagation Speed Artifact

Propagation speed artifacts occur when the medium through which the ultrasound beam passes does not propagate at 1540 meters per second, resulting in echoes that appear at incorrect depths on the monitor. An example of propagation speed artifact is the "bayonet artifact," which has been reported during an ultrasound-guided axillary brachial plexus block.[279] The shaft of the needle appeared bent when it accidentally traversed the axillary artery. This happens because of the difference in the velocity of sound between whole blood (1580 m/second) and soft tissue (1540 m/second).

Acoustic Shadowing

Acoustic shadow is an echo-free area behind surfaces that are highly reflective or attenuating, such as bone (see Fig. 40.12) or metallic implants. The implication for regional anesthesia is that tissues in the area of the shadow cannot be imaged.

SCANNING ROUTINE

Being able to consistently produce high-quality images of the area scanned is vital for safety and success during any ultrasound-guided regional anesthesia procedure. Without optimal images, it is not possible to accurately identify musculoskeletal structures or perform interventions with precision. We have found that following a "scanning routine," or a set of simple steps that are repeatable, is essential for optimal imaging; the routine that we follow is outlined in Table 40.6. Although the suggested routine may appear complicated at first, with repetition these steps are gradually internalized. Attaching a card with the scanning routine to the ultrasound machine facilitates easy recall.

Scout Scan

The aim of the scout scan, or the preintervention scan, as the name implies, is to examine the area of interest before the intervention.

TABLE 40.6	Scanning Routine
1.	Turn on the ultrasound machine.
2.	Select a scanning mode.
3.	Select an appropriate transducer.
4.	Dim the lights in the room.
5.	Assume a comfortable position.
6.	Apply liberal amount of ultrasound gel.
7.	Perform a scout scan.
8.	Orient the transducer and image.
9.	Select the appropriate ultrasound settings (preset, frequency—for broadband transducers, depth, gain, and focus point).
10.	Mark the position of the transducer on the patient's skin once an optimal image is obtained before the intervention.

This has also been referred to as a "mapping scan." During the scout scan, steps 8 and 9 described in Table 40.6 are performed, the sonoanatomy of the area is visualized, and the image is optimized. Once an optimal view with the target structure is obtained and the best possible site for needle insertion is determined, it is advisable to mark the position of the transducer on the patient's skin so the transducer can be returned to the same position after sterile preparations have been completed. It is common to diagnose anatomic variations during the scout scan.[280] The operator can then decide whether to continue with the block in the same location or to choose an alternative approach or technique that may be safer. This assessment of anatomic variation is one of the major benefits of using ultrasound for regional anesthesia.

General Considerations in Children

Preparations for an ultrasound-guided nerve block should begin during the preoperative visit by adequately explaining the technique, its benefits and risks, and, more importantly, the possibility of a failed block to the parents. In the event of failure, a contingency plan to quickly convert to general anesthesia or another form of postoperative analgesia must always be in place. In children, most regional anesthetic procedures are performed while the child is anesthetized. However, in a cooperative child or under special circumstances, such as in a child with difficult airway or a child predisposed to malignant hyperthermia, it is possible to perform the block after light sedation. We find that it is easy to explain the procedure to children who are older than 8 years of age. Some of them may even express a wish to stay awake and observe the ultrasound images during the block. To reduce needle-related pain, EMLA cream can be applied an hour before the procedure, or a J-tip can be used to anesthetize the skin over the area where the block needle and the intravenous catheter are to be inserted. Parental presence during the nerve block may also be helpful. In older children, allowing the child to listen to their favorite music through a personal stereo or watch a video, are useful distraction techniques that make the whole experience a more pleasant one for the child. We have connected a DVD player to our ultrasound machine, and this is used to play movies or cartoons through the monitor during the surgical procedure (E-Fig. 40.2).

Before any ultrasound-guided regional anesthesia procedure, intravenous access is established, standard monitoring is applied, and equipment and drugs appropriate for the child are prepared. Aseptic precautions and techniques are followed, and the skin over the needle puncture site is prepared with antiseptic solution in the usual fashion. The ultrasound probe is placed inside a custom-designed sterile transducer plastic cover.[281] When a catheter is to be placed, barrier drapes are recommended to avoid contaminating the catheter. A "time out" is performed to confirm the child's identity (name, medical record number), block type, laterality, presence of necessary equipment and drugs and to assure that the local anesthetic concentration and volume are within safe and effective limits for the patient.[282]

Tips and Tricks for Success

Certain steps are common to all ultrasound-guided procedures, and, if followed, they may increase success. The lights in the room must be dimmed to avoid any glare or reflection from the ultrasound monitor. The operator must assume a comfortable position (Fig. 40.16).[283] For upper extremity blocks, the operator sits at the ipsilateral head end of the child, and the ultrasound machine is placed directly in front. For lower extremity blocks, such as femoral nerve block, the operator stands on the ipsilateral side of the child, and the ultrasound machine is placed on the opposite side. For lower extremity or central neuraxial blocks in the lateral position, the operator sits behind the child, and the ultrasound machine is placed in front, with the monitor in the line of view of the operator. Because of the small muscle bulk in young children, the nerves are relatively superficial and can most frequently be easily visualized using high-frequency linear transducers. The exact choice of transducer depends on the area scanned, but a high-frequency linear transducer with a small footprint (13-6 MHz, 25-mm footprint) is particularly suited for young children. The 15-6–megahertz broadband linear-array transducer is also useful for most blocks in young children. In older children, a 10-7–megahertz broadband linear-array transducer, which allows greater flexibility with the depth of scan, is adequate for most procedures. Low-frequency (5-2 MHz) curved-array transducers are rarely used in children but are useful for imaging deeper structures such as the lumbar plexus and sciatic nerve in older children.

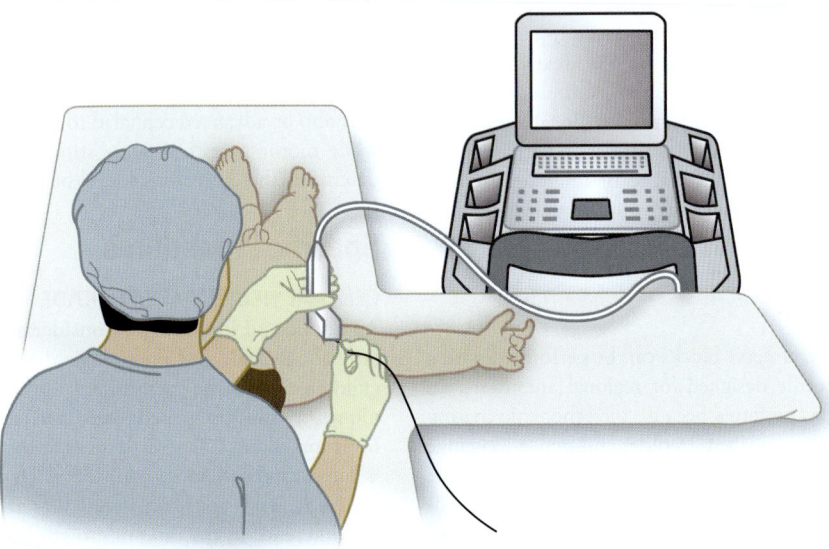

FIGURE 40.16 Position of the child, anesthesiologist, and ultrasound machine during an ultrasound-guided regional anesthesia procedure.

To improve dexterity, hold the transducer with the nondominant hand and perform interventions with the dominant hand. Holding the transducer steady for even short periods can be quite trying. We have found that gently resting the hand that is holding the transducer on the child during a block helps to keep the transducer steady (see Fig. 40.16). It is important to maintain light contact between the transducer and the skin because excessive pressure will cause the veins to collapse or distort the anatomy of the area of interest. Always apply liberal amounts of ultrasound gel to maintain adequate acoustic coupling between the skin and the transducer because even small amounts of air trapped between the two can result in artifacts. We use sterile ultrasound gel from single-use sachets for all ultrasound-guided peripheral nerve blocks. At any given time during an ultrasound-guided intervention, either the transducer or the needle must be moved. It is impossible to maintain the needle within the plane of imaging if both are moving, a common error by novices. This results in an inability to visualize the needle. If the needle is not visible in the ultrasound image, a good strategy is to keep the needle steady and manipulate the transducer (slide, tilt, or rotate) until the needle becomes visible on the monitor. Thereafter the transducer should be held steady, and the needle should be gently advanced to the target nerve, maintaining it in the imaging plane. When the angle of insertion of the needle is steep (>60 degrees), it is preferable to introduce the needle in the short axis using the out-of-plane technique. However, if the in-plane approach is used for all ultrasound-guided interventions, as in our case, inserting the needle a few centimeters away from the edge of the transducer may improve needle visibility by decreasing the angle between the needle and the imaging plane.

Injecting air into the area of the intervention must be avoided because air bubbles will degrade the image. We routinely purge the block needle with saline solution or local anesthetic to remove air before proceeding with the block. An assistant aids with the injection. When the needle tip is close to the target nerve, the assistant gently aspirates to exclude unintended intravascular placement. The assistant must avoid generating excessive negative pressure because small blood vessels are prone to collapse. A short length of extension tubing attached between the needle and the local anesthetic syringe allows the operator to hold the needle steady while the assistant performs the injection.[284] We routinely perform a test injection with 0.5 to 1 milliliters of saline solution or 5% dextrose (when nerve stimulation is also used)[260] and visualize the distribution of the injectate in real time before injecting the local anesthetic. Failure to visualize the injectate in the ultrasound image indicates that the needle is not in the plane of imaging, or it is intravascular until proven otherwise. No further injection should be made until the needle is repositioned and the distribution of the injectate is confirmed.

Ancillary Equipment

Most single-shot peripheral nerve blocks can be performed with a standard short-bevel needle designed for regional anesthesia; an echogenic block needle is preferred because the echogenic coating allows it to be more easily identified. In older children, a 22-gauge block needle is a good choice. Most block needles also allow the use of peripheral nerve stimulation together with ultrasound guidance. Indwelling catheters also can be placed under ultrasound guidance. A standard continuous peripheral nerve block kit (stimulating catheter with echogenic introducing needle) of an appropriate size can be used for catheter placement.

Use of a Nerve Stimulator

The use of a peripheral nerve stimulator is an alternative safe and effective method to locate the nerve to be blocked. Despite the nearly ubiquitous use of ultrasound, some anesthesiologists still use nerve stimulation to verify the position of the tip of the needle when ultrasound is not available, or in combination with ultrasound, particularly for paravertebral blocks. A nerve stimulator is not a substitute for anatomic knowledge, but it is a useful adjunct that allows the performance of the block in an unconscious or uncooperative heavily sedated child. It avoids the need to seek sensory paresthesias or to rely purely on anatomic landmarks. The tiny amount of current flowing from the uninsulated needle tip stimulates the nerve and produces a motor response when the needle is in close proximity to the nerve. The nerve stimulator is attached to the child as shown in E-Fig. 40.3. The cathode (negative pole) cable is attached to the low-output terminal of the nerve stimulator at one end and to the proximal (uninsulated) shaft of a Teflon-insulated needle via a sterile alligator clip, or to the plug-in lead of a specially designed block needle at the other end (the child). The anode (positive lead) cable is attached to the high-output terminal of the stimulator at the one end and to the child, distant to the block site, via an ECG electrode at the other end.[285,286] The needle is advanced in the appropriate anatomic direction, and when it appears to be in the correct position, the nerve stimulator is adjusted to approximately 0.5 mA with repetitive single-pulse output at 1-second intervals. Local muscle contraction should be minimal at this setting, although direct muscle stimulation can occur and must be distinguished from neural stimulation. The area innervated by the nerves to be blocked is observed for the appropriate muscle contractions. As the uninsulated needle tip approaches the nerve, the muscle contractions will increase in intensity and become weaker as the needle tip moves away from the nerve. One should be able to decrease the current to approximately 0.2 mA with continued elicitation of easily perceptible muscle contraction to ensure that the needle tip is correctly positioned, but stimulation at currents below this value raise the concern of intraneural needle placement. It should be noted that the injection of even a very small volume of local anesthetic will ablate or dramatically attenuate responses produced by the low current of the nerve stimulator, so the needle position should be optimized before injection (Video 40.1). The responses to stimulation of the radial, median, ulnar, and musculocutaneous nerves are shown in Fig. 40.17. An insulated epidural catheter may also be advanced cephalad to the abdominal and thorax levels while motor paresthesias are stimulated using a low current to determine the dermatomal level of the tip of the catheter.[287,288]

Specific Procedures

CENTRAL NEURAXIAL BLOCKADE

Anatomic and Physiologic Considerations

Several anatomic and physiologic differences between adults and children affect the performance of regional anesthetic techniques.[289] The conus medullaris (the terminus of the spinal cord) in neonates and infants is located at the L3 vertebral level, which is more caudal than in adults.[289,290] It does not reach the adult level at L1 until approximately 1 year of age (Fig. 40.18) owing to the difference in the rates of growth between the spinal cord and the bony vertebral column. Thus, lumbar puncture for subarachnoid block in neonates and infants should be performed at the L4–5 or L5–S1 interspace to avoid needle injury to the spinal

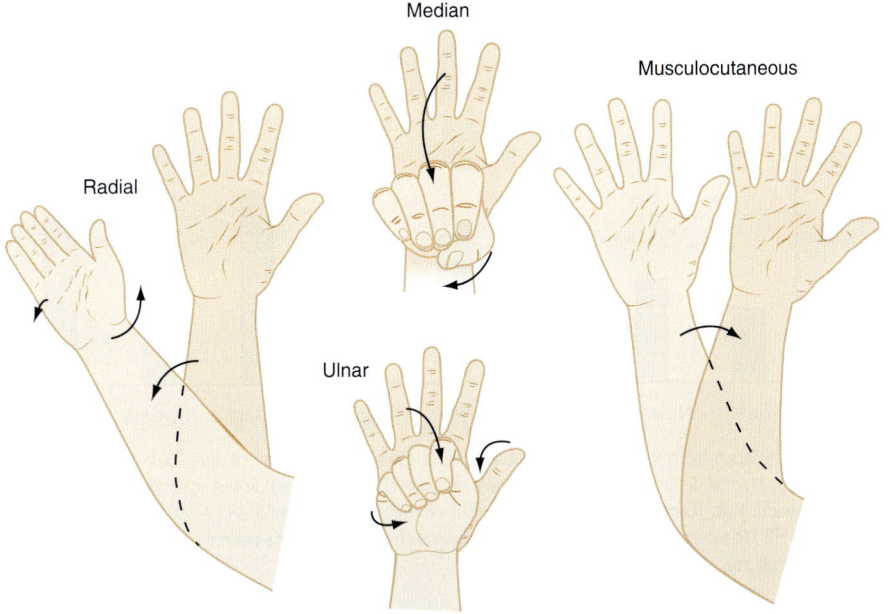

Median

Musculocutaneous

Radial

Ulnar

FIGURE 40.17 Characteristic movements of the fingers, wrist, and elbow in response to nerve stimulation of four specific nerves (Modified from Cousins MJ, Bridenbaugh PO, eds. *Neural Blockade in Clinical Anesthesia and Management of Pain*. 2nd ed. Philadelphia: JB Lippincott; 1988:406.)

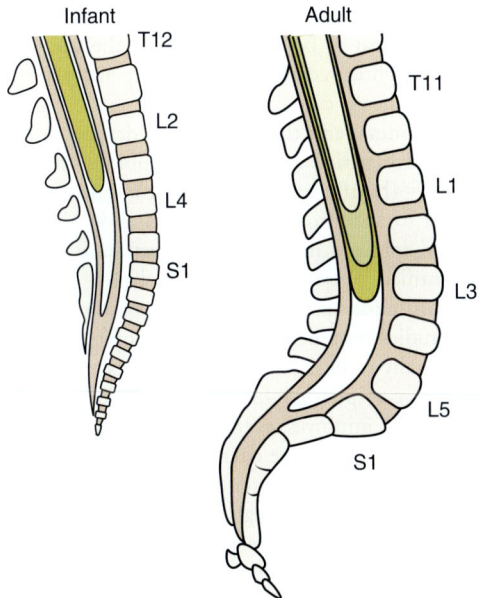

Infant   Adult

FIGURE 40.18 Anatomic differences between adults and children that affect the performance of spinal and epidural anesthesia; an infant's sacrum *(left)* is flatter and narrower than an adult's *(right)*. Note that the tip of the spinal cord in a neonate ends at L3 and does not achieve the normal adult position (L1–L2) until approximately 1 year of age. The relative location of the spinal cord with growth to adulthood is illustrated on the *right* as different shades of yellow, the darkest being neonates and the lightest being the final adult configuration.

cord. The vertebral laminae are poorly calcified at this age, so a midline approach is preferable to a paramedian one in which the needle is "walked off" the laminae. Another anatomic difference is that the neonate's sacrum is narrower and flatter than in adults (see Fig. 40.18). Thus, the dura can be breached and the subarachnoid space inadvertently entered with relative ease via the caudal canal. To avoid dural puncture, the needle for a caudal block must not be advanced deeply in neonates.[291] The presence of a deep sacral dimple may be associated with spina bifida occulta, greatly increasing the possibility of dural puncture; a caudal block may be contraindicated in these children; ultrasound imaging may help to rule out spinal cord abnormalities.[292]

The distance from the skin to the subarachnoid space is small in neonates (~14 mm) and increases progressively with age (Fig. 40.19).[293] The ligamenta flava are much thinner and less dense in infants and children than in adults, which makes the engagement of the epidural needle more difficult to detect and the likelihood of unintended dural puncture during epidural catheter placement increased. Cerebrospinal fluid (CSF) volume as a percentage of body weight is greater in infants and young children than in adults (E-Fig. 40.4)[294–298]; this may contribute in part to the comparatively larger doses of local anesthetics required for surgical anesthesia with subarachnoid block in neonates and young infants. The rate of turnover of CSF in infants and children is also greater than that in adults, accounting in part for the much briefer duration of subarachnoid block. These anatomic differences necessitate meticulous attention to detail to achieve successful and uncomplicated spinal or epidural anesthesia.

In contrast to older children and adults, subarachnoid and epidural blockade in infants and small children is characterized by hemodynamic stability, even when the level of the block reaches the upper thoracic dermatomes.[299–301] Although heart rate variability, as determined by spectral analysis, is less, the heart rate is preserved, because the parasympathetic activity modulating the heart rate appears to be attenuated in infants who receive spinal anesthesia.[302] This attenuated vagal tone allows the heart rate to compensate for changes in peripheral vascular tone, an effect that may be the most important factor in preserving hemodynamic stability compared with other factors, such as the relatively small venous capacitance in the lower extremities and the relative lack of resting sympathetic peripheral vascular tone in infants.[303] Very high levels of spinal

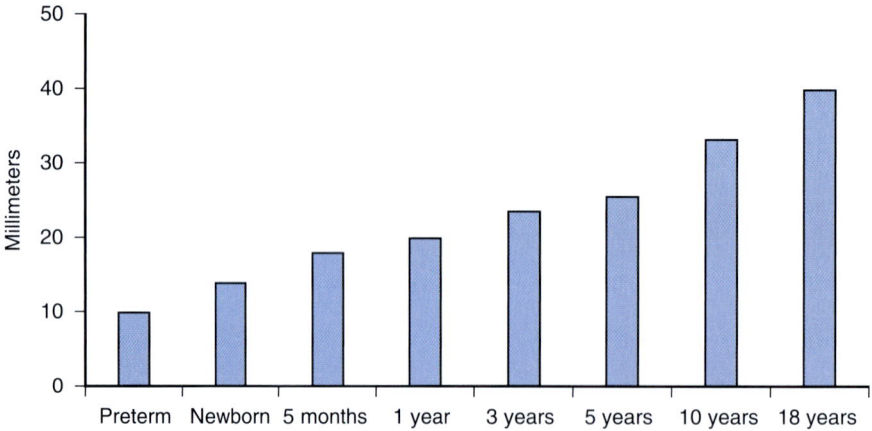

FIGURE 40.19 Distance from the skin to the subarachnoid space as a function of age. (Data from Bonadio WA, Smith DS, Metrou M, et al. Estimating lumbar puncture depth in children. *N Engl J Med.* 1988;319[14]:952-953; Kosaka Y, Sato K, Kawaguchi R. [Distance from the skin to the epidural space in children.] *Masui.* 1974;23[9]:874-875 [in Japanese]; Lau HP. [The distance from the skin to the epidural space in a Chinese patient population.] *Ma Tsui Hsueh Tsa Chi.* 1989;27:261-264.)

anesthesia can still cause bradycardia that may require treatment with a vagolytic.[304] Nonetheless, data suggest that alterations in vascular resistance and blood flow to some vascular beds may occur, at least under certain conditions, in infants. In former preterm infants who received isobaric bupivacaine for subarachnoid block, cerebral blood flow decreased concomitant with changes in systemic blood pressure, although the conditions under which the baseline pressures were measured were not clear.[305] In a study in which changes in regional temperature were used as a surrogate sign of sympathetic activity, extremity but not truncal temperature increased during subarachnoid block, together with small insignificant changes in blood pressure.[306] Our experience has been that clinically significant systemic blood pressure changes do not occur in young infants after a subarachnoid block.[304]

Central neuraxial blockade can affect the respiratory mechanics of the chest wall and diaphragm by diminution in intercostal muscle activity. This may be particularly relevant in infants and young children, whose chest walls are very compliant because the ribs are minimally ossified.[307] Infants rely more on excursions of the diaphragm to maintain tidal volume to a greater extent than older children and adults.[307] Paradoxical movement of the chest wall—that is, inward displacement of the rostral edge of the rib cage even in the absence of airway obstruction—occurs during inspiration in healthy infants during deep sleep. This paradoxical chest wall motion increases as the force of diaphragmatic excursion increases during rapid eye movement (REM) and deep sleep.[308] In a similar fashion, suppression of intercostal muscle activity decreases the contribution of the rib cage to ventilation in infants during spontaneous respiration under anesthesia.[307,309] Using respiratory inductance plethysmography to study the contributions of the rib cage and diaphragm to breathing in former preterm infants under high thoracic (T2–4) levels of motor blockade spinal anesthesia,[307] outward motion of the lower rib cage decreased and paradoxical motion of the lower rib cage increased in more than half of the infants. The contribution of the diaphragm to respiration, as estimated by abdominal displacement, was increased in all infants. This suggests a shift in the respiratory workload from rib cage to diaphragm to compensate for the loss of the intercostal muscles to breathing. Other factors, such as an altered conformation of the diaphragm relative to the chest wall, with concomitant

changes in the size of the zone of apposition (the portion of the anterior diaphragm that lies against the lower rib cage), may also contribute. These measurements were compared within each infant to their awake measurements before spinal anesthesia, not during deep sleep. Whether these findings would be unchanged with a different baseline measurement remains unclear. Nonetheless, these changes appear to be well-tolerated in the vast majority of infants as the diaphragm can adequately compensate for the loss of contribution of the rib cage to breathing.

Upper abdominal and thoracic surgery depress respiration in the postoperative period by neurally inhibiting diaphragmatic function.[310–312] The afferent pathways that induce this inhibition are presumed to arise from the chest and abdominal walls and possibly the diaphragm itself, although they have not been conclusively identified.[313] Contrary to popular belief, pain itself is not a major contributor to postoperative respiratory dysfunction. Numerous studies have demonstrated that opioids administered either parenterally or in the central neuraxis exert limited impact on postoperative respiratory function.[314–316] Regional blockade, on the other hand, improves several indices of postoperative respiratory function.[21,311,317] These data suggest that regional anesthesia has an important role in attenuating diaphragmatic dysfunction postoperatively. Although the mechanism for this improvement has been attributed to blockade of the putative inhibitory neural pathways, other data suggest that alterations in respiratory mechanics, in particular an increase in the resting length of the diaphragm to its control value and a shift in the workload from the rib cage to the diaphragm, may contribute to a far greater extent.[20] These data also suggest that the beneficial effects of regional anesthesia on postoperative respiratory function may, in part, be related to the degree of motor blockade. In terms of timing, it is not known whether a preoperative regional block preserves or enhances respiratory function to a greater extent than a block applied postoperatively, as has been postulated in "preemptive analgesia."

Spinal Anesthesia

Successful spinal anesthesia has been reported in children since 1900[289,318–321] and administered for a variety of surgical procedures in infants.[322–325] Ultrasound-guided spinal anesthesia is a recent refinement to the technique.[326] Reports of postanesthetic apnea in former preterm infants after general anesthesia led to a resurgence of this technique in former preterm infants to potentially reduce the incidence of perioperative apnea, particularly for herniorrhaphy.[327–332,333] However, when the spinal anesthetic was supplemented with ketamine, the incidence of postoperative apnea was even greater than with general anesthesia.[334] A Cochrane review on the risk of apnea after spinal or general anesthesia in former preterm infants undergoing inguinal hernia surgery concluded that spinal anesthesia reduced the risk of a postoperative apnea with a number needed to treat of 4 compared with general anesthesia.[335] As a secondary outcome from the GAS study (a randomized trial that investigated neurocognitive outcomes after spinal or general anesthesia), the incidence of apnea in the first 12 hours after surgery with the two techniques was similar, 3% and 4% respectively, although the incidence of early apneas (defined as an apnea within the first 30 minutes after anesthesia) was reduced but not eliminated after spinal anesthesia, whereas the frequency of late apneas (from 30 minutes to 12 hours) was similar in both groups.[336] These apnea rates after sevoflurane anesthesia compare favorably with the rates reported in the mid-1990s, when halothane was the primary general anesthetic.[329,337] Caution continues to be advised; all former preterm infants less than approximately 60 weeks postconceptional age should be monitored for postoperative apneas, irrespective of the anesthetic technique.[338–341] We believe, however, that regional anesthesia offers advantages in former preterm infants for whom it would provide adequate operating conditions.

Epidural anesthesia has also been reported for lower extremity and abdominal surgery in former preterm infants. Continuous epidural anesthesia and even continuous spinal anesthesia, for surgeries that outlast the duration of a "single-shot" subarachnoid block are alternative strategies that can achieve the same goals as single-injection subarachnoid block. The risk of LAST with a continuous caudal epidural blockade in this population must be recognized; with some recommending 2,3-chloroprocaine as the most prudent agent in this situation.[342] For cardiac surgery, high spinal anesthesia with tetracaine (2.4 mg/kg) has been used for ligation of the patent ductus arteriosus. Because spinal anesthesia in infants is associated with hemodynamic stability, it has been advocated as an ideal anesthetic for cardiac catheterization in infants with congenital heart defects and has been used, in conjunction with a light general anesthetic, for cardiac surgery.[323,343–346] Those infants whose tracheas were intubated for surgery were successfully extubated immediately after the operation. Hemodynamic stability was maintained without the use of inotropic agents in most children. Spinal anesthesia has also been reported in a series of infants who underwent successful gastroschisis closures and open pyloromyotomies.[325,343]

Concerns regarding the potential for adverse neurodevelopmental sequelae of general anesthetics administered to infants has led to additional interest in spinal anesthesia even in term infants. The most recent studies, including one large prospective, randomized controlled trial, concluded that for procedures lasting an hour or less there is no difference in neurodevelopmental outcome between spinal and general anesthesia (see Chapter 23).[347–349]

When an effective block[35,340,350–353] is achieved, most neonates fall asleep, a phenomenon attributed to *deafferentation*, which is a reduced level of consciousness arising from diminished sensory input to the reticular activating system from the periphery. This mechanism has been confirmed in an animal model using spectral edge frequency analysis.[354] Sedation levels have been measured using bispectral index and spectral edge frequency analysis in infants undergoing spinal anesthesia without adjunctive sedatives.[355] The investigators found a decrease in bispectral index, from 97 to 66.5 after 30 minutes, and in spectral edge frequency, from 26.1 to 9.9. These data indicate that sedation with dense regional blockade is a real physiologic phenomenon; they also suggest that if sedation is administered to these infants, smaller doses than usual should be considered to avoid oversedation. Other investigators suggested that the adult algorithms used in these devices may have overestimated the depth of sedation in infants.[356]

Spinal Ultrasonography

Spinal ultrasonography has been used as a diagnostic screening tool in neonates and infants suspected of having a spinal dysraphism and for detecting spinal tumors, vascular malformations, and trauma.[292,357–362] Spinal ultrasonography is possible in neonates and infants because the incomplete ossification of the predominantly cartilaginous posterior spinal elements creates an acoustic window that allows the transmission of the ultrasound beam. The overall visibility of neuraxial structures decreases with increasing age. Neuraxial structures are best visualized in neonates and infants younger than 3 months of age; progressive ossification of the posterior spinal elements makes detailed sonographic evaluation of the spine increasingly difficult beyond 6 months of age unless the child has a persistent posterior spinal defect. The overall visibility of neuraxial structures also decreases as one progresses cephalad, with the best visibility in the sacral level followed by the lumbar and thoracic.

Spinal ultrasound is most frequently performed with the child positioned in the lateral decubitus position. Because the neuraxial structures are relatively superficial, they are best visualized using high-frequency (10-5 MHz) transducers, which also produce better images than sector transducers. Scans are obtained in both the transverse (axial) and longitudinal (sagittal) axes and performed either through the midline or parallel and lateral (paramedian) to the spinous processes. The paramedian scan is preferable in older children because it avoids the ossified spinous processes that can interfere with ultrasound transmission. In neonates and young infants, the spinal canal can be scanned with the transducer placed directly over the spinous processes (i.e., a median longitudinal scan). Beyond this age group a paramedian longitudinal scan provides the best overall view of neuraxial structures.

On a longitudinal sonogram, the neonatal spinal cord is seen as a hypoechoic tubular structure with hyperechoic anterior and posterior walls. A thin strip of variable intense echo, "the central echo complex" (Fig. 40.20A), extends longitudinally through the center of the spinal cord and represents the area between the myelinated ventral white commissure and the central portion of the anterior median fissure. This produces the "triplet echoes" that are characteristic of the spinal cord at all levels (Fig. 40.20B). The diameter of the spinal cord varies, being largest in the cervical and lumbar regions and smallest at the thoracic region. Anterior and posterior to the spinal cord are two well-defined linear and hyperechoic echoes that represent the arachnoid-dural layer (see Fig. 40.20A). The ligamentum flavum, which is relevant for epidural access, is also readily visualized in young children and appears less echogenic than the dura (see Fig. 40.20B). The dural layers taper distally to close the thecal sac at the S2 level. The epidural space is the hypoechoic area between the dura and the ligamentum flavum (see Fig. 40.20B) and arterial pulsations also may be visible on ultrasound between these two layers. The CSF surrounds the spinal cord as an anechoic layer between the dura

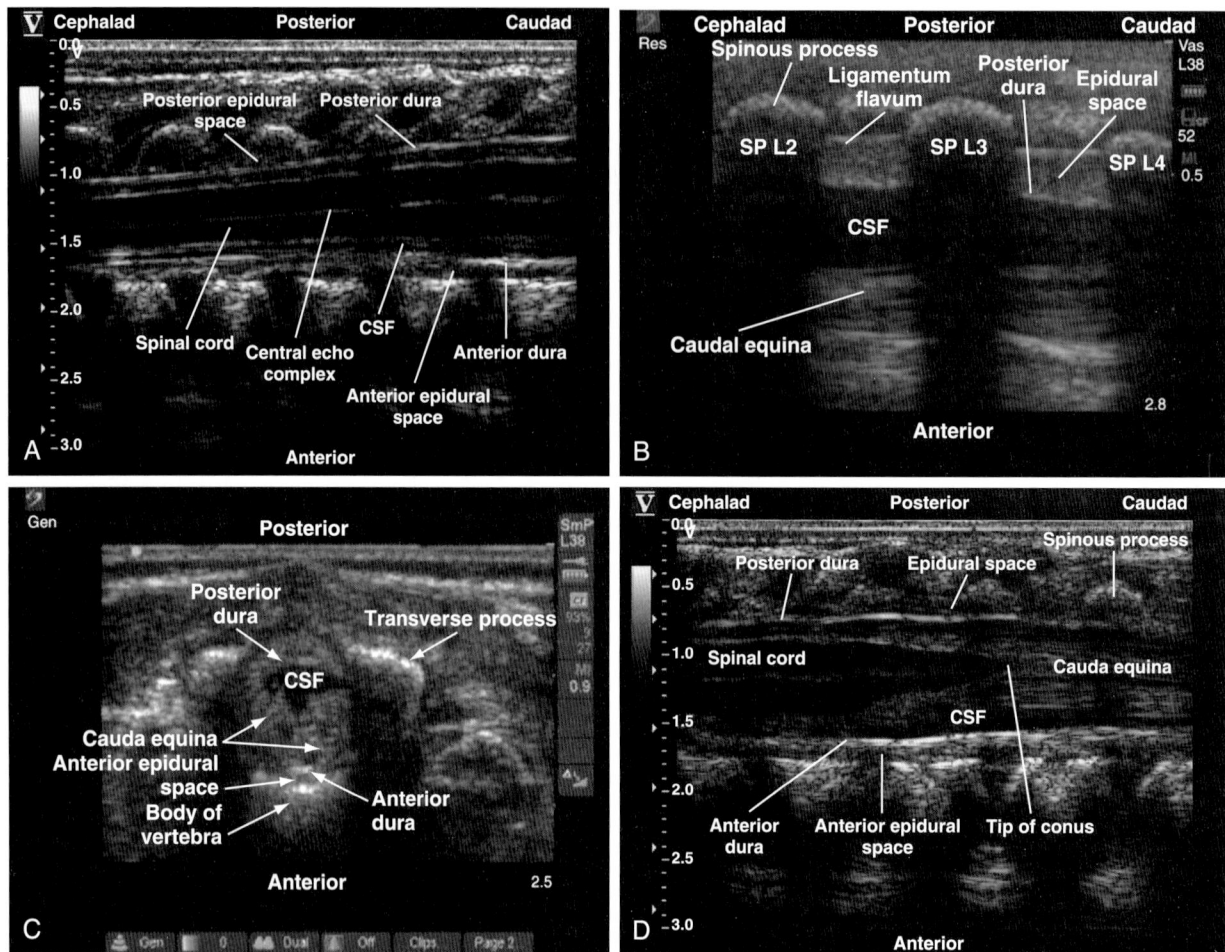

FIGURE 40.20 A, Longitudinal paramedian sonogram of the thoracic spine in a neonate. **B,** Longitudinal midline sonogram of the lumbar spine in a neonate. **C,** Transverse sonogram of the lumbar spine in a neonate showing the cauda equina. **D,** Longitudinal paramedian sonogram of the thoracolumbar spine in a neonate showing the termination of the spinal cord. *CSF,* Cerebrospinal fluid; *SP L2,* spinous process of L2; *SP L3,* spinous process of L3; *SP L4,* spinous process of L4.

and spinal cord (Fig. 40.20C). The vertebral bodies are seen as echogenic structures anterior to the spinal cord. The spinal cord tapers distally to form the conus medullaris (Fig. 40.20D) at the level of the first and second lumbar vertebral bodies. The conus medullaris is continuous with the filum terminale, which extends into the sacral canal as a hyperechoic structure. It is surrounded by the roots of the cauda equina, which appear as multiple parallel echogenic lines surrounding the filum terminale (Fig. 40.21A). Differentiation of the filum terminale from the roots of the cauda equina can sometimes be difficult. The cauda equina typically lies in the anterior half of the spinal canal when the child is in the prone position, but it moves freely within the CSF with change in position and with crying. Slight anteroposterior movement of the spinal cord, superimposed on the arterial pulsations, is commonly seen during real-time imaging.

On a transverse (axial) sonogram, the spinal cord is seen as a round or oval hypoechoic structure, with its bright central echo complex (Fig. 40.21B). The spinal cord is fixed laterally by the dentate ligament (see Fig. 40.21B), which represents the transversely oriented, echogenic arachnoid duplications that are seen in parts of the thoracic spinal canal. Paired (ventral and dorsal) echogenic nerve roots are seen below the L2 level. Farther caudally

in the lumbar region, a transverse scan shows the filum terminale surrounded by the nerve roots of the cauda equina (Fig. 40.21C). The arachnoid–dura mater complex is hyperechoic and forms the anterior and posterior border of the subarachnoid space in the lumbar region (see Fig. 40.21C). The vertebral bodies are the hyperechoic structures anterior to the spinal canal. The vertebral arches are also echogenic and cast an acoustic shadow anteriorly (see Fig. 40.21C). The paraspinal muscles appear hypoechoic on ultrasound.

Ultrasonographic- or Landmark-Guided Technique

After routine monitors (ECG, blood pressure cuff, pulse oximeter, and precordial stethoscope) are affixed, the child is placed in a sitting or lateral decubitus position.[363] For neonates and infants, care must be taken to avoid flexion of the neck because this position may obstruct the airway (Fig. 40.22A).[364,365] The sitting position may aid in recognizing successful dural puncture by increasing CSF hydrostatic pressure, which increases flow through the spinal needle. The skin is infiltrated with a minute quantity of 1% lidocaine (<0.2 mL is sufficient; the authors use a 30-gauge needle on an insulin syringe); alternatively, a small amount of EMLA or other transcutaneous local anesthetic

40

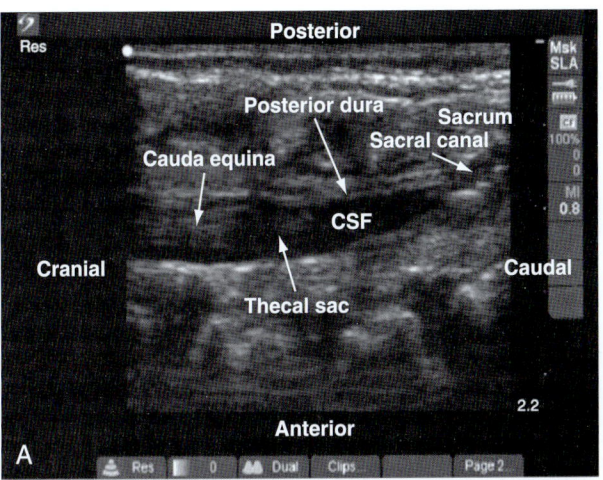

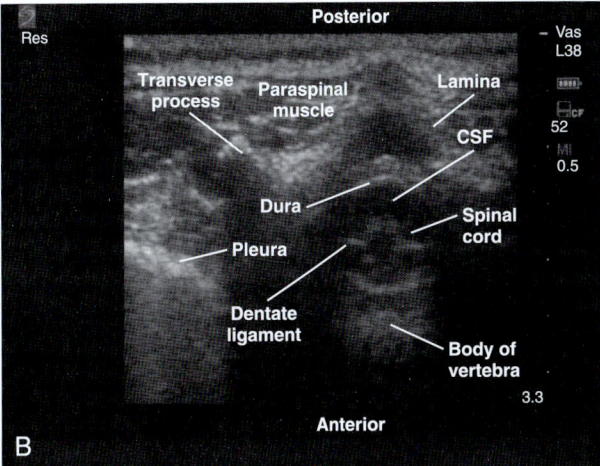

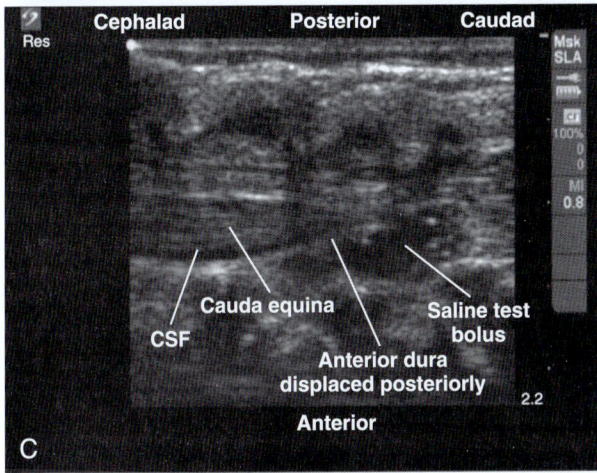

FIGURE 40.21 A, Longitudinal sonogram of the sacrum showing the tapered end of the thecal sac. **B,** Transverse sonogram of the thoracic spine in a neonate. **C,** Longitudinal sonogram of the sacrum after a test bolus injection of saline solution through an indwelling caudal catheter during a single-shot caudal epidural injection. Note the displacement of the dura. *CSF,* Cerebrospinal fluid.

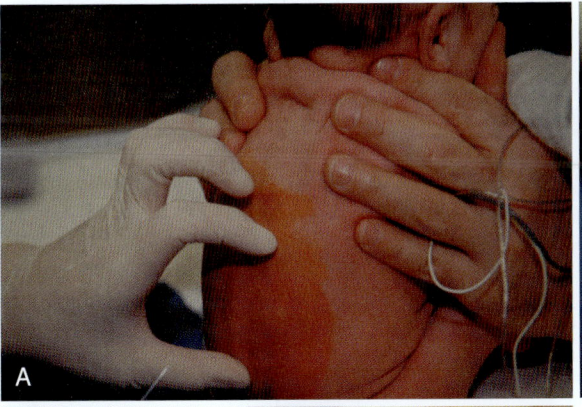

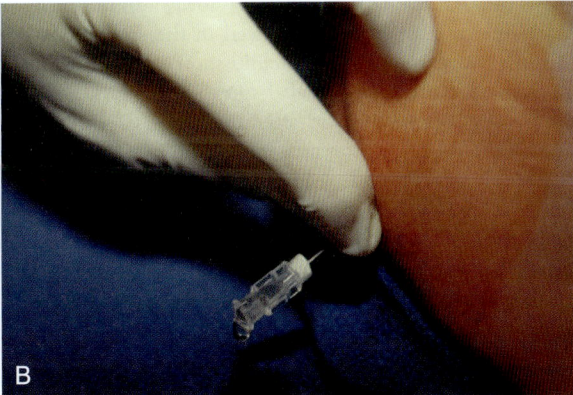

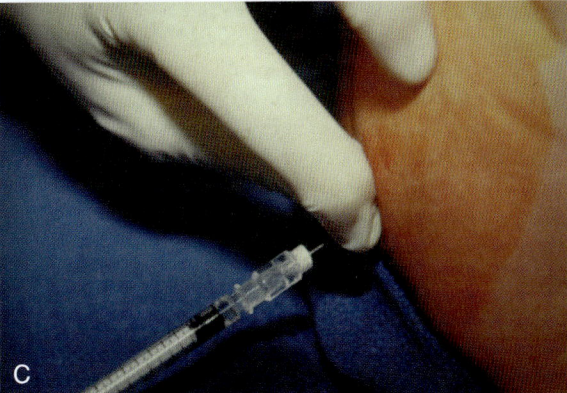

FIGURE 40.22 A, Lumbar puncture in a neonate or infant is generally performed with the child in the sitting position. Note that the head is maintained in the neutral position to prevent airway obstruction. **B,** After local infiltration of 1% lidocaine with a 25- to 30-gauge needle, lumbar puncture is performed with a 22-gauge, 1.5-inch styletted needle at the L4–L5 or L5–S1 interspace. Entrance into the subarachnoid space is confirmed by free flow of cerebrospinal fluid. **C,** Local anesthetic is injected with a tuberculin syringe. Care must be taken not to inject rapidly or a high level of blockade might result.

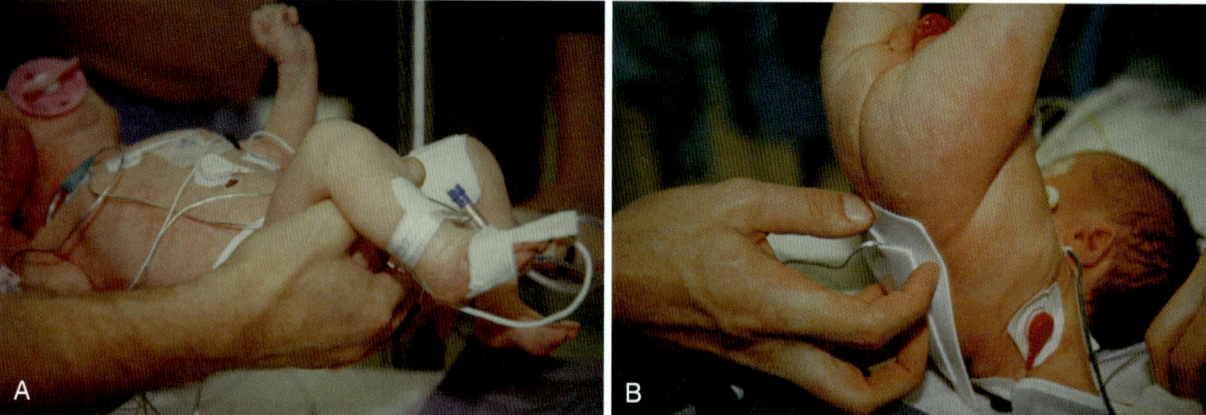

FIGURE 40.23 A, The proper method of applying an electrocautery pad; the infant's entire body is elevated while maintaining the horizontal position or the infant is log-rolled along its long axis to avoid excessively high spread of subarachnoid blockade. **B,** Improper method of applying an electrocautery pad in a neonate after subarachnoid administration of local anesthetic; the legs should never be elevated as this may lead to a high or total spinal block.

cream is applied to the infant's lumbar area at least 1 hour before spinal placement. The lumbar puncture is performed using a midline approach with a 22-gauge, 1.5-inch styletted spinal needle (Fig. 40.22B,C). We do not routinely use a 25-gauge spinal needle because of the time delay between entering the subarachnoid space and the appearance of CSF in the needle hub. Whitacre, Sprotte, Marx, and other "pencil-point" needles are available in pediatric sizes.[366,367] Lumbar puncture is performed only at the L4–5 or L5–S1 interspaces, for reasons described previously. The subarachnoid space in infants less than 60 weeks postconception age is approximately 1.5 centimeters from the skin (see Fig. 40.19); care must be taken not to pass the needle beyond the subarachnoid space.[293] When the subarachnoid space is located, the local anesthetic is slowly administered. Immediately thereafter, the child is placed in the supine position. Once the block is in place, the child should remain completely horizontal to preclude cephalad spread of the local anesthetic. If the legs are raised soon after the block is placed, a "total" spinal anesthetic may occur (see Fig. 40.23A,B).[368] The grounding pad is best applied by lifting the entire infant while maintaining the body in the horizontal plane or simply log-rolling the infant, or the pad can be affixed to the anterior thigh if sufficient space and muscle mass are available. *The legs should never be raised above the torso once the spinal block is in place as this may produce a high spinal block.*

Because spinal anesthesia maintains remarkable hemodynamic stability in infants, some pediatric anesthesiologists advocate starting the IV after the onset of lower extremity analgesia. Although this may be relatively safe in this setting, if a "total spinal" occurred and the airway had to be instrumented or resuscitation drugs had to be administered, having IV access before the spinal block would be important. In addition, should IV access prove difficult, valuable operating time and spinal block time would be lost while searching for a suitable vein. Applying the pulse oximeter to a toe of one leg and the blood pressure cuff to the thigh of the other allows the neonate to remain undisturbed during the surgical procedure (e.g., inguinal herniorrhaphy) (E-Fig. 40.5).

Because the addition of sedatives during spinal anesthesia has been associated with postanesthetic apnea with an incidence at least as great as that of general anesthesia, we try to avoid all sedatives, especially ketamine.[334] Most neonates fall asleep once the

block has set, which obviates the need for sedatives. A pacifier dipped in 50% dextrose will also help keep the infant quiet and still. Gentle restraint with soft cuffs applied to the wrists is advisable to prevent movement of the arms. In some cases, particularly during the most stimulating phase of the operation, when traction is applied to the hernia sac, irritation is transmitted to the peritoneum. It is particularly important for the infant to be still and not bear down when the hernia sac is dissected to avoid both tearing the sac and extruding abdominal contents through the open hernia. Should the infant become agitated or unsettled at this point, one should administer inhalational anesthesia by mask or a small dose of propofol until the stimulation abates, allowing the operation to proceed without difficulty.

Selection of Drug for Neonates and Infants

The proportional dose requirement of local anesthetic for spinal anesthesia in neonates when calculated on a per-kilogram basis[369] is greater than that required in adults to achieve a similar dermatomal distribution. In addition, the duration of the block lasts about one-third to one-half of that in the adult. This is due in part to the greater volume of CSF per kilogram and to the more rapid turnover of CSF in neonates. Hyperbaric bupivacaine (0.75 mg/kg of 0.75% bupivacaine in 8.25% dextrose), isobaric bupivacaine (0.5–1.0 mg/kg of a 0.5% solution), isobaric levobupivacaine (1 mg/kg of 0.5% levobupivacaine).[370] Tetracaine (0.75-1.0 mg/kg, with 0.01 mg/mL of epinephrine (1:100,000) was commonly used in the past and is still a viable option, but the hyperbaric preparation is no longer available, and it has largely been supplanted by the options discussed above.[294,371–375] Isobaric and hyperbaric bupivacaine have a duration similar to that of tetracaine, although the duration of action of the isobaric solution is slightly greater than for the hyperbaric solution.[374–376] Epinephrine prolongs the duration of a tetracaine spinal by more than 30%[377] but does not prolong the duration of a bupivacaine spinal.[377] These doses usually provide adequate analgesia for inguinal hernia repair with a duration of motor block of 70 to 90 minutes and a dermatome height in the mid to upper thoracic region. For surgeries of limited duration that involve a lower extremity, smaller doses (0.5–0.6 mg/kg) may be used. A dose-ranging study reported that the addition of clonidine (1 μg/kg) prolonged the duration of blockade from a mean of 67 minutes (plain bupivacaine) to 111

TABLE 40.7	Local Anesthetics for Spinal Anesthesia in Neonates and Infants	
Anesthetic Drug	Usual Dose (mg/kg)	Range (mg/kg)
1% Tetracaine in 10% dextrose	0.75	0.75–1
0.5% Bupivacaine (isobaric)	0.8	0.5–1
0.75% Bupivacaine in 8.25% dextrose	0.75	0.5–1

minutes.[378] The use of larger doses of clonidine (2 μg/kg), however, caused transient hypotension and apnea, which required treatment with caffeine. Although lidocaine (2 mg/kg) is useful for a block of brief duration, such as for a muscle biopsy of the lower extremity, the duration of block is only approximately 30 minutes. In light of concerns regarding lidocaine in the subarachnoid space, we no longer recommend its use in infants.[379–381] A summary of doses for commonly used local anesthetics for subarachnoid block in neonates and infants is provided in Table 40.7.

Selection of Drug for Children

There is little information regarding the dose of local anesthetics for spinal anesthesia in children, as subarachnoid block is much less commonly used beyond infancy. When a neuraxial regional technique is desirable in children, an epidural or caudal block together with a "light" general anesthetic is often preferred. For spinal anesthesia, 0.3 to 0.5 mg/kg of bupivacaine (5 mg/mL concentration) may be used in children 2 months to 18 years of age[367]; there was no difference in one study between hypobaric and isobaric approaches.[382,383] Doses of 0.3 to 0.4 mg/kg tetracaine have been used for subarachnoid block in children between 12 weeks and 2 years of age, and 0.2 to 0.3 mg/kg in children older than 2 years of age.[384–386] Tetracaine dosing data are based on hyperbaric tetracaine which is no longer available; these limited and largely anecdotal data suggest that the dose requirement for spinal anesthesia decreases with increasing age.

Complications

Complications of spinal anesthesia include block failure, total spinal anesthesia, post–dural puncture headache, backache, neurologic sequelae, and the risk of lumbar epidermoid tumors if nonstyletted needles are used for subarachnoid puncture.[366–368,387–393]

Block failure is a risk with any regional anesthetic technique. The General Anesthesia Compared to Spinal Anesthesia Study (GAS) consortium reported that fewer than 10% of patients in that trial required conversion from spinal to general anesthesia, and just 6.8% required a brief period of sedation. Nonetheless, the overall failure rate for spinal anesthesia was approximately 19%.[336,341,370]

Total spinal anesthesia has been reported in neonates. It is most commonly manifested by apnea with no change in systemic blood pressure or heart rate, although should pronounced bradycardia occur, a reduction in cardiac output is likely and should be treated aggressively.[304,368,394] It can occur after a dose of as little as 0.6 mg/kg of tetracaine.[368] Alteration in position, particularly by raising the lower body above the level of the head or thorax, may be the most common cause of a high spinal block. Although the rate of administration of the local anesthetic does not appear to affect the level of spinal anesthesia in adults, similar studies have not been conducted in neonates or infants.[395] It is possible that

factors, such as the use of a relatively large-bore needle (22-gauge) and a tuberculin syringe providing the means for injecting with high pressure, along with the small distance between vertebrae, combines to make the rate of injection an important consideration in neonates and infants by producing unintended barbotage. We have observed this complication with rapid drug administration. Management consists of assisted or controlled ventilation until the return of spontaneous respiratory function.

The incidence of post–dural puncture headache appears to be infrequent in infants and children, although the incidence in preverbal children is unknown. An early study reported an incidence of spinal headache of approximately 2% using 20- to 22-gauge needles in children 2 to 17 years of age.[386] However, no details were provided about the distribution of headache with respect to age. Other studies reported a 5% incidence of headaches in children ranging from 2 months to nearly 10 years of age, but again, no age distribution was cited.[366,367] A prospective study of pediatric oncology patients undergoing a lumbar puncture with a 20-gauge needle reported that post–dural puncture headache was relatively rare in children younger than 13 years of age.[388] In most instances, the headaches were mild and resolved spontaneously. It is not entirely clear why young children have a very low incidence of post–dural puncture headache. Several possible reasons include reduced CSF pressure,[389] the increased rate of CSF production, and hormonal changes with age.[388] Pencil-point style spinal needles, now available for children, may further reduce this problem.

Backache is a frequent postoperative complaint after both general and regional anesthesia in adults. It is thought to occur because of flattening of the normal lordotic lumbar curve secondary to muscle and ligament relaxation that occurs with spinal anesthesia. The incidence in children is unknown. Neurologic sequelae after spinal anesthesia are exceedingly rare. There are no reports in the literature of permanent neurologic injury caused by subarachnoid block, but data in children remain limited. There have been no cases detected in more than 1700 consecutive spinal anesthetics at the University of Vermont Medical Center, in another large series from Schneider Children's Medical Center (Petah Tikva, Israel), or in the 260 subarachnoid blocks in infants in the PRAN database.[15,160,394]

Epidural Anesthesia

Epidural anesthesia administered by the caudal, lumbar, or thoracic route can be used for the same types of surgical procedures and indications as spinal anesthesia. The most common indication, however, is for augmentation of general anesthesia and for postoperative pain management. The details of postoperative epidural infusions are discussed in Chapter 41.

Caudal Epidural Anesthesia

Although epidural use was first described in 1933,[396] it was not until the early 1960s that caudal anesthesia gained any degree of popularity.[396–411] Improvements in catheter material, the availability of pediatric-sized needles and catheters, and the growing recognition of the benefits and safety of regional analgesia have increased the interest in this technique for children.[412] Even as pediatric peripheral and plexus blockade is increasingly used, the single-injection caudal block remains the most frequently used regional anesthetic technique in children. It is almost always used in combination with general anesthesia for surgery involving the lower thoracic, lumbar, and sacral dermatomes.[413–415] In a prospectively collected cohort of more than 18,000 children, the PRAN investigators detected no sequelae after caudal blockade,[416] but more recent data from PRAN, which includes over 38,000 caudal blocks reported three cases of local anesthetic systemic toxicity, including two cases of cardiac arrest. These were presumably from accidental intravascular or intramedullary injection, as doses were 1.5 mg/kg of bupivacaine equivalents or less, and all patients were rapidly resuscitated and recovered without sequelae.[109] A prospective analysis found that ultrasound guidance for caudal block improved success and detected unsuspected needle misplacement.[417]

Several methods are used to perform a caudal epidural injection. Detecting the characteristic pop or give as the needle traverses the sacrococcygeal ligament to enter the caudal epidural space is by far the most commonly used method in children. However, even in experienced hands it can result in failure, as the overall failure rate varies between 2.8% and 11%. Ultrasound has been used to guide caudal epidural injection in children,[418–420] confirmed either by visualizing correct needle or catheter positioning in the sacral canal or caudal epidural space, or by observing dural displacement after a saline solution test bolus (1–3 mL) injection.

Ultrasonographic Guided-Caudal Epidural

The anesthetized child is positioned in the lateral position with the knee and hips flexed. The operator sits or stands behind the child, and the ultrasound machine is positioned directly in front. A linear-array transducer (13-10 MHz) is used to image the sacrum. A transducer with a wide footprint is preferable because it allows a greater length of the spine to be examined in a single view. The transducer is initially positioned directly over the sacral cornua in the transverse axis (Fig. 40.24A). On a transverse sonogram at the level of the sacral hiatus, the sacral cornua are seen as two hyperechoic reverse U-shaped structures, one on either side of the midline. Connecting the two sacral cornua and deep to the skin and subcutaneous tissue is a hyperechoic band, the sacrococcygeal ligament (see Fig. 40.24A). Anterior to the sacrococcygeal ligament is another linear hyperechoic structure, which represents the posterior surface of the sacrum. The hypoechoic area between the sacrococcygeal ligament and the bony posterior surface of the sacrum is the sacral hiatus. The two sacral cornua and the posterior surface of the sacrum produce an ultrasound image that we refer to as the "frog-eye sign" because of its resemblance to the eyes of a frog. On a longitudinal sonogram of the sacrum, the sacrococcygeal ligament, the base of the sacrum, and the sacral hiatus can be clearly seen (Fig. 40.24B). In neonates and young infants, the

tapered end of the thecal sac with CSF, the anterior and posterior epidural space filled with fat, and the cauda equina may be visualized in the sacral canal (see Fig. 40.24B; Video 40.2).

For ultrasound-guided caudal epidural injection, either the in-plane or out-of-plane technique can be used. We prefer the in-plane approach, and the needle is advanced under real-time guidance into the sacral canal through the sacrococcygeal ligament. During insertion, the needle is maintained at an angle (approximately 20 degrees) so that it is parallel to the posterior surface of the sacrum. Correct position of the needle in the caudal epidural space is confirmed objectively by performing a test bolus injection of saline solution and observing the real-time displacement of the dura (Fig. 40.25; Video 40.3). Anterior displacement of the posterior dura is more frequently seen than posterior displacement of the anterior dura. If dural displacement is not seen in the ultrasound image, it implies that the needle or catheter is not in the correct position, the needle or catheter is not in the plane of ultrasound imaging, or the needle is intravascular. The needle should be withdrawn and the procedure repeated until the typical dural displacement is visualized. The calculated dose of local anesthetic is then injected in aliquots. The cephalad spread of the local anesthetic within the epidural space also can be visualized in real time.[421] Depending on the volume of local anesthetic injected, progressive widening of the epidural space and a resultant compression of the thecal sac occur (see Fig. 40.25). These changes are visualized in the sacral canal and at the lumbar and thoracic levels. In some cases, the thecal sac is almost completely obliterated in the sacral and lumbar region. Because the compression and obliteration of the thecal sac occurs in a caudal-to-cranial direction, it indicates that there is a net cranial displacement of CSF (Video 40.4). It is important to note that the initial vertebral level that the injection reaches cannot be used as a measure of the final height that the block will reach, as hysteresis occurs as the compliance of the epidural and subarachnoid spaces comes to equilibrium. As this equilibration occurs, and CSF volume rebounds, driving the local anesthetic volume in the epidural space cephalad.[422] Thus, the final level at which the volume of injectate settles is somewhat higher that initially visualized.

Ultrasound guidance during a caudal epidural injection in children provides real-time images that are easy to interpret; and, unlike the nerve-stimulation technique, is not affected by the use of neuromuscular blocking drugs or epidural local anesthetics. Moreover, ultrasound can demonstrate the underlying caudal anatomy, which is useful in children with cutaneous markers of

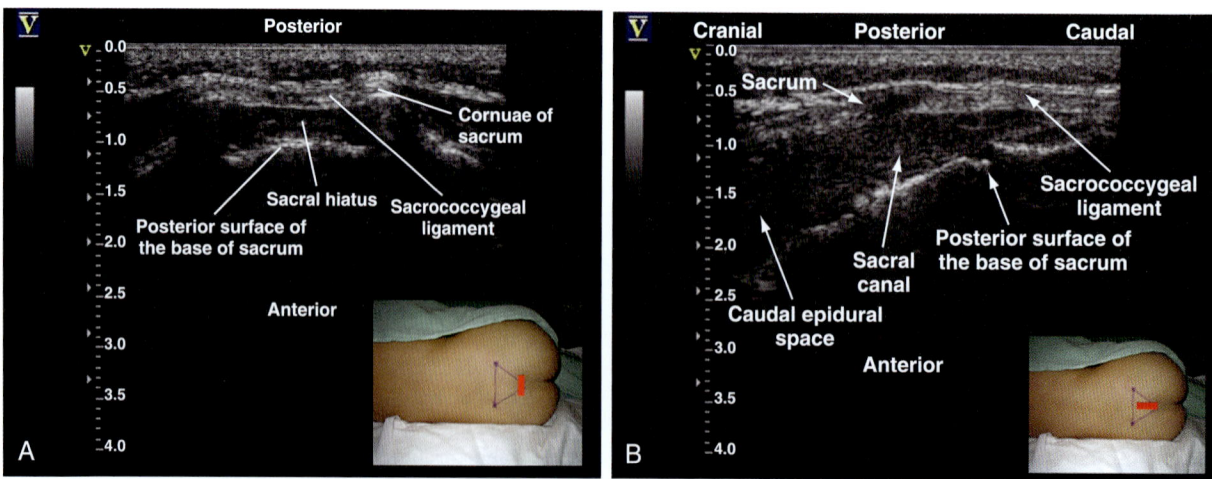

FIGURE 40.24 A, Transverse sonogram of the sacrum ("frog-eye sign"). **B,** Longitudinal sonogram of the sacrum. The red bar indicates the orientation of the ultrasound transducer.

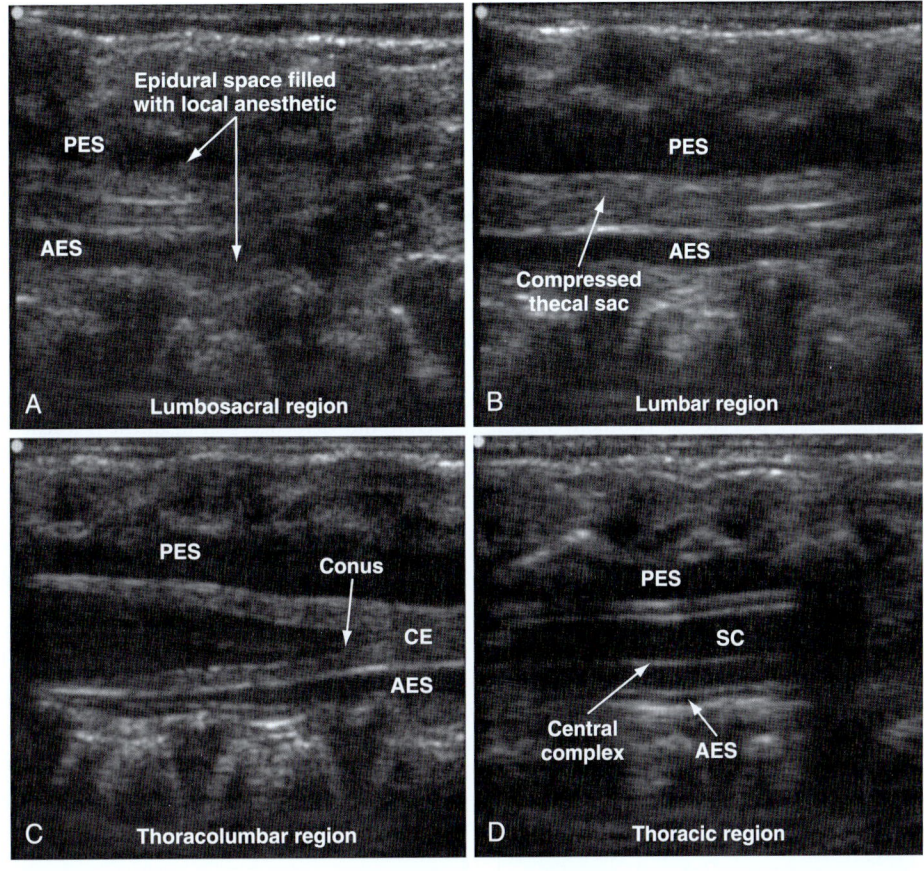

FIGURE 40.25 Longitudinal sonogram of the spine after a single-shot caudal epidural injection at the **A,** lumbosacral, **B,** lumbar, **C,** thoracolumbar, and **D,** thoracic levels. Note the displacement of the anterior and posterior dura, widening of the epidural space, and the compression of the thecal sac at the various levels. *AES,* Anterior epidural space; *CE,* cauda equina; *PES,* posterior epidural space; *SC,* spinal cord.

dysraphism when it can be used to screen the underlying spinal anatomy. Children who may have otherwise been excluded from a caudal block can benefit from its effects.

Ultrasonographic-Guided Epidural Catheterization
Compared with the traditional loss-of-resistance method, when epidural catheterization is performed using the loss-of-resistance method in conjunction with ultrasound guidance, fewer bony contacts occur during the procedure, and the time required for catheter placement is reduced.[423–425] The spread of local anesthetic in the epidural space can also be visualized in real time. In addition, the underlying anatomy and the depth from the skin to the ligamentum flavum, dura, and epidural space can be assessed before needle insertion. However, epidural catheterization under ultrasound guidance requires two anesthesiologists who are familiar with epidural anesthesia and spinal sonography in children. The first anesthesiologist performs the scan in the longitudinal paramedian axis and maintains a steady image while the second anesthesiologist performs the needle insertion through the midline. Entry of the needle into the epidural space is confirmed by the loss of resistance to saline solution and observing the local sonographic changes resulting from the saline solution injection (i.e., anterior displacement of the posterior dura, widening of the epidural space, and compression of the thecal sac). Ultrasound-guided epidural catheterization in young children should be undertaken only by those with adequate training and skill in ultrasound-guided regional anesthesia.

Landmark-Guided Lumbar and Thoracic Epidural Anesthesia
It may be preferable to place epidural catheters at a lumbar or thoracic interspace when the area of operation is innervated by higher dermatomes. Advantages include less risk of contamination by stool and urine, closer proximity to the desired tip location, and smaller volume of drug required for a more cephalad dermatomal level (if the caudal catheter is not threaded cephalad). Both lumbar and thoracic epidural catheters may be safely placed in anesthetized infants and children by experienced anesthesiologists.[426]

The technique for both lumbar and thoracic epidural catheter placement is similar to that in adults, with several important differences. The midline approach is most commonly used, for the same reasons cited earlier regarding subarachnoid block. The ligamenta flava are considerably thinner and less dense in infants than in older children and adults. This makes recognition of engagement in a ligament more difficult and requires both extra care and slower, more deliberate passage of the needle to avoid subarachnoid puncture. It takes experience to perceive the more subtle differences in "feel" that are characteristic of the tissue planes in small children. The angle of approach to the epidural space is slightly more perpendicular to the plane of the back than in older children and adults, owing to the orientation of the spinous processes in infants and small children. We believe the loss-of-resistance technique should be used with saline solution, not air. There are several reports of venous air embolism in infants and children when air was used to test for loss of resistance.[427–429] Some experts suggest putting a small air bubble (that is not injected) in the fluid to improve the feel of compression of the syringe. Another method used to identify the epidural space is to attach an IV infusion chamber with a minidrip or other free-flowing fluid delivery device to the epidural needle; commencement of dripping identifies entry into the epidural space.[424,430,431] We use a short (5-cm) 18-gauge Tuohy needle and a 20- or 21-gauge catheter in infants and children. The shorter length offers much better control than an adult-length (9- to 10-cm) needle. These catheters have fewer problems than the 24-gauge catheters, which are prone to kinking, resulting in very high resistance to injecting the solution. Epidural kits specifically for infants and children are available, but aside from the substitution of a shorter needle, they are identical to the adult sets.

The child is placed either in the lateral decubitus or prone position with a small roll beneath the anterior iliac crests. The cornua of the sacral hiatus are most easily palpated as two bony ridges, about 0.5 to 1.0 centimeter apart, when the examiner moves their finger in a medial-to-lateral direction (Fig. 40.26A). When the sacral cornua are not prominent or easily appreciated, it may prove easier to locate the space by palpating the L4–L5 intervertebral space in the midline and then palpate moving caudally until the sacral hiatus is reached. Because the space between the sacrum and coccyx may be mistaken for the sacral hiatus, the latter technique may make identification of the landmarks easier. The proper location is often, but not always, located just at the beginning of the

crease of the buttocks. A short-bevel styletted needle, 22-gauge, should be used because a long-bevel needle may increase the risk of intravascular injection.[415] Some practitioners believe that a styletted needle avoids the possibility of introducing a dermal plug into the caudal space, whereas others recommend puncturing the skin and subcutaneous tissues with an 18-gauge needle *a priori*, an IV catheter can be inserted without entraining dermis and displacing it to the subarachnoid space. Fears of translocating epidermal tissue to the caudal/epidural space with a hollow bore needle may be unfounded because an epidermal tumor has yet to be reported.[432,433]

For caudal blocks, the IV catheter is directed cephalad at a 45- to 75-degree angle to the skin until it "pops" through the sacrococcygeal ligament (Fig. 40.26B) into the caudal canal, which is contiguous with the epidural space. If bone is encountered before the sacrococcygeal ligament is reached, the needle should be withdrawn 1 to 2 millimeters, the angle with the skin decreased to approximately 30 degrees, and the needle again should be advanced in a cephalad direction until the sacrococcygeal ligament is pierced (Fig. 40.26C). As the needle is advanced slightly farther, bone (the anterior table of the sacrum) may be encountered. The needle should then be oriented parallel to the plane of the child's back before it is advanced, parallel to the plane of the child's back. The needle should then be advanced into the caudal epidural space with the needle advanced only a few millimeters. Advancing

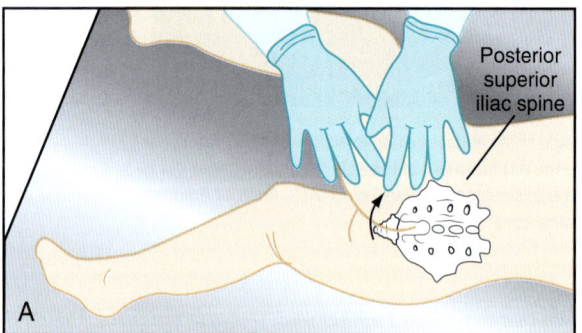

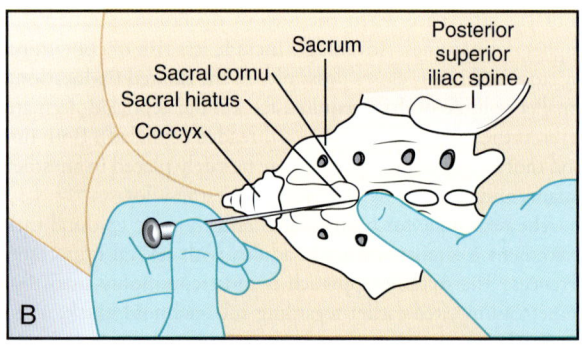

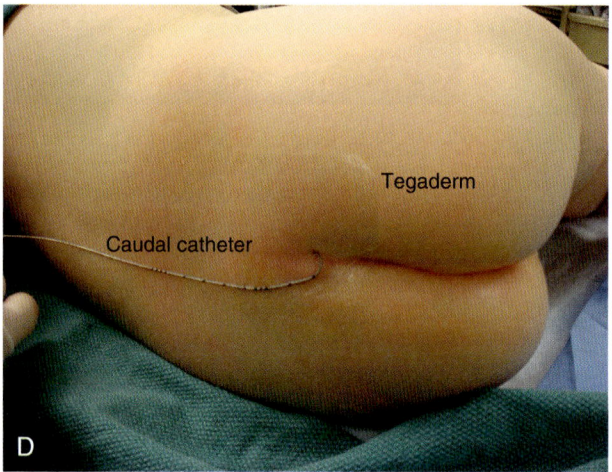

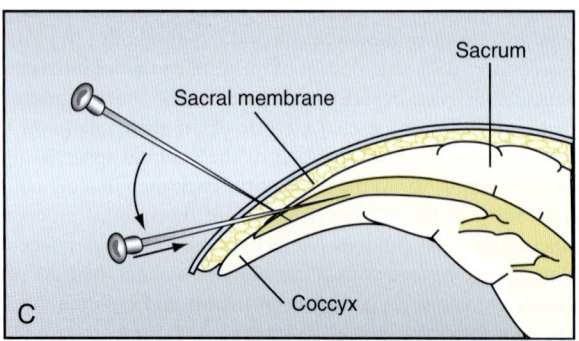

FIGURE 40.26 Performing a caudal block. **A,** The child is placed in a lateral decubitus position. **B,** The posterior superior iliac spines are located and the sacral cornu is palpated; an intravenous needle, an intravenous catheter, or a Crawford needle of appropriate size is advanced at an angle of approximately 45 degrees until a distinct "pop" is felt as the needle pierces the sacrococcygeal ligament. **C,** The angle of the needle with the skin is reduced parallel to the sacrum, and the needle or intravenous catheter is advanced into the caudal canal. **D,** If a continuous technique is used, the caudal catheter is advanced to the midlevel of the surgical incision (it usually readily passes in children younger than 5 years of age) and the introducing needle or catheter is withdrawn. The catheter is secured with benzoin and an occlusive dressing.

the needle any further should not be attempted because the dural sac lies relatively caudad in infants and may be entered at a very short distance from the ligament (Video 40.5).[291,434] It has been suggested that if an IV catheter is used for caudal blocks, the catheter should be advanced with the bevel facing down because sliding the IV catheter off the needle without resistance or buckling implies the catheter is within the caudal canal and not bone. Although advancing the cannula off the stylet smoothly and easily is not a completely reliable sign that the catheter is correctly placed, it is certainly unlikely to be within bone.

Once it is confirmed that neither blood nor CSF has been aspirated or flows passively back, a test dose of local anesthetic (1–2 mL in volume) is administered. If ECG changes are not evident after the test dose, the remainder of the dose of local anesthetic should be slowly injected in an incremental fashion over 1 to 2 minutes while observing the ECG for peaked T waves and changes in heart rate and/or blood pressure. We strongly recommend the use of a test dose, even with single-shot caudal anesthesia. In addition to the risk of intravascular injection, it is also possible that the needle could be misplaced in the intramedullary cavity of the sacrum. Intraosseous injection of drugs results in very rapid uptake, similar to direct IV injection. The authors are aware of at least one case of circulatory collapse that occurred from this complication when a test dose was not used.

The block may be placed before the onset of surgery without a significant decrement in duration of postoperative analgesia for short surgical procedures.[435] This has the advantage of reducing the amount of general anesthesia needed, resulting in a more rapid recovery. In addition, there is adequate time for the block to "set up," improving the chances of a pain-free awakening.

Inserting a catheter for a continuous caudal block follows a similar procedure (Video 40.6). First, one should determine the length of catheter that should be inserted into the caudal space by measuring the distance from the sacral hiatus to the desired site where the catheter tip will be positioned. Instead of a small-gauge needle or catheter, an 18-gauge IV catheter[436] or an 18-gauge Crawford needle is used to enter the epidural space (Fig. 40.26D). Because the internal diameters of IV cannulae vary, it is advisable to test that the epidural catheter easily passes through the IV catheter before puncturing the sacrococcygeal membrane. Once the epidural space has been accessed, the IV catheter and needle are advanced several millimeters. The catheter is then advanced off the needle several millimeters. Localization of the IV catheter tip in the epidural space is confirmed by lack of resistance to the injection of a small volume of saline solution and the absence of CSF or blood, or by ultrasound visualization of saline (see earlier). During injection, the area of the back overlying the IV catheter tip should be palpated; swelling or a fullness on injection of local anesthetic indicates a subcutaneous (SC) rather than an epidural catheter placement. The epidural catheter is advanced through the IV catheter and the IV catheter is withdrawn. After confirming the presence of neither blood nor CSF, a test dose of local anesthetic containing 1:200,000 epinephrine may be administered (see earlier). Test doses should be repeated each time a catheter is reinjected with a bolus dose of local anesthetic.

For those younger than 5 years of age, the catheter can often be advanced to any level desired without exiting a dural sleeve or becoming tangled or knotted, although catheter misplacements that were not suspected clinically have been identified using epidurograms.[35,437] It is prudent to use some method of localization when a catheter is threaded cephalad more than several centimeters. Epidurograms are easily performed when the catheter is placed; a small (0.5 to 2 mL maximum) volume of iopamidol is injected and imaged using fluoroscopy. A characteristic "bubbly" pattern in the midline is diagnostic of proper placement (Fig. 40.27). In addition to confirming placement in the epidural space and the location of the catheter tip, spread of the contrast may give a sense of how much volume is needed to cover the desired dermatomes. Besides epidurography, there are two other useful localizing techniques. The Tsui stimulating catheter, a catheter with an electrode at its uninsulated proximal end that is connected to a low-voltage nerve stimulator, produces motor twitches in the myotome at the catheter's tip.[231,438,439] One can mark the catheter's advance by watching the motor paresthesias move up the legs, abdomen, and thorax. For infants who weigh less than 5 kilograms, successful catheter advancement may be less reliable than in older children, and an epidurogram, ultrasound, or use of a stimulating catheter may be needed to confirm proper placement of the catheter tip if the catheter is not radiopaque.[440] An epidurogram can be useful in any situation in which the catheter is threaded or when there is concern for proper catheter position, although the routine use of an epidurogram is not standard practice. We usually strive to place the catheter tip at a level near or at the midpoint of the dermatomes encompassing the surgical incision. This position allows a more specific site of administration for both intraoperative anesthesia and continuous infusions for postoperative pain management, with the attendant advantage of being able to use reduced doses of medication. If the catheter does not pass easily to the desired level, it should

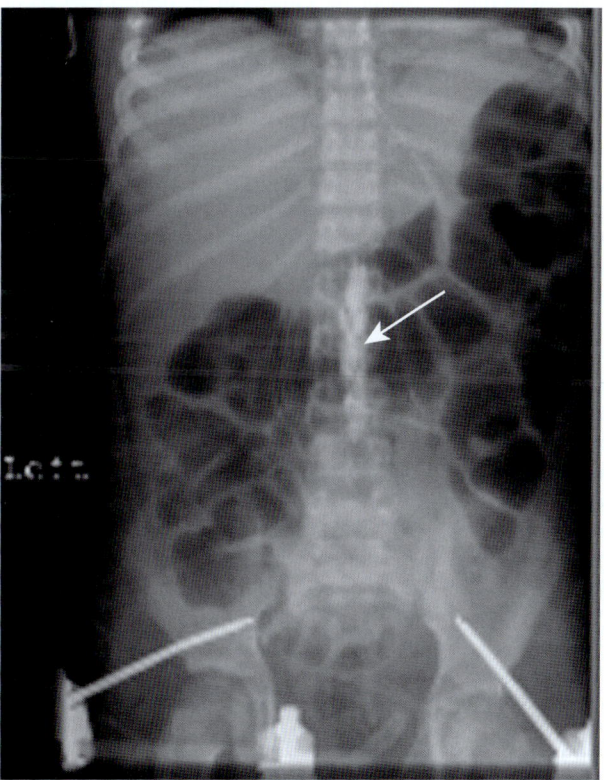

FIGURE 40.27 Epidurogram, performed with 0.5 to 2 milliliters (maximum) of iopamidol nonionic contrast agent, demonstrating the "bubbly" appearance of contrast in the epidural space *(arrow)*. Note the central localization of contrast within the borders bounded by the vertebral bodies. On occasion, contrast may be seen only on one side of the epidural space, with a sharp line of demarcation in the midline. This usually results in unilateral blockade, and is theorized to result from septation or some other impediment to bilateral spread of anesthetic within the epidural space.

be withdrawn several millimeters and a localizing technique used to ascertain its location. The catheter should never be forced or advanced against resistance.

Because caudal catheters are at greater risk of contamination from feces in infants and children who wear diapers or who are not yet toilet trained, meticulous attention to the dressing is necessary. Our practice is to apply Mastisol (Ferndale Pharma Group, Ferndale, MI) or tincture of benzoin to secure the catheter to the skin with several layers of an adherent clear dressing, such as Tegaderm (3M, St. Paul, MN) or OpSite (Smith & Nephew, Andover, MA), to affix the dressing in the crease of the buttocks (Video 40.7). With this transparent dressing, the insertion site can be clearly observed, which is essential because this is the most likely source of infection (see later). A piece of single adhesive-edged plastic drape (e.g., Steri-Drape 1010; 3M, St. Paul, MN) can be affixed just caudad to the lower edge of the dressing in a similar manner; this helps prevent direct soiling of the dressing. If there is any question of contamination, the catheter should be promptly removed.

In an observational study of 307 neonates with caudal or epidural catheters, catheter malfunction was the primary complication (4.8%).[441] The catheter was contaminated in 2.9% of infants requiring premature removal, which contributed to an overall complication rate of 13.3% (95% CI 9.8%–17.4%).

Assessment of Indwelling Epidural Catheters

For optimal epidural anesthesia or analgesia, the epidural catheter tip must be located in the correct dermatomal level. This is often achieved by directly placing the catheter in the desired level via the lumbar or thoracic route. Even with this approach, and in particular when loss of resistance is used to locate the epidural space, it is not possible to determine with certainty the exact location of the catheter tip. It is possible to use ultrasound to confirm the injection and cannula in the epidural space[442] and to visualize the catheter in the epidural space, although this technique may be technically difficult in children older than 6 months of age.[443,444] Epidurography can locate the catheter tip, but this exposes the child to radiation and the risk of anaphylaxis from the contrast medium (Fig. 40.27).[445,446] An epidural catheter inserted via the caudal route can be advanced to the lumbar or thoracic epidural space. However, this is technically difficult in children older than 1 year of age, and even in children younger than 6 months of age, the catheter can be misplaced in the sacral, lumbar, and even the cervical region. Greater success has been reported with styletted catheters.[447] Even if a catheter is successfully advanced to the thoracic epidural space, an x-ray can confirm the position of the catheter tip.[445,446] Electric nerve stimulation through an indwelling styletted epidural catheter and observation of myotomal contractions have been used to locate the position of the catheter tip.[438] In experienced hands this technique has a success rate of ~89%. However, this test cannot be performed if neuromuscular blocking drugs or local anesthetics have been administered. Epidural electrocardiography also can be used to locate the position of a thoracic epidural catheter and is not affected by the use of neuromuscular blocking drugs or local anesthetics in the epidural space.[448] This method relies on matching the evolving ECG recorded from the tip of a specially adapted epidural catheter, as it is advanced, to the surface ECG recorded at the target vertebral level. However, this method is not specific because even a subcutaneous electrocardiographic electrode at the same position relative to the heart will produce a similar electrocardiographic pattern.

Ultrasound has been used to directly visualize the position of epidural catheters in children (see Fig. 40.28).[444,449] Ultrasound localization noninvasively provides real-time images of the catheter during

placement. However, not all epidural catheters or their tips can be identified using ultrasound, and it may be limited by the acoustic window available for scanning in children of different ages. Gently jiggling the catheter and observing tissue movement within the epidural space also has been used to facilitate epidural catheter localization. Injecting saline solution with air bubbles may improve catheter localization using ultrasound, but the use of air in the injectate can lead to inadvertent air embolism or a patchy block.[450] A small volume of contrast material may be injected under x-ray guidance as well to localize the tip of the catheter. Therefore, it is suggested that observing surrogate markers such as the widening of the epidural space, dural displacement, and compression of the thecal sac, after a saline solution test injection, may be more accurate in locating the position of the tip of an epidural catheter in children (Video 40.8).

Selection of Drugs

The drug dose required for epidural blockade to reach a given dermatomal level depends on the volume (not the concentration) of the local anesthetic and the volume and capacitance of the epidural space, which changes with age. The greater the volume of local anesthetic, the more rostral the level of block achieved. In two studies, the height of the block achieved when local anesthetic was administered caudal epidurally varied inversely with age using ultrasound to detect the spread; for example, the maximum spinal level of local anesthetic in infants younger than 1 year of age was one to two levels more cephalad than in those older than 1 year.[421,442] This effect of age on the spread of local anesthetic, however, has been disputed.[421,451] Numerous studies investigated the doses of local anesthetic drugs used for caudal anesthesia in children.[396,398–400,402,403,405–411,421,451] The volumes of local anesthetic reported to block from a T4 to a T10 dermatome level span a 5-fold range. In our experience, the volume of local anesthetic required is 0.05 mL/kg per dermatome to be blocked.[403] However, it is important to note that there are wide variations in dosing that have been used. An analysis from the PRAN found that such variability does not appear to be based on experimentally confirmed evidence, but rather on institutional custom or tradition.[143] Thus, in a 10-kilogram child in whom we wish to produce a T10 dermatome level, we would use a volume of (0.05 mL/kg per dermatome) × (10 kg) × (12 dermatomes) = 6 mL.

Another simple method is to administer 1 mL/kg (up to 20 mL) of local anesthetic (usually 0.125% bupivacaine with

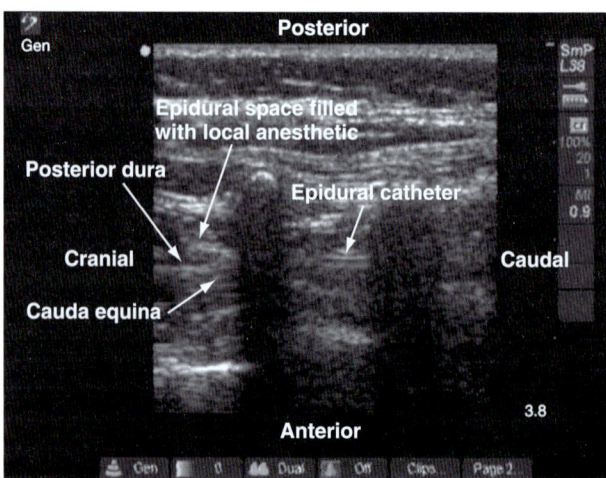

FIGURE 40.28 Longitudinal paramedian sonogram of the lumbar spine demonstrating an indwelling epidural catheter.

1:200,000 epinephrine). This generally provides a sensory block with minimal motor block up to the T4–6 level; this volume limits the potential for toxicity for children older than 6 months of age and is on the border for younger infants. If repeated doses are anticipated, or in infants younger than 6 months of age, it is prudent to reduce the concentration or volume to avoid the risk of drug accumulation and development of drug toxicity.

A third simple regimen for a caudal block used in the United Kingdom and Australasia is that of Armitage[410]: 0.5 mL/kg for lumbosacral, 1 mL/kg for thoracolumbar, and 1.25 mL/kg for midthoracic. If the total volume is less than 20 mL, then use bupivacaine 0.25%. If the volume exceeds 20 mL, then use bupivacaine 0.125%.

Because the level of the block depends on the volume of drug administered, the concentration of the local anesthetic should be based on the desired density of the block (less dense for postoperative analgesia, more dense for intraoperative anesthesia) and on the risk of toxicity.

Continuous Epidural Infusions

Although intermittent doses of local anesthetic are often used to maintain epidural anesthesia during a prolonged surgical procedure, it is also common practice to initiate continuous infusions of local anesthetics during surgery. Continuous infusions maintain the block at a constant level, assuming that the infusion rate is appropriate. This obviates the need for repetitive test dosing. Theoretically, fewer entries into the epidural catheter may reduce the risk of infection and the risk of accidental administration of the wrong drug. Strict attention to the total drug administered per hour (i.e., the drug concentration and infusion rate) is required to preclude potentially toxic drug doses. We recommend that the same dosing guidelines for postoperative infusion rates be followed intraoperatively: *a maximum of 0.4 mg/kg per hour of bupivacaine after the initial block is established, with this dose reduced by approximately 30% for infants younger than 6 months of age.*[56] The concentration of local anesthetic solution depends on the age of the child, the surgical procedure, and the extent of the area that needs to be blocked. When a denser block is required in a small infant, it may be beneficial to use 2,3-chloroprocaine because its action is terminated by ester hydrolysis and has a minimal risk of accumulation compared with amide local anesthetics. A denser block with a more concentrated solution may then be achieved. The amides ropivacaine and levobupivacaine, because they are levorotary enantiomers and carry reduced risks of toxicity, may also successfully address the toxicity issues, and allow the administration of more concentrated agents to produce denser blockade with less potential for adverse effects. In a study of children 1 to 9 years of age, infusion rates of up to 0.4 mg/kg per hour of ropivacaine that followed a 2-mg/kg bolus were found to result in stable concentrations of unbound ropivacaine in plasma, all well below the toxic threshold; clearance did not differ with age.[452]

Epidural Opioids

Epidural opioids can be safely used to augment intraoperative anesthesia in children, as well as to provide postoperative analgesia. Their use is discussed in detail in Chapter 41. If extubation of the trachea is expected at the end of the surgical procedure, one must account for both the systemic and the central neuraxial opioid doses to avoid excessive respiratory depression.

Adjunctive Drugs

Numerous non-opioid agents have been injected into the epidural space in attempts to prolong analgesia, to improve the quality of analgesia while reducing the dose of opioid and local anesthetic, or to replace the local anesthetic or opioid with a drug that may have fewer adverse effects. It is concerning, however, that several of these agents have neither undergone exhaustive neurotoxicity testing nor are prepared or labeled for neuraxial use.[453] In the United States, the only adjunctive drug accepted for epidural administration is clonidine, an α_2-adrenoceptor agonist. The effect of clonidine to prolong the duration of epidural analgesia remains controversial. Several studies, including a meta-analysis, reported clonidine prolonged the duration of analgesia by 2 hours, as measured by the time to first supplemental analgesic.[453–457] In contrast, other investigators found no increase in the duration of analgesia, including one double-blind, randomized trial.[458,459] In neonates, neuraxial clonidine at doses of 2 µg/kg or greater has been associated with apnea.[460] Increased sedation has been reported after epidural clonidine in older infants and children at the same doses. We recommend limiting the dose of neuraxial clonidine to 1 µg/kg, especially in ambulatory patients.

Complications

Complications after epidural anesthesia or analgesia include cardiac arrest from an intravascular or intraosseous injection, hematoma, neural injury, and infection. E-Fig. 40.6 illustrates sites of unintended needle placement during the performance of a caudal epidural block. Injection of local anesthetic into an epidural blood vessel or intraosseous injection into the marrow cavity may result in a rapid increase in the blood concentration of the local anesthetic and a toxic reaction as discussed previously. It is also possible to pass the needle through the sacrum and perforate bowel or the pelvic organs, particularly in infants in whom ossification of the sacrum is incomplete.

Several large-scale prospective audits have examined the incidence and nature of complications in regional anesthetics in children. The prospective audit from the United Kingdom and Ireland is the largest and most carefully described study on complications of epidural anesthesia in pediatrics to date.[461] A total of 10,633 cases were accrued over a period of 5 years, and all complications were reviewed and categorized by severity and type. Only five complications were graded as serious, and of these only one, the result of a drug error, had lasting sequelae. The French-Language Society of Pediatric Anesthesiologists (ADARPEF) published a follow-up prospective study on regional anesthetics in children in which they reported on 10,098 epidural blocks without a single child sustaining permanent sequelae.[462] The PRAN consortium in the United States reported data from their first prospective cohort in which 9073 epidural and caudal blocks were accrued: 6127 single-injection (mostly caudal) and 2946 continuous caudal or epidural anesthesia events.[15] In this study there were no complications of any kind that lasted more than 3 months. The most common complication was catheter displacement or malfunction in the postoperative period in continuous blocks. Caudal safety was further supported in a subsequent PRAN analysis of 18,650 single-injection caudal epidurals, which detected an overall incidence of complications of 1.9% (95% CI 1.7%–2.1%) and no instances of temporary or permanent sequelae, calculated as 0.005% (95% CI 0% to 0.03%).[416]

Infection is of grave concern when it occurs in either the subarachnoid or the epidural space.[463,464] A study of 1620 children over a 6-year period reported a zero frequency of epidural abscess.[465] Catheters remained in situ for a mean of 2 days (maximum 8 days). The adult literature also suggests that infection is an uncommon complication.[466,467] However, both superficial and deep abscesses may rarely occur, particularly in those children with immunodeficiency syndromes or cancer who are receiving long-term infusions.[468] Epidural abscess and meningitis are the most potentially serious complications.[463,469] The development of an epidural abscess is a surgical emergency because failure to treat it promptly can lead to a permanent neurologic injury. The signs and symptoms (Table 40.8) are the same as those for epidural hematomas, although fever, increased erythrocyte sedimentation rate, and increased leukocyte count with a leftward shift are also often present. Surgical drainage may be necessary. In a British audit, three serious infections (two epidural abscesses and one case of meningitis) were noted. These infections were all related to infections at the insertion site. All cultures grew *Staphylococcus aureus*. Twenty-five local infections were reported, mostly *S. aureus*, and 80% were associated with catheters left in place more than 48 hours. Of note is that some localized infections that developed at the catheter insertion site only became apparent several days after the catheter had been removed. Similar findings were reported in the PRAN study. In the British report, one case progressed to an epidural abscess. Whether these infections developed while the catheter was in place, leaving bacteria to track through the open site in the skin after the catheter was removed, or by hematologic spread is unknown, although the former etiology is most frequently cited. Infants and toddlers who are in diapers require meticulous management of these catheters and their insertion site. A mild erythema occasionally occurs at the site of catheter insertion when children have indwelling catheters in place for several days, and this must be distinguished from a cellulitis (see Fig. 41.9). In most cases these superficial infections resolve with removal of the catheter and local care. On occasion, these superficial infections may require treatment with a systemic antibiotic. If there is any question that the site is infected, the catheter should be removed. Although no serious systemic infection occurred in a prospective study of 210 children with 170 caudal catheters (age 3 ± 1 years) and 40 lumbar epidural catheters (age 11 ± 3 years) that were in place for 3 ± 1 days, 35% were colonized with

bacteria.[470] This rate of colonization was similar with both caudal (25%) and lumbar epidural (23%) approaches. These results suggest that colonization is not synonymous with infection and that caudal catheters are not necessarily associated with greater infectious risk than lumbar epidural catheters. The factors that transform colonization into infection remain unknown. An MRI examination seems to provide the best method for assessment.[471]

It is common to have a small amount of epidural fluid leak at the insertion site of caudal epidural catheters, especially in the presence of presacral edema. If an indwelling caudal epidural catheter is in place when a child develops a fever of unknown origin, the catheter should be removed because it may be causing the infection or become seeded by the infection (see Chapter 41).

Epidural hematoma is also a rare complication after epidural blockade. Optimal outcome depends on rapid diagnosis and prompt treatment and decompression. Signs and symptoms are presented in Table 40.8. The presence of clinically important coagulopathy or thrombocytopenia is an unacceptable risk for developing an epidural hematoma and is a contraindication to central neuraxial blockade. Guidelines for the conduct of neural blockade in the anticoagulated patient have been published by the ASRA.[472,473] Of particular note is that there is a difference in the management of the patient who is receiving conventional (unfractionated) heparin and low–molecular-weight heparins, such as enoxaparin. Guidelines for the management of patients who are anticoagulated are shown in Table 40.9.[472]

Postoperatively, *urinary retention* has been associated with the presence of both epidural and spinal anesthesia. In this regard, it is important to distinguish between the effects of local anesthetics and central neuraxial opioids in the blocks. There is scant evidence that neuraxial anesthesia with local anesthetics alone causes urinary retention, and, indeed, there are data to the contrary. In a prospective study of infants and children undergoing inguinal herniorrhaphy or orchiopexy, caudal blockade, ilioinguinal-iliohypogastric nerve block by the surgeon, or a control consisting of caudal injection of 1:200,000 epinephrine (no local anesthetic) yielded similar times to voiding postoperatively.[474] In a retrospective study of 326 children undergoing inguinal herniorrhaphy and urologic surgery, 237 received a caudal block and 66 received local anesthesia by the surgeon. The incidence of urinary retention was similar for the two groups, with the type of surgery being the primary determinant of urinary retention.[475]

The epidural and subarachnoid use of opioids, however, is associated with an increased incidence of urinary retention. Epidural morphine in a dose of 70 μg/kg (a dose that would now be considered excessive) was associated with a 50% incidence of urinary retention[476]; 70% of those with urinary retention required treatment. Another study reported an incidence of urinary retention of 27% after caudally administered morphine, 33 to 100 μg/kg, although most of the children had urinary catheters.[477] Finally, 50 μg/kg diacetylmorphine was associated with an 11% incidence of urinary retention.[478] A dose of 33 μg/kg epidural morphine is most commonly recommended in current practice.

Data from the large prospective databases indicate that the incidence of *neural injury* after epidural blockade is very small and that long-term neurologic sequelae of neuraxial blockade is rare. One must slightly temper these conclusions, however, based on the limited follow-up of children in these studies who did not have problems reported within the immediate time frame of the block. A prospective study of more than 2500 infants and children who received epidural blocks demonstrated no evidence of neurologic complications, although a retrospective review of the

TABLE 40.8	Signs and Symptoms of Epidural Hematoma and Abscess
Abscess	**Hematoma**
Fever	Afebrile
± Increased WBC	WBC normal
± Increased sedimentation rate	Sedimentation rate normal or slightly increased
± Left WBC shift	
Localized back pain	Localized back pain
Radicular pain	Radicular pain
Paraplegia	Paraplegia
Sensory loss	Sensory loss
Urinary and fecal retention	Urinary and fecal retention
Incontinence	Incontinence
Local tenderness	Local tenderness
Defect on myelography	Defect on myelography
Localized lesion on magnetic resonance imaging	Localized lesion on magnetic resonance imaging

WBC, White blood cell count.

TABLE 40.9	Guidelines for the Use of Regional Anesthesia in the Anticoagulated Patient			
Drug (Generic)	Common Trade Names	Interval for Catheter Placement After Last Dose	Interval for Catheter Removal After Most Recent Dose	Time Interval to Restart Anticoagulant After Catheter Is Removed
Enoxaparin[a] (therapeutic)	Lovenox (>60 mg daily or 1 mg/kg BID or 1.5 mg/kg daily)	24 hours	Catheter should be removed before first dose. If medication given, wait >24 hours	2–4 hours after catheter removed
Enoxaparin[a] (prophylactic)	Lovenox (≤60 mg per day)	12 hours	12 hours	2–4 hours
Heparin SC BID	Heparin	No significant risk at dose of 5000 units BID		
Heparin SC tid	Heparin	Unknown risk at 5000 units tid: suggest check PTT. 10,000 units tid: check PTT		
Heparin IV	Heparin	2–4 hours, PTT <35 seconds	2–4 hours, PTT <35 seconds	2 hours
NSAID, ASA	Celebrex, Motrin, Naprosyn, and so on	No significant risk		
Streptokinase	Streptase	10 days	10 days	Uncertain; at least 24 hours
Warfarin	Coumadin	3–5 days, INR ≤1.5	If >24 hours, check INR ≤1.5	Same day

[a]Note for low–molecular-weight heparin: Prophylactic dosing may be started 6 to 8 hours postoperatively. Therapeutic dosing or BID dosing should be started at least 24 hours postoperatively. Epidural catheters should be removed before initiation of therapy.
ASA, Acetylsalicylic acid; INR, international normalized ratio; IV, intravenous; NSAID, nonsteroidal antiinflammatory drug; PTT, partial thromboplastin time; SC, subcutaneous.
Modified from the guidelines of the Massachusetts General Hospital Department of Anesthesia, Critical Care and Pain Medicine, 2011.

first ADARPEF data determined that 1 in 5000 infants younger than 3 months of age had neurologic complications with MRI evidence of spinal cord ischemia.[134,479] In four of the five cases reported in that study, the epidural space was identified using loss of resistance to air (in the fifth case, the technique was not specified) and the authors concluded that the etiology of the neurologic injury was an air embolus. Based on these data, the use of air for loss of resistance in infants and children has been strongly discouraged, using saline solution instead. However, this reasoning has been questioned. The use of loss of resistance to saline solution with an air bubble has been advocated by some experts.[171] In the follow-up ADARPEF study there were no cases of neurologic injury.[462] The British epidural audit found six cases of neural injury in 10,633 (1:1770) children in that prospective study. Of particular note was the delay in recognition of the injury, as no cases were discovered before 2 days had elapsed from the time the block was placed, and some diagnoses were not made for 10 days after the block. All children had complete resolution of their symptoms within 1 year. Two children were referred to a chronic pain service and treated with gabapentin, and one child developed a common peroneal nerve injury that was attributed to malpositioning of the leg during surgery. In our experience, one child who developed symptoms of complex regional pain syndrome after common peroneal nerve injury from positioning in the postoperative period sustained persistent motor block, which emphasizes (1) the importance of early recognition of motor blockade as a potential for injury after surgery and (2) the critical importance of positioning and nursing care in preventing pressure injuries. There were no cases of persistent neurologic injury in the PRAN data cohort. In young rabbits , decreased spinal cord blood flow was detected using colored microspheres coincident with a

fall in blood pressure during lidocaine epidural anesthesia.[480] The addition of epinephrine to the local anesthetic solution did not increase the incidence of ischemia. These studies suggest that it may be particularly important to take care positioning the patient, maintaining adequate systemic blood flow during "combined technique" anesthesia in infants and children, and treating hypotension promptly. Because blood pressure changes caused by neuraxial blockade are uncommon in infants and small children, hypotension in these patients is most likely to be due to other causes and should prompt an assessment of intravascular filling pressures, inotropic state, and the depth of general anesthesia.

PERIPHERAL NERVE BLOCKS

Peripheral nerve blocks are useful adjuvants to general anesthesia. These blocks are also useful as a means for providing postoperative pain relief. Peripheral nerve blocks differ from central neuraxial blocks in several respects:

- A targeted area is anesthetized.
- Adverse effects, such as weakness of extremities, are minimal.
- The dose of local anesthetic is reduced.
- There is no risk of an unintended spinal anesthetic.
- There is no risk of urinary retention.
- Peripheral blocks can be used in areas where a central neuraxial block is not possible (e.g., face and scalp).

There are many peripheral nerve blocks that can be used in the practice of pediatric anesthesia and many are described in the following text (Table 40.10).

Selection of a Local Anesthetic

Local anesthetics commonly used for peripheral blocks in children include lidocaine, mepivacaine, bupivacaine, levobupivacaine, and

TABLE 40.10	Peripheral Nerve Blocks
Head and Neck	
Supraorbital and supratrochlear nerves	
Infraorbital nerve	
Greater occipital nerve	
Great auricular nerve	
Chest Wall	
Intercostal nerve	
Upper Extremity	
Brachial plexus	
Elbow blocks (ulnar, radial, and median nerves)	
Wrist blocks (ulnar, radial, and median nerves)	
Digital	
Abdomen and Genitalia	
Ilioinguinal nerve	
Penile	
Rectus sheath	
Lower extremity	
Femoral nerve	
Lateral femoral cutaneous nerve	
Fascia iliaca	
Sciatic nerve	
Classic approach	
Lateral approach (popliteal fossa)	
Ankle	
Digital nerves	

TABLE 40.11	Suggested Dosing for Local Anesthetic Volumes for Common Peripheral Nerve Blocks	
Technique		**Dose (mL/kg)**
Head and neck blocks		0.05
Brachial plexus blocks		0.2–0.3
Ilioinguinal nerve block		0.075
Rectus sheath block		0.1
Femoral nerve block		0.2–0.3
Sciatic nerve block		0.2–0.3
Digital nerve block		0.05

ropivacaine.[85,88,481] Long acting agents such as ropivacaine or bupivacaine are especially preferable when the block is placed at the beginning of surgery so that its full effect is in place and persists after emergence. Lidocaine can be combined with bupivacaine to provide both a rapid onset and a long duration of action, although evidence for the efficacy of this practice is mostly anecdotal. If this is done, one must be careful to calculate the doses of the two drugs properly to avoid toxicity. Alternatively, the addition of sodium bicarbonate (1 mEq of bicarbonate/10 mL of local anesthetic [lidocaine]) can speed the onset and reduce the pain of injection of the block by increasing the pH of the solution.[482–485] This alters the pK_a of the solution, increasing the active cationic form of the local anesthetic in the solution.[486] Bicarbonate should be added to the local anesthetic solution immediately before administration because precipitation of the local anesthetic and therefore loss of bioavailability increases over time (it should be administered within 10 minutes after alkalinization).[487] This is particularly a problem with mepivacaine, bupivacaine, and ropivacaine in which the addition of 0.1 mL of 8.4% bicarbonate precipitates the anesthetic within 10 minutes.[486,487] The total drug dose administered should not exceed the recommended maximum recommended dose per kilogram (see Table 40.2). The addition of epinephrine (1 : 200,000) may decrease both the vascular absorption and the potential for toxicity; for some local anesthetics the addition of epinephrine will also extend the duration of the block. The exact dose of local anesthetic in terms of volume or concentration needed for most peripheral blocks in children has not been adequately studied. Similar to

caudal block dosing, a prospective observational study from the PRAN of local anesthetic dosing in pediatric peripheral blocks found very high degrees of dosing variability that was mostly related to the institution where the block was performed. Such variability is largely unwanted, as it is based on local custom, not on evidence, and may pose a risk of either suboptimal block efficacy (too little drug) or to local anesthetic systemic toxicity (too much).[144] Most blocks performed in children are based on adult experience. Suggested dosing for common peripheral blocks based on volume per kilogram and our experience is presented in Table 40.11, although these doses are usually reduced with ultrasound guidance.

HEAD AND NECK BLOCKS

Peripheral nerve blocks for postoperative pain relief for the head and neck can be performed with the child under general anesthesia.[488] These blocks can also be used for the provision of pain relief in children with chronic painful problems, such as headaches. Anatomically, two major nerves, the ophthalmic division (V_1) of the trigeminal nerve and the branches of the cervical root C2, supply the sensory innervations of the face and scalp (Fig. 40.29). These blocks do not generally require ultrasound guidance.[489]

Supraorbital and Supratrochlear Nerve Block
Anatomy
The supraorbital and supratrochlear are the end branches of the ophthalmic division (V_1) of the trigeminal nerve. The supraorbital nerve, the terminal branch of V_1, exits the supraorbital foramen to supply the scalp anterior to the coronal suture. The supratrochlear nerve exits the orbit between the trochlea and the supraorbital foramen and innervates the lower part of the forehead (Fig. 40.30A). We use this combined block to provide pain relief in children undergoing frontal craniotomies[490] and in children undergoing frontal ventriculoperitoneal shunt revisions. The technique can be used as the sole anesthetic in very sick neonates,[491] and to both avoid opioids and control postoperative pain in children undergoing excision of scalp lesions.[492]

Technique
With the child supine and the head in the neutral position, the supraorbital notch is palpated by running a finger from the midline laterally along the eyebrow (the supraorbital notch is usually located in line with the pupil with the eye in midline position). The skin is prepared with povidone-iodine or chlorhexidine, taking care to avoid spilling chlorhexidine into the eye as corneal damage is possible.[493] A 27-gauge needle is inserted in the proximity of the supraorbital notch; 0.5 to 1.0 milliliter of bupivacaine (0.25% with epinephrine 1 : 200,000) is injected into the space after careful

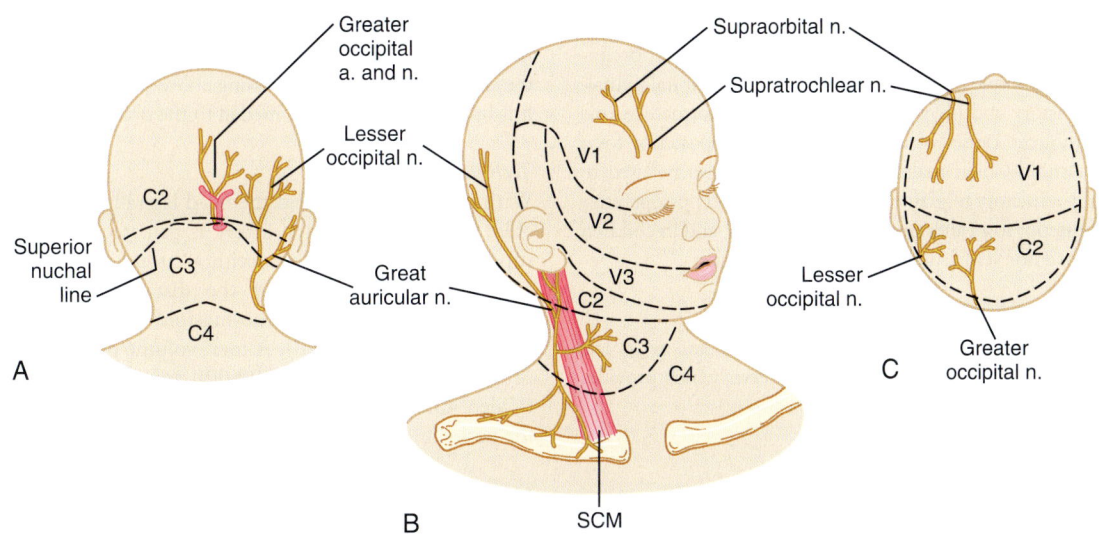

FIGURE 40.29 Dermatomal innervation of head and neck. Sensory and dermatomal innervation of greater and lesser occipital nerves and the innervation of the anterior head by the first division of the trigeminal nerve. Note the sensory innervation anterior to the coronal suture is from the first division of the trigeminal nerve (supraorbital and supratrochlear nerves) and posterior to the coronal suture is from branches of C2 (greater and lesser occipital nerves). These nerves can be blocked individually and in combination to provide postoperative analgesia for a wide variety of procedures; see text for details. **A,** Posterior view. **B,** Anterolateral view. **C,** Axial view. *a.,* Artery; *C2, C3, C4,* cervical sensory branches of the nerve roots; *n.,* nerve; *SCM,* sternocleidomastoid muscle; *V₁, V₂, V₃,* branches of the trigeminal nerve.   (Modified from Brown DL, Wong GY. Occipital nerve block. In: Waldman S, Winnie AP, eds. *Interventional Pain Management.* Philadelphia: WB Saunders; 1996:227.)

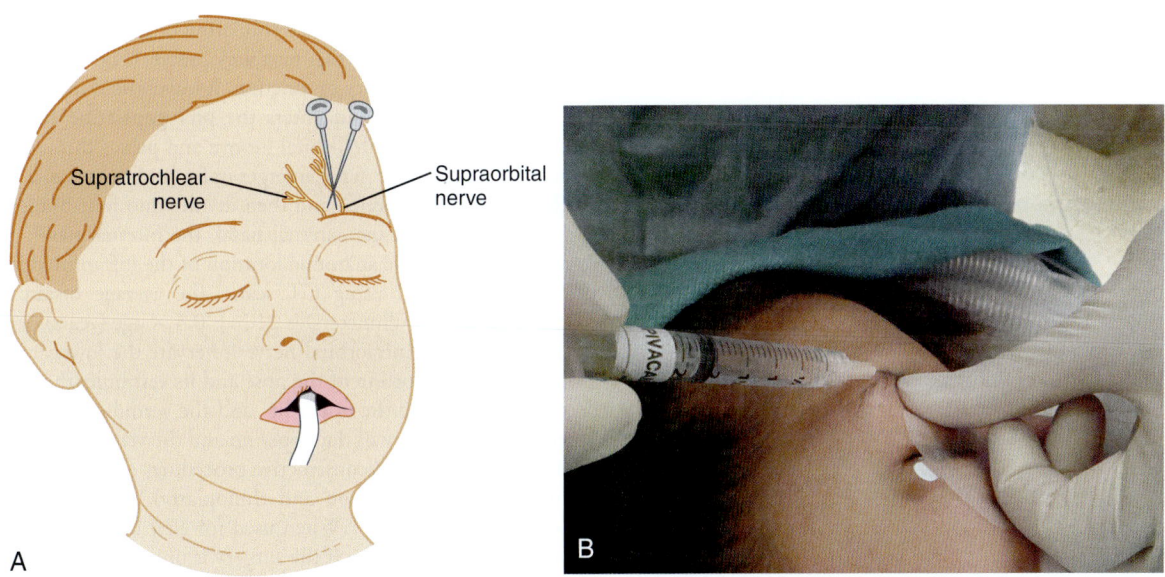

FIGURE 40.30 A, Supraorbital and supratrochlear nerve block. The supraorbital notch is palpated by running a finger from the midline laterally along the eyebrow. **B,** A 27-gauge needle is inserted into the supraorbital notch perpendicularly; bupivacaine (1 mL, 0.25% with 1:200,000 epinephrine) is injected into the space after careful aspiration. To block the supratrochlear nerve, the needle is withdrawn to skin level and then directed medially several millimeters toward the apex of the nose; bupivacaine (1 mL, 0.25% with 1:200,000 epinephrine) is injected. This block provides postoperative pain relief for children undergoing frontal craniotomies or frontal ventriculoperitoneal shunt insertion.

aspiration to prevent intravascular placement (Fig. 40.30B). To block the supratrochlear nerve, the needle is withdrawn to the skin level and then directed and advanced several millimeters medially toward the apex of the nose; 0.5 to 1.0 milliliters of bupivacaine (0.25% with epinephrine 1:200,000) is injected (Video 40.9).

Complications

Because of the loose adventitious tissue of the eyelid, gentle pressure should be applied to the supraorbital area; this prevents local anesthetic from dissecting into the eyelid and supraorbital tissue and may reduce the potential for ecchymosis and/or hematoma.

Greater Occipital Nerve Block

The greater occipital nerve block is used to diagnose and treat occipital pain. If this technique is used for the diagnosis of occipital neuralgia, a careful history and physical examination is performed to rule out other pathologic causes of headaches, including posterior fossa tumors and Arnold-Chiari malformation.[494] It can also be used to treat medically refractory migraine headaches[495–497] and postoperative pain in the posterior fossa after posterior fossa surgery, and in children undergoing posterior ventriculoperitoneal shunt revisions.[498]

Anatomy

The cervical spinal nerves innervate the posterior head and neck. The dorsal rami of C2 end in the greater occipital nerve, which provides the cutaneous innervation to the major portion of the posterior scalp (Fig. 40.31A). The nerve becomes subcutaneous slightly inferior to the superior nuchal line by passing above the aponeurotic sling; here it is in close proximity and medial to the occipital artery.

Technique

With the child supine and the head laterally rotated or with the child prone, the occipital artery is palpated at the level of the superior nuchal line. The occipital artery is usually located at approximately one-third of the distance from the external occipital protuberance to the mastoid process on the superior nuchal line (Fig. 40.31B). A total volume of 2 milliliters of bupivacaine (0.25% with 1:200,000 epinephrine) is injected SC (Video 40.10). Ultrasound guidance has been used in children for performing occipital nerve blocks.[499]

Complications

It is rare to see complications with this block because of the superficial location of the nerve. One must bear in mind the close proximity to the spinal canal, particularly in children who have had surgery in the area. Thus, the needle must remain just beneath the skin during injection of local anesthetic. It is more difficult to perform this block at the C2 nerve root without the aid of either ultrasonography or fluoroscopy and hence it cannot cover the entire distribution of the greater occipital nerve. Intravascular injection may be avoided with incremental injection and frequent aspiration.

Infraorbital Nerve Block

Anatomy

The infraorbital nerve is the termination of the second division of the trigeminal nerve, the maxillary nerve (Fig. 40.32A). This nerve is entirely sensory in function. It leaves the skull through the foramen rotundum and enters the pterygopalatine fossa. From there it enters the infraorbital groove and passes through the infraorbital canal. The nerve emerges in front of the maxilla through the infraorbital foramen and then divides into four branches: the inferior palpebral, the external nasal, the internal nasal, and the superior labial. The anatomic location of the infraorbital foramen has been studied using CT scans: the average distance from the midline (in millimeters) is $21.3 + 0.5 \times$ age (years).[500,501] The branches of the infraorbital nerve innervate the lower eyelid, the lateral inferior portion of the nose and its vestibule, the upper lip, the mucosa along the upper lip, and the vermilion. This block is effective for surgery of the upper lip and the vermilion after a cleft lip repair,[502,503] for reconstructive procedures on the nose (including septal reconstruction and rhinoplasty),[504,505] and for endoscopic sinus surgery.[506] When used for cleft lip repair, both sides should be blocked even if the surgery is unilateral because there is almost always some dissection across the midline. There are two approaches to the infraorbital nerve: intraoral and extraoral.

Intraoral Approach

The intraoral approach is our preferred method for this block. The infraorbital foramen is located by palpation of the infraorbital notch. After folding back the upper lip, a 27-gauge needle is inserted through the buccal mucosa approximately parallel to the maxillary second molar and passed SC with the tip of the needle directed toward the infraorbital foramen. It is important to place a finger over the infraorbital foramen so as to palpate the progress of the needle beneath the skin and prevent unintended passage of the needle into the orbit. With the tip of the needle at the level of the infraorbital foramen and after careful aspiration, 0.5 to 1.0 milliliters of local anesthetic is injected (Fig. 40.32B and Video 40.11).

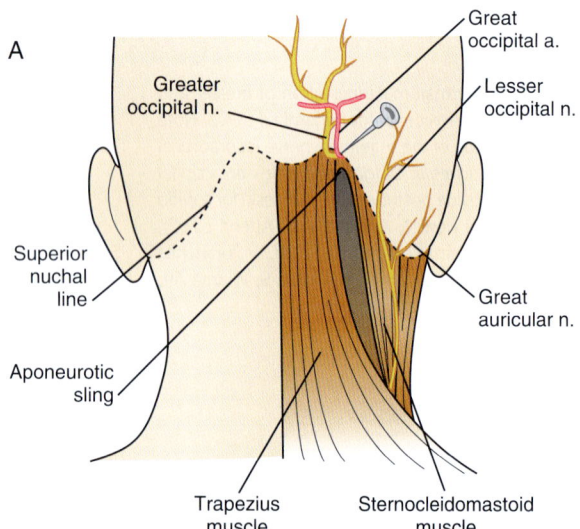

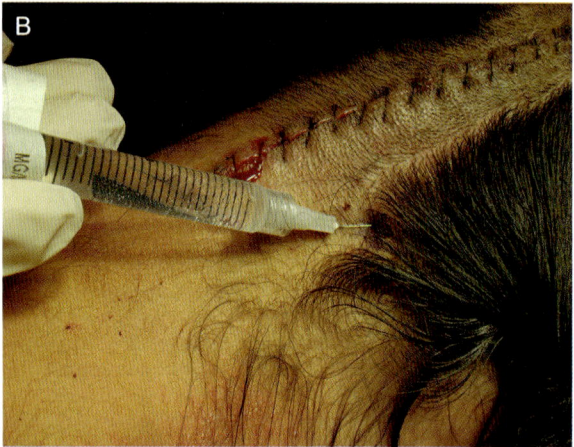

FIGURE 40.31 **A,** Greater occipital nerve and site of block. **B,** With the patient supine and with the head turned to one side or with the patient prone, the occipital artery is palpated at the level of the superior nuchal line. The occipital artery is located about one-third of the distance from the external occipital protuberance (dashed line, part **A**) to the mastoid process on the superior nuchal line. A total volume of 2 mL of bupivacaine (0.25% with 1:200,000 epinephrine) is injected subcutaneously to form a skin wheal. Frequent aspiration and incremental injection may avoid intravascular injection. This block is used to diagnose occipital neuralgia and as a means for providing postoperative pain relief for children undergoing posterior fossa tumor resection or posterior ventriculoperitoneal shunt insertion. a., Artery; n., nerve. (Modified from Brown DL, Wong GY. Occipital nerve block. In: Waldman S, Winnie AP, eds. Interventional Pain Management. Philadelphia: WB Saunders; 1996:228.)

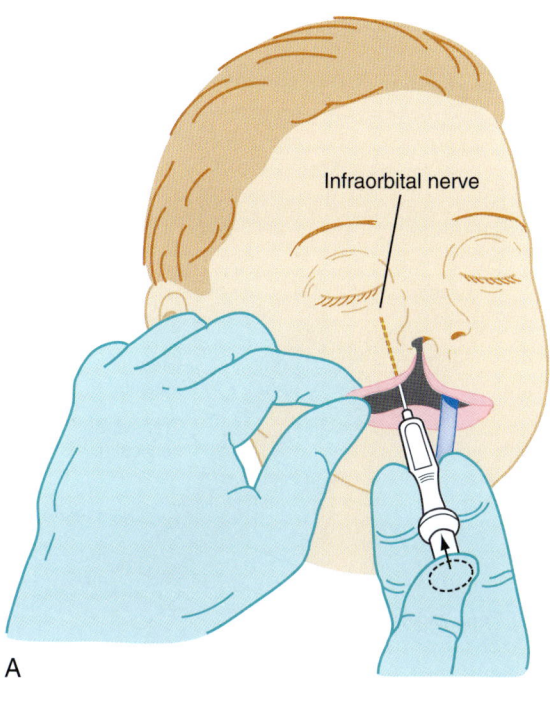

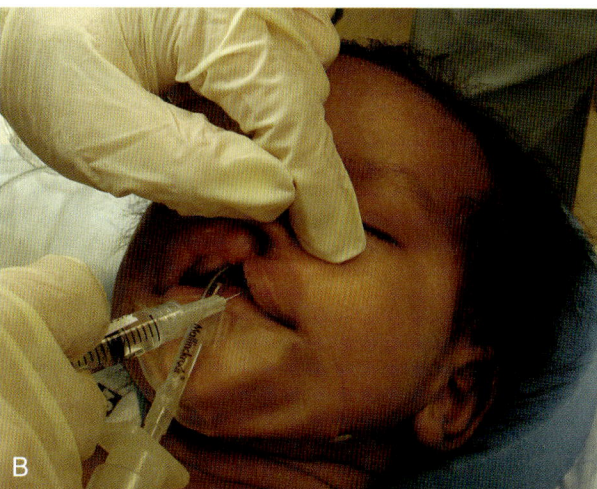

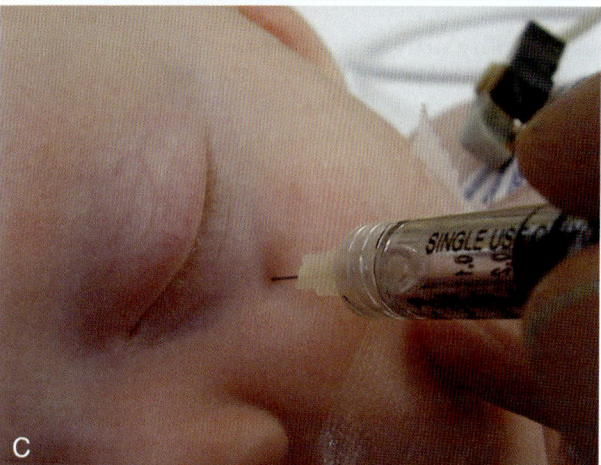

FIGURE 40.32 A, Infraorbital block (intraoral approach): The infraorbital foramen is located by palpation of the infraorbital notch (right-sided block). **B,** The lip is folded back and a 27-gauge needle is inserted through the buccal mucosa approximately parallel to the maxillary second molar. The tip of the needle is directed toward the infraorbital foramen. A finger is placed over the infraorbital foramen to track the progress of the needle tip and to avoid accidental placement of the needle into the orbit. After careful aspiration to avoid intravascular injection, 0.5 to 1.0 mL of bupivacaine (0.25% with 1:200,000 epinephrine) is injected (left-sided block). **C,** For the extraoral approach (left-sided block) the infraorbital ridge of the maxillary bone should be identified and the infraorbital foramen is palpated. A 27-gauge needle is advanced toward the foramen at a 45-degree angle to the maxilla (midpupillary point). After careful aspiration, 0.5 to 1.0 mL of bupivacaine (0.25% with epinephrine 1:200,000) is injected. This block is used to provide postoperative pain relief for children undergoing upper lip or cleft lip repair, reconstructive procedures of the nose (e.g., rhinoplasty), and endoscopic sinus surgery.

Bupivacaine (0.25% with epinephrine 1:200,000) provides prolonged postoperative analgesia with this block.

Extraoral Approach
The infraorbital ridge of the maxillary bone should be identified and the infraorbital foramen palpated. A 27-gauge needle is advanced toward the foramen at a 45-degree angle to the maxilla (Fig. 40.32C). After careful aspiration, 0.5 to 1.0 milliliters of bupivacaine (0.25% with epinephrine 1:200,000) is injected. We recommend *not* attempting to enter the foramen with the needle out of concern for injuring the nerve itself in a tightly confined space. Ultrasound may be used to assist with this block.[507]

Complications
Because of the loose adventitious tissue of the eyelid, children can develop ecchymosis and swelling. Pressure should be applied to the infraorbital area to retain the solution within the infraorbital foramen, prevent dissection of the local anesthetic into the periorbital area, and reduce the potential for the formation of a hematoma or ecchymosis. Care should be taken to avoid direct injection into the orbit or eye. Intravascular injection may be avoided with incremental injection and frequent aspiration. This block can be achieved with low volumes in infants and toddlers; hence every attempt should be made to decrease the volume of the local anesthetic solution. Using other additives, including clonidine, may be helpful, although there are no randomized controlled trials to demonstrate the improved efficacy of this block using additives.

Suprazygomatic Approach to the Maxillary Nerve
The suprazygomatic approach to the maxillary division of the maxillary nerve provides analgesia for cleft palate,[508–510] cleft lip, and endoscopic sinus surgery.[511,512] The nerve is located in close proximity to the maxillary artery in the infraorbital location between the ethmoid and the zygomatic arch.

Technique

This nerve can be blocked by palpating the zygomatic arch, and inserting a needle above the superior edge of the zygomatic arch and posterior to the lateral rim of the orbit in an inferior medial direction for about 2 centimeters to reach the greater sphenoid wing using ultrasound guidance.[508,513] After hitting bone, the needle is withdrawn slightly and reoriented toward the nasolabial fold in an ~20-degree forward and ~10-degree inferior direction and advanced 3 to 4 centimeters toward the pterygopalatine fossa. Before injecting local anesthetic, aspirate to preclude an intravascular injection. Bupivacaine 0.25% or ropivacaine 0.2% in a volume of 0.15 mL/kg bilaterally is effective in reducing postoperative pain with a duration of block of ~12 hours[513]; if dexmedetomidine (0.5 µg/kg) is added to the injection, the duration of the block may be extended by an additional 60% to ~24 hours.[514] Ultrasound further confirms appropriate spread of the local anesthetic.[514]

Complications

With the maxillary artery located close to the nerve, it is imperative to aspirate before injection of local anesthetic to ensure that it is not intravascular. The block will render the upper lip numb, so caution should be exercised to ensure that the child does not bite their upper lip and disrupt the surgical site or cause bleeding.

Great Auricular Nerve Block

The great auricular nerve supplies the sensory innervation to the mastoid area and the external ear. It is a branch of the superficial cervical plexus. Cervical plexus blocks were first performed by Halstead in 1884. This block has been used to provide postoperative analgesia in children undergoing otoplasty repair,[515] as well as in tympanomastoid surgery.[516] We found that the great auricular nerve block decreases the incidence of nausea and vomiting, which is a major morbidity associated with tympanomastoid surgery.[516] It provides surface analgesia but not muscle relaxation and hence can be used for intraoperative analgesia despite the need for facial nerve monitoring in children undergoing tympanomastoid procedures.

Anatomy

The cervical plexus is formed by the anterior primary division of the anterior and posterior roots of cervical nerves C2–4. The great auricular nerve is derived from C3, which was described by McKinney. The anatomic location of the nerve for blockade has been described as the McKinney point.[517] The great auricular nerve wraps around the belly of the sternocleidomastoid muscle at the level of the cricoid cartilage and emerges to supply the area of the mastoid and external ear (Fig. 40.33A).

Technique

With the child under general anesthesia, the cricoid cartilage is identified. A line is drawn from the superior margin of the cricoid cartilage laterally to the posterior border of the sternocleidomastoid muscle (McKinney point). Bupivacaine (2–3 mL, 0.25% with epinephrine 1:200,000) is injected superficially at this point (Fig. 40.33B and Video 40.12).

Complications

Deep rather than superficial injection can result in a deep cervical plexus block and the risk of Horner syndrome, phrenic nerve block, or unintended central neuraxial blockade. A small erythematous area may be seen at the site of the needle injection.

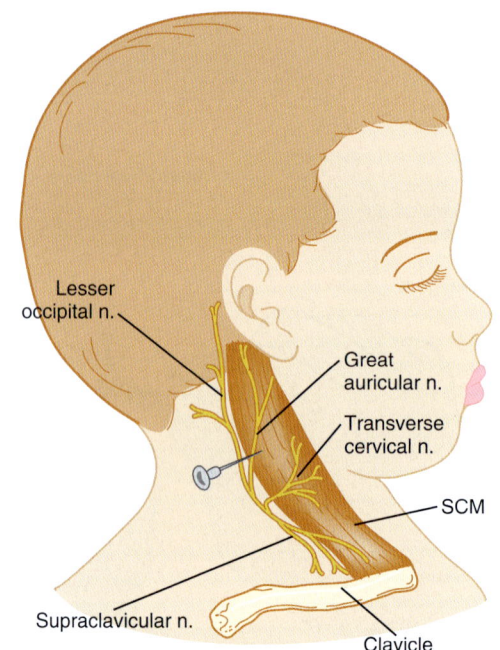

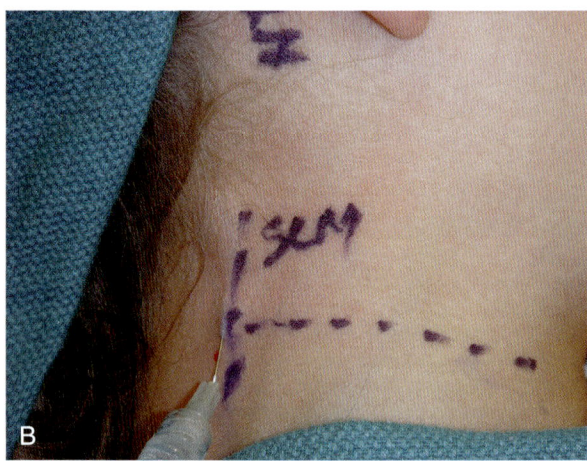

FIGURE 40.33 A, Great auricular nerve block. The cricoid cartilage is identified. **B,** A broken line drawn from the superior border of the cricoid cartilage laterally to the posterior border of the sternocleidomastoid *(SCM)* (McKinney point) is identified; bupivacaine (2–3 mL, 0.25% with 1:200,000 epinephrine) is injected subcutaneously at this point. Gentle massage after the injection allows spread of the local anesthetic in the injected site. This block is used to provide postoperative analgesia for children undergoing tympanomastoid surgery or otoplasty. *n.*, Nerve. (Modified from Brown DL, ed. *Atlas of Regional Anesthesia.* Philadelphia: WB Saunders; 1999:185.)

Intravascular injection may be avoided by incremental injection of the solution and frequent aspiration.

Nerve of Arnold (Auricular Branch of Vagus)

The auricular branch of the vagus supplies the sensory nerve that supplies the innervation to the auditory canal, as well as the inferior portion of the tympanic membrane. This is useful for providing analgesia to the tympanic membrane after myringotomy and tube placement, as well as for tympanoplasty surgery. In a randomized controlled trial, intranasal fentanyl and blockade of the auricular branch of the vagus provided equivalent analgesia without adverse effects.[518]

Indications

This block is used to provide analgesia for myringotomy and tube placement, and for tympanoplasty.

Technique

After induction of anesthesia, and with the child turned to one side, the tragus is cleaned and reflected laterally, a 30-gauge needle is inserted into the tragus to pierce the cartilage; after aspiration, 0.2 milliliters of local anesthetic solution is injected (Video 40.13). Mild pressure is applied to prevent any bleeding following the procedure.

Complications

It is rare to see complications, although occasionally there can be some brisk bleeding from the needle entry site, which can be off-set by applying pressure.

TRUNCAL BLOCKS

Truncal blocks are performed in children for a variety of different surgical procedures. The most common blocks include intercostal blocks,[58] ilioinguinal blocks, penile blocks, rectus sheath blocks, and paravertebral blocks. Also included in this category are fascial plane blocks, in which local anesthetic is injected into the con-fined space bound by layers of fascia through which nerves course, rather than targeting a specific nerve. These blocks are particularly useful in providing analgesia of small nerves or collections of nerves that may be difficult or impossible to visualize without ul-trasound, but where ultrasound imaging can easily identify the target tissue plane itself. More recently introduced blocks of this type include erector spinae blocks, quadratus lumborum blocks and pectointercostal plane blocks. These blocks are far more reli-able when placed using ultrasound guidance; landmark-guided approaches carry an increased risk of needle misplacement in the wrong tissue plane.

Intercostal Nerve Block

Intercostal blocks after thoracotomy are useful in reducing opioid requirements, optimizing respiratory mechanics, and encouraging early ambulation.[58,519,520] Their major disadvantage is the limited duration of analgesia. Currently, we more commonly use epidural blockade or various fascial plane blocks for this purpose. There are, however, still situations in which intercostal blocks are useful, par-ticularly when analgesic needs are of relatively short duration.[521,522] Cryoablation, a technique where a probe cooled to -50 to $-70\,°C$ is applied by the surgeon to intercostal nerves, has also proven to be an alternative effective and durable analgesic modality for thora-cotomy but is beyond the scope of this chapter.[523]

The uptake of local anesthetic after intercostal blocks is the most rapid of all sites of regional anesthesia, yielding the greatest plasma concentrations of local anesthetics when compared with any other regional block. Furthermore, plasma concentrations in children increase more rapidly than after identical blocks in adults.[524] For this reason, epinephrine ($1:200,000$) should always be added to reduce the absorption of local anesthetic. We com-monly use 1 to 5 milliliters of 0.25% bupivacaine with epineph-rine to block each intercostal nerve, depending on the size of the child and the number of ribs to be blocked. A maximum of 2 mg/kg of bupivacaine is used, although this amount should be reduced by about 30% for infants younger than 6 months of age. The con-centration of bupivacaine should be decreased to provide adequate volume for the desired number of intercostal blocks while avoiding the risk of systemic toxicity.

Anatomy

The intercostal nerves are derived from the ventral rami of the first through the twelfth thoracic nerves. There are four branches. The first branch is the gray rami communicans, which goes to the sympathetic ganglion. The second branch arises as the posterior cutaneous branch, which supplies the skin in the paravertebral area. The third branch, the lateral cutaneous branch, arises ante-rior to the midaxillary line and sends subcutaneous branches both anteriorly and posteriorly. The final branch provides cutaneous innervation to the midline of the chest and abdomen. The dura mater and the arachnoid membrane fuse with the epineurium as they exit the vertebral foramen. This could lead to subarachnoid block if the posterior paravertebral approach is used.

Ultrasound-Guided Intercostal Nerve Block

A simple approach to the intercostal nerve is using ultrasound guidance. The advantage of ultrasound guidance is clearly the avoidance of the pleura. In addition, presence of lung sliding and B-lines on M-mode ultrasound is assurance that a pneumothorax was not created during performance of the block. While imaging, the innermost and inner intercostal muscle can be identified and injection of 0.5 to 2 milliliters of local anesthetic can provide ad-equate analgesia.

Landmark-Guided Intercoastal Nerve Block

The site of injection may be either paravertebral or in the midaxil-lary line. The lower rib margin is located, and the skin is retracted cephalad (Fig. 40.34A). The needle is inserted perpendicular to the skin over the rib and advanced until the rib is encountered (Fig. 40.34B). The skin through which the needle is passed is al-lowed to retract caudally, and the needle is then walked off the lower edge of the rib for a distance of 2 to 3 millimeters (Fig. 40.34C). This method may reduce the potential for pneu-mothorax because the needle strikes the rib and is not advanced more than half of the thickness of the rib. A distinct pop may be felt as the needle enters the neurovascular sheath. After negative aspiration for blood, an appropriate volume of anesthetic is in-jected. With the use of ultrasound guidance, we can avoid punc-turing the pleura because it can be adequately visualized while performing the block (E-Fig. 40.7).

Complications

Pneumothorax has been reported after intercostal blockade, with an incidence of approximately 0.07% in adults.[525] However, the majority of the blocks in that study were performed by residents in training. If a small pneumothorax occurs, reabsorption is fa-cilitated with the use of oxygen. Placement of a chest tube is indi-cated only if breathing is compromised. A more important com-plication is the toxic effect of absorbed local anesthetic drugs. Using smaller volumes of more dilute local anesthetic may reduce the risk of achieving toxic plasma concentrations. The risk of in-travascular injection may be reduced with incremental injection and frequent aspiration. A third complication is a high subarach-noid block, usually associated with the posterior paravertebral approach.

Inguinal Block (Ilioinguinal and Iliohypogastric Nerves)

Inguinal block, supplemented by wound infiltration, is sometimes used in adult patients undergoing inguinal hernia repair. However, in children, an inguinal nerve block is used almost exclusively as an adjunct to general anesthesia and to provide analgesia after ingui-nal hernia repair, orchidopexy, or hydrocele surgery, and it offers

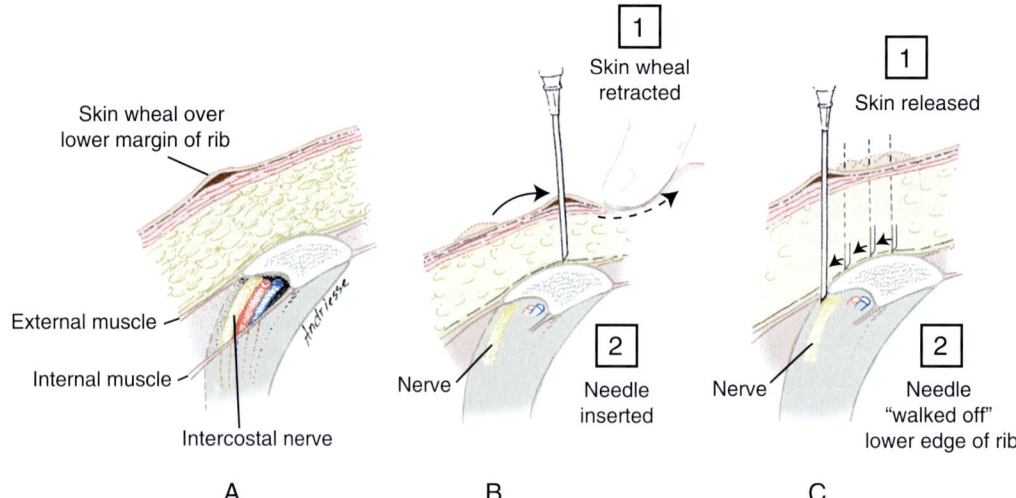

FIGURE 40.34 Intercostal block. **A,** A skin wheal is inserted on the lower rib margin. **B,** The skin wheal is retracted over the body of the rib, and a needle is inserted until contact is made with the rib. **C,** The skin is released, and the needle is carefully "walked" off the edge of the rib margin. After negative aspiration for blood, the appropriate volume of drug is injected. This block is used for postoperative analgesia for thoracotomy or chest tube insertion (see also E-Fig. 40.7).

the advantage of not affecting micturition after surgery, making it ideal for an outpatient procedure. This block is as effective as caudal anesthesia for inguinal repairs.[526,527] Blockade of the ilioinguinal and iliohypogastric has few associated complications, although injection into the femoral vessels and potential femoral nerve block are possible adverse outcomes.[528,529] The risks of toxicity from excessive drug doses may be greater than previously recognized, but ultrasound guidance has demonstrated adequate analgesia with reduced doses of local anesthetic solution because the drug is placed in the optimal location.[235] This block may be (and commonly is) performed in conjunction with infiltration of the wound; pain relief has been shown to be superior with a nerve block rather than simple wound infiltration.[530,531] The use of ultrasound may also avoid the risk of bowel perforation.[532,533]

Anatomy
The inguinal area is innervated by the subcostal nerve (T12) and the iliohypogastric and ilioinguinal nerves (L1) which lie in close proximity to each other medial and superior to the anterior superior iliac spine (ASIS) (Fig. 40.35). After piercing the internal oblique 2 to 3 centimeters medial to the anterior superior iliac spine, the nerve then lies between the internal oblique and the external oblique aponeurosis. Here it accompanies the spermatic cord (in males) to the genital area. The *iliohypogastric nerve* is situated superior to the ilioinguinal nerve. It continues inferomedially for a short distance, then the ventral rami traverse the internal oblique muscle to lie between the internal and external oblique muscles, before giving off branches that pierce the external oblique muscle to provide cutaneous sensation to the skin over the inguinal region. The *ilioinguinal nerve* continues anteroinferiorly with the spermatic cord or the round ligament in the inguinal canal and becomes superficial by emerging through the superficial inguinal ring to innervate the skin of the upper medial aspect of the thigh and either the skin of the upper part of the scrotum and the root of the penis or the skin covering the labia majora and mons pubis.

Ultrasound-Guided Ilioinguinal/Iliohypogastric Nerve Block
When anatomic landmarks and tactile sensations are relied upon to perform this block, failure may be seen in up to 20% to 30% of cases. Ultrasound-guided ilioinguinal/iliohypogastric nerve block has been compared with the traditional landmark-based method; an ultrasound ilioinguinal/iliohypogastric nerve block is more accurate, uses smaller volumes of local anesthetic, and has a greater success rate.[235] One study demonstrated more prolonged analgesia with caudal blocks compared with ultrasound-guided nerve blocks,[534] whereas another found the reverse.[535,536] A systematic review found a reduced incidence of complications with ultrasound-guided blocks compared with landmark-guided blocks.[537]

A linear-array transducer (13-10 MHz) is used for imaging the ilioinguinal and iliohypogastric nerves, which are best visualized close to the ASIS.[235,538,539] The operator stands on the ipsilateral side to be blocked, and the ultrasound machine is positioned directly opposite on the contralateral side. The transducer is positioned close to the ASIS and parallel to a line joining the ASIS and the umbilicus (Fig. 40.36). The ilioinguinal and iliohypogastric nerves are identified as two small, rounded structures lying side by side between the internal oblique and transversus abdominis muscle (see Fig. 40.36). The external oblique is frequently identified only as a hyperechoic aponeurotic layer at the point of needle insertion. Deep to the transversus abdominis muscle, the peritoneum and the bowel are also visualized (see Fig. 40.36).

The block needle is inserted in the long axis (in-plane) of the ultrasound beam in a medial-to-lateral direction (Fig. 40.37). We prefer this orientation because it facilitates visualization of the needle (in-plane) and, in the event that the needle is inadvertently inserted too deep, further passage is obstructed by the iliac bone, thus reducing the potential for a major complication such as bowel perforation.[533] When the tip of the needle is close to the two nerves, a test injection is performed with 0.5 to 1 milliliters. Correct position of the needle tip is confirmed by observing the widening of the tissue plane between the internal oblique and

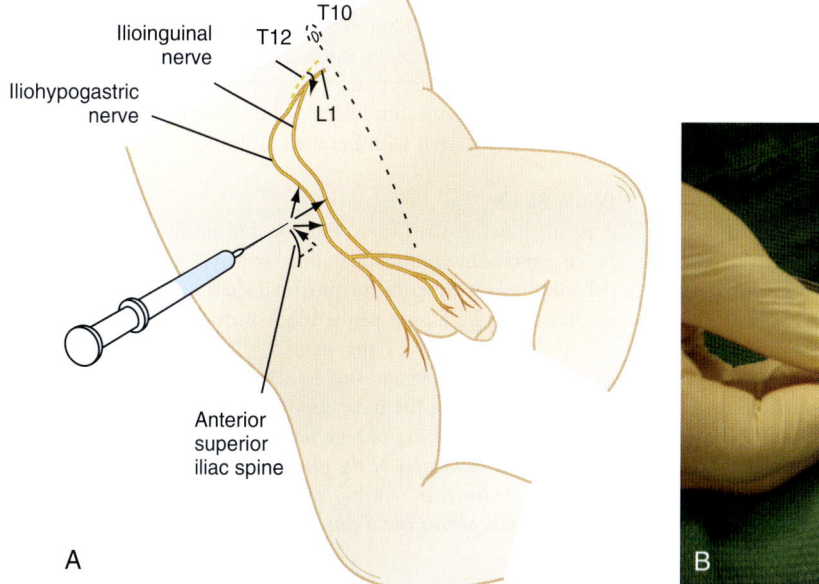

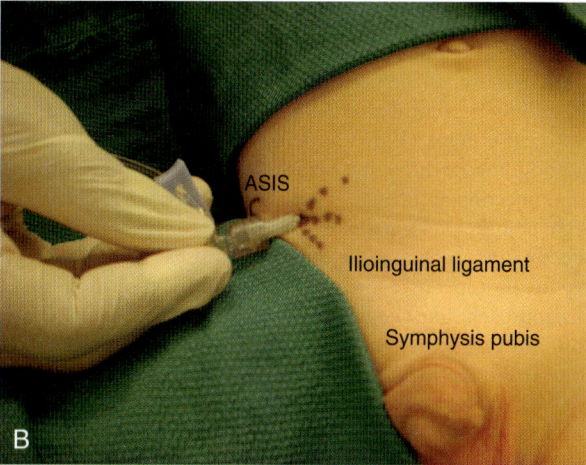

FIGURE 40.35 Ilioinguinal and iliohypogastric nerve blocks. **A** and **B,** The anterior superior iliac spine *(ASIS)* is palpated, and a point 1.0 to 1.5 cm cephalad and toward the midline is located *(dashed line)*. A 22-gauge needle is passed through the external and internal oblique muscles, and 1.0 to 5.0 mL of local anesthetic is deposited in a fan-like fashion cephalad toward the umbilicus, medially, and caudad toward the groin *(solid arrows)*. Just before removal from the skin, another 0.5 to 1.0 mL of local anesthetic is injected subcutaneously to block the iliohypogastric nerve. Blockade of these nerves provides postoperative analgesia for inguinal hernia and orchidopexy procedures.

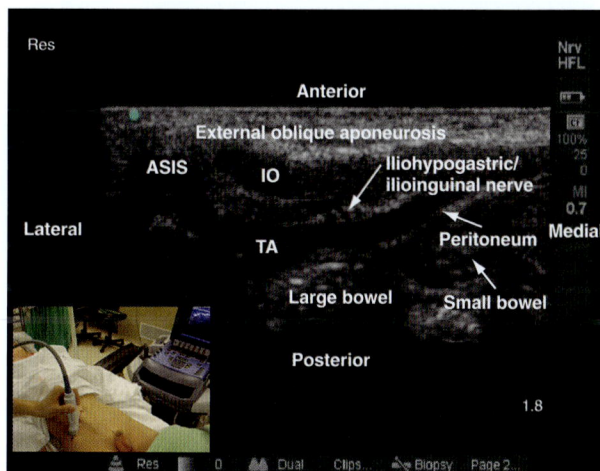

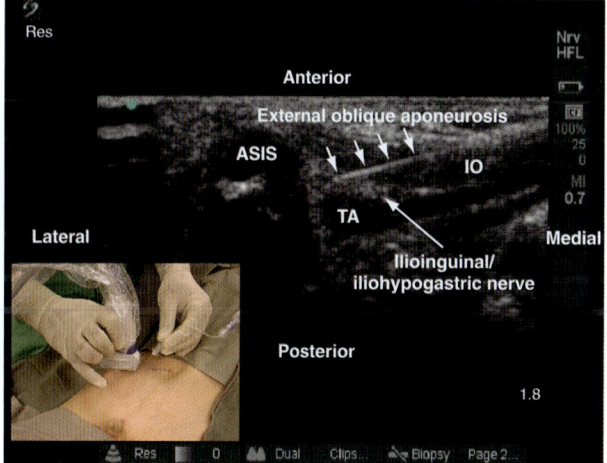

FIGURE 40.36 Transverse sonogram of the inguinal region showing the ilioinguinal and iliohypogastric nerves and its relation to the abdominal musculature. *ASIS,* Anterior superior iliac spine; *IO,* internal oblique; *TA,* transversus abdominis.

FIGURE 40.37 Ilioinguinal-iliohypogastric nerve block. The in-plane needle insertion technique. *ASIS,* Anterior superior iliac spine; *IO,* internal oblique; *TA,* transversus abdominis

transversus abdominis muscles. A calculated dose of a long-acting local anesthetic (e.g., 0.4 mL/kg) is then injected and the spread of local anesthetic to both nerves visualized (Video 40.14).

Landmark-Guided Technique

The block may be performed either at the beginning of surgery or before the end of general anesthesia. If bupivacaine is used, a minimum of 15 minutes is usually required from the completion of the block until maximal analgesia is obtained. Thus, blocks placed at the beginning of the surgical procedure (or at least 15–30 minutes before the patient awakens) may provide

superior postoperative analgesia than those performed at the end of surgery. Blocks performed before skin incision may also provide "preemptive analgesia," although the evidence for this is still under debate and somewhat conflicting.[540–543] The duration of postoperative analgesia is minimally affected by the timing of placing the block at the beginning of the procedure, assuming that the surgical procedure takes less than 1 hour. A short-bevel 27-gauge needle is inserted at a 45-degree angle at a point one-quarter of the way toward the midline along a line drawn from the ASIS to the umbilicus (1.0–1.5 cm cephalad and toward the midline from the anterior superior iliac spine in a 10- to 15-kg child). As the needle is advanced through the external and internal oblique muscles (see Fig. 40.35B), two pops are elicited and provide useful guides of proper needle placement. Negative aspiration should be confirmed several times during the incremental injection of local anesthetic. A volume of 0.3 mL/kg of local anesthetic solution is injected in a fan-like fashion, cephalad toward the umbilicus, caudad toward the groin, and medially. Before removal of the needle from the skin, an additional 0.5 to 1.0 milliliters of local anesthetic is injected SC to block the iliohypogastric nerve (Video 40.15). Care must be taken to avoid entering the peritoneum, which has been reported after the blind injection approach.[532] For inguinal herniorrhaphy, orchiopexy, or other inguinal procedures, local anesthetic deposited directly into the wound before it is closed has also proved effective for postoperative analgesia.[527] The volume of drug used by this approach, like the volume of drug used for wound infiltration, must be accounted for when calculating the maximal dose of local anesthetic that can be used. It is important to note that this block will not provide pain relief for scrotal procedures because this area is supplied by the genitofemoral nerve; hence it is important to have the surgeon infiltrate the scrotum for complete pain relief after orchiopexy or any other scrotal procedures. As mentioned earlier, an ultrasound-guided technique may be easier to perform and is associated with fewer complications (E-Fig. 40.8).[235]

Complications

Complications are rare but needle injury can lead to issues such as partial femoral nerve block causing leg weakness,[528] pelvic hematoma, and bowel perforation.[533] Care should be taken not to enter the peritoneal cavity. Intravascular injection may be avoided by incremental injection with frequent aspiration.

Penile Block

A penile block is used for anesthesia and postoperative analgesia for circumcision, urethral dilatation, and hypospadias repair. Caudal anesthesia is superior for proximal shaft or penoscrotal hypospadias repair because a penile block provides analgesia only for the distal two-thirds of the penis.[407,544,545] The block is easily performed with very good success. Bupivacaine, levobupivacaine, and ropivacaine are the most useful agents because of their prolonged duration of action. *Epinephrine is avoided for this block because the dorsal artery of the penis is an end artery and, although definitive evidence is lacking, there are concerns that vasospasm caused by epinephrine could cause necrosis.*

Anatomy

The nerve supply of the penis is from the pudendal nerve and the pelvic plexus (Fig. 40.38A). Along the dorsal artery to the penis are two dorsal nerves that separate at the level of the symphysis pubis; they supply the sensory innervation to the penis.

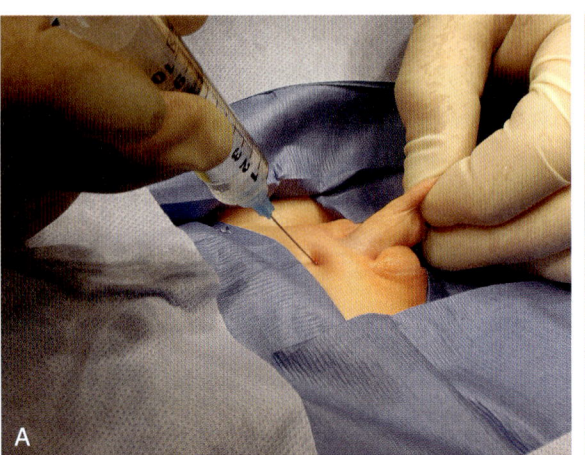
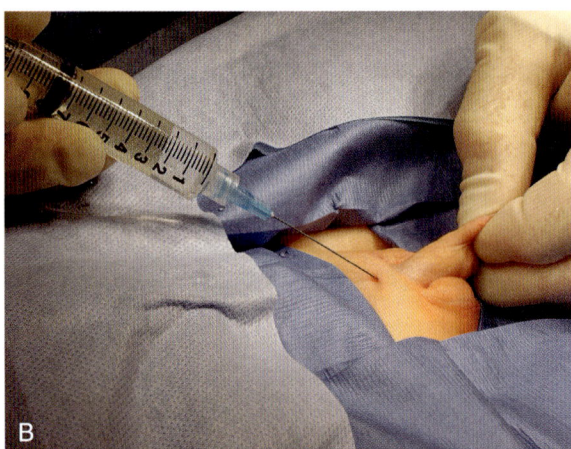
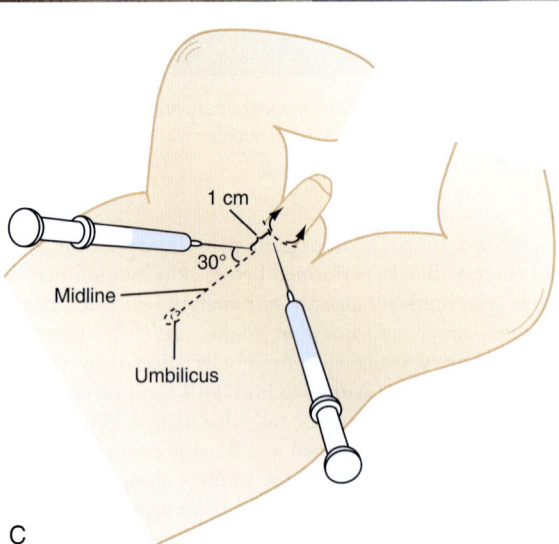

FIGURE 40.38 Penile block. **A,** Dorsal nerve block: a 27- or 25-gauge needle is inserted in the midline, 1 cm above the symphysis pubis at an angle of 30 degrees from the plane of the abdominal wall and directed caudad. **B,** After piercing the penile fascia (0.5–1.0 cm) and negative aspiration for blood, 1.0 to 4.0 mL of local anesthetic without epinephrine is injected. **C,** Ring block: a 25-gauge needle is inserted at the base of the penis at a 45-degree angle, and a ring of local anesthetic is deposited *(curved arrows).* This may be done through a single needle placement by redirecting the needle. This block may be used in children in whom a caudal block is contraindicated.

Technique

There are two commonly used techniques for penile block: (1) a ring block and (2) blockade of the dorsal nerve. One investigation compared the efficacy of these techniques and concluded that the ring block provided analgesia of prolonged duration, although both techniques provided analgesia superior to EMLA cream.[546] The ring block is performed by inserting a 27-gauge needle at the base of the penis and, after negative aspiration, injecting the local anesthetic without epinephrine in a ring-shaped pattern around the base of the penile shaft. The needle may be inserted once in the midline and then redirected to each side (Fig. 40.38B). The alternate dorsal nerve block is performed with a 27-gauge needle inserted 1 centimeter above the symphysis pubis, in the midline, at a 30-degree angle and directed caudally (Fig. 40.38C). The needle is advanced 1 centimeter after it pierces the penile fascia. After negative aspiration for blood, 1 to 4 milliliters of local anesthetic *without epinephrine* is injected slowly. There is a small risk of injury to the adjacent neurovascular structures. Ultrasound guidance can be used but is generally not indicated for this block.[547]

Complications

The major complication is compromise of organ blood flow.[548] *Most, but not all, believe that vasoconstrictors, such as epinephrine, must never be used for this block.* There is also a case report suggesting that the vasoconstrictive properties of more concentrated ropivacaine might also be a risk.[549] Applying pressure after the injection may minimize hematoma formation. Intravascular injection may be avoided with incremental injection and frequent aspiration. A literature review found 47 cases of LAST and 23% were associated with penile blocks.[108,550–552] In order to avoid such complications, one institution initiated the following measures: (1) injection of no more than 0.5 mL/kg of 0.25% bupivacaine (1.25 mg/kg) at any one time; (2) injection can only be repeated once, 30 minutes after the initial dose; and (3) penile block injections must all be directed laterally, away from midline, to cover the anatomic location of the two penile nerves and to avoid the midline venous plexus.[553]

FASCIAL PLANE BLOCKS

The advent of ultrasound guidance has allowed refinement of preexisting blocks and creation of new techniques to deposit local anesthetics adjacent to the course of target nerves through tissue planes. Fascial plane blocks are a class of regional anesthesia techniques wherein the target of needle insertion and local anesthetic injection is a compartment (the "plane") between two anatomically separate layers of fascia and there is no attempt to locate individual nerves. They can be broadly categorized into thoracic and abdominal fascial plane blocks. In the past decade fascial plane blocks have garnered a lot of enthusiasm as an alternative or replacement for neuraxial (epidural) blocks. However, high-quality data supporting their site of action, block quality, efficacy, and reproducibility are limited.[554] Although neuraxial blocks continue to be the gold standard, as they comprehensively cover somatic, visceral, and autonomic components of pain, these newer fascial plane blocks deserve description even while we wait on further validation and reports describing their efficacy and safety. It should be noted that most blocks in this class only lend themselves to ultrasound guidance and not landmark-guided approaches.

Erector Spinae Block

This block was first reported in 2016 to manage thoracic neuropathic pain in a patient with metastatic disease of the ribs and rib fractures.[555] Local anesthetic is injected in the plane between the erector spinae muscles and the transverse process. Subtle variations on this block have been described. In a retrolaminar block, local anesthetic is injected in the plane between the erector spinae muscles and the lamina. For an intertransverse process block the anesthetic is injected in the tissue between the two transverse processes, posterior to the superior costotransverse ligament, or in the space halfway between the posterior aspect of the transverse process and the pleura.[556] Both single-injection and continuous catheter techniques have been described.[557,558] It is hypothesized that a multidermatomal sensory block is achieved by blocking the dorsal and ventral rami of the thoracic and abdominal spinal nerves[555] to achieve diminished sensation over anterior, posterior, and lateral thoracic and abdominal walls. However, Lönnqvist et al., in a well-researched dissenting discourse, write that for an erectae spinae block to be of value for procedures involving the anterior torso is merely wishful thinking.[559] They suggest that evidence indicates that local anesthetic deposition at this site blocks only the posterior rami of the spinal nerves over several adjacent spinal levels, therefore back and spine surgery may prove to be its primary useful indication.[556]

Rectus Sheath Block

Although reported almost 30 years ago,[560] this block has slowly become popular for children undergoing repair of an umbilical or paraumbilical hernia.[561–565] We have also found it to be useful for analgesia after laparoscopic procedures in children in whom the port insertion sites are close to the midline. Local anesthetic is injected into the potential space between the rectus muscle and the posterior rectus sheath. The rectus sheath contains the ventral rami of the intercostal nerves as they traverse the rectus muscle to supply the skin of the anterior abdominal wall on either side of the midline. These thoracic intercostal nerves (T10) can thus be blocked at the paraumbilical area using a small volume of local anesthetic solution. Because the seventh and eighth intercostal nerves also provide motor innervation to the rectus abdominis muscle, a rectus sheath block at this level should also produce relaxation of the muscle.

Anatomy

The rectus abdominis muscle arises as two tendinous heads from the lateral part of the pubic crest and the anterior pubic ligament. The fibers run vertically upward and are inserted to the front of the chest wall through the xiphoid process and the fifth, sixth, and seventh costal cartilages. The muscle is enclosed in a fibrous aponeurotic sheath, the rectus sheath, which is formed by the aponeurosis of the external oblique, internal oblique, and transversus abdominis muscles. The anterior rectus sheath is complete and covers the muscle from end to end. However, the posterior rectus sheath is incomplete, being deficient above the costal cartilage and below the arcuate line (or the fold of Douglas), which is located midway between the umbilicus and the pubic symphysis. The rectus sheath on both sides is held together in the midline by a raphe, the linea alba, which is formed by the fusion of the fibers of the three aponeuroses that form the rectus sheath. The ventral rami of the seventh to twelfth intercostal nerves pass anteriorly and downward from the intercostal spaces and pierce the posterolateral aspect of the rectus sheath before passing anteriorly through the muscle to supply the skin of the anterior abdominal wall. Three transverse fibrous bands (tendinous insertions)—one at the level of the umbilicus, one at the level of the xiphoid process, and one midway between the two—divide the rectus muscle into three smaller parts. These fibrous bands are adherent to the anterior rectus sheath and traverse only the anterior half of the rectus muscle. Therefore, a potential space exists between the rectus muscle and the posterior rectus sheath that communicates from the xiphisternum to the pubic crest. Local anesthetic injected into this space can spread up and down the sheath and is the basis of a rectus sheath block.

Ultrasound-Guided Rectus Sheath Block

Use of ultrasound will facilitate performing this block[565–567] A linear-array transducer (13-10 MHz) with a small footprint (25 mm) is used for imaging in children (Fig. 40.39). The operator stands or sits on one side of the anesthetized child, and the ultrasound machine is positioned directly opposite on the contralateral side. The transducer is positioned in the longitudinal axis midway between the umbilicus and the xiphisternum. The rectus muscle is seen as a hypoechoic structure between the hyperechoic anterior and posterior rectus sheath (see Fig. 40.39). Deep to the posterior rectus sheath, the hyperechoic peritoneum can be recognized by its typical peritoneal sliding movement and the comet-tail artifacts produced. The fibrous bands (tendinous insertions) in the rectus sheath can also be recognized in the longitudinal sonogram as hyperechoic areas on the anterior surface of the hypoechoic muscle that do not traverse the whole muscle belly.[563,566,568] The linea alba can be recognized on a transverse sonogram, and the posterior deficiency of the rectus sheath is also readily recognized below the level of the arcuate line.

The block needle is inserted using the in-plane technique in a caudal-to-cranial direction (Fig. 40.40A,B). When the tip of the needle is visualized in the potential space between the rectus muscle and the posterior rectus sheath, a test injection of saline solution (1–2 mL) is performed to confirm the longitudinal spread of the injectate between the muscle and the rectus sheath and the widening of the space (Fig. 40.40C,D, Video 40.29). Injection into the muscle will offer resistance to injection and is readily recognized in the sonogram. The needle should be repositioned, and the typical spread of the test injection under the rectus muscle should be confirmed before a calculated dose of the local anesthetic is injected.[569] For umbilical hernia surgery, bilateral rectus sheath blocks are performed just above the umbilicus on either side.

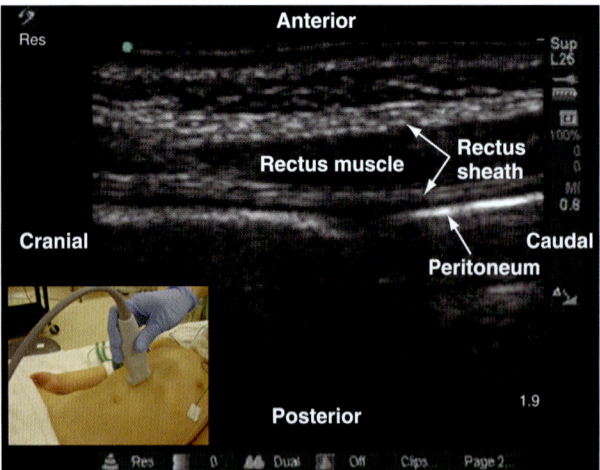

FIGURE 40.39 Longitudinal sonogram of the rectus muscle showing the anterior and posterior rectus sheath.

Landmark-Guided Rectus Sheath Block

On either side of the umbilicus, about 1 centimeter from the midline, a needle is inserted into the rectus sheath (Fig. 40.41). A pop can be felt as the needle advances beyond the anterior rectus sheath, through the rectus abdominis muscle, and then just anterior to the posterior rectus sheath. After aspiration, a volume of 0.1 mL/kg of local anesthetic solution is injected. This provides excellent analgesia for most umbilical area surgery, including laparoscopic surgery.

Transversus Abdominis Plane Block

Anatomy

The sensory supply of the abdominal wall is provided by the anterior rami of the T7–L1 thoracolumbar nerves. Dermatomes T7–T9 innervate the skin above the umbilicus, T10 innervates the skin around the umbilicus, and T11, T12 (cutaneous branches of the subcostal nerve), and L1 (iliohypogastric and ilioinguinal nerves) innervate the skin below the umbilicus. These nerves pass inferoanteriorly in a plane between the internal oblique and transversus abdominis muscles, also known as the transversus abdominis plane (TAP). The lateral cutaneous branch is given off at the midaxillary line and innervates the abdominal wall up to the lateral edge of the rectus abdominis muscle. The segmental nerve then courses anteriorly and medially toward the midline in the TAP to penetrate the lateral margin of the rectus sheath and emerge anteriorly through the rectus muscle as the anterior cutaneous branch. The lateral and anterior cutaneous branches of the thoracolumbar nerves supply the skin from the midline to the anterior axillary line. The thoracolumbar nerves, as they course through the TAP, also supply muscular branches to the abdominal musculature.

Local anesthetic injected into the TAP plane produces sensorimotor blockade (segmental) of the abdominal wall. TAP block techniques can be classified according to the site of needle insertion (i.e., the posterior, lateral, and subcostal TAP blocks).[570] The posterior TAP block is discussed together with the quadratus lumborum block (QLB) in the next section. For the lateral TAP block, local anesthetic is injected in the TAP plane between the iliac crest and the costal margin at the midaxillary line; for a subcostal TAP block the local anesthetic is injected into the TAP plane just below the costal margin at the midclavicular line.[571] Anesthesia and analgesia produced by a TAP block is unilateral; thus it is useful for surgical procedures (e.g., orchidopexy, herniotomy, appendectomy) in which the incision does not cross the midline. Bilateral TAP blocks are indicated for abdominal surgical procedures in which the surgical incision is in the midline or crosses the midline. It is also the authors' practice to perform bilateral TAP blocks for laparoscopic procedures.[572–574] However, since TAP blocks do not produce visceral analgesia, they should be used as part of a multimodal analgesic regimen for perioperative analgesia. TAP blocks may be useful as an alternative when central neuraxial blocks are contraindicated (e.g., in children with underlying coagulopathy or spinal dysraphism). The ideal local anesthetic dose for this block remains unresolved; two prospective randomized studies of relatively small cohorts investigated the relationship between administered dose and quality and duration of analgesia. Although one study found no difference between high concentration/low volume and low concentration/high volume blocks,[575] a second found longer duration of analgesia when greater concentrations of local anesthetic were administered.[576]

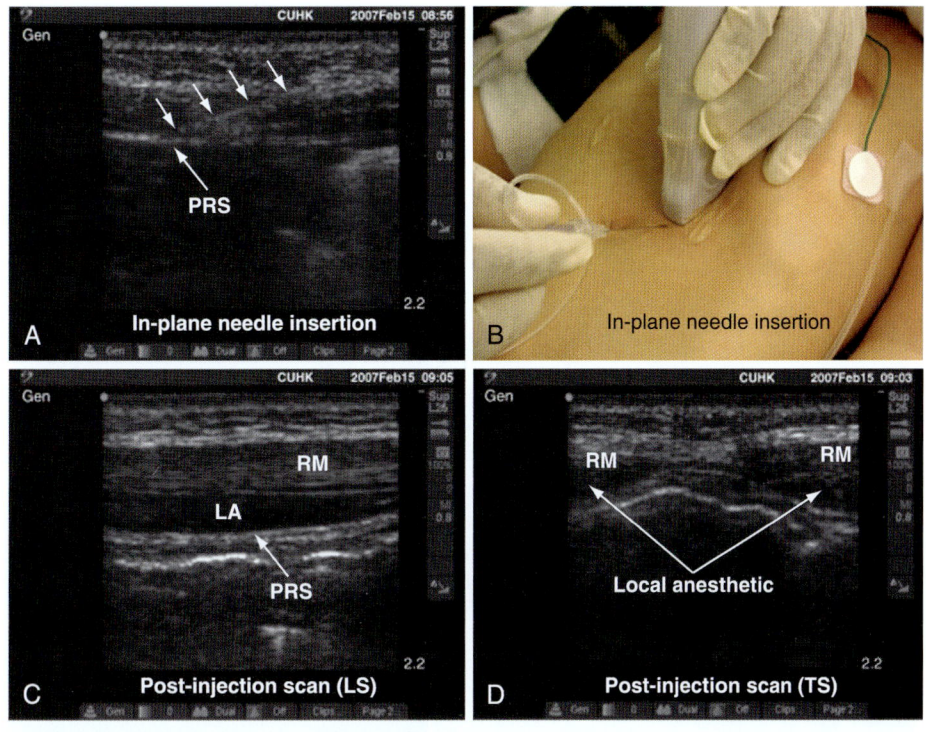

FIGURE 40.40 Rectus sheath block. The in-plane needle insertion technique. *LA*, Local anesthetic; *LS*, longitudinal sonogram; *PRS*, posterior rectus sheath; *RM*, rectus muscle; *TS*, transverse sonogram.

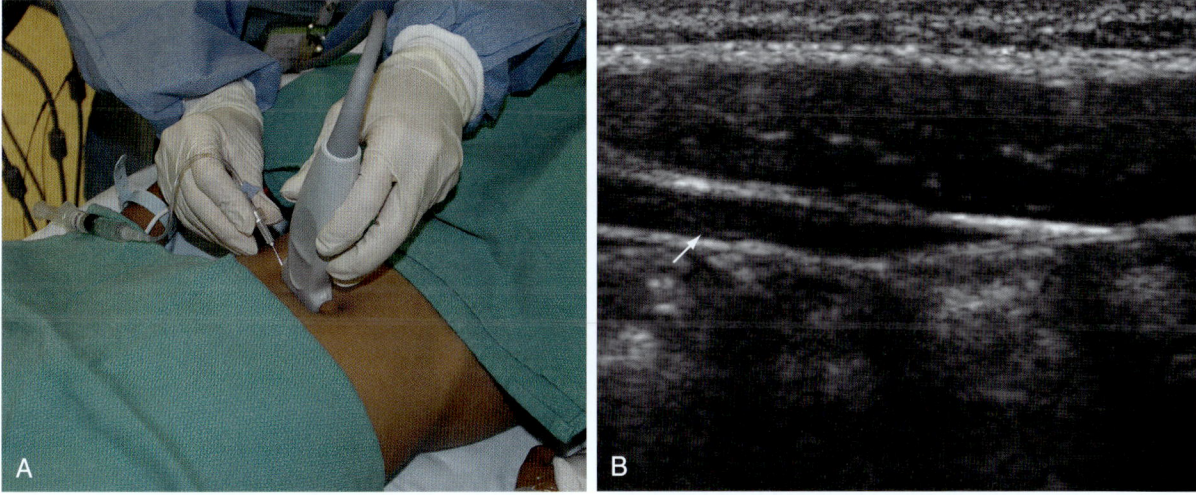

FIGURE 40.41 Rectus sheath block. The rectus sheath is encompassed between the rectus abdominis muscle anteriorly and the posterior rectus sheath. **A,** A linear ultrasound probe is placed lateral to the umbilicus, and the anterior rectus sheath, the rectus abdominis muscle, and the posterior rectus sheath are identified. **B,** With the use of an in-plane approach, a 27-gauge needle is inserted through the rectus abdominis muscle anterior to the posterior rectus sheath and 0.1 mL/kg of local anesthetic solution is injected *(arrow)*.

Ultrasound-Guided Transversus Abdominis Plane Block

For a lateral TAP block, a high-frequency linear-array transducer (15-7 MHz) is placed midway between the iliac crest and the costal margin along the midaxillary line (Fig. 40.42). For infants and young children, a linear transducer with a small footprint (25 mm) is preferred. The operator stands or sits on one side of the child, and the ultrasound machine is positioned directly opposite on the contralateral side. The various layers of the abdominal wall are identified on the sonogram (see Fig. 40.42B). From superficial to deep, they include a layer of subcutaneous tissue and fat and the three abdominal muscles with their fascial layers (i.e., the external oblique, internal oblique, and the transversus abdominis muscles, respectively). Deep to the transversus abdominis muscle the hypoechoic peritoneum is also visualized (see Fig. 40.42B). The block needle (50 mm) is inserted 1 to 2 centimeters medial to the medial edge of the ultrasound transducer (see Fig. 40.42C) in the plane of the ultrasound beam. Because the abdominal wall in infants and young children is relatively thin, and to avoid inadvertent deep

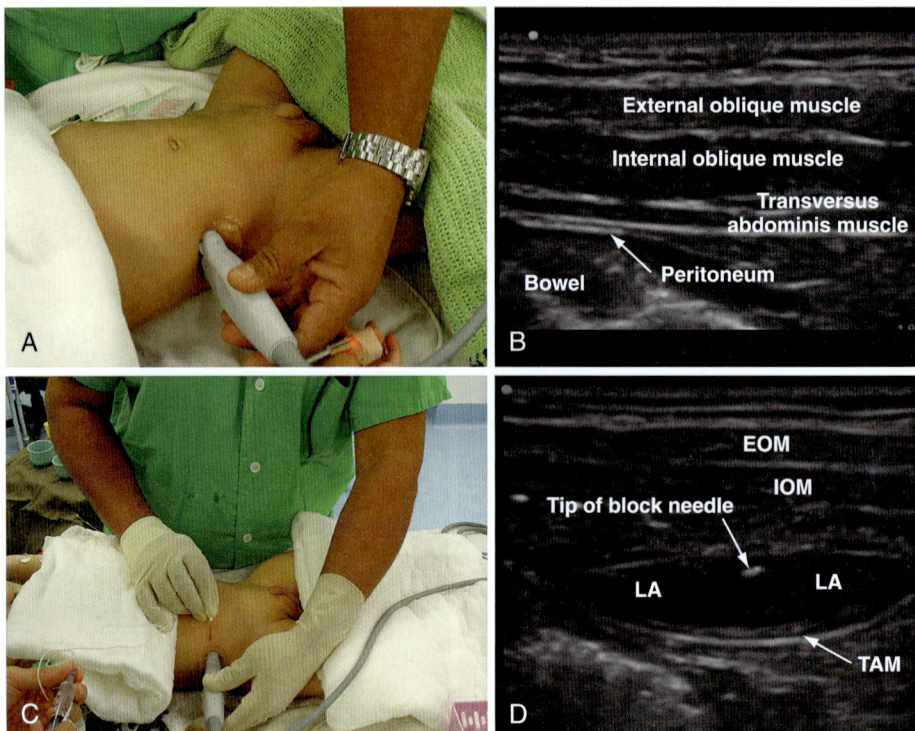

FIGURE 40.42 Posterior transverse abdominis plane (TAP) block. **A,** Note how the ultrasound transducer is positioned between the iliac crest and the costal margin along the midaxillary line. **B,** The three layers of the abdominal musculature. **C,** In-plane needle insertion during a posterior TAP block. **D,** Distention of the TAP by the injected local anesthetic *(LA)*. *EOM,* External oblique muscle; *IOM,* internal oblique muscle; *TAM,* transversus abdomen muscle.

needle insertion and visceral puncture, it is the authors' practice to initially insert the block needle directed toward the ultrasound transducer rather than in an anteroposterior direction. Once the needle tip penetrates the skin and enters the abdominal muscles, it is redirected and slowly advanced under direct vision through the external oblique and internal oblique muscles. The TAP is identified between the internal oblique and transversus abdominis muscles. A test injection (1 mL) of saline solution is performed to confirm correct needle placement in the TAP, which is indicated by distention of the TAP by the hypoechoic fluid. A long-acting local anesthetic is then injected, while distention of the TAP by the injection is visualized in real time (see Fig. 40.42D; Video 40.16).

For a subcostal TAP block, a high-frequency linear-array transducer (15-6 MHz) is placed immediately below the costal margin along the midclavicular line and the block needle (50–80 mm) is inserted in the plane of the ultrasound beam and from a medial-to-lateral direction until the tip is identified to be in the TAP. 1 to 2 milliliters of saline or local anesthetic is injected to confirm correct needle placement in the TAP. A calculated dose of local anesthetic is then injected, and as the local anesthetic hydrodissects the TAP plane, the block needle is advanced posteriorly in the TAP to improve spread of the local anesthetic. Bilateral subcostal TAP blocks are indicated for midline upper abdominal incisions. Currently, published data on the use of subcostal TAP blocks in children are limited, and its role in children is still not defined.

Quadratus Lumborum Block
Anatomy
The QLB is an abdominal wall field block in which the local anesthetic is injected into a fascial plane located deep to the fascia transversalis (the deep fascia of the abdominal wall) and on the anterolateral aspect of the quadratus lumborum muscle (Fig. 40.43).[577–581] The fascia transversalis of the abdominal wall blends medially with the anterior layer of the quadratus lumborum fascia and the psoas fascia (psoas sheath) (see Fig. 40.43). The subcostal (T12), iliohypogastric (L1), and ilioinguinal (L1) nerves course anterior to and in close contact with the quadratus lumborum muscle and the lateral femoral cutaneous nerve of the thigh (L2, L3) crosses the lateral border of the psoas muscle at the level of the inferior border of the L4 vertebra in this fascial plane. The point of injection is believed to approximate the landmark-based technique of performing a posterior TAP block at the lumbar triangle of Petit.[582,583] Several ultrasound-guided techniques for QLBs or their variations have been described in the literature: QLB-I, QLB-II, and transmuscular QLB (Fig. 40.44), but the optimal technique or the best site of injection remains unclear.[584–586]

There are limited data on QLBs in children,[578,579,581,587] but studies in adults show that a QLB produces multidermatomal ipsilateral anesthesia of the thoracolumbar nerves. A bilateral single-injection QLB (20 mL of 0.375% ropivacaine on each side) produces loss of sensation to cold from (T7–L1),[577] compared with bilateral lateral TAP blocks (T10–T12).[584–586] Also the duration of analgesia after a bilateral QLB in adults is greater (attributed to paravertebral spread of local anesthetic) than that produced by bilateral lateral TAP blocks.[577] QLB may also produce ipsilateral sympathetic blockade since paravertebral spread of contrast has been demonstrated. Therefore, a QLB may be effective in relieving sympathetic-mediated visceral pain that is otherwise not affected by a lateral TAP block. However, since there is a paucity of data on the use of bilateral QLBs for major abdominal

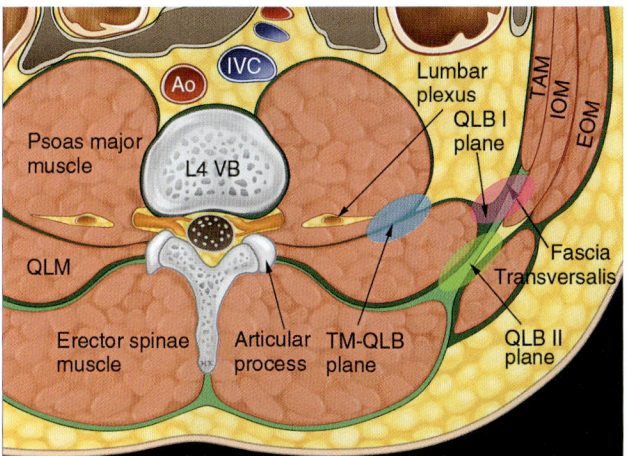

FIGURE 40.43 Cross-sectional anatomy at the L4 level illustrating the anatomy relevant for quadratus lumborum block *(QLB)*. The QLB-I block involves injecting the local anesthetic at the anterolateral aspect of the quadratus lumborum muscle *(pink region)*. QLB-II involves injection posterior to the quadratus lumborum muscle *(green region)*. QLB III block, also known as transmuscular QLB *(TM-QLB)*, involves advancing the needle through the quadratus lumborum muscle and injecting the local anesthetic between the quadratus lumborum and psoas muscle *(blue region)*. *Ao,* Aorta; *EOM,* external oblique muscle; *IOM,* internal oblique muscle; *IVC,* inferior vena cava; *QLM,* quadratus lumborum muscle; *TAM,* transversus abdominis muscle; *VB,* vertebral body.

surgery in children, no recommendations can be made at this time, but QLBs hold promise as a technique for perioperative pain management.

Ultrasound-Guided Quadratus Lumborum Block

A QLB is performed with the child in the lateral or supine position (see Fig. 40.44). The lateral position is preferable for unilateral QLB because the transmuscular approach can be easily

performed. For bilateral QLBs the child is placed in the supine position (see Fig. 40.44). The abdomen is exposed between the costal margin and the iliac crest. The operator stands on one side of the subject, and the ultrasound machine is placed directly opposite on the contralateral side. A high-frequency (13-8 MHz) linear-array transducer is used in young children; a curved-array transducer (5-1 MHz), which produces a wider field of view, may be used in older or obese children. The transducer is placed in the transverse orientation on the flank immediately above the iliac crest. The operator then gently slides the transducer posteriorly, aiming to identify the anterolateral surface of the vertebral body and the transverse process in the transverse sonogram. Once the transverse process is located and the relevant anatomy is identified, the operator tilts or slides the transducer slightly caudally to perform the transverse scan through the intertransverse space (ITS). The acoustic shadow of the transverse process will now no longer be visible and will be replaced by the hyperechoic articular process. On the transverse sonogram the vertebral body and transverse process of the vertebra appear as hyperechoic structures with a corresponding acoustic shadow (see Fig. 40.44). The psoas major, quadratus lumborum, and erector spinae muscles are easily recognized surrounding the transverse process. Also, depending on the side scanned, the inferior vena cava (on the right) and aorta (on the left) are visualized anterolateral to the vertebral body. The arrangement of the three muscles around the transverse process— that is, the psoas muscle lying anterior, the erector spinae muscle lying posterior, and the quadratus lumborum muscle lying at the apex—produces a sonographic pattern that has been likened to a "shamrock" with the muscles representing the three leaves.[588] Superficial and anterior to these three muscles, the external oblique, internal, and transversus abdominis muscles are identified. In the transverse sonogram through the lumbar intertransverse space, the acoustic shadow of the transverse process is no longer visualized, and the intervertebral foramen and spinal canal may also be visualized in addition to the psoas major, quadratus lumborum, and erector spine muscles (Fig. 40.45).

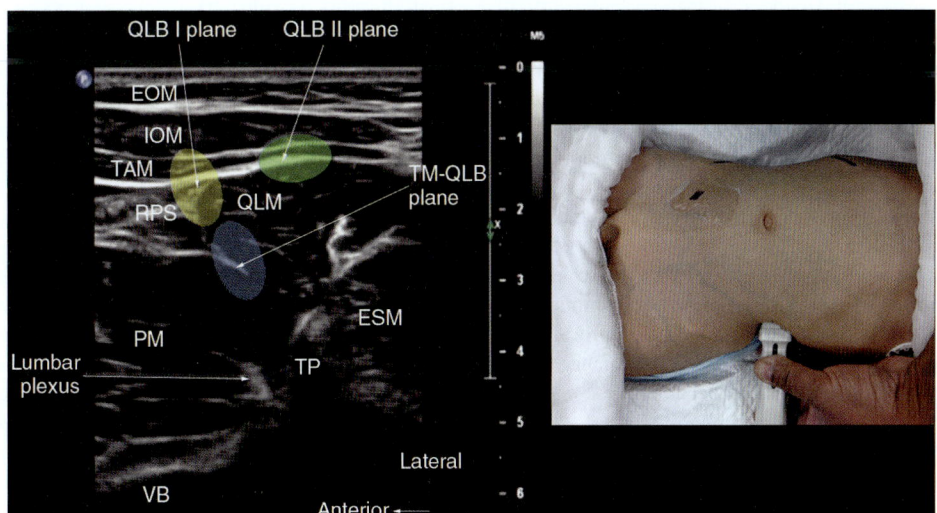

FIGURE 40.44 Quadratus lumborum block in a child. Note how the ultrasound transducer is positioned in the posterior flank immediately above the iliac crest. Transverse sonogram demonstrating the relevant sonoanatomy and the anatomic planes for local anesthetic injection during a quadratus lumborum block. *EOM,* External oblique muscle; *ESM,* erector spinae muscle; *IOM,* internal oblique muscle; *PM,* psoas major; *QLM,* quadratus lumborum muscle; *RPS,* retroperitoneal space; *TAM,* transversus abdominis muscle; *TM-QLB,* transmuscular quadratus lumborum block; *TP,* transverse process; *VB,* vertebral body.

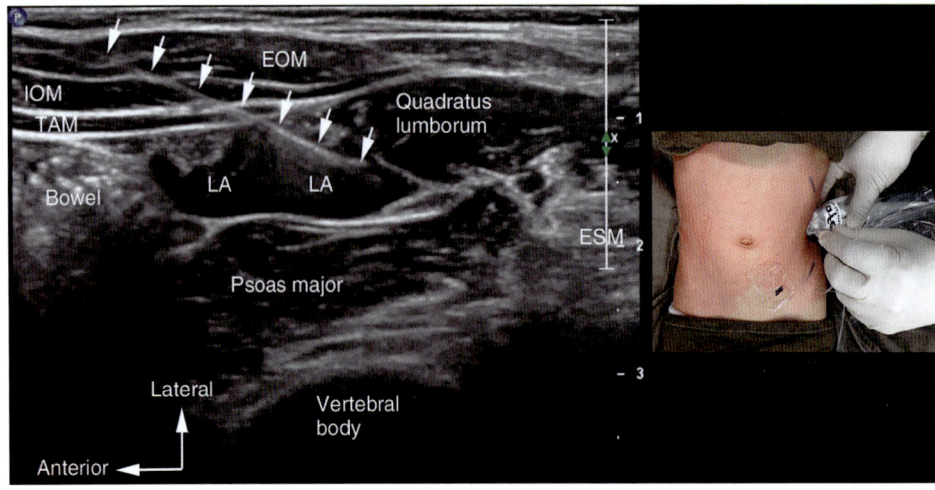

FIGURE 40.45 Quadratus lumborum block II with the patient in the supine position. Note the needle is inserted in-plane *(arrows)* and advanced into a fascial plane deep to the fascia transversalis and on the anterolateral aspect of the quadratus lumborum muscle. *EOM,* External oblique muscle; *ESM,* erector spinae muscle; *IOM,* internal oblique muscle; *LA,* local anesthetic; *TAM,* transversus abdominis muscle.

A 22-gauge (50- to 80-mm) nerve block needle is inserted in-plane from the anterior to posterior direction, and the needle tip is positioned between the anterior border of QLM and its fascia (QLB-I) (see Figs. 40.43–40.45). Correct needle tip position is confirmed by injection of 1 to 2 millilters of normal saline solution and observing the spread of the injectate in relation to the quadratus lumborum muscle (see Fig. 40.45). After negative aspiration, a calculated dose of local anesthetic (e.g., 0.2–0.3 mL/kg per side) is injected. It is prudent to identify the lower pole of the kidney and the limits of the peritoneal cavity during the scout scan to avoid deep needle insertion and visceral injury (Video 40.17).

Paravertebral Block (Thoracic Paravertebral Block)

This block is gaining in popularity for use in children for abdominal and thoracic procedures.[589–593] Although landmark and nerve stimulator techniques are well described, real-time, in-plane ultrasound-guided paravertebral catheter placement in young infants and children is both feasible and beneficial.[594–597] Deposition of local anesthetics in the paravertebral space will produce ipsilateral, segmental, somatic, and sympathetic nerve blockade that is effective for relieving unilateral postoperative pain following thoracic or abdominal surgical procedures (Fig. 40.46). These blocks are often used in patients where a thoracic epidural block is not indicated but involves major thoracic or abdominal procedures. In a study of 2390 thoracic paravertebral blocks (TPVBs; 625 of which included catheter placement); there was one major complication which was a brief seizure following a test dose of chloroprocaine.[598] These blocks are also gaining popularity for fast-track management for children undergoing cardiac surgical procedures.[599,600]

Anatomy

The paravertebral space is a triangular wedge-shaped area situated in the angle between the lateral border of the vertebral body and the anterior surface of the transverse process (Fig. 40.47). The paravertebral space exists only between T1 and T12. Below T12 the space is sealed off by the origin of the psoas muscle from the vertebral body and the transverse process.[601] Cranially the space appears to communicate with fascial planes in the neck, because an upper thoracic paravertebral block may cause Horner syndrome.

The communication of different thoracic levels of the paravertebral space is the foundation for spread of local anesthetic to multiple segments (see Fig. 40.46). The medial boundary of the paravertebral space is the lateral part of the vertebral body and disk, the dorsal limitation is the transverse process and costotransverse ligament, and the anterolateral boundary is the parietal pleura. Structures that pass through the paravertebral space include the spinal nerve root–intercostal nerve, the sympathetic chain, and the intercostal vessels. The paravertebral space is not like the epidural space, because the pleura are very adhesive to the other structures; it should instead be viewed as a "potential space." This accounts for the slight difficulty in introducing a percutaneous catheter into the paravertebral space. In the lumbar region, a paravertebral block is still possible but each individual space must be blocked separately because there are no communications between adjacent lumbar levels, limiting its utility. Three approaches to perform a paravertebral block in children have been described: loss of resistance, nerve stimulator, and ultrasound. Additionally, a hybrid *ultrasound-aided approach* may be employed. With the aid of ultrasound, the position of the transverse processes and the depth to the paravertebral space can be determined, and ultrasound is very helpful even when a loss-of-resistance– or nerve-stimulator–guided technique is used.

Ultrasound-Guided Paravertebral Block

Ultrasound-guided thoracic paravertebral block (TPVB) is performed with the child in the lateral position and with the side to be blocked uppermost (Fig. 40.48). The operator sits or stands behind the child, and the ultrasound machine is positioned directly in front on the opposite side of the operating table. In most children a 15-6 or 13-8 megahertz linear-array transducer is adequate for imaging the paravertebral anatomy. However, a high-frequency linear-array transducer with a small footprint (25 mm) is ideal for ultrasound-guided TPVB in neonates and young infants.

The thoracic paravertebral region can be imaged in the transverse or sagittal axis. We prefer the transverse axis, and the ultrasound scan is performed by sequentially imaging three contiguous sites at the target thoracic level (Fig. 40.49). Each of the three transverse ultrasound scan windows produces a very distinct sonogram, reflecting the different osseous (Fig. 40.50A–C) and musculoskeletal structures that are visualized in the sonograms. On a transverse sonogram with the ultrasound beam insonated over the ipsilateral spinous process, lamina, transverse process, and the rib (position 1, Fig. 40.50A), the hyperechoic outlines of the osseous structures with their corresponding acoustic shadows are clearly delineated from a medial-to-lateral direction. This ultrasound window does not demonstrate the paravertebral anatomy per se but is the initial ultrasound window that one should acquire after which identification of the transverse sono-anatomy of the paravertebral region becomes relatively simple. From position 1, one can gently slide or tilt the transducer caudally until the acoustic shadow of the rib is no longer visualized (position 2) (see Fig. 40.49), and the hyperechoic outline of the lamina and transverse process with their acoustic shadow are seen (see Fig. 40.50B). Lateral to the transverse process the hyperechoic pleura and lung are visualized anteriorly, the hyperechoic internal intercostal membrane (IICM) posteriorly, and a hypoechoic triangular space that represents the apex of the thoracic paravertebral space (TPVS) is interposed between the two (see Fig. 40.50B). If one now gently slides or tilts the ultrasound transducer slightly more caudally (position 3) (see Fig. 40.49), the acoustic shadow of the transverse process disappears and the hyperechoic inferior articular process is visualized medially (see Fig. 40.50C). The thick superior costotransverse ligament (SCTL), parietal pleura, lung, and the apical part of the paravertebral space are also delineated. Continuation of the SCTL to the IICM laterally can also be delineated in some children (see Fig. 40.50C). However, since the acoustic shadow of the transverse process is no longer visualized, outlines of the entire TPVS can now be seen (see Fig. 40.50C). The location of the intervertebral foramen, which lies anteromedial to the inferior articular process, can also be defined (Video 40.18).

Currently the majority of the published data on ultrasound-guided TPVB in children exclusively use the transverse axis, and the scan is performed at the level of the transverse process (position 2, see Fig. 40.49 and Fig. 40.50B).[589,590] There are no data describing the use of the transverse ultrasound scan window at the level of the articular process for TPVB. The latter is our preferred ultrasound window for imaging and needle insertion during ultrasound-guided TPVB because it not only delineates the entire TPVS but there is also less bony obstruction during needle insertion. One can also accurately define the location of the intervertebral foramen, "a no-go zone" during TPVB (position 3) (see Fig. 40.49 and Fig. 40.50C).

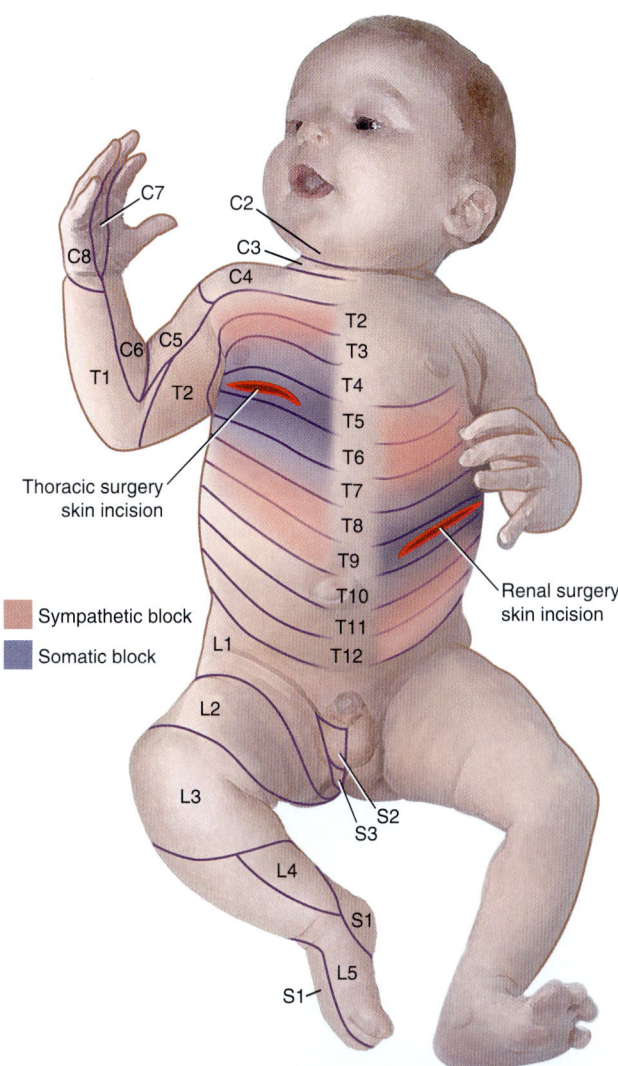

FIGURE 40.46 Distribution of somatic and sympathetic blockade after thoracic paravertebral blocks. *Blue shading* indicates the approximate spread of somatic blockade and *pink shading* indicates the approximate extent of sympathetic blockade. (See text for details.) (From Lönnqvist PA, Richardson J. Use of paravertebral blockade in children. *Tech Region Anesth Pain Manage.* 1999;3[3]:184-188.)

Labels in figure 40.46:
C7, C2, C8, C3, C4, C5, C6, T1, T2 (on arm)
T2, T3, T4, T5, T6, T7, T8, T9, T10, T11, T12
Thoracic surgery skin incision
Renal surgery skin incision
Sympathetic block
Somatic block
L1, L2, L3, L4, L5
S1, S2, S3

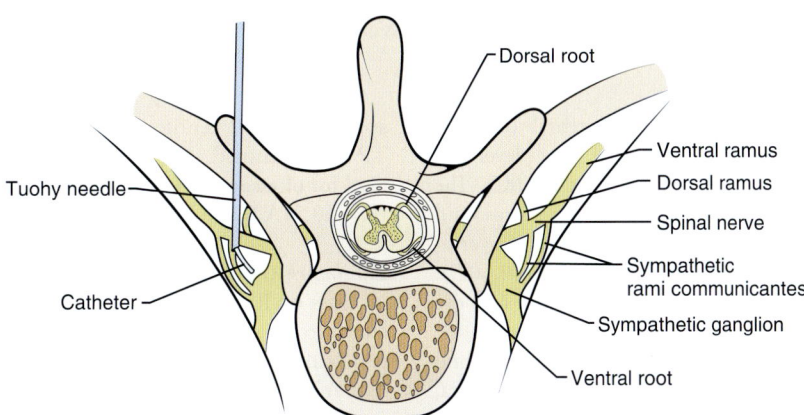

FIGURE 40.47 Anatomic relationship of the paravertebral block and correct position of Tuohy needle and catheter. (From Lönnqvist PA, Richardson J. Use of paravertebral blockade in children. *Tech Region Anesth Pain Manage.* 1999;3[3]:184-188.)

Labels in figure 40.47:
Dorsal root
Ventral ramus
Dorsal ramus
Spinal nerve
Sympathetic rami communicantes
Sympathetic ganglion
Ventral root
Tuohy needle
Catheter

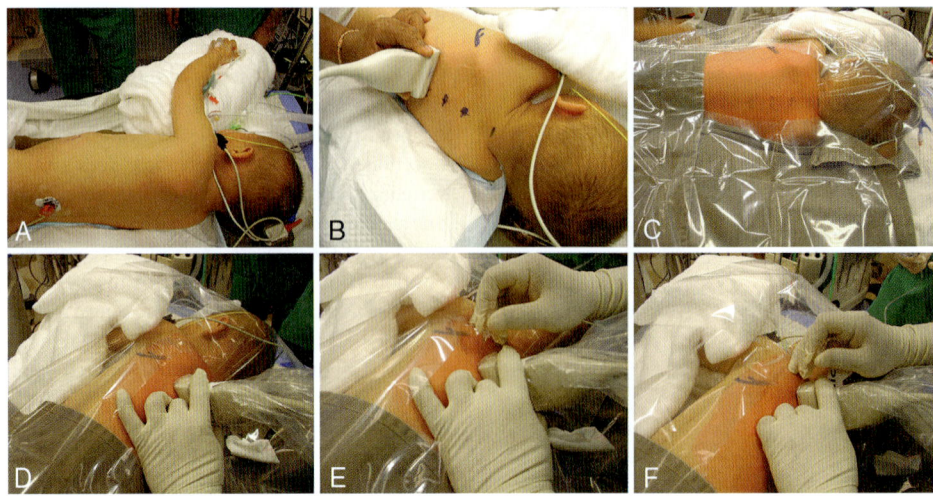

FIGURE 40.48 Ultrasound-guided thoracic paravertebral block in a child. **A,** The child is positioned in the lateral position with the side to be blocked uppermost. **B,** Transverse scan using a 13-8 MHz linear-array transducer. **C,** Aseptic precautions. **D,** The ultrasound transducer is placed inside a sterile cover. **E,** In-plane needle insertion. **F,** Local anesthetic is injected by an assistant.

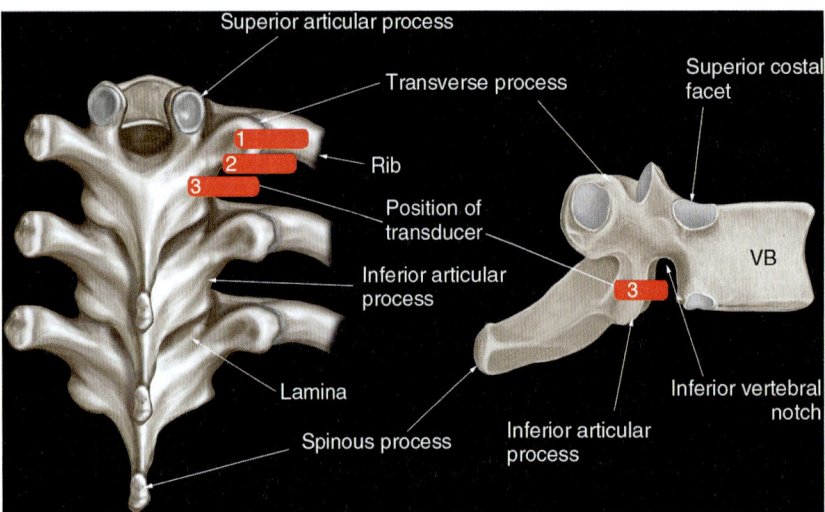

FIGURE 40.49 Schematic diagram showing the positions of the ultrasound transducer at the three contiguous sites over the paravertebral region relevant for thoracic paravertebral block. *Position 1,* The ultrasound transducer is placed over the ipsilateral spinous process, lamina, transverse process, and the rib. *Position 2,* The ultrasound transducer is placed over the ipsilateral lamina and transverse process. *Position 3,* From position 2 the ultrasound transducer is gently slid or tilted caudally until the inferior articular process of the vertebral body is visualized medially.

For an ultrasound-guided thoracic paravertebral block, a transverse view of the paravertebral space at the target level and at the articular process level, is obtained (see Fig. 40.50C). The block needle (50 mm) is inserted lateral to the ultrasound transducer and advanced toward the apical part of the paravertebral space in the plane of the ultrasound beam (see Fig. 40.50D). The advancing needle is visualized in real time, and entry into the TPVS is confirmed using a test bolus injection (1 mL) of saline solution. Correct placement of the needle in the paravertebral space is indicated by anterior displacement of the parietal pleura, distention of the paravertebral space, and increased echogenicity of the parietal pleura (see Fig. 40.50D). A calculated dose of local anesthetic (e.g., 0.4 mL/kg) is then injected with the needle in situ before a catheter is inserted through the needle, leaving

approximately 2 centimeters of catheter in situ if a continuous TPVB is planned. The technique described above can also be used for ultrasound-guided TPVB in young infants and neonates (Fig. 40.51A,B and Video 40.19).

Landmark-Guided Paravertebral Block

LOSS-OF-RESISTANCE TECHNIQUE.[601] The skin is punctured lateral to the spinous process and the needle is advanced in a perpendicular manner until contact is made with the transverse process. A Tuohy needle (19- to 20-gauge if the child is younger than 1 year of age, 18-gauge if older than 1 year of age) is then "walked" below (underneath) the transverse process and by means of a loss-of-resistance technique the costotransverse ligament is pierced and the paravertebral space located. Alternatively, the

40

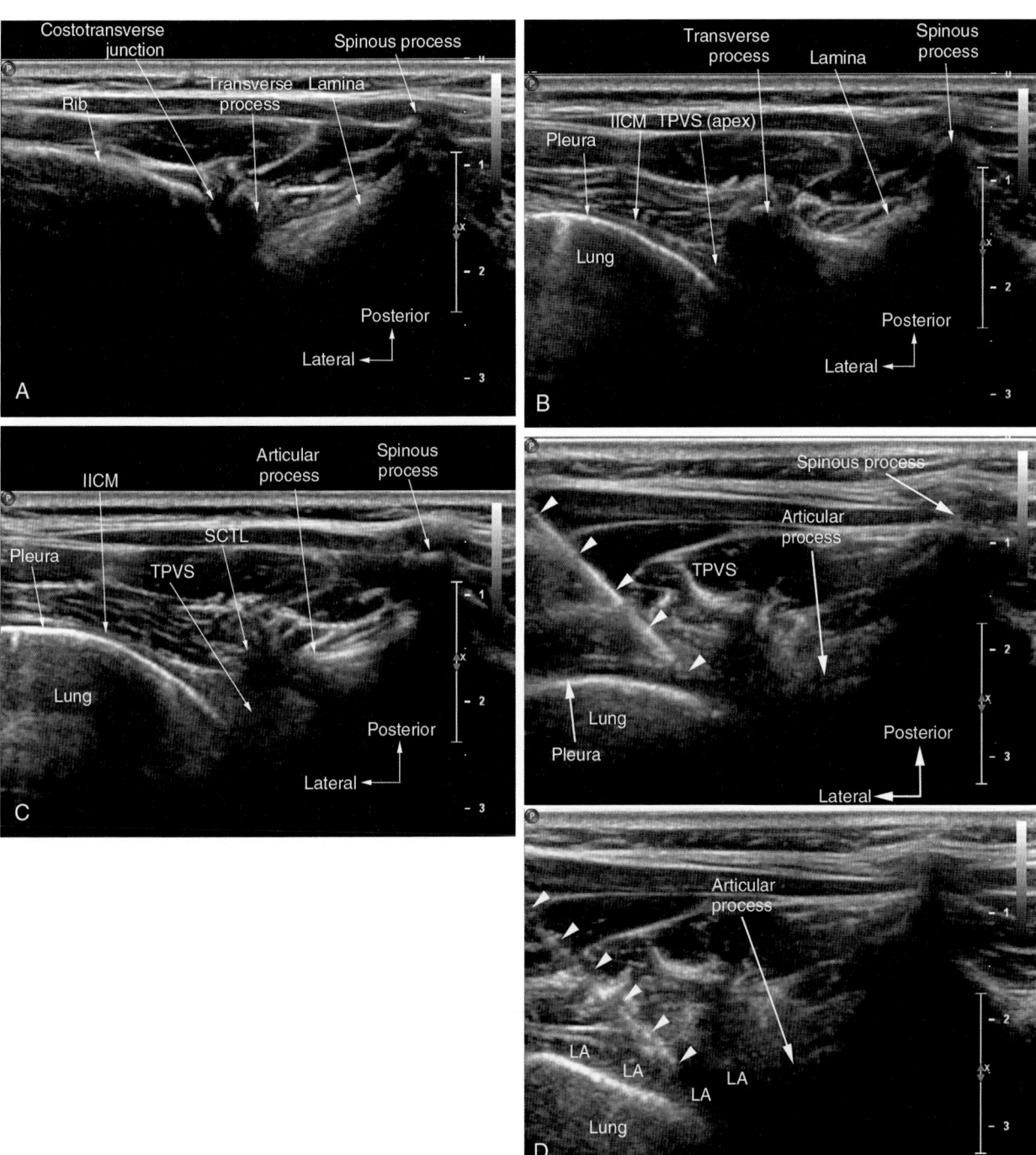

FIGURE 40.50 A, Transverse sonogram of thoracic paravertebral region at the T5 level with the ultrasound transducer placed over position 1 (see Fig. 40.49). The hyperechoic outlines of the ipsilateral spinous process, lamina, transverse process, and the rib with their corresponding acoustic shadow anteriorly are clearly delineated from a medial-to-lateral direction. **B,** Transverse sonogram of thoracic paravertebral block region at the T5 level with the ultrasound transducer placed over position 2 (see Fig. 40.49). The hyperechoic outline of transverse process and the lamina with their acoustic shadow are visualized medially. **C,** Transverse sonogram of thoracic paravertebral block region at T5 level with the ultrasound transducer placed over position 3 (see Fig. 40.49). Note the acoustic shadow of the transverse process is no longer visualized and the hyperechoic inferior articular process is visualized medially. The outlines of the thoracic paravertebral space are also clearly delineated. **D,** Ultrasound-guided thoracic paravertebral block with the block needle being inserted in-plane and at the level of the articular process in the transverse sonogram; *arrowheads* indicate the path of the needle. Note the anterior displacement of the parietal pleura and distention of the paravertebral space after the local anesthetic *(LA)* injection. *IICM,* Internal intercostal membrane; *SCTL,* superior costotransverse ligament; *TPVS,* thoracic paravertebral space.

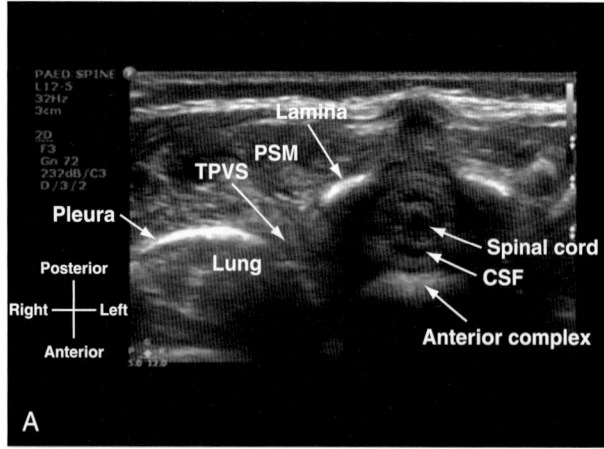
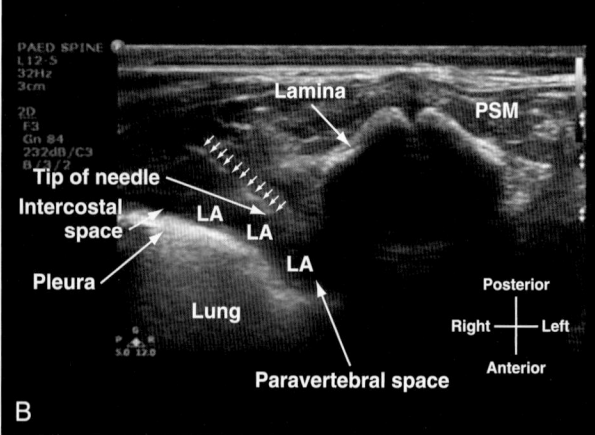

FIGURE 40.51 **A,** Transverse sonogram demonstrating the sonoanatomy of the right thoracic paravertebral region in a neonate. Note the hyperechoic pleura anteriorly and the hypoechoic apical part of the thoracic paravertebral space *(TPVS)* posterior to the pleura. Also note the large acoustic window resulting from incomplete ossification of the posterior spinal elements that allows visualization of the neuraxial structures within the spinal canal. **B,** Transverse sonogram of the right thoracic paravertebral region in a neonate after an ultrasound-guided thoracic paravertebral block. Note the direction of needle insertion *(small arrows)* and distention of the right thoracic paravertebral and intercostal spaces, adjacent to the level of injection, with the local anesthetic *(LA)*. *CSF,* Cerebrospinal fluid; *PSM,* paraspinal muscles.

needle can be "walked" above (over the top of) the transverse process, but by using this approach, there is the risk of striking the neck of the rib before entering the paravertebral space. Occasionally this will redirect the needle, making it virtually impossible to obtain access to the paravertebral space. The approach from below the transverse process is clearly advantageous.

Once in the paravertebral space, the bolus dose of local anesthetic can be injected after careful aspiration to exclude the presence of blood or air. If a continuous technique is preferred, a catheter can be introduced 1 to 2 centimeters into the paravertebral space through the Tuohy needle. The insertion of the catheter frequently needs manipulation of the Tuohy needle to be successful, and occasionally one will have to use the injection of the bolus dose to "open up" or "create" a space to allow catheter insertion. One should not insert more than 1 to 2 centimeters of the catheter into the paravertebral space because further advancement may cause the catheter to migrate into the spinal canal through the intervertebral foramen (causing an epidural distribution of the block) or to go laterally, following the path of the intercostal nerve (giving a dense block of only one dermatome).

An estimate of the distance from the spinous process to the skin puncture site (spinous process to paravertebral space distance) and the distance from the skin to the paravertebral space can be approximated by the equations[602,603]:

Spinous process to paravertebral space distance (mm) = 0.12 × kg + 10.2
Skin to paravertebral space distance (mm) = 0.53 × kg + 21.2.

The level of the puncture depends on the surgical intervention, but for a thoracotomy, the puncture is best performed at T5–T6 and for renal surgery at T9–T10.

NERVE-STIMULATOR–GUIDED TECHNIQUE.[604] The intervertebral lines corresponding to the specific dermatomes are determined by manual palpation. The site of injection is marked 1 to 2 centimeters laterally from the midline on the intervertebral line according to the child's weight. A 21-gauge insulated needle of appropriate length, attached to a nerve stimulator (initial stimulating current: 2.5–5 mA, 1 Hz), is introduced perpendicular to the skin in all planes. A contraction of the paraspinal muscles is initially observed, and the needle is advanced until the costotransverse ligament is reached. At this point the contraction of the paraspinal muscles will disappear. After piercing the costotransverse ligament, muscle contractions of the corresponding level are sought, and the needle tip is manipulated into a position allowing continued muscular contractions while reducing the stimulating current from 1.0 mA to 0.4–0.6 mA. The desired local anesthetic dose and volume is injected. Manipulation of the needle tip within the paravertebral space is not an "in and out" movement but is rather an angular manipulation and circumferential rotation around the axis of the needle to reach an optimal position of the needle tip regarding the nerve within the paravertebral space.

Selection of Drug

After a negative aspiration test and administration of a test dose, 0.4 to 0.5 mL/kg of the local anesthetic is injected in toddlers and older children. This dose will usually spread to cover at least five dermatomes. A typical distribution of the block will be unilateral analgesia of the trunk ranging from T4 to T12 (see Fig. 40.46). In neonates and infants, slightly modified dosage regimens are recommended[595,605,606]; these dosages have been found to be both effective and associated with acceptable plasma concentrations of bupivacaine.[605]

Complications

The use of a percutaneous loss-of-resistance technique in a mixed adult and pediatric population was found to be associated with an overall failure rate of approximately 10%, and the complications experienced were hypotension (5%; only adults), vascular puncture (4%), pleural puncture (1%), and pneumothorax (0.5%).[607] The risk for block failure is reduced to less than 5% when a nerve-stimulator–guided technique is used, and this technique also appears to be associated with a reduced risk for complications.[604,608] Total spinal,[609] pulmonary hemorrhage,[610] and a variety of unintended nerve blocks have been rarely reported.[611–613] Use of ultrasound guidance may further improve success while reducing complications.

UPPER EXTREMITY BLOCKS

Brachial Plexus Block

Of the four techniques used to block the brachial plexus (axillary, infraclavicular, supraclavicular, and interscalene), the axillary approach is most commonly used in children when using nerve-stimulation or landmark approaches.[614] Advantages include ease of insertion, a high rate of success in experienced hands, and low morbidity. The block is also well suited for orthopedic or plastic surgical repairs on the hand or forearm in a child with a full stomach.[615,616] In the latter situation, the child is at greater risk for aspiration of gastric contents with deeper levels of sedation, an intravascular injection, or a drug overdose. Because it is unnecessary to elicit a sensory paresthesia, the block can also be performed in an anesthetized child for postoperative pain management.

With the use of ultrasound guidance, infraclavicular, supraclavicular, and interscalene blocks have largely supplanted the axillary block in children. The infraclavicular or supraclavicular blocks are our preferred technique for the placement of a continuous catheter in the postoperative period. Unintentional block of the phrenic and recurrent laryngeal nerves is much more common in young children because these nerves are close to the site of injection, especially with an interscalene block. Data suggest that some degree of phrenic nerve blockade is present with every interscalene block.[617,618] Phrenic nerve blockade may cause respiratory failure in very young children whose breathing depends almost completely on the diaphragm, whereas blockade of the recurrent laryngeal nerve will paralyze the vocal cords and increase airway resistance. The risk of pneumothorax is greater because the apex of the lung is situated more rostral in infants and small children, especially on the left side. Total spinal anesthesia is also more likely with the interscalene approach to brachial plexus blockade.[619] An ultrasound may also be used in conjunction with a nerve stimulator to further improve the localization of each nerve bundle (Figs. 40.52–40.55).[616] Because assessments of neurological function may be needed following some operations of the upper extremity, it is a advisable to check with the surgeon about whether an upper extremity block is contraindicated.

Anatomy

The brachial plexus arises in the neck from spinal nerves C5, C6, C7, C8, and T1, passes between the clavicle and first rib, and extends into the axilla. At that point, the axillary artery is surrounded by a narrow fascial sheath that contains the median nerve anteriorly, the ulnar nerve posteriorly, and the radial nerve on the posterolateral aspect (see Fig. 40.52). In children, the axillary artery and, at times, the axillary sheath itself may be palpable.

Ultrasound-Guided Axillary Brachial Plexus Block

Ultrasound-guided axillary brachial plexus block is typically performed with the child in the supine position.[620–622] The arm is abducted (to 90 degrees) and externally rotated so that the palm of the hand is facing up. The operator sits at the ipsilateral head end of the child, and the ultrasound machine is positioned directly in front (see Fig. 40.16). Because the nerves of the brachial plexus are relatively superficial in the axilla, a high-frequency linear-array transducer (13-6 MHz) is used. During the scout scan, the transducer is positioned just below the lateral border of the pectoralis major muscle, with its orientation marker directed laterally (see Fig. 40.52). The resultant image on the monitor is a transverse scan of the axillary structures. The pulsatile vessel in the image is the axillary artery. The axillary vein is medial to the artery; it is common to see more than one vein (Fig. 40.53).

At this level, the three major nerves of the brachial plexus (the median, ulnar, and radial nerves) lie very close to the axillary artery. In adults, when the arm is abducted and externally rotated, the median nerve is located on the anterior or anterolateral side of the axillary artery (97.9%), the ulnar nerve is located on the anteromedial side of the artery (91.3%), and the radial nerve is located posterior to the axillary artery (89.9%)[623] (see Fig. 40.54). To accurately identify these three nerves, it may be necessary to trace the nerve distally along its course. The musculocutaneous nerve frequently courses between the coracobrachialis and the biceps muscle or within the substance of the coracobrachialis muscle (see Fig. 40.54).[624,625] Occasionally, the musculocutaneous nerve also may be located very close to the median nerve, and local anesthetic injected close to the median nerve may affect the musculocutaneous nerve. The shape of the musculocutaneous nerve varies along its course, and it may appear oval, round, elliptical, or even triangular.

We prefer the in-plane approach for needle insertion during axillary brachial plexus block in both sedated and anesthetized children. The block needle is inserted from the lateral to the medial side of the arm, keeping it within the plane of the ultrasound imaging. A subtle pop is often felt when the tip of the needle traverses the epimysium of the biceps muscle and enters the fascial plane containing the neurovascular bundle. Multiple injections are required to block the median, radial, and ulnar nerves. The objective is to produce a circumferential spread of local anesthetic around the artery (i.e., "the doughnut sign" in the ultrasound image). To achieve this, local anesthetic is injected close to the anterior (12-o'clock position), posterior (6-o'clock position), and lateral (9-o'clock position) aspects of the axillary artery. The musculocutaneous nerve is then identified and selectively blocked using a few milliliters of local anesthetic. We have found this approach to be technically simple, safe, and effective in producing brachial plexus blockade in children (Video 40.20).

Landmark-Guided Axillary Brachial Plexus Block

Several techniques can be used to establish that the needle is within the axillary sheath. The first is by eliciting a sensory paresthesia with the needle, but this has little application in pediatric practice, particularly in young children and in those who are anesthetized. The use of a nerve stimulator allows precise placement of the needle in the neurovascular sheath without either the cooperation of the child or the need for painful sensory paresthesias (see Fig. 40.17). In thin children, the sheath can often be palpated as a cord-like structure inferior to the coracobrachialis muscle, allowing the placement of the needle in the sheath by "feel." A transarterial approach can also be used.[626] With all techniques, it is useful to attach a short piece of extension tubing between the needle and syringe to facilitate precise handling during needle placement, aspiration, and drug injection.

The use of a nerve stimulator for the axillary approach to the brachial plexus is best accomplished by abducting the arm to 90 degrees (see E-Fig. 40.3). Care should be taken not to hyperabduct the arm and obscure the axillary pulse. The artery is palpated in the axilla, and a short-beveled needle is advanced toward it (see Fig. 40.52B,C). When using a nerve stimulator, a distal motor response is elicited in the distribution of the radial, ulnar, or median nerves at a threshold of less than 0.2 mA (see E-Fig. 40.3). If one is not using a nerve stimulator, the needle is advanced until a distinct pop is felt as the needle pierces the axillary sheath. The axillary sheath may be divided into fascial compartments for each nerve, and these may limit the spread of local anesthetic within the

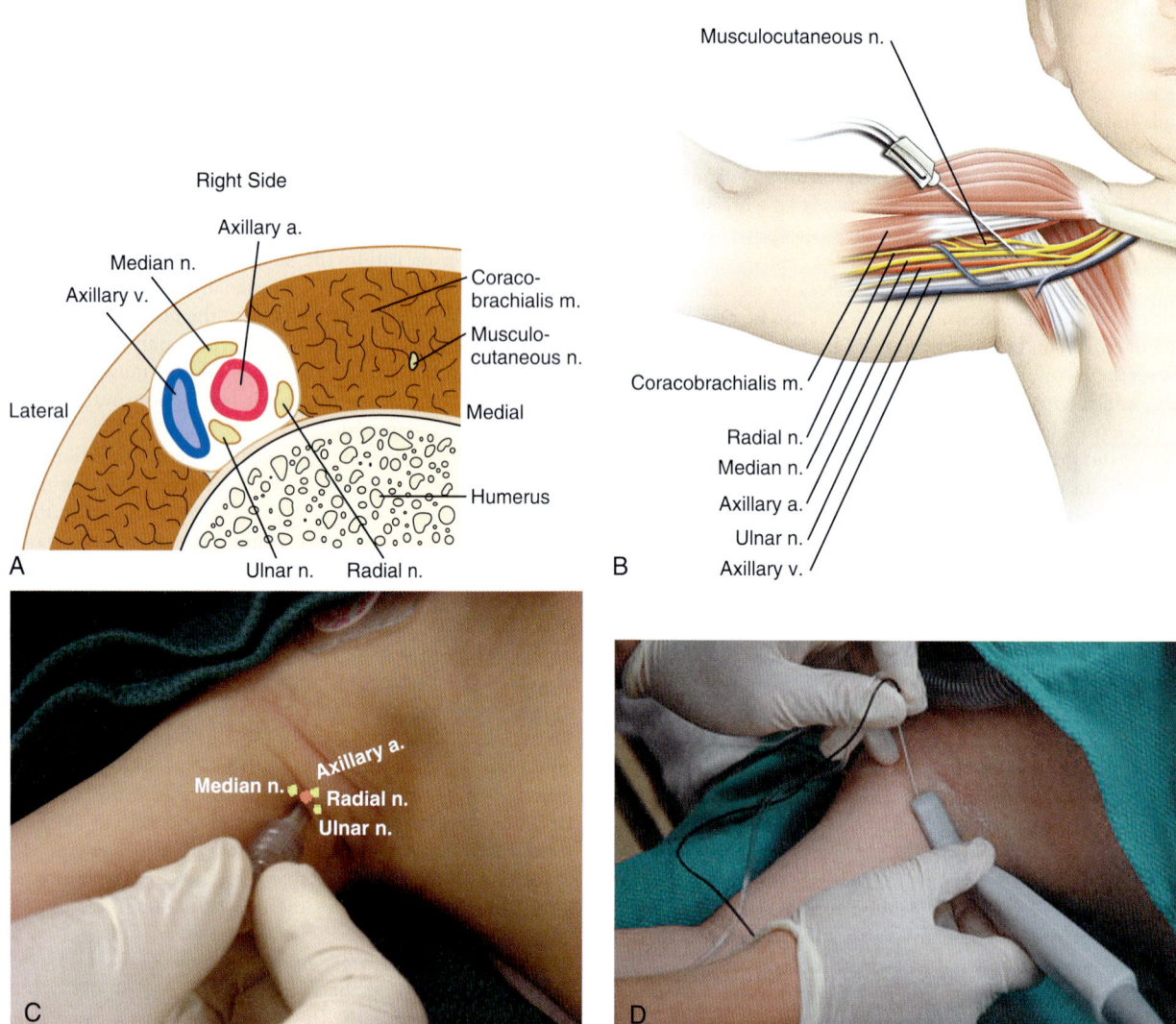

FIGURE 40.52 A and **B,** The anatomic relationships of the brachial plexus are presented. Note that the fascial sheath envelops the nerves and the axillary artery and vein; the musculocutaneous nerve lies within the body of the coracobrachialis muscle. Local anesthetic injected within the sheath (on either side of the axillary artery) produces a satisfactory block. There may be septation within the sheath in some individuals (not pictured). **C,** The axillary artery is palpated with the arm in abduction in the axilla. A needle is introduced superior to the pulsation to block the median nerve. If a nerve stimulator is used, opposition of the thumb can be elicited as the median nerve is stimulated. The needle is then gently positioned below the artery; the ulnar nerve can be blocked in this position. If a nerve stimulator is used, flexion of the fifth finger is elicited. For blocking the radial nerve situated posterior to the artery, it may be necessary to pass the needle posterior to the artery while constantly aspirating to avoid intravascular placement. If the needle does encounter the axillary artery, continue to advance the needle so that the aspirate is negative while the needle is situated posterior to the artery. If a nerve stimulator is used, biceps flexion may be observed. A total volume of 0.1 to 0.15 mL/kg in divided doses between all three nerves will provide an adequate blockade of the nerves. If the axillary artery is encountered while accessing the radial nerve, it is imperative to apply pressure after the block is placed to avoid hematoma formation. **D,** An ultrasound is particularly useful for successful placement of an axillary block. A linear ultrasound probe or a hockey stick probe is placed on the axilla. With the use of an in-plane approach, the median nerve (located anterior to the artery), then the radial nerve (located posterior to the axillary artery), and then the ulnar nerve (located below the artery) are blocked individually. Careful aspiration before injection may prevent intravascular injection. *a.,* Artery; *m.,* muscle; *n.,* nerve; *v.,* vein.

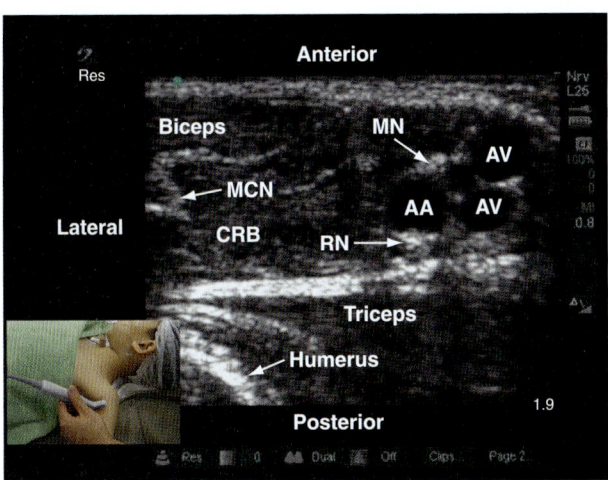

FIGURE 40.53 Transverse sonogram of the left axilla. *AA,* Axillary artery; *AV,* axillary vein; *CRB,* coracobrachialis muscle; *Res,* resolution; *RN,* radial nerve.

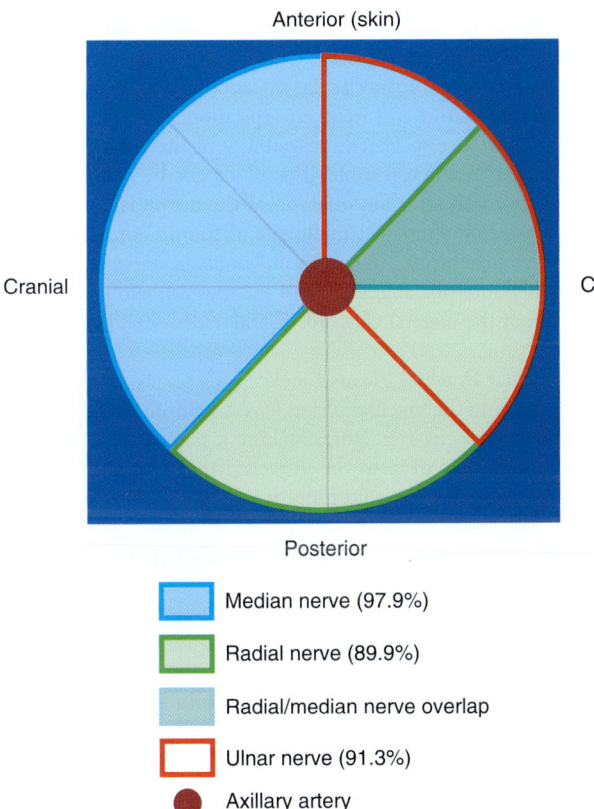

Median nerve (97.9%)

Radial nerve (89.9%)

Radial/median nerve overlap

Ulnar nerve (91.3%)

Axillary artery

FIGURE 40.54 Schematic diagram showing the positions of the three main nerves (median, radial, and ulnar) of the brachial plexus in relation to the axillary artery, as identified on transverse ultrasonography, in the axilla.

axillary sheath. Although distinct paresthesias to the distribution of all three nerves may be elicited with the nerve stimulator, and divided doses of anesthetic may be administered to each of those locations, in practice it becomes extremely difficult to find the second and third motor paresthesia after the administration of even a very small amount of local anesthetic with the first injection (Video 40.21). Alternatively, the transarterial technique, which involves direct puncture of the axillary artery, allows deposition of

local anesthetic at two sites within the sheath. The needle is aimed directly toward the axillary pulse. As soon as blood is aspirated, the needle is advanced through the posterior wall of the artery. When blood can no longer be aspirated, half of the dose of local anesthetic is deposited posterior to the artery. The needle is withdrawn through the anterior wall of the artery, and the remainder of the dose is deposited anterior to the artery after reconfirming a negative aspiration for blood. Regardless of technique, the local anesthetic is administered in incremental quantities with intermittent aspiration to confirm that the needle is still outside the artery. It is sometimes difficult to block the musculocutaneous nerve, which carries sensory fibers to the radial aspect of the forearm, because it exits the brachial plexus proximal in the axillary fossa. Therefore, some practitioners advocate applying a tourniquet distal to the site where the block is to be performed. Applying a tourniquet promotes proximal spread of local anesthetic and enhances the chances of a successful block of this nerve. Alternatively, the musculocutaneous nerve may be blocked by infiltrating 1 to 3 milliliters (proportional to the size of the child) of local anesthetic into the body of the coracobrachialis muscle. Regardless of the technique chosen, an additional 1 to 3 milliliters of local anesthetic is deposited as a subcutaneous cuff to block the intercostobrachial nerve and its communications with the musculocutaneous nerve. These additional quantities of local anesthetic must be accounted for when calculating the total drug dose.

Supraclavicular Brachial Plexus Block

This is an easy approach to the brachial plexus in children and can be readily performed, particularly with the aid of ultrasound guidance. The risk of performing this procedure without ultrasound guidance is the potential for injection into the vertebral artery. It can be used for most procedures performed on the upper arm and forearm. The cervical pleura is also located close to the supraclavicular plexus; caution should be exercised while performing this block. The entire brachial plexus, including the musculocutaneous and the axillary nerves, is located lateral to the artery. Occasionally, the suprascapular nerve may leave the upper trunk more cranially.

Indications

This block is used for analgesia or anesthesia for upper arm surgery and can be performed with either a single-injection or catheter technique.

Ultrasound-Guided Supraclavicular Brachial Plexus Block

In the era before ultrasound-guided blocks, the supraclavicular brachial plexus block in children[627] was rarely used because of fear of pleural puncture and pneumothorax. However, ultrasound-guided supraclavicular brachial plexus block has been performed in children younger than 6 years of age, and it and infraclavicular blocks are now the most common pediatric upper extremity blocks.[628] Even though the brachial plexus and cervical pleura are clearly delineated using ultrasound in the supraclavicular fossa, this technique should be performed by experienced operators because of the close proximity between the cervical pleura and the brachial plexus.

The child's head rests on a head ring and is slightly turned to the contralateral side, and a small roll is placed between the scapula. For a right-sided block, a right-handed operator stands or sits at the head end of the child, and the ultrasound machine is placed directly in front on the ipsilateral side (see Fig. 40.16). The position of the operator and ultrasound machine is reversed for a left-sided block.

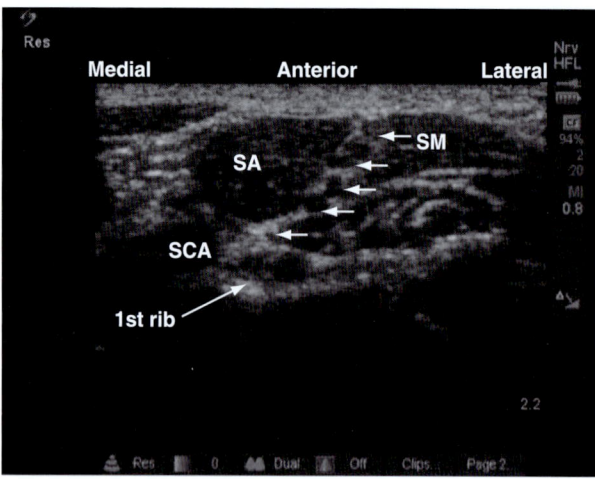

FIGURE 40.55 Sonographic appearance of the brachial plexus *(white arrows)* in the supraclavicular fossa. *SA,* Scalenus anterior; *SCA,* subclavian artery; *SM,* scalenus medius.

In the supraclavicular fossa, the subclavian artery lies on top of the first rib. The trunks and divisions of the brachial plexus are superficial and lateral to the subclavian artery and sandwiched between the scalenus anterior and scalenus medius muscle (see Fig. 40.55). A linear-array transducer (13-10 MHz) is used to perform the block; the hockey stick probe or a linear-array transducer with a small footprint (25 mm) is particularly suited for this block.

During the scout scan, the transducer is positioned parallel to and against the clavicle and the subclavian artery is identified. The trunks and divisions of the brachial plexus often resemble a bunch of grapes on the superficial and lateral aspect of the subclavian artery (see Fig. 40.55). The cervical pleura and lung are deep to the first rib. The operator should bear in mind that the acoustic shadow of the first rib can obscure the view of the pleura and lung. The block needle is inserted in the long axis (in-plane) of the transducer in a lateral to medial direction, keeping the pleura in view. A test injection with saline solution is performed to ensure optimal needle position, after which the calculated dose of local anesthetic is injected in aliquots. We have been able to decrease the dose of local anesthetic solution to 0.15 to 0.2 mL/kg, allowing visualization of the "doughnut" of injectate to guide the necessary volume, although missing the musculocutaneous nerve might be a consequence of low drug volumes.

Landmark-Guided Supraclavicular Brachial Plexus Block
Owing to the considerations noted above, the nerve-stimulating landmark technique should be used with considerable caution, and ultrasound guidance is the preferred method for blocking the supraclavicular plexus. The supraclavicular plexus is located above the clavicle and is approximately at the middle of the sternocleidomastoid. A stimulating needle (1 mA) is passed above the clavicle lateral to the arterial pulsation and close to the inferior margin of the anterior scalene. The plexus is located superficially and can be easily stimulated as soon as the skin is pierced. Any movement of the child's fingers or arm is accepted as an adequate stimulation to the plexus. The energy is reduced to 0.4 mA and, if continued response to the stimulation is observed, 0.15 to 0.2 mL/kg of local anesthetic solution is injected in graduated doses after careful aspiration (Video 40.22; see also Fig. 40.55).

Selection of Drug
Local anesthetics commonly used in our practice include ropivacaine and bupivacaine (see Table 40.2). Although block of the musculocutaneous nerve can be more effective with large volumes (0.5 mL/kg), separate ultrasound targeting of that nerve can also be performed.[625] One report of ultrasound-guided blocks found that the median effective volume of 0.2% ropivacaine was 0.15 mL/kg.[629] Care must always be taken not to exceed the maximal allowable doses of bupivacaine on a milligram per kilogram basis (2.5 mg/kg).[630] Adding epinephrine (1:200,000) may decrease vascular absorption and the potential for toxicity. Sodium bicarbonate (1 mEq/10 mL of local anesthetic) added to the local anesthetic will speed the onset of blockade by increasing the pH of the solution; this is particularly the case with the premixed anesthetic-epinephrine formulations that have a reduced pH.

Complications
Pleural puncture (pneumothorax) and intravascular injection can occur from misplacement of the needle. All the nerves of the brachial plexus occupy a neurovascular bundle and hence are prone to unintended injection into a blood vessel. A hematoma may form at the site of injection. If it is large enough, the hematoma may compress the neurovascular bundle, rendering the limb ischemic. It is important to know the child's coagulation status before attempting the block. Intravascular injection may be avoided with incremental injection and frequent aspiration. Practitioners may feel the importance to check the viability of the radial, median, and ulnar nerves when feasible. This block can be carried out in the recovery room after the function of the nerves is determined in cooperative children. A simple rule of thumb is to check the radial nerve (extension of the thumb), median nerve (flexion of the proximal interphalangeal joint of the thumb), and ulnar nerve (scissoring of the fingers) (Fig. 40.17 and Video 40.23).[631]

Infraclavicular Brachial Plexus Block
This approach to the brachial plexus is very helpful, particularly in children who may have fractures making it painful to abduct the arm. A vertical approach to the infraclavicular brachial plexus is performed using the coracoid process as a landmark to access the nerve.[632] We routinely use this technique in children who require continuous infusions of local anesthetic solution in the postoperative period.

Ultrasound-Guided Infraclavicular Brachial Plexus Block
Ultrasound-guided infraclavicular brachial plexus block is performed with the child in the supine position. The block can be performed with the arms by the side, but it is preferable to abduct the arm (to 90 degrees) whenever possible because it elevates the lateral part of the clavicle, which makes more space available below the clavicle for transducer placement. The operator sits at the ipsilateral head end of the child, and the ultrasound machine is positioned directly in front. Because the cords of the brachial plexus are relatively superficial in the infraclavicular fossa in children, a linear-array transducer (13-10 MHz in young children and 10-7 MHz in the older child) is used to perform the block. The transducer is positioned in the sagittal plane over the deltopectoral region, medial and inferior to the coracoid process, with its orientation marker directed cephalad.

During the scout scan, the second part of the axillary artery and the axillary vein are identified deep to the pectoral muscles (Fig. 40.56). The axillary artery is located superior to the vein, and the cords of the brachial plexus are closely related to the axillary

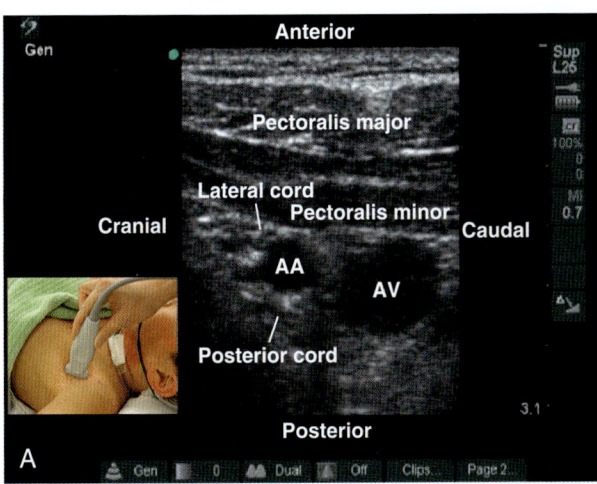
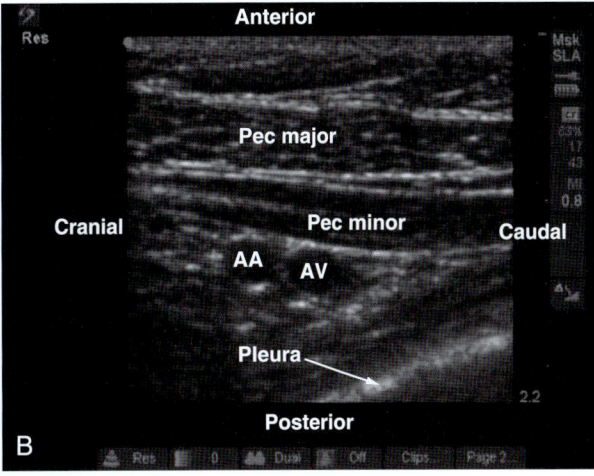

FIGURE 40.56 A, Sagittal sonogram of the left infraclavicular fossa. **B,** Sagittal sonogram of the infraclavicular fossa with the transducer positioned medially. Note the hyperechoic pleura in the lower right corner of the image *(arrow). AA,* Axillary artery; *AV,* axillary vein; *Pec,* pectoralis

artery at this level. The medial cord is situated caudal to the axillary artery, often between the axillary artery and vein, whereas the posterior and lateral cords are posterior and cephalad to the artery, respectively (see Fig. 40.56A). Despite this relation, in most cases it is not easy to identify all three cords of the brachial plexus in a single plane of imaging. If the transducer is moved medially, the pleura usually comes into view (see Fig. 40.56B). In infants and young children, the margin of safety between the cords of the brachial plexus and the pleura is relatively small and pleural puncture is a risk if the block is performed in this medial position. Therefore, we recommend that the infraclavicular brachial plexus block be performed laterally where the pleura is not visible in the ultrasound image.

We prefer to perform multiple injections targeting the areas where the three cords of the brachial plexus are located. The aim is to produce a circumferential spread of the local anesthetic around the axillary artery, the "doughnut sign" (Fig. 40.57), which correlates well with successful brachial plexus anesthesia. This perivascular injection technique is best visualized by imagining the transverse image of the axillary artery as a clock face with its 12-o'clock position in its anterior aspect and the 6-o'clock position in the posterior aspect of the artery (Fig. 40.58). The block needle is inserted in-plane and from a cranial to caudal direction (see Fig. 40.58) and one-third of the total dose of local anesthetic is injected close to each of the posterior (6-o'clock position), lateral (9-o'clock position), and medial (3-o'clock position) cords.[633–639] Because the angle of needle insertion is fairly steep with this approach, the needle is rarely seen on the ultrasound image, and the operator has to gently jiggle the needle to locate the needle tip. A subtle pop may be felt as the needle tip traverses the epimysium of the pectoralis minor muscle. A test injection with 1 milliliter of saline solution should be performed before the local anesthetic injection to ensure optimal needle position and distribution of the injectate (Video 40.24) (see also Fig. 40.52 for landmark-guided techniques).

Landmark-Guided Infraclavicular Brachial Plexus Block

Ultrasound guidance is preferred for this block. With the arm in abduction, the acromial process is palpated. A line drawn 2 centimeters below and medial to the coracoid process is usually where the needle is introduced (Fig. 40.59A). At this level, the pleura is not usually

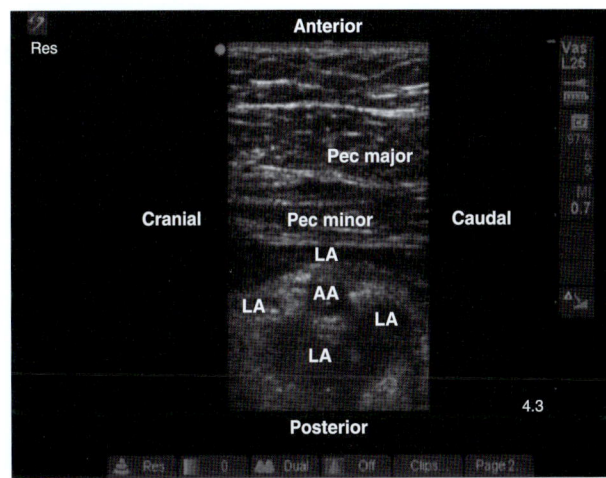

FIGURE 40.57 Infraclavicular brachial plexus block. Sagittal sonogram of the infraclavicular fossa after local anesthetic injection demonstrating the circumferential spread of local anesthetic around the axillary artery—the "doughnut sign." *AA,* Axillary artery; *LA,* local anesthetic; *Pec,* pectoralis.

affected. A sheathed needle with a nerve stimulator is introduced, and the nerve is stimulated at about 1 mA then reduced to 0.4 mA to confirm proximity to the nerve. Any stimulation other than forearm flexion is taken as a positive stimulation of the brachial plexus. Forearm flexion denotes stimulation of the musculocutaneous nerve. The needle should then be directed medial to provide a blockade of the cords of the brachial plexus (Fig. 40.59B).

Complications

There is the potential for intrapleural injection and pneumothorax, especially if the needle is directed medially. Because of the proximity of the plexus to the subclavian vein and artery, it is imperative that the procedure not be attempted on children who have coagulation abnormalities.

Interscalene Approach to the Brachial Plexus

The main indication for this technique is for children undergoing shoulder surgery; this approach is generally reserved for the older teenager or young adult.

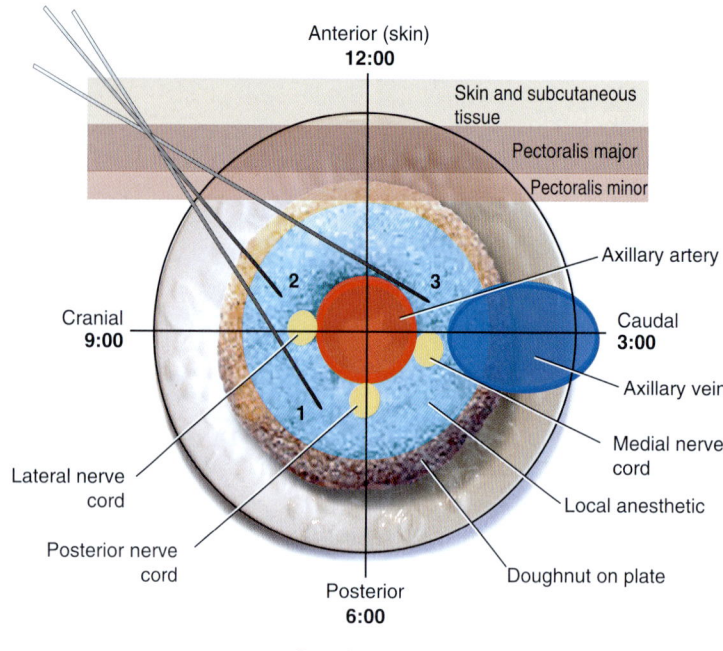

Doughnut sign

FIGURE 40.58 Infraclavicular brachial plexus block (oriented as with a wall clock). Schematic diagram showing the positions of the cords of the brachial plexus and the sites at which the local anesthetic is injected: *(1)* posterior cord, *(2)* lateral cord, and *(3)* medial cord.

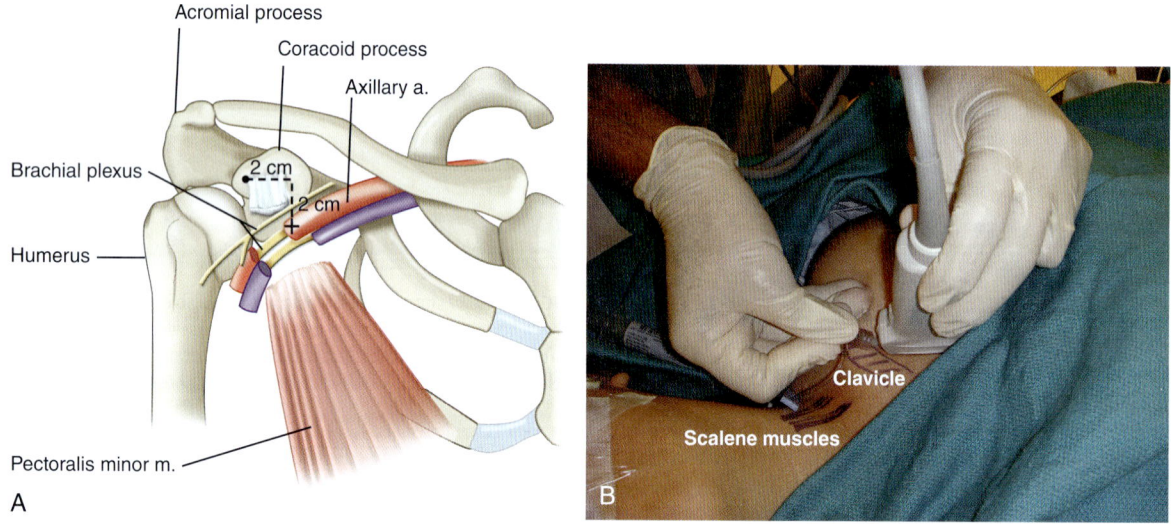

FIGURE 40.59 A, Anatomic landmarks for the infraclavicular approach to the brachial plexus. Note that the arm is in an abducted position, which may be quite useful for children with fractures. **B,** The coracoid process is palpated. With the arm abducted, a needle is inserted 2 cm medial and inferior to the coracoid process. A nerve stimulator is used, and stimulation is initiated at 1 mA and then decreased to 0.4 mA as the nerve is accessed. Elicitation of hand flexion or extension is used as an indicator of being close to the nerve. After aspiration, 0.2 mL/kg of local anesthetic solution is injected. Use of ultrasound may also improve the success of this block. *a.,* Artery; *m.,* muscle. (Modified from Wilson JL, Brown DL, Wong GY, et al. Infraclavicular brachial plexus block: parasagittal anatomy important to the coracoid technique. *Anesth Analg.* 1998;87[4]:870-873.)

Anatomy

The interscalene groove is formed by the anterior and middle scalene muscles and is located in most children at the lateral border of the sternocleidomastoid muscle (Fig. 40.60A). The upper three nerve roots are superficial, whereas the lower two roots are in a deeper position. In children the lower nerve roots are close to the pleura, which may increase the potential for a pneumothorax especially on the left side. The phrenic nerve is also close to the nerve roots and is always unintentionally blocked to some degree on the ipsilateral side. Therefore, this block is clearly avoided in children who may have a compromised pulmonary system. However, a study in adults has shown that employing lower doses, facilitated by ultrasound guidance, can reduce the incidence or severity of phrenic nerve blockade which

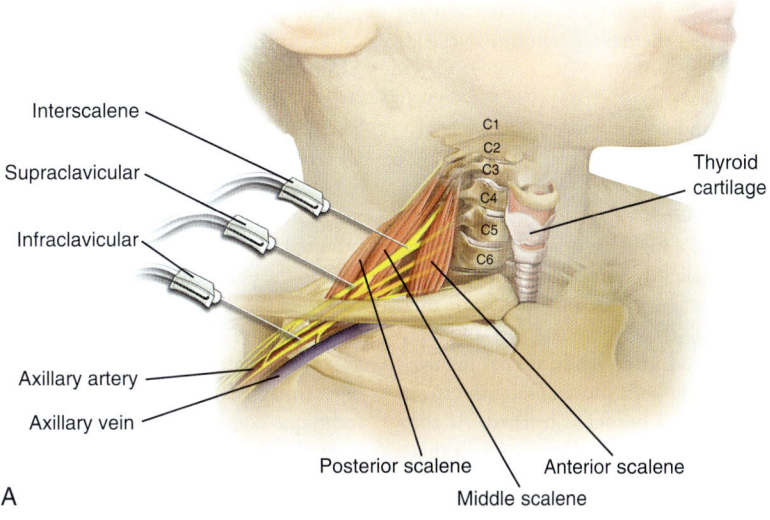

Interscalene

Supraclavicular

Infraclavicular

Axillary artery

Axillary vein

C1
C2
C3
C4
C5
C6

Thyroid cartilage

Posterior scalene

Middle scalene

Anterior scalene

A

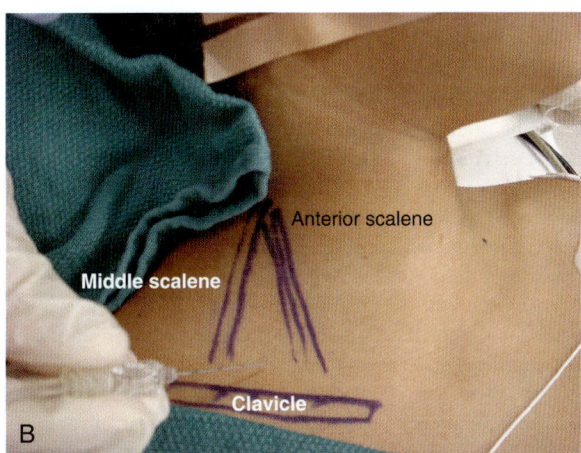

Anterior scalene

Middle scalene

Clavicle

B

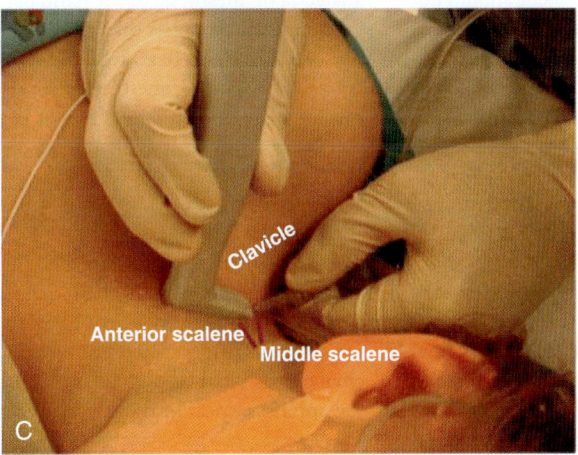

Clavicle

Anterior scalene

Middle scalene

C

FIGURE 40.60 A right-sided supraclavicular block (landmark technique): The supraclavicular block is used frequently in children for most procedures on the hand and elbow. **A,** The divisions and cords are located around the carotid artery cephalad to the clavicle at the inferior margins of the scalene muscles. **B,** A stimulating needle, using 0.5 mA of energy, is introduced at the inferior border of the anterior scalene muscle. Any movement of the patient's fingers (including flexion or extension) suggests adequate positioning of the needle. After aspiration to avoid intravascular injection, 0.15 mL/kg of local anesthetic solution is injected. **C,** Supraclavicular block with ultrasound guidance. A linear ultrasound probe or a hockey stick probe is placed lateral to the suprasternal notch and above the clavicle. The carotid artery is identified. The supraclavicular plexus is located around the carotid artery at this location like a "bunch of grapes." A needle is placed in an in-plane approach (along the axis of the probe), and the plexus is penetrated. Injection of local anesthetic solution will be seen as a hypoechoic spread around the plexus.

can be beneficial in all patients.[639a] The vertebral artery is located in close proximity to the lower nerve roots (C7) and hence it is important to aspirate and ensure that the needle is not in a vessel.

Indications
Shoulder and upper arm surgery and ensuing postoperative analgesia can be provided with this block.

Ultrasound-Guided Interscaline Block
To visualize the anatomic structures, a high-frequency linear probe is used. The process is facilitated by slightly turning the child's head to the contralateral side. The probe should be oriented from the medial to the lateral aspect. Medially, the thyroid gland and the major vessels in the neck area (carotid artery and internal jugular vein) are easily identified. Then the probe is moved along the sternocleidomastoid muscle until its lateral border is reached. At the same time, the transducer is moved in a caudal direction such that the posterior scalene gap and the upper anterior roots (C5–C7) of the brachial plexus become visible between the anterior and medial scalene muscles. In very small children, all roots of the brachial plexus (C5–T1) can be simultaneously visualized. The puncture is performed in a tangential direction relative to the neck above the transducer. The C5 nerve root will be encountered superficially, within a few millimeters. As a rule, the needle should be oriented lateral to the C7 root, which will ensure that the neck vessels remain at an adequate distance from the needle insertion site. As soon as the local anesthetic has been injected, it will spread toward the C5 root, which can be visualized in the ultrasound image. Depending on the blockade required, the needle can be advanced to a deeper level for injection after the deep roots (C8 and T1) have been visualized. If the local anesthetic fails to spread adequately in a medial direction, the needle is retracted toward the subcutaneous level and is then repositioned on the medial side of the posterior scalene gap in the area of the C7 root. In most cases, however, the local anesthetic will spread in an adequate manner even when the needle is in a lateral position. The injected volume of local anesthetic should not exceed the amount necessary to fully cover the root surfaces. It is, therefore, inappropriate to recommend a specific volume. In general, however, complete blockade via the interscalene route can be expected with local anesthetic volumes of 0.15 to 0.25 mL/kg.

Landmark-Guided Interscaline Block
Dalens and associates reported a technique of parascalene brachial plexus blockade for pediatric shoulder surgery using an extended head position and placing the puncture between the lower and middle thirds of the line extending from the center of the clavicle to the C6 transverse process (Chassaignac tubercle; see Fig. 40.60A).[640] The rationale for selecting this puncture site was to avoid the vertebral artery and pleura. With the use of a perpendicular needle orientation, the lower roots (C8 and T1) are not blocked at all or require very large amounts of local anesthetic to be successfully blocked. Ultrasound guidance is greatly advantageous in this situation because it highlights the way for safe blockade of both roots (C8 and T1). With the use of a nerve stimulator, diaphragmatic stimulation may be observed as a result of ventromedial needle position (the phrenic nerve runs ventral to the body of the anterior scalene muscle).

Complications
Pneumothorax, intravascular injection, and temporary phrenic nerve injury are risks of this block. Although performing this block has traditionally been proscribed in patients under general anesthesia, a prospective observational study in children and adolescents found no differences in safety, and we perform this block under general anesthesia when indicated.[641] This prospective study reported one vascular puncture and one postoperative infection in 518 interscalene blocks, 88% of which were ultrasound guided.[641]

SELECTIVE PERIPHERAL NERVE BLOCKS OF THE UPPER EXTREMITY
Selective blockade of the nerves of the upper extremity can be used to rescue incomplete or partial brachial plexus block or provide analgesia or anesthesia over a specific dermatome.[642] It has been successfully used in the emergency department for pain control and interventions involving the hand after trauma.[643] We have also found it to be useful for ultrasound-guided differential nerve blockade in children undergoing ambulatory hand surgery, although more commonly these blocks may be placed by the surgeon under direct vision. Another technique combines an axillary brachial plexus block with a short-acting local anesthetic agent such as lidocaine and a peripheral nerve block (e.g., a median or ulnar nerve block, depending on the dermatomes involved) in the forearm using a long-acting drug (bupivacaine or ropivacaine). Because of the shorter duration of action of lidocaine compared with bupivacaine or ropivacaine, the child regains protective motor function of the elbow fairly quickly after surgery (2 to 4 hours) while still enjoying prolonged postoperative analgesia from distal nerve blockade. All the major nerves of the upper extremity (median, ulnar, and radial) can be identified using high-frequency linear-array transducers (13-10 MHz), and it is possible to selectively block these nerves at various sites along their course with only 1 to 2 milliliters of local anesthetic. In an adult study, the mean 95% effective dose (ED95) of 1% mepivacaine to block the ulnar nerve at the forearm is only 0.7 milliliters.[644] We prefer the in-plane needle insertion technique and use a short-beveled nerve-block needle.

Peripheral Blocks at the Elbow
There is usually no great advantage to blocking the peripheral nerves at the elbow compared with blocking them at the wrist for analgesia or anesthesia of the hand because the forearm is supplied by cutaneous branches that originate in the upper arm. However, on some occasions (e.g., to avoid injections into surgical fields or areas of infection), anesthesia of the hand may be achieved by blocking the appropriate nerves at the elbow because the cutaneous nerve supply to the hand arises at the elbow.

Radial Nerve
Anatomy
The radial nerve supplies the radial side of the dorsum of the hand and the proximal parts of the radial three-and-a-half digits. Block at the elbow is useful for the provision of anesthesia for an arteriovenous fistula. It is also useful to supplement an inadequate brachial plexus block at the axillary level. The radial nerve passes over the anterior aspect of the lateral epicondyle (Fig. 40.61A).

Technique
The intercondylar line is marked. After identification of the biceps tendon, a 27-gauge needle is inserted directly toward the lateral margin of the lateral epicondyle of the humerus. 2.0 to 5.0 milliliters (depending on the child's weight) of bupivacaine (0.25% with epinephrine 1:200,000) is injected into the area (Fig. 40.61B). Ultrasound helps to identify the exact location of the nerves in the forearm.

Ultrasonography
Proximally, the radial nerve is posterior to the brachial artery. It then diverges from the artery to enter the radial (spiral) groove on the

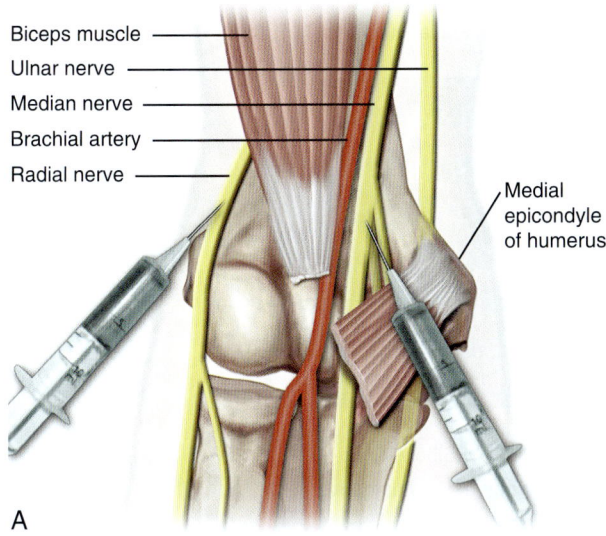

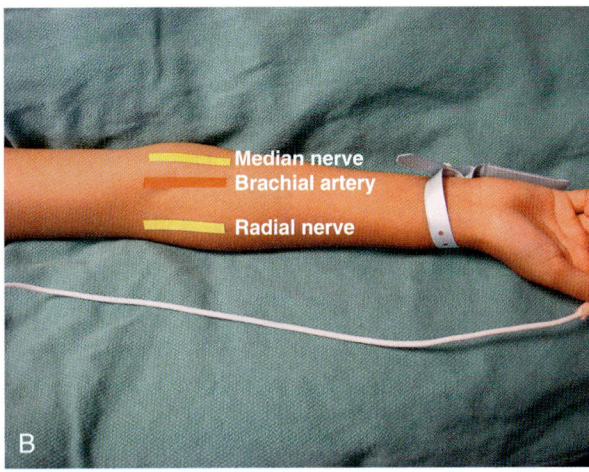

FIGURE 40.61 **A,** Anatomic relationship of the nerves around the elbow. **B,** Radial nerve block: the intercondylar line is marked. After identification of the biceps tendon, a 27-gauge needle is inserted directly toward the bone of the lateral epicondyle toward the lateral margin; 2.0 to 5.0 mL (depending on the patient's weight) of bupivacaine (0.25% with epinephrine 1:200,000) is injected into the area. To block the median nerve, the brachial artery is palpated at the elbow crease. The median nerve is located immediately medial to the brachial artery. A nerve stimulator is used, and flexion of the patient's fingers denotes adequate localization of the nerve.

back of the arm, where it is accompanied by the profunda brachii artery. In the distal arm the radial nerve pierces the lateral intermuscular septum and enters the anterior compartment. In the antecubital fossa it is lateral to the biceps tendon and lies in an intermuscular gap between the brachialis (medially), the brachioradialis, and the extensor carpi radialis longus (laterally) (Fig. 40.62). At the level of the lateral epicondyle, the radial nerve gives off the posterior interosseous nerve (deep branch of the radial nerve), which leaves the fossa by piercing the supinator muscle. In the forearm, the radial nerve (superficial branch of the radial nerve) continues as a pure cutaneous nerve and supplies the radial half of the dorsum of the hand and the proximal parts of the dorsal surfaces of the thumb and index finger. The radial nerve is best blocked before its division in the antecubital fossa.[642]

Complications
Intravascular injection and intraneural injections are potential complications. The use of a nerve stimulator or ultrasound can reduce unintended intraneural injection. Intravascular injection may be avoided with incremental injection and frequent aspirations.

Median Nerve
Anatomy
This nerve supplies the radial side of the palm and the three-and-a-half digits of the palmar aspect (see Fig. 40.61A). It accompanies the brachial artery in its course down the arm. It is initially lateral and then crosses the ventral side of the artery and eventually lies medial to the artery at the bend of the elbow. It is deep to the bicipital fascia and superficial to the brachialis muscle.

Technique
The arm is abducted and the forearm supinated. After marking the intercondylar line between the medial and the lateral epicondyle of the humerus, the brachial artery is palpated (see Fig. 40.61A). A 27-gauge needle is inserted just medial to the artery and directed perpendicular to the skin; 2.0 to 5.0 milliliters (depending on the child's weight) of bupivacaine (0.25% with epinephrine 1:200,000) is injected into the site. Caution must be exercised to avoid the artery because it lies close to the nerve. Surface mapping using a nerve stimulator probe generating 5 mA or greater can locate the nerve in the forearm if it proves difficult to palpate the artery (see Fig. 40.61A).[645]

Ultrasonography
The median nerve is closely related to the brachial artery throughout its course in the arm. Proximally, it is lateral to the artery; in the middle of the upper arm, it crosses to the medial side, and then distally, it continues medially distal to the elbow. In the antecubital fossa, the median nerve lies medial to the brachial artery, behind the bicipital aponeurosis, and in front of the brachialis muscle (see Fig. 40.62A). In the forearm, the median nerve is deep to the flexor digitorum superficialis and on the surface of the flexor digitorum profundus (see Fig. 40.62B) and accompanied by the median artery that is a branch of the anterior interosseous artery. Pulsations of the latter can occasionally be observed on the ultrasound image. A few centimeters proximal to the wrist, the median nerve becomes superficial and lies between the tendon of the flexor carpi radialis (laterally) and the flexor digitorum superficialis (medially) and may also be overlapped by the tendon of the palmaris longus. Because the nerve is superficial at this level and it can be difficult to differentiate the nerve from the tendons, we prefer to perform median nerve block at the midforearm, where it is clearly delineated (Video 40.25).

Complications
Intravascular injection and intraneural injections are potential complications. The use of a nerve stimulator can prevent unintended intraneural injection. Intravascular injection may be avoided with incremental injections and frequent aspirations.

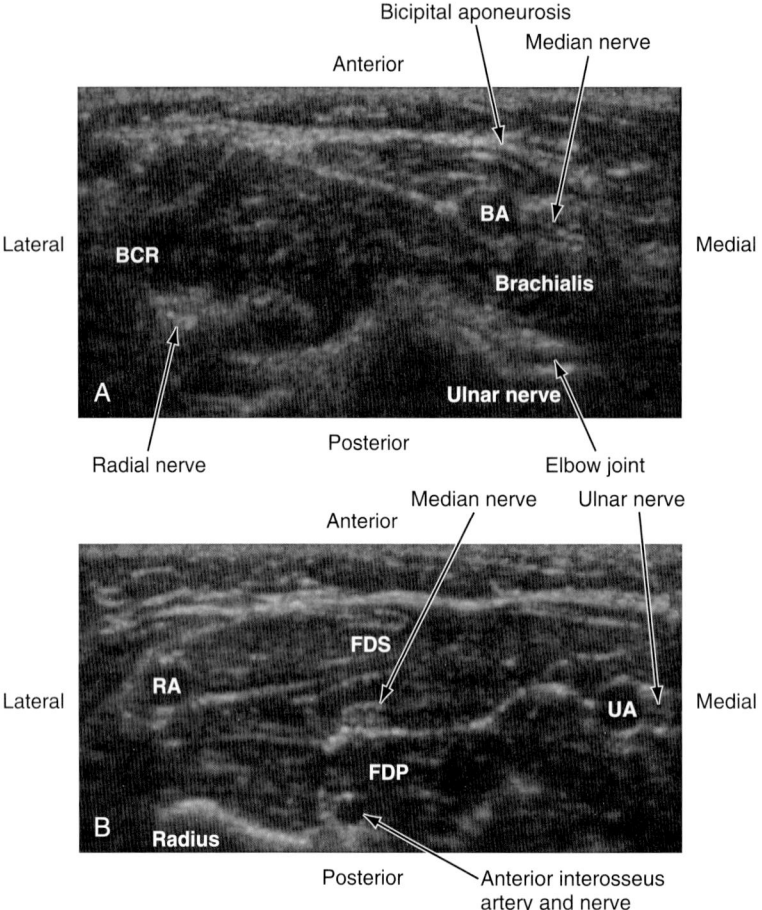

FIGURE 40.62 A, Transverse sonogram of the cubital fossa. **B,** Transverse sonogram of the forearm. *BA,* Brachial artery; *BCR,* brachioradialis; *FDP,* flexor digitorum profundus; *FDS,* flexor digitorum superficialis; *RA,* radial artery; *UA,* ulnar artery.

Ulnar Nerve

Anatomy

The ulnar nerve is the superficial nerve to the arm and the ulnar side of the forearm and the hand. It is the terminal continuation of the medial cord of the brachial plexus. At the elbow, it pierces the medial intermuscular septum and follows along the medial head of the triceps to the groove between the olecranon and the medial epicondyle of the humerus. It is covered only by skin and fascia and can be easily palpated and blocked at this level (see Figs. 40.61 and 40.63).

Ultrasound-Guided Ulnar Nerve Block at the Elbow

Proximally, the ulnar nerve runs medial to the brachial artery to about the midhumeral level or the insertion of the coracobrachialis muscle, where it pierces the medial intermuscular septum and enters the posterior compartment of the arm. At the elbow, it passes behind the medial epicondyle to enter the ulnar nerve sulcus. Although the nerve is palpable and superficial at the sulcus, it is often difficult to visualize using ultrasound because of bony and contact artifacts. The ulnar nerve then enters the proximal forearm and runs between the flexor digitorum profundus (posterior) and the flexor digitorum superficialis (laterally) muscles, and in the distal forearm it is accompanied by the ulnar artery (lateral) (see Fig. 40.62B). Close to the wrist, the ulnar nerve is lateral to the flexor carpi ulnaris muscle. The ulnar artery may be used as a

reference to locate the ulnar nerve. Once the artery is located, the nerve is traced backward and the local anesthetic injected away from the artery (see Video 40.25).[646]

Landmark-Guided Ulnar Nerve Block at the Elbow

With the child supine, the elbow is flexed. The medial epicondyle and the ulnar groove are palpated (see Fig. 40.63). A 27-gauge needle is advanced perpendicular to the skin along the line of the nerve; 1 to 3 milliliters (depending on the child's weight) of bupivacaine (0.25% with epinephrine 1:200,000) is injected into the area. An ultrasound-guided technique may also be used for this block (see Fig. 40.62).

Complications

Intravascular injection and intraneural injections are potential complications. Because this is a very superficial nerve, injection just after the skin is pierced in the area of the ulnar nerve usually produces a good block. Intravascular injection may be avoided with incremental injection and frequent aspiration.

Wrist Blocks

Blocking the median, radial, and ulnar nerves at the wrist can be easily achieved without the aid of ultrasound. These blocks provide very good analgesia and, because they are easy to perform, they generally have a predictable successful outcome.

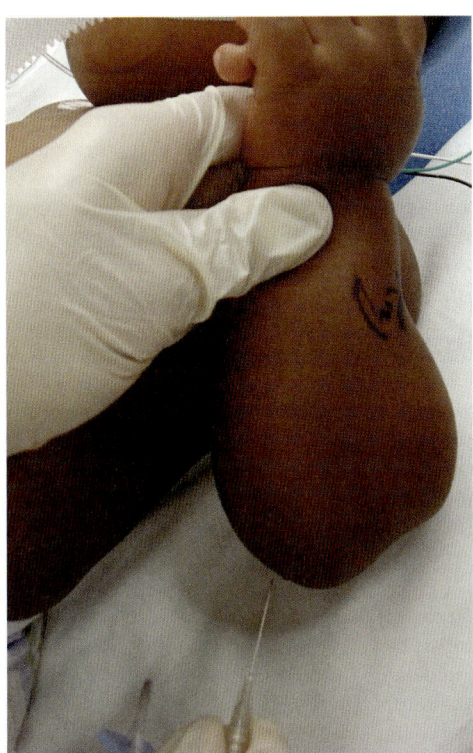

FIGURE 40.63 Ulnar nerve block at the elbow. The olecranon process is palpated. The ulnar nerve is located in the olecranon groove; after aspiration, 1 to 3 mL of local anesthetic solution is injected. It is important not to deposit the local anesthetic deep into the olecranon groove because the nerve is superficial and can be easily blocked by a subcutaneous injection.

Radial Nerve at the Wrist

The cutaneous branches of the radial nerve supply the radial side of the dorsum of the hand and the proximal parts of the radial three-and-a-half digits.

ANATOMY. The superficial branch of the radial nerve runs along the lateral border of the forearm under the brachioradialis muscle. In the distal third of the forearm, it angles dorsally under the tendon of the brachioradialis toward the dorsum of the wrist. It pierces the deep fascia and divides into two branches: (1) the lateral branch supplies the radial side and the tip of the thumb, and (2) the medial branch communicates with the dorsal branch of the ulnar nerve. This then divides into the four digital nerves that supply the ulnar side of the thumb, the radial side of the index finger, and the space between the index finger and thumb. A communicating branch with the ulnar nerve supplies the adjacent sides of the middle and ring finger.

TECHNIQUE. This is essentially a field block of the superficial terminal branches. An attempt to make the "anatomic snuffbox" prominent by extension of the thumb before anesthesia is desirable (Fig. 40.64A). The extensor pollicis and brevis tendons are marked. A 27-gauge needle is inserted close to the dorsal radial tubercle over the extensor longus tendon, and 2.0 milliliters of bupivacaine (0.25% with epinephrine 1:200,000) is injected SC. An attempt to fan the local anesthetic in the anatomic snuffbox helps to distribute the local anesthetic over the radial nerve (Fig. 40.64B).

COMPLICATIONS. Intravascular injection may be avoided with incremental injection and frequent aspiration. Post–nerve block dysesthesia may be occasionally experienced with a radial nerve block and is usually self-limited.

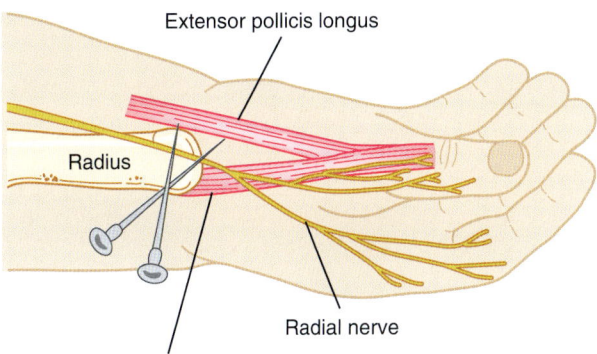

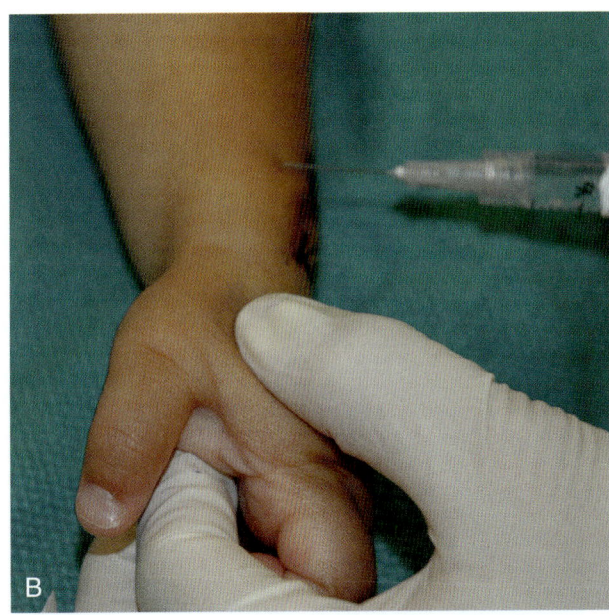

FIGURE 40.64 Wrist block: radial nerve. **A,** This is a superficial block of the terminal branches of the radial nerve. An attempt to make the "anatomic snuffbox" prominent by extension of the thumb before anesthesia is desirable. The extensor pollicis and brevis tendons are marked. **B,** A 27-gauge needle is inserted close to the dorsal radial tubercle over the extensor longus tendon; bupivacaine (2 mL, 0.25% with 1:200,000 epinephrine) is injected subcutaneously. Fanning the local anesthetic in the anatomic snuffbox helps to distribute the local anesthetic over the radial nerve. (Modified from Raj P, Pai U. Techniques of nerve blocking. In: Raj P, ed. *Handbook of Regional Anesthesia*. New York: Churchill Livingstone; 1985:185.)

Median Nerve at the Wrist

ANATOMY. In the palm of the hand, the median nerve is very superficial and is covered only by skin and the palmar aponeurosis and rests on the tendons of the flexor muscles. It emerges from under the retinaculum and splits into muscular and digital branches. The muscular division of the median nerve supplies the muscles of the thenar eminence. The palmar digital nerve supplies the thumb, index finger, middle finger, and ring finger. These nerves also supply the lumbricals (Fig. 40.65A).

TECHNIQUE. The palmaris tendon is identified. This may be done before general anesthesia by asking the child to flex the wrist against resistance. The radial border of the tendon is identified. Cutaneous landmarks include both distal wrist skin creases. A 27-gauge needle is inserted at the level of the second skin crease (1–1.5 cm proximal to the distal crease in teenagers) perpendicular to the skin. The nerve is at a depth of less than 1 centimeters

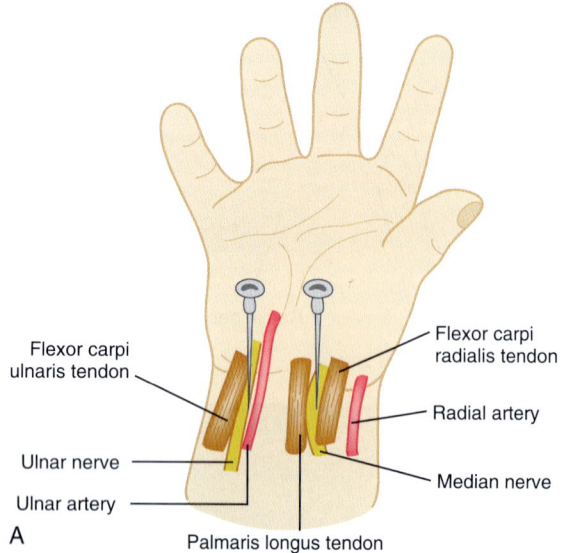

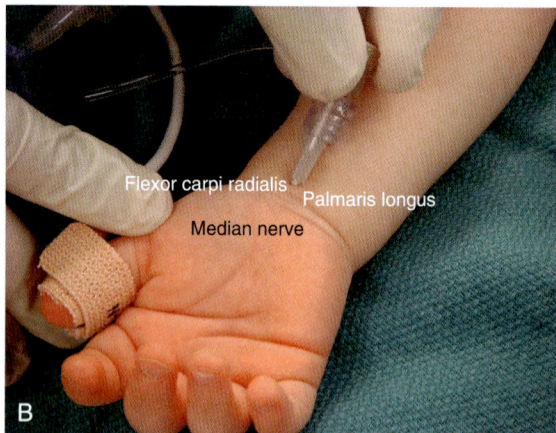

FIGURE 40.65 Wrist block: median and ulnar nerves. **A,** Median nerve: identify the palmaris tendon by asking the child to flex the wrist against resistance. Distal skin creases are identified. **B,** A 27-gauge needle is inserted at the level of the distal skin crease perpendicular to the skin. The nerve is at a depth of less than 1 cm in teenagers and less than that in younger children; 1.0 to 2.0 mL of bupivacaine (0.25% with 1:200.000 epinephrine) is injected in the area. If the child is awake, it is better to elicit paresthesias because the needle may be anterior to the neurovascular bundle, which can be missed altogether. Ulnar nerve: identify the flexor carpi ulnaris tendon, which lies proximal to the pisiform bone. A 27-gauge needle is inserted just proximal to the pisiform bone and directed radially a distance of approximately 0.5 cm. Bupivacaine (2–3 mL, 0.25% with epinephrine 1:200,000) is injected. (Modified from Raj P, Pai U. Techniques of nerve blocking. In: Raj P, ed. *Handbook of Regional Anesthesia.* New York: Churchill Livingstone; 1985:185.)

in the teenager and less in younger children; 1.0 to 2.0 milliliters of bupivacaine (0.25% with epinephrine 1:200,000) is injected into the area (see Fig. 40.26B). If the child is awake, it is better to elicit paresthesias because the needle may be anterior to the neurovascular bundle and the nerve could be missed altogether.

COMPLICATIONS. Intravascular placement should be avoided by repeated aspiration before injection.

Ulnar Nerve at the Wrist

ANATOMY. The palmar cutaneous branch of the ulnar nerve arises near the middle of the forearm and accompanies the ulnar artery into the hand (see Fig. 40.65A). It then perforates the flexor

retinaculum and ends in the skin of the palm communicating with the palmar branch of the median nerve. There are two dorsal digital nerves and a metacarpal communicating branch. The more medial digital nerve supplies the ulnar side of the little finger, and the digital branch supplies the adjacent sides of the little and ring finger. The palmar or the terminal portion of the ulnar nerve crosses the ulnar border of the wrist in company with the ulnar artery.

TECHNIQUE. Blocking the ulnar nerve at the wrist is easier than at the elbow. The nerve is blocked at the wrist, where it lies under cover of the flexor carpi ulnaris tendon just proximal to the pisiform bone. The best way to access the nerve is to approach it from the ulnar side of the tendon. A 27-gauge needle is inserted just proximal to the pisiform bone and directed radially a distance of approximately 0.5 centimeters; 2.0 to 3.0 milliliters of bupivacaine (0.25% with epinephrine 1:200,000) is injected (see Fig. 40.65A).

COMPLICATIONS. The ulnar artery runs in close proximity to the ulnar nerve; every possible effort should be made to avoid intravascular placement. Intravascular injection may be avoided with incremental injection with frequent aspiration.

Digital Nerve Blocks: Hand
Digital nerve blocks are useful for providing pain relief to children who are undergoing procedures to individual fingers. These are useful for postoperative analgesia in procedures, such as trigger finger release, and also for the provision of pain relief in children undergoing laser therapy for warts on their fingers.[647]

Anatomy
The common digital nerves are derived from the median and ulnar nerves and divide in the palm to volar digital nerves that supply the fingers. All digital nerves are usually accompanied by digital vessels. There are three digital nerves derived from the median nerve. The first common digital nerve divides into three palmar digital nerves that supply the sides of the thumb; the second common digital nerve supplies the web between the index and middle finger; and the third common palmar digital nerve communicates with a branch of the ulnar nerve and supplies the web space between the middle and ring fingers. These common digital nerves then become the proper digital nerves (digital collaterals) that supply the skin of the palmar surface and the dorsal side of the terminal phalanx of their respective digits. All digital nerves ultimately terminate in two branches: one ramifies in the skin of the fingertips and the other ends in the pulp under the nail. Smaller digital nerves are derived from the radial and ulnar nerves and supply the back of the fingers. These tend to lie on the dorsolateral aspect of the finger. There are four dorsal digital nerves: (1) ulnar side of the thumb; (2) radial side of the index finger; (3) adjacent sides of index and middle fingers; and (4) communication to the adjacent sides of middle and ring finger.

Technique
There are two techniques for blockade of the digital nerves.

For blockade at the base of the thumb (Fig. 40.66A,B), with the thumb extended, on the palmar surface of the hand, a 27-gauge needle is inserted into the web space between the index finger and thumb. The needle is advanced to the junction of the web space and the palmar skin of the hand, a distance of about 1 centimeter; 0.5 milliliters of bupivacaine *without epinephrine* is injected. A second needle is inserted into the thenar eminence on the radial aspect of the thumb; 1.0 milliters of bupivacaine *without epinephrine* is injected. Caution must be exercised if the child has collagen vascular disease, because this may precipitate acute vascular spasm that may not be relieved.

40

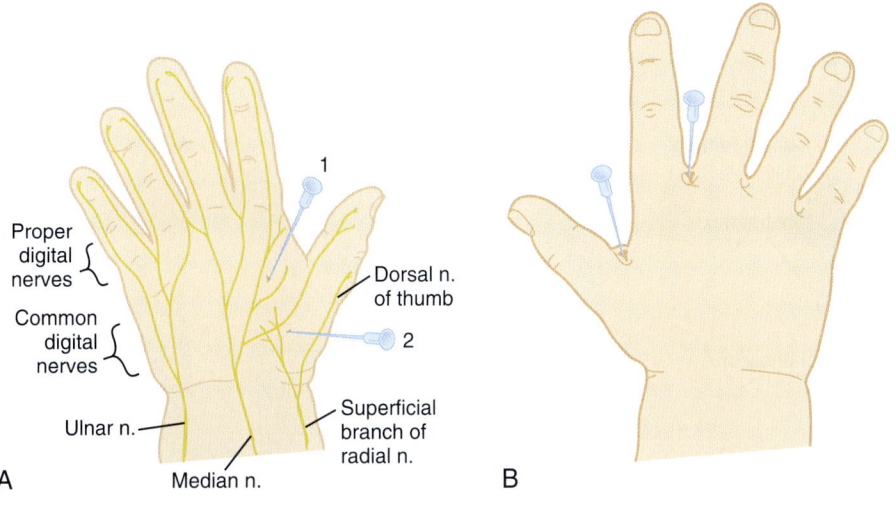

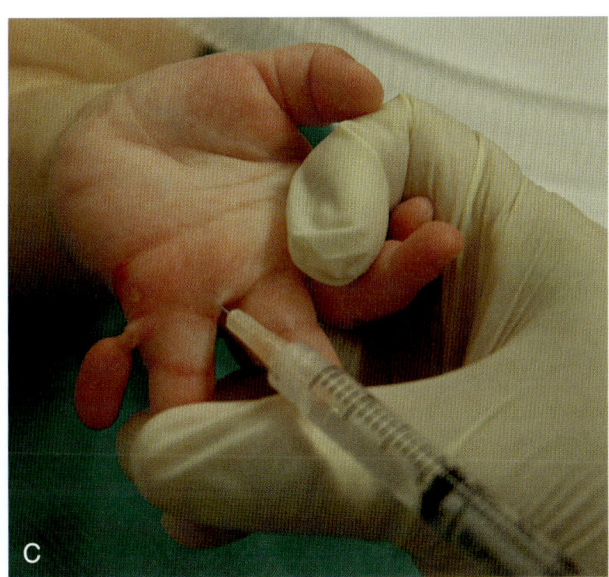

FIGURE 40.66 Digital nerve blocks. **A,** Blockade of the thumb: with the thumb extended, on the palmar surface of the hand, a 27-gauge needle is inserted into the web space between the index finger and thumb *(1)*. The needle is advanced to the junction of the web space and the palmar skin of the hand a distance of about 1 cm; bupivacaine (0.5 mL, *without epinephrine*) is injected. A second needle is inserted into the thenar eminence on the radial aspect of the thumb, and 1.0 mL of bupivacaine *without epinephrine* is injected *(2)*. Caution must be exercised if the patient has collagen vascular disease because this may precipitate acute vascular spasm that may not be relieved. **B,** Blockade of other digits: blockade of the other fingers is accomplished at the bifurcation between the metacarpal heads. With the fingers widely extended, a 27-gauge needle is inserted into the web about 3 mm proximal to the junction between the web and the palmar skin; bupivacaine (1.0 to 2.0 mL, *without epinephrine*) is injected. **C,** This can be performed either from a dorsal approach or a volar approach. The web on either side will have to be blocked to provide analgesia for each finger to be anesthetized. *n.,* Nerve.

Blockade of the other fingers is accomplished at the bifurcation between the metacarpal heads (Fig. 40.66B,C). With the fingers extended, a 27-gauge needle is inserted into the web about 3 millimeters proximal to the junction between the web and the palmar skin; 1.0 to 2.0 milliliters of bupivacaine *without epinephrine* is injected. This can be performed either from a dorsal approach or a volar approach.

Complications

Large volumes of local anesthetic are contraindicated because of the possibility of pressure and vascular compromise. Vasoconstrictors are generally avoided because they may cause necrosis of the digit. The use of dilute epinephrine concentrations (1 : 100,000–1 : 200,000) in digital nerve blocks may be undergoing a renaissance as epinephrine with local anesthetics have been used in almost 3000 digital blocks without sequelae.[648] Intravascular injection may be avoided with incremental injection and frequent aspiration.

LOWER EXTREMITY BLOCKS

The major use of nerve blocks of the lower extremity in children is for managing postoperative pain and as an adjunct to general anesthesia. When considering the sensory and cutaneous innervation of the lower extremity (Fig. 40.67), it is not surprising that few surgical procedures can be accomplished under single nerve

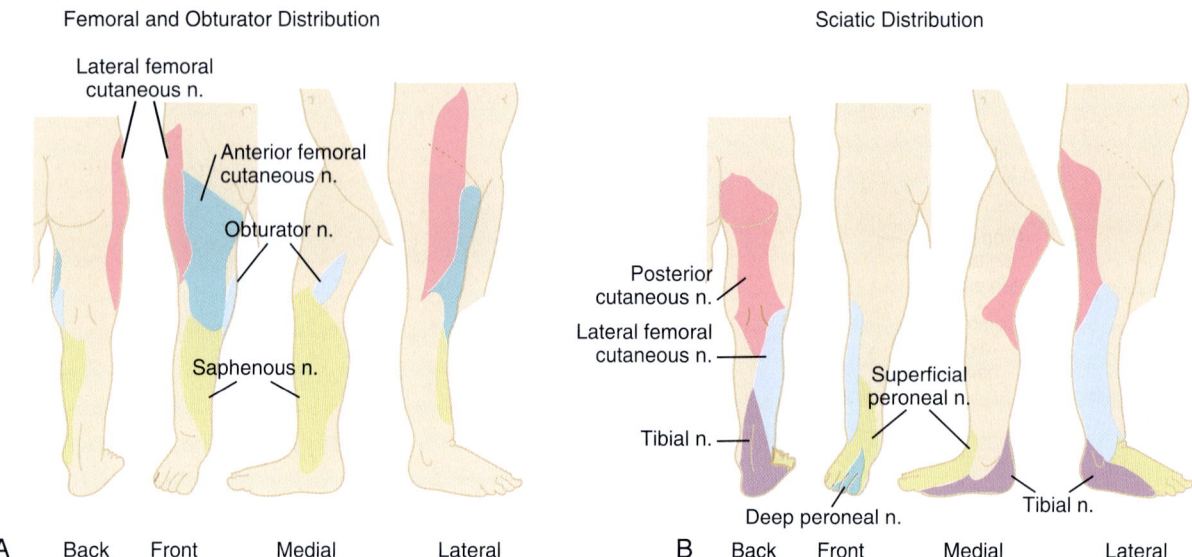

FIGURE 40.67 The sensory innervation of the lower extremity is presented. Note that anesthesia of the lower extremity requires a block of the femoral nerve **(A)** (and its branches), as well as the sciatic nerve **(B)**. *n.*, Nerve.

blocks. However, combinations of sciatic, femoral, and lateral femoral cutaneous blockade can provide both excellent postoperative analgesia and surgical anesthesia for selected operations; the fascia iliaca block produces anesthesia of multiple nerves with a single injection, and the lumbar plexus block is useful for operations of the hip and anterior thigh. Continuous peripheral nerve blocks extend the duration of postoperative analgesia with a good safety profile. In a large review of peripheral nerve blocks, with lower extremity blocks accounting for 85% of blocks, the incidence of complications and adverse events was 12.1% (95% CI 10.7%–13.5%), the vast majority of which were catheter malfunction or block failure; superficial infection, and vascular puncture were less common, and there were no reports of persistent neurologic problems, catheter malfunctions, or toxicity.[238]

Lumbar Plexus Block
Anatomy
The lumbar plexus, as the name suggests, is a confluence of nerves derived from the anterior rami of lumbar nerve roots L1–L4, with variable contributions from T12 and L5. These roots divide into anterior and posterior divisions within the psoas major muscle. They join to form six major motor and sensory nerves that supply the lower limb: the iliohypogastric, ilioinguinal, genitofemoral, femoral, obturator nerves, and the lateral cutaneous nerve of the thigh. The obturator nerve emerges on the medial border of the psoas muscle, the genitofemoral nerve emerges on the anterior surface, and the remaining nerves run along the lateral border of the psoas muscle.[649,650] Blocking the nerves of this plexus provides anesthesia and analgesia for hip, proximal femur, and anterior thigh surgery. When combined with a sciatic nerve block, complete anesthesia of the lower limb can be achieved. The psoas muscle compartment is a highly vascular noncompressible space; therefore, the lumbar plexus block is considered a "deep" peripheral nerve block, and anticoagulation guidelines and restrictions similar to those for neuraxial blocks apply.[27] This block can be performed both by using landmark/nerve-stimulation techniques and ultrasound guidance.[651] Sonoanatomic views may be challenging given the depth of the neural elements and poorly defined echotexture of the nerves at that depth. The depth of the plexus

varies with patient weight, and besides being more superficial, the less fibrous psoas muscle in children lends itself to better sonoanatomic views than in adults.[652,653] Hence, a combined approach using real-time ultrasound for needle advancement and nerve stimulation for plexus localization is recommended.[654]

The lumbar plexus lies within the "psoas compartment", which is a deep fascial plane in the posterior one-third of the psoas muscle. The lateral cutaneous nerve of the thigh and the femoral nerve are also located in the psoas muscle compartment. The obturator nerve has a variable location, and may lie in a different intramuscular fold, separated from the lateral cutaneous nerve of the thigh and the femoral nerve. The obturator nerve is spared in approximately 10% of lumbar plexus blocks, and this is likely due to its variable location. Anatomically, the psoas muscle is anterior to the transverse processes of the lumbar vertebrae. The kidney is located anterior and lateral to the psoas muscle, usually at the L2–L3 level but may be lower, at the L4–L5 level in young children, infants, and those with significant curvature of the thoracolumbar spine. The dorsal branch of the lumbar artery is located between the psoas muscle and the transverse process, and the psoas compartment itself contains a network of arteries and veins.

Ultrasound-Guided Lumbar Plexus Block
A linear-array transducer (10-5 MHz) is adequate for imaging in young children, whereas in the older child (>6 to 8 years of age) a curved-array transducer (8-5 or 5-2 MHz) is required. The shamrock method first described in 2013 by Sauter is the most commonly performed technique for ultrasound-guided lumbar plexus blocks.[588,655,656] Other techniques have also been described including the trident technique by Karmakar et al.[654] and the paramedian transverse oblique method.[653,657,658]

For the shamrock technique, the patient is placed in the lateral decubitus position with the nonoperative side dependent, a bump is placed below the dependent flank to open up the space between the ribs and iliac crest, and hips and knees flexed. A pillow between the legs helps align the hips and spine. The anterior thigh is exposed to visualize quadriceps muscle contraction with peripheral nerve stimulation.

Position the curvilinear transducer adjacent to the iliac crest to visualize a transverse view of the intraabdominal structures. The psoas major, erector spinae, and quadratus lumborum muscles are arranged in the shape of a shamrock with the psoas major muscle anterior, the erector spinae muscle posterior, and the quadratus lumborum muscle at the apex of the transverse process. The lumbar plexus lies in the posterior third of the psoas muscle. The needle insertion point can be decided by an ultrasonographical estimation of the distance from the bottom of the transducer to the posteromedial quadrant of the psoas major muscle, where the lumbar plexus is expected to be located. The needle is advanced anteriorly in-plane under dual ultrasound- and nerve-stimulator–guidance until the needle tip reaches the lumbar plexus and elicits muscle twitches in the quadriceps muscle between 0.3 and 0.6 mA of current. Contractions elicited at <0.3 mA indicate an intraneural needle placement, and the needle should be withdrawn until optimal stimulation is elicited.

In a variation of this technique, the ultrasound transducer is positioned approximately 2 to 3 centimeters lateral to the lumbar spine at the L3–L4 vertebral level, with its orientation marker directed laterally. Align the transducer slightly medially to produce a paramedian oblique transverse scan (PMOTS) of the lumbar paravertebral region.[652,659–662] During a PMOTS of the lumbar paravertebral region, the ultrasound beam can be insonated either at the level of the transverse process (PMOTS-TP, Fig. 40.68A) or through the gap between the two adjacent transverse processes (i.e., the intertransverse space), producing a PMOTS-ITS scan (Fig. 40.68B). In a typical PMOTS-ITS sonogram of the lumbar paravertebral region, the erector spinae muscle, the vertebral body, the psoas major muscle, the quadratus lumborum muscle, and the anterolateral surface of the vertebral body are clearly visualized (see Fig. 40.68B). The inferior vena cava (on the right side) and the aorta (on the left side) are also identified anterior to the vertebral body. The lower pole of the kidney is closely related to the anterior surfaces of the quadratus lumborum and psoas muscle and is seen as an oval structure that moves with respiration in the retroperitoneal space. The lumbar plexus is not sonographically visualized in

all patients, but when it is visualized, it appears as an oval hyperechoic structure in the posterior part of the psoas muscle (see Fig. 40.68B) and close to the intervertebral foramen. In contrast, because the acoustic shadow of the transverse process obscures the posterior part of the psoas muscle and the area close to the intervertebral foramen during a PMOTS-TP, the lumbar plexus is rarely visualized in this ultrasound scan window (see Fig. 40.68A). Therefore, if a transverse scan is performed during an ultrasound-guided lumbar plexus block, the PMOTS-ITS may provide better acoustical windows.[662]

For the trident technique, a sagittal scan of the lumbar paravertebral region is utilized, and the ultrasound transducer is positioned approximately 2 to 3 centimeters lateral and parallel to the lumbar spine, with its orientation marker directed cranially. In a typical sagittal sonogram of the lumbar paravertebral region, the L2, L3, and L4 transverse processes with their acoustic shadow produce what we refer to as the "trident sign" (Fig. 40.69) because of its similarity to the trident that is often associated with Poseidon (the god of the sea in Greek mythology) and the trishula of the Hindu god Shiva.[658] The hypoechoic psoas muscle is seen between the transverse processes, and the lumbar plexus is identified as hyperechoic longitudinal striations within the posterior aspect of the muscle. A laterally positioned transducer will produce a suboptimal scan without the trident, and the lower pole of the kidney, which can reach the L4–L5 level in young children, will come into view.

Once an optimal image of the lumber paravertebral region is obtained, the insulated block needle is inserted in the plane of the ultrasound beam. The needle is inserted from the medial side of the transducer when a PMOTS-ITS is used or from the caudal end of the transducer when a sagittal scan is used. The needle is slowly advanced under ultrasound guidance to the posterior part of the psoas muscle, and the correct position of the needle tip close to the lumbar plexus is confirmed by observing ipsilateral quadriceps muscle contraction.

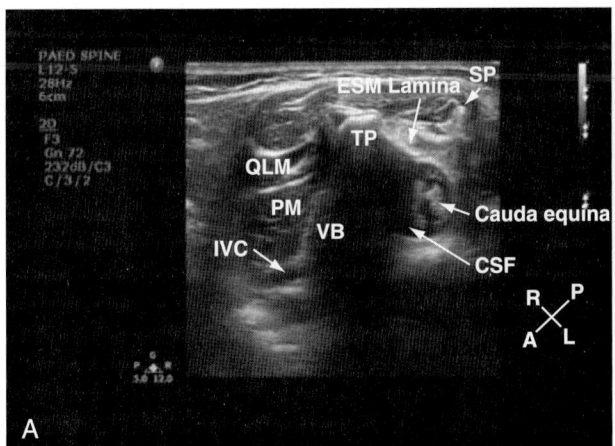 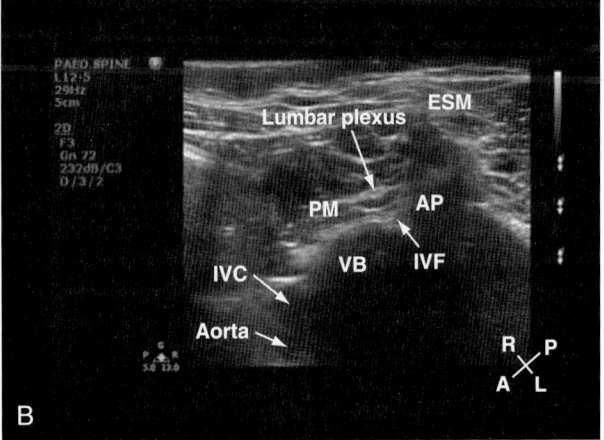

FIGURE 40.68 A, Paramedian oblique transverse scan of the right lumbar paravertebral region at the level of the transverse process (PMOTS-TP) in an 11-month-old infant. Note how the acoustic shadow of the transverse process (TP) obscures the posterior part of the psoas muscle (PM) and how parts of the spinal canal and neuraxial structures (dura, intrathecal space, and cauda equina) are seen through the interlaminar space. **B,** Paramedian oblique transverse scan of the right paravertebral region through the gap between two adjacent transverse processes (PMOTS-ITS) in a 14-month-old child. Note the intervertebral foramen (IVF), articular process (AP), and the lumbar plexus in the posterior part of the PM. A, Anterior; CSF, cerebrospinal fluid; ESM, erector spinae muscle; IVC, inferior vena cava; L, left; P, posterior; PM, psoas muscle; QLM, quadratus lumborum muscle; R, right; SP, spinous process; VB, vertebral body.

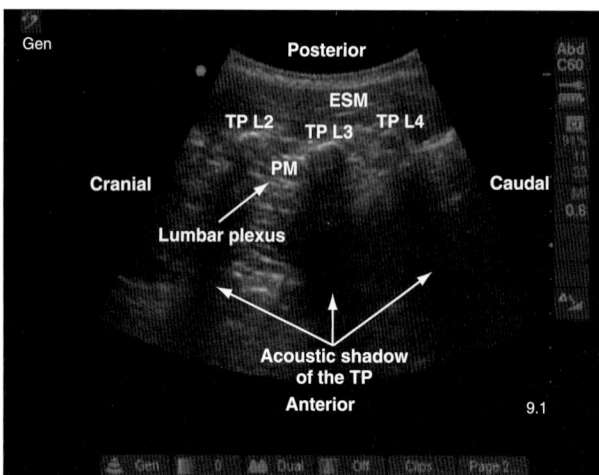

FIGURE 40.69 Longitudinal sonogram of the lumbar paravertebral region showing the lumbar plexus. *ESM*, Erector spinae muscle; *PM*, psoas muscle; *TP*, transverse process ("trident sign").

Selection of Drug

Lumbar plexus block should be dosed as a fascial plane block. After maximum dose for weight is calculated, bolus volumes of 0.3 mL/kg to 0.5 mL/kg can be administered. Typical continuous catheter infusion rates are 0.2 mL/kg per hour for 0.2% ropivacaine or 0.4 mL/kg per hour for 0.1% ropivacaine.

Complications

Complications with a lumbar plexus block can occur from needle trauma, intravascular injection of medications, or improper injection site (failed block). A needle inserted too medially may result in injury to vascular structures like the aorta, lumbar arteries, kidney, bowel, and produce retroperitoneal hematomas. Intravascular injections or large volume local anesthetic absorption might lead to LAST; slow incremental injection with ECG monitoring and observation of the injection target is always indicated. A misdirected needle tip can lead to epidural or intrathecal injections with neuraxial effects.

Sciatic Nerve Block

Anatomy

The sciatic nerve is the largest mixed nerve in the body, arising from the L4–S3 roots of the sacral plexus, and passes through the pelvis, and becomes superficial at the lower margin of the gluteus maximus muscle. It then descends into the lower extremity in the posterior aspect of the thigh, supplying sensory innervation to the posterior thigh, as well as to the entire leg and foot below the level of the knee, except for the medial aspect, which is supplied by the femoral nerve (see Fig. 40.67B). The sciatic nerve block is used for operations on the foot and lower leg, such as clubfoot repair or triple arthrodesis, and in children having knee surgery, particularly when combined with a femoral nerve block.[663] The adductor canal approach has the advantage of relatively preserving hamstring function and allows early ambulation with crutches.

Sciatic Nerve Block at the Subgluteal Space

ANATOMY. The sciatic nerve exits the pelvis through the greater sciatic foramen, between the piriformis and the superior gemelli muscles, and enters the subgluteal space below the piriformis muscle. It then descends over the dorsum of the ischium, lying on the dorsal surface of the superior gemellus muscle, tendon of obturator

internus, inferior gemellus muscle, and quadratus femoris muscle (in a cranial to caudal relation) before it enters the hollow between the greater trochanter and the ischial tuberosity and then goes on to the posterior compartment of the thigh. The anterior surface of the gluteus maximus covers the upper part of the sciatic nerve; immediately distal to its lower border (infragluteal position), the sciatic nerve is fairly superficial. In between the greater trochanter and the ischial tuberosity, the sciatic nerve lies in the subgluteal space, which is a well-defined anatomic space between the anterior surface of the gluteus maximus and the posterior surface of the quadratus femoris muscle (Fig. 40.70).[664] Other structures present in the subgluteal space include the posterior cutaneous nerve of the thigh, the inferior gluteal vessels and nerve, the nerve to the short and long head of the biceps femoris, the comitans artery and vein of the sciatic nerve, and the ascending branch of the medial circumflex artery (Fig. 40.71). Local anesthetic injected into the subgluteal space blocks the sciatic nerve and the posterior cutaneous nerve of the thigh, which is useful when anesthesia over the posterior aspect of the thigh is needed.

Ultrasound-Guided Sciatic Nerve at Subgluteal Space Block

Ultrasound-guided sciatic nerve block at the subgluteal space is performed with the child in the lateral position. The side to be anesthetized is placed uppermost, and the hip and knees are flexed (Fig. 40.72). The operator sits or stands behind the child, and the ultrasound machine is positioned directly in front. In young children, a linear-array transducer (10-5 MHz) is adequate for imaging the sciatic nerve; in children older than 6 to 8 years of age, the sciatic nerve can also be imaged using a curved linear-array transducer (8-5 or 5-2 MHz) (preferred) because the increased depth of scan required (as a result of increased muscle bulk) limits the field of vision when a linear transducer is used.

The greater trochanter and the ischial tuberosity are identified, and a line is drawn between these two landmarks. The ultrasound transducer is placed parallel to this line, with its orientation marker directed toward the greater trochanter to obtain a transverse scan of the sciatic nerve and the subgluteal space.[664–666] It may be necessary to slide the transducer slightly cephalad or caudad before an optimal image of the sciatic nerve in the subgluteal space can be obtained. On a transverse sonogram, the subgluteal space is seen as a hypoechoic area between the hyperechoic epimysium of the gluteus maximus and quadratus femoris muscle (see Fig. 40.72), extending from the greater trochanter laterally to the ischial tuberosity medially. The subgluteal space is not so well delineated in young children and is better visualized in older children. The sciatic nerve is seen as an oval or triangular hyperechoic structure within the subgluteal space (see Fig. 40.72). The medial limit of the space is obscured by the attachments of the semimembranosus, semitendinosus, and biceps femoris muscles to the ischial tuberosity. Pulsations of the inferior gluteal artery often can be detected medial to the sciatic nerve on the sonogram.

The block needle is inserted using an in-plane technique from the ischial tuberosity side and advanced slowly toward the sciatic nerve.[664,667] Once the block needle is deemed to be in the subgluteal space, the position is confirmed by injecting 1 to 2 milliliters of saline solution and observing a distention of the subgluteal space (i.e., separation of the epimysium of the gluteus maximus and quadratus femoris muscle) on the ultrasound image (Fig. 40.73). However, if the test injection of saline solution spreads posterior to the epimysium of the gluteus maximus muscle, it indicates that the tip of the needle is not in the subgluteal space. The needle should be reoriented and advanced a little farther until the typical distention

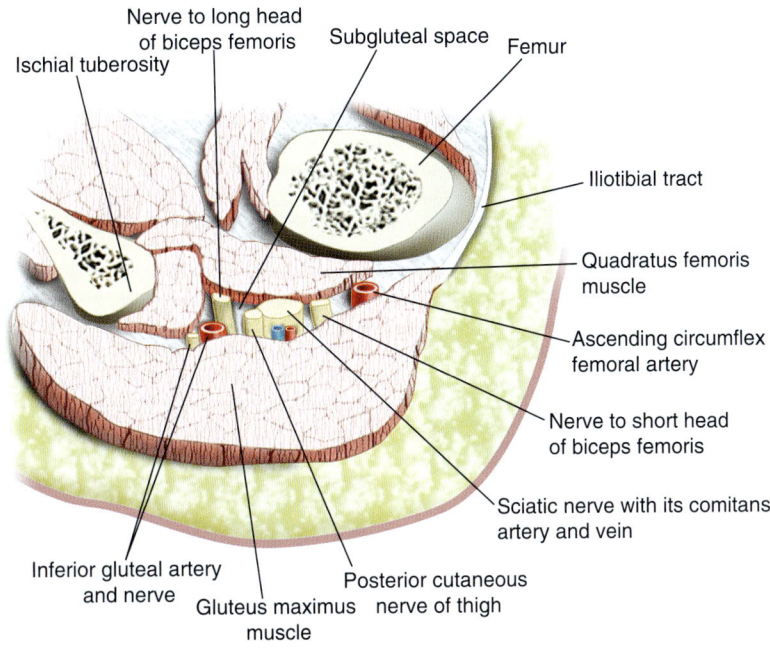

FIGURE 40.70 Transverse section through the gluteal region at the level of the quadratus femoris muscle showing the subgluteal space and its contents.

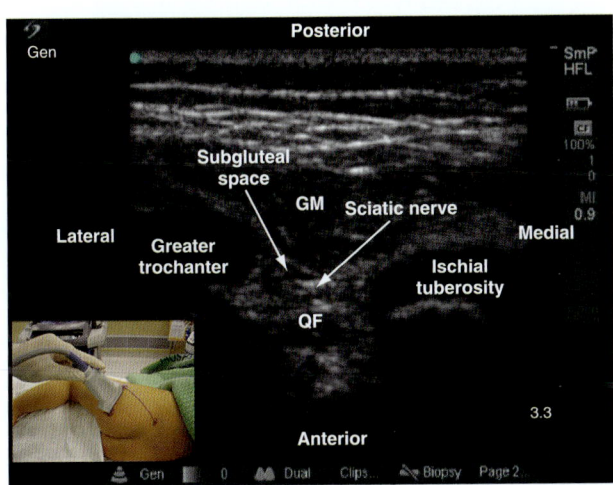

FIGURE 40.71 Transverse sonogram between the greater trochanter and the ischial tuberosity showing the hypoechoic subgluteal space between the hyperechoic perimysium of the gluteus maximus and the quadratus femoris muscle. The sciatic nerve is seen as a hyperechoic structure in the medial aspect of the subgluteal space. *GM*, Gluteus maximus; *QF*, quadratus femoris.

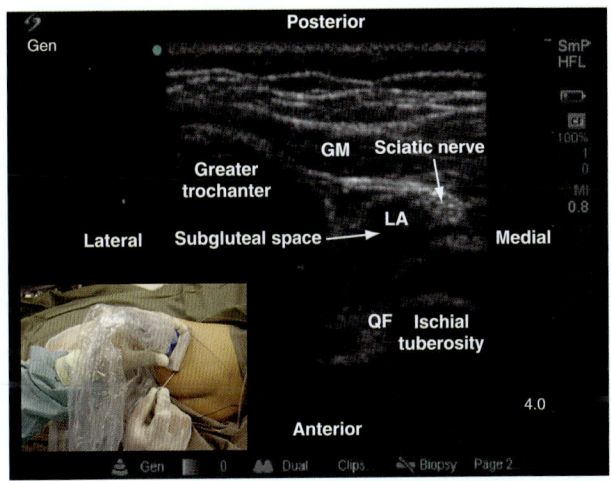

FIGURE 40.72 Transverse sonogram of the sciatic nerve at the subgluteal space after local anesthetic injection. Note the distention of the subgluteal space caused by the local anesthetic and the distribution of local anesthetic around the sciatic nerve. *GM;* Gluteus maximus; *LA,* local anesthetic; *QF,* quadratus femoris.

of the subgluteal space to the saline solution test injection is seen. Occasionally, a subtle pop is felt when the needle tip traverses the epimysium of the gluteus maximus muscle and enters the subgluteal space. Local anesthetic is then injected in aliquots over 2 to 3 minutes while observing for the distention of the subgluteal space and the spread of local anesthetic in relation to the sciatic nerve. It is also easy to pass a catheter into the subgluteal space when a continuous sciatic nerve block is planned. Because the catheter is inserted into an anatomic space, the catheter is also more likely to stay in situ (Video 40.26).

Landmark Approach of Labat (Posterior Approach) to Sciatic Nerve

The child is placed in the lateral decubitus position lying on the nonoperative leg. The leg to be blocked is flexed and the lower leg is extended (Fig. 40.74A). A line is drawn from the posterior superior iliac spine to the greater trochanter of the femur. Another line is drawn from the greater trochanter to the coccyx. The first line is bisected, and a perpendicular line is drawn from that point to the second line; the point at which it intersects the second line is the site of needle insertion (Fig. 40.74B). A 22-gauge insulated

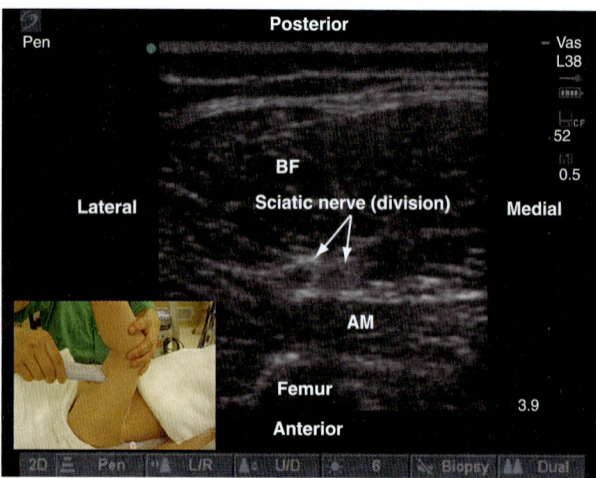

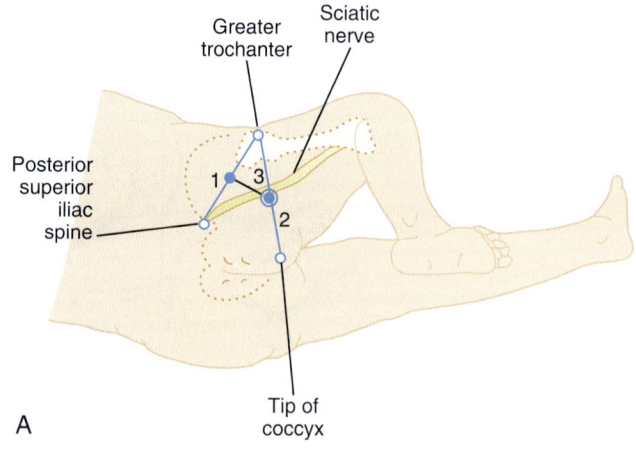

FIGURE 40.73 Popliteal sciatic nerve block. Transverse sonogram of the sciatic nerve at the apex of the popliteal fossa. *AM*, Adductor magnus; *BF*, biceps femoris.

needle is advanced in the perpendicular plane until it strikes bone. It is possible for the needle to pass through the sciatic notch without either encountering bone or causing a paresthesia. In that case, the needle is redirected in a cephalad direction until bone is encountered. A motor paresthesia is then sought using an organized grid-like approach, fanning medially to laterally.

Landmark-Guided Anterior Approach to Sciatic Nerve

As the sciatic nerve emerges from the lower border of the gluteus maximus to extend down the thigh, it passes medial and deep to the lesser trochanter of the femur (Figs. 40.75A, 40.76, 40.77).

With the child in the supine position, a line is drawn from the anterior superior iliac spine to the pubic tuberosity. The greater trochanter is then located, and another line is drawn parallel to the first line (see Fig. 40.75B); at the medial one-third of the first line, a perpendicular is dropped to the second line. The point of intersection with the line originating at the greater trochanter marks the point of needle entry. The needle is inserted in a perpendicular plane until bone is encountered. It is then partially withdrawn and redirected medially. When the needle is posterior to the medial margin of the femur, ease of injection is determined after negative aspiration for blood. This approach carries a greater risk of unintended puncture of the femoral vessels, and repeated negative aspirations must precede incremental injection. If the needle is in muscle or a fascial bundle, resistance to injection will be felt. In this case, the needle is advanced until minimal resistance to injection is felt. Motor paresthesia is a helpful indicator.

For the previous two techniques, a dose of 0.2 mL/kg of bupivacaine (0.25% with epinephrine 1:200,000) is the dose usually administered for children older than 6 months of age. If the sciatic nerve block is used in conjunction with a femoral nerve block, consideration should be given to diluting the local anesthetic concentration further to limit the total injected dose to 2.5 mg/kg of bupivacaine.[668]

Landmark-Guided Infragluteal-Parabiceps Sciatic Nerve Block

This approach is a simple way to access the sciatic nerve.[669] It offers an advantage over the popliteal fossa technique because the posterior cutaneous nerve supplying the posterior portion of the thigh can be blocked with this approach.

Technique. The child is placed in the supine position or a lateral position to perform this block. The biceps femoris tendon

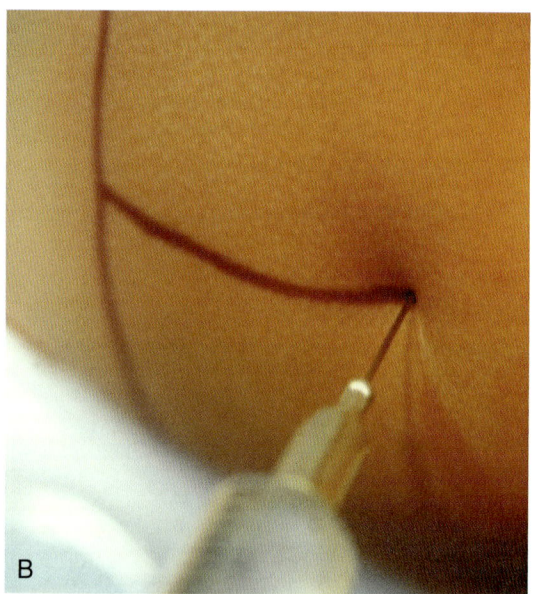

FIGURE 40.74 A, Sciatic nerve block (approach of Labat). The patient is placed in a lateral position with the lower leg extended and the upper leg, the one to be blocked, flexed; a line is drawn from the greater trochanter of the femur to the posterior superior iliac spine *(blue line 1)*. A second line is drawn from the greater trochanter to the coccyx *(blue line 2)*. Line 1 is bisected, and a perpendicular line is drawn from that point to line 2 *(black line 3)*; the point at which the perpendicular broken line intersects line 2 *(encircled dot)* is the point of needle insertion. **B,** A 22-gauge needle is advanced perpendicular to the skin until it strikes bone or, if the child is awake, a paresthesia is elicited. Use of a nerve stimulator will produce either plantar flexion or dorsiflexion of the foot.

is palpated and traced cephalad to the distal crease of the buttocks (see Fig. 40.77). A stimulating needle is then inserted perpendicular to the femoral shaft, along the biceps femoris tendon (parabiceps) until a twitch is obtained (see Fig. 40.76B). Either inversion or eversion of the foot is a reasonable response for localization of the nerve. Next, 0.2 mL/kg of local anesthetic solution is injected into the area (Video 40.27). An ultrasound-guided approach may facilitate this block (see also Figs. 40.75–40.79).[670]

Complications. Profound motor block can be seen in most children after a subgluteal (infragluteal) parabiceps sciatic nerve block. If the child is discharged home, caution should be exercised because of the motor weakness produced. More recently, we have used continuous catheters in hospitalized children having major lower extremity surgical procedures, with very good results.[671]

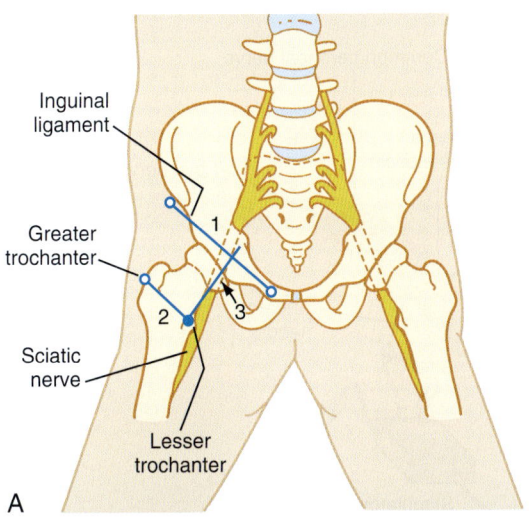

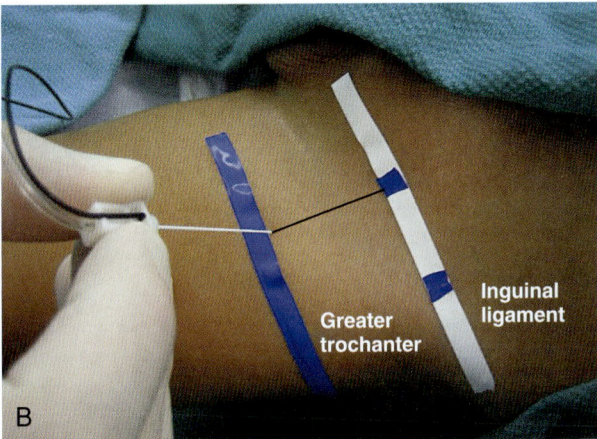

FIGURE 40.75 A, Sciatic nerve block (anterior approach). With the patient supine, a line is drawn from the anterior iliac spine to the pubic tuberosity *(line 1).* The greater trochanter is located, and another line is drawn parallel to the first *(line 2).* A perpendicular line is drawn from line 1 at a point one-third the distance laterally from the pubic tuberosity to the anterior iliac spine *(line 3).* **B,** Left sciatic nerve block. A needle is inserted at the intersection of line 2 and the perpendicular line (in **A,** *solid circle*) until bone is encountered. The needle is redirected off the edge of the femur to the approximate posterior margin of the femur and, after negative aspiration for blood, ease of injection is ascertained. Resistance to injection indicates that the needle is within muscle or fascial bundle; the needle should be advanced until there is minimal resistance to injection or until a paresthesia is elicited.

Ultrasound-Guided Sciatic Nerve Block at the Popliteal Fossa

The sciatic nerve block at the popliteal fossa is the preferred approach for children undergoing foot surgery. The popliteal fossa is a diamond-shaped space lying behind the knee joint, the lower part of the femur, and the upper part of the tibia. It is bound superolaterally by the biceps femoris tendon, superomedially by the semitendinosus and the semimembranosus tendons, inferolaterally by the lateral head of the gastrocnemius, and inferomedially by the medial head of the gastrocnemius. The sciatic nerve enters the posterior aspect of the thigh at the lower border of the gluteus maximus and runs vertically downward to the apex of the superior triangle of the popliteal fossa, where it terminates by dividing into the tibial and the common peroneal nerve, usually 3 to 7 centimeters above the popliteal crease in adults.[672–675] The division of the sciatic nerve into its terminal branches may, however, take place

anywhere above this level. This accounts for the occasional sparing of either division of the sciatic nerve after distal sciatic nerve block techniques using nerve stimulation.

The child is positioned supine with the leg elevated by an assistant or a bolster (Fig. 40.80). During ultrasound-guided popliteal sciatic nerve block the operator sits on the ipsilateral side facing the head of the patient, and the ultrasound machine is positioned directly in front of the operator on the contralateral side of the patient. In young children, a linear-array transducer (10-5 MHz) is adequate for imaging the sciatic nerve in the popliteal fossa; in the adolescent child or children with muscular thighs, a curved-array transducer (8-5 MHz) may be preferable. The transducer is positioned just above the apex of the upper triangle of the popliteal fossa in the transverse axis (see Fig. 40.76). It may be necessary to first scan for the sciatic nerve in the middle of the thigh and then trace it distally to the popliteal fossa, where the sciatic nerve is seen as a round, hyperechoic structure. Division of the sciatic nerve into the tibial and common peroneal nerves varies widely but can be visualized in children.[676] In the popliteal fossa and proximal to the popliteal crease, the tibial and common peroneal nerves are seen as hyperechoic structures superficial and lateral to the popliteal artery.

The block needle is inserted using in-plane technique from the lateral aspect of the thigh with its point of entry being anterior to the tendon of the biceps femoris (if it is palpable). This places the needle in the same orientation as for the lateral approach to the sciatic nerve at the popliteal fossa. The exact point of needle entry will depend on where the sciatic nerve is best visualized. The needle is gradually advanced under ultrasound guidance, and the tip is positioned just posterior to the sciatic nerve. This is confirmed by injecting 1 to 2 milliliters of saline solution through the needle, after which half of the calculated dose of local anesthetic is injected. The same process is repeated by repositioning the tip of the needle anterior to the sciatic nerve. This ensures that the local anesthetic spreads optimally around the sciatic nerve.

Landmark-Guided Sciatic Nerve Block at the Popliteal Fossa

There are multiple approaches to the sciatic nerve: anterior, transgluteal, infragluteal, lateral, posterior subgluteal, proximal thigh (adductor canal), or at the popliteal fossa.[677] All blocks in the absence of ultrasound guidance are performed with the aid of a nerve stimulator to elicit a motor paresthesia in the foot, and, if the block is performed in a lightly sedated trauma victim, the approach that places the child in a greater position of comfort should be chosen. Ultrasound guidance improves the performance of the nerve block and should always be utilized if available.[561–563,664–667,672–676] The lateral approach via the popliteal fossa offers the additional advantage of being able to provide the block in the supine position and is most commonly used (see Fig. 40.76), often in combination with block of the saphenous nerve. An infragluteal-parabiceps approach is another easy method of providing a sciatic nerve block in children.[669]

Saphenous Nerve Block

The saphenous nerve, a branch of the femoral nerve, provides sensory innervation to the medial aspect of the leg and foot. When blocked in the thigh, as it courses through the adductor canal, it provides excellent analgesia after operations on the knee without weakness of the quadriceps muscle produced by a femoral nerve block (Video 40.28).[678] Thus, early ambulation is easily achieved.

Anatomy

The saphenous nerve is the terminal sensory branch of the anterior division of the femoral nerve and supplies the skin on the

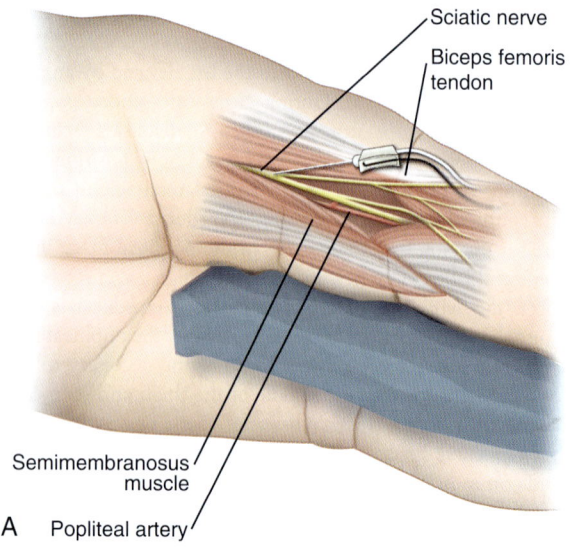

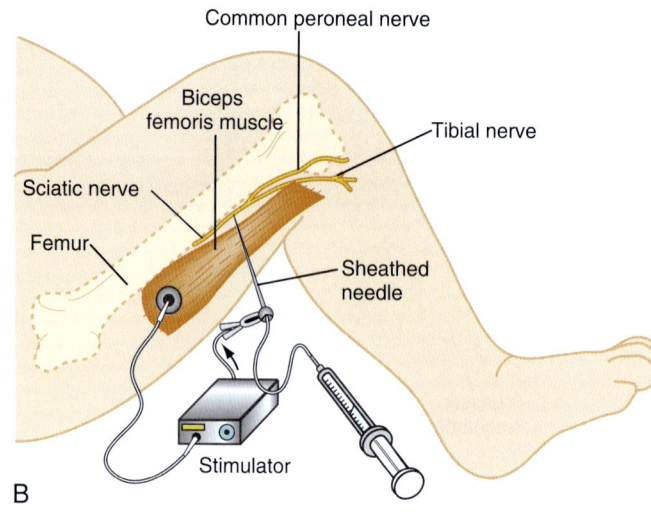

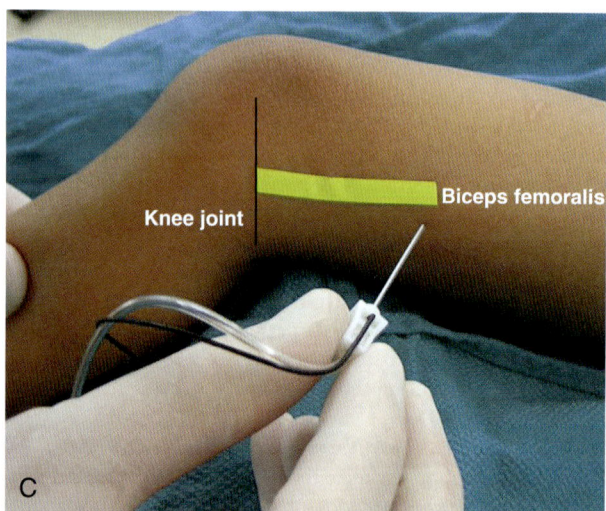

FIGURE 40.76 Lateral popliteal sciatic nerve block. **A,** Anatomy for lateral popliteal approach to the sciatic nerve. The calf is elevated on a pillow and the biceps femoris tendon is palpated. The tendon is traced proximally for 3 to 5 cm. **B,** A 22-gauge insulated needle is inserted anterior to the tendon in a horizontal plane with a cephalad angulation. A nerve stimulator is attached to the needle and with low-current stimulation (0.2–0.5 mV), the foot is observed for plantar flexion or dorsiflexion. With injection of the test dose of 1.0 mL of bupivacaine (0.25% with 1 : 200,000 epinephrine), the twitching is abolished. This confirms the correct placement of the needle. **C,** Then 5 to 10 mL of additional local anesthetic is injected.

medial aspect of the leg and foot up to the ball of the big toe. In the thigh, the saphenous nerve is located in the subsartorial (adductor) canal, and local anesthetic injected into this intramuscular space produces a saphenous nerve block. The subsartorial canal is also referred to as the adductor canal or Hunter canal and is situated on the medial side of the middle one-third of the thigh and extends from the apex of the femoral triangle, above, to the tendinous opening in the adductor magnus muscle, below. The canal is triangular in cross-section. Its anterior wall is formed by the vastus medialis muscle, the posterior wall or floor is formed by the adductor longus, and the medial wall or roof is formed by a strong fibrous membrane that is overlapped by the sartorius muscle (see Fig. 40.78). The subsartorial canal contains: the femoral artery and vein, saphenous nerve, nerve to vastus medialis, and the two divisions of the obturator nerve. The femoral vein lies posterior to the artery in the upper part and lateral to the artery in the lower part of the canal. The saphenous nerve crosses the femoral artery anteriorly from the lateral to the medial side in the canal.[679–682]

Ultrasound-Guided Subsartorial (Adductor Canal) Saphenous Nerve Block

A high-frequency (13-6 MHz) linear-array probe is used to scan the saphenous nerve in the subsartorial canal with the child the supine position.[683] The ipsilateral lower limb is slightly abducted and externally rotated, and the knee is also slightly flexed. For a right-sided block, a right-handed operator stands on the right side of the patient, and the ultrasound machine is positioned directly in front on the contralateral side. The transducer is positioned in the transverse axis over the middle one-third of the thigh. The triangular subsartorial canal can be identified between the epimysium of the vastus medialis (closely related to the femur), the adductor longus, and the sartorius muscles. The pulsatile femoral artery lies anterior to the vein in the canal, and the saphenous nerve is seen as a round or oval hyperechoic structure anterior to the artery (12-o'clock position). Because the saphenous nerve is a small nerve, it may not always be visible on ultrasound imaging in children. However, owing to the close relation of the saphenous nerve

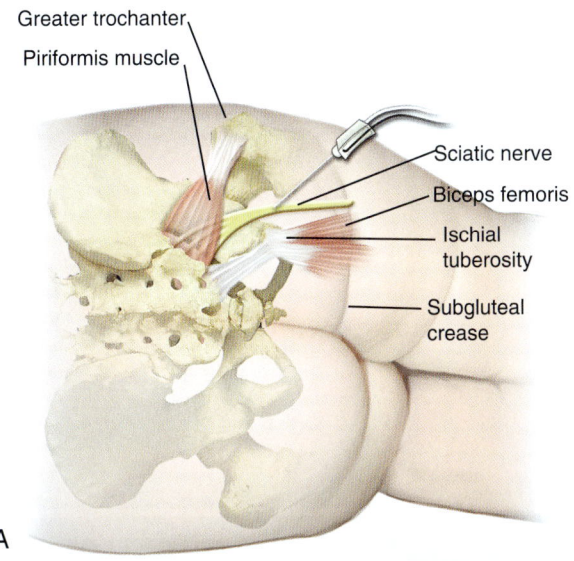

Greater trochanter
Piriformis muscle
Sciatic nerve
Biceps femoris
Ischial tuberosity
Subgluteal crease

A

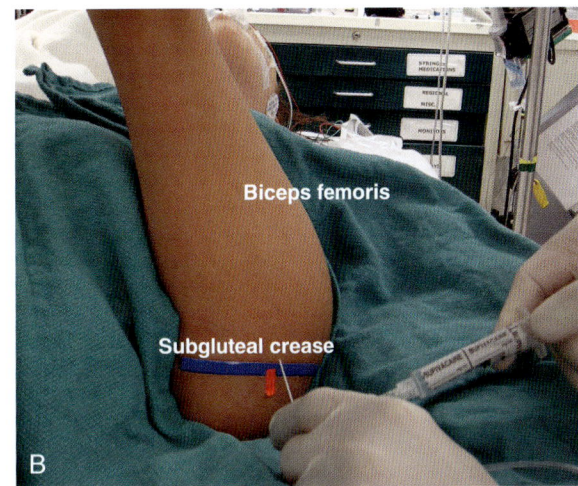

Biceps femoris
Subgluteal crease

B

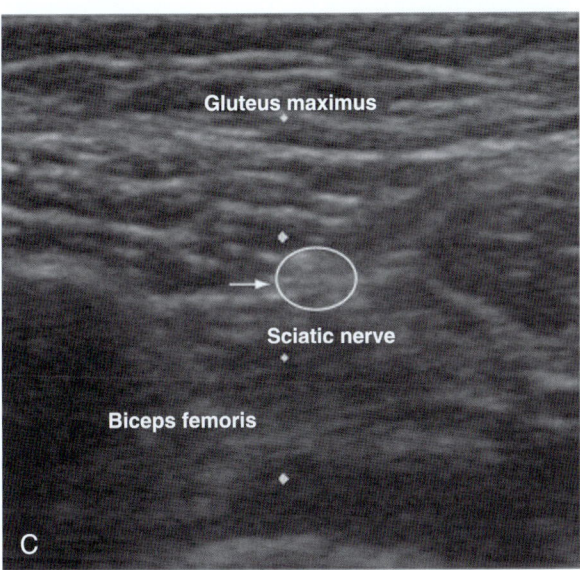

Gluteus maximus

Sciatic nerve

Biceps femoris

C

FIGURE 40.77 A, Anatomy of the infragluteal-parabiceps approach to the sciatic nerve block. **B,** The gluteal crease is identified (left leg) in the prone or supine position. The biceps femoris muscle is identified (distal portion not illustrated) and followed cephalad to the gluteal crease. A stimulating needle is inserted at the level of the gluteal crease along the medial border of the biceps femoris muscle *(blue line);* with stimulation at 0.5 mA, plantar flexion or extension or inversion or eversion denotes adequate positioning of the needle. After aspiration to rule out intravascular injection, 0.2 mL/kg of local anesthetic solution is injected to provide an adequate blockade of the sciatic nerve. **C,** An ultrasound technique may also be used. A linear ultrasound probe is placed along the inferior border of the gluteus maximus along the gluteal crease. The biceps femoris muscle and the semitendinosus muscle are identified. The sciatic nerve is seen as a hyperechoic shadow *(arrow).* In this location, the nerve may be isoechoic. This may require mild rotation or movement of the ultrasound probe to recognize the nerve completely. With the use of an in-plane approach, the needle is advanced close to the sciatic nerve. After aspiration, 0.2 mL/kg of local anesthetic solution is injected. A "doughnut sign" is seen as the nerve is surrounded by the local anesthetic solution.

to the femoral artery in the subsartorial canal, a perivascular (arterial) injection in the canal will produce a saphenous nerve block. The block needle is inserted in the long-axis (in-plane) of the ultrasound transducer from the medial-to-lateral side and is directed to the anterior aspect of the femoral artery. A test injection of saline solution (1 mL) is performed to confirm that the tip of the needle is in the canal, after which the local anesthetic is injected.

Lateral Popliteal Sciatic Nerve Block

This approach to the sciatic nerve can be performed with the child in the supine position.[684]

ANATOMY. The popliteal fossa is a diamond-shaped area located behind the knee. It is bordered by the biceps femoris laterally, medially by the tendons of the semitendinosus and semimembranosus muscles, and inferiorly by the heads of the gastrocnemius muscle. The sciatic nerve, after its formation from L4–S5, innervates all areas of the leg and foot below the knee except the anteromedial cutaneous areas of the leg and foot, which are supplied by the femoral nerve. The sciatic nerve divides into two branches; the larger tibial

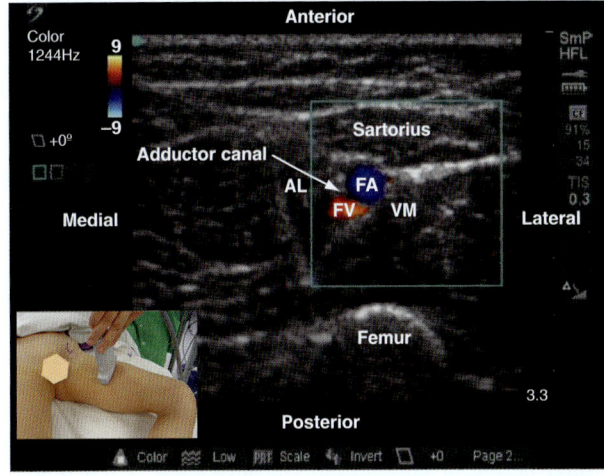

FIGURE 40.78 Transverse sonogram of the thigh showing the adductor canal. *AL,* Adductor longus; *FA,* femoral artery; *FV,* femoral vein; *VM,* vastus medialis.

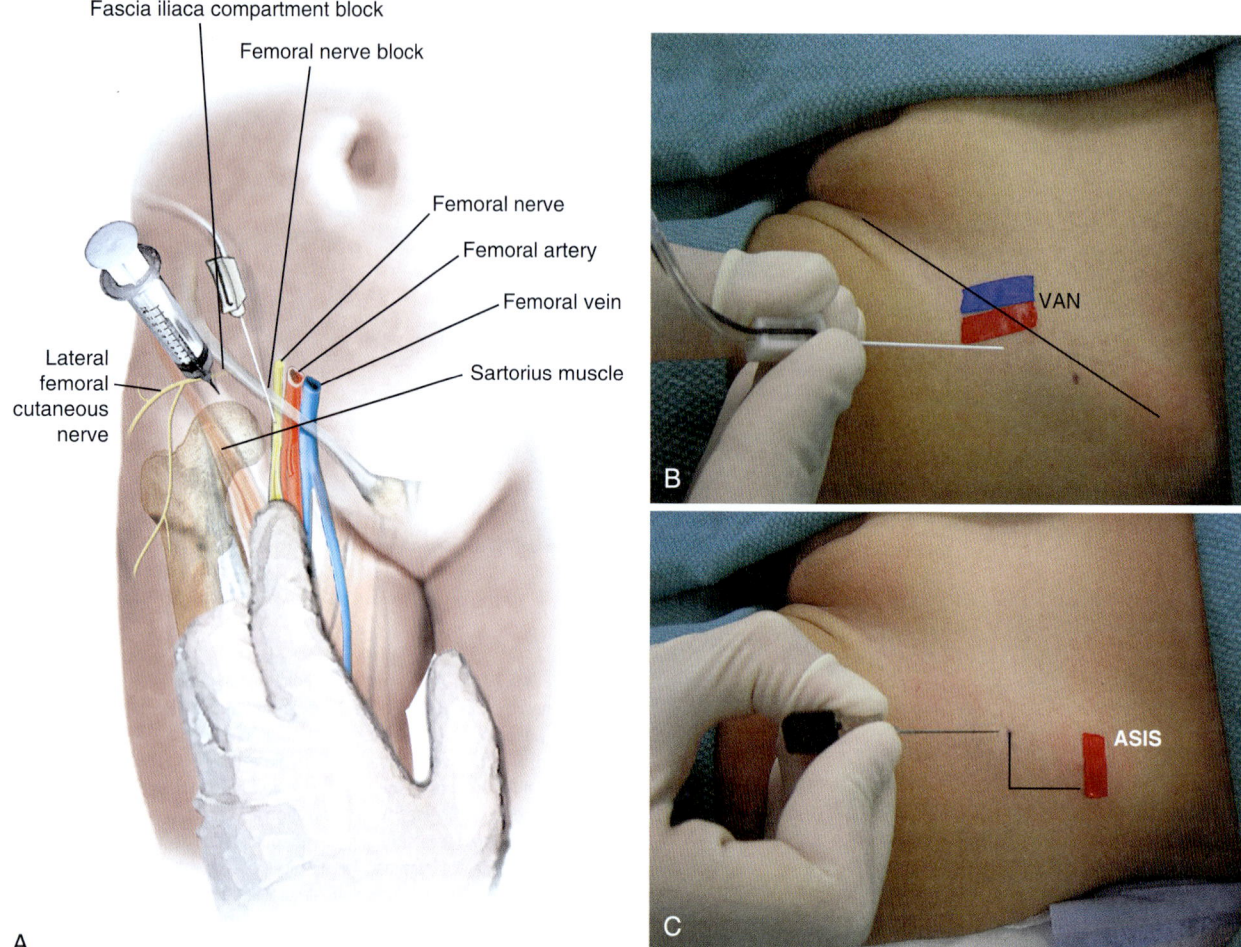

Fascia iliaca compartment block

Femoral nerve block

Femoral nerve

Femoral artery

Femoral vein

Sartorius muscle

Lateral femoral cutaneous nerve

VAN

ASIS

A

B

C

FIGURE 40.79 A, Right femoral nerve block and fascia iliaca compartment block. Note that the femoral nerve lies lateral to the femoral artery. The appropriate dose of local anesthetic is administered while maintaining pressure on the nerve sheath distal to the site of injection just below the inguinal ligament; local anesthetic is thus forced proximally. **B,** For a left femoral nerve block, the point of injection is lateral to the pulse, over the site of the nerve (A, Femoral artery; N, femoral nerve; V, vein) (*black line* indicates inguinal ligament). **C,** The left lateral femoral cutaneous nerve is blocked by injecting 1.0 to 2.0 mL of local anesthetic 1 to 2 cm medial and caudal to the anterior superior iliac crest *(ASIS)*. A caudal needle is used to better feel the "pop" through tissue planes. For the fascia iliaca block, the point of injection is just lateral to the site depicted for the femoral nerve block, 1 cm inferior to the lateral and middle thirds of the inguinal ligament. An injection at this location will bathe all three nerves in the compartment, resulting in blockade with a single injection.

nerve located medially, and the common peroneal nerve located laterally. The nerves are together at the apex of the popliteal fossa, where they are in close proximity to each other and are enclosed in a connective tissue sheath for a few more centimeters before dividing into the component nerves (see Fig. 40.76A).

Ultrasound-Guided Lateral Popliteal Sciatic Nerve Block.
After induction of general anesthesia, the calf is elevated on a pillow. The biceps femoris tendon is palpated. The tendon is then traced upward for 3 to 5 centimeters. A 22-gauge insulated needle is inserted anterior to the tendon in a horizontal plane with a cephalad angulation (see Fig. 40.76B). A nerve stimulator is attached to the sheathed needle and the foot is observed for plantar flexion or dorsiflexion. On injection of a test dose of 1 milliliter of bupivacaine (0.25% with epinephrine 1 : 200,000), the twitching is abolished. This confirms the correct placement of the needle (see Fig. 40.76C); 5 to 10 milliliters of additional local anesthetic is then injected. In adult studies, it has been shown that the sciatic nerve block is longer lasting than an ankle block or subcutaneous infiltration, and it provides excellent postoperative analgesia.[684] Continuous catheter techniques can be used to provide effective analgesia in children in the postoperative period.[685]

COMPLICATIONS. Intraneural injection must be avoided. Using a low-voltage nerve stimulator ensures the proper placement of the needle. It is rare to see intravascular placement of the needle with this approach. Intravascular injection may be avoided with incremental injections and frequent aspirations.

Femoral Nerve Block
A femoral nerve block is particularly useful in children with a fractured femoral shaft so that transport, radiographic, and other manipulations are not painful.[686–688] This block provides analgesia and relieves muscle spasms around the fracture site.

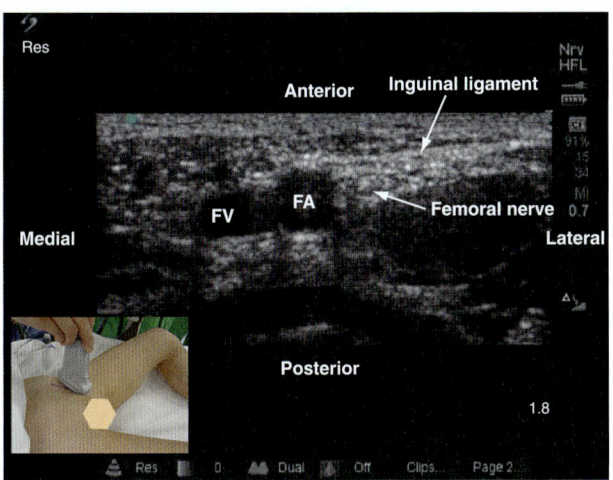

FIGURE 40.80 Transverse sonogram of the inguinal region showing the femoral nerve and its relations. *FA,* Femoral artery; *FV,* femoral vein.

Anatomy

The femoral nerve is located immediately lateral to the femoral artery and deep to both the fascia lata and fascia iliaca (see Fig. 40.79A). It is the largest branch of the lumbar plexus and is the major nerve of the anterior (extensor) compartment of the thigh. It is formed by the dorsal division of the anterior primary rami of spinal nerves L2, L3, and L4 and exits the pelvis and enters the femoral triangle in the thigh by passing under the inguinal ligament just lateral to the femoral artery. In the thigh it lies in the groove between the iliacus and the psoas major muscle, outside the femoral sheath, and lateral to the femoral artery. A femoral nerve block is used to provide postoperative analgesia after femoral fractures or surgery.[689] Depending on the operation, it may be performed in combination with a sciatic block.

Ultrasound-Guided Femoral Nerve Block

The block is performed with the child in the supine position. A high-frequency (13-10 MHz) linear-array transducer is used to scan the femoral nerve. On a transverse sonogram the femoral nerve is seen as an oval or triangular hyperechoic structure lateral to the femoral artery (see Fig. 40.80). The femoral nerve exhibits marked anisotropy, and it may be necessary to tilt or rotate the transducer during the scan before it can be visualized.[262] In young children one must avoid exerting too much pressure during the scan because it is easy to compress the femoral vein. The ipsilateral lower limb is slightly abducted and externally rotated, and the knee is also slightly flexed. A right-handed operator stands on the right side of the child, and the ultrasound machine is positioned directly in front on the contralateral side. The sides of the operator and the ultrasound machine are reversed for a left-handed operator. The scout scan is performed with the transducer positioned parallel and just below the inguinal ligament. This ensures that the femoral nerve is scanned before its division. Once an optimal view of the femoral nerve is obtained, the block needle is inserted in the long axis (in-plane) of the ultrasound transducer from the lateral to medial side and directed to the lateral aspect of the femoral nerve.[262,690] A test injection with saline solution is performed before the local anesthetic is injected to confirm that the needle is deep to the fascia iliaca and to observe the distribution of the injectate in relation to the femoral nerve (see also Fig. 40.77 for landmark-guided techniques).

Landmark-Guided Femoral Nerve Block

A 22-gauge blunt B-bevel needle is advanced lateral to the pulsation of the femoral artery. Two fascial planes can be located by the distinct pop that is felt as the needle traverses these fascial tissues. The nerve is blocked by depositing an appropriate volume (5–10 mL) of local anesthetic lateral to the femoral pulse and deep to the fascia iliaca. The needle is advanced in a perpendicular plane (see Fig. 40.79B and Video 40.30). It is not necessary to elicit a motor paresthesia, provided that the two fascial planes are penetrated. Performance of this block may, on occasion, produce a fascia iliaca block. Repeated aspiration and incremental injection should be used to avoid injection into the femoral artery. A catheter can be placed to provide continuous analgesia in the postoperative period.[686]

Complications

It may be preferable to avoid this technique in children who are taking anticoagulants or who may have blood dyscrasias, owing to the proximity of the nerve to the femoral artery. Intravascular injection may be avoided with incremental injection and frequent aspiration.

Lateral Femoral Cutaneous Nerve
Anatomy

The lateral femoral cutaneous nerve arises from the L2 and L3 roots of the lumbar plexus. It emerges from the lateral border of the psoas muscle and passes obliquely under the fascia iliaca to enter the thigh 1 to 2 centimeters medial to the anterior superior iliac crest (see Fig. 40.79A). The nerve innervates the lateral aspect of the thigh. One of its anterior branches forms part of the patellar plexus; thus it must be blocked for regional anesthesia of the knee. Blockade is also indicated for supplementation of femoral and sciatic nerve blocks to provide relief of tourniquet pain. It is also suitable for anesthetizing the lateral aspect of the thigh as a donor site for small skin grafts, fascia iliaca grafts, or muscle biopsy for muscular disorders.[691,692] This block can also be used for both diagnostic and therapeutic purposes in treating meralgia paresthetica, a condition that leads to chronic pain along the lateral aspect of the thigh.[693-695] In most cases, a fascia iliaca block will block this nerve along with the femoral and obturator nerves, thus obviating the need for performing an isolated lateral femoral cutaneous block.

Landmark-Guided Lateral Femoral Cutaneous Nerve Block

A point approximately 2 centimeters caudal and 2 centimeters medial to the anterior superior iliac spine is located (see Fig. 40.79C). A blunt needle is then advanced through the skin and then through the fascia lata. A distinct pop is felt at this point. The fascia lata and fascia iliaca compartments are entered as two distinct pops can be felt as the needle advances into the fascia iliaca compartment. Between 2 and 10 mL of local anesthetic, depending on the size of the child, is deposited in a fan-like fashion (Video 40.31). Recently, we have used an ultrasound-guided technique[683] that allows us to visualize the fascia iliaca compartment as it fills up with the local anesthetic solution on injection.

Complications

It is rare to see any complications associated with a lateral femoral cutaneous nerve block. However, care must be taken to avoid an intraneural placement of the local anesthetic solution. Intravascular injection may be avoided with incremental injection and frequent aspiration.

Fascia Iliaca Block

This block is particularly useful in children to provide unilateral anesthesia or analgesia of the lower extremity. The block has been reported to be less reliable in adults than in children.[696] It produces blockade of the femoral, lateral femoral cutaneous, and obturator nerves with a single injection of local anesthetic. It has the advantage of producing blockade without requiring the needle to be in close proximity to any major nerves or blood vessels. One study reported a greater than 90% success rate and found it far superior in children to the "3 in 1" block described by Winnie.[696] The ultrasound-guided suprainguinal fascia iliaca block, described by Hebbard in 2011, built on earlier anatomic discoveries to more reliably anesthetize the three nerves.[697] Suprainguinal placement of the fascia iliaca block results in better anesthesia of anterior hip nerves, at least in part due to more reliable obturator blockade compared to landmark techniques.[651]

Anatomy

The compartment is bounded superficially by the fascia iliaca and iliacus muscle, superiorly by the iliac crest, and deeply by the psoas muscle (see Fig. 40.79A).

Ultrasound-Guided Fascia Iliaca Block

The anatomical orientation begins in the same manner as the femoral nerve block: identifying the femoral artery at the level of the inguinal crease and then retracing superiorly and laterally to where the anterior inferior iliac spine is seen as a protuberance toward the probe on the ilium. With the probe in this location, small maneuvers of tilt are performed to optimize the visualization of the fascia iliaca. The deep circumflex iliac artery may be identified between the internal oblique and fascia iliaca and serves as both a landmark and a "stop sign" to stop further needle advancement. An echogenic needle is inserted in-plane from the inferior aspect of the probe. Both Hebbard and Desmet described entering skin just inferior to the inguinal ligament[697,698] and reaching the fascia iliaca roughly at the level of the ligament, or just superior to the ligament.[697,699] Hydrodissection with saline can be used to define the plane to confirm spread between the hyperechoic fascia iliaca and the more heterogeneous iliacus muscle beneath it. With appropriate spread, the needle is further advanced into the pocket of local anesthetic, moving in the cephalad direction as the iliacus muscle is hydrodissected away from the overlying fascia iliaca. Catheters can be deployed in this space after creating a pocket. A volume of 0.5 to 0.7 mL/kg can be injected, limited by the maximum allowed local anesthetic dose.

Landmark-Guided Facia Iliaca Block

The injection is made approximately 1 centimeter inferior to the junction of the outer and middle thirds of the inguinal ligament (see Fig. 40.79A). As the needle is inserted at a perpendicular angle of about 75 degrees to the skin, two characteristic pops are felt as the needle pierces the fascia lata and then the fascia iliaca. Slight pressure on a fluid-filled syringe attached to the needle may aid in placement of the block by producing a subtle loss of resistance when the fascia iliaca compartment is entered. The angle of needle insertion is decreased and directed cephalad, and the local anesthetic is incrementally injected. One should feel little resistance to injection. Digital pressure is exerted distally to the site during the injection and for a short time afterward, and the swelling produced in the groin by the volume of local anesthetic is massaged to promote proximal flow of the drug. A long-acting local anesthetic, such as bupivacaine, ropivacaine, or levobupivacaine, is usually chosen so that postoperative blockade can provide prolonged analgesia. A volume of 0.3 to 0.5 mL/kg is sufficient in most cases.

Complications

Because of the larger volume required to provide an adequate block, care must be taken to not exceed the maximum dosage of the local anesthetic. Intravascular injection may be avoided with incremental injection and frequent aspiration.

Ankle Blocks

Block of the nerves of the foot at the ankle is a technique that is valuable to produce both surgical anesthesia and postoperative analgesia for procedures on the foot. These blocks are commonly performed without ultrasound guidance.

Anatomy

Three nerves can be blocked from the dorsal aspect of the foot. The deep peroneal nerve (L4, L5, S1, and S2) innervates the web space between the great and second toes. This nerve extends down the anterior aspect of the leg medial to the extensor hallucis longus and lateral to both the anterior tibial muscle and the anterior tibial artery. It is blocked at the level of the ankle crease in the lower part of the leg by inserting a 25-gauge needle through the skin until it contacts the tibia (Fig. 40.81A). 2 to 3 milliliters of local anesthetic are injected, and then an additional amount as the needle is being withdrawn. The superficial peroneal nerve (L4, L5, S1, and S2) innervates the medial and lateral aspects of the dorsum of the foot. Its anatomic course passes through the crural fascia on the anterior aspect of the distal two-thirds of the leg and subcutaneously along the lateral aspect of the foot. It is blocked immediately above the talocrural joint. It can be blocked by subcutaneous infiltration of local anesthetic from the anterior border of the tibia to the lateral malleolus. The last nerve that lies on the dorsal aspect of the foot is the saphenous nerve, which innervates the skin over the medial malleolus. It is blocked by subcutaneous infiltration around the great saphenous vein at the level of the medial malleolus. The tibial and sural nerves are blocked using a posterior approach. The tibial nerve (L4, L5, S1, S2, and S3) lies posterior to the posterior tibial artery and divides into the medial and lateral plantar branches, which innervate their respective aspects of the sole of the foot. It is blocked at the level of the posterior medial malleolus.

Technique

It is not necessary to elicit paresthesias, and an ankle block can be satisfactorily performed in sedated children without the use of a nerve stimulator. Five principal nerves must be blocked to provide analgesia to the entire foot: (1) the deep peroneal, (2) superficial peroneal, (3) saphenous, (4) tibial, and (5) sural nerves (see Fig. 40.81). The technique is the same as in the adult. It should be noted that there might be some variation in the precise distribution of distal innervation from child to child. A 25-gauge needle is inserted at a 90-degree angle to the posterior aspect of the tibia and is directed lateral to the posterior tibial artery until the tibia is contacted. Several milliliters of local anesthetic are deposited at this level and several more are injected as the needle is withdrawn. The sural nerve innervates the heel. It is blocked by subcutaneous infiltration of local anesthetic from the Achilles tendon to the lateral malleolus (see Fig. 40.81B). The deep peroneal nerve is located next to the extensor hallucis longus tendon, usually located by palpating the dorsalis pedis artery. The needle is inserted lateral to the extensor hallucis longus tendon and is advanced until it meets the periosteum of the metatarsal. It is then withdrawn a few millimeters. After careful aspiration, a volume of 2 to

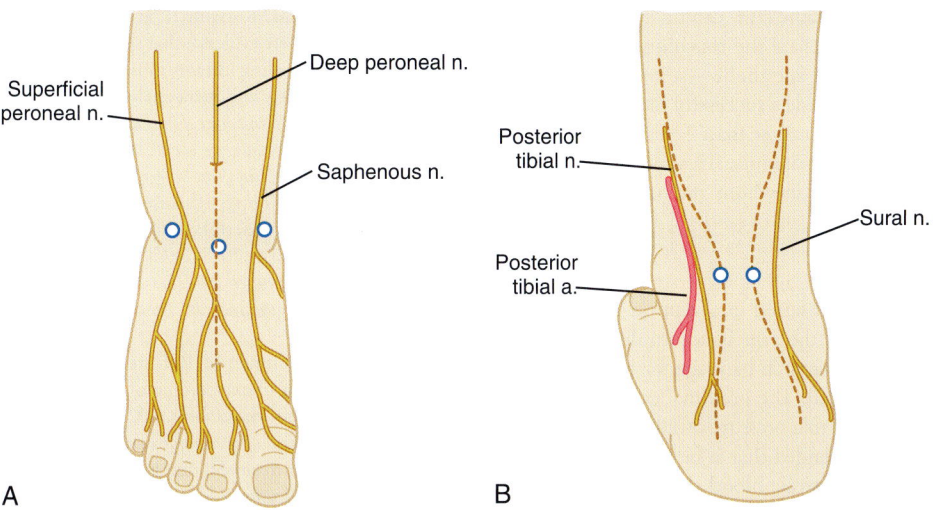

FIGURE 40.81 Ankle block. Block of the ankle generally requires five separate nerves to be blocked. Three nerves can be blocked from the dorsal aspect of the foot **(A)** and two on either side of the Achilles tendon **(B)**. Sites of injection are indicated by the *circles. a.,* Artery; *n.,* nerve.

3 milliliters of local anesthetic is injected. The superficial peroneal nerve is located under the dorsum of the foot. A superficial injection from the lateral malleolus to the extensor hallucis longus tendon area blocks all the branches of the superficial peroneal nerve.

Complications

It is very rare to see complications from an ankle block. However, the use of vasoconstrictors can theoretically cause necrosis of the toes. Care should be taken to avoid the use of an ankle block in children who may have compromised blood flow to the lower extremity.

Digital Nerve Blocks: Foot

This is an easy block to perform and is useful for surgeries that include trauma to the nails and toes, ingrown toenail surgery, and laser treatment of warts.[647]

Anatomy

The digital nerves of the foot are derived from the plantar cutaneous branches of the tibial nerve. The proper digital nerve of the great toe pierces the plantar aponeurosis posterior to the tarsal-medial joint and supplies the medial side of the great toe. The three common digital nerves pass between the divisions of the plantar aponeurosis and split into two proper digital nerves each. The first supplies the adjacent areas of the great and second toes; the second supplies the adjacent sides of the second and third toes; the third supplies the adjacent sides of the third and fourth toes. Each proper digital nerve gives off cutaneous and articular filaments that terminate at the tip of the toe. The superficial peroneal nerve gives off branches that supply the dorsum of the foot. They are derived from two nerves: (1) the dorsal cutaneous divides into two branches, a medial one that supplies the great toe and a lateral one that supplies the adjacent sides of the second and third toes; and (2) the intermediate dorsal cutaneous nerve, which passes along the lateral part of the foot supplying the lateral part of the dorsum of the foot and communicating with the sural nerve. This latter nerve terminates by dividing into two dorsal digital branches, one of which supplies the adjacent sides of the third and fourth toes and another one that supplies the adjacent sides of the fourth and little toes.

Landmark-Guided Foot Blocks

Placement of the needle for this block can be initially difficult owing to the thickness of the overlying skin. We prefer using an approach in which we access the nerve from the web space or at the dorsolateral aspect of the toe. Bupivacaine *without epinephrine* is injected (1–2 mL) after aspiration to rule out intravascular placement. These blocks should be avoided in children with already compromised blood flow to the toes.

Complications

Large volumes of local anesthetic are contraindicated because this may cause pressure and vascular compromise. *Vasoconstrictors should be avoided because this may cause necrosis of the digit.*[648] Intravascular injection may be avoided with incremental injection with frequent aspiration.

Intravenous Regional Anesthesia

Intravenous regional anesthesia was first described in 1908 by August Bier and is frequently referred to as the Bier block.[700] Although infrequently performed in children, this technique has been advocated for upper extremity procedures lasting 30 to 60 minutes because of its rapid onset of anesthesia and its ease of performance.[701,702]

Only dilute lidocaine (0.25% or 0.5%) should be used because of the risk of local anesthetic toxicity, particularly if the tourniquet is deflated early or inadvertently. This can be a useful block for upper extremity fracture reduction[703,704] or suture of a large laceration in children with a full stomach cared for in the emergency room. It is also helpful for chronic painful conditions, including complex regional pain syndrome type 1 in children and adolescents, and other agents have been injected along with local anesthetics for this purpose.[705] The exsanguination and manipulation of the limb before administering the local anesthetic may prove to be unduly painful for children with a fracture, and many children may not tolerate the discomfort of the tourniquet without significant sedation. Another disadvantage is the possibility of toxic reactions in the event of tourniquet failure. Strict attention to detail—elevation or exsanguination of the extremity to be blocked, proper application of a double pneumatic cuff, careful attention to anesthetic dose, and care not to deflate the tourniquet until 30 minutes after injection of the local anesthetic—is important to avoid serious complications and provide a successful block. This block is unsuitable for infants (those younger than 1 year of age) because of the risk of toxic reactions in infants. This technique may also be contraindicated in children in whom the prolonged use of a tourniquet is inadvisable.

TECHNIQUE

A small-gauge IV cannula is inserted in a vein on the dorsum of the hand. Exsanguination of the arm is accomplished either by wrapping the limb with an Esmarch bandage, or by elevating the limb if wrapping is too painful. The proximal compartment of a double tourniquet is inflated to a pressure of 200 to 250 mm Hg, although some have recommended that it be inflated to 150 mm Hg greater than the child's systolic blood pressure. If tourniquet pain develops during the procedure, the distal cuff may be inflated, followed by deflation of the proximal cuff. The tourniquet must remain inflated for a minimum of 30 minutes to prevent a rapid IV infusion of lidocaine and sequelae. It is best to deflate the tourniquet incrementally. Because no residual blockade persists after the tourniquet is released, supplementary analgesia must be considered (e.g., IV opioids, local infiltration with a long-acting local anesthetic).

SELECTION OF DRUGS

Use 1 mL/kg of *preservative-free* 0.25% to 0.5% lidocaine without epinephrine for this block because the duration of the block is limited by the tourniquet time and because of the greater potential for cardiac toxicity with longer-acting agents. A very low dose of a nondepolarizing neuromuscular blocking agent such as rocuronium (0.03 mg/kg) may improve the quality of the motor blockade.[706–708]

COMPLICATIONS

Unintended deflation of the tourniquet results in release of drug into the intravascular compartment; hence, only a short-acting local anesthetic, such as lidocaine, should be used. *Bupivacaine should never be used for this block because of concerns around cardiotoxicity.*

Acknowledgment

The authors wish to thank Per-Arne Lönnqvist, MD, DEAA, FRCA, PhD, for his generous contribution to the paravertebral block section of this chapter and Wing H Kwok, MB, ChB, FANZCA for his contributions to the ultrasound-guided portions of this chapter from the previous edition. Figures, sonograms, and videos in this chapter were reproduced with permission from https://www.aic.cuhk.edu.hk/usgraweb or created and generously shared by Rani Sunder, MD and Corrie Anderson, MD, FAAP.

ANNOTATED REFERENCES

Adler AC, Belon CA, Guffey DM, Minard CG, Patel NV, Chandrakantan A. Real-time ultrasound improves accuracy of caudal block in children. *Anesth Analg.* 2020;130(4):1002-1007.

In this prospective study the authors suggest that caudal blockade, long considered a landmark-guided technique, might also be better performed with ultrasound guidance.

Dohms K, Hein M, Rossaint R, et al. Inguinal hernia repair in preterm neonates: is there evidence that spinal or general anaesthesia is the better option regarding intraoperative and postoperative complications? A systematic review and meta-analysis. *BMJ Open.* 2019;9(10):e028728.

This meta-analysis found that spinal anesthesia had both fewer intraoperative and postoperative adverse events compared with general anesthesia, albeit with a 7% conversion rate to general anesthesia.

Guay J, Suresh S, Kopp S. The use of ultrasound guidance for perioperative neuraxial and peripheral nerve blocks in children. *Cochrane Database Syst Rev.* 2019;2019(2):CD011436.

This is the most updated evidence-based review article to support the use of ultrasound guidance in neuraxial and peripheral nerve blocks for children.

Macfarlane AJR, Gitman M, Bornstein KJ, El-Boghdadly K, Weinberg G. Updates in our understanding of local anaesthetic systemic toxicity: a narrative review. *Anaesthesia.* 2021;76(S1):27-39.

An up-to-date review of the major concepts in understanding local anesthetic toxicity and its treatment and prevention. The senior author is one of the primary investigators who developed lipid rescue therapy.

Marhofer P, Frickey N. Ultrasonographic guidance in pediatric regional anesthesia Part I: theoretical background. *Pediatr Anesth.* 2006;16(10):1008-1018.

In this review article, Marhofer and Frickey, from Vienna, Austria, discuss the basic principles of ultrasound that are a prerequisite for the safe application of ultrasound for regional anesthesia in children.

Masaracchia MM, Sunder RA, Polaner DM. Error traps in pediatric regional anesthesia. *Pediatr Anesth.* 2021;31(11):1161-1169.

A review of some of the heuristic errors that can lead to failure, complications, or suboptimal performance of regional anesthetics in children, along with ways to avoid them.

Rosenberg PH, Veering BT, Urmey WF. Maximum recommended doses of local anesthetics: a multifactorial concept. *Reg Anesth Pain Med.* 2004;29(6):564-575, discussion 524.

A scientific and pharmacologic approach to local anesthetic toxicity that explains the important concept that a simple dose per kilogram is insufficient to determine how much drug is safe to administer.

Taenzer AH, Hoyt M, Krane EJ, et al. Variation between and within hospitals in single injection caudal local anesthetic dose: a report from the Pediatric Regional Anesthesia Network. *Anesth Analg.* 2020;130(6):1693-1701.

Of direct impact on LAST risk, this study, and a companion study on peripheral nerve blockade (Taenzer AH, Herrick M, Hoyt M, et al. Variation in pediatric local anesthetic dosing for peripheral nerve blocks: an analysis from the Pediatric Regional Anesthesia Network (PRAN). Regional Anesthesia and Pain Medicine. 2020;45(12):964-969.) found large amounts of unwarranted variability in local anesthetic dosing.

Taenzer AH, Walker BJ, Bosenberg AT, et al. Asleep versus awake: does it matter? Pediatric regional block complications by patient state: a report from the Pediatric Regional Anesthesia Network. *Reg Anesth Pain Med.* 2014;39(4):279-283.

A landmark study that presents the first prospective data that administering regional blocks in children under general anesthesia does not increase risk. Previous admonitions about the risk of this practice were based on a few case reports. These data show that administering regional anesthesia in anesthetized pediatric patients is at least as safe, and possibly safer, than in awake or sedated children.

Walker BJ, Long JB, De Oliveira GS, et al. Peripheral nerve catheters in children: an analysis of safety and practice patterns from the Pediatric Regional Anesthesia Network (PRAN). *Br J Anaesth.* 2015;115(3):457-462.

Peripheral nerve catheters are being increasingly used for ambulatory surgery of the extremities. These catheters can be safely managed at home if well-designed follow-up systems are in place. Accidental catheter dislodgment remains the primary problem.

Walker BJ, Long JB, Sathyamoorthy M, et al. Complications in pediatric regional anesthesia: an analysis of more than 100,000 blocks from the Pediatric Regional Anesthesia Network. *Anesthesiology.* 2018;129(4):721-732.

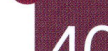

This is a follow-up to the original paper from the Pediatric Regional Anesthetic Network (Polaner DM, Taenzer AH, Walker BJ, et al. Pediatric Regional Anesthesia Network (PRAN): a multiinstitutional study of the use and incidence of complications of pediatric regional anesthesia. Anesth Analg. 2012;115(6):1353-1364) with a huge cohort of close to 10 times the original population. It is the most comprehensive prospective analysis of regional anesthesia practice in the United States and confirms a very low incidence of adverse events and complications.

A complete reference list can be found online at Elsevier eBooks+.

40

41 Acute Pain

JARED R. E. HYLTON, BENJAMIN WALKER, AND DAVID M. POLANER

Developmental Neurobiology of Pain
Pain Assessment
Self-Report Measures
Observational-Behavioral Measures
Limitations of Pain Assessment
Special Considerations for the Cognitively
Impaired Child
Strategies for Pain Management
Surgical Considerations

Pharmacologic Treatment of Pain
Nonopioid Analgesics
Selection of Opioids for Parenteral Use
Regional Blockade and Analgesia
Pain Management in the Cognitively Impaired Child
Opioid Analgesics
Nonopioid Analgesics
Epidural and Regional Analgesia

THE PRACTICE OF PAIN MANAGEMENT in children continues to advance. Since the early 1980s, clinicians have recognized that neonates and infants experience pain and process those learned experiences. There are long-term adverse consequences of unrelieved pain, including harmful neuroendocrine responses, disrupted eating and sleep cycles, and increased pain perception during subsequent painful experiences.[1–3] Adequate pain control is second only to correct diagnosis for parents who were surveyed about their priorities and concerns surrounding hospital admission.[4] Disparities in pain treatment led organizations, such as the Agency for Healthcare Research and Quality (AHRQ) and the Society for Pediatric Pain Medicine (SPPM) (https://pedspainmedicine.org), to provide guidelines and the Joint Commission (formerly the Joint Commission on Accreditation of Healthcare Organizations) to issue mandates that further enhanced pediatric pain management.[5–7] The availability of reliable and valid pain assessment tools for children and governmental incentives encouraged the inclusion of children in analgesic drug trials.[8] Many children's hospitals have dedicated multidisciplinary teams that manage acute and chronic pain. The increasing use of regional analgesia techniques led to the development of the Pediatric Regional Anesthesia Network, a registry of practice patterns and complications of regional anesthetics in children.[9] An enormous expansion of opioid-sparing multimodal analgesic regimens and regional anesthetic techniques for acute pain management in children, the establishment of pediatric pain services, and the development of pediatric-specific enhanced recovery after anesthesia (ERAS) protocols,[7,10–12] all attest to the importance accorded to this aspect of perioperative care.

Developmental Neurobiology of Pain

Nociceptive pathways in the periphery, spinal cord, and brain develop in a series of stages through the second and third trimester in humans. By 26 weeks postconceptional age, peripheral and spinal afferent transmissions have matured sufficiently for the late-gestation fetus or preterm neonate to respond to tissue injury or inflammation with withdrawal reflexes, autonomic arousal, and hormonal metabolic stress responses. There are also changes in responsiveness after injury or repetitive stimulation indicative of central sensitization. In general, preterm neonates have reduced thresholds for withdrawal to noxious thermal and mechanical stimuli and immature descending inhibitor pathways that are necessary for modulating the pain response compared with older infants and children. One mechanism that may contribute to these low-threshold responses involves projections of low-threshold peripheral afferents to superficial as well as deep laminae in the spinal dorsal horn; later in development these afferents project only to deeper dorsal horn laminae. Most of the neural pathways that conduct nociception from the periphery through the central nervous system (CNS) are present and functional at 24-weeks gestational age, although the central connections, particularly in the thalamocortical pathways that are involved in the integration and perception of conscious pain, are not as well developed.[8,12–17] Controversy remains as to the meaning and implications of this neural immaturity. Opioid receptors and responses are present in the spinal cord at the time of birth, although spinal glial inflammatory mechanisms are immature. Because these latter mechanisms are central to the cyclooxygenase (COX-1 and COX-2) responses, this may imply that there is limited or no analgesic response to nonsteroidal antiinflammatory drugs (NSAIDs) and COX inhibitors in preterm infants or neonates, although clinical studies do not support this hypothesis. Opioid responses, however, are active.

Gamma-aminobutyric acid (GABA) receptors and associated pathways, which play an important role in the effects of analgesics and anesthetics, can be either excitatory or inhibitory, depending on the stage of development.[18] The neuroplasticity that is characteristic of these infants may be a double-edged sword. Animal models and some clinical evidence suggest that repeated noxious stimuli may result in heightened sensitivity to nociceptive input and adverse behavioral sequelae.[2,18–20] On the other hand, nerve injury in infant animals may result in less pain than in older animals.[21,22] In humans, for example, the neural injury to the brachial plexus after shoulder dystocia during delivery rarely results in chronic pain. It may be that there are both vulnerable periods and periods of greater resiliency during development, so that the consequences of pain in young children may not be easily predictable.

Investigators have examined indices suggestive of cortical activation, including near-infrared spectroscopy[2,23] and electroencephalography,[22,24] in response to noxious events. Using near-infrared spectroscopy, a unilateral heel stick (performed for clinical purposes) produces signal changes suggestive of contralateral cortical activation.[21,25–27] Despite these lines of evidence, the nature of pain in neonates, viewed as conscious suffering, continues to be an active area of investigation. Another area of interest is how pain experienced during the neonatal period can influence neurodevelopmental outcomes and either the somatosensory or emotional components of subsequent pain responses later in life. The developing nervous system is vulnerable to alterations in activity. Noxious stimuli influence neurodevelopmental outcomes, and intervention with analgesics likely modulates the potential long-term effects of acute pain within the neonatal period.[25] It is recognized that the specific long-term effects of pain are difficult to study and distinguish from other comorbidities in neonates.[28] The most immature and clinically complex neonates may require numerous procedures and have other confounding factors such as infection, physiologic instability, environmental factors, and pharmacologic exposures. It is known that surrogates for pain exposure within the neonatal period are associated with poorer cognitive, motor, and behavioral neurodevelopmental outcomes in infancy.[27] Given this evolving information, many clinicians and investigators have adopted the view that, in the absence of better information about either the nature of suffering experienced by neonates or the potential adverse long-term consequences of pain, caregivers should err on the side of providing adequate analgesia for acute pain.[29] Although this is a compelling perspective, it is important to highlight three concerns: (1) in general, available studies have had difficulty showing effects of routine administration of analgesia (e.g., morphine infusions) on immediate behavioral indexes of distress in neonates undergoing intensive care[26]; (2) repeated or prolonged administration of anesthetics and sedatives in animal models have been shown to have deleterious effects on brain development,[30,31] although human studies have not corroborated these findings,[32,33] and the implications of these animal studies remain unclear at this time[34,35] (see also Chapter 23); and (3) as detailed later, younger organisms develop tolerance to opioids and benzodiazepines more rapidly than older organisms, so that the management of tolerance and withdrawal has now become a nearly universal consequence of prolonged administration of these medications to critically ill neonates, infants, and children.

A review of data regarding the development of consciousness in the fetus concluded that *"it is rather unlikely that the infant can be seen as a conscious human before 24 weeks of gestational age, thus before all the thalamocortical connections are established."*[36] Another review states that *"the fetus processes sensory stimuli at a cortical level, including painful stimulus, from about 25 weeks of gestation onwards."*[37] It is clear that there is much more work needed to separate reflex withdrawal from a painful stimulus and cognition of that stimulus as pain.

Pain Assessment

The International Association for the Study of Pain has defined *pain* as an unpleasant sensory and emotional experience associated with actual or potential tissue damage or *described* in terms of such damage. This definition was expanded in 2020 to include six key notes[38]:

- Pain is always a personal experience that is influenced to varying degrees by biological, psychological, and social factors.

- Pain and nociception are different phenomena. Pain cannot be inferred solely from activity in sensory neurons.
- Through life experiences, individuals learn the concept of pain.
- A person's report of an experience as pain should be respected.
- Although pain usually serves an adaptive role, it may have adverse effects on function and social and psychological well-being.
- Verbal description is only one of several behaviors to express pain; inability to communicate does not negate the possibility that a human or a nonhuman animal experiences pain.

The International Association for the Study of Pain and others have acknowledged that the inability to communicate verbally, as in the preverbal, nonverbal, or the cognitively impaired, does not preclude the possibility that an individual is experiencing pain and is in need of appropriate pain management.[39,40] Table 41.1 summarizes other pain assessment tools categorized in terms of appropriate age, target population, ease of use, and practicality. Commonly used scales are discussed in more detail later.

Consensus guidelines have been published with recommendations for appropriate tools to use for research studies, many of which are simple to apply in routine clinical settings.[8,41] It should be emphasized that pain intensity is only one of a multitude of factors that should be considered when performing a global pain assessment. Other factors of a biopsychosocial approach to pain assessment should include functional recovery, patient satisfaction, perception of care, adverse effects, emotional recovery, and economic factors. The Revised American Pain Society Patient Outcomes Questionnaire (APS-POQ-R) consists of 12 questions pertaining to multiple pain outcomes.[42] A pediatric version for children <12 years of age[43] and adolescents[44] revealed excellent feedback from parents regarding the quality and improvement of pain management.[39,45] This questionnaire was easy to administer and understandable by both pediatric patients and their parents. The domains of pain intensity, functional interference, emotional response, side effects, perceptions of care and usual pain allow greater individualized management of hospitalized children. It likely holds the greatest utility for quality improvement purposes.

SELF-REPORT MEASURES

Self-report metrics in which a patient is asked to quantify the severity of the pain between 0 (no pain) and 10 (maximum severe pain) most accurately reflect acute pain because pain is a subjective experience. Because many children lack the cognitive skills to use such scales, pain assessment metrics have been developed to include developmentally appropriate self-report tools, behavioral-observational tools, and physiologic-biologic measures (see Table 41.1).[46–49] Therefore, regardless of the metric used, it must be emphasized that a complete pain assessment is more than just a number attempting to quantify the severity of pain, which is why these metrics must not be used as an independent indicator to prescribe or dose pharmacotherapy. Estimating the impact of pain on the suffering and the quality of the individual's life and recovery process, targeting appropriate therapeutic metrics, and evaluating the efficacy and side effects of such measures are additional key components of a global and ongoing pain assessment and treatment strategy.

For children to use numeric scales, they must understand the concepts of magnitude and ordinal position—that is, they must be able to identify which of different-sized objects is bigger and place them in order from smallest to largest. They must also be able to arrange geometric figures or numbers in a series *(seriation)*. These skills are typically not present until about 7 years of age;

TABLE 41.1	Other Appropriate Pain Assessment Measures by Age Group: Self-Report, Observational/Behavior, and for the Cognitively Impaired	
Self-Report Tools	**Appropriate Age Groups**	**Comments**
Faces Pain Scale	3–18 years	Simple and quick to use; extensively validated in healthy school children with postoperative and cancer pain
Oucher	3–18 years	Photographic for ≥3-year-olds, numeric 0–10 scale for ≥6-year-olds; less clinical utility and feasibility compared with other faces scales
Manchester Pain Scale	3–18 years	Panda bear faces eliminate gender and ethnic bias; tested in emergency department setting
Computer Face Scale	4–18 years	Offers option for continuous rather than categorical format; good construct validity; preferred by children over the Wong-Baker Faces Scale; further testing needed
Sydney Animated Facial Expression Scale (SAFE)	4–18 years	Animated version of Faces Pain Scale; rated by children as easiest to use; no psychometric advantage compared with other scales
Visual Analog Scale[54]	6–18 years	Simple and quick to use; requires the concepts of order, magnitude, and seriation (the ability to place or visualize in series); widely used across settings; preferred to other self-report tools by children ≥8 years old and adolescents
Numeric Rating Scale (NRS)	7–18 years	Simplest and most commonly used in clinical as well as research settings
Observational/Behavioral Measures		
Comfort Scale	0–18 years	Developed for use in intensive care settings; useful in mechanically ventilated children and in the postoperative setting
Face, Legs, Activity, Cry, Consolability (FLACC)	2 months–7 years	Excellent pragmatic and psychometric qualities; widely adopted in clinical and research settings; has been translated into several languages other than English
Children's Hospital of Eastern Ontario Pain Scale (CHEOPS)	1–7 years	Good psychometric properties; lengthy with inconsistent scoring among categories; cumbersome; extensively used both in clinical and research settings
Cognitively Impaired Children		
Revised FLACC	All ages	Allows for scoring individualized pain behaviors; good psychometric properties; highest clinical utility compared with the Non-Communicating Children's Pain Checklist–Postoperative Version (NCCPC-PV) and Nursing Assessment of Pain Intensity (NAPI)
Non-Communicating Children's Pain Checklist (NCCPC)	All ages	Requires 5-minute observation period; comprehensive but cumbersome; used in clinical and research setting
University of Wisconsin Pain Scale	All ages	Inconsistent scoring style compared with other clinical scoring systems; scoring style may permit flexibility but limits precision
The Pain Indicator for Communicatively Impaired Children	All ages	Useful for pain assessment in cognitively impaired children in the home setting

thus, pain assessment tools that use graphic facial displays representing different degrees of pain expression are often used to facilitate self-report of pain in young children.

Faces Pain Scales

Faces pain scales consist of a series of line diagrams of faces with expressions of increasing distress.[48–54] Some versions have a smiling face, whereas others, notably the Faces Pain Scale and Faces Pain Scale-Revised (FPS-R), have a neutral face to represent the "no pain" end of the scale (Fig. 41.1).[52,54,55] Unlike the numeric scales, the faces scales do not require the concept of magnitude or seriation and can therefore be used by preschool-aged children. The Wong-Baker Faces Pain Scale has been extensively studied and its reliability and validity confirmed in children 3 to 18 years of age. Strong correlations have been reported between the Wong-Baker Scale scores and other faces scales, the Visual Analog Scale,[54] as well as nurses' ratings based on behavior.[55–58] Versions with the smiling face at the no-pain end of the spectrum, such as the Wong-Baker Scale, may overestimate pain because children without pain, but

with distress from other sources, may be reluctant to choose the smiling face.[54] The Wong-Baker Scale was preferred by children to the numeric rating scale, the graphic rating scale, and the Color Analog Scale.[49,53,54,56,58] Overall, the FPS-R is the faces scale with the largest support for its validity.[59] The International Association for the Study of Pain (IASP) has the FPS-R available in dozens of languages on its website (http://www.iasp-pain.org/education). An electronic version using a hand-held device is also available.

Visual Analog Scale

Several versions of the visual analog scale (VAS) are available, including horizontal and vertical lines, word anchors representing extremes of pain, and lines with divisions and numeric values (Fig. 41.2). When using the vertical versions of this scale, the severity of the pain increases as one ascends the ladder. Although moderate to strong correlations have been reported between the VAS, faces pain scales, the Oucher (E-Fig. 41.1), and ethnic versions of the Oucher (E-Fig. 41.2),[60–62] the effect of user age on VAS ratings are conflicting.

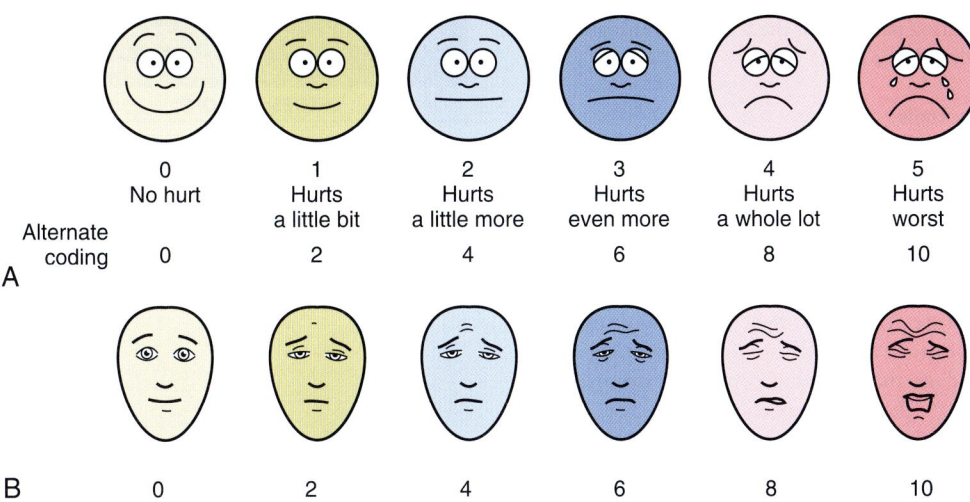

FIGURE 41.1 A, The Wong-Baker Faces Pain Scale. **B,** The Bieri Faces Pain Scale. (**B** modified from Bieri D, Reeve RA, Champion GD, et al. The Faces Pain Scale for the self-assessment of the severity of pain experienced by children: development, initial validation, and preliminary investigation for ratio scale properties. *Pain.* 1990;41(2):139-150.)

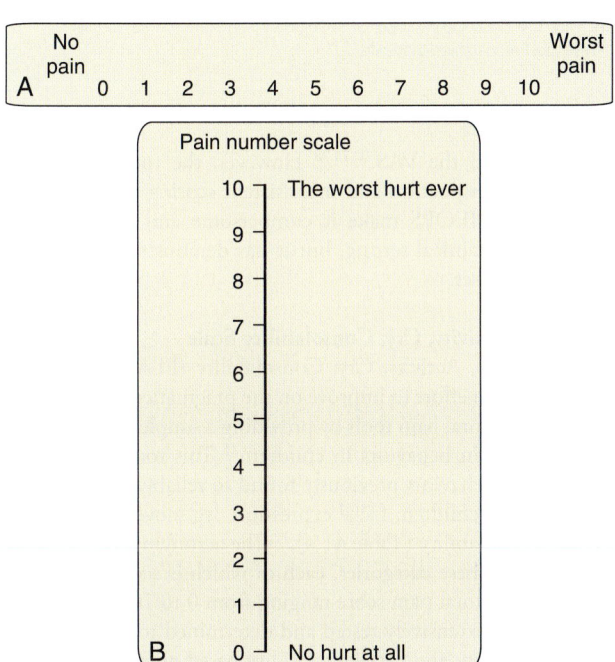

FIGURE 41.2 Numerical self-report scales. **A,** Horizontal Visual Analog Scale. **B,** Vertical Visual Analog Scale.

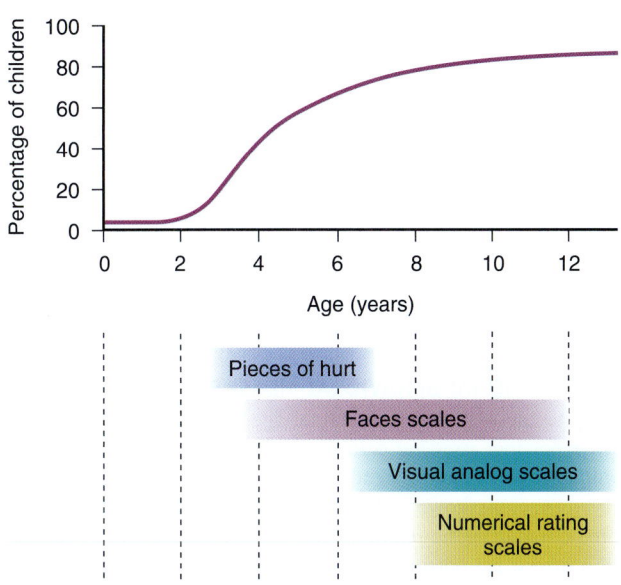

FIGURE 41.3 Self-report tools most appropriate for different age ranges. The percentage of children at different ages who can self-report their pain is shown in the upper panel. The lower panel shows suitable pain measures for different ages.

Numeric Rating Scale

The numeric rating scale (NRS) is the simplest and most commonly used scale. The child rates the pain from 0 (no pain) to 10 (worst pain). Its validity has been established with good correlations between NRS and FPS-R scores in children 7 to 17 years of age and NRS and VAS scores in children 9 to 17 years of age.[59,63] The NRS also correlates well with perceived need for analgesia, pain relief, and patient satisfaction in children.[64]

Selection Criteria

Selection of a self-report tool for a child requires careful consideration of the age and cognitive and developmental level. Fig. 41.3

depicts the percentages of children of different ages who can self-report their pain and the tools most appropriate for various age ranges. Children who are unable to use a self-report tool may be able to report their pain intensity using simple words, such as "small," "medium," and "big." However, self-reports of pain are subject to the modulating influences of many factors, including the child's previous pain experience and response to treatment, psychosocial factors, and parental preferences and influences. Consequently, in many cases, it may be necessary to complement self-reported pain scores with behavioral observations, particularly in preschool-aged children. Regardless of the tool selected, assessment of postoperative pain is greatly facilitated by the introduction of the concept of rating pain and of the tool itself during the preoperative preparation of the child.

Novel Self-Report Tools

These self-report tools use a categorical format and the static faces do not allow for "fine-tuning" of the ratings before a final assessment regarding the severity of pain is reached.[62,65] In recent years, there has been interest in developing computer-based self-report assessment tools that use a continuous rather than categorical format.[66]

The Computer Face Scale allows the child to adjust the shape of the mouth of a cartoon face from smiling to frowning and simultaneously to adjust the eyes from completely open to completely closed.[64,65,67,68] The suggested benefits of this scale include increased sensitivity (given the ability to select from a wide range of faces) and computerized storage of the results, with ready access and data display; this scale has demonstrated its construct validity, and it was preferred by children over the Wong-Baker Faces Scale.[65,66]

The Sydney Animated Facial Expression Scale (SAFE) is an animated version of the Faces Pain Scale[65,69] and consists of a series of 101 faces. To administer this scale, the child pushes the left or right arrow key on a computer, causing the expression of the single face to change until it corresponds with the child's pain intensity. At this point, a keystroke records a score between 0 and 100. The SAFE scale was rated to be easiest to use by children aged 4 to 16 years compared with other scales, including the Faces Pain Scale, the Color Analog Scale, and Pieces of Hurt,[67,70] although it offered no psychometric advantage over the other scales. Further research with this tool is needed before its role can be clearly defined. A systematic review concluded that by balancing feasibility and psychometric properties, the Faces Pain Scale-Revised is recommended for self-assessment taking into account feasibility and psychometric properties.[71]

OBSERVATIONAL-BEHAVIORAL MEASURES

Despite the availability of several age-appropriate methods for self-reporting, assessing pain in children who are unable or unwilling to self-report depends on observations of their behaviors. Five behaviors shown to be reliable, specific, and sensitive when predicting analgesic requirements are facial expression, vocalization or cry, leg posture, body posture, and motor restlessness.[72] Variations in these behaviors have been used in several observational pain tools. Table 41.2 describes the content validity of some commonly used observational tools. Behavior checklists provide a list of pain behaviors that are marked as present or absent, and the extent of pain is estimated on the basis of the number of behaviors present at the time of the assessment.[69,70,73,74] Behavior rating scales also incorporate a rating of the intensity or frequency and duration of each behavior.[75] Global rating scales provide a rating of the observer's overall impression of the child's pain. These scales require further validation in preverbal and early verbal children.[76]

Children's Hospital of Eastern Ontario Pain Scale

The Children's Hospital of Eastern Ontario Pain Scale (CHEOPS), one of the earliest behavioral rating scales (Table 41.3),[77] incorporates six categories of behavior scored individually from 0 to 2 or 1 to 3 and then sums them to provide a pain score ranging from 4 to 13. Scores of 6 or less indicate no pain. Its validity and reliability for brief painful events and for postoperative pain has been well established, with good to excellent correlations with faces

TABLE 41.2	Content Validity of Behavioral Pain Tools: Categories of Behavior in Pain Assessment Tools			
FLACC	**CHEOPS**	**OPS**	**TPPPS**	**Büttner/Finke**
Face	Facial expression		Facial pain expression	Facial expression
Legs	Leg movement	Movement		Leg position
Activity	Torso movement	Agitation	Bodily pain expression	Position of torso
				Motor restlessness
Cry	Cry	Cry	Vocal pain expression	Cry
Consolability	Touching of the wound	Blood pressure		Consolability
	Verbal report of pain	Verbal complaint and body language		

CHEOPS, Children's Hospital of Eastern Ontario Pain Scale; *FLAAC*, Face, Legs, Activity, Cry, Consolability scale; *OPS*, Objective Pain Scale; *TPPPS*, Toddler Preschool Preoperative Pain Scale.

pain scales and the VAS.[62,74,78] However, the time required to complete the evaluation and inconsistent scoring among categories of the CHEOPS make it cumbersome and impractical to use in a busy clinical setting, but it has demonstrated utility for research purposes.

Face, Legs, Activity, Cry, Consolability Scale

The Face, Legs, Activity, Cry, Consolability (FLACC) scale was developed in an effort to improve on the pragmatic qualities of the existing behavioral pain tools by providing a simple framework for quantifying pain behaviors in children.[75] This tool includes five categories of behaviors previously found to reliably correlate with pain in young children: facial expression, leg movement, activity, cry, and consolability (Table 41.4).[72] The acronym FLACC facilitates recall of these categories, each of which is scored from 0 to 2 to provide a total pain score ranging from 0 to 10. The FLACC tool has been extensively tested and determined to have good interrater reliability and excellent validity based on changes in pain scores from before to after analgesic administration and excellent correlation with the Objective Pain Scale (OPS), the CHEOPS, the Toddler Preschool Preoperative Pain Scale (TPPPS), and good correlation with self-reported pain scores using faces pain scales.[72,78–80] The FLACC scale has been translated into several languages, including Spanish, Chinese, Swedish, French, Italian, Portuguese, Norwegian, and Thai. A systematic review of 201 papers reported that the FLACC scale, the revised FLACC scale, and the Pediatric Pain Profile were the recommended observation tools for their specific age groups.[71]

COMFORT Scale

The COMFORT scale (Table 41.5), developed for use in an intensive care setting, consists of six behavioral and two physiologic measures, each of which has five response categories, thereby allowing detection of subtle changes in the child's distress.[78,81] Initial evaluation of the COMFORT scale found acceptable interrater reliability and

41

TABLE 41.3	Children's Hospital of Eastern Ontario Pain Scale (CHEOPS)[a]		
Item	**Behavioral**	**Score**	**Definition**
Cry	No cry	1	Child is not crying.
	Moaning	2	Child is moaning or quietly vocalizing silent cry.
	Crying	2	Child is crying, but the cry is gentle or whimpering.
	Scream	3	Child is in a full-lunged cry; sobbing; may be scored with complaint or without complaint.
Facial	Composed	1	Child has neutral facial expression.
	Grimace	2	Score only if definite negative facial expression.
	Smiling	0	Score only if definite positive facial expression.
Child Verbal	None	1	Child is not talking.
	Other complaints	1	Child complains, but not about pain, e.g., "I want to see mommy" or "I am thirsty."
	Pain complaints	2	Child complains about pain.
	Both complaints	2	Child complains about pain and about other things, e.g., "It hurts; I want my mommy."
	Positive	0	Child makes any positive statement or talks about other things without complaint.
Torso	Neutral	1	Body (not limbs) is at rest; torso is inactive.
	Shifting	2	Body is in motion in a shifting or serpentine fashion.
	Tense	2	Body is arched or rigid.
	Shivering	2	Body is shuddering or shaking involuntarily.
	Upright	2	Child is in a vertical or in upright position.
	Restrained	2	Body is restrained.
Touch	Not touching	1	Child is not touching or grabbing at wound.
	Reach	2	Child is reaching for but not touching wound.
	Touch	2	Child is gently touching wound or wound area.
	Grab	2	Child is grabbing vigorously at wound.
	Restrained	2	Child's arms are restrained.
Legs	Neutral	1	Legs may be in any position but are relaxed; includes gentle swimming or discrete movements.
	Squirming/kicking	2	Definitive uneasy or restless movements in the legs and/or striking out with foot or feet.
	Drawn up/tensed	2	Legs tensed and/or pulled up tightly to body and kept there.
	Standing	2	Standing, crouching, or kneeling.
	Restrained	2	Child's legs are being held down.

[a]Recommended for children 1 to 7 years old; a score greater than 6 indicates pain.

TABLE 41.4	The FLACC Behavioral Pain Scale		
	SCORING		
Categories	**0**	**1**	**2**
Face	No particular expression or smile	Occasional grimace or frown, withdrawn, disinterested	Frequent to constant frown, clenched jaw, quivering chin
Legs	Normal position or relaxed	Uneasy, restless, tense	Kicking, or legs drawn up
Activity	Lying quietly, normal position, moves easily	Squirming, shifting back and forth, tense	Arched, rigid, or jerking
Cry	No cry (awake or asleep)	Moans or whimpers, occasional complaint	Crying steadily, screams or sobs, frequent complaints
Consolability	Content, relaxed	Reassured by occasional touching, hugging, or being talked to, distractible	Difficult to console or comfort

Each of the five categories, (F) Face; (L) Legs; (A) Activity; (C) Cry; (C) Consolability, is scored from 0 to 2, which results in a total score between 0 and 10.
©2002, The Regents of the University of Michigan. All rights reserved.

TABLE 41.5	Comfort Scale				
	1	2	3	4	5
Alertness	Deeply asleep	Lightly asleep	Drowsy	Fully awake and alert	Hyper-alert
Calmness or Agitation	Calm	Slightly anxious	Anxious	Very anxious	Panicky
Respiratory Response	No coughing and no spontaneous respirations	Spontaneous respiration with little or no response to ventilation	Occasional cough or resistance to ventilator	Actively breathes against ventilator or coughs regularly	Fights ventilator; coughing or choking
Physical Movement	No movement	Occasional, slight movement	Frequent slight movement	Vigorous movement limited to extremities	Vigorous movement including torso and head
Blood Pressure	Less than baseline	Consistently at baseline	Infrequent increases of 15% or more (1–3 episodes during observation period)	Frequent increases of 15% or more (>3 episodes)	Sustained increase >15%
Muscle Tone	Muscles totally relaxed; no muscle tone	Reduced muscle tone	Normal muscle tone	Increased muscle tone and flexion of fingers and toes	Extreme muscle rigidity and flexion of fingers and toes
Facial Tension	Facial muscles totally relaxed	Facial muscle tone normal; no facial muscle tension evident	Tension evident in some facial muscles	Tension evident throughout facial muscles	Facial muscles contorted and grimacing
Heart Rate	Below baseline	Consistently at baseline	Infrequent elevations of 15% or more above baseline	Frequent elevations of 15% or more above baseline	Sustained elevation of 15% or more above baseline

good correlations with VAS scores in 37 mechanically ventilated infants.[81] Further study has evaluated the reliability and validity of the COMFORT scale as a postoperative pain instrument in children after thoracic or abdominal surgery.[82] That study found good to excellent interrater agreement for all categories except respiratory response, for which there was moderate agreement. Additionally, strong correlations between COMFORT and VAS pain scores support the use of the COMFORT scale as a postoperative pain assessment instrument in children; a systematic review reported adequate reliability regarding distress, pain, and sedation.[83]

After a systematic review of observational pain measures, the FLACC and CHEOPS[77] scales were recommended for assessment of pain associated with medical procedures, the FLACC for postoperative pain, and the Comfort scale for pain in children in critical care.[46] Despite the extensive science supporting the use of behavioral tools, it may be difficult to separate behaviors caused by pain from those caused by other sources of distress in some children.[84] Accurate pain assessment therefore requires careful consideration of the context of the behaviors. Input from the parents or caregivers may be valuable as proxy measures, although some parents may lose objectivity in such a situation. Similarly, a regular caregiver may best assess older children with significant developmental delay. When in doubt regarding the source of distress, a trial of analgesics is appropriate and may be both diagnostic and therapeutic. It also should be emphasized that the total score must be calculated by rating each category individually and never by simply assigning a total "gestalt" score.

Parents' Postoperative Pain Measure

The Parents' Postoperative Pain Measure (PPPM) is a 15-item yes/no questionnaire that is completed by a parent/caregiver and designed specifically for use at home without involvement of a health professional (E-Table 41.1). A score of 6 or greater correlates with clinically significant pain. This tool has been validated for children 2 to 12 years old[46,74,85] and is useful for research and quality improvement projects, especially as more operations are done on an outpatient basis.[84,86] A recent study of 319 children, 2 to 12 years of age, who underwent adenotonsillectomy, assessed pain scores using the PPPM scale in comparison with FLACC for children 2 to 3 years of age and FPS-R for children 4 to 12 years of age, confirmed the validity of the PPPM for children as young as 2 years old.[87]

LIMITATIONS OF PAIN ASSESSMENT

It remains unclear whether integration of routine pain assessment into clinical practice improves patient outcomes. A critical review of the studies that addressed this question determined that in two of six studies, children experienced a reduction in pain intensity when a standardized pain assessment tool was used; in two studies there was no change in pain intensity; and in two studies pain intensity decreased when pain assessment was combined with pain management interventions.[74,88] Studies that examined sustainability of the benefits over time yielded conflicting results, with most studies reported to have major methodologic problems.[85,89,90] Additional investigation is required to determine whether routine assessment of pain has any effect on pain outcomes.

Despite the large body of evidence supporting the psychometric properties of numerous structured pain assessment tools, there remains considerable variability in the interpretation of the clinical relevance of pain scores.[48,88] Attempts have been made to define what range of pain scores is associated with a perceived need for medicine or what magnitude of change in pain score is associated with a perception of better or worse pain.[48,64,91,92] A survey of 6- to 16-year-old hospitalized children found that a median pain score of 3 on a 0-to-6 Faces Pain Scale was associated with the child's perceived need for medicine.[91] Others have reported that a 10-mm change in a 0-to-100-mm VAS score was the minimum difference whereby children in the emergency department perceived their pain to be slightly better or slightly worse.[92] In the postoperative period, children with a median pain score of 6 on a 0-to-10 NRS scale perceived the need for an analgesic, whereas those with a score of 3 felt there was "no need" for treatment.[64] In addition, children felt "a little better" or "worse" if the NRS scale changed by at least 1. Adult patients perceived a change of 1.65 points on NRS and 16.55 on VAS in their pain severity as meaningful.[93] Despite these findings, there was large variability and overlap in scores associated with these outcomes.

Evaluations of the effectiveness of pain treatment algorithms based on numerical pain scores have yielded conflicting results. One study reported increased prescription of opioid and nonopioid analgesics, an increased administration of nonopioids, and reduced pain scores in children who received postoperative pain treatment based on a pain score–based algorithm.[94] Children whose pain management was algorithm-based experienced more nausea, but no other adverse effects. In contrast, hospitalized adults whose pain management was based on a numerical pain treatment algorithm experienced a 2-fold increase in episodes of oversedation and a 49% increase in opioid-related adverse drug events.[95] This latter study highlights the potential for harm when numeric pain scores alone are used to guide decisions regarding pain treatment. Combined self-reporting and behavioral observations are recommended to make decisions regarding the optimal pain treatment.[8,96] The pediatric Core Outcome Domains and Measures for Pediatric Acute and Chronic/Recurrent Pain Clinical Trials (PedIMMPACT) recommendations summarized the available validity and feasibility of many pain assessment tools and should be used as a guide for further pediatric pain studies.[41]

The over prescription of analgesics and sedatives has been attributed in part, to the widespread adoption of pain as the fifth vital sign.[97] National survey data demonstrate that approximately 276,000 adolescents in the United States abused prescription pain relievers in 2015, second only to marijuana. Prescription use of opioids in the teenage years has even been identified as an independent risk factor for nonmedical use of opioids in early adulthood.[98] Adult data show that many patients use only a fraction of their prescribed opioids after common outpatient procedures.[99] Quality improvement data from one hospital showed that children used only 10% to 20% of the opioid prescribed to them after tonsillectomy, and data from other institutions demonstrate that opioids are prescribed irrespective of the patient's age or weight.[100] Overprescribing of opioids is compounded by numerous studies that show that most families fail to properly dispose of unused opioids, leading to the inappropriate availability of opioids and risk of their abuse by the patient or other members of the household.[98]

State legislative efforts that limit the quantity of pediatric opioid prescriptions from practitioners in one state reported a ~24% decrease in morphine equivalent prescriptions, which should translate into a reduced risk of residual unused opioids available for later abuse.[101] A systematic review of opioid-reducing legislation in 24 states, with most limiting to 7-day limits, as well as several similar institution-based guidelines, found that such policies were effective in reducing postoperative opioid prescriptions in adults.[102]

These data highlight the need for procedure-specific opioid prescribing guidelines for children, as well as the importance of patient and family education regarding proper use, storage, and disposal of prescription opioids.

SPECIAL CONSIDERATIONS FOR THE COGNITIVELY IMPAIRED CHILD

Children who are cognitively impaired experience pain more frequently than cognitively intact children because of many inherent conditions, such as spasticity, muscle spasms, the need for assistive devices for positioning and mobility, and the need for invasive surgical procedures. Indeed, as many as 60% of children with cerebral palsy undergo orthopedic surgery by 8 years of age, and many of them require repeated procedures.[103] Yet both children and adults who are cognitively impaired receive fewer analgesics than those who are cognitively intact with similar painful conditions.[104,105] Barriers to effective pain management in the cognitively impaired include the complexity of pain assessment in those who cannot verbalize their pain, outdated beliefs that these children have altered or blunted pain perception, limited evidence for the safety and efficacy of analgesic regimens, and an exaggerated concern regarding opioid adverse effects, particularly respiratory depression. Although there is also evidence that cognitive impairment is an independent risk factor for rescue intervention when patient-controlled analgesia (PCA) by proxy is used,[106] this may reflect challenges in thoroughly assessing these patients rather than inherent differences in pain tolerance or opioid metabolism. Difficulties with pain assessment have led to the virtual exclusion of these children from clinical drug trials, leading to deficits in our knowledge of how to effectively manage their pain. A survey of clinicians who treat children who are cognitively impaired identified inadequate pain assessment tools and inadequate training and knowledge by clinicians as important barriers to providing effective pain relief, despite the respondents' beliefs that children who are cognitively impaired perceive pain to a similar extent as cognitively intact children.[104,107]

Revised Face, Legs, Activity, Cry, Consolability Observational Tool

Initial evaluation of the FLACC tool in children with cognitive impairment found a good correlation between scores assigned independently by different observers and by parent global ratings of pain.[108] Although measures of exact agreement between observers were acceptable for the face, cry, and consolability categories, measure of agreement for the legs and activity categories were less acceptable, likely because of coexisting motor impairments such as spasticity. The FLACC tool was therefore revised to incorporate additional descriptors of behaviors most consistently associated with pain in children with cognitive impairment (Table 41.6).[109] Interrater reliability for the total FLACC scores, as well as for each of the categories, improved when the evaluation included the revised FLACC (r-FLACC) in 52 cognitively impaired children. Also, good correlation among r-FLACC, parent, and child scores supported its criterion validity. The r-FLACC scores decreased after an opioid was administered, supporting the construct validity of the tool. The pragmatic attributes of the r-FLACC were compared with those of the Nurses' Assessment of Pain Intensity (NAPI) and the Non-Communicating Children's Pain Checklist-Postoperative Version (NCCPC-PV) (E-Tables 41.2 and 41.3).[107,110] Clinicians using these tools to score pain rated the complexity as less and the relative advantage and overall clinical utility of the FLACC and the NAPI

TABLE 41.6	Revised FLACC for Pain Assessment in the Cognitively Impaired[a]		
	0	**1**	**2**
Face	No particular expression or smile	Occasional grimace/frown; withdrawn or disinterested (Appears sad or worried)	Consistent grimace or frown; frequent/constant quivering chin, clenched jaw (Distressed-looking face; expression of fright or panic)
Legs	Normal position or relaxed	Uneasy, restless, tense (Occasional tremors)	Kicking, or legs drawn up (Marked increase in spasticity, constant tremors, or jerking)
Activity	Lying quietly, normal position, moves easily	Squirming, shifting back and forth, tense (Mildly agitated [e.g., head back and forth, aggression]; shallow, splinting respirations, intermittent sighs)	Arched, rigid, or jerking (Severe agitation head banging; shivering [not rigors]; breath-holding, gasping or sharp intake of breath; severe splinting)
Cry	No cry (awake or asleep)	Moans or whimpers, occasional complaint (Occasional verbal outburst or grunt)	Crying steadily, screams, or sobs; frequent complaints (Repeated outbursts, constant grunting)
Consolability	Content, relaxed	Reassured by occasional touching, hugging, or "talking to"; distractible	Difficult to console or comfort (Pushing away caregiver, resisting care or comfort measures)

[a]Revised descriptors for children with disabilities shown in parentheses.

to be greater compared with the NCCPC-PV, suggesting that these tools may be more readily adopted into clinical practice.

Strategies for Pain Management

Pain is a complex phenomenon that occurs via the transmission of nociceptive stimuli from the peripheral nervous system through the spinal cord to the cerebral cortex. Pain perception is further influenced by emotions, behavior, and previous pain experiences via multiple synapses in the limbic system, frontal cortex, and thalamus. Given the complexity of the pain experience, effective treatment optimally requires the use of multimodal therapies that target multiple sites along neural pathways that transmit and modulate pain sensation, as illustrated in Fig. 41.4. Multimodal treatment includes many nonpharmacologic techniques that are used more commonly for brief procedures (e.g., comfort position, cold/vibration, distraction) in addition to pharmacologic interventions (see further). *The primary goal of this approach is to minimize opioid needs and opioid-related adverse effects.*

Analgesics with additive or synergistic activity and different adverse effect profiles should be selected so that adequate analgesia can be provided with fewer adverse consequences. Thus, pain can be treated at the peripheral level using local anesthetics, peripheral nerve blockade, NSAIDs, antihistamines, or opioids. At the spinal cord level, pain can be treated with local anesthetics, neuraxial opioids, α_2-adrenoceptor agonists, and N-methyl-D-aspartate (NMDA) receptor antagonists. Finally, at the cortical level systemic opioids, α_2-agonists, and voltage-gated calcium channel $\alpha_2\delta$ proteins (targets for anticonvulsants) can be used.[111] Acetaminophen, a cornerstone of most opioid-sparing multimodal regimens, appears to exert its effects peripherally through the peroxidase (POX) site of prostaglandin H2 synthase (PGHS) enzyme, with mild inhibition of cyclooxygenase pathways peripherally and a more pronounced effect centrally.[112] There is also a possible central effect mediated through activation of descending inhibitory serotonergic pathways as well as modulation of the central endogenous cannabinoid receptor system.[109] Acetaminophen has a ceiling analgesic effect of approximately 5 to 6 out of 10 (VAS 0–10)[113]; most cases of moderate to severe pain are best treated with a multimodal approach.

The strategy for postoperative pain management is an integral part of the preanesthetic plan, so that informed consent for procedures, such as placement of peripheral or regional blocks, can be obtained (see Chapter 40). Additionally, appropriate parental teaching of techniques such as PCA should begin in the preoperative period. A discussion with the child and parents and/or guardians that, although some discomfort is inevitable, every effort will be made to minimize pain after surgery; such discussions decrease anxiety related to the perioperative experience. This, together with the use of nonpharmacologic techniques, may even reduce the need for opioids and other analgesics. Selection of an analgesic regimen requires careful consideration of many factors, including scope of the surgical procedure, age and cognitive abilities of the child, underlying medical conditions that might alter the response to pain medications, and child and family preferences. The goal should be for the child to emerge from anesthesia in reasonable comfort because it is generally easier to maintain analgesia in a pain-free child than to achieve analgesia in a child with severe pain. Fig. 41.5 presents a flowchart describing strategies to assess and manage acute postoperative pain in a child.

Poor perioperative pain control can contribute to the development of chronic postsurgical pain, which has been estimated to occur in 10% to 20% of children. Other risk factors include preexisting pain before surgery, greater patient and parent anxiety, and child pain coping efficacy.[110,111] Efforts should be undertaken to minimize these risk factors when formulating a postoperative pain regimen for complex operations.[114]

Many institutions have implemented some type of enhanced recovery after surgery (ERAS) protocols for high volume procedures such as spinal fusion or pectus excavatum repair.[10,11,115,116] These programs are designed to optimize pain control and functional recovery to reduce hospital length of stay and associated costs. It is important that all stakeholders (surgery, anesthesia, nursing, pharmacy, physical therapy, etc.) provide input toward formulating these care pathways, and that clear preoperative education is provided to patients about the expected recovery course for these operations.

Special consideration should be given to children with a history of chronic pain. Potentiation of peripheral nociceptors, spinal cord reorganization of pain pathways, and alterations in connectivity of brain areas including the nucleus accumbens, amygdala,

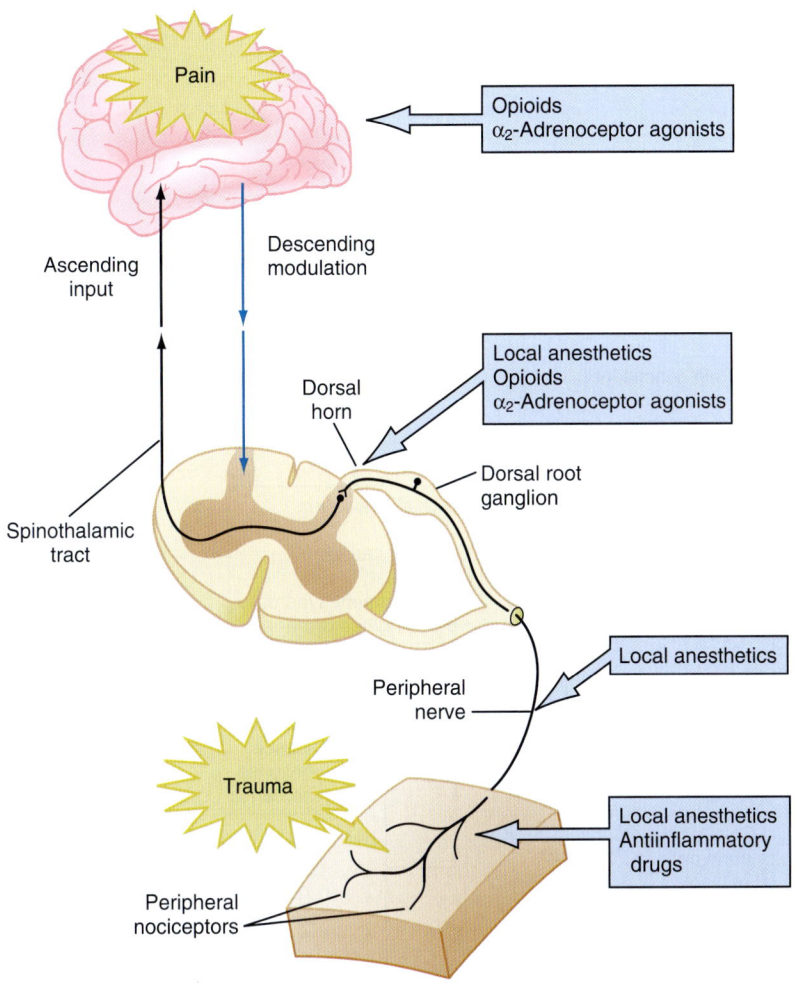

FIGURE 41.4 Schematic diagram of the pain pathways and multimodal measures to provide pain relief. (From Kehlet H, Dahl JB. The value of "multimodal" or "balanced analgesia" in postoperative pain treatment. *Anesth Analg.* 1993;77:1049.)

and prefrontal cortex, may predispose pediatric chronic pain patients to an exaggerated pain response after surgery.[117] Chronic opioid use and tolerance, although less common in pediatric patients with chronic pain compared with adult patients, may also complicate postoperative analgesia. It is imperative that a postoperative analgesic plan is formulated in advance with input from the patient, parents, and surgeon. A preemptive multimodal strategy that includes the use of opioids, regional anesthesia, opioid-sparing adjuvants, and nonpharmacologic therapies can help decrease peripheral and central sensitization to uncontrolled pain. An individualized plan is likely the best approach, as a standard treatment algorithm may not be appropriate for the specific needs of these complex patients.

SURGICAL CONSIDERATIONS

The scope and requirements of the surgical procedure, as well as specific postoperative issues, should be discussed with the surgical team before choosing an analgesic regimen, particularly if a regional technique is planned. For example, the location of an epidural catheter or truncal fascial plane catheter and the choice of the local anesthetic solution differ in a child with a vertical midline incision compared with one with a transverse suprapubic incision. With certain procedures, a nerve block catheter may intrude into

the surgical field or access to the catheter site in the postoperative period may be obscured by a cast or dressing. In such cases, the catheter may be tunneled subcutaneously away from the surgical field. Alternatively, to avoid inadvertent manipulation or dislodgement of the catheter during surgery, the catheter can be placed at the end of the surgical procedure before emergence from anesthesia. Placement of nerve block catheters by the surgeon under direct visualization into the surgical field have been described, such as one or more epidural catheters placed under direct vision by the surgeon at the end of the procedure (e.g., spinal fusion or selective dorsal rhizotomy).[118] Postoperative pain is managed using an infusion of local anesthetic with or without opioids or other adjunctive medication solutions through the catheter.[119,120] Painful muscle spasms after certain procedures are often ameliorated by continuous regional analgesia.[118,119,121,122] Regional anesthetic techniques often do not adequately cover the pain from severe or recurrent postoperative skeletal or bladder muscle spasms and supplemental antispasmodic medications are often needed.[121] This phenomenon depends in part on the density of blockade and type of regional anesthetic used. Oral or parenteral supplemental antispasmodic medications such as benzodiazepines, tizanidine, or cyclobenzaprine can be added if the block alone is inadequate. It is important to be mindful of the sedative adverse effect profile of

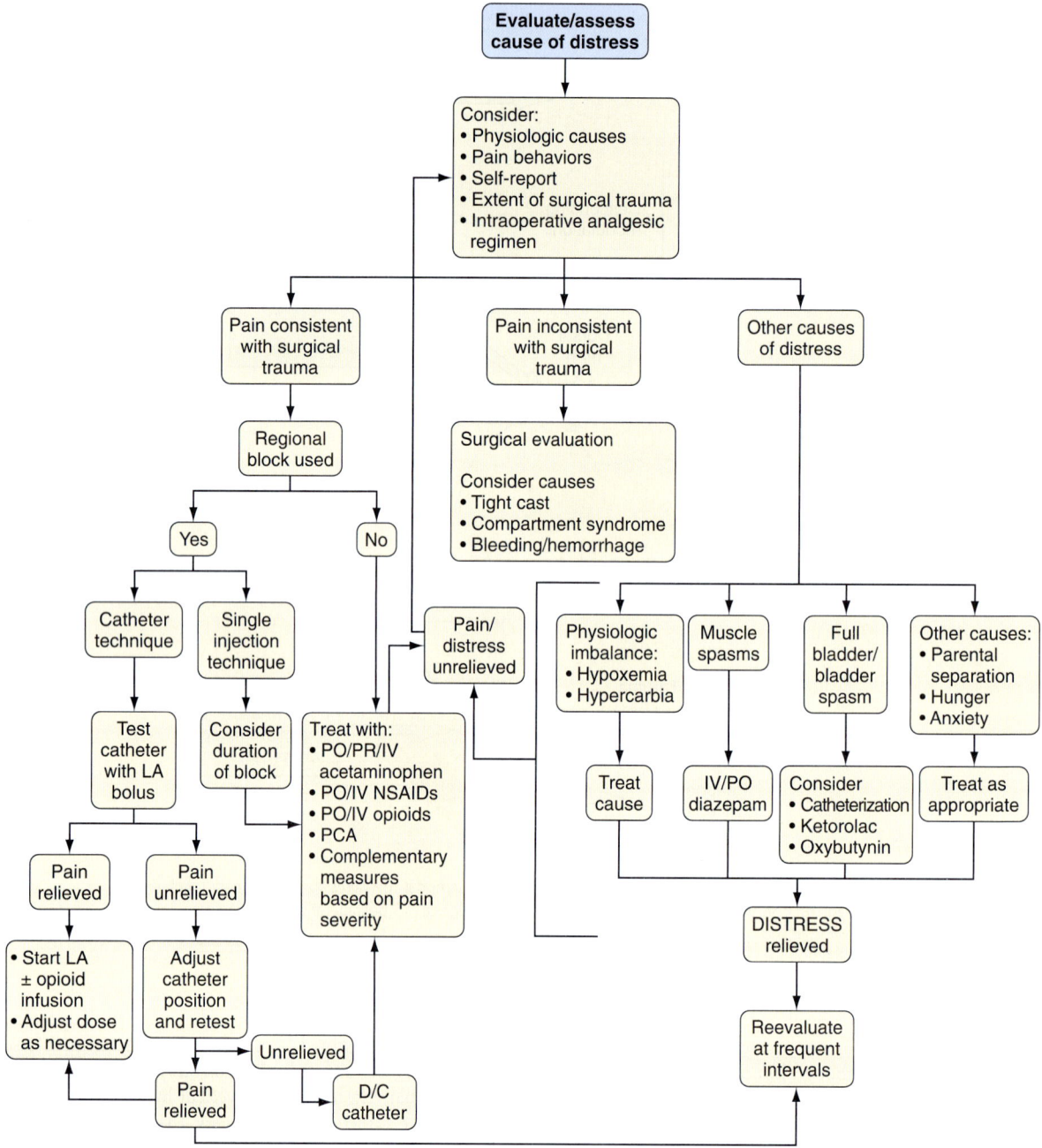

FIGURE 41.5 Flowchart for assessment and management of acute postoperative pain in a child. *D/C,* Discontinue; *IV,* intravenous; *LA,* local anesthetic; *NSAIDs,* nonsteroidal antiinflammatory drugs; *PCA,* patient-controlled analgesia; *PO,* orally; *PR,* per rectum.

these medications and possible synergistic interactions with other sedating medications such as opioids. Refractory spasms of the bladder, which can be quite problematic after some surgeries (e.g., ureteral reimplantation), can also be effectively treated with NSAIDs or anticholinergics.[123] Intravesical bupivacaine has also been used to manage bladder spasm in children based on clinical experience.[124] In a study of adults in whom bupivacaine 60 mL of 0.25% was instilled in the bladder, the blood concentration 1-hour postinstillation was <0.1 µg/mL in 3 patients and undetectable levels in the remaining 19 samples.[124] Based on the serum concentrations of lidocaine after intravesical instillation in adults 400 mg for 1 or 2 hours (levels were low except for 1 patient after 2 hours

with a level of 1.5 µg/mL),[125] clinicians in several countries, including New Zealand, use this approach to treat bladder spasm assuming peak serum concentrations are small in children, although comparable data have not been forthcoming.[121,126,127] Nonetheless, the possibility of local anesthetic toxicity should be considered in children for several hours after intravesical instillation.

Epidural blockade may favorably alter diaphragmatic mechanics after thoracotomy and upper abdominal surgery. This effect likely results from the motor blockade of the intercostal muscles and alteration in the resting length of the diaphragm and is not solely a result of reversal of diaphragmatic inhibition.[128–131]

However, it remains uncertain whether analgesia alone, achieved by systemic opioids or central neuraxial blockade, diminishes postoperative diaphragmatic inhibition or significantly improves postoperative pulmonary function.[129,130,132,133] Effective analgesia, however, does improve child compliance with measures such as deep breathing and early mobilization, thereby reducing the incidence of postoperative complications.[131,134]

Child-Related Considerations
Age and Cognitive Abilities
Analgesic techniques, such as infiltration of the wound with local anesthetics, peripheral nerve blocks, or regional blockade that minimize the use of opioids and central respiratory depressants, may be ideal for preterm or very young infants with impaired central respiratory drive.[133,135,136] Historical dogma had held that pain perception was immature in premature infants and acted as a rationale for inadequate analgesia.[29] A more thorough understanding of neonatal development found that the immaturity of the central nervous system mainly affects descending pain inhibitory pathways that modulate connections within the dorsal horn of the spinal cord. These inhibitory mechanisms do not fully develop until the 32nd week of gestation and thus the immaturity of the premature neonatal nervous system may predispose these neonates to heightened responses to painful stimuli.[15,16,134]

Acetaminophen is the foundation of most acute pain regimens; when used within its recommended dose range, it has a large therapeutic window with few untoward effects. Although the judicious use of opioids is not contraindicated, preterm infants <1 month of age or term neonates who receive these medications require careful observation and monitoring to diagnose respiratory depression.[137] The use of local anesthetics in infants younger than 6 months of age also requires careful attention to the dose used because decreased protein binding, immature hepatic oxidation and reduction pathways, and reduced clearance of local anesthetics increases their risk for local anesthetic toxicity.[138] The local anesthetic 2-chloroprocaine is rapidly metabolized at all ages by plasma cholinesterases and has gained popularity as an attractive alternative for continuous epidural infusions in neonates, especially if concomitant liver impairment is present or large infusion rates are needed to achieve analgesia.[17] Age-related differences in anatomy must also be considered. For example, the epidural space in infants has increased vascularity, less surface area for absorption of local anesthetics, and less fat compared with older children and adults. In addition, the vertebral column in infants less than

6 months old remains cartilaginous, and epidural or caudal catheters can be visualized with ultrasonography.

Older infants and toddlers who are expected to experience moderate to severe pain may be adequately treated with liquid formulation oral opioids when oral intake resumes. Alternatively, low-dose continuous opioid infusions, nurse-controlled analgesia,[139] PCA by proxy, or regional blockade may be required in those undergoing extensive surgery. Nonpharmacologic techniques that focus on distraction, such as child-life therapy, play, and the presence of a comforting parent, can augment the analgesic therapy.

Preschool- and school-aged children have greater fears and better understanding of the postoperative experience than do their younger counterparts. Most cognitively intact children 7 years of age or older are able to understand the concept of PCA, which may help to give a sense of control back to the child during a period in which all other aspects of control are removed.[140] Such issues of control and dependency assume even greater importance in adolescents; allowing them to participate in decision making will contribute to the success of any analgesic technique.[140] Regional techniques are excellent for providing analgesia in all age groups and are associated with a reduced incidence of adverse effects compared with systemic opioids (e.g., nausea, vomiting, excessive sedation, dysphoria, and respiratory depression).

Regardless of the child's age, a detailed history regarding the child's previous pain experience, analgesic history, response to treatment, and adverse effects from previous analgesic regimens should be carefully considered when selecting a pain management technique. As the use of genomic testing becomes more available and clinically feasible, identification of target polymorphisms, particularly in the cytochrome P450 enzyme system, may be used to tailor drug selection and dosing.

Pharmacologic Treatment of Pain

NONOPIOID ANALGESICS
Nonopioid analgesics are used as sole agents for mild pain and as important adjuncts for multimodal treatment of moderate to severe pain.[139] Although most nonopioid analgesics produce dose-dependent responses, they are limited by a ceiling effect in the analgesia achieved; that is, larger doses of the medication provide no additional analgesia. Hence, more severe pain is resistant to therapy from these medications alone.[141] Not all nonopioid analgesics are appropriate for all types of pain (e.g., neuropathic pain). Ideally, nonopioid medications (Table 41.7)

TABLE 41.7 Oral Dosing Guidelines for Commonly Used Nonopioid Analgesics

Medication	Individual Dose for Children <60 kg (mg/kg)	Individual Dose for Children ≥60 kg (mg)	Dosing Interval (hours)	Maximum Daily Dose for Children <60 kg (mg/kg)	Maximum Daily Dose for Children ≥60 kg (mg)
Acetaminophen	10–15	650–1000	4–6	75[a]	3000
Ibuprofen	5–10	400–600	6	40	2400
Naproxen	5–6	250–375	12	10	1000
Diclofenac	1	50	8	3	150
Ketorolac[b]	0.5	30	6–8	2	120
Tramadol	1–2	50	6	8	400

[a]See text for new age-related dosing.
[b]Ketorolac should be administered for a maximum of 5 days or 20 doses up to 15 mg per dose for children <60 kg or 30 mg per dose for children >60 kg.
Modified from Berde CB, Sethna NF. Analgesics for the treatment of pain in children. *N Engl J Med.* 2002;347(14):1094-1103; and World Health Organization. *World Health Organization Guidelines on the Pharmacological Treatment of Persisting Pain in Children with Medical Illnesses.* WHO: Geneva, Switzerland; 2012.

are delivered on a scheduled basis for at least the first few days postoperatively, whereas opioids are available pro re nata (PRN) for breakthrough pain.

Acetaminophen

Acetaminophen is the most common antipyretic and nonopioid analgesic used in children. Despite years of study, the predominant mechanism of its analgesic action remains unclear. It may exert its analgesic effects by blocking central and peripheral prostaglandin synthesis, reducing substance P–induced hyperalgesia, and modulating the production of hyperalgesic nitric oxide in the spinal cord.[141–144] In addition, acetaminophen might produce analgesia via activation of descending serotonergic pathways.[112,145,146] One putative site of action may be to inhibit prostaglandin H2 synthetase at the peroxidase site.[112,145] Evidence supports that acetaminophen weakly inhibits peripheral cyclooxygenase enzymes and modulates the endogenous cannabinoid receptor system.[147] Effective analgesia and antipyresis have been described with plasma concentrations of 5 to 20 µg/mL[146–151]; a target effect-site (similar to cerebrospinal fluid) concentration of 10 µg/mL reduces pain after tonsillectomy by 3.6/10 pain units.[152] The total daily dose of acetaminophen via any route is age- and weight-based, but doses of 75 mg/kg for children, 60 mg/kg for neonates 32 to 44 weeks postconception age, and 40 mg/kg for preterm neonates 28 to 32 weeks[150] postconception are currently suggested.

Acetaminophen has a wide margin of safety when administered in the recommended therapeutic dose range. However, hepatotoxicity has been reported with doses only slightly exceeding the recommended dose when administered over 3 days continuously, suggesting that acetaminophen may have a narrow therapeutic index in some children.[153,154] Acetaminophen is available in a wide variety of formulations, alone or in combination with decongestants, for oral use in a variety of cold remedies, and with opioids for the treatment of moderate to severe pain. There are currently more than 600 over-the-counter acetaminophen-containing products, increasing the risk of an overdose because children may take more than one formulation that contains the drug.[155] Frequent review of medications and parental education is needed to minimize the risk of overdose. In the past, pediatric liquid formulations of acetaminophen as in infant drops were commonly supplied in larger concentrations than that in elixirs, resulting in dosing errors. As a result, the 80-mg/mL concentration has been removed from the US market by the manufacturer, and liquid formulations have been standardized to 32 mg/mL. This concentration equals approximately 0.5 mL/kg of acetaminophen if given as a 15-mg/kg dose. Since both gastric fluid volume and pH are unchanged after liquid acetaminophen (40 mg/kg of a 50 mg/mL elixir, 0.8 mL/kg) administered orally 90 minutes before induction of anesthesia, it is feasible to use this preoperatively. These results are applicable to acetaminophen that is administered closer to the time of induction with a small drink of water, independent of the fasting regimen for clear liquids.[156]

Intravenous acetaminophen is available as a 10-mg/mL solution and should be infused over ~15 minutes in a dose of 12.5 mg/kg every 4 hours or 15 mg/kg every 6 hours, with a total daily limit of 75 mg/kg (max 4000 mg/day). In neonates between 32 and 44 weeks postconception age, a loading dose of 20 mg/kg should be followed by 10 mg/kg every 6 hours (every 12 hours in neonates 28 to 31 weeks postconception age).[157] Each dose of IV acetaminophen must be documented in a timely manner to avoid overdoses from multiple dosing; several cases of frank overdoses have occurred in young infants who received excessive doses of IV acetaminophen on the ward, although no cases have been reported in the past decade as more health care providers have become familiar with the drug.[148,154,157–161] Dosing recommendations for premature and full-term neonates continues to be an active area of research[162]; weight is a reasonable predictor of individual pharmacokinetics (PK) in this narrow cohort.[159,163,164]

After IV administration of acetaminophen, the onset of analgesia can be expected within 15 minutes and antipyresis within 30 minutes.[165,166] Intravenous acetaminophen rapidly penetrates the blood-brain barrier, yielding detectable concentrations in the cerebrospinal fluid (CSF) within 5 minutes of administration, and peak CSF concentrations within 57 minutes after injection (compared with 2 to 3 hours after rectal or oral administration).[167–169] The CSF is not the effect compartment, but serves as a proxy for the effect compartment with a similar equilibration half time.[152,163] A controlled randomized trial reported that both rectal acetaminophen, 40 mg/kg, and IV acetaminophen, 15 mg/kg, administered after induction of anesthesia in children undergoing adenotonsillectomy provided good analgesia for the first 6 hours after surgery.[170] However, children who received acetaminophen rectally had a greater duration of analgesia and did not require rescue analgesia as early as those in the IV group.[170] This is attributable to the slow absorption of rectal acetaminophen, causing sustained effective concentrations (see also E-Fig. 2.6).[171] When compared with oral acetaminophen, there was evidence of reduced intraoperative opioid requirements (attributable to differing time to peak effect-site concentration), but no difference in postoperative opioid consumption in young children undergoing cleft palate repair when children received scheduled acetaminophen via the oral or IV route.[170,172] The analgesic effect of acetaminophen is concentration rather than formulation dependent, and clinical experience reflects the paucity of evidence that IV acetaminophen is superior to PO acetaminophen. Oral acetaminophen has high bioavailability. The quality of analgesia and opioid-sparing characteristics of IV and oral acetaminophen are equivalent.[147,170]

Absorption of acetaminophen is slow and unpredictable after rectal administration, with peak concentrations reached between 60 and 180 minutes (see E-Fig. 2.6).[150,172–176] This unpredictability was illustrated in a series of studies from the same group of investigators examining opioid-sparing with rectal and IV acetaminophen in infants undergoing major abdominal and thoracic surgery. In a rectal study, an opioid-sparing effect was not detected, although plasma concentrations of acetaminophen varied 50-fold among patients.[150] In a follow-up study in the same population using IV acetaminophen, opioid consumption was reduced by 60% and the frequency of apnea was also reduced.[177] In children undergoing orthopedic surgery, a loading dose of 40 mg/kg rectal acetaminophen followed by 20 mg/kg every 6 hours yielded serum concentrations of 10 to 20 µg/mL in half of the patients, with no evidence of accumulation over a 24-hour period.[174] This dosing scheme is now the one most commonly recommended when the rectal route is used, but it should be noted that scheduled dosing with this scheme would result in a dose of 80 mg/kg per day (or 100 mg/kg on the first day with the loading dose). Contrary to previous assumptions, acetaminophen is relatively evenly distributed in most suppositories, allowing them to be split to achieve a desired dose, although accuracy of dosing is problematic.[178]

In conclusion, acetaminophen has opioid-sparing potential with very few adverse effects and a low risk of toxicity if appropriate dosing is followed. Its analgesic effect is concentration-dependent, oral bioavailability is high, and the oral and IV routes provide equivalent analgesia when differences attributable to enteral absorption are considered. The rectal route is the least favored because of unpredictable and slow absorption. Financial considerations (drug cost and intravenous delivery systems) have limited the routine use of IV acetaminophen at many centers in the United States.[179]

Nonsteroidal Antiinflammatory Drugs

NSAIDs provide good analgesia for mild to moderate pain resulting from surgery, injury, and disease. There are few concentration-response relationships described in children; those for ibuprofen and diclofenac suggest a ceiling analgesic effect similar to that of acetaminophen (5–6, VAS 0–10).[180,181] Their principal mechanism of action is via inhibition of the enzyme prostaglandin H2 synthase at the COX site, reducing production of prostaglandins at the site of tissue injury and attenuation of the inflammatory cascade. In addition to their peripheral effects, the NSAIDs have also been shown to exert a direct spinal action by blocking the hyperalgesic response induced by activation of spinal glutamate and substance P receptors.[182] Decreased production of leukotrienes, activation of serotonin pathways, and inhibition of excitatory amino acids, NMDA-mediated hyperalgesia, and central inhibition of prostaglandin biosynthesis have been proposed as additional mechanisms of action.[183,184] The COX-1 enzyme is present in the brain, gastrointestinal tract, kidneys, and platelets and is expressed constitutively. It preserves gastric mucosal integrity and function, platelet aggregation, and renal perfusion. COX-2 expression is induced by inflammation or tissue injury. Most NSAIDs exist on a spectrum of selectivity with regard to the relative inhibition of the COX-1 versus COX-2 enzymes. For example, ketorolac is skewed toward more COX-1 selectivity whereas ibuprofen and naproxen are more balanced with relatively equal COX-1 and COX-2 inhibition.[182] Selective COX-2 inhibitors reduce inflammation but have less effect on gastric mucosal function and have fewer effects on platelet aggregation, thereby resulting in fewer adverse effects. Their deleterious effects on renal perfusion, however, are no different than the nonselective COX drugs, because COX-2 is constitutively expressed in renal tissues and may be involved in prostaglandin-dependent renal homeostatic processes.[185] The risks of renal toxicity increase in the presence of hypovolemia, cardiac failure, preexisting renal dysfunction, or with the concurrent use of other nephrotoxic drugs. Reports of thrombotic cardiovascular and CNS events after both long-term and short-term use in adults led to withdrawal of two of the COX-2 inhibitors, rofecoxib and valdecoxib, from the market[186–188]; the risk of these agents causing thrombotic complications in children remains unknown. Most pediatric studies have evaluated the use of nonselective COX medications. In adult studies, COX-2 inhibitors have generally, but not always, produced analgesia roughly equivalent to that of traditional NSAIDs. Selective COX-2 inhibitors, such as celecoxib, have not been well studied in children within the perioperative setting. Celecoxib has been shown to modestly reduce the mean greatest pain scores within a 24-hour period and acetaminophen consumption in children undergoing elective adenotonsillectomy when compared with placebo.[189,190] There are no meaningful comparisons within the pediatric perioperative literature with regard to comparisons between nonselective NSAIDs and COX-2 inhibitors.

Ibuprofen, one of the oldest orally administered NSAIDs, has been used extensively for treatment of fever and pain related to surgery, trauma, arthritis, menstrual cramps, and sickle cell disease. A large, controlled, randomized, double-blind study reported a greater decrease in VAS pain scores with ibuprofen than with acetaminophen or codeine in children presenting to the emergency department with acute pain after musculoskeletal trauma.[191] Additionally, more children who received ibuprofen had VAS scores less than 30 on a 0-to-100-mm VAS scale than in the other two groups. The recommended dose of ibuprofen is 5 to 10 mg/kg every 6 hours. Like acetaminophen, ibuprofen is available in a variety of formulations and concentrations, placing children at risk for an overdose. For pediatric use, ibuprofen is available as:

- Concentrated drops containing 50 mg ibuprofen in 1.25 mL.
- Oral suspension containing 100 mg of ibuprofen in 5 mL.
- Junior strength chewable tablets or caplets containing 100 mg of ibuprofen each.

Diclofenac provides effective analgesia after minor surgical procedures in children. It is available only as an oral tablet in the United States. Relative bioavailabilities were 0.36, 0.63, and 0.35 for suspension, suppository, and dispersible tablets.[192] The pediatric dose of diclofenac is 1 mg/kg every 8 hours orally, 0.5 mg/kg rectally, and 0.3 mg/kg IV to yield a similar area under the curve to 50 mg in adults.[192–195] Children who received diclofenac experienced analgesia comparable to those who received caudal bupivacaine or IV ketorolac for inguinal hernia repair.[194,196–198] In children undergoing tonsillectomy and/or adenoidectomy, diclofenac yielded superior analgesia with less supplemental opioid dosing, less nausea and vomiting, and earlier resumption of oral intake compared with acetaminophen.[199,200] A Cochrane review found that NSAIDs did not increase the risk of post-tonsillectomy bleeding that required a return to the operating room for children.[200] Recent evidence indicates that ketorolac does not increase the risk of bleeding after tonsillectomy.[201–204] Overall, there was less nausea and vomiting with NSAIDs compared with alternative analgesics, suggesting their benefits outweigh their negative aspects. A prospective, randomized trial assigned 91 children with sleep-disordered breathing to acetaminophen with ibuprofen or morphine for analgesia after tonsillectomy. There was an almost 4-fold increase in the number of desaturation events (from preoperative levels) during the first postoperative night in the morphine group, and a decrease in the number of desaturation events during the same period in the ibuprofen group. Overall, the pain scores in the morphine group were slightly less, but there was neither a statistically nor clinically significant difference between the groups. The study was terminated early as a result of preliminary results and an incident of respiratory depression at home, resulting in admission to the pediatric intensive care unit in the morphine group.[205]

Ketorolac, indomethacin, and ibuprofen are the only injectable NSAIDs available in the United States. Intravenous parecoxib (prodrug for valdecoxib),[206] ketoprofen, and diclofenac are available in some countries. Indomethacin is an NSAID commonly used for closure of patent ductus arteriosus in preterm neonates. A large multicenter study compared the risks of serious adverse events from IV ketorolac, ketoprofen, and diclofenac in more than 11,000 adults undergoing major surgery.[207] The results indicated that 1.4% of adults experienced a serious adverse outcome, including surgical site bleeding (1%), death (0.17%), severe allergic reactions (0.12%), renal failure (0.09%), and gastrointestinal bleeding (0.04%), with no differences in outcomes among the groups. In a systematic review and meta-analysis of adults and children undergoing adenotonsillectomy, IV ketorolac increased the risk of post-tonsillectomy bleeding in adults by 5-fold but had no effect on the risk of bleeding in children.[201] In a systematic review of ibuprofen, 5 or 10 mg/kg orally, in children undergoing adenotonsillectomy compared with NSAID controls, neither dose affected the risk of post-tonsillectomy bleeding.[208] In a retrospective study of 1046 children undergoing tonsillectomy who received 7.5 mg/kg oral ibuprofen, 3.1% developed secondary post-tonsillectomy bleeds.[208] In a placebo-controlled study of 161 children undergoing tonsillectomy, IV ibuprofen (10 mg/kg IV) was opioid-sparing without increasing secondary bleeding,[209] consistent with the findings of larger reviews.[204] Interestingly, the risk of bleeding after tonsillectomy appears to be much lower in children than in adults.[207]

Ketorolac has been shown to provide postoperative analgesia similar to opioids in children of all ages.[210–213] Its benefits include lack of opioid adverse effects (respiratory depression, sedation, nausea, and pruritus), making it an attractive choice for the treatment of postoperative pain. However, in common with all NSAIDs, it carries risks of platelet dysfunction, gastrointestinal bleeding, and renal dysfunction. When ketorolac (1 mg/kg) given to 18 preterm and term neonates undergoing painful procedures in the operating room or the neonatal ICU,[211] pain scores (Neonatal Infant Pain Scale) were reduced with no incidents of systemic or local bleeding and no hematologic, hepatic, or renal complications (note that this dose is twice the usually recommended dose of 0.5 mg/kg). Similarly, no adverse effects on surgical drain output, renal or hepatic function tests, or oxygen saturation after major surgery were noted in 37 infants and toddlers between 6 and 18 months of age.[214] Children in that study received continuous morphine infusions postoperatively, confounding the evaluation of the analgesic efficacy of ketorolac. In single dose studies, the PK of ketorolac in infants and small children (2–18 months of age) appear to be homogeneous and show a relatively rapid elimination of the analgesic S enantiomer, with slower clearance of the R enantiomer.[214,215] Finally, ketorolac has been used to supplement opioid analgesia, with no increase in renal or bleeding complications in infants and children after open heart surgery.[216–218] Nonetheless, many limit the course of treatment to 48 to 72 hours because ketorolac reduces renal blood flow. It is also prudent to check renal function if a treatment course exceeds 72 hours.[214,215]

Another contentious issue regarding NSAIDs relates to their effects on bone healing and their use in children undergoing spinal fusion. Prostaglandins play an integral role in bone metabolism and significantly influence bone resorption and formation; however, their effects on bone formation predominate. NSAIDs inhibit the formation of prostaglandins, thereby raising the concern that they could promote nonunion after spinal fusion. Studies in rabbits and some studies in adult humans have reported a greater incidence of nonunion or pseudarthrosis, particularly with the use of large doses of ketorolac.[219,220] However, no differences in curve progression, hardware failure, pseudarthrosis, or need for reoperation have been found in children and adolescents who received ketorolac in the immediate postoperative period compared with those who did not.[221–223] Of note, the majority of the pediatric data are from otherwise healthy children with idiopathic scoliosis; it is unknown if one can extrapolate these data to children with comorbidities or those with neuromuscular scoliosis. There is no unique advantage of the IV route with NSAIDs. There is also no evidence that IV ketorolac is a more potent analgesic than comparable (i.e., equipotent) doses of a number of other NSAIDs administered by oral or rectal routes.[224]

A metanalysis of the use of NSAIDs for postoperative pain that included 27 studies compared 567 children who received NSAIDs with 418 children who did not.[225] The coadministration of NSAIDs and opioids during the perioperative period decreased opioid requirement in the postanesthesia care unit (PACU) and the first 24 hours after surgery, decreased pain intensity in the PACU, and reduced postoperative nausea and vomiting (PONV) during the first 24 hours postoperatively. Although NSAIDs appear to be more effective than acetaminophen for acute pain,[226] combination therapy prolongs the duration of analgesia of both drugs.[180,181,224,227] Scheduled combination therapy in children performs better than either drug alone.[228,229] Therefore these two medications are part of the World Health Organization global guidelines on treating pain in children[230] and should serve as the foundation of a safe, effective, and opioid-sparing analgesic regimen.

The question often arises regarding the youngest age that NSAIDs can safely be administered. Limited data exist for safety and beneficial analgesic effects of numerous different NSAIDs for use in children under 6 months of age. The main theoretical concern is whether young infants are more susceptible to renal toxicity given that glomerular and tubular maturation continues through 18 to 24 months of age. As discussed previously, numerous reports in the literature illustrate the safe and efficacious use of NSAIDs in infants and neonates. For example, several studies have reported no increase in renal dysfunction after administration of ketorolac to young infants.[231,232] At our institution (JH), NSAIDs are administered within the perioperative period to neonates greater than 40 weeks postmenstrual age without evidence of renal dysfunction or coagulopathy.

It is prudent to note that the available literature on this topic is limited to mostly small, retrospective studies, and offers little consensus on the risk of renal injury or bleeding dysfunction in neonates or young infants. Some pediatric centers are more conservative in their approach and do not administer NSAIDs to infants under 6 months of age.

Tramadol

Tramadol is a synthetic analog of codeine that exerts its analgesic properties by two complementary mechanisms. One of its metabolites has a weak affinity for the μ opioid receptor with no affinity for the δ or the κ receptors. In addition to its mild opioid effects, it also inhibits serotonin and norepinephrine uptake. Based on tramadol's metabolism via the CYP2D6 pathway, there are concerns that "ultra-metabolizers" could produce excessive amounts of the potent O-desmethyltramadol metabolite, a metabolite with 200-fold greater affinity for μ receptors than tramadol.[205,233] Toxicity occurs after administration of 7 to 10 mg/kg of tramadol.[234] Other adverse effects associated with its use include nausea and vomiting (9%–10% of cases), pruritus (7%), and rash (4%).[235] Its use has also been associated with seizures. Tramadol is available only in tablet form alone or in combination with acetaminophen in the United States. However, it is available in a liquid formulation, as a suppository, and as an injectable solution in other countries.

Tramadol has been used for postoperative pain treatment in children undergoing ambulatory surgery and has also been used when transitioning from IV opioids to oral analgesics. Tramadol, 2 mg/kg IV, produced similar analgesia and sedation with fewer episodes of oxygen desaturation compared with morphine 0.1 mg/kg IV in children with obstructive sleep apnea undergoing adenotonsillectomy.[236] Tramadol has also been found to produce a similar analgesic effect as that of ilioinguinal and iliohypogastric nerve blocks in children undergoing herniorrhaphy[237]; the tramadol group, however, experienced a greater incidence of nausea and vomiting.

Tramadol has also been effective when administered via the neuraxial route. Caudal tramadol (2 mg/kg) produced reliable postoperative analgesia comparable with that produced by caudal morphine (30 μg/kg) in children undergoing inguinal hernia repair.[238] No additional pain medications were required in the first 24 hours in more than 90% of children in each group. Rigorous drug-specific neurotoxicity studies, however, are lacking, and therefore this route of administration is not recommended until such data are available and confirmed. Overall, tramadol appears to be an analgesic of mild to medium potency that has been used alone and in combination with other analgesics for mild to moderate pain.

Despite the evidence in support of tramadol for acute pain and postoperative analgesia, safety concerns have emerged regarding its use for pediatric patients. Adverse events related to tramadol, including deaths, have been reported in children.[233] These appear related to use of concentrated adult liquid formulations in children resulting in inadvertent overdose rather than "ultra-metabolism."[239,240] However, the Food and Drug Administration (FDA) has issued a US block box warning for tramadol use in pediatric patients that states *"tramadol use should be avoided in all pediatric patients less than 12 years and all pediatric patients undergoing tonsillectomy or adenoidectomy. Additionally, tramadol should be avoided in patients 12 to 18 years who are obese or have conditions such as obstructive sleep apnea or severe lung disease, which may increase the risk of serious breathing problems."* Other contraindications listed for tramadol include patients at elevated risk from respiratory depression, and recent monoamine oxidase inhibitor (MAOI) therapy within the prior 14 days. Given these issues as well as tramadol's overall weak analgesic effect, its use has largely fallen out of favor for use in children.

Ketamine

Ketamine is an NMDA-receptor antagonist used in the treatment of both chronic and acute pain. Its professed benefits include an opioid-sparing effect, avoidance of opioid tolerance, prevention of central sensitization and wind-up, mitigation of opioid-induced hyperalgesia, and provision of synergistic analgesia in multimodal regimens by virtue of its own antinociceptive properties. Case series in children with intractable pain resulting from advanced stages of cancer have reported reduction in opioid requirement, decreased opioid adverse effects, improvement in pain control and function, and increased ability to interact with their families.[241–243] Ketamine is also very popular as a single agent for both analgesia and sedation for burn care.[244]

Studies evaluating the use of ketamine alone or in combination with opioids for acute postoperative pain in children have yielded equivocal results. In one study, children undergoing tonsillectomy who received IV ketamine 0.5 mg/kg after induction or at the end of surgery experienced reduced pain scores and required fewer rescue analgesics compared with those who received placebo.[245] All children in this study received a standardized analgesic regimen, including rectal diclofenac before the start of surgery and oral acetaminophen at scheduled intervals postoperatively. Another study reported reduced pain scores and reduced requirement for rescue analgesics in children who received ketamine as a bolus dose and by infusion that began before the start of a tonsillectomy, compared with those who received a single bolus dose of

ketamine at the end of surgery.[246] Intramuscular (IM) ketamine 0.5 mg/kg has also produced equivalent analgesia in terms of similar pain scores and need for rescue analgesics compared with IM morphine 0.1 mg/kg as sole analgesics for tonsillectomy.[247] Other studies have found no such benefits when ketamine was compared with placebo for tonsillectomy, urologic, and orthopedic surgery.[248–251]

A meta-analysis of 35 randomized controlled trials compared 567 children who received ketamine as an adjuvant analgesic by a variety of routes for a variety of surgical procedures with 418 who did not receive ketamine.[252] Although the use of ketamine was associated with reduced pain intensity in the PACU and there was a reduced need for nonopioids, there was no opioid-sparing effect. A systematic review of 37 studies included 4 in children, 2 of which demonstrated beneficial effects of ketamine administered as an adjuvant analgesic and 2 of which found no benefits.[253] The investigators could draw no conclusions regarding the use of ketamine as an adjuvant analgesic. The use of ketamine in all the previous studies was associated with only a few mild and self-limiting adverse effects. Dysphoria, a well-known adverse effect of ketamine when used as a primary anesthetic, appears to be common with much larger doses than those employed for analgesia in children, although the published data are of poor quality. Intraoperative low-dose S-ketamine had no effect on morphine consumption during the first 72 hours after surgery in children. The differences in pain intensity and time to first PCA use probably reflect additional sedation and antinociceptive effects of S-ketamine rather than a true "prevention" of pain.[251] Ketamine was associated with decreased PACU postoperative pain intensity and nonopioid analgesic requirement. However, ketamine failed to exhibit a postoperative opioid-sparing effect.[252]

It is difficult to draw concrete conclusions from these reviews and meta-analyses as they compile data from studies that are disparate in study design and vary widely in the administration protocol for ketamine. For example, some studies include intraoperative bolus dosing with a continuous infusion, whereas others only feature bolus doses of ketamine, and the doses used on a weight basis vary widely among papers. Despite these limitations, ketamine is likely a safe and effective opioid-sparing analgesic adjunctive medication that could be considered as part of a perioperative analgesic plan for specific patients and procedures. Further investigation is needed to evaluate the benefits of low-dose ketamine for acute postoperative pain before its routine use can be broadly recommended. We recommend analgesic bolus doses of 0.5 mg/kg or less, and infusion rates of 0.25 mg/kg per hour or less to avoid dysphoria.

Gabapentin

Gabapentin is an anticonvulsant that exhibits an analgesic effect through binding to presynaptic calcium channels and modulating the release of glutamate and other excitatory neurotransmitters. It is available in 100-, 300-, 600-, and 900-mg tablets as well as a 50-mg/mL oral solution. Although it has been studied most extensively for chronic neuropathic pain, there is some evidence in adults for its analgesic effects on acute pain,[254] and it is also useful in preventing PONV.[255] There is comparatively less evidence for its benefit in pediatric acute pain. A prospective, randomized study of children undergoing posterior spinal fusion demonstrated a reduction in morphine consumption in the early postoperative period when given as a preoperative loading dose of 15 mg/kg followed by 5 mg/kg 3 times daily.[256] Another study using only a single preoperative dose did not have an opioid-sparing effect.[257] Gabapentin does not cause respiratory depression, but sedation is a common adverse effect, which may confound patient assessment when co-administered with opioids. Gabapentinoids prescribed together with opioids have led to increased rates of adverse events.[255] More recent data in adult patients have cast doubt on the analgesic efficacy for gabapentin for acute pain.[256] Similar findings from a recent systematic review also found a lack of efficacy for use of gabapentin for acute pain in pediatric patients.[257] These emerging data are not surprising given that when prescribed for chronic neuropathic pain, a clinically significant analgesic effect for gabapentin is typically not seen until after 2 weeks. It is also not surprising given that most acute pain is not neuropathic in origin. We believe that the most recent and best critical evidence argues against gabapentin as an acute pain analgesic.

Pregabalin

Pregabalin is an anticonvulsant and anxiolytic medication that has been used to manage epilepsy, restless leg syndrome, neuropathic pain, and generalized anxiety disorder. Similar to gabapentin, pregabalin is a gabapentinoid that exerts its effect through binding to the alpha-2-delta subunit of voltage-gated calcium channels within the CNS and modulates calcium influx at nerve terminals. This inhibits excitatory neurotransmitter release. Pregabalin may also play a role in modulating descending noradrenergic and serotonergic pain transmission pathways between the brainstem and spinal cord. It comes in tablet (multiple dosages available), extended-release tablet, and 20 mg/mL oral solution formulations. Pregabalin has been used to treat pediatric patients with complex regional pain syndrome (CRPS) and fibromyalgia with questionable efficacy for these indications. As with gabapentin, there is little evidence in the literature to support the use of pregabalin for acute pain. Perioperative pregabalin did not reduce postoperative opioid consumption or the development of chronic postoperative pain following posterior spinal fusion in children.[258]

Dexamethasone

Dexamethasone is commonly used for postoperative nausea and vomiting, and the analgesic and opioid-sparing properties of it have also been examined for pediatric acute pain. Most of the work in this area has centered on postoperative analgesia for children undergoing tonsillectomy and/or adenoidectomy. One meta-analysis that pooled data from 8 randomized controlled trials concluded that a single dose of dexamethasone (0.4–1 mg/kg) significantly reduced postoperative pain scores in children after tonsillectomy.[259] In a study of children undergoing tonsillectomy who were randomized to low (0.15 mg/kg) or high dose (0.5 mg/kg) dexamethasone or placebo,[260] early severe postoperative pain did not differ among the groups, whereas the incidence of severe pain on postoperative day 2 was significantly less in both dexamethasone groups. Pain scores in the two dexamethasone groups were similar. Interestingly, most studies that examined the effectiveness of dexamethasone for postoperative analgesia did not compare the opioid or other analgesic requirements between the groups. In another double-blind randomized study of 105 children undergoing adenotonsillectomy, pain scores and postoperative nausea and vomiting were reduced for seven postoperative days compared with the placebo group.[261] Overall, dexamethasone appears to have a modest analgesic effect and reduces acute pain scores in children postoperatively after tonsillectomy and/or adenoidectomy surgery. Further research is needed to confirm opioid-sparing properties and validation of these data for other types of surgeries.

Beyond systemic use, dexamethasone has also been utilized as an adjunct to local anesthetic solutions for both caudal and peripheral nerve blocks. A meta-analysis of randomized trials in adult studies reported that combining dexamethasone with local anesthetic solutions prolonged the duration of the peripheral nerve blocks (mean difference of 351 minutes), compared with the local anesthetic alone.[262] Dexamethasone added to local anesthetic solution in caudal blocks for children may double or triple the duration of action of the block relative to plain local anesthetic.[263,264]

A meta-analysis of 35 trials with 2702 patients 15 to 78 years of age undergoing upper or lower limb surgery reported that both perineural and intravenous dexamethasone may prolong the duration of the block but that pediatric evidence was lacking.[265] There has been considerable debate within the literature regarding the efficacy of perineural versus systemic dexamethasone for regional anesthetic techniques, with some authors advocating for one approach over another. For pediatric patients, the data addressing this question are evolving but one large-scale systematic review suggests that both perineural and systemic dexamethasone are equally efficacious in prolonging regional anesthetic techniques in pediatric patients.[266] Overall, there is moderate-quality evidence for efficacy for both perineural and systemic dexamethasone as an adjunct to prolong caudal and peripheral nerve blocks.[262]

Clonidine

Clonidine activates inhibitory neural pathways within the CNS via stimulation of alpha-2 adrenoceptors. Clonidine has weak alpha-1 receptor agonist activity, it is primarily an alpha-2 selective agonist. When acting centrally in the brain stem, this results in reduced sympathetic outflow from the CNS, which leads to decreased peripheral resistance, renal vascular resistance, heart rate, and blood pressure. These properties have led to its use as an antihypertensive agent. When used as an adjunct for epidural analgesia, clonidine is thought to exert its analgesic properties at spinal presynaptic and postjunctional alpha-2 adrenoreceptors by decreasing ascending transmission of pain signals. Available formulations include immediate-release tablet, extended-release tablet, transdermal-patch, and a preservative-free solution that is primarily utilized as an adjunct to potentiate and prolong the action of epidural analgesia and peripheral nerve blocks.

There has been considerable interest in the use of systemic clonidine as an agent for acute pain in pediatric patients. One systematic review explored clonidine premedication for pediatric patients undergoing ophthalmic surgery and its effects on postoperative pain and vomiting.[267] When compared with placebo or benzodiazepine, children receiving clonidine premedication were found to have better postoperative pain scores and less analgesic requirements. Another meta-analysis examined perioperative clonidine and its effects on postoperative pain for children undergoing adenotonsillectomy, ventriculoperitoneal shunt insertion, ophthalmologic, urologic, general surgical, and other minor surgical procedures.[267,268] The studies included in this analysis exhibited significant heterogeneity with regard to comparison groups and surgical procedures but these data suggest that "high-dose" (4 µg/kg) clonidine reduces the number of patients that need additional postoperative analgesics as well as providing better pain scores. The opioid-sparing effect should be quantified, and optimal dosing regimen clarified in future studies. It is important to note that in all available studies, clonidine was explored as an adjunct to other traditional systemic analgesics, such as opioids, and does not appear to have any utility as a stand-alone acute pain analgesic. Its analgesic properties are likely weak to moderate.

Clonidine appears to be well-tolerated within the pediatric population with few reported side effects or adverse events.

Clonidine may be one of the most-studied adjuvants for caudal and peripheral blocks in the pediatric population. The interest and reported efficacy to prolong regional blocks in both adults and pediatrics is perplexing given the fact that peripheral nerves do not express alpha-2 adrenoceptors.[265] Despite this fact, animal models have shown that alpha-2 agonists are capable of significant interference with the hyperpolarization-activated cation current (H-current). The H-current is an inward current generated by the hyperpolarization-activated cyclic nucleotide-gated (HCN) cation channels that plays an essential role in regulating normal neuronal properties and is necessary for the return of normal conductivity after depolarization of a peripheral nerve.

The adult literature generally supports using clonidine as an adjunct for peripheral nerve blocks, but the pediatric literature can be conflicting.[269,270] However, the pediatric clinical literature generally supports using clonidine as an adjunct to extend the duration of action of caudal blocks.[271–274] A review of 20 randomized trials in children that compared the duration of caudal blockade with or without clonidine reported a longer duration of analgesia and fewer patients that required rescue analgesics; there was a small incidence of respiratory depression.[268,270,275] Most studies report a perineural dose of clonidine of 1 µg/kg.

Dexmedetomidine

Like clonidine, dexmedetomidine is a selective alpha-2 adrenergic receptor agonist but it has an alpha-2 to alpha-1 selectivity ratio of 1620:1, reportedly making it eight times more selective for the alpha-2 receptor compared to clonidine.[275,276] It has been investigated as a perioperative opioid-sparing and analgesic in both pediatric and adult patients. In one meta-analysis, the efficacy of perioperative IV dexmedetomidine on postoperative pain, rescue analgesia, and adverse effects was examined in 11 randomized controlled clinical trials that included pediatric patients undergoing otolaryngology procedures, appendectomies, and other outpatient procedures.[275] A wide range of bolus and intraoperative infusion dosing regimens were reported. Compared with placebo and fentanyl, postoperative pain scores and opioid consumption decreased in patient groups that received dexmedetomidine intraoperatively. Another meta-analysis that examined the effects of intraoperative IV dexmedetomidine on postoperative pain for pediatric patients undergoing adenotonsillectomy, ophthalmologic surgery, and other outpatient surgeries, also reported an opioid-sparing effect within the postoperative period.[277] Subgroup analysis revealed that bolus doses of ≥0.5 µg/kg reduced postoperative opioid consumption and pain scores, irrespective of the use of a continuous infusion. In a study of anesthetic techniques to spare or eliminate opioids for adenotonsillectomy, a dose of 1 µg/kg was effective.[278]

The available data support the use of a single intraoperative intravenous bolus dose of dexmedetomidine to reduce opioid consumption and pain scores in the postoperative period for outpatient pediatric surgeries. The ideal dose and timing of administration is unclear. The most common reported adverse effects are sedation,[279] bradycardia,[280] and hypotension.[281] Although some clinicians have the belief that dexmedetomidine is a "safer" sedative and analgesic with minimal effect on respiratory function, they may be operating under false assumptions. Dexmedetomidine causes dose-dependent sedation that can synergistically act with other sedating medications (i.e., opioids) to increase the risk of airway relaxation and collapse in patients who are at risk of airway obstruction. In pediatric patients, dexmedetomidine was found to cause the same degree of airway collapse as propofol when both were compared during deep sedation for children undergoing MRI scanning procedures.[282] Evidence suggests that intraoperative dexmedetomidine prolongs PACU length of stay in a dose-dependent fashion in adults[283] but heterogeneity of current available studies complicates comparisons within the pediatric literature. Patients that receive dexmedetomidine as part of their anesthetic should be monitored closely in the recovery period.

Dexmedetomidine has also been examined as an adjunct to local anesthetics in caudal blocks, peripheral nerve blocks,[284] and fascial plane blocks in children. There is some conflicting evidence and the literature is in its early stages regarding this topic, but initial studies have reported benefit in terms of prolongation of sensory blockade, decreased postoperative opioid consumption, and reduced pain scores, and time to first rescue analgesic with use of dexmedetomidine as a perineural adjunct for a variety of regional anesthetic techniques.[285–289] Perineural may be superior to systemic administration; however, further research is warranted before definitive conclusions are made.[286] Whether perineural dexmedetomidine offers any advantages over perineural clonidine is not known. Studied doses have ranged from a total of 0.3 to 1 µg/kg.

Lidocaine

Perioperative continuous intravenous infusions of lidocaine have been used as an opioid-sparing multimodal analgesic for a variety of surgical procedures. Within the adult literature, the majority of studies investigated patients undergoing either open or laparoscopic abdominal surgical procedures.[290] There is low to moderate level evidence from adults to support that perioperative intravenous lidocaine infusions reduce pain scores in the early postoperative period (<24 hours) but not in the later periods.[291] This analysis also found low to moderate evidence for reducing the time to first flatus and bowel movement, decreased length of hospital stay, decreased postoperative nausea, and decreased intraoperative and postoperative opioid consumption. The optimal dose and timing of administration is unclear. There is a paucity of data that compares epidural analgesia and intravenous lidocaine.

As with many topics within acute pediatric pain, the pediatric data for continuous intravenous lidocaine infusions are less evolved compared with adult data. One study examined 50 pediatric patients who received a lidocaine infusion for postoperative pain after a variety of procedures that included Nuss procedure, spinal fusion,[292] laparoscopic procedures,[293] and nephrectomy. Twenty-four percent of the infusions were associated with adverse effects,[292] the most common being neurologic side effects including paresthesias in the upper extremities and visual disturbances. This led to the discontinuation of some of the infusions, but others were managed with dose reduction; no patients experienced systemic toxicity.

Systemic intravenous lidocaine has been compared with placebo in 66 children undergoing laparoscopic inguinal hernia repair.[293] Study patients received a 1mg/kg IV bolus of lidocaine at initiation of therapy followed by a continuous infusion of 1.5 mg/kg per hour. There was no difference in their primary endpoint (i.e., the number of patients needing rescue analgesia in the PACU) between those treated with lidocaine and controls. Pain scores in the lidocaine group were significantly lower than those in the control group, a difference that persisted for up to 48 hours after surgery. Furthermore, they reported no adverse events.

A systematic review that included 45 trials (2802 patients) examined the safety and efficacy of intravenous lidocaine for postoperative pain in pediatric patients.[290] The patient population included children undergoing a wide variety of surgical procedures including open or laparoscopic abdominal surgery, cardiac, thoracic, extremity, and other minor surgical procedures. The results indicated that perioperative lidocaine infusions were associated with lower pain scores within the first 24 hours but not at 48 hours after surgery. Subgroup analysis revealed that the most benefit with regard to level of analgesia and duration of pain relief was with laparoscopic abdominal surgery followed by open abdominal surgery. They also found that opioid consumption and postoperative nausea and vomiting after perioperative systemic lidocaine were reduced. Postoperative ileus occurred in a greater percent of control patients. Systemic lidocaine significantly decreased the time to first flatus but not the time to first defecation. Perioperative systemic lidocaine also reduced length of hospital stay by about 8 hours.

When considered in aggregate, the pediatric and adult data present an argument for the use of systemic lidocaine as an opioid-sparing adjunct for acute surgical pain in the immediate postoperative period. There is little evidence to guide use for other types of nonsurgical acute pain. Systemic lidocaine appears to provide the most utility for laparoscopic and open abdominal surgeries with less evidence for efficacy for other types of surgical procedures. There are few if any comparisons of systemic lidocaine to regional anesthetic techniques or other multimodal therapies. Systemic lidocaine may have a role as an opioid-sparing adjunct for patients undergoing abdominal surgery that have a contraindication to continuous epidural analgesia or an abdominal fascial plane regional anesthetic approach.

Other Nonopioid Analgesics

Several other agents with widely varying pharmacology and mechanisms of action have been examined for use as analgesics for pediatric acute pain including magnesium, amantadine, esmolol, caffeine, and dextromethorphan. Although some initial results may be promising, the data for these agents are evolving and incomplete at this time.

Opioid Analgesics

Opioids are indicated for moderate to severe pain after surgery or trauma, for acute painful crises such as in sickle cell disease, as well as for chronic painful conditions such as cancer. Opioids mimic the effects of endogenous ligands known as endorphins, exerting their effects by binding to specific opioid receptors located at presynaptic and postsynaptic sites in the brain, spinal cord,[294] and peripheral nerve cells. There are four opioid receptors in the central nervous system: μ, κ, δ, and σ.[294–296] When these receptors are activated, they inhibit neurons by decreasing the release of excitatory neurotransmitters from presynaptic terminals. The μ receptors are further subdivided into μ_1 receptors, responsible for supraspinal analgesia and physical dependence; and μ_2 receptors, responsible for respiratory depression, bradycardia, physical dependence, and gastrointestinal dysmotility.[295] Activation of the κ receptors causes analgesia without significant respiratory depression, whereas activation of the σ receptors causes dysphoria, tachycardia, tachypnea, hypertonia, and mydriasis. The δ receptors modulate the activity of the μ receptors.

Drugs that exert their effects on opioid receptors are classified as agonists, antagonists, partial agonists, and mixed agonist-antagonists. The mixed agonist-antagonist drugs act as agonists at certain opioid receptors and antagonists at others. E-Table 41.4 depicts the various opioid receptors, their effects, as well as the drugs that exert activity on each of them. The opioids that are used most commonly to manage pain are the μ-receptor agonists, which include morphine, hydromorphone, fentanyl, methadone, hydrocodone, and oxycodone. Of these, morphine is the prototypic opioid used as first-line therapy for moderate to severe pain in children and, consequently, is the agent with which pediatric

TABLE 41.8	Opioid Analgesics: Relative Potency and Initial Dosing Guidelines[a]			
Analgesic	Conversion Factor (Convert to Morphine Equivalents)	Intravenous Dose	Oral Dose	Additional Routes of Administration
Morphine	1	Bolus: 0.05–0.1 mg/kg q 2–4 hours Infusion: 0.01–0.03 mg/kg per hour	0.3 mg/kg q 3–4 hours	Intrathecal, Epidural, intramuscular
Hydrocodone	1–1.5	N/A	0.1–0.2 mg/kg q 4–6 hours	N/A
Oxycodone	1–1.5	N/A	0.1–0.2 mg/kg q 4–6 hours	N/A
Tapentadol	0.3	N/A	50–100 mg q 4–6 hours	N/A
Codeine	0.1–0.15	N/A	0.5–1 mg/kg q 4–6 hours	N/A
Fentanyl	80–100	Bolus: 0.5–1 μg/kg q 0.5–2 hours Infusion: 0.5–2 μg/kg per hour	N/A	Intrathecal, epidural, transdermal, intranasal
Hydromorphone	4–7	5–10 μg/kg q 2–4 hours	0.04–0.08 mg/kg q 3–4 hours	Intrathecal, epidural
Methadone[b]	4–12	0.05–0.2 mg/kg	0.1–0.2 q 6–12 hours	N/A
Sufentanil[c]	800–1000	Bolus: 0.05–0.1 μg/kg Infusion: 0.05–0.15 μg/kg per hour	NR	Intrathecal, epidural, transmucosal, intranasal
Diamorphine	2	Bolus: 0.1–0.2 mg/kg q 2–4 hours Infusion: 0.02–0.05 mg/kg per hour	NA	Nasal[d]
Nalbuphine	0.8–1	N/A	50–100 μg/kg q 3–6 hours	N/A

NR, not recommended.
[a]Recommended doses are general starting dose guidelines for infants and children >6 months of age.
[b]Methadone has a highly variable and potentially long half-life that depends on both dose and timing of repeat administration, with risk of delayed sedation or respiratory depression. Caution should be taken with initial weight-based dosing as well as dosing interval. If sedation or respiratory depression occurs, additional doses should be withheld until the respiratory depression resolves and the medication restarted at a lower dose.
[c]Sufentanil is a highly potent opioid with few dosing conversion studies with respect to morphine.
[d]intravenous morphine: intranasal diamorphine 1:1; oral morphine: intranasal diamorphine 3:1.

clinicians have the most experience. Table 41.8 lists the relative potencies and suggested initial doses of the opioids in common clinical use. The Society for Pediatric Anesthesia also convened a task force to develop guidelines for the use of opioids during the perioperative period.[297] Developmental pharmacology, pharmacokinetics, and side effects of opioids are discussed in depth in Chapter 5.

Oral Administration

Oral opioids are well tolerated and suited for children with mild to moderate pain, for those who undergo outpatient surgery, or as adjuncts to regional anesthetics. For those who receive regional anesthetics, oral administration of an opioid just before the block is expected to wear off may provide a smooth transition and more stable and satisfactory analgesia. In most cases, oral opioids are better tolerated after resumption of oral intake.

Hydrocodone and oxycodone are two of the most commonly prescribed oral opioids. Hydromorphone and morphine also come in oral formulations. Morphine elixir is commonly used in children, but serum concentrations are variable.[298] Hydrocodone and oxycodone are available in a variety of formulations either alone or in combination with acetaminophen. Both hydrocodone and oxycodone are available in liquid form, making them easy to prescribe for infants and young children. Oxycodone is available in 1-mg/mL and 20-mg/mL strengths. Oxycodone PK and dosing (IV, IM, buccal, nasogastric) to a specific target concentration have been described in children.[299,300] Although the different formulations allow flexibility in dosing, extreme caution is required in prescribing and dispensing the correct concentration to avoid a potentially lethal overdose.

There are many combination products that contain oral opioids and a nonopioid adjuvant, such as acetaminophen. Although the primary advantage of these combinations is to reduce the number of tablets needed, this is outweighed by the disadvantage of a potential overdose of acetaminophen, and can result in suboptimal dosing (i.e., PRN) when scheduled dosing of adjuvant medications results in the greatest amount of opioid sparing. Therefore, we discourage the use of combination products and encourage the practice of scheduled dosing of nonopioids complemented by as-needed dosing of opioids for breakthrough pain. *Indeed, this strategy is an important trend in the contemporary use of opioids for acute pain that can ameliorate the problems of opioid adverse effects and overuse. A multimodal analgesic approach, which leverages the synergistic interactions between nonopioid and opioid analgesics, can result in enhanced analgesia with fewer untoward effects and reduced opioid requirements.*[301–303] Although randomized controlled trials are still limited in infants and children, we believe that the preponderance of evidence and clinical experience support a multimodal strategy as logical and clinically beneficial to children and should be used as the principal approach to treating most acute pain.

It should be noted that many oral opioids (oxycodone, hydrocodone, codeine) undergo metabolism via the CYP2D6 pathway (see Chapters 5 and 6). Hydrocodone and oxycodone have intrinsic analgesic properties, but codeine is the only prodrug that requires conversion to active metabolites, morphine via demethylation. There are significant genetic polymorphisms that affect the relative production of active metabolites of these drugs (oxymorphone, hydromorphone, and morphine, respectively). These differences result in individuals who are poor-, rapid-, or ultra-metabolizers of 2D6 substrates, depending on the number of functional copies of CYP2D6 alleles that are present, and they account for considerable variability in the response to these drugs. Ineffective conversion of codeine to morphine may be

present in up to 7% to 10% of White children. Another polymorphism, present in about 0.5% of children, results in rapid demethylation of codeine to morphine, producing exaggerated conversion to morphine and excessive sedation and respiratory depression when codeine is administered to children with this polymorphism.[304,305] These incidences are genetically influenced, with a significantly greater incidence of polymorphisms in North African descendants.[304,306–309] Numerous case reports have described severe and sometimes fatal respiratory depression in ultra-metabolizers who were prescribed codeine, most often in children with obstructive sleep apnea.[304] These reports have prompted the FDA to issue a black box warning for codeine and tramadol in children undergoing tonsillectomy*[307] and has further contraindicated use in children† <18 years of age.[309] To minimize the risk of complications from codeine and other opioids due to polymorphisms, several guidelines, including one published by the Clinical Pharmacogenetics Implementation Consortium regarding CYP2D6 genotypes, have been developed with a summary of current evidence and therapeutic recommendations.[310,311]

Therefore, because of both its lack of effect in some children (poor-metabolizers) and an exaggerated effect in others (ultra-metabolizers), we strongly discourage the use of codeine unless the recipient's polymorphisms have been characterized.[311] When 2D6 polymorphisms were identified in a group of children with pain from sickle cell crisis, those with usual 2D6 polymorphisms exhibited a normal response to codeine dosing, whereas those with poor and ultrarapid metabolizer polymorphisms received a substitute (noncodeine) opioid for analgesia.[312] All children, those who received codeine and those who did not, responded with excellent analgesia to the opioids administered and did so without complications. Tailoring opioid treatment to the 2D6 polymorphisms of patients ensures effective and safe opioid treatments. It is also important to note that active metabolites of codeine are excreted in breast milk, and there is a report of an opioid overdose in a neonate who was breastfed by a mother who was an ultra-metabolizer.[313] Mothers taking oxycodone while breastfeeding reported similar rates of infant sedation as those taking codeine.[314] Other oral opioids metabolized by CYP2D6 have also resulted in serious and fatal complications as a result of polymorphisms.[233,310,313,315] Thus all opioids, including oxycodone, hydrocodone, and tramadol, are theoretically at risk for similar complications associated with polymorphisms as codeine, albeit these complications are mostly associated with tramadol and codeine. Alternatively, if pain is of moderate or lower intensity, another class of analgesics (e.g., NSAIDs, ketamine, or dexmedetomidine) may be substituted.

Methadone is a synthetic opioid with a very prolonged elimination half-life (mean of 19 hours) in children between 1 and 18 years of age, and a large bioavailability (approximately 90%) after oral administration.[316] Oral or IV methadone has been considered a good alternative to the use of continuous opioid infusions because repeated dosing at intervals of every 6 to 12 hours can achieve relatively stable plasma drug concentrations.[317,318] Although it is used most frequently to facilitate weaning of opioid-tolerant children, it has also been recommended for postoperative analgesia after major surgery (e.g., Nuss procedure, posterior spinal fusion)[319] and may have an overall opioid-sparing effect when compared with regimens that

---

*https://www.fda.gov/downloads/Drugs/DrugSafety/UCM339116.pdf
†(https://www.fda.gov/Drugs/DrugSafety/ucm549679.htm)

utilize other opioids such as morphine.[318,320–322] Methadone is especially useful for children with cancer, burns, or other serious illnesses who require a long-acting oral opioid because it is available in an elixir formulation. Methadone should be thought of as virtually a combination analgesic. It is supplied as a racemic mixture. The *l*-isomer acts as a μ opioid, whereas the *d*-isomer acts as an antagonist at the NMDA subclass of excitatory amino acid receptors. Action at NMDA receptors makes methadone uniquely effective in the treatment of neuropathic pain. This NMDA-blocking action, and a differential activation of receptor-mediated endocytosis versus protein kinase activation,[323,324] may lead to a relatively slower rate of development of tolerance for methadone compared with some other opioids.

Advocates note that methadone is very underused as an intraoperative opioid for long major operations.[325] It has many characteristics that make it desirable for this purpose: rapid onset, prolonged analgesia, and a PK profile that, for operations of moderate to long duration, results in a blood level below the threshold of respiratory depression before emergence. A PK study of a single intraoperative dose of 0.1, 0.2, or 0.3 mg/kg methadone in adolescents undergoing posterior spinal fusion found similar kinetics to adults.[322] There was no difference in adverse events, including respiratory depression, compared with controls who did not receive methadone in any of the dose cohorts. Opioid consumption postoperatively was not decreased in that study.

Despite the advantages of methadone, it requires careful titration and repeated reassessment to avoid delayed oversedation when used for repeated dosing. This challenge in methadone dosing is due, in part, to its slow and widely variable clearance, as well as to its effects on NMDA antagonism, generating incomplete cross tolerance on conversion to methadone from other opioids. In opioid-naive subjects, a single dose of IV morphine is roughly equipotent to a single dose of methadone. Although morphine has active metabolites, the slower clearance of methadone compared with morphine translates, in opioid-naive subjects, into daily IV methadone requirements that are roughly one-third those of morphine. *However, in the setting of marked opioid tolerance, such as in the case of children with advanced cancer or in the setting of intensive care, the equipotent daily dose of IV methadone may be as small as one-tenth the preceding daily dose of IV morphine.*[151,317,322,326–329] A convenient web-based calculation tool‡ has synthesized the information from these and other studies to aid in opioid conversions in both opioid-naive and opioid-tolerant subjects. In our practice, this calculation tool appears quite useful, although it must be noted that it has not been independently assessed for use in children. Smartphone applications for multiple platforms are also available.

Intravenous Administration

Intermittent IV injections with opioids of short or moderate duration administered on an as-needed basis (PRN) do not achieve stable blood concentrations and predispose to cyclical periods of excessive sedation alternating with periods of inadequate analgesia as the drug level fluctuate. Yet this arguably inappropriate technique persists as the most common method of treating postoperative pain in many centers. A partial solution to this problem is to prescribe the opioid at closer intervals (such as 2 hourly) and then use a "reverse-PRN" schedule, in which the medication is offered at the prescribed interval, but the child can choose to take it or refuse it. Children should be assessed frequently, with the goal of administering the next dose before

moderate to severe pain recurs. The use of a long-acting opioid, such as methadone, has been recommended to provide more prolonged and stable periods of analgesia than could be achieved with shorter-acting opioids, approaching the efficacy of continuous infusions.[330] However, careful titration of dosing and frequent assessment of the child are required because of methadone's slow and variable clearance.

Continuous IV opioid infusions are an excellent means of providing analgesia to children with moderate to severe pain who are unable to use PCA, such as infants, young children, and those who are cognitively impaired or physically disabled.[331] Once a therapeutic blood concentration of the opioid is achieved by administering an initial loading dose, an infusion rate can be selected to maintain that concentration without excessive fluctuations. Additionally, rescue doses of IV opioids may be required for breakthrough pain. Opioids, however, cause a dose-dependent respiratory depression by shifting the CO_2 response curve, reduce peripheral and central chemoreceptor responsiveness to plasma CO_2 levels, and decrease the hypoxic ventilatory response. Residual and synergistic effects of sedatives and hypnotics in the early postoperative period further increase the risk of opioid-induced respiratory depression. This is particularly true in preterm and term infants because of age-related differences in elimination and clearance of opioids and other sedating medications (see also Chapter 5). This is of particular concern with the use of continuous opioid infusions because inappropriate dosing, prolonged elimination, and considerations related to the context-sensitive half-life may lead to drug accumulation, placing infants at great risk for side effects. In a prospective audit of 10,726 opioid infusions in the United Kingdom and Ireland, the overall risk of permanent harm was found to be 1 in 10,000 cases, and serious events without permanent harm 1 in 383, with half of the serious events being respiratory depression.[332] Therefore, the rate of the infusion should be carefully selected, based on the child's age, comorbidities, and clinical condition. In addition, children who receive opioid infusions should be monitored and assessed frequently for depth of sedation and respiratory rate. *The onset of sedation and bradypnea is an important clinical index of incipient respiratory depression* and should alert the nursing staff and physicians to decrease the infusion rate and observe the child more closely. Continuous pulse oximetry is widely recommended during continuous opioid infusions, especially in opioid-naive children and other children at increased risk for respiratory depression, but it is a surrogate measure of ventilation. If supplementary oxygen is administered, then detection of respiratory depression becomes hindered, rendering desaturation a late metric of respiratory depression, which could result in a fatal outcome outside of critical care monitored settings.[333,334] Capnography or other techniques in development (such as temperature based, piezoelectric, or bioimpedance detectors for respiratory depression) that identify changes in respiratory patterns instantly warrant consideration but must overcome known weaknesses that include false-positive alarms, disposable costs, and others.[334–337]

Another method of IV opioid delivery is via PCA (see further). With any infusion technique, scrupulous attention must be paid to protocols for checking pump settings to avoid errors. Pump programming errors, none of which caused serious harm, but which had the potential to do so, occurred in 17 instances in the UK audit, all from a single center, highlighting the critical importance of system safeguards to prevent patient harm.[332] "Smart" infusion pumps which utilize preprogrammed drug libraries with set drug concentrations and dosage limits can be an aid in reducing programming errors.

---

‡https://www.globalrph.com/narcoticonv.htm

Intramuscular and Subcutaneous Routes

Intermittent IM and subcutaneous injections of opioids are generally obsolete because they are frightening and unpleasant for children and are often perceived as worse than the pain for which they are administered.[338] Additionally, they have the PK disadvantage of unpredictable and erratic uptake if regional blood flow is impaired, and they produce pronounced wide swings in blood concentrations. The goal of maintaining an even level of analgesia is thus nearly impossible to achieve with these routes of administration. An important exception is the use of indwelling subcutaneous catheters for continuous infusions and PCA as in palliative care.

Intranasal Route

Fentanyl is generally the most common opioid used for the intranasal (IN) route in pediatrics. At reported doses between 1 and 2 μg/kg in children weighing more than 10 kilograms, it can be a useful technique to provide initial sedation or analgesia to a child who does not yet have IV access or for a child who has difficulties with oral medications. This is most commonly used in the emergency department or preoperative area, but has also been used for analgesia after myringotomy and tympanostomy tube placement.[339,340]

Diamorphine (diacetylmorphine, heroin) is a strong opioid with rapid onset of action when given by intravenous, intramuscular, and transmucosal routes. It is used for burns and fracture reduction in the acute setting and in palliative care for breakthrough pain in children with life-limiting conditions.[341–343] Drug use for these indications is limited to the United Kingdom.[344] The intranasal route is used for acute pain in the emergency room (0.1 mg/kg) for bone fracture reduction.[345,346]

SELECTION OF OPIOIDS FOR PARENTERAL USE

Morphine is the opioid most used for postoperative analgesia and has been extensively studied in all pediatric age groups. After major abdominal, thoracic, and orthopedic surgery, children who received continuous morphine infusions had reduced pain scores compared with those who received intermittent IM or IV injections.[332,347,348] However, other investigators were only able to demonstrate reduced pain scores with continuous morphine infusions compared with intermittent IV injections of morphine in children between 1 and 3 years of age, and not in infants in the first year of life.[349,350] Similarly, evidence of the beneficial effects of opioid analgesia in ameliorating the postoperative response to surgical stress is conflicting. A reduction in serum β-endorphin concentrations has been reported in neonates after the initiation of a continuous infusion of postoperative morphine.[351] In neonates whose lungs were mechanically ventilated, both epinephrine and norepinephrine concentrations decreased after the initiation of morphine or fentanyl infusions.[352] However, β-endorphin concentrations decreased only in the children who received fentanyl. When the effects of continuous infusions of morphine were compared with those of intermittent IV injections of morphine on the stress response in children between 1 and 3 years of age, reduced glucose concentrations in the continuous infusion group suggested only a modest ablation of the stress response in this age group.[349] It should be noted that these older studies were performed in neonates receiving mechanical ventilation and not experiencing postoperative pain, so these results might not be directly extrapolated to the perioperative setting.

Several studies have described the PK of morphine administered as a continuous infusion and evaluated the pharmacodynamic effects of morphine on respiratory indexes in neonates, infants, and children after various surgical procedures. In children 14 months to 17 years of age who underwent cardiac surgery,[348] morphine infusions were adjusted between 10 and 50 μg/kg per hour to minimize discomfort and avoid excessive sedation. Supplemental boluses of 100 μg/kg morphine were administered for breakthrough pain. Steady-state morphine concentrations were achieved in 4 hours. Those children who could self-report their pain reported good analgesia with morphine concentrations more than 12 ng/mL. Morphine infusions of 10 to 30 μg/kg per hour yielded mean serum concentrations between 10 and 22 ng/mL with less than 2% experiencing evidence of respiratory depression (partial pressure of carbon dioxide [$PaCO_2$] >50 mm Hg). Furthermore, children who received morphine infusions of 10 to 30 μg/kg per hour breathed spontaneously after extubation of the trachea, and those who were weaned from assisted to spontaneous ventilation maintained a normal $PaCO_2$. On the other hand, 60% (three of five children) who received a greater infusion rate of morphine, 40 to 50 μg/kg per hour, experienced hypercarbia ($PaCO_2$ 48–66 mm Hg). A subsequent study by the same investigators evaluated the severity of respiratory depression in infants and children aged 2 days to 18 months treated with morphine. Of those whose morphine concentrations exceeded 20 ng/mL, approximately 70% experienced respiratory depression ($PaCO_2$ >55 mm Hg and/or a depressed slope of the CO_2 response curve) compared with 15% to 28% of those whose concentrations were less than 20 ng/mL.[353] The investigators proposed a steady-state morphine concentration of 20 ng/mL as the threshold concentration beyond which respiration may be depressed in this age group.

Previous studies determined that the clearance of morphine is impaired in preterm infants and that clearance increases with postmenstrual age (see Fig. 5.12).[354] Additionally, morphine clearance is immature in infants up to 1 to 2 months of postmenstrual age.[137,355] Clearance maturation is complete within the first 2 postnatal years.[356,357] Preterm and full-term neonates, therefore, have a narrower therapeutic window for morphine analgesia compared with older children. These young infants have reduced morphine requirements postoperatively, requiring fewer rescue doses of morphine when receiving continuous infusions or intermittent bolus doses.[358] Therefore, opioids should be carefully titrated in infants in a monitored environment with significantly reduced continuous infusion rates. Based on PK modeling and morphine clearance predictions, a target morphine concentration of 10 ng/mL can be achieved with morphine infusions ranging from 5 μg/kg per hour in term neonates to 16 μg/kg per hour in 1- to 3-year-old children (see Chapter 5).[357] In addition, reduced clearance in patients with renal insufficiency can result in accumulation of the potent morphine-6-glucuronide metabolite, which can cause delayed respiratory depression, so morphine should be avoided in these patients.[359]

Pharmacodynamic differences between infants and children have been postulated as the mechanism responsible for the greater sensitivity of infants (compared with older children) to the respiratory depressant effects of opioids. However, this may not be the case. Although rodent data suggest that opioid brain concentrations in immature rodents are greater than in their mature counterparts at similar serum concentrations,[360] these findings may not be applicable to humans.[358] Neonatal rats have a relatively immature brain and a far more permeable blood-brain barrier than that in human infants. Consequently, the rodent may not be an appropriate model to depict the human condition.[360] It appears that the "increased sensitivity" is related, at least in part, to PK variables, perhaps in some measure as a result of a neonate's decreased conjugating ability.[361]

Regardless of the mechanism, respiratory depression remains the most feared adverse effect of opioids administered by any route. Current monitoring technologies have numerous advantages and disadvantages (see the section "Monitoring the Child Using PCA"). Neonates and infants younger than 6 months of age are at greater risk for opioid-induced respiratory depression because the ventilatory responses to airway obstruction, hypoxemia, and hypercapnia are immature at birth and mature over the first several months of life in preterm as well as full-term infants (see also Figs. 2.12 and 2.13). Indeed, there was a 4.5% incidence of failure to wean from the ventilator and a 13.5% incidence of apnea (30 seconds or more that required intervention) or severe respiratory depression in spontaneously breathing neonates who received opioids for postoperative pain.[359,362] Another report of a 3-year surveillance period for adverse drug reactions described 15 children aged 2 days to 17 years who experienced opioid-induced respiratory depression.[363] Respiratory depression in the latter study was defined as apnea, hypoxemia, cyanosis, a marked decrease in respiratory rate, or a need for naloxone. Although this study was unable to define the incidence of respiratory depression because the denominator was unknown, it did identify several predisposing factors, including age younger than 1 year (7 of 15 children), drug errors (including prescription and administration errors; 6 of 15 children), concurrent medical problems (diminished respiratory reserve, hepatic, and/or renal impairment), and concurrent sedative drugs. A prospective UK audit found 14 cases of respiratory depression (out of 10,726 total infusions, or 0.13%), 10 with nurse-controlled analgesia, 2 with continuous infusions, and 2 with PCA; programming or prescribing errors accounted for 17 incidents.[332] Potentially contributing risk factors in half of the cases included very young age and neurodevelopmental, respiratory, or cardiac disease. In contrast to the earlier studies, no case of respiratory depression was reported in 110 children older than 3 months of age who received opioid infusions postoperatively.[364] Interpretation of this literature is confounded by different monitoring techniques and different definitions of respiratory depression. For instance, in the latter study, a 4.5% incidence of clinically significant hypoxemia was reported but was not included in their definition of respiratory depression. Additionally, children in that study were monitored with hourly documentation of respiratory rate, but oxygen saturation was not monitored after discharge from the PACU, thereby reducing the ability to detect more subtle episodes of respiratory depression. In summary, the results of these studies suggest that children who receive opioids require careful monitoring for respiratory depression, with appropriate age-based reduction of dosage, particularly for neonates and infants younger than 6 months of age.

The most common adverse effect of opioid therapy is nausea and vomiting. One study reported nausea and vomiting in 34 of 80 children (42.5%) who received postoperative morphine infusions. These were well managed with antiemetic therapy in all but two children who required discontinuation of the opioids.[364] In the same study, the incidence of pruritus and urinary retention was 13% for both and that of dysphoria was 7%. Seizures have been reported in two neonates who received bolus doses of morphine followed by infusions of 32 and 40 µg/kg per hour and whose serum morphine concentrations were 61 and 90 ng/mL, respectively.[365] Irregular jerking movements, as well as one case of a generalized seizure, have been reported in children 1 to 15 years of age receiving postoperative morphine infusions.[347] Intravenous

metoclopramide (100–150 µg/kg) is an effective antiemetic but may also cause extrapyramidal symptoms (9%), diarrhea (6%), and sedation (6%).[366] The serotonin-receptor antagonist antiemetics, such as ondansetron, have the advantage of virtually eliminating the risk of dystonic or oculogyric reactions that occur with phenothiazines, butyrophenones, and metoclopramide. However, headaches occur in a small number of those who receive serotonin-receptor antagonists. A "microdose" naloxone infusion (0.25–1.0 µg/kg per hour) reverses the incidence of both nausea and pruritus after opioids without affecting the analgesia or opioid consumption.[364,365,367,368] A dose-escalation study demonstrated that doses of 1 to 1.65 µg/kg per hour resulted in greater efficacy in reducing adverse effects, particularly pruritus, without degrading analgesia.[368] It is likely that these results may be generalized to other routes of opioid administration. Agonist-antagonists such as nalbuphine have also been found effective for nausea, pruritis, and other opioid-induced side effects.[369]

Opioid-induced bowel dysfunction, reported in more than 90% of patients receiving opioid therapy, occurs by blocking propulsive peristalsis, inhibiting secretion and increasing reabsorption of intestinal fluids, and decreasing the activity of excitatory and inhibitory neurons in the myenteric plexus. Bowel dysfunction manifests as abdominal distention and bloating, delayed gastric emptying, and constipation. Aggressive prophylactic measures, including osmotic, lubricant, or stimulant laxatives, should be prescribed early during treatment. Naloxone as well as the selective gastrointestinal peripheral µ-opioid receptor antagonist, methylnaltrexone,[370,371] have shown similar efficacy.[370–373]

Fentanyl may be a useful substitute for morphine in children with hemodynamic instability, in whom a decrease in peripheral vascular tone is undesirable, and in whom histamine release caused by morphine is not well tolerated. Additionally, its rapid onset of analgesia makes it ideal for children with severe escalating pain who require urgent pain relief. Fentanyl is metabolized by the liver into an inactive metabolite, norfentanyl, which is excreted via the kidneys. It is 80 to 100 times more potent than morphine. Although its elimination half-life is significantly less than that for morphine, its context-sensitive half-life during chronic infusion increases as a result of peripheral compartment accumulation (see Fig. 5.29). Like morphine, clearance in neonates is immature, predisposing them to a greater risk for accumulation with repeat dosing compared with older infants.[374,375] For a given bolus of fentanyl, plasma concentrations in infants between 3 months and 1 year of age are less than those in older children and adults because volume of distribution is increased.[376] This finding is consistent with the almost 2-fold greater clearance of fentanyl in children compared with neonates. In children 18 days to 14 years of age who were mechanically ventilated, the clearance (L/kg per hour) of fentanyl was age related yet quite variable, with the slowest clearance occurring in infants younger than 6 months of age and the most rapid in those between 6 months and 6 years of age.[377] The clearance of fentanyl is further reduced in preterm infants, and although clearance correlates with the postmenstrual age, the clinical impact of postnatal age remains uncertain.[378,379]

Fentanyl causes all the adverse effects reported with opioids, including pruritus, nausea, vomiting, constipation, and sedation, but does not release histamine. Respiratory depression and chest wall and glottic rigidity, however, are its most concerning adverse effects. One study compared the incidence of respiratory depression in full-term and former preterm infants and young infants receiving 2-µg/kg bolus doses of fentanyl every 2 hours or

41

a continuous infusion of 1 µg/kg per hour after abdominal or thoracic surgery.[380] Randomization was terminated prematurely because of a 6-fold greater incidence of apnea that required intervention in the bolus dose group compared with the continuous infusion group (89% vs. 14%). The continuous infusion arm was continued for another 20 children, resulting in a 25% incidence of apnea in this group. In contrast, the incidence of respiratory depression (based on transcutaneous $PaCO_2$ measurements and the incidence of apnea) for a given plasma fentanyl concentration in infants 1 to 12 months of age and children 1 to 5 years of age was less than that in adults undergoing hernia repair or other peripheral surgery.[381] Differences in surgical procedures and the inclusion of preterm infants in the former study may account for the significant difference in the incidence of apnea found in these two studies.

Although chest wall and glottic rigidity usually occurs after the rapid bolus administration of high-dose fentanyl, it has also been reported in an infant after a low-dose continuous infusion of fentanyl. Chest wall rigidity was reported in 9% of preterm and full-term neonates who received an average of 4.9 µg/kg over a 2- to 3-minute period for a procedure or for perioperative analgesia.[382] In every case, naloxone reversed the chest wall rigidity. Additionally, a case of chest wall rigidity has been reported in a preterm neonate after high-dose fentanyl was administered to the parturient before a cesarean section.[383] Although administration of naloxone has been used successfully to treat cases of chest wall rigidity, severe cases associated with rapid oxygen desaturation may require the use of neuromuscular blocking drugs and mechanical ventilation.

The use of continuous fentanyl infusions in infants and children has been associated with a rapid development of tolerance, as indicated by a steady increase in infusion rate to maintain the desired effect[384,385] and a large incidence of opioid withdrawal syndrome after termination of the infusion.[385,386] The incidence of opioid withdrawal is directly related to the total dose administered and the duration of infusion.[385,386] Iatrogenic opioid withdrawal was reported in 21 of 37 neonates (57%) after continuous fentanyl infusions during extracorporeal membrane oxygenation.[385] Both a cumulative fentanyl dose greater than 1.6 mg/kg and extracorporeal membrane oxygenation that lasted more than 5 days were predictors of opioid withdrawal. A similar incidence has been reported in 23 children 1 week to 22 months of age who received continuous fentanyl infusions during mechanical ventilation.[386] This study also found that a cumulative dose of 1.5 mg/kg of fentanyl over 5 days was associated with a greater than 50% incidence of withdrawal symptoms. Furthermore, a cumulative dose of 2.5 mg/kg as a continuous infusion over 9 days was 100% predictive of the occurrence of withdrawal. Finally, movement disorder and irritability have been reported after withdrawal of fentanyl infusion in five infants who were mechanically ventilated.[387] None of the infants who developed the movement disorder had received another opioid after withdrawal of fentanyl, whereas five of eight controls who did not develop withdrawal during the same period had received a substitute opioid. These data suggest that opioid withdrawal occurs earlier and with greater frequency after fentanyl infusions compared with other opioids. Therefore, it seems prudent to use fentanyl infusions for pain relief during periods of hemodynamic instability, such as in the early postoperative period, and to transition to another opioid, such as morphine, hydromorphone, or methadone, as soon as the child is stabilized. Children who require fentanyl infusions for 5 days or more should undergo a slow taper (e.g., 10% decrease every 12 hours) or be transitioned to another parenteral or oral opioid regimen.

Hydromorphone has a spectrum of action similar to that of morphine. Adult opioid equipotency data suggest that it is 3.5 to 7 times as potent as morphine.[388-391] In a study of children with mucositis pain after bone marrow transplant, a conversion ratio of morphine to hydromorphone, 7:1, underestimated the hydromorphone requirements by 27%.[392] These data suggest that a 5:1 conversion ratio may be more appropriate, particularly in children with chronic pain. Despite its widespread use, very few studies have evaluated the use of hydromorphone in children. One small pediatric study that randomized patients to morphine or hydromorphone PCA (5:1 ratio) showed no difference in analgesia or side effects.[393] A meta-analysis of adult studies showed very similar analgesia and side effect profiles, although methadone does not cause histamine release.[394] Overall, morphine and hydromorphone are very similar for most outcomes. Because adverse effect profiles for each drug may differ within an individual patient, it remains common practice to prescribe a trial of hydromorphone in children who experience unacceptable adverse effects with morphine (or vice versa). Hydromorphone does have more rapid effect-site equilibration compared with morphine,[394] so there is a theoretical risk of dose stacking and subsequent respiratory depression with morphine compared with hydromorphone, but the requisite large studies needed to examine the clinical importance of this risk have not been done. It should be noted that the analogous hydromorphone-3-glucuronide has been associated with dose-dependent neuroexcitatory effects in hospice patients with renal insufficiency, but no cases have been reported in children. Therefore, hydromorphone (or fentanyl or methadone) is a preferential choice in patients with kidney disease.[395] Although hydromorphone has an active glucuronide metabolite that is cleared by the kidney, it is considered intermediate in risk, better than morphine, but worse than fentanyl and methadone, for patients with renal failure.

Meperidine (pethidine), used clinically for many years,[396] is approximately one-tenth as potent as morphine. Accumulation of normeperidine, its active metabolite (which has CNS stimulant properties), after repeated doses places children at risk for seizures.[397] Therefore, its use has been restricted to the treatment of postoperative shivering[398,399] or rigors after amphotericin. However, there are a number of alternative options for management of postoperative shivering (e.g., opioids, ketamine, dexmedetomidine, tramadol)[400] that can replace meperidine for this indication.[401] Although its short-term use continues by a small number of clinicians for procedural sedation and analgesia, other analgesics are preferable choices. Meperidine is not recommended for PCA or as a continuous infusion and has been removed from the formulary of many children's hospitals.

Patient-Controlled Analgesia

PCA was first studied in adults in 1965. The initial interest with this technique was as a research tool for the study of pain. By the early 1970s, it was identified as an excellent strategy for treating pain in the clinical setting, with studies demonstrating that pain relief was achieved by PCA with relatively smaller doses of opioids and with greater patient satisfaction than with conventional methods.[402] However, it was not until the late 1980s that PCA was studied in children.[403] Since that time, it has become the preferred method for opioid delivery in children older than 6 to 7 years of age (depending on their level of understanding) for acute pain, as well as chronic pain associated with cancer or sickle cell disease.[403-406] The primary benefit of PCA is that it allows children to titrate the analgesic to the extent of their pain. The goal is for the child to self-regulate a blood opioid concentration within the therapeutic range. Most children strike a balance between adequate pain relief on the one hand and adverse effects of the drug on the other. This approach, which grants the child some degree of autonomy, is the rationale given since pain is an entirely subjective and individual experience and that opioid metabolism and pain perception varies among individuals. It also reduces the apprehension of older children and adolescents regarding pain relief because they can control it and they can tailor the opioid delivery to the extent of pain they have at a given time, for example, before physical therapy, removal of tubes or drains, dressing changes, or getting out of bed. Additionally, the use of PCA avoids delays in administration of analgesics associated with standard "as-needed" orders of IV opioids and allows smaller doses of opioids to be delivered more frequently without increasing nursing workload. Therefore, PCA is thought to provide more consistent pain relief with less total opioid dosing, resulting in fewer adverse effects, such as sedation, nausea, and vomiting. Purportedly, children using PCA report better analgesia and reduced pain scores compared with children who must rely on the nursing staff to administer analgesics when they are in pain. These and other benefits of PCA have been extensively touted in the medical literature,[406–408] as well as in the lay press.[409] Recently, however, risks associated with PCA use have also been highlighted and are discussed later.[410–412] Recognition of these risks has led to recommendations for careful dosing and monitoring of all children who are receiving opioids, particularly those receiving continuous infusions and those with specific risk factors.[413,414]

Child training is a necessary part of PCA, because successful use of PCA requires that both the child and family understand how it works.[415] The instructions should be clear that the pump should be activated whenever the child feels pain, that children cannot give themselves "too much medication" because of the pump lockout interval, that the child should not wait for severe pain to activate the pump, and that a dose can also be given in anticipation of painful stimuli, such as ambulation or chest physiotherapy. Most importantly, PCA does not mean *parent*-controlled analgesia, and parents should never activate the pump unless specifically authorized to do so by the primary care or pain service physician (see the "Nurse-/Caregiver-Controlled Analgesia" section later in this chapter).[413]

Choice of Drug and Drug Dosages

Morphine remains the most common opioid administered via PCA in many centers, although hydromorphone is an increasingly common first-line option, especially for patients with renal disease or a history of intolerance to morphine. Fentanyl is also used, but the disadvantage is a more rapid development of tolerance. Suggested initial dosages for opioids via PCA for opioid-naive children are presented in Table 41.8. Children with opioid tolerance require adjustments to these settings, considering the previous opioid history and the opioid doses that the child was receiving before the acute painful stimulus. For example, one study reported that children with sickle cell disease self-administered more than double the dose of morphine via PCA, required more nonopioid adjuvant analgesics, reported greater pain scores, and stayed in the hospital for twice the duration compared with non–sickle cell disease–affected children after laparoscopic cholecystectomy.[416]

Fentanyl PCA has been used with success as a first-line and a secondary drug in children with cancer pain, as well as acute postoperative pain.[408,417] Most of the adverse effects, including nausea and pruritus, were mild and easily managed. However,

some reported an overall incidence of apnea and hypoxemia of 3.5% in 212 children receiving PCA, of whom 144 had received fentanyl.[408] Concerns related to the context-sensitive half-life and potential rapid development of tolerance suggest that fentanyl should not be considered the first-line choice for PCA. The benefits that hydromorphone PCA offers over morphine PCA in the chronic and acute pain settings require further investigation.

Pump Settings

Most PCA pumps have five settings to adjust:

- A *loading dose* of opioid ranging from 0.025 to 0.1 mg/kg of morphine divided into incremental doses is usually given to establish adequate analgesia before therapy is turned over to the child, because self-administered doses with this technique are generally small. A sufficient interval between incremental doses must be allowed, so that the drug achieves its peak effect before the next dose, thereby avoiding an overdose. If PCA is started in the PACU, opioid doses administered during surgery must be considered before prescribing a loading dose. Additionally, it may be desirable to administer the loading dose via the PCA pump so that it is included in the initial 4-hour or hourly limit of the PCA since children who receive IV-PRN doses of opioids in the PACU, followed by initiation of PCA, may be at risk for oversedation and respiratory depression from opioid stacking. Children who have received opioids toward the end of surgery, those who awaken in comfort, or those who receive nerve blocks may not need a loading dose and may start to use the demand doses as needed on awakening.
- A *patient bolus dose*—that is, the dose that will be administered with each child's activation of the pump—must be prescribed. These small boluses are usually in the range of 0.01 to 0.02 mg/kg of morphine in opioid-naive subjects.
- A *registered nurse bolus dose* may be ordered to allow the bedside nurse to administer an additional dose of opioid analgesic for severe breakthrough pain that is not being managed by the patient bolus dose. This dose is typically 1 to 2 times the patient dose and is ordered to be allowed once every 30 to 60 minutes.
- A *lockout interval* of usually 5 to 15 minutes prevents a child from activating the pump until the full effect from the previous bolus is achieved, and it should correspond to the time from IV injection to the peak effect of the drug.
- A *continuous basal infusion* ranging from 0.00 to 0.02 mg/kg per hour of morphine (or more, in opioid-tolerant subjects) may be used in selective cases (see later text).
- A *maximum hourly dose or a 4-hour limit* may be chosen to limit the cumulative amount of drug a child can administer. Once this limit is reached, the child cannot activate the pump until the 4-hour limit has passed. Four-hour limits allow for increased flexibility in dosing over greater periods of time and pain intensity. Typically, the maximum hourly dose ranges from 0.05 to 0.1 mg/kg and 4-hour limits from 0.25 to 0.4 mg/kg of morphine in opioid-naive subjects. This amount may be chosen based on the average hourly use of morphine during the past 24 hours or, in children started on PCA immediately after surgery, at the reduced range of the dosage scale. Fig. 41.6 presents sample PCA orders, including choice of drugs, dosing, and suggested monitoring.

Continuous Basal Infusions

The use of a continuous basal infusion of the opioid to supplement child-administered doses remains a subject of controversy. The primary benefit of a continuous basal infusion is improved

41

Pediatric Acute Pain Service (APS)	BIRTHDATE

Pediatric Acute Pain Service (APS)

Patient Controlled Analgesia (PCA) Initial Orders

BIRTHDATE

NAME

Reg. No.

Date: _____   Time: _____

Clerk's Initials: _____   Unit: _____

No other OPIOIDS or SEDATIVES to be administered while on PCA unless Pain Service has ordered them or been notified.
Please page Pain Service before discontinuing PCA at pager xxxx.

AGE: _____ months/year   WEIGHT: _____ kg

MODE: ☐ PCA ONLY
 ☐ PCA & Continuous
 ☐ Nurse Controlled
 ☐ Continuous
 ☐ Other: _____

Select drug to be used	☐ Morphine		☐ Hydromorphone		☐ Fentanyl _____
Drug Concentration	☐ 1 mg/mL	☐ 100 µg/mL (3000 µg/30 mL use for pts ≤10 kg)	☐ 0.5 mg/mL (use only for pts requiring excessive dosing)	☐ 100 µg/mL (3000 µg/30 mL)	20 µg/mL
PCA Dose	_____ mg 0.01-0.03 mg/kg	_____ µg 10-30 µg/kg	_____ mg 0.002-0.006 mg/kg	_____ µg 2-6 µg/kg	_____ µg 0.2-0.5 µg
Lockout Interval	_____ minute 8-15 minutes	_____ minute 8-15 minutes	_____ minute 8-15 minutes	_____ minute 8-15 minutes	_____ minute 8-15 minutes
Continuous Infusion Rate	_____ mg/h 0.01-0.02 mg/kg/h	_____ µg/h 10-20 µg/kg/h	_____ mg/h 0.002-0.004 mg/kg/h	_____ µg/h 2-4 µg/kg/h	_____ /h 0.1-0.5 µg/kg/h
4-Hour Limit	_____ mg 0.25-0.4 mg/kg	_____ µg 250-400 µg/kg	_____ mg 0.05-0.08 mg/kg	_____ µg 50-80 µg/kg	_____ 7-10 µg/kg
Double-check	Double-check pump settings against the order. Document double-check on the PCA/Epidural Flowsheet.				
Emergency Measures	**For sedation score >2 or respiratory rate < _____ :** Hold PCA and page Pain Service **For sedation score = 4 or respiratory rate < _____ :** Hold PCA, give Naloxone and STAT page Primary Service **FIRST**, then Pain Service **Naloxone Dose:** Under 10 kg _____ mg IV STAT (0.01 mg/kg/dose, maximum of 0.1 mg), may repeat every 2 minutes × 2 Over 10 kg 0.1 mg IV STAT, may repeat every 2 minutes × 2 For O₂ Saturation < _____ : (Consider baseline saturation) Stimulate patient and encourage deep breathing Administer O₂ by face mask or nasal cannula and page the Primary Service and Pain Service				
Antipruritic	☐ Naloxone (Narcan) 0.25 µg/kg/h. Add 0.25 mg to 100 mL normal saline (0.1 mL/kg/h = 0.25 µg/kg/h) to be infused at 0.1 mL/h × weight (kg) = _____ mL/h or Nalbuphine 0.05 mg/kg = _____ mg IV every 4 hours				
Antiemetic	☐ Ondansetron (Zofran)_____ mg IV every 6 hours PRN (0.1 mg/kg/dose up to 4 mg) MAX single dose: 4 mg ☐ Per Primary Service ☐ Other: _____				
Other	☐ Other: _____				

1. Monitoring:

Continuous pulse oximetry while on PCA except while patient is out of bed. Record pulse oximetry readings at same frequency as respiratory rate. Respiratory rate and sedation level:

Initiation of therapy: every 30 minutes × 1 hour and then every 2 hours for the first 24 hours and then every 4 hours
Transfer to a new unit: every 30 minutes × 1 hour then either every 2 or 4 hours (depends upon start of PCA therapy)
With loading dose and increases in doses, infusions, limits: every 30 minutes × 2 then every 2 or 4 hours (depends upon start of PCA therapy)
Regularly scheduled Day/Night changes: every 4 hours if therapy has been initiated longer than 24 hours.

Pain Scores:
every 2 hours × 8 hours, then every 4 hours. If pain not controlled after 1 hour, page xxxx or xxxx

2. The Acute Pain Service (APS) nurse may change PCA orders by increasing or decreasing pump settings by 20% and stop the continuous infusion.
3. Any order changes in #2 must be documented on a subsequent PCA order form.

Verbal   ☐
Telephone ☐   Print name/title of person giving order   Signature/title of person taking order   Date   Time

Physician Signature   Dr. #   Date   Time

FIGURE 41.6 Sample patient-controlled analgesia orders. *IV,* Intravenous; *MAX,* maximum; *PCA,* patient-controlled anesthesia; *PRN,* as needed; *STAT,* immediately. (Modified from the University of Michigan Hospitals & Health Centers.)

A

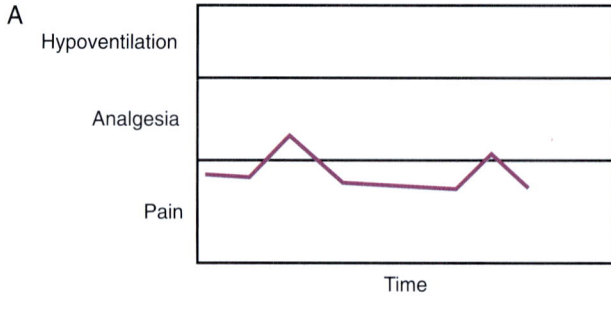

B

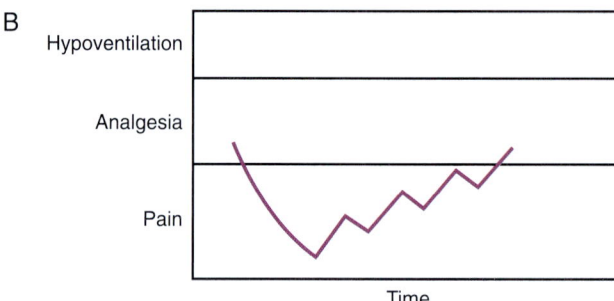

C

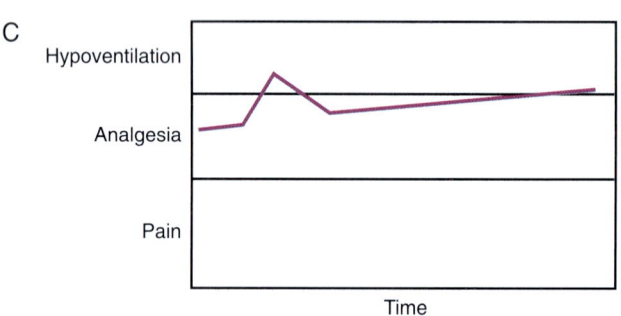

FIGURE 41.7 Patient-controlled analgesia (PCA) with an appropriate dose of continuous basal infusion. **A,** Use of an appropriate dose of continuous basal infusion maintains near-therapeutic plasma opioid concentrations during sleep with rapid increase to analgesic concentrations as soon as the child awakens and activates the PCA button. **B,** Chart depicts plasma opioid concentrations in a child who is receiving PCA bolus doses only, with no continuous basal infusion. Plasma concentrations decrease significantly when the child is asleep, necessitating multiple doses to achieve analgesic concentrations. **C,** An excessive dose continuous basal infusion results in opioid accumulation with delayed hypoventilation even when the PCA button is not activated. (Reproduced with permission from Berde CB, Solodiuk J. Multidisciplinary programs for management of acute and chronic pain in children. In: Schecter NL, Berde CB, Yaster M, eds. *Pain in Infants, Children and Adolescents.* 2nd ed. Philadelphia: Lippincott Williams and Wilkins; 2003:476.)

quality of sleep[418] as near-therapeutic plasma opioid concentrations are maintained (Fig. 41.7A). On the other hand, as depicted in Fig. 41.7B, a child who receives only PCA bolus dosing with no continuous basal infusion is likely to awaken with unrelieved pain that may require multiple doses to again achieve adequate pain relief. Decreased nocturnal awakenings secondary to pain, improved restfulness, or sleep patterns, reduced total opioid consumption, fewer adverse effects, and improved analgesic effectiveness are all potential reasons for using continuous basal infusions. However, the use of a continuous basal infusion commits the child to receiving a fixed dose of opioid regardless of the level of sedation, and has the theoretical potential for overriding one of the inherent safety features of PCA, that is, an excessively sedated or somnolent child is unlikely to push the button and therefore receives no additional opioid but, with a fixed infusion, drug may accumulate (Fig. 41.7C), with the potential for hypoventilation.[419] It has also been argued that programming errors with continuous basal infusions can lead to more serious adverse events because the opioid medication is delivered regardless of the child's level of sedation.[420,421] These concerns highlight the need for strict attention to detail when ordering a continuous basal infusion for pediatric patients as well as superb communication with nursing staff and appropriate monitoring modalities.

Continuous basal infusions may have limited efficacy and are associated with a greater incidence of adverse opioid effects, including respiratory depression.[422–424] Studies in children, however, have yielded conflicting results.[405,406,422,424–429] Children 7 to 19 years of age who received PCA with a continuous basal infusion after orthopedic surgery reported better pain scores compared with those who received PCA boluses alone or IM morphine.[406] There were no differences in morphine consumption or in opioid adverse effects among the three groups, with no incidents of respiratory depression. Notably, child satisfaction was greatest in the PCA with the continuous basal infusion group. Similar pain scores with improved sleeping patterns have also been reported with the use of PCA with a continuous basal infusion, compared with those who received PCA alone, on the first two postoperative nights in children after abdominal surgery. No incidents of respiratory depression or excessive sedation were reported in either group.[405] Children who received a continuous basal infusion with PCA or nurse-controlled analgesia in one study had slightly reduced pain scores without differences in morphine use or adverse effects after spine fusion surgery compared with those who received PCA or nurse-controlled analgesia alone.[429] In contrast, others have reported greater morphine use and a greater incidence of hypoxemia with similar pain scores in children who received PCA plus a continuous basal infusion after surgery compared with those who received PCA alone.[426,428] A subsequent study found that children who received PCA with a continuous basal infusion of low-dose morphine (4 μg/kg per hour) experienced fewer adverse effects and less hypoxemia than children who received PCA with higher dose continuous basal infusion (10 to 20 μg/kg per hour) or those who received PCA bolus doses alone, noting similar pain scores in all three groups.[427] Both of the PCA with continuous basal infusion groups reported better sleep at night than did the PCA alone group.

A meta-analysis of data from the previously mentioned studies found no difference in pain scores or opioid consumption between children who received a continuous basal infusion and those who received a bolus-only PCA. Improved sleep quality was reported in three of the four studies that examined this outcome. Although there was a 4.6% incidence of excessive sedation (a marker of respiratory depression risk) in the continuous basal infusion groups as opposed to none in the bolus-only group, this difference was not statistically significant. Overall, the pooled studies had significant heterogeneity and small sample sizes (and thus lower-quality evidence). Therefore, the authors concluded that further large-scale randomized trials are necessary.[418]

Based on these studies and our own experience, we hold the view that continuous basal infusions may benefit some children, although it requires careful selection of dose, based on the surgical severity and the child's comorbid conditions, and vigilant monitoring to ensure safety. A continuous basal infusion should be used as a routine for most children with pain resulting from cancer, for most children with mucositis resulting from cancer treatment or bone marrow transplantation, and for a large number of children with sickle cell vasoocclusive episodes. A sensible compromise may be to use a continuous basal infusion at night with the goal of improved sleep quality and allow patients to self-regulate during daytime hours.[428] At our institutions, the standard practice is to use continuous basal infusions, unless limited by somnolence or hypoventilation, for the first night in most children after selected major painful surgeries, such as scoliosis surgery, pelvic osteotomies, and thoracotomies, unless concomitant regional analgesia techniques or other protocols involving long-acting opioids (e.g., methadone) are used.

Nurse-/Caregiver-Controlled Analgesia

Activation of the PCA pump by the bedside nurse, a parent, or a guardian (such as a grandparent) has been used with success in children who are unable to push the button because of young age or because of physical or cognitive impairments.[106,407,408,418,429,430] In much of the literature, and in some policy statements by the Joint Commission and other organizations, there is, in our view, too little distinction between activation of PCA pumps by nurses and activation by nonclinician surrogates. The term *caregiver* is used variably in this literature; here it is used to mean nonclinician surrogates. In pediatrics, this means primarily parents or other family members.

A small study of 12 children who received nurse-controlled analgesia after spine fusion surgery reported adequate analgesia, parent and nurse satisfaction, and no complications.[429] Children who received nurse-controlled analgesia received smaller total morphine doses compared with those who could use the PCA device themselves, likely because of the tendency for nurses to underestimate their patients' pain. A larger observational study of 212 children who received parent- or nurse-controlled analgesia with morphine, fentanyl, or hydromorphone reported effective analgesia (observational pain scores 3/10 or 2/5 or below) in more than 80% of children.[408] Pruritus occurred in 8% and vomiting in 15% of the children on the first day of treatment. 9 children (4.2%) required naloxone for: apnea (n = 4), hypoxemia (n = 1), excessive sedation (n = 3), or to facilitate extubation (n = 1). Six of these children had major comorbid conditions, and five received additional sedatives. These investigators emphasized the importance of close monitoring to minimize risk and permit early intervention when using nurse-/caregiver-controlled analgesia (nurse-controlled analgesia/CCA).

Another study found that the incidence of overall adverse events in opioid-naive children who received nurse-controlled analgesia was similar to that in children who received PCA after surgery (22% and 24%, respectively).[106] However, children who were able to self-administer PCA required only minor interventions (stimulation, reduction in opioid dosage, or supplemental oxygen), whereas those who received nurse-controlled analgesia were more likely to require more aggressive interventions, such as opioid reversal, airway management, or escalation of care. They found that cognitive impairment and opioid dose on the first postoperative day independently predicted adverse events. Although the mean time to the occurrence of adverse events was 16 to 27 hours, some events occurred during the third postoperative day, suggesting that monitoring, including continuous pulse oximetry, should be continued as long as the PCA is used and highlights two risk factors: the possibility of drug accumulation when context-sensitive half-life is not considered, and the possibility of decreasing opioid requirements as recovery proceeds. In a study of

children with cancer, five respiratory and/or neurologic serious adverse effects were reported, with one child requiring naloxone during the 576 days of treatment with nurse-controlled analgesia/caregiver-controlled analgesia.[430] In that study, pulse oximetry was used only at the discretion of the clinician, perhaps reducing the investigator's ability to recognize hypoxemia in some children. Furthermore, the reduced incidence of adverse events may be explained by the fact that most children in that study were not opioid naive and may have developed some degree of opioid tolerance.

A study of 10,000 pediatric patients who received nurse-controlled analgesia further confirms the safety and tolerability of this delivery method.[139] For infants younger than 1 year of age, few studies have examined the role of nurse-controlled analgesia. In one study of almost 800 infants, nurse-controlled analgesia with fentanyl, morphine, or hydromorphone all provided similar analgesia, although rapid response team calls (total of 39) were significantly more frequently associated with morphine than with fentanyl use.[431] Only one rapid response call was for apnea.

For safety reasons, however, it is important to distinguish between authorized and unauthorized use of the PCA button by an individual other than the child. Several reports describe serious adverse events, including excessive sedation, severe respiratory depression, respiratory arrest, and death, attributed to unauthorized activation of the PCA device by parents, spouses, other family members, and health care providers.[106,139,431–435] The practice of PCA by proxy has come under scrutiny and its safety questioned by the Joint Commission and the Institute for Safe Medication Practices (ISMP).[436–438] In 2004, the Joint Commission issued a sentinel event alert based on PCA errors reported to the US Pharmacopeia. Of 460 errors that resulted in death or some level of harm to the patient, 15 resulted from PCA by proxy, including 12 attributed to family members, 2 to a nurse, and 1 to a pharmacist.[436] In interpreting this report and other reports, it should be emphasized that most do not cite denominator data (total numbers of patients receiving PCA vs. nurse-controlled analgesia/caregiver-controlled analgesia), so the relative or absolute risks of these techniques is unknown. Recognition of these risks has led the Joint Commission and ISMP to strongly recommend that specific policies and procedures be developed and implemented related to the use of PCA by individuals other than the child. Such policies must address the following issues:

- Appropriate selection of children. Many pediatric centers restrict parent-controlled analgesia to children with chronic pain, those who require palliative care, and in special circumstances for children who undergo repeated and extensive surgery. In pediatric centers worldwide, nurse-controlled analgesia is increasingly being used, with appropriate observation, for both opioid-naive and opioid-tolerant children.
- The specific process of identifying suitable caregivers who will be allowed to activate the PCA button.
- Communication among clinicians, including the primary service physician, the pain service team, and the primary bedside nurse, regarding the suitability of caregiver-controlled analgesia.
- An educational plan for clinicians involved in the decision making.
- Education of caregivers, including pain assessment, recognition of opioid adverse effects, and scenarios when not to activate the PCA button (e.g., when the child is asleep or somnolent). The caregiver should be encouraged to call the nursing staff when in doubt.

■ Monitoring protocols, including assessment of sedation depth, respiratory status, and pain assessment at regular intervals. It must be emphasized that the primary responsibility for monitoring the safety and effectiveness of analgesia remains with the nursing staff. Electronic monitoring, including pulse oximetry, is widely used in this setting.

With carefully defined policies and procedures, adequate education of clinicians and caregivers, prevention of unauthorized dosing, and vigilant monitoring, it may be possible to reduce the frequency of adverse events from PCA, nurse-controlled analgesia, and, especially, caregiver-controlled analgesia. However, large outcomes studies are needed after implementation of such policies to confirm the safety and efficacy of practice based on these recommendations. Our view is that proxy-administered PCA by properly trained caregivers is a well-established practice and should be encouraged as a generally safe and effective means for delivering opioids to children who are unable to self-administer.

Risks and Adverse Events With Patient-Controlled Analgesia

Despite its numerous benefits, the use of PCA has been associated with a wide range of adverse effects, adverse events, and unfavorable outcomes in adults.[410,411,433,439–442] Although some adverse effects from PCA therapy may be attributed to the opioid drugs themselves or to patient comorbidities, a significant number of harmful effects occur as a result of human error, with incorrect prescribing, dispensing, administration, or equipment failure. E-Table 41.5 describes the causes of PCA medication errors as identified by the ISMP.[437,438,440,443] Increasing awareness of preventable adverse events from PCA has led to improved pump technology directed at minimizing the likelihood of programming errors, including integrated drug libraries and the development of smart PCA pumps that use bar-coded syringes and an integral bar-code reader to prevent incorrect programming of drug concentration. Potential PCA pump errors have been reduced with "smart pumps."[444] Children are at greater risk for medication-related adverse events resulting from calculation errors in drug doses (because all doses are based on body weight or body surface area) and to developmental differences in PK.[414] However, data for PCA-related adverse events in children are limited.[412,445–447] The reported incidence of respiratory depression in children receiving PCA ranges from 0% to 25%.[106,445,446,448,449] Risk factors for respiratory depression identified by these studies include cumulative opioid dose, use of basal infusions, concomitant administration of sedatives, and comorbid conditions, including renal failure and cognitive impairment. Recognition of the risks from PCA[450,451] has led organizations, such as the ISMP, to emphasize the importance of monitoring children who use PCA and of the need for detailed child and staff education regarding its use.[452]

Monitoring the Child Using Patient-Controlled Analgesia

Despite the recommendation from the ISMP that practitioners should identify children at risk for opioid-related respiratory depression and define the appropriate level of monitoring, there remains no consensus regarding the risk/benefit ratio and effectiveness of any specific forms of monitoring for children receiving PCA, nurse-controlled analgesia, or caregiver-controlled analgesia. No monitor in widespread use today detects respiratory depression in all circumstances, so nursing staff are the frontline personnel for detection. Extensive nursing education and standard monitoring protocols are essential to the safe use of PCA (especially with a continuous basal infusion).

The Anesthesia Patient Safety Foundation (APSF) recommended the use of continuous respiratory monitoring (minimally pulse oximetry and a continuous measure of respiratory rate) for children receiving PCA, neuraxial, or serial doses of parenteral opioids.[453] Additionally, the Anesthesia Patient Safety Foundation recommended that reliable alerting methods, such as audible alarms, central stations, or pagers, be implemented to ensure timely and appropriate clinician response to deteriorating respiratory status of those receiving opioid therapy. The impact of implementing such technology on the incidence of PCA-related adverse events requires investigation. *It must be emphasized that pulse oximetry can detect hypoventilation only if the child is breathing room air.*[454] Oximetry is *not* a measure of ventilation but rather of oxygenation. The use of supplemental oxygen interferes with the ability of pulse oximetry to detect respiratory depression by delaying the onset of desaturation.[454,455] Any patient who requires supplemental oxygen while using a PCA should have additional measures in place to detect hypoventilation. Additionally, respiratory monitoring that uses impedance changes across electrocardiogram leads to detect chest wall movement will not detect partial upper airway obstruction and does not ensure that ventilation is adequate as it only measures ventilatory effort and not effective gas exchange.

Side stream sampling of end-tidal carbon dioxide ($ETCO_2$) via a nasal cannula or noninvasive capnography detects respiratory depression earlier and more frequently than does pulse oximetry or periodic checks of respiratory rate in adults who are receiving opioids via PCA, or for procedural sedation/analgesia.[456,457] A systematic review and metanalysis of adult postsurgical patients revealed a 6-fold greater odds-ratio for detecting respiratory depression with capnography compared with pulse oximetry use (11.5% vs. 2.8%).[458] Although similar data for children receiving PCA therapy are not available, studies in children undergoing procedural sedation in the emergency department and ICU have reported that capnography detected respiratory events that would not have been recognized as quickly if using pulse oximetry, periodic respiratory rate monitoring, and/or clinical examination.[459–462] Thus capnography or an alternate monitor that is capable of measuring the respiratory rate may provide the earliest warning of impending respiratory compromise and may alert clinicians to carefully evaluate the children under their care and adjust opioid doses accordingly. Conversely, in real-world practice, capnography cannulas can be difficult to maintain in proper position in children on a busy postoperative ward, readings can be influenced by mouth breathing, with the potential for false-positive and false-negative conclusions.[463] Nasal canulae may not be tolerated by children due to age-related or developmental factors.

Acoustic impedance (usually on the neck) is better tolerated than nasal capnography by children,[464] and has the advantage over chest wall impedance of detecting upper airway obstruction. However, it is not 100% sensitive, and episodes of oxygen desaturation are not always correlated to a low respiratory rate.[465]

Newer technology incorporates a fully integrated PCA system with modules for continuous monitoring of oxygen saturation and $ETCO_2$.[458,463,466,467] Some of these pumps also have a feature that shuts off PCA delivery if preset threshold parameters for oxygen saturation and $ETCO_2$ are reached. Studies evaluating the benefits of such technology in reducing PCA-related adverse events in children are needed. Although electronic monitoring has an important role in patient safety, all currently available methods are imperfect and it is likely that any technology can only augment, not supplant, vigilance by a skilled nurse. Moreover, they generate frequent false alarms that annoy children and families, disturb the restorative sleep of both children and parents, and contribute to desensitization of nurses' vigilance. Despite these limitations of electronic monitoring, it has been reported that the use of computerized physician order entry and involvement of dedicated pediatric pain teams improved compliance with routine monitoring and increased the likelihood of early identification of adverse events.[468]

REGIONAL BLOCKADE AND ANALGESIA

The use of local anesthetics for neuraxial and peripheral regional anesthesia, both with and without the addition of adjunct medications, offers many advantages for postoperative analgesia. The exploration of new regional anesthetic approaches, including head and neck blocks, and fascial plane blocks, has rapidly expanded within pediatric anesthesiology. Blockade with long-acting local anesthetic or continuous peripheral nerve blockade with infusion of local anesthetic via catheters and elastomeric infusion pumps can provide postoperative analgesia for outpatient surgery such that a child can be discharged home in comfort. Reducing or eliminating the need for systemic analgesics diminishes the potential for side effects or adverse events associated with their use. Relevant to pediatric anesthesiology, regional blockade affords the ability to provide excellent analgesia to children who might otherwise not tolerate large doses of opioids. This group includes neonates, especially preterm and former preterm infants who are at risk for apnea; children with problems of central ventilatory control, respiratory disease, or precarious airways; or those who risk obstruction with sedation (e.g., children with obstructive sleep apnea). Epidural analgesia that covers thoracic dermatomes improves resolution of ileus and return to normal feeding after major abdominal surgery.[469,470] This section will provide a brief overview of recent advances and information specific to pediatric regional anesthesiology as it relates to the practice of acute pain (see Chapter 40).

There are few absolute contraindications to regional blockade. Anatomic anomalies, such as myelodysplasia, sacral dysgenesis, and other abnormalities, either disrupting the epidural space or making access to it impossible, may prevent the performance of a caudal or epidural block. A report of epidural analgesia in children with myelodysplasia, however, suggests that catheters may be used safely in these children when placed at a level above the anatomic neural abnormality.[471] In cases involving these types of anatomic anomalies, we encourage consultation with experts in pediatric regional anesthesia, prior review of imaging studies, and consideration of fluoroscopic guidance. Active infection at or near the site of injection is a contraindication to block placement. Children with burn injuries may be candidates for continuous regional techniques, provided the burned area is distant from the catheter insertion site (see Chapter 34).[472,473]

Sepsis or bacteremia presents a similar problem. In general, it is not advisable to place caudal or epidural catheters in children with sepsis for fear of seeding the epidural space during a period of bacteremia. Peripheral nerve, plexus, or fascial plane catheters may pose less of a problem in this regard, but there are no data to provide guidance regarding this issue. Coagulopathy and thrombocytopenia are relative contraindications to regional anesthesia, with mild abnormalities in hemostasis not necessarily precluding a regional block. Peripheral or truncal fascial plane block types can be subdivided into "superficial" versus "deep" blocks with deep blocks theoretically having a higher risk of

complications if bleeding were to occur, although no data exist to confirm this hypothesis. When considering the risk of hematoma, it is safer to place a catheter in a site that can be compressed (e.g., femoral) as opposed to a site that cannot (e.g., epidural, paravertebral). In unusual cases, and with proper consideration of risk/benefit issues, fresh frozen plasma, cryoprecipitate, or platelets can be infused at the time of a regional procedure to provide temporary correction of coagulopathy. The considerations regarding regional anesthesia, coagulopathy, and anticoagulation are complex and have been reviewed extensively for adults and children by consensus groups from the American and European Societies of Regional Anesthesia.[474–476] We recommend that clinicians review these adult and pediatric publications for guidance in how to manage these special populations.[477] When placing a catheter for continuous blockade, consideration of the state of coagulation must include the time of catheter withdrawal as well as placement.

There is no consensus on the timing of a regional block (at the beginning or end of the surgical procedure). Placing a single-injection caudal block before incision confers a similar duration of postoperative analgesia, after a surgical procedure of 1 hour or less, as placing it at the end of surgery. For example, the times from recovery until the first request for analgesics after caudal blocks placed before incision or after surgery for inguinal herniorrhaphy were similar.[478] For more prolonged procedures, the block may be renewed with a second caudal injection before emergence or a catheter placed and repeat dose at appropriate intervals (usually approximately 1.5 hours). A volume of half of the original dose is usually sufficient if less than 2 hours have elapsed. A reduced concentration of local anesthetic is usually effective for postoperative analgesia. Adjunctive additives, such as clonidine, have also been shown in some studies to prolong the action of "single-shot" central neuraxis and some peripheral blocks (see later discussion), permitting a single-injection block placed before the incision to augment both intraoperative and postoperative analgesia for longer operations. In cases of major surgery on the extremities and shoulders, placement of indwelling plexus or peripheral nerve catheters can be considered for local anesthetic infusions for several days.[479–484] An audit of the Pediatric Regional Anesthesia Network database of 2074 peripheral catheter blocks ranging from 1 to 7 days of placement found an overall complication rate of ~12%.[485] There were no serious infections, persistent neurologic issues, or patients with systemic local anesthetic toxicity; complications in children were similar to that reported in adults. Infections were correlated to duration of insertion. Many pediatric specialty centers send select patients home with peripheral nerve block catheters and elastomeric pain pumps for prolonged analgesia for between 2 and 5 days.[480,486,487]

Evidence suggests that placing a regional block at the beginning of surgery may offer several potential advantages.[488,489] Although preemptive or preventive analgesia is a reproducible phenomenon in laboratory studies, the results in humans have been conflicting.[490] For example, initial studies in adults demonstrated a dramatic decrease in the incidence of phantom limb pain when an epidural block was administered before an amputation, although subsequent studies did not consistently reaffirm the initial observations.[491–494] Similarly, children who receive intraoperative neural blockade may experience less postoperative pain than those managed with general anesthesia alone, with the duration of analgesia in some cases lasting beyond the pharmacologic action of the block. On the other hand, a blinded study of postoperative analgesia in children who received a caudal block either before or after circumcision or inguinal hernia repair reported similar levels of analgesia with both.[478,495]

It is theorized that interruption of nociceptive impulses at the spinal cord level attenuates imprinting of painful stimuli on the sensory cortex or forestalls the development of spinal cord hyperexcitability and "wind-up," thereby reducing the neural input and persistent postoperative pain.[493,496–499] It has also become increasingly evident, however, that if preemptive or preventive analgesia is to have a beneficial effect, other conditions must be met: the block must be of sufficient duration in relation to the nociceptive stimulus, it must extend into the postoperative period, and it must be effective at preventing central transmission of the nociceptive signals.[488] This third requirement suggests that a multimodal analgesic approach may offer the greatest benefit. The presence of poorly controlled preoperative pain may sensitize the CNS, rendering pain difficult to control via intraoperative or postoperative interventions because hyperexcitability and wind-up have already occurred.[500,501] Additionally, epidural opioids have been shown to reduce the inflammatory response after surgery in adults, as indicated by interleukin-2 concentrations, suggesting that attenuating the stress response to surgery may improve postoperative analgesia.[502]

Further evidence suggests that local anesthetic infiltration of the incision site, especially when performed in conjunction with a regional anesthetic technique, may be an effective means of providing prolonged analgesia after surgery.[503,504] This simple and effective approach can be used before or at the end of virtually any surgical procedure.

Peripheral nerve and plexus blocks tend to provide blocks of greater duration than do central neuraxial blocks, the former lasting 8 to 12 hours, and on occasion exceeding 24 hours. Depending on the nature of the surgery, this may permit the child to transition to nonopioid analgesics at the time the block wears off, thereby eliminating or reducing the use of opioids and their potential untoward effects. Children undergoing outpatient surgery may be discharged after a single-injection regional block, but follow-up the next day with the family is necessary to ensure that the block has receded, and no complications have developed. This is especially the case after peripheral nerve blocks. Parents must further be cautioned that there may be some degree of motor blockade present, and that the blocked limb must be protected from injury. If a lower extremity is blocked, assistance with ambulation is mandatory.

Choice of Local Anesthetics, Additives, and Dosing

Dilute long-acting local anesthetics, such as bupivacaine 0.125% to 0.25% or ropivacaine 0.1% to 0.2%, are the most commonly used local anesthetics for regional blockade. Epinephrine (1 : 200,000 to 1 : 400,000) is often added to bupivacaine to decrease systemic absorption and increase duration of action, although *caution is advised when a digital or penile block is performed, because of the theoretic risk of inducing ischemia by direct vasoconstriction.*[505–508] These concerns are historical and relate to preparations with larger epinephrine concentrations (e.g., 1/80,000); however, there is probably little advantage to adding epinephrine to the local anesthetic in continuous infusions, since prolonging the block effect is not a consideration. Further, ropivacaine has inherent vasoconstrictive properties, rendering any additional benefits from adding epinephrine to the solution moot.

Initial studies concluded that the optimal concentration of bupivacaine that provides maximum sensory blockade without motor blockade for caudal analgesia was 0.125%,[509] although subsequent studies demonstrated that the optimal concentration was actually 0.175% (7 mL of 0.25% bupivacaine combined with 3 mL of saline solution).[510] More concentrated solutions of bupivacaine (0.2% to 0.25%) may be used for blocks that do not significantly affect motor function, such as for an ilioinguinal-iliohypogastric nerve block after herniorrhaphy or in infants whose ability to stand or walk is not a prerequisite for discharge from the hospital or ambulatory surgery after a caudal or epidural block.

Block duration correlates most closely with total local anesthetic dose. The use of a greater concentration such as 0.5%, as is common in adult practice, will produce a block with a duration that is 40% greater than that with an equal volume of 0.25%.[511] This will, of course, increase the incidence of motor blockade. Supraclavicular brachial plexus block using a combination of perineural 0.5% ropivacaine and dexamethasone or IV dexamethasone produces a block with an average duration of 25 hours, ensuring a first postoperative night with an excellent analgesia.[512] Pediatric peripheral nerve blockade can be extended with the addition of α_2-adrenoreceptor agonists (9.75 vs. 3.75 hours) although α_2-adrenoreceptor agonists are not FDA approved for use in the neural canal in the United States.[513]

Ropivacaine, an *l*-enantiomer amide local anesthetic, is widely used in children, particularly in neonates and infants.[514,515] In both pediatric and adult studies, the duration of analgesia after ropivacaine is similar to that after bupivacaine, although motor block occurs more frequently with bupivacaine.[516] Ropivacaine is less cardiotoxic than bupivacaine, but it is also less potent in adult studies than bupivacaine,[517] although similar results are obtained with larger doses of ropivacaine.[518] Ropivacaine causes less motor blockade than bupivacaine, an effect that has been attributed to the reduced lipophilicity of the former, thus reducing its penetration into large motor fibers. Similarly, ropivacaine causes less cardiac toxicity than bupivacaine possibly also due to its reduced lipophilicity.[519] The toxic thresholds for both CNS and cardiovascular toxicity based on animal studies are 20% to 30% greater with ropivacaine in both adults and infants, although seizures can still occur with ropivacaine if the dose exceeds the toxic threshold.[520] Although the recommended dose limits are similar for ropivacaine and bupivacaine (2.5 mg/kg bolus, 0.4–0.5 mg/kg per hour infusion), PK modeling suggests that larger doses of ropivacaine are likely safe.[521]

Some authors recommend using a levorotatory enantiomer (levo-enantiomer), such as ropivacaine, in preference to the racemic mixture, bupivacaine, in infants younger than 6 months of age because of the potential increased margin of safety.[520,522] Another option for continuous infusion is chloroprocaine, which undergoes rapid ester metabolism in the bloodstream, and thus has a small risk of toxicity. Because of chloroprocaine's favorable therapeutic margin in infants, larger volumes can be infused to achieve adequate spread of blockade, an important consideration with epidural analgesia after extensive intraabdominal or intrathoracic operations.[523–525]

In the quest for a longer-acting local anesthetic and prolonged analgesia, the development of a suspension of biodegradable polymer microspheres or lipospheres that contain bupivacaine has been approved for local wound infiltration in patients 6 years and older, and interscalene nerve block in adults. After injection, these microspheres release bupivacaine in a controlled manner for periods of 2 to 6 days, depending on dose, formulation, and site of injection.[526–529] Despite considerable initial enthusiasm in adults, the clinical utility of this formula has produced mixed results in the literature and has not definitively been proven to provide extended analgesia[530] in adults compared with conventional bupivacaine.[531–533] A systematic review of 27 prospective randomized studies in adults undergoing orthopedic procedures reported inconsistent prolonged pain relief or reduction in opioid use. The authors concluded that there was no support for the routine use of liposomal bupivacaine compared with other local anesthetics.[534] Another review of 76 adult trials that compared liposomal bupivacaine with plain bupivacaine concluded that *"the preponderance of evidence fails to support the routine use of liposomal bupivacaine over standard local anesthetics."*[535]

In 2021, the FDA approved bupivacaine liposome injectable suspension for wound infiltration for pediatric surgical patients ages 6 years old and above but it has not been approved for specific peripheral nerve blocks in children. A multicenter study evaluated the PK of liposomal bupivacaine (2 or 4 mg/kg) via local infiltration in 95 children (6 to <17 years of age) undergoing spine or cardiac surgical procedures and concluded that the plasma concentrations remained below the toxic threshold; peak blood levels were ~1.5 times higher in the bupivacaine groups compared with the liposomal bupivacaine groups.[536]

Although the pediatric data are evolving, there are no high-quality direct comparisons of liposomal bupivacaine versus conventional bupivacaine in children. One study failed to show any difference in pain scores or opioid consumption in pediatric patients undergoing posterior spinal fusion when surgical wound infiltration with liposomal bupivacaine was compared with a multimodal analgesic regimen.[529] Another study of pediatric spine surgery patients compared 47 children who received liposomal bupivacaine and 94 children who did not receive this formulation in a nonrandomized matched cohort study; there was no associated reduction in postoperative opioid use.[537] Plasma bupivacaine concentrations were consistently below the toxic threshold with a wound infiltration dose of liposomal bupivacaine of ≤4 mg/kg in children between the ages of 6 months and 17 years undergoing posterior spinal fusion or cardiac surgery.[532] At present, we cannot advocate the use of liposomal bupivacaine in children given the lack of evidence of analgesic benefit beyond conventional bupivacaine as well as the increased cost relative to conventional bupivacaine. Further large-scale comparison data are needed.[530,531,533]

Additives and Adjuvants

Opioids have been injected in the epidural and intrathecal spaces for analgesia in children, both with and without local anesthetics. Central neuraxial opioids have been used for more than 2 decades to produce effective analgesia in children. However, opioids administered into the central neuraxis have the potential to cause delayed respiratory depression and are generally avoided in the outpatient setting to ensure the safety of children after discharge (see further).[538] Neuraxial and intrathecal opioids are also associated with pruritus and urinary retention at fairly high rates, which can prove rather bothersome to some.

Adjuvant drugs have been added to the local anesthetic administered for caudal blockade to prolong the duration of the sensory block, an obviously desirable attribute for a single-injection block. However, their use is not without controversy. Many drugs have been injected into the epidural space with only limited laboratory evidence for safety and lack of neurotoxicity; therefore, some caution is necessary.[539,540] Clonidine, 0.5 to 2 µg/kg, has been shown to lack evidence of neurotoxicity.[540] It increases the duration of analgesia after bupivacaine in caudal blocks by approximately

3 hours, with insignificant hemodynamic effects, mild sedation, and no delay in recovery times.[273,541–546] A metanalysis of 15 randomized controlled pediatric caudal block trials reported that clonidine, when combined with other anesthetics, had equal efficacy as other additives but with fewer complications. However, the details of the other adjuvants (opioids, dexmedetomidine, epinephrine, midazolam, ketamine, and neostigmine) and what they defined as a complication were poorly described.[547] Despite these reported beneficial effects of clonidine, several studies have questioned the increased duration of the caudal block. A double-blind investigation of IV and caudally administered clonidine, 2 µg/kg, as an adjunct to caudal blocks with bupivacaine yielded no differences the duration of analgesia.[269] Another study compared 1, 2, or 3 µg/kg in 0.165% bupivacaine with a similar concentration of plain bupivacaine in 80 children undergoing hypospadias repair and reported no difference in morphine consumption among the four groups.[548] A study comparing caudal blockade with plain bupivacaine, bupivacaine with clonidine (2 µg/kg) and plain bupivacaine co-administered with IV clonidine (2 µg/kg) detected no difference in analgesic duration between the caudal and systemic clonidine administration.[549] In contrast, when clonidine was administered caudally with levobupivacaine, the need for rescue analgesia was delayed and pain scores were reduced compared with those who received IV clonidine, suggesting the prolonged analgesia occurred at a spinal cord site of action[272,274,545] and/or that absorption of amide local anesthetics from the caudal space is delayed when combined with clonidine.[550] Caudal clonidine produces less nausea, itching, ileus, and urinary retention than opioid additives, although it may increase postoperative somnolence or respiratory depression at doses in excess of 1 µg/kg, particularly in the neonate.[271,545,551,552] The clearance of clonidine in infants is approximately one-third that of older children.[271,553] The preponderance of evidence[275,547] supports the use of clonidine to prolong the analgesic effect of central neuraxial blocks, but we caution against the use of more than 1 µg/kg for outpatient procedures, especially in younger infants, because of an increased risk of respiratory depression.

The clinical use of adjuvant caudal dexmedetomidine 1 µg/kg, another α_2-adrenoreceptor agonist, is increasing. However, it has not been clearly established if dexmedetomidine lacks toxicity on the myelin sheath.[553,554] Sensory block duration is reported to increase by 8.21 hours (95% confidence interval 5.02, 11.40 hours).[288] Perineural dexmedetomidine significantly prolongs block duration and is associated with faster onset of sensory blockade compared with IV dexmedetomidine.[288] Dexmedetomidine has been studied in both perineural and systemic administration with results similar to clonidine. For caudal block, both perineural and IV dexmedetomidine (0.5 mg/kg) provide improved quality and duration of analgesia. A systematic review of 13 trials involving almost 800 children reported that the addition of dexmedetomidine (1–2 µg/kg) to caudal bupivacaine prolonged postoperative analgesia compared with plain bupivacaine, reduced intraoperative sevoflurane requirements and provided prolonged postoperative sedation.[555] A review of 21 pediatric publications reported that dexmedetomidine (1–2 µg/kg) added to caudal local anesthetics provided postoperative analgesia for a greater duration than either 1 µg/kg of fentanyl or 30 µg/kg of morphine used as adjuncts to caudal local anesthetics, and a 2- to 3-fold greater duration than local anesthetics without adjuncts; there was no difference between clonidine or dexamethasone as adjuncts.[556] In a randomized study of 60 children, the duration of ilioinguinal-iliohypogastric blockade with ropivacaine (0.2%) used with dexmedetomidine (1 µg/kg) was double that of plain ropivacaine (970 ± 47 vs. 419 ± 61 minutes).[557] A review of eight pediatric randomized trials found significant prolongation of analgesia for up to 8 hours postoperatively.[558] Adult data in some studies show equivalence between perineural and IV dexmedetomidine,[512] although a systematic review of 10 adult studies reported perineural dexmedetomidine provided analgesia of greater duration and faster onset than with IV dexmedetomidine.[286] There is increased potential for neurotoxicity with any adjuvant compared with local anesthetic alone. In most cases data are lacking regarding potential neuronal injury when drugs approved for intravenous administration are applied directly to nerve tissues; using IV rather than adding unapproved agents to the local anesthetic to prolong blockade is likely the safest approach until adequate safety data regarding the drugs and their preservatives[559] are performed.[560,561]

When performing a regional block, the total safe dose of local anesthetic should be calculated first and the volume and concentration of the solution adjusted if necessary to avoid administering a toxic dose. Most peripheral blocks can be performed with 0.2 to 0.3 mL/kg of local anesthetic, but single-injection caudal blocks require 0.75 to 1.25 mL/kg. Since a larger volume equates to a greater risk of administering a toxic dose, more dilute concentrations should be used. This is particularly important when performing blocks in infants. For example, a 7-kilogram infant has a maximal allowable dose of 17.5 mg of bupivacaine (or 2.5 mg/kg). If a 0.25% solution (2.5 mg/mL) were administered, the total volume would be limited to 7 mL. The maximum dose should probably be slightly more restrictive in infants younger than 6 months of age. At this age, a cautious approach is to further reduce the allowable dose by 25% to 30%, particularly if an infusion is to be used following the initial bolus. For example, a 4-kilogram, 2-month-old infant would be permitted to receive 2.7 mL (6.6 mg) of the same solution. A simple rule of thumb for calculating the maximum bolus dose of bupivacaine and ropivacaine in children older than 6 months is 1 mL/kg of 0.25% or 0.5 mL/kg of a 0.5% solution. For most circumstances, there is little benefit in using a 0.5% concentration. Use of different concentrations increases the odds of a dose calculation error. To prevent this type of error, some hospitals have standardized dosing for infiltration and boluses to a single concentration, namely, 0.2% for ropivacaine or 0.25% for bupivacaine. It is also important to keep in mind that the success of some regional anesthetic techniques, particularly fascial plane blocks (e.g., transversus abdominis plane block), requires higher volumes to ensure adequate spread over the targeted sensory nerves. Careful attention to local anesthetic concentration and total dose must be considered in these situations, and toxicity considerations may limit the use of some blocks that require large volumes, particularly in younger children and when bilateral approaches are considered.

Choice of Regional Anesthetic Approach

Single-Injection Techniques

There are many circumstances in which the simplicity and duration of action of a single-injection block is desirable. The caudal block remains the most common technique in pediatric regional anesthesia. It provides analgesia of the lower extremity and lower abdomen and is easily and rapidly performed in most infants and children (see Chapter 40). When an operation is performed on both legs, caudal injection or bilateral lower extremity blocks can be considered.

With advances in ultrasound technology and nerve block techniques, the use of ultrasound is arguably the gold standard for identification of plexuses and peripheral nerves in an anesthetized child. Despite this, nerve stimulation techniques still likely play a role in optimizing the safety and efficacy of nerve blocks, especially when utilized concurrently with ultrasound guidance.[562] Nerve stimulation techniques should continue to be taught to anesthesiology residents. To precisely position the needle in the target area and avoid piercing adjacent structures, one must develop skill in coordinating its trajectory with the ultrasound image so that the needle tip does not pass out of the plane of view. Although it remains unknown whether ultrasound and more precise needle placement will reduce nerve injury, there is evidence that it reduces the volume of local anesthetic needed to produce an effective block and preinjection visualization aids in more precise drug administration.[563–566] Ultrasound visualization of the local anesthetic surrounding a nerve or plexus provides reliable confirmation that a block will be successful. Nerve blocks of the lower extremity can often be used instead of caudal blockade (see Chapter 40). The primary disadvantage is that multiple blocks (i.e., femoral and sciatic) are needed to cover the entire extremity. They provide a field of analgesia limited to the operative site, but they have a prolonged duration of analgesia (usually at least twice that of caudal block) and eliminate some of the potential undesirable effects of central neuraxis blockade, such as urinary retention (and need for a urinary catheter) or unintentional unilateral blockade (of the nonoperative leg). Blockade of the femoral nerve, the sciatic nerve, and the nerves of the ankle is easily performed in children by using similar techniques to those in adults (see Chapter 40). Regional blockade of the upper extremity may involve an interscalene, supraclavicular, infraclavicular, or axillary block, or less commonly, blockade of the individual nerves at the level of the arm or wrist. Unlike the lower extremity, a single block of the brachial plexus can provide anesthesia to the entire extremity. Paravertebral blocks may be used in lieu of an epidural after thoracic or upper abdominal surgery. This block may be considered for procedures of limited scope, such as open-lung biopsy or thoracostomy for drainage, but the duration of blockade is limited to several hours. Placement of paravertebral catheters for continuous infusion can provide longer duration of analgesia for thoracic and upper abdominal surgery.[567–571] For open-chest procedures, intercostal blocks by the surgeon pose a low risk and may be indicated, although their effectiveness is limited by their short duration. Epinephrine is commonly included in the local anesthetic for these blocks to limit the rate of uptake. More extensive surgery anticipated to cause postoperative pain of longer duration may be best managed with a catheter continuous infusion technique.

An ilioinguinal-iliohypogastric nerve block provides excellent postoperative analgesia for inguinal herniorrhaphy, a common outpatient procedure in children (see Chapter 40). It appears similar in efficacy to a caudal block, with a duration of analgesia of at least 4 hours when bupivacaine with epinephrine is used. For orchiopexy, an ilioinguinal nerve block has been found to be as effective as caudal blockade to the T10 level in a randomized and blinded investigation.[572] In our experience, however, postoperative analgesia for procedures that involve considerable manipulation and traction on the spermatic cord and testis may be better managed with caudal blockade in younger children. Penile block is effective for both circumcision and distal, simple hypospadias repair. More extensive procedures on the penis, especially repair of penile-scrotal hypospadias, require a caudal or pudendal block, rather than a penile block, to produce effective analgesia.[573-576] Some concerns have been raised regarding an association between caudal block and postoperative wound healing complications in pediatric patients that have undergone hypospadias repair surgery,[577] but the literature is conflicting with mostly low-quality, retrospective data[578]; one literature review found no association with postoperative complications and caudal blocks.[579] Bilateral pudendal nerve blocks are likely superior to caudal block for pediatric penile surgery (e.g., hypospadias repair) with increased duration of analgesia, decreased length of stay in recovery area, and lack of lower extremity motor block.[573,580]

The use of single-injection neuraxial opioids is an additional technique that can provide longer-lasting analgesia, but must be used in inpatients only because of the need for respiratory monitoring. Intrathecal morphine has been administered to infants and children for several decades and provides long-acting analgesia (up to 24 hours) after a single injection.[581,582] It is essential that only preservative-free preparations of the drug be used because preservative-containing solutions may result in injury to the central neuraxis. Intrathecal morphine doses ranging from 4 to 10 µg/kg are usually chosen. Because of the hydrophilicity of this agent, respiratory monitoring is mandated. Respiratory depression, as well as pruritus, nausea, and urinary retention, are reported after intrathecal morphine. The drug can be administered by the surgeon under direct vision of the dura, but if administered at the beginning of the case, it has been reported to reduce intraoperative blood loss by up to 40%.[583,584] This route of administration has also been used before cardiac surgery.[585] The effective intrathecal dose of opioid is roughly one-fifth to one-tenth that of the epidural dose, and the duration of action, especially with morphine, is significantly prolonged. Therefore, observation in a monitored setting must be continued for 24 hours or until no further evidence of respiratory compromise exists (without the use of naloxone).

Catheter Techniques

A catheter placed in the epidural space or adjacent to a nerve or plexus can be used to provide continuous uninterrupted analgesia for prolonged periods after surgery. These catheters are commonly used for about 3 days but may be used for more prolonged periods in selected situations. However, the risk of infection does increase when catheters are left in place for more than 3 days.[485] If necessary, catheters tunneled under the skin may be left in situ for more than 7 days,[586-588] and they have been left in place for longer periods without infectious complications in palliative care patients.[589]

Continuous regional blockade is remarkably effective and safe, although as with any technique, monitoring for untoward effects is necessary to prevent complications. New technology for the delivery of drugs to peripheral nerves and plexuses has made it possible for children to receive the benefits of continuous neural blockade after discharge from the hospital or day surgery unit.[479] Catheters may deliver local anesthetics and other medications via controlled infusion devices that use a pressurized elastomer-bulb reservoir that controls the infusion rate with a flow limiter (ON-Q pump, I-Flow LLC, Lake Forest, CA; Infusor, Baxter Healthcare Corporation, Deerfield, IL; Accufuser, Moog Medical Devices, Salt Lake City, UT; Easypump, B Braun Melsungen AG, Melsungen, Germany; and others) (E-Fig. 41.3). These devices can be used at home after discharge, for infusion of medication into a tissue plane to provide a continuous field blockade or a continuous peripheral nerve block. As the use of peripheral nerve blocks continue to increase, we believe that these techniques may eventually become more common than neuraxial analgesia for suitable indications.

Infusion of local anesthetics in the subcutaneous (SC) tissues at the incision site or into the surgical plane using these devices provides prolonged analgesia in both adults and children. Several types of these infusion systems are available, including ones that have options for fixed, variable, or continuous infusion rates with a bolus option. The latter two must be used with caution in smaller children in whom local anesthetic toxicity from excessive dosage may be a risk; we generally use the fixed-rate devices. When continuous peripheral nerve or plexus blocks are used for outpatients, a carefully designed system must be in place to follow-up with these children to avoid complications and achieve early detection of adverse events. Patient and family education to recognize potential complications, along with telephone follow-up, are necessary to ensure safe use of catheters at home. Cases have been reported of possible excessive doses of local anesthetic from a continuous infusion pump used at home, although no catastrophic events have been reported.[590]

CAUDAL AND EPIDURAL CATHETERS. With experience and proper equipment, the lumbar or thoracic routes are feasible at any age, but specific pediatric expertise is required for neonates, infants, and toddlers. Regardless of the level of insertion, the goal should be to place the tip of the catheter as close as possible to the dermatome(s) most affected by the operation.

For caudal catheter placement, epidurography has been used to confirm the position of the catheter tip. In one series of 20 preterm infants, epidurography revealed misplaced catheters in three infants or 15%.[591] New data suggest that misplacement of threaded catheters in all ages may be more common than is generally recognized.[592] In this series of 724 epidurograms, unexpected misplacement was detected in 11 or 1.5%, including three intravascular catheters, despite negative test doses; two intrathecal without cerebrospinal fluid aspiration; four that were intraperitoneal; and one each in the rectum and psoas compartments.[593] These authors recommended epidurography in all cases, although this is not the current standard of practice and must be weighed against the risks of radiation exposure in young children. If specific dermatomal placement of a catheter is sought, one should consider obtaining an imaging study to confirm the dermatomal level of the tip of the catheter, and the aforementioned data suggest that imaging might be advisable whenever a catheter is advanced to a level substantially more rostral than its insertion level.

As an alternative to epidurography, ultrasound is especially useful in infants weighing less than 10 kilograms. Ultrasound can be used to estimate the skin–ligamentum flavum distance to aid in placement, as well as imaging proper catheter placement. In general, it is more difficult to image the actual catheter but local anesthetic spread can be easily visualized with anterior depression of the dura on injection.[594,595]

Nerve-stimulating catheters present another alternative, which allow real-time monitoring of the location of the tip of the catheter as it is advanced cephalad.[596,597] If a stimulating catheter is not available, a saline solution–filled catheter can serve in its stead. The technique requires the use of saline loss-of-resistance and avoiding air bubbles in the epidural space or in the catheter-connector-injection system, because air impedes electrical conduction. With either system, neuromuscular blockade must be avoided because it abolishes the motor response. Used in conjunction with a nerve stimulator set to very low milliamperage (approximately 6 mA), the muscles supplied by a nerve root will twitch as the catheter approaches the segments that supply that dermatome, thereby confirming the catheter tip's location. Specifically, twitches in the feet and ankles occur with catheter tips around L5 to S1, hip flexion occurs with catheter tips around T12 to S1, abdominal muscle twitches without hip flexion imply thoracic positioning above T12, and intercostal muscle twitches imply midthoracic tip positioning. Finger twitches would imply advancement to around T1. This technique can also be used to detect catheter malposition. Bilateral twitching at a current less than 0.6 mA generally implies subarachnoid positioning. Unilateral twitches in a narrow motor distribution at a current less than 1 mA may suggest advancement out a root foramen. Unilateral twitches at a current less than 1 mA in a very broad motor distribution may indicate subdural positioning. Absence of twitches as the current is increased to about 15 mA (in the absence of air bubbles or neuromuscular blockade) generally indicates that the epidural catheter is not in the epidural space (Table 41.9). Our experience is that the use of one of these confirmatory techniques when catheters are threaded cephalad can help avoid problems with failed or incomplete blocks in the postoperative period.

The choice of drugs for epidural infusions depends on several factors, including site of surgery, site of the epidural catheter tip, and child risk factors. Local anesthetics, lipophilic opioids, and, to some extent, clonidine all have more restricted cephalad distribution of action during infusions compared with hydrophilic opioids, such as hydromorphone or morphine. Consequently, optimal positioning of the catheter tip during insertion can improve the analgesic action postoperatively. Experience in adults suggests that when local anesthetics are used, analgesia is optimized when the tip of the epidural catheter is positioned at or slightly above the dermatomal levels involved in the surgery. This effect may be more pronounced when children are moving than when they are at rest. Positioning at levels slightly above the dermatomal levels involved in surgery is more relevant for surgery in lumbosacral dermatomes compared with upper thoracic dermatomes because of the greater distance between root level and dorsal horn level in these two circumstances.[598]

Placement of catheters at thoracic levels requires consideration of risk/benefit trade-offs. Therefore, if a catheter tip is at the lumbar or caudal level and the surgery is in thoracic and upper abdominal dermatomes, continuous infusions containing local anesthetics alone or with lipophilic opioids, such as fentanyl, are likely to be ineffective. Increasing the infusion volume is limited by the maximum allowable systemic local anesthetic concentrations. In this circumstance, a reasonable alternative is to administer hydrophilic opioids (e.g., morphine or hydromorphone) through lumbar or caudal catheters. Repeated caudal-catheter administered morphine has been used to provide analgesia in neonates after abdominal surgery.[599] Such a technique, however, precludes the optimal use of local anesthetics and the considerable benefit that may accrue from a multimodal approach to regional analgesia. An epidural catheter can be placed in an awake, sedated, or anesthetized child. A prospective analysis of data from the

Pediatric Regional Anesthesia Network database found that the risk of inserting an epidural catheter in an anesthetized child by an experienced clinician is not greater and may be less than attempting such placement in an awake adult. It also is uncertain that a child can accurately report sensations of paresthesia or differentiate the discomfort of needle passage from more ominous pain.[138,600,601] There is a perception that placing an epidural in the thoracic region is more dangerous than in other spinal levels, but current data do not support this. In the UK epidural audit, serious (grade 1) complications were independent of the level of insertion.[601] Overall, there was a greater risk of all types of complications in thoracic epidurals placed in neonates and infants, but half of these complications were of the less severe grade 3 variety. Similar data have been reported by Pediatric Regional Anesthesia Network, where no serious complications were reported in 4400 thoracic epidural blocks. Risk is likely more related to the age of the patient rather than level of insertion.[9,138] In a report of four cases of neurologic complications in children with epidurals, three of four catheters were at T11 level or lower.[602] We believe that data and experience support the safety of placement of epidural catheters in anesthetized children by anesthesiologists trained and experienced in this procedure, although the tolerances for error in infants are smaller than in adults and older children.[138,601,603,604]

It is extremely important to secure caudal catheters to the skin with a clear occlusive dressing to avoid contamination or dislodgment and to allow daily inspection of the site. In addition, tincture of benzoin or other adhesive solution reduces the incidence of catheter and dressing displacement. For a caudal catheter, the use of an adhesive-edged plastic drape, covering the area from the gluteal crease over the dressing, also helps prevent fecal soiling of the dressing by children who are in diapers. Another option is to tunnel the caudal catheter in a cephalad-lateral direction, which decreases colonization rates to that seen with epidural catheters.[587] Despite the above precautions, if a dressing becomes detached and the insertion site is contaminated, it is prudent to remove the catheter. The use of lumbar or thoracic catheters removes the insertion site from the diaper area and thereby further reduces the potential for contamination of the catheter and the insertion site.

Successful management of children with an epidural catheter requires carefully coordinated monitoring protocols, nursing management, and medical management of drug selection and dosing. As with PCA or continuous-infusion opioids, the orders should be standardized and written in consultation with the nursing staff, so that misinterpretations are less likely to occur (Fig. 41.8). Because the single most sensitive monitor of children receiving epidural opioids is the nurse, rather than a mechanical or electronic device, education of the nursing staff is of paramount importance to ensure safety. Nursing staff can also assess the adequacy of analgesia and thereby help to titrate the drug dose. Catheter insertion sites should be inspected at least once daily by the pain service, both for the integrity of the dressing and for any evidence of erythema or skin infection (Fig. 41.9). *When continuous infusions are used, the tubing connecting the infusion*

TABLE 41.9	Patient-Controlled Analgesia Dosing Guidelines			
Drug	Demand Dose (µg/kg)	Lockout Interval (minutes)	Continuous Basal Infusion (µg/kg per hour)	4-Hour Limit (µg/kg)
Morphine	10–30	8–15	0–20	250–400
Hydromorphone	2–6	8–15	0–4	50–80
Fentanyl	0.5	5–10	0–0.5	7–10

41

Child's weight: _____ kg
Allergies: _____

Continuous regional analgesia via (check appropriate modality)
☐ Caudal epidural ☐ Lumbar epidural ☐ Thoracic epidural ☐ Plexus or peripheral nerve catheter (specify)

_____

The catheter is _____ cm at the skin. Loss of resistance (for lumbar and thoracic epidurals) was at _____ cm.

Infusion:
(Choose one only) ☐ Bupivacaine ☐ Ropivacaine ☐ Chloroprocaine
(Concentration) ☐ 0.075% ☐ 0.1% ☐ 0.2% ☐ 1% (chloroprocaine only)

Additives (caudal and epidural only):
Opioid (choose one only) ☐ Fentanyl ☐ Hydromorphone ☐ Morphine
Concentration (µg/mL): ☐ 1 ☐ 2 ☐ 3 ☐ 5 (hydromorphone and morphine only) ☐ 7 (morphine only)
☐ 10 (morphine only)
☐ Clonidine Concentration (µg/mL): ☐ 0.5 ☐ 1

Infusion rate: Start at _____ mL/h. Range: _____ to _____ mL/h. This is a maximum of _____ mg/kg/h of local anesthetic and _____ µg/kg/h of opioid.

Dosing guidelines for regional anesthesia/analgesia solution

	Local anesthetics		Opioids			
	Bupivacaine or ropivacaine	Chloroprocaine	Fentanyl	Hydromorphone	Morphine	Clonidine
Concentration	0.05%-0.1% (0.5-1 mg/mL) May use up to 0.2% for ropivacaine	1%-1.5% (10-15 mg/mL)	1-3 µg/mL	3-7 µg/mL	5-10 µg/mL	0.5-1 µg/mL
Suggested dose	Less than 6 months of age: 0.2 mg/kg/h; Maximum dose: 0.2 mg/kg/h 6 months of age or older: 0.2-0.4 mg/kg/h Maximum dose: 0.4–0.5 mg/kg/h	0.2-0.8 mL/kg/h (neonates)*	0.3-1 µg/kg/h	1-2.5 µg/kg/h	1-5 µg/kg/h	0.1-0.2 µg/kg/h

*Note that the concentration of additives must be proportionally reduced with chloroprocaine if higher infusion rates are administered to avoid overdose.

Treatment of side effects:
Respiratory depression: For RR < _____ BPM, immediately stop epidural infusion and call acute pain service STAT. Administer O_2, ensure clear airway, and assist ventilation if necessary.
☐ Naloxone (Narcan) 1 µg/kg IV = _____ µg, repeat q1min as needed

Nausea and vomiting: ☐ Ondansetron 0.1 mg/kg (4 mg maximum) = _____ mg IV q6h
☐ Metoclopramide 0.1 mg/kg (10 mg maximum) = _____ mg IV q6h

Pruritus: ☐ Nalbuphine 0.05 mg/kg = _____ mg IV q4h

☐ *For any of above,* begin naloxone infusion at 0.25 µg/kg/h = _____ µg/h

Adjunctive medications: ☐ Acetaminophen 10 mg/kg PO q4h for 24 hours then q4h prn
Inadequate analgesia: ☐ Morphine 0.05-0.1 mg/kg IV = _____ mg q3-4h prn for pain
☐ Ketorolac 0.5 mg/kg IV = _____ mg q6h prn for pain (up to 15 mg ≤ 50 kg; up to 30 mg > 50 kg)
Muscle spasms: ☐ Diazepam 0.05-0.1 mg/kg IV = _____ mg q6h prn

Monitoring and equipment: *must choose for patients receiving epidural opioids*
☐ Continuous pulse oximetry and respiratory monitoring
☐ O_2 and bag/mask delivery system, suction at the bedside

Nursing orders:
VS: ☐ q4h: temp, HR, RR, BP, pain score
☐ Dermatome level for caudal and epidural
☐ Spo2 and sedation score (required if opioids are used). Call acute pain service for RR < _____ bpm.
☐ Record Bromage score q8hr; call acute pain service if 4 or less (choose for children receiving local anesthetics).

Call acute pain service for any questions or problems: inadequate analgesia despite intervention, loose or contaminated dressing, catheter disconnect, sedation score >3, increased somnolence, confusion, agitation, dizziness, tinnitus, hypotension, bradycardia, fever >38.2°C; inflammation, tenderness, or swelling at catheter site; Bromage score >0.

Maintain IV access.

For epidural or peripheral nerve block of lower extremity: Ambulate with assistance only with order from primary service and Bromage score of 0. Pad block extremities and elevate heels off of bed.

FIGURE 41.8 Sample Epidural Orders. *BP,* Blood pressure; *BPM,* breaths per minute; *HR,* heart rate; *RR,* respiratory rate; *PO,* orally; *prn,* as needed; *Spo₂,* oxygen saturation measured by pulse oximetry; *STAT,* immediately; *VS,* vital signs. (Modified from the University of Michigan Hospitals & Health Centers.)

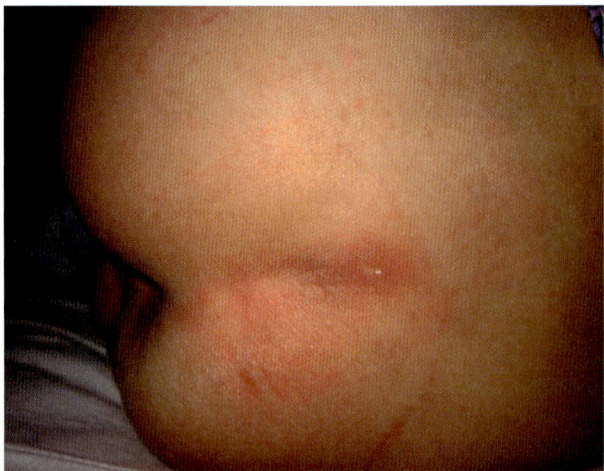

FIGURE 41.9 Superficial skin infection at the site of an epidural catheter insertion. The catheter was withdrawn, and the problem resolved with local skin care only.

TABLE 41.10	Estimated Dermatomal Level With Epidural Catheter Advancement	
Amperage (mA)	Estimated Dermatomal Level	Twitch Response Level
6	L5–S1	Feet and ankles
6	T12–S1	Hip flexors
6	Above T12	Abdominal muscle without hip flexion
6	Midthoracic	Intercostal muscles
6	T1	Fingers
<0.6	Subarachnoid malposition	Bilateral motor response
<1	Nerve root	Unilateral
<1	Subdural	Unilateral but broad motor distribution
15	Out of epidural space	No twitches observed

pump to the catheter should not have any injection ports and it should be clearly labeled as an epidural catheter to preclude unintended epidural administration of drugs intended for IV use. The advent of the new International Standardization Organization ISO80369 standard for regional block connectors is expected to reduce the likelihood of these potentially catastrophic errors from occurring.[603,605,606] A specific modification (ISO 80369-6 NRFit) requires a different connector diameter incompatible with standard Luer Lok devices and are specific for epidural catheters but at this time only California mandates its use.[607] These catheters and corresponding syringes are also either yellow in color or have a yellow line to indicate a difference from other infusion lines and syringes.[608]

A variation of traditional epidural analgesia and PCA is the technique of patient-controlled epidural analgesia.[609–613] With this variation of traditional PCA, children are generally maintained with an infusion of epidural analgesics (frequently opioid alone or an opioid–local anesthetic mixture) and have the capability of self-administering supplemental doses when required. When using this technique, the background infusion is used to provide the majority of the analgesia and the child can add to this when needed. It must be emphasized that the time needed for a bolus dose to effect a change with epidural administration is more prolonged than it is with IV agents. Therefore, with patient-controlled epidural analgesia, lockout intervals are greater (often 15 to 30 minutes) than with PCA.[609,614,615] The considerations one would use for choosing this technique include the same child-monitoring factors for IV PCA and epidural analgesia, and maximum local anesthetic doses must be carefully calculated to cover the contingency of the greatest possible activation of the patient-controlled epidural analgesia demand doses. Smart pump technology has been demonstrated to improve safety of this technique.[444,616]

SELECTION OF DRUGS AND DOSES. Local anesthetics, opioids, and adjuvant agents were discussed previously; this section addresses the specifics of drug choices for continuous infusion through indwelling catheters. Many drugs and combinations have been administered via continuous infusion to the epidural space to provide postoperative analgesia.[545] The most common choices involve mixtures of local anesthetics and opioids, such as bupivacaine and fentanyl, although increasingly, clonidine is being added (Table 41.10). Continuous infusions for peripheral nerve and plexus blocks are generally limited to local anesthetics, as adjuvants are generally utilized primarily for single-shot techniques.

The choice of drug is based on several factors: the age and size of the child, the operation, and the underlying medical conditions that may decrease the margin of safety of one of the agents. The volume of solution required to fill the epidural space on a milliliter-per-kilogram basis appears to decrease with age; therefore, older children and adolescents may require less volume than infants and young children, based on weight. In children older than 1 year of age, continuous infusions of ropivacaine up to 0.4 mg/kg per hour for up to 72 hours produced stable blood concentrations of unbound ropivacaine without evidence of accumulation or toxicity.[617,618] In very young or preterm infants, clearance is slower and the risk of accumulation of the amino-amide local anesthetics during infusion, and thus the potential for toxicity, is particularly problematic.[619,620] Neonates are at increased risk for local anesthetic toxicity because of decreased protein binding (resulting in increased unbound drug) and immature drug metabolism. The manifestations of local anesthetic toxicity in infants and neonates may be more difficult to recognize than in adults. Hence, we recommend a conservative maximum infusion dose for ropivacaine of 0.2 mg/kg per hour for infants younger than 6 months, which produces stable plasma levels for up to 72 hours.[621] Bupivacaine remains in common use despite its lower therapeutic index; the same reduced maximal dose limits apply (i.e., <0.2 mg/kg per hour).[619,622] Of the five cases of local anesthetic toxicity reported to the Pediatric Regional Anesthesia Network, four were in infants 3 months of age or younger, highlighting the greater risk in this age group.[9,138] Because safe infusion rates of ropivacaine in the neonate frequently provide insufficient analgesia when wide dermatomal coverage is needed, the amino-ester local anesthetic chloroprocaine may be used in an epidural infusion instead.[523–525,571,623,624] Although the amino-amide local anesthetics are slowly cleared in neonates and young infants, the amino-ester chloroprocaine is cleared extremely rapidly via ester hydrolysis even in preterm infants with an elimination half-life of several minutes.[623] This permits large doses and infusion rates with a reduced risk for systemic toxicity. Case reports of chloroprocaine toxicity in infants are rare, generally short-lived (<1 minute), and self-limiting owing to its rapid metabolism.[625,626] Previous concerns regarding neurotoxicity after chloroprocaine involved a succession of formulations with preservatives, including metabisulfite, methylparaben, and ethylenediaminetetraacetic acid, although the current formulation is preservative-free. An epidural solution of 1% to 1.5% chloroprocaine can be infused at rates of 0.2 to 1 mL/kg per hour.

When a block is not previously established in the operating room, it is useful to dose through catheters with local anesthetic (without opioids) at a volume of 0.05 mL/kg per spinal segment or between 0.5 and 1 mL/kg of local anesthetic, not to exceed 5 mg/kg of lidocaine, or 2.5 mg/kg of bupivacaine or ropivacaine. Some clinicians administer a loading dose of opioid as well, such as 1 to 3 μg/kg of hydromorphone. Bupivacaine infusion rates should not exceed 0.4 mg/kg per hour (e.g., 0.4 mL/kg per hour for 0.1% bupivacaine) for children because toxicity may result.[627] If epidural local anesthetic infusions are begun without either opioids or clonidine (e.g., 0.0625%–0.125% bupivacaine) and inadequate analgesia occurs at infusion rates of 0.3 to 0.4 mL/kg per hour (a maximum dosage of 0.4 mg/kg per hour), bolus doses or further increases in the local anesthetic infusion rate or concentration should be avoided. Instead, correct placement of the catheter should be confirmed (e.g., with an epidurogram or chloroprocaine/lidocaine test dose) if dermatomal levels cannot be unequivocally determined. If the catheter is properly located, an epidural opioid or clonidine can be added to the local anesthetic infusion. It is imperative to confirm that an epidural catheter is properly functioning immediately after an infant or child arrives in the PACU or if there is any question of its proper location later. If an amino-amide local anesthetic has been given during or after surgery as an initial bolus followed by a continuous infusion, then use of a repeat bolus dose of these amino amides may result in a "stair casing" of plasma concentrations (i.e., accumulation), with a risk for systemic toxicity. Although administration of epidural or systemic opioids may provide analgesia, they may not clarify the site of the epidural catheter tip. For this reason, confirmation of the catheter location is imperative whenever the clinical picture is not clear. Several means of accomplishing this are described later.

Local anesthetic and opioid combinations (e.g., 0.1% bupivacaine or 0.1% to 0.2% ropivacaine with hydromorphone 3 to 5 μg/mL at infusion rates of 0.2 to 0.4 mL/kg per hour) via lumbar epidural catheters or caudal catheters advanced to a lumbar position, provide adequate analgesia in most children undergoing lower abdominal or lower extremity surgery. Fentanyl alone (0.3 μg/kg per hour) has been shown to provide 90% effective postoperative analgesia after a levobupivacaine block was established during surgery.[628] However, the blood concentrations achieved with epidural fentanyl have been shown to be in the therapeutic range, suggesting that much of the therapeutic effect is due to systemic absorption, not entirely surprising with a highly lipophilic agent.[629] We do not recommend the use of epidural fentanyl for this reason. Epidural opioids should be used with great caution, or at considerably reduced doses, in children at risk for apnea or hypoventilation (e.g., former preterm infants, children with chronic respiratory failure or disorders of central control of ventilation, or those with obstructive sleep apnea). In very young infants, epidural infusions of both local anesthetics and opioids and other adjuvants can be used safely, but they require increased surveillance and reduced initial infusion rates. This is because (1) drug clearance may be reduced[627]; (2) protein binding, which is decreased, may increase the free serum drug concentrations; and (3) titration to clinical end points (e.g., pain scoring) is less precise. A double-blind

randomized study demonstrated that the combination of 0.1% bupivacaine with 1 μg/mL of fentanyl provided superior analgesia compared with local anesthetic alone, with no increase in adverse effects, when infused through thoracic catheters after thoracotomy in infants younger than 6 months of age.[630] In contrast, another study found no incremental benefits in children after abdominal surgery from the addition of fentanyl to epidural catheters with greater local anesthetic concentrations (e.g., 0.125% bupivacaine at 0.3 mL/kg per hour).[628,631] The use of fentanyl as an adjunct may increase nausea and vomiting.[631] In some centers, application of epidural infusions, especially with opioids, for children younger than 3 to 6 months of age is restricted to intensive care areas. Some centers avoid the use of epidural opioids altogether and instead use clonidine (0.5–1 μg/mL) as the preferred adjunct. Acetaminophen or NSAIDs should be administered if additional analgesia is needed.

If the catheter tip is positioned at the thoracic dermatomes, bupivacaine or ropivacaine with opioid may be used for thoracic and upper abdominal surgery.[122,134,631–635] Infusion rates may need to be decreased for thoracic catheters compared with lumbar catheters because the capacitance or volume of the epidural space appears to be less than in lumbar regions. Using hydromorphone may be of benefit in these instances, as its greater hydrophilicity results in wider spread. We rarely use epidural morphine and prefer a continuous epidural infusion of hydromorphone when greater spread is desired, as its adverse effect profile appears to be preferable. Studies in adults suggest an epidural potency ratio of between 2:1 and 3:1, compared with 5:1 for systemic morphine.[636] When mixed with a local anesthetic for lumbar epidural infusion, concentrations of 3 to 5 μg/mL of hydromorphone yield a solution that results in an appropriate infusion rate of both drugs. Hydrophilic opioids, especially when administered by infusion, require prolonged careful observation (see later discussion). If somnolence, shallow breathing, or hypopnea occurs, the infusion must be stopped, not simply decreased, until these effects subside, and appropriate therapy is instituted (Table 41.11). Common epidural infusions and alternative modalities for pain management of sample cases are provided in Appendix 41.1.

Adjuvant agents, particularly clonidine, can be administered continuously via epidural catheter, most commonly in combination with or in place of local anesthetics and opioids. The primary analgesic effect appears to be via an α-adrenergic mechanism. Although epidural clonidine has been found to be less potent in terms of analgesic efficacy compared with epidural opioids, such as fentanyl, it has occasionally been substituted for neuraxial opioids because it is associated with a smaller incidence of untoward effects, such as respiratory depression, nausea, and pruritus.[637–640] This also suggests that the combination of all three agents, each at smaller concentrations than required individually, might be beneficial at reducing the incidence of adverse effects while optimizing analgesia, but carefully controlled studies have yet to be performed.

Risks and Untoward Effects

Adverse effects associated with regional analgesia can be grouped according to those caused by the technique (e.g., the catheter) and those related to the medications (e.g., local anesthetics, opioids, other adjuvants). A number of large prospective studies have confirmed the safety of regional anesthetics in children, detecting only very small complication rates.[9,138,601,603]

Local anesthetics in the dilute concentrations used for postoperative analgesia have a very small incidence of untoward effects.

TABLE 41.11 | Commonly Used Medications for Epidural Administration

	Dose Range	Untoward Effects	Comments
Local Anesthetics			
Bupivacaine	0.2–0.4 mg/kg per hour	Motor block	Maximum dose 0.2 mg/kg per hour for infants <6 months
Ropivacaine	0.2–0.5 mg/kg per hour	Motor block	Levo-enantiomer; 20%–30% less toxicity than racemic
Levobupivacaine	0.2–0.5 mg/kg per hour	Motor block	amino amides. Maximum dose 0.2 mg/kg per hour for infants <6 months
Chloroprocaine	1%–1.5%; 0.2–0.8 mL/kg per hour (neonates)	Motor block	
Opioids		Respiratory depression, sedation, pruritus, urinary retention	
Fentanyl	0.3–1 µg/kg per hour		Lipophilic; high rate of systemic absorption
Hydromorphone	1–3 µg/kg per hour	Delayed respiratory depression from rostral spread	Hydrophilic; use when surgery is more extensive. Hydromorphone recommended over morphine due to less rostral spread
Morphine	1–5 µg/kg per hour		
Adjuncts			
Clonidine	0.1–0.2 µg/kg per hour	Sedation, respiratory depression at greater doses, hypotension (possibly postural) at high doses	Increased risk of apnea with high doses in neonates

TABLE 41.12 | Treatment of Untoward Effects of Epidural Opioids

Adverse Effect	Treatment	Infusion Rate
Pruritus	Naloxone, 0.5–1 µg/kg IV or infusion at 0.25–1 µg/kg per hour	No change, or decrease opioid concentration, or remove opioid if pruritis persists
	Nalbuphine, 0.025–0.05 mg/kg IV every 6 hours	
Nausea and vomiting	NPO for 24 hours	Decrease opioid concentration or decrease rate by 10%–20% or remove opioid if nausea persists
	Naloxone, 0.5 µg/kg IV or infusion at 0.25–1 µg/kg per hour	
	Ondansetron 0.1 mg/kg (maximum 4 mg) IV every 6 hours	
	Metoclopramide, 0.1–0.15 mg/kg IV every 6–8 hours	
Urinary retention	Bladder catheterization (one time; some institutions keep urinary catheters in these children routinely)	Decrease opioid concentration
	Naloxone, 0.5 µg/kg IV or infusion at 0.25–1 µg/kg per hour	
	Indwelling urinary catheter	
Respiratory depression[a]; child unarousable, hypoxemic, hypercarbic, or apneic	Oxygen by mask; assisted ventilation if needed	Discontinue infusion; consider possibility of intrathecal catheter migration (check by aspirating)
	Naloxone, 5–10 µg/kg IV	
	Transfer child to monitored setting until episode is fully resolved.	
	Consider naloxone infusion (0.25–1 µg/kg per hour)	
	Consider naloxone infusion (0.25–1 µg/kg per hour)	

IV, Intravenous; *NPO*, nothing by mouth.
[a]Stop infusion until the child is alert, if using morphine or hydromorphone.

Motor blockade occurs less frequently with dilute concentrations but can be observed even with small concentrations of bupivacaine, such as 0.1%. As discussed earlier, children with neuromuscular disorders causing motor weakness are especially at risk and should be observed carefully for exacerbation of their motor weakness. Motor weakness and blockade can result in several problems. Inability or difficulty in ambulation may impede recovery. The inability of a child to move a limb can result in skin breakdown or peripheral nerve compression injuries, especially if meticulous attention to frequent repositioning does not occur. We are aware of a case of complex regional pain syndrome in the distribution of the peroneal nerve that arose in this manner. Motor blockade should be avoided, and frequent examinations can quantify motor function using the Bromage score (Tables 41.12 and 41.13). At our institutions, motor function is assessed every 8 hours along with the other vital signs pertinent to regional blockade. If motor blockade occurs, the clinician should (1) reduce the dose (volume or concentration) of local anesthetic,[9] (2) pay strict attention to padding and to frequent repositioning of the extremity involved, and (3) consider stopping the infusion until motor function returns. *Rapid onset of more profound motor block during epidural infusion should raise immediate concern about erosion of the catheter*

TABLE 41.13 | Bromage Score[a] for Assessment of Motor Function of the Legs

Full motor function: can flex hip, knee, and ankle	0
Can't flex hip (unable to perform straight-leg lift)	1
Can't flex hip or knee	2
Can't flex hip, knee, or ankle	3

[a]Note that alternative scoring schemes for the Bromage scale exist that range from 1 to 4 (sometimes denoted I–IV) that directly correspond to the 0–3 scale depicted here.

41

into the subarachnoid space. Motor blockade may occur more frequently with peripheral nerve or plexus analgesia than with epidural blocks and is subject to the same precautions. When children are discharged home with a peripheral nerve catheter, it is particularly important to teach the parents how to deal with motor blockade and to protect the extremity from unintended injury.

The PK of bupivacaine have been studied in infants and children after both single-injection doses[641,642] and continuous infusions.[622] Reduced protein binding increases circulating unbound bupivacaine after administration, which increases the risk of bupivacaine toxicity.[642] Neonates and infants with immature clearance may be at particular risk for unbound bupivacaine accumulation with infusion.[622] Seizures and cardiac arrest have been reported when large doses of bupivacaine have been administered, usually after excessive infusion rates or unintended intravascular injection. Limited information is available regarding extended administration over days; total bupivacaine concentration may increase because alpha 1-acid-glycoprotein (AAG, an amide anesthetic binding protein) is a reactive protein that increases after surgery; unbound concentrations, however, remain at steady state.[619,643]

The *l*-enantiomers of amino amides (ropivacaine and levobupivacaine) have toxic thresholds that are greater than that of bupivacaine by as much as 30%, and such drugs should be considered in smaller children and for blocks that require greater infusion rates and for greater durations. A particular "hidden" risk occurs when a block is functioning less than optimally, and bolus doses are administered in an attempt to broaden the dermatome level. Even though the infusion rate is kept within the recommended range, the bolus doses can raise the blood concentration above the toxic threshold.[644] *Whenever a local anesthetic is administered by continuous infusion, nursing and medical staff must be aware of the signs and symptoms of local-anesthetic toxicity, be vigilant in monitoring for the early detection of those signs, and be familiar with the use of lipid rescue protocols to treat toxicity if it occurs.* The use of lipid emulsion for treating local anesthetic toxicity is discussed in detail in Chapter 40.

Tachyphylaxis during prolonged administration of local anesthetics is a theoretic consideration, although no systematic studies have addressed this phenomenon in children. In animal models, tachyphylaxis is accelerated by hyperalgesia and prevented by agents that prevent hyperalgesia at spinal sites. One rationale for coadministration of opioids or clonidine in epidural infusions may be to reduce the incidence or severity of tachyphylaxis. As discussed in Chapter 40, hemodynamic stability is maintained in children younger than 6 years of age during spinal or epidural blockade, even with extensive sympathetic blockade. As children approach school age, however, rapid position changes may produce

hemodynamic responses after extensive sympathetic blockade, and this must be considered in children who receive continuous epidural blockade. Orthostatic changes may be exacerbated when epidural clonidine is infused, and extra caution should be taken.

Neuraxial opioids confer several potential adverse effects, including respiratory depression, nausea, urinary retention, and pruritus. Indeed, despite their proven analgesic efficacy, not all practitioners are proponents of their use because of these effects, preferring other adjuvants instead.[645] The most effective means of treating or preventing the adverse effects is the use of opioid antagonists or mixed agonist-antagonists. This approach directly targets the etiology of the signs rather than simply treating their manifestations. Low-dose naloxone infusions, which have been shown to be effective in children receiving parenteral opioids, are also effective for treating the adverse effects of neuraxial opioids, although pediatric data are lacking.[367,368,646–650] We have used rates similar to those shown effective in the PCA studies, beginning at 0.25 µg/kg per hour.[367,368] This infusion rate can be titrated upward as needed to 1 µg/kg per hour without adversely affecting analgesic efficacy.[368]

The most worrisome and dangerous complication is respiratory depression. The lipophilic agents (fentanyl and sufentanil) have the widest therapeutic indexes. This results from greater receptor binding in the substantia gelatinosa of the spinal cord adjacent to the area of drug administration, thus limiting the rostral spread of the drug, but systemic absorption is considerably greater, resulting in risk of respiratory depression owing to greater blood concentrations. Even though the hydrophilic opioids, hydromorphone and morphine, pose a risk for respiratory depression, the incidence remains small when prudent dosing is followed. Nevertheless, reports of respiratory depression after epidural administration of morphine demonstrate that vigilance in monitoring is mandatory.[538,651,652] *The hallmark of impending overdose of central neuraxial opioids is increasing sedation and decreasing DEPTH AND RATE of respiration. It is important to recognize that the depth of respiration must be assessed, not just the rate, because children frequently develop decreased tidal volume before the respiratory rate decreases, leading to alveolar hypoventilation and the potential for hypercarbia and hypoxemia.*[653] Monitoring patients receiving neuraxial opioids entails considerations similar to those with systemic opioids as discussed earlier. As previously noted, pulse oximetry becomes a poorly sensitive monitor for hypoventilation if the child is using supplemental oxygen, and capnographic techniques are plagued by a high rate of false alarms and not well tolerated by children; no monitor can replace vigilance and frequent clinical assessment.

Oversedation, diminished respiratory depth, and slowing of the respiratory rate are treated by decreasing the rate of opioid administration and, if necessary, administering small incremental doses of naloxone (0.5–1 µg/kg) every few minutes until the adverse effects are reversed (see earlier discussion). A continuous low-dose infusion of naloxone, as described earlier (0.25 to 1 µg/kg per hour), may need to be started. More profound respiratory depression, including inability to arouse the child and apnea, must be treated more aggressively. *The new development of respiratory depression in a child receiving what appears to be an appropriate opioid dose should always raise the question of catheter migration into the subarachnoid space. Whenever central neuraxial opioids are administered, facilities must be immediately available at the child's bedside for resuscitation, in the unlikely event of respiratory depression.* It is recommended that emergency equipment, including a bag-valve device, appropriate sizes of masks and airways, and suction, be at the child's bedside or in a "code cart" that is accessible within seconds, should the need arise. Naloxone should similarly be immediately available, without the need to obtain the drug from the pharmacy. All children receiving continuous regional analgesia should also have an IV line (a heparin lock is adequate in those children not requiring IV fluids).

Pruritus is a common adverse effect associated with epidural or intrathecal opioid use, occurring in as many as 30% to 70% of children. Antihistamines are less effective antipruritics in this situation, because the primary mechanism is a central opioid, not a histamine effect. Thus opioid antagonists, used in small doses, are most effective. Again, low-dose infusions of naloxone can be administered with good results.[368,646,647,649,650,653] Some practitioners have found low-dose nalbuphine to be effective to antagonize pruritus (25 to 50 µg/kg every 6 hours PRN).[647,648] In a pediatric study of nalbuphine, it was no better than placebo; however, the placebo arm had a remarkable efficacy of 58% (nalbuphine 57%).[654]

Nausea and vomiting can also occur in association with opioids (both systemic and neuraxial) and may be more common with morphine than with fentanyl. Children who are fasted during the first 24 hours after surgery do not vomit excessively, even when given caudal morphine.[655] As with all other opioid adverse effects, nausea and vomiting respond to the previously mentioned doses of naloxone or mixed agonist-antagonists, such as nalbuphine. Some antiemetics, such as antihistamines and butyrophenones, may cause sedation and should be used with caution. Serotonin-receptor antagonists, such as ondansetron (0.1–0.15 mg/kg, maximum 4 mg) or dolasetron (0.35 mg/kg, maximum 12.5 mg), may be effective and not cause sedation.[656] It is sometimes prudent to decrease the infusion rate of the epidural (if the block level permits) or the opioid concentration in the infusate, or substitute clonidine for the opioid altogether, when untoward opioid effects require treatment (see Table 41.11).

Urinary retention is a relatively common complication of neuraxial opioids. Studies of single-injection caudal blocks have found that this complication does not occur when epidural local anesthetics are used, only when neuraxial opioids are added.[657] Neuraxial opioids depress detrusor contractility in a dose-dependent manner, and this effect may actually outlast the analgesic effect of the drug by hours.[658,659] Different approaches have been used for this problem, including indwelling urinary catheterization and the use of opioid antagonists.[660]

Concerns have been raised that regional analgesia could mask or delay the detection of compartment syndrome of an extremity because of the intensity or quality of analgesia produced by neural blockade.[661] Although there are several case reports in adults, this problem appears to be limited primarily to high velocity traumatic fractures and to fractures of the tibia, conditions where compartment syndrome may be more common. It is also not clear from most reports if warning signs such as breakthrough pain, were adequately heeded. Indeed, the opposite has been observed, that the onset of pain in a patient with previously adequate analgesia from an epidural or nerve block is an early warning sign that may herald the onset of compartment syndrome.[662,663] The concentration of local anesthetics used for postoperative analgesia appears to be inadequate to mask the intensity of ischemic pain caused by compartment syndrome.[664,665] The loss of effective analgesia in a child at risk of compartment syndrome should raise suspicion and prompt urgent investigation before any changes are made to the analgesic regimen and lead to early detection, rather than obscuring the diagnosis of compartment syndrome (see also Chapter 30).[662]

Catheter-Related Complications

Catheter-related complications are common, with an incidence of around 5% in most studies.[9,485] Although they are generally minor, a nonfunctioning catheter usually results in premature discontinuation of the infusion and a reliance on opioids for analgesia. Inadequate analgesia must prompt an examination of the child and a review of the operative procedure and the analgesic technique. The dermatome level should be determined using differentiation between cold and warm sensation in children who are cognitively and developmentally able to cooperate. The presence of a dermatome level suggests a successful block of inadequate height. No demonstrable blockade suggests a primary malfunction, although low concentrations of local anesthetic may make differentiation of the level difficult in some children. If there were difficulties during catheter placement coupled with a lack of effective analgesia when the child emerges from general anesthesia, the catheter is likely mispositioned. We often use epidurography in this situation to determine whether the catheter is in the epidural space. Misplacement in various locations has been reported, including the subdural space, paravertebral space, tissue planes adjacent to the spine, and even in an epidural blood vessel after a negative test dose.[9,588,593,666–668] The catheter's location can be easily visualized on a plain radiograph (or with fluoroscopy in the operating room) after the injection of a small volume of nonionic contrast agent. Contrast agent in the epidural space has a characteristic "bubbly" appearance, with the contrast agent centrally located over the spinal column (Fig. 41.10). The existence of a median raphe in the epidural space has been postulated and may be the cause of unilateral multi-dermatome blockade.[669] This has been demonstrated on epidurography when unilateral blockade has occurred (Fig. 41.11). A single unilateral dermatomal band of analgesia or temperature-sensation change may indicate that the catheter has passed through a spinal foramen. In some cases,

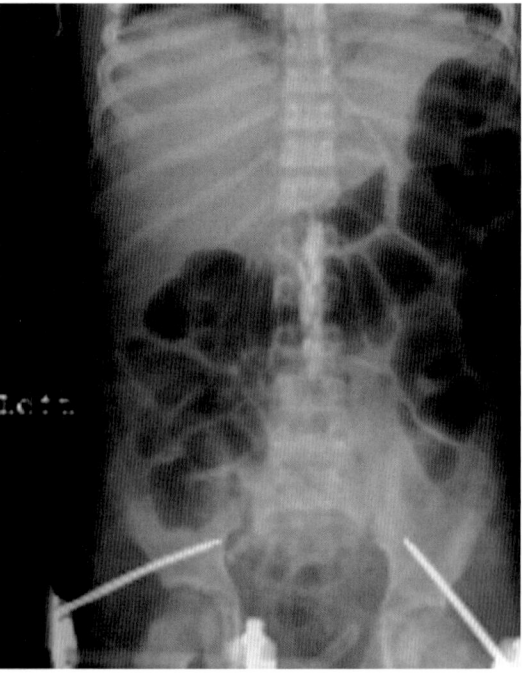

FIGURE 41.10 An epidurogram shows the appearance of the contrast agent centered in the spinal column and also the bubbly appearance of the contrast agent, presumably produced by the epidural fat and plexus.

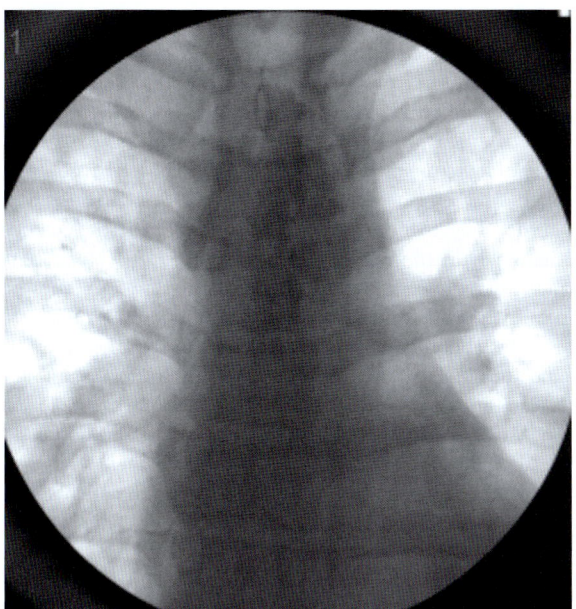

FIGURE 41.11 Epidurogram taken with fluoroscopy demonstrating unilateral spread of contrast agent. The contrast agent appears to have a very sharp edge precisely in the center of the spinal column, demarcating one side of the epidural space from the other.

simply withdrawing the catheter 1 or 2 cm may allow proper repositioning within the epidural space. A functional, rather than anatomic, method of confirming epidural placement is the "chloroprocaine test," which has the advantage of both providing rapid analgesia (with a properly located catheter) and confirming the site of placement. A chloroprocaine test is presented in Fig. 41.12.

The catheter site should be inspected daily to ensure that the dressing is intact and to assess for the presence of infection. Infections are exceedingly rare, perhaps in part because of the bactericidal properties of the local anesthetics themselves.[670] Although colonization of catheters (usually with *Staphylococcus epidermidis* and other Gram-positive organisms) appears common, adult and pediatric studies have shown that this is not associated with neuraxial infection.[9,671,672] In the UK epidural audit, there were three cases of deep tissue infection and 25 local infections reported out of 10,660 epidural catheters,[601] and longitudinal data from a single institution showed similar rates of infection.[671,672] The Pediatric Regional Anesthesia Network reported one epidural abscess in a 2-month old and 92 local cutaneous infections in 18,065 continuous catheter placements; cutaneous infection was associated with longer median catheter insertion duration.[588] Tunneling a catheter subcutaneously may reduce the risk of bacteriologic contamination and permit the use of a catheter for a greater period of time.[586,587] A study of the microbiology of the infusion fluids and delivery systems has demonstrated that catheter-related

PROCEDURE FOR THE CHLOROPROCAINE TEST

An anesthesiologist is present for the procedure with use of standard monitors and supplies for providing respiratory or hemodynamic support.

1. A loading dose of chloroprocaine 3% is divided in five equal increments, each given at 1- to 2-minute intervals (over 5-10 minutes total) according to weight approximately as follows: (doses may be adjusted according to clinical circumstances)

Weight Group	Increment Volume	Total Volume
0-10 kg	0.125 mL/kg	0.6 mL/kg
10-20 kg	0.1 mL/kg	0.5 mL/kg
20-35 kg	2.5 mL (fixed volume)	12.5 mL (fixed volume)
35-60 kg	3 mL (fixed volume)	15 mL (fixed volume)
≥60 kg	3.5 mL (fixed volume)	17.5 mL (fixed volume)

2. Incremental dosing is stopped before giving the full dose if there are clear signs of bilateral lower extremity sensory or motor block, or a very definite reduction in heart rate (e.g., 30 beats/min) and blood pressure (e.g., 25-mm Hg drop in systolic pressure). In most cases, because you are performing this test because of signs of pain, there is some tachycardia and hypertension relative to baseline values at the start of the test. Transient cessation of crying in an infant or toddler is not a sufficiently specific positive response to warrant interruption of the test.

3. A catheter positioned in the **thoracic** epidural space will generally not show lower extremity sensory or motor block with the chloroprocaine test, but should give a very clear drop in heart rate and blood pressure, as well as a clear and persistent reduction in pain reports or pain behaviors.

4. If the chloroprocaine test is positive (i.e., confirms epidural placement), this implies that a stronger or different epidural solution is needed for steady-state pain relief. Because hydromorphone is sufficiently hydrophilic to spread from lumbar to thoracic spinal levels, **switching the solution from bupivacaine-fentanyl to bupivacaine-hydromorphone will provide good steady-state pain relief in >90% of these cases**. A typical loading dose of hydromorphone of 2 μg/kg (0.002 mg/kg) will provide analgesia within 30 minutes in most cases.

If the chloroprocaine test fails to confirm epidural placement, the catheter is repositioned, removed, or replaced according to clinical circumstances.

FIGURE 41.12 Chloroprocaine test to determine regional catheter function as performed at Children's Hospital, Boston. (Personal communication, C. Berde.)

infections of the deep tissues, including epidural abscess, appear to have their origin in local skin infections that track along the catheter's path or via a bacteremia.[673] *Any sign of local infection is cause for immediate catheter removal.* Epidural abscess is a catastrophic complication that can be generally avoided if the catheter is removed early, when only a localized cutaneous infection is present.[674] Clinical signs include fever, malaise, and back pain. Specific neurologic signs, paresthesia, and motor symptoms (e.g., flaccid paralysis as cord compression develops, eventually progressing to spasticity) may occur late in the course if early warning signs are not heeded but may progress rapidly once established. Children who develop fever or sepsis need to be evaluated on an individual basis. If a clear source for the fever is found, it is acceptable to leave the catheter in place with regular and frequent observation and reassessment, although we remove it if a child is overtly septic or if the situation is unclear.

Plexus and Peripheral Nerve Catheters

Catheters may be placed adjacent to upper and lower extremity plexuses or adjacent to individual nerves. When major analgesic needs are not expected to exceed 24 hours, the prolonged duration of analgesia after a single-injection plexus block reduces the need for an indwelling catheter in many instances, and duration of action can be further prolonged by the adjunctive use of dexamethasone.[512] A systematic review of 29 randomized adult trials involving 1695 patients receiving various nerve blocks concluded that dexamethasone (4 or 8 mg) added to the local anesthetic shortened the time of onset and prolonged the duration of both the sensory and the motor block with no serious adverse events.[266] Specialized kits for peripheral nerve and plexus cannulation are commercially available. These catheters are inserted using the same ultrasound landmarks and techniques as for placing a single-injection block. After initial dosing, 0.125% bupivacaine or 0.2% ropivacaine at 0.1 to 0.2 mL/kg per hour may be infused. Potential complications of continuous plexus or peripheral nerve blockade include infection and nerve injury, although these are quite rare, and no persistent neurologic deficits have been reported in major pediatric databases.[485,590]

Infusions can be delivered with conventional infusion pumps or disposable elastomeric controlled infusion devices described earlier. Although conventional infusion pumps can be used for inpatients owing to reduced cost and to the increased safety that may be inherent in the familiarity of the inpatient nurses with such systems, initiating the infusion with the elastomeric pump is now more commonly done, which eliminates tubing reconnections and the risk of infection and connection error, and increases simplicity. The disposable devices permit the child to be discharged home and still receive long-lasting analgesia with a regional anesthetic. Most commonly, 0.2% ropivacaine is used at rates of 0.1 to 0.2 mL/kg per hour.[485] An organized system of daily follow-up by telephone or visiting nurses is essential for safety and efficacy of such a service, but both limited published and anecdotal experience suggests that ambulatory analgesia with peripheral neural blockade can be an effective modality in pediatric outpatients.[485,590] Catheters with multiple side holes can be placed in a fascial plane or wound bed by the surgeon at the time of closure and local anesthetics are infused over several days for postoperative analgesia. There are now increasing numbers of pediatric studies that have reported successful responses when dexamethasone is added to local anesthetics.[122,134,485,590,631–635,675,676] Infusion rates and volumes of 2 to 5 mL/hour of 0.2% ropivacaine are most commonly used, infused via the elastomeric pumps.

Fascial Plane Catheters

Fascial plane regional anesthetic techniques have garnered extensive interest over the past decade. These techniques, including the quadratus lumborum block (QLB),[677] transversus abdominis plane block (TAP),[482,678–680] and erector spinae block,[681–683] target local anesthetic deposition into muscle interfascial tissue planes through which distal sensory nerves traverse and then travel to reach their targets for sensory innervation of a specific cutaneous dermatomal distribution. For example, the TAP block is performed with ultrasound guidance by depositing local anesthetic solution within the tissue plane between the interior oblique and transversus abdominis muscles and provides sensory blockade to cutaneous branches of the ventral rami of the thoracoabdominal intercostal nerves. Within the pediatric literature, the majority of comparison studies for fascial plane nerve block techniques use single-shot injections. Although continuous catheters have been used for prolonged analgesia for pediatric surgical patients in case reports and case series, large-scale comparison data are lacking.[675] Despite the lack of large-scale efficacy data, initial reports are promising and these techniques continue to be used as options for advanced analgesia for specific clinical scenarios.

Removal of Catheters and Transition to Oral Analgesics

The transition from continuous regional blockade to oral analgesics should ideally be achieved without a decrement in the quality of pain relief for the child and should permit the clinician to revert to more aggressive modalities, should the decision prove to be premature. The duration of continuous blockade is dependent on the type of operation and the underlying medical and/or surgical problems of the child. Some children do well with transition to oral analgesics on the morning after surgery. For more painful procedures, such as Nuss bar placement for pectus excavatum in an adolescent, strong analgesics will be required for a longer duration. The norm in this situation is up to 3 days. We find it most effective to begin the transition from regional analgesia to oral therapy early in the morning. As soon as the regional infusion is discontinued, a dose of oral analgesic, usually an oral opioid, is administered. In addition, by this time the child should already be receiving scheduled nonopioid oral adjuvants (i.e., NSAID, acetaminophen). This ensures that the oral agents have provided their full effect before the block recedes. The catheter is not removed until the child has demonstrated that the oral agents provide adequate comfort without any residual analgesia from the block, so that blockade can be reestablished if transition fails. For children who have undergone extensive or multiple surgical procedures or those with a history of underlying chronic pain, they may need to be transitioned to scheduled or long-acting opioids (e.g., methadone) to provide sustained analgesia after catheter removal. Weaning of the opioid regimen can be accomplished over days to weeks and should be tailored to the specific needs and clinical situation of each child.

Children who are anticoagulated require special consideration before removing epidural catheters. Although there are no specific pediatric data, the recommendations of the consensus panel of the American Society of Regional Anesthesia and Pain Medicine (ASRA), last published in 2018, as well as those from several other societies are generally accepted.[474,475,477] The American Society of Regional Anesthesia and Pain Medicine report notes *"the initiation of systemic therapeutic heparin therapy for medical or surgical indications in the presence of a neuraxial catheter potentially increases the risk of hematoma formation during catheter removal."* Recommendations regarding how long to withhold heparin therapy before removing the catheter and how long to wait before restarting heparin vary based on whether the patient is receiving subcutaneous prophylactic doses (withhold 4–6 hours before removing the catheter and restart immediately after removing it) or a therapeutic IV infusion (withhold 2–4 hours before removing the catheter, restart the infusion 1 hour after removal). Fractionated or low–molecular-weight heparins pose a risk as well, compounded by several different regimens in common clinical use (once-a-day vs. twice-a-day dosing), differences between different agents, and the inability to assess the degree of anticoagulation with commonly available tests of coagulation (prothrombin time and partial thromboplastin time). The consensus panel recommends that catheters should be removed no sooner than 10 to 12 hours after the last dose of low–molecular-weight heparin with once-a-day administration, and dosing should resume no sooner than 4 hours after the catheter's removal. The use of continuous regional techniques is not recommended when twice-a-day administration is used. Many national societies have also published evidence-based guidelines that can assist in decision making, and the American Society of Regional Anesthesia and Pain Medicine has developed a smartphone app on this subject.

Pain Management in the Cognitively Impaired Child

The goals of pain management in the child who is cognitively impaired are the same as for those who are not impaired: to minimize discomfort, maximize function, and improve the quality of life. However, cognitively impaired children can pose a challenge in terms of assessing a child's pain, so it is important to use guardian and nursing input to synthesize a global assessment of the level of pain and the effect of interventions.[684] With these goals in mind, the child's pain management plans should include multimodal pharmacologic and nonpharmacologic strategies tailored to the severity and etiology of pain. The World Health Organization's analgesic guideline[230] provides a framework for decision making related to analgesic use based on severity and persistence of pain.

OPIOID ANALGESICS

The use of opioids in children with cognitive impairment has been limited by concerns regarding potential adverse effects and a perceived reduced margin of safety because of diminished cardiorespiratory reserve and neurologic impairment. Indeed, one study identified that cognitive impairment was an independent predictor of adverse events from PCA/nurse-controlled analgesia.[106] Therefore, it is necessary to carefully balance the goals of providing adequate analgesia while minimizing adverse events related to analgesic treatments. For moderate to severe pain, scheduled nonopioid analgesics combined with judicious use of opioids titrated to effect is a suitable option. Children with cognitive impairment may lack the cognitive and motor skills to use PCA devices successfully. In these children, nurse-controlled analgesia or caregiver-controlled analgesia permits titration of small amounts of opioids to effect, without significantly increasing nursing workload.[685] A study of children whose postoperative pain was managed by parent- or nurse-controlled analgesia reported low pain scores and modest opioid requirements, with the use of basal infusions in addition to bolus dosing, in the majority of children.[686] Adverse effects included nausea and vomiting, and pruritus requiring treatment in 14% and 32% of children, respectively. Supplemental oxygen was required in 79% of the children,

and naloxone was required in 2.8% for respiratory depression. The management of two children was remarkable, in that one had received an average morphine dose of 0.045 mg/kg per hour and four concomitant sedatives, including diphenhydramine, diazepam, droperidol, and chloral hydrate, and the second had received only a small dose of morphine and no other sedatives, but the basal infusion of morphine was implicated as the cause of respiratory depression. Both recovered without sequelae. The studies noted previously highlight the importance of frequent and careful assessment of pain, depth of sedation, and respiratory status (using continuous pulse oximetry and/or noninvasive capnography) to ensure the safety and comfort of children who are cognitively impaired and receiving opioid therapy.

NONOPIOID ANALGESICS

Nonopioid adjuvants, such as acetaminophen, NSAIDs, or other adjuncts (e.g., ketamine, gabapentin), should be added to provide synergistic multimodal analgesia and to reduce opioid requirements. They may be administered orally or via gastrostomy tubes or IV if necessary. Intravenous ketorolac provides excellent analgesia in children who have not initiated oral intake after surgery, although the risks of platelet dysfunction must be considered if ongoing bleeding is an issue. The α_2-agonist clonidine has also been used for its synergistic analgesic effects in these patients. However, it has the potential to cause sedation and hypotension with doses larger than 1 to 2 µg/kg.

Muscle spasms and clonus are an ongoing source of pain that may be difficult to differentiate in children who are cognitively impaired, and may be exacerbated after surgical procedures, particularly orthopedic and neurosurgical procedures. Pain related to skeletal muscle spasm can often be identified by its episodic and severe qualities. Caregivers will often describe their child as having episodes of sudden, severe pain, seemingly unprovoked, and this may resolve after seconds to minutes or persist for longer. Diazepam, baclofen, and tizanidine all effectively treat acute painful muscle spasms after surgery in children with spasticity, but all of these medications have sedative effects, which can confound patient assessments when used with opioids. Benzodiazepines in particular have synergistic respiratory depressant effects when used in conjunction with opioids, so judicious use is essential.

EPIDURAL AND REGIONAL ANALGESIA

Epidural analgesia has been used with success in children who are cognitively impaired who are undergoing lower extremity orthopedic procedures, selective dorsal rhizotomy, and Nissen fundoplication.[119,687] Epidural catheters may be technically difficult to place in some of these children because of contractures and spine deformities. However, when feasible, this technique provides excellent analgesia, reduces muscle spasms, and promotes overall child comfort, with a small incidence of sedation and respiratory depression. Some children will still experience muscle spasms and will require intermittent benzodiazepines. Epidurals have been compared with systemic opioids in children with cerebral palsy undergoing selective dorsal rhizotomy.[119,688] Epidural catheters were placed under direct visualization by the neurosurgeon at the end of surgery. Both studies showed improved analgesia in the epidural groups, and one study demonstrated a smaller incidence of desaturation in the epidural group, which allowed patients in this group to go directly to the general ward (instead of the pediatric ICU).[688] In summary, these studies support the attributes and safety of epidural analgesia in children who are cognitively impaired.

Children with cerebral palsy who received continuous infusion of local anesthetics via catheters tunneled into the incision site following orthopedic surgery experienced better pain scores and required less oral analgesics on the first two postoperative days, compared with controls who received oral analgesics alone.[675] Although data related to peripheral and plexus blocks in cognitively impaired children are limited, our experience suggests that these, too, are safe and effective in this population and can contribute to reducing the reliance on systemic analgesics and, thereby, their adverse effects.

Emerging data must be used to guide treatment plans and protocols that incorporate frequent evaluation and careful monitoring of children who are cognitively impaired. A multidisciplinary pain team led by an anesthesiologist with expertise in postoperative pain management and that includes a primary care clinician, psychologist, nurse, physical therapist and occupational therapist is required to provide the expertise needed to care for these children with special needs.[689]

ANNOTATED REFERENCES

Berde CB, Sethna NF. Analgesics for the treatment of pain in children. *N Engl J Med.* 2002;347(14):1094-1103.

This authoritative reference provides a succinct yet complete review of the pharmacology of effective analgesic regimens in children.

Eccleston C, Fisher E, Howard RF, et al. Delivering transformative action in paediatric pain: a Lancet Child & Adolescent Health Commission. *Lancet Child Adolesc Health.* 2021;5:47-87.

This reference reviews current knowledge concerning pediatric pain and sets out to discuss how we further answer that which remains unknown. It is a roadmap to guide future acute and chronic pain research.

Llewellyn N, Moriarty A. The national pediatric epidural audit. *Paediatr Anaesth.* 2007;17(6):520-533.

The largest prospective study on epidural anesthesia to date followed patients into the postoperative period and highlights the incidence and nature of complications and adverse events, which were rare. This should be read in conjunction with the French-Language Society of Paediatric Anaesthesiologists study[603] and the Pediatric Regional Anesthesia Network studies.

Lynn AM, Nespeca MK, Opheim KE, Slattery JT. Respiratory effects of intravenous morphine infusions in neonates, infants, and children after cardiac surgery. *Anesth Analg.* 1993;77(4):695-701.

This old but important study identified the threshold serum morphine concentration for respiratory depression in neonates, infants, and children receiving continuous morphine infusions following heart surgery to be 20 ng/mL and, as such, provides a framework to guide appropriate dosing of morphine in these populations. The authors recommended careful observation of all children receiving morphine because of the wide variability in the CO_2 response slope seen in their subjects.

Malviya S, Voepel-Lewis T, Burke C, et al. The revised FLACC observational pain tool: improved reliability and validity for pain assessment in children with cognitive impairment. *Pediatr Anesth.* 2006;16: 258-265.

The FLACC tool was revised to incorporate behavioral descriptors consistently associated with pain in cognitively impaired children. This paper describes the development of the Revised Face, Legs, Activity, Cry, Consolability (r-FLACC) scale and demonstrates its reliability and validity in assessing pain in this vulnerable population.

Maxwell LG, Kaufmann SC, Bitzer S, et al. The effects of a small-dose naloxone infusion on opioid-induced side effects and analgesia in children and adolescents treated with intravenous patient-controlled analgesia: a double-blind, prospective, randomized, controlled study. *Anesth Analg.* 2005;100(4):953-958.

This study demonstrated that a low-dose naloxone infusion significantly reduced the incidence and severity of opioid-induced adverse effects, including pruritus and nausea, without affecting opioid-induced analgesia. These data address the important clinical problem of opioid-induced adverse effects that frequently limits the utility of opioids in the treatment of pain.

Michelet D, Andreu-Gallien J, Bensalah T, et al. A meta-analysis of the use of nonsteroidal anti-inflammatory drugs for pediatric postoperative pain. *Anesth Analg.* 2012;114:393-406.

This meta-analysis shows that perioperative NSAID administration reduces opioid consumption and PONV during the postoperative period in children. In 27 randomized controlled trials, perioperative administration of NSAIDs reduced opioid requirement in the postanesthesia care unit (PACU), and for the first 24 hours after surgery, decreased pain intensity in the PACU and PONV. Results from this study suggest that multimodal analgesia should be used in an effort to reduce opioid consumption and adverse effects in children undergoing surgery.

Morton NS, Errera A. APA national audit of pediatric opioid infusions. *Paediatr Anaesth.* 2010;20:119-125.

This very large prospective audit of opioid infusions of all types (continuous, PCA, nurse-controlled analgesia) confirmed the safety of these techniques, but highlights the potential complications and pitfalls that are always present. Respiratory depression and pump programming errors each occurred in about 1 of 766 cases and 1 of 631 cases, respectively, and there was one permanent injury (1 of 10,000 cases).

Polaner DM, Taenzer AH, Walker BJ, et al. Pediatric Regional Anesthesia Network: a multi-institutional study of the use and incidence of complications of pediatric regional anesthesia. *Anesth Analg.* 2012;115(6): 1353-1364.

This is the first report from this network in the United States that prospectively examined the incidence of adverse events and complications in nearly 15,000 regional blocks in children. There were no permanent complications detected. The Pediatric Regional Anesthesia Network now has over 140,000 cases accrued. These data provided similar results to those reported in the French study.[603]

Voepel-Lewis T, Burke CN, Jeffreys N, et al. Do 0–10 numeric rating scores translate into clinically meaningful pain measures for children? *Anesth Analg.* 2011;112:415-421.

This study provides important information regarding the clinical interpretation of NRS pain scores in children. Ten NRS scores were found to be reliably associated with the child's perceived need for medicine, perceived pain relief, and satisfaction with pain treatment. However, a significant overlap in scores associated with these outcomes suggests that the use of specific cutoff scores to guide treatment decisions would be inappropriate in children.

von Baeyer CL, Spagrud LJ. Systematic review of observational (behavioral) measures of pain for children and adolescents aged 3 to 18 years. *Pain.* 2007;127(1-2):140-150.

This is a comprehensive review of the numerous behavioral-observational measures of pain for children and identifies the most appropriate tools for assessing pain in various settings, including the postoperative period and in critical care.

A complete reference list can be found online at Elsevier eBooks+.

Appendix 41.1   Clinical Examples of Postoperative Analgesic Management Strategy

41

Case 1

A 2-year-old child, ASA 1 (American Society of Anesthesiologists physical status classification system, category 1) presented for inguinal hernia repair, weight 15 kg.

CONSIDERATIONS

- Mildly painful surgery
- Outpatient setting—avoidance of nausea and oversedation is helpful

ALTERNATIVES

1. Ilioinguinal nerve block: bupivacaine 0.25% with epinephrine 1:200,000, 0.2 to 0.3 mL/kg × 15 kg = 3 to 5 mL (3.75 mL on each side) or similar volume of ropivacaine 0.2%. Either can be administered in conjunction with IV dexamethasone to prolong block duration.
2. Wound infiltration with bupivacaine 0.25% with epinephrine 1:200,000, 0.5 mL/kg × 15 kg = 7.5 mL (3.75 mL on each side).
3. Caudal block using bupivacaine 0.125% to 0.25% with epinephrine 1:200,000, 0.5 to 0.75 mL/kg × 15 kg = 7 to 11 mL.
4. Add acetaminophen, 10 to 15 mg/kg every 4 to 6 hours (oral), or ibuprofen, 5 to 10 mg/kg every 6 hours.
5. Consider adding IV ketorolac 0.5 mg/kg to intraoperative management at conclusion of surgery and consultation with surgeon.

Case 2

A 6-month-old, 6-kg child, ASA 1, presented for ureteral reimplantation.

CONSIDERATIONS

- Moderately painful surgery, bladder spasms
- Urinary retention is not an issue
- Pain assessment using behavioral tools such as the *Face, Legs, Activity, Cry, Consolability (FLACC) scale*

ALTERNATIVES

1. Epidural analgesia
   - For caudal approach, need to cover approximately 10 dermatomes (5 sacral, 5 lumbar); initial bolus, 10 × 0.05 mL/kg per dermatome × 6 kg = 3.0 mL. May reduce bolus dose to 0.3 to 0.5 mL/kg for direct lumbar placement.
   - Bupivacaine 0.1% with hydromorphone, 3 μg/mL, starting at 0.2 mL/kg per hour × 6 kg = 1.2 mL/hour, or similar volume of ropivacaine 0.1% with clonidine 0.5 μg/mL.
   - Apnea monitoring, pulse oximetry, and frequent observation.
   - Add scheduled acetaminophen, 10 to 15 mg/kg every 4 to 6 hours (oral) or 15 mg/kg every 6 hours (IV), or 35 to 40 mg/kg initial dose (rectal) followed by 20 mg/kg every 6 hours (rectal) not to exceed 100 mg/kg per day (rectal).
   - Add ketorolac 0.5 mg/kg every 6 hours for 48 hours for bladder spasms.

2. Continuous IV morphine infusion
   - Loading dose of up to 0.075 to 0.1 mg/kg × 6 kg = 0.45 to 0.6 mg in incremental doses if needed.
   - Infusion starting at 0.02 mg/kg per hour (20 μg/kg per hour) × 6 kg = 0.12 mg/hour.
   - Apnea monitoring, continuous pulse oximetry, and frequent observation.
   - Add scheduled acetaminophen and NSAID if possible.
3. Nurse-controlled analgesia (NCA) with morphine
   - Loading dose 0.05 to 0.1 mg/kg × 6 kg = 0.3 to 0.6 mg administered via patient-controlled anesthesia (PCA) pump in the postanesthesia care unit (PACU).
   - Continuous basal infusion of 0.01 to 0.02 mg/kg per hour.
   - Bolus dose of 0.02 to 0.03 mg/kg.
   - Lockout interval: 8 to 15 minutes.
   - 4-hour limit of 0.25 to 0.3 mg/kg.
   - Apnea monitoring, continuous pulse oximetry, and frequent observation.
   - Add scheduled acetaminophen and NSAID if possible.

Case 3

A 6-week-old, 3-kg child, ASA 3, presented for thoracoabdominal incision for excision of a Wilms tumor.

CONSIDERATIONS

- Painful surgery.
- Pain assessment using behavioral tools such as FLACC.
- Impairment of respiration.
- Many dermatomes involved.
- Bladder catheter warranted.

ALTERNATIVES

1. A continuous epidural infusion (direct placement at T8–T9 or inserted through the caudal approach and threaded to the mid-portion of the surgical incision)
   - For caudal approach, need to cover approximately 16 dermatomes (5 sacral, 5 lumbar, 6 thoracic): Initial bolus 16 × 0.05 mL/kg per dermatome × 3 kg = 2.4 mL loading dose. May reduce bolus dose to 0.3 to 0.5 mL/kg for direct thoracic placement. The infusion could be chloroprocaine 1.5% at 0.2 to 0.3 mL/kg per hour or ropivacaine 0.1% to 0.2% at a dose not exceeding 0.2 mg/kg per hour.
   - Add scheduled acetaminophen if possible.
   - PRN IV opioid should be available.
   - Apnea monitoring, continuous pulse oximetry, and frequent observation.
2. Nurse-controlled analgesia with morphine
   - Loading dose of 0.05 to 0.1 mg/kg × 6 kg = 0.3 to 0.6 mg administered via PCA pump in the PACU.
   - Continuous basal infusion of 0.01 to 0.02 mg/kg per hour.
   - Bolus dose of 0.02 to 0.03 mg/kg.
   - Lockout interval: 8 to 15 minutes.
   - 4-hour limit of 0.25 to 0.3 mg/kg.

- Apnea monitoring, continuous pulse oximetry, and frequent observation.
- Add acetaminophen 10 to 15 mg/kg every 4 hours (oral) or 35 to 40 mg/kg initial dose (rectal) followed by 20 mg/kg every 6 hours (rectal) not to exceed 100 mg/kg per day. IV acetaminophen 15 mg/kg every 6 hours may be used instead.

Case 4

An 8-year-old, 18-kg girl with cerebral palsy, severe cognitive impairment, ASA 3, presented for femoral osteotomy.

CONSIDERATIONS
- Painful surgery.
- Altered/individual pain behaviors: use specific tools for pain assessment such as r-FLACC.
- Potential for altered pain perception.
- Increased risk of opioid-induced respiratory depression.
- May need benzodiazepines for muscle spasms.

ALTERNATIVES
1. Continuous epidural analgesia
   - For caudal approach, need to cover approximately 10 dermatomes (5 sacral, 5 lumbar); initial bolus, 10 × 0.05 mL/kg per dermatome × 18 kg = 9 mL. May reduce bolus to 0.3 to 0.5 mL/kg for direct lumbar placement.
   - Bupivacaine 0.1% with hydromorphone 3 µg/mL, starting at 0.2 mL/kg per hour × 18 kg = 3.6 mL/hour.
   - Apnea monitoring, pulse oximetry, and frequent observation.
   - Add acetaminophen scheduled, 10 to 15 mg/kg every 4 hours (oral) or 35 to 40 mg/kg initial dose (rectal) followed by 20 mg/kg every 6 hours (rectal), not to exceed 100 mg/kg per day (rectal). IV acetaminophen 15 mg/kg every 6 hours may also be added.
   - Add scheduled NSAID if possible.

2. Femoral nerve, fascia iliaca, or lumbar plexus block
   - There is the need to block the distribution of the femoral, lateral femoral cutaneous, and obturator nerves.
   - Single-injection block of the peripheral nerves will provide analgesia for 8 to 16 hours; a continuous catheter technique will provide greater duration of analgesia.
   - Blockade of just the upper leg is provided without risks of urinary retention or motor block of the contralateral leg.
   - 0.2% ropivacaine or 0.125% to 0.25% bupivacaine; initial dose of 0.3 mL/kg = 5.4 mL, followed by infusion of 0.2 mL/kg per hour = 3.6 mL/hour.
   - Add scheduled acetaminophen and NSAID if possible, and diazepam as needed for muscle spasms.

3. Continuous IV morphine infusion
   - Loading dose of up to 0.05 to 0.1 mg/kg × 18 kg = 0.9 to 1.8 mg in incremental doses if needed.
   - Infusion starting at 0.02 mg/kg per hour (20 µg/kg per hour) × 18 kg = 0.36 mg/hour.
   - Apnea monitoring, continuous pulse oximetry, and frequent observation.
   - Add scheduled acetaminophen and NSAID if possible.
   - Consider IV/PO diazepam, 0.05 to 0.1 mg/kg, for muscle spasms.

4. Nurse-controlled analgesia with morphine
   - Loading dose 0.05 to 0.1 mg/kg × 18 kg = 0.9 to 1.8 mg administered via PCA pump in PACU.
   - Continuous basal infusion of 0.01 to 0.02 mg/kg per hour.
   - Bolus dose of 0.02 to 0.03 mg/kg.
   - Lockout interval: 8 to 15 minutes.
   - 4-hour limit of 0.25 to 0.3 mg/kg.
   - Apnea monitoring, continuous pulse oximetry, and frequent observation.
   - Add scheduled acetaminophen and NSAID if possible.
   - Consider IV/oral diazepam, 0.05 to 0.1 mg/kg, for muscle spasms.

Chronic Pain 42

ALEXANDRA SZABOVA, KENNETH GOLDSCHNEIDER, AND MOTAZ AWAD

Chronic Pain in Children
The Multidisciplinary Approach
The Pain Physician
The Psychologist
The Physical Therapist
The Nurse
The Consultant
General Approach to Management
History
Physical Examination
Ancillary Data
Patient and Family Education
Chronic Pain Conditions

Abdominal Pain
Headache
Complex Regional Pain Syndrome
Musculoskeletal Pain
Rheumatologic and Musculoskeletal Pain
Pain in Sickle Cell Disease, Trait, and Variants
Pain Pharmacotherapy
Acetaminophen
Nonsteroidal Antiinflammatory Drugs
The "Opioid Epidemic" and Pain Management
Adjuvant Drugs
Complementary Therapies

AS THE PRACTICING PEDIATRIC ANESTHESIOLOGIST, you will encounter chronic pain in one of three main settings: a child presenting to the operating room, when providing care for a child referred from a colleague of another specialty, or during rounds on the acute pain service. In this chapter we focus on the essential approaches to children with chronic pain and provide some guidelines to assist in helping the patient and colleagues who request your assistance.

Chronic Pain in Children

Chronic pain affects large numbers of children.[1] Back pain has been reported in up to 50% of children by the mid-teens,[2] and abdominal pain occurs weekly in up to 17%.[3] Other commonly encountered conditions include headaches, chronic regional pain syndrome (CRPS), fibromyalgia, limb pain, chest pain, and joint pain.

Pain can also be related to several chronic medical conditions. Such forms of pain can be complex and blur the boundaries between acute and chronic pain treatment. These conditions include sickle cell disease, cystic fibrosis,[4] epidermolysis bullosa,[5] inflammatory bowel disease,[6] chronic pancreatitis,[7] and cancer. Individuals with these diseases are predisposed to pain and may require more hospitalizations than those with many other conditions. At times, the severity of pain can be substantial. Given that these children present with pain in the hospital, medical care is often guided by the model for acute pain treatment, with pharmacotherapy as the basis. Psychosocial factors heavily influence the child's ability to cope and can either improve or worsen the child's suffering, depending on personal and family factors.[8,9] Therefore, it is appropriate to involve psychology, child life, and physical therapy consultations as part of the therapeutic plan. The ultimate plan for these medical conditions is to stabilize the patient's condition and return the child home. After discharge, the patient remains vulnerable to enduring pain and dysfunction. Therefore, discharge planning may need to integrate treatment of acute pain with management of long-term symptoms and impairment as well as potential weaning from opioids.

The Multidisciplinary Approach

The model of care that appears to work optimally for children with chronic pain is one in which there are multiple disciplines involved in developing a coordinated care plan.[10,11] In the outpatient setting, there is a pain physician, a psychologist, nurses, and a physical therapist. At times, a neurologist or physiatrist may be involved. If, as an anesthesiologist, you are consulted to care for a child with chronic pain, it will be useful to keep these disciplines in mind and include them in your recommendations for care. Advocating for involvement of other therapies will be an advance in the patient's care over simply suggesting a regional block or medication.

THE PAIN PHYSICIAN

As a consulting anesthesiologist in an inpatient setting, you may be called to provide care for one of three reasons. First, you may be asked to perform a regional nerve block, such as an epidural steroid injection for magnetic resonance imaging-confirmed discogenic pain or epidural catheter placement to assist physical therapy. This consult is fairly straightforward and is an extension of basic regional anesthesia principles. Second, a child may present to the hospital on chronic opioids or other medications that have implications for anesthesia or postoperative pain management. This situation requires checking for drug interactions and chronic medications; this is an extension of basic perioperative anesthesia skills. Third, your input may be requested regarding assessing and diagnosing the source of pain. This last scenario is the most complex, requires taking a detailed history and performing a physical examination, and will most likely require multidisciplinary care from the initial evaluation and extending into treatment.

THE PSYCHOLOGIST

Pain is more than just a physical phenomenon. It can cause and be worsened by stress, suffering, family tension and dysfunction, anxiety, and depression.[12,13] Pain can disrupt almost any aspect of a child's and the family's life. Family and school problems can worsen a painful condition and dramatically reduce a child's level of function. The family is always involved in the child's suffering and should therefore be included in the pain evaluation process. Thus, psychological assessment is a central component in the evaluation and treatment of chronic painful conditions.

Often, families are wary at the thought of seeing a psychologist and afraid of being stigmatized. They must be judiciously counseled to disavow this concern. It is important to address and validate the child's pain and suffering, regardless of whether an obvious organic cause is identified. The child must be treated as a person, not just as a painful body part; this principle should be emphatically described to the child's family.

Psychology-based therapy includes relaxation training, biofeedback, hypnotherapy, coping skills training, and psychotherapy. Biofeedback is a modality that trains the child to become more aware of their body, enhancing the sense of control over it. Therapies aimed at parental and familial aspects of the child's pain include teaching strategies for behavioral interventions (e.g., distraction), activity pacing, consistent discipline, coaching skills training, stress management, and occasionally family therapy.

THE PHYSICAL THERAPIST

Physical therapy is a crucial component of evaluating and treating chronic pain. Painful conditions can cause loss of muscle strength and range of motion. Alterations in the use of a limb affect the biomechanics and activities of daily function. Children can become deconditioned and require a reconditioning program to restore lost strength and stamina. These changes may not only affect the original pain site but also generate secondary pain problems that will also need to be addressed.

Importantly, physical therapy can benefit many painful conditions (e.g., myofascial pain improves with stretching and range-of-motion exercises) and also be the cornerstone of treatment for others (e.g., CRPS).[14] Emphasizing self-reliance and responsibility for their own care is an important aspect of caring for adolescents. However, one cannot expect young children, or older ones in pain, to work aggressively at home without beginning with a structured program. Parental involvement is especially important for younger children, but one must be careful to position them to be encouraging and supportive while not making them their child's taskmasters.

Rehabilitative therapies include stretching, strengthening, and reconditioning programs; range-of-motion exercises and endurance training are important. Aquatic therapy is very useful for those children who are non–weight-bearing or have limited range of motion or strength. Massage, heat, and cold therapies are helpful adjuncts to increase functioning and enhance other physical therapy modalities.

Transcutaneous electrical nerve stimulation (TENS) is an effective, low-risk, analgesic therapy that is usually provided under the guidance of a physical therapist.[15] TENS is excellent for localized pain. The fact that it is portable, can be used discreetly, and has few side effects makes it attractive for use at school. Tolerance to TENS can develop with prolonged use, so children need to limit use to no longer than 2 hours at a time. They can take a break for an equal amount of time to that which they used the TENS, then restart it.

THE NURSE

Pain nurses play a major role in hospital-wide education of floor nurses regarding assessment and treatment of pain, including the use of epidural and patient-controlled analgesia (PCA) pumps. If you are asked to start seeing chronic pain patients, your first personnel request should be for an advanced practice nurse who can be trained to triage and perform the initial evaluation and intake assessment as well as assist with all subsequent pain-related issues that do not require the direct input of a physician.

THE CONSULTANT

Being cognizant of our limitations should lead to judicious use of consultants to help make or confirm diagnoses and fashion the best treatment plan for a variety of painful conditions. Neurologists are generally well versed in headache management, including use of the many medications indicated for neuropathic pain. They can help with the diagnosis of peripheral neuropathies. Physical medicine and rehabilitation specialists can assist in structuring a treatment plan for a variety of musculoskeletal pains and are facile in the treatment of spasticity.

General Approach to Management

Most children with chronic, noncancer pain are adolescents who require a number of special considerations regarding both history and physical examination. First, adolescent behavior can fluctuate as they transition from childhood to adulthood. It is important to always ask questions directly to them, but also involve the parents to the extent needed to obtain the relevant and complete history. A very useful approach is to refer to older pediatric patients as "young adults" instead of "children" when talking with the child and family, because even 12- and 13-year-olds like to think they are no longer children. Do not try to be "cool" with the adolescent patient, because teenagers tend to find that condescending and will respond negatively, even if you mean well. Thus, it is most useful to "play it straight"; and if patients seem uneasy with the questions, acknowledge their feelings and reassure them you are asking only what is needed in order to help them. Often you can find a point of common interest and use that to establish a greater rapport. Adolescents tend to be very image conscious. They may or may not want to discuss body functions such as defecation or menstruation, especially in the presence of their parents, even when these functions are directly relevant to the problem.

HISTORY

The basic history focuses on the pain: location, duration, quality, intensity, aggravating and alleviating factors, associated symptoms, what therapies have been tried, and what tests have been performed and by whom. Pain intensity is often assessed via a 0 to 10 numeric rating scale for children older than approximately 8 years of age. The child must be asked about the current pain level and the "best" and "worst" pain levels to obtain an idea of

TABLE 42.1	Principles of Pain Education

Goals

1. Pain as experience, not just as nociception; understanding the role of pain and how it is altered in chronic pain
2. Understand chronic pain as no longer a signal of harm (pain is real but nonprotective)
3. Reduce anxiety and catastrophic thinking
4. Facilitate a more active coping strategy
5. Challenge (in nonthreatening manner) existing knowledge and how they think about pain and how they can incorporate new knowledge about it

Tools/Approaches

1. Ask the patient what they understand, what they have been told in the past, and what their concerns are
2. Use methods that play to patient learning styles:
   a. Visual – drawings, photos, online images
   b. Aural – stories, explanations, analogies
   c. Kinesthetic – hands-on demonstrations, workshops, interactive activities
3. Stop periodically and ask how they are understanding what you are trying to communicate
4. Learn and employ what motivates them

Roadblocks

1. Use of jargon and intimidating terms
2. Talking without listening
3. Failing to take enough time
4. Ignoring patient beliefs, motivations, culture, concerns

TABLE 42.2	"Red Flag" Signs and Symptoms for Abdominal Pain

- Persistent right upper or right lower quadrant pain
- Dysphagia
- Persistent or cyclic vomiting
- Gastrointestinal blood loss
- Family history of inflammatory bowel disease, celiac disease, or peptic ulcer disease
- Pain that wakes the child from sleep
- Arthritis
- Nocturnal diarrhea
- Involuntary weight loss
- Deceleration of linear growth
- Delayed puberty
- Unexplained fever
- Hepatosplenomegaly, masses, perianal lesions
- Bilious emesis
- Costovertebral angle tenderness

TABLE 42.3	"Red Flag" Signs and Symptoms for Secondary Headache

- Persistent vomiting
- Focal neurologic signs
- Meningeal signs
- Unexplained fever
- Increased intracranial pressure
- Changes in behavior or mental status
- Sudden onset of severe headache
- Morning headaches
- Headaches awakening the child from sleep

the pattern of pain and when it peaks. Quality descriptors include "burning," "sharp," "aching," "throbbing," "tingling," "numb," "weird," and others, each of which may give a clue as to the type of pain the child is experiencing. Odd descriptors, burning, and tingling suggest neuropathic pain; sharp, tight, and aching may indicate bony or muscular causes; throbbing suggests a vascular component; cramping or pain that comes in waves often suggests spasm of muscle or hollow viscus. It is also useful to ask what their understanding of the pain is, and what they have been told in the past. This information will provide context for your educational approach (see later).

A vital part of the chronic pain evaluation process is to look for "red flags." These are signs or symptoms that may indicate a serious illness. Some of the "red flag" signs and symptoms for major pain types can be found in Tables 42.1, 42.2, and 42.3. For example, a child with back pain who also has weak legs and incontinence may have a tethered spinal cord. A recurring headache that is worse in the morning and associated with vomiting suggests increased intracranial pressure. Back pain with loss of ankle jerk suggests compression of the S1 nerve root.

A complete pain evaluation comprises further history regarding medications, allergies, family history, and a thorough review of systems. Certain painful conditions have a genetic basis, such as migraine headaches,[16] fibromyalgia,[17] irritable bowel syndrome,[18] and sickle cell disease. Knowing the family history can assist in making the diagnosis. At times, the child may model their behavior after a family member. For example, if a parent has a "bad back" and is functionally compromised by that, then the child may complain of back pain as well. This does not mean the child is faking the complaints but simply patterning the behavioral response to

pain after a model that they understand. Treatment would include reassurance, cognitive behavioral therapy, and gentle physical therapy to restore the child's functional ability and help them with any underlying issues. Therefore, family and social histories can be useful in fashioning a treatment plan, in conjunction with the general history, physical examination, and relevant testing.

PHYSICAL EXAMINATION

The physical examination should focus on the area of interest, but a brief, general examination is also important. A full screening examination (including neurological exam) takes only a few minutes and can be combined with the social history. Note that there will be times when a systemic illness manifests as a localized complaint. For instance, diabetes can manifest as abdominal pain, leukemia as focal bone pain, and metabolic derangements as back, extremity, or abdominal pain.

When examining a child of the opposite sex, you should have a nonfamily observer of the same sex as the child present. Some children will be very conscious of their body and may consider routine examination maneuvers as invasions of their privacy. The occasional child will have a history of being abused and can be further traumatized by even a standard examination. A useful approach is to demonstrate examination techniques on yourself that may make the child uneasy. For example, a pinprick examination requires a needle or sharp object; touch your own skin with the probe first, to demonstrate that you will not be drawing blood. One of the authors uses the tips of a newly fractured wooden tongue depressor, which he finds to be less intimidating to kids than a needle or pin. Children are often fascinated by the deep tendon reflexes and vibration exams, so they may have fun with the examination. Often for children who have had many examinations, doing something a little different or "fun" can help them accept your examination and enhance rapport.

ANCILLARY DATA

Most often, by the time chronic pain patients have reached a pain clinic they have undergone a series of investigative tests, which must be reviewed. On the other hand, once it becomes clear that there is no life-threatening illness, the focus should shift away from further testing. This can be a hard transition for families and children to accept, especially if no concrete diagnosis has been made to explain the pain. It is a challenge for them to embrace the thought that the pain itself is the disease rather than it being a surrogate for something more sinister lurking, undiagnosed, in the shadows. So, if you believe that a study would help explain the pain, or make a diagnosis that had not been entertained, you should certainly recommend it. However, the drawback in pursuing tests and imaging in an unfocused manner is not only a waste of resources but a delay in treatment while the family holds out for a diagnosis. Until the child wholeheartedly endorses the treatment plan, and becomes active in it, the child or adolescent's chronic pain will continue unabated.

PATIENT AND FAMILY EDUCATION

Perhaps the corner piece of chronic pain treatment is educating the patient and family regarding the nature of the pain and the basis for the course of treatment. Once a tentative diagnosis has been established, the pain physician should explain the patient's chronic pain, an already complex and vague phenomenon, and make it more relatable to the patient and family. This involves discussing the suspected mechanisms mediating pain and dysfunction, specific factors contributing to the patient's state, and the basis for the proposed course of treatment. Failure to provide education in a clear and concrete manner may cause further confusion and distress to the patient and family. They may feel reluctant to comply with treatment, or simply seek a second opinion. A variety of terms for this process can be found in the literature: "explaining pain," "therapeutic neuroscience education," "pain neuroscience education," "pain biology education." Some basic principles to guide how to optimally educate the patient with pain are listed in Table 42.4. Introducing the concept that *pain is an experience* and not only a sensation and describing pain through the lens of the biopsychosocial model can be very helpful, providing the premise for addressing pain from many aspects.

Examples of educational videos that target families of children with pain can be found on the author's hospital website (https:// www.cincinnatichildrens.org/service/p/pain/pain-management-center/patient-resources). Explanations and descriptions of images

TABLE 42.4	"Red Flag" Signs and Symptoms for Back Pain

- Unexplained fever
- Night sweats
- Weight loss
- Night pain
- Constant pain
- Bowel function changes
- Urinary retention
- Neurologic changes in legs: Trouble walking, footdrop, weakness, loss of reflexes, sensory changes

must be provided in a manner that the layperson will understand, regardless of their socioeconomic status or educational background. Thus, jargon is the enemy of communication with families and patients; language should be as simple as possible while remaining accurate. Practitioners will find it useful to build a small collection of images and analogies to use that are accurate but flow naturally in conversation and are relevant to the majority of patients in that locale.[19–23]

Chronic Pain Conditions

Any part of the body can hurt, but in practical terms there are several diagnostic clusters that represent the majority of pediatric pain conditions. The frequency and intensity of the pain can be striking. One study on the 3-month prevalence, characteristics, consequences, and provoking factors of chronic pain in children and adolescents described the experience of 749 children and adolescents in one elementary and two secondary schools: 83% experienced pain during the preceding 3 months.[24] The leading sources of pain were headaches (60.5%, also perceived as most bothersome), abdominal pain (43.3%), extremity pain (33.6%), and back pain (30.2%). More than one-half of the children and adolescents with pain reported associated sleep problems, restriction in hobbies, and eating issues. School absenteeism reached 48.8% in the population with pain; children with abdominal pain and headache reported the greatest school absenteeism, whereas children with back pain reported the least. The utilization of health care resources by children and adolescents with pain was extensive: 50.9% visited the physician's office, and 51.5% reported using pain medications.

ABDOMINAL PAIN

Abdominal pain is a major source of distress in children and invites a large amount of testing and anxiety. This painful condition is no longer referred to as recurrent abdominal pain and is currently described as functional gastrointestinal disorders (FGIDs).[25] Specific criteria exist for the major categories so that FGIDs are no longer considered diagnoses of exclusion. There are four subtypes of FGID that feature pain prominently: (1), functional dyspepsia; (2), irritable bowel syndrome (IBS); (3), abdominal migraine; and (4), functional abdominal pain syndrome. It is thought that the pain is caused by abnormal interactions between the enteric and central nervous systems.[26,27] Research suggests that peripheral sensitization (by transient receptor potential vanilloid receptor [TRPV] 1)[27] and abnormal central processing of afferent signals at the level of the central nervous system play roles in the pathophysiology of visceral hyperalgesia decreasing the threshold for pain in response to changes in intraluminal pressure.[28] These disorders usually affect patients 4 years of age and older. The history and physical examination should focus on excluding warning signs and symptoms of underlying disease (see Table 42.4).[25,29] The role for testing, endoscopy, and radiographic evaluation is limited.

Visceral hyperalgesia can be secondary to prior ongoing or recurrent gastrointestinal inflammation as seen in inflammatory bowel disease or chronic pancreatitis. The distinction between acute and chronic pain can become challenging as patient-reported quality and intensity of pain often remain the same. During the acute phase, multimodal analgesia, including brief use of opioids if needed, is warranted. If the pain continues despite improved clinical, laboratory, imaging, or invasive studies beyond the usual time frame for recovery, the focus of treatment should shift toward treatment of FGID and an opioid wean. Patient and family education about differences between acute and chronic pain and explanation of visceral hyperalgesia are essential for successful management.

Treatment

The treatment of FGIDs requires a multidisciplinary approach that includes medication, psychological interventions, and education. The most important part of the approach is to establish realistic goals, which frequently means return of function rather than complete elimination of pain. Although the literature for treatment is sparse, tricyclic antidepressants such as amitriptyline, nortriptyline, or doxepin have been used effectively for FGID-related pain. Another useful drug group is the anticonvulsants, which modify nerve conductivity and transmission.

Symptomatically, antacids, antispasmodic agents, smooth muscle relaxants, laxatives, and antidiarrheal agents can be added. Peppermint oil capsules are a food supplement that may be useful for IBS, although gastroesophageal reflux can be a limiting side effect.[30] Children with functional bowel disorders can develop abnormal bowel reactivity in response to physiologic stimuli, noxious stressful stimuli, or psychological stimuli (parental separation, anxiety). Children benefit from cognitive behavioral therapy, coping skill development, biofeedback, hypnosis, and relaxation techniques.[31,32] Ongoing education and reassurance of the family and child is necessary (see Table 42.5 for Care Pathway).

HEADACHE

Headaches can be divided into primary and secondary headaches.[33] Primary headaches include migraine headache, tension-type headache, cluster headache, and trigeminal neuralgia. Secondary headaches are attributable to head and neck traumas; muscle spasms; vascular disorders; nonvascular intracranial disorders; infection; eye, ear, cranium, nose, sinuses, temporomandibular joint and teeth/mouth diseases; homeostasis disturbances; and psychiatric disorders.[34] To investigate for secondary headache syndromes in children, the pneumonic **SNOOPPPY** was created: **(S)**ystemic symptoms, abnormal **(N)**eurologic signs, acute **(O)**nset, **(O)**ccipital, **(P)**recipitated by Valsalva, **(P)**ositional, **(P)**rogressive, **(P)**arents-lack of family history, and **(Y)**ears for <6 years.[35] Headaches represent one of the more poorly tolerated types of chronic pain, with generally greater medication use than in other types of chronic pain. The long-term prognosis for headache pain overall is that 27%

| TABLE 42.5 | Care Pathway for Abdominal Pain |

Evaluation

- Medical
- Behavioral medicine
- Review of records, treatments, history, physical findings
- Consult with Pediatrics/Surgery/Gastroenterology as indicated by presence of "red flags"—potentially including laboratory testing, ultrasound, computed tomography/magnetic resonance imaging, endoscopy, lactose testing

Treatment of Functional Gastrointestinal Disorders

- Medications: tricyclic antidepressants; consider selective serotonin reuptake inhibitors or serotonin-norepinephrine reuptake inhibitors; peppermint oil
- Behavioral medicine: very important and effective—demedicalize: deemphasize testing and search for organic diagnoses. Redirect focus to treatment and improved function
- Physical therapy: not usually involved; trial of transcutaneous electrical nerve stimulation (TENS), if abdominal wall origin found
- Other:
  Blocks are rare, unless palliative situation; celiac plexus with local anesthetic and steroid; epidural
  Trigger point injections if abdominal wall trigger point(s) found
  Acupuncture
  Hypnosis
  Meditation
  Dietary management

become headache-free in a 20-year follow-up with 66% reporting improvement in the pain.[36] In young children (before 6 years of age) who developed migraines, a similar long-term follow-up showed that migraines resolved in one-third of the children although 69% had persistent pain and 56% developed cranial autonomic symptoms.[37]

Migraines (especially migraine without aura) and tension-type headaches are the most common pediatric headaches. The prevalence of migraine ranges from 2.7% to 10%.[38] These headaches are more frequent in boys than girls between 4 and 7 years of age, but that frequency equalizes between 7 and 11 years of age. After 11 years of age, the female:male ratio changes to 3:1.[39,40] Studies are not routinely recommended in the absence of focal neurologic findings. However, the practitioner must be alert to "red flag" signs and symptoms that warrant imaging and laboratory studies that might be indicated to rule out an underlying condition as a cause of the headaches (see Table 42.2). There is a genetic component to migraine and chronic tension headaches; 50% to 77% of children with migraine have a positive family history for migraine, especially on the maternal side. The clearest genetic link has been established for familial hemiplegic migraine.[16] Children with frequent headaches often suffer from medication overuse headaches due to chronic or repeated use of over-the-counter analgesics. If possible, patients need to be weaned off analgesics gradually.

Treatment

Treatments of migraine and tension-type headaches overlap greatly. Start with the basics and educate the patient about headache healthy habits. Hydration with water, 1 oz/lb of weight, up to 120 oz/day, avoidance of caffeine, regular meals to minimize fluctuations in blood glucose levels, consuming one serving of green vegetables a day, daily aerobic activity for 30 minutes, and daily routine with sufficient length of sleep (9 hours) are important initial steps in effective symptom control.[34,41] The second step is a consultation with a pain psychologist to work on pain coping skills and stress management. The third step is a pharmacologic intervention. Unfortunately, this approach is not particularly effective, although for those significantly disabled by the headache pain, it is a reasonable option. These interventions can be divided into two types[34]: (1) abortive treatment, which focuses on stopping the acute headache (e.g., nonsteroidal antiinflammatory drugs [NSAIDs] and acetaminophen)[38] and (2) prophylactic therapy to prevent the occurrence of headaches if they occur more frequently than twice per month, if the headaches are severe, and/or for frequent headaches that are poorly responsive or unresponsive to treatment medication (Table 42.6).[42] Triptans are a new category of treatments for migraines, based on 5HT-1$_{B/D}$ receptor agonists.[38,41] Gepants and ditans have recently been approved for the treatment of migraines. Early formulations of gepants were withdrawn due to increased liver enzymes and hepatic toxicity, but the current formulations of ubrogepant and rimegepant do not cause similar changes. The ditans are serotonin 5-HT$_{1F}$ receptor agonists, the first released is lasmiditan, which caused lethargy, fatigue, somnolence, and nausea. The gepants and ditans are not approved for use in children and adolescents.[41]

Older medications that have been used successfully for prophylactic treatment of headaches in adolescents are amitriptyline and trazodone; both tend to make children drowsy, so these medications are usually administered 30 to 60 minutes before bedtime. Younger children appear to respond well to the antihistamine cyproheptadine. Selective serotonin reuptake inhibitors (SSRIs) have proven to be no more effective than placebo in prophylaxis of migraine in adults, so they are unlikely to be effective in children or adolescents. In tension-type headache, SSRIs were less effective than tricyclic antidepressants (TCAs). However, the incidence of adverse effects was greater with TCAs.[43] Overall, few recommendations can be made as randomized controlled trials in children are lacking.[44] A major randomized controlled trial (known as CHAMP-Childhood and Adolescent Migraine Prevention) of 328 children 8 to 17 years of age with at least a 5-year history of migraine headaches was designed to compare the frequency and severity of the headaches after treatment with amitriptyline, topiramate (a carbonic anhydrase inhibitor) or placebo over a 28 day period. However, the trial was terminated prematurely due to a lack of difference among the interventions.[45] The authors concluded that there was no consensus reached on which drugs to treat with or when to initiate treatment for migraines in children. In a follow-up study of 205 patients who completed the CHAMP trial, the frequency and severity of migraine headaches were recorded up to 3 years after stopping the CHAMP trial.[46] The frequency of headache days and disability continued to improve during the 3-year follow-up, without specific treatment (including placebo), leading the authors to conclude that after a brief treatment for migraines, these headaches continue to improve over the subsequent 3 years without further treatment in children and adolescents.[46] The anesthesiologist may be called to provide a greater occipital nerve block for patients with cervicogenic headaches, occipital neuralgia, or postconcussive headaches, which may have some common elements. Evidence for this intervention is modest but it is a low-risk procedure and neurology colleagues may consult an anesthesiologist for assistance in performing this block.[47–49]

COMPLEX REGIONAL PAIN SYNDROME

There are two categories of CRPS (type I and type II). They differ only in the presence of a documented nerve injury in type II (formerly causalgia). The presence of pain is obligatory, often alongside allodynia or hyperalgesia. There must be evidence at some time (not necessarily at the time of diagnosis) of edema, changes in skin blood flow, or abnormal sudomotor activity in the region of pain. There are often features of motor disorder, such as tremor, dystonia, and weakness, sometimes leading to loss of joint mobility. Nail and hair growth can also be affected. In the past, there were three distinct "stages" described; however, it is postulated that there are phenotypic subtypes instead of stages.[50]

From a clinical standpoint, the typical pediatric CRPS patient is older than 10 years of age, White, female, and very active/high achiever from an active family and presents with lower extremity pain. A genetic predisposition is suggested by the clinical observation that CRPS is rare in the African-American population. Furthermore, the rarity of CRPS in preadolescent children suggests a developmental aspect to its etiology.[51,52]

On evaluation, it is important to take a detailed history of the mechanism of trauma and the signs and symptoms.[53] One should specifically look for pain, allodynia, hyperalgesia, and hyperpathia. Edema, cyanosis, mottling, and other color changes may also be observed (Fig. 42.1). A complete neurologic examination includes testing the muscle strength, reflexes, sensory testing (cold, touch, pinprick), capillary refill, temperature, and color differences. One should also examine the child for deep tissue hyperalgesia. On occasion, noninvasive or invasive testing may be helpful but not sensitive or specific. This may include an electromyogram with nerve conduction velocity (EMG/NCV),

TABLE 42.6	Care Pathway for Headaches

Evaluation

- Medical
- Behavioral medicine
- Physical therapy if neck or upper back tightness is present
- Review of records, treatments, history, physical findings
- Magnetic resonance imaging and neurology consultation as indicated by presence of "red flags"

Treatment

- Medications: tricyclic antidepressants, topiramate, trazodone, cyproheptadine
- Behavioral medicine: biofeedback, relaxation, coping and pacing skills
- Physical therapy: transcutaneous electrical nerve stimulation (TENS) unit on shoulders, posterior neck; stretching
- Other:
  Yoga
  Acupuncture
  Meditation
  Occasional neck trigger point injection or occipital nerve block

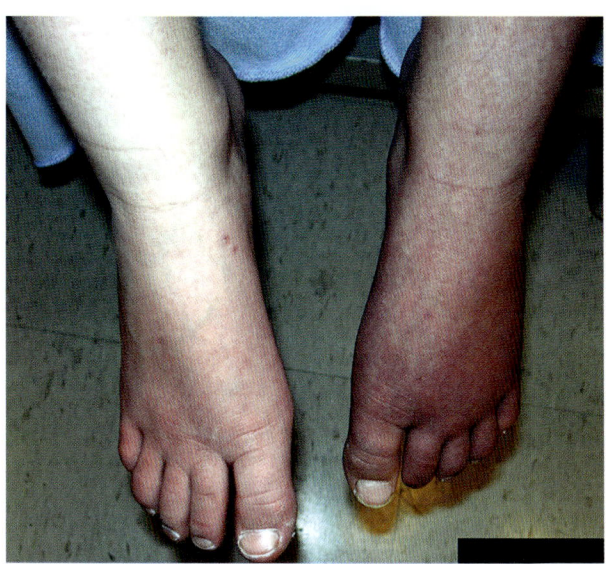

FIGURE 42.1 Left foot/ankle complex regional pain syndrome. Note cyanosis and mottling. Foot was cool, and allodynia was prominent. Left foot toenails had not been trimmed in 3 months.

TABLE 42.7	Care Pathway for Complex Regional Pain Syndromes (CRPS)

Evaluation

- Medical
- Behavioral medicine
- Physical therapy
- Review of records, treatments, history, physical findings, radiographic studies

Treatment

- Medications: tricyclic antidepressants, gabapentin, oxcarbazepine
- Physical therapy: activate, range of motion, desensitization, strength training. Structured home program extremely important. May use transcutaneous electrical nerve stimulation (TENS) unit.
- Behavior medicine: very important, especially in refractory cases
- Other:
  Consider intravenous regional block for hand or foot
  Consider lumbar sympathetic block catheter and admission for structured program for lower extremity CRPS that is refractory despite best efforts of patient and family
  Consider high thoracic epidural or continuous brachial plexus catheter for upper extremity CRPS.

quantitative sensory testing (QST), and quantitative sudomotor axon reflex testing (QSART) to detect small fiber dysfunction, thermography, and bone scan.[54] Sympathetic ganglion blocks are not considered necessary for diagnosis, but they may be part of the therapeutic approach.

Treatment

The therapeutic goal in CRPS is restoration of function. It may seem simple, but in daily practice this may represent the biggest challenge for the physician and the child. The therapeutic approach to the child with CRPS is multidisciplinary, with focus on the psychosocial and physical aspects of the disease[55,56] (Table 42.7). Education is important, and the information available on the internet is ubiquitous, often discouraging, and often not applicable to pediatric CRPS. No single treatment technique has been found helpful for this condition.[57] Children and physicians should follow an algorithm and adjust the therapeutic strategy every 4 weeks if the patient does not respond satisfactorily to chosen measures.

The mainstay of treatment in CRPS is physical therapy. However, the pain can be severe and disabling enough to prevent active participation by the child in the physical therapy program. Pharmacologic therapy is often initiated along with behavioral strategies to facilitate physical therapy.[58] Medications for neuropathic pain (see later) take time to titrate to effect. Therefore, it is reasonable to use NSAIDs and opioids for a short time until the primary medications take effect. Psychosocial issues must be aggressively addressed.[59] The psychology team must play an active role in the overall treatment program. With the three components of physical therapy, psychology, and medications, most patients achieve good results with resolution of their disease.

Interventional Therapy

The role of interventional therapy in the treatment of CRPS is to alleviate the pain and provide the child with the opportunity to tolerate and advance in physical therapy. Sympathetic nerve blocks are widely used in adults[60] though recent systematic

reviews revealed a lack of randomized controlled trials to confirm efficacy of this approach in short- and long-term pain relief.[61–63] In addition, interventional therapies can be a double-edged sword, representing an "easy solution" which can demotivate the child from taking an active role in their physical therapy. On the other hand, pain may be too severe to allow physical therapy and thereby accelerate loss of function. There are several techniques that are popular with pediatric pain specialists. For isolated distal limb CRPS, intravenous regional blockade with local anesthetic and adjuncts such as clonidine, dexmedetomidine, ketamine, or ketorolac can be performed.[64] General anesthesia or deep sedation is frequently required because placement of intravenous catheters in the affected limb and inflation of the tourniquet are poorly tolerated. More invasive alternatives would be placement of a lumbar sympathetic plexus catheter (Fig. 42.2) or a tunneled epidural catheter in the upper thoracic or lumbar areas. Peripheral catheters have been placed to facilitate inpatient, intensive rehabilitation with some success.[65,66] The duration of infusion ranges from 3 to 5 days to as long as 4 to 6 weeks and can require extensive logistical support. Spinal cord or direct nerve stimulation[67–69] and intrathecal drug delivery are used very rarely in pediatric CRPS. Reasons include the overall good prognosis with more conservative treatment as well as the continued growth of the skeleton, which would change the area of paresthesia in the case of spinal cord stimulators.

MUSCULOSKELETAL PAIN

Musculoskeletal pain in children and adolescents is a recognized problem, with back pain being a common issue in adolescents.[70–73] Though many potential factors are blamed for musculoskeletal pain (heavy backpacks, participation in sports, sedentary lifestyle, presence of scoliosis, and increased body mass index), only a limited number have been proven to contribute to musculoskeletal pain. According to one of the reviewed studies, in more than one-half of the cases the cause

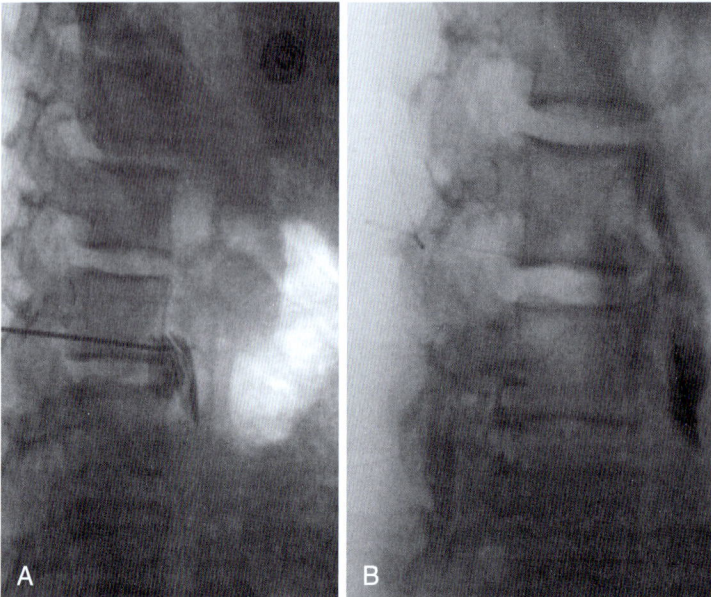

FIGURE 42.2 Lumbar sympathetic block. **A,** Lateral view. Tuohy needle is in proper position. Note pre-psoas spread of contrast agent. **B,** Catheter in situ. Note dye spread and clearing due to injection of local anesthetic through catheter. Catheter is tunneled and can be left in place for a week.

could not be identified and only a minority of children had an underlying disease process (spondylolysis, infection, tumor, disk problem). Radiologic studies correlated poorly with the pain and failed to distinguish between individuals with and without pain. Selected "red flags" for back pain are presented in Table 42.3. A care pathway for the evaluation and treatment of back pain in children and adolescents is presented in Table 42.8.

RHEUMATOLOGIC AND MUSCULOSKELETAL PAIN

A special group of children with musculoskeletal pain are those with rheumatologic diseases. The majority of children referred to the rheumatologist's office complain of musculoskeletal pain. Only a portion of these are diagnosed with the true rheumatologic diseases of which juvenile idiopathic arthritis is the most frequent. Besides pain, the diseases often manifest as morning stiffness, fatigue, and sleep problems. The process may progress and cause joint deformities and destruction due to osteoporosis, with resulting growth abnormalities and functional disability. Management is a combination of pharmacologic and nonpharmacologic interventions. The mainstay of therapy is to prescribe NSAIDs, acetaminophen, and, rarely, opioids for severe breakthrough pain. The rheumatologist may prescribe agents such as methotrexate, cyclophosphamide, or systemic corticosteroids for severe flareups. Splints, physical therapy, and psychological intervention such as cognitive behavioral therapy are also commonly used.[74] We have found that some children with Ehlers-Danlos syndrome or other connective tissue disorders suffer from unstable joints that become very painful from repeated dislocations and mechanical stress.

A fair number of young women will present with fatigue, poor sleep, and pain or unusual tenderness in multiple sites. Fibromyalgia is more commonly seen in adolescents than generally appreciated and can be a significant problem. Depression and suicidal ideation is common; one study found more than

TABLE 42.8	Care Pathway for Back Pain

Evaluation

- Medical
- Behavior medicine
- Physical therapy
- Review of records, treatments, history, physical findings
- Consult orthopedics; magnetic resonance imaging/computed tomography, as indicated by history and examination findings

Treatment

- Medications:
  Tricyclic antidepressants
  Muscle relaxants (e.g., baclofen, cyclobenzaprine)
  Anticonvulsant (if radicular component)
  Nonsteroidal antiinflammatory drug of choice
  Cyclooxgenase-2 inhibitor if gastrointestinal/bleeding issues
  If disk disease with radicular pain is documented, up to three epidural steroid injections may be helpful.

- Behavior medicine: biofeedback, coping skills, and relaxation techniques

- Physical therapy:
  Stretching, postural rehabilitation, general reconditioning, lifting techniques
  Limit bed rest; reactivate
  Transcutaneous electrical nerve stimulation (TENS)
  Exercise program

- Other:
  Acupuncture
  Yoga
  Chiropractic (older patients, lumbar only)
  Massage
  Trigger point injections
  Additional modalities for specific indications include back bracing, surgery, bisphosphonate therapy

25% of 31 subjects 12 to 17 years of age had such tendencies.[75] Therapy includes education,[76] general restorative therapy, with a focus on aerobic reconditioning,[77] and medications. Traditionally, TCAs and cyclobenzaprine have been used. Duloxetine and milnacipran are more recent additions,[78] but have been shown to be only modestly helpful in a minority of adults, with little to no data in pediatric patients.[79] One placebo controlled study of 184 teenagers (13–17 years of age) found a 30% to 50% reduction in pain.[80] As with many chronic pain conditions, cognitive behavioral approaches such as relaxation, hypnosis, biofeedback, and coping skills training[81] are valuable components of treatment.[82]

One patient population for whom musculoskeletal pain is a particularly difficult problem is the group of children with cerebral palsy.[83,84] Spasticity itself can be painful, and certainly the daily stretching exercises are reported to be painful by many patients. Additionally, a subgroup of children with cerebral palsy are nonverbal, making assessments very difficult. The parents or guardians can provide information regarding how their child displays pain and how the pain manifests itself during daily life. Musculoskeletal and abdominal pain are most common and sometimes relieved by changes in position or massage.[84] If diaper changes seem to hurt, then one should suspect hip or perineal pain. Pain after eating or a history of hard stools may point toward constipation-based abdominal pain. A careful, sometimes multistaged, examination is required. A thoughtful, empirical approach to therapy and judicious use of radiologic, laboratory evaluations, and occasionally select nerve blocks, Botox injections,[85] or surgical interventions (rhizotomy),[86] can often lead to diagnosis and successful treatment to improve their lifestyle (Table 42.9).

PAIN IN SICKLE CELL DISEASE, TRAIT, AND VARIANTS

Sickle cell disease is a hereditary disorder characterized by the presence of abnormal hemoglobin S (with valine substitution for glutamic acid on the β-globulin chain) (see Chapter 8). The homozygous form presents as a hemolytic anemia with unique vasoocclusive features. The heterozygous form is milder and presents as a borderline anemia (sickle cell trait) and rarely with vasoocclusive features. Hemoglobin SC is another variant, whose clinical presentation is similar to HbSS but whose vasoocclusive episodes are fewer and usually less intense. About 8% of Black Americans carry the sickle gene. From a pain management perspective, the homozygous HbSS genotype manifests as either acute pain attacks (pain crisis, vasoocclusive episodes, acute chest syndrome) or as underlying chronic pain with acute exacerbations (avascular necrosis, vertebral collapse, joint involvement). Treatment frequently is multidisciplinary with close cooperation between hematologist, psychologist, and pain physician.[87,88] Most of the episodes can be managed at home with NSAIDs or acetaminophen, supplemented with opioids such as morphine, hydrocodone, oxycodone, or tramadol. In severe cases, patients are often hospitalized and treated with intravenous opioids and gradually weaned off as the primary process improves. For episodes of localized, hard-to-control pain, or if acute chest syndrome develops, epidural analgesia can provide excellent relief.[89] Rarely, children require opioid maintenance with long-acting preparations of morphine sulfate, oxycodone, or methadone (Table 42.10). The presence of hyperalgesia over the affected area suggests either peripheral or central sensitization, although the role for neuropathic medications is undefined.

| TABLE 42.9 | Care Pathway for Nonverbal Patients |

Evaluation

- Medical: often tricky; go slowly
  May need more than one visit to complete the examination
  Try to isolate body part during examination, to avoid generalized effect
  Watch facial/vocal and parent reaction to each examination maneuver

- Behavioral medicine (often not possible)

- Physical therapy (often already engaged in therapy)

- Review of records, treatments, history, physical findings

- Video: the parent may be able to capture pain behaviors for you to view

Treatment

- Medications: often on multiple agents at baseline
  Coordination with other practitioners is important
  Use general principles when choosing medications
  Sometimes a long-acting opioid is beneficial for refractory musculoskeletal pain
  Watch for worsening of constipation

- Physical therapy: often already engaged
  If not, then engage for musculoskeletal pain or help therapist focus efforts on a particular region of the body

- Behavioral medicine: often not possible if patient's cognitive ability is too low
  However, sometimes the family can benefit because they carry a large burden when caring for patients with multiple medical problems

- Other:
  Nerve blocks can be used to identify painful areas, if more than one seems active
  Rarely, a patient needs to be brought to the operating suite for an infusion of remifentanil to identify opioid responsiveness versus potentially centralized or behavioral pain phenomena
  The latter may respond to anticonvulsant therapy
  Intrathecal baclofen (and occasionally morphine)
  Surgical therapy for select conditions

Cautions

- Site of pain is often unclear

- Do not forget to look in the ears

- If patient is spastic, strongly consider hip pathology (e.g., subluxation, bursitis, infection)

- Constipation, gallbladder pain, and gastroesophageal reflux are all possible

- These patients often require more testing than verbal patients

- Be careful with use of nonsteroidal antiinflammatory drugs because gastroesophageal reflux can be a problem and reporting abdominal pain as a signal of gastrointestinal side effects may not be possible

Pain Pharmacotherapy

Pain treatment has received less study in children than adults, as it is true for much pediatric pharmacologic therapy. In the absence of US Food and Drug Administration (FDA)–approved indications and experimental data, off-label use of many medications used to treat chronic pain is common.[90] In this situation, the decision to use a particular medication is most often based on extrapolation from adult literature, expert consensus, applied theory, and clinical judgment (see Chapter 5).

TABLE 42.10	Care Pathway for Sickle Cell Disease

Evaluation

- Medical

- Behavioral medicine (may be limited to social support in acute setting)

- Review of records, treatments (need opioid exposure history for dosing), history

- Hematology almost always directly involved, with focused evaluation

Treatment of Vasoocclusive Episodes

- Medications: opioid (often requires basal infusion for the first days) Nonsteroidal antiinflammatory drug Consider neuropathic medication if hyperalgesia is present

- Behavioral medicine: can be helpful, although learning techniques in the acute setting may be difficult Introducing this modality early in life may be more helpful

- Physical therapy: transcutaneous electrical nerve stimulation for localized pain

- Other: Regional anesthesia may be helpful Strongly consider thoracic epidural for acute chest crisis

Treatment of Chronic Problems

- Medications: may involve chronic opioids; otherwise follows treatment of particular pain condition

- Behavioral medicine: as per particular pain condition Early involvement may reduce need for hospitalizations

- Physical therapy: as per particular pain condition May have joint, bone, and deconditioning issues from recurrent vasoocclusive episodes

Knowledge about the safety or efficacy of pharmacological medicines in children and adolescents with chronic pain is scant, despite their common use. There are no randomized controlled trials in reviews relating to reducing pain in children suffering chronic regional pain syndromes. There is no evidence from randomized controlled trials for pharmacological interventions in children with cancer-related pain, yet individual children cannot be denied access to potential pain relief.[91]

Three categories of medications are available for consideration: nonopioid analgesics (NSAIDs and acetaminophen), opioid analgesics, and a broad spectrum of adjuvant analgesics (including anticonvulsants, antidepressants, muscle relaxants, local anesthetics, N-methyl-D-aspartate [NMDA]-receptor antagonists, α_2 agonists, and corticosteroids).

ACETAMINOPHEN

Acetaminophen remains the most common analgesic given to children (see Chapter 5). There is no evidence that acetaminophen is useful in treating adults with cancer pain, either alone or in combination with an opioid. Nor is there evidence to disprove that it is useful. Similarly, there are no robust studies that have evaluated the efficacy of acetaminophen to manage cancer pain.[92] Furthermore, there are no randomized controlled trials that support or refute a role for acetaminophen in the treatment of chronic noncancer pain in children and adolescents. Although acetaminophen is widely used in chronic pain conditions, its efficacy or harm in the treatment of chronic pain in children and adolescents remains unproven.[93]

NONSTEROIDAL ANTIINFLAMMATORY DRUGS

NSAIDs come from various chemical groups (salicylates, propionic acid, oxicams, naphthylalkalones, fenamates). The mechanism of action is inhibition of cyclooxygenases (COX), COX-1 (constitutive, always present) and COX-2 (inducible, produced in the body under proper conditions). NSAIDs differ in their selectivity for COX-1 or COX-2, with selective COX-2 inhibitors having predominant action on inducible COX-2. The benefit of selective blockade is decreased risk of gastrointestinal bleeding. Celecoxib is the only selective COX-2 inhibitor currently available for use in the United States. The analgesic and antiinflammatory actions of NSAIDs exhibit a dose-dependent response until they reach a maximum effect, beyond which there is no further benefit of increasing the dose (also known as the ceiling effect). In contrast to opioids, NSAIDs do not develop either a physical dependence or tolerance. The choice of NSAID is empirical and based on clinical judgment. If the child provides a history of good response to a particular NSAID, we tend to continue the same medication and/or adjust the dose. If the response is inadequate, we select a different medication until we find one that is effective. In children with a history of gastrointestinal side effects, we prescribe combination preparations with protective agents (e.g., misoprostol) or a histamine-2 or proton pump inhibitor, or switch to selective COX-2 inhibitor. Preexisting renal disease and disorders that reduce actual or effective intravascular volume vastly increase the risk for renal toxicity; NSAIDs must be used cautiously in these situations.

There is no high-quality evidence to prove that NSAIDs are useful in treating adults with cancer pain. Nor is there evidence to disprove that they are useful. There is very low-quality evidence that shows that some people with moderate or severe cancer pain experience a marked reduction in their pain within 1 or 2 weeks following treatment with NSAIDS.[94] Similarly there is no evidence (e.g., no randomized controlled trials) that NSAIDs reduce either cancer or chronic non–cancer-related pain in children and adolescents.[95,96]

THE "OPIOID EPIDEMIC" AND PAIN MANAGEMENT

In the 1990s, the use of opioids for both acute and chronic pain increased because of several concurrent factors. There was a global increase in advocacy for patients in pain[97] and increased understanding of how to prescribe them and an increasing number of formulations,[98] but there were also advertising campaigns and incomplete data that promoted the increased use of opioids.[99] As a result of the rapid and generalized use of opioids, overdoses and misuse became more frequent and the term "opioid epidemic" gained popularity as a shorthand label for the problem. In the pediatric realm, prescribing opioids to children and adolescents confers an increased risk for prescription opioid abuse.[100] A prospective study demonstrated that any legitimate opioid use in high school seniors was associated with a 33% increased risk of future opioid misuse.[101] Further compounding this problem was a national survey that reported that 21% of adolescents used prescription opioids in the preceding year.[102]

In lieu of these events, the use of opioids in chronic nonmalignant pain has been associated with many challenges. Their use in the past was reserved for children with acute and cancer-related pain. However, in carefully selected cases, opioids can improve quality of life and functional capacity without significant risk of addiction, tolerance, and toxicity. Screening patients for "red flags" for opioid prescribing such as history of substance abuse (in adolescent and young adult populations) and/or a family member with substance abuse, a dysfunctional social situation can help risk stratification and guide proper monitoring.

TABLE 42.11 | Opioid Side Effects With Chronic Usage

With Development of Tolerance

Sedation

Miosis

Respiratory depression

Itching

Nausea

Urinary retention

Cognitive impairment

Prolonged reaction time

Without Development of Tolerance

Constipation

Side Effects Associated With Long-Term Use

Hypogonadism

Immunosuppression

Pure opioid agonists morphine, oxycodone, and hydromorphone are used almost exclusively, tapentadol has been more recent option; however, agents such as tramadol have also gained some popularity in off-label use among practitioners due to overall safety[74] and an assumed decreased effect on GI motility, despite an FDA boxed warning against using it in patients under the age of 12 years for any reason and under 18 years for certain situations wherein airway compromise might be encountered (e.g., tonsillectomy).[103,104] The utility of agonist-antagonists is diminished by their analgesic ceiling effect and difficulty in using them outside the realm of intravenous administration. We typically use opioids in two chronic pain scenarios. The first features opioids as a bridge while titrating other classes of medications to effect or while awaiting physical therapy or an intervention to exert their effect. In the second scenario, we use opioids as maintenance analgesics in carefully selected children (e.g., for chronic musculoskeletal pain in a child with cerebral palsy or in children with juvenile rheumatoid arthritis or avascular necrosis in patients who received high-dose steroids). Medication is titrated in increments toward the main goal of optimal (although rarely complete) pain relief, improved function, and minimal side effects. Escalations are seen usually with exacerbations of the primary disease process. Common opioid side effects and their time courses can be found in Table 42.11.

A special medication within this group is methadone, which has been gaining increasing interest among pain practitioners because of its unique properties.[105] Besides being an opioid agonist, methadone also has some effect in controlling neuropathic components of pain.[106,107] There are a few caveats with its use. It has a long half-life and presents a risk of accumulation leading to sedation and respiratory depression. The "usual" 1 : 1 methadone : morphine equianalgesia ratio does not work for dose conversion. The greater the dose of opioid being converted, the more skewed the conversion ratio; in one study this conversion ratio, methadone : morphine ratio ranged from 1 : 2.5 to 1 : 14.3.[108] Because of the long half-life, no dose adjustments should be made more frequently than every 5 days. A unique side effect of methadone among opioids is its potential to prolong the QT interval on the ECG, which can cause serious arrhythmias.[109,110] However, one study of 51 PICU patients found no change in QT interval in children without structural heart disease; the only children who experienced a 40 milliseconds or longer corrected QT interval also had structural heart disease.[111] Another study of methadone in 44 preterm infants found no prolongation of the corrected QT interval.[112]

When a child who is prescribed long-term opioids presents to the operating room, a thorough medication history is essential for appropriate perioperative pain management. If the child is prescribed traditional opioid and has not taken a morning dose due to NPO concerns, that dose should be replaced via the intravenous route to avoid withdrawal. It is essential to convert the home medication into morphine equivalents and the daily dose of home opioids should be provided as a baseline, with all further dosing being in addition to the baseline, to avoid pain at the time of emergence. Because of tolerance to long-term opioids, larger doses than usual may be required, and it is advisable (as in all children) to titrate to comfort in the immediate postoperative period and use the amount required to achieve optimal analgesia.

Abuse-Deterrent Opioid Formulations

Practitioners may occasionally encounter a pediatric or adolescent patient who is being prescribed abuse-deterrent opioid formulations (ADFs) as part of medication-assisted treatment of addiction. Medications in this class are modifications of prescribed opioids designed to resist manipulation and drug abuse.[113] To date, the FDA has approved the designation of ADF status to 10 new formulations.[114] The basis for ADFs largely rests on technologies that make adapting the oral medication for alternate routes of administration difficult or that incorporate antagonists (i.e., naloxone) in ways in which they are innocuous when the medication is taken as intended, but with which opioids become active in situations of misuse. Although exciting in theory, ADFs have generated concerns about cost and safety and they are not entirely effective in preventing diversion and abuse.[115,116] Further, ADFs do not prevent abuse by ingestion by taking increased quantities, which is the most common form of misuse.[117,118] The current consensus is that prescribing ADFs instead of non–ADF opioids would not produce a net health benefit.[115,118] Currently, more cost-effective measures exist, such as increasing preventive and therapeutic resources for addiction, informing prescribers about multimodal analgesia and the dangers of over-prescription, and educating patients on their pain management plan and opioid-related risks.[113]

Medically, pediatric chronic pain practice has not required the same magnitude of change as in adult practice, as the emphasis has been on multidisciplinary care from the outset. However, on the acute side, there have been changes going as far as proposals for "opioids-free" anesthesia and analgesia.[119–121] The relative merits of such approaches run beyond the scope of this chapter. At a minimum, practitioners are advised to become familiar with the controlled-substance related laws in their state and the rules of their specific institution as prescribing of the ADF drugs may require additional training and licensure.

Buprenorphine in the Perioperative Arena

On occasion, buprenorphine (with or without naloxone) is used to manage pediatric chronic pain; however, it has a larger role in the management of opioid addiction.[122,123] Infrequently, such patients may be encountered in the perioperative area or admitted for acute illness. The consultant should have basic knowledge and understanding of the mechanism of action of buprenorphine to appropriately treat the patient.[124] Buprenorphine exhibits a greater affinity to the mu-receptor and slower association and dissociation with the receptor than other opioids and naloxone. It also has antagonism at kappa and delta opioids receptors.[122,125] Therefore, traditional opioids can be presumably less effective in the face of buprenorphine therapy, making perioperative opioid therapy tricky.[126] Guidelines for care in this situation are limited by a lack of evidence. Recommended options for managing buprenorphine include its discontinuation, reducing the dose, substitution with traditional opioids, substituting methadone in advance, or continuation throughout the perioperative period.[124,126] Administering perioperative opioids with high mu-receptor affinity (sufentanil, hydromorphone) is another recommended option.[127–129] It is imperative in situations such as this to coordinate care planning with the prescribing physician. One needs to expect that opioid needs may be greater in these patients and pain control postoperatively may be more difficult to achieve. A multimodal approach is recommended, with reliance on regional anesthesia and nonopioids being prominent. A transition plan for how the patient will resume their baseline regimen needs to be designed with the prescribing physician.

ADJUVANT DRUGS
Anticonvulsants

This group of medications has been widely used in the pharmacologic treatment of chronic pain since the 1960s. Often referred to as membrane stabilizers, anticonvulsants work on neural receptors, ion channels, and nerve conductivity. They modify the level of excitatory and inhibitory neurotransmitters and activation of nerve cells. They are most effective in controlling neuropathic pain. The first generation of agents (e.g., carbamazepine) are being prescribed less often due to significant adverse effects, and replaced by the second-generation drugs with better adverse-effect profiles. Therapeutic effect is achieved with all membrane stabilizers by gradually titrating the dose to the response. The purpose is twofold: (1) to avoid adverse effects by allowing enough time for the child to develop tolerance (mainly to sedation) and (2) to find the smallest effective dose for a given child. The treatment course usually lasts from 3 to 6 months. At the end of the course, the patient is gradually weaned off in reverse order as the medication was titrated in. Although weaning is not necessary to prevent seizures, rapid termination in therapy may result in pain, sleep, or mood disturbance. A gradual weaning will allow rapid reescalation, in case the pain begins to return, in children for whom the pain has been controlled but not completely eliminated. In that case, one would determine the child's minimal effective dose. If pain recurs, then we continue medication for 3 to 6 months longer.

Although the use of anticonvulsants for pain in children represents an "off-label" use, without support from clinical studies (often even in adults),[130] this class of medications is a mainstay of therapy for select pain conditions in children. The choice of the drug is based on thoughtful consideration and expert consensus, as with all therapies for which randomized, controlled trials are lacking.[131]

Gabapentin and Pregabalin

Gabapentin is an anticonvulsant with a complex mechanism of action. Its name is deceiving; gabapentin does not interact with the γ-aminobutyric (GABA)–ergic system. It binds to the α_2-delta subunit of the voltage-dependent calcium channel and reduces release of glutamate in the dorsal horn of the spinal cord. This leads to decreased production of substance P, less activation of α-amino-3-hydroxy-5-methylisoxazole-4-propionate (AMPA) receptors on noradrenergic synapses, decreased transmitter release, and, finally, decreased neuronal activity.[132] This mechanism is shared by both gabapentin and pregabalin. As mentioned earlier, gabapentin is usually the first drug of choice owing to its tolerance, minimal side effects, and positive clinical experiences. Besides sedation, patients can retain sodium and water, develop peripheral edema, and gain weight. In teenagers, gabapentin can cause mood swings, irritability, and suicidality. Despite these concerns, we use gabapentin frequently, after detailed explanation and discussion with the patient and parents. Patients and parents are instructed to call our office and discontinue the medication if side effects occur. We use two titration schedules: (1) for younger children the target dose is 10 to 15 mg/kg per dose three times per day; (2) in older children weighing more than 60 kilograms, we use "adult" titration to effect. Gabapentin does not have to be adjusted in patients with liver failure because it is metabolized extra-hepatically; however, the dose needs to be adjusted in children with impaired renal function. Pregabalin is chemically related to gabapentin but has fewer side effects and a significantly faster titration schedule. Currently, it is approved for postherpetic neuralgia, diabetic neuropathy, and fibromyalgia in adults; experience with the drug in children is growing.[133,134]

Oxcarbazepine

This is the second-generation relative of carbamazepine and has potential for the treatment of neuropathic pain states, though data are not strong at this time.[135] Although rare, Stevens-Johnson syndrome can occur with oxcarbazepine, as with a number of other anticonvulsants. Hyponatremia can also occur, in addition to side effects common to anticonvulsants (sedation, difficulty concentrating, ataxia, mood instability).

Carbamazepine, Valproic Acid, Phenytoin

A summary of effectiveness of these drugs has been presented. Carbamazepine[136] has proven effective in the treatment of trigeminal neuralgia, spasticity in multiple sclerosis, and spinal cord injury (in comparison with tizanidine). Phenytoin has been used in cancer pain, either by itself or in combination with buprenorphine, and provided good pain relief in more than 60% of patients. Despite their effectiveness, the use of these medications is limited owing to potentially serious side effects. For carbamazepine and phenytoin, these include liver and renal toxicity (regular laboratory tests are necessary), aplastic anemia, Stevens-Johnson syndrome, and a syndrome of inappropriate secretion of antidiuretic hormone (SIADH)-like picture. Valproate lacks renal side effects but can cause pancreatitis.

Antidepressants

Two major groups of antidepressants are used in the treatment of chronic pain: TCAs (amitriptyline, nortriptyline, desipramine, doxepin, imipramine) and newer SSRIs (fluoxetine, paroxetine) and serotonin-norepinephrine reuptake inhibitors (SNRIs) (venlafaxine, duloxetine). The efficacy of TCAs in the treatment of neuropathic pain has been confirmed in meta-analyses,[136,137] although a recent Cochrane review of antidepressants for chronic noncancer pain in children and adolescents identified only a small number of studies with insufficient data to draw meaningful conclusions.[133]

The doses required to control chronic pain are usually less than those used in the treatment of depression. The efficacy of antidepressants has been demonstrated in neuropathic as well as nonneuropathic pain (such as fibromyalgia and low back pain).[78,137,138] When prescribing antidepressants, we recommend vigilance about the potential increase in suicidal ideation and attempts in adolescents and young adults. We inform patients and families in detail, to ensure that they would communicate such ideation with us. We refer patients at greater risk for psychiatric comorbidity to a psychologist for evaluation before prescribing this class of medications. It is important to note that although antidepressants are commonly used for chronic pain in children, further studies are needed to thoroughly examine their efficacy.[133]

Tricyclic Antidepressants

The major limiting factor in prescribing TCAs is their adverse effects. Onset of side effects can be reduced by slow dose escalation, as with the anticonvulsants. The most frequent adverse effect is sedation, which is often beneficial in chronic pain patients who have difficulties sleeping; we prescribe the drug to be taken at bedtime. It is important to monitor the child in the mornings for carryover sedation. In such cases, it is reasonable either to decrease the dose or encourage the child to take the medication earlier in the evening. Because of the anticholinergic effects of TCAs, children will often notice a dry mouth and may experience constipation, urinary retention, or weight gain. TCAs are known to prolong the cardiac QT interval, which can cause a lethal arrhythmia. We take a careful history of cardiac symptoms and conduction abnormalities in the child and family members.[139] Guidelines are lacking, but it is a good practice to order a baseline electrocardiogram to rule out congenital prolonged QT interval before initiation of therapy. Concomitant use of SSRIs, serotonin-norepinephrine reuptake inhibitors, or tramadol can decrease the seizure threshold in children with a seizure disorder; therefore, their simultaneous use is discouraged. Amitriptyline and nortriptyline are the most commonly used medications of this group. The usual starting dose is 5 to 10 mg orally at night, increased to 20 or 25 mg at night 1 week later. The dose can be escalated up to 1 mg/kg, although a dose this high is rarely required in chronic pain patients. Analgesic effects can be seen in 1 to 3 weeks, as with antidepressant effects. Nortriptyline is a metabolite of amitriptyline, with similar utility for pain but less sedation. The dosing schedule is the same as for amitriptyline. If top-range dosing is required, periodic electrocardiographic monitoring for QTc changes is suggested.

Selective Serotonin (and Norepinephrine) Reuptake Inhibitors

Venlafaxine's starting dose is 37.5 mg/day in adults, which can be increased by 37.5 mg every week up to 300 mg/day. Adverse effects include headaches, nausea, sweating, sedation, hypertension, and seizures. If the dose is below 150 mg/day, the effects are mostly serotoninergic. If it is above 150 mg/day, the effects are mixed serotoninergic and noradrenergic. Duloxetine has antidepressant effects as well as analgesic effects for neuropathic pain, fibromyalgia, and back pain.[78,138,140] It is usually started at 20 to 30 mg daily to a maximum dose of 120 mg/day. The major side effects are nausea, dry mouth, constipation, dizziness, and insomnia. Use of both drugs in children is off-label and best left to those who prescribe them frequently as dosing and efficacy have not been well established in the pediatric age group.[141]

Muscle Relaxants

Muscle relaxants are commonly used as an adjunct to other medications (mostly NSAIDs) in patients with myofascial pain.

Cyclobenzaprine

Cyclobenzaprine is a centrally acting muscle relaxant. Its major side effects are somnolence, dizziness, and asthenia. The usual starting dose is 5 mg at nighttime, which can be increased to 10 mg after 5 to 7 days unless the child has difficulties awakening in the morning. The dose can be escalated up to 10 mg three times a day.

Baclofen

Baclofen is one of the most powerful centrally acting muscle relaxants. It interacts with the GABA(b) receptor subtype. It is usually indicated in patients with spasticity such as cerebral palsy or multiple sclerosis. In children 2 to 7 years old, the dose is 10 to 15 mg/day, divided in two to three doses. The dose can be escalated every 3 days by 5 mg to a maximum dose of 40 mg/day. In children older than 8 years of age, the maximum dose is 60 mg/day. Baclofen is one of a few medications approved for intrathecal administration via implanted pumps in children with spasticity (e.g., cerebral palsy, spinal cord injury).[142]

Tizanidine

Tizanidine has been shown to reduce pain associated with myofascial pain. It tends to be sedating and can improve sleep, making it a reasonable choice for patients with muscle spasms and difficulty with sleep onset. Tizanidine is a centrally acting alpha-2 adrenergic agonist. In children aged 2 to 10 years old, the starting dose is 1 mg at bedtime. For older children, the dose is 2 mg at bedtime. The dose can be titrated to a higher dose by 1 or 2 mg increments if needed.[143,144]

Methocarbamol

Methocarbamol is muscle relaxant that is generally less sedating than other muscle relaxants. The general dose is 10 mg/kg up to three times a day, but for severe muscle spasm and tetanus, it can be used at 15 mg/kg three times a day for shorter periods of time.[143,144]

Corticosteroids, Local Anesthetics, NMDA Receptor Antagonists, Capsaicin, α2-Adrenergic Receptor Agonist

There are many drugs utilized in the treatment of chronic pain, with a wide array of mechanisms of action. Oral medications with local anesthetic properties such as mexiletine have been used in the treatment of neuropathic pain in CRPS. The α_2 receptor agonist clonidine finds its application in the same arena. It is used orally or added to local anesthetic solutions in intravenous regional techniques. The major limiting factor in the use of these drugs is their side effect profile, which includes hypotension, sedation, bradycardia, and nausea (especially with mexiletine). In contrast to its use in adults, the experience in pediatrics is limited. α_2-Adrenergic agonist blocking properties are also part of the mechanism of action of the muscle relaxant tizanidine. The topical agent capsaicin, originating from hot chili peppers, is also helpful in neuropathic pain, but its application can cause a burning sensation where applied, which is often poorly tolerated. The topical lidocaine patch has been proven effective in controlling symptoms of postherpetic neuralgia and has also been used for localized myofascial pain, hyperpathia, and allodynia in other

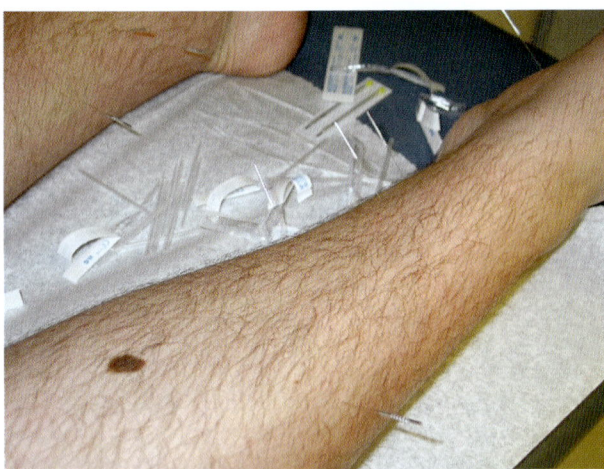

FIGURE 42.3 Acupuncture needles in situ.

neuropathic conditions.[145] Pharmacokinetic studies in adults have found minimal lidocaine blood levels, suggesting a large margin of safety, although similar studies have not been carried out in children.[146] We believe that this is a safe adjunct to symptomatic treatment of chronic pain. NMDA receptor antagonists such as ketamine, amantadine, or dextromethorphan have anecdotal evidence supporting their utility in the treatment of neuropathic pain. It is also thought that NMDA receptor antagonists exert an opioid-sparing effect. An important limiting factor of the broader use of ketamine in the treatment of chronic pain symptoms is the potential for psychotropic side effects.

Complementary Therapies

Alternative therapies have held appeal to patients for a long time. Given that "traditional" medical therapies have a high failure rate, patients will continue to search for other possible treatments. There are a variety of treatments that are useful in the treatment of chronic pain. As a consultant, one should consider suggesting some of these therapies in situations where they seem appropriate. TENS and biofeedback have been discussed earlier.

Acupuncture (and its derivative, acupressure) originated in China and is an important part of traditional Chinese medicine (Fig. 42.3). In acupuncture, the body energy or qi (pronounced "chi") circulates in body meridians and collaterals. Meridians and collaterals are pathways that represent body organ systems called the Zang-Fu organs. In Chinese medicine, pain is caused by obstruction in the circulation of qi in these channels due to multiple causes. Acupuncture has been utilized in acute and chronic pain conditions such as neck and back pain, dental pain, musculoskeletal and arthritic pain, CRPS, migraine, facial pain, and fibromyalgia.[147] The data from randomized controlled trials are controversial or insufficient to support or deny efficacy of acupuncture.[148,149]

ANNOTATED REFERENCES

Eccleston C, Fisher E, Howard RF, et al. Delivering transformative action in paediatric pain. *Lancet Child Adolesc Health.* 2021;5:47-87.

The authors outline the poor current treatment of pain in children. Four transformative goals that will improve the lives of children and adolescents with pain and their families are presented: make pain matter, make pain understood, make pain visible, make pain better. This commissioned manuscript reviews current and future study and direction for pain management.

FDA Drug Safety Communication: FDA restricts use of prescription codeine pain and cough medicines and tramadol pain medicines in children; recommends against use in breastfeeding women.

Practitioners should be aware of changes in FDA labeling of medications. The science behind limitations in codeine restrictions is good, the science behind the restrictions in tramadol is not. This underscores a reason to be aware of the science, and to not simply follow edicts without consideration of the data.

Powers SW, Coffey CS, Chamberlin LA, et al., Trial of amitriptyline, topiramate, and placebo for pediatric migraine. *N Engl J Med.* 2017; 376(2):115-124.

Excellent example of a study that was stopped at midpoint due to lack of efficacy of active intervention versus placebo. Lessons to be learned are not that the active intervention failed, but that the placebo worked as well; this is why the investigative process has checkpoints throughout the study.

Stanton-Hicks M, Baron R, Boas R, et al. Complex regional pain syndromes: guidelines for therapy. *Clin J Pain.* 1998;14:155-166.

Outlines the multidisciplinary approach to complex regional pain syndromes.

Wilder RT, Berde CB, Wolohan M, et al. Reflex sympathetic dystrophy in children. Clinical characteristics and follow-up of seventy patients. *J Bone Joint Surg Am.* 1992;74:910-919.

The classic paper describing CRPS/RSD in children, its treatment, and outcome. Its observations hold up today.

A complete reference list can be found online at Elsevier eBooks+.

SPECIAL TOPICS

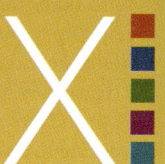

Anesthesia Outside the Operating Room $\quad$ 43

VANESSA A. OLBRECHT, JOSEPH P. CRAVERO, AND MARY LANDRIGAN-OSSAR

Standards and Guidelines
Off-Site Anesthesia: Structure
Personnel Requirements
Specific Environmental Requirements
Quality Assurance of Anesthesia Services and Outcome in the Off-Site Areas
Anesthetic Risk in Non–Operating Room Anesthesia
Logistics of Managing Acute Emergencies and Cardiopulmonary Arrest Outside the Operating Room
Emergencies in the MRI Scanner
Anesthetic Options for Non–Operating Room Procedures and Tests in Children

Difficult Airway Management in the Non–Operating Room (Off-Site) Environment
Specific Locations for Non–Operating Room Anesthesia
Computed Tomography
Magnetic Resonance Imaging
Magnetoencephalography
Nuclear Medicine
Stereotactic Radiosurgery
Radiation Therapy
Interventional Radiology
Endoscopic Procedures

THE APPROACH TO PROVIDING ANESTHESIA outside the operating room (also known as "non–operating room anesthesia" [NORA] or "off-site anesthesia") for children varies greatly among health care organizations and even from one anesthesia provider to another. Approximately 23% of pediatric anesthesia practice occurs in non–operating room venues.[1] Given the variety of environments and types of procedures, NORA practice is neither as standardized as anesthesia delivered in the operating room nor is it as well studied or reported, although advances in large database studies are beginning to close that knowledge gap. As such, it is a difficult topic to review using an evidence-based approach. Nonetheless, issues that may contribute to adverse events such as inadequate lighting, cramped work space, noise, and older equipment are now recognized and should be addressed.[2] The anesthetic plan for delivering anesthesia to a 2-year-old child undergoing an inguinal hernia repair is relatively standardized, whereas the anesthetic plan for anesthetizing a child for a magnetic resonance imaging (MRI) scan holds much more variability (in terms of drugs used, airway management techniques, and general organization of care). These issues are made even more confusing by the fact that NORA procedures may be performed with deep sedation in one institution and with general anesthesia and tracheal intubation in another. Furthermore, a procedure that is performed using deep sedation provided by an *anesthesiologist* in one institution may be performed using sedation provided by a specialist *other* than an anesthesiologist at another.[3]

The discussion of anesthesia services outside the operating room must also include the recognition that the level of sedation or anesthesia for a given child at any moment during a procedure is often a matter of some conjecture. Almost any procedure that involves pain, or absolute movement control in a child, necessitates deep sedation or general anesthesia. The distinction between these two states of anesthesia (defined by the presence or absence of movement in reaction to painful stimuli) is often unclear.[4] For anesthesiologists, the difference is more of semantic interest than practical importance since anesthesia outside the operating room often involves children with major comorbidities undergoing routine procedures. Many of these children would be managed with moderate to deep sedation by other specialists were it not for the complexity of the child's underlying illness(es). Comorbid conditions that require referral to an anesthesiologist vary among institutions but common (generally accepted) examples include[5]:

1. Extremely young age, including healthy children younger than 2 months of age.
2. History of prematurity (<37 weeks gestational age at birth) and postmenstrual age less than 60 weeks.
3. History of ongoing apnea and bradycardia episodes.
4. Craniofacial anomalies or any known difficult functional or anatomic airway problem.
5. Cyanotic congenital heart disease or cardiomyopathy.
6. Any serious coexisting disease such as sickle cell disease, obstructive sleep apnea, a known difficult airway (syndrome), or muscular dystrophy that would qualify a patient as American Society of Anesthesiologists (ASA) status III to IV.

7. Procedures that require elective airway control (intubation) or respiratory control such as breath-holding.

With these considerations in mind, this chapter focuses on issues specifically related to the delivery of anesthesia and deep sedation outside the operating room *provided by anesthesiologists*. Issues concerning the nuances of minimal, moderate, and deep sedation, as well as issues involving care by specialists other than anesthesiologists, are reviewed in Chapter 44.

Standards and Guidelines

Administration of anesthesia is influenced by a number of standards and regulations. Specifically, the Center for Medicare's (CMS) *Conditions for Participation* for hospitals are enforced by The Joint Commission (TJC) in the United States, regardless of location of care. The *Conditions for Participation for Anesthesia Services* are principles that are articulated to surveyors as instructions in the Interpretive Guidelines* published in January 2023. These guidelines describe appropriate training, credentialing, and oversight of sedation and anesthesia providers and some of the specific requirements for care documentation. NORA services must be organized in such a way as to meet the *Conditions for Participation* (and thus TJC) standards, just as they are met in the operating room. Depending on how NORA is organized in a particular institution, this can be challenging. The departments that require anesthesia services must appreciate the need to meet these standards and provide the infrastructure needed to meet or exceed them, particularly regarding the preanesthetic assessment and postanesthetic follow-up requirements.

The ASA has developed templates for these required policies that help institutions meet the standards of the Interpretive Guidelines. These resources can be downloaded from the ASA website.† With reference to NORA, there are several notable templates:

1. Preanesthesia Evaluation Policy, Form, and Note:

On the day of the procedure, a qualified practitioner must perform a preanesthetic evaluation of the child that includes, at a minimum: (1) a review of the medical history including previous anesthetics and complications, drugs, and allergies, and (2) an interview regarding the child's medical conditions with a parent present as indicated, and (3) physical examination emphasizing the airway, and the respiratory and cardiovascular systems. In addition, the following must be reviewed and updated before anesthesia:

   a. Notation of the anesthesia risk.
   b. Identification of potential anesthesia problems.
   c. Updated preanesthesia data and additional information, if applicable and as required in accordance with standard practice before administration of anesthesia (e.g., laboratory test results, physiological assessments).
   d. Development of the plan for the patient's anesthesia care, including the type of medications for induction, maintenance, and postoperative care and discussion with the patient (parents) of the risks and benefits of the delivery of anesthesia.
   e. Written informed consent for deep sedation/general anesthesia is required in many jurisdictions. Although MRI scanning itself does not require consent from the parents as the risks are considered negligible, the administration of

general anesthesia together with the administration of intravenous contrast are considered risks and written consent regarding the perianesthetic risks must be obtained (based on local requirements).

2. Intraoperative record policy: Standard data elements and times must be included in the intraoperative record, just as in the operating room. The intraoperative electronic record should ideally be accessible from all NORA locations within an institution, but where that is not feasible, a written anesthesia record should be completed and scanned afterwards into the electronic record.

3. Postanesthesia Evaluation Policy, Note, and Form (template): Although many procedures are performed in NORA sites on an ambulatory basis, a postanesthesia note must be completed within 48 hours of the anesthetic for all in-patients. The person completing the evaluation does not have to be the person who delivered the anesthetic. The elements of the postanesthesia note include assessment of:

   a. Respiratory function
   b. Cardiovascular function
   c. Mental status
   d. Temperature
   e. Pain
   f. Nausea and vomiting
   g. Postoperative hydration
   h. Complications

Off-Site Anesthesia: Structure

There is a paucity of literature concerning the organization of pediatric anesthesia services outside the operating room. Based on information available from the Pediatric Sedation Research Consortium (PSRC), we know *some* institutions organize these services through an off-site anesthesia unit that can be used for general anesthesia or sedation cases, in some institutions coordinating care with non–anesthesia trained sedation specialists.[6] Anesthesia-run units have the advantage of providing all anesthesia-related care through one location that can access the personnel and equipment required to provide the anesthesia care, resulting in the ability to provide all levels of sedation during each encounter. Ideally, these units are self-contained, providing a location for direct admission to the unit, preanesthesia assessment, induction, procedure location, and recovery. Children may have to be transported to remote locations when equipment (such as MRI scanners) cannot be brought to the sedation unit. The advantages of this organizational scheme include a uniform environment that maximizes the consistency in equipment and personnel who interact with children and their families and thus increased safety, efficiency, parent satisfaction, and effectiveness of care. Specialty teams or microsystems to provide NORA are coordinated groups of professionals who deliver a specific service that achieve the best possible outcomes by developing reliable, efficient, and responsive processes.[7] They meet the individual needs of each child,[8] continually improving care for the next child, and create a user-friendly work environment. The NORA microsystem should be made up of pediatric anesthesiologists, nurses, and technical and administrative personnel who are familiar with the off-site service and dedicated to this practice venue.[9,10] As members gain expertise and comfort with the off-site environment, their care becomes consistent and reproducible, leading to less confusion with other services. Such systems of care improve the effectiveness of the sedation (decreasing failed anesthesia and sedation cases) and improved patient, family, and staff satisfaction.[11–14]

---

*Guidelines available at https://www.cms.gov/files/document/medicare-ncci-policy-manual-2023-chapter-2.pdf
†https://www.asahq.org

Another option for the organization of NORA is the use of standard operating room same-day unit admission services and postanesthesia care unit recovery capability while providing induction and procedural anesthesia at the site of the procedure (e.g., endoscopy suite or hematology and oncology unit). This organizational paradigm uses existing anesthesia ancillary services and almost always requires patient transport before and after the procedure itself.

Finally, anesthesia services outside the operating room may be primarily organized at the site of procedural care (e.g., in radiology departments or gastrointestinal [GI] procedure suites). For this organizational setup, the procedure unit itself may be outfitted for admission and preanesthesia assessment and recovery of children is accomplished in a space contiguous with the procedural location. This kind of organization is most common in children's hospitals, where high volumes of procedures are performed in a given location such as the MRI scanner or the endoscopy suite.[15]

PERSONNEL REQUIREMENTS

Inadequate experience or familiarity with equipment/monitoring devices, poor communication with team members, production pressure, inattention, carelessness, and fatigue are critical contributors to the incidence of anesthesia-related adverse events.[16] The environment and the demands of providing anesthesia outside the operating room are unique regardless of the specific organizing strategy. To create a functional and efficient anesthesia microsystem, several common themes lead to optimal safety and effectiveness of care[17]:

1. Anesthesia providers should rotate on this service with a frequency that allows them to develop a working relationship among the anesthesiologists, anesthesia extenders, the proceduralists including radiologists, gastroenterologists, oncologists, respirologists, and others, respiratory therapists, registered nurses, patient care technicians, biomedical engineers, and child-life specialists. This familiarity should be based on a common understanding of the routines and protocols for standard procedures and a common agreement on the goals of the service.

2. Effective and efficient communication among personnel is critical to optimize outcomes. In day-to-day operations a "point person" who can act as a subject matter expert for their anesthesiologist colleagues and a point of contact for the radiologist or proceduralist will help ensure the seamless care of more complex patients. In urgent situations, an explicit chain of communication must be established such that in the event of an emergency there is no confusion about how outside resources (additional anesthesia assistance from main operating room, hospital code team) will be activated when necessary. The use of cell phones, Internet phones, "stat buttons,"[18] or other devices to optimize communication in NORA locations is often helpful in ensuring a quick response to a critical event (ideally within 3 to 4 minutes).

3. The ancillary personnel in each location must be familiar with the needs and processes of providing anesthesia to children and should be ready to assist in crisis events.[19] *In situ* simulation of the response to critical events is becoming increasingly accessible, and allows teams to practice the technical and communication skills that are necessary in an emergency.[20–22] High fidelity human patient simulation training is particularly useful in the NORA setting when additional anesthesia staff who can respond to an emergency may be some distance away.

4. Equipment and monitoring standards should mimic those in the operating room. Anesthesia carts, machine preparation, and setup should mirror the operating room environment as much as possible to maximize the similarity to the most common workspace.[23] It is critical to use a system that ensures supplies are restocked and anesthesia carts are secured in all off-site locations with the same level of scrutiny as in the operating room. All off-site carts should include a full range of drugs, intravenous (IV) equipment, fluids, and age and size appropriate airway equipment such as tracheal tubes, supraglottic devices, laryngoscopes, oral and nasal airways, masks, and suction equipment.[4]

5. Scheduling off-site anesthesia resources is complex and time-consuming. Timing for some procedures is inexact. In addition, anesthesia time requirements can vary with the child and the associated pathology. Success is enhanced by focusing the task of scheduling NORA procedures with one individual (or a small group) who intimately understands the process involved in anesthesia. This type of organization allows the NORA service to have one focal point for communication between the individuals who perform procedures and the anesthesia service, thus maximizing communication and minimizing incorrect assumptions of staffing or timing for procedures.[24]

6. Successful off-site anesthesia is maximized when arrangements are made for anesthesiologists to be integrated with other sedation/anesthesia providers in a way that allows them to transfer care for those who are *not* successfully sedated, and convert to anesthesia care as needed.[11,25]

SPECIFIC ENVIRONMENTAL REQUIREMENTS

Equipment and monitoring standards must meet those of the main operating room environment. The ASA requires that remote locations must have two sources of oxygen (preferably a central source of piped oxygen and a backup E cylinder), an anesthesia workstation if administering inhalational anesthetics, a scavenging system for waste anesthetic gases, suction, a self-inflating hand resuscitator bag able to deliver 95% oxygen and positive-pressure ventilation, standard of care monitors and equipment,[14,15] and sufficient electrical outlets, illumination, and space. The ASA Standards for Basic Anesthetic Monitoring include:

- Pulse oximetry with audible pulse tone and low-threshold alarm.
- Adequate illumination and exposure of the patient to assess color.
- Anesthesia machine with oxygen analyzer.
- Continuous end-tidal carbon dioxide ($ETCO_2$) analysis with an audible alarm.
- Continuous electrocardiogram (ECG).
- Arterial blood pressure and heart rate every 5 minutes or more frequently as indicated.
- Temperature monitor where clinically significant changes in body temperature are possible.

In addition, it is important to make further adaptations (e.g., duplicates of critical equipment, such as laryngoscope handles and blades) to enhance patient safety and quality of care. In the MRI unit, it is essential to have MRI-compatible laryngoscope blades and handles, compatible monitoring devices, and MRI-compatible portable oxygen tanks. Each site should be carefully evaluated for important items such as wall-delivered gases (oxygen, nitrous oxide, and air), the location of suction equipment, and an Ambu bag (Ambu, Copenhagen, Denmark). Every site must have backup gas supplies. If pipeline oxygen is not available, oxygen should be drawn from H cylinders (6600 L) rather than the smaller E tanks (659 L), and oxygen reserves should be checked prior to each use. All equipment for monitoring and resuscitation should be up to date and standardized to that used in the operating rooms.

MRI suites designed for general anesthesia include walled gas lines (oxygen, air, and nitrous oxide) and suction. For older MRI suites such as those designed without general anesthesia in mind, a suction canister can be mounted with 30 feet of suction tubing threaded through a hole in the console wall in the MRI suite. If walled gas lines were not included in the original MRI unit design, they cannot be retrofitted to service an existing MRI suite in most instances. In such cases, MRI-compatible E tanks for gases can be mounted on an MRI-compatible anesthesia workstation if one is available. If an MRI-compatible workstation is not available, anesthesia will have to be induced outside the operating room. To maintain anesthesia in these cases, either the anesthesia circuit with extensions or tubing to deliver a total intravenous anesthesia (TIVA) anesthetic is passed through a hole in the wall of the scanner while the anesthesia workstation or syringe pump remain outside the scanner room.[26]

Scavenging systems should be available in all NORA locations. When passive scavenging is not possible, active scavenging may be developed by using the wall-source vacuum or wall suction canisters. A scavenging system dedicated solely to waste gases should be present if inhalational anesthetics are used.[27] Where scavenging systems are not available, TIVA is the preferred anesthetic of choice.

Electrical circuitry in off-site locations must meet operating room standards. Specifically, although the outlets tend to be grounded and hospital grade, plug and outlet incompatibility may be present. Adapters and conversion plugs must be readily available. Although off-site locations tend not to have as great of a risk of electrical shock or electrocution to the child as in the operating room, these sites do not have line-isolation monitors. In the event of excessive leakage of current, the anesthesiologist would not be warned that a shock is imminent. The National Electrical Code no longer requires line-isolation monitors in nonflammable anesthetizing locations; however, it is strongly recommended for areas with multiple power sources. To ensure child and health care personnel safety, biomedical engineers must be attentive to the safe maintenance of all electrical equipment.

NORA locations may pose specific challenges when considering specific infectious risks and the need for isolation of patients and special precautions for providers. Infection control measures need to be addressed and designed with each unique off-site environment in mind.[28]

In most NORA settings, the physical environment and practice patterns are typically that of another medical specialty. It should be noted that these other specialties practice under standards developed by their own professional organizations that apply to the procedures within their locations and to different procedure goals. The varying specialties involved include (but are not limited to) gastroenterology, dentistry, cardiology, oncology, intensive care, emergency medicine, and radiology.[12] Anesthesia providers who work in these environments are well served by familiarizing themselves with the standards for the given specialty area in which they are working as well as those published for the various professional organizations.

Hypothermia is a risk in NORA settings, particularly in infants in MRI suites where forced air warming blankets are incompatible with the strong magnetic field.[29,30] Forced air warming devices can be used in many NORA sites including the cardiac catheterization laboratory where procedures are commonly prolonged. Temperature decreases in the MRI scanner depend in part on the type of anesthesia and the duration of the scan. Post-MRI temperatures averaged 35.5°C in 250 children after TIVA anesthesia, with the decrement in temperature being similar for 1.5T and 3T scanners.[31] Under light sedation, the child's temperature may actually slightly increase after MRI.

Quality Assurance of Anesthesia Services and Outcome in the Off-Site Areas

It is important to develop a strategy to track all clinically important complications associated with NORA, as we do in the operating room. Each department can set its own thresholds for review; however, certain incidents require a full inquiry[32]:

- Aspiration
- Respiratory arrest or need for airway rescue, e.g., emergent intubation
- Cardiac arrest
- Cardiovascular or respiratory compromise that requires assistance from an outside rescue team or leads to a "call for help"
- Unscheduled admissions to the hospital as a direct result of the sedation (i.e., because of protracted emesis, prolonged sedation, respiratory or cardiac complication)
- Medication errors that led to or could have led to patient harm
- Procedures that could not be completed because of inadequate or problematic anesthesia or sedation

Many institutions choose to follow outcomes such as prolonged nausea and vomiting after anesthesia or oxygen desaturation events after anesthesia.[33] The frequency of emergency calls for help in NORA are less than in the operating room although contributing factors including age <1 year, prematurity, and ASA Physical Status ≥III are similar for both sites.[18,34] Regardless of the data that the quality improvement (QI) committee chooses to review, the process should include anesthesiologists and anesthesia extenders, nurses, and other technical personnel who are routinely involved in sedation/anesthesia care and support. It is particularly important to note that in the case of NORA sites, it is critical to include members of the departments (other than anesthesiology) to review cases. The timing of quality improvement meetings depends on the number and acuity of the NORA cases provided at a given institution. Review committee meetings should be considered not just an opportunity to evaluate complications but also a forum for exchange of ideas, expertise, and information that can lead to improvements in the systems of patient care. It is important for the anesthesia service to not be viewed as "sedation police," but rather to be constructive members of the team designed to improve safety, outcomes, and efficiency of patient throughput.

Anesthetic Risk in Non–Operating Room Anesthesia

Despite the many challenges to safe practice in off-site locations, anesthesia in these locations is safer than one might expect. The traditional understanding was that the risks of providing anesthesia services in NORA were greater than those in the operating room based on an analysis of early closed claim data. These data showed a 2-fold greater incidence of death in NORA when compared with comparable cases in the operating room, although these data were biased toward settled malpractice judgments without a denominator.[35] More recently, "big data" from several large sources have changed this understanding. The ASA Anesthesia Quality Institute's National Anesthesia Clinical Outcomes Registry (NACOR) compiled data from more than 3 million cases. These data confirm closed claims data that off-site anesthesia locations involved older patients, a greater proportion of whom who were ASA Physical Status ≥III, a greater rate of emergent procedures, a greater complication rate in cardiology and radiology locations, and more anesthetics that were started after elective work hours.[36] However, even with these potential negatives, NACOR data failed to demonstrate that off-site anesthesia as a whole is associated with increased morbidity and mortality compared with operating-room-based anesthesia. Analysis of other databases such as the PSRC and the Wake Up Safe project, focused on pediatric anesthesia adverse events, reiterated the same results.[37,38] PSRC and the Wake Up Safe project found an increased risk associated with procedures performed in interventional radiology and the cardiac catheterization areas. The most recent analysis of the closed claims data supports the findings of these databases that cardiac catheterization and radiology suites are areas of increased risk and this is almost certainly due to the underlying pathology of the patients involved in these procedures or specific procedures themselves that put these patients at increased risk for adverse events (e.g., stent placement, balloon dilation procedures, valve and closure device placements).[39,40]

Logistics of Managing Acute Emergencies and Cardiopulmonary Arrest Outside the Operating Room

Although the actual management of a cardiopulmonary arrest should not vary between the operating room and NORA sites, the logistics of performing a resuscitation in these remote locations may be challenged by unanticipated factors, such as personnel who may not be familiar with code situations, the distance additional anesthesia personnel may have to travel to provide assistance, an environment that poses challenges to performing a resuscitation, or equipment that may be unsafe if used in the particular location (e.g., the MRI environment). It is important that all personnel in the off-site location be familiar with the location and operation of the code cart. The anesthesia cart and the code cart in the off-site location should be stocked identically to all others throughout the hospital and operating rooms. Standardizing the code carts throughout the hospital ensures that all ancillary personnel can quickly locate critical items. If the code cart is kept locked, the key or access code must be readily accessible and in a location that is known to all essential personnel. A hard board on which chest compressions may be performed should also be readily available. Each off-site location should have an identified and rehearsed routine for announcing a code situation and summoning aid. Responders to a code must be assured of access to the location to which they are called; in the current age of card-key access, this should be simple but needs to be verified in advance of an actual code. The use of patient simulation may help to evaluate the response of a team to critical events. Simulators can be used in place in off-site locations to replicate critical events and evaluate the ability of the care team and backup systems to resuscitate a patient. This methodology has documented significant variation in the ability of rescuers to resuscitate children from sedation or anesthesia critical events in locations outside the operating room.[41,42]

EMERGENCIES IN THE MRI SCANNER

Of all the non–operating room environments in which anesthesiologists are asked to provide care, the MRI scanner poses a unique challenge for cardiopulmonary resuscitation. The MRI environment is divided into four zones that correlate with the intensity of the magnetic field and the risk to children and health care providers. These zones are delineated in Table 43.1.

The American College of Radiology provides the industry standard on safety in MRI.[43] The ASA published an updated practice advisory report in 2015.[44,45] These documents advise that in the case of a medical emergency within the scanner, the anesthesia

TABLE 43.1	Descriptions of the American College of Radiology's Four Zones in the Magnetic Resonance Imaging Suite	
ACR Zones	**Occupants**	**Hazards**
Zone I	General public	Negligible
Zone II	Unscreened MRI patients	Immediately outside area of hazard
Zone III	Screened MRI patients and personnel	Potential biostimulation interference, access to magnet room
Zone IV	Screened MRI patients under constant direct supervision of trained MRI personnel	Biostimulation interference, radiofrequency heating, missile effect, cryogens

ACR, American College of Radiology; *MRI*, magnetic resonance imaging.
From American College of Radiology Manual on MR Safety. American College of Radiology; 2020.

providers should (1) initiate cardiopulmonary resuscitation while the patient is immediately evacuated from zone IV, (2) call for help, and (3) transport the patient to a previously designated safe location near the MRI suite. This designated location should contain a defibrillator, vital signs monitors, and a code cart with all resuscitation drugs, airway equipment, oxygen, and suction. Other acute emergencies that are unique to the MRI environment include a "quench" in the scanner.[44,45] Quenching occurs when the liquid that cools the magnet boils off rapidly allowing helium to escape from the cryogen bath. The magnetic field decreases rapidly thereafter because the coils in the magnet cease to be superconducting and become resistive. In addition to performing the institution's protocol in reaction to either of these events, the ASA consultants involved in writing the advisory agree that in the event of a quench (1) the child should be removed from zone IV immediately, (2) oxygen should be administered immediately, and (3) emergency response personnel should be restricted from entering zone IV because of the potential for a residual powerful magnetic field even after a quench.

Anesthetic Options for Non–Operating Room Procedures and Tests in Children

Anesthesiologists can provide any level of sedation or anesthesia for procedures outside the operating room. The choice of whether to deliver general anesthesia with a secured airway (tracheal tube or supraglottic device) using potent inhalational anesthetics, deep sedation with face mask oxygen and propofol ± dexmedetomidine infusion, or moderate or minimal sedation supplemented by Child Life or electronic device distractions depends on many factors.[46,47] These include the child's comorbidities, the procedure, and the experience and comfort level of the anesthesia provider[48]; specific options for various NORA locations are discussed later.

Many techniques have been reported as effective and safe outside the operating room; there are few data that demonstrate that one technique is superior to another. Recognizing this fact, it is appropriate to carefully evaluate the nature of the sedation/anesthesia provided in the NORA setting, consider the possible implications of a given technique for each patient, and proceed with the technique that best meets the intended goals. For instance, how efficient and effective is the care provided? How well does that care meet the requirements of the procedure in terms of movement/behavior control and prevention of pain, and how can this be best assessed?[49] How rapid is the emergence from sedation or anesthesia with a given technique? Do the short-term or long-term complications differ? What approach best meets the needs for the proceduralist while optimizing patient safety, rapidity of recovery, and safe discharge? Only after careful analysis can location- and institution-specific guidelines be established for the optimal technique for a given procedure.[50]

When delivering general anesthesia to children outside the operating room, the risks/benefits of instrumenting the airway must be carefully evaluated. In healthy children, deep sedation is appropriate (e.g., for an MRI scan); it often includes a propofol infusion or dexmedetomidine supplemented with another adjunct, an optimally positioned upper airway (with a roll under the cervical spine and the neck extended), and noninvasive monitoring (nasal capnometry supplemented with oximetry, an ECG, and noninvasive blood pressure monitoring).[51] The majority of children do not require an airway during deep sedation for medical tests. However, in some (e.g., those with sialorrhea, obstructive sleep apnea, morbid obesity, or congenital airway anomaly such as midfacial hypoplasia), interventions may be required to relieve airway obstruction: (1) reposition the airway; (2) perform a jaw thrust; (3) insert an oral or nasal airway;[52,53] (4) consider calling for help; (5) if obstruction persists, place a supraglottic device; and (6) if the supraglottic device fails to provide adequate gas exchange and oxygenation, place a tracheal tube using standard direct visualization, video scope, or fiberoptic techniques, or if all of these maneuvers fail; (7) perform a surgical airway.[54]

Difficult Airway Management in the Non–Operating Room (Off-Site) Environment

Two potential difficult airway scenarios may occur in non–operating room locations: the child with a known difficult airway and the child with an unrecognized difficult airway. There is little peer-reviewed literature that addresses these scenarios, but logic dictates that children who are identified as having potentially difficult airways should have their airways secured in a controlled environment such as the operating room. With the trachea intubated, the child may be safely transported to the off-site location for subsequent care. Regardless of an anesthesiologist's comfort level and familiarity with the intended off-site environment, the critical backup personnel and the full array of airway equipment[55] are not generally available in remote locations, hence the recommendation to secure the airway first in a location with ample support help and then proceed to the NORA site.

It is important to note that a fiberoptic bronchoscope and light source and most video laryngoscopes are not MRI-compatible, although an MRI-compatible video laryngoscope is available (Tru-MR [Truphatek International Ltd., Netanya, Israel]). The advent of advanced video laryngoscopes has supplanted flexible fiberoptic bronchoscopes as the first choice to secure the difficult airway (see also Chapter 12).[56,57] This equipment should be readily available in NORA locations for any child with a proven or suspected difficult laryngoscopy (before and during the procedure). The ASA task force on care in the MRI recommends complex airway management should be performed in a controlled environment outside zone IV.[45]

The more difficult scenario is that of the unrecognized difficult airway[58]; this situation may best be handled by establishing a local management protocol that can be activated when the situation arises. Each institution has particular equipment, space, and personnel resources. NORA leaders should establish a local protocol for management of the unanticipated difficult airway in an off-site location. In some cases, this might involve bringing advanced airway management equipment to the location in a rapid, organized manner. In other cases, the best option would include "temporizing" management with alternative airway devices and transporting the child to a location where a definitive airway can be placed in a controlled manner. For this reason, it is important to have alternative airway devices such as supraglottic devices stocked in all anesthesia carts that are designated for off-site locations. In the event that the lungs cannot be ventilated or the trachea intubated, the supraglottic device has a proven track record for providing a lifesaving temporary airway until more definitive action can be taken.[59–61]

Specific Locations for Non–Operating Room Anesthesia

COMPUTED TOMOGRAPHY

Specific considerations for computed tomography (CT) include the use of ionizing radiation, the need for brief immobility, administration of intravenous contrast with the potential for contrast reactions, and oral contrast with the potential for aspiration. CT provides a good modality for differentiating between high-density (calcium, iron, bone, contrast-enhanced vascular and cerebrospinal fluid [CSF] spaces) and low-density (air, fat, CSF, muscle, white matter, gray matter, and water-containing lesions) structures. To reduce occupational exposure, the anesthesia team is generally not present in the room during a scan. Scan time with current scanners continues to decrease with actual imaging time ranging from 5 to 50 seconds for image acquisition. A new generation of high-speed CT scanners obtains images in as little as 0.3 seconds, which should allow even more images to be acquired without sedation and with less exposure to radiation.[62] It should be noted that radiologists and surgeons will (at times) request an MRI scan instead of a CT scan for a given patient due to the perceived risk of ionized radiation involved in CT scanning. In fact, the risk from radiation in these cases is extremely low and must be balanced against the fact that many CT scans can be performed without anesthesia, whereas MRI scans will almost certainly require anesthesia (which carries its own short- and [potentially] long-term risks). The risk calculation in these cases should take into account the number of scans required, the underlying comorbidities of the patient involved, and other issues such as the fasting status.[63]

The use of intravascular contrast media is ubiquitous in CT, interventional radiology, and cardiac catheterization. It is important that the anesthesiologist is aware of the risks and potential adverse effects of these agents.[64,65] Reactions to iodinated contrast material in patients under anesthesia range from rash to bronchospasm to a diffuse anaphylactoid reaction[66] that can be life-threatening. These reactions are divided temporally into immediate (1 to 6 hours after administration) and delayed (>6 hours after administration). Immediate reactions result from both IgE (in a minority of cases) and non–IgE-mechanisms including complement activation and direct mediator release, and present with symptoms that range from urticaria, pruritus, and gastrointestinal manifestations (vomiting and cramps) to anaphylaxis.[67,68] In contrast, delayed reactions often begin as a maculopapular rash but in some, may progress to Steven-Johnson syndrome or toxic epidermal necrolysis.[68] The pathophysiology of immediate reactions is primarily mediated through the release of histamine and tryptase from basophils and mast cells, whereas the pathophysiology of delayed reactions is usually T-cell medicated.

The incidence of both mild and life-threatening acute hypersensitivity reactions to contrast media has decreased with the advent of low-osmolality nonionic contrast media.[69,70] The overall frequency of hypersensitivity reactions after iodinated contrast material in adults is estimated at 0.2% to 12% of patients, with anaphylactic (severe) reactions accounting for 0.01% to 0.2% of all reactions.[68,71] This overall frequency is 3- to 4-fold greater than the overall frequency of reactions with noniodinated contrast material, 0.05% to 3%.[72] In children, hypersensitivity reactions to contrast material occur less frequently than in adults.[73,74] The risk of a fatal outcome after a hypersensitivity reaction is estimated to occur in 1:170,000, a rate much improved from that reported in the 1970s of 1:30,000.[65] This reduction in fatal adverse reactions is due to the use of newer noniodinated contrast media and improved recognition and treatment of reactions. Anaphylactic shock is the most worrisome of all contrast reactions and may occur at any time after the contrast material, from 1 minute until several hours afterwards. Although adverse reactions to intravascular contrast media are unpredictable, some children may be at increased risk: those with a prior reaction to contrast material, those who suffer from allergies or an atopic disease; asthma (a 6-fold increased risk for a repeat hypersensitivity reaction if asthma is not well-controlled), hypothyroid disease due to congenital hypothyroidism, cancer, or treated Graves disease (due to up to 150-fold greater daily intake of iodine in children 1 to 8 years of age with iodinated contrast), and contrast-induced nephropathy leading to acute kidney injury.[64,67] Some recommend withholding metformin before giving iodinated contrast because metformin is excreted via the kidney and may cause lactic acidosis if it is accumulated due to reduced kidney function.[67] The need for gadolinium should be reevaluated in children with nephrogenic systemic fibrosis and chronic kidney disease.[67] Furthermore, properties of the contrast material that are known to increase the risk of reactions include the osmolality, size, and complexity of the iodinated contrast material itself. Children who have been identified as being at increased risk for a reaction to contrast material should be premedicated with corticosteroids (in a total dose equivalent to 25 to 125 mg prednisolone) and antihistamines[67,68]; one retrospective study reported a 21% incidence of breakthrough reactions despite this premedication regimen.[75–78] In NORA settings where contrast media is routinely given, protocols should be in place to administer prophylaxis in children who have experienced a prior reaction to contrast material as well as to identify and treat a de novo reaction should it occur.

The effect of contrast media on renal function must also be considered.[53] The mechanisms underlying renal injury from contrast media are complex and not fully characterized.[79] Direct renal tubular injury as well as renal hypoperfusion seem to play a role.[77] The trend toward low- and iso-osmolar contrast has reduced renal damage from contrast. Nonetheless, in patients at high risk for renal injury, such as those with preexisting renal insufficiency (serum creatine ≥1.5 mg/dL), diabetes mellitus, dehydration, cardiovascular disease, hypertension, and hyperuricemia, good hydration and careful follow-up of renal function must be maintained.[80] In some institutions, a protocol of prehydration and posthydration with alkalinized IV fluids is used to help reduce the risk of renal injury from contrast agents. A retrospective study of 19,377 scans in 10,407 children reported an incidence of acute kidney injury of 1.6% but interestingly the incidence was greater in those with an estimated glomerular filtration rate ≥60 mL/minute per 1.73 m² compared with those with a lower glomerular filtration rate (1.3% vs. 8.5%). The authors concluded that exposure to contrast material did not increase the risk of acute kidney injury consistently in children and that this incidence was less than that reported in adults.[79,81]

Perhaps the most controversial issue facing anesthesiologists regarding CT scans is the issue of oral contrast for CT and its effect on nil per os (NPO) status. Because children lack abundant retroperitoneal fat, they do not have the natural contrast needed to adequately visualize many abdominal structures and/or pathology. Thus, children are often required to ingest radiopaque agents such as diatrizoic acid (Gastrografin) (Bracco Diagnostics, Monroe Township, NJ) to opacify the stomach and bowel orally or via nasogastric tube. Oral contrast is useful in the identification of an intraabdominal abscess, mass, fluid collection, bowel injury, pancreatic injury, or other traumatic injury. Oral contrast, sold commercially as Gastrografin, 3% concentration, is hypertonic (2200 mOsm/L) and can cause pulmonary edema, pneumonitis, osmotic effusions, and death if aspirated.[61,82] Gastrografin is recommended to be diluted with water to a 1:1.5% concentration (1 part agent, 3 parts water), which is thought to be much less dangerous if aspirated.[83] The volume of oral contrast that is administered can be quite large due to dilution with water. Neonates typically receive 60 to 90 mL; infants between 1 month and 1 year of age may receive up to 240 mL; and children between the ages of 1 and 5 years receive between 240 and 360 mL. Risk is introduced when these children require anesthesia within 30 minutes to 1 hour after receiving the contrast, the optimal window after ingestion to enhance visualization. By most fasting guidelines (NPO), Gastrografin consumption within 1 to 2 hours of an anesthetic or sedation does not fall within the usual NPO guidelines. On the other hand, the scan must be completed while the Gastrografin is present in the GI tract.

Two studies provide our only guidance on the rate of gastric emptying after the ingestion of oral iodinated contrast in children. In the first study, contrast was aspirated from the stomachs of 6 children within 2 hours after ingesting iodinated contrast[84]; the authors concluded that oral contrast remained in the stomach at least 50 minutes after ingestion of the contrast. The second study was conducted on 101 children who ingested contrast before CT scans.[85] Using a Kaplan-Meier analysis to determine the rate of oral contrast emptying from the stomach, the authors recommended waiting 3 hours after oral contrast to empty the stomach of contrast.

A review of the pediatric and adult literature confirms that over the past 35 years and hundreds of thousands of contrast GI CT scans, only a few case reports have been published of aspiration syndrome attributed to oral contrast, and all of these events occurred in extremely high-risk patients with issues such as bowel obstruction or acute abdomen.[61,82,86] In one study, a cohort of 50 children who received oral contrast after blunt abdominal trauma were evaluated for radiologic evidence of aspiration pneumonia or clinical complications of aspiration.[87] Some received general anesthesia and some were neurologically impaired, including several with increased intracranial pressure. In this very high-risk group, only one child was thought to have possibly aspirated based on a chest radiograph after the CT scan but failed to develop pulmonary symptoms. Another study evaluated the volume of gastric contents of 365 children undergoing deep sedation or general anesthesia for abdominal CT scans. Omnipaque 3 mL was diluted 50-fold to a volume of 150 mL and given to children younger than 1 year of age and a volume of 600 mL was given to teenagers; starting 2 hours before the scheduled scan and ending 1 hour before general anesthesia ($N = 207$) or sedation ($N = 158$); all were elective scans with standard fasting times. The authors note that gastric contents exceeded 0.4 mL/kg in 49% of those who received gastric contrast[87] although the threshold gastric fluid volume needed to produce symptomatic aspiration is likely closer to 0.8 mL/kg.[88] Two cases of vomiting were recorded. None of the children in the study developed clinical evidence of aspiration. The incidence of vomiting from two retrospective studies of children who ingested oral contrast within 2 hours of sedation was 18% after ketamine sedation and 1% after propofol sedation in 22 and 85 children, respectively.[89,90] In those same two reports, there were no instances of pulmonary aspiration. When dilute Gastrografin is used, the risks associated with pulmonary aspiration appear to be small, even in children who are moderately to deeply sedated.[91]

Despite this evidence, cohort studies with sufficient power to determine the actual incidence of aspiration in this setting have not been performed. Therefore, *no* accepted standard of care for the airway management of these children has been determined. Some anesthesiologists induce anesthesia with an IV or inhalational technique and maintain the anesthetic without securing the airway with a tracheal tube, whereas others perform rapid-sequence induction and tracheal intubation (Fig. 43.1). The lack

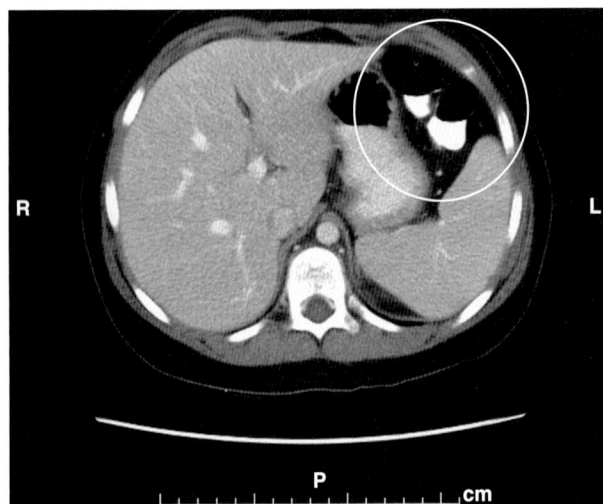

FIGURE 43.1 Four hours after ingestion of Gastrografin, oral contrast is still present in the stomach and small intestine. Although dilute Gastrografin is still frequently present in the stomach at the time of CT, there are no case reports validating an increase in risk of pulmonary aspiration to date.

of consensus among anesthesiologists and the absence of evidence precludes clear and consistent recommendations for managing the airway in these children. Common sense would lead one to conclude that a rapid-sequence induction with tracheal intubation/general anesthesia would be most appropriate for children with bowel pathology that interferes with gastric emptying.

CT scans that involve airway imaging are another challenge for anesthesiologists.[92,93] Traditionally, although these scans are brief, they require breath-holding to capture images of sufficient quality to be of diagnostic use. Appropriate apnea intervals can be obtained under anesthesia with tracheal intubation with or without neuromuscular blockade, or by placing a supraglottic device, providing moderate hyperventilation, and a bolus of propofol when apnea is required. The current generation of "flash" CT technology with ultra-fast image capture is diminishing the need for breath-holding with these studies and may further decrease the need for sedation or anesthesia for many CT studies in children of any age.[62]

Anesthesia or sedation is required for children who are unable to cooperate by lying still for a scan, due to factors such as cognitive impairment or young age. Some CT units are particularly concerned about children moving when contrast is injected; because of dose restrictions the contrast injection cannot be repeated, and they therefore request anesthesia services for any child they cannot confidently predict will stay motionless for the study. Other indications for anesthesia for CT scans include emergent evaluation of head trauma, unstable respiratory status in need of a pulmonary diagnosis, unexplained changes in mental status, neoplasm workup, or radiation therapy planning. Anesthesia management is also necessary in patients with a potentially unstable airway (peritonsillar abscess, anterior mediastinal mass, craniofacial anomaly, tracheoesophageal fistula, uncontrolled vomiting, or gastroesophageal reflux). It is also required if a child cannot cooperate with necessary breath-holding during acquisition of images (three-dimensional dynamic airway studies or certain pulmonary scans) (Figs. 43.2 and 43.3). In certain situations, such as those at increased risk for aspiration or when periods of

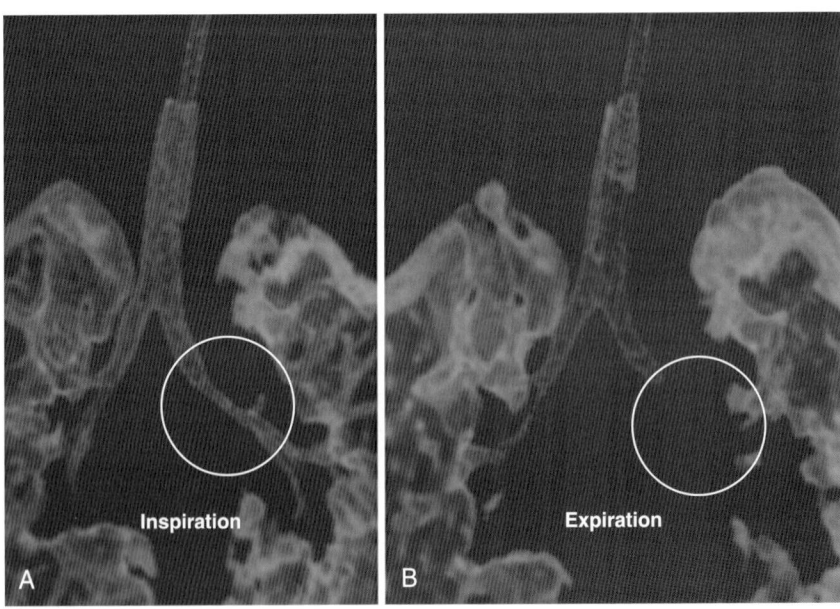

FIGURE 43.2 Three-dimensional dynamic computed tomography scan demonstrating change in caliber of left main-stem bronchus *(circle)* in an intubated child at end-inspiration (pressure held at 15–18 mm Hg) **(A)** versus end-expiration **(B)**.

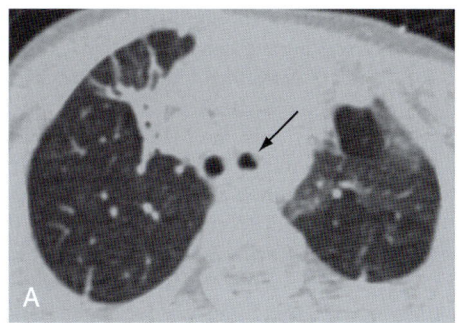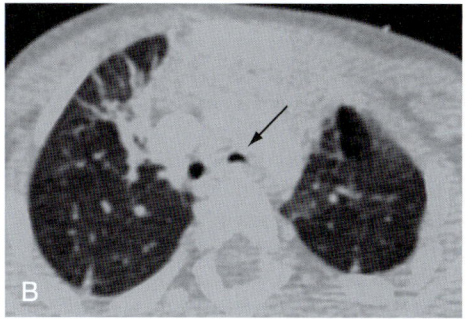

FIGURE 43.3 Three-dimensional CT scan demonstrating change in caliber of left main-stem bronchus *(arrows)* on inspiration **(A)** versus expiration **(B)**.

apnea are required for the scan, tracheal intubation may be required. But in the majority of sedations or anesthetics for CT scans, short acting oral, intranasal, or intravenous agents and an airway that is not instrumented are usually sufficient.[94]

MAGNETIC RESONANCE IMAGING

Specific considerations for MRI include the accommodations necessary for safe practice in the magnetic field: the need for specialized MRI-compatible monitoring equipment and pumps, injury to patients due the action of the magnetic field on implanted medical devices, intravenous contrast with the potential for hypersensitivity reactions, the need for prolonged immobility, and the long distance between the child relative to the anesthesia team.[95–97]

MRI, magnetic resonance spectroscopy (MRS), magnetic resonance angiography (MRA), and magnetic resonance venography (MRV) are used to evaluate neoplasms, nonhemorrhagic trauma, vascular, cardiac, orthopedic (including joint disorders, osteomyelitis), central nervous system and spinal cord lesions, craniofacial disorders, as well as identification of the cause of developmental delay, behavioral disorders, seizures, failure to thrive, apnea, cyanosis, and hypotonia, and to workup mitochondrial and metabolic diseases.[98–102] MRA and MRV are especially helpful in evaluating blood flow, oftentimes replacing invasive angiography in follow-up evaluations of vascular malformations,[103,104] interventional therapy, or radiotherapy.[105,106] All of these imaging modalities are essentially equivalent in terms of the requirements to provide anesthesia or sedation and thus can be considered equivalent to MRI scanning.

Most MRI systems are superconducting magnets set up in a horizontal configuration within the bore so that the magnetic field is directed lengthwise to the child. The magnet is cooled by liquid helium to a temperature of approximately −268°C. The strength of the magnetic field in these scanners is described in units called tesla (T) that range from 0.5 to 3.0 T. To put this into perspective, a 1.5-T magnet is the equivalent to 30,000 times the earth's magnetic field.

The foremost complications in the MR environment relate to the risks of burns[107] and projectile injuries from ferromagnetic objects attracted to the magnetic core of the MRI scanner that can result in injury and mortality to both the children and health care personnel (Fig. 43.4). A review of 1.3 million patient exposures in the United Kingdom reported an incidence of ~1:2000 safety-related events.[107] A 10-year review of 1568 adverse events reported to the US Food and Drug Administration (FDA) revealed 906 thermal injuries (59%) and 133 related to projectile events (9%); acoustic injury was reported in 86 patients.[108] Numerous injuries, including death, have been reported from objects accidentally

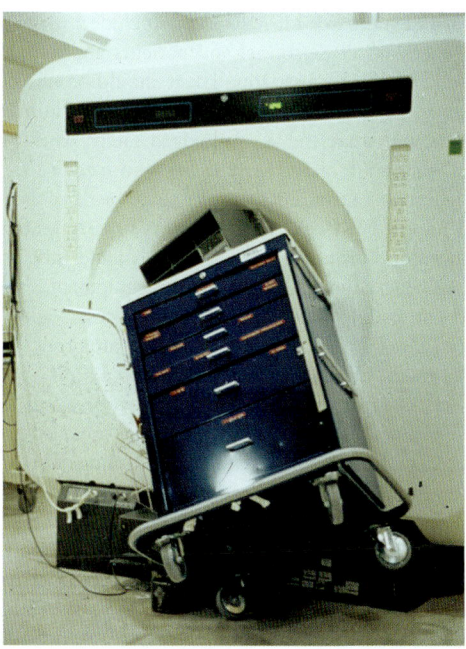

FIGURE 43.4 Magnetic resonance imaging cart that is not compatible inadvertently brought into scanner room. To extricate the cart, the magnet had to be quenched, incurring a cost in excess of $20,000 USD.

attracted to the MRI magnet. Objects reported to have propelled into an MRI magnet include: an anesthesia cart, a metal fan, a floor polisher, walkers, wheelchairs, a pulse oximeter, shrapnel, a cigarette lighter, a stethoscope, a pager, a hearing aid, a vacuum cleaner, a calculator, a hair pin, an oxygen tank, a prosthetic limb, a pencil, an insulin infusion pump, an IV pole, gas cylinders, ventilator, keys, watches, scissors, clipboards, steel-toe or steel-heeled shoes, ferrous jewelry, and even a concealed police revolver.[108–110] It should be noted that a loaded handgun may be triggered, resulting in fragments or direct patient or technician injury and death.[108,111] Mortality can result from projectile disasters, as in the case of a ferrous oxygen tank that was "pulled" from the hands of the respiratory therapist into the magnet, crushing the skull of the child in the scanner.[112] It is absolutely mandatory to check whether the patient has in or on them ferromagnetic objects, as 69% of the causes of accidents in adults resulted from a failure to check the patient for ferromagnetic and implanted devices (notably pacemaker, oxygen cylinder, and IV splint to name several).[113] It is essential to assure that all equipment entering zone IV, including anesthesia machines and monitors, medication pumps, and portable oxygen tanks, are MRI-compatible and that anesthesia carts are not brought into the area.

A thorough review of safety issues with respect to MRI can be found in the American College of Radiology safety manual.[43] All individuals who work in the MRI environment should be familiar with the primary recommendations in this report. The FDA has terminology for designating objects in terms of their safety in the MRI environment. *MRI-safe* is defined as not posing any known hazard in any MR environment. *MRI-conditional* refers to objects that may or may not be safe, depending on the specific conditions that are present. *MRI-unsafe* means the object should never be brought into the MRI environment because it poses a potential or realistic risk or hazard.[‡] All objects or medical devices should be referenced and vetted for safety prior to being brought into zone IV. Some devices are compatible with 1.5-T but not with 3.0-T units. Current standards for MRI safety include a magnetic metal detector check of all personnel and patients and/or family each time they enter the scanner zone III; it should be noted that the magnet may not detect all implanted ferromagnetic materials.[114] MRI technologists are the acknowledged safety experts and final arbiter of what equipment is safe to bring into zone IV.

MRI-compatible equipment continues to be developed and improved. Multiple MRI-compatible anesthesia machines (with ventilators), monitors (including wireless models), and infusion pumps are now available, although the cost for this equipment is substantial: an MRI-compatible anesthesia machine costs approximately $60,000 to $80,000 USD; MRI-compatible monitors range up to $140,000, and compatible infusion pumps cost $12,000 to $18,000.

MRI-safe stethoscopes, stylets, laryngoscopes, and flashlights should be available. If they are not available, standard equipment can be used with some modification and testing. The only component of the laryngoscope that is usually *not* MRI-safe is the battery. Replacing the standard battery with a lithium battery may be a simple, safe, and less expensive alternative to purchasing a marketed MRI-compatible laryngoscope. Before introducing any equipment into the MRI environment, a rudimentary safety check should be performed by first passing a handheld magnet over the object to confirm that there is no ferrous material within. As a final safety check, an MRI safety expert should carefully introduce the object into the scanner to confirm safety.

Another major risk related to the magnetic field in MRI scanning results from MRI interactions with implanted devices (e.g., cardiac pacemakers, orthodontic and orthopedic hardware, vagal and spinal cord stimulators, programmable ventriculoperitoneal shunts, and cochlear implants) that may malfunction in the powerful magnetic field of the MRI scanner and result in injury.[115] These injuries are most often caused by inappropriate patient screening or unfamiliarity with a particular implant's MRI compatibility.[113]

All implanted objects should be carefully evaluated before a patient or health care provider enters the MRI suite. The website http://www.MRIsafety.com is a useful resource for identifying the MRI safety of various objects. Note that stainless steel or surgical stainless objects may interact with the external magnetic field, potentially resulting in translational (attractive) and rotational (torque) forces. Special attention should be paid to older intracranial aneurysm clips (may move and potentially dislodge), vascular stents,[116,117] cochlear and stapedial implants (some may be safe, check before scanning; some develop pain, or the internal magnet becomes dislocated),[118–120] shrapnel,[121] intraorbital metallic

bodies, and prosthetic limbs.[115] In fact, some eye make-up and tattoos may contain metallic dyes[122,123] and are at risk of causing skin, ocular, periorbital, and cutaneous irritation and burning.[116,117,124] Importantly, tracheostomy tubes should be checked before children enter the MRI scanner. It is generally advised to switch a child's tracheostomy tube to a cuffed tracheal tube for MRI scanning to ensure a secure airway during the scan. Currently, small-diameter cuffed tracheostomy tubes (Bivona) from Smiths Medical (Minneapolis, MN) are considered MRI-conditional.[§] Although they are acceptable for use during the scan, the pilot balloon must be taped out of the way during the scan.

Cardiac pacemaker compatibility has been a matter of some debate in the past 2 decades.[125,126] Historically, having an implanted pacemaker was considered by the FDA to be a contraindication to have an MRI scan. The evolution of pacemakers and cardiac implanted devices from MRI-unsafe to MRI-conditional during the past 2 decades paralleled our understanding of the causes of the problems and strategic changes in the design of these devices to minimize the adverse events. The hazards associated with these implanted devices stemmed from the formation of (1) magnetic fields and (2) radiofrequency pulses.[127] The magnetic fields induced a torque effect (movement resulting in dislodgement of part of the devices (e.g., wire), electric currents (causing burns), or Reed switch activation (which may deactivate the implanted device). The replacement of the Reed switch with a Reed sensor precluded potentially deactivating the device.[128] The radiofrequency pulse potentially induced heat from an antenna effect or induced electric currents. In 2017, a review of 2103 MRIs using a 1.5-T magnet and legacy (defined by the FDA as MRI-conditional) "pacemakers" concluded that "no long-term clinically significant adverse events" were detected.[129] In at least two known cases, patients with legacy pacemakers died from cardiac arrest while in the MRI scanner.[130] Adverse events associated with legacy pacemakers in the MRI scanner include ventricular fibrillation, rapid atrial pacing, asynchronous pacing, inhibition of pacing output, and movement of the device.[131,132] In the past 2 decades, the changes in the electronics of pacemakers have included reduced ferromagnetic content and increased the sophistication of the computer capabilities, which in aggregate have dramatically reduced the risks of implanted devices in the MRI scanners. Since 2004, multiple studies have reported no serious changes in pacemaker capabilities or adverse outcomes in several thousand patients with cardiac implanted devices after 1.5-T MRI and more recently, after 3-T MRI.[125,129,133–137] There are few data for children with pacemakers or implanted defibrillators who underwent MRI scans with respect to scanners with 3-T field strength but one study found no changes in pacemaker function, even those with epicardial leads, during 44 1.5-T scans in children.[138] No deaths or serious adverse events were reported in this study, and the authors echoed the sentiments that MRI scans should only be performed after consultation with experts and even then, only if the benefits outweigh potential risks. It appears that with modern implantable cardiac devices, MRI scans may be safely performed following published algorithms for the type of device,[139] provided a cardiologist or a consultant from the device manufacturer has been consulted both pre- and post-scan to ensure that the settings are unchanged and the device remains fully operational.

Adverse auditory responses related to loud banging sounds and vibrations produced as the forces generated within the gradient

---

[‡]https://www.fda.gov/media/74201/download

[§]www.MRIsafety.com, search for the MRI-compatible object to determine MRI compatibility coils of the MRI scanner cause the gradient coils to vibrate may occur. The noises generated range from 65 to 95 dB in a 1.5-T magnet. Tinnitus, temporary, and permanent hearing loss after an MRI scan have been reported.[108,140] These reports suggest that earplugs are essential; earplugs or MRI-compatible headphones should be routinely used in children undergoing MRI scans.

Temperature regulation for infants and children during sedation or anesthesia is of particular concern. Cool temperatures and humidity are required to maintain optimal magnet function, which augment a child's radiant and convective heat losses, particularly since anesthesia limits intrinsic thermoregulation. However, heat losses to the environment may be offset by the radiofrequency radiation that is absorbed by the child during the MRI scan.

The specific absorption rate, measured in watts per kilogram, is used to follow the effects of radiofrequency heating. The FDA allows a specific absorption rate of 0.4 W/kg averaged over the whole body.[141] Early data suggested that children can increase their core body temperature by 0.5°C during an MRI of less than 1-hour duration in a 1.5-T environment, although in a study of 200 children, more than half became hypothermic after their scans, whereas in another study of 74 children, temperature increased ≥0.5°C in only 7%.[142–145] The temperature of infants who underwent MRI scans of the brain increased 0.2°C with a 1.5-T scanner and 0.5°C with a 3-T scanner, with minimal efforts to prevent passive heat loss.[146] Given the cool environment needed to operate the MRI scanner, few measures are available to preserve the child's temperature within the scanner, such as covering the children with warm blankets.

Focal heating remains a concern with respect to monitoring equipment in the MRI scanner.[108] For example, the ECG leads should not have frays or exposed wires; *any coils or loops in a conductor such as ECG wires or a pulse oximeter probe can cause tissue burns* (Fig. 43.5). Cases of first-, second-, and third-degree burns after MRI have been reported.[147,148] To avoid patient injury, the following precautions should be undertaken: (1) avoid creating a conductive loop between the child and a conductor (ECG monitoring or gating leads, plethysmographic gating wire, and fingertip

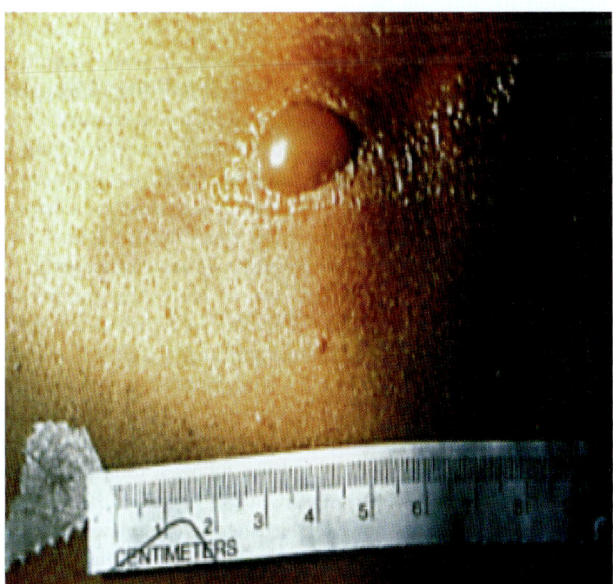

FIGURE 43.5 MRI-induced burn at site of electrocardiogram pad from a frayed lead.

attachment); (2) do not leave any unconnected imaging coils in the magnet during imaging; and (3) prevent all exposed wires or conductors from touching the child's skin during the scan. Objects reported to be associated with thermal injuries include: MR coils, ECG leads, patient clothing,[149] pulse oximeters, tattoos, headphones, dermal patches, and jewelry.[108]

Many MRI scans require contrast administration. Gadolinium (gadopentetate dimeglumine) is an FDA-approved contrast agent that is intravascularly administered for MRI enhancement. Approved for use in 1998, gadolinium provides greater contrast between normal and abnormal tissues throughout the body. Gadolinium forms a complex with chelating agents that facilitates biodistribution to the extracellular compartment and excretion via the kidneys. Unlike iodinated contrast agents, gadolinium complexes do not present a significant osmotic load and are safer than iodine agents with respect to adverse reactions. It is reportedly easily removed with dialysis.[150] On the other hand, warnings from the FDA suggest that gadolinium-containing contrast agents may be associated with the development of nephrogenic systemic fibrosis or nephrogenic fibrosing dermopathy in patients with moderate to end-stage kidney disease.[151] No cases of nephrogenic systemic fibrosis have been reported in children with normal renal function. A literature review of 4931 adults with stage 4 or 5 chronic kidney disease found that the risk for developing nephrogenic systemic fibrosis was "likely <0.07%" and that the risk from withholding indicated gadolinium-based contrast agents may "outweigh the risk of nephrogenic systemic fibrosis."[152] The FDA suggests that gadolinium be administered only if necessary in children with advanced kidney failure and that prompt dialysis should be considered after gadolinium administration for MRA studies.

The incidence of severe anaphylactic or anaphylactoid reactions to gadolinium (0.01% to 0.0003%) is less than that of iodine-based contrast media.[153,154] Another concern regarding gadolinium stems from evidence that increased uptake and deposition of gadolinium in the dentate nucleus and globus pallidus in normal brain tissue was found at autopsy after repeated scans.[155] Given the lack of long-term follow-up, this has raised safety concerns and prompted some countries to eliminate its availability[156] and many centers in the United States to change from using gadolinium to gadoterate meglumine (Dotarem)[157] or other contrast agents.[156,158] These latter contrast agents may not accumulate in the brain,[157] although this remains the subject of ongoing investigation.[159–161] In a multicentered observational study of more than 1600 children who received gadoterate meglumine for MRI contrast (SECURE trial), this agent yielded only one child who vomited after the scan and no other adverse events including follow-up for nephrogenic systemic fibrosis from 3 months to 2 years.[157]

Anesthetic management of children in the MRI suite depends to a large extent on the availability of support personnel and equipment, the anesthesiologist's personal anesthetic practice, institutional practices, and the child's medical history. Airway management may include a natural airway, a supraglottic device, or a tracheal tube. With a supraglottic device or tracheal tube, either inhalational or IV anesthesia may be used.[15,20,162–167] ETCO₂ should be monitored in any patient receiving moderate or deep sedation[54]; in the case of nasal prongs, a septate design that delivers oxygen (2 to 4 L/minute) through one nostril while aspirating gas for carbon dioxide (CO_2) (capnometry) through the other allows for continuous assessment of respirations during spontaneous ventilation.[168] Alternatively, a face mask of oxygen can be used

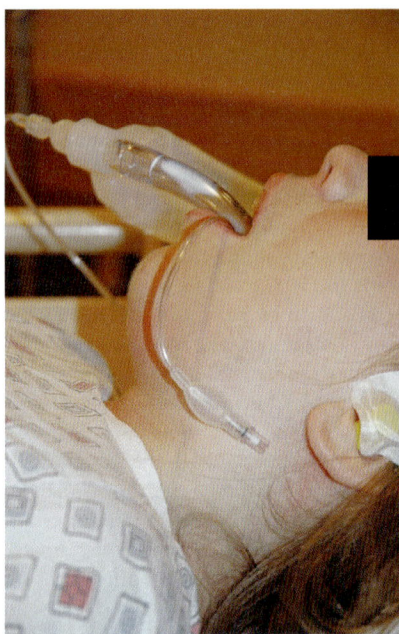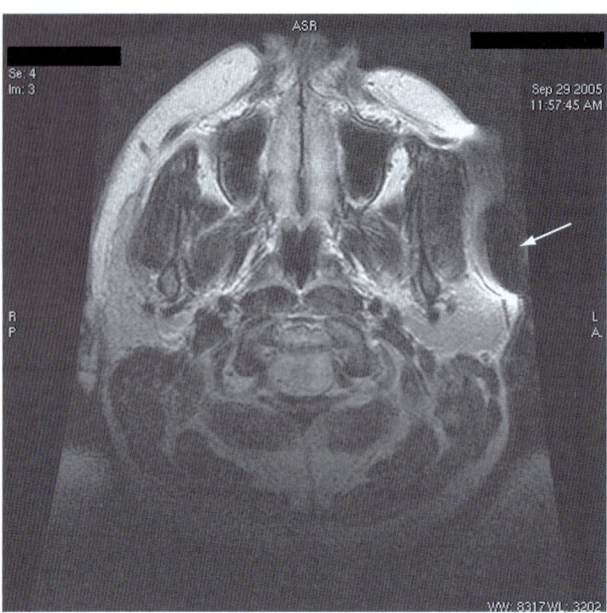

FIGURE 43.6 **(A)** Laryngeal mask airway with pilot balloon left adjacent to face; such positioning could cause MRI artifact. We recommend taping to the Y-piece. **(B)** MRI scan of the patient in **A** demonstrating artifact *(arrow)* created by ferrous material in pilot balloon.

with a sidestream CO_2 monitor placed near the nose or mouth. If respiratory problems occur during the scan, immediate access to the airway is not possible while the child is in the bore of the scanner; for this reason, some anesthesiologists prefer to insert a supraglottic device or tracheal tube in all children. This is extraordinarily rare during a TIVA anesthetic with a shoulder roll to maintain a patent upper airway. Most supraglottic devices are MRI-compatible, although the pilot balloon should be taped to the circuit tubing when imaging the head or neck because it may create imaging artifacts (Fig. 43.6).

Propofol deep sedation with a natural airway has been the most commonly used technique and has been suggested as a safe and effective option in children with airway pathologic conditions or who are premature or very young.[169,170] For generally healthy children undergoing MRI scans, adverse events were reportedly less common when deep sedation/anesthesia with propofol and a natural airway were used compared with inhaled anesthesia through a supraglottic device.[171] The same report noted that recovery was faster after propofol (alone) compared with inhalational anesthesia. According to the largest retrospective assessment of trends in anesthesia used for pediatric MRI at a single institution, there has been a notable decrease in "propofol-only" anesthesia and a rise in the use of combination propofol plus dexmedetomidine.[170] According to this same study, reports of major adverse events were rare. Of note, there was a significant increase in desaturation in children who received volatile agents.[170] Propofol has been found to be more effective and efficient than dexmedetomidine when used alone or in combination with other agents.[51,172] However, intranasal dexmedetomidine (4 µg/kg followed by a second dose of 2 µg/kg as needed) is used by radiologists for sedation for MRI when anesthesia providers are not available, with 93% of studies successfully completed.[173] Heart rates were <60 bpm in one infant 3 to 6 months of age and seven children 3 to 8 years of age before discharge; these episodes of bradycardia were not treated.

Few studies have directly compared general anesthesia with a controlled airway to IV sedation or general anesthesia techniques during MRI. One randomized study of 200 children demonstrated no difference in airway complications between the 2 groups. However, more pauses occurred during scans (for movement) with propofol sedation, but much less agitation was experienced on emergence after the scan.[174] To ensure MRI scans occur without interruption in most children, many practitioners begin with an inhalational induction with 8% sevoflurane and transition to a propofol infusion (200 to 250 µg/kg per minute) while nasal prongs are applied to deliver oxygen and sample carbon dioxide and a shoulder roll is placed to ensure a patent upper airway. Thereafter the infusion rate is maintained at the same rate or tapered up to 25% as the procedure proceeds.[175,176] For younger children, including infants, and children with severe cognitive dysfunction, infusion rates 20% to 50% greater than 250 µg/kg per minute may be required initially to prevent movement during MRI scans but the rate can be adjusted down once the child is no longer likely to move. The addition of remifentanil to propofol using a TIVA technique often smooths sedation (see Chapter 6). Target controlled infusion pumps simplify management by allowing practitioners to target an effective concentration[177,178] rather than using an empiric infusion rate, but these pumps are not available in North America. Other studies documented agitation[179] and prolonged nausea and vomiting[180] after MRI scans performed under general anesthesia with inhalation agents. If the child's airway remains partially obstructed despite an adequate shoulder roll and sponges around the head such that the scout scans are blurry, an algorithm should be followed to clear the upper airway and prevent head movement beginning with inserting an oral airway, if that is not effective, then a nasal airway, and finally, if necessary, a supraglottic airway. Some MRI scans (cardiac, thoracic, or abdominal) require breath-holding to obtain adequate images. In such cases, it is usually necessary to control the airway with a supraglottic device or tracheal tube and deliver a general anesthetic. After reviewing the literature, insufficient evidence exists to recommend a particular anesthetic technique for MRI scans and the favored techniques have evolved over time. Anesthesiologists must still consider their own practice environment and expertise, the demands of the scan itself, and the comorbidities of the particular child when selecting an anesthetic technique, particularly for children undergoing a cardiac MRI.

This cost of MRI-compatible anesthesia equipment may be overwhelming for some institutions, especially in facilities with limited financial resources or limited need for MRI anesthetics. If patient volume is insufficient or financial backing to support such an investment is lacking, then special planning may be instituted to deliver anesthesia without a full complement of MRI-compatible equipment. Specifically, a non–MRI-compatible anesthesia machine could be used in the following manner: the machine is positioned outside the MRI suite, and 30 feet of airway circuit extension tubing is threaded through the wall of the scanner to the child within. Alternatively, IV sedation or anesthesia can be delivered using MRI-compatible infusion pumps and oxygen can be delivered using a face mask or nasal cannula. If an MRI-compatible $ETCO_2$ monitor is not available, a conventional CO_2 monitor may be situated outside the MRI room in a similar fashion.[146] If tracheal intubation or a supraglottic device is required without an MRI-compatible anesthesia machine, it is safer to anesthetize the child outside the scanner with the anesthesia circuit threaded through the console wall and then back out the entrance door to an induction area, secure the airway, and then move the child into the scanner. Similarly, if propofol sedation is intended, the propofol infusion pump can also be situated outside the scanner and equipped with 30 feet of IV infusion tubing. It is important to determine whether the pump can infuse accurately through the resistance of the long tubing and that the caliber of the tubing is sufficiently large that the length of tubing required does not trigger the pump's high-pressure alarm. An Ambu bag or Mapleson circuit (Mercury Medical, Clearwater, FL) must always be situated in the MRI suite and connected directly to an oxygen source to allow quick provision of positive-pressure ventilation should the need arise. This ability is critical, especially when the anesthesia machine is far from the child.

MAGNETOENCEPHALOGRAPHY

Magnetoencephalography, a noninvasive imaging technique that records the magnetic fields created by the brain's electrical activity, is increasingly being used to evaluate patients with a history of intractable seizures to help pinpoint seizure foci in preparation for surgical resection.[181] Magnetoencephalography scans are often used in conjunction with MRI to create a precise spatial map of epileptogenic foci in the brain. These scans are performed in a special chamber which is magnetically shielded to prevent or minimize any interference of other magnetic fields in the environment created by other electronic objects.[182] Although most children are able to undergo this scan without sedation, younger children or those with developmental disability will require individualized sedation for successful completion.

Specific considerations for magnetoencephalography are very similar to those for MRI and include the accommodations necessary for safe practice in the magnetic field and the remote location of the patient relative to the anesthesia team. In addition, some consideration must be given to choosing an anesthetic that will not interfere with the detection of epileptiform activity in the patient's brain. Like proton therapy and MRI, this anesthetizing location poses challenges to the anesthesiologist because the

patient is in a different room and the patient's head is positioned inside the scanner, limiting access to both the patient and the airway. An additional unique challenge to magnetoencephalography scans is the impact of anesthetics on imaging quality. Before 2009, the literature supported premedication with chloral hydrate and a propofol infusion.[181] However, chloral hydrate is no longer available in some countries and propofol infusions have been shown to influence the quality of scan.[182,183] Dexmedetomidine-based protocols for anesthesia in the magnetoencephalography scan provide both reliable sedation and a high success rate for the scan as it causes few interictal artifacts and negligible impacts on epileptiform spike frequency.[184]

NUCLEAR MEDICINE

Specific considerations for nuclear medicine scans differ from most other radiology areas in that the source of radiation in these cases is the patient themselves. Other challenges are the length of scan, the need for immobility during the scan, and the necessary exclusion of glucose ingestion and administration.

Nuclear medicine is one of the oldest functional imaging disciplines and these scans are useful for identification of the extent of disease for many neoplasms.[185] They can also be used to detect epileptic foci in refractory epilepsy, evaluate cerebrovascular disease (e.g., Moyamoya disease) and cognitive and behavior disorders, and detect and delineate renal function and disease, including detection of reflux and acute pyelonephritis.[186] Improvements in the hardware for nuclear imaging have greatly decreased scan time, although with the advent of two-level emission and transmission scans and combined CT imaging, some of the scans can still last 2 hours or more.

The equipment in nuclear medicine imaging emits no ionizing radiation; rather, the radiation is contained within the child and is of very low energy levels. Depending on the nature of the study, patients require IV access for administration of the nuclear tracer well in advance of the scan and therefore usually have IV access in situ for the anesthesia or sedation. Many nuclear scans also require an empty bladder to avoid interference from concentrated tracer in an enlarged bladder. Accordingly, the bladder is often catheterized after anesthesia is induced and the radioactive urine that is collected is disposed of in a radioactive-safe manner.

Two nuclear scans that involve anesthesia (and present challenges) are single-photon emission computed tomography (SPECT) and positron emission tomography (PET) scans. Both of these scans can be combined with a CT scan for optimal imaging.[187,188] SPECT scans involve the use of radiolabeled technetium-99m (half-life of 6 hours), which undergoes extensive first-pass extraction and intracellular trapping in proportion to regional cerebral blood flow. This scan is useful for localizing seizure foci. It appears to be as accurate as invasive direct cortical mapping in this regard.[189] Injection of the radionuclide proximate to the time of a seizure will tag areas of increased cerebral blood flow and localize the seizure foci. The patient should be scanned within 1 to 6 hours of the seizure and injection of the tracer. This technique poses some obvious logistical challenges since there is no way to predict (exactly) when a seizure will occur. The anesthesiology service must be flexible in order to provide anesthetic services within the window of time allowed to complete the test whenever the next seizure occurs.

PET scans use radionuclide tracers of metabolic activity such as oxygen usage and glucose metabolism. Radionuclide tracers of glucose may be useful when seeking seizure foci or tumor recurrence.[185,190–192] Unlike SPECT scans, PET scans require a seizure-free period of at least 2 hours. Tracer is then injected, and the scan is performed after 30 to 45 minutes. In some centers, glucose-containing fluids are avoided so that the tracer is more efficiently taken up by the cells in the seizure focus.[193] Outpatient scans may be scheduled but are canceled if a seizure occurs. Inpatient scans required for children who have frequent seizures can be extremely difficult to schedule and must be coordinated between the neurology and anesthesiology services.

Both SPECT and PET scan techniques are noninvasive. Although the noise level with both is minimal, and there are no electromagnetic fields produced as in the MRI scanner, patients must hold very still in a specific position with the detector unit very close to their face/head. These requirements obviate the use of digital movies for distraction, although music can be used, and parents can be present if the patient is awake. Anesthesia/sedation is required for those children who cannot hold still for the time periods required for the scans, which can range from 10 minutes for a PET/CT of the head to 2 hours for SPECT scanning of the body.[185] When there are no concerns for respiratory decompensation, these scans are commonly performed with deep sedation with an infusion of propofol with or without dexmedetomidine and a natural airway.

STEREOTACTIC RADIOSURGERY

Specific considerations for stereotactic radiosurgery are in large part related to the length of the procedure and the need for transportation from one area of the hospital to another while under anesthesia, as well as remoteness of the patient from the anesthesia team while in the linear accelerator.

Stereotactic radiosurgery (gamma knife) is a major advance in the treatment of selected malignant tumors (e.g., ependymoma, glioblastomas), vascular malformations,[194,195] acoustic neuromas, and pituitary adenomas in children.[196,197] Radiosurgery is indicated, especially for those children with a tumor located deep in the brain,[198] in an area that could put the child at surgical risk (e.g., speech, motor, cerebellum, brainstem areas), or for the recurrent brain tumor that has failed prior treatment. Radiosurgery involves the use of a single large fraction of radiation that is directed at a specific target with minimal radiation exposure to the surrounding normal tissues. Optimal results are achieved with small tumor volumes (≤ 14 cm^3).[199]

Stereotactic radiosurgery requires the coordination of the departments of radiology, radiation therapy, and anesthesiology. The procedure averages 9 hours but can take up to 15 hours or more, with several transports from one area to another. The stereotactic portion of the procedure begins in the morning in a CT scanner. A stereotactic head frame is applied after induction of general anesthesia and tracheal intubation.[200] Although some older children can tolerate the application of the head frame with local anesthesia alone, they may develop anxiety because of the pressure sensation produced by the head frame. Most children require general anesthesia with a tracheal tube for application of the frame and subsequent imaging and surgery. When the head frame is in place, the key to unlock and remove it should be taped to the frame itself in the event of a situation necessitating its emergent removal (e.g., vomiting, airway obstruction, or accidental tracheal extubation). For smaller children, nasal intubation may provide better stability during transport from the radiology suite to the operating room. After the head frame is in place and the imaging study is complete, the child is transported while still intubated, sedated, and appropriately monitored to the postanesthesia care unit while the radiologists and neurosurgeons review the images

and plan radiosurgery. The postanesthesia care unit stay can range from 3 to 5 hours, during which time these children require continued anesthesia/sedation and appropriate physiologic monitoring.

After the images are reviewed and the radiosurgery planning is complete, the child is transported to the stereotactic radiosurgery linear accelerator for treatment. The treatment room is equipped with an anesthesia machine and monitors. To minimize radiation exposure to health care personnel, only the child remains in the scanner area during treatment. The child is observed at a distance with video cameras that are focused on both the child and the physiologic monitors. Treatment usually lasts about 1 hour.

After radiosurgery is completed, the child is returned to the postanesthesia care unit where the trachea is extubated under controlled conditions. Risks are inherent with this prolonged anesthesia, which requires multiple transports between sites. Open communication and coordination between the anesthesia team and the staff of all areas involved in the case are essential to reduce risk and delays in care. Four potentially serious anesthesia-related events were reported in 68 radiosurgery procedures in 65 children who received general anesthesia for these cases.[201] Serious complications included obstruction of the tracheal tube while in the head frame and lobar collapse requiring prolonged mechanical ventilation.

RADIATION THERAPY

Specific considerations for radiation therapy include the need for absolute patient immobility during repeated sessions, remote location of most radiation therapy units from the hospital proper, and the remote placement of the patient in a separate room during treatment.

Radiation therapy for children uses ionizing photons to destroy lymphomas, acute leukemias, Wilms tumor, retinoblastomas, and tumors of the central nervous system. Improved three-dimensional imaging and enhanced computing power have allowed radiation oncologists to conform radiation dose to the shape of the tumor and minimize radiation to the surrounding tissues.[202] Although most children receive standard x-ray therapy, specific lesions may respond better to bombardment with electron, proton, or neutron beam therapy. Radiation therapy involves "fractionated" exposure and thus repeat sessions are typical. The child must remain motionless throughout each treatment to precisely target malignant cells and reduce damage to surrounding tissues. Radiation therapy is typically administered by dividing the total radiation therapy course among daily or twice-daily sessions. In general, most treatment sessions last between 15 and 30 minutes, and the planning simulation session may take as long as 2 hours, depending on the nature and location of the target lesion or area for therapy. For children who require neuraxial treatments for spinal metastases, as many as four fields may be irradiated with the child in both the supine and prone positions. Dividing the total radiation therapy course into discrete daily sessions allows normal tissue repair between sessions while the tumor burden is lessened or destroyed.

The anesthetic considerations are identical regardless of the type of therapy in this respect and a systematic review of anesthetic-related complications reported an incidence similar to that observed in the operating room.[203,204] A planning session in a simulator is typically scheduled before the initiation of radiation therapy to map the fields that require irradiation while the child is in a fixed position. For proton beam treatments, a planning session is performed in a CT scanner. A fiberglass immobilization mask of the head is made while the child is sedated/anesthetized with propofol, optimizing the head position to allow unobstructed

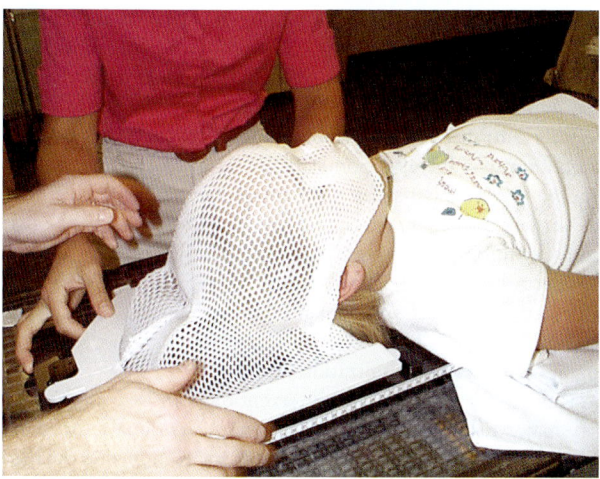

FIGURE 43.7 Child in fiberglass mask for radiation treatment of a cerebral neoplasm.

spontaneous respirations during future treatment sessions (Fig. 43.7). This cast allows secure positioning to ensure that the child does not move during treatment; considerable care is required to configure the mask for optimal airway patency while ensuring proper windows for treatments. Once the mask is completed, if the potential use of an oral airway or supraglottic device has not been factored in, its use is not possible as these maneuvers will alter the head position and thus the direction of the radiation beam.[48]

These children are optimally managed via central venous access that obviates the need for repeated venipunctures. Unless there is a specific airway anomaly, daily anesthetic management typically consists of deep sedation using a propofol infusion (with or without midazolam pretreatment),[205] blow-by oxygen via nasal cannula or face mask, and spontaneous ventilation monitored with $ETCO_2$. Tachyphylaxis to propofol does not appear to be an issue even with multiple, frequent treatments.[206] A global survey conducted in six continents reported that ~70% of children received TIVA without intubation for all radiation treatments in both supine and prone positions.[207] Inhalational anesthetics with laryngeal mask airways were used in ~20% of cases in all continents except Australia/Oceania, where 80% used this regimen and 0% used TIVA. Given all the challenges, it is somewhat surprising that these treatments have not been associated with an increased rate of adverse events. One retrospective review of 177 patients undergoing 3833 radiation treatments documented a 1.3% complication rate,[208] which compares favorably with the rate of complications for children without cancer undergoing propofol-based anesthesia.[209]

Dexmedetomidine sedation has been increasingly used for radiation therapy, but its use has not become widespread, most likely because of the need for a 10-minute loading dose,[210] relatively frequent need for repeated boluses at the doses that have so far been studied, the need for escalation of dose as the session progressed, the need to use larger than recommended doses, and the frequency of unpredictable wake-up.[211,212] IV ketamine 0.5 to 0.8 mg/kg provides effective initial sedation, albeit with more movement, and an increased rate of adverse events on emergence (e.g., vomiting) than propofol; ketamine combined with propofol is another option.[213–215]

One exceptional case in radiation therapy is retinoblastoma. In this case, the eye must be completely immobile during the treatment. General anesthesia or deep propofol sedation is required to ensure appropriate irradiating conditions; ketamine, with its side effect of lateral nystagmus, is not appropriate for these children (see Video 5.1).

The logistics of anesthesia and sedation for radiation therapy are complex, even though the treatments themselves are not challenging. First, only the child remains in the room during treatment. Monitoring must be performed using video observation. For this reason, radiation therapy units are equipped with multiple video monitors adjusted to allow viewing of both the child from several views and the physiologic monitors. Second, children are often moved to allow different angles of access for the radiation treatment. This movement must be taken into consideration when positioning monitors and power cords. Third, many cases of spinal irradiation require the child to be prone with the head at a specific angle with respect to the back. Often several adjustments to the head position are required to maintain a patent airway with the tight-fitting mask and monitoring of expired carbon dioxide is therefore essential.

Most children undergoing radiation therapy are also receiving chemotherapy. As the treatment progresses, nausea, vomiting, and respiratory illness stemming from local radiation effects and chemotherapy can create deteriorating conditions for spontaneous, natural airway ventilation. Psychological factors associated with the illness and its management can also influence anesthesia plans. It is important to work with the child's oncologist to manage symptoms and complete the treatment series as close to the planned treatment regimen as possible as this is critical to the child's survival and quality of life.

INTERVENTIONAL RADIOLOGY

Specific considerations for interventional radiology include radiation risk for patients and staff, contrast reactions (discussed earlier), adverse effects from sclerosants, potentially lengthy procedures, and a high proportion of urgent/emergent add-on procedures. A wide variety of cases with unique anesthetic needs are performed in the interventional radiology suite, and the anesthesia team must be familiar with this range.

Interventional radiology has evolved greatly and the trend is for increased use of interventional radiology both as a replacement to and in conjunction with surgical interventions.[216,217] Many interventional radiology procedures are minimally invasive and not particularly painful, although most children require sedation somewhere between moderate sedation and general anesthesia to complete their procedure. Procedures vary widely in terms of the level of stimulation, postprocedure pain, emergence agitation, and requirements in terms of apnea and positioning. Familiarity with interventional radiology procedures and their anesthetic and postoperative requirements is essential for efficient functioning in this area.[217,218] As a large number of cases in interventional radiology are scheduled on an urgent or emergent basis, it is vital that anesthesiologists in this area have a well-established habit of mutually respectful communication with the interventional radiology team to coordinate patient triage and ensure that cases proceed safely and expeditiously.

Radiation safety in interventional radiology is of paramount concern and may be underappreciated by anesthesiologists.[219] In pediatric settings, we are aided by the "Image Gently" campaign to reduce doses for pediatric patients,[220] but it is ultimately our responsibility to reduce our lifelong exposure to ionizing radiation with its attendant long-term health consequences.[221] Appropriate use of portable lead shields, lead aprons (preferably wraparound), thyroid shields, and lead glasses is crucial, as is increasing one's distance from the radiation source when possible and leaving the room for angiographic "runs." Portable dosimeters should be worn and monitored in compliance with local regulations.

Diagnostic Angiography

Diagnostic angiography of the brain or of the periphery requires absolute control of movement, often with intermittent breath-holding to acquire clear images. For pediatric patients, this implies general anesthesia with a tracheal tube. Mature older children who can cooperate with instructions may be able to tolerate a short diagnostic angiogram with nothing more than minimal sedation, but care should be exercised that they do not become disinhibited or so somnolent that they cannot cooperate with breath-holding. Diagnostic angiography usually takes about 1 hour to complete and requires arterial access (usually of the femoral artery). Once access is obtained, the procedure is not stimulating. During these cases, orogastric and nasogastric tubes, esophageal stethoscopes, and esophageal temperature probes should be used with caution because they may cause artifacts on the angiographic images; consultation with the interventional radiology nurses and technologists is recommended to determine where lines and monitors will be least obtrusive. After any femoral arterial access, patients must lie still for a period of time after the procedure to reduce the risk of complications at the sheath site.[222]

Cerebral angiography may be indicated in the workup or postoperative follow-up of vascular malformation or tumor resections, stroke, hemorrhagic events, vascular disease, and unexplained mental status changes. Hypercarbia to an $ETCO_2$ of ~50 mm Hg may promote vasodilation to allow better access and visualization of cerebral vasculature (E-Fig. 43.1) but should only be employed after consultation with the neurointerventional radiologist. Although MRA studies continue to improve, catheter angiography remains the gold standard for delineating vascular structures in the brain.

Any child who requires a study for the potential or confirmed diagnosis of vasculopathies such as Moyamoya disease should be treated with utmost caution. These children should have an anesthetic that minimizes the risk of transient ischemic attacks and stroke during the procedure.[163] Anesthetic care should ideally begin with the preinduction administration of 10 mL/kg of IV fluid to minimize the risk of hypotension and potential cerebral ischemia on induction of anesthesia. Sedating the child before starting the IV decreases crying and hyperventilation that can lead to cerebral ischemia. Gentle mask induction with close attention to blood pressure has also been used in our institution with success. Blood pressure should be carefully maintained, avoiding hypotension with its potential for cerebral hypoperfusion. Vasoactive drugs are rarely necessary in pediatric patients with these conditions but should be available. Intraarterial blood pressure monitoring for these short procedures is rarely necessary. Hypocarbia should be avoided throughout. In the event of vasospasm or difficult access of small, tortuous vessels, locally administered vasodilators such as nitroglycerin or calcium channel blockers through the catheter in small doses may facilitate visualization and access. Although often effective for discretely vasodilating specific areas, these small doses will generally not have a clinically important systemic effect on blood pressure. Specific protocols have been suggested for minimizing perioperative strokes in these children.[164] Close attention to postoperative pain control can similarly improve outcomes (see Chapters 40 and 41).

Peripheral diagnostic angiography is less common but may be useful before complex surgical or orthopedic procedures to delineate arterial anatomy. Angiography of the abdomen and pelvis has unique considerations. Nitrous oxide can diffuse into the bowel, causing distention and potential distortion of the vasculature of interest; it should be used with caution. In addition, the interventional radiologist may request that the anesthesiologist administer IV glucagon, usually in 0.25-mg increments. Glucagon reduces peristalsis and, as a consequence, reduces motion artifact during image acquisition.[223] However, it may cause nausea, vomiting, hyperglycemia, depression of clotting factors, and electrolyte disturbances[162]; close monitoring is warranted, particularly in neonates and small infants.

Angiography With Embolization

Intracranial angiography with interventions can be complex and carry major risks. Indications for neurointerventional procedures include embolization of intracranial vascular anomalies such as arteriovenous malformations (AVMs), arteriovenous fistulae or aneurysms, targeted injection of intraarterial chemotherapy for tumors, and presurgical embolization of AVMs or tumors of the head and neck.[224] These procedures can take up to 10 to 12 hours, and complete immobility is required. Patient padding and positioning must be meticulous for such a long procedure, as moving the patient once catheters are deployed may be impossible.

Invasive arterial blood pressure monitoring is usually necessary during the treatment of intracranial AVMs. A maximal acceptable blood pressure should be determined with the radiologist because of the risk of hemorrhage as flow through the AVM is altered by embolization.[225] For the same reason, close blood pressure control immediately after the procedure is essential. Low dose dexmedetomidine infusion overnight in the ICU may aid in maintaining a calm child with fewer elevations in blood pressure. In infants presenting in heart failure from high-flow AVMs such as vein of Galen malformations,[226] immediate improvements in hemodynamics have been described as high-flow AVMs are closed.[227]

Good IV access is necessary for hydration; the chance of noteworthy blood loss is extremely small. Euvolemia to slight hypervolemia is recommended to offset the osmotic diuretic effect of contrast.[228] Note that a continuous infusion of heparinized saline solution is instilled via the femoral sheath to reduce the risk of microemboli.[229] This can result in a considerable volume of fluid delivered to the patient by the neuroradiologist.

Many agents are used for embolization, including various types of glue, metal coils, or polyvinyl alcohol particles.[230] It should be noted that children can become intoxicated if excessive ethanol is used (E-Fig. 43.2). Embolization of brain AVMs carries the risk that perfusion to surrounding normal brain tissue may be compromised with a concomitant loss of function. Although there are descriptions of assessment of adult patients' motor, language, or visual function during test injections of agents such as amobarbital before definitive closure of a feeder vessel, this requires an awake cooperative patient and few descriptions of this technique exist in children.[231,232] The goal in treatment of intracranial AVMs in children is to obliterate the lesion. Surgical resection when possible usually preceded by embolization for better localization and hemostasis has been suggested as the standard of care in pediatric cerebral AVM.[233–235]

Injection of intraarterial chemotherapy carries some unique challenges for the anesthesiologist. Accessing the ophthalmic artery for injection of chemotherapeutic drug in retinoblastoma has considerable risk of bronchospasm and bradycardia.[236] Agents such as albuterol (salbutamol) or anticholinergics are often administered preemptively just before chemotherapy instillation.[237]

Postprocedure nausea and vomiting is possible due to adverse effects of the chemotherapy; aggressive antiemetic prophylaxis is encouraged to prevent a child with a femoral puncture from vomiting.

Embolization of peripheral AVMs also has the potential to be of prolonged duration because in many cases the lesion is quite complex. The natural history of AVMs, like all vascular malformations, is to grow over time, with acceleration of growth during puberty[238]; the end stage is tissue destruction and high-output cardiac failure (E-Fig. 43.3). Blood loss is rarely a risk during these minimally invasive procedures, but excellent hydration is necessary both to offset the diuretic effect of the contrast load and to counteract the hemolyzing effect of sclerosing agents (see later discussion). Although complete cure is rare, embolization combined with surgical resection in some cases can keep AVM symptoms manageable.[239]

Embolization for hemorrhage has a long track record of success in cases of trauma, allowing for less insensible fluid loss and no disruption of tamponade.[240] The greatest predictor of success is the volume of blood resuscitation needed before embolization; a larger requirement presages a worse outcome. Anesthetic management for these children is similar to that of any massive transfusion case (see Chapter 10).

Catheter-based embolization of pulmonary vessels for hemoptysis presents several challenges for the anesthesiologist. Embolization is effective for gaining short-term control of hemoptysis, even massive hemoptysis, while not affecting the overall disease course in the case of cystic fibrosis.[241] Massive hemoptysis often necessitates single-lung ventilation and transfusion, coupled with the challenge of securing the airway in the face of ongoing blood loss from the trachea. A gray area exists for more stable patients. Some reports have suggested that positive-pressure ventilation may itself be detrimental in cystic fibrosis patients, and that sedation at most is preferable.[242] This must be weighed against a child's ability to lie flat while in a state of respiratory compromise for a potentially prolonged procedure. With any patient undergoing bronchial embolization, clear communication with the patient and family about goals of care in the event of catastrophe is recommended.

Sclerotherapy of Venous and Lymphatic Malformations

Children may present shortly after birth with vascular malformations that arise from *PIK3CA*-associated overgrowth syndromes such as CLOVES (**C**ongenital, **L**ipomatous, **O**vergrowth, **V**ascular malformations, **E**pidermal nevi, and **S**pinal/skeletal anomalies and/or scoliosis [Fig. 43.8]) or Klippel-Trénaunay syndrome,[243] or they may present later in life with isolated lesions that, while present at birth, may have not been recognized. The natural history of venous and lymphatic malformations is to grow steadily with the child, expand rapidly, and accelerate in size with puberty.[244,245] One review reported that only 18% of patients with lesions presented before 15 years of age.[165] This rapid proliferative phase may occur in response to hormonal changes (pregnancy, puberty), trauma, or other stimuli. Vascular malformations may be classified as high-flow or low-flow lesions, depending on which vessels are involved.[246] High-flow lesions may include arteriovenous fistulas, some large hemangiomas, and AVMs. Low-flow lesions consist of venous, lymphatic, and capillary malformations (Fig. 43.9). The mainstay of treatment for many high-flow and low-flow vascular anomalies is chemical sclerotherapy, possibly combined with surgical resection; many lesions are inaccessible surgically or have a poor result from primary surgical resection alone.[247,248]

Sclerotherapy of vascular malformations usually requires a general anesthetic to ensure motionless conditions, especially

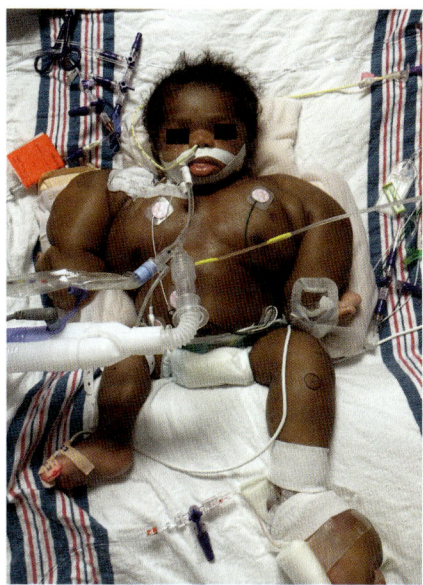

FIGURE 43.8 Neonate with severe CLOVES syndrome, a *PIK3CA*-associated overgrowth syndrome.[258] *CLOVES*, **C**ongenital, **L**ipomatous, **O**vergrowth, **V**ascular malformations, **E**pidermal nevi, and **S**pinal/skeletal anomalies and/or scoliosis.

during complex prolonged procedures that involve injection of potentially painful sclerosants. These procedures require careful planning and discussion between the interventional radiologist and the anesthesiologist for safe airway management, intraprocedural and postprocedural care, and postprocedure disposition.

The anesthesiologist should be familiar with the mechanism of action and potential risks associated with the various agents used for sclerotherapy (Table 43.2). All sclerosants act by inducing a local tissue reaction that ideally scars closed abnormal vascular channels. Pain and swelling are a result with all sclerosants, to varying degrees. Ethanol and sodium tetradecyl sulfate produce hemolysis when administered into the vascular bed. They cause hemoglobinuria in a dose-dependent manner that can result in renal injury, necessitating generous hydration and alkalinization of urine to mitigate damage to the kidneys (Fig. 43.10).[249] Hemoglobinuria may not occur until the end of the procedure, sometimes after a large dose of sclerosant has been administered or the tourniquet (if used) has been released. Ethanol in large doses has been associated with complications, which has caused its use to fall out of favor as a primary agent in many institutions.[250] The most infrequent but serious risk is cardiovascular collapse, which is generally preceded by hypoxemia and bradycardia.[251] Most reported cases of cardiovascular collapse involved lower extremity malformations[252] after release of tourniquets in extremities that had been injected with ethanol. An ethanol gel formulation has been used for treatment of low-flow lesions with apparent success and a low incidence of complications.[253–256]

Children with vascular malformations that result in stagnant flow (especially venous malformations) can have preexisting coagulation disturbances that resemble disseminated intravascular coagulation.[257] This is particularly true for patients with *PIK3A*-associated overgrowth syndromes as this syndrome is associated with huge ectatic veins with slow flow. Children with laboratory indexes consistent with preexisting consumptive coagulopathy, particularly low fibrinogen, should have a hematology consultation for initiation of anticoagulation before and after the procedure to

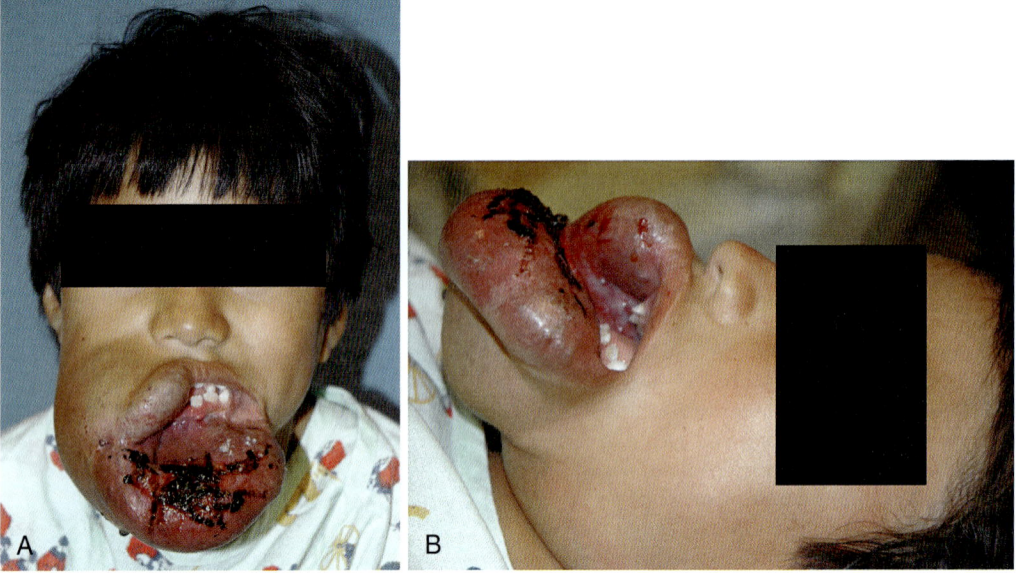

FIGURE 43.9 Venous malformation of the face with patient sitting upright **(A)** and supine **(B)**.

TABLE 43.2	Sclerosants Used for Treatment of Vascular Anomalies[218]			
Agent	**Indications**	**Swelling**	**Pain**	**Complications**
Sodium tetradecyl sulfate	LM, VM	Moderate	Moderate	Hemoglobinuria, skin blistering
Ethanol	LM, VM	Marked	Marked	Nausea, hemoglobinuria, skin blistering, ethanol intoxication, nerve injury, cardiovascular collapse
Doxycycline	LM	Marked	Marked	Minimal
Bleomycin	LM, VM primarily cervicofacial	Moderate	Moderate	Transient fever
				Concern for pulmonary fibrosis, never described after sclerotherapy
OK-432	LM	Marked	Marked	Not FDA-approved for use in USA

FDA, US Food and Drug Administration; *LM*, lymphatic malformations; *VM*, vascular malformations.

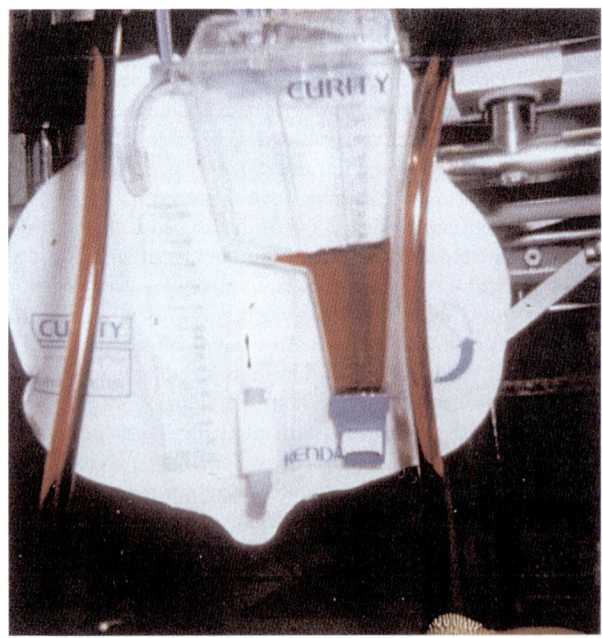

FIGURE 43.10 Hemoglobinuria after ethanol embolization.

reduce the chance of a catastrophic periprocedure thromboembolic event.[258]

Vascular malformations that involve the airway are particularly challenging (see Fig. 43.9). The anesthesiologist and radiologist should review the imaging studies (preferably MRI) before the procedure. If there is any question of malformation involvement of the oropharynx or nasopharynx, evaluation by an otorhinolaryngologist familiar with vascular anomalies is essential before proceeding with anesthetic induction; nasal fiberoptic endoscopy will provide very useful information and can be performed in the office. Most interventional radiology suites are not situated in the operating room. If there is potential for airway compromise, difficulty in attaining a mask airway, or failure to intubate, the airway should be secured in the operating room before transport to the radiology suite.

If postsclerotherapy edema and vascular congestion involving the airway structures are anticipated, the child's trachea should be intubated nasally and remain intubated for 48 hours or until the swelling subsides. Nasal intubation is preferred to minimize the risk of dislodging the tracheal tube or premature extubation. The decision to have the child remain intubated after the procedure is usually made after the anesthesiologist and radiologist review the MR images. If the patient remains intubated after the procedure, they should be extubated in the intensive care unit after an air leak around the tracheal tube is confirmed or a flexible nasal fiberoptic view of the airway can be performed at the bedside. If there is any doubt about the patency or self-sufficiency of the airway following extubation, these children should be transferred to the operating room for extubation in a controlled setting with an otorhinolaryngologist present.

Venous malformations involving the head, neck, or airway structures typically swell with dependency or Valsalva maneuver (e.g., crying). Before extubation, these children should be positioned head-up to promote venous drainage and reduce swelling and efforts should be made to minimize coughing. In the event of respiratory compromise, venous malformations can enlarge when the child coughs, increasing intrathoracic pressure and/or the use of accessory muscles. Attempts at reintubation, cricoid pressure, head extension, and mask ventilation can further enlarge the malformation. Mask ventilation can be challenging, and sometimes impossible, if the malformation is swollen and firm. Achieving an occlusive mask seal is particularly difficult when there is swelling of the cheek, tongue, lip, chin, or nares. Venous malformations of the lips and tongue, because of their blue color, can make it difficult to assess the child for hypoxemia in the event of respiratory distress. Reintubation can become impossible in these situations because all the maneuvers to achieve a mask seal increase venous pressure and swelling. When attempting to reintubate a child with intraoral or pharyngeal malformations, special care should be taken to avoid damaging the malformation: even a small nick can create significant bleeding. In the event of oropharyngeal bleeding and inability to mask ventilate and/or intubate, it is critical to have alternative airway devices immediately available. Supraglottic airway devices, in particular those with high occluding pressures such as the ProSeal LMA (Teleflex Medical Inc., Research Triangle Park, NC), can be lifesaving. Proper insertion and inflation of a supraglottic device can secure an airway and, more importantly, tamponade bleeding. However, because the supraglottic airway rests above the vocal cords, it does not protect the airway from pulmonary aspiration.

ENDOSCOPIC PROCEDURES

Before anesthesiologists became involved in sedation for endoscopic procedures, gastroenterologists directed/performed intravenous sedation as well as the endoscopies. When propofol was introduced, anesthesiologists became involved in sedation for endoscopy, with a focus on delivering deep sedation for the brief period of the endoscopy and monitoring the child's vital signs. It was imperative to appreciate these procedures occurred in a setting of a shared airway and in children at risk for pulmonary aspiration because of an unprotected airway and gastroesophageal reflux.

A range of sedation and anesthesia options have been used for both simple[259–261] and more complex procedures, such as foreign body removal, endoscopic retrograde cholangiopancreatography (ERCP), and percutaneous gastrostomy placement.[262] The choice of deep sedation versus general anesthesia (with or without tracheal intubation) depends on the medical condition of the child, the risks associated with the specific procedure, and the anticipated duration of the case.

Upper GI endoscopies have the inherent risk of apnea, laryngospasm, bronchospasm, and airway obstruction. Most problems resolve after withdrawal of the endoscope and positive-pressure ventilation with a face mask.[263] Apart from the need to intubate the trachea to prevent upper airway stridor from the pediatric

endoscope compressing the trachealis muscle in young children (<10 kg), tracheal intubation is rarely required to complete a GI procedure or resolve an airway issue. Little published evidence exists on which to base age-related practice in endoscopy sedation and analgesia. Within institutions, the sedation regimen varies among anesthesiologists.[237] Upper airway stridor after passage of the pediatric size endoscope has led many practitioners to electively intubate the trachea in infants up to 10 kilograms because stridor occurs during the procedures and respiratory complications may occur afterwards.[259,260] Before extubating these infants, remind the gastroenterologist to empty the stomach of all residual air to avoid limiting effective ventilation and causing desaturation or oxygen dependence in the recovery room.

Few large studies have reported outcomes after pediatric GI endoscopy. The Clinical Outcomes Research Initiative (CORI) is a national registry of endoscopic procedures started in 1995. The PEDS-CORI is the pediatric component started in 1999. A 2007 report collected the complications from pediatric upper endoscopy involving 10,236 encounters from 13 different institutions over 4 years.[264] Overall, there was a 2.3% incidence of complications of any kind. Of these, 79.9% were cardiopulmonary, 18% were GI, and 5.9% were "other" complications, including prolonged sedation, drug reactions, or rash. Not surprisingly, children who developed complications were younger and had a greater ASA physical status. General anesthesia was associated with a reduced overall complication rate (1.2%) compared with IV sedation (3.7%). Although these data were not controlled or randomized, they do shed some insight into the complication rates associated with pediatric sedation outside the operating room. Data from closed claims analysis confirm the risk associated with endoscopic procedures in children. Half of NORA closed claims involved the GI unit, 25% involved the diagnostic imaging department, and 25% involved cardiac procedures.[35]

Many techniques may be used to maintain adequate conditions for upper and lower GI endoscopy. Although all anesthesia-delivery areas must meet ASA standards, scavenging and ventilation in endoscopy suites may not always be up to standard to ensure the safe use of inhalational anesthetics. In these cases, total IV anesthesia can substitute for inhalational anesthetics.[265–268] As a general rule, propofol is used either alone,[269] in combination with an opioid (fentanyl or remifentanil),[270,271] or with ketamine.[272,273] Recently, a randomized clinical trial demonstrated that the addition of low dose dexmedetomidine to propofol allowed for the successful completion of upper and lower endoscopies while decreasing the total propofol dose provided to children and showing a trend toward faster discharge.[268] In another study where a direct comparison was made between the techniques for GI procedures, recovery was more rapid and agitation less common after a propofol-based sedation technique rather than an inhaled anesthesia-based anesthetic technique.[265]

Acknowledgment

We wish to thank Charles J. Coté for his prior contributions to this chapter.

ANNOTATED REFERENCES

Coté CJ, Wilson S, American Academy of Pediatrics, American Academy of Pediatric Dentistry. Guidelines for monitoring and management of pediatric patients before, during, and after sedation for diagnostic and therapeutic procedures. *Pediatrics.* 2019;143(6):e20191000.

This is the most recent American Academy of Pediatrics sedation guideline, jointly published with the American Academy of Pediatric Dentistry. This continually-updated set of recommendations for safe practice acts as the gold standard. This most recent update specifies safe staffing for sedation in addition to best-practice recommendations for room setup, monitoring, and sedation management.

Cravero JP, Beach ML, Blike GT, et al. The incidence and nature of adverse events during pediatric sedation/anesthesia with propofol for procedures outside the operating room: a report from the Pediatric Sedation Research Consortium. *Anesth Analg.* 2009;108(3):795-804.

This is the largest study to date that examines the side effects and adverse events associated with the use of propofol for sedation of children during procedures outside the operating room.

Kanal E, Borgstede JP, Barkovich AJ, et al. American College of Radiology White Paper on MR Safety: 2004 update and revisions. *AJR Am J Roentgenol.* 2004;182(5):1111-1114.

Updated paper details the standards and recommendations for providing safe patient care in the MR environment.

Shellock FG, Crues JV. MR procedures: biologic effects, safety, and patient care. *Radiology.* 2004;232(3):635-652.

This detailed article reviews the biologic effects and important safety issues in delivering safe patient care in the MR environment.

A complete reference list can be found online at Elsevier eBooks+.

Sedation for Diagnostic and Therapeutic Procedures Outside the Operating Room

VANESSA A. OLBRECHT, CHARLES J. COTÉ,
JOSEPH P. CRAVERO, AND MARY LANDRIGAN-OSSAR

The Evolution of Pediatric Sedation and the Anesthesiologist's Role
Sedation Depth
The Concept of Levels of Sedation
Sedation Scoring Systems
Sedation Depth Versus Sedation Risk
The Concept of "Safety"
Guidelines
American Academy of Pediatrics Guidelines
American Society of Anesthesiologists Guidelines
American College of Emergency Physicians Guidelines
Joint Commission on Accreditation of Healthcare Organizations Guidance
Goals of Sedation
Training and System Issues for Pediatric Procedural Sedation

Documentation
Specific Sedation Techniques
Local Anesthetics
Anxiolytics and Sedatives
Barbiturates
Opioids
A_2-Adrenoceptor Agonist: Dexmedetomidine
Ketamine
Propofol
Nitrous Oxide
Etomidate
Future of Pediatric Sedation

PERHAPS MORE THAN EVER, the care of children in the hospital setting requires the provision of safe and effective sedation in a timely manner. Many children who require an imaging procedure or invasive test before surgery will not tolerate the procedure without sedation. In addition, children with neurologic, gastroenterologic, or oncologic (medical) illnesses require repeat tests and procedures for a single course of treatment that may be uncomfortable or invasive. In some, sedation is required because of age, anxiety, or developmental delay. A responsive and accommodating sedation service that helps accomplish these procedures in a safe, efficient, and effective manner is an indispensable component of a functional hospital or health system.

The Evolution of Pediatric Sedation and the Anesthesiologist's Role

Sedation of children undergoing diagnostic tests and procedures outside the operating room continues to evolve. Forty years ago, physical restraint without sedating or analgesic medications to complete these procedures was common. It is now clear that physical and psychological stresses in early life[1–5] can lead to long-term behavioral challenges and responses to pain later in life[6–10]; therefore, it is essential to provide sedation/analgesia in an atmosphere of respect and safety on par with the quality of care provided to children undergoing surgery. With this evolution in care, however, we must recognize that the sheer number of children who require sedation/analgesia exceeds the capacity of pediatric anesthesiologists to provide all of this care. Partnership with other types of properly trained and credentialed physicians and nurses, who are capable and willing to deliver pediatric procedural sedation, is required. Furthermore, economic pressures in medicine

demand systems that optimize efficiency, throughput, and effectiveness of the care provided. Understanding the environment, guidelines, and organizational issues involving sedation practice for ourselves and our partners is critical if we are to improve the overall delivery of this care to children globally.

Sedation/analgesia for painful procedures performed outside the operating room (e.g., bone marrow aspiration, lumbar puncture, repair of minor surgical wounds, insertion of arterial or venous catheters, burn dressing changes, fracture reduction, bronchoscopy, and endoscopy) requires the same attention to detail as for procedures performed in the operating room because the level of sedation needed is usually deep sedation or general anesthesia, particularly for children 6 years of age and younger, as well as for those at any age with developmental delay. Children undergoing diagnostic studies (e.g., computed tomography [CT], magnetic resonance imaging [MRI], positron emission tomography [PET], electroencephalography [EEG], electromyography) and those who require high doses of ionizing radiation require deep levels of sedation or general anesthesia because they must remain absolutely motionless (sometimes with breath-holding).[11] Given these requirements, a coordinated team approach is required to provide safe, optimal conditions for these procedures.

The need for sedation services goes beyond the very young and developmentally challenged patients usually associated with this requirement. Older children and adolescents without developmental delay may also require sedation to undergo a procedure/investigation in a confined space (e.g., MRI scans) because of claustrophobia. Other procedures, such as sexual abuse examinations or urinary catheterization, evoke more emotion than pain. Nonetheless, these children still require sedation to control anxiety and fear, that if inadequately addressed, can ultimately lead to long-term emotional/psychological harm. Furthermore, a child's emotional state may be worsened by parental anxiety, separation from parents, and the pain (or anticipation of pain) from the procedure (see Chapter 2). Child-Life professionals, distraction, guided imagery, and the use of videos and music have proven beneficial in this respect, although they may be insufficient to provide the conditions needed to complete all procedures in their entirety.[12–19]

The pharmacologic armamentarium for sedation for diagnostic and therapeutic procedures has greatly expanded over the past several decades to include potent sedative hypnotics, new opioids, and dissociative agents. Determining which medications physicians can use and what qualifications they must have to provide deep sedation/anesthesia has been the subject of considerable debate. Although the final determination of how this care will be provided remains contentious, the trend is toward liberalizing the use of drugs such as propofol, dexmedetomidine, remifentanil, and ketamine for physicians and providers with the appropriate competence in their use and the skills to rescue the patient should an adverse event occur.[20,21] One driving force for this change is the demand for efficient sedation and analgesia services outside the operating room. Pressure comes from many sources including hospital administrators, insurance companies, medical specialists, and families because failures and missed appointments increase hospital costs and frustrate families.[22] Failed sedations for diagnostic or therapeutic procedures is no longer tolerated or accepted as part of the sedation process; the use of more potent medications decreases the risk of failures. All these factors have led to the "professionalization" of pediatric sedation with the creation of pediatric sedation services, many of which are led by pediatricians, hospitalists, emergency medicine physicians, intensivists, and dentists.

Examples of the changing landscape of sedation abound. A 2005 survey of pediatric sedation practice in 116 children's hospitals in the United States and Canada[23] reported that anesthesiologists exclusively provided the sedation in 26% of institutions. Similarly, the Pediatric Sedation Research Consortium, a collaborative of hospitals heavily committed to improving pediatric sedation, noted that most sedation in the participating institutions (over 100,000 encounters) was delivered by organized sedation services of which only 19% of the sedation encounters involved anesthesiologists, with the balance provided by an increasing number of pediatric subspecialists.[24–26] In the case of propofol, the Pediatric Sedation Research Consortium reported that anesthesiologists were involved

in only 10% of the 50,000 encounters it reviewed.[27] Despite this changing landscape of sedation, anesthesiologists are still charged by the federal government and the Joint Commission on Accreditation of Healthcare Organizations (JCAHO) in the United States to exercise oversight of sedation practices.[28] To provide effective leadership, anesthesiologists must have a full appreciation of the issues involved in this dynamic area of practice.

Sedation Depth

THE CONCEPT OF LEVELS OF SEDATION

The levels of sedation from the American Academy of Pediatrics (AAP), the American Society of Anesthesiologists (ASA), JCAHO, and the American Academy of Pediatric Dentistry (AAPD) are the most frequently cited and agreed-upon position statements.[21–23,29–34] These organizations define sedation and analgesia for procedures in terms of a continuum, including minimal sedation (anxiolysis), moderate sedation (whereby the patient interacts throughout), deep sedation, and general anesthesia (Fig. 44.1). The definitions that follow are taken from JCAHO (2010)[35] and are consistent with the current AAP, AAPD, and ASA definitions[21,29–31,36]:

- *Minimal sedation (anxiolysis):* "A drug-induced state during which patients respond to verbal commands. Although cognitive function and coordination may be impaired, cardiorespiratory functions are unaffected" (Video 44.1).
- *Moderate sedation* (previously called "conscious sedation" or sedation/analgesia): "A drug-induced depression of consciousness during which patients respond purposefully to verbal commands, either alone or accompanied by light tactile stimulation. No interventions are required to maintain a patent airway, and spontaneous ventilation is adequate. Cardiovascular function is usually maintained" (Video 44.2).
- *Deep sedation:* "A drug-induced depression of consciousness during which patients cannot be easily aroused but respond purposefully after repeated or painful stimuli. (*Note: reflex withdrawal from a painful stimulus is not considered a purposeful response.*) The ability to independently maintain respiratory homeostasis may be impaired. Patients may require assistance in maintaining a patent airway and spontaneous ventilation may be inadequate. Cardiovascular function is usually maintained" (Video 44.3).
- *General anesthesia:* "A drug-induced loss of consciousness during which patients are not arousable, even to painful stimuli. The ability to independently maintain respiratory homeostasis

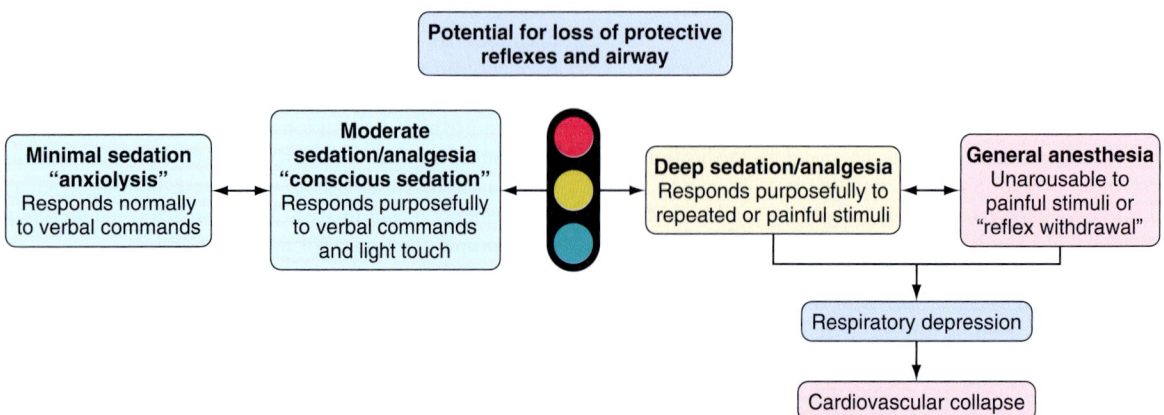

FIGURE 44.1 The sedation continuum. A patient may readily pass from a light level of sedation to deep sedation or general anesthesia. Health care providers must be prepared to increase vigilance and intensity of monitoring consistent with the depth of sedation.

is often impaired. Patients often require assistance in maintaining a patent airway, and positive-pressure ventilation may be required because spontaneous ventilation is depressed or neuromuscular function is compromised. In addition, cardiovascular function may be impaired" (Video 44.4).

In clinical practice, procedures that require sedation are rarely performed in children under true "moderate sedation," a term which is often used inappropriately when describing pediatric sedation. Theoretically, a child who is moderately sedated responds to touch or firm rubbing by an appropriate response, such as saying "ouch," pushing your hand away, or pulling up the covers. *The lack of a purposeful response is a sign that the child has progressed to a deeper sedation level and should lead to an escalation of monitoring and personnel.*[37–40] In point of fact, children often require deep sedation or general anesthesia for pain control (e.g., bone marrow biopsies) or movement control (e.g., MRI scans). In general, it is not feasible to accurately describe the depth of sedation based on the child's responses to stimulation (Fig. 44.2) because stimulating the child may defeat the entire sedation process.

All of the definitions described earlier are created with the appreciation that a child's depth of sedation may easily pass from one level to another and without easily identifying signs of any change in the child's condition.[21,41] Not surprisingly, an audit in a large pediatric hospital reported that their target level of either moderate or deep sedation was achieved in only 50% to 75% of patients; an awake state was achieved in 12% to 28% of the children, and general anesthesia was achieved in 35% of children.[41]

SEDATION SCORING SYSTEMS

There are several validated scoring systems available for assessing sedated patients and grading their level of sedation. The Ramsay scale was developed[42] in 1974 for the purpose of monitoring sedation with alphaxalone-alphadolone (Table 44.1). It continues to be the most widely used scale for assessing and monitoring sedation.[43] It spans the continuum of sedation but does not clearly separate purposeful from nonpurposeful responses. The Ramsey scale has been modified from 6 to 8 categories of alertness to more clearly coincide with the AAP and JCAHO guidelines (Table 44.2): a score of 2 to 3 is anxiolysis, 4 to 5 is consistent with moderate sedation, 6 is deep sedation, and 7 to 8 is general anesthesia.

The Observer's Assessment of Alertness/Sedation (OAA/S) scale[44] is often used as a scale for sedation. It is scored as: 1, no response to shaking; 2, responds to mild prodding; 3, responds to name called loudly; 4, lethargic response to name; and 5, readily

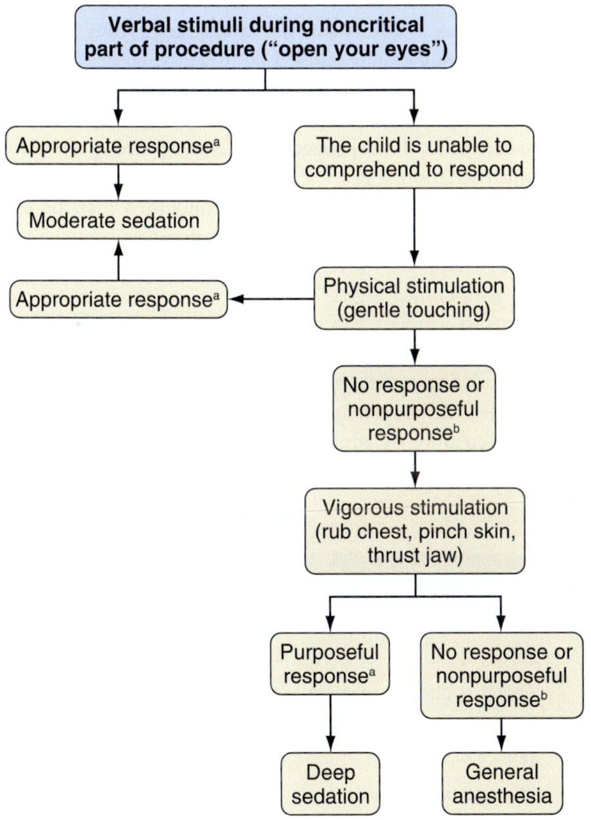

44

FIGURE 44.2 Sedated children must be continuously evaluated for depth of sedation and appropriateness of response. As diagrammed here, sedation is a continuum. Note that a purposeful response to voice or light touch is consistent with moderate sedation. A purposeful response to pain is consistent with deep sedation. A nonpurposeful response to pain is consistent with general anesthesia. However, such stimulation often defeats the purpose of the sedation, thus rendering these assessments less helpful unless patient movement is acceptable. None of the current sedation guidelines require such assessments.
[a]*Purposeful:* opens eyes, talks back, pushes you out of the way.
[b]*Nonpurposeful:* winces, shrugs shoulders, nonspecific withdrawal to pain.

TABLE 44.1	Ramsay Scale
Level	**Characteristics**
1	Patient awake, anxious, agitated, or restless
2	Patient awake, cooperative, orientated, and tranquil
3	Patient drowsy, with response to commands
4	Patient asleep, brisk response to glabella tap or loud auditory stimulus
5	Patient asleep, sluggish response to stimulus
6	Patient has no response to firm nail-bed pressure or other noxious stimuli

TABLE 44.2	Modified Ramsay Sedation Scale
Score	**Characteristics**
1	Awake and alert, minimal or no cognitive impairment
2[a]	Awake but tranquil, purposeful responses to verbal commands at conversation level
3[a]	Appears asleep, purposeful responses to verbal commands at conversation level
4[b]	Appears asleep, purposeful responses to verbal commands but at louder than usual conversation level or requiring light glabellar tap
5[b]	Asleep, sluggish purposeful responses only to loud verbal commands or strong glabellar tap
6[c]	Asleep, sluggish purposeful responses only to painful stimuli
7[d]	Asleep, reflex withdrawal to painful stimuli only (no purposeful responses)
8[d]	Unresponsive to external stimuli, including pain

[a]Minimal sedation.
[b]Moderate sedation.
[c]Deep sedation.
[d]General anesthesia.

TABLE 44.3 | University of Michigan Sedation Scale (UMSS)

Score	Characteristics
0	Awake and alert
1	Minimally sedated: tired/sleepy, appropriate response to verbal conversation and/or sound
2	Moderately sedated: somnolent/sleeping, easily aroused with light tactile stimulation or a simple verbal command
3	Deeply sedated: deep sleep, arousable only with significant physical stimulation
4	Unarousable

responds to name. Its inability to clearly categorize deep levels of sedation and lack of a clear differentiation between purposeful and nonpurposeful responses limit its usefulness, particularly for non-verbal children. A more clinically useful scale is the University of Michigan Sedation Scale (UMSS).[45] It has been validated against the OAA/S scale and other scales of sedation (Table 44.3). This scale has proven particularly useful for children with learning impairment and delays[43,46]; it separates patients into the sedation categories in line with those defined by the AAP, ASA, and JCAHO.

These responsiveness-based assessment tools require intermittently stimulating the child during the procedure to categorize the level of sedation. Unfortunately, poking or prodding the child to determine the depth of sedation defeats the purpose of sedation in many situations (e.g., infants, developmentally delayed children, or procedures requiring immobility). Guidelines that reference levels of sedation do not require frequent testing of sedation depth. Rather the responsiveness-based definitions are meant to provide a road map for safety that bases the depth of sedation on the behavior of the patient in response to the procedure itself, with the understanding that a nonresponding child is deeply sedated and requires an increased level of vigilance.[21,22] Unfortunately, infrequent testing leaves the sedation provider uncertain about the depth of sedation for considerable periods of time during a test or intervention. Concerns regarding these types of assessment tools have led to the suggestion by some experts that there is a need to revise the sedation continuum and to use other monitoring parameters (such as physiologic status) to assess the

depth of sedation.[47] Others have suggested that the use of an observational scale that simply codifies the "state" of the child at any time during the sedation/procedure is more useful than stimulation (Table 44.4).[48,49]

For many years, the "holy grail" of sedation has been the non-invasive sedation monitor that would accurately detect and record the depth of sedation without stimulating the child or interfering with a procedure. Several monitors have been developed to assess the depth of sedation or anesthesia in a nonstimulating, continuous manner including the bispectral index (BIS) monitor (Medtronic/Covidien, Minneapolis, MN); Sedline (Masimo, Neuchatel, Switzerland); Narcotrend monitor (Narcotrend-Gruppe, Hannover, Germany); Danmeter AEP monitor/2 (Danmeter DK-5000, Odense C, Denmark); Patient State Monitor (PSA-4000, Pfizer/Hospira, Lake Forest, IL), the Cerebral State Monitor (Danmeter DK-5000, Odense C, Denmark); and the Entropy module (GE Healthcare/Datex-Ohmeda, Chicago, IL). Although each of these has shown some level of utility, the most broadly applied (and thoroughly studied) of these is the BIS monitor,[50] which uses a proprietary method for processing the EEG signal and converting that reading into a number between 0 and 100, which has been correlated with the depth of sedation. The BIS was derived from empirically estimating processed EEG parameters that best predicted OAA/S scale levels in adult volunteers receiving a wide variety of anesthetics, analgesics, and sedatives.[51] BIS values in adults who are awake range from 95 to 100; when lightly to moderately sedated 70 to 95; when deeply sedated with a small probability of explicit recall 60 to 70; and general anesthesia, 40 to 60.[52–54] A systematic review of studies in adult intensive care units (ICUs) suggest moderate to strong correlation with clinical sedation scales.[55] However a Cochrane review of 52 studies involving 41,331 adult patients concluded that the effectiveness of using BIS to guide anesthetic depth is imprecise and there was low-certainty of reduced awareness and rapid recovery compared with clinical signs.[56]

Attempts to correlate BIS values with the depth of sedation in children have also met with varying success, particularly when attempting to distinguish moderate from deep sedation.[57–60] In part, these difficulties relate to two factors: (1) the algorithms have been validated only in adults, and (2) many of the anesthetics and drugs used to anesthetize and sedate children have not been

TABLE 44.4 | The Dartmouth Operative Conditions Scale (DOCS)

Patient State	Observed Behaviors			
Pain/Stress	(0)	(1)	(2)	
	Eyes closed or calm expression	Grimace or frown	Crying, sobbing, screaming	
Movement	(0)	(1)	(2)	(3)
	Still	Random little movement	Major purposeful movement	Thrashing, kicking, biting
Consciousness	(0)	(−1)	(−2)	
	Eyes open	Ptosis, uncoordinated, "drowsy"	Eyes closed	
Sedation Side Effects	(−1)	(−1)	(−1)	(−1)
	SpO_2 <92%	Noise with respiration	Respiratory pauses >10 seconds	BP decrease of >50% from baseline

Patients are scored in four state categories at any one time during sedation for a procedure. The sum of the scores in all four categories is used to determine the DOCS score for any discrete point during a sedation encounter.
BP, Blood pressure; *SpO_2*, oxygen saturation as measured by pulse oximetry.

adequately studied with the BIS monitor, even in adults. Other issues with the use of the BIS in children include:

1. BIS values are not age specific and are relatively inaccurate in children younger than 1 year of age.[61,62]
2. BIS readings may differ from one side of the head to the other.[63]
3. BIS readings are diminished in developmentally delayed children.[64]
4. BIS is drug specific; it is inaccurate with ketamine sedation because of ketamine-induced or nitrous oxide-induced central excitation.[65–67] BIS readings correlate reasonably well with dexmedetomidine sedation scores in adults,[68] but do not correlate well in children.[69]

Additionally, practical problems with the use of BIS-type monitoring include:

1. It is not feasible for many procedures, such as MRI scans.
2. BIS is not applicable for procedures involving the mouth and airway (endoscopy, dental, bronchoscopy), because the monitor creates artifacts or is in the way of the proceduralist.
3. Muscular activity around the head creates artifacts.

Overall, the lack of specificity for levels of sedation, low quality of BIS data, and the lack of information for different age groups or specific drugs preclude recommendation of the BIS for use in procedural sedation in children.[53] Similar limitations exist for the other monitors of sedation/anesthesia depth. Although they may be helpful in specific instances or clinical situations, their general use is not advised.

SEDATION DEPTH VERSUS SEDATION RISK

Sedation scales and sedation depth monitors quantify the depth of sedation but do not directly measure the risk of sedation. The sedative drug prescription, intended procedure, and patient's medical conditions all impact the risk of a procedure for each patient. Although the depth of sedation is defined by their responses to stimulation, the *important assessment of the child is not the response to stimulation, but rather the ability to protect and maintain their airway and to initiate rescue interventions as indicated*.[21,70,71] Sedative drugs or a particular dose of a drug may provide pain relief or hypnosis, but may also obstruct the airway or depress ventilation. For example, propofol is a potent, effective sedative that confers no analgesia but has marked effects on the airway tone and depresses the respiratory drive,[72] whereas dexmedetomidine provides less intense sedation than propofol, but modest pain relief with minimal compromise of airway morphology and minimal depression of respiration.[73] Midazolam causes limited sedation but may also lead to airway obstruction by causing a loss of pharyngeal patency, which is especially noted in children with enlarged tonsils.[74,75] In contrast, ketamine produces intense analgesia and decreases the responses to stimulation, but rarely obstructs the airway or depresses respiratory effort (even at very large doses) because it maintains upper airway dilator muscle function (Table 44.5).[76–79]

There are also aspects of the *patient* that affect the risks for airway-related adverse events as much as the depth of sedation. For instance, a child with obstructive sleep apnea (OSA) or obesity is much more likely to obstruct their airway during deep sedation than one without this comorbidity.[80–82] A history of prematurity increases the risks associated with sedation even throughout childhood and adolescence.[83] Other comorbidities such as congenital heart disease, airway anomalies, lower respiratory tract disease, and upper respiratory tract infection increase the risk of general anesthesia. One might also expect that these

TABLE 44.5	Examples of Sedative Drugs That Have Varying Effects on Response to Pain and Airway Protection

RESPONSE TO PAIN DOES NOT PREDICT AIRWAY MAINTENANCE
ALL DRUG EFFECTS ARE DIFFERENT

	Response to Pain	Airway Maintenance
Fentanyl	↓↓	↓
Propofol	±	↓
Ketamine	↓	±
Dexmedetomidine	↓	+

↓↓, Large decrease in response to pain or large effect on airway patency; ↓, some decrease in response to pain or some effect on airway patency; ±, minimal to no effect on response to pain or effect on airway patency; +, no effect on airway patency.

comorbidities would also increase the risk of sedation.[84–86] Similarly, the *procedure itself* can increase the risk for a child. A bronchoscopy or upper gastrointestinal endoscopy carries a much greater risk of airway-related events than a noninvasive diagnostic test.[87] The environment of the procedure can also increase risk. The MRI scanner (where the observer is remote from the airway during the scan and ferromagnetic objects are forbidden) is a more difficult environment than one where the sedation provider can be positioned adjacent to the airway and the monitors and rescue equipment are immediately available (as per standard routine). In summary, when assessing the risk of sedation, one must consider the multidimensional aspects of sedation that include the planned level of sedation, existing comorbidities in the child, the procedure to be performed, and the environment in which the procedure will be performed.

The safety of sedation must also focus on appropriate discharge readiness and the subtle differences in recovery from sedation. Adverse events, including deaths, have occurred after premature discharge following procedural sedation.[70,71] These events were most often associated with sedating medications with a prolonged duration of effect such as chloral hydrate (Fig. 44.3).[70,71] Accordingly, a simple "maintenance of wakefulness" score (infants had to stay awake for at least 15 to 20 consecutive minutes in a quiet environment before discharge) ensured that more than 90% of children had returned to baseline levels of consciousness compared with only 55% of children assessed as "street ready" according to usual hospital discharge criteria.[88]

The Concept of "Safety"

"Safety" in pediatric sedation is multidimensional. Although the adverse events related to the airway hold the greatest risk to cause immediate harm to the child, several additional risks should also be considered.

Since the early 2000s, concern has increased about the effect of drugs used for sedation or anesthesia on the developing brain and the possible association with neuroapoptosis and/or subsequent learning/behavioral deficiencies[89–95] (this topic is covered in detail in Chapter 23). The US Food and Drug Administration (FDA) has been particularly concerned about this issue, warning in editorials in 2011 and again in 2015 of the uncertain effects of sedatives and anesthetics on the developing brain.[96,97] Specific advisories on the use of anesthesia in young children have been vague and generally recommend that the use of anesthesia for procedures in the first 3 years after birth should be based on a

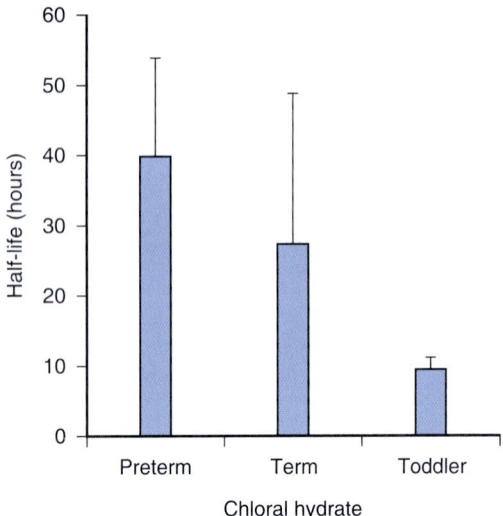

FIGURE 44.3 β-Elimination half-life of the active metabolite of chloral hydrate, trichloroethanol, in preterm infants, term infants, and toddlers. Note the extremely prolonged half-lives and the large standard deviations in all age groups. Although often thought of as a short-acting sedative, chloral hydrate can have profoundly long sedative effects, with a real possibility of resedation after a procedure when the child is left undisturbed. It is for this reason that we recommend a longer period of observation in a step-down area before discharge or avoiding its use.

balance of the known risks of delaying the procedure versus the uncertain risk of harm from anesthetics on the developing brain in humans. The FDA Advisory Committee Background Document to the Anesthetic and Life Support Drugs Advisory Committee issued a caveat that exposure to anesthesia drugs should be avoided for purely elective procedures in children younger than 3 years of age.[96] However in December 2016, the FDA rescinded their warning about anesthesia in children younger than 3 years of age, stating that *recent human studies suggest that a single, relatively short exposure to these drugs in infants or toddlers is unlikely to have negative effects on behavior or learning*.[98] Subsequent follow-up human studies have failed to demonstrate long-term sequelae after single exposures to anesthesia.[99–102] The 2017 update states that *exposure to these medicines for lengthy periods of time or over multiple surgeries or procedures may negatively affect brain development in children younger than 3 years*.[99–103]

Practitioners who deliver sedation must balance the risks of inadequate versus excessive sedation. Adverse events related to inadequate sedation are more difficult to track than the immediate risk of oversedation; however, this issue should not be discounted. Several studies have associated untreated procedural pain with long-term adverse behaviors in animals and children. Specifically, painful experiences in childhood have been linked to excessive pain responses and behaviors later in life.[6–10,104–106] In addition, a stressful anesthesia induction has been associated with greater maladaptive behaviors for up to 2 weeks after the experience; a similar response may be expected after sedation/anesthesia for a diagnostic procedure.[107] The incidence of these behaviors decreases with the use of appropriate preoperative sedation. Sequelae have also been reported after repeated invasive procedures in pediatric ICUs.[108] Such data suggest that "less sedation" is not a solution to concerns regarding possible apoptosis with current sedative drugs in neonates and infants.

The risks and markers associated with adverse sedation events have been the subject of multiple studies. A retrospective review of 95 cases of sedation-related deaths and critical incidents derived from the FDA adverse drug event reporting system, the US Pharmacopeia, and a survey of pediatric specialists in 2000[70,71] revealed that the overwhelming majority of critical events were preventable and resulted from operator error or lack of robust rescue systems rather than by the drugs themselves. Drug interactions were the most common causative factor, followed by drug overdose, inadequate monitoring, inadequate cardiopulmonary resuscitation skills, inadequate evaluation before sedation, and premature discharge from medical supervision.[70,71] The reports emphasize that most sedation complications are related to adverse respiratory events (80%); a majority progressed to cardiac arrest, indicating a lack of rescue skills on the part of the practitioners. A disproportionately large number of severe complications and deaths occurred when sedation was performed in offices outside hospitals (29/60 deaths or neurologic injury occurred during dental procedures), pointing to inadequate rescue planning and training. Most adverse sedation events in children were related to inadequate skills to rescue a nonbreathing child or to successfully manage airway obstruction. There was no relationship with class of drug or route of administration, although there was a positive correlation with complications when three or more sedating medications (pointing to drug interactions) were administered.[71]

Another method for analyzing sedation safety is the review of cases performed in a single institution using a particular drug or technique. The literature on pediatric sedation includes a large number of these studies reporting relatively small numbers of patients ($n < 200$) receiving a variety of sedative medications in a number of settings. Almost all these reports end with the conclusion that the described technique resulted in successful completion of the procedures, no fatalities, and to be "safe and effective."[109–121] Negative trial results are almost never published. Most studies are retrospective and describe different frequencies of transient airway obstruction or oxygen desaturation. In sum, these trials indicate that young age, increased ASA status, and certain procedures such as endoscopy and bronchoscopy have greater rates of adverse events. The sample size of some older studies limits their external validity to evaluate major adverse events or critical incidents, although more recent evidence is more heartening.[122] Accordingly, single-institution trials offer information on sedation techniques but infrequently provide robust evidence on risk and outcomes compared with multicentered, comprehensive studies and databases.[25,120,123–125]

Simulation may be used to test the abilities of practitioners to diagnose and treat low-frequency adverse effects that occur during pediatric sedation and the ability of systems to rescue patients.[126–128] In one of these studies, a simulated scenario of laryngospasm was programmed so that the physiologic variables either degraded with time after the event if inappropriate interventions were undertaken, or, improved with time if an effective intervention was performed. The event was videotaped in three different sedation locations. Hypoxia and hypotension lasted less than 90 seconds in the postanesthesia care unit but more than 360 seconds in the emergency department and radiology (CT scanner) settings.[129] Such studies demonstrate that analysis of simulated low-frequency adverse events can identify areas and practitioners within the hospital that need to improve their rescue systems to improve patient safety.

The advent of the electronic medical record and improved data sharing has allowed the capture of data from large numbers of pediatric sedation encounters that can lead to an enhanced understanding of the nature and frequency of adverse sedation events. The Pediatric Sedation Research Consortium consists of a group of more than 50 institutions in North America that shares prospective data on pediatric sedation.[24] Analysis of the first 30,000 records identified demographics, procedures, sedation techniques, outcomes, and adverse events:

1. There were no deaths and only one cardiac arrest.
2. Unanticipated admission occurred infrequently, 1 per 1500 sedations.
3. Vomiting occurred in 1 per 200 sedations, including one aspiration.
4. Stridor, laryngospasm, wheezing, and apnea occurred in 1 per 400 procedures.
5. Airway or ventilatory manipulations were required in 1 per 100 sedations.[129]

Risk factors for adverse events included age younger than 3 months, ASA physical status 3 or greater, and multiple drug combinations for sedation. The Pediatric Sedation Research Consortium has also reviewed the incidence of adverse events in 49,386 propofol sedation and/or anesthesia encounters for procedures outside of the operating room.[27] Propofol was delivered by multiple providers (anesthesiologists, intensivists, emergency medicine physicians, pediatricians, and radiologists). No deaths were recorded although cardiopulmonary resuscitation was required in two children and aspiration occurred in four others. The most common adverse event was related to the airway, which occurred with a frequency of 1:65 sedations; 1 in 70 children required airway rescue. Desaturation (<90% for more than 30 seconds) occurred 154 times per 10,000 sedations; central apnea or obstruction occurred 575 times per 10,000 sedations, and unexpected admissions occurred 7 times per 10,000 sedations. When all possible adverse events were considered according to the provider of the sedation, anesthesiologists reported fewer events than other medical specialists, with an odds ratio of 1.38 (95% confidence interval, 1.21 to 1.57, $P <0.001$).[27] An outcome analysis of major complications failed to identify any difference among providers. These data indicate that propofol sedation and/or anesthesia when provided by structured sedation services with well-trained providers (i.e., following the AAP sedation guidelines)[21] can provide effective sedation with an acceptable (low) incidence of severe adverse events. The safety of this practice depends on the ability to quickly and safely rescue patients from impending serious events.

An analysis of the complications from 437,842 pediatric sedations yielded similar findings to previous data with a greater incidence of complications in children with a history of prematurity, upper respiratory infection, reactive airway disease, developmental delay, or OSA undergoing dental or gastrointestinal procedures. The complications included 6805 instances of airway obstructions, 1112 laryngospasms, 210 unplanned hospital admissions, 52 emergency anesthesia consultations, 47 aspirations, 13 cardiac arrests, and no deaths, leading clinicians to conclude that with the right safety measures and training, sedation can be safely provided by nonanesthesiologists.[25]

Guidelines

AMERICAN ACADEMY OF PEDIATRICS GUIDELINES

Multiple organizations have produced guidelines for the conduct of sedation in children based on the definitions of the depth of sedation. The first sedation guideline was published in 1985 from the Committee on Drugs and the Section on Anesthesiology of the AAP.[130] The guideline emphasized systems issues pioneered in anesthesiology such as the need for informed consent, fasting before sedation, frequent measurement and charting of vital signs, the availability of age- and size-appropriate equipment, the use of continuous physiologic monitoring (pulse oximetry), the need for basic life support skills in the providers, as well as proper recovery and discharge procedures. This guideline was updated in 1992[131] and amended in 2002.[132] This amendment eliminated the use of the confusing term *conscious sedation* and replaced it with the term *moderate sedation.* The AAP's guideline was updated again in 2006,[22] 2016,[133] and 2019.[21,29] These revisions have unified the definitions of sedation depth used by the ASA and the JCAHO and emphasized further refinements of a systematic approach to sedation that included:

- No administration of sedative medications without the safety net of medical supervision (i.e., no sedative medications given at home).
- Careful presedation evaluation to include review of pertinent medical and surgical conditions.
- Careful history for ingestion of nutraceuticals and other medications that may alter drug metabolism and prolong sedation.
- Appropriate fasting guidelines for elective and urgent procedures. There should be a balance between the depth of sedation and the risk for those who are unable to fast because of the urgent nature of the procedure.
- Focused airway examination with particular attention to anatomic airway abnormalities and enlarged tonsils.
- Understanding the pharmacokinetic and pharmacodynamic effects of sedation medications and drug interactions.
- Appropriate training and skills in airway management for sedation providers to allow for rescue. Deep sedation requires training in Pediatric Advanced Life Support (PALS) or Advanced Pediatric Life Support (APLS).
- Immediate availability of size- and age-appropriate airway, monitoring, and resuscitation equipment.
- Appropriate emergency medications and reversal agents, available for sedation in all cases.
- Sufficient personnel to carry out the procedure *and* monitor the child; for moderate sedation this observer can assist with interruptible tasks but for deep sedation the observer's only responsibility is to monitor the patient and to help manage emergency events.
- Appropriate physiologic monitoring during and after the procedure; use of capnography is encouraged for moderate sedation but is now required for deep sedation.
- A "time-out" should be performed before sedation.
- Recovery personnel, monitoring, and discharge criteria with return to baseline condition before discharge.
- Continuous quality improvement to track common markers of potential safety issues, such as desaturation events, airway obstructions, laryngospasm, unplanned hospital admission, unsatisfactory sedation, and medication errors.
- Use of simulators to practice management of rare adverse events.
- Assume that all children younger than 6 years of age will be deeply sedated for painful procedures or those that are not painful but prolonged.

The 2016 update of the AAP guidelines[134] unified recommendations for pediatric medical and dental practitioners. The 2019 revision[21] clarified safety concerns for pediatric dental procedures with deep sedation or general anesthesia. Some dentists practice where the same individual performs the procedure and directs the sedation/anesthesia concurrently (the single-provider model). This dangerous practice has been associated with a number of deaths; when an emergency occurred, there was only one medically trained person present, the dentist.[135–141] The oral surgeons have developed a program to train dental anesthesia assistants (Dental Anesthesia Assistant National Certification [DAANCE])[142] who assume the role of the independent observer.[21] A 36-hour internet self-study course with no advanced educational requirements cannot replace what was intended to be the role of an independent observer in the AAP guideline. The 2019 AAP guideline now specifies that for dental procedures, the independent observer's *"sole responsibility is to administer drugs and constantly observe the patient's vital signs, depth of sedation, airway patency, and adequacy of ventilation. The independent observer must, at a minimum, be trained in PALS (or APLS) and capable of managing any airway, ventilatory, or cardiovascular emergency event resulting from the deep sedation and/or general anesthesia. The independent observer must be trained and skilled to establish intravenous access and draw up and administer rescue medications. The independent observer must have the training and skills to rescue a nonbreathing child; a child with airway obstruction; or a child with hypotension, anaphylaxis, or cardiorespiratory arrest, including the ability to open the airway, suction secretions, provide CPAP, insert supraglottic devices (oral airway, nasal trumpet, or laryngeal mask airway), and perform successful bag-valve-mask ventilation, tracheal intubation, and cardiopulmonary resuscitation. **The independent observer in the dental facility, as permitted by state regulation, must be 1 of the following: a physician anesthesiologist, a certified registered nurse anesthetist, a second oral surgeon, or a dentist anesthesiologist."***

The dental provider must have current PALS certification. A dental anesthesia assistant cannot supplant the independent observer. Three decision trees that guide the management of airway obstruction, laryngospasm, and apnea were also added. This most recent guideline further emphasized:

- *Patient Evaluation.* Clinicians should be familiar with the sedation-related aspects of the patient's medical history. These include (1) abnormalities of major organ systems; (2) previous adverse effects with sedation and general anesthesia; (3) drug allergies, current medications, nutraceuticals, and drug interactions; (4) time and nature of oral intake; and (5) history of tobacco, alcohol, or substance abuse. (6) A focused physical examination, including auscultation of the heart and lungs, and the airway, as well as a review of the vital signs, is recommended.

- *Preprocedural Preparation.* Patients and the parents/guardians should be informed of and agree to the sedation including its risks, benefits, limitations, and alternatives. All children should be fasted as per the ASA guidelines: minimum fasting intervals of 2 hours after clear liquids, 4 hours after breast milk, 6 hours after infant formula, nonhuman milk, or a light meal (dry toast, tea without milk), and 8 hours after fatty food.[143] If urgent, emergent, or other situations impair gastric emptying, the potential for pulmonary aspiration of gastric contents must be considered when determining the target level of sedation, delay of the procedure/investigation, or the need to secure the airway (e.g., tracheal intubation).

- *Monitoring Level of Consciousness.* Monitoring of verbal commands should be routine during moderate sedation, i.e., the patient should be interactive, with the exception of young children and those who are developmentally impaired, uncooperative patients, or when the response would be detrimental.

- *Physiologic Monitoring.* All patients undergoing sedation/analgesia should be monitored by pulse oximetry with appropriate alarms. In addition, respiration should be continuously monitored by observation or auscultation. End-tidal carbon dioxide ($ETCO_2$) is encouraged for children who are moderately sedated and is required for all those are who are deeply sedated and for those whose ventilation could not be directly observed during moderate sedation as per AAP guidelines.[21] The ASA standards for basic monitoring were amended in 2012 to include $ETCO_2$ monitoring for those sedated at moderate and deeper levels of sedation and reaffirmed in 2020.[134,144] In addition, the guidelines recommended that blood pressure should be determined before sedation/analgesia is initiated where possible and at regular intervals during the procedure, unless such monitoring interferes with the procedure (e.g., pediatric MRI, in which stimulation from the blood pressure cuff could arouse an appropriately sedated child). Electrocardiographic (ECG) monitoring should also be used in all children during deep sedation, and during moderate sedation, in those with significant cardiovascular disease, or those who are undergoing procedures in which dysrhythmias are anticipated.

- *Recording of Monitored Parameters.* For both moderate and deep sedation, the child's level of consciousness, respiratory status, and hemodynamic variables should be assessed and recorded at a frequency commensurate with the type and amount of medication administered, the duration of the procedure, and the medical condition of the child. At a minimum, this should be (1) before the beginning of the procedure; (2) after administration of sedative/analgesic agents; (3) at regular intervals during the procedure; (4) during initial recovery; and (5) immediately before discharge. If recording is performed automatically, device alarms should be set to alert the care team to critical changes in patient status.

- *Availability of an Appropriately Trained and Skilled Individual Responsible for Patient Monitoring.* A designated individual, other than the practitioner performing the procedure, should be present to monitor the child throughout procedures performed with sedation/analgesia. During deep sedation, this individual should have no other responsibilities. However, during moderate sedation, this individual may assist with minor, interruptible tasks once the patient's level of sedation/analgesia and vital signs have stabilized, provided that adequate monitoring for the child's level of sedation is maintained.

- *Training of Personnel.* Individuals responsible for children who receive sedation/analgesia should understand the pharmacology of the medications that are administered, as well as the role of pharmacologic antagonists for opioids and benzodiazepines. Individuals who monitor children receiving sedation/analgesia should be able to recognize the associated complications. At least one individual capable of establishing a patent airway and positive-pressure ventilation, as well as a means for summoning additional assistance, should be present whenever sedation/analgesia is administered as described earlier.

- *Availability of Emergency Equipment.* Antagonists for sedatives and opioids, as well as appropriately sized equipment for establishing a patent airway and providing positive-pressure ventilation with supplemental oxygen, should be present whenever sedation/analgesia is administered. Suction, advanced airway equipment, and resuscitation medications should be immediately available and in good working order. A functional defibrillator should be immediately available whenever deep sedation is administered and when moderate sedation is administered to those with mild or severe cardiovascular disease.

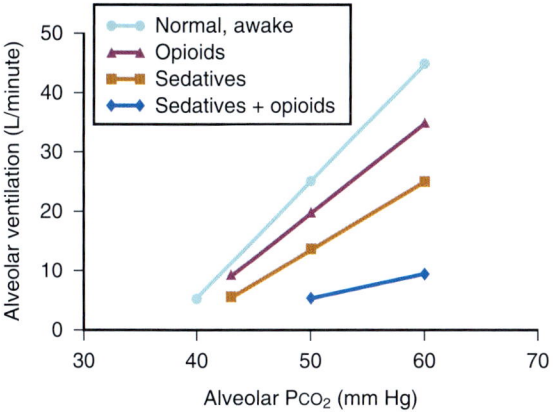

FIGURE 44.4 Relationship between ventilation and carbon dioxide is represented by a family of curves. Each curve has two parameters: an *x*-intercept and a slope. Sedatives and opioids increase the intercept and decrease the slope. The combination of sedatives and opioids produce the most profound effect. (From Yaster M, Nichols DG, Deshpande JK, Wetzel RC. Midazolam-fentanyl intravenous sedation in children: case report of respiratory arrest. *Pediatrics.* 1990;86(3):463-467.)

■ *Use of Supplemental Oxygen.* Equipment to administer supplemental oxygen should be present when sedation/analgesia is administered. Supplemental oxygen should be considered for moderate sedation and should be administered for deep sedation unless specifically contraindicated for a particular child or procedure. If hypoxemia is anticipated or develops during sedation/analgesia, supplemental oxygen should be administered.

■ *Combinations of Sedative/Analgesic Agents.* Combinations of sedative and analgesic agents may be administered as indicated for the procedure being performed and the condition of the child. Ideally, each component should be administered individually to achieve the desired effect (e.g., additional analgesic medication to relieve pain; additional sedative medication to decrease awareness or anxiety). The propensity for combinations of sedative and analgesic agents to cause respiratory depression and airway obstruction emphasizes the need to appropriately reduce the dose of each component, as well as the need to continually monitor respiratory function (Fig. 44.4). It is vital to wait appropriate intervals between drug administration so as to not "stack" dosing and cause respiratory depression.

■ *Recovery Care.* After sedation for diagnostic and therapeutic procedures, the children should be observed in an appropriately staffed and equipped area until they are near their baseline level of consciousness and are no longer at increased risk for cardiorespiratory depression. Oxygenation should be monitored periodically until they are no longer at risk for hypoxemia. Ventilation and circulation should be monitored at regular intervals until the children are suitable for discharge. Discharge criteria should be designed to minimize the risk of central nervous system (CNS) or cardiorespiratory depression after discharge from observation by trained personnel. This is particularly important for children who have OSA or are cognitively impaired.

■ *Consultation and Availability of an Anesthesiologist.* Whenever possible, appropriate medical specialists should be consulted before sedating children with comorbidities. The choice of specialists depends on the nature of the underlying condition and the urgency of the situation. For severely compromised or medically unstable children (e.g., anticipated difficult airway, severe

TABLE 44.6	Guidelines for the Consultation of an Anesthesiologist

1. Medical Problems
   - ASA physical status III or IV
   - Pulmonary: airway obstruction (tonsils/adenoids)—loud snoring, obstructive sleep apnea. Poorly controlled asthma, congenital or acquired anomalies of the airway or face (Trisomy 21, Pierre Robin syndrome, Treacher Collins syndrome, Crouzon disease, tracheomalacia)
   - Morbid obesity (≥2 times ideal body weight, BMI >30 kg/m²)
   - Cardiovascular: cyanosis, repaired or unrepaired congenital heart disease with significant symptoms of cyanosis or congestive heart failure
   - Prematurity: less than 60 weeks postconception age at time of sedation
   - Residual pulmonary, cardiovascular, gastrointestinal, neurologic problems
   - Neurologic: developmental disabilities, poorly controlled seizures, central apnea
   - Gastrointestinal: uncontrolled gastroesophageal reflux
   - Severe liver or renal disease
2. Procedures requiring deep sedation in patients with a full stomach
   - Emergency procedures
3. Management problems
   - Severe developmental delay
   - Patients who are difficult to control
   - Severe attention-deficit disorder (paradoxically, the child may develop increased agitation during or after the procedure)
4. History of failed sedation
   - Oversedation (loss of airway reflexes)
   - Inability to adequately sedate
   - Hyperactive (paradoxical) response to sedatives

ASA, American Society of Anesthesiologists; BMI, body mass index.

obstructive pulmonary disease, or congestive heart failure), practitioners who are not trained in the administration of general anesthesia should consult an anesthesiologist (Table 44.6).

AMERICAN SOCIETY OF ANESTHESIOLOGISTS GUIDELINES

The ASA has numerous statements and guidelines for sedation by physicians other than anesthesiologists. The "Practice Guidelines for Sedation and Analgesia by Non-Anesthesiologists" was last updated in 2002 and for moderate sedation in 2018,[30,34] in many respects, these guidelines are in concert with the AAP guideline.[21] The ASA currently has many statements discussing sedation guidelines available through their website (https://www.asahq.org). Some statements specifically address questions related to the provision of moderate and deep sedation by nonanesthesiologists as well as the use of medications such as propofol by nonanesthesiologists. Most pertinent of these is the 2022 document "Statement on Granting Privileges for Deep Sedation to Non-Anesthesiologist Sedation Practitioners."[145] This document provides guidance to assist the chief of anesthesia and hospital administrators in granting privileges consistent with JCAHO recommendations, focusing on three topics:

EDUCATION AND TRAINING

1. *The qualified non-anesthesia professional must have satisfactorily completed a formal training program in (1) the safe administration of sedative and analgesic drugs used to establish a level of deep sedation and (2) rescue of patients who exhibit adverse physiologic consequences of a deeper-than-intended level of sedation.*

44

- *This training includes the didactic and performance concepts obtained through part of a recently completed Accreditation Council for Graduate Medical Education (ACGME) residency or fellowship training (e.g., within two years), or may be a separate deep sedation educational program that is accredited by Accreditation Council for Continuing Medical Education (ACCME), or equivalent, for dentists, oral surgeons, or podiatrists.*
- *The content required must include all appropriate ASA Statements and Guidelines, identification of procedural or patient considerations that make performance by qualified anesthesia personnel essential, and the pharmacology of all appropriate pharmaceuticals.*

2. *A knowledge-based test is necessary to demonstrate the knowledge of concepts required to obtain privileges in an objective manner.*

3. *A skills-based test is necessary to demonstrate competency in airway management skills necessary to rescue a patient from a deeper than intended level of sedation.*

PERFORMANCE EVALUATION

1. *Before granting initial privileges to administer or supervise the administration of sedative and analgesic drugs to establish a level of deep sedation, a process will be developed to evaluate the applicant's performance and competency. For recent graduates (e.g., within two years), this may be accomplished through letters of recommendation from directors of residency or fellowship training programs that include deep sedation as part of the curriculum. For those who have been in practice since the completion of their training, performance evaluation may be accomplished through specific documentation of performance evaluation data transmitted from department heads or supervisors at the institution where the individual previously held privileges to administer deep sedation. Alternatively, the non-anesthesiologist applicant could be proctored or supervised by a qualified person privileged to administer sedative and analgesic agents to provide deep sedation. The Director of Anesthesia Services, with oversight by the facility governing body, will determine the number of cases that need to be performed and the threshold for quality metrics to determine competency in deep sedation.*

2. *Before granting ongoing privileges to administer or supervise the administration of sedative and analgesic drugs to establish a level of deep sedation, a process will be developed to re-evaluate the practitioner's performance at regular intervals. Re-evaluation of competency in airway management will be part of this performance evaluation. For example, the applicant's performance could be reviewed by a qualified person who is currently privileged to administer deep sedation. The facility will establish an appropriate number of procedures that will be reviewed.*

PERFORMANCE IMPROVEMENT

Privileging for the administration of sedative and analgesic drugs to establish a level of deep sedation will require active participation in an ongoing process that evaluates the qualified person's clinical performance and patient care outcomes through a formal facility program of continuous performance improvement. The facility's deep sedation performance improvement program will be developed with oversight by the Director of Anesthesia Services."

Separate privileging is required for the care of children. The exact nature of these requirements is not specified, but pediatric sedation training over and above baseline competencies is advised.

AMERICAN COLLEGE OF EMERGENCY PHYSICIANS GUIDELINES

Other organizations, notably the American College of Emergency Physicians (ACEP), have published their own sedation guidelines and clinical practice advisories for sedation.[146–150] These guidelines are distinguishable from the AAP and ASA guidelines in several respects, including the definition of the continuum of sedation. The ACEP guideline prefers the term "procedural sedation." It is defined *"as a technique of administering sedatives, analgesics, dissociative agents, alone or in combination to induce a state that allows the child to tolerate unpleasant procedures while maintaining cardiopulmonary function."* It is intended to result in a depressed level of consciousness but one that allows the child to *"independently and continuously"* control their own airway. They have an additional level of sedation called "dissociative sedation":

Dissociative sedation is a trance-like cataleptic state characterized by profound analgesia and amnesia, with retention of protective airway reflexes, spontaneous respirations, and cardiopulmonary stability. In the emergency department, ketamine is commonly administered to evoke dissociative levels of sedation. Dissociative state can facilitate moderate to severely painful procedures, as well as procedures requiring immobilization in uncooperative patients.[149]

This guideline was updated in 2014 and 2018 to address several issues with the recommendations[149,151]:

1. Do not delay procedural sedation in adults or children in the emergency department based on fasting time. Preprocedural fasting for any duration has not reduced the risk of emesis or aspiration when administering procedural sedation and analgesia.

2. Capnography may be used as an adjunct to pulse oximetry and as a clinical tool to detect hypoventilation and apnea earlier than pulse oximetry and/or clinical assessment alone in children undergoing procedural sedation and analgesia in the Emergency Department. Patient responsiveness to stimulation is now viewed as counterproductive and imprecise; ventilatory adequacy and cardiovascular stability should be the focus, not the specific drugs used for sedation.[151]

3. During procedural sedation and analgesia, a nurse or other qualified individual (respiratory therapist) should be present to continually observe and monitor the patient, in addition to the provider performing the procedure. Physicians who are working or consulting in the emergency department should coordinate procedures requiring procedural sedation and analgesia with the emergency department staff.

4. Ketamine and etomidate can be safely administered individually to children and propofol can be administered to both children and adults for procedural sedation and analgesia in the emergency department. A combination of propofol and ketamine can be safely administered to children and adults for procedural sedation and analgesia.

5. ACEP opposes credentialling based on short courses such as ACLS or PALS as a requirement since their training is more extensive than that provided by these courses.[151]

The ACEP suggests a very different clinical practice advisory for the fasting interval before sedation based on analysis of reports from the sedation literature and expert consensus. The suggested time frames for fasting start with a 3-hour baseline and vary based on the urgency of the procedure and the planned depth of sedation. In addition, the practitioner can be directing the sedation and performing the procedure, and there is vague language regarding the nurse observer. The result is a strategy that differs significantly from the standard recommendations from the AAP and ASA.[152]

JOINT COMMISSION ON ACCREDITATION OF HEALTHCARE ORGANIZATIONS GUIDANCE

It is mandatory that sedation policies used in hospitals conform to JCAHO standards that have been derived from the Department of Health and Human Services (DHHS) Centers for Medicare & Medicaid Services (CMS). These requirements are consistent with the AAP/ASA guidelines but are more explicit in terms of the oversight of sedation services. The standards require documentation (e.g., medical history, physical status, and record-keeping during the procedure and the recovery from the procedure), a fasting protocol, and informed consent procedures that are mandatory for all those undergoing sedation, regardless of the nature, duration, patient's history, and location of the procedure. Similarly, the sedation personnel, monitoring equipment, and recovery facilities must meet uniform standards within an institution. Hospitals risk losing federal funding if they fail to comply. As of the CMS regulations published in 2011,[28] the leadership and responsibilities for the delivery of deep sedation are assigned to a *"qualified doctor of medicine or osteopathy who leads the department of anesthesia services."* This would logically fall under the purview of the chair of the department of anesthesiology in most cases; however, there are many small or unique hospitals where such a position does not exist. In such cases, the hospital administration must designate a physician who will fill this role and meet these qualifications (Fig. 44.5).

Under the CMS directives, deep sedation is placed under anesthesia services and *subject to the anesthesia administration requirements at 42 CFR 482.52(a):* whereas *minimal and moderate sedation* are placed under analgesia/sedation and therefore not subject to anesthesia administrative requirements.[28] To ensure continuity and equanimity of sedation care, CMS states that there should be one anesthesia service that has responsibility for oversight of all anesthesia services. Anesthesia must be administered by a (1) qualified anesthesiologist; (2) certified registered nurse anesthetist (CRNA) or anesthesiologist assistant (AA) with appropriate supervision; (3) doctor of medicine or osteopathy (other than an anesthesiologist); and (4) dentist, oral surgeon, or podiatrist who is qualified to administer anesthesia under state regulations. Credentialing and privileging must be done per hospital policy **and is the responsibility of the hospital's director of anesthesia services (or his/her designee).** The appropriateness and quality of anesthesia, including sedation, must be reviewed and approved by the director of anesthesia services. The standards for sedation require that each hospital develop specific appropriate protocols for patients receiving sedation, but these guidelines offer little detail on the exact content of the protocols (those are left to the individual organizations). These protocols must include delineation of:

1. Qualified individuals in sufficient numbers to perform and monitor patients during and after the procedure. A registered nurse must supervise perioperative nursing care.
2. Competency-based education, training, and experience in evaluating patients. These must include:
   a. Evaluating patients before the sedation.
   b. Performing moderate and deep sedation, including rescuing patients who slip into a deeper than desired level of sedation. These include:
      i. Moderate sedation—personnel are qualified to rescue patients from deep sedation and are competent to manage a compromised airway and to provide adequate oxygenation and ventilation.

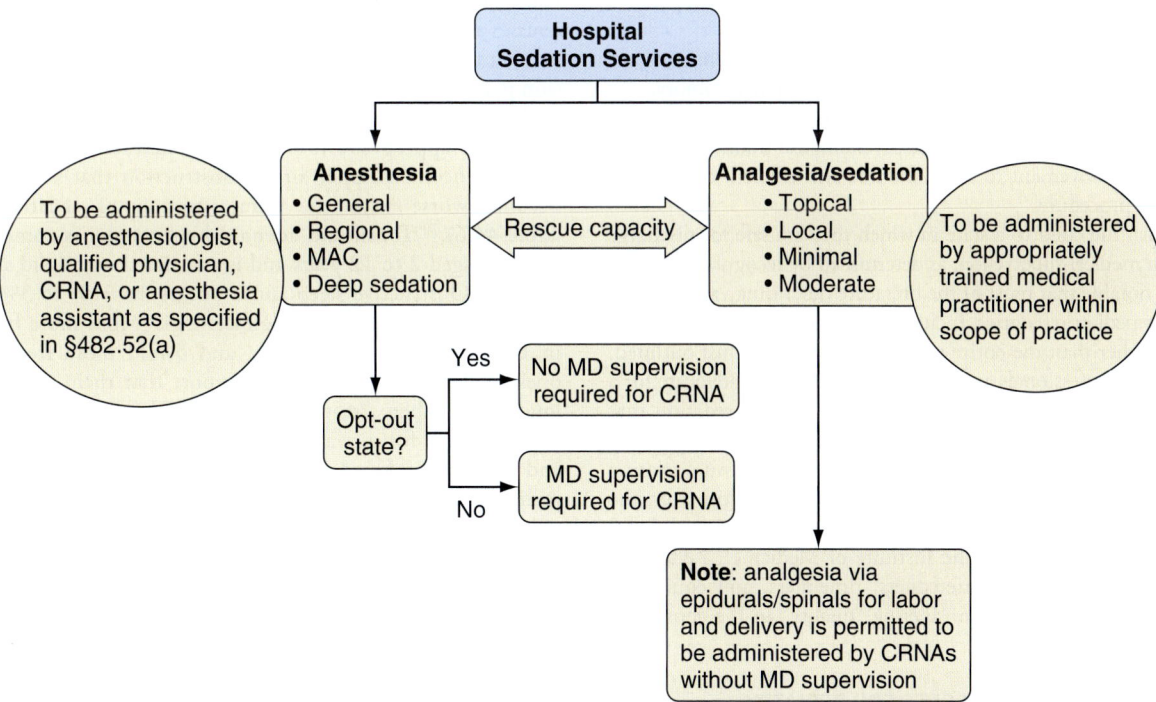

FIGURE 44.5 Centers for Medicare & Medicaid Services organizational chart showing deep sedation under the category of "Anesthesia" and supervised by "Hospital Sedation Services." *CRNA,* Certified registered nurse anesthetist; *MAC,* monitored anesthesia care; *MD,* physician.

    ii. Deep sedation—personnel are qualified to rescue patients from general anesthesia and are competent to manage an unstable cardiovascular system, as well as a compromised airway and inadequate oxygenation and ventilation.

3. Appropriate equipment for care and resuscitation.
4. The following must occur before moderate or deep sedation:
   a. Appropriate needs of the patient are assessed.
   b. Preprocedural education is provided to the patient according to a plan of care.
   c. A time-out is conducted immediately before starting, as described in universal protocol.
   d. A licensed independent practitioner plans or concurs with the planned procedure.
5. Appropriate monitoring of vital signs during and after the procedure, including, but not limited to, heart rate and oxygenation using pulse oximetry, respiratory frequency and adequacy of pulmonary ventilation, monitoring of blood pressure at regular levels, and cardiac monitoring (by ECG or use of a continuous cardiac monitoring device) in patients with significant cardiovascular disease or when dysrhythmias are anticipated or detected.
6. Documentation of care before, during, and after the procedure.
7. Monitoring of outcomes. In particular, analysis of data is performed on adverse events or patterns of adverse events during moderate or deep sedation.

The guidelines for sedation are actually quite similar among the various organizations and government entities that are responsible for these standards. It is critical that anesthesiologists who oversee and coordinate this care be familiar with the various guidelines and help their colleagues meet or exceed them.

Goals of Sedation

The goals of pediatric sedation are similar to the goals of operative anesthesia[29,40]:

- Guard the child's safety and welfare. This includes ensuring appropriate airway maintenance and cardiovascular stability.
- Minimize physical discomfort and pain.
- Control anxiety and minimize psychological trauma.
- Control movement to allow the safe and efficient completion of the procedure.
- Return the child to a state in which they are safe for discharge from medical supervision, as determined by recognized criteria.

It is notable that most of the literature describing various strategies for pediatric sedation focuses on the completion of the procedure rather than the entire spectrum of the goals just outlined. Anesthesia professionals are in a unique position to advocate for a more complete appreciation of the overall goals of sedation that should meet the high standards that have been set in the operating room environment. To this end, a useful analysis of issues relating to overall "quality" of sedation is provided by a report from the Society for Pediatric Sedation in which sedation quality is placed in the context defined by the Institute of Medicine[153]: effectiveness, efficiency, family centeredness, timeliness, and equity (in addition to safety) when considering "quality" in the context of sedation practices.

TRAINING AND SYSTEM ISSUES FOR PEDIATRIC PROCEDURAL SEDATION

Education is vital to maintain safety. Institution-wide ongoing educational programs on sedation, emphasizing physician (and dentist) responsibility, nursing responsibility, guidelines, and the pharmacology of drugs, should be readily available to all individuals who care for children requiring sedation/analgesia. Teaching modules, videos, handouts, simulations, and hands-on supervision have been used to supplement such programs.[122] Most institutions have adopted a computerized teaching module that includes a review of hospital policy, equipment, personnel, pharmacology of drugs used, rescue from deeper levels of sedation and management of airway-related adverse events such as obstruction, laryngospasm, or apnea. Usually, a quiz must be successfully completed at the end of the computerized teaching module. These modules are part of the orientation and hospital privileging procedure for each physician and nurse and must be successfully completed before they can administer sedation; the modules must be reviewed and successfully completed every 2 years. Staff privileging requirements should include training in PALS or equivalent because this is now a requirement of the 2019 AAP sedation guideline.[21] Further information on the nature of training required for sedation credentialing is sparse. One survey reported that 51% of institutions provided a specific training packet for sedation, whereas 59% depended on sedation training during fellowships, and 49% documented a specific number of procedural sedation encounters.[154]

Specialty organizations are also becoming involved in training sedation providers. The Society for Pediatric Sedation provides an extensive "primer" on pediatric sedation on its website.* This organization also provides a credentialing course for pediatric sedation that uses a test of knowledge based on its written materials (see previous discussion) and the completion of a full-day "Sedation Provider Course," which includes lectures, interactive sessions, and human patient simulation sessions (developed from data relating to pediatric sedation adverse events) to teach and test core competencies. Hands-on simulation-based courses such as this have been shown to improve provider confidence and perceived ability to care for pediatric procedural sedation patients.[155]

Education should also emphasize the limits of sedation and when it is appropriate to consult an anesthesiologist. Of particular concern is upper airway obstruction that would likely become worse with the administration of sedatives (see Table 44.6).[70] Tonsil and adenoid hypertrophy is common in children aged 2 to 12 years and is associated with loud snoring or OSA. Obstructive sleep apnea occurs in ~1% to 3% of all children, in up to 12% of adolescents, is 3-fold more frequent in Black than White children, and 5-fold more frequent in obese children.[156] Parents often report that their child snores loudly and then "stops breathing." These children are at increased risk for airway obstruction and opioid sensitivity[157] and should be referred to an airway specialist (anesthesiologist, pediatric intensivist, pediatric emergency medicine specialist) if sedation is required for their procedures. They may also require overnight admission and monitoring (see also Chapters 2 and 31).[158–162] Children with developmental disabilities should raise concern for sedation because they are at increased risk for airway obstruction during sedation and anesthesia.[163] Problems for which consultation with an anesthesiologist or other expert is suggested are listed in Table 44.6.

---

*https://learnpedsedation.org/

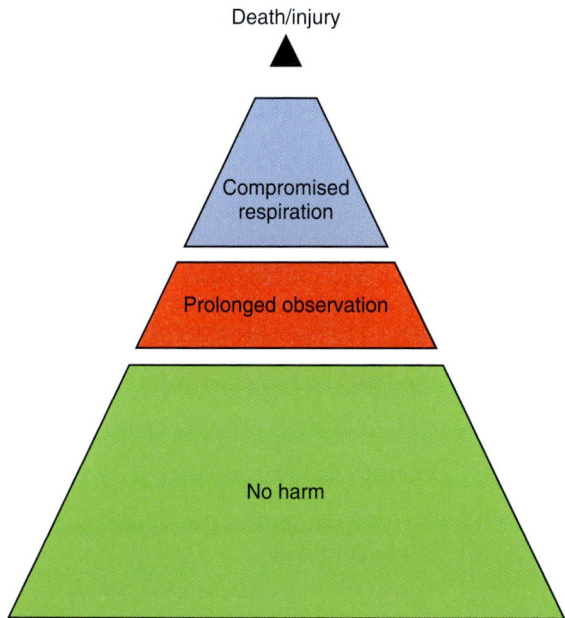

Death/injury

Compromised respiration

Prolonged observation

No harm

FIGURE 44.6 The sedation accident pyramid. The majority of adverse sedation events result in no harm. A smaller number result in no harm but require prolonged observation. An even smaller number result in the need for some intervention, usually related to respiration (repositioning the head, a jaw thrust, bag-mask respirations, or intubation). A very small number result in injury or death because the sentinel event was missed or inadequately treated. The latter cases are the types that occasionally are reported in newspapers, but in general go unreported. The reported cases likely represent just the tip of the pyramid in terms of events that could have indicated a developing problem.

The importance of nursing in the provision of safe and effective sedation for children cannot be overemphasized.[164] Nurses are the "front line" in sedation safety and frequently are the part of the sedation team that identifies variation in policy compliance. Their support and education is mandatory. In addition, state nursing restrictions on nurses administering certain drugs (such as propofol and ketamine) must be taken into consideration.

Quality improvement is a critical piece in ensuring optimal training and sedation system functioning. Compliance can be monitored by the medical and dental office staff or the department of nursing, as well as a committee charged with the responsibility of continuing quality improvement regarding sedation services. Nursing and medical staff offices should monitor compliance with educational certification for appropriate credentialing. It is the responsibility of the department chairperson and nursing supervisors to ensure individual staff within their department's compliance. Finally, variance reports should be generated when sedation policy is not followed or when a critical incident occurs; the appropriate institutional committee should review each incident for possible remedial measures. The committee should review system problems and recommend fixes for organizational issues that contribute to sedation care inefficiencies and failures. (e.g., inadequate presedation assessment, inadequate monitoring leading to delay in problem recognition, or inadequate recovery procedures). Tracking common problems, such as the need for bag-mask ventilation, apnea, desaturation,

unplanned hospital admissions, or unsatisfactory sedation, can provide direction for developing changes in policy and training that will prevent more severe but much less frequent events (e.g., cardiac arrest) from occurring (Fig. 44.6). This type of critical incident analysis provides the basis for recommendations to reduce or prevent future adverse events.[165–168]

DOCUMENTATION

A single documentation interface, as recommended by JCAHO, that is used wherever sedation is delivered within an institution provides uniformity of care and compliance with sedation policies. The sedation interface should be organized such that practitioners have a readily apparent guide to sedation policies. The very act of following and completing the sedation record ensures compliance with hospital policy (E-Fig. 44.1). The near-universal application of electronic medical records now allows demographic, allergy, and comorbidity data to be gathered from other areas of the electronic medical record and automatically adds vital signs before and during the intervention (Video 44.5). Appropriate electronic record documentation for sedation generally includes a variety of dropdown menus, which allow the practitioner to access drug dosing, rating scale information, and automatically enter vital signs (see Video 44.5).

To be in line with standard guidelines on sedation, the documentation should include:

- *Presedation responsibilities.* During this time, the responsibilities of the registered nurse include evaluation of the child to include learning assessment, NPO (nothing by mouth) status, allergies, current medications, and review of medical problems. The licensed independent practitioner verifies this information with particular emphasis on assessing the airway. A sedation plan is identified and informed consent is obtained. The practitioner assigns an ASA physical status and reassesses the child immediately before the procedure.

- *Presedation pause.* A time-out should be performed immediately before sedation medications are given. The time-out includes a process of verbal confirmation of the patient and procedure identification, verification of informed consent, as well as ASA physical status and confirmation of the procedure and site of the procedure. **No medications are administered without completion of the time-out.** One advantage of the electronic record is that it forces the practitioner to verify the time-out before it allows further access to the rest of the sedation flow sheet.

- *During sedation.* The time-based flow sheet identifies the depth of sedation, which monitors should be used, and how frequently the vital signs should be recorded for both moderate and deep sedation. Table 44.7 summarizes monitoring, documentation, personnel, and equipment during sedation as recommended by the AAP sedation guideline.[21]

- *Postsedation.* The criteria for discharge from the sedation area, pain score, and disposition of the child, as well as discharge teaching, are specified. This includes documentation and signature by the practitioner and nurse. Space is given for additional documentation and medications given.

Most importantly, both the paper and electronic record forms have critical parts of the sedation policy for immediate bedside review. This includes pain assessment scales, NPO guideline variations, reassessment by the licensed practitioner before sedation, and the opioid medication order verification. A table that defines the levels of sedation, required monitors, and frequency

44

TABLE 44.7	Recommended Intensity of Monitoring, Documentation, Personnel, and Equipment for Different Levels of Sedation[21]	
	Moderate Sedation	**Deep Sedation**
Monitoring	Pulse oximetry ECG recommended Heart rate Blood pressure Respiration Capnography recommended	Pulse oximetry ECG required Heart rate Blood pressure Respiration **Capnography required**
Documentation	Name, route, site, time of administration, and dosage of all drugs administered Continuous oxygen saturation, heart rate, and ventilation (capnography recommended) Parameters recorded q10 minutes	Name, route, site, time of administration, and dosage of all drugs administered Continuous oxygen saturation, heart rate, and ventilation (capnography required) Parameters recorded at least q5 minutes
Personnel	An observer who will monitor the patient but who may also assist with interruptible tasks—trained in pediatric advanced life support (PALS)	An independent observer whose only responsibility is to continuously monitor the patient—trained in PALS **and capable of assisting with any emergency event**
Responsible practitioner	Skilled to rescue a child with apnea, laryngospasm, and/or airway obstruction including the ability to open the airway, suction secretions, provide continuous positive airway pressure (CPAP), perform successful bag-valve-mask ventilation. Recommended that at least one practitioner should be skilled in obtaining vascular access in children	**Skilled to rescue a child with apnea, laryngospasm, and/or airway obstruction including the ability to open the airway, suction secretions, provide CPAP, perform successful bag-valve-mask ventilation, tracheal intubation, and cardiopulmonary resuscitation; training in PALS required.** At least one practitioner skilled in obtaining vascular access in children immediately available
Equipment	Pulse oximeter, blood pressure device, ECG (recommended), stethoscope, capnometer (recommended) Rescue cart and equipment immediately available properly stocked with rescue drugs and age- and size-appropriate equipment required	Pulse oximeter, blood pressure device, stethoscope, **ECG monitor (required), capnometer (required)** Rescue cart and equipment immediately available properly stocked with rescue drugs and age- and size-appropriate equipment required
Other Equipment	Suction equipment Adequate oxygen source/supply	Suction equipment Adequate oxygen source/supply **Defibrillator required**
Emergency checklists	Recommended	Recommended
Dedicated recovery area: With a rescue cart properly stocked with rescue drugs and age- and size-appropriate equipment with dedicated recovery personnel and adequate oxygen supply	Recommended Initial recording of vital signs may be needed at least every 10 minutes until the child begins to awaken, then recording intervals may be increased	Recommended Initial recording of vital signs may be needed at least 5-minute intervals until the child begins to awaken, then recording intervals may be increased to 10–15 minutes

of monitoring is also present. This, in addition to the online availability of the hospital policies, ensures that sedation practitioners have all information available to comply and to safely and successfully sedate children.

Sedation services, how ever they are configured, may find it helpful to create information sheets on presedation assessment, telephone interviews, and postsedation follow-up. Examples of a radiology-nursing database that consists of presedation telephone information, presedation instructions, NPO guidelines, health history, and postexamination telephone call information are shown in E-Figs. 44.2 and 44.3. Samples of presedation and

postsedation instruction sheets for pediatric dentistry are shown in E-Figs. 44.4 and 44.5. It is helpful if such forms are available in Spanish and other common languages and explained using interpreters if necessary.

Specific Sedation Techniques

A *sedation treatment plan* that addresses the requirements for analgesics, anxiolytics, or both is necessary for each child, according to the procedure being performed and the anxiety of the child and family. Psychological techniques to allay anxiety and distract children's attention from the procedural environment (e.g., iPad, games/movies, virtual reality, cuddling, parental support, child life specialists, guided imagery techniques, warm blankets, a gentle reassuring voice, and hypnosis) are extraordinarily useful adjuncts to the sedation plan.[12–19] Certified child life specialists play an important role in assessment and provision of comfort and distraction during procedures. At times, distraction techniques alone can suffice to produce conditions amenable to accomplishing a simple nonpainful procedure.[17,169]

Many of the drugs used for sedation and analgesia in children are not approved by the FDA for use in children under certain ages (e.g., fentanyl <2 years; morphine <18 years; bupivacaine <12 years; propofol <2 months; and dexmedetomidine <1 month of age). Although midazolam is approved in the United States even in preterm infants, the reversal agent flumazenil is *not* approved in children younger than 1 year of age. The lack of "approval" by the FDA does not imply that a drug can/should not be used; rather, it only means that the manufacturer did not conduct studies to garner FDA approval.[37,170–173] A number of legislative changes have improved drug research and labeling in children; however,[174–176] some drugs are no longer under patent protection, and there is no motivation for drug companies to study their use in children (see also Chapter 5).[177–179]

It is important to review the child's presedation medications, particularly chronic opioid or benzodiazepines; tolerance can significantly increase the doses to achieve the desired depth of sedation and analgesia. On the other hand, protease inhibitors, used for HIV and coronavirus therapy,[180] can be both inhibitors (e.g., nelfinavir, ritonavir, saquinavir, delavirdine, amprenavir, indinavir)[181] and inducers (e.g., nevirapine, efavirenz) of the cytochrome P450 CYP3A metabolic pathway.[182–184] Inhibition of this pathway, which is responsible for the metabolism of many sedatives, including midazolam, may markedly prolong its duration of action and lead to life-threatening respiratory depression. Erythromycin, grapefruit juice,[185] some neutraceuticals, and calcium channel blockers[186] may also inhibit the cytochrome system and delay metabolism of midazolam.[187–189]

Sedation medications can also interact with other classes of drugs. Dexmedetomidine should not be combined with digoxin (or other atrioventricular node conduction blockers) in infants because severe bradycardia may result.[190] Although not always appreciated as the source of potent interactions, herbal medicines can enhance or abbreviate sedative medication activity.[191–195] Herbal medicines (e.g., St. John's wort or echinacea) may alter drug metabolism by inhibiting the cytochrome P450 system, prolonging drug effects and altered (increased or decreased) blood drug concentrations. Kava may augment the effects of sedatives, and valerian may itself produce sedation (see also E-Table 2.5).[196–199]

Several drug classes need to be considered when formulating a plan for procedural sedation. The needs of the procedure and the child will affect the exact choice of drugs in each case. Paramount among the considerations is the issue of whether the procedure is accompanied by significant pain. If it is painful (e.g., bone marrow biopsy, central line placement), some form of analgesia (with local anesthetics or a systemic drug that offers analgesia) is indicated to achieve all of the goals for the procedural sedation. If the procedure strictly requires sedation and motion control (e.g., MRI scans, CT scans), a pure sedative approach is usually sufficient and preferable.

LOCAL ANESTHETICS

Local anesthetics play a critical role in analgesia for painful procedures and greatly reduce requirements for systemic opioids. Unlike most drugs used in medicine, local anesthetics must be physically deposited at their site of action to produce their effect. For most blocks and local skin infiltration, epinephrine (1 : 200,000 [5 μg/mL]) is used as a vasoconstrictor to increase the duration of blockade, decrease bleeding, and reduce systemic toxicity by decreasing vascular uptake. *Historically, the combination of local anesthetics and epinephrine has NOT been advised for digits or the penis. Today the combination is considered safe as long as the concentration of epinephrine is ≤1 : 200,000.*[200–202] No more than the maximum allowable dose (mg/kg) should be prepared in the syringe to minimize the risk of an accidental overdose (see Table 40.2). Local anesthetics can be extremely useful in obtunding airway reflexes when sprayed in the oropharynx or glottis before bronchoscopy or gastrointestinal endoscopy.

Local anesthetics can be administered in the sedated child by subcutaneous (SC) infiltration, field blocks, ultrasound-guided nerve blocks, and IV regional anesthesia. A discussion of these topics and treatment of local anesthetic use and toxicity is found in Chapters 40, 41, and 42. Topical local anesthetics facilitate painless venous access before sedation. A eutectic mixture of local anesthetics (EMLA) cream (lidocaine 2.5% and prilocaine 2.5%) (AstraZeneca Pharmaceuticals LP, Wilmington, DE) provides analgesia when placed on the skin for 40 to 60 minutes[203,204]; it is useful for reducing the pain of skin incision, IV cannula insertions, lumbar punctures, and circumcision.[205–207] Because EMLA contains prilocaine, excessive absorption can cause methemoglobinemia if applied in large doses, for prolonged periods, or on mucosal surfaces.[40] For children weighing <10 kilograms, apply to a maximum of approximately 100 square centimeters surface area; for those 10 to 20 kilograms, apply to a maximum of approximately 600 square centimeters surface area; and for those >20 kilograms, apply to a maximum of approximately 2000 square centimeters surface area. EMLA cream can cause blanching of the skin and local vasoconstriction, which can make IV access difficult.

Other topical anesthetics include ELA-Max and LMX4 (Ferndale Healthcare, Ferndale, MI); these are 4% liposomal lidocaine preparations with onset within 30 minutes. Skin penetration is slightly deeper than with EMLA cream.[208] The S-Caine Patch (ZARS, Inc., Salt Lake City, UT) is a eutectic mixture of 70 milligrams of lidocaine and 70 milligrams tetracaine in a bioadhesive layer that contains a heating element. A 20-minute application is effective in lessening pain from venipuncture procedures.[209] Amethocaine (Ametop) is a topical cream of 4% tetracaine (40 mg tetracaine base per gram of gel) that anesthetizes the skin in 20 to 30 minutes without causing vasoconstriction or other sequelae. It is available internationally in the United Kingdom, Canada, Australia, as well as in several other countries (from Smith & Nephew Canada, Mississauga, Ontario) but not in the United States. A systematic review of amethocaine versus EMLA cream yielded a weak endorsement of amethocaine over EMLA cream for first-time IV cannulation.[210] As with EMLA cream, attention must be paid to size-appropriate dosing to avoid toxicity.

ANXIOLYTICS AND SEDATIVES

Chloral hydrate has historically been a widely used sedative. It is currently not commercially available in the United States but continues to be used internationally and in some US hospitals where it is compounded, although its use over time is decreasing as reported by the Pediatric Sedation Research Consortium (Table 44.8).[25,211–214] Its most common use is as a sedative to facilitate nonpainful diagnostic procedures, such as EEG, CT, or MRI.[213] It is rapidly and completely absorbed when given orally. Rectal absorption is erratic and not recommended. The onset of sedation is 30 to 60 minutes, and the usual clinical duration is 1 hour. Although it has a long history of successful use, it can cause respiratory depression and airway obstruction. Deaths have

TABLE 44.8	Sedation Regimens for Children			
Drug Regimen	**Dose/Route**	**Onset (minutes)**	**Duration (minutes)**	**Comments**
Pentobarbital	4–6 mg/kg IV or PO	IV: 2–5 PO: 20–60	IV: 15–45 PO: 60–240	Long history of safety Slow onset Prolonged emergence May have paradoxical excitement Half-life increased by valproic acid and MAO inhibitors Contraindicated in porphyria
Midazolam	0.25–0.75 mg/kg PO 0.05 mg/kg IV 0.2 mg/kg intranasal 0.1–0.15 mg/kg IM	15–30 1–3 10–15 10–15	60–90 60–90 45–60	Paradoxical response infrequent Intranasal route very irritating Increased respiratory depression when used with opioids; reduce midazolam dose by 25% Prolonged duration with protease inhibitors Antagonist: flumazenil
Chloral hydrate	50–100 mg/kg PO (maximum not to exceed 2 grams)	30–60	60–120	Very popular for nonpainful radiologic procedures in small children when IV not available Effects unreliable over 1–2 years of age Prolonged sedation and paradoxical responses noted Respiratory depression and obstruction reported with tonsil hypertrophy and anatomic abnormalities Moderate sedation guidelines required Markedly prolonged half-life in neonates may require extended observation Contraindicated in porphyria
Etomidate	0.1–0.4 mg/kg IV	<1	5–15	No analgesic effect Larger doses cause general anesthesia, respiratory depression, and loss of airway Stable cardiovascular profile Few data in children Must be credentialed for deep sedation/anesthesia No reversal drug Causes adrenal suppression ~12 hours
Methohexital	0.25–0.50 mg/kg IV 20–25 mg/kg rectal 10 mg/kg IM	<1 10–15 10–15	10–20 30–60 30–60	Avoid if temporal lobe epilepsy or porphyria IV doses quickly lead to general anesthesia Rectal doses may cause apnea and should be administered with caution Deep sedation/anesthesia credentialing Contraindicated in children <3 months of age, psychosis, stimulation of oropharynx, increased intracranial pressure, head injury, glaucoma
Dexmedetomidine	IV: 1–2 µg/kg bolus (over 10 minutes) Infusion: 1–2 µg/kg per hour	10	Clinical 30 minutes to 1 hour; half-life 1.5–3 hours	Mimics natural sleep Rapid bolus may cause hypertension Minimal respiratory depression Dose-dependent hypotension and bradycardia Use with caution with digitalis medications Glycopyrrolate treatment of bradycardia may induce sustained hypertension of unknown mechanism
Fentanyl with propofol	Fentanyl 1–2 µg/kg IV with propofol 50–150 µg/kg per minute infusion IV	1–2	30–60	Child may rapidly become anesthetized with loss of airway Advanced airway management skills required, with appropriate credentialing
Midazolam with fentanyl	Midazolam 0.02 mg/kg IV with fentanyl 1–2 µg/kg IV	2–3	45–60	Commonly used for painful procedures Careful titration needed to avoid deep sedation/anesthesia with apnea and hypoxia Reduce dose of fentanyl when combined with benzodiazepine Reduce dose with protease inhibitors

TABLE 44.8	Sedation Regimens for Children—Cont'd			
Drug Regimen	**Dose/Route**	**Onset (minutes)**	**Duration (minutes)**	**Comments**
Ketamine	3–4 mg/kg IM 1–2 mg/kg IV 4–6 mg/kg PO	5 1 10–20	30–60 30–60 30–90	Nausea and vomiting common after procedure Laryngospasm, apnea, agitation, hallucinations reported but uncommon Midazolam may not prevent emergence delirium Larger doses can produce state of general anesthesia Usually causes tachycardia, hypertension, and bronchodilatation Paradoxical hypotension in critically ill patients No antagonist available Advanced airway management skills required, with appropriate credentialing
Propofol	Bolus 1–2 mg/kg Infusion 50–250 µg/kg per minute	30 seconds	5–15 minutes after discontinuation	Profound, dose-related respiratory depressant Assume deep sedation/anesthesia when using in children Infusions >5 hours may cause propofol infusion syndrome Caution when used in mitochondrial myopathies Pain on injection mitigated by IV lidocaine Advanced airway management skills required, with appropriate credentialing
Remifentanil	0.1–0.25 µg/kg per minute	1	10–15 minutes after discontinuation	Difficulty in titration frequently leads to apnea and general anesthesia Few studies in children Exclusively used by anesthesiologists
Nitrous oxide	50% in 50% oxygen for "minimal sedation"; up to 70% used by some for moderate sedation	<5	On discontinuing	Requires specialized equipment for delivery, monitoring, and scavenging Use alone (50% in oxygen or less) or with local anesthesia is considered "minimal sedation" Greater doses or addition of other sedatives/analgesics require a minimum of "moderate sedation" guidelines Contraindications include respiratory failure, altered mental status, otitis media, bowel obstruction, and pneumothorax No antagonist available
Opioid antagonist: naloxone	0.01–0.1 mg/kg IV or IM Max 2 mg/dose May repeat every 2 minutes	1–2	IV: 20–40 IM: 60–90	Specifically antagonizes opioid effects Should not be used for routine reversal of opioid effect Adverse reactions: nausea, vomiting, tachycardia, hypertension, delirium, pulmonary edema Reversal after long-term opioid use may lead to acute withdrawal Children may renarcotize 1 hour after IV dosing
Benzodiazepine antagonist: flumazenil	IV 0.01–0.02 mg/kg May repeat every 1 minute to 1 mg	1–2	30–60	Specific benzodiazepine antagonist Does not antagonize opioids or other sedatives Resedation may occur in 1 hour Prolonged observation (2 hours) required Not for routine sedation reversal Children using benzodiazepine to control seizures or drug dependency may have exacerbations with flumazenil

IM, Intramuscularly; *IV*, intravenously; *MAO*, monoamine oxidase; *PO*, by mouth.
Data modified from Cravero JP, Burke GT. A review of pediatric sedation. *Anesth Analg.* 2004;99(5):1355-1364; Krauss B, Green SM. Procedural sedation and analgesia in children. *Lancet.* 2006;367(9512):766-780.

been associated with its use as a sole sedative agent and when combined with other sedatives, particularly for dental procedures[71,215]; it is particularly problematic in situations where the drug was administered in an unmonitored setting (such as a car seat).[70,161,215–219] One large series showed a 0.6% incidence of respiratory depression, especially at larger doses (75–100 mg/kg).[220] Chloral hydrate acts primarily through its active metabolite trichloroethanol, which is formed in the liver and erythrocytes.[221] Trichloroethanol has a half-life of 10 hours in toddlers, 18 hours in term infants, and 40 hours in preterm infants (see Fig. 44.3).[222]

Agitation and restlessness of more than 6 hours in one-third of children sedated with chloral hydrate has been reported, 5% of whom did not return to baseline activity for 2 days after the procedure![88,223]

Benzodiazepines are commonly used for pediatric sedation. They provide anxiolysis, amnesia, and sedation with anticonvulsant activities. Their high lipid solubility at physiologic pH accounts for the rapid CNS effects. As opposed to diazepam, midazolam is delivered in a water-soluble form (pH 3.5), which markedly decreases the incidence of pain on injection and thrombophlebitis.[221]

Time to Peak EEG Effect

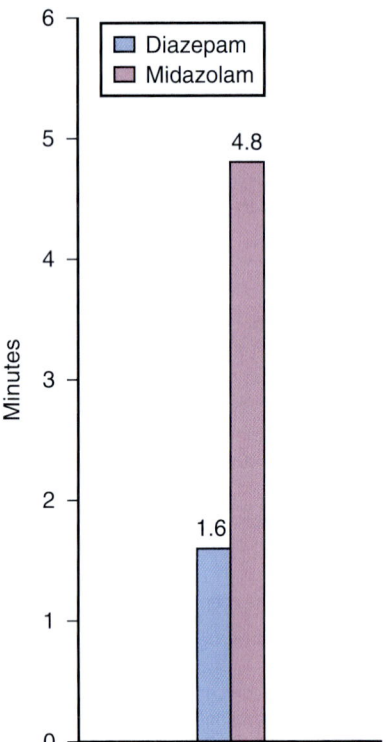

FIGURE 44.7 Time to peak electroencephalographic *(EEG)* effect of diazepam versus midazolam in adults. Note that it takes nearly three times longer to achieve a peak EEG effect after intravenous (IV) midazolam than after IV diazepam. This is likely caused by the difference in fat solubility; because midazolam is less fat-soluble than diazepam, midazolam does not cross biologic membranes as easily. The clinical importance of this observation is the need to wait 3 to 5 minutes between IV doses of midazolam to avoid stacking of doses and excessive drug effect. (Data from Bührer M, Maitre PO, Crevoisier C, Stanski DR. Electroencephalographic effects of benzodiazepines: II. Pharmacodynamic modeling of the electroencephalographic effects of midazolam and diazepam. *Clin Pharmacol Ther.* 1990;48(5):555-567.)

However, the resulting decrease in fat solubility delays transport into the CNS (peak EEG effect 4.8 minutes for midazolam vs. 1.6 minutes for diazepam in adults; Fig. 44.7).[224,225] Benzodiazepines exert their effects by occupying the benzodiazepine receptor that modulates γ-aminobutyric acid (GABA), the major inhibitory neurotransmitter in the brain. The clearance of benzodiazepines is decreased in neonates and in older children by liver enzyme inhibition that occurs during concomitant use of erythromycin, cimetidine, grapefruit juice, or protease inhibitors.[185,188]

When administered at the recommended doses, benzodiazepine-sedated patients become compliant but do not lose consciousness (minimal to moderate sedation). This level of sedation has limited application for achieving ideal procedural conditions for most interventions. Benzodiazepines provide no analgesia; analgesic medications must be added for painful procedures. A systematic review and other studies have found that benzodiazepines have the advantage of providing potent anterograde but not retrograde amnesia[226] that in some cases seems to correlate with the onset of slurred speech.[227,228] Midazolam is the preferred drug for pediatric sedation because of its brief and more consistent half-life compared with diazepam.[229–234] The time to

peak effect after IV administration of midazolam may be faster in children than adults (2 to 4 minutes), with a duration of 45 to 60 minutes. Midazolam can be given IV, intranasally (IN), sublingually, orally, or rectally (see Table 44.8). Nasal administration is well documented and can be very effective; however, it causes nasopharyngeal burning[235]; prior administration of intranasal lidocaine can decrease the irritation.[236] A meta-analysis of nasal midazolam versus nasal ketamine for pediatric sedation found a more rapid onset and recovery with midazolam.[237] Rectal administration is usually well tolerated in children who have not been toilet trained, but absorption may be irregular owing to many factors, including superior versus inferior hemorrhoidal vein absorption within the rectum.

Benzodiazepines produce mild respiratory depression and upper airway obstruction.[238–240] Small doses of oral midazolam (0.3 mg/kg) that produce minimal sedation were associated with a 6.5% decrease in functional residual capacity and a 7.4% increase in respiratory resistance.[241] Respiratory depression may become marked in children who are neurologically impaired or in children with OSA, although premedication with oral midazolam (0.25 to 0.5 mg/kg) carries an extremely small risk of transient hemoglobin desaturation.[242] The combination of benzodiazepines and opioids can produce a "super-additive effect" on respiratory depression where the total depressant effect from the combination of drugs is much greater than the sum of their anticipated individual effects.[243–246]

Benzodiazepines may have a paradoxical effect in 1% to 15% of children depending on age and personality, rendering the child combative rather than cooperative.[247–249] A history of this type of paradoxical response should be elicited before administering a benzodiazepine.

Flumazenil is a specific benzodiazepine-receptor antagonist that rapidly reverses the sedative, paradoxical,[250] and respiratory effects of benzodiazepines.[251–256] Children who take benzodiazepines for seizures or drug dependency may experience symptoms rapidly if flumazenil is given.[257] It should also be used with caution in children with increased intracranial pressure and in those taking drugs that decrease the seizure threshold (e.g., cyclosporine, theophylline, and lithium). Because of these concerns, flumazenil should not be administered for the routine reversal of the sedative effects of benzodiazepines but should be reserved for emergency reversal of respiratory depression. The recommended dose of flumazenil is 10 micrograms per kilogram up to 200 micrograms every minute to a maximum cumulative dose of 1 milligram IV. Antagonism begins within 1 to 2 minutes after administration and lasts approximately 1 hour.[256] Because recrudescence of sedation after 1 hour may occur, any child who receives flumazenil must be carefully monitored for at least 2 hours. It should be noted that flumazenil does not antagonize respiratory depression induced by opioids.[258] The pharmacokinetics and pharmacodynamics of anxiolytics, opioids, and sedatives are described in Chapter 5.

BARBITURATES

Pentobarbital is an intermediate-acting barbiturate that is now infrequently used. It provides excellent sedation, hypnosis, and amnesia without analgesia. The onset of sedation is 3 to 5 minutes with a peak effect by approximately 10 minutes and duration of action of 1 to 2 (or more) hours after intravenous administration. Respiratory obstruction, transient desaturation, and hypotension occur infrequently.[259,260] Barbiturates reduce the threshold for pain in children, so it is best avoided in painful procedures. Recovery after pentobarbital is often protracted, leaving children in a disinhibited state for extended periods. This may lead to a prolonged recovery and, in some cases, the need for restraint (see Table 44.8).[212] Oral pentobarbital is a suitable replacement for chloral hydrate in children younger than 3 years of age undergoing radiologic procedures[261]; it has also been successfully used to sedate children younger than 4 years of age for echocardiograms.[262]

Methohexital is a short-acting oxybarbiturate that is rapidly metabolized and redistributed, and has a rapid recovery (see Table 44.8).[263] Loss of consciousness occurs with IV doses of 1 to 2 milligrams per kilogram. Apnea, hiccups, and methohexital-induced seizures in children with temporal lobe epilepsy have been reported.[264] IM methohexital has been used in doses of 8 to 10 milligrams per kilogram, but the onset of sedation is slow,[265] and it is not generally recommended. Rectal methohexital (20–25 mg/kg [from a 100-mg/mL solution]) can induce deep sedation in 7 to 11 minutes[266-268] with a duration of action of ~30 to 45 minutes.[266,268] Absorption through the rectal route is erratic.[267] The variability of absorption, tendency to deep sedation, possible induced defecation, and airway problems have decreased the use of methohexital in favor of newer drugs administered by other routes. This medication should be used only by individuals with advanced airway skills, because upper airway obstruction and apnea may readily occur.[269]

OPIOIDS

Opioid analgesics are rarely effective sedatives in isolation, but their use is essential to manage painful diagnostic and therapeutic procedures. Opioids confer a degree of sedation, but the sedation is usually inadequate to perform procedures in children; they are usually combined with sedatives (see Fig. 44.1).[243,270] Combinations require particular caution in infants and children with upper airway obstruction (e.g., tonsil and/or adenoid hypertrophy, OSA, trisomy 21, mucopolysaccharidosis). The use of opioids as part of total intravenous anesthesia or sedation is discussed in Chapter 6.

Morphine may be used for painful procedures with prolonged duration or when pain is expected after the procedure.[271] Morphine may be given orally (0.2–0.5 mg/kg), IV (0.05–0.1 mg/kg [maximum 0.3 mg/kg]), or IM (0.1–0.2 mg/kg), and diamorphine may be given nasally.[272-274] Times to peak effect for oral, IV, and IM administration are 60 minutes, 1 to 2 minutes, and 10 to 30 minutes, respectively.

Fentanyl is the opioid of choice for sedation/analgesia for most procedures in children because of its brief duration of action. It may be given IV, IN, or IM.[275-279] IV fentanyl is approximately 50 to 100 times more potent an analgesic than morphine but without amnesic properties. Its high lipid solubility allows for a rapid onset of action (within 30 seconds) and time to peak effect, 2 to 3 minutes. It has a brief clinical duration of 20 to 40 minutes when given in small doses, owing to its rapid redistribution to skeletal muscle, fat, and other inactive sites. Unlike morphine, it has no active metabolites. Fentanyl is frequently used in combination with a short-acting anxiolytic (e.g., midazolam). IV doses of fentanyl usually begin at 0.5 to 1 microgram per kilogram. Serial doses may be titrated every 5 to 10 minutes to effect, to a maximum dose not exceeding 5 micrograms per kilogram.[280] Fentanyl can also be administered IN at a dose of 1.5 micrograms per kilogram; it has been effective at this dose for emergency department procedures.[275,277-279] When carefully titrated and appropriately

monitored, fentanyl has few adverse effects. Chest wall rigidity[270] is a centrally mediated idiosyncratic reaction that can interfere with breathing but can be antagonized with either naloxone or muscle relaxants[281]; it is rarely observed in sedation practice.[282-284] Other adverse reactions from fentanyl include bradycardia, dysphoria, delirium, nausea, vomiting, pruritus, urinary retention, hypotension, and smooth muscle spasm. Close postprocedural observation is required because respiratory depression can outlast analgesia (see Table 44.8).

Remifentanil, an ultrashort-lived, rapid-acting, potent, lipophilic opioid that is metabolized by plasma and tissue esterases, must be administered as a continuous infusion. It has a context-sensitive half-life of 3 to 6 minutes that is independent of the duration of infusion. Remifentanil has been used for intraoperative and procedural sedation by anesthesiologists and in intubated children in the ICU.[285-290] If postoperative pain is anticipated, another analgesic or local anesthetic nerve block should be administered before stopping the infusion. Children develop a degree of opioid tolerance after several hours of infusing remifentanil, although this adverse effect remains controversial.[291-293] Accordingly, provision for pain control after procedures must be anticipated and instituted before emergence from sedation/anesthesia. Remifentanil is also associated with a substantial incidence of apnea, hypoxemia, and chest wall and glottic rigidity, and is not recommended as a sole agent for pediatric sedation (see Table 44.8).[287,289,294] Remifentanil may be administered together with propofol to provide total intravenous anesthesia and sedation (see Chapters 5 and 6).

Opioid antagonists reverse the respiratory and analgesic effects of opioids and should be readily available when opioids are used (see Table 44.8). Naloxone (Narcan) is the most commonly used antagonist[295] and may be given IV, IM, IN (resulting in greater peak concentrations in children than in adults),[296,297] or SC.[298] The initial dose for respiratory depression is 10 micrograms per kilogram titrated to effect every 2 to 3 minutes. A dose of 10 to 100 micrograms per kilogram up to 2 milligrams may be required for respiratory arrest. Adverse reactions from the rapid reversal of opioid effects include nausea, vomiting, tachycardia, hypertension, delirium, and pulmonary edema.[299-301] Children who have been receiving long-term opioid therapy should be given opioid reversal agents in small doses and with extreme caution because withdrawal seizures, sympathetic overdrive, and delirium may occur. Children given a single dose of IV naloxone may have a recrudescence of the respiratory depression 1 hour later. It is for this reason that the same effective IV dose is then administered IM; *the child should be observed for a minimum of 2 hours after the IV naloxone.* Nasal naloxone spray is approved for the emergency treatment of known or suspected opioid overdose.[302] Nalmefene (Revex), like naltrexone, is a μ-receptor antagonist and weak κ- agonist that boasts a greater half-life (~10 hours) than naloxone.[303] Although experience in children is limited, it accelerates recovery from sedation.[304] Because of its relatively long half-life, it outlasts the effects of fentanyl and may oppose pain treatment for several hours; it is currently approved for nasal administration in children 12 years of age or older.[305]

A₂-ADRENOCEPTOR AGONIST: DEXMEDETOMIDINE

Dexmedetomidine is highly lipid soluble and rapidly crosses the blood-brain barrier. Its mechanism of action in the CNS is via stimulating receptors in the medullary vasomotor center, which decreases sympathetic tone.[306] It also stimulates central parasympathetic outflow and decreases sympathetic outflow from the locus coeruleus of the brainstem. The decreased outflow from the locus coeruleus increases activity of the inhibitory GABA neurons, which cause sedation and analgesia.[307,308] The concentration-response relationship has a steeper slope than that described for clonidine (see Fig. 5.7),[68,309] consistent with better sedation at moderate doses. Dexmedetomidine is approved by the FDA for procedural sedation in children 1 month to 17 years of age.[310] In addition to its IV use, it has been administered via the buccal, IN, and IM routes in children.[311–316] A meta-analysis and systematic review concluded that IN dexmedetomidine was safe and effective for procedural sedation, that the optimal IN dose was ~2 micrograms per kilogram and that IN dexmedetomidine had a greater sedation success rate than IN midazolam.[317,318] Another meta-analysis of 19 trials with 2137 children examined IN dexmedetomidine alone and when combined with other sedating medications for nonpainful procedures (e.g., MRI echo, ophthalmologic examination, auditory brainstem response testing).[319] Doses ranged from 1 to 4 micrograms per kilogram; the incidence of bradycardia was 2.2% when just dexmedetomidine was administered, hypotension 1.2%, and desaturation 0.5%, which was similar to the incidence in those who received dexmedetomidine combined with other sedating medications.

When administered in clinical doses, dexmedetomidine causes limited depression of ventilation and may mimic natural rapid-eye-movement sleep; however, it does have cardiovascular effects that may be profound.[308,320–323] Because rapid IV boluses can cause transient systemic hypertension, the initial loading dose must be given as a 10-minute infusion and may be followed by a continuous infusion. When given in the recommended fashion, it decreases blood pressure and heart rate in a dose-dependent manner. It should be used with caution in children with preexisting bradycardia, atrioventricular conduction defects, hypotension, and decreased cardiac output.[324–327] It has been associated with severe bradycardia in infants receiving digoxin and β-blockers, and those with preexisting atrioventricular nodal conduction delays.[190] Caution is advised in children with known congenital heart disease, as dexmedetomidine depresses sinus and atrioventricular node function and may pose an increased risk for children prone to bradycardia.[328–332] Several brief episodes of asystole have been reported during dexmedetomidine sedation, anecdotally. In the first case, transient asystole developed in an 8-week-old in the ICU with bronchiolitis who was sedated with 0.7 micrograms per kilogram per hour. The heart rate was restored spontaneously without intervention. In the second case, a 27-month-old with moderate pulmonary hypertension sedated after surgery for diaphragmatic hernia with 1.2 micrograms per kilogram per hour developed asystole. Heart rate was restored after chest compressions.[333] A meta-analysis in 2017 reported a 3% frequency of bradycardia in infants and children sedated with dexmedetomidine (with a range of 0% to 22%).[327] The minimum heart rate during dexmedetomidine sedation correlated only with the baseline heart rate, and not with age, weight, or the dexmedetomidine dose. In a systematic review of dexmedetomidine for MRI sedation, of 6204 children, 4626 received only dexmedetomidine for sedation.[334] Adverse events occurred in 15% of sedations; hypotension occurred in 8.7%, bradycardia in 10%, and desaturation in only 1.2%. The frequency of treatment for hypotension and bradycardia was not reported. In a retrospective review of 39 premature and full-term neonates sedated with dexmedetomidine for MRI, sedation was successful in all infants, although 38.5% developed bradycardia, one-third of whom required atropine.[335]

Dexmedetomidine has seen a rapid increase in pediatric sedation over the past 10 years largely owing to its lack of respiratory depressant effects.[25,334–339] Dexmedetomidine does not cause neuroapoptosis (unlike all other sedatives). However, there is evidence that dexmedetomidine has neuroprotective properties[308,340–342] and may hold a unique advantage for sedation in young children when these effects are of greatest concern. Sedation after IV administration has a relatively rapid onset of 10 minutes and a half-life of 1.5 to 3 hours. Its minimal effect on respiration has led to its use alone for nonpainful procedures (e.g., EEG, CT, and MRI), in children with Down syndrome and children with OSA.[306,308] It has also been used in combination with ketamine and propofol for painful procedures (e.g., cardiac catheterizations and complex regional pain syndrome).[328,329]

When analyzed by MRI, the dose-response effects of dexmedetomidine (1 to 2 μg/kg per hour) on the morphology of the upper airway in children[308,343,344] revealed minimal changes in the dimensions of the upper airway. Infants and children 5 months to 16 years of age also show minimal effects on respiration.[73] These characteristics make dexmedetomidine a popular choice for children with OSA.[308,343,344]

Dexmedetomidine has intermediate potency when compared with other sedatives such as etomidate or propofol and has limited efficacy as a sole agent for longer sedations. Studies investigating the dose of dexmedetomidine for pediatric patients to successfully complete MRI scans demonstrated the need for high doses (3 μg/kg loading dose with a 2 μg/kg per hour infusion), which resulted in significant bradycardia, transient hypertension, and delayed postanesthesia care unit discharge secondary to prolonged drowsiness.[345,346] It should be noted that caution must be used when administering glycopyrrolate to treat the bradycardia from dexmedetomidine because severe and sustained hypertension after traditional doses of 5 micrograms per kilogram glycopyrrolate have occurred (e.g., blood pressure 161/113 mm Hg in a 3-year-old).[347]

An alternative approach to improving success with dexmedetomidine is to combine dexmedetomidine with other sedative medications.[348] A loading dose of 1 microgram per kilogram dexmedetomidine over 10 minutes followed by an infusion of 0.5 micrograms per kilogram per hour plus a 0.1-milligram per kilogram bolus of midazolam. With this regimen, sedation was very successful with only small changes in ETCO$_2$ and minimal hemodynamic effects. A propofol/dexmedetomidine combination has also proven to be a very effective sedative regimen, associated with few adverse effects.[349,350] Other investigators reported that the combination of ketamine, propofol, and dexmedetomidine was very effective for sedation in the cardiac catheterization laboratory.[351] Combination regimens provide very successful sedation with few adverse events, although there are insufficient data to recommend a specific regimen to maximize the sedation with dexmedetomidine.

KETAMINE

Ketamine, available since the 1960s, is one of the few sedatives that produces sedation, amnesia, and analgesia.[352] The clinical appearance is that of a child who has open eyes (usually with horizontal nystagmus)(see Video 5.1) but does not respond to pain; the "dissociative" state.[352,353] Ketamine preserves cardiovascular function and exerts limited effects on respiratory mechanics, allowing spontaneous respirations in most children.[352,354] Although it is certainly not a new drug, ketamine has experienced a resurgence in popularity for procedural sedation, particularly in the emergency department.[355] Clinical practice guidelines from American College of Emergency Physicians proposed a distinct classification of sedation for ketamine, "Dissociative Sedation,"[356,357] because it has unique properties that do not neatly fit into the current definitions of sedation or anesthesia.[357–360] To date, this reclassification has not been accepted by the AAP, ASA, AAPD, or regulatory agencies. Interestingly the Royal College of Emergency Physicians recommends that three individuals are required for dissociative sedation: (1) one performing the procedure, (2) a second undertaking the sedation, and (3) a third to monitor the child; this differs from the recommendations of the American College of Emergency Physicians.[151,361]

IM and IV ketamine (with and without midazolam) are frequently used for closed fracture reductions and other painful minor procedures in the emergency department (see Table 44.8).[360,362–365] Two studies of adverse events after ketamine for procedural sedation in the emergency department reported adverse event rates of 0.9% to 13.3%.[364,365] A systematic review of 41 publications in which ketamine was used for procedural sedation in children (13,876 sedations) in the emergency department, adverse events were infrequent. The most common adverse events were vomiting and agitation, with frequencies of 55 and 18/1000 sedations, respectively.[366] Hypoxia occurred in 1.5% of sedations, apnea in 0.7%, laryngospasm in 0.3%, and 0 case of aspiration. Another review of 8282 emergency department sedations with ketamine reported a similar incidence of laryngospasms (~0.3%).[358] In a retrospective review of 173 children younger 2 years of age who were sedated for minor procedures in the emergency department with ketamine/midazolam or morphine/midazolam, for the majority of cases, the frequency of complications was 6%, of which all but one was related to ketamine/midazolam. Most were considered minor in severity (three desaturated, four vomited, one developed stridor, two failed sedation), although one infant (2 months of age) developed bradycardia necessitating tracheal intubation.[367] In a prospective study by the Pediatric Sedation Research Consortium of more than 22,000 sedations in children (median age 5 years, range <1 month to 22 years) with ketamine in radiology and sedation suites, 7.3% experienced adverse events and 1.8% experienced serious adverse events.[368] Two patients with cardiac arrests were successfully resuscitated. Risk factors for adverse events included cardiac and gastrointestinal diseases, lower respiratory tract infections, and co-administration of propofol and anticholinergics.

Ketamine (1 to 3 mg/kg IV) has also been studied in children undergoing gastroendoscopy procedures, with transient laryngospasm occurring in 8.2%, emesis in 4.1%, emergence agitation in 2.4%, partial airway obstruction in 1.3%, apnea and respiratory depression in 0.5%, and excessive salivation in 0.3%.[116] This greater incidence of laryngospasm compared with the previously referred to studies suggests that this complication is more likely when the procedure involves the airway.

Ketamine has also been successfully combined with propofol for endoscopic procedures.[369–371] This combination has been given the name "ketofol" with excellent sedation for painful procedures in the emergency department and for other procedures requiring sedation and analgesia.[370,372] The drugs may be given separately or mixed in a 1:1 ratio then titrated to effect.[373,374] A systematic review found weak evidence in reducing recovery time and moderate evidence that this combination reduces the incidence of hypotension compared with other drug combinations (see Chapter 5).[375]

The analgesic effects of ketamine make it very appealing for use during burn dressing changes.[376] In one study, 4.9% of the ketamine sedations resulted in adverse outcomes, of which 2.9% required an intervention. Eight events were related to the airway.[377] Ketamine sedation/analgesia has a very long history of safety, perhaps offering advantages over other sedation regimens, although these studies indicate that potentially life-threatening events can and do occur even with ketamine sedation. Ketamine is also associated with nonpurposeful motion, which limits its usefulness when immobility is necessary (e.g., use during MRI scans).

Ketamine is contraindicated in several clinical scenarios. Human studies support a trend to increase global and regional cerebral blood flow in healthy patients[378] and warrant a relative contraindication for this drug in children with significantly increased intracranial pressure, particularly without controlled respirations. Similarly, ketamine is contraindicated in those with head injury, open globe injury, hypertension, and psychosis. Although it does not directly decrease the ventilatory drive, ketamine decreases the ventilatory response to hypercarbia. Although anticholinergics have been recommended when ketamine was used for procedural sedation in the emergency department,[379] studies from the emergency department have not only refuted the need for anticholinergics during ketamine sedation but also suggested that the use of anticholinergics may actually increase the odds of adverse events.[368,380,381] It is unclear how the use of an anticholinergic could increase the number of adverse events. No antagonist to ketamine is available. Recovery from ketamine is notable for a greater incidence of emesis and agitation than other sedatives.[366,382,383]

Typical starting doses[384] of ketamine are 3 to 4 milligrams per kilogram IM, 0.25 to 1.0 milligrams per kilogram IV, and 4 to 6 milligrams per kilogram orally.[385–387] The onset after IM injection is 2 to 5 minutes, with a peak at approximately 20 minutes; duration can be 30 to 120 minutes. Onset after IV administration occurs in less than 1 minute, with a peak effect in several minutes and duration of action of approximately 15 minutes. Oral doses of 4 to 6 milligrams per kilogram are usually combined with atropine and have an effect in 30 minutes and last up to 120 minutes.[40] In a dose-ranging study of ketamine in the emergency department, doses of 1.5 to 2 milligrams per kilogram IV provided similar sedation and satisfaction after the procedures.[388]

PROPOFOL

Propofol is widely used for pediatric sedation and anesthesia with an onset within 30 seconds.[389] It has no analgesic properties, but it does have antiemetic and antipruritic properties. Although small doses of propofol (25 to 50 µg/kg per minute) can provide moderate sedation in adults, children require much larger doses to prevent movement (150 to 250 µg/kg per minute) with starting infusions in infants and cognitively impaired children even greater. It is generally best administered by titration with an infusion pump. Adverse reactions include increased salivary and tracheobronchial secretions, myoclonic movements, anaphylactic reactions, and bacterial contamination. Pain on injection can be lessened by several strategies, although the two most effective strategies are pretreatment with nitrous oxide (N_2O) by inhalation, or a mini-Bier block with 1 milligram per kilogram lidocaine applied for 1 minute.[390,391] Hypotension is mild and usually not clinically significant.

Case reports of fatal metabolic acidosis, myocardial failure, and lipemic serum have been reported in children who received propofol infusions (propofol infusion syndrome) for more than 48 hours at doses exceeding 5 milligrams per kilogram per hour (83 µg/kg per minute) although biochemical abnormalities consistent with an infusion syndrome have appeared after only 5 to 6 hours in some instances.[392–399] Some have speculated that the syndrome was triggered by an underlying mitochondrial disorder, although evidence of such a relationship has not been forthcoming.[399,400] Unexplained metabolic acidosis, progressive myocardial failure (arrhythmias and hypotension), and rhabdomyolysis are key features; continuous hemofiltration and partial exchange blood transfusion have been effective reversing the syndrome.[401,402]

Propofol is also a profound respiratory depressant that may cause apnea. Respiratory complications have been reported in 8% to 30% of children.[403] In a study of propofol sedation (2.5 to 3 mg/kg IV loading dose with an infusion up to 200 micrograms per kilogram per minute) in 105 painful procedures in the pediatric ICU, 21% of the children required airway repositioning, 17% had apnea, 5% had hypotension, and 45% had events that required intervention.[119] In the emergency department, propofol was administered to 113 children in an average dose of 4.5 milligrams per kilogram in addition to fentanyl 1 to 2 micrograms per kilogram[404] that proved to be sufficient to ensure that the fractures could be successfully reduced. The net effect was an incidence of desaturation of 31%, laryngospasm in 1%, and a supplemental oxygen requirement in 25%. In a study of sedation by nonanesthesiologists for bone marrow procedures, lumbar punctures, and esophagoscopies titrated propofol to a target of "not arousable"; 21 children from 27 weeks to 18 years of age were studied. Propofol at doses of 520 micrograms per kilogram per minute conferred 100% sedation with BIS readings of 45 or less (consistent with general anesthesia).[405] These responses to stimulation, effects on the airway, doses of propofol, and BIS levels are beyond the range of deep sedation and more in keeping with the definition of general anesthesia, with the inherent risk of loss of the airway. More recent studies that reviewed large numbers of sedation encounters involving propofol sedation by a variety of physicians (working in elective sedation services) document that propofol can be used with much fewer severe adverse outcomes (and much smaller doses) than previously reported.[27,125,406,407] In these studies of more than 100,000 total propofol encounters, the rate of noteworthy airway events was less than 2.5%.[121,125]

There has been increasing use of a combination of ketamine (10 mg/mL) with propofol (10 mg/mL), so-called ketofol, for painful procedures in the emergency department and for oncology patients.[408–413] This combination is administered in incremental doses of 0.5 milligrams per kilogram of each drug at approximately 1-minute intervals. Other mixture proportions of these two drugs have also been investigated[414] and a better ratio of racemic ketamine to propofol may be 1:3 for brief procedures (5 to 20 minutes).[414,415] Although experience with this combination of drugs is growing, the limited number of prospective studies at this point preclude assessment of safety and efficacy (see also the section on ketamine earlier in the text).[412]

NITROUS OXIDE

N_2O is a potent inhalation analgesic with a peak effect in 3 to 5 minutes and very rapid return to baseline when discontinued (see Table 44.8). A premixed tank of no more than 50% N_2O is available (Entonox). Administration of N_2O can be used for "minimal sedation" under AAP guidelines:

1. N_2O can be used only in ASA physical status I or II patients.
2. Only 50% N_2O or less is used; no other sedating medications are administered.

3. Inhalation equipment must have the capacity to deliver 100% oxygen and never less than 25% oxygen.
4. A calibrated oxygen analyzer must be used. The child is able to maintain verbal communication throughout the procedure.

Although 50% N_2O in oxygen usually produces "minimal" sedation, the addition of any sedative or hypnotic may rapidly produce a deeper level of sedation and require increased monitoring and vigilance.[218,238] N_2O is frequently used by dentists for sedation and by physicians in the emergency department for laceration closure and closed fracture reductions.[416] The results of a survey of dentists who performed treatments on patients under sedation during their training found that the majority used N_2O sedation.[417,418] Adverse reactions, drug interactions, and special concerns are listed in Table 44.8. The use of nitrous oxide for sedation or procedural pain on the ward requires a dedicated room with scavenging requirements consistent with local regulations.[419]

ETOMIDATE

Etomidate is a carboxylated imidazole that is primarily used as an induction agent for anesthesia. Its mechanism is thought to be potentiation of GABA inhibitory neurotransmission via alteration of chloride conductance. Loss of consciousness occurs in 15 to 20 seconds. Recovery results from redistribution within 5 to 10 minutes. It is hydrolyzed in the liver to inactive metabolites and excreted (90%) in the urine.[221] Etomidate produces sedation, anxiolysis, and amnesia similar to the barbiturates and propofol. Its major advantage is its lack of adverse cardiovascular effects. It has been used in adults and children for procedural sedation, although the endpoint of sedation is not well described and often is a state of general anesthesia.[112] Etomidate has been compared with pentobarbital for CT sedation. Adverse events were more common with pentobarbital (4.5%) than etomidate (0.9%).[420] Etomidate with fentanyl has been compared with ketamine with midazolam for reduction of limb fractures in children in the emergency department. The combination of etomidate and fentanyl led to a more rapid recovery but was less effective in reducing observed patient distress than midazolam and fentanyl.[421,422] Transient adrenal suppression can occur after etomidate,[148,423–426] which is why it is infrequently used in acutely ill children.[427]

Future of Pediatric Sedation

Pediatric sedation has evolved from a clinical "orphan," with few champions and almost no formal organization, to a well-documented field with clear standards and guidelines for practice. Appropriately, procedural sedation is expected to provide the same level of safety and effectiveness associated with the operating room. At the same time, anesthesiologists must recognize that the literature is replete with reports of *other* pediatric specialists working in sedation systems that provide care with potent medications and excellent outcomes.[336,428–436] Anesthesiologists will continue to provide the ultimate "back-up" for these services and take on the most challenging sedation cases, while recognizing the capabilities of other professionals. Anesthesiologists must explore ways to collaborate with these other specialists so as to provide the best possible sedation results for all patients undergoing sedation for procedures and tests.

Acknowledgment

The authors would like to thank Richard F. Kaplan for his contribution to prior versions of this chapter.

ANNOTATED REFERENCES

Brown R, Coté CJ, Mason LJ, Lalwani K, Fukami C, Kost SA. Joint Statement from the American Society of Anesthesiologists, the Society for Pediatric Anesthesia, the American Society of Dentist Anesthesiologists, and the Society for Pediatric Sedation Regarding the Use of Deep Sedation/General Anesthesia for Pediatric Dental Procedures Using the Single-Provider/Operator Model. Available at: https://www.asahq.org/advocacy-and-asapac/advocacy-topics/office-based-anesthesia-and-dental-anesthesia/joint-statement-pediatric-dental-sedation.

This joint statement swas published as a result of the dangerous practice by some dental practitioners who use the "single-provider model" of practice whereby the dental practitioner simultaneously performs the procedure and directs the anesthesia or deep sedation that use a dental assistant as the monitor. "With the single-provider/operator practice model, crucial monitoring of the child's vital signs may be left primarily to a dental assistant who is not medically trained and is incapable of assisting with a life-threatening medical emergency (e.g., laryngospasm, apnea, seizure, anaphylactic reaction)." The statement concluded that "The model that the AAOMS continues to embrace does not ensure an appropriately qualified, dedicated monitor who is prepared to meaningfully help in the event of a patient emergency. ASA, the Society for Pediatric Anesthesia (SPA), the ASDA, and the Society for Pediatric Sedation (SPS) in the interest of safe oral surgery/dental care for all children, endorse the highest standards for procedural monitoring, administration of sedating drugs, and resuscitation by trained professionals independent of the operating surgeon/dentist, as clearly stated in the revised AAP guidelines. The use of a second oral surgeon to manage sedation, monitoring and rescue would be entirely consistent with this standard. The standards that continue to be espoused by the AAOMS are wholly inconsistent with the standards of practice for any clinician under any circumstance involving elective pediatric care, including those of the World Health Organization."

Coté CJ, Notterman DA, Karl HW, et al. Adverse sedation events in pediatrics: a critical incident analysis of contributory factors. *Pediatrics.* 2000;105(4 Pt 1):805-814.

Landmark study that collated severe adverse outcomes from multiple sources and allowed the identification of sedation practices that led to injury and death. In particular, it highlighted the need for appropriate personnel, monitors, and rescue capability to ensure safety.

Coté CJ, Wilson S, American Academy of Pediatrics, American Academy of Pediatric Dentistry. Guidelines for monitoring and management of pediatric patients before, during, and after sedation for diagnostic and therapeutic procedures. *Pediatrics.* 2019;143(6):e20191000.

These are the most recent American Academy of Pediatrics Sedation Guidelines that now require the use of capnography for all deeply sedated children and encourage its use for moderately sedated children. Important changes are that the responsible practitioner for moderate sedation must have the skills to rescue a child with apnea, laryngospasm, and airway obstruction, and perform successful bag-mask ventilation. The practitioner who practices deep sedation must have these same skills and be able to perform tracheal intubation and cardiopulmonary resuscitation. For children undergoing dental procedures with deep sedation of general anesthesia, a trained anesthesia provider must be the independent observer (physician anesthesiologist, dental anesthesiologist, certified registered nurse anesthetist, or a second oral surgeon).

Cravero JP, Beach M, Gallagher SM, et al. The incidence and nature of adverse events during pediatric sedation/anesthesia for procedures with propofol outside the operating room: report from the Pediatric Sedation Research Consortium. *Anesth Analg.* 2009;108(3):795-804.

A review of nearly 50,000 sedation encounters using propofol by a variety of sedation providers. The participating providers were highly trained members of organized sedation services with advanced airway education and ongoing quality improvement efforts. Adverse events and requirements for airway interventions are analyzed. The information is useful in understanding the critical competencies necessary for the safe use of this drug.

Cravero JP, Blike GT, Beach M, et al. Incidence and nature of adverse events during pediatric sedation/anesthesia for procedures outside the operating room: report from the Pediatric Sedation Research Consortium. *Pediatrics.* 2006;118(3):1087-1096.

A review of more than 30,000 sedation cases from the Pediatric Sedation Research Consortium. This study is useful as it supplements anecdotal information on sedation complications and aids in understanding the nature and frequency of adverse events in a large group of patients cared for by a variety of sedation providers.

A complete reference list can be found online at Elsevier eBooks+.

44

45 The Post Anesthesia Care Unit and Beyond

TIMOTHY M. EARLEY, JEANA E. HAVIDICH, AND ANDREAS H. TAENZER

Perioperative Environment
Transport to the Care Unit
Arrival in the Care Unit
Central Nervous System
Pharmacodynamics of Emergence
Emergence Agitation and Delirium
Respiratory System
Criteria for Extubation
Extubation in the Operating Room or Postanesthesia Care Unit
High Care Need After Tonsillectomy
Hypoxemia
Hypoventilation
Airway Obstruction
Respiratory Effort
Discharge of Preterm Infants From the Postanesthesia Care Unit

Cardiovascular System
Bradycardia
Tachycardia
Other Arrhythmias
Blood Pressure Control
Renal System
Gastrointestinal System
Postoperative Nausea and Vomiting
Postoperative Care and Discharge
Pain Management in the Postanesthesia Care Unit
Temperature Management
Discharge Criteria
Beyond PACU: Postoperative Monitoring in the General Care Setting

EMERGENCE FROM ANESTHESIA IN CHILDREN differs substantially when compared with emergence in adults. The process is multifaceted, and depends on the nature and duration of the surgery, the patient characteristics, and the type of anesthetic administered. Younger children rapidly emerge from inhalational agents because of their increased minute ventilation, increased blood flow to the vessel-rich group (see Chapter 5), decreased anesthetic solubilities in blood and tissues, and decreased total body muscle and fat stores, whereas emergence from intravenous (IV) agents may be delayed even in neonates and infants because of immature clearance pathways.

One important aspect to appreciate is the rapidity with which serious complications can develop in the postoperative period. Neonates, infants, and young children have less cardiopulmonary reserve compared with adults, resulting in a more rapid physiologic deterioration should airway obstruction, bleeding or surgical complications occur. Vigilant and frequent monitoring by pediatric postanesthesia care nurses and anesthesiologists is essential for appropriate postoperative care as well as to prevent and treat adverse events. Parents or primary caregivers should be considered active partners in the postoperative care of the child. Those who routinely provide comfort and care for the child are essential for the child's sense of well-being. In addition, caregivers should alert medical professionals to changes in the child's status that may require urgent medical attention.

Perioperative Environment

A well-designed, safe perioperative environment is essential for the delivery of high-quality pediatric anesthetic and surgical care as recommended by the American Academy of Pediatrics (AAP), which published a policy statement in 2015 delineating the critical elements of the perioperative environment.[1] The recommendations focus on the patient care facility and medical policies, including staff credentialing and necessary supportive services. This document was developed to complement the Society for Pediatric Anesthesia (SPA) statement on the provision of pediatric anesthesia care.[2] Institutions that desire verification by the American College of Surgeons Children's Surgery Verification Program must include a designated postanesthetic care unit (PACU) with appropriately credentialed staff and supportive resources.[3] These guidelines acknowledge that the perioperative environment can be challenging and that health care facilities must understand these challenges and be prepared to manage children and family members throughout this difficult process. Policies and procedures based on recommendations from national organizations were developed with input from all stakeholders, including physicians, nurses, family members, and child-life specialists to comprise the foundation for a safe, patient- and family-centered perioperative environment.

The ideal perioperative environment should also combine ergonomics with safety. The family and patient experience starts with the admission process and concludes with the discharge to home or the hospital ward. Familiarity with personnel and surroundings reduces stress for patients and families while fostering trust and comfort. Ideally, a child should be under the care of the same team throughout the perioperative period. For example, the child and family benefit if the admitting nurse later cares for the child and the family in the PACU or day-stay unit (the phase 2 or stepdown unit prior to discharge home). This may be achieved by creating an integrated perioperative environment, in

TABLE 45.1	Suggested Essential Bedside Equipment

Oxygen supply with regulated flows

Oxygen face masks and face tents for spontaneous ventilation (various sizes)

Oxygen nebulizers for administration of albuterol and racemic epinephrine

Stethoscope

Resuscitation bags, self-inflating (Ambu)

Anesthesia facemasks for positive-pressure ventilation (pediatric sizes: 0, 1, 2, 3; adult sizes: small, medium, large)

Oral airways (sizes 00, 0, 1–5)

Nasal airways (sizes 12Fr–36Fr)

Suction and appropriate suction catheters (sizes 6.5Fr–14Fr); tonsil-type (Yankauer)

IV supplies: needles, syringes, saline flushes, alcohol wipes, Betadine solution, gauze pads, Tegaderm dressings (3M, Minneapolis, MN), tourniquets, tape

Nonlatex gloves (various sizes)

Pulse oximeter and sensors (size appropriate, stick-on type preferred to clip-on type)

Electrocardiograph, monitor, and pads

Manual and automated blood pressure devices

All sizes of blood pressure cuffs

TABLE 45.2	Suggested Emergency Supplies for a Crash Cart or Central Location

Cognitive aids for resuscitation (weight-based pediatric advanced life support cards) (e.g., Broselow tapes [see E-Figs. 37.1 to 37.3])

Laryngoscopes with blades: Miller 0, 1, 2, 3; Macintosh 2, 3, 4; extra laryngoscope bulbs and batteries

Endotracheal tubes, sizes 2.0-mm internal diameter (ID) through 8-mm ID; cuffed and uncuffed tubes for all sizes when available

Stylet appropriate for each endotracheal tube size

Syringe for endotracheal cuff inflation

End-tidal carbon dioxide monitor or portable detector

Tape and liquid adhesive for endotracheal tube fixation

Intravenous catheter (14 gauge) with 3-mm ID endotracheal tube adapter for emergency cricothyroidotomy

Backup resuscitation bags and masks and oral airways for each bedside

Jet-Ventilation-Catheters 13 gauge (adult), 14 gauge (child), and 16 gauge (infant).

Nasogastric tubes

Intravenous infusion solutions, tubing, drip chambers

Supplies for intravenous cannulation, catheter sizes 24 to 14 gauge

Cutdown tray, tracheostomy, and suture sets

Central venous catheter insertion sets (3Fr–7Fr, single- and multiple-lumen)

Tube thoracotomy set and system for suction and underwater seal

Automated electric defibrillator or defibrillator (adult, child paddles)

Electrocardiograph

Pressure transducer system and oscilloscope monitor

Sterile gowns, gloves, masks, towels, drapes

Urinary catheters of appropriate pediatric size

Bed board for cardiopulmonary resuscitation

which children are admitted, prepared, and allowed to recover in the same space, with the same nurses and child-life specialist.

Privacy and shelter from noise can be important aspects of the patient and family experience. The ability to spend time with the child without being disturbed is something that many families appreciate, and this may help the child cope with the stress of a strange environment. Many PACUs contain individual patient rooms or cubicles for preoperative and postoperative care.

Equipment (Table 45.1) and available medications (Tables 45.2 and 45.3) should be standardized throughout the unit. All monitors should be compatible with transport monitors and other devices used in the medical facility (e.g., pediatric intensive care unit [PICU]). Cognitive aids such as preprinted emergency drug cards may be useful.[1] This important safety measure may reduce the risk of drug errors in emergency situations. These rapid reference sheets may be attached to each child's bed or chart on admission so that a quick dosing guide is readily available. Alternatively, the electronic record should have precalculated emergency drug doses for each child.

All PACU providers must be competent in neonatal and pediatric advanced life support. Team training, including mock codes and the use of enhanced communication techniques, improves outcomes.[4–8] Continuous medical education in the provision of pediatric care is often required by hospital credentialing committees as well as institutions requesting American College of Surgeons verification.[3]

TRANSPORT TO THE CARE UNIT

The PACU should be located near operating or procedural rooms to decrease transport time and increase operating room efficiency. If transporting a sedated patient from a remote location, the patient's vital signs and a metric of respiration should be monitored along the route. Appropriate airway equipment and drugs should be immediately available. Transport from the operating room to the PACU should be carried out under the direct supervision of a trained expert. The security and patency of the airway, IV and arterial lines, drains, chest tubes, and urinary catheters should be checked before transport. Children should be covered during transport to maintain normothermia and a presentable appearance. Children suffering infectious diseases (e.g., COVID-19–positive patients) require special considerations during transport, in the operating room, and in the PACU (see Chapter 47).

Unless there is a contraindication, children who are sedated or emerging from anesthesia should be transported in the lateral position (known as the recovery or "tonsil" position) to decrease the likelihood of airway obstruction and/or aspiration. To assess ventilation and maintain a patent airway with the child in the decubitus position, we recommend applying the thumb to the forehead to extend the neck and holding the fingers (the fingertips are the most sensitive part of the hand) over the mouth (or nose) to feel for exhalation. The presence of "misting" or "fogging" in an oxygen mask also confirms airway patency. If there is concern about airway patency, a transport capnogram can be used to monitor the adequacy of ventilation during this period. A precordial stethoscope placed over the trachea may also be used to auscultate respirations. If the child is breathing room air, a pulse oximeter can serve as a crude metric of ventilation because desaturation will occur quickly if hypopnea develops. However, if

TABLE 45.3 | Suggested Recovery Room Medications

Suggested Emergency Medications on Crash Cart[a]

Albuterol (also known as salbutamol outside the United States)
Amiodarone
Atropine
Calcium chloride or gluconate
Dextrose
Diphenhydramine
Dopamine
Epinephrine
Etomidate
Flumazenil
Furosemide
Hydrocortisone, dexamethasone, methylprednisolone
Lidocaine (intravenous and topical)
Naloxone
Neostigmine
Norepinephrine
Physostigmine
Propranolol, atenolol, esmolol, labetalol
Sodium bicarbonate
Sodium nitroprusside
Succinylcholine and rocuronium
Sugammadex
Propofol
Verapamil
For inhalation: racemic epinephrine (2.25% at 0.05 mL/kg, common in the United States) *or* epinephrine 1:1000 (0.1%), 0.5 mL/kg, maximum of 5 mL

Medications to Be Kept Under Lock[a]

Diazepam
Fentanyl
Ketamine
Meperidine
Midazolam (intravenous and oral)
Morphine
Potassium chloride

Other Medications for Central Location[a]

Acetaminophen (oral, rectal, and intravenous)
Antibiotics
Antiemetics (e.g., 5-HT$_3$-antagonist, promethazine, metoclopramide)
Dantrolene
Digoxin
Heparin
Insulin
Mannitol
Potassium chloride
Protamine
Ketorolac
Dexmedetomidine

[a]Alternative or additional medications may be needed.

oxygen is delivered, desaturation will be delayed in the setting of apnea or hypopnea,[9] and ventilation should be monitored by close observation, a precordial stethoscope, capnography, or ideally, by a combination of these monitors.

We recommend that children in a potentially unstable condition be transported with a pulse oximeter, capnography, an electrocardiographic (ECG) monitor, and a blood pressure cuff or transduced arterial line. The monitoring lines, IV drips, epidural or regional catheters, infusion pumps, and other equipment should be clearly labeled and simplified before transport. Airway equipment and emergency medications should be readily available, especially when children are transported to or from remote locations.

A child often appears awake after the stimulation of tracheal extubation and transfer to the stretcher but may subsequently become obtunded and obstruct the airway during transit to the PACU or PICU. Just as frequently, a child may become restless during transit. Although restless behavior has many causes, hypoxia should be foremost in our mind to rule out or treat. The guard rails on the stretcher should always be raised and padded when the child is in it to prevent injury. Most importantly, the anesthesiologist should remain at the head of the stretcher during transport to maintain vigilance of the child and the monitors throughout the transfer. Ideally, two individuals should be present to transport the child to PACU.

ARRIVAL IN THE CARE UNIT

The transfer of care from the operating room personnel to the PACU or PICU is a crucial element of quality patient care that deserves considerable focus. Its importance cannot be overemphasized. Ideally, it is a stepwise process following an institutional protocol that begins in the operating or procedural room with communication to the receiving unit before the end of surgery or the procedure. Information should include a brief report, including patient information and required equipment or medication that will be needed in the PACU. On arrival in the PACU, a rapid assessment of the child should be undertaken to ensure that the child has a patent airway and vital signs are stable; transfer to each monitor is made in a step-by-step manner to avoid a gap in monitoring. Once the child has been properly assessed, vital signs including an admission heart rate, oxygen saturation, respiratory rate, blood pressure, and temperature should be recorded. Supplemental oxygen should be administered as indicated, recognizing the limitations of the monitors to detect hypoventilation in such cases. Many children object to having an oxygen mask fixed to their faces; a funnel-type mask or open hose with large flow rates may be less objectionable (although also less optimal); nasal prongs may be an alternative oxygen source. In the healthy child, if the child is awake enough to object to a mask on their face, more often than not, the child does not require supplemental oxygen (although the combative, hypoxic child will require not only oxygen but establishment of a patent airway as well).

Numerous patient safety organizations and health care institutions have devoted considerable time and resources to improve patient transfer processes with the primary objective to improve safety, increase the quality of care, and decrease health care costs. Education of health care personnel about the importance of this endeavor is the first step to implementing effective transfers of care; several methods have been suggested.[4,10–16] A standardized handoff that contains a validated checklist and protocol is essential so that the PACU team is fully informed of all issues related to the child, their anesthetic, and their surgery. However, no validated handover checklist has been forthcoming for infants and children, resulting in incomplete handover of material to the PACU team.[17] In institutions with effective and organized handoff systems, the number of medical errors decreased and patient outcomes improved.[6,18–23]

Surgeons, anesthesia providers, and intensive care physicians involved in the care of the child should be present and actively participate during the transfer of care from the operating room to the PACU or PICU. Specific circumstances including language barriers, developmental delay, or family issues should be conveyed to members of the team accepting care of the child. Since cultures vary within and among different institutions, we recommend developing a formalized transfer of care process that focuses on critical aspects of patient care, including pertinent patient information and history, surgical procedures, type of anesthesia administered, airway management, medications and fluids administered, hemodynamics, estimated blood loss, unexpected events, anticipated patient progress, pain management strategies, possible complications, and information that needs to be relayed to parents or hospital staff in the event the patient is being admitted. Any unanticipated or serious events, such as unanticipated difficult airway, hemodynamic instability, or surgical complications, should be clearly communicated. If continuous infusions of local anesthetics are administered (e.g., epidural catheter infusion), the dose, concentration, rate, and maximum infusion rate should be conveyed. Tasks that need to be completed in the near future should be discussed with the team accepting the care of the patient. All stakeholders should have the opportunity to ask questions and confirm the transfer of information before concluding the handoff.

The anesthesia team must remain with the child until vital signs are stable and the PACU or PICU team is comfortable and ready to assume responsibility for the child. Physicians who will provide care for the child in the PACU or PICU after the anesthesia team leaves must be clearly identified by name, and methods to contact them (e.g., pager number) must be given to surgeons, anesthesiologists, and regional block and pain services. It is important to understand that barriers may exist at several levels that preclude the effective transfer of care. Such circumstances frequently implicated include: external distractions, noisy environments, shift changes, and differences in culture and priorities between individuals providing and accepting care of the child.[15,24–27]

Ideally, nurses taking care of the child postoperatively are already familiar with the child and family from the preoperative setting. The nurse/patient ratio should be 1:1 for sick children or children whose airway remains intubated and 1:2 or 1:3 for routine cases. Staffing ratios, nursing surveillance techniques, and vigilant monitoring of patients in the PACU by pediatric-trained nursing staff improve patient outcomes.[28–31] Available staffing and resources in the PACU or PICU should be in place before transporting the child from the operating room.

All children should be monitored continuously in the PACU. At the very least, this should include continuous pulse oximetry, respiratory rate, intermittent noninvasive blood pressure, and temperature monitoring. Most PACUs monitor the electrocardiogram continuously, although some limit this to children with cardiac disease or complex multiple-organ disease. During emergence, many children can be quite active, and it is impossible to maintain the monitoring devices in place. If the child is not hypoxic and is sufficiently awake to remove the monitors, they probably do not require the monitors any longer. If the child falls back to sleep, then a pulse oximeter probe should be reapplied, particularly for at-risk children such as those with obstructive sleep apnea (OSA).[32] For a child who is physically or mentally challenged, it may be necessary to apply light restraints until they are oriented and awake.

Central Nervous System

PHARMACODYNAMICS OF EMERGENCE

Emergence from anesthesia is a complex process that depends on the dose and types of medications administered, the age of the

child, and their physiologic status. The age of the child exerts a minimal influence on the wash-out of inhalational anesthetic agents and has little impact on the rapidity of emergence, although age may be a factor for infants younger than 1 year.[33] However, the overall clinical implications of age-related differences in emergence are exceedingly difficult to detect.[34] The speed of emergence correlates closely with the duration of anesthesia: that is, the greater the duration of anesthesia, the more the tissue compartments become filled with anesthetics and the more time it takes to eliminate the anesthetics during recovery. For example, emergence from 30 minutes of sevoflurane anesthesia is faster than emergence from 2 hours of sevoflurane anesthesia, which is more rapid than from 8 hours of sevoflurane anesthesia.[35] This relationship between emergence time and the duration of anesthesia holds to a lesser extent for less soluble agents, (e.g., desflurane) because redistribution to "deep" compartments is diminished compared with more soluble agents (e.g., sevoflurane).[36–38]

The quality and rapidity of emergence after IV anesthetic agents compared with inhalation agents differs.[39,40] For outpatient surgery, emergence after propofol anesthesia is as rapid as that after sevoflurane but with far less agitation and pain behaviors.[41] The recovery characteristics of propofol with remifentanil (total IV anesthesia [TIVA]; see Chapter 6) have been compared with those after desflurane inhalational anesthesia. Recovery is as rapid as that after desflurane with nitrous oxide, with a similar or reduced incidence of nausea and vomiting but with much less agitation.[42,43] Time to recovery after propofol infusion mirrors changes in context-sensitive half-time with age, the target concentration used for anesthesia, adjuvant drug use, and the child's clinical status.[44]

Although rarely used for maintenance of anesthesia, midazolam is often used as an oral or IV premedication for anxiolysis and amnesia in the preinduction period in children. The addition of midazolam before an inhalational or propofol anesthetic may delay early emergence after brief anesthesia. However, this delay is attenuated as the duration of anesthesia increases and when only late emergence is considered.[45] Midazolam has yielded inconsistent effects on the incidence of emergence delirium; as an oral or rectal premedication, midazolam does not diminish the incidence of emergence delirium after sevoflurane anesthesia in children, whereas a single IV dose of midazolam at the end of surgery diminishes the incidence (see later).[46–48]

EMERGENCE AGITATION AND DELIRIUM

Emergence agitation and emergence delirium are disruptive behaviors that occur postoperatively and may result in injury to the patient, family members, and staff. Emergence delirium was first described in a large cohort of postsurgical patients over 60 years ago but still remains poorly understood.[49] From a clinical perspective, it may be difficult to differentiate pure agitation from delirium, which may account for these terms to be used interchangeably.[50] Moreover, clinically differentiating emergence delirium from pain may be exceedingly difficult, particularly since most analgesics confer sedation as well as analgesia, which further blurs the distinction. For the purpose of this discussion, the term emergence agitation is defined as an unpleasant state of extreme arousal, that may be manifested by verbal aggression, excessive motor activity, and maladaptive or regressive behaviors.[51,52] Emergence delirium is a disturbance in attention and awareness, where the child appears to have a change in cognition and fails to interact appropriately with caregivers and family members (Videos 45.1 and 45.2).[53–55] In addition, delirium is categorized into three subtypes, hyperactive, hypoactive, and mixed. The hyperactive subtype is the most easily recognizable; children may be inconsolable, incoherent, fail to make eye contact, appear agitated, and display excessive motor activity. Children with hypoactive delirium appear withdrawn, quiet, or apathetic.[56,57] The hypoactive form of delirium may be underdiagnosed because the child appears well behaved and changes may only be noticeable to a family member or close caregiver. Children who display a continuum of both hypoactive and hyperactive delirium are classified as manifesting mixed delirium.[51,52]

The true incidence of emergence delirium is unknown but is reported to range from 2% to 80% of children. It is usually self-limiting although long-term maladaptive behaviors in children who experience emergence agitation or emergence delirium are increasingly reported.[37,52,58-63] Several authors have recommended evaluating every patient for the development of agitation or delirium, to improve patient/parental satisfaction and decrease the possibility of potential serious complications.[64,65]

It is imperative to have a working differential diagnosis when examining the child who may appear to be experiencing agitation or delirium (Table 45.4) It is important to remember life-threatening events, such as hypoxemia, sepsis, or a drug reaction can mimic emergence agitation and delirium and should be ruled out first. The mechanism of emergence delirium in children has not been completely elucidated, but differences in the frontal lobe electroencephalogram[66,67] and locus coeruleus[68] compared with children without delirium suggest potential sources within the brain. Evidence also points to differences in central nervous system metabolites in the parietal cortex that may contribute to delirium; brain injury markers, lactic acid concentrations, and other metabolites after sevoflurane in children correlated with greater Pediatric Anesthesia Emergence Delirium (PAED) scale values than those after propofol.[69,70] To aid in the prevention and diagnosis of emergence agitation or emergence delirium, it is helpful to identify associated risk factors. Published risk factors include: age less than 7 years, parental stress/anxiety, developmental age of the child, communication abilities, previous hospitalizations, prolonged fasting, trauma, coping skills, socioeconomic status, ethnicity, use of inhalation agents, the temperament of the child, and rapid emergence in a hostile or unfriendly environment.[39,42,58,65,71-75] Certain surgeries have also been associated with a greater incidence of emergence delirium, although in most, pain was inadequately or incompletely controlled, precluding differentiating pain from emergence delirium.[76] Surgery is not a cause of emergence delirium in and of itself; in contrast, inhalation anesthesia in the absence of surgery is an unequivocal cause of delirium.[77]

Several scales have been developed to assess emergence delirium, although only the PAED scale has been validated for this purpose in the postoperative period.[78-80] Tables 47.5 and 47.6 present two scoring systems that have been used to evaluate emergence behaviors in children. In evaluating emergence delirium with the PAED scale after anesthesia, preliminary evidence suggested that values greater than 10 or possibly greater than 12 were consistent with emergence delirium.[81-83] In the PICU, evidence suggests that a PAED score greater than 8 predicts emergence delirium.[79] The literature regarding postoperative delirium in children is quite confusing, in part because many studies used nonvalidated, unproven scales in children whose pain was not controlled, leaving the cause of the behavior attributable to delirium, pain, or both. This explains in part why the type of surgery has been reported as a risk factor for emergence delirium. During radiological investigations, the incidence of emergence delirium in both the control and treated (with sevoflurane) groups were dramatically less than those during surgeries.[77]

Our understanding of emergence delirium continues to evolve. Delirium occurs after surgical procedures and after procedures that are pain-free, such as magnetic resonance imaging (MRI).[77,84-86] Although some claim that there is a greater incidence of emergence delirium after certain painful surgeries, in most of these

TABLE 45.4	Differential Diagnosis of Pediatric Agitation and Delirium
Differential Diagnosis of Emergence Delirium	
Airway obstruction	Malignant Hyperthermia
Hypoxemia	Metabolic acidosis
Hypotension	Stroke
Cardiac Dysfunction	Catatonia
Hemorrhage	Hypoglycemia
Electrolyte imbalances	Sepsis
Allergic reaction	Drug reaction
Acute organ failure	Surgical complications
Substance abuse disorder	Post traumatic stress disorder

TABLE 45.5	Pediatric Anesthesia Emergence Delirium Scale				
	SCORING				
Scored Factor	**0**	**1**	**2**	**3**	**4**
Child makes eye contact with caregiver	Extremely	Very much	Quite a bit	Just a little	Not at all
Child's actions are purposeful	Extremely	Very much	Quite a bit	Just a little	Not at all
Child is aware of surroundings	Extremely	Very much	Quite a bit	Just a little	Not at all
Child is restless	Not at all	Just a little	Quite a bit	Very much	Extremely
Child is inconsolable	Not at all	Just a little	Quite a bit	Very much	Extremely
Total score[a]					

[a]Preliminary evidence suggested that a total pediatric anesthesia emergence delirium score greater than 10 defined emergence delirium, but later evidence suggested that a total score greater than 12 might be more specific.
Modified from Sikich N, Lerman J. Development and psychometric evaluation of the pediatric anesthesia emergence delirium scale. *Anesthesiology.* 2004;100:1138-1145.

TABLE 45.6	Postanesthesia Behavior Assessment Scale

Perceptual Disturbances (Maximal Score 3)[a]

0 None evident
1 Feelings of depersonalization (says that situation is not real, comments on "out of body" feelings)
2 Visual illusions or misperceptions (misidentifies objects, such as urinates in trash can)
3 Markedly confused about external reality (misidentifies self or surroundings, such as being at school)

Hallucination Type (Maximal Score 6)[a]

0 None evident
1 Auditory hallucinations only (responds to questions not asked)
2 Visual hallucinations or misperceptions (responds to things only the child can see)
3 Tactile, olfactory (responds to sensations not obvious to others, such as a bug crawling on the leg)

Psychomotor Behavior (Maximal Score 3)[a]

0 No significant agitation
1 Mild restlessness, tremulousness, or anxiety
2 Moderate agitation with pulling at intravenous lines
3 Severe agitation, needs to be restrained, combative

[a]A larger postanesthesia behavior assessment score is associated with a greater degree of postanesthetic distress.
From Przybylo HJ, Martini DR, Mazurek AJ, Bracey E, Johnsen L, Coté CJ. Assessing behaviour in children emerging form anaesthesia: can we apply psychiatric diagnostic techniques? *Pediatr Anesth.* 2003;13:609-616.

TABLE 45.7	Prophylactic Measures to Prevent Emergence Delirium

Prophylactic Measure	Timing
Propofol (IV)	TIVA,[41,312] a brief infusion of 3 mg/kg over 3 minutes after sevoflurane,[96] a single dose at the end of anesthesia (1 mg/kg IV)[88,90,93,313,314]
Opioid (IV)	Meta-analysis[315] of fentanyl, remifentanil, sufentanil, alfentanil[230,316]; nalbuphine (0.1 mg/kg)[317]
Midazolam	
(IV)	0.03–0.05 mg/kg at end of anesthesia[48,318]
(PO)	0.2–0.5 mg/kg[319]; 0.5 mg/kg with parental presence[320]
α₂-Agonist (IV) (caudal)	Clonidine 2 µg/kg at induction[319,321,322]; dexmedetomidine 0.3–1 µg/kg at emergence[87,323–326] Meta-analysis of dexmedetomidine demonstrates effectiveness[87,327] Dexmedetomidine 1 µg/kg followed by 1 µg/kg per hour[328] Clonidine 1 µg/kg[329]
Ketamine (IV)	Ketamine 1 mg/kg followed by 1 mg/kg per hour[328] or 0.25 mg/kg[317]
Melatonin (PO)	0.25 or 0.5 mg/kg premedication[330]
Tropisetron (IV)	0.1 mg/kg at induction[331]
Magnesium sulfate (IV)	30 mg/kg followed by 10 mg/kg per hour[332]
Regional anesthesia	Infraorbital block,[38,333] fascia iliaca block[334]
Acupuncture	Heart 7 site bilaterally during surgery[335]

IV, Intravenous; *PO*, oral; *TIVA*; total intravenous anesthesia.

instances this cannot be proven as pain was not controlled and a nonvalidated metric of delirium was used.[60]

Several strategies have been used to prevent and treat emergence delirium (Table 45.7). Effective regional analgesia, dexmedetomidine, opioids, ketamine, melatonin, midazolam, magnesium, and propofol have been used with success.[58,87–91] Fentanyl (2 to 2.5 µg/kg intranasally or 1 to 2 µg/kg IV) decreases the duration and intensity of emergence delirium,[92] even in the absence of painful stimuli, most likely because of its sedating effect.[74] Administration of propofol by continuous infusion or by bolus (1 to 3 mg/kg) at the end of surgery appears to be preventive, although these findings have not been consistent.[82,93] A dose of propofol at induction of anesthesia does not prevent postoperative emergence delirium.[94] A meta-analysis of 12 randomized controlled studies reported reduced PAED scores in those who received propofol compared with those who did not.[95] A TIVA anesthetic is superior to inhalational agents in the prevention of emergence delirium.[40,42,86]

When emergence delirium does occur, it is important to explain to the parents that most cases are self-limiting. Whether to terminate the delirium pharmacologically or let it resolve without intervention should be discussed with the parents. Many parents prefer to avoid administering additional medications, knowing that the delirium will abate spontaneously after several minutes and that their child will recover to their normal disposition soon. Treatment of ongoing delirium has not been widely studied, but current strategies include propofol (1 to 3 mg/kg) as a bolus dose or as a longer infusion,[96] fentanyl (1 to 2 µg/kg), or dexmedetomidine (0.3 µg/kg).[97] Most use an initial small dose and titrate to effect.

Discharge from the PACU may be delayed while waiting for the agitation or delirium to wane or for the effects of the interventional drugs to dissipate. Injury to the child who is delirious, to the site of surgery, or to a parent is a concern, as is pulling out a drain, dressing, IV, or self-extubation. Parental satisfaction decreases when severe emergence delirium occurs. Although the impact of extreme delirium is not fully known, evidence suggests that the incidence of postoperative maladaptive behaviors is greater among children who experience marked emergence delirium.[98]

Respiratory System

CRITERIA FOR EXTUBATION

Very little evidence exists regarding the optimal timing for tracheal extubation in infants and children, leaving clinicians to use their clinical judgment to determine when to extubate and minimize the risks of laryngospasm, desaturation, breath-holding, and vomiting.[99] To answer when should the tracheal tube be removed, we need to know which recovery indices should be present to increase the probability that tracheal extubation with be both successful and safe. In a study of infants and children <7 years of age, the authors reported five criteria that were associated with a successful extubation after inhalational anesthesia: conjugate gaze, facial grimace, eye opening, purposeful movement, and tidal volume >5 mL/kg.[100] The practice at some institutions is to extubate the trachea when a child is awake and demonstrating eye opening, conjugate gaze, and purposeful movements, whereas at others, the practice is to extubate while the child is deeply anesthetized and breathing spontaneously such that removal of the tracheal tube does not impact the child's respiratory status or trigger upper airway reflex responses. The frequencies of respiratory complications with both approaches when they are done properly are rare and mild in severity.[101,102] In the case of extubating laryngeal mask airways (LMAs), a systematic review found an overall reduction in airway complications (cough, desaturation), when the laryngeal mask airways were removed during "deep" inhalational anesthesia, although extubation during deep anesthesia was associated with an increased risk of airway obstruction; the incidence of laryngospasm or breath-holding was similar.[103] In contrast, a randomized trial in 106 children whose laryngeal mask airway was removed during deep anesthesia or when awake reported no statistically significant difference in adverse respiratory events.[104] Most clinicians agree that extubating the trachea or removing a supraglottic airway during a very light plane of anesthesia (stage 2), is when laryngospasm is more likely and vomiting may occur while protective reflexes are impaired. Regardless of the approach taken, consideration should be given to draining stomach contents prior to extubation.

EXTUBATION IN THE OPERATING ROOM OR POSTANESTHESIA CARE UNIT

In most cases, tracheal extubation may be safely performed in the operating room after elective surgery. However, a child's condition may necessitate that extubation be delayed. For example, there is widespread agreement that children who have been anesthetized with a full stomach, children at risk for airway obstruction, those with difficult airways, premature infants, and other infants predisposed to apnea should be awake before extubation is attempted.

The "just in time" algorithm that highlights the key elements required for a successful extubation as described by Veyckemans begins with pharyngeal suctioning during deep level of anesthesia, preoxygenation, and then discontinuing the anesthetic.[105] When spontaneous respiration has resumed, the following clinical signs should be anticipated before considering to extubate the airway: absence of thoracoabdominal asynchrony, adequate respiratory rate, presence of adequate pharyngeal tone, conjugate gaze, and optimal head and neck position,[105] criteria that are similar to those included in the Templeton review.[100] Another important caveat is to perform a lung inflation maneuver with 100% oxygen rather than suctioning the tracheal tube as the final step, immediately before extubation. The former maneuver prolongs the time to desaturate <92% after extubation by more than 3-fold, from 25 seconds to 85 seconds, compared with the latter maneuver.[106] Furthermore, the immediate application of 100% oxygen in the form of a facemask with continuous positive airway pressure (CPAP) while performing a jaw thrust (to stimulate the child to take breaths) ensures that ventilation and oxygenation indices will be maintained and minimizes the risks of airway obstruction, laryngospasm, and vomiting. Transporting the child from the operating room should not begin until the airway is stable and patent, and oxygenation and ventilation are confirmed. Placing the child in the lateral decubitus position before extubation maintains a patent airway and facilitates drainage of oropharyngeal secretions and blood if present out of the mouth and away from the glottic opening, thereby preserving spontaneous respiration.[107]

In some institutions where children undergo elective ambulatory procedures, the trachea may be extubated in the PACU to increase operating room efficiency.[108,109] In these studies, the time spent in the operating room was less when the trachea was extubated in the PACU than it was when extubation occurred in the operating room.[108,109] Interestingly, the incidence of adverse events in PACU was similar to those that occurred during extubation in the operating room. However, for this practice to be a successful program, the PACU nurses must be properly trained and locally certified to be competent to manage the airway and to perform tracheal extubation. Once the child is extubated, the nurses must be competent to diagnose and treat acute airway obstruction and know when to call for help. These patients may spend more time in the PACU (an amount similar to the time needed to extubate), although this has been debated. What we know is once the child is in PACU with an instrumented airway, the nurses are under no pressure to hasten tracheal extubation, ensuring the children are clearly and optimally recovered to achieve a successful extubation without adverse events. Given the enormous difference in the cost per unit time in the operating room and PACU, it is reasonable for the child to spend more time in PACU to avoid delaying operating room throughput. Conversely, some children present with conditions that contraindicate tracheal extubation in the PACU. Such conditions include former premature infants, infants and children <2 years of age, those with dysmorphic facies or difficult intubations, those with neuromuscular or myopathic disorders, and those with severe pulmonary or cardiac disorders that would warrant additional expertise in the immediate postextubation period. Importantly, the presence of an anesthesiologist with advanced pediatric airway skills is recommended in this model to ensure rapid assessment and management of airway complications.[108]

For children whose tracheas are extubated in the PACU, airway obstruction and desaturation are the most worrisome and frequent complications. However, the evidence presented to date argues that the incidence of adverse events after extubation in the operating room and PACU are equal. The reasons have been cited above. Respiratory insufficiency represents approximately two-thirds of critical perioperative events when it occurs during emergence from anesthesia.[110] Respiratory insufficiency may be manifested by difficulty breathing, anxiety, unresponsiveness, tachycardia, bradycardia, hypertension, arrhythmia, or seizures with cardiac arrest as a late manifestation. When any of these conditions are present, respiratory insufficiency must be considered as the root cause. Hypoxemia, hypoventilation, and upper airway obstruction are the three most common adverse respiratory events that occur in children in the PACU.[111] Such events can increase health care costs considerably.[112] This is particularly true for children after tonsillectomy complicated by obesity and possible OSA and for those who have undergone diagnostic bronchoscopy.[32,113]

HIGH CARE NEED AFTER TONSILLECTOMY

Consensus statements have been published to help clinicians identify those children who may be at increased risk for respiratory complications after tonsillectomy. The criteria include age younger than 2 years, weight less than 15 kg, failure to thrive, obesity (body mass index >2.5 standard deviation or >99th centile), severe OSA, and significant comorbidities (neuromuscular, craniofacial, respiratory, cardiac).[114] These children are considered at increased risk for respiratory complications following tonsillectomy and should be admitted overnight. In addition to admitting these children, they should be monitored with oximetry if supplemental oxygen is not given and with capnography as well as oximetry if supplemental oxygen is supplied because the sensitivity of an oximeter to detect an apnea or obstructed airway in the presence of supplemental oxygen is reduced.

Preoperative indices for admission to PICU after adenotonsillectomy have remained elusive, leaving the decision to admit to PICU to the discretion of the clinician.[115,116] Clinical judgment is most often sufficient to detect complicated patients with OSA who may require PICU after tonsillectomy[117]; a retrospective review from England of 1328 children of whom 814 had formal polysomnography studies found that ~1.6% had planned PICU admission but 1.2% had unplanned PICU admission. The majority of these patients had severe OSA (22/37) and the majority (78%) were classified as ASA class ≥3; the need for a nasopharyngeal airway was associated with PICU admission.[118] In another retrospective review of 195 children <3 years of age with polysomnography-proven OSA, most children recovered after adenotonsillectomy without developing adverse respiratory events; however, 65 patients were monitored in the PICU, 92% of whom had severe OSA.[119] Children with severe OSA were more likely to require respiratory intervention postoperatively in the PICU (CPAP, intubation, or >2L/minute of oxygen) had an apnea-hypopnea index >13.6 events/hour, hypopneas >19.5/hour, and an oxygen saturation (SaO_2) nadir <67.15%. Several studies identified a number of variables that are associated with an increased risk for postoperative intensive care monitoring. Comorbidities including preoperative home CPAP, the presence of a neuromuscular disorder, and an oxygen saturation nadir <80%, increased the risk that the child may require more intensive care monitoring postoperatively.[120] In a retrospective review of 278 children with severe OSA and/or PICU admission, end-tidal CO_2 ≥60 mm Hg during polysomnography, the presence of a neuromuscular disorder, and intraoperative airway complications (hypoxia, difficult airway) during adenotonsillectomy pointed to an increased need for perioperative airway management and prolonged hospital stay.[121] In the most recent retrospective review of 1774 children postpolysomnography undergoing adenotonsillectomy, it was found that those with an apnea-hypopnea index ≥30 or an SaO_2 <70% and major medical comorbidity warrant being considered for a PICU admission.[122] This current evidence suggests that severe OSA with respiratory indices during polysomnography (SaO_2 <80% or end-tidal partial pressure of carbon dioxide [PCO_2] ≥60 mm Hg) and the presence of comorbidities (craniofacial anomaly, morbid obesity, neuromuscular disorders) should raise an index of suspicion that a PICU bed may be warranted following tonsillectomy.

Many selected posttonsillectomy patients may not require routine admission for intensive care if they have had an incident-free period in PACU, even if they were deemed to be high-risk in the preoperative assessment.[123–125] The level of care they require in PACU will usually reflect the level of care required on the ward or in PICU. The decision to admit patients to PICU or the ward should remain flexible. A postoperative PACU assessment is just as important as a preoperative assessment to provide an appropriate level of care for the child with OSA after adenotonsillectomy.[126,127]

HYPOXEMIA

Hypoxemia may result from hypoventilation, upper airway obstruction, bronchospasm, aspiration, pulmonary edema, pneumothorax, atelectasis, cardiac shunting, pulmonary embolism, or rarely from postobstructive pulmonary edema.[119] Hypoxia occurs more rapidly and may be more profound during emergence from general anesthesia because general anesthesia inhibits the hypoxic and hypercapnic ventilatory drive, reduces functional residual capacity, and alters hypoxic pulmonary vasoconstriction. Hypoxia

may also develop rapidly if the clinician suctioned the tracheal tube immediately before extubation without performing an alveolar recruitment with 100% oxygen to prevent desaturation.[106] Shivering may further increase oxygen consumption by a factor of 2- to 5-fold[128,129] and exacerbate the rate of developing and severity of hemoglobin desaturation.

Postoperative hemoglobin desaturation is more common in children with or recovering from an active upper respiratory tract infection owing to increased airway reactivity, atelectasis, and increased secretions than in children without a history of upper respiratory tract infection.[130–132] In neonates, hypoxia *increases* ventilation for approximately 1 minute but then *depresses* the respiratory drive (i.e., respiratory rate and tidal volume).[133] The normal ventilatory response to hypoxia is delayed for several months in former premature nursery graduates with severe bronchopulmonary dysplasia, placing them at particular risk for desaturation in the perioperative period.[134]

HYPOVENTILATION

Severe hypoventilation causes respiratory acidosis, hypoxemia, carbon dioxide narcosis, and apnea. Hypoventilation may result from a decrease in ventilatory drive, muscle weakness, or mechanical effects. Inhalational anesthetics, opioids, benzodiazepines, and other sedating medications (except α_2-agonists) decrease the ventilatory drive in children in a dose-dependent manner (see Figs. 2.13 and 2.14). At particular risk for postoperative hypoventilation are children with underlying disturbances in respiration, such as infants with apnea of prematurity (formerly preterm infants of less than 60 weeks postconception age [PCA]) (see Fig. 2.12); those with central nervous system injury such as head injury, strokes, and intracranial surgery; obese children; and those with OSA. These children may require prolonged observation in a setting with continuous monitoring capabilities.

Muscular weakness may contribute to respiratory insufficiency. Preexisting muscular disorders (e.g., muscular dystrophy) and inadequate antagonism of neuromuscular blockade, electrolyte abnormalities, neurologic disorders, drugs, infection, hypothermia, and endocrine disease may impair the respiratory effort sufficiently to cause hypoventilation and respiratory insufficiency.[135] Inadequate analgesia can lead to splinting and hypoventilation, which may in turn increase ventilation-perfusion mismatch and decrease the oxygen saturation.

AIRWAY OBSTRUCTION

Among the most common and serious problems in the PACU is upper airway obstruction. Airway obstruction is a feature in children with known airway problems resulting from congenital anomalies of the face (particularly those with midfacial hypoplasia as in trisomy 21, achondroplasia, and Crouzon disease), micrognathia (as in Pierre Robin sequence), and obese children with a history of OSA. Clinical hallmarks of airway obstruction include hemoglobin desaturation, inspiratory stridor, inspiratory retraction, and paradoxical chest wall motion. Auscultation of either the lungs or the trachea is a quick and effective method of detecting the presence or absence of air movement. If there is any doubt about the patency of a patient's airway, auscultation can be performed in a matter of seconds. Common interventions for the child who is attempting to breathe but remains obstructed include stimulating the child, repositioning, suctioning, performing a jaw thrust, insertion of an oral or nasal airway, and application of positive end-expiratory pressure (PEEP) (see Figure 31.8). If the child is unconscious, strategies should be undertaken to restore consciousness and spontaneous respirations. If these measures fail, patency of the upper and lower airways should be considered because gas exchange may be compromised by laryngospasm, subglottic narrowing as the result of edema, bronchospasm, atelectasis, or tracheal secretions. Incomplete recovery from general anesthesia or neuromuscular blockade,[136] a neck wound hematoma (such as after a thyroidectomy), and vocal cord paralysis may also lead to upper airway obstruction. If the airway is not cleared by any of the previously described maneuvers, oxygen should be administered by mask with continuous positive airway pressure along with the medications necessary to intubate the trachea.

Postobstructive pulmonary edema is a complication of acute upper airway obstruction and after relief of chronic airway obstruction following tonsillectomy.[137] The mechanism appears to be generation of extreme negative intrathoracic pressure against a closed glottis or obstructed airway and its sudden release, resulting in a dramatic increase in pulmonary blood flow that leads to noncardiogenic or neurogenic pulmonary edema.[138,139] This complication should be suspected when hypoxia, persistent tachypnea, or tachycardia follows a prolonged episode of laryngospasm, airway obstruction, or tonsillectomy and the child has pink, frothy secretions emanating from the airway. Treatment of noncardiogenic pulmonary edema includes tracheal intubation, positive-pressure ventilation with PEEP, 100% oxygen to maintain an adequate oxygen tension, furosemide, and morphine. Furosemide 0.5 to 1 mg/kg IV should be given intravenously; its immediate effects to clear the lungs are mediated by venodilation (decreasing preload) and improving the translocation of fluids out of the airspaces via the alveolar epithelium, and later by diuresis.[140–143]

Postintubation croup or subglottic edema has been associated with factors such as traumatic intubation, tight-fitting tracheal tubes, multiple intubation attempts, coughing with an in situ tracheal tube, a change in the child's position during surgery, prolonged duration of intubation, surgery of the head and neck, and a history of prematurity (with neonatal intubation), Down syndrome, or croup.[144,145] If the symptoms do not abate, nebulized epinephrine (0.5 mg/kg up to a maximum of 5 mg, or 0.25 to 0.75 mL of 2.25% racemic epinephrine) should be administered, although its effects are temporary.[146] Repeated use of epinephrine may cause rebound laryngeal edema.[145] If nebulized epinephrine is used, a prolonged period of observation is mandated. Outpatients may require overnight hospital admission or observation in the unit for an extended period. Steroids (e.g., dexamethasone 0.6 mg/kg) are effective for reducing mucosal edema but maximum response is delayed (approximately 6 hours).[147]

RESPIRATORY EFFORT

If the airway is patent, attention turns to the adequacy of ventilatory effort. Residual neuromuscular blockade can be assessed qualitatively (i.e., the patient's ability to lift extremities against gravity or perform a sustained head lift) and quantitatively using a peripheral nerve stimulator. Depending on the severity and the clinical situation, this condition may be treated with supplemental doses of reversal agents (unless sugammadex had been used to restore neuromuscular function) or ventilatory assistance.[148] If the respiratory rate is slow, suggesting opioid-induced respiratory depression, titrated incremental doses of naloxone (0.01 to 0.1 μg/kg) to antagonize the respiratory depression without precipitating acute anxiety, pain, or pulmonary edema is indicated. Risk factors

for opioid-induced respiratory depression include age less than 1 year, OSA, obesity, prematurity, and developmental delay.[149] If naloxone is effective, continuous monitoring of respiratory status is advised because naloxone has a short half-life of approximately 20 minutes. The same effective total dose of naloxone that restored respiration may be given intramuscularly to prevent a recrudescence of the opioid-induced respiratory depression. Alternately, nalmefene (Revex), a congener of naltrexone with a half-life of 10 hours, may be used to reverse the opioid-induced respiratory depression (see Chapter 5); its use is primarily for opioid overdose rather than antagonism of anesthesia-associated respiratory depression.[150] Residual sedation or paradoxical excitation[151,152] after benzodiazepines may be antagonized with flumazenil but may require an additional 2 hours of observation to ensure that sedation does not recur after reversal.[153]

Children who have an adequate airway and adequate muscular strength may experience difficulty breathing because of pain, restriction from bandages or casts, abdominal distention, pneumothorax, atelectasis, aspiration pneumonitis, or cardiogenic or postobstructive pulmonary edema. In most cases, the history and physical examination focus on the differential diagnosis, and when necessary, investigations that include a chest radiograph, blood gas analysis, and possibly invasive hemodynamic monitoring can identify the underlying cause and guide effective treatment.

DISCHARGE OF PRETERM INFANTS FROM THE POSTANESTHESIA CARE UNIT

Preterm infants (<37 weeks gestation) are at risk for apnea after sedation, spinal,[154,155] or general anesthesia; however, the risk decreases as infants age and the risk for early apnea is more common following general anesthesia, whereas late apnea (after PACU discharge) occurs with both spinal and general anesthesia.[156–158] Guidelines for monitoring after the administration of sedation or anesthesia have been suggested, but it should be noted that preterm and former preterm children are considered to be a heterogeneous population with various comorbidities and the decision on the length and extent of monitoring should be individualized for each patient.[159–161] However, it is recommended that formerly preterm infants who are 55 to 60 weeks PCA and who are not anemic and not experiencing apnea be observed for an extended period and, if stable, later discharged. Infants younger than 55 weeks PCA, those who are anemic (hematocrit <30%), and those with ongoing apnea should be admitted for monitoring.[155,156,161–163] Prophylactic administration of caffeine (10 mg/kg IV or orally) may reduce the risk of apnea after general anesthesia for infants at high risk, although it should not supplant postoperative admission and monitoring.[156,159,164,165] Former preterm infants younger than 55 weeks PCA, those with anemia, or those with major cardiorespiratory or neurologic disorders should be admitted and monitored for at least 12 apnea-free hours after general anesthesia, regional anesthesia, or sedation (see Chapter 2).[159,162,164]

It has been suggested that preterm infants who undergo surgery with spinal anesthesia are at low risk for the development of adverse events compared with those undergoing general anesthesia; however, it should be noted these infants remain at risk for late apnea, whereas those receiving general anesthesia are at risk for early apnea.[166–170] Similarly, caudal anesthesia has been reported as an effective alternative to spinal anesthesia in preterm infants undergoing herniotomy.[171–175] Despite evidence of a reduced risk of apnea after regional anesthesia and no discharge complications on the day of surgery in some institutions, there is insufficient evidence to make general recommendations regarding this practice. Our recommendation is to admit and monitor these infants regardless of the type of anesthesia administered.

Full-term neonates typically have a reduced risk of apnea and bradycardia after general anesthesia compared with preterm infants. Opinions vary on the minimum PCA for ambulatory surgery in infants 44 to 50 weeks PCA. Many children's hospitals admit all full-term neonates (<28 days of age) for overnight monitoring after general anesthesia, although this is not evidence-based practice. All full-term infants with a history of apnea and bradycardia or those who have siblings with sudden infant death syndrome[176] should be observed for an extended period or admitted for overnight monitoring after general anesthesia since their risk for sudden death appears to be 10-fold greater than children without this family history.[177]

Cardiovascular System

BRADYCARDIA

Bradycardia is the most common dysrhythmia in children and requires immediate attention because of its association with decreased cardiac output. *Until proven otherwise, the most common cause of bradycardia in infants and children is hypoxemia.* Other possible causes for bradycardia include vagal responses (e.g., passage of a nasogastric tube, laryngoscopy), medications (e.g., neostigmine, β-adrenergic blockade, $α_2$-agonists, opioids such as fentanyl), increased intracranial pressure, and high neuraxial anesthetic block. The definition of bradycardia depends on the age of the child; the incidence decreases with increasing age (see Chapter 2).

Treatment is directed at correcting the underlying cause, including the administration of oxygen, ensuring a patent airway, and if necessary, with ventilation. If these interventions do not immediately restore the heart rate, atropine (0.02 mg/kg) should be administered; if no response is observed within 30 seconds, administration of epinephrine (2 to 10 μg/kg) is indicated. For symptomatic bradycardia (e.g., hypotension, decreased level of consciousness), immediate administration of epinephrine is indicated. If there is no response to epinephrine, chest compressions should be instituted, and standard cardiopulmonary resuscitation algorithms followed (see Chapter 38).

TACHYCARDIA

Tachycardia is an important postoperative sign that is a marker for one of several disorders, such as inadequate cardiac output or oxygen delivery, a response to pain or a direct drug effect (e.g., epinephrine, atropine). Tachycardia may occur in response to hypoxemia, hypercarbia, hypovolemia, hypervolemia, emergence delirium, anxiety, sepsis, fever, a full bladder, a previously unrecognized cardiac conduction abnormality (see Chapters 14 and 16), heart failure, or malignant hyperthermia. The threshold for diagnosing tachycardia decreases with the age of the child.

Treatment is directed at correcting the underlying cause. Occasionally, children present with a sustained tachycardia unrelated to the previously described conditions that is refractory to the usual therapy. A cardiac consultation is required to investigate and identify uncommon causes, such as an aberrant conduction system or ectopic foci, as a source of supraventricular tachycardia (SVT). Supraventricular tachycardia, which is defined as more than 220 beats/minute in infants and more than 180 beats/minute in children, may be treated with adenosine when there are no other symptoms. The initial dose should be 100 μg/kg IV in children and 150 to 200 μg/kg IV in infants.[178] It should be noted that for adenosine to be effective, it must be manually flushed through the IV and into the circulation as rapidly as possible, otherwise its efficacy will be compromised. Most supraventricular tachycardias require more than one dose of adenosine to break the tachycardia. In a retrospective study of 44 episodes of supraventricular tachycardia, 30% of the tachyarrhythmias resolved with a single dose, 41% resolved with two doses, and 24% required a third dose, for an average dose of 173 μg/kg.[179] If the initial dose is unsuccessful after 1 to 2 minutes or there is a recrudescence of the tachycardia, the dose should be doubled with most arrhythmias resolving with ≤400 μg/kg.[178,180] However, supraventricular tachycardia with accompanied hypotension or decreased level of consciousness may require cardioversion. Children who have had prior cardiac surgery are particularly at risk.

OTHER ARRHYTHMIAS

Except for bradycardia and tachycardia, postoperative arrhythmias are rare in children. Isolated premature ventricular or atrial beats may be observed in the PACU and, unless they progress, are unimportant. Multifocal premature ventricular beats are uncommon in children. They may occur because of inadequately treated pain, a structural cardiac or cardiac conduction defect, or in rare instances, may be a harbinger of malignant hyperthermia (see Chapters 14, 16, and 39) with acute rhabdomyolysis and possible hyperkalemia. Electrolyte and arterial blood gas status should be checked. Children with known congenital heart disease should have continuous ECG monitoring in the PACU (see Chapters 14 and 16); all arrhythmias should be recorded, and a cardiologist consulted because this may be the first manifestation of a developing ectopic focus.

BLOOD PRESSURE CONTROL

Hypotension

The anesthesiologist should be familiar with the normal blood pressure ranges[181] of infants and children (see Chapter 2). The measurement should be obtained with an appropriately sized blood pressure cuff; the width of the cuff should be two-thirds of the length of the upper arm. An improperly sized cuff produces spurious readings. Small cuffs may overestimate the blood pressure, whereas large cuffs may underestimate it. The American Heart Association has published guidance regarding cuff sizes.[182] Evidence from adults indicates that inaccurate noninvasive blood pressure readings result from improperly sized cuffs and not improperly positioned cuffs.[183,184] A study in which upper arm and calf measurements were compared using invasive arterial blood pressures reported that noninvasive measurements deviate from invasive mean arterial blood pressure assessments (7 ± 7 mm Hg arm vs 8 ± 8 mm Hg calf, respectively) with a greater frequency of deviations of mean arterial pressure >10 mm Hg in the calf measurements.[185] Noninvasive upper arm and calf systolic blood pressures are similar in infants <6 months of age; however in infants >6 months and children of all ages, calf systolic blood pressures exceed the arm pressures.[186,187]

The most common cause of hypotension in children is hypovolemia, which arises from inadequate replacement of blood and fluids lost during the surgical procedure or ongoing blood loss. Clinical hallmarks of hypovolemia are hypotension, tachycardia, urine output of less than 0.5 to 1 mL/kg per hour, slow capillary refill (>3 seconds), and narrowing of the pulse pressure. If the hematocrit is adequate, hypovolemia may be treated with an initial bolus of 10 to 20 mL/kg of isotonic crystalloid solution or 5% albumin. This may be repeated until the blood pressure is normalized. If the hematocrit is inadequate, packed red blood cells (PRBCs) or whole blood should be administered. In this case, a rough guide for the volume of blood required is 4 mL/kg of packed cells or 6 mL/kg of whole blood to raise the hemoglobin 1 g/dL in children and adults (see Chapters 8 and 10). To achieve a desired hematocrit more precisely, the volume of PRBCs may be estimated as:

$$\frac{(\text{Desired hematocrit} - \text{present hematocrit}) \times \text{estimated blood volume}}{\text{The hematocrit in the PRBCs}}$$

If the child does not respond to volume expansion, other causes for the hypotension need to be considered, such as occult blood loss (e.g., intrabdominal, retroperitoneal, intrathoracic [blocked chest tube], cardiac tamponade), sepsis, or other disorders. Any factor that interferes with venous return can cause hypotension, including positive-pressure ventilation, auto-PEEP, tension pneumothorax, pericardial tamponade, and compression of the inferior vena cava.

Large end-tidal concentrations of inhalational anesthetics, local anesthetics, or opioids and interactions between benzodiazepines and opioids may produce hypotension through vasodilation (i.e., relative hypovolemia) and direct myocardial depression. However, these factors are rarely important in the PACU. Uncommon causes include anaphylaxis (e.g., latex allergy, antibiotics), transfusion reaction, adrenal insufficiency, systemic inflammation, infection, severe liver failure, and administration of antihypertensive, antidysrhythmic, and anticonvulsant medications. Increased body temperature may cause vasodilation and a relative hypovolemia. The increased metabolic demands of fever may compromise an already stressed myocardium. If a child arrives in the PACU requiring vasopressors and subsequently develops hypotension, consider mechanical causes such as a disconnect or kink in the vasopressor infusion, disruption of the IV access, disruption of the carrier infusion, a disconnect from the pump, or pump failure.

Vasodilation caused by sympathetic blockade associated with regional anesthesia occasionally causes hypotension, especially with a high-level blockade and restricted fluid intake. However, this is quite uncommon in children younger than 6 years of age. Because of the developmental changes in the sympathetic nervous system, most children younger than 6 years of age are normally peripherally vasodilated and therefore have little response to further vasodilation with a regional block.[188,189]

Decreased inotropy, dysrhythmia, cardiomyopathy, calcium channel blockers, sepsis, hypothyroidism, negative inotropic agents, and congestive heart failure are uncommon causes of hypotension in children. Treatment is directed at the underlying cause, such as correcting hypovolemia with volume loading, treating the allergic reaction, or treating the sepsis. Decreased cardiac contractility may be treated by diuresis and the administration of inotropic agents that also decrease the afterload (i.e., inodilators).

Hypertension

Postoperative hypertension in children is less common than hypotension and most often reflects an inaccurate measurement or pain. A blood pressure cuff that is too small may overestimate the blood pressure and should be one of the first considerations in the differential diagnosis, especially if the child has no other symptoms consistent with pain.[182] Additional factors that may cause hypertension include hypervolemia, preexisting hypertension (e.g., renal disease), distended bladder, hypercarbia, hypoxemia, agitation and delirium, increased intracranial pressure, drug error and exogenous vasoactive drugs (e.g., epinephrine).

Renal System

Complications related to the renal system are rare in the postoperative period. The most likely cause of low urine output (<0.5 to 1 mL/kg per hour) is hypovolemia (e.g., postoperative hypotension). Mechanical obstruction downstream from the kidneys may result from direct surgical interference or a misplaced or dysfunctional urinary catheter (i.e., blood clot or kink). If the child has regional (spinal or epidural) anesthesia that includes an opioid and there is no urinary catheter in place, placement of a Foley or straight catheter may be indicated. Renal failure is a rare possibility in children who have had major operations or have systemic inflammatory disease. If screening tests such as blood urea nitrogen, serum creatinine, and urine analysis suggest renal insufficiency, a pediatric nephrologist should be consulted (see also Chapter 26).

Gastrointestinal System

POSTOPERATIVE NAUSEA AND VOMITING

Postoperative nausea and vomiting (PONV) are two of the most bothersome adverse effects of anesthesia and surgery. Unlike adults, most children are unfamiliar with and have never experienced nausea. Hence, PACU personnel should not expect that children will complain of nausea after surgery. The Baxter Retching Faces (BARF) scale was introduced to assess the presence and severity of nausea in children >6 years of age.[190] A score ≥4 was associated with treatment with an antiemetic, although children were often not treated for nausea unless it was accompanied by emesis. In children, vomiting and complaining about a "sore tummy" are typically the first and only manifestations of gastrointestinal upset. Among children, PONV is inversely related to age.[191] The incidence of PONV is small in very young children, increases throughout childhood, and reaches a zenith in adolescents, for whom the incidence exceeds that for adults.[191,192]

The type of surgery influences the incidence of PONV. The incidence of PONV in children is greatest after tonsillectomy, strabismus repair, hernia repair, orchiopexy, microtia, and middle ear procedures.[191,193] Before puberty, there are no gender-related differences in PONV; after puberty, girls experience greater PONV than boys.[191] The medical complications of PONV include pulmonary aspiration, dehydration, electrolyte imbalance, fatigue, wound disruption, and esophageal tears. PONV can produce psychological effects that may produce anxiety in the children and parents and lead them to avoid further surgery. The cost implications of PONV can be major because of delayed recovery and discharge, increased medical care, and reoperation. Although these problems are seldom life-threatening, the cumulative costs in terms of prolonged PACU stays, unplanned admissions, and patient dissatisfaction are serious.[194]

Evidence-Based Consensus Management of PONV

Management of PONV is complex, and many treatment strategies have been formulated (Fig. 45.1). The superiority of some treatments over others has not been established, in part because of study design flaws such as inadequate dosing, small sample sizes, or varying periods of observation and data collection; some studies monitored PONV only during the first few hours after surgery, whereas others monitored the children for 24 to 48 hours after

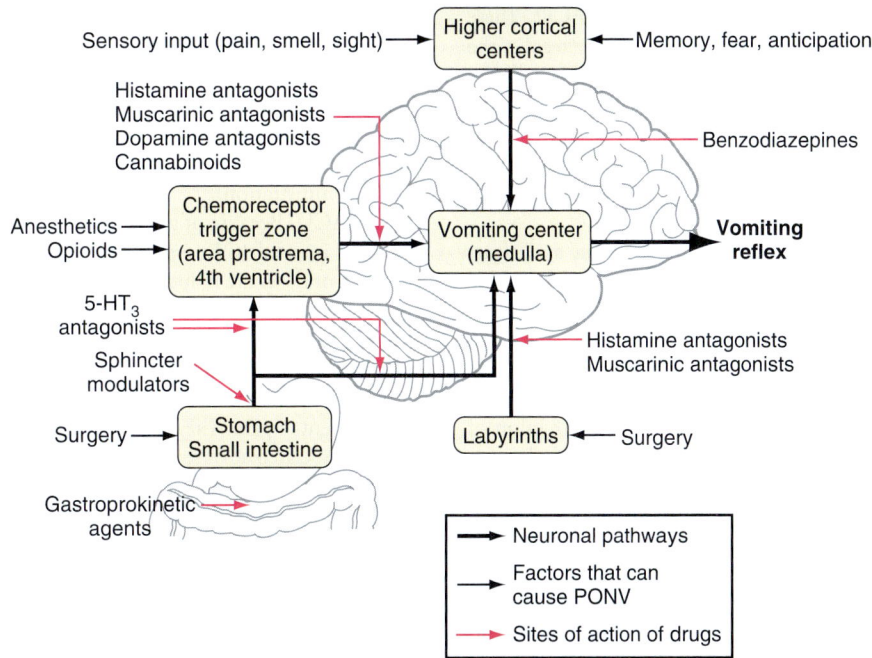

FIGURE 45.1 Treatment strategies for postoperative nausea and vomiting *(PONV)*.

surgery. To make sense of the conflicting data that exist, consensus-based management strategies for the prevention and management of PONV have been suggested.[192,195,196] These guidelines advise to first identify the children at major risk for developing PONV as outlined earlier and to then administer prophylaxis in that patient population. Studies frequently focus on postoperative vomiting as the primary outcome because nausea may be difficult to identify in children.

The consensus guidelines recognize that the choice of anesthetic can influence the incidence of PONV in children. Propofol-based anesthesia during operations associated with a large incidence of PONV dramatically reduces the incidence of PONV compared with inhalational anesthesia.[42,197,198] Similarly, multimodal therapy (i.e., a combination of PONV treatment strategies) is more effective than a single-treatment strategy.[199–201] Some advocate avoiding nitrous oxide to prevent PONV, although the evidence in favor of this position is weak and of limited clinical significance for ambulatory and most pediatric surgeries of less than 2 hours duration.[42,199,202,203] In a meta-analysis that examined perioperative PONV when nitrous oxide was avoided, the investigators reported a 2% incidence of awareness when nitrous oxide was omitted from the anesthetic regimen.[202] Additionally, in a comprehensive large study of PONV in adults given up to three antiemetics in the presence of inhaled agents, nitrous oxide and/or propofol, the reduction in PONV observed in the absence of nitrous oxide when two antiemetics (ondansetron and dexamethasone) were administered was <10%.[204]

Other prophylactic strategies recommended to decrease the rate of PONV include the use of the smallest dose of opioids that still provides adequate pain control and the use of regional anesthesia if possible.[205] TIVA is associated with reduced PONV (Chapter 6). The use of nonopioids such as acetaminophen, dexmedetomidine, ketamine, and ketorolac should be considered.[203,205] Adequate parenteral hydration and avoidance of early postoperative fluid ingestion can reduce the incidence of PONV (see Chapter 2).

Prophylactic Therapy

Ondansetron has been studied extensively as a prophylactic measure for PONV in children undergoing a range of surgeries.[206] It decreases both early and late PONV at doses of 50 to 150 μg/kg.[195,207] Because the 5-HT$_3$-receptor antagonists as a group have greater efficacy in the prevention of vomiting than nausea, they are the drugs of first choice for prophylaxis in children. Dexamethasone also is effective in decreasing PONV.[195,201,203,208] When administered in combination, the preponderance of evidence supports 100 μg/kg IV of both ondansetron and dexamethasone, the former 20 minutes before the end of surgery and the latter after induction of anesthesia.[206] Administration of dexamethasone alone or in combination with other antiemetics can extend the period of effective treatment up to 24 hours. Before the black box warning was added for droperidol, it was also recommended for prophylaxis of PONV in the United States[209]; however, for medicolegal reasons alone, it is no longer a first-tier antiemetic. Droperidol is commonly used in low doses, which limit extrapyramidal and sedation side effects. Adequate fluid resuscitation also plays in important role in PONV prevention,[210] for example, children given 10 mL/kg of lactated Ringer solution during strabismus correction had more PONV than those given 30 mL/kg (54% vs. 22%).[199,211,212]

The most effective prophylaxis strategy in children at moderate or high risk for PONV is to use combination therapy that includes hydration, a 5-HT$_3$-receptor antagonist, and a second drug such as dexamethasone.[213] Antiemetic rescue therapy should be administered to children who vomit after surgery. Although some guidelines advise against repeating the dose of 5-HT$_3$-receptor antagonist in PACU if a dose had been given intraoperatively, the possibility exists that the early onset of vomiting resulted from a single-nucleotide polymorphism in either the CYP450 2D6 isoenzyme that rapidly destroyed the 5-HT$_3$-receptor antagonist or the cassette transporter gene (*ABCB1*) that removes xenobiotics by rapidly transporting them across the blood-brain barrier and out of the brain.[214,215] Until routine perioperative identification of polymorphisms for these two genes is available, a second dose of a 5-HT$_3$-receptor antagonist could be given in PACU. These antiemetics have a low risk of complications and may resolve the vomiting if the cause was an unrecognized polymorphism.[216] An emetic episode more than 6 hours postoperatively can be treated with any of the drugs used for prophylaxis except dexamethasone and transdermal scopolamine.[195,217]

Alternative Treatments

Alternative antiemetic techniques for the prevention and treatment of PONV that have been reported to be successful include acupuncture, electroacupuncture, transcutaneous electrical nerve stimulation, and acupoint stimulation; however, these have not been shown to be effective consistently in children.[218–223] There are reports of the use of acupuncture (PC6) to prevent and treat PONV in children especially when provided before induction of anesthesia.[205,224–226] The primary advantage of this technique is that it is cost effective and low risk.

Postoperative Care and Discharge

PAIN MANAGEMENT IN THE POSTANESTHESIA CARE UNIT

Acute postoperative pain management strategies are discussed in detail in Chapter 41. A child's level of pain (or the perception of pain) changes more rapidly in the PACU than in any other unit of the hospital. Frequent and consistent use of pain scores for children of all ages, including those with developmental disabilities, is essential. Many pain scales have been validated for use in children. More important than the specific scale used, the scale should be used consistently and follow simple principles. For instance, children who are verbal and developmentally appropriate should be encouraged to describe their pain using a self-report scale (e.g., Oucher scale, or a numeric rating scale).[227] Young children or those without verbal skills should be assessed using an objective pain behavior scale (e.g., **F**ace, **L**egs, **A**ctivity, **C**ry, **C**onsolability [FLACC] scale).[228,229] Equally as important is the consistent application of protocols to treat pain; treatment of a given pain level should not vary from shift to shift or from one nurse to another.[230]

As with other areas of pediatric pain control, a multimodal approach to postoperative pain is recommended. A plan for pain management should be discussed among the family, surgical team, and anesthesia team before surgery. Depending on the surgery, the plan may include any or all: acetaminophen, nonsteroidal agents, local anesthesia, nerve blocks, regional anesthesia, α_2-agonists, opioids, patient-controlled analgesia, and patient-controlled epidural analgesia.

Acetaminophen and nonsteroidal antiinflammatory drugs (NSAIDs) act through inhibition of prostaglandins and their metabolites.[231] Many of these drugs can be given orally in the preoperative period or intravenously (acetaminophen ketorolac, parecoxib) during the surgery to be effective in the PACU. Occasionally, they may be indicated in the PACU if they were not administered before arrival. Oral acetaminophen (15 mg/kg) or ibuprofen (10 mg/kg) has been shown to decrease opioid requirements by 20% to 30% after a number of surgical procedures.[232,233] Intravenous acetaminophen has become a popular analgesia for mild to moderate pain in the PACU and as an opioid-sparing drug.[234–237] The IV dose of 10 mg/kg every 6 hours is recommended for patients weighing less than 50 kilograms and should be administered over 15 minutes.[238] Although instances of hepatotoxicity have been reported[232,239–242] in neonates, these are invariably attributed to overdose and not associated with routine care.[243,244] Acetaminophen is effective for the treatment of mild to moderate pain or fever[245,246] and concentration-response relationships in both children and neonates have been described.[247,248]

Acetaminophen 35 to 45 mg/kg can also be given rectally as a preoperative loading dose[249]; however, because absorption varies and is delayed (i.e., peak concentration at 60 to 180 minutes after rectal administration)[250–252] this route is not recommended for use in the PACU. Because of the pharmacokinetics of the rectal route, a greater interval (6 hours) between doses is recommended, and subsequent doses are reduced (20 mg/kg) so that the total dose per 24 hours does not exceed 100 mg/kg.[253] If a child has received rectal acetaminophen, the first oral dose should be delayed until 6 hours after the rectal dose.[254]

Acetaminophen and NSAIDs are often given together for the management of pain. They can be safely combined without increases in their associated adverse effect profiles. Combined acetaminophen and ibuprofen therapy for postoperative pain management[255] is supported over acetaminophen alone for tonsillectomy pain in children and following tooth extraction. Concentration-response relationships for acetaminophen, when combined with diclofenac or ibuprofen have been reported.[256–258] These response relationships generally show a maximal analgesic effect (Visual Analog Scale 5/10 to 6/10) common to both drugs, but that effect is achieved with lower doses of the drugs when combined. Bigger doses do not achieve better analgesia, but that analgesia is sustained for a longer duration than seen in single drug therapy.[256]

Simulation for a 20 kilogram child showed the addition of acetaminophen to ibuprofen doses of less than 5 mg/kg was effective; acetaminophen had minimal effect when given with ibuprofen at doses greater than 5 mg/kg in the immediate postoperative period. A more sustained analgesic effect was noted at 4 to 8 hours after combination dosing.[256,258] Similar responses have been reported in children given acetaminophen-diclofenac combinations. Combination therapy of acetaminophen 300 mg and diclofenac 20 mg was equally effective as acetaminophen 600 mg alone after adenotonsillectomy in a 5-year-old child.[257]

The NSAID ketorolac can decrease opioid requirements by approximately 30%. The recommended dosage is 0.2 to 0.5 mg/kg IV (up to 15 mg for children <50 kg and up to 30 mg for children >50 kg) every 6 hours.[259] Caution is warranted in postoperative children with significant bleeding or a history of renal insufficiency. The use of ketorolac is controversial in the pediatric orthopedic surgical literature because the drug has been linked to adverse outcomes including increased bleeding and nonunion of fractures; however, other researchers have suggested it does not negatively impact patient outcomes.[260–262] Similar considerations may also apply to parecoxib,[263] but animal models have found no negative effects on fracture healing.[264]

Opioids are indicated during the immediate postoperative period for any procedure in which moderate or severe pain is not being managed by other means. Morphine, fentanyl, oxycodone,[265,266] and hydromorphone have a long history of safe use for infants and children in the PACU when vital signs are monitored appropriately. Meperidine is only recommended for shivering in children because of the potential for seizures from epileptogenic metabolites (e.g., normeperidine) if repeat doses are administered.[267] Opioid dosing should be initiated according to body weight, physiologic development, underlying medical or surgical conditions, coadministered medications, and severity of pain. The goal should be effective and rapid pain relief. Subsequent dosing of the medications should be titrated based on response to the initial dose. Administration of multiple, small, ineffective doses results in prolongation of pain, stress, and anxiety without improving the safety of care provided. With this caveat in mind, patient-controlled analgesia and patient-controlled epidural analgesia (see Chapters 40 and 41) may be used in the PACU environment, but either intervention should be started only after acute pain has been adequately treated. It is essential to reduce opioid dosing by 33% to 50% in those children at risk for OSA due to their known opioid sensitivity.[32,268] In this population, pulse oximetry must be maintained at all times and deaths in PACU have occurred when monitoring was discontinued due to patient upset treated with sedatives or opioids and monitors not reapplied (see also Chapter 31).[269]

Regional analgesia is a common mode of intraoperative pain control in the child that extends into the PACU (see Chapters 40 to 42). The PACU personnel should be competent in assessing the adequacy of the block trouble shooting epidural or other catheter infusions, and familiar with the use and programming of the administration pumps.

Evidence that the regional block is effective should first be detected during surgery because the anesthetic requirements for successful surgical completion are reduced. The addition of hydrophilic opioids or clonidine may extend the level and duration of analgesia to some extent over the course of several hours; however, a block many dermatome segments away from the site of the surgical incision is unlikely to remain adequate for very long. The addition of opioids to an epidural or spinal block increases the risk of pruritus, urinary retention, and emesis. Similarly, visceral pain such as bladder spasms (which have thoracic innervation) or sore throat after intubation are not attenuated by a lumbar epidural catheter and must be managed by other measures.

The anesthesiologist must verify that the catheter is properly located in the epidural space. Older children can be questioned about their sensation level using ice or another cold sensation to determine the level of sympathectomy. Preverbal or developmentally disabled children require some other objective form of confirmation. Previous reports have focused on electrical stimulation through the epidural catheter at the time of catheter placement to determine the level of the catheter tip.[270,271] Ultrasound methods for detecting epidural catheter placement have been described.[272–275] Perhaps the most practical method may be radiographic confirmation of the dermatome level of the tip of the catheter, often with the use of an appropriate contrast material (i.e., epidurogram) to ensure appropriate placement in the epidural space. A small amount (<1 mL) of contrast (e.g., Omnipaque 180 or 240) can be infused into the catheter while a radiograph is taken to confirm placement (see Figs. 41.10 and 41.11).[276]

TEMPERATURE MANAGEMENT

Intraoperative normothermia is key to maintaining a normal temperature postoperatively. Hypothermia is associated with discomfort, bleeding, infections, altered metabolism of drugs, delayed return of cognitive functions, and prolonged recovery.[277–281] Because about 90% of heat loss occurs through the skin, only heat exchange through the skin in the PACU provides an adequate way of warming children. This method of warming is enhanced by the vasodilation properties of most anesthetic agents. Forced-air warming blankets are effective as the sole method for maintaining normothermia in children.[282–284] Given the vasoconstriction that occurs after anesthesia, attempts at warming are less effective postoperatively than intraoperatively, and most of the detrimental physiologic changes have already taken place.

Infants and children may suffer burns from overly aggressive rewarming measures.[285–287] This is particularly true for nonverbal children, children who are somnolent, and children who have decreased sensation owing to disease or use of regional anesthesia techniques.

DISCHARGE CRITERIA

The recovery process and discharge criteria vary from institution to institution. Some institutions require an assessment by a physician before discharge for all patients, but others require an evaluation only if routine discharge criteria are not met. The modified Aldrete scale is the most common system used to assess discharge readiness, but specific criteria depend on the particular situation or environment to which the child will be discharged.[288–290] For example, a child with a slight degree of postextubation croup or stridor may be discharged for monitoring on a pediatric floor or ICU, but the same child is not discharged to parental care and a 2-hour drive home. The criteria for discharge of children to a general inpatient setting are summarized in Table 45.8. For outpatients, these criteria hold, and the additional criteria outlined in Table 45.9 usually must be met before discharge.

TABLE 45.8	Discharge Criteria for Inpatients
1. Recovery of airway and respiratory reflexes adequate to support gas exchange and to protect against aspiration of secretions, vomitus, or blood
2. Stability of circulation and control of any surgical bleeding
3. Absence of anticipated instability in criteria 1 and 2
4. Reasonable control of pain and vomiting
5. Appropriate duration of observation after opioid or naloxone flumazenil administration (minimum of 60 minutes after intravenous naloxone and up to 2 hours after flumazenil)
6. Return to baseline level of consciousness unless transfer is to an intensive care unit environment

TABLE 45.9	Discharge Criteria for Outpatients
All Criteria in Table 45.8, Plus:
1. Cardiovascular function and airway patency are satisfactory and stable
2. The child is easily rousable, and protective reflexes are intact
3. The child can talk (if age appropriate)
4. The child can sit up unaided (if age appropriate)
5. For a very young or disabled child, who is incapable of the usually expected responses, the preanesthetic level of responsiveness or a level as close as possible to the normal level for that child should be achieved unless the child is to be transferred to another monitored location
6. The state of hydration is adequate
7. It may be permissible for parents to carry their children without full recovery of gait (parents must be advised that the child is at risk of injury if improperly supervised)
8. Control of pain should be achieved to permit adequate analgesia by the oral route thereafter
9. Control of nausea and vomiting should be achieved to allow for oral hydration (see "Discharge Criteria" in text)

Traditionally, children have been allowed to recover in a first-stage recovery unit until the airway is stable, consciousness is regained, baseline motor activity is confirmed, vital signs are stable, and oxygen saturation values are stable in room air (or at baseline) without respiratory support (unless needed at baseline). Pain should be well controlled. Children then can be transferred to a second-stage recovery unit, where more complete recovery takes place with a reduced nurse/child ratio, until children have met criteria for adequate hydration, minimal emesis, appropriate wound status, stable vital signs, and appropriate ambulation and mental status.

The requirements for children to eat, drink, and void before leaving the secondary recovery area delay discharge. Efforts should be made to reinstate volume homeostasis during surgery, negating any physiologic imperative for oral intake in the immediate postoperative period. Postoperative maintenance fluids should consist of isotonic rather than hypotonic solutions for those expected to remain as inpatients to reduce the risk of hyponatremia (see also Chapter 7).[291-294] Other than children who are at high risk for urinary retention (e.g., history of urinary retention, urethral surgery), there is little evidence that discharge before voiding results in readmission for voiding problems. In fact, this requirement is no longer part of standard discharge criteria.[295] Children who have received a caudal block for surgery are likewise at low risk for urinary retention as long as opioids have not been added to the caudal medication.[290]

Although there are few data on the current status of recovery processes across the United States, there appears to be a trend toward one-stage (fast-track) recovery for pediatric outpatients, even in those undergoing cardiac interventions.[296] This process allows selected children to bypass the first-stage recovery and go directly to the second-stage unit based on an appropriate level of consciousness, physical activity, vital signs, respiratory status, and pain control (Table 45.10). This approach has proved successful and quite safe, although appropriate attention to issues such as pain control must be addressed when initiating such a program.

Beyond PACU: Postoperative Monitoring in the General Care Setting

The transition of children from the operating room and the PACU to the general care setting goes along with a dramatic change in monitoring. Continuous, automated monitoring of multiple vital signs is replaced with spot checks of vital signs, often with hours in between. Furthermore, older children wearing smart watches have vital signs ranging from heart rate, oxygen saturation, ECG to heart rate variability readily available, while general care monitoring is often the same it was decades ago.[297] This discrepancy can be difficult to understand for patients, families, and even health care professionals.

Adult postoperative patients who are taking opioids are a subset of the inpatient population at particular risk for failure-to-rescue because of respiratory depression[298]; postoperative respiratory failure represents nearly 11% of all inpatient safety events[299] and has the greatest mortality rate per 100 discharges of all classified safety events.[300] A study in adult, noncardiac surgical patients who were continuously monitored with pulse oximetry found that 21% had oxyhemoglobin saturation (SpO_2) of 90% for an average of $\geq$10 minutes per hour and 8% had average of $\geq$20 minutes/hour, and 8% had SpO_2 <85% for $\geq$5 minutes/hour. A further 3% of postsurgical patients had SpO_2 less than 80% for 30 minutes or

TABLE 45.10	Discharge Criteria for Fast Tracking
Criteria	**Score**
Level of Consciousness	
Aware and oriented	2
Arousable with minimal stimulation	1
Responsive only to tactile stimulation	0
Physical Activity	
Able to move all extremities on command	2
Some weakness in movement of extremities	1
Unable to voluntarily move extremities	0
Hemodynamic Stability	
Blood pressure <15% of baseline MAP value	2
Blood pressure 15%–30% of baseline MAP value	1
Blood pressure >30% of baseline MAP value	0
Respiratory Stability	
Able to breathe deeply	2
Tachypneic with good cough	1
Dyspneic with weak cough	0
Oxygen Saturation Status	
Maintains value >95% on room air	2
Requires supplemental oxygen (nasal prongs)	1
Saturation <90% with supplemental oxygen	0
Postoperative Pain Assessment	
None or mild discomfort	2
Moderate to severe pain controlled with intravenous analgesics	1
Persistent, severe pain	0
Postoperative Emetic Symptoms	
None or mild nausea with no active vomiting	2
Transient vomiting or retching	1
Persistent, moderate to severe nausea and vomiting	0
Total[a]	14

[a]Pediatric patients must score 14 to bypass the phase 1 (PACU) recovery unit to be admitted directly to the stepdown care unit.
MAP, Mean arterial pressure; PACU, postanesthesia care unit.
From White PF, Song D. New criteria for fast-tracking after outpatient anesthesia: a comparison with the modified Aldrete's scoring system. *Anesth Analg.* 1998; 88:1069-1072.

longer.[301] This increased risk prompted the Anesthesia Patient Safety Foundation to advocate continuous electronic physiologic monitoring for all inpatients receiving postoperative opioids.[302] Adult respiratory monitoring with a threshold of 8 breaths per minute in PACU has become statutory care. Although equivalent data or recommendations for the pediatric population are missing, there is little reason to assume that similar considerations should be different in children.

Historically, the selective monitoring of children perceived to be at an increased risk for adverse events ("condition monitoring") because of comorbidities, surgical procedures, or opioid use has mostly failed. Recent research in pharmacogenomics as well as error analysis has provided more insight as to why condition monitoring is an inadequate approach to address the problem. Clinicians have been aware of interindividual variation in response to opioids, and advances in pharmacogenetics have provided the scientific background for these variations. The FDA has proscribed the use of codeine and codeine-containing cough suppressants in children after tonsil and adenoidectomies as a result of the single-nucleotide polymorphisms (SNPs) in cytochrome P450 2D6, in whom ultrarapid metabolizers experience greater morphine conversion and greater plasma concentrations in patients under the age of 18 years.[303,304] The estimated prevalence of ultrarapid metabolizers varies from 1% to 29%, depending on ethnicity and only 1.6% of patients have been reported as poor metabolizers (see Chapters 4 and 5).[304,305] Many other genetic variations are yet to be discovered but probably contribute to unanticipated adverse events.

According to The Joint Commission's Sentinel Event Database (2004–2011), 47% of respiratory depression events were wrong-dosing medication errors, 29% were related to improper monitoring of the patient, and 11% were related to other factors, including excessive dosing, medication interactions, and adverse drug reactions.[306] These data provide some insight into why risk stratification and selective, individual monitoring has failed. Future mitigation of drug errors by bar coding medication[307] and their administration as well as medication reconciliation efforts may minimize adverse respiratory events and make selected monitoring a viable option in the future.

There have been some successful implementations of surveillance systems to dramatically reduce inpatient adverse events by using pulse oximetry–based surveillance reaching back over a decade.[308] However, the understanding of surveillance monitoring and its approach of applying principles of population health medicine to hospital wards is still in its infancy.[309–311] Using a pulse oximetry surveillance system in an orthopedic inpatient unit, a research group at Dartmouth (Lebanon, NH) decreased unanticipated ICU transfers by 50% and activations of the rapid response by 65%. Using a static alarm–based threshold system for heart rate and oxygen saturation, the system redirects attention of nursing staff to these physiologic deteriorations via a paging system, prompting early intervention.[309] Routine surveillance using pulse oximetry for all inpatients on general care units has been institutional policy at Dartmouth since 2009 for adults and since 2012 for children. Because of the physiologic developmental changes in heart rate in children, creating static alarm triggers is more complex in children than in adults. Table 45.11 shows the alarm thresholds used at Children's Hospital at Dartmouth. Strategies to manage alarm fatigue and alerting for actionable events have been described for adults, but they apply equally for children.[309,310] The introduction of pediatric patient surveillance at

Dartmouth has decreased the use of the rapid response team because of earlier detection of physiologic deterioration, similar to that in adults.

The role and importance of surveillance monitoring and the needed expertise of pediatric anesthesiologists and intensivists is likely to expand in the future. With the rapid adoption of telemedicine, surveillance monitoring of pediatric patients is likely to exponentially grow not only in the inpatient general care setting, but also is likely to expand to the home setting as length of stay in the hospital will continue to decline.

ANNOTATED REFERENCES

American Academy of Pediatrics Statement: Critical elements for the pediatric perioperative anesthesia environment. *Pediatrics.* 2015; 136(6):1200-1205.

Society for Pediatric Anesthesia Policy Statement on Provision of Pediatric Anesthesia Care. http://www.pedsanesthesia.org/about/society-for-pediatric-anesthesia-policy-statement-on-provision-of-pediatric-anesthesia-care/.

American College of Surgeons. Optimal Resources for Children's Surgical Care; 2021. https://www.facs.org/quality-programs/accreditation-and-verification/childrens-surgery-verification/standards/standards-and-resources/.

The above citations outline the standards for the perioperative care of children.

Boat AC, Spaeth JP. Handoff checklists improve the reliability of patient handoffs in the operating room and postanesthesia care unit. *Paediatr Anaesth.* 2013;23(7):647-654.

The authors demonstrate improvement in effective communication through the implementation of checklists in the postoperative period.

Choong K, Arora S, Cheng J, et al. Hypotonic versus isotonic maintenance fluids after surgery for children: a randomized controlled trial. *Pediatrics.* 2011;128:857-866.

This important paper addresses the issue of postoperative hyponatremia in children. The authors randomly assigned 258 children to 2 groups receiving isotonic or hypotonic maintenance solutions. Children in the isotonic group had hyponatremia at a rate of 22.7% (vs. 40.8%), with no increased risk for hypernatremia.

Coté CJ, Posner KL, Domino KB. Death or neurologic injury after tonsillectomy in children with a focus on obstructive sleep apnea: Houston, we have a problem! *Anesth Analg.* 2014;118(6):1276-1283.

This paper reported 16 children who died or suffered neurologic injury within 24 hours of their tonsillectomy. Thirteen died at home, one on the ward that evening, but most importantly two died in PACU after monitors were removed; one in his father's lap and the other in bed next to mom. These cases illustrate the insidious nature of obstructive sleep apnea and why such children require the utmost attention to opioid dosing and monitoring with a need for postoperative admission and monitoring for those with severe obstructive sleep apnea.

Coté CJ, Zaslavsky A, Downes JJ, et al. Postoperative apnea in former preterm infants after inguinal herniorrhaphy. A combined analysis. *Anesthesiology.* 1995;82(4):809-822.

Data presented by the authors are frequently used for admission requirements of formerly preterm neonates.

Cravero JP, Beach M, Thyr B, Whalen K. The effect of small dose fentanyl on the emergence characteristics of pediatric patients after sevoflurane anesthesia without surgery. *Anesth Analg.* 2003;97:364-367.

The authors performed a prospective, randomized, blinded trial in which they studied patients undergoing magnetic resonance imaging with general inhaled sevoflurane anesthesia through a laryngeal mask airway. They concluded that small doses of opioids decrease emergence agitation without increasing unwanted side effects.

Hannam JA, Anderson BJ, Potts A. Acetaminophen, ibuprofen, and tramadol analgesic interactions after adenotonsillectomy. *Pediatr Anesth.* 2018;28:841-851.

The authors explored analgesic concentration-relationships for combination acetaminophen-ibuprofen mixes. Ibuprofen had an EC50 for analgesia in

TABLE 45.11	Patient Surveillance Alarm Thresholds	
Age	Heart Rate (beats/minute)	Oxygen Saturation (%)
0–6 months	80–235	80
6–12 months	70–220	80
1–5 years	60–200	80
5–12 years	55–180	80
>12 years	50–140	80

A pulse oximetry–based system used at the Children's Hospital at Dartmouth.

children similar to that of adults (3.95 mg/L; 95%CI 2.57–7.53, vs. 5–10 mg/L adults). The maximum effect from combination therapy (i.e., 65% reduction in pain score) achieved satisfactory analgesia with commonly used doses; increased dose adds little additional benefit, although duration of effect was increased. The addition of tramadol to this analgesic mixture also prolonged analgesia duration.

Hicks CW, Rosen M, Hobson DB, et al. Improving safety and quality of care with enhanced teamwork through operating room briefings. *JAMA Surg.* 2014;149(8):863-868.

The authors describe methods to improve operating room communication and provide examples of successful methods.

Jung H, Kim HJ, Lee YC, Kim HJ. Comparison of lateral and supine positions for tracheal extubation in children. *Anaesthesist.* 2019; 68(5):303-308.

The authors demonstrated that compared to supine extubation, deep extubation in the lateral decubitus position decreases the incidence of airway obstruction and improves oxygen saturation during emergence from anesthesia. Reasons include improved patency of noncartilaginous airway structure and decreased incidence of pulmonary aspiration.

Kain ZN, Caldwell-Andrews AA, Maranets I, et al. Preoperative anxiety and emergence delirium and postoperative maladaptive behaviors. *Anesth Analg.* 2004;99:1648-1654.

This study is extremely unusual in its ability to correlate perioperative anxiety with the incidence of emergence agitation. Preoperative anxiety is significantly related to the incidence of emergence agitation, and the incidence of agitation is related to the rate of postoperative maladaptive behaviors. This study argues strongly for identifying children at risk for emergence agitation and provides some evidence for why it is worth the effort to prevent or ameliorate this phenomenon.

Morrison C, Wilmshurst S. Postoperative vomiting in children. *BJA Education.* 2019;19:329-333.

Most pediatric anesthesia societies or associations have produced guidelines for the management of postoperative nausea and vomiting. This review article looks at the rationale behind causes, groups at risk, drug choices, combinations, prevention, and active management.

Oviedo P, Engorn B, Carvalho D, Hamrick J, Fisher B, Gollin G. The impact of routine post-anesthesia care unit extubation for pediatric surgical patients on safety and operating room efficiency. *J Pediatr Surg.* 2022;57(1):100-103.

The authors demonstrated that routinely extubating patients in the postanesthesia care unit increases operating room efficiency, potentially reduces costs, and does not compromise safety. The presence of a pediatric anesthesiologist is essential to manage any respiratory events.

Taenzer AH, Pyke JB, McGrath SP. A review of current and emerging approaches to address failure-to-rescue. *Anesthesiology.* 2011;115(2): 421-431.

The authors describe and review the current state of failure-to-rescue for inpatients and discuss strategies to mitigate adverse events.

A complete reference list can be found online at Elsevier eBooks+.

Procedures for Vascular Access

PEGGY YIP AND CHARLES J. COTÉ

46

Infection Control Practice	**Arterial Cannulation**
Safety Measures	Umbilical Artery
Venous Cannulation	Radial Artery
Peripheral Intravenous Cannulation	Brachial Artery
Establishing a Large Intravenous Catheter in Small Patients	Axillary Artery
Intraosseous Infusion	Temporal Artery
Central Venous Catheterization	Femoral Artery
Central Vein Cannulation Sites	Dorsalis Pedis and Posterior Tibial Artery
Vascular Access Specialist Team	

VASCULAR CANNULATION IS AN IMPORTANT PROCEDURE in the anesthetic and perioperative management of children. Establishing vascular access is one of the most common procedures performed by anesthesiologists and we encounter many different types of vascular access devices in our clinical practice.

The indications for vascular access are to provide routes to administer fluids, drugs, and blood products, monitor cardiopulmonary function, and access blood for laboratory testing. Pediatric vascular access can be challenging and complex especially in infants with chronic illness. The field of vascular access specialty has been expanding with an increasing amount of evidence-based literature.[1] Use of current evidence-based literature can improve success rate and safety profile and reduce complications. This chapter will describe approaches to enhance pediatric vascular access practice.

Infection Control Practice

The Centers for Disease Control (CDC) and the National Institute for Occupational Safety and Health (IOSH) recommended and published Universal Precautions for Preventing the Transmission of Bloodborne Infections for healthcare workers.* They recommend using gloves as a standard when performing a vascular access procedure. Catheter-related blood stream infections are associated with increased morbidity, mortality, and health costs. Appropriate use of hand hygiene, skin asepsis and maximum barrier precaution (sterile gloves, long-sleeved gowns, full-size drapes, and a nonsterile mask and cap) as components of the Universal Precautions are effective at preventing infections, especially in central venous cannulation (see Chapter 47).[2,3] An aseptic no-touch technique with an emphasis of keeping the key venipuncture site sterile after skin asepsis is used for peripheral cannulation. The practice of aseptic no-touch technique is also recommended for peripheral arterial cannulations and accessing injection ports

for these catheters after insertion.[4] Chlorhexidine has persistent bactericidal activity after application and when combined with alcohol, it speeds up antimicrobial activity.[5] A systematic review found that a 1% chlorhexidine solution offers greater protection from catheter-related infection than a 0.5% chlorhexidine solution or a 10% povidine solution.[6] Povidone iodine with 70% alcohol or aqueous povidone iodine preparations can be used as alternatives if chlorhexidine is contraindicated. Neonates, particularly those who are premature and have very low birth weight, are prone to skin reaction and systemic absorption of skin antiseptic agents; burns, dermatitis, and hypothyroidism are reported. Aqueous chlorhexidine preparations are currently used for skin decontamination in premature neonates.[7]

All intravascular catheters should be covered with transparent semipermeable dressings to allow regular clinical assessment of exit site and prevent contamination.[8] To maintain sterility and avoid cross-contamination, ultrasound probes should be covered with a sterile cover for venipuncture under real-time ultrasound guidance in all but emergency situations for vascular access insertions.

Safety Measures

1. Devices with standardized secure (e.g., Luer-Lok) add-on fittings should be used when available; they reduce the risk of disconnection leading to blood loss, failure to administer therapy, and air embolus.[9]
2. A calibrated burette limits the total infusion and provides a means to titrate fluids accurately in infants and young children.
3. A flow-limiting infusion pump is advised for neonates.
4. Flow rates may be altered by catheter brand, tubing type, and addition of extensions and stopcocks.
5. One-way valves in the intravenous tubing prevent backflow of drugs or infusions.
6. Air filters are useful for children at risk for paradoxical gas embolization.

---

*www.cdc.gov/niosh/topics/bbp/universal.html

Venous Cannulation

PERIPHERAL INTRAVENOUS CANNULATION

Indications
Peripheral intravenous (IV) access is commonly used for the administration of perioperative IV therapy that is nonirritant and nonvesicant to peripheral veins.

Practical Suggestions
Preparations
Peripheral IV cannulation can be challenging and anxiety provoking in children and for caregivers. Meta-analyses support the use of sucrose in neonates, topical anesthesia agents (e.g., EMLA, Ametop) and vapocoolants to reduce pain during cannulation in children.[10–12] Localized warming, premedication, comfort holding, swaddling, and distraction techniques can assist in securing vascular access prior to general anesthesia in some cases.[13] Common venous sites to secure access using the palpation method include dorsum of hand and foot, antecubital fossa (basilic or cephalic vein), medial malleolus of the ankle (saphenous vein), and the scalp in neonates, although complications occur more frequently when access is sited in the antecubital fossa (e.g., interstitial cannulation).[14] Prefilling the cannula with saline solution may reduce meniscus tension and allow a more rapid blood flashback. First-attempt success rates for venous canulation with the palpation technique in the emergency department range from 68% to 75% and with any technique in the operating room, 73% to 81%.[15,16] In pediatric clinical practice, three variables predicted the likelihood of failing to secure IV access on the first attempt: veins that are not palpable, veins that are not visible, and children who are younger than 12 months of age.[17,18] In the operating room, four variables predicted difficult IV access: infant age, obesity, American Society of Anesthesiologists (ASA) physical status (PS) 3 and 4, and emergency surgery.[19] Two additional variables, being of Black non-Hispanic race and Down syndrome, have also been associated with difficult IV access.[20,21] Ultrasound, transillumination, and infrared technology are available to aid cannulation.[22]

Saphenous Vein Cannulation
The saphenous vein is often a reliable point for IV access in infants and children that may be directly visualized or cannulated with a "blind" technique (Fig. 46.1). The size of the canula should be appropriate for the child's age: a 22-gauge catheter in infants, a 20-gauge in toddlers, and an 18-gauge in children >8 years of age. It is consistently found lateral to the medial malleolus of the ankle one-half to one fingerbreadth over the anterior quadrant.

1. Apply a tourniquet to the bottom third of the lower extremity below the knee. In general, the closer the tourniquet is to the vein to be canulated, the larger the vein will appear as the volume of veins below the tourniquet is smaller.
2. Laterally rotate the ankle while abducting the leg 30 degrees and repeatedly squeeze the heel and soft tissues of the foot to fill the veins with blood from the muscles.
3. Enter the skin at a 30-degree angle at the expected site of the saphenous vein at the level of the medial malleolus, with the tip of the needle directed toward the upper two-thirds of the calf. If no evidence of venipuncture is seen on insertion, slowly withdraw the needle because the flash of blood often occurs while exiting the vein.
4. If unsuccessful on the first attempt, fan medially and then laterally from the same insertion point, slowly advancing and

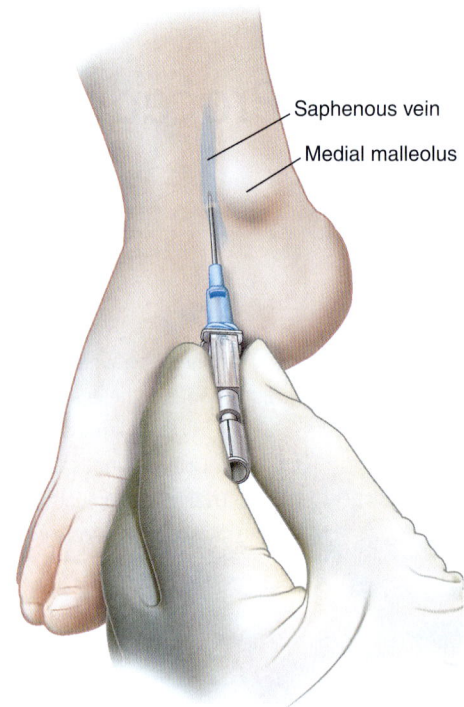

FIGURE 46.1 Long saphenous vein cannulation.

withdrawing the catheter until blood return is obtained. An aid to cannulation may be warranted if the vein is not easily accessed.

5. Once a flashback is identified, gently advance the entire unit 2 to 3 mm into the lumen before twisting and advancing the catheter off the needle.

Ultrasound-Guided Cannulation
Pediatric ultrasound-guided cannulation improves first-attempt success rate in children with difficult IV access, may reduce the number of attempts and lessens procedural time in the hands of experienced operators.[23–26] High frequency (6–13 MHz) linear ultrasound probes with small foot prints are commonly used to visualize superficial vessels in children. Vessel assessment prior to insertion aids cannulation. Vessels that are small (under 0.4 cm in diameter), too superficial (under 0.3 cm deep from skin) or too deep (over 1.5 cm deep) are more difficult to cannulate using ultrasound guidance in adults but this remains poorly defined in pediatric practice.[27] Ultrasound-guided saphenous and cephalic vein cannulation has a greater success rate compared with the dorsum of hands.[28] Long axis in-plane and dynamic needle tip positioning and short axis out-of-plane ultrasound-guided approaches are used during venipuncture to track needle tip movement during cannulation (Fig 46.2).[29] These techniques may reduce trauma to the posterior wall of vessels and guide intravascular placement of cannula. Such techniques could improve the longevity of peripheral venous cannulas.[15]

Dwell time of peripheral IV catheters was found to be greater with smaller diameter catheters and forearm insertion sites.[30] Complication rates from peripheral venous catheters may be reduced by using the smallest cannula diameter that is clinically indicated, ensuring over 65% of the cannula is intravascular, and

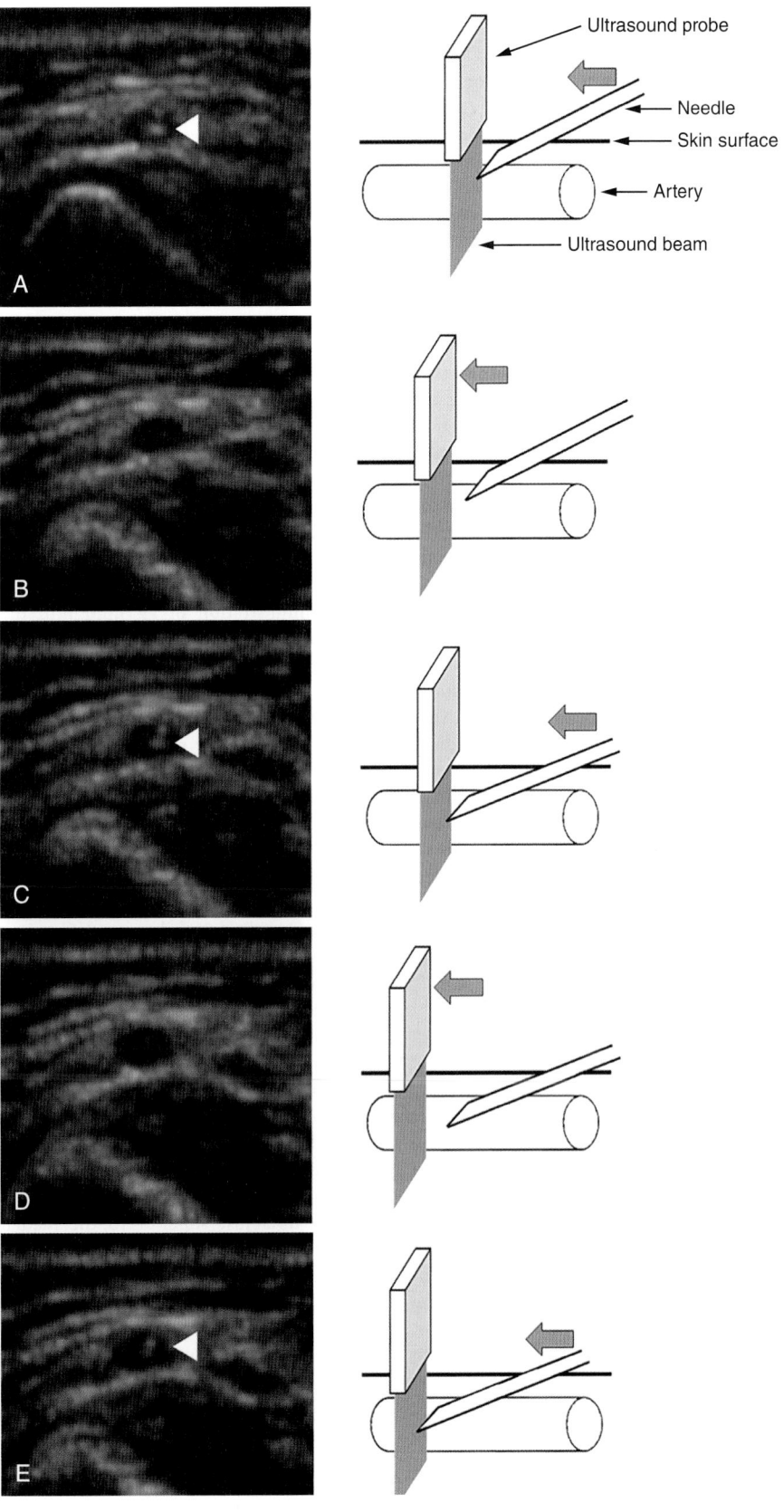

FIGURE 46.2 Dynamic needle tip positioning technique. **A,** Confirmation of initial blood return and needle tip visualization of the vessel on ultrasound screen *(arrowhead)*. **B,** The probe is advanced forward slightly until the needle tip disappears from the screen. **C,** The needle tip is advanced further slightly with a reduced puncture angle until it appears on the screen *(arrowhead)*. **D,** The probe is advanced further until the needle tip disappears from the screen. **E,** The needle tip is advanced further until it reappears on the screen *(arrowhead)*, and the entire tip of the outer catheter is advanced into the vessel.[29]

avoiding inserting the cannula over a joint to reduce catheter movement.[9] The US Food and Drug Administration (FDA) has approved the use of midline catheters for IV therapy for up to 30 days in adults. A midline catheter is a long peripheral catheter inserted in the upper arm vein with the tip located just below the axilla. Extended dwell catheter (long peripheral venous catheters or midline catheters) are being used in some pediatric centers.[31] Their extended dwell time could be related to optimizing catheter to vein ratio, ultrasound-guided cannulation, and a longer portion of the cannula residing within the lumen. Evidence is scant in children; further study is required to guide clinical use.[32]

Complications

Peripheral IV catheters are commonly used in the operating room and in the rest of the hospital. However, insertion failure rate and complications after insertion are high.[33] Complications seen in the operating room tend to be self-limiting and usually resolve with remediation (e.g., hematoma, dislodgement). Other complications like phlebitis, infiltration, and extravasation injury can lead to notable morbidity. The severity of extravasation injuries depends on many factors, including pH, osmolarity, diluent, vasoactive, or cytotoxic properties. The treatment of extravasation injuries varies with the extent of the injury from simple cessation of the IV solution and removal of the IV catheter while aspirating as much infiltrate as possible, to limb elevation, application of heat or cold packs, saline washout, topical treatments or injections (topical lidocaine, prilocaine, nitroglycerine, antimicrobials, subcutaneous or intradermal hyaluronidase, phentolamine, sodium thiosulfate or dexamethasone), assessment of compartment pressures, escharotomy, and in some cases, skin grafting.[34–38] Sepsis from peripheral IV catheters is rare but can cause serious patient harm.

Failure due to catheter occlusion can be due to mechanical obstruction or be thrombotic or medication related. There are insufficient data to support the routine use of heparin to prolong the patency of peripheral IV catheters in neonates and children.[39]

ESTABLISHING A LARGE INTRAVENOUS CATHETER IN SMALL PATIENTS

Indications

The following procedure is used for any child in whom there is the potential for massive, rapid hemorrhage:

1. Prepare and drape the appropriate area using an aseptic no-touch technique.
2. Perform a standard IV cannulation of an antecubital, saphenous, or external jugular vein with a small IV catheter (e.g., 22-gauge).
3. If ultrasound technology is available, preinsertion assessment and real-time guidance is recommended; this improves the success rate and reduces the complication rates.
4. Pass a small, flexible guidewire (e.g., 0.018 inch) through the IV catheter, remove the catheter, and with a No. 11 blade, make a small incision at the skin entry point of the wire.
5. Pass the next larger size IV catheter over the wire to dilate the vein and leave in place; stiff IV catheters are more effective. An alternative is to use a small dilator from a pulmonary artery catheter introducer and leave the sheath in place. The wire is removed, and the next larger size wire is inserted (0.025 inch). The catheter (or sheath) is removed, leaving this larger wire within the vein. This process may be repeated with larger catheters and wires until the desired size cannula or sheath is reached.

Rapid Infusion Catheters and Introducer Sheaths

Special rapid volume catheters (6 Fr and larger; Arrow International, Reading, PA) allow venipuncture with a needle or small IV catheter, passage of a guidewire, and then introduction of a dilator and sheath, with fewer steps required.

Intravenous Cutdown

Indications

- Percutaneous cannulation is unsuccessful.
- Percutaneous cannulation is tenuous.
- The catheter in place is inadequate for the planned surgical procedure.

The most common sites for insertion are the saphenous vein at the medial malleolus and the brachiocephalic vein at the antecubital fossa. This procedure may require considerable time to perform and has limited utility for emergent access.[40,41]

Complications

An IV cutdown has a high incidence of infection, and therefore should be used only on a short-term basis.

INTRAOSSEOUS INFUSION

The administration of IV fluid into the medullary cavity of long bones is a proven method for volume resuscitation in a hypovolemic child, and works even in teenagers.[42–49] This method can effectively deliver drugs to the central circulation as quickly as using peripheral IV infusion sites.[50] It is a particularly valuable emergency route of drug administration, even in the hands of emergency medical technicians[51–53] and as part of emergency department resuscitation of pediatric trauma patients.[46,54] Complications such as cellulitis, abscess, fractures, and osteomyelitis have been reported in less than 1% of cases, and this technique does not appear to affect later growth of the tibia with proper insertion technique,[55–57] but the time required for bone healing is unknown.[58] Compartment syndrome may occur if the needle is misplaced. These complications relate in part to duration of infusion, underlying medical conditions, and aseptic technique. The major difficulties with this technique are due to failure to adhere to proper landmarks[59] and bending and clotting of the needle. One should remove an intraosseous needle as soon as practical.[60] This technique is used in an emergency situation even in neonates[61] if several attempts at peripheral or central venous cannulation have failed, which generally means after three attempts or 90 seconds.[62,63] Sites for insertion include the upper medial tibia just below the tibial tuberosity, the lower medial tibia just superior to the medial malleolus (to avoid growth plates), the lower femur, and the anterior iliac crest. Intraosseous infusions are discontinued once an alternative IV infusion site has been secured. This technique has been successfully used for resuscitation of burn victims.[64,65] Intraosseous devices should not be used in a fractured leg. For the most recent, complete information, please refer to a review directed to the anesthesiologist caring for pediatric patients.[66]

Technique

1. Palpate the tibial tuberosity and prepare skin with antiseptic solution and sterile gloves. Infiltrate site with local anesthesia if required.
2. Locate a point on the medial surface of the tibia at least 1 to 2 cm below and medial to the tibial tuberosity for the site of needle puncture, because the mantle of the tibia is thin at this location (Fig. 46.3A).

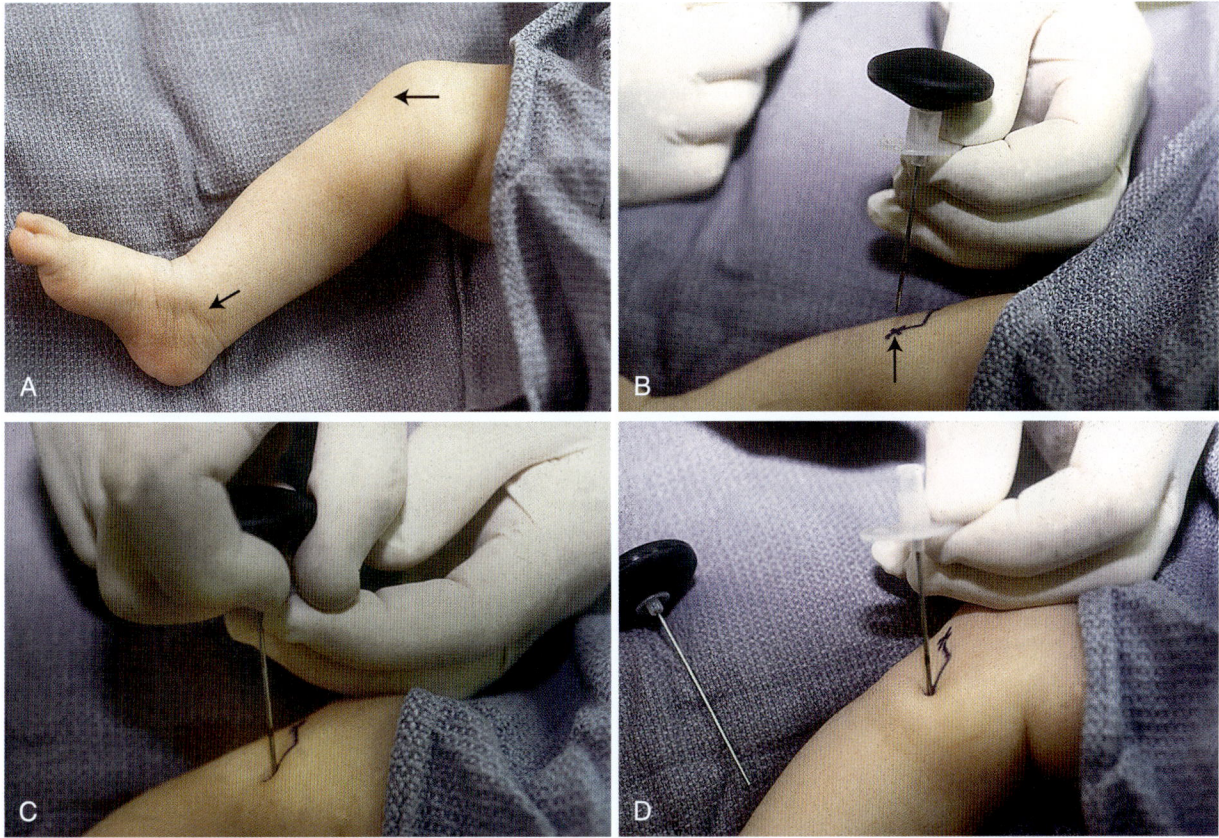

FIGURE 46.3 A, The intraosseous needle may be inserted in either of two locations: at a point 1 to 2 cm below and medial to the tibial tuberosity or at the medial malleolus *(arrows).* **B** and **C,** The leg is prepared, and the intraosseous needle punctures the skin (note the *X mark (arrow)* connecting the tibial tuberosity with the point of needle insertion); the needle is advanced with a twisting motion in a caudal direction. **D,** The stylet is removed, and the selected solution is infused.

3. Use a special short needle with a stylet to puncture the mantle of the tibia at a 75-degree angle directed toward the feet to avoid the epiphyseal plate (see Fig. 46.3B and C). A stylet spinal needle also may be used.
4. The appropriate position is readily achieved with the loss of resistance; take care to avoid advancing the needle too far (i.e., out the opposite side or against the opposite mantle of the tibia). The needle is usually quite stable if properly positioned.
5. Attach standard IV infusion equipment. Fluid should flow freely without extravasation (see Fig. 46.3D).

A mechanical handheld, battery-powered intraosseous needle insertion device that works much like an electric drill (Fig. 46.4) is the EZ-IO (Teleflex Medical Inc., Research Triangle Park, NC). Several sizes of intraosseous needles (depth of insertion) are available to limit the depth of insertion (determined by patient weight); we recommend that this device be immediately available in all emergency rooms,[67] operating rooms,[68] and neonatal and pediatric intensive care units,[61,69] because this is the simplest and easiest means for establishing emergent intraosseous access (even in out of hospital venues).[70–75] A simulation study found a very high success rate (27/30) with no difference between experienced emergency medical technicians or emergency room nurses.[76] The specially designed IV fluid low-profile adapter (already primed with IV fluid) is then attached to the sheath, providing clear access for drugs, fluid, or blood administration.

CENTRAL VENOUS CATHETERIZATION
Short-Term Central Venous Access
Indications
The common sites for central venous cannulation are the external and internal jugular veins, the subclavian, brachiocephalic veins, infraclavicular axillary veins, the femoral vein in infants and children, and the umbilical vein in neonates. Common indications for these central venous devices are for blood sampling and for generating cardiovascular parameters and surrogates for monitoring in the perioperative and intensive care setting. They also provide secure means to administer fluid and drugs that are sclerosing to peripheral veins and on rare occasions aspirating air emboli from the heart. They are not suitable for long-term use and are often removed after 7 to 10 days. However, if there is no sign of infection and IV access is still clinically indicated, there is no need for catheter replacement if the catheter lumens are patent.

Complications
- Arrhythmia
- Air embolus
- Local hematoma
- Pneumothorax
- Inadvertent arterial puncture
- Venous or arterial vessel wall trauma
- Cardiac tamponade

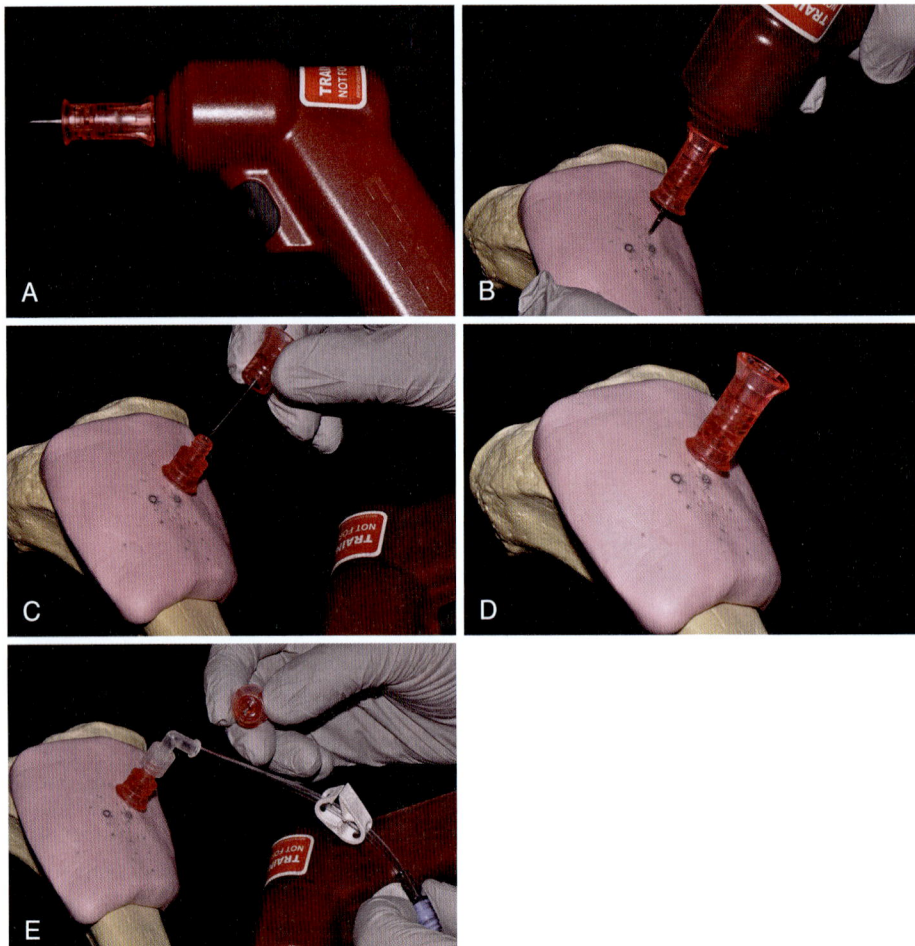

FIGURE 46.4 A, The EZ-IO (Teleflex Medical Inc., Research Triangle Park, NC) is a battery-powered intraosseous needle insertion device that works much like an electric drill. **B,** After appropriate preparation of the skin, at a point 1 to 2 cm below and medial to the tibial tuberosity, the intraosseous needle is directed down and away from the epiphyseal plate. **C,** After successful insertion of the needle and its sheath, the needle is removed, leaving the tip of the metal sheath lodged within the bone marrow cavity. **D,** The intraosseous system is ready for connection and use. **E,** The specially designed intravenous fluid adapter (already primed with intravenous fluid) is then attached to the sheath, providing clear access for drugs, fluid, or blood administration. (Courtesy Charles J. Coté, MD.)

- Thoracic duct injury
- Hemothorax
- Malposition
- Soft tissue infection around insertion site
- Central venous catheter–associated blood stream infection
- Vessel thrombosis
- Wire retention or embolus

Risk Mitigating Strategies

Maximum Barrier Precaution and Securement

Strict infection control practice must be followed during central venous catheter insertion and future access unless in life-threatening situations. Risk of infection can be further reduced by avoiding areas of skin injury or contamination and opting for the smallest caliber catheters with the minimum number of lumens as clinically indicated. Once insertion is completed, catheters should be secured to avoid dislodgement; the most common method is suturing. The insertion site should be covered with a transparent occlusive dressing to avoid contamination. The use of a chlorhexidine-impregnated dressing may be indicated for patients who are at greater risk of infection (Fig. 46.5). However, dermatitis related to chlorhexidine can limit the use in neonates.[77,78]

Ultrasound Guidance

Ultrasound-guided access assists successful cannulation of the internal jugular vein,[79] the infraclavicular axillary vein,[80] brachiocephalic vein,[81,82] and the subclavian vein.[83,84] Some international guidelines recommend the use of ultrasound prior to and during venipuncture to assess the vessel, identify anatomical variation, pathology, and surrounding structures.[85,86] When real-time ultrasound guidance is used, strict aseptic technique using a sterile probe cover and sterile ultrasound gel is mandatory except in life-threatening situations. Ultrasound training with good hand-eye coordination, equipment ergonomics, and a thorough knowledge of anatomy are essential for the safety and reliability of this

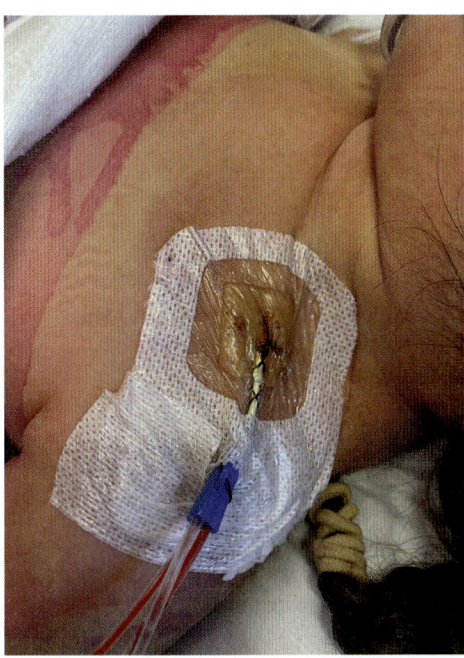

FIGURE 46.5 Chlorhexidine-impregnated clear transparent dressing covering left-sided brachiocephalic venous catheter.

technique.[86] The small size of neonates can make ultrasound probe placement and visualization difficult. Ultrasound guidance, pressure-waveform analysis, or electrocardiographic guidance may help verification of needle tip and guidewire placement and prevent complications related to central catheter placement.[79,80] Approaches such as the subclavian and brachiocephalic veins should be used with extreme caution in the presence of a bleeding diathesis because hemostasis may be difficult.

Use of Seldinger and Modified Seldinger Technique

The Seldinger technique and the modified Seldinger technique describe venipuncture using a small gauge needle or catheter over needle, respectively. The needle or catheter is used as a conduit for introducing a guide wire into the vein. Introducing a large catheter through the small venipuncture site minimizes the chances of hematoma formation even after systemic heparinization, and the procedure often can be accomplished when access is required emergently (Fig. 46.6).[87,88] The wire should advance easily. However, if the wire cannot be advanced, the needle has passed out of the vessel lumen or its tip rests against the vessel wall. In this situation, the wire and needle should be withdrawn simultaneously to avoid shearing the wire. If the wire passes without difficulty, then cannulation proceeds as demonstrated in Figs. 46.5A–C. The ultrasound-guided percutaneous approach to central venous cannulation is most successful using a modified Seldinger technique in neonates.[89]

Verification of Intravenous Location of Guide Wire Before Dilatation

Verification of the location of the guide wire before dilatation within the vein is recommended to avoid venous injury. Other methods of verification include ultrasound imaging, manometry, pressure-waveform analysis, or venous blood gas measurement. Blood color or absence of pulsatile flow are not reliable parameters.[8,90]

Catheter Tip Location Optimization

Whenever a central line is inserted into the heart from above, care must be taken to ensure that the catheter tip is positioned at the junction of the superior vena cava and the right atrium because that site marks the upper end of the pericardium (thus reducing the risk of causing pericardial tamponade should a perforation occur); other positions have been associated with perforation of large vessels and the myocardium, (Fig. 46.7A–H) and with triggering of ventricular arrhythmias.[91] Cannulation of the right side of the neck virtually ensures a central location of the catheter tip because the internal jugular vein, the superior vena cava, and the right atrium are in a straight line.[87] Cannulation of the left side risks possible pneumothorax because the apex of the lung is more cephalad on the left. Thoracic duct damage is rarely reported.[92] In addition, if the catheter is inserted on the left side and is too short to reach the heart, the tip may rest against the wall of the superior vena cava, be position dependent, and possibly erode through the wall of the vessel. Fig. 46.6A–H illustrates desirable and less desirable sites for catheter tips that may avoid or result in perforation. The optimal length of a catheter varies with insertion sites and the use of anatomical versus ultrasound techniques.[93]

The most common method of confirming central venous catheter tip location is to perform a chest radiograph or fluoroscopy after insertion. These techniques will also diagnose a pneumothorax if one is present. Radiographically, the tip should be visualized at the level of the T6 vertebral body, approximately one vertebra below the level of the carina and the lower border of the right main bronchus.[94,95] Other methods using transthoracic or transesophageal echocardiography, intracavitary electrocardiography, and computed tomography have been described to confirm correct positioning of the catheter tip, but they are less commonly available.[93,96,97]

CENTRAL VEIN CANNULATION SITES

External Jugular Vein Catheterization

1. Position the child in the Trendelenburg position with the head turned 45 degrees away from the side of cannulation. Locate the apex of a triangle formed by the two bellies of the sternocleidomastoid muscle. This point is usually where the external jugular vein crosses the sternocleidomastoid muscle. The external jugular vein lies in the superficial fascia of the neck crossing the sternocleidomastoid muscle obliquely.

2. Place a pillow or rolled sheet under the shoulders to extend the head and allow complete access to the neck. A J-wire is usually more useful to circumvent the plexus of veins at the clavicle.[98,99]

3. Many catheters will not pass beyond the clavicle or will pass into the axillary vein; success is generally more often attained on the right side.[100,101] If a shorter catheter is used, infusion and pressure monitoring will depend on the position of the head.[102] Continuous free-flowing infusion is best maintained with the head turned away from the side of catheter insertion. This vein is particularly valuable in children with difficult peripheral venous access and in an emergent situation that suddenly develops intraoperatively that requires additional and large gauge IV access. In this situation, a short but larger gauge catheter will be more valuable than a longer but smaller diameter catheter that passes centrally.

Internal Jugular Vein Catheterization

Numerous approaches and techniques are used for internal jugular vein cannulation.[87,103–106] A high approach using the apex

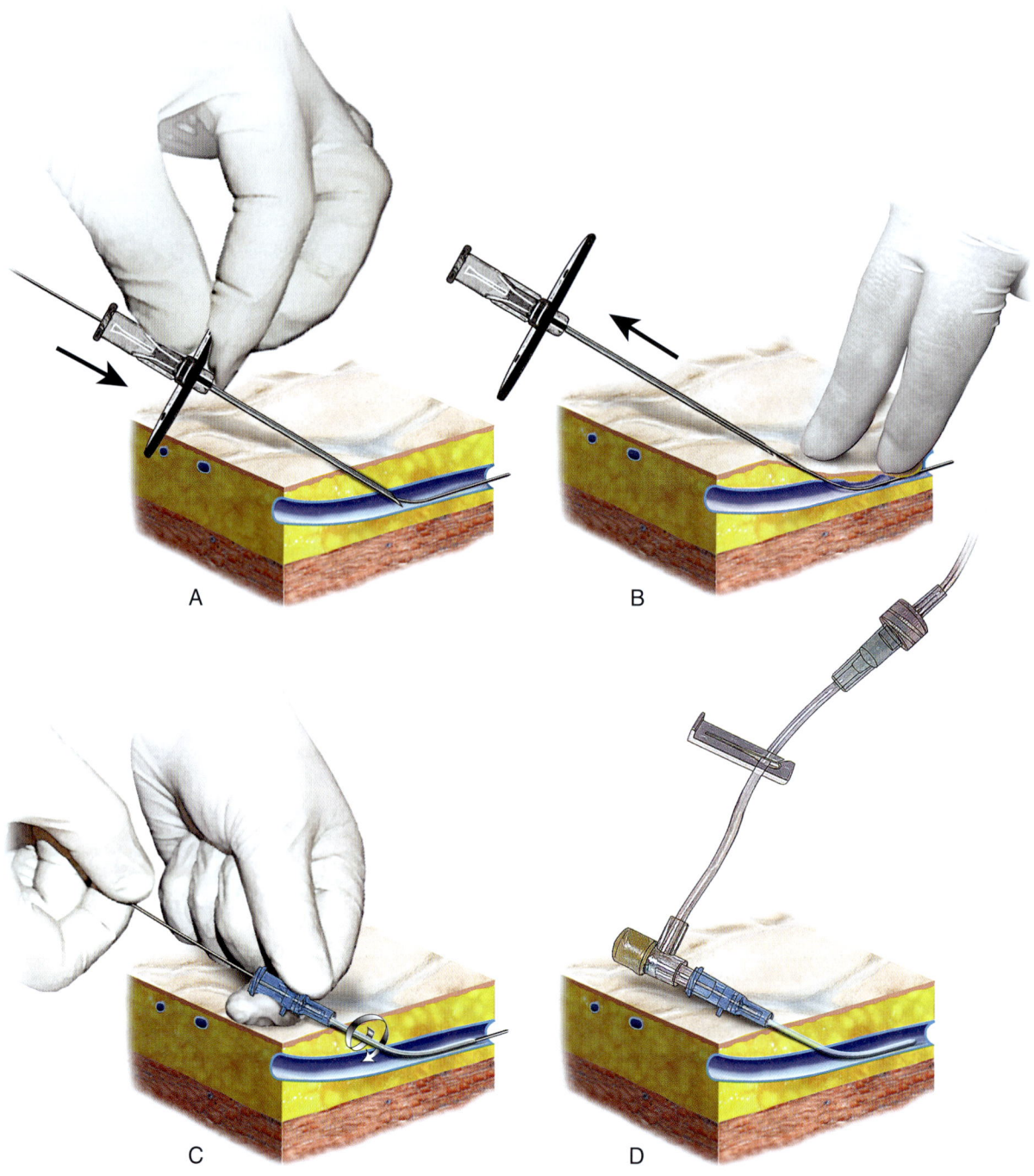

FIGURE 46.6 A, Seldinger technique for catheter placement. The needle is inserted into the target vessel, and the flexible end of the guidewire is passed freely into the vessel. **B,** The needle is then removed, leaving the guidewire in place. **C,** The catheter is advanced with a twisting motion into the vessel. **D,** The wire is removed, and the catheter is connected to an appropriate infusion or monitoring device. (Redrawn with permission from Schwartz AJ, Coté CJ, Jobes DR, et al. Central venous catheterization in pediatrics. Scientific exhibit, American Society of Anesthesiologists, New Orleans, 1977.)

of a triangle formed by the two bellies of the sternocleidomastoid muscle and the clavicle may be used as a landmark for insertion (Fig. 46.7A–C).[87] It is easily compressible in case of hematoma formation after accidental puncture in patients with a bleeding diathesis. The Seldinger technique without ultrasound use had a success rate, even in neonates, that approached 75% on the first attempt and 90% to 95% on the second attempt.[87] The principal advantage of the high approach is that the most common complication (arterial puncture in approximately 10% of cases) is easily recognized and treated successfully. A simulated Valsalva maneuver (positive inspiratory pressure of 25 mm Hg for 10 seconds), liver compression, and Trendelenburg position individually or in

46

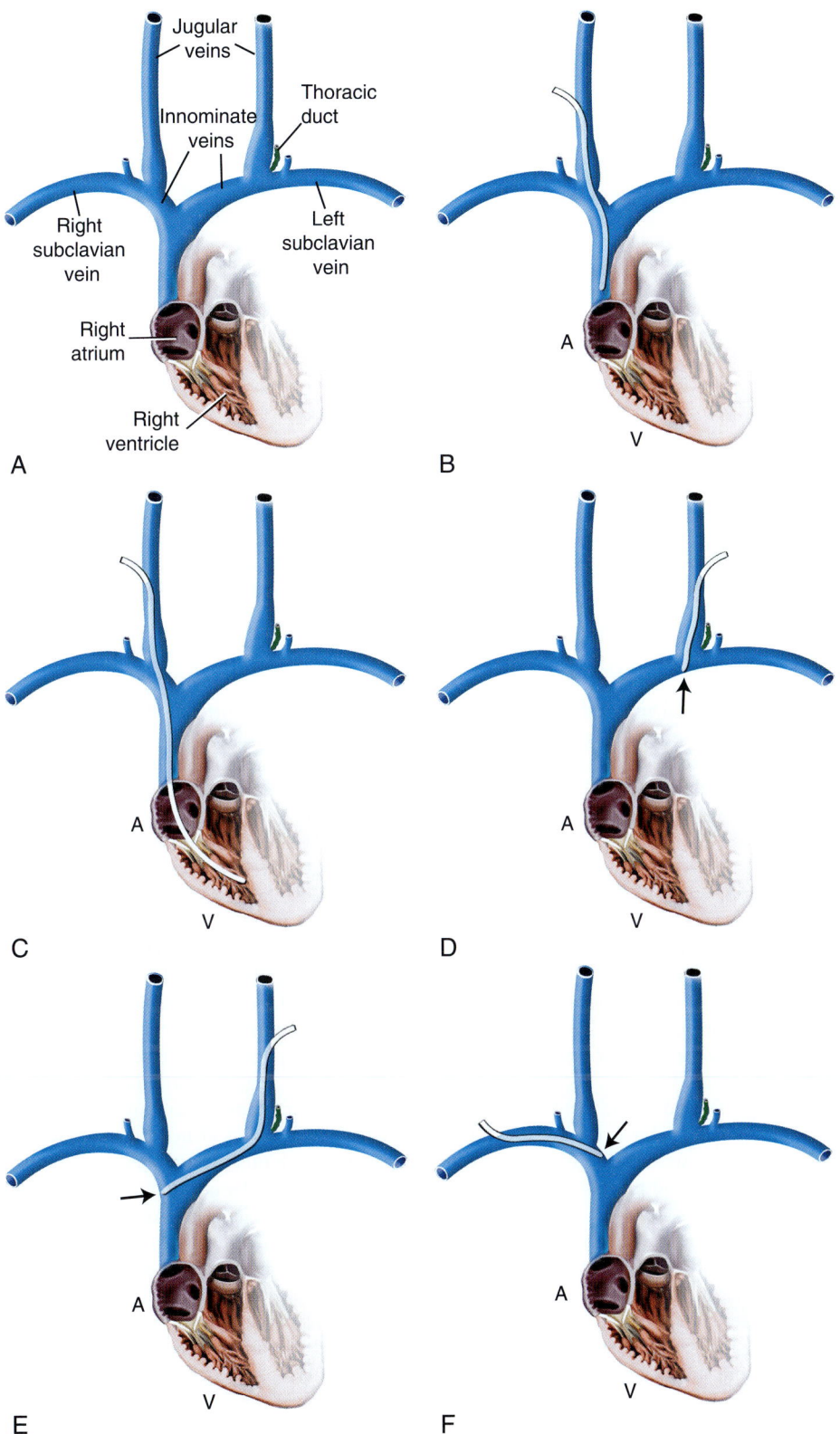

FIGURE 46.7 Proper and improper central venous pressure catheter placement. **A,** Normal vascular anatomy. **B,** Proper location for right internal jugular catheter (i.e., high right atrium or superior vena cava). **C,** Ventricular location of any catheter is dangerous and contraindicated. **D,** A short left-sided internal jugular catheter may erode through the innominate vein *(arrow)*. **E,** A left-sided internal jugular catheter striking the lateral wall of the superior vena cava *(arrow)* may erode through it and must be partially withdrawn or advanced. **F,** A short right subclavian catheter may strike the lateral wall of the innominate vein *(arrow)* and erode through it; this catheter should be advanced or withdrawn. *Continued*

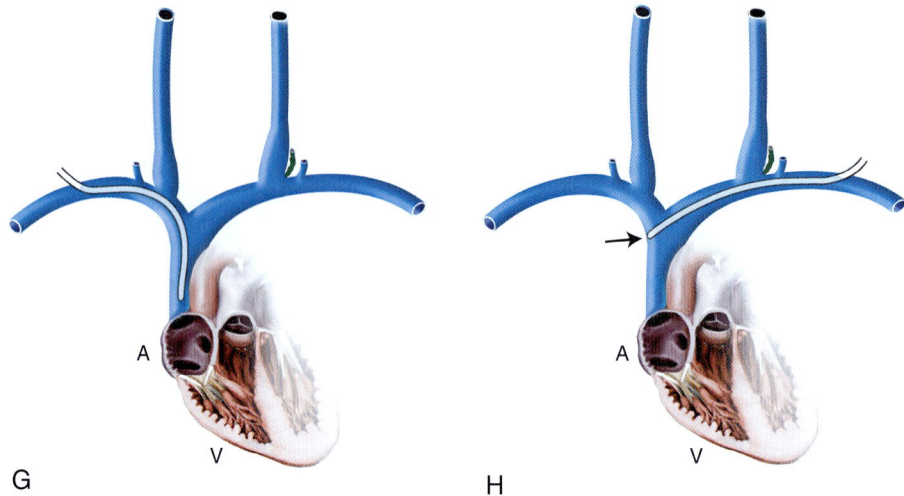

FIGURE 46.7, cont'd G, Proper location for a right subclavian line. **H,** A short left subclavian line may erode through the superior vena cava *(arrow)*; this catheter should be advanced or withdrawn. The optimal length of a catheter varies with insertion sites and the use of anatomical versus ultrasound technique. When inserting multi-lumen catheters with staggered orifices, one needs to ensure that the proximal lumen orifice is located within the intravascular space to avoid drug or fluid extravasation leading to infiltration injury and swelling. Most central venous catheters are 5 cm, 8 cm. *A,* Atrium; *V,* ventricle.

combination increase the cross-sectional area of the right internal jugular vein.[107] For neonates, a study using skin traction in infants weighing less than 5 kilograms showed that a technique using tape for skin traction combined with ultrasound guidance increased internal jugular cross-sectional area and decreased the time to place the catheter.[108–110]

TECHNIQUE

1. Position the child as for external jugular vein cannulation but with a rolled towel under the center of the back to allow the head to be slightly extended (see Fig. 46.8A–C) for positioning and the use of ultrasound to guide insertion). The head is turned 40 degrees from the side of insertion; *turning the head too far to the side may compress the vein and move the vein in closer proximity to the carotid artery.*[111,112]

2. Locate the apex of a triangle formed by the two bellies of the sternocleidomastoid muscle. This point is usually where the external jugular vein crosses the sternocleidomastoid muscle or the midpoint between the mastoid process and the sternal notch.

3. When using a landmark technique, palpate the carotid artery. Introduce the needle just lateral to the artery at an angle of 30 degrees to the skin surface and direct the tip of the needle toward the ipsilateral nipple (see Fig. 46.8A). If the internal jugular vein is superficial, a less acute angle may be indicated. While continuously aspirating, advance the needle toward the ipsilateral nipple a distance of no more than 2.5 cm. If no blood is freely obtained, slowly withdraw the needle while maintaining aspiration. In some circumstances the needle can compress the vessel on entry, and it straightens during withdrawal, allowing free aspiration of blood.

4. When using an ultrasound-guided technique, position the ultrasound screen in the line of sight of the inserter. For right side insertion, the inserter should stand at the head of the bed. (Fig 46.9).

5. Place the ultrasound probe over the apex of a triangle formed by the two bellies of the sternocleidomastoid muscle to visualize the transverse short axis view of the internal jugular vein and carotid artery. Use the "out-of-plane dynamic needle tip positioning" technique to track needle tip movement during venipuncture.

Subclavian Vein Catheterization

The subclavian vein is a site frequently used for central vein cannulation.[113,114] Success rates greater than 80% have been reported even in neonates.[115–118] The advantages include fixed landmarks, ease of securing the line to children for long-term management, and patient comfort. Disadvantages include pneumothorax, hemothorax, and the site is not physically compressible to reduce the risk of hematoma in patients with a bleeding diathesis.[119,120] A chest radiograph should be taken after the catheter is inserted and before surgery begins to preclude an unrecognized intraoperative tension pneumothorax. Early introduction of the Seldinger technique reduced the incidence of damage to intrathoracic structures compared with other techniques. In a comparison of neutral versus lowered shoulder position in 361 adult patients, neutral position reduced the incidence of misplacement of the catheter tip (ipsilateral internal jugular or brachiocephalic vein) with no difference in the rate of arterial puncture or pneumothorax.[121]

Historically, the internal jugular approach was associated with a greater incidence of positive catheter tip culture results (22% vs. 3.4%) and bloodstream infection (6.9% vs. 0%) compared with the subclavian approach.[122] There was no difference in first-attempt success (64% vs. 69%), although the frequency of arterial punctures was greater with the internal jugular vein approach (8% vs. 2%), and catheter malposition was greater with the subclavian approach (17% vs. 1%). A Cochrane review of 13 studies with 2360 procedures compared ultrasound cannulation of femoral or subclavian access with landmark techniques and found no difference in complications or success rate, although the experience of the clinicians was not examined.[123] Ultrasound-guided infraclavicular approaches for the subclavian/axillary vein are described in adult patients and used clinically (see Fig. 46.10).[124] Safety and risk profile is yet be elucidated in pediatric practice.[125,126]

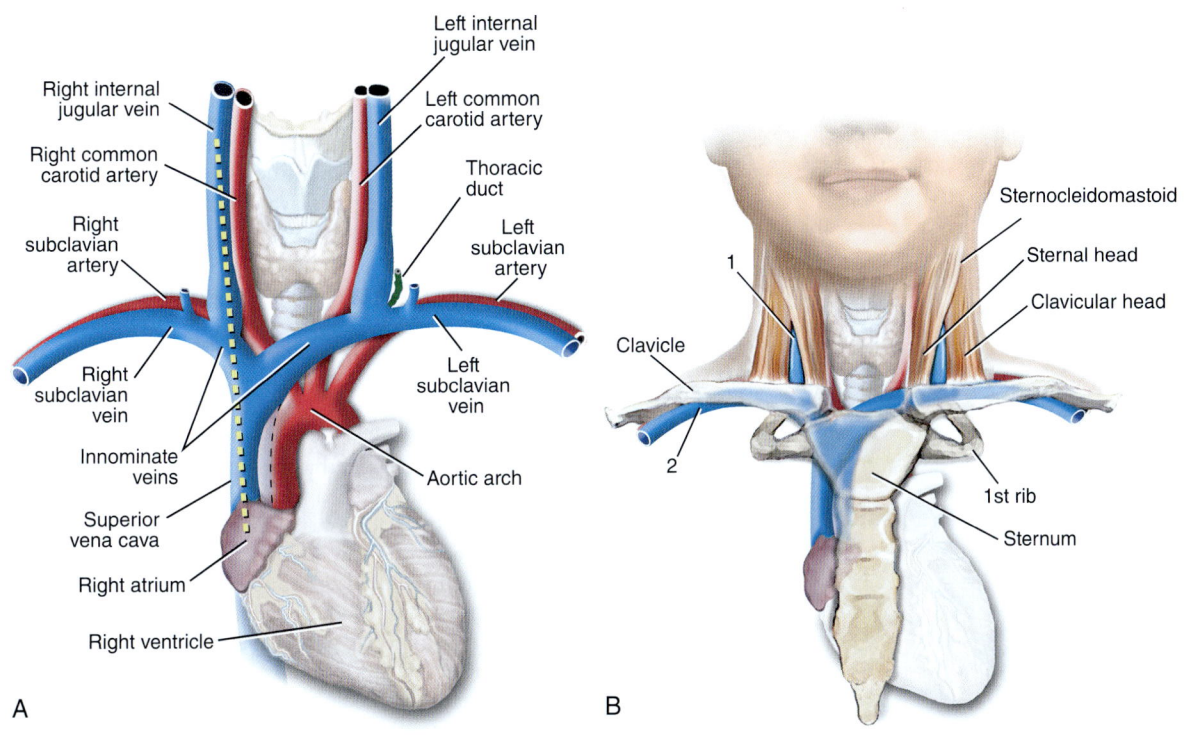

A

B

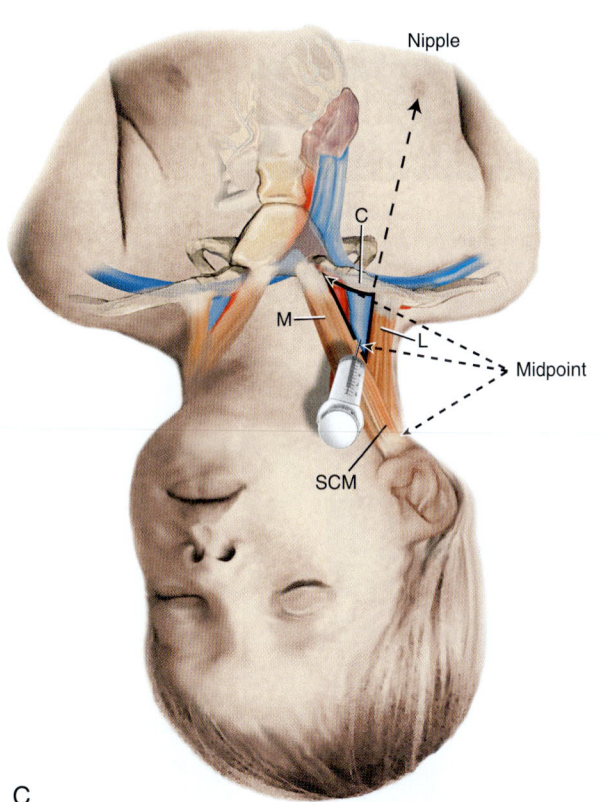

C

FIGURE 46.8 A, The anatomic relationships of major chest and neck structures. Note how the internal jugular vein is in close proximity to the carotid artery. Also, note that a nearly straight line is formed by the internal jugular vein, innominate vein, superior vena cava, and right atrium *(yellow dashed line)*; it is rare for a right internal jugular catheter to migrate anywhere but to the right atrium. **B,** The relationship of external anatomic landmarks to the anatomy illustrated in **A**. Note the triangle formed by the two bellies of the sternocleidomastoid muscle and the clavicle. *1,* The preferred point of needle insertion at the apex of this triangle for internal jugular vein puncture. *2,* The point of needle insertion for subclavian vein puncture. **C,** The anatomic landmarks as they would appear to an anesthesiologist. The needle is introduced at the apex of the triangle outlined in **C** and is directed at an angle of 30 degrees to the skin toward the ipsilateral nipple. This point of entry is generally half the distance between the mastoid process and the sternal notch. *C,* Clavicle; *M* and *L,* medial and lateral bellies of the sternocleidomastoid muscle *(SCM).*

TECHNIQUE
1. Prepare and position the child as previously described for external jugular vein puncture.
2. Insert a needle immediately inferior to the clavicle at a point one-half to two-thirds its length from the sternoclavicular junction; while "hugging" the undersurface of the clavicle, the needle is directed toward the suprasternal notch while continuously aspirating.

If the child's ventilation is controlled, the risk of pneumothorax may be decreased by momentarily ceasing ventilation so that the apex of the lung is away from the needle tip while probing for the subclavian vein. Once successful venipuncture has been achieved, maintaining positive end-expiratory pressure reduces the possibility of air embolism.

Supraclavicular Ultrasound-Guided Brachiocephalic Vein (Innominate) Catheterization

Longitudinal view of the brachiocephalic vein at the junction of internal jugular vein and subclavian vein can be visualized with ultrasound (Videos 46.1 and 46.2). A case series of 141 infants weighing between 0.7 and 10 kilograms[127] reported a first-attempt successful puncture rate for the left brachiocephalic vein of 82.9% using an in-plane ultrasound-guided technique. The right brachiocephalic first-attempt success rate was significantly lower. The length of the right brachiocephalic vein is much shorter than the left and it takes a sharp angled and caudad turn to enter the heart, whereas the left vein runs in a more horizontal and less caudad direction.

Real-time ultrasound guidance is mandatory for this technique. The advantages of this technique are that it allows good in-plane visualization of the needle trajectory and pleura during venipuncture and the intrathoracic location of the vessel helps to maintain the caliber of vessel (see Videos 46.1 and 46.2). The exit site of the brachiocephalic catheter is located just above the clavicle. This can facilitate more secure positioning, care, and maintenance compared with the internal jugular vein. Additionally, the catheter moves less with changes in the neck position, which cause the catheter to dislodge and increase the risk of infection. (Fig 46.5).

TECHNIQUE
1. Prepare and position the child as previously described for internal jugular vein puncture and keep the ipsilateral shoulder adducted.

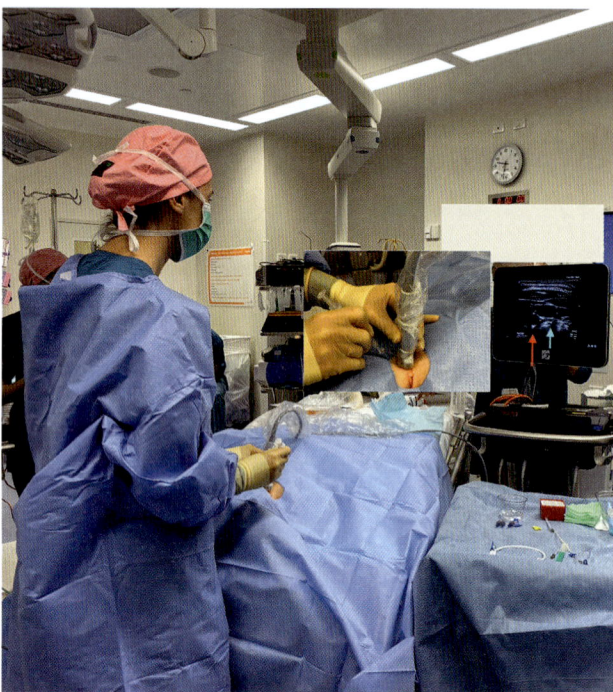

FIGURE 46.9 Position the ultrasound machine in line of sight of inserter to visualize internal jugular vein *(blue arrow)* and artery *(red arrow)*. Sternocleidomastoid muscle can be seen superficial to vessels. *Insert* demonstrating placement of ultrasound probe with sterile covering.

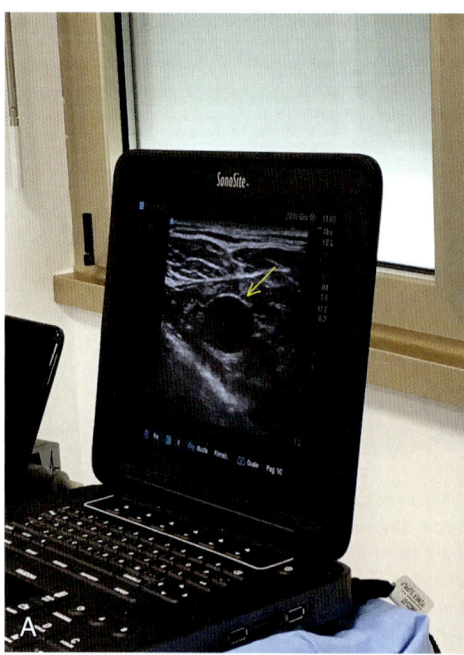
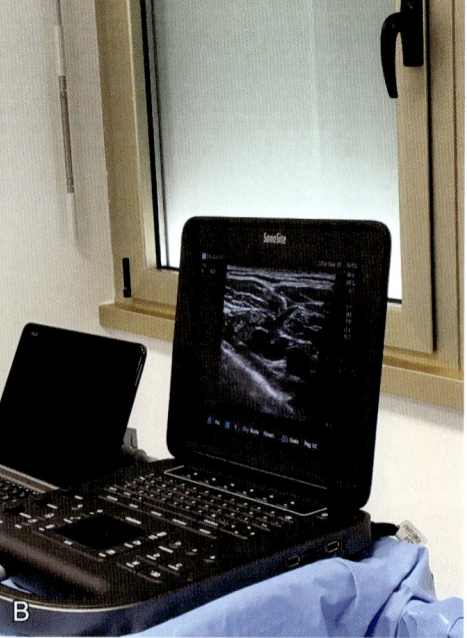

FIGURE 46.10 Infraclavicular approach to subclavian vein. **A,** Out of plain view of subclavian vein *(arrow)* and artery. **B,** Real-time ultrasound guidance of subclavian venipuncture.

2. For left-sided insertion, stand on the left side of the bed next to the patient's torso. Place the ultrasound probe between the two heads of the sternocleidomastoid muscle to visualize the internal jugular vein and carotid artery. With the probe just adjacent to the clavicle, follow the course of the internal jugular vein until it joins the subclavian vein, usually indicated by the presence of a valve at the base of the internal jugular vein. Then rotate the probe caudally to aim the ultrasound beam under the clavicle. A longitudinal image of the brachiocephalic vein will come into view (see Videos 46.1 and 46.2).

3. For right-sided insertion, the same ergonomic approach applies as for a right-sided internal jugular cannulation.

Femoral Vein Catheterization

The femoral vein may also be used for access to the central circulation.[128] Although the catheter tip should be sited in the thorax to provide accurate measurements of the cardiac filling pressures, there is a reasonable correlation with central filling pressures even when the catheter tip rests within the abdomen.[129] Occasionally, the catheter is inadvertently advanced into a vertebral vein; this can be confirmed with a lateral radiograph. One advantage of this route is that the vein is large and presents easy access distant from the vital intrathoracic structures (Fig. 46.11). Disadvantages of femoral venous canulation include difficulty in securing the catheter to the child, kinking of the catheter with hip flexion, and problems in maintaining sterility at the insertion site. Short-term catheterization can provide large-bore venous access for the duration of a procedure with expected large and rapid blood loss if other veins are not accessible. Surprisingly, this site is not associated with a greater incidence of catheter-related sepsis compared with other insertion sites.[130,131] However, this site is associated with a greater incidence of venous thromboembolism compared with internal jugular and subclavian sites.[132] This site is inappropriate for resuscitation and volume replacement if blood flow in the inferior vena cava could be disrupted or occluded (e.g., Wilms tumor resection with invasion of the inferior vena cava, abdominal trauma). The tip of the catheter should be located either low in the atrium or inferior to the level of the diaphragm but superior to the level of the renal veins to reduce the potential for renal vein thrombosis. Use of this technique also has been reported to be safe in infants weighing less than 1000 grams with the added caution to avoid cardiac perforation when the catheter is threaded cephalad.[133]

TECHNIQUE

1. Prepare and drape the groin using an aseptic technique with the legs at 40 to 60-degree angles ("frog-leg position") (see Fig. 46.11B).[134] Place a roll under the hips, thereby slightly elevating the hip, to provide optimal conditions.

2. Palpate the femoral artery at a point midway between the pubic tubercle and the anterior superior iliac spine (see Fig. 46.11A). Using the Seldinger technique, enter the vein at a point just medial to the femoral artery and 1 to 2 cm below the inguinal ligament. Insert a catheter as in Fig. 46.5.

3. 30-degree reverse Trendelenburg position and compression 1 to 2 cm above the inguinal ligament can increase the femoral venous diameter.[135] As with many vascular access methods, ultrasound guidance can be quite useful to identify the vein and adjacent structures.[136–139] One study in 84 children under the age of 9 years demonstrated that 12% of the femoral arteries overlap the femoral vein.[140]

4. The saphenous vein may be cannulated by direct venous cutdown at its junction with the femoral vein if percutaneous techniques are unsuccessful.

Umbilical Vein Catheterization

Indications

The umbilical vein provides convenient access to the central circulation of a neonate to restore blood volume and to administer glucose and drugs. In neonates, the umbilical vein joins the portal vein to form the ductus venosus, which runs directly to the inferior vena cava. This procedure is often carried out blindly. An anteroposterior and lateral abdominal and chest radiograph or ultrasonography are used to confirm correct position at the level of T9 just distal to the right atrium. A large fraction of catheters are initially malpositioned, which if unrecognized, can lead to life-threatening complications.[141–145] Placement under electrocardiogram (ECG) guidance may be helpful to avoid entry into the atrium, but a sterile ECG lead and training are required for success; this technique is limited to neonates who are in sinus rhythm and have normal QRS complexes.[141] A change in the configuration of the ECG suggests that a small QRS complex reflects catheter position below the diaphragm; a normal-sized QRS complex with a small P wave was associated with location within the inferior vena cava at the thoracic level; and the appearance of a tall P wave indicated positioning within the right atrium.[141] Umbilical vein catheterization also provides a route for the procedure of exchange transfusion and for measuring central venous pressure.

EQUIPMENT

- Umbilical artery catheter sizes 3.5 Fr and 5 Fr
- Scalpel and blade
- Fine-curved forceps
- Mosquito hemostats
- Umbilical tape
- Scissors
- Sutures with needle (3-0 silk)
- Antiseptic solutions
- Three-way stopcocks
- 10-mL syringe
- Sterile drapes
- Infusion solution of 10% dextrose in water, with 1 to 2 units of heparin per milliliter at 1 mL/hour
- Calibrated transducer/monitoring system if used for central venous pressure measurement

TECHNIQUE

1. Prepare and drape the umbilicus with sterile technique; cut the cord approximately 1 cm above the umbilicus. The umbilical vein orifice is more patulous and thinner walled than the two umbilical arteries (Fig. 46.12).

2. Holding the catheter filled with heparinized solution 2 cm from the tip, gently introduce it into the vein. In some situations, forceps can aid in directing the catheter. Traction of the umbilical stump *caudad* may help to advance the catheter (see Fig. 46.12). The catheter is passed a distance that approximates the length between the umbilical stump and the right atrium. Blood should freely aspirate into a syringe. Inability to withdraw blood may occur if the tip of the catheter is resting against a vessel wall or if a clot is present within the catheter lumen. At times, the catheter may fail to traverse the ductus venosus and become wedged in the liver. This position is potentially

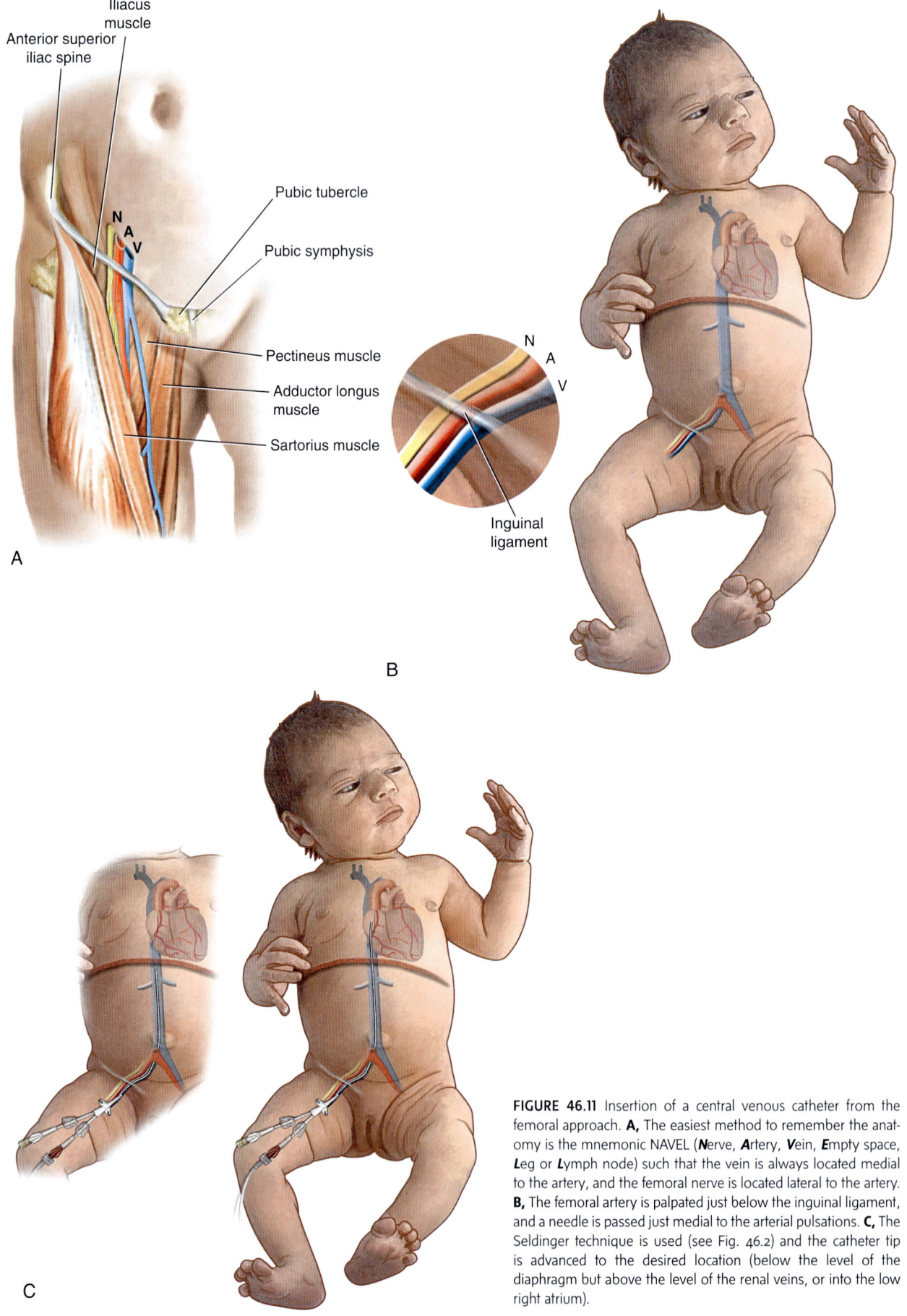

FIGURE 46.11 Insertion of a central venous catheter from the femoral approach. **A,** The easiest method to remember the anatomy is the mnemonic NAVEL (**N**erve, **A**rtery, **V**ein, **E**mpty space, **L**eg or **L**ymph node) such that the vein is always located medial to the artery, and the femoral nerve is located lateral to the artery. **B,** The femoral artery is palpated just below the inguinal ligament, and a needle is passed just medial to the arterial pulsations. **C,** The Seldinger technique is used (see Fig. 46.2) and the catheter tip is advanced to the desired location (below the level of the diaphragm but above the level of the renal veins, or into the low right atrium).

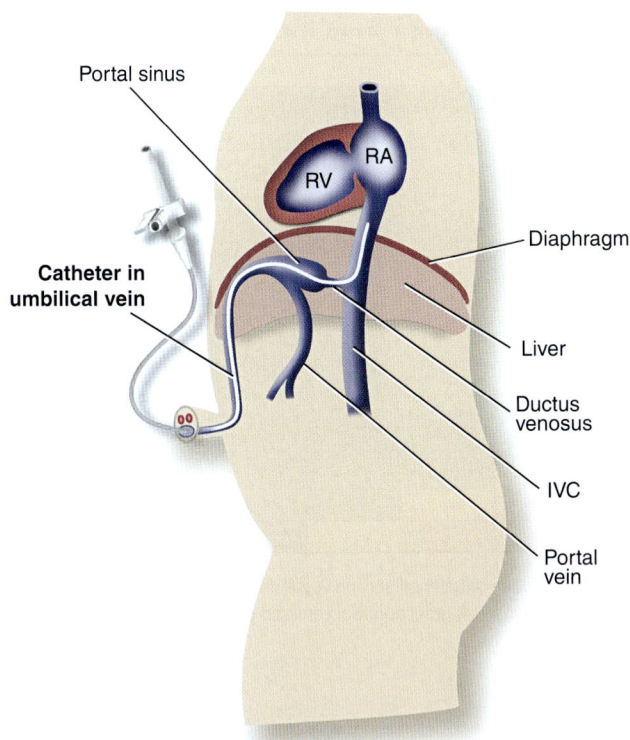

Portal sinus

RA

RV

Catheter in
umbilical vein

Diaphragm

Liver

Ductus
venosus

IVC

Portal
vein

FIGURE 46.12 Umbilical vein catheterization. The umbilical vein is thin walled and patulous, whereas umbilical arteries are thicker walled and of smaller diameter. *Caudal* traction on the umbilical stump may facilitate catheter advancement. The catheter should be advanced through the liver into the central circulation within the low right atrium *(RA)* before administration of any medications. *IVC,* Inferior vena cava; *RV,* right ventricle.

dangerous because portal necrosis and subsequent cirrhosis may result should hyperosmolar or sclerosing solutions be injected (calcium, sodium bicarbonate, 25%–50% glucose).[145–147] A caudal position might be acceptable for short-term use if it is not possible to pass the catheter centrally, but the distance of insertion should be no more than 3 to 4 cm or just until blood is freely aspirated.

3. Suture the catheter in place, cover the insertion site with antibiotic ointment, and tape it to the abdominal wall. The catheter is then connected to a constant-infusion system and should be removed as soon as the indications for its insertion have passed. Complications appear to relate in part to the duration of insertion.[143,145,148]

COMPLICATIONS
- Thrombosis of portal or mesenteric veins[145,149]
- Infection (septicemia)[143]
- Endocarditis
- Pulmonary infarction (misplacement of the catheter into the pulmonary vein through a patent foramen ovale)
- Portal cirrhosis and esophageal varices later in life[150–153]
- Cardiac tamponade[154]
- Liver abscess and subcapsular hematoma[142,155]

Medium Term Central Venous Access
If central venous access is required for IV treatment for a longer duration (2 weeks to 6 months), a peripherally inserted central

venous catheter or a tunneled uncuffed central venous catheter should be considered. These can provide central venous access for weeks or months. They are not suitable for administration of a rapid and large bolus of fluid or drugs in an emergency setting. Surgically placed central venous access (e.g., implanted subcutaneous central venous device or tunneled cuffed central venous catheter) is more suitable for longer term use.[32]

Peripherally Inserted Central Venous Catheter
These are long catheters that are inserted into peripheral veins in the upper limbs (basilic, brachial, or cephalic) and the greater saphenous vein of the leg. The tip of the catheter is advanced to the cavoatrial junction for upper limb peripherally inserted central venous catheter (PICC) and to the inferior vena cava for lower limb PICC.

Even though the insertion site is remote from the thorax, PICCs are not free of risks and complications. Infection like other central venous devices can lead to morbidity and mortality. Deep vein thrombosis can develop if tip position, care, and maintenance are not optimized. Complications can potentially lead to permanent damage to blood vessels. This can have a major impact on children having life-preserving treatment via the venous route (e.g., chronic lung disease requiring frequent IV antibiotics therapy and those requiring long-term IV nutrition).

Careful assessment of vessel caliber, choice of catheter size to keep catheter to vein ratio to under 45%, limiting the number of lumens to a minimum, ultrasound-guided insertion, optimizing insertion site to avoid the catheter running over a joint, evidence-based care, and maintenance practice focusing on aseptic nontouch and pulsatile flushing technique, are all important factors to improve longevity of PICCs and prevent complications (Fig 46.13).[156]

Tunneled Uncuffed Central Venous Catheter
In neonates and small infants, the limb vessels are often too small for insertion of a 3 Fr PICC. Small caliber neonatal (1.9 Fr, 2.6 Fr) PICCs are available but they are prone to occlusion with blood sampling and continuous infusion is required to maintain patency. Tunneling of central venous access and moving the catheter exit site from supraclavicular region to infraclavicular region or from groin to upper thigh region can increase the longevity of these central venous catheters from days to months (Fig 46.14).[157] This allows a 3 Fr catheter to be inserted as it is more versatile for blood sampling and only requires intermittent flushing to maintain patency. A cuffed catheter will increase the longevity of venous access, but sedation or general anesthesia is usually required for removal.

Vascular Access Specialist Team

There are increasing numbers of vascular access devices and evidence to support their clinical use has evolved over time. The establishment of vascular access specialist teams provides advanced knowledge to guide the clinical use and placement of vascular access devices. There are few published reports to support improved outcomes but one institution's study seems to support reduced complications and high success rate of insertion.[158,159] However, shared responsibilities among various medical and nursing teams regarding assessment, insertion, care, intervention, and removal can lead to disjointed care and increase risk of complications.[160]

A collaborative approach across different disciplines and initiation of evidence-based best practices will result in improved outcomes.[159]

46

Vessel size	1 mm	1.5 mm	2 mm	2.25 mm	2.5 mm	2.75 mm	3 mm	3.5 mm	4 mm	4.5 mm	5 mm
Catheter size											
24G	×										
22G	×	~									
20G	×	×									
18G	×	×	~	~							
16G	×	×	×	×	×	~	~				
1 Fr											
2 Fr	~										
3 Fr	×	~									
4 Fr	×	×	~	~							
4.5 Fr	×	×	×	~	~						
5 Fr	×	×	×	×	~	~					
5.5 Fr	×	×	×	×	×	~					
6 Fr	×	×	×	×	×	×	~				
7 Fr	×	×	×	×	×	×	×	~			
8 Fr	×	×	×	×	×	×	×	×	~		

LEGEND
- ≥45%
- 44–34%
- ≤33%

FIGURE 46.13 Catheter to vessel ratio table demonstrating relationship between catheter caliber and vessel diameter.[156] From Spencer TR, Mahoney KJ. Reducing catheter-related thrombosis using a risk reduction tool centered on catheter to vessel ratio. *J Thromb Thrombolysis* 2017; 44: 427-434, with permission.

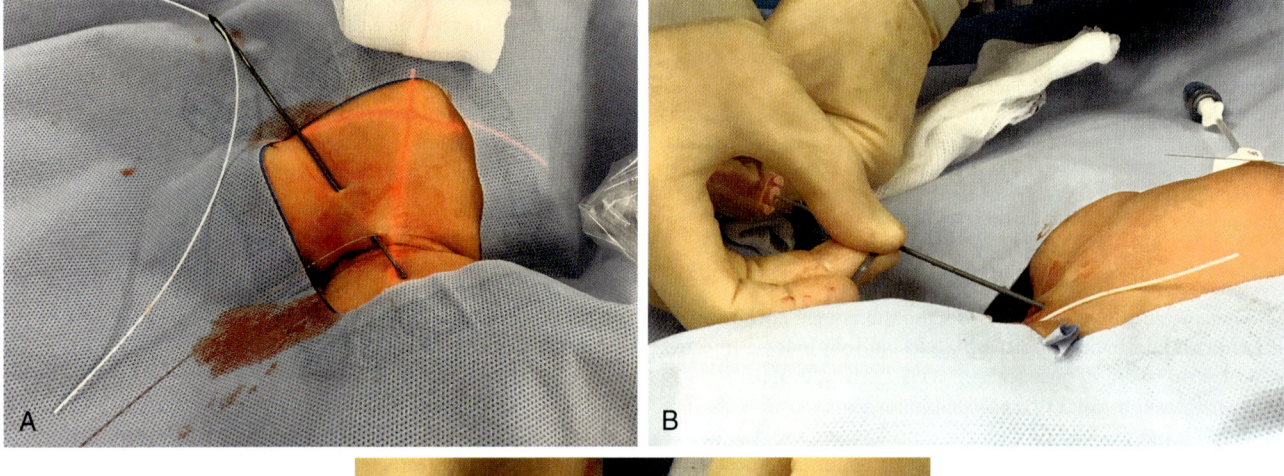

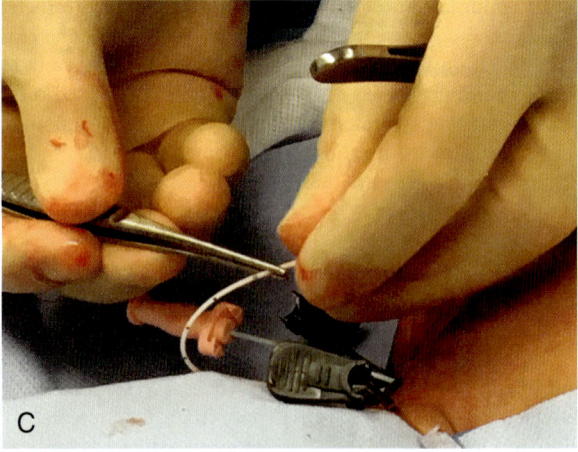

FIGURE 46.14 Tunneling of catheter moves the exit site to optimize securement, care, and maintenance. **A,** Guide wire was introduced into left brachiocephalic vein. The venous catheter is tunneled through the subcutaneous space created by a blunt metal introducer. **B,** A dilator with peel-away sheath is advanced into the vein. **C,** The catheter is threaded into the vein via the peel-away sheath.

Vessel health preservation frameworks can guide the development of these guidelines.[1] This can include clinical pathways to manage difficult vascular access and to guide the choice of vascular access devices. One report found a median rate of catheter-related blood-stream infection per 100 catheter days decreased from 2.7 infections at baseline to 0 at 3 months after implementation of evidence-based interventions for infection control.[2]

Individual institutions all have different resource constraints. Hospital-based guidelines can be useful to guide clinicians to choose the most appropriate vascular access device based on patient characteristics, treatment requirements, and institutional resources availability (Fig. 46.15).

Arterial Cannulation

Arterial cannulation is commonly used for continuous arterial blood pressure monitoring and frequent blood sampling for monitoring patients who are critically unwell or having surgery with cardiovascular, respiratory, neurological, and metabolic challenges. Major complications associated with arterial cannulation are uncommon but can lead to acute interruption of arterial blood supply leading to infection or permanent ischemia of limb and vital organs. Complications are more commonly related to femoral artery cannulation and in younger children.[161] A careful risk benefit assessment together with real-time ultrasound guidance can improve success rate and potentially minimize vessel injury. Other risk mitigating strategies include cannulating large caliber vessels, reducing catheter to artery ratio, cannulating distal arteries with collaterals rather than proximal end arteries, and active decision making to remove cannula at the earliest possible time.[162–166]

UMBILICAL ARTERY

The umbilical artery in a neonate is a convenient site for monitoring arterial blood pressure, blood gases, and pH. It provides emergency access to an infant's circulation for restoration of blood volume and administration of glucose and drugs.[167–170] Continuous monitoring of arterial O_2 saturation is also possible.[171]

Equipment

The materials used for cannulation are identical to those described for umbilical venous catheterization. Equipment is required for continuous monitoring of blood pressure. *End-hole rather than side-hole catheters may have a smaller incidence of thrombosis or associated ischemic events.*[172]

Technique

1. Prepare and drape the area with sterile technique; cut the umbilical cord approximately 1 cm above the umbilicus. The two umbilical arteries are identified (Fig. 46.16). The cut vessel ends have thicker walls, are smaller than the vein, and are usually in spasm. The artery is entered in the manner described for umbilical vein catheterization, except that *cephalad* traction is applied to the umbilical stump (see Fig. 46.16A) to encourage *caudal* direction of the catheter. The catheter should course through the umbilical artery into the iliohypogastric artery and then into the descending aorta. Proper positioning of the catheter tip is crucial. If the catheter is advanced too far up the aorta, it may pass through the ductus arteriosus and into the pulmonary artery. If this situation is

not recognized, blood pressure and blood gas measurements may be misleading. Care should be taken to ensure the placement of the catheter tip in the descending aorta (at T7 to T9). Early reports suggested that a cephalad position, at or above the level of the diaphragm, is easier to maintain but predisposes infants to increased risk of embolization to renal or mesenteric vessels (see Fig. 46.16B).[163–166] However, positioning just above the bifurcation of the descending aorta, that is, at L3 to L5 (see Fig. 46.16A) (below the origin of the renal arteries and visceral branches of the aorta), has not been supported by a Cochrane review; a cephalad position is recommended.[173] The caudad position is difficult to maintain, and the catheter tip may slip into one of the iliac arteries, resulting in tissue ischemia (see Fig. 46.16C).

2. Confirm the position radiographically. Once the catheter is properly positioned, the system is connected to a constant-infusion pump and heparinized fluids (10% dextrose in water or normal saline solution) are infused. Suture and tape the catheter and apply antibiotic ointment as for umbilical vein catheters. A Cochrane review of the use of heparin suggested that low-dose heparinization of the infusate (0.25 unit/mL) reduces the likelihood of catheter occlusion compared with intermittent flushing with heparinized solutions.[174]

Complications

Using the umbilical artery as a source for blood pressure monitoring and blood gas analysis only and reserving alternative sites for glucose and drug administration may minimize complications. Changes in cerebral blood flow are associated with intraventricular hemorrhage and have been documented to occur with umbilical artery blood sampling; fewer changes in cerebral blood flow occur with low-positioned catheters.[175] The incidence of documented intraventricular hemorrhage appears to have a stronger relation with age than with catheter position and is not associated with the use of low-dose heparin.[174,176] The use of an alternate site for monitoring may reduce complications.[177] Other complications are:

- Accidental disconnection of stopcocks and catheters or vessel perforation can lead to potentially dangerous exsanguination.[178]
- Blood clots may embolize retrograde or, more likely, distally, leading to ischemia or infarction of the infant's gut, kidneys, or lower limbs (see Fig. 46.16C).[179]
- Vascular spasm is usually transitory and may be resolved by withdrawal of the catheter. Several cases of flaccid paraplegia have been reported resulting from spasm or embolic phenomena.[180]
- The infant is always at risk for sepsis; clear indications for the insertion of this catheter are mandatory. The catheter should be removed at the earliest possible time. A Cochrane review failed to establish a role for prophylactic antibiotics in reducing catheter-related infections.[181]
- Hypertension as a result of renal artery emboli may cause ischemia and infarction of the kidney.[166,182]
- Aortic thrombosis may occur.[183]

RADIAL ARTERY

Radial artery cannulation is a reasonable alternative to umbilical artery cannulation in a neonate and is the primary site of arterial cannulation in infants and children in most pediatric institutions. Percutaneous radial artery cannulation is widely practiced, with minimal morbidity.[143,184–189] The right radial artery is preferred in neonates because it is representative of preductal blood flow. It is

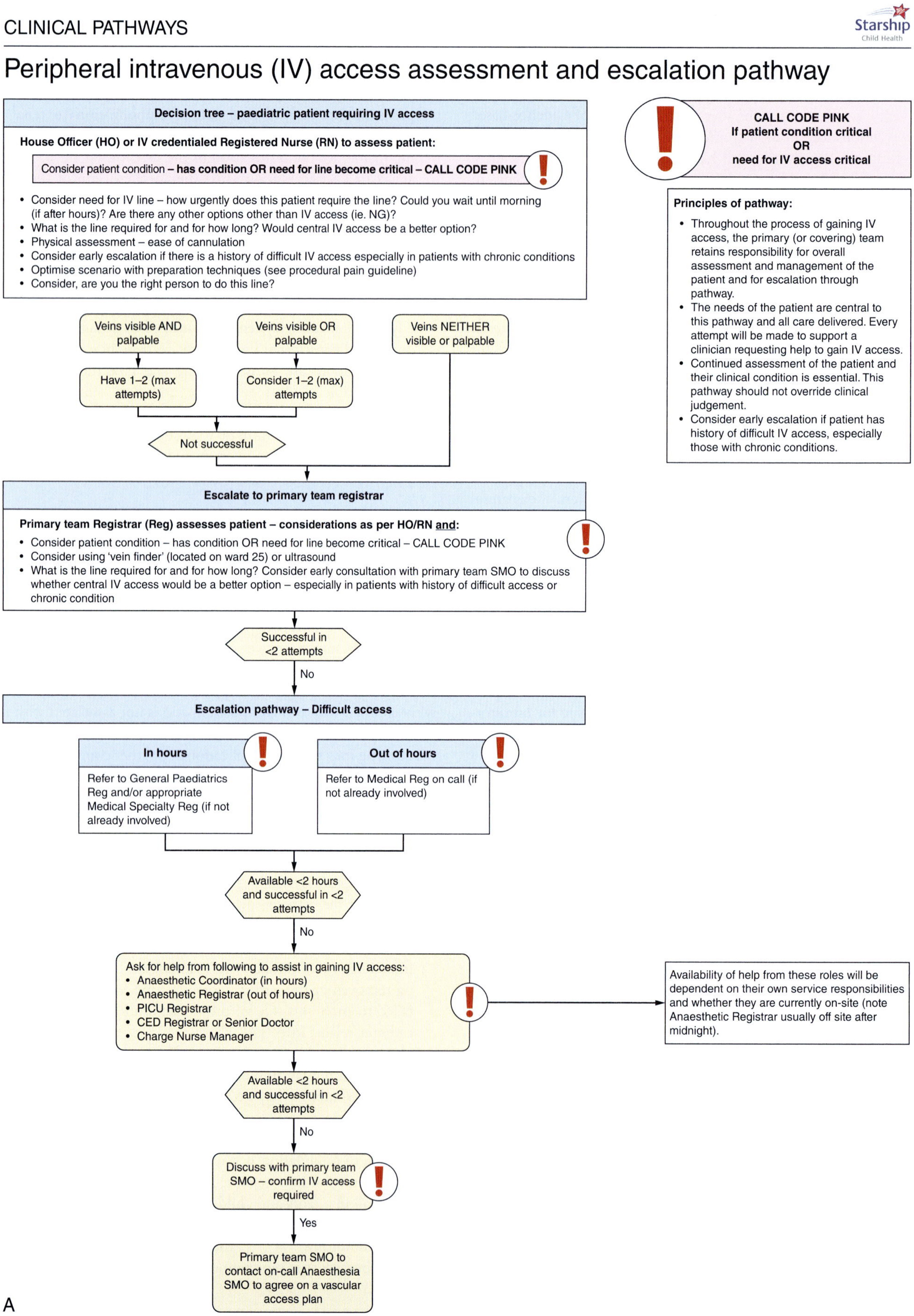

CLINICAL PATHWAYS

Starship
Child Health

Peripheral intravenous (IV) access assessment and escalation pathway

Decision tree – paediatric patient requiring IV access

House Officer (HO) or IV credentialed Registered Nurse (RN) to assess patient:

Consider patient condition – **has condition OR need for line become critical – CALL CODE PINK** !

- Consider need for IV line – how urgently does this patient require the line? Could you wait until morning (if after hours)? Are there any other options other than IV access (ie. NG)?
- What is the line required for and for how long? Would central IV access be a better option?
- Physical assessment – ease of cannulation
- Consider early escalation if there is a history of difficult IV access especially in patients with chronic conditions
- Optimise scenario with preparation techniques (see procedural pain guideline)
- Consider, are you the right person to do this line?

CALL CODE PINK
If patient condition critical
OR
need for IV access critical

Principles of pathway:
- Throughout the process of gaining IV access, the primary (or covering) team retains responsibility for overall assessment and management of the patient and for escalation through pathway.
- The needs of the patient are central to this pathway and all care delivered. Every attempt will be made to support a clinician requesting help to gain IV access.
- Continued assessment of the patient and their clinical condition is essential. This pathway should not override clinical judgement.
- Consider early escalation if patient has history of difficult IV access, especially those with chronic conditions.

Veins visible AND palpable → Have 1–2 (max attempts)

Veins visible OR palpable → Consider 1–2 (max) attempts

Veins NEITHER visible or palpable

Not successful

Escalate to primary team registrar

Primary team Registrar (Reg) assesses patient – considerations as per HO/RN and:
- Consider patient condition – has condition OR need for line become critical – CALL CODE PINK
- Consider using 'vein finder' (located on ward 25) or ultrasound
- What is the line required for and for how long? Consider early consultation with primary team SMO to discuss whether central IV access would be a better option – especially in patients with history of difficult access or chronic condition

Successful in <2 attempts — No

Escalation pathway – Difficult access

In hours !
Refer to General Paediatrics Reg and/or appropriate Medical Specialty Reg (if not already involved)

Out of hours !
Refer to Medical Reg on call (if not already involved)

Available <2 hours and successful in <2 attempts — No

Ask for help from following to assist in gaining IV access:
- Anaesthetic Coordinator (in hours)
- Anaesthetic Registrar (out of hours)
- PICU Registrar
- CED Registrar or Senior Doctor
- Charge Nurse Manager

Availability of help from these roles will be dependent on their own service responsibilities and whether they are currently on-site (note Anaesthetic Registrar usually off site after midnight).

Available <2 hours and successful in <2 attempts — No

Discuss with primary team SMO – confirm IV access required — Yes

Primary team SMO to contact on-call Anaesthesia SMO to agree on a vascular access plan

A

FIGURE 46.15 Examples of clinical pathways. **A,** Management of pediatric difficult venous access. (Courtesy Starship Children's Hospital, with permission).

Flow chart for paediatric vascular access requests

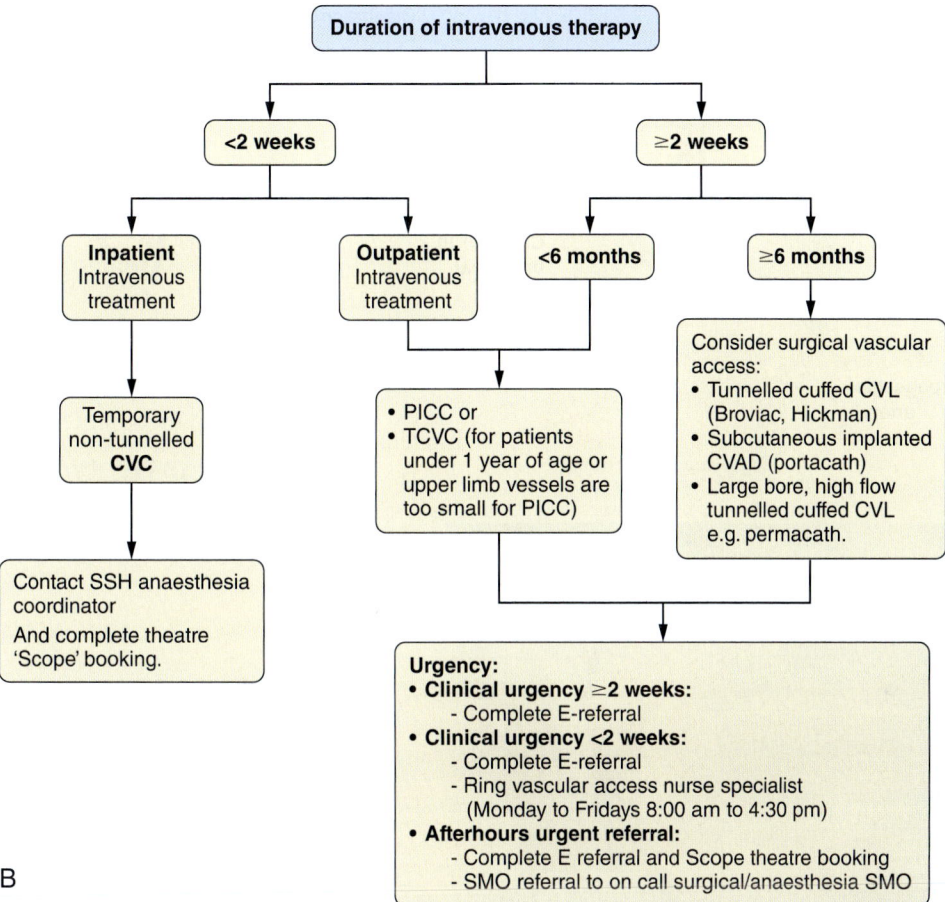

Establishing need for central venous access
- Primary team SMO/fellow approval for referral
- Pharmacist can advise on extravasation risk or refer to 'Guardrail'
- Senior nurse can guide safe infusion practice
- Other subspecialties can optimise choice of intravenous therapy. E.g., Infectious disease, cardiology, cardiac surgeon, gastroenterology.
- Community and social support can influence choice of intravenous therapy
- Vascular access nurse specialist can advise on the appropriate choice of device

Duration of intravenous therapy

<2 weeks   ≥2 weeks

Inpatient Intravenous treatment   **Outpatient** Intravenous treatment   <6 months   ≥6 months

Temporary non-tunnelled **CVC**

- PICC or
- TCVC (for patients under 1 year of age or upper limb vessels are too small for PICC)

Consider surgical vascular access:
- Tunnelled cuffed CVL (Broviac, Hickman)
- Subcutaneous implanted CVAD (portacath)
- Large bore, high flow tunnelled cuffed CVL e.g. permacath.

Contact SSH anaesthesia coordinator
And complete theatre 'Scope' booking.

Urgency:
- **Clinical urgency ≥2 weeks:**
  - Complete E-referral
- **Clinical urgency <2 weeks:**
  - Complete E-referral
  - Ring vascular access nurse specialist (Monday to Fridays 8:00 am to 4:30 pm)
- **Afterhours urgent referral:**
  - Complete E referral and Scope theatre booking
  - SMO referral to on call surgical/anaesthesia SMO

B

FIGURE 46.15, cont'd B, Guideline for choice of pediatric vascular access devices demonstrating multidisciplinary team approach.

relatively superficial, the average depth is 2.3 mm in children.[190] One study reported a mean radial artery diameter less than 0.7 mm in a prospective cohort of 50 infants under 6 months of age before induction.[162] The use of ultrasound improves first-attempt success rate and reduces the risk of hematoma formation.[191,192] Ultrasound can be used to assess the relative size and depth of radial and ulnar arteries before catheter insertion (Video 46.3). Some believe the ulnar artery should never be used for cannulation. If the radial artery is damaged, then the ulnar artery remains available for hand perfusion.[193]

Children with Down syndrome (trisomy 21) have abnormal radial vessels (both size and location, 16% to 19%), which can make arterial cannulation particularly difficult; some children with Down syndrome have a single median artery.[21,194,195] The ulnar artery also has been used as an alternative site for arterial

catheterization when attempts at insertion in other locations have been unsuccessful. Once an attempt at cannulation of the radial artery is made, the ipsilateral ulnar artery should not be instrumented to ensure adequate perfusion of the entire hand.[196] Strict indications for inserting radial artery catheters are necessary, and their removal must be considered at the earliest possible time.[163–166]

Technique

1. Confirm the adequacy of ulnar artery collateral flow by the modified Allen test (Fig. 46.17A). The color of the hand is noted. The hand is passively clenched, and the radial and ulnar arteries are simultaneously compressed at the wrist (see Fig. 46.17B). The ulnar artery is then released, and flushing (reperfusion) of the blanched hand is noted (see Fig. 46.17C). If the entire hand is well perfused while the radial artery

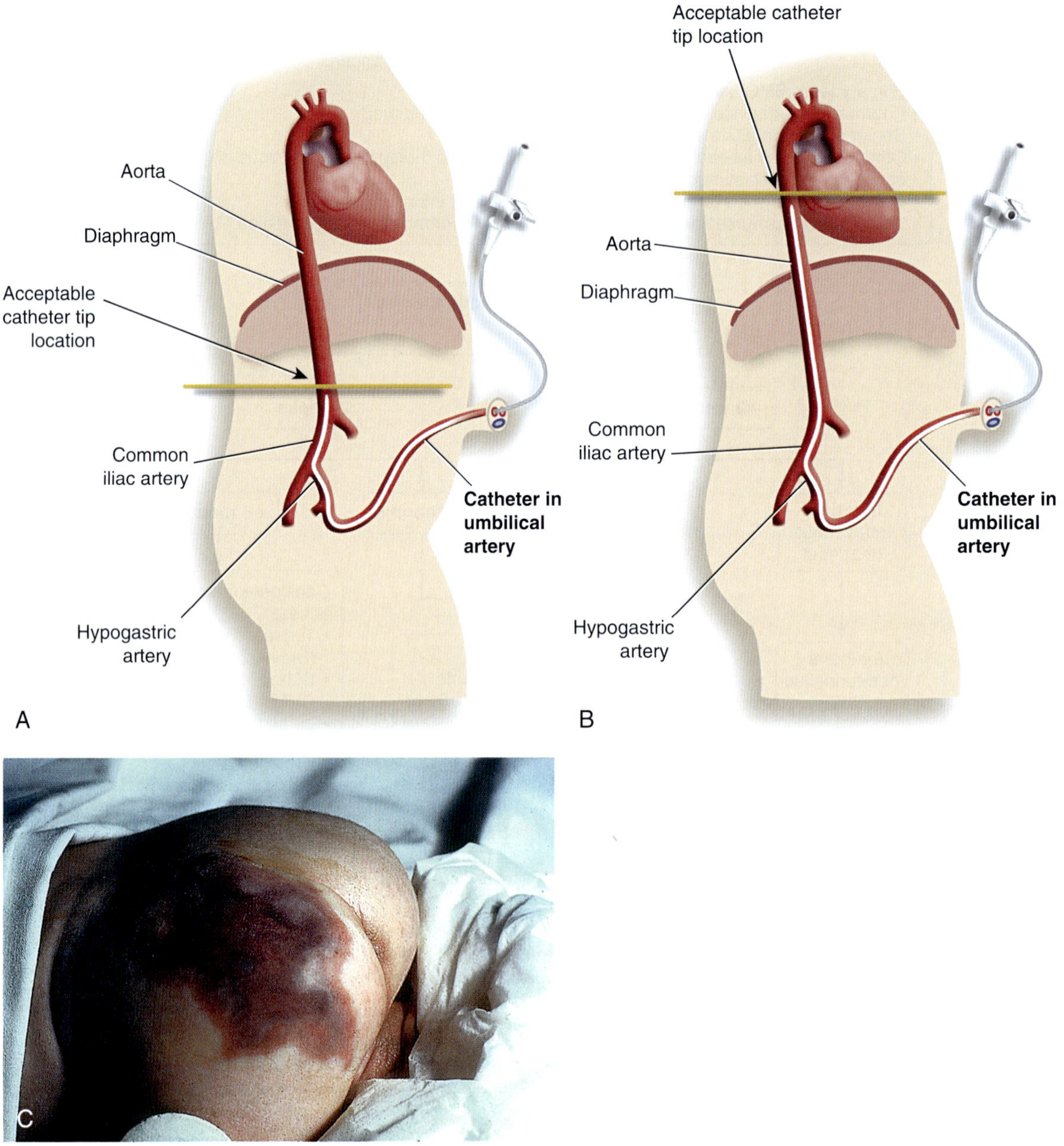

Acceptable catheter tip location

Aorta

Diaphragm

Acceptable catheter tip location

Common iliac artery

Catheter in umbilical artery

Hypogastric artery

A

Acceptable catheter tip location

Aorta

Diaphragm

Common iliac artery

Catheter in umbilical artery

Hypogastric artery

B

C

FIGURE 46.16 Umbilical artery catheterization. *Cephalad* traction on the umbilical stump may facilitate catheter advancement. **A,** The catheter tip at L3–L4 just above the aortic bifurcation and below the renal arteries is one acceptable location *(arrow to yellow line).* **B,** An alternative acceptable location is in the descending aorta between T7 and T9 *(arrow to yellow line).* **C,** An area of necrosis in the left buttock that resulted from a catheter migrating into the internal iliac vessel, occluding one of its branches.

remains occluded, indicating adequate collateral flow, catheterization of the radial artery is performed. Note that the sensitivity of the Allen test is only 73%, with a specificity of 97%.[197–199] Many have abandoned the Allen test because its sensitivity to predict an ischemic hand after radial artery canulation is poor[200] if the test failed and they simply avoid cannulating the ulnar artery.

2. Secure the hand using an arm board with slight extension of the wrist to avoid excessive median nerve stretching. The fingertips should be left exposed when the hand is taped down so that any peripheral ischemic changes from spasm, clot, or air can be observed.

3. The radial artery on the dorsal aspect of the wrist within the anatomic snuff box may be used as an alternative site.[201] The use of ultrasound improves first-attempt success rate and reduces the risk of hematoma formation.[191] Dorsiflexion of the wrist up to 45 degrees reduces the depth of radial artery without affecting the vessel diameter (Fig 46.18).[202]

4. Select a 24-, 22- or 20-gauge IV catheter or a Seldinger kit to canulate the artery at an angle of 15 to 20 degrees or on withdrawing the cannula after transfixion of the artery (Fig. 46.18A to C) (Video 46.3). Some have recommended approaching the artery (as well as a vein) with the bevel of the canula facing downward to ensure the leading edge of the

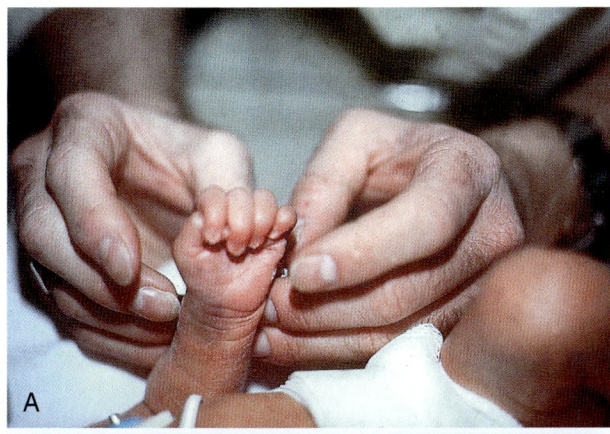

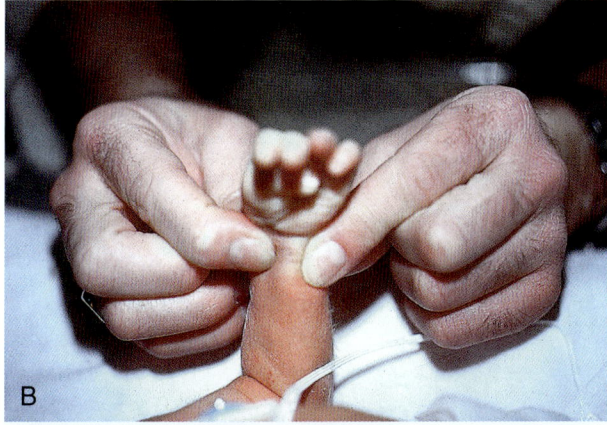

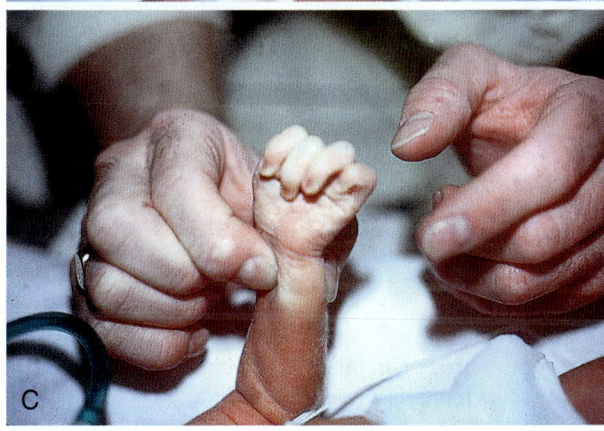

FIGURE 46.17 Modified Allen test. **A,** Color and perfusion of the hand are noted. **B,** The hand is first passively clenched, and then both radial and ulnar vessels are occluded. **C,** The ulnar artery is released while the radial artery remains occluded. If flow through the ulnar artery and collateral arch in the hand is adequate, the color and perfusion should rapidly return. If not adequate, then simply do not cannulate the radial artery.

needle is within the lumen when the flash of blood is identified and to ensure the catheter slides off the needle into the lumen (rather than into the back wall of the artery if the needle tip had inadvertently entered the back wall of the artery).[203] A 0.018 inch wire may be used as an aid to advance 22-gauge catheters; a 0.015 inch wire can be used for 24-gauge catheters.

5. Attach the catheter firmly to a T-connector or a three-way stopcock to permit continuous infusion of isotonic saline solution (heparin 1 unit/mL) at the rate of 1 to 2 mL/hour via a constant-infusion pump (see Fig. 46.18D). The catheter

is securely taped or sutured in place. A pressure transducer is connected to allow continuous arterial pressure monitoring. To ensure accurate blood pressure measurement, it is essential that the transducer is calibrated to the neonate's or child's heart level, that all air bubbles are removed from the tubing and transducer, and that no more than 3 feet of tubing is used between the neonate or child and the transducer to minimize artifacts caused by the tubing (under and over damping).[204,205]

6. Obtain blood samples by clamping off the distal end of the T-connector, cleaning the injection port of the T-connector with antiseptic solution, introducing a 22-gauge needle, and withdrawing 1 mL of blood. A sample of blood is obtained by heparinized syringe, with minimal blood loss and minimal manipulation of the system.[184,206] An alternative is the use of a 3-mL syringe on a three-way stopcock: aspirate 2 to 3 mL, clamp the system, and then take the sample of blood from the T-connector as just described. After sampling, the clamp is released, the aspirated blood is readministered, and continuous infusion is resumed or flush is run into the 3-mL syringe and then the system is gently manually flushed intermittently with a syringe, which is changed once per 24 hours. This method of sampling maintains a closed system with reduced potential for sources of infection. Bolus flushes should be very brief or a slow infusion because prolonged flushing in neonates and infants may flush a crystalloid solution retrograde to the brain and cause a stroke. Disastrous results may occur if an air bubble or blood clot should accompany a bolus flush.[207–211] *All arterial lines must be clearly identified (red tape) to avoid accidental infusion of hypertonic solutions and sclerosing medications.*

Complications

- Infection at the site of the catheter insertion, with possible septicemia.
- Arterial thrombus formation. This depends on the size of catheter inserted, the material of which it is constructed, the technique of insertion, and the duration of cannulation.
- Emboli. A blood clot or air may embolize to the digits, resulting in arteriolar spasm or more serious ischemic necrosis.
- Disconnecting the catheter from the infusion system. Blood loss may be life-threatening, especially in an infant.
- Ischemia. The radial artery cannula should be withdrawn if ischemic changes develop.
- Vasospasm. Usually transient but requires careful observation.

BRACHIAL ARTERY

The brachial artery is an alternative vessel but is less frequently used than the radial artery because of the absence of collateral flow. The median nerve is prone to damage as it runs medially alongside the brachial artery. A retrospective study in a single center reviewed 1574 arterial catheter insertions for pediatric cardiac surgery from 1998 to 2003 and reported no complications in 386 brachial arterial catheters in neonates and infants. In that study, the brachial artery was the next alternative after failed radial arterial cannulation attempts; ultrasound guidance should improve accuracy and reduce insertion complications.[212]

AXILLARY ARTERY

Axillary arterial cannulation has been used in children for monitoring when radial or lower extremity access failed; there are few studies specifically related to the risks and benefits of axillary

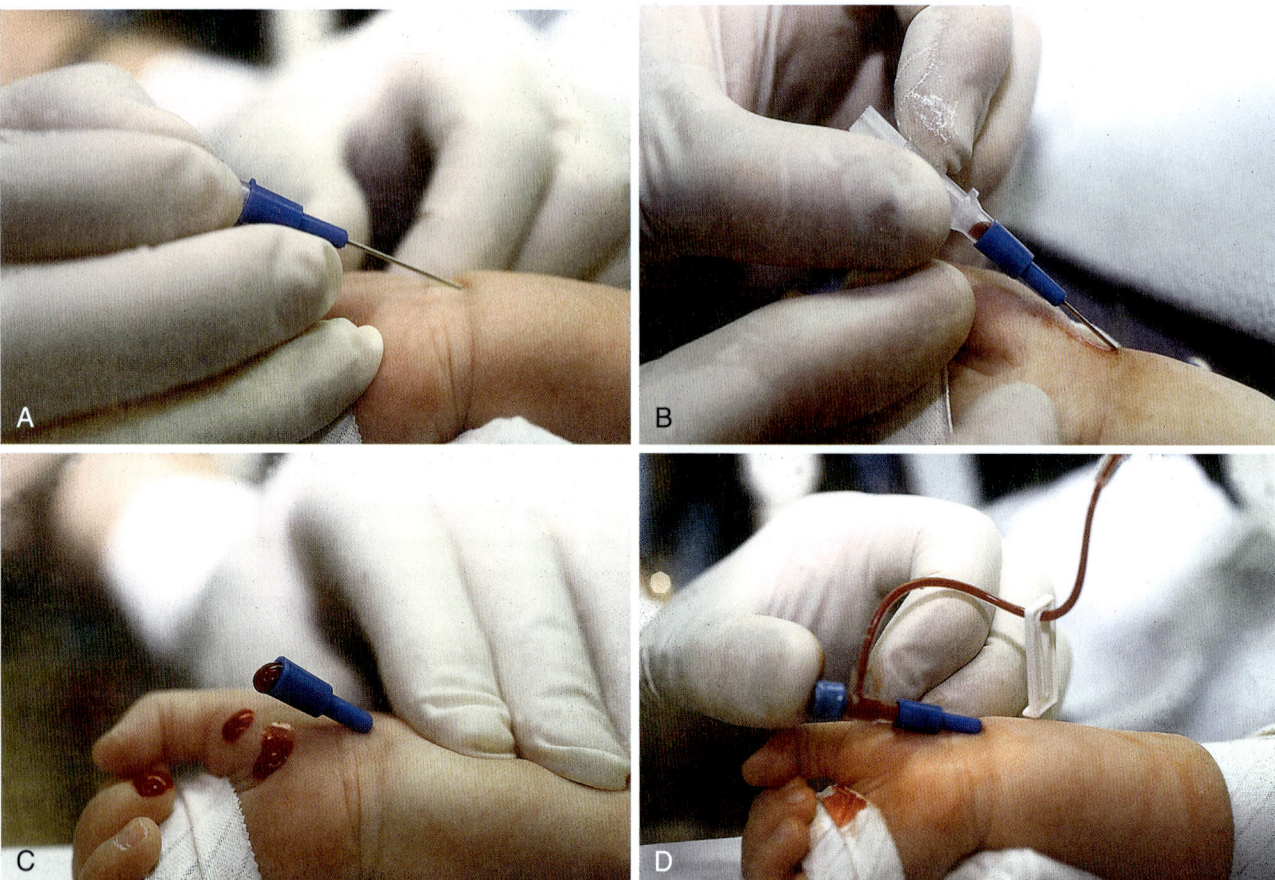

FIGURE 46.18 A, After adequate collateral circulation has been ensured, the radial artery is palpated and the appropriate catheter is advanced into the vessel. **B,** After blood return is noted, the catheter is threaded over the needle and into the artery. **C,** Pulsatile back bleeding confirms intraarterial position. **D,** A T-connector with appropriate flush solution is connected; the catheter is aspirated to clear air bubbles and then gently flushed. Antibiotic ointment and benzoin are applied. The injection port should be clearly marked as "arterial" to minimize accidental drug administration into the artery. A Luer-Lok connection is preferred to prevent accidental disconnection.

access. One publication reported the use of axillary arterial monitoring in pediatric patients with no major complications in 16 children.[213] Another group reported axillary cannulation in 62 neonates with birth weights that ranged from 750 to 3800 grams without complications.[214] In general, an ultrasound-guided technique is highly recommended to minimize damage to surrounding structures (brachial plexus).

TEMPORAL ARTERY
When the radial artery has been previously cannulated or is inaccessible, the temporal artery may be used.[215] Cerebral infarction has been described as a complication of this technique. It appears to be related to retrograde embolization of air or a blood clot.[216] Case reports of selective use of temporal artery cannulation described the use for monitoring during repair of coarctation of the aorta or administration of anterograde cerebral perfusion in patients having associated aberrant origin of the right subclavian artery.[217] Both catheters were removed on the same day and no complications were reported; as with other locations ultrasound guidance might be helpful in improving successful insertion.

FEMORAL ARTERY
Femoral catheterization in infants and children includes a greater risk of vascular injury or thrombosis resulting in ischemia[218] and is not recommended if other peripheral sites are available. In situations in which peripheral arterial cannulation is impossible (e.g., in burned patients, children with poor peripheral perfusion, children with congenital heart disease), the remote possibility of a complication must be balanced versus a greater likelihood of life-threatening complications owing to less than ideal monitoring.[219]

Technique
1. Locate the femoral artery by palpation at the groin; this can be confirmed with ultrasound guidance. Anatomically, it is situated midway between the anterior superior iliac spine and the pubic tubercle (see Fig. 46.11).
2. After sterile preparation of the skin, insert a catheter of appropriate size into the femoral artery using the Seldinger technique. The artery is entered at the point of maximal pulsation, approximately 1 cm below the line joining the anterior superior iliac spine and the pubic tubercle.

3. After cannulation, connect the catheter to a continuous-flow system and pressure transducer. The catheter is sutured in place, the insertion site is covered, and an occlusive dressing is applied. The possibility of fecal and urinary contamination makes this last step particularly important.

Complications

- Infection.
- Emboli of clot and air, leading to ischemic necrosis of the lower limb.
- Poor arterial puncture technique, leading to osteoarthritis of the hip joint; severe trauma to the femoral artery has resulted in gangrene of the lower limb, retroperitoneal hemorrhage, and arteriovenous fistula formation.[220–222] The potential for these complications would be reduced by using an ultrasound guided technique. Up to approximately 24% of children will have no resolution of thrombosis and approximately 1% may have partial arrest of bone growth, likely as a result of thrombus formation.[223,224]
- Vasospasm is usually transient but requires careful observation for resolution.

DORSALIS PEDIS AND POSTERIOR TIBIAL ARTERY

The dorsalis pedis and posterior tibial arteries are additional sites for arterial cannulation in children when more desirable locations are inaccessible. Collateral circulation should always be checked. If cannulation is attempted or performed in one artery in the foot, the ipsilateral artery should not be instrumented to ensure adequate collateral blood flow. Ultrasound guidance may be helpful.[225] One study performed ultrasound assessment and cannulation of 234 children under the age of 2 years.[202] The posterior tibial artery was found to be comparable in size to the radial artery and the dorsalis pedis artery is comparatively smaller. The posterior tibial artery is approximately 3 to 4 mm deep from skin surface compared with the radial artery which is 2.5 to 3 mm deep. It can be located between the medial malleolus and the Achilles tendon. Ankle dorsiflexion and eversion reduces the depth and may facilitate cannulation of the posterior tibial artery.[190,202]

Technique

The artery is cannulated in the same manner as the radial artery at a point of maximal pulsation. An understanding of the anatomy of the dorsalis pedis and posterior tibial arteries before attempting this procedure is important. If percutaneous cannulation is impossible, ultrasound guidance can improve success rate[202]; however, a cutdown technique may be required. The complications are similar to other arterial line sites of insertion.

Acknowledgment

We wish to thank Samuel H. Wald, Julianne Mendoza, and Frederick G. Mihm for prior contributions to this chapter.

ANNOTATED REFERENCES

Camkiran Firat A, Zeyneloglu P, Ozkan M, Pirat A. A randomized controlled comparison of the internal jugular vein and the subclavian vein as access sites for central venous catheterization in pediatric cardiac surgery. *Pediatr Crit Care Med.* 2016;17:e413-e419.

This randomized, prospective study compared the success rate for placement of central venous catheters via the internal jugular route with subclavian routes in 280 children scheduled for cardiac surgery. There was no significant difference in the success rate at first attempt (64% vs. 69%), but the rate of arterial puncture was significantly higher in the internal jugular group (8% vs. 2%) and success rate overall was greater in the subclavian group (91% vs. 82%). However, catheter malposition was greater with the subclavian route (17% vs. 1%). Overall, the risk of catheter-associated infection complications was greater with the internal jugular route (22% vs. 3.6%).

Carter JH, Langley JM, Kuhle S, Kirkland S. Risk factors for central venous catheter-associated bloodstream infection in pediatric patients: a cohort study. *Infect Control Hosp Epidemiol.* 2016;37(8):939-945.

This was a within-institution study reviewing their experience from 1995 to 2013 involving 5648 patients that revealed a central line–associated bloodstream infection rate of 3.87/1000 in-hospital line days. Over time there was an 84% reduction in these infections that was primarily related to a vigorous hand hygiene campaign.

Gleich SJ, Wong AV, Handlogten KS, Thum DE, Nemergut ME. Major short-term complications of arterial cannulation for monitoring in children. *Anesthesiology.* 2021;134(1):26-34.

This is a retrospective cohort of 5142 arterial cannulations and postoperative complications in 4178 elective pediatric surgical patients from 2006 to 2016. The most common sites for complications were the radial (n=3395, 66%) and femoral (n=1528, 29%) arteries. There were 11 major complications, all in femoral arterial lines in children younger than 5 years old: 8 vascular and 3 infections. The overall incidence is 2 per 1000 lines (95% CI 1–4). The majority of femoral lines were placed for cardiac procedures. Infants and neonates had the greatest complication rates, 16 and 11 per 1000 lines, respectively (95%CI 7–34 and 3–39, respectively).

Siddik-Sayyid SM, Aouad MT, Ibrahim MH, et al. Femoral arterial cannulation performed by residents: a comparison between ultrasound-guided and palpation technique in infants and children undergoing cardiac surgery. *Paediatr Anaesth.* 2016;26(8):823-830.

This was a randomized prospective study that compared ultrasound-guided with palpation-guided placement of femoral arterial lines in 106 pediatric patients. The number of successful cannulations of first attempt was greater in the ultrasound group (24/5 vs. 13/53), and the time to successful cannulation was also shorter (301 ± 234 seconds versus 420 ± 248 seconds). The ultrasound-guided technique when used by residents was superior to the palpation-guided technique.

Song IK, Kim EH, Lee JH, Jang YE, Kim HS, Kim JT. Seldinger vs. modified Seldinger techniques for ultrasound-guided central venous catheterization in neonates: a randomized controlled trial. *Br J Anaesth.* 2018;121(6):1332-1337.

This randomized controlled trial of 120 neonates younger than 1 month of age compared the Seldinger to the modified Seldinger technique in internal jugular catheterization. The incidence of successful catheterization on the first attempt was higher in the modified Seldinger group (83% vs. 65%).

A complete reference list can be found online at Elsevier eBooks+.

46

47 Infectious Disease Considerations for the Operating Room

ANDRE L. JAICHENCO, SR., LUCIANA CAVALCANTI LIMA, AND JOHN C. WELCH

Causative Agent

Host

Methods of Transmission

Air Transmission

Contact Transmission

Accidents With Cutting or Piercing Devices

Coronavirus and Future Pandemics

Preparation

Preoperative Covid-19 Testing and Timing of Procedures after Covid-19 Infection

Induction and Airway Management

Regional Anesthesia

Emergence and Extubation

Specific Pediatric Anesthesia Considerations

Cardiac Arrest

Equipment Decontamination and Room Turnover

Summary on COVID-19 Care

Strategy for Preventing Infection Transmission in Health Care Institutions

Measures for Prevention of Infection Transmission in the Operating Room

Prevention of Airborne Pathogen Transmission

Standard Precautions

Antimicrobial Prophylaxis

"Clean hands are the single most important factor in preventing the spread of pathogens and antibiotic resistance in healthcare settings" (Center for Disease Control and Prevention).

"Clean Care is Safer Care is not a choice, but a basic right. Clean hands prevent patient suffering and save lives" (World Health Organization).

Health-care–associated infections are often preventable, and they affect hundreds of millions of people each year around the world. The prevalence of health-care–associated infections in low- and middle-income countries is about 2 to 20 times higher than in high-income countries.[1] Basic knowledge in infection control is essential for anesthesiologists.

- On average, 1 in 10 patients per year are affected by a health-care–associated infection; ~7% in developed countries and ~15% in developing countries.[2,3]
- In the United States, 2 million hospitalized patients develop health-care–associated infections per year, of whom 90,000 will die.[4]
- In 2021, 1 in 31 hospitalized patients in the United States developed a health-care–associated infection[5]; more than 722,000 cases of infections were attributed to poor infection control practices in health centers, generating 400,000 extra days of hospitalization at an additional cost of 28 to 33 billion dollars. These infections resulted in approximately 75,000 deaths.[2,6]
- In low- or middle-income countries, ~11% of patients who undergo surgery develop infections. In Africa, up to 20% of women undergoing cesarean section contract a surgical site infection, compromising their well-being and ability to care for their children.[2]
- No one should become ill while seeking medical attention. However, each year millions of people around the world are affected by health-care–associated infections, many of which are preventable. There is no country or health system that is free from health-care–associated infections.[2]

The consequences of health-care–associated infections are profound and include increased costs, selection for drug-resistant organisms, patient and family dissatisfaction, and major morbidity and mortality. The source of these health-care–associated infections is multifactorial, but a large fraction of these infections originate in the operating room and routine anesthetic practices can contribute to these infections. Although the environment around the patient can be an important source of infection, contaminated hands of anesthesiologists are also sources of bacterial transmission through an intravenous (IV) line, with consequent increased patient mortality. The incidence of bloodstream infections related to the IV has been reported as ~0.18%; prolonged insertion time and emergent placement increase the risk.[7] The perioperative environment poses a risk for cross-transmission of infectious organisms. This risk is in part, related to the activation of the cytokine system in response to surgical stress and the effects of anesthetic agents (e.g., inhalation agents, opioids) on immune cellular responses.[8] These factors may also serve as important source of infections in the operating room.

Anesthesiologists have long been advocates of patient safety, so it is not surprising that anesthesiologists have assumed increasing responsibility for preventing health-care–associated infections including surgical site infections and ventilator-associated infections. Anesthesia providers practice in a nonsterile environment within the operating room (OR) touching parts of the body that are known to be contaminated such as the axilla, nares, and pharynx. Hand hygiene, wearing gloves, and proper skin preparation are strategies known to reduce the risk of transmitting infections, although these are haphazardly followed at times.[9,10]

Bacterial contamination of drugs and syringes during routine preparation in the operating room has occurred in up to 6% of instances from a variety of sources, including drawing air into vials to facilitate drug withdrawal or inserting a needle through a nonsterile or contaminated rubber stopper on a vial that had not been wiped with alcohol.[11] In more than 6% of 300 cases where microbial filters were used when drugs were administered intravenously, *Staphylococcus, Corynebacterium, Micrococcus,* and *Bacillus* species were cultured from the filters. Equally alarming, 2.4% of residual fluid samples in syringes at the end of these surgical cases demonstrated the presence of other bacteria.[12] A similar study of IV fluid bags has also demonstrated bacterial contamination in a simulated study (5/38 bags).[13] These studies highlight the importance of disinfecting catheter ports with alcohol-based disinfectants before each use.[14]

The environmental contamination of the anesthesia workspace has been characterized according to rate and time using video observation during patient care. Anesthesia induction and awakening were identified as key moments in which environmental contamination reached a predetermined threshold to increase the likelihood of contamination. This study suggests that environmental cleanup strategies may be more effective if implemented during these moments.[15] Trained housekeeping staff were superior to anesthesia staff for cleaning anesthesia work spaces after procedures.[16] A Society for Healthcare Epidemiology of America panel recommended that the World Health Organization's (WHO's) five moments of hand hygiene be followed[17]: (1) when entering or exiting the operating room, (2) before aseptic tasks (e.g., IV, central line placement), (3) after removing gloves, (4) when hands are soiled, and (5) before touching contents of the anesthesia cart.[14]

As anesthesiologists, the two greatest contributors to healthcare–associated infections are right in front of us: *our hands.* Interactions between anesthesiologists and operating room equipment (the anesthesia machine, monitor surfaces, computers and keyboards, drawers, vascular catheters, stopcocks, IV catheters, and many others) were documented during 8 hours of observation.[18] Anesthesiologists touched these surfaces 1132 times, touched stopcocks 66 times, and inserted 4 vascular catheters. Unfortunately, proper hand hygiene occurred in only 13 instances and failed after exposures to blood, and before and after procedures (e.g., IV placement, and alcohol cleaning of stopcocks occurred in only 10 of 66 exposures).[18,19] Another study used a fluorescent dye technique to illustrate how anesthetists' gloved hands contaminate anesthesia work surfaces within 6 minutes after a routine anesthetic induction and tracheal intubation. Of particular concern, there was 100% contamination of the IV hub, anesthesia circuit, and anesthesia cart. Furthermore, compelling evidence demonstrated that even syringes that were not used in the work environment became contaminated.[20] Without encouragement, anesthesiologists perform hand hygiene less frequently than once per hour during a case, but with reminders, the rate of hand hygiene is more frequent. Improved hand hygiene reduces contamination of the work area and IV access ports from 32% to 8%, which in turn may reduce health-care–associated infections.[21,22]

Surgical site infections are especially relevant because they account for 20% or more of all health-care–associated infection cases. In fact, surgical site infections affect 1% to 3% of all surgical patients, increasing the length of hospital stay and increasing mortality.[4] Surgical site infections are just one of the four most common types of health-care–associated infections, which include catheter-associated urinary tract infection, catheter-associated bloodstream infection (27,021 reported in 2021),[5] and ventilator-associated pneumonia.[5] Overuse or misuse of antibiotics constitutes an additional risk factor for all infections.[23,24] Transport from the floor to the operating room (intensive care unit or ward) is also an independent risk factor for catheter-associated bloodstream infection.[25]

Anesthesiologists are uniquely challenged to manage the patient's airway, placing IV catheters, and administering medications while balancing the need to maintain aseptic techniques.[26] The human mouth is home to over 500 different types of bacteria, some of which are essential for normal oral health and some that have the potential to cause disease. Bacteria such as staphylococci and streptococci normally colonize the oral cavity and nasopharynx and are also identified as flora in health-care–associated infections. Airway management during mask ventilation or placement of oral airways, laryngeal mask airways, or tracheal tubes increase the potential for bacterial contamination. In contrast to the practice of anesthesia in adults where intravenous access and drug administration are usually performed by individuals other than the anesthesiologist before the airway is manipulated, the practice of pediatric anesthesia often involves induction of anesthesia using a face mask and manipulating the airway before or while venous access is established and drugs are administered, which can further increase the risk of contamination.[27]

New strategies have been suggested to address this dilemma: (1) the double-glove technique,[14] in which contaminated outer gloves are removed immediately after airway management; (2) minimizing the number and location of intravenous access points; (3) the physical separation of "clean spaces" for drug preparation and administration; and (4) designating a "dirty space" for immediate evacuation of contaminated supplies.[28]

The transmission of infection depends on the presence of three interconnected elements: a causative agent, a source, and a mode of transmission (Fig. 47.1). Understanding the characteristics of each element provides the practicing anesthesiologist with methods to protect susceptible patients and themselves and avoid spreading infection.[29]

There has always been concern about the transmission of infectious agents to the patient from the anesthesiologist and vice versa.[30] In addition, there are many sites within the hospital environment where moist or desiccated organic material that can host potentially pathogenic microbes may survive for extended periods of time (Table 47.1)[31,32]; some pathogens may even resist the

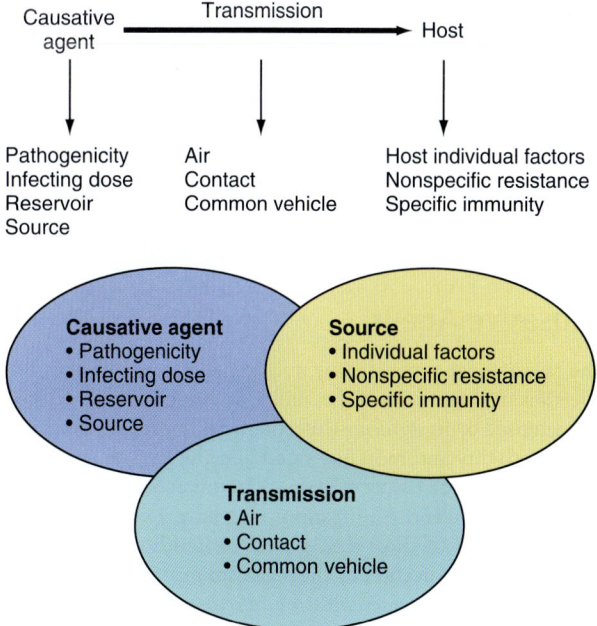

FIGURE 47.1 Elements of chain of infection.

TABLE 47.1   Nosocomial Pathogens and Survival

Pathogen	Organism Survival Time
Influenza virus	24–48 hours on nonporous surfaces, 8–12 hours on clothing[308]
Parainfluenza virus	10 hours on nonporous surfaces; 4 hours on clothes[309]
Norovirus	20 days on wood, 137 hours on plastic, 92 hours stainless steel, and may remain on food-contact surfaces up to 28 days[310]
Hepatitis B virus	7 days[311]
Human immunodeficiency virus	Plastic >7 days, glass 5 days[312]
SARS-CoV-2	3 to >8 days stainless steel[312]
Candida	3 days for Candida albicans and 14 days for Candida parapsilosis[313]
Clostridium difficile	5 months on hospital floors[314]
Pseudomonas aeruginosa	6–7 hours on glass or stainless steel[315]
Acinetobacter baumannii	Up to 4 months under dry conditions[316]
Staphylococcus aureus including methicillin resistant	≤58 days on working surfaces,[317] up to 5 years on dry surfaces, 60–72 days on clothing[318]
Escherichia coli	1.5 hours to 16 months[319]
Enterococcus	5 days to 4 months[319]
Haemophilus influenzae	12 days[319]
Klebsiella	2 hours to >30 months[319]
Mycobacterium tuberculosis	1 day to 4 months[319]
Neisseria gonorrhoeae	1–3 days[319]
Streptococcus pneumoniae	1–20 days[319]
Adenovirus	>8 weeks, 7–60 days on aluminum, china, latex[312]
Vancomycin-resistant Enterococcus	5 days to 5 years on dry surfaces, 21 days on floor and clothing[318]
Serratia marcescens	3 days to 2 months, 5 weeks on dry floor[319]
Rotavirus	2–12 days stainless steel[312]

usual cleaning and disinfection techniques.[33] Their transmission from the source to the host may occur via indirect nonapparent mechanisms (e.g., most commonly through hand contact).[29]

Causative Agent

The causative agent may be any microorganism capable of causing infection. Pathogenicity is the ability to induce disease, which is characterized by its *virulence* (infection severity, determined by the germ morbidity and mortality rates) and the level of *invasiveness* (capacity to invade tissues). There are no microorganisms that are completely avirulent. An organism may have a very low level of virulence, but if the host (i.e., patient or health care provider) is very susceptible, infection by the organism may cause disease. The risk of infection increases with the *infecting dose* (the number of organisms available to induce disease), the *reservoir* (the site where the organisms reside and multiply), and the *infection source*

(the site from which the pathogen is transmitted to a susceptible host either directly or indirectly through an intermediary object). The infectious source may be a symptomatic or asymptomatic human (e.g., health care providers, parents, children, visitors, housekeeping personnel) during the incubation period. The source may also be temporarily or permanently colonized (the most frequently colonized tissues are the skin, digestive system, nares, and respiratory tracts).[29]

Host

The presence of a susceptible host is a fundamental element in the infection chain. Host susceptibility is determined by specific and nonspecific defense mechanisms. Nonspecific defense mechanisms involve the skin, mucous membranes, ciliary activity, normal bacterial flora, secretions (saliva, bronchial secretion, mucin, gastric fluid), the cough reflex, enzymatic activity, inflammatory response, acute phase proteins, hormonal responses, nutritional status, and genetic factors. Specific defense mechanisms involve antibodies against particular antigens that may be acquired in response to infection, vaccination, toxins, or transplacental transmission,[34] breast milk, or exogenous immunoglobulins.[35] Neonates are at particular risk of contracting infectious diseases because they have an immature immune system,[35] and the normal flora are not yet developed. Prematurity is associated with a greater immune deficit and the need for invasive procedures, mechanical ventilation, or parenteral nutrition.[36] The risk of infections in surgical patients is further increased by factors such as immunosuppression associated with surgical trauma and invasive procedures that damage protective barriers (e.g., skin, mucous membranes, lungs, intestinal and genitourinary tracts, intravascular access), facilitating the entry of microorganisms into the body, as well as long pre- and postoperative hospitalization times.[37]

Methods of Transmission

Microorganisms are transmitted in the hospital environment through several different routes, and the same microorganism may be transmitted via more than one route. In the operating room, the two main routes of transmission are through the air and contact (direct and indirect).

AIR TRANSMISSION

Respiratory infectious agents are transmitted from their natural reservoir to a susceptible person primarily through droplet and aerosol transmission.[38] In general, the infected person distributes the pathogen when talking, breathing, coughing, and crying, or during procedures such as laryngoscopy, bronchoscopy, or aspiration of secretions. Infectious agents may also emerge enclosed in a capsule of urine, saliva, or water. The fate of these bacterial capsules in the environment depends mainly on their size. Larger particles fall quickly before evaporating as droplets, whereas smaller particles evaporate quickly, forming aerosols that remain suspended in the air for a prolonged period allowing them to spread further than droplets.[39] Respiratory transmission can be classified as droplet or aerosol depending on the size of the particle and its consequent aerodynamic characteristics. Particles that are less than 5 to 10 micrometers in diameter can aerosolize in the environment and be transmitted long distances, whereas particles that are less than 5 micrometers in diameter enter the airway as far as the alveolus. Particles less than 10 micrometers in diameter can enter through the glottis. The airborne ability and small size of bioaerosols necessitate health care providers to use personal protective equipment (PPE) that is well-sealed around the airway. Large particles (greater than 10 to 20 μm) follow a ballistic trajectory due to the influence of gravity, traveling a distance ≤1 meter. Particles larger than 10 micrometers do not penetrate into the lower respiratory tract, but instead impact the upper respiratory tract. A standard surgical mask acts as a physical barrier to drops 10 to 20 micrometers in diameter and should effectively protect against transmission of such upper respiratory pathogens.[40]

For protection against smaller particles, especially during manipulation of the airway such as tracheal intubation, the use of an N95 (where N refers to non-oil, and 95 to 95% efficiency in blocking particles, US standard) mask is recommended. Wearing a properly fitted N95 mask should prevent ~95% of particles ≥0.3 micrometers in diameter from reaching the person's airway.[41] Even a loose-fitting N95 mask will filter out ~90% of these particles; KN95 (K=Korea, China standard) masks are much less efficient (53% to 85%) than N95 masks, whereas a standard surgical mask has filtering efficiency of 37% to 69%.[42] Particles <10 micrometers in diameter present a different degree of risk than larger particles due to two fundamental characteristics: the time the particles are suspended in the air and the ability of the particles to reach the airway. Environmental conditions such as air currents, ventilation systems, and others can facilitate large particles remaining suspended in the air for prolonged periods and traveling further. Consequently, the actual suspension times of large particles may be greater in a hospital environment where currents are generated due to opening and closing of doors, bed and equipment movement, room air ventilation turnover, and the intermittent movement of personnel.[40] Noninvasive ventilation and respiratory physiotherapy are droplet-generating procedures (not aerosols), generating droplets >10 micrometers in diameter that will land on surfaces in the immediate vicinity (i.e., less than 1 meter away from where they originated) (E-Fig. 47.1).[40] Nebulization, intubation, extubation, bronchoscopy, and open airway aspiration are aerosol-generating procedures and use of PPE is especially important during these events.[43] In addition, patients who are known to carry respiratory pathogens should wear a mask to protect any personnel with whom they come in contact.[44]

CONTACT TRANSMISSION

Direct and indirect contact are the most frequent methods of hospital infection transmission.

Direct Contact

This type of disease transmission involves direct physical contact between two individuals. The physical transfer of microorganisms from an infected or colonized person to a susceptible host may occur from a child to a health care provider or vice versa during patient care procedures (e.g., venous cannulation, laryngoscopy, burn care, or suction of secretions). Health care providers who work in the operating room may be exposed to body fluids (saliva, vomitus, blood, abscess fluids) by skin contamination. This is an issue of grave concern because of the potential exposure of health care providers to patients with unrecognized infections, especially hepatitis B virus (HBV), hepatitis C virus (HCV), and human immunodeficiency virus (HIV). HBV is a highly infectious virus that requires only a small amount of blood (10^{-7} to 10^{-9} mL) to transmit the disease.

The incidence of skin contamination of anesthesiologists and related personnel by blood and saliva is substantial. In a study that examined 270 anesthetic procedures during 7 consecutive days,

the blood of 35 patients (14%) contaminated the skin of 65 anesthesiologists in 46 incidents. Of these contamination events, 28 (61%) occurred during venous cannulation. Of the anesthesiologists who had been contaminated by blood, 5 of 65 (8%) had cuts in the skin of their hands.[45] The importance of this observation is that seroconversion of health care providers has been reported after skin contamination by infected blood from HIV carriers,[46] and HBV infection after blood splashed into health care workers' eyes.[47] Scabies, pediculosis, and herpes simplex are among the diseases most frequently transmitted by direct contact.[48–56] Meticulous hand washing before and after every patient contact and routine use of barriers such as gloves and eye protection are essential basic methods for protecting ourselves even during routine procedures such as starting an IV line or performing laryngoscopy.[2,22]

Regarding HIV vertical transmission (mother to baby), the virus is highly transmissible from untreated mothers to their infants, at rates between 25% and 42%. However, if the mother has been treated prophylactically, the risk of transmission is reduced to ≤1%.[57] For HBV, vertical transmission is the main mechanism of transmission with ~2 million children <5 years of age at risk of infection worldwide, at rates of 70% to 90%. To reduce this very high transmission rate, vaccination and hepatitis B immunoglobulin are essential.[58] Approximately 150 million people are infected with HCV worldwide, with a prevalence of 0.05% to 0.36% of children in medically advanced countries versus 1.8% to 5% in less advanced countries.[59] The main route of infection in childhood is through vertical transmission, at a rate of 3% to 10%.[60]

Indirect Contact

Indirect contact involves transmitting microorganisms from a source (animate or inanimate) to a susceptible host by means of a vehicle (e.g., an intermediary object) contaminated by body fluids. E-Tables 47.1 and 47.2 provide examples of diseases associated with bodily fluids to which health care workers may be exposed. The vehicle for transmission may be the hands of a health care provider who is not wearing gloves or a provider who fails to wash their hands after providing care to a child.[9,21,51,60–62] This type of contact can also come from health care providers who touch (with or without gloves) contaminated monitoring or other patient-care devices (e.g., blood pressure cuffs, stethoscopes, electrocardiographic cables, or ventilation systems [respirators, corrugated tubes, Y-pieces, valves]) that are used without proper cleaning or disinfection between each use.[63–65]

Knowledge about the transmission of bacteria from patients to health care workers' hands and to the hospital environment (Fig. 47.2) has driven many interventions that have succeeded

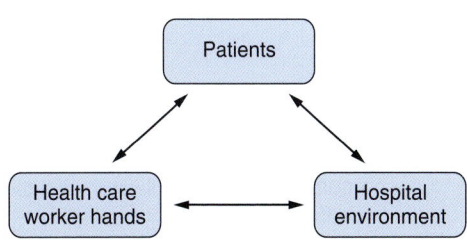

FIGURE 47.2 Epidemiologic links for transmission of multidrug-resistant organisms. (From Munoz-Price LS, Weinstein RA. Fecal patina in the anesthesia work area. *Anesth Analg.* 2015;120(4):703-705.)

in reducing patient risks for developing health-care–associated infections.[19]

Studies on vancomycin-resistant enterococci established the importance of a domino effect of contamination in ICUs and inpatient wards: vancomycin-resistant enterococci that colonized patient gastrointestinal tracts ("rectal carriage") spread to the patient's skin, then to the hospital environment, to the hands of health care workers, and then to other patients. The skin contamination of patients with enteric organisms inspired the rather graphic description, the patient's "fecal patina"[66] (also referred to as a "stool veneer"). This coating with enteric organisms is not limited to a patient's skin; it also extends to surfaces in the surrounding environment that are touched, and thereby contaminated, by patients and by health care workers. The environmental contamination spreads out from the patient in a target-like concentric pattern, with the densest contamination closest to the rectum of patients who have rectal carriage of the index bacteria. This interplay among organisms on patients' body surfaces, hospital environment, and health care workers' hands constitutes the foundation for the development of infection control interventions.[19]

The transmission of frequently encountered Gram-negative bacteria in the anesthesia work area environment[67] demonstrates that spread follows an epidemiologic pattern similar to that seen in ICUs and inpatient wards: from patient, to the environment and health care workers' hands, and to other patients (Fig. 47.3). In this report, provider hands were less likely to serve as a vehicle to transmit infection than contaminated environmental or patient skin surfaces. These findings hold clinical implications for the risk of colonization and subsequent pathology (e.g., surgical site infections). Reports such as these call attention to the need to develop and enforce strict hand hygiene guidelines for personnel who are providing anesthesia care, and more importantly, the need to increase compliance with environmental disinfection of the operating room (between cases and terminal cleaning), and to further study the directions of the spread of pathogens in the operating room and anesthesia work areas. This study unequivocally underscores our need to improve cleaning procedures in the operating room and equipment surfaces to reduce infection transmission risk.[14,16,29,44]

There are also reports of equipment, fomites, and drugs (mainly propofol) that have resulted in hospital-acquired infections.[53,68–86]

More than 50 years ago, Spaulding devised a rational disinfection and sterilization system for the elements and equipment used in surgical-anesthetic procedures.[87] This classification is so logical and clear that it is still currently used, with some modifications, to divide the elements into three risk categories of medical equipment decontamination (Table 47.2).[88,89]

In addition to the indirect transmission of infectious agents described above, transmission may also occur via drug administration procedures. For example, early propofol preparations were found to be favorable for bacterial growth (*Staphylococcus aureus*, *Escherichia coli*, *Pseudomonas aeruginosa*, and *Candida albicans*), thus leading to infection due to contamination, which in turn led to the addition of antimicrobial preservatives (e.g., ethylenediaminetetraacetic acid [EDTA] or sodium metabisulfite) to current formulations.[90,91] These preservatives inhibit the rate of bacterial growth for up to 12 hours.[92] Despite the presence of antibacterial preservatives, contamination of the vial of propofol remains a concern in the clinical setting. Horizontal transmission occurred due to anesthesiologists using the same vial on multiple patients or leaving vials open to room air.[91] Hence, the current recommendation is to wipe the vial cap clean with alcohol and to use each vial for only one patient.[92,93] Intralipids and other intravenous fat emulsions that do not contain preservatives may also promote bacterial growth and are therefore associated with the risk of infection. Patient colonization may also occur due to contamination at the IV hub after administering either propofol or intralipid, as well as at stopcocks.[94] Flushing the hub and changing stopcocks are recommended to reduce the potential for bacterial contamination.[92,94,95]

Due to its ubiquitous presence on human skin and its ability to form biofilms on instruments, *S. epidermidis* is among the most frequent causative agent involved in infections from long-term medical devices (including peripheral or central IV catheters). Several studies examined interventions to arrest bacterial growth in propofol. Curiously, both diphenhydramine and ketamine individually inhibited bacterial growth (e.g., *S. aureus*, *P. aeruginosa*)

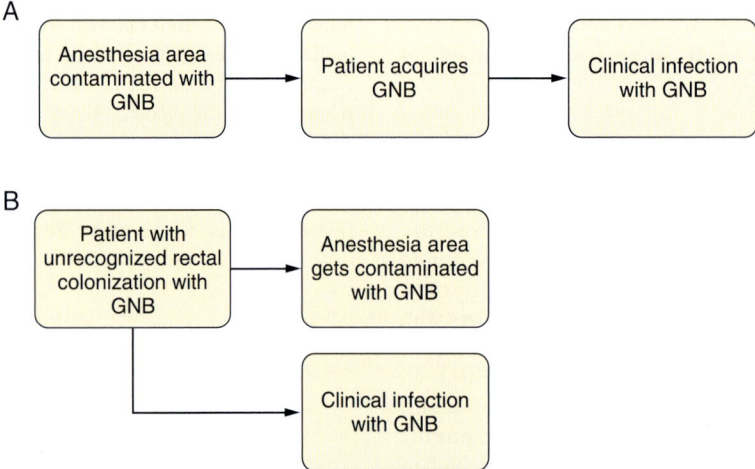

FIGURE 47.3 Possible explanations of subsequent clinical infections caused by the same organism cultured in the anesthesia work area. **A,** Contaminated environment exposes patient to Gram-negative bacilli *(GNB)* with the subsequent development of a clinical infection. **B,** Patient with unrecognized rectal colonization undergoes surgery, contaminating the anesthesia area with their endogenous GNB, and later develops a clinical infection with the same organism. (Data from Loftus RW, Brown JR, Patel HM, et al. Transmission dynamics of Gram-negative bacterial pathogens in the anesthesia work area. *Anesth Analg.* 2015;120(4):819-826.)

TABLE 47.2 | Risk Categories for Medical Decontamination and Common Methods

Grade	Definition	Microbicidal Action Level	Decontamination Method	Common Items/Equipment Examples
High (critical)	Medical devices that penetrate the skin, mucous membranes, or sterile body cavities	Eliminates all microorganisms	Sterilization by heat (if it is stable at high temperatures), or chemical	Surgical instruments, implants, prostheses, urinary catheters, needles, syringes, sutures, vascular catheters, etc.
Intermediate (semicritical)	Medical devices in contact with mucous membranes or nonintact skin	Eliminates all microorganisms, except large numbers of bacterial spores	High level of heat or chemical disinfection (under controlled conditions with minimal toxicity to humans)	Respiratory therapy and anesthetic equipment, flexible endoscopes, vaginal specula, etc.
Low (noncritical)	Items in contact with intact skin	Eliminates vegetative bacteria, fungi, and lipid viruses	Low level of disinfection (cleanliness)	Pressure cuffs, stethoscopes, ECG cables, etc. Environmental surfaces, including cart and anesthesia workstation surfaces

in propofol in a dose-dependent manner, and were more effective than lidocaine.[96–98] Although some studies observed that fentanyl and remifentanil also inhibited bacterial growth in propofol (but less so with *E. coli and C. albicans*)[99], one study concluded that fentanyl, like propofol, actually supported bacterial growth (including *P. aeruginosa and S. aureus*) and that lidocaine exerted antibacterial effects.[100]

Other indirect sources that may contribute to infection include:

- Up to 40% of anesthetic equipment in direct or indirect contact with a child (blood pressure cuffs, cables, oximeters, laryngoscopes, monitors, respirator settings, and horizontal and vertical surfaces) may be contaminated with blood because of inadequate cleansing procedures between uses.[19,20,31,32,63,101,102]
- In some institutions, up to 8% of the Bain circuits that were reused without previous sterilization were contaminated.[103]
- Syringe contents have been found to be contaminated with glass particles. Presumably, when an ampule was opened, glass particles were introduced to the solution; this in turn may have compromised the sterility of the contents, presumably because of the passage of bacteria contained on glass particles spilling into the solution.[104–106]
- IV tubing can have both direct blood contamination and contamination by blood from syringes used to inject medications. These can occur with the absence of visible blood reflux in the tubing or syringe. Simply replacing the needle on a syringe that will be reused is ineffective in preventing cross-infection; it is essential to not use the same syringe or vial in multiple patients.[107,108]
- Refilling syringes (both glass and plastic) several times has also been shown to result in contamination of the syringe contents; single use is therefore recommended.[107–110]
- Some drug formulations can sustain bacterial growth under certain conditions. Thus great care should be given to aseptic technique when transferring drugs from the vial to a syringe and to use the contents of the syringe within 4 hours.[111–115] Propofol vials should not be used for multiple patients because of concerns for cross-contamination, particularly since not all countries have added antimicrobial preservatives to the propofol emulsion.[116,117]
- Needles that have been used for spinal or epidural anesthesia were contaminated with coagulase-negative staphylococci (15.7%), yeasts (1.5%), enterococci (0.8%), pneumococci (0.8%), and micrococci (0.8%), suggesting that there may be needle contamination despite standard skin preparation and cleansing.[118] It is unclear whether these skin organisms can be transmitted and cause an infection during administration of a neuraxial block. Spinal and epidural needles should only be used on one patient.

- Blood and saliva frequently contaminate the skin of anesthetic personnel during routine anesthetic practice; wearing gloves is essential to minimize contamination.[21]
- Violations of contemporary guidelines for preventing infections (e.g., washing hands, wearing gloves, surgical masks, ocular protection, scrubs, or reusing syringes) by anesthesiologists are frequent. Anesthesia staff are aware that they work in a potentially infectious environment, but they commonly do not adopt appropriate protective measures to reduce infections in both themselves and their patients (11% to 99%).[63,119–121]

ACCIDENTS WITH CUTTING OR PIERCING DEVICES

Occupational exposure to bloodborne pathogens through needlestick or other sharps injuries is a serious but frequently preventable problem. According to a 2002 report from the WHO, there are approximately 2 million occupational exposures to bloodborne pathogens per year out of an estimated 35 million health workers in the world.[122] Fortunately, this incidence has rapidly declined over the past 30 years.[123]

Percutaneous Contamination

Percutaneous contamination from a cutting or piercing accident is the most effective means to transmit bloodborne pathogens. Evidence suggests that this is the main route of HIV, HBV, and HCV infection,[124–126] especially if the injury is caused by hollowbore needles that were used to draw blood or establish IV access.[127,128] Over 20 other bloodborne pathogens have been transmitted by this means, including those causing herpes, malaria, and tuberculosis.[129] The risk of exposure to blood and bloodborne pathogens is greater for health care personnel than for people who do not work around blood. An exposure to infected blood, tissue, or other potentially infectious body fluids can occur by percutaneous injury, nonintact skin, or contact with mucous membranes. The risk of infection after an exposure depends on a number of variables and appears to be greater with exposure to a larger quantity of blood or other infectious fluid; prolonged or extensive exposure of nonintact skin or mucous membrane to blood or other infectious fluid or concentrated virus in a laboratory setting; exposure to the blood of a patient in an advanced disease stage or with a higher HIV viral load; a deep percutaneous injury; a procedure wherein the sharp was in

TABLE 47.3	Circumstances Associated With Accidents With Hollow-Bore Needles (n=10,239) (1995–2003) Reported to Centers for Disease Control and Prevention
Circumstance of Hollow-Bore Needle Injury	**Percent**
Manipulating needle in patient	28
During sharps disposal	13
Collision with coworker or needle	10
Improper disposal	9
During cleanup	9
Recapping needle	6
Passing equipment to colleague	6
Accessing IV line	5
Transferring or processing specimen	5
Other	5
In transit to disposal	4

From https://www.cdc.gov/sharpssafety/part1TEXTONLY.html

the vein or artery of an infected source patient; an injury with a hollow-bore, blood-filled needle; and limited or delayed access to postexposure prophylaxis.[123]

The Center for Disease Control examined the circumstances of 10,239 hollow-bore needle injuries in 2003 (Table 47.3); at that time 64% were determined to be preventable, 18% nonpreventable, and the remainder undetermined.[130] It should be noted, however, that the vast majority of such injuries do not result in infection; the major factor determining infection development is the availability of postexposure prophylaxis.[123] After exposure, the risk of infection varies for specific bloodborne pathogens. For HBV, if the source patient has active HBV and the health care provider does not already have immunity, the risk for infection after percutaneous injury is between 1% and 30%. However, recent data suggest that the rate of infection has dramatically fallen (500 health care workers in 1997 to 13 in 2009) due to improved safety practices and the availability of HBV vaccine.[123] If the source patient has active HCV, the risk of hepatitis C transmission is approximately 1.8% (range 0% to 7%) after a percutaneous injury and such cases represent 2% to 4% of total HCV disease.[123] If the source patient has HIV infection, the risk of HIV transmission is approximately 0.3% after a percutaneous exposure and 0.09% after a mucous membrane exposure.[123] Fortunately, due to the availability of postexposure prophylaxis, there were only 57 cases reported in exposed workers from 1981 to 2010 and this number is likely even lower in current day practice.[123] The risk of HIV transmission for an exposure with nonintact skin has not been determined and is estimated to be less than the risk after a mucous membrane exposure.[131]

Preventing Accidental Punctures With Sharps

In 1981, the characteristics of percutaneous accidents in hospital personnel were described including housekeeping and nursing assistants injured by needles left in bed linen or disposed into regular trash bins, and recommended a series of prevention strategies, including educational programs, the proscription on replacing needle caps, and better disposal systems (tamper-evident plastic boxes).[132] In 1987, the US Centers for Disease Control and Prevention (CDC) published universal precautions that included

guides for percutaneous accident prevention focusing on the careful handling and disposal of needles. During the subsequent years, the improved design of safety intravenous catheters and containers for the safe disposal of sharps and needles as well as educational programs have greatly improved health care worker safety.[133–136] New needle stick regulations include the need for engineering and work place controls to prevent needle sticks and a requirement to keep a log of employee needle stick injuries (USA Occupational Safety Hazard Administration Regulation for *General Industry (29 CFR 1910.*1030).

Universal precautions focus on personal protection elements (e.g., camisole, mask, goggles, gloves, etc.) and control of correct practices (e.g., not recapping needles, rigid discard containers, etc.); these best practices have demonstrated effectiveness in preventing exposure to blood and/or biological fluids of the skin and mucous membranes[137]; however, most of the protective equipment is easily pierced by sharp elements. These needle puncture events can be drastically reduced with the use of needle-free drug administration, although a recent meta-analysis revealed that the quality of the scientific evidence showing that these devices reduce needle stick injuries is moderate, and they also may increase exposure to blood.[138,139] One study demonstrated that the use of IV catheters with a retractable needle generated a greater number of splashes with blood toward the health care provider and patients than common catheters, and suggested that the use of this technology should be left to the choice of the user trained in these devices.[140]

Should such an accident occur (e.g., needle puncture, exposure to nonintact skin, or mucous membrane exposure), there are now specific recommendations regarding immediate assessment of the risk of the exposure source (chart review, inform the patient that an accident has occurred, and ask permission to determine HBV, HCV, and HIV serologic status), and rapid initiation of appropriate antiviral treatment (postexposure prophylaxis) of the health care worker.[141] It is advised to obtain as much information regarding the patient as possible. If the patient is possibly infected: (1) obtain a sample of blood from the patient for determination of potential carrier state (Table 47.4) and (2) report to the health service for immediate institution of prophylaxis and follow-up (E-Table 47.3), especially for HIV, HVB, and HVC exposure (E-Tables 47.4 and 47.5). Since successful HIV treatment is related to rapid initiation of postexposure prophylaxis (best within 2 hours of exposure), this should be started without delaying to assess the source; prophylaxis can be stopped if the source tests negative.[142]

Coronavirus and Future Pandemics

The coronavirus disease 2019 (COVID-19) pandemic unveiled numerous important considerations at the intersection of infectious disease and anesthesiology. The rapid spread of the severe acute respiratory syndrome-coronavirus-2 (SARS-CoV-2) virus around the world brought a collective awareness of the threats of emerging infectious diseases and the challenges of maintaining essential health services during a global pandemic. At the time of this writing, nearly 771 million cases of COVID-19 have been reported in the United States, with a mortality approaching 1%, or just under 6.9 million deaths.[143] Some regions of the world have ample experience responding to dangerous epidemics such as cholera or Ebola, while continuing to provide safe surgical and anesthesia care.[144–146] This section will review some of the important lessons learned during the COVID-19 pandemic and provide general recommendations for providing anesthesia care during any pandemic.

TABLE 47.4   Guide to Postexposure Prophylaxis and Prevention of Infection Transmission

Step 1: Treat Exposure Site

- Use soap and water to wash areas exposed to potentially infectious fluids as soon as possible after exposure.
- Flush exposed mucous membranes with water.
- Flush exposed eyes with water or saline solution.
- Do NOT apply caustic agents or inject antiseptics or disinfectants into the wound.

Step 2: Report and Document

- Date and time of exposure.
- Details of the incident: where and how the exposure occurred, exposure site(s) on HCP's body; if related to sharp device, the type and brand of device.
- Details of the exposure: type and amount of fluid or material, severity of exposure.
- Documentation of counseling following exposure and postexposure management plan.
- Details about the exposure source: if the source patient is known or unknown; whether the source material contained HIV, HBV, or HCV; if the source patient is HIV-infected, determine stage of disease, CD4 cell count, HIV viral load, history of antiretroviral therapy, and antiretroviral resistance information as available.
- Details about the exposed HCP: hepatitis B vaccination and vaccine-response status (HBsAb titer); other medical conditions that may influence choice of prophylactic agent(s) if needed; current medications, and drug allergies; pregnancy status or lactation status.

Step 3: Evaluate the Exposure

- The exposure should be evaluated for the potential to transmit HBV, HCV, or HIV based on the type of body substance involved, the route, severity, and frequency of exposure.
- Significant exposures to any of the following may pose a risk for bloodborne pathogen transmission and require further evaluation: blood, semen, vaginal secretions, cerebrospinal fluid, synovial fluid, pleural fluid, peritoneal fluid, pericardial fluid, amniotic fluid.
- Body fluids that do NOT pose a risk of bloodborne pathogen transmission unless visibly contaminated with blood include: urine, stool, tears, saliva, gastric secretions or vomitus, sweat, nonpurulent sputum, nasal discharge.

Step 4: Evaluate the Exposure Source
When source patient is known:

- Test source patient for HBsAg, HCV antibody, and HIV antibody.
  - Use a rapid HIV antibody test. Use of fourth-generation HIV antigen/antibody testing is recommended if available.
  - HIV viral load assessment for routine screening of source patient is NOT recommended.
  - If the source person is NOT infected with a bloodborne pathogen, further follow-up testing of the exposed HCP is not necessary. Follow state regulations related to informed consent and confidentiality.
- For patients who cannot be tested, consider medical diagnoses, clinical symptoms, and history of risk behaviors.

When source patient is NOT known/unable to be tested immediately:

- Evaluate the likelihood of high-risk exposure:
  - Consider the likelihood of bloodborne pathogen infections among patients in the exposure setting: what is the community infection rate? Does the clinic/hospital unit care for a large number of HIV-, HBV-, or HCV-infected or at-risk patients?
  - Is there a high suspicion for HIV infection and the patient is unable to be tested immediately?
- Do not test discarded needles for bloodborne pathogens; the reliability of these findings is not known.

The "window period":

- To date, there has not been a documented case of occupational HIV transmission from a source patient with a negative HIV antibody test result with risk factors for HIV acquisition.
- Postexposure prophylaxis should be considered only if the source patient has risk factors and has been determined to have symptoms consistent with acute HIV infection.

HBV, Hepatitis B virus; *HBsAg,* hepatitis B surface antigen; *HCV,* hepatitis C virus; *HCP,* health care personnel; *HIV,* human immunodeficiency virus.
From Mountain Plains AIDS Education and Training Center. PEP Steps, A Quick Guide to Postexposure Prophylaxis in the Health Care Setting (April 2006); PEP Steps: A Quick Guide to Postexposure Prophylaxis in the Health Care Setting (March 2014).

The most important practice consideration during an active infectious disease outbreak is to protect health care providers from acquiring the infection. This is particularly challenging for novel infections whose mechanisms and dynamics of disease transmission and incubation time, and level of PPE required, are unknown or poorly understood during the acute phase of the pandemic. Shortages of PPE and continually evolving infection prevention and control guidance further compound the complexities providers face. The discovery that COVID-19 could spread through respiratory droplets that could be easily aerosolized[147] was a particular concern for anesthesia providers. Rapid innovation occurred early in the COVID-19 pandemic to protect anesthesia providers while emergency cases persisted.[148,149] Providers were often redeployed to airway management teams. Recommendations have been compiled (see later) for those caring for patients suspected or confirmed of having COVID-19. Despite

the fact that these guidelines have been effective for other novel respiratory viruses, one should always consult the most up-to-date recommendations from the CDC or the WHO. Adopting guidelines from such organizations and implementing appropriate prevention and control measures allows anesthesia providers to ensure the safety of their patients while protecting themselves from infection.

PREPARATION

A preoperative huddle among operating room staff, anesthesia team, nursing staff, and surgeon improves safety and efficiency for managing COVID-19 cases.[150,151] The preoperative huddle should discuss risk for contamination, choice of PPE, transport plans, anesthesia plans, recovery plans, and other risk mitigation strategies.[150] The operating room to be used for a COVID-19 case should be clearly labeled with a sign to prevent inadvertent exposure of operating room staff not properly outfitted with PPE. If possible, the room should be switched from positive pressure to negative pressure.[152] If a negative pressure operating room is not available, it may be beneficial to perform the induction and intubation in a negative pressure room elsewhere in the hospital when possible.[151] The location where the patient will be met, interviewed, examined, and consented should be determined before bringing the patient to the operating room. These preliminary steps are ideally completed in an isolation room in the preoperative area, the patient's hospital room, the emergency department, or in the operating room itself. The surgical team should agree on the appropriate patient movements through the perioperative area as well as postoperatively to limit the exposure of hospital personnel and other patients to the virus. The anesthesia team should properly don appropriate PPE before contact with the patient to reduce their risk of acquiring COVID-19 or other viruses[153]:

- Perform hand hygiene
- Hair covering
- Fit-tested N95 respirator or powered air-purifying respirator (PAPR) with hood
- Eye protection or face shield (placed before a PAPR & hood combination)
- Isolation gown
- Gloves (some providers wear two layers of gloves to remove the outer gloves after airway management and remain protected)

Visual aids are important to ensure that providers wear all the pieces of PPE. Relying on a colleague to double check the PPE list is always wise (E-Fig. 47.2).[151]

Although most PPE is disposable and designed for single use, critical shortages of certain elements of PPE may occur during a pandemic. The US Occupational Safety and Health Administration (OSHA), for example, recommends that an N95 respirator mask may be reused up to five times.[154,155] Care must be taken, however, to avoid contamination when reusing PPE as the outermost layers may become contaminated.[156] If decontamination of PPE is employed (e.g., by steam), providers should take particular care in assessing the PPE fit before a patient is contacted as repeated use and sterilization may degrade the equipment. The design, manufacturer, local policies, and costs will ultimately dictate the PPE used and protocol for safe donning, doffing, decontamination, and disposal thereof.

If a COVID-19–positive patient must be transported through the hospital to the operating room, care should be taken to avoid contamination and infectious transmission enroute. The risk of transmission to providers and casual contacts during transport can be mitigated by having those infected patients who are spontaneously breathing wear an N95 mask, discontinuing all aerosol-generating treatments for transport, using high-efficiency particulate (HEPA) filters with patients whose airways are intubated,[157] restricting public access to patient transport routes, and ensuring all providers who are in the vicinity of or in contact with the infected patient wear appropriate PPE. Droplets may persist in enclosed spaces such as hospital elevators. Many modern elevators automatically discontinue air exchange when idle for more than several minutes. To reduce the risk of viral transmission in elevators, the ventilation providing air exchange should be maximized and maintained continuously. A study mimicking droplet dissemination and dissipation in hospital elevators found that holding elevator doors open for 3 to 5 minutes reduced the concentration of aerosolized particles by 100-fold versus 24 to 30 minutes when the doors were closed.[158]

All airway management materials including laryngoscope blades and handles, video laryngoscopes, supraglottic devices, tracheal tubes, oropharyngeal airways, and masks should be assembled and tested before the patient is brought into the operating room. Institutions that routinely provide anesthesia for "crash" cases like trauma, cesarean deliveries, and other emergent cases should consider establishing protocols to maintain COVID-19 airway management supplies always at-the-ready and tested periodically. Despite the advances in rapid testing for COVID-19, testing may need to be delayed or foregone for the most urgent cases. In such a situation, it is reasonable for providers to treat the patient as if they were COVID-19–positive.

Modifications to the anesthesia machine to accommodate COVID-19 patients are minimal but should include a HEPA filter between the tracheal tube and Y-piece of the breathing circuit. HEPA filters are designed to capture at least 99.97% of particles that are 0.3 micrometers or larger, which includes most viruses.[159] The filter media is made of a mat of randomly arranged fibers composed of fiberglass with diameters between 0.5 and 2.0 microns. The fibers are coated with a resin binder to increase their strength and durability.[151] An additional HEPA filter can be placed between the breathing hose set and expiratory port to avoid contaminating the anesthesia machine. The gas sample port must be placed on the device side of the viral filter to prevent contaminating the gas sampling system. Some filters have gas sample ports incorporated for ease-of-use (Fig. 47.4).[159]

PREOPERATIVE COVID-19 TESTING AND TIMING OF PROCEDURES AFTER COVID-19 INFECTION

Recommendations for routine preoperative testing in nonurgent and elective cases continue to evolve. Anesthesia personnel should consult the most up-to-date CDC and ASA recommendations on perioperative testing. It appears that COVID-19 has become endemic, and, in this case, anesthesia providers can be guided by levels of community transmission to determine a preoperative testing strategy. A COVID-19 Data Tracker is available from the CDC that simply requires state or county to provide immediate community or state updates: https://covid.cdc.gov/covid-data-tracker/#datatracker-home. The ASA suggests the following strategy using community transmission risk to guide perioperative testing strategies[160]:

- *Low to moderate community transmission: If the patient is asymptomatic, is up-to-date in vaccination, and is having a lower-risk procedure, facilities could consider a more permissive approach to perioperative testing. Those facilities should consider if preoperative testing may still inform such infection prevention decisions such as room assignment/cohorting after surgery.*
- *Substantial or high community transmission: Facilities should continue preprocedural testing using nucleic acid amplification testing (NAAT).*

It is also important to note that preprocedural testing is not a panacea; therefore, particularly during times of widespread community transmission, facilities might consider universal use of N95 or higher respirators for perioperative care.[160]

INDUCTION AND AIRWAY MANAGEMENT

Although airway instrumentation may increase the risk of viral aerosolization, the clinical needs and status of the patient, the procedure, and patient safety should drive the anesthetic plan. Provider safety underpins the *execution* of the best anesthetic plan for every patient. For this reason, there is no single best anesthetic plan for all COVID-19 cases. Nevertheless, the use of appropriate

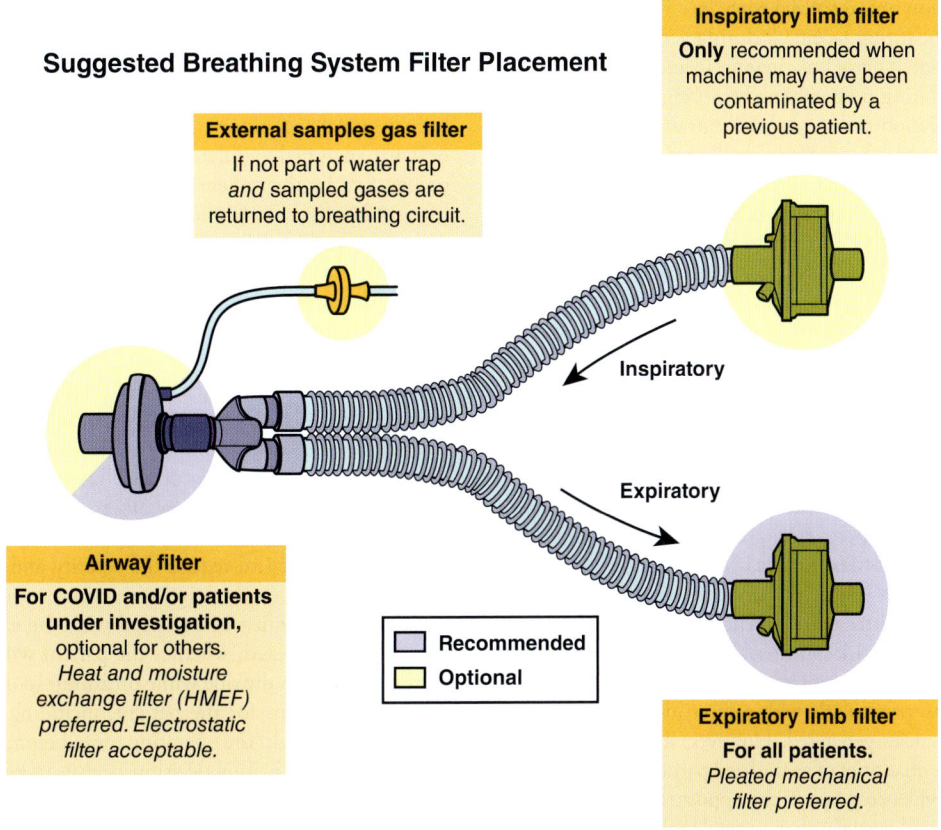

Suggested Breathing System Filter Placement

Inspiratory limb filter
Only recommended when machine may have been contaminated by a previous patient.

External samples gas filter
If not part of water trap *and* sampled gases are returned to breathing circuit.

Inspiratory

Expiratory

Airway filter
For COVID and/or patients under investigation, optional for others. *Heat and moisture exchange filter (HMEF) preferred. Electrostatic filter acceptable.*

Recommended
Optional

Expiratory limb filter
For all patients. *Pleated mechanical filter preferred.*

FIGURE 47.4 Suggested breathing system filter placement. (Taken from: https://www.apsf.org/faq-on-anesthesia-machine-use-protection-and-decontamination-during-the-covid-19-pandemic/.)

PPE, HEPA filters, and regional anesthesia techniques have been found to reduce the risk of COVID-19 transmission during surgery and anesthesia.[161,162] At the outset of the COVID-19 pandemic in December 2019, authorities had minimal understanding of how the virus was spread and therefore how to prevent its spread, particularly when anesthetizing patients and managing the airway. Consequently, the recommendations that were forthcoming were empirical and overly conservative, and most patients who required intubation were extremely sick.[163,164] The optimal management eschewed face mask ventilation and the use of supraglottic devices in favor of tracheal intubation with cuffed tracheal tubes. However, in the intervening years, evidence has clarified the risks associated with the unprotected and instrumented airway such that the initial recommendations were nullified. In the discussion that follows, we present an evidence-based approach to airway management in COVID-19 patients and alert the reader that some of the recommendations that follow will conflict with known published guidelines. However, since this is a subject of intense research and discovery, practice changes should be expected to evolve with the evidence.

Intubation boxes, tents, and plastic sheeting are used to isolate the head and neck of the patient and reduce the risk of viral transmission to the intubator during tracheal intubation. There is limited research on the efficacy of such devices in the context of COVID-19; although several studies concluded that these devices may effectively reduce the risk of transmission to the intubator, others suggested that they also increased the difficulty of tracheal intubation.[165–171] One study suggested that these devices reduced provider exposure to droplets but there may be a greater concentration

of viral aerosol within the device itself.[166] The addition of a vacuum suction device within the tent or box may reduce this risk.[167] Another study suggested reduction in exposure to aerosolized virus, but providers later contaminated themselves during the PPE doffing process,[165] suggesting that safe doffing procedures are essential to prevent viral spread. Video laryngoscopy has been employed more frequently during the pandemic to distance the face of the intubator from the patient's airway during laryngoscopy and reduce the risk of aerosol exposure. This approach may also be critical when an intubation box or tent is used, not because the success rate for intubation differed between direct and video laryngoscopy, but because the time to secure the airway was prolonged when paramedics used these boxes in simulated airway scenarios with manikins.[172] In addition, the glottic aperture may be difficult to view by direct vision from outside the box, so visualizing the airway on the monitor of the video laryngoscope can facilitate tracheal intubation.[173–175] More research is needed to fully understand the benefits and risks of intubation boxes, tents, and other barriers but they do appear to effectively reduce provider exposure to viral droplets and aerosols when used correctly. The use of vacuum suction within these barriers, as well as proper PPE doffing procedures, also reduce the risk of viral exposure.

From a practical perspective, evidence supports the order of the risk of exposure to aerosols in the perioperative period to be: EXTUBATION > BEFORE induction of anesthesia (while the patient is breathing spontaneously or coughing) > TRACHEAL INTUBATION.[176,177] Continuous positive airway pressure masks with an exhalation port filter yield less aerosol than speaking and coughing without a face mask. Of these, coughing yielded the greatest concentration of aerosolized particles.[178] Aerosolized virus released from a tight-fitting facemask during gentle manual ventilation, even with a small mask leak present, in anesthetized patients is much less than during tidal volume breathing and coughing.[177] In fact, when respiration ceases, the concentration of aerosol particles around the patient's head diminishes as evidenced by the low concentration of aerosol particles during tracheal intubation.[176]

Bag-mask ventilation should be minimized as much as possible in patients with COVID-19 to reduce aerosolization of viral particles, although the risk is low even with a small leak around the face mask.[177] The induction technique that will minimize the exposure to aerosol is a modified rapid sequence induction (RSI). This should be performed by an experienced intubator, particularly for acutely ill patients with moderate to severe COVID-19.[157,161,162,164,174,179] When bag-mask ventilation cannot be avoided (usually due to rapid desaturation), the provider should make every attempt to maintain a tight mask seal, minimize the fresh gas flow, ensure that all health care workers in the room are wearing properly fitting N95 respirators and other appropriate PPE, and ventilate for the briefest amount of time.[164]

In children with COVID-19, the airway is typically secured using tracheal intubation with a cuffed tracheal tube to adequately seal the airway and reduce the risk of aerosolizing virus. Debate continues regarding the efficacy of supraglottic airway devices (SGA) in COVID-19 patients, particularly with respect to the magnitude of aerosolized viral particles generated. However, the perception that SGAs generate large quantities of aerosolized particles is not evidence based. In fact, the evidence supports the opposite; that SGAs generate no more aerosolized particles than normal shallow breathing and <4% of a volitional cough.[180] The importance of retaining SGAs in COVID-19 relates to their importance in the difficult airway algorithm and the likelihood that moderate to severe COVID-19 patients may require ventilation between intubation attempts.[164] There is a theoretical risk of an air leak around the cuff and therefore viral exposure to the providers, though the exposure is less than it is with face mask ventilation.[181] If a SGA is used, it should accommodate the exchange of a tracheal tube over a bronchoscope, which is not significantly aerosol-generating technique in an apneic patient.[181] If the patient's airway will be managed with just a SGA, then it is preferable to allow the patient to breathe spontaneously without positive pressure or pressure support to reduce the air leak and viral aerosolization.[181] Evidence suggests that it is reasonable to consider a SGA in carefully selected patients if the device is well-seated, has an adequate seal, and has a small leak at reasonable peak inspiratory pressures. A second-generation SGA that provides minimal leak up to ≥20 cm H_2O peak inflation pressure (e.g., ProSeal) may be more advantageous.[182]

REGIONAL ANESTHESIA

Early in the pandemic there was enthusiasm for the use of regional anesthesia to avoid mask ventilation, intubation, and mechanical ventilation given the concern for viral aerosolization.[183] At the outset of the pandemic as transmission dynamics were studied, airway management protocols were developed and PPE was in high demand. It was reasonable to make every effort to avoid airway instrumentation. An early analysis of COVID-19 deaths among health care providers in the United Kingdom, however, suggested that there was not a greater mortality rate for those who were exposed to aerosol-generating procedures frequently, perhaps because these providers were proficient and rigorous in their use of PPE.[184]

The counter to this argument is that, in skilled hands with a patient who does not cough at the time of intubation or extubation,

an intubated COVID-19 patient may pose less transmission risk than one who is spontaneously breathing with a regional technique. Proper PPE and placing a mask on those patients who can tolerate it will mitigate these transmission risks. It is likely that both regional techniques and general anesthesia are equally safe, or with marginally different risk profiles. Providers should be guided first by the patient's condition, procedure, provider comfort, and patient preference over their COVID-19 status alone. A survey concluded that regional anesthesia can be safely used in COVID-19 patients, although a comparative pediatric study has not been conducted. A single study indicated that the frequency of use of regional anesthesia in children did not change before or after the pandemic.[185,186]

EMERGENCE AND EXTUBATION

Emergence and extubation carries the greatest risk of aerosolization and viral transmission of all phases of the perioperative period. As such, all health care workers must don full PPE. It may be reasonable to plan to extubate the trachea while the patient is deeply anesthetized to reduce the severity and amount of coughing, bucking, and further viral spread in the room. The benefits of deep extubation must be balanced with the ease with which the patient was intubated, whether the patient will tolerate a modest increase in carbon dioxide while breathing spontaneously, and the postoperative plans for the patient, including where the trachea will be extubated: in the operating room before transport to recovery or in the ICU. This decision is also affected by the location where the patient will recover; that is, in some institutions COVID-19 patients are recovered in the operating room to minimize exposure of other health care workers or families.

For those patients who are not candidates for deep extubation, other transmission mitigation strategies should be considered. These include techniques to reduce airway irritation and coughing during emergence, such as administration of intravenous opioids, lidocaine, or dexmedetomidine. The same barrier device used for intubation, such as an intubation box or tent, is also effective during extubation.[187] A very simple technique to minimize the risk of aerosolizing virus during extubation is to extubate the trachea by pulling the tracheal tube through an anesthesia face mask applied to the face (Video 47.1). It is important to thread the pilot balloon tube through the stem of the anesthesia face mask to deflate the cuff before extubating the trachea. To avoid emergency airway interventions on a COVID-19 patient outside of the controlled, negative pressure environment of the operating room, patients should be extubated in the operating room and fully awake. A period of observation before leaving the operating room is prudent to ensure that spontaneous and effective respiratory effort can be maintained in children with COVID-19.

SPECIFIC PEDIATRIC ANESTHESIA CONSIDERATIONS

At the time of this writing, the number of COVID-19 cases in the United States in those under 18 years of age exceeded 16 million, including 1642 deaths as of June 2023*.[183] Case fatality for children has remained low and asymptomatic infection is common. Therefore, it is important for pediatric anesthesia providers to closely follow all previously described recommendations as well as those from public health officials to establish perioperative testing schemes, risk mitigation strategies, and surveillance for providers to prevent provider infection.

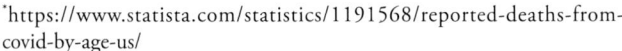

*https://www.statista.com/statistics/1191568/reported-deaths-from-covid-by-age-us/

In institutions where providers may have previously embraced parental presence at induction of anesthesia, such an approach will need to be modified for several reasons.[151] First, parents accompanying their children for surgery (often limited to one parent per child in the preoperative area during COVID-19) are not tested for COVID-19. Accordingly, they should not be permitted into the induction area or operating room. Second, the additional stress of inducing anesthesia in a child who is COVID-19–positive is compounded by presence of the parent.[151] Lastly, quickly proceeding to securing the airway to minimize the time interval of particulate aerosolization might prove very destressing to a parent. It is recommended that pediatric providers strongly consider substituting a premedication for parental presence in the operating room to facilitate safe and calm separation of the child from their parents.

Evidence presented earlier suggests that the combination of intubation boxes or barriers and video laryngoscopes may reduce the risk of provider exposure to COVID-19 during induction of anesthesia. Furthermore, apnea should be achieved as quickly as possible, whether using a combination of intravenous and inhalational agents and/or a muscle relaxant, as the absence of breathing dramatically reduces the concentration of aerosol around the head. Airway management in small children might complicate these recommendations[170,171]; therefore, the most experienced airway provider should make the first intubation attempt, assisted by a second experienced provider. If a difficult airway is anticipated, a third experienced provider should be dressed in PPE and waiting just outside the room to assist.[151] It is also important to avoid contamination of clean equipment and materials, particularly during times of pandemic as supply chain shortcomings limit available stock. A nursing assistant or anesthesia technician should be made available to pass clean materials to the airway team.

The pediatric considerations for emergence and extubation should focus on those high risks of any pediatric case; however, amplified vigilance is prudent given the transmission risks associated with emergent reintubation, aggressive mask ventilation, and excessive coughing. Children have greater risks of laryngospasm and secretions that can easily block smaller diameter endotracheal tubes. Such factors should be considered in deciding on deep versus awake extubation, as well as using additional techniques previously described to reduce coughing.

CARDIAC ARREST

Very little data exist regarding the success rates of cardiac arrest in children during the COVID-19 pandemic. In one retrospective study, cardiopulmonary resuscitation (CPR) was conducted with similar efficiency in children with and without COVID-19 with survival to discharge, ~29%, better than that reported in adults, but poorer compared with the benchmark cohort of unaffected children, 45%.[188] Protection of the operators during CPR is critically important when resuscitating patients who are COVID-19–positive. Simulated studies demonstrated that N95 masks may not provide optimal protection during vigorous movement such as in performing CPR in up to 18% of cases because of leaks arising from the face straps slipping.[189] The authors recommended powered air-purifying respirators in these cases as they are 2.5 to 100 times better than N95 masks at reducing aerosol contamination. The downside of using these respirators, however, includes requiring more training, greater noncompliance, less ready availability, and greater donning and doffing times that may delay the onset of CPR.

EQUIPMENT DECONTAMINATION AND ROOM TURNOVER

Anesthesia providers should consult their local infection prevention and control teams for specifics of equipment decontamination procedures. In general, reusable equipment, such as laryngoscopes and video laryngoscope blades, should be placed in a sealed container and clearly marked that they are COVID-19 contaminated. Procedures should be established to communicate with processing teams that COVID-19–contaminated equipment is incoming and how that equipment should be received. All disposable equipment should be properly discarded in biohazard containers. The usual cleaning practices and solutions should be used according to local protocol; hospital grade cleaning solutions are effective in COVID-19 decontamination.

An important consideration in case turnover is the time necessary for airborne contaminant removal. After caring for a COVID-19 patient in the operating room, the space should be taken offline to allow for air change and virus removal. Table 47.5 describes the number of air changes per hour and the time necessary to remove 99% and 99.9% of airborne contaminants.[190] Providers should consult their facilities engineers to verify the number of exchanges per hour the air handling system can provide. After leaving the room, clear signage should be posted to notify all staff of the time when the room may be entered for terminal cleaning according to local protocol before commencing the next case.

SUMMARY ON COVID-19 CARE

Rapid evolution of care and innovation was required at the outset of the COVID-19 pandemic to reduce transmission to anesthesia providers. Since then, various recommendations have been made on best practice and are summarized above. As the pandemic evolves, immunizations continue, and additional therapeutics are developed, our collective understanding of best practice will also evolve. The key to success is to understand the risks of contamination and infection and to take the appropriate steps to mitigate them. These efforts mimic some foundations of anesthesia practice: vigilance, communication, careful planning, risk mitigation, and redundancy. Providers should always refer to the most updated recommendations from the CDC, WHO, the Anesthesia Patient Safety Foundation, and other professional organizations to develop policies.[5,17,160,191,192] These principles of practice and procedures will certainly be applicable during future pandemics or for patients with other highly contagious diseases presenting for our care.

TABLE 47.5	Air Exchanges per Hour and Time for Removal of Airborne Contaminants	
Air Changes per Hour	Time to 99% Removal (minutes)	Time to 99.9% Removal (minutes)
2	138	207
4	69	104
6	46	69
8	35	52
10	28	41
12	23	35
15	18	28
20	14	21
50	6	8

(From: https://www.cdc.gov/infectioncontrol/guidelines/environmental/appendix/air.html#tableb1)

Strategy for Preventing Infection Transmission in Health Care Institutions

Institutional administrative measures aimed at developing, implementing, and monitoring specifically designed accident prevention policies and procedures are important for reducing and preventing transmission of infectious agents in health care centers. To this end, centers should consider[129,193,194]:

- Include infection control as a major goal in the organizational mission statement and implement safety programs for patients and health care workers.
- Provide sufficient administrative and financial support to carry out this mission.
- Provide sufficient administrative and financial support for the microbiology laboratory and implement an infection surveillance plan, especially for postsurgical infections.
- Establish a multidisciplinary cross-discipline team (e.g., a team manager, an epidemiologist, a representative from industrial health, and a person trained in quality control) to identify health and safety issues within the institution, analyze trends, assess outcomes, implement interventions, and make recommendations to other members of the organization.
- Provide sufficient administrative and financial support to develop and implement education programs for health care providers, patients, and their families.
- Provide health care workers with hepatitis A and B vaccines and document that an appropriate immunologic response was achieved. Provide hepatitis A and B immune globulins (HAIG, HBIG) for those exposed who do not have established immunity.[23]
- Provide a health care service for employees for counseling and postexposure prophylaxis should an exposure to HIV occur.[195]
- Provide regular surveillance of health care workers to determine established immunity to infectious diseases such as coronavirus, tuberculosis, measles, mumps, rubella, and chickenpox. Lack of immunity may require immunization based upon the need to prevent risk to their own safety, and there is also an ethical issue to reduce risk to their patients.[196] Several studies have demonstrated the cost-effectiveness of immunization (to prevent disease) versus the cost to replace health care workers who have become infected.[125,197–202]

Measures for Prevention of Infection Transmission in the Operating Room

Awareness of the situation is the first step in taking aggressive preventive behaviors; emphasis should be placed on modifiable risk factors.[203]

PREVENTION OF AIRBORNE PATHOGEN TRANSMISSION

Airborne pathogens may be transmitted through the operating room heating, ventilation, and air conditioning systems. It is vital to have in place proper systems to (1) remove contaminated air, (2) facilitate air management requirements to protect susceptible health care providers and children against hospital-related airborne pathogens, and (3) minimize the risk of airborne pathogens being transmitted by children.[5] Many regulatory institutions, such as the National Institute for Occupational Safety and Health; the American Society of Heating, Refrigerating and Air-Conditioning Engineers,[204] the CDC, and the American Institute of Architects, have developed standards and guidelines for operating room ventilation

systems. As in any other environment, ventilation in the operating room is an important issue to control infection from microbiologic pollutants.[205] Most wound contamination in the operating room is the result of the patient's skin flora and bacteria shed on airborne particles from the operating room personnel. Room ventilation affects the distribution of these airborne particles in four ways: total ventilation (dilution), air distribution (directional airflow), room pressurization (filtration barrier), and filtration (contaminant removal).[204] As the air flows of the room increase, the greater the dilutional effect on airborne particles. Balancing this phenomenon is important because although increased flow increases the effectiveness of air exchange, the resultant turbulent flow increases microbial distribution throughout the room. Low-velocity unidirectional flow minimizes the spread of microbes in the room. Directional flow can be inward, from the outside into the operating room (negative pressure), or outward, from the operating room to the outside (positive pressure). Negative-pressure ventilation is used for highly infective rooms in the hospital (e.g., isolation rooms for tuberculosis patients), and positive-pressure ventilation is used for protective environments (e.g., operating rooms and rooms with immunocompromised patients). Most hospital operating rooms are currently designed with HEPA filtration systems to maximize removal of airborne contaminants.[204] Operating room ventilation systems should operate at all times, except during maintenance. During unoccupied hours, air exchange can be reduced if positive pressure is maintained in each operating room. Air is delivered to each operating room from the ceiling, with downward movement toward several exhaust or return ducts near the floor. This design helps provide steady movement of clean air through the breathing and working zones.

The American Institute of Architects has specific guidelines for the location of outside fresh air inlets to minimize contamination from exhaust systems and noxious fumes. A greater air inflow rate and a larger air-inlet area are desirable for contaminant control, but these approaches are detrimental to the thermal comfort of the staff and patient.[206] The American Institute of Architects recommends an air-change rate in an operating room of 20 to 25 air changes per hour for ceiling heights between 9 feet (2.74 meters) and 12 feet (3.66 meters). Some controversy exists between engineers and clinicians over the need for laminar airflow ventilation in the operating room to further minimize airborne infection; mathematical analyses of airflow suggest that laminar airflow is not necessary and clinical studies are confirmatory.[207–209] Similarly, the use of ultraviolet (UV) light to cleanse the room air has been shown to be effective but is no longer recommended due to concerns about exposure of skin to UV light.[204,205,210–212] Table 47.6 shows the 2003 Healthcare Infection Control Practices Advisory Committee and CDC general recommendations for ventilation system specifications for the operating room.[213] Children with tuberculosis require special consideration because of the high risk of occupational transmission of *Mycobacterium tuberculosis*,[214,215] especially after the emergence of multidrug-resistant strains (E-Tables 47.6 and 47.7). An easy preventive measure is to screen all children before coming to the operating room to determine recent exposure to infectious disease such as measles, mumps, rubella, and chickenpox because these infections can pose a risk to unimmunized health care workers and patients, especially those who are immunocompromised.[127,201] Another potential source for airborne spread of pathogens is through the anesthesia circuit; this may be reduced by the use of circuit filters (Fig. 47.4).

However, at present there are no regulatory requirements to use such devices, and performance characteristics vary widely.[64,65,216–220]

TABLE 47.6	Ventilation System Specifications for the Operating Room

- Minimize the circulation of people during surgeries. It has been proved that the level of microbes in the operating room air is directly proportional to the number of people moving inside the room.
- Maintain humidity under 68% and temperature control to prevent environmental conditions that favor the development of germs.
- Maintain positive pressure compared with corridors and surrounding areas to prevent microorganisms from entering the operating room.
- Provide at least 15 air changes per hour in the operating room, 20% of which should be fresh air. Air should be recirculated through a high-efficiency particulate air (HEPA) filter.
- Air should be introduced at ceiling level and disposed of at ground level.

From Centers for Disease Control and Prevention. Guidelines for environmental infection control in health-care facilities: recommendations of CDC and the Healthcare Infection Control Practices Advisory Committee (HICPAC). *MMWR Recommendations and Reports.* 2003;52(RR10):1-42. Available at https://www.cdc.gov/mmwr/preview/mmwrhtml/rr5210a1.htm.

These filters are rated according to "viral filter efficiency"; a rating of 99.99% means that only one virus particle in 10,000 will pass the filter.[159] A summary of performance characteristic of heat and moisture exchange filters, airway filters without humidification, breathing circuit filters, and water trap filters by manufacturer from the Anesthesia Patient Safety Foundation is available.[†]

STANDARD PRECAUTIONS

Standard precautions[191] assume that any person or patient is potentially infected or colonized by microorganisms that could be transmitted and cause an infectious process. Standard precautions must be implemented with all patients and include:

- *Universal precautions—blood and body fluid precautions*, developed to reduce bloodborne pathogen transmission.
- *Body substance isolation*, designed to reduce the risk of pathogen transmission by moist body substances.

Standard precautions are used to reduce the transmission of all infectious agents from one person to another, thus protecting health care providers and children against exposure to the most common microorganisms. Standard precautions are implemented for any contact with blood and body fluids, secretions, and excretions (except sweat), whether or not they contain visible blood, as well as for any contact with nonintact skin, mucous membranes, and intact skin that is visibly soiled with blood and/or body fluids. *Prevention is primary.* All health care providers should be familiar with standard precautions: wash hands frequently and thoroughly before and after patient care; use PPE: gloves, gowns, boots, shoe covers, eyewear, masks, and shields, as appropriate for the patient care situation; gloves must be worn when any kind of venous or arterial access is being performed; use sharps with caution: plan ahead (use sharps in a safe environment with a sharps disposal container nearby), dispose of used sharps in puncture-proof receptacles immediately after use, do not recap needles, and use safety devices if available. All health care providers should be vaccinated with the HBV vaccine series and should be tested for antibodies to HBV after completing the vaccine series to document their

presence. Employees who have not gone through the vaccination series previously should be offered the HBV series through their employer at no cost.[221] Summaries of standard precautions, droplet precautions, airborne precautions, and contact precautions are available online. [192,222,223]

Hand Washing

With the recent adoption of alcohol-based gel for hand decontamination, "Hand Hygiene" should now refer to using gel or washing hands with soap and water. Bacteria counts on hands range from 40,000 to 4 million colony forming units per square centimeter.[224] These organisms consist of resident and transient flora; transient flora are responsible for most health-care–associated infections.[225] Transmission occurs when a health care worker's hands come into contact with organisms directly on a patient or when organisms spread on inanimate objects in the vicinity of a patient. If the organism is able to survive for at least a few minutes on the professional's hands, and if hand hygiene is inadequate, the caregiver will contaminate the physical environment and other patients, repeating the cycle.[88]

Why is routine hand hygiene so critical? Bacterial contamination of anesthesia providers has been directly linked to high-risk bacterial transmission events to IV stopcocks and 30-day postoperative infections.[60] Overall hand hygiene compliance across health care providers ranges from 5% to 89%, with the average, 40% to 50%,[17,225] with anesthesia providers identified as a particularly noncompliant group (with a compliance rate of only 23% in one study).[226,227]

The vast majority of surgical site infections are caused by *Staphylococcus aureus*. Transmission of specific staphylococcal phenotypes within and between patients is a major contributing factor to surgical site infections and health-care–associated infections.[2,9,228] The role of the anesthesia provider in transmitting *Enterococcus* via hand contamination to the workstation and patient biome is a concern, although there are no reports of clinical infections arising from anesthesiologists as the bacterial vector. Nonetheless, with the steadily increasing rates of antibiotic-resistant organisms and the observation that *Enterococcus* is becoming a more prevalent pathogen, anesthesiologists must become more compliant with hand washing and general hygiene.[2,67] Two approaches have been proposed to address this issue: improve methods to decontaminate the patient and develop more effective and frequent provider hand cleansing. Hand hygiene is a well-known and effective solution to the problem of bacterial transmission within and between patients. Compliance with the current "5 moments" WHO guidelines could have a profound effect to reduce provider hand and workspace contamination:

Moment 1 = before entering a patient room (treatment zone), after touching the door handle and before touching the patient; Moment 2 = after touching a patient and before touching a critical site (e.g., inspecting a wound or IV); Moment 3 = immediately after accessing a critical site (e.g., a surgical incision), and before touching anything else; Moment 4 = when leaving the treatment zone and before touching anything else; Moment 5 = after touching anything in the treatment zone and before touching anything else.[199]

One study found that only 20% of anesthesia providers demonstrated complete knowledge regarding WHO hand hygiene guidelines.[229] Failure of providers to recognize prior contact with environmental surfaces and prior contact with the patient's skin surfaces as hand hygiene opportunities contributed to this low

---

[†](https://www.apsf.org/wp-content/uploads/patient-safety-resources/covid-19/Breathing-Circuit-Filters.pdf.)

percent of compliance.[229] Because alcohol is not effective in inactivating spores, soap and water (or antimicrobial soap) should be used if hands are suspected of being contaminated with spores, for example, *Clostridium difficile* or *Bacillus anthracis*.[230]

Health care providers are a leading source of hospital-acquired infections[2,60,231]; the average frequency of hand hygiene episodes fluctuates with the method used for monitoring and the setting where the observations are conducted.[232] Hand washing per hour may vary over 30-fold. The number of opportunities for hand hygiene depends largely on the process of care provided[233]; revision of protocols for patient care may reduce unnecessary contacts and, consequently, improve hand hygiene opportunities. In 11 observational studies, the duration of hand cleansing episodes by health care workers ranged from 6.6 seconds to 30 seconds.[17,225] In addition to washing their hands for very brief periods, health care workers often failed to cover all surfaces of their hands and fingers thus even if the hand hygiene compliance rate were high, the cleansing technique may be inadequate.

The risk of pathogen transmission via the hands is proportional to the number of times a child is touched.[234] Efforts to stop this cycle of contamination have provided impetus for WHO to make hand hygiene a top priority since 2009 and are the focus of WHO's First Global Patient Safety Challenge: "Clean Care is Safer Care."[17,221] Both the CDC[235] and the WHO[17,221] have published hand hygiene protocols. Most hospital systems adopt some variant of these two protocols, which are considered functionally comparable. Table 47.7 presents a summary of the indications for and the strength of supporting evidence for hand washing and antisepsis.[221] WHO recommendations for surgical hand preparation are presented in Table 47.8.[221] Readers are referred to an excellent summary of hand cleaners at https://www.cdc.gov/mmwr/PDF/rr/rr5116.pdf.[225] At present, alcohol-based handrubs are the only known means for rapidly and effectively inactivating a wide array of potentially harmful microorganisms on hands. Alcohol-based products have a rapid disinfecting onset and readily kill Gram-positive/Gram-negative bacteria, mycobacteria, viruses, and fungi (the notable exception is spore-forming pathogens such as *Clostridium difficile*). However, these products have no persistent activity and must be reapplied to maintain effectiveness. The WHO recommends alcohol-based handrubs based on the following factors: evidence-based, intrinsic advantages of fast-acting and broad-spectrum microbicidal activity with a minimal risk of generating resistance to antimicrobial agents; suitability for use in resource-limited or remote areas with lack of accessibility to sinks or other facilities for hand hygiene (including clean water, towels, and so on); capacity to promote improved compliance with hand hygiene by making the process faster and more convenient; economic benefit by reducing annual costs for hand hygiene; minimization of risks from adverse events because of increased safety associated with better acceptability and tolerance than other products.[221]

The prevalence of skin problems and complaints in health care professionals after repeated use of alcohol-based products may be as great as 40%. Although previous research has suggested that the irritant potential of alcohol commonly used in hand sanitizers is generally low, the incidence of irritant contact dermatitis following the WHO hand hygiene protocol is unknown. A study with volunteers who applied alcohol-based solutions to their hands every 15 minutes for 8 hours, repeated for 5 days for a total of 160 exposures, with independent verification of compliance showed that after critical evaluation at the beginning and end of the study period, nearly two-thirds of them felt discomfort with the process and 80% of the volunteers reported that the frequency of hand hygiene interfered with other tasks.[236] After hand washing, it is very important to dry the hands properly with appropriate paper towels, hot air flow, or both, because the level of pathogen transmission from a health care worker's hands to a patient is greatly increased if the hands are wet.[237] Clinicians may have misplaced concerns about the potential flammability of alcohol-based solutions used in the operating room environment. The Federal Aviation Administration examined the general flammability characteristics of these solutions also used in commercial airline

---

TABLE 47.7 | Indications for Hand Hygiene

1. Wash hands with soap and water when visibly dirty or visibly soiled with blood or other body fluids (IB) or after using the toilet (II).
2. If exposure to potential spore-forming pathogens is strongly suspected or proven, including outbreaks of *Clostridium difficile*, hand washing with soap and water is the preferred means (IB).
3. Use an alcohol-based handrub as the preferred means for routine hand antisepsis in all other clinical situations described in terms 4(a) to 4(f) listed below, if hands are not visibly soiled (IA). If alcohol-based handrub is not obtainable, wash hands with soap and water (IB).
4. Perform hand hygiene:
   a. before and after touching the patient (IB);
   b. before handling an invasive device for patient care regardless of whether or not gloves are used (IB);
   c. after contact with body fluids or excretions, mucous membranes, nonintact skin, or wound dressings (IA);
   d. if moving from a contaminated body site to another body site during care of the same patient (IB);
   e. after contact with inanimate surfaces and objects (including medical equipment) in the immediate vicinity of the patient (IB);
   f. after removing sterile (II) or nonsterile gloves (IB).
5. Before handling medication or preparing food, perform hand hygiene using an alcohol-based handrub or wash hands with either plain or antimicrobial soap and water (IB).
6. Soap and alcohol-based handrub should not be used concomitantly (II).

Category IA. Strongly recommended for implementation and strongly supported by well-designed experimental, clinical, or epidemiologic studies.
Category IB. Strongly recommended for implementation and supported by some experimental, clinical, or epidemiologic studies and a strong theoretical rationale.
Category IC. Required for implementation, as mandated by federal and/or state regulation or standard.
Category II. Suggested for implementation and supported by suggestive clinical or epidemiologic studies or a theoretical rationale or a consensus by a panel of experts.

Adapted from *WHO Guidelines on Hand Hygiene in Health Care: First Global Patient Safety Challenge Clean Care Is Safer Care*. Geneva: World Health Organization; 2009: 152.

TABLE 47.8 | World Health Organization Recommendations for Surgical Hand Preparation[221]

A Remove rings, wrist-watch, and bracelets before beginning surgical hand preparation (II). Artificial nails are prohibited (IB).

B Sinks should be designed to reduce the risk of splashes (II).

C If hands are visibly soiled, wash hands with plain soap before surgical hand preparation (II). Remove debris from underneath fingernails using a nail cleaner, preferably under running water (II).

D Brushes are not recommended for surgical hand preparation (IB).

E Surgical hand antisepsis should be performed using either a suitable antimicrobial soap or suitable alcohol-based handrub, preferably with a product ensuring sustained activity, before donning sterile gloves (IB).

F If quality of water is not assured (as described in Table I.11.3) in the operating theater, surgical hand antisepsis using an alcohol-based handrub is recommended before donning sterile gloves when performing surgical procedures (II).

G When performing surgical hand antisepsis using an antimicrobial soap, scrub hands and forearms for the length of time recommended by the manufacturer, typically 2–5 minutes. Long scrub times (e.g., 10 minutes) are not necessary (IB).

H When using an alcohol-based surgical handrub product with sustained activity, follow the manufacturers' instructions for application times. Apply the product to dry hands only (IB). Do not combine surgical hand scrub and surgical handrub with alcohol-based products sequentially (II).

I When using an alcohol-based handrub, use sufficient product to keep hands and forearms wet with the handrub throughout the surgical hand preparation procedure (IB).

J After application of the alcohol-based handrub as recommended, allow hands and forearms to dry thoroughly before donning sterile gloves (IB).

The consensus recommendations are categorized according to the CDC/HICPAC system, as outlined in Table 47.7.

Modified from the *WHO Guidelines on Hand Hygiene in Health Care First Global Patient Safety Challenge Clean Care is Safer Care;* 2009: 152-153.

47

lavatories and found that "*burning hand sanitizer presents no significant risk to commercial transport aircraft fire safety.*"[238] The National Fire Protection Association (NFPA) in 2018 published Codes and Standards, which specifically address the proper use and placement of dispensers of solutions to mitigate the potential for flammability.[239] A review of fires related to the use of alcohol-based solutions found seven nonserious incidents in 25,038 hospital-years of use. All incidents were caused "*by individual human actions and not by technical failure,*" reinforcing the safety of using alcohol-based solutions in hospitals.[240] The WHO reports only seven nonsevere fire incidents during ~35 million liters of such solutions used worldwide.[241] Therefore, solutions must be available inside and immediately outside every operating room and anesthesia site.[240] A prospective observational study found that the use of a personalized, body-worn alcohol dispenser was associated with increased hand decontamination events per hour, reduced contamination of intravenous connections, and reduced environmental contamination.[3] Use of the same personalized alcohol-based cleanser device was also associated with a reduction in ventilator-associated pneumonia (from 6.9 to 3.7 events/1000 ventilation days).[22]

Gloves

As described earlier, wearing clean or sterile gloves while caring for children is an effective means of reducing health-care–associated infections. Gloves remain a supplementary barrier to infection that should not replace proper hand hygiene. Gloves protect patients by reducing health care provider hand contamination and the subsequent transmission of pathogens to other children, provided the gloves are discarded after each use. Additionally, when the use of gloves is combined with CDC standard precautions, they protect the health care provider against exposure to blood-borne infections or infections transmitted by any other body fluids, such as excretions, secretions (except sweat), mucous membranes, and nonintact skin. Examination gloves are single-use and usually nonsterile. Sterile surgical gloves are required for surgical interventions. Some nonsurgical care procedures, such as central vascular catheter insertion, also require surgical glove use.

During shortages of PPE during the COVID-19 epidemic, some considered that gloves could be reused if cleansed with hand sanitizers. However, the durability of commonly used nitrile gloves after multiple applications of alcohol-based solutions to the gloves themselves rather than replacing gloves has provided mixed results. Repeated application of disinfectant to gloves (instead of hands) 15 times over 2 hours did not disrupt the structural or tactile integrity of the nitrile gloves.[236] Conversely, breakdown in the integrity of nitrile gloves with bleach-containing solutions was worse than with alcohol-based solutions, but both reduced the "breaking load."[242] Thus, it seems that cleansing gloves with disinfectant is a potentially risky practice. The WHO strongly discourages glove reprocessing.[17]

Double gloving for laryngoscopy and intubation and then removing the outer glove reduces environmental contamination.[27] As contamination of the intraoperative environment has been identified as a potent transmission vehicle for intravascular devices, a double-glove technique may also serve as a mechanism to reduce contamination of intravascular devices[20,27]; several systematic reviews have confirmed that this safety practice also reduces the blood exposure of surgical and nursing personnel to glove perforations or failures.[243–246]

The use of gloves in situations when their use is not indicated represents a waste of resources without necessarily reducing cross-transmission. The wide-ranging recommendations for glove use have led to frequent and inappropriate use. Indications for gloving and glove removal are shown in Table 47.9. Situations that require and that do not require glove use are presented in Fig. 47.5.

Ranked consensus recommendations for the use of gloves include[221,247,248]: (1) Gloves should be worn in case of contact with blood or any other potentially infecting body fluid, such as excretions, secretions (except sweat), mucous membranes, and nonintact skin. (2) Gloves should be removed immediately after providing care to a child. Staff should not wear the same pair of gloves to take care of more than one child, nor should they touch the surfaces of any equipment, monitoring devices, or even light switches. Contaminated gloves can pass blood or other body fluids to working surfaces and are vectors for hepatitis transmission.[124]

(3) Gloves should be changed when taking care of a child if you must move from a contaminated to a clean body site. Hand hygiene measures should be applied immediately after removing the gloves because hands may get contaminated through small (microscopic) holes in the gloves.[231,249–251] (4) Gloves should be removed by using an appropriate technique (so as not to contaminate your hands with the contaminated surface of the gloves). Alcohol-based handrub dispensers and clean glove boxes (at least two sizes) should be in place near every patient care site (e.g., on top of every anesthesia cart, medication cart, or in the nursing station). (5) Disposable gloves should not be washed, resterilized, or disinfected. (6) Since sterile gloves are much more expensive than disposable gloves, they should only be used for procedures, such as when hands are in contact with normally sterile body areas or when inserting intravascular or urinary catheters. (7) Clean gloves should be used during any other procedure, including wound dressing changes. (8) Latex-free gloves should be worn when caring for children at risk for latex allergy.

ANTIMICROBIAL PROPHYLAXIS

Surgical antimicrobial prophylaxis is an essential tool to help combat perioperative complications and specifically, surgical site infections, which occur in 0.5% to 3% of adult patients, prolong hospital stay 7 to 11 days, and incur between 3.5 and 10 billion US dollars annually in additional health care costs.[252,253] Approximately 2% to 4% of children require readmission after surgical discharge, with surgical site infections accounting for about 25% of these.[254] However, a systematic review and meta-analysis of studies of antimicrobial prophylaxis to prevent surgical site infections in children failed to prove a direct benefit from the antimicrobials in the pediatric age range, and actually recommended avoiding antimicrobials in children with procedures classified as surgical wound class 1 (clean).[255] Others have also challenged the need to give antimicrobial prophylaxis in infants and children undergoing "clean" surgeries as the frequency of surgical site infections is exceedingly small, 0.56%.[256] In the case of pyloromyotomy in one study and all nonemergent surgeries in another, not only is the incidence of surgical site infections small, but the rates of surgical infections were similar whether antimicrobials were given or not.[257,258] Interestingly, antimicrobial prophylaxis is but one of a number of strategies that is used in the perioperative period to minimize surgical site infections and in neonates, infants and children, it may not be the most consequential factor.[252,253,259]

TABLE 47.9   Indications for Gloving and Glove Removal

Indication
Glove Use

1. Before a sterile condition
2. Anticipation of a contact with blood or another body fluid, regardless of the existence of sterile conditions and including contact with non-intact skin and mucous membrane
3. Contact with a patient (and their immediate surroundings) during contact precautions

Glove Removal

1. As soon as gloves are damaged (or nonintegrity suspected)
2. When contact with blood, another body fluid, nonintact skin, and mucous membrane has occurred and has ended
3. When contact with a single patient and their surroundings, or a contaminated body site on a patient has ended
4. When there is an indication for hand hygiene

From *WHO Guidelines on Hand Hygiene in Health Care. First Global Patient Safety Challenge Clean Care Is Safer Care.* Geneva: World Health Organization; 2009: 137.

STERILE GLOVES INDICATED

Any surgical procedure; vaginal delivery; invasive radiological procedures; performing vascular access and procedures (central lines); preparing total parental nutrition and chemotherapeutic agents.

EXAMINATION GLOVES INDICATED IN CLINICAL SITUATIONS

Potential for touching blood, body fluids, secretions, excertions, and items visibly soiled by body fluids

DIRECT PATIENT EXPOSURE: contact with blood; contact with mucous membrane and with nonintact skin; potential presence of highly infectious and dangerous organism; epidemic; or emergency situations; IV insertion and removal; drawing blood; discontinuation of venous line; pelvic and vaginal examination; suctioning nonclosed systems of endotracheal tubes.

INDIRECT PATIENT EXPOSURE: emptying emesis basins; handling/cleaning instruments; handling waste; cleaning up spills of body fluids.

GLOVES NOT INDICATED (except for CONTACT precautions)

No potential for exposure to blood or body fluids, or contaminated environment

DIRECT PATIENT EXPOSURE: taking blood pressure; temperature and pulse; performing SC and IM injections; bathing and dressing the patient; transporting patient; caring for eyes and ears (without secretions); any vascular line manipulation in absence of blood leakage.

INDIRECT PATIENT EXPOSURE: using the telephone, writing the patient's chart; giving oral medications; distributing or collecting patient dietary trays; removing and replacing linen for patient bed; placing noninvasive ventilation equipment and oxygen cannula; moving patient furniture.

FIGURE 47.5 Situations requiring and not requiring glove use. *IM,* Intramuscular; *SC,* subcutaneous. (Adapted from *WHO Guidelines on Hand Hygiene in Health Care: First Global Patient Safety Challenge Clean Care Is Safer Care.* Geneva: World Health Organization; 2009.)

For example, the evidence for the optimal skin antiseptic for use in neonates, infants, and children in the perioperative period is sparse, with most recommendations simply adopted from studies in adults without validation.[260,261] Where anesthesiologists may have the greatest impact is in the timing and dosing of prophylactic antibiotics.[262,263] The purpose of preoperative antibiotics is to achieve plasma and tissue concentrations that exceed the minimum inhibitory concentration for those infectious bacteria that are most likely to cause an infection. This will reduce the microbial load in the perioperative period; but it is not intended to cover all possible pathogens because this can lead to drug-resistant bacteria. Continued use of antibiotic prophylaxis postoperatively is not evidence based in terms of reducing wound infections.[264]

There have been several studies regarding the effectiveness of prophylactic antimicrobials to prevent surgical site infections in children.[265–268] Currently, prophylactic antibiotic guidelines exist for some subsets of the pediatric surgical population and surgeries,[269] but there are no global recommendations, and the guidelines that exist are for the most part, based on studies from adults or from expert opinion. A retrospective study suggested that the appropriate use of antibiotic prophylaxis was a vital modifiable risk factor and may be one of the easiest factors to influence. Primary failure to administer the correct dose of antibiotics at the appropriate time resulted in an almost 2-fold increase in the risk of developing a surgical site infection. However, quality assurance measures can optimize the timing of administration and procedure specific antibiotic selection.[270] The importance of correct antibiotic usage and dosing plays a major role in decreasing risk of surgical site infections in children. Recommendations are provided for adult (age ≥19 years) and pediatric (age 1 to 18 years) patients. The guidelines do not specifically address premature and full-term infants (Table 47.10).[271]

TABLE 47.10	Antimicrobial Prophylaxis Dosing Recommendations	
Antimicrobial	Pediatric Recommended Dose[a]	Recommended Redosing Interval (From Initiation of Preoperative Dose) (hours[b])
Ampicillin-sulbactam	50 mg/kg of the ampicillin component (up to 3 grams)	2
Ampicillin	50 mg/kg (up to 2 grams)	2
Aztreonam	30 mg/kg (up to 2 grams)	4
Cefazolin	30 mg/kg (up to 2 grams, 3 grams if >120 kg)	4
Cefuroxime	50 mg/kg (up to 1.5 grams)	4
Cefotaxime	50 mg/kg (up to 1 gram)	3
Cefoxitin	40 mg/kg (up to 2 grams)	2
Cefotetan	40 mg/kg (up to 2 grams)	6
Ceftriaxone	50–75 mg/kg (up to 2 grams)	N/A
Ciprofloxacin[c]	10 mg/kg (up to 400 mg)	N/A
Clindamycin	10 mg/kg (up to 900 mg)	6
Ertapenem	15 mg/kg (up to 1 gram)	N/A
Fluconazole	6 mg/kg (up to 400 mg)	N/A
Gentamicin[d]	2.5 mg/kg based on dosing weight	N/A
Levofloxacin[c]	10 mg/kg (up to 500 mg)	N/A
Metronidazole	15 mg/kg (up to 500 mg) Neonates weighing <1200 grams should receive a single 7.5-mg/kg dose	N/A
Moxifloxacin[c]	10 mg/kg (up to 400 mg)	N/A
Piperacillin-tazobactam	Infants 2–9 months of age: 80 mg/kg of the piperacillin component (up to 3.375 grams) Children >9 months of age and ≤40 kg: 100 mg/kg of the piperacillin component	2
Vancomycin	15 mg/kg	N/A
Oral Antibiotics for Colorectal Surgery Prophylaxis (Used in Conjunction With a Mechanical Bowel Preparation)		
Erythromycin base	20 mg/kg (up to 1 gram)	N/A
Metronidazole	15 mg/kg (up to 1 gram)	N/A
Neomycin	15 mg/kg (up to 1 gram)	N/A

[a]The maximum pediatric dose should not exceed the usual adult dose.
[b]For antimicrobials with a short half-life (e.g., cefazolin, cefoxitin) used before long procedures, redosing in the operating room is recommended at an interval of approximately two times the half-life of the agent in patients with normal renal function. Recommended redosing intervals marked as "not applicable" (N/A) are based on typical case length; for unusually long procedures, redosing may be needed.
[c]Although fluoroquinolones have been associated with an increased risk of tendinitis/tendon rupture in all ages, use of these agents for single-dose prophylaxis is generally safe.
[d]In general, gentamicin for surgical antibiotics prophylaxis should be limited to a single dose given preoperatively. Dosing is based on the patient's actual body weight. If the patient's actual weight is more than 20% above ideal body weight (IBW), the dosing weight (DW) can be determined as follows: DW = IBW + 0.4 (actual weight − IBW).
Adapted from Bratzler DW, Dellinger EP, Olsen KM, et al. Clinical practice guidelines for antimicrobial prophylaxis in surgery. *Am J Health Syst Pharm.* 2013;70(3):195-283.

Selection of an Antimicrobial Agent

Although pediatric-specific prophylaxis data are sparse, available data have been evaluated for specific procedures. Selection of antimicrobial prophylactic agents mirrors that in adult guidelines, with the agents of choice being first- and second-generation cephalosporins, reserving the use of vancomycin and clindamycin for patients with verified β-lactam allergies. Although the use of a penicillin with a β-lactamase inhibitor in combination with cefazolin or vancomycin and gentamicin has also been studied in pediatric patients, the number of patients included in these evaluations remains small. As with adults, there is little evidence supporting the use of vancomycin, alone or in combination with other antimicrobials, for routine perioperative antimicrobial prophylaxis in institutions that have a high prevalence of methicillin-resistant S. aureus (MRSA). Vancomycin may be considered in children who have or had MRSA to decrease MRSA infections.[272]

Fluoroquinolones (e.g., ciprofloxacin) should not be routinely used for surgical prophylaxis in pediatric patients because of the potential for toxicity. There are sufficient pharmacokinetic studies of most agents to recommend pediatric dosages that provide adequate systemic exposure and, presumably, efficacy comparable to that demonstrated in adults. Therefore, the pediatric doses recommended in guidelines are based largely on pharmacokinetic data and the extrapolation of adult efficacy data to pediatric patients. Because few clinical trials have been conducted in pediatric surgical patients, strength of evidence criteria has not been applied to these recommendations. With few exceptions (e.g., aminoglycoside dosages), pediatric doses should not exceed the maximum adult recommended dosages. Generally, if a dose is calculated on a milligram-per-kilogram basis for children weighing more than 40 kilograms, the calculated dosage will likely exceed the maximum recommended dose for adults; adult dosages should therefore be used for larger children.[201,273]

The Timing of Antibiotic Prophylaxis

The risk of surgical site infections is reduced with appropriate timing and dosage of preoperative antimicrobials irrespective of the wound class and type of surgery, with a relative risk reduction of 18% to 78%.[274] One of the most studied strategies to reduce the risk of surgical site infection is the administration of preoperative antibiotics that reduce the bacterial load present during surgery. Interventions to increase compliance with the timing and recommended dose of antibiotics should be encouraged in all institutions.[270,275] The optimal time for administration of surgical antibiotic prophylaxis is important. The American Society of Hospital Pharmacists[273] and the WHO[1] recommend administration of prophylaxis between 0 and 60 minutes before surgical incision, which also holds true for children. However, in the case of children, in whom >80% are ambulatory, IV access is often not established until after induction of anesthesia. The risk of a surgical site infection is almost doubled if the antibiotic is given AFTER skin incision (odds ratio 1.89) and 5-fold greater (odds ratio 5.25) if it is given >2 hours before skin incision.[274] Hence, timely administration of antimicrobial prophylaxis is a goal in the perioperative period, although the significance of the timing was challenged in a study of more than 30,000 predominantly elderly, male patients.[276] They concluded that the duration of surgery and the choice of antibiotic were the two most important covariates in predicting the risk of a surgical site infection. A second intraoperative dose is indicated if the duration of the procedure exceeds two half-lives of the drug or if there is excessive blood loss during the procedure.

Allergy to β-Lactams

The prevalence of penicillin allergy in the general population is ~8% to 15%, and ~5% in children, although up to 95% test negative when they are investigated for penicillin allergy.[277,278] Children <4 years of age who are commonly treated with β-lactams frequently develop maculopapular and urticarial rashes that are not reproduced with subsequent drug challenges.[279] In fact, <7% react upon rechallenging them with the same medication. Nonetheless, a growing cohort of children who are labeled as "penicillin allergic," unlikely to experience an adverse reaction if challenged with a β-lactam, and will almost certainly receive a substitute antimicrobial at the time of surgery because of the allergy label. The use of broad-spectrum substitute antimicrobials increases the odds ratio of a surgical site infection by ~50% in adults, contributes to antibiotic resistance, increases the duration of hospital stay, and increases health care costs.[280,281] In contrast to data in adults, the incidence of surgical site infections in children with and without penicillin allergy label was similar, 1.8% and 1.9%.[282] Hence, the use of substitute antimicrobials in children do not appear to increase the risk of a surgical site infection or antibiotic resistance.

Only 5.5% of children who reported allergies to medications including antimicrobials had follow-up to confirm their β-lactam allergy according to their parents.[283] Of a cohort of 1001 children, only 0.4% reported confirmed sensitivities/allergy to medications that would lead the practitioner to a substitute medication in their anesthetic prescription.[283] Although surgical site infections may not differ in children with and without penicillin allergy, there are several additional reasons cited above to use penicillin and avoid broad-spectrum substitute antimicrobials, providing the decision to administer a β-lactam antimicrobial is judicious and sensible.

The basis for most reports of "penicillin allergy" is weak and likely erroneous for several reasons, including that the reaction was not temporally related to receiving the antibiotics, the rash was primarily maculopapular, the child had a coincidental viral infection, the airway and remote organ systems (e.g., kidneys) were not involved, and there was no follow-up to confirm the sensitivity. In a study of 191 children with histories of allergy to penicillin, 72% had developed signs of a reaction within 1 hour of taking the penicillin and 28% within 1 to 6 hours. A multivariate analysis pointed to a history of urticaria with angioedema (odds ratio 28) and anaphylaxis (odds ratio 52) as the primary predictors of true penicillin allergy, which were verified in 18.8% of children using diagnostic testing.[284] Unfortunately, unconfirmed diagnoses of allergy to β-lactams or penicillin and misperceptions that these cross-react with cephalosporins has led to many children receiving an inferior, possibly more dangerous (e.g., vancomycin) and more expensive antimicrobials for surgical wound prophylaxis.[285,286]

After completing a careful history of the purported allergy along with associated events and timing, many clinicians assert that β-lactam antimicrobials could be given to 90% to 95% of these children without fear of an anaphylactic or other systemic and life-threatening reaction.[281,283] Hence, there has been a growing shift in management away from skin testing of patients for allergies to antimicrobials to direct drug challenges known as drug provocation testing, particularly in those whose past exposure resulted in mild reactions that were nonanaphylactic and not severe to confirm which patients can tolerate the drug.[287] In two studies of almost 1000 children who were labeled "penicillin allergic" based on a previous reaction, drug provocation testing was determined to be safe as they resulted in 2.1% to 2.6% of the children developing an immediate reaction that was deemed to be mild, cutaneous, and self-resolving.[288,289] In addition, the positive predictive value of skin testing that was performed in 783 children who carried a label of "penicillin allergy" was only 22%, less than half the positive predictive value of drug provocation testing, which was 55.6%, with a final result of 90% unlikely react to a further challenge with a β-lactam.[290] Given these data, several national organizations have recommended "delabeling" those with a label of "penicillin allergy" and either testing them or rechallenging them in a β-lactam drug provocation test, depending on the duration and severity of the original reaction.[291,292] Most drug provocation testing involves the oral form of the antibiotic; a consensus panel found no agreement on whether the IV route was more appropriate for patients scheduled to receive IV penicillin during surgery and did not recommend the IV route.[281] Some institutions have implemented quality improvement and educational strategies that included a multidisciplinary team of surgeons, anesthesiologists, pharmacists, and nurses to screen children with labels of "penicillin allergy" who present for surgery to identify those who are candidates to receive cephalosporins.[293] The percent of children who received cephalosporins increased from 34% to >80%.

Most find it easy to diagnose the extremes of reactions, low or no risk (no reaction to an antimicrobial) or very high risk (anaphylaxis, Steven Johnson syndrome). However, most children fall in between these two extremes, making it difficult to quantify their risk of reacting to a penicillin challenge. Although it may be difficult to label a child as low or very low risk for a β-lactam allergic reaction, the signs with which they presented during their initial reaction speak to the low risk of an immunologic reaction: a macular, maculopapular, or urticarial rash, onset >1 hour after the dose, absence of progression to involving skin, arthritis, mucous membranes, lymph nodes, or systemic involvement (renal or hepatic).[280,294] Those children are very low risk and may be prescribed a β-lactam. However, those who exhibited signs and symptoms consistent with a high risk of reaction to β-lactams are those with an IgE-mediated reaction within 1 hour of administration including urticaria, angioedema, wheezing, hypotension, and anaphylaxis may be allergic and should not be rechallenged with the antimicrobial.[280] This electronic algorithm to stratify the risk of penicillin allergy shows great promise. For the average practitioner, a decision-making algorithm provides the most useful metric to determine whether administering a β-lactam antimicrobial is low or very low risk. In a study of >600 adults, the PEN-FAST mnemonic was developed: **PEN**icillin allergy, **F**ive or fewer years ago (2 points), **A**naphylaxis/Angioedema (2 points), **S**evere cutaneous adverse reaction (SCAR) (2 points) and **T**reatment required (1 point) with a total of <3 points signifying a low risk of a penicillin allergy within the study and with external validation[295]; a similar mnemonic and evaluation in children has not been forthcoming.

The cross-reactivity between penicillin and cephalosporin allergy has been 8% to 10%, although more recently, the true cross-reactivity has waned and stabilized at ~2%.[296] In adults, the frequency of anaphylaxis with penicillin is ~2:1000, whereas the frequency with cephalosporins is ~16:100,000.[297,298] In children, allergic reactions including IgE-mediated reactions fade within 8 to 10 years such that the children can be rechallenged with a penicillin antibiotic without fear of triggering an allergic reaction.[277,296] Approximately 90% to 95% of children with a previous history of allergy to β-lactams could safely receive β-lactam antibiotics after evaluation by a specialist and negative testing.[299]

Although there is some concern among professionals about the use of cephalosporins in patients "labeled" allergic to penicillin, cephalosporins have been used safely in the perioperative period.[273,300] The risk for a cross allergic reaction to penicillin allergic patients with the third and fourth-generation cephalosporins appears to be negligible[301]; the avoidance of cefazolin when there is a vague family history of allergy to penicillin should be reconsidered.[300]

Patients who have a "penicillin allergy" label should be stratified to determine whether they will likely tolerate first generation cephalosporins using the following list[277]:

Low risk: Penicillin reactions that were gastrointestinal, neurologic, or musculoskeletal, with clinical findings that were non-urticaria, angioedema and urticaria, reaction was >5 to 10 years ago, or an unknown allergy.

Moderate risk: Reaction was a hypersensitivity reaction, angioedema or urticaria, difficulty breathing, and occurred <5 years ago. These patients should undergo allergy testing (e.g., skin testing) and receive clindamycin or vancomycin.

Severe risk: Reaction to penicillin included toxic epidermolysis necrolysis or Stevens Johnson syndrome or multiorgan involvement. The frequency of severe risk is <0.5%. Antimicrobial prophylaxis should include clindamycin or vancomycin.

If the surgical procedure indicates prophylaxis against Gram-positive cocci and the patient is tested allergic to β-lactams (cephalosporins), vancomycin or clindamycin is warranted.[302]

Indications for Prophylactic Antibiotics

Surgical wounds are classified into four categories (E-Table 47.7). The use of antibiotic prophylaxis for postoperative infections is well established for clean-contaminated procedures. Within the clean category, prophylaxis has been traditionally reserved for surgical procedures involving a foreign body implantation or for surgical procedures where a surgical site infection would be catastrophic (e.g., cardiac surgery or neurosurgical procedures). However, there is evidence that postoperative infections resulting from procedures not involving prosthetic elements are underreported; estimates show that more than 50% of all complications occur after the patient is discharged and are thus unrecognized by the surgical team. Therefore, antibiotic prophylaxis is also recommended for specific procedures.[158,303] In the case of contaminated or dirty procedures, bacterial contamination or infection is established before the procedure begins. Accordingly, the perioperative administration of antibiotics is a therapeutic, not a prophylactic, measure. The use of antibiotics in children has implications not only for the response to the current treatment but also to future treatments. Thus, all medical professionals are jointly responsible for the rational use of antibiotics. Protocols, although effective, require continuous feedback on their acceptance and surgical site infection results.[304] No surgical protocol can replace the judgment of the medical professional; clinical reasoning must be tailored to the individual circumstances. Finally, children with congenital heart disease and a subgroup of those with repaired congenital heart disease may require bacterial endocarditis prophylaxis (see also Tables 14.2 and 14.3).[305] A summary of the prophylactic antibiotic doses is described in Table 47.10.

Other recommendations by the WHO to prevent surgical site infections include[1]:

- Perioperative discontinuation of immunosuppressive agents: Discontinuation of immunosuppressive treatment may reduce the risk for surgical site infections; however, the WHO panel suggests not discontinuing immunosuppressive medication before surgery to prevent surgical site infections.[1] The decision to discontinue immunosuppressive medication must be made individually and involve the prescribing physician, patient, and surgeon.

- Nutritional support: Patients' nutritional status can lead to changes in host immunity that can make them more susceptible to postoperative infections. Nutritional support should not delay surgery and evidence for such support reducing surgical site infections is uncertain.[2]

- Preoperative bath: Full body bath before the operation is considered good clinical practice to ensure that the skin is as clean as possible before surgery and to reduce bacterial load, especially at the incision site. In general, an antiseptic soap is used in environments where it is available and accessible. A simple soap can also be used for this purpose. Care should be taken with low-birth-weight infants due to the risk of contact dermatitis or absorption of chlorhexidine by immature skin.

- Decolonization with mupirocin ointment with or without chlorhexidine gel for body wash in nasal carriers of *Staphylococcus aureus* undergoing surgery: The WHO panel recommends that patients known to be nasal carriers of *S. aureus*, receive perioperative intranasal applications of 2% mupirocin ointment with or without a combination of liquid soap and chlorhexidine gluconate; no guidance was provided for pediatric patients.[306] However this treatment has been successfully used in the neonatal population to eradicate *S. aureus*, but those who remained hospitalized became recolonized.[307]

- Surgical site skin preparation: The panel recommends alcohol-based antiseptic solutions that are based on chlorhexidine gluconate for surgical site skin preparation.[1] Alcohol-based solutions should not be used on neonates or come into contact with mucous membranes or eyes. Chlorhexidine gluconate solutions can cause skin irritation and should not come into contact with the brain, meninges, eyes, or middle ear. Notably, alcohol-based solutions can be difficult to acquire and expensive in low-income countries, particularly when combined with an antiseptic compound. Local production may be a more affordable and viable option in these environments, provided there are adequate quality controls in place.

- Maintain normal body temperature (normothermia): Hypothermia leads to vasoconstriction, which lowers the oxygen tension in the tissues, increasing the risk of developing infection.[1] Neonates are especially vulnerable to heat loss. The panel suggests the use of heating devices in the operating room and during the surgical procedure to warm the patient's body with the aim of reducing surgical site infections. In developing countries, heating equipment costs represent a substantial financial burden, and availability and procurement are additional issues. The best methods for keeping patients warm include forced-air blankets, warm IV fluids, and increased ambient operating room temperature. Blankets can be considered an effective, low-cost option in low-resource settings.

- Adequate maintenance of blood volume (normovolemia): The panel suggests the use of goal-directed fluid therapy intraoperatively to reduce the risk of surgical site infection.[1] Adequate intravascular volume is an essential component of tissue perfusion and an important aspect of tissue oxygenation. In imbalance (hypovolemia and hypervolemia) tissue oxygenation is compromised and may increase the risk of a surgical site infection.

- Drapes and gowns: The panel suggests that both sterile surgical drapes and gowns (disposable or reusable fabric) be used during surgical operations for the purpose of prevention, including possible availability and cost issues in resource-poor settings and the ecological effect.[1]

- The panel suggests that either sterile disposable nonwoven or sterile reusable woven drapes and surgical gowns be used during surgical operations for the purpose of preventing surgical site infection; plastic adhesive incise drapes with or without antimicrobial properties should not be used (conditional recommendation, low to very low quality of evidence).

- Incisional wound irrigation: The panel suggests considering the use of incisional wound irrigation with an aqueous solution of povidone-iodine prior to closure; however, incisional wound irrigation with antibiotics before closure should not be performed; this practice is associated with an unnecessary risk of antimicrobial resistance.[1]

ANNOTATED REFERENCES

Fernandez PG, Loftus RW, Dodds TM, et al. Hand hygiene knowledge and perceptions among anesthesia providers. *Anesth Analg.* 2015;120(4):837-843.
Anesthesiologists have long been patient safety advocates. It is not surprising that anesthesia providers have taken on increasing responsibility for preventing health-care–associated infections. However, the overall hand hygiene compliance across health care providers remains less than 50%, with anesthesia providers identified as a particularly noncompliant group. In this paper, the authors identified risk factors for knowledge deficits among anesthesia providers and characterized anesthesia provider perceptions, attitudes, awareness of individual group performance, workload and type, and accessibility of hand hygiene agents.

Loftus RW, Brown JR, Koff MD, et al. Multiple reservoirs contribute to intraoperative bacterial transmission. *Anesth Analg.* 2012;114(6):1236-1248.
Bacterial cross-contamination is thought to play an important role in the development of health-care–associated infections, but the relative importance of the known hospital bacterial reservoirs (health care providers' hands, patient, and environment, including health care equipment) in this process is unknown. A better understanding of how bacterial cross-contamination occurs can provide the basis for the development of evidence-based preventive measures. This paper examined the relative contributions of anesthesia providers' hands, the patient, and the patient environment to stopcock contamination.

Odor PM, Neun M, Bampoe S, et al. Anaesthesia and COVID-19: infection control. *Br J Anaesth.* 2020;125(1):16-24.
This article presents a summary of learning points in epidemiological infection control from the COVID-19 epidemic, alongside a review of evidence connecting current understanding of the virologic and environmental contamination properties of SARS-CoV-2. Suggestions are made for how personal protective equipment policies relate to the viral pandemic context and how the risk of transmission by and to anesthetic practitioners, intensivists, and other health care workers can be minimized.

Rizzo M. Striving to eliminate catheter-related bloodstream infections: a literature review of evidence-based strategies. *Semin Anesth Perioper Med Pain.* 2005;24(4):214-225.
This paper reviews and emphasizes the need for preventive measures that could help to avoid or reduce most nosocomial catheter-related infections. The use of evidence-based standardized protocols will result in "best practices" and markedly reduce such infections.

Sagoe-Moses CH, Pearson R, Perry J, Jagger J. Risks to health care workers in developing countries. *N Engl J Med.* 2001;345(7):538-541.
Protecting health care workers in developing countries from exposure to bloodborne pathogens will involve some cost. Health care workers are a crucial resource in the health care systems of developing nations. In many countries, including those in sub-Saharan Africa, workers are at increased risk for preventable, life-threatening occupational infections. This paper expands on the need for improved support of health care workers throughout the world with appropriate supplies of gloves, barriers, sharps disposal, and the need for accident education programs.

A complete reference list can be found online at Elsevier eBooks+.

Pediatric Anesthesia in Developing Countries

48

ADRIAN T. BÖSENBERG

The Child
Children and War
Pain
Human Resources
Pathology
COVID-19 Pandemic
Human Immunodeficiency Virus Infection and
Acquired Immunodeficiency Syndrome
Tuberculosis

Malaria
Cardiac Disease
Tetanus
Drugs
Blood Safety
Equipment
Drawover Anesthesia
Oxygen Concentrators
Visiting Providers

THE POPULATION IN THE DEVELOPING WORLD continues to grow while world demographics trend toward an aging population in an urbanized, developed world.

Children, many orphaned by the ravages of war, human immunodeficiency virus (HIV) infection,[1] and famine, constitute more than one-half of the population in many of these low and middle income countries (LMIC).[2] Eighty-five percent will require surgery before their 15th birthday.[3] The burden of surgical disease requires safe anesthesia,[4,5] but provision of safe pediatric anesthesia[6] and intensive care[7–9] in the developing world presents serious challenges.[10–12] Recognition of the surgical burden of disease as a global public health problem has been slow. Few of these countries have adopted the World Health Organization (WHO) drive for safe surgery. Safe anesthesia and surgical care are not available when needed for over 5 billion of the world's 8 billion people.

Poverty, poor educational standards, and limited health resources characterize the developing world.[5,6,13] Debt repayment, housing, education, social services, and health care provision are near-impossible tasks for most governments of these countries. Of the world's poorest countries, 70% are in sub-Saharan Africa; they are ravaged by HIV, malaria, Ebola virus, and tuberculosis, and desperately short of health care providers.[4,5] The COVID-19 pandemic has stressed the health care systems worldwide, but none more so than those in low- and middle-income countries.

Pediatric anesthesia in low-income countries cannot keep pace with the advances made in developed countries.[4] International standards for the safe practice of anesthesia, adopted by the World Federation of Societies of Anaesthesiologists (WFSA), are seldom met.[14–24] In one survey, only 13% of anesthesiologists were able to provide safe anesthesia for children.[3] Consequently, perioperative morbidity and mortality rates are high by developed world standards.[5,17–23,25–30] One study of pediatric surgical cases from 24 government hospitals in Kenya found the pediatric perioperative mortality rate to be 100-fold greater than in high-income countries.[31] Notwithstanding, local expectations are commensurate with the available facilities and quality of care.

This chapter outlines some of the many challenges that anesthesiologists face when providing anesthesia for children in low- and middle-income countries. Different countries have different problems, requiring different solutions. The problems faced in many tropical countries,[8–13] for example, are completely different from those on a tropical island in the South Pacific[29] or West Indies,[32,33] at altitude in Nepal[34] and Afghanistan,[35] or in the humidity of sub-Saharan Africa.[2,3,26,36–39] These diverse situations necessitate that generalizations be made. The main differences among these sites are related to the personnel, the spectrum and nature of the disease, the facilities and equipment available, and a tenuous supply of cheap, generic, and perhaps outdated drugs.[10,40]

The Child

Children of the developing world are, for the most part, victims of circumstance: natural disasters, war, social unrest,[41] and economic crises. For many, medical care or timely access to care can be a remote or nonexistent possibility.[10,34,39,42,43] Fear, superstition, poor understanding of medical problems, and poor education often result in delayed presentation. Frequently, prior visits to well-meaning traditional healers expose the child to additional risks caused by potions that may be hepatic or nephrotoxic or enemas that can lead to bowel perforation.[44] Further delays occur when children need to undertake long journeys to reach the hospital and if the initial diagnosis is incorrect, tertiary referral is often made only when complications occur (Fig. 48.1).[10,39,45,46]

A typical example is acute appendicitis, a relatively uncommon condition in the developing world, where many other causes for a change in bowel habit are initially suspected.[46,47] Most children present for surgery with generalized peritonitis, and perforation is common. In the developing world, the prospect of providing emergent anesthesia for a toxic, acidotic, and dehydrated child is daunting.

Another example is infantile hypertrophic pyloric stenosis, also uncommon in developing countries, where symptoms other than the classic triad of bile-free vomiting, visible peristalsis, and a palpable pyloric tumor are more likely. The unsuspecting anesthesiologist, who may have no access to a laboratory[2,13–15] and is limited in the choice of fluid for resuscitation, would be challenged to correct the metabolic derangements in these infants.

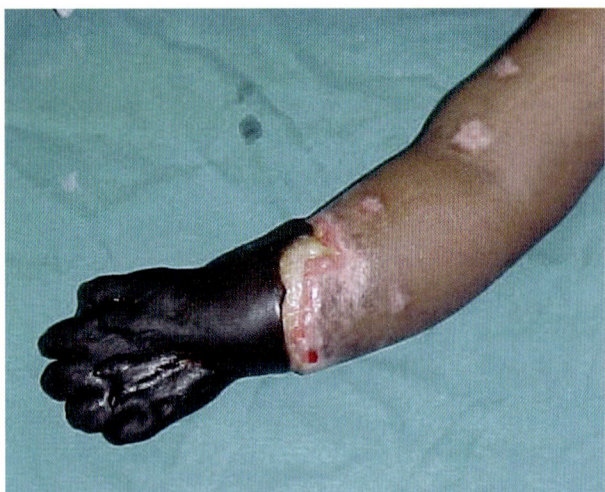

FIGURE 48.1 Peripheral gangrene of the hand. Severe dehydration in this infant was caused by severe gastroenteritis. Dehydration associated with delayed presentation, hypernatremia, herbal medications, and pneumonia are common contributors to this disastrous outcome.

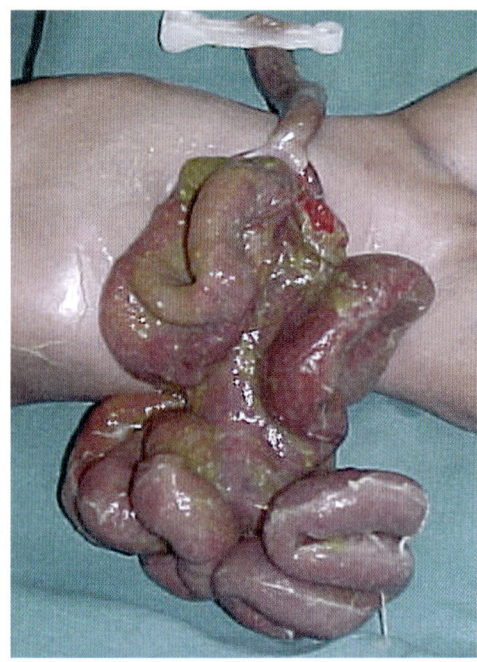

FIGURE 48.2 Gastroschisis is a major problem in the developing world. The outcome is poor because of a paucity of facilities for neonates. This defect was not diagnosed antenatally, and the patient presented late for closure, which proved difficult. Ventilatory support was not available, and a silo was fashioned. Unfortunately, the child died of overwhelming sepsis a week later.

Superstition plays a role in compounding the anesthetic risk. For example, rural Vietnamese believe that it is not good to die with an empty stomach. Parents consider surgery to be an enormous risk, so they feed their children beforehand. In these circumstances where aspiration risk is high, passage of a nasogastric tube before induction is routine, although it is very unlikely that the stomach can be emptied of solids.[33]

Perinatal mortality in some parts of the developing world is 10 times greater than those in developed countries.[5,48–50] The common denominators are early childbearing, poor maternal health, and lack of appropriate and quality medical services. Although lifesaving practices for most infants have been known for decades, one-third of pregnant women still have no access to medical services during pregnancy, and almost 50% do not have access to medical services for childbirth.[39,43,50] Most parturients give birth at home or in rural health centers,[43] where basic neonatal resuscitation equipment is deficient or nonexistent.[39] Those who require surgery may need to be transferred, but specialized transport teams rarely exist.

In some hospitals, neonates are not candidates for surgery because mortality rate is high; "they always die,"[51] whereas in others, they undergo surgery without anesthesia[32] because "it's safer" and because some still believe that neonates do not feel pain. When neonates undergo surgery, there are additional challenges, particularly in emergency situations.[32] Appropriately sized equipment is lacking,[45] and it may be extremely difficult to maintain normothermia even in relatively warm climates without improvisation. Regional anesthesia can play an important role in neonatal anesthesia[39,45,52] and in some centers may be the only choice for anesthesia.[43,53] Apart from providing analgesia without respiratory depression, the need for postoperative ventilatory support for conditions such as esophageal atresia,[54] congenital diaphragmatic hernia,[55] and abdominal wall defects can be reduced by continuous epidural analgesia (Fig. 48.2).

Regrettably, even neonates who receive skilled anesthesia and surgery may die because of inadequate postoperative care.[53] Overwhelming infection, sepsis, respiratory insufficiency, and surgical complications are the main causes of morbidity and mortality.[39,43] The development of highly specialized neonatal anesthesia and surgical services,[7,49–51] essential for a good outcome after neonatal surgery,[39,43,45] is a low priority.

Although the burden of disease is dominated by infections and malnutrition,[4,5] pediatric trauma has a low level of advocacy and is given scant attention.[39,45,56] Socioeconomic advances introduce a new danger in the form of faster, more powerful vehicles without the necessary maintenance culture or road discipline. Road traffic accidents are inevitable, and effective systems to handle the polytrauma victims that result are hard to find.[45]

Even simple bone fractures may have disastrous outcomes. Inappropriate management by traditional bonesetters frequently results in compartment syndromes or gangrene.[56] Trauma prevention strategies are given low priority despite the acknowledged impact of trauma on the economy of any country. Many developing countries are at war, and this has led to massive trauma and injuries to children who may be either participants in the fighting or innocent bystanders.

CHILDREN AND WAR

Children may be victims of all aspects of violence. They face an intense struggle for survival manifesting in displacement, separation from or loss of parents, poverty, hunger, and disease. Children are vulnerable to the abuse of abandonment, abduction, rape, and forced soldiering. An estimated 300,000 children are used as child soldiers in more than 30 countries.[57] Many sustain physical injuries and permanent disabilities, and a large number acquire sexually transmitted disease, including HIV and AIDS. These HIV-positive child soldiers then become vectors in communities where they are deployed.[58]

For many of these children, acts of violence become their form of normality, and former victims become the perpetrators.[41] Survivors are subjected to the total collapse of economic, health,

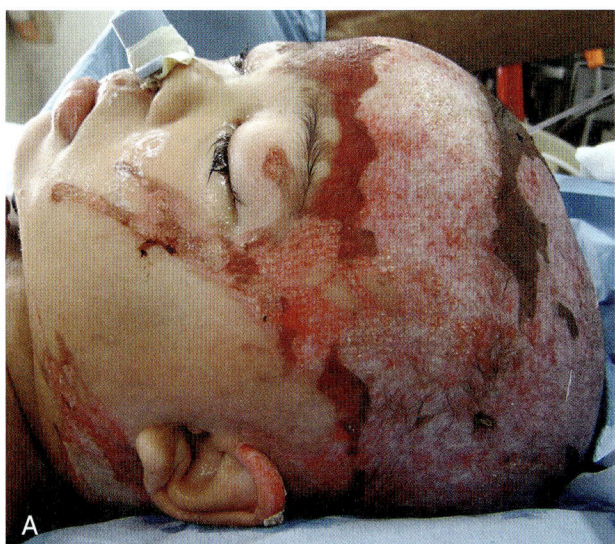

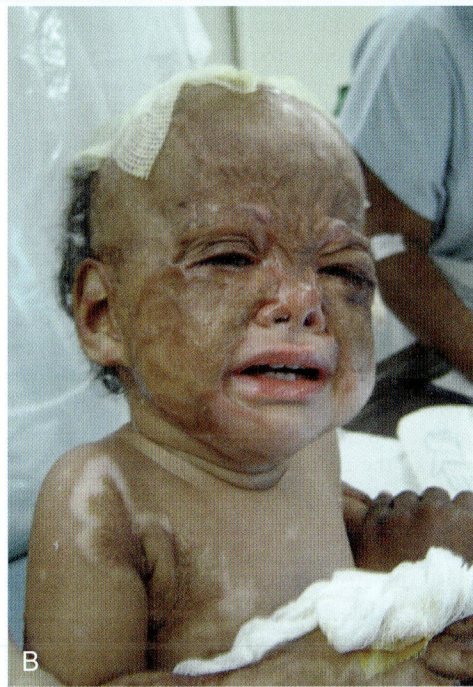

FIGURE 48.3 Facial burn injuries are common in the developing world, and these children may require multiple episodes of anesthesia. **A**, Flame burns of the face are invariably associated with inhalation injuries that may necessitate ventilatory support in intensive care facilities, which are not readily available. **B**, Pain management and pain assessment are challenging. The pained expression on this child's face is one of fear (and possible indignation about having the photograph taken) rather than actual pain.

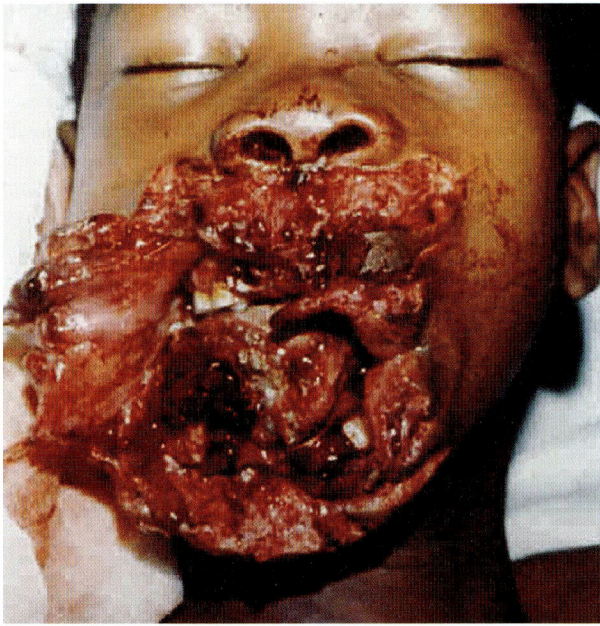

FIGURE 48.4 Children fare poorly in war. This 8-year-boy bit a detonator he found while playing. Endotracheal intubation proved a major challenge without a fiberoptic laryngoscope, which is a luxury in the developing world.

social, and educational infrastructures. Lost and abandoned children sleep on the streets and are forced to beg for food while trying to find their families. Many become child laborers or turn to crime or prostitution for survival.[59]

Children in war-torn areas sustain bullet, machete, or shrapnel injuries, and others are burned. They can sustain mutilating injuries (Figs. 48.3 and 48.4) that are not commonly seen in civilians.[60] Land mines are responsible for killing or maiming an estimated 12,000 civilians per annum. In Angola, a country with the greatest incidence of amputees in the world, there were an estimated 5.5 land mines for every child; continuing land mine

explosions remain a legacy of this conflict.[60] These blast injuries leave children without feet or lower limbs and with genital injuries, blindness, and deafness; a pattern of injury that has become a post–civil war syndrome encountered by surgeons worldwide.[60] Although the war in Angola is over, the cost of mine removal is beyond the means of local governments. Ironically, artificial limb manufacture has become a developing industry.[60] Tragedies such as these are likely to be repeated in the ongoing conflicts and ethnic violence in Afghanistan, the "Tigray war" in Ethiopia, "Drug wars" in Mexico and Central America, Mali, Mozambique, South Sudan, Somalia, and Yemen (Fig 48.5D).

The terrible psychological effects of war persist even though the armed conflict may be over. Mental and psychiatric disorders with all the ramifications of posttraumatic stress disorder are almost inevitable among child survivors and refugees. Refugees face new challenges in their adoptive countries where the health care providers have little experience with their language, customs, beliefs, and superstitions.

PAIN

Pain management in children of the developed world is vastly different from that available to practitioners with limited resources.[61] Attempts to apply similar standards are fraught with difficulty. Illiteracy, malnutrition, poor cognitive development, different coping strategies, altitude (e.g., chronic hypoxia),[62] and pharmacogenetic, cultural, and language differences all contribute to the complexity of the problem.[63]

Children of the developing world cope with vastly different problems. Victims of poverty, malnutrition, and violence (e.g., war, trauma, abuse), their attitudes toward pain, and pain tolerance, are diverse. These children seem more stoic and indifferent even to severe pain. After cardiac surgery, for example, some appear to need very little pain relief and are easily soothed by lollipops or play therapy.[42] Many walk from the intensive care unit to the general ward on the first postoperative day.

Pain assessment of children from an impoverished background is difficult (see Fig. 48.3B).[64] Many children in acute pain do not show facial expressions. Is this stoicism or simply a reflection of malnutrition, lack of social stimulation, severity of illness, or even cultural attitude? Language difficulties, cultural barriers, unwillingness to share information, emotional expressiveness, and outdated attitudes of the caregiver may underpin this quandary. Some cultures convey pain readily, but others teach that expression of pain is inappropriate. Although many pain assessment instruments are available, few have been validated in the developing world.[64–67]

There is a definite need to develop pain treatment strategies applicable to children of the developing world.[67] Local conditions dictate their use and applicability. Simple pain management strategies may produce the best results with the least risk, whereas more complex techniques, offering greater benefit, require minimum standards of monitoring and regular reassessment to titrate analgesia to the needs of the individual. These devices and the necessary trained personnel are seldom available. The final choice is therefore dictated by economic pressures or by the facilities available rather than what would be considered best for the child.

Human Resources

Anesthesia does not enjoy a high profile and lacks the voice to demand access to basic resources in most developing countries. The critical shortage of manpower is a barrier to progress.[5,8,18,22] Anesthesia is frequently delivered by nonphysicians,[3,6,68,69] a reality that has remained constant over many decades. Many anesthetics are still administered by nurses or unqualified personnel[70,71] who have little medical background and are "trained on the job."[3,45] In many African[5,72] and Asian countries,[5,73] the ratio of doctors to patients is so small that the ideal of employing a physician specifically to provide routine anesthesia is out of the question.[5,74,75] Salaries are not sufficient to attract suitably trained and qualified practitioners for more than short periods. Emigration of trained personnel to developed countries in search of better salaries and improved lifestyles exacerbates these human resource shortfalls.[5,10,68,74–77]

Anesthesia is not perceived as an attractive career for many undergraduates,[76] who receive little or no exposure to the specialty during their training.[77] In some countries, surgery has been performed without the "luxury" of anesthesia.[78] Few developing countries can afford specialist anesthesiologists, with the possible exception of the principal hospitals. Supervision of "nonphysician anesthesiologists" is invariably inadequate.[74] Access to textbooks, journals, or other medical literature is limited.

Internet access is invaluable but is dependent on a reliable electrical supply, a telecommunications network, and a computer.[79,80] In October 2018, a pediatric anesthesia collaborative chat group was launched. Individuals with WhatsApp, Wi-Fi, and internet access can seek advice or help with challenging cases and other information from a variety of sources: (PedsAnesthesia.Net [https://www.pedsanesthesia.net/] SPA Global Ped Anesthesia [https://spaglobal.pedsanesthesia.org/] and PeDi chat [https://www.pediatricchat.com/]).

Despite these challenges, many individuals provide high-quality anesthesia for a limited range of surgical procedures. Few receive formal training in pediatric or neonatal anesthesia. Inadequately trained anesthesiologists tend to shy away from children, particularly neonates and infants, because of the perceived

difficulty or fear. This is understandable in view of the lack of supervision, the severity of the child's condition, and with equipment that is more suited to adults.[71] Invariably, the "pediatric anesthetist" is someone who may simply have an interest in or affinity for children or is allocated to pediatric anesthesia for the day because there is no one else. A genuine pediatric trained anesthesiologist is a luxury.

The WHO has recognized that surgery is a public health issue and has launched the Safe Surgery Saves Lives campaign.[5,16,17,75,81] International standards for safe anesthetic care have been developed by the WFSA and the WHO. The WHO has emphasized that safe surgery does not exist without safe anesthesia.[10,11,16,17] The WFSA anesthesia facility assessment tool can be used to assess each facility for infrastructure, service delivery, workforce, medications, equipment, and monitoring practices.[22,23] Many facilities to this day still fall short on all facets of anesthesia facility assessment tool.[22,82] A study in East Africa, with a total population of 142.9 million, reported that there were only 237 anesthesiologists, with a workforce density of 0.08 in Uganda, 0.39 in Kenya, 0.05 in Tanzania, 0.13 in Rwanda, and 0.02 anesthesiologists in Burundi per 100,000 population in each country.[83]

Training anesthesiologists in the skills required for pediatric anesthesia is a slow process. Hopefully the WFSA fellowship programs,[6,15,81,83–90] including those in East Africa, will continue to develop so that children undergoing surgery in developing countries will reap the benefit.

Pathology

Many pathologic conditions seldom seen in industrialized countries are more prevalent in developing countries because of poor health education, malnutrition, the proximity of livestock to humans, earth-floored homes, poor sanitation, and contaminated water supplies (Fig. 48.5). Some conditions prevalent worldwide and relevant to the anesthesiologist are considered in the next sections.

COVID-19 PANDEMIC

Since early 2020, the COVID-19 pandemic has been a harsh reminder of the global inequity in health in low- and middle-income countries. Diversion of resources from child health to address the pandemic among adults impacts the care of children. The indirect effects of the pandemic on child health are of considerable concern.[90,91] These include increasing poverty levels, disrupted schooling, lack of access to school feeding schemes, reduced access to health facilities, and interruptions in vaccinations and other child health programs.

Additional challenges in these countries include the inability to implement effective public health measures such as social distancing, hand hygiene, timely identification of infected people with self-isolation, and universal use of masks. Lack of adequate personal protective equipment, especially N95 masks, is a key concern for health care worker protection. Although continued schooling is crucial for children in low- and middle-income countries, provision of safe environments is particularly challenging in overcrowded resource-constrained schools.

Poor living conditions in these low- and middle-income countries including lack of sanitation, running water, and overcrowding, may facilitate transmission of SARS-CoV-2. The risk of coronavirus disease (COVID-19) in populations with high prevalence of comorbidities, the impact on health and economies, and

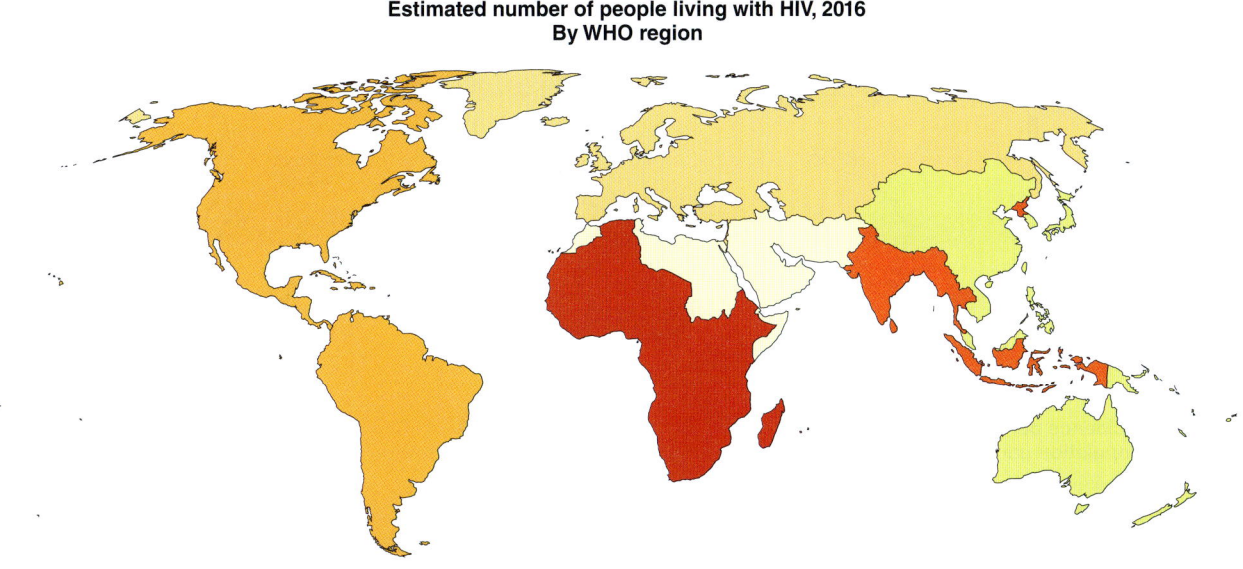

**Estimated number of people living with HIV, 2016
By WHO region**

Number of people, by WHO region

☐ Eastern Mediterranean: 360,000 (290,000–500,000) ☐ Americas: 3,300,000 (2,900,000–3,800,000) **Total: 36,700,000**
☐ Western Pacific: 1,500,000 (1,200,000–2,000,000) ☐ Southeast Asia: 3,500,000 (2,500,000–8,200,000) **(30,800,000–42,900,000)**
☐ Europe: 2,400,000 (2,300,000–2,600,000) ☐ Africa: 25,600,000 (22,900,000–28,600,000)

A

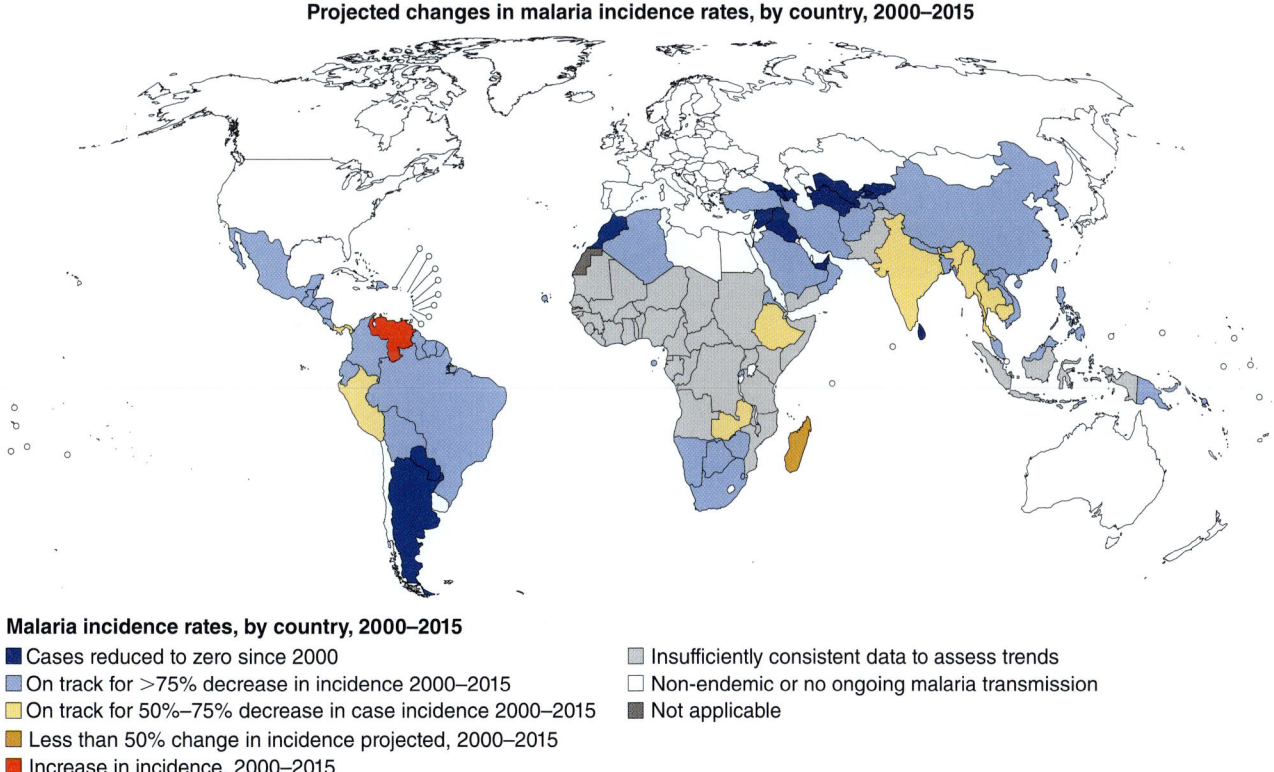

Projected changes in malaria incidence rates, by country, 2000–2015

Malaria incidence rates, by country, 2000–2015

■ Cases reduced to zero since 2000
☐ On track for >75% decrease in incidence 2000–2015
☐ On track for 50%–75% decrease in case incidence 2000–2015
■ Less than 50% change in incidence projected, 2000–2015
■ Increase in incidence, 2000–2015

☐ Insufficiently consistent data to assess trends
☐ Non-endemic or no ongoing malaria transmission
■ Not applicable

B

FIGURE 48.5 A, Global distribution of human immunodeficiency virus infection and acquired immunodeficiency syndrome (HIV/AIDS). Developing countries, particularly sub-Saharan Africa, carry the greatest health burden with the poor resources. **B,** Changes in the malaria incidence since 2015. Distribution of malaria is remarkably similar to that of HIV/AIDS. Blood products in these regions carry an enormous risk, even if family members act as donors.

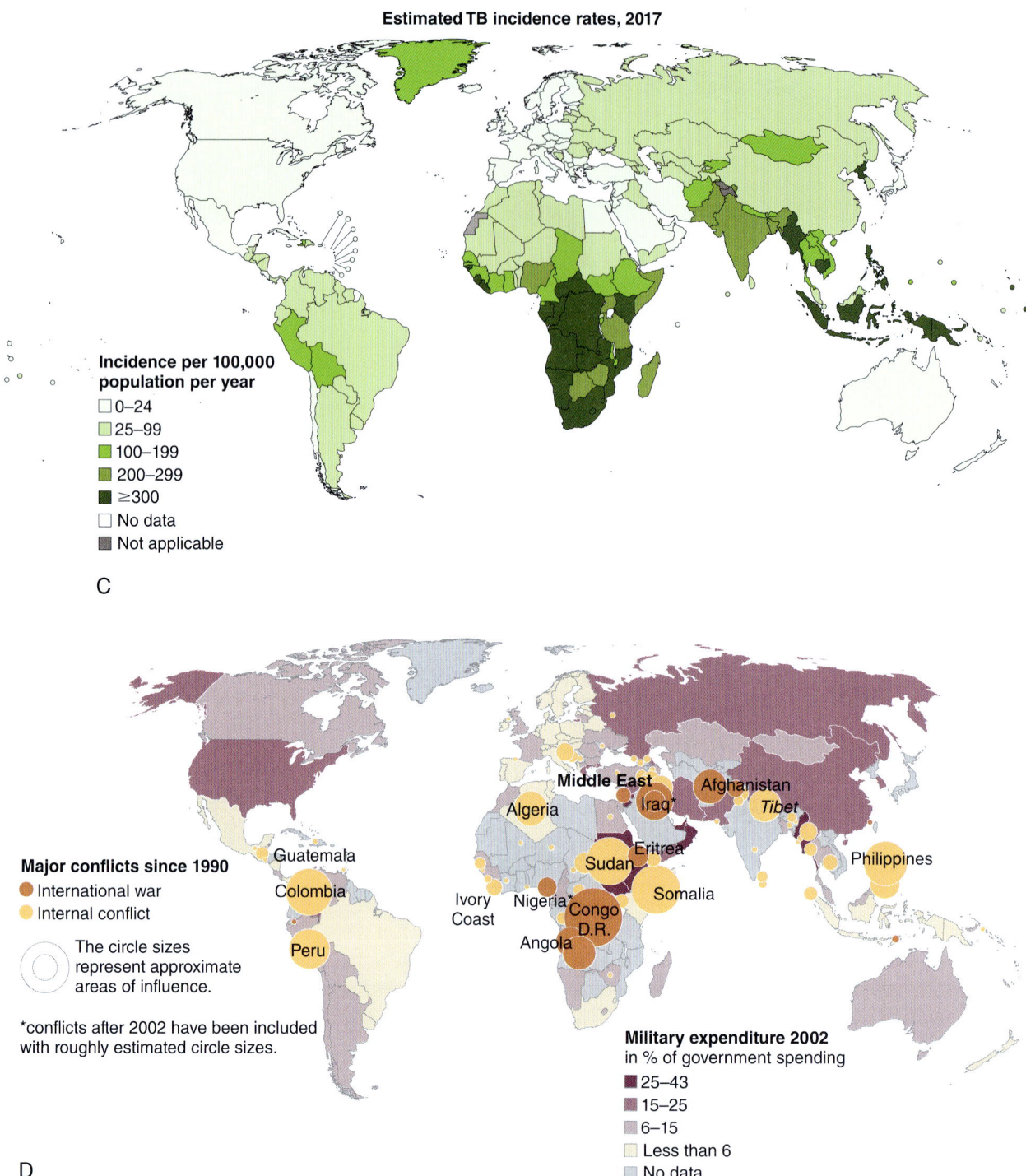

Estimated TB incidence rates, 2017

Incidence per 100,000 population per year
- ☐ 0–24
- 25–99
- 100–199
- 200–299
- ≥300
- ☐ No data
- Not applicable

C

Major conflicts since 1990
- ● International war
- ● Internal conflict

The circle sizes represent approximate areas of influence.

*conflicts after 2002 have been included with roughly estimated circle sizes.

Military expenditure 2002
in % of government spending
- 25–43
- 15–25
- 6–15
- Less than 6
- No data

D

FIGURE 48.5, cont'd C, Global distribution of tuberculosis (*TB*) in 2005. **D,** Major areas of conflict worldwide since 1990 (All maps sourced from WHO Map gallery website who.int).

the capacity of existing health systems to manage the additional burden of COVID-19 has taxed already depleted health care systems. Vaccination rates in these countries are low.

Children make up a larger proportion of the population in low- and middle-income countries. The direct effects of COVID-19 were initially of less concern in children, who seem to be either largely asymptomatic or afflicted with a mild illness. Risk factors for severe lower respiratory infection such as HIV, tuberculosis, or malnutrition are more prevalent. Mutations and spreading

variants, such as Delta, Omicron, and other variants have affected more children and the prevalence continues to climb.[90,91]

HUMAN IMMUNODEFICIENCY VIRUS INFECTION AND ACQUIRED IMMUNODEFICIENCY SYNDROME

Although the world has committed to ending the AIDS epidemic by 2030, an estimated 37.7 million people are living with HIV, 16% of whom do not know their HIV status. Seventy-five percent of those who knew their HIV status in 2020 were able to access

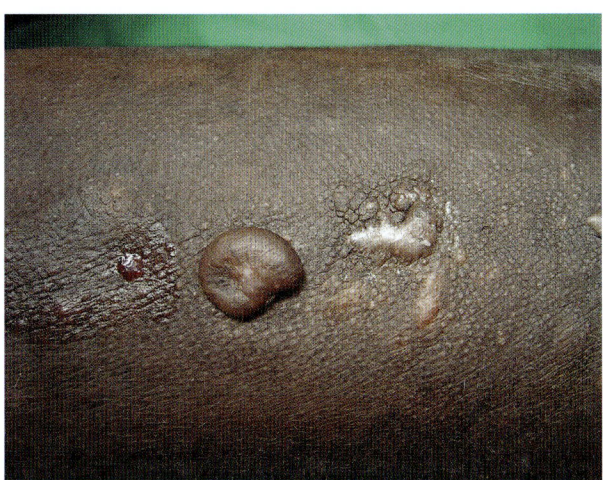

FIGURE 48.6 Human immunodeficiency virus infection and acquired immunodeficiency syndrome (HIV/AIDS) is a serious problem in developing countries, particularly in sub-Saharan Africa. The skin manifestations in this 8-year-old boy indicate Kaposi sarcoma, an AIDS-defining tumor.

antiretroviral therapy. Most cases occur in the developing world (90%), with sub-Saharan Africa (24.7 million) and Southeast Asia (4.8 million) making up two-thirds of the global total; approximately 8% are children (see Fig. 48.5A).[92] More than 35 million have died of HIV-related diseases since the start of the epidemic in 1981, and as a consequence, there are an estimated 15 million orphans in sub-Saharan Africa alone.[92] Worldwide, more than 500 children were newly infected with HIV each day in 2016 (down from 1000 each day in 2010); most of these children are in sub-Saharan Africa (Fig. 48.6).[93] The prevalence of HIV seropositivity varies from one country to another. In these clinical situations, anesthesiologists and surgeons[94] should assume a positive status for every patient they serve until proven otherwise.[45]

Some success has been achieved in slowing the transmission of HIV in developed countries.[94-100] In sub-Saharan Africa today, 90% of those who know their HIV status have received treatment and 76% have achieved viral suppression. Numerous barriers exist for the treatment of HIV-infected children.[92] Treatment has lagged behind that of adults primarily as a result of poor human resources and infrastructure for administration of antiretroviral treatment,[101] but also because of the expense and the lack of pediatric drug formulations.[97] Only an estimated 25% of children infected with HIV receive treatment.[92]

Children are infected by vertical transmission from the mother (>90%) or when sexually abused (≈2%) by an infected adult.[102] Transmission through blood products remains a risk, but with the global trend toward volunteer donors and more sophisticated testing of donated blood, this risk is diminishing.

Vertical transmission can occur in utero, during labor and delivery, or postnatally. Risk factors include maternal viral load and breastfeeding.[93,99] Mixed feeding (i.e., breastfeeding with other oral foods and liquids) is associated with the greatest risk of transmission.[103] Perinatal transmission rates are dramatically reduced by universal HIV testing of pregnant women, provision of antiretroviral therapy (when needed for maternal health); or prophylaxis, elective cesarean delivery, and avoidance of breastfeeding.[93,99] Highly active antiretroviral therapy, the triple antiretroviral therapy, has changed HIV from a fatal illness to a chronic disease with decreased mortality rates and improved quality of life.[99] However, these strategies require resources.

In practical terms, it is difficult to differentiate infants who are infected by vertical transmission from those who are not infected because differentiating between actively or passively acquired antibodies is virtually impossible in low-income countries. All children born to HIV-positive mothers have acquired HIV antibodies for the first 6 to 18 months. Only 30% to 40% of the infants who are infected develop AIDS. The presence of HIV antibody is therefore not a reliable indicator of infection. More sophisticated and expensive tests have been developed but are not widely available. All children born to HIV-positive mothers should be considered infected; if antibody persists beyond 15 months, infection should be assumed.

Progression of the disease depends on the mode of transmission; vertically acquired infection is more aggressive than other forms. Between 20% and 30% of untreated HIV-infected children will develop profound immunodeficiency and AIDS-defining illnesses within a year, whereas two-thirds will have a slowly progressive disease. The course of the disease depends on a variety of factors, including timing of infection in utero, the viral load, the mother's stage of the disease, and whether the mother is receiving antiretroviral therapy. Treatment of children depends on clinical category, CD4 T-cell cell count, viral load, and age at the time of diagnosis. According to the current state of knowledge, after highly active antiretroviral therapy is started, it must be carried on lifelong. This implies great challenges for adherence to avoid development of resistance and to evade long-term adverse effects of HIV therapy. Emerging drug resistance in children in low- and middle-income countries has necessitated new treatment strategies.[97,100]

The clinical manifestation of HIV in infants and children depends on whether they have been managed with antiretroviral drugs or not.[94,97,100] Most have asymptomatic infections, and the presentation may be subtle, such as failure to thrive, lymphadenopathy, hepatosplenomegaly, interstitial pneumonia, chronic diarrhea, or persistent oral thrush. Some present for the first time with life-threatening disease.

Chronic diarrhea, wasting, and severe malnutrition predominate in Africa, whereas systemic and pulmonary pathologies are more common in the United States and Europe. Recurrent bacterial infections, chronic parotid swelling, lymphocytic interstitial pneumonitis, and early onset of progressive neurologic deterioration are characteristic of children with AIDS.

Pulmonary disease remains the leading cause of morbidity and mortality.[104-106] Bacterial pneumonia, viral pneumonia, and pulmonary tuberculosis are common, and the course of these infections is more fulminant when associated with HIV infection.[107] As the CD4 T-cell count falls, acute opportunistic infections occur, including: *Pneumocystis carinii* (PCP) now called *Pneumocystis jiroveci* pneumonia (PJP), cytomegalovirus infection, and the more typical *Haemophilus influenzae, Streptococcus pneumoniae,* and respiratory syncytial virus (RSV) infections.[104,105,107] The classic presentation of pneumocystis carinii/jiroveci is fever, tachypnea, dyspnea, and marked hypoxemia, but in some children, the presentation is more indolent, with hypoxemia preceding clinical or radiologic changes.[108]

Lymphocytic interstitial pneumonitis is a slowly progressive, chronic form of lung disease found in older children that can lead to an insidious onset of dyspnea, cough, and chronic hypoxia with normal auscultatory findings but with pulmonary lymphoid hyperplasia in AIDS patients. In contrast to adults, lymphocytic interstitial pneumonitis in children may cause acute respiratory failure that is treated with steroids and bronchodilators. Clinical manifestations may present as signs and symptoms recognized

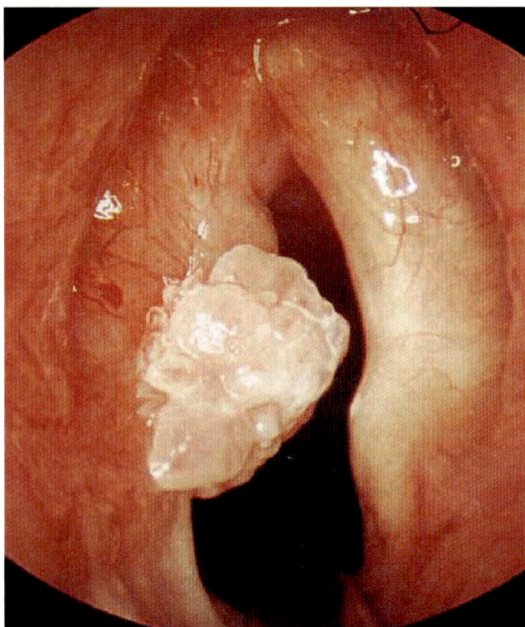

FIGURE 48.7 Laryngeal papilloma. Papillomata, caused by the human papillomavirus, are prevalent in low socioeconomic groups and have the highest incidence in the 2- to 5-year-old age group. This age distribution is changing in the populations exposed to human immunodeficiency virus. Even in well-equipped institutions, anesthesia for these patients can be challenging.

principally by otolaryngologists[109] or dental surgeons.[110] Management of the upper airway may be difficult in the presence of stomatitis and gingival disease. Intubation can be difficult in the presence of acute (i.e., candida infection) or chronic epiglottitis (i.e., lymphoid hyperplasia), necrotizing laryngotracheitis, Kaposi sarcoma (Fig. 48.6), or Kaposi sarcoma laryngeal papillomas (Fig. 48.7). These comorbid respiratory disorders challenge even the most experienced pediatric anesthesiologist (Fig. 48.8).

Cardiac disease is being diagnosed with increasing frequency in children with HIV. The pathogenesis of cardiomyopathy is multifactorial, including pulmonary insufficiency, anemia, nutritional deficiencies, specific viral infections, and drug therapy. Left and right ventricular dysfunction, arrhythmias, and pericardial effusions occur, but pulmonary hypertension is rare.[111] HIV may directly infect the myocardium, leading to early electrocardiogram changes and abnormal echocardiograms showing hyperdynamic left ventricular dysfunction or evidence of diminished contractility (e.g., dilated cardiomyopathy, myocarditis).

The gastrointestinal tract is commonly involved,[112] particularly in those living in tropical countries. Affected children show evidence of malabsorption (i.e., "slim"), chronic recurrent diarrhea, dysphagia, failure to thrive, or enteric infection requiring diagnostic endoscopy. From the anesthesiologist's point of view, there is an increased risk of reflux owing to esophagitis caused by infection (e.g., *Candida*, cytomegalovirus) or drugs (e.g., zidovudine). Pseudobulbar palsy, a manifestation of central neurologic involvement, or esophageal strictures may occur.

Nausea and vomiting may have a neurologic, infectious, or drug-related cause. Pancreatitis, lymphomas, or smooth muscle tumors may delay gastric emptying. Hepatomegaly is invariably present, but severe hepatocellular dysfunction is seldom a major problem unless the patient has chronic hepatitis (e.g., hepatitis B

or C, cytomegalovirus). Cholestasis and fluctuating transaminase levels may be caused by HIV infection, poor nutrition, or drugs. In theory, hepatic enzyme dysfunction caused by antiretroviral therapy should affect the metabolism and pharmacokinetics of some anesthetic agents, although there has been a paucity of research on this subject.

Medications used to manage HIV are involved in drug interactions on several levels.[113] The reverse transcriptase inhibitors (e.g., zidovudine) are excreted by the kidneys, and drugs that affect renal clearance reduce excretion. Reverse transcriptase inhibitors may induce CYP3A4 (e.g., nevirapine) or inhibit CYP3A4 (e.g., delavirdine) and affect the clearance of other drugs (e.g., midazolam, levobupivacaine, ketamine, methadone). Prolonged sedation may occur with midazolam and simultaneous administration of protease inhibitors.[114] Protease inhibitors are also substrates and inhibitors of P-glycoprotein transporters. Coagulation status with the concomitant use of warfarin, which is metabolized by CYP2C9, may be altered by enzyme induction (e.g., ritonavir) or competition for clearance pathways (e.g., efavirenz, nelfinavir).[115]

Protease inhibitors also can inhibit specific uridine 5'-diphosphoglucuronosyltransferase (UGT) pathways. This accounts for the increase in bilirubin concentration (i.e., UGT1A1 glucuronidates bilirubin) observed in some patients, although UGT1A6 (i.e., acetaminophen glucuronidation) and UGT2B7 (i.e., morphine glucuronidation) are unaffected.[116] Gastric motility changes related to opioids (e.g., methadone) reduce absorption of some reverse transcriptase inhibitors.

HIV, a neurotrophic virus, can have a devastating effect on the immature brain, which can be further compromised by opportunistic infections or neoplasms that occur as a consequence of the associated immunosuppression.[117] Neurologic impairment is observed in most symptomatic HIV-infected children, commonly as a progressive encephalopathy with developmental delay, progressive motor dysfunction, and behavioral changes. Craniofacial dysmorphic features have been described. Hematologic abnormalities can reflect depression of all cell lines. Anemia may be caused by primary marrow failure, malnutrition, or drugs, whereas thrombocytopenia may reflect an autoimmune disorder.

Universal precautions should be strictly applied for all anesthesia procedures. Extra care should be taken when anesthetizing an HIV-infected child. Precautions should be taken to prevent contamination of the anesthetic circuits; disposable equipment, bacterial filters, and disposable circuits are recommended. The prohibitive cost of disposables limits their use in most institutions in developing countries. Reusable equipment must be cleaned, sterilized, and decontaminated according to the manufacturer's instructions; HIV is sensitive to a wide range of disinfectants.[118]

TUBERCULOSIS

Tuberculosis remains an important cause of morbidity and mortality.[45,119–124] The epidemiology of pediatric tuberculosis is shaped by risk factors such as age, race, immigration, poverty, overcrowding, and prevalence of HIV/AIDS (see Fig. 48.5C).[123,124] HIV and tuberculosis form a dangerous synergy that is difficult to manage because of drug interactions between the antituberculosis and antiretroviral agents.[92,120,125] Even bacillus Calmette-Guérin (BCG) vaccinations can cause complications in immunocompromised HIV patients.[120] The emergence of drug-resistant tuberculosis adds to the burden and is a constant danger to health care workers in general and anesthesiologists in particular.

Primary tuberculosis infection usually does not produce clinical illness in well-nourished, immunized children, whereas reactivated

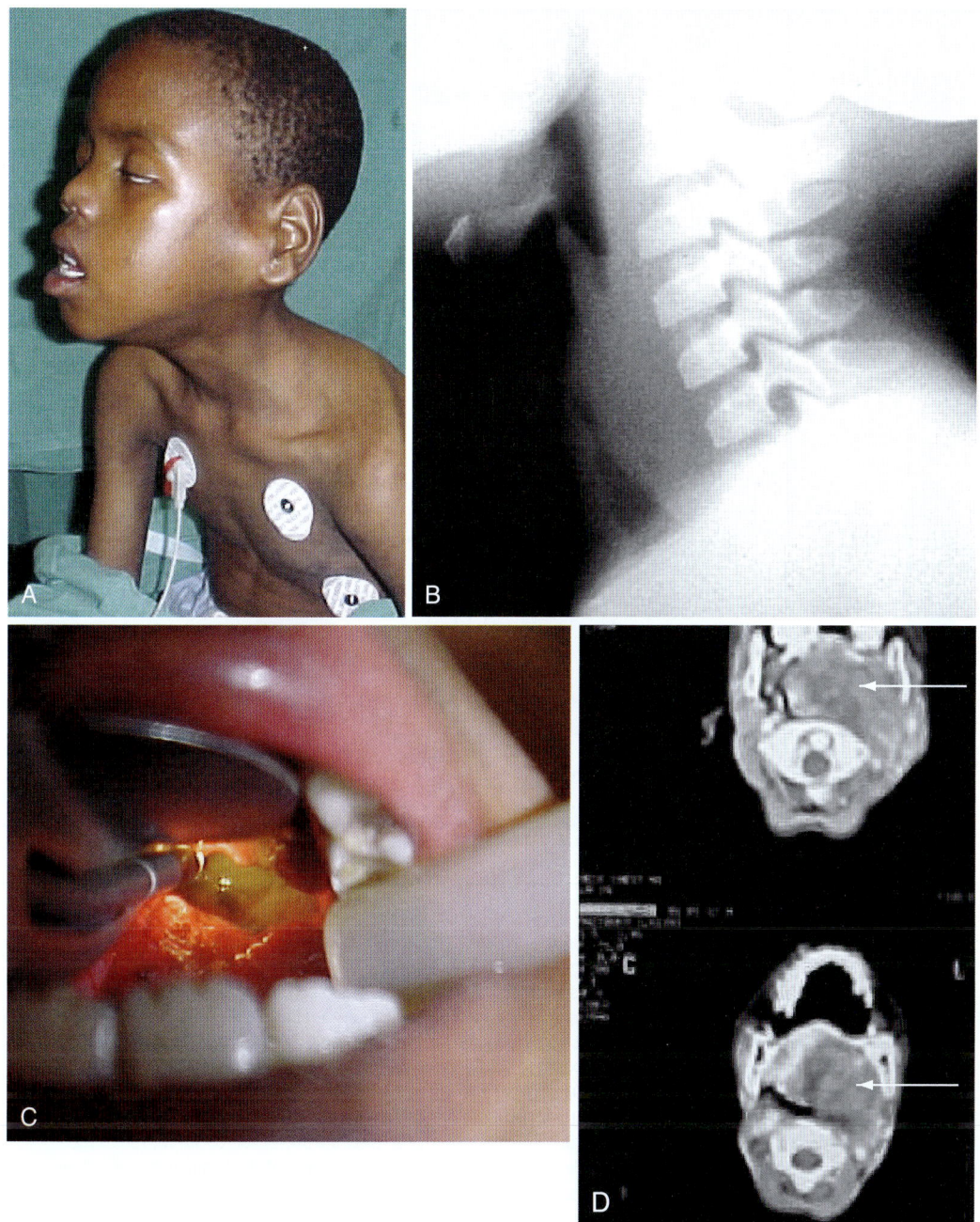

FIGURE 48.8 Kaposi sarcoma is a marker for acquired immunodeficiency syndrome (AIDS). **A,** AIDS was previously considered rare in children, but it may affect the airway at different levels, as shown in this 12-year-old girl. She is clearly fatigued from the respiratory distress caused by Kaposi sarcoma at three levels: base of the tongue, tonsil, and trachea. She also has an underlying pneumonia. Significant supraclavicular recession suggests upper airway obstruction. **B,** The Kaposi sarcoma of the base of the tongue, tonsil, and trachea is shown on a poor-quality, lateral neck radiograph, which illustrates one of the many difficulties faced in remote areas: the lack of high-quality imaging. **C,** Laryngoscopic view of the Kaposi sarcoma at the base of the tongue and the tonsil. **D,** Computed tomography shows a large retropharyngeal Kaposi sarcoma *(arrows)* obstructing the upper airway. The poor quality of the scan reflects inexperienced radiographers using the poor-quality equipment commonly found in developing countries.

pulmonary tuberculosis is a chronic or subacute disease that may present a variety of challenges for the anesthesiologist, including preventing transmission by contamination of the anesthetic circuits and the risks associated with pleural effusions, pulmonary cavitation, or bronchiectasis.[106,108] Mediastinal and hilar lymphadenopathy may severely compromise the airway.

Primary tuberculosis and its complications are more common in children than in adults. After young children are infected, they are at increased risk for progression to extrapulmonary disease.[123,124] *Mycobacterium tuberculosis* infection can cause symptomatic disease in any organ of the body and is usually a reactivation of a latent site of infection. The most common sites of

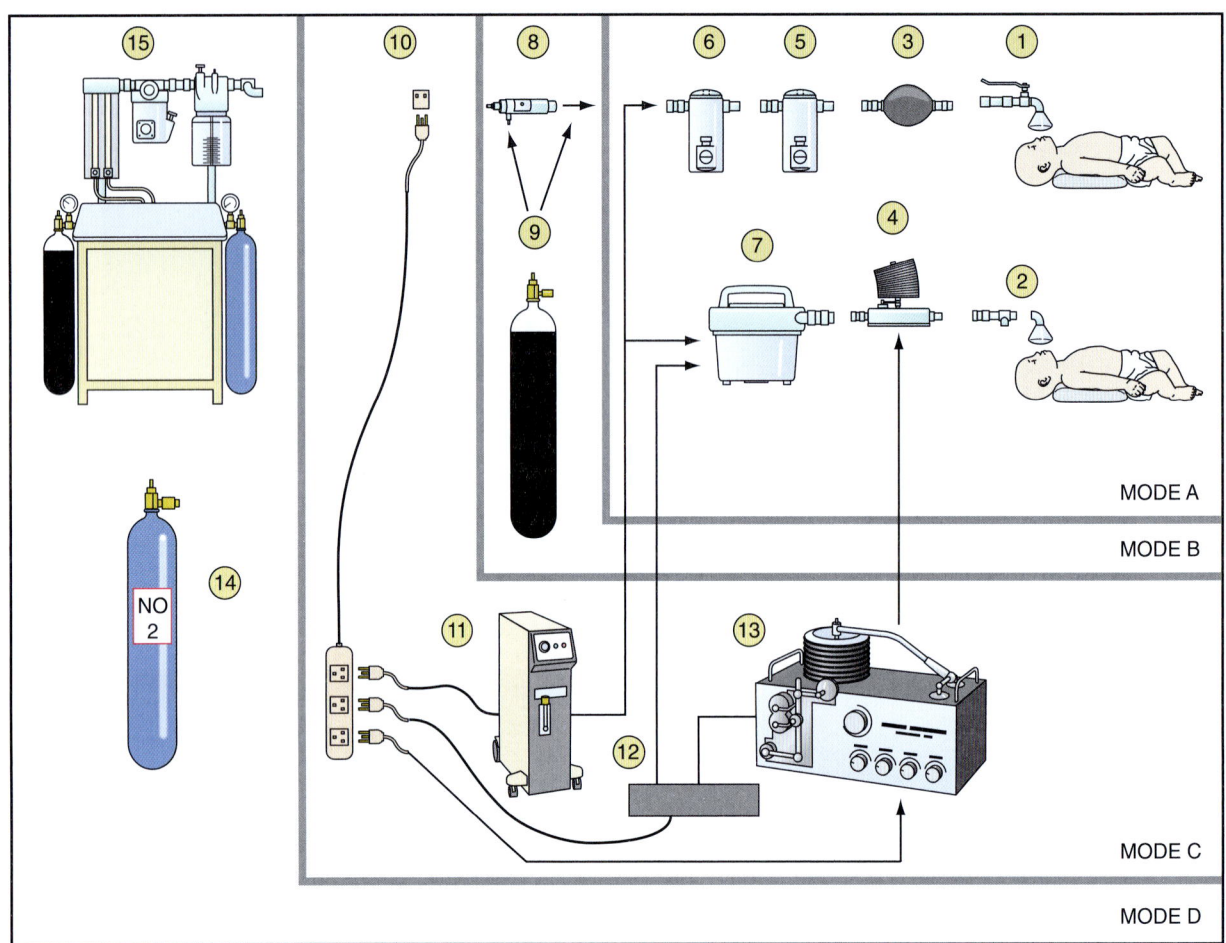

FIGURE 48.9 The schematic diagram shows the use of anesthetic systems, depending on available resources. **Mode A** provides basic inhalational anesthesia with air, spontaneous ventilation, or self-inflating bags. Drawover vaporizers are required. **Mode B** provides oxygen enrichment but requires the availability of oxygen cylinders. Plenum vaporizers can be used. **Mode C** requires electricity to power the oxygen concentrator, air compressor, and ventilator. A mechanical ventilator (e.g., Manley) does not require electrical power. **Mode D** requires a Boyle machine and nitrous oxide cylinders. **1,** T-piece with reservoir tube and face mask. **2,** Ambu Pedi valve. **3,** Self-inflating bag (Ambu). **4,** Oxford Inflating Bellows (OIB). **5,** Oxford Miniature Vaporizer (OMV) with halothane. **6,** OMV with trichloroethylene. **7,** Epstein, Macintosh, Oxford (EMO) vaporizer with ether. These circuits and manual ventilators are interchangeable, and ether, halothane, and trichloroethylene can be used on their own or in series. Farman entrainer (**8**) with an oxygen cylinder (**9**) can be used to supplement oxygen, or an electrical power source (**10**) with an oxygen concentrator (**11**), air compressor (**12**), or Manley ventilator (**13**). Nitrous oxide (**14**) and Boyle apparatus (**15**) allow anesthesia practice equivalent to that of developed countries.

reactivation are lymph nodes, bones, joints, and the genitourinary tract. Less frequently, the disease may involve the gastrointestinal tract, peritoneum, pericardium, or skin. Tuberculosis meningitis and miliary tuberculosis, both more common in children, carry a high mortality rate.[123] In view of the high prevalence of HIV infection among tuberculous children, HIV testing should be performed in all children with tuberculosis; conversely, tuberculosis should be sought in all HIV-positive children. Tuberculosis is, however, difficult to diagnose in young children, and the search for affordable, more sensitive tests continues.[119]

MALARIA

Malaria (see Fig. 48.5B) is a febrile, flu-like illness caused by one of four species of malaria parasites: *Plasmodium falciparum, Plasmodium vivax, Plasmodium ovale,* and *Plasmodium malariae.* Effective and safe prophylaxis against malaria has become

increasingly difficult because the species that causes the most severe illness, *P. falciparum,* has become widely resistant to chloroquine and to other antimalarial drugs in some areas.[124] Severe malaria, even when optimally treated, carries a mortality rate of 10% to 25%.[124,126,127]

Prompt diagnosis and early treatment is an important determinant of outcome. Uncomplicated malaria usually manifests as fever, headache, dizziness, and arthralgia. Gastrointestinal symptoms may predominate and include anorexia, nausea, vomiting, and abdominal discomfort or pain mimicking appendicitis. In children, malaria can manifest with an acute, life-threatening disease or run a chronic course with acute exacerbations. The acute manifestations include three overlapping syndromes: respiratory distress as the result of a severe underlying metabolic acidosis (pH <7.3), usually a lactic acidemia; severe anemia (hemoglobin <5 g/dL) with hypovolemia[128] and thrombocytopenia; or neurologic impairment as a manifestation of cerebral malaria.[126–129] Seizures are an important presenting feature in 60% to 80% of cases. Prolonged seizures refractory to treatment and those that occur on antimalarial treatment are ominous signs that are commonly associated with neurologic sequelae or death.[128] Cerebral malaria may also manifest as a prolonged postictal state, status epilepticus, severe metabolic derangement (i.e., hypoglycemia and metabolic acidosis), or a primary neurologic syndrome, ranging from diffuse cortical involvement to brainstem abnormalities.

Children with chronic malaria adjust physiologically to low hemoglobin concentrations but may decompensate rapidly when challenged with a febrile illness or surgery. The characteristic physical findings in children with severe anemia are respiratory distress and a hyperdynamic circulation. Blood transfusion may be administered rapidly in children with metabolic acidosis because most have a depleted intravascular volume.

Although controversial, exchange transfusion has been advocated for severe malaria, particularly for those with cardiorespiratory compromise, hyperparasitemia, or cerebral malaria. The rationale is to remove harmful metabolites, toxins, and cytokines; decrease the parasite load; remove deformed red blood cells; and restore normal red blood cell mass, platelets, and other clotting factors.[128] Unfortunately, many malaria-endemic areas also have a high prevalence of HIV, adding significantly to the risk of blood transfusions.

Chronic recurrent malarial infections may manifest with splenic enlargement. This may cause delayed gastric emptying and pose an aspiration risk on induction of anesthesia. The spleen may enlarge acutely or rupture spontaneously during coughing, vomiting, or defecation. Rupture during external cardiac massage has also been described. Malaria may cause bloody diarrhea with massive fluid loss resembling dysentery in children.

CARDIAC DISEASE

In general, pediatric cardiac services are too expensive for most developing countries, and the increasing economic divide threatens the services that do exist.[130,131] In North America, each cardiac center serves 120,000 people; by contrast, one center serves 16 million people in Asia and 33 million in Africa.[74] Despite the need, few developing-world units can treat the required volume of cases.[132] Unless families have the financial means to travel to a developed country, the options for diagnostic or therapeutic cardiac procedures remain poor.[42,130,131,133] Medical missions may provide immediate help, but their impact on a developing country is short-term and potentially disruptive. These visiting teams ultimately have little effect on the complex socioeconomic and sociopolitical problems that exist.[131]

Rheumatic heart disease is more common than congenital heart disease in many developing countries,[130,131,133] reflecting the socioeconomic problems of poverty, overcrowding, malnutrition, and lack of antibiotics. Children often present late with life-threatening symptoms as the result of repeated infections and superimposed endocarditis. The acute deterioration precipitated by endocarditis may be the factor that prompts the search for medical attention. Valve replacement can be lifesaving,[134] but long-term follow-up of anticoagulant therapy is often not feasible.

Congenital heart disease is an additional challenge, and it is common to see congenital heart defects in adults in developing countries. Those who have survived without the benefit of palliative or corrective surgery may present with pulmonary hypertension or endocarditis. Total correction of these defects is usually not feasible, and palliative surgery may be the more effective

alternative. Excellent palliation with reasonable quality of life can be achieved relatively cheaply.[131]

TETANUS

Tetanus is caused by the exotoxin of *Clostridium tetani*, an organism that is ever present in the soil and contaminated wounds.[135] Tetanus is prevalent in countries where children are not routinely immunized. In contrast, it is rarely reported in developed countries. Tetanus neonatorum carries a high mortality rate and is still encountered in areas where it is customary to apply feces to the umbilical cord to stop bleeding.

The exotoxin produced by *Clostridium tetani* is a potent neurotoxin, tetanospasmin, that forms at the site of the injury and enters lower motor neurons, responsible for voluntary muscle activity and then into the spinal cord and brainstem. The neurotoxin can block acetylcholine causing flaccid paralysis or block inhibitory neurotransmitter release resulting in painful tonic muscle spasms, hyperreflexia, and autonomic instability.[135] The injury itself may be trivial, even overlooked at the time of presentation. Thus, the clinical manifestations of the disease do not result from invasive tissue injury. The incubation period is inversely related to the distance between the site of the injury and the central nervous system, usually within 14 days of the injury.

Trismus is the presenting sign in most cases, and sustained trismus produces a characteristic sardonic smile (i.e., risus sardonicus). Persistent contraction of the chest and back muscles is manifested as opisthotonus. Restlessness and irritability may be followed by tetanic seizures, often precipitated by trivial stimuli (e.g., touch, noise). Glottic or laryngeal spasm can cause sudden death. Late deaths may be caused by nosocomial infection, renal failure, sudden cardiac arrest, or cerebral hemorrhage secondary to the autonomic instability.[135]

Treatment consists of surgical debridement of the wound, administration of human tetanus immunoglobulin, antibiotic therapy, and intensive supportive medical care. Ventilatory support is invariably necessary because the frequent spasms impair ventilation already compromised by sedative therapy. Benzodiazepines and opioids are the mainstay of treatment, but numerous protocols have been studied.[135] Magnesium sulfate effectively reduces spasms as well as circulating catecholamines,[136] whereas clonidine does not.[137] Nondepolarizing neuromuscular blocking drugs remove trismus as an obstacle for tracheal intubation. Since the neurotoxin blocks lower motor neurons, succinylcholine is contraindicated in these patients as hyperkalemia may occur.

Pain management should also be considered, and the use of continuous epidural analgesia for these children is encouraging. Further advantages of epidural analgesia include good control of autonomic instability, earlier weaning from ventilatory support, and possible reduction in the complication rate.[135]

Drugs

The supplies of anesthetic gases and drugs for rural medical facilities are erratic and unreliable.[3,8] The cost of many drugs, particularly those used in modern anesthesia, has increased alarmingly above and beyond the reach of most health care budgets. Accordingly, anesthesiologists in developing countries must use less expensive older anesthetics or generic medications.

Halothane and isoflurane are the most widely available inhalational anesthetics in developing countries; the former remains the mainstay of inhalational anesthesia although it has been supplanted by sevoflurane and desflurane in developed countries for several decades.[2,3,10,40,138] As demand for the less expensive agents halothane and isoflurane has waned, some manufacturers seeking profitability have threatened their withdrawal. Although this may make commercial business sense, these agents sustain the anesthesia services for millions of patients in the developing world[2] and their loss would be tragic.

Ketamine is probably the most commonly used intravenous (IV) anesthetic.[3,78,138] Ketamine is simple to use, effective, and relatively safe when used as a sole agent for brief procedures, used in combination with neuromuscular blocking drugs, or to supplement general anesthesia for major surgery. It should be used with midazolam to reduce the psychotomimetic effects and nightmares observed after ketamine use. Benzodiazepines, however, are not always available. Morphine and other opioids may not be permitted in some cultures or even available in some institutions. It is sobering to realize that only 6% of the morphine consumption worldwide is used in the low- and middle-income countries that are home to 80% of the world's population.[61]

The choice of neuromuscular blocking drugs is limited. Succinylcholine, gallamine, curare, alcuronium, and pancuronium are the usual options, with the selection of which one dictated by their availability or the availability of agents to antagonize the neuromuscular blockade. For this reason, neuromuscular blocking drugs are not commonly used.

Nitrous oxide is infrequently used because it is expensive to purchase and store, delivery is erratic, and oftentimes budget constraints are restrictive.[139,140] Closed or semiclosed anesthetic systems are considered dangerous in an environment where the oxygen supply is erratic,[140] agent monitors are seldom available,[34] and the supply of soda lime and compressed gas cylinders is erratic. These eliminate any potential benefits and cost savings from low-flow anesthesia.[140,141]

Regional anesthesia has many benefits in terms of safety, cost savings, and immediate postoperative analgesia.[2,32,39,43,45,52,142–144] Children in developing countries usually are very accepting of this form of analgesia. However, there seems to be a general reluctance to perform regional anesthesia in children,[38,45] even in some institutions in the developed world. Possible reasons include lack of training or expertise, fear of failure, and the unavailability of drugs, disposables, and other ancillary equipment such as ultrasound.

Improvisation may be the key. In the absence of appropriate equipment, access to the epidural space can be achieved by using a technique first described before the introduction of pediatric epidural needles into clinical practice. A catheter can be threaded through an IV cannula into the epidural space through the sacral hiatus in neonates and small infants.[144] Cheap, uninsulated needles can be used for peripheral nerve blocks when more expensive, insulated needles are not available.[145]

Blood Safety

An estimated 70% of all blood transfusions in Africa are given to children with severe anemia caused by malaria. Blood transfusion services, when they exist, provide a lifesaving service by ensuring an adequate supply of safe blood.[146–148] Patients, particularly children, in developing countries, face the greatest risks from unsafe blood and blood products.[147–150]

Fewer than 39% of developing countries have a nationally coordinated blood transfusion service. Many do not perform the most rudimentary tests for diseases such as HIV or hepatitis B and C because of economic constraints.[150] Even limited testing

doubles the basic cost of a unit of blood. It is estimated that only 76% of blood products undergo basic screening in low income countries and 83% in low-middle income countries and these countries account for over 71 million donations. Many of these transfusions (40%) go to children younger than 5 years of age.[150]

Many countries still rely on paid donors or family members to donate blood before surgery.[150] In Argentina, for example, up to 92% of the blood supply is derived from family members. Although voluntary, unpaid blood donation has increased to 20% in the past 5 years in Pakistan; family donors represented 70% and paid donors 10% of the blood donors in 2004.[148] Public education about the value of blood transfusion is vital to improve supply.[146,147] Through concerted efforts by the WHO to improve blood safety worldwide over the past decade, the number of voluntary, unpaid donors has increased considerably. For example, voluntary blood donation in China increased from 45% of donations in 2000 to 90% in 2004. Similarly, the rate of voluntary, unpaid donations in Bolivia increased from 10% in 2002 to 50% in 2005. Malaysia, China, and India reached 100% screening of donated blood for HIV by the year 2000.[149]

There are risks in any system.[146,147] Family and paid donors may hide aspects of their health and lifestyle that could make the blood unsafe for different reasons. Family members may feel pressured to donate, whereas paid donors are driven by need and avoid important details about their health status that would negate the transaction. The commercial plasma industry and blood trade can fuel the transmission of HIV. In 1999, for example, 26 million liters of plasma were fractionated for global use,[150] and the major source was paid donors from developing countries. Voluntary, unpaid donors have a greater sense of responsibility to their community and keep themselves healthy to be able to continue giving safe blood. South Africa has had 100% voluntary, unpaid donations since it established a national blood service. With HIV prevalence approaching 30% among the adult population of Africa, only 0.02% of its regular blood donors in South Africa have contracted HIV.

Storage of blood is difficult considering the unreliable and unpredictable electricity supply in many developing countries. To obviate the risk of transmission of malaria, HIV, and other infectious diseases, blood should be transfused only when absolutely necessary. In sophisticated blood transfusion units, the use of predonated autologous blood is an option.[151,152] In poorer countries, this is not practical because malnutrition and chronic anemia are common. There is often a lack of appropriate equipment, and cost is prohibitive. Similarly, intraoperative blood salvage and cell savers for use in children are not available. Recombinant factor VIIa, for example, that is being used increasingly to reduce blood use by those who can afford it,[151] is beyond the scope (and cost) of practice in many countries.[152]

Equipment

Electricity is unreliable in many hospitals in the developing world. In some, particularly in rural areas, neither power-line electricity nor a reliable functional backup generator is available.[3,4] Even though recycling disposable equipment such as endotracheal tubes is considered normal practice in many countries, general facilities for infection control, such as running water, disinfectants, or gloves, are also unreliable.[2]

Essential equipment to provide safe anesthesia for children and particularly for neonates is in short supply.[3,34,39,45] Neonatal or pediatric ventilators are virtually nonexistent outside the main centers.[39,71] Small IV cannulas are a precious commodity, and butterfly needles are still used. Syringe pumps and other control devices are impractical in environments with an erratic electricity supply. Metal or plastic laryngoscopes for children may be available but not well maintained. Batteries may be in short supply and light bulbs unreliable. A full range of pediatric endotracheal tubes is considered a luxury. Laryngeal mask airways in pediatric sizes are usually unavailable. IV fluids are very expensive if not manufactured locally, and many developing countries do not have local production facilities.[10] The choice of IV fluid is therefore limited and in short supply.

Monitoring is very basic: a precordial stethoscope and a finger on the pulse.[2,11] Electrocardiogram monitoring is used when available but depends on a continuous electricity supply, battery backup, and proper maintenance. Appropriately sized blood pressure cuffs are scarce. Pulse oximetry has been the most useful monitor and should be available in all centers where pediatric surgery is performed.[2,34] Unfortunately, this ideal is far from reality, but it is hoped that the global pulse oximetry project will be rewarded with universal quality improvement.[17]

Anesthetic machines in developing countries fall into two categories: modern, sophisticated machines and simple, low-maintenance equipment. The electronic machines provided by well-meaning donors have a poor track record in austere environments. Sophisticated equipment needs to be understood and maintained, but operating manuals printed in foreign languages are not helpful. Sophisticated machines require ongoing maintenance, but individuals trained to repair such equipment are seldom available. Service contracts are not viable. Unfortunately, these machines are invariably discarded when the first fault occurs, because guarantees are unlikely to be honored and faults are considered too expensive to repair. Poorly maintained equipment becomes hazardous and potentially life-threatening in untrained hands.

Simplicity and safety have long been the keys to anesthetic equipment in developing countries.[2–4,153] Ideally, a suitable anesthetic machine should be inexpensive, versatile, robust, and able to withstand extreme climatic conditions; able to function even if the supply of cylinders or electricity is interrupted; easy to understand and operate by those with limited training; economical to use; and easily maintained by locally available skills.[153–155] The cheapest, most practical, and most widely used method is inhalational anesthesia administered through an Epstein Macintosh Oxford (EMO) drawover vaporizer (Penlon Ltd., Oxford, UK; Glostavent Penlon Ltd.), or Oxford Miniature Vaporizer (OMV, Penlon Ltd.). Oxygen concentrators supplement oxygen delivery and eliminate the need for expensive oxygen cylinders, whose reducing valves are often faulty or destroyed in these situations. The most appropriate ventilator is the Manley Multivent Ventilator (Penlon Ltd.), which essentially functions like a mechanical version of the Oxford inflating bellows (OIB) and can be used with a drawover system.[155]

A general scheme for inhalational anesthesia, which was first proposed by Ezi-Ashi and colleagues in 1983,[141] for use in developing countries is shown in Fig. 48.9.[153] Applying this scheme, four different modes can be used and modified according to the available supplies and services. The basic mode A is used when there is no electricity and no supply of compressed gases. The apparatus consists of a low-resistance vaporizer linked by valves to the child to act as a drawover system with room air as the carrier gas. The self-inflating bag or hand bellows makes it possible to provide artificial ventilation while the vaporizer remains as a drawover device. The addition of low-flow oxygen to the inspired gas in mode B depends on the availability of an oxygen cylinder.

The addition of a length of reservoir tubing to the circuit enables oxygen to be stored on expiration and to be used on the next inspiration, substantially improving its economy.

When electricity is available, (mode C), operation of the anesthetic apparatus can be extended by permitting the use of an air compressor to provide continuous gas flow (allowing use of a Boyle apparatus and plenum vaporizer), an oxygen concentrator, and ventilators. When nitrous oxide is available (mode D), all types of inhalational anesthesia available in developed countries can be practiced. When services and supplies are interrupted even briefly, it is possible to change from one mode to another without requiring other anesthetic apparatuses.

These techniques may be of little interest to the anesthesiologist working comfortably in the well-maintained, sophisticated environment of developed nations. Their roles, however, are essential in field situations (e.g., war, natural disasters), and all anesthesiologists should be acquainted with their functioning in this unpredictable world (Videos 48.1 and 48.2).

DRAWOVER ANESTHESIA

Drawover anesthesia enables inhalational anesthesia to be administered using atmospheric air as the carrier gas. The essential features of this system consist of a calibrated vaporizer with sufficiently low resistance (i.e., EMO and OMV) to allow the negative pressure created by the child's inspiratory effort to draw room air through the vaporizer during spontaneous ventilation. Positive-pressure ventilation can be provided by means of a self-inflating bag or bellows (OIB), using a valve to prevent the gas mixture from reentering the vaporizer and a unidirectional valve at the child's airway to direct expired gases to the atmosphere, preventing rebreathing (see mode A, Fig. 48.9). In this way, an anesthetic can be administered in the absence of compressed gases. The vaporizer has an inlet for supplementary oxygen that can be attached to the oxygen output tube of an oxygen concentrator or oxygen cylinder when available (see modes B and C, Fig. 48.9).

The EMO and OMV are the more commonly used low-resistance vaporizers. The EMO is calibrated only for ether, but its performance is linear for other agents. The OMV is calibrated for a variety of agents,[51,154–156] and despite the lack of temperature compensation, its performance is stable under most conditions. Both vaporizers have been used successfully in pediatric anesthetic practice,[42] but it is recommended that they be converted to form a T-piece for greater safety.

The OMV has been evaluated as a simple drawover system for pediatric anesthesia. Wilson and Bem[52] showed that when a self-inflation bag is used in a drawover mode, more efficient vaporization occurs despite vaporizer cooling. However, the respiratory efforts of neonates or weak infants are insufficient to operate the valve mechanisms of the self-inflating bag (e.g., Ambu bag), necessitating continuous assisted ventilation even in the presence of ether, which stimulates ventilation.

DiaMedica Therapeutics markets a variety of devices specifically designed for use in austere environments where oxygen supply and electricity are unreliable. Examples include a portable anesthesia machine using drawover, which weighs 9.5 kilograms (Fig. 48.10; Video 48.3) that may be used with or without oxygen, and the vaporizer may be used with halothane, isoflurane, or sevoflurane (E-Fig. 48.1). It allows for both spontaneous and controlled ventilation. A portable ventilator (pediatric or adult) may be used with the portable anesthesia machine (Fig. 48.11); the bellows tidal volume is adjusted by the turn of a screw (E-Fig. 48.2). The ventilator is equipped with an internal

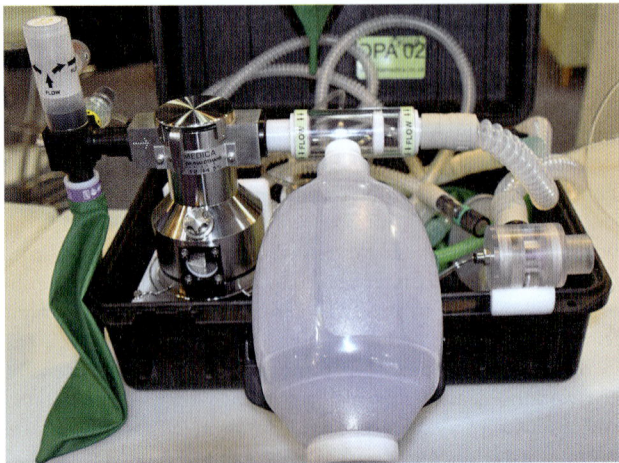

FIGURE 48.10 This portable drawover anesthesia machine weighs 9.5 kg and has a vaporizer capable of delivering halothane, isoflurane, or sevoflurane, packed in a shockproof and waterproof box (47 × 35 × 17 cm). It can work with supplemental oxygen or room air. It may also be used with a portable ventilator for children or adults (see Fig. 48.11). (With permission from DiaMedica Ltd., UK.)

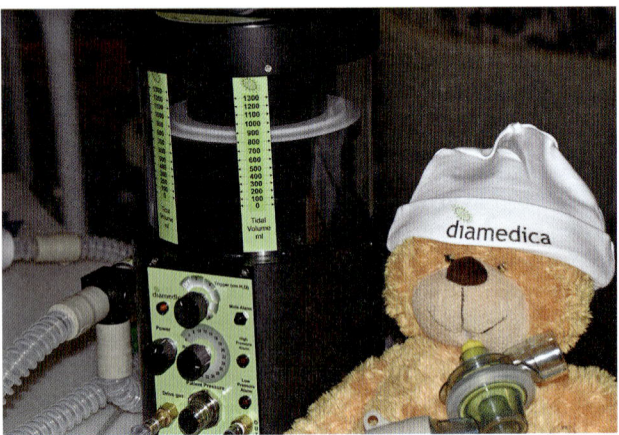

FIGURE 48.11 This is a portable anesthesia ventilator for children or adults. The bellows tidal volume is adjusted by the turn of a screw (see E-Fig. 48.2). The ventilator is equipped with an internal battery, which remains charged for approximately 100 hours without recharge and can be recharged from 100/240-V electrical sources or a 12-V charger. This is a gas-driven ventilator that may be used with an oxygen concentrator, or if no oxygen source is available, a portable battery power pump can run the ventilator using room air. This has a battery life of approximately 20 hours. (See text for further details and video links.) (With permission from DiaMedica Ltd., UK.)

battery, which remains charged for approximately 100 hours without recharge and can be recharged from a 100/240-V electrical source or a 12-V charger. This is a gas-driven ventilator (Video 48.4), which may be used with an oxygen concentrator; or if no oxygen source is available, a portable battery power pump can run the ventilator using room air. This has a battery life of approximately 20 hours. The full-size machine (Glostavent Helix; E-Fig. 48.3) with all four components—(1) low-resistance drawover vaporizer, (2) gas-driven ventilator, (3) oxygen concentrator (E-Fig. 48.4), and (4) power supply with battery backup—is shown in E-Fig. 48.5 (Videos 48.5 and 48.6).

OXYGEN CONCENTRATORS

Improved oxygen availability, independent of compressed gas and electrical power supply, can be provided by linking oxygen concentrators[157,158] to a drawover anesthetic apparatus as first described by Fenton.[140] Maintenance requirements are low, and servicing is recommended only after approximately 10,000 hours of usage. The benefits are enormous, but a reliable electricity supply is critical.

The concentrator functions by using a compressor to pump ambient air alternately through one of two canisters containing a molecular sieve of zeolite granules that reversibly absorbs nitrogen from compressed air.[138,153,157] The controls are simple and consist of an on/off switch for the compressor and a flow-control knob to deliver 0 to 5 L/minute. Flow of oxygen continues uninterrupted as the canisters are alternated automatically so that oxygen from one canister is available while the other regenerates. A warning light on a built-in oxygen analyzer illuminates if the oxygen concentration is less than 85%, and the concentrator switches off automatically when the oxygen concentration is less than 70%. This action is heralded by visual and audible alarms. Air is then delivered as the effluent gas. Modern machines are relatively silent.

The oxygen output of the concentrator depends on the size of the unit, the inflow of oxygen, the minute volume, and pattern of ventilation. The addition of dead space (or oxygen economizer tube) at the outlet improves the performance, and predictable concentrations of more than 90% oxygen can be obtained with flows between 1 and 5 L/minute, independent of the pattern of ventilation. Much lower concentrations and less predictability were observed when the dead-space tubing was omitted.[159] An example of a ventilator (mode C, Fig. 48.9) that can use a concentrator for gas supply is shown in E-Fig. 48.6. The possible hazards of oxygen concentrators are few if they are positioned in the operating room so that the in-draw area is free from pollutants. Failure of the power supply or failure of the zeolite canisters results in the delivery of ambient air. A bacterial filter at the outlet combined with the use of dust-free zeolite should prevent contamination of the delivered gas. Dirty internal air filters may produce lower oxygen concentrations and must be checked. An oxygen storage tank and booster pumps afford protection against the vagaries in electrical supply.

Visiting Providers

Personality traits compatible with survival have been suggested as a prerequisite for working in the developing world. These traits include an almost pathologic desire for work, a willingness to merge or at least sympathize with different cultures, patience in relating to and teaching people sometimes far removed educationally, the ability to withstand prolonged periods of cultural isolation, and mostly a never-failing ability to improvise and make the best of a bad situation.[160–164] There is no place for risk-taking "cowboy anesthesiologists."[156,164]

International travel, particularly visits to many parts of the developing world, needs careful preparation and planning, whether the anesthesiologist is part of a volunteer organization[42,162–165] or traveling as an individual.[163] Detailed advice[161–166] is beyond the scope of this chapter, but some generalizations are made based on personal experience and that of colleagues. Changing political climates and international health guidelines dictate visa and vaccination requirements. Expert advice should be sought to tailor the traveler's needs according to the individual's medical and immunization history, the duration of stay, and proposed itinerary.

Physical acclimatization to jet lag, altitude sickness, and heat or sun exposure is necessary, as is adjustment to the local culture and cuisine. Social graces acceptable in a Western culture may be deemed offensive in some other cultures. An interpreter is an important ally. The inability to understand a language or the local dialect places a visiting anesthesiologist at a serious disadvantage, particularly when dealing with children. Children often use subtle ways to describe their feelings that even a skilled interpreter may fail to convey.

The hospital environment may be disconcerting for some. In contrast to the familiar comforts of a clean, child-friendly hospital, the visitor may be struck by the relatively shabby, bland appearance of many hospitals in developing countries. The buildings may not have received a coat of paint since they were built, and broken windowpanes provide the only air conditioning. Children are often cared for in adult wards.

In the operating room, the visitor may be faced with anesthetic equipment barely recognizable from its original manufacture or in a state of disrepair with nonstandard improvisations to make it functional. The choice of drugs may be limited, and the names of locally manufactured generic drugs and the presentation of IV solutions may add to the perplexity. Surgical safety may be the next issue. Informed consent as we know it is unlikely, and identification of the child in the absence of parents may not be obvious to the newcomer. A local or itinerant surgeon may suggest an extensive procedure on a malnourished child without consideration for monitoring, blood transfusion, or availability of intensive care or postoperative analgesia in an unmonitored environment. The anesthesiologist is obligated to consider the risks and benefits carefully in such circumstances.

Anesthesiologists from high-income countries who work on a temporary basis with teams in developing countries should routinely and critically self-analyze their personal and institutional motivations. Short-term surgical teams typically do not engage in developing sustainable medical systems that are required to improve surgical access in some very big low- and middle-income countries. Such teams achieve minimal long-term benefit for most patients and some have suggested that the enormous cost of these missions could be better spent on training locals and establishing a local infrastructure that might lead to independence from "short-term 11 day missions" and that might benefit a population into the future.[167]

Different standards of care may emerge from different parts of the world. These standards need not necessarily be considered inferior but may open the way for the assimilation of new ideas.[166] The nuances of practice in different communities inevitably vary and may challenge some fondly held beliefs in pediatric anesthesia. A safe anesthetic is not necessarily the most expensive one.[168] It is usually not the agents that we use but the skill with which we use them that determines outcome. It should never be necessary to depart from the dictum *primum non nocere*. Simplicity may be the key, but there is no place for double standards. Guidelines that have evolved over time in the United Kingdom, United States, and Australasia may be untenable in many parts of the world,[164] but every attempt should be made to exercise the same standard of care as expected in developed countries.[169] Our children deserve no less.

ANNOTATED REFERENCES

Chikumbanje S, Bell GT, Kapatuka K, Pollach G. Continuous flow using an entrainer and T-piece vs draw over apparatus for inhalational induction of anesthesia in children. *Paediatr Anaesth.* 2014;24(11):1169-1173.

There are few studies in modern literature that compare circuits that are no longer in use in developed countries. The authors from Malawi compare inhalation induction in children using a Farnham entrainer with the Ayres T-piece (Mapleson F) and a drawover system. There was no difference in oxygen saturation measured by oximetry (SpO₂) recordings, but induction times were slightly (but not clinically significant) longer with the drawover system.

Ekenze SO, Ajuzieogu OV, Nwomeh BC. Challenges of management and outcome of neonatal surgery in Africa: a systematic review. *Pediatr Surg Int.* 2016;32(3):291-299.

This study reviews publications on neonatal surgery from 11 countries in Africa over the past 20 years. Although the overall mortality rate has improved in the past decade, it remains high, around 30%. Although each country has its own problems, delayed presentation, inadequate facilities, a dearth of trained personnel, major neonatal surgery, and an absence of intensive care were the common denominators contributing to this poor outcome.

Hodges SC, Mijumbi C, Okello M, et al. Anaesthesia services in developing countries: defining the problems. *Anaesthesia.* 2007;62(1):4-11.

This paper identifies the difficulties of providing anesthesia in Uganda. The disturbing result was that only 23% of anesthesiologists have the facilities to provide safe anesthesia to adults, 13% for a child, and only 6% for cesarean section.

Walker IA, Merry AF, Wilson IH, et al. Global oximetry: an international anaesthesia quality improvement project. *Anaesthesia.* 2009;64(1):1051-1060.

This paper describes the initial quality assurance program for pulse oximetry in four pilot studies of pulse oximetry in Uganda, Vietnam, India, and the Philippines. The studies determined that formal training in pulse oximetry needed to be a central part of the WHO Safe Surgery Saves Lives project.

Walker IA, Newton M, Bösenberg AT. Improving surgical safety globally: pulse oximetry and the WHO Guidelines for Safe Surgery. *Paediatr Anaesth.* 2011;21(7):825-828.

This paper describes the fact that approximately 78,000 operating rooms worldwide lack pulse oximetry. It discusses the WHO Safe Surgery Saves Lives Program as well as the Global Pulse Oximetry Program.

Zoumenou E, Gbenou S, Assouto P, et al. Pediatric anesthesia in developing countries: experience in the two main university hospitals of Benin in West Africa. *Paediatr Anaesth.* 2010;20(8):741-747.

This article describes anesthesia in Benin. Cardiac arrests occurred at a rate of 156 per 10,000 cases with a mortality rate of approximately 60%, even in two university hospitals. The authors are to be congratulated for studying this issue to gain more financial support from their government for better equipment and monitoring.

A complete reference list can be found online at Elsevier eBooks+.

49 Pediatric Equipment and Monitoring

JUSTIN J. SKOWNO AND CHARLES J. COTÉ

Heating and Cooling Systems
Patient Warming
Forced Air Warmers
Warming Blankets
Radiant Warmers
Passive Heat and Moisture Exchangers
Heated Humidifiers
Fluid and Blood Warmers
Controlling Exposure
Intravenous Therapy
Maintenance Fluids
Resuscitation
Total Intravenous Anesthesia and Vasoactive Medications
Luer Adapters
Airway Apparatus
Masks
Oropharyngeal Airways
Nasopharyngeal Airways
Laryngeal Mask Airways
Endotracheal Tubes
Intubation Equipment
Laryngoscopes
Suction Devices
Anesthesia Workstation
Scavenging Systems
Carbon Dioxide Absorption

Humidification
Mechanical Ventilation
Equipment Cart
Defibrillator and External Pacemakers
Ultrasound for Regional Anesthesia and Vascular Cannulation
Monitoring Equipment
The Anesthesia Record
Drug Errors, Bar Coding, and Integration
Precordial and Esophageal Stethoscopes
Noninvasive Blood Pressure Monitoring
Electrocardiogram
Oxygen Monitors
Temperature Monitors
Noninvasive Oxygen Saturation Monitors
Reflectance Oximetry
Near-Infrared Spectroscopy
Carbon Dioxide Analyzers
Transcutaneous Carbon Dioxide Measurement
Blood Loss Monitors
Neuromuscular Transmission Monitors
Processed Electroencephalogram Monitors
Nociception Monitoring
Cardiac Output Monitoring
Ultrasound Determination of Cardiac Output
Purchasing Anesthesia Equipment

Heating and Cooling Systems

The operating room environment is a compromise between the ideal environment for the patient, and the ideal for the operating room staff.

Consider the anesthetized infant in a standard operating room at a standard temperature of 20°C. From the moment the infant enters the operating room, they are partially if not completely uncovered. With a very high surface area to body mass ratio, the infant loses heat primarily through two primary mechanisms: radiation and convection. Consider then the surgeon, in a sterile airtight gown, under operating room lights for several hours; eventually they will overheat, unless they can be in a cooler environment. Thus the infant needs a warm operating room, but their scrub staff and surgeon need a cool operating room.

Patients lose heat through four mechanisms: radiation (39%), convection (34%), evaporation (24%), and conduction (3%).[1] Radiation heat loss is the transfer of energy via electromagnetic waves to solid surfaces such as cold walls. Convection heat loss is the transfer of energy from the child to the gas or liquid surrounding them. Convection heat loss can be passive, as in still air, or active when air flows past the infant. Evaporative heat loss is the energy that is lost when a liquid vaporizes into gas, known as the heat of vaporization. This typically results when alcohol evaporates from the skin during sterilization but can also occur when major wounds are exposed to the ambient air. Conduction heat transfer is the transfer of energy by direct contact from one object to another, whether in the solid, liquid, or gas states.

Several strategies help us deal with this problem, and offset heat loss from the child. Before the child enters the operating room, the room should be warmed (to >25°C) or as much as tolerable to minimize radiation and convective heat losses. The child should be placed on a forced air warming blanket that is preheated to 43°C before the child is unclad. Preferably, inhaled gases and intravenous (IV) fluids should be warmed throughout the surgery, although their contributions are generally considered minor unless major transfusions and crystalloid volumes are infused.

Hypothermia, a core temperature <35°C, is classified in four stages: mild, 32°C to 35°C; moderate, 28°C to 32°C; severe, 24°C to 28°C; and profound <24°C.[2] In some cases, hypothermia is induced deliberately to improve patient outcomes. For example, hypothermia is a necessity for cardiopulmonary bypass[3,4] and continues to be studied to ameliorate the sequelae from neonatal asphyxia,[5–7] although it has not conferred any benefit after pediatric cardiac arrest or head injury.[8–10] Other than in these specific circumstances, normothermia should be the goal for our patients. Mild to moderate hypothermia may cause apnea in infants, alter the pharmacokinetics of medications, decrease blood clotting, and increase surgical site infections,[11] among other complications.[12,13] Conversely, iatrogenic hyperthermia with active warming may increase the metabolic rate and heart rate, introducing concerns of a malignant hyperthermia reaction, thyrotoxicosis, and other metabolic and drug-related disorders. Basic strategies to maintain normothermia and temperature monitoring should be provided for every patient who undergoes general anesthesia, except for those having very brief procedures.

Patient Warming

FORCED AIR WARMERS

Forced air warming devices remain one of the most common and effective strategies to maintain and increase the child's temperature in the OR. These devices consist of a central unit that regulates the air temperature and forces heated air through a hose to a disposable perforated blanket that can be placed underneath or on top of the child or around the child's head. The device must be used in accordance with the manufacturer's instructions to minimize the risk of thermal injury.[14,15] These devices maintain the child's temperature very effectively through the combination of active convection and a plastic wrap or blanket that eliminates radiation and evaporative heat losses. Concerns have been raised regarding internal accumulation of microbes,[16] disruption of laminar airflow in the OR,[17,18] and surgical site infections including infections of implanted material.[17] However, most recent evidence does not support the early infection risks associated with forced air warmers, including a greater rate of surgical site infections and periprosthetic joint infections.[19–22] Forced air warmers continue to be used in children without reports of increased surgical site infection rates. Nonetheless, some surgeons prefer that forced air warmers be powered on only after the child has been prepped and draped (e.g., ventriculoperitoneal catheter insertion), a practice that has been applied to many other surgeries without evidence. The Asian Pacific Society of Infection Control published recent guidelines to reduce surgical site infections; maintaining normothermia using forced air warming prevents surgical infections.[23] Several manufacturers produce forced air warmers and blankets. The devices all operate in a similar manner and may be considered equivalent in effectiveness: 3M (St. Paul, MN), Celsius Medical (Madrid, Spain), Stryker (Kalamazoo, MI), and Medical Solutions, Inc. (Omaha, NE).

WARMING BLANKETS

Warming blankets include circulating water mattresses placed underneath the child and electrical heat-generating conductive blankets that can be placed either underneath or on top of the child. However, they are ineffective at maintaining or increasing a patient's temperature during anesthesia. When placed underneath the child, these devices contact the entire undersurface of the child's torso and legs, transferring heat by conduction, but this only accounts for 4% of perioperative heat loss. Since these devices are in direct contact with the child and have a greater thermal density, care must be taken to avoid surface burns at high temperature settings. In contrast to forced air warmers, warming blankets do not change the airflow in the OR. Typically, these devices are also reusable and require wipe-down disinfection. Circulating water blankets include the Blanketrol by Cincinnati Sub-Zero (Cincinnati, OH), and the Medi-Therm III by Gaymar Industries (Orchard Park, NY). Manufacturers of non-water–based blankets include Augustine Biomedical (Eden Prairie, MN), Inditherm (Rotherham, United Kingdom), and Novamed USA (Elmsford, NY).

RADIANT WARMERS

Overhead radiant heating units, sometimes referred to as "French fry lights or warmers," are less commonly used in the OR since the introduction of forced air warmers, although they remain in use in the neonatal intensive care unit (NICU) and are built into many NICU beds. These devices include a skin temperature sensor that supplies feedback to a servomechanism to adjust the heat output. Without this feedback or if the heating element is placed too close to the patient, particularly to a neonate, there is a risk of skin burns to the patient and nearby staff.

PASSIVE HEAT AND MOISTURE EXCHANGERS

Heat and moisture exchangers (HMEs) are reflective filters interposed between the tracheal tube and the ventilator circuit to preserve the child's temperature and airway humidity. Under the correct circumstances, these devices may maintain body temperature[24] but they cannot directly increase body temperature. During anesthesia they provide inadequate humidity and heat in children but they may conserve heat loss and humidity.[25] They are less effective at maintaining temperature compared with heated humidifiers in the airway circuit. Even the smallest exchanger can increase the airway dead space and resistance, particularly in neonates,[26] blunting the capnogram until it is almost uninterpretable. A Cochrane review found that HMEs and heated humidifiers were equally effective at preventing pneumonia and mortality in ventilated adults and children.[27] However, these exchangers are effective and useful for preventing the contamination of devices attached to the airway such as pulmonary function testing equipment.

HEATED HUMIDIFIERS

Heated humidifiers or heated breathing circuits are typically a sealed heated wire within one limb of the breathing circuit. Sterile water is introduced into the circuit and the servomechanism-controlled heater maintains temperature. These devices are prone to hazards, such as overheating, condensation, changes in the compressible volume of the circuit, leaks in the tubing, and obstruction, if they are not connected correctly. They are superior to any other device for preventing the secretions in the airway from drying out and are universally used with ICU ventilators. However, as the circle breathing circuit supplanted the Mapleson F circuit (Jackson-Rees modification of the Ayre T-piece) (E-Fig 49.1) in clinical anesthesia care globally, heated humidifiers became anachronistic as it could be difficult to adapt them to the circle circuit. The additional cost and complications of these devices also limit their use except for anesthesia cases of prolonged duration. Manufacturers include Armstrong Medical (Lincolnshire, IL), CareFusion (Becton Dickinson, Franklin Lakes, NJ), Dräger (Telford, PA), Fisher & Paykel (Irvine, CA), Philips Healthcare (Bothell, WA), Teleflex (Morrisville, NC), and Westmed Inc. (Tucson, AZ), among others.

FLUID AND BLOOD WARMERS

When large volumes of IV fluid are infused at a rapid rate, the child's core temperature may decrease precipitously unless a fluid warmer is used. In contrast, when IV fluid is infused at a maintenance or small flow rates, heated IV fluids cool when they pass through noninsulated tubing to the child rendering heating IV fluids under these circumstance ineffective.[28] To offset the heat loss while in transit from the heater to the child, the IV tubing was coiled under a water warming mattress. Using age-appropriate infusion rates, a warming mattress improved core temperature compared with a fluid warming system although fluid warmers should be one of several strategies to increase core temperature.[29] One strategy to deliver warmed IV fluid is to warm the IV fluid bags using blanket warmers already in use in the ORs or with specialized warmers such as the ivNow fluid warmer by Enthermics (Menomonee Falls, WI). The IV fluid bags should be used within a week or two to prevent degradation of the plastic bags. Individuals have warmed IV fluid bags in a standard microwave oven, but this practice is not recommended because hot spots, overheating, or deterioration of the container might develop. Using a mathematical model and thermodynamic equations to simulate the effects of infusion of crystalloid at 4°C, 20°C, or 42°C and the specific heat of crystalloid solutions in 70 kilograms adults, core temperature was calculated at these temperatures.[30] In a mildly hypothermic patient, 42°C crystalloid will increase the core temperature 0.2°C to 0.8°C for every 30 mL/kg of administered crystalloid, whereas 20°C crystalloid will cool a mildly hyperthermic patient 0.6°C to 0.9°C for every 30 mL/kg crystalloid administered. This model predicts very modest effects of crystalloid infusions on core temperature.

In general, blood products are stored in refrigerated coolers. When the products are selected for use, they are warmed before they are administered to the child. Fluid warmers currently marketed are designed to warm crystalloid solutions and blood products. The two main designs for these fluid warmers are a water bath and dry heat. The Level 1 Hotline device (Smiths Medical, Dublin, OH) uses a heated water bath and specialized tubing with a sterile inner lumen. Warmed water circulates in the outer lumen, increasing the temperature of the fluid. The Level 1 can deliver warmed fluids with a gravity flow rate up to 83 mL/ minute. The dry heat designs use either standard IV tubing or proprietary tubing sets. These are placed in contact with a heat exchanger usually made of metal because of its conductive properties. The device warms the tubing and the fluid as it passes through the tubing. The designs vary in their priming volume, flow rates, portability, and the distance they can be placed from the patient. The greater the distance between the device and the patient, the greater the cooling of the fluid before it reaches the patient. Both pressurized and nonpressurized warmers can deliver large fluid flow rates that are commonly necessary for trauma and transplantation surgeries. Nonpressurized warmers that use proprietary tubing sets include the enFlow by CareFusion (Becton Dickinson, Franklin Lakes, NJ) with a 4-mL priming volume and a flow rate up to 200 mL/minute; the Medi-Temp by Stryker

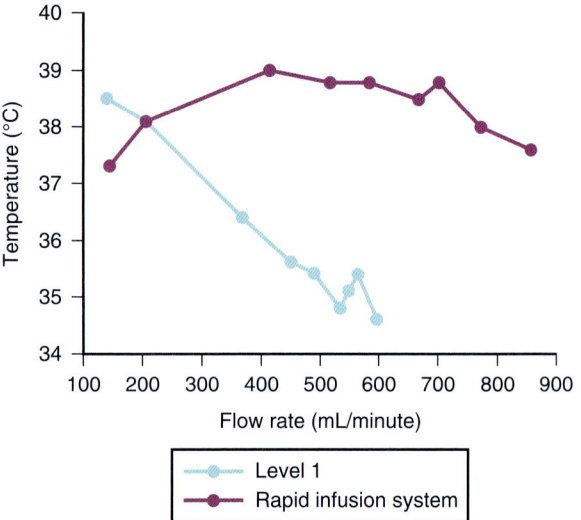

FIGURE 49.1 This figure plots the mean temperature of the fluid at the end of two 2-liter infusions of crystalloid for the Level 1 versus the Rapid Infusion System (RIS). Note that both devices have equivalent warming capacities with flow rates of 200 mL or less per minute, but there is markedly less warming capacity with the Level 1 system at higher flow rates. Note that the RIS was the precursor to the Belmont Rapid Infuser, so the warming characteristics would be similar to those of the RIS. (From Barcelona SL, Vilich F, Coté CJ. A comparison of flow rates and warming capabilities of the Level 1 and Rapid Infusion System with various-size intravenous catheters. *Anesth Analg.* 2003;97[2]:358-363.)

(Kalamazoo, MI) with a flow rate up to 500 mL/minute; and the Ranger by 3M (St. Paul, MN) with a flow rate up to 500 mL/ minute. Some nonpressurized warmers that adapt to standard IV tubing sets manufactured in Germany include the Nuova/05 by Nuova GmbH (23909 Ratzeburg, Germany) and the Astoflo Plus by Stihler Electronic GmbH (Germany). For massive transfusion of blood, pressurized fluid warmers are used. The Belmont Rapid Infuser RI-2 (Belmont Medical, Billerica, MA) uses electromagnetic induction heating, has an optional blood reservoir, and infuses the warmed fluid with a rapid roller pump. This device can deliver more than 750 mL/minute of warmed blood. The Level 1 H-1200 Fast Flow Fluid Warmer (Smiths Medical, Dublin, OH) uses an aluminum heat exchanger, a countercurrent water bath, has two chambers for fluid bags, and uses pressurized air to compress the IV bags and infuse fluids at flows of up to 600 mL/minute, although at the greater rates, the temperature of the IV fluid is not sustained (Fig. 49.1). The flow rate of these devices is limited by the size (E-Fig. 49.2) and length of the inserted venous catheter and, to a lesser extent, by the length of the tubing before the patient. These devices have integrated air and pressure detectors that will automatically stop the infusion if a breech is detected. Even with the air detector, it is important to eliminate all air from the bags to avoid the possibility of infusing air into the circulation.

CONTROLLING EXPOSURE

Body temperature can be preserved if the child is covered to reduce the major sources of heat loss: radiant and convective losses. Covering the infant's head is an important strategy to prevent heat loss since the infant's head has a large body surface area/volume ratio. Reflective aluminized Mylar blankets are also very effective but more expensive. Using a blanket warmer and uncovering only the necessary small portions of the child during induction and IV placement attenuates heat loss. If the child must be uncovered at any time, warming the air temperature within the OR is effective as it reduces both radiation and convective heat losses. In one study of neonatal and maternal hypothermia, fewer hypothermic neonates ($<36°C$) were identified when room temperature was $23°C$ compared with a room temperature of $20°C$ (5% vs. 19%).[31] Once the neonate has been covered, the room temperature can be reduced.

Intravenous Therapy

The basis for determining the adequacy of IV access is Poiseuille law, which is embodied by the equation for laminar flow:

$$Q = \frac{\pi R^4 (P_2 - P_1)}{8 \eta L}$$

Here, the volumetric flow rate (Q) of the fluid is directly related to the fourth power of the radius of the catheter lumen (R) and the pressure difference across the tubing ($P_2 - P_1$) and inversely related to the viscosity of the fluid (η) and the length of the tubing (L). Increasing the radius of the catheter increases the fluid flow rate by the fourth power. However, for long catheters such as central venous lines or peripherally inserted percutaneous intravenous central catheters (PICC), additional length and fluid viscosity (as in changing from crystalloid to packed red blood cells [PRBCs]) can substantially increase the resistance to flow and thereby dramatically reduce fluid flow rates, even when the fluid bag is pressurized.

The fluid drip rate from a 500-mL solution bag ranges from a macrodrip (10–20 drops/mL) to a microdrip (60 drops/mL). The microdrip set may contain a Buretrol (Baxter International, Deerfield, IL) to finely control the volume of fluid infused and prevent an overdose of IV fluids in neonates and infants. Extension tubing may be small bore in caliber with a small priming volume of 1 to 2 mL or large bore with a larger priming volume of 6 to 10 mL. The latter is recommended as it offers less resistance to flow when fluid resuscitation or blood must be administered. The small-caliber tubing may be inserted ("Y'd") into the IV set close to the cannula site to administer drugs to small infants without large volumes of crystalloid. For most neonates and infants, 24-gauge catheters are used, although 22-gauge may be sited in larger veins such as the saphenous. In toddlers and older children undergoing noncomplex surgery, a 22-gauge IV catheter is preferred and for older children to adults 16- to 20-gauge catheters or larger are usually placed. Caution must be used if the caliber of extension tubing is downsized to a small caliber as it may restrict the ability to rapidly transfuse fluids. A three-way stopcock or an access port permits needleless injections of medications into the IV tubing.

Fluid can be administered via gravity flow, via mechanical pump, or via an external pressure bag. The addition of a 5-μm bacterial filter increases the resistance to flow and decreases the flow rate. Additionally, antireflux valves further increase the resistance to flow. However, these valves are essential when infusing fluids or drugs as these may flow (unnoticed) retrograde in the tubing if an antireflux valve is not in-line. Each medication access point such as the stopcock or needleless hub is a site where air can be introduced; care should be taken to aspirate all air from IV access points (e.g., stopcocks and Luer locks) in all infants and children. The components of the IV set—the tubing, extensions,

connectors, and a method of delivery appropriate for the size of the child and the procedure—are determined by individual preferences. There is slight variation among manufacturers, but general flow rates by gravity for IV catheters and central venous lines are listed in Table 49.1; the larger the catheter, the greater the flow rates (E-Fig. 49.3). This information is also printed on the catheter packages.

TABLE 49.1	Intravenous Catheter Flow Rate by Gauge and Length[a]	
Gauge	**Length (inches)**	**Flow Rate (mL/minute)**
Peripheral IV		
24	0.75	20
22	1.0	37
20	1.0	63
20	1.16	61
20	1.88	54
18	1.16	95
18	1.88	87
16	1.16	193
16	1.77	185
14	2.0	295
Central Venous Line		
4F Double Lumen		
20		23
22		12
5F Double Lumen		
20		15
20		20
5F Triple Lumen		
18		20
23		2
23		2
7F Triple Lumen		
16		49
18		20
18		20
8F Cordis (4-inch)[b]		133
Percutaneous Intravenous Central Catheters (PICC)		
4F Single lumen		21.2
5F Single lumen		20
5F Dual (each lumen)		9.6
6F Dual (each lumen)		12.5

Information regarding central venous catheters was abstracted from Cook Medical "Quick Reference Guide for Spectrum" catheters (https://www.cookmedical.com/data/resources/4%20CC-BM-ABRMQR-EN-201111.pdf). PICC line information is for the PowerPICC Catheter from Bard Access Systems (Salt Lake City, UT).
[a]The standard by which flow rate is measured (by gravity) is that the intravenous bag of crystalloid is suspended 1 meter above the height of measurement.
[b]Cordis (Milpitas, CA).

MAINTENANCE FLUIDS

For neonates, preterm infants, and chronically ill infants in whom there is risk of hypoglycemia, a dextrose-containing fluid should be used. If the child is receiving 10% dextrose or a similar infusion from the NICU, this can be continued at the same infusion rate during anesthesia and surgery, although evidence supports the safe practice of halving the infusion rate during general anesthesia to avoid hyperglycemia.[32] Risk factors for hyperglycemia in the first 4 hours after surgery are two-fold: the glucose infusion rate and the neonate's gestational age.[33] Hyperglycemia increases morbidity and mortality in neonates with necrotizing enterocolitis.[34] Hence, the practice of halving the dextrose infusion rate during surgery seems beneficial. If the dextrose infusion rate is decreased, ideally the serum dextrose concentration should be measured periodically during surgery, although this may be challenging in neonates under the drapes. To prevent fluid overload, consider the use of a pump to control the infusion of IV fluids, with a stopcock close to the cannula to infuse medications. Some have recommended in-line filters in IV lines to prevent morbidity and mortality in neonates associated with contamination of the infusions (bacteria, endotoxins, and others). However, a Cochrane review concluded that there was insufficient evidence to recommend in-line filters in neonates to reduce morbidity and mortality.[35] If vasoactive medications and maintenance fluids are infusing and a separate IV catheter is present, the medications should be flushed as close to the patient as possible in the second IV in order to minimize the risk of injecting boluses of vasoactive medications.

RESUSCITATION

If there is an anticipated need for large volume fluid resuscitation, the largest IV that can be easily placed should be used, recognizing that attempting to place a catheter that is too large may result in failure. It is better to have two working 22-gauge IVs rather than multiple puncture sites from failed attempts with an 18- or 20-gauge IV. Table 49.1 indicates that a shorter catheter delivers a greater flow rate than a longer catheter and that a central venous catheter, which is often a long catheter, is usually limited to infuse low fluid flow rates because of resistance caused by their length. PICC lines cannot be used for resuscitation (and may prevent the rapid administration of a bolus of propofol) because of their narrow caliber and extra length (see Table 49.1).

Large-bore tubing used for blood transfusion or resuscitation has the best flow characteristics. There are multiple strategies to increase the IV flow rate, including using a pressure bag placed around the fluid bag, IV tubing sets with integrated bulb pumps, use of a large (60-mL) syringe[36] and a stopcock to create a pull-push system or large prefilled syringes,[37] and a purpose-built device such as the Level 1 H-1200 Fast Flow Fluid Warmer (Smiths Medical Dublin, OH) or Belmont Rapid Infuser RI-2 (Belmont Instrument, Bellerica, MA). If a 20-gauge or larger catheter is already in place, it may be exchanged for an Arrow rapid infusion catheter (Teleflex, Morrisville, NC) that is typically a 7F or 8.5F (internal diameter) 2-inch-long catheter. Fluid resuscitation is limited with the commercially available IV pumps to their maximum flow rates, 999 mL/hour or 16.6 mL/minute. If a pressure infusion bag is used, the IV bag should be de-aired to prevent air from being pumped into the circulation, creating an air embolism, as the bag empties.

The temperature and viscosity of IV fluids greatly affect the infusion rate. Less viscous fluids are infused more rapidly than more viscous fluids (e.g., colloid solutions). Crystalloid solutions are the least viscous fluids followed by colloids, whole blood, and

PRBCs. PRBCs may be diluted with normal saline solution to reduce viscosity, improve flow characteristics, and decrease the risk of hemolysis during a rapid infusion.[38]

TOTAL INTRAVENOUS ANESTHESIA AND VASOACTIVE MEDICATIONS

If total IV anesthesia (TIVA) or the use of vasoactive medications is necessary, they are ideally infused through dedicated venous access. Guidelines on the safe provision of TIVA have been published, and emphasize the risks of delivery level issues, with processes and equipment to mitigate these risks (see Chapter 6).[39,40]

The speed at which the medication is administered depends on the location of the access point in the infusion line, how much priming volume is present in the tubing, and the speed at which the fluids are infusing (Fig. 49.2).[41,42] A carrier solution on a

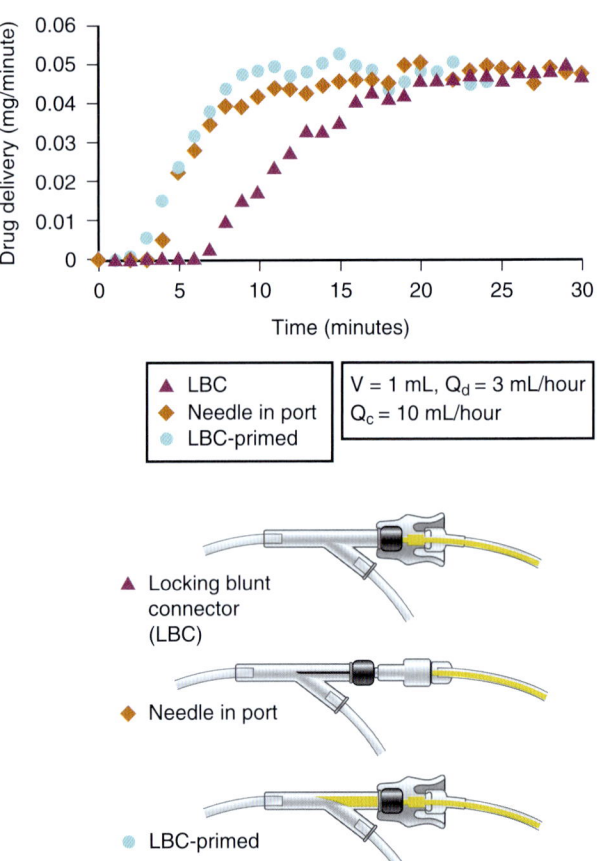

FIGURE 49.2 The time delay in onset of drug delivery to steady-state drug delivery as affected by a needle in an injection port and a locking blunt connector (LBC) or "priming" of the dead space of the injection port are illustrated. Note that the time to initiate drug delivery is delayed by several minutes and the time to achieve a steady-state rate of drug administration may be delayed by 10 minutes or longer when the dead space is not primed or a needle is not used to bypass the dead space of the injection port (in this example, the parameters were: carrier rate $[Q_c]$, 10 mL/hour, drug flow rate $[Q_d]$, 3 mL/hour, dead-space volume $[V]$, 1 mL). This concept has important implications regarding drug delivery to all patients, but it is particularly important in infants and neonates in whom small volumes of drug may be administered into a relatively large dead space that must be filled before any drug enters the flow of the intravenous fluid and the hourly rate of the carrier is low. (From Lovich MA, Doles J, Peterfreund RA. The impact of carrier flow rate and infusion set dead-volume on the dynamics of intravenous drug delivery. *Anesth Analg.* 2005;100[4]:1048-1055.)

pump should be infused at a baseline rate because most vasoactive medications are piggy-backed into the tubing at slow infusion rates. The carrier solution should be adjusted to the child's maintenance infusion rate and the other IV fluids reduced accordingly. Multiple stopcock manifolds allow for the connection of multiple infusions as well as the carrier solution. Fig. 49.3 shows various multiple-drug infusion systems, each of which has slightly different priming volumes, which in turn affect the speed at which medications are infused, particularly through central venous access.[41–43] Many practitioners prime their medications and then initiate the pumps to run the fluids to the end of the manifold. When connected directly to an IV line, medications should be delivered without delay provided the carrier fluid rate is maintained at the same rate.

LUER ADAPTERS

Luer-Lok adapters allow for the rapid and secure connection of syringes and IV fluid lines to catheters. This has particular significance in the OR as access to the arterial or venous lines are remote from the caregiver and hidden under the drapes. However, the Luer-Lok adapter is also interchangeable with epidural, spinal and nerve block catheters, feeding tubes, total parenteral nutrition lines, and even sidestream carbon dioxide

(CO_2) connectors.[44–46] All of these have the identical six-degree Luer-Lok taper that allows them to be connected interchangeably.[47] This universal connection has led to the accidental injection of drugs not meant for the neuraxial space into epidural catheters,[48–50] parenteral chemotherapy (vincristine) given intrathecally (more than 30 times since 1968),[51] local anesthetics (e.g., bupivacaine) injected intravenously,[52,53] a blood pressure (BP) cuff attached to a Hep-Lock IV set (Baxter Healthcare), gastric feeds, and breast milk infused through a central venous catheter,[54] causing significant morbidity and mortality.[55] Labeling of all catheters at the hub, color-coding, and vigilance have been effective, in part, to reduce this risk. However, to address this risk formally, an international, multidisciplinary team convened in 2007 to draft a standard by which Luer-Lok connectors will be modified such that a unique Luer-Lok design will be available for each type of Luer-Lok connection (e.g., IV, gastrointestinal, genitourinary, neurologic, anesthesia breathing circuits, and hemodynamic monitoring [BP cuffs]) that will also prevent cross-connection of tubing meant for different uses.[50,56] This meeting resulted in publication of ISO-80369 standard, which after several iterations, is being implemented.[57] This new standard modifies the six-degree Luer-Lok taper to preclude cross-connection of tubing intended for differences

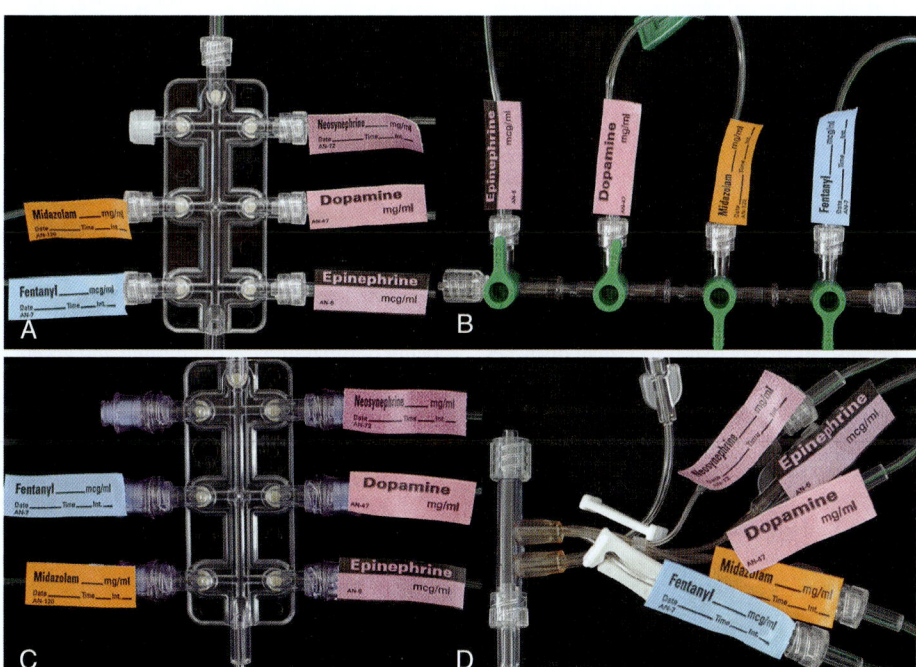

FIGURE 49.3 Several multiple-drug and fluid administration systems are illustrated. Note the wide variation in dead-space volume among the screw-in connectors **(A)**, simple stopcocks **(B)**, screw-in connectors with one-way valves **(C)**, and multiple short tubing connections **(D)**. To avoid variations in rate of drug delivery, it is advised to use a dedicated carrier on a pump. To ensure that the initiation of drug delivery is timely, the following steps are necessary: (1) each dead-space port must be flushed and primed with the desired infusion as it is attached to the delivery manifolds; (2) after priming, the stopcock is turned to the off position or the tubing is clamped; (3) the carrier portion of the system is then run through or flushed with the carrier intravenous fluid; and (4) the system is attached to the patient with just the carrier ensuring a constant flow to the patient. When the drug infusion is initiated, the stopcock is turned to the on position or the tubing unclamped, and each drug infusion pump turned on at the desired rate. This ensures that no drug is accidentally administered and reduces the time to initial drug delivery by priming the dead space of the system for each drug infusion. It should be borne in mind that this system should be connected as closely as possible to the intravenous catheter to avoid further delay in drug delivery because of the need to fill the dead space between the multiple-drug manifolds and the entry into a vein. The use of a pump for the carrier solution also prevents retrograde drug infusion.

uses by creating non–Luer-Lok connectors for non–IV equipment larger or smaller than the standard Luer-Lok connections. A multicenter clinical simulation evaluation of ISO 80369-6 for neuraxial and regional anesthesia non-Luer connectors (known as NRFit connectors) prevented misconnecting errors from occurring.[58] The roll out of these modified connectors continues slowly worldwide.

Airway Apparatus

MASKS

Transparent disposable plastic (latex-free) face masks are available in a wide variety of sizes for children of all ages, to deliver oxygen as well as induce and maintain inhalational anesthesia. These air-filled cushioned masks, which can be inflated to fill the cuff (except for the smallest infant sizes), replaced the old Rendell-Baker/Soucek face masks, which had a very small dead space but often failed to seal completely on some children. With the wide variability in the morphology of children's faces, especially those who are syndromic, the anesthesiologist should prepare cushioned masks that are smaller and larger than the size chosen for the child. The selected mask should maintain a tight mask seal on the face with the least amount of dead space. Masks vary according to the manufacturer; however, there are few features that would lead us to recommend one over another. Some masks can be purchased already flavored (with fruit such as strawberry), although most anesthesiologists prefer to offer their own flavors (e.g., watermelon or strawberry lip balms) to engage the child. They choose the preferred flavor and apply it to the mask either in the preoperative holding area or in the OR. Specialized masks with a built-in port for endoscopy or fiberoptic intubation are also available for specific indications (see E-Fig. 12.14).

OROPHARYNGEAL AIRWAYS

Oropharyngeal airways are hard, nonlatex plastic that are preformed in different sizes from 40 mm (infant) to 100 mm (large adult). Care should be taken to choose an airway that is the correct size for the child because an airway that is too small displaces the posterior portion of the tongue or too long displaces the epiglottis into the glottic opening, causing upper airway obstruction. If the oropharyngeal airway is very large, it may cause damage to laryngeal structures, resulting in swelling and potential postoperative obstruction (see Fig. 12.16).

Accurately predicting the correct size oropharyngeal airway has remained somewhat elusive. Some estimate the airway size using the distance from the corner of the mouth to the ramus of the mandible by holding the airway next to the child's cheek. However, this distance has proven inaccurate as the airway may be oversized by ≥1 cm in almost 30% of children but also under-sized by 0.5 cm in others.[59] In a magnetic resonance imaging (MRI) study to predict the size, the distance from the lips to the prevertebral pharyngeal space was used to create algorithms for age, weight, and sex in children 0 to 17 years of age. The equation to estimate the size was: Oropharyngeal airway size = 5.51 ± 0.25 × Age (years) − 0.01 × Age^2 (years) + 0.02 (weight [kg]) + 0.12 (for males).[60] Obviously this equation is far too complex to be useful in daily clinical practice. A nomogram that estimated the correct size oral airway for boys based on their age and weight recommended a 7 cm airway for 1- to 2-year-olds, 8 cm for 3- to 8-year-olds, and 9 cm for 9- to17-year-olds. More recently, the size of the oral airway was predicted using the distance determined with a Miller blade from the mouth to the vallecula.[59] This

method is also impractical as an oral airway is most commonly placed prior to laryngoscopy.[59] A nomogram was created for age (months) versus mouth to mandible distance (cm) which yield similar results. For practical purposes, the starting size based on the above equation is: 7 cm airway for 1- to 2-year-olds, 8 cm for 3- to 8-year-olds, and 9 cm for 9- to 17-year-olds.

An oral airway should always be placed midline, without rotating it as it is inserted as is commonly done in adults, since toddlers often have loose primary teeth that could be dislodged. Misplaced oral airways that obstruct venous and/or lymphatic drainage of the tongue can precipitate acute macroglossia.[61] Additional causes of acute macroglossia include retained throat packs,[62] surgical positioning,[63] and the presence of transesophageal echocardiography (TEE) probes.

NASOPHARYNGEAL AIRWAYS

Nasopharyngeal airways are an additional adjunct to reduce or prevent upper airway obstruction.[64,65] Latex-free, soft nasal airways are available in sizes from 12F to 36F. By lubricating the tip of the airway and spraying the nostril with oxymetazoline, the soft texture of the nasopharyngeal airway minimizes injury to the mucosa or the risk of dissecting adenoidal tissue. Hence bleeding and aspirating adenoidal tissue are infrequent when they are used. Selecting the correct diameter and length of the airway is important because an overly wide airway could damage the ala of the nose, while an excessively long airway may trigger laryngeal reflexes or enter the esophagus, leading to insufflation of the stomach.[66] Some nasal airways have a movable flange to prevent them from being inserted too deeply. The flange should be adjusted before it is inserted. The correct size for the nasal airway has been estimated to be the distance from the nares to the angle of the jaw or the earlobe.[67] In neonates to 12-year-olds, the "nares to earlobe distance minus 10 mm" provided the most accurate estimate of the airway size compared with other estimates and thus is recommended until a better estimate becomes available.[67] In children, the distance from the "nares to the tragus − 10 mm" provided a valid estimate of the correct size of the nasopharyngeal airways, being optimal in 37% of children and acceptable in 75% of those tested.[68] If an appropriately sized nasal airway was not present, an alternative nasal airway could be fashioned from the distal end of an appropriately sized tracheal tube (with the Murphy eye) cut to an appropriate length.[69] Note that a cut tracheal tube is stiffer than a commercially available nasal airway and has a greater potential for injury. Prewarming the tracheal tube using hot water may soften the tube but may not significantly reduce the severity of nasal bleeding.[70] The most effective means to reduce nasal bleeding when inserting a nasotracheal tube is to pass a soft catheter with the tracheal tube telescoped in the flange.[70] The lumen of any nasal airway is limited and can be occluded with secretions and/or blood. Therefore, they should be removed as quickly as possible if airway obstruction is diagnosed.

LARYNGEAL MASK AIRWAYS

In 1983, Dr Archibald Brain designed and marketed the reusable (Classic) Laryngeal Mask Airway (LMA, Teleflex) a supraglottic airway device (SGA) developed to replace the facemask in adults. Reusable models of the LMA are still available, although most SGAs currently marketed are single-use devices. Supraglottic airway devices can be classified into two generations.[71] The first generation are simple airway tubes that include the classic LMA (cLMA), flexible LMA (fLMA) (soft, malleable wired neck), Unique LMA (ULMA)(used in emergency setting), and the

Cobra perilaryngeal airway (CobraPLA). The second generation are SGAs with a drainage tube that include the ProSeal LMA (PLMA)(with a second channel to direct gastric contents away from the airway), I-gel (noninflatable cuff), Laryngeal tube, the LMA Supreme (the ProSeal with a built-in bite block), and the Streamlined Liner of the pharyngeal airway (SLIPA). These devices are available in a variety of sizes from neonates to adults. Several meta-analyses and reviews have summarized the advantages and disadvantages of the devices in children.[72–78] The SGA is a lifesaving airway adjunct that should be used to establish ventilation when either ventilation by face mask or tracheal intubation is difficult or impossible. These devices are usually easy to place by displacing the tongue cephalad using a tongue depressor and then inserting the SGA directly into the hypopharynx. Some prefer to rotate the SGA 90 degrees during insertion so that the bowl faces the laryngeal opening when seated.[79] Occasionally, the LMA will not advance past the posterior pharynx, especially if the bowl has been deflated. This may occur if there is a step-up in the alignment of the mucosa over the vertebral bodies against which the tip of the LMA abuts or if the tip of the bowl has flipped backward, toward the nasopharynx, during insertion. To advance the LMA in these circumstances, the tip of the bowl should be lifted using a finger and the LMA then advanced. The bowl should be inflated until there is no air audible leak at ~16 to 20 cm H_2O peak inspiratory pressure. These airways can be used as the sole airway during anesthesia or as a conduit for bronchoscopy or fiberoptic intubation. There are several manufacturers with small to moderate differences among these devices (see also Figs. 12.21 to 12.24). For routine use in children with normal airways these small differences may not matter; some are specifically designed as a conduit for intubation. Supraglottic devices may have either one or two lumens. Dual-lumen SGAs are placed blindly into the oropharynx. They have two separate cuffs that can be inflated to allow isolation of the trachea (see E-Fig. 12.2). The dual-lumen devices are more typically used for prehospital providers during resuscitation and are not discussed further here. A typical single-lumen SGA is also readily placed blindly into the hypopharynx and makes a nonocclusive seal with the larynx. Single-lumen SGAs have a variety of additional features and design elements, such as nonferrous valves for use in MRI; spiral reinforced and flexible, containing a thermoplastic cuff that molds to the airway; drains or sites for drainage of gastric contents; curvature to facilitate fiberoptic intubation; internal bars to prevent the epiglottis from obstructing the lumen; devices specifically designed to facilitate blind endotracheal intubation; and modifications that allow greater airway occlusive pressures during positive-pressure ventilation.

Success rates for inserting the LMA on the first attempt are very high in most age groups, although in neonates and infants the success rates are only moderate (~80%).[80] In most infants and children, the epiglottis lies within the bowl of the LMA, without evidence of upper airway obstruction.[81,82] In neonates and infants, it behooves the anesthesiologist to maintain very close vigilance of oxygenation and ventilation as the airway may become compromised quite suddenly and rescue measures must be adopted quickly.[83–85]

Most SGAs are inserted during general anesthesia using sevoflurane and their success rates are cited above. A single dose of propofol (1–2 mg/kg IV) could be added to ensure an adequate depth of anesthesia to facilitate insertion of the airway, although transient apnea may ensue. One study compared the ease of insertion of an SGA and the complications after induction with intravenous agents, in children premedicated with midazolam and glycopyrrolate and in the case of ketamine, the airways were sprayed with lidocaine 1 minute before inserting the SGA. The success rates for insertion and upper airway irritability with ketamine and propofol up to 4 mg/kg IV were similar.[86] The difference in the success rate may be attributed to the profound relaxation of the oropharyngeal muscles with propofol and not as much with other IV induction agents.

ENDOTRACHEAL TUBES

Endotracheal tubes (ETT) are polyvinyl chloride in composition, implant tested (based on Z79 standards in rabbits), and nonreusable. Endotracheal tube sizes range from 2 to 10 mm inner diameter (ID). There are small differences in wall thickness among manufacturers, although the variability is generally less than that of the anatomy of the upper airway in children of the same age. Additional differences include the bevel angle, tip design, and presence of a Murphy eye. Uncuffed ETTs were the standard in pediatric anesthesia in infants and children up to 8 years of age for decades, but practice has shifted toward the use of cuffed tracheal tubes. The primary reason for this shift in practice has been the documented safety of cuffed tubes; that is, the incidence of postextubation stridor and glottic edema after using cuffed tubes is no greater and possibly less than it is after using uncuffed tubes.[87–93] Other benefits from using modern cuffed tracheal tubes include the high-volume, low-pressure cuffed ETTs (likely less injurious than low volume high pressure cuffs), cylindrically-shaped cuffs (that are more likely to mimic tracheal anatomy),[94] reduced OR contamination,[95,96] reduced fresh gas flow (less atmospheric pollution),[95] and a reduced need to reintubate the airway due to a large gas leak[93]; several ICU studies have documented the safety of prolonged tracheal intubation with cuffed tracheal tubes.[97–99] However, Microcuff ETTs completely redesigned the ETT for children, introducing an elliptically shaped cuff that is positioned more distal on the tube, a thinner compliant cuff, and removing the Murphy eye (see Fig. 12.18).[94] The cuff seals at a low pressure (10–12 cm H_2O), is permeable to nitrous oxide (N_2O), and is distal along the shaft of the ETT.[100] Proper positioning is recommended using the markings and visual inspection on the shaft of the tube such that the cuff is beyond the cricoid inlet, rather than relying upon the number of centimeters at the mandibular gumline.[101–103]

Several formulas have been developed to predict the ID of the ETT for each age group. The metric most widely used to select the diameter of the ETT is age. In the case of uncuffed ETTs, Cole originally published his formula in 1957[104] in French catheter gauge, which was subsequently modified by Morgan and Steward in 1982 to:

Uncuffed ETT size (mm ID) = age (years)/4 + 4 for children 2 years and older.[105]

For infants and children younger than 2 years, most recommend 2.5-mm ID ETT in infants weighing less than 1500 grams, 3.0-mm ID for infants 1500 to 3000 grams, and 3.5 mm for those who weigh more than 3000 grams and full-term.[106]

For cuffed ETTs, Khine[96] published in 1997 that the correct size is:

Cuffed ETT size (mm ID) = age (years)/4 + 3.

Other authors have modified Khine's formula to the size (mm ID) as (age (years)/4 + 3.5) for children older than 1 year.[107] The use of cuffed tubes in neonates <3 kilograms has been explored in a retrospective study, which showed that the majority of patients weighing >2700 grams could be safely intubated with a 3.0 Microcuff tube.[108]

49

The outer diameter of cuffed ETTs is larger than their un-cuffed counterparts, with substantial variability between manufacturers, particularly for those made of polyvinylchloride compared with polyurethane.[109,110] One may choose to use the modified Cole formula for the initial ETT size for both cuffed and uncuffed ETTs and subtract 0.5 for the size of the cuffed ETT. Others developed formulas for selecting ETT size based on the child's height.[111,112] Age-based formulas are more accurate than direct comparison with the child's finger width.[113] A number of studies have assessed the accuracy of these formulas,[107,114] but this is a moot point as they should simply be considered a starting point for selecting the correct ETT size. Given the physiologic variability among children, ETT sizes smaller and larger should always be immediately available in the unlikely event that subglottic stenosis is diagnosed, or a large trachea is uncovered and the predicted tube size for the child's age is erroneous (see Table 12.2). Some have advocated the use of ultrasound to assess the tracheal dimensions before selecting a tracheal tube to improve the accuracy of the ETT size predicted.[115] In specific populations such as congenital heart disease where the data are available, 3D printed airway models can be used to assist in prediction of EET size.[116]

A number of criteria have been proposed to confirm the appropriate fit and placement of the ETT in children. The ETT should pass through the vocal cords and subglottic space without meeting resistance. If resistance is felt, an ETT 0.5-mm ID smaller should be used. Once positioned, many recommend listening for an audible leak between peak inspiratory pressures of 15 and 30 mm H_2O. This pressure range is consistent with the peak inflation pressure for ventilation in most healthy children and maintains mucosal perfusion while avoiding a large gas leak and polluting the OR.[117] The simplest way to test for a leak is to slowly close the adjustable pressure limiting valve until the desired pressure is reached and either listening or placing a stethoscope over the larynx for a leak. However, the leak test is subject to a number of confounding variables, including the head position of the patient and the presence of neuromuscular blockade.[118] If a cuffed ETT is used and there is a substantial leak with the cuff uninflated, then small amounts of air should be injected into the cuff until the leak disappears, or the cuff is inflated to 15 to 20 mm H_2O. It is important to assure a leak at no more than 30 cm H_2O even with cuffed tracheal tubes. If N_2O is used, it can diffuse into the cuff and increase the cuff volume (and pressure) over time. The absence of an initial leak with a cuffed ETT even with the cuff deflated has been associated with postextubation stridor[119] and warrants exchange to the next smaller size ETT. Cuff pressure should be monitored periodically throughout the period of intubation.

A number of specialty ETTs are available, including those for single-lung ventilation, those with preformed curves, for laser surgery near the airway, microlaryngeal tubes for airway surgery, with spiral reinforcement, for neuromonitoring, and with sampling or suction ports (see also Chapters 12, 13, and 31). A preformed oral or nasal Ring, Adair, and Elwyn (RAE) tube allows surgeons to work on the face or in the mouth without the ETT obscuring their view or being at risk for damage or kinking. They are also useful in head and neck surgery to keep the anesthesia circuit out of the field. It should be noted that the preformed curve has a specific length based on the ETT size predicted from average children. Securing the ETT with the angle of the curve well seated in the mouth or nares may cause the tip of the ETT to be either high or endobronchial, depending on the anatomy of the child. It is essential to pay special attention to the equality of

breath sounds after the ETT is taped and the child placed in the position for surgery. Cuffed nasal RAE ETTs begin at 5.0-mm ID, are more difficult to suction through, and more prone to kinking than non–RAE ETTs. Manufacturers of the cuffed oral and nasal RAE ETT aligned the distance from the bend to the tip with an adult-sized ETT of the corresponding diameter rather than pediatric, resulting in longer distances from the bend than corresponds to the distance in the child's airway.[120] This may result in an endobronchial intubation if these ETTs are inserted until the bend is fully inserted into the nares or on the lower lip for the nasal and oral RAE tubes, respectively. As a result of needing to pull back slightly before taping, the bend in these cuffed RAE tubes may sit in the surgical field when the tip of the ETT is properly positioned in the trachea and therefore at risk for kinking (see Chapter 12 for a more in-depth discussion).

For these reasons, smaller versions of these ETTs are not always acceptable for long-term ventilation in the pediatric ICU (PICU); it is worth having this discussion before initiating anesthesia. For example, children undergoing complex craniofacial reconstructions in which the upper airway may swell postoperatively will likely remain intubated for several days, requiring frequent suctioning while daily assessing for the presence of a leak. Preformed ETTs may impede the ability to suction effectively.

Laser airway surgery places the child at risk for an airway fire. The polyvinylchloride (PVC) of a normal ETT can be damaged by the laser, resulting in mucosal injury or an airway fire. Oxygen and N_2O should both be reduced as much as possible as these are more flammable than air. Designs of specialty ETTs for laser surgery include a flexible stainless steel body, an ETT wrapped in an aluminum material, and rubber tubes with or without metallic wrapping. The use of true natural rubber may put some patients with latex allergies at risk. Previously some institutions have wrapped normal ETTs in metallic tape to reduce the risk of damage to the PVC, but the rough edges of the tape may injure the mucosa. Microlaryngeal ETTs are longer regular ETTs and have a larger cuff providing more space in the airway for surgery; for example, a size 5.0-mm ID microlaryngeal ETT has the length of a 7.0-mm ID ETT. The trade-off is more room for surgical exposure versus a limited increase in airway resistance.

Reinforced ETTs have a wire wrapped in a spiral fashion throughout the PVC wall of the ETT. They are often used in circumstances where kinking of the ETT is a risk. A slightly smaller-sized ETT than expected should be selected as reinforced ETTs have a larger outer diameter than the comparable standard ETT of the same size. In addition, a stylet is often needed to manipulate the floppy tube through the larynx. Once in place, a bite block is often used to stabilize the tube.

Another ETT useful in head and neck surgery is the electromyographic ETT that permits neuromonitoring of the recurrent laryngeal nerve during neck dissection or thyroidectomy.[121] This type of specialty ETT is not available in sizes smaller than 5.0-mm ID.[122]

Finally, there are uncuffed ETTs with an extra internal lumen that allows monitoring of airway pressure or exhaled gases (Mallinckrodt Inc., St. Louis, MO).

Endotracheal tubes have been developed that are designed to reduce ventilator-associated pneumonia in children in the ICU. One such ETT has a suction port that allows continuous aspiration of secretions, whereas another takes advantage of a cone-shaped ETT cuff to prevent microaspiration of airway secretions around the ETT. Evidence for their effectiveness, however, remains weak.[123,124]

Intubation Equipment

LARYNGOSCOPES

A full range of straight (Miller, Wis-Hipple) and curved (Macintosh, MacIntosh or Mac) laryngoscope blades for direct laryngoscopy should be available. It is quite possible in a typical pediatric anesthesia practice to use both a Miller 00 and a Mac 4 blade in the same day. Both small and large laryngoscope handles are available to accommodate differences in body habitus among children. The blade and handle combinations should be tested before anesthesia is induced. Backup blades and handles should be immediately available; additional batteries and light bulbs should be in stock. The light source for laryngoscopes has changed over time from a simple light bulb at or near the tip of the blade powered by two D cell batteries to a fiberoptic channel powered by a rechargeable battery that lights a xenon bulb near the tip of the blade. This latter advance has increased the brightness of laryngoscopes and reduced the frequency of bulb changes; however, visual acuity does not appear to improve once illuminance exceeds 700 lux.[125] Disposable laryngoscope handles and blades have also been developed for use on code carts, during transport, and with highly infectious patients. The price of this equipment can be cost-effective if used only occasionally, although in some institutions with large volumes the cost of single-use devices is lower than the need for replacement of lost or stolen handles and blades. MRI-compatible laryngoscopes are also available but are extremely expensive; most use standard laryngoscope handles equipped with non-ferromagnetic batteries for use in 2-Tesla magnets, but their use is restricted to the side of the magnetic core in zone 4. Laryngoscope blades with a supplemental oxygen channel are available; these delay the time to desaturation in spontaneously breathing infants (see E-Fig. 12.3).[126–129] This same effect has also been demonstrated with the addition of nasal cannula oxygen during intubation.[130]

A difficult airway cart with all needed equipment should be present in the OR complex (see Table 12.9). These carts should contain fiberoptic bronchoscopes in the three major sizes as well as other airway adjuncts such as LMAs, bougies, and indirect laryngoscopes that use prisms, fiberoptics, or video devices (see also Chapter 12). Video laryngoscopy has rapidly become a mainstream aid to intubation in some developed world centers; the unit cost, ease of use, and availability have all greatly improved their cost effectivness.[77]

Suction Devices

Suction devices include a container for waste and a regulator to control the degree of suction. Although regulators can provide low intermittent suction, systems used in anesthesia are not usually set up this way. Injury to the gastric mucosa can occur if continuous suction is applied to a nasogastric or orogastric tube. Vented tubes (e.g., Salem Sump, Sherwood Medical, St. Louis, MO) in a variety of sizes should be available for continuous gastric drainage. If low intermittent suction cannot be provided, we prefer to leave the open end of these tubes sealed in a glove. Suction catheters with a thumb-controlled side port in sizes from 6 Fr to 14 Fr should be available to suction ETTs. Yankauer tip suction devices are available in small and large sizes and are more effective at clearing material compared with the thumb-controlled catheters. They may be metal or plastic; the latter material is preferable to limit the risk of damaging teeth. Yankauer suction devices should never be inserted into the mouth between the central incisors because

the child may bite down on it and break or dislodge teeth. Rather, the devices should be inserted along the inside of the cheek, reaching the hypopharynx behind where the molars or bicuspids will be growing. The small size Yankauer works well in infants, limiting damage to the oropharynx. However, if a large amount of material must be cleared, the larger Yankauer is more effective. If there is the potential for a very large volume to be suctioned (e.g., gastric bleeding), it is prudent to have two separate suction devices and parallel systems available.

Anesthesia Workstation

An anesthesia machine is a device that allows for mechanical or electronic control of gas titration (O_2, N_2O, and air), titration of anesthetic vapor, and manual or mechanical ventilation. It is also an ergonomically designed workstation that includes storage; a place for computer or hand charting; a work surface for drugs and intubation equipment and patient and machine monitoring; a reservoir bag for hand ventilation with an adjustable pressure limit (APL) valve; a means of scavenging anesthesia and waste gas; and an absorber for CO_2 removal. It is also advisable to have a self-inflating bag readily available should a power failure occur, or a patient develop malignant hyperthermia. The anesthesia machine has had a unique role in improving patient safety in the OR. Modern machines cannot deliver a hypoxic gas mixture; they monitor inspired and expired oxygen and anesthesia gases; use an index system to prevent connection of wrong gas lines; and monitor airway pressure and alarms for high pressure, disconnections, high or low minute ventilation, and apnea. The current anesthesia system is a marvel of design that is a very long way from the nonrebreathing open anesthesia systems of the past.

Current anesthesia machines are unidirectional semiclosed circuits in which fresh gas is added to the circle breathing circuit and a means of removing CO_2 is present. These systems contaminate the environment with anesthetic gases less than the open systems, as well as retain the airway gas temperature and humidity better than the open systems. In the following text we describe the key components of the system with specific highlights to pediatrics when applicable, including scavenging systems, CO_2 absorption, humidification, and mechanical ventilation.

SCAVENGING SYSTEMS

Scavenger systems are a necessary part of an anesthesia machine to prevent contamination of the OR with waste anesthesia gases. Scavenging systems are either open or closed and movement of waste gas can be either active or passive. An open system uses a reservoir to collect waste gas, which is then actively suctioned from the reservoir. The reservoir in these open systems communicates with the atmosphere, thereby avoiding either positive or negative pressure transmission to the airway. A closed system is not connected to the atmosphere of the OR, but waste gas exits the machine and then the OR through a series of valves. In a closed system, scavenging can be either active via means of suction or passive, relying on heavier-than-air anesthesia gases and pressure to move waste gas to evacuation. These systems must have both positive- and negative-pressure relief valves to prevent pressure from being transmitted to the airway. Scavenger systems are necessary and helpful means to reduce the contamination of the OR.[131] In addition, anesthesiologists can also contribute substantively to reducing OR contamination if: fresh gas flows are not increased until the patient is ready for induction of anesthesia, a tight mask fit is maintained, the leak around the ETT is minimal, and fresh gas flow rates are reduced or turned off before disconnecting the anesthesia circuit to move or position the child.

The carbon footprint of volatile anesthesia gases is substantial.[132] Concerns regarding ozone depletion and greenhouse warming have encouraged using low fresh gas flows and avoiding or minimizing the use of nitrous oxide and desflurane.[133–136] The ability to scavenge, collect, and reuse volatile agents such as sevoflurane and desflurane is under active exploration using a range of techniques.[137]

CARBON DIOXIDE ABSORPTION

CO_2 absorption or the removal of CO_2 from the breathing circuit makes a circle system possible. This allows for the rebreathing of exhaled gases and inhalational agents, which reduces waste, pollution of the OR and the environment, and retention of heat and humidity within the circuit. All the materials that absorb CO_2 are chemicals that react with CO_2, converting it to stable compounds, hardeners to prevent obstruction of the canister, and dye indicators that identify when the absorption material is expended and should be changed. Soda lime, one typical CO_2 absorbent, contains approximately 80% calcium hydroxide ($Ca(OH)_2$), 15% water (H_2O), 4% sodium hydroxide (NaOH), and 1% potassium hydroxide (KOH). The chemical reactions can be described as a strong alkali with metal hydroxide functioning as a catalyst in the presence of water to convert CO_2 into calcium carbonate. The equations are:

1. $CO_2 + H_2O \rightleftharpoons H_2CO_3$
2. $H_2CO_3 + 2NaOH$ (or KOH) $\rightleftharpoons Na_2CO_3$ $(K_2CO_3) + 2H_2O +$ Heat
3. Na_2CO_3 $(K_2CO_3) + Ca(OH)_2 \rightleftharpoons CaCO_3 + 2NaOH$ (or KOH)

A number of sequelae occur when potent inhalational anesthetic interacts with these absorbents; in the presence of desiccated soda lime, ether anesthetics can degrade to carbon monoxide and in the case of sevoflurane, to compound A,[138–142] a vinyl compound known to cause renal injury in rats.[143,144] In the presence of favorable conditions, carbon monoxide production follows the order desflurane > isoflurane > sevoflurane > halothane.[145] Extreme heat and fire have been associated with the absorbent, Baralyme, which contained barium hydroxide. The reaction of sevoflurane with desiccated Baralyme created such a severe exothermic reaction that it has caused acute respiratory distress syndrome (ARDS),[146] fires,[147] and explosions[148,149] in the OR (Fig. 49.4). Both carbon monoxide poisoning and fires typically occurred on a Monday morning after a weekend during which the fresh gas flow had been left running through the anesthesia machine without a reservoir bag, desiccating the absorbent. Baralyme was voluntarily withdrawn from the market in 2004 to prevent additional human injuries; further experiments showed that increased temperatures could occur with desiccated soda lime.[150] These events emphasize that we must remain vigilant and turn off the fresh gas flows between cases, ensure a reservoir bag is in place in the circuit and replace desiccated CO_2 absorbents with fresh absorbent. Concerns about degradation of inhaled anesthetics to carbon monoxide and compound A[151,152] led to the development of several CO_2 absorbents that do not contain the strong alkali agents NaOH or KOH and are inert to the ether anesthetics. These include Amsorb Plus (Armstrong Medical Limited, Coleraine, Northern Ireland), Lithely (Allied Healthcare Products, St. Louis, MO), Sodasorb LF (Smiths Medical), and Yabashi Lime-f (Yabashi Holdings Co., Akasaka, Japan). There are also absorbents that contain a reduced amount of NaOH, including Spherasorb (Intersurgical Ltd., Berkshire, United Kingdom), and Drägersorb 800 Plus (Dräger). In addition, the risk of developing renal injury is related to the dose exposure of compound A and not just to sevoflurane.[153] However, this risk is far less likely than originally thought and now likely eliminated with the newer absorbents.[154–156] However, in a conservative fashion the US Food and Drug Administration in the January 2010 Prescribing Information for Ultane (sevoflurane) recommends: *"To minimize exposure to Compound A, sevoflurane exposure should not exceed 2 MAC·hours at flow rates of 1 to <2 L/min. Fresh gas flow rates, 1 L/min are not recommended"*; in the absence of any ill effects of compound A reported in humans, it is unclear if this recommendation is necessary (see also Chapter 5).

CO_2 absorbents must also include color indicators to identify when the capacity of the absorbent has been exhausted. Ethyl violet is one indicator, which changes from colorless to violet when the pH of the absorbent decreases. Exposure to fluorescent lights can decrease the concentration of functioning ethyl violet.[157] In addition, if consumed absorbent material is left unused for a period of time, it is possible for the color indicator to revert to white or colorless. This can occur when NaOH or KOH regenerates in the absorbent material with a subsequent increase in pH. This does not occur with absorbents that are NaOH- or KOH-free.

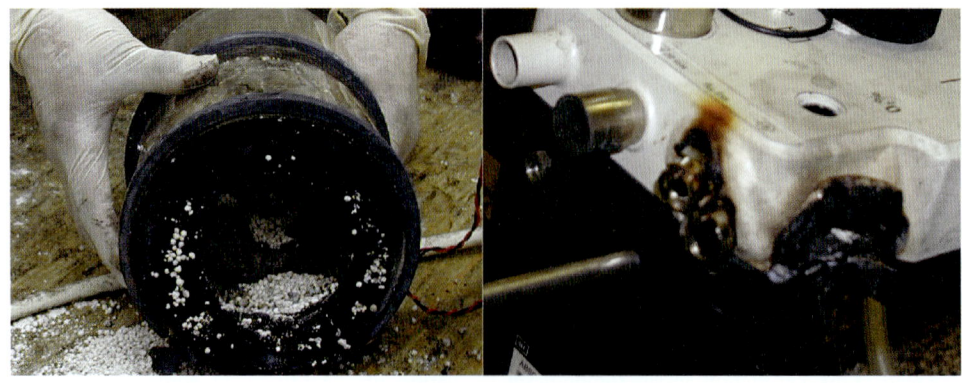

FIGURE 49.4 Sevoflurane/Baralyme interaction produced this fire in an anesthesia machine. (Courtesy Mr. A. Rich.)

HUMIDIFICATION

Oxygen, N_2O, and air from tanks and connecting lines contain no humidity and are room temperature or cold compared with the patient. Warming and humidifying inspired gases help to maintain body temperature and prevent the drying of secretions, improve mucociliary function,[158,159] and reduce the inflammatory response.[160]

A small amount of heat is produced during the exothermic reaction that occurs when CO_2 is removed from the breathing circuit. However, the amount of heat produced is insufficient to maintain a child's temperature. The use of small fresh gas flows increases the humidity relative to high fresh gas flows.[161] However, small fresh gas flows do not increase the humidity sufficiently to preserve mucociliary function. Further, there was no difference in airway temperature between small and large fresh gas flows.[161] Clinicians may choose to use passive humidification with an HME. The passive HMEs have a reflective filter or membrane that retains heat and moisture on the patient side of the circuit. HMEs increase the temperature and heat of the inspired gases to the point that they approach physiologic levels.[162] The best results are achieved when an HME is used in conjunction with small fresh gas flows. The downside to using HMEs is that they increase the dead space and can increase the partial pressure of CO_2 (PCO_2) if the minute ventilation is not increased.[163] Humidification of airway gases can also be active with systems that include heated wires within the breathing circuit or reservoirs for sterile water connected to the breathing circuit that can be heated. These systems are very effective at maintaining temperature and humidity but have some drawbacks. Active humidification systems are prone to condensation or "rain out" on the inside of the breathing circuit that can lead to obstruction of the airway, obstruction of the CO_2 gas sampling line, and inaccurate measurement of airway pressure and gas flow. Active humidification systems increase the resistance to gas flow and can alter the compliance and compression volume if they are not in line and warm when the machine check is performed. Finally, if active humidification systems are set incorrectly or malfunction, they can overheat and cause damage to the airway and trachea. The decision to use active or passive systems should be based on factors such as the size of the patient, duration of the case, and difficulty in maintaining an increased minute ventilation.

MECHANICAL VENTILATION

In addition to delivering anesthetic gases and oxygen and eliminating CO_2, one of the primary purposes of the anesthesia workstation is to ventilate the lungs. The complexity of this task is compounded in small infants and children in whom an inaccuracy of 20 mL might double the delivered tidal volume.[164] The determinants of the delivered tidal volume include the compliance of the anesthesia breathing circuit, the fresh gas inflow, the means of delivering the breath, the gas flows, the inspired to expired ratio, and the dead space of airway circuit.[165] Additionally, mechanical ventilation should aim to avoid atelectasis using strategies such as PEEP and recruitment manoeuvres.[166]

Modern anesthesia machines use internal electronics to address all of these components except dead space and to compensate for changes in these variables to estimate the minute ventilation[167] and their detailed use is well reviewed elsewhere.[168,169]

The electronics of modern anesthesia workstations compensates for the compliance and compression volume of both the gases delivered and the tubing of the breathing circuit. Breathing circuits are either parallel or coaxial and can be smooth or, more commonly, corrugated. Corrugated breathing circuits come in a variety of sizes to accommodate the patient's size. Larger lumens have reduced resistance to air flow but a greater increase in volume when pressure is applied to the circuit.[170] Compensation calibration can be performed with modern anesthesia workstations to accommodate for the change in volume as the circuit expands under pressure. However, if the circuit and tubing are not fully expanded before commencing the machine check, the compliance estimate of the corrugated circuit tubing is reduced, and therefore the ventilator compensation underestimated.[171] The end of the breathing circuit should be occluded and the compensation test performed before use; the workstation increases the volume in the occluded circuit while pressure is being measured. The compliance factor of that breathing circuit is automatically entered into the ventilation system memory and used to compensate for the volume of expansion. This test is specific to the circuit in its current state. If the circuit size is changed or if the corrugated circuit's length is altered, the compliance factor will be inaccurate and therefore the delivered tidal volume will be inaccurate. If either of these changes occur, the compensation test should be repeated to ensure that the displayed respiratory indices are accurate.

One concern with the first generation of anesthesia ventilators was that changing the fresh gas flow could alter the tidal volume delivered to the lungs. The volume of gas set to be delivered entered the bellows mechanism of the ventilator during inspiration, augmenting or diminishing the intended tidal volume with the volume-controlled mode. The most recent generation of anesthesia ventilators does not have this limitation.[167] The mechanism by which this is accomplished varies among manufacturers. One design is to incorporate a valve that shuts off fresh gas flow during the delivery of the inspired breath. Another design is to measure the amount of fresh gas flow and adjust the volume in the bellows, piston, or turbine used to deliver the dialed tidal volume. The ability to measure gas flow very accurately throughout the anesthesia workstation allows for this type of adjustment as well as circuit compensation. Real-time monitoring extends to the ventilation system of the newest generation of anesthesia machines regardless of whether this is accomplished by pneumatics, piston, or turbine.

Modern anesthesia machines provide multiple modes of mechanical ventilation. These include pressure-controlled ventilation (PCV), volume-controlled ventilation (VCV), and volume-guaranteed ventilation (VGV). These modes can be set as intermittent mechanical ventilation (IMV), or synchronized intermittent mechanical ventilation (SIMV), in which the child's effort to breathe can trigger the ventilator to deliver a breath. Additionally, the ventilator can deliver pressure support (PS) above PEEP. PCV has historically been the predominant mode chosen for controlled ventilation in pediatric anesthesia, but the evolution of the anesthesia ventilator is changing this. This preference may have developed from a time when the measurement of tidal volume with the ventilator was less accurate. For PCV, the clinician sets a positive inspiratory pressure (PIP) level, PEEP level, inspiratory:expiratory (I:E) ratio, and respiratory rate. The adequacy of ventilation is determined by observing the chest rise, auscultating breath sounds, monitoring the end-tidal CO_2 (ETCO$_2$), and intermittent blood gases as indicated. The ventilator delivers a breath with a very fast initial flow, which decreases as the target pressure is achieved. This is known as a decelerating flow pattern. The pressure in the airway is constant throughout the inspiratory breath and forms a square wave. In PCV mode, the tidal volume delivered depends on the compliance of the ventilator circuit and the respiratory system. One disadvantage of this mode of ventilation is that with a decrease in compliance (e.g., surgeon leaning on the infant's chest), the delivered tidal volume decreases. Alternatively, in a VCV mode, the clinician sets a tidal volume to be delivered, PEEP level, rate, and I:E ratio. The adequacy of ventilation is determined in the same manner. The inspiratory pressure required to deliver the tidal volume depends on the compliance of the ventilator circuit and respiratory system as well as the time over which the breath is delivered. This inspiratory time is determined by the rate and the I:E ratio. In a VCV mode of ventilation, the rate of air flow is constant throughout the entire inspiratory cycle and forms a square wave. However, the pressure in the airway increases throughout the inspiratory time.

As a consequence of the differences in the air flow patterns between PCV and VCV modes, a greater pressure is required to achieve the same tidal volume as in the VCV mode. For most children with normally compliant lungs, this difference is negligible. VGV modes of ventilation have different names based on the manufacturer and combine pressure and volume control strategies into one mode. The clinician sets a required tidal volume while the ventilator measures the pressure in the airway over several breaths as it adjusts to deliver the desired tidal volume. Then, in an iterative manner, the ventilator uses pressure to achieve that set volume. The goal is to use the minimum pressure to deliver the prescribed tidal volume. The air flow pattern used is a decelerating waveform and the pressure is constant throughout the inspiratory breath. This would seem like the best of both worlds as this mode can be used for children who are receiving muscle relaxants or are deeply anesthetized.

The respiratory management of children with acute lung injury or ARDS requires specific barotrauma-sparing ventilator strategies. The newest generation of anesthesia machine ventilators can measure and deliver tidal volumes accurately enough to target 6 to 8 mL/kg. Compared with the overall population of patients, only a small number of children with ARDS come to the OR. Therefore, with the current state-of-the-art anesthesia ventilators, there may not be a significant benefit to bringing an ICU ventilator into the OR even for children with poor respiratory compliance. The current anesthesia machines include all the modes of ventilation that are generally used in an ICU setting. In addition, a significant advantage to using an anesthesia machine is the ability to rapidly deepen the depth of anesthesia with inhalational anesthetics. Further, if the APL valve is set to the same value as PEEP, the clinician can switch back and forth between mechanical and hand ventilation without altering PEEP. With an ICU ventilator, the patient is disconnected from the circuit to be hand ventilated; PEEP may be lost, potentially reducing lung recruitment.

For support of spontaneous ventilation in children, previously done with T-Piece or Mapleson D circuits (Fig. 49.5) with no mechanical assistance, modern ventilators allow clinicians to provide inspiratory pressure support with PEEP during spontaneous ventilation. Pressure support mode provides additional airway pressure when the patient triggers a breath either by negative pressure on the ventilator circuit or altering the airflow. Sensitivity triggers can be adjusted such that most children are able to initiate PS. If the triggers are set very low, it is possible for "autocycling" to occur. Autocycling occurs when PS breaths are triggered by changes in pressure or flow within the ventilator circuit owing to leaking around an ETT or other non–patient-initiated mechanisms. This

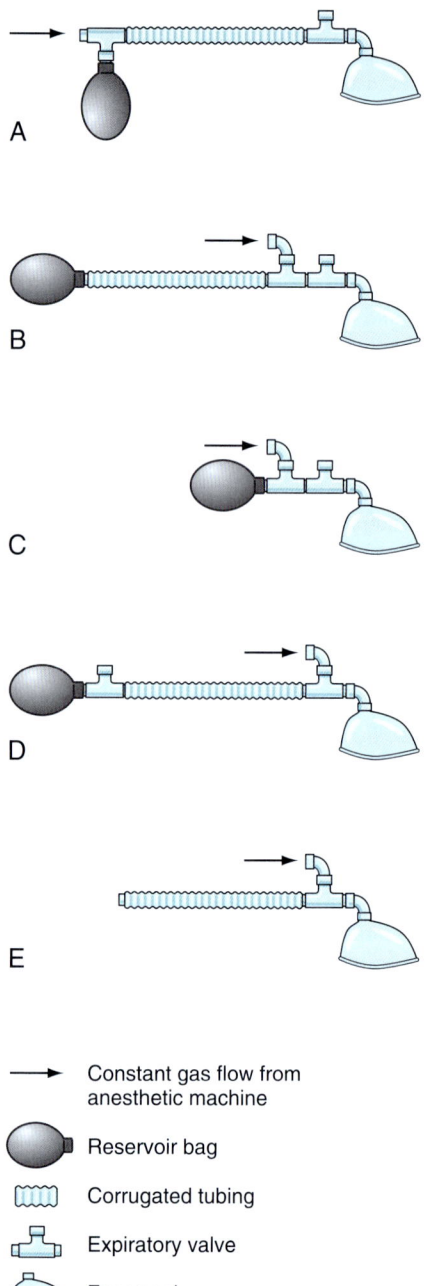

→	Constant gas flow from anesthetic machine
(bag)	Reservoir bag
(tubing)	Corrugated tubing
(valve)	Expiratory valve
(mask)	Facemask

FIGURE 49.5 The Mapleson categories of breathing circuits (Mapleson configurations A to E). The most commonly used circuit for infants is the Mapleson D configuration **(D)**. (From Mapleson WW. The elimination of rebreathing in various semi-closed anaesthetic systems. *Br J Anaesth.* 1954; 26[5]:323-332.)

can generally be identified by a very rapid ventilator rate with very small tidal volumes.

There are several benefits to PS ventilation. For children who are not receiving neuromuscular blocks drugs (NMBDs), PS allows them to set their own ventilator rate. This allows the clinician to use respiratory rate as a measure for depth of anesthesia as well as for titration of opioid pain medications. PS may also provide increased minute ventilation at the end of the procedure compared with spontaneous ventilation, which might decrease the time for emergence. As stated earlier, the conducting portion or shaft of an LMA can substantively increase the mechanical dead space in infants and small children. At times, the patient's tidal volume can be small enough that dead space cannot be overcome. The use of PS and PEEP can assist the child to overcome this dead space and maintain a normal CO_2 level.

In earlier anesthesia machines, the constant fresh gas flow would generate small amounts of PEEP. Modern anesthesia ventilators can accurately deliver a set PEEP value using an interruption in fresh gas flow such that tidal volume is neither altered by nor dependent on the fresh gas flow. With the current ventilators, it is possible to provide anesthetics with zero PEEP. We can think of very few circumstances (possibly increased intracranial pressure or single-lung ventilation) where even a small amount of PEEP is not beneficial. Even high levels of PEEP do not decrease cardiac output in children who have an adequate intravascular volume.[172,173] Rather than increasing the inspired fraction of oxygen (FiO_2) in response to decreasing saturations, the clinician should perform an alveolar recruitment maneuver followed by the addition of PEEP to keep the alveoli open.[174] Recruitment maneuvers can be automated on some workstations, and procedures to identify optimal PEEP levels using manual, and in future, automated processes, are possible.[175]

Anesthesia machines can monitor pressure and flow in the airway. Further, they monitor the inspired and expired concentration of gases from the elbow of the breathing circuit. These monitors increase patient safety and provide immediate feedback regarding the adequacy of ventilation and the depth of anesthesia. The anesthesia machine can detect increased airway pressure, indicating obstruction of the airway or bronchospasm, airway disconnection, apnea, high and low pressures, as well as minute ventilation, low inspired FiO_2, high anesthesia concentrations, increased inspired CO_2, and increased expired CO_2. Further, continuous CO_2 waveforms and pressure-flow and pressure-volume loops can provide a great deal of information about the respiratory system.

One aspect of monitoring airway gases is that there must be a Luer connection to tightly connect the gas sampling line to the anesthesia machine. Mechanical dead space begins at the Y piece of the anesthesia breathing circuit and extends distally. This includes the elbow itself, HMEs, flexible airway connections or accordion, and the connecting area of the LMA. All of these items can increase the dead space significantly for small children; items with minimum internal volume should be used when possible, particularly in neonates and infants.

It should be noted that anesthesia machines have no means to automatically increase the tidal volume to compensate for a leak around the ETT; larger tidal volumes can be used to compensate for leaks.

Equipment Cart

It is advantageous to use mobile, lockable, multidrawer carts to stock the wide range and sizes of items necessary to care for the full spectrum of infants and children. The drawers should be organized for ease of use: airway equipment, drugs, IV supplies, monitoring equipment, circuits, and suction catheters, separated into appropriately labeled drawers. To facilitate efficient and safe delivery of anesthesia, it is prudent to design and stock each cart identically. Because pediatric anesthesia is often administered outside the OR suite, these mobile carts simplify the safe practice of anesthesia and guarantee the availability of all necessary equipment in these remote locations for children of all sizes (Table 49.2).

Defibrillator and External Pacemakers

Every OR facility should be equipped with a direct-current defibrillator. It is not necessary to have a unit specifically for use with children provided the energy range may be adjusted to the appropriate levels (e.g., 2 joules/kg) and pediatric paddles are immediately available. Ideally, the design should incorporate all controls in the paddles, facilitating use without leaving the child's side. A sensing circuit that provides the capacity for synchronous defibrillation is desirable. External defibrillators with disposable pads applied to the front and back or right chest and left lateral chest of the child have improved the rapidity of response in some circumstances. These can be placed on high-risk children (e.g., cardiac surgery, cardiomyopathy, atrioventricular conduction defects) before induction of anesthesia.[114,176-180] Similar devices that allow for external cardiac pacing represent a major new advance for high-risk infants and children (see also Chapter 38).[181-183]

Ultrasound for Regional Anesthesia and Vascular Cannulation

The application of ultrasound to anesthesia practice has been rapid and widespread. It is used to assist with venous and arterial cannulation, and regional nerve blocks,[184-187] but is increasingly used as a general purpose tool in many clinical situations including airway assessment, respiratory complications, cardiovascular assessment, and others. Improved success and safety have been reported with ultrasound for vascular access (see Chapter 46)[185,188-191] and for regional anesthesia if the practitioner is experienced (see Chapter 40).[184,192-194]

Most anesthesiologists can use ultrasound to obtain two-dimensional (2D) images but may not be aware of all the features of their ultrasound machines. These allow the clinician to freeze the image, measure distances, zoom into an area, increase the gain of the image, interrogate a color Doppler signal, print, and transmit images. Color Doppler is the use of a color-coded representation of velocity of the reflecting tissue put on top of the 2D image. Typically blood flow is depicted in red when the flow is directed away from the transducer and in blue when it is directed toward the transducer. The use of color Doppler can improve identification of arterial versus venous vessels, thus improving patient safety.

The physics of ultrasound favor the pediatric patient. Probes that operate at higher frequencies offer better spatial resolution but with a limited depth of penetration of the image, whereas those that operate at lower frequencies penetrate to identify deeper structures but have decreased resolution. Small children and infants, therefore, have excellent acoustic windows and structures that can easily be identified because the structures are more superficial than in adults (see Chapter 40). Needles can be difficult to visualize with ultrasound[195] because they do not enter the ultrasound field of view parallel to the transducer. The steeper the angle of the needle, the less reflection and therefore the less the ultrasound waveform. Further, soft tissue is a mix of fluid, fat, connective tissue, and muscle, each with different impedance, which creates difficulty in distinguishing the needle from background material.[196] Manufacturers have addressed this issue in two separate ways: by increasing the echogenicity of the needle and by electronically manipulating the ultrasound signal to enhance the needle-tissue interface. Manufacturers such as Havel's

TABLE 49.2 | **Suggested Pediatric Equipment Cart Inventory**

Drawer Contents	Drawer Contents
Drawer 1 — Laryngoscope handles (functioning) (2) Laryngoscope blades (functioning) Miller: 0 (2); 1 (2); 2 (2); 3 (2) Macintosh: 1 (2); 2 (2); 3 (2) Wis-Hipple: 1.5 (2) Magill forceps: 1 pediatric, 1 adult 1-inch tape (4) 0.5-inch waterproof tape (4) Tourniquets of nonlatex material: 4 each 0.75-inch and 0.25-inch Scissors Flashlight Extra batteries for laryngoscope handle	**Drawer 4—cont'd** — Diphenhydramine 50 mg (2) Calcium chloride 10% (4) Calcium gluconate 10% (4) Sterile water Lidocaine 1% (5) Phenylephrine (5) Neostigmine 1:2000 (10) Ephedrine (5) Atropine (10) Isoproterenol (1) Furosemide (3) Epinephrine 1:1000 (10) Succinylcholine (1) Rocuronium (1) Dexamethasone 4 mg/mL (2) Dopamine (2) Ondansetron (10) Propofol (10)
Drawer 2 — Masks Neonate (3) Infant (3) Toddler (3) Child (3) Medium adult (3) Large adult (3) Airways 3.5 cm (5) 5.0 cm (5) 6.0 cm (5) 7.0 cm (5) 8.0 cm (5) 9.0 cm (5)	**Drawer 5** — Pediatric uncuffed endotracheal tubes: 2.5 (6); 3.0 (6); 3.5 (6); 4.0 (6); 4.5 (6); 5.0 (6); 6.0 (6) Pediatric cuffed endotracheal tubes: 5.0 (3); 5.5 (3) Adult cuffed endotracheal tubes: 2 each of 6.0; 6.5; 7.0 Stylets in various appropriate sizes
	Drawer 6 — Pediatric and adult esophageal stethoscopes (6) Adult electrocardiography pads (10) Pediatric electrocardiography pads (10) 6.5 Fr suction catheters (6); 10 of each size 8 Fr and 14 Fr Pediatric and adult Yankauer suction devices (10 each)
Drawer 3 — Gauze sponges (sterile and nonsterile) Double-stick disks Rubber bands Adhesive bandages Alcohol swabs Antibiotic ointment Water-soluble surgical lubricant Lidocaine ointment 5% Bulldog clips Safety pins Corneal lubricant Pediatric blood tubes (blue, red, purple, and green) Eye patches	**Drawer 7** — Syringes: 60-mL (2); 20-mL (6); 12-mL (10); 6-mL (10); 3-mL (20); 3-mL (20); 1-mL with 27-gauge needle (20); a variety of needles to facilitate drug withdrawal (18-, 20-, 22-, 25-gauge)
	Drawer 8 — Intravenous catheters: 24-gauge; 22-gauge; 20-gauge; 18-gauge; 16-gauge; 14-gauge Pediatric intravenous boards: 2 sizes (4) T-connectors Three-way stopcocks, multiple stopcock manifolds, claves, Luer connectors, small volume (0.5–1 mL) drug administration tubing
Drawer 4 — Adult sodium bicarbonate (2) Pediatric sodium bicarbonate 8.4% (2) Infant sodium bicarbonate 4.2% (2) Cardiac lidocaine 100 mg (2) Dextrose 50% (1) Mannitol 25% (1)	**Drawer 9** — Pediatric and adult intravenous sets (6) Pediatric Buretrol (2) Intravenous extension sets (2) Lactated Ringer solution 250 mL 0.9 normal saline solution (5) Air trap filters (6) Head strap Blood pressure cuffs (2 each size), 1 adult size with stethoscope Oximeter sensors for infants and children

NOTE: These are only suggested equipment cart materials. Each hospital should alter the order of drawers and their contents to suit its particular needs and for convenience.

Incorporated (Cincinnati, OH), Pajunk (Norcross, GA), B. Braun Medical (Bethlehem, PA), and others have adapted the sides of the needle to increase its echogenicity. There are multiple manufacturers of ultrasound equipment for anesthesia. These manufacturers have enhanced software to improve our ability to visualize the needle. BK Ultrasound (Peabody, MA) calls its feature "X-Shine"; GE Healthcare (Little Chalfont, United Kingdom) calls its feature LOGIQ-e; Mindray Zonare (Mountain View, CA) calls its feature "iNeedle"; Philips (Foster City, CA) calls its feature "Needle Visualization"; FujiFilm SonoSite (Bothell, WA) calls its feature "Advanced Needle Visualization (AVN)"; and Toshiba Medical Systems (Otawara, Tochigi Prefecture, Japan) calls its feature

"Biopsy Enhancement Auto Mode (BEAM)." There are numerous ultrasound workshops each year at various medical society meetings to train practitioners to use ultrasound for vascular access and regional anesthesia.

Monitoring Equipment

THE ANESTHESIA RECORD

Anesthesia **I**nformation **M**anagement **S**ystems (AIMS) are rapidly becoming ubiquitous in anesthesia practice, in parallel with adoption of hospital-wide electronic health records (EHR). AIMS can be stand-alone products but are more often an integrated component of the hospital EHR itself. These systems are expensive, requiring sizable hardware and software investments, and hospital administrators usually decide which systems to purchase with advice from their Informatics and Anesthesiology departments.[197–199] An effective AIMS replaces the paper chart and reduces the workload of anesthesiologists, integrating information from the anesthesia machine, physiologic monitors, other equipment, and the EHR (Fig. 49.6). Additional functions include automatically calculating cumulative totals for intakes, outputs, and drug infusions, documenting compliance with regulatory requirements such as "time-outs" and administering "antibiotics before surgical incision."[200,201] Whether these functions will reduce perioperative morbidity and mortality remains unclear.[202,203]

The automatic recording of physiologic variables may improve accuracy of data but are not without errors.[204,205] For example, a pulse oximeter signal may be altered by the presence of a tourniquet at the time of IV cannulation, electrocautery may temporarily interfere with both electrocardiographic and temperature readings, and arterial BP readings will be interrupted by blood draws for periodic lab testing. These values can be annotated but most anesthesia providers either miss or disregard these erroneous or absent readings, leaving unusual or missing data in the electronic record. Such errors may have medicolegal implications as well as quality assurance questions.[206]

There are many reasons to use the same manufacturer for AIMS and EHR. However, most of these systems were designed by engineers, not anesthesiologists, with clumsy user interfaces and workflow patterns. The workflow can initially be very taxing and quite different than using paper records. Before these systems are purchased, they should be evaluated under real-world conditions to determine their suitability. With regard to data, the accuracy of the information that one can extract from the AIMS is directly reflected by the accuracy of its input.[204] If data are easy to input and flow directly from the EHR and the OR monitors, the data may be more accurate. Unfortunately, the manufacturers of most AIMS are concerned with replacing a paper record, providing regulatory compliance, and integrating with the EHR and less focused on the need to extract data for research or quality improvement projects. We encourage the adoption of AIMS that record physiologic data such as heart rate, respiratory rate, expired and inspired gases, and CO_2 and oxygen saturation at 10-second intervals for research purposes and for medicolegal defense.

DRUG ERRORS, BAR CODING, AND INTEGRATION

Studies of adult and pediatric patients[207] suggest that medication errors are common in the OR.[208,209] A pediatric systematic review of several million anesthetics across 10 countries reported medication errors in 1/1250 anesthetics, which is lower than in adult studies but most frequent in children <1 year of age.[210] Medication errors are a major concern in pediatric practice and one of the

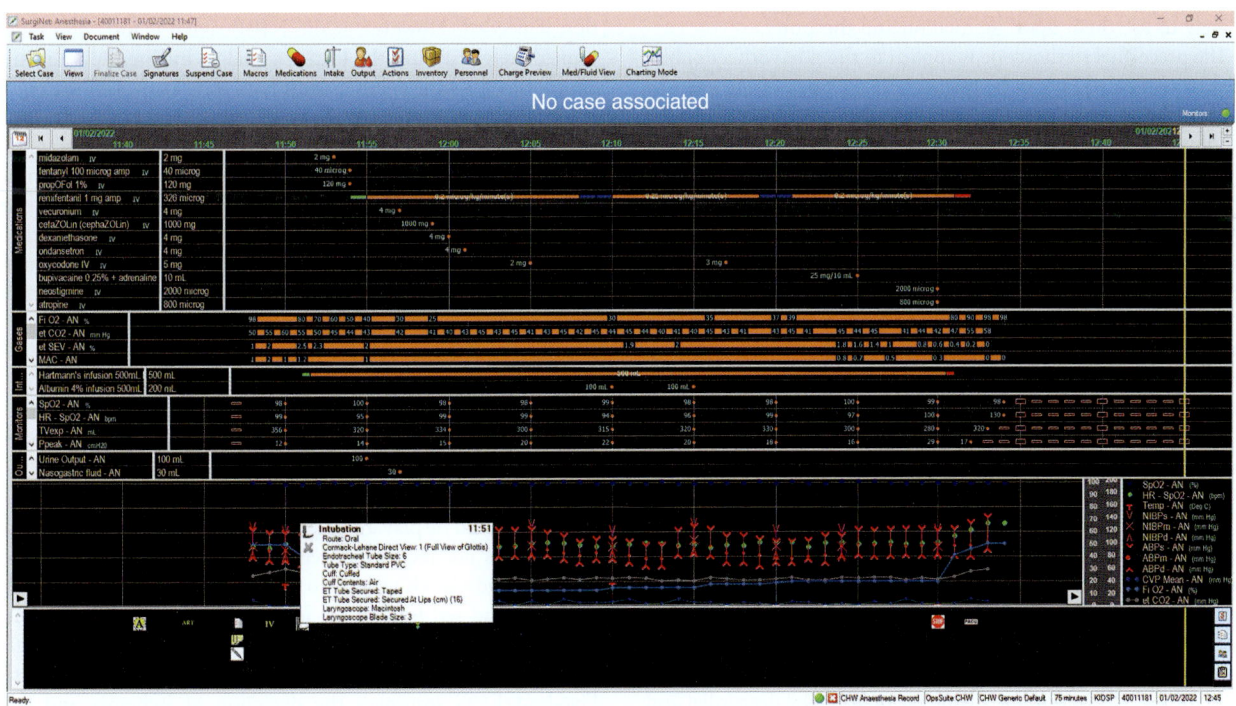

FIGURE 49.6 A modern Anesthesia Information Management System fully integrated with the hospital-wide Electronic Medical Record. This is the anesthesiologist's customized access to the entire patient record, with automated monitoring, medications, and alerts. (Simulated patient data, courtesy of Dr. Stuart Ross, The Children's Hospital at Westmead, Australia, using Cerner Surginet Anaesthesia.)

focuses of the Wake Up Safe Quality Improvement campaign.[211] These include wrong drug, wrong dose, wrong route, incorrect dilution, and wrong patient errors; errors most commonly involve antibiotics and opioids.[212] The process of labeling a medication syringe offers multiple opportunities for medication errors by the person drawing up the wrong drug, mislabeling the syringe, and mislabeling the concentration.[213] Medication errors that result in administration of the wrong drug may be reduced by color-coded labels (e.g., red for NMBDs, blue for opioids, yellow for induction drugs) but advanced technology allows us to consider implementing bar code confirmation of a particular drug.[214] Such systems provide accurate labeling of syringes (date, time, concentration, and initials of provider) and have had great success in reducing medication errors both in and out of the OR.[208,215–219] It does not yet appear that there is significant integration of this technology in pediatric anesthesia.[220] In a 2014 study,[221] none of 34 children's hospitals across the United States used bar code technology to identify medications. Bar code labeling can easily be integrated into the AIMS; it can be used to label individual syringes and verify that the correct drug is being administered. We encourage the adoption of this safety feature by all pediatric anesthesiologists, a change we expect will be universal in the future.

PRECORDIAL AND ESOPHAGEAL STETHOSCOPES

Precordial and esophageal stethoscopes offer the opportunity for an experienced practitioner to detect cardiac arrhythmias, obstruction of the endotracheal tube, wheezing, airway obstruction, laryngospasm, and decreases in BP compared with baseline (softening of heart tones), among other critical events. Unfortunately, the use of precordial stethoscopes to monitor children in the OR has decreased during the past few decades in a trend that appears to be continuing with each successive generation of anesthesiologists. This problem is underscored by the fact that if clinicians do not use precordial stethoscopes during their training, they are very unlikely to use them upon graduation and thereafter.

The precordial stethoscope is applied to the skin with a double-sided adhesive disk. It can be placed near the apex of the heart to best hear heart sounds, at the suprasternal notch to best hear the combination of heart and breath sounds, or in the left axilla if there is a chance of inadvertent right mainstem intubation (e.g., tracheoesophageal fistula repair). Nonferrous versions may be available for use in MRI, but practically speaking, practitioners are more likely to monitor the exhaled CO_2 tension than use a precordial stethoscope.

Disposable esophageal stethoscopes, often combined with a temperature probe, have supplanted precordial stethoscopes as cardiothoracic monitors. The integrated probes are bigger than a simple temperature probe, so they are preferred in children 2 years of age and older. These probes are ideally positioned in a retrocardiac manner by passing the probes down the esophagus until the volume of the auscultated heart sounds is maximized.

Several technologic advances to both the precordial and esophageal stethoscopes have reached the commercial market. A wireless version of these monitors transforms the audio signal into digital data so the "sound" is transmitted wirelessly to a receiver worn by the anesthesiologist.[222] This allows the anesthesiologist to move about in the OR and not be tethered to the short stethoscope tubing. An important advantage of both the precordial and esophageal stethoscopes rests with the fact that they transmit sound waves mechanically and equipment malfunctions are less likely. Even when combined with pulse oximetry and capnography, the stethoscope provides great reassurance that the patient has a BP and cardiac output. *If both the noninvasive blood pressure (NIBP) monitor and the oximeter fail, but the child has strong heart tones, a technical problem likely exists with the former two monitors. However, if the NIBP and pulse oximeter fail and the heart tones are very weak, then cardiac output may be compromised, and attention should be immediately focused on resolving that problem rather than troubleshooting the monitors.*

NONINVASIVE BLOOD PRESSURE MONITORING

NIBP monitoring is a mainstay of clinical care. BP cuffs should be available in all age-appropriate sizes. The BP cuff should cover approximately two-thirds of the upper arm length. Many practitioners recommend similar-sized BP cuffs on the calf of the lower leg and the upper arm, but there is little evidence to support this recommendation.[223,224] Some individuals may choose to use the thigh to measure BP when the arms are not available, but this is less common. As a result of the propagation of the arterial waveform throughout the body, a BP obtained on the calf may have a slightly greater systolic and lesser diastolic pressures compared with the same values in the upper arm.[223,225] Automatic NIBP units use an oscillatory means to detect the BP. These units are capable of frequent and accurate measurements. To prevent injury to the patient it is important that the NIBP units are set to the correct size (neonate, child, adult). The correct setting will ensure that the range of inflation pressures and deflation time do not cause venous stasis or nerve compression damage. Most devices have two sets of connecting tubing: one for children and adults and one for neonates. Neonatal tubing has different connectors and complementary BP cuffs; they are not interchangeable with adult tubing. Neonatal BP cuffs typically are sized 1 through 5 and fit approximately the same number as the infant's weight in kilograms; the monitor must be set to the correct patient and tubing size for the algorithms to produce accurate information. Backup equipment should be available to obtain BP by auscultation if needed. However, if the NIBP signal is lost, one should immediately attribute the loss of signal to hypotension and treat appropriately (with volume and/or vasopressors) until the equipment is assessed.

Noninvasive continuous blood pressure measurements are possible using finger cuffs, and a technique utilizing volume clamping and photoplethysmography.[226] Initial pediatric experience using this technique shows promise, with excellent agreement with invasive arterial pressures.[227] Studies in adults and in obese patients suggest a better correlation with mean rather than systolic arterial pressure[228–230]; further pediatric studies are needed before routine adoption of this technology.

ELECTROCARDIOGRAM

The electrocardiogram (ECG) is a mainstay of clinical care. For general pediatric anesthesia, three-lead monitoring of the ECG is usually sufficient to detect arrhythmias and the basic heart rate. A monitor should display a single waveform (commonly lead II) and usually does not require ST-segment analyses. The typical placement of leads is white lead to right shoulder, black lead to left shoulder, and red lead to the left flank. Further, lead placement often gets changed slightly based on the surgical field. For pediatric cardiac anesthesia five-lead monitoring of the ECG is used. Five-lead ECG improves the detection of ischemia and three waveforms are usually monitored. Lead placement for a five-lead ECG is the same as three with the addition of a green lead to right flank and a brown lead (V1) to the fourth intercostal space on the right side of the chest. Detection of the QRS is automatic.

Automated ST and QT segment analysis are standard features in several monitoring systems and are useful in specific patients. Signaling of the QRS tone can be set on the monitor to come from either ECG, pulse oximetry, or arterial waveform if present. The choice depends on the surgical type as electrocautery interferes with the ECG signal. Special nonferrous ECG leads and monitors are necessary for use in MRI. Most problems with ECG monitoring occur because of poor contact of the leads with the patient. This can sometimes be improved by cleaning the skin first with alcohol and placing new leads. Given the interference during electrocautery and during MRI, the heart rate is best determined from the pulse oximeter.

OXYGEN MONITORS

Sensors that monitor the FiO_2 are built into every modern anesthesia machine. This is in addition to fail-safe devices that detect a decrease in the pressure in the oxygen line. Oxygen monitors with alarms are necessary to prevent the delivery of an hypoxic gas mixture, but they can also be set to alarm for a high FiO_2 as well. Low FiO_2 can be an unintentional consequence of very low flow anesthesia with air-oxygen blends in a closed circle system. However, there are several circumstances when a low FiO_2 is intentional and desirable: (1) a reduced FiO_2 may be necessary in some children with congenital heart disease to reduce the oxygen saturation to balance the pulmonary and systemic blood flows, (2) during airway surgery to reduce the risk of airway fires, and (3) in infants and neonates to reduce the risk of retinopathy of prematurity (see Chapter 32).[231–233] It is not the FiO_2 but the child's arterial partial pressure of oxygen (PaO_2) that is important regarding retinopathy of prematurity. It is common practice to reduce the FiO_2, if otherwise safe for the neonate, to the point where the oxygen saturation measured by pulse oximetry (SpO_2) is between 91% and 95% to minimize the risk of oxygen toxicity without increasing perioperative mortality (see Chapter 35). Monitoring of FiO_2 can be combined with that of expired oxygen concentrations (FeO_2) to estimate oxygen uptake on a breath by breath or minutely basis. Acute changes in delta O_2 ($FiO_2 - FeO_2$) along with tachycardia, and hypercarbia, are one of the earliest signs of malignant hyperthermia; temperature elevation is a late sign (see Chapter 39).[234–236]

TEMPERATURE MONITORS

The child's temperature should be monitored throughout anesthesia to prevent hypothermia or hyperthermia. Hypothermia was a very common problem in pediatric anesthesia, particularly in neonates and infants, that has been resolved to a large extent with the adoption of forced air warmers. Hyperthermia most commonly occurs because of iatrogenic overheating and failure to decrease the temperature of the exogenous heat source in the face of an increasing body temperature. Other causes of hyperthermia include malignant hyperthermia, thyrotoxicosis, sepsis, drug overdose (cocaine, monoamine oxidase inhibitors, and meperidine), and in children with arthrogryposis or osteogenesis imperfecta. In a child with malignant hyperthermia, fever is a late sign preceded by other factors, including an increase in end-tidal carbon dioxide tension ($PETCO_2$), increased oxygen uptake (delta O_2), tachypnea, and tachycardia.[234–236] Temperature can be monitored in the axilla, nasopharynx, esophagus, rectum, tympanic membrane, and the skin. Core temperature is most reliably measured on the tympanic membrane or in the esophagus. Rectal temperature is unpredictable as the tip of the probe may be lodged in stool and buffered from the true body temperature. Bladder temperature

may be measured via a Foley catheter that has an integrated temperature monitor, but these catheters are sized only for older children. Skin temperature often slowly responds to changes in body temperature and is well known to underestimate the body temperature. The axillary temperature often underestimates the body temperature because the probe tip is not positioned within the axilla. In such a case, the probe measures the ambient temperature, which may be room air or the temperature from a forced air warmer (as great as 43°C). A properly placed axillary temperature probe may detect an increase in temperature that results from malignant hyperthermia because the deltopectoral triangle is the largest muscle group whose venous blood can be sensed with a probe in the axilla.

NONINVASIVE OXYGEN SATURATION MONITORS
Pulse Oximetry

Pulse oximetry is a mainstay of clinical care in pediatric anesthesia, mandated for routine use in every anesthetic in most jurisdictions. Sensors are typically placed on the fingers and toes but can be applied to the ears or other body parts. When pulse oximeters were first introduced, clinicians needed proof that pulse oximetry was better than clinical judgment in detecting oxygen desaturations.[237,238] This notion is now uniformly accepted (E-Figs. 49.4, 49.5, and 49.6).

Pulse oximetry provides clinicians with two forms of physiological information: oximetry itself and pulse plethysmography. Both rely on the absorbance of light between 660 and 940 nm as it passes through tissue and blood. The presence of two sensors allows the unit to identify blood that is moving (arterial) as opposed to the background oxygen saturation of the tissue. The wavelengths are chosen to take advantage of the differences in the absorption of light between oxygenated and deoxygenated hemoglobin at these various wavelengths, allowing calculation of arterial hemoglobin oxygenation.[239] Pulse plethysmography is obtained from this light absorption signal as well, giving us the familiar plethysmograph trace, with its heart rate data, waveform shape, and perfusion-related data. Thus, the pulse oximeter recording provides a large amount of useful physiological data (Fig. 49.7).[240]

The plethysmographic data allow clear identification of arterial pulsation, hence the name "pulse oximeter." The ratio of absorbance of light at these different wavelengths is converted into arterial oxygen saturation using an algorithm that is proprietary to each of the manufacturers; that is, their combination of LED lights and detectors produces a certain ratio or signal, and it is their own algorithm that produces the saturation value that is displayed. These algorithms are generated by producing various degrees of desaturation in adult volunteers while receiving a hypoxic gas mixture through a face mask. Arterial saturation values from 70% and greater with their paired pulse oximeter ratios are used to calibrate the algorithm. However, the algorithms were created with adult volunteers and then applied to children.

So how accurate are pulse oximeters? The largest prospective study published comparing the SpO_2 values with SaO_2 values measured from arterial samples with co-oximetry in children had 225 subjects and 1980 samples.[241] The bias or the difference between SpO_2 and SaO_2 varied depending on the range of the saturations. SpO_2 values between 90% and 97% exceeded the SaO_2 by only 1%. However, SpO_2 values that were less than 90% exceeded the SaO_2 by 5% (with greater differences as the SpO_2 decreased). More recently, a very large scale pediatric critical caredatabase exploration of $SpO_2 - SaO_2$ correlations in 112,101 samples showed SpO_2 overestimating SaO_2 by 4% to 5% over a wide range of values.[242]

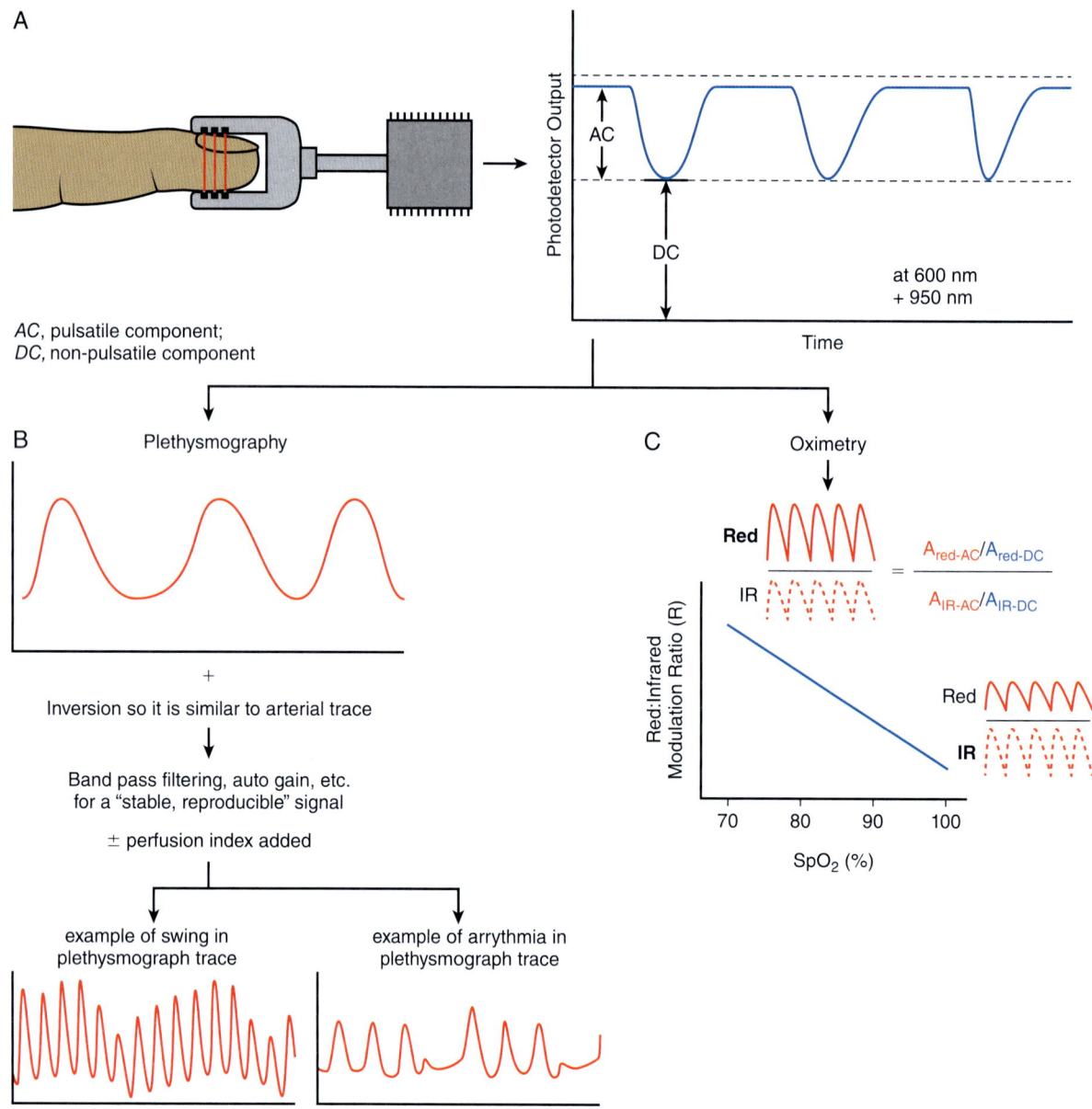

FIGURE 49.7 Pulse oximetry and plethysmography. **A,** Red and near-infrared light is shone through tissue. Detected light is used for two purposes, plethysmography and oximetry. **B,** The plethysmograph is the familiar waveform provided on most monitors, with its shape similar to an invasive arterial line waveform. The waveform can be used to look for "swing"(evidence of reduced preload, arrhythmias, and other physiological phenomena.) **C,** Hemoglobin saturation is calculated using the differential absorbance of red and near-infrared light by oxy and deoxy hemoglobin. Sp_{O_2}, Oxygen saturation measured by pulse oximetry. (Modified diagram from Alian AA, Shelley KH. Photoplethysmography. *Best Pract Res Clin Anaesthesiol.* 2014;28:395-406.)

However, the accuracy of pulse oximeters in infants and children whose SpO_2 is less than 90% (e.g., in cyanotic heart disease or during laryngospasm) is of greater concern as palliative surgeries or the decision to intervene during an acute event is often based on the pulse oximeter saturation reading much less than 90%. Sensors specifically calibrated for cyanotic patients (Masimo Blue, Irvine, CA) have shown improved accuracy and precision compared with standard probes, but still show increasing disagreement with SaO_2 below 75%.[243]

The beat-to-beat variability in the plethysmograph signal can be large and is dealt with using averaging of the signal over 5 to 15 second time windows, which will introduce a slight delay in the response to actual desaturation events. The significance of this averaging must be understood by the clinician during episodes of desaturation or hypoxia. For example, with difficult intubations or laryngospasm, the pulse oximeter signal will lag the desaturation event. This also means that an improvement in saturation will always take longer than anticipated after an open airway and ventilation have been reestablished. A study of continuous cardiac output in anesthetized children found that stroke index decreased with the severity of desaturation, but this was accompanied by a compensatory increase in heart rate with maintained cardiac output; it appears that bradycardia is a relatively late sign of cardiac hypoxemia.[244]

Manufacturers are continually working to improve the algorithms and equipment to eliminate artifacts that may be introduced by movement, variable skin color, poor perfusion, hypothermia, or increased ambient light. Improved algorithms and filtering have resulted in significant reductions in movement artifacts. Low perfusion and hypoxemic states provide ongoing challenges for pulse oximeter technology and some manufacturers have generated specific units and sensors to address these issues.

Pulse oximeter manufacturers have moved in various directions to improve the accuracy of their devices. Masimo Corporation (Masimo Corporation, Irvine, CA) has developed pulse oximeters using multiple wavelength technology: the Masimo Rainbow Pulse Co-oximeters, which can provide much more information beyond oxygen saturation. The presence of additional wavelengths allows the oximeter to provide continuous readings for hemoglobin, carboxyhemoglobin, and methemoglobin. Validation of the hemoglobin measurements in various populations has been studied with varied success in adults,[245-249] but with poor accuracy and precision in children with congenital heart disease.[250] Although these devices might not be absolutely accurate, the ability to follow them as a trend monitor during surgery may offer promise.

Any abnormal value and a suspected clinical scenario with a normal result (false negative) should be assessed with a confirmatory test. The presence of abnormal hemoglobin beyond carboxyhemoglobin and methemoglobin can, in theory, affect the accuracy of pulse oximeters,[251] although the most common types of abnormal hemoglobin (fetal and sickle cell) do not have an impact on pulse oximetry.[252-254] It should be further noted that these specialized oximeter probes are quite expensive (three to four times the cost of a normal probe) and thus have a limited role in routine pediatric care. Another advance relates to signal processing, or as Masimo termed it, Signal Extraction Technology (SET). For some manufacturers, the pulse oximeter waveform or plethysmograph (commonly referred to as "pleth") is stylized and not an actual reflection of the strength of the arterial waveform. For other manufacturers, the pleth is reflective of the degree of perfusion. During inspiration, there is an increase in the venous return to the heart; during exhalation, there is a decrease in venous return. This periodic variation in venous return with respiration translates to subtle changes in the arterial pulse wave height. This effect (pulsus paradoxus) is more pronounced when there is a decrease in the central venous filling pressure (hypovolemia) or if there is a significant increase in the inspiratory force (upper airway obstruction). The newest generation of pulse oximeters has signal processing technology that can detect these variations. Hypovolemia, vasoconstriction, and decreased cardiac output can also lead to the loss of the pleth signal.[255,256] In addition to providing a visual representation of perfusion, the processing that identifies the pleth can be used to estimate respiratory rate. Taking this a step further with the Masimo SET, the Pleth Variability Index (PVI) is an algorithm used to predict patients whose cardiac output might benefit from fluid boluses. The PVI technology has been investigated and the results show promise in adults[257-260] and children,[261] although there remains some uncertainty in this regard particularly in neonates where the pleth has been shown to vary by extremity[262] and even on the same extremity.

Covidien (Boulder, CO) have taken their Nellcor pulse oximeters in a different direction to improve the accuracy of their devices. Rather than producing multiple wavelengths of light, with its OxiMax technology Nellcor has embedded a digital memory chip onto the sensor. This chip contains the calibration and operating characteristics of that sensor that should in turn improve the accuracy. There is some variability in the wavelength of light produced by any light-emitting diode (LED). This chip allows the specific wavelength information to be stored and relayed to the device to use the most accurate algorithm. Nellcor pulse oximeters have respiratory rate monitoring, but they do not appear to yet have an algorithm to assess fluid responsiveness.

REFLECTANCE OXIMETRY

Reflectance oximetry was first created to improve oxygen saturation data in difficult clinical conditions, such as decreased perfusion, movement, and conditions in which optimal sites for standard transmission oximetry probes may not exist (e.g., burns). The technology behind reflectance oximetry involves the emission of multiple wavelengths of red and infrared light that are sensed in two or more photodetectors located a distance away from the diodes on the same probe sensor (Fig. 49.8). These devices measure reflected rather than transmitted light. The technology used to create these oximeter probes permits usage on a flat surface such as the forehead and on the fetal scalp. The forehead devices have had the largest use among pediatric anesthesiologists. Studies of reflectance oximeters in general demonstrate that these devices are more susceptible to erratic measurements when the probe is placed directly over an artery and vein.[263,264] Some potential advantages to using reflectance oximetry on the forehead include better signals during conditions of poor perfusion, lack of motion, artifacts and faster response time than conventional peripheral oximeter probes.[265,266] However, possible disadvantages include a high signal dropout rate (no measurable signal) and poor accuracy, often measuring lower than finger transmission oximetry, particularly in cases of venous congestion (e.g., Trendelenburg position or situations that impede venous return). Several studies report good correlation between concurrent measurements of oxygen saturation comparing reflectance oximetry on the forehead[267,268] and around the chest of premature infants[269] with extremity pulse oximetry and arterial co-oximetry measurements; these studies also report a clear dropout rate.

The Lifebox Monitoring Initiative

We have long recognized the improvement in patient safety with the use of pulse oximetry technology, and its use is ubiquitous in developed nations. Unfortunately, in developing countries the availability of pulse oximetry during general anesthesia cannot be guaranteed (see Chapter 48). In fact, it is estimated that 5 billion of the world's 8.1 billion people do not have access to safe surgery with approximately 70,000 ORs without basic anesthesia equipment and a shortage of 1 million surgeons, anesthesiologists, and obstetricians worldwide.[270,271] The anesthesia-related death rate is 100 to 1000 times greater than in developed countries.[272-275] Pulse oximetry is now part of the Safe Surgery Saves Lives project from the World Health Organization.[273,276,277]

Lifebox was founded in 2011 as a global patient safety initiative to provide pulse oximeters and education to low- and middle-income countries.[278] The device has been shown to be accurate in healthy volunteers[279] and it has improved safety under anesthesia for thousands of individuals.[272,280,281] A donation of $250 USD to Lifebox will purchase one device for donation, which includes a universal age probe, a pediatric probe for neonates, a multicountry charger, and links to educational resources; further information is available at www.lifebox.org. As of the end of 2023, more than 33,400 oximeters have been deployed worldwide.

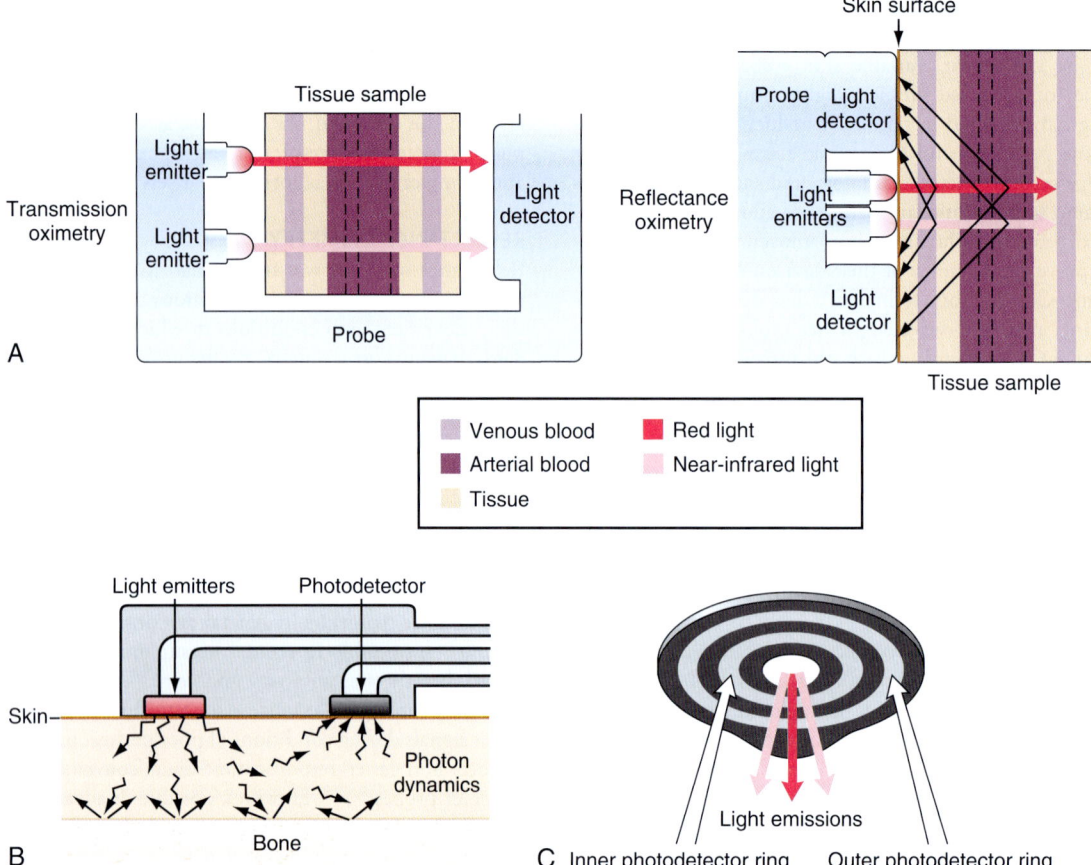

FIGURE 49.8 A, Comparison of conventional transmission pulse oximetry with reflectance oximetry. Note that with conventional oximetry the light detector is located directly opposite on the other side of a digit and detects light transmitted through the digit; with reflectance oximetry the light detector is located next to the light emitters and detects the light reflected back through and from the tissues. **B,** The typical configuration of a reflectance oximeter. **C,** Another configuration, in which several light detectors are located at different distances from the light emitters. In addition, reflectance oximeters may emit light in more than just 2 wavelengths, which is typical of conventional transmission pulse oximeters. (Modified from Kugelman A, Wasserman Y, Mor F, et al. Reflectance pulse oximetry from core body in neonates and infants: comparison to arterial blood oxygen saturation and to transmission pulse oximetry. *J Perinatol.* 2004;24[6]:366-371; and Keogh BF, Kopotic RJ. Recent findings in the use of reflectance oximetry: a critical review. *Curr Opin Anesth.* 2005;18[6]:649-654.)

NEAR-INFRARED SPECTROSCOPY

Near-infrared spectroscopy (NIRS) is a noninvasive, optical technology very similar to pulse oximetry in its basic principles of operation (E-Fig. 49.7). Oxyhemoglobin and deoxyhemoglobin absorb light at different frequencies, and the use of a probe that emits and detects different frequencies of near-infrared light can be used to estimate tissue hemoglobin oxygenation. NIRS is much less susceptible to motion artifact than pulse oximetry, but is affected by ambient light, although software algorithms have significantly decreased this source of error. The NIRS device functionally measures the oxygenation of hemoglobin in the underlying tissues, including blood in the arterioles, capillaries, and venules. The majority (approximately 85%) of the signal originates from the venules.[282] Skin and bone and extracranial blood absorb only limited amounts of light, which is subtracted from the signal and does not have a significant impact on the measurement in infants and children. In cerebral oximetry, the oxygen saturation of the blood in the tissue (i.e., between the sending and emitting probe) depends on factors that affect oxygen transport, including cerebral blood flow (arterial partial pressure of carbon dioxide [$PaCO_2$]), hemoglobin saturation, hemoglobin–oxygen binding affinity, central venous pressure, and oxygen saturation in the arterial blood. Therapies aimed at improving oxygen delivery or decreasing oxygenation consumption by the brain will potentially increase cerebral oxygenation.[283]

In pediatric anesthesia, NIRS has been widely used to measure "regional" cerebral oxygen saturation (rSO_2) for children undergoing and following congenital heart surgery.[284–291] It is also used in this same population to detect renal perfusion[292] and has been shown to predict the development of acute kidney injury.[293,294] NIRS has also been used to detect ischemia in neurosurgery,[295] spine surgery,[296] kidney transplant,[297,298] and tissue free flaps.[299] Although mild desaturations were noted to be common in a recent large observational study of 453 infants <6 months of age undergoing anesthesia, severe desaturation ($rSO_2 < 50\%$, or a decline of >30% from baseline) was uncommon (2%) and not closely linked to hypotension.[300] NIRS may have applications in an ICU setting,[301] following brain injury,[302] and during the use of therapeutic hypothermia.[303]

There are several cerebral oximeters on the market: Equanox (Nonin Medical, Plymouth, MN); Fore-Sight (Casmed, Branford, CT); Invos (Medtronic, Fridley MN); Masimo O3 (Masimo, Irvine, CA); and NIRO-200NX (Hamamatsu Photonics, Hamamatsu City, Japan). The performance of these NIRS devices has been reviewed[304]; they are able to detect episodes of desaturation but their accuracy may vary widely. In turn, they may be better suited to monitor trends in cerebral and tissue oxygenation. All manufacturers now offer sensors for infants and children. Normal rSO2 in awake adults is ~51% to 82%, mean ~66%.[283] Although no similar pediatric studies in children exist, normal values for term and preterm neonates is reported to be 65% to 70%.[305,306] During anesthesia in children the normal range is believed to be between 60% and 80%.[283,307] The range of rSO2 has been shown to vary in infants and children with congenital heart disease based on their anatomic lesion as well as their arterial saturations[308,309] but rSO2 is within the normal range in those with adequately compensated hypoxemia.[310] In controlled hypoxic-ischemic states in animals, electroencephalogram (EEG) slowing and increased tissue lactic acid levels occur at rSO2 between 40% and 45%. The EEG becomes flat at rSO2 between 30% and 35%, and if the cerebral ischemia is protracted, it may be associated with tissue infarction.[311] One other point that requires emphasis is that rSO2 for cerebral oximetry can be greatly influenced by $PaCO_2$[312]; thus, emphasis should be on interpreting values only during steady-state ventilation.

The current generation of commercial NIRS devices has important limitations. They are relatively simple, cheap, and robust optical instruments, operating as continuous-wave devices, using a few discrete wavelengths. They are unable to measure scattering and absorption coefficients, photon time-of-flight, or the presence or influence of other chromophores.[313] These monitors measure only the saturation in tissue 0.5 to 3 cm below the probes, which reflects focal tissue oxygenation or ischemia. If the probe is placed on the forehead, it will reflect the state of the tissue in the frontal cortex and not necessarily other areas of the brain. The same would be true of renal oxygen saturations. Although the kidney is the organ in the flank with the greatest oxygen extraction, all the tissue in that area contributes to the signal. We cannot therefore interpret all decreases in "renal" NIRS as reflecting a global acute kidney injury.[314] One final issue remains with NIRS monitoring. We had hoped that NIRS would provide real-time guidance of regional tissue oxygenation and permit study of the effectiveness of interventions to improve brain oxygenation. Research has shown a potential association between reduced saturations and outcomes. However, there is limited information linking any interventions to outcomes. As suggested by recent review articles,[283,315,316] further research and improvements in NIRS technology are needed to clarify the role of regional tissue oximetry in pediatric patient management. Advances in instrumentation are proceeding rapidly, with cerebral autoregulation metrics, time domain NIRS, broadband NIRS, and diffuse correlation spectroscopy-based flow measurements all seeing substantial progress toward clinical use. Hybrid instruments combining the best of these systems may offer the greatest promise.[317]

CARBON DIOXIDE ANALYZERS
Mainstream and Sidestream Analyzers
The most commonly used gas monitor is the infrared CO_2 monitor. This monitor is particularly useful in teaching about ventilation, CO_2 elimination from alveoli, and airway and ventilator management. Two configurations of infrared CO_2 monitors are

available. They differ only in the location of the CO_2 analysis: (1) the sidestream analyzer, in which expired gas is aspirated from the anesthesia circuit and analyzed remotely; and (2) a mainstream analyzer, in which the gas is analyzed by an optical sensor within a cuvette just proximal to the elbow of the breathing circuit. Sidestream analyzers are lighter and less cumbersome than mainstream analyzers because the former involves no additional pieces to be inserted into the breathing circuit. Sidestream analyzers aspirate gas through a narrow-gauge flexible tube connected to the breathing circuit at the elbow. The gas sampling line and water trap can become obstructed with water or secretions, requiring replacement of the parts. Mainstream gas analyzers are less often obstructed with secretions, but the analyzers are heavy, and if a small-ID tracheal tube is used, the analyzer may kink the tracheal tube, resulting in acute airway obstruction. Most OR monitors today use sidestream sampling, whereas most ICU monitors use mainstream sampling. The current generation of sidestream monitors has improved precision that reduces the gas sampling rate to just 50 mL/minute and excellent accuracy even with small rapid tidal volumes.

The presence of CO_2 is the gold standard to ensure that the tracheal tube has been inserted within the trachea. In the OR this is generally achieved using capnography but during code situations, this is achieved using litmus color-changing devices (see E-Fig. 37.4). If no expired CO_2 is detected after a presumed tracheal intubation, one must assume that the tracheal tube is in the esophagus, or during a code it is presumed that there is inadequate CO_2 in the exhaled breath because of inadequate chest compressions or esophageal intubation. One should consider that the lack of CO_2 detected may be due to equipment malfunction such as obstruction of the sampling line[316] or severe bronchospasm (Fig. 49.9). However, the prudent course of action is to first reexamine the glottis with a laryngoscope to determine whether the tube appears to pass through the cords and if it does, consider alternative explanations for the lack of CO_2. This would be particularly wise if the intubation had been difficult in the first place. Alternately, some remove the tracheal tube without reexamining the airway, mask ventilate the lungs, and reassess the situation. It is possible to have CO_2 present on capnography for one or two breaths if the tracheal tube was inserted into the esophagus. This can occur if the stomach had been distended by manual ventilation or crying before tracheal intubation, or if carbonated soft drinks were present in the stomach, CO_2 could be transiently detected immediately after an esophageal intubation.[318,319] If there is expired CO_2 detected after an esophageal intubation, the CO_2 peak tension will be very low and will decrease rapidly with successive breaths. Although it is beyond the scope of this chapter, it should be noted that the ETCO2 value can be an indicator of effective cardiopulmonary resuscitation and correlates with outcome (see Chapters 37 and 38).[320-322]

Measurement of expired CO_2 tension is also helpful in detecting other clinical problems.[323] Clinically important air embolism causes a transient but marked reduction in CO_2 excretion because the lungs are ventilated but not perfused; hence dead space is suddenly increased (see Figs. 24.6 and 24.7). Quantitative measurement allows detection of the change in circuit flows, disconnections, tracheal tube kinking, or accidental extubations.[323,324] Rising end-tidal CO_2 with stable minute ventilation is an early clinical sign of an acute malignant hyperthermia reaction and the effectiveness of treatment (see Fig. 39.3).[324-326] The CO_2 waveform may also assist when diagnosing other types of respiratory

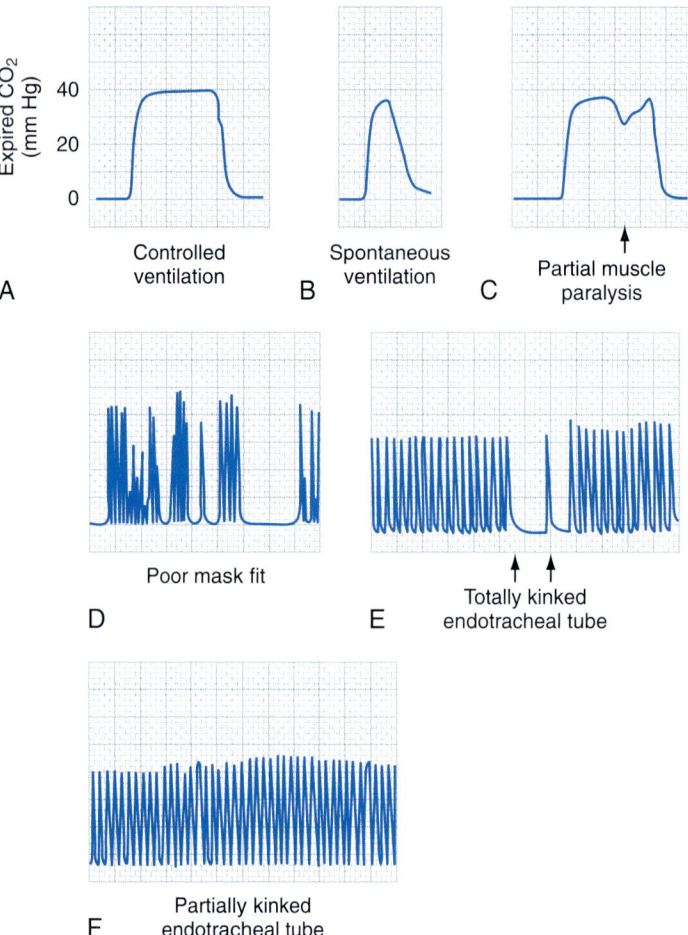

FIGURE 49.9 Expired carbon dioxide *(CO₂)* tracings (**A, B, C** = rapid recording; **D, E, F** = trend recording). **A,** Normal waveform with a long alveolar plateau indicating good alveolar gas sampling during controlled ventilation. **B,** Spontaneous ventilation with rapid respiratory rate; minimal alveolar plateau. **C,** Patient with partial muscle paralysis; note the change in the CO_2 waveform *(arrow)* during inspiration, which took place during the ventilator expiration. **D,** Poor mask fit with many periods when no CO_2 was detected; this also results in many false alarms. **E,** A totally kinked endotracheal tube was detected by the absence of a CO_2 waveform *(between arrows)*; a similar trace could result in a circuit disconnect, esophageal intubation, or a simple pause in respiration. **F,** A partially kinked endotracheal tube may result in a slow change in peak expired CO_2; a similar change could be noted with an unrecognized endobronchial intubation, change in pulmonary compliance, circuit leak, or increase in metabolic rate. The reverse would occur with air embolism, hypothermia (decreased metabolic rate), improved compliance, or, increased fresh gas flow without compensatory change in ventilator settings. (From Coté CJ, Liu LM, Szyfelbein SK, et al. Intraoperative events diagnosed by expired carbon dioxide monitoring in children. *Can Anaesth Soc J.* 1986;33[3 Pt 1]:315-320.)

difficulties (see Fig. 49.9).[327] Bronchospasm and its response to treatment may be identified by changes in the CO_2 waveform; bronchospasm causes an increasing slope of the plateau during expiration, and resolution of the bronchospasm restores the plateau to the horizontal (see Fig. 11.9). Routine use of $ETCO_2$ graphic trending on the anesthesia monitor is particularly useful in diagnosing small circuit leaks, partially kinked tracheal tubes, and rebreathing.[323] In children free from pulmonary shunts, the arterial and alveolar CO_2 values ($PaCO_2$ and $PACO_2$ [as reflected by a true end-expired sample]) should be within 2 to 3 mm Hg. The severity of a shunt or the diagnosis of a shunt may be made if this difference is greater than 5 mm Hg and if the CO_2 sensor is properly calibrated. Children with major pulmonary problems such as inhalation injury may have larger differences between arterial and expired CO_2 values. In such cases, expired CO_2 monitoring

may be used only for trending and as a disconnect alarm.[328] Expired CO_2 will be more accurate in assessing the adequacy of ventilation in children whose trachea is intubated compared with airway management with a facemask. However, even with a facemask the presence of bronchospasm and airway obstruction can be identified. During mechanical ventilation with an LMA, the accuracy of $ETCO_2$ monitoring approaches that of an endotracheal tube.[329] In very premature infants, the dead space imposed by the endotracheal tube and HME can markedly alter $ETCO_2$ traces due to inadequate alveolar gas sampling. In these patients, placing the sampling port as close to the ETT as possible, removing any unnecessary connectors, and considering using alternative humidification and filtering options to a standard HME are all important steps in retaining the utility of $ETCO_2$ monitoring in this particularly vulnerable population. This dead space can easily exceed the child's tidal volume, and lead to both substantial over- and underventilation.

TRANSCUTANEOUS CARBON DIOXIDE MEASUREMENT

Transcutaneous partial pressure of CO_2 ($PtcCO_2$) monitoring has been available for many years for use in preterm and full-term neonates but never achieved widespread acceptance in pediatric anesthesia. The monitor includes a heating element and a variant of the Severinghaus-type CO_2 electrode. Heating the skin increases capillary blood flow as well as the PCO_2 and oxygen. The skin becomes more permeable to diffusion of gas, and the gas tensions are measured by the sensors. CO_2 is calculated using a change in the pH sensed by the electrode. In turn, pH is proportional to the logarithm of the change in CO_2. Previously, transcutaneous monitoring was limited because of difficulties preparing and fixing the sensor, preparing the skin, needing to rotate the sensor to prevent burns, calibration time, and concerns for reliability. New transcutaneous monitors have eliminated some of the earlier technical difficulties. These newer versions can limit the temperature so they are less likely to burn children's skin[330]; they remain calibrated for greater intervals, and they appear to be more accurate. One study comparing expired CO_2 values versus transcutaneous CO_2 values in newborns without significant lung diseases who weighed 1000 to 3000 grams found greater precision and accuracy with expired CO_2 monitoring.[331] Another study reported an acceptable correlation with arterial CO_2 among several models[332]: TCM5 (Radiometer, Copenhagen, Denmark), and SenTec (Therwil, Arlesheim, BL, Switzerland). Because the skin must be heated, the CO_2 values are greater than the local arterial values owing to increased local metabolic production; these systems correct for this increase.

The most common use for transcutaneous monitoring has been in intubated premature neonates and small infants because the dead space of a mainstream CO_2 cuvette greatly increases the dead space for these small infants. Another circumstance for which transcutaneous monitors are used is for those who require high-frequency oscillatory ventilation.[333] In this case, it is not possible to monitor $ETCO_2$. There are also some clinical conditions in which $ETCO_2$ monitoring can be inaccurate and a transcutaneous monitor may be helpful.[334] These include uncuffed tracheal tubes with a large gas leak, high respiratory rates, significant cardiopulmonary disease associated with increased dead space and/or right-to-left shunt, conditions of frequent movement, and airway surgery requiring a shared airway approach. One clear disadvantage of $PtcCO_2$ is the lack of breath-to-breath monitoring capability for apnea and disordered breathing provided by end-tidal capnography.[335] $PtcCO_2$ monitoring may have a role in anesthetized children with severe pulmonary disease or other pathology that prevents accurate $ETCO_2$ measurement. These devices work less well where there is thickened skin or significant subcutaneous edema. There may be a role for these devices in the monitoring of nonintubated patients who are receiving sedation. However, nasal cannula sidestream CO_2 monitoring will provide more immediate identification of apnea or obstruction.

BLOOD LOSS MONITORS

Close observation of the surgical field is the best single monitor of blood loss. A small-volume trap on the suction line before the major evacuation trap is particularly useful to quantify blood loss in small children. Surgical sponges are often weighed on a dietary scale immediately after they come off the surgical field, assuming that 1 gram of weight is equivalent to 1 mL of blood, to assess the blood soaked up by the sponges. This minimizes the evaporative losses from the sponges. Point-of-care testing devices such as the HemoCue (HemoCue America, Brea, CA) and the i-STAT (Abbott Point of Care Inc., Princeton, NJ) rapidly assess hemoglobin values but each may underestimate the hematocrit at lower values. In addition to point-of-care testing, many ORs have blood gas analyzers such as the GEM Premier 3000 (Instrumentation Laboratory, Bedford, MA) that can provide hemoglobin measurements. One study that compared the two GEM Premier 3000 blood gas analyzers (BG-A & BG-B) and the HemoCue found that all three devices underestimated the hemoglobin values (when the hemoglobin was 6–10 g/dL), but that the HemoCue provided more reliable measurements than the other two point of care devices.[336] The accuracy of all of these devices is likely sufficient to follow trends and make decisions about the potential need for transfusion.[337,338] Noninvasive hemoglobin measurements using multiwavelength pulse oximetry in general may be useful only for trend monitoring.[245-248] Overall, these noninvasive devices underestimate hemoglobin values and may err up to 1 g/dL, thus limiting their value during rapid blood loss where more accurate measurements are essential.

NEUROMUSCULAR TRANSMISSION MONITORS

Clinical monitoring of the neuromuscular junction has been possible since the 1970s, with the development of the train of four (TOF) ratio by Hassan Ali, and has been thoroughly reviewed.[339] It is based on the comparison of the amplitude or magnitude of the first to the fourth stimulus applied to a nerve-muscle combination such as the ulnar nerve and thumb adductor pollicis. Ratios of >0.7 were previously thought to be associated with full recovery of muscle strength, but more recent evidence suggests a TOF ratio of >0.9 or even >0.95 is more closely associated with complete recovery of neuromuscular function in adults.[340] Residual or incomplete reversal of neuromuscular blockade is a common reason that adult patients are delayed in leaving the OR, may have prolonged postanesthesia care unit (PACU) recovery times, and develop respiratory complications in the early postoperative period.[341-345] Evidence confirms that even experienced anesthesiologists cannot assess the decrement in the TOF accurately without some other monitor. Clinical signs (e.g., sustained head lift) are often difficult to perform in younger children but even if they are, they may fail to uncover significant residual blockade, introducing the potential for respiratory complications.[342,343] In neonates and infants, flexion of the hips is analogous to the clinical signs of recovery of neuromuscular blockade in adults.[346]

The advent of sugammadex based reversal of aminosteroid neuromuscular blockade has resulted in changes in practice regarding monitoring of the neuromuscular junction and its reversal that are important to note.[347,348] A systematic review of 20 randomized clinical trials suggests that sugammadex is superior to neostigmine for reversal of neuromuscular blockade with rocuronium or vecuronium.[349] A systematic review of pediatric patients using sugammadex involving 10 studies with 580 patients found that sugammadex provided a more rapid reversal and lower incidence of bradycardia than neostigmine but no difference in residual blockade.[350] However, it is clear that routine use of neuromuscular junction monitoring in pediatric anesthesia is not very common, that the types of TOF monitors vary, and that the routine use of sugammadex is affected by its availability. Several types of neuromuscular monitoring devices are available for clinical use. Quantitative devices include mechanomyography, acceleromyography, and electromyography, together with variants of these based upon physical approaches (kinemyography, cuff-based techniques). Mechanomyography models use constant current nerve stimulation of a nerve together with measurement of the isometric force applied by the associated muscle, most often the adductor pollicis. These devices self-calibrate and then deliver a constant stimulus (30–70 mA) to the skin regardless of other influences. Failure to deliver a supramaximal stimulus may result in overestimation of twitch suppression. Acceleromyography uses a piezoelectric sensor to quantify the acceleration (proportional to force) of the thumb and converts it to an electrical signal. There is considerable disagreement in the published literature as to which of these devices is most accurate.[351–353] Monitors based on acceleromyography are becoming more commonly available and some consider these to be more accurate than mechanomyography-based TOF monitors. However, these monitors are not user-friendly and difficult to use in infants because of the small arc of the displaced thumb. Acceleromyography may generate TOF ratios of greater than 100% prior to administration of neuromuscular blockade, and thus correction for this baseline is required for an accurate assessment during the reversal phase.[354,355] This requirement for a baseline prior to administration of neuromuscular agent is practically difficult in the clinical environment, and thus a target TOF ratio of 1.0 is suggested when baselines are not obtained using acceleromyography monitoring.

Others regard mechanomyography as more accurate because it is less influenced by external disturbances; that is, it does not go out of calibration.[356] Mechanomyography is currently the simplest and most useful clinical monitor to assess the degree of paralysis when using NMBDs in infants and children (see also E-Figs. 5.15, 5.16 and 5.18). The TOF does not require recording capability or baseline measurement because it compares only the fourth twitch with its own internal standard, the first twitch.[357] The unit may also be used with depolarizing NMBDs, monitoring only the first twitch amplitude. A significant decrement ($>50\%$) between the first and fourth twitch in this context suggests phase II blockade (see E-Fig. 5.18).[358]

Electromyography utilizes measurement of the compound muscle action potentials following neural stimulation and this type of monitor is incorporated into some modern anesthesia workstations. It does not require the free movement of any muscle and can thus be used in many scenarios where direct physical transduction is difficult.

Needle electrodes should not be used in children because they may cause bleeding, infection, burns, or nerve injury; current density may be very high owing to the limited contact surface and the resistance of surrounding skin. Self-adhesive electrodes designed specifically for twitch monitors are available, but they are unnecessary, expensive, and tend to be too large for infants and small children. A reasonable alternative is a pair of infant-sized ECG electrodes. The choice of monitoring location depends on the nature of the surgery. It is preferable to select a site where a motor nerve is close to the body surface and its associated muscle group is available for observation. The most common site is the ulnar nerve in the forearm, observing the thumb movement (adductor pollicis brevis); this is the standard site for most research reports. Quantitating the response of other motor nerves is less reliable. Using the facial nerve may result in false-positive responses because the muscles may be directly stimulated, potentially leading to an overdose of NMBDs.

PROCESSED ELECTROENCEPHALOGRAM MONITORS

Accurately monitoring the depth of anesthesia during general anesthesia and sedation in children has been an elusive goal.

Clinically, we use endpoints such as loss of the eyelash reflex, loss of consciousness, and absence of limb movement in unparalyzed children as metrics of depth of anesthesia, but these are gross endpoints that do not measure potential awareness or other brain functionalities. Electroencephalogram (EEG), MRI, and functional Near-Infrared Spectroscopy (fNIRS) all quantify neural information but the processed EEG (pEEG) has advanced the most in this respect.[359,360] The EEG data displayed by our various monitors contain a large amount of information, including the raw EEG waveforms, spectral edge frequencies, EMG data, and other metrics. The processed numeric depth of hypnosis measurement (e.g., BIS/PSI/Narcotrend) serves to summarize this complex information in a single numeric for clinician use. Several devices have been developed to compile pEEG data for the clinician including the Bispectral Index monitor (BIS Brain Monitoring System, Covidien, Boulder, CO), the SedLine Brain Function Monitor (Masimo, Irvine, CA), Narcotrend (Narcotrend-Gruppe, Hannover, Germany), and the Entropy Module (GE Healthcare, USA). For each monitor, a sensor that detects EEG signals from the frontal lobe and motor cortex is placed on the forehead. These raw EEG (and EMG data in the case of Entropy) data are processed yielding a dimensionless number between 0 and 100 where 0 represents electroencephalographic silence or complete (isoelectric) suppression and 100 represents a patient who is fully awake. Each device uses a different proprietary algorithm,[361,362] that is based on a wide variety of signal processing and approaches over the past 3 decades in adults using isoflurane, but none included sevoflurane or children. More recently the algorithms were tested successfully with propofol. Although the pEEG sensors are available in pediatric sizes, the EEG changes with both age and development, especially in infants and neonates[363,364]; however, these developmental changes were not included in the algorithms.

Using the pEEG monitors in infants and children has presented a number of challenges. One study documented marked developmental changes in EEG patterns in children 0 to 3 years of age under anesthesia.[365] This undermines the reliability of these values in children, particularly in infants younger than 1 year of age.[365–370] The pEEG values in children are also reduced in children with developmental delay[371,372]; are greater with halothane than sevoflurane at equipotent MAC concentrations; paradoxically increase with values of expired sevoflurane concentrations greater than 3%;[373–376] and vary with adjuvant drugs such as opioids and benzodiazepines.[377,378] N_2O paradoxically increases the BIS value when added to equi-MAC concentrations of both sevoflurane and desflurane in adults,[379] but not during intravenous sedation.[380] Although nitrous oxide is partially additive to the MAC of desflurane and sevoflurane in children, N_2O actually increases the value in some devices. Loss of consciousness with dexmedetomidine during propofol sedation occurs at greater BIS values than during propofol alone[381]; ketamine also paradoxically increases the BIS value.[382] Curiously, NMBDs directly interfere with the BIS readings in adults; that is, both succinylcholine and rocuronium decreased the BIS immediately from values in the mid-90s to mid-80s and 70s and then after about 4 minutes to the 40s and 50s.[383] Comparable data in children are lacking. In summary, pEEG signal profiles differ in children according to age and the anesthetics administered, rendering interpretation of this metric more challenging and less reliable than in adults.

Apart from the processed numeric value representing anesthesia depth (BIS, PSI, State Entropy, etc.), EEG signals can be displayed in varying ways that may have clinical utility. Basic presentation of the raw EEG signals from one or more channels can be combined with use of a density spectral array to better comprehend changes in the frequency content of the EEG signals. Fig. 49.10 illustrates a density spectral array, or spectrograms of right and left brain activity and four channels of the bilateral EEG waveforms. The pEEG monitor from Narcotrend (Narcotrend-Gruppe, Hannover, Germany) shows the raw EEG, a letter A to E indicating the stage of anesthesia, a dimensionless number, and a cerebrogram. The Response and State Entropy monitor from General Electric (GE Healthcare, Helsinki, Finland) integrates the frontal EEG and electromyography signals to produce its value, which is loosely based on the concept of entropy being a measure of disorder or information content in a physical system.[362] With anesthesia, the EEG and motor activity decrease and the entropy decreases in parallel.

To recommend the use of pEEG monitoring for most pediatric anesthetic cases, we must be able to demonstrate that such use is reliable, predictable, and associated with a significant benefit or a reduction in adverse events. A number of outcomes have been studied in children and adults. In theory, by using pEEG monitoring, the aim is to prevent excessive anesthesia depth during surgery; the tangible benefits are a reduction in the time to emergence, extubation, PACU stay, and the amount of anesthetic agent used. In addition, such monitoring may indirectly decrease postoperative nausea and vomiting (PONV) rates given the dose-response relationship between volatile dose and PONV rates observed in adults.[384,385] Adult studies have also focused on the potential for reduction in delirium and cognitive decline.[386] Alternatively, the use of pEEG monitoring would ensure a sufficient depth of anesthesia to prevent the possibility of intraoperative awareness. Thus, on the one hand, an adequate depth of anesthesia is achieved, whereas on the other, a more rapid emergence may be established. pEEG monitoring has been used to decrease the time to emergence in adults[387] and children.[388,389]

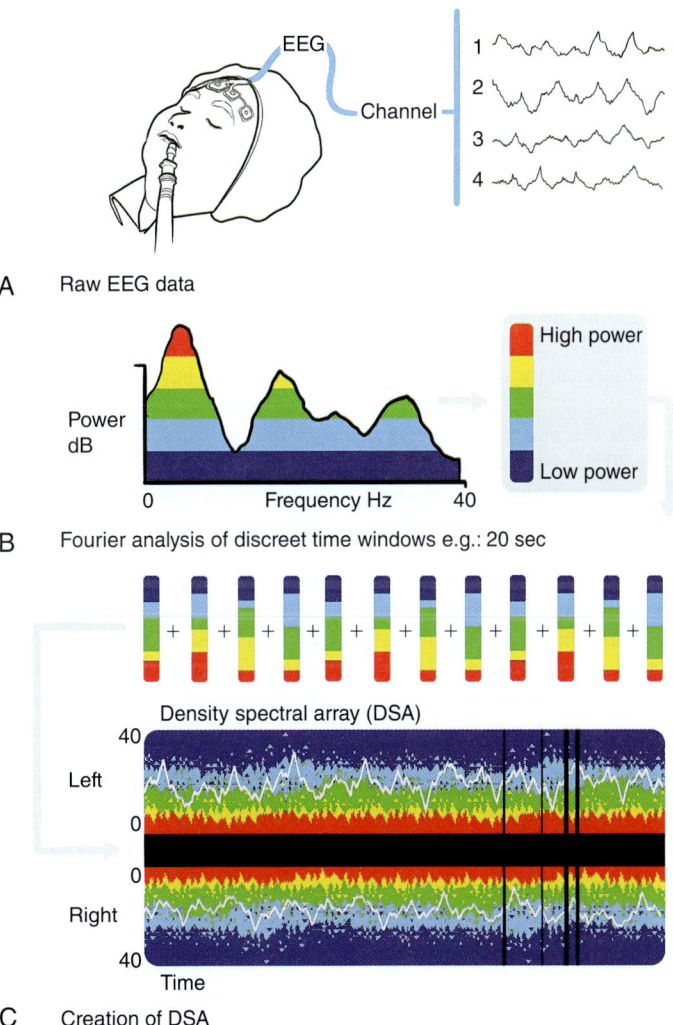

FIGURE 49.10 Density Spectral Array (DSA). **A,** Frontocortical electrodes collect raw EEG data on 1 to 4 channels. **B,** Fourier analysis of data transforms it into the frequency domain, allowing assessment of the relative contributions from different frequency bands (Delta=0–4 Hz, Theta=4–7 Hz, Alpha=7–12 Hz, Beta 12–30 Hz, Gamma=30–100 Hz). These are then color coded according to power (relative contribution). **C,** Each discrete analysis is then converted into a single strip with frequency along the y-axis, and color representing relative contribution. These strips are then linked together to create the DSA itself. This visually shows changes in frequency content of the EEG over time in a human readable format.

In adults, pEEG monitoring has decreased PONV[385]; no similar studies have been forthcoming in children. A meta-analysis showed a modest reduction in the consumption of anesthetic, PONV risk, and PACU time for adult ambulatory surgery but the cost savings were not greater than the electrodes and the monitors.[390] One additional issue that affects whether pEEG monitoring shows benefit is the type of anesthetic delivered; the only drug whereby pEEG provides consistent proven relationships with depth of anesthesia is propofol.[391–394] pEEG monitoring may have its greatest value as a monitor of depth of anesthesia during TIVA, for which an end-tidal anesthetic concentration for propofol is not currently available, although this may change in the future.[395,396] It remains unclear if this is true in younger children but certainly it may provide value in teenagers undergoing spinal instrumentation when motor evoked potential monitoring is required.

The use of cerebral monitoring to prevent intraoperative awareness in adults has been studied in several trials. The B-AWARE Trial (2004) showed a decrease in awareness in adults with the use of pEEG monitoring.[397] The B-Unaware Trial failed to find a decrease in frequency of awareness.[398] The BIS or Anesthesia Gas to Reduce Explicit Recall Clinical Trial (BAG-RECALL, 2008) also failed to confirm the superiority of the BIS over end-tidal anesthetic concentrations to prevent awareness.[399] The Michigan Awareness Control Study (MACS) (2012) was stopped for futility.[400] The TIVA Trial (2011) was intended to demonstrate the differences between inhaled anesthetics and TIVA, wherein you can monitor depth of anesthesia reasonably well with end-tidal anesthetic gas concentrations. The TIVA Trial (2011) concluded that BIS monitoring prevents awareness during TIVA,[401] but a secondary analysis of the data showed that there was an effect of midazolam on the participants (amnesia of the operating room in the B-Unaware and BAG-RECALL trials).[402] In hospitals where patients receive midazolam in the holding area, the majority do not remember events in the OR.

A smaller body of literature regards the risk of awareness for children undergoing anesthesia. In 2011, a secondary analysis of five pediatric cohort studies[403] was published investigating awareness.[404–408] The multivariable regression analysis showed that maintenance of anesthesia with N_2O and the use of a tracheal tube were independently associated with awareness, both curious findings since the former confers some amnesia and the latter implies use of an inhalational anesthetic. Interestingly, the incidence of awareness in these cohort studies averaged 0.74%, a frequency that exceeded the 0.1% to 0.2% reported in adults by severalfold.[409,410] In contrast to the adults who experienced awareness, none of the children in the earlier cohorts who had awareness reported distress, although 50% reported distress in the 5th National Audit Project (NAP5).[404,411–413] More recently, data from the Wake Up Safe collaborative[414] over a 10-year period reported 14 cases of self-reported awareness out of 555,360 cases (age 5–20 years), for an incidence of 1:40,000. This is substantially less that that from the previously mentioned cohort studies with different methodology, and is also less than the NAP5 reported overall incidence of accidental awareness of 1:19,600 (adults and children). Whether this represents a true lower rate of accidental awareness in pediatrics, or underreporting due to young patient age, immaturity, reluctance to report, or lack of comprehension of what an awareness episode means is unclear.

There is no evidence that pEEG devices decrease the frequency of awareness in children as 70% of the events in one report occurred at induction or emergence when the depth of anesthesia may not have stabilized.[413] The adult literature would indicate that there might still be a role for monitoring of pEEG in patients who are at high risk for recall (e.g., trauma patients and obstetric patients who require general anesthesia). A case could be made for their use in pediatrics, (e.g., for adolescents undergoing posterior spine fusion with a TIVA anesthetic that the clinician must often adjust during the case). In most instances, these patients are unparalyzed and monitored with motor evoked potentials, which requires deep levels of IV anesthesia to prevent movement. By the completion of surgery, recovery may be protracted because of the large amount of propofol infused, unless the dose was adjusted based on a pEEG monitor. Alternately, the anesthetic may need to be adjusted to perform a wake-up test and this too may be protracted if excess anesthesia had been administered. The use of pEEG monitoring or direct feedback from a skilled neurophysiologist who was monitoring the child can provide an indication of the depth of anesthesia. Other potential uses for pEEG monitoring may include neuroanesthesia and otorhinolaryngology. Finally, placement of the sensors on the forehead could interfere with the surgical site or sterile prep in some procedures involving the forehead and face.

Several other issues raised in an editorial identified the need for more specific outcomes after pEEG monitoring to clarify the potential benefits in children.[415] Currently, it appears that our outcomes focus on the times to removal of a tracheal tube, discharge from the PACU, or the frequency of adverse events. The numbers of children needed to study or treat to prevent an adverse outcome that is extremely rare are exceedingly large, rendering these studies unfeasible. Similarly, if we wish to monitor brain function during anesthesia, we may prefer to monitor an index of nociception.[416] The pEEG devices available today are limited to monitoring the frontal EEG and to detecting motor movement but not to detect nociception. New devices under development will monitor the entire brain, but they remain experimental at this time.

A more recent use of pEEG monitoring is to prevent "overdosing" of anesthetic.[417] In the context of concerns about the potential neurodevelopmental consequences of anesthesia at an early age (see Chapter 23) high degrees of EEG suppression are assumed to reflect very deep planes of anesthesia, perhaps too deep. Cornelissen et al. published a small single center observation of the incidence of discontinuity/isoelectricity noted in infants under GA,[369] noting an incidence of 51%. A large multinational observational study of the incidence of isoelectricity during pediatric anesthesia included 648 infants and showed a wide range of incidences (range 9% to 88%) with an average of 32%. They conclude that isoelectricity was common in young children undergoing anesthesia, and was associated with age and hypotension during anesthesia.[418] However, there is no evidence yet directly linking high degrees of isoelectricity in the EEG during noncardiac anesthesia with adverse outcomes, although that evidence does exist for isoelectricity associated with cardiac surgery in children.[419]

NOCICEPTION MONITORING

The monitoring of nociception during anesthesia has been limited to assessment of standard clinical measures such as heart rate, blood pressure, and respiratory rate; cortical assessment of the EEG is not capable of assisting with assessing adequate blockade of nociception. The subcortical structures involved in nociception link intimately with the autonomic nervous system, and it is the assessment of autonomic response to nociception via several techniques that has us closest to a "pain monitor."[420,421] These include skin conductance, heart rate variability, frequency domain analysis, photoplethysmography amplitude changes, and pupillary diameter changes.[422] Several of these have been assessed in children and adults[423–428] and although clear evidence of postoperative benefits are still to be found, early decreases in opiate usage and stress hormone levels have been shown. Their basic mode of operation is conceptually similar; variations in autonomic tone induced by painful stimuli are sensed using the above mentioned modalities, and a nociception index generated to summarize these changes for the clinician.[429] In addition to the signal transduction component, complex signal processing, exploration techniques are being used to assess these signals for useful nociception-related features, including deep learning networks and other machine learning approaches.[430]

CARDIAC OUTPUT MONITORING

Cardiac output monitoring for anesthesia and critical care has great potential value. We routinely consider the impact of various actions on cardiac output, but without an easy clinical ability to measure it. Multiple physiologic, pathophysiologic, and critical events and surgical interventions can affect preload, afterload, cardiac contractility, and heart rate and therefore decrease cardiac contractility and cardiac output (CO). Physicians have few monitors at their disposal to measure CO or systemic vascular resistance noninvasively.[431–433] The ideal device would be accurate for both individual and trend measurements compared with a gold standard, would be minimally or noninvasive, cheap, portable, and independent of operator technique and experience. Ideally, the accuracy of the device should be unaffected by changes in patient age and size, developmental physiology, position, or nature of the procedure (preterm infants to teenagers). Most current continuous CO monitors do not fulfill these criteria. Several techniques may be used to measure CO: indicator dilution, evaluation of the arterial pressure waveform, ultrasound, direct or indirect Fick method, and variations of bioimpedance.[434–438] These multiple different technologies provide CO measurements evaluated initially in adults and later in children. In some instances, this has been easily accomplished, whereas in others physiology and size vary so dramatically that they cannot be used in infants or small children.

The classic gold standard for the measurement of CO in humans is the direct Fick method. In this method, oxygen consumption ($\dot{V}O_2$) must be measured directly. The oxygen saturations of arterial and venous blood are measured to calculate arterial oxygen content (CaO_2) and venous oxygen content (CvO_2), respectively. CO is calculated using the formula:

$$CO = \dot{V}O_2/(CaO_2 - CvO_2)$$

Measurement of oxygen consumption at the bedside is still difficult, though modern infrared gas analyzers are rapidly approaching the accuracy of older mass spectrometers. The patient's trachea must be intubated without an air leak around the ETT.

A second gold standard for the measurement of CO is the pulmonary artery thermodilution (PAT) catheter. This method requires a catheter placed from a central venous location through the right atrium and ventricle into a pulmonary artery. Successful placement can be technically difficult, is associated with risks (embolism, pneumothorax, hemothorax, chylothorax, cardiac tamponade), and is infrequently used in the PICU. Pediatric use is now confined to limited cardiac surgical populations and during cardiac catheterization. Because of the limited use of Fick dilution in children, studies have compared a new method to measure CO with another new technique, which is not a gold standard; such comparisons limit the validity of the new techniques.[439] For devices that may be used for neonates, the accuracy of the CO monitors is usually confirmed in animal studies using ultrasonic flow probes placed around the pulmonary artery. These flow probes are very accurate and reproducible. However, the applicability of data from animal models to humans is fraught with pitfalls. With these limitations, pediatric studies of new devices include small sample sizes and are often not tested in children in whom the data would be of greatest value (e.g., those in shock [septic, hypovolemic, cardiogenic]).

Indicator Dilution (Cold Saline) Method

This technique is based on the Stewart-Hamilton equation, where flow is proportional to the amount of dye injected divided by the area under the concentration-time curve as the dye passes a detector. This is the principle used by PAT CO monitors to estimate CO. Cold saline solution may also be used as the indicator; it is injected into a proximal port of the catheter and then the temperature change is detected using a thermistor at the tip of the catheter. This is an invasive device as the catheter must be placed into the pulmonary artery. Furthermore, 5 to 10 mL of cold saline solution is used for each measurement, which is performed in triplicate. For repeated measurements, the fluid load can be substantial, particularly in neonates, infants, and critically ill patients who require fluid restriction. One means to eliminate or reduce the cold saline solution boluses is by using a thermal filament that intermittently heats the blood (Vigilance [Edwards Lifescience, Irvine, CA], Opti-Q [Abbott, Abbott Park, IL], truCCOMS [Omega Critical Care, East Kilbride, GB]).[440] With these devices the saline injectate is replaced by thermal energy as an indicator as the filament intermittently heats and cools. These catheters are also able to perform PAT measurements in the usual manner. However, even the size of the smallest catheters are so large that their use is limited to adolescents or adults.

Another strategy to reduce the fluid boluses is to use another means of CO measurement between calibrations (that may use cold saline solution) as in both the PiCCO (Pulsion Medical Systems, Munich, Germany) and the LiDCO systems (LiDCO, London, United Kingdom). The PiCCO system uses a combination of central venous and arterial access. Cold saline solution is injected in the central venous line and the dilution curve is measured from the arterial line. This technique is also referred to as transpulmonary thermodilution (TPTD) as the cold injectate traverses the right heart, lungs, and left heart before being measured, but their accuracy may depend in part on the size and locations of the catheter (central or peripheral).[441,442] The PiCCO devices also measure continuous CO using the arterial pressure-based continuous cardiac output technique (APCCO) (described later). The intermittent injections of cold saline solution are used to calibrate the APCCO measurements. TPTD systems are considered less invasive compared with PAT as they are typically performed with femoral central venous access and peripheral arterial access and do not require a catheter to transverse the heart. Furthermore, the arterial catheter can be used for normal BP monitoring and laboratory testing. However, the arterial catheter required is specific to the device manufacturer, which adds cost to the system. The TPTD technique has been validated in an animal model compared with perivascular flow probes as accurate and capable of tracking CO changes.[443] The TPTD technique using an earlier version of a Pulsion Medical System device (COLD Z-021, Pulsion Medical Systems) has been validated in children compared with the direct Fick method.[444,445] There is some evidence that TPTD can measure CO in subjects with left to right shunting. However, for the moment this appears to have been demonstrated only in animals. The LiDCO system uses a similar basic principle of operation but substitutes a small dose of lithium chloride as the indicator.

There is an additional CO monitoring device that uses an indicator dilution method but does not also incorporate APCCO. The Costatus Monitor from Transonic (Transonic, Ithaca, NY) uses an ultrasound dilution method to measure CO. The system connects the patient's existing arterial and central venous lines with an extracorporeal customized tubing set. During measurement, a pump circulates blood through the arterial to venous tubing loop. Ultrasound measurements are taken of the arterial to venous tubing loop and a bolus of warmed saline solution is given to the patient. The saline solution bolus will dilute the blood in the arterial to venous tubing loop, changing the velocity of the ultrasound signal. The ultrasound velocity of blood is 1560 to 1590 m/second depending on blood protein concentration. The ultrasound velocity of saline solution is 1533 m/second. The difference between the two values creates a conventional indicator dilution curve. The saline solution bolus given is diluted as it transverses the right heart, lungs, and left heart in the same manner as a TPTD measurement. The benefits of this device are the use of a low volume of warmed saline solution, reducing the risk for temperature changes and volume overload. A further advantage is that this system uses standard central venous and arterial catheters that may already be in place. The accuracy of the device has been demonstrated in animal models[446] and in children.[447–449] This device has been shown to be accurate in the detection of intracardiac shunts as a result of the characteristic changes that occur in the ultrasound dilution curve.[225,449,450] The device is limited to children with central venous and arterial catheters limiting its utility for the general population of anesthetized children. One concern, however, is that it requires recalibration during states of vasoconstriction or vasodilation, perhaps limiting its value when most needed.[451]

Arterial Pressure-Based Continuous Cardiac Output Monitors
This broad approach is based upon the work and formulas of the renowned physicist Karel H. Wesseling beginning in the mid-1970s.[452] When the heart contracts, the arterial pressure wave created by the stroke volume (SV) exiting the aortic valve is transmitted through the arterial tree, with the precise shape of the resulting pressure waveform affected by the characteristics of the vascular system at that point (total peripheral vascular resistance, aortic impedance, and compliance, etc.). Reversing this process, one can in principle calculate the stroke volume from a measured arterial waveform, by making assumptions about the same characteristics of the vascular system. These parameters of the vascular system such as aortic compliance changes not only with age but also with blood pressure and other factors. The arterial pressure waveform changes its morphology as it is transmitted from the aorta to the periphery, further complicating arterial pressure-based methods. Other influences include vasoactive medications, patient temperature, and volume status on vascular tone. From a pediatric standpoint, we must consider that these formulas or algorithms were generated in adults and then applied to children. The specific physiologic changes as a child grows and develops will likely change their accuracy and therefore their validity. The systems available can be divided into the those employing a separate technique to calibrate the system (PiCCO, LiDCOplus), with the aim of increased accuracy and precision, and those that do not employ calibration (LiDCOrapid, Flowtrac [Edwards Lifescience, Irvine, CA], PRAM [MostCare, Vytech, Padova, Italy]). For the

PiCCO system there has been some support that the accuracy of the device is sufficient for use in children,[453,454] although other investigators reported a large interindividual variability in the measurements obtained.[455] These conflicting results suggest that further studies are needed to validate the accuracy of this device in children. The LiDCO system refers to their APCCO method as PulseCO and the majority of validation studies have been in adults; only one pediatric study has demonstrated PulseCO to be accurate compared with PAT.[456] Two studies in children that compared FloTrac with PAT and the Fick technique respectively concluded that the FloTrac was inaccurate in children, with substantial overreading that worsened as CO increased.[457,458] The MostCare PRAM device has been shown to be accurate in children, though with weight-based influences in younger and older children.[459–462] As is common with these devices, accuracy and precision are higher in bigger, healthier children, and lower in sicker, smaller infants and neonates.

ULTRASOUND DETERMINATION OF CARDIAC OUTPUT
Ultrasound determination of CO includes 2D transthoracic evaluation of the size and flow through the aortic valve to determine stroke volume (SV), transesophageal ultrasound of the descending aorta to determine blood velocity, and transthoracic continuous-wave Doppler of the aortic or pulmonary valve determines velocity through the valve to determine SV. Transthoracic 2D echocardiography is frequently obtained for clinical needs. The cross-sectional area of the aortic valve is measured and the velocity of blood through the valve is recorded and then integrated as the velocity time integral (VTI). The area of the valve multiplied by VTI is the SV, and SV multiplied by heart rate is CO. Echocardiography as a technique to estimate CO has been extensively reviewed[463] and deemed to be sufficiently accurate that it is frequently used as the reference standard to compare with other methods of CO determination.[459,464–468] This technique requires considerable expertise and can only be applied intermittently. However, it does provide additional details of the structure and function of the heart, particularly in an ICU setting and the OR.

The velocity of blood moving in the descending aorta can be measured with an ultrasound probe that is positioned in the mid-esophagus. Once in place, the probe is directed to produce the maximum Doppler signal. If the cross-sectional area of the descending aorta is obtained from a nomogram, then the SV of blood flow to the lower half of the body is known. Calculations are made to adjust for the percentage of blood flow to the upper and lower portions of the body (crucial in younger patients) and the entire SV and then CO can be measured. Alternatively, without using the cross section of the descending aorta the VTI alone can be used. One system, EDM+ (Deltex Medical, Greenville, SC), has a pediatric probe for use in children who weigh 3 kilograms or more, are 50 cm or more in height, and younger than 16 years of age. The measurement of CO in children has been shown to be accurate[463,469,470] and predict fluid responsiveness.[471] Further studies have suggested measuring the velocity of blood flow in the descending aorta to improve accuracy. It appears that small changes in the angle between the ultrasound probe head and the descending aorta substantively change the VTI, thus requiring frequent adjustments to improve the measurements. The large size of the probe prevents it from being left in small children for a prolonged period. In addition, the presence of a nasogastric tube in the esophagus may alter the measurement. When properly used, this technique does seem to be accurate, although it requires frequent repositioning and is limited to intubated children.

Velocity through the aortic or pulmonary valve can also be measured with a continuous-wave Doppler and then VTI calculated from the output. The Ultrasonic Cardiac Output Monitor (USCOM 1A model) (USCOM, Sydney, Australia) is a portable device that uses a small continuous-wave Doppler probe to measure VTI through either the aortic or pulmonary valve. The USCOM software uses the patient's height to determine the area of the aortic or pulmonary valve from a nomogram. The valve area is multiplied by the VTI to SV and SV multiplied by heart rate to give CO. The device was demonstrated to be accurate in animal studies compared with ultrasonic flow probes[472]; it also was inaccurate compared with PAT in children with intracardiac shunting.[471] One study in neonates found an ~8 ± 7% difference between USCOM and echocardiography assessments.[473] Our experience differed in that we found that the device is accurate when compared with PAT in children without atrial or ventricular septal defects.[474,475] We found that the measurement technique was easy to learn with good interobserver variability. However, the measurements are intermittent, and the clinician must have access to the neck or thorax. Further studies will be needed to demonstrate the response to changes in CO to determine whether the USCOM can be used as a trending device.

Direct and Indirect Fick Measurement of Cardiac Output

CO can be calculated directly using the Fick equation:

$$CO = \text{Oxygen consumption}/(\text{Arterial oxygen content} - \text{Venous oxygen content})$$
$$\text{Oxygen content} = (\text{Saturation of oxygen} \times \text{Hemoglobin} \times 1.34 + [0.003 \times PaO_2])$$

During cardiac catheterization, samples of blood are drawn for arterial and mixed venous saturations and can be used to measure direct Fick CO. However, most catheterization laboratories do not measure oxygen consumption. Rather, they use a nomogram or formula to estimate oxygen consumption.[476,477] Oxygen consumption can be measured with a respiratory mass spectrometer,[478] which can produce extremely precise results. These mass spectrometers are exceedingly expensive and not widely available. Oxygen can also be measured using a photoacoustic infrared gas analyzer such as the Innocor monitor from Innovision (Innovision ApS, Glamsbjerg, Denmark). Oxygen consumption can be calculated breath by breath by measuring the difference between inspired and exhaled oxygen. Further, this same device has a system for inert gas rebreathing as a means of determining CO. If a patient has both arterial and venous access to measure oxygen content, CO can be measured directly. If the patient does not have these catheters, CO can be measured indirectly. During an inert gas rebreathing test the patient breathes from a rebreathing bag for approximately 5 breaths or 15 seconds. In the rebreathing bag is a known, measured, starting concentration of N_2O and sulfur hexafluoride. The N_2O is rapidly taken up by the blood and its rate of decrease in the bag is proportional to the blood flow to the lung. The blood flow to the lung is the effective pulmonary blood flow and in the absence of significant intrapulmonary shunt is equal to CO. The sulfur hexafluoride is not taken up in the blood and the change in its concentration in the bag is measured to determine the lung volume from which the N_2O was taken up. The oxygen consumption technique in the Innocor device yielded excellent correlations with the gold standard of measurement using a Douglas bag method[479] in children weighing more than 15 kilograms whose

airways were intubated.[480] Additionally, the dead space of the equipment is large for infants and small children, which could limit the ability to perform the test. Although it is a noninvasive technique, a further limitation is that the inert gas rebreathing technique is intermittent, and it requires an intubated patient.

CO can be measured indirectly by using a modification of the Fick equation. In this case, partial rebreathing of CO_2 is used in place of oxygen consumption.

$$CO = VCO_2/(CvCO_2 = CcCO_2)$$

In brief, the amount of oxygen entering the lungs is directly proportional to the pulmonary blood flow. In the same way, the amount of CO_2 leaving the lungs is proportional to pulmonary blood flow. If there is limited intrapulmonary shunting, then the amount of pulmonary blood flow equals CO. During a measurement with the NICO device the dead space of the breathing circuit is temporarily increased. During that period, there is a change in the elimination of CO_2 ($\Delta\dot{V}CO_2$) and a rise in the $PETCO_2$. Pulmonary blood flow is calculated from the above formula.

A newer approach to CO_2 based CO monitoring (called dynamic capnography) utilizes similar basic methods to the aforementioned, estimating $CcCO_2$ from exhaled CO_2 analysis with VCO_2 and $CvCO_2$ largely constant during the short window of measurement. Measurements of $CcCO_2$ are done during stable ventilation for 6 breaths at an I:E ratio of 1:2, and then repeated during 3 breaths with an extended respiratory pause. This acute but short change in alveolar ventilation allows calculation of CO from the solution of the differential Fick equation.[481] Dynamic capnography has been validated in an animal model using flow probes and pulmonary artery thermodilution, showing excellent agreement and trending,[482] and shows promise in infants in clinical situations.[483]

Bioimpedance, Electrical Cardiometry, and Bioreactance

Thoracic electrical bioimpedance (TEB) is a means of using the changes in electrical conductivity of the blood flow in the aortic arch to determine SV and in turn CO. A low-amplitude, high-frequency alternating electrical current is passed through the thorax and the impedance is measured. Small changes in the volume of the aorta within the thorax during the cardiac cycle results in a change in impedance, allowing calculation of SV using some assumptions. The theory and technique is several decades old[484] and had many problems that led to inaccuracies. There have been marked improvements in bioimpedance measurements and are referred to as electrical cardiometry (or as electrical velocimetry). Electrical cardiometry also uses skin sensors to impart high-frequency current into the thorax and measure the change in impedance. This system takes advantage of the difference in thoracic impedance that occurs owing to the arrangement of red blood cells during the cardiac cycle. During diastole, the red blood cells in the heart and aorta are in a random orientation (chaotically oriented) and the electrical resistance is increased. During systole, the red blood cells are in motion and are therefore aligned (parallel oriented) and the electrical resistance is lower. The computer algorithms derive peak acceleration of blood in the aorta, the duration of left ventricular ejection, and then the velocity of blood flow, which then determines the SV. The Osypka Medical Company (Osypka Medical Inc., La Jolla, CA) has two products that measure CO through electrical cardiometry. The Icon model is a handheld, battery-operated, portable monitor. The Aesculon model incorporates the electrical cardiometry measurement but is a complete hemodynamic monitoring system; common settings are to record measurements at 10 second intervals that average the prior 20 heart beats. The Aesculon incorporates pulse oximetry, noninvasive BP, and so on, and provides data storage for research. In several studies using either the Icon or the Aesculon to measure CO, the latter was shown to be accurate compared with Fick determinations and PAT even in neonates.[465,485–487] In children after a Fontan palliation for congenital heart disease[488,489] and in a general OR setting,[244,490] the Aesculon provided valuable clinical information. The unique value of the device is that it requires application of only four standard ECG electrodes and no other special equipment (Figs. 49.11 and 49.12). This device is approved for use even in neonates.

Bioreactance is another noninvasive technology that measures CO (Nicom [Cheetah Medical, Newton Center, MA]). This device also passes an electrical current through the thorax; it evaluates the phase shifts that occur as the resistance and reactance of the thorax change during the cardiac cycle. Phase shifts or time delays between the applied current and measured voltage occur as a result of the pulsatile blood flow in the larger arteries of the thorax. The phase shifts are used to estimate SV and therefore CO. The accuracy of the Nicom model has been demonstrated in adults[491,492] and neonates,[467] but the pediatric trials have limitations. One study[493] showed that the CO measurements were in a range appropriate for the patients being studied, although no reference standard for CO was included. Studies have been conflicting regarding whether Nicom could predict fluid responsiveness.[494,495] One pediatric study (mean age of ~5 years, weight 17 kilograms) compared this device with transesophageal Doppler; they concluded that "bioreactance cannot be considered suitable for monitoring pediatric patients."[496] This device is not approved for use in children, although studies are ongoing.

Purchasing Anesthesia Equipment

With the increasing sophistication of monitoring and life support equipment, purchasing decisions are no longer intuitive. A complete grounding in the underlying engineering concepts would probably require an advanced degree in engineering, but a reasonable working knowledge of the operating principles, advantages, and special hazards of the various types of apparatus is relatively easy to obtain. Most hospitals now have a full-time biomedical professional staff, who often have considerable engineering and practical experience to assist in the purchasing, maintenance, and safety of all the equipment and systems used in the hospital setting. The biomedical professionals should be closely integrated into the purchasing, maintenance, and ongoing safety monitoring of all devices. Although vendors are pleased to promote a product, the manufacturer's information literature should be obtained from an unbiased source such as the equipment periodical *Health Devices*, published by ECRI (formerly Emergency Care Research Institute, Plymouth Meeting, PA). The biomedical or hospital safety office of each hospital usually subscribes to this periodical.

Another useful source of information is the specialty pediatric hospital. Whether through inquiry at medical meetings or by direct solicitation, practitioners at these unique resource institutions are often willing to share their special expertise.

The following are useful principles for any equipment purchase:

1. New purchases should interface with equipment that is already present. Considerable cost savings can occur if the same or compatible equipment is used in all the perioperative areas, including the OR, PACU, PICU, and NICU. Another issue to consider is how the equipment will interface with automated record-keeping systems and other hospital information systems if they are present. If an automated recording device is a possible, plan for the future; the equipment should be evaluated for how well it will interface with systems that will possibly be purchased. Another compatibility issue to carefully review is the software required to use the equipment. Review the product information carefully to identify the need for software upgrades and compatibility, which can be important for safety and cost-effectiveness.

2. Recognize that the salesperson is inherently biased.

3. Always test proposed equipment in the environment in which it will be used, with the personnel who will be using it. What appears attractive in a display as presented by a salesperson may not function well in practice. It is also important to test the device in unusual circumstances to see how well it performs. The use of simulation is becoming an important modality to test devices under normal and unusual circumstances. Human

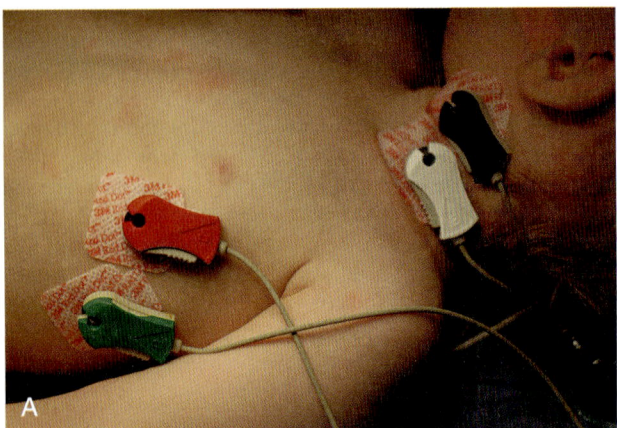
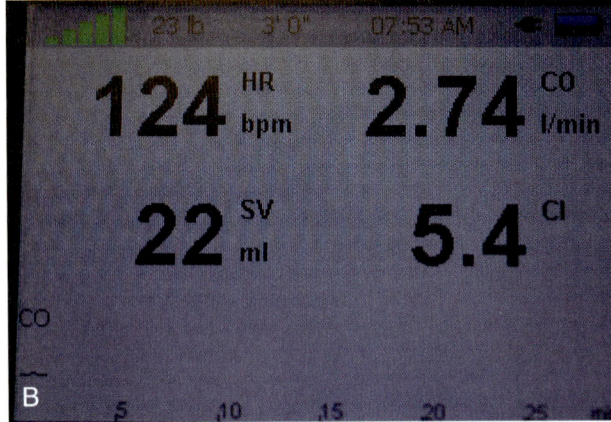

FIGURE 49.11 A, Cardiotronic Icon cardiac output device. The only additional equipment is four standard electrocardiogram (ECG) pads placed according to the manufacturer's instructions (Adult: two on left side at the level of xiphoid depression; two on the left neck over the carotid artery; Neonate: one on the left cheek or forehead, one over the left carotid artery, one on the left side at level of xiphoid depression, and the fourth on the left leg). **B,** Electrical cardiometry continuously estimates cardiac output (*CO*), cardiac index (*CI*), stroke volume (*SV*), stroke index, and a variety of other parameters through quantitation of changes in impedance associated with changes in the orientation of red blood cells. During diastole, red blood cells are organized chaotically, but during systole they assume a position parallel to the direction of blood flow. Thus thoracic electrical bioimpedance relates to changes in thoracic aortic blood flow, and by using refined algorithms noninvasive measurement of continuous cardiac output with four ECG pads is achieved. *bpm,* Beats per minute; *HR,* heart rate.

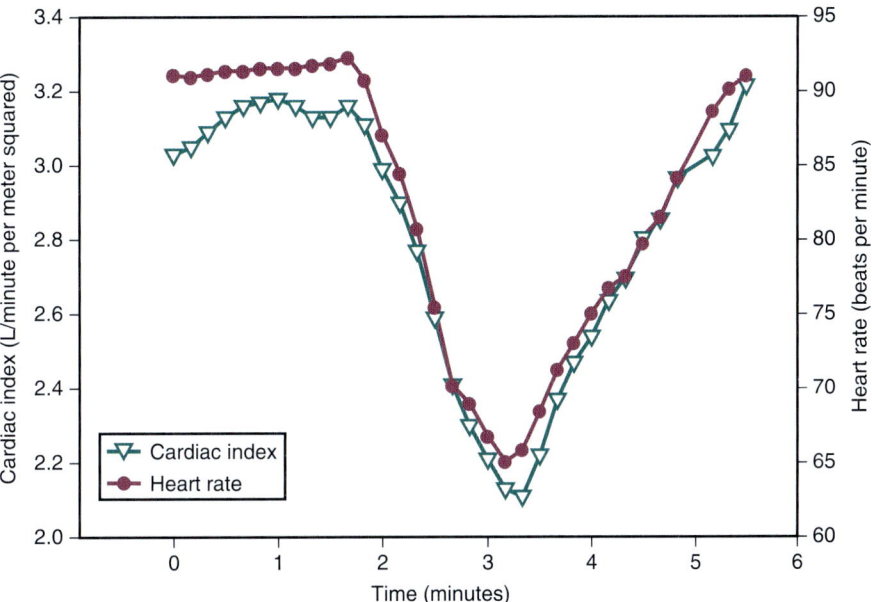

FIGURE 49.12 This graph plots the continuous cardiac index versus heart rate in a 6-year-old child undergoing a posterior fossa procedure. The bradycardia occurred with surgical brainstem irrigation with saline solution that was not adequately warmed. The Icon model averages data from the prior 20 heart beats and records this every 10 seconds. Data plotted here are the average for the six values during each minute of the event. In this case, we asked the surgeon to stop irrigating and administered atropine (0.02 mg/kg). Note how the Icon immediately tracked the improved cardiac index as the atropine took effect.

factors must be considered, such as how easy it is to use the equipment clinically (i.e., the user interface), and equally important, the safety of the equipment or product. Evaluate systems issues that could lead to error or misuse. Software-driven products are harder to test for potential failures when they are connected to existing systems and products in your workstations; always test new equipment in the environment where it will be used.

4. Do not use equipment for any purpose other than that for which it has been designed.

5. Have your hospital biomedical staff be intimately involved with the safety issues of your systems and periodically check for electrical leakage and other safety issues.

6. Decide explicitly how the product will be maintained. Will the biomedical professionals perform the necessary calibration, testing, and repair of the equipment, or will a member of your department assume this role? Spend the necessary resources to properly maintain the product; this is typically on the order of 10% of the cost of the device per year. Consider a maintenance contract, if available. Ask the company to ensure the future availability of parts and the compatibility of subsequent modifications or design evolutions with your equipment.

7. Consider the cost of disposable components; this can significantly impact costs.

8. If two products are comparable but one has local service facilities, that one may be the better choice.

9. If areas of special needs have been recognized, be as detailed as possible with specifications. For example, if a monitor is to be used strictly in the OR, it may be reasonable to operate it from wall power. Conversely, if the monitor is to serve in the OR and for transport between the OR and the recovery room or ICU, it must have internal battery backup.

The more precisely needs can be defined, the more accurate the comparisons will be between the bids of rival vendors. Note that any given piece of equipment will occasionally be out of service, whether for regular preventive maintenance or for some unanticipated repair. Given this fact, in this era of cost containment it is often difficult to convince the hospital administration of a need for additional spare units.

ANNOTATED REFERENCES

Cook TM, Wilkes A, Bickford Smith P, et al. Multicentre clinical simulation evaluation of the ISO 80369-6 neuraxial non-Luer connector. *Anaesthesia.* 2019;74(5):619-629.

The introduction of new connectors (epidural, etc.) in anesthesia is underway, and this article describes the evaluation of the neuraxial connector, in a series of simulations across several different procedures in anesthesia. It clearly describes the neuraxial connectors, and their assessment, and is an excellent resource for departments beginning this transition.

McGain F, Muret J, Lawson C, Sherman JD. Environmental sustainability in anaesthesia and critical care. *Br J Anaesth.* 2020;125(5): 680-692.

The disproportionately high carbon footprint of anesthesia is increasingly clear, and this review provides an excellent introduction to the field. It addresses the unique contributions of the volatile agents and nitrous oxide to the problem, covers the topic of life cycle assessments as a tool to understand and quantify the ecological footprint of various aspects of anesthesia, and provides the reader with a clear background as to how these are important to effective action in this area.

Murphy GS, Brull SJ. Quantitative neuromuscular monitoring and postoperative outcomes: a narrative review. *Anesthesiology.* 2022; 136(2):345-361.

Renew JR, Tobias JD, Brull SJ. The time to seriously reassess the use and misuse of neuromuscular blockade in children is now. *Anesth Analg.* 2021;132(6):1514-1517.

These two articles, one specific to pediatrics, present a very thorough and up-to-date summary of the monitors themselves, the clinical issues they address, and modern conundrums related to using reversal agents such as sugammadex.

Navaratnam M, Dubin A. Pediatric pacemakers and ICDs: how to optimize perioperative care. *Paediatr Anaesth.* 2011;21(5):512-521.

Unless one works in cardiac anesthesia routinely, exposure to pacemakers and ICDs is usually very intermittent, and this practical article is a great single point resource to assist pediatric anesthesiologists with these cases.

Stein ML, Park RS, Kovatsis PG. Emerging trends, techniques, and equipment for airway management in pediatric patients. *Paediatr Anaesth.* 2020;30(3):269-279.

This review article covers the current cutting edge of equipment and procedures related to difficult airway management in pediatrics, including video laryngoscopy, hybrid approaches to difficult airways, use of supraglottic airways, and methods of oxygen delivery including passive oxygenation.

Weber F, Scoones GP. A practical approach to cerebral near-infrared spectroscopy (NIRS) directed hemodynamic management in noncardiac pediatric anesthesia. *Paediatr Anaesth.* 2019;29(10):993-1001.

Exactly how to properly use NIRS requires that clinicians have some degree of experience. This pragmatic and clear guide to its use in pediatrics provides beginners and more experienced users with a focused approach template.

A complete reference list can be found online at Elsevier eBooks+.

Simulation in Pediatric Anesthesia

50

A. REBECCA L. HAMILTON, JEFFREY B. COOPER, AND CHRISTINE L. MAI

Simulation-Based Training in Anesthesia
What Is Simulation?
Technologies Used in Simulation
Partial Task Trainers
Human Patient Simulators
Standardized Patients
Hybrid Simulation
Screen-Based Simulator: Virtual
Reality and Immersive Environments
Sites for Simulation

Applications of Simulation in Perioperative Pediatric Education
**Comparing Traditional Learning with Simulation-Based
Learning**
Aspects of a High-Fidelity Simulation
What is a Debriefing?
Using Simulation for Evaluation
Simulation for Other Uses
Challenges in Using Simulation
Future of Simulation

THE FIELD OF PEDIATRIC anesthesiology has become increasingly subspecialized, with unique challenges for medical educators to provide high-quality, consistent clinical instruction. Teaching and training sessions traditionally held in the operating room (OR) have expanded to out-of-OR locations in parallel with the advent of technology and minimally invasive procedures. Furthermore, growing case volumes and fast turn-over requirements create time pressure, which results in limited didactic opportunities. This certainly applies to the field of pediatric anesthesiology, which has seen a steady rise in procedural sedation cases in remote locations such as the intensive care unit, endoscopy, and interventional radiology suites, locations where critical events are more frequently encountered than in the main OR.[1,2] Additionally, tertiary pediatric services are often centralized to academic centers, decreasing the exposure to clinical educational opportunities, challenging cases, and pediatric emergencies during anesthesiology training.[3,4]

As a response to these challenges, medical simulation programs have provided an experiential learning paradigm for training and assessment since the first practical computer-controlled mannequin was introduced in 1990.[5–8] Anesthesiologists were pioneers in adopting this new technology and developing this field of simulation education, providing opportunities to improve medical knowledge, strengthening communication skills, and enhancing clinical decision making for common as well as rare events.[9–11] Simulation programs have since become an integral part of anesthesiology training and continuing education in the United States and around the world. Simulation societies such as the American Society of Anesthesiologists (ASA) Simulation Education Network* promote the exchange of knowledge and implementation experiences in education, as well as other purposes such as health systems evaluations and interdisciplinary team building.[12] Simulation training played an important role for pandemic preparedness during the COVID-19 pandemic,

demonstrating that experiential learning provided valuable opportunities for emergency preparation.[13–15]

Medical simulation programs can play a central role in anesthesiology training, whether in the OR, in remote locations, or preparing for emergency scenarios. Because crises in pediatric anesthesia are relatively rare and unpredictable, simulation education is valuable in filling the need for deliberate practice and addressing performance gaps specific to pediatric patients.[16] In this chapter, we review how simulation is applied in pediatric anesthesiology by describing its key technologies, its uses for learning and practicing clinical skills, performance evaluation, teaching approaches, and other applications.

Simulation-Based Training in Anesthesia

Interest in simulation in health care derived from the historic utility of simulation for training in nonmedical industries, such as commercial aviation, nuclear power production, and the military.[17] Similar to health care, these industries are known to be associated with hazards and complexities that benefit from simulation training. Many of the concepts in health care simulation education, including systematic training, rehearsals, performance assessment, situational awareness, and team interactions, have been adopted from the aviation industry and its work with flight simulators.

Gaps in decision making and crisis management during anesthesia training were identified and diagnostic decisions were found to be inflexible relative to the clinical context over 35 years ago.[18,19] To reconcile this schism, Gaba and colleagues at Stanford University developed the *anesthesia crisis resource management* (ACRM) program based on the commercial aviation model, crew resource management (CRM).[20,21] A framework was created to train anesthesiologists in individual and team leadership skills and the use of effective communication practices. In its early years, ACRM focused on providing anesthesia trainees with tools that were similar to those that made the complex dynamic world of aviation safer via CRM. The development of anesthesia simulators and simulated clinical settings became critical in the implementation and growth of ACRM as trainees were exposed to cases that

*(https://www.asahq.org/education-andcareer/educational-and-cme-offerings/simulation-education)

challenged them in diagnostic problem solving, fixation errors, and teamwork.[20]

ACRM was an outgrowth of the patient safety movement that began in anesthesiology in the United States in the early 1980s. In the late 1980s, research funding from the Anesthesia Patient Safety Foundation (APSF) supported the development of several forms of human patient simulators (HPS). Further publicity and advocacy from the APSF propelled anesthesiology to the forefront of specialties in the application and adoption of simulators, with strong patient safety implications through education (residents attempting new skills for the first time on a mannequin), training (teamwork, critical event management, and situational awareness), and research (human performance).[22] Today, simulation in anesthesiology is a global endeavor, with emphasis not only on medical knowledge and skills training, but also on ACRM, disaster training, debriefing, and other patient safety applications. To become a board-certified anesthesiologist in the United States, candidates are now required to pass a simulation-based Objective Structured Clinical Examination (OSCE). To maintain their certification over time, US anesthesiologists are required to complete the Maintenance of Certification in Anesthesia (MOCA) program. A simulation-based course at a simulation center that is endorsed by the American Society of Anesthesiologists or an online simulation requirement are two key options to fulfill that requirement.[5] In some institutions, such training is required as a condition of credentialing for practice and insurance coverage.

What Is Simulation?

Simulation is a *technique* to replace or amplify real experiences with guided experiences that evoke or replicate aspects of the real world. Simulation is enabled by a diverse set of emergent *technologies*.[17] The application of simulation in health care is focused primarily, but not exclusively, on education and training of clinicians. *Education* emphasizes knowledge, skills, and introduction to the actual work. *Training* emphasizes the actual tasks and work to be performed.[17] The term "simulator" is used in health care to refer to a device that replicates many features of a patient and interacts appropriately in response to the actions of the learner. In aviation, pilots are trained in a full feature simulator while seated in the cockpit of a flight simulator. Likewise, in health care, clinicians are in a simulated OR, emergency room, or health care setting, providing care for a simulated "patient" experiencing a critical event or simply providing routine patient care.

Participants in a simulation are "immersed" into a task or setting to the extent necessary to achieve the learning objectives.[23] This may be conducted in a normal classroom or in an environment that extensively replicates the real world. When the learning objectives require it, the instructor prepares an engaging simulation scenario and the participant attempts to care for the "patient" as if it were a real person.[22] This is best enabled by having trainees enter into a "fiction contract" with the simulation instructor, agreeing to accept that they will act as best they can as if the situation were real. Most importantly, it is incumbent on those who create and implement the simulation to create sufficient *realism* to enable the learner to feel the authenticity of the situation and respond accordingly.[22,24]

Participants in a simulation scenario experience *realism* in three distinct domains: *physical, conceptual, and emotional*.[22] Simulations that address all three domains are more likely to instill the intended learning objectives. The level of realism needed in each domain should be appropriate to the specific learning objectives; too little simulation for objectives where it is called for may prevent sufficient

learner engagement; too much realism, such as engaging emotions when teaching basic skills, can be distracting.

The *physical* properties of the simulator (the patient) such as weight, flexibility, tensile strength, and color, are important for developing kinesthetic awareness and muscle memory. For example, the weight of the head and force required to effectively perform laryngoscopy are important for teaching tracheal intubation, whereas the rubbery feel of the mannequin skin is not. *Conceptual realism* refers to the causal relationships observed in the scenario, such as a decrease in oxygen saturation during a period of apnea or the resolution of hypotension after an appropriate intravenous fluid bolus. High conceptual reality enhances clinical reasoning and decision making. Finally, *emotional* and *experiential* fidelity is achieved when participants experience familiar and authentic feelings, such as "emotional activation," anxiety, stress, fear, or excitement. Ultimately, realism in simulation is perceived as "an exciting simulation that captures the imagination, triggering physiological responses and execution of ingrained clinical algorithms."[22] Although realism is important, it has been said that, *"when learning is the focus, the flawless recreation of the real world is less important"*[24]; it is necessary to find circumstances that help participants learn, rather than circumstances that exactly mimic a clinical situation.[24] The degree of realism desired for a successful simulation education program is an amount sufficient to achieve the intended learning outcomes.

Technologies Used in Simulation

PARTIAL TASK TRAINERS

Partial task trainers are mannequins or models designed to allow participants to practice clinical skills and tasks (Fig. 50.1). They should be reliable, robust, and medically meaningful. They usually represent a portion of a person rather than the whole. Although many are simple devices designed for learning or practicing a specific procedure (e.g., suturing, IV insertion, arterial line placement, laryngoscopy, cricothyrotomy, or intraosseous access), some are coupled with computers, robotic interphases, and digital graphics to provide sophisticated partial task simulators designed for learning or practicing more involved procedures (e.g., bronchoscopy and endoscopy, endovascular catheterization, or laparoscopic skills). These models are particularly useful for teaching invasive, risky, and rare procedures (e.g., emergency cricothyrotomy, transvenous pacing, or pericardiocentesis), complex psychomotor skills requiring repetitive training (e.g., ultrasound-guided central venous catheterization), or those that are safe, but create increased anxiety for either the learner or the patient and their family (e.g., urethral catheterization, caudal block, IV insertion, or arterial puncture).

Task trainers are frequently used in pediatrics to practice pediatric endotracheal intubation, lumbar puncture, caudal block placement, and neonatal cardiopulmonary resuscitation (CPR) (see Fig. 50.1).[25,26] The use of partial task trainers in a simulation environment is conducive for coaching and deliberate practice[27] with an increased knowledge-acquisition in these simulation-enhanced training models.[28] Curricula that use these types of devices focus on skills training at varying levels of skill-oriented goals, rather than a particular situation. For example, cricothyrotomy training on a partial task simulator aims to teach the procedure, regardless of the indication (e.g., angioedema, burns, obstructing mass, or hemorrhage; see Video 50.1). In the context of skills training, there is evidence that Simulation-Based Mastery Learning can improve patient outcomes.[7] Although there are partial task trainers commercially available for many invasive

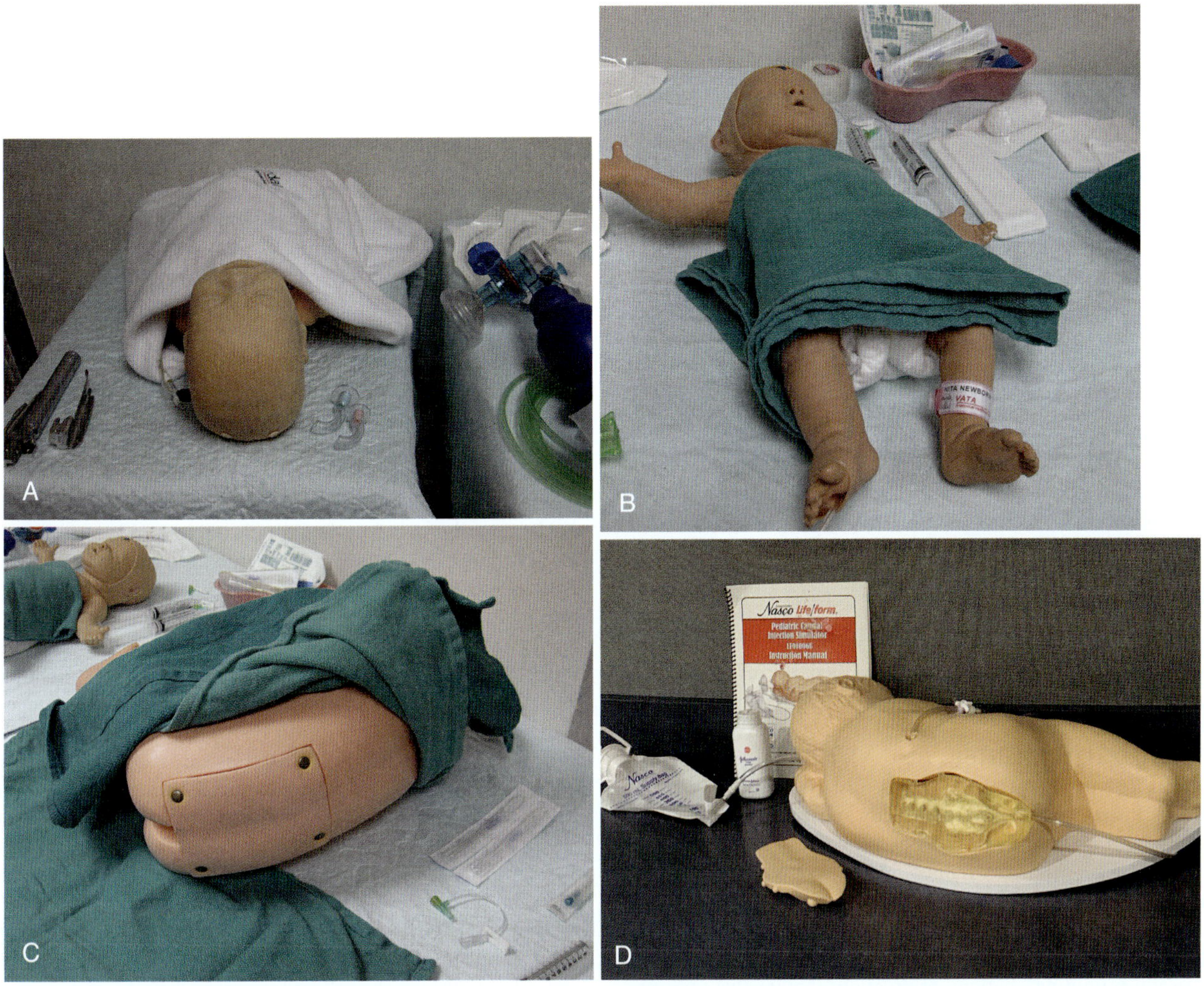

FIGURE 50.1 Examples of partial task trainers to practice intubation in neonates **(A)** (Laerdal SimNewB, Laerdal Medical, Stavanger, Norway), peripheral intravenous placement **(B)** (Nita Newborn Model #1800 Infant Venous Access Simulator, VATA, Canby, OR), lumbar puncture **(C)** (M43C Pediatric LP Simulator, Kyoto Kagaku, Kyoto, Japan) caudal injection **(D)** (Nasco Life/Form Pediatric Caudal Injection Simulator, Fort Akinson, WI).

procedures, simulation education faculty and operations specialists may sometimes design and produce more cost-efficient models to teach practice procedures, such as neonatal intubation models in rural medical education,[29] postpartum hemorrhage models in low-resource settings,[30] or even the use of meat glue to create inexpensive nerve block models for trainees.[31,32]

HUMAN PATIENT SIMULATORS

An HPS is a representation of the human body constructed on a mannequin, typically made of plastic and metal, without a bony skeletal frame. Although popularized in the 1990s, the first mannequin-based simulator (SimOne) was developed at University of Southern California in the 1960s and was intended to facilitate medical education and training.[33] Adult HPSs became commercially available in the early 1990s; the first high-fidelity pediatric simulator was introduced in 1999. This was followed by the METI PediaSIM (CAE Healthcare, Sarasota, FL) representing a child between 5 and 7 years of age; two models of integrated infant HPS eventually became available in 2005: the METI BabySIM and the Laerdal SimBaby (Laerdal Medical, Stavanger, Norway) (Fig. 50.2). Both models exhibited standard vital signs and variable airway

features (e.g., tongue swelling and laryngospasm), breathing patterns and sounds (e.g., to illustrate upper airway obstruction, wheezing and pneumothorax), cardiovascular features (e.g., heart sounds and peripheral pulses [diminished or absent]), and others (e.g., abdominal sounds and distension, fontanelle bulging). Both infant simulators produce a variety of monitor signals and allow extensive treatment interventions (e.g., intubation, laryngeal mask and nasogastric tube insertion, chest compressions, intravenous and intraosseous cannulation, and thoracocentesis).[34]

Incorporated into the clinical setting or in a simulation room outfitted with biomedical equipment and teams of health care providers, the high-fidelity HPS can provide a higher degree of clinical authenticity compared to its predecessors (see Video 50.1). Today's HPS models are highly advanced compared with the original SimOne, offering a range of physical features that mirror complex clinical encounters. Some models are preprogrammed to react to certain types of treatment whereas others are remotely controlled for interactive simulation scenarios.[35] In pediatrics, the most commonly used HPSs are designed to provide an accurate anatomical representation of the pediatric population at different ages, from premature neonates to adolescents,

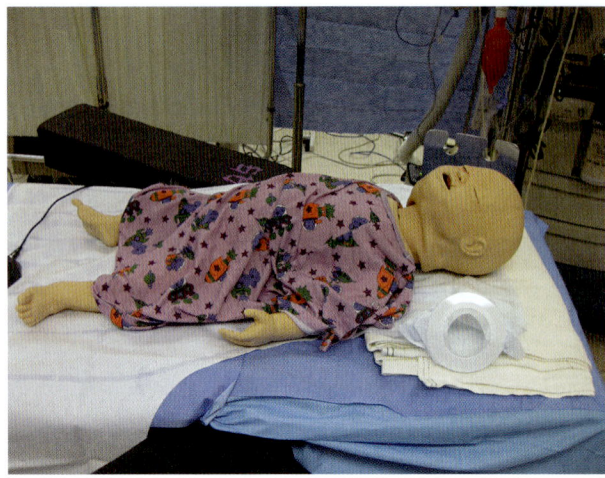

FIGURE 50.2 An infant human patient simulator (Laerdal SimBaby Laerdal Medical, Stavanger, Norway) exhibits standard vital signs, variable airway features (tongue swelling, laryngospasm), breath sounds (retraction, wheezing), cardiovascular features (palpable pulses, heart sounds), and others (abdominal sounds, bulging fontanelle).

and the simulation scenarios are designed to reflect realistic clinical challenges encountered both in and outside the OR.[36]

STANDARDIZED PATIENTS

Standardized patients (referred to as SPs; the term "embedded simulated participants" [ESPs], formerly known as "confederates," has also been used for some types of roles that SPs play) are amateur or professional actors trained to represent a patient's condition (e.g., symptoms or social situation) and may also be trained to provide informative feedback. Standardized patients are commonly used for scenarios that involve interviewing, counseling, physically examining a patient, or situations that involve emotionally charged challenges such as giving bad news or de-escalating an upset family member. In pediatrics, SPs may include pediatric patients, parents, extended family, other pediatric professional consultants, social workers and more, simulating the complex care team involved in the care of children.[37,38]

These SPs can also play the role of parents or other team members such as nurses, surgeons, or even students, sometimes for the purpose of teaching supervision skills to trainees[39] (see Video 50.1). SPs are commonly used in OSCEs found in the curricula of many undergraduate and graduate medical education programs. Since 2005, a required portion of the US medical licensing exam (USMLE Step II Clinical Skills) includes a series of standardized patient cases. Over the past 2 decades, OSCEs have also been incorporated into the national board certification exams for Anesthesiology in Israel, the United Kingdom, and the United States, among many others.[40]

HYBRID SIMULATION

Hybrid simulation refers to a technique of combining any of the above simulators into a single activity. For instance, in the OR, the simulation scenario may take shape using a combination of three elements: an HPS, to provide the representation of the patient and clinical feedback in the form of the physiologic variables that can be measured and monitored; a partial task simulator deployed to integrate a surgical skill that allows cutting and suturing of tissue; and an actor trained to represent the patient's parent and enact family presence during resuscitation. Hybrids have been used successfully to assess professional, communication, and technical skills.[41]

Hybrid learning (also known as *blended learning*) refers to the combination of web-based instruction incorporated with physical skills practice. As the field of simulation education has matured, it has become clear that learning with simulation should not be isolated. Integration of simulation into course curricula has given way to hybrid learning techniques. For example, clinicians may complete online precourse material to strengthen or activate prior knowledge in the days leading up to a simulation session. This model allows participants to obtain background knowledge to assist them with understanding the planned simulated procedural skills, which can save time and resources when conducting a training course for many clinicians (e.g., Neonatal Resuscitation Program [NRP]†).

SCREEN-BASED SIMULATOR: VIRTUAL REALITY AND IMMERSIVE ENVIRONMENTS

Virtual reality (VR) offers a simulated environment using two- or three-dimensional models on a screen where learners maneuver through clinical scenarios or perform a task. Initially, VR was used primarily for screen-based task trainers and simple patient models; however, after improvements in technology and cost-efficient development programs stemming from the computer gaming industry, VR programs today offer learners an immersive reality that aims to develop both technical and nontechnical skills.[42] For example, the American Heart Association uses a screen-based simulation model to teach and assess knowledge on Pediatric Advanced Life Support (PALS) as a part of their online credentialing courses.‡[43] VR programs can also be incorporated into OSCE training when standardized patients are not available, a strategy employed by the American Board of Anesthesiology (ABA) for the anesthesiology board certification process during the COVID-19 pandemic when national lock-down strategies prevented in-person examinations.

Immersive environments, such as Advanced Disaster Management Simulator (Environmental Tectonics Corp., Orlando, FL) and other multiuser virtual environments, have been designed to teach disaster management using interactive virtual simulation systems.[44] Other user examples include Gas Man (Med Man Simulations, Inc., Boston, MA) for teaching, simulating, and experimenting with the uptake and distribution of inhalational anesthetics, and a VR simulator for training in regional anesthesia such as online modules offered by Ultrasound for Regional Anesthesia (USRA).[45,46] The American Society of Anesthesiologists now offers high-fidelity online simulation training addressing anesthesia emergencies and other anesthesia-specific modalities are under development. Completing modules from these online trainings§ qualifies for credit toward MOCA, and the SimSTAT is currently the most popular choice for completing MOCA part IV. Finally, a novel yet rapidly expanding field in anesthesia simulation is the use of VR in patient care, where it has been shown to reduce perioperative pain and anxiety in surgical patients.[47,48] For instance, the Childhood Anxiety Reduction through Innovation and Technology (CHARIOT) program at Stanford provides VR games and immersive environment to alleviate perioperative anxiety for young patients undergoing surgery. Although this field is still in its early development stages (and not without

---

†https://cpr.heart.org/en/resuscitation-science/cpr-and-eccguidelines/neonatal-resuscitation] online course via the American Heart Association [AHA]
‡https://www.acls.net/signup
§https://www.asahq.org/education-and-career/educational-and-cme-offerings/simulation-education/anesthesia-simstat?gclid5CjwKCAjw7rWKBhAtEiwAJ3CWLJc8IQYCqfLAf4IfAGGJQaQHATYLGQUnzxVGVb_3qnzxVQP24JOvYhoCPh4QAvD_BwE

controversy), it may offer new opportunities for incorporating simulation as a part of high-quality anesthesia care in the future.

SITES FOR SIMULATION

The number of simulation education centers has increased exponentially since the mid-1990s. Although there is no exact count, these centers are incorporated worldwide within medical schools and residency training programs in hospital settings,[16] as well as nursing schools, and allied health professions' colleges.[49,50] The Society for Simulation in Healthcare (SSiH◆), a growing multidisciplinary society of educators and researchers dedicated to providing technical and political leadership to the global simulation community, has nearly 850 member programs listed in its directory. Different settings of simulation education centers include hospital-based or medical school-based simulation centers, freestanding simulation facilities, and in-situ simulation located within the actual clinical work environment (Fig. 50.3). Dedicated simulation facilities, either within an existing medical institution or a freestanding center, have been constructed across the world to house high-technology simulator equipment, such as mannequins, laparoscopic surgical equipment, robotics, and audiovisual laboratories. The Managing Emergencies in Paediatric Anaesthesia (MEPA◊) collaborative, for example, operates at over 60 centers worldwide, providing insight on simulation experiences and the effectiveness of learner-based models between collaborating institutions.[11] Other models include mobile simulation programs which, although still relatively uncommon, offer simulation training to locations that may otherwise not have the resources to implement their own training programs.[51]

◆https://www.ssih.org/
◊https://mepa.org.uk/

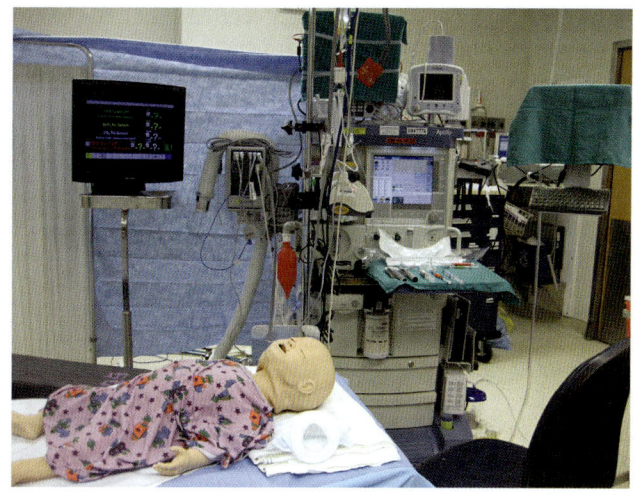

FIGURE 50.3 Simulation in-situ setup in an operating room. A human patient simulator (Laerdal SimBaby, Laerdal Medical, Stavanger, Norway) is used in this setting.

Although simulation education centers can be expensive to maintain and do require manpower to operate, they may serve to replace some traditional forms of clinical education for many of the reasons that simulation has generally become more accepted (e.g., patient safety, clinical production efficiency, and lack of standardized curricula in the apprenticeship model). An in-situ simulation location involves setting up the simulator equipment, trainers, and trainees within the actual work environment, such as the OR, emergency room, or intensive care unit. The benefits of an in-situ simulation include imitation of the work environment with equipment, personnel, and surroundings that are real and familiar to the trainee.[52] Disadvantages of in-situ simulation

TABLE 50.1	Features of Simulation-Based Education by Location			
	Distance	**Features**	**Limitations**	**Operations**
Hospital Simulation Center	*Pro*: Trainees available before, during, and after clinical duties. Other disciplines and professions available. *Con*: Interruptions may occur. Risk of simulation equipment or medication leakage back to clinical environment.	Multimodal education possible (human patient simulators, task trainer, standardized patients, hybrids). Hospital name, numbers, and infrastructure preserved.	Clinical environment may not be accurately represented (outdated equipment, medications not real).	Real estate might be at premium. Equipment and supplies must be ordered separately.
Freestanding Simulation Center	*Pro*: Greatest separation between working and learning environment. Psychological safety and confidentiality are easier to preserve *Con*: Environment and equipment may be significantly different from clinical practice.	Audio and video recording without compromising patient confidentiality. Ability to recreate different clinical environments.	Generic features required to represent multiple hospital systems may lead to environments that are significantly different from the clinical environment.	Must fund and staff independent organization. May need to pay for transportation. Equipment and supply chain not readily available.
In-situ Simulation	*Pro*: Shortest distance to travel. Participants present for work. *Con*: Interruptions are frequent. Family and other practitioners may be disturbed or bothered. Risk of simulation equipment or medication leakage back to clinical environment.	Ability to train in the intended environment enables evaluation of system-level safety features. Findings are readily applicable.	High acuity or census may lead to cancellation of sessions. Emergency equipment may go out of service (MH cart). Equipment may be used for clinical practice during the session (bronchoscope or GlideScope). Difficult to obtain video recording and guarantee patient confidentiality.	Low facility cost (If not charged). Training at work requires no overtime. Disposable material and restocking, including medications, time, and effort to transport equipment to location.

MH, Malignant hyperthermia.

involve challenges in accessing clinical locations and sudden loss of accessibility due to patient care demands, setup of simulation equipment to locations not designed to accommodate it, greater manpower to help with setup and relocation, and especially safety considerations (Table 50.1).[53]

However, novel virtual simulation modalities have become increasingly available over the past decade, expanding the access to simulation training beyond the reach of large academic medical centers in high-income countries. In an effort to address the need for anesthesia providers worldwide, bilateral virtual simulation education models have been successful in enhancing clinical training for anesthesia providers in low-resource settings with otherwise limited educational resources.[54] This development has been propelled forward by the COVID-19 pandemic, prompting an introduction of more accessible and interactive online simulation curricula and training programs reaching trainees and practitioners well beyond traditional academic institutions.[55–57]

Applications of Simulation in Perioperative Pediatric Education

Neonatal and infant emergencies are rare events that may not be encountered during training. Simulation education fills this void by offering trainees simulated scenarios where they manage a variety of pediatric-specific conditions, such as neonatal cardiac arrest and airway emergencies. Newer infant simulators can generate a wide range of pediatric case scenarios, and are mobile and wireless for in-situ simulation in the OR and intensive care unit. Some examples of simulation-based curricula developed for pediatric critical-care medicine include postcongenital heart surgery (using a 3-D printed cardiac model),[58] cardiac pulmonary resuscitation skills,[59–62] neonatal resuscitation,[63] and specific critical-care scenarios including mechanical ventilation of the critically ill patient.[64] Training and managing low-frequency, high-risk cases have been demonstrated in high-fidelity multi-institutional simulation "boot-camps" in both the pediatric intensive care unit[65] and pediatric anesthesia fellowships.[66] Partial task trainers can be used to teach airway management skills such as difficult airway and neonatal intubation,[67] as well as regional techniques.[68–70] High-fidelity simulations have been used in interprofessional health education to improve patient safety, surgical and anesthesia team communication, patient handovers, and patient-caregiver interactions,[71–73] and recently served as metrics of residents' Accreditation Council for Graduate Medical Education milestone competencies.[74]

Comparing Traditional Learning With Simulation-Based Learning

The medical learner at each level of higher education (i.e., undergraduate, graduate, postgraduate) is an adult, who learns by divergent methods for different reasons at various stages in their education.[75] Adult learning theory suggests that active learning with simulation is an effective way to prepare for the dynamic clinical environment.[75] Five adult learning principles that help guide medical learners have been described (Table 50.2).[75,76]

Traditional medical education emphasizes learning and mastering cognitive skills based on textbook readings, lectures, and small group discussions. Evaluation of medical knowledge relies mainly on written or oral examinations. Training models are

TABLE 50.2	Five Adult Learning Principles That Apply to the Medical Learner
1. Adult learners need to know why they are learning
2. Adult learners are motivated by the need to solve problems
3. The previous experiences of adult learners must be respected and built upon
4. The educational approach should match the diversity and background of adult learners
5. Adult learners need to be involved actively in the process

Modified from Okuda Y, Bryson E, Demaria S. The utility of simulation in medical education: what is the evidence? *Mt Sinai J Med.* 2009;76:330-343; Bryan R, Kreuter M, Brownson R. Integrating adult learning principles into training for public health practice. *Health Promot Pract.* 2009;10:557-563.

isolated and sometimes described as being within a "silo," in an insular environment where nurses train with nurses, doctors with doctors, or pharmacists with pharmacists. Retention and transfer are weak when passive learning models are employed. According to Kolb's Experiential Learning Theory, simulation-based training allows for active learning, whereby participants are immersed into clinical scenarios and are able to experience how behaviors, interactions, and communication among multidisciplines affect patient care and potentially, patient outcomes.[77] The more realistic the simulation case scenario, environment, and actors are, the more those participating are able to become immersed in the task and engaged in the clinical scenario. Although learning benefits may be reaped from observing simulated scenarios, the learning experience and knowledge retention is enhanced when trainees play an active role in high-fidelity simulation scenarios. This engagement with an authentic clinical problem and the need to resolve it as a team serves as the foundation for the debriefing that follows a simulation scenario.[78]

Aspects of a High-Fidelity Simulation

High-fidelity simulation requires considerable manpower and preparation. A typical simulation consists of the following: a team leader, actors and/or standardized patients, high-fidelity mannequin, a simulation room, audiovisual equipment, learners, and one or more debriefers.[79] Team leaders may be compared with film directors; they are responsible for the smooth execution of the case scenario, from assigning and delegating roles to team members and directing the evolving scenario (usually from a control room), to handling unexpected problems and situations that may arise during the simulation. This position may be the same or different from an "operator" who is responsible for operating the mannequin behind the scenes in the console room. Actors are responsible for creating the emotional realism of the case. They may take roles, e.g., nurses, physicians, technicians, or administrative staff, so the participants will act and interact in a way that is clinically familiar and realistic. A challenge for actors is to maintain their simulated character and to interact with participants, often in a scripted way, to elicit behaviors as part of the learning objectives. They must do this without overt interference with the clinical decisions and management. Communication between actors and the control room personnel using wireless audio devices is helpful in guiding the actors' responses in a manner that maintains conceptual fidelity and smooth flow of the scenario. The clinician caring for the patient or leading a clinical team within a simulated setting is frequently said to be "in the hot seat" because, during the scenario, the clinician preforms and makes critical decisions that influence the care of the patient. During the debriefing, one or more designated debriefers work with the team to aid in transforming the clinical experience into a learning opportunity.

The simulation room, whether physical or virtual, is ideally a flexible setting that can be converted into a range of patient care environments, such as an OR, emergency department or obstetric ward treatment room, a cafeteria or other public place; anywhere an anesthesia team might be called to respond. Elaborate scenery, anesthesia and surgical equipment used in everyday work, and moulage (e.g., simulated blood and vomitus) may create realistic scenarios. The rooms may be equipped with medical air, oxygen, and vacuum suction capabilities to run the high-fidelity mannequins and to provide for their use in the scenario.[79] Audiovisual equipment, such as cameras and microphones, are strategically placed so as to not be obvious to the participants, whose actions are followed in the simulation for debriefing and feedback. The debriefer is responsible for observing the simulation scenario, and to stimulate learning and discussion in a nonthreatening and organized way at the end of the event. The debriefer identifies elements of the simulation that possess educational value pertinent to the learning objectives of the course and facilitates the discussion of these learning nuggets (e.g., point out where communication broke down or where situational awareness was lost) (see Video 50.2).

What Is a Debriefing?

A debriefing is a "conversation between two or more people to review a real or simulated event in which participants analyze their actions and interactions, and reflect on the roles of thought processes, psychomotor skills, and emotional states, to improve or sustain performance in the future."[80,81] Debriefing is considered the most important component of simulation-based education; it is the time when learning is embedded.[82] As such, it has been explored through different timing (during or after simulation), conversation facilitation techniques, and conversation structure with different process elements such as scripts, co-debriefers, and the use of video of the simulation session.[83] The debriefing usually follows each simulation case scenario; however, there are other techniques utilized such as "pause-and-discuss" where the instructor interjects during pauses in a scenario[84] and "rapid cycle deliberate practice" debriefing, both of which have been shown to be effective.[85] Team-based debriefings, as proposed in the TeamGAINS debriefing method, have been shown to increase collective orientation compared with individual problem-oriented debriefings.[86] Often perceived as a stressful situation for the learner, there is some support for the use of relaxation techniques before debriefing to enhance the learning experience and improve knowledge retention.[86,87]

Many simulation centers offer audio and video capture mechanisms, which can be used to review portions of the scenario during a debriefing. Debriefers can show trainees key moments, clarify recall discrepancies, and offer a global view of the room to participants who might have been focused on a task or fixated on a portion of the action. Although many instructors use video during debriefing to present learners with the opportunity to see what they could not appreciate during the simulation, there are limited published data on the specific value of this technique.[84]

There are numerous styles and methods of debriefing in health care simulation. Some of the published debriefing methods are: Structured and Supported Debriefing,[88] TeamGAINS,[89] PEARLS,[90]

SAiL Diamond,[91] and Debriefing with Good Judgment.[92] Here, we describe one method that is commonly used in our institution: Debriefing with Good Judgment. Like most debriefing methods, there are three phases to this debriefing technique: *reactions, understanding,* and *summary*.[80,81,93] The *reactions phase* asks participants to share how they felt, allowing the participants to vent and deactivate from the heightened emotional state that participating in a simulation provokes. The debriefer leads the group through a description of the facts of the case, to ensure that everyone understands the clinical scenario before tackling the learning objectives. The *understanding phase* is the richest and longest phase, intended to help participants analyze and apply what happened and explore deeper meaning of the interactions. Discussion and teachings are involved in this phase to help simulation participants gain new perspectives and insights into group dynamics and communication. Lessons learned during the simulation can be generalized and applied to the real world, preparing participants to transfer new knowledge into their clinical practice. In the *summary phase*, participants share lessons learned, including individual and group behaviors (both positive and negative), skills, and thinking patterns that they wish to improve, as well as those that were productive and they wish to retain for future performance.[80,81,93]

To become an effective debriefer requires training and practice to acquire skills that are not taught in traditional health care educational programs. Instructors and facilitators are encouraged to learn about the principles of effective debriefing via the literature, formal courses, and mentoring.[94–97] The Debriefing Assessment for Simulation in Healthcare (DASH#) is an example of a testing instrument that was developed to assess and improve debriefing skills.[80]

Theories on debriefing, along with other aspects of simulation education, have been a central focus of simulation educator programs providing training platforms for professional clinical instructors in simulation. These programs have developed as a subspeciality in clinical education, with training programs, fellowships, and even formal accreditation programs increasingly available at academic centers around the world.[98,99] A list of endorsed simulation centers in the US can be found on the American Society of Anesthesiologists' education center webpage.[Δ 100]

USING SIMULATION FOR EVALUATION

Although patient simulators are well accepted as a core component of crisis resource management and other areas of clinical training, their acceptance as assessment tools for clinical performance is not yet fully established. However, some scoring systems for simulator-based performance assessments have been developed, such as the Anaesthetists' Non-Technical Skills (ANTS) system.[34,101] Recent studies have demonstrated that simulation-based assessments can be undertaken with sufficient reliability to be used for testing (e.g., reproducible scenarios can be created and implemented, raters can be trained to assign reproducible scores of performance, and critical clinical skills can be simulated).[102,103] Main challenges in evaluating participants of standardized simulation scenarios include accounting for the speed and sequence of events rather than the events themselves. Therefore, prioritizing

---

#https://harvardmedsim.org/debriefing-assessment-for-simulation-in-healthcare-dash/

Δhttps://education.asahq.org/mod/page/view.php?id=20716&_ga=2.14781942.1751507722.1638196977-1943946361.1633632325

several shorter scenarios rather than a few long ones has been proposed to increase reliability and reproducibility of such evaluations.[104] Multiscenario, simulation-based assessment has the potential to assess performance of pediatric anesthesia skills for residents and fellows; however, further measures of validity, including correlations with direct measures of clinical performance, are needed to establish the true utility and validity of these simulations as assessment tools.[105,106]

Simulation is widely thought to be effective for improving clinical skills in a way that is safer than the traditional apprentice model of training.[72] Although there is not yet a large body of evidence regarding the effectiveness of simulation or the cost relative to its benefit, there is substantial literature that documents its utility. A meta-analysis has established the overall effectiveness of simulation-based training.[5] Furthermore, simulation-based training has improved patient outcomes, specifically in the survival of children after cardiopulmonary resuscitation.[107]

SIMULATION FOR OTHER USES

Simulation has been used for other purposes in health care in general and specifically in pediatric anesthesia. Simulation can be highly effective for research using various methods and to study a broad range of questions, for patient safety and quality assurance and improvement, and for teamwork training of nonclinical health care teams. For example, the Validate Anesthesia Simulation in Error Research (VASER) study employed a simulation trial to determine the effects on medication administration errors, concluding that the results were comparable to a traditional clinical trial.[108] Simulation settings also offer opportunities for medical education research, especially when focused toward sustained, thematic, and theory-based programs utilizing standardized material.[109] As a response to the rapidly expanding field of simulation-based research, the International Network for Simulation-based Pediatric Innovation, Research, and Education (INSPIRE) has proposed a set of reporting guidelines as a quality measure and to unify a broad field of research.[110] More recently, translational simulation has been proposed as an intervention strategy for health service institutions to target specific health care outcomes through directed education and training aimed at health systems, rather than traditional case-specific training.[111] Translational simulation offers a functional alignment with quality improvement activities in health care institutions, aiming to improve patient care within health care systems while maintaining an education-based learning platform to enhance practice behavior and patient outcomes.[112,113]

CHALLENGES IN USING SIMULATION

Although simulation centers are increasingly popular worldwide, there are many challenges to establishing and maintaining a simulation program. There are relatively few educators formally trained to use simulation. The time demands of clinical care and increasing cost pressures make it difficult for faculty to acquire time to become trained themselves and even when they are, to devote time to develop curricula and routinely run simulation sessions.[114] Similarly, challenges of time and resource constraints apply to residency and fellowship trainees as well, where simulation programs compete with clinical experience and other didactic programs over a limited period of training.

In institutions where a freestanding simulation center is not feasible, establishing in-situ simulations using existing hospital facilities, remodeling old facilities into a simulation room, or having mobile units that contain simulation equipment have been successfully implemented. The Managing Emergencies in Paediatric Anaesthesia course, initiated by the Royal College of Anaesthetists in the United Kingdom, allows for sharing of simulation scenarios in pediatric anesthesia and is now offered at over 60 locations worldwide.[11] The course content has been adapted to telesimulation modules that are offered to residents and other trainees in remote locations.[115] In countries where lack of funding, poor infrastructure, and limited manpower may impede structuring local simulation centers, this "telesimulation" model promotes sharing of knowledge and opportunities for simulation education worldwide.[115]

FUTURE OF SIMULATION

Simulation-based education in pediatric anesthesia provides many opportunities for curriculum development for training programs as well as faculty participating in continuing education. Simulation models offer creative strategies to enhance and supplement clinical experiences such as practicing technical skills, managing infrequent critical events, strengthening multidisciplinary team building, and developing communication skills. Simulation models have also been used to reinforce educational curricula in remote and under-resourced settings in the United States and abroad. Today, a wide network of global societies and multinational collaboratives promote the use of simulation in medical education across a wide range of clinical specialties. In addition to providing training opportunities, simulation-based programs are increasingly used in medical education research, health system evaluations, and translational research. Although the long-term benefits remain to be established, early studies have indicated a potential use of simulation in direct patient care to address perioperative anxiety and pain management.

Medical simulation is rapidly evolving and increasingly accepted as a central component of anesthesia training. This was clearly demonstrated during the COVID-19 pandemic where simulation programs were swiftly constructed and implemented for pandemic preparedness exercises. Although the many national and international simulation societies reflect this growing interest for simulation in medical education, the full potential of simulation in pediatric anesthesia remains to be explored. Perhaps the Improving Pediatric Acute Care Through Simulation (ImPACTS) group, which uses simulation to advance the field of pediatric emergency medicine by sharing knowledge, experiences and resources in a collaborative network of academic centers and community hospitals, may offer some inspiration for a potential model in pediatric anesthesia.[116] A national, or international, collaborative on actively driving advances in medical management, research, and patient care using simulation as a unifying platform could further promote the role of simulation in pediatric anesthesia practices in the United States and elsewhere. More research is required to fully determine the long-term impact of simulation on quality of pediatric anesthesia care, patient safety, and health care outcomes, but the positive trajectory holds much promise for the future.

ANNOTATED REFERENCES

Ambardekar AP, Singh D, Lockman JL, et al. Pediatric anesthesiology fellow education: is a simulation-based boot camp feasible and valuable? *Paediatr Anaesth.* 2016;26(5):481-487.

A simulation-based boot camp was developed for pediatric anesthesiology fellows to assess learner perceptions of boot camp activities. Learners reported improved knowledge, self-confidence, technical skills, and clinical performance after completing the course.

Andreatta P, Saxton E, Thompson M, Annich G. Simulation-based mock codes significantly correlate with improved pediatric patient cardiopulmonary arrest survival rates. *Pediatr Crit Care Med.* 2011; 12(1):33-38.

A longitudinal, mixed-method research design evaluating the viability and effectiveness of a simulation-based mock code program on patient outcomes as well as residents' confidence in performing resuscitations. The results suggest that a simulation-based mock code program may significantly benefit pediatric patient outcomes as well as improve learner perceived value and increase learner confidence.

Blum RH, Boulet JR, Cooper JB, Muret-Wagstaff SL. Simulation-based assessment to identify critical gaps in safe anesthesia resident performance. *Anesthesiology.* 2014;120:1-13.

Valid methods are needed to identify anesthesia residents' performance gaps early in training. However, many assessment tools in medicine have not been properly validated. In this study, a behaviorally anchored scale was designed for use in simulation-based assessment and tested to identify high- and low-performing residents with regard to domains of concern to expert anesthesiology faculty. The study provides initial evidence to support the validity of a simulation-based performance assessment tool.

Fehr JJ, Boulet JR, Waldrop WB, Snider R, Brockel M, Murray DJ. Simulation-based assessment of pediatric anesthesia skills. *Anesthesiology.* 2011;115(6):1308-1315.

The purpose of this study was to develop a set of relevant simulated pediatric perioperative scenarios and to determine their effectiveness in the assessment of anesthesia residents and fellows. The study showed that the simulation content was relevant, and raters could reliably score the scenarios.

MaGaghie WC, Issenberg SB, Petrusa ER, Scalese RJ. A critical review of simulation-based medical education research: 2003–2009. *Med Educ.* 2010;44:50-63.

This review article presents a qualitative synthesis of historical and contemporary research on simulation-based medical education from 2003 to 2009.

Rudolph JW, Simon R, Dufresne RL, Raemer D. There's no such thing as "non-judgmental" debriefing: a theory and method for debriefing with good judgment. *Simul Healthc.* 2009;1:49-55.

The authors describe an approach to debriefing known as "debriefing with good judgment" which emphasizes disclosing instructors' judgment and eliciting trainees' assumptions about the situation and their reasoning for acting as they did. This approach draws on theory and empirical findings from a 35-year research program in the behavioral sciences on how to improve professional effectiveness through "reflective practice."

Soneru CN, Fernandez AM, Bradford V, et al. A survey of the global impact of COVID-19 on the practice of pediatric anesthesia: a study from the pediatric anesthesia COVID-19 Collaborative Group. *Paediatr Anaesth.* 2021;31(6):720-729.

Sixty-three institutions participating in the Pediatric Anesthesia COVID-19 Collaborative were surveyed on four major domains concerning testing, safety, clinical management/policy and economics related to pediatric anesthesia care during the COVID-19 pandemic. 65% of participating institutions were from the United States, 35% were from other countries. Structured simulation training aimed at improving COVID-19 safety and patient care was implemented at 62% of institutions.

Weinstock PH, Kappus LJ, Kleinman ME, Grenier B, Hickey P, Burns JP. Toward a new paradigm in hospital-based pediatric education: the development of an onsite simulator program. *Pediatr Crit Care Med.* 2005;6:635-641.

This is a descriptive study looking at how an onsite, comprehensive pediatric simulation program in the Pediatric Intensive Care Unit can serve as a cost-effective method to enhance the frequency and breadth of critical-incident training and education.

A complete reference list can be found online at Elsevier eBooks+.

A

ABCB1, 90
ABCC3, 90
Abdominal compartment syndrome, 747–748, 941–942
Abdominal injury, intraoperative management of, 1013
Abdominal pain, 1183t, 1184–1185, 1185t
Abdominal surgery, 745–767. *see also* Urologic surgery
  abdominal compartment syndrome and, 747–748
  anesthetic in, 748
  fluid balance in, 747
  laboratory testing before, 748
  monitoring requirements in, 748
  Nissen fundoplication and, 755
  in pectus excavatum, 755–756
  preoperative nasogastric tube placement in, 746–747
  pulmonary aspiration of gastric contents in, 745
  rapid-sequence induction in, 745–746
  spinal anesthesia in, 1075
  succinylcholine for, 746
Abdominal trauma, 1009–1011, 1011t
Aberrant subclavian artery, 407, 408f
AbioMed. *see* Impella
Ablation catheters, 577
Abnormal airway, 349–369
  cervical spine anomalies, 350t
  classification of, 349–350, 350t
  documentation of, 354
  extubation of, 354–356, 356.e1–356.e2f, 356.e3f
  intubation techniques, 359–369
    air-Q Mask Laryngeal Airway in, 347, 349f
    Airtraq optical laryngoscope in, 365–366, 366f
    Bullard laryngoscope in, 363–364, 363.e1f
    flexible fiberoptic bronchoscope used in retrograde manner, 368
    flexible laryngoscopy in, 360–363
    GlideScope in, 364–365, 364.e1f
    lighted stylet in, 363, 363.e1f
    MultiView Scope in, 365, 365.e2f
    optical laryngoscopes in, 365–367
    retrograde light-guided laryngoscopy, 368–369
    retrograde wire and flexible intubation scope, 368
    retrograde wire-guided intubation in, 364
    rigid laryngoscopy and flexible fiberoptic bronchoscope, 368
    rigid laryngoscopy in, 359–360
    Shikani optical stylet in, 367, 367.e1f
    Storz Bonfils optical stylet in, 367, 367.e2f
    Storz Video Laryngoscope in, 365, 365.e1f
    supraglottic airway as conduit for, 367–368, 368.e1f
    Truview EVO2 infant device in, 366–367, 366.e1f
    video and indirect intubating devices for, 364–367
    video laryngoscopy and flexible intubation scope, 368

Abnormal airway *(Continued)*
  management principles, 350–356, 351t, 352f, 353.e1f
  pathology related to anatomic site, 350t
  unexpected difficult intubation and, 354, 355f
  ventilation techniques, 356–359
    anterior commissure scope and rigid ventilating bronchoscope, 359
    multi-handed mask ventilation, 356, 356f
    percutaneous needle cricothyroidotomy, 357–359, 357f, 358f, 358.e1f, 359.e1f, 359.e2f
    supraglottic airways, 356, 356.e1–356.e2f, 356.e3f
ABO compatibility of blood components, 282t
Abortion, 69
Abscess, peritonsillar, 871–872, 872f
Absorption, drug, 112–113
  enteral administration of, 112
Absorptive atelectasis, 766, 972
Acceleromyography, 149, 1337–1338
Accidental punctures, with sharps, prevention of, 1284, 1285t, 1284.e1t, 1284.e2t
ACE inhibitors. *see* Angiotensin-converting enzyme inhibitors
Acetaminophen, 173–175, 173f, 174f, 1250
  for bone and joint infections, 835
  genetics and, 93
  liver failure caused by, 776
  metabolism of, 84
  for myringotomy, 842
  for orthopedic and spine surgery, 810
  pain management using
    description of, 1145t, 1146–1147
    postoperative, 1250
  pharmacokinetics of, 173–175
  rectal administration of, 1250
Acetylation reactions, hepatic metabolism of, 771
Acetylcholine, 658, 907t
Acetylcholine receptors, 149, 944
Acetylcysteine, 934–935
Achondroplasia, 340t, 1245–1246
α_1-acid glycoprotein, 109–110, 1055, 1057
Acid-base abnormality
  in dehydration, 229–230
  during liver transplantation, 783
Acid-base balance
  evaluation of, 229
  massive blood transfusion and, 298
  renal regulation of, 730–731
Acidosis
  lactic, 711
  metabolic, 229f
    in chronic renal failure, 737
    in malignant hyperthermia, 1039
  respiratory, in malignant hyperthermia, 1039
Acinus, 8
Acoustic shadowing, 1070
Acquired heart disease, 395–402
  cardiac tumors, 401–402
  cardiomyopathy, 395–398, 395f, 396f, 397f
  infective endocarditis, 399–400, 400t, 401t
  Kawasaki disease, 400–401, 401f

Acquired heart disease *(Continued)*
  myocarditis, 398–399, 398f
  rheumatic fever and rheumatic heart disease, 399
Acquired immunodeficiency syndrome, 1303–1304f, 1304–1306, 1305f
Acquired laryngeal stenosis, 889
Acquired subglottic stenosis, 895
Acquired upper airway obstruction, 889
ACT. *see* Activated clotting time
Actin, 656
ACTION. *see* Advanced Cardiac Therapies Improving Outcomes Network
Activated agents, 540–541
Activated clotting time (ACT), 436, 509, 563
  in cardiopulmonary bypass, 436
  hemodialysis monitoring, 735
  heparin and, 535
Activated partial thromboplastin time (aPTT), 236, 533, 535, 920
  in bleeding disorders, 249
  values at different ages, 237t
  in von Willebrand disease, 250
Active compression-decompression, in cardiopulmonary resuscitation, 1028
Acupuncture, 866, 1194, 1194f
Acute bacterial endocarditis, 399
Acute chest syndrome (ACS), 243, 322
Acute emergencies, managing of, outside operating room, 1199
Acute epiglottitis, 883–885, 883.e1f, 884f, 885f
Acute kidney injury, 731–736, 731t
  after cardiopulmonary bypass, 739
  causes of, 732t
  diagnostic procedures of, 733–734
  etiology and pathophysiology of, 731–732
  hemodialysis in, 735
  therapeutic interventions for, 734–736, 735f
Acute lung injury, 1326
Acute lymphoblastic leukemia (ALL), 253–255, 256t, 261
Acute malignant hypertension, management of, 743t
Acute motor and sensory axonal neuropathy, 634
Acute motor axonal neuropathy, 634
Acute myelogenous leukemia (AML), 255–257
Acute normovolemic hemodilution
  in craniosynostosis surgery, 920
  for Jehovah's Witnesses, 511
Acute pain, 1134–1180
  acetaminophen for, 1146–1147
  assessment of. *see* Pain assessment
  burn injuries as cause of, 942f, 950–952, 951f, 952t
  in developing countries, 1301–1302
  developmental neurobiology of, 1134–1135
  ketamine for, 1149
  limitations of, 1140–1141
  nonsteroidal antiinflammatory drugs for, 1147–1148
  opioid analgesics for, 1152–1153, 1152t
    in cognitively impaired child, 1177
    epidural administration of, 1172t
    intramuscular and subcutaneous routes for, 1155

Acute pain *(Continued)*
    intranasal route, 1155
    intravenous administration of, 1154
    nurse-/caregiver-controlled analgesia and, 1161–1162
    oral administration of, 1153–1154
    patient-controlled analgesia in, 1157–1161
    relative potency of, 1152t
  pharmacologic treatment of, 1145–1177
  in postanesthesia care unit, 1148, 1250–1251
  strategies for, 1142–1145
  tramadol for, 1148–1149
Acute promyelocytic leukemia (APL), 257, 271–272
Acute renal failure, 733f
Acute respiratory distress syndrome (ARDS)
  after cardiopulmonary bypass, 522, 1324, 1326
  pulmonary ultrasound for, 387
Acute tubular necrosis (ATN), 731, 780
Acyclovir, 731–732
Addiction, 92
Adductor pollicis brevis, 1338
Adenocard. *see* Adenosine
Adenoidectomy, 846
Adenoscan. *see* Adenosine
Adenosine, 499t, 502–503
  for supraventricular tachycardia, 1027
Adenotonsillar hyperplasia, 847
  obstructive sleep apnea and, 850
Adenotonsillectomy, 85–87, 845–872
  admission policies for, 863, 863f, 864f
  adverse respiratory events in, 858–859, 859f
  airway control in, 859–860
  anesthetic choice for, 860–861, 860f, 860.e1t
  anesthetic considerations for, 857, 857t
  complications of, 866–867, 867t
  emergence and recovery in, 867–869
  extubation in, 867, 867f
  indications for, 845–846, 845t, 854–855, 854f
  neuromuscular compromise in, 867
  obstructive sleep apnea and, 57, 57t, 846–851
  perioperative considerations for, 857–858
  perioperative pain in, 862–863, 862.e1t
  peritonsillar abscess and, 871–872, 872f
  postoperative adenotonsillectomy adverse events in, 869
  postoperative admission guidelines for, 868–869, 868.e1f, 869f, 870t
  postoperative considerations for, 858–863
  postoperative nausea and vomiting in, 861–862, 861f, 868
  posttonsillectomy hemorrhage and, 847.e1t, 870–871, 871f
  preoperative evaluation in, 850.e1t, 851–854
    drug-induced sleep endoscopy in, 854
    identification of at-risk children, 851
    overnight pulse oximetry in, 852–854, 853f
    physical assessment in, 852
    polysomnogram in, 852, 852.e1–852.e2f
    questionnaires in, 851–852
  recurrent tonsillitis and, 846

Adenotonsillectomy *(Continued)*
  respiratory events in, 868
  risk stratification for perioperative
    adverse events in, 855–857, 855t,
    855.e1f
  sleep-disordered breathing and,
    845–846
  surgical approach in, 846
Adjunctive drugs, for epidural anesthesia,
  1085
Adolescent
  abortion and, 69
  confidentiality for, 69
  idiopathic scoliosis in, 816
  informed consent, 66, 66t
  pregnancy in, 69
  refusal of emergency treatment by, 70
Adoptive T-cell therapies, 264
Adrenal crisis, 320
Adrenal endocrinopathies, 722–724
  adrenal insufficiency and, 722–723, 722f
  hypercortisolism in, 723–724
  perioperative management of, 723
  physiology of, 722
  testing for, 723
Adrenal gland, tumor of, 760
Adrenal insufficiency, 722–723, 722f
Adrenaline, 1023–1024
α₂-Adrenergic agonists
  for blunt reflex bronchoconstriction,
    860.e1t
  effects on evoked potentials, 831
  ophthalmic uses of, 907t
  pain management using, 1142
  premedication, 36t
  preoperative, 38–39
  for sedation, 1233–1234
β-Adrenergic blockers, 491–492,
    501, 646t
  acute hyperkalemia, 232
  atenolol, 491
  carvedilol, 491–492
  esmolol, 491
  eye surgery uses of, 907–908
  for hyperthyroid crisis, 720t
  ivabradine, 492
  labetalol, 491
  for pheochromocytoma, 725
  propranolol, 491
Adrenocorticotropic hormone, 722
Advanced Cardiac Therapies Improving
    Outcomes Network (ACTION), 550
Adverse childhood experiences, 77
African Americans, 97
Afterload, in Fontan circulation, 480
Age
  blood pressure and, 12, 12t
  body water and, 6t
  fine motor/adaptive milestones, 19t
  glomerular filtration rate and,
    109.e1f, 115
  heart rate and, 12, 12t
  language milestones to, 19t
  motor milestones based on, 19t
  pain management based on, 1145
  personal-social milestones to, 19t
  respiratory variables with, 10t
  weight and, 6t
Age-appropriate pain assessment tools,
  1015t
Agitation, emergence, 1241–1243,
    1242t, 1243t
β₂-Agonists, for asthma exacerbations,
    318, 318.e1f, 319.e2–319.e3t
Air aspiration, from central venous
    catheter, 690
Air embolism, 1335
  cardiac catheterization and, 579
  neurosurgical procedures and, 689–690,
    690f
  noncardiac surgery in congenital heart
    disease and, 613
  venous, 921–922
Air transmission, of infectious disease,
    1280–1281, 1281.e1f

Airborne pathogen, prevention of
    transmission, 1287f, 1290–1291,
    1290.e1t, 1291t
Air-Q Mask Laryngeal Airway, 347, 349f
Airtraq optical laryngoscope, 365–366,
    366f
Airway, 324–369
  abnormal. *see* Abnormal airway
  developmental anatomy of, 324–328
    epiglottis, 325, 327f
    larynx, 324–325, 325f, 326f
    subglottis, 325–328, 328f, 329f
    tongue, 324
    vocal folds, 325
  difficult. *see* Difficult airway
  distribution of resistance in, 11
  dynamic collapse of, 331, 332f
  evaluation of, 333–336
    diagnostic testing in, 336
    medical history in, 334
    physical examination in, 335–336,
      335f
    in trauma patient, 1006–1007
  inspiratory and expiratory flow
    limitation in, 11
  intubation techniques, 359–369
    air-Q Mask Laryngeal Airway in,
      347, 349f
    Airtraq optical laryngoscope in,
      365–366, 366f
    Bullard laryngoscope in, 363–364,
      363.e1f
    flexible fiberoptic bronchoscope used
      in retrograde manner, 368
    flexible laryngoscopy in, 360–363
    GlideScope in, 364–365, 364.e1f
    lighted stylet in, 363, 363.e1f
    MultiView Scope in, 365, 365.e2f
    retrograde light-guided laryngoscopy,
      368–369
    retrograde wire and flexible
      intubation scope, 368
    retrograde wire-guided intubation
      in, 364
    rigid laryngoscopy and flexible
      fiberoptic bronchoscope, 368
    rigid laryngoscopy in, 359–360
    Shikani optical stylet in, 367, 367.e1f
    Storz Bonfils optical stylet in, 367,
      367.e2f
    Storz Video Laryngoscope in, 365,
      365.e1f
    supraglottic airway as conduit for,
      367–368, 368.e1f
    Truview EVO2 infant device in,
      366–367, 366.e1f
    video and indirect intubating devices
      for, 364–367
    video laryngoscopy and flexible
      intubation scope, 368
  larynx, 328–331
    blood supply of, 330
    function of, 330–331
    histology of, 329–330
    sensory and motor innervation
      of, 330
    structure of, 328–329, 329f, 330f
  mask ventilation and, 336–337, 336f
  nasopharyngeal, 337
  neonatal surgical emergencies
      involving, 966–968, 967t, 968f
  normal, 336–349
  oropharyngeal, 337, 338f
  physiology of, 331–333
    airway obstruction during
      anesthesia, 333
    obligate nasal breathing and, 331
    tracheal and bronchial function in,
      331, 332f
    work of breathing and, 332–333,
      333f
  regulation of breathing and, 11–12
  resistance and conductance of, 11
  supraglottic, 343–349, 345f, 1005
    insertion technique for, 347–349

Airway *(Continued)*
  for resuscitation, 349
  styles of, 345–347, 346f, 346t, 347t,
    347.e1f, 348f, 348t
  surgical, 359
  surgical repair of, 893, 893t
  tracheal intubation, 337–343
    complications of, 342–343
    continuous waveform capnography
      for, 342
    distance to insert tracheal tube and,
      341–342, 342t, 343f
    laryngoscope blade for, 340, 340t
    laryngotracheal stenosis and, 343, 344f
    postintubation croup and, 342–343
    technique in, 337–340, 339f, 337.e1f
    tubes in, 340–341, 341f, 341t
    video laryngoscopy in, 340
  trauma to, 893–894
  tumors of, 265
  upper, 8f
  ventilation techniques, 356–359
    anterior commissure scope and rigid
      ventilating bronchoscope, 359
    multi-handed mask ventilation,
      356, 356f
    percutaneous needle
      cricothyroidotomy, 357–359,
      357f, 358f, 358.e1f, 359.e1f,
      359.e2f
    supraglottic airways, 356,
      356.e1–356.e2f, 356.e3f
Airway apparatus, 1320–1322
Airway compression, 267
Airway control, in adenotonsillectomy,
    859–860
Airway edema
  airway resistance and, 326, 329f
  prone position and, 687
Airway exchange catheter, 945, 945.e1f
Airway management
  in burn injuries, 938–939, 938f,
    947–949, 949f
  in cardiopulmonary resuscitation,
    1017–1018
  COVID-19 and, 1286–1288
  in craniosynostosis surgery, 919, 919.e1
  in hemifacial dysostosis surgery, 924–925
  in laparoscopic surgery, 752–753
  in liver disease, 779
  in neurosurgical procedures, 684–685
  in orthognathic surgery, 925
  in trauma, 1005–1006, 1010f
Airway obstruction
  after burn injury, 933–934, 938
  during anesthesia, 333
  in cervical teratoma, 996
  in laryngeal papillomatosis, 847–848
  postoperative, 1245–1246
Airway patency, 859
Airway resistance, 333
ALARA mnemonic, 580
ALARP mnemonic, 580
Albumin, 773
  burn injury and, 933
  transfusion, 288
Albuterol, 737t
  for asthma exacerbations, 319.e2–319.e3t
Alcuronium, 1310
Aldosterone, 234, 722
Alfaxalone, 148
Alfentanil, 168, 169–170
  infusion schemes, 197t
  propofol and, 195
ALL. *see* Acute lymphoblastic leukemia
Allergy
  allogenic. *see* Allogenic blood
    components, exposure to
  to latex, 621, 749
Allodynia, 1186
Allogenic blood components, exposure to,
    301–304
  autotransfusion for, 301–302
  controlled hypotension in, 302–303
  erythropoietin for, 301

Allogenic blood components *(Continued)*
  intraoperative blood recovery and
    reinfusion for, 301–302
  normovolemic hemodilution for,
    303–304
  preoperative autologous blood donation
    for, 301
Allometry, 106
Allopurinol, 448–449
All-trans retinoic acid, 271–272
Alobar holoprosencephaly, 624
Alpers-Huttenlocher syndrome, neuronal
    degeneration, 637t
α–stat management, 514
Alpha-fetoprotein, 14–15
Alport syndrome, 903
Alveolar to venous partial pressure
    gradient, 123
Alveolar ventilation, 10t
Alveolar ventilation/functional residual
    capacity, 108f, 121
Alveoli, 8
Amblyopia, 912
Ambrisentan, 497
Ambu bag, 1207
American Academy of Pediatrics, sedation
    guidelines, 1221–1223, 1223t
American College of Emergency
    Physicians (ACEP), sedation
    guidelines, 1224–1225
American College of Surgeons National
    Quality Improvement Program, 281
American Society of Anesthesiologists (ASA),
    sedation guidelines, 1223–1224
Amethocaine, 1056
Amides, 1054–1055
  bupivacaine in, 1054
  lidocaine in, 1055
  ropivacaine in, 1055
α-amino-3-hydroxy-5-methyl-4-isoxazole-
    propionic acid (AMPA), 658
γ-aminobutyric acid (GABA), 81, 652,
    656–657, 658, 1134
ε-Aminocaproic acid (EACA), 508, 508t
  for blood loss in craniosynostosis
    surgery, 920
  in cardiac surgery, 438
  dosing of, 546
  fibrinolysis inhibition using, 116
Aminophylline, 319
Amiodarone, 499t, 501, 646t
  for cardiopulmonary resuscitation,
    1025–1026
Amitriptyline, 1192
AML. *see* Acute myelogenous leukemia
Amlodipine, 477t
Ammonia, hepatic encephalopathy
    and, 779
Amniotic band syndrome, 983t
Amoxicillin, 400, 401t
Ampicillin, 400, 401t
Amplatzer Duct Occluder, 576f
Amrinone, 484–485t, 488
Anaesthesia Practice in Children
    Observational Trial (APRICOT),
    333–334
Analgesia
  acetaminophen for, 1146–1147
  in burn injuries, 949–950, 950f
  developing countries and, 1302
  epidural
    after scoliosis surgery, 826
    in cognitively impaired child,
      1177–1178
    for postoperative pain, 1250–1251
    for tetanus, 1309
  ketamine for, 1149
  for neuroendocrine stress, 708
  nonsteroidal antiinflammatory drugs,
    1147–1148
  opioid analgesics for, 1152t
  patient-controlled, 1157–1161
    adverse events with, 1162, 1162.e1t
    continuous basal infusions in,
      1158–1161, 1160f

Analgesia (Continued)
dosing guidelines, 1168t
drug and drug dosages for, 756, 1158
equipment for, 1162
monitoring of, 1162–1163
pain nurse administration of, 1182
pump settings in, 1158, 1159f
risks associated with, 1162, 1162.e1t
pharmacogenomics of, 85–87
pharmacologic treatment, 1145–1177
in postanesthesia care unit, 1148, 1250
regional. see Regional analgesia
strategies for, 1142–1145, 1143f, 1144f
age and cognitive abilities in, 1145
surgical considerations in, 1143–1145
tramadol for, 1145t, 1148–1149
Anaphylactic reaction, 508
Anaphylactic shock, to contrast media, 1200–1201
Anaphylaxis
cardiopulmonary resuscitation in, 1027
cause of, 1248
latex, 34
Anaplastic astrocytoma, 626t
Anaplastic large cell lymphoma, 258
Anasarca, 226
Anatomic shunts, 475–476
Ancestry information markers, 96–97
Anchoring, 353
Andexanet alfa, 536
Anemia
in cancer patients, 276
in chronic renal failure, 741
in liver transplantation, 780
physiologic, of infancy, 53
sickle cell, 242
Anemia of prematurity, 17
Anencephaly, 622
Anesthesia, 650–677
on cardiopulmonary bypass, 519–520
pharmacodynamics, changes in, 520
pharmacokinetics, changes in, 519
in chronic kidney disease, 741–743
COVID-19 and, 1288–1289
in developing countries, 1299–1313
blood safety and, 1310
cardiac disease and, 1309
childhood diseases in, 1299–1302, 1300f
COVID-19 pandemic and, 1302–1304
drawover anesthesia and, 1311–1312, 1312f
drugs in, 1309–1310
equipment in, 1308f, 1310–1312
human immunodeficiency virus
infection and acquired
immunodeficiency syndrome
and, 1303–1304f, 1304–1306,
1305f
human resources and, 1302
malaria and, 1308–1309
oxygen concentrators and, 1311,
1312, 1312.e1f
pain management and, 1301–1302
tetanus and, 1309
tuberculosis and, 1306–1308
visiting providers and, 1312–1313
war and, 1300–1301, 1301f
in epileptic patients, 646–648, 647t
immunosuppression after, 277
long-term outcome in children exposed
to, 668–674
anesthetic neurotoxicity, 668–669
data linkage studies, 669–671
GAS, MASK, and PANDA
studies, 673
longitudinal cohort and registry
datasets, 671–672
major surgery in neonatal
period, 668
prenatal exposure, 674
prospective cohort studies with
children, 672–673
randomized trials, 673

Anesthesia (Continued)
neurotoxicity of
anesthetic exposure effects on,
developing brain and, 651f,
652–656
anesthetic neuroprotection and, 662
animal studies in, 663–668
barbiturates, 659
benzodiazepines, 659
chloral hydrate, 652.e1–652.e11t, 659
deleterious effects of untreated pain
and stress, 661
dexmedetomidine, 652.e1–652.e11t,
660
exposure time, dose, and anesthetic
combinations, 660–661
future research in, 675–676
inhaled anesthetics, 658–659
ketamine, 652.e1–652.e11t, 657–658
limitations of available clinical
studies in, 674–675
nitrous oxide, 652.e1–652.e11t, 659
normal brain development, 651–652
opioid analgesics, 660
potential alleviating strategies for,
661–662
propofol, 652.e1–652.e11t, 659–660
putative mechanisms for, 656–657
recommendations for clinical
practice in, 676
xenon, 652.e1–652.e11t, 659
non-operating room, 1195
anesthetic risk in, 1198–1199
angiography with embolization and,
1210.e1f, 1211.e1f, 1210–1211
computed tomography and,
1200–1203, 1202f
diagnostic angiography and, 1210.e1f,
1210
difficult airway management and, 1200
emergencies in MRI scanner in, 1199
endoscopic procedures in, 1213
interventional radiology and,
1209–1213
magnetic resonance imaging and,
1203–1207, 1203f, 1205f, 1206f
magnetoencephalography in, 1207
nuclear medicine in, 1207–1208
personnel requirements for, 1197
procedures in, 1199–1200
quality assurance of, 1198
radiation therapy and, 1208–1209,
1209f
sclerotherapy of venous and lymphatic
malformations in, 1211–1213,
1211f, 1212f, 1212t
specific locations for, 1200–1213,
1202f, 1203f
standards and guidelines in, 1196
stereotactic radiosurgery and, 1208
off-site. see Off-site anesthesia
outside of operating room and,
outcome after exposure to, 674
past medical history and, 32
pharmacogenetics that affect, 94–96
simulation in, 1347–1356
applications of, 1352
challenges in, 1354
debriefing in, 1353–1354
definition of, 1348
future of, 1354
high-fidelity, 1352–1353
human patient simulators in,
1349–1350, 1350f
hybrid simulation in, 1350
partial task trainers in, 1348–1349,
1349f
simulation-based training in,
1347–1348
sites for, 1351–1352, 1351f, 1351t
standardized patients, 1350
traditional learning versus, 1352, 1352t
use in evaluation, 1353–1354
virtual reality and immersive
environments, 1350–1351

Anesthesia carts, 1197
Anesthesia crisis resource management
(ACRM) program, 1347–1348
Anesthesia information management
systems, 1329, 1329f
Anesthesia machine, 1207, 1323–1327
circuits of, 1326f
humidifier of, 1325
scavenger system of, 1323–1324
ventilator of, 1325–1327
Anesthesia Patient Safety Foundation, 1348
Anesthesia record, 1329, 1329f
Anesthesia workstation (AWS), patient
evaluation and preparation, 1034–1035
Anesthesiologists' Non-Technical Skills
(ANTS), 1353–1354
Anesthetic crisis resource management
(ACRM), 1038
Anesthetic depth control, of inhalation
anesthetic agents, 110f, 124–126, 124t
Anesthetic neuroprotection, 662
Anesthetic risk, in non-operating room
anesthesia, 1198–1199
Angiography
description of, 426–429, 427f, 428f
with embolization, 1210–1211,
1210.e1f, 1211.e1f
Angiotensin I, 218, 722, 739
Angiotensin II, 218, 722, 739
Angiotensin-converting enzyme (ACE)
inhibitors, 495, 566, 602, 740, 749
Anisotropy
musculoskeletal ultrasound imaging,
1066–1067, 1067f
Ankle block, 1130–1131, 1131f
Ankle clonus test, 820
Anomalous origin of left coronary artery
from pulmonary artery, 395, 411–412,
597
Anomalous pulmonary venous
connection, 458, 459f
Anoplasty, 976
Antacids, 43, 43t
Antagonists, 188–189
5-hydroxytryptamine type 3-receptor,
185–186
flumazenil, 189
methylnaltrexone, 189
naloxone, 188
naltrexone, 188–189
physostigmine, 189
Anterior chamber paracentesis, 911
Anterior commissure scope, rigid
ventilating bronchoscope and, 359
Anterior cricoid split, 895–896, 896f
Anterior fontanel, 6
Anterior horn cell, disorders of, 632–633
Anterior ischemic optic neuropathy, 922
Anterior mediastinal mass, 255, 267,
267t, 268t, 275, 384, 385f
Anthracycline chemotherapeutics, 262
Antiarrhythmic agents, 498–503, 499t
adenosine, 502–503
amiodarone, 501
atenolol, 501
β-blockers, 501
class III agents, 501–502
digoxin, 503
dofetilide, 502
dronedarone, 501–502
esmolol, 501
flecainide, 500–501
ibutilide, 502
lidocaine, 500
magnesium sulfate, 503
phenytoin, 500
procainamide, 498–499
propafenone, 500–501
propranolol, 501
sotalol, 502
Vaughan Williams classification of, 498t
verapamil, 502
Antibiotics
after tourniquet, 829
for bone and joint infections, 835

Antibiotics (Continued)
endocarditis prophylaxis uses of,
400, 401t
neuromuscular depressing properties
of, 157
preoperative, 42, 43t
prophylactic uses of, 400, 401t
Anticholinergics, 187–188
for asthma exacerbations,
319.e2–319.e3t
preoperative, 39
Anticoagulation
hemodialysis uses of, 735
noncardiac surgery in congenital heart
disease and, 613
protamine reversal of, 535
Anticonvulsants
for intracerebral hematomas, 696
perioperative management in
epilepsy, 647t
Antidiuretic hormone, 217, 217.e1f, 715
dysregulation of, 221t
serum osmolality regulation by, 730
syndrome of inappropriate antidiuretic
hormone secretion and, 232,
715–716, 716t
Antiemetics, 185–187
for postoperative nausea and vomiting,
910t
preoperative, 42
Antiepileptic drugs, 644, 645t, 646t
Antifibrinolytics, 507, 542–545, 542f
for cardiac surgery, 438, 543–544,
543f, 546
in cardiopulmonary bypass, 508
for craniosynostosis surgery, 547, 920
dosing of, 545–546
for other types of major surgery,
546–547
recommendations for, 547
in scoliosis surgery, 828–829
trauma and, 547
Antihistamines, 185
cimetidine, 185
diphenhydramine in, 185
famotidine, 185
ranitidine, 185
Antihypertensives, 492–493t
Antiinsulin effect of anesthesia, 773
Antimicrobial prophylaxis, 1294–1298,
1295t
indications for, 1290.e1t, 1297–1298
β-lactams allergy in, 1296–1297
selection of, 1296
timing of, 1296
Antireflux valves, 1317
Antisialagogues, 888
Antithrombin (AT), 530, 534–535
Antithrombin III
deficiency, 509
deficiency of, 563
source of, 238
Anus, imperforate, 976
Anxiolytics, for sedation, 1229–1232,
1230–1231t, 1232f
Aortic aneurysms, 593
Aortic balloon valvuloplasty, 576
Aortic cross-clamp, in cardiopulmonary
bypass, 514
Aortic dissection, in Marfan syndrome, 406
Aortic root replacement, in Marfan
syndrome, 406
Aortic stenosis, 404–405, 405f, 463–464,
576, 592, 983t
Aortopulmonary window, 451–452, 452f
Aortoventriculoplasty, 430–431t
Apert syndrome
airway difficulties in, 340t
congenital hand anomalies in, 928
craniosynostosis in, 917–918
midface procedures in, 922–923
orbital hypertelorism in, 922, 922f
Apidra, 706
APL. see Acute promyelocytic leukemia
Aplastic crises, 240

Apnea
  defined, 846
  perioperative, 1074–1075
  postoperative
    in formerly preterm infant, 59–61,
      60f, 60.e1f, 61f, 62f
    in micropremie, 956, 957t
    in premature/preterm infant, 12, 1246
  of prematurity, 12
Apnea hypopnea index (AHI), 852
Apneic technique, 888–889
Apology of medical errors, 68–69
Apoptosis, 19
  normal brain development and, 651
Apoptotic cell death, 652–654,
  652.e1–652.e11t, 653f, 654f
Apoptotic neurodegeneration, 688
Apparent volume of distribution,
  103–104
Appendectomy, laparoscopic, 750f
Apraclonidine, 907t
Aprepitant, 186
Apresoline. see Hydralazine
APRICOT. see Anaesthesia Practice in
  Children Observational Trial
Aprotinin, 507–508
  adverse effects of, 544
  in cardiac surgery, 438
  dosing of, 546
  in scoliosis surgery, 828–829
  secondary benefits of, 544–545
  for stress response after cardiac
    surgery, 448
  use of, 543
aPTT. see Activated partial thromboplastin
  time
Aqueous humor, 904–905
Arachidonic acid, 145f
Arachnoid cysts, 699.e1f
Argatroban, 508–509, 564
Arginine vasopressin, 218, 712–713, 730
Argon, 752
Arndt Emergency Cricothyrotomy Set,
  359, 359.e1f
Arrhythmias, 414–420
  acute management of, 412–420
  atrioventricular block, 410–411, 411f,
    415–416t
  bundle branch block, 411, 415–416t
  halothane-induced, 135
  hyperkalemia and, 641–642
  in interventional cardiology, 579
  junctional rhythm, 415t, 417f
  long QT syndrome, 418–420, 419f
  during neurosurgery, 694
  noncardiac surgery in congenital heart
    disease and, 613
  postoperative, 1247
  premature atrial contractions or
    beats, 414
  premature ventricular contractions or
    beats, 418
  sinus, 413–414, 414f, 415t
  sinus bradycardia, 415t
  sinus rhythm, 415t, 418f
  sinus tachycardia, 415t, 416f
  succinylcholine-related, 152
  supraventricular tachycardia, 414–418,
    418f
  ventricular fibrillation, 420
  ventricular tachycardia, 418–420, 419f
Arterial blood gases, in malignant
  hyperthermia, 1032, 1032t
Arterial cannulation, 1271–1277
  axillary artery catheterization,
    1275–1276
  in burn injury, 944
  dorsalis pedis and posterior tibial artery
    catheterization, 1277
  femoral artery catheterization, 1276–1277
  radial artery catheterization, 1271–1275,
    1275f, 1276f
  temporal artery catheterization, 1276
  umbilical artery catheterization, 1271,
    1274f

Arterial carbon dioxide tension
  (PaCO2), 474
  age-dependent variables of, 10t
Arterial catheter
  for craniotomies, 683
  in thoracic surgery, 370
Arterial line
  in abdominal surgery, 748
  in cardiopulmonary bypass, 440
  in massive blood transfusion, 303
  in trauma patient, 1013
Arterial occlusion, cardiac catheterization
  and, 578
Arterial oxygen tension (PaO2), 474
  age-dependent variables of, 10t
Arterial pressure
  continuous cardiac output technique
    based on, 1342
  fluid management and, 216–218,
    218f
Arterial saturation (SaO2), 477
Arterial switch operation, 430–431t,
  455, 457f, 508, 595
Arterial thrombosis, cardiac
  catheterization and, 578
Arterial-venous ECMO
  (AV ECMO), 555
Arteriovenous malformation (AVM),
  695–696
  in cystic hygromas, 927
  in non-operating room anesthesia,
    1211, 1211.e1f
Artery of Adamkiewicz, 818
Arthrogryposis, 1331
Arthrogryposis multiplex congenita, 340t
  orthopedic surgery in, 839
Artifacts, 1070
ASD. see Atrial septal defect
Aseptic necrosis, 723
Aseptic technique, in central venous
  catheterization, 1260–1261, 1262f
Aspirated foreign bodies, endoscopy for,
  866.e1f, 877–881, 878f, 879f, 879t,
  880.e1f, 880.e1t
Aspirin, 536, 613
  for Kawasaki disease, 401
  respiratory disease and, 176
Asthma, 316–320
  adenotonsillectomy and, 856
  assessment of, 317.e2t
  classification of, 317.e1t,
  development of, 316
  diagnosis of, 311, 316
  exacerbations, 319t, 319.e1f,
    319.e2–319.e3t
  intraoperative bronchospasm in,
    318, 318f
  treatment of, 317, 317.e3f, 318.e1f
Astigmatism, 912
Astrocytoma, 269–270, 625, 695
Asymptomatic cardiac murmur, 58, 59t
Ataxia telangiectasia, 904
Ataxic cerebral palsy, 620t
Atelectasis
  absorption, 766
  after scoliosis surgery, 816, 816t
  postoperative, 1245
  regional, 522
  in sickle cell disease, 323
Atenolol, 491, 501
Atlantooccipital dislocations, 693
Atlanto-associated wheezers, 316
ATP-binding cassette proteins, 111
Atracurium, 154, 155, 646t, 742
  effective doses of, 128t
  in liver transplantation, 782
Atrial arrhythmias, 596
Atrial myxomas, 401
Atrial natriuretic peptide, 218
Atrial pressure, 429
Atrial septal defect (ASD)
  closure of, 574, 574f
  description of, 391–392, 450, 451f,
    588–590, 589t
Atrial septostomy, 557, 561, 573–574

Atrioventricular block, 410–411, 411f,
  415–416t
  during cardiac catheterization, 579
Atrioventricular canal defect, 394, 450
Atrioventricular canal repair, 430–431t
Atrioventricular (AV) dissociation, 418
Atrioventricular septal defect (AVSD),
  450–451, 452f
  complete form of, 591
  description of, 450, 451f, 452t
  noncardiac surgery in congenital heart
    disease and, 589t, 591
  partial form of, 591
  repair, 430–431t
  transitional or intermediate forms of, 591
Atropine, 187, 907t
  for bradycardia, 1247
  for cardiopulmonary resuscitation, 1024
  emergency surgery in trauma patient
    using, 1009t
  oculocardiac reflex and, 905
  for postoperative adenotonsillectomy, 867
  preoperative, 685
Auricular branch of vagus nerve block,
  1092–1093
Autism spectrum disorder, 51–53, 52t
Autoimmune adrenal insufficiency, 723
Autologous blood donation, 304
Autologous predonation, in scoliosis
  surgery, 828
Automated external defibrillation, 1021
Autonomic hyperreflexia, 694
Autophagy, 652–653, 655
Autosomal dominant congenital muscular
  dystrophy, 639t
Autosomal recessive congenital muscular
  dystrophy, 639t
Autotransfusion, 301–302
AV ECMO. see Arterial-venous ECMO
AVSD. see Atrioventricular septal defect
Awake craniotomy, 697
Awake intubation, 340
Axillary artery, catheterization of,
  1275–1276
Axis of intervention, in musculoskeletal
  ultrasound imaging, 1065–1066,
  1067f
Axis of scan, musculoskeletal ultrasound
  imaging, 1065
Axonal disorders, 633–634
Azathioprine, 635
  in liver transplant, 787
  in lung and heart-lung transplantation,
    800
Azithromycin, 400, 401t

B
Back pain
  causes of, 1187–1188
  chronic, 1181, 1184t
Baclofen, 621, 1193
Bacterial infection
  in infective endocarditis, 399–400,
    400t, 401t
  in rheumatic fever and rheumatic heart
    disease, 399
Bag-mask ventilation, 1288
Bag-valve-mask ventilation, 1018
Balloon angioplasty, 465
Balloon atrial septostomy, 427, 455, 595
Balloon valvuloplasty, 578
  aortic, 576
  percutaneous, 592, 593
Balloon-tipped bronchial blockers, for
  single-lung ventilation, 373–376,
  374f, 375f, 375t
Bar coding, 1329–1330
Baralyme, 1324
Barbiturates, 140–141
  methohexital, 140
  neurotoxicity of, 659
  for sedation, 1230–1231t, 1232–1233
  thiopental, 140–141
Bariatric surgery, 763–767
Barium esophagram, 423, 423f

Baroreceptor reflex response, 131–132
Barotrauma, 938–939
Barrel chest, 972–973
Base excess, 229–230
Basilar skull fractures, 692
"Bat ears," 928
Battery unit, 1312.e1f
Battle sign, 692
"Batwing" sign, 386–387, 386f
BCPA. see Bidirectional cavopulmonary
  anastomosis
Becker muscular dystrophy (BMD),
  550–551, 639t, 640, 838
Beckwith-Wiedemann syndrome, 269,
  340t, 760–761, 978
Behavior rating scales, 1138
Behavioral interventions
  parental presence during induction of
    anesthesia and, 28–29, 30f
  pharmacologic interventions, 29
  preoperative preparation on, 27–28,
    27.e1t
Benzodiazepine sedatives, 178–180
Benzodiazepines
  emergency procedures application, 1012
  in extremely premature infant, 965–966
  for lidocaine-induced seizures, 1026
  neurophysiologic effects of, 688t
  neurotoxicity of, 659
  noncardiac surgery in congenital heart
    disease using, 608–609
  pharmacogenetics of, 95
  premedication uses of, 1059
  preoperative, 36–37
  for sedation outside operating room,
    1231–1232
Beraprost, 497
Berlin Heart EXCOR, 552t, 559, 559f,
  562f
Bernoulli equation, 424
Best interests standard, informed
  permission and, 66–67
Best Pharmaceuticals for Children Act,
  75, 119–120
Betapace. see Sotalol
Betaxolol, 907–908, 907t
Bevacizumab, 907t, 908, 912, 981
Bicarbonate, 230
  in body fluids, 227t
  kidney regulation of, 730–731
Bicaval cannulation, 514
Bicuspid aortic valve, 463, 592
Bidirectional cavopulmonary anastomosis
  (BCPA), 598
Bidirectional Glenn operation, 460
Bier block, 1131
Bile ducts, 14
Bilevel positive airway pressure therapy, 863
Biliary atresia, 776
Biliary reconstruction, 785
Biliary stones, 243
Biliary tract growth and development, 14
Bilirubin, 773
Bioavailability, 113
Bioimpedance, 1343–1344, 1344f
Biolung, 571
Bio-Medicus BP-50 (Medtronic), 552t,
  557–558
Bioreactance, 1343–1344, 1344f
Biotransformation, alterations in,
  115–116
Biphasic kinetics, 103, 103f
Biphasic stridor, 877–878
Birth, hemodynamic changes at, 470.e1t,
  471
Bispectral index, 108f, 117, 190–191, 1338
  in scoliosis surgery, 830
Bisphosphonates, 722
Bitolterol, for asthma exacerbations,
  319.e2–319.e3t
BiVAD. see Biventricular ventricular assist
  device
Bivalirudin, 509
Biventricular ventricular assist device
  (BiVAD), 551, 570

Bivona Pedia-Trake percutaneous tracheostomy device, 359, 359.e2f
Bladder exstrophy, 762–763, 762f
Blalock-Taussig shunt, 430–431t, 434, 455, 460, 461f, 598
Bleeders, 249
Bleeding
  cardiac surgery-related, 438, 537t
  in chronic renal failure, 741
  coagulation tests for, 534
  genetics of, 533
  in heart-lung transplantation, 804
  hemostatic medications for, 529
  in middle ear and mastoid surgery, 843
  perioperative, 96
  in rhinologic procedures, 844
  surgical, human factors for, 534
Bleeding risk, 236–237
Bleeding time, 236–237, 237t
Blended learning, 1350
Bleomycin, 262, 268–269, 1212t
Blood coagulation, 525–526
Blood flow
  in cardiopulmonary resuscitation, 1018–1019, 1019f
  pulmonary
    obstruction of, in congenital heart disease, 394, 394t
    shunting and, 475
  renal
    description of, 729
    developmental issues in, 13
Blood loss
  in craniosynostosis surgery, 919–921
  estimated predicted, during surgery, 280, 280t
  in interventional cardiology, 578–579
  monitoring of, 1337
  during neurosurgical anesthesia, 688–689
  in orthognathic surgery, 925
  physiologic derangement associated with, 534
  in scoliosis surgery
    managing, 829–830
    minimizing, 827–829
Blood pressure
  cerebrovascular autoregulation and, 680–681, 681f
  control of, in postanesthesia care unit, 1247–1248
  dexmedetomidine and, 181f
  equilibrium point of, 217–218, 218f
  inhaled anesthetics and, 131
  in noncardiac surgery in congenital heart disease, 604–605
Blood pressure cuffs, 1330
Blood pressure device, 1330
Blood products, 537–538
  albumin, dextrans, starches, and gelatins in, 288
  allogenic, reduce patient exposure to, 301–304
    autotransfusion in, 301–302
    controlled hypotension in, 302–303
    erythropoietin in, 301
    intraoperative blood recovery and reinfusion in, 301–302
    normovolemic hemodilution in, 303–304
    preoperative autologous blood donation in, 301
  in chronic kidney disease, 741
  cryoprecipitate, 282t, 285–286, 534, 538
  desmopressin, 288
  fractionated human, 538–541
  fresh frozen plasma, 281, 282t, 286f, 534, 538
  plasma-derived factor concentrates, 287
  platelets, 282t, 283–284
    activation of, 531
    after cardiac bypass, 537
  red blood cell substitutes in, 288–289
  red blood cell-containing components, 281–283, 281t
  in scoliosis surgery, 828–829

Blood products (Continued)
  special processing of cellular blood components in, 284–285, 285.e1t
  in transfusion therapy, 278–306
Blood resuscitation, 1011
Blood safety, in developing countries, 1310
Blood transfusion, 278–306, 279t
  allogenic blood components, reduce patient exposure to, 301–304
    autotransfusion in, 301–302
    controlled hypotension in, 302–303
    erythropoietin in, 301
    intraoperative blood recovery and reinfusion in, 301–302
    normovolemic hemodilution in, 303–304
    preoperative autologous blood donation in, 301
  avoidance of, 529
  blood components and alternatives in, 281–289
    albumin, dextrans, starches, and gelatins in, 288
    cryoprecipitate in, 282t, 285–286
    desmopressin in, 288
    pathogen inactivation/reduction in, 286–287
    plasma in, 282t, 285, 286f
    plasma-derived factor concentrates in, 287
    platelets in, 282t, 283–284
    prothrombin complex concentrates in, 287–288, 288t
    recombinant factors in, 287
    red blood cell substitutes in, 288–289
  in cancer patients, 276–277
  in developing countries, 1309
  in hematologic disorders, 237–239
  intraperitoneal, 983
  massive transfusion in, 289–300, 289e
    acid-base balance in, 298
    citrate toxicity in, 296–298, 298f
    coagulopathy in, 289–291, 290f, 291f
    dilutional thrombocytopenia in, 291–292, 292f, 293f
    disseminated intravascular coagulation in, 294
    factor deficiency in, 292–294, 294t
    fibrinolysis in, 294
    hyperkalemia in, 295–296, 295f, 295.e1t
    hypocalcemia in, 296–298, 298f
    hypothermia in, 298
    infectious disease considerations in, 300
    monitoring during, 298–300, 298.e1f, 299f, 300f
  during neurosurgical procedures, 688–689
  in scoliosis surgery, 830
  in sickle cell disease, 245, 322
Blood urea nitrogen (BUN), 733
Blood vessels
  choice of access, in interventional cardiology, 577
  ultrasound of, 1068–1069
Blood volume
  cardiopulmonary bypass prime and, 507
  circulating, 218–219
    in extremely premature infant, 957t
  developmental issues in, 17
  fluid management and, 219f, 219t
  in transfusion therapy, 279–281, 280t
Blood warmer, 1316, 1316f, 1316.e1f
Blood-brain barrier, 216, 688
Blood-brain barrier transporter, 92
Bloom syndrome, 254
Blunt reflex bronchoconstriction, anesthetic agents for, 860.e1t
B-mode (brightness) ultrasound, 1062
BNP. see B-type natriuretic peptide
Body composition, drug distribution and, 110–111, 110f
Body fluid(s)
  compartments, 219t
  composition of, 227t

Body mass index, 764
Body piercings, 25, 25.e1t
Body plethysmography, 311
Body substance isolation, 1291
Body surface area, 932–933, 933f
Body temperature
  in cardiopulmonary bypass, 439
  in cardiopulmonary resuscitation, 1023
  monitoring of
    in magnetic resonance imaging, 1205
    in malignant hyperthermia, 1036
    in scoliosis surgery, 827
  in neurosurgical procedures, 684–685
  postoperative, 1251
  premature infant and, 966
  preservation of, 1316–1317
  tourniquet-related, 834
Body water
  age and, relationship between, 6t
  electrolyte distribution and, 218, 219f, 219t
  normal losses of, 221t
  regulatory mechanisms of, 216–218, 216.e1f
Body weight
  gestational age and, 5, 5t
  maintenance fluid requirements and, 221t
  total body water and, 218, 219f
Bohr equation, 966
Bone, ultrasound of, 1068, 1068f
Bone and joint infections, 834–835
  anesthesia considerations for, 835
  clinical presentation of, 835
  pain management for, 835
  pathophysiology of, 834–835
  treatment options for, 835
Bone marrow aspiration procedures, 274
Bone morphogenetic protein-7 (BMP-7), 740–741
Bone-anchored hearing aids, 843, 844t
Bosentan, 497, 958
Botulinum toxin, 621
Boyle apparatus, 1311
Brachial plexus block, 1107–1109, 1108f, 1109f, 1110f
  dosing for, 1088t
  infraclavicular, 1110–1111, 1111f, 1112f, 1113f
  interscalene, 1111–1114, 1113f
  supraclavicular, 1109–1110, 1110f
Brachial plexus injury, during cardiac catheterization, 580
Brachial plexus surgery, 928
Brachiocephalic vein catheterization, 1266–1267, 1266f
Bracing, for scoliosis, 811
Bradycardia
  dexmedetomidine as cause of, 182–183
  dexmedetomidine-induced, 608
  fetal, 985–986
  hypoxemia as cause of, 1247
  inhaled anesthetics and, 131
  ketorolac as cause of, 181
  in neonate, 131
  postoperative, 1247
  postoperative apnea and, 956
  reflex, 907
  sevoflurane causing, 443
  spinal anesthesia as cause of, 1079
  succinylcholine-related, 152
Bradykinin, 506
Brain
  anesthetic exposure effects on, 651f, 652–656
    abnormal reentry into cell cycle in, 656
    apoptotic cell death and, 652–654, 652.e1–652.e11t, 653f, 654f
    dendritic architecture alterations, 655
    destabilization of cytoskeleton in, 656
    developing spinal cord and, 656
    genomic, proteomic, and epigenetic alterations, 656

Brain (Continued)
  long-term brain cellular viability, neurologic function, and behavior in, 654–655
  mitochondria degeneration, 655
  neurogenesis and gliogenesis, 655
  trophic factors, 655
  development of, 651–652
  growth and development of, 18
  immature, 650–677, 958–960
Brain injury, intraoperative management of, 1012
Brain tumors, 694–695, 695f, 695.e1f
  primary, 625–627, 628t
Brain-derived neurotrophic factor (BDNF), 655
Brainstem gliomas, 625, 694
Breast milk, preoperative fasting and, 23, 23f, 25.e1t
Breast reduction surgery, 930
Breath-hold/breath-holding, 1202
Breath-holds, 583
Breathing, cardiopulmonary resuscitation and, 1018, 1018t
Breathing circuits, 1323, 1325
Breathing mechanics, 9–11
  airway dynamics in, 11–12
  chest wall and respiratory muscles in, 9
  closing capacity and, 11
  elastic properties of lung and, 9
  functional residual capacity and, 11, 11f
  regulation of breathing in, 11–12
  static lung volumes and, 10, 10t
  total lung capacity and, 10, 10f
Breathing system filter placement, 1287f
Brevibloc. see Esmolol
Brimonidine, 907t
British Committee for Standards in Haematology (BCSH), 237–238
Brody disease, 639t
Bromage score, 1173t
2-Bromochloroethylene, 138
Bronchial obstruction, types of, 879t
Bronchial smooth muscle tone, anesthetic agents for, 860.e1t
Bronchial stenosis, 806
Bronchoalveolar lavage, 806
Bronchogenic cysts, 380
Bronchomalacia, 316
Bronchopneumonia, after burn injury, 934–935
Bronchopulmonary dysplasia, 62–63
  in extremely premature infant, 955, 955t
Bronchopulmonary fistula, 973
Bronchoscopy
  diagnostic, 872–873, 873t, 874f
  direct, 872–881
  fiberoptic, in double-lumen tubes, 377
Bronchospasm, 1335
  intraoperative, in asthma, 318, 318f
Brooke formula, for burns, 939–940, 940t
Brown fat, 961
Brown-Roberts-Wells stereotactic head frame, modified, 695.e1f
Brugada syndrome, 96
B-type natriuretic peptide (BNP), 490–491, 550
Bullard laryngoscope, 363–364, 363.e1f
Bundle branch block, 411, 415–416t
Bupivacaine, 96
  after thoracic surgery, 370
  asystole induced by, 1060
  epidural, 1171, 1172t
  epinephrine with, 1056–1057, 1056f
  hyperbaric, 1078–1079
  infusion dose of, 1057
  intravesical, 1143–1144
  pharmacokinetics of, 1054
Buprenorphine, 772, 1191–1192
  neurotoxicity of, 652.e1–652.e11t
Burkitt lymphoma, 258
Burn injuries, 932–952
  airway control in, 947–949, 949f
  anesthetic management in, 943–952, 943t, 945f, 946f

Burn injuries (Continued)
  awakening and, 949
  blood loss monitoring and, 946–947,
    946f, 948f
  calcium homeostasis in, 936–937,
    937.e1f
  carbon monoxide poisoning, 934,
    939, 939.e1f
  cardiac issues in, 933
  central nervous system issues in,
    935, 943t
  endocrine issues in, 936
  gastrointestinal issues in, 936
  hematologic issues in, 935–936, 943t
  hepatic issues in, 935, 943t
  hyperalimentation and, 949
  maintenance of anesthesia in, 945,
    945.e1f, 946.e1f
  mediators released from, 932–933
  metabolic issues in, 936, 943t
  methemoglobinemia and, 947
  mortality rate for, 932
  neuropsychiatric issues in, 937
  pain management and postoperative
    care in, 942f, 950–952, 951f, 952t
  pathophysiology of, 932–937, 933f
  pharmacology considerations in, 937–938
  pulmonary issues in, 933–935, 934f,
    943t
  renal issues in, 935, 943t
  resuscitation and initial evaluation in,
    938–942
    airway and oxygenation in, 938–939,
      938f
    associated injury in, 940
    carbon monoxide and cyanide
      poisoning in, 939, 939.e1f
    circumferential burns and, 940–941,
      941f
    electrical burns and, 941, 941f, 945f
    volume resuscitation in, 939–940,
      940f, 940t, 940.e1f
  skin issues in, 932–933, 936, 943t
  succinylcholine-related hyperkalemia
    in, 160
  tracheal tube size in, 947
  ultrasound-guided vascular access,
    regional analgesia, and
    cardiovascular assessment in,
    949–950
Butorphanol, 170–171
Butyrylcholinesterase (BChE),
  95–96, 116
Bypass circuit, 505, 506t

C

C5, 1031–1032
CACNA1A, 94
Caffeine, 60, 81, 902, 956–957, 1246
Caffeine-halothane contracture test
  (CHCT), 1032, 1049f
Calabadion, 159
Calan. *see* Verapamil
Calcineurin phosphatase inhibitors, 787
Calcitonin, 722
Calcitriol, 720–721
Calcium, 489
  cardiac, 116–117
  for cardiopulmonary resuscitation,
    1025
  citrate toxicity and, 296, 298f
  homeostasis of
    burn injury effects on, 936–937,
      937.e1f
    physiology of, 720–721
  hypercalcemia and, 721–722
  hypocalcemia and, 721
  ionized, 439, 962
  malignant hyperthermia and,
    1039, 1045f
  monitoring concentrations during
    cardiac surgery, 439
Calcium channel antagonists, 646t
Calcium channel blockers, 725
  in scoliosis surgery, 828

Calcium chloride, 484–485t
  for cardiopulmonary bypass, 519
  for cardiopulmonary resuscitation, 1025
  citrate toxicity and, 296
  for hyperkalemia, 737, 737t
  for hypocalcemia, 721, 947
Calcium gluconate, 484–485t
  for cardiopulmonary resuscitation, 1025
  citrate toxicity and, 296
  for hyperkalemia, 737, 737t
  for hypocalcemia, 721, 947
Calcium homeostasis, 962
Calcium-sensing receptor, 720–721
Calcium-sensitizing agents, 490
Cancer, 261
  airway tumors, 265
  anemia and, 276
  anterior mediastinal mass, 267, 267t,
    268f, 275
  blood transfusion for, 276–277
  cardiac tumors, 265–267
  children with, 273–275, 274f, 275f
  coagulation disorders, 270–271
  coagulation factor deficiency in, 276–277
  coagulopathy in, 273t
  gastrointestinal tumors, 269
  hematologic malignancies, 271, 273t
  hematopoietic stem cell transplant,
    272–273
  hepatic tumors, 269
  immunomodulation, 277
  incidence of, 262t
  neurocognitive impairments in, 271
  pain and, 271
  perioperative considerations for, 273–276
  preoperative laboratory testing and
    evaluation, 273, 273t
  red blood cell transfusion for, 276
  renal tumors, 269
  retinoic acid syndrome, 271–272
  surgical interventions for, 275
  thrombocytopenia in, 276
  tumor lysis syndrome, 271
Cancer therapy
  chemotherapy, 262, 263t
  principles of, 261–265
  radiation therapy, 264–265
  targeted antitumor agents, 263–264
Cannizzaro reaction, 138
Cannon *a* waves, 417f
Cannulas, 504–506, 506t
Cannulation, of cardiopulmonary
  bypass, 514
Capillary leak, 227
Capnography, 1239–1240
  for cardiopulmonary resuscitation
    monitoring, 1023
  for malignant hyperthermia, 1036
  in noncardiac surgery in congenital
    heart disease, 605
Capoten. *see* Captopril
Captopril, 495
Capoten. *see* Captopril
Carbachol, 907t
Carbamazepine, 645t, 1192
Carbapenem, 646t
Carbohydrate metabolism, disorders
  of, 630
Carbohydrates, 773
Carbon dioxide (CO_2)
  in cerebral blood flow, 681–682, 681f
  description of, 579, 599
  pneumoperitoneum uses of, 751–752
  ventilatory response to, in micropremie,
    956
Carbon dioxide absorbents, 124t
Carbon dioxide absorption, 1324, 1324f
Carbon dioxide analyzers, 1335–1337,
  1336f
Carbon monoxide
  detection of, 137–138
  inhaled anesthesia breakdown and,
    124t, 138
Carbonic acid, 730–731
Carbonic anhydrase, 730–731
Carboxyhemoglobin, 26, 1333

Cardene. *see* Nicardipine
Cardiac allograft vasculopathy, 483
Cardiac arrest
  after extubation, 1244
  causes of, 593
  COVID-19 and, 1289
  diagnosis of, 1017
  epidemiology and outcome of,
    1016–1017
  extracorporeal membrane oxygenation
    for, 570
  hyperkalemic, 295, 1027, 1031
  non-operating room anesthesia and, 1198
  perioperative, 1026–1027
  post-resuscitation stabilization in,
    1028–1029
  simulation applications for, 1352
Cardiac arrhythmias, 414–420
  acute management of, 412–420
  atrioventricular block, 410–411, 411f,
    415–416t
  bundle branch block, 411, 415–416t
  junctional rhythm, 415t, 417f
  long QT syndrome, 418–420, 419f
  premature atrial contractions or
    beats, 414
  premature ventricular contractions
    or beats, 418
  sinus, 413–414, 414f, 415t
  sinus bradycardia, 415t
  sinus rhythm, 415t, 418f
  sinus tachycardia, 415t, 416f
  supraventricular tachycardia, 414–418,
    418f
  ventricular fibrillation, 420
  ventricular tachycardia, 418–420, 419f
Cardiac calcium, 116–117
Cardiac catheterization, 426–429, 427f,
  428f
  complications and limitations of,
    577–581
    arterial thrombosis and occlusion, 578
    blood loss, 578–579
    cardiac perforation and
      tamponade, 578
    cardioversion, 579
    contrast toxicity, 579–580
    damage or dysfunction of valve, 578
    desaturation, 579
    dysrhythmias, 579
    embolization, 579
    endocarditis, 581
    hypothermia and hyperthermia, 581
    morbidity, 577–578
    mortality, 577–578
    neurologic events, 580
    overcoming of, 581
    radiation exposure, 580–581
    venous thrombosis and occlusion, 578
    vessel rupture, perforation, and
      dissection, 578
  hemodynamic calculations using, 584f
  interventional procedures of, 573–576
    angioplasty and stenting, 575–576
    aortic balloon valvuloplasty, 576
    atrial septal defect closure, 574, 574f
    atrial septostomy, 573–574
    diagnostic catheterization in, 573, 574t
    electrophysiologic catheterization
      in, 577
    patent ductus arteriosus closure, 575,
      575f, 576f
    percutaneous pulmonary valve
      replacement, 576
    ventricular septal defect closure,
      574–575, 575f
  liver disease and, 779
  spinal anesthesia for, 1075
  vessel access in, 577
Cardiac chambers, measurements of, 425
Cardiac disease, anesthesia for VAD
  patient with, 566–567
Cardiac disturbances, in liver disease, 778
Cardiac fibroma, 402
Cardiac implantable electronic device, 421

Cardiac index, 753
Cardiac murmur, 409
Cardiac output
  after burn injury, 933
  determination of, 429
  developmental issues in, 13
  in extremely premature infant, 957
  fetal, 470–471, 470.e1t
  Fick measurement of, 1343
  in Fontan circulation, 480
  inhalation anesthetics uptake from
    lung, 108f, 121–122
  monitoring of, 1341–1342
  neuromuscular blocking drugs and, 150
Cardiac pacing, transcutaneous, 1021–1022
Cardiac pump mechanism, 1018–1019
Cardiac rhabdomyoma, 401–402, 402f
Cardiac surgery, 433–467
  anesthetic drugs used in, 443–446
    etomidate, 444–445
    fentanyl, 445
    halothane, 443–444
    isoflurane, 443
    ketamine, 444
    long-term neurocognitive-
      developmental outcomes
      associated with, 446
    nitrous oxide, 444
    pancuronium, 445
    propofol, 445
    remifentanil, 445
    sevoflurane, 443
    sufentanil, 445
  antifibrinolytics for, 543–544, 543f, 546
  in aortic stenosis, 463–464
  cardiopulmonary bypass in, 438–443
    induction of anesthesia, 440–441
    institution and separation from
      bypass, 442–443
    maintenance of anesthesia, 441–442
    monitoring in, 438–440
  in coarctation of aorta, 464–465
  congenital heart disease and, 449t
  fast tracking in, 447
  hemostatic alterations during, 534–536
    failure of hemostasis in, 536, 536t
    routine anticoagulation, 534–535
  in interrupted aortic arch, 465, 465f
  long-term neurocognitive-
    developmental outcomes
    associated with, 446
  pancuronium for, 156
  pediatric intensive care unit, transport
    and transfer to, 466
  perioperative challenges in cardiac
    anesthesia in, 435–438
    cyanosis in, 435–436
    impaired hemostasis in, 436–438
    intracardiac shunting in, 436
  preoperative evaluation in, 433–435, 435t
  pulmonary vascular resistance in, 443
  regional anesthesia in, 446–447
  in simple left-to-right shunts, 449–453,
    449t
    aortopulmonary window, 451–452,
      452f
    atrial septal defect, 450, 451f
    atrioventricular septal defect,
      450–451, 451f, 452f, 452t
    patent ductus arteriosus, 452–453,
      453f
    ventricular septal defect, 450
  in simple right-to-left shunts, 453–455
    anomalous pulmonary venous
      connection, 458, 459f
    hypoplastic left heart syndrome,
      459–463, 460f
    tetralogy of Fallot, 453–455, 454f
    transposition of great arteries,
      455–456, 456f, 457f
    truncus arteriosus, 456–458, 458f
  stress response to, 447–449
  systemic vascular resistance in, 443
  thrombosis and, 536–537
Cardiac tamponade, 578

Cardiac transplantation, 553, 791–800
  anesthesia and, 799–800
  for congenital heart disease, 792–793
  contraindications to, 793
  demographics and epidemiology of,
    791–792, 792f
  for dilated cardiomyopathy, 793
  for hypertrophic cardiomyopathy, 793
  immediate postoperative management
    in, 797–799, 798f
  intraoperative problems and
    management in, 796–797, 797t
  myocarditis indications for, 398
  noncardiac surgery in congenital heart
    disease and, 614
  pathophysiology of disease in, 792
  preoperative evaluation in, 794–795,
    795t
  repeat transplantation, 793
  for restrictive cardiomyopathy, 793
  surgical technique in, 795–796
  survival and quality of life in, 799,
    799f, 800f, 800t, 801f
  waitlist and donor selection in, 793–794,
    794t
Cardiac tumors, 265–267, 401–402
CardiacAssist. see TandemHeart
Cardiology, essentials of, 391–432
Cardiomuscular glycogen storage disease,
    340t
Cardiomyopathy, 395–398, 395f, 396f,
    397f
  in dystrophinopathies, 640
  portal hypertension with, 778
  surveillance recommendation for
    childhood cancer survivors, 273t
Cardioplegia, in cardiopulmonary bypass,
    442
Cardioplegia solution, 513t
Cardiopulmonary arrest, outside operating
    room, 1199
Cardiopulmonary bypass (CPB), 438–443,
    504–528
  acute kidney injury after, 739–740
  anesthesia on, 519–520
    pharmacodynamics, changes in, 520
    pharmacokinetics, changes in, 519
  basic aspects of, 504–508, 505f, 506t
    cardiopulmonary bypass prime,
      506–508, 506t
    cardiopulmonary bypass pumps, 506
    circuit and cannulas, 504–506, 506t
  conventional ultrafiltration and
    modified ultrafiltration during,
      518–519
  deep hypothermic circulatory arrest in,
    520–521, 520f, 521f
  effects of, 522–526
    cardiac, 522
    coagulation, 525–526, 526f
    endocrine system, 527
    gastrointestinal, 526–527
    hepatic, 526–527
    immune system, 527
    neurologic monitoring, 524–525
    pulmonary, 522, 523f
    pulmonary vasculature, 522
    renal, 526–527
    systemic vasculature, 522
  failure to wean from, 551–553
  fast tracking and recovery, 527
  flow rates on, 517–518
  in heart transplantation, 796
  hematocrit on, 517
  hemostasis impairments during, 436
  heparin for, 534–535
  induction of anesthesia, 440–441
  institution and separation from bypass,
    442–443
  intensive care unit transport, 527
  in Jehovah's Witnesses, 511–512
  maintenance of anesthesia, 441–442
  monitoring in, 438–440
  myocardial protection in, 512, 513t
  pediatric versus adult, 506t

Cardiopulmonary bypass (Continued)
  phases of, 512–515
    aortic cross-clamping and
      intracardiac repair phase in, 514
    cannulation and initiation of bypass
      in, 514
    checklist for bypass management
      and, 515t
    cooling phase in, 514
    deep hypothermic circulatory arrest
      or selective cerebral perfusion
      phase in, 514
    heparin and coagulation
      management in, 513–514
    postbypass period in, 515, 515t
    prebypass period in, 512
    removal of aortic cross-clamp and
      rewarming phase in, 514
    separation from bypass in, 514–515
  pH-stat versus α-stat management,
    515–517, 516f
  prebypass anesthetic management in, 519
  regional cerebral perfusion in, 521–522,
    521f
  sickle cell disease and, 246
  special coagulation and hematologic
    problems of, 508–511
    antithrombin III deficiency, 509
    desmopressin, 510
    fibrinogen concentrate, 509–510
    heparin-induced thrombocytopenia,
      508–509
    prothrombin complex concentrate,
      510
    recombinant factor VIIa for massive
      hemorrhage, 509
    sickle cell disease, 510–511
  stress response to, 448–449
  systemic inflammatory response
    syndrome and, 523f, 525
  temperature monitoring during, 439
Cardiopulmonary bypass prime, 506–508,
    506t
Cardiopulmonary bypass pumps, 506
Cardiopulmonary resuscitation (CPR),
    1016–1029
  active compression-decompression in,
    1028
  in anaphylaxis, 1027
  COVID-19 and, 1289
  defibrillation and cardioversion in,
    1020–1022
    automated external defibrillation, 1021
    electric countershock in, 1020, 1020f
    open-chest, 1021
    transcutaneous cardiac pacing in,
      1021–1022
  diagnosis of cardiac arrest and, 1017
  epidemiology and outcome of in-
    hospital cardiopulmonary arrest,
    1016–1017
  extracorporeal, 553
  extracorporeal membrane oxygenation
    for, 1028
  historical background of, 1016
  in hyperkalemic cardiac arrest, 1027
  mechanics of, 1017–1020
    airway management in, 1017–1018
    breathing in, 1018, 1018t
    circulation in, 1018–1020, 1019f
    rate and duty cycle in, 1019–1020
  medications used during, 1023–1026
    amiodarone, 1025–1026
    calcium, 1025
    epinephrine, 1023–1024
    glucose, 1025
    lidocaine, 1026
    sodium bicarbonate, 1024–1025
    vasopressin, 1024
  monitoring during, 1022–1023
  open-chest, 1028
  in perioperative cardiac arrest, 1026–1027
  post-resuscitation stabilization in,
    1028–1029
  in pulseless electrical activity, 1028

Cardiopulmonary resuscitation (Continued)
  in supraventricular tachycardia,
    1027–1028
  2020 AHA pediatric advanced life
    support guidelines update, 1029
  vascular access in, 1022–1023
    intraosseous, 1022
    intravenous, 1022
Cardiovascular assessment
  in burn injury, 949–950
  in scoliosis surgery, 824
Cardiovascular disease. see Heart disease
Cardiovascular pharmacology, 483–503
  antiarrhythmic agents, 498–503, 499t
    adenosine, 502–503
    amiodarone, 501
    atenolol, 501
    β-blockers, 501
    class III agents, 501–502
    digoxin, 503
    dofetilide, 502
    dronedarone, 501–502
    esmolol, 501
    flecainide, 500–501
    ibutilide, 502
    lidocaine, 500
    magnesium sulfate, 503
    phenytoin, 500
    procainamide, 498–499
    propafenone, 500–501
    propranolol, 501
    sotalol, 502
    Vaughan Williams classification
      of, 498t
    verapamil, 502
  β-blocking agents, 491–492
    atenolol, 491
    carvedilol, 491–492
    esmolol, 491
    ivabradine, 492
    labetalol, 491
    propranolol, 491
  B-type natriuretic peptide, 490–491
  calcium, 489
  calcium-sensitizing agents, 490
    levosimendan, 490
    nesiritide, 490–491
    triiodothyronine, 489
  vasoactive drugs, 483–484
    amrinone, 488
    digoxin, 484–485t, 488–489
    dobutamine, 486
    dopamine, 485–486
    enoximone, 488
    epinephrine, 486
    isoproterenol, 486
    milrinone, 488
    norepinephrine, 486–487
    phenylephrine, 487
    phosphodiesterase inhibitors, 487–488
    practical considerations for, 484–485
    vasopressin, 487
  vasodilators, 492–493t, 492–498
    ambrisentan, 497
    angiotensin-converting enzyme
      inhibitors, 495
    beraprost, 497
    bosentan, 497
    captopril, 495
    clevidipine, 494
    enalapril, 495
    endothelin-receptor antagonists, 497
    epoprostenol, 496
    hydralazine, 495
    iloprost, 497
    inhaled nitric oxide, 495–496
    lisinopril, 495
    losartan, 495
    macitentan, 497
    nicardipine, 494
    nitroglycerin, 493–494
    phenoxybenzamine, 494–495
    phentolamine, 494–495
    prostaglandin E₁, 495
    prostanoids, 473f, 477t, 496–497

Cardiovascular pharmacology (Continued)
  selexipag, 497
  sildenafil, 497–498
  sodium nitroprusside, 493
  treprostinil, 496
Cardiovascular physiology, 468–474
  congenital heart disease
    exercise physiology in the child with
      repaired, 476t, 478–479
    incidence and prevalence of,
      474–475, 474t, 475.e2f
    pathophysiologic classification of,
      475–478
  fetal, 989–991, 990f
  fetal circulation and, 468–471, 470.e1t,
    475.e2f, 480.e1f
  Fontan physiology and, 479–480,
    480f, 480.e1f, 481f, 482f
  neonatal cardiovascular system and,
    471–472, 471t, 473f, 480.e1f
  pulmonary vascular physiology and,
    471t, 472–474, 474f, 474t
  transitional circulation and, 470.e1t, 471
  of transplanted heart, 480–483
    denervated heart and, 482–483,
      483f, 483t
  transplant morbidity and, 483
Cardiovascular system
  associated with childhood obesity, 55t
  growth and development of, 12–13
    blood pressure and, 12, 13t
    cardiac output and, 13
    heart rate and, 12, 12t
    normal electrocardiographic
      findings, 13
  inhaled anesthetics and, 130–133
  laparoscopic surgery effects on, 753
  prematurity and, 957–958, 957t
  toxicity of local anesthetics and, 1056
Cardioversion, 579, 1020–1022
Careload. see Beraprost
Carpal tunnel syndrome, 634
Carpenter syndrome, 918
Carteolol, 907t
Carvedilol, 402–403, 491–492
Caspases, 652–653
Casting, for scoliosis, 811
Catabolism, 631
CATCH-22 association, 405, 452
Catecholamines
  halothane and, 132
  in pain perception, 87
Catechol-O-methyltransferase (COMT), 87
Catheters
  central venous, 439, 725, 1318
  complete heart block induced by, 579
Caudal anesthesia
  in preterm infants, 1246–1247
  urinary retention and, 1252
Caudal epidural anesthesia, 1079–1080,
    1080f, 1081f
Caudal morphine, 446
Causalgia, 1186
Cavopulmonary connection, 407, 430–431t
CBC. see Complete blood count
Cefazolin, for endocarditis prophylaxis,
    400, 401t
Ceftriaxone, 400, 401t
Celecoxib, 93, 1190
Celiac syndrome, 320
Cell salvage device, for Jehovah's
    Witnesses, 511
Cellular blood components, special
    processing of, 284–285, 285.e1t,
Central alveolar hypoventilation, 927
Central core disease, 636, 1049–1050
Central diabetes insipidus, 712–713
Central hypoventilation syndrome, 760–761
Central line-associated bloodstream
    infection, 1264
Central nervous system (CNS), 650
  burn injury effects on, 935, 943t
  cerebral palsy in, 621
  congenital anomalies of, 700–702, 701f

Central nervous system *(Continued)*
  inhaled anesthetics and, 128–130
  interventional cardiology and, 580
  laparoscopic surgery effects on, 753–754
  local anesthetic toxicity and, 1056
  malformations of, 622–624, 624t
  tumors of, 269–270
Central neuraxial blockade, 1072–1087
  anatomic and physiologic
      considerations in, 1072–1074,
      1072.e1f, 1073f, 1074f
  epidural, 1079–1087
      adjunctive drugs in, 1085
      caudal, 1079–1080, 1080f, 1081f
      complications of, 1078.e1f,
          1085–1087, 1086t
      opioids for, 1085
  spinal, 1074–1079, 1076f, 1077f
      complications of, 1079
      drug selection for, 1079
Central pontine myelinolysis, 231, 716, 780
Central sensitization, 1149
Central shunt, 430–431t
Central venous cannulas, in burn
      injury, 944
Central venous catheter, 725, 1318
  during massive blood transfusion, 280
Central venous catheterization, 1259–1261
  in abdominal surgery, 748
  aseptic technique in, 1260–1261, 1262f
  brachiocephalic vein and, 1266–1267,
      1266f
  in cardiopulmonary bypass, 439
  complications of, 1259–1260
  external jugular vein and, 1261
  femoral vein and, 1267, 1268f
  indications for, 1259
  internal jugular vein and, 1261–1267,
      1263–1264f, 1265f
  in neurosurgery, 690
  Seldinger technique in, 1261, 1261f
  subclavian vein and, 1264–1266, 1266f
  in urologic surgery, 750
Central venous pressure (CVP), 226, 561
Centrifugal pump, 557–558, 557f
CentriMag (Thoratec), 552t, 558
Cerebellar astrocytomas, 694
Cerebellar herniation, 679
Cerebral aneurysms, 593
Cerebral angiography, 1210, 1210.e1f
Cerebral blood flow (CBF)
  dexmedetomidine effects on, 183
  increased intracranial pressure and,
      679f, 680
  inhaled anesthetics and, 128
Cerebral blood volume, 680
Cerebral cortex, malformations of, 625
Cerebral edema, 735, 935
  liver disease and, 779
Cerebral ischemia, 678–679, 679f
Cerebral metabolic rate, for oxygen
      consumption, 680
Cerebral metabolic rate for oxygen
  inhaled anesthetics and, 128
Cerebral metabolic rate for oxygen
      consumption (CMRO₂), 302
Cerebral near-infrared spectroscopy, 510
Cerebral oxygen saturation, 754
Cerebral palsy, 19, 620–622, 620t, 621t,
      623t
  comorbidities in, 621–622
  minimum alveolar concentration
      affected by, 127
  musculoskeletal pain in, 1184t,
      1187–1188, 1188t, 1189
  orthopedic surgery in, 835–836
  pain in, 1189t
  scoliosis in, 817
Cerebral perfusion pressure
  description of, 1011
  increased intracranial pressure and,
      679f, 680
  liver transplantation and, 779–780
Cerebral salt wasting, 234, 921
Cerebrospinal fluid (CSF), 678

Cerebrovascular autoregulation, 680–682
Cervical spine
  anomalies, 350t
  evaluation of, 1008f
  injury, 693
  injury of, 1006
  instability of, 903
  teratoma of, 996, 996f
Chain of communication, 1197
Charcoal filters, in malignant
      hyperthermia, 125–126, 1038–1039,
      1038.e1f
Charcot-Marie-Tooth disease, 633
CHARGE association, 452
CHARGE syndrome, 406, 969
CHD. *see* Congenital heart disease
CHD7 gene, 406
Chemotherapy, 262, 263t, 269
Cherubism, 340t
Chest
  anatomic relationship with neck,
      1263–1264f
  circumferential burn of, 940–941, 941f
Chest cage disruption, 817
Chest compressions, 1018t, 1247
Chest radiography
  in heart disease, 422, 423f
  in noncardiac surgery in congenital
      heart disease, 602
Chest trauma, 1007–1009, 1011t
  intraoperative management of, 1013
Chest wall
  breathing mechanics and, 9
  fentanyl, 167
Chest-encircling method for cardiac
      compressions, 1019f
Chewing gum, preoperative fasting and, 23
Chiari malformations, 624, 624t, 701–702,
      701t, 702f, 703f
Child
  circulating blood volume, 219t
  growth and development of
      airway dynamics in, 11–12
      blood volume, 12, 12t
      cardiac output, 13
      cardiovascular system, 12–13
      chest wall and respiratory muscles, 9
      closing capacity and, 11
      elastic properties of lung, 9
      face, 6
      functional residual capacity and,
          11, 11f
      gastrointestinal tract, 16
      heart rate and, 12, 12t
      hematopoietic and immunologic
          system, 17–18
      hepatic system, 14–15
      neurologic and cognitive issues,
          18–20, 19t
      normal electrocardiographic
          findings, 13
      pancreas, 16–17
      regulation of breathing in, 11–12
      renal system, 13–14, 14f
      respiratory system, 6–12
      static lung volumes and, 10, 10t
      teeth, 6
      total lung capacity, 10
      upper airway, 6–12, 8f
  head circumference and, 5–6
  in informed consent, 65, 66t
  intrathoracic lesions in, 384–386, 385f,
      386f
  normal and abnormal, 1, 2t
  perioperative behavioral stress in
      health care provider intervention
      in, 29
  single-lung ventilation, 373–379
Child abuse, 77
Child maltreatment, 77
Child soldiers, 1300
Childhood Adenotonsillectomy Trial
      (CHAT), 850
Children's Hospital of Eastern Ontario
      Pain Scale, 1136t, 1138, 1139t

Children's Hospital of Wisconsin Sedation
      Scale, 117
Child-Turcotte-Pugh (CTP) score, 776–777
Chin lift, 333
Chloral hydrate, 184–185, 1230–1231t
  neurotoxicity of, 652.e1–652.e11t, 659
  sedation outside operating room,
      1229–1231
Chloramphenicol, 84
Chlorhexidine, 1260
Chloride
  in body fluids, 227t
  neurotoxicity of anesthetics and, 656–657
Chloroprocaine, epidural, 1172t
Chloroprocaine test, 1175f
Chlorpromazine, 518
Choanal atresia, 922–923, 969
Cholecystectomy, 244
Cholestatic liver disease, 776
Cholinesterase deficiency, 80, 151–152
Chordee, 756
Choreoathetoid cerebral palsy, 620t
Choroid plexus papillomas, 695
Choroidal blood volume, 901
Christmas disease, 250–251
Chromaffin tumors, 724
Chromatin immunoprecipitation (ChIP), 80
Chromosomal syndromes, 404
Chromosome 22q11.2 deletion
      syndrome, 405
  DiGeorge syndrome and, 405, 962
Chronic hemolytic anemia, 243
Chronic inflammatory demyelinating
      polyneuropathy, 634
Chronic kidney disease, 736–739
  cardiovascular complications in, 738–739
  causes of, 739, 739t
  hematologic problems in, 738
  management of, 741
  postoperative concerns of, 740–741
  prevention of, 740–741
  risk factors of, 739–740
Chronic otitis media, myringotomy with
      tube insertion and, 842
Chronic pain, 1181–1194
  abdominal, 1183t, 1184–1185, 1185t
  ancillary data in, 1184
  complementary therapies for, 1194
  in complex regional pain syndrome,
      1186–1187, 1187f, 1187t
  genetics of, 93–94
  headache, 1182, 1183t, 1185–1186,
      1186t
  history in, 1182–1183, 1183t, 1184t
  multidisciplinary approach to,
      1181–1182
  musculoskeletal, 1184t, 1187–1188,
      1188t
  pharmacotherapy for, 1189–1194
      acetaminophen in, 1190
      adjuvant drugs in, 1192–1194
      anticonvulsants in, 1192
      antidepressants in, 1192–1193
      corticosteroids, local anesthetics,
          NMDA receptor antagonists,
          capsaicin, α2-adrenergic
          receptor agonist, 1193–1194
      muscle relaxants in, 1193
      nonsteroidal antiinflammatory drugs
          in, 1190
      opioids and pain management in,
          1190–1192, 1191t
Chronic renal failure
  causes of, 739t
  urologic surgery in, 749
Chronic sinusitis, rhinologic procedures
      for, 843–844
Cidofovir, 731–732
Cimetidine, 185, 646t
Cineangiography, 427
Ciprofol, 144
Circuit surfaces, biocompatibility of, 506
Circuits
  for anesthesia machine, 1326f
  cardiopulmonary bypass, 504–506, 506t

Circulating blood volume, 218–219
  estimation of, in transfusion therapy,
      279–281, 280t
  in extremely premature infant, 957t
  fluid management and, 219t
Circulation, fetal, 468–471, 470.e1f,
      475.e2f, 480.e1f
Circulatory arrest
  deep hypothermic, 448–449
  safe duration of, 520f
Circulatory support, mechanical, 549–572
  complications of, 570–571
  contraindications for, 554
  criteria for, 551t
  devices for, 552t, 554
  future directions in, 571
  indications for, 550–554, 550t
  initiation for, 551–553
  learning systems and databases of, 550
  organ transplantation and, 568
  outcomes of, 567–570
  perioperative management of, 561–567
      anesthetic considerations, 564–567,
          565t
      hematologic considerations, 562–564
      hemodynamics, 561–562, 562f, 563f
      prevention of infection in, 564
      respiratory considerations, 562
  single ventricle physiology and, 555–556,
      569–570
  ventricular assist devices for, 557–560,
      567
      biventricular, 551, 570
      centrifugal pump, 557–558, 557f
      continuous flow pumps, 560
      extracorporeal membrane
          oxygenation, 549–550, 552t,
          554–557
      history of, 549
      immunologic complications of, 571
      implantation of, 570
      left, 551, 557
      long-term devices, 559–560
      pulsatile pumps, 559–560, 559f
      short-term devices, 557–559
  on wait-list survival, effect of, 568–569
Circumcision, 756
Circumferential burns, 933, 940–941, 941f
Circumferential technique for cardiac
      compressions, 1018, 1019f
Circumoral paresthesia, 1056
Cisatracurium, 155, 646t, 742, 963
  effective doses of, 128t
  in liver transplantation, 782
Cisplatin, 262, 269
Citrate toxicity, 296–298, 298f
Citrate-phosphate-dextrose, 507
Clarithromycin, 400, 401t
Classic hemophilia, 250–251
Clearance
  in children, 106
  creatinine, 13, 107
  "perfusion limited," 113
Cleft lip and palate, 914–917, 914.e1,
      915f, 915t, 916.e1
Clevidipine, 494
Cleviprex. *see* Clevidipine
Clindamycin, 400, 401t
Clinical Croup Score, 890t
Cloacal exstrophy, 757, 762–763, 762f
Clonazepam, 645t
  neurotoxicity of, 652.e1–652.e11t, 659
Clonidine, 38, 180–181, 866, 1187
  effects on evoked potentials, 831
  epidural, 1085, 1172t
  for pain, 1150–1151
  preoperative, 36t
  regional anesthesia and, 1251
Clopidogrel, 536
Closing capacity, 11
Closing volume, 11
Clostridium botulinum, 636
Clostridium difficile, 571
Clot inhibition, 531
Clotting factor enzyme complexes, 290f

Clotting profile, 537
CLOVES syndrome, 1211, 1211f
CNS. *see* Central nervous system
Coagulation, 270–271, 1306
  cardiopulmonary bypass and, 525–526, 526f
  developmental, 533
  physiology of, 530–532
    amplification in, 531, 531f
    clot inhibition in, 531
    fibrinolysis in, 531–532, 532f
    initiation in, 530, 530f
    propagation in, 531, 531f
Coagulation cascade, 288
Coagulation disorders, 249–253
  hemophilia, 250–252, 251t, 252t
  hypercoagulability, 252–253
  platelet disorders, 248
  screening for, 249
  von Willebrand disease, 250, 251t
Coagulation factors, deficiency of, 276–277
Coagulopathy
  after heart surgery, 536
  in cancer patients, 273t
  in craniosynostosis surgery, 919–921
  desmopressin for, 288
  in inborn errors of metabolism, 632
  major surgery and, 533–534
  massive blood transfusion and, 289–291, 290f, 291f
Coarctation of aorta, 464–465, 589t, 593
Coarctation repair, 430–431t
Cobb method, 810, 810f
Cocaine, 907t
  intoxication, malignant hyperthermia *versus*, 1033t
  topical, 908
Cochlear implants, 843, 844t
Codeine, 85t, 87–89, 162t, 171–172, 772
  dosing guidelines for, 1152t
  for opioid-induced respiratory depression, 865
  pharmacokinetics of, 87–89, 88f
Coercion, 67–68
Cognition, pain management strategies and, 1135
Cognitive behavioral therapy, 1185
Cognitive biases, 353
Cognitive frame, 353
Cognitively impaired child
  pain assessment in, 1135–1142
    Face, Legs, Activity, Cry, Consolability Observational Tool in, 1136t, 1138, 1138t
    Non-Communicating Children's Pain Checklist in, 1136t, 1141.e1t
    Pain Indicator for Communicatively Impaired Children in, 1136t, 1141.e1t
    University of Wisconsin Pain Scale in, 1136t
Cold blood cardioplegia, 512
Cold steel technique, in adenotonsillectomy, 846
COLDS scoring tool, 858
Cole formula, 1322
Colloid oncotic pressure, 216
Colloids
  in abdominal surgery, 747
  after burn injury, 940
Color Analog Scale, 1136
Color flow Doppler techniques, 424
Comfort Scale, 1136t, 1138–1140, 1140t
Common arterial outlet, 456–458
Common atrium, 450, 588
Communicating hydrocephalus, 699
Communication
  in neurologic disorders, 620
  in pediatric intensive care unit, 67, 67t, 72, 73t
Compartment syndrome, 809–810, 930
Complete blood count (CBC), 254–255
Complete heart block, catheter-induced, 579
Complete tracheal rings, 896–897

Complex regional pain syndrome (CRPS), 1186–1187, 1187f, 1187t
Complex shunts, 476, 477t
Compound A, 138, 1324
Compound B, 138
Compound imaging, 1069, 1069f
Compound muscle action potential (CMAP), 821
Compression atelectasis, 974
Computed tomography (CT)
  heart disease applications of, 426, 426f, 427t
  for non-operating room anesthesia, 1200–1203, 1202f, 1203f
Computer Face Scale, 1136t, 1138
Conal defects, in ventricular septal defect, 590
Conceptual realism, 1348
Concussion, 694
Conditions for Participation for Anesthesia Services, 1196
Conducting research, 75
Conduction, 1315
Conduction disorders, 414, 415–416t
Conduction disturbances, noncardiac surgery in congenital heart disease and, 613
Conductive blankets, 1315
Confidentiality, for adolescents, 69
Conflicts of interest, 75–76
Congenital adrenal hyperplasia, 722
Congenital anomalies of coronary arteries, 597
Congenital cystic adenomatoid malformation, 983t
Congenital cystic lesions, 380
Congenital diaphragmatic hernia, 380–381, 382f, 972–973, 972.e1, 983t, 986–987
Congenital glaucoma, 905
Congenital goiter, 997
Congenital heart disease (CHD), 391–395, 985–986, 986f
  adenotonsillectomy and, 856
  cardiac surgery for, 433–467
    in anomalous pulmonary venous connection, 458, 459f
    in aortic stenosis, 463–464
    in aortopulmonary window, 451–452, 452f
    in atrial septal defect, 450, 451f
    in atrioventricular septal defect, 450–451, 451f, 452f, 452f
    cardiopulmonary bypass in, 438–443
    in coarctation of aorta, 464–465
    control of systemic and pulmonary vascular resistance in, 443
    cyanosis in, 435–436
    etomidate in, 444–445
    failure of hemostasis in, 436
    fast tracking in, 447
    fentanyl in, 445
    halothane in, 443–444
    in hypoplastic left heart syndrome, 459–463, 460f
    in interrupted aortic arch, 465, 465f
    intracardiac shunting in, 436
    isoflurane in, 443
    ketamine in, 444
    long-term neurocognitive-developmental outcomes associated with, 446
    nitrous oxide in, 444
    pancuronium in, 445
    in patent ductus arteriosus, 452–453, 453f
    preoperative evaluation in, 433–435, 435t
    propofol in, 445
    regional anesthesia in, 446–447
    remifentanil in, 445
    sevoflurane in, 443
    stress response to, 447–449
    sufentanil in, 445
    in tetralogy of Fallot, 453–455, 454f

Congenital heart disease *(Continued)*
    transport and transfer to pediatric intensive care unit in, 466
    in transposition of great arteries, 455–456, 456f, 457f
    in truncus arteriosus, 456–458, 458f
    in ventricular septal defect, 450
  cardiac transplantation for, 792–793
  classification of, 449t
  congenital lobar emphysema and, 973–974, 974f
  defined, 474–475
  in developing countries, 1309
  eye surgery and, 901
  grown-up, 433–434
  heparin for, 534–535
  incidence and prevalence of, 391–392, 392f, 474–475, 474t, 475.e2f
  noncardiac surgery in, 587–618
    altered respiratory mechanics and, 611
    ancillary studies and laboratory data in, 601–602
    anesthesia technique in, 607
    anticoagulation and, 613
    arrhythmias and, 613
    arterial blood pressure assessment in, 604–605
    in atrial septal defects, 588–590, 589t
    capnography in, 605
    cardiac transplantation and, 614
    conduction disturbances and, 613
    in congenital anomalies of coronary arteries, 597
    cyanosis and, 609–610
    Eisenmenger syndrome and, 590, 612–613
    electrocardiography in, 605
    emergence from anesthesia in, 609
    emergency drugs in, 604
    endocarditis prophylaxis and, 611
    fasting guidelines in, 602
    Fontan procedure and, 599
    Glenn anastomosis and, 598–599
    heart failure and, 610
    Hemi-Fontan procedure and, 598–599
    history and physical examination in, 601
    hypotension and, 609
    increase perioperative risk in, 600t
    induction of anesthesia in, 604
    informed consent in, 602
    inhalational agents in, 607
    intraoperative management in, 603–609
    intravenous access in, 604
    intravenous agents in, 607–609
    maintenance of anesthesia in, 606–609
    mechanical circulatory support devices and, 614
    medications in, 602, 603f
    monitoring in, 604–606
    myocardial ischemia and, 596, 611
    nerve palsies and, 614
    Norwood procedure and, 598
    outcomes of, 589t, 615–616
    pacemakers and implantable cardioverter-defibrillators and, 613
    perioperative problems and special considerations in, 609–615
    perioperative stress response and, 614–615
    postoperative care in, 609
    premedication in, 603
    pulmonary artery banding and, 598
    pulmonary hypertension and, 611–612, 612.e1f
    pulse oximetry in, 605
    risk analysis in, 615–616
    systemic air embolization and, 613
    systemic-to-pulmonary artery shunt and, 598
    temperature monitoring in, 605
    types of, 615

Congenital heart disease *(Continued)*
    urinary output measurements in, 605
    ventricular dysfunction and, 610
    ventricular pressure overload and, 611
    in ventricular septal defects, 589t, 590–591
    ventricular volume overload and, 610
  pathophysiologic classification of, 475–478
    intercirculatory mixing in, 474f, 476–477, 477f
    shunting in, 475–476, 476f, 476t, 477t
    single ventricle physiology in, 477–478, 478t
  physiologic classification of, 394–395, 394t
  prior repair, 432
  repaired, exercise physiology in the child with, 476t, 478–479
  segmental approach to diagnosis of, 392–393, 392f, 393f
  selected, 588–600, 589t
  surgical procedures in, 430–431t
Congenital high airway obstruction syndrome, 996
Congenital hypothyroidism
  airway difficulties in, 340t
  in Down syndrome, 903
Congenital laryngeal webs, 883.e1f, 889
Congenital lobar emphysema, 380, 381f, 973–974, 974f
Congenital muscular dystrophies, 639t, 641
Congenital myasthenic syndromes, 635
Congenital myopathies, 636, 636t
Congenital pulmonary lesions, 987
Congenital scoliosis, 811–813, 812t
Congenital tracheal stenosis, 380
Congenital upper airway obstruction, 889
Congenitally corrected transposition of great arteries, 589t, 595–596
Congestive heart failure, 222
Conjugation, 769
Conotruncal malformations, 407
Consultant, on pain management team, 1182
Consumptive coagulopathy, 1211–1212
Contact artifact, 1070
Contact transmission, of infectious disease, 1281–1283
Context-sensitive half-time
  after short duration infusion, in total intravenous anesthesia, 205f, 206f
  of desflurane, 766
  of fentanyl, 167, 167f
  of inhalation anesthetics, 126
  of opioids, 205t
  of remifentanil, 169–170
Continuous flow pumps, 560, 563f
Continuous glucose monitor, 707
Continuous murmurs, 409
Continuous positive airway pressure (CPAP)
  in mediastinal mass, 384–385
  for obstructive sleep apnea, 858
  for pharyngeal airway obstruction, 333
Continuous renal replacement therapy, 736
Continuous subcutaneous insulin infusion, 710–711, 710f
Continuous venovenous hemodiafiltration (CVVHDF), 734
Continuous venovenous hemodialysis (CVVHD), 734
Continuous venovenous hemofiltration (CVVH), 734
Continuous waveform capnography, 342
Continuous-wave Doppler imaging, 424
Contractility, 1341
  in Fontan circulation, 480
Contracture testing, in malignant hyperthermia, 1048, 1049f
Contrast media nephrotoxicity, 580
Contrast toxicity, in interventional cardiology, 579–580

Controlled hypotension, 302–303
  after scoliosis surgery, 827
  anesthetic management during, 303
  aneurysms and, 696
  contraindications of, 303
  nitroglycerin for, 302
  remifentanil for, 302–303
Conus medullaris, 966, 1072–1073
Convection, of heat, 1314
Conventional ultrafiltration, during
    cardiopulmonary bypass, 518–519
Cook 5 Fr endobronchial catheter,
    375, 375f
Cook airway exchange catheter with Rapi-
    Fit adapter, 356, 356.e1–356.e2f
Cooley anemia, 340t
Cooling phase, in cardiopulmonary
    bypass, 514
Cooperative Study of Sickle Cell
    Disease, 244
Cor pulmonale, 689
Cordarone. see Amiodarone
Cordemcura. see Amrinone
Coreg. see Carvedilol
Corlanor. see Ivabradine
Cormack and Lehane laryngoscopic
    grading system, 335f
Cornelia de Lange syndrome, 340t
Coronary sinus, 407–409, 408f
Coronary sinus atrial septal defect, 450
Coronary sinus defects, 588
Coronavirus disease 2019 (COVID-19),
    1284–1289
  cardiac arrest and, 1289
  emergence and extubation in, 1288
  equipment decontamination and room
    turnover and, 1289, 1289t
  induction and airway management in,
    1286–1288
  preoperative testing for, 1286
  preparation for, 1285–1286, 1286.e1f,
    1287f
  regional anesthesia in, 1288
  specific pediatric anesthesia
    considerations in, 1288–1289
  summary on, 1289
Corpus callosotomy, 698
"Correction factor," for hyperglycemia, 709
Cortical development disorders, 625
Cortical oxygen saturation (So2),
    during deep hypothermic circulatory
    arrest, 521f
Corticosteroids, 646t
  during anesthesia, 708
  for chronic inflammatory demyelinating
    polyneuropathy, 634
  for laryngotracheobronchitis, 886
  in neurosurgery, 682, 691t
  preoperative, 42
  for renal disease, 749–750
  for spinal injury, 693–694
  for stress response after cardiac
    surgery, 448
  for systemic inflammatory response
    syndrome, 525
  urologic surgery and, 749–750
Cortisol, 936
  adrenal insufficiency and, 723
  hypercortisolism, 723–724
  response to surgery, 708
Cortisone, 723t
Corvert. see Ibutilide
Cosmetic procedures, 930
Cosyntropin, 723
Cosyntropin stimulation, 723
Cotrel-Dubousset instrumentation, 810
Cough, asthma and, 316–317
Cough reflex, 805
Coumadin. see Warfarin
Covera. see Verapamil
COVID-19. see Coronavirus disease 2019
COX-1, 93, 175
COX-2, 93
COX-2 inhibitors, 862, 1147
Cozaar. see Losartan

CPAP. see Continuous positive airway
    pressure
CPB. see Cardiopulmonary bypass
Cranial dysraphism, 622–624
Cranial molding, 6
Cranial vault reconstruction, in
    craniosynostosis, 918, 918f, 918.e1
Craniofacial dysostosis of Crouzon, 340t
Craniofacial syndromes, 904, 905.e1f
Craniopharyngioma, 233–234, 270, 625,
    626t, 694, 713
Craniosynostosis, 917–922, 917f,
    917t, 917.e1
  airway management in, 919, 919.e1
  blood loss, coagulopathy, and
    hyponatremia in, 919–921
  classification of, 917t
  cranial vault reconstruction in, 918.e1
  increased intracranial pressure in,
    917–918
  venous air embolism in, 921–922
Craniotomy, 694–699
  in arteriovenous malformations,
    695–696
  awake, 697
  in brain tumors, 694
  in seizure surgery, 697–699, 698.e1f
Creatine kinase
  in muscular dystrophies, 638
  succinylcholine-related increase of, 153
Creatinine clearance, 13, 107
Creatinine concentration, serum, 729
Cricoid cartilage, 325
Cricoid pressure, 49, 50t, 745–746, 1014
Cricoid split procedure, 380
Cricothyroidotomy, 693
Crigler-Najjar syndrome, 773
Crisis management, 1347–1348
Critical aortic stenosis, 592
Croup, 885–887, 885t, 886f, 886.e1f
  postintubation, 342–343, 1246
Crouzon syndrome, 1245–1246
  airway difficulties in, 340t
  craniosynostosis in, 918
  midface procedures in, 922
CRPS. see Complex regional pain
    syndrome
Cryoprecipitate, 238, 285–286, 437,
    509–510, 534, 538, 564
  for hematologic disorders, 238
  initial doses of, 282t
Cryotherapy, for retinopathy of
    prematurity, 981
Cryptorchidism, 757–758, 757f
Crystalloid(s), 224
  abdominal surgery applications
    of, 747
  in blood and fluid management,
    688–689
  for cardiovascular toxicity to local
    anesthetics, 1060
  in craniosynostosis surgery, 919
Crystalloid cardioplegia, 511–512
Cuffed tracheal tubes, 341, 341t,
    859–860, 1322
Curare, 1310
Curling ulcers, 936
Cushing syndrome, 723–724
Cutting accidents, 1283–1284
CVP. see Central venous pressure
Cyanide toxicity, 493, 939, 939.e1f
Cyanosis, 592
  in cardiac surgery, 435–436
  in interventional cardiology, 579
  in noncardiac surgery in congenital
    heart disease, 609–610
  in tetralogy of Fallot, 454
Cyclic guanosine monophosphate (GMP)
    pathway, 518
Cyclobenzaprine, 1193
Cyclooxygenase, 1134
Cyclopentolate hydrochloride, 907, 907t
Cyclophosphamide, 265–266, 635
Cycloplegia, 905
Cycloplegic agents, topical, 907

Cyclosporine, 646t
  liver disease and, 778
  in lung and heart-lung transplantation,
    806
CYP isozymes, 114, 114t, 133
CYP1A2, 81–83, 82t, 96
CYP2A6, 94–95
CYP2B6, 82t, 86t
CYP2C9, 82t, 83, 93
CYP2C19, 82t, 95
CYP2D6, 82t, 83–84, 85t, 87, 181–182,
    769, 1153
  for opioid-induced respiratory
    depression, 865
CYP2E1, 82t, 84, 93
CYP3A, 83
CYP3A4, 81, 82t, 90, 96, 168
CYP3A4.5, 82t
CYP3A5, 770
CYP3A7, 82t, 96, 770
Cystic adenomatoid
    malformations, 380
Cystic fibrosis, 16, 976
  in lung and heart-lung
    transplantation, 801
Cystic hygroma
  description of, 926
  EXIT procedure for, 996, 996f
  illustration of, 926f
Cysts
  arachnoid, 699.e1f
  bronchogenic, 380
  dermoid, 380
Cytochrome P-450 (CYP) enzyme
    system, 81, 82t, 113–114, 114t,
    770–771, 770t
Cytokine-release syndrome, 264
Cytokines
  in burn injury, 932–933
  in cardiopulmonary bypass-induced
    lung injury, 522
Cytomegalovirus infection, blood
    transfusion and, 285, 285e
Cytomegalovirus-seronegative red blood
    cells, 238–239, 239t
Cytoskeleton, destabilization
    of, 656

D
Dabigatran, 536
Dacryocystorhinostomy, 911f, 911–912,
    911.e1f
Dactylitis, 243
Damage control, 289
Damus-Kaye-Stansel procedure,
    430–431t
Dantrium, 1040t
Dantrolene
  dosing of, 1040
  for malignant hyperthermia, 1031f,
    1033t, 1036f, 1039–1041,
    1039.e1f, 1040f, 1040t
  molecular mechanisms and physiologic
    effects of, 1046f, 1047–1048,
    1047f, 1048f
  pharmacokinetics of, 1040, 1040f
  toxicity, 1041
Dapiprazole, 907t
Dartmouth Operative Conditions Scale
    (DOCS), 1218t
DDAVP. see Desmopressin acetate
Dead space/tidal volume, 10t
Deafferentation, 1075
Debriefing, 1353–1354
Debriefing Assessment for Simulation in
    Healthcare (DASH), 1353
Debrisoquine, 85–87
Deep hypothermic circulatory arrest
  in cardiopulmonary bypass, 448–449,
    514, 520–521, 520f, 521f
  neurologic monitoring for, 524
Deep sedation, 1216, 1228t
  during cardiac catheterization, 583
Deep vein thrombosis,
    tourniquet-related, 834

Defibrillation and cardioversion, 421–422,
    1020–1022
  automated external defibrillation, 1021
  electric countershock in, 1020, 1020f
  open-chest, 1021
  paddles in, 1020
  practical aspects of, 1020–1021, 1021f
  transcutaneous cardiac pacing in,
    1021–1022
  for ventricular fibrillation, 421–422
Defibrillator, 1327
Deflazacort, 640
Dehydration, 228–230, 229f, 229t
  in children, 229
  hypertonic, 229
  hypotonic, 229
  induction, in neurosurgery, 689
Delta opioid receptors, 1152, 1152.e1t
Denervated heart, physiology, 482–483,
    483f, 483t
Dental mirror, 360
Dental procedures, infective endocarditis
    prophylaxis in, 400
Denver Developmental Screening, 19
Dependent shunting, during cardiac
    anesthesia, 436
Depressed skull fractures, 692, 692f
Dermoid cysts, 380
Dermoid tracts, 702
1-Desamino-8-D-arginine, 541–542
Desaturation, in interventional
    cardiology, 579
Desflurane
  for blunt reflex bronchoconstriction,
    860.e1t
  context-sensitive half-time of, 766
  contraindications for, 964
  in eye surgery, 909
  hepatic effects of, 782
  inhalation induction with, 46
  minimum alveolar concentration
    of, 128t
  neurophysiologic effects of, 688t
  neurotoxicity of, 652.e1–652.e11t, 658
  physiochemical properties of, 114t
  remifentanil versus, 1241
  respiratory depression and, 133
Desipramine, 1192
Desmopressin, 541–542
  cardiopulmonary bypass and, 510
  for clot formation promotion after
    cardiac surgery, 438
  for coagulopathy, 438
  for diabetes insipidus, 691, 714
  in hemophilia, 287
  intranasal, 288
  in scoliosis surgery, 829
  transfusion, 288
  for von Willebrand disease, 238, 288
Desmopressin acetate (DDAVP), 541–542
Developing countries, 1299–1313
  blood safety in, 1310
  cardiac disease in, 1309
  child soldiers in, 1300
  COVID-19 pandemic in, 1302–1304
  diseases in child and, 1299–1302, 1300f
  drawover anesthesia in, 1311–1312,
    1312f
  drugs in, 1309–1310
  equipment in, 1308f, 1310–1312
  human immunodeficiency virus
    infection and acquired
    immunodeficiency syndrome in,
    1303–1304f, 1304–1306, 1305f
  human resources in, 1302
  malaria in, 1308–1309
  oxygen concentrators in, 1311, 1312,
    1312.e1f
  pain management in, 1301–1302
  perinatal mortality in, 1300
  tetanus in, 1309
  tuberculosis in, 1306–1308
  visiting providers in, 1312–1313
  war and, 1300–1301, 1301f
Developmental coagulation, 533

Developmental disabilities, 960
Developmental issues
    in cardiac anesthesia, 446
    in coagulation, 18–20
Dexamethasone, 186–187, 723
    after scoliosis surgery, 825
    for bronchopulmonary dysplasia, 955
    bupivacaine and, 1055
    for croup, 886
    for pain, 1150
    postoperative
        for adenotonsillectomy, 862–863, 862.e1t
        for nausea and vomiting, in adenotonsillectomy, 861, 861f, 862.e1t
        for opioid-induced respiratory depression, 866
    for postoperative nausea and vomiting, 1249
    steroid equivalency ratios and doses of, 723t
Dexamethasone suppression test, 723
Dexmedetomidine, 181–184, 181f, 182f, 1230–1231t, 1233–1234, 1243
    for abnormal airway, 352–353
    after myringotomy with tube insertion, 842
    after scoliosis surgery, 826
    bradycardia, 182
    burn injury effects on, 937
    cardiac catheterization uses of, 583
    effects on evoked potentials, 831
    emergence delirium from, 1243
    metabolism of, 84
    neurophysiologic effects of, 687–688, 688t
    neurotoxicity of, 652.e1–652.e11t, 660
    noncardiac surgery in congenital heart disease using, 608
    for opioid-induced respiratory depression, 866
    for pain, 1151
        after adenotonsillectomy, 866
        after burn injury, 942f, 950–951
    pharmacogenetics of, 94–95
    for pharyngeal airway obstruction, 333
    preoperative, 38
    sedation, in non-operating room anesthesia, 1209
Dextrans, 288
Dextrocardia, 392, 392f
Dextrose, cardiopulmonary bypass prime and, 507
Dextrose-containing solutions, 225
Diabetes insipidus, 233–234, 691, 712–715
    central, 712–713
    diagnosis of, 713
    major procedures and, 714
    minor procedures and, 713–714, 713f, 714t
    neurogenic, 712–713
    new perioperative diagnosis of, 714–715
    postoperative management of, 715
    transient medication-induced, 715
    triple-phase response in, 713
Diabetes mellitus, 61–62, 705–712
    anesthesia in, metabolic response to, 708
    classification of, 705–706, 706t
    cystic fibrosis-related, 320
    epidemiology of, 705–706, 706t
    glucose monitoring for, 710
    hyperglycemia and, 708
    insulin administration, methods of, 710–711
    intraoperative management of, 710–711
    intravenous fluids for, 710
    intravenous insulin infusions for, 711, 711f
    major surgery in, 711, 712f
    malignant hyperthermia-like syndrome in, 1050
    management principles for, 706–707, 706t
    postoperative management of, 711–712

Diabetes mellitus (Continued)
    premedication and, 42
    preoperative consultation of, 708–709, 709f
    preoperative management of, 709, 710f
    special surgical situations in, 712, 712f
    surgery in, metabolic response to, 708
    type 1, 705
    type 2, 705–706, 707, 711
    urgent surgery and, 712
Diabetic ketoacidosis (DKA), 712, 1050
Diagnostic angiography, 1210, 1210.e1f
Diagnostic catheterization, 573, 574t
Diagnostic laryngoscopy and bronchoscopy, 872–873, 873t, 874f
Dialysis
    perioperative, 735–736
    in renal disease, 749
    urologic surgery and, 749
DiaMedica drawover vaporizer, 1311–1312, 1311.e1f
Diamorphine, 162
Diaphragm, work of breathing and, 333, 333f
Diaphragmatic palsy, 928
Diastematomyelia, 702
Diastolic dysfunction, 454–455, 610
Diastolic murmur, 409
Diazepam, 81, 180
    in micropremie, 965–966
    neurotoxicity of, 652.e1–652.e11t, 659
    pharmacogenetics of, 95
Dibenzyline. see Phenoxybenzamine
DIC. see Disseminated intravascular coagulation
Diclofenac, 93, 909, 1145t
Difficult airway. see also Abnormal airway
    in cleft lip and palate repair, 915
    extubation of child with, 354–356. 356.e1–356.e2f, 356.e3f
    in non-operating room anesthesia, 1200
    in orbital hypertelorism, 924
    syndromes and disease processes with associated, 340t
Diffuse astrocytoma, 626t
Diffuse intrinsic pontine glioma (DIPG), 626t
DiGeorge syndrome, 405, 452t, 454, 596, 609, 721, 962
    chromosome 22q11.2 deletion syndrome and, 405, 962
Digestive system, growth and development of, 14–17
Digital block
    dosing for, 1088t
    of foot, 1131
    of hand, 1118–1119, 1119f
Digitek. see Digoxin
Digox. see Digoxin
Digoxin, 484–485t, 488–489, 499t, 503, 1028
1, 25-Dihydroxyvitamin D, 720–721
Dilantin. see Phenytoin
Dilated cardiomyopathy, 265–266, 395, 395f
    cardiac transplantation for, 793
    in developing countries, 1306
    in Duchenne muscular dystrophy, 815
Diltiazem, 477t
Dilutional coagulopathy, 299, 920
Dilutional thrombocytopenia, 284, 291–292, 299
Dipeptidyl peptidase-intravenous inhibitors, 707
Diphenhydramine, 39, 185
2, 3-Diphosphoglycerate, 435
Dipivefrin, 907t
Direct contact transmission, 1281
Direct laryngoscopy, 872–881, 1323
Disaster training, 1348
Discharge, from postanesthesia care unit
    criteria for, 1251–1252, 1251t, 1252t
    preterm infant and, 1246–1247
Disclosure, informed consent and, 68
Disequilibrium syndrome, 735

Disseminated intravascular coagulation, 270–271, 291, 532
    D-dimer test for, 294
    in malignant hyperthermia, 1031t, 1041
    massive blood transfusion and, 294
    in micropremie, 963–964
Dissociative anesthesia, 584
Distal hereditary motor neuropathy, 633
Distraction, 1142
Distraction osteogenesis, mandibular, 924
Diuretics, for acute renal failure, 733
DNA methylation, 81
"Do Not Resuscitate," 70
Dobutamine, 484–485t, 486
Dobutrex. see Dobutamine
Documentation, of sedation, 1227–1228, 1227.e1f, 1228t, 1228.e1f, 1228.e3f, 1228.e4f, 1228.e5f
Dofetilide, 502
Dolasetron, 185–186
Donation after cardiac death, 72, 73t
Donation after circulatory death (DCD) donors, 802–803
Donor blood, cellular blood component processing, 284–285, 285.e1t,
Dopamine, 484–485t, 485–486
    for acute renal failure, 734
Doppler tissue imaging, 424
Doppler ultrasound, 1062–1063, 1062f
Dorsalis pedis catheterization, 1277
Dosimeters, 581
Double discordance, 596
"Double-bubble" sign, 976, 976f
Double-glove technique, 1279
Double-lumen tubes, for single-lung ventilation, 376–378, 376f, 377t
Double-switch procedure, 456, 596
Doubly committed defect, in ventricular septal defect, 590
Down syndrome, 404
    aberrant subclavian artery in, 407
    airway difficulties in, 340t
    bradycardia in, 132
    eye surgery in, 903
    postintubation croup in, 1246
Down syndrome, pulmonary hypertension in, 591
Doxacurium, 771–772
Doxepin, 1192
Doxorubicin, 762
Doxycycline, 1212t
Drawover anesthesia, 1312–1313, 1312f
Drawover system, 1311
DRD1, 92
Dressing change, in burn injury, 951
Dronedarone, 501–502
Droperidol, 1249
    neurophysiologic effects of, 688t
Drug allergies, 682
Drug approval process, 119–120
Drug distribution, 109–111
    protein binding and, 102f, 103f, 109–110, 109f, 110f
Drug errors, 1329–1330
Drug interactions, 118–119, 118f
Drug labeling, 119–120
Drug metabolism and excretion, 113–116
    biotransformation alterations and, 115–116
    cytochrome P-450, 81, 113–114, 114t
    extrahepatic routes of metabolic clearance and, 116
    hepatic, 104f, 113
    phase I reactions in, 81, 113–114, 114t
    renal, 107t, 115f, 116, 116f
Drug package insert, 119–120
Drug research, 76t
Drug therapy
    absorption and, 112–113, 112f
    central nervous system effects of, 128–130
    development of, for bleeding, 547–548
    drug approval process, package insert, and drug labeling, 119–120
    drug distribution and, 109–111

Drug therapy (Continued)
    body composition in, 110–111, 110f
    protein binding in, 102f, 103f, 109–110, 109f, 110f
    drug interactions and, 118–119, 118f
    linking pharmacokinetics with pharmacodynamics in, 109
    metabolism and excretion, 113–116
        biotransformation alterations and, 115–116
        cytochrome P-450, 113–114, 114t
        extrahepatic routes of metabolic clearance and, 116
        kidney and, 115f, 116, 116f
        liver and, 104f, 113
        phase I reactions in, 113–114, 114t
        phase II reactions in, 84
    pharmacodynamic models in, 107–108
        logistic regression model in, 108
        sigmoid E_{max} model in, 107–108, 108f
    pharmacodynamics of, 116–118
    pharmacokinetic principles and calculations in, 101–105
        apparent volume of distribution, 103–104
        first-order kinetics in, 101–102
        first-order multiple-compartment kinetics in, 102–103, 103f
        first-order single-compartment kinetics in, 102
        half-life in, 102
        loading dose, 105
        repetitive dosing and drug accumulation in, 105
        steady state in, 105
        zero-order kinetics, 103, 104f
Drug-induced liver injury, 773
Drug-Induced Liver Injury Network, 773
Drug-induced sleep endoscopy, for obstructive sleep apnea, 854
Dry weight, 738–739
D-TGA. see D-transposition of great arteries
D-transposition of great arteries (D-TGA), 573–574, 589t, 595
Dubowitz scoring system, 2
d-tubocurarine, 150–151, 156
Duchenne muscular dystrophy (DMD), 547, 550–551, 639t, 640, 1037–1038
    dilated cardiomyopathy in, 815
    neuromuscular blocking drugs and, 153
    neuromuscular scoliosis in, 815
    orthopedic surgery in, 838–839
Ductus arteriosus, 470
    patent, 452–453, 453f, 902–903, 957–958
        closure of, 575, 575f, 576f
        ligation of, 430–431t, 980
        noncardiac surgery in congenital heart disease and, 589t, 591–592
        transcatheter occlusion of, 980
Ductus venosus, 14, 468–469, 768
Duke criteria, for infectious endocarditis, 399
Duodenal atresia, 976, 976f
Duplicated thumb, 928
Duty cycle
    in cardiopulmonary resuscitation, 1019–1020
    in chest compressions, 1019
Dynamic airway collapse, 331
Dysfibrinogenemia, cryoprecipitate for, 285–286
Dyskinetic cerebral palsy, 620t
Dysraphism, 700
Dysrhythmias, 579
    in heart-lung transplantation, 807
Dystrophin, 640, 640f
Dystrophinopathies, 639t, 640–641
Dystrophy, 638

E

EACA. see ε-Aminocaproic acid
Ear, gestational age assessment, 5t
Early-onset scoliosis, 811–813
    postoperative complications in, 816

Ebstein anomaly, 589t, 596–597
Ecarin clotting time, 509
Echinacea, 32, 32.e1t
Echocardiography, 423–425, 423t, 424f
  cardiac output monitoring using, 1342
  noncardiac surgery in congenital heart
    disease, 605
Echogenicity, musculoskeletal ultrasound
    imaging, 1065
Echothiophate, 907t, 908
ECMO. *see* Extracorporeal membrane
    oxygenation
ECPR. *see* Extracorporeal
    cardiopulmonary resuscitation
Edema
  fluid overload and, 222, 228, 228t
  pulmonary, 228
    fluid overload and, 222
    in infants, 946–947
    noncardiogenic, 1246
    postobstructive, 1246
    postoperative fluid management
      and, 228
Edrophonium, 157, 482
Edwards syndrome, 404–405
Eectroencephalogram (EEG), for depth of
    anesthesia monitoring, 196
Effective blood flow, 475
Effect-site target concentration, 117
Ehlers-Danlos syndrome
  eye surgery in, 903–904
  pain management in, 1188
Eisenmenger syndrome, 449–450
  noncardiac surgery in congenital heart
    disease and, 590, 612–613
Ejection fraction, 425
Elbow, nerve blocks of, 1114
  at median nerve, 1115
  at radial nerve, 1114–1115, 1115f
  at ulnar nerve, 1116, 1117f, 1118f
Electric countershock in cardiac arrest,
    1020, 1020f
Electrical burns, 941, 941f, 945f
Electrical cardiometry, 1343–1344, 1344f
Electrical circuitry, non-operating room
    anesthesia, 1198
Electrocardiogram (ECG), 409–412, 410f,
    411f, 412f, 413f, 1017, 1330–1331
  in noncardiac surgery in congenital
    heart disease, 605
  normal findings, 13
Electrocautery, 1078f
Electrocorticography, for epilepsy, 698
Electroencephalography
  cortical activity and, 1135
  halothane anesthesia monitoring uses
    of, 128
Electrolyte(s)
  in body fluid compartments, 219t
  distribution of, 218, 218.e1f, 219f, 219t
  renal regulation of, 730, 730t
Electrolyte balance, in chronic kidney
    disease, 736–737
Electrolyte disturbances, 216
  fluid overload and edema, 228, 228t
  hyperchloremic acidosis, 234
  hyperkalemia, 231–232, 232f, 233f
  hypernatremia, 230–231
  hypochloremic metabolic alkalosis, 234
  hypokalemia, 232
  hyponatremia, 230–231
    in preterm infant, 220
Electromyographic endotracheal
    tube, 1322
Electromyography, 635
  for spinal surgery, 819.e1t
  triggered, 819.e1t, 822
Electrophysiologic catheterization, 577
Elimination half-life, 102
Embedded simulation participants, 1350
Embolic stroke, 580
Embolism
  air, 1335
    cardiac catheterization and, 579
    in craniosynostosis surgery, 921–922

Embolism *(Continued)*
  neurosurgical procedures and,
    689–690, 690f
  tourniquet-related, 834
Embolization
  angiography with, 1210–1211,
    1210.e1f, 1211.e1f
  cardiac catheterization and, 579
Emergence, from anesthesia
  COVID-19 and, 1288
  inhalation anesthetic agents and,
    125–126, 136
  in neurosurgical procedure,
    690–691, 691t
  pharmacodynamics of, 1241
Emergence delirium, 136–137, 1241–1243,
    1242f, 1243t
  propofol and, 143
Emergency department, trauma
    evaluation and management in,
    1006–1011, 1007f
Emergency drugs, in noncardiac surgery
    in congenital heart disease, 604
Emergency intubation cart, 351t
Emergency surgery, ophthalmologic,
    908–909
Emergency Transtracheal Airway Catheter,
    357–358, 358.e1f
Emery-Dreifuss muscular dystrophy,
    639t, 641
Emicizumab, 541
  for hemophilia A, 287
Enalapril, 495
Enalaprilat, 492–493t
Encephalocele, 622, 700, 701f
Encephalotrigeminal angiomatosis, 904
Endocardial cushion defect, 450
Endocardial fibroelastosis, 793
Endocarditis
  cardiac catheterization and, 581
  prophylaxis for, 611
Endocrine disorders
  associated with childhood obesity, 55t
  diabetes insipidus, 233–234
  diabetes mellitus, 61–62
Endocrine system
  burn injury effects on, 936
  cardiopulmonary bypass effects on, 527
  growth and development of, 14–17, 15t
Endocrine tumors, 270
Endocrinology, 705–728
  adrenal endocrinopathies, 722–724
    adrenal insufficiency and, 722–723
    hypercortisolism, 723–724
    perioperative management of, 723
    physiology of, 722
  diabetes insipidus, 712–715
    central, 712–713
    diagnosis of, 713
    major procedures and, 714
    minor procedures and, 713–714,
      713f, 714t
    neurogenic, 712–713
    new perioperative diagnosis of,
      714–715
    postoperative management of, 715
    transient medication-induced, 715
    triple-phase response in, 713
  diabetes mellitus, 705–712
    anesthesia in, metabolic response
      to, 708
    classification and epidemiology of,
      705–706, 706t
    general management principles for,
      706–707, 706t
    hyperglycemia and, 708
    intraoperative management of,
      710–711
    major surgery and intravenous
      insulin infusions in, 711,
      711f, 712f
    postoperative management of,
      711–712
    preoperative consultation of,
      708–709, 709f

Endocrinology *(Continued)*
  preoperative management of, 709
  special surgical situations in,
    712, 712f
  surgery in, metabolic response to, 708
  type 1, 705
  type 2, 711
  urgent surgery and, 712
  parathyroid and calcium disorders,
    720–722
    hypercalcemia in, 721–722
    hypocalcemia in, 721
    physiology of calcium homeostasis
      and, 720–721
  syndrome of inappropriate antidiuretic
    hormone secretion, 715–716, 716t
  thyroid disorders, 716–720
    hyperthyroidism, 718–720, 720t
    hypothyroidism, 716–718
End-of-life ethical issues, 70–72
  communication in pediatric intensive
    care units and, 72, 73t
  donation after cardiac death and, 72, 73t
  life-sustaining medical therapy and,
    70–72, 71t
Endomyocardial biopsy, 799
Endophthalmitis, 908
End-organ dysfunction, obstructive sleep
    apnea and, 849.e1t
Endoscopic procedures, for non-operating
    room anesthesia, 1213
Endoscopic sinus surgery, 1090
Endoscopic strip craniectomy, 918
Endoscopy, 872–883
  anesthetic plan for, 874–876, 875.e1t,
    876t
  for aspirated foreign bodies, 866.e1f,
    877–881, 878f, 879f, 879t,
    880.e1f, 880.e1t
  complications from, 877, 877t
  diagnostic laryngoscopy and
    bronchoscopy in, 872–873,
    873t, 874f
  direct laryngoscopy and bronchoscopy
    in, 872–881
  drug-induced sleep, 854
  high-flow nasal oxygenation and, 877
  indications for, 873–874, 873.e1t, 875t
  jet ventilation and, 876–877, 876.e1t
Endothelin-1, 518, 754
Endothelin-receptor antagonists, 497
Endotoxins, 932–933
Endotracheal tube exchanger,
    356.e1–356.e2f
Endotracheal tubes, 1321–1322
  for upper respiratory tract infection,
    318, 318f
End-tidal carbon dioxide
  during cardiopulmonary bypass, 439
  laparoscopic surgery and, 751–752
  in malignant hyperthermia,
    1031–1032, 1036
  in neonatal surgical emergencies, 966
End-tidal gas tension, monitoring of,
    689–690
Enflurane
  minimum alveolar concentration
    of, 126t
  neurophysiologic effects of, 688t
  neurotoxicity of, 652.e1–652.e11t, 658
  physiochemical properties of, 114t
  seizure activity and, 129
Enk Oxygen Flow Modulation set,
    356, 356.e3f
Enoximone, 488
Enteral feeding, after burn injury, 936
Enucleation, 912
Epaned. *see* Enalapril
Ependymoma, 269–270, 626t, 627, 694
Ephedra, 32.e1t
Epidermoid tumors, 1079
Epidermolysis bullosa, 340t
Epidural administration
  of fentanyl, 168
  of ketamine, 146

Epidural analgesia
  after scoliosis surgery, 826
  in cognitively impaired child, 1177–1178
  patient-controlled, 826
  for postoperative pain, 1250–1251
  for tetanus, 1309
Epidural anesthesia, 1079–1087
  adjunctive drugs for, 1085
  caudal, 1079–1080, 1080f, 1081f,
    1084f
  complications of, 1078.e1f, 1085–1087,
    1086f
  continuous, 1085
  lumbar and thoracic, 1081–1084,
    1082f, 1083f
  opioids for, 1086
  for thoracic surgery, 371t
Epidural fat, 1054
Epidural hematoma, 692, 692f, 1086,
    1086t, 1087f
Epidural monitors, 679
Epidural space, 1054, 1251
Epidurogram, 1083–1084, 1251
Epigenetics, 81, 113
Epiglottis, 325, 327f
Epiglottitis, 329–330
  acute, 883.e1f, 884f, 885f, 885t,
    883–885
Epilepsy, 642–648, 643f, 644t
  in cerebral palsy patient, 621
  neurosurgical procedure for, 697
  perioperative management of, 648t
  surgery in, 644–646
Epinephrine, 484–485t, 486, 907t,
    946–947, 1078–1079
  for asthma exacerbations, 319.e2–319.e3t
  for bleeding in burn injury, 946–947,
    946f, 948t
  for bradycardia, 1247
  bupivacaine with, 1056–1057, 1056f
  for cardiopulmonary resuscitation,
    1024
  concentration and dilution of, 1058,
    1059t
  glucagon production affected by, 708
  nebulized, for croup, 886
  oculocardiac reflex and, 905–906
  response to surgery, 708
Epispadias, 763
Epoprostenol, 496, 958
Epstein Macintosh Oxford drawover
    vaporizer, 1311
Epstein-Barr virus-related adenotonsillar
    hypertrophy, 791
Equipment, 1314–1346
  airway apparatus, 1320–1322
  anesthesia machine, 1323–1327
    circuits of, 1326f
    humidifier of, 1325
    scavenger system of, 1323–1324
    ventilator of, 1325–1327
  defibrillator and external pacemakers,
    1327
  in developing countries, 1308f,
    1310–1312
  heating and cooling systems,
    1314–1315
  intravenous therapy, 1317.e1f,
    1317–1320, 1317t
  intubation, 1323
  Luer adapters, 1319–1320
  monitoring, 1329–1344
    anesthesia record in, 1329, 1329f
    for blood loss, 1337
    blood pressure device in, 1330
    for cardiac output monitoring,
      1341–1342
    drug errors, bar coding, and
      integration in, 1329–1330
    electrocardiogram in, 1330–1331
    for neuromuscular transmission,
      1337–1338
    noninvasive oxygen saturation
      monitors in, 1331–1333
    oxygen monitors in, 1331

Equipment *(Continued)*
  precordial and esophageal
    stethoscopes in, 1330
  for processed electroencephalogram,
    1338–1340, 1339f
  temperature monitors in, 1331
  peripheral intravenous cannulation,
    1256–1258
  in postanesthesia care unit, 1239, 1239t
  purchasing of, 1344–1345
  regional anesthesia, 1060–1064, 1061f,
    1327–1329
  suction devices, 1323
  ultrasound for regional anesthesia and
    vascular cannulation in, 1327–1329
  umbilical artery catheterization, 1271,
    1274f
  umbilical vein catheterization in,
    1267–1269, 1269f
  warming devices in, 1315–1317
    fluid and blood warmers in, 1316,
      1316f, 1316.e1f
    forced air warming devices in, 1315
    heated humidifiers in, 1315–1316,
      1315.e1f
    passive heat and moisturizer
      exchangers in, 1315
    radiant warmers in, 1315
    warming blankets in, 1315
    wrapping in, 1315
Equipment cart, 1327, 1328t
Equipment decontamination, COVID-19
  and, 1289, 1289t
Erb palsy, 634
Erector spinae plane (ESP) block, for
  thoracic surgery, 371t
Erythrocytes, 241
Erythropoietin, 920
  for chronic renal failure, 738
  red blood cell transfusion and, 301
Escharotomy, 940–941, 941f
Esmolol, 491, 492–493t, 499t, 501,
  594–595
  for hyperthyroid crisis, 720t
  in neurosurgery, 690
Esophageal atresia, 382–383, 383f,
  971–972, 971f
Esophageal stethoscopes, 1330
Esophagoscopy, for foreign bodies, 881–883
Esters, 1055–1056
Estradiol, 659, 662
Ethanol, 1212t
Ethical issues
  end-of-life, 70–72
    communication in pediatric intensive
      care units and, 72, 73t
    donation after cardiac death and,
      72, 73t
    life-sustaining medical therapy and,
      70–72, 71t
  ethics consultation service and, 77–78
  informed consent, 65–70
    adolescent abortion and, 69
    confidentiality for adolescent and, 69
    disclosure and, 68
    emergency care and, 70
    impaired parent and, 70
    informed permission and best
      interests standard in, 66–67
    informed refusal and, 67–68
    Jehovah's Witnesses and, 69–70
    medical errors and, 68–69
    role of patient, 65–66, 66t
  in pediatric anesthesiology, 65–78
  pediatric research, 72–75
    conflicts of interest and, 75–76
    imperative for pharmacologic
      research and, 74–75
    interaction with industry and,
      75–76, 76t
    minimal risks and, 73–74
    minor increase over minimal risk
      and, 74
    socioeconomic concerns and
      distribution of risk and, 74

Ethical issues *(Continued)*
    in physician obligations, advocacy, and
      good citizenship, 76t
Ethics consultation service, 77–78
Ethnicity, 96–97
  adenotonsillectomy and, 856
Ethyl chloride, 40
Etomidate, 147–148
  blood flow affected by, 443
  in cardiac surgery, 444–445
  effects on evoked potentials, 831
  emergency surgery in trauma patient
    using, 1009t
  intravenous administration of, 147
  intravenous induction of, 48–49
  molecular structures of, 147f
  neurophysiologic effects of, 684, 688t
  noncardiac surgery in congenital heart
    disease using, 608
  for sedation, 1230–1231t, 1236
  in VAD patient, 566
European Malignant Hyperthermia
  Group (EMHG) test, 1048
Eutectic mixture of local anesthetics
  (EMLA), 40, 440, 1055–1056
  adverse reactions to, 241–242, 440,
    1055–1056
Euthyroidism, 997
Evaporation, 1314
Examination under anesthesia in eye
  disorders, 900
Exchange transfusion, for malaria, 1309
Excision, of full-thickness burn, 947
Excitation-contraction coupling, in
  malignant hyperthermia,
    1044–1045, 1045f, 1046f
Exenatide, 707
Exercise physiology, in repaired congenital
  heart disease, 476t, 478–479
Exhalation, laryngeal function during, 330
EXIT procedure, 984f, 995–998, 995f
  for cervical teratoma, 995f, 996, 996f
  for congenital goiter, 997
  for congenital high airway obstruction
    syndrome, 996
  for cystic hygroma, 996, 996f
  extracorporeal membrane oxygenation
    and, 995, 997
  intraoperative considerations, 997–998
  for laryngeal atresia, 889
  for microretrognathia, 997
  postoperative considerations, 998
  preoperative considerations, 997
  to resection, 997
  to separation, 997
External cardiac massage, 1016
External cooling measures, in malignant
  hyperthermia, 1039
External jugular vein catheterization, 1261
External pacemaker, 1327
Extracellular fluid
  composition of, 219t
  in preterm neonates, 150
Extracorporeal cardiopulmonary
  resuscitation (ECPR), 553, 556f
Extracorporeal membrane oxygenation
  (ECMO), 549–550, 552t, 554–557,
    995
  arterial-venous, 555
  for cardiac arrest, 570
  for cardiopulmonary resuscitation, 1028
  circuit configurations of, 554–557
  EXIT procedure and, 997
  in neonates, 553
  persistent pulmonary hypertension
    applications of, 958
  preoperative, 551
  schematic diagram of, 555f
  venoarterial, 554–555, 555f
  venovenous, 555, 555f
Extrahepatic routes, of metabolic
  clearance, 116
Extramedullary hematopoiesis, 247
Extraoral approach, in infraorbital nerve
  block, 1091

Extremely premature infant, 953–981
  anesthetics and, 964–966
    inhalational anesthetics, 964
    intravenous anesthetics, 964–966
  definition of, 953
  fentanyl affected by, 964
  neurologic development, 958–961
    immature brain and, 958–960
  physiology of prematurity related to
    anesthesia, 953–964
    cardiovascular system, 957–958, 957t
    glucose in, 962–963
    hematologic function, 963–964
    intraventricular hemorrhage and,
      960–961
    neurologic development and, 958–961
    renal and metabolic function, 961–963
    respiratory control and, 956–957, 956f
    respiratory system and, 953–954,
      954f, 954t
    temperature regulation and, 961
Extubation
  in adenotonsillectomy, 867, 867f
  after cardiac surgery, 446–447
  COVID-19 and, 1288
  of difficult airway, 354–356,
    356.e1–356.e2f, 356.e3f
  in operating room, 1244
  in postanesthesia care unit, 1244
Eye surgery, 909
  in Alport syndrome, 903
  anterior chamber paracentesis, 911
  cataract, 911, 911f
  common diagnoses requiring, 901, 901t
  in craniofacial syndromes, 904, 905.e1f
  dacryocystorhinostomy, 911–912, 911f,
    911.e1f
  in Down syndrome, 903
  elective, 908–909
  emergent, 908–909
  in Ehlers-Danlos syndrome, 903–904
  in homocystinuria, 903–904, 903.e1f
  in Marfan syndrome, 903–904, 903.e1f
  in mucopolysaccharidoses, 904
  ophthalmologic medications and, 910t
  ophthalmologic pharmacotherapeutics
    and systemic implications, 906–908,
    907t, 907.e1f
  ophthalmologic physiology and, 904
    intraocular pressure in, 904–905, 904f
    oculocardiac reflex in, 905–906, 906f
  in phakomatoses, 904
  postoperative nausea and vomiting
    in, 910t
  preoperative evaluation in, 900–901
  ptosis repair in, 912
  in retinopathy of prematurity, 901
  strabismus repair, 910–911, 910f
  urgent, 908–909
Eyelash reflex, 144
EZ-IO, 1022, 1259, 1260f

F

Face, growth and development of, 6
Face, Legs, Activity, Cry, Consolability
  Observational Tool, 1136t, 1138,
    1138t, 1139t
Faces pain scales, 1136, 1136t, 1137f
Facial hemangioma, 926–927, 927f
Facioscapulohumeral muscular dystrophy,
  639t, 641
Factor deficiency
  after cardiopulmonary bypass, 539–540
  massive blood transfusion and, 292–294,
    294t
Factor eight inhibitor bypassing activity
  (FEIBA), 541
Factor IX, 531
  deficiency of, 250
  for hemophilia B, 287
Factor VIIa, recombinant, 530, 540–541,
  540f
Factor VIII, 533
  concentrate, 287
  deficiency of, 250–251

Factor VIIIa, 531
Factor X deficiency, 292
Factor Xa, 530
Factor XIII
  deficiency of, 539–540
  description of, 509–510
Factor XIII deficiency, cryoprecipitate for,
  285–286
"Failing the Fontan" procedure, 792–793
False vocal cords, 329
Familial amyloid polyneuropathy, 633
Familial hyperkalemic periodic
  paralysis, 642
Familial hypokalemic periodic
  paralysis, 642
Familial renal-retinal dystrophy, 903
Family history, 35
Famotidine, 185
Fanconi syndrome, 269
Farnesyl transferases, 263–264
Fascia, ultrasound of, 1068
Fascia iliaca block, 949–950, 1130
Fascial plane catheters, 1176
Fasciculations, succinylcholine-related, 153
Fasciotomy, 941
Fast tracking, in cardiac surgery, 447
Fasting, 22–24, 24f, 25f, 25t, 745
  intraoperative fluid management and,
    225–226
  in noncardiac surgery in congenital
    heart disease, 602
Fat, ultrasound of, 1068
Fat mass, 765
Fat-free mass, 765
Fatty acid amide hydrolase (FAAH), 92
Fatty acid metabolism disorders,
  malignant hyperthermia and,
    1050–1051
Fatty acid oxidation, disorders of, 630
Fava beans, 241
Favism, 241
FDA Modernization Act, 75
Fearful child, 51
Feedback responses, to inhalation
  anesthetic agents, 110f, 124
FEIBA. *see* Factor eight inhibitor
  bypassing activity
Felbamate, 645t
Felodipine, 646t
Female genitalia, 5t
Femoral artery catheterization, 1276–1277
Femoral nerve block, 1127f, 1128–1129,
  1128f, 1129f
  dosing for, 1088t
  lateral femoral cutaneous nerve, 1129
Femoral vein catheterization, 1267,
  1268f
Fenoldopam, 741
Fentanyl, 162t, 165–168, 167f, 1230–1231t
  for blunt reflex bronchoconstriction,
    860.e1t
  for cardiac surgery, 445
  for cardiopulmonary bypass, 445
  dosing guidelines for, 1152t
  emergence delirium uses of, 1243
  emergency surgery in trauma patient
    using, 1009t
  epidural, 1172t
  in extremely premature infant, 964
  for general anesthesia, 687–688
  infusion schemes, 197t
  intranasal, after myringotomy with
    tube insertion, 842
  intravenous, emergence and, 690
  in liver transplantation, 782
  neurotoxicity of, 652.e1–652.e11t
  pancuronium and, 445
  pharmacokinetics of, 772
  preoperative, 37
  for sedation outside operating
    room, 1233
Fentanyl transdermal therapeutic system
  (TTS), 167–168
Fetal airway compression, 983t
Fetal anemia, 983t

Fetal circulation, 468–471, 470.e1t, 475.e2f, 480.e1f
   neonatal circulation transition from, 957
Fetal coagulation factors, 533
Fetal heart rate (FHR), 990
Fetal hemoglobin, 17, 242–243
Fetal hydrops, 996
Fetal intervention
   anesthetic considerations, 993–995
      intraoperative, 993–994
      minimally invasive procedures, 993
      open fetal procedures, 993–994, 994f
      postoperative, 995
      preoperative, 993
   in congenital diaphragmatic hernia, 983t, 986–987
   in congenital heart defects, 985–986, 986f
   in congenital pulmonary lesions, 987
   EXIT procedure and, 995–998, 995f
   indications for, 983–988
   in lower urinary tract obstruction, 983t, 985
   maternal physiology, 988–989
      cardiovascular considerations, 988–989, 989t
      pharmacologic consequences of pregnancy, 989, 989t
      respiratory and airway considerations, 988, 988t
   in myelomeningocele, 988
   physiology and monitoring, 989–993
      fetal cardiovascular physiology, 989–991, 990f
      fetal central and peripheral nervous system, 991–992
      fetal monitoring, 992–993
      fetal oxygenation, 991, 991f, 992f
      pain perception, 991–992
   in sacrococcygeal teratoma, 987–988, 987f
   in twin reversed arterial perfusion sequence, 983t, 984–985
   in twin-twin transfusion syndrome, 983–984, 984f, 984t
Fetal thrombocytopenia, 983t
Fetoscopic myelomeningocele repair, 988
Fetus
   bradycardia, 985–986
   pulmonary vasculature of, 471t, 472–473
   transition to air breathing, 8
Fever
   before elective surgery, 59, 59.e1f
   ibuprofen for, 1145t
   in malignant hyperthermia, 1036
Fever of unknown origin, 400
FFP. see Fresh frozen plasma
FGIDs. see Functional gastrointestinal disorders
Fiberoptic bronchoscopy, in double-lumen tubes, 377
Fiberoptic intubation, 948, 949f, 1320
Fibrillin 1 gene (FBN1), 903
Fibrin, 531–532
Fibrin sealants, 438
Fibrin split products, 935–936
Fibrinogen, 531–532, 538
   age-based values of, 237t
   deficiency of, 292
   hematologic disorders, 236
Fibrinogen concentrate, 539, 539t
   cardiopulmonary bypass and, 509–510
Fibrinolysis, 531–532, 532f
   after reperfusion, 785
   massive blood transfusion and, 294
Fibroblast growth factor receptor, 917
Fibroblast growth factor receptor 2 gene (FGFR2), 904
Fibroma, cardiac, 402
Fibromyalgia, 1188–1189
Fibrous dysplasia of jaw, 340t
Fick method, 13, 429, 1341
First-degree atrioventricular block, 410–411, 415–416t
First-order kinetics, 101–102

First-order multiple-compartment kinetics, 102–103, 103f
First-pass effect, 112
Fistula
   tracheocutaneous, 892
   tracheoesophageal, 382–383, 383f, 971–972, 971f
Fixed infusion rate, in total, intravenous anesthesia, 200
Flecainide, 500–501, 1028
Flexible bronchoscopy, 873.e1t
Flexible fiberoptic bronchoscope, 368
   in retrograde manner, 368
Flexible fiberoptic endoscopy, 336
Flexible intubation scope, 368
Flexible laryngoscopy, 360–363
   ancillary equipment for, 361–362
   direct technique for, 362, 362f
   equipment for, 361
   staged techniques of, 362–363
"Flip-flop" circulation, 9
Flolan. see Epoprostenol
Flow rates, on cardiopulmonary bypass, 517–518
Flow-volume loop, 311
Fludrocortisone, 723
Fluid(s), requirements for, 220–222, 220f, 221t
Fluid administration devices, 222–223
Fluid and blood warmers in, 1316, 1316f, 1316.e1f
Fluid balance, in chronic kidney disease, 737, 741
Fluid management, 216, 221t
   in abdominal surgery, 747
   body water and electrolyte distribution and, 218, 218.e1f, 219f, 219t
   circulating blood volume and, 218–219, 219t
   in diabetes mellitus, 710
   fluid and electrolyte requirements and, 220–222, 220f, 221t
   fluid volume, osmolality, and arterial pressure in, 216–218, 216.e1f, 217f, 217.e1f, 218f
   homeostatic mechanisms and, 218–220
   intraoperative, 222–227
      fasting recommendations and, 225–226
      hyperalimentation and, 225, 225t
      intravascular volume, assessment of, 226–227
      intravenous fluids in, 223–224, 223t
      ongoing losses and third-spacing, 226
   intraosseous access for, 1022
   intravenous access and fluid administration devices in, 222–223
   in laparoscopic surgery, 754
   neonatal, 222
   in neurosurgical procedures, 688–689
   pathophysiologic states and, 228–234
      dehydration in, 228–230, 229f, 229t
      diabetes insipidus in, 233–234
      fluid overload and edema in, 228, 228t
      hyperchloremic acidosis in, 234
      hyperkalemia, 231–232, 232f, 233f
      hypernatremia in, 230–231
      hypochloremic metabolic alkalosis in, 234
      hypokalemia, 232
      hyponatremia, 230–231
      syndrome of inappropriate antidiuretic hormone secretion, 232–233
   postoperative, 227–228
      general approach to, 227, 227t
      hyponatremia and, 227–228
      pulmonary edema and, 228
   in renal disease, 741
Fluid overload and edema, 228, 228t
Fluid replacement, in burn injury, 939–940, 940t
Fluid shift, in burn injury, 932

Fluid volume, 216–218, 216.e1f, 217f, 217.e1f
Flumazenil, 189, 1232, 1246
Fluoroquinolones, 1296
Fluoroscopy, in cardiac catheterization, 427
Focal heating, MRI and, 1205, 1205f
Fogarty embolectomy catheter, 373, 374f
Fontan circulation, 435
Fontan physiology, 479–480, 480f, 480.e1f, 481f, 482f, 555–556, 570, 750–751
   laparoscopic surgery and, 750–751
Fontan procedure, 430–431t, 439, 599
Fontanelles, 679
Food, Drug, and Cosmetic Act, 119
Food allergies, 682
Food and Drug Administration
   description of, 119–120
   Modernization Act, 75
   Safety and Innovation Act, 75
Foot
   digital nerve block of, 1131
   gestational age assessment and, 5t
Foramen of Bochdalek, 380–381
   hernia, 972
Foramen of Monro, 683
Foramen ovale, patent, 450, 588, 689
Forced air warming, 689, 1251, 1315
Forced glottic closure, of larynx, 330–331
Forced vital capacity (FVC)
   after scoliosis, 813–814, 816t
   in respiratory system, 309, 310f
Foreign bodies
   aspirated, 866.e1f, 877–881, 878f, 879f, 879t, 880.e1f, 880.e1t
   esophagoscopy for, 881–883
   lithium (button) batteries as, 881–883, 882f
   swallowed objects as, 878f, 881
Fosaprepitant, 186
Fossa ovalis defects, 588
Fractional excretion of sodium, 220, 733
Fractionated human blood products, 538–541
Frank-Starling mechanism, 482
Frank-Starling response, 296
Freeman-Sheldon syndrome, 340t
Freestanding simulation center, 1351t
Frei endoscopy mask, 361, 361.e1f
Fresh frozen plasma (FFP), 276–277, 281, 286f, 534, 538, 554, 947
   in craniosynostosis surgery, 920
   for hematologic disorders, 238
   for hypocalcemia after burn injury, 947
   initial doses of, 282t
Frontonasal dysplasia, 624
Fukuyama congenital muscular dystrophy, 639t, 641
Full stomach
   liver transplantation and, 782
   pulmonary aspiration of gastric contents risks, 745
   rapid-sequence induction and, 49–51, 49t, 51f
Full-term neonate, 2, 5t
   circulating blood volume of, 219t
   growth curve for, 5f
   oxygen consumption of, 332
Fulminant hepatic failure, 779
Functional endoscopic sinus surgery (FESS), 843–844
   for chronic sinusitis, 843–844
Functional gastrointestinal disorders (FGIDs), 1184–1185
Functional residual capacity
   inhalation anesthetics to lung and, 108f, 121
   transitional circulation and, 471
Furosemide, 737t, 955

G

G6PD. see Glucose-6-phosphate dehydrogenase deficiency
GABA. see γ-aminobutyric acid

Gabapentin, 1192
   for acute pain, 1149–1150, 1177
   after scoliosis surgery, 825
   for opioid-induced respiratory depression, 866
Gadolinium, for MRI enhancement, 1205
Gadoterate meglumine, for MRI enhancement, 1205
Gallamine, 1310
Gallstones, 240–241
Ganglioneuroma, 760
Gantacurium, 155
Gardos channel, 510
Garlic, 32, 32.e1t
Gas dilution, 311
Gas emboli, 752
Gastric bypass surgery, 766–767
Gastric emptying, 745
Gastroesophageal reflux, 621, 55, 766
Gastroesophageal reflux disease, 806–807
Gastrografin, 1201
Gastrointestinal system
   associated with childhood obesity, 55t
   burn injury effects on, 936
   cardiopulmonary bypass effects on, 526–527
   cerebral palsy in, 621
   neonatal surgical emergencies involving, 974–980
Gastrointestinal tract complications, after scoliosis surgery, 817
Gastrointestinal transit time, 16
Gastrointestinal tumors, 269
Gastroparesis, 806–807
Gastroschisis, 978–980, 978t, 978.e1, 1300f
Gastrostomy, 632–633
Gelatins, 288
Gene silencing, in malignant hyperthermia, 1044
General anesthesia, 1216–1217
   during cardiac catheterization, 583–585
   regional anesthesia and, 1053–1054
   spinal anesthesia conversion to, 1079
General care setting, postoperative monitoring in, 1252–1253
General surgery, 749–750
   bladder and cloacal exstrophy, 762–763, 762f
   chordee, 756
   circumcision, 756
   corticosteroid medications and, 749–750
   hypospadias, 756, 757f, 757.e1f
   infection or sepsis in, 750
   monitoring requirements in, 750
   nephrectomy in, 760
   neuroblastoma, 760–761
   posterior urethral valves, 758
   pyeloplasty in, 760
   reduced renal function and, 749
   systemic hypertension and, 749
   ureteral reimplantation, 759–760, 760f
   Wilms tumor, 761–762, 761f, 762f
Genetic considerations
   acetaminophen, 93
   nonsteroidal antiinflammatory drugs, 93
Genetic counseling, 97
Genetic research studies, 97
Genetic testing, in malignant hyperthermia, 1048–1049
Genetics, of bleeding, 533
Genitalia, gestational age assessment, 5t
Genome-wide association study, 96
Genomic prescribing system (GPS), 97–98
Genomics, of drug metabolism, exposure, and effects, 84–85, 86t
Genotyping methods
   common, 97
   current costs of, 97
Gestational age
   assessment of, 5t
   probability of apnea by, 60f, 60.e1f
Gilbert syndrome, 773
Ginkgo biloba, 32, 32.e1t
Ginseng, 32, 32.e1t
Glanzmann thrombasthenia, 540

Glasgow Coma Scale (GCS), 1004–1005, 1004t
Glaucoma, 905
Glenn anastomosis, 430–431t, 598–599
Glenn shunt, 435, 460
GlideScope, 364–365, 364.e1f
Glioblastoma, 695
Gliogenesis, 655
Glioma, 269–270, 695
Glomerular filtration rate
after burn injury, 935
age and, 109.e1f, 115
arginine vasopressin and, 218
in children, 107
in chronic renal failure, 736–737
description of, 729
developmental issues in, 13
in neonate, 220
time course of, 84
Glomerulonephritis, acute, 731
Glossopharyngeal nerve blocks, 866
Glossoptosis, 914–915
Glostavent Helix machine, 1312.e1f
Gloves, 1293–1294, 1294f, 1294t
Glucagon, 708
diagnostic angiography and, 1210
Glucagon response to surgery, 708
Glucagon-like peptide-1, 707
Glucocorticoids
for adrenal insufficiency, 723
adrenal suppression and, 270
for Duchenne muscular dystrophy, 640
for intraventricular hemorrhage, 961
Gluconeogenesis, 14, 222
Glucose
administration of, during cardiopulmonary resuscitation, 1025
carbohydrates and, 773
for hyperkalemia, 737t
neonatal
brain requirements, 960
fluid management and, 222
serum levels, 222
prematurity and, 962–963
Glucose monitoring, for diabetes, 710
Glucose-6-phosphate dehydrogenase (G6PD) deficiency, 241–242, 241t, 242t
Glucose-dependent insulinotropic polypeptide, for type 2 diabetes, 707
Glucose-insulin and potassium, 449
Glucuronidation, 115, 771
Glucuronosyltransferase, 84
Glucuronyl transferase, deficiency of, 773
Glutathione S-transferases, 771
Glycemic control, 707
Glycogen storage disorders, prevention of, 631
Glycogenolysis, 222
Glycopyrrolate, 187–188, 905
for dexmedetomidine-induced bradycardia, 608
emergency surgery in trauma patient using, 1009t
Goldenhar syndrome, 923–925, 923.e1, 924f
airway difficulties in, 340t
eye surgery in, 904
G proteins, 182
Gracilis muscle transplantation, in Möbius syndrome, 927, 927.e1
Graft-versus-host disease (GVHD)
chronic, 272–273
description of, 272–273
in hematopoietic stem cell transplantation, 275–276, 276t
transfusion-related, 285, 285.e1t, 797
Gram-negative bacteria, 947
Granisetron, 185–186
Grasp reflex, 5t, 19
Graves disease, 718, 719f
Gray baby syndrome, 84, 114–115
Great auricular nerve block, 843, 1092, 1092f

Greater occipital nerve block, 687, 1090, 1090f
Grown-up congenital heart disease, 433–434
Growth and development, 1–21, 3f, 4f
breathing mechanics, 9–11
airway dynamics, 11–12
chest wall and respiratory muscles in, 9
closing capacity, 11
elastic properties of lung and, 9
static lung volumes and, 10, 10t
total lung capacity and, 10, 10f
cardiovascular system, 12–13
blood pressure and, 12, 13t
cardiac output and, 13
heart rate and, 12, 12t
normal electrocardiographic findings, 13
chronic kidney disease and, 738
definition of, 1
face, 6
gastrointestinal tract, 16
gestational age assessment and, 2–6, 2t, 5t
head circumference and, 5–6
hematopoietic system, 17–18
hepatic system, 14–15, 15t
immunologic system, 17–18
interactions with the external world during, 19–20
length assessment, 5
neurologic and cognitive issues in, 18–20
normal and abnormal, 1–2
pancreas, 16–17
pharmacokinetic considerations and, 106–107
child size in, 106, 106f
maturation in, 106–107, 107f
organ function in, 107
renal system, 13–14, 14f
respiratory system, 7–8, 9f
teeth, 6
transition to air breathing, 8–9
upper airway, 6–7
weight assessment, 5
Growth curve, 5f
Growth hormone, 708
Growth retardation, renal disease and, 788
Guedel airways, 361–362
Guillain-Barré syndrome, 634
Gum elastic bougie, 360, 360.e1f

H
H1N1 pandemic, 556–557
Haemophilus influenzae
in bone and joint infections, 835
epiglottitis, 883
Hairy pigmented nevus, 929–930, 929f, 929.e1
Half-life, 102, 102f
Hallermann-Streiff syndrome, 340t
Hallow-bore needles, accidents with, 1284, 1284t
Halothane
baroreceptor reflex response in, 131–132
in cardiac surgery, 443–444
degradation of, 138
in developing countries, 1309–1310
hepatitis, 95, 134
hypotension and, 131
inhalation induction with, 46
malignant hyperthermia caused by, 1043, 1043.e1f
minimum alveolar concentration of, 126t
myocardial effects of, 131
neurophysiologic effects of, 688t
neurotoxicity of, 652.e1–652.e11t, 658
physiochemical properties of, 114t
problems during induction with, 121t
succinylcholine after, 159
Hand, congenital anomalies of, 928, 928.e1
Hand hygiene, 1292t
Hand washing, 1291–1293, 1292t, 1293t

Handoff systems, 1240
Haplotypes, 92
Harm threshold standard, 66–67
Harrington rod system, 810
Hashimoto thyroiditis, 718
Head and neck nerve blocks, 1088–1093, 1088t, 1089f
great auricular, 1092, 1092f
greater occipital, 1090, 1090f
greater occipital nerve, 1090, 1090f
infraorbital nerve, 1090–1091, 1091f
nerve of Arnold, 1092–1093
supraorbital and supratrochlear nerves, 1088–1089, 1089f
Head circumference, 5–6, 7f
Head injury, 691, 1000, 1007
Head trauma, 1007
Headache, 1183t, 1185–1186, 1186t
chronic, 1183t
medication-overuse, 1185
post-dural puncture, 1079
Health-care-associated infections, 1278
Heart
burn injury effects on, 933, 943t
fetal, 957
laparoscopic surgery effects on, 753
physiology of, 468–474
congenital heart disease
exercise physiology in the child with repaired, 476t, 478–479
incidence and prevalence of, 474–475, 474t, 475.e2f
pathophysiologic classification of, 475–478
fetal circulation and, 468–471, 470.e1t, 475.e2f, 480.e1f
Fontan physiology and, 479–480, 480f, 480.e1f, 481f, 482f
neonatal cardiovascular system and, 471–472, 471t, 473f, 480.e1f
pulmonary vascular physiology and, 471t, 472–474, 474f, 474t
transitional circulation and, 470.e1t, 471
of transplanted heart, 480–483
denervated heart and, 482–483, 483f, 483t
transplant morbidity and, 483
Heart disease, 433–467
acquired, 395–402
cardiac tumors, 401–402
cardiomyopathy, 395–398, 395f, 396f, 397f
infective endocarditis, 399–400, 400t, 401t
Kawasaki disease, 400–401, 401f
myocarditis, 398–399, 398f
rheumatic fever and rheumatic heart disease, 399
aortic stenosis, 404–405, 405f, 463–464
arrhythmias, 414–420
acute management of, 412–420
atrioventricular block, 410–411, 411f, 415–416t
bundle branch block, 411, 415–416t
junctional rhythm, 415t, 417f
long QT syndrome, 418–420, 419f
premature atrial contractions or beats, 414
premature ventricular contractions or beats, 418
sinus, 413–414, 414f, 415t
sinus bradycardia, 415t
sinus rhythm, 415t, 418f
sinus tachycardia, 415t, 416f
supraventricular tachycardia, 414–418, 418f
ventricular fibrillation, 420
ventricular tachycardia, 418–420, 419f
cardiac murmur in, 409
CHARGE syndrome in, 406
chronic renal failure-related complications of, 739
congenital, 391–395

Heart disease (Continued)
incidence and prevalence of, 391–392, 392f, 474–475, 474t, 475.e2f
pathophysiologic classification of, 475–478
intercirculatory mixing in, 474f, 476–477, 477f
shunting in, 475–476, 476f, 476t, 477t
single ventricle physiology in, 477–478, 478t
physiologic classification of, 394–395, 394t
prior repair, 432
repaired, exercise physiology in the child with, 476t, 478–479
segmental approach to diagnosis of, 392–393, 392f, 393f
surgical procedures in, 430–431t
in developing countries, 1309
diagnosis of, 422–429, 422t
barium esophagram for, 423, 423f
cardiac catheterization and angiography for, 426–429, 427f, 428f
chest radiography for, 422, 423f
computed tomography for, 426, 426f, 427t
echocardiography for, 423–425, 423t, 424f
magnetic resonance imaging for, 425–426, 426t
DiGeorge and velocardiofacial syndrome in, 405
Down syndrome in, 404
electrocardiogram in, 409–412, 410f, 411f, 412f, 413f
heart failure in, 402–403, 402t
anesthetic considerations in, 403
clinical features of, 402
definition of, 402
etiology of, 402
pathophysiology of, 402
treatment strategies for, 402–403, 403f
Marfan syndrome in, 406, 406f
Noonan syndrome in, 405
pacemaker therapy in, 420–422, 421t
perioperative considerations in, 429–432
signs and symptoms of, 59t
syndromes, associations, and systemic disorders associated with, 403–407
trisomy 13 in, 404
trisomy 18 in, 404
tuberous sclerosis in, 401–402, 407
Turner syndrome in, 404
VACTERL association in, 406–407
vascular anomalies in, 407–409
aberrant subclavian artery, 407, 408f
Williams syndrome in, 404–405, 405f
Heart failure, 402–403, 402t, 403f
anesthetic considerations in, 403
clinical features of, 402, 450t
definition of, 402
etiology of, 402
mechanical circulatory support for, indications for, 550–551, 550t
noncardiac surgery in congenital heart disease and, 610
pathophysiology of, 402
treatment strategies for, 402–403, 403f
Heart murmur, 409
Heart rate
developmental issues in, 12, 12t
dexmedetomidine and, 182
in Fontan circulation, 480
inhaled anesthetics and, 132
succinylcholine and, 151
Heart rhythm, in Fontan circulation, 480
Heart-lung transplantation, 553, 800–807
bilateral sequential, 804
contraindications to, 802
cystic fibrosis in, 801
demographics and epidemiology of, 800–801

Heart-lung transplantation (Continued)
immediate postoperative management of, 805
intraoperative problems and management in, 803–805
long-term concerns in, 805–807, 805t
pathophysiology of disease in, 801, 802t
preoperative evaluation of, 803
pulmonary hypertension in, 801–802
surgical technique in, 803
survival and quality of life in, 807, 808f
waitlist and donor selection in, 802–803
HeartMate 3, 552t, 560
HeartWare HVAD, 552t, 560
HeartWare Ventricular Assist System, 560
Heat and moisturizer exchangers, 1315, 1325
Heat loss, 1315
Heat stroke
classic, 1042–1043
dantrolene for, 1043
malignant hyperthermia and, 1033t, 1042–1043
Heated humidifiers, 1315–1316, 1315.e1f
Heating and cooling systems, 1314–1315
Heinz bodies, 241
Helium, 752
Hemangioma
facial, 926–927, 926.e1, 927f
subglottic, 970
Hematocrit, 279–280
age-related values of, 237t
on cardiopulmonary bypass, 517
Hematologic disorders, 236–260
coagulation disorders, 249–253
hemophilia, 250–252, 251t, 252t
hypercoagulability, 252–253
screening for, 249
von Willebrand disease, 250, 251t
diagnostic tests in, 236–237, 237t
hemolytic anemias, 239–242
glucose-6-phosphate dehydrogenase (G6PD) deficiency, 241–242, 241t, 242t
hereditary spherocytosis, 239–241, 240t
idiopathic thrombocytopenic purpura, 248–249, 249t
sickle cell disease, 242–246, 245t
laboratory values in, 236–237, 237t
platelet disorders and bleeding, 248
transfusion guidelines for, 237–239, 238t
Hematologic function, in extremely premature infant, 963–964
Hematologic malignancies, 253–260, 253t, 254f, 271
acute lymphoblastic leukemia, 253–255, 256t
acute myelogenous leukemia, 255–257
Hodgkin lymphoma, 257–258
Langerhans cell histiocytosis, 259
myelodysplastic disorders, 259–260
myeloproliferative disorder, 259–260
non-Hodgkin lymphoma, 258–259
Hematologic system
burn injury effects on, 935–936, 943t
hematologic values at different ages, 237t
mechanical circulatory support and, 562–564
prematurity and, 963–964
Hematopoiesis, 14–15, 768
Hematopoietic stem cell transplantation (HSCT), 236, 272–273, 275–276
Hematopoietic system, growth and development of, 17–18
Hematuria, 733
Hemidiaphragmatic paralysis, pulmonary ultrasound for, 387, 388f
Hemifacial microsomia, 923–925, 924f
Hemi-Fontan procedure, 460, 598–599
Hemiplegia, 580
Hemithorax, 380–381, 382f
Hemivertebra, 811
Hemodialysis, 735
Hemodilution, in scoliosis surgery, 828

Hemodynamic instability, 693
Hemodynamic response, 96
Hemodynamics
changes at birth, 470.e1t, 471
mechanical circulatory support and, 561–562, 562f, 563f
Hemoglobin
developmental issues in, 17
fetal, 17
in hematologic disorders, 237t
pulse oximetry of, 1331, 1333
values at different ages, 237t
Hemoglobin A, 242
Hemoglobin electrophoresis, 510
Hemoglobin F, 242
Hemoglobin S, 242, 322
Hemoglobin SC, sickle cell disease and, 1189
Hemoglobin-based oxygen carriers, 288–289
Hemoglobinopathies, 242–248
sickle cell disease, 64, 242–246
thalassemias, 246–248
Hemoglobinuria, after ethanol embolization, 1212f
Hemolytic anemias, 239–242
glucose-6-phosphate dehydrogenase (G6PD) deficiency, 241–242, 241t, 242t
hereditary spherocytosis, 239–241, 240t
sickle cell disease, 242–246, 245t
thalassemia, 246–248, 248t
Hemolytic uremic syndrome, 731
Hemopericardium, 578
Hemophilia, 250–252, 251t, 252t
Hemophilia A, 533
Hemophilia B, 287
Hemophilia C, 250–251
Hemoptysis, 1211
Hemorrhage
embolization for, 1211
massive, recombinant factor VIIa, 509
mechanical circulatory support and, 564
posttonsillectomy, 847.e1t, 870–871, 871f
Hemorrhagic cystitis, 272
Hemorrhagic pulmonary edema, protamine and, 535
Hemostasis
alterations in, during pediatric cardiac surgery, 534–536
failure of hemostasis in, 536, 536t
routine anticoagulation, 534–535
cardiac surgery-related alterations/impairments in, 436–438
medications for, 529–547
antifibrinolytics, 542–545, 542f
blood products, 537–538
coagulopathy and major surgery, 533–534
Hemothorax, 578
Heparin
adverse effects of, 534–535
in cardiopulmonary bypass, 442, 513–514
low-molecular-weight, 560, 564
in pulmonary inhalation injury, 934–935
regional anesthesia and, 1086, 1087t
unfractionated, 563
Heparin cofactor II (HCII), 531
Heparinase-assisted thromboelastography, 515
Heparin-induced thrombocytopenia, cardiopulmonary bypass and, 508–509
Hepatectomy, 783–784, 784f
Hepatic acinus, 768
Hepatic artery reconstruction, 785
Hepatic drug metabolism, 104f, 113, 769–771
cytochrome P-450 activity in, 770–771, 770f
phase I reactions in, 113–114, 114t, 769–770, 770t
phase II reactions in, 84, 114–115, 114t, 771
Hepatic encephalopathy, 779

Hepatic system
anatomy of, 768–769, 769f
associated with childhood obesity, 55t
burn injury effects on, 935, 943t
cardiopulmonary bypass effects on, 526–527
growth and development of, 14–15, 15t
inhaled anesthetics and, 134
Hepatitis B virus, blood transfusion transmission of, 279t, 300
Hepatitis C virus, blood transfusion transmission of, 279t, 300
Hepatocytes, 90
Hepatopulmonary syndrome, 773–774, 778
Hepatorenal syndrome, 780
Hepatotoxicity, of anesthetic agents, 773
Hepcon system, 513
Hep-Lock IV set, 1319–1320
Herbal diuretics, 32.e1t
Herbal remedies, 31–32, 32.e1t
Hereditary neuralgic amyotrophy, 633
Hereditary neuropathies, 633–634
Hereditary sensory and autonomic neuropathy, 633
Hereditary spherocytosis (HS), 239–241, 240t
Hering-Breuer reflexes, 308
Hernia
congenital diaphragmatic, 380–381, 382f, 972–973, 972.e1
foramen of Bochdalek, 972
inguinal, 757, 976–977
Morgagni, 972
umbilical, 758
Herniation syndromes, 679
Heroin, neurotoxicity of, 652.e1–652.e11t
Heterotaxy syndromes, 392–393
High-fidelity mannequins, 1353
High-fidelity simulation, 1352–1353
High-flow nasal oxygenation, 877
High-frequency oscillatory ventilation, 1337
High-grade gliomas (HGG), 626t
Highly active antiretroviral therapy (HAART), 835, 1305
High-molecular-weight kininogen (HMWK), 531
Hill equation, 192–193
Hippocrates, 80
Hirschsprung disease, 16, 760–761, 979–980
Hispanic Americans, 97
Histidine-imidazole, 512
Histiocytes, 259
Histiocytoses, 253
Histone deacetylation, 81
History of present illness, 30–31, 31t, 31.e1t
HIV. see Human immunodeficiency virus
HLHS. see Hypoplastic left heart syndrome
HMWK. see High-molecular-weight kininogen
Hodgkin disease, 384
Hodgkin lymphoma, 257–258
Holoprosencephaly, 404, 624
Holt-Oram syndrome, 928
Homatropine, 907t
Homeostasis
body water and electrolyte distribution, 218–220, 219f, 219t
circulating blood volume, 218–219, 219t
mechanisms of, maturation of, 218–220
neonatal fluid management, 222
Homocystinuria, 903–904, 903.e1f
Hopkins telescope, in airway endoscopy, 877
Hormones, stress response to cardiac surgery and, 447
Horner syndrome, 908, 928, 1092
Horseshoe kidneys, 761–762
Hospital simulation center, 1351t
HPS haplotype, 87
HSCT. see Hematopoietic stem cell transplantation
5-HT₃. see Serotonin

H-type tracheoesophageal fistula, 384, 972.e1
Humalog, 706
Human factors, for surgical bleeding, 534
Human Genome Project, 79, 98
Human immunodeficiency virus (HIV)
blood transfusion transmission of, 300
in developing countries, 1303–1304f, 1304–1306, 1305f
transmission of, from blood transfusion, 529–530
Human patient simulators (HPS), 1349–1350, 1350f
Humidification, 1325
Humidifiers, heated, 1315–1316, 1315.e1f
Humidity, during sedation, 1205
Hunter syndrome, 340t
Hurler syndrome, 340t
Hurler-Scheie syndrome, 340t
Hybrid closed-loop systems, 707
Hybrid learning, 1350
Hybrid procedures, 427–429, 573, 576–577, 581
Hybrid simulation, 1350
Hydralazine, 492–493t, 495
Hydraulic model, for total intravenous anesthesia, 200
Hydrocele, 757, 757.e1f
Hydrocephalus, 624, 699–700, 699.e1f, 700f
Hydrocodone, 89–90, 164–165, 865
dosing guidelines for, 1152t
Hydrocortisone, 723
steroid equivalency ratios and doses of, 723t
Hydrogen cyanide, 934
Hydromorphone, 163
dosing guidelines for, 1152t
epidural, 1172t
Hydroxocobalamin, in cyanide toxicity, 939
Hydroxyamphetamine, 907t
Hydroxyethyl starches, 224, 288
Hydroxylation, 769
5-Hydroxytryptamine type 3-receptor antagonists, 185–186
Hydroxyurea, 243
Hydroxyzine, 39
Hyperalgesia, 1186
opioid-induced, 1149
Hyperalimentation, 61
burn injury and, 949
intraoperative fluid management and, 225, 225t
Hyperammonemia, prevention of, 631
Hyperbaric oxygen therapy, 939
Hyperbilirubinemia, 15, 15t, 240
Hypercalcemia, 721–722
description of, 412, 721
electrocardiographic findings, 412
Hypercalciuria, 955
Hypercapnia, 751–752
Hypercarbia, in malignant hyperthermia, 1031–1032
Hyperchloremic acidosis, 234
Hypercoagulability, 252–253, 949
Hypercortisolism, 723–724
Hypercyanotic episodes, in tetralogy of Fallot, 454, 579, 594
Hyperfibrinolysis, 532
Hyperglycemia, 708
after burn injury, 936
in hepatic failure, 780
maternal, 16
in newborn, 16, 222
preoperative management of, 709
stress-induced, in cardiac surgery, 448
wound healing affected by, 708
Hyperglycemic hyperosmotic nonketotic syndrome (HHNS), 1050
Hyperkalemia, 231–232, 232f, 233f, 271
arrhythmias and, 641–642
cardiac arrest caused by, 1027, 1031
causes of, 730t
in chronic kidney disease, 737, 737t
in chronic renal failure, 742

Hyperkalemia (Continued)
  electrocardiographic findings, 413f
  in hepatectomy, 785
  massive blood transfusion and,
    295f, 295.e1t
  in renal transplantation, 790–791
  rhabdomyolysis with, 1247
  succinylcholine-related, 152–153,
    685, 746
Hyperkalemic cardiac arrest, 1027
Hyperleukocytosis, 254–255, 270
Hypermetabolic state
  after burn injury, 933
  in malignant hyperthermia, 1032
Hypernatremia, 230–231
Hyperosmolality, 224–225
Hyperosmolar hyperglycemic nonketotic
    coma, 940
Hyperoxia, 981
  in extremely premature infant, 955–956
Hyperparathyroidism, 721, 955
Hypersensitivity reactions, to contrast
    media, 1200–1201
Hypersensitivity to local anesthetics, 1060
Hypersplenism, 240
Hypertension
  after burn injury, 933
  in chronic kidney disease, 738–739
  dexmedetomidine as cause of, 183
  intracranial
    in hydrocephalus, 699
    intracranial compliance and, 679
    in liver disease, 779
    monitoring of, 679
  paroxysmal, rhinologic procedures and,
    844–845
  in pheochromocytoma, 724
  postoperative, 1248
  urologic surgery and, 749
Hyperthermia, 1315
  in arthrogryposis multiplex
    congenita, 839
  cardiac catheterization and, 581
Hyperthyroidism, 718–720, 720t
  malignant hyperthermia versus, 1033t
Hypertonic dehydration, 229
Hypertonic saline solution, 940
Hypertonic solution, 216
Hypertrophic cardiomyopathy, 395–396,
    397f, 554, 577–578, 955
  cardiac transplantation for, 793
Hypertrophic pyloric stenosis,
    974–976, 975f
Hyperventilation, 684
Hyperviscosity syndrome, 17, 435–436
Hypnotic induction, 46–47
Hypnotics, neurophysiologic effects of, 688t
Hypoalbuminemia, 741, 962
Hypocalcemia, 271, 721
  after burn injury, 947
  citrate-induced, 297–298
  electrocardiographic findings, 412
  ionized, 947, 1025
  massive blood transfusion and,
    296–298, 298f
  in premature infants, 962
Hypocarbia, 1210
Hypochloremic metabolic alkalosis, 234
Hypocoagulability, 224
Hypofibrinogenemia, cryoprecipitate for,
    285–286
Hypoglycemia
  cardiopulmonary resuscitation in
    patients with, 1025
  definition of, 962
  in hepatic failure, 780
  maintenance fluids for, 1318
  in newborn, 222, 1318
  prevention of, 631
  reactive, 726
  rebound, 949
Hypokalemia, 232
  alkalosis causing, 1024–1025
  causes of, 730t
  electrocardiographic findings, 412

Hypomagnesemia
  amiodarone contraindications in, 1026
  electrocardiographic findings, 412
Hyponatremia, 220, 230–231, 715
  adrenocorticotropic hormone deficiency
    and, 722
  during craniosynostosis surgery, 919–921
  postoperative fluid management and,
    227–228, 1252
Hyponatremic encephalopathy, 716
Hypoosmolality, 715
Hypopharyngeal patency, 337–339
Hypoplastic left heart syndrome (HLHS),
    592, 598, 792–793
  description of, 443, 750–751
  for fetal intervention, 985
Hypopnea event, 846
Hypospadias, 756, 757f, 757.e1f
Hypotension
  amiodarone causing, 501
  arginine vasopressin and, 217
  controlled, 302–303
    after scoliosis surgery, 827
    anesthetic management during, 303
    contraindications of, 303
    nitroglycerin for, 302
    remifentanil for, 302–303
  dexmedetomidine as cause of, 184
  esmolol causing, 491
  flecainide causing, 500–501
  halothane and, 132
  hepatectomy and, 784
  induced, for blood loss, in
    craniosynostosis surgery, 920
  intraabdominal pressure and, 748
  midazolam causing, 965
  in noncardiac surgery in congenital
    heart disease, 609
  pheochromocytoma and, 726
  physiologic responses to, 218f
  postoperative, 1247–1248
Hypotensive anesthesia, 303
Hypothermia, 514
  after burn injury, 936
  cardiac catheterization and, 581
  during cardiac surgery, 520–521
  causes of, 1331
  during craniosynostosis surgery, 922
  in extremely premature infant, 961
  intraoperative, 836
  massive blood transfusion and, 298
  neuromuscular blocking drugs and, 157
  in non-operating room anesthesia, 1198
  symptoms of, 1251
  therapeutic, 1029, 1315
Hypothyroidism, 716–718, 903
  biochemical tests of thyroid function, 717
  classification of, 716–717
  clinical manifestations of, 717
  congenital, 717, 717f
  epidemiology of, 716–717
  neonatal, 717
  preoperative management of, 718
  primary, 716–717
  sick euthyroid syndrome and, 718
  treatment of, 717
Hypotonic dehydration, 229
Hypotonic fluids, 223
Hypoventilation, postoperative, 1245
Hypovolemia, 217, 226, 585, 1247–1248
Hypovolemic shock, 1007
Hypoxemia, 165–166, 543–544, 1245
  bradycardia and, 1247
  postoperative, 1245
Hypoxia, in liver disease, 778
Hypoxic encephalopathy, 935
Hysteresis loop, 193–194
Hyvan anaesthesia machine, 1312.e1f

I
Iatrogenic adrenal insufficiency, 723
Ibuprofen, 175, 980, 1145t, 1147
Ibutilide, 502
ICE blocks mnemonic, 1058
Ideal body weight, 765

Idiopathic scoliosis, 812t, 813–814, 814f
  long-term changes in, 817–818
  postoperative complications in, 816
Idiopathic thrombocytopenic purpura,
    248–249, 249t
Ifosfamide, 262, 269
I-gel supraglottic device, 347, 348f, 348t
Iliohypogastric nerve block, 1093–1096,
    1095f, 1096.e1f
Ilioinguinal nerve block, dosing for, 1088t
Iloprost, 497, 958
Imipramine, 1192
Immune system, cardiopulmonary bypass
    effects on, 527
Immunomodulation, 277
Immunosuppression, 798
Immunotolerance, 787
Impaired parent, informed consent and, 70
Impedance cardiometry, for continuous
    cardiac output assessment, 130–131
Impella (AbioMed), 552t, 557–559, 558f
Imperforate anus, 976
Implantable cardioverter-defibrillators,
    422, 613
In situ simulation, 1351t
  in non-operating room anesthesia, 1197
In vitro contracture test, in malignant
    hyperthermia, 636, 1048
Inborn errors of metabolism (IEM),
    627–632, 629–630t
Incisional pain, 754
Incontinentia pigmenti, 904
Increased intracranial pressure (ICP), 1001
  intracranial compliance and,
    679–680, 680f
  laparoscopic surgery in patients
    with, 753
  monitoring of, 679
  signs of, 679
Incretins, 707
Inderal. see Propranolol
Indirect contact transmission, 1281–1283,
    1281f, 1281.e1t, 1282f, 1283t
Indirect intubating devices, 364–367
Indomethacin, 1147–1148
  for intraventricular hemorrhage, 961
  for patent ductus arteriosus, 980
Induction of anesthesia, 43–51, 44f, 44.e1f
  in adenotonsillectomy, for obstructive
    sleep apnea, 870–871, 871f
  in anterior mediastinal masses, 384–385
  aspiration during, 225–226
  in cardiopulmonary bypass, 440–441
  in cleft lip and palate repair, 915
  in COVID-19, 1286–1288
  in emergency surgery in trauma
    patient, 1012
  in eye surgery, 909–910
  full stomach and rapid-sequence
    induction and, 49–51, 49t, 51f
  inhalation, 45–48, 45f, 45.e1f, 123–124
  intramuscular, 49
  intravenous, 48–49, 48t
  in mechanical circulatory support, 566
  in neurosurgical procedures, 684
  parental presence during, 27
Infant. see also Full-term neonate; Preterm
    infant
  circulating blood volume of, 219t
  intrathoracic lesions, 379–384, 381f,
    382f, 383f
  single-lung ventilation, 373–379
  spinal anesthesia for, 1073–1074, 1079t
  total lung capacity, 10, 10f
  vasoactive infusion, 485
Infant of a diabetic mother, 16
Infantile myopathy and lactic acidosis, 637t
Infantile scoliosis, 811–813, 813f
Infection
  after heart-lung transplantation, 807
  after renal transplantation, 791
  after ventricular assist device placement,
    570–571
  chain of, 1279f
  in cystic fibrosis, 320

Infection (Continued)
  epidural anesthesia-related, 1085–1086,
    1086t
  in infective endocarditis, 399–400,
    400t, 401t
  in myocarditis, 398–399, 398f
  prevention of, in mechanical circulatory
    support, 564
  in rheumatic fever and rheumatic heart
    disease, 399
  in sickle cell disease, 243
  transmission of, 1279, 1279f
  urologic surgery and, 750
Infection control practice, 1255
Infectious disease, considerations, for
    operating room, 1278–1298,
    1279f, 1280t
  antimicrobial prophylaxis for,
    1294–1298, 1295t
    indications for, 1290.e1t, 1297–1298
    β-lactams allergy in, 1296–1297
    selection of, 1296
    timing of, 1296
  causative agent in, 1280
  coronavirus in, 1284–1289
    cardiac arrest and, 1289
    emergence and extubation in, 1288
    equipment decontamination and
      room turnover and, 1289, 1289t
    induction and airway management
      in, 1286–1288
    preoperative testing for, 1286
    preparation for, 1285–1286,
      1286.e1f, 1287f
    regional anesthesia in, 1288
    specific pediatric anesthesia
      considerations in, 1288–1289
    summary on, 1289
  host of, 1280
  methods of transmission of, 1280–1284
    accidents with cutting or piercing
      devices in, 1283–1284
    air transmission, 1280–1281, 1281.e1f
    contact transmission, 1281–1283
    percutaneous contamination,
      1283–1284, 1284t
  prevention of transmission of,
    1290–1298
    airborne, 1287f, 1290–1291,
      1290.e1t, 1291t
    in health care institutions, 1290
    standard precautions in, 1291–1294
Infectious tuberculosis, precautionary
    procedures for, 1290.e1t
Infective endocarditis, 399–400, 400t,
    401t, 835
Inflammatory mediators, in
    cardiopulmonary bypass-induced
    lung injury, 522
Informed consent, 27
  adolescent abortion and, 69
  confidentiality for adolescent and, 69
  disclosure and, 68
  emergency care and, 70
  ethical issues regarding, 67
  impaired parent and, 70
  informed permission and best interests
    standard in, 66–67
  informed refusal and, 67–68
  Jehovah's Witnesses and, 69–70
  liability in, 68
  malpractice, 68
  medical errors and, 68–69
  in noncardiac surgery in congenital
    heart disease, 602
  patient's role in, 65–66, 66t
  physician judgment and, 68
  psychological preparation and, 27
  role of patient, 65–66, 66t
  surrogate, 66
Informed refusal, 67–68
Infracardiac total anomalous pulmonary
    venous connection, 458
Infraclavicular brachial plexus block,
    1110–1111, 1111f, 1112f, 1113f

Infragluteal-parabiceps approach, in lower extremity nerve blocks, 1124, 1125f, 1127f
Infraorbital nerve block, 1090–1091, 1091f
  bilateral, 916
Infundibular spasm, 594
Infusion rate, in total intravenous anesthesia
  bolus and variable rate, 200–204, 204f, 207f
  fixed, 200
Inguinal block, 1093–1096, 1095f
Inguinal hernia, 757, 976–977
Inhalation anesthetic agents, 95, 120–139
  breakdown products of, 124t, 126t, 137–138
  for cardiac surgery, 443–444
  clinical effects of, 134–138
    induction techniques and, 121t, 134–136
  effects on evoked potentials, 830
  emergence delirium and, 136–137, 136t
  emergence from, 136, 1241
  environmental impact of, 139
  in extremely premature infant, 964
  hepatic metabolism of, 771
  for liver transplantation, 782
  malignant hyperthermia and, 137
  mitochondrial disorders and, 637–638
  neuromuscular junction and, 137
  neurophysiologic effects of, 688t
  nitrous oxide in, 138–139
  noncardiac surgery in congenital heart disease using, 607
  oxygen and, 139–140
  pharmacodynamics of, 126–134
    cardiovascular system and, 130–133
    central nervous system and, 128–130
    hepatic system and, 134
    minimal alveolar concentration and, 126–128, 126t, 127f
    renal system and, 120t, 133–134
    respiratory system and, 133
  pharmacokinetics of, 114t, 120–124, 121f
    alveolar to venous partial pressure gradient and, 123
    alveolar ventilation/functional residual capacity, 108f, 121
    cardiac output, 108f, 121–122
    control of anesthetic depth and, 110f, 124–126, 124t
    induction and, 123–124
    second gas effect and, 123
    shunts and, 124–125, 125f
    solubility and, 109f, 110f, 122–123
    washout and emergence and, 125–126
  physiochemical properties of, 114t, 120
  for thoracic surgery, 370
  wash-in, 108f, 120t, 121f, 121t
Inhalation induction, of anesthesia, 45–48, 45f, 45.e1f
  total intravenous anesthesia after, 210–211
Inhalational injury, 893–894
Inhaled anesthetics, neurotoxicity of, 658–659
Inhaled nitric oxide, 495–496, 958, 960f
Inlet defects, in ventricular septal defect, 590
In-line filters, 1318
Innocent murmurs, 58, 409
InnoPran. see Propranolol
Inocor. see Amrinone
Inomax. see Inhaled nitric oxide
Inotropics, 484–485t
INR. see International normalized ratio
Inspiration
  accessory muscles of, 9
  laryngeal function during, 330
Inspiratory stridor, 334, 883
Insulin
  carbohydrates and, 773
  "correction factor" for, 709
  diabetes mellitus and

Insulin (Continued)
  intraoperative management of, 710–711
  intravenous infusions in major surgery and, 711, 711f, 712f
  postoperative management of, 711–712
  preoperative management of, 709
  urgent surgery and, 712
  "1800 rule" for, 709
  "1500 rule" for, 709
  for hyperkalemia, 737t
  intermediate-acting, 710
  pharmacokinetic profiles of, 706t
  preoperative, 42
  response to surgery, 708
Insulin injection, subcutaneous, 710, 710f
Insulin pump, 707
Insulin resistance, 55, 709, 936
Intact atrial septum, 983t
Intensive care unit transport, cardiopulmonary bypass and, 527
Interagency Registry for Mechanically Assisted Circulatory Support (INTERMACS), 550
INTERCEPT system, 286–287
Intercirculatory mixing, 474f, 476–477, 477f
Intercostal nerve block, 1085.e1f, 1093, 1094f, 1094.e1f
  for thoracic surgery, 371t
Interleukin-6, 94
INTERMACS. see Interagency Registry for Mechanically Assisted Circulatory Support
Intermediate-acting neuromuscular blocking drugs, 156
Intermediate-acting nondepolarizing neuromuscular blocking drugs, 154–156
Intermittent mechanical ventilation, 1325–1326
Internal jugular vein catheterization, 1261–1267, 1263–1264f, 1265f
International normalized ratio (INR), 236, 533, 773
International Society for Pediatric and Adolescent Diabetes (ISPAD) Clinical Practice Consensus Guidelines, 708
International Society on Thrombosis and Haemostasias, 250
Interrupted aortic arch, 465, 465f, 589t, 597
Interventional cardiology, 573–586
  anesthesia in, 581–586
    aims of, 581
    anatomy and function in, 582
    cardiac catheterization, environment and, 582, 582f
    choice of, 582–585
    future of, 586
    general anesthesia and, 583–585
    preprocedural assessment and management in, 581–582
    principles of technique in, 585
    sedation and, 583
  angioplasty and stenting, 575–576
  aortic balloon valvuloplasty, 576
  atrial septal defect closure, 574, 574f
  atrial septostomy, 573–574
  choice of vessel access in, 577
  diagnostic catheterization, 573, 574t
  electrophysiologic catheterization in, 577
  patent ductus arteriosus closure, 575, 575f, 576f
  percutaneous pulmonary valve replacement, 576
  procedures in, 573–577
  ventricular septal defect closure, 574–575, 575f
Interventional radiology, for non-operating room anesthesia, 1209–1213

Intraabdominal pressure, 978–979
  abdominal compartment syndrome and, 747
  laparoscopic surgery and, 751
Intraarterial chemotherapy, injection of, 1210–1211
Intraatrial baffles, 456
Intracapsular tonsillectomy, 846
Intracardiac electrograms, 577
Intracardiac repair phase, in cardiopulmonary bypass, 514
Intracardiac shunting, 436
Intracerebral hematoma, 693
Intracranial aneurysms, 696
Intracranial compartments, 678
Intracranial compliance, 680f
Intracranial hypertension
  in hydrocephalus, 699
  intracranial compliance and, 679
  in liver disease, 779
  monitoring of, 679
  thiopental for, 141
Intracranial pressure (ICP), 624, 678–680, 679f
  increased, 678–680
    in craniosynostosis, 917–918
    intracranial compliance in, 679, 680f
    ketamine-related, 146
    in liver transplantation, 779
    monitoring, 679
    signs of, 679
  laparoscopic surgery in patients with, 753
Intracranial venous sinuses, 689
Intralipid rescue, from local anesthetic toxicity, 1060
Intramuscular injection, opioids, 1155
Intraocular pressure
  description of, 904–905, 904f
  ketamine-related, 146
  succinylcholine-related increase of, 153
Intraoperative blood recovery and reinfusion, 301–302
Intraoperative fluid management, 222–227
  fasting for, 225–226
  hyperalimentation and, 225, 225t
  intravascular volume, assessment of, 226–227
  intravenous access and fluid administration devices in, 222–223
  intravenous fluids in, 223–224, 223t
  ongoing losses and third-spacing in, 226
Intraoperative magnetic resonance imaging, 703, 703.e1f
Intraoperative record policy, 1196
Intraoperative salvage of shed blood, in scoliosis surgery, 829
Intraosseous access, in cardiopulmonary resuscitation, 1022
Intraosseous infusion, 1257f, 1258–1259, 1259f, 1260f
Intrathoracic trachea, 331
Intravascular fluid volume, 217–218, 226–227
Intravenous access
  in cardiopulmonary resuscitation, 1022
  for intraoperative fluid management, 222–223
  in noncardiac surgery in congenital heart disease, 604
Intravenous anesthesia, 48–49, 48t, 140–148
  emergence from, 1241
  in endoscopy, 875, 875.e1t
  etomidate in, 147–148
  in extremely premature infant, 964–966
  ketamine in, 144–147, 145f, 145t
  methohexital, 140
  in mitochondrial disorders, 637–638
  propofol for, 115f, 141–144
  target concentration, 192–193, 198–208, 198f, 199f, 200f, 200t, 201–203f
  thiopental for, 140–141
  total, 190–215, 687–688

Intravenous anesthesia (Continued)
  after inhalational induction, 211
  bispectral index monitoring in, 1340
  bolus and variable rate infusion in three-compartment model in, 200–204, 204f
  depth of anesthesia monitoring in, 196–197, 1340
  drug delivery in, 208, 209t
  for emergence delirium, 1243
  in epilepsy, 647–648, 647t
  fixed infusion rate and three-compartment model in, 198f, 199f, 200
  indications for, 190
  infusion schemes, 197t
  during malignant hyperthermia, 1034–1035
  manual infusion schemes for, 204f
  in muscular dystrophy, 641
  in myasthenia gravis patients, 635–636
  in obese child, 212–214, 213f, 214f
  pharmacodynamics of, 190–194
  pharmacokinetics of, 190–194
  postoperative nausea and vomiting and, 1249
  principles of, 190–194, 191f
  propofol and, 205f
  target-controlled infusion in, 204–208, 205t, 206t, 207f
  vasoactive medications and, 1318–1319, 1318f, 1319f
Intravenous cutdown, 1258
Intravenous drug dosing, 55–56
Intravenous fluid therapy, 223, 223t
  for diabetes, 710
  for postoperative nausea and vomiting, 910
Intravenous immunoglobulin, 401
Intravenous induction agents, for cardiac surgery, 444–445
Intravenous regional anesthesia, 1131–1132
Intravenous therapy, equipment of, 1317–1320, 1317t, 1317.e1f
Intraventricular hemorrhage
  eye surgery and, 903
  prematurity and, 960–961
Intrinsic myocardial disorders, 394t, 395
Introducer sheaths, 1258
Intubation
  abnormal airway, 359–369
    air-Q Mask Laryngeal Airway in, 347, 349f
    Airtraq optical laryngoscope in, 365–366, 366f
    Bullard laryngoscope in, 363–364, 363.e1f
    flexible fiberoptic bronchoscope used in retrograde manner, 368
    flexible laryngoscopy in, 360–363
    GlideScope in, 364–365, 364.e1f
    lighted stylet, 363, 363.e1f
    MultiView Scope in, 365, 365.e2f
    retrograde light-guided laryngoscopy, 368–369
    retrograde wire and flexible intubation scope, 368
    retrograde wire-guided intubation in, 364
    rigid laryngoscopy and flexible fiberoptic bronchoscope, 368
    rigid laryngoscopy in, 359–360
    Shikani optical stylet in, 367, 367.e1f
    Storz Bonfils optical stylet in, 367, 367.e2f
    Storz Video Laryngoscope in, 365, 365.e1f
    supraglottic airway as conduit for, 367–368, 368.e1f
    Truview EVO2 infant device in, 366–367, 366.e1f
    video and indirect intubating devices for, 364–367

Intubation (Continued)
    video laryngoscopy and flexible
        intubation scope, 368
    in acute epiglottitis, 883
    in burn injury, 938, 938f, 948
    in cleft lip and palate repair, 915
    equipment for, 1323
    in hemifacial dysostosis, 925f
    in neurosurgical procedures, 684–685
    tracheal, 337–343
        complications of, 342–343
        continuous waveform capnography
            for, 342
        CPR medication administration
            via, 1022
        distance to insert tracheal tube and,
            341–342, 342t, 343f
        laryngoscope blade for, 340, 340t
        laryngotracheal stenosis and, 343, 344f
        postintubation croup and, 342–343
        technique in, 337–340, 337.e1f, 339f
        tubes in, 340–341, 341f, 341t
        video laryngoscopy in, 340
    in tracheotomy, 890
Iodine, for hyperthyroid crisis, 720t
Iodine deficiency, 716–717
Ion channel muscle diseases, 639t, 642
Ion channelopathies, 395
Ionized calcium, 439, 936–937, 962
Ionized hypocalcemia, 947, 1025
Ipratropium bromide, for asthma
    exacerbations, 319.e2–319.e3t
Irritable bowel syndrome, 1183
Isaacs syndrome, 639t
Ischemia, tourniquet and, 833
Ischemic bowel, 747
Ischemic conditioning, tourniquet and, 833
Ischemic optic neuropathy, 827
Ischemic preconditioning, for stress
    response after cardiac surgery, 449
Isoboles, 194
Isobolographic analysis, 118
Isoflurane
    for cardiac surgery, 443
    in developing countries, 1309–1310
    in eye surgery, 909
    hyperglycemia caused by, 708
    metabolism of, 81, 771
    minimum alveolar concentration of,
        124, 124t
    neurophysiologic effects of, 688t
    neurotoxicity of, 652.e1–652.e11f, 658
    physiochemical properties of, 114t
Isoproterenol, 484–485t, 486
Isoptin. see Verapamil
Isotonic salt solution, 221–222
Isotonic solutions, 225
Isovolumic reduction, of hemoglobin,
    acute, 511
ISPAD. see International Society for
    Pediatric and Adolescent Diabetes
Isuprel. see Isoproterenol
Ivabradine, 492
Ivacaftor, 321

J
Jackson frame, 826f
Janeway lesions, 399
Jatene procedure, 430–431t, 595
Jaundice, physiologic, 15, 15t
Jaw thrust, 333
Jehovah's Witnesses
    and cardiopulmonary bypass, 511–512
    children of, 69–70
    informed consent in, 69–70
    transfusion therapy in, 304
Jervell and Lange-Nielsen syndrome, 418
Jet ventilation
    in endoscopy, 876–877, 876.e1t
    transtracheal, 359
Jet Ventilation Catheter, 357, 358f
Joint Commission on Accreditation
    of Healthcare Organizations
    (JCAHO), sedation guidelines,
    1225–1226, 1225f

Joint contractures
    in muscular dystrophy, 641
    in spinal muscular atrophy, 632–633
Jones criteria, for rheumatic fever, 399
Jostra RotaFlow (Maquet), 552t, 558
Judicial bypass, 69
Jugular venous bulb oxygen
    saturation, 524
Junctional ectopic tachycardia, 441–442
Junctional rhythm, 415t, 417f
Juvenile idiopathic scoliosis, 813
Juvenile laryngeal papillomatosis, 887
Juvenile myasthenia gravis, 635
Juvenile rheumatoid arthritis, 925
Juvenile scoliosis, 811–813

K
Kallikrein, 506
Kallikrein system, 532
Kallikrein-kinin (contact) system, 543
Kaplan-Meier analysis, 1201
Kaposi sarcoma, 1307f
Kappa opioid receptors, 1152, 1152.e1t
Kataria model, 191, 209
Kataria system, 206–207, 206t
Kava, 32.e1t
Kawasaki disease, 400–401, 401f
Kayexalate, 737t
Kearns-Sayre syndrome, 637t
Kefauver-Harris Amendment, 119
Kenny-Caffey syndrome, 721
Kernicterus, 15, 963
Ketamine, 144–147, 145f, 145t
    for abnormal airway, 352–353
    adverse effects of, 145–146
    after scoliosis surgery, 825
    for asthma, 317–318
    blood flow affected by, 443
    for blunt reflex bronchoconstriction,
        860.e1t
    for bone marrow aspiration
        procedures, 274
    for burn injury pain, 945
    for cardiac catheterization, 583
    for cardiac surgery, 444
    for cardiopulmonary bypass, 441
    for caudal epidural analgesia, 146
    in developing countries, 1310
    dissociative anesthesia caused by, 584
    effects on evoked potentials, 831
    emergence delirium reduction
        using, 1243
    emergency surgery in trauma patient
        using, 1009t, 1013
    in extremely premature infant, 965
    hepatic metabolism of, 769–770
    hypotension caused by, 566
    infusion schemes, 197t
    intracranial pressure affected by, 146
    intramuscular, 38
    intranasal, 38
    intraocular pressure affected by, 146
    intravenous induction of, 49
    in micropremie, 965
    midazolam and, 352–353, 945
    nasal administration of, 145
    neurophysiologic effects of, 688t
    neurotoxicity of, 652.e1–652.e11t,
        657–658
    noncardiac surgery in congenital heart
        disease using, 608
    oculocardiac reflex and, 909
    oral, 38
    for pain management, 1193–1194
        description of, 146, 1149
        postoperative, 146
    premedication of autistic child
        using, 36
    preoperative uses of, 38
    racemic, 657
    for sedation, 1230–1231t, 1234–1235
Ketogenic diet, 63t, 64, 644
Ketone bodies, disorders of, 630
Ketones, 710

Ketorolac, 93, 175, 176–177, 908, 1250
    after myringotomy with tube
        insertion, 842
    age-related pharmacokinetic changes,
        145t, 175t
    oral dosing guidelines for, 1145t
    for pain management, 1187, 1250
Kidney
    burn injury effects on, 935, 943t
    drug metabolism, 107f, 115f, 116, 116f
    growth and development of, 13
    inhaled anesthetics and, 121t, 134
    nephrogenesis, 13
    physiology of, 729–731
        acid-base balance, 730–731
        fluids and electrolytes and, 730, 730t
        intraoperative management in,
            739–743
        maintenance of phosphate and, 738
    prematurity and, 961
    tumors of, 269
King-Denborough syndrome, 1049–1050
Klippel-Feil syndrome, 914–915, 914.e1
Klumpke palsy, 634, 928
Klumpke's palsy, 634
Konno procedure, 597
Konno-Rastan procedure, 430–431t
Krabbe disease, 633–634
Kugelberg-Welander disease, 633
Kyphoscoliosis, 837
Kyphosis, 810

L
Labetalol, 491, 492–493t
    in neurosurgery, 690
Laboratory data
    in abdominal surgery, 748
    in neurosurgery, 682
    in noncardiac surgery in congenital
        heart disease, 601–602
    preoperative preparation and, 35
Lacosamide, 645t
β-Lactams allergy, 1296–1297
Lactated Ringer's solution, 223t
Lactic acidosis, 711
Lamotrigine, 645t
Laminar flow, 1317
Land mines, 1301
Langerhans cell histiocytosis, 259
Lanoxicaps. see Digoxin
Lanoxin. see Digoxin
Lantus, 706
Laparo-endoscopic single site surgery, 751
Laparoscopic surgery, 615, 750–754,
    750f, 751f
    appendectomy, 750f
    cardiovascular effects of, 753
    central nervous system effects of,
        753–754
    fluid requirements in, 754
    pain management after, 754
    pyloromyotomy, 975.e1
    renal effects of, 754
    respiratory effects of, 752–753
    vertical sleeve gastrectomy, 764,
        766–767
Laryngeal atresia, 889
Laryngeal cartilages, 328, 329f
Laryngeal clefts, 894–895, 894f
Laryngeal mask airway (LMA), 337,
    368.e1f, 1320–1321
    for cardiopulmonary resuscitation,
        1017–1018
    eye surgery uses of, 911–912
    for myringotomy, 841
    prehospital trauma airway management
        using, 1012
Laryngeal Mask Airway Classic, 346, 359
Laryngeal Mask Airway Fastrach, 346
Laryngeal Mask Airway Supreme, 346, 346f
Laryngeal papilloma, 1306f
Laryngeal papillomatosis, 887–889, 887f,
    888f, 888.e1f
Laryngeal stenosis, acquired, 889
Laryngeal Tube, 346–347, 347t, 347.e1f
Laryngeal web, 969f

Laryngeal webs, congenital, 883.e1f, 889
Laryngomalacia, 883
Laryngoscope
    in airway endoscopy, 877
    Bullard, 363–364, 363.e1f
    optical, 365–367
        Airtraq optical laryngoscope,
            365–366, 366f
        Truview EVO2 infant device,
            366–367, 366.e1f
    video, 364–365
        GlideScope, 364–365, 364.e1f
        MultiView Scope, 365, 365.e2f
        Storz Video Laryngoscope,
            365, 365.e1f
Laryngoscope blade, 340, 340t, 1197, 1323
Laryngoscopy, 340
    diagnostic, 872–873, 873t, 874f
    direct, 872–881, 1323
    flexible, 360–363
    retrograde light-guided, 368–369
    rigid, 359–360
        dental mirror in, 360
        flexible fiberoptic bronchoscope
            and, 368
        intubation guides, 360, 360.e1f
        lateral approach to, 360, 361f
        optimal external laryngeal
            manipulation in, 360
        paraglossal approach to, 360, 361f
        retromolar approach to, 360, 361f
Laryngospasm, 314–315, 1243–1244
    in adenotonsillectomy, 858, 859f
    glottic closure during, 330–331
Laryngotracheal edema, 226
Laryngotracheal injury, 893
Laryngotracheal reconstruction, 895–897
    anesthetic considerations for, 897,
        897f, 898t
    surgical approach on, 895–897,
        896f, 897f
Laryngotracheal stenosis, 343, 344f
Laryngotracheitis, 885–886
Laryngotracheobronchitis, 329–330,
    885–887, 885t
Laryngotracheoplasty, 380
Larynx, 324–325, 328–331
    blood supply of, 330
    developmental anatomy of, 324–325,
        325f, 326f
    function of, 330–331
    growth and development of, 8f
    histology of, 329–330
    obstruction of, 969–970, 969f, 970f
    pathology related to, 350t
    sensory and motor innervation of, 330
    structure of, 328–329, 329f, 330f
Laser interstitial thermal therapy
    (LITT), 698
L-Asparaginase, 270
Lateral approach, to rigid laryngoscopy,
    360, 361f
Lateral decubitus position, 371, 379f
Lateral femoral cutaneous nerve block,
    949–950, 1129
Lateral popliteal sciatic nerve block,
    1126f, 1127–1128
Lateral position, modified, in
    neurosurgery, 687
Latex allergy, 33–34, 749
    cerebral palsy in, 621
Laudanosine, 155
Leber hereditary optic neuropathy, 637t
LeFort procedures, 923f, 925
Left superior vena cava to coronary sinus,
    persistent, 407–409, 408f
Left ventricular assist device (LVAD), 551,
    557, 567
Left ventricular failure, 739
Left ventricular outflow tract obstructions,
    589t, 592–593
Left-to-right shunts, 124, 436, 449–453,
    449t
    aortopulmonary window in,
        451–452, 452f

Left-to-right shunts (Continued)
  atrial septal defect, 450, 451f
  atrioventricular septal defect in,
      450–451, 451f, 452f, 452t
  patent ductus arteriosus in, 452–453,
      453f
  simple, 449–453, 449t
    aortopulmonary window in,
      451–452, 452f
    atrial septal defect, 450, 451f
    atrioventricular septal defect in,
      450–451, 451f, 452f, 452t
    patent ductus arteriosus in,
      452–453, 453f
    ventricular septal defect, 450
  ventricular septal defect, 450
Leigh encephalomyeloneuropathy, 637t
Length assessment, 5, 6t
Lenke classification system, 811, 811.e1f
Lepirudin, 508–509
Letairis. see Ambrisentan
Leukemia
  acute lymphoblastic, 253–255, 256t
  acute myelogenous, 255–257
  Hodgkin lymphoma, 257–258
Leukemia cutis, 256
Leukocyte-reduced red blood cells, for
    hematologic disorders, 248t
Leukocytes, 17
  cardiopulmonary bypass and, 527
Leukodystrophies, 633–634
Leukoreduction, 277
Levalbuterol, for asthma exacerbations,
    319.e2–319.e3t
Level of consciousness, monitoring, in
    sedation, 1222
Levemir, 706
Levetiracetam, 645t
Levobunolol, 907t
Levobupivacaine, 1054, 1172t
Levocardia, 392, 392f
Levophed. see Norepinephrine
Levosimendan, 490
Levothyroxine, 717
Lid reflex, after thiopental, in burn injury,
    944, 944.e1f
LiDCO systems, 1341–1342
Lidocaine, 96, 499t, 500
  after scoliosis surgery, 825–826
  for blunt reflex bronchoconstriction,
    860.e1t
  for cardiopulmonary resuscitation, 1026
  emergency surgery in trauma patient
    using, 1009t
  infusion dose of, 1057
  intravenous regional anesthesia uses
    of, 1114
  for intubation, 690
  oculocardiac reflex and, 908
  for pain, 1151–1152
  pharmacokinetics of, 1055
  topical, after adenotonsillectomy,
    866, 866.e1f
  toxicity of, 1057
Lifebox Foundation, 1333
Life-sustaining medical treatment
  barriers to honoring preferences for
    resuscitation in, 71–72
  definition of, 70–72, 71t
  physician orders for, 72
Lighted stylet, for difficult airway,
    363, 363.e1f
Lignocaine. see Lidocaine
Limb girdle muscular dystrophy, 639t, 641
Limb hemangioma, 926–927
Line-isolation monitors, 1198
Lipid emulsion, 1059–1060
Lipid metabolism, disturbances of, 633–634
Lipid solubility, 769
Lipomeningoceles, 702
Lipomyelomeningoceles, 702
Liposuction, 930
Lisinopril, 495
Lissencephaly, 625
Lithium, 659–660, 662

Lithium (button) batteries, 881–883, 882f
Liver, 768–774
  anatomy of, 768–769, 769f
  burn injury effects on, 935, 943t
  cellular function in, anesthetic effects
    on, 773
  drug metabolism by, 104f, 113,
    769–771
    cytochrome P-450 activity, 770–771,
      770f
    phase I reactions, 81–83, 769–770
    phase II reactions, 771
  growth and development of, 14
  inhalational anesthetics and, 134, 771
  lobule of, 768
  neuromuscular blocking drugs and,
    771–772
  opioids and, 772
  sedatives and, 772
  tumors of, 269
Liver disease
  cardiac considerations in, 778
  hematologic considerations in, 780
  metabolic considerations in, 780
  neurologic considerations in, 779–780
  opioids metabolism and, 772
  pathophysiology of, 778–780
  perioperative considerations in, 773–774
  pulmonary considerations in, 778–779
  renal manifestations in, 780
Liver transplantation, 775–787
  anhepatic stage in, 784–785
  biliary and hepatic artery
    reconstruction in, 785
  epidemiology and demographics of,
    776–778, 776f, 777t
  hepatectomy in, 783–784, 784f
  immediate postoperative care for,
    786–787
  indications for, 776
  intraoperative care in, 782–783
  living-donor, 785–786
  long-term issues of, 787
  orthotopic, 775
  outcomes of, 786
  pathophysiology of liver disease,
    778–780
  preoperative evaluation in,
    780–782, 781t
  reperfusion period in, 785
  split liver techniques in, 785–786
  surgical technique in, 783–786
Living-donor liver transplants, 785–786
LMWH. see Low-molecular-weight
    heparin
Loading dose, 110, 197
Lobar holoprosencephaly, 624
Lobectomy, 698
Local anesthetics
  eye surgery uses of, 908
  for neurosurgical procedures, 687
  for pain management, 1143f, 1164–1165,
    1170–1171, 1172t
  peripheral nerve blocks using,
    1087–1088, 1088t
  pharmacogenetics of, 96
  pharmacology and pharmacokinetics of,
    1054–1060, 1054t, 1054.e1f
    amides, 1054–1055
    bupivacaine, 1054–1055
    esters, 1055–1056
    hypersensitivity, 1060
    intralipid rescue for toxicity, 1060
    lidocaine, 1055
    ropivacaine in, 1055
    toxicity and, 1056–1057, 1056f,
      1058t
    treatment of systemic toxic reactions
      and, 1059–1060
  for sedation, 1229
  tonsillar infiltration, 866, 866.e1f
Logistic regression model, 108
Long QT syndrome, 418–420, 419f
Long-acting nondepolarizing
    neuromuscular blocking drugs, 156

Loop of Henle, 730
Lorazepam, 84
Lordosis, 810
Losartan, 495
Loss aversion, 353
Loss of consciousness, 1338
Loss-of-resistance technique, in
    paravertebral block, 1104–1106
Low-birth-weight infant, 2
  blood volume, 218–219
  jaundice in, 15
Lower esophageal sphincter, 16
Lower extremity nerve blocks, 1119–1131,
    1120f
  ankle, 1130–1131, 1131f
  digital foot, 1131
  fascia iliaca, 1130
  femoral nerve block, 1129
  infragluteal-parabiceps approach in,
    1124, 1125f, 1127f
  lateral popliteal sciatic nerve, 1126f,
    1127–1128
  lumbar plexus, 1120–1122, 1121f,
    1122f
  sciatic nerve, 1122–1125, 1123f, 1124f
Lower motor neuron, 632f
Lower respiratory tract infections, in
    adenotonsillectomy, 856
Lower urinary tract obstruction,
    983t, 985
Low-flow hypothermic bypass, neurologic
    monitoring for, 524
Low-grade gliomas, 626t
Low-molecular-weight heparin (LMWH),
    560, 564
LPS haplotype, 87
Luer adapters, 1319–1320
Lugol solution, 719–720
Lumbar plexus block, 1120–1122, 1121f,
    1122f
Lumbar puncture, 274, 1077f
Lumbar sympathetic block, 1188f
Lung
  abnormalities of, 972–974, 972.e1
  development of, 307, 308f
  elastic properties of, 9
  of extremely premature infant,
    954–956
  inhalation anesthetic delivery to, factors
    affecting, 108f, 121–123
  pulmonary vascular physiology of,
    471t, 472
Lung disease
  cystic fibrosis and, 320
  in sickle cell disease, 322
Lung volumes, 474
  static, 10, 10t
LV hypertrophy, 593
LVAD. see Left ventricular assist device
Lymphatic malformations, sclerotherapy
    of, 1211–1213, 1211f, 1212f, 1212t
Lymphoblastic lymphoma, 384
Lymphocytic interstitial pneumonitis,
    1305–1306
Lymphoma
  Hodgkin, 257–258
  non-Hodgkin, 258–259
Lysine analogues, 508
  adverse effects of, 544
  synthetic, 542–543, 542f
Lysosomal storage disease, 629–630t,
    630–631

M
Ma huang, 32.e1t
Macitentan, 497
Macrocephaly, 625
Macrodrip, 1317
α2-Macroglobulin, 531–532
Macroglossia, 717, 948, 1320
Macrolides, 646t
Magnesium sulfate, 499t, 503
  for opioid-induced respiratory
    depression, 866
  for torsades de pointes, 420

Magnetic resonance angiography (MRA),
    for non-operating room anesthesia,
    1203
Magnetic resonance imaging (MRI)
  for cleft lip and palate, 914
  heart disease evaluations, 425–426, 426t
  neurosurgical anesthesia and, 703
  for non-operating room anesthesia,
    1203–1207, 1203f, 1205f, 1206f
Magnetic resonance spectroscopy
    (MRS), for non-operating room
    anesthesia, 1203
Magnetic resonance venography
    (MRV), for non-operating room
    anesthesia, 1203
Magnetoencephalography, for non-
    operating room anesthesia, 1207
Mainstream carbon dioxide analyzers,
    1335–1337
Maintenance fluids, 220
Maintenance of anesthesia
  in bladder and cloacal exstrophy, 763
  in burn injury, 945, 945.e1f, 946.e1f
  in cardiopulmonary bypass, 441–442
  in eye surgery, 909–910
  in neurosurgical procedures,
    687–688, 688t
  in noncardiac surgery in congenital
    heart disease, 606–609
  in renal transplantation, 790–791
Maintenance of Certification in
    Anesthesia (MOCA), 1348
Malaria, 1308–1309
Male genitalia, gestational age
    assessment, 5t
Malformations
  of cortical development, 625
  of nervous system, 622–624, 624t
Malignancy, after renal transplantation, 791
Malignant hyperthermia (MH), 1030–1052,
    1031f, 1247, 1315
  caffeine-induced contractures in, 137
  clinical presentation of, 1031–1033,
    1031t, 1032t, 1033t, 1034t
  congenital myopathy, 1049–1050
  congenital myopathy and, 636
  contracture testing in, 1048, 1049f
  dantrolene for, 1031f, 1036f, 1039–1041,
    1039.e1f, 1040f, 1040t
  molecular mechanisms and
    physiologic effects of, 1046f,
    1047–1048, 1047f, 1048f
  diagnosis of, 752
  diagnostic muscle biopsy in, 1041–1042
  differential diagnosis of, 1033t
  disseminated intravascular coagulation
    in, 1031t, 1041
  evaluation and preparation of patient
    in, 1034–1036, 1035t
  excitation-contraction coupling in,
    1044–1045, 1045f, 1046f
  fatality rate in, 1031f
  fatty acid metabolism disorders and,
    1050–1051
  fulminant, 1030
  genetic investigation in, 1042, 1042.e1f
  genetic testing in, 1048–1049
  genetics of, 97, 1043–1044, 1043.e1f,
    1044t
  grading scale, 1033, 1034t
  halothane causing, 1043, 1043.e1f
  historical description of, 80
  incidence of, 1030
  inhalation anesthetic agents and, 137
  intermediate, 1038–1039, 1038t,
    1038.e1f
  laboratory diagnosis of, 1048–1049
  laboratory testing of, 1036–1038,
    1036f, 1036.e1f
  late complications in, 1041
  malignant hyperthermia–like syndrome
    in diabetes mellitus and, 1050
  management of, 1038–1042
  MedicAlert bracelets for, 1038
  mimics, 1050–1051

Malignant hyperthermia *(Continued)*
  in Möbius syndrome, 927
  monitoring in, 1036
  myopathic syndromes and, 1049–1050
  neuroleptic malignant syndrome
      and, 1051
  noninvasive testing of, 1049
  notification in, 1042
  pathophysiology of, 1036–1038, 1036f,
      1036.e1f, 1045–1047, 1046f
  patient evaluation and preparation and,
      1034–1036
  physiology of, 1044–1048
  postreaction follow-up in, 1041–1042
  recrudescence of, 1041
  rhabdomyolysis *versus*, 641–642,
      1037–1038, 1037t
  screening for, 1042
  stress-triggered, 1042–1043
  succinylcholine and, 159, 1030
  thyroid storm *versus*, 720
Malignant hyperthermia-like syndrome
    (MHLS), 1050
Malnutrition
  cerebral palsy in, 621
  cystic fibrosis and, 320
Malocclusion surgery, 925
Malpractice, 68
Malrotation, 979
Managing Emergencies in Paediatric
    Anaesthesia, 1354
Manchester Pain Scale, 1136t
Mandible
  hypoplasia of, 324–325, 915
  limited excursion, 1032t
  pathology related to, 350t
Mannequins, 1348, 1349f
Manual infusion schemes, for total
    intravenous anesthesia, 197t,
    198f, 204f
Mapleson circuit, 1207, 1326, 1326f
Maquet. *see* Jostra RotaFlow
Marfan syndrome, 406, 406f
  airway difficulties in, 340t
  eye surgery in, 903–904, 903.e1f
Marsh model, 191–192
MASK study. *see* Mayo Anesthesia Safety
    in Kids study
Mask ventilation, 336–337, 336f, 338f
Masks, 1320
Mass casualty disaster management plan,
    1003–1004
Masseter muscle spasm, in malignant
    hyperthermia, 1030, 1033t
Massive blood transfusion, 289–300, 289e
  acid-base balance in, 298
  citrate toxicity in, 296–298, 298f
  coagulopathy and, 289–291, 290f, 291f
  dilutional thrombocytopenia in, 291–292,
      292f, 293f
  disseminated intravascular coagulation
      in, 294
  factor deficiency in, 292–294, 294t
  fibrinolysis in, 294
  hyperkalemia in, 295–296, 295f, 295.e1t
  hypocalcemia in, 296–298, 298f
  hypothermia in, 298
  infectious disease considerations in, 300
  monitoring during, 298–300, 298.e1f,
      299f, 300f
  protocol for, 289
  in scoliosis surgery, 830
Mastoid surgery, 842–843, 844t
Mastoidectomy, 842–843
Maturity-onset diabetes of the young, 706
Maxilla
  osteotomy of, 915
  pathology related to, 350t
Mayfield head holder, 685
Mayo Anesthesia Safety in Kids (MASK)
    study, 672
McCune-Albright syndrome,
    hyperthyroidism associated with, 718
McGill oximetry score, 852, 853f
MDR-1, 93

Mean arterial pressure, regulation of, 680
Mechanical circulatory support, 549–572
  complications of, 570–571
  contraindications for, 554
  criteria for, 551t
  devices for, 552t, 554
  future directions in, 571
  in heart transplantation, 795
  indications for, 550–554, 550t
  initiation for, 551–553
  learning systems and databases of, 550
  noncardiac surgery in congenital heart
      disease and, 614
  organ transplantation and, 568
  outcomes of, 567–570
  perioperative management of, 561–567
    anesthetic considerations,
        564–567, 565t
    hematologic considerations, 562–564
    hemodynamics, 561–562, 562f, 563f
    prevention of infection in, 564
    respiratory considerations, 562
  single ventricle physiology and, 555–556,
      569–570
  ventricular assist devices for,
      557–560, 567
    biventricular, 551, 570
    centrifugal pump, 557–558, 557f
    continuous flow pumps, 560
    extracorporeal membrane oxygenation,
        549–550, 552t, 554–557
    history of, 549
    immunologic complications of, 571
    implantation of, 570
    left, 551, 557
    long-term devices, 559–560
    pulsatile pumps, 559–560, 559f
    short-term devices, 557–559
  on wait-list survival, effect of, 568–569
Mechanical dead space, 1327
Mechanical insufflation-exsufflation, 816
Mechanomyography, 1337–1338
Meconium, 16, 963
Meconium ileus, 976, 976f
Median effective dose, 220
Median nerve block, 1117–1118, 1118f
Mediastinal masses
  anterior, 384, 385f
  posterior, 385–386, 386f
Medical decontamination, risk categories
    for, 1283t
Medical errors, 68–69, 77
Medical history
  airway evaluation and, 334
  in chronic pain, 1182–1183, 1183t
  past, 31–35, 31.e1t
    allergies to medications and latex in,
        32–35, 34t
    family history in, 35
MedicAlert bracelets, 1038
MedicAlert Foundation, 354
Medication-overuse headache, 1185
Medications
  allergies to, 32–35, 34t
  cardiopulmonary resuscitation,
      1023–1026
    adrenergic agonists, 1023
    amiodarone, 1025–1026
    atropine, 1024
    calcium, 1025
    epinephrine, 1024
    glucose, 1025
    lidocaine, 1026
    sodium bicarbonate, 1024–1025
    vasopressin, 1024
  in postanesthesia care unit, 1239,
      1239t, 1240t
  premedication uses, 36–43
    α_2-agonists, 38–39
    antacids, H_2-receptor antagonists,
        and gastrointestinal motility
        drugs, 43, 43t
    antibiotics, 42, 43t
    anticholinergic drugs, 39
    antiemetics, 42

Medications *(Continued)*
    antihistamines, 39
    benzodiazepines, 36–37, 36t, 37.e1f
    corticosteroids, 42
    insulin, 42
    ketamine, 38
    nonbarbiturate sedatives, 37
    nonopioid analgesics, 41–42, 41f
    opioids, 37
    topical anesthetics, 39–40, 40t
  total intravenous anesthesia, 190–215
Medtronic. *see* Bio-Medicus BP-50
Medulloblastoma, 625, 626t, 694
Mee shunt, 430–431t
Meissner plexus, 16, 979–980
Melanocortin-1 receptor, 95, 127
Melatonin
  description of, 662
  emergence delirium reduction
      using, 1243
Mendel, Gregor, 80
Meningomyelocele, 700
Meperidine, 162–163, 162t, 163f, 772
Mesenchymal scoliosis, 812t
Mesocardia, 392, 392f
Messenger RNA (mRNA), 80
Metabolic acidosis, 229f
  in chronic kidney disease, 737
  in malignant hyperthermia, 1039
  prevention of, 631
Metabolic alkalosis, hypochloremic, 234
Metabolic myopathies, 636–637, 637t
Metabolic system, burn injury effects on,
    936, 943t
Metabolism, drug, 113–116
  cytochromes P-450, 81–83
  extrahepatic routes of metabolic
      clearance and, 116
  kidney and, 107f, 115f, 116, 116f
  liver and, 104f, 113
  phase I reactions in, 81, 113–114,
      114t
  phase II reactions in, 84
Metabolomics, 80–81
Metaiodobenzylguanidine, 724–725
Metanephrine, 724
Metaraminol, 594–595
Metastatic carcinoid, malignant
    hyperthermia *versus*, 1033t
Metformin, 707
Methadone
  description of, 162t, 165, 166f
  dosing guidelines for, 1152t
  neurotoxicity of, 652.e1–652.e11t
  pharmacokinetics of, 90–91
  for scoliosis surgery, 825
Methemoglobin, 241–242, 1333
Methemoglobinemia, 958
  burn injury and, 947
  glucose-6-phosphate dehydrogenase
      deficiency and, 241–242
Methimazole, 719–720
Methocarbamol, 1193
Methohexital, 140, 1230–1231t, 1233
  intravenous induction of, 48
  rectal, 140
Methotrexate, 270, 635, 1188–1189
Methoxamine, 1023
Methoxyflurane, 122
Methyl transferases, 84
Methylene blue, 241–242
Methylnaltrexone, 189
Methylprednisolone
  for asthma exacerbations, 319.e2–319.e3t
  for spinal injury, 693–694
Methylxanthines, 319, 956–957
Metipranolol, 907t
Metoclopramide, 43, 185
Metoprolol, 646t
Michaelis-Menten kinetics, 103, 104f
Microangiopathic hemolytic anemia, 935
Microcephaly, 625
Microcolon, 976
MICROCUFF endotracheal tube (MET),
    341, 341f, 947

Microcuff endotracheal tubes, 1321
Microdrip, 223, 1317
Micrognathia, 404, 914–915, 927
Microlaryngeal tubes, 1322
Micropremies, 2
Microretrognathia, 997
Microstomia, 997
Midazolam, 147f, 178–180, 179f, 179t,
    646t, 1230–1231t
  for abnormal airway, 352–353
  for asthma, 317–318
  for burn injury pain, 950f
  for cardiac catheterization, 583
  in cardiac surgery, 435
  effects on evoked potentials, 831–832
  emergence delirium reductions
      using, 1241
  emergency procedures application, 1012
  emergency surgery in trauma patient
      using, 1009t
  in extremely premature infant, 965–966
  hepatic metabolism of, 772
  infusion schemes, 197t
  ketamine and, 352–353, 945
  for local anesthetic toxicity, 1059–1060
  in micropremie, 965–966
  in neurosurgery, 683
  neurotoxicity of, 652.e1–652.e11t, 659
  in noncardiac surgery in congenital
      heart disease, 608–609
  opioids combined with, 37
  pharmacogenetics of, 36–37, 36t, 95
Middle ear surgery, 842–843, 843–e, 844t
Midface hypoplasia, 324–325, 325f
Midface procedures, 922–923, 922.e1
Midfacial hypoplasia, 918–919
Midgut volvulus, 979
Migraine, 1185
Miliary tuberculosis, 1307–1308
Miller blade, 337–339
Miller Fisher syndrome, 634
Milrinone, 462, 484–485t, 488, 958
Mineral bone disorder, in chronic kidney
    disease, 737–738
Minimal residual disease (MRD), 255
Minimal sedation, 1216
Minimum alveolar concentration (MAC),
    107, 220
  definition of, 964
  in extremely premature infant, 964
  inhaled anesthetics, 112f, 120
  in neonate, 116
  quantal effect model of
      pharmacodynamics and, 108
Minute ventilation, age-dependent
    variables of, 10t
Mirror image artifact, 1070
Mitochondrial cocktail, 637
Mitochondrial disorders underlying
    myopathies, 637, 637t, 638t
Mivacurium, 646t, 772
Mixed-effects models, 105
M-mode imaging, 423–424, 424f
M-mode (motion) ultrasound, 1062
Möbius syndrome, 927, 927.e1
Model for End-Stage Liver Disease
    (MELD), 776–777
Moderate sedation, 1216, 1228t
Modified Allen test, 1275f
Modified Blalock-Taussig shunt, 455
Modified Duke criteria, for infective
    endocarditis, 399
Modified lateral position, in neurosurgery,
    687
Modified Ramsay Sedation Scale, 1217t
Modified single-breath induction, of
    anesthesia, 47–48, 47f
Modified ultrafiltration, during
    cardiopulmonary bypass, 518–519
Moe method, 811
Monitoring
  abdominal surgery, 748
  blood loss during surgery, 280t
  burn injury, 944
  cardiopulmonary bypass, 438–440

Monitoring *(Continued)*
cardiopulmonary resuscitation, 1022–1023
increased intracranial pressure, 679
intracranial hypertension, 679
malignant hyperthermia and, 1036
massive blood transfusion, 298–300, 298.e1f, 299f, 300f
in noncardiac surgery in congenital heart disease, 604–606
for patent ductus arteriosus, 453
Monitoring equipment, 1329–1344
anesthesia record in, 1329, 1329f
for blood loss, 1337
blood pressure device in, 1330
for cardiac output monitoring, 1341–1342
drug errors, bar coding, and integration in, 1329–1330
electrocardiogram in, 1330–1331
for neuromuscular transmission, 1337–1338
noninvasive oxygen saturation monitors in, 1331–1333
multiple wavelength pulse oximetry, 1333
near infrared spectroscopy, 1334–1335, 1334.e1f
pulse oximetry, 1331–1333, 1331.e1f, 1332f
reflectance oximetry, 1333, 1334f
oxygen monitors in, 1331
precordial and esophageal stethoscopes in, 1330
for processed electroencephalogram, 1338–1340, 1339f
temperature monitors in, 1331
in urologic surgery, 750
Monoclonal antibodies, 263
Monogenic diabetes, 706t
Monro-Kellie hypothesis, 678, 845
MOR1K, 91–92
Moro reflex, gestational age assessment and, 5t
Morphine, 160–162, 161f, 162t
in adenotonsillectomy, for obstructive sleep apnea, 864f, 865
after scoliosis surgery, 825
for blunt reflex bronchoconstriction, 860.e1t
for bone and joint infections, 835
for burn injury pain, 950f
caudal, 446
in developing countries, 1310
dosing guidelines for, 1152t
epidural, 1172t
in extremely premature infant, 965
intrathecal, 824, 828
metabolism of, 84, 772
neurotoxicity of, 652.e1–652.e11t
in noncardiac surgery in congenital heart disease, 608–609
pharmacokinetics of, 90
preoperative, 37
relative potency for, 155
respiratory depression caused by, 160
for sedation outside operating room, 1233
Morphine-6-glucuronide (M6G), 90
Morquio syndrome, 340t
Morse model, 192, 192f
Motor evoked potentials
effects of anesthetics on, 830–832, 832t
myogenic, 830
during spinal surgery, 819.e1t
in spinal surgery, 819.e1t, 820f, 821.e1–821.e2f, 821–822, 822–823f
Motor innervation, of larynx, 330
Motor milestones, 19t
Motor neuron, 632f
Mouth-to-mouth resuscitation, 1016
Moyamoya disease, 696–697, 697f, 1210
MRD. *see* Minimal residual disease
MRI-safe, defined, 1204
MRI-unsafe, defined, 1204
Mu opioid receptors, 1152, 1152.e1t

Mucociliary transport, 805
Mucopolysaccharidoses, 634
airway difficulties in, 340t
eye surgery in, 904
Muenke syndrome, 918
Multaq. *see* Dronedarone
Multi-handed mask ventilation, 356, 356f
Multiple congenital contractures, 340t
Multiple endocrine neoplasia, 721
Multiple wavelength pulse oximetry, 1333
MultiView Scope, 365, 365.e2f
Muscle, ultrasound of, 1068
Muscle biopsy, diagnostic, in malignant hyperthermia, 1033t, 1041–1042
Muscle damage, tourniquet-related, 833
Muscle fibers, disorders of, 636–642
Muscle relaxants
effective doses for, 128t
long-acting nondepolarizing neuromuscular blocking drugs, 156
neuromuscular blocking drugs in, 148–151
antagonism, 156–159
increased sensitivity in neonates, 116
neuromuscular junction and, 149–150
neuromuscular monitoring of, 121f, 125f, 148–149
pharmacodynamics of, 150, 150f
pharmacokinetics of, 150–151
special situations for, 159–160
succinylcholine in, 151–154, 151t
Muscle-eye-brain disease, 639t, 641
Muscular defects, in ventricular septal defect, 590
Muscular dystrophy, 638–642, 639t
neuromuscular blocking drugs and, 159
Musculoskeletal deformities, cerebral palsy in, 621
Musculoskeletal pain, 1184t, 1187–1188, 1188t
Musculoskeletal ultrasound imaging, 1065–1067, 1066f
Mustard procedure, 430–431t, 456, 595
Myasthenia gravis, 634–636, 635t
Myasthenia-like syndrome, 636
Mycophenolate mofetil, 635
Mydriatic agents, topical, 907
Myelination, 18
Myelodysplasia, 700–701
Myelodysplastic syndrome, 259–260
Myelomeningocele, 983t
Myeloproliferative disorder, 259–260
Myelosuppression, 270
Myocardial contractility, inhaled anesthetics and, 131
Myocardial fibrosis, 593
Myocardial fibrosis, radiation-related, 266
Myocardial ischemia, 596, 611
Myocardial protection, in cardiopulmonary bypass, 512, 513t
Myocarditis, 398–399, 398f, 1306
Myocardium, 471f
Myogenic motor evoked potentials, 830
Myoglobinemia, succinylcholine-related, 153
Myonecrosis, 941
Myopathic syndromes, malignant hyperthermia and, 1049–1050
Myopathies, 636–638
congenital, 636, 636t
in malignant hyperthermia, 1049–1050
mitochondrial disorders underlying, 637, 637t
undiagnosed, 642
Myotonic dystrophy, 638–640, 639t
Myringotomy, with tube insertion, 841–842, 842f
Myxedema coma, 717

N

N95 mask, 1281
N-acetyl procainamide (NAPA), 498–499
N-acetyl-p-benzoquinone imine (NAPQI), 93, 174
N-acetyltransferase, 114, 114t, 771

Nadir saturation (nSAT), 852–853
Nager syndrome, 340t
Nalbuphine, 170–171
dosing guidelines for, 1152t
Nalmefene, 1233, 1246
Naloxone, 188
Naltrexone, 188–189, 1246
Naphazoline, 907t
Naproxen, 1145t
Narcotrend monitor, 1338–1339
Nasal capnography, 868
Nasal fractures, 893
Nasal intubation, 362
in neurosurgery, 684–685
Nasal polypectomy, 321
Nasal sufentanil, 169
Nasogastric tube, in abdominal surgery, 746–747
Nasolacrimal duct obstruction, 912
Nasopharyngeal airway, 337
after cleft lip and palate repair, 916, 916f
description of, 1320
Nasopharynx, pathology related to, 350t
Nasotracheal intubation, in neurosurgery, 684–685
Nasotracheal tubes, 684–685
NAT1, 771
Natrecor. *see* Nesiritide
Natriuresis, 217–218
Natriuretic peptide receptors, 490
Nausea and vomiting
antiemetics for, 185–186
postoperative, 900, 1248–1250, 1249f
5-HT 3 receptor antagonists for, 185–186
in adenotonsillectomy, 861–862
after middle ear surgery, 843
alternative treatments of, 1250
emergence and recovery, 868
evidence-based consensus management of, 1248–1249, 1249f
inhalational anesthetics and, 139
multimodal therapy for, 1239
in myringotomy, 842
pharmacogenomics of, 96
prophylactic therapy for, 1249–1250
rescue therapy for, 1249–1250
Near-infrared spectroscopy (NIRS), 440, 598, 605, 606f, 683–684, 754, 1135, 1334–1335, 1334.e1f
Necrosis, 652–653
Necrotizing enterocolitis, 16, 977–978, 977f, 978f
Needle cricothyroidotomy, percutaneous, 357–359, 357f, 358f, 358.e1f, 359.e1f, 359.e2f
Needle electrodes, 1338
Needle visibility, musculoskeletal ultrasound imaging, 1066
Needle-free pressurized delivery systems, 40
Needleless hub, 1317
Negative-feedback response to inhalation anesthetic agents, 110f, 124
Negative-pressure pulmonary edema, 885
Neitlich variant, 95–96
Neoaortic root, 595
Neonatal transient myasthenia gravis, 635
Neonate. *see* Newborn
Neonate and Children Audit of Anaesthesia Practice in Europe (NECTARINE) study, 333–334
Neostigmine, 158, 482
Neosynephrine. *see* Phenylephrine
Nephrectomy, 760
Nephrocalcinosis, 955
Nephrogenesis, 13
Nephrogenic fibrosing dermopathy, 1205
Nephrogenic systemic fibrosis, 1205
Nephrology, essentials of, 729–744
Nephrotoxicity
of chemotherapeutic agents, 269
of inhaled anesthetics, 133–134
Nerve block, 1054
peripheral, 1087–1088, 1088t
head and neck, 1088–1093, 1089f

Nerve block *(Continued)*
lower extremity, 1119–1131, 1120f
selection of local anesthetic for, 1087–1088, 1088t
truncal, 1093–1097
upper extremity, 1107–1114
Nerve growth factor-β (NGFB), 87
Nerve injuries, tourniquet-related, 833
Nerve of Arnold nerve block, 1092–1093
Nerve palsies, 634–642
noncardiac surgery in congenital heart disease and, 614
Nerve stimulator
description of, 1071.e1f, 1072, 1073f
paravertebral block guided using, 1107–1109
Nerves, 1067–1068, 1068f
Nesiritide, 402–403, 490–491
Neural injury, after epidural anesthesia, 1086–1087
Neural tube defects, 622–624
Neuraxial blockade, central, 1072–1087
anatomic and physiologic considerations in, 1072–1074, 1072.e1f, 1073f, 1074f
epidural anesthesia in, 1079–1087
spinal, 1074–1079, 1076f, 1077f
Neuraxial regional anesthesia, 446
Neuroapoptosis, 652
Neuroblastoma, 269, 760–761
Neurocognitive impairment, 271, 654, 661
Neuroectodermal tumors, 269–270
Neurofibromatosis, 260, 625, 760–761, 904
Neurogenesis, 655
Neurogenic diabetes insipidus, 712–713
Neurokinin 1, 186
Neuroleptic malignant syndrome (NMS), 720, 1033t, 1051
Neurologic development, 958–961
Neurologic disorders, 619–649
associated with childhood obesity, 55t
cerebral palsy, 620–622, 620t, 621t, 623t
comorbidities in, 621–622
Chiari malformations, 624, 624t
chronic inflammatory demyelinating polyneuropathy, 634
congenital myasthenic syndromes, 635
congenital myopathies, 625, 636, 636t
cortical development disorders, 625
epilepsy, 642–648, 643f, 644t
in cerebral palsy patient, 621
perioperative management of, 648t
surgery in, 644–646
general considerations in, 619–620
Guillain-Barré syndrome, 634
hereditary neuropathies, 633–634
hydrocephalus, 624
inborn errors of metabolism, 627–632, 629–630t
metabolic myopathies, 636–637, 637t
mitochondrial disorders underlying myopathies, 637, 637t, 638t
muscular dystrophy, 638–642, 639t
myasthenia gravis, 634–636, 635t
myasthenia-like syndrome, 636
neural tube defects, 622–624
poliomyelitis, 633
primary brain tumors, 625–627, 626t
spinal muscular atrophy, 632–633
syringomyelia, 624
undiagnosed myopathy, 642
Neurologic events, interventional cardiology and, 580
Neurologic system
burn injury effects on, 935, 943t
cardiac anesthesia and, 446
growth and development of, 18–20
liver disease and, 779–780
Neuromuscular blocking drugs, 148–151, 566
for airway obstruction, 351–352
antagonism of, 156–159
for blunt reflex bronchoconstriction, 860.e1t
for burn injury, 944, 945f, 946f

Neuromuscular blocking drugs (Continued)
for cardiac surgery, 445–446
in developing countries, 1310
effects on evoked potentials, 832
emergence and, 690–691
hepatic metabolism of, 771–772
increased sensitivity in neonates, 116
monitoring of, 121f, 125f, 148–149
in neonates, 116
neuromuscular junction and, 149–150
neuromuscular monitoring of, 121f, 125f, 148–149
neurosurgical procedures using, 685
noncardiac surgery in congenital heart disease using, 609
nondepolarizing, 635, 746, 839, 937
pharmacodynamics of, 150, 150f
pharmacogenetics of, 95–96
pharmacokinetics of, 150–151
rapid sequence induction uses of, 746
recovery from, 944–945
for renal insufficiency, 742
special situations for, 159–160
succinylcholine, 151–154, 151t
Neuromuscular compromise, in adenotonsillectomy, 867
Neuromuscular disorders, 619–634, 632f
chronic inflammatory demyelinating polyneuropathy, 634
congenital myasthenic syndromes, 635
congenital myopathies, 636, 636t
epilepsy, 642–648, 643f, 644t
in cerebral palsy patient, 621
perioperative management of, 648t
surgery in, 644–646
Guillain-Barré syndrome, 634
hereditary neuropathies, 633–634
metabolic myopathies, 636–637, 637t
mitochondrial disorders underlying myopathies, 637, 637t, 638t
muscular dystrophy, 638–642, 639t
myasthenia gravis, 634–636, 635t
myasthenia-like syndrome, 636
poliomyelitis, 633
spinal muscular atrophy, 632–633
undiagnosed myopathy, 642
Neuromuscular junction
disorders, 634–636
inhalation anesthetic agents and, 137
Neuromuscular monitoring, of
neuromuscular blocking drugs, 121f, 125f, 148–149
Neuromuscular scoliosis, 812t, 814–815
long-term changes in, 818
postoperative complications in, 816–817, 816t
postoperative ventilation for, 824
Neuromuscular transmission monitoring, 1337–1338
Neuronal apoptosis, 446
Neurons, 632f, 665
Neuropathic pain, 1182–1183
Neuropathies, hereditary, 633–634
Neuroplasticity, 1134
Neuroprotection, maneuvers of, 691t
Neuroradiologic procedure, 703–704, 703.e1f
Neurosurgical anesthesia, 678–704
airway management and intubation in, 684–685
in aneurysms, 696
apoptotic neurodegeneration and, 688
in arteriovenous malformations, 695–696
blood and fluid management in, 688–689
blood pressure in, effects of, 680–681, 681f
carbon dioxide in, effects of, 681–682, 681f
cerebral blood flow and, 679f, 680
cerebral blood volume in, 680
cerebral perfusion pressure and, 680

Neurosurgical anesthesia (Continued)
cerebrovascular autoregulation and, 680–682
in Chiari malformations, 701–702, 701t, 702f, 703f
in concussion, 694
in congenital anomalies, 700–702, 701f
in craniotomy, 694–699
diabetes insipidus and, 691, 694–695, 713
emergence from, 690–691, 691t
in encephalocele, 700, 701f
in epidural hematoma, 692, 692f
in epilepsy, 697
equipment and monitoring issues in, 703–704
in head injury, 691
in herniation syndromes, 679
in hydrocephalus, 699–700, 699.e1f, 700f
in increased intracranial pressure, 679
induction of, 684
in intracerebral hematoma, 693
in intracranial aneurysms, 696
intracranial compartments and, 678
intracranial pressure and, 678–680, 679f
intracranial compliance and, 679–680, 680f
monitoring of, 679
signs of increased in, 679
local anesthesia in, 687
maintenance of, 687–688, 688t
management of, 682–691
modified lateral position in, 687
monitoring in, 683–684
in Moyamoya disease, 696–697, 697f
in myelodysplasia, 700–701
neuromuscular blocking drugs in, 685
neuroradiologic procedures of, 703–704, 703.e1f
oxygen in, effects of, 681, 681f
pathophysiology of, 678–682
patient positioning in, 704
positioning in, 685–687, 686f
premedication and, 683
preoperative evaluation in, 682
prone position in, 685–687, 686f
in scalp injuries, 691–694
in seizure surgery, 697–699, 698.e1f
sitting position in, 687
in skull fractures, 692, 692f
special situations in, 691–704
in spinal defects, 702
in spinal injury, 693–694
in subdural hematoma, 692–693
temperature control in, 689
in trauma, 691–694
in tumors, 694–695, 695f, 695.e1f
in vascular anomalies, 695–697
venous air emboli and, 689–690, 690f
Neurotoxicity, of anesthesia
anesthetic exposure effects on, developing brain and, 651f, 652–656
anesthetic neuroprotection and, 662
animal studies in, 663–668
anesthetic doses and, 664, 664f
assessing neurobehavioral or cognitive outcomes in, 665–666
comparative brain development and, 665, 666f, 667f
duration of exposure and, 663–664, 663f
experimental versus clinical conditions and, 664–665
nonhuman primate studies in, 666–668
barbiturates, 659
benzodiazepines, 659
chloral hydrate, 652.e1–652.e11t, 659
deleterious effects of untreated pain and stress, 661
dexmedetomidine, 652.e1–652.e11t, 660
exposure time, dose, and anesthetic combinations, 660–661

Neurotoxicity, of anesthesia (Continued)
future research in, 675–676
inhaled anesthetics, 658–659
ketamine, 652.e1–652.e11t, 657–658
limitations of available clinical studies in, 674–675
nitrous oxide, 652.e1–652.e11t, 659
normal brain development, 651–652
opioid analgesics, 660
potential alleviating strategies for, 661–662
propofol, 652.e1–652.e11t, 659–660
putative mechanisms for, 656–657
recommendations for clinical practice and, 676
xenon, 652.e1–652.e11t, 659
Neurotrophic tyrosine kinase receptor type 1 gene, 87
Neutral protamine Hagedorn, 706
Neutrophils, 17
Newborn
age-dependent respiratory variables of, 10t
asphyxia in, 1315
awake intubation in, 340
body water of, gestational age and, 6t
calcium administration in, 489
cardiovascular system of, 471–472, 471t, 473f, 480.e1f
circulation transition from fetal circulation, 957
coarctation of aorta repair in, 464–465
with combined anesthesia and regional blockade, 214
encephalopathy in, 627–628
equipment setup, 967, 967t, 968f
extracorporeal membrane oxygenation in, 553
fluids and medication, 967–968
hepatic metabolism in, 963
hypocalcemia in, 721
hypothyroidism in, 717, 717f
monitoring in, 966–968
nature of pain in, 1135
operating room for, 966
physiologic anemia in, 963
polycythemia in, 18
preparation for surgery, 966
problems related to weight and gestation, 5t
propofol and, 146
regional anesthetics, 966
sickle cell screening in, 242–243
subglottic hemangioma, 970
subglottic stenosis, 969–970
surgical emergencies in
bedside procedures, 968
choanal atresia, 969
congenital bronchogenic and pulmonary cysts, 973
congenital diaphragmatic hernia, 972–973, 972.e1
congenital lobar emphysema, 973–974, 974f
duodenal atresia, 976, 976f
esophageal atresia, 971–972, 971f
family considerations, 968
gastrointestinal, 974–980
gastroschisis, 978–980, 978t, 978.e1
Hirschsprung disease, 979–980
hypertrophic pyloric stenosis, 974–976, 975f
imperforate anus, 976
inguinal hernia, 976–977
laryngeal obstruction, 969–970, 969f, 970f
laryngeal webs, 969f
lung abnormalities, 972–974, 972.e1
malrotation, 979
meconium ileus, 976, 976f
midgut volvulus, 979
necrotizing enterocolitis, 977–978, 977f, 978.e1
omphalocele, 978–980, 978t, 978.e1, 979f

Newborn (Continued)
patent ductus arteriosus ligation, 980
respiratory, 969
retinopathy of prematurity, 980–981
tracheoesophageal fistula, 971–972, 971f
thrombocytopenia in, 18
transient tachypnea of, 8–9
transition to air breathing, 8–9
ventilator for, 967
weight of, gestational age and, 5t
"Next-generation sequencing," of malignant hyperthermia, 1048–1049
Nicardipine, 492–493t, 494
Nicotine, 26
Nifedipine, 477t, 646t
Nikaidoh procedure, 430–431t
Nil per os status, 225–226
Nimodipine, 646t
Nipride. see Sodium nitroprusside
NIRS. see Near-infrared spectroscopy
Nissen fundoplication, 753, 755
Nitric oxide (NO), 282, 562, 754
inhaled, 495–496, 958, 960f
Nitric oxide synthase, 959f
Nitro-Bid. see Nitroglycerin
Nitrogen dioxide, 934
Nitroglycerin, 302, 492–493t, 493–494
in cardiopulmonary bypass, 518
Nitronal. see Nitroglycerin
Nitropress. see Sodium nitroprusside
Nitroprusside, in cardiopulmonary bypass, 518
Nitrous oxide, 138–139, 579
for cardiac surgery, 444
diagnostic angiography and, 1210
effects on evoked potentials, 830
environmental impact of, 139
in liver transplantation, 782
in middle ear and mastoid surgery, 843
minimum alveolar concentration of, 128–129
negative inotropic effects of, 444
neurophysiologic effects of, 687, 688t
neurotoxicity of, 652.e1–652.e11t, 659
pharmacogenetics of, 95
properties of, 120
for sedation, 1230–1231t, 1236
NKCC1, 655
NMDA. see N-methyl-D-aspartate
N-methyl-D-aspartate (NMDA), 652, 656–657, 658, 1025
Nocturnal hypoxia, 88–89
Nonaccidental trauma, 692, 1001–1002, 1001f, 1002–1003f
Nonalcoholic fatty liver disease, 773
Nonalcoholic steatohepatitis, 773
Non-atopic wheezers, 316
Noncardiac surgery, anesthesia for VAD patient for, 567
Noncardiogenic pulmonary edema, 868
Non-Communicating Children's Pain Checklist, 1136t, 1141.e1t
Noncommunicating hydrocephalus, 699
Non-Hodgkin lymphoma, 258–259, 384
Noninvasive oxygen saturation monitors, 1331–1333
multiple wavelength pulse oximetry, 1333
near infrared spectroscopy, 1334–1335, 1334.e1f
pulse oximetry, 1331–1333, 1331.e1f, 1332f
reflectance oximetry, 1333, 1334f
Noninvasive positive-pressure ventilation (NPPV), 815
Noninvasive testing, of malignant hyperthermia, 1049
Non-malignant hyperthermia syndrome, malignant hyperthermia versus, 1033t
Nonobstructive hydrocephalus, 699
Non-operating room anesthesia (NORA), 1195
anesthetic risk in, 1198–1199
angiography with embolization and, 1210–1211, 1210.e1f, 1211.e1f

Non-operating room anesthesia
    (Continued)
    computed tomography and, 1200–1203,
        1202f
    diagnostic angiography and, 1210,
        1210.e1f
    difficult airway management and, 1200
    emergencies in MRI scanner in, 1199
    endoscopic procedures in, 1213
    interventional radiology and, 1209–1213
    magnetic resonance imaging and,
        1203–1207, 1203f, 1205f, 1206f
    magnetoencephalography in, 1207
    nuclear medicine in, 1207–1208
    personnel requirements for, 1197
    procedures in, 1199–1200
    quality assurance of, 1198
    radiation therapy and, 1208–1209, 1209f
    sclerotherapy of venous and lymphatic
        malformations and, 1211–1213,
        1211f, 1212f, 1212t
    specific locations for, 1200–1213,
        1202f, 1203f
    standards and guidelines in, 1196
    stereotactic radiosurgery and, 1208
Nonopioid analgesics, 1145–1155, 1145t
    acetaminophen, 1145t, 1146–1147
    clonidine, 1150–1151
    dexamethasone, 1150
    dexmedetomidine, 1151
    gabapentin, 1149–1150
    ketamine, 1149
    lidocaine, 1151–1152
    nonsteroidal antiinflammatory drugs,
        1147–1148
    pregabalin, 1150
    preoperative, 41–42
    tramadol, 1148–1149
Nonrestrictive shunts, 476t
Nonshivering thermogenesis, 961
Nonsteroidal antiinflammatory drugs
        (NSAIDs), 175–177, 175f, 1250
    for acute pain, 1147–1148
    genetic considerations and, 93
    for headaches, 1185–1186
    for musculoskeletal pain, 1188t
    ocular uses of, 908
    for orthopedic and spine surgery, 810
    for pain
        after adenotonsillectomy, 862
        postoperative, 1250
    for scoliosis surgery, 825
Noonan syndrome, 340t, 405, 757, 926
Noradrenaline. see Norepinephrine
Norepinephrine, 89, 484–485t, 486–487,
        594–595, 724
Norketamine, 145
Normal perfusion pressure
        breakthrough, 696
Normal saline, 223t
Normeperidine, seizures and, 162–163
Normetanephrine, 724
Normocapnia, 696–697
Normodyne. see Labetalol
Normothermia, 514, 947, 1315
Normovolemic hemodilution, 303–304
    acute, 511
    advantages of, 304
    complications in, 304
    contraindications in, 304
    indications in, 304
    Jehovah's Witnesses and, 304
    technique and key concepts in, 304
Noroxycodone, 90
Nortriptyline, 1192
Norwood procedure, 430–431t, 443, 460,
        461f, 462f, 551–553
    in cardiopulmonary bypass, 518
    noncardiac surgery in congenital heart
        disease and, 598
Nosocomial pathogens, 1280t
NovoLog, 706
Nuclear medicine, for non-operating
        room anesthesia, 1207–1208
Nucleosomes, 81

Numeric Rating Scale, for pain,
        1136t, 1137
Nurse, on pain management team, 1182
Nurse-/caregiver-controlled analgesia,
        1161–1162
Nurses' Assessment of Pain Intensity,
        1141–1142
Nuss procedure, 755–756
Nu-Trake, 359
Nutrition, chronic kidney disease and, 738

O
Obesity
    anesthesia-induced liver injury and, 773
    anesthetic implications of, 764–767, 766t
    bariatric surgery for, 763–764, 764t
    description of, 54–56, 55t, 56t
    laparoscopic vertical sleeve gastrectomy
        for, 764, 766–767
    liver injury and, 773
    obstructive sleep apnea and, 766,
        848–849, 849f
    organ disorders associated with, 764
    total intravenous anesthesia in child
        with, 212–214, 213f, 214f
Objective Pain Scale, 1138
Obligate nasal breathing, 331
Obstructive hydrocephalus, 699, 903
Obstructive sleep apnea (OSA), 56–58,
        57t, 58t
    adenotonsillectomy for, 846–851
    in Apert syndrome, 917–918
    complications of, 850, 850.e2t
    endotypes of, 847, 847t
    incidence of, 846–847
    mechanisms of, 847
    obesity causing, 55, 766
    opioid-induced respiratory depression
        in, 863–866, 864f
        avoidance of opioids in, 865–866
        codeine for, 865
        CYP2D6 for, 865
        dose titration in, 865
    pathophysiology of, 847–850, 847.e1t,
        848f, 849f, 849.e1t
    pharyngeal airway obstruction in, 333
    risk factors for, 56–57, 59t
    signs and symptoms of, 56, 845t
    surgery indication for, 850–851
    treatment thresholds of, 850
Obstructive sleep-disordered breathing,
        adenotonsillectomy and, 846
Oculoauriculovertebral syndrome, 340t
Oculocardiac reflex (OCR), 901, 905–906,
        906f, 922
Oculomandibulodyscephaly, 340t
Odontoid displacement, 693
OELM. see Optimal external laryngeal
        manipulation
Off-label drugs, 74
Off-site anesthesia, 1196–1198
    acute emergencies and cardiopulmonary
        arrest in, 1199, 1199t
    computed tomography and, 1200–1203,
        1202f
    difficult airway management and, 1200
    endoscopic procedures in, 1213
    interventional radiology and, 1209–1213
    magnetic resonance imaging and,
        1203–1207, 1203f, 1205f, 1206f
    nuclear medicine and, 1207–1208
    personnel requirements for, 1197
    quality assurance of, 1198
    specific locations for, 1200–1213,
        1202f, 1203f
    standards and guidelines for, 1196
    stereotactic radiosurgery and, 1208
OK-432, 1212t
Oliceridine, 162, 164f
Omeprazole, 646t
Omnipaque, 1251
Omphalocele, 978–980, 978t, 978.e1, 979f
Oncology, 261–277
Ondansetron, 185–186, 1249
Open globe injury, 900

Open Payments program, 75
Open-chest cardiopulmonary
        resuscitation, 1028
Open-chest defibrillation, 1021
Operant Test Battery (OTB), 666–668
Ophthalmology, 900
    in Alport syndrome, 903
    anterior chamber paracentesis, 911
    common diagnoses requiring, 901, 901t
    in craniofacial syndromes, 904, 905.e1f
    in Down syndrome, 903
    in Ehlers-Danlos syndrome, 903–904,
        903.e1f
    elective, 908–909
    emergent, 908–909
    in homocystinuria, 903–904, 903.e1f
    induction and maintenance of
        anesthesia in, 909–910
    in Marfan syndrome, 903–904, 903.e1f
    in mucopolysaccharidoses, 904
    ophthalmologic medications and, 910t
    ophthalmologic pharmacotherapeutics
        and systemic implications,
        906–908, 907t, 907.e1f
    ophthalmologic physiology and, 904
        intraocular pressure in, 904–905, 904f
        oculocardiac reflex in, 905–906, 906f
    in phakomatoses, 904
    preoperative evaluation in, 900–901
    in retinopathy of prematurity, 901
    strabismus repair, 910–911, 910f
    urgent, 908–909
Opioid(s), 85–87, 160–173, 646t
    after scoliosis surgery, 824–825
    for blunt reflex bronchoconstriction,
        860.e1t
    cannabinoid system and, 92
    for cardiac surgery, 445
    context-sensitive half-time of, 205t
    effects on evoked potentials, 831
    epidural anesthesia uses of, 1085
    for general anesthesia, 584
    hepatic metabolism of, 772
    hyperalgesia induced by, 1149
    infusion schemes, 197t
    neurophysiologic effects of, 688t
    neurotoxicity of, 660
    noncardiac surgery in congenital heart
        disease using, 608–609
    overprescribing of, 1141
    for pain management, 1152–1153,
        1152t, 1190–1192, 1191t
        abuse-deterrent opioid formulations
            in, 1191
        buprenorphine in perioperative
            arena, 1191–1192
        in burn injury, 950, 951f
        choice of drug and drug dosages
            in, 1158
        continuous basal infusions
            for, 1158–1161, 1160f
        epidural administration of, 1172t
        intramuscular and subcutaneous
            route of, 1155
        intranasal route, 1155
        intravenous administration, 1154
        nurse-/caregiver-controlled analgesia
            in, 1161–1162
        oral administration, 1153–1154
        patient-controlled analgesia in,
            1157–1161
        postoperative, 1250–1251
        pump settings in, 1158, 1159f
    for parenteral use, 1155–1163
    pharmacodynamics of, 91–92
    pharmacokinetics of, 87–91
    respiratory depression caused by, 160
    for sedation, 1216f, 1230–1231t, 1233
    for stress response after cardiac
        surgery, 448
Opioid antagonists, for sedation, 1233
Opioid receptors, 91–92, 772, 1152,
        1152.e1t
Opioid-cannabinoid system interactions, 92
OPRM1, 92, 97

Opsumit. see Macitentan
Optic pathway gliomas, 625, 626t
Optical laryngoscopes, 365–367
    Airtraq optical laryngoscope, 365–366,
        366f
    Truview EVO2 infant device, 366.e1f,
        366–367
Optical spectrophotometry, 440
Optical stylets, 367
Optimal external laryngeal manipulation
        (OELM), 360
Oral breathing, 331
Oral cavity, growth and development of, 6
Oral contrast, 1201
Oral fluids, for diabetes insipidus, 714
Oral intubation, in neurosurgery, 684–685
Oral transmucosal fentanyl, 167
OraVerse. see Phentolamine
Orbital hypertelorism, 922, 922f
Orchiopexy, 757, 1095–1096
Organ donation after cardiac death, 72, 73t
Organ toxicity, of chemotherapeutic
        agents, 277.e1–277.e3t
Organ transplantation, 775–808
    cardiac, 791–800
        anesthesia and, 799–800
        for congenital heart disease, 792–793
        contraindications to, 793
        demographics and epidemiology of,
            791–792, 792f
        for dilated cardiomyopathy, 793
        for hypertrophic cardiomyopathy, 793
        immediate postoperative
            management in, 797–799, 798f
        intraoperative problems and
            management in, 796–797, 797t
        pathophysiology of disease in, 792
        preoperative evaluation in, 794–795,
            795t
        repeat transplantation, 793
        for restrictive cardiomyopathy, 793
        surgical technique in, 795–796
        survival and quality of life in, 799,
            799f, 800f, 800t, 801f
        waitlist and donor selection in,
            793–794, 794t
    liver, 775–787
        anhepatic stage in, 784–785
        biliary and hepatic artery
            reconstruction in, 785
        epidemiology and demographics of,
            776–778, 776f, 777t
        hepatectomy in, 783–784, 784f
        immediate postoperative care for,
            786–787
        indications for, 776
        intraoperative care in, 782–783
        living-donor, 785–786
        long-term issues of, 787
        orthotopic, 775
        outcomes of, 786
        pathophysiology of liver disease,
            778–780
        preoperative evaluation in,
            780–782, 781t
        reperfusion period in, 785
        split liver techniques in, 785–786
        surgical technique in, 783–786
    lung and heart-lung, 800–807
        bilateral sequential, 804
        contraindications to, 802
        cystic fibrosis in, 801
        demographics and epidemiology of,
            800–801
        immediate postoperative
            management of, 805
        intraoperative problems and
            management in, 803–805
        long-term concerns in, 805–807, 805t
        pathophysiology of disease in,
            801, 802t
        preoperative evaluation of, 803
        pulmonary hypertension in, 801–802
        surgical technique in, 803
        survival and quality of life in, 807, 808f

Organ transplantation (*Continued*)
  waitlist and donor selection in, 802–803
  renal, 787–791, 789f, 790t
    anesthetic induction in, 790
    anesthetic management of, 788–791
    immediate postoperative management of, 791
    long-term issues in, 791
    maintenance of anesthesia in, 790–791
    monitors and vascular access in, 790
    pathophysiology of, 788
    preoperative evaluation of, 788
    surgical technique in, 788
Organic cation transporters (OCT), 90
Organogenesis, 14
Oropharyngeal airways, 337, 338f, 1320
Orthognathic surgery, 925
Orthopedic surgery, 809–840
  in acute bone and joint infections, 834–835
  in arthrogryposis multiplex congenita, 839
  associated with childhood obesity, 55t
  in cerebral palsy, 621, 835–836
  in Duchenne muscular dystrophy, 838–839
  history in, 810–811
  in osteogenesis imperfecta, 837–838
  in scoliosis, 810–815
    anesthetic and intraoperative management in, 826–832
    anesthetic drugs and techniques in, 832
    cardiovascular assessment in, 824
    classification of, 811, 812t, 811.e1f
    complications in the early postoperative period, 815–817, 815f, 816t
    congenital, 811–813
    decreasing transfusion requirements in, 827–829
    definition of, 810
    early-onset, 811–813
    idiopathic, 813–814
    improving outcome from surgical intervention in, 815–818
    infantile, 811–813, 813f
    juvenile, 811–813
    long-term changes in, 817–818, 817f
    minimizing blood loss in, 827–829
    natural history of, 811–815
    neuromuscular, 814–815
    pain management for, 824–826
    pathophysiology of, 811–815, 813f
    patient monitoring in, 827
    positioning in, 826–e, 826–827, 826f
    postoperative planning for, 823–824
    postoperative ventilatory support for, 824
    preoperative assessment in, 823–824
    respiratory assessment in, 824
    respiratory function in, 815–817
    risk minimization in, 815–818
    somatosensory evoked and motor evoked potentials, effects of anesthetics on, 830–832
    temperature regulation in, 827
  in spina bifida, 836–837
  spinal cord injury during, 818–822
    etiology of, 818, 819f
    monitoring of, 819, 819.e1t, 819f
    risk of, 819
  surgical development in, 810–811, 810f
  terminology in, 810–811
  tourniquets in, 832–834
Orthopedic trauma, intraoperative management of, 1013–1014
Orthotopic liver transplantation (OLT), 775
Osler nodes, 399
Osmolality, 216–218, 227t
Osmolyte, 217
Osmotic diuretic, 580
Osmotic fragility (OF), 240

Osteogenesis imperfecta, 1331
  orthopedic surgery in, 837–838
Osteomyelitis, 834
Ostium primum defects, 588
Ostium secundum defects, 588
OTB. *see* Operant Test Battery
Otitis media, chronic, myringotomy with tube insertion and, 842
Otologic procedures, 841–843
  bone-anchored hearing aids in, 843, 844t
  cochlear implants in, 843, 844t
  mastoid surgery in, 842–843, 844t
  middle ear surgery in, 842–843, 843–e, 844t
  myringotomy in, 841–842, 842f
  otoplasty in, 928, 928.e1
  tube insertion in, 841–842, 842f
Otomandibular dysostosis, 923
Otoplasty, 928, 928.e1, 1092
Otorhinolaryngologic procedures, 841–899
  adenotonsillectomy in, 845–872
    admission policies for, 863, 863f, 864f
    adverse respiratory events in, 858–859, 859f
    airway control in, 859–860
    anesthetic choice for, 860–861, 860f, 860.e1t
    anesthetic considerations for, 857, 857t
    complications of, 866–867, 867t
    emergence and recovery in, 867–869
    extubation in, 867, 867f
    indications for, 845–846, 845t, 854–855, 854f
    neuromuscular compromise in, 867
    obstructive sleep apnea and, 846–851
    perioperative considerations for, 857–858
    perioperative pain in, 862–863, 862.e1t,
    peritonsillar abscess and, 871–872, 872f
    postoperative adenotonsillectomy adverse events in, 869
    postoperative admission guidelines for, 868–869, 868.e1f, 869f, 870f
    postoperative considerations for, 858–863
    postoperative nausea and vomiting in, 861–862, 861f, 868
    posttonsillectomy hemorrhage and, 847.e1t, 870–871, 871f
    recurrent tonsillitis and, 846
    respiratory events in, 868
    risk stratification for perioperative adverse events in, 855–857, 855t, 855.e1f
    sleep-disordered breathing and, 845–846
    surgical approach in, 846
  in airway trauma, 893–894
  endoscopy, 872–883
  laryngotracheal reconstruction, 895–897
    anesthetic considerations for, 897, 897f, 898t
    surgical approach on, 895–897, 896f, 897f
  otologic procedures in, 841–843
    bone-anchored hearing aids in, 843, 844t
    cochlear implants in, 843, 844t
    mastoid surgery in, 842–843, 844t
    middle ear surgery in, 842–843, 843–e, 844t
    myringotomy in, 841–842, 842f
    tube insertion in, 841–842, 842f
  rhinologic procedures in, 843–845
  tracheotomy, 883.e1f, 889–892, 889.e1t, 891f
    complications associated with, 890t
    indications and contraindications for, 889.e1t
    management of, 891–892, 892t, 892.e1t
    tracheocutaneous fistula after, 892

Otorhinolaryngologic procedures (*Continued*)
  for upper airway obstruction, 883–889
    acquired laryngeal and subglottic stenosis, 874f, 889
    acute epiglottitis in, 883–885, 883.e1f, 884f, 885f
    congenital and acquired, 889
    congenital laryngeal webs and, 883.e1f, 889
    croup and, 885–887, 885t, 886f, 886.e1f
    laryngeal atresia and, 889
    laryngeal papillomatosis and, 887–889, 887f, 888t, 888.e1f
    laryngomalacia in, 883
Otorrhea, 692
Oucher Pain Scale, 1136f, 1136.e1f
Oucher Scale, 1250
Overnight pulse oximetry
  for obstructive sleep apnea, 852–854, 853f
  for sleep-disordered breathing, 845–846
Overpressure technique, 124
Overventilation, during cardiopulmonary resuscitation, 1018
Oxcarbazepine, 645t, 1192
Oxford Miniature Vaporizer, 1311
Oxycodone, 90, 162t, 163–164, 865, 1152t
Oxygen
  in cerebral blood flow, 681, 681f
  inhalation anesthetic agents and, 139–140
  insufflation of, 378
  supplemental
    retinopathy of prematurity and, 139, 955
Oxygen concentrators, 1311, 1312, 1312.e1f
Oxygen consumption
  age-dependent variables of, 10t
  cerebral metabolic rate for, 680
  in child with repaired congenital heart disease, 478
  of full-term infant, 332
  neonatal, 472
  in neonate, 954t
Oxygen monitors, 1331
Oxygen pulse, 479
Oxygen saturation, 478, 902
Oxygenation
  fetal, 991, 991f, 992f
  issues in, in burn injuries, 938–939, 938f
Oxyhemoglobin dissociation curve, 12
Oxymetazoline, 314–315, 685, 844
Oxyscope, 353, 353.e1f

P

Pacemaker, 420–422, 421t
  magnetic resonance imaging and, 1204
  noncardiac surgery in congenital heart disease and, 613
Pacerone. *see* Amiodarone
Packed red blood cells (PRBCs), 237–238, 554, 920, 1247–1248
  cardiopulmonary bypass prime and, 507
  for hematologic disorders, 237–238
  initial doses of, 282t
  transfusion of, 281–283, 281t, 282t, 529
PACU. *see* Postanesthesia care unit
Paedfusor pharmacokinetic data set
  Kataria system *versus*, 207t
  in target-controlled infusion, 206–207, 206f, 207f, 207t, 208f
Pain
  acute. *see* Acute pain
  cancer-related, 271
  chronic, 1181–1194
    abdominal, 1183t, 1184–1185, 1185t
    ancillary data in, 1184
    complementary therapies for, 1194
    in complex regional pain syndrome, 1186–1187, 1187f, 1187t
    headache, 1183t, 1185–1186, 1186f

Pain (*Continued*)
    history in, 1182–1183, 1183t, 1184t
    multidisciplinary approach to, 1181–1182
    musculoskeletal, 1184t, 1187–1188, 1188t
    pharmacotherapy for, 1189–1194
    physical examination in, 1183–1184
    in sickle cell disease, trait, and variants, 1189, 1190t
  deleterious effects of untreated, 661
  in developing countries, 1301–1302
  emergence and, 691
  neuropathic, 1182–1183
  perception of, 87
  perioperative, in adenotonsillectomy, 862–863, 862.e1t
  pharmacogenomics of, 85–87
  rheumatologic and musculoskeletal, 1188–1189, 1189t
  tourniquet-related, 833–834
Pain assessment, 1135–1142, 1136t
  in cognitively impaired child, 1141–1142
    Non-Communicating Children's Pain Checklist, 1136t, 1141.e1t
    Pain indicator for Communicatively Impaired Children in, 1136t, 1141.e1t
    revised Face, Legs, Activity, Cry, Consolability Observational Tool in, 1141–1142, 1142t
  intensity of pain, 1182–1183
  limitations of, 1140–1141
  observational-behavioral measures in, 1138–1140, 1138t
    Children's Hospital of Eastern Ontario Pain Scale, 1136t, 1138, 1139t
    Comfort Scale, 1136t, 1138–1140, 1140t
    Face, Legs, Activity, Cry, Consolability Observational Tool, 1136t, 1138, 1138t, 1139t
  selection criteria for, 1137–1138, 1137f
  self-report metrics in, 1135–1138
    Computer Face Scale in, 1138
    faces pain scales in, 1136, 1136t, 1137f
    Numeric Rating Scale, for pain, 1136t, 1137
    Oucher Pain Scale in, 1136, 1136.e1f
    Sydney Animated Facial Expression Scale, 1136t, 1138
    Visual Analog Scale in, 1136, 1137f
Pain indicator for Communicatively Impaired Children, 1136t, 1141.e1t
Pain management
  acetaminophen for, 1145t, 1146–1147
  in burn injury, 942f, 950–952, 951f, 952t
  in cognitively impaired child, 1177–1178
  in developing countries, 1301–1302
  ketamine for, 1149
  nonsteroidal antiinflammatory drugs for, 1147–1148
  opioid analgesics for, 1152–1153, 1152t
    in cognitively impaired child, 1177
    epidural administration of, 1172t
    intramuscular and subcutaneous routes for, 1155
    intranasal route, 1155
    intravenous administration of, 1154
    nurse-/caregiver-controlled analgesia and, 1161–1162
    oral administration of, 1153–1154
    patient-controlled analgesia in, 1157–1161
    relative potency of, 1152t
  pharmacologic treatment in, 1145–1177
  in postanesthesia care unit, 1250–1251
  strategies for, 1142–1145, 1143f, 1144f
    age and cognitive abilities in, 1145
    surgical considerations in, 1143–1145
  tramadol for, 1148–1149

Pain physician, 1181–1182
Palliative care, in congenital heart disease, 615–616
Palonosetron, 96
Pamidronate, 722, 936–937
Pancreatic autoimmunity, 705–706
Pancuronium, 156, 646t, 1310
 for cardiac surgery, 445–446
 effective doses of, 128t
 fentanyl and, 445
Pancytopenia, 270
PANDA study. see Pediatric Anesthesia and Neurodevelopment Assessment study
Panel reactive antibodies, in cardiac transplantation, 794–795
Panoramic imaging, 1069, 1070f
Papilledema, 1001
Papillomatosis, laryngeal, 340t, 887–889, 887f, 888t, 888.e1f,
Paracetamol, 980
Paradoxical aciduria, 974–975
Paragangliomas, 724
Paraglossal approach, to rigid laryngoscopy, 360, 361f
Parallel circulation, in congenital heart disease, 394, 394t
Paraplegia, 465, 818
Parathyroid and calcium disorders, 720–722
 calcium homeostasis and, 720–721
 hypercalcemia, 721–722
 hypocalcemia, 721
Parathyroid hormone, 720–721
Parathyroid hormone-related protein, 721–722
Parathyroid hyperplasia, 722
Parathyroidectomy, 722
Paravertebral block, 371t, 1102–1106, 1103f, 1104f, 1105f, 1106f
Paravertebral space, 1102
Parecoxib, 177
Parent(s)
 communication in ICU and, 72, 73t
 impaired, informed consent and, 70
Parenteral nutrition
 after burn injury, 936
 liver disease associated with, 773–774
 solution for, 225, 225t
Parents' Postoperative Pain Measure, 1140, 1140.e1t
Parkland formula, for burns, 939–940, 940t
Paroxysmal hypertension, rhinologic procedures and, 844–845
Partial pressure of arterial carbon dioxide
 cerebral blood flow and, 680–681, 681f
 laparoscopic surgery and, 754
Partial pressure of arterial oxygen, cerebral blood flow and, 681f
Partial task trainers, 1348–1349, 1349f
Partial thromboplastin times (PTT), 290–291
Passive heat and moisturizer exchangers, 1315
Past medical history, 31–35, 31.e1t,
 allergies to medications and latex in, 32–35, 34t
 family history in, 35
Patau syndrome, 404
Patent ductus arteriosus (PDA), 452–453, 453f, 957–958
 closure of, 575, 575f, 576f
 ligation of, 430–431t
 noncardiac surgery in congenital heart disease and, 589t, 591–592
 transcatheter occlusion of, 980
Patent foramen ovale (PFO), 450, 588, 689, 957
Pathogen inactivation/reduction, 286–287
Pathogenicity, 1280
Patient positioning
 in laparoscopic surgery, 754
 in middle ear and mastoid surgery, 843, 843–e

Patient positioning (Continued)
 in neurosurgical procedures, 704
 in scoliosis surgery, 826–e, 826–827, 826f
 in thoracic surgery, 371
Patient State Index, 1338–1339
Patient-controlled analgesia, 1157–1161
 adverse events with, 1162, 1162.e1t
 after scoliosis surgery, 826
 continuous basal infusions in, 1158–1161, 1160f
 dosing guidelines, 1168t
 drug and drug dosages for, 756, 1158
 equipment for, 1162
 monitoring of, 1162–1163
 pain nurse administration of, 1182
 pump settings in, 1158, 1159f
 risks associated with, 1162, 1162.e1t
Patil-Syracuse endoscopy mask, 361
PCC. see Prothrombin complex concentrates
PDA. see Patent ductus arteriosus
Pectoralis block, for thoracic surgery, 371t
Pectus excavatum, 755–756
PediaSIM, 1349
Pediatric Advanced Life Support (PALS), 230, 1000
Pediatric Anesthesia and Neurodevelopment Assessment (PANDA) study, 672
Pediatric Anesthesia Emergence Delirium, 136t, 1242, 1242t, 1243t
Pediatric anesthesiology, ethical issues in, 65–78
 end-of-life, 70–72
 ethics consultation service, 77–78
 informed consent, 65–70
 pediatric research, 72–75, 74t
 physician obligations, advocacy, and good citizenship, 76–77, 76t
Pediatric Difficult Intubation (PeDI), 352
Pediatric End-Stage Liver Disease (PELD), 776–777
Pediatric intensive care unit
 communication in, 72, 73t
 transport and transfer to, after cardiac surgery, 466
Pediatric Perioperative Cardiac Arrest Registry, 432
Pediatric Regional Anesthesia Network, 1134
Pediatric research, 72–75, 74t
 conflicts of interest and, 75–76
 imperative for pharmacologic research and, 74–75
 interaction with industry and, 75–76, 76t
 minimal risks and, 73–74
 minor increase over minimal risk and, 74
 socioeconomic concerns and distribution of risk and, 74
Pediatric Research Equity Act (PREA), 75, 119–120
Pediatric sleep questionnaire-sleep-related breathing disorder subscale (PSQ-SRBD), 851
Pediatric Trauma Score, 1004–1005, 1005t, 1008t
Pedicle screw, for scoliosis surgery, 810–811, 817
PediMag (Thoratec), 552t, 558
Pedunculated papillomas, 887, 887f
Penicillin
 allergy, 1296
 prophylactic uses of, 240
Penile block, 1096–1097, 1096f
Pentazocine, 95
Pentobarbital, 1230–1231, 1232–1233
Pentobarbital, neurotoxicity of, 652.e1–652.e11t, 659
Percutaneous balloon valvuloplasty, 592, 593
Percutaneous central venous cannulation, 683

Percutaneous contamination, 1283–1284, 1284t
Percutaneous intravenous central catheters, 1318
Percutaneous needle cricothyroidotomy, 357–359, 357f, 358f, 358.e1f, 359.e1f, 359.e2f
Percutaneous pulmonary valve replacement (PPVR), 576
Perfan. see Enoximone
Perfluorocarbon liquids, 908
Perfusion, during thoracic surgery, 370–371
Pericardial tamponade, 690
Pericardiectomy, 739
Pericardiocentesis, 739
Pericarditis, 739
Perimembranous defects, 590
Perinatal asphyxia, 13
Perinatal mortality, 1300
Periodic breathing, 12
Perioperative adverse events, risk stratification for, 855–857, 855t, 855.e1f
Perioperative behavioral stress, pharmacologic interventions for, 29–30
Perioperative cardiac arrest, 1026–1027
Perioperative dialysis, 735–736
Perioperative evaluation, in mechanical circulatory support, 565
Periorbital ecchymoses, 692
Peripheral diagnostic angiography, 1210
Peripheral intravenous cannulation, 1256–1258
Peripheral nerve blocks, 1087–1088, 1088t
 head and neck, 1088–1093, 1089f
  great auricular, 1092, 1092f
  greater occipital, 1090, 1090f
  infraorbital, 1090–1091, 1091f
  nerve of Arnold, 1092–1093
  supraorbital and supratrochlear nerves, 1088–1089, 1089f
 lower extremity, 1119–1131, 1120f
  ankle, 1130–1131, 1131f
  digital foot, 1131
  fascia iliaca, 1130
  femoral nerve, 1127f, 1128–1129, 1128f, 1129f
  infragluteal-parabiceps approach, 1124, 1125f, 1127f
  lateral femoral cutaneous nerve, 1129
  lateral popliteal sciatic nerve, 1126f, 1127–1128
  lumbar plexus, 1120–1122, 1121f, 1122f
  sciatic nerve, 1122–1125, 1123f, 1124f
 selection of local anesthetic for, 1087–1088, 1088t
 truncal, 1085.e1f, 1093–1097, 1094.e1f
  inguinal, 1093–1096, 1095f
  intercostal, 1085.e1f, 1093, 1094f, 1094.e1f
  paravertebral, 1102–1106, 1103f, 1104f, 1105f, 1106f
  penile, 1096–1097, 1096f
  quadratus lumborum, 1100–1102, 1101f, 1102f
  rectus sheath, 1097–1098, 1098f, 1099f, 1100f
 upper extremity, 1107–1114
  brachial plexus, 1107–1109, 1108f, 1109f, 1110f
  digital hand, 1118–1119, 1119f
  at elbow, 1114
  intravenous, 1131–1132
  median nerve, 1117–1118, 1118f
  radial nerve, 1114–1115, 1115f, 1116f
  ulnar nerve, 1118, 1118f
  at wrist, 1118
Peripheral nerves
 acquired disorders of, 634
 palsies, 634

Peripheral nervous system, interventional cardiology and, 580
Peripherally inserted central catheter (PICC), 222, 399, 949, 1269, 1270f
Peritonsillar abscess, 871–872, 872f
Periventricular white matter, 958–960
Permanent cardiac pacing, 420–422
Permissive hypercapnia, 378, 955
Permissive hypercarbia, 938–939
Peroxisomal disorders, 631
Persistent fetal circulation, 472–473
Persistent left superior vena cava to coronary sinus, 407–409, 408f
Persistent pulmonary hypertension, 958, 960f
Personal protective equipment (PPE), 1286, 1286.e1f
Personalized medicine, 80
Personnel requirements, on off-site anesthesia, 1197
Persuasion, 67–68
Pertrach system, 359, 359.e2f
Pfeiffer syndrome, 904
 craniosynostosis in, 918
 hemifacial microsomia in, 922.e1
 midface procedures in, 922
PFO. see Patent foramen ovale
P-glycoprotein (P-gp), 92
pH
 age-dependent variables of, 10t
 of body fluids, 227t
 in breathing regulation, 11
 in pulmonary vascular physiology, 474
PHACES syndrome, 970
Phakomatoses, 904
Pharmacodynamics, 116–118
 cardiopulmonary bypass and, 520
 inhalation anesthetic agents, 126–134
  cardiovascular system and, 130–133
  central nervous system and, 128–130
  hepatic system and, 134
  minimal alveolar concentration and, 126–128, 126t, 127f
  renal system and, 120t, 133–134
  respiratory system and, 133
 interaction models, 194–196
 models, 107–108
  logistic regression model, 108
  quantal effect model, 108
  sigmoid E_{max} model in, 107–108, 108f
 of neuromuscular blocking drugs, 150, 150f
 pharmacokinetics and, 109
 response surface mode, 195–196, 196f
Pharmacogenetics, 80
 anesthesia affected by, 94–96
 of benzodiazepines, 95
 definition of, 80, 1252–1253
 genetic counseling, 97
 genotyping methods, 97
 hepatic metabolism and, 81–84
 of local anesthetics, 96
 of midazolam, 95
 of neuromuscular blocking drugs, 95–96
 of nitrous oxide, 95
 of propofol, 94–95
Pharmacogenomics, 79–99
 of analgesia, 85–87
 basic concepts of, 80–81
 definition of, 80
 methods, 97
 nomenclature associated with, 80–81
 of pain, 85–87
 resources for, 98t
Pharmacokinetics, 101
 apparent volume of distribution, 103–104
 burn injury effects on, 937, 943t
 cardiopulmonary bypass and, 519
 first-order kinetics in
  description of, 101–102
  half-life in, 102
  multiple-compartment, 102–103, 103f
  single-compartment, 102

Pharmacokinetics (Continued)
inhalation anesthetic agents, 114t,
120–124, 121f
alveolar ventilation/functional
residual capacity, 108f, 121
cardiac output and, 108f, 121–122
control of anesthetic depth and,
110f, 124–126, 124t
induction and, 123–124
second gas effect and, 123
shunts, 124–125, 125f
solubility and, 109f, 110f, 122–123
washout and emergence and, 125–126
linkage with pharmacodynamics, 109
loading dose in, 105
local anesthetics of, 1054t, 1054.e1f,
1054–1060
amides, 1054–1055
esters, 1055–1056
hypersensitivity, 1060
lidocaine, 1055
ropivacaine in, 1055
toxicity and, 1056–1057, 1056f, 1058t
treatment of toxic reactions and,
1059–1060
neuromuscular blocking drugs, 150–151
pediatric considerations in, 106–107
child size in, 106, 106f
maturation in, 106–107, 107f
organ function and, 107
remifentanil, 169–170, 169f, 170t
repetitive dosing and drug
accumulation in, 105
zero-order kinetics in, 103, 104f
Pharmacologic armamentarium, for
sedation, 1216
Pharmacologic research, 74–75
Pharyngoplasty, 914
Pharyngoplasty surgery, 917
Pharynx, pathology related to, 350t
Phase reversal, 695
Phenobarbital, 81, 645t
neurotoxicity of, 652.e1–652.e11t, 659
Phenoxybenzamine, 494–495, 518, 725
Phentolamine, 492–493t, 494–495, 518
Phenylalanine, 87
Phenylephrine, 314–315, 484–485t, 487,
609, 685, 907, 907t, 1023
Phenytoin, 81, 499t, 500, 645t, 1192
Pheochromocytoma, 721, 724–726, 1033t
Phlebotomy, 610
Phonation, 331
Phosphodiesterase inhibitors, 487–488
Phototherapy, 15
Phrenic nerve block, 1107
pH-stat versus α-stat management, 515–517,
516f
Physical examination
in airway evaluation, 335–336, 335f
in chronic pain, 1183–1184
in neurosurgery, 682
in noncardiac surgery in congenital
heart disease, 601
Physical therapist, 1182
Physical therapy, in complex regional pain
syndrome, 1187
Physician
informed consent and, 68
obligations, advocacy, and good
citizenship, 76–77, 76t
pain physician, 1181–1182
Physician orders, for life-sustaining
treatment, 72
Physiologic anemia
of infancy, 17
of newborn, 963
Physiologic jaundice, 15, 15t
Physiologic murmurs, 409
Physiologic shunting, 475
Physostigmine, 189, 907t
PICC. see Peripherally inserted central
catheter
PiCCO system, 1341–1342
Piercing devices, accidents with, 1283–1284
Pierre Robin syndrome

Pierre Robin syndrome (Continued)
airway difficulties in, 340t
airway evaluation in, 334
cleft lip and palate in, 914–915, 914.e1
eye surgery in, 904
tracheotomy in, 888.e1f
PIK3CA-associated overgrowth syndrome,
1211, 1211f
Pilocarpine, 907t, 908
Pilocytic astrocytoma, 625, 626t
Pirbuterol, for asthma exacerbations,
319.e2–319.e3t
Pitressin, 714
Pituitary adenomas, 270, 694
Placental gas exchange, 468–469
Plasma, 285
Plasma butyrylcholinesterase, 116
Plasma protein binding, 109, 109f,
110f, 1057
Plasma thromboplastin antecedent
deficiency, 250–251
Plasma-derived factor concentrates, 287
Plasma-Lyte, 223t
Plasmapheresis, 634
Plasmin, 531–532
α2-plasmin inhibitor (α2-PI), 531–532
Plasminogen, 236, 531–532, 544
Plasminogen activator inhibitor-1
(PAI-1), 96, 531–532
Plastic surgery, 914–931
brachial plexus surgery in, 928
in cleft lip and palate, 914–917,
914.e1, 915f, 915t, 916.e1
in congenital hand anomalies, 928,
928.e1, 929f
cosmetic procedures in, 930
in craniosynostosis, 917–922, 917f,
917t, 917.e1
airway management in, 919
blood loss, coagulopathy, and
hyponatremia in, 919–921
classification of, 917t
cranial vault reconstruction in, 918,
918f, 918.e1
midface procedures in, 922–923, 922.e1
prolonged surgery in, 922
venous air embolism in, 921–922
in hairy pigmented nevus, 929–930,
929f, 929.e1
in hemifacial microsomia, Treacher
Collins syndrome, and Goldenhar
syndrome, 923–925, 923.e1,
924f, 924.e1
in Möbius syndrome, 927, 927.e1
in orbital hypertelorism, 922, 922f
orthognathic surgery in, 925
otoplasty in, 928, 928.e1
tissue expanders in, 929, 929f, 929.e1
in trauma, 930
Platelet(s), 248
activation of, 531
after cardiac bypass, 537
description of, 17–18
dysfunction of, 276
in hematologic disorders, 238, 238t
hemostasis, 290
transfusion of, 282t, 283–284
Platelet count, 249, 507
in renal disease, 738
values at different ages, 237t
Platelet disorders, 248
Platelet function analyzer (PFA-100), 237
Platinum chemotherapeutic agents, 270
Plenum vaporizer, 1311
Pleura, ultrasound of, 1069
Pleural effusion, pulmonary ultrasound
for, 387
Pneumatocele, 835
Pneumatosis intestinalis, 977
Pneumomediastinum, 753
Pneumonia, after scoliosis surgery, 816t
Pneumoperitoneum, 615, 751–752
Pneumothorax, 753, 888–889, 1093, 1107
after scoliosis surgery, 816t
pulmonary ultrasound for, 387

Poikilothermia, 940
Point person, 1197
Point-of-care testing, 237
Point-of-care ultrasound (POCUS),
386–389
for acute respiratory distress
syndrome, 387
for hemidiaphragmatic paralysis,
387, 388f
introduction to, 386–388, 386f
in noncardiac surgery in congenital
heart disease, 605, 606f
for pleural effusion, 387
for pneumothorax, 387
tracheal diameter for tracheal tube
sizing, 388–389, 389f
tracheal tube positioning with, 389, 390f
Poiseuille law, 1317
Poland syndrome, 928
Poliomyelitis, 633
Polycystic kidney disease, 696
Polycythemia, 18, 543–544, 609–610, 762
Polyhydramnios, 972–973
Polymicrogyria, 625
Polysomnogram
for obstructive sleep apnea, 850,
852, 852.e1–852.e2f
in sleep-disordered breathing, 845
Polyuria, 233, 713
Polyvinyl alcohol particles, 1210
Pompe disease, 340t, 397f, 411–412, 636
Population modeling, 105
Porcine stress syndrome, malignant
hyperthermia and, 1042
Porphyria, 80
Portal hypertension
cardiomyopathy and, 778
in liver disease, 778, 780
Portal vein, 768, 769f
Portoacaval shunt, 784–785
Portopulmonary hypertension, 779
Positioning
in laparoscopic surgery, 754
in middle ear and mastoid surgery, 843,
843–e
in neurosurgical procedures, 685–687,
686f
in scoliosis surgery, 826–e, 826–827,
826f
Positive end-expiratory pressure, 690, 747
Positive-feedback cardiovascular response,
124, 124t
Positron emission tomography (PET),
1207–1208
Postanesthesia apnea, in formerly preterm
infant, 59–61, 60f, 60.e1f, 61f, 62f
Postanesthesia behavior assessment scale,
1243t
Postanesthesia care unit (PACU), 714,
1238–1254
airway obstruction and, 1245–1246
arrhythmias and, 1247
arrival in, 1240–1241
bradycardia and, 1247
discharge criteria for, 1251–1252,
1251t, 1252t
discharge of preterm infant from,
1246–1247
emergence agitation or delirium and,
1241–1243, 1242t, 1243t
hypertension and, 1248
hypotension and, 1247–1248
hypoventilation and, 1245
hypoxemia and, 1245
pain management in, 1250–1251
perioperative environment and,
1238–1241, 1239t, 1240t
pharmacodynamics of emergence
and, 1241
postoperative nausea and vomiting and,
1248–1250, 1249f
renal system considerations in, 1248
tachycardia and, 1247
temperature management in, 1251
transport to, 1239–1240

Postanesthesia evaluation policy, 1196
Postbypass period, in cardiopulmonary
bypass, 515, 515t
Post-dural puncture headache, 1079
Posterior cerebral artery, 695
Posterior fossa, tumor of, 626t
Posterior fossa surgery, 685–686
Posterior mediastinal masses, 385–386, 386f
Posterior scalp, 1090
Posterior spinal fusion, 546–547, 810
Posterior tibial artery catheterization, 1277
Posterior urethral valves, 758
Postintubation croup, 342–343, 1246
Postligation cardiac syndrome, 980
Postoperative apnea
in formerly preterm infant, 59–61,
60f, 60.e1f, 61f, 62f
in micropremie, 956
Postoperative care
after cardiopulmonary resuscitation,
1028–1029
in burn injury, 942f, 950–952, 951f, 952t
in cardiac transplantation, 797–799, 798f
in fluid management, 227–228
general approach to, 227, 227t
hyponatremia and, 227–228
pulmonary edema and, 228
in heart-lung transplantation, 805
in liver transplantation, 786–787
monitoring in general care setting,
1252–1253
in noncardiac surgery in congenital
heart disease, 609
Postoperative nausea and vomiting
(PONV), 900, 1248–1250, 1249f
5-HT 3 receptor antagonists for,
185–186
in adenotonsillectomy, 861–862, 861f
after middle ear surgery, 843
alternative treatments of, 1250
emergence and recovery, 868
evidence-based consensus management
of, 1248–1249, 1249f
in eye surgery, 910
inhalational anesthetics and, 139
multimodal therapy for, 1239
in myringotomy, 842
pharmacogenomics of, 96
prophylactic therapy for, 1249–1250
rescue therapy for, 1249–1250
Postoperative pain management
incisional pain, 754
in laparoscopic surgery, 754
for scoliosis surgery, 824–826
Postrenal renal failure, 732t
Post-resuscitation stabilization, 1028–1029
Postsedation, 1227
Post-term neonate, 2, 2t
Posttonsillectomy hemorrhage, 847.e1t,
870–871, 871f
Post-tourniquet syndrome, 833
Posttransplant lymphoproliferative
disorder (PTLD)
in heart-lung transplantation, 807
in renal transplantation, 791
Posttransplant renal failure, 797–798
Potassium, 217
in body fluids, 227t
dehydration states and, 230
homeostasis, 230
hyperkalemia and, 231–232, 232f, 233f
hypokalemia and, 232
kidney regulation of, 730, 730t
serum concentrations of, 153
Potassium channels, 1056
Potassium hydroxide, 134
Potassium iodide, 720t
Potts shunt, 430–431t
Povidone iodine, 1255
PPVR. see Percutaneous pulmonary valve
replacement
PR interval, 410–411
Prader-Willi syndrome, 757
Pralidoxime, 908
Pramlintide acetate, 707

PRBCs. *see* Packed red blood cells
Preanesthesia evaluation policy, 1196
Prebypass anesthetic management, in cardiopulmonary bypass, 519
Prebypass period, in cardiopulmonary bypass, 512
Precordial stethoscope, 1239–1240, 1330
Prednisolone, 319.e2–319.e3t, 723t
Prednisone, 319.e2–319.e3t, 723t
Pregabalin, 645t, 1192
  after scoliosis surgery, 825
  for pain, 1150
Pregnancy
  informed consent and, 69
  pharmacologic consequences of, 989, 989t
  testing, 35–36
Prehospital care in trauma, 1002–1006, 1004t
Prekallikrein, 531
Preload, in Fontan circulation, 480
Premature atrial contractions or beats, 414
Premature suture closure, 917
Premature ventricular beats, 1247
Premature ventricular contractions or beats, 418
Prematurity, 2, 953–964
  apnea of, 12
  complications of, 960–961
  hematologic function and, 963–964
  intraventricular hemorrhage and, 960–961
  neurologic development and, 958–961
  postintubation croup in, 1246
  respiratory control and, 956
Premedication, 22–43, 36t
  α_2-agonists, 38–39
  antacids, H_2-receptor antagonists, and gastrointestinal motility drugs, 43, 43t
  antibiotics, 42, 43t
  anticholinergic drugs, 39
  antiemetics, 42
  antihistamines, 39
  benzodiazepines, 36–37, 36t, 37.e1f
  during bronchoscopy, 875
  in cardiac surgery, 435
  corticosteroids, 42
  emergency procedures application, 1012
  insulin, 42
  ketamine, 38
  in neurosurgical procedures, 683
  nonbarbiturate sedatives, 37
  in noncardiac surgery in congenital heart disease, 603
  nonopioid analgesics, 41–42, 41f
  opioids, 37
  topical anesthetics, 39–40, 40t
Preoperative cardiopulmonary stabilization, 551
Preoperative evaluation
  in adenotonsillectomy, 850.e1t, 851–854
  airway evaluation in, 333–336
    diagnostic testing in, 336
    medical history in, 334
    physical examination in, 335–336, 335f
  in anterior mediastinal masses, 384
  in cardiac surgery, 433–435, 435t
  in cardiac transplantation, 794–795, 795t
  in craniosynostosis, 927
  in diabetes mellitus, 708–709, 709f
  in eye surgery, 900–901
  in liver transplantation, 780–782, 781t
  in neurosurgical procedures, 682
  in noncardiac surgery in congenital heart disease, 600–603, 600t
  of respiratory system, 309
  in spinal surgery, 823–824
  in trauma, 1011–1012, 1012t
Preoperative preparation, 22–36
  behavioral interventions, 27–28, 27.e1t
  child development, 27–28, 27.e1t
  fasting, 22–24, 24f, 25f, 25t
  health care provider intervention in, 29

Preoperative preparation (*Continued*)
  laboratory data and, 35
  past medical history and, 31–35, 31.e1t
    allergies to medications and latex in, 32–35, 34t
    family history in, 35
    pregnancy testing, 35–36
    preoperative anxiety, 27–28, 27.e1t
    primary and secondary smoking and, 25–26
    psychological preparation in, 27
Preprocedural preparation, in sedation, 1222
Prerenal azotemia, 733, 780
Prescription Drug User Fee Act, 119
Presedation pause, 1227
Presedation responsibilities, 1227
Pressure diuresis, 217–218
Pressure gradients, 429
Pressure support ventilation, 600, 1325–1326
Pressure-controlled ventilation, 1325–1326
Preterm infant, 2, 5t
  airway management in eye surgery, 903
  apnea in, 12, 60
  blood pressure of, 12t
  blood volume, 218–219
  circulating blood volume of, 219t
  discharge from postanesthesia care unit, 1246–1247
  drug distribution in, 110
  drug metabolism in, 113
  growth curve for, 6f
  heart rate of, 12t
  jaundice in, 15
  laryngeal position in, 325f
  postanesthesia apnea in, 59–61, 60f, 60.e1f, 61f, 62f
  postanesthesia apnea in former, 59–61, 60f, 60.e1f, 61f, 62f
  retinopathy of prematurity in, 901
Primacor. *see* Milrinone
Primary brain tumors, 625–627, 626t
Primary smoking, 25–26, 25f
Primary survey in trauma, 1006t
Prime volume (cardiac bypass), 436
Primum atrial septal defect, 450, 451f
Prinivil. *see* Lisinopril
Probe, musculoskeletal ultrasound imaging, 1065
Procainamide, 498–499, 499t
Procedural sedation, training and system issues for, 1226–1227, 1227f
Processed electroencephalogram monitors, 1338–1340, 1339f
Production pressure, 76
Programmed cell death, normal brain development and, 651
Progressive encephalopathy, 1306
Progressive neurologic disorders, 625–632
  inborn errors of metabolism in, 627–632, 629–630t
  primary brain tumors in, 625–627, 626t, 628t
Proinflammatory cytokines, 708
Prone position, in neurosurgical procedures, 685–687, 686f
Pronestyl. *see* Procainamide
Propafenone, 500–501
Propagation, 531, 531f
Propagation speed artifact, 1070
Proparacaine, 908
Prophylaxis, for endocarditis, 400, 400t
Propofol, 115f, 141–144, 646t, 1051, 1241, 1282
  alfentanil and, 195
  anaphylactoid reactions with, 144
  bispectral index and, 193f
  for blunt reflex bronchoconstriction, 860.e1t
  for bone marrow aspiration procedure, 274
  cardiac catheterization uses of, 583
  for cardiac surgery, 445
  deep sedation, 1206

Propofol (*Continued*)
  dosing of, 193t
  effects on evoked potentials, 830–831
  egg allergy and, 144
  emergence and, 690
  emergence delirium from, 1243
  emergency surgery in trauma patient using, 1009t
  equilibration rate constant of, 194f
  in extremely premature infant, 964–965
  eye surgery uses of, 909
  eyelash reflex and, 141–142
  hepatic metabolism of, 772
  infusion rates of, 194t
  infusion schemes, 197t, 205f
  intravenous induction of, 48
  for laryngospasm, 909
  in lipid emulsion, 1059–1060
  for local anesthetic toxicity, 1059–1060
  manual infusion of, 208–210, 209f, 210f, 210t
  metabolism of, 80
  in micropremie, 965
  in mitochondrial disorders, 638
  in neonates, 144
  in neurosurgery, 687–688
  neurophysiologic effects of, 688t
  neurotoxicity of, 652.e1–652.e11t, 659–660
  noncardiac surgery in congenital heart disease using, 607
  pain associated with, 210–211
  pharmacogenetics of, 94–95
  pharmacokinetics of, 191t
  for postoperative nausea and vomiting, 1239
  proteomics and, 80
  remifentanil and, 170, 195–196
  for renal insufficiency, 740–741
  for sedation, 1230–1231t, 1235–1236
  soy allergy and, 144
  target-controlled infusion of, 191, 191f, 191t
  time-concentration profile for, 191t, 193f, 195f
Propofol infusion syndrome, 159, 190, 445, 638, 965, 1051
Propranolol, 491, 492–493t, 501, 646t, 933, 935
  for hyperthyroid crisis, 720t
  for retinopathy of prematurity, 140
  for subglottic hemangiomas, 970
Propylthiouracil, 720t
ProSeal laryngeal mask airway, 345–346
Prostaglandins
  E$_1$, 492–493t, 495, 536, 595, 597
  H2 synthetase, 1146
  I$_2$, 729
Prostanoids, 473f, 477t, 496–497
Protamine
  reactions, 515
  reversal of anticoagulation with, 535
  titration, 535
Protamine sulfate, 797
Protein
  binding of, in drug distribution, 102f, 103f, 109–110, 109f, 110f
  metabolism, disorders of, 627
  synthesis of, anesthetic effects on, 773
Protein C, 531
Protein kinase C, 449
Protein S, 531
Protein-losing enteropathy, 599
Proteinuria, 733
Proteolytic enzymes, 544–545
Proteomics, 80
Prothrombin complex concentrates (PCCs), 287–288, 288t, 538–539
  cardiopulmonary bypass and, 510
Prothrombin time (PT), 18, 236, 533, 535, 773
  massive blood transfusion and, 282t, 285
  values at different ages, 237t
Proton radiation therapy, 264–265, 266f, 275f
Protruding ears, 928, 928.e1

Prune-belly syndrome, 758–759, 759f, 759.e1f
Pseudoaneurysm, 578
Pseudocholinesterase, 151, 1055
Pseudocholinesterase deficiency, 84, 95
Pseudohypoparathyroidism, 721
Psychological preparation of child for anesthesia, 27
Psychologist, 1182
PT. *see* Prothrombin time
PTT. *see* Partial thromboplastin times
Pulmonary arterial catheters, 439
Pulmonary arterial hypertension, 473
Pulmonary artery banding, 430–431t, 598
Pulmonary artery pressure, 429
Pulmonary artery thermodilution, 1341
Pulmonary aspiration of gastric contents
  preoperative fasting, 23
  risk in abdominal surgery, 745
Pulmonary atresia, 983t
Pulmonary blood flow
  obstruction of, in congenital heart disease, 394, 394t
  shunting and, 475
Pulmonary complications
  after burn injury, 933–935, 934f, 943t
  in cerebral palsy, 621
  in liver disease, 778–779
  in neuromuscular scoliosis, 816t
Pulmonary disease
  asthma. *see* Asthma
  in developing countries, 1305
Pulmonary edema, 227t
  fluid overload and, 222
  in infants, 946–947
  negative-pressure, 885
  noncardiogenic, 868, 1246
  postobstructive, 1246
  postoperative fluid management and, 228
Pulmonary embolism, 1018
Pulmonary exacerbations, 320
Pulmonary fibrosis, 267–268
Pulmonary function tests, 309–311, 310f, 310t, 311f, 311.e1f, 312f, 313f
Pulmonary hypertension, 553
  cardiac catheterization in, 577–578
  in congenital diaphragmatic hernia, 381
  in Down syndrome, 591
  eye surgery and, 902
  in lung and heart-lung transplantation, 801–802
  mediastinal radiation causing, 266
  medications for, 473f, 477t
  noncardiac surgery in congenital heart disease and, 611–612, 612t
  paradoxical, 458
  persistent, 958, 960f
  postoperative, 449–450
  protamine and, 535
  rebound, 958
Pulmonary inhalation injury, 934–935
Pulmonary malignancies, 267
Pulmonary oxygen toxicity, 139
Pulmonary regurgitation, 454–455
Pulmonary sequestrations, 380
Pulmonary steal phenomenon, 591
Pulmonary stretch receptors, 308
Pulmonary system, cardiopulmonary bypass effects on, 522, 523f
Pulmonary to systemic blood flow (Q_{pulm}/Q_{sys}), ratio of, 478
Pulmonary valve
  dysplasia of, in Noonan syndrome, 405
  replacement of, percutaneous, 576
Pulmonary vascular disease, 455–456
Pulmonary vascular resistance (PVR), 472, 551, 582, 598–599
  in cardiac transplantation, 793
  control in cardiac surgery, 435, 443
  manipulations of, 474t
  transitional circulation and, 8
Pulmonary vasculature
  cardiopulmonary bypass effects on, 522
  physiology of, 471t, 472–474, 474f, 474t

Pulmonary venous drainage obstruction, 474
Pulmonary venous saturation ($S_{pulm}vO_2$), 478
Pulmonary vessels, 8
Pulmonology, 307–323
  perioperative etiology and epidemiology in, 312–323
    asthma. see Asthma
    cystic fibrosis, 320–322, 321t, 321.e1f
    lower respiratory tract infection in, 315–320
    sickle cell disease in, 322–323
    upper respiratory tract infection in, 312–315, 314t, 315f, 315t
  preoperative assessment in, 309
  pulmonary function tests in, 309–311, 310f, 310t, 311f, 311t, 311.e1f, 312f, 313f
  respiratory physiology, 307–309, 308f
Pulsatile pumps, 559–560, 559f
Pulse oximetry, 683, 1331–1333, 1331.e1f, 1332f
  alarm thresholds, 1253, 1253t
  cardiac arrest diagnosis using, 1023
  in malignant hyperthermia, 1036
  multiple wavelength, 1333
  in neonatal surgical emergencies, 966
  in noncardiac surgery in congenital heart disease, 605
  postoperative monitoring in general care setting using, 1253
Pulse wave amplification, 429
Pulsed-Doppler imaging
  cardiac output determinations using, 13
  description of, 424
Pulseless electrical activity, 1028
Pulseless ventricular tachycardia, 1021
Pulsus paradoxus, 1333
Purchasing of anesthesia equipment, 1344–1345
PVR. see Pulmonary vascular resistance
P wave, 409–410
Pyeloplasty, 760
Pyloric stenosis, hypertrophic, 974–976, 975f
Pyloromyotomy, laparoscopic, 975.e1
Pyridostigmine, 635
Pyruvate dehydrogenase complex, 637

Q

Q wave, 411–412
Qbrelis. see Lisinopril
QRS axis, 409–410
QRS complex, 409–410
QT interval, 412
QT prolongation
  amiodarone causing, 1026
  liver disease and, 778
Quadratus lumborum block, 1100–1102, 1101f, 1102f
Quality assurance, in non-operating room anesthesia, 1198
Quality improvement, 77, 1227
Quantal effect model, 108
Quantitative sensory testing, 1186–1187
Quantitative sudomotor axon reflex testing, 1186–1187
Quenching of MRI magnet, 1199
Questionnaires, for obstructive sleep apnea, 851–852
QuickTrach Emergency Cricothyrotomy Device, 358–359, 359.e1f
Quinsy tonsillectomy, 872

R

Race, 96–97
Racemic ketamine, 657
Rachischisis, 700
Radial artery catheterization, 1271–1275, 1275f, 1276f
Radial nerve, anesthetic block of, 1117, 1117f
Radiant warmers, 1315
Radiation, of heat, 1314

Radiation exposure, in interventional cardiology, 580–581
Radiation therapy
  for cancer, 264–265
  duration of, 274
  late effects of, 265t
  mediastinal, 266
  for non-operating room anesthesia, 1208–1209, 1209f
  proton, 264–265, 266f, 275f
  simulation for, 274
Radioactive iodine therapy, 719
Radiofrequency ablation, 585
Radionuclide angiography, 794
Radionuclide tracers, of glucose, 1207–1208
Radiosurgery, stereotactic, 1208
Ramsay Scale, 1217t
Ranitidine, 185
Rapid infusion catheters, introducer sheaths and, 1258
Rapid-sequence induction (RSI), 974
  in abdominal surgery, 745–746
  controlled, 746
  succinylcholine for, 908
Rastelli operation, 430–431t, 456
Reactive hypoglycemia, 726
Rebound hypoglycemia, 949
Rebound pulmonary hypertension, 958
Recombinant erythropoietin, 935
Recombinant factor VII (rFVIIa), 292
Recombinant factor VIIa (rFVIIa), 293–294, 509, 530, 540–541, 540f
Recombinant human granulocyte-macrophage colony-stimulating factor, 270
Reconstructive surgery, 914–931
  brachial plexus surgery in, 928
  in cleft lip and palate, 914–917, 914.e1, 915f, 915t, 916.e1
  in congenital hand anomalies, 928, 928.e1, 929f
  cosmetic procedures in, 930
  in craniosynostosis, 917–922, 917f, 917t, 917.e1
    airway management in, 919
    blood loss, coagulopathy, and hyponatremia in, 919–921
    classification of, 917t
    cranial vault reconstruction in, 918, 918f, 918.e1
    midface procedures in, 922–923, 922.e1
    prolonged surgery in, 922
    venous air embolism in, 921–922
  in cystic hygromas and hemangiomas, 926, 927f
  in hairy pigmented nevus, 929–930, 929f, 929.e1
  in hemifacial microsomia, Treacher Collins syndrome, and Goldenhar syndrome, 923–925, 923.e1, 924f, 924.e1
  in Möbius syndrome, 927, 927.e1
  in orbital hypertelorism, 922, 922f
  orthognathic surgery in, 925
  otoplasty in, 928, 928.e1
  tissue expanders in, 929, 929f, 929.e1
  in trauma, 930
Recovery care, in sedation, 1223
Rectal administration, of methohexital, 140
Rectus sheath block, 1088t, 1097–1098, 1098f, 1099f, 1100f
Recurrent abdominal pain, 1184–1185
Recurrent croup, 886
Recurrent laryngeal nerve, 330, 1107
Recurrent respiratory papillomatosis, 887
Red blood cell substitutes, 288–289
Red blood cell transfusion, 543
  in cancer patients, 276
  in hematologic disorders, 237–238
Red blood cell-containing components in transfusion therapy, 281–283, 281t
Reed-Sternberg cells, 257
Reflectance oximetry, 1333, 1334f
Reflex bradycardia, 907

Refractory seizures, 648
Refsum disease, 633–634
Regional analgesia, 1163–1177
  additives and adjuvants, 1165–1166
  catheter techniques in, 1167–1171, 1167.e1f, 1168t, 1169f, 1170f, 1170t, 1172t
  catheter-related complications, 1174–1176, 1174f, 1175f
  fascial plane catheters, 1176
  for intraoperative pain, 1251
  local anesthetics, additives, and dosing in, 1164–1165
  plexus and peripheral nerve catheters, 1176
  risks and untoward effects of, 1171–1174, 1172t, 1173t
  single-injection techniques in, 1166–1167
  transition to oral analgesics, 1176–1177
Regional anesthesia, 1053–1133
  in abdominal surgery, 748
  in burn injury, 949–950
  in cardiac surgery, 446–447
  central neuraxial blockade in, 1072–1087
    anatomic and physiologic considerations in, 1072–1074, 1072.e1f, 1073f, 1074f
    epidural anesthesia in, 1079–1087
    spinal, 1074–1079, 1076f, 1077f
  COVID-19 and, 1288
  equipment for, 1060–1064, 1061f
    nerve stimulator in, 1071.e1f, 1072, 1073f
    ultrasound, 1060–1064, 1061f, 1327–1329
  lower extremity nerve blocks, 1119–1131, 1120f
    ankle, 1130–1131, 1131f
    digital foot, 1131
    fascia iliaca, 1130
    infragluteal-parabiceps approach in, 1124, 1125f, 1127f
    lateral popliteal sciatic nerve, 1128
    sciatic nerve, 1122–1125, 1123f, 1124f
  neuraxial, 446
  in noncardiac surgery in congenital heart disease, 607
  in orthopedic and spine surgery, 810
  peripheral nerve blocks in, 1088t
    brachial plexus, 1107–1109, 1108f, 1109f, 1110f
    digital hand, 1118–1119, 1119f
    at elbow, 1114–1115, 1115f
    femoral, 1127f, 1128–1129, 1128f, 1129f
    great auricular nerve, 1092, 1092f
    greater occipital nerve, 1090, 1090f
    infraorbital nerve, 1090–1091, 1091f
    inguinal, 1093–1096, 1095f
    intercostal, 1085.e1f, 1093, 1094f, 1094.e1f
    intravenous, 1131–1132
    lateral popliteal sciatic nerve block, 1126f, 1127–1128
    median nerve block, 1117–1118, 1118f
    nerve of Arnold, 1092–1093
    paravertebral, 1102–1106, 1103f, 1104f, 1105f, 1106f
    penile, 1096–1097, 1096f
    radial nerve, 1114–1115
    rectus sheath, 1088t, 1097–1098, 1098f, 1099f, 1100f
    ulnar nerve, 1118, 1118f
    at wrist, 1118
  pharmacology and pharmacokinetics of local anesthetics, 1054–1060, 1054t, 1054.e1f
    amides, 1054–1055
    bupivacaine, 1054
    esters, 1055–1056

Regional anesthesia (Continued)
    hypersensitivity and, 1060
    lidocaine, 1055
    prevention of toxicity and, 1057–1059, 1058t
    ropivacaine and, 1055
    toxicity and, 1056–1057, 1056f, 1058t
    treatment of toxic reactions and, 1059–1060
  for postoperative apnea in formerly preterm infant, 60–61
  selection of local anesthetic for, 1088t
  supraorbital and supratrochlear, 1088–1089, 1089f
Regional cerebral oxygen saturation (rSO2), 683
Regional cerebral perfusion
  in cardiopulmonary bypass, 521–522, 521f
  neurologic monitoring for, 524–525
Regional nerve block, 1181–1182
Regitine. see Phentolamine
Rejection
  after heart-lung transplantation, 806
  after liver transplantation, 787
Remifentanil, 169–170, 169f, 170t, 302–303, 909, 1241
  for cardiac surgery, 445
  desflurane versus, 1241
  in extremely premature infant, 965
  infusion schemes, 197t
  pharmacokinetics of, 772
  propofol and, 195–196
  in scoliosis surgery, 828
  for sedation outside operating room, 1233
  target-controlled infusion of, 191, 192
  tolerance to, 170
  total intravenous anesthesia uses, 210, 211f
Remimazolam, 180
Remodulin. see Treprostinil
Remote ischemic preconditioning, 449
Renal blood flow
  description of, 729
  developmental issues in, 13
Renal disease, 731
  in dehydration states, 230
  in sickle cell disease, 244
Renal failure, 116
  anesthesia concerns in patients presenting with, 741
  cardiopulmonary bypass effects on, 526–527
  intrinsic, 732t
  in liver disease, 780
Renal function
  after burn injury, 935
  contrast media and, 1201
  laparoscopic surgery and, 754
  urologic surgery and, 749
Renal function curve, 217–218
Renal insufficiency, 741, 750, 903
Renal osteodystrophy, 737
Renal output curve, 218f
Renal plasma flow, 220
Renal protection, strategies for, 739
Renal replacement therapy, 566–567
Renal system
  burn injury effects on, 935, 943t
  growth and development of, 13–14, 14f
  inhaled anesthetics and, 120t, 133–134
Renal transplantation, 787–791, 789f, 790t
  anesthetic induction in, 790
  anesthetic management of, 788–791
  immediate postoperative management of, 791
  long-term issues in, 791
  maintenance of anesthesia in, 790–791
  monitors and vascular access in, 790
  pathophysiology of, 788
  preoperative evaluation of, 788
  surgical technique in, 788
Renal tumors, 269, 761
Renin, 219–220, 739

Renin-angiotensin system, 218, 723
Reperfusion, 732
  after burn injury, 935
  in heart-lung transplantation, 805
  in liver transplantation, 785
  tourniquet-related, 833
Reperfusion syndrome, 785
Repetitive dosing, drug accumulation
    and, 105
Reptilase, 541
Residual neuromuscular blockade, 867
Residual obstructive sleep-disordered
    breathing, 869
Respiratory acidosis, in malignant
    hyperthermia, 1039
Respiratory depression
  opioid-induced, 863–866, 864f
    avoidance of opioids in, 865–866
    codeine for, 865
    CYP2D6 for, 865
    dose titration in, 865
    postoperative in formerly preterm
      infant, 60
    remifentanil-related, 170
    inhaled anesthetics and, 133
Respiratory distress syndrome, 954
Respiratory disturbance index, 852
Respiratory effort, postoperative, 1246
Respiratory events, in adenotonsillectomy,
    868
Respiratory exchange ratio (RER), 479
Respiratory failure, 693
  extracorporeal membrane oxygenation
    for, 553
Respiratory fatigue, 333
Respiratory insufficiency, 1244
Respiratory muscles, 9
Respiratory system
  associated with childhood obesity, 55t
  burn injury effects on, 933–935, 934f
  cerebral palsy in, 621
  inhaled anesthetics and, 133
  in mechanical circulatory support, 562
  physiology of, 307–309, 308f, 331–333
    airway obstruction during
      anesthesia, 333
    obligate nasal breathing and, 331
    tracheal and bronchial function in,
      331, 332f
    work of breathing and, 332–333, 333f
  prematurity and, 953–957, 954f, 954t
  preoperative assessment of, 309
Responsiveness-based assessment tools, 1218
Restrictive cardiomyopathy, 265–266,
    396–398, 411f
  cardiac transplantation for, 793
Restrictive intracardiac shunting, during
    cardiac surgery, 436
Restrictive lung disease, 311
Restrictive shunts, 476t
Resuscitation, in burn injuries, 938–942
  airway and oxygenation in,
    938–939, 938f
  associated injury in, 940
  carbon monoxide and cyanide
    poisoning in, 939, 939.e1f
  circumferential burns and, 940–941, 941f
  electrical burns and, 941, 941f, 945f
  volume resuscitation in, 939–940,
    940f, 940t, 940.e1f
Reticulocyte count, 240
Retinal hemorrhages, 1001
Retinoblastoma, 900, 912, 912f
  radiation therapy and, 1209
Retinoic acid syndrome, 271–272
Retinopathy of prematurity (ROP),
    901, 902f
  supplemental oxygen and, 139, 955
  treatment, 913
Retrobulbar block, 905
Retrograde light-guided laryngoscopy,
    368–369
Retrograde wire and flexible intubation
    scope, 368
Retrograde wire-guided intubation, 364

Retromolar approach, to rigid
    laryngoscopy, 360, 361f
Return of spontaneous circulation, 1023
Reverberation artifact, 1070
Reverse transcriptase inhibitors, 1306
Review of systems, 31t
Revonto, 1040, 1040t
Rewarming phase, in cardiopulmonary
    bypass, 514
Reynolds number, 328
Rhabdomyolysis, 1247
  Alport syndrome and, 903
  anesthesia-induced, 1037–1038, 1037t
  malignant hyperthermia versus, 641–642
  prevention of, 631
  succinylcholine-related, 153
Rhabdomyomas, 401–402, 402f
Rh(D) compatibility of blood
    components, 282t
Rheumatic fever, 399
Rheumatic heart disease, 399, 1309
Rheumatoid arthritis, 340t
Rheumatologic pain, 1188–1189, 1189t
Rhinologic procedures, 843–845
Rhinoplasty, 914, 1090
Rhinorrhea, 692
Right to self-determination, 66
Right ventricular dysfunction, 454–455
Right ventricular outflow tract
    obstructions, 589t, 592
Right-to-left shunts, 124, 453–455,
    472–473, 562
  anomalous pulmonary venous
    connection, 458, 459f
  hypoplastic left heart syndrome,
    459–463, 460f
  inhalation anesthetic agents and, 124,
    125f
  simple, 453–455
  tetralogy of Fallot, 453–455, 454f
  transposition of great arteries,
    455–456, 456f, 457f
  truncus arteriosus, 456–458, 458f
Rigid bronchoscopy, 873, 873.e1t
Rigid laryngoscopy, 359–360
  dental mirror in, 360
  flexible fiberoptic bronchoscope and, 368
  intubation guides, 360, 360.e1f
  lateral approach to, 360, 361f
  optimal external laryngeal manipulation
    in, 360
  paraglossal approach to, 360, 361f
  retromolar approach to, 360, 361f
Rigid ventilating bronchoscope, 359
Ring-Adair-Elwyn (RAE) tube, 1322
  in cleft lip and palate repair, 915–916
  description of, 909
Rippling muscle disease, 639t
Risus sardonicus, 1309
Rituximab, 635
Robin syndrome, 340t
Robot-assisted surgery, 244, 754–755, 755t
Rocuronium, 154–155, 646t, 685
  effective doses of, 128t
  emergency surgery in trauma patient
    using, 1009t
  eye surgery uses of, 905
  rapid-sequence intubation using,
    746, 909
  reversal of, 136t
Rocuronium, hepatic metabolism of, 772
Romano-Ward syndrome, 418
Room turnover, COVID-19 and,
    1289, 1289t
Ropivacaine, 1164
  epidural, 1172t
  pharmacokinetics of, 1055
Rosenthal syndrome, 250–251
Rosiglitazone, for type 2 diabetes, 707
Ross operation, 593
Ross-Konno operation, 597
Rotational thromboelastometry
    (ROTEM), 237, 299, 525–526
ROTEM. see Rotational thromboelastometry

Roth spots, 399
Roux-en-Y procedure, 764
Rubinstein-Taybi syndrome, 340t
Rufinamide, 645
Ryanodex, 1040t
Ryanodine receptor
  in malignant hyperthermia, 1048
  secondary dysfunction of, 640
Rythmol. see Propafenone

S

S100B protein, 518
Sacrococcygeal teratoma, 983t, 987–988,
    987f
Safe Surgery Saves Lives campaign, 1302
Safety, in sedation, 1219–1221
Safety intravenous catheter, 1258
Salbutamol
  for acute hyperkalemia, 232
  for asthma exacerbations, 319.e2–319.e3t
Sanfilippo syndrome, 340t
Sano modification, of Norwood
    procedure, 430–431t, 598
Saphenous vein cannulation, 1256, 1256f
Scalp injury, 691–692
Scanning routine, 1070–1072, 1070t, 1071f
Scavenger system, 1323–1324
Scavenging systems, 1198
Schaefer-Fuhrman laryngeal injury
    classification, 893t
Scheduling, on off-site anesthesia, 1197
Schwartz-Jampel syndrome, 639t
Sciatic nerve block, 1122–1125, 1123f,
    1124f
  anterior approach in, 1124, 1124f,
    1125f
  approach of Labat in, 1123–1124,
    1124f
  lateral popliteal sciatic nerve, 1128
  suggested dosing for, 1088t
Scleral buckle surgery, 981
Scleroderma, 340t
Sclerosants, 1211, 1212t
Sclerotherapy, of venous and lymphatic
    malformations, 1211–1213, 1211f,
    1212f, 1212t
SCN9A, 87
Scoliosis, 621, 810–815
  anesthetic and intraoperative
    management of, 826–832
  anesthetic drugs and techniques in,
    832, 832t
  cardiovascular assessment in, 824
  classification of, 811, 811.e1f, 812t
  complications in the early postoperative
    period, 815–817, 815f, 816t
  congenital, 811–813
  decreasing transfusion requirements in,
    827–829
  definition of, 810
  early-onset, 811–813
  idiopathic, 813–814, 814f
  improving outcome from surgical
    intervention in, 815–818
  infantile, 811–813, 813f
  juvenile, 811–813
  long-term changes in, 817–818, 817f
  minimizing blood loss in, 827–829
  in muscular dystrophy, 641
  natural history of, 811–815
  neuromuscular, 814–815
  pain management for, 824–826
  pathophysiology of, 811–815, 813f
  patient monitoring in, 827
  positioning in, 826–e, 826–827, 826f
  postoperative planning for, 823–824
  postoperative ventilatory support for, 824
  preoperative assessment in, 823–824
  respiratory assessment in, 824
  respiratory function in, 815–817
  risk minimization in, 815–818
  somatosensory evoked and motor
    evoked potentials, effects of
    anesthetics on, 830–832, 832t
  temperature regulation in, 827

Scoop and run, 1002–1003
Scopolamine, 187, 907t, 1249–1250
Scout scan, 1070–1071
Screen-based simulator, 1350–1351
Screening for bleeding disorders, 249
Scrotal hypospadias, 757f
Second gas effect, of inhalation anesthetic
    agents, 123
Secondary hyperparathyroidism, 737
Secondary smoking, 25–26
Second-degree atrioventricular block,
    415–416t
Secundum atrial septal defect, 450, 451f
Sedation, outside operating room,
    1215–1237
  anesthesiologist's role in, 1215–1216
  anxiolytics and sedatives for, 1229–1232,
    1230–1231t, 1232f
  barbiturates for, 1230–1231t, 1232–1233
  dexmedetomidine for, 1233–1234
  documentation in, 1227–1228,
    1227.e1f, 1228t, 1228.e1f,
    1228.e3f, 1228.e4f, 1228.e5f
  etomidate for, 1236
  evolution of, 1215–1216
  future of, 1236
  goals of, 1226–1228
  guidelines for, 1221–1226
    American Academy of Pediatrics,
      1221–1223, 1223t
    American College of Emergency
      Physicians, 1224–1225
    American Society of
      Anesthesiologists, 1223–1224
    Joint Commission on Accreditation
      of Healthcare Organizations,
      1225–1226, 1225f
  ketamine for, 1230–1231t, 1234–1235
  levels of, 1216–1217, 1216f, 1217f
  local anesthetics for, 1229
  nitrous oxide for, 1230–1231t, 1236
  opioids for, 1216f, 1230–1231t, 1233
  propofol for, 1235–1236
  safety in, 1219–1221
  scoring systems, 1217–1219, 1217t,
    1218t, 1223t
  sedation depth, 1216–1219, 1219t, 1220f
  sedation risk, 1219, 1219t, 1220f
  specific techniques in, 1228–1236
  training and system issues for,
    1226–1227, 1227f
  treatment plan, 1228–1236
Sedatives
  hepatic metabolism of, 772
  nonbarbiturate, 37
  premedication uses of
    in interventional cardiology, 581
    in neurosurgery, 683
  for sedation, 1229–1232, 1230–1231t,
    1232f
Segmental gracilis muscle transplantation,
    927
Seizure, 63–64
  definition of, 642
  enflurane and, 129
  in epilepsy, 642, 643f
  in inborn errors of metabolism, 632
  refractory, 648
  surgery, 697–699, 698.e1f
  synthetic lysine analogs and, 544
Seldinger technique, 359, 1261, 1261f
Selective cerebral perfusion phase, in
    cardiopulmonary bypass, 514
Selective fetoscopic laser photocoagulation
    (SFLP), 984
Selexipag, 497
Self-determination, right to, 66
Self-report metrics, in pain assessment,
    1135–1138
  Computer Face Scale, 1136t, 1138
  faces pain scales in, 1136, 1137f
  Numeric Rating Scale, for pain, 1136t,
    1137
  Oucher Pain Scale in, 1136, 1136.e1f
  selection criteria for, 1137–1138, 1137f

Self-report metrics, in pain assessment (Continued)
  Sydney Animated Facial Expression Scale, 1136t, 1138
  Visual Analog Scale, 1136, 1137f
Semilobar holoprosencephaly, 624
Senning operations, 595
Senning procedure, 430–431t, 456
Sensor-augmented pump therapy, 707
Sensory innervation, of larynx, 330
Separation, from cardiopulmonary bypass, 514–515
Sepsis
  abdominal surgery and, 747
  malignant hyperthermia versus, 1033t
  in micropremie, 972
  urologic surgery and, 750
Septal defect closure, 430–431t
Septic arthritis, 834–835
Septic shock, 230
Septo-optic dysplasia, 723
Serine protease inhibitors, 507
Serotonergic toxicity, malignant hyperthermia versus, 1033t
Serotonin (5-HT₃), 658
Serotonin (and norepinephrine) reuptake inhibitors, selective, 1193
Serratus anterior plane (SAP) block, for thoracic surgery, 371t
Serum osmolality, 217
SEVENFACT, for hemophilia, 287
Severe cognitive impairment, 127
Sevoflurane
  awareness during, 129–130
  bradycardia caused by, 443
  for cardiac surgery, 443
  for cardiopulmonary bypass, 441
  in children, 684
  degradation of, 138
  emergence delirium with, 136
  eye surgery uses of, 909
  heart rate effects of, 126
  hepatic effects of, 134
  hepatic metabolism of, 773
  inhalation induction with, 782
  inhalation with, 46
  minimum alveolar concentration of, 128t, 441
  neurophysiologic effects of, 688t
  neurotoxicity of, 652.e1–652.e11t, 658
  physiochemical properties of, 114t
  proteomics and, 80
  respiratory depression and, 133
Shaken baby syndrome, 692
Sharp foreign bodies, 881
Sharps, prevention of transmission, 1284, 1284.e1t, 1284.e2t, 1285t
Shikani optical stylet, 367, 367.e1f, 367.e2f
Shivering, 180, 1245
Shone complex, 592
Short bowel syndrome, 774
Short-acting neuromuscular blocking drugs, 156
Shortening fraction, 425
Shprintzen-Goldberg syndrome, 918
Shunt
  calculations of, 429
  for congenital heart disease, 475–476, 476f, 476t, 477t
  inhalation anesthetic agents and, 124–125, 125f
  ventriculoperitoneal, 622–624, 682, 753, 903
  vesicoamniotic, 758
Shunt orifice, 475–476, 476t
SIADH. see Syndrome of inappropriate antidiuretic hormone secretion
Sick euthyroid syndrome, 718
Sickle cell anemia, 242
Sickle cell disease (SCD), 64, 242–246, 245t, 1183
  cardiopulmonary bypass and, 510–511
  perioperative considerations in, 246
  tourniquet-related, 834
  trait, and variants, pain in, 1189, 1190t

Sickle cell lung disease (SCLD), 322
Sickle cell trait (HbAS), 242
Sickle cell/β-thalassemia (HbSβ-thalassemia), 242
Sidestream carbon dioxide analyzers, 1335–1337
Sievert, 581
Sigma opioid receptors, 1152, 1152.e1t
Sigmoid Emax model, 107–108, 108f
Silastic pouch, 978
Sildenafil, 497–498, 958
Silicone oils, 908
Silo pouch, 973
Simdax. see Levosimendan
Simendan. see Levosimendan
SimOne, 1349
Simple left-to-right shunts, 449–453, 449t
  aortopulmonary window in, 451–452, 452f
  atrial septal defect, 450, 451f
  atrioventricular septal defect in, 450–451, 451f, 452f, 452t
  patent ductus arteriosus in, 452–453, 453f
  ventricular septal defect, 450
Simple right-to-left shunts, 453–455
  anomalous pulmonary venous connection, 458, 459f
  hypoplastic left heart syndrome, 459–463, 460f
  tetralogy of Fallot, 453–455, 454f
  transposition of great arteries, 455–456, 456f, 457f
  truncus arteriosus, 456–458, 458f
Simple shunts, 475–476
Shunt orifice, 475–476, 476t
Simulation, in pediatric anesthesia, 1347–1356
  applications of, 1352
  based training in, 1347–1348
  challenges in, 1354
  debriefing in, 1353–1354
  definition of, 1348
  future of, 1354
  high-fidelity, 1352–1353
  human patient simulators in, 1349–1350, 1350f
  hybrid simulation in, 1350
  partial task trainers in, 1348–1349, 1349f
  sites in, 1351–1352, 1351f, 1351t
  standardized patients, 1350
  technologies used in, 1348–1352
    human patient simulators in, 1349–1350, 1350f
    partial task trainers in, 1348–1349, 1349f
  traditional learning versus, 1352, 1352t
  use in evaluation, 1353–1354
  virtual reality and immersive environments, 1350–1351
Single lung transplantation, 803
Single lung ventilation, 804
Single ventricle, 394–395, 394t
  description of, 589t, 597–600
  mechanical circulatory support and, 555–556, 569–570
  physiology, 477–478, 478t
Single-gene defects, 405–406
Single-incision laparoscopic surgery, 751
Single-incision multiport laparoscopy (SIMPL), 751, 751.e1f
Single-lumen endotracheal tube, 373, 373f
Single-lung ventilation, 373–379
  balloon-tipped bronchial blockers for, 373–376, 374f, 375f, 375t
  double-lumen tubes for, 376–378, 376f, 377t
  general considerations in, 378–379, 379f, 380t
  single-lumen endotracheal tube for, 373, 373f
  in thoracic surgery, 1322
  Univent tube for, 376, 376f, 376t
Single-nucleotide polymorphism (SNP), 80, 1252–1253

Single-photon emission computed tomography (SPECT), 1207
Single-stage laryngotracheal reconstruction, 895
Single-twitch stimulation, 149
Sinus arrhythmia, 413–414, 414f, 415t
Sinus bradycardia, 415t
Sinus tachycardia, 415t, 416f
Sinus venosus atrial septal defect, 451f
Sinus venosus defects, 588
Sinusitis, chronic, rhinologic procedures for, 843–844
Sinusoidal obstruction syndrome, 269
Sinusoids, 768
Sirolimus, 806
Sitting position, in neurosurgery, 687
Situs ambiguous, 392–393, 393f
Situs inversus, 392–393, 393f
Situs solitus, 392–393, 393f
Skeletal muscle, excitation-contraction coupling in, 1044–1045, 1045f
Skin
  burn injury effects on, 932–933, 936, 943t
  gestational age assessment and, 5t
  growth and development of, 20–21, 20f
Skin safety, tourniquet-related, 833
Skull fractures, 692, 692f
Sleep endoscopy, drug-induced, for obstructive sleep apnea, 854
Sleep-disordered breathing, 845–846, 845t
Sleep-related breathing disorder subscale (SRBD), 851
Slide tracheoplasty, 896–897, 897f
Slit ventricle syndrome, 699–700
Small-for-gestational-age (SGA), 14
SmartTots, 676
Smith-Lemli-Opitz syndrome, 340t
Smoke inhalation injury, 939
Smoking, primary, 25–26, 25f
Sniffing position, 333
Society for Pediatric Anesthesia, 1238
Socioeconomic concerns in pediatric research, 74
Soda lime, 1324
Sodium, in body fluids, 227t
Sodium bicarbonate
  for cardiopulmonary resuscitation, 1024–1025
  for hyperkalemia, 737t
Sodium bicarbonate, for acidosis, 231–232
Sodium channel gene, 96
Sodium hydroxide, 134
Sodium nitroprusside, 302, 465, 492–493t, 493
Sodium polystyrene sulfonate, 232, 737t
Sodium tetradecyl sulfate, 1212t
Sodium thiopental, noncardiac surgery in congenital heart disease using, 608
Sodium valproate, 645t
Somatic oximetry, 527
Somatosensory evoked potentials, 820–821
  effects of anesthetics on, 830–832, 832t
  in spinal surgery, 819.e1t, 820–821, 820f
Sonoclot, 237
Sonorheometry, 299
Sorine. see Sotalol
Sotalol, 502
Sotylize. see Sotalol
Soy protein allergy and propofol, 144
Sparteine, 85–87
Spastic cerebral palsy, 620t
Sphenopalatine nerve block, 916
Spina bifida, 622, 700
  orthopedic surgery in, 836–837
Spina bifida aperta, 836
Spina bifida cystica, 622
Spina bifida occulta, 622, 836
Spinal anesthesia, 583, 1074–1079, 1076f, 1077f
  complications of, 1079
  drug selection for, 1074.e1f, 1078–1079, 1079t
  in preterm infants, 1246–1247
Spinal canal, tumor of, 626t

Spinal cord, tumor of, 625
Spinal cord injury, 693–694
  during orthopedic surgery, 818–822
  etiology of, 818, 819f
  monitoring of, 819, 819.e1t
  risk of, 819
  without radiologic abnormality, 1014
Spinal cord stimulation, 1187
Spinal cord surgery, 685
Spinal defects, 702
Spinal dysraphism, 622–624
Spinal fusion, 1148
Spinal muscular atrophy (SMA), 632–633
Spinal shock, 693
Spine, cervical
  anomalies, 350t
  evaluation of, 1008f
  injury of, 1006
  instability of, 903
Spine surgery, 809–840
  in acute bone and joint infections, 834–835
  in arthrogryposis multiplex congenita, 839
  in cerebral palsy, 835–836
  congenital anomalies of, 811
  in Duchenne muscular dystrophy, 838–839
  history in, 810–811
  in osteogenesis imperfecta, 837–838
  in scoliosis, 810–815
    anesthetic and intraoperative management of, 826–832
    anesthetic drugs and techniques in, 832
    cardiovascular assessment in, 824
    classification of, 811, 811.e1f, 812t
    complications in the early postoperative period, 815–817, 815f, 816t
    congenital, 811–813
    decreasing transfusion requirements in, 827–829
    definition of, 810
    early-onset, 811–813
    idiopathic, 813–814
    improving outcome from surgical intervention in, 815–818
    infantile, 811–813, 813f
    juvenile, 811–813
    long-term changes in, 817–818, 817f
    minimizing blood loss in, 827–829
    in muscular dystrophy, 641
    natural history of, 811–815
    neuromuscular, 814–815
    pain management for, 824–826
    pathophysiology of, 811–815, 813f
    patient monitoring in, 827
    positioning in, 826–e, 826–827, 826f
    postoperative planning for, 823–824
    postoperative ventilatory support for, 824
    preoperative assessment in, 823–824
    respiratory assessment in, 824
    respiratory function in, 815–817
    risk minimization in, 815–818
    somatosensory evoked and motor evoked potentials, effects of anesthetics on, 830–832
    temperature regulation in, 827
  in spina bifida, 836–837
  spinal cord injury during, 818–822
    etiology of, 818, 819f
    monitoring of, 819, 819.e1t
    risk of, 819
  surgical development in, 810–811, 810f
  terminology in, 810–811
  tourniquets in, 832–834
Spirometry, 311
Spironolactone, 737
Splenectomy
  in hereditary spherocytosis, 240
  in idiopathic thrombocytopenic purpura, 248
  pneumococcal vaccination and, 247

Splenectomy (Continued)
  prophylactic antibiotics and, 247
  in thalassemia, 247
Splenomegaly, 239–240, 270–271
Splinter hemorrhages, 399
Split liver techniques, in liver
    transplantation, 785–786
SPLIT registry, 786
Split-mixed insulin regimens, 710
Spring-assisted cranioplasty, 918
St. John's wort, 32, 32.e1t
ST segment, 412
Standard precautions, for operating room,
    1291–1294
Staphylococcus aureus
  in epidural anesthesia-related infection,
    1085–1086
  in osteomyelitis, 834
Starches, 288
Starling equation, 216, 216.e1f
Starling equilibrium, 216
Static lung volumes, 10, 10t
Static neurologic disorders, 620–625
  cerebral palsy, 620–622, 620t, 621t, 623t
  comorbidities in, 621–622
  cortical development disorders, 625
  nervous system malformations,
    622–624, 624t
  ventral induction disorders, 624–625
Status asthmaticus, 319
Status epilepticus, 648
Stay and play approach to trauma,
    1003–1004
Steady state, 105
Stents, 575–576
Stereotactic biopsies, 695
Stereotactic electroencephalography
    (SEEG), 698
Stereotactic radiosurgery, for non-
    operating room anesthesia, 1208
Steroid equivalency ratios and doses, 723t
Steroids, for spinal cord injury, 693–694
Stethoscope, precordial, 1330
Stevens-Johnson syndrome, 340t
Still murmurs, 409
STOP-BANG questionnaire, 851
Stopcocks, 300, 1317
Storz Bonfils optical stylet, 367, 367.e2f
Storz Video Laryngoscope, 365, 365.e1f
Strabismus surgery, 910–911, 910f
Straight blade, 360
Strangulated bowel, 747
Stress, deleterious effects of untreated, 661
Stress hormones, 708
  burn injury and, 936
Stress response
  to cardiac surgery, 447–449
  perioperative, 614–615
Stress ulcers, after burn injury, 936
Stress-induced hyperglycemia, in cardiac
    surgery, 448
Stress-triggered malignant hyperthermia,
    1042–1043
Stridor, 872–873, 873t
  inspiratory, 334
Stroke
  embolic, 580
  mechanical circulatory support as cause
    of, 570
  in sickle cell disease, 244, 323
Stroke volume variation, 1343–1344
Sturge-Weber syndrome, 904
Stylet
  lighted, 363, 363.e1f
  Shikani optical stylet, 367, 367.e1f
  Storz Bonfils optical stylet, 367, 367.e2f
Subacute bacterial endocarditis, 399
Subarachnoid block, 1072–1073
Subarachnoid bolts, 679
Subarterial defects, 590
Subclavian artery, aberrant, 407, 408f
Subclavian vein catheterization,
    1264–1266, 1266f
Subcutaneous injection, opioids, 1155
Subdural hematoma, 692–693

Subendocardial ischemia, 464, 592
Subglottic area, 325
Subglottic edema, postintubation, 1246
Subglottic hemangioma, 970
Subglottic jet ventilation, 876–877,
    876.e1t
Subglottic stenosis, 62–63, 343, 344f,
    379–380, 874f, 889, 954
Subglottis, developmental anatomy of,
    325–328, 328f, 329f
Subvalvar aortic stenosis, 592
Succinylcholine, 151–154, 151t, 685,
    937, 1310
  adverse effects of, 152–153
  arrhythmias caused by, 152
  biochemical changes caused by, 153
  in burn injury patients, 944
  cholinesterase deficiency and, 151–152
  clinical uses of, 153–154
  contraindications for, 633, 944
  effective doses of, 128t
  emergency surgery in trauma patient
    using, 1009t
  fasciculations caused by, 153
  hepatic metabolism of, 771
  hyperkalemia, 685
  hyperkalemia and, 152–153, 160,
    746, 1027
  intramuscular administration of, 151
  intraocular pressure affected by, 905
  jaws of steel, 152, 1031–1032, 1032f
  malignant hyperthermia and, 1030
  for myasthenia gravis, 635
  myoglobinemia caused by, 153
  myotonic dystrophy and, 639
  rapid-sequence intubation using,
    746, 909
  rhabdomyolysis caused by, 143, 153
  temporomandibular joint stiffness
    caused by, 152
Sucking reflex, 5t
Suction catheters, 1323
Suction devices, 1323
Sudden cardiac death, 395–396, 597
Sufentanil (Sufenta), 127f, 168–169
  for cardiac surgery, 445
  infusion schemes, 197t
  nasal, 169
  neurotoxicity of, 652.e1–652.e11t
  pharmacokinetics of, 772
Suffering, 77
Sugammadex, 157–159, 158f, 482, 905,
    1009t
Sulfation, 771
Sulfonylureas, 707
Sulfotransferase, 82t, 93, 114t, 115, 771
Sulfur dioxide, 934
Sulfur hexafluoride, 908
Sunshine Act, 75
Superior laryngeal nerve, 330
Superior vena cava, persistent left superior
    vena cava to coronary sinus and,
    407–409, 408f
Superior vena cava syndrome, 267
Superstition, 1300
Supplemental oxygen
  retinopathy of prematurity and, 139, 955
  for sedation outside operating room, 1223
Supraclavicular plexus, 1110
Supracristal defects, in ventricular septal
    defect, 590
Supraglottic airway, 343–349, 345f, 1005,
    1213, 1320–1321
  as conduit for intubation, 367–368
    368.e1f
  insertion technique for, 347–349
  for resuscitation, 349
  styles of, 345–347, 346f, 346t, 347t,
    347.e1f, 348f, 348t
Supraglottic jet ventilation, 888–889
Supraglottoplasty, 883
Supraorbital nerve block, 687, 1088–1089
Supratentorial compartment, tumor
    of, 626t
Supratentorial tumors, 694

Supratrochlear nerve block, 687,
    1088–1089, 1089f
Supravalvar aortic stenosis, 592
Supraventricular arrhythmias, 414–418
Supraventricular tachycardia, 414–418,
    418f, 596, 1027–1028, 1247
Surch-Lite Lighted Intubation Stylet,
    363, 363.e1f
Surface-active enzyme complexes, 290–291
Surfactant, 555
Surgery, 650–677
  long-term outcome in children exposed
    to, 668–674
    anesthetic neurotoxicity, 668–669
    data linkage studies, 669–671
    GAS, MASK, and PANDA studies, 673
    longitudinal cohort and registry
      datasets, 671–672
    major surgery in neonatal period, 668
    prenatal exposure, 674
    prospective cohort studies with
      children, 672–673
    randomized trials, 673
Surgical airway, 359
Surgical hand preparation, 1293t
Surgical site infections, 1279
  after scoliosis surgery, 817
Surrogate consent, 66
Suxamethonium, hepatic metabolism
    of, 771
SVR. *see* Systemic vascular resistance
Swallowed objects, 878f, 881
Swallowing
  development of, 16
  laryngeal function during, 331
Sydney Animated Facial Expression Scale,
    1136t, 1138
Sympathetic nervous system, stimulation
    of, 474
Synaptogenesis, 652
SynCardia Total Artificial Heart, 552t,
    560, 561f
Synchronized direct current
    cardioversion, 414
Synchronized intermittent mechanical
    ventilation, 1325–1326
Syndactyly, 928, 928.e1, 929f
Syndrome of inappropriate antidiuretic
    hormone secretion (SIADH),
    232–233, 269, 715–716, 716t
Syntelencephaly, holoprosencephaly
    and, 624
Synthetic lysine analogs, 542–543, 542f
  adverse effects of, 544
Syringobulbia, 624
Syringomyelia, 624
Systemic analgesics, after scoliosis
    surgery, 825
Systemic blood flow obstruction, in
    congenital heart disease, 394, 394t
Systemic corticosteroids, for asthma
    exacerbations, 319.e2–319.e3t
Systemic inflammatory response
    syndrome (SIRS), and
    cardiopulmonary bypass, 523f, 525
Systemic vascular resistance (SVR)
  in cardiac surgery, 443
  description of, 561, 1341
Systemic vasculature, cardiopulmonary
    bypass effects on, 522
Systemic venous saturation ($S_{sys}vO_2$), 478
Systemic-to-pulmonary shunt, 455

T

T3. *see* Triiodothyronine
T4. *see* Thyroxine
Tachycardia
  junctional ectopic, 441–442
  in malignant hyperthermia, 1031–1032
  postoperative, 1247
  sinus, 415t, 416f
  supraventricular, 414–418, 418f, 596,
    1027–1028, 1247
  volume status and, 226
Tachyphylaxis, 493

TACO. *see* Transfusion-associated
    circulatory overload
Tacrolimus, 635
  in cardiac transplantation, 806
  liver disease and, 778
Tadalafil, 498
TAFI. *see* Thrombin-activated fibrinolysis
    inhibitor
TA-GVHD, Transfusion-associated graft-
    versus-host disease
TAH. *see* Total Artificial Heart
Tambocor. *see* Flecainide
TandemHeart (CardiacAssist), 552t,
    558, 558f
Tapentadol, 172–173
Target concentration, 117, 192–193,
    198–208, 198f, 199f, 200f, 200t,
    201–203f
Target effect, 117
Target-controlled infusion, 204–208,
    205t, 207f, 208f
  hydraulic model of, 201–203f
  Paedfusor pharmacokinetic data set for,
    206t, 207f
  pediatric, 191–192
  pharmacodynamics of, 190–194
  pharmacokinetics of, 190–194
  target concentration, 192–193, 198–208,
    201–203f
Targeted antitumor agents, 263–264
T-cell therapies, 264
TEE. *see* Transesophageal
    echocardiography
Teeth, 6
TEG. *see* Thromboelastography
Telesimulation, 1354
Temperature
  in malignant hyperthermia, 1030, 1031t
  monitoring of
    during cardiopulmonary bypass, 439
    during cardiopulmonary
      resuscitation, 1023
    in noncardiac surgery in congenital
      heart disease, 605
    during non-operating room
      anesthesia, 1205
    in scoliosis surgery, 827
  postoperative, 1251
  premature infant and, 961
Temperature control, in neurosurgical
    procedures, 689
Temperature monitors, 1331
Temporal artery catheterization, 1276
Temporal lobe epilepsy, 140
Temporomandibular joint stiffness,
    succinylcholine-related, 152
Tendons, ultrasound of, 1068
Tenormin. *see* Atenolol
TENS. *see* Transcutaneous electrical nerve
    stimulation
Tension-type headache, 1185
Terbutaline, for asthma exacerbations,
    319.e2–319.e3t
Term infant
  drug distribution in, 109, 110f
  renal excretion of drugs in, 115f,
    116, 116f
Testis
  intraabdominal, 757f
  torsion of, 758, 758f
Tet spells, 453–454, 594
Tetanic stimulation, 116f, 118f, 148–149
Tetanospasmin, 1309
Tetanus, 1309
Tethered spinal cord, 702
Tetracaine, 908
Tetrahydrobiopterin, 87
Tetrahydrozoline, 907t
Tetralogy of Fallot (TOF), 391–392, 435,
    453–455, 454f, 546
  anatomy of, 392f
  hypercyanotic episode in, 454, 579, 594
  noncardiac surgery in congenital heart
    disease and, 589t, 593–595
  repair of, 430–431t

TF. *see* Tissue factor
TFPI. *see* Tissue factor pathway inhibitor
TGA. *see* D-transposition of great arteries
Thalassemia, 246–248, 248t
α–thalassemia, 247
β–thalassemia, 247
Thalassemia major, 340t
Theophylline, 81, 902, 956–957
Therapeutic orphans, 119
Thermal ablation, 698
Thermodilution cardiac output, 429
Thermoregulation
  growth and development of, 20–21, 20f
  tourniquet-related, 834
Thiazolidinedione, 711
Thioamides, 719
Thiopental, 140–141
  for blunt reflex bronchoconstriction, 860.e1t
  clearance, 84
  in extremely premature infant, 965
  for intracranial hypertension, 141
  intravenous induction of, 48
  mechanism of action, 659
  in micropremie, 965
  neurophysiologic effects of, 688t
  neurotoxicity of, 652.e1–652.e11t, 659
  noncardiac surgery in congenital heart disease using, 607
  tolerance to, 140–141
Thiopentone, 646t
Third-degree atrioventricular block, 415–416t, 417f
Third-space fluid, 754
Third-spacing, 226
Thoracic electrical bioimpedance, 1343–1344
Thoracic epidural anesthesia, 1081–1084, 1082f, 1083f
Thoracic pump, 1019
Thoracic surgery, 370–390
  general perioperative considerations in, 370–372, 371t
  point-of-care ultrasound pulmonary exam in, 386–389
    for acute respiratory distress syndrome, 387
    for hemidiaphragmatic paralysis, 387, 388f
    introduction to, 386–388, 386f
    for pleural effusion, 387
    for pneumothorax, 387
    tracheal diameter for tracheal tube sizing, 388–389, 389f
    tracheal tube positioning with, 389, 390f
  single-lung ventilation in, 373–379
    balloon-tipped bronchial blockers for, 373–376, 374f, 375f, 375t
    double-lumen tubes for, 376–378, 376f, 377t
    general considerations in, 378–379, 379f
    single-lumen endotracheal tube for, 373, 373f
    Univent tube for, 376, 376f, 376t
  surgical lesions of the chest, 379–386
    in childhood, 384–386, 385f, 386f
    in neonates and infants, 379–384, 381f, 382f, 383f
  thoracoscopy in, 371–372, 372f, 372t, 373f
  ventilation and perfusion during, 370–371
Thoratec. *see* CentriMag; PediMag
Three-axis theory, 339–340
Three-compartment model, 198, 198f
Three-dimensional conformal radiotherapy, 264
Thrombin, 530, 530f, 539
Thrombin-activated fibrinolysis inhibitor (TAFI), 531–532
Thrombocytopenia, 248–249, 292
  after burn injury, 935–936
  in cancer patient, 276

Thrombocytopenia *(Continued)*
  dilutional, 284
  in extremely premature infant, 977
  in idiopathic thrombocytopenic purpura, 248–249
  in liver transplantation, 781
  massive blood transfusion and, 289–300
  in platelet disorders and bleeding, 248
Thrombocytosis, 240
  in burns, 935–936
Thromboelastography (TEG), 514, 525–526, 533, 560, 920
  clot elasticity properties, 537
  in massive blood transfusion, 284, 299
  in scoliosis surgery, 830
Thromboelastometry, 509–510
Thrombomodulin (TM), 531
Thrombosis
  heart surgery and, 536–537
  prevention of, 530
  recombinant factor VIIa and, 541
Thymic hypoplasia, 405
Thyroid disorders, 716–720
  Graves disease in, 718, 719f
  hyperthyroidism in, 718–720, 720t
  hypothyroidism, 716–718
  thyroiditis in, 718–719
Thyroid dysgenesis, 717
Thyroid function tests, 718
Thyroid hormones, 716
Thyroid replacement, for hypothyroidism, 717
Thyroid storm, 719
Thyroidectomy, 719
Thyroiditis, 718–719
Thyroid-stimulating hormone, 717
Thyrotropin-releasing hormone, 716
Thyroxine (T4), 716
Thyroxine globulin deficiency, 717
Tiagabine, 645t
Tidal volume, 10t, 1325
Tikosyn. *see* Dofetilide
Time to peak effect (T$_{PEAK}$), 105
Timolol, 907–908, 907t
Timothy syndrome, 928
Tissue damage, effect of, 534
Tissue expanders, in plastic and reconstructive surgery, 929, 929f. 929.e1
Tissue factor (TF), coagulation initiation, 530, 530f
Tissue factor pathway inhibitor (TFPI), 530
Tissue harmonic imaging, 1069, 1069f
Tissue plasminogen activator (tPA), 506, 531–532, 785
Tizanidine, 1193
TM. *see* Thrombomodulin
TODAY. *see* Treatment Options for Type 2 Diabetes in Adolescents and Youth
Toddler Preschool Preoperative Pain Scale, 1138
TOF. *see* Tetralogy of Fallot
Tongue
  developmental anatomy of, 324, 327f
  pathology related to, 350t
Tonsillectomy, 1246
  high care need after, 1244–1245
  obstructive sleep apnea and, 57
Tonsillitis, recurrent, 846
Topical agents, for clot formation promotion after cardiac surgery, 438
Topiramate, 645t, 1186
Torsades de pointes, 420, 1026
Total Artificial Heart (TAH), 560, 561f
Total blood flow, 475
Total body water
  body weight and, 218, 219f
  in preterm neonates, 150
Total body weight, 765
Total intravenous anesthesia (TIVA), 190–215, 687–688, 1012
  after inhalational induction, 211
  bispectral index monitoring in, 1340

Total intravenous anesthesia *(Continued)*
  bolus and variable rate infusion in three-compartment model in, 207f
  depth of anesthesia monitoring in, 196–197, 1340
  drug delivery in, 208, 209t
  for emergence delirium, 1243
  in endoscopy, 875.e1t
  in epilepsy, 647–648, 647t
  fixed infusion rate and three-compartment model in, 198f, 200
  indications for, 190
  infusion schemes, 197t
  in malignant hyperthermia, 1034–1035
  in muscular dystrophy, 644
  in myasthenia gravis patients, 635–636
  in obese child, 212–214, 213f, 214f
  pharmacodynamics of, 190–194
  pharmacokinetics of, 190–194
  postoperative nausea and vomiting and, 1249
  practical approach in children, 208–212
  principles of, 190–194, 191f
  propofol and, 204–205, 205f
  ready mixes of, 212, 212f, 213f
  remifentanil with, 210, 211f
  spontaneously breathing with, 211
  target concentration, 192–193, 198–208, 201–203f
  target-controlled infusion in, 204–208, 205t, 206f, 207f, 208f
  vasoactive medications and, 1318–1319, 1318f, 1319f
Total lung capacity of infant, 10, 10f
Total parenteral nutrition (TPN), 61, 519, 774
Total sodium deficit, 231
Tourniquets, 832–834
  complications of, 833–834
  indications and design of, 832–833
  physiology of, 833
  recommended cuff pressures, 834
Toxic megacolon, 980f
Toxicity, of local anesthetics, 1056–1057, 1056f, 1058f
  prevention of, 1057–1059, 1058t
    alteration in toxic threshold and, 1059
    rate of uptake and, 1058, 1058t
    site of injection and, 1058
    technique of administration and, 1059
    total drug dose and, 1058
tPA. *see* Tissue plasminogen activator
Trachea
  dynamic collapse of, 11
  function of, 331, 332f
  pathology related to, 350t
  stenosis of, 379–380, 954
Tracheal intubation, 337–343
  in cardiac arrest, 1017
  complications of, 342–343
  continuous waveform capnography for, 342
  CPR medication administration via, 1022
  distance to insert tracheal tube and, 341–342, 342t, 343f
  in laryngeal papillomatosis, 888–889, 888t
  laryngoscope blade for, 340, 340t
  in laryngotracheal reconstruction, 895
  laryngotracheal stenosis and, 343, 344f
  in laryngotracheobronchitis, 886–887
  postintubation croup and, 342–343
  prehospital, in trauma patients, 1005
  technique in, 337–340, 337.e1f, 339f
  tubes in, 340–341, 341f, 341t
  video laryngoscopy in, 340
Tracheal rings, complete, 896–897, 897f
Tracheal tube, 1321–1322
  insertion distance for, 341–342, 342t, 343f
  in tracheal intubation, 340–341, 341f, 341t
Tracheobronchial foreign body aspiration, 877–878, 877t

Tracheobronchomalacia, 954
Tracheocutaneous fistula, after tracheotomy, 892
Tracheoesophageal fistula, 382–383, 383f, 971–972, 971f
Tracheomalacia, 316
Tracheostomy
  for abnormal airways, 359
  after burn injury, 938–939
  after scoliosis surgery, 824
Tracheotomy, 883.e1f, 889–892, 889.e1t, 891f
  complications associated with, 890t
  indications and contraindications for, 889.e1
  management of, 892.e1t, 891–892, 892t
  tracheocutaneous fistula after, 892
Trachlight stylet, 363.e1f
Trachlite, 363, 363.e1f
Tracleer. *see* Bosentan
Train-of-four stimulation, 127f, 149, 1337
TRALI. *see* Transfusion-related acute lung injury
Tramadol, 172
  pain management, 1145t, 1148–1149
  pharmacokinetics of, 89, 89f
  preoperative, 37
Trandate. *see* Labetalol
Tranexamic acid (TXA), 508
  for blood loss, in craniosynostosis surgery, 920
  for cardiac surgery, 438
  dosing of, 545–546, 545t
  in scoliosis surgery, 828–829
Transcranial Doppler (TCD) ultrasonography, 524
Transcranial motor evoked potentials (tcMEP), for spinal surgery, 819.e1t
Transcription, 80
Transcriptomics, 80
Transcutaneous carbon dioxide measurement, 1337
Transcutaneous cardiac pacing, 421–422, 1021–1022
Transcutaneous electrical nerve stimulation (TENS), 1182
Transcutaneous partial pressure of carbon dioxide, 1337
Transcutaneous ultrasound, 872
Transesophageal echocardiography (TEE), 434, 566
  for cardiac catheterization, 585
  for cardiopulmonary bypass, 439–440
  in children, 130–131
  for liver transplantation, 783, 783.e1f
  in noncardiac surgery in congenital heart disease, 605
Transfer, to pediatric intensive care unit, 466
Transfusion therapy, 247, 278–306, 279t
  allogenic, reduce patient exposure to, 301–304
    autotransfusion in, 301–302
    controlled hypotension in, 302–303
    erythropoietin in, 301
    intraoperative blood recovery and reinfusion in, 301–302
    normovolemic hemodilution in, 303–304
    preoperative autologous blood donation in, 301
  avoidance of, 529
  blood components and alternatives in, 281–289
    albumin, dextrans, starches, and gelatins in, 288
    cryoprecipitate in, 282t, 285–286
    desmopressin in, 288
    fresh frozen plasma in, 281, 282t, 286f
    plasma-derived factor concentrates in, 287
    platelets in, 282t, 283–284
    red blood cell substitutes in, 288–289
    red blood cell-containing components in, 281–283, 281t, 282t

Transfusion therapy (Continued)
  special processing of cellular blood components in, 284–285, 285.e1t
  whole blood in, 283
blood volume and, 279–281, 280t
complications of, 279t
fresh frozen plasma, 281, 282t, 286f
for hematologic disorders, 237–239, 238t
  for cytomegalovirus transmission reduction, 239t
  for irradiation of cellular blood components, 238–239, 239t
  for leukocyte reduction of RBC units, 238–239, 238t
massive blood transfusion, 289–300, 289e
  acid-base balance in, 298
  citrate toxicity in, 296–298, 298f
  coagulopathy and, 289–291, 290f, 291f
  dilutional thrombocytopenia in, 291–292, 292f, 293f
  disseminated intravascular coagulation in, 294
  factor deficiency in, 292–294, 294t
  fibrinolysis in, 294
  hyperkalemia in, 295–296, 295f, 295.e1t
  hypocalcemia in, 296–298, 298f
  hypothermia in, 298
  infectious disease considerations in, 300
  monitoring during, 298–300, 298.e1f, 299f, 300f
Transfusion threshold, 237
Transfusion-associated circulatory overload (TACO), 278
Transfusion-associated graft-versus-host disease (TA-GVHD), 277, 285, 797
Transfusion-related acute lung injury (TRALI), 278
Transient ischemic attacks, 1210
Transient receptor potential vanilloid, type 1, 87
Transient tachypnea of newborn, 8–9
Transient wheezers, 316
Transition
  to air breathing, 8–9
  from fetal to neonatal circulation, 957
Translation, 80
Transplantation, 775–808
  cardiac, 791–800
    anesthesia and, 799–800
    for congenital heart disease, 792–793
    contraindications to, 793
    demographics and epidemiology of, 791–792, 792f
    for dilated cardiomyopathy, 793
    for hypertrophic cardiomyopathy, 793
    immediate postoperative management in, 797–799, 798f
    intraoperative problems and management in, 796–797, 797f
    noncardiac surgery in congenital heart disease and, 614
    pathophysiology of disease in, 792
    preoperative evaluation in, 794–795, 795t
    repeat transplantation, 793
    for restrictive cardiomyopathy, 793
    surgical technique in, 795–796
    survival and quality of life in, 799, 799f, 800f, 800t, 801f
    waitlist and donor selection in, 793–794, 794t
  liver, 775–787
    anhepatic stage in, 784–785
    biliary and hepatic artery reconstruction in, 785
    epidemiology and demographics of, 776–778, 776f, 777t
    hepatectomy in, 783–784, 784f
    immediate postoperative care for, 786–787
    indications for, 776

Transplantation (Continued)
    intraoperative care in, 782–783
    living-donor, 785–786
    long-term issues of, 787
    orthotopic, 775
    outcomes of, 786
    pathophysiology of liver disease, 778–780
    preoperative evaluation in, 780–782, 781t
    reperfusion period in, 785
    split liver techniques in, 785–786
    surgical technique in, 783–786
  lung and heart-lung, 800–807
    bilateral sequential, 804
    contraindications to, 802
    cystic fibrosis in, 801
    demographics and epidemiology of, 800–801
    immediate postoperative management of, 805
    intraoperative problems and management in, 803–805
    long-term concerns in, 805–807, 805t
    pathophysiology of disease in, 801, 802t
    preoperative evaluation of, 803
    pulmonary hypertension in, 801–802
    surgical technique in, 803
    survival and quality of life in, 807, 808f
    waitlist and donor selection in, 802–803
  organ, mechanical circulatory support and, 568
  renal, 787–791, 789f, 790t
    anesthetic induction in, 790
    anesthetic management of, 788–791
    immediate postoperative management of, 791
    long-term issues in, 791
    maintenance of anesthesia in, 790–791
    monitors and vascular access in, 790
    pathophysiology of, 788
    preoperative evaluation in, 788
    surgical technique in, 788
Transplanted heart
  morbidity, 483
  physiology of, 483f
Transport
  to pediatric intensive care unit, 466
  to postanesthesia care unit, 1239–1240
Transposition of great arteries, 392f, 394, 455–456, 456f, 457f
Transpulmonary flow, 480, 482f
Transpulmonary pressure, 333
Transpulmonary thermodilution, 1341–1342
Transsphenoidal surgery, tumors and, 695
Transtentorial herniation, 679
Transtracheal jet ventilation, 359, 876–877
Transtracheal kink-resistant catheter, 358.e1f
Transvenous intracardiac echocardiography, 689
Transversus abdominal plane blocks, 949.e1f
Trauma, 1000–1015
  abdominal, 1009–1011
  anesthesia management in
    airway management in, 1009t, 1010f
    antifibrinolytics and, 547
    cricoid pressure in, 1014
    emergency department evaluation and management in, 1006–1011, 1006t, 1007f
    epidemiology of, 1000–1001, 1001t
    future directions in, 1015
    mass casualty events, 1014
    in neurosurgery, 691–694
    nonaccidental, 1001–1002, 1001f, 1002–1003f
    pain management, 1015
    plastic and reconstructive surgery for, 930
    prehospital care in, 1002–1006, 1004t

Trauma (Continued)
    primary survey in, 1006t
    systems, 1002–1005
Trauma systems, 1004
Trauma-informed care, 77
Treacher Collins syndrome, 923–925, 923.e1, 924f, 924.e1
  airway difficulties in, 340t
  cleft lip and palate in, 915
  eye surgery in, 904
  larynx position in, 324–325, 325f
Treatment Options for Type 2 Diabetes in Adolescents and Youth (TODAY) trial, 707
Treprostinil, 496
Tresiba, 706
T-REX study, 676
Trichloroethanol, 184–185
  sedation outside operating room, 1229–1231
Tricuspid regurgitation, 596
Tricyclic antidepressants
  for chronic pain, 1193
  for functional gastrointestinal disorders, 1185t
Triggered electromyography, 819.e1t, 822
Triiodothyronine (T3), 489, 716
Triple-phase response, in diabetes insipidus, 713
Triptans, for headache, 1185–1186
Trismus
  following succinylcholine, 152
  in peritonsillar abscess, 872, 872f
  in tetanus, 1309
Trisomy 13, 404
Trisomy 18, 404, 759
Trisomy 21, 404, 716–717, 976, 1245–1246. see also Down syndrome
Tromethamine, 512
Tropicamide, 907, 907t
Tropisetron, 185–186
Troponin C, 490
Troponin T, 441
True vocal cords, 329
Truncal nerve blocks, 1093–1097
  inguinal, 1093–1096, 1095f
  intercostal, 1085.e1f, 1093, 1094f, 1094.e1f
  paravertebral, 1102–1106, 1103f, 1104f, 1105f, 1106f
  penile, 1096–1097, 1096f
  rectus sheath, 1088t, 1097–1098, 1098f, 1099f, 1100f
Truncus arteriosus, 406, 430–431t, 456–458, 458f, 589t, 596
Truview EVO2 infant device, 366–367, 366.e1f
Tube insertion, myringotomy with, 841–842, 842f
Tuberculosis, 1306–1308
Tuberculosis meningitis, 1306
Tuberous sclerosis, 401–402, 407, 625, 904
Tumor(s)
  airway, 265
  cardiac, 265–267, 401–402
  central nervous system, 269–270
  endocrine tumors, 270
  hepatic, 269
  renal, 269
Tumor lysis syndrome, 256–257, 271, 731–732
Tunneled uncuffed central venous catheter, 1269, 1270f
Turner syndrome, 340t, 404, 926
T waves, 412, 1059
Twin reversed arterial perfusion sequence, 983t, 984–985
Twin-twin transfusion syndrome, 983–984, 983t, 984f, 984t
Two-compartment kinetics, 103, 103f
Two-dimension echocardiography, 130–131
Two-dimension mode ultrasound, 1062
TXA. see Tranexamic acid
Tympanomastoid surgery, 1092
Tympanoplasty, 842–843

Type 1 diabetes mellitus, 706
Type 2 diabetes mellitus, 711

U
Ulnar nerve block, 1118, 1118f
"Ultra-fast" tracking, 447
Ultrafiltration
  cardiac surgery using, 438
  during cardiopulmonary bypass, 518–519
"Ultra-metabolizers," 1148
Ultrasound
  cardiac output determinations using, 1342–1344
  equipment for, 1060–1064, 1061f
  modes of, 1062–1063
  principles of, 1061, 1061t
  use of, 1060–1061
Ultrasound machine, 1063–1064, 1063f, 1064f, 1065f
Ultrasound-guided regional anesthesia, equipment for, 1327–1329
Ultrasound-guided vascular access
  in burn injury, 949–950
  equipment for, 1327–1329
Umbilical artery catheterization, 1271, 1274f
Umbilical hernia, 758
Umbilical vein, catheterization of, 1267–1269, 1269f
Uncuffed tracheal tubes, 341, 341t
Undiagnosed myopathy, 642
Unfractionated heparin, 563
Univent tube, 376, 376f, 376t
Universal precautions, 1291, 1306
University of Michigan Sedation Scale (UMSS), 1218t
University of Wisconsin Pain Scale, 1136t
Unrestrictive intracardiac shunting, during cardiac surgery, 436
Upper airway development, 6–7
Upper airway inhalational injury, 894
Upper airway obstruction, 883–889
  acquired laryngeal and subglottic stenosis, 874f, 889
  acute epiglottitis in, 883–885, 883.e1f, 884f, 885f
  congenital and acquired, 889
  congenital laryngeal webs and, 883.e1f, 889
  croup and, 885–887, 885t, 886f, 886.e1f
  in hemifacial dysostosis, 925
  laryngeal atresia and, 889
  laryngeal papillomatosis and, 887–889, 887f, 888t, 888.e1f
  laryngomalacia in, 883
  laryngotracheobronchitis and, 885–887, 885t
Upper extremity nerve blocks, 1107–1114
  brachial plexus, 1107–1109, 1108f, 1109f, 1110f
  digital hand, 1118–1119, 1119f
  at elbow, 1114
  intravenous, 1131–1132
  median nerve, 1117–1118, 1118f
  radial nerve, 1114–1115
  ulnar nerve, 1118
  at wrist, 1118
Upper respiratory tract infection, 53–54, 53t, 54t, 312–315, 314t, 315f, 315t, 1245
  in adenotonsillectomy, 856
  cardiac surgery and, 435, 435t
Upshaw-Schulman syndrome, 285–286
Uptravi. see Selexipag
Urea cycle defects, 627–628
Uremia, 738
Ureteral reimplantation, 759–760, 760f
Urethral hypoplasia, 757.e1f
Uridine diphosphoglucuronosyltransferases, 82t, 84, 114–115, 114t
Urinary catheter, in abdominal surgery, 748
Urinary retention
  description of, 1252
  epidural analgesia-related, 1086

Urine
  alkalization of, 941
  in utero production of, 13–14
Urine output, 605, 750
Urologic surgery, 749–750
  bladder and cloacal exstrophy, 762–763, 762f
  chordee, 756
  circumcision, 756
  corticosteroid medications and, 749–750
  hypospadias, 756, 757f, 757.e1f
  infection or sepsis in, 750
  monitoring requirements in, 750
  nephrectomy in, 760
  neuroblastoma, 760–761
  posterior urethral valves, 758
  pyeloplasty in, 760
  reduced renal function and, 749
  systemic hypertension and, 749
  ureteral reimplantation, 759–760, 760f
  Wilms tumor, 761–762, 761f, 762f

V

V1 receptor, 1024
V2 receptor, 1024
VA ECMO. see Venoarterial extracorporeal membrane oxygenation
Vaccination, past medical history and, 32
VACTERL association, 406–407, 971
VACTERL complex, 382–383, 451
VADs. see Ventricular assist devices
Vagal nerve stimulator, 644, 699
Vagal reflex, 1027
Vagus nerve
  auricular branch block of, 1092–1093
  in innervation of larynx, 330
Valdecoxib, 177
Valerian, 32.e1t
Valproic acid, 1192
Valve replacement, 430–431t
Valvectomy, 430–431t
Valvotomy, 430–431t
Valvuloplasty, 430–431t
Vaping, primary, 25–26, 25f
Vascular access, 1255–1277
  arterial cannulation in, 1271–1277
    axillary artery catheterization, 1275–1276
    dorsalis pedis and posterior tibial artery catheterization, 1277
    femoral artery catheterization, 1276–1277
    radial artery catheterization, 1271–1275, 1275f, 1276f
    temporal artery catheterization, 1276
    umbilical artery catheterization, 1271, 1274f
  cardiopulmonary resuscitation, 1022–1023
    intravenous access in, 1022
  infection control practice in, 1255
  in renal transplantation, 790
  safety measures for, 1255
  specialist team, 1269–1271, 1272–1273f
  venous cannulation in, 1256–1269
    central venous catheterization, 1259–1261
    intraosseous infusion in, 1257f, 1258–1259, 1259f, 1260f
    peripheral intravenous cannulation in, 1256–1258
    peripherally inserted central venous catheter in, 1269, 1270f
    tunneled uncuffed central venous catheter in, 1269, 1270f
    umbilical vein catheterization in, 1267–1269, 1269f
Vascular anomalies, 695–697
  aberrant subclavian artery, 407, 408f
  in heart disease, 407–409
  persistent left superior vena cava to coronary sinus, 407–409, 408f
Vascular damage, tourniquet-related, 833

Vascular malformations, sclerotherapy of, 1211
Vascular resistance, 429
Vasoactive drugs, 483–484
  amrinone, 488
  digoxin, 484–485t, 488–489
  dobutamine, 486
  dopamine, 485–486
  enoximone, 488
  epinephrine, 486
  isoproterenol, 486
  milrinone, 488
  norepinephrine, 486–487
  phenylephrine, 487
  phosphodiesterase inhibitors, 487–488
  practical considerations for, 484–485
  total intravenous anesthesia and, 1318–1319, 1318f, 1319f
  vasopressin, 487
Vasoconstriction, during cardiopulmonary bypass, 518
Vasodilatation, 226
Vasodilators, 492–493t, 492–498
  ambrisentan, 497
  angiotensin-converting enzyme inhibitors, 495
  beraprost, 497
  bosentan, 497
  captopril, 495
  for child, on ventricular assist device, 561–562
  clevidipine, 494
  enalapril, 495
  endothelin-receptor antagonists, 497
  epoprostenol, 496
  hydralazine, 495
  iloprost, 497
  inhaled nitric oxide, 495–496
  lisinopril, 495
  losartan, 495
  macitentan, 497
  nicardipine, 494
  nitroglycerin, 493–494
  phenoxybenzamine, 494–495
  phentolamine, 494–495
  prostaglandin E₁, 495
  prostanoids, 473f, 477t, 496–497
  in pulmonary vascular physiology, 474
  selexipag, 497
  sildenafil, 497–498
  sodium nitroprusside, 493
  treprostinil, 496
Vasomotor paralysis, 682
Vasoocclusive episodes, 243
Vasopressin, 217, 484–485t, 487, 594–595
  for cardiopulmonary resuscitation, 1024
  for diabetes insipidus, 714
Vasopressors, 484–485t, 726
Vasotec. see Enalapril
VATER association, 406–407
Vaughan Williams classification, of antiarrhythmic agents, 498t
Vecuronium, 155–156, 646t, 742
  effective doses of, 128t
  pharmacodynamics of, 150
Vegetable allergies, latex allergy, 33–34
Vegetations, cardiac, 399
Vein of Galen, 695
Veletri. see Epoprostenol
Velocardiofacial syndrome, 405
Velopharyngeal incompetence, 914
Venlafaxine, 1193
Venoarterial extracorporeal membrane oxygenation (VA ECMO), 554–555, 555f
Venous air embolism, 921–922
  neurosurgical procedures and, 689–690, 690f
Venous cannulation, 1256–1269
  central venous catheterization in, 1259–1261
    aseptic technique in, 1260–1261, 1262f
    brachiocephalic vein and, 1266–1267, 1266f

Venous cannulation (Continued)
    complications of, 1259–1260
    external jugular vein and, 1261
    femoral vein and, 1267, 1268f
    indications for, 1259
    internal jugular vein and, 1261–1267, 1263–1264f, 1265f
    Seldinger technique in, 1261, 1261f
    subclavian vein and, 1264–1266, 1266f
  intraosseous infusion in, 1257f, 1258–1259, 1259f, 1260f
  peripheral intravenous cannulation in, 1256–1258
  peripherally inserted central venous catheter in, 1269, 1270f
  tunneled uncuffed central venous catheter in, 1269, 1270f
  umbilical vein catheterization in, 1267–1269, 1269f
Venous malformations, sclerotherapy of, 1211–1213, 1211f, 1212f, 1212t
Venous occlusions, cardiac catheterization and, 578
Venous thromboembolism, 271
Venous thrombosis, 835
  cardiac catheterization and, 578
Venovenous ECMO (VV ECMO), 555, 555f
Ventavis. see Iloprost
Ventilation
  for abnormal airway, 356–359
    anterior commissure scope and rigid ventilating bronchoscope, 359
    multi-handed mask ventilation, 356, 356f
    percutaneous needle cricothyroidotomy, 357–359, 357f, 358f, 358.e1f, 359.e1f, 359.e2f
    supraglottic airways, 356, 356.e1–356.e2f, 356.e3f
  during thoracic surgery, 370–371
Ventilation system, for operating room, 1291t
Ventilation-perfusion mismatch, 439, 1245
  in thoracic surgery, 371
Ventilator, anesthesia machine, 1325–1327
Ventilatory anaerobic threshold (VAT), 479
Ventral induction disorders, 624–625
Ventricular arrhythmias, 418
Ventricular assist devices (VADs), 557–560, 567, 568
  biventricular, 551
  centrifugal pump, 557–558, 557f
  continuous flow pumps, 560
    hemodynamics with, 563f
  extracorporeal membrane oxygenation, 549–550, 552t, 554–557
    arterial-venous, 555
    for cardiac arrest, 570
    circuit configurations of, 554–557
    in neonates, 553
    preoperative, 551
    schematic diagram of, 555f
    venoarterial, 554–555, 555f
    venovenous, 555, 555f
  history of, 549
  immunologic complications of, 571
  implantation of, 570
  left, 551, 557, 567
  long-term devices, 559–560
  pulsatile pumps, 559–560, 559f
  short-term devices, 557–559
Ventricular catheters, 679
Ventricular compliance, 472
Ventricular dysfunction, 593, 610
Ventricular dysrhythmias, 1056
Ventricular fibrillation, 579
  defibrillation in, 1021
  description of, 420
Ventricular function assessment, 425
Ventricular pressure, 429
Ventricular pressure overload, 611

Ventricular septal defects (VSDs), 450, 589t, 590–591
  closure of, 574–575, 575f
  description of, 391–392, 450
Ventricular tachycardia, 418–420, 419f, 579
  defibrillation in, 1021
  pulseless, 1021
Ventricular volume overload, 610
Ventriculoperitoneal shunt, 622–624, 682, 753, 903, 1088
Ventriculostomy, 699
Verapamil, 499t, 502, 646t
Verelan. see Verapamil
Vertebral artery, 1112–1114
Vertebral fracture, 641
Vertical expandable prosthetic titanium rib (VEPTR), 811
Very low-birth-weight infant, 6
  fluid management in, 222
Vesicoureteral reflux, 759
Vessel dimensions, measurements of, 425
Viagra. see Sildenafil
Video and indirect intubating devices, 364–367
  video laryngoscopes, 364–365
    GlideScope, 364–365, 364.e1f
    MultiView Scope, 365, 365.e2f
    Storz Video Laryngoscope, 365, 365.e1f,
Video laryngoscopes, 364–365
  GlideScope, 364–365, 364.e1f
  MultiView Scope, 365, 365.e2f
  Storz Video Laryngoscope, 365, 365.e1f
Video laryngoscopy, 368
Video laryngoscopy in Small Infants (VISI) trial, 340
Video-assisted thoracoscopic surgery, for scoliosis surgery, 817
Vigabatrin, 645t
Vincristine, 274
Viral filter efficiency, 1290–1291
Viral infection, in myocarditis, 398–399, 398f
Viral laryngotracheitis, 885–886
Virtual reality, in simulation, 1350–1351
Visceroatrial situs, 392–393, 393f
Visceromegaly, 340t
Viscoelastic tests, 237
Viscoelastography, for clot formation, 299
Visual Analog Scale, 1136, 1137f
Vital capacity, age-dependent variables of, 10t
Vitamin B12, 95
Vitamin C, 920
Vitamin K, 536
  deficiency, 693
  in newborn, 18, 285
Vitamin K-dependent coagulation factors, 436
Vitamin K-dependent factors, 18, 236, 533
Vitrectomy, 913, 981
Vitreous humor, 904–905
Vocal cord paralysis, 701–702
Vocal folds, 325
Volatile agents, for blunt reflex bronchoconstriction, 860.e1t
Volume expansion, in SIADH, 715
Volume of distribution
  of amides, 1057
  apparent, 103–104
  in obese patients, 765
  at steady state, 105, 198
Volume overload
  description of, 394, 394t, 585, 738–739
  ventricular, 610
Volume resuscitation, 1318
  in burn injury, 939–940, 940f, 940t, 940.e1f
Volume-controlled ventilation, 1325–1326
Volumetric chamber, 223
Volutrauma, 973
Vomiting. see also Nausea and vomiting
  antiemetics for, 185–186
  propofol and, 143

von Willebrand disease, 250, 251t, 287, 762
von Willebrand factor (vWF), 224, 236, 437, 531, 533
VSDs. *see* Ventricular septal defects
VV ECMO. *see* Venovenous ECMO
vWF. *see* von Willebrand factor

W

Wake Up Safe Quality Improvement campaign, 1329–1330
Wake-up test, 819–820, 819.e1t
Walker-Warburg syndrome, 639t, 641
War, in developing countries, 1300–1301, 1301f
Warfarin (Coumadin), 564, 613
Warming blankets, 1315
Warming devices, 1315–1317
    fluid and blood warmers in, 1316, 1316f, 1316.e1f
    forced air warming devices in, 1315
    heated humidifiers in, 1315–1316, 1315.e1f

Warming devices *(Continued)*
    passive heat and moisturizer exchangers in, 1315
    radiant warmers in, 1315
    warming blankets in, 1315
    wrapping in, 1315
Wash-in, 108f, 120t, 121f, 121t
Washout, of inhalation anesthetic agents, 125–126
Water bath, 1316
Water mattresses, 1315
Water restriction, for SIADH, 716
Waterston shunt, 430–431t
Weight
    gestational age and, 5
    maintenance fluid requirements, 221t
    total body water and, 218, 219–220, 219f
Werdnig-Hoffmann disease, 632
Wheezing, 316t
Whistling face, 340t

White blood cell count
    developmental issues in, 17
    values at different ages, 237t
Whole blood (WB), 281, 291–292
Whole-exome sequencing (WES), 97
Williams syndrome, 404–405, 405f, 592, 721–722
Williams-Beuren syndrome, 404–405, 577–578, 592
Wilms tumor, 269, 761–762, 761f, 762f
Wincoram. *see* Amrinone
Wind-up, 1149
Wolff-Chaikoff effect, 719–720
Wolff-Parkinson-White syndrome, 410–411, 411f, 596
Wong-Baker Faces Pain Scale, 1136, 1137f
Wood units, 429
Work of breathing, 312, 332–333, 333f
World Health Organization, 1302
Wound classification system, 1290.e1t
Wrapping, 1315
Wrist, nerve blocks of
    at median nerve, 1117–1118, 1118f

Wrist, nerve blocks of *(Continued)*
    at radial nerve, 1117, 1117f
    at ulnar nerve, 1118

X

Xanthine oxidase, 448–449
Xenobiotics, 768
Xenon, 656–657
    advantages of, 133
    induction with, 135
    minimum alveolar concentration of, 133
    neurotoxicity of, 652.e1–652.e11t, 659
    physiochemical properties of, 114t
X-linked muscular dystrophy, 639t, 640

Y

Yankauer tip suction devices, 1323
Yasui operation, 430–431t

Z

Zero-order kinetics, 103, 104f
Zestril. *see* Lisinopril
Zonisamide, 645t

AAGBI Safety Guideline

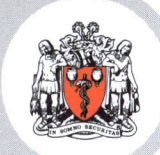

Management of Severe Local Anaesthetic Toxicity

1 Recognition

Signs of severe toxicity:
- Sudden alteration in mental status, severe agitation or loss of consciousness, with or without tonic-clonic convulsions
- Cardiovascular collapse: sinus bradycardia, conduction blocks, asystole and ventricular tachyarrhythmias may all occur
- Local anaesthetic (LA) toxicity may occur some time after an initial injection

2 Immediate management

- Stop injecting the LA
- Call for help
- Maintain the airway and, if necessary, secure it with a tracheal tube
- Give 100% oxygen and ensure adequate lung ventilation (hyperventilation may help by increasing plasma pH in the presence of metabolic acidosis)
- Confirm or establish intravenous access
- Control seizures: give a benzodiazepine, thiopental or propofol in small incremental doses
- Assess cardiovascular status throughout
- Consider drawing blood for analysis, but do not delay definitive treatment to do this

3 Treatment

IN CIRCULATORY ARREST
- Start cardiopulmonary resuscitation (CPR) using standard protocols
- Manage arrhythmias using the same protocols, recognising that arrhythmias may be very refractory to treatment
- Consider the use of cardiopulmonary bypass if available

GIVE INTRAVENOUS LIPID EMULSION

(following the regimen overleaf)

- Continue CPR throughout treatment with lipid emulsion
- Recovery from LA-induced cardiac arrest may take >1 h
- Propofol is not a suitable substitute for lipid emulsion
- Lidocaine should not be used as an anti-arrhythmic therapy

WITHOUT CIRCULATORY ARREST
Use conventional therapies to treat:
- hypotension,
- bradycardia,
- tachyarrhythmia

CONSIDER INTRAVENOUS LIPID EMULSION

(following the regimen overleaf)

- Propofol is not a suitable substitute for lipid emulsion
- Lidocaine should not be used as an anti-arrhythmic therapy

4 Follow-up

- Arrange safe transfer to a clinical area with appropriate equipment and suitable staff until sustained recovery is achieved
- Exclude pancreatitis by regular clinical review, including daily amylase or lipase assays for two days
- Report cases as follows:

  in the United Kingdom to the National Patient Safety Agency (via **www.npsa.nhs.uk**)

  in the Republic of Ireland to the Irish Medicines Board (via **www.imb.ie**)

  If Lipid has been given, please also report its use to the international registry at **www.lipidregistry.org**. Details may also be posted at **www.lipidrescue.org**

Your nearest bag of Lipid Emulsion is kept ....

IMMEDIATELY

Give an initial intravenous bolus injection of 20% lipid emulsion

1.5 ml.kg⁻¹ over 1 min

AND

Start an intravenous infusion of 20% lipid emulsion at **15 ml.kg⁻¹.h⁻¹**

AFTER 5 MIN

Give **a maximum of two** repeat boluses (same dose) if:

- cardiovascular stability has not been restored **or**

- an adequate circulation deteriorates

Leave **5 min** between boluses

A maximum of **three** boluses can be given (including the initial bolus)

AND

Continue infusion at same rate, but:

Double the rate to **30 ml.kg⁻¹.h⁻¹** at any time after 5 min, if:

- cardiovascular stability has not been restored or

- an adequate circulation deteriorates

Continue infusion until stable and adequate circulation restored or maximum dose of lipid emulsion given

Do not exceed a maximum cumulative dose of 12 ml.kg⁻¹

An approximate dose regimen for a 70-kg patient would be as follows:

IMMEDIATELY

Give an initial intravenous bolus injection of 20% lipid emulsion 100 ml over 1 min

AND

Start an intravenous infusion of 20% lipid emulsion at 1000 ml.h⁻¹

AFTER 5 MIN

Give a **maximum of two** repeat boluses of 100 ml

AND

Continue infusion at same rate but **double** rate to 2000 ml.h⁻¹ if indicated at any time

Do not exceed a maximum cumulative dose of 840 ml

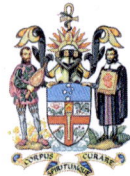

This AAGBI Safety Guideline was produced by a Working Party that comprised:
Grant Cave, Will Harrop-Griffiths (Chair), Martyn Harvey, Tim Meek, John Picard, Tim Short and Guy Weinberg.

This Safety Guideline is endorsed by the Australian and New Zealand College of Anaesthetists (ANZCA).